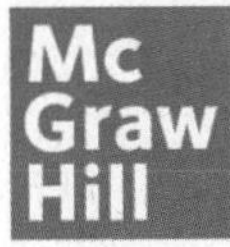
Mc
Graw
Hill

M000199135

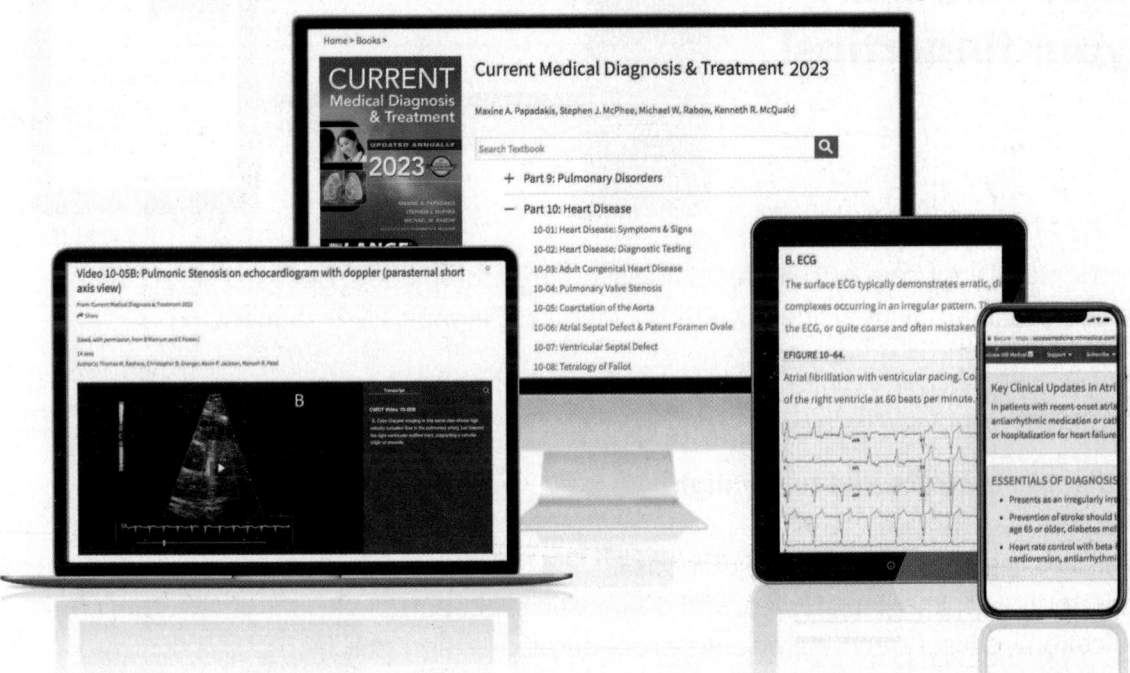

a LANGE medical book

2023 CURRENT Medical Diagnosis & Treatment

SIXTY-SECOND EDITION

Edited by

Maxine A. Papadakis, MD
Professor of Medicine, Emeritus
Department of Medicine
University of California, San Francisco

Stephen J. McPhee, MD
Professor of Medicine, Emeritus
Division of General Internal Medicine
Department of Medicine
University of California, San Francisco

Michael W. Rabow, MD
Professor of Medicine and Urology
Division of Palliative Medicine
Department of Medicine
University of California, San Francisco

Associate Editor

Kenneth R. McQuaid, MD
Professor of Medicine
Department of Medicine
University of California, San Francisco

With Contributing Authors

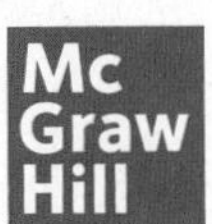

New York Chicago San Francisco Athens London Madrid Mexico City
Milan New Delhi Singapore Sydney Toronto

Current Medical Diagnosis & Treatment 2023, Sixty-Second Edition

1 2 3 4 5 6 7 8 9 0 LWI 27 26 25 24 23 22

ISBN 978-1-2646-8734-3
MHID 1-2646-8734-6
ISSN 0092-8682

Notice

Medicine is an ever-changing science. As new research and clinical experience broaden our knowledge, changes in treatment and drug therapy are required. The authors and the publisher of this work have checked with sources believed to be reliable in their efforts to provide information that is complete and generally in accord with the standards accepted at the time of publication. However, in view of the possibility of human error or changes in medical sciences, neither the authors nor the publisher nor any other party who has been involved in the preparation or publication of this work warrants that the information contained herein is in every respect accurate or complete, and they disclaim all responsibility for any errors or omissions or for the results obtained from use of the information contained in this work. Readers are encouraged to confirm the information contained herein with other sources. For example and in particular, readers are advised to check the product information sheet included in the package of each medication they plan to administer to be certain that the information contained in this work is accurate and that changes have not been made in the recommended dose or in the contraindications for administration. This recommendation is of particular importance in connection with new or infrequently used medications.

This book was set in Minion Pro by KnowledgeWorks Global Ltd.
The editors were Kay Conerly and Jennifer Bernstein.
The production supervisor was Jeffrey Herzich.
Project management was provided by Nitesh Sharma at KnowledgeWorks Global Ltd.
The copyeditor was Allison Scerbo.
Design modified from original by Alan Barnett.
The index was prepared by Kathrin Unger.

This book is printed on acid-free paper.

Contents

Authors v
Preface xiii
Dedication xvii

Year in Review: Key Clinical Updates in *CMDT* 2023

1. Disease Prevention & Health Promotion 1

Michael Pignone, MD, MPH, & René Salazar, MD

2. Common Symptoms 15

Paul L. Nadler, MD, & Ralph Gonzales, MD, MSPH

3. Preoperative Evaluation & Perioperative Management 42

Hugo Q. Cheng, MD

4. Geriatric Disorders 52

Leah J. Witt, MD, Rossana Lau-Ng, MD, & G. Michael Harper, MD

5. Palliative Care & Pain Management 69

Michael W. Rabow, MD, Steven Z. Pantilat, MD, Ann Cai Shah, MD, Lawrence Poree, MD, MPH, PhD, & Raj Mitra, MD

6. Dermatologic Disorders 101

Kanade Shinkai, MD, PhD, & Lindy P. Fox, MD

7. Disorders of the Eyes & Lids 168

Jacque L. Duncan, MD, Neeti B. Parikh, MD, & Gerami D. Seitzman, MD

8. Otolaryngology Disorders 204

Elliott D. Kozin, MD, & Lawrence R. Lustig, MD

9. Pulmonary Disorders 244

Meghan E. Fitzpatrick, MD, Niall T. Prendergast, MD, & Belinda Rivera-Lebron, MD, MS, FCCP

10. Heart Disease 323

Todd Kiefer, MD, Christopher B. Granger, MD, & Kevin P. Jackson, MD

11. Systemic Hypertension 442

Michael Sutters, MD, MRCP (UK)

12. Blood Vessel & Lymphatic Disorders 473

Warren J. Gasper, MD, James C. Iannuzzi, MD, MPH, & Meshell D. Johnson, MD

13. Blood Disorders 500

Lloyd E. Damon, MD, & Charalambos Babis Andreadis, MD, MSCE

14. Disorders of Hemostasis, Thrombosis, & Antithrombotic Therapy 546

Andrew D. Leavitt, MD, & Erika Leemann Price, MD, MPH

15. Gastrointestinal Disorders 579

Kenneth R. McQuaid, MD

16. Liver, Biliary Tract, & Pancreas Disorders 674

Lawrence S. Friedman, MD

17. Breast Disorders 737

Armando E. Giuliano, MD, FACS, FRCSEd, & Sara A. Hurvitz, MD, FACP

18. Gynecologic Disorders 763

Jill Brown, MD, MPH, MHS, FACOG, & Katerina Shvartsman, MD, FACOG

19. Obstetrics & Obstetric Disorders 794

Vanessa L. Rogers, MD, & Scott W. Roberts, MD

20. Rheumatologic, Immunologic, & Allergic Disorders 819

Rebecca L. Manno, MD, MHS, Jinoos Yazdany, MD, MPH, Teresa K. Tarrant, MD, & Mildred Kwan, MD, PhD

21. Electrolyte & Acid-Base Disorders 875

Nayan Arora, MD, & J. Ashley Jefferson, MD, FRCP

22. Kidney Disease 903

Tonja C. Dirkx, MD, & Tyler B. Woodell, MD, MCR

23. Urologic Disorders 943

Mathew Sorensen, MD, MS, FACS, Thomas J. Walsh, MD, MS, & Brian J. Jordan, MD

24. Nervous System Disorders 970

Vanja C. Douglas, MD, & Michael J. Aminoff, MD, DSc, FRCP

25. Psychiatric Disorders 1046

Kristin S. Raj, MD, Nolan R. Williams, MD, & Charles DeBattista, DMH, MD

26. Endocrine Disorders 1099

Paul A. Fitzgerald, MD

27. Diabetes Mellitus & Hypoglycemia 1195

Umesh Masharani, MB, BS, MRCP (UK)

28. Lipid Disorders 1239

Michael J. Blaha, MD, MPH

29. Nutritional Disorders & Obesity 1250

Katherine H. Saunders, MD, & Leon I. Igel, MD, FACP, FTOS

30. Common Problems in Infectious Diseases & Antimicrobial Therapy 1270

Monica Fung, MD, MPH, Peter V. Chin-Hong, MD, B. Joseph Guglielmo, PharmD, & Katherine Gruenberg, PharmD

31. HIV Infection & AIDS 1311

Monica Gandhi, MD, Matthew A. Spinelli, MD, MAS, & Mitchell H. Katz, MD

32. Viral & Rickettsial Infections 1353

Christine Akamine, MD, Eva Clark, MD, PhD, & Wayne X. Shandera, MD

33. Bacterial & Chlamydial Infections 1440

Bryn A. Boslett, MD, & Rachel Bystritsky, MD

34. Spirochetal Infections 1480

Susan S. Philip, MD, MPH

35. Protozoal & Helminthic Infections 1496

Philip J. Rosenthal, MD

36. Mycotic Infections 1534

Stacey R. Rose, MD, FACP, FIDSA, & Richard J. Hamill, MD

37. Disorders Related to Environmental Emergencies 1548

Jacqueline A. Nemer, MD, FACEP, & Marianne A. Juarez, MD

38. Poisoning 1564

Craig Smollin, MD

39. Cancer 1594

Sunny Wang, MD, Tiffany O. Dea, PharmD, BCOP, Lawrence S. Friedman, MD, Carling Ursem, MD, Kenneth R. McQuaid, MD, & Marc A. Dall'Era, MD

40. Genetic & Genomic Disorders 1658

Reed E. Pyeritz, MD, PhD

41. Orthopedic Disorders & Sports Medicine 1675

Anthony Luke, MD, MPH, & C. Benjamin Ma, MD

42. Sexual & Gender Minority Health 1709

Patricia A. Robertson, MD, Nicole Rosendale, MD, Kevin L. Ard, MD, MPH, Kenneth H. Mayer, MD, Mitzi Hawkins, MD, MAS, & Madeline B. Deutsch, MD, MPH

The following chapters are available online without subscription at www.accessmedicine.com/CMDT

e1. Anti-Infective Chemotherapeutic & Antibiotic Agents Online*

Katherine Gruenberg, PharmD, & B. Joseph Guglielmo, PharmD

e2. Diagnostic Testing & Medical Decision Making Online*

Chuanyi Mark Lu, MD

e3. Information Technology in Patient Care Online*

Russ Cucina, MD, MS

e4. Integrative Medicine Online*

Darshan Mehta, MD, MPH

e5. Podiatric Disorders Online*

Monara Dini, DPM, & Charles B. Parks, DPM

e6. Women's Health Issues Online*

Brigid M. Dolan, MD, MEd, & Judith Walsh, MD, MPH

e7. Appendix: Therapeutic Drug Monitoring, Laboratory Reference Intervals, & Commonly Used Blood Specimen Collection Tubes Online*

Chuanyi Mark Lu, MD

Index 1731

Authors

Christine Akamine, MD
Assistant Professor of Medicine, Section of Infectious Diseases, Department of Medicine, Baylor College of Medicine, Houston, Texas
akamine@bcm.edu
Viral & Rickettsial Infections

Michael J. Aminoff, MD, DSc, FRCP
Distinguished Professor and Endowed Chair in Parkinson's Disease Research, Department of Neurology, University of California, San Francisco; Attending Physician, University of California Medical Center, San Francisco
michael.aminoff@ucsf.edu
Nervous System Disorders

Charalambos Babis Andreadis, MD, MSCE
Professor of Clinical Medicine, Division of Hematology/ Oncology, Department of Medicine, University of California, San Francisco
Charalambos.Andreadis@ucsf.edu
Blood Disorders

Kevin L. Ard, MD, MPH
Faculty, Division of Infectious Diseases, Massachusetts General Hospital; Medical Director, National LGBTQIA+ Health Education Center, Fenway Institute; Assistant Professor of Medicine, Harvard Medical School, Boston, Massachusetts
kard@mgh.harvard.edu
Sexual & Gender Minority Health

Nayan Arora, MD
Assistant Professor, Division of Nephrology, Department of Medicine, University of Washington, Seattle, Washington
narora@uw.edu
Electrolyte & Acid-Base Disorders

David M. Barbour, PharmD, BCPS
Pharmacist, Denver, Colorado
dbarbour99@gmail.com
Drug References

Michael J. Blaha, MD, MPH
Professor of Medicine, Division of Cardiology, Department of Medicine; Director of Clinical Research, Ciccarone Center for the Prevention of Cardiovascular Disease; Johns Hopkins University School of Medicine, Baltimore, Maryland
mblaha1@jhmi.edu
Lipid Disorders

Bryn A. Boslett, MD
Associate Clinical Professor, Division of Infectious Diseases, Department of Medicine, University of California, San Francisco
Bryn.Boslett@ucsf.edu
Bacterial & Chlamydial Infections

Jill Brown, MD, MPH, MHS, FACOG
Medical Officer, Contraceptive Development Program, National Institute of Child Health and Human Development, Bethesda, Maryland
Jilleb75@yahoo.com
Gynecologic Disorders

Rachel Bystritsky, MD
Assistant Professor, Division of Infectious Diseases, Department of Medicine, University of California, San Francisco
Rachel.Bystritsky@ucsf.edu
Bacterial & Chlamydial Infections

Hugo Q. Cheng, MD
Clinical Professor of Medicine, Division of Hospital Medicine, Department of Medicine, University of California, San Francisco
quinny.cheng@ucsf.edu
Preoperative Evaluation & Perioperative Management

Peter V. Chin-Hong, MD
Professor of Medicine, Division of Infectious Diseases, Department of Medicine, University of California, San Francisco
peter.chin-hong@ucsf.edu
Common Problems in Infectious Diseases & Antimicrobial Therapy

Eva Clark, MD, PhD
Assistant Professor, Department of Medicine (Section of Infectious Diseases) and Department of Pediatrics (Section of Tropical Medicine), Baylor College of Medicine, Houston, Texas
eva.clark@bcm.edu
Viral & Rickettsial Infections

Russ Cucina, MD, MS
Professor of Hospital Medicine, Department of Medicine; Vice President, Genetic and Genomic Services and Chief Health Information Officer, UCSF Health System; University of California, San Francisco
russ.cucina@ucsf.edu
CMDT Online—Information Technology in Patient Care

Rand Dadasovich, MD, MS
Clinical Education Fellow, Division of Infectious Diseases, University of California, San Francisco
References

Marc A. Dall'Era, MD
Professor of Urology, Department of Urology, UC Davis Health, University of California, Davis
mdallera@ucdavis.edu
Genitourinary Cancers (in Chapter 39)

Lloyd E. Damon, MD
Professor of Clinical Medicine, Division of Hematology/ Oncology, Department of Medicine; Director of Quality for the Adult Hematologic Malignancies and Blood and Marrow Transplantation Program, University of California, San Francisco
lloyd.damon@ucsf.edu
Blood Disorders

Tiffany O. Dea, PharmD, BCOP
Oncology Pharmacist, Veterans Affairs Health Care System, San Francisco, California; Adjunct Professor, Thomas J. Long School of Pharmacy and Health Sciences, Stockton, California
tiffany.dea@va.gov
Cancer

Charles DeBattista, DMH, MD
Professor of Psychiatry and Behavioral Sciences, Department of Psychiatry and Behavioral Sciences; Director, Depression Clinic and Research Program; Director of Medical Student Education in Psychiatry, Stanford University School of Medicine, Stanford, California
debattista@stanford.edu
Psychiatric Disorders

Madeline B. Deutsch, MD, MPH
Associate Professor of Clinical Family & Community Medicine, Department of Family & Community Medicine; Medical Director, UCSF Gender Affirming Health Program, University of California, San Francisco
Madeline.Deutsch@ucsf.edu
Sexual & Gender Minority Health

Chukwuka A. Didigu, MD, PhD
Clinical Fellow, Division of Hematology & Medical Oncology, Department of Medicine, University of California, San Francisco
References

Monara Dini, DPM
Associate Clinical Professor of Orthopedics, Department of Orthopedic Surgery, University of California, San Francisco
monara.dini@ucsf.edu
CMDT Online—Podiatric Disorders

Tonja C. Dirkx, MD
Chief, Nephrology Section, Veterans Affairs Portland Health Care System; Associate Professor of Medicine, Division of Nephrology, Department of Medicine, Oregon Health & Science University, Portland, Oregon
dirkxt@ohsu.edu
Kidney Disease

Brigid M. Dolan, MD, MEd
Associate Professor of Medicine and Medical Education, Division of General Internal Medicine, Department of Medicine, Northwestern University Feinberg School of Medicine
brigid.dolan@northwestern.edu
CMDT Online—Women's Health Issues

Vanja C. Douglas, MD
Sara & Evan Williams Foundation Endowed Neurohospitalist Chair, Professor of Clinical Neurology, Department of Neurology, University of California, San Francisco
Vanja.Douglas@ucsf.edu
Nervous System Disorders

Jacque L. Duncan, MD
Professor of Clinical Ophthalmology, Department of Ophthalmology, University of California, San Francisco
jacque.duncan@ucsf.edu
Disorders of the Eyes & Lids

Neela Easwar, MD
Resident Physician, Department of Medicine, Weill Cornell Medicine, New York, New York
References

Sarah Adler Fink, RD, CDN, CNSC
Senior Clinical Dietitian, Department of Food and Nutrition, New York-Presbyterian Hospital/Weill Cornell Medical Center, New York, New York
Saa9108@nyp.org
Nutritional Support (in Chapter 29)

Paul A. Fitzgerald, MD
Clinical Professor of Medicine, Division of Endocrinology, Department of Medicine, University of California, San Francisco
paul.fitzgerald@ucsf.edu
Endocrine Disorders

Meghan E. Fitzpatrick, MD
Assistant Professor of Medicine, Division of Pulmonary and Critical Care Medicine, Department of Medicine, University of Pittsburgh School of Medicine, Pittsburgh, Pennsylvania
fitzpatrickme2@upmc.edu
Pulmonary Disorders

Lindy P. Fox, MD
Professor of Dermatology, Department of Dermatology, University of California, San Francisco
Lindy.Fox@ucsf.edu
Dermatologic Disorders; Callosities & Corns of Feet or Toes (CMDT Online—Podiatric Disorders)

Lawrence S. Friedman, MD
Professor of Medicine, Harvard Medical School; Professor of Medicine, Tufts University School of Medicine, Boston, Massachusetts; The Anton R. Fried, MD, Chair, Department of Medicine, Newton-Wellesley Hospital, Newton, Massachusetts; Assistant Chief of Medicine, Massachusetts General Hospital, Boston
lfriedman@partners.org
Liver, Biliary Tract, & Pancreas Disorders; Hepatobiliary Cancers (in Chapter 39)

Monica Fung, MD, MPH
Assistant Professor, Division of Infectious Diseases, Department of Medicine, University of California, San Francisco
Monica.Fung@ucsf.edu
Common Problems in Infectious Diseases & Antimicrobial Therapy

Monica Gandhi, MD, MPH
Professor, Division of HIV, ID, and Global Medicine, Zuckerberg San Francisco General Hospital; University of California, San Francisco
Monica.Gandhi@ucsf.edu
HIV Infection & AIDS

Warren J. Gasper, MD
Associate Professor of Clinical Surgery, Division of Vascular and Endovascular Surgery, Department of Surgery, University of California, San Francisco
warren.gasper@ucsf.edu
Blood Vessel & Lymphatic Disorders

Armando E. Giuliano, MD, FACS, FRCSEd
Professor of Surgery, Linda and Jim Lippman Chair in Surgical Oncology; Director, Surgical Oncology; Associate Director, Cedars-Sinai Cancer Center, Los Angeles, California
armando.giuliano@cshs.org
Breast Disorders

Ralph Gonzales, MD, MSPH
Professor of Medicine, Division of General Internal Medicine, Department of Medicine; Associate Dean, Clinical Innovation and Chief Innovation Officer, UCSF Health; University of California, San Francisco
ralph.gonzales@ucsf.edu
Common Symptoms

Matthew Gorgone, DO, FACP
Pulmonary and Critical Care Fellow, Department of Medicine, University of Pittsburgh Medical Center
References

Christopher B. Granger, MD
Professor of Medicine, Division of Cardiology, Department of Medicine; Director, Cardiac Care Unit, Duke University Medical Center, Duke Clinical Research Institute, Durham, North Carolina
christopher.granger@dm.duke.edu
Heart Disease

Katherine Gruenberg, PharmD
Assistant Professor, School of Pharmacy, University of California, San Francisco
Katherine.Gruenberg@ucsf.edu
Common Problems in Infectious Diseases & Antimicrobial Therapy; CMDT Online—Anti-Infective Chemotherapeutic & Antibiotic Agents

B. Joseph Guglielmo, PharmD
Professor and Dean Emeritus, School of Pharmacy, University of California, San Francisco
BJoseph.Guglielmo@ucsf.edu
Common Problems in Infectious Diseases & Antimicrobial Therapy; CMDT Online—Anti-Infective Chemotherapeutic & Antibiotic Agents

Richard J. Hamill, MD
Professor of Medicine, Division of Infectious Diseases, Departments of Medicine and Molecular Virology & Microbiology, Baylor College of Medicine, Houston, Texas; Staff Physician, Infectious Diseases Section, Michael E. DeBakey Veterans Affairs Medical Center
rhamill@bcm.edu
Mycotic Infections

G. Michael Harper, MD
Professor, Division of Geriatrics, Department of Medicine, University of California, San Francisco School of Medicine; San Francisco Veterans Affairs Health Care System, San Francisco, California
Michael.Harper@ucsf.edu
Geriatric Disorders

Mitzi Hawkins, MD, MAS
Assistant Professor, Obstetrics, Gynecology & Reproductive Sciences, University of California, San Francisco; Chief, Division of Gynecology, San Francisco Veteran Affairs Health System
Mitzi.Hawkins@ucsf.edu
Sexual & Gender Minority Health

Sara A. Hurvitz, MD, FACP
Professor of Medicine; Division of Hematology/Oncology, Department of Internal Medicine; Director, Breast Oncology Program, University of California, Los Angeles
shurvitz@mednet.ucla.edu
Breast Disorders

James C. Iannuzzi, MD, MPH
Assistant Professor of Surgery, Division of Vascular and Endovascular Surgery, Department of Surgery, University of California, San Francisco
james.iannuzzi@ucsf.edu
Blood Vessel & Lymphatic Disorders

Leon I. Igel, MD, FACP, FTOS
Assistant Professor of Clinical Medicine, Division of Endocrinology, Diabetes and Metabolism, Department of Medicine, Weill Cornell Medical College, New York, New York
lei9004@med.cornell.edu
Nutritional Disorders & Obesity

Kevin P. Jackson, MD
Associate Professor of Medicine, Division of Cardiology, Department of Medicine; Director of Electrophysiology, Duke Raleigh Hospital, Duke University Medical Center, Durham, North Carolina
k.j@duke.edu
Heart Disease

J. Ashley Jefferson, MD, FRCP
Professor of Medicine, Division of Nephrology, Department of Medicine; Section Head, Nephrology, University of Washington Medical Center, Seattle, Washington
jashleyj@uw.edu
Electrolyte & Acid-Base Disorders

Jane Jih, MD, MPH, MAS
Associate Professor of Medicine, Division of General Internal Medicine, Department of Medicine, University of California, San Francisco
References

Meshell D. Johnson, MD
Professor of Medicine, Chief, Division of Pulmonary, Critical Care, and Sleep Medicine, San Francisco Veterans Affairs Health Care System; Associate Chair for Diversity, Equity, and Inclusion, Department of Medicine, University of California, San Francisco
meshell.johnson@ucsf.edu
Blood Vessel & Lymphatic Disorders; Alcohol Use Disorder (Alcoholism) (in Chapter 25)

Brian J. Jordan, MD
Assistant Professor, Department of Urology, University of Washington, Seattle
bjordan2@uw.edu
Urologic Disorders

Marianne A. Juarez, MD
Associate Clinical Professor, Department of Emergency Medicine, University of California, San Francisco
Marianne.Juarez@ucsf.edu
Disorders Related to Environmental Emergencies

Sakeen Kashem, MD, PhD
Resident, Department of Dermatology, University of California, San Francisco
References

Mitchell H. Katz, MD
President and Chief Executive Officer of NYC Health + Hospitals, New York, New York
mitchell.katz@nychhc.org
HIV Infection & AIDS

Todd Kiefer, MD
Associate Professor of Medicine, Division of Cardiology, Duke University Medical Center, Durham, North Carolina
todd.kiefer@duke.edu
Heart Disease

Whitney Kleinmann, MD
Maternal Fetal Medicine Fellow, Department of Obstetrics & Gynecology, UT Southwestern, Dallas, Texas
References

Elliott D. Kozin, MD
Assistant Professor of Otolaryngology - Head and Neck Surgery, Harvard Medical School, Boston, Massachusetts; Physician and Surgeon, Massachusetts Eye and Ear, Boston, Massachusetts
Elliott_Kozin@meei.harvard.edu
Otolaryngology Disorders

Mildred Kwan, MD, PhD
Assistant Professor of Medicine, Division of Rheumatology, Allergy & Immunology, Department of Medicine, University of North Carolina School of Medicine, Chapel Hill, North Carolina
mildred_kwan@med.unc.edu
Allergic & Immunologic Disorders (in Chapter 20)

Rossana Lau-Ng, MD
Assistant Professor, Section of Geriatrics, Department of Medicine, Boston University School of Medicine, Boston, Massachusetts
rossana.lau-ng@bmc.org
Geriatric Disorders

Andrew D. Leavitt, MD
Professor, Departments of Medicine (Hematology) and Laboratory Medicine; Medical Director, UCSF Adult Hemophilia Treatment Center, University of California, San Francisco
andrew.leavitt@ucsf.edu
Disorders of Hemostasis, Thrombosis, & Antithrombotic Therapy

Chuanyi Mark Lu, MD
Professor and Vice Chair, Department of Laboratory Medicine, University of California, San Francisco; Chief, Lab Medicine Service, Veterans Affairs Health Care System, San Francisco, California
chuanyi.lu@ucsf.edu
Selected Pharmacogenetic Tests: Clinical Relevance (in Chapter 40); CMDT Online—Diagnostic Testing & Medical Decision Making; CMDT Online—Appendix: Therapeutic Drug Monitoring, Laboratory Reference Intervals, & Commonly Used Blood Specimen Collection Tubes

Anthony Luke, MD, MPH
Benioff Distinguished Professor in Sports Medicine, Department of Orthopaedics; Director, UCSF Primary Care Sports Medicine; Director, Human Performance Center at the Orthopaedic Institute, University of California, San Francisco
anthony.luke@ucsf.edu
Orthopedic Disorders & Sports Medicine

Lawrence R. Lustig, MD
Howard W. Smith Professor and Chair, Department of Otolaryngology—Head & Neck Surgery, Columbia University Irving Medical Center & New York Presbyterian Hospital, New York, New York
lrl2125@cumc.columbia.edu
Otolaryngology Disorders

C. Benjamin Ma, MD
Professor and Vice Chairman of Adult Clinical Operations, Department of Orthopaedic Surgery, University of California, San Francisco
MaBen@orthosurg.ucsf.edu
Orthopedic Disorders & Sports Medicine

Rebecca L. Manno, MD, MHS
Adjunct Assistant Professor, Division of Rheumatology, Johns Hopkins University School of Medicine, Baltimore, Maryland
rmanno3@jhmi.edu
Rheumatologic, Immunologic, & Allergic Disorders

Umesh Masharani, MB, BS, MRCP (UK)
Professor of Medicine, Division of Endocrinology and Metabolism, Department of Medicine, University of California, San Francisco
umesh.masharani@ucsf.edu
Diabetes Mellitus & Hypoglycemia

Kenneth H. Mayer, MD
Professor of Medicine, Harvard Medical School; Co-Chair and Medical Research Director, The Fenway Institute; Director of HIV Prevention Research, Beth Israel Deaconess Medical Center, Boston, Massachusetts
kmayer@fenwayhealth.org
Sexual & Gender Minority Health

Kenneth R. McQuaid, MD
Professor of Medicine, Marvin H. Sleisenger Endowed Chair and Vice-Chairman, Department of Medicine, University of California, San Francisco; Chief, Medical Service, San Francisco Veterans Affairs Medical Center
Kenneth.McQuaid@ucsf.edu
Gastrointestinal Disorders; Alimentary Tract Cancers (in Chapter 39)

Darshan Mehta, MD, MPH
Assistant Professor of Medicine, Harvard Medical School; Medical Director, Benson-Henry Institute for Mind-Body Medicine, Massachusetts General Hospital; Director, Office for Well-Being, Center for Faculty Development, Massachusetts General Hospital; Director of Education, Osher Center for Integrative Medicine, Harvard Medical School and Brigham and Women's Hospital; Boston, Massachusetts
dmehta@partners.org
CMDT Online—Integrative Medicine

Raj Mitra, MD
Senator Robert J. Dole Professor and Chair, Department of Rehabilitation Medicine, University of Kansas Medical Center, Kansas City, Kansas
rmitra@kumc.edu
Opioids (in Chapter 5, Palliative Care & Pain Management)

Paul L. Nadler, MD
Clinical Professor of Medicine; Division of General Internal Medicine, Department of Medicine; Director, UCSF Adult Urgent Care; University of California, San Francisco
Paul.Nadler@ucsf.edu
Common Symptoms

Anand Narayanan, MD
Clinical Fellow, Endocrinology, Department of Medicine, University of California, San Francisco
References

Jacqueline A. Nemer, MD, FACEP
Professor of Emergency Medicine; Department of Emergency Medicine; Director of Value; Medical Director, Clinical Documentation Integrity, Department of Quality, University of California, San Francisco
jacqueline.nemer@ucsf.edu
Disorders Related to Environmental Emergencies

Akinyemi Oni-Orisan, PharmD, PhD
Assistant Professor, Department of Clinical Pharmacy University of California, San Francisco
akinyemi.oni-orisan@ucsf.edu
Unconscious Bias Reviewer

Steven Z. Pantilat, MD
Professor of Medicine, Department of Medicine; Kates-Burnard and Hellman Distinguished Professor of Palliative Care; Chief, Division of Palliative Medicine, University of California, San Francisco
steve.pantilat@ucsf.edu
Palliative Care & Pain Management

Neeti B. Parikh, MD
Assistant Professor of Ophthalmology, Department of Ophthalmology, University of California, San Francisco
Neeti.Parikh@ucsf.edu
Disorders of the Eyes & Lids

Charles B. Parks, DPM
Associate Clinical Professor, Chief of Podiatric Surgery Division, Department of Orthopedic Surgery, University of California, San Francisco
Charles.Parks@ucsf.edu
CMDT Online—Podiatric Disorders

Susan S. Philip, MD, MPH
Assistant Clinical Professor, Division of Infectious Diseases, Department of Medicine, University of California, San Francisco; Disease Prevention and Control Branch, Population Health Division, San Francisco Department of Public Health, San Francisco, California
susan.philip@sfdph.org
Spirochetal Infections

Michael Pignone, MD, MPH
Professor of Medicine; Chair, Department of Medicine, Dell Medical School, The University of Texas at Austin
pignone@austin.utexas.edu
Disease Prevention & Health Promotion

Lawrence Poree, MD, MPH, PhD
Professor of Anesthesia and Pain Medicine, Department of Anesthesia & Perioperative Care, University of California, San Francisco
Lawrence.Poree@ucsf.edu
Palliative Care & Pain Management

Niall T. Prendergast, MD
Fellow, Division of Pulmonary, Allergy and Critical Care Medicine, Department of Medicine, University of Pittsburgh School of Medicine, Pittsburgh, Pennsylvania
niall.prendergast@gmail.com
Pulmonary Disorders

Erika Leemann Price, MD, MPH
Clinical Professor, Department of Medicine, University of California, San Francisco Hospitalist, San Francisco Veterans Affairs Health Care System
erika.price@ucsf.edu
Disorders of Hemostasis, Thrombosis, & Antithrombotic Therapy

Reed E. Pyeritz, MD, PhD
William Smilow Professor of Medicine and Genetics, Emeritus, Raymond and Ruth Perelman School of Medicine of the University of Pennsylvania, Philadelphia
reed.pyeritz@pennmedicine.upenn.edu
Genetic & Genomic Disorders

Michael W. Rabow, MD
Professor of Clinical Medicine and Urology, Division of Palliative Medicine, Department of Medicine; Helen Diller Family Chair in Palliative Care; Director, Symptom Management Service, Helen Diller Family Comprehensive Cancer Center, University of California, San Francisco
Mike.Rabow@ucsf.edu
Palliative Care & Pain Management

Kristin S. Raj, MD
Clinical Associate Professor of Psychiatry, Department of Psychiatry and Behavioral Sciences, Stanford University School of Medicine, Stanford, California
kraj@stanford.edu
Psychiatric Disorders

Belinda Rivera-Lebron, MD, MS, FCCP
Associate Professor of Medicine, Division of Pulmonary, Allergy and Critical Care Medicine, Department of Medicine, University of Pittsburgh School of Medicine, Pittsburgh, Pennsylvania
riveralebronbn@upmc.edu
Pulmonary Disorders

Scott W. Roberts, MD
Professor of Obstetrics and Gynecology, Department of Obstetrics and Gynecology, University of Texas Southwestern Medical Center, Dallas, Texas
scott.roberts@utsouthwestern.edu
Obstetrics & Obstetric Disorders

Patricia A. Robertson, MD
Professor of Obstetrics and Gynecology, Department of Obstetrics, Gynecology, and Reproductive Sciences, University of California, San Francisco
Patricia.Robertson@ucsf.edu
Sexual & Gender Minority Health

Vanessa L. Rogers, MD
Professor of Obstetrics and Gynecology, Department of Obstetrics and Gynecology; Chief, Division of Education and Faculty Development, University of Texas Southwestern Medical Center, Dallas, Texas
vanessa.rogers@utsouthwestern.edu
Obstetrics & Obstetric Disorders

Stacey R. Rose, MD, FACP, FIDSA
Assistant Professor of Internal Medicine, Division of Infectious Diseases, Department of Medicine; Associate Dean of Curriculum, Baylor College of Medicine, Houston, Texas
srrose@bcm.edu
Mycotic Infections

Nicole Rosendale, MD
Assistant Professor of Neurology, Neurohospitalist Division, Department of Neurology, University of California, San Francisco
nicole.rosendale@ucsf.edu
Sexual & Gender Minority Health

Philip J. Rosenthal, MD
Professor of Medicine, Department of Medicine, University of California, San Francisco; Associate Chief, Division of HIV, Infectious Diseases, and Global Medicine, Zuckerberg San Francisco General Hospital
philip.rosenthal@ucsf.edu
Protozoal & Helminthic Infections

René Salazar, MD
Professor of Internal Medicine and Medical Education, Department of Medicine, Dell Medical School, The University of Texas at Austin
rene.salazar@austin.utexas.edu
Disease Prevention & Health Promotion

Katherine Sanders, MD
Research Resident, Department of Surgery, University of California, San Francisco
References

Katherine H. Saunders, MD
Assistant Professor of Clinical Medicine, Division of Endocrinology, Diabetes and Metabolism, Department of Medicine, Weill Cornell Medicine, New York, New York
kph2001@med.cornell.edu
Nutritional Disorders & Obesity

Gerami D. Seitzman, MD
Associate Professor of Ophthalmology, Department of Ophthalmology, Francis I. Proctor Foundation, University of California, San Francisco
gerami.seitzman@ucsf.edu
Disorders of the Eyes & Lids

Ann Cai Shah, MD
Assistant Clinical Professor of Anesthesia and Pain Medicine, Department of Anesthesia and Perioperative Care, University of California, San Francisco
ann.shah@ucsf.edu
Palliative Care & Pain Management

Wayne X. Shandera, MD
Associate Professor of Medicine, Department of Medicine, Baylor College of Medicine, Houston, Texas
shandera@bcm.tmc.edu
Viral & Rickettsial Infections

Kanade Shinkai, MD, PhD
Professor of Dermatology, Department of Dermatology, University of California, San Francisco
Kanade.Shinkai@ucsf.edu
Dermatologic Disorders; Callosities & Corns of Feet or Toes (CMDT Online—Podiatric Disorders)

Katerina Shvartsman, MD, FACOG
Associate Professor of Obstetrics and Gynecology, Department of Obstetrics and Gynecology, Uniformed Services University, Bethesda, Maryland
Gynecologic Disorders

Craig Smollin, MD
Professor of Emergency Medicine, Department of Emergency Medicine, University of California, San Francisco; Medical Director, California Poison Control System—San Francisco Division
Craig.Smollin@ucsf.edu
Poisoning

Mathew Sorensen, MD, MS, FACS
Associate Professor of Urology, Department of Urology, University of Washington, Seattle; Residency Program Director, Department of Urology; Director, Comprehensive Metabolic Stone Clinic, Puget Sound Veterans Affairs Health Care System
mathews@uw.edu
Urologic Disorders

Matthew A. Spinelli, MD, MAS
Assistant Professor, Division of HIV, ID, and Global Medicine, Zuckerberg San Francisco General Hospital; University of California, San Francisco
Matthew.Spinelli@ucsf.edu
HIV Infection & AIDS

Gaelen Stanford-Moore, MD, MPhil
Resident Physician, Otolaryngology/Head and Neck Surgery University of California, San Francisco
References

Michael Sutters, MD, MRCP (UK)
Attending Nephrologist, Virginia Mason Medical Center, Seattle, Washington
michael.sutters@commonspirit.org
Systemic Hypertension

Teresa K. Tarrant, MD
Associate Professor, Department of Medicine, Division of Rheumatology and Immunology, Duke University Health System, Durham, North Carolina
teresa.tarrant@duke.edu
Allergic & Immunologic Disorders (in Chapter 20)

Philip Tiso, MFA
Principal Editor, Division of General Internal Medicine, University of California, San Francisco
References

Carling Ursem, MD
Assistant Professor, Division of Hematology and Oncology, Department of Medicine, University of California, San Francisco; Staff Physician, Veterans Affairs Health Care System, San Francisco
Carling.Ursem@ucsf.edu
Alimentary Tract Cancers (in Chapter 39)

Jonathan A. Waitman, MD
Assistant Professor of Medicine, Division of Endocrinology, Diabetes and Metabolism, Department of Medicine, Weill Cornell Medicine, New York, New York
jaw2016@med.cornell.edu
Nutritional Support (in Chapter 29)

Judith Walsh, MD, MPH
Professor of Clinical Medicine, Division of General Internal Medicine, Women's Health Center of Excellence, University of California, San Francisco
Judith.Walsh@ucsf.edu
CMDT Online—Women's Health Issues

Thomas J. Walsh, MD, MS
Professor of Urology, Department of Urology, University of Washington School of Medicine, Seattle, Washington
walsht@uw.edu
Urologic Disorders

Sunny Wang, MD
Professor of Clinical Medicine, Division of Hematology/Oncology, University of California, San Francisco; Chief of Hematology/Oncology, San Francisco Veterans Affairs Health Care System
sunny.wang@ucsf.edu
Cancer

Nolan R. Williams, MD
Assistant Professor of Psychiatry and Behavioral Sciences, Department of Psychiatry; Director of Brain Stimulation Laboratory, Stanford University School of Medicine, Stanford, California
nolanw@stanford.edu
Psychiatric Disorders

Leah J. Witt, MD
Assistant Professor, Division of Geriatrics and Division of Pulmonary, Critical Care, Allergy and Sleep Medicine, Department of Medicine, University of California, San Francisco
Leah.Witt@ucsf.edu
Geriatric Disorders

Tyler B. Woodell, MD, MCR
Assistant Professor of Medicine, Division of Nephrology-Hypertension, Department of Medicine, University of California, San Diego
twoodell@ucsd.edu
Kidney Disease

Jinoos Yazdany, MD, MPH
Alice Betts Endowed Professor, Department of Medicine, University of California, San Francisco; Chief of Division of Rheumatology, Zuckerberg San Francisco General Hospital
Jinoos.Yazdany@ucsf.edu
Rheumatologic, Immunologic, & Allergic Disorders

Preface

Current Medical Diagnosis & Treatment 2023 (CMDT 2023) is the 62nd edition of this single-source reference for practitioners of adult medicine in both hospital and ambulatory settings. The book emphasizes the practical features of clinical diagnosis and patient management in all fields of internal medicine and in specialties of interest to primary care practitioners and to subspecialists who provide general care.

With a growing recognition of systemic racism and other biases in institutions across our societies, including the institution of medicine (https://www.mdcalc.com/race), the editors of *CMDT,* with humility, have committed to a thorough examination of our content to remove biased language, research, and recommendations. Since 2020, we have been pursuing an ongoing, formal process of review and revision in an effort to recognize and correct biases and to promote equity in our book and the practice of medicine. While we, the editors, take this on as our responsibility, we also invite readers to share with us any *CMDT* content that they find problematic or biased.

We have tried to describe populations used in the studies that form the basis of the information in *CMDT,* use appropriate language where we can (eg, persons of sub-Sahara African descent, rather than African-Americans), and use the gender-neutral term Latinx. We acknowledge that, like others,[1] we find this an imperfect solution. We continue, however, to use terms from original sources when study populations are broad.

INTENDED AUDIENCE FOR *CMDT*

House officers, medical students, and all other health professions students will find the descriptions of diagnostic and therapeutic modalities, with citations to the current literature, of everyday usefulness in patient care.

Internists, family physicians, hospitalists, nurse practitioners, physician assistants, and all primary care providers of adult medicine will appreciate *CMDT* as a ready reference and refresher text. Physicians in other specialties, pharmacists, and dentists will find the book a useful basic medical reference text. Nurses, nurse practitioners, and physician assistants will welcome the format and scope of the book as a means of quickly referencing medical diagnosis and treatment modalities.

Patients and their family members who seek information about the nature of specific diseases and their diagnosis and treatment may also find this book to be a valuable resource.

NEW IN THIS EDITION OF *CMDT*

- INNOVATIVE TABLE highlighting the **"Year in Review: Key Clinical Updates in *CMDT 2023*,"** individually listed with page numbers and reference citations, for easy access to significant changes in this edition
- Ongoing concerted effort to address and remove unconscious bias
- List of Common Abbreviations used in *CMDT* can be found on the inside of the front cover
- New section on opioids for pain management
- Overhauled organization of Dermatology chapter to better reflect categorization of conditions and lesions
- Expanded section of interventional therapies to manage chronic pain
- Updated USPSTF lung cancer screening recommendations using low-dose CT
- New prognostic systems for primary myelofibrosis: GIPSS and MIPSSv2
- Discussion of the use of DOACs in patients with morbid obesity who require antithrombotic therapy
- Updated section on osmotic laxatives to treat chronic constipation
- Ozanimod approved for the treatment of moderate to severe ulcerative colitis
- Landmark change in staging female breast carcinoma modifying anatomic stage and adding prognostic stage
- New medications for treating metastatic breast cancer (olaparib, talazoparib, palbociclib, ribociclib, and abemaciclib)
- New recommendations on treating cholestasis of pregnancy
- Updated criteria for diagnosing systemic lupus erythematosus to include antinuclear antibody measurement
- New medications for active lupus nephritis, including voclosporin used with mycophenolate mofetil as well as belimumab
- Anifrolumab is approved for nonrenal lupus when standard therapies fail

[1]April 2021 Annals of Internal Medicine: A Comprehensive Policy Framework to Understand and Address Disparities and Discrimination in Health and Health Care: A Policy Paper From the American College of Physicians. Appendix 2: Glossary.

- New guidelines for diagnosing polyarteritis nodosa
- New American College of Rheumatology/Vasculitis Foundation recommendations for the treatment of granulomatosis with polyangiitis
- A newly described genetic syndrome, VEXAS (vacuoles, E1 enzyme, X-linked, autoinflammatory, somatic) in the differential diagnosis of relapsing polychondritis
- Discussion of the role of left atrial appendage closure in preventing stroke and systemic embolization
- Aducanumab (anti-amyloid therapy) is approved by the US FDA for the treatment of Alzheimer disease
- Extensive revision of the Thyroiditis section in Endocrine Disorders chapter
- Substantial revision of the Nutritional Support section in the Nutritional Disorders & Obesity chapter
- Substantial revision in the HIV Infection & AIDS chapter, including updates in the available therapeutic regimens
- Rewritten SARS-CoV-2 section and inclusion of SARS-CoV-2 information relevant to specific chapters throughout the textbook
- Extensive revision of Sexual & Gender Minority Health chapter, including sections on family planning and health care for transgender and gender diverse persons

OUTSTANDING FEATURES OF *CMDT*

- Medical advances up to time of annual publication
- Detailed presentation of internal medicine disciplines, plus primary care topics in gynecology, obstetrics, dermatology, ophthalmology, otolaryngology, psychiatry, neurology, toxicology, urology, geriatrics, orthopedics, women's health, sexual and gender minority health, preventive medicine, and palliative care
- Concise format, facilitating efficient use in any practice setting
- More than 1000 diseases and disorders
- Specific disease prevention information
- Easy access to medication dosages, with trade names indexed and current costs updated in each annual edition
- Recent references, with unique identifiers (PubMed, PMID numbers) for rapid downloading of article abstracts and, in some instances, full-text reference articles

E-CHAPTERS, *CMDT ONLINE*, & AVAILABLE APPS

Seven ***e-chapters*** listed in the Table of Contents can be accessed at **www.AccessMedicine.com/CMDT.** These online-only chapters (available without need for subscription) include

- Anti-Infective Chemotherapeutic & Antibiotic Agents
- Diagnostic Testing & Medical Decision Making
- Information Technology in Patient Care
- Integrative Medicine
- Podiatric Disorders
- Women's Health Issues
- Appendix: Therapeutic Drug Monitoring, Laboratory Reference Intervals, & Commonly Used Blood Specimen Collection Tubes

Institutional or individual subscriptions to AccessMedicine also have full electronic access to *CMDT 2023*. Subscribers to ***CMDT Online*** receive full electronic access to *CMDT 2023* as well as

- An expanded, dedicated media gallery; new to this edition are educational videos and printable protocols in the Orthopedic Disorders & Sports Medicine chapter
- ***Quick Medical Diagnosis & Treatment***—a concise, bulleted version of *CMDT 2023*
- ***Guide to Diagnostic Tests***—for quick reference to the selection and interpretation of commonly used diagnostic tests
- ***CURRENT Practice Guidelines in Primary Care***—delivering concise summaries of the most relevant guidelines in primary care
- ***Diagnosaurus***—consisting of 1000+ differential diagnoses

CMDT 2023, QMDT, Guide to Diagnostic Tests, and *Diagnosaurus* are also available as individual apps for your smartphone or tablet and can be found in the Apple App Store and Google Play.

SPECIAL RECOGNITION: MITCHELL H. KATZ, MD

With this 2023 edition of *CMDT*, we express our immense gratitude and say goodbye to Mitchell H. Katz, MD as he transitions away from his 30+ years as author of Chapter 31 "HIV Infection & AIDS."

A graduate of Yale College and Harvard Medical School, Dr. Katz completed his residency in the UCSF Primary Care General Internal Medicine Residency, and then trained as a Robert Wood Johnson Clinical Scholar.

Dr. Katz has spent the bulk of his career in public service. He began his work in 1991 in the San Francisco Department of Public Health, ultimately being appointed Director and Health Officer of the Department of Health. He was probably best known for funding San Francisco's successful needle exchange program; for creating its "Healthy San Francisco" Program as the first comprehensive municipal health care and financing system in the United States; for outlawing the sale of tobacco at pharmacies; and for winning ballot measures funding the replacement of the City's 780-bed nursing home, the Laguna Honda Hospital & Rehabilitation Center, and for rebuilding its 386-bed public "safety net" hospital, the Zuckerberg San Francisco General Hospital.

In 2010, Dr. Katz was appointed the Director of the Los Angeles County Department of Health Services (DHS), the second largest public safety net system in the U.S. While in L.A., he created an ambulatory care network that empaneled over 350,000 patients in a primary care home and that transitioned over 4000 medically complex patients from care at hospitals and emergency departments into independent housing, effectively eliminating unnecessary and expensive hospital care and giving these patients the dignity of their own home.

Moving to New York City in 2018, Dr. Katz became President and CEO of NYC Health and Hospitals, the largest municipal health system in the U.S. He is the architect of NYC Care, a health access program that provides comprehensive health care to New Yorkers regardless of income or immigration status. In the spring of 2019, Dr. Katz steered the municipal health system through the worst of the COVID-19 outbreak when NYC was the epicenter of the U.S. pandemic. In a 6-week period, he tripled the number of ICU beds to care for acutely ill patients.

Dr. Katz is an elected member of the National Academy of Sciences and is the Deputy Editor of *JAMA Internal Medicine*. He has published extensively in the areas of HIV epidemiology and health care access. He practices as a primary care physician at Gouverneur Health in Manhattan. Mitch and his partner, Rabbi Igael Gurin-Malous, have two children, Maxwell and Roxie, who were adopted from an orphanage in Vietnam.

As Mitch's editors, we are particularly thankful for his expert annual submissions, providing us a precis about the care of patients with HIV infection/AIDS. We are immensely grateful for his friendship and look forward to hearing about the next chapters in his amazing career of service.

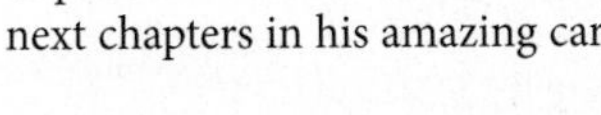

ACKNOWLEDGMENTS

We wish to thank our authors for participating once again in the annual updating of this important book. We are especially grateful to N. Franklin Adkinson, Jr., MD, Antoine Azar, MD, Thomas M. Bashore, MD, C. Seth Landefeld, MD, Manesh R. Patel, MD, George R. Schade, MD, Joshua S. Schindler, MD, and Scott Steiger, MD who are leaving *CMDT* this year. We have all benefited from their clinical wisdom and commitment.

With enormous gratitude and respect, we dedicate this 62nd edition of *Current Medical Diagnosis & Treatment* to all health care professionals and staff who have cared for patients with COVID-19. We honor their competence, their humanity, and their bravery. We also wish to extend our heartfelt gratitude to Eva Clark, MD, PhD, and to Wayne Shandera, MD, for coauthoring (along with Christine Akamine, MD) the authoritative section on COVID-19 (SARS-CoV-2) in the Viral chapter of the print edition of *CMDT* and for providing ongoing, current, and expert updates on this topic in *CMDT Online*.

Many students and physicians have contributed useful suggestions to this and previous editions, and we are grateful. We continue to welcome comments and recommendations for future editions in writing or via electronic mail. The editors' e-mail addresses are below, and author e-mail addresses are included in the Authors section.

Maxine A. Papadakis, MD — Maxine.Papadakis@ucsf.edu
Stephen J. McPhee, MD — Stephen.McPhee@ucsf.edu
Michael W. Rabow, MD — Mike.Rabow@ucsf.edu
Kenneth R. McQuaid, MD — Kenneth.McQuaid@ucsf.edu

San Francisco, California

Dedication

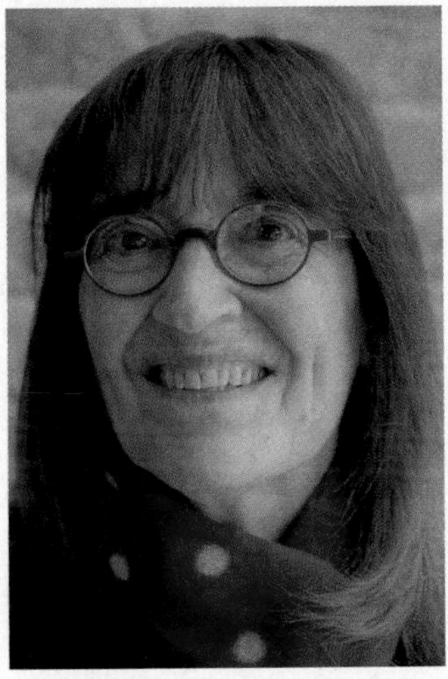

Harriet Lebowitz

The editors and publishers of *Current Medical Diagnosis & Treatment* (*CMDT*) wish to dedicate this 62nd edition of *CMDT* to Harriet Lebowitz, in recognition of her more than 20 years of service as our Senior Project Development Editor. Harriet, who is retiring with this edition, has been the major organizing force responsible for the annual production of *CMDT*.

In particular, we would like to express our gratitude to Harriet for her dedication in making *CMDT* the world's number one best-selling annually updated medical textbook in print, online, app, and abbreviated formats (*Quick Medical Diagnosis & Treatment*). Among other innovations that Harriet has contributed, she most recently envisioned and helped create *CMDT's* "Year in Review: Key Clinical Updates" feature.

Throughout many changes over the years, Harriet has been a constant positive presence. Her familiarity with the text, editors, and authors as well as all the arcane details of publishing helped guide our journey to an on-time publication each year. We will all miss working with Harriet very much and wish her the absolute best in her retirement.

Dedication

YEAR IN REVIEW: KEY CLINICAL UPDATES IN CMDT 2023

Topic	Page Number	Key New Advances Affecting Clinical Practice*
CHAPTER 2: COMMON SYMPTOMS		
Dyspnea	19	• Point-of-care ultrasonography (POCUS) consistently improved the sensitivities of standard diagnostic pathways to detect heart failure, pneumonia, PE, pleural effusion, or pneumothorax. Specificities increased in most, but not all, studies; in-hospital mortality and length of hospital stay, however, did not differ significantly between patients who did or did not receive POCUS in addition to standard diagnostic tests. *Gartlehner G et al. Ann Intern Med. [PMID: 33900798]*
Dysuria	41	• A systematic review and meta-analysis found D-mannose protective against recurrent UTIs. *Lenger SM et al. Am J Obstet Gynecol. [PMID: 32497610]*
Fatigue & Systemic Intolerance Disease (Chronic Fatigue Syndrome)	34	• Pitolisant, a selective histamine H3-receptor antagonist with wake-promoting effect, may reduce daytime sleepiness in patients with moderate to severe obstructive sleep apnea who do not want continuous positive airway pressure treatment. *Dauvilliers Y et al. Am J Respir Crit Care Med. [PMID: 31917607]*
CHAPTER 4: GERIATRIC DISORDERS		
Dementia	55	• Aducanumab, a monoclonal antibody that targets amyloid-beta protein and promotes its clearance from the brain, became the first new drug approved by the FDA for the treatment of Alzheimer disease since 2003. However, its role in routine clinical care remains unclear. *Lin GA et al. https://icer.org/assessment/alzheimersdisease-2021/*
CHAPTER 7: DISORDERS OF THE EYES & LIDS		
Optic Neuritis	194	• Newer therapies include monoclonal antibodies against immune cells and cell-based therapies to deplete or modulate T- and B-cell responses. *Derdelinckx J et al. Int J Mol Sci. [PMID: 34360690]*
CHAPTER 8: OTOLARYNGOLOGY DISORDERS		
Bacterial Rhinosinusitis	220	• Dupilumab, a monoclonal antibody with inhibition of IL-4 and IL-13, is FDA-approved for patients with chronic sinusitis with nasal polyposis. *Hoy SM. Drugs. [PMID: 32240527]*
Sensorineural Hearing Loss	212	• There is emerging evidence that conventional audiometry may not fully capture hearing loss (known as "hidden hearing loss"). Many patients may have subclinical hearing loss. *Drennan WR. Audiol Neurootol. [PMID: 34727540]*
CHAPTER 9: PULMONARY DISORDERS		
Allergic Bronchopulmonary Aspergillosis	266	• For patients with frequent exacerbations, the use of biologic agents, such as anti-IgE (omalizumab), anti-IL-5 (mepolizumab, benralizumab), or anti-IL4 receptor (dupilumab), has been shown to improve outcomes. *Koutsokera A et al. J Cyst Fibros. [PMID: 31405730]*
Bronchial Carcinoid Tumors	291	• The aggressiveness of bronchial carcinoid tumors is determined by the cell histology, with "typical carcinoid," a low-grade tumor, demonstrating a more indolent and favorable course than "atypical carcinoid," an intermediate-grade tumor. Bronchial carcinoid tumor staging follows the same TNM classification as other lung cancers. *Singh S et al. J Thorac Oncol. [PMID: 32663527]*

*See chapter for further details and references.

(continued on following page)

Topic	Page Number	Key New Advances Affecting Clinical Practice*
Screening for Lung Cancer	289	• The USPSTF updated its recommendation for low-dose CT screening. Annual low-dose CT screening for lung cancer is recommended for those at high risk; with high-risk criteria including age 50–80 years, at least a 20 pack-years smoking history, and either current smoking or quit date within past 15 years. Screening should be stopped once 15 years have elapsed since quitting smoking, or if a comorbid condition renders the benefits of screening null. Simulation models developed for the purposes of informing this recommendation found yearly screening with these parameters to be the most efficient in reducing lung-cancer related deaths, although more false-positive test results are expected compared with the original recommendation. *Krist AH et al. JAMA. [PMID: 33687470]*
CHAPTER 10: HEART DISEASE		
Chronic Stable Angina Pectoris (Chronic Coronary Syndromes)	361	• CT-functional fractional reserve (CT-FFR) is approved for clinical use and is endorsed with a level IIa recommendation for intermediate-risk patients with chest pain and no prior history of CAD with a 40–90% stenosis on CT imaging to guide need for revascularization. *Writing Committee Members; Gulati M et al. J Am Coll Cardiol. [PMID: 34756653]*
Heart Failure	408, 409	• The FDA approved sacubitril/valsartan in patients with heart failure and preserved LVEF, particularly for patients with an EF less than 50%, including patients with a mildly reduced EF of 41–49%. • Empagliflozin has been FDA-approved to treat heart failure with reduced LVEF, with or without diabetes; it is the only therapy shown to reduce cardiovascular death or heart failure hospitalization in this population. *McDonagh TA et al. Eur J Heart Fail. [PMID: 35083827]* *Bozkurt B et al. J Card Fail. [PMID: 33663906]*
Infectious Myocarditis	414	• Myocarditis following infection with SARS-CoV-2 infection and following vaccination have been reported in the medical literature. In both scenarios, younger male patients seem to be at highest risk for this overall rare event. *Boehmer TK et al. MMWR Morb Mortal Wkly Rep. [PMID: 34473684]* *Witberg G et al. N Engl J Med. [PMID: 34614329]*
Primary & Secondary Prevention of CHD	358	• The USPSTF issued new guidance on the use of aspirin for primary prevention of cardiovascular events; patients aged 40–49 years should have a shared decision-making conversation regarding the potential risks and benefits of initiating aspirin therapy for primary prevention, and patients aged 60 years or older should not initiate aspirin for primary prevention of CVD. *USPSTF.* *https://www.uspreventiveservicestaskforce.org/uspstf/sites/default/files/file/supporting_documents/aspirin-cvd-prevention-final-rec-bulletin.pdf*
CHAPTER 11: SYSTEMIC HYPERTENSION		
Systemic Hypertension	465	• Most guidelines now recommend the use of home blood pressure monitors in the diagnosis of hypertension. The availability of blood pressure profiles generated from multiple home-gathered data points over continuous intervals allows more precise control of the overall hypertensive burden. *Milani RV et al. Curr Opin Cardiol. [PMID: 33871402]*
CHAPTER 12: BLOOD VESSEL & LYMPHATIC DISORDERS		
Aortic Dissection	487	• For patients who cannot tolerate a beta-blocker or who need a second agent to control hypertension, intravenous calcium channel blocker infusions such as nicardipine are an alternative. Start nicardipine 5 mg/hour intravenously and titrate the infusion to the desired effect. *Bossone E et al. Nat Rev Cardiol. [PMID: 33353985]*
Occlusive Disease: Femoral & Popliteal Arteries	475	• Dual treatment with rivaroxaban 2.5 mg orally twice daily and aspirin 81 mg orally daily has been shown to reduce limb-related events, major amputation, and cardiovascular events in patients with femoral and popliteal artery atherosclerosis. *Bauersachs RM et al. J Am Coll Cardiol. [PMID: 34010631]*

*See chapter for further details and references.

Topic	Page Number	Key New Advances Affecting Clinical Practice*
CHAPTER 13: BLOOD DISORDERS		
Plasma Cell Myeloma	538	• For patients with multi-agent refractory disease, chimeric antigen receptor T-cell therapy targeting the early plasma cell antigen BCMA has shown response rates exceeding 70% and median duration of response of over 11 months. *van de Donk NWCJ et al. Lancet Haematol. [PMID: 34048683]*
CHAPTER 14: DISORDERS OF HEMOSTASIS, THROMBOSIS & ANTITHROMBOTIC THERAPY		
Antithrombotic Therapy	563	• For patients with morbid obesity, standard doses of apixaban or rivaroxaban should be chosen rather than using dabigatran or edoxaban. • DOACs are not recommended for VTE treatment in the acute setting following bariatric surgery but can be considered for ongoing treatment after the initial 4 weeks of therapy.
	571	• Heparins may be preferable as initial therapy in hospitalized patients with clinical instability and fluctuating renal or hepatic function, when bleeding risk is high, or when there is concern that thrombolysis may be required. *Stevens SM et al. Chest. [PMID: 34352278]*
Primary VTE Prevention & Treatment in Severe COVID-19	578	• Therapeutic dosing of anticoagulation may benefit some patients who are hospitalized in the acute care setting with COVID-19, who have very elevated D-dimer values and require supplemental oxygen, and who have low bleeding risk. • Patients who are critically ill in ICUs have not been shown to benefit from therapeutic dosing of anticogulation. • There is no clear benefit from VTE prophylaxis for patients with COVID-19 who do not require hospitalization. *ATTACC Investigators; ACTIV-4a Investigators; REMAP-CAP Investigators; Lawler PR et al. N Engl J Med. [PMID: 34351721]* *REMAP-CAP Investigators; ACTIV-4a Investigators; ATTACC Investigators; Goligher EC et al. N Engl J Med. [PMID: 34351722]* *Spyropoulos AC. JAMA Intern Med. [PMID: 34617959]*
CHAPTER 15: GASTROINTESTINAL DISORDERS		
Acute Diarrhea	591	• Immune checkpoint inhibitor therapy for malignancies may cause mild to severe GI side effects in 8–27% of patients. *Dougan M et al. Gastroenterology. [PMID: 33080231]* *Siciliano V et al. Rev Recent Clin Trials. [PMID: 32598272]*
	592	• Patients with severe diarrhea or dysentery and a known history of IBD or prior immune checkpoint inhibitor therapy require expedited evaluation with stool studies and possible sigmoidoscopy or colonoscopy with biopsy to exclude infection prior to therapy with intravenous corticosteroids. • Shiga-toxin–producing *Escherichia coli* infection should not be treated with antibiotics due to an increased risk of hemolytic-uremic syndrome, especially in children. *Dougan M et al. Gastroenterology. [PMID: 33080231]* *Siciliano V et al. Rev Recent Clin Trials. [PMID: 32598272]*
Anorectal Infections	670	• Nucleic acid amplification testing for gonorrhea and chlamydia has excellent sensitivity and specificity and is preferred in most clinical settings. *Workowski KA et al. MMWR Recomm Rep. [PMID: 34292926]*
Chronic Diarrhea	594	• Elevated fasting levels (> 48 ng/mL) of the bile acid precursor 7αC4 are strongly predictive of bile acid diarrhea. *Borup C et al. Am J Gastroenterol. [PMID: 32740083]*
Gastrointestinal Hemorrhage	630	• Endoscopic application of a topical hemostatic powder (Hemospray) may provide temporary hemostasis for up to 24 hours in patients with massive bleeding that interferes with effective application of thermocoagulation or endoclip placement. *Hussein M et al. Endoscopy. [PMID: 32459010]*
Inflammatory Bowel Disease	651	• Ozanimod is FDA-approved for the treatment of moderate to severe ulcerative colitis. *Sandborn WJ et al. N Engl J Med. [PMID: 34587385]*

*See chapter for further details and references.

(continued on following page)

Topic	Page Number	Key New Advances Affecting Clinical Practice*
Irritable Bowel Syndrome (IBS)	646	• Peppermint oil may be useful to relieve global IBS symptoms and abdominal pain. *Lacy BE et al. Am J Gastroenterol. [PMID: 33315591]*
	647	• Probiotics are not recommended for IBS treatment. *Lacy BE et al. Am J Gastroenterol. [PMID: 33315591]*
Other Primary Esophageal Motility Disorders	620	• Opioids may exacerbate esophageal dysmotility and should be discontinued, if possible. No medications have been shown to improve symptoms in patient with esophageal hypomotility. *DeLay K et al. Clin Gastroenterol Hepatol. [PMID: 34405804]*
Peptic Ulcer Disease	627	• Commercial laboratories now offer culture-based and molecular-based susceptibility testing for *Helicobacter pylori*, which may be helpful for patients who have failed an initial empiric course of treatment. *Graham DY. Gastroenterology. [PMID: 33647279]*
Zenker Diverticulum	615	• Minimally invasive intraluminal approaches that use flexible endoscopes or rigid esophagoscopes are preferred when symptomatic patients require cricopharyngeal myotomy. *Jirapinyo P et al. Gastrointest Endosc. [PMID: 33926711]*
CHAPTER 16: LIVER, BILIARY TRACT, & PANCREAS DISORDERS		
Cirrhosis	702	• In patients with clinically significant portal hypertension, carvedilol, a nonselective beta-receptor antagonist with alpha-1 blocking activity, appears to reduce the frequency of decompensating events, although it may lead to hypotension particularly in patients with decompensated cirrhosis. *Tandon P et al. Clin Gastroenterol Hepatol. [PMID: 33221550]*
	703	• Vancomycin should be added in patients with prior bacterial peritonitis or a positive surveillance swab for methicillin-resistant *Staphylococcus aureus*. Daptomycin should be added in patients with a positive surveillance swab for vancomycin-resistant enterococcus. Meropenem can be used in patients with current or recent exposure to piperacillin-tazobactam. *Biggins SW et al. Hepatology. [PMID: 33942342]*
Hemochromatosis	710	• Serum biomarkers of fibrosis may be an alternative to liver biopsy for identifying advanced fibrosis. *Chin J et al. Clin Gastroenterol Hepatol. [PMID: 32745684]*
Nonalcoholic Fatty Liver Disease	698	• Noninvasive approaches to the assessment of fibrosis are now preferred, with liver biopsy reserved when results of noninvasive testing are inconclusive. The FIB-4 score is often used particularly to exclude advanced fibrosis because of its simplicity. It is based on age, platelet count, and serum AST and ALT levels. *Younossi ZM et al. Am J Gastroenterol. [PMID: 33284184]*
Primary Biliary Cholangitis	708	• Obeticholic acid, a farnesoid X receptor agonist, can cause serious liver injury in patients with advanced cirrhosis, and its use in these patients has been restricted by the FDA. *Lleo A et al. Lancet. [PMID: 33308474]*

*See chapter for further details and references.

Topic	Page Number	Key New Advances Affecting Clinical Practice*
CHAPTER 17: BREAST DISORDERS		
Carcinoma of the Female Breast	752	• Olaparib has been shown to reduce the relative risk of an invasive recurrence for *BRCA1/2* carriers with high-risk disease; abemaciclib has been shown to improve the invasive disease-free survival for those with high-risk HR-positive disease; pembrolizumab has been shown to improve the event-free survival for patients with stage II or greater triple-negative breast cancer. *Schmid P et al; KEYNOTE-522 Investigators. N Engl J Med. [PMID: 32101663]* *Tutt ANJ et al; OlympiA Clinical Trial Steering Committee and Investigators. N Engl J Med. [PMID: 34081848]*
	754	• Hormonally driven breast cancer may be particularly sensitive to inhibition of cell cycle regulatory proteins, called cyclin dependent kinases 4 and 6 (CDK 4/6). Three oral CDK4/6 inhibitors—palbociclib, ribociclib, and abemaciclib—are FDA-approved for treatment of HR-positive, HER2-negative metastatic breast cancer. • Two poly(ADP-ribose) polymerase (PARP) inhibitors (olaparib and talazoparib) are FDA-approved for the treatment of BRCA-associated metastatic breast cancer. The NCCN guidelines include adjuvant olaparib for select patients and recommend germline genetic testing for any patient who may be a candidate for adjuvant olaparib. *Schmid P et al; KEYNOTE-522 Investigators. N Engl J Med. [PMID: 32101663]* *Tutt ANJ et al; OlympiA Clinical Trial Steering Committee and Investigators. N Engl J Med. [PMID: 34081848]*
CHAPTER 18: GYNECOLOGIC DISORDERS		
Intrauterine Devices	778	• The levonorgestrel 52-mg intrauterine device can be inserted within 5 days following a single episode of unprotected midcycle coitus as a postcoital contraceptive. *Turok DK et al. N Engl J Med. [PMID: 33503342]*
Pelvic Inflammatory Disease (Salpingitis, Endometritis)	786	• The recommended outpatient regimen is ceftriaxone (500 mg intramuscularly; 1 g for persons who weigh 150 kg or greater) plus doxycycline (100 mg orally twice a day for 14 days) with metronidazole 500 mg orally twice a day or a single dose of cefoxitin (2 g intramuscularly) with probenecid (1 g orally) plus doxycycline (100 mg orally twice daily for 14 days) and metronidazole 500 mg orally twice daily for 14 days. *Workowski KA et al. MMWR Recomm Rep. [PMID: 34292926]*
CHAPTER 19: OBSTETRICS & OBSTETRIC DISORDERS		
Cholelithiasis & Cholecystitis	817	• The most common cause of acute pancreatitis in pregnancy is gallstone disease. The diagnosis can be confirmed with an appropriate history and an elevated serum amylase or lipase. Management is conservative, including bowel rest, intravenous fluids, supplemental nutrition if necessary, and analgesics. CT imaging should be avoided unless severe complications are suspected. *Abushamma S et al. Obstet Gynecol. [PMID: 34011887]*
Immunizations During Pregnancy	795	• Vaccination against COVID-19 is recommended for women who are pregnant, trying to get pregnant or may become pregnant, and who are breastfeeding. The CDC has determined that the benefits of vaccination outweigh any risks. There is no evidence that vaccination causes problems with fertility in men or women. Pregnant women who have been vaccinated may receive the COVID-19 booster shot. There have been rare reports of thrombosis with thrombocytopenia syndrome in women younger than 50 years old who received the Johnson and Johnson's Janssen vaccine. This risk has not been found with the Pfizer-BioNTech and Moderna vaccines; women younger than 50 years old with access to multiple vaccines may want to factor this into their decision-making process. *CDC. https://www.cdc.gov/coronavirus/2019-ncov/vaccines/recommendations/pregnancy.html*
Maternal Hepatitis B & C Carrier State	816	• Universal screening for hepatitis C virus in pregnancy is recommended. Direct-acting antiviral regimens should only be initiated during pregnancy if in the setting of a clinical trial. Cesarean section is not recommended solely for a maternal history of hepatitis C. During labor, early rupture of membranes and placement of a fetal scalp electrode should be avoided if safe to do so. *Dotters-Katz SK et al. Am J Obstet Gynecol. [PMID: 34116035]*

*See chapter for further details and references.

(continued on following page)

Topic	Page Number	Key New Advances Affecting Clinical Practice*
Preterm Labor	805	• The recommended regimen for antimicrobial prophylaxis against group B streptococcus is penicillin G, 5 million units intravenously as a loading dose and then 2.5–3 million units intravenously every 4 hours until delivery. In penicillin-allergic patients not at high risk for anaphylaxis, 2 g of cefazolin can be given intravenously as an initial dose and then 1 g intravenously every 8 hours until delivery. In patients at high risk for anaphylaxis, vancomycin, 20 mg/kg intravenously every 8 hours until delivery, can be used. Clindamycin, 900 mg intravenously every 8 hours until delivery, can also be used after a group B streptococcal isolate has been confirmed to be susceptible to clindamycin. *American College of Obstetricians and Gynecologists. Obstet Gynecol. [PMID: 34794160]*
CHAPTER 20: RHEUMATOLOGIC, IMMUNOLOGIC, & ALLERGIC DISORDERS		
Complex Regional Pain Syndrome	867	• Vitamin C supplementation may have a role in preventing the development of complex regional pain syndrome following surgical procedures known to be a risk factor. *Jacques H et al. Int Orthop. [PMID: 33438072]*
Gonococcal Arthritis	863	• The treatment of disseminated gonorrhea is parenteral ceftriaxone. Once susceptibility testing has been obtained, 24–48 hours after clinical improvement the antibiotic regimen can be changed to an oral agent to complete a 7-day course. *CDC. https://www.cdc.gov/std/treatment-guidelines/gonorrhea-adults.htm*
Granulomatosis with Polyangiitis	853	• American College of Rheumatology/Vasculitis Foundation recommendations favor rituximab as first-line induction therapy. Cyclophosphamide may also be used for induction therapy. Avacopan is FDA-approved as add-on treatment for severe ANCA-associated vasculitis induction therapy in combination with rituximab or cyclophosphamide plus corticosteroids. • For nonsevere disease without life- or organ-threatening manifestations, methotrexate up to 25 mg oral or subcutaneous weekly plus corticosteroids may be effective induction therapy. • Rituximab, dosed at a fixed interval of 1 g every 6 months or 500 mg every 4 months, is favored as first-line maintenance treatment. *Chung SA et al. Arthritis Rheumatol. [PMID: 34235894]* *Jayne DRW et al; ADVOCATE Study Group. N Engl J Med. [PMID: 33596356]*
Polyarteritis Nodosa	851	• High-dose pulse methylprednisolone is recommended as the initial treatment for severe polyarteritis nodosa. *Chung SA et al. Arthritis Rheumatol. [PMID: 34235883]*
Relapsing Polychondritis	856	• A newly described genetic syndrome, VEXAS (vacuoles, E1 enzyme, X-linked, autoinflammatory, somatic), is caused by somatic mutations in *UBA1* in hematopoietic progenitor cells. Clinical features include hematologic manifestations (cytopenias, bone marrow failure) and a spectrum of inflammatory features such as chondritis, vasculitis, fever, and arthritis. This rare syndrome (predominately in males because it is X-linked) should be considered in the differential diagnosis of chondritis especially in the presence of an unexplained macrocytosis and evidence of systemic inflammation (ie, high ESR/CRP). *Ferrada MA et al. Arthritis Rheumatol. [PMID: 33779074]*
Rheumatoid Arthritis	831	• Because rituximab reduces the humoral immune response, it should be used with caution during the COVID-19 pandemic as multiple studies suggest a higher risk of mortality from COVID-19 in patients using this medication. *Fraenkel L et al. Arthritis Care Res (Hoboken). [PMID: 34101387]*
Systemic Lupus Erythematosus	835–836	• Belimumab is FDA-approved for the treatment of active lupus nephritis. • Anifrolumab, a type 1 interferon receptor antagonist, is FDA-approved to treat non-renal lupus that has not responded to standard therapies. • Voclosporin, a novel calcineurin inhibitor, is FDA-approved to treat active lupus nephritis when used in combination with mycophenolate mofetil. • Evidence increasingly suggests that renal response can be enhanced with combination immunosuppressive therapy. *Morand EF et al; TULIP-2 Trial Investigators. N Engl J Med. [PMID: 31851795]* *Rovin BH et al. Lancet. [PMID: 33971155]*

*See chapter for further details and references.

Topic	Page Number	Key New Advances Affecting Clinical Practice*
Systemic Sclerosis (Scleroderma)	841	• Tocilizumab, an IL-6 inhibitor, slows the rate of decline in pulmonary function and may be used as an alternative for patients who cannot tolerate mycophenolate mofetil. Azathioprine is an additional option for treatment of systemic sclerosis–associated lung disease. *Khanna D et al; focuSSced Investigators. Lancet Respir Med. [PMID: 32866440]*
CHAPTER 21: ELECTROLYTE & ACID-BASE DISORDERS		
Hyperkalemia	886	• Small studies have suggested the utility of patiromer and sodium zirconium cyclosilicate in acute hyperkalemia; if administered for hyperkalemic emergency, sodium zirconium cyclosilicate is preferred due to its more rapid onset of action. *Rafique Z et al. Acad Emerg Med. [PMID: 31599043]* *Peacock WF et al. Acam Emerg Med. [PMID: 32149451]*
CHAPTER 22: KIDNEY DISEASE		
Diabetic Nephropathy	935	• Mineralocorticoid receptor antagonism can be considered for blood pressure and proteinuria management in type 2 diabetes mellitus with careful monitoring for hyperkalemia. *Hahr AJ et al. Am J Kidney Dis. [PMID: 34600745]*
IgA Nephropathy	927	• SGLT2-inhibitors may be added to standard care in the well-selected patient. There are conflicting data regarding the efficacy of corticosteroids for reducing proteinuria and slowing progression; however, they may be considered for patients with GFR greater than 30 mL/ minute/1.73 m^2 and persistent proteinuria greater than 1 g/day despite maximal ACE inhibitor or ARB. *Cheung CK et al. J Clin Med. [PMID: 34200024]*
CHAPTER 24: NERVOUS SYSTEM DISORDERS		
Dementia	1016	• Aducanumab was approved by the FDA despite mixed results in clinical trials. Its use is limited to patients with mild cognitive impairment or mild dementia and amyloid pathology proven by amyloid PET. The ultimate role of this medication is still being debated.
Idiopathic Intracranial Hypertension (Pseudotumor Cerebri)	1005	• Weight loss is important: bariatric surgery led to a decrease in both intracranial pressure and weight at 2 years compared with a community weight management program in a randomized trial and may be considered in patients with a BMI of 35 or greater. *Mollan SP et al. JAMA Neurol. [PMID: 33900360]*
Metastatic Intracranial Tumors	1001	• Memantine (5 mg once daily orally titrated by 5 mg weekly to 10 mg twice daily) reduced cognitive toxicity associated with whole-brain radiotherapy in a randomized trial and is recommended; this effect can be augmented through intensity modulated radiation therapy with hippocampal avoidance. *Brown PD et al. J Clin Oncol. [PMID: 32058845]*
Muscular Dystrophies	1044	• Casimersen is FDA-approved for treatment of Duchenne muscular dystrophy; it shows benefit in patients with a mutation amenable to exon 45 skipping.
Transient Ischemic Attack (TIA)	987	• Dual antiplatelet therapy with aspirin and clopidogrel is recommended for 90 days after a TIA or stroke due to 70–99% stenosis of an intracranial artery. • The left atrial appendage is the source of embolism in most patients with atrial fibrillation. Several randomized trials showed percutaneous left atrial appendage closure was equivalent to anticoagulation in preventing stroke and systemic embolization, and several devices are approved for this indication in the United States and Europe. The procedure should be considered in patients with a contraindication to long-term anticoagulation, although short-term anticoagulation (45 days) followed by dual antiplatelet therapy (4.5 months) and then indefinite aspirin monotherapy is usually necessary after device placement. *Kleindorfer DO et al. 2021 Stroke. [PMID: 34024117]*
CHAPTER 25: PSYCHIATRIC DISORDERS		
Psychosexual Disorders	1059	• Bremelanotide is FDA-approved for the treatment of hypoactive sexual desire disorder in premenopausal women; however, the mechanism of action is unclear and subjective improvement is low. *Wheeler LJ et al. Obstet Gynecol. [PMID: 32541291]*

*See chapter for further details and references.

(continued on following page)

Topic	Page Number	Key New Advances Affecting Clinical Practice*
Somatic Symptom Disorders (Abnormal Illness Behavior)	1055	• Physical-based therapies such as speech/occupational/physical have strong evidence for improving symptoms in those suffering from functional neurologic disorder. *Gilmour GS et al. J Neurol. [PMID: 32193596]*
Trauma & Stressor-related Disorders	1048	• MDMA (methylenedioxymethamphetamine, also called ecstasy) significantly enhanced the treatment effects associated with manualized therapy for severe PTSD. *Mitchell JM et al. Nat Med. [PMID: 33972795]*
CHAPTER 28: LIPID DISORDERS		
Treatment of High LDL Cholesterol	1247	• The FDA approved the novel PCSK9 inhibitor inclisiran, which uses silencing RNA technology to reduce liver production of PCSK9 protein by approximately 80%. Twice-yearly dosing is novel for lipid-lowering therapy; inclisiran enables new delivery strategies, including in-clinic administration. *Raal FJ et al; ORION-9 Investigators. N Engl J Med. [PMID: 32197277]* *Ray KK et al; ORION-10 and ORION-11 Investigators. N Engl J Med. [PMID: 32187462]*
CHAPTER 29: NUTRITIONAL DISORDERS & OBESITY		
Obesity	1257	• Semaglutide, a GLP-1 receptor agonist, is FDA-approved for the treatment of obesity. *Wilding JPH et al. N Engl J Med. [PMID: 33567185]*
CHAPTER 30: COMMON PROBLEMS IN INFECTIOUS DISEASES & ANTIMICROBIAL THERAPY		
Infections in the Immunocompromised Patient	1276	• While the traditional approach was to continue antibiotics until resolution of neutropenia, current evidence supports earlier discontinuation of antibiotics in the neutropenic patient who becomes afebrile for 72 hours, if no signs or symptoms of infection persist.
CHAPTER 31: HIV INFECTION & AIDS		
HIV Infection & AIDS	1329	• In the ANCHOR study, which involved nearly 4500 individuals with anal high-grade squamous intraepithelial lesions (HGSIL), nine patients who were assigned to aggressive therapy (mostly office-based electrocautery) developed anal cancer compared with 21 of those in an active monitoring group, representing a 57% decrease in relative risk over the median 25.8-month follow-up period. This pivotal study will change care toward more aggressive screening for HGSIL and treatment to prevent progression to anal cancer. *Palefsky J et al. CROI 2022 (special session).*
	1332	• Cabotegravir was FDA-approved for use as preexposure prophylaxis as an injectable medication, every 8 weeks. This medication has been shown to be superior to oral tenofovir disoproxil fumarate/emtricitabine in preventing HIV infection among men who have sex with men, transgender women who have sex with men, and cisgender women in sub-Saharan Africa.
	1337	• Prophylaxis against *Mycobacterium avium* complex is no longer recommended in most individuals who are initiating antiretroviral therapy (ART), including in those with CD4+ counts less than 50 cells/mcL. The incidence of *M avium* complex infection is very low among those on ART.
	1338	• The TEMPRANO trial showed that individuals immediately initiating ART versus delaying treatment for CD4 count to fall below 500 cells/mcL had lower rates of severe illness.

*See chapter for further details and references.

Topic	Page Number	Key New Advances Affecting Clinical Practice*
CHAPTER 32: VIRAL & RICKETTSIAL INFECTIONS		
Ebola Viral Disease	1390	• The World Health Organization recommends automated or semi-automated nucleic acid tests (NATs) of EDTA-anticoagulated whole blood from symptomatic patients for routine diagnostic management, and rapid antigen detection tests in areas where NATs are not available. Oral fluid can be used for diagnostics when blood collection is not possible. *Choi MJ et al. MMWR Recomm Rep. [PMID: 33417593]*
Japanese Encephalitis	1382	• At least eight effective types of vaccine against Japanese encephalitis are available worldwide, including live attenuated and inactivated vaccines. *Kwak BO et al. Vaccine. [PMID: 33712352]*
Poliomyelitis	1375	• A novel oral polio vaccine type 2 (nOPV2) has been developed in response to the ongoing circulating vaccine-derived type 2 poliovirus outbreaks and has been shown to be safe and immunogenic in previously immunized adults. Studies have shown that nOPV2 is more genetically stable than the mOPV2 and therefore less prone to reverting to neurovirulence. The nOPV2 was recommended for initial use under the World Health Organization's Emergency Use Listing Procedure in November 2020. *Coster ID et al. Lancet. [PMID: 33308429]*
Severe Acute Respiratory Syndrome—COVID-19 (SARS-COV-2)	1401	• *CMDT* updates the ever-evolving knowledge of SARS-CoV-2 and the related disease online at www.accessmedicine.com
Tick-borne Encephalitis (TBE)	1383	• TicoVac (known as FSME-Immun in Europe) was FDA-approved. The vaccine is indicated for those residing and traveling to endemic areas (and the disease is now extending to higher altitudes with climate change). *Ličková M et al. Ticks Tick Borne Dis. [PMID: 32173297]*
CHAPTER 34: SPIROCHETAL INFECTIONS		
Lyme Disease (Lyme Borreliosis)	1493	• When assessing for CNS Lyme disease in an appropriate clinical syndrome, serum antibody testing is recommended over cerebrospinal fluid serology or PCR. • While serology is recommended to diagnose Lyme arthritis, PCR can be done on synovial fluid or tissue if needed to confirm the diagnosis and guide treatment. *Lantos PM et al. Clin Infect Dis. [PMID: 33417672]*
CHAPTER 35: PROTOZOAL & HELMINTHIC INFECTIONS		
African Trypanosomiasis (Sleeping Sickness)	1497	• Fexinidazole is recommended by the World Health Organization as first-line therapy and is FDA-approved for treatment of early and advanced (CNS) West African disease. *Hidalgo J et al. Cureus. [PMID: 34513456]*
Leishmaniasis	1501	• Alternative therapies increasingly used to treat cutaneous leishmaniasis are miltefosine, which benefits from oral dosing and relatively little toxicity, and amphotericin B, which is widely available. *Machado PRL et al. Clin Infect Dis. [PMID: 32894278]*
Malaria	1507	• Artemisinin resistance is mediated by any of a series of mutations in the *Plasmodium falciparum* kelch (K13) gene; of great concern, these same mutations and evidence for delayed clearance after treatment with artemisinins were reported in East Africa in 2021. *Balikagala B et al. N Engl J Med. [PMID: 34551228]*
CHAPTER 36: MYCOTIC INFECTIONS		
Candidiasis	1535	• Oral ibrexafungerp, a highly bioavailable glucan synthase inhibitor, may be used to treat vulvovaginal candidiasis from any disease-causing *Candida* strains, including azole-resistant pathogens. *Gold JAW et al. Clin Infect Dis. [PMID: 34079987]*

*See chapter for further details and references.

(continued on following page)

Topic	Page Number	Key New Advances Affecting Clinical Practice*
CHAPTER 38: POISONING		
Marijuana & Synthetic Cannabinoids	1585	• Cannabidiol (CBD) is a constituent of Cannabis that does not produce THC-like intoxication. CBD extracts are available over the counter and via the internet for a variety of proposed effects (anti-inflammatory, antioxidant, anxiolysis) and by prescription for some pediatric seizure disorders. Overdoses are typically not dangerous. *Alves VL et al. Crit Rev Toxicol. [PMID: 32530350]*
Theophylline & Caffeine	1592	• Hemodialysis has been used in patients with caffeine overdose. • Extracorporeal membrane oxygenation has been used successfully in hemodynamic collapse after caffeine overdose. *Ou HC et al. Am J Emerg Med. [PMID: 34922795]* *Yasuda S et al. Acute Med Surg. [PMID: 33532077]*
CHAPTER 39: CANCER		
Bladder Cancer	1644	• Pembrolizumab is FDA-approved for patients with high-risk, non–muscle invasive bladder cancers who have failed intravesical bacillus Calmette–Guérin therapy. Nivolumab has also been approved in the adjuvant setting after radical cystectomy or nephroureterectomy for urothelial carcinoma at high risk for recurrence. • The fibroblast growth factor receptor inhibitor erdafitinib is approved after initial therapy for patients with progressive metastatic urothelial carcinoma whose tumors harbor these mutations with expected response rates of up to 40%. • Enfortumab vedotin is the first antibody-drug conjugate approved for advanced and metastatic urothelial carcinoma. The antibody targets Nectin-4 and demonstrates a 44% response rate (including 12% complete response) in patients who have progressed after multiple other lines of therapy. *Bajorin DF et al. N Engl J Med. [PMID: 34077643]* *Balar AV et al. Lancet Oncol. [PMID: 34051177]* *Rosenberg JE at al. J Clin Oncol. [PMID: 31356140]*
Bronchogenic Carcinoma	1606–1607	• The FDA approved sotorasib (AMG 510) for the treatment of *KRAS* G12C mutated lung cancers after progression on first-line treatment. • Atezolizumab (PD-L1 inhibitor) can be given for 1 year post–adjuvant chemotherapy for resected stage II to IIIA NSCLC, based on a phase 3 trial showing improvement in disease-free survival compared with adjuvant chemotherapy without atezolizumab. For stage III NSCLCs, a phase 3 trial has shown improved survival outcomes by adding durvalumab (PD-L1 inhibitor) as consolidation therapy post–definitive chemoradiation. • Five-year follow-up data for patients with 50% or greater PD-L1 expression show that patients who received pembrolizumab versus chemotherapy alone had improved median overall survival of 26 months versus 13 months. *Skoulidis F et al. N Engl J Med. [PMID: 34096690]* *Reck M et al. J Clin Oncol. [PMID: 33872070]* *Felip E et al. Lancet. [PMID: 34555333]*
Colorectal Cancer (CRC)	1630	• For the 50% of patients with metastatic CRC who have *KRAS/NRAS/BRAF* wild-type tumors, cetuximab and panitumumab (monoclonal antibodies to the epithelial growth factor receptor), in combination with chemotherapy, can extend median survival by 2 to 4 months compared with chemotherapy alone. For the 5% to 10% with BRAF V600E sequence variations, targeted combination therapy with BRAF and EGFR inhibitors extend overall survival to 9.3 months, compared with 5.9 months for those receiving standard chemotherapy.
	1633	• In four randomized clinical trials (n = 458,002), intention to screen with 1- or 2-time flexible sigmoidoscopy versus no screening was associated with a significant decrease in CRC–specific mortality. *National Comprehensive Cancer Network. https://www.nccn.org/professionals/physician_gls/pdf/colon.pdf* *National Comprehensive Cancer Network. https://www.nccn.org/professionals/physician_gls/pdf/rectal.pdf* *Shaukat A et al. Am J Gastroenterol. [PMID: 33657038]*

*See chapter for further details and references.

Topic	Page Number	Key New Advances Affecting Clinical Practice*
Esophageal Cancer	1618	• For patients who complete neoadjuvant chemoradiation and undergo a complete resection but are found to have residual cancer in the resection specimen, a year of adjuvant immunotherapy with nivolumab is recommended. *Ahmed O et al. Clin Gastroenterol Hepatol. [PMID: 33813072]*
Gastric Adenocarcinoma	1621	• Triplet chemotherapy for resectable gastric cancer is recommended for patients who are fit but is associated with more toxicity than doublet chemotherapy.
	1622	• The development of immunotherapy represents a promising strategy in a selected patients with locally advanced and metastatic gastric cancer. Testing for microsatellite instability-high (MSI-H), mismatch repair deficiency (dMMR), PD-1, and PD-L1 is recommended in advanced disease to identify tumors that may respond to immunotherapy. *ASGE Standards of Practice Committee; Jue TL et al. Gastrointest Endosc. [PMID: 33168194]* *de Steur WO et al; CRITICS investigators. Ann Oncol. [PMID: 33227408]* *Kawazoe A et al. Jpn J Clin Oncol. [PMID: 33241322]* *Ng SP et al. Ann Surg Oncol. [PMID: 33689079]*
Malignancies of the Small Intestine	1625	• For advanced/unresectable disease, first-line doublet chemotherapy is standard. Two trials suggest value from adding bevacizumab to chemotherapy. Pembrolizumab is an accepted treatment modality for mismatch repair-deficient tumors. *National Comprehensive Cancer Network.* *https://www.nccn.org/professionals/physician_gls/pdf/small_bowel.pdf*
Prostate Cancer	1635	• Multiparametric MRI (mpMRI) has emerged as the imaging study of choice for localized prostate cancer detection and characterization. Suspicious prostatic lesions may then be sampled via MRI-guided needle biopsy or via MR Fusion (in which prostate MRI images are fused in real-time with images from an ultrasound-guided needle biopsy). Such an approach may improve discovery of potentially life-threatening disease while limiting over-detection of indolent prostate cancer or unnecessary prostate biopsies. *Kovac E et al. JAMA Netw Open. [PMID: 31940039]*
	1637	• NCCN guidelines recommend considering germline genetic testing in men presenting with localized high-risk, regionally advanced, or metastatic disease. Commercially available cancer tissue RNA-based assays are available for further risk assessment after prostate cancer diagnosis; these may help determine the need for and timing of prostate cancer treatment as well as treatment intensity. *Kovac E et al. JAMA Netw Open. [PMID: 31940039]*
	1637	• A secondary data analysis from the Prostate, Lung, Colorectal, and Ovarian trial demonstrated that baseline PSA for younger men in their 50s can predict long-term risk of prostate cancer and can be used to tailor PSA screening intervals. *Kovac E et al. JAMA Netw Open. [PMID: 31940039]*
	1638	• Active surveillance is now the preferred initial treatment recommendation for men with well-differentiated prostate cancer and low-risk clinical features. *Kovac E et al. JAMA Netw Open. [PMID: 31940039]*
	1641	• Results from the PEACE-1 trial demonstrate that a three-drug regimen, with androgen deprivation therapy, docetaxel and abiraterone acetate used together, provides the best survival outcome for men with hormone-naïve metastatic cancer. With this regimen, the median survival for men with de novo metastatic prostate cancer is now expected to be 5 years. *Kovac E et al. JAMA Netw Open. [PMID: 31940039]*
	1641	• Poly(ADP-ribose) polymerase (PARP) inhibitors represent a novel class of anticancer agents with some activity against prostate cancer, particularly those harboring mutations in genes important for homologous recombination such as *BRCA1*, *BRCA2*, and *ATM*. There are two FDA-approved PARP inhibitors available for men with metastatic castrate-resistant prostate cancer with these genetic alterations. *Kovac E et al. JAMA Netw Open. [PMID: 31940039]*

*See chapter for further details and references.

(continued on following page)

Topic	Page Number	Key New Advances Affecting Clinical Practice*
Renal Cell Carcinoma	1646	• For patients with von Hippel-Lindau disease and renal cell carcinoma, belzutifan, a HIF2a inhibitor, leads to dramatic size reductions in both renal and non-renal neoplasms and offers a new treatment option. • Pembrolizumab is FDA-approved for adjuvant treatment after surgical resection of renal cell carcinoma in patients at high risk for disease recurrence. • The SURTIME randomized trial compared immediate versus deferred cytoreductive nephrectomy in patients with metastatic renal cell carcinoma treated with sunitinib and showed an overall survival advantage with the deferred approach. This may serve to identify patients who respond the best to systemic therapy prior to undergoing removal of the primary tumor. *Bex A et al. JAMA Oncol. [PMID: 30543350]* *Jonasch E et al. N Engl J Med. [PMID: 34818478]* *Rini BI et al; KEYNOTE-426 Investigators. N Engl J Med. [PMID: 30779529]*
Toxicity & Dose Modification of Chemotherapeutic Agents	1657	• The main toxicities of immune checkpoint inhibitors involve immune-related adverse events which occur via the same mechanisms as their antitumor effects (ie, self-reactive T-cells escaping central tolerance). The combination of PD-1 or PD-L1 inhibitors with CTLA-4 inhibitors results in higher rates of grade 3 or higher and all grades of immune-related adverse events. *Brahmer JR et al. J Immunother Cancer. [PMID: 34172516]*
CHAPTER 41: ORTHOPEDIC DISORDERS & SPORTS MEDICINE		
Dupuytren Contracture	1691	• Some evidence suggests superior clinical outcomes of percutaneous needle aponeurotomy for Dupuytren Contracture compared with collagenase *Clostridium histolyticum* (CCH) injections and a higher minor complication rate with CCH. *Hirase T et al. J Hand Microsurg. [PMID: 34511831]*
Low Back Pain	1685	• Heat treatments have shown to have short-term benefits for acute low back pain. • There is good evidence that spinal manipulation and acupuncture provide short-term improvement compared with usual care alone. • Intra-articular steroid injections and cooled radiofrequency ablation of the sacral lateral branch nerves and dorsal ramus of L5 can be considered for patients with persistent sacroiliac joint pain. There is fair evidence that thermal radiofrequency ablation of the facet joints improves pain for at least 6 months. *Kreiner DS et al. Spine J. [PMID: 32333996]*
CHAPTER 42: SEXUAL, GENDER, & MINORITY HEALTH		
Health Care for Lesbian & Bisexual Women	1718	• One study of 150 lesbian, bisexual, and queer women offered preliminary evidence that social support, resilience, and self-esteem help foster body appreciation, which might be protective against mental health concerns and disordered eating.
	1714	• A report demonstrated significantly better reproductive outcomes after reciprocal in vitro fertilization (IVF), with a clinical pregnancy rate of 60% compared with 40% after autologous IVF, and live birth rate of 57.1% in reciprocal IVF versus 29.8% in autologous IVF. However, both partners of the couple need to be willing to participate in reciprocal IVF. *Burnette CB et al. Health Equity. [PMID 31289784]* *Núñez A et al. LGBT Health. [PMID: 34061679]*

*See chapter for further details and references.

Disease Prevention & Health Promotion

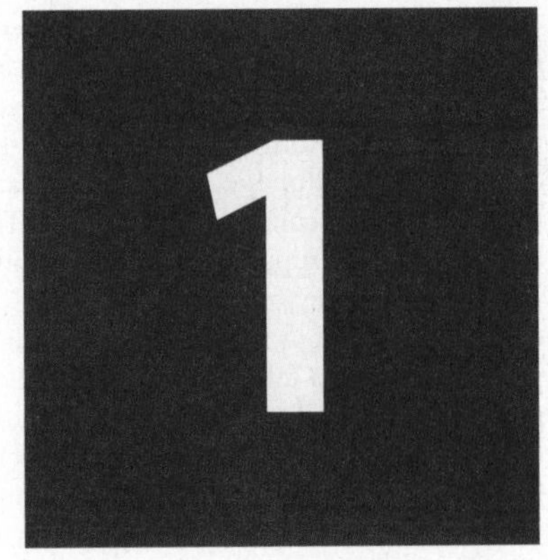

Michael Pignone, MD, MPH[1]
René Salazar, MD

GENERAL APPROACH TO THE PATIENT

The medical interview serves several functions. It is used to collect information to assist in diagnosis (the "history" of the present illness), to understand patient values, to assess and communicate prognosis, to establish a therapeutic relationship, and to reach agreement with the patient about further diagnostic procedures and therapeutic options. It also serves as an opportunity to influence patient behavior, such as in motivational discussions about smoking cessation or medication adherence. Interviewing techniques that avoid domination by the clinician increase patient involvement in care and patient satisfaction. Effective clinician-patient communication and increased patient involvement can improve health outcomes.

Patient Adherence

For many illnesses, successful prevention and treatment depends on difficult fundamental behavioral changes, including altering diet, taking up exercise, giving up smoking, cutting down drinking, wearing masks to prevent infection, and adhering to medication regimens that are often complex. Adherence is a problem in every practice; up to 50% of patients fail to achieve full adherence, and one-third never take their medicines. Many patients with medical problems, even those with access to care, do not seek appropriate care or may drop out of care prematurely. Adherence rates for short-term, self-administered therapies are higher than for long-term therapies and are inversely correlated with the number of interventions, their complexity and cost, and the patient's perception of overmedication.

As an example, in HIV-infected patients, adherence to antiretroviral therapy is a crucial determinant of treatment success. Studies have unequivocally demonstrated a close relationship between patient adherence and plasma HIV RNA levels, CD4 cell counts, and mortality. Adherence levels of more than 95% are needed to maintain virologic suppression. However, studies show that 40% of patients are less than 90% adherent and that adherence tends to decrease over time.

Patient reasons for suboptimal adherence include simple forgetfulness, being away from home, being busy, and changing daily routine. Other reasons include psychiatric disorders (depression or substance misuse), uncertainty about the effectiveness of treatment, lack of knowledge about the consequences of poor adherence, regimen complexity, and treatment side effects. The rising costs of medications, including generic drugs, and the increase in patient cost-sharing burden, have made adherence even more difficult, particularly for those with lower incomes.

Patients seem better able to take prescribed medications than to adhere to recommendations to change their diet, exercise habits, or alcohol intake or to perform various self-care activities (such as monitoring blood glucose levels at home). For short-term regimens, adherence to medications can be improved by giving clear instructions. Writing out advice to patients, including changes in medication, may be helpful. Because low functional health literacy is common (almost half of English-speaking US patients are unable to read and understand standard health education materials), other forms of communication—such as illustrated simple text, videotapes, or oral instructions—may be more effective. For non–English-speaking patients, clinicians and health care delivery systems can work to provide culturally and linguistically appropriate health services.

To help improve adherence to long-term regimens, clinicians can work with patients to reach agreement on the goals for therapy, provide information about the regimen, ensure understanding by using the "teach-back" method, counsel about the importance of adherence and how to organize medication-taking, reinforce self-monitoring, provide more convenient care, prescribe a simple dosage regimen for all medications (preferably one or two doses daily), suggest ways to help in remembering to take doses (time of day, mealtime, alarms) and to keep appointments, prescribe lower-cost generic medications when available, and provide ways to simplify dosing (medication boxes). Single-unit doses supplied in foil wrappers can increase adherence but should be avoided for patients who have difficulty opening them. Medication boxes with

[1]Dr. Pignone is a former member of the US Preventive Services Task Force (USPSTF). The views expressed in this chapter are his and Dr. Salazar's and not necessarily those of the USPSTF.

compartments (eg, Medisets) that are filled weekly are useful. Microelectronic devices can provide feedback to show patients whether they have taken doses as scheduled or to notify patients within a day if doses are skipped. Reminders, including cell phone text messages, are another effective means of encouraging adherence. The clinician can also enlist social support from family and friends, recruit an adherence monitor, provide a more convenient care environment, and provide rewards and recognition for the patient's efforts to follow the regimen. Collaborative programs in which pharmacists help ensure adherence are also effective. Motivational interviewing techniques can be helpful when patients are ambivalent about their therapy.

Adherence is also improved when a trusting doctor-patient relationship has been established and when patients actively participate in their care. Clinicians can improve patient adherence by inquiring specifically about the behaviors in question. When asked, many patients admit to incomplete adherence with medication regimens, with advice about giving up cigarettes, or with engaging only in "safer sex" practices. Although difficult, sufficient time must be made available for communication of health messages.

Medication adherence can be assessed generally with a single question: "In the past month, how often did you take your medications as the doctor prescribed?" Other ways of assessing medication adherence include pill counts and refill records; monitoring serum, urine, or saliva levels of drugs or metabolites; watching for appointment nonattendance and treatment nonresponse; and assessing predictable drug effects, such as weight changes with diuretics or bradycardia from beta-blockers. In some conditions, even partial adherence, as with drug treatment of hypertension and diabetes mellitus, improves outcomes compared with nonadherence; in other cases, such as HIV antiretroviral therapy or tuberculosis treatment, partial adherence may be worse than complete nonadherence.

Guiding Principles of Care

Ethical decisions are often called for in medical practice, at both the "micro" level of the individual patient-clinician relationship and at the "macro" level of allocation of resources or the adoption of infection-reducing public health interventions. Ethical principles that guide the successful approach to diagnosis and treatment are honesty, beneficence, justice, avoidance of conflict of interest, and the pledge to do no harm. Increasingly, Western medicine involves patients in important decisions about medical care, eg, which colorectal screening test to obtain or which modality of therapy for breast cancer or how far to proceed with treatment of patients who have terminal illnesses (see Chapter 5).

The clinician's role does not end with diagnosis and treatment. The importance of the empathic clinician in helping patients and their families bear the burden of serious illness and death cannot be overemphasized. "To cure sometimes, to relieve often, and to comfort always" is a French saying as apt today as it was five centuries ago—as is Francis Peabody's admonition: "The secret of the care of the patient is in caring for the patient." Training to improve mindfulness and enhance patient-centered communication increases patient satisfaction and may also improve clinician satisfaction.

Daliri S et al. Medication-related interventions delivered both in hospital and following discharge: a systematic review and meta-analysis. BMJ Qual Saf. 2021;30:146. [PMID: 32434936]

Foley L et al. Prevalence and predictors of medication non-adherence among people living with multimorbidity: a systematic review and meta-analysis. BMJ Open. 2021;11:e044987. [PMID: 34475141]

Peh KQE et al. An adaptable framework for factors contributing to medication adherence: results from a systematic review of 102 conceptual frameworks. J Gen Intern Med. 2021;36:2784. [PMID: 33660211]

HEALTH MAINTENANCE & DISEASE PREVENTION

Preventive medicine can be categorized as primary, secondary, or tertiary. Primary prevention aims to remove or reduce disease risk factors (eg, immunization, giving up or not starting smoking). Secondary prevention techniques promote early detection of disease or precursor states (eg, routine cervical Papanicolaou screening to detect carcinoma or dysplasia of the cervix). Tertiary prevention measures are aimed at limiting the impact of established disease (eg, partial mastectomy and radiation therapy to remove and control localized breast cancer).

Tables 1–1 and 1–2 give leading causes of death in the United States for 2020 and recent estimates of deaths from preventable causes from 2019. The 2020 data demonstrate the large impact of COVID-19 on mortality and continue to show increased mortality rates, generally driven by the effects of COVID-19 as well as increases in deaths from

Table 1–1. Leading causes of death in the United States, 2020.

Category	Estimate
All causes	**3,358,814**
1. Diseases of the heart	690,882
2. Malignant neoplasms	598,932
3. COVID-19	345,323
4. Unintentional injuries	192,176
5. Cerebrovascular diseases	159,050
6. Chronic lower respiratory diseases	151,637
7. Alzheimer disease	133,382
8. Diabetes mellitus	101,106
9. Influenza and pneumonia	53,495
10. Nephritis, nephrotic syndrome, and nephrosis	52,260
11. Intentional self-harm (suicide)	44,834

Data from National Center for Health Statistics, 2021.

Table 1–2. Leading preventable causes of death in the United States, 2019.

Category	Estimate
Tobacco	546,401
High blood pressure	495,201
High fasting plasma glucose	439,212
Dietary risks	418,350
High BMI	392,352
High LDL cholesterol	226,343
Impaired kidney function	214,740
Alcohol use	136,866
Non-optimal temperature	126,623
Drug use	104,141

Data from the US Burden of Disease Collaborators, 2021.

heart disease, unintentional injuries (including overdoses), and Alzheimer disease.

Many effective preventive services are underutilized, and few adults receive all of the most strongly recommended services. Several methods, including the use of provider or patient reminder systems (including interactive patient health records), reorganization of care environments, and possibly provision of financial incentives to clinicians (though this remains controversial), can increase utilization of preventive services, but such methods have not been widely adopted.

Ahmad FB et al. The leading causes of death in the US for 2020. JAMA. 2021;325:1829. [PMID: 33787821]
Levine DM et al. Quality and experience of outpatient care in the United States for adults with or without primary care. JAMA Intern Med. 2019;179:363. [PMID: 30688977]
US Burden of Disease Collaborators. The state of US health, 1990–2016: burden of diseases, injuries, and risk factors among US states. JAMA. 2018;319:1444. [PMID: 29634829]
Woolf SH et al. Life expectancy and mortality rates in the United States, 1959–2017. JAMA. 2019;322:1996. [PMID: 31769830]

PREVENTION OF INFECTIOUS DISEASES

Much of the historic decline in the incidence and fatality rates of infectious diseases is attributable to public health measures—especially immunization, improved sanitation, nonpharmacologic interventions (eg, mask-wearing to prevent respiratory-transmissible conditions), and better nutrition. This observation has been reinforced by the experience during the global COVID-19 pandemic.

Immunization remains the best means of preventing many infectious diseases. Recommended immunization schedules for children and adolescents can be found online at http://www.cdc.gov/vaccines/schedules/hcp/child-adolescent.html, and the schedule for adults is at http://www.cdc.gov/vaccines/schedules/hcp/adult.html (see also Chapter 30 and Chapter 32). In addition to the severe toll in morbidity and mortality from COVID-19, substantial morbidity and mortality continues to occur from vaccine-preventable diseases, such as hepatitis A, hepatitis B, influenza, and pneumococcal infections. The high incidence and mortality rates from COVID-19 and other recent outbreaks of vaccine-preventable diseases in the United States highlight the need to understand the association of vaccine hesistancy or refusal and disease epidemiology and methods for overcoming it.

The Advisory Committee on Immunization Practices recommendations for the following vaccines appears in Table 1–3: influenza; measles, mumps, and rubella; 23-valent pneumococcal polysaccharide vaccine; tetanus, diphtheria, and acellular pertussis; hepatitis B; and HPV.

Persons traveling to countries where infections are endemic should take the precautions described in Chapter 30 and at https://wwwnc.cdc.gov/travel/destinations/list. Immunization registries—confidential, population-based, computerized information systems that collect vaccination data about all residents of a geographic area—can be used to increase and sustain high vaccination coverage.

Globally, **COVID-19** has resulted in over 5 million deaths. COVID-19 is caused by SARS-CoV-2. The impact on frontline workers, including health care workers, has been substantial, and the pandemic has revealed profound inequities in health and health care. In the United States, the COVID-19 mortality rates are higher in Black, Latinx, and Native American people compared to White people. Three COVID-19 vaccines are currently approved or authorized in the United States (Pfizer-BioNTech/Comirnaty, Moderna, and Janssen [Johnson & Johnson]). Currently, the CDC recommends everyone ages 5 and older get a COVID-19 vaccine to help protect against COVID-19 (see Chapter 32). Recent guidance has recommended third-dose boosters to be administered 6 months after primary series completion for individuals receiving Pfizer and Moderna mRNA-vaccines and 2 months after those receiving the Janssen adenovirus vector vaccine.

The USPSTF recommends behavioral counseling for adolescents and adults who are sexually active and at increased risk for **sexually transmitted infections.** Sexually active women aged 24 years or younger and older women who are at increased risk for infection should be screened for chlamydia and gonorrhea. Screening HIV-positive men or men who have sex with men for syphilis every 3 months is associated with improved syphilis detection.

The CDC recommends universal HIV screening of all patients aged 13–64, and the USPSTF recommends that clinicians screen adolescents and adults aged 15–65 years. Clinicians should integrate biomedical and behavioral approaches for HIV prevention. In addition to reducing sexual transmission of HIV, initiation of antiretroviral therapy reduces the risk for AIDS-defining events and death among patients with less immunologically advanced disease.

Daily **preexposure prophylaxis (PrEP)** with the fixed-dose combination of tenofovir disoproxil 300 mg and emtricitabine 200 mg (Truvada) should be considered for people who are HIV-negative but at substantial risk for HIV infection. Studies of men who have sex with men suggest that PrEP is very effective in reducing the risk of

Table 1–3. Advisory Committee on Immunization Practices vaccine recommendations, 2021.

Vaccine	Recommendation	Comment
Influenza	Routine vaccination for all persons aged 6 months and older, including all adults An alternative high-dose inactivated vaccine is available for adults aged 65 years and older	When vaccine supply is limited, certain groups should be given priority, such as adults aged 50 years and older, individuals with chronic illness or immunosuppression, and pregnant women
MMR	Two doses for adults at high risk for exposure and transmission (eg, college students, health care workers); otherwise, one dose for adults aged 18 years and older	Physician documentation of disease is not acceptable evidence of MMR immunity
PPSV23	Adults aged 65 and older If PPSV23 was administered prior to age 65 years, administer one dose PPSV23 at least 5 years after previous dose A shared clinical decision-making approach is recommended for use of PCV13 in average-risk individuals aged 65 and older	
Tdap	Routine use of a single dose of for adults aged 19–64 years	Replaces the next booster dose of Td
Hepatitis B	Three-dose series is recommended for all children aged 0–18 years and high-risk individuals (ie, health care workers, injection drug users, people with ESKD) Recommended for diabetic patients aged 19–59 years Should be considered in diabetic persons age 60 and older	Prevents chronic hepatitis B and cirrhosis and their predispositions to HCC
HPV VLP	Routine HPV vaccination for children and adults aged 9–26 years Shared decision-making is recommended for some individuals between 27 and 45 years of age (vaccine is not licensed for adults older than 45 years)	Prevents persistent HPV infections effectively and thus may impact the rate of CIN II–II

CIN, cervical intraepithelial neoplasia; HCC, hepatocellular carcinoma; HPV VLP, human papillomavirus virus-like particle vaccine; MMR, measles, mumps, and rubella vaccine; PCV13, 13-valent pneumococcal conjugate vaccine; PPSV23, 23-valent pneumococcal polysaccharide vaccine; Td, tetanus and diphtheria toxoids vaccine; Tdap, tetanus, diphtheria, and five-component acellular pertussis vaccine.

contracting HIV. Patients taking PrEP should be encouraged to use other prevention strategies, such as consistent condom use to maximally reduce their risk. **Postexposure prophylaxis (PEP)** with combinations of antiretroviral drugs is widely used after occupational and nonoccupational contact and may reduce the risk of transmission by approximately 80%. PEP should be initiated within 72 hours of exposure.

Herpes zoster, caused by reactivation from previous varicella zoster virus infection, affects many older adults and people with immune system dysfunction. The ACIP recommends the herpes zoster subunit vaccine (HZ/su; Shingrix) be used for the prevention of herpes zoster and related complications in immunocompetent adults age 50 and older and in individuals who previously received Zostavax.

Centers for Disease Control and Prevention (CDC). COVID-19, 2021. https://www.cdc.gov/coronavirus/2019-ncov/index.html

Centers for Disease Control and Prevention (CDC). About COVID-19 vaccines (updated January 21, 2022). https://www.cdc.gov/coronavirus/2019-ncov/vaccines/about-vaccines/index.html

Centers for Disease Control and Prevention (CDC). Pneumococcal vaccination. https://www.cdc.gov/vaccines/schedules/hcp/imz/adult.html

Centers for Disease Control and Prevention (CDC). Recommended adult immunization schedule for ages 19 years or older, United States, 2020. https://www.cdc.gov/vaccines/schedules/hcp/imz/adult.html

Chou R et al. Epidemiology of and risk factors for coronavirus infection in health care workers: a living rapid review. Ann Intern Med. 2020;173:120. [PMID: 32369541]

PREVENTION OF CARDIOVASCULAR DISEASE

CVDs, including CHD and stroke, represent two of the most important causes of morbidity and mortality in developed countries. Several risk factors increase the risk for coronary disease and stroke. These risk factors can be divided into those that are modifiable (eg, lipid disorders, hypertension, cigarette smoking) and those that are not (eg, age, sex, family history of early coronary disease). Impressive declines in age-specific mortality rates from heart disease and stroke have been achieved in all age groups in North America from 1980 to 2015, in large part through improvement of modifiable risk factors: reductions in cigarette smoking, improvements in lipid levels, and more aggressive detection and treatment of hypertension. However, the past several years have seen a disturbing increase in cardiovascular deaths in the United States and leveling off of the reduction in cardiovascular mortality rates. This section considers the role of screening for cardiovascular risk and the use of effective therapies to reduce such risk. Key recommendations for cardiovascular prevention are shown in Table 1–4. Guidelines encourage regular assessment of global cardiovascular risk in adults 40–79 years of age without known CVD, using standard

Table 1–4. Expert recommendations for cardiovascular risk prevention methods: USPSTF.[1]

Prevention Method	Recommendation/[Year Issued]
Screening for AAA	Recommends one-time screening for AAA by ultrasonography in men aged 65–75 years who have ever smoked. (B) Selectively offer screening for AAA in men aged 65–75 years who have never smoked. (C) Current evidence is insufficient to assess the balance of benefits and harms of screening for AAA in women aged 65–75 years who have ever smoked or have a family history of AAA. (I) Recommends against routine screening for AAA in women who have never smoked and have no family history of AAA. (D) [2019]
Aspirin use	Recommends initiating low-dose aspirin use for the primary prevention of cardiovascular disease (CVD) and colorectal cancer (CRC) in adults aged 50–59 years who have a 10% or greater 10-year CVD risk, are not at increased risk for bleeding, have a life expectancy of at least 10 years, and are willing to take low-dose aspirin daily for at least 10 years. (B) The decision to initiate low-dose aspirin use for the primary prevention of CVD and CRC in adults aged 60–69 years who have a 10% or greater 10-year CVD risk should be an individual one. Persons who are not at increased risk for bleeding, have a life expectancy of at least 10 years, and are willing to take low-dose aspirin daily for at least 10 years are more likely to benefit. Persons who place a higher value on the potential benefits than the potential harms may choose to initiate low-dose aspirin. (C) The current evidence is insufficient to assess the balance of benefits and harms of initiating aspirin use for the primary prevention of CVD and CRC in adults younger than 50 years or older than age 70. (I) [2016]
Blood pressure screening	Recommends screening for hypertension in adults 18 years or older with office blood pressure measurement. Recommends obtaining blood pressure measurements outside of the clinical setting for diagnostic confirmation before starting treatment. (A) [2021]
Serum lipid screening and use of statins for prevention	Recommends that adults without a history of CVD use a low- to moderate-dose statin for the prevention of CVD events and mortality when all of the following criteria are met: (1) they are aged 40–75 years; (2) they have one or more CVD risk factors (ie, dyslipidemia, diabetes mellitus, hypertension, or smoking); and (3) they have a calculated 10-year risk of a cardiovascular event of 10% or greater. Identification of dyslipidemia and calculation of 10-year CVD event risk requires universal lipids screening in adults aged 40–75 years. See the "Clinical Considerations" section of the USPSTF recommendations[1] for more information on lipids screening and the assessment of cardiovascular risk. (B) Concludes that the current evidence is insufficient to assess the balance of benefits and harms of initiating statin use for the primary prevention of CVD events and mortality in adults aged 76 years and older without a history of heart attack or stroke. (I) [2016]
Counseling about healthful diet and physical activity for CVD prevention	Recommends offering or referring adults with cardiovascular disease risk factors to behavioral counseling interventions to promote a healthy diet and physical activity. (B) [2020] Recommends that primary care professionals individualize the decision to offer or refer adults without obesity who do not have hypertension, dyslipidemia, abnormal blood glucose levels, or diabetes to behavioral counseling to promote a healthful diet and physical activity. (C) [2017]
Screening for diabetes mellitus	The USPSTF recommends screening for prediabetes and type 2 diabetes in adults aged 35–70 years who have overweight or obesity. Clinicians should offer or refer patients with prediabetes to effective preventive interventions. (B) [2021]
Screening for smoking and counseling to promote cessation	Recommends that clinicians ask all adults about tobacco use, advise them to stop using tobacco, and provide those who use tobacco behavioral interventions, and prescribe US FDA–approved pharmacotherapy to nonpregnant adults. (A) [2021]

USPSTF recommendations available at http://www.uspreventiveservicestaskforce.org/BrowseRec/Index/browse-recommendations.
Recommendation A: The USPSTF strongly recommends that clinicians routinely provide the service to eligible patients. (The USPSTF found good evidence that the service improves important health outcomes and concludes that benefits substantially outweigh harms.)
Recommendation B: The USPSTF recommends that clinicians routinely provide the service to eligible patients. (The USPSTF found at least fair evidence that the service improves important health outcomes and concludes that benefits substantially outweigh harms.)
Recommendation C: The USPSTF makes no recommendation for or against routine provision of the service.
Recommendation D: The USPSTF recommends against routinely providing the service to asymptomatic patients. (The USPSTF found at least fair evidence that the service is ineffective or that harms outweigh benefits.)
Recommendation I: The USPSTF concludes that the evidence is insufficient to recommend for or against routinely providing the service.

cardiovascular risk factors. The role of nontraditional risk factors for improving risk estimation remains unclear.

Cho L et al. Summary of updated recommendations for primary prevention of cardiovascular disease in women: JACC State-of-the-Art Review. J Am Coll Cardiol. 2020;75:2602. [PMID: 32439010]
Roth GA et al. Global burden of cardiovascular diseases and risk factors, 1990–2019: update from the GBD 2019 study. J Am Coll Cardiol. 2020;76:2982. [PMID: 33309175]

Abdominal Aortic Aneurysm

One-time screening for AAA by ultrasonography is recommended by the USPSTF (B recommendation) in men aged 65–75 years who have ever smoked. One-time screening for AAA is associated with a relative reduction in odds of AAA-related mortality over 12–15 years (OR, 0.65 [95% CI 0.57–0.74]) and a similar reduction in AAA-related ruptures (OR, 0.62 [95% CI 0.55–0.70]). Women who have never smoked and who have no family history of AAA do not appear to benefit from such screening (D recommendation); the current evidence for women who have ever smoked or who have a family history of AAA is insufficient to assess the balance of risks versus benefits (I recommendation) (Table 1–4).

Guirguis-Blake JM et al. Primary care screening for abdominal aortic aneurysm: updated evidence report and systematic review for the US Preventive Services Task Force. JAMA. 2019;322:2219. [PMID: 31821436]
US Preventive Services Task Force, Owens DK et al. Screening for abdominal aortic aneurysm: US Preventive Services Task Force Recommendation Statement. JAMA. 2019;322:2211. [PMID: 31821437]
Ying AJ et al. Abdominal aortic aneurysm screening: a systematic review and meta-analysis of efficacy and cost. Ann Vasc Surg. 2019;54:298. [PMID: 30081169]

Cigarette Smoking

Cigarette smoking remains the most important cause of preventable morbidity and early mortality. In 2019, there were an estimated 7.69 million deaths in the world attributable to smoking and tobacco use (13.6% of all deaths worldwide); smoking is the second leading cause of disability-adjusted life-years lost overall and leading cause among men. Cigarettes are responsible for one in every five deaths in the United States, or over 480,000 deaths annually. Annual cost of smoking-related health care is approximately $130 billion in the United States, with another $150 billion in productivity losses. Fortunately, US smoking rates have been declining; in 2015, 15.1% of US adults were smokers, and by 2018, 13.7% were smokers. Global direct health care costs from smoking in 2012 were estimated at $422 billion, with total costs of over $1.4 trillion.

Over 1.3 million deaths worldwide are attributed to secondhand smoke in 2019.

Although tobacco use constitutes one of the most serious common medical problems, it is undertreated. Almost 40% of smokers attempt to quit each year, but only 4% are successful. Persons whose clinicians advise them to quit are 1.6 times as likely to attempt quitting. Over 70% of smokers see a physician each year, but only 20% of them receive any medical quitting advice or assistance.

Factors associated with successful cessation include having a rule against smoking in the home, being older, and having greater education. Several effective clinical interventions are available to promote smoking cessation, including counseling, pharmacotherapy, and combinations of the two.

Helpful counseling strategies are shown in Table 1–5. Additionally, a system should be implemented to identify smokers, and advice to quit should be tailored to the patient's level of readiness to change. All patients trying to quit should be offered pharmacotherapy (Table 1–6) except those with medical contraindications, women who are

Table 1–5. Inquiries to help in support of smoking cessation.

Component	Helpful Clinician Statements and Inquiries
Communicate your caring and concern	"I am concerned about the effects of smoking on your health… • and want you to know that I am willing to help you quit." • and so how do you feel about quitting?" • do you have any fears or ambivalent feelings about quitting?"
Encourage the patient to talk about the quitting process	"Tell me… • why do you want to quit smoking?" • when you tried quitting smoking in the past, what sort of difficulties did you encounter?" • were you able to succeed at all, even for a while?" • what concerns or worries do you have about quitting now?"
Provide basic information about smoking (eg, its addictive nature) and successful quitting (eg, nature and time course of withdrawal)	"Did you know that… • the nicotine in cigarette smoke is highly addictive?" • within a day of stopping, you will notice nicotine withdrawal symptoms, such as irritability and craving?" • after you quit, any smoking (even a single puff) makes it likely that you will fully relapse into smoking again?"
Encourage the patient to make a quit attempt	"I want you to reassure you that… • as your clinician, I believe you are going to be able to quit." • there are now available many effective smoking cessation treatments." • more than half the people who have *ever* smoked have now successfully quit."

Table 1–6. Medications for tobacco dependence and smoking cessation.

Drug	Some Formulations	Usual Adult Dosage[1,2]	Cost 30/days
Nicotine Replacement Therapies (NRTs)			
Nicotine transdermal patch[3] – generic (NicoDerm CQ)	7, 14, 21 mg/24-h patches	1 patch/day[4]	$51.40
Nicotine polacrilex gum[3] – generic (Nicorette gum)	2, 4 mg/pieces	8–24 pieces/day[4,5,6]	$63.12
Nicotine polacrilex lozenge[3,7] – generic (Nicorette lozenge)	2, 4 mg/lozenges	8–20 lozenges/day[4,5,8]	$66.24
Nicotine oral inhaler – Nicotrol	10 mg cartridges[9]	4–16 cartridges/day[4]	$578.66
Nicotine nasal spray – Nicotrol NS	200 sprays/10 mL bottles (0.5 mg/spray)	2 sprays 8–40×/day (max 10 sprays/h)[3]	$607.60 (4-bottle package)
Dopaminergic-Noradrenergic Reuptake Inhibitor			
Bupropion SR – generic	100, 150, 200 mg SR tablets[10]	150 mg orally once daily × 3 days, then 150 mg orally twice daily	$112.80
Nicotinic Receptor Partial Agonist			
Varenicline tartrate – Chantix	0.5, 1 mg tablets	0.5 mg orally once daily × 3 days, then 0.5 mg twice daily on days 4–7, then 1 mg twice daily	$603.41

SR, sustained-release.
[1]Dosage reductions may be needed for liver or kidney impairment.
[2]Patients should receive a minimum of 3–6 months of effective therapy. In general, the dosage of NRTs can be tapered at the end of treatment; bupropion SR and varenicline can usually be stopped without a gradual dosage reduction, but some clinicians recommend a taper.
[3]Available over the counter for persons ≥ 18 years old.
[4]See expanded table for dosage titration instructions, available at: medicalletter.org/TML-article-1576c.
[5]Avoid eating or drinking within 15 minutes of using a gum or lozenge.
[6]A second piece of gum can be used within 1 hour. Continuously chewing one piece after another is not recommended.
[7]Also available in a mini-lozenge.
[8]Maximum of 5 lozenges in 6 hours or 20 lozenges/day. Use of more than 1 lozenge at a time or continuously using one after another is not recommended.
[9]Each cartridge delivers 4 mg of nicotine.
[10]Only the generic 150-mg SR tablets are FDA-approved as a smoking cessation aid.
Reprinted with special permission from The Medical Letter on Drugs and Therapeutics, July 15, 2019; Vol. 61 (1576):106.
Average wholesale price (AWP, for AB-rated generic when available) for quantity listed. Source: IBM Micromedex® Red Book (electronic version). IBM Watson Health, Greenwood Village, Colorado, USA. Available at https://www-micromedexsolutions-com.proxy.hsl.ucdenver.edu (cited: March, 11, 2022). AWP may not accurately represent the actual pharmacy cost because wide contractual variations exist among institutions.

pregnant or breast-feeding, and adolescents. Weight gain occurs in most patients (80%) following smoking cessation. Average weight gain is 2 kg, but for some (10–15%), major weight gain—over 13 kg—may occur. Planning for the possibility of weight gain, and means of mitigating it, may help with maintenance of cessation.

Several pharmacologic therapies shown to be effective in promoting cessation are summarized in Table 1–6. Nicotine replacement therapy doubles the chance of successful quitting. The nicotine patch, gum, and lozenges are available over the counter and nicotine nasal spray and inhalers by prescription. The sustained-release antidepressant drug bupropion (150–300 mg/day orally) is an effective smoking cessation agent and is associated with minimal weight gain, although seizures are a contraindication. It acts by boosting brain levels of dopamine and norepinephrine, mimicking the effect of nicotine. Varenicline, a partial nicotinic acetylcholine-receptor agonist, has been shown to improve cessation rates; however, its adverse effects, particularly its effects on mood, are not completely understood and warrant careful consideration. No single pharmacotherapy is clearly more effective than others, so patient preferences and data on adverse effects should be taken into account in selecting a treatment. Combination therapy is more effective than a single pharmacologic modality. The efficacy of e-cigarettes in smoking cessation has not been well evaluated, and some users may find them addictive. Recent reports of "vaping-related" lung disease should prompt additional caution in the use of unregulated nicotine delivery devices for smoking cessation (see Chapter 9).

Clinicians should not show disapproval of patients who fail to stop smoking or who are not ready to make a quit attempt. Thoughtful advice that emphasizes the benefits of cessation and recognizes common barriers to success can increase motivation to quit and quit rates. An upcoming medical procedure or intercurrent illness or hospitalization may motivate even the most addicted smoker to quit.

Individualized or group counseling is very cost effective, even more so than treating hypertension. Smoking cessation counseling by telephone ("quitlines") and text messaging–based interventions have both proved effective. An additional strategy is to recommend that any smoking take place outdoors to limit the effects of passive smoke on housemates and coworkers. This can lead to smoking reduction and quitting.

Public policies, including higher cigarette taxes and more restrictive public smoking laws, have also been shown to encourage cessation, as have financial incentives directed to patients.

Anonymous. Drugs for smoking cessation. Med Lett Drugs Ther. 2019;61:105. [PMID: 31381546]

Black N et al. Behaviour change techniques associated with smoking cessation in intervention and comparator groups of randomized controlled trials: a systematic review and meta-regression. Addiction. 2020;115:2008. [PMID: 32196796]

Centers for Disease Control and Prevention (CDC). Current cigarette smoking among adults in the United States. 2020 December 10. https://www.cdc.gov/tobacco/data_statistics/fact_sheets/adult_data/cig_smoking/index.htm

Hollands GJ et al. Interventions to increase adherence to medications for tobacco dependence. Cochrane Database Syst Rev. 2019;8:CD009164. [PMID: 31425618]

Tibuakuu M et al. National trends in cessation counseling, prescription medication use, and associated costs among US adult cigarette smokers. JAMA Netw Open. 2019;2:e194585. [PMID: 31125108]

Villanti AC et al. Smoking-cessation interventions for U.S. young adults: updated systematic review. Am J Prev Med. 2020;59:123. [PMID: 32418800]

Lipid Disorders

Higher LDL cholesterol concentrations and lower HDL levels are associated with an increased risk of CHD (see Chapter 28). Measurement of total and HDL cholesterol levels can help assess the degree of CHD risk. The best age to start screening is controversial, as is its frequency. Cholesterol-lowering therapy reduces the relative risk of CHD events, with the degree of reduction proportional to the reduction in LDL cholesterol achieved, at least at initial LDL levels greater than 100 mg/dL. The absolute benefits of screening for—and treating—abnormal lipid levels depend on the presence and level of other cardiovascular risk factors, including hypertension, diabetes mellitus, smoking, age, and sex. If other risk factors are present, atherosclerotic CVD risk is higher and the potential benefits of therapy are greater. Patients with known CVD are at higher risk and have larger benefits from reduction in LDL cholesterol. The optimal risk threshold for initiating statins for primary prevention remains somewhat controversial, although most guidelines now suggest statin therapy when the 10-year atherosclerotic cardiovascular risk is greater than 10%. Use of a cardiovascular risk calculator can help inform decision making for primary prevention.

Evidence for the effectiveness of statin-type drugs is better than for the other classes of lipid-lowering agents or dietary changes specifically for improving lipid levels. Multiple large, randomized, placebo-controlled trials have demonstrated important reductions in total mortality, major coronary events, and strokes with lowering levels of LDL cholesterol by statin therapy for patients with known CVD. Statins also reduce cardiovascular events for patients with diabetes mellitus. For patients with no previous history of cardiovascular events or diabetes, meta-analyses have shown important reductions of cardiovascular events.

Newer antilipidemic monoclonal antibody agents (eg, evolocumab and alirocumab) lower LDL cholesterol by 50–60% by binding proprotein convertase subtilisin kexin type 9 (PCSK9), which decreases the degradation of LDL receptors. PCSK9 inhibitors also decrease Lp(a) levels. These newer agents are very expensive so are often used mainly in high-risk patients when statin therapy does not reduce the LDL cholesterol sufficiently at maximally tolerated doses or when patients are intolerant of statins. So far, few side effects have been reported with PCSK9 inhibitor use.

Guidelines for statin and PCSK9 therapy are discussed in Chapter 28.

Lloyd-Jones DM et al. Use of risk assessment tools to guide decision-making in the primary prevention of atherosclerotic cardiovascular disease: a special report from the American Heart Association and American College of Cardiology. Circulation. 2019;139:e1162. [PMID: 30423392]

Mortensen MB et al. Elevated LDL cholesterol and increased risk of myocardial infarction and atherosclerotic cardiovascular disease in individuals aged 70–100 years: a contemporary primary prevention cohort. Lancet. 2020;396:1644. [PMID: 33186534]

Navarese EP et al. Association between baseline LDL-C level and total and cardiovascular mortality after LDL-C lowering: a systematic review and meta-analysis. JAMA. 2018;319:1566. [PMID: 29677301]

Hypertension

According to the American Heart Association, over 133 million US adults have hypertension, of which approximately 83 million are eligible for pharmacologic treatment. Of these 83 million, hypertension is treated in only about 66% and well controlled in only about 30% (see Chapter 11). In every adult age group, higher values of systolic and diastolic blood pressure carry greater risks of stroke and heart failure. Systolic blood pressure is a better predictor of morbid events than diastolic blood pressure. Home monitoring is better correlated with target organ damage than clinic-based values. Clinicians can apply specific blood pressure criteria, such as those of the Joint National Committee or American Heart Association guidelines, along with consideration of the patient's cardiovascular risk and personal values, to decide at what levels treatment should be considered in individual cases.

Primary prevention of hypertension can be accomplished by strategies aimed at both the general population and special high-risk populations. The latter include persons with high-normal blood pressure or a family history of hypertension, Blacks, and individuals with various behavioral risk factors, such as physical inactivity; excessive consumption of salt, alcohol, or calories; and deficient intake of potassium. Effective interventions for primary prevention of hypertension include reduced sodium and alcohol consumption, weight loss, and regular exercise. Potassium supplementation lowers blood pressure modestly, and a diet high in fresh fruits and vegetables and low in fat, red meats, and sugar-containing beverages also reduces blood pressure. Interventions of unproven efficacy include pill supplementation of potassium, calcium, magnesium, fish oil, or fiber; macronutrient alteration; and stress management.

Improved identification and treatment of hypertension has been a major cause of the decline in stroke deaths as well as the reduction in incidence of heart failure–related hospitalizations; more recently, stalled progress in control of hypertension has led to slowing of improvements in cardiovascular outcomes. Because hypertension is usually asymptomatic, screening is strongly recommended to identify patients for treatment. Elevated office readings should be confirmed with repeated measurements, ideally from ambulatory monitoring or home measurements. Despite strong recommendations in favor of screening and treatment, hypertension control remains suboptimal. An intervention that included both patient and provider education was more effective than provider education alone in achieving control of hypertension, suggesting the benefits of patient participation; another trial found that home monitoring combined with telephone-based nurse support was more effective than home monitoring alone for blood pressure control. Pharmacologic management of hypertension is discussed in Chapter 11.

Bundy JD et al. Comparison of the 2017 ACC/AHA Hypertension Guideline with earlier guidelines on estimated reductions in cardiovascular disease. Curr Hypertens Rep. 2019;21:76. [PMID: 31473837]

Centers for Disease Control and Prevention (CDC). Million Hearts 2022: estimated hypertension prevalence, treatment, and control among U.S. adults. https://millionhearts.hhs.gov/data-reports/hypertension-prevalence.html

Muntner P et al. Trends in blood pressure control among US adults with hypertension, 1999–2000 to 2017–2018. JAMA. 2020;324:1190. [PMID: 32902588]

US Preventive Services Task Force. Screening for hypertension in adults: US preventive services task force reaffirmation recommendation statement. JAMA. 2021;325:1650. [PMID: 33904861]

Chemoprevention

Regular use of low-dose aspirin (81–325 mg) can reduce cardiovascular events but increases GI bleeding and hemorrhagic stroke. The potential benefits of aspirin may exceed the possible adverse effects among middle-aged adults who are at increased cardiovascular risk, which can be defined as a 10-year risk of greater than 10%, and who do not have an increased risk of bleeding. A newer trial in older healthy adults did not find clear benefit from aspirin for reduction of cardiovascular events and saw an increase in all-cause mortality with aspirin. Therefore, aspirin should not be routinely initiated in healthy adults over age 70.

NSAIDs may reduce the incidence of colorectal adenomas and polyps but may also increase heart disease and GI bleeding, and thus are not recommended for colon cancer prevention in average-risk patients.

Antioxidant vitamin (vitamin E, vitamin C, and beta-carotene) supplementation produced no significant reductions in the 5-year incidence of—or mortality from—vascular disease, cancer, or other major outcomes in high-risk individuals with CAD, other occlusive arterial disease, or diabetes mellitus.

Gaziano JM. Aspirin for primary prevention: clinical considerations in 2019. JAMA. 2019;321:253. [PMID: 30667488]

Huang WY et al. Frequency of intracranial hemorrhage with low-dose aspirin in individuals without symptomatic cardiovascular disease: a systematic review and meta-analysis. JAMA Neurol. 2019;76:906. [PMID: 31081871]

Marquis-Gravel G et al. Revisiting the role of aspirin for the primary prevention of cardiovascular disease. Circulation. 2019;140:1115. [PMID: 31545683]

Patrono C et al. Role of aspirin in primary prevention of cardiovascular disease. Nat Rev Cardiol. 2019;16:675. [PMID: 31243390]

Zheng SL et al. Association of aspirin use for primary prevention with cardiovascular events and bleeding events: a systematic review and meta-analysis. JAMA. 2019;321:277. [PMID: 30667501]

PREVENTION OF OSTEOPOROSIS

See Chapter 26.

Osteoporosis, characterized by low bone mineral density, is common and associated with an increased risk of fracture. The lifetime risk of an osteoporotic fracture is approximately 50% for women and 30% for men. Osteoporotic fractures can cause significant pain and disability. As such, research has focused on means of preventing osteoporosis and related fractures. Primary prevention strategies include calcium supplementation, vitamin D supplementation, and exercise programs. The effectiveness of calcium and vitamin D for fracture prevention remains controversial, particularly in noninstitutionalized individuals.

Screening for osteoporosis on the basis of low bone mineral density is recommended for women over age 65, based on indirect evidence that screening can identify women with low bone mineral density and that treatment of women with low bone density with bisphosphonates is effective in reducing fractures. However, real-world adherence to pharmacologic therapy for osteoporosis is low: one-third to one-half of patients do not take their medication as directed. Screening for osteoporosis is also recommended in younger women who are at increased risk. The effectiveness of screening in men has not been established. Concern has been raised that bisphosphonates may increase the risk of certain uncommon atypical types of femoral fractures and rare osteonecrosis of the jaw, making consideration of the benefits and risks of therapy important when considering osteoporosis screening.

US Preventive Services Task Force. Screening for osteoporosis to prevent fractures: US Preventive Services Task Force recommendation statement. JAMA. 2018;319:2521. [PMID: 29946735]

US Preventive Services Task Force. Vitamin D, calcium, or combined supplementation for the primary prevention of fractures in community-dwelling adults: US Preventive Services Task Force recommendation statement. JAMA. 2018;319:1592. [PMID: 29677309]

Yedavally-Yellayi S et al. Update on osteoporosis. Prim Care. 2019;46:175. [PMID: 30704657]

PREVENTION OF PHYSICAL INACTIVITY

Lack of sufficient physical activity is the second most important contributor to preventable deaths, trailing only tobacco use. The US Department of Health and Human Services and the CDC recommend that adults (including older adults) engage in 150 minutes of moderate-intensity (such as brisk walking) or 75 minutes of vigorous-intensity (such as jogging or running) aerobic activity or an equivalent mix of moderate- and vigorous-intensity aerobic activity each week. In addition to activity recommendations, the CDC recommends activities to strengthen all major muscle groups (abdomen, arms, back, chest, hips, legs, and shoulders) at least twice a week.

Patients who engage in regular moderate to vigorous exercise have a lower risk of MI, stroke, hypertension, hyperlipidemia, type 2 diabetes mellitus, diverticular disease, and osteoporosis. Regular exercise may also have a positive effect on executive function in older adults.

In longitudinal cohort studies, individuals who report higher levels of leisure-time physical activity are less likely to gain weight. Conversely, individuals who are overweight are less likely to stay active. However, at least 60 minutes of daily moderate-intensity physical activity may be necessary to maximize weight loss and prevent significant weight regain. Moreover, adequate levels of physical activity appear to be important for the prevention of weight gain and the development of obesity.

Physical activity can be incorporated into any person's daily routine. The basic message should be the more the better, and anything is better than nothing.

When counseling patients, clinicians should advise patients about both the benefits and risks of exercise, prescribe an exercise program appropriate for each patient, and provide advice to help prevent injuries and cardiovascular complications.

Although primary care providers regularly ask patients about physical activity and advise them with verbal counseling, few providers provide written prescriptions or perform fitness assessments. Tailored interventions may potentially help increase physical activity in individuals. Exercise counseling with a prescription, eg, for walking at either a hard intensity or a moderate intensity with a high frequency, can produce significant long-term improvements in cardiorespiratory fitness. To be effective, exercise prescriptions must include recommendations on type, frequency, intensity, time, and progression of exercise and must follow disease-specific guidelines. Several factors influence physical activity behavior, including personal, social (eg, family and work), and environmental (eg, access to exercise facilities and well-lit parks) factors.

Chen FT et al. Effects of exercise training interventions on executive function in older adults: a systematic review and meta-analysis. Sports Med. 2020;50:1451. [PMID: 32447717]

Jeong SW et al. Mortality reduction with physical activity in patients with and without cardiovascular disease. Eur Heart J. 2019;40:3547. [PMID: 31504416]

PREVENTION OF OVERWEIGHT & OBESITY

Obesity is now a true epidemic and public health crisis that both clinicians and patients must face. Normal body weight is defined as a BMI of less than 25, overweight is defined as a BMI of 25.0–29.9, and obesity as a BMI greater than 30.

Risk assessment of the overweight and obese patient begins with determination of BMI, waist circumference for those with a BMI of 35 or less, presence of comorbid conditions, and a fasting blood glucose and lipid panel. Obesity is clearly associated with type 2 diabetes mellitus, hypertension, hyperlipidemia, cancer, osteoarthritis, cardiovascular disease, obstructive sleep apnea, and asthma.

Obesity is associated with a higher all-cause mortality rate. Data suggest an increase among those with grades 2 and 3 obesity (BMI more than 35); however, the impact on all-cause mortality among overweight (BMI 25–30) and grade 1 obesity (BMI 30–35) is questionable. Persons with a BMI of 40 or higher have death rates from cancers that are 52% higher for men and 62% higher for women than the rates in men and women of normal weight.

Prevention of overweight and obesity involves both increasing physical activity and dietary modification to reduce caloric intake. Adequate levels of physical activity appear to be important for the prevention of weight gain and the development of obesity. Physical activity programs consistent with public health recommendations may promote modest weight loss (~2 kg); however, the amount of weight loss for any one individual is highly variable.

Clinicians can help guide patients to develop personalized eating plans to reduce energy intake, particularly by recognizing the contributions of fat, concentrated carbohydrates, and large portion sizes (see Chapter 29). Patients typically underestimate caloric content, especially when consuming food away from home. Providing patients with caloric and nutritional information may help address the current obesity epidemic.

Commercial weight loss programs are effective in promoting weight loss and weight loss management. A randomized controlled trial of over 400 overweight or obese women demonstrated the effectiveness of a free prepared meal and incentivized structured weight loss program compared with usual care.

Weight loss strategies using dietary, physical activity, or behavioral interventions can produce significant improvements in weight among persons with prediabetes and a significant decrease in diabetes incidence. Lifestyle interventions including diet combined with physical activity are effective in achieving weight loss and reducing cardiometabolic risk factors among patients with severe obesity.

Bariatric surgical procedures, eg, adjustable gastric band, sleeve gastrectomy, and Roux-en-Y gastric bypass, are reserved for patients with morbid obesity whose BMI exceeds 40, or for less severely obese patients (with BMIs between 35 and 40) with high-risk comorbid conditions such as life-threatening cardiopulmonary problems or severe diabetes mellitus. In selected patients, surgery can produce substantial weight loss (10–159 kg) over 1–5 years, with rare but sometimes severe complications. Nutritional deficiencies are one complication of bariatric surgical procedures and close monitoring of a patient's metabolic and nutritional status is essential.

Finally, clinicians seem to share a general perception that almost no one succeeds in long-term maintenance of weight loss. However, research demonstrates that approximately 20% of overweight individuals are successful at long-term weight loss (defined as losing 10% or more of initial body weight and maintaining the loss for 1 year or longer).

Ryan DH et al. Guideline recommendations for obesity management. Med Clin North Am. 2018;102:49. [PMID: 29156187]

Wadden TA et al; STEP 3 Investigators. Effect of subcutaneous semaglutide vs placebo as an adjunct to intensive behavioral therapy on body weight in adults with overweight or obesity: the STEP 3 randomized clinical trial. JAMA. 2021;325:1403. [PMID: 33625476]

Walsh K et al. Health advice and education given to overweight patients by primary care doctors and nurses: a scoping literature review. Prev Med Rep. 2019;14:100812. [PMID: 30805277]

CANCER PREVENTION

Primary Prevention

Persons who engage in regular physical exercise and avoid obesity have lower rates of breast and colon cancer. Chemoprevention has been widely studied for primary cancer prevention without clear evidence of benefits (see earlier Chemoprevention section and Chapter 39). Use of tamoxifen, raloxifene, and aromatase inhibitors for breast cancer prevention is discussed in Chapters 17 and 39. Hepatitis B vaccination can prevent HCC. Screening and treatment of hepatitis C is another strategy to prevent HCC (see Chapter 16); new recommendations have extended the population eligible for screening. HPV virus-like particle (VLP) vaccine is recommended to prevent cervical cancer (Table 1–3). HPV vaccines may also have a role in the prevention of HPV-related head and neck and possibly anal cancers. The USPSTF recommends genetic counseling and, if indicated after counseling, genetic testing for women whose family or personal history is associated with an increased risk of harmful mutations in the *BRCA 1/2* gene. Guidelines for optimal cancer screening in adults over the age of 75 are unsettled; thus, an individualized approach that considers differences in disease risk rather than chronological age alone is recommended.

Athanasiou A et al. HPV vaccination and cancer prevention. Best Pract Res Clin Obstet Gynaecol. 2020;65:109. [PMID: 32284298]

US Preventive Services Task Force; Owens DK et al. Risk assessment, genetic counseling, and genetic testing for *BRCA*-related cancer: US Preventive Services Task Force Recommendation Statement. JAMA. 2019;322:652. [PMID: 31429903]

Screening & Early Detection

Screening prevents death from cancers of the breast, colon, and cervix. Current cancer screening recommendations from the USPSTF are available online at https://www.uspreventiveservicestaskforce.org/BrowseRec/Index/browse-recommendations. Despite an increase in rates of screening for breast, cervical, and colon cancer over the last decade, overall screening for these cancers is suboptimal.

Though breast cancer mortality is reduced with mammography screening, screening mammography has both benefits and downsides. Clinicians should discuss the risks and benefits with each patient and consider individual patient preferences when deciding when to begin screening (see Chapters 17 and e6).

Screening for testicular cancers among asymptomatic adolescent or adult males is not recommended by the USPSTF. Prostate cancer screening remains controversial, since no completed trials have answered the question of whether early detection and treatment after screen detection produce sufficient benefits to outweigh harms of treatment. For men between the ages of 55 and 69, the decision to screen should be individualized and include a discussion of its risks and benefits with a clinician. The USPSTF recommends against PSA-based prostate cancer screening for men older than age 70 years (grade D recommendation).

The USPSTF recommends colorectal cancer screening for adults aged 45–75 years and selectively screening adults aged 76–85 years (considering the patient's overall health, prior screening history, and patient's preferences).

Annual or biennial fecal occult blood testing reduces mortality from colorectal cancer. Fecal immunochemical tests (FIT) are superior to guaiac-based fecal occult blood tests (gFOBT) in detecting advanced adenomatous polyps and colorectal cancer, and patients are more likely to favor FIT over gFOBT. CT colonography (virtual colonoscopy) is a noninvasive option in screening for colorectal cancer. It has been shown to have a high safety profile and performance similar to colonoscopy.

The USPSTF recommends screening for cervical cancer in women aged 21–65 years with a Papanicolaou smear (cytology) every 3 years or, for women aged 30–65 years who desire longer intervals, screening with cytology and HPV testing every 5 years. The American Cancer Society recommends screening for people aged 25–65 years with primary HPV testing every 5 years. The USPSTF recommends against screening in women younger than 21 years of age and average-risk women over 65 with adequate negative prior screenings. Receipt of HPV vaccination has no impact on screening intervals.

Women whose cervical specimen HPV tests are positive but cytology results are otherwise negative should repeat co-testing in 12 months (option 1) or undergo HPV-genotype–specific testing for types 16 or 16/18 (option 2). Colposcopy is recommended in women who test positive for types 16 or 16/18. Women with atypical squamous cells of undetermined significance (ASCUS) on cytology and a negative HPV test result should continue routine screening as per age-specific guidelines.

The USPSTF recommends offering annual lung cancer screening with low-dose CT to current smokers aged 50 to 80 years and 20-pack-year smoking history or to smokers who quit within the past 15 years. Screening should stop once a person has not smoked for 15 years or a health problem that significantly limits life expectancy has developed. Screening should not be viewed as an alternative to smoking cessation but rather as a complementary approach.

Fontham ETH et al. Cervical cancer screening for individuals at average risk: 2020 guideline update from the American Cancer Society. CA Cancer J Clin. 2020;70:321. [PMID: 32729638]

Jonas DE et al. Screening for lung cancer with low-dose computed tomography: updated evidence report and systematic review for the US Preventive Services Task Force. JAMA. 2021;325:971. [PMID: 33687468]

Qaseem A et al. Screening for breast cancer in average-risk women: a guidance statement from the American College of Physicians. Ann Intern Med. 2019;170:547. [PMID: 30959525]

US Preventive Services Task Force; Curry SJ et al. Screening for cervical cancer: US Preventive Services Task Force recommendation statement. JAMA. 2018;320:674. [PMID: 30140884]

US Preventive Services Task Force. Screening for colorectal cancer: US Preventive Services Task Force recommendation statement. JAMA. 2021;325:1965. [PMID: 34003218]

US Preventive Services Task Force; Grossman DC et al. Screening for prostate cancer: US Preventive Services Task Force recommendation statement. JAMA. 2018;319:1901. [PMID: 29801017]

US Preventive Services Task Force; Krist AH. Screening for lung cancer: US Preventive Services Task Force recommendation statement. JAMA. 2021;325:962. [PMID: 33687470]

PREVENTION OF INJURIES & VIOLENCE

Injuries remain the most important cause of loss of potential years of life before age 65. Homicide and motor vehicle accidents are a major cause of injury-related deaths among young adults, and accidental falls are the most common cause of injury-related death in older adults. Approximately one-third of all injury deaths include a diagnosis of traumatic brain injury, which has been associated with an increased risk of suicide. Although motor vehicle accident deaths per miles driven have declined in the United States, there has been an increase in motor vehicle accidents related to distracted driving (using a cell phone, texting, eating).

Men ages 16–35 are at especially high risk for serious injury and death from accidents and violence, with Black and Latino men at greatest risk. Deaths from firearms have reached epidemic levels in the United States. Having a gun in the home increases the likelihood of homicide nearly threefold and of suicide fivefold. Educating clinicians to recognize and treat depression as well as restricting access to lethal methods have been found to reduce suicide rates.

Clinicians have a critical role in the detection, prevention, and management of intimate partner violence (see Chapter e6). The USPSTF recommends screening women of childbearing age for intimate partner violence and providing or referring women to intervention services when needed. Inclusion of a single question in the medical history—"At any time, has a partner ever hit you, kicked you, or otherwise physically hurt you?"—can increase identification of this common problem. Assessment for abuse and offering of referrals to community resources create the potential to interrupt and prevent recurrence of domestic violence and associated trauma. Clinicians should take an active role in following up with patients whenever possible, since intimate partner violence screening with passive referrals to services may not be adequate.

Physical and psychological abuse, exploitation, and neglect of older adults are serious, underrecognized problems; they may occur in up to 10% of elders. Risk factors for elder abuse include a culture of violence in the family; a demented, debilitated, or depressed and socially isolated victim; and a perpetrator profile of mental illness, alcohol or drug abuse, or emotional and/or financial dependence on the victim. Clues to elder mistreatment include the patient's ill-kempt appearance, recurrent urgent-care visits, missed appointments, suspicious physical findings, and implausible explanations for injuries.

Cimino-Fiallos N et al. Elder abuse—a guide to diagnosis and management in the emergency department. Emerg Med Clin North Am. 2021;39:405. [PMID: 33863468]

Kirk L et al. What barriers prevent health professionals screening women for domestic abuse? A literature review. Br J Nurs. 2020;29:754. [PMID: 32649247]

Mercier É et al. Elder abuse in the out-of-hospital and emergency department settings: a scoping review. Ann Emerg Med. 2020;75:181. [PMID: 31959308]

PREVENTION OF SUBSTANCE USE DISORDER: ALCOHOL & ILLICIT DRUGS

Unhealthy alcohol use is a major public health problem in the United States, where approximately 51% of adults 18 years and older are current regular drinkers (at least 12 drinks in the past year). The spectrum of alcohol use disorders includes alcohol dependence, harmful pattern use of alcohol, and entities such as alcohol intoxication, alcohol withdrawal, and several alcohol-induced mental disorders. The ICD-11 includes a new category: hazardous alcohol use. Categorized as a risk factor, hazardous alcohol use is a pattern of alcohol use that appreciably increases the risk of physical or mental health harmful consequences to the user.

Underdiagnosis and undertreatment of alcohol misuse is substantial, both because of patient denial and lack of detection of clinical clues.

As with cigarette use, clinician identification and counseling about unhealthy alcohol use are essential. The USPSTF recommends screening adults aged 18 years and older for unhealthy alcohol use. The National Institute on Alcohol Abuse and Alcoholism recommends the following single-question screening test (validated in primary care settings): "How many times in the past year have you had X or more drinks in a day?" (X is 5 for men and 4 for women, and a response of more than 1 time is considered positive.)

Those who screen positive on the single-item questionnaire should complete the Alcohol Use Disorder

Identification Test (AUDIT), which consists of questions on the quantity and frequency of alcohol consumption, on alcohol dependence symptoms, and on alcohol-related problems (Table 1–7).

Clinicians should provide those who screen positive for hazardous or risky drinking with brief behavioral counseling interventions to reduce alcohol misuse. Use of screening procedures and brief intervention methods (see Chapter 25) can produce a 10–30% reduction in long-term alcohol use and alcohol-related problems. Those whose AUDIT scores suggest alcohol use disorder (AUDIT > 12) should undergo more extensive evaluation and potential referral for treatment.

Deaths due to opioid overdose have dramatically increased. Opioid risk mitigation strategies include use of risk assessment tools, treatment agreements (contracts), and urine drug testing. Additional strategies include establishing and strengthening prescription drug monitoring programs, regulating pain management facilities, and establishing dosage thresholds requiring consultation with pain specialists. Medication-assisted treatment, the use of medications with counseling and behavioral therapy, is effective in the prevention of opioid overdose and substance abuse disorders. Methadone, buprenorphine, and naltrexone are FDA approved for use in medication-assisted treatment. Buprenorphine has potential as a medication to ameliorate the symptoms and signs of withdrawal from opioids and is effective in reducing concomitant cocaine and opioid abuse. The FDA supports greater access to naloxone and is currently exploring options to make naloxone more available to treat opioid overdose. (See Chapter 5.)

Use of illegal drugs—including cocaine, methamphetamine, and so-called designer drugs—either sporadically or episodically remains an important problem. Lifetime prevalence of drug abuse is approximately 8% and is generally greater among men, young and unmarried individuals, Native Americans, and those of lower socioeconomic status. As with alcohol, drug abuse disorders often coexist with personality disorders, anxiety disorders, and other substance abuse disorders.

Clinical aspects of substance abuse are discussed in Chapter 25.

Chou R et al. Interventions for unhealthy drug use—supplemental report: a systematic review for the U.S. Preventive Services Task Force [Internet]. Rockville (MD): Agency for Healthcare Research and Quality (US); 2020 Jun. Report No.: 19-05255-EF-2. https://www.ncbi.nlm.nih.gov/books/NBK558205/ [PMID: 32550674]

Table 1–7. Screening for alcohol abuse using the Alcohol Use Disorder Identification Test (AUDIT).

(Scores for response categories are given in parentheses. Added together, Total Scores range from 0 to 40, with scores of 1 to 7 suggesting low-risk drinking; 8 to 14, hazardous or harmful drinking; and >15, alcohol dependence.)				
1. How often do you have a drink containing alcohol?				
(0) Never	(1) Monthly or less	(2) Two to four times a month	(3) Two or three times a week	(4) Four or more times a week
2. How many drinks containing alcohol do you have on a typical day when you are drinking?				
(0) 1 or 2	(1) 3 or 4	(2) 5 or 6	(3) 7 to 9	(4) 10 or more
3. How often do you have six or more drinks on one occasion?				
(0) Never	(1) Less than monthly	(2) Monthly	(3) Weekly	(4) Daily or almost daily
4. How often during the past year have you found that you were not able to stop drinking once you had started?				
(0) Never	(1) Less than monthly	(2) Monthly	(3) Weekly	(4) Daily or almost daily
5. How often during the past year have you failed to do what was normally expected of you because of drinking?				
(0) Never	(1) Less than monthly	(2) Monthly	(3) Weekly	(4) Daily or almost daily
6. How often during the past year have you needed a first drink in the morning to get yourself going after a heavy drinking session?				
(0) Never	(1) Less than monthly	(2) Monthly	(3) Weekly	(4) Daily or almost daily
7. How often during the past year have you had a feeling of guilt or remorse after drinking?				
(0) Never	(1) Less than monthly	(2) Monthly	(3) Weekly	(4) Daily or almost daily
8. How often during the past year have you been unable to remember what happened the night before because you had been drinking?				
(0) Never	(1) Less than monthly	(2) Monthly	(3) Weekly	(4) Daily or almost daily
9. Have you or has someone else been injured as a result of your drinking?				
(0) No		(2) Yes, but not in the past year		(4) Yes, during the past year
10. Has a relative or friend or a doctor or other health worker been concerned about your drinking or suggested you cut down?				
(0) No		(2) Yes, but not in the past year		(4) Yes, during the past year

Reproduced with permission from Babor TF, Higgins-Biddle JC, Saunders JB, Montiero MG. AUDIT. *The Alcohol Use Disorders Identification Test. Guidelines for use of primary health care*, 2nd ed. Geneva, Switzerland: World Health Organization; 2001.

Fairbanks J et al. Evidence-based pharmacotherapies for alcohol use disorder: clinical pearls. Mayo Clin Proc. 2020;95:1964. [PMID: 32446635]

Hepner KA et al. Rates and impact of adherence to recommended care for unhealthy alcohol use. J Gen Intern Med. 2019;34:256. [PMID: 30484101]

Higher-dose naloxone nasal spray (Kloxxado) for opioid overdose. JAMA. 2021;326:1853. [PMID: 34751711]

Mekonen T et al. Treatment rates for alcohol use disorders: a systematic review and meta-analysis. Addiction. 2021;116:2617. [PMID: 33245581]

Patel AK et al. JAMA Patient Page. Treatment of alcohol use disorder. JAMA. 2021;325:596. [PMID: 33560323]

Patnode CD et al. Screening for unhealthy drug use in primary care in adolescents and adults, including pregnant persons: updated systematic review for the U.S. Preventive Services Task Force [Internet]. Rockville (MD): Agency for Healthcare Research and Quality (US); 2020 Jun. Report No.: 19-05255-EF-1. https://www.ncbi.nlm.nih.gov/books/NBK558174/ [PMID: 32550673]

Saunders JB et al. Alcohol use disorders in ICD-11: past, present, and future. Alcohol Clin Exp Res. 2019;43:1617. [PMID: 31194891]

Substance Abuse and Mental Health Services Administration (SAMHSA). Medication-Assisted Treatment (MAT). https://www.samhsa.gov/medication-assisted-treatment

Common Symptoms

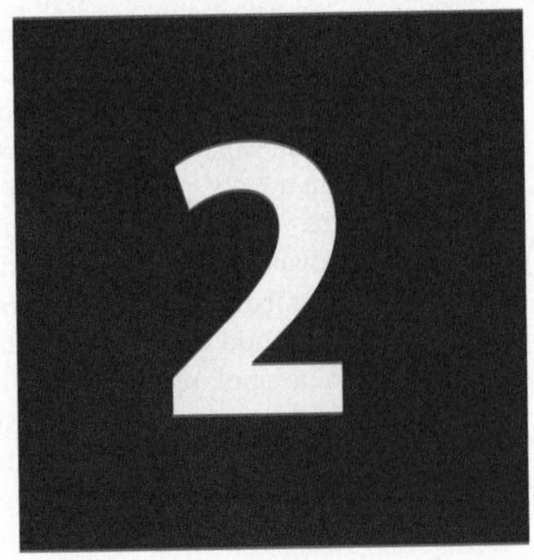

Paul L. Nadler, MD
Ralph Gonzales, MD, MSPH

COUGH

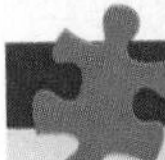

ESSENTIAL INQUIRIES

- Age, occupational history, environmental exposures, risk of infection with SARS-CoV-2, and duration of cough.
- Use of tobacco, cannabis, e-cigarettes (vaping).
- Dyspnea (at rest or with exertion).
- Vital signs (heart rate, respiratory rate, body temperature); pulse oximetry.
- Chest examination.
- Chest radiography, especially when unexplained cough lasts > 3–6 weeks.

General Considerations

Cough is the most common symptom for which patients seek medical attention. Cough results from stimulation of mechanical or chemical afferent nerve receptors in the bronchial tree. Effective cough depends on an intact afferent–efferent reflex arc, adequate expiratory and chest wall muscle strength, and normal mucociliary production and clearance.

Clinical Findings

A. Symptoms

Distinguishing **acute** (less than 3 weeks), **persistent** (3–8 weeks), and **chronic** (more than 8 weeks) cough illness syndromes is a useful first step in evaluation. Postinfectious cough lasting 3–8 weeks has also been referred to as **subacute** cough to distinguish this common, distinct clinical entity from acute and chronic cough.

1. Acute cough—In healthy adults, most acute cough syndromes are due to viral respiratory tract infections. Additional features of infection such as fever, nasal congestion, and sore throat help confirm this diagnosis. Dyspnea (at rest or with exertion) may reflect a more serious condition, and further evaluation should include assessment of oxygenation (pulse oximetry or arterial blood gas measurement), airflow (peak flow or spirometry), and pulmonary parenchymal disease (chest radiography). The timing and character of the cough are not very useful in establishing the cause of acute cough syndromes, although cough-variant asthma should be considered in adults with prominent nocturnal cough, and persistent cough with phlegm increases the likelihood of COPD. The presence of posttussive emesis or inspiratory whoop in adults modestly increases the likelihood of pertussis, and the absence of paroxysmal cough and the presence of fever decrease its likelihood. Loss of smell or taste accompanying a new cough illness is specific but not sensitive for COVID-19 infection. Uncommon causes of acute cough should be suspected in those with HF or hay fever (allergic rhinitis) and those with occupational risk factors (such as farmworkers).

2. Persistent and chronic cough—Cough due to acute respiratory tract infection resolves within 3 weeks in more than 90% of patients. Pertussis should be considered in adolescents and adults who have persistent or severe cough lasting more than 3 weeks, who have not been adequately boosted with Tdap, and who have been exposed to a person with confirmed pertussis. It should also be considered in geographic areas where the prevalence of pertussis approaches 20% (although its exact prevalence is difficult to ascertain due to the limited sensitivity of diagnostic tests).

When ACE inhibitor use, acute respiratory tract infection, and chest radiographic abnormalities are absent, most cases of persistent and chronic cough are related to postnasal drip (upper airway cough syndrome), cough-variant asthma, or GERD, or some combination of these three entities. Approximately 10% of cases are caused by nonasthmatic eosinophilic bronchitis. A history of nasal or sinus congestion, wheezing, or heartburn should direct subsequent evaluation and treatment, though these conditions frequently cause persistent cough in the absence of typical symptoms. Dyspnea at rest or with exertion is not commonly reported among patients with persistent cough;

dyspnea requires assessment for chronic lung disease, HF, anemia, PE, or pulmonary hypertension.

Bronchogenic carcinoma is suspected when cough is accompanied by unexplained weight loss, hemoptysis, and fevers with night sweats, particularly in persons with significant tobacco or occupational exposures (asbestos, radon, diesel exhaust, and metals). Persistent and chronic cough accompanied by excessive mucus secretions increases the likelihood of COPD, particularly if there is a history of cigarette smoking, or of bronchiectasis if accompanied by a history of recurrent or complicated pneumonia; chest radiographs are helpful in diagnosis. Chronic cough with dry eyes may represent Sjögren syndrome. A chronic dry cough may be the first symptom of idiopathic pulmonary fibrosis.

B. Physical Examination

Pneumonia is suspected when acute cough is accompanied by vital sign abnormalities (tachycardia, tachypnea, fever). Findings suggestive of airspace consolidation (crackles, decreased breath sounds, fremitus, egophony) are significant predictors of community-acquired pneumonia but are present in a minority of cases. Purulent sputum is associated with bacterial infections in patients with structural lung disease (eg, COPD, cystic fibrosis), but it is a poor predictor of pneumonia in the otherwise healthy adult. Wheezing and rhonchi are frequent findings in adults with acute bronchitis and do not indicate consolidation or adult-onset asthma in most cases.

Examination of patients with persistent cough should include a search for chronic sinusitis, which may contribute to postnasal drip syndrome or to asthma. Physical examination may help distinguish COPD from HF. In patients with cough and dyspnea, a normal match test (ability to blow out a match from 25 cm away) and maximum laryngeal height greater than 4 cm (measured from the sternal notch to the cricoid cartilage at end expiration) substantially decrease the likelihood of COPD. Similarly, normal jugular venous pressure and no hepatojugular reflux decrease the likelihood of biventricular HF.

C. Diagnostic Studies

1. Acute cough—Chest radiography should be considered for any adult with acute cough whose vital signs are abnormal or whose chest examination suggests pneumonia. The relationship between specific clinical findings and the probability of pneumonia is shown in Table 2–1. A large, multicenter randomized clinical trial found that elevated serum CRP (levels greater than 30 mg/dL) improves diagnostic accuracy of clinical prediction rules for pneumonia in adults with acute cough; serum procalcitonin had only marginal utility in outpatient management (in contrast with severe pneumonia requiring hospital care). A meta-analysis found that lung ultrasonography had better accuracy than chest radiography for the diagnosis of adult community-acquired pneumonia. Lung ultrasonography had a pooled sensitivity of 0.95 and a specificity of 0.90. Chest radiography had a pooled sensitivity of 0.77 and a specificity of 0.91. In patients with dyspnea, pulse oximetry

Table 2–1. Positive and negative likelihood ratios of history, physical examination, and laboratory findings for the diagnosis of pneumonia.

Finding	Positive LR	Negative LR
Medical history		
Fever	1.7–2.1	0.6–0.7
Chills	1.3–1.7	0.7–0.9
Physical examination		
Tachypnea (respiratory rate > 25 breaths/min)	1.5–3.4	0.8
Tachycardia (> 100 beats/min in two studies or > 120 beats/min in one study)	1.6–2.3	0.5–0.7
Hyperthermia (> 37.8°C)	1.4–4.4	0.6–0.8
Chest examination		
Dullness to percussion	2.2–4.3	0.8–0.9
Decreased breath sounds	2.3–2.5	0.6–0.8
Crackles	1.6–2.7	0.6–0.9
Rhonchi	1.4–1.5	0.8–0.9
Egophony	2.0–8.6	0.8–1.0
Laboratory findings		
Leukocytosis (> 11,000/mcL [11×10^9/L] in one study or ≥ 10,400/mcL [10.4×10^9/L] in another study)	1.9–3.7	0.3–0.6

and peak flow help exclude hypoxemia or obstructive airway disease. However, a normal pulse oximetry value (eg, greater than 93%) does not rule out a significant alveolar–arterial (A–a) gradient when patients have effective respiratory compensation. During documented outbreaks, clinical diagnosis of influenza has a positive predictive value of ~70%; this usually obviates the need for rapid diagnostic tests.

2. Persistent and chronic cough—Chest radiography is indicated when ACE inhibitor therapy–related and postinfectious cough are excluded. If pertussis is suspected, PCR testing should be performed on a nasopharyngeal swab or nasal wash specimen—although the ability to detect pertussis decreases as the duration of cough increases. When the chest film is normal, postnasal drip, asthma, or GERD are the most likely causes. The presence of typical symptoms of these conditions directs further evaluation or empiric therapy, though typical symptoms are often absent. Definitive tests for determining the presence of each are available (Table 2–2). However, empiric treatment with a maximum-strength regimen for postnasal drip, asthma, or GERD for 2–4 weeks is one recommended approach since documenting the presence of postnasal drip, asthma, or GERD does not mean they are the cause of the cough. Alternative approaches to identifying patients who have corticosteroid-responsive cough due to asthma include examining induced sputum for increased eosinophil counts

Table 2–2. Empiric therapy or definitive testing for persistent cough.

Suspected Condition	Step 1 (Empiric Therapy)	Step 2 (Definitive Testing)
Postnasal drip	Therapy for allergy or chronic sinusitis	Sinus CT scan; otolaryngologic referral
Asthma	Beta-2-agonist	Spirometry; consider methacholine challenge if normal
GERD	Lifestyle and diet modifications with or without PPIs	Esophageal pH monitoring

(greater than 3%) or providing an empiric trial of prednisone, 30 mg daily orally for 2 weeks.

Nonasthmatic eosinophilic bronchitis can be diagnosed by finding eosinophils with induced sputum analysis after the exclusion of other causes for chronic cough by clinical, radiologic, and lung function assessment. The cough usually responds well to inhaled corticosteroids.

Spirometry may help measure large airway obstruction (eg, foreign body or cancer) in patients who have persistent cough and wheezing and who are not responding to asthma treatment. When empiric treatment trials are not successful, additional evaluation with pH manometry, endoscopy, barium swallow, sinus CT, or high-resolution chest CT may identify the cause.

Differential Diagnosis

A. Acute Cough

Acute cough may be a symptom of acute respiratory tract infection, COVID-19, asthma, allergic rhinitis, HF, and ACE inhibitor therapy, as well as many less common causes.

B. Persistent and Chronic Cough

Causes of persistent cough include environmental exposures (cigarette smoke, air pollution), occupational exposures, pertussis, postnasal drip, asthma (including cough-variant asthma), GERD, COPD, chronic aspiration, bronchiectasis, nonasthmatic eosinophilic bronchitis, tuberculosis or other chronic infection, interstitial lung disease, and bronchogenic carcinoma. COPD is a common cause of persistent cough among patients older than 50 years who have been cigarette smokers. Persistent cough may also be due to somatic cough syndrome or tic cough, or vocal fold dysfunction.

C. Cough in the Immunocompromised Patient

The evaluation of cough in immunocompromised patients is the same as in immunocompetent patients but with an increased concern for tuberculosis (regardless of radiographic findings) as well as fungi, cytomegalovirus, varicella, herpesvirus, and *Pneumocystis jirovecii*.

Treatment

A. Acute Cough

Treatment of acute cough should target the underlying etiology of the illness, the cough reflex itself, and any additional factors that exacerbate the cough. Cough duration is typically 1–3 weeks, yet patients frequently expect cough to last fewer than 10 days. Limited studies on the use of dextromethorphan suggest a minor or modest benefit. Honey may provide symptomatic benefit.

When influenza is diagnosed (including H1N1 influenza), oral oseltamivir or zanamivir or intravenous peramivir are equally effective (1 less day of illness) when initiated within 30–48 hours of illness onset; treatment is recommended regardless of illness duration when patients have severe, complicated, or progressive influenza and in patients requiring hospitalization. In *Chlamydophila*- or *Mycoplasma*-documented infection or outbreaks, first-line antibiotics include erythromycin or doxycycline. Antibiotics do not improve cough severity or duration in patients with uncomplicated acute bronchitis. In patients with bronchitis and wheezing, inhaled beta-2-agonist therapy reduces severity and duration of cough. In patients with acute cough, treating the accompanying postnasal drip (with antihistamines, decongestants, saline nasal irrigation, or nasal corticosteroids) can be helpful. Two studies (n = 163 total patients) found codeine to be no more effective than placebo in reducing acute cough symptoms.

B. Persistent and Chronic Cough

Evaluation and management of persistent cough often require multiple visits and therapeutic trials, which frequently lead to frustration, anger, and anxiety. When pertussis infection is suspected early in its course, treatment with a macrolide antibiotic (see Chapter 33) is appropriate to reduce organism shedding and transmission. When pertussis has lasted more than 7–10 days, antibiotic treatment does not affect the duration of cough, which can last up to 6 months. Early identification, revaccination with Tdap, and treatment are encouraged for adult patients who work or live with persons at high risk for complications from pertussis (pregnant women, infants [particularly younger than 1 year], and immunosuppressed individuals).

Table 2–2 outlines empiric treatments for persistent cough. There is no evidence to guide how long to continue treatment for persistent cough due to postnasal drip, asthma, or GERD. Studies have not found a consistent benefit of inhaled corticosteroid therapy in adults with persistent cough.

There is insufficient evidence to recommend the routine use of any pharmacologic treatments (antibiotics, bronchodilators, mucolytics) as a means of relieving cough for adult patients with chronic cough due to stable chronic bronchitis.

When empiric treatment trials fail, consider other causes of chronic cough such as obstructive sleep apnea, tonsillar or uvular enlargement, and environmental fungi (see Chapter 36). The small percentage of patients with idiopathic chronic cough should be managed in consultation with an otolaryngologist or a pulmonologist; consider a high-resolution CT scan of the lungs. Treatment options include nebulized lidocaine therapy and morphine sulfate, 5–10 mg orally twice daily. Sensory dysfunction of the laryngeal branches of the vagus nerve may contribute to persistent cough syndromes and may help explain the effectiveness of gabapentin in patients with chronic cough. Baclofen may have similar neuromodulatory action and benefit as gabapentin.

Speech pathology therapy combined with pregabalin has some benefit in chronic refractory cough. In patients with cough hypersensitivity syndrome, therapy aimed at shifting the patient's attentional focus from internal stimuli to external focal points can be helpful. PPIs are not effective when used in isolation for treating chronic cough due to gastroesophageal reflux; most benefit appears to come from lifestyle modifications and weight reduction.

When to Refer

- Failure to control persistent or chronic cough following empiric treatment trials.
- Patients with recurrent symptoms should be referred to an otolaryngologist, pulmonologist, or gastroenterologist.

When to Admit

- Patient at high risk for tuberculosis for whom compliance with respiratory precautions is uncertain.
- Need for urgent bronchoscopy, such as suspected foreign body.
- Smoke or toxic fume inhalational injury.
- Gas exchange is impaired by cough.
- Patients at high risk for barotrauma (eg, recent pneumothorax).

Kardos P et al. German Respiratory Society guidelines for diagnosis and treatment of adults suffering from acute, subacute and chronic cough. Respir Med. 2020;170:105939. [PMID: 32843157]

Malesker MA et al; CHEST Expert Cough Panel. Chronic cough due to stable chronic bronchitis: CHEST Expert Panel Report. Chest. 2020;158:705. [PMID: 32105719]

Smith MP et al; CHEST Expert Cough Panel. Acute cough due to acute bronchitis in immunocompetent adult outpatients: CHEST Expert Panel Report. Chest. 2020;157:1256. [PMID: 32092323]

DYSPNEA

ESSENTIAL INQUIRIES

- Fever, cough, risk of COVID-19, and chest pain.
- Vital sign measurements; pulse oximetry.
- Cardiac and chest examination.
- Chest radiography and arterial blood gas measurement in selected patients.

General Considerations

Dyspnea is a subjective experience or perception of uncomfortable breathing. The relationship between level of dyspnea and the severity of underlying disease varies widely among individuals. Dyspnea can result from conditions that increase the mechanical effort of breathing (eg, asthma, COPD, restrictive lung disease, respiratory muscle weakness), alveolar lung disease (pulmonary edema, pneumonia, alveolar proteinosis), conditions that produce compensatory tachypnea (eg, hypoxemia, acidosis), primary pulmonary vasculopathy (pulmonary hypertension), or psychogenic conditions.

Clinical Findings

A. Symptoms

The duration, severity, and periodicity of dyspnea influence the tempo of the clinical evaluation. Rapid onset or severe dyspnea in the absence of other clinical features should raise concern for pneumothorax, PE, or increased left ventricular end-diastolic pressure (LVEDP).

Spontaneous pneumothorax is usually accompanied by chest pain and occurs most often in thin, young males and in those with underlying lung disease. PE should always be suspected when a patient with new dyspnea reports a recent history (previous 4 weeks) of prolonged immobilization or surgery, estrogen therapy, or other risk factors for DVT (eg, previous history of thromboembolism, cancer, obesity, lower extremity trauma) and when the cause of dyspnea is not apparent. Silent MI, which occurs more frequently in persons with diabetes and women, can result in increased LVEDP, acute HF, and dyspnea.

Accompanying symptoms provide important clues to causes of dyspnea. When cough and fever are present, pulmonary disease (particularly infection) is the primary concern; myocarditis, pericarditis, and septic emboli can also present in this manner. Chest pain should be further characterized as acute or chronic, pleuritic or exertional. Although acute pleuritic chest pain is the rule in acute pericarditis and pneumothorax, most patients with pleuritic chest pain in the outpatient clinic have pleurisy due to acute viral respiratory tract infection. Periodic chest pain that precedes the onset of dyspnea suggests myocardial ischemia or PE. Most cases of dyspnea associated with wheezing are due to acute bronchitis; however, other causes include new-onset asthma, foreign body, and vocal fold dysfunction. Interstitial lung disease and pulmonary hypertension should be considered in patients with symptoms (or history) of connective tissue disease. Pulmonary lymphangitic carcinomatosis should be considered if a patient has a malignancy, especially breast, lung, or gastric cancer.

When a patient reports prominent dyspnea with mild or no accompanying features, consider noncardiopulmonary causes of impaired oxygen delivery (anemia, methemoglobinemia, cyanide ingestion, carbon monoxide poisoning), metabolic acidosis, panic disorder, neuromuscular disorders, and chronic PE.

Platypnea-orthodeoxia syndrome is characterized by dyspnea and hypoxemia on sitting or standing that improves in the recumbent position. Hyperthyroidism can cause dyspnea from increased ventilatory drive, respiratory muscle weakness, or pulmonary hypertension. Patients in whom moderate to severe SARS-CoV-2 disease develops typically have 4–10 days of upper respiratory infection symptoms followed by a precipitous increase in dyspnea. Patients who recover from their initial COVID-19 infection may have persistent dyspnea as part of the "long COVID" syndrome.

B. Physical Examination

A focused physical examination should include evaluation of the head and neck, chest, heart, and lower extremities. Visual inspection of the patient can suggest obstructive airway disease (pursed-lip breathing, use of accessory respiratory muscles, barrel-shaped chest), pneumothorax (asymmetric excursion), or metabolic acidosis (Kussmaul respirations). Patients with impending upper airway obstruction (eg, epiglottitis, foreign body) or severe asthma exacerbation sometimes assume a tripod position. Focal wheezing raises the suspicion for a foreign body or other bronchial obstruction. Maximum laryngeal height (the distance between the top of the thyroid cartilage and the suprasternal notch at end expiration) is a measure of hyperinflation. Obstructive airway disease is virtually nonexistent when a nonsmoking patient younger than age 45 years has a maximum laryngeal height greater than 4 cm.

Factors increasing the likelihood of obstructive airway disease (in patients without known obstructive airway disease) include patient history of more than 40 pack-years smoking (adjusted LR+ 11.6; LR– 0.9), patient age 45 years or older (LR+ 1.4; LR– 0.5), and maximum laryngeal height greater than or equal to 4 cm (LR+ 3.6; LR– 0.7). With all three of these factors present, the LR+ rises to 58.5 and the LR– falls to 0.3.

Absent breath sounds suggest a pneumothorax. An accentuated pulmonic component of the second heart sound (loud P_2) is a sign of pulmonary hypertension and PE.

Clinical predictors of increased LVEDP in dyspneic patients with no prior history of HF include tachycardia, systolic hypotension, jugular venous distention, hepatojugular reflux, bibasilar crackles, third heart sound, lower extremity edema, and chest film findings of pulmonary vascular redistribution or cardiomegaly. When none is present, there is a very low probability (less than 10%) of increased LVEDP, but when two or more are present, there is a very high probability (greater than 90%) of increased LVEDP.

C. Diagnostic Studies

Causes of dyspnea that can be managed without chest radiography are few: anemia, carbon monoxide poisoning, and ingestions causing lactic acidosis and methemoglobinemia. The diagnosis of pneumonia should be confirmed by chest radiography in most patients, and elevated blood levels of procalcitonin or CRP can support the diagnosis of pneumonia in equivocal cases or in the presence of interstitial lung disease. Conversely, a low procalcitonin can help exclude pneumonia in dyspneic patients presenting with HF.

Chest radiography is fairly sensitive and specific for new-onset HF (represented by redistribution of pulmonary venous circulation) and can help guide treatment of patients with other cardiac diseases. NT-proBNP can assist in the diagnosis of HF (see below). End-expiratory chest radiography enhances detection of small pneumothoraces. A systematic review of five randomized controlled trials and 44 prospective cohort-type studies in patients with acute dyspnea assessed point-of-care ultrasonography (POCUS) as a diagnostic tool to determine the underlying cause of dyspnea. When added to a standard diagnostic pathway, POCUS led to statistically significantly more correct diagnoses in patients with dyspnea than the standard diagnostic pathway. POCUS consistently improved the sensitivities of standard diagnostic pathways to detect HF, pneumonia, PE, pleural effusion, or pneumothorax. Specificities increased in most studies; in-hospital mortality and length of hospital stay, however, did not differ significantly between patients who did or did not receive POCUS in addition to standard diagnostic tests.

A normal chest radiograph has substantial diagnostic value. When there is no physical examination evidence of COPD or HF and the chest radiograph is normal, the major remaining causes of dyspnea include PE, *P jirovecii* infection (the initial radiograph may be normal in up to 25%), upper airway obstruction, foreign body, anemia, and metabolic acidosis. If a patient has tachycardia or hypoxemia but a normal chest radiograph and ECG, then tests to exclude pulmonary emboli, anemia, or metabolic acidosis are warranted. High-resolution chest CT is particularly useful in the evaluation of interstitial and alveolar lung disease. Helical ("spiral") CT is useful to diagnose PE since the images are high resolution and require only one breath-hold by the patient, but to minimize unnecessary testing and radiation exposure, the clinician should first consider a clinical decision rule (with or without D-dimer testing) to estimate the pretest probability of a PE. It is appropriate to forego CT scanning in patients with very low probability of pulmonary embolus when other causes of dyspnea are more likely (see Chapter 9).

Laboratory findings suggesting increased LVEDP include elevated serum BNP or NT-proBNP levels. BNP has been shown to reliably diagnose severe dyspnea caused by HF and to differentiate it from dyspnea due to other conditions.

Arterial blood gas measurement may be considered if clinical examination and routine diagnostic testing are equivocal. With two notable exceptions (carbon monoxide poisoning and cyanide toxicity), arterial blood gas measurement distinguishes increased mechanical effort causes of dyspnea (respiratory acidosis with or without hypoxemia) from compensatory tachypnea (respiratory alkalosis with or without hypoxemia or metabolic acidosis) and from psychogenic dyspnea (respiratory alkalosis). Carbon monoxide and cyanide impair oxygen delivery with minimal alterations in Po_2; percent carboxyhemoglobin identifies carbon monoxide toxicity. Cyanide poisoning should be considered in a patient with profound lactic acidosis following exposure to burning vinyl (such as a theater fire or industrial accident). Suspected carbon monoxide poisoning or methemoglobinemia can also be confirmed with venous carboxyhemoglobin or methemoglobin levels. Venous blood gas testing is also an option for assessing acid-base and respiratory status by measuring venous pH and Pco_2 but is unable to provide information on oxygenation status. To correlate with arterial blood gas values, venous pH is typically 0.03–0.05 units lower, and venous Pco_2 is typically 4–5 mm Hg higher than arterial samples.

Because arterial blood gas testing is impractical in most outpatient settings, pulse oximetry has a central role in the office evaluation of dyspnea. Oxygen saturation values above 96% almost always correspond with a Po_2 greater than 70 mm Hg, whereas values less than 94% may represent clinically significant hypoxemia. Important exceptions to this rule include carbon monoxide toxicity, which leads to a normal oxygen saturation (due to the similar wavelengths of oxyhemoglobin and carboxyhemoglobin), and methemoglobinemia, which results in an oxygen saturation of about 85% that fails to increase with supplemental oxygen. Pulse oximetry to detect occult hypoxia is less accurate in Black patients (OR, 2.57) compared to White patients. A delirious or obtunded patient with obstructive lung disease warrants immediate measurement of arterial blood gases to exclude hypercapnia and the need for intubation, regardless of the oxygen saturation. If a patient reports dyspnea with exertion, but resting oximetry is normal, assessment of desaturation with ambulation (eg, a brisk walk around the clinic) can be useful for confirming impaired gas exchange. Persons with COVID-19 may have low oxygen saturation with minimal dyspnea and profound desaturation with minimal exertion.

A study found that for adults without known cardiac or pulmonary disease reporting dyspnea on exertion, spirometry, NT-proBNP, and CT imaging were the most informative tests.

Episodic dyspnea can be challenging if an evaluation cannot be performed during symptoms. Life-threatening causes include recurrent PE, myocardial ischemia, and reactive airway disease. When associated with audible wheezing, vocal fold dysfunction should be considered, particularly in a young woman who does not respond to asthma therapy. Spirometry is very helpful in further classifying patients with obstructive airway disease but is rarely needed in the initial or emergent evaluation of patients with acute dyspnea.

Differential Diagnosis

Urgent and emergent conditions causing acute dyspnea include pneumonia, COPD, asthma, pneumothorax, PE, cardiac disease (eg, HF, acute MI, valvular dysfunction, arrhythmia, intracardiac shunt), pleural effusion, COVID-19, diffuse alveolar hemorrhage, metabolic acidosis, cyanide toxicity, methemoglobinemia, and carbon monoxide poisoning. Chronic dyspnea may be caused by interstitial lung disease, pulmonary hypertension, or pulmonary alveolar proteinosis.

Treatment

The treatment of urgent or emergent causes of dyspnea should aim to relieve the underlying cause. Pending diagnosis, patients with hypoxemia should be immediately provided supplemental oxygen unless significant hypercapnia is present or strongly suspected pending arterial blood gas measurement. Dyspnea frequently occurs in patients nearing the end of life. Opioid therapy, anxiolytics, and corticosteroids can provide substantial relief independent of the severity of hypoxemia. However, inhaled opioids are not effective.

Oxygen therapy is most beneficial to patients with significant hypoxemia (Pao_2 less than 55 mm Hg) (see Chapter 5). In patients with severe COPD and hypoxemia, oxygen therapy improves exercise performance and mortality. Pulmonary rehabilitation programs are another therapeutic option for patients with moderate to severe COPD or interstitial pulmonary fibrosis. Noninvasive ventilation may be considered for patients with dyspnea caused by an acute COPD exacerbation.

When to Refer

- Following acute stabilization, patients with advanced COPD should be referred to a pulmonologist, and patients with HF or valvular heart disease should be referred to a cardiologist.
- Cyanide toxicity or carbon monoxide poisoning should be managed in conjunction with a toxicologist.
- Lung transplantation can be considered for patients with advanced interstitial lung disease.

When to Admit

- Impaired gas exchange from any cause or high risk of PE pending definitive diagnosis.
- Suspected cyanide toxicity or carbon monoxide poisoning.

Corson-Knowles DR et al. In outpatients, low or moderate clinical pretest probability with probability-defined D-dimer cut points ruled out PE. Ann Intern Med. 2020;172:JC47. [PMID: 32311731]

Gartlehner G et al. Point-of-care ultrasonography in patients with acute dyspnea: an evidence report for a clinical practice guideline by the American College of Physicians. Ann Intern Med. 2021;174:967. [PMID: 33900798]

Valbuena VSM et al. Racial bias in pulse oximetry measurement among patients about to undergo ECMO in 2019–2020, a retrospective cohort study. Chest. 2021 Sep 27. [Epub ahead of print] [PMID: 34592317]

HEMOPTYSIS

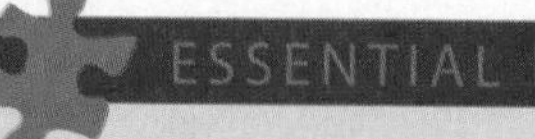

ESSENTIAL INQUIRIES

- Fever, cough, and other symptoms of lower respiratory tract infection.
- Smoking history.
- Nasopharyngeal or GI bleeding.
- Chest radiography and CBC (and, in some cases, INR).

General Considerations

Hemoptysis is the expectoration of blood that originates below the vocal folds. It is commonly classified as trivial, mild, or massive—the latter defined as more than 200–600 mL (about 1–2 cups) in 24 hours. Massive hemoptysis can be usefully defined as any amount that is hemodynamically significant or threatens ventilation. Its in-hospital mortality was 6.5% in one study. The initial goal of management of massive hemoptysis is therapeutic, not diagnostic.

The causes of hemoptysis can be classified anatomically. Blood may arise from the upper airway due to malignant invasion or foreign body; from the airways in COPD, bronchiectasis, bronchial Dieulafoy disease, and bronchogenic carcinoma; from the pulmonary vasculature in LV failure, mitral stenosis, PE, pulmonary arterial hypertension, telangiectasias, arteriovenous malformations, and multiple pulmonary artery aneurysms; from the systemic circulation in intralobar pulmonary sequestration, aortobronchial fistula; or from the pulmonary parenchyma in pneumonia, fungal infections, inhalation of crack cocaine, granulomatosis with polyangiitis, or Takayasu arteritis with pulmonary arteritis. Hemoptysis can be caused by the parasitic diseases paragonimiasis (most common cause worldwide) and human echinococcosis (also called hydatid disease). Diffuse alveolar hemorrhage—manifested by alveolar infiltrates on chest radiography—is due to small vessel bleeding usually caused by autoimmune or hemostatic disorders, or rarely precipitated by hypertensive emergency or anticoagulant therapy. Most cases of hemoptysis presenting in the outpatient setting are due to infection (eg, acute or chronic bronchitis, pneumonia, tuberculosis, infection with *Mycobacterium avium* complex, aspergillosis). Hemoptysis due to lung cancer increases with age, causing up to 20% of cases among older adults. Pulmonary venous hypertension (eg, mitral stenosis, PE) causes hemoptysis in less than 10% of cases. Most cases of hemoptysis that have no visible cause on CT scan or bronchoscopy will resolve within 6 months without treatment, with the notable exception of patients at high risk for lung cancer (patients who smoke cigarettes and are older than 40 years). Iatrogenic hemorrhage may follow transbronchial lung biopsies, anticoagulation, or pulmonary artery rupture due to distal placement of a balloon-tipped catheter. Obstructive sleep apnea with elevated pulmonary arterial pressure may be a risk factor for hemoptysis. Amyloidosis of the lung can cause hemoptysis, as can endometriosis. No cause is identified in up to 15–30% of cases.

Clinical Findings

A. Symptoms

Blood-tinged sputum in the setting of an upper respiratory tract infection in an otherwise healthy, young (age under 40 years) nonsmoker does not warrant an extensive diagnostic evaluation if the hemoptysis subsides with resolution of the infection. However, hemoptysis is frequently a sign of serious disease, especially in patients with a high prior probability of underlying pulmonary pathology. Hemoptysis is the only symptom found to be a specific predictor of lung cancer. It portends a high risk of mortality in COVID-19 infection. There is no value in distinguishing blood-streaked sputum and cough productive of blood during evaluation; the goal of the history is to identify patients at risk for one of the disorders listed earlier. Pertinent features include duration of symptoms, presence of respiratory infection, and past or current tobacco use. Nonpulmonary sources of hemorrhage—from the sinuses or the GI tract—must be excluded.

B. Physical Examination

Elevated pulse, hypotension, and decreased oxygen saturation suggest large-volume hemorrhage that warrants emergent evaluation and stabilization. The nares and oropharynx should be carefully inspected to identify a potential upper airway source of bleeding. Chest and cardiac examination may reveal evidence of HF or mitral stenosis.

C. Diagnostic Studies

Diagnostic evaluation should include a chest radiograph and CBC. Kidney function tests, UA, and coagulation studies are appropriate in specific circumstances. Hematuria that accompanies hemoptysis may be a clue to anti-basement membrane antibody disease or vasculitis. Flexible bronchoscopy reveals endobronchial cancer in 3–6% of patients with hemoptysis who have a normal (non-lateralizing) chest radiograph. Nearly all these patients are cigarette smokers over the age of 40, and most will have had symptoms for more than 1 week. High-resolution chest CT scan complements bronchoscopy; it can visualize unsuspected bronchiectasis and arteriovenous malformations and will show central endobronchial cancers in many cases. It is the test of choice for suspected small peripheral malignancies. Helical pulmonary CT angiography is the initial test of choice for evaluating patients with suspected PE, although caution should be taken to avoid large contrast loads in patients with even mild CKD (serum creatinine greater than 2.0 g/dL or rapidly rising creatinine in normal range). Helical CT scanning can be avoided in patients who are at "unlikely" risk for PE using the Wells score or PERC (Pulmonary Embolism Rule-Out Criteria) rule for PE and the sensitive D-dimer test (see Chapter 9). Echocardiography may reveal evidence of HF or mitral stenosis. Multidetector CT angiography is the study of choice to determine the location, etiology, and mechanism of the bleeding.

Treatment

Management of mild hemoptysis consists of identifying and treating the specific cause. Massive hemoptysis is life-threatening. The airway should be protected with endotracheal intubation, ventilation ensured, and effective circulation maintained. If the location of the bleeding site is known, the patient should be placed in the decubitus position with the involved lung dependent. Uncontrollable hemorrhage warrants rigid bronchoscopy and surgical consultation. In stable patients, flexible bronchoscopy may localize the site of bleeding, and angiography can embolize the involved bronchial arteries. Embolization is effective initially in 85% of cases, although rebleeding may occur in up to 20% of patients during the following year. The anterior spinal artery arises from the bronchial artery in up to 5% of people, and paraplegia may result if it is inadvertently cannulated and embolized.

One double-blind, randomized controlled trial compared treatment with inhalations of tranexamic acid (an antifibrinolytic drug) versus placebo (normal saline) in patients hospitalized with mild hemoptysis (less than 200 mL of expectorated blood per 24 hours). Compared to patients receiving placebo (normal saline), more patients treated with tranexamic acid experienced resolution of hemoptysis within 5 days of admission (96% versus 50%). In addition, mean hospital length of stay was shorter for the tranexamic acid group, and fewer patients required invasive procedures (interventional bronchoscopy, angiographic embolization) to control the hemorrhage. Another randomized study found that compared to the control group, patients given tranexamic acid on admission had significantly lower in-hospital mortality (11.5% versus 9.0%).

When to Refer

- Refer to a pulmonologist when bronchoscopy of the lower respiratory tract is needed.
- Refer to an otolaryngologist when an upper respiratory tract bleeding source is identified.
- Refer to a hematologist when severe coagulopathy complicates management.

When to Admit

- To stabilize bleeding process in patients at risk for or experiencing massive hemoptysis.
- To correct disordered coagulation (using clotting factors or platelets, or both) or to reverse anticoagulation.
- To stabilize gas exchange.

Davidson K et al. Managing massive hemoptysis. Chest. 2020;157:77. [PMID: 31374211]

Kinoshita T et al. Effect of tranexamic acid on mortality in patients with haemoptysis: a nationwide study. Crit Care. 2019;23:347. [PMID: 31694697]

CHEST PAIN

- Pain onset, character, location/size, duration, periodicity, and exacerbators; shortness of breath.
- Vital signs; chest and cardiac examinations.
- ECG and biomarkers of myocardial necrosis in selected patients.

General Considerations

Chest pain (or chest discomfort) can occur as a result of cardiovascular, pulmonary, pleural, or musculoskeletal disease; esophageal or other GI disorders; herpes zoster; cocaine use; or anxiety states. The frequency and distribution of life-threatening causes of chest pain, such as acute coronary syndrome (ACS), pericarditis, aortic dissection, vasospastic angina, PE, pneumonia, and esophageal perforation, vary substantially between clinical settings.

SLE, rheumatoid arthritis, reduced eGFR, and HIV infection are conditions that confer a strong risk of CAD. Precocious ACS (occurring in patients aged 35 years or younger) may represent acute thrombosis independent of underlying atherosclerotic disease. Risk factors for precocious ACS are obesity, hyperlipidemia, and smoking.

Although ACS presents with a broader range of symptoms in women than men, specific chest pain characteristics of acute MI do not differ in frequency or strength between men and women.

Because PE can present with a wide variety of symptoms, consideration of the diagnosis and rigorous risk factor assessment for venous thromboembolism (VTE) is critical. Classic VTE risk factors include cancer, trauma, recent surgery, prolonged immobilization, pregnancy, oral contraceptives, and family history and prior history of VTE. Other conditions associated with increased risk of PE include HF and COPD. Sickle cell anemia can cause acute chest syndrome. Patients with this syndrome often have chest pain, fever, and cough.

Clinical Findings

A. Symptoms

Myocardial ischemia is usually described as a dull, aching sensation of "pressure," "tightness," "squeezing," or "gas," rather than as sharp or spasmodic. Pain reaching maximum intensity in seconds is uncommon. Ischemic symptoms usually subside within 5–20 minutes but may last longer. Progressive symptoms or symptoms at rest may represent unstable angina. Up to one-third of patients with acute MI do not report chest pain. Chest pain is present in more than 90% of patients having a STEMI who are under age 65 but in only 57% of patients having a STEMI who are over age 85.

Continuous chest pain lasting 24 hours or longer is unlikely due to an acute MI (LR, 0.15). However, chest pain lasting 1 minute or less does not exclude MI (LR, 0.95). When present, pain due to myocardial ischemia is commonly accompanied by a sense of anxiety or uneasiness. The location is usually retrosternal or left precordial. Because the heart lacks somatic innervation, precise localization of pain due to cardiac ischemia is difficult; the pain is commonly referred to the throat, lower jaw, shoulders, inner arms, upper abdomen, or back. Ischemic pain may be precipitated or exacerbated by exertion, cold temperature, meals, stress, or combinations of these factors and is usually relieved by rest. However, many episodes do not conform to these patterns, and a broader range of symptoms of ACS are more common in older adults, women, and persons with diabetes mellitus. Other symptoms that are associated with ACS include shortness of breath; dizziness; a feeling of impending doom; and vagal symptoms, such as nausea and diaphoresis. In older persons, fatigue is a common presenting complaint of ACS.

The presenting symptoms of acute MI in young patients are different in men and women. Women are more likely than men to present with three or more associated symptoms (eg, epigastric symptoms; palpitations; and pain or discomfort in the jaw, neck, arms, or between the shoulder blades; 61.9% for women versus 54.8% for men). In adjusted analyses, women with an acute STEMI were more likely than men to present without chest pain (OR, 1.51). In comparison with men, women were more likely to perceive symptoms as stress/anxiety (20.9% versus 11.8%) but less likely to attribute symptoms to muscle pain (15.4% versus 21.2%).

One analysis found the following clinical features to be associated with acute MI: chest pain that radiates to the left, right, or both arms (LR, 2.3); diaphoresis (LR, 2.0); nausea and vomiting (LR, 1.9); third heart sound (LR, 3.2); systolic blood pressure less than or equal to 80 mm Hg (LR, 3.1); pulmonary crackles (LR, 2.1); any ST-segment elevation greater than or equal to 1 mm (LR, 11.2); any ST depression (LR, 3.2); any Q wave (LR, 3.9); any conduction defect (LR, 2.7); and new conduction defect (LR, 6.3).

A meta-analysis found the clinical findings and risk factors most suggestive of ACS were prior abnormal stress test (specificity, 96%; LR, 3.1), peripheral arterial disease (specificity, 97%; LR, 2.7), and pain radiation to both arms (specificity, 96%; LR, 2.6). The ECG findings associated with ACS were ST-segment depression (specificity, 95%; LR, 5.3) and any evidence of ischemia (specificity, 91%; LR, 3.6). Risk scores derived from both the HEART trial (https://www.mdcalc.com/heart-score-major-cardiac-events) and TIMI trial (https://www.mdcalc.com/timi-risk-score-ua-nstemi#use-cases) performed well in detecting ACS (LR, 13 for HEART score of 7–10, and LR, 6.8 for TIMI score of 5–7).

Hypertrophy of either ventricle or aortic stenosis may also give rise to chest pain with less typical features. Pericarditis produces pain that may be greater when supine than upright and increases with breathing, coughing, or swallowing. Pleuritic chest pain is usually not ischemic, and pain on palpation may indicate a musculoskeletal cause. Aortic dissection classically produces an abrupt onset of tearing pain of great intensity that often radiates to the back; however, this classic presentation occurs in a small proportion of cases. Anterior aortic dissection can also lead to myocardial or cerebrovascular ischemia.

In PE, chest pain is present in about 75% of cases. The chief objective in evaluating patients with suspected PE is to assess the patient's clinical risk for VTE based on medical history and associated symptoms and signs (see above and Chapter 9). Rupture of the thoracic esophagus iatrogenically or secondary to vomiting is another cause of chest pain.

B. Physical Examination

Findings on physical examination can occasionally yield important clues to the underlying cause of chest pain; however, a normal physical examination should never be used as the sole basis for ruling out most diagnoses, particularly ACS and aortic dissection. Vital signs (including pulse oximetry) and cardiopulmonary examination are always the first steps for assessing the urgency and tempo of the subsequent examination and diagnostic workup. Although chest pain that is reproducible or worsened with palpation strongly suggests a musculoskeletal cause, up to 15% of patients with ACS will have reproducible chest wall tenderness. Pointing to the location of the pain with one finger has been shown to be highly correlated with nonischemic chest pain.

Aortic dissection can result in differential blood pressures (greater than 20 mm Hg), pulse amplitude deficits, and new diastolic murmurs. Although hypertension is considered the rule in patients with aortic dissection, systolic blood pressure less than 100 mm Hg is present in up to 25% of patients.

A cardiac friction rub represents pericarditis until proven otherwise. It can best be heard with the patient sitting forward at end-expiration. Tamponade should be excluded in all patients with a clinical diagnosis of pericarditis by assessing pulsus paradoxus (a decrease in systolic blood pressure greater than 10 mm Hg during inspiration) and inspection of jugular venous pulsations. Subcutaneous emphysema is common following cervical esophageal perforation but present in only about one-third of thoracic perforations (ie, those most commonly presenting with chest pain).

The absence of abnormal physical examination findings in patients with suspected PE usually serves to *increase* its likelihood, although a normal physical examination is also compatible with the much more common conditions of panic/anxiety disorder and musculoskeletal disease.

C. Diagnostic Studies

Unless a competing diagnosis can be confirmed, an ECG is warranted in the initial evaluation of most patients with acute chest pain to help exclude ACS. When compared with White patients, Black patients who came to the emergency department with chest pain were less likely to have an ECG ordered (adjusted OR = 0.82). In a study of 11 emergency departments in Italy, 67% of patients with confirmed ACS had new-onset alterations of the ECG (compared with only 6.2% among non-ACS patients). ST-segment elevation is the ECG finding that is the strongest predictor of acute MI; however, up to 20% of patients with ACS can have a normal ECG.

In the emergency department, patients with suspected ACS can be safely removed from cardiac monitoring if they are pain-free at initial physician assessment and have a normal or nonspecific ECG. This decision rule had 100% sensitivity for serious arrhythmia. Clinically stable patients with CVD risk factors, normal ECG, normal cardiac biomarkers, and no alternative diagnoses (such as typical GERD or costochondritis) should be followed up with a timely exercise stress test that includes perfusion imaging. However, more than 25% of patients with stable chest pain referred for noninvasive testing will have normal coronary arteries and no long-term clinical events. The ECG can also provide evidence for alternative diagnoses, such as pericarditis and PE. Chest radiography is often useful in the evaluation of chest pain and is always indicated when cough or shortness of breath accompanies chest pain.

Findings of pneumomediastinum or new pleural effusion are consistent with esophageal perforation. Stress echocardiography is useful in risk stratifying patients with chest pain, even among those with significant obesity.

Diagnostic protocols using a single high-sensitivity troponin assay combined with a standardized clinical assessment are an efficient strategy to rapidly determine whether patients with chest pain are at low risk and may be discharged from the emergency department. A study of the modified HEART score using a single blood draw of either high-sensitivity troponin (3.9 ng/L), high-sensitivity troponin I (0.9 ng/L) or conventional troponin I (0.0 ng/L) at presentation had a sensitivity of 100% for 30-day major adverse cardiac events. Point-of-care troponin testing during ambulance transport to the emergency department has been found to have good specificity and positive predictive value (99.2% and 85.7%) but poor sensitivity (26.5%).

Six established risk scores are (1) the modified Goldman Risk Score, (2) TIMI Risk Score, (3) Global Registry of Acute Cardiac Events Risk Score, (4) HEART Risk Score, (5) Vancouver Chest Pain Rule, and (6) the European Society of Cardiology (ESC) 0/1-h algorithm. A study comparing these risk scores (not including the ESC algorithm) for predicting acute MI within 30 days reported a sensitivity of 98% (which correlates with a negative predictive value of greater than or equal to 99.5%). Patients eligible for discharge (about 30%) were those with a TIMI score of less than or equal to 1, modified Goldman score of less than or equal to 1 with normal high-sensitivity troponin T, TIMI score of 0, or HEART score of less than or equal to 3 with normal high-sensitivity troponin I. In Black patients with average cardiovascular risk, HEART score is a better predictive tool for 6-week major adverse cardiac events when compared to TIMI score. Six-week major adverse cardiac events among patients with a low-risk HEART score (0–3) was 0.9–1.7%. The HEART score performs poorly in stratifying risk from cocaine-associated chest pain.

The Emergency Department Assessment of Chest Pain Score identified more patients as low-risk compared to the Heart Pathway (58.1% to 38.4%), but major adverse cardiac events occurred in 0.4% of Heart Pathway patients compared to 1.0% of the Emergency Department Assessment of Chest Pain Score identified patients.

While some studies of high-sensitivity cardiac troponin suggest that it may be the best cardiac biomarker, it may not outperform conventional troponin assays if an appropriate cutoff is used.

Patients who arrive at the emergency department with chest pain of intermediate or high probability for ACS without electrocardiographic or biomarker evidence of an MI can be safely discharged from an observation unit after stress cardiac MRI. Sixty-four–slice coronary CT angiography is an alternative to stress testing in the emergency department for detecting ACS among patients with normal or nonspecific ECG and normal biomarkers. A meta-analysis of nine studies found CT angiography had an estimated sensitivity of 95% for ACS and specificity of 87%, yielding an a negative LR of 0.06 and a positive LR of 7.4.

Functional testing appears to be the best initial noninvasive test in symptomatic patients with suspected CAD. CT-derived fractional flow reserve in acute chest pain has higher specificity for anatomic and physiologic assessment of coronary artery stenosis compared with coronary CT angiography. Coronary CT angiography applied early in the evaluation of suspected ACS does not identify more patients with significant CAD requiring coronary revascularization, shorten hospital stay, or allow for more direct discharge from the emergency department compared to high-sensitivity troponins. CT angiography is an option for patients who do not have access to functional testing.

A minimal-risk model developed by the PROMISE investigators includes 10 clinical variables that correlate with normal coronary CT angiography results and no clinical events: (1) younger age; (2) female sex; (3) racial or ethnic minority; (4–6) no history of hypertension, diabetes, or dyslipidemia; (7) no family history of premature CAD; (8) never smoking; (9) symptoms unrelated to physical or mental stress; and (10) higher HDL cholesterol level. In the PROMISE trial, women had higher rates of normal noninvasive testing compared with men, but women with abnormalities on such testing were less likely to be referred for catheterization or to receive statin therapy.

In the evaluation of PE, diagnostic test decisions and results must be interpreted in the context of the clinical likelihood of VTE. A negative D-dimer test is helpful for excluding PE in patients with low clinical probability of VTE (3-month incidence = 0.5%); however, the 3-month risk of VTE among patients with intermediate and high risk of VTE is sufficiently high in the setting of a negative D-dimer test (3.5% and 21.4%, respectively) to warrant further imaging given the life-threatening nature of this condition if left untreated. CT angiography has replaced ventilation-perfusion scanning as the preferred initial diagnostic test, having approximately 90–95% sensitivity and 95% specificity for detecting PE (compared with pulmonary angiography). However, for patients with high clinical probability of VTE, lower extremity ultrasound or pulmonary angiogram may be indicated even with a normal helical CT.

Panic disorder is a common cause of chest pain, accounting for up to 25% of cases that present to emergency departments and a higher proportion of cases presenting in primary care office practices. Features that correlate with an increased likelihood of panic disorder include absence of CAD, atypical quality of chest pain, female sex, younger age, and a high level of self-reported anxiety. Depression is associated with recurrent chest pain with or without CAD (OR, 2.11).

Treatment

Treatment of chest pain should be guided by the underlying etiology. The term "noncardiac chest pain" is used when a diagnosis remains elusive after patients have undergone an extensive workup. Almost half of patients with noncardiac chest pain reported symptom improvement with high-dose PPI therapy. Relief of constipation may be therapeutic in PPI refractory noncardiac chest pain. A meta-analysis of 15 trials suggested modest to moderate benefit for psychological (especially cognitive-behavioral) interventions. It is unclear whether tricyclic or SSRI antidepressants have benefit in noncardiac chest pain. Hypnotherapy may offer some benefit.

When to Refer

- Refer patients with poorly controlled, noncardiac chest pain to a pain specialist.
- Refer patients with angina that is poorly controlled using maximal medical therapy to a cardiologist.
- Refer patients with sickle cell anemia to a hematologist.

When to Admit

- Failure to adequately exclude life-threatening causes of chest pain, particularly MI, dissecting aortic aneurysm, PE, and esophageal rupture.
- Patients with high-risk of complications from PE, or when PE is likely despite negative spiral CT.
- TIMI score of 1 or more, HEART score greater than 3, abnormal ECG, and abnormal 0- and 2-hour troponin tests.
- Pain control for rib fracture that impairs gas exchange.

Gulati M et al. 2021 AHA/ACC/ASE/CHEST/SAEM/SCCT/SCMR guideline for the evaluation and diagnosis of chest pain: a report of the American College of Cardiology/American Heart Association Joint Committee on Clinical Practice Guidelines. Circulation. 2021;144:e368. [PMID: 34709879]

Meyer MR. Chronic coronary syndromes in women: challenges in diagnosis and management. Mayo Clin Proc. 2021;96:1058. [PMID: 33814074]

Mukhopadhyay A et al. Racial and insurance disparities among patients presenting with chest pain in the US: 2009–2015. Am J Emerg Med. 2020;38:1373. [PMID: 31843328]

Smith LM et al. Identification of very low-risk acute chest pain patients without troponin testing. Emerg Med J. 2020;37:690. [PMID: 32753395]

Stepinska J et al. Diagnosis and risk stratification of chest pain patients in the emergency department: focus on acute coronary syndromes. A position paper of the Acute Cardiovascular Care Association. Eur Heart J Acute Cardiovasc Care. 2020;9:76. [PMID: 31958018]

Tan JWC et al. Performance of cardiac troponins within the HEART score in predicting major adverse cardiac events at the emergency department. Am J Emerg Med. 2020;38:1560. [PMID: 31493982]

Zitek T et al. The association of chest pain duration and other historical features with major adverse cardiac events. Am J Emerg Med. 2020;38:1377. [PMID: 31843326]

PALPITATIONS

ESSENTIAL INQUIRIES

- Forceful, rapid, or irregular beating of the heart.
- Rate, duration, and degree of regularity of heartbeat; age at first episode.
- Factors that precipitate or terminate episodes.
- Light-headedness or syncope; neck pounding.
- Chest pain; history of MI or structural heart disease.

General Considerations

Palpitations are defined as an unpleasant awareness of the forceful, rapid, or irregular beating of the heart. They are the primary symptom for approximately 16% of patients presenting to an outpatient clinic with a cardiac complaint. In an observational cohort study of palpitations at an outpatient cardiac unit, cardiac arrhythmias were the cause of palpitations in 81% of cases. Palpitations represent 5.8 of every 1000 emergency department visits, with an admission rate of 24.6%. While palpitations are usually benign, they are occasionally the symptom of a life-threatening arrhythmia. To avoid missing a dangerous cause of the patient's symptom, clinicians sometimes pursue expensive and invasive testing when a conservative diagnostic evaluation is often sufficient. The converse is also true. Table 2–3 lists history, physical examination, and ECG findings suggesting a cardiovascular cause for the palpitations.

When assessing a patient with palpitations in an urgent care setting, the clinician must ascertain whether the symptoms represent (1) a significant CVD, (2) a cardiac manifestation of a systemic disease such as thyrotoxicosis, (3) an arrhythmia that is minor and transient, or (4) a benign somatic symptom that is amplified by the patient's underlying psychological state.

Etiology

Patients with palpitations who seek medical attention in an emergency department instead of a medical clinic are more likely to have a cardiac cause (47% versus 21%), whereas psychogenic causes are more common among those who seek attention in office practices (45% versus 27%). In a study of patients who went to a university medical clinic with the chief complaint of palpitations, causes were cardiac in 43%, psychogenic in 31%, and miscellaneous in 10%.

Cardiac arrhythmias that can result in symptoms of palpitations include sinus bradycardia; atrial fibrillation or flutter; sinus, supraventricular, and ventricular tachycardia; premature ventricular and atrial contractions; sick sinus syndrome; and advanced atrioventricular block.

Cardiac structural causes of palpitations include valvular heart diseases, such as aortic regurgitation or stenosis, atrial or ventricular septal defect, cardiomyopathy, congenital heart disease, pericarditis, arrhythmogenic RV cardiomyopathy, and atrial myxoma. Mitral valve prolapse is not associated with arrhythmic events, but ventricular arrhythmias are frequent in mitral annulus disjunction.

Pericardial or myocardial infection with SARS-CoV-2, tuberculosis, and *Trypanosoma cruzi* (Chagas disease) can cause palpitations.

The most common psychogenic causes of palpitations are anxiety and panic disorder. The release of catecholamines during a significant stress or panic attack can trigger an arrhythmia. Asking a single question, "Have you experienced brief periods, for seconds or minutes, of an overwhelming panic or terror that was accompanied by racing heartbeats, shortness of breath, or dizziness?" can help identify patients with panic disorder.

Other causes of palpitations include fever, dehydration, hypoglycemia, anemia, thyrotoxicosis, mastocytosis, and pheochromocytoma. Drugs (such as cocaine, alcohol, caffeine, pseudoephedrine, cannabis, and illicit ephedra), prescription medications (including digoxin, amitriptyline, erythromycin, methylphenidate) as well as other drugs that prolong the QT interval, class 1 antiarrhythmics, dihydropyridine calcium channel blockers, phenothiazines, theophylline, and beta-agonists can precipitate palpitations.

Clinical Findings

A. Symptoms

Guiding the patient through a careful description of their palpitations may indicate a mechanism and narrow the differential diagnosis. Pertinent questions include the age at first episode; precipitants; and rate, duration, and degree of regularity of the heartbeat during the subjective palpitations. Palpitations lasting less than 5 minutes and a family history of panic disorder reduce the likelihood of an arrhythmic cause (LR+ = 0.38 and LR+ = 0.26, respectively). To better understand the symptom, the examiner can ask the patient to "tap out" the rhythm with his or her fingers. The circumstances associated with onset and termination can also be helpful in determining the cause. Palpitations that start and stop abruptly suggest supraventricular or ventricular tachycardias. Termination of palpitations using vagal maneuvers (eg, Valsalva maneuver) suggests supraventricular tachycardia.

Three common descriptions of palpitations are (1) "flip-flopping" (or "stop and start"), often caused by premature contraction of the atrium or ventricle, with the perceived "stop" from the pause following the contraction, and the "start" from the subsequent forceful contraction; (2) rapid "fluttering in the chest," with regular "fluttering" suggesting supraventricular or ventricular arrhythmias (including sinus tachycardia) and irregular "fluttering" suggesting atrial fibrillation, atrial flutter, or tachycardia with variable block; and (3) "pounding in the neck" or neck pulsations, often due to "cannon" A waves in the jugular venous pulsations that occur when the right atrium contracts against a closed tricuspid valve.

Palpitations associated with chest pain suggest ischemic heart disease, or if the chest pain is relieved by leaning forward, pericardial disease. Palpitations associated with light-headedness, presyncope, or syncope suggest hypotension and may signify a life-threatening cardiac arrhythmia. Palpitations that occur regularly with exertion suggest a rate-dependent bypass tract or hypertrophic cardiomyopathy as well as silent ischemia. If a benign etiology cannot be ascertained at the initial visit, then ambulatory monitoring or prolonged cardiac monitoring in the hospital might be warranted.

Noncardiac symptoms should also be elicited since the palpitations may be caused by a normal heart responding to a metabolic or inflammatory condition. Weight loss suggests hyperthyroidism. Palpitations can be precipitated by vomiting or diarrhea causing electrolyte disorders and hypovolemia. Hyperventilation, hand tingling, and nervousness are common when anxiety or panic disorder is the cause of the palpitations. Palpitations associated with flushing, episodic hypertension, headaches, anxiety, and diaphoresis may be caused by a pheochromocytoma or paraganglioma.

A family history of palpitations or sudden death suggests an inherited etiology such as long QT syndrome or Brugada syndrome. Chagas disease may cause palpitations and acute myocarditis. Younger patients should be asked about consumption of "energy drinks." Finally, dual use of cigarettes and e-cigarettes may cause palpitations.

B. Physical Examination

Careful cardiovascular examination can find abnormalities that can increase the likelihood of specific cardiac arrhythmias. The midsystolic click of mitral valve prolapse can suggest the diagnosis of a supraventricular arrhythmia. The harsh holosystolic murmur of hypertrophic cardiomyopathy, which occurs along the left sternal border and increases with the Valsalva maneuver, suggests atrial fibrillation or ventricular tachycardia. A crescendo mid-diastolic murmur may be caused by an atrial myxoma. The presence of dilated cardiomyopathy, suggested on examination by a displaced and enlarged cardiac point-of-maximal impulse, increases the likelihood of ventricular tachycardia and atrial fibrillation. In patients with chronic atrial fibrillation, in-office exercise (eg, a brisk walk in the hallway) may reveal an intermittent accelerated ventricular response. The clinician should also look for signs of hyperthyroidism (eg, tremulousness, brisk deep tendon reflexes, or fine hand tremor) or signs of stimulant drug use (eg, dilated pupils or skin or nasal septal perforations). Visible neck pulsations (LR+, 2.68) in association with palpitations increase the likelihood of atrioventricular nodal reentry tachycardia.

C. Diagnostic Studies

1. ECG—A 12-lead ECG should be performed on all patients reporting palpitations, although in most instances, a specific arrhythmia will not be detected. Evidence of prior MI on ECG (eg, Q waves) increases the patient's risk of nonsustained or sustained ventricular tachycardia. Ventricular preexcitation (Wolff-Parkinson-White syndrome) is suggested by a short PR interval (less than 0.20 ms) and delta waves (upsloping PR segments). The presence of left atrial enlargement as suggested by a terminal P-wave force in V1 more negative than 0.04 msec and notching in lead II reflects an increased risk of atrial fibrillation. A prolonged QT interval and abnormal T-wave morphology suggest the long QT syndrome, and an increased risk of ventricular tachycardia.

2. Monitoring devices—For high-risk patients (Table 2–3), further diagnostic studies are warranted. A stepwise approach has been suggested—starting with ambulatory monitoring devices (ambulatory ECG monitoring if the palpitations are expected to occur within the subsequent 72-hour period, event monitoring if less frequent). An implantable loop recorder can be used for extended monitoring if clinical suspicion is high, especially if there is syncope. A single-lead, lightweight, continuously recording ambulatory adhesive patch monitor (Zio Patch)

Table 2–3. Palpitations: Patients at high risk for a cardiovascular cause.

Historical risk factors
Family history of significant arrhythmias
Personal or family history of syncope or resuscitated sudden death
History of MI
Palpitations that occur during sleep
Anatomic abnormalities
Structural heart disease such as dilated or hypertrophic cardiomyopathies
Valvular disease (stenotic or regurgitant)
ECG findings
Long QT syndrome
Bradycardia
Second- or third-degree heart block
Sustained ventricular arrhythmias

worn for 14–21 days increases diagnostic yield while reducing cost of diagnosis in patients with recurrent unexplained palpitations. Inpatient continuous monitoring is indicated if serious arrhythmias are strongly suspected despite normal findings on the ambulatory monitoring; invasive electrophysiologic testing should be done if the ambulatory or inpatient monitor records a worrisome arrhythmia.

In patients with a prior MI, ambulatory cardiac monitoring or signal-averaged ECG is an appropriate next step to help exclude ventricular tachycardia. ECG exercise testing is appropriate in patients with suspected CAD and in patients who have palpitations with physical exertion. Echocardiography is useful when physical examination or ECG suggests structural abnormalities or decreased ventricular function.

Treatment

After ambulatory monitoring, most patients with palpitations are found to have benign atrial or ventricular ectopy or nonsustained ventricular tachycardia. In patients with structurally normal hearts, these arrhythmias are not associated with adverse outcomes. Abstention from caffeine and tobacco may help. Often, reassurance suffices. If not, or in very symptomatic patients, a trial of a beta-blocker may be prescribed. A three-session course of cognitive-behavioral therapy that includes some physical activity has proven effective for patients with benign palpitations with or without chest pain. For treatment of specific atrial or ventricular arrhythmias, see Chapter 10.

When to Refer

- For electrophysiologic studies.
- For advice regarding treatment of atrial or ventricular arrhythmias.

When to Admit

- Palpitations associated with syncope or near-syncope, particularly when the patient is aged 75 years or older and has an abnormal ECG, hematocrit less than 30%, shortness of breath, respiratory rate higher than 24/min, or a history of HF.
- Patients with risk factors for a serious arrhythmia.

Francisco-Pascual J et al. Diagnostic yield and economic assessment of a diagnostic protocol with systematic use of an external loop recorder for patients with palpitations. Rev Esp Cardiol (Engl Ed). 2019;72:473. [PMID: 29805092]

Pasha AK et al. Cardiovascular effects of medical marijuana: a systematic review. Am J Med. 2021;134:182. [PMID: 33186596]

Weinstock C et al. Evidence-based approach to palpitations. Med Clin North Am. 2021;105:93. [PMID: 33246525]

LOWER EXTREMITY EDEMA

ESSENTIAL INQUIRIES

- History of VTE.
- Symmetry of swelling.
- Pain.
- Change with dependence.
- Skin findings: hyperpigmentation, stasis dermatitis, lipodermatosclerosis, atrophie blanche, ulceration.

General Considerations

Acute and chronic lower extremity edema present important diagnostic and treatment challenges. **Chronic venous insufficiency** is by far the most common cause, affecting up to 2% of the population, and the incidence of venous insufficiency has not changed over the past 25 years. Venous insufficiency is a common complication of DVT; however, only a small number of patients with chronic venous insufficiency report a history of this disorder. Venous ulceration commonly affects patients with chronic venous insufficiency, and its management is labor-intensive and expensive. Normal lower extremity venous pressure (in the erect position: 80 mm Hg in deep veins, 20–30 mm Hg in superficial veins) and cephalad venous blood flow require competent bicuspid venous valves, effective muscle contractions, normal ankle range of motion, and normal respirations. When one or more of these components fail, venous hypertension may result. Chronic edema increases the risk of cellulitis, with risk increasing as the stage of edema increases.

Clinical Findings

A. Symptoms and Signs

1. Unilateral lower extremity edema—Among common causes of unilateral lower extremity swelling, DVT is the most life-threatening. Clues suggesting DVT include a history of cancer, recent limb immobilization, or confinement to bed for at least 3 days following major surgery within the

Table 2–4. Risk stratification of adults referred for ultrasound to rule out DVT.

Step 1:		
Score 1 point for each		
Untreated malignancy		
Paralysis, paresis, or recent plaster immobilization		
Recently bedridden for > 3 days due to major surgery within 4 weeks		
Localized tenderness along distribution of deep venous system		
Entire leg swelling		
Swelling of one calf > 3 cm more than the other (measured 10 cm below tibial tuberosity)		
Ipsilateral pitting edema		
Collateral superficial (nonvaricose) veins		
Previously documented DVT		
Step 2:		
Subtract 2 points if alternative diagnosis has equal or greater likelihood than DVT		
Step 3:		
Obtain sensitive D-dimer for score ≥ 0		
Score	D-Dimer Positive[1]	D-Dimer Negative
0–1	Obtain ultrasound	Ultrasound not required
≥ 2	Obtain ultrasound	

[1]"Positive" is above local laboratory threshold based on specific test and patient age.

past month (Table 2–4). Adults with varicose veins have a significantly increased risk of DVT. Lower extremity swelling and inflammation in a limb recently affected by DVT could represent anticoagulation failure and thrombus recurrence but more often are caused by **postphlebitic syndrome** with valvular incompetence. Other causes of a painful, swollen calf include cellulitis, musculoskeletal disorders (Baker cyst rupture ["pseudothrombophlebitis"]), gastrocnemius tear or rupture, calf strain or trauma, and left common iliac vein compression (May-Thurner syndrome), as well as other sites of nonthrombotic venous outflow obstruction, such as the inguinal ligament, iliac bifurcation, and popliteal fossa.

2. Bilateral lower extremity edema—Bilateral involvement and significant improvement upon awakening favor systemic causes (eg, venous insufficiency) and can be presenting symptoms of volume overload (HF, cirrhosis, kidney disease [eg, nephrotic syndrome]). The most frequent symptom of chronic venous insufficiency is the sensation of "heavy legs," followed by itching. Chronic exposure to elevated venous pressure accounts for the brawny, fibrotic skin changes observed in patients with chronic venous insufficiency as well as the predisposition toward skin ulceration, particularly in the medial malleolar area. Pain, particularly if severe, is uncommon in uncomplicated venous insufficiency.

Lower extremity swelling is a familiar complication of therapy with calcium channel blockers (particularly felodipine and amlodipine), pioglitazone, gabapentin, and minoxidil. Prolonged airline flights (longer than 10 hours) are associated with edema even in the absence of DVT.

B. Physical Examination

Physical examination should include assessment of the heart, lungs, and abdomen for evidence of pulmonary hypertension (primary or secondary to chronic lung disease), HF, or cirrhosis. The skin findings related to chronic venous insufficiency depend on the severity and chronicity of the disease, ranging from hyperpigmentation and stasis dermatitis to abnormalities highly specific for chronic venous insufficiency: lipodermatosclerosis (thick, brawny skin; in advanced cases, the lower leg resembles an inverted champagne bottle) and atrophie blanche (small, depigmented macules within areas of heavy pigmentation). The size of both calves should be measured 10 cm below the tibial tuberosity and pitting and tenderness elicited. Swelling of the entire leg or of one leg 3 cm more than the other suggests deep venous obstruction. The left calf is normally slightly larger than the right as a result of the left common iliac vein coursing under the aorta.

A shallow, large, modestly painful ulcer located over the medial malleolus is a hallmark of chronic venous insufficiency, whereas small, deep, and more painful ulcers are more apt to be due to arterial insufficiency, vasculitis, or infection. Diabetic vascular ulcers, however, may be painless. When an ulcer is on the foot or above the mid-calf, causes other than venous insufficiency should be considered.

The physical examination is usually inadequate to distinguish lymphedema from venous insufficiency. Only the Kaposi-Stemmer sign (the inability to pinch or pick up a fold of skin at the base of the second toe because of its thickness) was a significant predictor of lymphedema (OR, 7.9; $P = 0.02$).

C. Diagnostic Studies

Patients without an obvious cause of acute unilateral lower extremity swelling (eg, calf strain) should have an ultrasound performed, since DVT is difficult to exclude on clinical grounds. A prediction rule allows a clinician to exclude a lower extremity DVT in patients without an ultrasound if the patient has low pretest probability for DVT and a negative sensitive D-dimer test (the "Wells prediction rule") (https://www.mdcalc.com/wells-criteria-pulmonary-embolism) (Chapter 9).

The diagnostic study of choice to detect chronic venous insufficiency due venous incompetence is duplex ultrasonography. Assessment of the ankle-brachial pressure index is important in the management of chronic venous insufficiency since peripheral arterial disease may be exacerbated by compression therapy. Caution is required in interpreting the results of ankle-brachial pressure index in older patients and diabetic patients due to the decreased compressibility of their arteries. A urine dipstick test that is strongly positive for protein can suggest nephrotic syndrome, and a serum creatinine can help estimate kidney function. Measuring serum albumin can be considered to further evaluate suspected nephrotic syndrome or when chronic liver disease is suspected. Lymphoscintigraphy can be used to confirm a clinical suspicion of lymphedema.

Treatment

See relevant chapters for treatment of edema in patients with HF (Chapter 10), nephrosis (Chapter 22), cirrhosis (Chapter 16), and lymphedema and venous stasis ulcers (Chapter 12). Edema resulting from calcium channel blocker therapy responds to concomitant therapy with ACE inhibitors or ARBs.

In patients with chronic venous insufficiency without a comorbid volume overload state (eg, HF), it is best to avoid diuretic therapy. These patients have relatively decreased intravascular volume, and administration of diuretics may first enhance sodium retention through increased secretion of renin and angiotensin and then result in AKI and oliguria. Instead, the most effective treatment involves (1) leg elevation, above the level of the heart, for 30 minutes three to four times daily, and during sleep; (2) compression therapy; and (3) ambulatory exercise to increase venous return through calf muscle contractions.

A wide variety of stockings and devices are effective in decreasing swelling and preventing ulcer formation and reducing the risk of cellulitis. They should be put on with awakening before hydrostatic forces result in edema. To control mild edema, 20–30 mm Hg compression is usually sufficient, whereas 30–40 mm Hg compression is usually required to control moderate to severe edema associated with ulcer formation. To maintain improvement, consider switching from an elastic stocking to one made of inelastic grosgrain material. Patients with decreased ankle-brachial pressure index should be managed in concert with a vascular surgeon. Compression stockings (12–18 mm Hg at the ankle) are effective in preventing edema and asymptomatic thrombosis associated with long airline flights in low- to medium-risk persons, and compression therapy decreases recurrence of cellulitis among patients with chronic venous insufficiency. Support stockings are recommended for pregnant women during air travel. For lymphedema, bandaging systems applied twice weekly can be effective. Multi-component compression bandaging may offer additional benefit. Short-term manual lymphatic drainage treatment may improve chronic venous insufficiency severity, symptoms, and quality of life. For patients with reduced mobility and leg edema, intermittent pneumatic compression treatment can reduce edema and improve ankle range of motion.

Liposuction, suction-assisted lipectomy, and subcutaneous drainage may have treatment benefit if conservative measures fail in treatment of lymphedema.

When to Refer

- Refer patients with chronic lower extremity ulcerations to wound care specialist.
- Refer patients with nephrotic syndrome to a nephrologist.
- Refer patients with coexisting severe arterial insufficiency (claudication) that would complicate treatment with compression stockings to a vascular surgeon.

When to Admit

- Pending definitive diagnosis in patients at high risk for DVT despite normal lower extremity ultrasound.
- Severe, acute swelling raising concern for an impending compartment syndrome.
- Severe edema that impairs ability to ambulate or perform activities of daily living.

Chopard R et al. Diagnosis and treatment of lower extremity venous thromboembolism: a review. JAMA. 2020;324:1765. [PMID: 33141212]

Webb E et al. Compression therapy to prevent recurrent cellulitis of the leg. N Engl J Med. 2020;383:630. [PMID: 32786188]

FEVER & HYPERTHERMIA

ESSENTIAL INQUIRIES

- Age; injection substance use.
- Localizing symptoms; weight loss; joint pain.
- Immunosuppression or neutropenia; history of cancer, risk of COVID-19.
- Medications.
- Travel.

General Considerations

The average normal oral body temperature taken in midmorning is 36.7°C (range 36–37.4°C). This range includes a mean and 2 standard deviations, thus encompassing 95% of a normal population (normal diurnal temperature variation is 0.5–1°C).

The normal rectal or vaginal temperature is 0.5°C higher than the oral temperature, and the axillary temperature is 0.5°C lower. However, a normal body temperature based on a peripheral thermometer (tympanic membrane, temporal artery, axillary, oral) does not always exclude the presence of a fever. To exclude a fever, a rectal temperature is more reliable than an oral temperature (particularly in patients who breathe through their mouth, who are tachypneic, or who are in an ICU setting where a rectal temperature probe can be placed to detect fever).

Fever is a regulated rise to a new "set point" of body temperature in the hypothalamus induced by pyrogenic cytokines. These cytokines include interleukin-1 (IL-1), tumor necrosis factor, interferon-gamma, and interleukin-6 (IL-6). The elevation in temperature results from either increased heat production (eg, shivering) or decreased heat loss (eg, peripheral vasoconstriction). **Hyperthermia**—not mediated by cytokines—occurs when body metabolic heat production (as in thyroid storm) or environmental heat load exceeds normal heat loss capacity or when there is impaired heat loss (eg, heat stroke). *Body temperature in cytokine-induced fever seldom exceeds 41.1°C unless there is structural damage to hypothalamic regulatory centers; body temperature in hyperthermia may rise to levels (more than 41.1°C) capable of producing irreversible protein denaturation and resultant brain damage; no diurnal variation is observed.*

Clinical Findings

A. Fever

Fever as a symptom provides important information about the presence of illness—particularly infections—and about changes in the clinical status of the patient. Fever may be more predictive of bacteremia in elderly patients. The fever pattern, however, is of marginal value for most specific diagnoses except for the relapsing fever of malaria, borreliosis, and occasional cases of lymphoma, especially Hodgkin disease. Furthermore, the degree of temperature elevation does not necessarily correspond to the severity of the illness. Fever with rash and eosinophilia defines the **d**rug **r**eaction with **e**osinophilia and **s**ystemic **s**ymptoms (DRESS) syndrome.

In general, the febrile response tends to be greater in children than in adults. In older persons, neonates, and persons receiving certain medications (eg, NSAIDs, corticosteroids), rather than a fever, a normal temperature or even hypothermia may be observed. Markedly elevated body temperature may result in profound metabolic disturbances. High temperature during the first trimester of pregnancy may cause birth defects, such as anencephaly. Fever increases insulin requirements and alters the metabolism and disposition of drugs used for the treatment of the diverse diseases associated with fever.

The source of fever varies by population and setting. In a study of 92 patients who underwent shoulder arthroplasty and developed fever, an infectious cause was found in only 6 patients. In the neurologic ICU, fever can occur directly from brain injury (called "central fever"). One model predicted "central fever" with 90% probability if a patient met all of the following criteria: (1) less than 72 hours of neurologic ICU admission; (2) presence of subarachnoid hemorrhage, intraventricular hemorrhage, or brain tumor; (3) absence of infiltrate on chest radiograph; and (4) negative cultures. Procalcitonin and CRP may have some utility in differentiating infectious and central fever in the ICU.

Fever may also be more common in patients with other forms of trauma. In a study enrolling 268 patients, including patients with multiple injuries (n = 59), isolated head injuries (n = 97), isolated body injuries (n = 100), and minor trauma (n = 12), the incidence of fever was similar in all groups irrespective of injury (11–24%). In all groups, there was a significant association between the presence of early fever and death in the hospital (6–18% versus 0–3%), as well as longer median ICU stays (3–7 days versus 2–3 days). Spinal cord injury may cause fever by the loss of supraspinal control of the sympathetic nervous system and defective thermoregulation due to loss of sensation.

Among pregnant women, the prevalence of intrapartum fever of 38°C or greater in pregnancies of 36 weeks' gestation or more is 6.8% (or 1 in 15 women in labor), but the neonatal sepsis rate among affected mothers is 0.24% (or less than 1 in 400 babies). This finding calls into question the need for universal laboratory work, cultures, and antibiotic treatment pending culture results for this newborn population.

Contrary to classical teaching, postoperative atelectasis probably does not cause fever. Febrile nonhemolytic transfusion reaction is common, occurring in about 1% of transfusion episodes, and is mediated by proinflammatory cytokines elaborated by donor leukocytes during storage.

B. Hyperthermia

Hyperthermia—not mediated by cytokines—occurs when body metabolic heat production (as in thyroid storm) or environmental heat load exceeds normal heat loss capacity or when there is impaired heat loss (eg, heat stroke).

Malignant catatonia is a disorder consisting of catatonic symptoms, hyperthermia, autonomic instability, and altered mental status.

Neuroleptic malignant syndrome, a variant of malignant catatonia, is a rare and potentially lethal idiosyncratic reaction to neuroleptic medications, particularly haloperidol and fluphenazine; however, it has also been reported with the atypical neuroleptics (such as olanzapine or risperidone) (see Chapter 25). **Serotonin syndrome** resembles neuroleptic malignant syndrome but occurs within hours of ingestion of agents that increase levels of serotonin in the CNS, including SSRIs, MAOIs, tricyclic antidepressants, meperidine, dextromethorphan, bromocriptine, tramadol, lithium, and psychostimulants (such as cocaine, methamphetamine, and MDMA) (see Chapter 38).

Clonus and hyperreflexia are more common in serotonin syndrome, whereas "lead pipe" rigidity is more common in neuroleptic malignant syndrome. Neuroleptic malignant and serotonin syndromes share common clinical and pathophysiologic features with **malignant hyperthermia of anesthesia** (see Chapter 38).

C. Fever of Undetermined Origin

See Fever of Unknown Origin, Chapter 30.

Treatment

Most fever is well tolerated. When the temperature is less than 40°C, symptomatic treatment only is required. The treatment of fever with antipyretics does not appear to affect mortality of critically ill patients or affect the number of ICU-free days. A temperature greater than 41°C is likely to be hyperthermia rather than cytokine-mediated fever, and *emergent management is indicated.* (See Heat Stroke, Chapter 37.)

A. General Measures for Removal of Heat

Regardless of the cause of the fever, alcohol sponges, cold sponges, ice bags, ice-water enemas, and ice baths will lower body temperature (see Chapter 37). They are more useful in hyperthermia since patients with cytokine-related fever will attempt to override these therapies.

B. Pharmacologic Treatment of Fever

1. Antipyretic drugs—Antipyretic therapy is not needed except for patients with marginal hemodynamic status. Early administration of acetaminophen to treat fever due to probable infection did not affect the number of ICU-free days. Aspirin or acetaminophen, 325–650 mg every 4 hours, is effective in reducing fever. These drugs are best administered around the clock, rather than as needed, since "as needed" dosing results in periodic chills and sweats due to fluctuations in temperature caused by varying levels of drug.

2. Prophylactic antimicrobial therapy—Antibacterial and antifungal prophylactic regimens are recommended only for patients expected to have less than 100 neutrophils/mcL for more than 7 days, unless other factors increase risks for complications or mortality.

3. Empiric antimicrobial therapy—Empiric antibiotic therapy is sometimes warranted. Even before infection can be documented, prompt broad-spectrum antimicrobials are indicated for febrile patients who have hemodynamic instability, severe neutropenia (neutrophils less than 500/mcL [0.5×10^9/L]), asplenia (surgical or from sickle cell disease), or immunosuppression (from HIV infection [see Chapter 31] or from medications such as systemic corticosteroids, azathioprine, cyclosporine) (Tables 30–4 and 30–5). Febrile neutropenic patients should receive initial doses of empiric antibacterial therapy within an hour of triage and should either be monitored for at least 4 hours to determine suitability for outpatient management or be admitted to the hospital (see Infections in the Immunocompromised Patient, Chapter 30). It is standard to admit patients to the hospital with febrile neutropenic episodes, although carefully selected patients may be managed as outpatients after systematic assessment beginning with a validated risk index (eg, Multinational Association for Supportive Care in Cancer [MASCC] score or Talcott rules). In the MASCC index calculation, low-risk factors include the following: age under 60 years (2 points), burden of illness (5 points for no or mild symptoms and 3 points for moderate symptoms), outpatient status (3 points), solid tumor or hematologic malignancy with no previous fungal infection (4 points), no COPD (4 points), no dehydration requiring parenteral fluids (3 points), and systolic blood pressure greater than 90 mm Hg (5 points). Patients with MASCC scores of 21 or higher or in Talcott group 4 (presentation as an outpatient without significant comorbidity or uncontrolled cancer), and without other risk factors, can be managed safely as outpatients.

The carefully selected outpatients determined to be at low risk by MASCC score (particularly in combination with a normal serum CRP level) or by Talcott rules can be managed with an oral fluoroquinolone plus amoxicillin/clavulanate (or clindamycin, if penicillin allergic), unless fluoroquinolone prophylaxis was used before fever developed. For treatment of fever during neutropenia following chemotherapy, outpatient parenteral antimicrobial therapy can be provided effectively and safely in low-risk patients with a single agent such as cefepime, piperacillin/tazobactam, imipenem, meropenem, or doripenem. High-risk patients should be referred for inpatient management with combination parenteral antimicrobial therapy based on specific risk factors such as pneumonia-causing pathogens or central line–associated bloodstream infections (see Infections in the Immunocompromised Patient and Table 30–5 in Chapter 30 and see Infections in Chapter 39).

If a fungal infection is suspected in patients with prolonged fever and neutropenia, fluconazole is an equally effective but less toxic alternative to amphotericin B.

C. Treatment of Hyperthermia

Discontinuation of the offending agent is mandatory. Treatment of neuroleptic malignant syndrome includes dantrolene in combination with bromocriptine or levodopa (see Chapter 25). Treatment of serotonin syndrome includes administration of a central serotonin receptor antagonist—cyproheptadine or chlorpromazine—alone or in combination with a benzodiazepine (see Chapter 38). In patients for whom it is difficult to distinguish which syndrome is present, treatment with a benzodiazepine may be the safest therapeutic option.

When to Admit

- Presence of additional vital sign abnormalities or evidence of end-organ dysfunction in clinical cases when early sepsis is suspected.
- Febrile neutropenic patients at high risk for clinical decompensation.
- For measures to control a temperature higher than 41°C or when fever is associated with seizure or other mental status changes.
- Heat stroke (see Chapter 37).
- Malignant catatonia; neuroleptic malignant syndrome; serotonin syndrome; malignant hyperthermia of anesthesia.

Bongers KS et al. Drug-associated hyperthermia: a longitudinal analysis of hospital presentations. J Clin Pharm Ther. 2020;45:477. [PMID: 31793011]

Douma MJ et al; First Aid Task Force of the International Liaison Committee on Resuscitation. First aid cooling techniques for heat stroke and exertional hyperthermia: a systematic review and meta-analysis. Resuscitation. 2020;148:173. [PMID: 31981710]

Guinart D et al. A systematic review and pooled, patient-level analysis of predictors of mortality in neuroleptic malignant syndrome. Acta Psychiatr Scand. 2021;144:329. [PMID: 34358327]

Lewis SR et al. Interventions to reduce body temperature to 35°C to 37°C in adults and children with traumatic brain injury. Cochrane Database Syst Rev. 2020;10:CD006811. [PMID: 33126293]

Long B et al. Oncologic emergencies: the fever with too few neutrophils. J Emerg Med. 2019;57:689. [PMID: 31635928]

Prakash S et al. Fatal serotonin syndrome: a systematic review of 56 cases in the literature. Clin Toxicol (Phila). 2021;5:89. [PMID: 33196298]

INVOLUNTARY WEIGHT LOSS

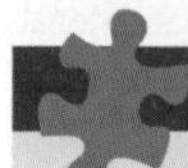

ESSENTIAL INQUIRIES

- Age; caloric intake; secondary confirmation (eg, changes in clothing size).
- Fever; change in bowel habits.
- Substance use.
- Age-appropriate cancer screening history.

General Considerations

Body weight is determined by a person's caloric intake, absorptive capacity, metabolic rate, and energy losses. Body weight normally peaks by the fifth or sixth decade and then gradually declines at a rate of 1–2 kg per decade. In NHANES II, a national survey of community-dwelling elders (aged 50–80 years), recent involuntary weight loss (more than 5% usual body weight) was reported by 7% of respondents, and this was associated with a 24% higher mortality. In postmenopausal women, unintentional weight loss was associated with increased rates of hip and vertebral fractures.

Etiology

Involuntary weight loss is regarded as clinically significant when it exceeds 5% or more of usual body weight over a 6- to 12-month period. It often indicates serious physical or psychological illness. Physical causes are usually evident during the initial evaluation. The most common causes are cancer (about 30%), GI disorders (about 15%), and dementia or depression (about 15%). Nearly half of patients with Parkinson disease have weight loss associated with disease progression. When an adequately nourished–appearing patient complains of weight loss, inquiry should be made about exact weight changes (with approximate dates) and about changes in clothing size. Family members can provide confirmation of weight loss, as can old documents such as driver's licenses. A mild, gradual weight loss occurs in some older individuals because of decreased energy requirements. However, rapid involuntary weight loss is predictive of morbidity and mortality. In addition to various disease states, causes in older individuals include loss of teeth and consequent difficulty with chewing, medications interfering with taste or causing nausea, alcohol use disorder, and social isolation. Among Black persons at an adult day health center, 65% had a significant nutritional disorder: 48.5% reported involuntary weight loss or gain, 21% ate fewer than two meals daily, and 41.2% had tooth loss or mouth pain.

Clinical Findings

Once the weight loss is established, the history, medication profile, physical examination, and conventional laboratory and radiologic investigations (eg, CBC, liver biochemical tests, kidney panel, serologic tests including HIV, TSH level, UA, fecal occult blood test, and chest radiography) usually reveal the cause. Age-appropriate cancer screening should be completed as recommended by guidelines (eg, Papanicolaou smear, mammography, fecal occult blood test/screening colonoscopy/flexible sigmoidoscopy, possibly PSA) (Chapter 1). Whole-body CT imaging is increasingly used for diagnosis; one study found its diagnostic yield to be 33.5%. When these tests are normal, the second phase of evaluation should focus on more definitive GI investigation (eg, tests for malabsorption, endoscopy). However, one prospective case study in patients with unintentional weight loss showed that colonoscopy did not find colorectal cancer if weight loss was the sole indication for the test.

If the initial evaluation is unrevealing, follow-up is preferable to further diagnostic testing. Death at 2-year follow-up was not nearly as common in patients with unexplained involuntary weight loss (8%) as in those with weight loss due to malignant (79%) and established nonmalignant diseases (19%). Psychiatric consultation should be considered when there is evidence of depression, dementia, anorexia nervosa, or other emotional problems. Ultimately, in approximately 15–25% of cases, no cause for the weight loss can be found.

Differential Diagnosis

Malignancy, GI disorders (poorly fitting dentures, cavities, swallowing or malabsorption disorders, pancreatic insufficiency), HF, HIV, tuberculosis, psychological problems (dementia, depression, paranoia), endocrine disorders (hyper-, hypothyroidism, hyperparathyroidism, hypoadrenalism), Whipple disease, eating problems (dietary restrictions, lack of money for food), social problems (alcohol use disorder, social isolation), and medication side effects are all established causes.

Treatment

Weight stabilization occurs in most surviving patients with both established and unknown causes of weight loss through treatment of the underlying disorder and caloric supplementation. Nutrient intake goals are established in relation to the severity of weight loss, in general ranging from 30 to 40 kcal/kg/day. In order of preference, route of administration options include oral, temporary nasojejunal tube, or percutaneous gastric or jejunal tube. Parenteral nutrition is reserved for patients with serious associated problems. A variety of pharmacologic agents have been proposed for the treatment of weight loss. These can be categorized into appetite stimulants (corticosteroids, progestational agents, cannabinoids, and serotonin antagonists); anabolic agents (growth hormone, ghrelin, and testosterone derivatives); and anticatabolic agents (omega-3 fatty acids, pentoxifylline, hydrazine sulfate, and thalidomide). There is no evidence that appetite stimulants decrease mortality, and they may have severe adverse side effects. The anabolic agent nandrolone decanoate reversed weight and lean tissue loss in women with HIV, and human growth hormone temporarily increased weight and walking speed in undernourished elderly people. Yet, studies have not consistently shown mortality benefit.

Exercise training may prevent or even reverse the process of muscle wasting in HF ("cardiac cachexia"). Protein supplementation combined with resistance exercise training and aerobic activity may prevent aging-related muscle mass attenuation and functional performance. Some patients with cancer-associated weight loss may benefit from nutritional assessment and intervention as decreased food intake may be playing a role. The effectiveness, acceptability, and safety of exercise training for adults with cancer cachexia has not been established.

When to Refer

- Weight loss caused by malabsorption.
- Persistent nutritional deficiencies despite adequate supplementation.
- Weight loss as a result of anorexia or bulimia.

When to Admit

- Severe protein-energy malnutrition, including the syndromes of kwashiorkor and marasmus.
- Vitamin deficiency syndromes.
- Cachexia with anticipated progressive weight loss secondary to unmanageable psychiatric disease.
- Careful electrolyte and fluid replacement in protein-energy malnutrition and avoidance of "re-feeding syndrome."

Grande AJ et al. Exercise for cancer cachexia in adults. Cochrane Database Syst Rev. 2021;3:CD010804. [PMID: 33735441]
Kabani A et al. The key role of nonpharmacologic management of cachexia in persons with advanced illness: a teachable moment. JAMA Intern Med. 2021;181:978. [PMID: 33900359]
Levy C et al. Cannabis for symptom management in older adults. Med Clin North Am. 2020;104:471. [PMID: 32312410]
Odio CD et al. Cryptic cachexia. N Engl J Med. 2020;383:68. [PMID: 32609985]
Valentova M et al. Cardiac cachexia revisited: the role of wasting in heart failure. Heart Fail Clin. 2020;16:61. [PMID: 31735316]

FATIGUE & SYSTEMIC INTOLERANCE DISEASE (Chronic Fatigue Syndrome)

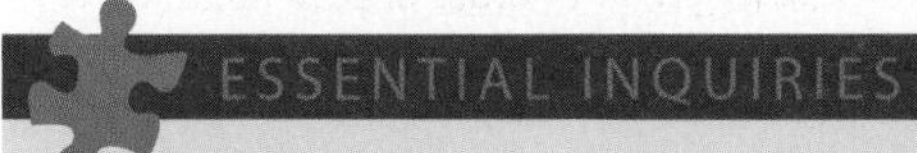

- Weight loss; fever.
- Sleep-disordered breathing.
- Medications; substance use.

General Considerations

Fatigue, as an isolated symptom, accounts for 1–3% of visits to generalists. The symptom of fatigue is often poorly described and less well defined by patients than symptoms associated with specific dysfunction of organ systems. Fatigue or lassitude and the closely related complaints of weakness, tiredness, and lethargy are often attributed to overexertion, poor physical conditioning, sleep disturbance, obesity, undernutrition, and emotional problems. A history of the patient's daily living and working habits may obviate the need for extensive and unproductive diagnostic studies.

Fatigue in older adults increases the risk of developing negative health outcomes (mortality OR, 2.14), the development of disabilities in basic activities of daily living (OR 3.22), or the occurrence of physical decline (OR, 1.42).

A working case definition of chronic fatigue syndrome indicates that it is not a homogeneous abnormality, there is no single pathogenic mechanism, and no physical finding or laboratory test can be used to confirm the diagnosis. The Institute of Medicine (now called the National Academy of Medicine) has recommended using the term **systemic exertion intolerance disease.** Other conditions identified as causing chronic fatigue include myalgic encephalitis and neurasthenia, each with specific diagnostic criteria creating inconsistent diagnoses and treatment plans.

Clinical Findings

A. Fatigue

Clinically relevant fatigue is composed of three major components: generalized weakness (difficulty in initiating activities); easy fatigability (difficulty in completing activities); and mental fatigue (difficulty with concentration and memory). Important diseases that can cause fatigue include hyper- and hypothyroidism, HF, infections (endocarditis, hepatitis), COPD, interstitial lung disease, ESKD, sleep apnea, anemia, autoimmune disorders, multiple sclerosis, IBS, Parkinson disease, cerebral vascular accident, and cancer. Solution-focused therapy has a significant initial beneficial effect on the severity of fatigue and quality of life in patients with quiescent IBD.

Alcohol use disorder, vitamin C deficiency (scurvy), side effects from medications (eg, sedatives and beta-blockers), and psychological conditions (eg, insomnia, depression, anxiety, panic attacks, dysthmia, and somatic symptom disorder [formerly called somatization disorder]) may be the cause. Common outpatient infectious causes include mononucleosis and sinusitis. These conditions are usually associated with other characteristic signs, but patients may emphasize fatigue and not reveal their other symptoms unless directly asked. The lifetime prevalence of significant fatigue (present for at least 2 weeks) is about 25%. Fatigue of unknown cause or related to psychiatric illness exceeds that due to physical illness, injury, alcohol, or medications.

Although frequently associated with Lyme disease, severe fatigue as a long-term sequela is rare.

B. Systemic Intolerance Disease (Chronic Fatigue Syndrome)

Diagnosis of systemic exertion intolerance disease requires the presence of all of the following three symptoms:

1. Substantial reduction or impairment in the ability to engage in pre-illness levels of occupational, educational, social, or personal activities that persists for more than 6 months and is accompanied by fatigue, which is often

profound, is of new or definite onset (not lifelong), is not the result of ongoing excessive exertion, and is not substantially alleviated by rest.

2. Postexertional malaise.
3. Unrefreshing sleep.

In addition, the patient must have at least one of the following two manifestations: (1) cognitive impairment or (2) orthostatic intolerance (lightheadedness, dizziness, and headache that worsen with upright posture and improve with recumbency).

The evaluation of systemic exertion intolerance disease includes a history and physical examination as well as CBC; ESR; kidney function; serum electrolytes, glucose, creatinine, calcium; liver biochemical tests and thyroid function tests; UA; tuberculin skin test; and screening questionnaires for psychiatric disorders. Other tests to be performed as clinically indicated are serum cortisol, antinuclear antibody, rheumatoid factor, immunoglobulin levels, Lyme serology in endemic areas (although rarely a long-term complication of this infection), and HIV antibody. More extensive testing is usually unhelpful, including antibody to Epstein-Barr virus. There may be an abnormally high rate of postural hypotension.

Treatment

A. Fatigue

Resistance training and aerobic exercise lessens fatigue and improves performance for a number of chronic conditions associated with a high prevalence of fatigue, including HF, COPD, arthritis, and cancer. Continuous positive airway pressure is an effective treatment for obstructive sleep apnea. Pitolisant, a selective histamine H_3-receptor antagonist with wake-promoting effect, may reduce daytime sleepiness in patients with moderate to severe obstructive sleep apnea who refuse continuous positive airway pressure treatment.

Psychostimulants such as methylphenidate have shown inconsistent results in randomized trials of treatment of cancer-related fatigue. Modafinil and armodafinil appear to be effective, well-tolerated agents in HIV-positive patients with fatigue and as adjunctive agents in patients with depression or bipolar disorder with fatigue. Testosterone replacement in hypoandrogenic men over age 65 had no significant benefits for walking distance or vitality, as assessed by the Functional Assessment of Chronic Illness Therapy-Fatigue scale. However, men receiving testosterone reported slightly better mood and lower severity of depressive symptoms than those receiving placebo. Methylphenidate, as well as cognitive-behavioral therapy, may improve mental fatigue and cognitive function in patients with traumatic brain injury. Vitamin D treatment significantly improved fatigue in kidney transplantation patients as well as in otherwise healthy persons with vitamin D deficiency. Internet-based cognitive-behavioral therapy is effective in reducing severe fatigue in breast cancer survivors. Therapeutic Care (a complementary medicine modality that uses acupressure) reduces fatigue in some patients with breast cancer receiving chemotherapy, while moderate intensity exercise did not. Six weeks of Swedish massage therapy reduced fatigue in female breast cancer survivors who had surgery plus radiation and/or chemotherapy/chemoprevention. There is limited and preliminary evidence that rasagiline, modafinil, and doxepin are associated with improvement of fatigue in Parkinson disease. Amantadine, modafinil, and methylphenidate were not found to be superior to placebo in improving fatigue associated with multiple sclerosis and caused more frequent adverse events.

The treatment of subclinical hypothyroidism is unlikely to benefit symptoms of fatigue. Oral melatonin does not improve fatigue in patients with advanced cancer. Exceeding the RDA for protein intake does not increase muscle or physical function, nor augment anabolic response to testosterone in older men, nor reduce muscle soreness or fatigue after prolonged moderate-intensity walking exercise.

B. Systemic Intolerance Disease

A variety of agents and modalities have been tried for the treatment of systemic intolerance disease without improvement in symptoms.

Some patients with postural hypotension report response to increases in dietary sodium as well as fludrocortisone, 0.1 mg orally daily. The immunomodulator rintatolimod improved some measures of exercise performance compared with placebo in two trials (with low strength of evidence). Low-dose naltrexone is being used off-label with anecdotal reports of benefit. There is very limited evidence that dietary modification is beneficial.

Patients with systemic intolerance disease have benefited from a comprehensive multidisciplinary intervention, including optimal medical management, treating any ongoing affective or anxiety disorder pharmacologically, and implementing a comprehensive cognitive-behavioral treatment program. At present, **cognitive-behavioral therapy** and **graded exercise** are the treatments of choice for patients with systemic intolerance disease.

When to Refer

- Infections not responsive to standard treatment.
- Difficult-to-control hyper- or hypothyroidism.
- Severe psychological illness.
- Malignancy.

When to Admit

- Failure to thrive.
- Fatigue severe enough to impair activities of daily living.

Kim DY et al. Systematic review of randomized controlled trials for chronic fatigue syndrome/myalgic encephalomyelitis (CFS/ME). J Transl Med. 2020;18:7. [PMID: 31906979]

Knoop V et al; Gerontopole Brussels Study group. Fatigue and the prediction of negative health outcomes: a systematic review with meta-analysis. Ageing Res Rev. 2021;67:101261. [PMID: 33548508]

Ten Haaf DSM et al. The impact of protein supplementation on exercise-induced muscle damage, soreness and fatigue following prolonged walking exercise in vital older adults: a randomized double-blind placebo-controlled trial. Nutrients. 2020;12:1806. [PMID: 32560436]

Wright A et al. Perfectionism, depression and anxiety in chronic fatigue syndrome: a systematic review. J Psychosom Res. 2021;140:110322. [PMID: 33278659]

ACUTE HEADACHE

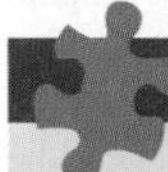

ESSENTIAL INQUIRIES

- Age > 40 years.
- Rapid onset and severe intensity (ie, "thunderclap" headache), trauma, onset during exertion.
- Fever, vision changes, neck stiffness.
- HIV infection.
- Current or past history of hypertension.
- Neurologic findings (mental status changes, motor or sensory deficits, loss of consciousness).

General Considerations

Approximately 90% of people in the United States experience a headache in their lifetime. A broad range of disorders can cause headache (see Chapter 24). This section deals only with acute nontraumatic headache in adults and adolescents. The challenge in the initial evaluation of acute headache is to identify which patients are presenting with an uncommon but life-threatening condition; approximately 1% of patients seeking care in emergency department settings and considerably less in office practice settings fall into this category.

Diminution of headache in response to typical migraine therapies (such as serotonin receptor antagonists or ketorolac) does not rule out critical conditions such as subarachnoid hemorrhage or meningitis as the underlying cause. A "sentinel headache" before a subarachnoid hemorrhage is a sudden, intense, persistent headache different from previous headaches; it precedes subarachnoid hemorrhage by days or weeks and occurs in 15–60% of patients with spontaneous subarachnoid hemorrhage.

Clinical Findings

A. Symptoms

A careful history and physical examination should aim to identify causes of acute headache that require immediate treatment. These causes can be broadly classified as (1) imminent or completed vascular events (intracranial hemorrhage, thrombosis, cavernous sinus thrombosis, vasculitis, malignant hypertension, arterial dissection, cerebral venous thrombosis, transient ischemic attack, or aneurysm; (2) infections (abscess, encephalitis, or meningitis), intracranial masses causing intracranial hypertension, preeclampsia; and (3) carbon monoxide poisoning and methemoglobinemia. Having the patient carefully describe the onset of headache can help diagnose a serious cause.

Report of a sudden-onset headache that reaches maximal and severe intensity within seconds or a few minutes is the classic description of a "thunderclap" headache; it should precipitate workup for subarachnoid hemorrhage, since the estimated prevalence of subarachnoid hemorrhage in patients with thunderclap headache is 43%.

Thunderclap headache during the postpartum period precipitated by the Valsalva maneuver or recumbent positioning may indicate reversible cerebral vasoconstriction syndrome or irreversible cerebral venous sinus thrombosis. Venous-specific imaging sequences may be needed for diagnosis. Other historical features that raise the need for diagnostic testing include headache brought on by cough, exertion, or sexual activity.

The medical history can also guide the need for additional workup. Under most circumstances (including a normal neurologic examination), new headache in a patient older than 50 years or with HIV infection warrants immediate neuroimaging (Table 2–5). When the patient has a history of hypertension—particularly uncontrolled hypertension—a complete search for other features of "malignant hypertension" is appropriate to determine the urgency of control of hypertension (see Chapter 11). Headache and hypertension associated with pregnancy may be due to preeclampsia. Episodic headache associated with the triad of hypertension, palpitations, and sweats is suggestive of pheochromocytoma. In the absence of thunderclap headache, advanced age, and HIV infection, a careful physical examination and detailed neurologic examination will usually determine acuity of the workup and need for further diagnostic testing. A history consistent with

Table 2–5. Clinical features associated with acute headache that warrant urgent or emergent neuroimaging.

Indications for neuroimaging prior to lumbar puncture
Abnormal neurologic examination (particularly focal neurologic deficits)
Abnormal mental status
Abnormal funduscopic examination (papilledema; loss of venous pulsations)
Meningeal signs
Indications for emergent neuroimaging completed prior to leaving office or emergency department
Abnormal neurologic examination
Abnormal mental status
"Thunderclap" headache
HIV-positive patients with new type of headache[1]
Indications for urgent neuroimaging scheduled prior to leaving office or emergency department
Age > 50 years (normal neurologic examination) with new type of headache

[1]Use CT with or without contrast or MRI if HIV positive.

Data from American College of Emergency Physicians. Clinical policy: critical issues in the evaluation and management of patients presenting to the emergency department with acute headache. Ann Emerg Med. 2008;52:407-436.

Table 2–6. Summary likelihood ratios for individual clinical features associated with migraine diagnosis.

Clinical Feature	LR+ (95% CI)	LR– (95% CI)
Nausea	19 (15–25)	0.19 (0.18–0.20)
Photophobia	5.8 (5.1–6.6)	0.24 (0.23–0.26)
Phonophobia	5.2 (4.5–5.9)	0.38 (0.36–0.40)
Exacerbation by physical activity	3.7 (3.4–4.0)	0.24 (0.23–0.26)

hypercoagulability is associated with an increased risk of cerebral venous thrombosis.

Symptoms can also be useful for diagnosing migraine headache in the absence of the "classic" migraine pattern of scintillating scotoma followed by unilateral headache, photophobia, and nausea and vomiting (Table 2–6). The presence of three or more of these symptoms (nausea, photophobia, phonophobia, and exacerbation by physical activity) can establish the diagnosis of migraine (in the absence of other clinical features that warrant neuroimaging studies), and the presence of only one or two symptoms (provided one is not nausea) can help rule out migraine. A systematic list called the SNNOOP10 has been developed as a screening method for secondary causes of headache (Table 2–7).

B. Physical Examination

Critical components of the physical examination of the patient with acute headache include vital signs, neurologic examination, and vision testing with funduscopic examination. The finding of fever with acute headache warrants additional maneuvers to elicit evidence of meningeal inflammation, such as Kernig and Brudzinski signs. The absence of jolt accentuation of headache cannot accurately rule out meningitis. Patients older than 60 years should be examined for scalp or temporal artery tenderness.

Careful assessment of visual acuity, ocular gaze, visual fields, pupillary defects, optic disks, and retinal vein pulsations is crucial. Diminished visual acuity is suggestive of glaucoma, temporal arteritis, or optic neuritis. Ophthalmoplegia or visual field defects may be signs of venous sinus thrombosis, tumor, or aneurysm. Afferent pupillary defects can be due to intracranial masses or optic neuritis. In the setting of headache and hypertension, retinal cotton wool

Table 2–7. SNNOOP10 list of "red" flags for secondary causes of headache.

Sign or Symptom	Related Secondary Headaches
Systemic symptoms[1]	Headache attributed to infection, nonvascular intracranial disorders, carcinoid, or pheochromocytoma
Neoplasm in history	Neoplasms of the brain; metastasis
Neurologic deficit/dysfunction	Headaches attributed to vascular, nonvascular intracranial disorders; brain abscess and other infections
Onset of headache is sudden or abrupt	Subarachnoid hemorrhage and other headache attributed to cranial or cervical vascular disorders
Older age (> 50 years)	Giant cell arteritis and other headache attributed to cranial or cervical vascular disorders; neoplasms and other nonvascular intracranial disorders
Pattern change or recent onset of headache	Neoplasms, headaches attributed to vascular, nonvascular intracranial disorders
Positional headache	Intracranial hypertension or hypotension
Precipitated by sneezing, coughing, or exercise	Posterior fossa malformations; Chiari malformation
Papilledema	Neoplasms and other nonvascular intracranial disorders; intracranial hypertension
Progressive headache and atypical presentations	Neoplasms and other nonvascular intracranial disorders
Pregnancy or puerperium	Headaches attributed to cranial or cervical vascular disorders; postdural puncture headache; hypertension-related disorders (eg, preeclampsia); cerebral sinus thrombosis; hypothyroidism; anemia; diabetes mellitus
Painful eye with autonomic features	Pathology in posterior fossa, pituitary region, or cavernous sinus; Tolosa-Hunt syndrome (severe, unilateral headaches with orbital pain and ophthalmoplegia due to extraocular palsies); other ophthalmic causes
Posttraumatic onset of headache	Acute and chronic posttraumatic headache; subdural hematoma and other headache attributed to vascular disorders
Immunosuppression, eg, HIV, immunosuppressive medications	Opportunistic infections
Painkiller overuse or new drug at onset of headache	Medication overuse headache; drug incompatibility

[1]"Orange" flag for isolated fever alone.

Reproduced with permission from Do TP et al. Red and orange flags for secondary headaches in clinical practice: SNNOOP10 list. Neurology. 2019;92(3):134–144. https://n.neurology.org/content/92/3/134.long.

spots, flame hemorrhages, and disk swelling indicate acute severe hypertensive retinopathy. Ipsilateral ptosis and miosis suggest Horner syndrome and in conjunction with acute headache may signify carotid artery dissection. Finally, papilledema or absent retinal venous pulsations are signs of elevated intracranial pressure—findings that should be followed by neuroimaging prior to performing lumbar puncture (Table 2–5). On nonmydriatic fundoscopy, up to 8.5% of patients who arrive at the emergency department complaining of headache had abnormalities; although few had other significant physical examination findings, 59% of them had abnormal neuroimaging studies.

Complete neurologic evaluations are also critical and should include assessment of mental status, motor and sensory systems, reflexes, gait, cerebellar function, and pronator drift. Any abnormality on neurologic evaluation (especially mental status) warrants emergent neuroimaging (Table 2–5).

C. Diagnostic Studies

Neuroimaging indications are summarized in Table 2–5. Under most circumstances, a noncontrast head CT is sufficient to exclude intracranial hypertension with impending herniation, intracranial hemorrhage, and many types of intracranial masses (notable exceptions include lymphoma and toxoplasmosis in HIV-positive patients, herpes simplex encephalitis, and brain abscess). When needed, a contrast study can be ordered to follow a normal noncontrast study. A normal neuroimaging study does not exclude subarachnoid hemorrhage and should be followed by lumbar puncture. One study supported a change of practice wherein a lumbar puncture can be withheld when a head CT scan was performed less than 6 hours after headache onset and showed no evidence of subarachnoid hemorrhage (negative predictive value 99.9% [95% CI, 99.3–100.0%]).

Based on one prospective study of 1536 emergency department patients, the yield for acute findings on head CT differed based on the indications for imaging and were 27% for seizures, 20% for confusion, 19% for syncope, 16% for focal neurologic deficit, 15% for head injury, 12% for headache, and 8% for dizziness.

In patients for whom there is a high level of suspicion for subarachnoid hemorrhage or aneurysm, a normal CT and lumbar puncture should be followed by angiography within the next few days (provided the patient is medically stable).

Lumbar puncture is also indicated to exclude infectious causes of acute headache, particularly in patients with fever or meningeal signs. Cerebrospinal fluid tests should routinely include Gram stain, WBC count with differential, RBC count, glucose, total protein, and bacterial culture. In appropriate patients, also consider testing cerebrospinal fluid for Venereal Disease Research Laboratory (syphilis), cryptococcal antigen (HIV-positive patients), acid-fast bacillus stain and culture, and complement fixation and culture for coccidioidomycosis. Storage of an extra tube with 5 mL of cerebrospinal fluid is prudent for conducting unanticipated tests in the immediate future. PCR tests for specific infectious pathogens (eg, herpes simplex 2) should also be considered in patients with evidence of CNS infection but no identifiable pathogen.

The Ottawa subarachnoid hemorrhage clinical decision rule had 100% sensitivity (and 13–15% specificity in different studies) in predicting subarachnoid hemorrhage. According to it, patients who seek medical attention in an emergency department complaining of an acute nontraumatic headache should be evaluated for subarachnoid hemorrhage if they have one or more of the following factors: age 40 years or older, neck pain or stiffness, witnessed loss of consciousness, onset during exertion, thunderclap headache (instantly peaking pain), or limited neck flexion on examination.

In addition to neuroimaging and lumbar puncture, additional diagnostic tests for exclusion of life-threatening causes of acute headache include ESR (temporal arteritis; endocarditis), UA (malignant hypertension; preeclampsia), and sinus CT (bacterial sinusitis, independently or as a cause of venous sinus thrombosis).

Treatment

Treatment should be directed at the cause of acute headache. In patients in whom migraine or migraine-like headache has been diagnosed, early treatment with ketorolac (oral, nasal, or intramuscular), dihydroergotamine, lasmiditan, ubrogepant, or triptans (oral, nasal, subcutaneous) can often abort or provide significant relief of symptoms (see Chapter 24). Intravenous prochlorperazine plus diphenhydramine was more effective for migraine pain relief than intravenous hydromorphone in the emergency department. Prochlorperazine appears to be superior to ketamine for the treatment of benign headaches (without signs or symptoms of serious intracranial pathology) in the emergency department. Sumatriptan may be less effective as immediate therapy for migraine attacks with aura compared to attacks without aura. Haloperidol (2.5 mg intravenously) given to patients in the emergency department with severe benign headache resulted in a significant reduction pain score compared with placebo. Although oral beta-blockers used for the prevention of migraine headache are not effective for the treatment of acute pain, timolol eye drops may be effective in the management of acute migraine pain.

There may be a role for oral corticosteroids to prevent rebound headache after emergency department discharge, but in one study, long-acting intramuscular methylprednisolone acetate did not decrease the frequency of post-emergency department discharge headache days compared with oral dexamethasone. Parenteral morphine and hydromorphone are best avoided as first-line therapy, although opioids are still prescribed to nearly half of all patients with acute migraine.

Subanesthetic ketamine infusions may be beneficial in individuals with chronic migraine and new daily persistent headache that has not responded to other aggressive treatments. Peripheral nerve blocks may be a safe and effective way to treat headaches in older adults. Surgical decompression of peripheral cranial and spinal nerves at trigger sites have been used to treat migraine. Noninvasive vagus nerve stimulation has shown promise in the management of migraine and acute cluster headaches.

High-flow oxygen therapy may also provide effective treatment for all headache types in the emergency department setting (eg, benefitting older patients with cluster headaches). Peripheral nerve blocks for treatment-refractory migraine may be an effective therapeutic option in pregnancy. The oral 5-HT_{1F} receptor agonist, lasmiditan, has been approved for the acute treatment of migraine with or without aura in adults. The calcitonin gene-related peptide antagonists ("gepants") rimegepant and atogepant and the monoclonal antibodies (erenumab, fremanezumab, galcanezumab) have been approved for prevention of migraine. Ubrogepant and rimegepant have been approved for the acute treatment of migraine. Galcanezumab has activity against cluster headache. Because triptans (and ergot derivatives) are contraindicated in patients with all forms of vascular disease, the calcitonin gene-related peptide antagonists and serotonin 5-HT_{1F}-receptor agonists "ditans" (lasmiditan) may be particularly helpful in treating migraine in older patients who have increased rates of contraindications to first-line therapy. Regular exercise may have a prophylactic effect on migraine frequency; however, new, intense exercise can trigger migraine.

When to Refer

- Frequent migraines not responsive to standard therapy.
- Migraines with atypical features.
- Chronic daily headaches due to medication overuse.

When to Admit

- Need for repeated doses of parenteral pain medication.
- To facilitate an expedited workup requiring a sequence of neuroimaging and procedures.
- To monitor for progression of symptoms and to obtain neurologic consultation when the initial emergency department workup is inconclusive.
- Pain severe enough to impair activities of daily living or impede follow-up appointments or consultations.
- Patients with subarachnoid hemorrhage, intracranial mass, or meningitis.

Bilello LA et al. Retrospective review of pregnant patients presenting for evaluation of acute neurologic complaints. Ann Emerg Med. 2021;77:210. [PMID: 32418678]
Burch R. Migraine and tension-type headache: diagnosis and treatment. Med Clin North Am. 2019;103:215. [PMID: 30704678]
Diamanti S et al. Leading symptoms in cerebrovascular diseases: what about headache? Neurol Sci. 2019;40:147. [PMID: 30891639]
Do TP et al. Red and orange flags for secondary headaches in clinical practice: SNNOOP10 list. Neurology. 2019;92:134. [PMID: 30587518]
McNeil M. Headaches in adults in primary care: evaluation, diagnosis, and treatment. Med Clin North Am. 2021;105:39. [PMID: 33246522]
Nesselroth D et al. Yield of head CT for acute findings in patients presenting to the emergency department. Clin Imaging. 2021;73:1. [PMID: 33246274]
Robbins MS. Diagnosis and management of headache: a review. JAMA. 2021;325:1874. [PMID: 33974014]
Sjulstad AS et al. What is currently the best investigational approach to the patient with sudden-onset severe headache? Headache. 2019;59:1834. [PMID: 31710108]
Soni PP et al. Recent advances in the management of migraine in older patients. Drugs Aging. 2020;37:463. [PMID: 32578024]
VanderPluym JH et al. Acute treatments for episodic migraine in adults: a systematic review and meta-analysis. JAMA. 2021;325:2357. [PMID: 34128998]
Wu WT et al. The Ottawa subarachnoid hemorrhage clinical decision rule for classifying emergency department headache patients. Am J Emerg Med. 2020;38:198. [PMID: 30765279]

DYSURIA

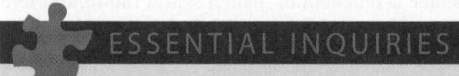

- Fever; new back or flank pain; nausea or vomiting.
- Vaginal discharge.
- Pregnancy risk.
- Structural abnormalities.
- Instrumentation of urethra or bladder.

General Considerations

Dysuria (painful urination) is a common reason for adults and adolescents to seek urgent medical attention.

An inflammatory process (eg, bacterial UTI, herpes simplex, autoimmune disorder) underlies most causes of dysuria. In women, cystitis is diagnosed in up to 50–60% of cases. Cystitis has an incidence of 0.5–0.7% per year in sexually active young women. The key objective in evaluating women with dysuria is to exclude serious upper urinary tract disease, such as acute pyelonephritis, and sexually transmitted diseases. In elderly men, dysuria may be a symptom of prostatitis. In contrast, in younger men, urethritis accounts for most cases of dysuria. Male cyclists have no worse sexual or urinary functions than swimmers or runners, but cyclists are more prone to urethral stricture.

Clinical Findings

A. Symptoms

Well-designed cohort studies have shown that some women can be reliably diagnosed with uncomplicated cystitis without a physical examination or UA, and randomized controlled trials show that telephone management of uncomplicated cystitis is safe and effective. An increased likelihood of cystitis is present when women report multiple irritative voiding symptoms (dysuria, urgency, frequency), fever, or back pain (positive LRs = 1.6–2.0). A cohort study found that the symptom of dysuria most reliably predicted a culture-positive UTI. Inquiring about symptoms of vulvovaginitis is imperative. When women report dysuria and urinary frequency, and deny vaginal discharge and irritation, the LR for culture-confirmed cystitis is 24.5. In contrast, when vaginal discharge or irritation is present, as well as dysuria or urinary frequency, the LR is 0.7. Gross hematuria in women with voiding symptoms usually represents hemorrhagic cystitis but can also be a sign of bladder cancer (particularly in older patients) or upper tract disease. Failure of hematuria to resolve with antibiotic treatment should prompt further evaluation of the bladder and kidneys. Chlamydial infection should be strongly considered among women aged 25 years or younger who are sexually active and seeking medical attention for a suspected UTI for the first time or who have a new partner.

Because fever and back pain as well as nausea and vomiting are clinical criteria for acute pyelonephritis, women with these symptoms should usually be examined before initiation of treatment to exclude coexistent urosepsis, hydronephrosis, or nephrolithiasis that would affect management decisions. Risk factors for acute pyelonephritis among women aged 18–49 years relate to sexual behaviors (frequent sexual intercourse [three times per week or more], new sexual partner in previous year, recent spermicide use), as well as diabetes mellitus and recent UTI or incontinence.

Finally, pregnancy, underlying structural factors (polycystic kidney disease, nephrolithiasis, neurogenic bladder), immunosuppression, diabetes mellitus, and a history of recent bladder or urethral instrumentation usually alter the treatment regimen (antibiotic choice or duration of treatment, or both) for cystitis. Presence of UTI during pregnancy is strongly associated with preeclampsia (particularly UTI during the third trimester).

B. Physical Examination

Fever, tachycardia, or hypotension suggests the possibility of urosepsis and potential need for hospitalization. A focused examination in women, in uncomplicated circumstances, could be limited to ascertainment of costovertebral angle tenderness as a finding for pyelonephritis and to a lower abdominal and pelvic examination if the history suggests vulvovaginitis or cervicitis.

C. Diagnostic Studies

1. Urinalysis—UA is probably overutilized in the evaluation of dysuria. The probability of culture-confirmed UTI among women with a history and physical examination compatible with uncomplicated cystitis is about 70–90%. UA is most helpful in atypical presentations of cystitis. Dipstick detection (greater than trace) of leukocytes, nitrites, or blood supports a diagnosis of cystitis. When both leukocyte and nitrite tests are positive, the LR is 4.2, and when both are negative, the LR is 0.3. The negative predictive value of UA is not sufficient to exclude culture-confirmed UTI in women with multiple and typical symptoms, and randomized trial evidence shows that antibiotic treatment is beneficial to women with typical symptoms and negative UA dipstick tests. Microscopy of unspun urine may also be helpful in diagnosis and reduces unnecessary use of antibiotics. The combination of urgency, dysuria, and pyuria assessed with the high-power (40×) objective for leukocytes (more than 1 leukocyte/7 high-power fields) had a positive predictive value of 71 and LR of 2.97. Urine samples produced at home rarely meet diagnostic standards.

2. Urine culture—Urine culture should be considered for all women with upper tract symptoms (prior to initiating antibiotic therapy), as well as those with dysuria and a negative urine dipstick test. In symptomatic women, a clean-catch urine culture is considered positive when 10^2–10^3 colony-forming units/mL of a uropathogenic organism are detected. The benefit of DNA next-generation sequencing and expanded quantitative urine culture is being studied, and in a recent study, multiplex polymerase chain reaction analysis was found to be as beneficial as a urine culture.

3. Renal imaging—When severe flank or back pain is present, the possibility of complicated kidney infection (perinephric abscess, nephrolithiasis) or of hydronephrosis should be considered. Renal ultrasound or CT scanning should be done to rule out abscess and hydronephrosis. To exclude nephrolithiasis, noncontrast helical CT scanning is more accurate than renal ultrasound and is the diagnostic test of choice. In a meta-analysis, the positive and negative LRs of helical CT scanning for diagnosis of nephrolithiasis were 23.2 and 0.05, respectively.

Differential Diagnosis

The differential diagnosis of dysuria in women includes acute cystitis, acute pyelonephritis, vaginitis (*Candida*, bacterial vaginosis, *Trichomonas*, herpes simplex), urethritis/cervicitis (*Chlamydia*, gonorrhea), and interstitial cystitis/painful bladder syndrome. Pelvic congestion syndrome (dilated and refluxing pelvic veins) may also cause dysuria and pelvic pain.

Nucleic acid amplification tests from first-void urine or vaginal swab specimens are highly sensitive for detecting chlamydial infection in men and women. Other infectious pathogens associated with dysuria and urethritis in men include *Mycoplasma genitalium* and Enterobacteriaceae.

Treatment

Definitive treatment is directed to the underlying cause of the dysuria. An evidence-informed algorithm for managing suspected UTI in women is shown in Figure 2–1. This algorithm supports antibiotic treatment of most women with multiple and typical symptoms of UTI without performing UA or urine culture. Telemedicine may be an appropriate technology to assess and manage uncomplicated UTI for average-risk patients who can self-diagnose. Antibiotic selection should be guided by local resistance patterns and expert-panel clinical practice guidelines; major options for uncomplicated cystitis include nitrofurantoin, cephalosporins, ciprofloxacin, fosfomycin, and trimethoprim-sulfamethoxazole. Five days of nitrofurantoin resulted in a significantly greater likelihood of clinical and microbiologic resolution than single-dose fosfomycin.

In a study of 47 patients with UTIs due to multidrug-resistant bacteria, treatment with fosfomycin resulted in clinical cure rates of 87% and 94% at 48 hours and 14 days, respectively.

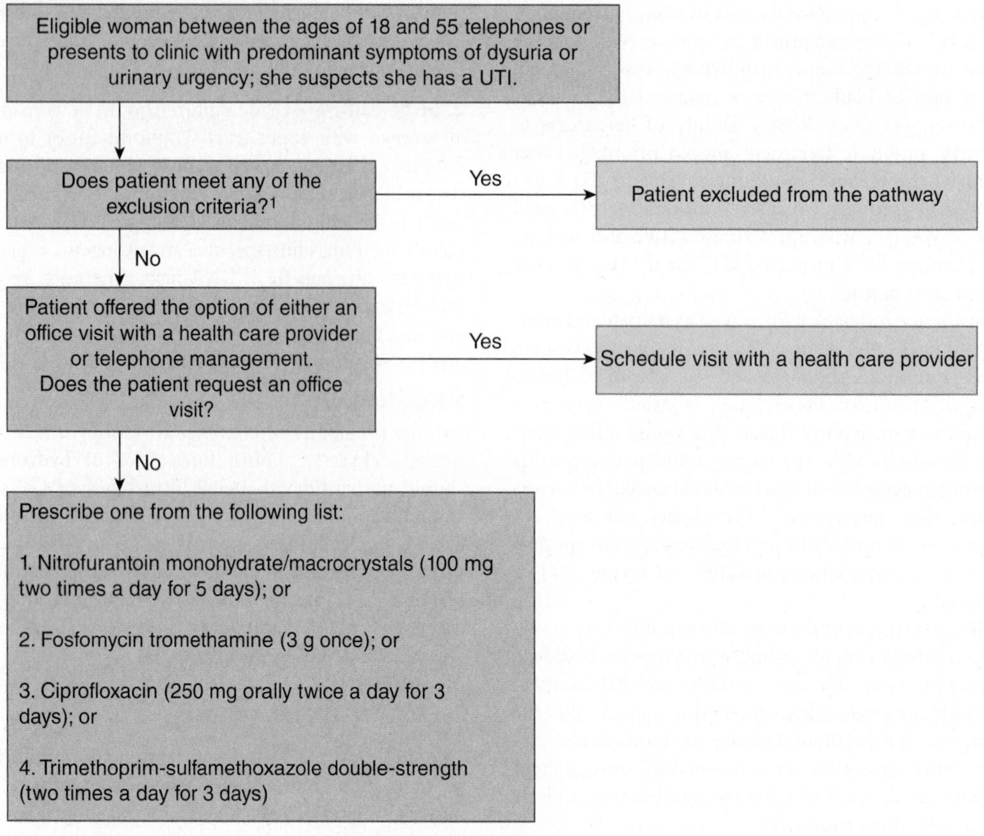
Eligible woman between the ages of 18 and 55 telephones or presents to clinic with predominant symptoms of dysuria or urinary urgency; she suspects she has a UTI.
Does patient meet any of the exclusion criteria?1
Yes
Patient excluded from the pathway
No
Patient offered the option of either an office visit with a health care provider or telephone management. Does the patient request an office visit?
Yes
Schedule visit with a health care provider
No
Prescribe one from the following list:
1. Nitrofurantoin monohydrate/macrocrystals (100 mg two times a day for 5 days); or
2. Fosfomycin tromethamine (3 g once); or
3. Ciprofloxacin (250 mg orally twice a day for 3 days); or
4. Trimethoprim-sulfamethoxazole double-strength (two times a day for 3 days)
1Primary exclusion criteria include documented fever 38°C; symptoms of dysuria or urgency ≥ 7 days; symptoms of vaginitis are present; abdominal pain, nausea, or vomiting; gross hematuria in patients older than 50 years; immunosuppression (eg, current use of chemotherapeutic agents); diabetes mellitus; known pregnancy; chronic renal or urologic abnormalities, other than stress urinary incontinence (eg, polycystic kidney disease, neurogenic bladder, renal failure); recent or persistent urinary stones; urinary catheterization or other urologic procedure ≤ 2 wk ago; discharge from hospital or nursing home ≤ 2 wk ago; treatment for UTI ≤ 2 wk ago; recurrent symptomatic UTI.

▲ **Figure 2–1.** Proposed algorithm for evaluating women with symptoms of acute UTI. (Data from Gupta K et al; Infectious Diseases Society of America; European Society for Microbiology and Infectious Diseases. International clinical practice guidelines for the treatment of acute uncomplicated cystitis and pyelonephritis in women: a 2010 update by the Infectious Diseases Society of America and the European Society for Microbiology and Infectious Diseases. Clin Infect Dis. 2011;52:e103.)

According to the American Academy of Pediatrics' Committee on Drugs, antibiotics that are usually acceptable when treating women who are breastfeeding include trimethoprim-sulfamethoxazole (unless G6PD deficiency is present), amoxicillin, nitrofurantoin, ciprofloxacin, and ofloxacin. Plazomicin, a novel neoglycoside, is FDA approved for the treatment of adults with complicated UTIs who have limited or no alternative treatment options.

In men, prolonged treatment of UTIs (more than 7 days) out of concern for delayed clearance of infection within the prostate does not appear to reduce early or late recurrences. A 5-day course of fluoroquinolones in outpatient men with UTI is as effective as a 10-day course. Among afebrile men with symptoms of UTI, treatment with ciprofloxacin or trimethoprim/sulfamethoxazole for 7 days was noninferior to 14 days regarding resolution of UTI symptoms.

Symptomatic relief can be provided with phenazopyridine, a urinary analgesic that is available over the counter; it is used in combination with antibiotic therapy (when a UTI has been confirmed) but for no more than 2 days. Patients should be informed that phenazopyridine will cause orange/red discoloration of their urine and other body fluids (eg, some contact lens wearers have reported discoloration of their lenses). Rare cases of methemoglobinemia and hemolytic anemia have been reported, usually with overdoses or underlying kidney dysfunction. NSAIDs have also been shown to be of symptomatic benefit, but less effective than antibiotic therapy. Although some women recover from uncomplicated UTI when treated with NSAIDs alone (53% in a Norwegian study), the rate of progression to pyelonephritis was substantial. Delayed antibiotic therapy in elderly patients with UTI leads to a substantially higher rate of bloodstream infections and all-cause mortality. If a broad-spectrum antibiotic was initially prescribed empirically for UTI and urine culture results return establishing efficacy of a narrow-spectrum antibiotic, treatment should be "de-escalated" to the narrow-spectrum antimicrobial. Among premenopausal women with recurrent UTIs, the group with increased daily water consumption had a lower mean number of cystitis episodes over a 12-month period of 1.7 compared with 3.2 in the control group and reduced number of antibiotic prescriptions (1.9 and 3.6, respectively). A systematic review and meta-analysis found D-mannose protective against recurrent UTIs. In patients with asymptomatic renal calculi and recurrent UTIs, stone extraction eliminated infections in 50% of women.

In cases of interstitial cystitis/painful bladder syndrome (see Chapter 23), patients will often respond to a multimodal approach that may include urethral/vesicular dilation, biofeedback, cognitive-behavioral therapy, antidepressants, dietary changes, vaginal emollients, and other supportive measures. Vaginal estrogen effectively relieves urinary urgency and frequency as well as recurrent UTIs related to vulvovaginal atrophy of menopause (also known as genitourinary syndrome of menopause).

A meta-analysis found that antibiotic treatment for most people with asymptomatic bacteriuria is not beneficial and may be harmful. Antibiotic treatment does benefit both pregnant women with asymptomatic bacteriuria as well as persons about to undergo urologic surgery. The USPSTF recommends screening pregnant women for asymptomatic bacteriuria by obtaining a urine culture (B recommendation). The USPSTF recommends against screening for asymptomatic bacteriuria in nonpregnant adults (D recommendation).

There were no differences in the prevalence of postoperative UTI in women who had mixed-flora on preoperative urine cultures compared to those with no growth on preoperative urine cultures.

When to Refer

- Anatomic abnormalities leading to repeated urinary infections.
- Infections associated with nephrolithiasis.
- Persistent interstitial cystitis/painful bladder syndrome.

When to Admit

- Severe pain requiring parenteral medication or impairing ambulation or urination (such as severe primary herpes simplex genitalis).
- Dysuria associated with urinary retention or obstruction.
- Pyelonephritis with ureteral obstruction.
- Symptoms and signs suggesting urosepsis.

Aslam S et al. Recurrent urinary tract infections in adult women. JAMA. 2020;323:658. [PMID: 31995139]

Colgan R et al. Asymptomatic bacteriuria. Am Fam Physician. 2020;102:99. [PMID: 32667160]

Henderson JT et al. Screening for asymptomatic bacteriuria in adults: updated evidence report and systematic review for the US Preventive Services Task Force. JAMA. 2019;322:1195. [PMID: 31550037]

Herness J et al. Acute pyelonephritis in adults: rapid evidence review. Am Fam Physician. 2020;102:173. [PMID: 32735433]

Hoffmann TC et al. Uncomplicated urinary tract infection in women. BMJ. 2021;372:n725. [PMID: 33785479]

Holm A et al. Diagnosis of urinary tract infection based on symptoms: how are likelihood ratios affected by age? A diagnostic accuracy study. BMJ Open. 2021;11:e039871. [PMID: 33419902]

Maki DG. USPSTF recommends screening for asymptomatic bacteriuria in pregnant women but not nonpregnant adults. Ann Intern Med. 2020;172:JC14. [PMID: 32066147]

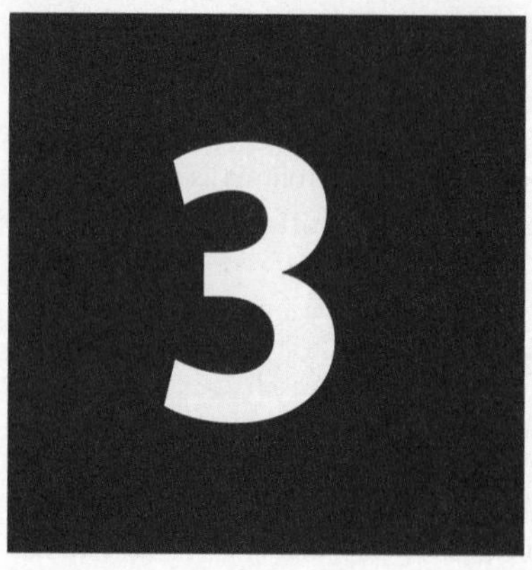

3 Preoperative Evaluation & Perioperative Management

Hugo Q. Cheng, MD

EVALUATION OF THE ASYMPTOMATIC PATIENT

Patients without significant medical problems—especially those under age 50—are at very low risk for perioperative complications. Their preoperative evaluation should include a history and physical examination; emphasis should be on a pharmacologic history and assessment of functional status, exercise tolerance, and cardiopulmonary status to look for unrecognized disease that may require further evaluation prior to surgery. In addition, a directed bleeding history (Table 3–1) should be taken to uncover coagulopathy that could contribute to excessive surgical blood loss. Routine preoperative laboratory tests in asymptomatic healthy patients under age 50 have *not* been found to help predict or prevent complications. Even elderly patients undergoing minor or minimally invasive procedures (such as cataract surgery) are unlikely to benefit from preoperative screening tests.

Siddaiah H et al. Preoperative laboratory testing: implications of "Choosing Wisely" guidelines. Best Pract Res Clin Anaesthesiol. 2020;34:303. [PMID: 32711836]

CARDIAC RISK ASSESSMENT & REDUCTION IN NONCARDIAC SURGERY

The most important perioperative cardiac complications are MI and cardiac death. Other complications include heart failure (HF), arrhythmias, and unstable angina. The principal patient-specific risk factor for cardiac complications is the presence of end-organ CVD. This includes not only CAD and HF but also CVD and CKD. Diabetes mellitus, especially if treated with insulin, is considered a CVD equivalent that increases the risk of cardiac complications. Major abdominal, thoracic, and vascular surgical procedures (especially AAA repair) carry a higher risk of postoperative cardiac complications. These risk factors were identified in a validated, multifactorial risk prediction tool: the Revised Cardiac Risk Index (RCRI) (Table 3–2). The American College of Surgeons' National Surgical Quality Improvement Program (NSQIP) risk prediction tool uses patient age, the location or type of operation, serum creatinine greater than 1.5 mg/dL (132.6 mcmol/L), dependency in activities of daily living, and the patient's American Society of Anesthesiologists physical status classification as predictors for postoperative MI or cardiac arrest. An online risk calculator using the NSQIP tool can be found at https://qxmd.com/calculate/calculator_245/gupta-perioperative-cardiac-risk. The American College of Cardiology and American Heart Association endorse both prediction tools. Patients with two or more RCRI predictors or a risk of perioperative MI or cardiac arrest in excess of 1% as calculated by the NSQIP prediction tool are deemed to be at elevated risk for cardiac complications.

Limited exercise capacity (eg, the inability to walk for two blocks at a normal pace or climb a flight of stairs without resting) also predicts higher cardiac risk. Emergency operations are also associated with greater cardiac risk but should not be delayed for extensive cardiac evaluation. Instead, patients facing emergency surgery should be medically optimized for surgery as quickly as possible and closely monitored for cardiac complications during the perioperative period.

Table 3–1. Directed bleeding history: Findings suggestive of a bleeding disorder.

Unprovoked bruising on the trunk of > 5 cm in diameter
Frequent unprovoked epistaxis or gingival bleeding
Menorrhagia with iron deficiency
Hemarthrosis with mild trauma
Prior excessive surgical blood loss or reoperation for bleeding
Family history of abnormal bleeding
Presence of severe kidney or liver disease
Use of medications that impair coagulation, including nutritional supplements and herbal remedies

Role of Preoperative Noninvasive Ischemia Testing

Most patients can be accurately risk-stratified by history and physical examination. A resting ECG should be obtained in patients with at least one RCRI predictor prior to major surgery but generally omitted in asymptomatic patients undergoing minor operations. Additional noninvasive ischemia

Table 3–2. Revised Cardiac Risk Index (RCRI).

Independent Predictors of Postoperative Cardiac Complications	
Intrathoracic, intraperitoneal, or suprainguinal vascular surgery	
History of ischemic heart disease	
History of heart failure	
Insulin treatment for diabetes mellitus	
Serum creatinine level > 2 mg/dL (> 176.8 mcmol/L)	
History of cerebrovascular disease	
Scoring (Number of Predictors Present)	**Risk of Major Cardiac Complications[1]**
None	0.4%
One	1%
Two	2.4%
More than two	5.4%

[1]Cardiac death, MI, or nonfatal cardiac arrest.
Data from Devereaux PJ et al. Perioperative cardiac events in patients undergoing noncardiac surgery: a review of the magnitude of the problem, the pathophysiology of the events and methods to estimate and communicate risk. CMAJ. 2005;173:627.

testing rarely improves risk stratification or management, especially in patients without CVD undergoing minor operations, or who have at least fair functional capacity. Stress testing has more utility in patients with elevated risk scores on clinical prediction tools, especially if they have poor functional status. In these patients, the absence of ischemia on dipyridamole scintigraphy or dobutamine stress echocardiography is reassuring; in contrast, extensive inducible ischemia predicts a high risk of cardiac complications, particularly with vascular surgery, which may not be modifiable by either medical management or coronary revascularization. The predictive value of an abnormal stress test result for nonvascular surgery patients is less well established. An approach to perioperative cardiac risk assessment and management in patients with known or suspected stable CAD is shown in Figure 3–1.

Role of Cardiac Biomarkers

Preoperative BNP or N-terminal fragment of proBNP (NT-proBNP) levels directly correlate with the risk for perioperative cardiac complications, and their measurement may improve risk assessment. A meta-analysis of 2179 patients found that BNP of 92 mg/L or higher or NT-proBNP of 300 ng/L or higher before noncardiac surgery were associated with a fourfold increase in 30-day mortality and MI. American and European cardiology society guidelines are equivocal about the use of biomarkers to enhance risk prediction; the Canadian Cardiovascular Society, however, strongly recommends measuring BNP or NT-proBNP levels prior to major noncardiac surgery in patients older than 65 years and younger patients with CVD or a RCRI score greater than or equal to 1.

Perioperative Management of Patients with Coronary Artery Disease

Patients with acute coronary syndromes require immediate management of their cardiac disease prior to any preoperative evaluation (see Chapter 10).

A. Medications

1. Antianginal medications—Preoperative antianginal medications, including beta-blockers, calcium channel blockers, and nitrates, should be continued throughout the perioperative period. Several trials have shown that initiation of beta-blockers before major noncardiac surgery reduces the risk of nonfatal MI. However, in the largest trial, a high, fixed dose of metoprolol succinate *increased* total mortality and the risk of stroke. Because of the uncertain benefit-to-risk ratio, initiation of perioperative beta-blockade should be considered only in patients with a high risk of cardiac complications. If used, beta-blockers should be started well in advance of surgery, to allow time to gradually titrate up the dose without causing excessive bradycardia or hypotension. They should not be started on the day of surgery. Possible indications and starting doses for prophylactic beta-blockade are presented in Table 3–3.

2. Statins—Several randomized trials found that HMG-CoA reductase inhibitors (statins) prevent MI in patients undergoing noncardiac surgery. Safety concerns, such as liver failure or rhabdomyolysis, have not materialized in these studies. It is unclear how far in advance of surgery statins must be started and what doses are needed to see benefits. However, based on treatment protocols used in clinical trials, at least a moderate statin dose (eg, atorvastatin 20 mg or fluvastatin 80 mg orally daily) should be considered in all patients undergoing vascular surgery and other patients deemed to be at high risk for cardiac complications, regardless of lipid levels, and initiated at least 30 days before surgery if possible. Patients already taking statins should continue these agents during the perioperative period.

3. Aspirin—In patients without coronary stents, initiation of aspirin therapy before noncardiac surgery is not recommended because it did not reduce cardiac risk and caused increased bleeding in a large, randomized trial. Holding long-term prophylactic aspirin therapy in such patients does not increase cardiac risk.

B. Coronary Revascularization

A trial that randomized over 500 patients with angiographically proven CAD to either coronary revascularization (with either coronary artery bypass grafting [CABG] or percutaneous coronary interventions [PCI]) or medical management alone before vascular surgery found no difference in postoperative MI, 30-day mortality, and long-term mortality. Thus, **preoperative CABG or PCI should be performed only when patients have guideline-concordant indications independent of the planned noncardiac operation.** In addition, surgical patients who have undergone recent coronary stenting are at high risk for stent thrombosis, especially if antiplatelet therapy is stopped prematurely. **Therefore, elective surgery should be**

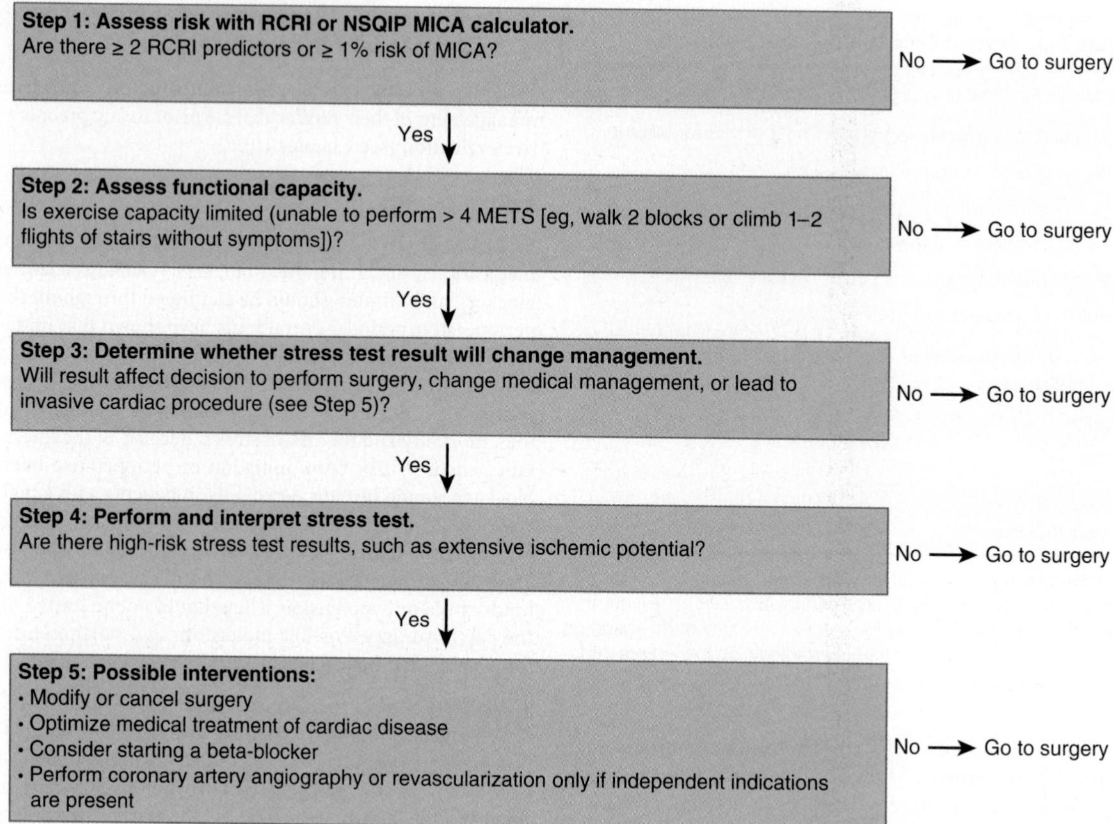

Step 1: Assess risk with RCRI or NSQIP MICA calculator.
Are there ≥ 2 RCRI predictors or ≥ 1% risk of MICA?
No → Go to surgery
Yes
Step 2: Assess functional capacity.
Is exercise capacity limited (unable to perform > 4 METS [eg, walk 2 blocks or climb 1–2 flights of stairs without symptoms])?
No → Go to surgery
Yes
Step 3: Determine whether stress test result will change management.
Will result affect decision to perform surgery, change medical management, or lead to invasive cardiac procedure (see Step 5)?
No → Go to surgery
Yes
Step 4: Perform and interpret stress test.
Are there high-risk stress test results, such as extensive ischemic potential?
No → Go to surgery
Yes
Step 5: Possible interventions:
• Modify or cancel surgery
• Optimize medical treatment of cardiac disease
• Consider starting a beta-blocker
• Perform coronary artery angiography or revascularization only if independent indications are present
No → Go to surgery
Notes:
Step 2: Reasonable to avoid stress test in patients with excellent functional capacity (> 10 METs) and not unreasonable to avoid stress test in patients with moderate or good functional capacity (4–10 METs); patients with unknown functional capacity should be considered unable to perform 4 METs.
Step 3: Regardless of decision to perform stress test, patients should receive optimal guideline-concordant medical therapy.
Step 4: Pharmacologic stress test preferred due to assumption of poor exercise capacity.
Step 5: Possible indications for beta-blockers include ≥ 3 RCRI predictors, ischemia on stress test, or indications independent of surgery.

▲ **Figure 3–1.** Approach to cardiac evaluation in stable patients undergoing major elective surgery. METs, metabolic equivalents; NSQIP MICA, National Surgical Quality Improvement Program Myocardial Infarction and Cardiac Arrest; RCRI, Revised Cardiac Risk Index.

Table 3–3. Indications for prophylactic perioperative beta-blockade.[1]

Strong indications	Patient already taking beta-blocker to treat ischemia, arrhythmia, or hypertension
Possible indications	Patient with myocardial ischemia detected on preoperative stress testing Patient has ≥ 3 Revised Cardiac Risk Index predictors (see Table 3–2)

[1]Initial dose recommendations: atenolol 25 mg orally daily, bisoprolol 2.5 mg orally daily, or metoprolol tartrate 25 mg orally twice daily. The dose of beta-blocker should be carefully titrated to keep heart rate < 70 beats per minute and systolic blood pressure > 100 mm Hg. Avoid initiating beta-blockade on the day of surgery.

deferred for at least 30 days after placement of a bare-metal stent and ideally for 6 months after placement of a drug-eluting stent. If this delay poses significant risks, such as in patients undergoing an operation for cancer, surgery could be considered 3 months after drug-eluting stent implantation. Antiplatelet agents should be continued perioperatively if possible or resumed as soon as possible after surgery. The patient, surgeon, anesthesiologist, and cardiologist should discuss risks and benefits of delaying surgery and management options for dual antiplatelet therapy.

Heart Failure & LV Dysfunction

Elective surgery should be postponed until decompensated HF (manifested by an elevated jugular venous

pressure, an audible third heart sound, or evidence of pulmonary edema) has been brought under control. In patients with compensated HF, the risk of perioperative cardiac complications is similar in patients with ischemic or nonischemic cardiomyopathy. HF with reduced EF likely confers more risk than HF with preserved EF. Guidelines recommend preoperative echocardiography to evaluate LV function in patients without known HF who have unexplained dyspnea and in patients with known HF with clinical deterioration.

Patients receiving diuretics and digoxin should have serum electrolyte and digoxin levels measured prior to surgery because abnormalities in these levels may increase the risk of perioperative arrhythmias. Clinicians must be cautious not to give too much diuretic, since the volume-depleted patient will be much more susceptible to intraoperative hypotension. The surgeon and anesthesiologist should be made aware of the presence and severity of LV dysfunction so that appropriate decisions can be made regarding perioperative fluid management and intraoperative monitoring.

Postoperative MI

In a large cohort study, postoperative MI (defined by a combination of ECG abnormality and cardiac enzyme elevation) typically occurred within 3 days of surgery and was asymptomatic in the majority of cases. Clinical findings that should prompt its consideration include unexplained hypotension, hypoxemia, and delirium. Postoperative MI is associated with increased mortality, even when asymptomatic. Elevated postoperative troponin levels correlate directly with mortality risk, even in patients without ECG abnormalities or other findings of myocardial ischemia. The Canadian Cardiovascular Society advocates routine postoperative screening of high-risk patients with troponin levels, while American and European guidelines remain equivocal. It remains unclear how asymptomatic postoperative MI or troponin elevation should be managed, but optimizing secondary cardiac risk reduction strategies is reasonable.

Valvular Heart Disease

If the nature or severity of valvular lesions is unknown, or if there has been a recent change in clinical status, echocardiography should be performed prior to noncardiac surgery. In addition, patients with known or suspected stenotic or regurgitant valvular disease that is moderately severe or worse should undergo echocardiography within 1 year before surgery. Candidates for valvular intervention independent of the planned noncardiac surgery should have the valve correction procedure performed first. Patients with uncorrected critical or symptomatic aortic stenosis are at particular risk for cardiac complications. They should undergo surgery only after consultation with a cardiologist and anesthesiologist. Patients with mitral stenosis require heart rate control to prolong diastolic filling time. Regurgitant valvular lesions are generally less problematic during surgery because the vasodilatory effect of anesthetics promotes forward flow. Patients with aortic or mitral regurgitation likely benefit from afterload reduction and careful attention to volume status, but negative chronotropes may worsen the regurgitant volume and should be avoided.

Arrhythmias

The finding of a rhythm disturbance on preoperative evaluation should prompt consideration of further cardiac evaluation, particularly when the finding of structural heart disease would alter perioperative management. **Patients with a rhythm disturbance without evidence of underlying heart disease are at low risk for perioperative cardiac complications.** While long-term antiarrhythmic medications should be continued perioperatively, there is no evidence that the use of medications to suppress an asymptomatic arrhythmia alters perioperative risk.

Patients with symptomatic arrhythmias should not undergo elective surgery until their cardiac condition has been addressed. Adequate rate control of atrial fibrillation or other supraventricular arrhythmias should be established prior to surgery. Symptomatic ventricular tachycardia must be thoroughly evaluated and controlled prior to surgery. Patients who have independent indications for a permanent pacemaker or implanted defibrillator should have it placed prior to noncardiac surgery. The anesthesiologist must be notified that a patient has an implanted pacemaker or defibrillator to prevent device malfunction from intraoperative electrocautery.

After major surgery, previously undiagnosed atrial fibrillation develops in approximately 1% of patients. Most episodes resolve spontaneously within hours to days. These patients, however, have an increased risk for subsequent atrial fibrillation and an elevated risk of stroke. Whether the same criteria for anticoagulation therapy should be used for patients undergoing surgery as for patients not undergoing surgery is unclear.

Hypertension

No evidence supports delaying surgery in order to better control mild to moderate hypertension (systolic blood pressure below 180 mm Hg and diastolic blood pressure below 110 mm Hg). Severe hypertension (systolic pressure greater than 180 mm Hg or a diastolic pressure greater than 110 mm Hg) appears to be an independent predictor of perioperative cardiac complications, including MI and HF. It is reasonable to consider delaying elective surgery in patients with such severe hypertension until blood pressure can be controlled, although it is not known whether the risk of cardiac complications is reduced with this approach.

Most medications for chronic hypertension should generally be continued up to and including the day of surgery. Cardiology societies' guidelines differ in their recommendation on whether to continue or hold ACE inhibitors and ARBs on the day of surgery. Continuation increases the risk of intraoperative and postoperative hypotension, whereas holding these agents increases postoperative hypertension. Diuretic agents are frequently held on the day of surgery to prevent hypovolemia and electrolyte disorders if they are not needed to control HF; however, the benefit of this practice is uncertain.

Patients without chronic hypertension may manifest hypertension after surgery, and patients being treated for hypertension often experience decreased control of their blood pressure. Potential causes include elevated sympathetic tone due to injury or pain, volume overload from intravenous fluids, hypercarbia, urine retention, and withholding long-term antihypertensive medications. Before initiating postoperative medical management of hypertension, reversible contributors should be addressed.

Fleisher LA et al. 2014 ACC/AHA guideline on perioperative cardiovascular evaluation and management of patients undergoing noncardiac surgery: a report of the American College of Cardiology/American Heart Association Task Force on Practice Guidelines. J Am Coll Cardiol. 2014;64:e77. [PMID: 25091544]

Hanley C et al. Perioperative risk assessment—focus on functional capacity. Curr Opin Anaesthesiol. 2021;34:309. [PMID: 33935179]

Smilowitz NR et al. Perioperative cardiovascular risk assessment and management for noncardiac surgery: a review. JAMA. 2020;324:279. [PMID: 32692391]

PULMONARY EVALUATION IN NON–LUNG RESECTION SURGERY

Pneumonia and respiratory failure requiring prolonged mechanical ventilation are the most important postoperative pulmonary complications. The occurrence of these complications has been associated with a significant increase in mortality and hospital length of stay. Pulmonary thromboembolism is another serious complication; prophylaxis against venous thromboembolic disease is detailed in Table 14–14.

Risk Factors for the Development of Postoperative Pulmonary Complications

Procedure-related risk factors for postoperative pulmonary complications include location of surgery (highest rates occur in cardiac, thoracic, and upper abdominal cases), prolonged anesthesia, and emergency cases. Operations not requiring general anesthesia tend to have lower rates of postoperative pulmonary complications; laparoscopic procedures tend to have lower risk than comparable open procedures.

A summary of patient-specific risk factors for pulmonary complications is presented in Table 3–4. Advanced age appears to confer increased risk. The presence and severity of systemic disease of any type is associated with pulmonary complications. In particular, patients with COPD or HF have at least twice the risk of postoperative pulmonary complications compared with patients without these conditions. As with preoperative cardiac risk assessment, physical debility and poor functional capacity predict higher risk of postoperative pulmonary complications. A risk calculator for predicting postoperative respiratory failure based on the NSQIP patient database is available (https://qxmd.com/calculate/calculator_261/postoperative-respiratory-failure-risk-calculator).

Table 3–4. Clinical risk factors for postoperative pulmonary complications.

Upper abdominal or cardiothoracic surgery
Prolonged anesthesia time (> 4 hours)
Emergency surgery
Age > 60 years
COPD
Heart failure
Severe systemic disease
Tobacco use (> 20 pack-years)
Impaired cognition or sensorium
Functional dependency or prior stroke
Preoperative sepsis
Low serum albumin level
Obstructive sleep apnea

Pulmonary Function Testing & Laboratory Studies

The main role for preoperative pulmonary function testing (PFT) is to identify pulmonary disease in patients with unexplained symptoms prior to major abdominal or cardiothoracic surgery. In patients with diagnosed lung disease, PFT often add little information above clinical assessment. Chest radiographs in unselected patients also rarely add clinically useful information. The benefit of polysomnography to diagnose obstructive sleep apnea prior to bariatric surgery is unproven. Arterial blood gas measurement is not routinely recommended except in patients with known lung disease and suspected hypoxemia or hypercapnia.

Preoperative Risk Reduction

Retrospective studies have shown that smoking cessation reduced the incidence of pulmonary complications, but only if it was initiated at least 1–2 months before surgery. A meta-analysis of randomized trials found that preoperative smoking cessation programs reduced both pulmonary and surgical wound complications, especially if smoking cessation was initiated at least 4 weeks prior to surgery. **The preoperative period may be an optimal time to initiate smoking cessation efforts.** A systematic review found that smoking cessation programs started in a preoperative evaluation clinic increased the odds of abstinence at 3–6 months by nearly 60%. Patients who have recovered from SARS-CoV-2 infection appear to have elevated surgical mortality up to 7 weeks after diagnosis. Increased mortality was observed even after mild or asymptomatic cases, and the risk persisted beyond 7 weeks in patients who were still symptomatic at that time. Elective surgery should not be scheduled within 7 weeks of SARS-CoV-2 infection for patients whose symptoms have resolved or longer while patients remain symptomatic.

Postoperative Risk Reduction

Postoperative risk reduction strategies have centered on promoting lung expansion through the use of incentive spirometry; deep breathing exercises; and in selected populations, continuous positive airway pressure (CPAP) or intermittent positive-pressure breathing (IPPB). Although trial results have been mixed, all these techniques have been shown to reduce the incidence of postoperative atelectasis and, in a few studies, to reduce the incidence of other postoperative pulmonary complications. In most comparative trials, these methods were equally effective. Given the higher cost of CPAP and IPPB, **incentive spirometry and deep breathing exercises are the preferred methods for most patients.** Multi-component respiratory care programs may be particularly beneficial. One program termed "I COUGH"—an acronym for *I*ncentive spirometry, *C*oughing and deep breathing, *O*ral care, *U*nderstanding (patient education), *G*et out of bed (early ambulation), and *H*ead of bed elevation—reduced the rates of pneumonia and unplanned intubation after general and vascular surgery.

Lumb AB. Pre-operative respiratory optimisation: an expert review. Anaesthesia. 2019;74:43. [PMID: 30604419]

Selzer A et al. Preoperative pulmonary evaluation. Med Clin North Am. 2019;103:585. [PMID: 30955524]

EVALUATION OF THE PATIENT WITH LIVER DISEASE

Patients with serious liver disease are at increased risk for perioperative morbidity, and decompensated liver disease is associated with an extremely high perioperative mortality. Appropriate preoperative evaluation requires consideration of the effects of anesthesia and surgery on postoperative liver function and of the complications associated with anesthesia and surgery in patients with preexisting liver disease.

Risk Assessment in Surgical Patients with Liver Disease

Screening unselected patients with liver biochemical tests has a low yield and is not recommended. Patients with suspected or known liver disease based on history or physical examination, however, should have measurement of liver enzyme levels as well as tests of hepatic synthetic function performed prior to surgery.

Elective surgery in patients with acute viral or alcoholic hepatitis should be delayed until the acute episode has resolved. In three small series of patients with acute viral hepatitis who underwent abdominal surgery, the mortality rate was roughly 10%. Similarly, patients with undiagnosed alcoholic hepatitis had high mortality rates when undergoing abdominal surgery. In the absence of cirrhosis or synthetic dysfunction, chronic viral hepatitis is unlikely to increase risk significantly. Similarly, nonalcoholic fatty liver disease without cirrhosis probably does not pose a serious risk in surgical patients.

In patients with cirrhosis, postoperative complication rates correlate with the severity of liver dysfunction. Traditionally, severity of dysfunction has been assessed with the Child-Pugh score (see Chapter 16). A conservative approach would be to avoid elective surgery in patients with Child-Pugh class C cirrhosis and pursue it with great caution in class B patients. The Model for End-stage Liver Disease (MELD) score, based on serum bilirubin and creatinine levels, and the prothrombin time expressed as the INR, also predicted surgical mortality and outperformed the Child-Pugh classification in some studies. A web-based risk assessment calculator incorporating age and MELD score can predict both perioperative and long-term mortality (https://www.mayoclinic.org/medical-professionals/model-end-stage-liver-disease/post-operative-mortality-risk-patients-cirrhosis). Generally, a MELD score less than 10 predicts low risk, whereas a score greater than 16 portends high mortality after elective surgery.

When surgery is elective, controlling ascites, encephalopathy, and coagulopathy preoperatively is prudent. Ascites is a particular problem in abdominal operations, where it can lead to wound dehiscence and hernias. Great care should be taken when using analgesics and sedatives, since these can worsen hepatic encephalopathy; in general, short-acting agents and lower doses should be used. Postoperative constipation should be aggressively treated because it can precipitate encephalopathy. Kidney function and volume status need to be closely monitored to prevent AKI and volume overload, which are common complications in these patients. Patients with coagulopathy should receive vitamin K and may need fresh frozen plasma transfusion at the time of surgery; however, transfusing to a specific INR target for cirrhosis is discouraged.

Northup PG et al. AGA Clinical Practice Update: surgical risk assessment and perioperative management in cirrhosis. Clin Gastroenterol Hepatol. 2019;17:595. [PMID: 30273751]

PREOPERATIVE HEMATOLOGIC EVALUATION

Three of the more common clinical situations faced by the medical consultant are the patient with anemia, the assessment of bleeding risk, and the perioperative management of long-term anticoagulation.

The main goals of the preoperative evaluation of the anemic patient are to determine the need for preoperative diagnostic evaluation and the need for transfusion. **When feasible, the diagnostic evaluation of the patient with previously unrecognized anemia should be done prior to surgery because certain types of anemia (particularly those due to sickle cell disease, hemolysis, and acute blood loss) have implications for perioperative management.** These types of anemia are typically associated with an elevated reticulocyte count. Given the prevalence of iron deficiency, excluding it as the cause of anemia is reasonable. However, the practice of administering intravenous iron to unselected anemic patients before elective surgery has not been proven beneficial. Preoperative anemia is associated with higher perioperative morbidity and mortality. Whether raising preoperative hemoglobin level to specific targets will improve postoperative outcomes is unknown. The clinician determining the need for preoperative transfusion in an individual patient must consider factors other than the absolute hemoglobin level, including

Table 3–5. Recommendations for perioperative management of DOACs.

Drug and Kidney Function	Last Dose Before Procedure	Resume Medication
Dabigatran with normal creatinine clearance (> 50 mL/min [0.83 mL/s]); rivaroxaban, apixaban, edoxaban	2 days before procedure with low risk of bleeding or 3 days before procedure with high risk of bleeding	If hemostasis adequate, resume 24 hours after procedure with low risk of bleeding or 48–72 hours after procedure with high risk of bleeding
Dabigatran with reduced creatinine clearance (30–50 mL/min [0.5–0.83 mL/s)	3 days before procedure with low risk of bleeding or 5 days before procedure with high risk of bleeding	

the presence of cardiopulmonary disease, the type of surgery, and the likely severity of surgical blood loss. The few studies that have compared different postoperative transfusion thresholds failed to demonstrate improved outcomes with a more aggressive transfusion strategy. Based on available evidence, the AABB (formerly American Association of Blood Banks) recommends transfusion for a hemoglobin level less than 8 g/dL (80 g/L) or for symptomatic anemia in patients undergoing orthopedic or cardiac surgery.

The most important component of the bleeding risk assessment is a directed bleeding history (see Table 3–1). Patients who provide a reliable history of no abnormal bleeding on directed bleeding history and have no suggestion of abnormal bleeding on physical examination are at very low risk for having an occult bleeding disorder. Laboratory tests of hemostatic parameters in these patients are generally not needed. When the directed bleeding history is unreliable or incomplete, or when abnormal bleeding is suggested, a formal evaluation of hemostasis should be done prior to surgery and should include measurement of the prothrombin time, activated partial thromboplastin time, and platelet count (see Chapter 13).

Patients receiving long-term oral anticoagulation are at risk for thromboembolic complications when an operation requires interruption of this therapy. However, "bridging anticoagulation," where unfractionated or low-molecular-weight heparin is administered parenterally while oral anticoagulants are held, has not been shown to be beneficial and can increase bleeding. A cohort study found that DOACs could be safely managed without bridging by using a protocol based on the patient's kidney function where the DOACs are withheld several days prior to surgery and restarted 24–48 hours after surgery if hemostasis appears adequate (Table 3–5). A randomized trial of bridging anticoagulation in surgical patients taking warfarin for atrial fibrillation demonstrated no difference in thromboembolism. Bleeding complications were twice as common in patients who received bridging anticoagulation. A trial of postoperative bridging anticoagulation that included patients with atrial fibrillation or mechanical prosthetic heart valves also found no benefit for stroke prevention. **Most experts recommend bridging therapy only in patients at high risk for thromboembolism.** An approach to perioperative anticoagulation management with warfarin is shown in Table 3–6, but the recommendations must

Table 3–6. Recommendations for management of perioperative anticoagulation with warfarin.

Thromboembolic Risk without Anticoagulation	Recommendation
Low (eg, atrial fibrillation with $CHADS_2$ score 0–4,[1] mechanical bileaflet aortic valve prosthesis, or single venous thromboembolism > 3 months ago without hypercoagulability condition[2])	Stop warfarin 5 days before surgery Measure INR the day before surgery to confirm that it is acceptable (< 1.6 for most operations) Resume warfarin when hemostasis permits No bridging with parenteral anticoagulants before or after surgery
High (eg, either atrial fibrillation or mechanical heart valve with stroke < 3 months prior, atrial fibrillation with $CHADS_2$ score 5 or 6, mechanical mitral valve prosthesis, caged-ball or tilting disk valve prosthesis, or venous thrombosis < 3 months ago or associated with hypercoagulability condition[2])	Stop warfarin 5 days before surgery Begin bridging with therapeutic dose UFH infusion or LMWH 2 days after stopping oral anticoagulation Administer last dose of LMWH 24 hours before surgery; discontinue UFH 4–6 hours before surgery Measure INR the day before surgery to confirm that it is acceptable (< 1.6 for most operations) Resume warfarin when hemostasis permits If hemostasis permits, consider bridging with therapeutic dose UFH infusion or LMWH beginning 48–72 hours after surgery and continuing until the INR is therapeutic

[1]1 point each for heart failure, hypertension, diabetes mellitus, and age > 75 years, and 2 points for stroke or transient ischemic attack.
[2]Patients should receive venous thromboembolism prophylaxis after surgery (see Chapter 14).
LMWH, low-molecular-weight heparin; UFH, unfractionated heparin.

be considered in the context of patient preference and hemorrhagic risk.

Douketis JD et al. Perioperative management of patients with atrial fibrillation receiving a direct oral anticoagulant. JAMA Intern Med. 2019;179:1469. [PMID: 31380891]
Kuo HC et al. Thromboembolic and bleeding risk of periprocedural bridging anticoagulation: a systematic review and meta-analysis. Clin Cardiol. 2020;43:441. [PMID: 31944351]
Shander A et al. How I treat anemia in the perisurgical setting. Blood. 2020;136:814. [PMID: 32556314]

NEUROLOGIC EVALUATION

Delirium can occur after any major operation but is particularly common after hip fracture repair and cardiovascular surgery, where the incidence is 30–60%. **Postoperative delirium has been associated with higher rates of major postoperative cardiac and pulmonary complications, poor functional recovery, increased length of hospital stay, increased risk of subsequent dementia and functional decline, and increased mortality.** The American Geriatrics Society recommends screening preoperative patients for these delirium risk factors: age greater than 65 years, chronic cognitive impairment or dementia, severe illness, poor vision or hearing, and the presence of infection. Patients with any of these risk factors should be enrolled in a multicomponent, nonpharmacologic delirium prevention program after surgery, which includes interventions such as reorientation, sleep hygiene, bowel and bladder care, mobilization and physical therapy, and the elimination of unnecessary medications. Moderate-quality evidence supports the use of these nonpharmacologic interventions.

Only a minority of patients with postoperative delirium will have a single, reversible etiology for their condition (see Delirium, Chapter 4). Evaluation of delirious patients should exclude electrolyte derangements, occult UTI, and adverse effects from psychotropic medications such as opioids, sedatives, anticholinergic agents, and antispasmodics. Conservative management includes reassuring and reorienting the patient; eliminating unneeded medications, intravenous lines, and urinary catheters; and keeping the patient active during the day while allowing uninterrupted sleep at night. Use of multimodal postoperative analgesic strategies can reduce or avoid the need for opioids. When agitation jeopardizes patient or provider safety, neuroleptic agents given at the lowest effective dose for the shortest duration needed are preferred over the use of benzodiazepines or physical restraints (Table 25–1).

Stroke complicates less than 1% of all surgical procedures but may occur in 1–6% of patients undergoing cardiac or carotid artery surgery. Most of the strokes in cardiac surgery patients are embolic in origin, and about half occur within the first postoperative day. A retrospective analysis found that patients who had previously suffered a stroke had an 18% risk of MI, recurrent stroke, or cardiac death if they underwent noncardiac surgery within 3 months of the stroke. This risk declined over time and reached its nadir 9 months after the stroke, suggesting a benefit to delaying elective surgery.

Symptomatic carotid artery stenosis is associated with a high risk of stroke in patients undergoing cardiac surgery. In general, patients with independent indications for correction of carotid stenosis should have the procedure done prior to elective surgery. In contrast, most studies suggest that asymptomatic carotid bruits and asymptomatic carotid stenosis are associated with little or no increased risk of stroke in surgical patients.

Benesch C et al. Perioperative neurological evaluation and management to lower the risk of acute stroke in patients undergoing noncardiac, nonneurological surgery: a scientific statement from the American Heart Association/American Stroke Association. Circulation. 2021;143:e923. [PMID: 33827230]
Jin Z et al. Postoperative delirium: perioperative assessment, risk reduction, and management. Br J Anaesth. 2020;125:492. [PMID: 32798069]

MANAGEMENT OF ENDOCRINE DISEASES

Diabetes Mellitus

The goal of management for all diabetic patients is the prevention of severe hyper- or hypoglycemia in the perioperative period. In addition, patients with type 1 diabetes are at risk for developing ketoacidosis. Increased secretion of cortisol, epinephrine, glucagon, and growth hormone during and after surgery causes insulin resistance and hyperglycemia in diabetic patients. Conversely, reduced caloric intake after surgery and frequent, unpredictable periods of fasting increase the risk for hypoglycemia. Thus, all surgical diabetic patients require frequent blood glucose monitoring. Ideally, patients with diabetes should undergo surgery early in the morning. The specific pharmacologic management of diabetes during the perioperative period depends on the type of diabetes (insulin-dependent or not), the level of glycemic control, and the type and length of surgery.

Poor preoperative glycemic control, as indicated by an elevated hemoglobin A_{1c} level, is associated with a greater risk of surgical complications, particularly infections. However, a strategy of delaying surgery until glycemic control improves has not been rigorously studied. The ideal postoperative blood glucose target is also unknown. Based on trials that showed increased mortality in hospitalized patients randomized to tight control, the American College of Physicians recommends maintaining serum glucose between 140 mg/dL and 200 mg/dL (7.8–11.1 mmol/L), whereas the British National Health Service guidelines recommend a range of 108–180 mg/dL (6–10 mmol/L).

A. Diabetes Controlled by Diet

For people with diabetes controlled with diet alone, no special precautions must be taken unless diabetic control is markedly disturbed by the procedure. If this occurs, small doses of short-acting insulin as needed will correct the hyperglycemia.

B. Diabetes Treated with Oral Hypoglycemic Agents

Most oral hypoglycemic agents should be held on the day of surgery. However, the sodium-glucose transporter 2 inhibitors (eg, canagliflozin) should be held for 3–4 days before surgery due to their long half-life and associated risk of ketoacidosis. Oral hypoglycemic agents should not be restarted after surgery until patients are clinically stable and oral intake is adequate and unlikely to be interrupted. Patients who experience significant hyperglycemia when oral agents are held should be treated in the same way as patients with type 2 diabetes who require insulin, as described below. Postoperative kidney function should be checked with a serum creatinine level prior to restarting metformin.

C. Diabetes Treated with Insulin

The protocol used to control glucose depends on (1) the kind of diabetes (type 1 or type 2); (2) whether it is minor surgery (lasting less than 2 hours and patient able to eat afterward) or major surgery (lasting more than 2 hours, with invasion of a body cavity, and patient not able to eat afterward); and (3) the preoperative insulin regimen (basal bolus or premixed insulin twice a day or premeal bolus only or regular insulin before meals and NPH at bedtime).

1. Preoperative insulin regimen—For patients with either type 1 or type 2 diabetes who are receiving insulin, a common practice is to reduce the last preoperative dose of long-acting, basal insulin by 30–50% and hold short-acting nutritional insulin.

2. Perioperative insulin regimen—Patients with type 1 diabetes must receive basal insulin to prevent the development of diabetic ketoacidosis. **Consultation with an endocrinologist or hospitalist should be strongly considered when a patient with type 1 diabetes mellitus undergoes major surgery.** Major surgical procedures in patients with type 1 diabetes lasting more than 2 hours usually require an insulin infusion. Some patients with type 2 diabetes who are taking insulin will also need insulin infusion to maintain adequate glycemic control. An insulin infusion is a complex procedure for a high-risk medication and involves extensive monitoring, dose titrations, and contingency plans. There are a number of algorithms available for insulin infusions (http://ucsfinpatientdiabetes.pbworks.com).

3. Postoperative insulin regimen—After surgery, when a patient with either type 1 or type 2 diabetes has resumed adequate oral intake, subcutaneous administration of insulin can be restarted. Intravenous administration of insulin and dextrose can be stopped 30 minutes after the first subcutaneous dose. Insulin needs may vary in the first several days after surgery because of continuing postoperative stresses and because of variable caloric intake. In this situation, multiple doses of short-acting insulin plus some long-acting basal insulin, guided by blood glucose determinations, can keep the patient in acceptable metabolic control. Use of correctional insulin only (without basal or nutritional insulin) after surgery is discouraged. A trial comparing correctional insulin with basal-bolus dosing found that the latter strategy led to fewer postoperative complications.

Glucocorticoid Replacement

Hypotension or shock resulting from primary or secondary adrenocortical insufficiency is rare, and the practice of administering supraphysiologic "stress-dose" glucocorticoid perioperatively has not been well studied. A guideline from rheumatology and orthopedic surgery societies recommends that patients taking glucocorticoids continue their regimen when undergoing arthroplasty and not receive "stress-dose" glucocorticoids. Another approach is to administer stress-dose glucocorticoids to any patient who has received the equivalent of at least 7.5 mg of prednisone daily for 3 weeks within the past year when they undergo major surgery. A commonly used stress-dose regimen is hydrocortisone 100 mg intravenously daily, divided every 8 hours, beginning before induction of anesthesia and stopped after 24 hours without tapering. Patients who have been taking less than 5 mg of prednisone daily and those receiving alternate-day glucocorticoid dosing are unlikely to require supplemental coverage.

Thyroid Disease

Severe symptomatic hypothyroidism has been associated with perioperative complications, including intraoperative hypotension, HF, cardiac arrest, and death. Elective surgery should be delayed in patients with severe hypothyroidism until adequate thyroid hormone replacement can be achieved. Patients with symptomatic hyperthyroidism are at risk for perioperative thyroid storm and should not undergo elective surgery until their thyrotoxicosis is controlled; an endocrinologist should be consulted if emergency surgery is needed. Patients with mild hypothyroidism (median TSH level 8.6 mIU/L) tolerate surgery well, with only a slight increase in the incidence of intraoperative hypotension; surgery need not be delayed for the month or more required to ensure adequate thyroid hormone replacement.

Chilkoti GT et al. Perioperative "stress dose" of corticosteroid: pharmacological and clinical perspective. J Anaesthesiol Clin Pharmacol. 2019;35:147. [PMID: 31303699]

Preiser JC et al. Perioperative management of oral glucose-lowering drugs in the patient with type 2 diabetes. Anesthesiology. 2020;133:430. [PMID: 32667156]

Simha V et al. Perioperative glucose control in patients with diabetes undergoing elective surgery. JAMA. 2019;321:399. [PMID: 30615031]

KIDNEY DISEASE

The development of AKI in patients undergoing general surgery is an independent predictor of mortality, even if mild or if kidney dysfunction resolves. The mortality associated with the development of perioperative AKI that requires dialysis exceeds 50%. Risk factors associated with postoperative deterioration in kidney function are shown in Table 3–7. Several medications, including "renal-dose" dopamine, mannitol, *N*-acetylcysteine, and clonidine, have not been proved effective in clinical trials to preserve kidney function during the perioperative period and should not be used for this indication. **Maintenance of adequate intravascular volume is likely to be the most effective**

Table 3–7. Risk factors for the development of AKI after general surgery.[1]

Age > 55 years
Male sex
CKD
Heart failure
Diabetes mellitus
Hypertension
Ascites
Intraperitoneal surgery
Emergency surgery

[1]Presence of 5 or more risk factors is associated with > 3% risk of creatinine elevation > 2 mg/dL (176.8 mcmol/L) above baseline or requirement for dialysis.

Reproduced with permission from Kheterpal S et al, Development and Validation of an Acute Kidney Injury Risk Index for Patients Undergoing General Surgery: Results from a National Data Set, Anesthesiology, 2009;110(3): 505–15. https://pubs.asahq.org/anesthesiology/article/110/3/505/10107/Development-and-Validation-of-an-Acute-Kidney.

method to reduce the risk of perioperative deterioration in kidney function. Exposure to renal-toxic agents, such as NSAIDs and intravenous contrast, should be minimized or avoided. ACE inhibitors and ARBs reduce renal perfusion and may increase the risk of perioperative AKI. Although firm evidence is lacking, it may be useful to temporarily discontinue these medications in patients at risk for perioperative AKI.

Although the mortality rate for elective major surgery is low (1–4%) in patients with dialysis-dependent CKD, the risk for perioperative complications, including postoperative hyperkalemia, pneumonia, fluid overload, and bleeding, is substantially increased. Patients should undergo dialysis preoperatively within 24 hours before surgery, and their serum electrolyte levels should be measured just prior to surgery and monitored closely during the postoperative period.

Gumbert SD et al. Perioperative acute kidney injury. Anesthesiology. 2020;132:180. [PMID: 31687986]

ANTIBIOTIC PROPHYLAXIS OF SURGICAL SITE INFECTIONS

Surgical site infection is estimated to occur in roughly 4% of general or vascular operations. Although the type of procedure is the main factor determining the risk of developing a surgical site infection, certain patient factors have been associated with increased risk, including diabetes mellitus, older age, obesity, smoking, heavy alcohol consumption, admission from a long-term care facility, and multiple medical comorbidities. **For most major procedures, the use of prophylactic antibiotics has been demonstrated to reduce the incidence of surgical site infections.** Substantial evidence suggests that a single dose of an appropriate intravenous antibiotic—or combination of antibiotics—administered 30–60 minutes prior to skin incision is as effective as multiple-dose regimens that extend into the postoperative period. For most procedures, a first-generation cephalosporin (eg, cefazolin 2 g intravenously) is as effective as later-generation agents.

Guidelines for antibiotic prophylaxis against infective endocarditis in patients undergoing invasive procedures are presented in Chapter 33. Given the lack of evidence for antibiotic prophylaxis against prosthetic joint infection before dental procedures, guidelines from the American Academy of Orthopedic Surgeons and the American Dental Association recommend against this practice.

Fields AC et al. Preventing surgical site infections: looking beyond the current guidelines. JAMA. 2020;323:1087. [PMID: 32083641]

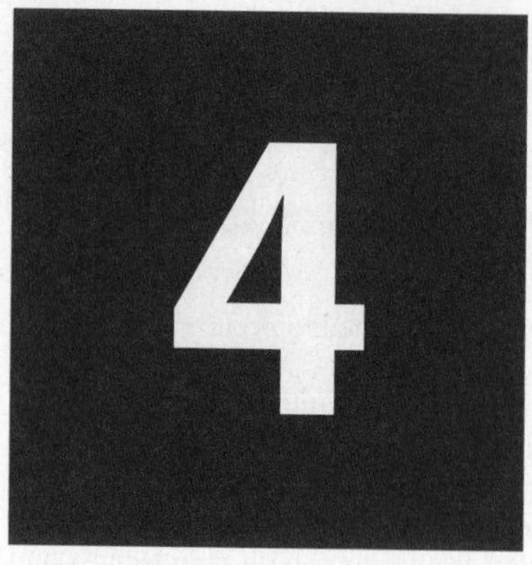

Geriatric Disorders

Leah J. Witt, MD
Rossana Lau-Ng, MD
G. Michael Harper, MD

GENERAL PRINCIPLES OF GERIATRIC CARE

The following principles help in caring for older adults:

1. Many disorders are multifactorial in origin and are best managed by multifactorial interventions.
2. Diseases often present atypically or with nonspecific symptoms (eg, confusion, functional decline).
3. Not all abnormalities require evaluation and treatment.
4. Complex medication regimens, adherence problems, and polypharmacy are common challenges.
5. Multiple chronic conditions often coexist and should be managed in concert with one another.

COMPREHENSIVE ASSESSMENT OF THE OLDER ADULT

In addition to conventional assessment of symptoms, diseases, and medications, comprehensive assessment addresses three topics: **prognosis, values and preferences,** and **ability to function independently.** Comprehensive assessment is warranted before major clinical decisions are made.

Assessment of Prognosis

When an older person's life expectancy is longer than 10 years (ie, 50% of similar persons live longer than 10 years), it is reasonable to consider effective tests and treatments much as they are considered in younger persons. When life expectancy is less than 10 years (and especially when it is much less), choices of tests and treatments should be made based on their ability to affect a clinical outcome that is valued by the patient in the context of their estimated life expectancy. The relative benefits and harms of tests and treatments often change as prognosis worsens, and net benefit (benefits minus harms) often worsens.

When an older patient's clinical situation is dominated by a single disease process (eg, lung cancer metastatic to brain), prognosis can be estimated well with a disease-specific instrument. Even in this situation, however, prognosis generally worsens with age (especially over age 90 years) and with the presence of serious age-related conditions, such as dementia, malnutrition, or functional impairment.

When an older patient's clinical situation is not dominated by a single disease process, prognosis can be estimated initially by considering basic demographic and health elements (Figure 4–1). For example, less than 25% of men aged 95 will live 5 years, whereas nearly 75% of women aged 70 will live 10 years. The prognosis for older persons living at home can be estimated by considering age, sex, comorbid conditions, and function. The prognosis is worse for older persons discharged from the hospital than for those living at home and can be estimated by considering sex, comorbid conditions, and function at discharge. A compilation of indices with online calculators that allow for estimating prognosis in multiple clinical settings can be found at ePrognosis (https://eprognosis.ucsf.edu).

Assessment of Values & Preferences

Although patients vary in their values and preferences, many frail older patients prioritize maintaining their independence over prolonging survival. Values and preferences are determined by speaking directly with a patient or, when the patient cannot express preferences reliably, with the patient's surrogate.

In assessing values and preferences (ie, what matters most to patients), it is important to keep in mind the following:

1. Patients are experts about their preferences for outcomes and experiences; however, they may not have adequate information to make and express informed preferences for specific tests or treatments.
2. Patients' preferences often change over time. For example, some patients find living with a disability more acceptable than they thought before experiencing it.

Assessment of Function

People often lose function in multiple domains as they age, with the result that they may not be able to do some activities as quickly or capably and may need assistance. Assessment of function improves prognostic estimates.

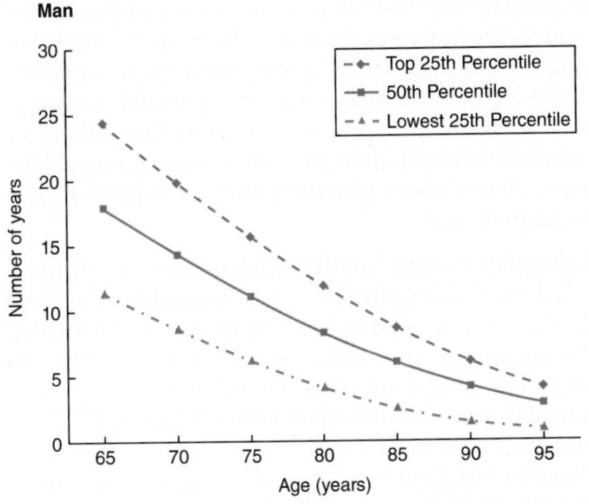

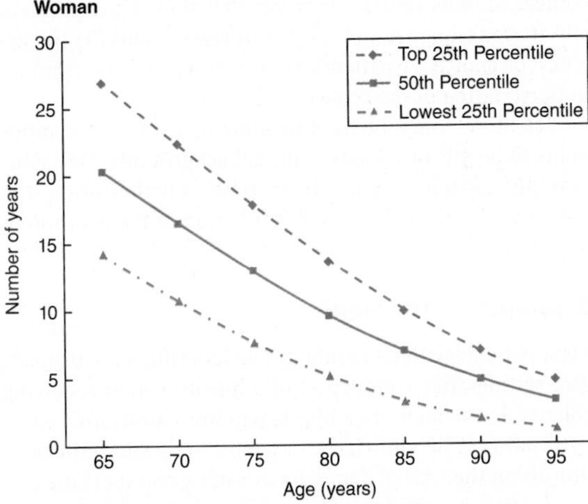

▲ **Figure 4–1.** Median life expectancy of older men and women. (Data derived from Arias E. United States Life Tables, 2011. Natl Vital Stat Rep. 2015;64(11):1–63.)

Assessment of function is essential to determine an individual's needs in the context of his or her values and preferences and the possible effects of recommended treatment.

About one-fourth of patients over age 65 and half of persons older than 85 need help performing their **basic activities of daily living (ADLs:** bathing, dressing, eating, transferring from bed to chair, continence, toileting) or **instrumental activities of daily living (IADLs:** transportation, shopping, cooking, using the telephone, managing money, taking medications, housecleaning, laundry).

Functional screening should include assessment of ADLs and IADLs and questions to detect weight loss, falls, incontinence, depressed mood, self-neglect, fear for personal safety, and common serious impairments (eg, hearing, vision, cognition, and mobility). Standard functional screening measures may not be useful in capturing subtle impairments in highly functional independent older adults. One technique for these patients is to identify and ask about a target routine activity, such as bowling or gardening. Difficulty with or discontinuation of the particular activity may indicate new or worsening impairment (such as cognitive impairment, urinary incontinence, or hearing loss). Additional gentle questioning or assessment may help uncover such changes.

Frailty

Frailty is a syndrome characterized by loss of physiologic reserve and dysregulation across multiple systems, ultimately resulting in greater risk of poor health outcomes. Estimates of its prevalence in community-dwelling older adults range from 5% to 17%. Elements of frailty include **weakness (grip strength), slow gait speed, decreased physical activity, weight loss,** and **exhaustion or low energy.** While there is not one universally agreed upon definition or assessment tool for frailty, generally an individual is defined as frail when three or more of the above features are present. Persons with frailty are at increased risk for falls, hospitalization, functional decline, poorer outcomes associated with medical interventions (eg, surgery, dialysis, chemotherapy), and death. **Exercise, particularly strength and resistance training, can increase walking speed and improve function.** There is evidence that optimal nutrition, particularly higher levels of protein intake, may be associated with reduced incidence of frailty. However, once frailty is established, the treatment is largely supportive, multifactorial, and individualized based on patient goals, life expectancy, and chronic conditions. Sometimes, transitioning a patient to a comfort-focused or hospice approach is the most appropriate clinical intervention when irreversible complications from frailty develop.

Garrard JW et al. Comprehensive geriatric assessment in primary care: a systematic review. Aging Clin Exp Res. 2020;32:197. [PMID: 30968287]

Pilotto A et al. A multidimensional approach to frailty in older people. Ageing Res Rev. 2020;60:101047. [PMID: 32171786]

MANAGEMENT OF COMMON GERIATRIC PROBLEMS

1. Dementia

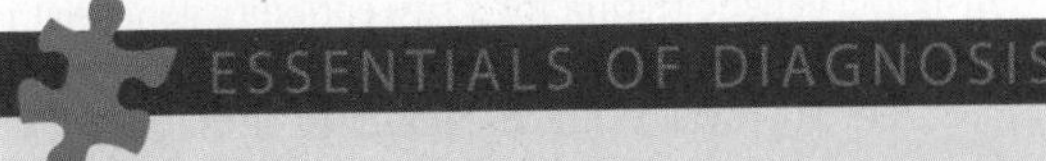

- Progressive decline of mental processes.
- Acquired cognitive deficits severe enough to impair function.
- Not due to delirium or another mental disorder.

General Considerations

Dementia is an acquired, persistent, and progressive impairment in mental processes, with compromise of one or more cognitive domains. *The Diagnostic and Statistical Manual of Mental Disorders,* 5th edition, identifies these domains (with example deficits) as: (1) **complex attention** (easily distracted, difficulty performing calculations), (2) **executive function** (poor abstraction, mental flexibility, planning, and judgment), (3) **learning and memory** (difficulty recalling items from a list, forgetting recent events), (4) **language** (word finding and object naming difficulty), (5) **perceptual-motor function** (difficulty navigating in known environments, copying a drawing), and (6) **social cognition** (change in personality, trouble reading social cues). The diagnosis of dementia requires a significant decline in function that is *severe enough to result in the loss of independence in IADLs.*

While dementia prevalence doubles every 5 years in the older population, reaching 30–50% at age 85, the prevalence among US adults 65 years or older has been declining. This improvement has been attributed to higher education levels and better control of cardiovascular risk factors. Alzheimer disease accounts for roughly two-thirds of dementia cases in the United States, with vascular dementia (either alone or combined with Alzheimer disease) and Lewy body dementia accounting for much of the rest.

Depression and delirium are also common in older adults, may coexist with dementia, and may also present with cognitive impairment. Major depressive disorder may occur in up to 20–50% of patients with dementia, and because they share common features, distinguishing the two can prove difficult. Delirium, characterized by acute confusion, occurs much more commonly in patients with underlying dementia.

Clinical Findings

A. Screening

1. Cognitive impairment—According to the USPSTF, there is insufficient evidence to recommend for or against screening all older adults for cognitive impairment. While there is logic in the argument that early detection may improve future planning and patient outcomes, empiric evidence that demonstrates a clear benefit for either patients or caregivers is lacking. It is important to note, however, that the Medicare Annual Wellness Visit mandates that clinicians assess patients for cognitive impairment based on the clinician's observations and reports from others.

At-home genetic testing for a susceptibility gene that is associated with late-onset Alzheimer disease (APOE-e4) has US FDA approval. While the presence of the APOE-e4 allele increases the risk of developing Alzheimer disease, quantifying such risk for an individual is difficult. Because it is possible to have one or two copies of the APOE-e4 allele and not develop Alzheimer disease or to have no copies and yet still become stricken, genetic testing is not widely recommended and, if considered, should not proceed without genetic counseling.

When there is suspicion of cognitive impairment, several cognitive tests have been validated for clinical use. The **mini-cog** is a combination of a three-item word recall with a clock drawing task, and it can be completed in 3 minutes. When a patient fails this simple test, further cognitive evaluation with a standardized instrument is warranted. The **Montreal Cognitive Assessment (MoCA©)** is a 30-point test that takes about 10 minutes to administer and examines several areas of cognitive function. A score below 26 has a sensitivity of 0.94 or more and a specificity of 0.60 or less. Free downloadable versions in multiple languages are available at https://www.mocatest.org. Completion of a training and certification program or signing a disclaimer if you choose not to take the training is required to gain access to the test.

2. Decision-making capacity—Older adults with cognitive impairment commonly face serious medical decisions, and the clinicians involved in their care must ascertain whether the capacity exists to make medical decisions. While no single test of capacity exists, the following five elements should be considered in a thorough assessment: (1) ability to express a choice; (2) understanding relevant information about the risks and benefits of the proposed intervention and the alternatives (including no intervention), in the context of one's values; (3) comprehension of the problem and its consequences; (4) ability to reason; and (5) consistency of choice. A patient's choice should follow from an understanding of the consequences.

Sensitivity must be used in applying these five components to people of various cultural backgrounds. Decision-making capacity varies over time. Furthermore, the capacity to make a decision is a function of the decision in question.

B. Symptoms and Signs

Most patients with dementia can be identified in a primary care setting after completion of a history (often requiring collateral information), a physical examination, and cognitive testing. The clinician can gather additional information about the type of dementia by asking about (1) the rate of progression of the deficits as well as their nature (including any personality or behavioral change); (2) the presence of other neurologic and psychiatric symptoms, particularly motor problems and psychotic symptoms; (3) risk factors for HIV; (4) family history of dementia; and (5) medications, with particular attention to recent changes.

Workup is directed at identifying any potentially *reversible* causes of dementia. However, such cases are rare. For a detailed description of the symptoms and signs of different forms of dementia, see Chapter 24.

C. Physical Examination

The neurologic examination emphasizes assessment of mental status but should also include evaluation for sensory deficits, previous strokes, parkinsonism, gait impairment, and peripheral neuropathy. The examination should focus on identifying comorbid conditions that may aggravate the individual's disability. For a detailed description of the neuropsychological assessment, see Chapter 24.

D. Laboratory Findings

Laboratory studies should include a CBC and serum electrolytes, calcium, creatinine, glucose, TSH, and vitamin B_{12} levels. While hypothyroidism or vitamin B_{12} deficiency may contribute to the cognitive impairment, treating these conditions typically does *not* reverse the dementia. HIV and rapid plasma reagin (RPR) tests, a heavy metal screen, and liver biochemical tests may be informative in selected patients but are not part of routine testing. For a detailed description of laboratory findings, see Chapter 24.

E. Imaging

The American Academy of Neurology recommends neuroimaging (noncontrast head CT or MRI) in all patients with dementia while other experts limit routine use of neuroimaging to those patients more likely to have a structural cause of dementia (eg, subdural hematoma, tumor, previous stroke, and hydrocephalus). Those who are younger; those who have focal neurologic symptoms or signs, seizures, or gait abnormalities; and those with an acute or subacute onset are most likely to have positive findings and most likely to benefit from MRI scanning. In older patients with a more classic picture of Alzheimer disease for whom neuroimaging is considered, a noncontrast CT scan is sufficient. For a detailed description of imaging, see Chapter 24.

Differential Diagnosis

Older individuals experience occasional difficulty retrieving items from memory (usually word-finding difficulty) and experience a slowing in their rate of information processing. In the amnestic type of **mild cognitive impairment (MCI)**, a patient complains of memory problems, demonstrates mild deficits (most commonly in short-term memory) on formal testing, but the impairment does not significantly impact function. Annual dementia conversion rates vary from less than 5% to 20%. No medications have been demonstrated to delay the progression of MCI to Alzheimer disease. An elderly patient with intact cognition but with severe impairments in vision or hearing may become confused in an unfamiliar medical setting and consequently may be falsely labeled as having dementia.

Delirium can be distinguished from dementia by its acute onset, fluctuating course, and deficits in attention rather than memory. Many medications have been associated with delirium and other types of cognitive impairment in older patients. Anticholinergic agents, hypnotics, neuroleptics, opioids, NSAIDs, antihistamines (both H_1- and H_2-antagonists), and corticosteroids are just some of the medications that have been associated with cognitive impairment in elders.

Treatment

Patients and families should be made aware of the Alzheimer's Association (http://www.alz.org) as well as the wealth of helpful community and online resources and publications available. Caregiver support, education, and counseling may prevent or delay nursing home placement. Education should include the manifestations and natural history of dementia as well as the availability of local support services, such as respite care. Exercise should be a component of treatment as evidence suggests physical activity may have beneficial effects on cognition and physical function.

A. Cognitive Impairment

1. Acetylcholinesterase inhibitors—Donepezil, galantamine, and rivastigmine are acetylcholinesterase inhibitors approved for the treatment of Alzheimer disease. These medications produce a modest improvement in cognitive function that is *not* likely to be detected in routine clinical encounters, and they have *not* convincingly been shown to delay functional decline or institutionalization. There is insufficient evidence to recommend their use in MCI to slow the progression toward dementia.

Starting (and maximum) doses are donepezil, 5 mg orally once daily (maximum 10 mg once daily); galantamine, 4 mg orally twice daily (maximum 12 mg twice daily); extended-release galantamine, 8 mg orally once daily (maximum 24 mg once daily); rivastigmine, 1.5 mg orally twice daily (maximum 6 mg twice daily); and rivastigmine transdermal patch, 4.6 mg/24 h (maximum 13.3 mg/24 h for severe disease). Dosages are increased as tolerated at no less than 4-week intervals. Donepezil is also available in a 23-mg tablet, but this higher dose is associated with greater frequency of side effects without appreciable increase in benefit. The most bothersome side effects of acetylcholinesterase inhibitors include diarrhea, nausea, anorexia, weight loss, and syncope. As dementia progresses, some patients with moderate to severe cognitive impairment may continue to experience subjective benefits from acetylcholinesterase inhibitors, but the medication should be discontinued in those patients who have had no apparent benefit, who experience side effects, or for whom the financial outlay is a burden. While there are no published guidelines that describe what constitutes an adequate treatment trial, evaluation after 2 months at the highest tolerated dose is reasonable.

2. Memantine—In clinical trials, patients with moderate to severe Alzheimer disease have been shown to have statistical benefit from the use of memantine (5 mg orally daily to 10 mg twice daily), an *N*-methyl-D-aspartate (NMDA) antagonist. Long-term and meaningful functional outcomes have yet to be demonstrated, and evidence suggests there is no clinically meaningful benefit to giving memantine in combination with an acetylcholinesterase inhibitor. Evidence does not support the use of memantine in other forms of dementia.

3. Aducanumab—In 2021, the FDA approved aducanumab, a monoclonal antibody that targets amyloid-beta protein and promotes its clearance from the brain, for the treatment of Alzheimer disease. Its approval was based mainly on the results of two identical phase 3 randomized clinical trials sponsored by the drug's manufacturer (ENGAGE and EMERGE) that enrolled participants aged 50–85 years with either MCI or early Alzheimer disease and amyloid-beta positive PET scans. Participants were randomized to either low- or high-dose aducanumab or placebo. The primary end point was the change in the mean score on the Clinical Dementia Rating Scale-Sum of Boxes (CDR-SB) at 18 months. Both studies were terminated early when they met prespecified criteria for futility. However, further data analysis of the high-dose arm in the EMERGE trial identified a statistically significant change in the CDR-SB score, but the difference was smaller than what would be considered clinically meaningful. Both studies found significant reduction in amyloid-beta plaque on PET imaging compared to placebo and yet the reasons for the divergent clinical outcomes are largely unexplained.

Roughly 40% of patients who received high-dose aducanumab in the two trials experienced amyloid-related imaging abnormalities, a known class effect of these drugs. While most cases were asymptomatic, about 25% experienced symptoms, such as headaches, confusion, or dizziness; these symptoms usually resolved with dose reduction or stopping the drug. The overall discontinuation rate in the high-dose group was 6.2% compared to 0.6% in the placebo group.

Before receiving approval, the FDA's scientific advisory panel voted nearly unanimously in recommending against aducanumab's approval, citing the lack of sufficient evidence demonstrating that it slowed cognitive decline. At an annual cost of $56,000 per year, aducanumab requires monthly intravenous infusions. Aducanumab should be restricted to patients with MCI or mild Alzheimer disease who demonstrate amyloid-beta protein on PET imaging and who can be monitored frequently for potential adverse effects.

B. Behavioral Problems

1. Nonpharmacologic approaches—Behavioral problems in patients with dementia are often best managed nonpharmacologically. Initially, it should be established that the problem is not unrecognized delirium, pain, urinary obstruction, or fecal impaction. Determining whether the caregiver or institutional staff can tolerate the behavior is also helpful, since it is often easier to find ways to accommodate to the behavior than to modify it. If not, the caregiver should keep a brief log in which the behavior is described along with antecedent events and consequences. This may uncover patterns that delineate precipitants of the behavior or perhaps that the behavior is somehow being rewarded. Caregivers are taught to use simple language when communicating with the patient, to break down activities into simple component tasks, and to use a "distract, not confront" approach when the patient seems disturbed by a troublesome issue. Additional steps to address behavioral problems include providing structure and routine, discontinuing all medications except those considered absolutely necessary, and correcting, if possible, sensory deficits.

2. Pharmacologic approaches—There is no clear consensus about pharmacologic approaches to the treatment of behavioral problems in patients who have not benefited from nonpharmacologic therapies. Pharmacologic treatment should be reserved for those patients who pose an imminent danger to others or themselves or when symptoms are substantially distressing to the patient.

Despite evidence of harm and recommendations against their use, antipsychotic medications have remained a mainstay for the treatment of behavioral disturbances, particularly agitation and aggression, largely because of the lack of alternatives. The atypical antipsychotic agents (eg, risperidone, olanzapine, quetiapine, aripiprazole) are increasingly becoming the first choice because of an overall better side-effect profile compared to typical agents (eg, haloperidol) but should be used with caution in patients with vascular risk factors due to an increased risk of stroke; they can also cause weight gain and are also associated with hyperglycemia in diabetic patients and are considerably more expensive. Both typical and atypical antipsychotics increase mortality compared with placebo when used to treat elderly patients with dementia and behavioral disturbances. Starting and target dosages should be much lower than those used in schizophrenia (eg, haloperidol, 0.5–2 mg orally; risperidone, 0.25–2 mg orally).

Citalopram at a dose of 30 mg daily may improve symptoms of agitation; however, according to the US FDA, the maximum recommended dose is 20 mg daily for patients older than 60 years because of the risk of QT prolongation and associated dysrhythmia. Thus, while citalopram may be used to treat agitation, safe and effective dosing for patients older than age 60 has not been established. In the specific instance of patients with Lewy body dementia, treatment with acetylcholinesterase inhibitors has been shown to improve behavioral symptoms. Valproate medications have been used in the treatment of agitated and physically aggressive behavior, but evidence demonstrates no identifiable benefit.

C. Driving

Although drivers with dementia are at an increased risk for motor vehicle accidents, many patients continue to drive safely well beyond the time of initial diagnosis, making the timing of when to recommend that a patient stop driving particularly challenging.

There is no clear-cut evidence to suggest a single best approach to determining an individual patient's capability, and there is no accepted "gold-standard" test. The result is that clinicians must consider several factors upon which to base their judgment. For example, determining the severity of dementia can be useful. Patients with very mild or mild dementia according to the Clinical Dementia Rating Scale were able to pass formal road tests at rates of 88% and 69%, respectively. Experts agree that patients with moderately severe or more advanced dementia should be counseled to stop driving. Although not well studied, clinicians should also consider the effects of comorbid conditions and medications and the role each may play in contributing to the risk of driving by a patient with dementia. Assessment of the ability to carry out IADLs may also assist in the determination of risk. Finally, in some cases of mild dementia, referral may be needed to a driver rehabilitation specialist for evaluation. Although not standardized, this evaluation often consists of both off- and on-road testing. Experts recommend such an evaluation for patients with mild dementia, for those with dementia for whom new impairment in driving skills is observed, and for those with significant deficits in cognitive domains, such as attention, executive function, and visuospatial skills.

Clinicians must also be aware of the reporting requirements in their individual jurisdictions. When a clinician has made the decision to report an unsafe driver to the Department of Motor Vehicles, he or she must consider the impact of a potential breach in confidentiality and must weigh and address, in advance when possible, the consequences of the loss of driving independence.

D. Advance Financial Planning

Difficulty in managing financial affairs often develops early in the course of dementia. Although expertise is not expected, clinicians should have some proficiency to address financial concerns. Just as clinicians counsel patients and families about advance care planning, the same should be done to educate about the need for advance financial planning and to recommend that patients complete a **durable power of attorney for finance matters (DPOAF)** while the capacity to do so still exists.

No gold-standard test is available to identify when a patient with dementia no longer has financial capacity. However, the clinician should be on the lookout for signs that a patient is either at risk for or actually experiencing financial incapacity. Because financial impairment can occur when dementia is mild, making that diagnosis should alone be enough to warrant further investigation. Questioning patients and caregivers about late, missed, or repeated bill payments, unusual or uncharacteristic purchases or gifts, overdrawn bank accounts, or reports of missing funds can provide evidence of suspected financial impairment. Patients with dementia are also at increased risk for becoming victims of financial abuse, and some answers to these same questions might also be signs of potential exploitation. When financial abuse is suspected, clinicians should be aware of the reporting requirements in their local jurisdictions.

Prognosis

Life expectancy after a diagnosis of Alzheimer disease is typically 3–15 years; it may be shorter than previously reported. Other neurodegenerative dementias, such as Lewy body dementia, show more rapid decline. Hospice care is often appropriate for patients with end-stage dementia.

When to Refer

Referral for neuropsychological testing may be helpful to distinguish dementia from depression, to diagnose dementia in persons of very poor education or very high premorbid intellect, and to aid diagnosis when impairment is mild.

Lin GA et al. Aducanumab for Alzheimer's disease: effectiveness and value; evidence report. Institute for Clinical and Economic Review, June 30, 2021. https://icer.org/assessment/alzheimersdisease-2021/.

Phillips NA et al. Special issues on using the Montreal Cognitive Assessment for telemedicine assessment during COVID-19. J Am Geriatr Soc. 2020;68:942. [PMID: 32253754]

Smith EE et al. Canadian Consensus Conference on Diagnosis and Treatment of Dementia (CCCDTD)5: guidelines for management of vascular cognitive impairment. Alzheimers Dement (N Y). 2020;6:e12056. [PMID: 33209971]

Tung EE et al. Approach to the older adult with new cognitive symptoms. Mayo Clin Proc. 2020;95:1281. [PMID: 32498781]

Zhuang L et al. Cognitive assessment tools for mild cognitive impairment screening. J Neurol. 2021;268:1615. [PMID: 31414193]

2. Depression

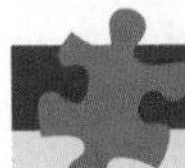

ESSENTIALS OF DIAGNOSIS

- May manifest in older adults as physical complaints (eg, fatigue, anhedonia) rather than complaints of depressed mood.
- Often undertreated in older adults. Approximately one-third of those treated with an antidepressant will achieve remission, and two-thirds will need additional treatment.

General Considerations

Major depressive disorder has prevalence rates of approximately 2% among community-dwelling adults aged 55 years and older. Prevalence rises with increasing age as well as conditions such as chronic illness, multimorbidity, cognitive impairment, and functional impairment. Major depressive disorder is less common in older adults than younger adults, but *depressive symptoms* (not meeting criteria for major depressive disorder) are common and present in up to 15% of older adults. Depression is more common among hospitalized and institutionalized elders. Older single men have the highest rate of completed suicides of any demographic group.

New incidence of depressive symptoms may be an early sign of cognitive impairment in older adults; therefore, evaluation of depression should include cognitive assessment. Older patients with depression and depressive symptoms who have comorbid conditions (eg, heart failure) are at higher risk for hospitalization, tend to have longer hospital stays, and have worse outcomes than patients without depression.

Clinical Findings

The **Patient Health Questionnaire-2 (PHQ-2)** is highly sensitive for detecting major depression in persons over age 65. Positive responses should be followed up with more comprehensive, structured interviews, such as the PHQ-9.

Evaluation of depression should include a careful review of substances that can contribute to depressive symptoms, such as medications (eg, benzodiazepines) and alcohol/illicit drugs. A thorough review of the medical history is critical, since many medical problems can cause fatigue, lethargy, or hypoactive delirium, all of which may be mistaken for depression.

Treatment

First-line treatment is the same for older adults as it is for younger adults; psychotherapy and SSRI medications are the mainstays of treatment. Adjunctive treatment may include psychosocial interventions, increased physical activity, reduction of substance use (eg, alcohol), reduction of potentially contributing medications, or electroconvulsive therapy. Depressed older adults may do better with a collaborative or multidisciplinary care model that includes socialization and other support elements. In older patients with depressive symptoms who do not meet criteria for major depressive disorder, nonpharmacologic treatments are indicated. Telehealth for mental health support is an important innovation in the field.

Choice of antidepressant agent is usually based on side-effect profile, cost, and patient-specific factors, such as presenting symptoms and comorbidities. SSRIs are used as first-line agents because they are relatively well-tolerated and have good evidence to support efficacy (see Table 25–6). Older adults are more susceptible to SSRI-induced hyponatremia, falls, and osteoporosis. SNRIs (eg, duloxetine and venlafaxine) lead to more adverse events versus placebo than do SSRIs. Regardless of the medication chosen, many experts recommend starting elders at a relatively low dose, titrating to full dose slowly, and continuing for a longer trial (at least 8 weeks) before trying a different medication. Titration to full dose is critical to achieve efficacy of treatment. Of note, the maximum citalopram dose for adults older than 60 years is 20 mg orally daily, due to dose-dependent QT prolongation.

One-third of older adults achieve remission after adequate treatment with first-line SSRI treatment. For the remainder, referral to a mental health specialist is indicated. For those who do not achieve remission, augmentation therapy (eg, with lithium, methylphenidate, or aripiprazole) can enhance clinical response. Esketamine, the S-enantiomer of ketamine, is approved for treatment-resistant depression, but studies of its safety and efficacy did not include adults older than age 65. For patients with severe or catatonic depression, electroconvulsive therapy has high rates of efficacy (60–80%) and should be considered.

Pharmacologic treatment for the first episode of depression should continue for 1 year after remission. Clinicians and patients should share in decision-making regarding maintenance therapy for depression since risk of major depressive disorder recurrence is high. This decision should weigh how long-term pharmacotherapy may contribute to polypharmacy and adverse effects in the landscape of their patient's comorbidities and medication regimen.

When to Refer

- Any patient who might be considered for electroconvulsive therapy should be referred for psychiatric evaluation.
- Consider referral for patients who have mania, psychosis, catatonia, or treatment-resistant depression.

When to Admit

Consider psychiatric evaluation and admission for patients who have psychosis, suicidality, homicidality, catatonia, grave disability, or self-neglect.

Choi NG et al. Effect of telehealth treatment by lay counselors vs by clinicians on depressive symptoms among older adults who are homebound: a randomized clinical trial. JAMA Network Open. 2020;3:e2015648. [PMID: 32865577]

Krishnamoorthy Y et al. Diagnostic accuracy of various forms of geriatric depression scale for screening of depression among older adults: systematic review and meta-analysis. Arch Gerontol Geriatr. 2020;87:104002. [PMID: 31881393]

Meyer JP et al. Electroconvulsive therapy in geriatric psychiatry: a selective review. Clin Geriatr Med. 2020;36:265. [PMID: 32222301]

Sobieraj DM et al. Adverse effects of pharmacologic treatments of major depression in older adults. J Am Geriatr Soc. 2019; 67:1571. [PMID: 31140587]

Zhang H et al. Comparison of the Geriatric Depression Scale-15 and the Patient Health Questionnaire-9 for screening depression in older adults. Geriatr Gerontol Int. 2020;20:138. [PMID: 31820572]

3. Delirium

ESSENTIALS OF DIAGNOSIS

- Rapid onset and fluctuating course.
- Primary deficit in attention rather than memory.
- May be hypoactive or hyperactive.
- Dementia frequently coexists.

General Considerations

Delirium is an acute, fluctuating disturbance of consciousness, associated with a change in cognition or development of perceptual disturbances (see also Chapter 25). It is the pathophysiologic consequence of an underlying general medical condition, such as infection, coronary ischemia, hypoxemia, or metabolic derangement. Delirium occurs in 29–64% of hospitalized older adults, persists in 25% or more, and is associated with worse clinical outcomes (higher in-hospital and post-discharge mortality, longer lengths of stay, delayed and limited recovery of physical function, greater probability of placement in a nursing facility).

Although the acutely agitated elderly patient often comes to mind when considering delirium **(hyperactive delirium)**, many episodes are subtler. Such **hypoactive delirium** may be suspected only if one notices new cognitive slowing or inattention.

Cognitive impairment is an important risk factor for delirium. Other risk factors include severe illness, polypharmacy, use of psychoactive medications, sensory impairment, depression, and alcoholism.

Clinical Findings

Several bedside instruments are available for the assessment of delirium (http://www.hospitalelderlifeprogram.org/delirium-instruments/). The **confusion assessment method (CAM)** requires (1) acute onset and fluctuating course and (2) inattention and *either* (3) disorganized thinking *or* (4) altered level of consciousness. The 3D CAM (3-minute diagnostic CAM) is particularly useful for clinical assessment of delirium.

A key component of a delirium workup is review of medications because polypharmacy, the addition of a new medication, an increase in dose of a medication, or the discontinuation of a medication known to cause withdrawal symptoms are all associated with the development of delirium. Medications that are particularly likely to increase the risk of delirium include sedative/hypnotics, anticholinergics, opioids, benzodiazepines, and H_1- and H_2-antihistamines.

Evaluation of most patients should include a CBC; BUN; serum electrolytes, creatinine, glucose, calcium, albumin, and liver biochemical tests; UA; and ECG. In selected cases, serum magnesium, medication levels, arterial blood gas measurements, blood cultures, chest radiography, urinary toxin screen, and lumbar puncture may be helpful. When delirium develops during a hospitalization in the absence of trauma or new localizing neurologic signs, a head CT is rarely revealing.

Prevention

The best evidence for prevention comes from nonpharmacologic multicomponent interventions. These components include improving cognition (frequent reorientation, activities, socialization with family and friends when possible), sleep (massage, noise reduction, minimizing interruptions at night), mobility (early initiation of rehabilitation services as appropriate), vision (visual aids and adaptive equipment), hearing (portable amplifiers or hearing aids, cerumen disimpaction), and hydration status (volume repletion). No medications, including antipsychotics, have been consistently shown to prevent delirium or improve outcomes such as length of stay or mortality should delirium develop.

Treatment

Management of established episodes of delirium combines the elements of preventive interventions with reassurance and reorientation, treatment of underlying causes, eliminating unnecessary medications, and avoidance of indwelling catheters and restraints. Antipsychotics, while still a mainstay of delirium treatment in hospitalized adults, offer little to no proven benefit and can cause harm. For example, haloperidol and second-generation antipsychotics have not been found to reduce delirium severity or duration, hospital length of stay, or mortality when compared to placebo. QT interval prolongation can occur and is a potential risk for serious dysrhythmias. Benzodiazepines should be avoided except in the circumstance of alcohol or benzodiazepine withdrawal. In ventilated patients in the ICU setting, dexmedetomidine or propofol (or both) may also be useful alternatives to antipsychotic therapy in patients with delirium.

Most episodes of delirium clear in a matter of days after correction of the precipitant, but some patients suffer episodes of much longer duration, and a significant percentage never return to their former baseline level of functioning.

When to Refer

If an initial evaluation does not reveal the cause of delirium or if entities other than delirium are in the differential diagnosis, referral to a geriatrician, neuropsychologist, neurologist, or geropsychiatrist should be considered.

When to Admit

Patients with delirium of unknown cause should be admitted for an expedited workup if consistent with the patient's goals of care.

Hshieh TT et al. Delirium in the elderly. Clin Geriatr Med. 2020;36:183. [PMID: 32222295]

Inouye SK. The importance of delirium and delirium prevention in older adults during lockdowns. JAMA. 2021;325:1779. [PMID: 33720288]

Kotfis K et al. COVID-19: ICU delirium management during SARS-CoV-2 pandemic. Crit Care. 2020;24:176. [PMID: 32345343]

Pereira JV et al. Delirium in older adults is associated with development of new dementia: a systematic review and meta-analysis. Int J Geriatr Psychiatry. 2021;36:993. [PMID: 33638566]

Salvi F et al. Non-pharmacological approaches in the prevention of delirium. Eur Geriatr Med. 2020;11:71. [PMID: 32297241]

4. Immobility

Mobility limitations are common in older adults and are associated with increased rates of morbidity, hospitalization, disability, and mortality. Hospital-associated bed rest is a common precipitant of immobility and functional decline. Among hospitalized medical patients over age 70, about 10% experience a decline in function, and those who experience critical illness are particularly at high risk.

The hazards of bed rest in older adults are multiple, serious, quick to develop, and slow to reverse. Within days of being confined to bed, deconditioning of the cardiovascular system occurs. This deconditioning causes fluid shifts, decreased cardiac output, decreased peak oxygen uptake, increased resting heart rate, and postural hypotension. More striking changes occur in skeletal muscle, resulting in loss of strength and function. Pressure injuries, venous thromboembolism, and falls are additional serious outcomes of immobility and deconditioning.

Prevention & Treatment

Physical activity should be encouraged for all elders, particularly sedentary elders. Physical activity is associated with a myriad of health benefits in older adults. Structured physical activity programs may help reduce mobility-related disability among community-dwelling elders.

When immobilization cannot be avoided, several measures can be used to minimize its consequences. To reduce the risks of contracture and weakness, range-of-motion and strengthening exercises should be started immediately and continued as long as the patient is in bed. Avoiding restraints and discontinuing intravenous lines and urinary catheters will increase opportunities for early mobility. Graduated ambulation should begin as soon as it is feasible. Among hospitalized elders, exercise protocols can improve functional outcomes. Prior to discharge, physical therapists can recommend appropriate exercises and assistive devices; after discharge, they can recommend home safety modifications and maintenance exercises. Severe functional disability impeding the ability to care for oneself independently often leads to discharge to an acute or subacute rehabilitation facility. Recovery from illness-related deconditioning takes weeks to months, and in many cases, full recovery to the pre-illness physical condition does not occur.

Flint LA et al. Rehabbed to death. N Engl J Med. 2019;380:408. [PMID: 30699322]
Martínez-Velilla N et al. Effect of exercise intervention on functional decline in very elderly patients during acute hospitalization: a randomized clinical trial. JAMA Intern Med. 2019;179:28. [PMID: 30419096]
Pahor M et al. Impact and lessons from the Lifestyle Interventions and Independence for Elders (LIFE) clinical trials of physical activity to prevent mobility disability. J Am Geriatr Soc. 2020;68:872. [PMID: 32105353]

5. Falls & Gait Disorders

Annually, about one-third of people over age 65 fall, and the frequency of falls increases markedly with advancing age. About 10% of falls result in serious injuries. Complications from falls (eg, hip fracture, subdural hematoma) are the leading cause of death from injury in persons over age 65, and fall-associated mortality is increasing.

Every older person should be asked about falls. Assessment of patients who fall should include postural blood pressure and pulse; cardiac examination; evaluations of strength, range of motion, cognition, and proprioception; and examination of feet and footwear. A thorough gait assessment should be performed in all older people. Gait and balance can be readily assessed by the **"Timed Up and Go Test,"** in which the patient is asked to stand up from a sitting position without use of hands, walk 10 feet/3 meters, turn around, walk back, and sit down. An older adult who takes 12.5 seconds or greater is considered at increased risk for falling. The ability to recognize common patterns of gait disorders is an extremely useful clinical skill to develop. Examples of gait abnormalities and their causes are listed in Table 4–1.

Causes of Falls

Balance and ambulation require a complex interplay of cognitive, neuromuscular, and cardiovascular function. With age, balance mechanisms can become compromised, reaction time slows, and postural sway increases. These changes predispose the older person to a fall when challenged by an additional insult to any of these systems.

Falls in older people are rarely due to a single cause, and effective intervention entails a comprehensive assessment of the patient's intrinsic deficits (eg, diseases and medications), the activity engaged in at the time of the fall, and environmental obstacles (Table 4–2).

Intrinsic deficits are those that impair sensory input, judgment, blood pressure regulation, reaction time, and balance and gait. Dizziness may be closely related to the deficits associated with falls and gait abnormalities. While it may be impossible to isolate a sole cause or a "cure" for falls, gait abnormalities, or dizziness, it is often possible to identify and ameliorate some of the underlying contributory conditions and improve the patient's overall function.

Medication use is one of the most common, significant, and reversible causes of falling. A meta-analysis found that sedative/hypnotics, antidepressants, and benzodiazepines were the classes of medications most likely to be associated with falling. The use of multiple medications simultaneously has also been associated with increased fall risk. Other often overlooked but treatable contributors include postural hypotension (including postprandial, which peaks 30–60 minutes after a meal), insomnia, use of multifocal lenses, and urinary urgency.

Since most falls occur in or around the home, a **home safety evaluation** by a visiting nurse, physical therapist, or health care provider may be beneficial in identifying environmental obstacles and is generally reimbursed by third-party payers, including Medicare.

Table 4–1. Evaluation of gait abnormalities.

Gait Abnormality	Possible Causes
Inability to stand without use of hands	Deconditioning Myopathy (hyperthyroidism, alcohol, statin-induced) Hip or knee pain
Unsteadiness upon standing	Orthostatic hypotension Balance problem (peripheral neuropathy, vision problem, vestibular, other CNS causes) Generalized weakness
Stagger with eyes closed	Often indicates that vision is compensating for another deficit
Short steps	Weakness Parkinson disease or related condition
Asymmetry	Cerebrovascular accident Focal pain or arthritis
Wide-based gait	Fear, balance problems
Flexed knees	Contractures, quadriceps weakness
Slow gait	Fear of falling, weakness, deconditioning, peripheral vascular disease, COPD, heart failure, angina pectoris

Table 4–2. Fall risk factors, targeted interventions, and best evidence for fall prevention.

To Consider for All Patients	
Exercise or physical therapy	Tai Chi, gait training, balance training, strength training
Multifactorial intervention	Home safety assessment, medication review, review of specific conditions (below), advice on appropriate footwear, vision check, adaptive aids as appropriate, physical therapy or exercise as appropriate
Condition	**Targeted Intervention**
Postural hypotension (> 20 mm Hg drop in systolic blood pressure, or systolic blood pressure < 90 mm Hg)	Behavioral recommendations, such as hand clenching, elevation of head of bed; discontinuation or substitution of high-risk medications
Use of benzodiazepine or sedative/hypnotic agent	Education about sleep hygiene; discontinuation or substitution of medications
Use of multiple prescription medications	Review of medications with a focus on discontinuation (deprescribing)
Environmental hazards	Removal or mitigation of hazards; installation of safety equipment (eg, grab bars)
Gait impairment	Gait training, assistive devices, balance or strengthening exercises
Impairment in transfer or balance	Balance exercises, training in transfers, environmental alterations (eg, grab bars)
Impairment in leg or arm muscle strength or limb range of motion	Exercise with resistance bands or putty, with graduated increases in resistance
Vision impairment	Cataract surgery or other interventions as appropriate (eg, corrective lenses)
Inability to get up after a fall	Medical alert system, physical therapy training for fall-prevention strategies
High-risk footwear	Education on appropriate footwear (eg, avoid slippers, high heels)
Osteoporosis	Bisphosphonate treatment to prevent first or recurrent fractures

Complications of Falls

The most common fall-related fractures are of the wrist, hip, and vertebrae. Osteoporosis significantly increases fracture risk, and unfortunately is vastly undertreated in older adults. Following hip fracture, elderly women experience a high mortality rate (approximately 20% in 1 year), particularly if they were debilitated prior to the time of the fracture. Fear of falling again is a common, serious, but treatable factor in the older person's loss of confidence and independence. Referral to a physical therapist for gait training with special devices is often all that is required.

Chronic subdural hematoma is an easily overlooked complication of falls that must be considered in any elderly patient presenting with new neurologic symptoms or signs, including evidence of new cognitive impairment. Headache and known history of trauma may both be absent.

Patients who are unable to get up from a fall are at risk for dehydration, electrolyte imbalance, pressure injuries, rhabdomyolysis, and hypothermia.

Prevention & Management

Exercise is the intervention that is most consistently reported to reduce the risk of falls. Balance focused exercises (eg, Tai Chi), gait, and strength training appear to be more effective for fall prevention than general exercise programs (Table 4–2).

Multifactorial interventions appear to have a small benefit in preventing falls. These interventions include an assessment of potentially modifiable risk factors and tailored interventions to reduce risk. Emphasis is placed on treating all contributory medical conditions, minimizing environmental hazards, and eliminating medications where the harms may outweigh the benefits (eg, sedative-hypnotics).

The USPSTF recommends *against* vitamin D supplementation to prevent falls in community-dwelling adults. Vitamin D supplementation might be considered for high-risk individuals (eg, institutionalized elders) on a case-by-case basis. High-dose vitamin D (60,000 IU per month) has been shown to *increase* the incidence of falls.

Osteoporosis treatment (both preventive and post-fracture) is essential to prevent first and recurrent fracture. First-line treatment with bisphosphonates is very effective; for example, alendronate significantly reduces the risk of hip, vertebral and nonvertebral fracture in people with osteoporosis. Unfortunately, less than 20% of people who sustain a fragility fracture receive osteoporosis treatment (this treatment failure is called the "osteoporosis care gap"; see Chapter 26 for more information).

Assistive devices, such as canes and walkers, are useful for many older adults but often are used incorrectly. Canes should be used on the "good" side. The height of walkers and canes should generally be at about the level of the wrist. Physical therapists are invaluable in assessing the need for an assistive device, selecting the best device, and training a patient in its correct use.

Eyeglasses, particularly bifocal or graduated lenses, may increase the risk of falls, particularly in the early weeks of use. Patients should be counseled about the need to take extra care when new eyeglasses are being used.

Patients with repeated falls are often reassured by the availability of telephones at floor level, a mobile telephone on their person, or a lightweight radio call system. Physical therapy should also include training in techniques for arising after a fall.

When to Refer

Patients with a recent history of falls should be referred for physical therapy, eye examination, and home safety evaluation.

When to Admit

Consider hospitalization for patients with new falls that are unexplained, particularly in combination with a change in the physical examination (eg, neurologic status) or with an injury/fracture requiring surgery.

Dautzenberg L et al. Interventions for preventing falls and fall-related fractures in community-dwelling older adults: a systematic review and network meta-analysis. J Am Geriatr Soc. 2021;69:2973. [PMID: 34318929]

Ganz DA et al. Prevention of falls in community-dwelling older adults. N Engl J Med. 2020;382:734. [PMID: 32074420]

Liu-Ambrose T et al. Effect of a home-based exercise program on subsequent falls among community-dwelling high-risk older adults after a fall: a randomized clinical trial. JAMA. 2019;321:2092. [PMID: 31162569]

Pahor M. Falls in older adults: prevention, mortality, and costs. JAMA. 2019;321:2080. [PMID: 31162553]

Silverstein WK et al. Closing the osteoporosis care gap: a teachable moment. JAMA Intern Med. 2021;181:1635. [PMID: 34661618]

6. Urinary Incontinence

ESSENTIALS OF DIAGNOSIS

- Involuntary loss of urine.
- *Stress* incontinence: leakage of urine upon coughing, sneezing, or standing.
- *Urge* incontinence: urgency and inability to delay urination.
- *Overflow* incontinence: variable presentation.

General Considerations

Urinary incontinence in older adults is common, and interventions can improve patients' quality of life. Many patients do not voluntarily disclose their experiences with urinary incontinence to their health care providers, possibly due to embarrassment or the belief that it is a normal part of aging. A simple question about involuntary leakage of urine is a reasonable annual screen: "Do you have a problem with urine leaks or accidents?"

Classification

A. Transient Causes

Use of the mnemonic "DIAPPERS" may be helpful in remembering the categories of "transient" urinary incontinence.

1. Delirium—A clouded sensorium impedes recognition of both the need to void and the location of the nearest toilet. Delirium is the most common cause of incontinence in hospitalized patients.

2. Infection—Symptomatic UTI can cause or contribute to urgency and incontinence. Asymptomatic bacteriuria does not.

3. Atrophic urethritis and vaginitis—Atrophic urethritis and vaginitis can usually be diagnosed presumptively by the presence of vaginal mucosal telangiectasia, petechiae, erosions, erythema, or friability. Urethral inflammation, if symptomatic, may contribute to incontinence in some women.

4. Pharmaceuticals—Medications are one of the most common causes of transient incontinence. Typical offending agents include potent diuretics, anticholinergics, psychotropics, opioid analgesics, alpha-blockers (in women), alpha-agonists (in men), and calcium channel blockers.

5. Psychological factors—Severe depression with psychomotor retardation may impede the ability or motivation to reach a toilet.

6. Excess urinary output—Excess urinary output may overwhelm the ability of an older person to reach a toilet in time. In addition to diuretics, common causes include excess fluid intake; metabolic abnormalities (eg, hyperglycemia, hypercalcemia, diabetes insipidus); and peripheral edema (when previously dependent legs assume a horizontal position in bed).

7. Restricted mobility—(See Immobility, above.) If mobility cannot be improved, access to a urinal or commode (eg, at the bedside) may improve continence.

8. Stool impaction—This is a common cause of urinary incontinence in hospitalized or immobile patients. Although the mechanism is still unknown, a clinical clue to its presence is the onset of both urinary and fecal incontinence.

B. Established Causes

Causes of "established" incontinence should be addressed after any "transient" causes have been managed appropriately.

1. Detrusor overactivity (urge incontinence)—Detrusor overactivity refers to uninhibited bladder contractions that cause leakage. It is the most common cause of established incontinence in older adults, accounting for two-thirds of cases. Women will complain of leakage associated with a strong and sudden urge to urinate that cannot be forestalled. In men, the symptoms are similar, but detrusor overactivity commonly coexists with urethral obstruction from benign prostatic hyperplasia. Because detrusor overactivity also may be due to bladder stones or tumor, the abrupt onset of otherwise unexplained urge incontinence—especially if accompanied by perineal or suprapubic discomfort or sterile hematuria—should be investigated by urine cytology and cystoscopy.

2. Urethral incompetence (stress incontinence)—Urethral incompetence is the second most common cause of established urinary incontinence in older women. In men, it commonly occurs after radical prostatectomy. Stress incontinence is characterized by instantaneous leakage of urine in response to an increase in intra-abdominal pressure. It can coexist with detrusor overactivity causing "mixed" incontinence. Typically, urinary loss occurs with laughing, coughing, or lifting heavy objects. To test for stress incontinence, have the patient relax the perineum and cough vigorously (a single cough) while standing with a full bladder. Instantaneous leakage indicates stress incontinence. A delay of several seconds or persistent leakage suggests that the problem is instead caused by an uninhibited bladder contraction induced by coughing.

3. Overflow incontinence—Urethral obstruction (due to prostatic enlargement, urethral stricture, bladder neck contracture, or prostatic cancer) is a common cause of established incontinence in older men but is rare in older women. It can present as dribbling incontinence after voiding, urge incontinence due to detrusor overactivity, or overflow incontinence due to urinary retention. Detrusor underactivity is less common but can also cause overflow incontinence. It may be idiopathic or have an identifiable cause including medications and sacral lower motor nerve dysfunction. When it causes incontinence, detrusor underactivity is associated with urinary frequency, nocturia, and frequent leakage of small volumes.

Treatment

A. Transient Causes

Each identified transient cause should be treated regardless of whether an established cause coexists. For patients with urinary retention induced by an anticholinergic agent, discontinuation of the medication should first be considered. If this is not feasible, substituting a less anticholinergic agent may be useful.

B. Established Causes

1. Detrusor overactivity—The cornerstone of treatment is **bladder training.** Patients start by voiding on a schedule based on the shortest interval recorded on a bladder record. They then gradually lengthen the interval between voids by 30 minutes each week using relaxation techniques to postpone the urge to void. Lifestyle modifications, including weight loss and caffeine reduction, may also improve incontinence symptoms. For cognitively impaired patients and nursing home residents who are unable to manage on their own, **timed and prompted voiding** initiated by caregivers is effective. **Pelvic floor muscle ("Kegel") exercises** can reduce the frequency of incontinence episodes when performed correctly and sustained.

If behavioral approaches prove insufficient, several FDA-approved **antimuscarinic agents** may provide additional benefit. Available regimens of these agents include short-acting tolterodine, 1–2 mg orally twice a day; long-acting tolterodine, 2–4 mg orally daily; short-acting oxybutynin, 2.5–5 mg orally twice or three times a day; long-acting oxybutynin, 5–15 mg orally daily; oxybutynin transdermal patch, 3.9 mg/day applied twice weekly; oxybutynin 10% transdermal gel, 100 mg applied daily; fesoterodine, 4–8 mg orally once daily; trospium chloride, 20 mg orally once or twice daily; long-acting trospium chloride, 60 mg orally daily; darifenacin, 7.5–15 mg orally daily; and solifenacin, 5–10 mg orally daily. All of these agents appear to have similar efficacy and side-effect profiles (eg, delirium/cognitive impairment, dry mouth, constipation, urinary retention). Long-acting and topical preparations are generally better tolerated.

The beta-3-agonists **mirabegron,** 25–50 mg orally daily, and vibegron, 75 mg orally once daily, are FDA approved for overactive bladder symptoms, which include urge urinary incontinence. In trials comparing mirabegron with antimuscarinic agents, the efficacy and safety profiles have been comparable, with less dry mouth reported in persons who received mirabegron. The experience accruing among adults over the age of 70 shows that adherence rates may be superior to the antimuscarinic medications.

An alternative to oral agents is an injection of **onabotulinum toxin A** into the detrusor muscle. While effective, it can lead to urinary retention and the need for self-catheterization.

The combination of behavioral therapy and antimuscarinics appears to be more effective than either alone, although one study in a group of younger women showed that adding behavioral therapy to individually titrated doses of extended-release oxybutynin was no better than with medication treatment alone.

In men with both benign prostatic hyperplasia and detrusor overactivity and with postvoid residual of 150 mL or less, an antimuscarinic agent added to an alpha-blocker may provide additional relief of lower urinary tract symptoms.

2. Urethral incompetence (stress incontinence)—**Lifestyle modifications,** including limiting caffeine and fluid intake, may be helpful for some women, particularly women with mixed stress/urge incontinence; strong evidence supports weight loss in obese women. **Pelvic floor muscle exercises** are effective for women with mild to moderate stress incontinence. Instruct the patient to pull in the pelvic floor muscles and hold for 6–10 seconds and to perform three sets of 8–12 contractions daily. Benefits may not be seen for 6 weeks. **Pessaries** or **vaginal cones** may be helpful in some women but should be prescribed only by providers who are experienced with using these modalities.

No medications are approved for the treatment of stress incontinence, and a clinical practice guideline from the American College of Physicians recommends against pharmacologic treatment. Although a last resort, **surgery** is the most effective treatment for stress incontinence; cure rates as high as 96% can result, even in older women.

3. Overflow incontinence—Most men with overflow incontinence from obstructive uropathy will first undergo bladder decompression with intermittent or indwelling catheterization followed by initiation of alpha-blocking agents (eg, terazosin, 1–10 mg orally daily; prazosin, 1–5 mg orally twice daily; or tamsulosin, 0.4–0.8 mg orally daily taken 30 minutes after a meal). Finasteride, 5 mg orally daily, can provide additional benefit in men with an enlarged prostate. If medical therapy fails to allow for adequate bladder emptying, surgical decompression can be an option. A variety of nonsurgical techniques make decompression feasible even for frail men. For the nonoperative candidate with urinary retention, intermittent or indwelling catheterization is used. For the patient with a poorly contractile bladder, augmented voiding techniques (eg, double voiding, suprapubic pressure) can prove effective. If further emptying is needed, intermittent or indwelling catheterization is the only option. Antibiotics should be used only for symptomatic UTI or as prophylaxis against recurrent symptomatic infections in a patient using intermittent catheterization; they should not be used as prophylaxis in a patient with an indwelling catheter.

When to Refer

- Men with urinary obstruction who do not respond to medical therapy should be referred to a urologist.
- Women who do not respond to medical and behavioral therapy should be referred to a urogynecologist or urologist.

Sung VW et al. Effect of behavioral and pelvic floor muscle therapy combined with surgery vs surgery alone on incontinence symptoms among women with mixed urinary incontinence: the ESTEEM randomized clinical trial. JAMA. 2019;322:1066. [PMID: 31529007]

Vaughan CP et al. Urinary incontinence in women. Ann Intern Med. 2020;172:ITC17. [PMID: 32016335]

7. Involuntary Weight Loss

General Considerations

Aging, even in the absence of disease, is associated with reduced appetite. Involuntary weight loss affects substantial numbers of older adults. Most studies of involuntary weight loss in community-dwelling older adults define it as loss of 5% of body weight in 6 months or 10% of body weight in 1 year.

Clinical Findings

The many potential causes of involuntary weight loss include **medical conditions** (60–70%; eg, cancer cachexia, chronic heart failure) and **psychiatric conditions** (10–20%; eg, depression), but in up to 25%, the cause of weight loss cannot be identified. **Social factors,** such as access to food and dental health, should be investigated. The clinical evaluation should search for symptoms and signs that could point to a potential cause (eg, abdominal pain to peptic ulcer disease; tachycardia to hyperthyroidism). When the history, physical examination, and basic laboratory studies do not suggest a possible diagnosis, additional evaluation (eg, total body CT scan) is usually low yield. When no other cause is identified, the frailty syndrome should be considered in the differential diagnosis.

Treatment

Initial treatment should focus on identifying medical causes of involuntary weight loss while also addressing and improving social barriers, such as social isolation and access to food. Social meals can improve intake and nutrition. Oral nutritional supplements of 200–1000 kcal/day can increase weight and improve outcomes in malnourished hospitalized older adults but have *not* been shown to have benefits in community-dwelling older adults. Sodium-containing flavor enhancers (eg, iodized salt) can improve food intake without adverse health effects when there is no contraindication to their use. Megestrol acetate as an appetite stimulant has *not* been shown to increase lean body mass or lengthen life among elders and has significant side effects. For those patients with advanced dementia, percutaneous liquid artificial nutrition ("tube feeding") is *not* recommended, but rather assiduous hand feeding may allow maintenance of weight and provide more comfort.

8. Pressure Injury

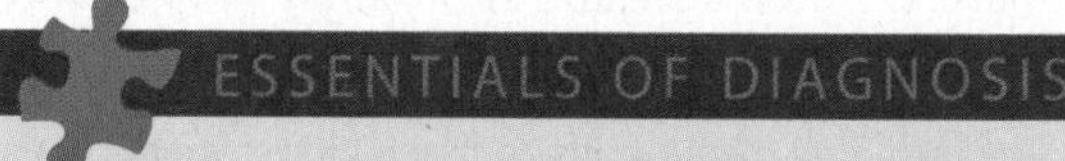

ESSENTIALS OF DIAGNOSIS

- Examine at-risk patients on admission to the hospital and daily thereafter.
- Pressure injury is classified into one of six categories:
  - Stage 1: Non-blanchable erythema of intact skin
  - Stage 2: Partial-thickness skin loss with exposed dermis
  - Stage 3: Full-thickness skin loss
  - Stage 4: Full-thickness skin and tissue loss
  - Unstageable: Obscured full-thickness skin and tissue loss
  - Deep tissue: Persistent non-blanchable, deep red, maroon, or purple discoloration

General Considerations

The National Pressure Injury Advisory Panel changed the term "pressure ulcer" to "pressure injury" to more accurately reflect the fact that stage 1 and deep tissue injury describe damage to intact skin, compared to the ulcers described in the other four stages. Deep tissue and unstageable pressure injury are included in the six pressure injury stages. An area of purple or maroon discolored intact skin or blood-filled blister is characteristic of deep tissue injury, sometimes preceded by tissue that is painful, firm, mushy, boggy, warmer, or cooler compared with adjacent tissue. Ulcers in which the base is covered by slough (yellow, tan, gray, green, or brown) or eschar (tan, brown, or black) are considered unstageable. Most pressure injuries develop during an acute illness. The primary risk factor for pressure injuries is immobility. Other contributing risk factors include reduced sensory perception, moisture (urinary and fecal incontinence), poor nutritional status, and friction and shear forces.

Older adults admitted to hospitals and nursing homes should be assessed for their risk of developing pressure injuries, and several risk assessment instruments can be used, including the Braden Scale and the Norton score. These tools should be used in conjunction with clinical judgment since each may cover a limited range of risk factors and each depends on the skills of examiner.

Prevention

Using specialized support surfaces (including mattresses, beds, and cushions), patient repositioning, optimizing nutritional status, reducing shear and friction forces, and moisturizing sacral skin are strategies that have been shown to reduce pressure injury. In general, advanced supportive surfaces are superior to standard hospital beds in preventing and managing pressure injuries, but there is no clear advantage of one support surface over another.

Evaluation

Evaluation of pressure injuries should include patient's risk factors and goals of care; injury stage, size, and depth; absence or presence (and type) of exudate; appearance of the wound bed and possible surrounding infection; and sinus tracking, or cellulitis.

Treatment

High-quality evidence that rigorously examines the effectiveness of various treatments remains limited. Clinicians should therefore focus on the principles of wound care, including pressure reduction, removing necrotic debris, and maintaining a moist wound bed that will promote healing and formation of granulation tissue. The type of dressing that is recommended depends on the location and depth of the wound, whether necrotic tissue or dead space is present, and the amount of exudate (Table 4–3). Pressure-reducing devices (eg, air-fluid beds and low-air-loss beds) are associated with improved healing rates. Although poor nutritional status is a risk factor for the development of pressure injury, the evidence that nutritional supplementation helps correct pressure injury is limited.

Providers can become easily overwhelmed by the array of products available for the treatment of established pressure injuries. Most institutions should designate a wound care expert or team to select a streamlined wound care product line that has simple guidelines. In a patient with end-stage disease who is receiving end-of-life care, appropriate treatment might be directed toward palliation only (including minimizing dressing changes and odors) rather than efforts directed at healing.

Complications

Bacteria contaminate all chronic pressure injuries with skin loss, but it can be difficult to identify those wounds that are infected. Suspicion for infection should rise if there is pain, increased or foul-smelling wound drainage, erythema of the skin around the wound, or if the wound will not heal. Fever and leukocytosis are other indicators of systemic infection but are not always present. Culture from a superficial swab adds little valuable diagnostic information. For nonhealing infected wounds without evidence of systemic involvement, topical antiseptics (eg, silver sulfadiazine) are recommended and may need to be accompanied by debridement of necrotic tissue. When systemic infections such as cellulitis and osteomyelitis are present, oral or parenteral antibiotics are warranted and medication choice should be guided by tissue culture, but obtaining this can be painful and it is not always readily available.

Table 4–3. Pressure injury dressings and other measures.

Injury Type	Dressing Type and Considerations
Stage 1	Polyurethane film Hydrocolloid wafer
Stage 2	Hydrocolloid wafers Semipermeable foam dressing Polyurethane film
Stages 3 and 4	For highly exudative wounds, use highly absorptive dressing or packing, such as calcium alginate Wounds with necrotic debris must be debrided Debridement can be autolytic, enzymatic, or surgical Shallow, clean wounds can be dressed with hydrocolloid wafers, semipermeable foam, or polyurethane film Deep wounds can be packed with gauze; if the wound is deep and highly exudative, an absorptive packing should be used
Heel injury	Do not remove eschar on heel pressure injury because it can help promote healing (eschar in other locations should be debrided)
Unstageable	Debride if appropriate before deciding on further therapy
Deep tissue injury	Offload pressure to the affected area

When to Refer

- Pressure injuries that are large or nonhealing should be referred to a plastic or general surgeon or dermatologist for biopsy, debridement, and possible skin grafting.
- For hospitalized patients or residents of skilled nursing facilities in whom pressure injuries develop, early involvement of a wound care specialist is crucial.

When to Admit

Patients with pressure injury should be admitted if the primary residence is unable to provide adequate wound care or pressure reduction, or if the wound is infected or requires complex or surgical care.

Gillespie BM et al. Repositioning for pressure injury prevention in adults. Cochrane Database Syst Rev. 2020;6:CD009958. [PMID: 32484259]

Hajhosseini B et al. Pressure injury. Ann Surg. 2020;271:671. [PMID: 31460882]

Moore Z et al. Prevention of pressure ulcers among individuals cared for in the prone position: lessons for the COVID-19 emergency. J Wound Care. 2020;29:312. [PMID: 32530776]

9. Pharmacotherapy & Polypharmacy

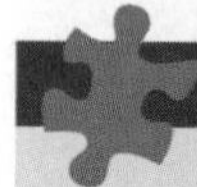

ESSENTIALS OF DIAGNOSIS

- Older adults experience more adverse drug events than younger patients. Evaluate for dose reduction or drug avoidance based on kidney function, comorbidities, and other medication use.
- The AGS Beers Criteria list is useful for identifying high-risk medications for older adults. Particular caution/avoidance should be used in prescribing benzodiazepines and other sedative-hypnotic medications.

General Considerations

Definitions of polypharmacy vary; it typically refers to the condition of taking or being prescribed a multitude of prescription and nonprescription medications. More adverse drug events occur in older adults compared to younger patients for many reasons, including changing drug metabolism in the kidney or liver or both, drug interaction with comorbid conditions, and interactions between multiple medications. Polypharmacy itself is associated with adverse health outcomes, including falls, impaired cognition, hospitalizations, and death.

Medication metabolism is often impaired in older adults due to decreased GFR, reduced hepatic clearance, and changes in body composition (eg, lean body mass). Most emergency hospitalizations for adverse medication events among older adults result from commonly prescribed medications used alone or in combination.

Precautions in Prescribing Medications

Most medications prescribed for chronic disease management should be initiated at the low end of the usual adult dosage range, with slow increases in dosage until a therapeutic level is reached or intolerable side effects develop. At the same time, it is imperative that a medication's therapeutic dose be achieved, since older adults are at risk for undertreatment of conditions such as depression, if the starting dose is not increased with careful monitoring.

Optimal medication adherence is less likely with increasing numbers of pills and doses, high cost, poor communication about medication changes as well as expected benefits and side effects; other factors affecting adherence include cognitive impairment, insurance issues, and psychosocial barriers. When possible, the clinician should simplify both dosing schedules with the fewest number of pills and doses (combination formulations can be useful in this regard, though perhaps complicating future dose adjustments) as well as modes of administration (eg, oral, ocular, transdermal, subcutaneous, inhalational). Other helpful medication management techniques include use of a single pharmacy, use of pillboxes or pharmacy-packaged medication sets, clarity about the prescriber of each medication (and ideally use of fewer prescribers), infrequent medication changes, and clear instructions about all medication changes using the "teach-back" method of patient communication. Clinicians should ask patients about their ability to afford their medications, and counsel patients about strategies for cost containment (eg, switching to a more affordable Medicare Part D plan during open enrollment and interrogating drug formularies for low-cost alternatives).

The patient or caregiver should bring in all medications at each visit in order to achieve an accurate **medication reconciliation** and reinforce reasons for medication use, dosage, frequency of administration, and possible adverse effects. Patients should also bring all supplements and over-the-counter medications used, including analgesics and sleep aids. Medication reconciliation is particularly important if the patient sees multiple clinicians. Clinicians should be aware of the "prescribing cascade" in which a medication is prescribed to counter the side effect of another medication.

The risk of toxicity goes up with the number of medications prescribed. Certain combinations of medications (eg, warfarin and many antibiotics, ACE inhibitors and NSAIDs, opioids and sedative-hypnotics) are particularly likely to cause drug-drug interactions and should be monitored carefully.

Trials of medication discontinuation (deprescribing) should be considered when the original indication is unclear or the patient is having side effects. Medication discontinuation is particularly important in patients with limited life expectancy who may be experiencing increasing burdens from polypharmacy and modest, if any, benefits from the medication (eg, bisphosphonates, antilipemics). Clinical tools such as "STOPP/START" and the AGS Beers Criteria can inform safe medication prescribing for older adults.

When to Refer

- Refer patients with polypharmacy or poor medication adherence to a clinical pharmacist, when available.
- Refer homebound patients with poor medication adherence and suboptimal chronic disease management to a home health nurse for medication reconciliation and teaching.

Fick DM et al. American Geriatrics Society 2019 Updated AGS Beers Criteria® for potentially inappropriate medication use in older adults. J Am Geriatr Soc. 2019;67:674. [PMID: 30693946]

Hoel RW et al. Polypharmacy management in older patients. Mayo Clin Proc. 2021;96:242. [PMID: 33413822]

Nicosia FM et al. What is a medication-related problem? A qualitative study of older adults and primary care clinicians. J Gen Intern Med. 2020;35:724. [PMID: 31677102]

Thevelin S et al. Potentially inappropriate prescribing and related hospital admissions in geriatric patients: a comparative analysis between the STOPP and START criteria versions 1 and 2. Drugs Aging. 2019;36:453. [PMID: 30694444]

10. Vision Impairment

Visual impairment due to age-related refractive error ("presbyopia"), macular degeneration, cataracts, glaucoma, or diabetic retinopathy is associated with several negative physical and mental health outcomes. These include falls, impaired mobility, and reduced quality of life. While the 2016 USPSTF guideline and 2018 Cochrane Review conclude that there is insufficient evidence for routine visual impairment screening, the American Academy of Ophthalmology recommends a complete eye examination every 1–2 years after age 65. Serious and correctable vision disorders are prevalent and morbid enough that it is reasonable for most elders to undergo a comprehensive eye examination by an ophthalmologist or optometrist every 1–2 years. Eye examinations should certainly be prioritized for patients with new or recurring falls, changes in vision, and conditions with risk of eye complications (eg, diabetes mellitus, thyroid disease). Patients with significant visual loss should be referred to low-vision community programs for support and assessment for assistive devices.

Assi L et al. A global assessment of eye health and quality of life: a systematic review of systematic reviews. JAMA Ophthalmol. 2021;139:526. [PMID: 33576772]

Ehrlich JR et al. Prevalence of falls and fall-related outcomes in older adults with self-reported vision impairment. J Am Geriatr Soc. 2019;67:239. [PMID: 30421796]

11. Hearing Impairment

Hearing loss in older adults is very common yet often undertreated. Over one-third of persons older than age 65 and half of those older than age 85 have some degree of hearing loss. Hearing loss is associated with social isolation, depression, disability, cognitive impairment and accelerated cognitive decline, hospitalization, and nursing home placement. Hearing loss is undertreated because it is underrecognized by clinicians and hearing assistive devices are expensive and not typically covered by insurance.

Although the USPSTF found insufficient evidence for routine hearing screening, clinicians should periodically ask patients about hearing loss and refer them to audiology if hearing loss is suspected. A reasonable clinical screen is to ask patients if they have noticed any hearing impairment. Those who answer "yes" should be referred for audiometry. For those who answer "no" but in whom hearing loss is still suspected, further in-office screening can be performed using the **whispered voice test.** To determine the degree to which hearing impairment interferes with functioning, the provider may ask patients if they become frustrated when conversing with family members, have challenges understanding conversations, are embarrassed when meeting new people, or have difficulty watching television. Caregivers or family members can provide important collateral information regarding potential hearing loss and the impact of hearing loss on social interactions.

Hearing loss assistive devices and technology include hearing aids, cochlear implants, sound amplification for telephones and televisions, speech to text software, smart phone applications, hearing loops, and alerting devices to inform hearing-impaired people of an event such as a fire alarm. Hearing amplification and cochlear implantation improve hearing-related quality of life and reduce depressive symptoms. Compliance with hearing amplification can be a challenge because of the high device cost, dissatisfaction with performance, and stigma associated with hearing aid use. Newer digital devices may perform better but are considerably more expensive. US federal law allows for the sale of over-the-counter devices that can be purchased directly without a prescription from a clinician. These devices are most appropriate for patients with mild to moderate hearing loss. Cochlear implantation is an underutilized treatment that is recommended for older adults with profound sensory hearing loss. It improves understanding of speech and quality of life. Portable hearing amplifiers (eg, "pocket talkers") are low-cost hand-held devices with a headset for the patient and microphone to amplify sound for the speaker. These devices are particularly useful to communicate with hearing-impaired patients in clinic and inpatient settings. In order to facilitate successful communication with hearing-impaired patients, providers should face toward patients when speaking, speak at a moderate pace and in a low tone, and practice the "teachback" method in order to assess that information was adequately transmitted.

Alattar AA et al. Hearing impairment and cognitive decline in older, community-dwelling adults. J Gerontol: Series A. 2020; 75:567. [PMID: 30753308]

Carlson ML. Cochlear implantation in adults. N Engl J Med. 2020;382:1531. [PMID: 32294347]

Feltner C et al. Screening for hearing loss in older adults: updated evidence report and systematic review for the US Preventive Services Task Force. JAMA. 2021;325:1202. [PMID: 33755082]

US Preventive Services Task Force; Krist AH et al. Screening for hearing loss in older adults: US Preventive Services Task Force Recommendation Statement. JAMA. 2021;325:1196. [PMID: 33755083]

12. Elder Mistreatment & Self-Neglect

Elder abuse is defined as "acts whereby a trusted person causes or creates risk of harm to an older adult." **Self-neglect** is the most common form of elder abuse and occurs among all demographic strata. In the United States, about 10% of adults over age 60 have experienced some sort of abuse or neglect in the previous year. Financial abuse is on the rise, and older adults with cognitive impairment are particularly vulnerable. Each year, at least 5% of elders are victims of financial abuse or scams.

Elder abuse risk factors include limited social support and poor physical health. Clues to the presence of elder mistreatment or self-neglect include observing that the patient's behavior changes in the presence of the caregiver, delays between injury occurrence and treatment seeking,

Table 4–4. Phrases and actions that may be helpful in situations of suspected abuse or neglect.

Questions for the Elder
1. Has anyone hurt you?
2. Are you afraid of anybody?
3. Is anyone taking or using your money without your permission?
Questions for the Caregiver
1. Are your relative's needs more than you can handle?
2. Are you worried that you might hit your relative?
3. Have you hit your relative?
If abuse is suspected
Tell the patient that you are concerned, want to help, and will call Adult Protective Services for further assistance
Document any injuries
Document the patient's words
Document whether the patient has decision-making capacity using a tool such as "Aid to Capacity Evaluation"

inconsistencies between an observed injury and its associated explanation, lack of appropriate clothing or hygiene, and unfilled prescriptions. Elder abuse and self-neglect can cause many health consequences, such as long-term care placement, anxiety, depression, and death.

While the USPSTF has not endorsed any screening tools to identify elder abuse, clinicians caring for older adults should maintain a high index of suspicion and meet with patients without the presence of caregivers on occasion. Vigilance for possible elder abuse is important across care settings including residential care facilities, ambulatory settings, and emergency departments. In these encounters, clinicians can ask questions about the caregiver relationship, and directly question about possible mistreatment and neglect, if suspected (Table 4–4).

When self-neglect is suspected, it is critical to establish whether a patient has decision-making capacity regarding the suspected neglectful behavior. A patient who has full decision-making capacity should be provided help and support but can choose to live in conditions of self-neglect, providing that the public is not endangered by their actions. In contrast, more aggressive intervention is recommended for a patient who lacks decision-making capacity and lives in conditions of self-neglect. Such interventions include reporting to Adult Protective Services and arranging in-home help, conservatorship, and placement in a supervised setting. Cognitive assessment may provide some insight into whether cognitive impairment is contributing to self-neglect, but these tools are not designed to assess decision-making capacity. A standardized tool, such as the "Aid to Capacity Evaluation," is easy to administer, has good performance characteristics for determining decision-making capacity, and is available free online at https://www.jcb.utoronto.ca/tools/documents/ace.pdf.

When to Refer

- Refer older adults suffering from suspected elder abuse or self-neglect to **Adult Protective Services**, as required by law in most states (consult the National Center on Elder Abuse at https://ncea.acl.gov/)
- Refer to a mental health professional and neurologist for evaluation of those cases in which decision-making capacity is unclear, neuropsychiatric testing would be useful, or if untreated mental illness is suspected to play a role in self-neglect.

When to Admit

- Admit older adults who would be unsafe in the community when an alternative plan cannot be put into place in a timely manner. In cases of self-neglect, surrogate decision-makers need to be identified and conservatorship may need to be pursued for safe discharge planning.

Cimino-Fiallos N et al. Elder abuse—a guide to diagnosis and management in the emergency department. Emerg Med Clin North Am. 2021;39:405. [PMID: 33863468]

DeLiema M et al. Financial fraud among older Americans: evidence and implications. J Gerontol B Psychol Sci Soc Sci. 2020;75:861. [PMID: 30561718]

Van Den Bruele AB et al. Elder abuse. Clin Geriatr Med. 2019;35:103. [PMID: 30390976]

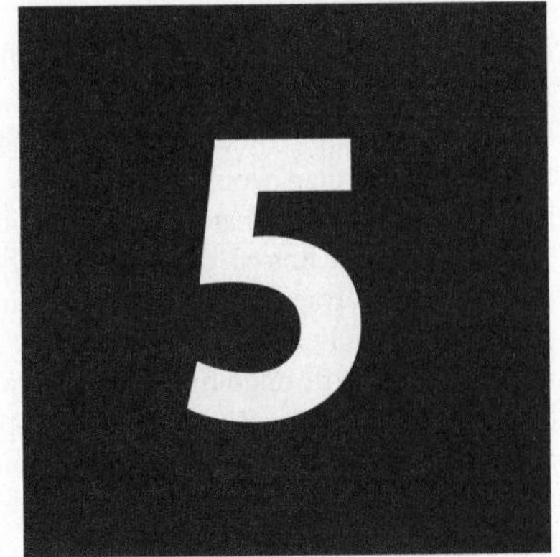

Palliative Care & Pain Management

Michael W. Rabow, MD
Steven Z. Pantilat, MD
Ann Cai Shah, MD
Lawrence Poree, MD, MPH, PhD
Raj Mitra, MD

PALLIATIVE CARE

DEFINITION & SCOPE

Palliative care is medical care focused on improving quality of life for people living with serious illness. Serious illness is defined as "a condition that carries a high risk of mortality, negatively impacts quality of life and daily function, and/or is burdensome in symptoms, treatments or caregiver stress." Palliative care addresses and treats symptoms, supports patients' families and loved ones, and through clear communication helps ensure that care aligns with patients' preferences, values, and goals. Near the end of life, palliative care may become the sole focus of care, but palliative care *alongside* cure-focused treatment or disease management is beneficial throughout the course of a serious illness, regardless of its prognosis. Randomized studies have shown that palliative care provided alongside disease-focused treatment can improve quality of life, promote symptom management, and even prolong life in some situations.

Palliative care includes management of physical symptoms, such as pain, dyspnea, nausea and vomiting, constipation, delirium, and agitation; emotional distress, such as depression, anxiety, and interpersonal strain; and existential distress, such as spiritual crisis. While palliative care is a medical subspecialty recognized by the American Board of Medical Specialties ("specialty palliative care") and is typically provided by an interdisciplinary team of experts, *all* clinicians should have the skills to provide "primary palliative care" including managing pain; treating dyspnea; addressing mood disorders; communicating about prognosis and patient preferences for care; and helping address spiritual distress. The fourth edition of the National Consensus Project's Clinical Practice Guidelines for Quality Palliative Care emphasizes that palliative care is the responsibility of all clinicians and disciplines caring for people with serious illness in all health care settings, including hospitals, primary care and specialty clinics, nursing homes, and the community. The scope of primary palliative care and the ideal timing to begin specialty palliative care for patients with different illnesses is an evolving area of practice.

As is true for clinicians of all medical specialties, palliative care clinicians and the systems of care for people with serious illness in the United States are influenced by systemic racial bias. Knowing that there are racial inequities in palliative care referral, pain management, communication, and outcomes, practitioners must work to identify and rectify injustice in how patient symptoms are assessed and treated and ensure equal access to palliative care services.

Fadul N et al. Integration of palliative care into COVID-19 pandemic planning. BMJ Support Palliat Care. 2021;11:40. [PMID: 32527790]

Kluger BM et al. Comparison of integrated outpatient palliative care with standard care in patients with Parkinson disease and related disorders: a randomized clinical trial. JAMA Neurol. 2020;77:551. [PMID: 32040141]

Mechler K et al. Palliative care approach to chronic diseases: end stages of heart failure, chronic obstructive pulmonary disease, liver failure, and renal failure. Prim Care. 2019;46:415. [PMID: 31375190]

Ornstein KA et al. Evaluation of racial disparities in hospice use and end-of-life treatment intensity in the REGARDS cohort. JAMA Netw Open. 2020;3:e2014639. [PMID: 32833020]

PALLIATION OF COMMON NONPAIN SYMPTOMS

GENERAL PRINCIPLES

During any stage of illness, patients should be screened routinely for symptoms. Any symptoms that cause significant suffering should be addressed quickly and aggressively with frequent elicitation, individualized treatment, and reassessment. While patients at the end of life may experience a host of distressing symptoms, pain, dyspnea, and delirium are among the most feared and burdensome.

DYSPNEA

Dyspnea is the subjective experience of difficulty breathing and may be characterized by patients as tightness in the chest, shortness of breath, breathlessness, or a feeling of suffocation. Up to half of people at the end of life may experience severe dyspnea.

Treatment of dyspnea is first directed at the cause (see Chapter 9) if a workup is consistent with the patient's goals. Dyspnea responds to opioids, which have been proven effective in multiple randomized trials. Starting doses are typically lower than would be necessary for the relief of moderate pain. Immediate-release morphine given orally (2–4 mg every 4 hours) or intravenously (1–2 mg every 4 hours) treats dyspnea effectively. Sustained-release morphine given orally at 10 mg daily is safe and effective for most patients with ongoing dyspnea. Many patients who become seriously ill with COVID-19 experience dyspnea and may require opioids as well as supplemental oxygen. Supplemental oxygen may be useful for the dyspneic patient *who is hypoxic* with any illness. Fresh air from a window or fan may provide relief for dyspneic patients who are not hypoxic. Judicious use of noninvasive ventilation (eg, high-flow oxygen via nasal cannula) as well as meditation and guided imagery may benefit some patients. Benzodiazepines may be useful for treatment of dyspnea-related anxiety.

NAUSEA & VOMITING

Nausea and vomiting are common and distressing symptoms. Management of nausea may be optimized by regular dosing and often requires multiple medications targeting one or more of the four major inputs to the vomiting center (see Chapter 15).

Vomiting associated with opioids is discussed below. Some patients with prolonged vomiting will require hospitalization. Nasogastric suction may provide rapid, short-term relief for vomiting associated with constipation (in addition to laxatives), gastroparesis, or gastric outlet or bowel obstruction. Metoclopramide (5–20 mg orally or intravenously four times a day) can be helpful in partial gastric outlet obstruction. Transdermal scopolamine (1.5-mg patch every 3 days) can reduce peristalsis and cramping pain, and H_2-blocking medications can reduce gastric secretions. High-dose corticosteroids (eg, dexamethasone, 20 mg orally or intravenously daily in divided doses) can be used in refractory cases of nausea or vomiting or when it is due to bowel obstruction or increased intracranial pressure. Malignant bowel obstruction in people with advanced cancer is a poor prognostic sign and surgery is rarely helpful.

Benzodiazepines (eg, lorazepam, 0.5–1.0 mg given orally every 6–8 hours) can be effective in preventing the *anticipatory* nausea and anxiety associated with chemotherapy. For emetogenic chemotherapy, treatment includes combinations of 5-HT_3-antagonists (eg, ondansetron, granisetron, or palonosetron), neurokinin-1 receptor antagonists (eg, aprepitant, fosaprepitant, or rolapitant), the N-receptor antagonist netupitant combined with palonosetron (NEPA), olanzapine, dexamethasone, or prochlorperazine. In addition to its effect on mood, mirtazapine, 15–45 mg orally nightly, may improve nausea and appetite. Finally, dronabinol (2.5–20 mg orally every 4–6 hours) can help with nausea and vomiting. Patients report relief from medical cannabis, although it is unclear which tetrahydrocannabinol (THC) or cannabidiol (CBD) strains are most effective.

CONSTIPATION

Given the frequent use of opioids, poor dietary intake, physical inactivity, and lack of privacy, constipation is a common problem in seriously ill and dying patients. Clinicians must inquire about any difficulty with hard or infrequent stools. Constipation is an easily preventable and treatable cause of discomfort, distress, and nausea and vomiting (see Chapter 15).

Constipation may be prevented or relieved if patients can increase their activity and intake of fluids. Provision of privacy, undisturbed toilet time, and a bedside commode rather than a bedpan, may be important for some patients.

A prophylactic bowel regimen with a stimulant laxative (senna or bisacodyl) should be started when opioid treatment is begun. Table 15–4 lists other agents (including **osmotic laxatives such as polyethylene glycol** and lactulose) that can be added as needed. Docusate, a stool softener, is *not* recommended because it does not add benefit beyond stimulant laxatives. Peripherally acting mu-receptor antagonists (including oral naloxegol and naldemedine, and subcutaneous methylnaltrexone) are recommended to treat laxative-refractory opioid-induced constipation. Evidence is insufficient to recommend lubiprostone or prucalopride. Patients who report being constipated and then have diarrhea typically are passing liquid stool around impacted stool. Such patients should have a rectal examination to assess for impaction; if it is present, disimpaction will be required.

FATIGUE

Fatigue is the most common complaint among people with cancer. Anemia, hypothyroidism, hypogonadism, cognitive and functional impairment, and malnutrition can contribute to fatigue and should be corrected if possible (and desired by the patient). Because pain and depression often coexist with fatigue as a "symptom cluster," they should be managed appropriately in fatigue. Fatigue from medication adverse effects and polypharmacy is common and should be addressed. For nonspecific fatigue, physical activity, rehabilitation, and exercise may be effective. Although psychostimulants, such as methylphenidate (5–10 mg orally in the morning and afternoon) or modafinil (100–200 mg orally in the morning), are commonly used for cancer-related fatigue, strong evidence for effectiveness is lacking. American ginseng (*Panax quinquefolius*) has been shown to be effective for cancer-related fatigue but may have an estrogenic effect. Corticosteroids may have a short-term benefit. Venlafaxine and buproprion tend to be activating. Caffeinated beverages can help.

DELIRIUM & AGITATION

Many patients die in a state of delirium—a waxing and waning in level of consciousness and a change in cognition that develops over a short time and is manifested by misinterpretations, illusions, hallucinations, sleep-wake cycle disruptions, psychomotor disturbances (eg, lethargy, restlessness), and mood disturbances (eg, fear, anxiety). Delirium may be hyperactive, hypoactive, or mixed. Agitated delirium at the end of life is also called **terminal restlessness.**

While some patients with delirium may appear "pleasantly confused," it is difficult to know what patients experience. In the absence of obvious distress in the patient, a decision by the patient's family and clinicians not to treat delirium may be prudent. Agitated delirium at the end of life, however, is often distressing to patient and family and requires treatment. Delirium may interfere with the family's ability to interact with the patient and may prevent a patient from being able to recognize and report important symptoms. Common reversible causes of delirium include urinary retention, constipation, pain, and anticholinergic medications; these should be addressed whenever possible. There is no evidence that dehydration causes or that hydration relieves delirium. Careful attention to patient safety and nonpharmacologic strategies to help the patient remain oriented (clock, calendar, familiar environment, reassurance and redirection from caregivers) may be sufficient to prevent or manage mild delirium. Benzodiazepines can worsen delirium and generally should be avoided, though they may be helpful in achieving sedation near the end of life. A randomized trial of placebo compared to risperidone or haloperidol in delirious patients demonstrated *increased* mortality with neuroleptics. Thus, **neuroleptic agents generally should be avoided.** When agitated delirium is refractory to other treatments and remains intolerable, however, especially at the end of life, neuroleptic agents (eg, haloperidol, 1–10 mg orally, subcutaneously, intramuscularly, or intravenously twice or three times a day, or risperidone, 1–3 mg orally twice a day) or frank sedation with barbiturates or benzodiazepines may be required (eg, midazolam, 0.5–5 mg/h subcutaneously or intravenously).

Davis MP et al. The benefits of olanzapine in palliating symptoms. Curr Treat Options Oncol. 2020;22:5. [PMID: 33244634]

Keeley P et al. Symptom burden and clinical profile of COVID-19 deaths: a rapid systematic review and evidence summary. BMJ Support Palliat Care. 2020;10:381. [PMID: 32467101]

Klasson C et al. Fatigue in cancer patients in palliative care—a review on pharmacological interventions. Cancers (Basel). 2021;13:985. [PMID: 33652866]

Sarrió RG et al; Working Group ActEIO Project. Delphi consensus on strategies in the management of opioid-induced constipation in cancer patients. BMC Palliat Care. 2021;20:1. [PMID: 33388041]

Verberkt CA et al. Effect of sustained-release morphine for refractory breathlessness in chronic obstructive pulmonary disease on health status: a randomized clinical trial. JAMA Intern Med. 2020;180:1306. [PMID: 32804188]

DECISION MAKING FOR PATIENTS WITH SERIOUS ILLNESS

Advance Care Planning & Advance Directives

The idea that patients must choose between quality and quantity of life is an outmoded concept that presents patients with a false choice. Clinicians should discuss with patients that an approach that provides *concurrent* palliative and disease-focused care is the one most likely to achieve improvements in both quality *and* quantity of life. Well-informed, competent adults have a right to refuse life-sustaining interventions, even if this would result in death. In order to promote patient autonomy, clinicians are obligated to inform patients about the risks, benefits, alternatives, and expected outcomes of medical interventions, such as CPR, mechanical ventilation, hospitalization and ICU care, and artificial nutrition and hydration.

Advance directives (ADs) are oral or written statements made by patients when they are competent that project their autonomy into the future. ADs are intended to guide care should patients lose the ability to make and communicate their own decisions. ADs are an important part of **advance care planning**, the goal of which is to help ensure that people receive medical care that is consistent with their values, goals and preferences during serious and chronic illness. ADs take effect when the patient can no longer communicate his or her preferences directly. While oral statements about these matters are ethically binding, they are not legally binding in all states. State-specific AD forms are available from a number of sources, including the National Hospice Palliative Care Organization (https://www.caringinfo.org/planning/advance-directives/) and Prepare for Your Care (prepareforyourcare.org).

Clinicians should address the core elements of advance care planning for all patients with serious illness—ideally, well before the end of life—to elicit their preferences, to appoint a surrogate, to talk to that person about their preferences, and to complete a formal AD. Most patients with a serious illness have already thought about end-of-life issues, want to discuss them with their clinician, want the clinician to bring up the subject, and feel better for having had the discussion. Patients who have such discussions with their clinicians are more satisfied with their clinician, are perceived by their family as having a better quality of life at the end of life, are less likely to die in the hospital, and are more likely to utilize hospice care. The loved ones of patients who engage in advance care planning discussions are less likely to suffer from depression during bereavement.

One type of AD is the **Durable Power of Attorney for Health Care (DPOA-HC)** that allows the patient to designate a surrogate decision maker. Identifying and documenting the surrogate decision maker may be the most important part of advance care planning. The DPOA-HC is particularly useful because it is often difficult to anticipate what specific decisions will need to be made. The responsibility of the surrogate is to provide "substituted judgment"—to decide as the *patient* would, not as the *surrogate* wants. Clinicians should encourage patients to talk with their surrogates about their preferences generally and about scenarios that are likely to arise, such as the need for mechanical ventilation in a patient with end-stage emphysema or in any patient with possible SARS-CoV-2 infection. In the absence of a designated surrogate, clinicians usually turn to family members or next of kin. In the United States, regulations require health care institutions to inform patients of their rights to formulate an AD. **Physician (or Medical) Orders for Life-Sustaining Treatment**

(**POLST or MOLST**) or **Physician (or Medical) Orders for Scope of Treatment (POST or MOST)** forms are clinician orders that document patient preferences and accompany patients wherever they are cared for—home, hospital, or nursing home. They are available in most states and used to complement ADs for patients approaching the end of life.

Gupta A et al. Value of advance care directives for patients with serious illness in the era of COVID pandemic: a review of challenges and solutions. Am J Hosp Palliat Care. 2021;38:191. [PMID: 33021094]

Hirakawa Y et al. Implementation of advance care planning amid the COVID-19 crisis: a narrative review and synthesis. Geriatr Gerontol Int. 2021;21:779. [PMID: 34318579]

Jones T et al. Advance care planning, palliative care, and end-of-life care interventions for racial and ethnic underrepresented groups: a systematic review. J Pain Symptom Manage. 2021;62: e248. [PMID: 33984460]

Do Not Attempt Resuscitation Orders

Because the "default" in US hospitals is that patients will undergo CPR in the event of cardiopulmonary arrest, clinicians should elicit patient preferences about CPR as a part of advance care planning. Most patients and many clinicians overestimate the chances of success of CPR. Only about 17% of all patients who undergo CPR in the hospital survive to hospital discharge and, among people with multisystem organ failure, metastatic cancer, or sepsis, the likelihood of survival to hospital discharge following CPR is virtually nil. Patients may ask their hospital clinician to write an order that CPR not be attempted should they experience cardiac arrest. Although this order initially was referred to as a **"DNR" (do not resuscitate)** order, many clinicians prefer the term **"DNAR" (do not attempt resuscitation)** to emphasize the low likelihood of success. Some clinicians and institutions use an order to **"Allow Natural Death"** for situations in which death is imminent and the patient wishes to receive only those interventions that will promote comfort.

For most patients at the end of life, decisions about CPR may not be about *whether* they will live but about *how* they will die. Clinicians should correct the misconception that withholding CPR in appropriate circumstances is tantamount to "not doing everything" or "just letting someone die." While respecting the patient's right to make the decision—and keeping in mind their own biases and prejudices—clinicians should offer explicit recommendations about DNAR orders and protect dying patients and their families from feelings of guilt and from the sorrow associated with vain hopes. Clinicians should discuss what interventions will be continued and started to promote quality of life rather than focusing only on what interventions will be stopped or not begun. For patients with implanted cardioverter defibrillators (ICDs), clinicians must also address the issue of turning off these devices, while leaving the pacemaker function on, as death approaches to prevent the uncommon but distressing situation of the ICD discharging during the dying process.

Kim C et al. The Do Not Resuscitate (DNR) order in the perioperative setting: practical considerations. Curr Opin Anaesthesiol. 2021;34:141. [PMID: 33630773]

CARE OF PATIENTS AT THE END OF LIFE

In the United States, more than 2.85 million people die each year. COVID-19 has emerged as a common cause of death both in the United States and around the world. Caring for patients at the end of life is an important responsibility and a rewarding opportunity for clinicians. From the medical perspective, the end of life may be defined as that time when death—whether due to terminal, acute or chronic illness—is expected within hours to months and can no longer be reasonably forestalled by medical intervention. Palliative care at the end of life focuses on relieving distressing symptoms and promoting quality of life, as it does in all other stages of illness. For patients at the end of life, palliative care may become the sole focus of care.

Prognosis at the End of Life

Clinicians must help patients understand when they are approaching the end of life. Most patients, and their family caregivers, want accurate prognostic information. This information influences patients' treatment decisions, may change how they spend their remaining time, and does *not* negatively impact patient survival. One-half or more of cancer patients do not understand that many treatments they might be offered are palliative and not curative.

While certain diseases, such as cancer, are more amenable to prognostic estimates, the other common causes of death—including heart disease, stroke, chronic lung disease, dementia, and COVID-19—have more variable trajectories and difficult-to-predict prognoses. Even for patients with cancer, clinician estimates of prognosis are often inaccurate and generally overly optimistic. The advent of new anticancer treatments including immunotherapy and targeted therapies has made prognosis more challenging in some cancers. Nonetheless, clinical experience, epidemiologic data, guidelines from professional organizations, and computer modeling and prediction tools (eg, the Palliative Performance Scale or http://eprognosis.ucsf.edu) may be used to offer patients more realistic estimates of prognosis. To determine whether a discussion of prognosis would be appropriate, clinicians can also ask themselves "Would I be surprised if this patient died in the next year?" If the answer is "no," then the clinician should initiate a discussion. Recognizing that patients may have different levels of comfort with prognostic information, clinicians can introduce the topic by simply saying, "I have information about the likely time course of your illness. Would you like to talk about it?"

Hui D et al. Prognostication in advanced cancer: update and directions for future research. Support Care Cancer. 2019;27:1973. [PMID: 30863893]

Wattanapisit S et al. Prognostic disclosure and quality of life in palliative care: a systematic review. BMJ Support Palliat Care. 2021;11:361. [PMID: 33257406]

Expectations About the End of Life

Death is often regarded by clinicians, patients, and families as a failure of medical science. This attitude can create or heighten a sense of guilt about the failure to prevent dying. Both the general public and clinicians often view death as an enemy to be battled furiously in hospitals rather than as an inevitable outcome to be experienced as a part of life at home. This idea contributes to the fact that most people in the United States die in hospitals or long-term–care facilities even though they may have wished otherwise. There is a trend of fewer deaths in hospitals and more deaths at home or in other community settings.

Relieving suffering, providing support, and helping the patient make the most of their life, or as a clinician might say to a patient, "helping you live as well as possible for as long as possible," should be foremost considerations, even when the clinician and patient continue to pursue cure of potentially reversible disease. Patients at the end of life and their families identify a number of elements as important to quality end-of-life care: managing pain and other symptoms adequately, avoiding inappropriate prolongation of dying, communicating clearly, preserving dignity, preparing for death, achieving a sense of control, relieving the burden on others, and strengthening relationships with loved ones.

Rosenberg A et al. Holding hope for patients with serious illness. JAMA. 2021;326:1259. [PMID: 34529011]

Communication & Care of the Patient at the End of Life

Caring for patients at the end of life requires the same skills clinicians use in other tasks of medical care: diagnosing treatable conditions, providing patient education, facilitating decision making, and expressing understanding and caring. Communication skills are vitally important and can be improved through training. Higher-quality communication is associated with greater satisfaction and awareness of patient wishes. Clinicians must become proficient at delivering serious news and then dealing with its consequences (Table 5–1). Smartphone and Internet communication resources are available to support clinicians (www.vitaltalk.org), and evidence suggests that communication checklists and guides can be effective. When the clinician and patient do not share a common language, the use of a professional interpreter is needed to facilitate clear communication and help broker cultural issues.

Table 5–1. Suggestions for the delivery of serious news.

Prepare an appropriate place and time.
Address basic information needs.
Be brief and direct; avoid jargon and euphemisms.
Allow for silence and expression of emotions.
Assess and validate patient reactions.
Respond to immediate discomforts and risks.
Listen actively and express empathy.
Achieve a common perception of the problem.
Reassure that care will continue.
Ensure follow-up and make specific plans for the future.

Three further obligations are central to the clinician's role at this time. First, he or she must work to identify, understand, and relieve physical, psychological, social, and spiritual distress or suffering. Second, clinicians can serve as facilitators or catalysts for hope. While hope for a particular outcome such as cure may fade, it can be refocused on what is *still* possible. Although a patient may hope for a "miracle," other more likely hopes can be encouraged and supported, including hope for relief of pain, for reconciliation with loved ones, for discovery of meaning, and for spiritual growth. With such questions as "What is still possible now for you?" and "When you look to the future, what do you hope for?" clinicians can help patients uncover hope, explore meaningful and realistic goals, and develop strategies to achieve them.

Finally, dying patients' feelings of isolation and fear demand that clinicians assert that they will care for the patient throughout the final stage of life. The *promise of nonabandonment* is the central principle of end-of-life care and is a clinician's pledge to serve as a caring partner, a resource for creative problem solving and relief of suffering, a guide during uncertain times, and a witness to the patient's experiences—no matter what happens. Clinicians can say to a patient, "I will care for you whatever happens."

Paladino J et al. Evaluating an intervention to improve communication between oncology clinicians and patients with life-limiting cancer: a cluster randomized clinical trial of the Serious Illness Care Program. JAMA Oncol. 2019;5:801. [PMID: 30870556]

Thodé M et al. Feasibility and effectiveness of tools that support communication and decision making in life-prolonging treatments for patients in hospital: a systematic review. BMJ Support Palliat Care. 2020 Oct 5. [Epub ahead of print] [PMID: 33020150]

Nutrition & Hydration

People approaching the end of life often lose their appetite and most stop eating and drinking in their last days. Clinicians should explain to families that the dying patient is not suffering from hunger or thirst; rather, the discontinuation of eating and drinking is part of dying, not its cause. The anorexia-cachexia syndrome frequently occurs in patients with advanced cancer, and cachexia is common and a poor prognostic sign in patients with heart failure. The associated ketonemia can produce a sense of well-being, analgesia, and mild euphoria. Although it is unclear to what extent withholding hydration at the end of life creates an uncomfortable sensation of thirst, any such sensation is usually relieved by simply moistening the dry mouth with ice chips, hard candy, swabs, or popsicles. Although this normal process of diminishing oral intake and accompanying weight loss is very common, it can be distressing to patients and families who may associate the offering of food with compassion and love and lack of eating with distressing images of starvation. In response, patients and families often ask about supplemental enteral or parenteral nutrition.

Supplemental artificial nutrition and hydration offer no benefit to those at the end of life and rarely achieve patient and family goals. The American Geriatrics Society recommends against artificial nutrition ("tube feeding") in people with advanced dementia because it does not provide any benefit. Furthermore, enteral feeding may cause nausea and vomiting in ill patients and can lead to diarrhea in the setting of malabsorption. Artificial nutrition and hydration may increase oral and airway secretions as well as increase the risk of choking, aspiration, and dyspnea; ascites, edema, and effusions may be worsened. In addition, artificial nutrition by nasogastric and gastrostomy tubes and parenteral nutrition impose risks of infection, epistaxis, pneumothorax, electrolyte imbalance, and aspiration—as well as the need to physically restrain the delirious patient to prevent dislodgment of tubes and catheters.

Individuals at the end of life have a right to voluntarily refuse all nutrition and hydration. Because they may have deep social and cultural significance for patients, families, and clinicians themselves, decisions about artificial nutrition and hydration are not simply medical. Eliciting perceived goals of artificial nutrition and hydration and correcting misperceptions can help patients and families make clear decisions.

Mayers T et al. International review of national-level guidelines on end-of-life care with focus on the withholding and withdrawing of artificial nutrition and hydration. Geriatr Gerontol Int. 2019;19:847. [PMID: 31389113]

Shih YA et al. Decision making of artificial nutrition and hydration for cancer patients at terminal stage—a systematic review of the views from patients, families, and healthcare professionals. J Pain Symptom Manage. 2021;62:1065. [PMID: 33933623]

Psychological, Social, & Spiritual Issues at the End of Life

Dying is not exclusively or even primarily a biomedical event. It is an intimate personal experience with profound psychological, interpersonal, and existential meanings. For many people at the end of life, the prospect of impending death stimulates a deep and urgent assessment of their identity, the quality of their relationships, the meaning and purpose of their life, and their legacy.

A. Psychological Challenges

Most patients at the end of life experience denial and isolation, anger, bargaining, depression, and acceptance but not in an orderly progression. In addition to these five reactions are the perpetual challenges of anxiety and fear of the unknown. Simple information, listening, assurance, and support may help patients with these psychological challenges. Patients and families rank emotional support as one of the most important aspects of good end-of-life care. Psychotherapy and group support may be beneficial as well.

Despite the significant emotional stress of facing death, clinical depression is *not* normal at the end of life and should be treated. Cognitive and affective signs of depression, such as feelings of worthlessness, hopelessness, or helplessness, may help distinguish depression from the low energy and other vegetative signs common with advanced illness. Although traditional antidepressant treatments such as SSRIs are effective, more rapidly acting medications, such as dextroamphetamine (2.5–7.5 mg orally at 8 AM and noon) or methylphenidate (2.5–10 mg orally at 8 AM and noon), may be particularly useful when the end of life is near or while waiting for another antidepressant medication to take effect. Ketamine is now approved, with restrictions, as a treatment for depression. Some research suggests a mortality benefit from treating depression in the setting of serious illness.

B. Social Challenges

At the end of life, patients should be encouraged to take care of personal, professional, and business obligations. These tasks include completing important work or personal projects, distributing possessions, writing a will, and making funeral and burial arrangements. The prospect of death often prompts patients to examine the quality of their interpersonal relationships and to begin the process of saying goodbye (Table 5–2). Concern about estranged relationships or "unfinished business" with significant others and interest in reconciliation may become paramount at this time.

C. Spiritual Challenges

Spirituality includes the attempt to understand or accept the underlying meaning of life, one's relationships to oneself and other people, one's place in the universe, one's legacy, and the possibility of a "higher power" in the universe. People may experience spirituality as part of or distinct from particular religious practices or beliefs.

The patient's spiritual concerns often require only a clinician's attention, listening, and witness. Clinicians can inquire about the patient's spiritual concerns and ask whether the patient wishes to discuss them. For example, asking, "How are you within yourself?" or "Are you at peace?" communicates that the clinician is interested in the patient's whole experience and provides an opportunity for the patient to share perceptions about his or her inner life. Questions that might constitute an existential "review of systems" are presented in Table 5–3. Formal legacy work and dignity therapy have been shown to be effective in improving quality of life and spiritual well-being.

Attending to the spiritual concerns of patients calls for listening to their stories. Storytelling may be facilitated by

Table 5–2. Five statements often necessary for the completion of important interpersonal relationships.

1. "Forgive me."	(An expression of regret)
2. "I forgive you."	(An expression of acceptance)
3. "Thank you."	(An expression of gratitude)
4. "I love you."	(An expression of affection)
5. "Goodbye."	(Leave-taking)

Source: Byock I. *Dying Well: Peace and Possibilities at the End of Life.* New York: Riverhead Books, an imprint of Penguin Group (USA) LLC, 1997.

Table 5–3. An existential review of systems.

Intrapersonal
"What does your illness/dying mean to you?"
"What do you think caused your illness?"
"How have you been healed in the past?"
"What do you think is needed for you to be healed now?"
"What is right with you now?"
"What do you hope for?"
"Are you at peace?"

Interpersonal
"Who is important to you?"
"To whom does your illness/dying matter?"
"Do you have any unfinished business with significant others?"

Transpersonal
"What is your source of strength, help, or hope?"
"Do you have spiritual concerns or a spiritual practice?"
"If so, how does your spirituality relate to your illness/dying, and how can I help integrate your spirituality into your health care?"
"What do you think happens after we die?"
"What do you think is trying to happen here?"

suggesting that the patient share his or her life story with family members, make an audio or video recording, assemble a photo album, organize a scrapbook, or write or dictate an autobiography.

The end of life offers an opportunity for psychological, interpersonal, and spiritual development and a chance to experience and achieve important goals. Individuals may grow—even experience a heightened sense of well-being or transcendence—in the process of dying. Through listening, support, and presence, clinicians may help foster this learning and be a catalyst for this transformation. Clinicians and patients may be guided by a developmental model of life that recognizes a series of lifelong developmental tasks and landmarks and allows for growth at the end of life.

Haufe M et al. How can existential or spiritual strengths be fostered in palliative care? An interpretative synthesis of recent literature. BMJ Support Palliat Care. 2020 Sep 14. [Epub ahead of print] [PMID: 32928785]

Lee W et al. Clinically significant depressive symptoms are prevalent in people with extremely short prognoses—a systematic review. J Pain Symptom Manage. 2021;61:143. [PMID: 32688012]

Cultural Issues

Various religious, ethnic, gender, class, and cultural traditions influence a patient's style of communication, comfort in discussing particular topics, expectations about dying and medical interventions, and attitudes about the appropriate disposition of dead bodies. While culture influences approaches to ADs, autopsy, organ donation, hospice care, and withdrawal of life-sustaining interventions, clinicians should be careful not to make assumptions about individual patients. Clinicians must appreciate that palliative care is susceptible to the same explicit and implicit biases documented in other medical disciplines. Being sensitive to a person's cultural beliefs and lived experiences and respecting traditions are important responsibilities of the clinician caring for a patient at the end of life. A clinician may ask a patient, "What do I need to know about you and your beliefs that will help me take care of you?" and "How do you deal with these issues in your family?"

Abdullah R et al. Preferences and experiences of Muslim patients and their families in Muslim-majority countries for end-of-life care: a systematic review and thematic analysis. J Pain Symptom Manage. 2020;60:1223. [PMID: 32659320]

De Souza J et al. Perspectives of elders and their adult children of Black and minority ethnic heritage on end-of-life conversations: a meta-ethnography. Palliat Med. 2020;34:195. [PMID: 31965907]

La IS et al. Palliative care for the Asian American adult population: a scoping review. Am J Hosp Palliat Care. 2021;38:658. [PMID: 32489147]

Wang SY et al. Racial differences in health care transitions and hospice use at the end of life. J Palliat Med. 2019;22:619. [PMID: 30615546]

Withdrawal of Curative Efforts

Requests from appropriately informed and competent patients or their surrogates for withdrawal of life-sustaining interventions must be respected. Limitation of life-sustaining interventions prior to death is common practice in ICUs in the United States. The withdrawal of life-sustaining interventions, such as mechanical ventilation, must be approached carefully to avoid patient suffering and distress for those in attendance. Clinicians should educate the patient and family about the expected course of events and the difficulty of determining the precise timing of death after withdrawal of interventions. Sedative and analgesic agents should be administered to ensure patient comfort even at the risk of respiratory depression or hypotension. While "death rattle," the sound of air flowing over airway secretions, is common in actively dying patients and can be distressing to families, it is doubtful that it causes discomfort to the patient. Turning the patient can decrease the sound of death rattle. Subcutaneous scopolamine butylbromide administered prophylactically can reduce death rattle. Suctioning should be avoided since it can cause patient discomfort.

McPherson K et al. Limitation of life-sustaining care in the critically ill: a systematic review of the literature. J Hosp Med. 2019;14:303. [PMID: 30794145]

van Esch HJ et al. Effect of prophylactic subcutaneous scopolamine butylbromide on death rattle in patients at the end of life: the SILENCE randomized clinical trial. JAMA. 2021;326:1268. [PMID: 34609452]

Hospice & Other Palliative Care Services

Hospice is a specific type of palliative care service that comprehensively addresses the needs of the dying, focusing on their comfort while not attempting to prolong their life or hasten their death. In the United States in 2018, 50.7% of people with Medicare who died used hospice, most at home or in a nursing home where they can be cared for by their family, other caregivers, and visiting hospice staff. Hospice care can also be provided in institutional residences and hospitals. As is true of all types of palliative care, hospice emphasizes individualized attention and human contact with appropriate precautions for COVID-19 and uses an interdisciplinary team approach. Hospice care can include arranging for respite for family caregivers and assisting with referrals for legal, financial, and other services. Patients in hospice require a physician, preferably their primary care clinician or specialist, to oversee their care.

Based on 2019 data, hospice care was used by 1.49 million US Medicare beneficiaries, about 30% of whom had cancer. Hospice is rated highly by families and has been shown to increase patient satisfaction and to decrease family caregiver mortality. In 2018, 51% of hospice patients died at home; 30% died in a skilled nursing facility. Despite evidence suggesting that hospice care does not shorten length of life, hospice care tends to be engaged very late, often near the very end of life. In 2018, the mean average length of stay in hospice care in the United States was 90 days, but the median length of stay was 18 days. Overall, 54% of patients died within 30 days of enrolling in a hospice, and 28% of patients died within 7 days of starting hospice.

In the United States, most hospice organizations require clinicians to estimate the patient's prognosis to be less than 6 months, since this is a criterion for eligibility under the Medicare hospice benefit and is typically the same for other insurance coverage. Many patients wait to enroll in hospice until they have decided with certainty that they no longer wish to pursue curative intent treatment. This approach contributes to late referrals and to many patients missing out on valuable hospice services. Patients can be encouraged to enroll in hospice while they are still deciding about further curative intent treatment and can disenroll if they decide to pursue it.

Tobin J et al. Hospice care access inequalities: a systematic review and narrative synthesis. BMJ Support Palliat Care. 2021 Feb 19. [Epub ahead of print] [PMID: 33608254]

Medical Aid in Dying

Medical aid in dying is the legally sanctioned process by which patients who have a terminal illness may request and receive a prescription from a physician for a lethal dose of medication that the patients can self-administer for the purpose of ending their own life. Terminology for this practice varies. "Medical aid in dying" is used here to clarify that a willing physician provides assistance in accordance with the law (by writing a prescription for a lethal medication) to a patient who makes a request for it and who meets specific criteria. Patients, family members, nonmedical and medical organizations, clinicians, lawmakers, and the public frequently use other terms, such as "physician-assisted death," "aid in dying," "death with dignity," or "physician-assisted suicide." Use of the latter term is discouraged because when this action is taken according to the law, it is not considered suicide and people who are actively suicidal are not eligible for this process.

Although public and state support for medical aid in dying has grown in the United States, this remains an area of debate. As of 2021, medical aid in dying has been legalized with specific procedures for residents in the District of Columbia and nine US states (Oregon, Washington, Vermont, Colorado, Hawaii, Maine, New Jersey, California, and Montana [the Supreme Court in Montana ruled that the state constitution does not bar medical aid in dying]. This means that medical aid in dying is currently available to about one-fifth of the US population. Medical aid in dying remains illegal in all other states. Internationally, medical aid in dying (and/or euthanasia, the administration a lethal dose of medication by a clinician) is legal in nine countries (the Netherlands, Belgium, Luxembourg, Switzerland, Colombia, Canada, Germany, Japan, and the Australian state of Victoria). Current US state laws permitting medical aid in dying generally require physician certification of a terminal disease with a prognosis of 6 months or less and require the patient be an adult resident of the state, be physically capable of self-administering the medication, and be capable of making and communicating their own health care decisions. Any clinician that participates in medical aid in dying should be familiar with the laws governing its use in their jurisdiction and seek recommendations and help with writing the appropriate prescription.

Most requests for medical aid in dying come from patients with cancer; US patients requesting it are usually male, White, college-educated, and receiving hospice care. Requests for medical aid in dying are relatively rare, and ultimately, use of the prescribed medication led to less than 0.5% of all deaths in the United States. In Oregon, the first US state to legalize medical aid in dying, approximately 0.39% of deaths in 2015 resulted from this practice. In California in 2017, just 0.21% of people who died did so through medical aid in dying. Patient motivations for medical aid in dying generally revolve around preserving dignity, self-respect, and autonomy (control), and maintaining personal connections at the end of life rather than experiencing intolerable pain or suffering. Some patients who have requested medication later withdraw their request when provided palliative care interventions.

Each clinician must decide his or her personal approach in caring for patients who ask about medical aid in dying. Regardless of the clinician's personal feelings about the process, the clinician can respond initially by exploring the patient's reasons and concerns that prompted the request. During the dialog, the clinician should inform the patient about palliative options, including hospice care; access to expert symptom management; and psychological, social, and spiritual support, as needed, and should provide reassurance and commitment to address future problems that may arise. For clinicians who choose not to participate in medical aid in dying, referral to another clinician may be necessary, may be required by law, and may help the patient avoid feeling abandoned. The clinician referred to must be willing to provide the prescription for lethal medication, to care for the patient until death, to sign the death certificate listing the underlying terminal condition as the cause of death, and in some jurisdictions to complete a mandatory follow-up form.

Barsness JG et al. US medical and surgical society position statements on physician-assisted suicide and euthanasia: a review. BMC Med Ethics. 2020;21:111. [PMID: 33143695]

Gruenewald DA et al. Options of last resort: palliative sedation, physician aid in dying, and voluntary cessation of eating and drinking. Med Clin North Am. 2020;104:539. [PMID: 32312414]

Madadin M et al. The Islamic perspective on physician-assisted suicide and euthanasia. Med Sci Law. 2020;60:278. [PMID: 32623956]

Patel T. Clinician responses to legal requests for hastened death: a systematic review and meta-synthesis of qualitative research. BMJ Support Palliat Care. 2021;11:59. [PMID: 32601150]

Ethical & Legal Issues at the End of Life

Clinicians' care of patients at the end of life is guided by the same ethical and legal principles that inform other types of medical care. Foremost among these are (1) truth-telling, (2) nonmaleficence, (3) beneficence, (4) autonomy, (5) confidentiality, and (6) procedural and distributive justice. Important ethical principles may come into conflict when caring for patients. For example, many treatments that promote beneficence and autonomy, such as surgery or bone marrow transplantation, may violate the clinician's obligation for nonmaleficence; thus, balancing the benefits and risks of treatments is a fundamental ethical responsibility. While in most cases clinicians and patients and families will agree on the appropriateness of decisions to withdraw life-sustaining interventions, in rare cases, clinicians may determine *unilaterally* that a particular intervention, such as CPR in multisystem organ failure, offers no possibility of benefit and thus need not be done. In such cases, the clinician's intention to withhold CPR should be communicated to the patient and family and documented, and the clinician must consult with another clinician not involved in the care of the patient. If differences of opinion persist about the appropriateness of particular care decisions, consultation with an institutional ethics committee should be sought. Because such unilateral actions violate the autonomy of the patient, clinicians should *rarely* resort to them. Studies confirm that most disagreements between patients and families and clinicians can be resolved with good communication. Although clinicians and family members often feel differently about withholding versus withdrawing life-sustaining interventions, there is consensus among ethicists, supported by legal precedent, of their ethical equivalence. Regarding the aggressive treatment of pain and other distressing symptoms at the end of life, the ethical principle of **"double effect"** argues that properly informed patients or their surrogates pursuing interventions, even with the potential to hasten imminent death, is acceptable if the negative outcome comes as the known but unintended consequence of a primary intention to provide comfort and relieve suffering.

Arantzamendi M et al. Clinical aspects of palliative sedation in prospective studies. A systematic review. J Pain Symptom Manage. 2021;61:831. [PMID: 32961218]

Chessa F et al. Ethical and legal considerations in end-of-life care. Prim Care. 2019;46:387. [PMID: 31375188]

Ciancio AL et al. The use of palliative sedation to treat existential suffering: a scoping review on practices, ethical considerations, and guidelines. J Palliat Care. 2020;35:13. [PMID: 30757945]

Caring for the Family of Patients at the End of Life

Clinicians must be attuned to the potential impact of illness on the patient's family, including greater physical caregiving responsibilities and financial burdens as well as higher rates of anxiety, depression, chronic illness, and even mortality. The threatened loss of a loved one may create or reveal dysfunctional or painful family dynamics. Family caregivers, most often women, commonly provide the bulk of care for patients at the end of life, yet their work is often not adequately acknowledged, supported, or compensated. Clinicians should recognize that in many cases patients and their families are the unit of care. Simply acknowledging and praising the caregiver can provide much needed and appreciated support.

Clinicians can help families confront the imminent loss of a loved one but often must negotiate amid complex and changing family needs. Identifying a spokesperson for the family, conducting family meetings, allowing all to be heard, and providing time for consensus may help the clinician work effectively with the family. Telemedicine allows family members to participate in medical visits even if they are far away and to communicate with a loved one who is hospitalized, including in the setting of visitation restrictions imposed by COVID-19. Providing good palliative care to the patient can reduce the risk of depression and complicated grief in loved ones after the patient's death. Palliative care support directly to caregivers can prevent or improve caregiver depression.

Durepos P et al. What does death preparedness mean for family caregivers of persons with dementia? Am J Hosp Palliat Care. 2019;36:436. [PMID: 30518228]

Soikkeli-Jalonen A et al. Supportive interventions for family members of very seriously ill patients in inpatient care: a systematic review. J Clin Nurs. 2021;30:2179. [PMID: 33616267]

Clinician Self-Care When Patients Die or Are Dying

Many clinicians find caring for patients at the end of life to be one of the most rewarding aspects of practice. However, working with the dying is also sad and can invoke feelings of grief and loss in clinicians. It has been overwhelming for many in the COVID-19 pandemic. Clinicians must be able to tolerate the uncertainty, ambiguity, and existential challenges of such caregiving. Clinicians also need to recognize and respect their own limitations, attend to their own needs, and work in sustainable health care systems in order to avoid being overburdened, overly distressed, or emotionally depleted.

Horn DJ et al. Burnout and self care for palliative care practitioners. Med Clin North Am. 2020;104:561. [PMID: 32312415]

Imbulana DI et al. Interventions to reduce moral distress in clinicians working in intensive care: a systematic review. Intensive Crit Care Nurs. 2021;66:103092. [PMID: 34147334]

Medisauskaite A et al. Reducing burnout and anxiety among doctors: randomized controlled trial. Psychiatry Res. 2019;274:383. [PMID: 30852432]

Zanatta F et al. Resilience in palliative healthcare professionals: a systematic review. Support Care Cancer. 2020;28:971. [PMID: 31811483]

TASKS AFTER DEATH

After the death of a patient, the clinician is called upon to perform a number of tasks, both required and recommended. The clinician must plainly and directly inform the family of the death, complete a death certificate, contact an organ procurement organization, and request an autopsy. Providing words of sympathy and reassurance, time for questions and initial grief and, for people who die in the hospital or other health care facility, a quiet private room for the family to grieve is appropriate and much appreciated.

The Pronouncement & Death Certificate

In the United States, state policies direct clinicians to confirm the death of a patient in a formal process called "pronouncement." The diagnosis of death is typically easy to make, and the clinician need only verify the absence of spontaneous respirations and cardiac activity by auscultating for each for 1 minute. A note describing these findings, the time of death, and that the family has been notified is entered in the patient's medical record. In many states, when a patient whose death is expected dies outside of the hospital (at home or in prison, for example), nurses may be authorized to report the death over the telephone to a physician who assumes responsibility for signing the death certificate within 24 hours. It is helpful to anticipate a death at home and inform families about what to do. They should be told that the death is not an emergency and that the family can spend time with their loved after death before calling a mortuary. For traumatic deaths, some states allow emergency medical technicians to pronounce a patient dead at the scene based on clearly defined criteria and with physician telephonic or radio supervision.

While the pronouncement may often seem like an awkward and unnecessary formality, clinicians may use this time to reassure the patient's loved ones at the bedside that the patient died peacefully and that all appropriate care had been given. Both clinicians and families may use the ritual of the pronouncement as an opportunity to begin to process emotionally the death of the patient.

Physicians are legally required to report certain deaths to the coroner and to accurately report the underlying cause of death on the death certificate. This reporting is important both for patients' families (for insurance purposes and the need for an accurate family medical history) and for the epidemiologic study of disease and public health. For example, it is important to understand the number of deaths due to COVID-19 and for clinicians to accurately report this cause of death. The physician should be specific about the major cause of death being the condition without which the patient would not have died (eg, "decompensated cirrhosis") and its contributory cause (eg, "hepatitis B and hepatitis C infections, chronic alcoholic hepatitis, and alcoholism") as well as any associated conditions (eg, "acute kidney injury")—and not simply put down "cardiac arrest" as the cause of death. In relevant cases, it is prohibited (in some jurisdictions) to list either "medical aid in dying" (or any synonymous term) or the medications used to accomplish it on the death certificate; instead, the clinician prescribing the lethal dose of medication for this purpose and following the patient until death must (in most jurisdictions) complete and submit a follow-up form and list the cause of death as the underlying condition that led to death.

Hatano Y et al. Physician behavior toward death pronouncement in palliative care units. J Palliat Med. 2018;21:368. [PMID: 28945507]

Autopsy & Organ Donation

Discussing the options and obtaining consent for autopsy and organ donation with patients prior to death is a good practice as it advances the principle of patient autonomy and lessens the responsibilities of distressed family members during the period immediately following the death. In the United States, federal regulations require that a designated representative of an organ procurement organization approach the family about organ donation because designated organ transplant personnel are more experienced and successful than treating clinicians at obtaining consent for organ donation from surviving family members. While most people in the United States support the donation of organs for transplants, organ transplantation is severely limited by the availability of donor organs. The families of donors experience a sense of reward in contributing, even through death, to the lives of others.

The results of an autopsy may help surviving family members and clinicians understand the exact cause of a patient's death and foster a sense of closure. Despite the use of more sophisticated diagnostic tests, the rate of unexpected findings at autopsy has remained stable, and thus, an autopsy can provide important health information to families. Pathologists can perform autopsies without interfering with funeral plans or the appearance of the deceased. A clinician–family conference to review the results of the autopsy provides a good opportunity for clinicians to assess how well families are grieving and to answer questions.

Madi-Segwagwe BC et al. Barriers and facilitators to eye donation in hospice and palliative care settings: a scoping review. Palliat Med Rep. 2021;2:175. [PMID: 34223518]

Follow-Up & Grieving

Proper care of patients at the end of life includes following up with surviving family members after the patient has died. Contacting loved ones by telephone or video telemedicine technology enables the clinician to assuage any guilt about decisions the family may have made, assess how families are grieving, reassure them about the nature of normal grieving, and identify complicated grief or depression. Clinicians can recommend support groups and counseling as needed. A card or telephone call from the clinician to the family days to weeks after the patient's death (and perhaps on the anniversary of the death) allows the clinician to express concern for the family and the deceased. For patients dying during the COVID-19 pandemic, physical closeness, leave-taking, and bereavement rituals have been constrained by the need for social distancing.

After a patient dies, clinicians also grieve. Although clinicians may be relatively unaffected by the deaths of some patients, other deaths may cause feelings of sadness, loss, and guilt. These emotions should be recognized as the first step toward processing and healing them. Each clinician may find personal or communal resources that help with the process of grieving. Shedding tears, sharing with colleagues, taking time for reflection, and engaging in traditional or personal mourning rituals all may be effective. Attending the funeral of a patient who has died can be a satisfying personal experience that is almost universally appreciated by families and that may be the final element in caring well for people at the end of life.

Johannsen M et al. Psychological interventions for grief in adults: a systematic review and meta-analysis of randomized controlled trials. J Affect Disord. 2019;253:69. [PMID: 31029856]

Rabow MW et al. Witnesses and victims both: healthcare workers and grief in the time of COVID-19. J Pain Symptom Manage. 2021;62:647. [PMID: 33556494]

Wallace CL et al. Grief during the COVID-19 pandemic: considerations for palliative care providers. J Pain Symptom Manage. 2020;60:e70. [PMID: 32298748]

PAIN MANAGEMENT

TAXONOMY OF PAIN

The International Association for the Study of Pain (IASP) defines **pain** as "an unpleasant sensory and emotional experience associated with, or resembling that associated with, actual or potential tissue damage." **Acute pain** resolves within the expected period of healing and is self-limited. **Chronic pain** persists beyond the expected period of healing and is itself a disease state. In general, chronic pain is defined as extending beyond 3–6 months, although definitions vary in terms of the time period from initial onset of nociception. **Cancer pain** is in its own special category because of the unique ways neoplasia and its therapies (such as surgery, chemotherapy, immunotherapy or radiation therapy) can lead to burdensome pain. Finally, related to cancer pain, there is **pain at the end of life,** for which measures to alleviate suffering may take priority over promoting restoration of function.

Pain is a worldwide burden; across the globe, one in five adults suffers from pain. In 2010, members from 130 countries signed the Declaration of Montreal stating that access to pain management is a fundamental human right. The first CDC guidelines on opioid prescribing for chronic pain, including chronic noncancer pain, cancer pain, and pain at the end of life, were published in March of 2016, and continue to be updated.

Centers for Disease Control and Prevention (CDC). Opioid Prescribing Guideline Resources. 2021 Feb 16. https://www.cdc.gov/opioids/providers/prescribing/index.html

Dowell D et al. No shortcuts to safer opioid prescribing. N Engl J Med. 2019;380:2285. [PMID: 31018066]

National Institutes of Health (NIH). National Institute on Drug Abuse. Opioid Overdose Crisis. 2021 Mar 11. https://nida.nih.gov/drug-topics/opioids/opioid-overdose-crisis

ACUTE PAIN

Acute pain resolves within the expected period of healing and is self-limited. Common examples include pain from dental caries, kidney stones, surgery, or trauma. Management of acute pain depends on comprehending the type of pain (somatic, visceral, or neuropathic) and on understanding the risks and benefits of potential therapies. At times, treating the underlying cause of the pain (eg, dental caries) may be all that is needed, and pharmacologic therapies may not be required for additional analgesia. On the other hand, not relieving acute pain can have consequences beyond the immediate suffering. Inadequately treated acute pain can develop into chronic pain in some patients. This transition from acute to chronic pain (so-called "chronification" of pain) depends on the pain's cause, type, and severity and on the patient's age, psychological status, and genetics, among other factors. This transition is an area of increasing study because chronic pain leads to significant societal costs beyond the individual's experiences of suffering, helplessness, and depression. Emerging studies have shown that increased intensity and duration of acute pain may be correlated with a higher incidence of chronic pain, and regional anesthesia, ketamine, gabapentinoids, and cyclooxygenase (COX) inhibitors may be helpful for prevention of chronic postsurgical pain. These approaches are particularly important given concerns that exposure to opioids in the perioperative period can lead to chronic opioid dependence.

The Oxford League Table of Analgesics is a useful guide; for example, it lists the number-needed-to-treat for specific doses of various medications to relieve acute pain. NSAIDs or COX inhibitors are at the top of the list, with the lowest number-needed-to-treat. These medications can be delivered via oral, intramuscular, intravenous, intranasal, rectal, transdermal, and other routes of administration. They generally work by inhibiting COX-1 and -2. The primary limitation of the COX inhibitors is their side effects of gastritis; kidney dysfunction; bleeding; hypertension; and cardiovascular adverse events, such as MI or stroke. Ketorolac is primarily a COX-1 inhibitor that has an analgesic effect as potent as morphine at the appropriate dosage. Like most pharmacologic therapies, the limitation of COX inhibitors is that they have a "ceiling" effect, meaning that beyond a certain dose, there is no additional benefit.

Acetaminophen (paracetamol) is effective as a sole agent, or in combination with a COX inhibitor or an opioid in acute pain. Its mechanism of action remains undetermined but is thought to act centrally through mechanisms such as the prostaglandin, serotonergic, and opioid pathways. It is one of the most widely used and best tolerated analgesics; its primary limitation is hepatoxicity when given in high doses or to patients with underlying impaired liver function.

Postoperatively, **patient-controlled analgesia (PCA)** with intravenous morphine, hydromorphone, or another opioid can achieve analgesia faster and with less daily medication requirement than with standard "as needed" or even scheduled intermittent dosing. PCA has been adapted for use with oral analgesic opioid medications and for neuraxial delivery of both opioids and local anesthetics in the epidural and intrathecal spaces. The goal of PCA is to maintain a patient's plasma concentration of opioid in the "therapeutic window," between the minimum effective analgesic concentration and a toxic dose.

In order to prevent opioid use disorder and prolonged inappropriate opioid use, multimodal analgesia (including regional anesthesia) has been employed to decrease the need for postoperative opioids. Patients may undergo either neuraxial anesthesia with an epidural catheter, for example, or regional anesthesia with a nerve block with or without a catheter. These techniques are effective for both intraoperative pain and postoperative pain management and can diminish the need for both intraoperative and postoperative opioids.

Glare P et al. Transition from acute to chronic pain after surgery. Lancet. 2019;393:1537. [PMID: 30983589]

Kandarian BS et al. Updates on multimodal analgesia and regional anesthesia for total knee arthroplasty patients. Best Pract Res Clin Anaesthesiol. 2019;33:111. [PMID: 31272649]

Small C et al. Acute postoperative pain management. Br J Surg. 2020;107:e70. [PMID: 31903595]

Tubog TD. Overview of multimodal analgesia initiated in the perioperative setting. J Perioper Pract. 2021;31:191. [PMID: 32508237]

CHRONIC NONCANCER PAIN

Chronic noncancer pain may begin as acute pain that then fails to resolve and extends beyond the expected period of healing or it may be a primary disease state, rather than the symptom residual from another condition. Common examples of chronic noncancer pain include chronic low-back pain and arthralgias (often somatic in origin), chronic abdominal pain and pelvic pain (often visceral in origin), and chronic headaches, peripheral neuropathy, and postherpetic neuralgia (neuropathic origin). Chronic noncancer pain is common, with the World Health Organization estimating a worldwide prevalence of 20%. In the United States, 11% of adults suffer from chronic noncancer pain.

Chronic noncancer pain requires interdisciplinary management. Generally, no one therapy by itself is sufficient to manage such chronic pain. Physical or functional therapy and cognitive behavioral therapy have been shown to be the most effective for treating chronic noncancer pain, but other modalities including pharmacologic therapy, interventional modalities, and complementary/integrative approaches are useful in caring for affected patients.

Chronic low-back pain, a common chronic noncancer pain, causes more disability globally than any other condition. Chronic low-back pain includes spondylosis, spondylolisthesis, spinal canal stenosis (Chapter 24), and the "failed back surgery syndrome". Also referred to as the post-laminectomy pain syndrome, it can affect 10–40% of patients after lumbar spine surgery.

Evidence-based practice does *not* support the use of prolonged opioid therapy for chronic low-back pain.

Qaseem A et al. Nonpharmacologic and pharmacologic management of acute pain from non-low back, musculoskeletal injuries in adults: a clinical guideline from the American College of Physicians and American Academy of Family Physicians. Ann Intern Med. 2020;173:739. [PMID: 32805126]

Treede RD et al. Chronic pain as a symptom or a disease: the IASP Classification of Chronic Pain for the International Classification of Disease (ICD-11). Pain. 2019;160:19. [PMID: 30586067]

Zhao L et al. Treatment of discogenic low back pain: current treatment strategies and future options—a literature review. Curr Pain Headache Rep. 2019;23:86. [PMID: 31707499]

CANCER PAIN

Cancer pain is unique in cause and in therapies. Cancer pain consists of both acute pain and chronic pain from the neoplasm itself and from the therapies associated with it, such as surgery, chemotherapy, radiation, and immunotherapy. In addition, patients with cancer pain may also have acute or chronic non–cancer-related pain.

Cancer pain includes somatic pain (eg, neoplastic invasion of tissue), visceral pain (eg, painful hepatomegaly from liver metastases), neuropathic pain (eg, neoplastic invasion of sacral nerve roots), or pain from a paraneoplastic syndrome (eg, peripheral neuropathy). Chemotherapy can cause peripheral neuropathies, radiation can cause neuritis or skin allodynia, surgery can cause persistent postsurgical pain, and immunotherapy can cause arthralgias.

Generally, patients with cancer pain may have multiple reasons for pain and thus benefit from a comprehensive and multimodal strategy. The WHO Analgesic Ladder, first published in 1986, suggests starting medication treatment with nonopioid analgesics, then weak opioid agonists, followed by strong opioid agonists. While opioid therapy can be helpful for a majority of patients living with cancer pain, therapy must be individualized depending on the individual patient, their family, and the clinician. For example, if one of the goals of care is to have a lucid and coherent patient, opioids may not be the optimal choice; interventional therapies such as implantable devices may be an option, weighing their risks and costs against their potential benefits. Alternatively, in dying patients, provided there is careful documentation of continued, renewed, or accelerating pain, use of opioid doses exceeding those recommended as standard for acute (postoperative) pain is acceptable.

One of the unique challenges in treating cancer pain is that it is often a "moving target," with disease progression and improvements or worsening pain directly stemming from chemotherapy, radiation, or immunotherapy. Therefore, frequent adjustments may be required to any pharmacologic regimen. Interventional approaches such as celiac plexus neurolysis and intrathecal therapy are well-studied and may be appropriate both for analgesia as well as reduction of side effects from systemic medications. Radiation therapy (including single-fraction external beam treatments) or radionuclide therapy (eg, strontium-89), which aims to decrease the size of both primary and metastatic disease, is one of the unique options for patients with pain from cancer.

Lau J et al. Interventional anesthesia and palliative care collaboration to manage cancer pain: a narrative review. Can J Anaesth. 2020;67:235. [PMID: 31571119]

Magee D et al. Cancer pain: where are we now? Pain Manag. 2019;9:63. [PMID: 30516438]

Swarm RA et al. Adult Cancer Pain, Version 3.2019, NCCN Clinical Practice Guidelines in Oncology. J Natl Compr Canc Netw. 2019;17:977. [PMID: 31390582]

PAIN AT THE END OF LIFE

Pain is what many people say they fear most about dying, and pain at the end of life is consistently undertreated. Up to 75% of patients dying of cancer, heart failure, COPD, AIDS, or other diseases experience pain. In the United States, the Joint Commission includes pain management standards in its reviews of health care organizations and, in 2018, it began mandating that each hospital have a designated leader in pain management.

The ratio of risk versus benefit changes in end-of-life pain management. Harms from the use of opioid analgesics, including death, eg, from respiratory depression (rare), are perhaps less of a concern in patients approaching the end of life. In all cases, clinicians must be prepared to use appropriate doses of opioids in order to relieve this distressing symptom for these patients. Typically, for ongoing cancer pain, a long-acting opioid analgesic can be given around the clock with a short-acting opioid medication as needed for "breakthrough" pain.

PRINCIPLES OF PAIN MANAGEMENT

The experience of pain is unique to each person and influenced by many factors, including the patient's prior experiences with pain, meaning given to the pain, emotional stresses, and family and cultural influences. A brief means of assessing pain and evaluating the effectiveness of analgesia is to ask the patient to rate the degree of pain along a numeric or visual pain scale (Table 5–4), assessing trends over time. Clinicians should ask about the nature, severity, timing, location, quality, and aggravating and relieving factors of the pain.

General guidelines for diagnosis and management of pain are recommended for the treatment of all patients with pain but clinicians must comprehend that such guidelines may not be suited for every individual. Because of pain's complexity, it is important to understand benefits and risks of treatment with growing evidence for each patient. Distinguishing between nociceptive (somatic or visceral) and neuropathic pain is essential to proper management.

In addition, while clinicians should seek to diagnose the underlying cause of pain and then treat it, they must balance the burden of diagnostic tests or therapeutic interventions with the patient's suffering. For example, single-fraction radiation therapy for painful bone metastases or nerve blocks for neuropathic pain may obviate the need for ongoing treatment with analgesics and their side effects. Regardless of decisions about seeking and treating

Table 5–4. Pain assessment scales.

A. Numeric Rating Scale Verbal Intensity		
No pain — Worst pain 0 1 2 3 4 5 6 7 8 9 10		None, mild, moderate, severe (0), (1–4), (5–6), (7–10)
B. Numeric Rating Scale Translated into Word and Behavior Scales		
Pain Intensity	**Word Scale**	**Nonverbal Behaviors**
0	No pain	Relaxed, calm expression
1–2	Least pain	Stressed, tense expression
3–4	Mild pain	Guarded movement, grimacing
5–6	Moderate pain	Moaning, restlessness
7–8	Severe pain	Crying out
9–10	Excruciating pain	Increased intensity of above

C. Wong-Baker FACES Pain Rating Scale[1]

0	1	2	3	4	5
No hurt	Hurts Little Bit	Hurts Little More	Hurts Even More	Hurts Whole Lot	Hurts Worst

[1]Especially useful for patients who cannot read English (and for pediatric patients).

Wong-Baker FACES Foundation (2015). Wong-Baker FACES® Pain Rating Scale. Retrieved with permission from http://www.WongBakerFACES.org.

the underlying cause of pain, every patient should be offered prompt pain relief.

The aim of effective pain management is to meet specific goals, such as preservation or restoration of function or quality of life, and this aim must be discussed between clinician and patient, as well as their family. For example, some patients may wish to be completely free of pain even at the cost of significant sedation, while others will wish to control pain to a level that still allows maximal cognitive functioning.

Whenever possible, the oral route of analgesic administration is preferred because it is easier to manage at home, is not itself painful, and imposes no risk from needle exposure. In unique situations, or near the end of life, transdermal, subcutaneous, rectal, and intravenous routes of administration are used; intrathecal administration is used when necessary.

Finally, pain management should not automatically indicate opioid therapy. While some individuals fare better with opioid therapy in specific situations, this does not mean that opioids are the answer for every patient. There are situations where opioids actually make the quality of life worse for individuals, due to a lack of adequate analgesic effect or due to their side effects.

Barriers to Good Care

One barrier to good pain control is that many clinicians have limited training and clinical experience with pain management and thus are reluctant to attempt to manage severe pain. Lack of knowledge about the proper selection and dosing of analgesic medications carries with it attendant and typically exaggerated fears about the side effects of pain medications. Consultation with a palliative care or a pain management specialist may provide additional expertise.

PHARMACOLOGIC PAIN MANAGEMENT STRATEGIES

Pain generally can be well controlled with nonopioid and opioid analgesic medications, complemented by nonpharmacologic adjunctive and interventional treatments. For mild to moderate pain, acetaminophen, aspirin, and NSAIDs (also known as COX inhibitors) may be sufficient. For moderate to severe pain, especially for those with acute pain, short courses of opioids are sometimes necessary; for those with cancer pain or pain from advanced, progressive serious illness, opioids are generally required and interventional modalities should be considered. In all cases, the choice of an analgesic medication must be guided by careful attention to the physiology of the pain and the benefits and risks of the particular analgesic being considered.

Acetaminophen, Aspirin, Celecoxib, & NSAIDs (COX Inhibitors)

Table 5–5 provides comparison information for acetaminophen, aspirin, the COX-2 inhibitor celecoxib and the NSAIDs. An appropriate dose of acetaminophen may be just as effective an analgesic and antipyretic as an NSAID but without the risk of GI bleeding or ulceration. Acetaminophen can be given at a dosage of 500–1000 mg orally every 6 hours, not to exceed 4000 mg/day maximum for short-term use. Total acetaminophen doses should not exceed 3000 mg/day for long-term use or 2000 mg/day for older patients and for those with liver disease. Hepatotoxicity is of particular concern because of how commonly acetaminophen is also an ingredient in various over-the-counter medications and because of failure to account for the acetaminophen dose in combination acetaminophen-opioid medications such as Vicodin or Norco. The FDA has limited the amount of acetaminophen available in some combination analgesics (eg, in acetaminophen plus codeine preparations).

Aspirin (325–650 mg orally every 4 hours) is an effective analgesic, antipyretic, and anti-inflammatory medication. GI irritation and bleeding are side effects that are lessened with enteric-coated formulations and by concomitant use of PPI medication. Bleeding, allergy, and an association with Reye syndrome in children and adolescents further limit its use.

NSAIDs are antipyretic, analgesic, and anti-inflammatory. Treatment with NSAIDs increases the risk of GI bleeding 1.5 times; the risks of bleeding and nephrotoxicity are both increased in elderly patients. GI bleeding and ulceration may be prevented with either the concurrent use of PPIs (eg, omeprazole, 20–40 mg orally daily) or the use of celecoxib (100 mg orally daily to 200 mg orally twice daily), the only COX-2 inhibitor available. Celecoxib and the NSAIDs can lead to fluid retention, kidney injury, and exacerbations of heart failure and should be used with caution in patients with that condition. Topical formulations of NSAIDs (such as diclofenac 1.3% patch or 1% gel), placed over the painful body part for treatment of musculoskeletal pain, are associated with less systemic absorption and fewer side effects than oral administration and are likely underutilized in patients at risk for GI bleeding.

Noori SA et al. Nonopioid versus opioid agents for chronic neuropathic pain, rheumatoid arthritis pain, cancer pain and low back pain. Pain Manag. 2019;9:205. [PMID: 30681031]

Opioids

A. Background

The 2019 National Health Interview Survey found that 20.5% of all Americans (50.2 million adults) suffer from chronic pain (defined as lasting 3 months or longer), with 11.2% of adults having daily pain. Roughly 20% of Americans who present to a primary care physician with noncancer pain receive a prescription for an opioid. There is moderate level randomized controlled trial evidence that opioids are effective in decreasing noncancer nociceptive pain lasting less than 3 months. However, there is no strong evidence to support use of opioids for management of chronic pain lasting longer than 3 months. The prevalence of opioid use is higher in men, those with chronic pain, those who are younger, and those with multiple prescription medications. One meta-analysis has estimated that in a cohort of patients utilizing opioids for chronic noncancer pain, one-third (36.3%) were doing so in a “problematic” fashion.

Table 5–5. Acetaminophen, aspirin, and useful NSAIDs and COX inhibitors.

Medication (Proprietary)	Usual Dose for Adults Based on Weight	Cost[1]	Comments[2]
Acetaminophen (Ofirmev)	*≥ 50 kg:* 1000 mg intravenously every 6–8 hours	*Per unit:* $24.00 per vial of 1000 mg *For 30 days:* $2880.00	
Acetaminophen or paracetamol[3] (Tylenol, Datril, etc)	*≥ 50 kg:* 325–500 mg orally every 4 hours or 500–1000 mg orally every 6 hours, up to 2000–4000 mg/day *< 50 kg:* 10–15 mg/kg every 4 hours orally; 15–20 mg/kg every 4 hours rectally, up to 2000–3000 mg/day	*Per unit:* $0.02/500 mg (oral) OTC; $0.43/650 mg (rectal) OTC *For 30 days:* $3.60 (oral); $77.40 (rectal)	Not an NSAID because it lacks peripheral anti-inflammatory effects. Equivalent to aspirin as analgesic and antipyretic agent. Limit dose to 4000 mg/day in acute pain, and to 3000 mg/day in chronic pain. Limit doses to 2000 mg/day in older patients and those with liver disease. Be mindful of multiple sources of acetaminophen from combination analgesics, cold remedies, and sleep aids.
Aspirin[4]	*≥ 50 kg:* 325–650 mg orally every 4 hours *< 50 kg:* 10–15 mg/kg every 4 hours orally; 15–20 mg/kg every 4 hours rectally	*Per unit:* $0.02/325 mg OTC; $1.46/300 mg (rectal) OTC *For 30 days:* $7.20 (oral); $525.60 (rectal)	Available also in enteric-coated oral form that is more slowly absorbed but better tolerated.
Celecoxib[3] (Celebrex)	*≥ 50 kg:* 200 mg orally once daily (OA); 100–200 mg orally twice daily (RA) *< 50 kg:* 100 mg orally once or twice daily	*Per unit:* $4.37/100 mg; $7.57/200 mg *For 30 days:* $227.10 OA; $454.20 RA	Cyclooxygenase-2 inhibitor. No antiplatelet effects. Lower doses for elderly who weigh < 50 kg. Lower incidence of endoscopic GI ulceration than NSAIDs. Not known if true lower incidence of GI bleeding. Celecoxib is contraindicated in sulfonamide allergy.
Diclofenac (Flector)	*≥ 50 kg:* 1.3% topical patch applied twice daily	*Per unit:* $14.92/patch *For 30 days:* $895.20	Apply patch to most painful area. Diclofenac 1% gel is available over the counter.
Diclofenac (Voltaren, Cataflam, others)	*≥ 50 kg:* 50–75 mg orally two or three times daily; 1% gel 2–4 g four times daily	*Per unit:* $0.95/50 mg; $1.14/75 mg; $0.52/g gel *For 30 days:* $85.50; $102.60; $249.60 gel	May impose higher risk of hepatotoxicity. Enteric-coated product; slow onset. Topical formulations may result in fewer side effects than oral formulations.
Diclofenac sustained release (Voltaren-XR, others)	*≥ 50 kg:* 100–200 mg orally once daily	*Per unit:* $2.70/100 mg *For 30 days:* $162.00	
Etodolac (Lodine, others)	*≥ 50 kg:* 200–400 mg orally every 6–8 hours	*Per unit:* $1.32/400 mg *For 30 days:* $158.40	
Ibuprofen (Caldolor)	*≥ 50 kg:* 400–800 mg intravenously every 6 hours	*Per unit:* $26.08/800 mg vial *For 30 days:* $3129.60	
Ibuprofen (Motrin, Advil, Rufen, others)	*≥ 50 kg:* 400–800 mg orally every 6 hours *< 50 kg:* 10 mg/kg orally every 6–8 hours	*Per unit:* $0.05/600 mg Rx; $0.02/200 mg OTC *For 30 days:* $6.00; $3.60	Relatively well tolerated and inexpensive.
Indomethacin (Indocin, Indometh, others)	*≥ 50 kg:* 25–50 mg orally two to four times daily	*Per unit:* $0.38/25 mg; $0.64/50 mg *For 30 days:* $45.60; $76.80	Higher incidence of dose-related toxic effects, especially GI and bone marrow effects.
Ketorolac tromethamine	*≥ 50 kg:* 10 mg orally every 4–6 hours to a maximum of 40 mg/day orally	*Per unit:* $2.16/10 mg *For 30 days:* Not recommended	Short-term use (< 5 days) only; otherwise, increased risk of GI side effects.
Ketorolac tromethamine[5]	*≥ 50 kg:* 60 mg intramuscularly or 30 mg intravenously initially, then 30 mg every 6 hours intramuscularly or intravenously	*Per unit:* $1.19/30 mg *For 30 days:* Not recommended	Intramuscular or intravenous NSAID as alternative to opioid. Lower doses for elderly. Short-term use (< 5 days) only.

(*continued*)

Table 5–5. Acetaminophen, aspirin, and useful NSAIDs and COX inhibitors. (continued)

Medication (Proprietary)	Usual Dose for Adults Based on Weight	Cost[1]	Comments[2]
Magnesium salicylate (various)	*≥ 50 kg:* 325–650 mg orally every 6 hours	*Per unit:* $0.25/325 mg OTC *For 30 days:* $60.00	
Meloxicam (Mobic)	*≥ 50 kg:* 7.5 mg orally every 12 hours	*Per unit:* $2.78/7.5 mg *For 30 days:* $166.80	Intermediate COX-2/COX-1 ratio similar to diclofenac.
Nabumetone (Relafen)	*≥ 50 kg:* 500–1000 mg orally once daily (max dose 2000 mg/day)	*Per unit:* $0.78/500 mg; $0.82/750 mg *For 30 days:* $46.80; $49.20	May be less ulcerogenic than ibuprofen, but overall side effects may not be less.
Naproxen (Naprosyn, Anaprox, Aleve [OTC], others)	*≥ 50 kg:* 250–500 mg orally every 6–8 hours *< 50 kg:* 5 mg/kg every 8 hours	*Per unit:* $1.26/500 mg Rx; $0.04/220 mg OTC *For 30 days:* $151.20; $3.60 OTC	Generally well tolerated. Lower doses for elderly.

OA, osteoarthritis; OTC, over the counter; RA, rheumatoid arthritis, Rx, prescription.
[1]Average wholesale price (AWP, for AB-rated generic when available) for quantity listed. Source: IIBM Micromedex® Red Book (electronic version). IBM Watson Health. Greenwood Village, Colorado, USA. Available at https://www-micromedexsolutions-com.proxy.hsl.ucdenver.edu/(cited March 11, 2022). AWP may not accurately represent the actual pharmacy cost because wide contractual variations exist among institutions.
[2]The adverse effects of headache, tinnitus, dizziness, confusion, rashes, anorexia, nausea, vomiting, gastrointestinal bleeding, diarrhea, nephrotoxicity, visual disturbances, etc, can occur with any of these drugs. Tolerance and efficacy are subject to great individual variations among patients. Note: All NSAIDs can increase serum lithium levels.
[3]Acetaminophen and celecoxib lack antiplatelet effects.
[4]May inhibit platelet aggregation for 1 week or more and may cause bleeding.
[5]Has the same gastrointestinal toxicities as oral NSAIDs.

Since its beginning in the 1990s, an epidemic of opioid use and opioid overdose deaths has emerged to be a critical public health crisis in the United States. Based on provisional data from the CDC's National Center for Health Statistics, there were an estimated 100,306 overdose deaths in the United States in the 12-month period preceding April 2021; of these, 78,673 were attributed to opioids. There was a roughly 28.5% increase in overdose deaths when compared to the previous year. Among patients who are prescribed long-term opioid therapy, between 2% and 6% develop a substance use disorder. Roughly 11.7% of patients over the age of 12 have used an illicit drug in the last month.

Interestingly, the contribution of opioids to overdose deaths has changed over time and has been characterized by three "waves." In 1999, most opioid-related overdose deaths were attributed to prescription opioids ("wave 1"), but in 2010 there was a marked increase in heroin-related deaths ("wave 2"), and finally in 2013 there was a dramatic increase in synthetic opioid-related deaths ("wave 3").

Since 2010, the percentage of opioid overdose deaths associated with opioid prescriptions has steadily declined, and in 2019, only 28% of all opioid overdose deaths were associated with prescriptions. Instead, a massive increase in the illicit production of synthetic fentanyl (fentanyl and fentanyl analogs—either prescribed or illicitly manufactured and sold as counterfeit tablets or heroin) largely contributed to the third wave. From 2013 to 2019, the CDC reported a 1040% increase in synthetic opioid involved death rate; roughly half of overdose deaths in 2019 were attributed to synthetic opioids.

Population-based studies have also demonstrated that a sharp increase in concurrent opioid and benzodiazepine use which has led to an increase in the overall risk of opioid overdose.

Sadly, a "fourth wave" of high opioid overdose–related mortality is anticipated, driven by a foundation of illicit synthetic fentanyl and synergized with increasing methamphetamine and cocaine use, as well as the psychosocial stress of the COVID-19 pandemic.

Centers for Disease Control and Prevention (CDC). National Center for Health Statistics. Illicit Drug Use. 2022 Jan 27. https://www.cdc.gov/nchs/fastats/drug-use-illicit.htm
Centers for Disease Control and Prevention (CDC). National Center for Health Statistics. Provisional Drug Overdose Death Counts. 2022 Feb 16. https://www.cdc.gov/nchs/nvss/vsrr/drug-overdose-data.htm
Centers for Disease Control and Prevention (CDC). Opioid Prescribing Guideline Resources. 2021 Feb 16. https://www.cdc.gov/opioids/providers/prescribing/index.html
Centers for Disease Control and Prevention (CDC). Prescription Opioid Overdose Death Maps. 2021 Mar 24. https://www.cdc.gov/drugoverdose/deaths/prescription/maps.html
Ciccarone D. The rise of illicit fentanyls, stimulants and the fourth wave of the opioid overdose crisis. Curr Opin Psychiatry. 2021;34:344. [PMID: 33965972]
Jantarada C et al. Prevalence of problematic use of opioids in patients with chronic noncancer pain: a systematic review with meta-analysis. Pain Pract. 2021;21:715. [PMID: 33528858]
Mattson CL et al. Trends and geographic patterns in drug and synthetic opioid overdose deaths—United States, 2013–2019. MMWR Morb Mortal Wkly Rep. 2021;70:202. [PMID: 33571180]
Yong RJ et al. Prevalence of chronic pain among adults in the United States. Pain. 2022;163:e328. [PMID: 33990113]

B. Opioid Metabolism

Opioid medications mimic the pharmacologic properties of endogenous opioid peptides and activate the primary opioid receptors (mu, delta, and kappa). Additionally, the different opioid medications activate the different opioid receptors to varying degrees. Any substance that causes analgesia via binding an opioid receptor and is reversed by naloxone is referred to as an "opioid." This broad class of drugs include alkaloids derived from the extract of a poppy plant (codeine and morphine) or synthetic peptides, both phenylpiperidines (eg, meperidine, fentanyl) and pseudopiperidines (eg, methadone).

Opioids are primarily metabolized by the liver via phase I (cytochrome P450 isoenzyme 3A4 and 2D6) and phase II (glucuronidation) processes. With advanced age, the following changes occur: hepatic blood flow decreases, systemic clearance of drugs decreases, elimination half-life increases, and the pharmacologic effect becomes longer. Such age-related changes in hepatic function predispose older individuals to adverse side effects from opioids, including delirium, falls, fractures, and respiratory depression. This predisposition seems to be dose-dependent—for example, individuals using greater than 50 oral morphine equivalents per day are twice as likely to suffer a fracture than those using less.

Opioid metabolism is also affected by kidney function. GFR typically decreases with age and a decrease in GFR can lead to an accumulation of active metabolites and consequent toxicity. For example, meperidine is metabolized to normeperidine and its accumulation results in neurotoxicity (seizures). Meperidine use should be avoided in older adults.

Therefore, clinicians should "start low and go slow," particularly in patients with older age, liver disease, decreased kidney function, and higher total body fat, when initiating opioid therapy. In addition, initially prescribing immediate-release opioid formulations is more desirable since these agents can be titrated down more rapidly in case of adverse reactions.

James A et al. Basic opioid pharmacology—an update. Br J Pain. 2020;14:115. [PMID: 32537150]

C. Principles of Opioid Management

Patients who suffer from opioid **addiction** continue to use the drug despite incurring harm. Often they are unable to fulfill work obligations or social roles yet they cannot control or decrease their opioid usage. Patients with opioid **pseudoaddiction** run out of their medication early and experience withdrawal symptoms. These patients are often undertreated but respond well to medication adjustment and typically do not require dose escalation once their medications are refilled on time correctly. Patients with opioid **dependence** have withdrawal symptoms with a rapid decrease or a stoppage of their opioid dosage. Patients afflicted with opioid **abuse** take the drug illicitly to obtain a "high" rather than for an analgesic or other medicinal purpose. Patients who have developed opioid **tolerance** have a decreased response to an opioid agonist with repeated use and will typically require increased dosages to achieve the same effect. Finally, utilization of high dosages of opioids over time can result in opioid-induced **hyperalgesia** (enhanced pain to noxious stimuli) and **allodynia** (pain from stimuli which typically do not provoke pain).

Once the decision has been made to prescribe an opioid, one of the initial challenges that a clinician may have is what dose to prescribe an opioid-naïve patient. Unlike most drugs, opioids have no ceiling effect for analgesia and a strategy for the management of future tolerance should be identified at the beginning. It is critical to calculate and understand the morphine milligram equivalent (MME) dose since adverse effects from opioids are dose-dependent (Table 5–6).

Table 5–6. Morphine milligram equivalent (MME) doses for commonly prescribed opioids.

Opioid	Conversion Factor
Morphine	1
Codeine	0.15
Fentanyl transdermal (in mcg/h)	2.4
Hydrocodone	1
Hydromorphone	4
Methadone	
1–20 mg/day	4
21–40 mg/day	8
41–60 mg/day	10
≥ 61–80 mg/day	12
Oxycodone	1.5
Oxymorphone	3

TO CALCULATE MMEs: Multiply the dose for each opioid by the conversion factor to determine the dose in MMEs. As an example: tablets containing hydrocodone 5 mg and acetaminophen 300 mg taken four times a day would contain a total of 20 mg of hydrocodone daily, equivalent to 20 × 1 = 20 MME daily. Or another example: Extended-release tablets containing oxycodone 10 mg taken twice a day contain a total of 20 mg of oxycodone daily, equivalent to 20 × 1.5 = 30 MME daily.

Note the following precautions: (1) All doses are in mg/day except for fentanyl, which is in mcg/hour. (2) Equianalgesic dose conversions are only estimates and cannot account for individual variability in genetics and pharmacokinetics. (3) Do not use the calculated dose in MMEs to determine the doses to use when converting one opioid to another; when converting opioids, the new opioid is typically dosed at a substantially lower dose than the calculated MME dose to avoid accidental overdose due to incomplete cross-tolerance and individual variability in opioid pharmacokinetics. (4) Use particular caution with methadone dose conversions because the conversion factor increases at higher doses. (5) Use particular caution with fentanyl because it is dosed in mcg/hour instead of mg/day, and its absorption is affected by heat and other factors.

From Dowell D et al. CDC guideline for prescribing opioids for chronic pain—United States, 2016. MMWR Recomm Rep. 2016;65(No. RR-1):1. [PMID: 26987082]. Adapted by the CDC from Von Korff M et al. De Facto long-term opioid therapy for noncancer pain. Clin J Pain. 2008;24:521 and Washington State Interagency Guideline on Prescribing Opioids for Pain. (http://www.agencymeddirectors.wa.gov/Files/2015AMDGO pioidGuideline.pdf) and from Yaksh T et al. Table 20-8. Opioids, Analgesia, and Pain Management. In: Brunton LL et al (editors). *Goodman & Gilman's: The Pharmacological Basis of Therapeutics, 13e.* McGraw Hill, 2018. Accessed November 22, 2021.

Adverse events are proportionately related to higher dosages. A population-based study that analyzed 607,156 patients prescribed opioids characterized the relationship between opioid dose and opioid overdose–related mortality. The adjusted OR for opioid overdose–related death increased from 1.32 (0.94–1.84) for patients prescribed between 20 and 50 MME/day to 1.92 (1.30–2.85) for those prescribed between 50 and 99 MME/day. In the same study, patients prescribed 200 MME/day or more had an OR of 2.88 (1.79–4.63) or a nearly threefold increase in the likelihood of death related to opioid overdose.

In other studies, rates of opioid abuse or dependence on long-term opioid therapy have ranged from 0.7% for patients prescribed 36 MME/day or less to 6.1% for those prescribed 120 MME/day or more. Prescribers must therefore remember that the risks of opioid overdose–related mortality substantially increases with dosages 50 MME/day or more. By contrast, studies have shown that initial opioid prescriptions for opioid-naïve patients of less than 50 MME/day have decreased risks of opioid overdose–related death. Recommended initial opioid dosing of selected opioid medications are shown in Table 5–7.

A particular challenge for clinicians is the management of the patient who presents in follow-up with inadequate pain control after the initial opioid prescription. Dose escalation performed within the first year of prescription has been associated with higher rates of substance abuse and more frequent non–face-to-face encounters. Men are at higher risk for dose escalation and opioid-related death than women. Dose escalation also increases the risk of overdose and subsequent development of opioid use disorder. Patients taking an MME dose of 200/day or more are at a particularly high risk for death from overdose.

Prescribers must therefore keep in mind that opioid overdose risk is dose dependent. Options for the patient with inadequate pain control after an initial opioid prescription include (1) increase the dosage, (2) use an extended-release version of the same drug with immediate-release medication for "breakthrough" pain, (3) add an adjuvant analgesic (eg, a muscle relaxant) or NSAID, (4) perform an opioid rotation, or (5) refer to a pain management specialist.

Once tolerance develops, clinicians who use only one opioid at a time (eg, morphine extended-release coupled with morphine immediate-release) can readily switch to an alternative opioid. In contrast, clinicians who use multiple different opioid agents (eg, morphine extended-release coupled with hydromorphone for breakthrough pain) have already used drugs targeting multiple opioid subreceptors at the same time and therefore have limited future possible opioid rotations once tolerance develops. Nonetheless, it is far more desirable to perform an opioid rotation than to escalate the dosage, which may result in adverse side effects (respiratory depression, constipation, urinary hesitancy, etc). Dose escalation is further undesirable as it may contribute to opioid-induced hyperalgesia, complicating future treatments and response to analgesics.

Clinicians must also carefully characterize the temporal patterns of pain when prescribing opioids. The astute clinician should discriminate between acute or "incident related" pain (pain experienced with activity but not at rest) and chronic pain (occurs at rest). Those with acute pain may be a better candidate for an immediate-release opioid formulation. Most opioid prescriptions (greater than 97%) are for immediate-release formulations; chronic pain patients are more likely to be prescribed extended-release formulations. However, patients who are prescribed extended-release opioids for their initial prescriptions have a higher risk of overdose compared to those prescribed immediate-release opioids.

Extended-release formulations offer a more convenient method of dosing, have a prolonged peak therapeutic drug range, less plasma level fluctuations, and improved compliance. Both extended- and immediate-release formulations pose significant risk of misuse and abuse. Reported immediate-release abuse has been linked to the perceived immediacy of relief. However, immediate-release formulations are easier to titrate and wean and seem a simpler choice when initiating an opioid prescription in opioid-naïve patients. Regardless of the final choice of agent, clinicians should characterize the temporal patterns of the pain and weigh the pros and cons of immediate- versus extended-release preparations. Key factors in the final choice include the length of the treatment plan, the minimally adequate MME dose, and the proposed length of opioid treatment.

Currently, there is no high-level evidence that supports the use of opioids in the long-term management of neuropathic pain. Instead, opioids have been found to have significantly more adverse effects when compared to neuropathic medications (Table 5–8).

Cuménal M et al. The safety of medications used to treat peripheral neuropathic pain, Part 2 (opioids, cannabinoids, and other drugs): review of double-blind, placebo-controlled, randomized clinical trials. Expert Opin Drug Saf. 2021;20:51. [PMID: 33103931]

Nalamachu SR et al. Abuse of immediate-release opioids and current approaches to reduce misuse, abuse, and diversion. Postgrad Med. 2018;1. [PMID: 30025214]

D. Adverse Effects of Opioids

Common adverse effects of opioids include constipation, nausea, sedation, pruritus, sexual dysfunction (especially hypogonadism in men), respiratory depression, and CNS depression. Core strategies to decrease adverse effects include performing an opioid rotation, dose reduction, change in route of administration (eg, from oral to transdermal), and symptom management.

Opioid-induced respiratory depression constitutes a medical emergency and must be managed appropriately. Though potentially fatal, it can be rapidly reversed by the opioid receptor antagonist, naloxone. There is moderate evidence that naloxone, when administered appropriately, can decrease opioid overdose–related mortality. However, out-of-hospital naloxone use is linked with opioid withdrawal syndrome. Naloxone-induced withdrawal can lead to cardiovascular events (increases in heart rate, mean arterial pressure, and cardiac index) as well as to pulmonary edema. Despite the risk, the CDC recommends coprescribing

Table 5–7. Opioids.

Medication (Proprietary)	Routes of Administration and Available Doses	Approximate Equianalgesic Dose (compared to morphine 30 mg orally or 10 mg intravenously/ subcutaneously)[1]	Usual Starting Dose in an Opioid-Naïve Patient Based on Weight	Cost
Opioid Agonists[2,3]				
Buprenorphine (Buprenex)[4]	*Parenteral* (intravenous, intramuscular)	300 mcg intravenously slowly once, may be repeated after 30–60 minutes once; or 600 mcg intramuscularly once	≥ *50 kg:* 300 mcg intravenously slowly once, may be repeated after 30–60 minutes once; or 600 mcg intramuscularly once	$14.77/300 mcg
Buprenorphine (Butrans)	*Transdermal:* 5, 7.5, 10, 15, and 20 mcg/h	Not available	≥ *50 kg:* Initiate 5 mcg/h patch for opioid-naïve patients (may currently be using nonopioid analgesics)	$114.77/10 mcg/h
Buprenorphine (Belbuca)	*Sublingual strips:* 75 mcg, 150 mcg, 300 mcg, 450 mcg, 600 mcg, 750 mcg, 900 mcg	Not available	≥ *50 kg:* In opioid-naive or opioid-intolerant patients, individualize dose every 12 h. Start: 75 mcg buccally every 12–24 hours for at least 4 days, then increase to 150 mcg buccally every 12 hours, then may increase by no more than 150 mcg buccally every 12 hours no more frequently than every 4 days. Maximum: 900 mcg/12 hours	$7.69/75 mcg
Fentanyl	*Parenteral* (intravenous, intramuscular): 50 mcg/mL	*Parenteral:* 100 mcg every hour	≥ *50 kg:* 50–100 mcg intravenously/intramuscularly every hour or 0.5–1.5 mcg/kg/h intravenous infusion < *50 kg:* 0.5–1 mcg/kg intravenously every 1–4 hours or 1–2 mcg/kg intravenously × 1, then 0.5–1 mcg/kg/h infusion	$0.80/100 mcg
Fentanyl (Actiq)	*Transmucosal strips:* 200 mcg, 400 mcg, 600 mcg, 800 mcg, 1200 mcg	Not available	*Initial dose:* ≥ *50 kg:* 200 mcg	$18.80/200 mcg
Fentanyl (Fentora)	*Buccal:* 100 mcg, 200 mcg, 400 mcg, 600 mcg, 800 mcg	Not available	*Initial dose:* ≥ *50 kg:* 100 mcg	$103.90/200 mcg
Fentanyl (Duragesic)	*Transdermal:* 12.5 mcg/h, 25 mcg/h, 37.5 mcg/h, 50 mcg/h, 62.5 mcg/h, 75 mcg/h, 87.5 mcg/h, 100 mcg/h	Conversion to fentanyl patch is based on total daily dose of oral morphine:[2] morphine 60–134 mg/day orally = fentanyl 25 mcg/h patch; morphine 135–224 mg/day orally = fentanyl 50 mcg/h patch; morphine 225–314 mg/day orally = fentanyl 75 mcg/h patch; and morphine 315–404 mg/day orally = fentanyl 100 mcg/h patch	*Initial doses:* ≥ *50 kg:* 12.5–25 mcg/h patch every 72 hours < *50 kg:* 12.5–25 mcg/h patch every 72 hours	$14.42/25 mcg/h

(*continued*)

Table 5–7. Opioids. (continued)

Medication (Proprietary)	Routes of Administration and Available Doses	Approximate Equianalgesic Dose (compared to morphine 30 mg orally or 10 mg intravenously/ subcutaneously)[1]	Usual Starting Dose in an Opioid-Naïve Patient Based on Weight	Cost
Hydromorphone[5] (Dilaudid)	*Oral:* 2 mg, 4 mg, 8 mg	*Oral:* 7.5 mg every 3–4 hours	*Oral:* ≥ *50 kg:* 1–2 mg every 3–4 hours < *50 kg:* 0.06 mg every 3–4 hours	$0.11/2 mg
	Parenteral (intravenous, intramuscular, subcutaneous): 0.5 mg/0.5 mL, 1 mg/mL, 2 mg/mL, 4 mg/mL	*Parenteral:* 1.5 mg every 3–4 hours	*Parenteral:* ≥ *50 kg:* 1.5 mg every 3–4 hours < *50 kg:* 0.015 mg/kg every 3–4 hours	$1.90/2 mg
Hydromorphone extended release	*Oral:* 8 mg ER, 12 mg ER, 16 mg ER, 32 mg ER	*Oral:* 45–60 mg ER every 24 hours	*Oral, initial dose:* ≥ *50 kg:* 8 mg ER every 24 hours	$9.24/8 mg
Levorphanol	*Oral:* 2 mg	*Oral:* 4 mg every 6–8 hours	*Oral, initial dose:* ≥ *50 kg:* 1–2 mg every 6–8 hours < *50 kg:* 0.04 mg/kg every 6–8 hours	$53.40/2 mg
Meperidine[6] (Demerol)	*Oral:* 50 mg, 100 mg	*Oral:* 300 mg every 2–3 hours; usual dose 50–150 mg every 3–4 hours	*Oral:* Not recommended	$5.22/100 mg
	Parenteral (intravenous, intramuscular, subcutaneous): 25 mg/mL, 50 mg/mL, 75 mg/mL, 100 mg/mL	*Parenteral:* 100 mg every 3 hours	*Parenteral:* ≥ *50 kg:* 50–100 mg every 3 hours; not to exceed 600 mg/24 h < *50 kg:* 0.75 mg/kg every 2–3 hours	$7.68/100 mg
Methadone (Dolophine, others)	*Oral:* 5 mg, 10 mg	*Oral:* 10–20 mg every 6–8 hours (when converting from < 100 mg long-term daily oral morphine[7])	*Oral, initial dose:* ≥ *50 kg:* 2.5–20 mg every 8–12 hours < *50 kg:* 0.2 mg/kg every 8–12 hours	$0.10/10 mg
	Parenteral: 10 mg/mL	*Parenteral:* 5–10 mg every 6–8 hours	*Parenteral:* ≥ *50 kg:* 2.5–10 mg every 6–8 hours < *50 kg:* 0.1 mg/kg every 6–8 hours	$21.00/10 mg
Morphine[5] immediate release (morphine sulfate, various)	*Oral:* 15 mg, 30 mg (tablets); 10 mg/5mL, 20 mg/5 mL, 100 mg/5 mL (solution) *Rectal:* 5 mg, 10 mg, 20 mg, 30 mg (suppositories)	*Oral:* 30 mg every 3–4 hours (around-the-clock dosing); 60 mg every 3–4 hours (single or intermittent dosing) *Rectal:* 10–20 mg per rectum every 4 hours	*Oral:* ≥ *50 kg:* 4–8 mg every 3–4 hours; used for breakthrough pain in patients already taking controlled-release preparations < *50 kg:* 0.3 mg/kg every 3–4 hours	$0.49/15 mg tablet; $0.84/20 mg oral solution
		Parenteral: 10 mg every 3–4 hours	*Parenteral:* ≥ *50 kg:* 10 mg every 3–4 hours < *50 kg:* 0.1 mg/kg every 3–4 hours	$4.89/10 mg
Morphine controlled release (MS Contin)	*Oral (tablets):* 15 mg ER, 30 mg ER, 60 mg ER, 100 mg ER, 200 mg ER	*Oral:* 90–120 mg ER every 12 hours	*Oral, initial dose:* ≥ *50 kg:* 15–60 mg ER every 8–12 hours	$0.73/30 mg
Morphine extended release (Kadian)	*Oral (capsules):* 10 mg ER, 20 mg ER, 30 mg ER, 40 mg ER, 50 mg ER, 60 mg ER, 80 mg ER, 100 mg ER, 200 mg ER	*Oral:* 180–240 mg ER every 24 hours	*Oral, initial dose:* ≥ *50 kg:* 30 mg ER every 24 hours	$5.69/30 mg

Oxycodone (Roxicodone, OXYIR)	*Oral:* *(capsules):* 5 mg IR *(tablets):* 5 mg IR, 10 mg IR, 15 mg IR, 20 mg IR, 30 mg IR	*Oral:* 20–30 mg every 3–4 hours	*Oral, initial dose:* ≥ *50 kg:* 5–10 mg every 3–4 hours < *50 kg:* 0.2 mg/kg every 3–4 hours	$0.08/5 mg
Oxycodone controlled release (Oxycontin)	*Oral:* *(tablets):* 10 mg ER, 15 mg ER, 20 mg ER, 30 mg ER, 40 mg ER, 60 mg ER, 80 mg ER *(solution):* 5 mg/mL, 100 mg/mL	*Oral:* 40 mg ER every 12 hours	*Oral, initial dose:* > *50 kg:* 10–40 mg ER every 12 hours	$10.43/20 mg
Oxycodone ER tamper-resistant capsules (Xtampza ER)	*Oral (capsules):* 9 mg ER, 13.5 mg ER, 18 mg ER, 27 mg ER, 36 mg ER	*Oral*: 36 mg every 12 hours	*Oral, initial dose:* 9 mg ER every 12 hours	$13.25/18 mg
Oxymorphone[5,8] oral, immediate release	*Oral (tablets):* 5 mg, 10 mg	*Oral:* 10 mg every 6 hours	*Oral, initial dose:* ≥ *50 kg:* 10–20 mg every 6 hours	$0.39/5 mg
Oxymorphone[5,8] oral, extended release	*Oral (tablets):* 5 mg ER, 7.5 mg ER, 10 mg ER, 15 mg ER, 20 mg ER, 30 mg ER, 40 mg ER	*Oral:* 30 mg every 12 hours	*Oral, initial dose:* ≥ *50 kg:* 5 mg ER orally every 12 hours	$14.88/20 mg
Combination Opioid Agonist–Nonopioid Preparations				
Codeine[9,10] (with acetaminophen or aspirin)	*Oral (tablets):* Acetaminophen with codeine phosphate (Tylenol #3) 300 mg/30 mg Acetaminophen with codeine phosphate (Tylenol #4) 300 mg/60 mg Aspirin 325 mg/codeine phosphate 30 mg Aspirin 325/codeine phosphate 60 mg	Not used secondary to acetaminophen or aspirin containing component	*Oral:* ≥ *50 kg:* 60 mg codeine phosphate every 4–6 hours < *50 kg:* 0.5–1 mg/kg every 3–4 hours	$0.64/60 mg
		Parenteral: 130 mg every 3–4 hours	*Parenteral:* ≥ *50 kg:* 60 mg codeine phosphate every 2 hours intramuscularly/subcutaneously; not available in the United States < *50 kg:* Not recommended	Not available in the United States
Hydrocodone[8] (with acetaminophen in Lortab)[11]	*Oral (solution):* 10 mg/300 mg per 15 mL *Oral (tablets):* 2.5 mg/325 mg, 5 mg/325 mg, 7.5 mg/325 mg, 10 mg/325 mg	Not used secondary to acetaminophen component	*Oral:* ≥ *50 kg:* 10 mg every 3–4 hours < *50 kg:* 0.2 mg/kg every 3–4 hours	$0.41/5 mg
Oxycodone (with acetaminophen)[10,11]	*Oral (tablets):* 2.5 mg/325 mg, 5 mg/325 mg, 7.5 mg/325 mg, 10 mg/325 mg	Not used secondary to acetaminophen component	*Oral, initial dose:* ≥ *50 kg:* 5–10 mg every 3–4 hours < *50 kg:* 0.2 mg/kg every 3–4 hours	$0.08/5 mg
Combination Opioid Agonist–Norepinephrine Reuptake Inhibitor Preparations				
Tapentadol (Nucynta)	*Oral (tablets):* 50 mg, 75 mg, 100 mg	Not available; use starting doses	*Oral, initial doses:* ≥ *50 kg:* Start 50–100 mg once, may repeat dose in 1 hour. Can increase to 50–100 mg every 4 hours. Maximum daily dose 600 mg	$14.36/100 mg

(*continued*)

Table 5–7. Opioids. (continued)

Medication (Proprietary)	Routes of Administration and Available Doses	Approximate Equianalgesic Dose (compared to morphine 30 mg orally or 10 mg intravenously/ subcutaneously)[1]	Usual Starting Dose in an Opioid-Naïve Patient Based on Weight	Cost
Tapentadol, extended release (Nucynta ER)	*Oral:* 50 mg ER, 100 mg ER, 150 mg ER, 200 mg ER, 250 mg ER	Not available; use starting doses	*Oral:* ≥ *50 kg:* Start 50 mg ER every 12 hours. Can increase by 50-mg increments twice daily every 3 days to dose of 100–250 mg ER twice daily	$16.71/100 mg
Tramadol	*Oral (tablets):* 50 mg, 100 mg	Not available	*Oral, initial dose:* ≥ *50 kg:* Start 25 mg orally daily. Can increase by 25 mg every 3 days to 25 mg orally 4 times daily, then may increase by 50 mg/day every 3 days to 100 mg orally 4 times daily. Limit of 300 mg/day in patients > 75 years old	$0.83/50 mg
Tramadol extended release (Conzip ER capsules)	*Oral (tablets):* 100 mg ER, 200 mg ER, 300 mg ER	Not available	*Oral, initial dose:* ≥ *50 kg:* 100 mg ER orally once daily, may titrate up by 100 mg increments every 5 days, max 300 mg	$19.35/200 mg

[1]Published tables vary in the suggested doses that are equianalgesic to morphine. Clinical response is the criterion that must be applied for each patient; titration to clinical efficacy is necessary. Because there is not complete cross-tolerance among these drugs, it is usually necessary to use a lower than equianalgesic dose initially when changing drugs and to retitrate to response.

[2]Conversion is conservative; therefore, do not use these equianalgesic doses for converting back from fentanyl patch to other opioids because they may lead to inadvertent overdose. Patients may require breakthrough doses of short-acting opioids during conversion to transdermal fentanyl.

[3]Several significantly more potent formulations of buprenorphine are available but generally reserved for the treatment of opioid use disorder with or without comorbid constant pain, most often by pain management specialists: a sublingual tablet (Subutex and others) or a sublingual film (Suboxone and others) in which the buprenorphine is combined with naloxone; a subdermal implant of buprenorphine alone (Probuphine); and a subcutaneous depot injection (Sublocade). Each of these is used in maintenance treatment to reduce problematic use of other opioids. See text.

[4]In opioid-experienced patients, taper current opioids to 30 mg/day oral morphine equivalent prior to starting buprenorphine. Thereafter, buprenorphine dosing schedule depends on prior current oral morphine equivalent:

< 30 mg/day, 75 mcg buccally every 12 hours;
30–89 mg/day, 150 mcg buccally every 12 hours;
90–160 mg/day, 300 mcg buccally every 12 hours;

In all patients, use same dose escalation and maximum dose as shown for opioid-naïve patients.

[5]*Caution:* For morphine, hydromorphone, and oxymorphone, rectal administration is an alternative route for patients unable to take oral medications. Equianalgesic doses may differ from oral and parenteral doses. A short-acting opioid should normally be used for initial therapy.

[6]Not recommended for chronic pain. Doses listed are for brief therapy of acute pain only. Switch to another opioid for long-term therapy.

[7]Methadone conversion varies depending on the equivalent total daily dose of morphine. Consult with a pain management or palliative care expert for conversion.

[8]*Caution:* Recommended doses do not apply to adult patients with kidney or liver impairment or other conditions affecting drug metabolism.

[9]*Caution:* Individual doses of codeine above 60 mg often are not appropriate because of diminishing incremental analgesia with increasing doses but continually increasing nausea, constipation, and other side effects.

[10]*Caution:* Doses of aspirin and acetaminophen in combination products must also be adjusted to the patient's body weight.

[11]*Caution:* Monitor total acetaminophen dose carefully, including any OTC use. Total acetaminophen dose maximum 3 g/day. If liver impairment or heavy alcohol use, maximum is 2 g/day. Available dosing formulations of these combination medications are being adjusted to reflect increased caution about acetaminophen toxicity. Acetaminophen doses in a single combination tablet or capsule will be limited to no more than 325 mg.

Note: Average wholesale price (AWP, generic when available) for quantity listed. Source: IBM Micromedex® Red Book (electronic version) IBM Watson Health. Greenwood Village, Colorado, USA. Available at https://www-micromedexsolutions-com.proxy.hsl.ucdenver.edu/ (cited March 15,2022). AWP may not accurately represent the actual pharmacy cost because wide contractual variations exist among institutions.

Table 5–8. Pharmacologic management of neuropathic pain.

Medication[1]	Starting Dose	Typical Dose
Antidepressants[2]		
Nortriptyline	10 mg orally at bedtime	10–150 mg orally at bedtime
Amitriptyline	10 mg orally at bedtime	10–150 mg orally at bedtime
Desipramine	12.5 mg orally at bedtime	12.5–250 mg orally at bedtime (can be divided into two doses)
Calcium Channel Alpha2-Delta Ligands		
Gabapentin[3]	100–300 mg orally once to three times daily	300–1200 mg orally three times daily
Pregabalin[4]	50 mg orally three times daily	50–150 mg orally three times daily
Selective Serotonin Norepinephrine Reuptake Inhibitors		
Duloxetine	30–60 mg orally daily or 20 mg orally twice daily in elders	60–120 mg orally daily
Venlafaxine[5]	75 mg orally daily divided into two or three doses	150–225 mg orally daily divided into two or three doses
Opioids	(see Table 5–7)	(see Table 5–7)
Topical and Other Medications		
Lidocaine transdermal	4% or 5% patch applied daily, for a maximum of 12 hours	1–3 patches applied daily for a maximum of 12 hours
Diclofenac transdermal	1.3% patch or 1% gel	Patch applied twice daily or gel applied three times daily
Tramadol hydrochloride[6]	50 mg orally four times daily	100 mg orally two to four times daily

[1]Begin at the starting dose and titrate up every 4 or 5 days. Within each category, drugs listed in order of prescribing preference.
[2]Begin with a low dose. Use the lowest effective dose. Pain relief may be achieved at doses below antidepressant doses, thereby minimizing adverse side effects. Do not combine with serotonin or norepinephrine reuptake inhibitors.
[3]Common side effects include nausea, somnolence, and dizziness. Must adjust dose for kidney impairment.
[4]Common side effects include dizziness, somnolence, peripheral edema, and weight gain. Must adjust dose for kidney impairment.
[5]*Caution:* Can cause hypertension and ECG changes. Consider obtaining baseline ECG and monitor.
[6]Tramadol is classified by the DEA as a Schedule IV controlled substance.

naloxone in patients who are receiving opioids of 50 MME/day or higher, who have a respiratory condition, who are concomitantly prescribed benzodiazepines, who have a history of substance abuse disorder, or who are otherwise at high risk for overdose.

Naloxone products approved by the US FDA include generic naloxone vials for injection and naloxone for intranasal administration.

Naloxone is typically administered intravenously; however, it can be administered subcutaneously, intramuscularly, or intranasally. The medication is titrated with the objective of improving the patient's respiratory function. Initial dosages usually range from 0.4 mg to 1.0 mg intravenously, though larger dosages (eg, 1.0 to 2.0 mg intravenously) may be used, even in patients without a history of opioid dependency. Apneic or cyanotic patients may require an even larger initial dosage. Naloxone generic is available in prefilled syringes containing 2 mg of naloxone per 2 mL for intramuscular, subcutaneous, or intravenous administration. The 2-mg dose is five times the original dosage when the medication was first approved; this is intended to counteract the effects of highly potent synthetic opioids. Narcan® Nasal Spray is now available in a prepackaged nasal spray with a 4 mg per actuation dosage; it is available in most US states for purchase directly from a pharmacist without a clinician's prescription. In addition, in 2021 the FDA approved Zimhi® 5 mg per 0.5 mL in prefilled syringes for injection. More recently in 2021, the FDA approved an even higher dosage (8 mg per actuation) of naloxone nasal spray (Kloxxado®) to combat overdose deaths related to the even more potent synthetic opioids.

Opioid-induced constipation is the most common adverse effect of opioids. Opioids bind to mu receptors in the GI tract and decrease bowel motility, secretions, and blood flow in a dose-related fashion. Ideally, patients treated with opioids will have a bowel movement at least every 24–48 hours. Initial recommendations for management of opioid-induced constipation should include patient education, increase in dietary fiber, adequate hydration, and regular physical activity. In addition, one successful approach combines laxatives (eg, Miralax®) along with a stimulant (eg, senna). Newer peripherally acting mu receptor antagonists (eg, naldemedine, naloxegol, and methylnaltrexone) block the GI actions of opioids without decreasing the opioid's analgesic effects. A recent meta- analysis has demonstrated promising effects, with a desired outcome of 3 or more bowel movements per week.

Roughly, 25% of patients prescribed opioids will develop nausea, likely secondary to direct stimulation of the chemoreceptor trigger zone, or to vestibular sensitivity, or to decreased GI motility. Management options include antipsychotics (eg, prochlorperazine or promethazine), prokinetic agents (eg, metoclopramide), serotonin antagonists (eg, ondansetron), or antihistamines (eg, diphenhydramine or meclizine). All these agents have side effects that must be carefully monitored.

Between 20% and 60% of patients treated with opioids report sedation or decreased cognition, most commonly with initiation of opioid therapy or with dose escalation. Nonpharmacologic management of minor sedation includes caffeinated beverages. Pharmacologic management options include methylphenidate; however, high-level evidence supporting its use for this indication is lacking. Cognitive impairment (delirium) may be managed with low-dose haloperidol, perhaps a first choice due to to its lower incidence of cardiovascular and anticholinergic effects.

Pruritus occurs in 2–10% of patients given opioids, likely secondary to peripheral histamine release. Management options include an opioid rotation, dose reduction, diphenhydramine, and cool compresses.

Centers for Disease Control and Prevention (CDC). Stop overdose: lifesaving naloxone. 2022 Feb 23. https://www.cdc.gov/stopoverdose/naloxone/

Lyden J et al. The United States opioid epidemic. Semin Perinatol. 2019;43:123. [PMID: 30711195]

Ouyang R et al. Efficacy and safety of peripherally acting mu-opioid receptor antagonists for the treatment of opioid-induced constipation: a Bayesian network meta-analysis. Pain Med. 2020;21:3224. [PMID: 32488259]

US Department of Health and Human Services. How to respond to an opioid overdose. 2020 Sep 25. https://www.hhs.gov/opioids/treatment/overdose-response/index.html

E. CDC Guidelines

In 2016, the CDC established guidelines for prescribing opioids for chronic pain. Nonpharmacologic therapy and nonopioid pharmacologic treatments should be undertaken prior to initiation of opioids. Then, only patients who benefit with improved pain and function outweighing the risks of opioids should be considered as candidates for ongoing opioids. Furthermore, nonopioid management options including physical therapy should be used concomitantly. Additionally, the patient's medication history should be reviewed through their state prescription drug monitoring program prior to the initial prescription and periodically thereafter.

Clinicians should avoid opioids, or cautiously titrate the opioid dosage in patients with a history of heart failure, obesity, COPD, or sleep apnea. In pregnant women, opioids can pose some risks to the mother and fetus, including poor fetal growth, stillborn delivery, birth defects, and neonatal withdrawal syndrome. It is highly recommended that appropriate referral to clinicians with expertise in pain management be made for these patients.

When initiating therapy for acute pain, the CDC recommends using immediate-release formulations, at the lowest effective dose, initially for a limited period of 3–7 days. Patients should have close follow-up after the initial prescription, typically within 4 weeks. Risks and benefits should be analyzed, particularly in patients prescribed greater than 50 MME/day. Patients who have risk factors for opioid overdose (eg, history of substance abuse or previous overdose, high opioid dose [greater than 50 MME/day], or current benzodiazepine dose) may also be offered naloxone. Patients should not be prescribed opioids and benzodiazepines concurrently. The CDC guidelines for prescribing opioids for chronic pain are summarized in Table 5–9.

Table 5–9. CDC guidelines for prescribing opioids for chronic pain.

	Guideline
Risk assessment	Nonpharmacologic and nonopioid pharmacologic therapy are preferred; weigh risks and benefits of opioids for pain and function Establish treatment goals and consider how opioids will be discontinued if benefits do not outweigh the risks Prior to starting opioid therapy, discuss risks, benefits, and responsibilities with the patient When starting opioid therapy, prescribe immediate-release opioids instead of extended release for acute (eg, "breakthrough") pain
Opioid selection and dosage	When starting opioids, prescribe the lowest effective opioid dose, carefully weigh risks if dose is > 50 MME/day and avoid doses > 90 MME/day For acute pain, prescribe the lowest effective dose, and limit duration: ≤ 3 days should be sufficient and > 7 days will rarely, if ever, be needed
Monitoring	Evaluate benefits and harms within 1–4 weeks of starting opioids or of any dose escalations, then again at least every 3 months (or sooner). If benefits do not outweigh harms, clinicians should lower dosages of opioids or taper to discontinue opioids Periodically evaluate risk factors for opioid-related harms; offer naloxone for patients with risk factors such as history of substance abuse or overdose, high opioid dose (> 50 MME/day) or concurrent benzodiazepine prescription Review the patient's history of controlled substance use through their state's prescription drug monitoring program Perform urine drug testing when initiating opioids and then periodically (randomly) during treatment Avoid prescribing opioids and benzodiazepines concurrently Manage or arrange treatment for opioid use disorder, typically with methadone or buprenorphine combined with behavioral therapy

Adapted from: Dowell D, Haegerich TM, Chou R. CDC Guideline for prescribing opioids for chronic pain—United States, 2016. MMWR Recomm Rep. 2016;65:1.

MME, morphine milligram equivalent.

Centers for Disease Control and Prevention (CDC). Urine drug testing factsheet. https://www.cdc.gov/opioids/providers/prescribing/pdf/Urine-Drug-Testing-508.pdf

Federal Register, Vol. 86, No. 121, June 28, 2021. Registration requirements for narcotic treatment programs with mobile components. https://www.federalregister.gov/documents/2021/06/28/2021-13519/registration-requirements-for-narcotic-treatment-programs-with-mobile-components.

F. Basics of Monitoring

Prior to the initial opioid prescription, it is prudent to clearly define the underlying condition, diagnostic workup, nonopioid therapeutic management plan and intended length of prescription. Ideally, the prescriber should determine how the opioid prescription fits into a broader comprehensive pain management plan. The Opioid Risk Tool (available at https://www.drugabuse.gov/sites/default/files/files/OpioidRiskTool.pdf) should be administered to understand the risk (low, moderate, or high) for future opioid abuse.

Standardized assessments such as the "PEG" scores may be used at initial and follow-up visits to gauge the efficacy of treatment (Table 5–10).

The primary goal of opioid monitoring initiatives is to improve patient compliance with the opioid prescription. Monitoring programs have been shown to improve compliance, reduce hospitalizations, and decrease specialty referrals. Although there is weak to moderate evidence to support the efficacy of opioid monitoring (urine drug testing and prescription drug monitoring programs) and treatment agreements, such interventions are considered to be standard care and to represent the best opioid prescription practices.

Most controlled substance agreements have integral components that address topics such as the goals of treatments, medical risks of opioid use, illicit use, polypharmacy, and diversion. Such agreements are ideally "patient-centric" and involve a mutual agreement between the clinician and the patient. Important topics such as safety, adverse side effects, dangers of polypharmacy, and concomitant alcohol or benzodiazepine use are typically reviewed. The prescribing clinician needs to assure that the patient understands and agrees to the agreement prior to prescribing the opioid. Potential risks of opioid use must be discussed and documented, including addiction, respiratory depression, overdose, and death.

Table 5–10. PEG score to gauge benefit from long-term opioid use.

During the past week:
1. What number best describes your *P*ain? 0 = no pain to 10 = worst pain imaginable
2. What number best describes how much your pain interfered with your *E*njoyment of life? 0 = no interference to 10 = complete interference
3. What number describes how much pain interfered with your *G*eneral activity? 0 = no interference to 10 = complete interference

To calculate PEG score, average scores from questions 1 through 3.
Source: https://www.cdc.gov/drugoverdose/pdf/pdo_checklist-a.pdf

The CDC recommends that all patients receiving long-term opioid therapy have periodic urine drug tests, at least annually. It is critical to convey to the patient that a urine drug test does not mean a lack of trust but is a standard safety measure for all patients who are prescribed long-term opioids. Patients should understand that urine drug tests may be conducted randomly and repeatedly during treatment. Immunoassays are less expensive and screen for a panel of drugs, but these tests do not differentiate between opioids, have low sensitivity, and typically miss semisynthetic opioids (eg, hydrocodone and oxycodone) and synthetic opioids (eg, fentanyl and tramadol). In contrast, although liquid chromatography/mass spectrometry tests are more expensive and must be performed in a laboratory, these tests are far more sensitive, differentiate between all opioids, and are more accurate for semisynthetic and synthetic opioids.

Finally, the treatment agreement also represents an ideal time to discuss the warning signs of overdose and what steps the patient must take if these were to occur. Although no formal guidelines for concomitant naloxone prescription have been established, an increasing number of clinicians are writing a naloxone prescription along with the opioid for patients who are deemed at high risk for accidental overdose.

Patients who are noncompliant with an agreed-upon opioid management schedule may eventually be good candidates for an opioid taper, but this must be done with caution and patience. Abrupt discontinuation of an opioid has been shown to have potential disastrous consequences, including withdrawal, suicide, and self-medication with illicit narcotics. It is critical to have a well thought out strategy for opioid reduction and cessation that uses a safe transition to nonopioid pain management techniques, including utilization of nonopioid analgesics, adjuvant analgesics, physical therapy, and mental health counseling.

Asamoah-Boaheng M et al. Interventions to influence opioid prescribing practices for chronic noncancer pain: a systematic review and meta-analysis. Am J Prev Med. 2021;60:e15. [PMID: 33229143]

Centers for Disease Control and Prevention (CDC). Urine Drug Testing Factsheet. https://www.cdc.gov/opioids/providers/prescribing/pdf/Urine-Drug-Testing-508.pdf

Covington EC et al. Ensuring patient protections when tapering opioids: consensus panel recommendations. Mayo Clin Proc. 2020;95:2155. [PMID: 33012347]

G. Management of Opioid Use Disorder

The FDA has approved several medications to manage opioid use disorder, including naltrexone, methadone, and buprenorphine. Naltrexone is an opioid antagonist that binds opioid receptors without activating them. Thus, use of naltrexone medication entails no risk of abuse or addiction. Naltrexone is prescribed orally or administered as an injectable to decrease the likelihood of relapse and to increase treatment retention. However, studies validating its efficacy have been mixed.

Methadone (a full opioid receptor agonist) and buprenorphine (a partial opioid receptor agonist) have long half-lives and have been shown to decrease withdrawal syndromes, decrease opioid cravings, decrease illicit drug use, and decrease all-cause mortality. Despite reasonable evidence for their efficacy, these medications are underutilized, possibly because of a lack of patient and clinician education, appropriate clinician training, or patient social stigma of being prescribed these drugs.

Both methadone and buprenorphine require special clinician training and certification to prescribe them for opioid use disorder. Recently, however, efforts have been made to improve access to them for patients. While both drugs carry a risk of abuse, buprenorphine is less addictive than methadone. The Drug Addiction Treatment Act of 2000 allows for waivered physicians to prescribe buprenorphine but despite this Act, less than half of the counties in rural areas of the United States have buprenorphine providers. In 2021, the US Drug Enforcement Administration (DEA) authorized preexisting DEA registrants to add a mobile component to allow for better access for patients in underserved and rural areas. As a result, narcotic treatment programs no longer need to have a separate registration at each principal place of business where substances are dispensed.

Federal Register, Vol. 86, No. 121, June 28, 2021. Registration requirements for narcotic treatment programs with mobile components. https://www.federalregister.gov/documents/2021/06/28/2021-13519/registration-requirements-for-narcotic-treatment-programs-with-mobile-components

Lyden J et al. The United States opioid epidemic. Semin Perinatol. 2019;43:123. [PMID: 30711195]

H. Weaning from Opioids

The goals of appropriately tapering opioids are to minimize symptoms and signs of opioid withdrawal while weaning. Common withdrawal symptoms and signs of withdrawal include anxiety, drug craving, tachycardia, vomiting, diarrhea, and mydriasis. Guidelines have suggested that a 10% decrease in opioid dosage per week is reasonable. However, a more rapid taper over 3 weeks may be appropriate in cases of adverse events such as overdose. Conversely, a slower wean of a 10% decrease in opioid dosage per month is also reasonable and may be better tolerated. Nonopioid management of pain (eg, by physical therapy, cognitive behavioral therapy, adjuvant analgesics, and nonopioid analgesics) should be maximized during the period of weaning.

Moss C et al. Weaning from long-term opioid therapy. Clin Obstet Gynecol. 2019;62:98. [PMID: 30601171]

Medications for Neuropathic Pain

When taking a patient's history, listening for pain descriptions such as "burning," "shooting," "pins and needles," or "electricity," and for pain associated with numbness is essential because such a history suggests neuropathic pain.

Table 5–11. Medications used for treatment of peripheral neuropathic pain.

Type of Medication	Numbers Needed to Treat (NNT) for Peripheral Neuropathies Compared to NSAIDs
Tricyclic antidepressants	2.1
Opioids	2.6
Cannabinoids	3.4
Pregabalin	4.5
Tramadol	4.9
Duloxetine	5.1
Capsaicin 0.04%	6.2
Gabapentin	6.5
SSRIs	6.8

Data from Moulin D et al; Canadian Pain Society. Pharmacological management of chronic neuropathic pain: revised consensus statement from the Canadian Pain Society. Pain Res Manag. 2014;19:328.

Studies are mixed with regard to efficacy of opioids for neuropathic pain. However, a number of nonopioid medications have also been found to be effective in randomized trials (Table 5–8). Successful management of neuropathic pain often requires the use of more than one effective medication. Since these medications bind to receptors on a large variety of neurons, they often have CNS side effects. These side effects often limit reaching therapeutic doses and may be the reason for higher numbers needed to treat (NNT 4–7) as compared to NSAIDs (NNT 2–4) (Table 5–11).

The calcium channel alpha2-delta ligands, gabapentin and pregabalin, are first-line therapies for neuropathic pain. Both medications have no significant medication interactions. However, they can cause sedation, dizziness, ataxia, and GI side effects. Both gabapentin and pregabalin require dose adjustments in patients with kidney dysfunction. Gabapentin should be started at low dosages of 100–300 mg orally once daily and titrated upward by 300 mg/day every 4–7 days by adding additional doses throughout the day with a typical effective dose of 1800–3600 mg/day in three divided doses. Pregabalin should be started at 40–150 mg/day in two or three divided doses. If necessary, the dose of pregabalin can be titrated upward to 300–600 mg/day in two or three divided doses. Both medications are relatively safe in accidental overdose and may be preferred over tricyclic antidepressants (TCAs) for a patient with a history of heart failure or arrhythmia or if there is a risk of suicide. Prescribing both gabapentin and an opioid for neuropathic pain may provide better analgesia at lower doses than if each is used as a single agent.

The SNRIs duloxetine and venlafaxine are also first-line treatments for neuropathic pain. Patients should be advised to take duloxetine on a full stomach because nausea is a common side effect. Duloxetine may provide increased benefit for neuropathic pain up to a total daily dose of

120 mg, beyond the 60-mg limit used for depression. Duloxetine generally should not be combined with other serotonin or norepinephrine uptake inhibitors, but it can be combined with gabapentin or pregabalin. Lower doses of venlafaxine have more serotonin than norepinephrine activity; therefore, higher doses may be required to treat neuropathic pain. Because venlafaxine can cause hypertension and induce ECG changes, patients with cardiovascular risk factors should be carefully monitored when starting this medication. Desvenlafaxine, the active metabolite of venlafaxine, is also available and may be tolerated better than venlafaxine.

TCAs are another class of medications for neuropathic pain that work through the norepinephrine and serotonin pathways. Among the TCAs that are effective for neuropathic pain, nortriptyline and desipramine are preferred over amitriptyline because they cause less orthostatic hypotension and have fewer anticholinergic effects. Start with a low dosage (10–25 mg orally daily) and titrate upward in 10-mg increments every 4 or 5 days aiming to use the lowest effective dose and to titrate up to a maximum of no greater than 100 mg daily. It may take several weeks for a TCA to have its full analgesic effect for neuropathic pain. Because TCAs and SNRIs both work through the serotonin and norepinephrine pathways, they generally should not be co-prescribed, particularly due to concerns for the serotonin syndrome.

Topical medications, such as lidocaine 5% patch and capsaicin 8% patches, are considered second-line therapies. The lidocaine 5% patch is particularly effective in postherpetic neuralgia and may be effective in other types of localized neuropathic pain. Due to its relatively minimal adverse effects, it is commonly used despite being considered second line. Topical lidocaine 4% patches and cream are available over the counter. Other medications effective for neuropathic pain include tramadol and tapentadol, both of which are opioids with norepinephrine activity. Medical cannabis strains high in cannabidiol have proven efficacy for some types of neuropathic pain.

Szok D et al. Therapeutic approaches for peripheral and central neuropathic pain. Behav Neurol. 2019;2019:8685954. [PMID: 31871494]

Adjuvant Pain Medications & Treatments

If pain cannot be controlled without intolerable medication side effects, clinicians should consider using lower doses of multiple medications, which is done commonly for neuropathic pain, rather than larger doses of one or two medications.

For metastatic bone pain, the anti-inflammatory effect of NSAIDs can be helpful. Furthermore, bisphosphonates (such as pamidronate and zoledronic acid) and receptor activator of NF-kappa-B ligand (RANKL) inhibitors (such as denosumab) may relieve such bone pain, although they are generally more useful for prevention of bone metastases than for analgesia.

Corticosteroids, such as dexamethasone, prednisone, and methylprednisolone, can be helpful for patients with headache due to increased intracranial pressure, pain from spinal cord compression, metastatic bone pain, and neuropathic pain due to invasion or infiltration of nerves by tumor. Because of the side effects of long-term corticosteroid administration, they are most appropriate for short-term use and in patients with end-stage disease. Low-dose intravenous, oral, buccal, and nasal ketamine has been used successfully for neuropathic and other pain syndromes refractory to opioids, although research data are limited.

PSYCHOLOGICAL, PHYSICAL, & INTEGRATIVE THERAPIES

Psychological Therapy

Nonpharmacologic and noninterventional therapies are valuable in treating pain. In fact, cognitive behavioral therapy and physical or functional therapy have been shown to be the most effective for management of chronic pain. In multiple randomized, controlled studies, cognitive behavioral therapy has been proven effective as a primary evidence-based treatment for chronic pain. Because mood and psychological issues play an important role in the patient's perception of and response to pain, psychotherapy, support groups, prayer, and pastoral counseling can also help in pain management. Depression and anxiety, which may be instigated by chronic pain or may alter the response to pain, should be treated aggressively with antidepressants and anxiolytics.

Urits I et al. An update on cognitive therapy for the management of chronic pain: a comprehensive review. Curr Pain Headache Rep. 2019;23:57. [PMID: 31292747]

Physical Therapy

Physical therapy is a mainstay of chronic pain management and encompasses several modalities, including strength training, manual therapy, and massage.

Physical therapy can be beneficial for a variety of types of chronic pain. For musculoskeletal pain, hot or cold packs, massage, and stretching (including traction) can be helpful.

But physical therapy can help not just musculoskeletal pain but also neuropathic pain. For example, if there is a cervical radiculopathy, the position and posture of individual neck muscles may exacerbate the narrowing of the neuroforamina; or nerves may become entrapped within hypertrophied muscles, leading to neuropathic pain. Therefore, functional rehabilitation through physical therapy may address multiple types of pain.

Physical therapy for management of low-back pain may involve "core stabilization." Bounded by the diaphragm and the pelvic floor, the body's "core" is composed of the abdominal muscles and back and gluteal muscles. Exercises can help stabilize the entirety of the core, so that the low back does not need to exert as much effort for movement, lifting, bending, etc. "Core stabilization" can thereby decrease low-back pain.

Because physical therapy has minimal potential harms associated with it, as opposed to pharmacologic or interventional approaches for pain management, it should be a key component in management of both acute and chronic pain. While physical therapy can be used on its own, it is often preferable to engage in it as part of a multidisciplinary approach to pain management (which may include psychological therapies).

Araujo FM et al. Physical therapy modalities for treating fibromyalgia. F1000Res. 2019;8:F1000. [PMID: 32047594]
Martin-Gomez et al. Motor control using cranio-cervical flexion exercises versus other treatments for non-specific chronic neck pain: a systematic review and meta-analysis. Musculoskelet Sci Pract. 2019;42:52. [PMID: 31030111]
Owen PJ et al. Which specific modes of exercise training are most effective for treating low back pain? Network meta-analysis. Br J Sports Med. 2020;54:1279. [PMID: 31666220]

Integrative Medicine Therapy

Integrative medicine therapies of acupuncture, chiropractic care, biofeedback, meditation, music therapy, guided imagery, cognitive distraction, and framing may be helpful in treating pain.

SELECTED INTERVENTIONAL MODALITIES FOR PAIN RELIEF

Pain management specialists are physicians who have completed a residency in anesthesiology, physical medicine and rehabilitation, neurology, internal medicine, emergency medicine, or psychiatry and usually also a fellowship in pain management to learn medication management and interventional techniques for acute, chronic, and cancer pain. Interventional pain management modalities performed by pain management specialists involve neuromodulation of specific targets to alleviate pain. The procedures they perform include percutaneous needle injection of local anesthetics or corticosteroids, radiofrequency (thermal) lesioning, cryotherapy, chemical neurolysis, or surgical implantation of intrathecal medication delivery pump systems or neurostimulation devices. While invasive procedures carry their own inherent risks such as bleeding or infection, they can drastically reduce or even obviate the need for conventional pharmacologic therapies that may have side effects or be burdensome to the individual.

For some patients, a nerve block, such as a celiac plexus block for pain from pancreatic cancer, can provide substantial relief. Intrathecal pumps may be most useful for patients with severe pain responsive to opioids but who require such large doses that systemic side effects (eg, sedation, urinary retention, and constipation) become limiting. In the palliative care setting, these pumps are appropriate when life expectancy is long enough to justify the discomfort and cost of surgical implantation.

Clinicians do not need to know all the details of interventional pain procedures but should consider referring their patients to pain management specialists if such procedures may be beneficial. For example, a common question is whether prolonged opioid therapy with its inherent risks is better than an injection or an implanted device. Beyond knowing the benefits and risks, fiscal considerations may be key.

Tables 5–12 and 5–13 list the procedures and the agents typically used in interventional pain modalities.

Table 5–12. Interventional techniques for chronic pain by anatomic location.

Neuraxial
Intrathecal
Epidural (caudal, lumbar, thoracic, cervical; interlaminar vs transforaminal)
Paraneuraxial (planar blockade)
Paravertebral (intercostal)
Transversus abdominis plane/quadratus lumborum
Pectoralis and serratus anterior
Peripheral nerve (perineural blockade)
Brachial plexus and branches
Lumbar plexus and branches
Joints
Intra-articular injections
Joint denervation procedures
Sympathetic ganglion
Gasserian ganglion
Sphenopalatine ganglion
Cervical sympathetic blockade (stellate ganglion)
Lumbar sympathetic blockade
Celiac plexus
Superior hypogastric plexus
Ganglion impar
Continuous neuraxial drug delivery
Epidural (tunneled catheter, port)
Intrathecal (implanted intrathecal pump)
Neurostimulation
Dorsal column stimulation (spinal cord stimulation)
Dorsal root ganglion stimulation
Peripheral nerve or field stimulation

INTRATHECAL DRUG DELIVERY SYSTEM

A. Indications

Intrathecal drug delivery therapy is indicated for patients with both malignant and nonmalignant pain and has been shown to be effective, cost-effective, and safe. It is generally accepted that intrathecal opioids have a 100- to 300-fold efficacy compared with oral opioids; therefore, the best candidates may be patients with good analgesic benefit from opioids but burdensome side effects. Common indications include cancer pain, chronic low-back pain (in particular, post-laminectomy syndrome), complex regional pain syndrome, and other causes of neuropathic pain. In a randomized controlled trial comparing intrathecal therapy with comprehensive medication management in cancer pain, intrathecal therapy was shown to be superior in analgesia and fewer side effects. Due to the cost of implanting the device as well as the recovery time needed from surgical implantation, it is recommended that patients have a life expectancy of at least 2–3 months.

Table 5–13. Agents used[1] in neuromodulatory therapies.

Voltage-gated sodium channel blockade—local anesthetics
Lidocaine
Mepivacaine
Bupivacaine
Ropivacaine
Corticosteroids
Triamcinolone
Methylprednisolone
Dexamethasone
Opioids
Morphine
Hydromorphone
Fentanyl
Adjuvants
Clonidine
Dexmedetomidine
Others
Chemical neurolysis
Alcohol
Phenol
Glycerol
Thermal neurolysis
Radiofrequency ablation
Cryoanalgesia
Neurostimulation
Various patterns, frequency, amplitude, pulse width

[1]Injected or applied.

List is not comprehensive but includes most commonly used agents.

B. Procedure

Intrathecal drug delivery systems consist of a pump with a drug reservoir, typically implanted in the abdominal wall, connected to a catheter that delivers medications into the intrathecal space. Initial percutaneous trialing is indicated for patients with noncancer or cancer pain; such percutaneous trialing may consist of either epidural or intrathecal delivery of bolus or continuous medication to determine efficacy and side effect profiles of planned therapeutic agent(s). Some cancer patients may not undergo a trial to avoid delaying final implantation. Subsequent implantation of an intrathecal drug delivery system involves two incisions: one in the spine to accommodate the catheter and anchor, and another in the lower abdominal region to create a pocket to hold the pump. The catheter is tunneled through the lower abdominal and flank subcutaneous tissues to connect to the pump. Both trial and implantation are typically performed under sedation with local anesthetic infiltration; spinal anesthesia delivered from the pump itself can also be utilized for pump implantation. Some patients may require general anesthesia to tolerate the implantation procedure.

C. Medications Used

According to the Polyanalgesic Conference Consensus (PACC) guidelines for both malignant and nonmalignant pain, first-line intrathecal delivery medications include monotherapy with either morphine or ziconotide, a calcium channel inhibitor. However, the PACC guidelines also state that de facto practice includes combination therapy with opioids (eg, fentanyl, hydromorphone) and local anesthetic (eg, bupivacaine) and may include other medications (eg, baclofen or clonidine). Respiratory depression and sedation are two of the most concerning side effects of many intrathecal medications. Ziconotide may cause myositis and polyarthralgias as well as psychiatric and neurologic adverse effects (it is contraindicated in patients with preexisting psychosis). Side effects of morphine and fentanyl include nausea, edema, constipation, urinary retention, and pruritus.

D. Advantages and Disadvantages

The main advantage of intrathecal delivery therapy is targeted delivery of medication to the spinal cord with increased efficacy and diminished side effects compared with systemic analgesic medications. Intrathecal therapy has been found to be effective with decreased side effects and improved analgesia in 80% of cancer patients. The increased efficacy is due to the 100- to 300-fold increased concentration of intrathecal drug compared with systemic medication. However, intrathecal therapy requires regular pump refills and may be complicated by infections, catheter or pump malfunctions requiring surgical revision, or development of catheter tip granulomas, potentially leading to inadequate analgesia or neurologic deficits. Pump batteries may last from 5 years to 10 years depending on usage. Fatalities surrounding intrathecal therapy have been linked to respiratory depression; patients must be monitored for respiratory depression or sedation when initiating or increasing intrathecal therapeutic agents. Some intrathecal pumps need to be emptied prior to MRI; due to the magnetic forces of the MRI, the entirety of the drug reservoir could inadvertently open. Therefore, it is critical that the type of pump is known prior to placing the patient and pump in an MRI machine. Additionally, anticoagulants and NSAIDs need to be stopped prior to pump implantation and need to be held briefly after the implantation as well; this temporary cessation imposes the risk of potentially causing blood clots.

E. Alternatives

For patients with limited life expectancy, continuous epidural drug delivery via an external pump or subcutaneous port may be more appropriate. Systemic medication delivered orally, intravenously, topically, or even by a subcutaneous infusion (as in palliative care settings) are alternatives to intrathecal therapy.

Abd-Elsayed A et al. Intrathecal drug delivery for chronic pain syndromes: a review of considerations in practice management. Pain Physician. 2020;23:E591. [PMID: 33185379]

Sindt JE et al. Initiation of intrathecal drug delivery dramatically reduces systemic opioid use in patients with advanced cancer. Neuromodulation. 2020;23:978. [PMID: 32459393]

Sindt JE et al. The rate of infectious complications after intrathecal drug delivery system implant for cancer-related pain is low despite frequent concurrent anticancer treatment or leukopenia. Anesth Analg. 2020;131:280. [PMID: 31990731]
Sommer B et al. Long-term outcome and adverse events of intrathecal opioid therapy for nonmalignant pain syndrome. Pain Pract. 2020;20:8. [PMID: 31291509]
Spiegel MA et al. Evaluation of an intrathecal drug delivery protocol leads to rapid reduction of systemic opioids in the oncological population. J Palliat Med. 2021;24:418. [PMID: 32640912]

SPINAL STIMULATION

A. Indications

Spinal stimulation targets neuropathic pain in the trunk and limbs, such as failed back surgery syndrome, complex regional pain syndrome, and radiculopathy. There is also growing literature around its use for neuropathic pain associated with cancer.

B. Procedure

Neurostimulation devices consist of an implantable pulse generator typically placed in the flank or abdomen just under the skin and an array of electrical contacts on small cylindrical or paddle leads placed in the epidural space. **Neurostimulation** devices transmit electrical pulses to the spinal cord or dorsal root ganglion to block pain transmission. Paddle leads require neurosurgical implantation with laminotomy (and general anesthesia), while percutaneous wire leads may be implanted under sedation. Patients undergo a 3- to 7-day trial during which the leads are attached to an external battery source and undergo programming with different pulse waveforms to assess therapeutic efficacy prior to surgical implantation of permanent leads and implantable pulse generator.

C. Frequencies Used

Traditional neurostimulation resulted in paresthesias that were used to mask pain. It was presumed that these paresthesias were the result of stimulation of the dorsal column axons. Recent studies have revealed that analgesia can be obtained independent of paresthesias by altering a variety of spinal cord stimulation parameters, including constant high-frequency stimulation and burst high-frequency stimulation. More recent double-blind, randomized, controlled trials have revealed that both functional status and pain scores could be significantly improved in spinal cord stimulation systems that were capable of adapting the output to the patient's individual neural response in a closed loop fashion. For more focal neuropathic pain conditions such as postoperative inguinal nerve injuries or thoracic post herpetic neuralgias, stimulation of the dorsal root ganglion is able to provide focal analgesia. These newer, more versatile systems deliver paresthesia-free analgesia with analgesic response rates that have steadily increased from about 50% with the traditional devices to about 80%. The newer devices also have greater longevity and most are MRI compatible.

D. Advantages and Disadvantages

Spinal cord stimulation is a reversible technology that may provide superior analgesic efficacy while eliminating the need for systemic medications. Current literature suggests spinal cord stimulation is efficacious in 80–90% of well-selected patients, such as those with neuropathic low-back pain due to post-laminectomy syndrome. In fact, spinal cord stimulation has now advanced to a higher position in the treatment continuum; it can be considered before using long-term moderate doses of systemic opioids. On the other hand, because it is a surgical procedure, it may be associated with complications, such as infection, lead migration, device malfunction, or neurologic deficits. While MRIs were contraindicated with some older systems, most newer systems allow for limited MRI imaging. Batteries may require daily charging but typically do not require replacement for 5–10 years. Similar to intrathecal pumps, anticoagulants and NSAIDs need to be stopped prior to implantation of spinal cord stimulation devices because of the potential risks (eg, bleeding). The implanting surgeon, prescribing physician, and patient need to discuss the benefits and risks before proceeding.

E. Alternatives

In addition to medication management for pain, two neuromodulatory techniques may serve as alternatives to dorsal horn and dorsal root ganglion stimulation. Peripheral nerve stimulation is an emerging technology; it targets peripheral nerves using a similar system of a lead connected to a pulse generator. It may be most appropriate when there is a very specific neurologic target. Transcutaneous electrical nerve stimulators (TENS) and systemic pharmacologic therapies are alternatives.

Deer TR et al. A systematic literature review of spine neurostimulation therapies for the treatment of pain. Pain Med. 2020;21:1421. [PMID: 32034422]
Hofmeister M et al. Effectiveness of neurostimulation technologies for the management of chronic pain: a systematic review. Neuromodulation. 2020;23:150. [PMID: 31310417]
Mekhail N et al. Long-term safety and efficacy of closed-loop spinal cord stimulation to treat chronic back and leg pain (Evoke): a double-blind, randomised, controlled trial. Lancet Neurol. 2020;19:123. [PMID: 31870766]
Mekhail N et al. Choice of spinal cord stimulation versus targeted drug delivery in the management of chronic pain: a predictive formula for outcomes. Reg Anesth Pain Med. 2020;45:131. [PMID: 31932490]
Moisset X et al. Neurostimulation methods in the treatment of chronic pain. J Neural Transm (Vienna). 2020;127:673. [PMID: 31637517]

CELIAC PLEXUS BLOCK & NEUROLYSIS

A. Indications

A celiac plexus block refers to injection of a long-acting anesthetic (eg, bupivacaine) with or without a corticosteroid (eg, methylprednisolone); with steroids, the block can provide relief for a few weeks to months. Celiac plexus neurolysis involves injection of a neurolytic agent (eg, alcohol or phenol); it may provide pain relief more consistently for 2–6 months. The most common indication is pancreatic cancer pain, but it can be used for pain from other malignancies (eg, stomach, liver, spleen, kidney, and GI tract) or from chronic pancreatitis. Multiple randomized controlled trials and meta-analyses have shown superiority of celiac plexus neurolysis to medication management for pancreatic cancer, but evidence of its efficacy for chronic pancreatitis is more mixed.

B. Procedure

The most common approach is a percutaneous posterior approach under fluoroscopy guidance, with bilateral needles targeted to the celiac plexus at the level of T12–L1. Alternatively, ultrasound, CT, or endoscopic guidance can be used. Minimal sedation is required for the percutaneous approaches, while heavy sedation or general anesthesia may be required for endoscopic guidance.

C. Medications Used

Chemical neurolysis with alcohol or phenol is used to extend the duration of the analgesia to 2 or more months compared to a block with local anesthetic (eg, bupivacaine) and corticosteroid (eg, methylprednisolone), which produces an analgesic duration of weeks to months. For chemical neurolysis, alcohol is used most often because it does not require compounding, and importantly has a lower chance of permanent neurologic damage compared with phenol; however, it is more painful on injection.

D. Advantages and Disadvantages

The primary advantage is improved analgesia without need for systemic medications and their untoward effects. Neurolytic celiac plexus blockade is effective in 70–80% of patients. Common side effects of celiac plexus interventions include transient hypotension and transient diarrhea. Transient or permanent spinal cord damage is rare, although there is an increased risk of its occurrence with plexus (chemical) neurolysis compared with plexus (anesthetic) block.

E. Alternatives

Standard pain management is with oral or transdermal systemic analgesic (eg, opioid) medication. Intrathecal therapy is also an alternative, especially for cancer pain.

Filippiadis DK et al. Percutaneous neurolysis for pain management in oncological patients. Cardiovasc Intervent Radiol. 2019;42:791. [PMID: 30783779]

Lau J et al. Interventional anesthesia and palliative care collaboration to manage cancer pain: a narrative review. Can J Anaesth. 2020;67:235. [PMID: 31571119]

Urits I et al. A comprehensive review of the celiac plexus block for the management of chronic abdominal pain. Curr Pain Headache Rep. 2020;24:42. [PMID: 32529305]

EPIDURAL CORTICOSTEROID INJECTION

A. Indications

Epidural corticosteroid injections are indicated for patients with chronic neck pain, low-back pain, and radicular pain resulting from central or neuroforaminal stenosis in the cervical, thoracic, or lumbosacral region. Both central and neuroforaminal stenosis may be caused by degenerative disk disease, disk herniation, or facet arthropathy. Epidural corticosteroid injections are relatively safe and are appropriate after conservative measures, such as physical therapy and analgesic medications, have been tried and found unsuccessful.

B. Procedure

Fluoroscopy is typically used to assist with visualizing the bony landmarks; either an interlaminar or a transforaminal approach can be used. Interlaminar access is obtained by placing a needle between the lamina of adjacent vertebral levels, whereas transforaminal access is obtained by inserting a needle through the neuroforamen to access the epidural space. These needle insertion procedures can be performed with topical local anesthetic or with minimal sedation.

C. Medications Used

Typically, a particulate corticosteroid such as methylprednisolone is used alone or in combination with a local anesthetic. For the transforaminal approach, where vascular access is more of a concern, a nonparticulate corticosteroid such as dexamethasone may be preferred.

D. Advantages and Disadvantages

Epidural corticosteroid injections are advantageous for patients who have not responded to conservative therapy, are not surgical candidates, or do not want surgery. The best evidence of the effectiveness of epidural corticosteroid injections is the short-term improvement of radiculopathy in both the lumbar and cervical regions. In a Cochrane analysis, side effects were noted in 10–24% of surgical cases but no side effects were reported for any conservative treatments. Disadvantages include possible postdural puncture headache, transient weakness, and, rarely, permanent neurologic deficits. Patients who are receiving systemic anticoagulation may need to hold their anticoagulants before receiving corticosteroid injections, which could increase their risk of cardiovascular events; these cases should be discussed with the clinician managing the anticoagulation prior to performing any epidural corticosteroid injections.

E. Alternatives

Alternatives include conservative therapy, such as oral analgesic medication management, physical therapy, pain psychology, acupuncture, and surgery.

Verheijen EJA et al. Epidural steroid compared to placebo injection in sciatica: a systematic review and meta-analysis. Eur Spine J. 2021;30:3255. [PMID: 33974132]

Yang S et al. Epidural steroid injection versus conservative treatment for patients with lumbosacral radicular pain. Medicine (Baltimore). 2020;99:e21283. [PMID: 32791709]

When to Refer

Patients should be referred to pain management specialists if they have:

- Pain that does not respond to opioids at typical doses or the opioids cause major adverse effects at typical doses.
- Pain that cannot be controlled expeditiously or safely by other clinicians.
- Neuropathic pain that does not respond to first-line treatments.
- Complex medication management that uses buprenorphine or methadone.
- Severe pain from malignancy, including primary disease (eg, pancreatic cancer) or metastatic disease (eg, bony metastases).

When to Admit

- Severe exacerbation of pain not responsive to previous stable oral opioids given around-the-clock plus breakthrough doses.
- Pain that is so severe that it cannot be controlled at home.
- Uncontrollable side effects from opioids, including nausea, vomiting, myoclonus, and altered mental status.
- Need for a surgical procedure, such as implantation of an intrathecal drug delivery pump or neurostimulation device.

Dermatologic Disorders

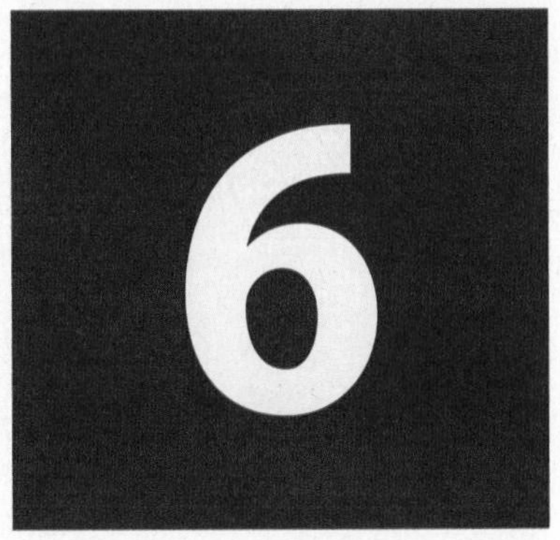

Kanade Shinkai, MD, PhD
Lindy P. Fox, MD

Dermatologic diseases are diagnosed by the types of lesions they cause. Identify the morphology of lesion(s) to establish a differential diagnosis (Table 6–1), and obtain the elements of the history, physical examination, and appropriate laboratory tests to confirm the diagnosis. Specific clinical situations, such as an immunocompromised or critically ill patient, lead to different diagnostic considerations.

PRINCIPLES OF DERMATOLOGIC THERAPY

Frequently Used Treatment Measures

A. Bathing

Soap should be used only in the axillae and groin and on the feet by persons with dry or inflamed skin. Soaking in water for 10–15 minutes before applying topical corticosteroids or emollient enhances their efficacy (Soak and Smear).

B. Topical Therapy

Nondermatologists should become familiar with a representative agent in each category for each indication (eg, topical corticosteroid, topical retinoid, etc).

1. Corticosteroids—Topical corticosteroid creams, lotions, ointments, gels, foams, and sprays are presented in Table 6–2. Topical corticosteroids are divided into classes based on potency. Agents within the same class are equivalent therapies; however, prices of topical corticosteroids vary dramatically. For a given agent, higher lipophilicity (greasiness) corresponds with increased potency; ie, triamcinolone 0.1% ointment is more potent than triamcinolone 0.1% cream which in turn is more potent than triamcinolone 0.1% lotion. The potency of a topical corticosteroid may be dramatically increased by occlusion (covering with a water-impermeable barrier) for at least 4 hours. Depending on the location of the skin condition, gloves, plastic wrap, moist pajamas covered by dry pajamas (wet wraps), or plastic occlusive suits for patients can be used. Caution should be used in applying topical corticosteroids to areas of thin skin (face, genitals, skin folds). Topical corticosteroid use on the eyelids may result in glaucoma or cataracts. One may estimate the amount of topical corticosteroid needed by using the "rule of nines" (as in burn evaluation; see Figure 37–2). Approximately 20–30 g is needed to cover the entire body surface of an adult. Systemic absorption does occur with topical corticosteroids, but complications of systemic corticosteroids are rare.

2. Emollients for dry skin ("moisturizers")—Dry skin is a result of abnormal function of the epidermis. Emollients restore the epidermis by promoting keratinocyte differentiation and by producing innate antimicrobials; some restore skin barrier lipids, including ceramides. Ointments and creams, rather than lotion, are the best moisturizers. **Emollients are most effective when applied to wet skin.** If the skin is too greasy after application, pat dry with a damp towel. Plain petrolatum is allergen-free and can be used if allergic contact dermatitis to topical products is suspected.

The scaly appearance of dry skin may be improved by emollients with concomitant use of keratolytics including urea, lactic acid, or glycolic acid–containing products provided no inflammation (erythema or pruritus) is present.

3. Drying agents for weepy dermatoses—If the skin is weepy from infection or inflammation, drying agents may be beneficial. The best drying agent is water, applied as repeated compresses for 15–30 minutes, alone or with aluminum salts (Burow solution, Domeboro tablets).

4. Topical antipruritics—Lotions that contain 0.5% each of camphor and menthol (Sarna) or pramoxine hydrochloride 1% (with or without 0.5% menthol, eg, Prax, PrameGel, Aveeno Anti-Itch lotion) are effective antipruritic agents. Hydrocortisone, 1% or 2.5%, may be incorporated for its anti-inflammatory effect (Pramosone cream, lotion, or ointment). Doxepin cream 5% reduces pruritus but may cause drowsiness. Pramoxine and doxepin are most effective when applied with topical corticosteroids. Topical capsaicin and lidocaine can be effective in some forms of neuropathic itch.

C. Systemic Antipruritic Drugs

1. Antihistamines and antidepressants—H_1-blockers are the agents of choice for pruritus due to histamine, such as urticaria. Otherwise, they appear to benefit itchy patients

Table 6–1. Morphologic categorization of skin lesions and diseases.

Pigmented	Freckle, lentigo, seborrheic keratosis, nevus, blue nevus, halo nevus, atypical nevus, melanoma, actinic keratoses, Bowen disease, Paget disease
Scaly	Psoriasis, dermatitis (atopic, stasis, seborrheic, chronic allergic contact or irritant contact), xerosis (dry skin), lichen simplex chronicus, tinea pedis/cruris/corporis, tinea versicolor, secondary syphilis, pityriasis rosea, discoid lupus erythematosus, exfoliative dermatitis, drug eruption
Vesicular	Herpes simplex, varicella, herpes zoster, pompholyx (vesicular dermatitis of palms and soles), vesicular tinea, autoeczematization, dermatitis herpetiformis, miliaria crystallina, scabies, photosensitivity, acute contact allergic dermatitis, drug eruption
Weepy or encrusted	Impetigo, acute contact allergic dermatitis, any vesicular dermatitis
Pustular	Acne vulgaris, acne rosacea, folliculitis, candidiasis, miliaria pustulosa, pustular psoriasis, any vesicular dermatitis, drug eruption
Figurate ("shaped") erythema	Urticaria, erythema multiforme, erythema migrans, cellulitis, erysipelas, erysipeloid, arthropod bites
Bullous	Impetigo, blistering dactylitis, pemphigus, pemphigoid, porphyria cutanea tarda, drug eruptions, erythema multiforme, toxic epidermal necrolysis
Papular	**Hyperkeratotic:** warts, corns, seborrheic keratoses **Purple-violet:** lichen planus, drug eruptions, Kaposi sarcoma, lymphoma cutis, Sweet syndrome **Flesh-colored, umbilicated:** molluscum contagiosum **Pearly:** basal cell carcinoma, intradermal nevi **Small, red, inflammatory:** acne, rosacea, miliaria rubra, candidiasis, scabies, folliculitis
Pruritus[1]	Xerosis, scabies, pediculosis, lichen planus, lichen simplex chronicus, bites, systemic causes, anogenital pruritus
Nodular, cystic	Erythema nodosum, furuncle, cystic acne, follicular (epidermal) inclusion cyst, metastatic tumor to skin
Photodermatitis	Drug eruption, polymorphic light eruption, lupus erythematosus
Morbilliform	Drug eruption, viral infection, secondary syphilis
Erosive	Any vesicular dermatitis, impetigo, aphthae, lichen planus, erythema multiforme, intertrigo
Ulcerated	Decubiti, herpes simplex, skin cancers, parasitic infections, syphilis (chancre), chancroid, vasculitis, stasis, arterial disease, pyoderma gangrenosum

[1]Not a morphologic class but included because it is one of the most common dermatologic presentations.

Table 6–2. Useful topical dermatologic therapeutic agents.[1]

Agent	Formulations, Strengths, and Prices[2]	Frequency of Application	Potency Class	Common Indications	Comments
Corticosteroids (Listed in Order of Increasing Potency)					
Hydrocortisone acetate	Cream 1%: $3.99/30 g Ointment 1%: $1.58/28 g Solution 1%: $7.34/44 mL	Twice daily	Low	Seborrheic dermatitis Pruritus ani Intertrigo	Not the same as valerate or hydrocortisone butyrate Not for poison oak OTC lotion (Aquanil HC), OTC solution (Scalpicin)
	Cream 2.5%: $9.66/28 g Ointment 2.5%: $11.00/28 g			As for 1% hydrocortisone	Perhaps better for pruritus ani Not clearly better than 1% More expensive Not OTC
Alclometasone dipropionate (Aclovate)	Cream 0.05%: $48.08/15 g Ointment 0.05%: $20.00/15 g	Twice daily	Low	As for hydrocortisone	More efficacious than hydrocortisone Perhaps causes less atrophy
Desonide	Cream 0.05%: $21.60/15 g Ointment 0.05%: $23.21/15 g Lotion 0.05%: $296.09/59 mL	Twice daily	Low	As for hydrocortisone For lesions on face or body folds resistant to hydrocortisone	More efficacious than hydrocortisone Can cause rosacea or atrophy Not fluorinated

(*continued*)

Table 6–2. Useful topical dermatologic therapeutic agents.[1] (continued)

Agent	Formulations, Strengths, and Prices[2]	Frequency of Application	Potency Class	Common Indications	Comments
Clocortolone (Cloderm)	Cream 0.1%: $322.47/45 g	Three times daily	Medium	Contact dermatitis Atopic dermatitis	Does not cross-react with other corticosteroids chemically and can be used in patients allergic to other corticosteroids
Prednicarbate (Dermatop)	Emollient cream 0.1%: $137.10/60 g Ointment 0.1%: $30.00/15 g	Twice daily	Medium	As for triamcinolone	May cause less atrophy No generic formulations Preservative-free
Triamcinolone acetonide	Cream 0.1%: $3.60/15 g Ointment 0.1%: $5.57/15 g Lotion 0.1%: $42.42/60 mL	Twice daily	Medium	Eczema on extensor areas Used for psoriasis with tar Seborrheic dermatitis and psoriasis on scalp	Caution in body folds, face Economical in 0.5-lb and 1-lb sizes for treatment of large body surfaces Economical as solution for scalp
	Cream 0.025%: $4.50/15 g Ointment 0.025%: $10.11/80 g	Twice daily	Medium	As for 0.1% strength	Possibly less efficacy and few advantages over 0.1% formulation
Fluocinolone acetonide	Cream 0.025%: $44.85/15 g Ointment 0.025%: $33.77/15 g	Twice daily	Medium	As for triamcinolone	
	Solution 0.01%: $90.00/60 mL	Twice daily	Medium	As for triamcinolone	
Mometasone furoate (Elocon)	Cream 0.1%: $29.16/15 g Ointment 0.1%: $25.92/15 g Lotion 0.1%: $57.04/60 mL	Once daily	Medium	As for triamcinolone	Often used inappropriately on the face or on children Not fluorinated
Desoximetasone	Cream 0.05%: $62.43/15 g Cream 0.25%: $40.00/15 g Gel 0.05%: $298.38/60 g Ointment 0.25%: $18.00/15 g	Twice daily	High	As for triamcinolone	Comparable potency to fluocinonide Suggested for use when allergic contact dermatitis to topical corticosteroid is suspected; ointment useful when allergic contact dermatitis to propylene glycol is suspected
Diflorasone diacetate	Cream 0.05%: $209.68/15 g Ointment 0.05%: $209.68/15 g	Twice daily	High	Nummular dermatitis Allergic contact dermatitis Lichen simplex chronicus	
Fluocinonide (Lidex)	Cream 0.05%: $45.55/15 g Gel 0.05%: $59.56/15 g Ointment 0.05%: $70.75/15 g Solution 0.05%: $84.00/60 mL	Twice daily	High	As for betamethasone Gel useful for poison oak	Economical generics Lidex cream can cause stinging on eczema Lidex emollient cream preferred
Betamethasone dipropionate (Diprolene)	Cream 0.05%: $44.00/15 g Ointment 0.05%: $50.45/15 g Lotion 0.05%: $43.19/60 mL	Twice daily	Ultra-high	For lesions resistant to high-potency corticosteroids Lichen planus Insect bites	Economical generics available

(continued)

Table 6–2. Useful topical dermatologic therapeutic agents.[1] (continued)

Agent	Formulations, Strengths, and Prices[2]	Frequency of Application	Potency Class	Common Indications	Comments
Clobetasol propionate (Temovate)	Cream 0.05%: \$127.10/15 g Ointment 0.05%: \$149.23/15 g Lotion 0.05%: \$288.96/59 mL	Twice daily	Ultra-high	As for betamethasone dipropionate	Somewhat more potent than diflorasone Limited to 2 continuous weeks of use Limited to 50 g or less per week Cream may cause stinging; use "emollient cream" formulation Generic available
Halobetasol propionate (Ultravate)	Cream 0.05%: \$39.60/15 g Ointment 0.05%: \$75.58/15 g	Twice daily	Ultra-high	As for clobetasol	Same restrictions as clobetasol Cream does not cause stinging Compatible with calcipotriene (Dovonex)
Flurandrenolide (Cordran)	Tape: \$857.28/24″ × 3″ roll Lotion 0.05%: \$360.00/120 mL	Every 12 hours	Ultra-high	Lichen simplex chronicus	Tape version protects the skin and prevents scratching
Nonsteroidal Anti-inflammatory Agents (Listed Alphabetically)					
Crisaborole (Eucrisa)	Ointment 2%: \$830.35/60 g	Twice daily	N/A	Atopic dermatitis	Steroid substitute not causing atrophy or striae May sting or burn on initial application
Pimecrolimus[3] (Elidel)	Cream 1%: \$608.71/60 g	Twice daily	N/A	Atopic dermatitis	Steroid substitute not causing atrophy or striae
Tacrolimus[3] (Protopic)	Ointment 0.1%: \$240.00/60 g Ointment 0.03%: \$168.01/60 g	Twice daily	N/A	Atopic dermatitis	Steroid substitute not causing atrophy or striae Burns in ≥ 40% of patients with eczema May cause flushing with ingestion of alcohol
Antibiotics (for Acne) (Listed Alphabetically)					
Clindamycin phosphate	Solution 1%: \$28.94/30 mL Gel 1%: \$54.00/30 mL Lotion 1%: \$115.38/60 mL Pledget 1%: \$50.58/60	Twice daily	N/A	Mild papular acne	Lotion is less drying than solution, gel, or pledgets for patients with sensitive skin Recommend use with benzoyl peroxide to avoid antibiotic resistance from monotherapy
Clindamycin/Benzoyl peroxide (BenzaClin)	Gel: \$90.00/25 g Gel: \$180.00/50 g	Twice daily	N/A	As for benzamycin	No generic More effective than either agent alone
Dapsone	Gel 5%: \$601.27/60 g	Once daily	N/A	Mild papulopustular acne	More expensive, well tolerated Recommend use with benzoyl peroxide to avoid antibiotic resistance from monotherapy

(*continued*)

Table 6–2. Useful topical dermatologic therapeutic agents.[1] (continued)

Agent	Formulations, Strengths, and Prices[2]	Frequency of Application	Potency Class	Common Indications	Comments
Erythromycin	Solution 2%: $47.63/60 mL Gel 2%: $60.48/30 g Pledget 2%: $92.65/60	Twice daily	N/A	As for clindamycin	Many different manufacturers Economical Recommend use with benzoyl peroxide to avoid antibiotic resistance from monotherapy
Erythromycin/ Benzoyl peroxide (Benzamycin)	Gel: $199.08/23.3 g Gel: $75.00/46.6 g	Twice daily	N/A	As for clindamycin Can help treat comedonal acne	No generic More expensive More effective than other topical antibiotics Main jar requires refrigeration
Minocycline	Foam: 4% $582.00/30 g	Once daily	N/A	As for clindamycin	No generic More expensive May cause skin yellowing (temporary, washes off)
Antibiotics (for Impetigo)					
Mupirocin (Bactroban)	Ointment 2%: $11.25/22 g Cream 2%: $245.16/15 g	Three times daily	N/A	Impetigo, folliculitis	Because of cost, use limited to tiny areas of impetigo Used in the nose twice daily for 5 days to reduce staphylococcal carriage
Retapamulin (Altabax)	Ointment 1%: $401.05/15 g	Twice daily	N/A	Impetigo	For *Staphylococcus aureus* or *Streptococcus pyogenes* infection Typically reserved for mupirocin-resistant infections
Ozenoxacin (Ozanex)	Cream 1%: $374.22/30 g	Twice daily (5 days)	N/A	Impetigo	Topical fluoroquinolone Activity against MRSA
Antifungals: Imidazoles (Listed Alphabetically)					
Clotrimazole	Cream 1%: $2.99/15 g OTC Solution 1%: $33.68/10 mL	Twice daily	N/A	Dermatophyte and *Candida* infections	Available OTC Inexpensive generic cream available
Econazole (Spectazole)	Cream 1%: $30.04/15 g	Once daily	N/A	As for clotrimazole	Somewhat more effective than clotrimazole and miconazole
Ketoconazole (Nizoral)	Cream 2%: $30.90/15 g	Once daily	N/A	As for clotrimazole	Somewhat more effective than clotrimazole and miconazole
Miconazole	Cream 2%: $2.99/28 g OTC	Twice daily	N/A	As for clotrimazole	As for clotrimazole
Oxiconazole (Oxistat)	Cream 1%: $614.73/30 g Lotion 1%: $771.91/30 mL	Twice daily	N/A	As for clotrimazole	
Sertaconazole (Ertaczo)	Cream 2%: $1079.41/60 g	Twice daily	N/A	Refractory tinea pedis	By prescription More expensive
Sulconazole (Exelderm)	Cream 1%: $72.38/15 g Solution 1%: $416.66/30 mL	Twice daily	N/A	As for clotrimazole	No generic Somewhat more effective than clotrimazole and miconazole

(continued)

Table 6–2. Useful topical dermatologic therapeutic agents.[1] (continued)

Agent	Formulations, Strengths, and Prices[2]	Frequency of Application	Potency Class	Common Indications	Comments
Other Antifungals (Listed Alphabetically)					
Butenafine (Mentax)	Cream 1%: $8.01/12 g OTC	Once daily	N/A	Dermatophytes	Fast response; high cure rate; expensive Available OTC
Ciclopirox (Loprox) (Penlac)	Cream 0.77%: $51.10/30 g Lotion 0.77%: $80.75/30 g Solution 8%: $60.18/6.6 mL	Twice daily	N/A	As for clotrimazole	No generic Somewhat more effective than clotrimazole and miconazole
Efinaconazole (Jublia)	Solution 10%: $818.69/4 mL	Once daily for 48 weeks	N/A	Onychomycosis	No generic; more effective than ciclopirox for nail disease
Naftifine (Naftin)	Cream 1%: $375.38/60 g Gel 1%: $522.38/60 mL	Once daily	N/A	Dermatophytes	No generic Somewhat more effective than clotrimazole and miconazole
Tavaborole (Kerydin)	Solution 5%: $616.42/4 mL	Once daily for 48 weeks	N/A	Onychomycosis	No generic available
Terbinafine (Lamisil)	Cream 1%: $8.72/12 g OTC	Once daily	N/A	Dermatophytes	Fast clinical response OTC
Antipruritics (Listed Alphabetically)					
Camphor/menthol (Sarna)	Lotion 0.5%/0.5%: $8.96/222 mL	Two to three times daily	N/A	Mild eczema, xerosis, mild contact dermatitis	
Capsaicin (various)	Cream 0.025%: $9.95/60 g Cream 0.075%: $10.39/56 g	Three to four times daily	N/A	Topical antipruritic, best used for neuropathic itching	Burning/stinging with initial application that subsides with consistent ongoing use
Doxepin (Zonalon)	Cream 5%: $802.56/45 g	Four times daily	N/A	Topical antipruritic, best used in combination with appropriate topical corticosteroid to enhance efficacy	Can cause sedation
Pramoxine hydrochloride (Prax)	Lotion 1%: $19.64/120 mL OTC	Four times daily	N/A	Dry skin, varicella, mild eczema, pruritus ani	OTC formulations (Prax, Aveeno Anti-Itch Cream or Lotion; Itch-X Gel) By prescription mixed with 1% or 2% hydrocortisone

[1]For a given agent, higher lipophilicity (greasiness) corresponds with increased potency; for example, triamcinolone 0.1% ointment is more potent than triamcinolone 0.1% cream, which in turn is more potent than triamcinolone 0.1% lotion.
[2]Average wholesale price (AWP, for AB-rated generic when available) for quantity listed. AWP may not accurately represent the actual pharmacy cost because wide contractual variations exist among institutions. IBM Micromedex ®Red Book (electronic version). IBM Watson Health, Greenwood Village, Colorado, USA. Available at: https://www-micromedexsolutions-com.proxy.hsl.ucdenver.edu/ (cited March 15, 2022).
[3]Topical tacrolimus and pimecrolimus should be used only when other topical treatments are ineffective. Treatment should be limited to an area and duration be as brief as possible. Use of these agents should be avoided in persons with known immunosuppression, HIV infection, bone marrow and organ transplantation, or lymphoma; those at high risk for lymphoma; and those with a history of lymphoma.
MRSA, methicillin-resistant *Staphylococcus aureus;* N/A, not applicable; OTC, over-the-counter.

only by their sedating effects. Hydroxyzine 25–50 mg orally at night is a typical dose. Sedating and nonsedating antihistamines are of limited value for the treatment of pruritus associated with inflammatory skin disease. Preferable agents include antidepressants (such as doxepin, mirtazapine, and paroxetine) and agents that act directly on the neurons that perceive or modulate pruritus (such as gabapentin, pregabalin, and duloxetine).

2. Systemic corticosteroids—(See Chapter 26.)

Andrade A et al. Interventions for chronic pruritus of unknown origin. Cochrane Database Syst Rev. 2020;1:CD013128. [PMID: 31981369]
Axon E et al. Safety of topical corticosteroids in atopic eczema: an umbrella review. BMJ Open. 2021;11:e046476. [PMID: 34233978]
Stacey SK et al. Topical corticosteroids: choice and application. Am Fam Physician. 2021;103:337. [PMID: 33719380]

Sunscreens

Protection from UV light reduces the incidence of sunburn, actinic keratoses, melanoma, and some nonmelanoma skin cancers when initiated at any age and in any skin type. The best protection is shade, but protective clothing, avoidance of direct sun exposure during the peak hours of the day, and daily use of sunscreens are important.

A broad-spectrum (protection against UVA and UVB) sunscreen should be used daily with a sun protective factor (SPF) of at least 30. Clinicians should reinforce regular sunscreen use and reapplication every few hours or more depending on exercise level and exposure to water. Health implications of systemic absorption of chemical sunscreens are unknown.

Lyons AB et al. Photoprotection beyond ultraviolet radiation: a review of tinted sunscreens. J Am Acad Dermatol. 2021;84:1393. [PMID: 32335182]
Matta MK et al. Effect of sunscreen application on plasma concentration of sunscreen active ingredients: a randomized clinical trial. JAMA. 2020;323:256. [PMID: 31961417]

Complications of Topical Dermatologic Therapy

Complications of topical therapy include allergy, irritation, and other side effects. Reactions may result from the active or inactive ingredients, including fragrances and preservatives.

A. Allergy

Of the topical antibiotics, neomycin and bacitracin have the greatest potential for sensitization. Diphenhydramine, benzocaine, vitamin E, aromatic oils, preservatives, fragrances, tea tree oil, and even topical corticosteroids can cause allergic contact dermatitis.

B. Irritation

Preparations of tretinoin, benzoyl peroxide, and other acne medications should be applied sparingly to the skin.

C. Other Side Effects

Topical corticosteroids may induce acne-like lesions on the face (steroid rosacea) and atrophic striae in body folds.

deGroot A. Allergic contact dermatitis from topical drugs: an overview. Dermatitis. 2021;32:197. [PMID: 34415695]

NEOPLASTIC LESIONS

PIGMENTED NEOPLASMS

BENIGN PIGMENTED LESIONS

1. Melanocytic Nevi (Normal Moles)

In general, a benign mole is a small (less than 6 mm) macule or papule with a well-defined border and homogeneous beige or pink to dark brown pigment. They represent benign melanocytic growths.

Moles have a typical natural history. Early in life, moles often appear as flat, small, brown lesions and are termed "junctional nevi" because the nevus cells are at the junction of the epidermis and dermis. Over time, these moles enlarge and often become raised, reflecting the appearance of a dermal component, giving rise to "compound nevi" (Figure 6–1). Moles may darken and grow during pregnancy. As White patients enter their eighth decade, most moles have lost their junctional component and dark pigmentation as a result of normal senescence. At every stage of life, normal moles should be well demarcated, symmetric, and uniform in contour and color. Regular mole screening is not an evidence-based recommendation for all adults, although rates of screening continue to rise.

Ko E et al. Pigmented lesions. Dermatol Clin. 2020;38:485. [PMID: 32892857]
Yeh I. New and evolving concepts of melanocytic nevi and melanocytomas. Mod Pathol. 2020;33:1. [PMID: 31659277]

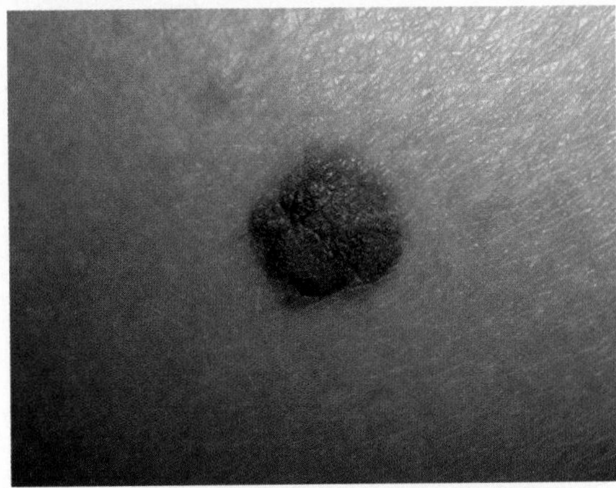

▲ **Figure 6–1.** Benign, compound nevus on the back. (Reproduced with permission from Richard P. Usatine, MD, in Usatine RP, Smith MA, Mayeaux EJ Jr, Chumley H. *The Color Atlas of Family Medicine*, 2nd ed. McGraw-Hill, 2013.)

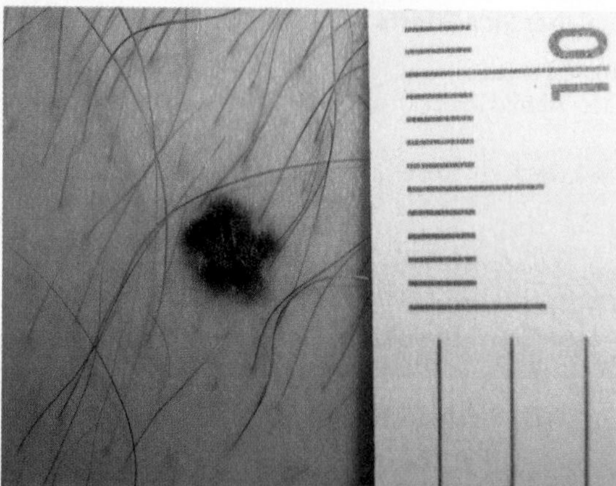

▲ **Figure 6–2.** Atypical (dysplastic) nevus on the chest. Note irregular border and variegation in color. (Reproduced with permission from Richard P. Usatine, MD, in Usatine RP, Smith MA, Mayeaux EJ Jr, Chumley H. *The Color Atlas of Family Medicine*, 2nd ed. McGraw-Hill, 2013.)

2. Atypical Nevi

The term "atypical nevus" or "atypical mole" has supplanted "dysplastic nevus." The diagnosis of atypical moles is made clinically, not histologically. Moles should be removed only if they are suspected to be melanomas. Dermoscopy by a trained clinician may be a useful tool in the evaluation of atypical nevi. Clinically, these moles are large (6 mm or more in diameter), with an ill-defined, irregular border and irregularly distributed pigmentation (Figure 6–2). An estimated 5–10% of the White population in the United States has one or more atypical nevi, for which recreational sun exposure is a primary risk. There is an increased risk of melanoma in patients with 50 or more nevi with one or more atypical moles and one mole 8 mm or larger and patients with any number of definitely atypical moles. These patients should be educated in how to recognize changes in moles and be monitored every 6–12 months by a clinician. Kindreds with familial melanoma (numerous atypical nevi and a family history of two first-degree relatives with melanoma) require closer attention since their risk of developing single or multiple melanomas approaches 50% by age 50.

Elder DE et al. The 2018 World Health Organization Classification of cutaneous, mucosal, and uveal melanoma: detailed analysis of 9 distinct subtypes defined by their evolutionary pathway. Arch Pathol Lab Med. 2020;144:500. [PMID: 32057276]

Fried L et al. Technological advances for the detection of melanoma: advances in diagnostic techniques. J Am Acad Dermatol. 2020;83:983. [PMID: 32348823]

3. Blue Nevi

Blue nevi are small, slightly elevated, blue-black lesions (Figure 6–3) that favor the dorsal hands. They are common in persons of Asian descent and may be single or multiple. If the lesion has remained unchanged for years, it may be considered benign, since malignant blue nevi are rare.

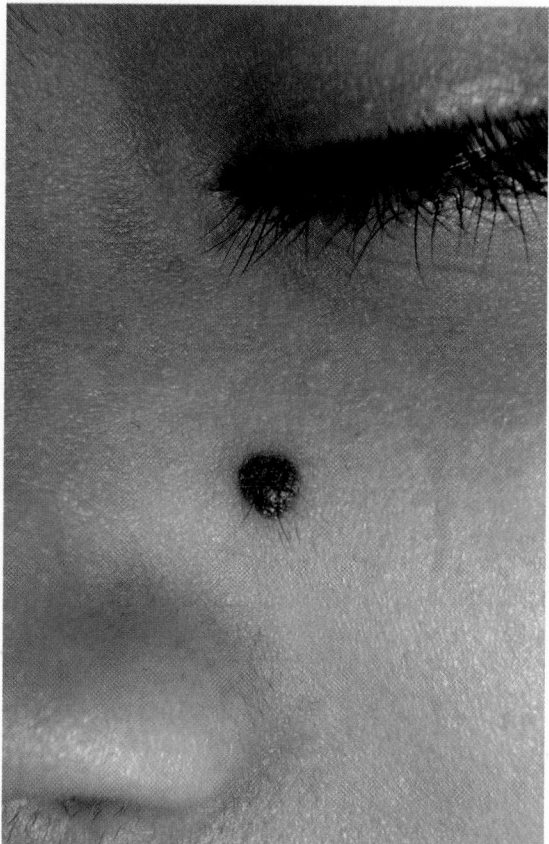

▲ **Figure 6–3.** Blue nevus on the left cheek, a darkly pigmented blue-black macule with some resemblance to a melanoma due to its dark pigmentation. (Reproduced with permission from Richard P. Usatine, MD, in Usatine RP, Smith MA, Mayeaux EJ Jr, Chumley H, Tysinger J. *The Color Atlas of Family Medicine*. McGraw-Hill, 2009.)

Blue-black papules and nodules that are new or growing must be evaluated to rule out nodular melanoma.

4. Freckles & Lentigines

Freckles (ephelides) and lentigines are flat brown macules, typically between 3 mm and 5 mm in diameter. Freckles first appear in young children, darken with UV exposure, and fade with cessation of sun exposure. They are determined by genetic factors. In adults, lentigines gradually appear in sun-exposed areas, particularly the face, dorsal hands, upper back, and upper chest, starting in the fourth to fifth decade of life, and are associated with photoaging as well as estrogen and progesterone use. They may have a very irregular border (ink spot lentigines). They do not fade with cessation of sun exposure. They should be evaluated like all pigmented lesions: if the pigmentation is homogeneous and they are symmetric and flat, they are most likely benign. They can be treated with topical retinoids such as 0.1% tretinoin or 0.1% adapalene, hydroquinone, laser/light therapy, or cryotherapy.

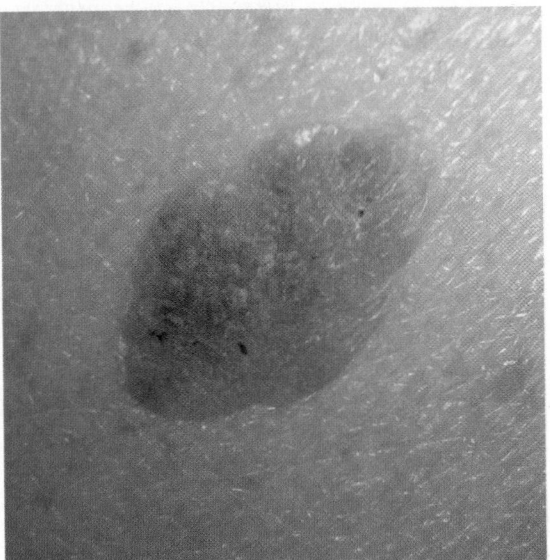

▲ **Figure 6–4.** Seborrheic keratosis with light pigmentation, with waxy, dry, "stuck-on," appearance. (Reproduced with permission from Richard P. Usatine, MD, in Usatine RP, Smith MA, Mayeaux EJ Jr, Chumley H. *The Color Atlas of Family Medicine*, 2nd ed. McGraw-Hill, 2013.)

5. Seborrheic Keratoses

Seborrheic keratoses are benign papules and plaques, beige to brown or even black, 3–20 mm in diameter, with a velvety or warty surface. They appear to be stuck or pasted onto the skin (Figure 6–4). They are extremely common—especially in older adults—and may be mistaken for melanomas or other types of cutaneous neoplasms. No treatment is needed. They may be frozen with liquid nitrogen or curetted if itchy or inflamed but usually recur after treatment.

Hruza GJ et al. Safety and efficacy of nanosecond pulsed electric field treatment of seborrheic keratoses. Dermatol Surg. 2020;46:1183. [PMID: 31809349]

MALIGNANT PIGMENTED LESIONS

1. Malignant Melanoma

ESSENTIALS OF DIAGNOSIS

- May be flat or raised with irregular borders.
- Examination may show varying colors, including red, white, black, and blue.
- Should be suspected in any pigmented skin lesion with recent change in appearance.
- Less than 30% develop from existing moles.

General Considerations

Malignant melanoma, the fifth most common of all cancers in the United States, is the leading cause of death due to skin disease and has doubled in incidence over the past 30 years. In 2021, approximately 106,110 new melanomas were diagnosed in the United States, with approximately 60% in men. In 2021, melanoma caused an estimated 7180 deaths (two-thirds in men). The lifetime risk of melanoma is 2% in White individuals and 0.1–0.5% in non-White persons. One in four cases occurs before age 40. Increased detection of early melanomas has led to increased survival, but fatalities continue to increase, especially in men older than 70 years.

Tumor thickness is the single most important prognostic factor. Ten-year survival rates related to melanoma thickness are less than 1 mm, 95%; 1–2 mm, 80%; and 2–4 mm, 55%. The 5-year survival rate is 62% with lymph node involvement and 16% with distant metastases.

Clinical Findings

Primary malignant melanomas may be classified into various clinicohistopathologic types, including lentigo melanoma (arising on chronically sun-exposed skin of older individuals); superficial spreading melanoma (two-thirds of all melanomas arising on intermittently sun-exposed skin); nodular melanoma; acral-lentiginous melanomas (arising on palms, soles, and nail beds); ocular melanoma; and melanomas on mucous membranes. Different types of melanoma appear to have distinct oncogenic mutations, which may be important in the treatment of patients with advanced disease. Less than 30% of melanomas develop from existing moles. Clinical features of pigmented lesions suspicious for melanoma are an irregular, notched border where the pigment appears to be spreading into the normal surrounding skin and irregular surface topography (ie, partly raised and partly flat) (Figure 6–5). Color variegation

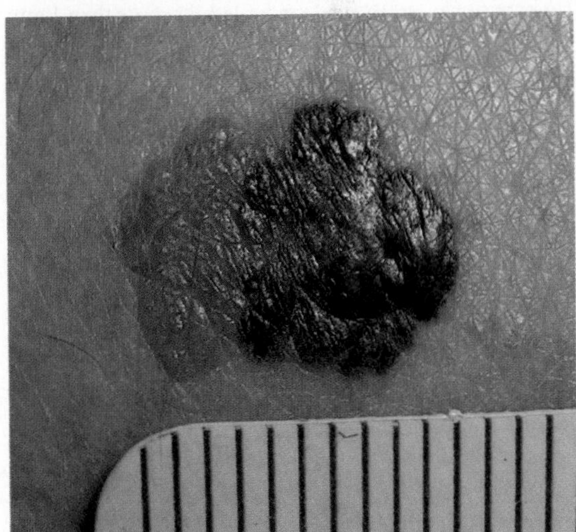

▲ **Figure 6–5.** Malignant melanoma. Note the classic "ABCDE" features: asymmetry, irregular border, multiple colors, diameter greater than 6 mm, and evolution or change. (Reproduced with permission from Richard P. Usatine, MD, in Usatine RP, Smith MA, Mayeaux EJ Jr, Chumley H. *The Color Atlas of Family Medicine*, 2nd ed. McGraw-Hill, 2013.)

is present and is an important indication for referral. A useful mnemonic is the ABCDE rule: Asymmetry, Border irregularity, Color variegation, Diameter greater than 6 mm, and Evolution. **The history of a changing mole (evolution, including bleeding and ulceration) is the single most important historical reason for close evaluation and possible referral.** A mole that appears distinct from the patient's other moles deserves special scrutiny—the "ugly duckling sign." A patient with a large number of moles is statistically at increased risk for melanoma and deserves annual total body skin examination by a primary care clinician or dermatologist, particularly if the lesions are atypical in appearance.

While superficial spreading melanoma is largely a disease of White individuals, persons with darker skin pigmentation are at risk for this and other types of melanoma, particularly acral lentiginous melanomas, for which UV exposure may not be a significant association. These occur as dark, irregularly shaped lesions on the palms and soles and as new, often broad and solitary, darkly pigmented, longitudinal streaks in the nails, typically with involvement of the proximal nail fold. Acral lentiginous melanoma may be a difficult or delayed diagnosis because benign pigmented lesions of the hands, feet, and nails occur commonly in more darkly pigmented persons, and clinicians may hesitate to biopsy these sites. Clinicians should give special attention to new or changing lesions in these areas.

Treatment

Treatment starts with complete excision of the melanoma with a normal margin. After histologic diagnosis, reexcision is recommended with margins dictated by the thickness of the tumor. Recommended surgical margins are 0.5–1 cm for melanoma in situ, 1 cm for lesions less than 1 mm in thickness, and 1–2 cm for lesions more than 1 mm in thickness.

Referral of intermediate-risk and high-risk patients to centers with expertise in melanoma is strongly recommended. Sentinel lymph node biopsy (selective lymphadenectomy) using preoperative lymphoscintigraphy and intraoperative lymphatic mapping is effective for staging melanoma patients with intermediate risk without clinical adenopathy and is recommended for all patients with lesions over 1 mm in thickness or with high-risk histologic features (ulceration). This procedure may not confer a survival advantage. Identifying the oncogenic mutations in patients with advanced melanoma may dictate targeted therapy, most commonly to specific BRAF mutations. Additionally, immunotherapy treatments directed toward immune costimulatory molecules such as PD-1 can activate systemic immune-directed destruction of metastatic melanoma.

Albittar AA et al. Immunotherapy for melanoma. Adv Exp Med Biol. 2020;1244:51. [PMID: 32301010]

Carr S et al. Epidemiology and risk factors of melanoma. Surg Clin North Am. 2020;100:1. [PMID: 31753105]

Swetter S et al. NCCN Guidelines® Insights: Melanoma: cutaneous, Version 2.2021. J Natl Compr Canc Netw. 2021;19:364. [PMID: 33845460]

NONPIGMENTED NEOPLASMS

BENIGN LESIONS

1. Epidermal Inclusion Cyst

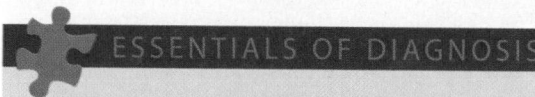

- Firm dermal papule or nodule.
- Overlying black comedone or "punctum."
- Expressible foul-smelling cheesy material.
- May become red and drain, mimicking an abscess.

General Considerations

Epidermal inclusion cysts (EICs) are common, benign growths of the upper portion of the hair follicle. They are common in Gardner syndrome and may be the first sign of the condition.

EICs favor the face and trunk and may complicate nodulocystic acne vulgaris. Individual lesions range in size from 0.3 cm to several centimeters. An overlying pore or punctum is characteristic. Dermoscopy can aid in observing a tiny punctum when not visible to the naked eye. Lateral pressure may lead to extrusion of a foul-smelling, cheesy material.

Differential Diagnosis

EICs are distinguished from lipomas by being more superficial (in the dermis, not the subcutaneous fat) and by their overlying punctum. Many other benign and malignant tumors may superficially resemble EICs, but all lack the punctum.

Complications

EICs may rupture, creating an acute inflammatory nodule very similar to an abscess. Cultures of the expressed material will be sterile.

Treatment

Treatment is not required if asymptomatic. Small (1–3 cm) lesions can be treated with a punch incision and removal of cystic contents. Inflamed lesions may be treated with incision and drainage or intralesional triamcinolone acetonide 5–10 mg/mL. For large or symptomatic cysts, surgical excision is curative.

MALIGNANT & PREMALIGNANT LESIONS

1. Actinic Keratoses

Actinic keratoses are small (0.2–0.6 cm) papules—flesh-colored, pink, or slightly hyperpigmented—that feel like sandpaper and are tender to palpation. They occur on sun-exposed parts of the body in persons of fair complexion.

Actinic keratoses are considered premalignant; 1:1000 lesions per year progress to squamous cell carcinoma.

Application of liquid nitrogen provides rapid eradication of lesions, which crust and disappear in 10–14 days. "Field treatment" with a topical agent can be considered in patients with multiple lesions in one region (eg, forehead, dorsal hands, etc). Fluorouracil cream is the most effective topical agent used for field treatment; imiquimod, ingenol mebutate, and photodynamic therapy are also effective. Combination therapy may be clinically beneficial. Any lesions that persist should be evaluated for possible biopsy.

Cornejo CM et al. Field cancerization: treatment. J Am Acad Dermatol. 2020;83:719. [PMID: 32387663]
Dianzani C et al. Current therapies for actinic keratosis. Int J Dermatol. 2020;59:677. [PMID: 32012240]
Willenbrink TJ et al. Field cancerization: definition, epidemiology, risk factors, and outcomes. J Am Acad Dermatol. 2020;83:709. [PMID: 32387665]

2. Squamous Cell Carcinoma

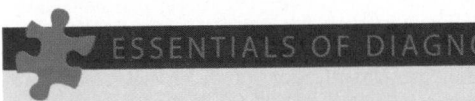

- Nonhealing ulcer or warty nodule.
- Skin damage due to long-term sun exposure.
- Common in fair-skinned organ transplant recipients.

Squamous cell carcinoma usually occurs subsequent to prolonged sun exposure on exposed parts in fair-skinned individuals who sunburn easily and tan poorly. It may arise from an actinic keratosis. The lesions appear as small red, conical, hard nodules that occasionally ulcerate (Figure 6–6). In actinically induced squamous cell cancers, rates of metastasis are estimated from retrospective studies to be 3–7%. Squamous cell carcinomas of the ear, temple, lip, oral cavity, tongue, and genitalia have much higher rates of recurrence or metastasis and require special management. Patients with multiple squamous cell carcinomas (especially more than 10) have higher rates of local recurrence and nodal metastases. Nicotinamide, 500 mg orally twice daily, can decrease the rate of development of squamous cell carcinomas by 30% in high-risk groups.

Squamous cell carcinoma in situ can be treated with imiquimod or 5-fluorouracil (in similar dosing as for superficial basal cell carcinoma) or curettage and electrodessication. The preferred treatment for invasive squamous cell carcinoma is excision or Mohs micrographic surgery. Mohs micrographic surgery is recommended for high-risk lesions (lips, temples, ears, nose), recurrent tumors, aggressive histologic subtypes (perineural or perivascular invasion), large lesions (greater than 1.0 cm on face, greater than 2.0 cm on trunk or extremities), immunosuppressed patients, lesions developing within a scar, and tumors arising in the setting of genetic diseases. Follow-up for squamous cell carcinoma must be more frequent and thorough than for basal cell carcinoma, starting at every 3 months, with careful examination of lymph nodes for 1 year, then twice yearly thereafter.

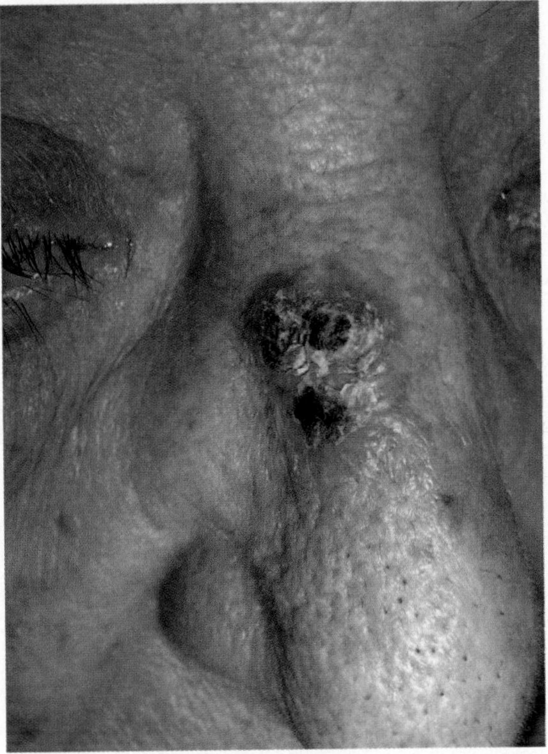

▲ Figure 6–6. **Squamous cell carcinoma: an irregular-shaped pink plaque with overlying hemorrhagic crust in a chronically sun-exposed area.** (Reproduced with permission from Richard P. Usatine, MD, in Usatine RP, Smith MA, Mayeaux EJ Jr, Chumley H. *The Color Atlas of Family Medicine*, 2nd ed. McGraw-Hill, 2013.)

Transplant patients with squamous cell carcinomas represent a highly specialized patient population. Biologic behavior of skin cancer in organ transplant recipients may be aggressive, and careful management is required. Multiple squamous cell carcinomas are very common on the sun-exposed skin of organ transplant patients. The tumors begin to appear after 5 years of immunosuppression. Regular dermatologic evaluation in at-risk organ transplant recipients is recommended. Other forms of immunosuppression, such as allogeneic hematopoietic stem cell transplants, chronic lymphocytic leukemia, HIV/AIDS, and chronic iatrogenic immunosuppression, may also increase skin cancer risk and be associated with more aggressive skin cancer behavior.

Cañueto J et al. Comparing the eighth and the seventh editions of the American Joint Committee on Cancer staging system and the Brigham and Women's Hospital alternative staging system for cutaneous squamous cell carcinoma: implications for clinical practice. J Am Acad Dermatol. 2019;80:106. [PMID: 30003984]
Firnhaber JM. Basal cell and cutaneous squamous cell carcinomas: diagnosis and treatment. Am Fam Physician. 2020;102:339. [PMID: 32931212]

3. Basal Cell Carcinoma

ESSENTIALS OF DIAGNOSIS

- Pearly papule, erythematous patch > 6 mm, or nonhealing ulcer in sun-exposed areas (face, trunk, lower legs).
- History of bleeding.
- Fair-skinned person with a history of sun exposure (often intense, intermittent).

General Considerations

Basal cell carcinomas are the most common form of cancer. They occur on sun-exposed skin in otherwise normal, fair-skinned individuals; UV light is the cause. Basal cell carcinomas can be divided into clinical and histologic subtypes, which determine both clinical behavior and treatment. The clinical subtypes include superficial, nodular, pigmented, and morpheaform. The histologic subtypes include superficial, nodular, micronodular, and infiltrative. Morpheaform, micronodular, and infiltrative basal cell carcinomas are not amenable to topical therapy or electrodesiccation and curettage and typically require surgical excision or Mohs micrographic surgery. Because a second basal cell carcinoma develops in up to half of patients, skin examination is required at least yearly to detect new or recurrent lesions. Nicotinamide, 500 mg orally twice daily, can decrease the rate of development of basal cell carcinomas by 20% in high-risk groups.

Clinical Findings

The most common presentation is a papule or nodule that may have a central scab or erosion. Occasionally the nodules have stippled pigment (pigmented basal cell carcinoma). Intradermal nevi without pigment on the face of older White individuals may resemble basal cell carcinomas. Basal cell carcinomas grow slowly, attaining a size of 1–2 cm or more in diameter, usually only after years of growth. There is a waxy, "pearly" appearance, with telangiectatic vessels easily visible (Figure 6–7). It is the pearly or translucent quality of these lesions that is most diagnostic, a feature best appreciated if the skin is stretched. On the back and chest, basal cell carcinomas appear as reddish, somewhat shiny, scaly thin papules or plaques. Morpheaform basal cell carcinomas are scar-like in appearance. Basal cell carcinomas are more common and more likely to recur in immunosuppressed patients, including those with non-Hodgkin lymphoma and those who have undergone solid organ or allogeneic hematopoietic stem cell transplantation.

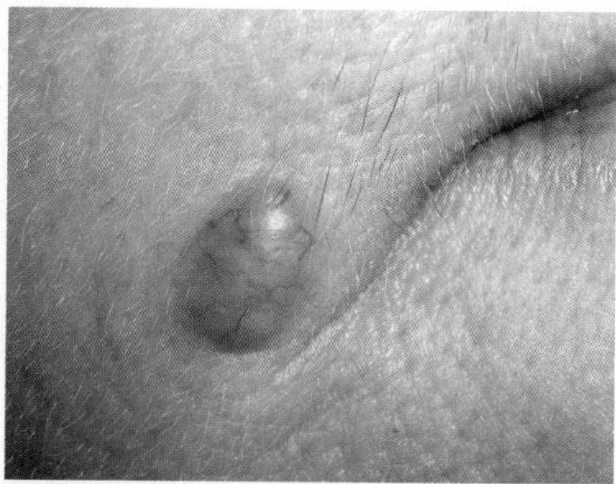

▲ Figure 6–7. **Pearly nodular basal cell carcinoma on the face of a 52-year-old woman present for 5 years.** (Reproduced with permission from Richard P. Usatine, MD, in Usatine RP, Smith MA, Mayeaux EJ Jr, Chumley H. *The Color Atlas of Family Medicine*, 2nd ed. McGraw-Hill, 2013.)

Treatment

Lesions suspected to be basal cell carcinomas should be biopsied by shave or punch biopsy. Therapy is then aimed at eradication with minimal cosmetic deformity. The histopathologic classification of basal cell carcinomas determines therapy. Imiquimod (applied topically 5 nights per week for 6–10 weeks depending on patient reaction) and 5-fluorouracil (applied topically twice daily for up to 12 weeks) may be appropriate for select patients with superficial basal cell carcinomas, but the treated area must be observed for evidence of complete cure. Superficial or nodular type lesions can be treated with curettage and electrodesiccation, excision, or Mohs micrographic surgery, while those that are classified as micronodular or infiltrative should be treated with excision or Mohs micrographic surgery depending on the size and location of the lesion.

Surgical excision has a recurrence rate of 5% or less. The technique of three cycles of curettage and electrodesiccation depends on the skill of the operator and is not recommended for head and neck lesions or basal cell carcinomas with morpheaform, infiltrative, or micronodular histopathology. After 4–6 weeks of healing, it leaves a broad, hypopigmented, at times hypertrophic scar.

Mohs micrographic surgery—removal of the tumor followed by immediate frozen section histopathologic examination of margins with subsequent reexcision of tumor-positive areas and final closure of the defect—gives the highest cure rates (98%) and results in least tissue loss. It is an appropriate therapy for tumors of the eyelids, nasolabial folds, canthi, external ear, and temple; for recurrent lesions; where tissue sparing is needed for cosmesis; and for those with morpheaform, infiltrative, or micronodular histopathology in certain locations.

Photodynamic therapy and topical application of a photosensitizing agent, followed by irradiation by a light source (typically blue or red), may be appropriate for some superficial and small nodular basal cell carcinomas.

Radiotherapy is effective and sometimes appropriate for older individuals (over age 65), but recurrent tumors after radiation therapy are more difficult to treat and may be more aggressive. Radiation therapy is the most expensive method to treat basal cell carcinoma and should be used only if other treatment options are not appropriate.

Hedgehog pathway inhibitors (vismodegib, sonidegib) are reserved for the treatment of advanced or metastatic basal cell carcinoma or in patients with extensive tumor burden (eg, basal cell nevus syndrome).

Firnhaber JM. Basal cell and cutaneous squamous cell carcinomas: diagnosis and treatment. Am Fam Physician. 2020; 102:339. [PMID: 32931212]

Peris K et al; European Dermatology Forum (EDF), the European Association of Dermato-Oncology (EADO) and the European Organization for Research and Treatment of Cancer (EORTC). Diagnosis and treatment of basal cell carcinoma: European consensus-based interdisciplinary guidelines. Eur J Cancer. 2019;118:10. [PMID: 31288208]

Thomson J et al. Interventions for basal cell carcinoma of the skin. Cochrane Database Syst Rev. 2020;11:CD003412. [PMID: 33202063]

4. Kaposi Sarcoma

General Considerations

Human herpes virus 8 (HHV-8), or Kaposi sarcoma–associated herpes virus, is the cause of all forms of Kaposi sarcoma. Kaposi sarcoma occurs in five forms. **Classic Kaposi sarcoma** occurs in older men, has a chronic clinical course, and is rarely fatal. **Endemic Kaposi sarcoma** occurs in an often aggressive form in young Black men of equatorial Africa. **Iatrogenic Kaposi sarcoma** occurs in patients receiving immunosuppressive therapy and improves upon decreasing immunosuppression. **Epidemic Kaposi sarcoma** is associated with HIV-associated immune deficiency. A fifth type is an indolent form of **Kaposi sarcoma** that occurs exclusively in HIV-negative men who have sex with men.

Red or purple plaques or nodules on cutaneous or mucosal surfaces are characteristic. Marked edema may occur with few or no skin lesions. Kaposi sarcoma commonly involves the GI tract and can be screened for by fecal occult blood testing. In asymptomatic patients, these lesions are not sought or treated. Pulmonary Kaposi sarcoma can present with shortness of breath, cough, hemoptysis, or chest pain; it may be asymptomatic, appearing only on chest radiograph. Bronchoscopy may be indicated. The incidence of AIDS-associated Kaposi sarcoma is diminishing. However, chronic Kaposi sarcoma can develop in patients with HIV infection, high CD4 counts, and low viral loads. In this setting, the Kaposi sarcoma usually resembles the endemic form, being indolent and localized. At times, however, it can be clinically aggressive. The presence of Kaposi sarcoma at the time of antiretroviral initiation is associated with Kaposi sarcoma–immune reconstitution inflammatory syndrome, which has an especially aggressive course in patients with visceral disease.

Treatment

For Kaposi sarcoma in elders, palliative local therapy with intralesional chemotherapy or radiation is usually all that is required. In the setting of iatrogenic immunosuppression, the treatment of Kaposi sarcoma is primarily reduction of doses of immunosuppressive medications. In AIDS-associated Kaposi sarcoma, the patient should first be given ART. Other therapeutic options include cryotherapy or intralesional vinblastine (0.1–0.5 mg/mL) for cosmetically objectionable lesions; radiation therapy for accessible and space-occupying lesions; and laser surgery for certain intraoral and pharyngeal lesions. Systemic therapy is indicated in patients with skin disease that is cosmetically unacceptable or those with advanced cutaneous, oral visceral, or nodal disease. ART plus chemotherapy appears to be more effective than ART alone (see Table 39–3). First-line systemic therapies include liposomal doxorubicin and paclitaxel. Other therapeutic options include pomalidomide, etoposide, gemcitabine, imatinib, interferon alpha-2b, thalidomide, vinorelbine, bleomycin plus vincristine, bevacizumab, lenalidomide, and immune checkpoint inhibitors.

Dupin N. Update on oncogenesis and therapy for Kaposi sarcoma. Curr Opin Oncol. 2020;32:122. [PMID: 31815777]

Reid E et al. AIDS-Related Kaposi Sarcoma, Version 2.2019, NCCN Clinical Practice Guidelines in Oncology. J Natl Compr Canc Netw. 2019;17:171. [PMID: 30787130]

5. Cutaneous T-Cell Lymphoma (Mycosis Fungoides)

ESSENTIALS OF DIAGNOSIS

- Localized or generalized erythematous patches that progress to scaly plaques and nodules.
- Sometimes associated with pruritus, lymphadenopathy.
- Distinctive histology.

General Considerations

Mycosis fungoides is a cutaneous T-cell lymphoma that begins on the skin and may remain there for years or decades. It may progress to systemic disease, including Sézary syndrome (erythroderma with circulating malignant T cells).

Clinical Findings

A. Symptoms and Signs

Localized or generalized erythematous patches or scaly plaques are present usually on the trunk. Plaques are almost always over 5 cm in diameter. Pruritus is a frequent complaint and can be severe. The lesions often begin as nondescript patches, and patients may have skin lesions for more than a decade before the diagnosis is confirmed. Follicular involvement with hair loss is characteristic of mycosis fungoides, and its presence should raise the suspicion of mycosis fungoides for any pruritic eruption. In more advanced cases, tumors appear. Local or diffuse lymphadenopathy may be due to benign expansion (dermatopathic lymphadenopathy) or involvement with mycosis fungoides.

B. Laboratory Findings

Diagnosis is based on skin biopsy though numerous biopsies may be required before the diagnosis is confirmed. In more advanced disease, circulating malignant T cells (Sézary cells) can be detected in the blood (T-cell gene rearrangement test). Eosinophilia may be present.

Differential Diagnosis

Mycosis fungoides may be confused with psoriasis, drug eruption, photoallergy, eczematous dermatitis, syphilis, or tinea corporis. Histologic examination can distinguish these conditions.

Treatment

The treatment of mycosis fungoides is complex. Early and aggressive treatment has not been proven to cure or prevent disease progression. Skin-directed therapies, including topical corticosteroids, topical mechlorethamine, bexarotene gel, and UV phototherapy, are used initially. If the disease progresses, PUVA plus retinoids, PUVA plus interferon, extracorporeal photopheresis, bexarotene, histone deacetylase inhibitors (romidepsin or vorinostat), targeted immunomodulators (brentuximab, mogamulizumab), and total skin electron beam treatment are used.

Prognosis

Mycosis fungoides is usually slowly progressive (over decades). Prognosis is better with patch or plaque stage disease and worse with erythroderma, tumors, and lymphadenopathy. Survival is not reduced in patients with limited patch disease. Elderly patients with limited disease commonly die of other causes. Overly aggressive treatment may lead to complications and premature demise.

Kempf W et al. Cutaneous T-cell lymphomas—an update 2021. Hematol Oncol. 2021;39:46. [PMID: 34105822]

Zinzani P et al. Critical concepts and management recommendations for cutaneous T-cell lymphoma: a consensus-based position paper from the Italian Group of Cutaneous Lymphoma. Hematol Oncol. 2021;39:275. [PMID: 33855728]

6. Bowen Disease & Paget Disease

Bowen disease (intraepidermal squamous cell carcinoma) can develop on sun-exposed and non–sun-exposed skin. The lesion is usually a small (0.5–3 cm), well-demarcated, slightly raised, pink to red, scaly plaque and may resemble psoriasis or a large actinic keratosis. Lesions may progress to invasive squamous cell carcinoma. Excision or other definitive treatment such as topical treatment (fluorouracil or imiquimod) or photodynamic therapy is indicated.

Extramammary Paget disease, a manifestation of intraepidermal carcinoma or underlying genitourinary or GI cancer, resembles chronic eczema and usually involves apocrine areas such as the genitalia. Mammary Paget disease of the nipple, a unilateral or rarely bilateral red scaling plaque that may ooze, is associated with an underlying intraductal mammary carcinoma (see Figure 17–3). While these lesions appear as red patches and plaques in fair-skinned persons, in darker-skinned individuals, hyperpigmentation may be prominent.

Morris CR et al. Extramammary Paget's disease: a review of the literature part ii: treatment and prognosis. Dermatol Surg. 2020;46:305. [PMID: 31688232]

Shim PJ et al. Photodynamic therapy for extramammary Paget's disease: a systematic review of the literature. Photodiagnosis Photodyn Ther. 2020;31:101911. [PMID: 32645437]

CUTANEOUS INFECTIONS, INFESTATIONS, & BITES

FUNGAL INFECTIONS

The diagnosis of fungal infections of the skin is based on the location and characteristics of the lesions and on the following laboratory examinations: (1) Direct demonstration of fungi in 10% KOH evaluation of suspected lesions. **"If it's scaly, scrape it" is a time-honored maxim** (Figure 6–8). (2) Cultures of organisms from skin scrapings. (3) Histologic sections of biopsies stained with periodic acid-Schiff technique may be diagnostic if scrapings and cultures are falsely negative.

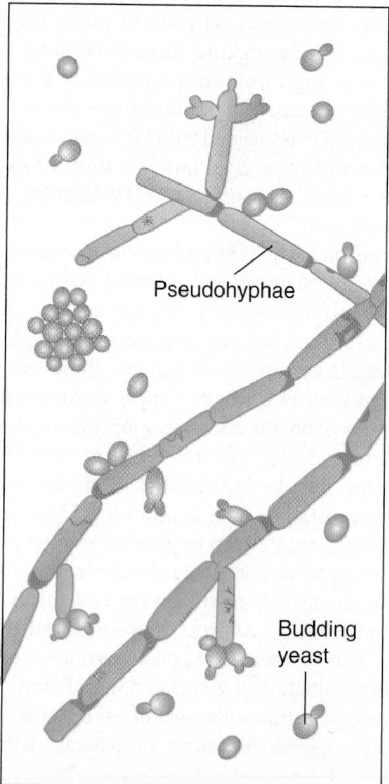

Figure 6–8. KOH preparation of fungus demonstrating pseudohyphae and budding yeast forms. (Reproduced, with permission, from Nicoll D et al. *Guide to Diagnostic Tests*, 7th ed. McGraw-Hill, 2017.)

Principles of Treatment

A diagnosis should always be confirmed by KOH preparation, culture, or biopsy. Many other diseases cause scaling, and use of an antifungal agent without a firm diagnosis makes subsequent diagnosis more difficult. In general, fungal infections are treated topically except for those with extensive involvement or involving the nails or hair follicles. In these situations, oral agents may be useful, with special attention to their side effects and complications, including hepatic toxicity.

General Measures & Prevention

Since moist skin favors the growth of fungi, dry the skin carefully after perspiring heavily or after bathing. The use of a hair dryer on a low setting may be helpful. Antifungal or drying powders may be useful with the exception of powders containing corn starch, which may exacerbate fungal infections. The use of topical corticosteroids for other diseases may be complicated by intercurrent tinea or candidal infection, and topical antifungals are often used in intertriginous areas with corticosteroids to prevent this.

TINEA CORPORIS OR TINEA CIRCINATA

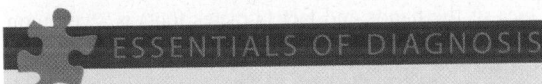

- Ring-shaped lesions with an advancing scaly border and central clearing or scaly patches with a distinct border.
- Microscopic examination of scrapings or culture confirms the diagnosis.

General Considerations

The lesions are often on exposed areas of the body such as the face and arms. A history of exposure to an infected pet (who may have scaly rash or patches of alopecia) may occasionally be obtained, usually indicating *Microsporum* infection. *Trichophyton rubrum* is the most common pathogen, usually representing extension onto the trunk or extremities of tinea cruris, pedis, or manuum.

Clinical Findings

A. Symptoms and Signs

Itching may be present. In classic lesions, rings of erythema have an advancing scaly border and central clearing.

B. Laboratory Findings

The diagnosis should be confirmed by KOH preparation or culture.

Differential Diagnosis

Positive fungal studies distinguish tinea corporis from other skin lesions with annular configuration, such as the annular lesions of psoriasis, lupus erythematosus, syphilis, granuloma annulare, and pityriasis rosea. Psoriasis has typical lesions on elbows, knees, scalp, and nails. Secondary syphilis is often manifested by characteristic palmar, plantar, and mucous membrane lesions. Tinea corporis rarely has the large number of symmetric lesions seen in pityriasis rosea. Granuloma annulare lacks scale.

Complications

Complications include extension of the disease down the hair follicles (which presents as papules and pustules and requires systemic antifungals to cure) and pyoderma.

Prevention

Treat infected household pets (*Microsporum* infections). To prevent recurrences, the use of foot powder and keeping feet dry by wearing sandals or changing socks can be useful.

Treatment

A. Local Measures

Tinea corporis responds to most topical antifungals, including terbinafine, butenafine, econazole, miconazole, and clotrimazole, most of which are available over the counter in the United States (see Table 6–2). Terbinafine and butenafine require shorter courses and lead to the most rapid response. **Treatment should be continued for 1–2 weeks after clinical clearing**. Betamethasone dipropionate with clotrimazole (Lotrisone) is not recommended. Long-term improper use may result in side effects from the high-potency corticosteroid component, especially in body folds.

B. Systemic Measures

Itraconazole as a single weeklong pulse of 200 mg orally daily is effective in tinea corporis. Terbinafine, 250 mg orally daily for 1 month, is an alternative.

Prognosis

Tinea corporis usually responds promptly to conservative topical therapy or to an oral agent within 4 weeks.

Preda-Naumescu A et al. Common cutaneous infections: patient presentation, clinical course, and treatment options. Med Clin North Am. 2021;105:783. [PMID: 34059250]

TINEA CRURIS (Jock Itch)

ESSENTIALS OF DIAGNOSIS

- Marked itching in intertriginous areas, usually sparing the scrotum.
- Peripherally spreading, sharply demarcated, centrally clearing erythematous lesions.
- May have associated tinea infection of feet or toenails.
- Laboratory examination with microscope or culture confirms diagnosis.

General Considerations

Tinea cruris lesions are confined to the groin and gluteal cleft. Intractable pruritus ani may occasionally be caused by a tinea infection.

Clinical Findings

A. Symptoms and Signs

Itching may be severe, or the rash may be asymptomatic. The lesions have sharp margins, cleared centers, and active, spreading scaly peripheries. Follicular pustules are sometimes encountered. The area may be hyperpigmented on resolution.

B. Laboratory Findings

Hyphae can be demonstrated microscopically in KOH preparations or skin biopsy. The organism may be cultured.

Differential Diagnosis

Tinea cruris must be distinguished from other lesions involving the intertriginous areas, such as candidiasis, seborrheic dermatitis, intertrigo, psoriasis of body folds ("inverse psoriasis"), and erythrasma (corynebacterial infection of intertriginous areas). Candidiasis is generally bright red and marked by satellite papules and pustules outside of the main border of the lesion. *Candida* typically involves the scrotum. Seborrheic dermatitis also often involves the face, sternum, axillae, and genitalia (but not the crural folds). Intertrigo tends to be less red, less scaly, and present in obese individuals in moist body folds with less extension onto the thigh. "Inverse psoriasis" is characterized by distinct plaques. Other areas of typical psoriatic involvement should be checked, and the KOH examination will be negative. Erythrasma is best diagnosed with Wood (UV) light—a brilliant coral-red fluorescence is seen.

Treatment

A. General Measures

Drying powder (eg, miconazole nitrate [Zeasorb-AF]) can be dusted into the involved area in patients with excessive perspiration or occlusion of skin due to obesity as a preventive measure but is less helpful for treatment.

B. Local Measures

Any of the topical antifungal preparations listed in Table 6–2 may be used. Terbinafine cream is curative in over 80% of cases after once-daily use for 7 days.

C. Systemic Measures

One week of either itraconazole, 200 mg orally daily, or terbinafine, 250 mg orally daily, can be effective.

Prognosis

Tinea cruris usually responds promptly to topical or systemic treatment but often recurs.

Preda-Naumescu A et al. Common cutaneous infections: patient presentation, clinical course, and treatment options. Med Clin North Am. 2021;105:783. [PMID: 34059250]

TINEA MANUUM & TINEA PEDIS (Tinea of Palms & Soles)

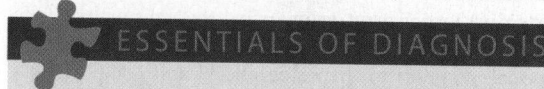

ESSENTIALS OF DIAGNOSIS

- Most often presents with asymptomatic scaling.
- May progress to fissuring or maceration in toe web spaces.
- May be a portal of entry for bacteria causing lower extremity cellulitis.
- Itching, burning, and stinging of interdigital web; scaling palms and soles; vesicles on soles in inflammatory cases.
- KOH preparation or fungal culture of skin scapings is usually positive.

General Considerations

Tinea of the hands and feet (athlete's foot) is a common acute or chronic dermatosis. Most infections are caused by *Trichophyton* species.

Clinical Findings

A. Symptoms and Signs

The presenting symptom may be itching, burning, or stinging. Pain may indicate secondary infection with complicating cellulitis. Interdigital tinea pedis is the most common predisposing cause of lower extremity cellulitis in healthy individuals. Regular examination of the feet of diabetic patients for evidence of scaling and fissuring and treatment of any identified tinea pedis may prevent complications. Tinea pedis has several presentations that vary with the location. On the sole and heel, tinea may appear as chronic noninflammatory scaling, occasionally with thickening and fissuring. This may extend over the sides of the feet in a "moccasin" distribution (Figure 6–9). The KOH preparation is usually positive. Tinea pedis often appears as a scaling or fissuring of the toe webs, often with maceration (Figure 6–10). As the web spaces become more macerated, the KOH preparation and fungal culture are less often positive because bacterial species begin to dominate. Finally, there may also be vesicles, bullae, or generalized exfoliation of the skin of the soles, or nail involvement in the form of discoloration, friability, and thickening of the nail plate.

B. Laboratory Findings

KOH and culture do not always demonstrate pathogenic fungi from macerated areas.

Differential Diagnosis

Another skin condition involving the same areas is interdigital erythrasma (use Wood light). Psoriasis may be a

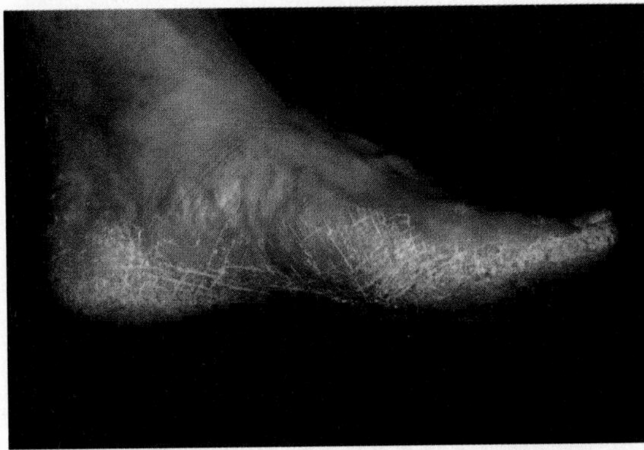

▲ **Figure 6–9.** Tinea pedis in the moccasin distribution. (Reproduced with permission from Richard P. Usatine, MD, in Usatine RP, Smith MA, Mayeaux EJ Jr, Chumley H. *The Color Atlas of Family Medicine*, 2nd ed. McGraw-Hill, 2013.)

cause of chronic scaling on the palms or soles and may cause nail changes. Repeated fungal cultures should be negative, and the condition will not respond to antifungal therapy. Contact dermatitis will often involve the dorsal surfaces and will respond to topical or systemic corticosteroids. Vesicular lesions should be differentiated from pompholyx (dyshidrosis) and scabies by proper scraping of the roofs of individual vesicles. Rarely, gram-negative organisms may cause toe web infections, manifested as an acute erosive flare of interdigital disease. This entity is treated with aluminum salts and imidazole antifungal agents or ciclopirox. *Candida* may also cause erosive interdigital disease.

Prevention

The essential factor in prevention is personal hygiene. Wear open-toed sandals if possible. Use of sandals in community showers and bathing places is often recommended, though the effectiveness of this practice has not been studied. Careful drying between the toes after showering is essential. A hair dryer used on cooler setting may be helpful. Socks should be changed frequently, and absorbent nonsynthetic socks are preferred. Apply dusting and drying powders as necessary. The use of powders containing antifungal agents (eg, Zeasorb-AF) or long-term use of antifungal creams may prevent recurrences of tinea pedis.

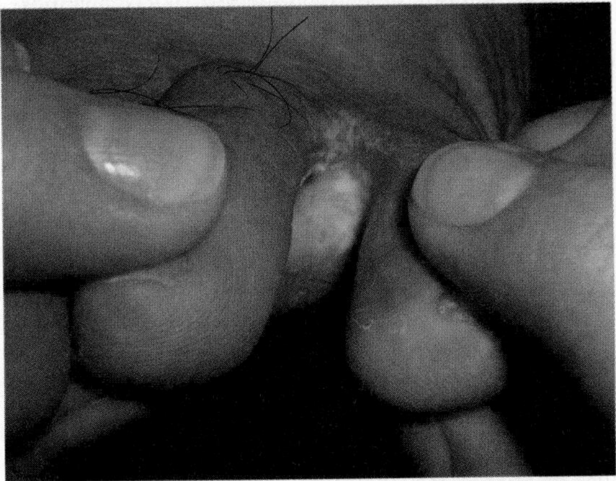

▲ **Figure 6–10.** Tinea pedis in the interdigital space between fourth and fifth digits. The differential diagnosis includes a bacterial primary or secondary infection with gram-negative organisms. (Reproduced with permission from Richard P. Usatine, MD, in Usatine RP, Smith MA, Mayeaux EJ Jr, Chumley HS. *The Color Atlas and Synopsis of Family Medicine*, 3rd ed. McGraw-Hill, 2019.)

Treatment

A. Local Measures

1. Macerated stage—Treat with aluminum subacetate solution soaks for 20 minutes twice daily. Broad-spectrum antifungal creams and solutions (containing imidazoles or ciclopirox) (Table 6–2) will help combat diphtheroids and other gram-positive organisms present at this stage and alone may be adequate therapy. If topical imidazoles fail, 1 week of once-daily topical allylamine treatment (terbinafine or butenafine) will often result in clearing.

2. Dry and scaly stage—Use any of the antifungal agents listed in Table 6–2. The addition of urea 10–20% lotion or cream may increase the efficacy of topical treatments in thick ("moccasin") tinea of the soles.

B. Systemic Measures

Itraconazole, 200 mg orally daily for 2 weeks or 400 mg daily for 1 week, or terbinafine, 250 mg orally daily for 2–4 weeks, may be used in refractory cases. If the infection is cleared by systemic therapy, the patient should be encouraged to begin maintenance with topical therapy, since recurrence is common.

Prognosis

For many individuals, tinea pedis is a chronic affliction, temporarily cleared by therapy only to recur. Treatment of tinea pedis or manuum without systemic treatment of affected nails may result in recurrent skin disease.

Foley K et al. Topical and device-based treatments for fungal infections of the toenails. Cochrane Database Syst Rev. 2020;1:CD012093. [PMID: 31978269]

TINEA VERSICOLOR (Pityriasis Versicolor)

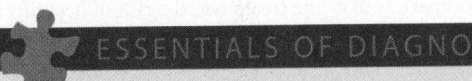

- Velvety, tan, pink, or white macules or white macules that do not tan with sun exposure.
- Fine scales that are not visible but are seen by scraping the lesion.
- Central upper trunk the most frequent site.
- Yeast and short hyphae observed on microscopic examination of scales.

General Considerations

Tinea versicolor is a mild, superficial *Malassezia* infection of the skin (usually of the upper trunk). This yeast is a colonizer of all humans, which accounts for the high recurrence rate after treatment. The eruption is often called to patients' attention by the fact that the involved areas will not tan, and the resulting hypopigmentation may be mistaken for vitiligo. A hyperpigmented form is not uncommon.

Clinical Findings

A. Symptoms and Signs

Lesions are asymptomatic, but a few patients note itching. The lesions are velvety, tan, pink, or white macules or thin papules that vary from 4 mm to 5 mm in diameter to large confluent areas. The lesions initially do not look scaly, but scales may be readily obtained by scraping the area. Lesions may appear on the trunk, upper arms, neck, and groin.

B. Laboratory Findings

Large, blunt hyphae and thick-walled budding spores ("spaghetti and meatballs") are seen on KOH. Fungal culture is not useful.

Differential Diagnosis

Vitiligo usually presents with larger periorificial and acral lesions and is also characterized by total (not partial) depigmentation. Vitiligo does not scale. Pink and red-brown lesions on the chest are differentiated from seborrheic dermatitis of the same areas by the KOH preparation.

Treatment & Prognosis

A. Initial Treatment

Topical treatments include selenium sulfide lotion, which may be applied from neck to waist daily and left on for 5–15 minutes for 7 days; this treatment is repeated weekly for a month. Ketoconazole shampoo, 1% or 2%, lathered on the chest and back and left on for 5 minutes may also be used weekly for treatment. Clinicians must stress to the patient that the raised and scaly aspects of the rash are being treated; the alterations in pigmentation may take months to fade or fill in.

A regimen of two doses of oral fluconazole, 300 mg, 14 days apart, is first-line treatment; the risk of hepatitis is minimal. Additional doses may be required in severe cases or humid climates. Ketoconazole is no longer recommended as first-line treatment because of the risk of drug-induced hepatitis.

B. Maintenance Therapy

Topical treatments as described above can be used for maintenance therapy. Selenium sulfide lotion should be used monthly, and ketoconazole shampoo, 1% or 2%, may be used to prevent recurrence. Imidazole creams, solutions, and lotions (eg, clotrimazole or miconazole) are quite effective for localized areas but are too expensive for use over large areas, such as the chest and back. Without maintenance therapy, recurrences will occur in over 80% of "cured" cases.

Bakr E et al. Adapalene gel 0.1% vs ketoconazole cream 2% and their combination in treatment of pityriasis versicolor: a randomized clinical study. Dermatol Ther. 2020;33:e13319. [PMID: 32182387]

MUCOCUTANEOUS CANDIDIASIS

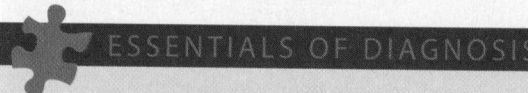

- Severe pruritus of vulva, anus, or body folds.
- Superficial denuded, beefy-red areas with or without satellite vesicopustules.
- Whitish curd-like concretions on the oral and vaginal mucous membranes.
- Yeast and pseudohyphae on microscopic examination of scales or curd.

General Considerations

Mucocutaneous candidiasis is a superficial fungal infection that may involve almost any cutaneous or mucous surface. It is particularly likely to occur in diabetic patients, during pregnancy, in obese persons, and in the setting of immunosuppression. Systemic antibiotics, oral corticosteroids, hormone replacement therapy, and oral contraceptive agents may be contributory. Oral and interdigital candidiasis may be the first sign of HIV infection (see Chapter 31). Denture use predisposes the elderly to infection. Abnormalities in the IL-17, IL-22, mannose-binding lectin, and toll-like receptors have all been implicated in predisposing patients to *Candida* infection of the skin and mucous membranes.

Clinical Findings

A. Symptoms and Signs

Itching may be intense. Burning is reported, particularly around the vulva and anus. The lesions consist of superficially denuded, beefy-red areas in the depths of the body folds, such as in the groin and the intergluteal cleft, beneath the breasts, at the angles of the mouth, in the webspaces of digits, and in the umbilicus. The peripheries of these denuded lesions are superficially undermined, and there may be satellite vesicopustules. Whitish, curd-like concretions may be present on mucosal lesions (Figure 6–11). Paronychia may occur.

B. Laboratory Findings

Clusters of budding yeast and pseudohyphae can be seen under high power (400×) when skin scales or curd-like

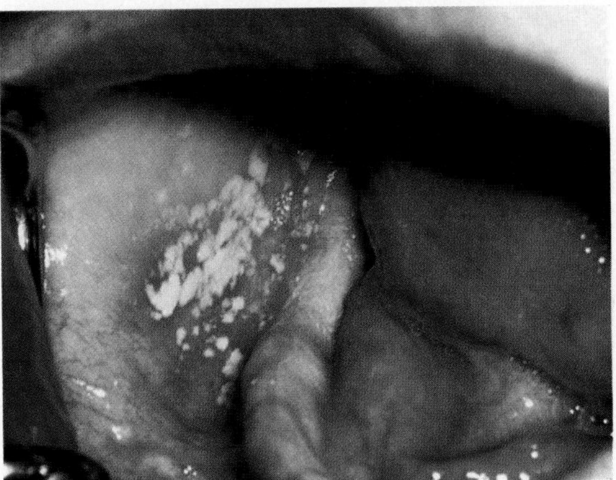

▲ **Figure 6–11.** Oral mucosal candidiasis. (Sol Silverman, Jr., D.D.S/Centers for Disease Control and Prevention.)

lesions are mounted in 10% KOH. Culture can confirm the diagnosis.

Differential Diagnosis

Intertrigo, seborrheic dermatitis, tinea cruris, "inverse psoriasis," and erythrasma involving the same areas may mimic mucocutaneous candidiasis.

Complications

Systemic invasive candidiasis with candidemia may occur in patients who are immunosuppressed or receiving broad-spectrum antibiotic or intravenous hypertonic glucose solutions (eg, hyperalimentation). There may or may not be clinically evident mucocutaneous candidiasis.

Treatment

A. General Measures

Affected parts should be kept dry and exposed to air as much as possible. Water immersion should be minimized and gloves should be worn for those with infected nails or digital skin. If possible, discontinue systemic antibiotics. For treatment of systemic invasive candidiasis, see Chapter 36.

B. Local Measures

1. Nails and paronychia—Apply clotrimazole solution 1% twice daily. Thymol 4% in ethanol applied once daily is an alternative.

2. Skin—Apply nystatin ointment or clotrimazole cream 1%, with hydrocortisone cream 1–2.5%, twice daily. Gentian violet 0.5% solution is economical and highly effective in treating mucocutaneous candidiasis, but the purple discoloration may represent a cosmetic issue. Severe or widespread cutaneous disease responds to fluconazole, 100–200 mg orally daily, for 1 week.

3. Vulvar and anal mucous membranes—For vaginal candidiasis, single-dose fluconazole (150 mg orally) is effective. Intravaginal clotrimazole, miconazole, terconazole, or nystatin may also be used. Long-term suppressive therapy may be required for recurrent or "intractable" cases. Non-albicans candidal species may be identified by culture in some refractory cases and may respond to oral itraconazole, 200 mg twice daily for 2–4 weeks.

4. Balanitis—This is most frequent in uncircumcised men, usually caused by *Candida*. Topical nystatin ointment is the initial treatment if the lesions are mildly erythematous or superficially erosive. Soaking with dilute 5% aluminum acetate for 15 minutes twice daily may quickly relieve burning or itching. Chronicity and relapses, especially after sexual contact, suggest reinfection from a sexual partner who should be treated. Severe purulent balanitis is usually due to bacteria. If it is so severe that phimosis occurs, oral antibiotics—some with activity against anaerobes—are required; if rapid improvement does not occur, urologic consultation is indicated.

5. Mastitis—Lancinating breast pain and nipple dermatitis in breast-feeding women may be a manifestation of *Candida* colonization/infection of the breast ducts. Topical nystatin cream and clotrimazole 0.1% cream are safe during lactation. Topical gentian violet 0.5% daily for 7 days is also useful. Oral fluconazole, 200 mg daily for 2 weeks, is effective and safe during lactation.

Prognosis

Cases of cutaneous candidiasis range from the easily cured to the intractable and prolonged.

Puel A. Human inborn errors of immunity underlying superficial or invasive candidiasis. Hum Genet. 2020;139:1011. [PMID: 32124012]

Yano J et al. Current patient perspectives of vulvovaginal candidiasis: incidence, symptoms, management and post-treatment outcomes. BMC Womens Health. 2019;19:48. [PMID: 30925872]

INTERTRIGO

Intertrigo is caused by the macerating effect of heat, moisture, and friction. It is especially likely to occur in obese persons and in humid climates. The symptoms are itching, stinging, and burning. The body folds develop fissures, erythema, maceration, and superficial denudation. Candidiasis may complicate intertrigo. "Inverse psoriasis," seborrheic dermatitis, tinea cruris, erythrasma, and candidiasis must be ruled out.

Maintain hygiene in the area and keep it dry. Compresses may be useful acutely. Hydrocortisone 1% cream plus an imidazole or clotrimazole 1% cream is effective. Recurrences are common.

Kottner J et al. Prevalence of intertrigo and associated factors: a secondary data analysis of four annual multicentre prevalence studies in the Netherlands. Int J Nurs Stud. 2020;104:103437. [PMID: 32105975]

VIRAL INFECTIONS

HERPES SIMPLEX (Cold or Fever Sore; Genital Herpes)

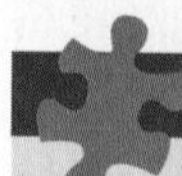

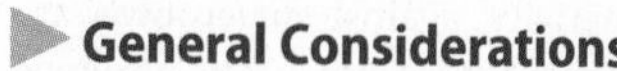

ESSENTIALS OF DIAGNOSIS

- Recurrent small grouped vesicles (especially orolabial and genital) on an erythematous base.
- May follow minor infections, trauma, stress, or sun exposure.
- Regional tender lymphadenopathy may occur.
- Direct fluorescent antibody tests are positive.

General Considerations

Over 85% of adults have serologic evidence of herpes simplex type 1 (HSV-1) infections, most often acquired asymptomatically in childhood. Occasionally, primary infections may be manifested as severe gingivostomatitis. Thereafter, the patient may have recurrent self-limited attacks, provoked by sun exposure, orofacial surgery, fever, viral infection, or immunosuppression.

About 25% of the US population has serologic evidence of infection with herpes simplex type 2 (HSV-2). HSV-2 causes lesions whose morphology and natural history are similar to those caused by HSV-1 but are typically located on the genitalia or buttocks of both sexes. The infection is acquired by sexual contact. In monogamous heterosexual couples where one partner has HSV-2 infection, seroconversion of the noninfected partner occurs in 10% over a 1-year period. Up to 70% of such infections appeared to be transmitted during periods of asymptomatic shedding. Genital herpes may also be due to HSV-1.

Clinical Findings

A. Symptoms and Signs

The principal symptoms are burning and stinging. Neuralgia may precede or accompany attacks. The lesions consist of small, grouped vesicles on an erythematous base that can occur anywhere but that most often occur on the vermilion border of the lips (Figure 6–12), the oral cavity, penile shaft, the labia, the perianal skin, and the buttocks. Any erosion or fissure in the anogenital region can be due to herpes simplex. Regional lymph nodes may be swollen and tender. The lesions usually crust and heal in 1 week. Immunosuppressed patients may have unusual variants, including verrucous or nodular herpes lesions at typical sites of involvement. Lesions of herpes simplex must be distinguished from chancroid, syphilis, lymphogranuloma venereum, pyoderma gangrenosum, or trauma.

B. Laboratory Findings

Direct fluorescent antibody slide tests offer rapid, sensitive diagnosis. Viral culture or PCR may also be helpful. Herpes

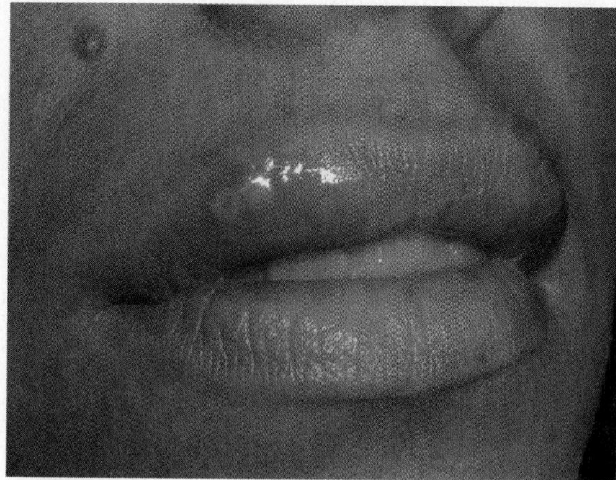

▲ **Figure 6–12.** Orolabial herpes simplex showing deroofed blisters (ulcer). (Reproduced with permission from Richard P. Usatine, MD, in Usatine RP, Smith MA, Mayeaux EJ Jr, Chumley H. *The Color Atlas of Family Medicine*, 2nd ed. McGraw-Hill, 2013.)

serology is not used in the diagnosis of an acute genital ulcer. Specific HSV-2 serology by Western blot assay or ELISA can determine who is HSV-infected and potentially infectious, but routine HSV-2 screening is not recommended by the USPSTF.

Complications

Complications include pyoderma, eczema herpeticum, herpetic whitlow, herpes gladiatorum (epidemic herpes transmitted by contact), proctitis, esophagitis, neonatal infection, keratitis, and encephalitis.

Treatment

A. Systemic Therapy

Three systemic agents are available for the treatment of acute herpes infections: acyclovir, valacyclovir, and famciclovir. All three agents are very effective, and when used properly, virtually nontoxic. Only acyclovir is available for intravenous administration. In the immunocompetent, with the exception of severe orolabial herpes, only genital disease is treated.

1. For first clinical episode—Recommended treatment for the first clinical episodes of herpes simplex includes acyclovir, 400 mg orally five times daily (or 800 mg three times daily); valacyclovir, 1000 mg orally twice daily; or famciclovir, 250 mg orally three times daily; treatment is for 7–10 days, depending on the severity of the outbreak.

2. For mild recurrences—Most cases do not require therapy. Pharmacotherapy of recurrent HSV is of limited benefit, reducing the average outbreak by only 12–24 hours. **To be effective, the treatment must be initiated by the patient at the first sign of recurrence**. If treatment is desired, recurrent genital herpes outbreaks may be treated with 3 days of valacyclovir, 500 mg orally twice daily, 5 days of acyclovir, 200 mg orally five times a day, or 5 days of famciclovir, 125 mg orally twice daily. Valacyclovir, 2 g twice daily for 1 day, and famciclovir, 1 g once or twice in 1 day, are equally effective short-course alternatives and can abort impending recurrences of both orolabial and genital herpes. The addition of a potent topical corticosteroid three times daily reduces the duration, size, and pain of orolabial herpes treated with an oral antiviral agent.

3. For frequent or severe recurrences—Suppressive treatment reduces recurrences by 85%, viral shedding by more than 90%, and the risk of transmission by 50%. The recommended suppressive doses, taken continuously, are acyclovir, 400 mg orally twice daily; valacyclovir, 500 mg orally once daily; or famciclovir, 125–250 mg orally twice daily. Pritelivir, 100 mg orally once daily, may have superior reduction of viral shedding in HSV-2 compared to valacyclovir, 500 mg orally once daily. Long-term suppression appears safe, and after 5–7 years a substantial proportion of patients can discontinue treatment.

Sunscreens are useful adjuncts in preventing sun-induced orolabial recurrences. A preventive antiviral medication should be started beginning 24 hours prior to UV light exposure, dental surgery, or orolabial cosmetic surgery. The use of latex condoms and patient education have proved effective in reducing genital herpes transmission in some but not all studies. No single or combination intervention absolutely prevents transmission.

B. Local Measures

Topical therapy has limited efficacy and is generally not recommended because evidence shows that it minimally reduces skin healing time.

Prognosis

Aside from the complications described above, recurrent attacks last several days, and patients recover without sequelae.

Damour A et al. Eczema herpeticum: clinical and pathophysiological aspects. Clin Rev Allergy Immunol. 2020;59:1. [PMID: 31836943]

HERPES ZOSTER (Shingles)

See Chapter 32.

MOLLUSCUM CONTAGIOSUM

Molluscum contagiosum, caused by a poxvirus, presents as single or multiple dome-shaped, waxy papules 2–5 mm in diameter that are umbilicated (Figure 6–13). Lesions at first are firm, solid, and flesh-colored but upon reaching maturity become soft, whitish, or pearly gray and may suppurate. The principal sites of involvement are the face, lower abdomen, and genitals.

The lesions are autoinoculable and spread by wet skin-to-skin contact. In sexually active individuals, they may be confined to the penis, pubis, and inner thighs and are considered a sexually transmitted infection.

Molluscum contagiosum is common in patients with AIDS, usually with a helper T-cell count less than 100/mcL (0.1×10^9/L). Extensive lesions tend to develop over the face and neck as well as in the genital area.

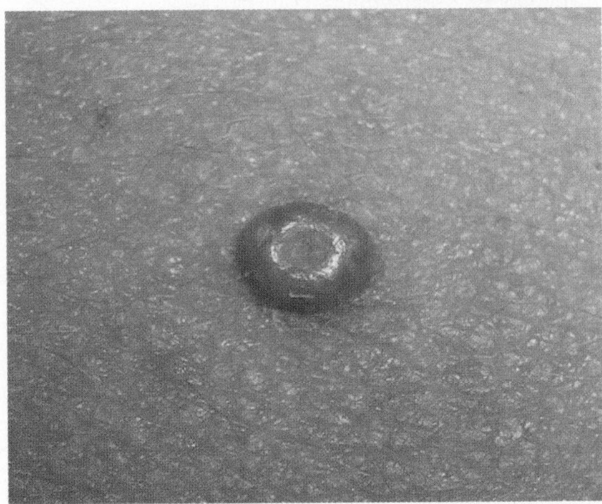

▲ **Figure 6–13. Umbilicated—molluscum.** (Reproduced with permission from Richard P. Usatine, MD, in Usatine RP, Smith MA, Mayeaux EJ Jr, Chumley H. *The Color Atlas of Family Medicine*, 3nd ed. McGraw-Hill, 2019.)

The diagnosis is easily established in most instances because of the distinctive central umbilication of the dome-shaped lesion. Estimated time to remission is 13 months. The best treatment is by curettage or applications of liquid nitrogen as for warts—but more briefly. When lesions are frozen, the central umbilication often becomes more apparent. Light electrosurgery with a fine needle is also effective. Cantharadin (applied in the office and then washed off by the patient 4 hours later) is a safe and effective option. Another treatment option is 10% or 15% potassium hydroxide solution applied twice daily until lesions clear. Salicylic acid, podophyllotoxin, tretinoin, imiquimod, and intralesional immunotherapy are additional treatment options. Physical destruction with pulsed dye laser or via extraction of molluscum bodies with a comedone extractor or currette is also effective. Lesions are difficult to eradicate in patients with AIDS unless immunity improves; however, with highly effective antiretroviral treatment, molluscum usually spontaneously clears.

Wells A et al. Intralesional immunotherapy for molluscum contagiosum: a review. Dermatol Ther. 2020;33:e14386. [PMID: 33044025]

WARTS

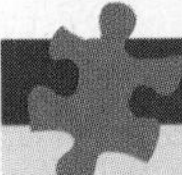

ESSENTIALS OF DIAGNOSIS

- Verrucous papules anywhere on the skin or mucous membranes, usually not > 1 cm in diameter.
- Prolonged incubation period (average 2–18 months).
- Spontaneous "cures" of common warts in 50% at 2 years.
- "Recurrences" (new lesions) are frequent.

General Considerations

Warts (common, plantar, and genital [condylomata acuminata]) are caused by HPVs. Typing of HPV lesions is not a part of standard medical evaluation except in the case of anogenital dysplasia.

Clinical Findings

There are usually no symptoms. Tenderness on pressure occurs with plantar warts; itching occurs with anogenital warts (Figure 6–14). Flat warts are most evident under oblique illumination. Periungual warts may be dry, fissured, and hyperkeratotic and may resemble hangnails. Plantar warts resemble plantar corns or calluses.

Differential Diagnosis

Some warty-looking lesions are actually seborrheic keratosis, hypertrophic actinic keratoses or squamous cell carcinomas. Some genital warty lesions are condylomata lata of secondary syphilis. Molluscum contagiosum lesions are pearly with a central dell. In AIDS, wart-like lesions may be caused by varicella zoster virus.

Prevention

Administration of a vaccine against certain anogenital HPV types (including 6, 11, 16, 18, 31, 33, 45, 52, and 58) can prevent infection with these wart types and reduce anogenital, oropharyngeal, and cervical cancer. It is recommended for teenagers and young adults, men who have sex with men, and immunocompromised patients (see Chapters 1 and 18). There may be a role for adjuvant vaccination in HPV-infected patients.

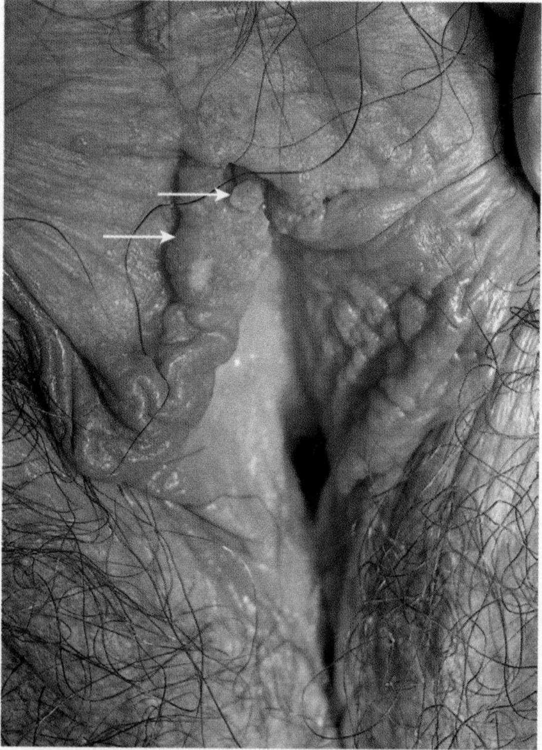

▲ **Figure 6–14.** Condylomata acuminata around the clitoris, labia minor, and opening of the vagina. (Reproduced with permission from Richard P. Usatine, MD, in Usatine RP, Smith MA, Mayeaux EJ Jr, Chumley H. *The Color Atlas of Family Medicine*, 2nd ed. McGraw-Hill, 2013.)

Treatment

Treatment is aimed at inducing "wart-free" intervals for as long as possible without scarring, since no treatment can guarantee a remission or prevent recurrences. In immunocompromised patients, the goal is to control the size and number of lesions present. Certain types (HPV 1) are more responsive to treatment than others (eg, HPV 2, HPV 27).

A. Treatment of Nongenital Warts

For common warts of the hands, patients are usually offered liquid nitrogen or keratolytic agents. The former may work in fewer treatments but requires office visits and is painful.

1. Liquid nitrogen—Liquid nitrogen cryotherapy is applied to achieve a thaw time of 30–45 seconds. Two freeze-thaw cycles are given every 2–4 weeks for several visits. Scarring will occur if it is used incorrectly. Liquid nitrogen may cause permanent depigmentation in darkly pigmented individuals.

2. Keratolytic agents and occlusion—Salicylic acid products may be used against common warts or plantar warts. They are applied, then occluded. Plantar warts may be treated by applying a 40% salicylic acid plaster after paring. The plaster may be left on for 5–6 days, then removed, the lesion pared down, and another plaster applied. Although it may take weeks or months to eradicate the wart, the method is safe and effective with almost no side effects. Chronic occlusion alone with water-impermeable tape (duct tape, adhesive tape) is less effective than cryotherapy.

3. Operative removal—Plantar warts may be removed by blunt dissection.

4. Laser therapy—The CO_2 laser can be effective for treating recurrent warts, periungual warts, plantar warts, and genital warts. It leaves open wounds that must fill in with granulation tissue over 4–6 weeks and is best reserved for warts resistant to all other modalities. Lasers with emissions of 585, 595, or 532 nm may also be used every 3–4 weeks to ablate common, plantar, facial, and anogenital warts but are not more effective than cryotherapy in controlled trials. Photodynamic therapy can be considered in refractory widespread flat warts.

5. Immunotherapy—Squaric acid dibutylester may be applied 1–5 times weekly in a concentration of 0.2–2% directly to the warts to induce a mild contact dermatitis. Between 60% and 80% of warts clear over 10–20 weeks. Injection of *Candida* antigen starting at 1:50 dilution and repeated every 3–4 weeks may be similarly effective in stimulating immunologic regression of common and plantar warts.

6. Other agents—Bleomycin (1 unit/mL), injected into common and plantar warts has been shown to have a high cure rate. It should be used with caution on digital warts because of the potential complications of Raynaud phenomenon, nail loss, and terminal digital necrosis. 5-Fluorouracil 5% cream applied once or twice daily, usually with occlusion, has similar efficacy to other treatment methods. Topical or intralesional cidofovir may be effective in treating recalcitrant lesions, especially in immunocompromised patients.

7. Physical modalities—Soaking warts in hot (42.2°C) water for 10–30 minutes daily for 6 weeks has resulted in involution in some cases.

B. Treatment of Genital Warts

1. Liquid nitrogen—Cryotherapy is first-line clinician-applied surgical treatment for genital warts. Liquid nitrogen cryotherapy is applied to achieve a thaw time of 30–45 seconds. Two freeze-thaw cycles are given every 2–4 weeks for several visits. Scarring will occur if it is used incorrectly. Liquid nitrogen may cause permanent depigmentation in pigmented individuals.

2. Podophyllum resin—For genital warts, the purified active component of the podophyllum resin, podofilox, is applied by the patient twice daily 3 consecutive days a week for cycles of 4–6 weeks. It is less irritating and more effective than "clinician-applied" podophyllum resin. After a single 4-week cycle, 45% of patients were wart-free but 60% relapsed at 6 weeks. Thus, multiple cycles of treatment are often necessary. Patients unable to obtain the take-home podofilox may be treated in the clinician's office by painting each wart carefully (protecting normal skin) every 2–3 weeks with 25% podophyllum resin (podophyllin) in compound tincture of benzoin.

3. Imiquimod—A 5% cream of this local interferon inducer has moderate activity in clearing external genital warts. Treatment is once daily on 3 alternate days per week. Response may be slow. Complete clearing of lesions occurs in 77% of women and 40% of men with 13% recurrences in the short term.

Although imiquimod is considerably more expensive than podophyllotoxin, it is the "patient-administered" treatment of choice for external genital warts in women due to its high response rate and safety. In men, podophyllin resin remains the preferred initial treatment due to its more rapid response, lower cost, and similar efficacy; imiquimod is used for recurrences or refractory cases. Imiquimod has no demonstrated efficacy for—and should not be used to treat—plantar or common warts.

4. Sinecatechins—Derived from green tea extract, sinecatechins (10% or 15%) is FDA approved for the treatment of anogenital warts. Application three times daily for 16 weeks achieves clearance rates from 40% to 81%, with the 15% formulation resulting in higher efficacy.

5. Operative removal—For pedunculated or large genital warts, snip biopsy (scissors) removal followed by light electrocautery is more effective than cryotherapy.

6. Laser therapy—See Treatment of Nongenital Warts, above. For genital warts, it has not been shown that laser therapy is more effective than electrosurgical removal. Photodynamic therapy can be considered in refractory genital warts.

Prognosis

There is a striking tendency to develop new lesions. Warts may disappear spontaneously or may be unresponsive to treatment. Combining therapies (eg, liquid nitrogen plus immunotherapy) may improve therapeutic response.

Anshelevich EE et al. Intralesional cidofovir for treatment of recalcitrant warts in both immunocompetent and immunocompromised patients: a retrospective analysis of 58 patients. J Am Acad Dermatol. 2021;84:206. [PMID: 32348821]

García-Oreja S et al. Topical treatment for plantar warts: a systematic review. Dermatol Ther. 2021;34:e14621. [PMID: 33263934]

Jung JM et al. Topically applied treatments for external genital warts in nonimmunocompromised patients: a systematic review and network meta-analysis. Br J Dermatol. 2020;183:24. [PMID: 31675442]

O'Mahony C et al. Position statement for the diagnosis and management of anogenital warts. J Eur Acad Dermatol Venereol. 2019;33:1006. [PMID: 30968980]

BACTERIAL INFECTIONS

IMPETIGO

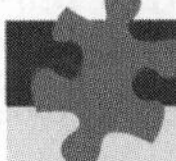

ESSENTIALS OF DIAGNOSIS

- Superficial blisters filled with purulent material that rupture easily.
- Crusted superficial erosions.
- Positive Gram stain and bacterial culture.

General Considerations

Impetigo is a contagious and autoinoculable infection of the skin (epidermis) caused by staphylococci or streptococci.

Clinical Findings

A. Symptoms and Signs

The lesions consist of macules, vesicles, bullae, pustules, and honey-colored crusts that when removed leave denuded red areas (Figure 6–15). The face and other exposed parts are most often involved. Ecthyma is a deeper form of impetigo caused by staphylococci or streptococci, with ulceration and scarring that occurs frequently on the extremities.

B. Laboratory Findings

Gram stain and culture confirm the diagnosis. In temperate climates, most cases are associated with *S aureus* infection. *Streptococcus* species are more common in tropical infections.

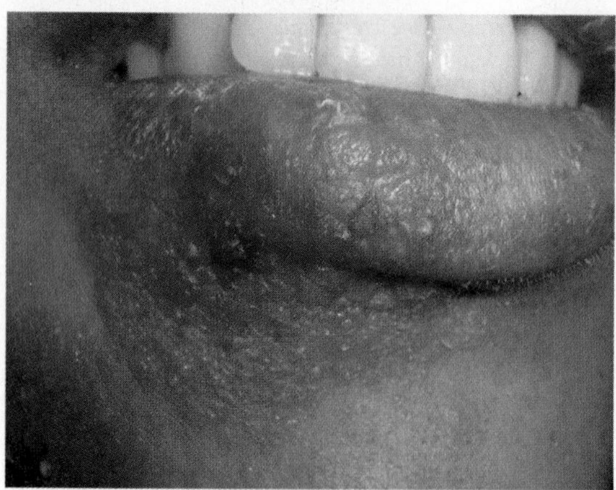

▲ **Figure 6–15.** Typical honey-crusted plaque on the lip of an adult with impetigo. (Reproduced with permission from Richard P. Usatine, MD, in Usatine RP, Smith MA, Mayeaux EJ Jr, Chumley HS. *The Color Atlas and Synopsis of Family Medicine*, 3rd ed. McGraw-Hill, 2019.)

Differential Diagnosis

The main differential diagnoses of honey-colored crusting are acute allergic contact dermatitis and herpes simplex. Contact dermatitis may be suggested by the history or by linear distribution of the lesions, and culture should be negative for staphylococci and streptococci. Herpes simplex infection usually presents with grouped vesicles or discrete erosions and may be associated with a history of recurrences. Viral cultures are positive.

Treatment

Soaks and scrubbing can be beneficial, especially in unroofing lakes of pus under thick crusts. Topical agents, such as mupirocin, ozenoxacin, and retapamulin, are first-line treatment options for infections limited to small areas. In widespread cases, or in immunosuppressed individuals, systemic antibiotics are indicated. Cephalexin, 250 mg orally four times daily, is usually effective. Community-associated methicillin-resistant *S aureus* (CA-MRSA) may cause impetigo, for which initial treatment may include doxycycline (100 mg orally twice daily) or trimethoprim-sulfamethoxazole (TMP-SMZ, double-strength tablet orally twice daily). Recurrent impetigo is associated with nasal carriage of *S aureus* and is treated with rifampin, 300 mg orally twice daily for 5 days. Intranasal mupirocin ointment twice daily for 14 days eliminates most MRSA strains. Bleach baths (¼ to ½ cup per 20 liters of bathwater for 15 minutes three to five times weekly) for all family members and the use of dilute household bleach to clean showers and other bath surfaces may help reduce the spread. Infected individuals should not share towels with household members. Among hospitalized patients colonized with MRSA, decolonization with chlorhexidine washes combined with nasal mupirocin for 5 days twice per month for 6 months resulted in 30% lower risk of MRSA infection than education alone.

Schachner LA et al. Treatment of impetigo and antimicrobial resistance. J Drugs Dermatol. 2021;20:366. [PMID:33852242]

FOLLICULITIS (Including Sycosis)

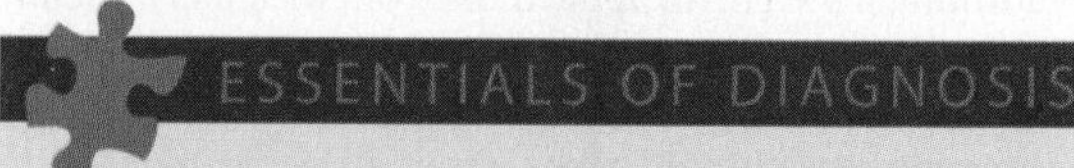

- Itching and burning in hairy areas.
- Pustule surrounding and including the hair follicle.

General Considerations

Folliculitis has multiple causes. It is frequently caused by staphylococcal infection and may be more common in the diabetic patient. When the lesion is deep-seated, chronic, and recalcitrant on the head and neck, it is called **sycosis.**

Gram-negative folliculitis, which may develop during antibiotic treatment of acne, may present as a flare of acne pustules or nodules. *Klebsiella, Enterobacter, Escherichia coli*, and *Proteus* have been isolated from these lesions.

Hot tub folliculitis (*Pseudomonas* folliculitis), caused by *Pseudomonas aeruginosa*, is characterized by pruritic or tender follicular, pustular lesions occurring within 1–4 days after bathing in a contaminated hot tub, whirlpool, or swimming pool. Flu-like symptoms may be present. Rarely, systemic infections may result. Neutropenic patients should avoid these exposures.

Nonbacterial folliculitis may also be caused by friction and oils. Occlusion, perspiration, and chronic rubbing (eg, from tight-fitting clothing or heavy fabrics on the buttocks and thighs) can worsen this type of folliculitis.

Steroid acne may be seen during topical or systemic corticosteroid therapy and presents as eruptive monomorphous papules and papulopustules on the face and trunk. It responds to topical benzoyl peroxide.

Eosinophilic folliculitis is a sterile folliculitis that presents with urticarial papules with prominent eosinophilic infiltration. It is most common in immunosuppressed patients, especially those with AIDS. It may appear first with institution of highly active antiretroviral therapy (ART) and be mistaken for a drug eruption.

Pseudofolliculitis is caused by ingrowing of tightly curled hairs in the beard area. In this entity, the papules and pustules are located at the side of and not in follicles. It may be treated by growing a beard, by using chemical depilatories, or by shaving with a foil-guard razor. Medically indicated laser hair removal is dramatically beneficial in patients with pseudofolliculitis and can be done on patients of any skin color.

Pityrosporum folliculitis presents as 1- to 2-mm pruritic pink papulopustules on the upper trunk, hairline, and arms. It is often pruritic and tends to develop during periods of excessive sweating. It can also occur in immunosuppressed patients.

Demodex folliculitis is caused by the mite *Demodex folliculorum*. It presents as 1–2 mm papules and pustules on an erythematous base, often on the background of

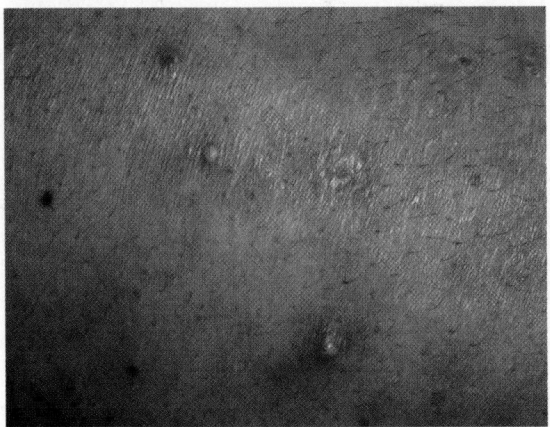

▲ **Figure 6–16.** Bacterial folliculitis. Hair emanating from the center of the pustule is the clinical hallmark of folliculitis. (Reproduced with permission from Richard P. Usatine, MD, in Usatine RP, Smith MA, Mayeaux EJ Jr, Chumley H. *The Color Atlas of Family Medicine*, 2nd ed. McGraw-Hill, 2013.)

rosacea-like changes, in patients who have not responded to conventional treatment for rosacea. It is more common in immunosuppressed patients. KOH from the pustules will demonstrate *Demodex folliculorum* mites.

Clinical Findings

The symptoms range from slight burning and tenderness to intense itching. The lesions consist of pustules of hair follicles (Figure 6–16).

Differential Diagnosis

It is important to differentiate bacterial from nonbacterial folliculitis. The history is important for pinpointing the causes of nonbacterial folliculitis, and a Gram stain and culture are indispensable. One must differentiate bacterial folliculitis from acne vulgaris or pustular miliaria (heat rash) and from other infections of the skin, such as impetigo or *Pityrosporum* folliculitis. Eosinophilic folliculitis in AIDS often requires biopsy for diagnosis.

Complications

Abscess formation is the major complication of bacterial folliculitis.

Prevention

Correct any predisposing local causes, such as oils or friction. Be sure that the water in hot tubs and spas is treated properly. If staphylococcal folliculitis is persistent, treatment of nasal or perineal carriage with rifampin, 600 mg daily for 5 days, or with topical mupirocin ointment 2% twice daily for 5 days, may help. Prolonged oral clindamycin, 150–300 mg/day for 4–6 weeks, or oral TMP-SMZ given 1 week per month for 6 months can be effective in preventing recurrent staphylococcal folliculitis and furunculosis. Bleach baths (¼ to ½ cup per 20 liters of bathwater for 15 minutes three to five times weekly) may reduce cutaneous staphylococcal carriage and not contribute to antibiotic resistance. Control of blood glucose in diabetes may reduce infections.

Treatment

A. Local Measures

Anhydrous ethyl alcohol containing 6.25% aluminum chloride, applied three to seven times weekly to lesions, may be helpful, especially for chronic frictional folliculitis of the buttocks. Topical antibiotics are generally ineffective if bacteria have invaded the hair follicle but may be prophylactic if used as an aftershave in patients with recurrent folliculitis after shaving.

B. Specific Measures

Pseudomonas folliculitis clears spontaneously in nonneutropenic patients if the lesions are superficial. It may be treated with ciprofloxacin, 500 mg orally twice daily for 5 days.

Systemic antibiotics are recommended for bacterial folliculitis due to other organisms. Extended periods of treatment (4–8 weeks or more) with antistaphylococcal antibiotics are required if infection involves the scalp or densely hairy areas, such as the axilla, beard, or groin (see Table 30–4).

Gram-negative folliculitis in acne patients may be treated with isotretinoin in compliance with all precautions discussed above (see Acne Vulgaris).

Eosinophilic folliculitis may be treated initially by the combination of potent topical corticosteroids and oral antihistamines. In more severe cases, treatment is with one of the following: topical permethrin (application for 12 hours every other night for 6 weeks); itraconazole, 200–400 mg orally daily; UVB or PUVA phototherapy; or isotretinoin, 0.5 mg/kg/day orally for up to 5 months. A remission may be induced by some of these therapies, but long-term treatment may be required.

Pityrosporum folliculitis is treated with topical sulfacetamide lotion twice a day, alone or in combination with oral itraconazole or fluconazole.

Demodex folliculitis can be treated until cleared with topical 5% permethrin applied every other night; oral ivermectin, 200 mcg/kg once weekly; oral metronidazole, 500 mg once daily or 250 mg three times daily; or topical ivermectin or metronidazole.

Prognosis

Bacterial folliculitis is occasionally stubborn and persistent, requiring prolonged or intermittent courses of antibiotics.

Chaitidis N et al. Oral treatment with/without topical treatment vs topical treatment alone in *Malassezia* folliculitis patients: a systematic review and meta-analysis. Dermatol Ther. 2020;33:e13460. [PMID: 32319163]

Lin HS et al. Interventions for bacterial folliculitis and boils (furuncles and carbuncles). Cochrane Database Syst Rev. 2021;2:CD013099. [PMID: 33634465]

FURUNCULOSIS (Boils) & CARBUNCLES

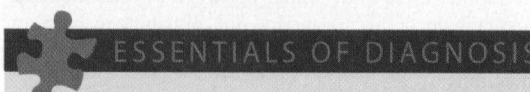

- Extremely painful inflammatory abscess based on a hair follicle.
- Coagulase-positive *S aureus* is the causative organism.
- Predisposing condition (diabetes mellitus, HIV disease, injection drug use) sometimes present.

General Considerations

A **furuncle (boil)** is a deep-seated infection (abscess) caused by *S aureus* that involves the hair follicle and adjacent subcutaneous tissue. The most common sites of occurrence are the hairy parts exposed to irritation and friction, pressure, or moisture. Because the lesions are autoinoculable, they are often multiple. Diabetes mellitus (especially if using insulin injections), injection drug use, allergy injections, and HIV disease all increase the risk of staphylococcal infections by increasing the rate of carriage. Certain other exposures including hospitalization, athletic teams, prisons, military service, and homelessness may also increase the risk of infection.

A **carbuncle** consists of several furuncles developing in adjoining hair follicles and coalescing to form a conglomerate, deeply situated mass with multiple drainage points.

Recurrent furunculosis (three or more episodes in 12 months) tends to occur in those with direct contact with other infected individuals, especially family members.

Clinical Findings

A. Symptoms and Signs

Pain and tenderness may be prominent. The abscess is either rounded or conical. It gradually enlarges, becomes fluctuant, and then softens and opens spontaneously after a few days to 1–2 weeks to discharge a core of necrotic tissue and pus. The inflammation occasionally subsides before necrosis occurs.

B. Laboratory Findings

There may be slight leukocytosis. Pus can be cultured to rule out MRSA or other bacteria. Culture of the anterior nares and anogenital area (including the rectum to test for GI carriage) may identify chronic staphylococcal carriage in cases of recurrent cutaneous infection.

Differential Diagnosis

The most common entity in the differential is an inflamed **epidermal inclusion cyst** that suddenly becomes red, tender, and expands greatly in size over one to a few days. The history of a prior cyst in the same location, the presence of a clearly visible cyst orifice, and the extrusion of malodorous cheesy material (rather than purulent material) helps in the diagnosis. Tinea profunda (deep dermatophyte infection of the hair follicle) may simulate recurrent furunculosis. Furunculosis is also to be distinguished from deep mycotic infections, such as sporotrichosis; from other bacterial infections, such as anthrax and tularemia (rare); from atypical mycobacterial infections; and from acne cysts. Hidradenitis suppurativa (acne inversa) presents with recurrent tender, sterile abscesses in the axillae and groin, on the buttocks, or below the breasts. The presence of old scars or sinus tracts plus negative cultures suggests this diagnosis.

Complications

Serious and sometimes fatal complications of staphylococcal infection such as septicemia can occur.

Prevention

Identifying and eliminating the source of infection is critical to prevent recurrences after treatment. The source individual may have chronic dermatitis or be an asymptomatic carrier of MRSA. Nasal carriage of MRSA and the number of children in a household are risk factors for transmission between household members. Local measures, such as meticulous handwashing; no sharing of towels, clothing, and personal hygiene products; avoiding loofas or sponges in the bath or shower; changing underwear, sleepwear, towels, and washcloths daily; aggressive scrubbing of showers, bathrooms, and surfaces with bleach; bleach baths (¼–½ cup per 20 liters of bathwater for 15 minutes three to five times weekly), 4% chlorhexidine washes, and isolation of infected patients who reside in institutions to prevent spread are all effective measures.

Treatment

A. Specific Measures

Incision and drainage are recommended for all loculated suppurations and are the mainstay of therapy. Systemic antibiotics are usually given. Patients who receive antibiotics (specifically, TMP-SMZ [160/800 or 320/1600 mg orally twice a day for 10 days or 7 days, respectively] or clindamycin [300 mg orally three times daily for 10 days]) at the time of drainage have higher cure and lower reinfection rates. Other oral antibiotic options include dicloxacillin or cephalexin, 1 g daily in divided doses for 10 days. For suspected MRSA, doxycycline 100 mg twice daily, TMP-SMZ double-strength one tablet twice daily, clindamycin 150–300 mg twice daily, and linezolid 400 mg twice daily for 7–10 days are effective. Recurrent furunculosis may be effectively treated with a combination of cephalexin (250–500 mg orally four times daily) or doxycycline (100 mg orally twice daily) for 2–4 weeks plus either rifampin (300 mg orally twice daily for 5 days) or long-term clindamycin (150–300 mg orally daily for 1–2 months). Shorter courses of antibiotics (7–14 days) plus longer-term daily 4% chlorhexidine whole body washing and intranasal, axilla, and anogenital mupirocin or retapamulin may also cure recurrent furunculosis. Oral vancomycin (1 g twice daily for 5 days) can treat GI carriage of *S aureus*. Family members, pets, and intimate contacts may need evaluation for staphylococcal carrier state and perhaps concomitant treatment. Stopping high-risk behavior, such as injection drug use, can also prevent recurrence.

B. Local Measures

Immobilize the part and avoid over-manipulation of inflamed areas. Use moist heat to help larger lesions "localize." Use surgical incision and drainage after the lesions are "mature."

Prognosis

Recurrent crops may occur for months or years.

Lin HS et al. Interventions for bacterial folliculitis and boils (furuncles and carbuncles). Cochrane Database Syst Rev. 2021;2:CD013099. [PMID: 33634465]

CELLULITIS

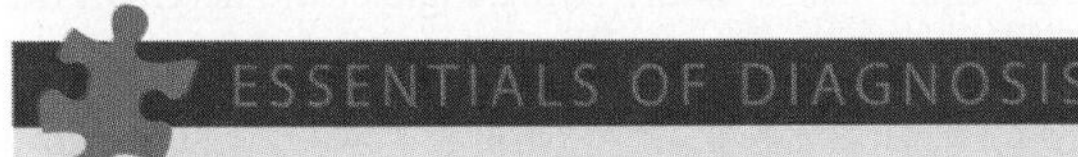

- Edematous, expanding, erythematous, warm plaque with or without vesicles or bullae.
- Lower leg is frequently involved.
- Pain, chills, and fever are commonly present.
- Septicemia may develop.

General Considerations

Cellulitis, a diffuse spreading infection of the dermis and subcutaneous tissue, is usually on the lower leg (Figure 6–17) and most commonly due to gram-positive cocci, especially group A beta-hemolytic streptococci and *S aureus*. Rarely, gram-negative rods or even fungi can produce a similar picture. In otherwise healthy persons, the most common portal of entry for lower leg cellulitis is interdigital tinea pedis with fissuring. Other diseases that predispose to cellulitis are prior episodes of cellulitis, chronic edema, venous insufficiency with secondary edema, lymphatic obstruction, saphenectomy, and other perturbations of the skin barrier. Bacterial cellulitis is almost never bilateral.

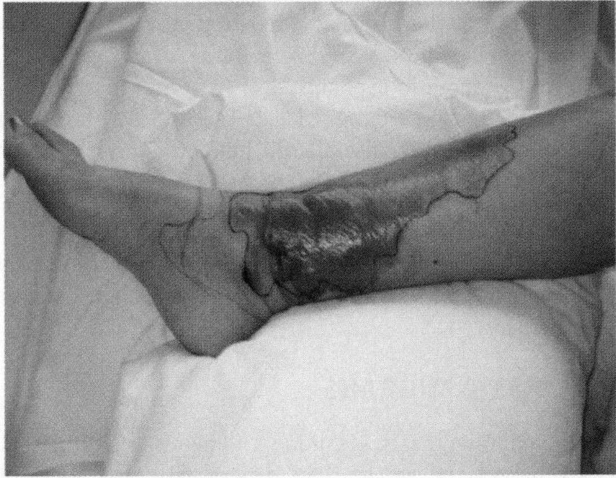

▲ **Figure 6–17.** Cellulitis. (Used, with permission, from Lindy Fox, MD.)

Clinical Findings

A. Symptoms and Signs

Cellulitis begins as a tender small patch. Swelling, erythema, and pain are often present. The lesion expands over hours, so that from onset to presentation is usually 6 to 36 hours. As the lesion grows, the patient becomes more ill with progressive chills, fever, and malaise. Lymphangitis and lymphadenopathy are often present. If septicemia develops, hypotension may develop, followed by shock.

B. Laboratory Findings

Leukocytosis or neutrophilia (left shift) may be present early in the course. Blood cultures are positive in only 4% of patients. If a central ulceration, pustule, or abscess is present, culture may be of value. Aspiration of the advancing edge has a low yield (less than 20%) and is usually not performed. In immunosuppressed patients, or if an unusual organism is suspected and there is no loculated site to culture, a full-thickness skin biopsy should be sent for routine histologic evaluation and for culture (bacterial, fungal, and mycobacterial). If a primary source for the infection is identified (wound, leg ulcer, toe web intertrigo), cultures from these sites isolate the causative pathogen in half of cases and can be used to guide antibiotic therapy.

Differential Diagnosis

Two potentially life-threatening entities that can mimic cellulitis (ie, present with a painful, red, swollen lower extremity) include DVT and necrotizing fasciitis. The diagnosis of necrotizing fasciitis should be suspected in a patient who has a toxic appearance, bullae, crepitus or anesthesia of the involved skin, overlying skin necrosis, and laboratory evidence of rhabdomyolysis (elevated creatine kinase) or disseminated intravascular coagulation. While these findings may be present with severe cellulitis and bacteremia, it is essential to rule out necrotizing fasciitis because rapid surgical debridement is essential. Other noninfectious skin lesions that may resemble cellulitis are termed "pseudocellulitis." Diseases in this differential include sclerosing panniculitis, an acute, exquisitely tender red plaque on the medial lower legs above the malleolus in patients with venous stasis or varicosities, and acute severe contact dermatitis on a limb, which produces erythema, vesiculation, and edema, as seen in cellulitis, but with itching instead of pain. Bilateral lower leg bacterial cellulitis is exceedingly rare, and other diagnoses, especially severe stasis dermatitis (see Figure 12–2), should be considered in this setting. Severe lower extremity stasis dermatitis usually develops over days to weeks rather than hours as with cellulitis. It is also not as tender to palpation as cellulitis. Cryptococcal cellulitis in the organ transplant recipient is often bilateral. The ALT-70 is a predictive model to diagnose cellulitis or a cellulitis mimic and to provide guidance about when a dermatology consultation is needed.

The ALT-70 variables are asymmetry (3 points), leukocytosis of 10,000/mcL (10×10^9/L) or more at presentation (2 points), tachycardia above 90 beats per minute (1 point), and age 70 years or older (1 point). An ALT-70 score above 5 points carries more than an 82% chance of a true cellulitis while a score below 2 points suggests a greater than 83% chance of a cellulitis mimicker.

▶ Treatment

Intravenous or parenteral antibiotics may be required for the first 2–5 days, with adequate coverage for *Streptococcus* and *Staphylococcus*. Methicillin-susceptible *S aureus* (MSSA) can be treated with nafcillin, cefazolin, clindamycin, dicloxacillin, cephalexin, doxycycline, or TMP-SMZ. If MRSA is suspected or proven, treatment options include vancomycin, linezolid, clindamycin, daptomycin, doxycycline, or TMP-SMZ. In mild cases or following the initial parenteral therapy, oral dicloxacillin or cephalexin, 250–500 mg four times daily for 5–10 days, is usually adequate. In patients in whom intravenous treatment is not instituted, the first dose of oral antibiotic can be doubled to achieve high blood levels rapidly. In patients with recurrent lower leg cellulitis (three to four episodes per year), oral penicillin 250 mg twice daily or oral erythromycin 250–500 mg twice daily can decrease the risk of recurrence. Prior episodes of cellulitis, lymphedema, chronic venous insufficiency, peripheral vascular disease, and DVT are associated with an increased risk of recurrent cellulitis. Additional measures to prevent recurrences include compression, treating toe web intertrigo and tinea pedis, and controlling venous insufficiency.

▶ When to Admit

- Severe local symptoms and signs.
- Signs of sepsis.
- Elevated WBC count of 10,000/mcL (10×10^9/L) or more with marked left shift. Failure to respond to oral antibiotics.

Klotz C et al. Adherence to antibiotic guidelines for erysipelas or cellulitis is associated with a favorable outcome. Eur J Clin Microbiol Infect Dis. 2019;38:703. [PMID: 30685804]

Rrapi R et al. Cellulitis: a review of pathogenesis, diagnosis, and management. Med Clin North Am. 2021;105:723. [PMID: 34059247]

Webb E et al. Compression therapy to prevent recurrent cellulitis of the leg. N Engl J Med. 2020;383:630. [PMID: 32786188]

ERYSIPELAS

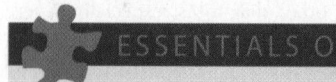

ESSENTIALS OF DIAGNOSIS

- Edematous, circumscribed, hot, erythematous area, with raised advancing border.
- Central face or lower extremity frequently involved.
- Pain and systemic toxicity may be striking.

▶ General Considerations

Erysipelas is a superficial form of cellulitis that is caused by beta-hemolytic streptococci.

▶ Clinical Findings

A. Symptoms and Signs

The symptoms are pain, malaise, chills, and moderate fever. A bright red spot appears and then spreads to form a tense, sharply demarcated, glistening, smooth, hot plaque. The sharp margin characteristically makes noticeable advances in days or even hours. The lesion is edematous with a raised edge and may pit slightly with the finger. Vesicles or bullae occasionally develop on the surface. The lesion does not usually become pustular or gangrenous and heals without scar formation. Breaks in the skin often provide a portal of entry for the organism. On the face, erysipelas begins near a fissure at the angle of the nose. On the lower extremity, tinea pedis with interdigital fissuring is a common portal of entry.

B. Laboratory Findings

Leukocytosis is almost invariably present; blood cultures may be positive.

▶ Differential Diagnosis

Erysipeloid is a benign bacillary infection by *Erysipelothrix rhusiopathiae* that produces cellulitis of the skin of the fingers or the backs of the hands in fishermen and meat handlers.

▶ Complications

Unless erysipelas is promptly treated, death may result from bacterial dissemination, particularly in older adults.

▶ Treatment

Intravenous antibiotics effective against group A beta-hemolytic streptococci and staphylococci should be considered, but outpatient treatment with oral antibiotics has demonstrated equal efficacy. Oral regimens include a 7-day course with penicillin VK (250 mg), dicloxacillin (250 mg), or a first-generation cephalosporin (250 mg) four times a day. Clindamycin (250 mg twice daily orally for 7–14 days) is an option for penicillin-allergic patients.

▶ Prognosis

With appropriate treatment, rapid improvement is expected. The presence of lymphedema carries the greatest risk of recurrence.

ERYTHEMA MIGRANS

Erythema migrans is a unique cutaneous eruption that characterizes the localized or generalized early stage of Lyme disease (caused by *Borrelia burgdorferi*) (Figure 6–18) (see also Chapter 34).

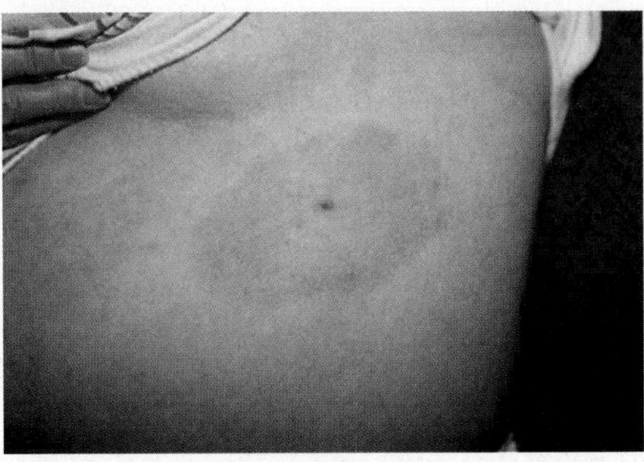

▲ **Figure 6–18.** Erythema migrans on trunk. Annular plaque with central clearing and central puncta from the bite. (Reproduced, with permission, from Soutor, Hordinsky MK. *Clinical Dermatology.* The McGraw-Hill Companies; 2013.)

PARASITIC INFESTATIONS

SCABIES

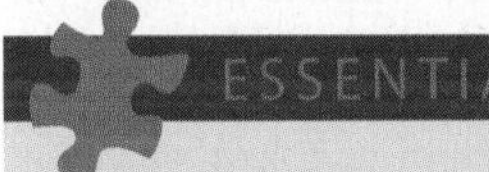

ESSENTIALS OF DIAGNOSIS

- Generalized very severe itching; infestation usually spares the head and neck.
- Burrows, vesicles, and pustules, especially on finger webs and in wrist creases.
- Mites, ova, and brown dots of feces (scybala) visible microscopically.
- Red papules or nodules on the scrotum and on the penile glans and shaft are pathognomonic.

General Considerations

Scabies is caused by infestation with *Sarcoptes scabiei*, affecting over 200 million people worldwide. Close physical contact for 15–20 minutes with an infected person is the typical mode of transmission. However, scabies may be acquired by contact with the bedding of an infested individual. Facility-associated scabies is common, primarily in long-term care facilities, and misdiagnosis is common. Index patients are usually elderly and immunosuppressed. When these patients are hospitalized, hospital-based epidemics can occur and are difficult to eradicate when health care workers become infected and spread the infestation to other patients.

Clinical Findings

A. Symptoms and Signs

Itching is almost always present and can be severe. The lesions consist of generalized excoriations with small pruritic vesicles, pustules, and "burrows" in the interdigital spaces of the hands and feet, on the heels of the palms, wrists, elbows, umbilicus, around the axillae, on or around the areolae (Figure 6–19), or on the penile shaft and scrotum in men. The burrow appears as a short irregular mark, 2–3 mm long and the width of a hair. Characteristic nodular lesions may occur on the scrotum or penis and along the posterior axillary line. The infestation usually spares the head and neck (though these areas may be involved in infants, older adults, and patients with AIDS).

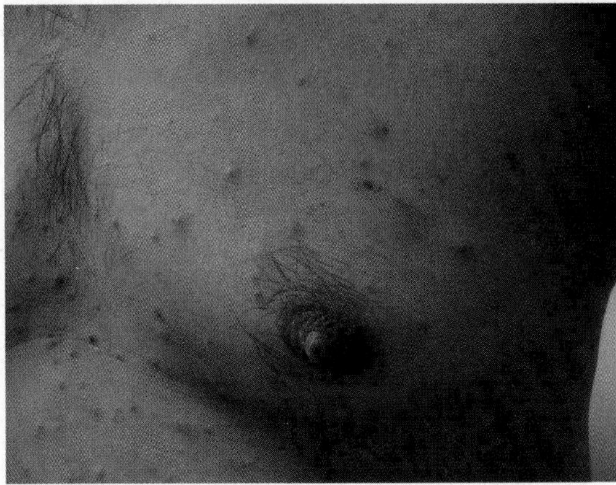

▲ **Figure 6–19.** Scabies. A polymorphic eruption of papulovesicles and excoriated papules scattered on the chest. (Used, with permission, from Kanade Shinkai, MD.)

Hyperkeratotic or crusted scabies presents as thick flaking scale. These areas contain millions of mites, and these patients are highly infectious. Pruritus is often absent. Patients with widespread hyperkeratotic scabies are at risk for superinfection with *S aureus*, which in some cases progresses to sepsis if left untreated. Crusted scabies is the cause of 83% of scabies outbreaks in institutions.

B. Laboratory Findings

The diagnosis should be confirmed by microscopic demonstration of the organism, ova, or feces in a mounted specimen, examined with tap water, mineral oil, or KOH. Best results are obtained when multiple lesions are scraped, choosing the best unexcoriated lesions from interdigital webs, wrists, elbows, or feet. A No. 15 blade is used to scrape each lesion until it is flat. Patients with crusted/hyperkeratotic scabies must be evaluated for immunosuppression (especially HIV and HTLV-1 infections) if no iatrogenic cause of immunosuppression is present. Patients with hyperkeratotic scabies and associated bacterial superinfection may have laboratory findings consistent with infection and, if severe, sepsis.

Differential Diagnosis

Scabies must be distinguished from the various forms of pediculosis, from bedbug and flea bites, and from other causes of pruritus.

Treatment & Prognosis

Treatment is aimed at killing scabies mites and controlling the dermatitis, which can persist for months after effective eradication of the mites. Bedding and clothing should be laundered or set aside for 14 days in plastic bags. High heat (60°C) is required to kill the mites and ova. Treatment is aimed at all infected persons in a family or institutionalized group. Otherwise, reinfestations will likely occur, which is why scabies in nursing home patients, institutionalized or mentally impaired patients, and AIDS patients may be much more difficult to treat.

1. Permethrin 5% cream—Treatment with permethrin, a highly effective and safe agent, consists of a single application from the neck down for 8–12 hours then washed off, repeated in 1 week. Patients often continue to itch for several weeks after treatment. Use of triamcinolone 0.1% cream helps resolve the dermatitis.

Pregnant patients should be treated only if they have documented scabies. Permethrin 5% cream once for 12 hours—or 5% or 6% sulfur in petrolatum applied nightly for 3 nights from the collarbones down—may be used.

Most failures in normal persons are related to incorrect use or incomplete treatment of the housing unit. In these cases, repeat treatment with permethrin once weekly for 2 weeks, with re-education regarding the method and extent of application, is suggested.

2. Ivermectin—In immunocompetent individuals, 200 mcg/kg orally is effective in about 75% of cases with a single dose and 95% of cases with two doses 2 weeks apart. Since the drug is not ovicidal, the second dose theoretically kills eggs that might have hatched after the first dose was given.

Ivermectin is often used in combination with permethrin. In immunosuppressed persons and those with crusted (hyperkeratotic) scabies, multiple doses of ivermectin (every 2 weeks for 2 or 3 doses) plus topical therapy with permethrin every 3 days to once weekly, depending on degree of involvement, may be effective when topical treatment and oral therapy alone fail. A topical keratolytic (urea) should be used to help remove the scale of hyperkeratotic scabies, thereby decreasing the mite load.

Ivermectin can be beneficial in mass treatment to eradicate widespread infection. In endemic areas, mass intervention with ivermectin is effective in controlling both scabies and associated bacterial infections.

If secondary pyoderma is present, it is treated with systemic antibiotics. Staphylococcal superinfection may lead to sepsis. In areas where nephritogenic streptococcal strains are prevalent, infestation with scabies or exposure to scabies-infested dogs may be followed by acute poststreptococcal glomerulonephritis.

Persistent pruritic post-scabietic papules may be treated with mid- to high-potency corticosteroids or with intralesional triamcinolone acetonide (2.5–5 mg/mL).

Engelman D et al. The public health control of scabies: priorities for research and action. Lancet. 2019;394(10192):81. [PMID: 31178154]

Engelman D et al. The 2020 International Alliance for the Control of Scabies consensus criteria for the diagnosis of scabies. Br J Dermatol. 2020;183:808. [PMID: 32034956]

Thomas C et al. Ectoparasites: scabies. J Am Acad Dermatol. 2020;82:533. [PMID: 31310840]

PEDICULOSIS

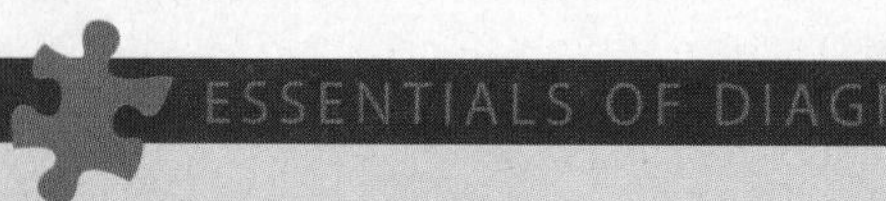

- Pruritus with excoriation.
- Nits on hair shafts; lice on skin or clothes.
- Occasionally, sky-blue macules (maculae ceruleae) on the inner thighs or lower abdomen in pubic lice infestation.

General Considerations

Pediculosis is a parasitic infestation of the skin of the scalp, trunk, or pubic areas. Body lice usually occur among people who live in overcrowded dwellings with inadequate hygiene facilities. Pubic lice may be sexually transmitted. Head lice may be transmitted by shared use of hats or combs. Adults in contact with children with head lice frequently acquire the infestation.

There are three different varieties (1) **pediculosis capitis,** caused by *Pediculus humanus* var *capitis* (head louse); (2) **pediculosis corporis,** caused by *Pediculus humanus* var *corporis* (body louse); and (3) **pediculosis pubis,** caused by *Phthirus pubis* (pubic louse, "crabs").

Head and body lice are 3–4 mm long and similar in appearance. The "body louse" can seldom be found on the body because it comes onto the skin only to feed; it must be looked for in the seams of the clothing. Trench fever, relapsing fever, and typhus are transmitted by the body louse in countries where those diseases are endemic. In the United States, *Bartonella quintana*, the organism that causes trench fever, has been found in lice infesting the homeless population.

Clinical Findings

In body lice infestations, itching may be very intense, and scratching may result in deep excoriations, especially over the upper shoulders, axillae, posterior flanks, and neck. In some cases, only itching is present, with few excoriations seen. Pyoderma (bacterial infection of the skin) may be the presenting sign. Diagnosis is made by examining the seams of clothing for nits and lice. Head lice presents as scalp pruritus often accompanied by erosions on the occipital scalp, posterior neck, and upper back. Diagnosis is made by finding lice on the scalp or small nits resembling pussy willow buds on the scalp hairs close to the skin. Nits are easiest to see above the ears and at the nape of the neck. Pubic lice infestations are occasionally generalized, particularly in hairy individuals; the lice may even be found on the eyelashes and in the scalp. Diagnosis is made by finding lice or nits on pubic hair, body hair, or eyelashes.

Differential Diagnosis

Head lice infestation must be distinguished from seborrheic dermatitis, body lice infestation from scabies and bedbug bites, and pubic lice infestation from anogenital pruritus and eczema.

Treatment

1. Pediculosis capitis—Permethrin 1% cream rinse (Nix) is a topical over-the-counter pediculicide and ovicide. It is applied to the scalp and hair and left on for 8 hours before being rinsed off. Although it is the treatment of choice for head lice, permethrin resistance is common. Malathion lotion 1% (Ovide) is very effective but highly volatile and flammable, so application must be done in a well-ventilated room or out of doors. Topical ivermectin 0.5% lotion, benzyl alcohol 5%, Oxyphthirine® lotion, spinosad 0.9% suspension, dimethicone, and abametapir 0.74% lotion are additional agents that have efficacy against pediculosis capitis; of these, topical ivermectin is the most effective. All infested persons in a household, school, or other facility should ideally be treated at the same time. Other than topical ivermectin, topical therapies should be repeated 7–9 days after the initial treatment. For involvement of eyelashes, petrolatum is applied thickly twice daily for 8 days and the remaining nits plucked off. Systemic treatment options, often used in combination with topical agents, are oral ivermectin (200 mcg/kg orally, repeated in 7 days) (for children older than 5 years and more than 15 kg) and oral TMP-SMZ (10 mg TMP/kg/day and 50 mg SMZ/kg/day divided twice daily for 10 days).

2. Pediculosis corporis—Body lice are treated by disposing of the infested clothing and addressing the patient's social situation.

3. Pediculosis pubis—Application of permethrin rinse 1% for 10 minutes or permethrin cream 5% for 8 hours to the pubis is effective. Sexual contacts should be treated. Clothes and bedclothes should be washed and dried at high temperature.

Coates SJ et al. Ectoparasites: pediculosis and tungiasis. J Am Acad Dermatol. 2020;82:551. [PMID: 31306729]
Gunning K et al. Lice and scabies: treatment update. Am Fam Physician. 2019;99:635. [PMID: 31083883]
Huntington MK et al. Infectious disease: bedbugs, lice, and mites. FP Essent. 2019;476:18. [PMID: 30615406]
Ogbuefi N et al. Common pediatric infestations: update on diagnosis and treatment of scabies, head lice, and bed bugs. Curr Opin Pediatr. 2021;33:410. [PMID: 34074914]

SKIN LESIONS DUE TO OTHER ARTHROPODS

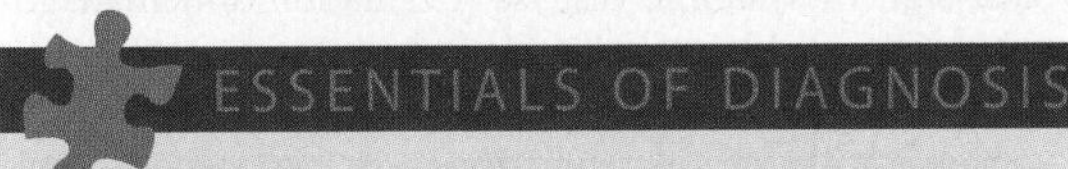

- Localized urticarial papules with pruritus.
- Lesions in linear groups of three ("breakfast, lunch, and dinner") are characteristic of bedbugs.
- Furuncle-like lesions containing live arthropods.
- Tender erythematous patches that migrate ("larva migrans").

General Considerations

Some arthropods (eg, mosquitoes and biting flies) are readily detected as they bite. Many others are not because they are too small, because there is no immediate reaction, or because they bite during sleep. Reactions are allergic and may be delayed for hours to days. Patients are most apt to consult a clinician when the lesions are multiple and pruritus is intense.

Many persons react most severely to their earliest contacts with an arthropod, thus presenting with pruritic lesions when traveling, moving into new quarters, etc. Body lice, fleas, bedbugs, and mosquitoes should be considered. Bedbug exposure typically occurs in hotels and in housing with inadequate hygiene but also occurs in stable domiciles. Spiders are often incorrectly believed to be the source of bites, but they rarely attack humans. However, the brown recluse spider (*Loxosceles laeta*, *L reclusa*) may cause severe necrotic reactions and death due to intravascular hemolysis, and the black widow spider (*Latrodectus mactans*) may cause severe systemic symptoms and death. (See also Chapter 38.) The majority of patient-diagnosed, clinician-diagnosed, and even published cases of brown recluse spider bites (or loxoscelism) are incorrect, especially if made in areas where these spiders are not endemic. Many of these lesions are actually due to CA-MRSA.

In addition to arthropod bites, the most common lesions are venomous stings (wasps, hornets, bees, ants, scorpions) or bites (centipedes), furuncle-like lesions due to fly maggots or sand fleas in the skin, and a linear creeping eruption due to a migrating larva.

Clinical Findings

The diagnosis may be difficult when the patient has not noticed the initial attack but suffers a delayed reaction. Individual bites are often in clusters and tend to occur either on exposed parts (eg, midges and gnats) or under clothing, especially around the waist or at flexures (eg, small mites or insects in bedding or clothing). The reaction is often delayed for 1–24 hours or more. Pruritus is almost always present and may be all but intolerable once the patient starts to scratch. Secondary infection may follow scratching. Urticarial wheals are common. Papules may become vesicular. The diagnosis is aided by searching for exposure to arthropods and by considering the patient's occupation and recent activities.

The principal arthropods are as follows:

1. **Fleas:** Fleas are bloodsucking ectoparasites that feed on dogs, cats, humans, and other species. Flea saliva produces papular urticaria in sensitized individuals. To break the life cycle of the flea, one must treat the home and pets, using quick-kill insecticides, residual insecticides, and a growth regulator.
2. **Bedbugs:** In crevices of beds or furniture; bites tend to occur in lines or clusters. Papular urticaria is a characteristic lesion of bedbug (*Cimex lectularius*) bites. Bedbugs are not restricted to any socioeconomic group and are a major health problem in some major metropolitan areas, especially in commercial and residential hotels.
3. **Ticks:** Usually picked up by brushing against low vegetation.

4. **Chiggers or red bugs:** These are larvae of trombiculid mites. A few species confined to particular regions and locally recognized habitats (eg, berry patches, woodland edges, lawns, brush turkey mounds in Australia, poultry farms) attack humans, often around the waist, on the ankles, or in flexures, raising intensely itching erythematous papules after a delay of many hours. The red chiggers may sometimes be seen in the center of papules that have not yet been scratched.
5. **Bird and rodent mites:** Larger than chiggers, bird mites infest birds and their nests. Bites are multiple anywhere on the body. Room air conditioning units may suck in bird mites and infest the inhabitants of the room. Rodent mites from mice or rats may cause similar effects. If the domicile has evidence of rodent activity, then rodent mite dermatitis should be suspected, as the mites are rarely found. Pet rodents or birds may be infested with mites, maintaining the infestation.
6. **Mites in stored products:** These are white and almost invisible and infest products, such as copra, vanilla pods, sugar, straw, cottonseeds, and cereals. Persons who handle these products may be attacked, especially on the hands and forearms and sometimes on the feet.
7. **Caterpillars of moths with urticating hairs:** The hairs are blown from cocoons or carried by emergent moths, causing severe and often seasonally recurrent outbreaks after mass emergence. The gypsy moth is a cause in the eastern United States.
8. **Tungiasis:** Tungiasis is due to the burrowing flea known as *Tunga penetrans* and is found in Africa, the West Indies, and South and Central America. The female burrows under the skin, sucks blood, swells to 0.5 cm, and then ejects her eggs onto the ground. Ulceration, lymphangitis, gangrene, and septicemia may result, in some cases with lethal effect. Simple surgical removal is usually performed.

Prevention

Arthropod infestations are best prevented by avoidance of contaminated areas, personal cleanliness, and disinfection of clothing, bedclothes, and furniture as indicated. Chiggers and mites can be repelled by permethrin applied to the head and clothing. (It is not necessary to remove clothing.) Bedbugs are no longer repelled by permethrin and can survive for up to 1 year without feeding. Aggressive cleaning, usually requiring removal of the affected occupant from the domicile, may be necessary to eradicate bedbug infestation in a residence.

Treatment

Living arthropods should be removed carefully with tweezers after application of alcohol and preserved in alcohol for identification. In endemic Rocky Mountain spotted fever areas, ticks should not be removed with the bare fingers.

Corticosteroid lotions or creams are helpful for the associated pruritus. Topical antibiotics may be applied if secondary infection is suspected. Localized persistent lesions may be treated with intralesional corticosteroids.

Stings produced by many arthropods may be alleviated by applying papain powder (Adolph's Meat Tenderizer) mixed with water, or aluminum chloride hexahydrate (Xerac AC).

Extracts from venom sacs of bees, wasps, yellow jackets, and hornets are available for immunotherapy of patients at risk for anaphylaxis.

Coates SJ et al. Ectoparasites: pediculosis and tungiasis. J Am Acad Dermatol. 2020;82:551. [PMID: 31306729]
Kamath S et al. Infestations, bites, and insect repellents. Pediatr Ann. 2020;49:e124. [PMID: 32155278]
Pace EJ et al. Tickborne diseases: diagnosis and management. Am Fam Physician. 2020;101:530. [PMID: 32352736]
Parola P et al. Bedbugs. N Engl J Med. 2020;382:2230. [PMID: 32492304]

INFLAMMATORY NODULES

ERYTHEMA NODOSUM

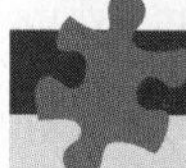

ESSENTIALS OF DIAGNOSIS

- Painful nodules without ulceration on anterior aspects of legs.
- Slow regression over several weeks to resemble contusions.
- Women are predominantly affected by a ratio of 10:1 compared to men.
- Some cases associated with infection, IBD, or medication exposure.
- Evaluation for underlying cause is essential.

General Considerations

Erythema nodosum is a symptom complex of panniculitis characterized by tender, erythematous nodules that appear most commonly on the extensor surfaces of the lower legs. It usually lasts about 6 weeks and may recur. Most cases are idiopathic in nature. However, erythema nodosum can be a skin sign of systemic disease. Evaluation and management include making the diagnosis, treating the symptoms, and searching for an underlying cause. The disease may be associated with various infections—streptococcosis, primary coccidioidomycosis, other deep fungal infections, tuberculosis, *Yersinia pseudotuberculosis* and *Y enterocolitica* infection, diverticulitis, or syphilis. It may accompany sarcoidosis, Behçet disease, and IBD. Erythema nodosum may be associated with pregnancy or with use of oral contraceptives. It may occur secondary to medications or, more rarely, an underlying malignancy.

Clinical Findings

A. Symptoms and Signs

The subcutaneous swellings are exquisitely tender and may be preceded by fever, malaise, and arthralgia. They are most often located on the anterior surfaces of the legs below the knees but may occur on the arms, trunk, and face. The lesions, 1–10 cm in diameter, are at first pink to red; with regression, all the various hues seen in a contusion can be observed (Figure 6–20) but, as a rule, the lesions do not ulcerate.

B. Laboratory Findings

Evaluation of patients presenting with acute erythema nodosum should include a careful history (including medication exposures) and physical examination. Significant findings include a history of prior upper respiratory infection, diarrheal illness, exposure to tuberculosis, or symptoms of any deep fungal infection endemic to the area. All patients should get a chest radiograph, a purified protein derivative or blood interferon gamma release assay (such as QuantiFERON) (see Pulmonary Tuberculosis in Chapter 9), and two consecutive ASO/DNAse B titers at 2- to 4-week intervals. Coccidioidomycosis should be looked for in patients from endemic areas. If no underlying cause is found, only a small percentage of patients will go on to develop a significant underlying illness (usually sarcoidosis) over the next year.

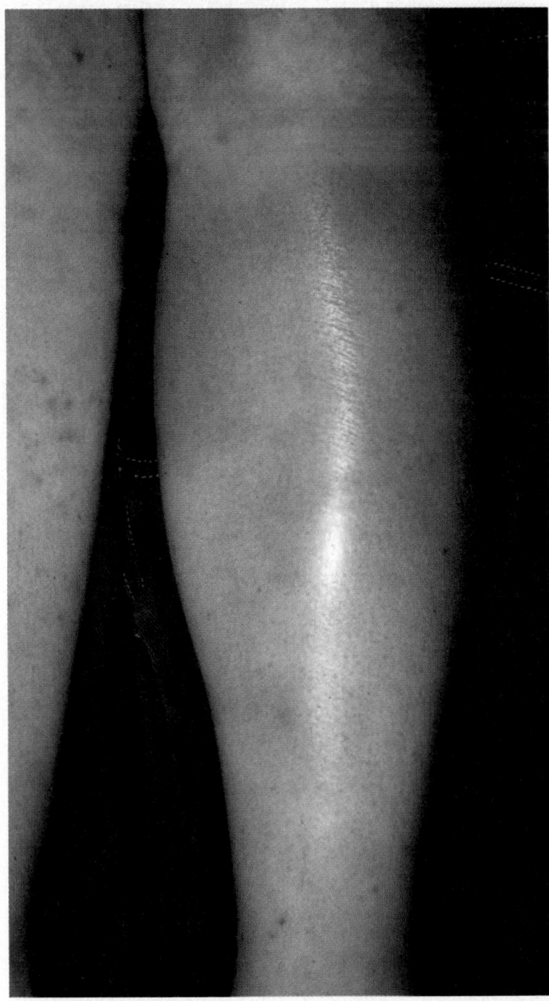

▲ **Figure 6–20.** Erythema nodosum. (Used, with permission, from TG Berger, MD, Dept Dermatology, UCSF.)

▶ Differential Diagnosis

Unlike other forms of panniculitis, a defining feature of erythema nodosum is that it does not ulcerate. Erythema induratum from tuberculosis is seen on the posterior surfaces of the legs and may ulcerate. Lupus panniculitis presents as tender nodules in fatty areas of the buttocks and posterior arms and heals with depressed scars. In polyarteritis nodosa, the subcutaneous nodules are often associated with fixed livedo reticularis. In its late stages, erythema nodosum must be distinguished from simple bruises and contusions.

▶ Treatment

The underlying cause should be identified and treated. Primary therapy is with NSAIDs in usual doses. Saturated solution of potassium iodide, 5–15 drops three times daily, results in prompt involution in many cases. Complete bed rest may be advisable if the lesions are painful. Systemic therapy directed against the lesions themselves may include corticosteroid therapy (see Chapter 26) (unless contraindicated by associated infection), dapsone, colchicine, or hydroxychloroquine.

▶ Prognosis

The lesions usually disappear after about 6 weeks but may recur.

Pérez-Garza DM et al. Erythema nodosum: a practical approach and diagnostic algorithm. Am J Clin Dermatol. 2021;22:367. [PMID: 33683567]

SCALING DISORDERS

ATOPIC DERMATITIS

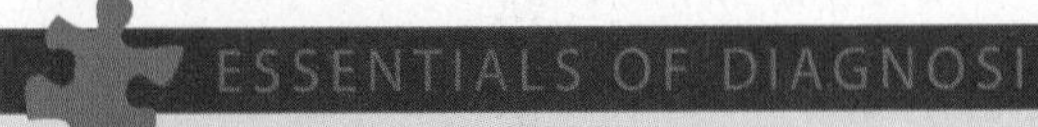

- Pruritic, xerotic, exudative, or lichenified eruption on face, neck, upper trunk, wrists, and hands and in the antecubital and popliteal folds.
- Personal or family history of atopy (eg, asthma, allergic rhinitis, atopic dermatitis).
- Tendency to recur.
- Onset in childhood most common; onset after age 30 is uncommon.

▶ General Considerations

Atopic dermatitis (also known as eczema) has distinct presentations in people of different ages and races. Diagnostic criteria for atopic dermatitis must include pruritus, typical morphology and distribution (flexural lichenification, hand eczema, nipple eczema, and eyelid eczema in adults), onset in childhood, and chronicity. Also helpful are (1) a personal or family history of atopy (asthma, allergic rhinitis, atopic dermatitis), (2) xerosis-ichthyosis, (3) facial pallor with infraorbital darkening, (4) elevated serum IgE, and (5) repeated skin infections.

Clinical Findings

A. Symptoms and Signs

Itching is a key clinical feature and may be severe and prolonged. Ill-defined, scaly, red plaques affect the face, neck, and upper trunk. The flexural surfaces of elbows and knees are often involved. In chronic cases, the skin is dry and lichenified. In patients with darker skin with severe disease, pigmentation may be lost in lichenified areas. During acute flares, widespread redness with weeping, either diffusely or in discrete plaques, is common. Virtually all patients with atopic dermatitis have skin disease before age 5; therefore, a new diagnosis of atopic dermatitis in an adult over age 30 should be made only after consultation with a dermatologist.

B. Laboratory Findings

Food allergy is an uncommon cause of flares of atopic dermatitis in adults. Eosinophilia and increased serum IgE levels may be present.

Differential Diagnosis

Atopic dermatitis must be distinguished from irritant or allergic contact dermatitis. Seborrheic dermatitis is less pruritic, with frequent scalp and central face involvement, greasy and scaly lesions, and responds quickly to therapy. Psoriasis is marked by sharply demarcated thickly scaled plaques on elbows, knees, scalp, and intergluteal cleft. Secondary staphylococcal or herpetic infections may exacerbate atopic dermatitis and should be considered during hyperacute, weeping flares. An infra-auricular fissure is a cardinal sign of secondary staphylococcal infection.

Treatment

Patient education regarding gentle skin care and proper use of medications is critical to successful management of atopic dermatitis.

A. General Measures

Atopic patients have hyperirritable skin. Anything that dries or irritates the skin may trigger dermatitis. Atopic individuals are sensitive to low humidity and often flare in the winter. Adults with atopic disorders should not bathe more than once daily. Soap should be confined to the armpits, groin, scalp, and feet. Washcloths and brushes should not be used. After rinsing, the skin should be patted dry (not rubbed) and then immediately—within minutes—covered with a thin film of an emollient or a corticosteroid as needed. Plain petrolatum can be used if contact dermatitis resulting from additives in medication is suspected. Skin may be irritated by rough fabrics, including wools and acrylics. Cottons are preferable, but synthetic blends also are tolerated. Other triggers may include sweating, ointments, and heat.

B. Local Treatment

Corticosteroids should be applied sparingly to the dermatitis once or twice daily and rubbed in well. Their potency should be appropriate to the severity of the dermatitis. In general, for treatment of lesions on the body (excluding genitalia, axillary or crural folds), one should begin with triamcinolone 0.1% or a stronger corticosteroid, then taper to hydrocortisone or another slightly stronger mild corticosteroid (alclometasone, desonide). **It is vital that patients taper off corticosteroids and substitute emollients as the dermatitis clears to avoid side effects of corticosteroids.** Tapering is also important to avoid dermatitis flares that may follow abrupt cessation. Tacrolimus ointment (Protopic 0.03% or 0.1%), pimecrolimus cream (Elidel 1%), and crisaborole (Eucrisa 2%) are nonsteroidal topical medications that may be effective in managing atopic dermatitis when applied twice daily. Burning with application occurs in about 50% of patients using Protopic and 10–25% using Elidel but may resolve with continued treatment. These noncorticosteroid medications prevent complications of long-term corticosteroid use, including atrophy or striae. They are safe for application on the face and eyelids but are more expensive than generic topical corticosteroids.

There is a US FDA black box warning for both topical tacrolimus and pimecrolimus due to concerns about the development of T-cell lymphoma. The agents should be used sparingly and only in locations where less expensive corticosteroids cannot be used. They should be avoided in patients at high risk for lymphoma (ie, those with HIV, iatrogenic immunosuppression, or prior lymphoma).

The treatment of atopic dermatitis is dictated by the pattern of the dermatitis—acute/weepy, subacute/scaly, or chronic/lichenified.

1. Acute weeping lesions—Staphylococcal or herpetic superinfection should be excluded by bacterial or viral culture, or both. Use water or aluminum subacetate solution (Domeboro or burow solution), or colloidal oatmeal as a bath or as wet dressings for 10–30 minutes two to four times daily. Lesions on extremities may be bandaged for protection at night. Use high-potency corticosteroids after soaking but spare the face and body folds. Tacrolimus is usually not tolerated at this stage. Systemic corticosteroids may be required. An allergic or irritating contactant should also be considered when acute weeping lesions are present, since contact dermatitis is more likely to develop in atopic patients.

2. Subacute or scaly lesions—The lesions are dry but still red and pruritic. Mid- to high-potency corticosteroids in ointment form should be continued until skin lesions are cleared and itching is decreased substantially. At that point, patients should begin a 2- to 4-week taper from twice-daily to daily dosing with topical corticosteroids to reliance on emollients, with occasional use of corticosteroids only to inflamed areas. It is preferable to switch to daily use of a low-potency corticosteroid instead of further tapering the frequency of usage of a more potent corticosteroid. Tacrolimus and pimecrolimus may be substituted if corticosteroids cannot be stopped completely.

3. Chronic, dry, lichenified lesions—Thickened and usually well demarcated, they are best treated with high-potency to ultra–high-potency corticosteroid ointments. Nightly occlusion for 2–6 weeks may enhance the initial response. Adding tar preparations, such as liquor carbonis detergens 10% in Aquaphor or 2% crude coal tar may be beneficial.

4. Maintenance treatment—Once symptoms have improved, constant application of effective moisturizers is recommended to prevent flares. In patients with moderate disease, use of topical anti-inflammatories only on weekends or three times weekly can prevent flares.

C. Systemic and Adjuvant Therapy

Systemic corticosteroids are indicated only for severe acute exacerbations. Oral prednisone dosages should be high enough to suppress the dermatitis quickly, usually starting with 1 mg/kg daily. The dosage is then tapered off over a period of 2–4 weeks. Owing to the chronic nature of atopic dermatitis and the side effects of long-term systemic corticosteroids, **ongoing use of these agents is not recommended for maintenance therapy.** Bedtime doses of hydroxyzine, diphenhydramine, or doxepin may be helpful via their sedative properties to mitigate perceived pruritus. Dupilumab is a targeted immunomodulator with minimal systemic adverse effects and requires minimal laboratory monitoring. Janus kinase (JAK) inhibitors (upadacitinib, abrocitinib), cyclosporine, mycophenolate mofetil, methotrexate, or azathioprine may also be used for the most severe and recalcitrant cases.

Complications of Treatment

The clinician should monitor for skin atrophy. Fissures, crusts, erosions, or pustules may indicate staphylococcal or herpetic infection clinically. Eczema herpeticum (herpes simplex superinfection) is manifested by monomorphic vesicles, crusts, or scalloped erosions superimposed on atopic dermatitis or other extensive eczematous processes and is treated with oral or intravenous acyclovir. Systemic antistaphylococcal antibiotics—such as a first-generation cephalosporin or doxycycline if methicillin-resistant *Staphylococcus aureus* is suspected—should be given only if indicated and guided by bacterial culture. Cultures to exclude methicillin-resistant *S aureus* are recommended. In this setting, continuing and augmenting the topical anti-inflammatory treatment often improves the dermatitis despite the presence of infection.

Prognosis

Atopic dermatitis runs a chronic or intermittent course. Affected adults may have only hand dermatitis. Prognostic factors for persistence into adulthood include generalized disease or onset early in childhood and asthma. Only 40–60% of these patients have lasting remissions.

Drucker AM et al. Systemic immunomodulatory treatments for patients with atopic dermatitis: a systematic review and network meta-analysis. JAMA Dermatol. 2020;156:659. [PMID: 32320001]

Lam M et al. Association between topical calcineurin inhibitor use and risk of cancer, including lymphoma, keratinocyte carcinoma, and melanoma: a systematic review and meta-analysis. JAMA Dermatol. 2021;157:549. [PMID: 33787818]

Langan SM et al. Atopic dermatitis. Lancet 2020;396:345. [PMID: 32738956]

LICHEN SIMPLEX CHRONICUS (Circumscribed Neurodermatitis)

ESSENTIALS OF DIAGNOSIS

- Chronic itching and scratching.
- Lichenified lesions with exaggerated skin lines overlying a thickened, well-circumscribed, scaly plaque.
- Predilection for nape of neck, wrists, external surfaces of forearms, lower legs, and genitals.

General Considerations

Lichen simplex chronicus represents a self-perpetuating scratch-itch cycle that is hard to disrupt.

Clinical Findings

Intermittent itching incites the patient to scratch the lesions and may interfere with sleep. Dry, hypertrophic, lichenified plaques appear on the neck, wrists, ankles, or perineum (Figure 6–21). The patches are rectangular, thickened, and hyperpigmented. The skin lines are exaggerated.

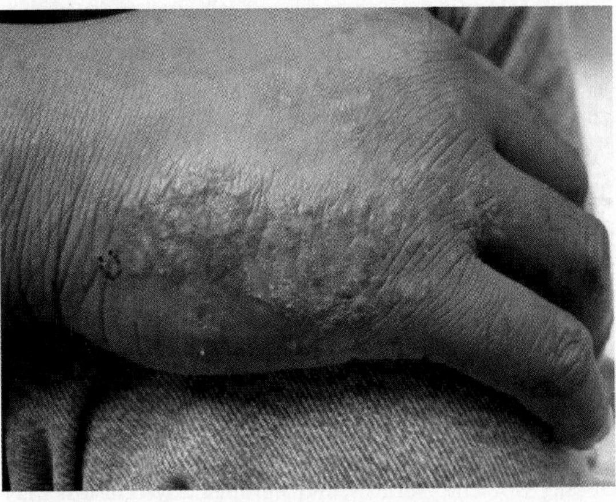

Figure 6–21. Lichen simplex chronicus on the hand. (Used, with permission, from Lindy Fox, MD.)

Differential Diagnosis

This disorder can be differentiated from plaque-like lesions such as psoriasis (redder lesions having whiter scales on the elbows, knees, and scalp and nail findings), lichen planus (violaceous, usually smaller polygonal papules), and nummular (coin-shaped) dermatitis. Lichen simplex chronicus may complicate chronic atopic dermatitis or scabetic infestation.

Treatment

For lesions in extragenital regions, ultra-high potency topical corticosteroids are effective, with or without occlusion, when used twice daily for several weeks (Table 6–2). In some patients, flurandrenolide (Cordran) tape may be effective, since it prevents scratching and rubbing of the lesion. The injection of triamcinolone acetonide suspension (5–10 mg/mL) into the lesions may occasionally be curative. Continuous occlusion with a flexible hydrocolloid dressing for 7 days at a time for 1–2 months may also be helpful. Dupilumab is a new treatment option for generalized disease or prurigo nodularis, its related condition. For genital lesions, see the section Pruritus Ani.

Prognosis

The disease tends to remit during treatment but may recur or develop at another site.

Calugareanu A et al; French Group of Research and Study in Atopic Dermatitis (Groupe de Recherche sur l'Eczéma Atopique, GREAT) from the French Society of Dermatology (SFD). Effectiveness and safety of dupilumab for the treatment of prurigo nodularis in a French multicenter adult cohort of 16 patients. J Eur Acad Dermatol Venereol. 2020;34:e74. [PMID: 31529718]

PSORIASIS

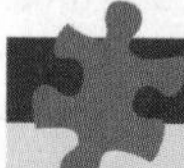

ESSENTIALS OF DIAGNOSIS

- Silvery scales on bright red, well-demarcated plaques, usually on the knees, elbows, and scalp.
- Nails: pitting and onycholysis (separation of the nail plate from the bed).
- Mild itching is common.
- May be associated with psoriatic arthritis.
- Histopathology helpful.

General Considerations

Psoriasis is a common benign, chronic inflammatory skin disease with both a genetic basis and known environmental triggers. Injury or irritation of normal skin tends to induce lesions of psoriasis at the site (Koebner phenomenon). Obesity worsens psoriasis, and significant weight loss may lead to substantial improvement. Psoriasis has several variants—the most common is the plaque type and hand involvement is also common. Eruptive (guttate) psoriasis consisting of numerous, smaller lesions 3–10 mm in diameter occurs occasionally after streptococcal pharyngitis. Rarely, life-threatening forms (generalized pustular and erythrodermic psoriasis) may occur.

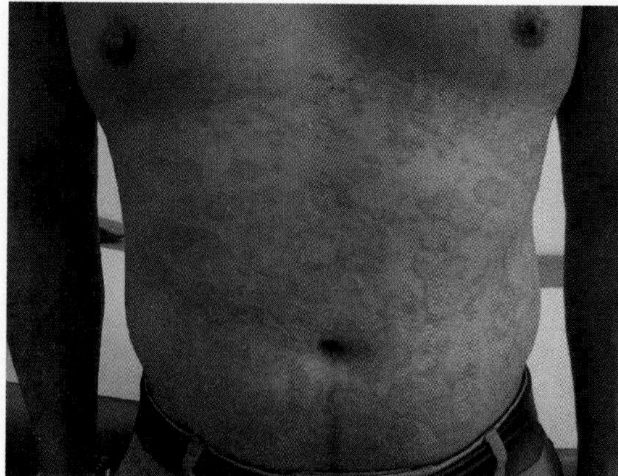

Figure 6–22. Extensive plaque psoriasis involving trunk of person with dark skin type. (Used, with permission, from Kanade Shinkai, MD.)

Clinical Findings

There are often no symptoms, but itching may occur and be severe. Favored sites include the scalp, elbows, knees, palms and soles, and nails. The lesions are red, sharply defined plaques covered with silvery scale (Figure 6–22). The glans penis and vulva may be affected. Occasionally, only the flexures (axillae, inguinal areas) are involved (termed inverse psoriasis). Fine stippling ("pitting") in the nails is highly suggestive of psoriasis (Figure 6–23) as is onycholysis. The combination of red plaques with silvery scales on elbows and knees, with scaliness in the scalp or

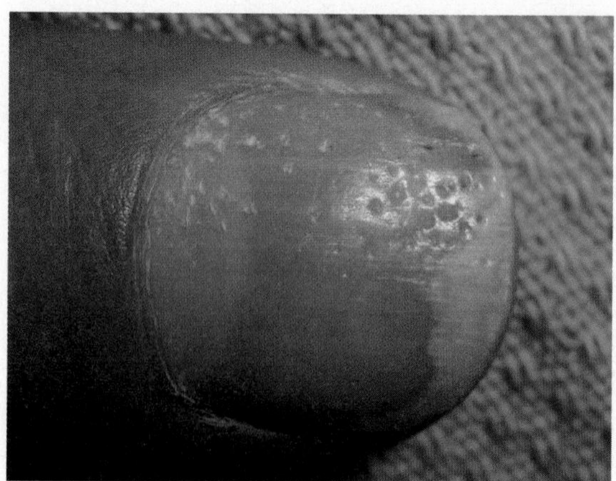

Figure 6–23. Nail pitting due to psoriasis in a patient with dark skin. (Reproduced with permission from Richard P. Usatine, MD, in Usatine RP, Smith MA, Mayeaux EJ Jr, Chumley H. *The Color Atlas of Family Medicine*, 2nd ed. McGraw-Hill, 2013.)

nail findings, is diagnostic. Patients with psoriasis often have a pink or red intergluteal fold. Not all patients have findings in all locations. Some patients have mainly hand or foot dermatitis with minimal findings elsewhere. There may be associated arthritis that is most commonly distal and oligoarticular, although the rheumatoid variety with a negative rheumatoid factor may occur. The psychosocial impact of psoriasis is a major factor in determining the treatment of the patient.

Differential Diagnosis

Psoriasis lesions are well demarcated and affect extensor surfaces—in contrast to atopic dermatitis, with poorly demarcated plaques in flexural distribution. In body folds, scraping and culture for *Candida* and examination of scalp and nails will distinguish inverse psoriasis from intertrigo and candidiasis. Dystrophic changes in nails may mimic onychomycosis, and a potassium hydroxide (KOH) preparation or fungal culture is valuable in diagnosis. The cutaneous features of reactive arthritis, pityriasis rosea, SLE, and syphilis mimic psoriasis.

Treatment

There are many therapeutic options in psoriasis to be chosen according to the extent (body surface area [BSA] affected) and the presence of other findings (for example, arthritis). Certain medications, such as beta-blockers, antimalarials, statins, lithium, and prednisone taper may flare or worsen psoriasis. Patients with moderate to severe psoriasis should be managed by or in conjunction with a dermatologist.

A. Limited Disease

For patients with large plaques and less than 10% of the BSA involved, the easiest regimen is to use a high-potency to ultra–high-potency topical corticosteroid cream or ointment. It is best to restrict the ultra–high-potency corticosteroids to 2–3 weeks of twice-daily use and then use them in a pulse fashion three or four times on weekends or switch to a mid-potency corticosteroid. Topical corticosteroids rarely induce a lasting remission. Initially, patients may be treated with twice-daily topical corticosteroids plus a vitamin D analog (calcipotriene ointment 0.005% or calcitriol ointment 0.003%) twice daily. This rapidly clears the lesions; eventually, the topical corticosteroids are stopped, and once- or twice-daily application of the vitamin D analog is continued long-term. Calcipotriene usually cannot be applied to the groin or face because of irritation. Treatment of extensive psoriasis with vitamin D analogs may result in hypercalcemia, so that the maximum dose for calcipotriene is 100 g/week and for calcitriol it is 200 g/week. Calcipotriene is incompatible with many topical corticosteroids (but not halobetasol), so if used concurrently, it must be applied at a different time. For patients with numerous small papules and plaques, such as guttate psoriasis, phototherapy is the best therapy.

For thick plaques on the scalp, start with a tar shampoo, used daily if possible. Additional treatments include 6% salicylic acid gel (eg, Keralyt), P & S solution (phenol, mineral oil, and glycerin), or fluocinolone acetonide 0.01% in oil (Derma-Smoothe/FS) under a shower cap at night, and shampoo in the morning. In order of increasing potency, triamcinolone 0.1%, fluocinolone, betamethasone dipropionate, amcinonide, and clobetasol are available in solution form for use on the scalp twice daily. Tacrolimus ointment 0.1% or 0.03% or pimecrolimus cream 1% may be effective in intertriginous, genital, and facial psoriasis, where potent corticosteroids are not recommended due to skin atrophy.

B. Moderate Disease

Psoriasis affecting 10–30% of the patient's BSA is frequently treated with UV phototherapy, either in a medical office or via a home light unit. Systemic agents listed below may also be used.

C. Moderate to Severe Disease

If psoriasis in a given location is severe or involves more than 30% of the body surface, it is difficult to treat with topical agents. These patients may be best managed in partnership with a dermatologist, especially when considering systemic therapy. The treatment of choice is outpatient narrowband UVB (NB-UVB) three times weekly. Clearing occurs in an average of 7 weeks, and maintenance may be required. Psoriatic arthritis may require distinct treatments, and benefits from management in partnership with a rheumatologist or dermatologist.

Methotrexate is effective for severe psoriasis in doses up to 25 mg once weekly according to published protocols. Long-term methotrexate use may be associated with cirrhosis. After receiving a 3.5–4-g cumulative dose, the patient should be referred to a hepatologist for evaluation. Administration of folic acid, 1–2 mg daily, can eliminate nausea caused by methotrexate without compromising efficacy.

Acitretin, a synthetic retinoid, is most effective for pustular psoriasis in oral dosages of 0.5–0.75 mg/kg/day. Liver enzymes and serum lipids must be checked periodically. Because acitretin is a teratogen and persists for 2–3 years in fat, women of childbearing age must wait at least 3 years after completing acitretin treatment before considering pregnancy. When used as single agents, retinoids will flatten psoriatic plaques, but will rarely result in complete clearing. Retinoids find their greatest use when combined with phototherapy—either UVB or PUVA, with which they are synergistic.

Cyclosporine dramatically improves psoriasis and may be used to control severe cases. Rapid relapse (rebound) frequently occurs after cessation of therapy, so another agent must be added if cyclosporine is stopped. The tumor necrosis factor (TNF) inhibitors etanercept (Enbrel), infliximab (Remicade), and adalimumab (Humira) are effective in pustular and chronic plaque psoriasis and are also effective for the associated arthritis. Infliximab provides the most rapid response and can be used for severe pustular or erythrodermic flares. Etanercept is used more frequently for long-term treatment at a dose of 50 mg subcutaneously twice weekly for 3 months, then 50 mg once weekly. All three TNF inhibitors can also induce or worsen psoriasis. IL-12/23 monoclonal antibodies (ustekinumab [Stelara], guselkumab, risankizumab), JAK inhibitors (tofacitinib, approved for use in rheumatoid arthritis but with strong data supporting its use in psoriasis), and IL-17 monoclonal antibodies (secukinumab, brodalumab, and ixekizumab) may be the most effective treatments among biologics. The oral phosphodiesterase 4 inhibitor apremilast is an approved option for plaque-type psoriasis and psoriatic arthritis with minimal immunosuppressive effects and requires no laboratory monitoring.

Prognosis

The course of psoriasis may be chronic and unpredictable, and it may be refractory to treatment. Patients (especially those older than 40 years) should be monitored for metabolic syndrome, which correlates with the severity of their skin disease. Complications of systemic therapy occur and active monitoring for infection is needed.

Armstrong AW et al. Comparison of biologics and oral treatments for plaque psoriasis: a meta-analysis. JAMA Dermatol. 2020;156:256. [PMID: 32022825]

Armstrong AW et al. Pathophysiology, clinical presentation, and treatment of psoriasis: a review. JAMA. 2020;323:1945. [PMID: 32427307]

Sbidian E et al. Systemic pharmacological treatments for chronic plaque psoriasis: a network meta-analysis. Update in: Cochrane Database Syst Rev. 2021;4:CD011535. [PMID: 31917873]

PITYRIASIS ROSEA

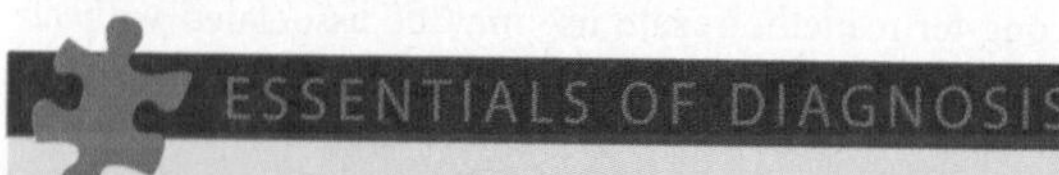

- Oval, fawn-colored, scaly eruption following cleavage lines of trunk.
- Herald patch precedes eruption by 1–2 weeks.
- Occasional pruritus.

General Considerations

Pityriasis rosea is a common mild, acute inflammatory disease that is 50% more common in females. Young adults are principally affected, mostly in the spring or fall. Concurrent household cases have been reported.

Clinical Findings

Itching is common but usually mild. The diagnosis is made by finding one or more classic lesions, such as oval, fawn-colored plaques up to 2 cm in diameter. The centers of a few lesions may have a characteristic crinkled or "cigarette paper" appearance and a collarette scale, ie, a thin bit of scale that is bound at the periphery and free in the center. Lesions follow cleavage lines on the trunk (so-called Christmas tree pattern, Figure 6–24), and the proximal portions of the extremities are often involved. A variant that affects the flexures (axillae and groin), so-called inverse pityriasis rosea, and a papular variant, especially in patients with more darkly pigmented skin types, also occur. An initial lesion ("herald patch") that is often larger than the later lesions often precedes the general eruption by 1–2 weeks. The eruption usually lasts 6–8 weeks and heals without scarring.

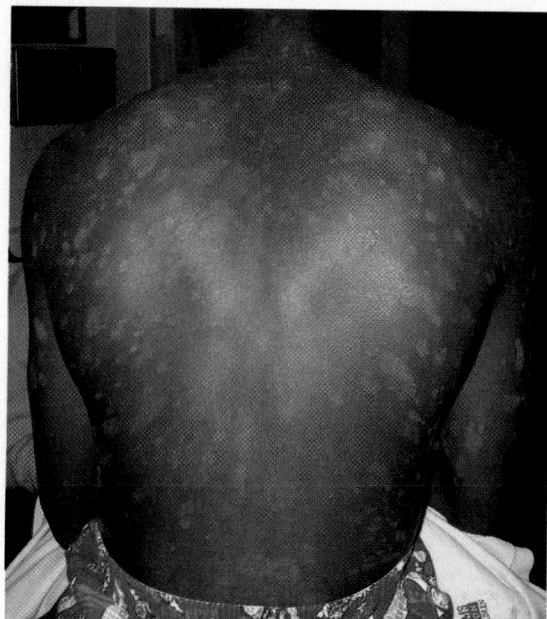

Figure 6–24. Pityriasis rosea with scaling lesions following skin lines and resembling a Christmas tree. (Used, with permission, from EJ Mayeaux, MD, in Usatine RP, Smith MA, Mayeaux EJ Jr, Chumley HS. *The Color Atlas and Synopsis of Family Medicine*, 3rd ed. McGraw-Hill, 2019.)

Differential Diagnosis

Serologic testing for syphilis should be performed if clinical risk factors are present. Palmar and plantar or mucous membrane lesions or adenopathy are features suggestive of secondary syphilis. Tinea corporis may present with a few red, slightly scaly plaques. Typically, the number of plaques of tinea corporis are significantly fewer than the number seen in pityriasis rosea. A potassium hydroxide examination should be performed to exclude a fungal cause. Seborrheic dermatitis on occasion presents on the body with poorly demarcated patches over the sternum, in the pubic area, and in the axillae. Tinea versicolor lacks the typical collarette rimmed lesions. Guttate or plaque psoriasis is an important diagnostic consideration and biopsy can help differentiate these from pityriasis rosea. Certain medications and immunizations rarely may induce a skin eruption mimicking pityriasis rosea. A pityriasis rosea–like eruption has been reported in association with SARS-CoV2 infection and COVID-19 vaccination.

Treatment

Pityriasis rosea often requires no treatment unless patients are symptomatic. In darker-skinned individuals, more aggressive management may be indicated because dyspigmentation of lesions may result. While well-designed clinical trials have not demonstrated highly effective treatments, most dermatologists recommend UVB treatments or a short course of prednisone for severe or severely symptomatic cases. For mild to moderate cases, topical corticosteroids of medium strength (triamcinolone 0.1%) and oral antihistamines may be used if pruritus is bothersome. The role of macrolide antibiotics is not evidence based.

Prognosis

Pityriasis rosea is usually an acute self-limiting illness that typically disappears in about 6 weeks, although prolonged variants have been reported.

Cohen L et al. Dermatologic problems commonly seen by the allergist/immunologist. J Allergy Clin Immunol Pract. 2020;8:102. [PMID: 31351991]

Freeman EE et al. The spectrum of COVID-19-associated dermatologic manifestations: an international registry of 716 patients from 31 countries. J Am Acad Dermatol.2020;83:1118. [PMID: 32622888]

Schwartzberg L et al. Cutaneous manifestations of COVID-19. Cutis. 2021;107:90. [PMID: 33891838]

SEBORRHEIC DERMATITIS

ESSENTIALS OF DIAGNOSIS

- Dry scales and underlying erythema.
- Scalp, central face, presternal, interscapular areas, umbilicus, and body folds.

General Considerations

Seborrheic dermatitis is an acute or chronic papulosquamous dermatitis that often coexists with psoriasis and is associated with inflammation due to *Malassezia* species.

Clinical Findings

The scalp, face, chest, back, umbilicus, eyelid margins, genitalia, and body folds have dry scales (dandruff) or oily yellowish scurf (Figure 6–25). Pruritus is a variable finding. Patients with Parkinson disease, HIV-infected patients, and patients who become acutely ill often have seborrheic dermatitis.

Differential Diagnosis

There is a spectrum from seborrheic dermatitis to scalp psoriasis. Extensive seborrheic dermatitis may simulate intertrigo in flexural areas, but scalp, face, and sternal involvement suggests seborrheic dermatitis.

Treatment

A. Seborrhea of the Scalp

Shampoos that contain zinc pyrithione or selenium are used daily if possible. These may be alternated with ketoconazole shampoo (1% or 2%) used twice weekly. A combination of shampoos is used in refractory cases. Tar shampoos are also effective for milder cases and for scalp psoriasis. Topical corticosteroid solutions or lotions are then added if necessary and are used twice daily. (See treatment for scalp psoriasis, above.)

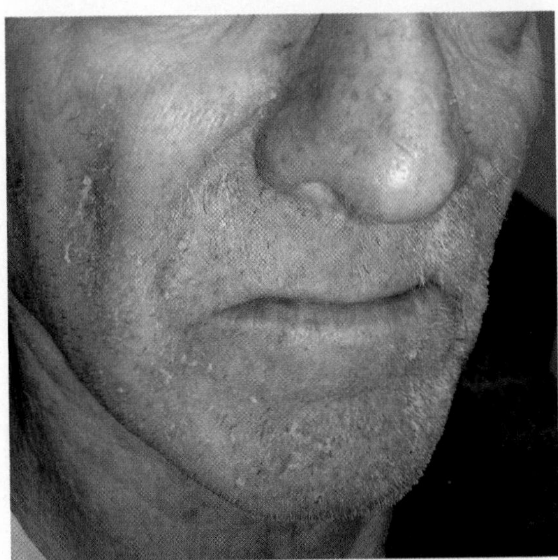

▲ **Figure 6–25. Close-up of seborrheic dermatitis showing flaking skin and erythema around the beard region.** (Reproduced with permission from Richard P. Usatine, MD, in Usatine RP, Smith MA, Mayeaux EJ Jr, Chumley H. *The Color Atlas of Family Medicine*, 2nd ed. McGraw-Hill, 2013.)

B. Facial Seborrheic Dermatitis

The mainstay of therapy is a mild corticosteroid (hydrocortisone 1%, alclometasone, desonide) used intermittently and not near the eyes. If the disorder cannot be controlled with intermittent use of a mild topical corticosteroid alone, ketoconazole 2% cream is added twice daily. Topical tacrolimus and pimecrolimus are steroid-sparing alternatives and may be more effective than antifungal therapy.

C. Seborrheic Dermatitis of Nonhairy or Intertriginous Areas

Low-potency corticosteroid creams—ie, 1% or 2.5% hydrocortisone, desonide, or alclometasone dipropionate—are highly effective when applied twice daily for 5–7 days and then once or twice weekly for maintenance as necessary. Selenium lotion, ketoconazole, or clotrimazole gel or cream may be a useful adjunct. Tacrolimus or pimecrolimus topically may avoid corticosteroid atrophy in chronic cases.

D. Involvement of Eyelid Margins

"Marginal blepharitis" usually responds to gentle cleaning of the lid margins nightly as needed, with undiluted baby shampoo or eyelid cleanser using a cotton swab.

Prognosis

The tendency is for lifelong recurrences. Individual outbreaks may last weeks, months, or years.

Joly P et al. Tacrolimus 0.1% versus ciclopiroxolamine 1% for maintenance therapy in patients with severe facial seborrheic dermatitis: a multicenter, double-blind, randomized controlled study. J Am Acad Dermatol. 2021;84:1278. [PMID: 33010323]
Piquero-Casals J et al. Non-steroidal topical therapy for facial seborrheic dermatitis. J Drugs Dermatol. 2020;19:658. [PMID: 32574015]

LICHEN PLANUS

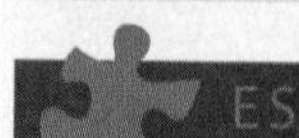

ESSENTIALS OF DIAGNOSIS

- Pruritic, violaceous, flat-topped papules with fine white streaks and symmetric distribution.
- Lacy or erosive lesions of the buccal, vulvar, and vaginal mucosa; nail dystrophy.
- Commonly seen along linear scratch marks (Koebner phenomenon) on anterior wrists, penis, and legs.
- Diagnostic histopathology.

General Considerations

Lichen planus is an inflammatory pruritic disease of the skin and mucous membranes characterized by distinctive papules with a predilection for the flexor surfaces and trunk. The three cardinal findings are typical skin lesions, mucosal lesions, and histopathologic features of band-like infiltration of lymphocytes in the upper dermis. Lichenoid drug eruptions can resemble lichen planus clinically and histologically. The most common medications include sulfonamides, tetracyclines, quinidine, NSAIDs, beta-blockers, and hydrochlorothiazide. Hepatitis C infection is found with greater frequency in lichen planus patients than in controls. Allergy to mercury and other metal-containing amalgams can trigger oral lesions identical to lichen planus.

Clinical Findings

The lesions are violaceous, flat-topped, angulated papules, up to 1 cm in diameter, discrete or in clusters (Figure 6–26), with very fine white streaks (Wickham striae) on the flexor surfaces of the wrists and ankles; on lower back; and on mucous membranes, including the penis, lips, tongue, buccal, vulvar, vaginal, esophageal, and anorectal mucosa. Itching is mild to severe. The papules may become bullous or eroded. The disease may be generalized. Mucous membrane lesions have a lacy white network overlying them that may be confused with leukoplakia. The presence of oral and vulvovaginal lichen planus in the same patient is common. Patients with both these mucous membranes involved are at much higher risk for esophageal lichen planus. Lichen planus is also a cause of alopecia and nail dystrophy. The Koebner phenomenon (appearance of lesions in areas of trauma) may be seen.

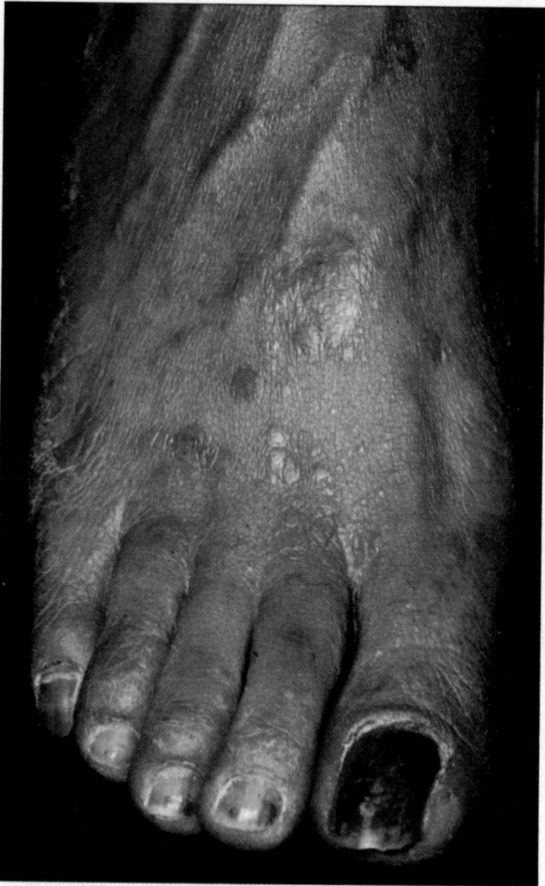

▲ **Figure 6–26.** Lichen planus. (Used, with permission, from TG Berger, MD, Dept Dermatology, UCSF.)

A special form of lichen planus is the erosive or ulcerative variety, a major problem in the mouth or genitalia. Squamous cell carcinoma develops in up to 5% of patients with erosive oral or genital lichen planus and may occur in esophageal lichen planus. There is also an increased risk of squamous cell carcinoma developing in lesions of hypertrophic lichen planus on the lower extremities.

Differential Diagnosis

Lichen planus must be distinguished from similar lesions produced by medications and other papular lesions, such as psoriasis, lichen simplex chronicus, graft-versus-host disease, and syphilis. Lichen planus on the mucous membranes must be differentiated from leukoplakia. Erosive oral lesions require biopsy and often direct immunofluorescence for diagnosis since lichen planus may simulate other erosive diseases, especially autoimmune blistering diseases that involve the oral mucosa.

Treatment

A. Topical Therapy

Superpotent topical corticosteroids applied twice daily are most helpful for localized disease in nonflexural areas.

Alternatively, high-potency corticosteroid cream or ointment may be used nightly under thin, pliable plastic film.

Topical tacrolimus appears effective in oral and vaginal erosive lichen planus, but long-term therapy is required to prevent relapse. If tacrolimus is used, lesions must be observed carefully for development of squamous cell carcinoma. Since absorption can occur through mucous membranes, serum tacrolimus levels should be checked at least once if widespread mucosal application (more than 5–10 cm^2) is used. If the erosive oral lichen planus lesions are adjacent to a metal-containing amalgam, removal of the amalgam may result in clearing of the erosions.

B. Systemic Therapy

NB-UVB, bath PUVA, oral PUVA, and the combination of an oral retinoid plus PUVA (re-PUVA) are all forms of phototherapy that can improve lichen planus. Hydroxychloroquine (5 mg/kg once daily), acitretin (10–25 mg orally daily), cyclosporine (3–5 mg/kg orally), and mycophenolate mofetil (1 g orally twice daily) can also be effective in mucosal and cutaneous lichen planus. Apremilast, 30 mg twice daily, has reported efficacy in case series. JAK inhibitors and anti-IL-12/23 and anti-IL-17 agents have also been used with success in refractory cases. Corticosteroids may be required in severe cases or in circumstances where the most rapid response to treatment is desired. Unfortunately, relapse almost always occurs as the corticosteroids are tapered, making systemic corticosteroid therapy an impractical option for the management of chronic lichen planus.

Prognosis

Lichen planus is a benign disease, but it may persist for months or years and may be recurrent. Hypertrophic lichen planus and oral lesions tend to be especially persistent, and neoplastic degeneration has been described in chronically eroded lesions.

Boch K et al. Lichen planus. Front Med (Lausanne). 2021;8:737813. [PMID: 34790675]

Li C et al. Global prevalence and incidence estimates of oral lichen planus: a systematic review and meta-analysis. JAMA Dermatol. 2020;156:172. [PMID: 31895418]

CUTANEOUS LUPUS ERYTHEMATOSUS

ESSENTIALS OF DIAGNOSIS

- Localized violaceous red plaques, usually on the head (discoid lupus erythematosus) or the trunk (chronic cutaneous lupus erythematosus).
- Scaling, follicular plugging, atrophy, dyspigmentation, and telangiectasia of involved areas.
- Photosensitivity.
- Distinctive histology.

General Considerations

Common forms of cutaneous lupus include chronic cutaneous lupus erythematosus (CCLE), typically chronic scarring (discoid) lupus erythematosus (DLE), and erythematous nonscarring red plaques of subacute cutaneous lupus erythematosus (SCLE). All occur most frequently in photoexposed areas. Permanent hair loss and loss of pigmentation are common sequelae of discoid lesions. SLE is discussed in Chapter 20. Patients with SLE may have DLE or SCLE lesions.

Clinical Findings

A. Symptoms and Signs

Symptoms are usually mild. In DLE, the lesions consist of violaceous red, well-localized, single or multiple plaques, 5–20 mm in diameter, usually on the face, scalp, and external ears (conchal bowl). In discoid lesions, there is atrophy, telangiectasia, central depigmentation or scarring, a hyperpigmented rim, and follicular plugging. On the scalp, significant permanent hair loss may occur. In SCLE, the lesions are erythematous annular or psoriasiform plaques up to several centimeters in diameter and favor the upper chest and back.

B. Laboratory Findings

In patients with DLE, SLE should be considered if the following findings are present: positive antinuclear antibody (ANA), other positive serologic studies (eg, anti-double-stranded DNA or anti-Smith antibody), high ESR, proteinuria, hypocomplementemia, widespread lesions (not localized to the head), nail fold changes (dilated or thrombosed nail fold capillary loops), or arthralgias with or without arthritis. Patients with marked photosensitivity and symptoms otherwise suggestive of lupus may have negative ANA tests but are positive for antibodies against Ro/SSA or La/SSB (SCLE).

Differential Diagnosis

The diagnosis is based on the clinical appearance confirmed by skin biopsy in all cases. In DLE, the scale is dry and "thumbtack-like" and thus distinguished from that of seborrheic dermatitis and psoriasis. Older lesions have hyperpigmented borders, depigmented central scarring, or areas of hair loss that also differentiate lupus from these diseases. Ten percent of patients with SLE have discoid skin lesions, and 5% of patients with discoid lesions have SLE. A number of medications may induce SCLE with a positive Ro/SSA.

Treatment

A. General Measures

Use photoprotective clothing and broad-spectrum sunblock of SPF of 30 or more daily. UVA coverage is essential in photosensitive patients. Avoid radiation therapy or medications that are potentially photosensitizing when possible.

B. Local Treatment

For limited lesions, the following should be tried before systemic therapy: high-potency corticosteroid creams applied each night and covered with airtight, thin, pliable plastic film (eg, Saran Wrap); Cordran tape; or ultra–high-potency corticosteroid cream or ointment applied twice daily without occlusion.

C. Local Infiltration

Triamcinolone acetonide suspension, 2.5–10 mg/mL, may be injected into DLE lesions once a month.

D. Systemic Treatment

1. Antimalarials—These medications should be used only when the diagnosis is secure because they have been associated with flares of psoriasis, which may be in the differential diagnosis.

A. HYDROXYCHLOROQUINE SULFATE—Daily dose of no more than 5 mg/kg orally (real-weight) for several months may be effective and is often used prior to chloroquine. A minimum 3-month trial is recommended. Screening for ocular toxicity is needed.

B. CHLOROQUINE SULFATE—250 mg orally daily may be effective in some cases when hydroxychloroquine is not.

2. Isotretinoin—Isotretinoin, 1 mg/kg/day orally, is effective in hypertrophic DLE lesions.

3. Thalidomide—Thalidomide is effective in refractory cases in doses of 50–300 mg orally daily. Monitor for neuropathy. Lenalidomide (5–10 mg orally daily) may also be effective with less risk for neuropathy.

Isotretinoin, thalidomide, and lenalidomide are teratogens and should be used with appropriate contraception and monitoring in women of childbearing age.

Prognosis

The disease is persistent but not life-endangering unless systemic lupus is present. Treatment with one or more antimalarials is effective in more than half of cases. Patients with cutaneous lupus erythematosus should be examined and tested annually (CBC and UA) to screen for early signs of systemic involvement. Although the only morbidity may be cosmetic, this can have significant quality of life impact in more darkly pigmented patients with widespread disease. Scarring alopecia can be prevented or lessened with close attention and aggressive therapy. Over years, DLE tends to become inactive. Drug-induced SCLE usually resolves over months when the inciting medication is stopped.

Fairley JL et al. Management of cutaneous manifestations of lupus erythematosus: a systematic review. Semin Arthritis Rheum. 2020;50:95. [PMID: 31526594]

Shi H et al. Treatment of cutaneous lupus erythematosus: current approaches and future strategies. Curr Opin Rheumatol. 2020;32:208. [PMID: 32141953]

VESICULAR & BLISTERING DERMATOSES

CONTACT DERMATITIS

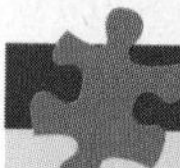

ESSENTIALS OF DIAGNOSIS

- Erythema and edema, with pruritus, vesicles, bullae, weeping, or crusting.
- **Irritant contact dermatitis:** occurs only in area of direct contact with irritant.
- **Allergic contact dermatitis:** extends beyond area of direct contact with allergen; positive patch test.

General Considerations

Contact dermatitis (irritant or allergic) is an acute or chronic dermatitis that results from direct skin contact with chemicals or allergens. Eighty percent of cases are due to excessive exposure to or additive effects of universal irritants (eg, soaps, detergents, organic solvents) and are called **irritant contact dermatitis**. The most common causes of **allergic contact dermatitis** are poison ivy or poison oak, topically applied antimicrobials (especially bacitracin and neomycin), anesthetics (benzocaine), preservatives, jewelry (nickel), rubber, essential oils, propolis (from bees), vitamin E, and adhesive tape. Occupational exposure is an important cause of allergic contact dermatitis.

Clinical Findings

A. Symptoms and Signs

1. Allergic contact dermatitis—The acute phase is characterized by intense pruritus, tiny vesicles, and weepy and crusted lesions (Figure 6–27). The lesions, distributed on exposed parts or in unusual asymmetric patterns, consist of erythematous macules, papules, and vesicles and may occur beyond the contact area, distinguishing it from irritant dermatitis. The affected area may also be edematous and warm with honey-colored crusting, simulating—and at times complicated by—bacterial or viral infection. The pattern of the eruption may be diagnostic (eg, typical linear streaked vesicles on the extremities in poison oak or ivy dermatitis). The location will often suggest the cause: scalp involvement suggests hair dyes or shampoos; face involvement suggests creams, cosmetics, soaps, shaving materials, nail polish; and neck involvement suggests jewelry, hair dyes. Reactions may not develop for 48–72 hours after exposure.

2. Irritant contact dermatitis—The rash is erythematous and scaly (but less likely vesicular) and occurs only in the direct sites of contact with the irritant. Resolving or chronic contact dermatitis presents with scaling, erythema, and possibly thickened skin. Itching, burning, and stinging may be severe in both allergic and irritant contact

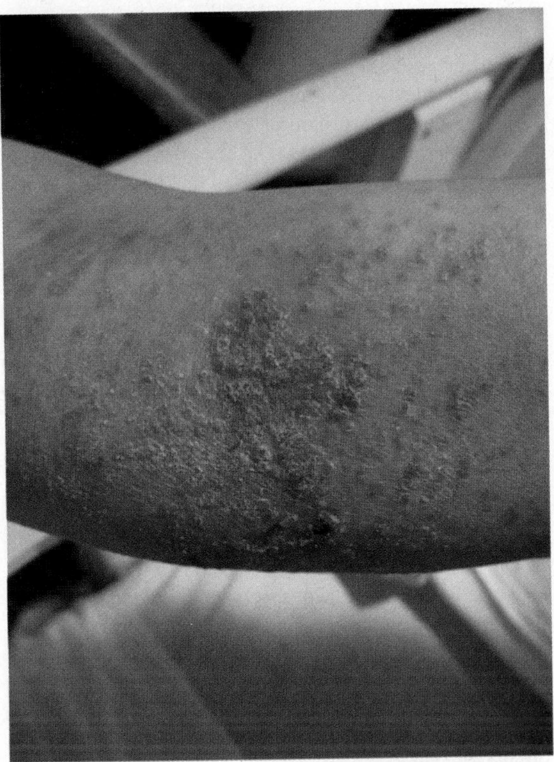

▲ **Figure 6–27.** Allergic contact dermatitis to an adhesive dressing in patient with darker skin. Key features are erythematous papules with impetigo-like honey-colored crusting. (Used, with permission, from Kanade Shinkai, MD.)

dermatitis. Reactions may develop within 24 hours of contact exposure.

B. Laboratory Findings

Gram stain and culture will rule out impetigo or secondary infection (impetiginization). After the episode of allergic contact dermatitis has cleared, patch testing may be useful if the triggering allergen is not known.

Differential Diagnosis

Asymmetric distribution, blotchy erythema around the face, linear lesions, and a history of exposure help distinguish acute contact dermatitis from other skin lesions. The most commonly mistaken diagnosis is impetigo, herpetic infection, or cellulitis. Chronic allergic contact dermatitis must be differentiated from scabies, particularly if itching is generalized; atopic dermatitis; and pompholyx.

Prevention

Removal of the causative oil by washing with liquid soap may be effective if done within 30 minutes after exposure to poison oak or ivy. Goop (oil remover) and Tecnu (chemical inactivator) are also effective but more expensive without increased efficacy. Over-the-counter barrier creams may be effective when applied prior to exposure and prevent/reduce the severity of the dermatitis.

The mainstay of prevention is identification of the agent causing the dermatitis and strict avoidance of exposure or use of protective clothing and gloves. Some allergens will transmit through latex gloves. In industry-related cases, prevention may require special accommodations or retraining the worker.

Treatment

A. Overview

Localized involvement (except on the face) can often be managed solely with topical agents. While local measures are important, severe or widespread involvement is difficult to manage without systemic corticosteroids because even the highest-potency topical corticosteroids seem not to work well on vesicular and weepy lesions. **Irritant contact dermatitis** is treated by protection from the irritant and use of topical corticosteroids as for atopic dermatitis (described above). The treatment of **allergic contact dermatitis** is detailed below.

B. Local Measures

1. Acute weeping dermatitis—Gentle cleansing and drying compresses (such as Domeboro) are recommended. Calamine lotion or zinc oxide paste may be used between wet dressings, especially for involvement of intertriginous areas or when oozing is not marked. Lesions on the extremities may be bandaged with wet dressings for 30–60 minutes several times a day. High-potency topical corticosteroids in gel or cream form (eg, fluocinonide, clobetasol, or halobetasol) may help suppress acute contact dermatitis and relieve itching. This treatment should be followed by tapering of the number of applications per day or use of a mid-potency corticosteroid, such as triamcinolone 0.1% cream, to prevent rebound of the dermatitis. A soothing formulation is 2 oz of 0.1% triamcinolone acetonide cream in 7.5 oz Sarna lotion (0.5% camphor, 0.5% menthol, 0.5% phenol) mixed by the patient.

2. Subacute dermatitis (subsiding)—Mid-potency (triamcinolone 0.1%) to high-potency corticosteroids (clobetasol, fluocinonide, desoximetasone) are the mainstays of therapy.

3. Chronic dermatitis (dry and lichenified)—High-potency to superpotency corticosteroids are used in ointment form. Occlusion may be helpful on the hands.

C. Systemic Therapy

For acute severe cases, prednisone may be given orally for 12–21 days. Prednisone, 60 mg for 4–7 days, 40 mg for 4–7 days, and 20 mg for 4–7 days, without a further taper is one useful regimen. The key is to use enough corticosteroid (and as early as possible) to achieve a clinical effect and to taper slowly over 2–3 weeks to avoid rebound.

Prognosis

Allergic contact dermatitis is self-limited if reexposure is prevented but often takes 2–3 weeks for full resolution. Removal of the causative agent is paramount to avoid recurrences.

Brar KK. A review of contact dermatitis. Ann Allergy Asthma Immunol. 2021;126:32. [PMID: 33091591]
Nassau S et al. Allergic contact dermatitis. Med Clin North Am. 2020;104:61. [PMID: 31757238]

POMPHOLYX

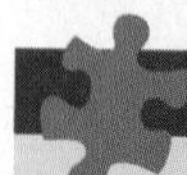

ESSENTIALS OF DIAGNOSIS

- Pruritic "tapioca" vesicles of 1–2 mm on the palms, soles, and sides of fingers.
- Vesicles may coalesce to form multiloculated blisters.
- Scaling and fissuring may follow drying of the blisters.
- Appearance in the third decade, with lifelong recurrences.

General Considerations

Pompholyx, or vesiculobullous dermatitis of the palms and soles, is formerly known as dyshidrosis or dyshidrotic eczema. About half of patients have an atopic background, and many patients report flares with stress. Patients with widespread dermatitis due to any cause may develop pompholyx-like eruptions as a part of an autoeczematization response.

Clinical Findings

Small clear vesicles resembling grains of tapioca stud the skin at the sides of the fingers and on the palms (Figure 6–28) and may also affect the soles, albeit less frequently. They may be associated with intense itching. Later, the vesicles dry and the area becomes scaly and fissured.

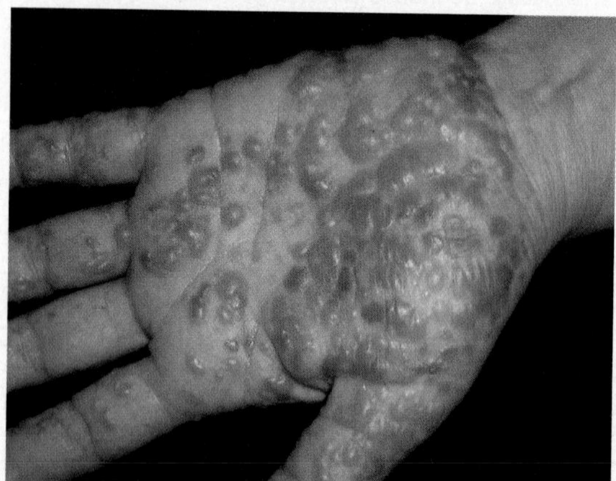

▲ **Figure 6–28.** Severe pompholyx. (Reproduced with permission from Richard P. Usatine, MD, in Usatine RP, Smith MA, Mayeaux EJ Jr, Chumley H. *The Color Atlas of Family Medicine*, 2nd ed. McGraw-Hill, 2013.)

Differential Diagnosis

Unroofing the vesicles and examining the blister roof with a KOH preparation will reveal hyphae in cases of bullous tinea. Patients with inflammatory tinea pedis may have a vesicular autoeczematization of the palms. NSAIDs may produce an eruption very similar to that of vesiculobullous dermatitis on the hands.

Prevention

There is no known way to prevent attacks if the condition is idiopathic. About one-third to one-half of patients with vesiculobullous hand dermatitis have a relevant contact allergen, especially nickel. Patch testing and avoidance of identified allergens can lead to improvement.

Treatment

Topical and systemic corticosteroids help some patients dramatically; however systemic corticosteroids are generally not appropriate therapy. A high-potency topical corticosteroid used early may help abort the flare and ameliorate pruritus. Topical corticosteroids are also important in treating the scaling and fissuring that are seen after the vesicular phase. Oral alitretinoin may be effective. It is essential that patients avoid anything that irritates the skin; they should wear cotton gloves inside vinyl gloves when doing dishes or other wet chores and use a hand cream after washing the hands. Patients respond to PUVA therapy and injection of botulinum toxin into the palms as for hyperhidrosis.

Prognosis

For most patients, the disease is an inconvenience. For some, vesiculobullous hand eczema can be incapacitating.

Agner T et al. Hand eczema: epidemiology, prognosis and prevention. J Eur Acad Dermatol Venereol. 2020;34:4. [PMID: 31860734]
Elsner P et al. Hand eczema: treatment. J Eur Acad Dermatol Venereol. 2020;34:13. [PMID: 31860736]

PORPHYRIA CUTANEA TARDA

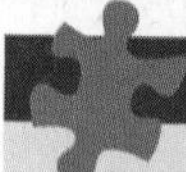

ESSENTIALS OF DIAGNOSIS

- Noninflammatory blisters on sun-exposed sites, especially the dorsal surfaces of the hands.
- Hypertrichosis, skin fragility.
- Associated liver disease.
- Elevated urine porphyrins.

General Considerations

Porphyria cutanea tarda is the most common type of porphyria. Cases are sporadic or hereditary. The disease is associated with ingestion of certain medications (eg, estrogens) and alcoholic liver disease, hemochromatosis, or hepatitis C.

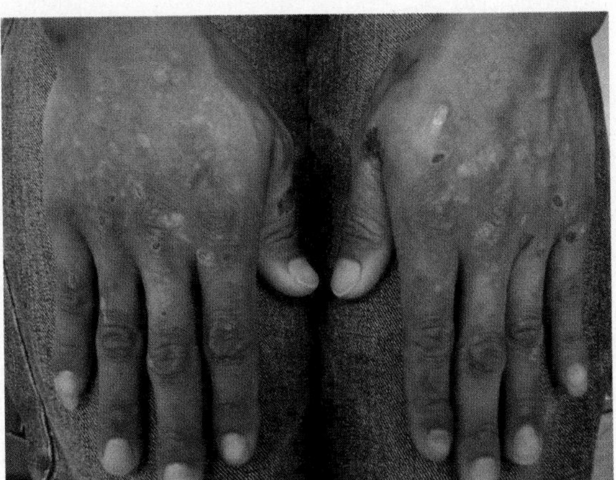

▲ **Figure 6–29.** Porphyria cutanea tarda of hands in patient with darker skin. (Used, with permission, from Kanade Shinkai, MD.)

Clinical Findings

A. Symptoms and Signs

Patients complain of painless blistering and fragility of the skin of the dorsal surfaces of the hands (Figure 6–29). Facial hypertrichosis and hyperpigmentation are common.

B. Laboratory Findings

Urinary uroporphyrins are elevated twofold to fivefold above coproporphyrins. Patients may also have abnormal liver biochemical tests, evidence of hepatitis C infection, increased liver iron stores, and hemochromatosis gene mutations.

Differential Diagnosis

Skin lesions identical to those of porphyria cutanea tarda may be seen in patients who undergo dialysis and in those who take certain medications (tetracyclines, voriconazole, and NSAIDs, especially naproxen). In this so-called pseudoporphyria, the biopsy results are the same as those associated with porphyria cutanea tarda, but urine porphyrins are normal.

Prevention

Barrier sun protection with clothing is required. Although the lesions are triggered by sun exposure, the wavelength of light triggering the lesions is beyond that absorbed by sunscreens.

Treatment

Stopping all triggering medications and substantially reducing or stopping alcohol consumption alone may lead to improvement in most cases. Phlebotomy at a rate of 1 unit every 2–4 weeks will gradually lead to improvement. Very low-dose antimalarial medication (as low as 200 mg of hydroxychloroquine orally twice weekly), alone or in combination with phlebotomy, increases porphyrin excretion and improves the skin disease. Deferasirox, an iron chelator, can also be beneficial. Treatment is continued until the patient is asymptomatic. Urine porphyrins may be monitored.

Prognosis

Most patients improve with treatment. Sclerodermoid skin lesions may develop on the trunk, scalp, and face.

Neeleman RA et al. Diagnostic and therapeutic strategies for porphyrias. Neth J Med. 2020;78:149. [PMID: 32641543]

DERMATITIS HERPETIFORMIS

Dermatitis herpetiformis is an uncommon disease manifested by intensely pruritic papules, vesicles, and papulovesicles mainly on the elbows, knees, buttocks, posterior neck, and scalp. It is associated with HLA antigens -B8, -DR3, and -DQ2. The histopathology is distinctive. Circulating antibodies to tissue transglutaminase are present in 90% of cases. NSAIDs may cause flares. Patients may have gluten-sensitive enteropathy. Three-fourths of patients have villous atrophy on small bowel biopsy; however, GI symptoms are subclinical in most. The prevalence of dermatitis herpetiformis to celiac disease is 1:8. Ingestion of gluten is the cause of dermatitis herpetiformis, and strict long-term avoidance of dietary gluten may eliminate the need for treatment or decrease the dose of dapsone (initial treatment dose is 100–200 mg orally daily) required to control the disease. Patients with dermatitis herpetiformis are at increased risk for GI lymphoma, and this risk is reduced by a gluten-free diet.

Reunala T et al. Dermatitis herpetiformis: an update on diagnosis and management. Am J Clin Dermatol. 2021;22:329. [PMID: 33432477]

Salmi T et al. Current concepts of dermatitis herpetiformis. Acta Derm Venereol. 2020;100:adv00056. [PMID: 32039457]

PEMPHIGUS

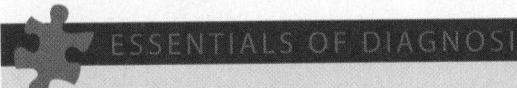

ESSENTIALS OF DIAGNOSIS

- Relapsing crops of bullae, often fragile and leading to erosions.
- Often preceded by mucous membrane bullae, erosions, and ulcerations.
- Superficial detachment of the skin after pressure or trauma variably present (Nikolsky sign).
- Acantholysis on biopsy.
- Immunofluorescence studies and serum ELISA for pathogenic antibodies are confirmatory.

General Considerations

Pemphigus is an uncommon intraepidermal blistering disease occurring on skin and mucous membranes.

It is caused by autoantibodies to adhesion molecules expressed in the skin and mucous membranes. The bullae appear spontaneously and are tender and painful when they rupture. Drug-induced pemphigus has been reported. There are several forms of pemphigus: pemphigus vulgaris and its variant, pemphigus vegetans; and the more superficially blistering pemphigus foliaceus and its variant, pemphigus erythematosus. All forms may present at any age but most commonly in middle age. The vulgaris form begins in the mouth in over 50% of cases. The foliaceus form may be associated with other autoimmune diseases or may be drug-induced. Paraneoplastic pemphigus, a unique form of the disorder, is associated with numerous benign and malignant neoplasms, most frequently chronic lymphocytic leukemia, Castleman disease, B cell lymphoma, plasmacytoma, and thymoma. Associated bronchiolitis obliterans is characteristic.

Clinical Findings

A. Symptoms and Signs

Pemphigus is characterized by an insidious onset of flaccid bullae, crusts, and erosions in crops or waves (Figure 6–30). In pemphigus vulgaris, lesions often appear first on the oral mucous membranes. These rapidly become erosive. The scalp is another site of early involvement. Rubbing a cotton swab or finger laterally on the surface of uninvolved skin may cause easy separation of the epidermis (Nikolsky sign). Downward pressure on a fresh bulla may cause lateral spread (Asboe-Hansen sign). Pemphigus vegetans presents as erosive vegetating plaques, most often in intertriginous areas. Pemphigus foliaceus is a superficial form of pemphigus where cutaneous lesions present as flaccid bullae that quickly evolve into superficial erosions and thin pink plaques with overlying scale. Mucosal lesions are rare in pemphigus foliaceus. Pemphigus erythematosus has overlapping features of pemphigus foliaceus and lupus erythematosus. It presents with flaccid bullae that develop overlying scale and crust in a photodistributed area. Again, mucosal lesions are rare. Paraneoplastic pemphigus is histologically and immunologically distinct from other forms of the disease. Oral lesions predominate and cutaneous erythematous plaques resembling erythema multiforme are characteristic. Survival rates are low because of the underlying malignancy.

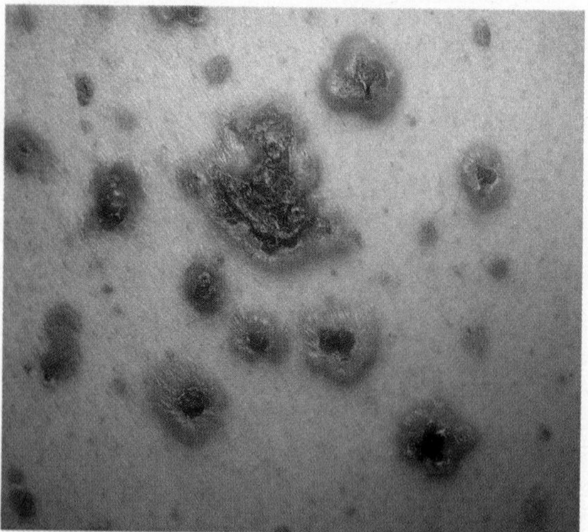

▲ **Figure 6–30. Pemphigus vulgaris on the back with crusted and intact bullae.** (Used, with permission, from Eric Kraus, MD, in Usatine RP, Smith MA, Mayeaux EJ Jr, Chumley HS. *The Color Atlas and Synopsis of Family Medicine*, 3rd ed. McGraw-Hill, 2019.)

B. Laboratory Findings

The diagnosis is made by light microscopy, direct and indirect immunofluorescence (IIF) microscopy, and ELISA assays to detect autoantibodies to intercellular adhesion molecules (desmoglien 3 and 1).

Differential Diagnosis

Blistering diseases include erythema multiforme, Stevens-Johnson syndrome (SJS)/toxic epidermal necrolysis (TEN), drug eruptions, bullous impetigo, contact dermatitis, dermatitis herpetiformis, and bullous pemphigoid, but flaccid blisters are not typical of these diseases, and acantholysis is not seen on biopsy. All these diseases have clinical characteristics and immunofluorescence test results that distinguish them from pemphigus. Pemphigus foliaceus must be distinguished from subacute cutaneous lupus erythematosus.

Complications

Secondary infection commonly occurs; this is a major cause of morbidity and mortality. Disturbances of fluid, electrolyte, and nutritional intake can occur as a result of painful oral ulcers.

Treatment

A. General Measures

Patients with severe disease should be hospitalized at bed rest and provided intravenous antibiotics and feedings as indicated. Anesthetic troches used before eating ease painful oral lesions.

B. Systemic Measures

Pemphigus requires systemic therapy as early in its course as possible. Initial therapy is with prednisone, 60–80 mg orally daily. In all but the mildest cases, a steroid-sparing agent is added from the beginning, since the disease course is long and the steroid-sparing agents take several weeks to exert their activity. Rituximab (1 g intravenously on days 1 and 15 as induction therapy followed by 500 mg intravenously every 6 months as maintenance therapy) is FDA approved for the treatment of pemphigus vulgaris, associated with induction of a complete remission, and considered by many experts to be first-line therapy. Repeated courses are efficacious and well tolerated in patients who do not achieve complete remission or relapse. Azathioprine (2–4 mg/kg orally daily) and mycophenolate mofetil (1–1.5 g orally twice daily) are other therapeutic options.

In refractory cases, monthly IVIG (2 g/kg intravenously over 3–4 days), pulse intravenous corticosteroids, cyclophosphamide, or plasmapheresis can be used.

C. Local Measures

In patients with limited disease, skin and mucous membrane lesions should be treated with topical corticosteroids. Complicating infection requires appropriate systemic and local antibiotic therapy.

Prognosis

Without antibiotic or corticosteroid treatment, the disease is fatal within 5 years. The course tends to be chronic in most patients; however, up to one-third experience remission. Infection is the most frequent cause of death, usually from *S aureus* septicemia.

Ellebrecht CT et al. Pemphigus and pemphigoid: from disease mechanisms to druggable pathways. J Invest Dermatol. 2022;142:907. [PMID: 34756581]

Lee MS et al. Network meta-analysis-based comparison of first-line steroid-sparing adjuvants in the treatment of pemphigus vulgaris and pemphigus foliaceus. J Am Acad Dermatol. 2021;85:176. [PMID: 32798583]

Werth VP et al; PEMPHIX Study Group. Rituximab versus mycophenolate mofetil in patients with pemphigus vulgaris. N Engl J Med. 2021;384:2295. [PMID: 34097368]

BULLOUS PEMPHIGOID

Bullous pemphigoid is a relatively benign pruritic disease characterized by tense blisters in flexural areas, usually remitting in 5 or 6 years, with a course characterized by exacerbations and remissions. Most affected persons are over the age of 60 and men are affected twice as frequently as women. The appearance of blisters may be preceded by pruritic urticarial or edematous lesions for months. Oral lesions are present in one-third. The disease may occur in various forms, including localized, vesicular, vegetating, erythematous, erythrodermic, and nodular. Drugs may induce bullous pemphigoid. The most common offender is furosemide. Immunotherapy for malignancies with PD-1 inhibitors can cause drug-induced bullous pemphigoid.

The diagnosis is made by biopsy with direct immunofluorescence examination and serum antibody testing. Light microscopy shows a subepidermal blister. With direct immunofluorescence, IgG and C3 are found at the dermal-epidermal junction. ELISA tests for bullous pemphigoid antibodies (BP 180 or BP 230) are 87% sensitive and 95% specific. If the patient has mild disease, ultrapotent topical corticosteroids may be adequate. Prednisone (0.75 mg/kg orally daily) is often used to achieve rapid control of more widespread disease. Tetracycline (500 mg orally three times daily) or doxycycline (100 mg orally twice a day), alone or combined with nicotinamide—not nicotinic acid or niacin—(up to 1.5 g orally daily), may control the disease in patients who cannot use corticosteroids or may allow for decreasing or eliminating corticosteroids after control is achieved. Dapsone (50–200 mg orally daily) is particularly effective in mucous membrane pemphigoid. If these medications are not effective, methotrexate (5–25 mg orally weekly), azathioprine (2–4 mg/kg orally daily), or mycophenolate mofetil (1–1.5 g orally twice daily) may be used as steroid-sparing agents. Intravenous immunoglobulin, rituximab, omalizumab, and dupilumab have been used with success in refractory cases.

Montagnon CM et al. Subepithelial autoimmune blistering dermatoses: Clinical features and diagnosis. J Am Acad Dermatol. 2021;85:1. [PMID: 33684496]

Tedbirt B et al. Mixed individual-aggregate data on all-cause mortality in bullous pemphigoid: a meta-analysis. JAMA Dermatol. 2021;157:421. [PMID: 33729430]

PUSTULAR DISORDERS

ACNE VULGARIS

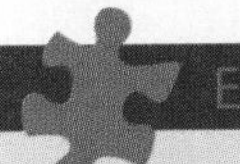

ESSENTIALS OF DIAGNOSIS

- Almost universal in puberty; may begin in premenarchal girls and present or persist into the fourth or fifth decade.
- Comedones are the hallmark. Severity varies from comedonal to papular or pustular inflammatory acne to cysts or nodules.
- Face, neck, and upper trunk may be affected.
- Scarring may be a sequela of the disease or picking by the patient.

General Considerations

Acne vulgaris is polymorphic. Open and closed comedones, papules, pustules, and cysts are found.

In younger persons, acne vulgaris is more common and more severe in males. Acne may persist into adulthood. Twelve percent of women and 3% of men over age 25 have acne vulgaris. This rate does not decrease until the fourth or fifth decade of life. The skin lesions parallel sebaceous activity. Pathogenic events include plugging of the infundibulum of the follicles, retention of sebum, overgrowth of the acne bacillus (*Cutibacterium acnes*) with resultant release of and irritation by accumulated fatty acids, and foreign-body reaction to extrafollicular sebum. Antibiotics may help control acne because of their antibacterial or anti-inflammatory properties.

Hyperandrogenism may be a cause of acne in women and may be accompanied by hirsutism or irregular menses. Polycystic ovary syndrome (PCOS) is the most common identifiable cause. Acne may develop in patients who use systemic corticosteroids or topical fluorinated corticosteroids on the face. Acne may be exacerbated or caused by cosmetic creams or oils as well as androgenic supplements or masculinizing hormone therapy in transgender individuals.

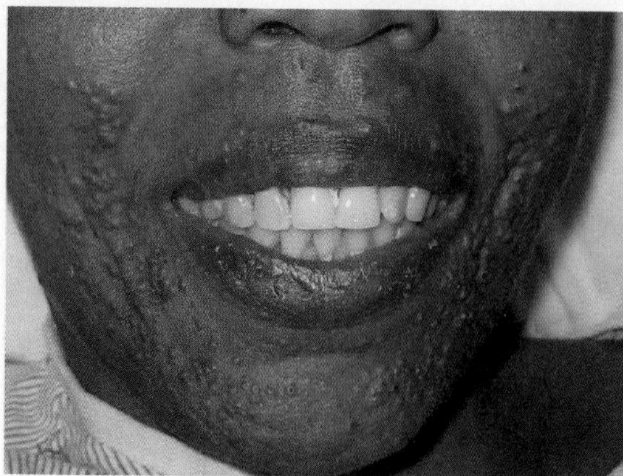

▲ **Figure 6–31.** Acne vulgaris. Extensive comedones and hyperpigmented macules are present in patient with dark skin. (Used, with permission, from Kanade Shinkai, MD.)

Clinical Findings

There may be mild tenderness, pain, or itching. The lesions occur mainly over the face, neck, upper chest, back, and shoulders. Comedones (tiny, flesh-colored, white or black noninflamed superficial papules that give the skin a rough texture or appearance) are the hallmark of acne vulgaris. Inflammatory papules, pustules, ectatic pores, acne cysts, and scarring are also seen (Figure 6–31).

Acne may have different presentations at different ages. Preteens often present with comedones as their first lesions. Inflammatory lesions in young teenagers are often found in the middle of the face, extending outward as the patient becomes older. Adult females may present with comedonal or papular lesions especially on the chin and jawline.

Differential Diagnosis

In adults, rosacea presents with papules and pustules in the middle third of the face, but absence of truncal involvement, telangiectasia, flushing, and the absence of comedones distinguish rosacea from acne vulgaris. A pustular eruption on the face in patients receiving antibiotics or with otitis externa should be investigated with culture to rule out a gram-negative folliculitis. Pustules on the face can also be caused by dermatophytic or demodex infection. Lesions on the back are more problematic. When they occur alone, staphylococcal folliculitis, miliaria ("heat rash") or, uncommonly, *Pityrosporum* folliculitis should be suspected. Bacterial culture, trial of an antistaphylococcal antibiotic, and observing the response to therapy will help in the differential diagnosis. In patients with HIV infection, folliculitis is common and may be either staphylococcal folliculitis or eosinophilic folliculitis (typically pruritic tumid papules on the face and neck).

Complications

Cyst formation, pigmentary changes, scarring, and poor quality of life may result.

Treatment

A. General Measures

1. Education of the patient—Education on proper use of medications and cosmetics is paramount. Because lesions take 4–6 weeks to improve, clinical improvement should be measured by the number of new lesions forming after 6–8 weeks of therapy. Additional time (3–4 months) will be required to see improvement on the back and chest, as these areas are slowest to respond. Avoid topical exposure to oils, cocoa butter (theobroma oil), and greases in cosmetics, including hair products. Scarring may occur with or without the patient manipulating the lesions. It is essential that the patient be educated in a supportive way about this complication. Anxiety and depression are common in patients with excoriated acne.

2. Diet—A low glycemic diet has been associated with improvement and lower incidence of acne. This improvement was associated with a reduction in insulin resistance. Hyperinsulinemia has also been associated with acne in both eumenorrheic women and individuals with PCOS.

B. Comedonal Acne

Treatment of acne is based on the type and severity of lesions. Comedones require treatment different from that of pustules and cystic lesions. In assessing severity, take the sequelae of the lesions into account. An individual who gets only a few new lesions per month that scar or leave postinflammatory hyperpigmentation must be treated much more aggressively than a comparable patient whose lesions clear without sequelae. Hygiene plays little role in acne treatment, and a mild soap is almost always recommended. The agents effective in comedonal acne are listed below in the order in which they should be tried.

1. Topical retinoids—Tretinoin is very effective for comedonal and papular acne, but its usefulness is limited by irritation. Start with 0.025% cream (not gel) and have the patient use it at first twice weekly at night, increasing frequency to nightly as tolerated. A few patients cannot tolerate this low-strength preparation more than three times weekly, which may still promote improvement. A lentil-sized amount is sufficient to cover the entire face. To avoid irritation, have the patient wait 20 minutes after washing to apply. For patients irritated by standard tretinoin preparations, other options are adapalene gel 0.1% and reformulated tretinoin (Renova, Retin A Micro, Avita). Although the absorption of tretinoin is minimal, its use during pregnancy is contraindicated. Patients should be warned that their acne may flare in the first 4 weeks of treatment.

2. Benzoyl peroxide—Benzoyl peroxide products are available in concentrations of 2.5%, 4%, 5%, 8%, and 10%, but 2.5% is as effective as 10% and less irritating. In general, water-based and not alcohol-based gels should be used to decrease irritation. Single formulations of benzoyl peroxide in combination with several other topical agents, including adapalene and topical antibiotics (erythromycin, clindamycin phosphate), are available.

C. Papular or Cystic Inflammatory Acne

Brief treatment (3 weeks to 3 months) with topical or oral antibiotics is the mainstay for treatment of inflammatory acne that does not respond to topical therapy with retinoids or benzoyl peroxide. Topical clindamycin phosphate and erythromycin are used only for mild papular acne or for patients who refuse or cannot tolerate oral antibiotics. To decrease resistance, benzoyl peroxide should be used in combination with the topical antibiotic.

1. Mild acne—The first choice of topical antibiotics in terms of efficacy and relative lack of induction of resistant *C acnes* is the combination of erythromycin or clindamycin with benzoyl peroxide topical gel or wash (Table 6–2). These may be used once or twice daily. The addition of tretinoin cream or gel at night may increase improvement since it works via a different mechanism. Topical retinoids should be used for long-term maintenance therapy.

2. Moderate acne—Common oral antibiotics used for acne include doxycycline (100 mg twice daily), minocycline (50–100 mg once or twice daily), TMP-SMZ (one double-strength tablet twice daily), or a cephalosporin (cefadroxil or cephalexin 500 mg twice daily), which should be used in combination with benzoyl peroxide to minimize development of antibiotic resistance. It may take 3 months or more for truncal acne to resolve with oral antibiotic treatment. In general, discontinuing antibiotics immediately without adjunctive topical therapy results in prompt recurrence. Topical retinoids are excellent for long-term maintenance following antibiotics. Subantimicrobial dosing of doxycycline (40–50 mg orally daily) can be used in patients who require long-term systemic therapy. Combination oral contraceptives or spironolactone (50–200 mg orally daily) are highly effective alternatives in women with treatment-resistant acne. Tetracycline, minocycline, and doxycycline are contraindicated in pregnancy, but certain oral erythromycins or cephalosporins may be used.

3. Severe acne—

A. ISOTRETINOIN—A vitamin A analog, isotretinoin is used for the treatment of severe acne that has not responded to conventional therapy. An oral dosage of 0.5–1 mg/kg/day for 20 weeks for a cumulative dose of at least 120 mg/kg is usually adequate for treating and preventing the recurrence of severe cystic acne. Patients should be offered isotretinoin therapy before they experience significant acne scarring. *Isotretinoin is absolutely contraindicated during pregnancy because of its teratogenicity.* Two forms of effective contraception must be used; abstinence is an acceptable alternative. Informed consent must be obtained before its use, and patients must be enrolled in a monitoring program (iPledge). In addition to its teratogenicity, isotretinoin has numerous side effects and should only be prescribed by clinicians well aware of these issues. Cheilitis, dry skin, and photosensitivity are almost universal side effects. Consider ordering laboratory tests, including total cholesterol levels, triglyceride levels, and liver enzyme tests (particularly ALT, which is the most liver-specific enzyme), in patients before treatment and after achieving therapeutic dosing; monitoring through the entire treatment may not be high value. Monthly pregnancy testing is required for premenopausal women.

Abnormal laboratory tests, especially elevated liver enzymes and triglyceride levels, return to normal quickly upon conclusion of therapy. The medication may induce long-term remissions in 40–60%, or acne may recur that is more easily controlled with conventional therapy. Occasionally, a second course is needed if acne does not respond or recurs.

B. INTRALESIONAL INJECTION—Intralesional injection of dilute suspensions of triamcinolone acetonide (2.5 mg/mL, 0.05 mL per lesion) will often hasten the resolution of deeper papules and occasional cysts.

C. SCAR REVISION—Cosmetic improvement may be achieved by excision and punch-grafting of deep scars and by physical or chemical abrasion of inactive acne lesions, particularly flat, superficial scars.

Prognosis

Acne vulgaris eventually remits spontaneously, but when this will occur cannot be predicted. The condition may persist throughout adulthood and may lead to severe scarring if left untreated. Patients treated with antibiotics continue to improve for the first 3–6 months of therapy. Relapse during treatment may suggest the emergence of resistant *C acnes*. The disease is chronic and tends to flare intermittently despite treatment. Remissions following systemic treatment with isotretinoin may be lasting in up to 60% of cases. Relapses after isotretinoin usually occur within 3 years and require a second course in up to 20% of patients.

Kurokawa I et al. Recent advances in understanding and managing acne. F1000Res. 2020;9:792. [PMID: 32765835]

Sadeghzadeh-Bazargan A et al. Systematic review of low-dose isotretinoin for treatment of acne vulgaris: focus on indication, dosage, regimen, efficacy, safety, satisfaction, and follow up, based on clinical studies. Dermatol Ther. 2021;34:e14438. [PMID: 33085149]

ROSACEA

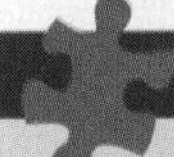

ESSENTIALS OF DIAGNOSIS

- A chronic disorder affecting the face.
- Neurovascular component: erythema and telangiectasis and a tendency to flush easily.
- Acneiform component: papules and pustules may be present.
- Glandular component: sebaceous hyperplasia and fibrosis of affected areas (eg, rhinophyma).

General Considerations

Rosacea is a common condition that presents in adulthood. The pathogenesis of this chronic disorder is not known.

Topical corticosteroids applied to the face can induce rosacea-like conditions.

Clinical Findings

Patients frequently report flushing or exacerbation of their rosacea due to heat, hot drinks, spicy food, sunlight, exercise, alcohol, emotions, or menopausal flushing. The cheeks, nose, chin, and ears—at times the entire face—may be affected. No comedones are seen. In its mildest form, erythema and telangiectasias are seen on the cheeks. Inflammatory papules may be superimposed on this background and may evolve to pustules (Figure 6–32). Associated seborrhea may be found. Some patients complain of burning or stinging with episodes of flushing and extremely cosmetic-intolerant skin. Patients may have associated ophthalmic disease, including blepharitis, keratitis, and chalazion, which often requires topical or systemic antibiotic or immunosuppressive therapy.

Differential Diagnosis

Rosacea is distinguished from acne by the presence of the neurovascular component and the absence of comedones. Lupus is often misdiagnosed, but the presence of pustules excludes that diagnosis.

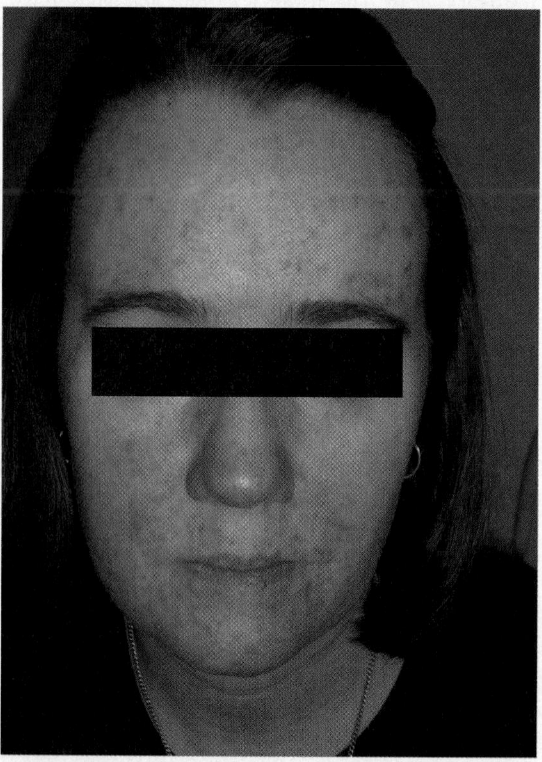

▲ **Figure 6–32.** **Rosacea in a 34-year-old woman showing erythema, papules, and pustules covering much of the face.** (Reproduced with permission from Richard P. Usatine, MD, in Usatine RP, Smith MA, Mayeaux EJ Jr, Chumley H. *The Color Atlas of Family Medicine*, 2nd ed. McGraw-Hill, 2013.)

Treatment

Educating patients to avoid the factors they know to produce exacerbations is important. Patients should wear a broad-spectrum mineral-based sunscreen; zinc- or titanium-based sunscreens are tolerated best. Medical management is most effective for the inflammatory papules and pustules and the erythema that surrounds them. Rosacea is usually a lifelong condition, so maintenance therapy is required. Most treatments target the papulopustular and cystic components. Only certain topical agents (brimonidine and oxymetazoline) and laser benefit erythema. Telangiectasias are benefited by laser therapy, and phymatous overgrowth of the nose can be treated by surgical reduction. Rhinophyma must be managed using surgical reduction.

A. Local Therapy

Avoidance of triggers (especially alcohol and spicy or hot foods) and drinking ice water may be effective in reducing facial erythema and flushing. Metronidazole (cream, gel, or lotion), 0.75% applied twice daily or 1% applied once daily, and ivermectin 1% cream applied once daily are effective topical treatments. Another effective treatment includes topical clindamycin (solution, gel, or lotion) 1% applied twice daily. Response is noted in 4–8 weeks. Sulfur-sodium sulfacetamide-containing topicals are helpful in patients only partially responsive to topical antibiotics. Topical retinoids or topical tacrolimus ointment (0.1%) can be carefully added for maintenance. Topical brimonidine tartrate gel 0.33% or oxymetazoline 1% cream can temporarily reduce the erythema, and laser treatment has longer-term benefit for erythema.

B. Systemic Therapy

Oral tetracyclines should be used when topical therapy is inadequate. Minocycline or doxycycline, 50–100 mg orally once or twice daily, is effective. Metronidazole or amoxicillin, 250–500 mg orally twice daily, or rifaximin, 400 mg orally three times daily (for 10 days), may be used in refractory cases. Side effects are few, although metronidazole may cause a disulfiram-like effect when the patient ingests alcohol and neuropathy with long-term use. Long-term maintenance with subantimicrobial dosing of minocycline or doxycycline is recommended once the initial flare of rosacea has resolved. Isotretinoin may succeed where other measures fail. A dosage of 0.5 mg/kg/day orally for 12–28 weeks is recommended, although very low-dose isotretinoin may also be effective. See precautions above.

Prognosis

Rosacea tends to be a persistent process. With the regimens described above, it can usually be controlled adequately.

Alexis AF et al. Global epidemiology and clinical spectrum of rosacea, highlighting skin of color: review and clinical practice experience. J Am Acad Dermatol. 2019;80:1722. [PMID: 30240779]

Tan J et al. Treating inflammation in rosacea: current options and unmet needs. J Drugs Dermatol. 2020;19:585. [PMID: 32574018]

MILIARIA (Heat Rash)

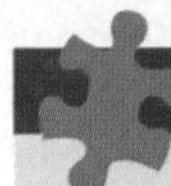

ESSENTIALS OF DIAGNOSIS

- Burning, itching, superficial aggregated small vesicles, papules, or pustules on covered areas of the skin, usually the trunk.
- More common in hot, moist climates.
- Rare forms associated with fever and even heat prostration.

General Considerations

Miliaria occurs most commonly on the trunk and intertriginous areas. A hot, moist environment is the most frequent cause. Occlusive clothing, fever while bedridden, and medications that enhance sweat gland function (eg, clonidine, beta-blockers, opioids) may increase the risk. Plugging of the ostia of sweat ducts occurs, with ultimate rupture of the sweat duct, producing an irritating, stinging reaction.

Clinical Findings

The usual symptoms are burning and itching. The histologic depth of sweat gland obstruction determines the clinical presentation: miliaria crystallina in the superficial (subcorneal) epidermis, miliaria rubra in the deep epidermis, and miliaria profunda in the dermis. The lesions consist of small (1–3 mm) nonfollicular lesions. Subcorneal thin-walled, discrete clear fluid-filled vesicles are termed "miliaria crystallina." When fluid is turbid and lesions present as vesicopustules or pustules, they are called miliaria pustulosa. Miliaria rubra (prickly heat) presents as pink papules. Miliaria profunda presents as nonfollicular skin-colored papules that develop after multiple bouts of miliaria rubra. In a hospitalized patient, the reaction virtually always affects the back.

Differential Diagnosis

Miliaria is to be distinguished from a drug eruption and folliculitis.

Prevention

Use of a topical antibacterial preparation, such as chlorhexidine, prior to exposure to heat and humidity may help prevent the condition. Frequent turning or sitting of the hospitalized patient may reduce miliaria on the back.

Treatment

The patient should keep cool and wear light clothing. A mid-potency corticosteroid (triamcinolone acetonide, 0.1%) in a lotion or cream may be applied two to four times daily. Secondary infections (superficial pyoderma) are treated with appropriate antistaphylococcal antibiotics. Anticholinergic medications (eg, glycopyrrolate 1 mg orally twice a day or topically applied) may be helpful in severe cases.

Prognosis

Miliaria is usually a mild disorder, but severe forms (tropical anhidrosis and asthenia) result from interference with the heat-regulating mechanism.

Rouai M et al. Miliaria crystallina in an intensive care patient. Clin Case Rep. 2021;9:e04665. [PMID: 34430023]

ERYTHEMAS

REACTIVE ERYTHEMAS

URTICARIA & ANGIOEDEMA

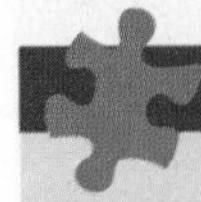

ESSENTIALS OF DIAGNOSIS

- Evanescent wheals or hives with or without angioedema.
- Intense itching; very rarely, pruritus may be absent.
- Urticaria is divided into acute and chronic forms.
- Most episodes are acute and self-limited (1–2 weeks).
- Chronic urticaria (lasting > 6 weeks) may have an autoimmune basis.

General Considerations

Urticaria involves hives, angioedema or both. It may be acute or chronic (more than 6 weeks' duration). Chronic urticaria is further divided into chronic spontaneous urticaria and chronic inducible urticaria. Chronic inducible urticaria is reproducibly triggered by specific exposures. Examples include cholinergic urticaria, solar urticaria, cold urticaria, dermatographism, and delayed pressure urticaria. True urticaria should be differentiated from diseases that present with similar lesions that are not true urticaria (eg, adult-onset Still disease, urticarial vasculitis, and cryopyrin-associated periodic syndromes). Some patients with chronic spontaneous urticaria demonstrate autoantibodies directed against mast cell IgE receptors.

Clinical Findings

A. Symptoms and Signs

Lesions are itchy, red swellings of a few millimeters to many centimeters (Figure 6–33). The morphology of the lesions may vary over a period of minutes to hours, resulting in geographic or bizarre patterns. Individual lesions in true urticaria last less than 24 hours and often only 2–4 hours. Angioedema is involvement of deeper subcutaneous tissue with swelling of the lips, eyelids, palms, soles, and genitalia.

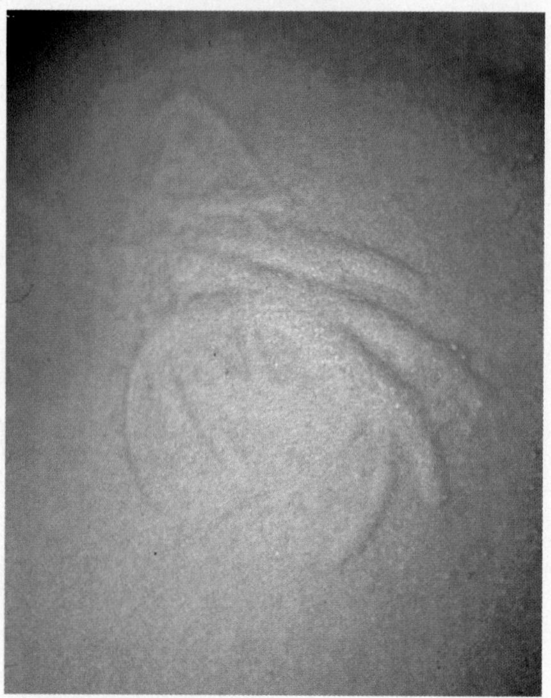

▲ **Figure 6–33.** Urticaria. (Used, with permission, from TG Berger, MD, Dept Dermatology, UCSF.)

Angioedema is no more likely than urticaria to be associated with systemic complications, such as laryngeal edema or hypotension. Dermatographism is induced by scratching and can be elicited during the clinic visit by scratching the patient's skin. The wheals of cholinergic urticaria are 2–3 mm in diameter with a large surrounding red flare.

B. Laboratory Findings

The most common causes of acute urticaria are foods, upper respiratory infections, and medications. The cause of chronic spontaneous urticaria is often not found. Although laboratory studies are not generally helpful in the evaluation of acute or chronic urticaria, a CBC with differential, ESR, CRP, TSH, and liver biochemical tests may be appropriate for some patients with chronic urticaria. Elevated inflammatory markers suggest an alternate diagnosis. In patients with individual lesions that persist past 24 hours, skin biopsy may confirm neutrophilic urticaria or urticarial vasculitis. A functional ELISA test looking for antibodies against the high-affinity receptor for IgE (Fc-Epislon RI) can detect patients with an autoimmune basis for their chronic urticaria.

Differential Diagnosis

Papular urticaria resulting from insect bites persists for days. A central punctum can usually be seen. Streaked urticarial lesions may be seen in the 24–48 hours before blisters appear in acute allergic plant dermatitis, eg, poison ivy, oak, or sumac. Urticarial responses to heat, sun, water, and pressure are quite rare. Urticarial vasculitis is defined as cutaneous vasculitis where the skin lesions clinically mimic urticaria. Lesions last longer than 24 hours and often sting or burn rather than itch. Patients do not respond to antihistamines. Urticarial vasculitis may be caused by viral hepatitis and may be seen as part of serum sickness. In hereditary angioedema, there is generally a positive family history and GI or respiratory symptoms. Wheals are not part of the syndrome, and lesions are not pruritic.

Treatment

A. General Measures

The etiology of acute urticaria is found in less than half of cases. The etiology of chronic urticaria is found in even fewer cases. In general, a careful history and physical examination are helpful but extensive costly workups for chronic spontaneous urticaria are not indicated. Patients with chronic autoimmune urticaria may have other autoimmune diseases and be more difficult to treat. In cases of chronic inducible urticaria, exposure to physical factors, such as heat, cold, sunlight, pressure, heat induced by exercise, excitement, and hot showers, should be modulated.

B. Systemic Treatment

The mainstay of treatment initially includes H_1-antihistamines, often starting with second-generation antihistamines. Second-generation H_1-antihistamines include fexofenadine (180 mg orally once daily) or cetirizine or loratadine (10 mg orally daily). Less than 40% of chronic urticaria cases respond to standard H_1-blockade, and higher doses of second-generation antihistamines (up to four times the standard recommended dose) increase the likelihood of response to therapy to 60%. Combining antihistamines (eg, fexofenadine plus cetirizine) at these higher doses can be done safely to achieve remission in refractory cases. First-generation H_1-antihistamines such as hydroxyzine, 10–25 mg orally two or three times daily, or as a single nightly dose of 25–75 may be added to this regimen.

Cyproheptadine, 4 mg orally four times daily, may be especially useful for cold urticaria.

Doxepin (a tricyclic antidepressant with potent antihistaminic properties), 10–75 mg orally at bedtime, can be very effective in chronic urticaria. It has anticholinergic side effects.

If a skin biopsy of a lesion of chronic urticaria identifies neutrophils as a significant component of the inflammatory infiltrate, dapsone or colchicine (or both) may be useful.

Although systemic corticosteroids in a dose of about 40 mg daily will usually suppress acute and chronic urticaria, corticosteroids are rarely indicated and, once withdrawn, urticaria virtually always returns. Therefore, consultation with a dermatologist or an allergist who has experience in managing severe urticaria is recommended before initiating systemic corticosteroid therapy. Omalizumab is approved for the treatment of refractory chronic urticaria and should be considered when severe chronic urticaria fails to respond to high-dose antihistamines.

C. Local Treatment

Local treatment is rarely rewarding.

Prognosis

Acute urticaria usually lasts only a few days to weeks. Half of patients whose urticaria persists for longer than 6 weeks will have it for years.

Agache I et al. Efficacy and safety of treatment with omalizumab for chronic spontaneous urticaria: a systematic review for the EAACI Biologicals Guidelines. Allergy. 2021;76:59. [PMID: 32767573]

Gonçalo M et al. The global burden of chronic urticaria for the patient and society. Br J Dermatol. 2021;184:226. [PMID: 32956489]

Kolkhir P et al. New treatments for chronic urticaria. Ann Allergy Asthma Immunol. 2020;124:2. [PMID: 31446134]

Maurer M et al. Biologics for the use in chronic spontaneous urticaria: when and which. J Allergy Clin Immunol Pract. 2021;9:1067. [PMID: 33685605]

Maurer M et al. Ligelizumab for chronic spontaneous urticaria. N Engl J Med. 2019;381:1321. [PMID: 31577874]

ERYTHEMA MULTIFORME/ STEVENS-JOHNSON SYNDROME/TOXIC EPIDERMAL NECROLYSIS

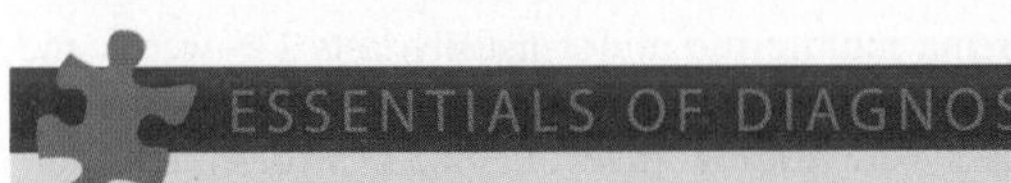

Erythema multiforme

- Herpes simplex is most common cause.
- Cutaneous lesions are true three ring targets.
- Presents on the extensor surfaces, palms, soles, or mucous membranes.
- Disease remains localized.

Stevens-Johnson syndrome and toxic epidermal necrolysis

- Stevens-Johnson syndrome: < 10% BSA detachment.
- Stevens-Johnson syndrome/toxic epidermal necrolysis overlap: 10–30% BSA detachment.
- Toxic epidermal necrolysis: > 30% BSA detachment.
- Medications are most common cause.
- Cutaneous lesions are targetoid but often not true three ring targets.
- Favors the trunk.
- Involves two or more mucous membranes.
- May progress to significant BSA involvement and may be life-threatening.

General Considerations

Erythema multiforme is an acute inflammatory skin disease that was traditionally divided into minor and major types based on the clinical findings. Approximately 90% of cases of erythema multiforme minor follow outbreaks of herpes simplex and is preferably termed "herpes-associated erythema multiforme." The term "erythema multiforme major" has largely been abandoned.

SJS is defined as atypical target lesions with less than 10% BSA detachment; TEN is defined as lesions with greater than 30% BSA detachment; and patients with SJS/TEN overlap have between 10% and 30% BSA detachment. The abbreviation SJS/TEN is often used to refer to these three variants of what is considered one syndrome. SJS/TEN is characterized by toxicity and involvement of two or more mucosal surfaces (often oral and conjunctival but can involve any mucosal surface, including respiratory epithelium). SJS/TEN is most often caused by oral or, less commonly, topical medications, especially sulfonamides, NSAIDs, allopurinol, and anticonvulsants. In certain races, polymorphisms of antigen-presenting major histocompatibility (MHC) loci increase the risk for the development of SJS/TEN. *Mycoplasma pneumoniae* may trigger a mucocutaneous reaction with skin and oral lesions closely resembling SJS in children/young adults, which tends not to progress to TEN-like disease and carries an overall good prognosis.

Clinical Findings

A. Symptoms and Signs

A classic target lesion, as in herpes-associated erythema multiforme, consists of three concentric zones of color change, most often on acral surfaces (hands, feet, elbows, and knees) (Figure 6–34). SJS/TEN presents with raised purpuric target-like lesions, with only two zones of color and a central blister, or nondescript reddish or purpuric macules favoring the trunk and proximal upper extremities (Figure 6–35). Pain on eating, swallowing, and urination can occur if relevant mucosae are involved.

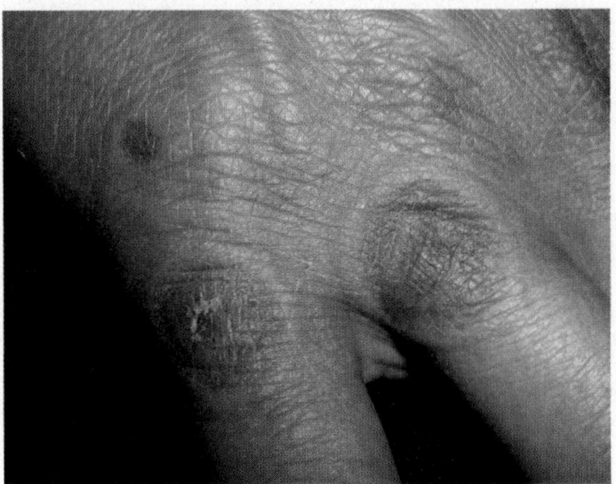

▲ **Figure 6–34.** Erythema multiforme with classic target lesions. Note the three zones of color change. (Reproduced with permission from Richard P. Usatine, MD, in Usatine RP, Smith MA, Mayeaux EJ Jr, Chumley H. *The Color Atlas of Family Medicine*, 2nd ed. McGraw-Hill, 2013.)

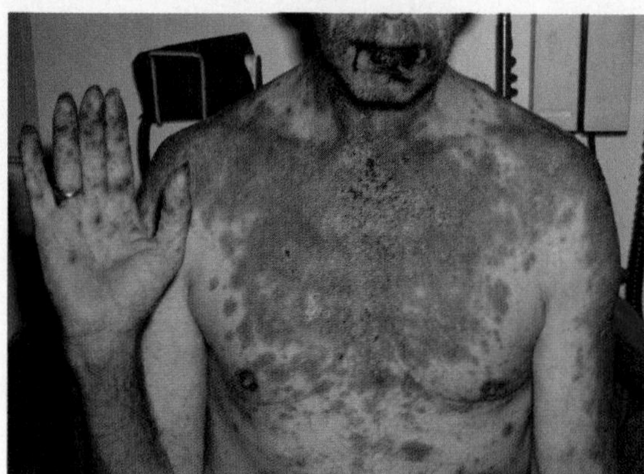

▲ **Figure 6–35.** Stevens-Johnson syndrome. (Used, with permission, from TG Berger, MD, Dept Dermatology, UCSF.)

B. Laboratory Findings

Skin biopsy is diagnostic. Direct immunofluorescence studies are negative. Blood tests are not useful for diagnosis.

Differential Diagnosis

Urticaria and drug eruptions are the chief entities that must be differentiated from erythema multiforme. In true urticaria, lesions are not purpuric or bullous, last less than 24 hours, and respond to antihistamines. Urticaria multiforme is a distinct eruption in infants and young children and presents with fever and targetoid urticarial plaques. The differential diagnosis of SJS/TEN includes autoimmune bullous diseases (eg, pemphigus vulgaris, bullous pemphigoid, and linear IgA bullous dermatosis), acute SLE, vasculitis, and Sweet syndrome. The presence of a blistering eruption requires biopsy and dermatologic consultation for appropriate diagnosis and treatment.

Complications

The tracheobronchial mucosa, conjunctiva, genital, and urethral mucosa may be involved and may result in scarring in severe cases. *Ophthalmologic consultation is required if ocular involvement is present because vision loss is the major consequence of SJS/TEN.*

Treatment

A. General Measures

Toxic epidermal necrolysis is best treated in an acute care environment, which may include an ICU or a burn unit. Patients should be admitted if mucosal involvement interferes with hydration and nutrition or extensive blistering develops. Open lesions should be managed like second-degree burns. Immediate discontinuation of the inciting medication (before blistering occurs) is a significant predictor of outcome. Delay in establishing the diagnosis and inadvertently continuing the offending medication results in higher morbidity and mortality.

B. Specific Measures

Oral and topical corticosteroids are useful in the oral variant of erythema multiforme. Oral acyclovir prophylaxis of herpes simplex infections may be effective in preventing recurrent herpes-associated erythema multiforme minor.

The most important aspect of treatment for SJS/TEN is to stop the offending medication and to move patients with greater than 25–30% BSA involvement to an appropriate acute care environment. Nutritional and fluid support and high vigilance for infection are the most important aspects of care. Reviews of systemic treatments for SJS and TEN have been conflicting. Some data support the use of high-dose corticosteroids. If corticosteroids are tried, they should be used early, before blistering occurs, and in high doses (prednisone, 1–2 mg/kg/day). Intravenous immunoglobulin (IVIG) (1 g/kg/day for 4 days) used early in the course has resulted in decreased mortality in some studies. Cyclosporine (3–5 mg/kg/day for 7 days) may also be effective. Etanercept is the treatment of choice in some centers.

C. Local Measures

Topical corticosteroids are not very effective in this disease (except the oral variant).

Prognosis

Erythema multiforme minor usually lasts 2–6 weeks and may recur. SJS/TEN may be serious with a mortality of 30% in cases with greater than 30% BSA involvement. The ABCD-10 and SCORTEN are severity of illness scales that predict mortality in SJS/TEN.

Grünwald P et al. Erythema multiforme, Stevens-Johnson syndrome/toxic epidermal necrolysis—diagnosis and treatment. J Dtsch Dermatol Ges. 2020;18:547. [PMID: 32469468]

Torres-Navarro I et al. Systemic therapies for Stevens-Johnson syndrome and toxic epidermal necrolysis: a SCORTEN-based systematic review and meta-analysis. J Eur Acad Dermatol Venereol. 2021;35:159. [PMID: 32946187]

Zhang S et al. Biologic TNF-alpha inhibitors in the treatment of Stevens-Johnson syndrome and toxic epidermal necrolysis: a systemic review. J Dermatolog Treat. 2020;31:66. [PMID: 30702955]

EXFOLIATIVE DERMATITIS (Exfoliative Erythroderma)

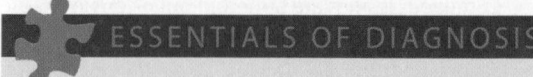

- Desquamation and erythema over most of the body.
- Itching, malaise, fever, chills, weight loss.

General Considerations

Erythroderma describes generalized redness and desquamation of more than 30% of the skin surface. A preexisting dermatosis is the cause of exfoliative dermatitis in two-thirds of cases, including psoriasis, atopic dermatitis, contact dermatitis, pityriasis rubra pilaris, and seborrheic dermatitis. Reactions to topical or systemic medications account for about 15% of cases, cancer (paraneoplastic symptom of lymphoma, solid tumors, and most commonly, cutaneous T-cell lymphoma) for 10%, and 10% are idiopathic. Widespread scabies is an important consideration since patients with erythrodermic presentation are highly contagious. At the time of acute presentation, without a clear-cut prior history of skin disease or medication exposure, it may be impossible to make a specific diagnosis of the underlying condition, and diagnosis may require continued observation.

Clinical Findings

A. Symptoms and Signs

Symptoms may include itching, weakness, malaise, fever, and weight loss. Chills are prominent. Erythema and desquamation are widespread. Loss of hair and nails can occur. Generalized lymphadenopathy may be due to lymphoma or leukemia or may be reactive. The mucosae are typically spared.

B. Laboratory Findings

A skin biopsy is required and may show changes of a specific inflammatory dermatitis or cutaneous T-cell lymphoma. Peripheral leukocytes may show clonal rearrangements of the T-cell receptor in Sézary syndrome.

Complications

Protein and electrolyte loss as well as dehydration may develop in patients with generalized inflammatory exfoliative erythroderma; sepsis may occur.

Treatment

A. Topical Therapy

Home treatment is with cool to tepid baths and application of mid-potency corticosteroids under wet dressings or with occlusion with plastic wrap. If the condition becomes unmanageable in an outpatient setting, the patient should be hospitalized.

B. Specific Measures

Stop all medications, if possible. Systemic corticosteroids may provide marked improvement in severe or fulminant exfoliative dermatitis but should be avoided long-term (see Chapter 26). For cases of psoriatic erythroderma and pityriasis rubra pilaris, acitretin, methotrexate, cyclosporine, or a TNF inhibitor may be indicated. Erythroderma secondary to lymphoma or leukemia requires specific topical or systemic chemotherapy. Suitable antibiotic medications with coverage for *Staphylococcus* should be given when there is evidence of bacterial infection.

Prognosis

Careful follow-up is necessary because identifying the cause of exfoliative erythroderma early in the course of the disease may be impossible. Most patients improve or recover completely but some require long-term therapy. Deaths are rare in the absence of cutaneous T-cell lymphoma. A minority of patients will suffer from undiminished erythroderma for indefinite periods.

Reynolds KA et al. A systematic review of treatment strategies for erythrodermic psoriasis. J Dermatolog Treat. 2021;32:49. [PMID: 31682547]

PHOTODERMATITIS

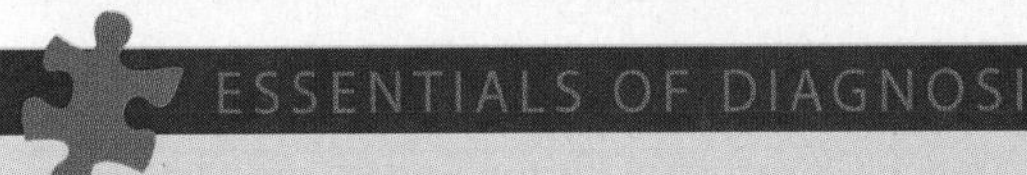

- Painful or pruritic erythema, edema, or vesiculation on sun-exposed surfaces (face, neck, hands, and "V" of the chest).
- Inner upper eyelids and area under the chin are spared.

General Considerations

Photodermatitis is a cutaneous reaction to UV radiation. It comprises four groups: (1) primary, idiopathic immunologically mediated photodermatoses; (2) drug- or chemical-induced photodermatoses; (3) dermatoses that are worsened or aggravated by UV exposure; and (4) genetic diseases with mutations predisposing to photodermatitis.

Primary photodermatoses include polymorphic light eruption, chronic actinic dermatitis, and actinic prurigo. Drug- or chemical-induced photodermatitis may be either exogenous or endogenous in origin. Porphyria cutanea tarda and pellagra are examples of endogenous phototoxic dermatoses. Exogenous drug- or chemical-induced photodermatitis manifests either as phototoxicity (a tendency for the individual to sunburn more easily than expected) or as photoallergy (a true immunologic reaction that presents with dermatitis). Drug-induced phototoxicity is triggered by UVA. Contact photosensitivity may occur with plants, perfumes, and sunscreens. The sunscreen oxybenzone (a benzophenone) is a common cause of photoallergic dermatitis. Dermatoses that are worsened or aggravated by UV exposure include SLE and dermatomyositis. Three percent of persons with atopic dermatitis, especially middle-aged women, are photosensitive.

Clinical Findings

A. Symptoms and Signs

The acute inflammatory phase of phototoxicity, if severe enough, is accompanied by pain, fever, GI symptoms, malaise, and even prostration. Signs include erythema, edema, and possibly vesiculation and oozing on exposed surfaces. Peeling of the epidermis and pigmentary changes often result. The key to diagnosis is localization of the rash to photoexposed areas, though eruptions may become generalized with time to involve photoprotected areas. The lower lip may be affected.

B. Laboratory Findings

Blood and urine tests are generally not helpful unless porphyria cutanea tarda is suggested by the presence of blistering, scarring, milia (white cysts 1–2 mm in diameter) and skin fragility of the dorsal hands, and facial hypertrichosis. Eosinophilia may be present in chronic photoallergic responses.

Differential Diagnosis

The differential diagnosis is long. If a clear history of the use of a topical or systemic photosensitizer is not available and if the eruption is persistent, then a workup including biopsy and light testing may be required. Photodermatitis must be differentiated from contact dermatitis that may develop from one of the many substances in sunscreens, as these may often have a similar distribution. Sensitivity to actinic rays may also be part of a more serious condition, such as porphyria cutanea tarda or lupus erythematosus. These disorders are diagnosed by appropriate blood or urine tests. The most common medications causing a phototoxic reaction are vemurafenib, NSAIDs, voriconazole, tetracyclines, quinolones, hydrochlorothiazide, amiodarone, and chlorpromazine. Other potent photosensitizers include TMP/SMZ, quinine or quinidine, griseofulvin, eculizumab, topical and systemic retinoids (tretinoin, isotretinoin, acitretin), and calcium channel blockers. Polymorphous light eruption (PMLE) is a common idiopathic photodermatitis and often has its onset in the third to fourth decades, except in Native Americans and Latinos, in whom it may present in childhood. PMLE is chronic in nature. Transitory periods of spontaneous remission do occur.

Complications

Some individuals continue to chronically react to light even when they no longer exposed to photosensitizing medications.

Prevention

While sunscreens are useful agents in general and should be used by persons with photosensitivity, patients may react to such low amounts of energy that sunscreens alone may not be sufficient. Sunscreens with an SPF of 30–60 and broad UVA coverage, containing dicamphor sulfonic acid (Mexoryl SX), avobenzone (Parasol 1789), titanium dioxide, and micronized zinc oxide, are especially useful in patients with photoallergic dermatitis. Photosensitivity due to porphyria is not prevented by sunscreens and requires barrier protection (clothing) to prevent outbreaks.

Treatment

A. Specific Measures

Medications should be suspected in cases of photosensitivity even if the particular medication (such as hydrochlorothiazide) has been used for months.

B. Local Measures

When the eruption is vesicular or weepy, treatment is similar to that of any acute dermatitis, using cooling and soothing wet dressings.

Sunscreens should be used as described above. Mid-potency to high-potency topical corticosteroids are of limited benefit in phototoxic reactions but may help in PMLE and photoallergic reactions. Since the face is often involved, close monitoring for corticosteroid side effects is recommended.

C. Systemic Measures

Aspirin may have some value for fever and pain of acute sunburn. Systemic corticosteroids in doses as described for acute contact dermatitis may be required for severe acute photosensitivity reactions. Otherwise, different photodermatoses are treated in specific ways.

Patients with chronic primary photodermatoses may require systemic treatment with hydroxycholoroquine (5 mg/kg once daily) or immunosuppressives, such as azathioprine (50–300 mg once daily) or cyclosporine (3–5 mg/kg once daily).

Prognosis

The most common phototoxic sunburn reactions are usually benign and self-limited. PMLE and some cases of photoallergy can persist for years.

Blakely KM et al. Drug-induced photosensitivity—an update: culprit drugs, prevention and management. Drug Saf. 2019;42:827. [PMID: 30888626]

Hinton AN et al. Feeling the burn: phototoxicity and photoallergy. Dermatol Clin. 2020;38:165. [PMID: 31753189]

Hofmann GA et al. Drug-induced photosensitivity: culprit drugs, potential mechanisms and clinical consequences. J Dtsch Dermatol Ges. 2021;19:19. [PMID: 33491908]

DRUG ERUPTION (Dermatitis Medicamentosa)

ESSENTIALS OF DIAGNOSIS

- Usually, abrupt onset of widespread, symmetric erythematous eruption.
- May mimic any inflammatory skin condition.
- Constitutional symptoms (malaise, arthralgia, headache, and fever) may be present.

General Considerations

Rashes are among the most common adverse reactions to medications and occur in 2–3% of hospitalized patients. There are multiple different types of cutaneous reactions to medications. Penicillins, cephalosporins, and NSAIDs are the most common cause of urticarial drug eruptions.

Antibiotics, anticonvulsants, allopurinol, and NSAIDs are common causes of maculopapular or morbilliform reactions. Drug-induced hypersensitivity reaction (DIHS) (also known as drug eruption with eosinophilia and systemic symptoms [DRESS]) is most often caused by anticonvulsants, allopurinol, and sulfonamides. SJS and TEN most commonly occur in response to antibiotics, sulfonamides, anticonvulsants, allopurinol, and NSAIDs. Phenolphthalein, pyrazolone derivatives, tetracyclines, NSAIDs, TMP-SMZ, and barbiturates are the major causes of fixed drug eruptions. Calcium channel blockers are a common cause of pruritus and eczemas in older adults.

Certain genetic polymorphisms of antigen-presenting major histocompatibility (MHC) loci increase the risk for the development of severe drug eruptions, including SJS/TEN and DIHS. Pharmacogenetic testing can help predict who is at risk for and therefore should avoid certain medication exposures.

Clinical Findings

A. Symptoms and Signs

Drug eruptions are generally classified as "simple" or "complex," referring to the risk of morbidity and mortality associated with the specific eruption. Simple morbilliform or maculopapular drug eruptions involve an exanthem, usually appear in the second week of medication therapy, and have no associated constitutional symptoms or abnormal laboratory findings. Complex drug eruptions include DIHS and SJS/TEN.

DIHS occurs later than the simple morbilliform drug eruptions with signs and symptoms developing 2–6 weeks after the medication has been started and has associated constitutional symptoms and abnormal laboratory findings. These may include fevers, chills, hematologic abnormalities (especially eosinophilia and atypical lymphocytosis), and abnormal liver or kidney function. Coexistent reactivation of certain viruses, especially HHV-6, but also Epstein-Barr virus, cytomegalovirus, HHV-7, and parvovirus B19, may be present and may be important in the pathogenesis of these complex drug eruptions. Table 6–3 summarizes the types of skin reactions, their appearance and distribution, and the common offenders in each case.

B. Laboratory Findings

Routinely ordered blood work is of no value in the diagnosis of simple drug eruptions, except upon initial evaluation to ensure that there is no systemic involvement. In complex drug eruptions, the CBC, liver biochemical tests, and kidney function tests should be monitored. Skin biopsies may be helpful in making the diagnosis. Serum PCR for HHV-6, HHV-7, Epstein-Barr virus, cytomegalovirus, and parvovirus B19 is performed in some centers.

Differential Diagnosis

Observation after discontinuation, which may be a slow process, helps establish the diagnosis. Rechallenge, though of theoretical value, may pose a danger to the patient and is best avoided.

Complications

Some cutaneous drug reactions may be associated with visceral involvement. The organ systems involved depend on the individual medication or drug class. Most common is an infectious mononucleosis-like illness and hepatitis associated with administration of anticonvulsants. Myocarditis may be a serious complication of drug-induced hypersensitivity syndrome and may present acutely or months after initial rash onset. Months after recovering from DIHS, patients may suffer hypothyroidism.

Treatment

A. General Measures

Systemic manifestations are treated as they arise (eg, anemia, icterus, purpura). Antihistamines may be of value in urticarial and angioneurotic reactions. Epinephrine 1:1000, 0.5–1 mL intravenously or subcutaneously, should be used as an emergency measure. In DIHS, corticosteroids are typically required; the most common regimen is oral prednisone, 1–1.5 mg/kg/day tapering slowly over a minimum of 6 weeks, since rapid taper leads to rebound and more recalcitrant disease. In the case of allopurinol-induced DIHS, starting a steroid-sparing agent (eg, mycophenolate mofetil) at the time of prednisone initiation is recommended because allopurinol-induced DIHS tends to rebound after corticosteroid discontinuation. Treatment in this special case often takes up to 12 months.

B. Local Measures

SJS/TEN with extensive blistering eruptions resulting in erosions and superficial ulcerations demands hospitalization and nursing care as for burn patients. See Erythema Multiforme/Stevens-Johnson Syndrome/Toxic Epidermal Necrolysis, above.

Prognosis

Drug rash usually disappears upon withdrawal of the medication and proper treatment. DIHS may be associated with autoimmune phenomena, including abnormal thyroid function. This can occur months after the hypersensitivity syndrome has resolved.

Cheraghlou S et al. Fixed drug eruptions, bullous drug eruptions, and lichenoid drug eruptions. Clin Dermatol. 2020;38:679. [PMID: 33341201]

Mockenhaupt M. Bullous drug reactions. Acta Derm Venereol. 2020;100:adv00057. [PMID: 32039459]

Noe MH et al. Diagnosis and management of Stevens-Johnson syndrome/toxic epidermal necrolysis. Clin Dermatol. 2020;38:607. [PMID: 33341195]

Owen CE et al. Recognition and management of severe cutaneous adverse drug reactions (including drug reaction with eosinophilia and systemic symptoms, Stevens-Johnson syndrome, and toxic epidermal necrolysis). Med Clin North Am. 2021;105:577. [PMID: 34059239]

Table 6–3. Skin reactions due to systemic medications.

Reaction	Appearance	Distribution and Comments	Common Offenders
Allergic vasculitis	The primary lesion is typically a 2–3 mm purpuric papule. Other morphologies include urticaria that lasts over 24 hours, vesicles, bullae, or necrotic ulcers.	Most severe on the legs.	Sulfonamides, phenytoin, propylthiouracil.
Drug exanthem	Morbilliform, maculopapular, exanthematous reactions.	The most common skin reaction to medications. Initially begins on trunk 7–10 days after the medication has been started. Spreads to extremities and begins to clear on the trunk over 3–5 days. In previously exposed patients, the rash may start in 2–3 days. Fever may be present.	Antibiotics (especially ampicillin and TMP-SMZ), sulfonamides and related compounds (including thiazide diuretics, furosemide, and sulfonylurea hypoglycemic agents), and barbiturates.
Drug-related subacute cutaneous lupus erythematosus (Drug-induced SLE rarely produces a skin reaction)	May present with a photosensitive rash, annular lesions, or psoriasis on upper trunk.	Less severe than SLE, sparing the kidneys and CNS. Recovery often follows medication withdrawal.	Diltiazem, etanercept, hydrochlorothiazide, infliximab, lisinopril, terbinafine.
Erythema nodosum	Inflammatory cutaneous nodules.	Usually limited to the extensor aspects of the legs. May be accompanied by fever, arthralgias, and pain.	Oral contraceptives.
Drug-induced hypersensitivity syndrome	Erythroderma	Entire skin surface. Typically associated with elevated liver biochemical tests, eosinophilia, and AKI. Eruption begins between 2 and 6 weeks after first dose of medication.	Allopurinol, sulfonamides, aromatic anticonvulsants, NSAID, dapsone, lamotrigine.
Fixed drug eruptions	Single or multiple demarcated, round, erythematous plaques that often become hyperpigmented.	Recur at the same site when the medication is repeated. Hyperpigmentation, if present, remains after healing.	Antimicrobials, analgesics (acetaminophen, ibuprofen, and naproxen), barbiturates, heavy metals, antiparasitic agents, antihistamines, phenolphthalein.
Lichenoid and lichen planus–like eruptions	Pruritic, erythematous to violaceous polygonal papules that coalesce or expand to form plaques.	May be in photo- or nonphotodistributed pattern.	Carbamazepine, furosemide, hydroxychloroquine, phenothiazines, beta-blockers, quinidine, quinine, sulfonylureas, tetracyclines, thiazides, and triprolidine.
Photosensitivity: increased sensitivity to light, often of UVA wavelengths, but may be due to UVB or visible light as well	Sunburn, vesicles, papules in photodistributed pattern.	Exposed skin of the face, the neck, and the backs of the hands and, in women, the lower legs. Exaggerated response to UV light.	Sulfonamides and sulfonamide-related compounds (thiazide diuretics, furosemide, sulfonylureas), tetracyclines, phenothiazines, sulindac, amiodarone, voriconazole, and NSAIDs.
Pigmentary changes	Flat hyperpigmented areas.	Forehead and cheeks (chloasma, melasma). The most common pigmentary disorder associated with drug ingestion. Improvement is slow despite stopping the medication.	Oral contraceptives are the usual cause. Diltiazem causes facial hyperpigmentation that may be difficult to distinguish from melasma.
	Blue-gray discoloration.	Light-exposed areas.	Chlorpromazine and related phenothiazines.

(*continued*)

Table 6–3. Skin reactions due to systemic medications. (continued)

Reaction	Appearance	Distribution and Comments	Common Offenders
	Brown or blue-gray pigmentation.	Generalized.	Heavy metals (silver, gold, bismuth, and arsenic).
	Blue-black patches on the shins.		Minocycline, chloroquine.
	Blue-black pigmentation of the nails and palate and depigmentation of the hair.		Chloroquine.
	Slate-gray color.	Primarily in photoexposed areas.	Amiodarone.
	Brown discoloration of the nails.	Especially in more darkly pigmented patients.	Hydroxyurea.
Pityriasis rosea–like eruptions	Oval, red, slightly raised patches with central scale.	Mainly on the trunk.	Barbiturates, bismuth, captopril, clonidine, methopromazine, metoprolol, metronidazole, and tripelennamine.
Psoriasiform eruptions	Scaly red plaques.	May be located on trunk and extremities. Palms and soles may be hyperkeratotic. May cause psoriasiform eruption or worsen psoriasis.	Antimalarials, lithium, beta-blockers, and TNF inhibitors.
SJS/TEN	Target-like lesions. Bullae may occur. Mucosal involvement.	Usually trunk and proximal extremities.	Sulfonamides, anticonvulsants, allopurinol, NSAIDs, lamotrigine.
Urticaria	Red, itchy wheals that vary in size from < 1 cm to many centimeters. May be accompanied by angioedema.	Chronic urticaria is rarely caused by medications.	Acute urticaria: penicillins, NSAIDs, sulfonamides, opioids, and salicylates. Angioedema is common in patients receiving ACE inhibitors and ARBs.

SJS/TEN, Stevens-Johnson syndrome/toxic epidermal necrolysis; TMP-SMZ, trimethoprim-sulfamethoxazole; TNF, tumor necrosis factor.

MISCELLANEOUS[1]

PRURITUS

Pruritus is the sensation that provokes a desire to scratch. Pruritus as a medical complaint is 40% as common as low back pain. Elderly Asian men are most significantly affected, with 20% of all health care visits in Asian men over the age of 65 involving the complaint of itch. The quality of life of a patient with chronic pruritus is the same as a patient undergoing hemodialysis. Better understanding of the role of pruritogens (interleukins-31, -4, -13 and thymic stromal lymphopoietin) in the pathophysiology of itch has enabled recent therapeutic advances.

Dry skin is the first cause of itch that should be sought since it is common and easily treated. The next step is to determine whether a primary skin lesion with associated pruritus is present. Examples of primary cutaneous pruritic diseases include scabies, atopic dermatitis, insect bites, pediculosis, contact dermatitis, drug reactions, urticaria, psoriasis, lichen planus, and fiberglass dermatitis, all of which have recognizable morphologies. The treatment of an underlying primary skin condition usually results in control of the associated pruritus.

Persistent pruritus not explained by cutaneous disease or association with a primary skin eruption should prompt a staged workup for systemic causes. Common causes of pruritus associated with systemic diseases include endocrine disorders (eg, hypo- or hyperthyroidism or hyperparathyroidism), psychiatric disturbances, lymphoma, leukemia, internal malignant disorders, iron deficiency anemia, HIV, hypercalcemia, cholestasis, and some neurologic disorders. Calcium channel blockers can cause pruritus with or without eczema, even years after they have been started, and it may take up to 1 year for pruritus to resolve after the calcium channel blocker has been stopped.

Treatment

The treatment of chronic pruritus can be frustrating. Most cases of pruritus are not mediated by histamine, hence the poor response of many patients to antihistamines. Emollients for dry skin are listed in Table 6–2. Emollient creams (preferred over lotions) should be generously applied from neck to toe immediately after towel drying and again one more time per day. Neuropathic pruritus responds to neurally acting agents, such as gabapentin (starting at 300 mg orally at around 4 PM and a second dose of 600 mg orally at bedtime) or pregabalin (150 mg orally daily).

[1]Hirsutism is discussed in Chapter 26.

Combinations of antihistamines, sinequan, gabapentin, pregabalin, mirtazapine, and opioid antagonists can be attempted in refractory cases. In cancer-associated and other forms of pruritus, aprepitant 80 mg orally daily for several days can be dramatically effective. Pruritus in conjunction with uremia and hemodialysis and to a lesser degree the pruritus of liver disease may be helped by phototherapy with UVB or PUVA. Gabapentin or mirtazapine may relieve the pruritus of CKD. Current trials are underway to study the inhibition of Il-31 (nemolizumab), Il-4 (dupilumab), IL-13 JAK (tofacitinib), opioid receptor, neurokinin, phosphodiesterase-4, and thymic stromal lymphopoietin in the treatment of chronic pruritus.

Prognosis

Elimination of external factors and irritating agents may give complete relief. Pruritus accompanying a specific skin disease will subside when the skin disease is controlled. Pruritus accompanying serious internal disease may not respond to any type of therapy.

Avila C et al. Cannabinoids for the treatment of chronic pruritus: a review. J Am Acad Dermatol. 2020;82:1205. [PMID: 31987788]
Kabashima K et al; Nemolizumab-JP01 Study Group. Trial of nemolizumab and topical agents for atopic dermatitis with pruritus. N Engl J Med. 2020;383:141. [PMID: 32640132]
Misery L et al. Chronic itch: emerging treatments following new research concepts. Br J Pharmacol. 2021;178:4775. [PMID: 34463358]
Sutaria N et al. Itch: pathogenesis and treatment. J Am Acad Dermatol. 2022;86:17. [PMID: 34648873]

Anogenital Pruritus

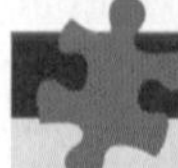

ESSENTIALS OF DIAGNOSIS

- Anogenital itching, chiefly nocturnal.
- Skin findings are highly variable, ranging from none to excoriations and inflammation of any degree, including lichenification.

General Considerations

Anogenital pruritus may be due to a primary inflammatory skin disease (intertrigo, psoriasis, lichen simplex chronicus, seborrheic dermatitis, lichen sclerosus), contact dermatitis (soaps, wipes, colognes, douches, and topical treatments), irritating secretions (diarrhea, leukorrhea, or trichomoniasis), infections (candidiasis, dermatophytosis, erythrasma), or oxyuriasis (pinworms). Erythrasma (Figure 6–36) is diagnosed by coral-red fluorescence with Wood light and cured with erythromycin. Squamous cell carcinoma of the anus and extramammary Paget disease are rare causes of genital pruritus.

In pruritus ani, hemorrhoids are often found, and leakage of mucus and bacteria from the distal rectum onto the perianal skin may be important in cases in which no other skin abnormality is found.

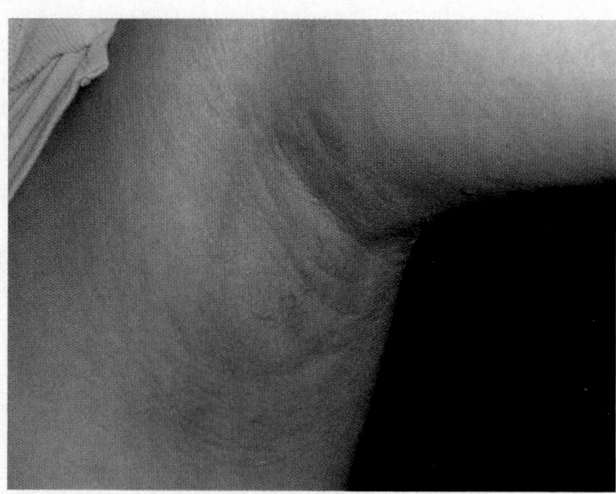

Figure 6–36. Erythrasma of the axilla. (Reproduced with permission from Richard P. Usatine, MD, in Usatine RP, Smith MA, Mayeaux EJ Jr, Chumley H. *The Color Atlas of Family Medicine*, 2nd ed. McGraw-Hill, 2013.)

Many women experience pruritus vulvae. Pruritus vulvae does not usually involve the anal area, though anal itching may spread to the vulva. In men, pruritus of the scrotum is most commonly seen in the absence of pruritus ani.

Up to one-third of unidentified causes of anogenital pruritus may be due to nerve impingements of the lumbosacral spine, so evaluation of lumbosacral spine disease is appropriate if no skin disorder is identified and topical therapy is ineffective.

Clinical Findings

A. Symptoms and Signs

The only symptom is itching. Physical findings are usually not present, but there may be erythema, fissuring, maceration, lichenification, excoriations, or changes suggestive of candidiasis or tinea.

B. Laboratory Findings

Microscopic examination or culture of tissue scrapings may reveal yeasts or fungi. Stool examination may show pinworms. Radiologic studies may demonstrate lumbar-sacral spinal disease.

Differential Diagnosis

The etiologic differential diagnosis consists of *Candida* infection, parasitosis, local irritation from contactants or irritants, nerve impingement, and other primary skin disorders of the genital area, such as psoriasis, seborrhea, intertrigo, or lichen sclerosus.

Prevention

Instruct the patient in proper anogenital hygiene after treating systemic or local conditions.

Treatment

Treating constipation, preferably with high-fiber management (psyllium), may help. Instruct the patient to use very soft or moistened tissue or cotton after bowel movements and to clean the perianal area thoroughly with cool water if possible. Women should use similar precautions after urinating. Patch testing reveals clinically relevant allergy in about 20% of patients, often to methylchloroisothiazolinone or methylisothiazolinone, preservatives commonly found in "baby wipes" and other personal care products.

Pramoxine cream or lotion or hydrocortisone-pramoxine (Pramosone), 1% or 2.5% cream, lotion, or ointment, is helpful for anogenital pruritus and should be applied after a bowel movement. Topical doxepin cream 5% is similarly effective but may be sedating. Topical calcineurin inhibitors (tacrolimus 0.03%) improve pruritus ani in patients with atopic dermatitis. Underclothing should be changed daily, and in men, the seam of their "boxers" should not rub against or contact the scrotum. Balneol Perianal Cleansing Lotion or Tucks premoistened pads, ointment, or cream may be very useful for pruritus ani. About one-third of patients with scrotal or anal pruritus will respond to capsaicin cream 0.006%. The use of high-potency topical corticosteroids should be avoided in the genital area.

Prognosis

Although benign, anogenital pruritus is often persistent and recurrent.

Cohee MW et al. Benign anorectal conditions: evaluation and management. Am Fam Physician. 2020;101:24. [PMID: 31894930]

Raef HS et al. Vulvar pruritus: a review of clinical associations, pathophysiology and therapeutic management. Front Med (Lausanne). 2021;8:649402. [PMID: 33898486]

ULCERS

Leg Ulcers Secondary to Venous Insufficiency

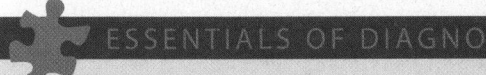

ESSENTIALS OF DIAGNOSIS

- History of varicosities, thrombophlebitis, or postphlebitic syndrome.
- Irregular ulceration, often on the medial lower legs above the malleolus.
- Edema of the legs, varicosities, hyperpigmentation, red and scaly areas (stasis dermatitis), and scars from old ulcers support the diagnosis.

General Considerations

Patients at risk may have a history of venous insufficiency, family history, varicosities, obesity, or genetic diseases that predispose to venous insufficiency (see Chronic Venous Insufficiency, Chapter 12). The left leg is usually more severely affected than the right.

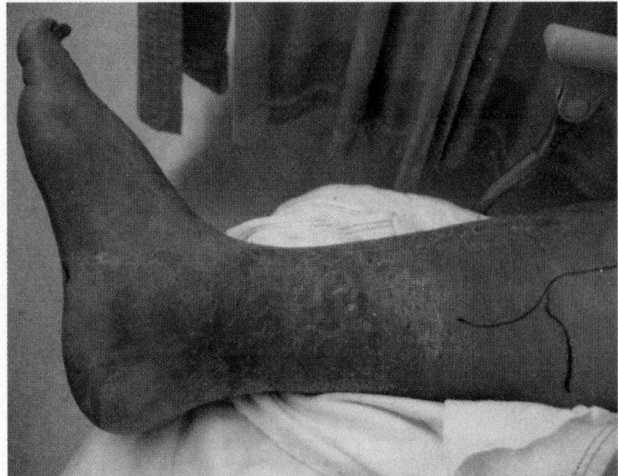

Figure 6–37. Venous stasis ulcer. (Used, with permission, from Lindy Fox, MD.)

Clinical Findings

A. Symptoms and Signs

Classically, chronic edema is followed by a dermatitis, which is often pruritic. These changes are followed by hyperpigmentation, skin breakdown, and eventually sclerosis of the skin of the lower leg (Figure 6–37). Red, pruritic patches of stasis dermatitis often precede ulceration (Figure 12–2). The ulcer base may be clean, but it often has a yellow fibrin eschar that may require surgical removal (Figure 6–38). Ulcers that appear on the feet, toes, or above the knees should be approached with other diagnoses in mind.

B. Laboratory Findings

Because venous insufficiency plays a role in 75–90% of lower leg ulcerations, testing of venous competence is a required part of a leg ulcer evaluation even without

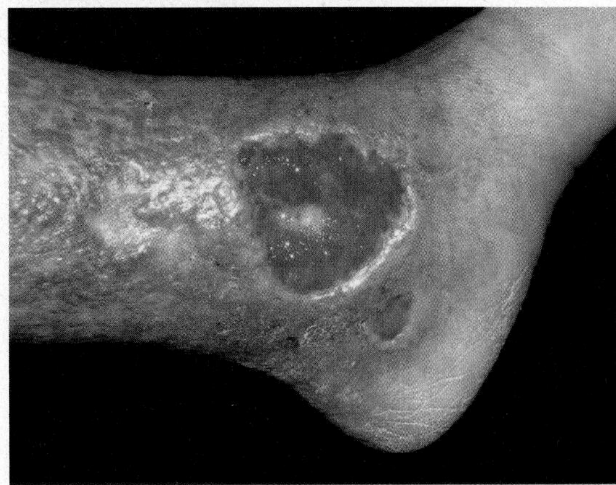

Figure 6–38. Ulcer—venous stasis ulcer. (Reproduced with permission from Richard P. Usatine, MD, in Usatine RP, Smith MA, Mayeaux EJ Jr, Chumley H. *The Color Atlas of Family Medicine*, 3rd ed. McGraw-Hill, 2019.)

changes of venous insufficiency (see Chapter 12). Doppler examination is usually sufficient (except in the diabetic patient) to evaluate venous competence. Arterial insufficiency may coexist with venous disease. An ankle/brachial index (ABI) less than 0.7 indicates the presence of significant arterial disease and requires vascular surgery consultation.

Differential Diagnosis

The differential includes vasculitis, pyoderma gangrenosum, arterial ulcerations, infection, trauma, skin cancer, arachnid bites, and sickle cell anemia. When the diagnosis is in doubt, a punch biopsy from the border (not base) of the lesion may be helpful.

Prevention

Compression stockings to reduce edema are the most important means of prevention. Compression should achieve a pressure of 30 mm Hg below the knee and 40 mm Hg at the ankle. The stockings should not be used in patients with arterial insufficiency with an ABI less than 0.7. Pneumatic sequential compression devices may be of great benefit when edema is refractory to standard compression dressings.

Treatment

A. Local Measures

Clean the base of the ulcer with saline or cleansers, such as Saf-Clens®. A curette or small scissors can be used to remove the yellow fibrin eschar; local anesthesia may be used if the areas are very tender.

Overall, there is little evidence to support topical antibiotics for the treatment of venous insufficiency ulcerations. Metronidazole gel is used to reduce bacterial growth and odor. Silver impregnated dressings may aid in healing. Red dermatitic skin is treated with a medium- to high-potency corticosteroid ointment such as triamcinolone acetonide 0.1% ointment. The ulcer is then covered with an occlusive hydroactive dressing (DuoDerm® or Cutinova®) or a polyurethane foam (Allevyn) followed by an Unna zinc paste boot. This is changed weekly. The ulcer should begin to heal within weeks, and healing should be complete within 4–6 months. If the patient has no history of skin cancer in the area, becaplermin (Regranex) may be applied to ulcers that are not becoming smaller or developing a granulating base. Some ulcerations require skin grafting.

No topical intervention has evidence to suggest that it will improve healing of arterial leg ulcers.

B. Systemic Therapy

Pentoxifylline, 400 mg orally three times daily administered with compression dressings, is beneficial in accelerating healing of venous insufficiency leg ulcers. Zinc supplementation is occasionally beneficial in patients with low serum zinc levels.

In the absence of cellulitis, there is no role for systemic antibiotics in the treatment of venous insufficiency ulcers. The diagnosis of cellulitis in the setting of a venous insufficiency ulcer can be very difficult. Surface cultures are of limited value. Cellulitis should be considered in the following settings: (1) expanding warmth and erythema surrounding the ulceration, with or without (2) increasing pain of the ulceration. The patient may also report increased exudate from the ulceration, but this without the other cardinal findings of cellulitis does not confirm the diagnosis of cellulitis. If cellulitis accompanies the ulcer, oral antibiotics are recommended: dicloxacillin, 250 mg four times a day, or levofloxacin, 500 mg once daily for 1–2 weeks, is usually adequate. Routine use of antibiotics and treating bacteria isolated from a chronic ulcer without clinical evidence of infection is discouraged. If the ulcer fails to heal or there is a persistent draining tract in the ulcer, underlying osteomyelitis should be sought.

Prognosis

The combination of limited debridement, compression dressings or stockings, and moist dressings will heal the majority of venous stasis ulcers within an average of 18 months. These modalities need to be applied at least 80% of the time to optimize ulcer healing. Topical growth factors, antibiotics, debriding agents, and xenografts and autografts can be considered in recalcitrant cases but are not required in most patients. Exercise in combination with compression therapy has an adjuvant role in promoting the healing of venous ulcerations. The failure of venous insufficiency ulcerations to heal is most often related to inconsistent use of basic treatment methods. Ongoing control of edema is essential to prevent recurrent ulceration. The use of compression stockings following ulcer healing is critical to prevent recurrence, with recurrence rates 2–20 times higher if patients do not comply with compression stocking use. Patients with an ABI below 0.5 or refractory ulcerations (or both) should be considered for surgical procedure (artery-opening procedures or ablation of the incompetent superficial vein). Early endovenous ablation has been shown to improve healing in patients with venous insufficiency ulcers.

Bowers S et al. Chronic wounds: evaluation and management. Am Fam Physician. 2020;101:159. [PMID: 32003952]

Schneider C et al. Lower extremity ulcers. Med Clin North Am. 2021;105:663. [PMID: 34059244]

PIGMENTARY DISORDERS

Although the color of skin may be altered by many diseases and agents, the vast majority of patients have either an increase or decrease in pigment secondary to an inflammatory disease, such as acne or atopic dermatitis.

Other pigmentary disorders include those resulting from exposure to exogenous pigments, such as carotenemia, argyria, and tattooing. Other endogenous pigmentary disorders are attributable to metabolic substances (eg, hemosiderin [iron]) in purpuric processes, to homogentisic acid in ochronosis, and bile pigments.

Classification

Disorders of hyper- or hypopigmentation may be considered to be primary or secondary to other disorders. Depigmentation, the absence of all pigment, should be differentiated from hypopigmentation, in which the affected skin is lighter than baseline skin color, but not completely devoid of pigment.

The evaluation of pigmentary disorders is helped by Wood light, which accentuates epidermal pigmentation in hyperpigmented disorders and highlights complete loss of pigment in depigmentating disorders. Depigmentation, as seen in vitiligo, enhances with Wood light examination, whereas postinflammatory hypopigmentation does not.

A. Primary Pigmentary Disorders

1. Hyperpigmentation—The disorders in this category are nevoid, congenital, or acquired. Nevoid and congenital disorders include pigmented nevi, mosaic hyperpigmentation, ephelides (juvenile freckles), and lentigines (senile freckles). Hyperpigmentation due to systemic diseases may be seen in in association with Addison disease, vitamin B_{12} deficiency, hemochromatosis, and Wilson disease. Melasma (chloasma) occurs as patterned hyperpigmentation of the face, most commonly as a direct effect of estrogens. It may occur during pregnancy, exposure to oral contraceptives, or be idiopathic. Although more common in women, melasma affects both sexes and all races.

2. Hypopigmentation and depigmentation—Depigmenting disorders in this category are vitiligo, albinism, and piebaldism. In vitiligo, pigment cells (melanocytes) are destroyed (Figure 6–39). Vitiligo, present in approximately 1% of the population, may be associated with other autoimmune disorders, such as autoimmune thyroid disease, pernicious anemia, diabetes mellitus, and Addison disease.

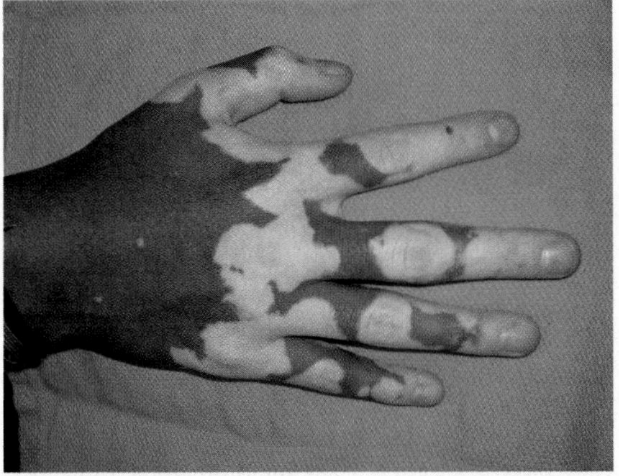

Figure 6–39. Depigmented—vitiligo. (Reproduced with permission from Richard P. Usatine, MD, in Usatine RP, Smith MA, Mayeaux EJ Jr, Chumley H. *The Color Atlas of Family Medicine*, 3rd ed. McGraw-Hill, 2019.)

B. Secondary Pigmentary Disorders

Any damage to the skin (irritation, allergy, infection, excoriation, burns, or dermatologic therapy, such as chemical peels and freezing with liquid nitrogen) may result in hyper- or hypopigmentation. Several disorders of clinical importance are described below.

1. Hyperpigmentation—The most common type of secondary hyperpigmentation occurs after another inflammatory dermatologic condition, such as acne, lichen planus, or eczema, and is most commonly seen in moderately complexioned persons (Asian, Latinx, and light-skinned Black individuals). It is called post-inflammatory hyperpigmentation. Hemosiderin deposition, as in stasis dermatitis, may lead to hyperpigmentation that is red-brown in color.

Pigmentation may be produced by certain medications, eg, chloroquine, chlorpromazine, minocycline (Figure 6–40), and amiodarone. Fixed drug eruptions to phenolphthalein (in laxatives), TMP-SMZ, NSAIDs, and tetracyclines also lead to hyperpigmentation, typically in annular patches.

2. Hypopigmentation—Hypopigmentation may complicate atopic dermatitis, lichen planus, psoriasis, discoid lupus, and lichen simplex chronicus. It may also be posttraumatic or iatrogenic (eg, due to the use of superpotent topical corticosteroids) or both. *Clinicians must exercise special care in using liquid nitrogen on any patients with*

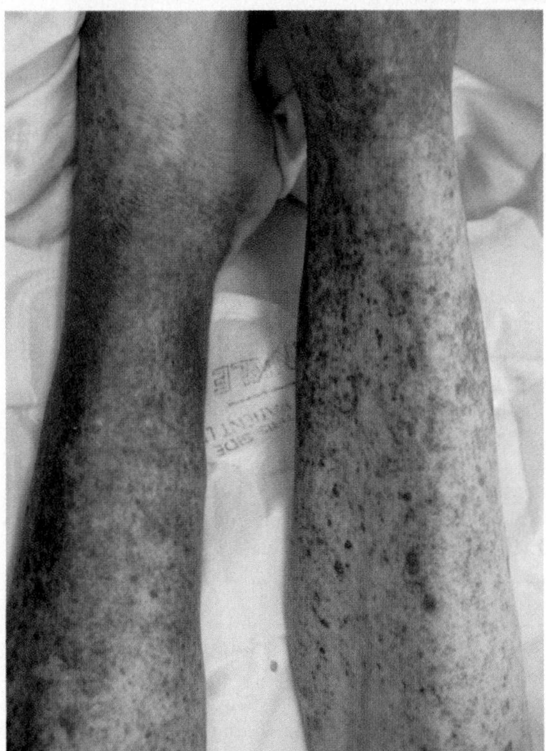

Figure 6–40. Minocycline hyperpigmentation. (Used, with permission, from Lindy Fox, MD.)

darker skin tones since doing so may result in hypopigmentation or depigmentation, at times permanent. Intralesional or intra-articular injections of high concentrations of corticosteroids may also cause localized temporary hypopigmentation. Vitiligo is a known complication of immune checkpoint inhibitor therapy for melanoma.

Complications

Actinic keratoses and skin cancers are more likely to develop in persons with vitiligo. Severe emotional trauma may occur in extensive vitiligo and other types of hypo- and hyperpigmentation, particularly in naturally dark-skinned persons.

Treatment & Prognosis

A. Hyperpigmentation

Therapeutic bleaching preparations generally contain hydroquinone. Hydroquinone has occasionally caused unexpected hypo- or hyperpigmentation, or even secondary ochronosis and pigmented milia, particularly with prolonged use.

The role of exposure to UV light cannot be overstressed as a factor promoting or contributing to most disorders of hyperpigmentation, and such exposure should be minimized. Melasma, ephelides, and postinflammatory hyperpigmentation may be treated with varying success with 4% hydroquinone and a sunscreen containing UVA photoprotectants (Avobenzone, Mexoryl, zinc oxide, titanium dioxide). Tretinoin cream, 0.025–0.05%, may be added. Adjuvant topical options for melasma include kojic acid, ascorbic acid, cysteamine, niacinamide, and azelaic acid. Superficial melasma responds well to topical therapy, but if there is predominantly dermal deposition of pigment (does not enhance with Wood light), the prognosis is poor. Response to therapy may take months and requires avoidance of sunlight. Hyperpigmentation often recurs after treatment if the skin is exposed to UV light. Tranexamic acid, 250 mg twice a day for 8–12 weeks, is an oral treatment for melasma. It should not be used in patients with hypercoagulability. Acne with postinflammatory hyperpigmentation responds well to azelaic acid and tretinoin, since both address acne and hyperpigmentation. Solar lentigines respond to liquid nitrogen application. Tretinoin 0.1% cream or tazarotene 0.1% used over 10 months can fade solar lentigines, facial hyperpigmentation, and postinflammatory hyperpigmentation. Lasers are available for the removal of epidermal and dermal pigment and should be considered for patients whose responses to medical treatment are inadequate.

B. Hypopigmentation

In secondary hypopigmentation, repigmentation may occur spontaneously. Cosmetics such as Covermark and Dermablend are highly effective for concealing disfiguring patches. Therapy of vitiligo is long and tedious, and the patient must be strongly motivated. If less than 20% of the skin is involved (most cases), topical tacrolimus 0.1% twice daily is the first-line therapy. A superpotent corticosteroid may also be used, but local skin atrophy from prolonged use may ensue. With 20–25% involvement, narrowband UVB or oral PUVA is the best option. Severe phototoxic response (sunburn) may occur with PUVA. The face and upper chest respond best, and the fingertips and the genital areas do not respond as well to treatment. Years of treatment may be required. Topical or systemic JAK inhibitors (tofactinib, ruxolitinib) may be effective in some patients with recalcitrant vitiligo.

Chang HC et al. The effectiveness of topical calcineurin inhibitors compared with topical corticosteroids in the treatment of vitiligo: a systematic review and meta-analysis. J Am Acad Dermatol. 2020;82:243. [PMID: 31408687]

Kubelis-López DE et al. Updates and new medical treatments for vitiligo (Review). Exp Ther Med. 2021;22:797. [PMID: 34093753]

McKesey J et al. Melasma treatment: an evidence-based review. Am J Clin Dermatol. 2020;21:173. [PMID: 31802394]

Wang Y et al. Clinical features, immunopathogenesis, and therapeutic strategies in vitiligo. Clin Rev Allergy Immunol. 2021; 61:299. [PMID: 34283349]

Zubair R et al. What's new in pigmentary disorders. Dermatol Clin. 2019;37:175. [PMID: 30850040]

ALOPECIA

Classification

Alopecias are divided into scarring and nonscarring forms. When evaluating a patient who complains of hair loss, it is most important to determine if follicular markings (the opening where hair exits the skin) are present or absent. Present follicular markings suggest a nonscarring alopecia; absent follicular markings suggest a scarring alopecia.

Nonscarring Alopecia

Nonscarring alopecia may occur in association with various systemic diseases, such as SLE, secondary syphilis, hyper- or hypothyroidism, iron deficiency anemia, vitamin D deficiency, and pituitary insufficiency. Prompt and adequate control of the underlying disorder usually leads to hair regrowth. Specific types of nonscarring alopecia are described below.

Androgenetic alopecia, the most common form of alopecia, is of genetic predetermination. In men, the earliest changes occur at the anterior portions of the calvarium on either side of the "widow's peak" and on the crown (vertex). The extent of hair loss is variable and unpredictable. Minoxidil 5% is available over the counter and can be recommended for persons with recent onset (less than 5 years) and smaller areas of alopecia. Approximately 40% of patients treated twice daily for a year will have moderate to dense growth. Finasteride (Propecia), 1 mg orally daily, has similar efficacy and may be additive to minoxidil.

Androgenetic alopecia also occurs in women. Classically, there is retention of the anterior hairline while there is diffuse thinning of the vertex scalp hair and a widening of the part. Treatment includes topical minoxidil (5% once daily) and, in women not of childbearing potential, finasteride at doses up to 2.5 mg/day orally. Spironolactone

50–200 mg daily may be used in premenopausal women. Low-dose oral minoxidil (0.25–1 mg daily in women and 2.5–5 mg daily in men) is also safe and effective. A workup consisting of determination of serum testosterone, DHEAS, iron, total iron-binding capacity, thyroid function tests, vitamin D level, and a CBC will identify most other causes of hair thinning in premenopausal women. Women who complain of thin hair but show little evidence of alopecia need follow-up, because more than 50% of the scalp hair can be lost before the clinician can perceive it.

Telogen effluvium is a transitory increase in the number of hairs in the telogen (resting) phase of the hair growth cycle. This may occur spontaneously; appear at the termination of pregnancy; be precipitated by severe illness, "crash dieting," high fever, stress from surgery, shock, malnutrition, or iron deficiency; or be provoked by hormonal contraceptives. Whatever the cause, telogen effluvium usually has a latent period of 4 months. The prognosis is generally good. The condition is diagnosed by the presence of large numbers of hairs with white bulbs coming out upon gentle tugging of the hair. Counts of hairs lost by the patient on combing or shampooing often exceed 150 per day, compared to an average of 70–100. If iron deficiency is suspected, a serum ferritin should be obtained, and any value less than 40 ng/mL followed with supplementation.

Alopecia areata is of unknown cause but is believed to be an immunologic process. Typically, there are patches that are perfectly smooth and without scarring. Tiny hairs 2–3 mm in length, called "exclamation hairs," may be seen. Telogen hairs are easily dislodged from the periphery of active lesions. The beard, brows, and lashes may be involved. Involvement may extend to all of the scalp hair (**alopecia totalis**) or to all scalp and body hair (**alopecia universalis**). Severe forms may be treated by systemic corticosteroid therapy, although recurrences follow discontinuation of therapy. Alopecia areata is occasionally associated with autoimmune disorders, including Hashimoto thyroiditis, pernicious anemia, Addison disease, and vitiligo. Additional comorbidities may include SLE, atopy, and mental health disease.

Intralesional corticosteroids are frequently effective for alopecia areata. Triamcinolone acetonide in a concentration of 2.5–10 mg/mL is injected in aliquots of 0.1 mL at approximately 1- to 2-cm intervals, not exceeding a total dose of 30 mg per month for adults. Alopecia areata is usually self-limiting, with complete regrowth of hair in 80% of patients with focal disease. Some mild cases are resistant to treatment, as are the extensive totalis and universalis types. Support groups for patients with extensive alopecia areata are beneficial. Oral JAK inhibitors (ruxolitinib, tofacitinib) are therapeutic options for patients with highly morbid disease, although relapse is the rule once the medication has been stopped. Efficacy of topical JAK inhibitors for alopecia areata is under investigation.

In **trichotillomania** (the pulling out of one's own hair), the patches of hair loss are irregular, with short, growing hairs almost always present, since they cannot be pulled out until they are long enough. The patches are often unilateral, occurring on the same side as the patient's dominant hand. The patient may be unaware of the habit. *N*-acetylcysteine (1200–2400 mg orally per day for 12 weeks) may be effective.

Scarring (Cicatricial) Alopecia

Cicatricial alopecia may occur following any type of trauma or inflammation that may scar hair follicles. Examples include chemical or physical trauma, bacterial or fungal infections, severe herpes zoster, chronic discoid lupus erythematosus (DLE), systemic sclerosis (scleroderma), and excessive ionizing radiation. The specific cause is often suggested by the history, the distribution of hair loss, and the appearance of the skin, as in DLE. Specific dermatologic diseases of the scalp that result in scarring alopecia include lichen planopilaris, frontal fibrosing alopecia, dissecting cellulitis of the scalp, and folliculitis decalvans. Biopsy is useful in the diagnosis of scarring alopecia, but specimens must be taken from the active border and not from the scarred central zone. Scarring alopecias are irreversible and permanent. It is important to diagnose and treat the scarring process as early in its course as possible.

Gao JL et al. Androgenetic alopecia in transgender and gender diverse populations: a review of therapeutics. J Am Acad Dermatol. 2021 Oct 28:S0190. [Epub ahead of print] [PMID: 34756934]

Hesseler MJ et al. Platelet-rich plasma and its utilities in alopecia: a systematic review. Dermatol Surg. 2020;46:93. [PMID: 31211715]

Jamerson TA et al. An approach to patients with alopecia. Med Clin North Am. 2021;105:599. [PMID: 34059240]

Meah N et al. The Alopecia Areata Consensus of Experts (ACE) study: results of an international expert opinion on treatments for alopecia areata. J Am Acad Dermatol. 2020;83:123. [PMID: 32165196]

Nestor MS et al. Treatment options for androgenetic alopecia: efficacy, side effects, compliance, financial considerations, and ethics. J Cosmet Dermatol. 2021;20:3759. [PMID: 34741573]

Randolph M et al. Oral minoxidil treatment for hair loss: a review of efficacy and safety. J Am Acad Dermatol. 2021;84:737. [PMID: 32622136]

NAIL DISORDERS

1. Morphologic Nail Abnormalities

Classification

Acquired nail disorders may be classified as local or associated with systemic or generalized skin diseases.

A. Local Nail Disorders

1. Onycholysis (distal separation of the nail plate from the nail bed, usually of the fingers) is caused by excessive exposure to water, soaps, detergents, alkalies, and industrial cleaning agents. Candidal infection of the nail folds and subungual area, nail hardeners, drug-induced photosensitivity, hyper- or hypothyroidism, and psoriasis may cause onycholysis.
2. Distortion of the nail, including nail splitting, occurs as a result of chronic inflammation or infiltration of the nail matrix underlying the eponychial fold.

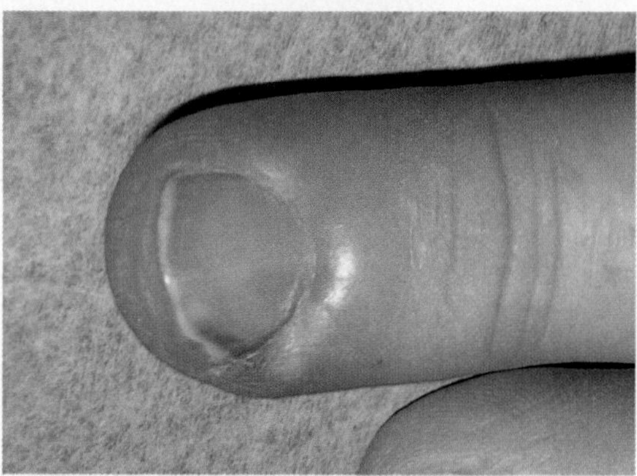

▲ **Figure 6–41.** Acute paronychia. (Used, with permission, from E.J. Mayeaux Jr, MD, in Usatine RP, Smith MA, Mayeaux EJ Jr, Chumley HS. *The Color Atlas and Synopsis of Family Medicine*, 3rd ed. McGraw-Hill, 2019.)

Such changes may be caused by impingement on the nail matrix by inflammatory diseases (eg, psoriasis, lichen planus, eczema), warts, tumors, or cysts.

3. Discoloration and crumbly thickened nails are noted in dermatophyte infection and psoriasis.
4. Allergic reactions (to resins in undercoats and polishes or to nail glues) are characterized by onycholysis or by grossly distorted, hypertrophic, and misshapen nails.
5. Paronychia is inflammation of the lateral or proximal nail folds. Acute paronychia presents as a painful erythematous papulonodule or frank abscess of the nail fold and is most commonly due to infection with *S aureus* (Figure 6–41). Chronic paronychia is most often caused by irritation from water or chemicals with resultant inflammation and possible *Candida* superinfection.

B. Nail Changes Associated with Systemic or Generalized Skin Diseases

1. Beau lines (transverse furrows) affect all nails and classically develop after a serious systemic illness.
2. Atrophy of the nails may be related to trauma or to vascular or neurologic disease.
3. Clubbed fingers may be due to the prolonged hypoxemia associated with cardiopulmonary disorders (Figure 6–42) (see Chapter 9).
4. Spoon nails may be seen in anemic patients.
5. Stippling or pitting of the nails is seen in psoriasis, alopecia areata, and hand eczema (Figure 6–23).
6. Nail hyperpigmentation may be caused by many chemotherapeutic agents, but especially the taxanes.

Differential Diagnosis

Onychomycosis may cause nail changes identical to those seen in psoriasis. Careful examination for more characteristic lesions elsewhere on the body is essential to the diagnosis of the nail disorders. Cancer should be suspected (eg, Bowen disease or squamous cell carcinoma) as the cause of any persistent solitary subungual or periungual lesion.

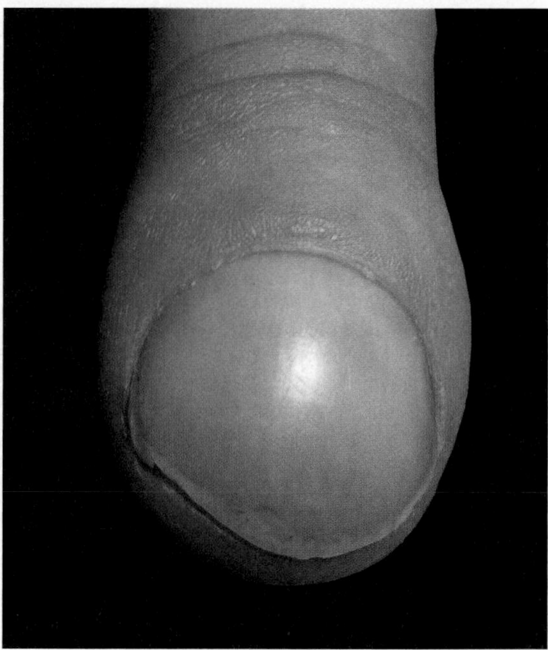

▲ **Figure 6–42. Clubbing of the finger in a 31-year-old man with congenital heart disease. Note the thickening around the proximal nail folds.** (Reproduced with permission from Richard P. Usatine, MD, in Usatine RP, Smith MA, Mayeaux EJ Jr, Chumley H. The Color Atlas of Family Medicine, 3rd ed. McGraw-Hill, 2019.)

Complications

Toenail changes may lead to an ingrown nail—in turn often complicated by bacterial infection and occasionally by exuberant granulation tissue. Poor manicuring and poorly fitting shoes may contribute to this complication. Cellulitis may result.

Treatment & Prognosis

Treatment consists usually of careful debridement and manicuring and, above all, reduction of exposure to irritants (soaps, detergents, alkali, bleaches, solvents, etc). Longitudinal grooving due to temporary lesions of the matrix, such as warts, synovial cysts, and other impingements, may be cured by removal of the offending lesion.

Acute paronychia is treated with topical antibiotics and drainage of the abscess, if present. To incise and drain an acute staphylococcal paronychia, insert a flat metal spatula or sharpened hardwood stick into the nail fold where it adjoins the nail. This will release pus from a mature lesion.

Treatment of chronic paronychia includes minimizing wetwork and toxic contactants, wearing gloves while performing tasks that expose the skin to water, minimizing trauma to the nail folds, and a combination of topical corticosteroids and an anticandidal twice daily to the affected area.

2. Tinea Unguium (Onychomycosis)

Tinea unguium is a trichophyton infection of one or more (but rarely all) fingernails or toenails. The species most commonly found is *T rubrum*. "Saprophytic" fungi may rarely cause onychomycosis (less than 5% of cases). Evidence supporting a genetic defect in the innate and adaptive immune system may explain why some people suffer from chronic tinea pedis and onychomycosis.

The nails are lusterless, brittle, and hypertrophic, and the substance of the nail is friable. Laboratory diagnosis is mandatory since only 50% of dystrophic nails are due to dermatophytosis. Portions of the nail should be clipped, digested with 10% KOH, and examined under the microscope for hyphae. Fungi may also be cultured from debris collected from underneath the nail plate. Periodic acid-Schiff stain of a histologic section of the nail plate also demonstrates the fungus readily. Each technique is positive in only 50% of cases so several different tests may need to be performed. Periodic acid-Schiff staining of nail plate coupled with fungal culture has a sensitivity of 96%.

Onychomycosis is difficult to treat because of the long duration of therapy required and the frequency of recurrences. Fingernails respond more readily than toenails. For toenails, treatment is indicated for patients with discomfort, inability to exercise, diabetes, and immune compromise.

In general, systemic therapy is required to effectively treat nail onychomycosis. Although historically topical therapy has had limited value, evidence suggests that efinaconazole 10% performs better than other topical treatment options. Tavaborole 5% solution is also approved for the treatment of onychomycosis, but its clearance rates do not appear to be as good as those of efinaconazole. Adjunctive value of surgical procedures is unproven, and the efficacy of laser treatments is lacking, especially with regard to long-term cures.

Fingernails can virtually always be cured, and toenails are cured 35–50% of the time and are clinically improved about 75% of the time. In all cases, before treatment, the diagnosis should be confirmed. The costs of the various treatment options should be known and the most cost-effective treatment chosen. Medication interactions must be avoided. Ketoconazole, due to its higher risk for hepatotoxicity, is not recommended to treat any form of onychomycosis. For fingernails, ultramicronized griseofulvin 250 mg orally three times daily for 6 months can be effective. Alternative treatments are (in order of preference) oral terbinafine, 250 mg daily for 6 weeks; oral itraconazole, 200–400 mg daily for 7 days each month for 2 months; and oral itraconazole, 200 mg daily for 2 months. Off-label use of fluconazole, 150–400 mg once weekly for 6–9 months, can also be effective, but there is limited evidence for this option. Once clear, fingernails usually remain free of disease for some years.

Onychomycosis of the toenails does not respond to griseofulvin therapy. The best treatment, which is also FDA approved, is oral terbinafine 250 mg daily for 12 weeks. Pulse terbinafine therapy with two cycles of 4 weeks on and 4 weeks off may be as efficacious as continuous oral therapy. Liver biochemical tests, CBC, and kidney function should be performed before oral therapy. Because the risk of idiosyncratic injury is very low (transaminitis occurs in less than 0.5% of patients) and the presentation of drug-induced liver injury is usually symptomatic (jaundice, malaise, abdominal pain), routine hepatic monitoring in healthy adults without known hepatic disease is not required. The dose might need adjustment in patients with reduced creatinine clearance. Itraconazole, 200 mg daily for 12 weeks, or pulse oral itraconazole, 200 mg twice daily for 1 week per month for 3 months, is inferior to standard terbinafine treatments, but it is an acceptable alternative for those unable to take terbinafine. The courses of terbinafine or itraconazole may need to be repeated 6 months after the first treatment cycle if fungal cultures of the nail are still positive. Fluconazole may be used off label at 150 mg weekly until the nail has grown out completely (12–18 month for toenails).

Treatment failures are multifactorial but may occur because of mixed infection with non-dermatophyte molds or reinfection. Culture of the nail to determine the organism responsible for infection is critical to choosing the correct therapy. In addition, part of the complete therapeutic regimen for onychomycosis should include replacing or sanitizing potential fungal reservoirs such as socks, shoes, and other textiles. Infected household members should also be treated. Shoes or sandals should be worn in high-risk areas (public showers or pools). Continued prophylactic therapy with topicals such as efinaconazole twice a week to nails and a topical antifungal cream to the feet should be continued for several years or longer after clearance of onychomycosis.

Bloom A et al. A review of nail dystrophies for the practitioner. Adv Skin Wound Care. 2020;33:20. [PMID: 31856029]

Frazier WT et al. Onychomycosis: rapid evidence review. Am Fam Physician. 2021;104:359. [PMID: 34652111]

Gupta AK et al. A paradigm shift in the treatment and management of onychomycosis. Skin Appendage Disord. 2021;7:351. [PMID: 34604322]

Gupta AK et al. A practical guide to curing onychomycosis: how to maximize cure at the patient, organism, treatment, and environmental level. Am J Clin Dermatol. 2019;20:123. [PMID: 30456537]

Gupta AK et al. Onychomycosis: a review. J Eur Acad Dermatol Venereol. 2020;34:1972. [PMID: 32239567]

Iorizzo M et al. Bacterial and viral infections of the nail unit. Dermatol Clin. 2021;39:245. [PMID: 33745637]

Maddy AJ et al. What's new in nail disorders. Dermatol Clin. 2019;37:143. [PMID: 30850036]

Ricardo JW et al. Safety of current therapies for onychomycosis. Expert Opin Drug Saf. 2020;19:1395. [PMID: 32990062]

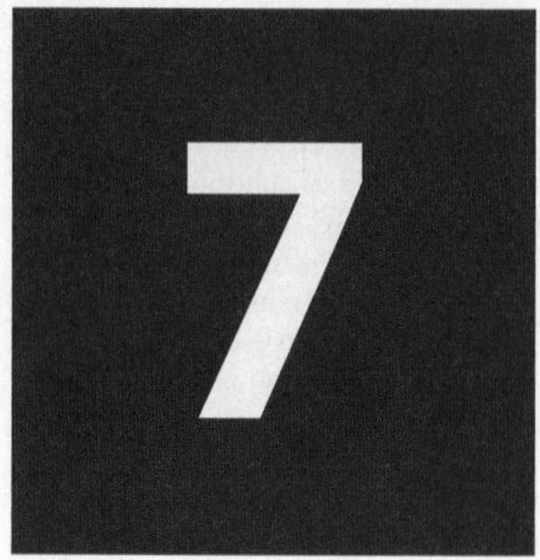

Disorders of the Eyes & Lids

Jacque L. Duncan, MD
Neeti B. Parikh, MD
Gerami D. Seitzman, MD

REFRACTIVE ERRORS

Refractive error is the most common cause of reduced clarity of vision (visual acuity).

Use of a pinhole will overcome most refractive errors and thus allows their identification as a cause of reduced visual acuity. Refractive error can be treated with glasses, contact lenses, or surgery.

Treatment

A. Contact Lenses

An estimated 40.9 million US adults wear contact lenses, mostly for correction of refractive errors, though decorative-colored contact lenses are used.

The major risk from contact lens wear is corneal infection, potentially a blinding condition. Such infections occur more often with soft lenses, particularly extended wear, for which there is at least a fivefold increase in risk of corneal infection compared with daily wear. Decorative contact lenses have a high prevalence of microbial contamination. Contact lens wearers should be made aware of the risks they face and ways to minimize them, such as avoiding overnight wear or use of lenses past their replacement date and maintaining meticulous lens hygiene, including not using tap water or saliva for lens cleaning. Contact lenses should be removed whenever there is ocular discomfort or redness.

Razmaria AA. JAMA patient page. Proper care of contact lenses. JAMA. 2015;314:1534. [PMID: 26462011]

B. Surgery

Various surgical techniques are available to reduce refractive errors, particularly nearsightedness. Laser corneal refractive surgery reshapes the middle layer (stroma) of the cornea with an excimer laser.

Other refractive surgery techniques are extraction of the clear crystalline lens with insertion of a single vision, multifocal, or accommodative intraocular lens as occurs after cataract extraction; insertion of an intraocular lens without removal of the crystalline lens (phakic intraocular lens); intrastromal corneal ring segments (INTACS); collagen cross-linking; laser thermal keratoplasty; and conductive keratoplasty (CK).

Wilkinson JM et al. Refractive eye surgery: helping patients make informed decisions about LASIK. Am Fam Physician. 2017;95:637. [PMID: 28671403]

C. Reduction of Rate of Progression of Nearsightedness

The rate at which nearsightedness progresses can be reduced by topical atropine and pirenzepine, a selective muscarinic antagonist; rigid contact lens wear during sleep (orthokeratology); and various types of soft contact lenses and spectacles, but their long-term efficacy and safety are uncertain.

When to Refer

Any contact lens wearer with an acute painful red eye must be referred emergently for ophthalmologic evaluation.

DISORDERS OF THE LIDS & LACRIMAL APPARATUS

1. Hordeolum

Hordeolum is an acute infection that is commonly due to *Staphylococcus aureus.* It is characterized by a localized red, swollen, acutely tender area on the upper or lower lid. Internal hordeolum is a meibomian gland abscess that usually points onto the conjunctival surface of the lid; external hordeolum, or stye, is usually smaller and on the lid margin and is an abscess of the gland of Zeis.

Warm compresses are helpful. Incision may be indicated if resolution does not begin within 48 hours. An antibiotic ointment (bacitracin or erythromycin) applied to the lid every 3 hours may be beneficial during the acute stage. Internal hordeolum may lead to generalized cellulitis of the lid.

2. Chalazion

Chalazion is a common granulomatous inflammation of a meibomian gland that may follow an internal hordeolum. It is characterized by a hard, nontender swelling on the upper or lower lid with redness and swelling of the adjacent conjunctiva. Initial treatment is with warm compresses. If resolution has not occurred by 2–3 weeks, incision and curettage is indicated. Corticosteroid injection may also be effective.

3. Blepharitis

Blepharitis is a common chronic bilateral inflammatory condition of the lid margins. **Anterior blepharitis** involves the lid skin, eyelashes, and associated glands. It may be ulcerative because of infection by staphylococci, or seborrheic in association with seborrhea of the scalp, brows, and ears. **Posterior blepharitis** results from inflammation of the meibomian glands. There may be bacterial infection, particularly with staphylococci, or primary glandular dysfunction, which is strongly associated with acne rosacea.

Clinical Findings

Symptoms are irritation, burning, and itching. In **anterior blepharitis,** the eyes are "red-rimmed" and scales or collerettes can be seen clinging to the lashes. In **posterior blepharitis,** the lid margins are hyperemic with telangiectasias, and the meibomian glands and their orifices are inflamed. The lid margin is frequently rolled inward to produce a mild entropion, and the tear film may be frothy or abnormally greasy.

Blepharitis is a common cause of recurrent conjunctivitis. Both anterior and, especially, posterior blepharitis may be complicated by hordeola or chalazia; abnormal lid or lash positions, producing trichiasis; epithelial keratitis of the lower third of the cornea; marginal corneal infiltrates; and inferior corneal vascularization and thinning.

Treatment

Anterior blepharitis is usually controlled by eyelid hygiene. Warm compresses help soften the scales and warm the meibomian gland secretions. Eyelid cleansing can be achieved by gentle eyelid massage and lid scrubs with baby shampoo or 0.01% hypochlorous acid. In acute exacerbations, an antibiotic eye ointment, such as bacitracin or erythromycin, is applied daily to the lid margins.

Mild **posterior blepharitis** may be controlled with regular meibomian gland expression and warm compresses. Inflammation of the conjunctiva and cornea is treated with long-term low-dose oral antibiotic therapy, eg, tetracycline (250 mg twice daily for 2–4 weeks), doxycycline (100 mg daily for 2–4 weeks), minocycline (50–100 mg daily for 2–4 weeks) erythromycin (250 mg three times daily for 2–4 weeks), or azithromycin (500 mg daily for 3 days in three cycles with 7-day intervals). Short-term (5–7 days) topical corticosteroids, eg, prednisolone, 0.125% twice daily, may also be indicated. Topical therapy with antibiotics, such as ciprofloxacin 0.3% ophthalmic solution twice daily, may be helpful but should be restricted to short courses of 5–7 days.

Amescua G et al; American Academy of Ophthalmology Preferred Practice Pattern Cornea and External Disease Panel. Blepharitis Preferred Practice Pattern®. Ophthalmology. 2019;126:P56. [PMID: 30366800]

4. Entropion & Ectropion

Entropion (inward turning of usually the lower lid) occurs occasionally in older people as a result of degeneration of the lid fascia or may follow extensive scarring of the conjunctiva and tarsus. Surgery is indicated if the lashes rub on the cornea. Botulinum toxin injections may also be used for temporary correction of the involutional lower lid entropion of older people.

Ectropion (outward turning of the lower lid) is common with advanced age. Surgery is indicated if there is excessive tearing, exposure keratitis, or a cosmetic problem.

5. Tumors

Lid tumors are usually benign. Basal cell carcinoma is the most common malignant tumor. Squamous cell carcinoma, meibomian gland carcinoma, and malignant melanoma also occur. Surgery for any lesion involving the lid margin should be performed by an ophthalmologist or suitably trained plastic surgeon to avoid deformity of the lid. Histopathologic examination of eyelid tumors should be routine, since 2% of lesions thought to be benign clinically are found to be malignant. Medications such as vismodegib (an oral inhibitor of the hedgehog pathway), imiquimod (an immunomodulator), and 5-fluorouracil occasionally are used instead of or as an adjunct to surgery for some basal and squamous cell carcinomas.

6. Dacryocystitis

Dacryocystitis is infection of the lacrimal sac usually due to congenital or acquired obstruction of the nasolacrimal system. It may be acute or chronic and occurs most often in infants and in persons over 40 years. It is usually unilateral. Infection is typically with *S aureus* and streptococci in acute dacryocystitis and *Staphylococcus epidermidis*, streptococci, or gram-negative bacilli in chronic dacryocystitis.

Acute dacryocystitis is characterized by pain, swelling, tenderness, and redness in the tear sac area; purulent material may be expressed. In chronic dacryocystitis, tearing and discharge are the principal signs, and mucus or pus may also be expressed.

Acute dacryocystitis responds well to systemic antibiotic therapy. To relieve the underlying obstruction, surgery is usually done electively but may be performed urgently in acute cases. The chronic form may be kept latent with systemic antibiotics, but relief of the obstruction is the only cure. In adults, the standard procedure is dacryocystorhinostomy, which involves surgical exploration of the lacrimal sac and formation of a fistula into the nasal cavity and, if necessary, supplemented by nasolacrimal intubation.

Congenital nasolacrimal duct obstruction is common and often resolves spontaneously. It can be treated by probing the nasolacrimal system, supplemented by nasolacrimal intubation or balloon catheter dilation, if necessary; dacryocystorhinostomy is rarely required.

CONJUNCTIVITIS

Conjunctivitis is inflammation of the mucous membrane that lines the surface of the eyeball and inner eyelids. It may be acute or chronic. Most cases are due to viral or bacterial (including gonococcal and chlamydial) infection. Other causes include keratoconjunctivitis sicca, allergy, chemical irritants, and trauma. The mode of transmission of infectious conjunctivitis is usually via direct contact of contaminated fingers or objects to the other eye or to other persons. It may also be spread through respiratory secretions or contaminated eye drops.

Conjunctivitis must be differentiated from acute uveitis, acute glaucoma, and corneal disorders (Table 7–1).

Varu DM et al; American Academy of Ophthalmology Preferred Practice Pattern Cornea and External Disease Panel. Conjunctivitis Preferred Practice Pattern®. Ophthalmology. 2019;126:P94. [PMID: 30366797]

1. Viral Conjunctivitis

Adenovirus is the most common cause of viral conjunctivitis. There is usually sequential bilateral disease with copious watery discharge and a follicular conjunctivitis. Infection spreads easily. Epidemic keratoconjunctivitis, which may result in decreased vision from corneal subepithelial infiltrates, is usually caused by adenovirus types 8, 19, and 37. The active viral conjunctivitis lasts up to 2 weeks, with the immune-mediated keratitis occurring later. Infection with adenovirus types 3, 4, 7, and 11 is typically associated with pharyngitis, fever, malaise, and preauricular adenopathy (pharyngoconjunctival fever). The disease usually lasts 10 days. Contagious acute hemorrhagic conjunctivitis (see Chapter 32) may be caused by enterovirus 70 or coxsackievirus A24, though etiologies vary globally. Viral conjunctivitis from herpes simplex virus (HSV) is typically unilateral and may be associated with lid vesicles.

Except for HSV infection for which treatment with topical (eg, ganciclovir 0.15% gel) and/or systemic (eg, oral acyclovir, valacyclovir) antivirals is recommended (Table 32–1), there is no specific treatment for contagious viral conjunctivitis. Artificial tears and cold compresses may help reduce discomfort. The use of topical antibiotics and steroids in the acute infection is discouraged. Frequent hand and linen hygiene is encouraged to minimize spread.

Kaur G, Seitzman GD et al. Keeping an eye on pink eye: a global conjunctivitis outbreak expert survey. Int Health. 2021 Aug 19. [Epub ahead of print] [PMID: 34409991]

2. Bacterial Conjunctivitis

The organisms isolated most commonly in bacterial conjunctivitis are staphylococci, including methicillin-resistant *S aureus* (MRSA); streptococci, particularly *Streptococcus pneumoniae*; *Haemophilus* species; *Pseudomonas;* and *Moraxella*. All may produce purulent discharge and eyelid matting. Blurring of vision and discomfort are mild. In severe (hyperpurulent) cases, examination of stained conjunctival scrapings and cultures is recommended, particularly to identify gonococcal infection that requires emergent treatment.

The disease is usually self-limited, lasting about 10–14 days if untreated. Most topical antibiotics hasten clinical remission.

Table 7–1. The inflamed eye: differential diagnosis of common causes.

	Acute Conjunctivitis	Acute Anterior Uveitis (Iritis)	Acute Angle-Closure Glaucoma	Corneal Trauma or Infection
Incidence	Extremely common	Common	Uncommon	Common
Discharge	Moderate to copious	None	None	Watery or purulent
Vision	No effect on vision	Often blurred	Markedly blurred	Usually blurred
Pain	Mild	Moderate	Severe	Moderate to severe
Conjunctival injection	Diffuse	Mainly circumcorneal	Mainly circumcorneal	Mainly circumcorneal
Cornea	Clear	Usually clear	Cloudy	Clarity change related to cause
Pupil size	Normal	Small	Moderately dilated	Normal or small
Pupillary light response	Normal	Poor	None	Normal
Intraocular pressure	Normal	Usually normal but may be elevated	Markedly elevated	Normal
Smear	Causative organisms	No organisms	No organisms	Organisms found only in corneal infection

This infection is typically self-limited, and no topical antibiotic has proven superiority over another.

A. Gonococcal Conjunctivitis

Gonococcal conjunctivitis, usually acquired through contact with infected genital secretions, typically causes copious purulent discharge. It is an ophthalmologic emergency because corneal involvement may rapidly lead to perforation. The diagnosis should be confirmed by stained smear and culture of the discharge. Systemic treatment is required with a single 500-mg dose of intramuscular ceftriaxone if the patient weighs less than 150 kg or 1-g dose if patient weighs more than 150 kg (see Chapter 33). Fluoroquinolone resistance is common. Eye irrigation with saline may promote resolution of conjunctivitis. Topical antibiotics such as erythromycin and bacitracin may be added. Other sexually transmitted diseases, including chlamydiosis, syphilis, and HIV infection, should be considered. Routine treatment for chlamydial infection is recommended.

Alsoudi AF... Seitzman GD. Purulent conjunctivitis and progressive corneal stromal necrosis. JAMA Ophthalmol. 2021;139:908. [PMID: 34081098]

B. Chlamydial Keratoconjunctivitis

1. Trachoma—Trachoma is the most common infectious cause of blindness worldwide, with approximately 40 million people affected and 1.2 million blind. Recurrent episodes of infection in childhood manifest as bilateral follicular conjunctivitis, epithelial keratitis, and corneal vascularization (pannus). Scarring (cicatrization) of the tarsal conjunctiva leads to entropion and trichiasis in adulthood with secondary central corneal scarring.

Immunologic tests or PCR on conjunctival samples will confirm the diagnosis but treatment should be started on the basis of clinical findings. A single 1-g dose of oral azithromycin is the preferred drug for mass treatment campaigns; improvements in hygiene and living conditions probably have contributed more to the marked reduction in the prevalence of trachoma during the past 30 years. Local treatment is not necessary. Surgical treatment includes correction of lid deformities and corneal transplantation.

Godwin W et al. Trachoma prevalence after discontinuation of mass azithromycin distribution. J Infect Dis. 2020;221:S519. [PMID: 32052842]

2. Inclusion conjunctivitis—The eye becomes infected after contact with genital secretions infected with chlamydia. The disease starts with acute redness, discharge, and irritation. Examination shows follicular conjunctivitis with mild keratitis. A nontender preauricular lymph node can often be palpated. Healing usually leaves no sequelae. Diagnosis can be rapidly confirmed by immunologic tests or PCR on conjunctival samples. Treatment is doxycycline, 100 mg orally twice a day for 7 days. All cases should be assessed for genital tract infection and other sexually transmitted diseases.

3. Dry Eyes

Dry eye, a common and chronic disorder, is an umbrella term that describes a condition of tear film instability and associated ocular and visual complaints. Dry eye is more common in women than men and increases with age. Hypofunction of the lacrimal glands, causing loss of the aqueous component of tears (keratoconjunctivitis sicca), may be due to aging, hereditary disorders, systemic disease (eg, Sjögren syndrome), or systemic drugs. Excessive evaporation of tears may be due to environmental factors (eg, excessive screen time, windy climate) or abnormalities of the lipid component of the tear film, as in blepharitis. Mucin deficiency may be due to vitamin A deficiency or conjunctival scarring from trachoma, Stevens-Johnson syndrome, mucous membrane pemphigoid, graft-versus-host disease, chemical burns, or topical drug toxicity.

▶ Clinical Findings

The patient complains of dryness, redness, foreign body sensation, and variable vision. In severe cases, there is persistent marked discomfort, with photophobia, difficulty in moving the lids, and excessive mucus secretion. In many cases, gross inspection reveals no abnormality, but on slit-lamp examination there are abnormalities of tear film stability and reduced tear volume. In more severe cases, damaged corneal and conjunctival cells stain with fluorescein and lissamine green. In the most severe cases, there is marked conjunctival injection, mucoid discharge, loss of the normal conjunctival and corneal luster, and epithelial keratopathy that stains with fluorescein and may progress to frank ulceration. The Schirmer test, which measures the rate of production of the aqueous component of tears, may be helpful.

▶ Treatment

Aqueous deficiency can be treated with artificial tears drops or ointments. The simplest preparations are physiologic (0.9%) or hypo-osmotic (0.45%) solutions of sodium chloride, which can be used as frequently as every half-hour, but in most cases are needed only three or four times a day. More prolonged duration of action can be achieved with drop preparations containing a mucomimetic such as hydroxypropyl methylcellulose (HPMC) or carboxymethylcelluose (carmellose).

Artificial tear preparations are generally safe and, in most cases, are used three or four times a day. However, preservatives included in some preparations to maintain sterility are potentially toxic and allergenic and may cause ocular surface toxicity in frequent users. Such reactions may be misinterpreted as a worsening of the dry eye state requiring more frequent use of the artificial tears and leading in turn to further deterioration, rather than being recognized as a need to change to a preservative-free preparation. Preservative-free preparations are recommended for any frequency of use greater than four times a day. Eye drops claiming to "get the red out" are not recommended as they cause toxicity and rebound hyperemia with prolonged use.

Dry eye is considered an inflammatory ocular surface disease. Accordingly, disease modification may require episodic treatment with low potency corticosteroid drops. All patients using topical corticosteroids should have their intraocular pressure monitored by eye care professionals. Corticosteroid-sparing anti-inflammatory drops such as the calcineurin inhibitor cyclosporine 0.05% ophthalmic emulsion (Restasis) and the integrin antagonist lifitegrast 5% are commonly used with no universal consensus of efficacy. Lacrimal punctal occlusion by canalicular plugs or cautery is useful in severe cases.

Blepharitis is treated as described above.

de Paiva CS et al. Topical cyclosporine A therapy for dry eye syndrome. Cochrane Database Syst Rev. 2019;9:CD010051. [PMID: 31517988]

Gonzales JA... Seitzman GD et al. Ocular clinical signs and diagnostic tests most compatible with keratoconjunctivitis sicca: a latent class approach. Cornea. 2020;39:1013. [PMID: 32251167]

4. Allergic Eye Disease

Allergic eye disease is common and takes a number of different forms, but all are expressions of atopy, which may also manifest as atopic asthma, atopic dermatitis, or allergic rhinitis.

▶ Clinical Findings

Symptoms include itching, tearing, redness, stringy discharge, and occasionally, photophobia and visual loss.

Allergic conjunctivitis is common. It may be seasonal (hay fever), developing usually during the spring or summer, or perennial. Clinical signs include conjunctival hyperemia and edema (chemosis), the latter at times being marked and sudden in onset. **Vernal keratoconjunctivitis** also tends to occur in late childhood and early adulthood. It is usually seasonal, with a predilection for the spring. Large "cobblestone" papillae are noted on the upper tarsal conjunctiva. There may be follicles at the limbus. **Atopic keratoconjunctivitis** is a more chronic disorder of adulthood. Both the upper and the lower tarsal conjunctivas exhibit a papillary conjunctivitis. Severe cases demonstrate conjunctival fibrosis, resulting in forniceal shortening and entropion with trichiasis. Corneal involvement, including refractory ulceration, is frequent during exacerbations of both vernal and severe atopic keratoconjunctivitis. The latter may be complicated by herpes simplex keratitis.

▶ Treatment

A. Mild and Moderately Severe Allergic Eye Disease

Topical anti-inflammatory agents include mast cell stabilizers and antihistamines (Table 7–2). Mast cell stabilization takes longer to act than antihistamines but can be useful for prophylaxis. Topical vasoconstrictors, such as ephedrine, naphazoline, tetrahydrozoline, and phenylephrine, alone or in combination with antihistamines, are available as over-the-counter medications and not typically used because of limited efficacy, rebound hyperemia, and follicular conjunctivitis. Systemic antihistamines (eg, loratadine 10 mg orally daily) may be useful in prolonged atopic keratoconjunctivitis. In allergic conjunctivitis, specific allergens may be avoidable.

B. Acute Exacerbations and Severe Allergic Eye Disease

Topical corticosteroids (Table 7–2) are essential to control acute exacerbations of both vernal and atopic keratoconjunctivitis. Corticosteroid-induced side effects should be monitored by eye care professionals and include cataracts, glaucoma, and exacerbation of herpes simplex keratitis. The lowest potency corticosteroid that controls ocular inflammation should be used. Topical cyclosporine or tacrolimus is also effective. Systemic corticosteroid or other immunosuppressant therapy may be required in severe atopic keratoconjunctivitis.

Beck KM, Seitzman GD et al. Ocular co-morbidities of atopic dermatitis. Part I: associated ocular diseases. Am J Clin Dermatol. 2019;20:797. [PMID: 31359350]

Beck KM, Seitzman GD et al. Ocular co-morbidities of atopic dermatitis. Part II: ocular disease secondary to treatments. Am J Clin Dermatol. 2019;20:807. [PMID: 31352589]

PINGUECULA & PTERYGIUM

Pinguecula is a yellowish, elevated conjunctival nodule in the area of the palpebral fissure. It is common in persons over age 35 years. Pterygium is a fleshy, triangular encroachment of the conjunctiva onto the cornea and is usually associated with prolonged exposure to wind, sun, sand, and dust. Pinguecula and pterygium are often bilateral and occur more frequently on the nasal side of the conjunctiva.

Pingueculae rarely grow but may become inflamed (pingueculitis). Pterygia become inflamed and may grow. Treatment is rarely required for inflammation of pinguecula or pterygium, and artificial tears are often beneficial.

The indications for excision of pterygium are growth that threatens vision by encroaching on the visual axis, marked induced astigmatism, or severe ocular irritation.

Shahraki T et al. Pterygium: an update on pathophysiology, clinical features, and management. Ther Adv Ophthalmol. 2021;13:25158414211020152. [PMID: 34104871]

CORNEAL ULCER

Corneal ulcers are most commonly due to infection by bacteria, viruses, fungi, or amoebas. Noninfectious causes—all of which may be complicated by infection—include neurotrophic keratitis (resulting from loss of

Table 7–2. Topical ophthalmic agents (selected list).

Agent	Cost/Size[1]	Recommended Regimen	Indications
Antibiotic Agents			
Amikacin 2.5% (fortified) solution	Compounding pharmacy		
Azithromycin (AzaSite)	$267.25/2.5 mL	1 drop two times daily for 2 days, then once daily for 5 days	Bacterial conjunctivitis
Bacitracin 500 U/g ointment (various)[2]	$118.44/3.5 g	Apply 0.5 inch into lower conjunctival sac or to eyelids three to four times daily for 7–10 days	Bacterial conjunctivitis, blepharitis, sty
Bacitracin/Polymyxin ointment (Polysporin, AK-Poly)	$25.70/3.5 g	Apply 0.5 inch into lower conjunctival sac and then three to four times daily, then as required	Corneal abrasion Following corneal foreign body removal
Besifloxacin ophthalmic suspension, 0.6% (Besivance)	$242.05/5 mL	1–2 drops every 2 hours while awake for 2 days, then every 4 hours for 5 days 1 drop every hour during the day and every 2 hours during the night for 48 hours, then gradually reduce	Bacterial conjunctivitis Bacterial keratitis
Ciprofloxacin HCl 0.3% solution (Ciloxan)	$11.09/5 mL	1–2 drops every 2 hours while awake for 2 days, then every 4 hours for 5 days 1 drop every hour during the day and every 2 hours during the night for 48 hours, then gradually reduce	Bacterial conjunctivitis Bacterial keratitis
Ciprofloxacin HCl 0.3% ointment	$257.23/3.5 g	Apply 0.5 inch into lower conjunctival sac three times daily for 2 days, then two times daily for 5 days	Bacterial conjunctivitis
Erythromycin 0.5% ointment (various)	$17.96/3.5 g	1-cm ribbon up to six times daily	Bacterial infection of the conjunctiva or lid margin
Fusidic acid 1% gel (Fucithalmic)	Not available in United States	1 drop two times daily	Bacterial conjunctivitis, blepharitis, sty, keratitis
Gatifloxacin 0.5% solution (Zymaxid)	$118.16/2.5 mL	1 drop every 2 hours while awake, up to eight times on day 1, then two to four times daily while awake, days 2–7 1 drop every hour during the day and every 2 hours during the night for 48 hours, then gradually reduce	Bacterial conjunctivitis Bacterial keratitis
Gentamicin sulfate 0.3% solution (various)	$19.18/5 mL	1–2 drops every 4 hours up to 2 drops every hour for severe infections	Ocular surface infection
Gentamicin sulfate 0.3% ointment (various)	$38.95/3.5 g	Apply 0.5 inch into lower conjunctival sac two to three times daily	Ocular surface infection
Gentamicin sulfate 1.5% (fortified preparation)	Compounding pharmacy	1 drop every hour during the day and every 2 hours during the night for 48 hours, then gradually reduce	Bacterial keratitis

(*continued*)

Table 7–2. Topical ophthalmic agents (selected list). (continued)

Agent	Cost/Size[1]	Recommended Regimen	Indications
Levofloxacin 0.5% solution (various)	$75.00/5 mL	1–2 drops every 2 hours while awake for 2 days (maximum eight times per day), then every 4 hours for 5 days (maximum four times per day) 1 drop every hour during the day and every 2 hours during the night for 48 hours, then gradually reduce	Bacterial conjunctivitis Bacterial keratitis
Moxifloxacin 0.5% solution (Vigamox)	$13.92/3 mL	1 drop three times daily for 7 days 1 drop every hour during the day and every 2 hours during the night for 48 hours, then gradually reduce	Bacterial conjunctivitis Bacterial keratitis
Neomycin/Polymyxin B/Gramicidin (Neosporin)	$61.26/10 mL	1–2 drops every 4 hours for 7–10 days or more frequently, as required	Ocular surface infection
Norfloxacin 0.3% solution	Not available in United States	1 drop every hour during the day and every 2 hours during the night for 48 hours, then gradually reduce	Ocular surface infection Bacterial keratitis
Ofloxacin 0.3% solution (Ocuflox)	$20.94/5 mL	1–2 drops every 2–4 hours for 2 days, then four times daily for 5 days 1 drop every hour during the day and every 2 hours during the night for 48 hours, then gradually reduce	Bacterial conjunctivitis Bacterial keratitis
Polymyxin B 10,000 U/mL/ Trimethoprim sulfate 1 mg/mL (Polytrim)[3]	$12.87/10 mL	1 drop every 3 hours for 7–10 days (maximum of 6 doses per day)	Ocular surface infection
Propamidine isethionate 0.1% solution	Not available in the United States	1–2 drops every 2–4 hours for 2 days, then four times daily for 5 days	Ocular surface infection (including *Acanthamoeba* keratitis)
Propamidine isethionate 0.1% ointment	Not available in the United States	Apply 0.5 inch into lower conjunctival sac up to four times daily	
Sulfacetamide sodium 10% solution (various)	$55.65/15 mL	1 or 2 drops every 2–3 hours initially; taper by increasing time intervals as condition responds; usual duration 7–10 days	Bacterial infection of the conjunctiva or lid margin
Sulfacetamide sodium 10% ointment (various)	$65.86/3.5 g	Apply 0.5 inch into lower conjunctival sac once every 3–4 hours and at bedtime; taper by increasing time intervals as condition responds; usual duration 7–10 days	Bacterial infection of the conjunctiva or lid margin
Tobramycin 0.3% solution (various)	$6.25/5 mL	1–2 drops every 4 hours for a mild to moderate infection or hourly until improvement (then reduce prior to discontinuation) for a severe infection	
Tobramycin 1.5% (fortified) solution	Compounding pharmacy	1 drop every hour during the day and every 2 hours during the night for 48 hours, then gradually reduce	Bacterial keratitis

(*continued*)

Table 7–2. Topical ophthalmic agents (selected list). (continued)

Agent	Cost/Size[1]	Recommended Regimen	Indications
Tobramycin 0.3% ointment (Tobrex)	$257.23/3.5 g	Apply 0.5 inch into lower conjunctival sac two to three times daily for a mild to moderate infection or every 3–4 hours until improvement (then reduce prior to discontinuation) for a severe infection	
Antifungal Agents			
Amphotericin 0.1–0.5% solution	Compounding pharmacy		Fungal blepharitis, conjunctivitis, keratitis
Natamycin 5% suspension (Natacyn)	$568.37/15 mL	1 drop every 1–2 hours initially	
Voriconazole 1% solution	Compounding pharmacy		
Antiviral Agents			
Acyclovir 3% ointment (Zovirax)	Not available in United States	Five times daily	Herpes simplex keratitis
Ganciclovir 0.15% gel (Zirgan)	$502.03/5 g	Five times daily	
Trifluridine 1% solution (Viroptic)	$178.28/7.5 mL	1 drop onto cornea every 2 hours while awake for a maximum daily dose of 9 drops until resolution occurs; then an additional 7 days of 1 drop every 4 hours while awake (minimum five times daily)	
Anti-Inflammatory Agents			
Antihistamines[4]			
Emedastine difumarate 0.05% solution (Emadine)	Not available in the United States	1 drop four times daily	Allergic eye disease
Levocabastine (Livostin)	Not available in United States	1 drop twice daily	
Mast cell stabilizers			
Cromolyn sodium 4% solution (Crolom)	$37.20/10 mL	1 drop four to six times daily	
Lodoxamide tromethamine 0.1% solution (Alomide)	$205.28/10 mL	1 or 2 drops four times daily (up to 3 months)	
Nedocromil sodium 2% solution (Alocril)	$269.41/5 mL	1 drop twice daily	
Pemirolast potassium 0.1% solution (Alamast)	Not available in the United States	1 drop four times daily	
Combined antihistamines and mast cell stabilizers			
Alcaftadine 0.25% ophthalmic solution (Lastacaft)	$283.99/3 mL	1 drop once daily	
Azelastine HCl 0.05% ophthalmic solution (Optivar)	$102.90/6 mL	1 drop two to four times daily (up to 6 weeks)	
Bepotastine besilate 1.5% solution (Bepreve)	$498.51/10 mL	1 drop twice daily	
Epinastine hydrochloride 0.05% ophthalmic solution (Elestat)	$106.95/5 mL	1 drop twice daily (up to 8 weeks)	
Ketotifen fumarate 0.025% solution (Zaditor)	OTC $7.79/5 mL	1 drop two to four times daily	
Olopatadine hydrochloride 0.1% solution (Patanol)	OTC $12.42/5 mL	1 drop twice daily	

(continued)

Table 7–2. Topical ophthalmic agents (selected list). (continued)

Agent	Cost/Size[1]	Recommended Regimen	Indications
Nonsteroidal anti-inflammatory agents			
Bromfenac 0.09% solution (Xibrom)	$213.69/1.7 mL	1 drop to operated eye twice daily beginning 24 hours after cataract surgery and continuing through 2 postoperative weeks	Treatment of postoperative inflammation following cataract extraction
Diclofenac sodium 0.1% solution (Voltaren)	$17.50/5 mL	1 drop to operated eye four times daily beginning 24 hours after surgery and continuing through 2 postoperative weeks	Treatment of postoperative inflammation following cataract extraction and laser corneal surgery
Flurbiprofen sodium 0.03% solution (various)	$51.50/2.5 mL	1 drop every half hour beginning 2 hours before surgery; 1 drop to operated eye four times daily beginning 24 hours after cataract surgery	Inhibition of intraoperative miosis; treatment of cystoid macular edema and inflammation after cataract extraction
Indomethacin 1% solution (Indocid)	Not available in United States	1 drop four times daily	Treatment of allergic eye disease, postoperative inflammation following cataract extraction and laser corneal surgery
Ketorolac tromethamine 0.5% solution (Acular)	$105.50/5 mL	1 drop four times daily	
Nepafenac 0.1% suspension (Nevanac)	$325.96/3 mL	1 drop to operated eye three times daily beginning 24 hours after cataract surgery and continuing through 2 postoperative weeks	Treatment of postoperative inflammation following cataract extraction
Corticosteroids[5]			
Dexamethasone sodium phosphate 0.1% solution (various)	$21.10/5 mL	1 or 2 drops as often as indicated by severity; use every hour during the day and every 2 hours during the night in severe inflammation; taper off as inflammation decreases	Treatment of steroid-responsive inflammatory conditions
Dexamethasone sodium phosphate 0.05% ointment	Compounding pharmacy	Apply thin coating on lower conjunctival sac three or four times daily	
Fluorometholone 0.1% suspension (various)[6]	$202.10/5 mL	1 or 2 drops as often as indicated by severity; use every hour during the day and every 2 hours during the night in severe inflammation; taper off as inflammation decreases	
Fluorometholone 0.25% suspension (FML Forte)[6]	$404.22/10 mL	1 drop two to four times daily	
Fluorometholone 0.1% ointment (FML S.O.P.)	$192.48/3.5 g	Apply thin coating on lower conjunctival sac three or four times daily	
Loteprednol etabonate 0.5% (Lotemax)	$450.67/10 mL	1 or 2 drops four times daily	
Prednisolone acetate 0.12% suspension (Pred Mild)	$384.97/10 mL	1 or 2 drops as often as indicated by severity of inflammation; use every hour during the day and every 2 hours during the night in severe inflammation; taper off as inflammation decreases	
Prednisolone sodium phosphate 0.125% solution	Compounding pharmacy		
Prednisolone acetate 1% suspension (various)	$105.60/10 mL	2 drops four times daily	
Prednisolone sodium phosphate 1% solution (various)	$63.25/10 mL	1–2 drops two to four times daily	

(continued)

Table 7–2. Topical ophthalmic agents (selected list). (continued)

Agent	Cost/Size[1]	Recommended Regimen	Indications
Immunomodulators			
Cyclosporine 0.05% emulsion (Restasis) 0.4 mL/container	$367.99/30 containers	1 drop twice daily	Dry eyes and severe allergic eye disease
Tacrolimus 0.1% ointment	$84.00/30 g tube	Apply to lower conjunctival sac twice daily	Severe allergic eye disease
Glaucoma and Ocular Hypertension Agents			
Sympathomimetics			
Apraclonidine HCl 0.5% solution (Iopidine)	$86.77/5 mL	1 drop three times daily	Reduction of intraocular pressure; expensive; reserve for treatment of resistant cases
Apraclonidine HCl 1% solution (Iopidine)	$33.27/unit dose	1 drop 1 hour before and immediately after anterior segment laser surgery	To control or prevent elevations of intraocular pressure after laser trabeculoplasty or iridotomy
Brimonidine tartrate 0.2% solution (Alphagan, Alphagan P [benzalkonium chloride-free])	$12.50/5 mL	1 drop two or three times daily	Reduction of intraocular pressure
Beta-adrenergic blocking agents			
Betaxolol HCl 0.5% solution (Betoptic) and 0.25% suspension (Betoptic S)[7]	0.5%: $117.91/10 mL 0.25%: $372.64/10 mL	1 drop twice daily	Reduction of intraocular pressure
Carteolol HCl 1% and 2% solution (various, Teoptic)[8]	1%: $40.10/10 mL	1 drop twice daily	
Levobunolol HCl 0.25% and 0.5% solution (Betagan)[9]	0.5%: $21.49/5 mL	1 drop once or twice daily	
Metipranolol HCl 0.3% solution (OptiPranolol)[9]	$29.67/5 mL	1 drop twice daily	
Timolol 0.25% and 0.5% solution (Betimol)[9]	0.5%: $182.83/5 mL	1 drop once or twice daily	
Timolol maleate 0.25% and 0.5% solution (Istalol, Ocudose [preservative-free], Timoptic) and 0.1%, 0.25%, and 0.5% gel (Timoptic-XE, Timoptic GFS)[9]	0.5% solution: $6.56/5 mL 0.5% gel: $217.27/5 mL	1 drop once or twice daily	
Miotics			
Pilocarpine HCl 1–4% solution[10]	1% solution: $92.73/15 mL	1 drop up to four times daily for elevated intraocular pressure	Reduction of intraocular pressure, treatment of acute or chronic angle-closure glaucoma, and pupillary constriction
Carbonic anhydrase inhibitors			
Brinzolamide 1% suspension (Azopt)	$366.01/10 mL	1 drop three times daily	Reduction of intraocular pressure
Dorzolamide HCl 2% solution (Trusopt)	$40.79/10 mL	1 drop three times daily	

(continued)

Table 7–2. Topical ophthalmic agents (selected list). (continued)

Agent	Cost/Size[1]	Recommended Regimen	Indications
Prostaglandin analogs			
Bimatoprost 0.03% solution (Lumigan)	$138.87/3 mL	1 drop once daily at night	Reduction of intraocular pressure
Latanoprost 0.005% solution (Xalatan, Monopost [preservative-free])	$27.26/2.5 mL (Monopost not available in United States)	1 drop once or twice daily at night	
Latanoprostene bunod 0.024% solution (Vyzulta)	$272.70/2.5 mL	1 drop daily at night	
Tafluprost 0.0015% solution (Saflutan [preservative-free], Taflotan, Zioptan [preservative-free])	$276.06/30 units (Saflutan not available in United States)	1 drop once daily at night	
Travoprost 0.004% solution (Travatan, Travatan Z [benzalkonium chloride-free])	$198.36/2.5 mL	1 drop once daily at night	
Unoprostone isopropyl 0.15% solution (Rescula)	$153.84/5 mL	1 drop twice daily	
Rho kinase inhibitor			
Netarsudil ophthalmic solution 0.02% (Rhopressa)	$356.52/2.5 mL	1 drop daily in the evening	Reduction of intraocular pressure
Combined preparations			
Bimatoprost 0.03% and timolol 0.5% (Ganfort)	Not available in United States	1 drop daily in the morning	Reduction of intraocular pressure
Brimonidine 0.2% and timolol 0.5% (Combigan)	$443.27/10 mL	1 drop twice daily	
Brimonidine 0.2% and brinzolamide 1% (Simbrinza)	$228.86/8 mL	1 drop three times a day	
Brinzolamide 1% and timolol 0.5% (Azarga)	Not available in United States	1 drop twice daily	
Dorzolamide 2% and timolol 0.5% (Cosopt, Cosopt PF [preservative-free])	$169.51/10 mL	1 drop twice daily	
Latanoprost 0.005% and timolol 0.5% (Xalacom)	Not available in United States	1 drop daily in the morning	
Tafluprost 0.0015% and timolol 0.5% (Taptiqom [preservative-free])	Not available in United States	1 drop daily	
Travoprost 0.004% and timolol 0.5% (DuoTrav)	Not available in United States	1 drop daily	

[1]Average wholesale price (AWP, for AB-rated generic when available) for quantity listed. IBM Micromedex Red Book (electronic version). IBM Watson Health, Greenwood Village, Colorado, USA. Available at: https://www-micromedexsolutions-com.proxy.hsl.ucdenver.edu/(cited March 15, 2022). AWP may not accurately represent the actual pharmacy cost because wide contractual variations exist among institutions.
[2]Little efficacy against gram-negative organisms (except *Neisseria*).
[3]No gram-positive coverage.
[4]May produce rebound hyperemia and local reactions.
[5]Long-term use increases intraocular pressure, causes cataracts, and predisposes to bacterial, herpes simplex virus, and fungal keratitis. These problems may be attenuated by the ester corticosteroid loteprednol.
[6]Less likely to elevate intraocular pressure.
[7]Cardioselective (beta-1) beta-blocker.
[8]Teoptic is not available in the United States.
[9]Nonselective (beta-1 and beta-2) beta-blocker. Monitor all patients for systemic side effects, particularly exacerbation of asthma.
[10]Decreased night vision and headaches possible.

corneal sensation), exposure keratitis (due to inadequate lid closure), severe dry eye, severe allergic eye disease, and inflammatory disorders that may be purely ocular or part of a systemic vasculitis. Delayed or ineffective treatment of corneal ulceration may lead to devastating consequences with corneal scarring and rarely intraocular infection. Prompt referral is essential.

Patients complain of pain, photophobia, tearing, and reduced vision. The conjunctiva is injected, and there may be purulent or watery discharge. The corneal appearance varies according to the underlying cause.

When to Refer

Any patient with an acute painful red eye and corneal abnormality should be referred emergently to an ophthalmologist. Contact lens wearers with acute eye pain, redness, and decreased vision should be referred immediately.

INFECTIOUS KERATITIS

1. Bacterial Keratitis

Risk factors for bacterial keratitis include contact lens wear—especially overnight wear—and corneal trauma, including refractive surgery. The pathogens most commonly isolated are staphylococci, including MRSA; streptococci; and *Pseudomonas aeruginosa, Moraxella* species, and other gram-negative bacilli. The cornea has an epithelial defect and an underlying opacity. Hypopyon may be present. Topical fluoroquinolones, such as levofloxacin 0.5%, ofloxacin 0.3%, norfloxacin 0.3%, or ciprofloxacin 0.3%, are commonly used as first-line agents as long as local prevalence of resistant organisms is low (Table 7–2). For severe central ulcers, diagnostic scrapings can be sent for Gram stain and culture. Treatment may include compounded high-concentration topical antibiotic drops applied hourly day and night for at least the first 48 hours. Fourth-generation fluoroquinolones (moxifloxacin 0.5% and gatifloxacin 0.3%) are also frequently used in this setting. Although early adjunctive topical corticosteroid therapy may improve visual outcome, it should be prescribed only by an ophthalmologist.

When to Refer

Any patient with suspected bacterial keratitis must be referred emergently to an ophthalmologist.

Lin A et al; American Academy of Ophthalmology Preferred Practice Pattern Cornea and External Disease Panel. Bacterial keratitis: Preferred Practice Pattern®. Ophthalmology. 2019; 126:P1. [PMID: 30366799]

2. Herpes Simplex Keratitis

Primary ocular herpes simplex virus infection may manifest as lid, conjunctival, or corneal ulceration. The ability of the virus to colonize the trigeminal ganglion leads to recurrences that may be precipitated by fever, excessive exposure to sunlight, or immunodeficiency. Herpetic corneal disease is typically unilateral but can be seen bilaterally in the setting of atopy or immunocompromise. The dendritic (branching) corneal ulcer is the most characteristic manifestation of herpetic corneal disease. More extensive ("geographic") ulcers also occur, particularly if topical corticosteroids have been used. The corneal ulcers are most easily seen after instillation of fluorescein and examination with a cobalt blue light. Resolution of corneal herpetic disease is hastened by treatment with topical antiviral agents (eg, trifluridine drops, ganciclovir gel, acyclovir ointment) or oral antiviral agents (eg, acyclovir, 400–800 mg five times daily or valacyclovir 500–1000 mg three times daily for 7–14 days). Topical antiviral agents may cause corneal toxicity after approximately 10–14 days of therapy and for that reason are not commonly used for long-term suppressive therapy.

Stromal herpes simplex keratitis produces increasingly severe corneal opacity with each recurrence. Antiviral agents alone are insufficient to control stromal disease, so topical corticosteroids are also used, but they may enhance viral replication and steroid dependence frequently occurs. **Caution:** *For patients with known or possible herpetic disease, topical corticosteroids should be prescribed only with ophthalmologic supervision.* Severe stromal scarring may require corneal transplantation; recurrence in the new cornea is common and long-term oral antiviral agents are required.

The rate of recurrent corneal herpetic disease is reduced by using long-term oral acyclovir, 400 mg twice daily; famciclovir, 250 mg once daily; or valacyclovir, 500 mg once daily. Long-term oral antiviral dosing may be adjusted if the disease breaks through suppressive dosing or if kidney dysfunction is present.

When to Refer

Any patient with a history of herpes simplex keratitis and an acute red eye should be referred urgently to an ophthalmologist.

Azher TN et al. Herpes simplex keratitis: challenges in diagnosis and clinical management. Clin Ophthalmol. 2017;11:185. [PMID: 28176902]

Poon SHL et al. A systematic review on advances in diagnostics for herpes simplex keratitis. Surv Ophthalmol. 2021;66:514. [PMID: 33186564]

3. Herpes Zoster Ophthalmicus

Herpes zoster frequently involves the ophthalmic division of the trigeminal nerve. It presents with malaise, fever, headache, and periorbital burning and itching. These symptoms may precede the eruption by a day or more. The rash is initially vesicular, quickly becoming pustular and then crusting. Involvement of the tip of the nose or the lid margin predicts involvement of the eye. Ocular signs include conjunctivitis, keratitis, episcleritis, and anterior uveitis, often with elevated intraocular pressure.

Recurrent anterior segment inflammation, neurotrophic keratitis, and posterior subcapsular cataract are long-term complications. Optic neuropathy, cranial nerve palsies, acute retinal necrosis, and cerebral angiitis occur infrequently. HIV infection is an important risk factor for herpes zoster ophthalmicus and increases the likelihood of complications.

High-dose oral acyclovir (800 mg five times a day), valacyclovir (1 g three times a day), or famciclovir (500 mg three times a day) for 7–10 days started within 72 hours after the appearance of the rash reduces the incidence of ocular complications but not of postherpetic neuralgia. Acute keratitis, or a "pseudo-dendrite," can be treated with a topical antiviral such as ganciclovir 0.15% gel, 1 drop five times daily until healing has occurred and then 1 drop three times daily for 1 more week. Anterior uveitis requires additional treatment with topical corticosteroids and cycloplegics. Topical corticosteroids, which promote viral replication, may have to be delayed until the keratitis has resolved. Neurotrophic keratitis is an important cause of long-term morbidity.

When to Refer

Any patient with herpes zoster ophthalmicus and ocular symptoms or signs should be referred urgently to an ophthalmologist.

Davis AR et al. Herpes zoster ophthalmicus review and prevention. Eye Contact Lens. 2019;45:286. [PMID: 30844951]

Vrcek I et al. Herpes zoster ophthalmicus: a review for the internist. Am J Med. 2017;130:21 [PMID: 27644149]

4. Fungal Keratitis

Fungal keratitis tends to occur after corneal injury involving plant material or in an agricultural setting, in eyes with chronic ocular surface disease, and in contact lens wearers. It may be an indolent process. The corneal infiltrate may have feathery edges and multiple "satellite" lesions. A hypopyon may be present. Unlike bacterial keratitis, an epithelial defect may or may not be present. Corneal scrapings should be cultured on media suitable for fungi whenever the history or corneal appearance is suggestive of fungal disease. Diagnosis is often delayed and treatment is difficult, commonly requiring 6 months or longer for severe disease. Natamycin 5%, amphotericin 0.1–0.5%, and voriconazole 0.2–1% are the most frequently used topical agents (Table 7–2). Systemic azoles are probably not helpful unless there is scleritis or intraocular infection. Corneal grafting is often required.

Donovan C et al. Fungal keratitis: mechanisms of infection and management strategies. Surv Ophthalmol. 2021 Aug 20. [Epub ahead of print] [PMID: 34425126]

5. Amoebic Keratitis

Amoebic infection, usually due to *Acanthamoeba*, is an important cause of keratitis. The two greatest risk factors in developed countries are contact lens wear and fresh-water or hot-tub exposure. Although severe pain with perineural and ring infiltrates in the corneal stroma is characteristic, it is not specific and earlier forms with changes confined to the corneal epithelium are identifiable. Diagnosis is facilitated by confocal microscopy and Giemsa staining of cornea smears. Culture requires specialized media. Intensive topical compounded biguanide (polyhexamethylene or chlorhexidine) is initiated immediately, and long-term treatment is required. Diamidine (propamidine or hexamidine) may be added. Oral miltefosine is FDA approved for the treatment of *Acanthamoeba* keratitis, but indications and efficacy have yet to be established. There should be close monitoring for systemic toxicity (vomiting, diarrhea, elevation of transaminases, and kidney function studies) during its use. Delayed diagnosis and prior treatment with topical corticosteroids adversely affect the visual outcome. Corneal grafting may be required after resolution of infection to restore vision. If there is scleral involvement, systemic anti-inflammatory and immunosuppressant medication is helpful in controlling pain, but the prognosis is poor.

Alsoudi AF...Seitzman GD et al. Comparison of two confocal microscopes for diagnosis of acanthamoeba keratitis. Eye (Lond). 2021;35:2061. [PMID: 32760010]

Carrijo-Carvalho LC et al. Therapeutic agents and biocides for ocular infections by free-living amoebae of *Acanthamoeba* genus. Surv Ophthalmol. 2017;62:203. [PMID: 27836717]

ACUTE ANGLE-CLOSURE GLAUCOMA

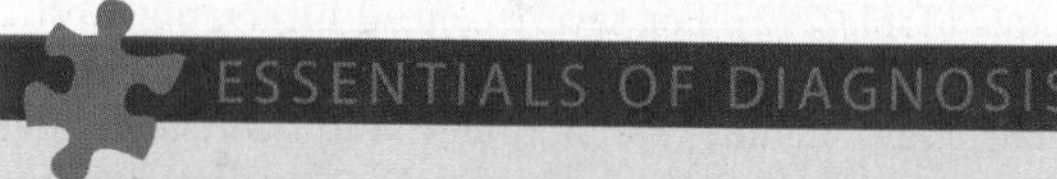

- Older age group, particularly farsighted individuals.
- Rapid onset of severe pain and profound visual loss with "halos around lights."
- Red eye, cloudy cornea, dilated pupil.
- Hard eye on palpation.

General Considerations

Primary acute angle-closure glaucoma (acute angle-closure crisis) results from closure of a preexisting narrow anterior chamber angle. The predisposing factors are shallow anterior chamber, which may be associated with farsightedness or a small eye (short axial length); enlargement of the crystalline lens with age; and inheritance, such as among Inuits and Asians. Closure of the angle is precipitated by pupillary dilation and thus can occur from sitting in a darkened theater, during times of stress, following nonocular administration of anticholinergic or sympathomimetic agents (eg, nebulized bronchodilators, atropine, antidepressants, bowel or bladder antispasmodics, nasal decongestants, or tocolytics), or, rarely, from pharmacologic mydriasis (see Precautions in Management of Ocular Disorders, below). Subacute primary angle-closure glaucoma may present as recurrent headache.

Secondary acute angle-closure glaucoma, for which the mechanism may differ between cases, does not require a preexisting narrow angle. Secondary acute angle-closure glaucoma may occur in anterior uveitis, with dislocation of the lens, with hemodialysis, or due to various drugs (see Adverse Ocular Effects of Systemic Drugs, below). The reduction in serum osmolarity that occurs with hemodialysis causes an osmotic gradient between the plasma and aqueous fluid, leading to a buildup of fluid in the aqueous compartment. Patients with a compromised outflow system (as with narrow angle) cannot accommodate the buildup and the intraocular pressure rises. Symptoms are the same as in primary acute angle-closure glaucoma, but differentiation is important because of differences in management.

Clinical Findings

Patients with acute glaucoma usually seek treatment immediately because of extreme pain and blurred vision, though there are subacute cases. Typically, the blurred vision is associated with halos around lights. Nausea and abdominal pain may occur. The eye is red, the cornea cloudy, and the pupil moderately dilated and nonreactive to light. Intraocular pressure is usually over 50 mm Hg, producing a hard eye on palpation.

Differential Diagnosis

Acute glaucoma must be differentiated from conjunctivitis, acute uveitis, and corneal disorders (Table 7–1).

Treatment

Initial treatment, regardless of mechanism, is reduction of intraocular pressure. A single 500-mg intravenous dose of acetazolamide, followed by 250 mg orally four times a day, together with topical medications that lower intraocular pressure is usually sufficient. Osmotic diuretics, such as oral glycerin and intravenous urea or mannitol—the dosage of all three being 1–2 g/kg—may be necessary if there is no response to acetazolamide. Definitive treatment depends on the mechanism.

A. Primary Angle-Closure Glaucoma

In primary acute angle-closure glaucoma, once the intraocular pressure has started to fall, topical 4% pilocarpine, 1 drop every 15 minutes for 1 hour and then four times a day, is used to reverse the underlying angle closure. The definitive treatment is cataract extraction, which is becoming more of a first-line treatment. Laser peripheral iridotomy is also still accepted as a first-line treatment.

All patients with primary acute angle closure should undergo prophylactic laser peripheral iridotomy to the unaffected eye, or early cataract extraction should be considered, unless that eye has already undergone cataract or glaucoma surgery.

B. Secondary Angle-Closure Glaucoma

In secondary acute angle-closure glaucoma, additional treatment is determined by the cause.

Prognosis

Untreated acute angle-closure glaucoma results in severe and permanent visual loss within 2–5 days after onset of symptoms. Affected patients need to be monitored for development of chronic glaucoma.

When to Refer

Any patient with suspected acute angle-closure glaucoma must be referred emergently to an ophthalmologist.

Prum BE Jr et al. Primary Angle Closure Preferred Practice Pattern(®) Guidelines. Ophthalmology. 2016;123:P1. [PMID: 26581557]

Tanner L et al. Has the EAGLE landed for the use of clear lens extraction in angle-closure glaucoma? And how should primary angle-closure suspects be treated? Eye (Lond). 2020;34:40. [PMID: 31649349]

CHRONIC GLAUCOMA

ESSENTIALS OF DIAGNOSIS

- Three types of chronic glaucoma: open-angle glaucoma, angle-closure glaucoma, and normal-tension glaucoma.
- No symptoms in early stages.
- Insidious progressive bilateral loss of peripheral vision resulting in tunnel vision; visual acuities preserved until advanced disease.
- Pathologic cupping of the optic disks.
- Intraocular pressure is usually elevated.

General Considerations

Chronic glaucoma is characterized by gradually progressive excavation ("cupping") of the optic disk with loss of vision progressing from slight visual field loss to complete blindness. In **chronic open-angle glaucoma,** primary or secondary, intraocular pressure is elevated due to reduced drainage of aqueous fluid through the trabecular meshwork. In **chronic angle-closure glaucoma,** which is particularly common in Inuits and eastern Asians, flow of aqueous fluid into the anterior chamber angle is obstructed. In **normal-tension glaucoma,** intraocular pressure is not elevated but the same pattern of optic nerve damage occurs.

Primary chronic open-angle glaucoma is usually bilateral. There is an increased prevalence in first-degree relatives of affected individuals and in diabetic patients. In Afro-Caribbean and African persons, and probably in Hispanic persons, it is more frequent, occurs at an earlier age, and results in more severe optic nerve damage. Secondary chronic open-angle glaucoma may result from ocular disease, eg, pigment dispersion, pseudoexfoliation, uveitis, or trauma; or corticosteroid therapy, whether it is intraocular, topical, inhaled, intranasal, or systemic.

In the United States, it is estimated that 2% of people over 40 years of age have glaucoma, affecting over 2.5 million individuals. At least 25% of cases are undetected. Over 90% of cases are of the open-angle type. Worldwide, about 45 million people have open-angle glaucoma, of whom about 4.5 million are bilaterally blind. About 4 million people, of whom approximately 50% live in China, are bilaterally blind from chronic angle-closure glaucoma.

Clinical Findings

Because initially there are no symptoms, chronic glaucoma is often first suspected at a routine eye test. Diagnosis requires consistent and reproducible abnormalities in at least two of three parameters—optic disk or retinal nerve fiber layer (or both), visual field, and intraocular pressure.

1. Optic disk cupping—Optic disk cupping is identified as an absolute increase or an asymmetry between the two eyes of the ratio of the diameter of the optic cup to the diameter of the whole optic disk (cup-disk ratio). (Cup-disk ratio greater than 0.5 or asymmetry between eyes of 0.2 or more is suggestive.) Detection of optic disk cupping and associated abnormalities of the retinal nerve fiber layer is facilitated by optical coherence tomography scans.

2. Visual field abnormalities—Visual field abnormalities initially develop in the paracentral region, followed by constriction of the peripheral visual field. Central vision remains good until late in the disease.

3. Intraocular pressure—The normal range of intraocular pressure is 10–21 mm Hg. In many individuals (about 4.5 million in the United States), elevated intraocular pressure is not associated with optic disk or visual field abnormalities (ocular hypertension). Monitoring for the development of glaucoma is required in all such cases; a significant proportion of eyes with primary open-angle glaucoma have normal intraocular pressure when it is first measured, and only repeated measurements identify the abnormally high pressure. In normal-tension glaucoma, intraocular pressure is always within the normal range.

Prevention

There are many causes of optic disk abnormalities or visual field changes that mimic glaucoma, and visual field testing may prove unreliable in some patients, particularly in the older age group. Hence, the diagnosis of glaucoma is not always straightforward and screening programs need to involve eye care professionals.

Although all persons over age 50 years may benefit from intraocular pressure measurement and optic disk examination every 3–5 years, screening for chronic open-angle glaucoma should be targeted at individuals with an affected first-degree relative, at persons who have diabetes mellitus, and at older individuals with African or Hispanic ancestry. Screening may also be warranted in patients taking long-term oral or combined intranasal and inhaled corticosteroid therapy. Screening for chronic angle-closure glaucoma should be targeted at Inuits and Asians.

Treatment

A. Medications

Medical treatment is directed toward lowering intraocular pressure, even with normal-tension glaucoma. Prostaglandin analog eye drops are commonly used as first-line therapy because of their efficacy, lack of systemic side effects, and convenient once-daily dose (except unoprostone) (see Table 7–2 for medications, doses, and side effects). All may produce conjunctival hyperemia, permanent darkening of the iris and eyebrow color, increased eyelash growth, and reduction of periorbital fat (prostaglandin-associated periorbitopathy). Latanoprostene bunod is metabolized into latanoprost and another component that releases nitric oxide, which increases trabecular outflow. Topical beta-adrenergic blocking agents may be used alone or in combination with a prostaglandin analog. They may be contraindicated in patients with reactive airway disease or heart failure. Cardioselective betaxolol is theoretically safer in reactive airway disease but less effective at reducing intraocular pressure. Brimonidine 0.2%, a selective alpha-2-agonist, and topical carbonic anhydrase inhibitors also can be used in addition to a prostaglandin analog or a beta-blocker or as initial therapy when prostaglandin analogs and beta-blockers are contraindicated. All three are associated with allergic reactions. Brimonidine may cause uveitis. Apraclonidine, 0.5–1%, another alpha-2-agonist, can be used to defer the need for surgery in patients receiving maximal medical therapy, but long-term use is limited by adverse reactions. It is more commonly used to control acute rise in intraocular pressure, such as after laser therapy. The topical agent netarsudil ophthalmic solution 0.02% (a Rho kinase inhibitor) increases aqueous fluid outflow through the trabecular meshwork. Pilocarpine 1–4% is rarely used because of adverse effects. Oral carbonic anhydrase inhibitors (acetazolamide, methazolamide, and dichlorphenamide) may be used on a long-term basis if topical therapy is inadequate and surgical or laser therapy is inappropriate.

Various eye drop preparations combining two agents (eg, prostaglandin analogs, beta-adrenergic blocking agents, brimonidine, and topical carbonic anhydrase inhibitors) are available to improve compliance when multiple medications are required. Formulations of one or two agents without preservative or not including benzalkonium chloride as the preservative are preferred to reduce adverse ocular effects for patients with allergies or severe dry eyes.

B. Laser Therapy and Surgery

1. Open-angle glaucoma—Laser trabeculoplasty is used as an adjunct to topical therapy to defer surgery for open-angle glaucoma; it is also advocated as primary treatment, especially when compliance with medications is an issue. Surgery is generally undertaken when intraocular pressure is inadequately controlled by medical and laser therapy, but it may also be used as primary treatment in advanced cases. Trabeculectomy remains the standard procedure. Adjunctive treatment with subconjunctival mitomycin or fluorouracil is used perioperatively or postoperatively in worse prognosis cases. A variety of less invasive procedures that avoid a full-thickness incision into the eye, called microinvasive glaucoma surgery, are appropriate for moderate glaucoma and are associated with fewer complications but can be more difficult to perform.

2. Angle-closure glaucoma—In chronic angle-closure glaucoma, laser peripheral iridotomy, surgical peripheral iridectomy, or cataract extraction may be helpful. In patients with asymptomatic narrow anterior chamber angles, which includes about 10% of Chinese adults, prophylactic laser peripheral iridotomy can be performed to reduce the risk of acute and chronic angle-closure glaucoma. However, there are concerns about the efficacy of such treatment and the risk of cataract progression and corneal decompensation. In the United States, about 1% of people over age 35 years have narrow anterior chamber angles, but acute and chronic angle closure are sufficiently uncommon that prophylactic therapy is not generally advised.

3. Normal-tension glaucoma—The goal of treatment for normal-tension glaucoma is reduction in intraocular pressure (even if it is in the normal range) to prevent progression. As with open-angle glaucoma, if intraocular pressure is not lowered with medical therapy alone, laser trabeculoplasty is used as an adjunct. Trabeculectomy is the standard surgical procedure if medical and laser therapy are inadequate.

Prognosis

Untreated chronic glaucoma that begins at age 40–45 years will probably cause complete blindness by age 60–65. Early diagnosis and treatment can preserve useful vision throughout life. In primary open-angle glaucoma and if treatment is required in ocular hypertension, the aim is to reduce intraocular pressure to a level that will adequately reduce progression of visual field loss. In eyes with marked visual field or optic disk changes, intraocular pressure must be reduced to less than 16 mm Hg. In normal-tension glaucoma with progressive visual field loss, it is necessary to achieve even lower intraocular pressure such that surgery is often required.

When to Refer

All patients with suspected chronic glaucoma should be referred to an ophthalmologist.

Jonas JB et al. Glaucoma. Lancet. 2017;390:2183. [PMID: 28577860]
Prum BE Jr et al. Primary open-angle glaucoma Preferred Practice Pattern(®) guidelines. Ophthalmology. 2016;123:P41. [PMID: 26581556]
Schehlein EM et al. New classes of glaucoma medications. Curr Opin Ophthalmol. 2017;28:161. [PMID: 27828896]
Stein JD et al. Glaucoma in adults—screening, diagnosis, and management: a review. JAMA. 2021;325:164. [PMID: 33433580]

UVEITIS

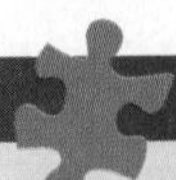

ESSENTIALS OF DIAGNOSIS

- Usually immunologic but possibly infective or neoplastic.
- Inflammation may be confined to the eye or may be systemic.
- **Acute anterior uveitis:** sudden redness and blurry vision often with photophobia.
- **Posterior uveitis:** gradual loss of vision, commonly with floaters, in a variably inflamed eye.

General Considerations

Intraocular inflammation (uveitis) is classified as acute or chronic and as nongranulomatous or granulomatous, according to the clinical signs, and by its involvement of the anterior, intermediate, posterior, or all (panuveitis) segments of the eye.

In most cases the pathogenesis of uveitis is primarily immunologic, but infection may be the cause, particularly in immunodeficiency states. The systemic disorders associated with acute nongranulomatous anterior uveitis are the HLA-B27-related conditions (ankylosing spondylitis, reactive arthritis, psoriasis, ulcerative colitis, and Crohn disease). Chronic nongranulomatous anterior uveitis occurs in juvenile idiopathic arthritis. Behçet syndrome produces both anterior uveitis, with recurrent hypopyon, and posterior uveitis, characteristically with branch retinal vein occlusions. Both herpes simplex and herpes zoster infections may cause nongranulomatous and granulomatous anterior uveitis as well as retinitis (acute retinal necrosis).

Diseases producing granulomatous anterior uveitis also tend to be causes of posterior uveitis. These include sarcoidosis, toxoplasmosis, tuberculosis, syphilis, Vogt-Koyanagi-Harada disease (bilateral uveitis associated with alopecia, poliosis [depigmented eyelashes, eyebrows, or hair], vitiligo, and hearing loss), and sympathetic ophthalmia that occurs after penetrating ocular trauma. In toxoplasmosis, there may be evidence of previous episodes of retinochoroiditis. Syphilis characteristically produces a "salt and pepper" fundus but may present with a wide variety of clinical manifestations. The principal pathogens responsible for ocular inflammation in HIV infection are cytomegalovirus (CMV), herpes simplex and herpes zoster viruses, mycobacteria, *Cryptococcus, Toxoplasma,* and *Candida.*

Retinal vasculitis and intermediate uveitis predominantly manifest as posterior uveitis with central or peripheral retinal abnormalities in retinal vasculitis and far peripheral retinal abnormalities (pars planitis) in intermediate uveitis. Retinal vasculitis can be caused by a wide variety of infectious agents and noninfectious systemic conditions but also may be idiopathic. Intermediate uveitis is often idiopathic but can be due to multiple sclerosis or sarcoidosis.

Clinical Findings

Anterior uveitis is characterized by inflammatory cells and flare within the aqueous. In severe cases, there may be hypopyon (layered collection of white cells) and fibrin within the anterior chamber. Cells may also be seen on the corneal endothelium as keratic precipitates. In granulomatous uveitis, there are large "mutton-fat" keratic precipitates, and sometimes iris nodules. In nongranulomatous uveitis, the keratic precipitates are smaller or absent with no iris nodules. The pupil is usually small, and with the development of posterior synechiae (adhesions between the iris and anterior lens capsule), it also becomes irregularly shaped and poorly reactive.

Nongranulomatous anterior uveitis tends to present acutely with unilateral pain, redness, photophobia, and visual loss. However, the ocular inflammation associated with juvenile idiopathic arthritis is frequently indolent, commonly asymptomatic initially, and carries a high risk of sight-threatening complications. Granulomatous anterior uveitis is also frequently chronic, recurrent, and indolent, causing blurred vision in a variably inflamed eye.

In **posterior uveitis,** there are cells in the vitreous and there may be inflammatory retinal or choroidal lesions. New retinal lesions are yellow with indistinct margins and there may be retinal hemorrhages. Older lesions have more defined margins and are commonly pigmented. Retinal vessel sheathing may occur adjacent to such lesions or more diffusely. In severe cases, vitreous opacity precludes visualization of retinal details.

Posterior uveitis can be unilateral or bilateral with symptoms of floaters and visual loss. Symptoms are commonly slower in onset, though acute presentations can occur. Visual loss may be due to vitreous haze and opacities, inflammatory lesions involving the macula, macular edema, retinal vein occlusion, or rarely, optic neuropathy.

Differential Diagnosis

Retinal detachment, intraocular tumors, and CNS lymphoma may all masquerade as uveitis.

Treatment

Anterior uveitis usually responds to topical corticosteroids. Occasionally, periocular or intraocular corticosteroid injections or even systemic corticosteroids are required. Dilation of the pupil is important to relieve discomfort and prevent permanent posterior synechiae. **Posterior uveitis** more commonly requires systemic, periocular, or intravitreal corticosteroid therapy. In chronic cases, systemic corticosteroid-sparing immunomodulatory therapy with agents such as azathioprine, cyclosporine, mycophenolate, methotrexate, tacrolimus, or sirolimus is commonly required. Biologic therapies are also often used. Pupillary dilation is not usually necessary.

If an infectious cause is identified, specific antimicrobial therapy is often needed. In general, the prognosis for anterior uveitis, particularly the nongranulomatous type, is better than for posterior uveitis.

When to Refer

- Any patient with suspected acute uveitis should be referred urgently to an ophthalmologist or emergently if visual loss or pain is severe.
- Any patient with suspected chronic uveitis should be referred to an ophthalmologist, urgently if there is more than mild visual loss.

When to Admit

Patients with severe uveitis, particularly those requiring intravenous therapy, may require hospital admission.

Al-Janabi A et al. Long-term outcomes of treatment with biological agents in eyes with refractory, active, noninfectious intermediate uveitis, posterior uveitis, or panuveitis. Ophthalmology. 2020;127:410. [PMID: 31607412]

Jabs DA. Immunosuppression for the uveitides. Ophthalmology. 2018;125:193. [PMID: 28942074]

Krishna U et al. Uveitis: a sight-threatening disease which can impact all systems. Postgrad Med J. 2017;93:766. [PMID: 28942431]

Rathinam SR et al; FAST Research Group. Effect of corticosteroid-sparing treatment with mycophenolate mofetil vs methotrexate on inflammation in patients with uveitis: a randomized clinical trial. JAMA. 2019;322:936. [PMID: 31503307]

Sève P et al. Uveitis: diagnostic work-up. A literature review and recommendations from an expert committee. Autoimmun Rev. 2017;16:1254. [PMID: 29037906]

CATARACT

ESSENTIALS OF DIAGNOSIS

- Gradually progressive blurred vision.
- No pain or redness.
- Lens opacities (may be grossly visible).

General Considerations

Cataracts are opacities of the crystalline lens and are usually bilateral. They are the leading cause of blindness worldwide. Age-related cataract is by far the most common cause. Other causes include (1) congenital (from intrauterine infections, such as rubella and CMV, or inborn errors of metabolism, such as galactosemia); (2) traumatic; (3) secondary to systemic disease (diabetes mellitus, myotonic dystrophy, atopic dermatitis); (4) topical, systemic, or inhaled corticosteroid treatment; (5) uveitis; or

(6) radiation exposure. Most persons over age 60 have some degree of lens opacity. Cigarette smoking increases the risk of cataract formation. Multivitamin/mineral supplements and high dietary antioxidants may prevent the development of age-related cataract.

Clinical Findings

The predominant symptom is progressive blurring of vision. Glare, especially in bright light or with night driving; change of focusing, particularly development of nearsightedness; and monocular double vision may occur.

Even in its early stages, a cataract can be seen through a dilated pupil with an ophthalmoscope or slit lamp. As the cataract matures, the retina will become increasingly difficult to visualize, until finally the fundus reflection is absent and the pupil is white.

Treatment

Functional visual impairment, specifically its effect on daily activities and increased risk of falls, is the prime criterion for surgery. The cataract is usually removed by one of the techniques in which the posterior lens capsule remains (extracapsular), thus providing support for a prosthetic intraocular lens. Ultrasonic fragmentation (phacoemulsification) of the lens nucleus and foldable intraocular lenses allow cataract surgery to be performed through a small incision without the need for sutures, thus reducing the postoperative complication rate and accelerating visual rehabilitation. The standard monofocal prosthetic intraocular lens can correct near or far vision. Premium intraocular lenses (multifocal, extended depth of focus, and accommodative) reduce the need for both distance and near vision correction. In the developing world, manual small-incision surgery, in which the lens nucleus is removed intact, is popular because less equipment is required. Additional laser treatment may be required subsequently (months to years after the initial cataract surgery) if the posterior capsule opacifies. The use of topical eye drops to dissolve or prevent cataracts has shown promising results in experimental models; surgery, however, is currently the only treatment option for a visually significant cataract.

Prognosis

Cataract surgery is cost-effective in improving survival and quality of life. In the developed world, it improves visual acuity in 95% of cases. In the other 5%, there is preexisting retinal damage or operative or postoperative complications. In less developed areas, the improvement in visual acuity is not as high, in part due to uncorrected refractive error postoperatively. A large number of drugs, such as alpha-adrenoreceptor antagonists for benign prostatic hyperplasia or systemic hypertension and antipsychotics, increase the risk of complications during surgery (floppy iris syndrome) and in the early postoperative period. Nasolacrimal duct obstruction increases the risk of intraocular infection (endophthalmitis).

The alpha-blocker tamsulosin has been shown to have the greatest risk of floppy iris syndrome. There is no consensus about whether to stop alpha-blockers before surgery because the effects of the drug on the iris can persist for months to years. The surgeon must know if the patient is taking an alpha-blocker to prepare for iris issues during surgery. If the patient has not yet started an alpha-blocker and is planning to have cataract surgery shortly, it is best to wait until after surgery to begin the medication, if possible.

When to Refer

Patients with cataracts should be referred to an ophthalmologist when their visual impairment adversely affects their everyday activities.

Enright JM et al. Floppy iris syndrome and cataract surgery. Curr Opin Ophthalmol. 2017;28:29. [PMID: 27653607]

Lian RR et al. The quest for homeopathic and nonsurgical cataract treatment. Curr Opin Ophthalmol. 2020;31:61. [PMID: 31770163]

Nanji KC et al. Preventing adverse events in cataract surgery: recommendations from a Massachusetts expert panel. Anesth Analg. 2018;126:1537. [PMID: 28991115]

Rampat R et al. Multifocal and extended depth-of-focus intraocular lenses in 2020. Ophthalmology. 2021;128:e164. [PMID: 32980397]

RETINAL DETACHMENT

ESSENTIALS OF DIAGNOSIS

- Loss of vision in one eye that is usually rapid, possibly with "curtain" spreading across field of vision.
- No pain or redness.
- Detachment seen by ophthalmoscopy.

General Considerations

Most cases of retinal detachment are due to development of one or more peripheral retinal tears or holes (rhegmatogenous retinal detachment). This usually results from posterior vitreous detachment, related to degenerative changes in the vitreous, and often occurs in persons over 50 years of age. Nearsightedness and cataract extraction are the two most common predisposing causes. It may also be caused by penetrating or blunt ocular trauma, sometimes years earlier.

Tractional retinal detachment occurs when there is preretinal fibrosis, such as in proliferative retinopathy due to diabetic retinopathy or retinal vein occlusion, or as a complication of rhegmatogenous retinal detachment. Exudative retinal detachment results from accumulation of subretinal fluid, such as in neovascular age-related macular degeneration or secondary to choroidal tumor.

Clinical Findings

Rhegmatogenous retinal detachment usually starts in the peripheral retina, spreading rapidly to cause visual field loss. Symptoms of the predisposing posterior vitreous

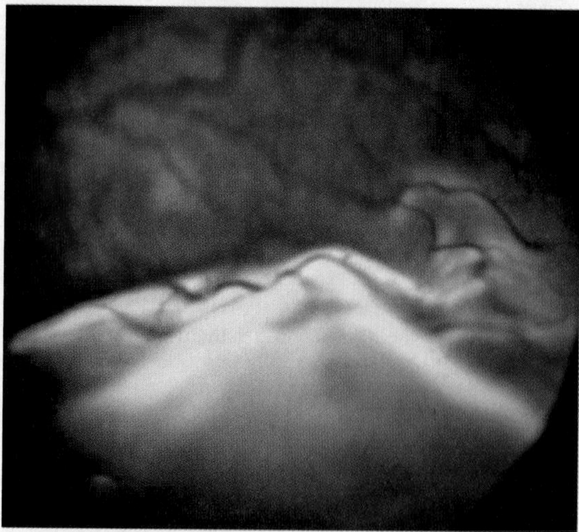

▲ **Figure 7–1.** Inferior retinal detachment as seen on direct or indirect ophthalmoscopy.

detachment with vitreo-retinal traction include recent onset of or increase in floaters (moving spots or strands like cobwebs in the visual field) and photopsias (flashes of light). Central vision remains intact until the central macula becomes detached. On ophthalmoscopic examination, the retina may be seen elevated in the vitreous cavity with an irregular surface (Figure 7–1). In tractional retinal detachment, there is irregular retinal elevation adherent to scar tissue on the retinal surface, sometimes extending into the vitreous. Exudative retinal detachments are dome-shaped and the subretinal fluid shifts position with changes in posture. Ocular ultrasonography assists the detection and characterization of retinal detachment.

Treatment

Treatment of rhegmatogenous retinal detachments requires closing all the retinal tears and holes by forming a permanent adhesion between the neurosensory retina, the retinal pigment epithelium, and the choroid with laser photocoagulation to the retina or cryotherapy to the sclera. Certain types of uncomplicated retinal detachment may be treated by pneumatic retinopexy, in which an expansile gas is injected into the vitreous cavity and the patient's head is positioned to facilitate apposition between the gas and the hole, which permits reattachment of the retina. Once the retina is reattached, the retinal defects are surrounded by laser photocoagulation or cryotherapy scars; these two methods are also used to seal retinal defects without associated detachment.

In complicated retinal detachments, particularly tractional retinal detachments, retinal reattachment can be accomplished only by vitrectomy, direct manipulation of the retina, and internal tamponade of the retina with air, expansile gas, or silicone oil. The presence of an expansile gas within the eye is a contraindication to air travel, mountaineering at high altitude, and nitrous oxide anesthesia, all of which can cause the gas to expand with severe increases in intraocular pressure. Such gases persist in the globe for weeks after surgery. (See Chapter 37.) Treatment of exudative retinal detachments is determined by the underlying cause.

Prognosis

About 90% of uncomplicated rhegmatogenous retinal detachments can be cured with one operation. The visual prognosis is worse if the macula is detached or if the detachment is of long duration.

When to Refer

All cases of retinal detachment must be referred urgently to an ophthalmologist, and emergently if central vision is good because this indicates that the macula has not yet detached. During transportation, the patient's head is positioned so that the retinal tear is placed at the lowest point of the eye to minimize extension of the detached retina. If the inferior retina is detached, the patient should keep the head upright so that the tear is located at the lowest point, whereas if the temporal retina is detached, the patient should keep the temporal side of the head down to reduce the chances that the fluid will extend beneath the central retina, causing the macula to detach. If vision is good and the macula is attached, patients should minimize eye motion; in some patients, patching both eyes can be helpful in preventing the eyes from moving rapidly around until surgery can be performed to repair the retinal detachment.

Lahham S et al. Role of point of care ultrasound in the diagnosis of retinal detachment in the emergency department. Open Access Emerg Med. 2019;11:265. [PMID: 32009820]

Sultan ZN et al. Rhegmatogenous retinal detachment: a review of current practice in diagnosis and management. BMJ Open Ophthalmol. 2020;5:e000474. [PMID: 33083551]

VITREOUS HEMORRHAGE

Patients with vitreous hemorrhage complain of sudden visual loss, abrupt onset of floaters that may progressively increase in severity, or occasionally, "bleeding within the eye." Visual acuity ranges from 20/20 (6/6) to light perception. The eye is not inflamed, red, or painful, and clues to diagnosis are inability to see fundus details or localized blood in the vitreous, in front of the retina. Causes of vitreous hemorrhage include retinal tear (with or without detachment), diabetic or sickle cell retinopathy, retinal vein occlusion, retinal vasculitis, neovascular age-related macular degeneration, retinal arterial macroaneurysm, blood dyscrasia, therapeutic anticoagulation, trauma, subarachnoid hemorrhage, and severe straining (Valsalva retinopathy).

When to Refer

All patients with suspected vitreous hemorrhage must be referred urgently to an ophthalmologist to determine the etiology. If the vitreous hemorrhage is caused by a retinal tear or detachment, it must be repaired urgently to prevent permanent vision loss.

Manandhar LD et al. Clinical profile and management of vitreous hemorrhage in tertiary eye care centre in Nepal. Nepal J Ophthalmol. 2020;12:99. [PMID: 32799245]

Propst SL et al. Ocular point-of-care ultrasonography to diagnose posterior chamber abnormalities: a systematic review and meta-analysis. JAMA Netw Open. 2020;3:e1921460. [PMID: 32074291]

AGE-RELATED MACULAR DEGENERATION

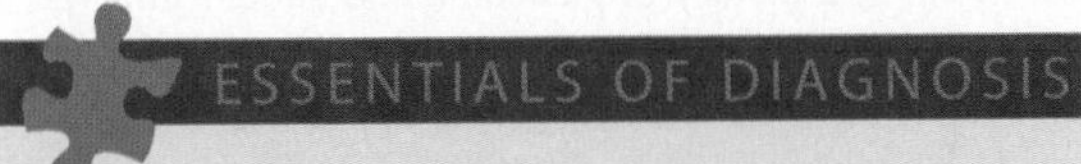

ESSENTIALS OF DIAGNOSIS

- Older age group.
- In one or both eyes; acute or chronic deterioration of central vision; distortion or abnormal size of images, sometimes developing acutely.
- No pain or redness.
- Classified as dry ("atrophic," "geographic") or wet ("neovascular," "exudative") macular degeneration.
- Macular abnormalities seen by ophthalmoscopy.

General Considerations

Age-related macular degeneration is the leading cause of permanent visual loss in the older population. Its prevalence progressively increases over age 50 years (to almost 30% by age 75). Its occurrence and response to treatment are likely influenced by genetically determined variations, many of which involve the complement pathway. Other associated factors are sex (slight female predominance), family history, hypertension, hypercholesterolemia, cardiovascular disease, farsightedness, light iris color, and cigarette smoking (the most readily modifiable risk factor).

Although both dry and wet age-related macular degeneration are progressive and usually bilateral, they differ in manifestations, prognosis, and management.

Clinical Findings

Drusen are the hallmark of age-related macular degeneration. Hard drusen appear ophthalmoscopically as discrete yellow subretinal deposits. Soft drusen are paler and less distinct. Large, confluent soft drusen are risk factors for neovascular (wet) age-related macular degeneration. Vision loss in age-related macular degeneration involves the central vision only in most patients. Peripheral fields, and hence navigational vision, are maintained, except in patients with severe neovascular age-related macular degeneration.

"Dry" age-related macular degeneration is characterized by gradually progressive bilateral visual loss due to geographic atrophy of the outer retina, the retinal pigment epithelium, and the choriocapillaris, which supplies blood to both the outer retina and the retinal pigment epithelium. In **"wet" age-related macular degeneration**, choroidal new vessels grow under either the retina or the retinal pigment epithelial cells, leading to accumulation of exudative fluid, hemorrhage, and fibrosis. The onset of visual loss is more rapid and more severe than in atrophic degeneration. The two eyes are frequently affected sequentially over a period of a few years. Although "dry" age-related macular degeneration is much more common, untreated "wet" age-related macular degeneration accounts for about 90% of all cases of legal blindness due to age-related macular degeneration.

Treatment

No dietary modification has been shown to prevent the development of age-related macular degeneration, but its progression may be reduced by oral treatment with antioxidants (vitamins C and E), zinc, copper, and carotenoids (lutein and zeaxanthin, rather than vitamin A [beta-carotene]). Oral omega-3 fatty acids do not provide additional benefit.

There is no specific treatment for dry age-related macular degeneration but, as for wet degeneration, rehabilitation including low-vision aids is important. In addition, patients should be advised to stop smoking and to take vitamin supplements as described above.

In wet age-related macular degeneration, inhibitors of vascular endothelial growth factors (VEGF), such as ranibizumab, bevacizumab, aflibercept, and brolucizumab, can cause regression of choroidal neovascularization with resorption of subretinal fluid and improvement or stabilization of vision. Long-term repeated intraocular injections are required and must be administered in the eye clinic several times a year, if not monthly. Treatment is well tolerated with minimal adverse effects, but there is a risk of infection (1/2000), retinal detachment (1/10,000), vitreous hemorrhage, and cataract. Brolucizumab has been associated with intraocular inflammation and occlusive retinal vasculitis resulting in irreversible vision loss in some patients. A certain percentage of patients do not respond to anti-VEGF injections and up to one-third of eyes lose vision despite regular treatment.

When to Refer

Older patients with sudden visual loss, particularly paracentral or central distortion or scotoma with preserved central acuity, should be referred urgently to an ophthalmologist.

Baumal CR et al. Retinal vasculitis and intraocular inflammation after intravitreal injection of brolucizumab. Ophthalmology. 2020;127:1345. [PMID: 32344075]

Cabral de Guimaraes TA et al. Treatments for dry age-related macular degeneration: therapeutic avenues, clinical trials and future directions. Br J Ophthalmol. 2022;106:297. [PMID: 33741584]

Plyukhova AA et al. Comparative safety of bevacizumab, ranibizumab and aflibercept for treatment of neovascular age-related macular degeneration (AMD): a systematic review and network meta-analysis of direct comparative studies. J Clin Med. 2020;9:1522. [PMID: 32443612]

CENTRAL & BRANCH RETINAL VEIN OCCLUSIONS

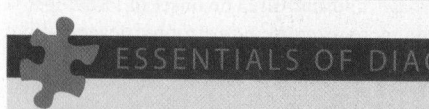

- Sudden monocular loss of vision.
- No pain or redness.
- Widespread or sectoral retinal hemorrhages.

General Considerations

Central and branch retinal vein occlusion are common causes of acute vision loss, with branch vein occlusions being four times more common. The major predisposing factors are the etiologic factors associated with arteriosclerosis, but glaucoma is also a major risk factor.

Clinical Findings

A. Symptoms and Signs

Ophthalmoscopic signs of **central retinal vein occlusion** include widespread retinal hemorrhages, retinal venous dilation and tortuosity, retinal cotton-wool spots, and optic disk swelling (Figure 7–2). Rarely, central retinal vein occlusion presents with severe vision loss and pain when neovascularization of the iris develops, usually about 90 days after a central retinal vein occlusion has caused severe retinal nonperfusion.

Branch retinal vein occlusion may present in a variety of ways. Sudden loss of vision may occur at the time of occlusion if the fovea is involved, or some time afterward from vitreous hemorrhage due to retinal new vessels. More gradual visual loss may occur with development of macular edema. In acute branch retinal vein occlusion, the retinal abnormalities (hemorrhages, microaneurysms, venous dilation and tortuosity, and cotton-wool spots) are confined to the area drained by the obstructed vein.

To assess for possible reversible risk factors, check blood pressure and ask about tobacco smoking in all patients, and ask women about estrogen therapy (including combined oral contraceptives). Patients should also be asked about a history of glaucoma and should undergo a comprehensive eye examination to check intraocular pressure and for signs of open- or narrow-angle glaucoma.

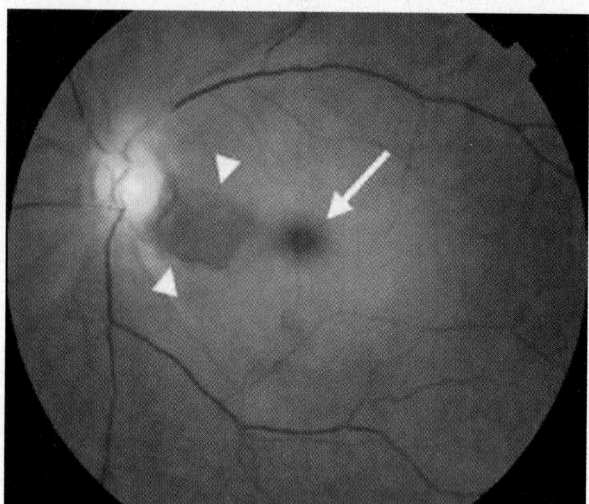

▲ **Figure 7–2.** Acute central retinal artery occlusion with cherry-red spot (arrow) seen at the fovea centered in macular loss of retinal transparency, and preserved retinal perfusion (arrowheads) adjacent to the optic disk due to macular cilioretinal artery supply. (Reproduced, with permission, from Riordan-Eva P, Augsburger JJ. *Vaughan & Asbury's General Ophthalmology*, 19th ed. McGraw Hill, 2018.)

B. Laboratory Findings

Obtain screening laboratory studies for diabetes mellitus, hyperlipidemia, and hyperviscosity (especially in simultaneous bilateral disease), including serum protein electrophoresis for paraproteinemia. Particularly in younger patients, consider obtaining antiphospholipid antibodies, lupus anticoagulant, tests for inherited thrombophilia, and plasma homocysteine levels.

Complications

If central retinal vein occlusion is associated with widespread retinal ischemia, manifesting as poor visual acuity (20/200 [6/60] or worse), florid retinal abnormalities, an afferent pupillary defect, and extensive areas of capillary closure on fluorescein angiography, there is a high risk of development of neovascular (rubeotic) glaucoma, typically within the first 3 months after the occlusion. Branch retinal vein occlusion may be complicated by peripheral retinal neovascularization or chronic macular edema.

Treatment

A. Macular Edema

Intravitreal injection of VEGF inhibitors, including ranibizumab, bevacizumab, or aflibercept, is beneficial in patients with macular edema due to either branch or central retinal vein occlusion. Intravitreal triamcinolone improves vision in chronic macular edema due to nonischemic central retinal vein occlusion, whereas an intravitreal implant containing dexamethasone is beneficial in both central and branch retinal vein occlusion. However, intraocular corticosteroids carry the risk of glaucoma in 20–65% of patients and will cause cataract in all patients who have not already had cataract surgery. Retinal laser photocoagulation may be indicated in chronic macular edema due to branch, but not central, retinal vein occlusion, but most patients are treated with VEGF inhibitor injections rather than laser.

B. Neovascularization

Eyes at risk for neovascular glaucoma following ischemic central retinal vein occlusion can be treated with panretinal laser photocoagulation prophylactically or as soon as there is evidence of neovascularization, with the latter approach necessitating frequent monitoring. Regression of retinal and iris neovascularization can be achieved with intravitreal injections of bevacizumab or other anti-VEGF agents. In branch retinal vein occlusion complicated by retinal neovascularization, the ischemic retina should be treated with laser photocoagulation.

Prognosis

In central retinal vein occlusion, severity of visual loss initially is a good guide to visual outcome. Initial visual acuity of 20/60 (6/18) or better indicates a good prognosis. Visual prognosis is poor for eyes with neovascular glaucoma. In branch retinal vein occlusion, visual outcome is determined by the severity of glaucoma and macular damage from hemorrhage, ischemia, or edema.

When to Refer

All patients with retinal vein occlusion should be referred urgently to an ophthalmologist.

Ang JL et al. A systematic review of real-world evidence of the management of macular oedema secondary to branch retinal vein occlusion. Eye (Lond). 2020;34:1770. [PMID: 32313172]

Hykin P et al; LEAVO Study Group. Clinical effectiveness of intravitreal therapy with ranibizumab vs aflibercept vs bevacizumab for macular edema secondary to central retinal vein occlusion: a randomized clinical trial. JAMA Ophthalmol. 2019;137:1256. [PMID: 31465100]

Scott IU et al. Month 24 outcomes after treatment initiation with anti-vascular endothelial growth factor therapy for macular edema due to central retinal or hemiretinal vein occlusion: SCORE2 Report 10: a secondary analysis of the SCORE2 randomized clinical trial. JAMA Ophthalmol. 2018;136:337. [PMID: 29476687]

Shalchi Z et al. Anti-vascular endothelial growth factor for macular oedema secondary to branch retinal vein occlusion. Cochrane Database Syst Rev. 2020;7:CD009510. [PMID: 32633861]

CENTRAL & BRANCH RETINAL ARTERY OCCLUSIONS

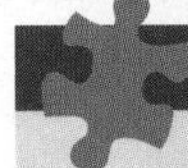

ESSENTIALS OF DIAGNOSIS

- Sudden monocular loss of vision.
- No pain or redness.
- Widespread or sectoral pale retinal swelling.

General Considerations

Acute retinal arterial ischemia, including central and branch retinal artery occlusion, is a true ocular and medical emergency. In patients 50 years of age or older with central retinal artery occlusion, giant cell arteritis must be considered (see Ischemic Optic Neuropathy and Chapter 20). Otherwise, even if no retinal emboli are identified on ophthalmoscopy, urgent investigation for carotid and cardiac sources of emboli must be undertaken in central and branch retinal artery occlusion so that timely treatment can be given to reduce the risk of stroke (see Chapters 12, 14, and 24). Diabetes mellitus, hyperlipidemia, and systemic hypertension are common etiologic factors. Migraine, oral contraceptives, systemic vasculitis, congenital or acquired thrombophilia, and hyperhomocysteinemia are also causes, particularly in young patients. Internal carotid artery dissection should be considered, especially when there is neck pain or a recent history of neck trauma.

Clinical Findings

A. Symptoms and Signs

Central retinal artery occlusion presents as sudden profound monocular visual loss. Visual acuity is usually reduced to counting fingers or worse, and visual field may be restricted to an island of vision in the temporal field. Ophthalmoscopy reveals pale swelling of the retina with a cherry-red spot at the fovea (Figure 7–2). Occasionally, emboli are seen in the central retinal artery or its branches. The retinal swelling subsides over a period of 4–6 weeks, leaving a pale optic disk with thinning of the inner retina on optical coherence tomography scans; these findings can help diagnose unexplained vision loss if the patient is not examined during the acute occlusive event.

Branch retinal artery occlusion may also present with sudden loss of vision if the fovea is involved, but more commonly sudden loss of a discrete area in the visual field in one eye is the presenting complaint. Fundus signs of retinal swelling and sometimes adjacent cotton-wool spots are limited to the area of retina supplied by the occluded artery.

The clinician should identify risk factors for cardiac sources of emboli including arrhythmia, particularly atrial fibrillation, and cardiac valvular disease, and check the blood pressure. Nonocular clinical features of giant cell arteritis are age 50 years or older, headache, scalp tenderness, jaw claudication, general malaise, weight loss, symptoms of polymyalgia rheumatica, and tenderness, thickening, or absence of pulse of the superficial temporal arteries. Table 20–12 lists the clinical manifestations of vasculitis.

B. Laboratory Findings

Giant cell arteritis should be considered in cases of central retinal artery occlusion without visible emboli. ESR and CRP are usually elevated in giant cell arteritis, but one or both may be normal (see Chapter 20). Consider screening for other types of vasculitis (see Table 20–11). Screen for diabetes mellitus and hyperlipidemia in all patients. Particularly in younger patients, consider testing for antiphospholipid antibodies, lupus anticoagulant, inherited thrombophilia, and elevated plasma homocysteine.

C. Imaging

A brain MRI with diffusion weighted imaging sequences should be obtained urgently to look for cerebral infarction, which is present in up to 31% of patients with branch or central retinal artery occlusion. Obtain duplex ultrasonography of the carotid arteries, ECG, echocardiography with transesophageal studies to identify carotid and cardiac sources of emboli, and CT or MR studies for internal carotid artery dissection, if necessary.

Treatment

Retinal artery occlusions require urgent referral to an emergency department for imaging and clinical assessment to prevent subsequent stroke. If the patient is seen within a few hours after onset, emergency treatment, comprising laying the patient flat, ocular massage, high concentrations of inhaled oxygen, intravenous acetazolamide, and anterior chamber paracentesis, may influence the visual outcome. Early thrombolysis, particularly by local intra-arterial injection but also intravenously, has shown good results in central retinal artery occlusion not due to giant cell arteritis. However, local intra-arterial injection of thrombolytic agents has a high incidence of adverse effects and may be difficult to accomplish quickly enough after the occlusion develops to prevent permanent vision loss due to inner retinal ischemia, which non-human primate studies suggest occurs within 90 minutes of occlusion.

In giant cell arteritis, there is risk of involvement of the other eye without prompt treatment. Recommended initial empiric treatment is intravenous methylprednisolone 1 g/day for 3 days. Whether oral methylprednisolone is similarly effective is unknown. All patients require subsequent long-term corticosteroid therapy (eg, oral prednisone); concomitant administration of long-term low-dose aspirin therapy is controversial. Tocilizumab, a monoclonal antibody against the receptor for interleukin-6, is also approved to treat adults with giant cell arteritis. There must be close monitoring to ensure that symptoms resolve and do not recur. Temporal artery biopsy should be performed promptly to confirm the diagnosis (see Polymyalgia Rheumatica & Giant Cell Arteritis, Chapter 20).

Patients with embolic retinal artery occlusion with 70–99% ipsilateral carotid artery stenosis, and possibly those with 50–69% stenosis, should be considered for carotid endarterectomy or possibly angioplasty with stenting to be performed within 2 weeks (see Chapters 12 and 24). Retinal embolization due to cardiac disease such as atrial fibrillation or a hypercoagulable state usually requires anticoagulation. Cardiac valvular disease and patent foramen ovale may require surgical treatment.

When to Refer

- Patients with retinal artery occlusions should be referred immediately to an emergency department to evaluate for stroke manifestations.
- Patients with central retinal artery occlusion should be referred emergently to an ophthalmologist.
- Patients with branch retinal artery occlusion should be referred urgently.
- Patients with suspected giant cell arteritis should be referred to a rheumatologist to guide management.

When to Admit

Patients with visual loss due to giant cell arteritis may require emergency admission for high-dose corticosteroid therapy and close monitoring to ensure adequate treatment.

Biousse V et al. Management acute retinal ischemia: follow the guidelines! Ophthalmology. 2018;125:1597. [PMID: 29716787]

Fallico M et al. Risk of acute stroke in patients with retinal artery occlusion: a systematic review and meta-analysis. Eye (Lond). 2020;34:683. [PMID: 31527762]

Flaxel CJ et al. Retinal and ophthalmic artery occlusions Preferred Practice Pattern®. Ophthalmology. 2020;127:P259. [PMID: 31757501]

Serling-Boyd N et al. Recent advances in the diagnosis and management of giant cell arteritis. Curr Opin Rheumatol. 2020;32:201. [PMID: 32168069]

TRANSIENT MONOCULAR VISUAL LOSS

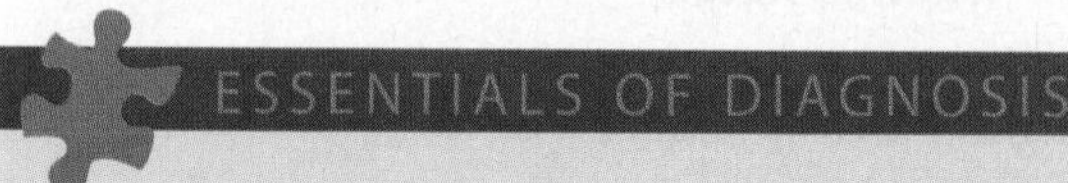

- Sudden-onset, monocular loss of vision usually lasting a few minutes with complete recovery.

Clinical Findings

A. Symptoms and Signs

Transient monocular visual loss ("ocular transient ischemic attack [TIA]") is usually caused by a retinal embolus from ipsilateral carotid disease or the heart. The visual loss is characteristically described as a curtain passing vertically across the visual field with complete monocular visual loss lasting a few minutes and a similar curtain effect as the episode passes (amaurosis fugax; also called "fleeting blindness"). An embolus is rarely seen on ophthalmoscopy. Other causes of transient, often recurrent, visual loss due to ocular ischemia are giant cell arteritis, hypercoagulable state (such as antiphospholipid syndrome), hyperviscosity, and severe occlusive carotid disease. More transient visual loss, lasting only a few seconds to 1 minute, usually recurrent, and affecting one or both eyes, occurs in patients with optic disk swelling, for example in those with raised intracranial pressure.

B. Diagnostic Studies

In most cases, clinical assessment and investigations are much the same as for retinal artery occlusion with emphasis on urgent neuroimaging to assess for cerebral infarction, as above, and identification of a source of emboli, since patients with embolic transient vision loss are at increased risk for stroke, MI, and other vascular events. Optic disk swelling requires different investigations (see Optic Disk Swelling, below).

Treatment

All patients with possible embolic transient visual loss should be treated immediately with oral aspirin (at least 81 mg daily), or another antiplatelet drug, until the cause has been determined. Affected patients with 70–99% (and possibly those with 50–69%) ipsilateral carotid artery stenosis should be considered for urgent carotid endarterectomy or possibly angioplasty with stenting (see Chapters 12 and 24). In all patients, vascular risk factors (eg, hypertension) need to be controlled. Retinal embolization due to cardiac arrhythmia, such as atrial fibrillation, or a hypercoagulable state usually requires anticoagulation. Cardiac valvular disease and patent foramen ovale may require surgical treatment.

When to Refer

In all cases of episodic visual loss, early ophthalmologic consultation is advisable.

When to Admit

Referral to a stroke center or hospital admission is recommended in embolic transient visual loss if there have been two or more episodes in the preceding week ("crescendo TIA") or the underlying cause is cardiac or a hypercoagulable state.

Biousse V et al. Management of acute retinal ischemia: follow the guidelines! Ophthalmology. 2018;125:1597. [PMID: 29716787]
Sharma RA et al. New concepts on acute ocular ischemia. Curr Opin Neurol. 2019;32:19. [PMID: 30461463]

RETINAL DISORDERS ASSOCIATED WITH SYSTEMIC DISEASES

1. Diabetic Retinopathy

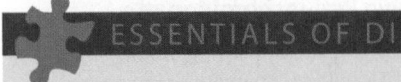

- Present in ~33% of all diagnosed diabetic patients.
- Present in ~20% of type 2 diabetic patients at time of diagnosis of diabetes.
- By 20 years after diagnosis of diabetes, 99% of type 1 diabetic patients and 60% of type 2 diabetic patients will have diabetic retinopathy.
- Nonproliferative diabetic retinopathy: can be mild, moderate, or severe. Microvascular changes are limited to the retina.
- Proliferative diabetic retinopathy: new blood vessels grow on the surface of the retina, optic nerve, or iris.
- Diabetic macular edema: central retinal swelling; can occur with any severity level of diabetic retinopathy; reduces visual acuity if the foveal center is involved.

General Considerations

Diabetic retinopathy is present in about one-third of patients in whom diabetes has been diagnosed, and about one-third of those have sight-threatening disease. In the United States, it affects about 4 million people; it is the leading cause of vision loss worldwide among adults aged 25–74 years; and the number of affected individuals aged 65 years or older is increasing. Worldwide, there are approximately 93 million people with diabetic retinopathy, including 28 million with vision-threatening disease. Retinopathy increases in prevalence and severity with increasing duration and poorer control of diabetes. In type 1 diabetes, retinopathy is not detectable for the first 5 years after diagnosis. In type 2 diabetes, about 20% of patients have retinopathy at diagnosis, likely because they had diabetes for a long time before diagnosis. Macular involvement is the most common cause of legal blindness in type 2 diabetes.

There are two main categories of diabetic retinopathy: nonproliferative and proliferative. Diabetic macular edema can occur at any stage. **Nonproliferative** (previously known as "background") **retinopathy** is subclassified as mild, moderate, or severe; **proliferative retinopathy** is less common but causes more severe visual loss.

Nonproliferative retinopathy represents the earliest stage of retinal involvement by diabetes. During this stage, the retinal capillaries leak proteins, lipids, or red cells into the retina. When this process occurs in the macula (clinically significant macular edema), visual acuity is affected; this is the most common cause of visual impairment in patients with type 2 diabetes.

Proliferative retinopathy involves the growth of new vessels and fibrous tissue on the surface of the retina, extending into the vitreous chamber. It is a consequence of capillary occlusion, which causes retinal ischemia and release of VEGF; this, in turn, stimulates new vessel growth.

Clinical Findings

Clinical assessment comprises visual acuity testing, stereoscopic examination of the retina, retinal imaging with optical coherence tomography, and sometimes fluorescein angiography.

Nonproliferative retinopathy manifests as microaneurysms, retinal hemorrhages, venous beading, retinal edema, and hard exudates. In mild nonproliferative diabetic retinopathy, there are mild retinal abnormalities without visual loss. Reduction of vision is most commonly due to diabetic macular edema, which may be focal or diffuse, but it can also be due to macular ischemia. Severe nonproliferative retinopathy is defined as having any one of the following: severe intraretinal hemorrhages and microaneurysms in four quadrants, venous beading in two or more quadrants, or intraretinal microvascular abnormalities in at least one quadrant.

Proliferative retinopathy is characterized by neovascularization, arising from either the optic disk or the retinal vascular arcades. Prior to proliferation of new capillaries, a preproliferative phase often occurs in which arteriolar ischemia is manifest as cotton-wool spots (small infarcted areas of retina). Vision is usually normal until macular edema, vitreous hemorrhage, or retinal detachment occurs. Proliferation into the vitreous of blood vessels, with associated fibrosis, may lead to vitreous hemorrhage (common) and tractional retinal detachment.

Diabetic retinopathy may worsen after bariatric surgery or in patients with long-standing hyperglycemia that is rapidly brought under tight control, such as after receiving an insulin pump with continuous glucose monitoring. It is believed that capillary endothelial cells retain "metabolic memory" of hyperglycemia and that epigenetic changes persist for several months after the hyperglycemia is corrected, sometimes causing retinopathy progression after intensive glycemic control is initiated; however, after the first 18–24 months, rates of progression are significantly lower in patients treated with intensive control compared to conventional regimens.

Screening

Visual symptoms and visual acuity are poor guides to the presence of diabetic retinopathy. Patients with diabetes mellitus should undergo regular fundus photography, which can be performed using telemedicine that may involve computer detection software programs, or dilated slit-lamp examination of the retina. Patients with type 1 diabetes mellitus should be screened 5 years after the diabetes is diagnosed. Patients with type 2 diabetes mellitus should be screened at or shortly after diagnosis of diabetes. More frequent monitoring is required in women with type 1 or 2 diabetes during pregnancy and in those planning pregnancy, and for the first 2 years after intensive glycemic control is initiated.

Treatment

Treatment includes optimizing blood glucose, blood pressure, kidney function, and serum lipids. When patients are initially brought into intensive glycemic control, they should be examined every 1–2 months so they can be treated if retinopathy progresses. Glycemic control is the most important modifiable factor in treating patients with diabetic retinopathy, but intensive blood pressure control and avoiding tobacco use also slow retinopathy progression.

Macular edema and exudates, but not macular ischemia, may respond to laser photocoagulation; to intravitreal administration of a VEGF inhibitor (ranibizumab, bevacizumab, aflibercept, or brolucizumab) or corticosteroid (triamcinolone, dexamethasone implant, or fluocinolone implant); or to vitrectomy. VEGF inhibitor therapy improves diabetic retinopathy severity in eyes at all levels of nonproliferative diabetic retinopathy and is the mainstay of treatment for diabetic macular edema.

In patients with **severe nonproliferative retinopathy,** fluorescein angiography can demonstrate the extent of retinal ischemia, which can help determine whether panretinal laser photocoagulation should be performed prophylactically. Vitrectomy is necessary to remove persistent vitreous hemorrhage, improve vision, allow panretinal laser photocoagulation, treat tractional retinal detachment involving the macula, and manage rapidly progressive proliferative disease.

Proliferative retinopathy is usually treated by intravitreal injection of a VEGF inhibitor or panretinal laser photocoagulation, preferably before vitreous hemorrhage or tractional detachment has occurred. Proliferative diabetic retinopathy, especially after successful laser treatment, is not a contraindication to treatment with thrombolytic agents, aspirin, or warfarin unless there has been recent intraocular hemorrhage.

When to Refer

- All diabetic patients with sudden loss of vision or retinal detachment should be referred emergently to an ophthalmologist.
- Proliferative retinopathy or macular involvement requires urgent referral to an ophthalmologist.
- Severe nonproliferative retinopathy or unexplained reduction of visual acuity requires early referral to an ophthalmologist.

Flaxel CJ et al. Diabetic Retinopathy Preferred Practice Pattern®. Ophthalmology. 2020;127:P66. [PMID: 31757498]

Gross JG et al; Diabetic Retinopathy Clinical Research Network. Five-year outcomes of panretinal photocoagulation vs intravitreous ranibizumab for proliferative diabetic retinopathy: a randomized clinical trial. JAMA Ophthalmol. 2018;136:1138. [PMID: 30043039]

Hutton DW et al; DRCR Retina Network. Five-year cost-effectiveness of intravitreous ranibizumab therapy vs panretinal photocoagulation for treating proliferative diabetic retinopathy: a secondary analysis of a randomized clinical trial. JAMA Ophthalmol. 2019;137:1424. [PMID: 31647496]

Wong TY et al. Strategies to tackle the global burden of diabetic retinopathy: from epidemiology to artificial intelligence. Ophthalmologica. 2020;243:9. [PMID: 31408872]

2. Hypertensive Retinochoroidopathy

Systemic hypertension affects both the retinal and choroidal circulations. The clinical manifestations vary according to the degree and rapidity of rise in blood pressure and the underlying state of the ocular circulation (see Chapter 11). The most florid ocular changes occur in young patients with abrupt elevations of blood pressure, such as may occur in pheochromocytoma, malignant hypertension, or preeclampsia-eclampsia.

Chronic hypertension accelerates the development of atherosclerosis. The retinal arterioles become more tortuous and narrower and develop abnormal light reflexes ("silver-wiring" and "copper-wiring") (Figure 11–2). There is increased venous compression at the retinal arteriovenous crossings ("arteriovenous nicking"), predisposing to branch retinal vein occlusions. Flame-shaped hemorrhages occur in the nerve fiber layer of the retina. Detection is aided by nonmydriatic fundus photography.

Acute elevations of blood pressure result in loss of autoregulation in the retinal circulation, leading to breakdown of endothelial integrity and occlusion of precapillary arterioles and capillaries that manifest as cotton-wool spots, retinal hemorrhages, retinal edema, and retinal exudates, often in a stellate appearance at the macula. Vasoconstriction and ischemia in the choroid result in exudative retinal detachments and retinal pigment epithelial infarcts that later develop into pigmented lesions that may be focal, linear, or wedge-shaped. The abnormalities in the choroidal circulation may also affect the optic nerve head, producing ischemic optic neuropathy with optic disk swelling. *Fundus abnormalities are the hallmark of hypertensive crisis with retinopathy (previously known as malignant hypertension) that requires emergency treatment* (see Chapter 11). Marked fundus abnormalities are likely to be associated with permanent retinal, choroidal, or optic nerve damage. Precipitous reduction of blood pressure may exacerbate such damage.

Chen X et al. Hypertensive retinopathy and the risk of stroke among hypertensive adults in China. Invest Ophthalmol Vis Sci. 2021;62:28. [PMID: 34283210]

Tsukikawa M et al. A review of hypertensive retinopathy and chorioretinopathy. Clin Optom (Auckl). 2020;12:67. [PMID: 32440245]

3. Blood Dyscrasias

Severe thrombocytopenia or anemia may result in various types of retinal or choroidal hemorrhages, including white-centered retinal hemorrhages (Roth spots) that occur in leukemia and other situations (eg, bacterial endocarditis). Involvement of the macula may result in permanent visual loss.

Sickle cell retinopathy is particularly common in hemoglobin SC disease but may also occur with other hemoglobin S variants. Manifestations include "salmon-patch" preretinal/intraretinal hemorrhages, "black sunbursts" resulting from intraretinal hemorrhage, and new vessels. Severe visual loss is rare with sickle cell retinopathy but more common in patients with pulmonary hypertension. Retinal laser photocoagulation reduces the frequency of vitreous hemorrhage from new vessels. Surgery is occasionally needed for persistent vitreous hemorrhage or tractional retinal detachment.

Alabduljalil T et al. Retinal ultra-wide-field colour imaging versus dilated fundus examination to screen for sickle cell retinopathy. Br J Ophthalmol. 2021;105:1121. [PMID: 32816790]

AlRyalat SA et al. Ocular manifestations of sickle cell disease in different genotypes. Ophthalmic Epidemiol. 2021;28:185. [PMID: 32757703]

4. HIV Infection/AIDS

See Chapter 31. **HIV retinopathy** causes cotton-wool spots, retinal hemorrhages, and microaneurysms but may also lead to reduced contrast sensitivity and retinal nerve fiber layer and outer retinal damage (HIV neuroretinal disorder).

CMV retinitis is less common since the availability of antiretroviral therapy (ART) but continues to be prevalent where resources are limited. It usually occurs when CD4 counts are below 50/mcL (0.05×10^9/L) and is characterized by progressively enlarging yellowish-white patches of retinal opacification and retinal hemorrhages, usually beginning adjacent to the major retinal vascular arcades. Patients are often asymptomatic until there is involvement of the fovea or optic nerve, or until retinal detachment develops. See Table 31–3 for initial therapeutic recommendations. Maintenance therapy can be achieved with lower-dose therapy or with intravitreal therapy. Systemic therapy has a greater risk of nonocular adverse effects but reduces mortality, incidence of nonocular CMV disease (but this is less common with ART), and incidence of retinitis in the other eye and avoids intraocular complications of intravitreal administration. In all patients with CMV retinitis, ART needs to be instituted or adjusted. This may lead to the immune reconstitution inflammatory syndrome (IRIS), which may lead to visual loss, predominantly due to cystoid macular edema. It may be possible to reduce the likelihood of IRIS by using immunomodulatory therapy to suppress the immune response causing the inflammation. If the CD4 count is maintained above 100/mcL (0.1×10^9/L), it may be possible to discontinue maintenance anti-CMV therapy.

Other ophthalmic manifestations of opportunistic infections occurring in AIDS patients include herpes simplex retinitis, which usually manifests as acute retinal necrosis; toxoplasmic and candidal chorioretinitis possibly progressing to endophthalmitis; herpes zoster ophthalmicus and herpes zoster retinitis, which can manifest as acute retinal necrosis or progressive outer retinal necrosis; and various entities due to syphilis, tuberculosis, or cryptococcosis. Kaposi sarcoma of the conjunctiva (see Chapter 31) and orbital lymphoma may also be seen on rare occasions.

Heiden D et al. Active cytomegalovirus retinitis after the start of antiretroviral therapy. Br J Ophthalmol. 2019;103:157. [PMID: 30196272]

Munro M et al. Cytomegalovirus retinitis in HIV and non-HIV individuals. Microorganisms. 2019;8:55. [PMID: 31905656]

Sudharshan S et al. Human immunodeficiency virus and intraocular inflammation in the era of highly active antiretroviral therapy—an update. Indian J Ophthalmol. 2020;68:1787. [PMID: 32823395]

Tang Y et al. Clinical features of cytomegalovirus retinitis in HIV infected patients. Front Cell Infect Microbiol. 2020;10:136. [PMID: 32318357]

ISCHEMIC OPTIC NEUROPATHY

ESSENTIALS OF DIAGNOSIS

- Sudden painless visual loss with signs of optic nerve dysfunction.
- Optic disk swelling in anterior ischemic optic neuropathy.

Anterior ischemic optic neuropathy—due to inadequate perfusion of the posterior ciliary arteries that supply the anterior portion of the optic nerve—produces sudden visual loss, usually with an altitudinal field defect and optic disk swelling. In older patients, it may be caused by giant cell arteritis (arteritic anterior ischemic optic neuropathy). The predominant factor predisposing to nonarteritic anterior ischemic optic neuropathy, which subsequently affects the other eye in around 15% of cases, is a congenitally crowded optic disk, compromising optic disk circulation. Other predisposing factors are systemic hypertension, diabetes mellitus, hyperlipidemia, systemic vasculitis, inherited or acquired thrombophilia, interferon-alpha therapy, and obstructive sleep apnea; hypotension and anemia during dialysis may cause bilateral anterior ischemic optic neuropathy. An association with phosphodiesterase type 5 inhibitors is controversial.

Posterior ischemic optic neuropathy, involving the retrobulbar optic nerve and thus not causing any optic disk swelling, may occur with severe blood loss; nonocular surgery, particularly prolonged lumbar spine surgery in the prone position with increased orbital pressure; severe burns; or in association with dialysis, as a consequence of profound hypotension and anemia. In all such situations, there may be several contributory factors.

Treatment

Arteritic anterior ischemic optic neuropathy necessitates emergency high-dose systemic corticosteroid treatment to prevent visual loss in the other eye. (See Central & Branch Retinal Artery Occlusions, above, and Polymyalgia Rheumatica & Giant Cell Arteritis, Chapter 20.) It is uncertain whether systemic or intravitreal corticosteroid therapy influences the outcome in nonarteritic anterior ischemic optic neuropathy or whether oral low-dose aspirin (~81 mg daily) reduces the risk of involvement of the other eye. In ischemic optic neuropathy after nonocular surgery or dialysis, treatment of marked anemia by blood transfusion may be beneficial.

When to Refer

Patients with ischemic optic neuropathy should be referred urgently to an ophthalmologist.

When to Admit

Patients with ischemic optic neuropathy due to giant cell arteritis or other vasculitis may require emergency admission for high-dose corticosteroid therapy and close monitoring to ensure that treatment is adequate.

Arora S et al. Sildenafil in ophthalmology: an update. Surv Ophthalmol. 2022;67:463. [PMID: 34175342]

Augstburger E et al. Acute ischemic optic nerve disease: pathophysiology, clinical features and management. J Fr Ophtalmol. 2020;43:e41. [PMID: 31952875]

OPTIC NEURITIS

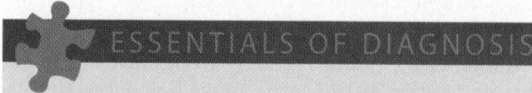

- Subacute, usually unilateral, visual loss.
- Pain exacerbated by eye movements.
- Optic disk is usually normal in acute stage but subsequently develops pallor.

General Considerations

Inflammatory optic neuropathy is strongly associated with demyelinating disease (typical optic neuritis), particularly multiple sclerosis, but it also occurs in acute disseminated encephalomyelitis; sarcoidosis; neuromyelitis optica spectrum disorder, which is characterized by serum antibodies to aquaporin-4; in association with serum antibodies to myelin oligodendrocyte glycoprotein; following viral infection (usually in children); in varicella zoster virus infection; in autoimmune disorders, particularly SLE and Sjögren syndrome; during treatment with biologics; and by spread of inflammation from the meninges, orbital tissues, or paranasal sinuses.

Clinical Findings

Optic neuritis in demyelinating disease is characterized by unilateral loss of vision developing over a few days. Visual acuity ranges from 20/30 (6/9) to no perception of light, with more severe visual loss being associated with low serum vitamin D. In almost all cases there is pain behind the eye, exacerbated by eye movements, central visual field loss, color vision loss, and a relative afferent pupillary defect. In about two-thirds of cases, the optic nerve is normal during the acute stage (retrobulbar optic neuritis). In the remainder, the optic disk is swollen (papillitis) with occasional flame-shaped peripapillary hemorrhages. Visual acuity usually improves within 2–3 weeks and returns to 20/40 (6/12) or better in 95% of previously unaffected eyes. Optic atrophy subsequently develops if there has been extensive optic nerve fiber damage. Any patient without a known diagnosis of multiple sclerosis in whom visual recovery does not occur, or if there is continuing deterioration of vision, or pain persisting after 2 weeks, should undergo MRI of the head and orbits to look for periventricular white matter demyelination or a lesion compressing the optic nerve.

Treatment

In acute demyelinating optic neuritis, intravenous methylprednisolone (1 g daily for 3 days followed by a tapering course of oral prednisolone) has been shown to accelerate visual recovery but not to improve final vision. However, in clinical practice, the oral taper is not often prescribed. Use in an individual patient is determined by the degree of visual loss, the state of the other eye, and the patient's visual requirements. Newer therapies include monoclonal antibodies against immune cells and cell-based therapies to deplete or modulate T and B cell responses.

Atypical optic neuritis due to sarcoidosis, neuromyelitis optica, herpes zoster, or SLE generally has a poorer prognosis, requires immediate and more prolonged corticosteroid therapy, may require plasma exchange, and may necessitate long-term immunosuppression.

Prognosis

Among patients with a first episode of clinically isolated optic neuritis, multiple sclerosis will develop in 50% within

15 years; however, the likelihood of developing multiple sclerosis ranges from 25% for patients without demyelinating lesions on brain MRI to 72% in patients with one or more demyelinating lesions. The major risk factors are female sex and multiple white matter lesions on brain MRI. Many disease-modifying drugs are available to reduce the risk of further neurologic episodes and disability, but each has adverse effects that in some instances are life-threatening. Retinal nerve fiber layer optical coherence tomography quantifies axonal damage that can be used to monitor disease progression.

When to Refer

All patients with optic neuritis should be referred urgently for ophthalmologic or neurologic assessment.

Derdelinckx J et al. Cells to the rescue: emerging cell-based treatment approaches for NMOSD and MOGAD. Int J Mol Sci. 2021;22:7925. [PMID: 34360690]
Graves JS. Optical coherence tomography in multiple sclerosis. Semin Neurol. 2019;39:711. [PMID: 31847042]

OPTIC DISK SWELLING

Optic disk swelling may result from any orbital or optic nerve lesion causing nerve compression, severe hypertensive retinochoroidopathy, or raised intracranial pressure, the last necessitating urgent imaging to exclude an intracranial mass, hemorrhage, infection, or cerebral venous sinus occlusion. Intraocular causes include central retinal vein occlusion, posterior uveitis, and posterior scleritis. Optic nerve lesions causing disk swelling include anterior ischemic optic neuropathy; optic neuritis; optic nerve sheath meningioma; and infiltration by sarcoidosis, leukemia, or lymphoma.

Papilledema (optic disk swelling due to raised intracranial pressure) is usually bilateral and most commonly produces enlargement of the blind spot without loss of acuity. Severe acute papilledema or chronic papilledema, as in idiopathic intracranial hypertension and cerebral venous sinus occlusion, may be associated with visual field and occasionally with profound visual acuity loss. All patients with chronic papilledema must be monitored carefully—especially their visual fields—and cerebrospinal fluid shunt or optic nerve sheath fenestration should be considered in those with progressive visual loss not controlled by medical therapy (weight loss where appropriate and usually acetazolamide in patients with idiopathic intracranial hypertension). In idiopathic intracranial hypertension, transverse venous sinus stenting is also an option.

Raoof N et al. Diagnosis and treatment of idiopathic intracranial hypertension. Cephalalgia. 2021;41:472. [PMID: 33631966]
Spiegel SJ et al. Neuro-ophthalmic emergencies. Neurol Clin. 2021;39:631. [PMID: 33896536]

CRANIAL NERVE PALSIES

A cranial nerve palsy of any of the three cranial nerves that supply the extraocular muscles can cause double vision.

In a complete **third nerve palsy,** there is ptosis with a divergent and slightly depressed eye (Figure 7–3). Extraocular movements are restricted in all directions except laterally (preserved lateral rectus function) (Figure 7–3E). Intact fourth nerve (superior oblique) function is detected by inward rotation on attempted depression of the eye. Pupillary involvement, manifesting as a relatively dilated pupil that does not constrict normally to light, usually

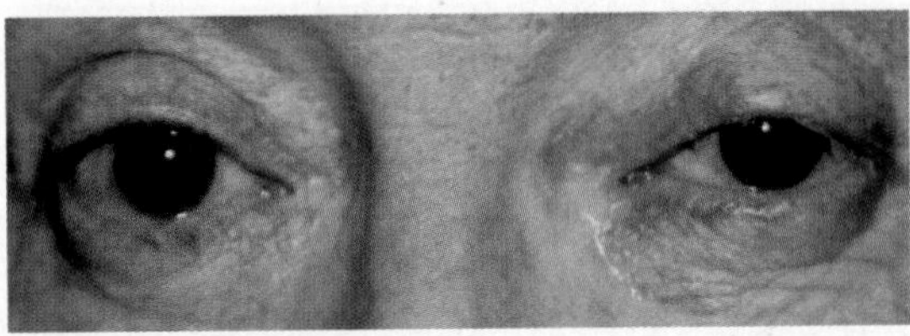
A

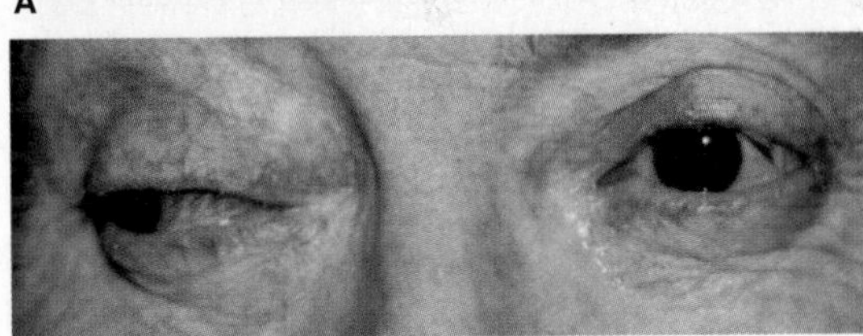
B

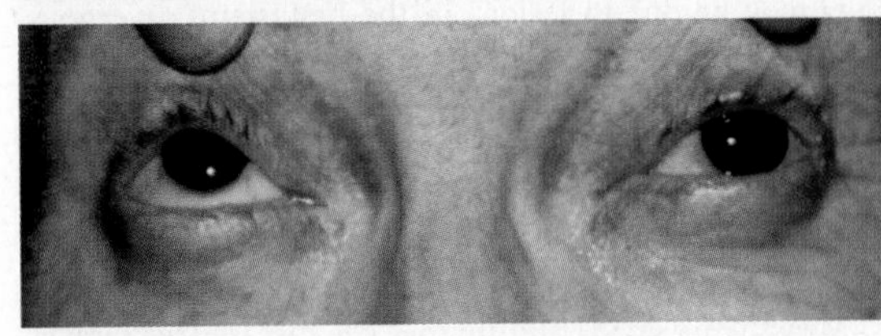
C

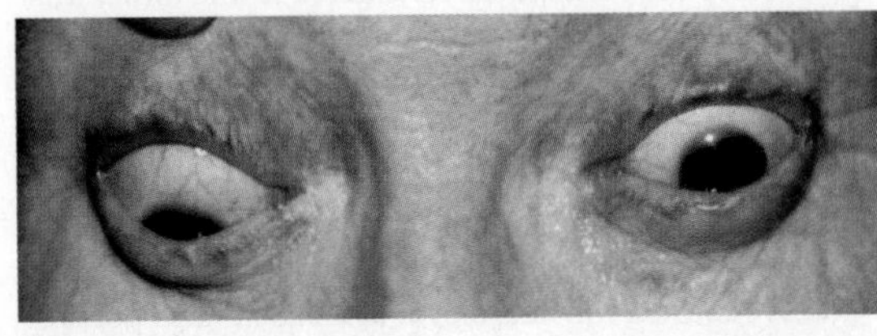
D

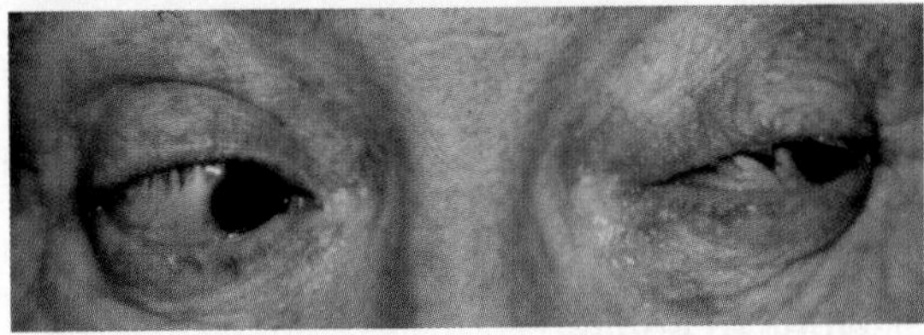
E

Figure 7–3. Left partial third nerve palsy with ptosis **(A),** reduced adduction **(B),** reduced elevation **(C),** and reduced depression **(D)** but normal abduction **(E)** of the left eye.

means compression, which may be due to aneurysm of the posterior communicating artery or uncal herniation due to a supratentorial mass lesion. In acute painful isolated third nerve palsy with pupillary involvement, posterior communicating artery aneurysm must be excluded. Pituitary apoplexy is a rarer cause. Causes of isolated third nerve palsy without pupillary involvement include diabetes mellitus, hypertension, giant cell arteritis, and herpes zoster.

Fourth nerve palsy causes upward deviation of the eye with failure of depression on adduction. In acquired cases, there is vertical and torsional diplopia that is most apparent on looking down. Trauma is a major cause of acquired—particularly bilateral—fourth nerve palsy, but posterior fossa tumor and medical causes, such as in third nerve palsy, should also be considered. Similar clinical features are seen in congenital cases due to developmental anomaly of the nerve, muscle, or tendon.

Sixth nerve palsy causes convergent squint in the primary position with failure of abduction of the affected eye, producing horizontal diplopia that increases on gaze to the affected side and on looking into the distance. It is an important sign of raised intracranial pressure and may also be due to trauma, neoplasms, brainstem lesions, petrous apex lesions, or medical causes (such as diabetes mellitus, hypertension, giant cell arteritis, and herpes zoster).

In an isolated cranial nerve palsy presumed to be due a medical cause, brain MRI is not always required initially, but it is necessary if recovery has not begun within 3 months.

A cranial nerve palsy accompanied by other neurologic signs may be due to lesions in the brainstem, cavernous sinus, or orbit. Lesions around the cavernous sinus involve the first and second divisions of the trigeminal nerve, the third, fourth, and sixth cranial nerves, and occasionally the optic chiasm. Orbital apex lesions involve the optic nerve and the three cranial nerves supplying the extraocular muscles.

Myasthenia gravis and thyroid eye disease (see Graves Ophthalmopathy) should be considered in the differential diagnosis of disordered extraocular movements.

When to Refer

- In recent-onset isolated third nerve palsy, especially if there is pupillary involvement or pain, immediate referral is required for neurologic assessment and possibly CT, MRI, or catheter angiography for intracranial aneurysm.
- All patients with recent-onset double vision should be referred urgently to a neurologist or ophthalmologist, particularly if there are multiple cranial nerve dysfunctions or other neurologic abnormalities.

When to Admit

Patients with double vision due to giant cell arteritis may require emergency admission for high-dose corticosteroid therapy and close monitoring to ensure that treatment is adequate. (See Central & Branch Retinal Artery Occlusions and Chapter 20.)

Prasad S. A window to the brain: neuro-ophthalmology for the primary care practitioner. Am J Med. 2018;131:120. [PMID: 29079403]

THYROID EYE DISEASE (Graves Ophthalmopathy)

See Hyperthyroidism (Thyrotoxicosis) in Chapter 26.

ORBITAL CELLULITIS

Orbital cellulitis is characterized by fever, proptosis, restriction of extraocular movements, and swelling with redness of the lids. Immediate treatment with intravenous antibiotics is necessary to prevent optic nerve damage and spread of infection to the cavernous sinuses, meninges, and brain. Infection of the paranasal sinuses is the usual underlying cause. Infecting organisms include *S pneumoniae*, the incidence of which has been reduced by the administration of pneumococcal vaccine; other streptococci, such as the anginosus group; *H influenzae*; and, less commonly, *S aureus* including MRSA. Penicillinase-resistant penicillin, such as nafcillin, is recommended, possibly together with metronidazole or clindamycin to treat anaerobic infections. If trauma is the underlying cause, a cephalosporin, such as cefazolin or ceftriaxone, should be added to ensure coverage for *S aureus* and group A beta-hemolytic streptococci. If MRSA infection is a concern, vancomycin or clindamycin may be required. For patients with penicillin hypersensitivity, vancomycin, levofloxacin, and metronidazole are recommended. The response to antibiotics is usually excellent, but surgery may be required to drain the paranasal sinuses or orbital abscess. In immunocompromised patients, zygomycosis must be considered.

When to Refer

All patients with suspected orbital cellulitis must be referred emergently to an ophthalmologist.

Tsirouki T et al. Orbital cellulitis. Surv Ophthalmol. 2018;63:534. [PMID: 29248536]

OCULAR TRAUMA

Ocular trauma is an important cause of avoidable severe visual impairment at all ages, and it is the leading cause of monocular blindness in young adult men in the United States. Thorough but safe clinical assessment, supplemented when necessary by imaging, is crucial to effective management. Ocular damage and the possible need for early assessment by an ophthalmologist need to be borne in mind in the assessment of any patient with midfacial injury.

1. Conjunctival & Corneal Foreign Bodies

If a patient complains of "something in my eye" and gives a consistent history, a foreign body is usually present on the cornea or under the upper lid even though it may not be visible. Visual acuity should be tested before treatment is instituted to assess the severity of the injury and as a basis for comparison in the event of complications.

After a local anesthetic (eg, proparacaine, 0.5%) is instilled, the eye is examined with a slit lamp or with a hand flashlight, using oblique illumination, and loupe. The instillation of sterile fluorescein may make corneal foreign bodies more apparent, which are then removed with a sterile wet cotton-tipped applicator or hypodermic needle. Bacitracin-polymyxin ophthalmic ointment should be instilled. It is not necessary to patch the eye. All patients need to be advised to return promptly for reassessment if there is any increase in pain, redness, or impairment of vision.

Iron foreign bodies usually leave a diffuse rust ring. This requires excision and is best done under local anesthesia using a slit lamp. **Caution:** Anesthetic drops should not be given to the patient for self-administration.

If there is no infection, a layer of corneal epithelial cells will line the crater within 24 hours. While the epithelium is defective, the cornea is extremely susceptible to infection. Early infection is manifested by a white necrotic area around the crater and a small amount of gray exudate.

In the case of a foreign body under the upper lid, a local anesthetic is instilled and the lid is everted by grasping the lashes gently and exerting pressure on the mid portion of the outer surface of the upper lid with an applicator. If a foreign body is present, it can easily be removed by passing a wet sterile cotton-tipped applicator across the conjunctival surface.

When to Refer

Refer urgently to an ophthalmologist if a corneal foreign body cannot be removed or if there is suspicion of corneal infection.

Fraenkel A et al. Managing corneal foreign bodies in office-based general practice. Aust Fam Physician. 2017;46:89. [PMID: 28260265]

2. Intraocular Foreign Body

An intraocular foreign body requires emergency treatment by an ophthalmologist. Patients giving a history of "something hitting the eye"—particularly while hammering on metal or using grinding equipment—must be assessed for this possibility, especially when no corneal foreign body is seen, a corneal or scleral wound is apparent, or there is marked visual loss or media opacity. Such patients must be treated as for open globe injury and referred without delay. Intraocular foreign bodies significantly increase the risk of intraocular infection.

When to Refer

Patients with suspected intraocular foreign body must be referred emergently to an ophthalmologist.

Loporchio D et al. Intraocular foreign bodies: a review. Surv Ophthalmol. 2016;61:582. [PMID: 26994871]

3. Corneal Abrasions

A patient with a corneal abrasion complains of severe pain and photophobia. There is often a history of trauma to the eye, commonly involving a fingernail, piece of paper, or contact lens. Visual acuity is recorded, and the cornea and conjunctiva are examined with a light and loupe to rule out a foreign body. If an abrasion is suspected but cannot be seen, sterile fluorescein is instilled into the conjunctival sac: the area of corneal abrasion will stain because fluorescein stains areas that are devoid of epithelium.

Treatment includes bacitracin-polymyxin ophthalmic ointment or drops, or a fluoroquinolone topical antibiotic in contact lens wearers, as prophylaxis against infection. A mydriatic (cyclopentolate 1%) and either topical or oral NSAIDs can be used for pain control. Patching the eye is probably not helpful for small abrasions. Corneal abrasions heal more slowly in persons who smoke cigarettes. Recurrent corneal erosion may follow corneal abrasions.

Although treatment of pain from a corneal abrasion with topical tetracaine for 24 hours has been reported, there is a risk of delayed healing and severe corneal disease from misuse of topical anesthetics, so it is not recommended.

Wakai A et al. Topical non-steroidal anti-inflammatory drugs for analgesia in traumatic corneal abrasions. Cochrane Database Syst Rev. 2017;5:CD009781. [PMID: 28516471]

4. Contusions

Contusion injury of the eye (closed globe injury) and surrounding structures may cause ecchymosis ("black eye"), subconjunctival hemorrhage, edema of the cornea, hemorrhage into the anterior chamber (hyphema), rupture of the root of the iris (iridodialysis), paralysis of the pupillary sphincter, paralysis of the muscles of accommodation, cataract, dislocation of the lens, vitreous hemorrhage, retinal hemorrhage and edema (most common in the macular area), detachment of the retina, rupture of the choroid, fracture of the orbital floor ("blowout fracture"), or optic nerve injury. Many of these injuries are immediately obvious; others may not become apparent for days or weeks. The possibility of globe injury must always be considered in patients with facial injury, particularly if there is an orbital fracture. Patients with moderate to severe contusions should be seen by an ophthalmologist.

Any injury causing hyphema involves the danger of secondary hemorrhage, which may cause intractable glaucoma with permanent visual loss. The patient should be advised to rest until complete resolution has occurred. Frequent ophthalmologic assessment is essential. Aspirin and any drugs inhibiting coagulation increase the risk of secondary hemorrhage and are to be avoided. Sickle cell anemia or trait adversely affects outcome.

▶ When to Refer

Patients with moderate or severe ocular contusion should be referred to an ophthalmologist, emergently if there is hyphema.

5. Lacerations

A. Lids

If the lid margin is lacerated, the patient should be referred for specialized care, since permanent notching may result. Lacerations of the lower eyelid near the inner canthus often sever the lower canaliculus, for which canalicular intubation is likely to be required. Lid lacerations not involving the margin may be sutured like any skin laceration.

Ko AC et al. Eyelid and periorbital soft tissue trauma. Facial Plast Surg Clin North Am. 2017;25:605. [PMID: 28941512]

B. Conjunctiva

In lacerations of the conjunctiva, sutures are not necessary. To prevent infection, topical sulfonamide or other antibiotic is used until the laceration is healed.

C. Cornea or Sclera

Patients with suspected corneal or scleral laceration or rupture (open globe injury) must be seen emergently by an ophthalmologist. Manipulation is kept to a minimum, since pressure may result in extrusion of intraocular contents. The eye is bandaged lightly and covered with a shield that rests on the orbital bones above and below. The patient should be instructed not to squeeze the eye shut and to remain still. If there may be a metallic intraocular foreign body, a radiograph or CT scan is obtained to identify and localize it. *MRI is contraindicated because of the risk of movement of any metallic foreign body but may be useful for non-metallic foreign body.* Endophthalmitis occurs in over 5% of open globe injuries.

▶ When to Refer

Patients with suspected open globe injury must be referred emergently to an ophthalmologist.

CHEMICAL CONJUNCTIVITIS & KERATITIS

Chemical burns are treated by copious irrigation of the eyes as soon as possible after exposure, with tap water, saline solution, or buffering solution if available. Neutralization of an acid with an alkali or vice versa may cause further damage. Alkali injuries are more serious and require prolonged irrigation, since alkalies are not precipitated by the proteins of the eye as are acids. It is important to remove any retained particulate matter, such as is typically present in injuries involving cement and building plaster. This often requires eversion of the upper lid. The pupil should be dilated with 1% cyclopentolate, 1 drop twice a day, to relieve discomfort, and prophylactic topical antibiotics should be started (Table 7–2). In moderate to severe injuries, intensive topical corticosteroids and topical and systemic vitamin C are also necessary. Complications include mucus deficiency, scarring of the cornea and conjunctiva, symblepharon (adhesions between the tarsal and bulbar conjunctiva), tear duct obstruction, and secondary infection. It is difficult to assess severity of chemical burns without slit-lamp examination.

Ahmmed AA et al. Epidemiology, economic and humanistic burdens of ocular surface chemical injury: a narrative review. Ocul Surf. 2021;20:199. [PMID: 33647471]

Sharma N et al. Treatment of acute ocular chemical burns. Surv Ophthalmol. 2018;63:214. [PMID: 28935121]

PRECAUTIONS IN MANAGEMENT OF OCULAR DISORDERS

1. Use of Local Anesthetics

Unsupervised self-administration of local anesthetics is dangerous because they are toxic to the corneal epithelium, delay healing, and the patient may further injure an anesthetized eye without knowing it.

Lee MD...Seitzman GD. Cornea specialists do not recommend routine usage of topical anesthetics for corneal abrasions. Ann Emerg Med. 2019;74:463. [PMID: 31445551]

2. Pupillary Dilation

Dilating the pupil can very occasionally precipitate acute glaucoma if the patient has a narrow anterior chamber angle and should be undertaken with caution if the anterior chamber is obviously shallow (readily determined by oblique illumination of the anterior segment of the eye). A short-acting mydriatic, such as tropicamide, should be used and the patient warned to report immediately if ocular discomfort or redness develops. Angle closure is more likely to occur if pilocarpine is used to overcome pupillary dilation than if the pupil is allowed to constrict naturally.

3. Corticosteroid Therapy

Comanagement with eye specialists is strongly recommended to monitor for ocular complications of corticosteroid therapy. Long-term use of local corticosteroids presents several hazards: ocular hypertension leading to open-angle glaucoma; cataract formation; and exacerbation of ocular infections, such as herpes simplex (dendritic) and fungal keratitis. Furthermore, perforation of the cornea may occur when corticosteroids are used indiscriminately for infectious keratitis. The potential for causing or exacerbating systemic hypertension, diabetes mellitus, gastritis, osteoporosis, or glaucoma must always be borne in mind when systemic corticosteroids are prescribed for such conditions as uveitis or giant cell arteritis.

4. Contaminated Eye Medications

Ophthalmic solutions are prepared with the same degree of care as fluids intended for intravenous administration, but once bottles are opened there is always a risk of contamination, particularly with solutions of tetracaine, proparacaine, fluorescein, and any preservative-free preparations. Single-use fluorescein eyedrops or sterile fluorescein filter paper strips are recommended for use in place of multiple-use fluorescein solutions.

Whether in plastic or glass containers, eye solutions should not remain in use for long periods after the bottle is opened. Four weeks after opening is the usual maximum time for use of a solution containing preservatives before discarding. Preservative-free preparations should be kept refrigerated and usually discarded within 1 week after opening. Single-use products should not be reused.

If the eye has been injured by accident or by surgical trauma, it is of the greatest importance to use freshly opened bottles of sterile medications or single-use products.

5. Toxic & Hypersensitivity Reactions to Topical Therapy

In patients receiving long-term topical therapy, local toxic or hypersensitivity reactions to the active agent or preservatives may develop (Figure 7–4), especially if there is inadequate tear secretion. Preservatives in contact lens cleaning solutions may produce similar problems. Burning and soreness are exacerbated by drop instillation or contact lens insertion; occasionally, fibrosis and scarring of the conjunctiva and cornea may occur. Preservative-free topical medications and contact lens solutions are available.

An antibiotic instilled into the eye can sensitize the patient to that drug and cause an allergic reaction upon subsequent systemic administration. Potentially fatal anaphylaxis is known to occur in up to 0.3% of patients after intravenous fluorescein for fluorescein angiography. Anaphylaxis also has been reported after topical fluorescein.

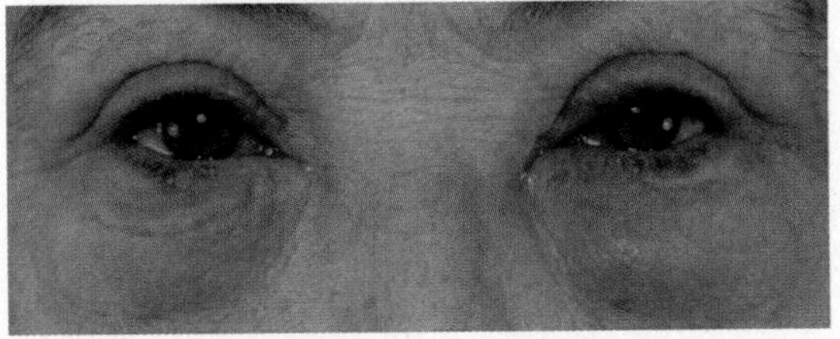

▲ **Figure 7–4.** Periocular contact dermatitis due to eye drop preservative.

6. Systemic Effects of Ocular Drugs

The systemic absorption of certain topical drugs (through the conjunctival vessels and lacrimal drainage system) must be considered when there is a systemic medical contraindication to the use of the drug. Ophthalmic solutions of the nonselective beta-blockers, eg, timolol, may worsen bradycardia, heart failure, or asthma. Phenylephrine eye drops may precipitate hypertensive crises and angina. Adverse interactions between systemically administered and ocular drugs should also be considered. Using only 1 or 2 drops at a time and a few minutes of nasolacrimal occlusion or eyelid closure ensures maximum ocular efficacy and decreases systemic side effects of topical agents.

ADVERSE OCULAR EFFECTS OF SYSTEMIC DRUGS

Systemically administered drugs produce a wide variety of adverse effects on the visual system. Table 7–3 lists the major examples. The likelihood of most complications is rare, but if visual changes develop while a patient is being treated with these medications, the patient should be referred to an eye care professional for an eye examination. Screening for toxic retinopathy is recommended at baseline in patients receiving long-term chloroquine or hydroxychloroquine therapy. If no baseline abnormalities are present, screening should be repeated annually beginning after 5 years. More frequent screening is necessary in patients treated with doses greater than 5.0 mg/kg real weight/day of hydroxychloroquine or greater than 2.3 mg/kg/day of chloroquine, in patients with kidney disease or in those taking tamoxifen.

Pentosan polysulfate (used to treat interstitial cystitis) has been associated with progressive vision loss due to maculopathy. Patients who receive pentosan polysulfate should be monitored with annual eye examinations, including color fundus photography, fundus autofluorescence, and optical coherence tomography images; irreversible progressive vision loss can occur after maculopathy develops.

Patients receiving long-term systemic corticosteroids are at increased risk for several ocular complications, including glaucoma, cataract, and central serous retinopathy. They should be referred to an eye care professional for an eye examination at baseline before starting corticosteroids and at any time if reduced or blurry vision develops.

An ophthalmologist should be informed whether a patient is taking or has ever taken alpha-adrenoreceptor antagonists (such as tamsulosin) before cataract surgery because these medications increase the risk of intraoperative floppy iris syndrome, which can make cataract surgery more challenging.

The chemotherapeutic MEK inhibitors are associated with ocular complications including serous retinal detachment,

Table 7–3. Adverse ophthalmic effects of systemic drugs (selected list).

Medications	Possible Ophthalmic Side Effects
Ophthalmic medications	
Carbonic anhydrase inhibitors (eg, acetazolamide, methazolamide)	Nearsightedness, angle-closure glaucoma due to ciliary body swelling
Beta-blockers (eg, timolol, betaxolol, levobunolol, metipranolol)	Bradycardia, arrhythmias, syncope, hypotension, bronchoconstriction
Respiratory medications	
Anticholinergic bronchodilators (eg, ipratropium)	Angle-closure glaucoma due to mydriasis, blurring of vision due to cycloplegia, dry eyes
Sympathomimetic bronchodilators (eg, salbutamol) and decongestants (eg, ephedrine)	Angle-closure glaucoma due to mydriasis
Cardiovascular system medications	
Amiodarone	Corneal deposits (vortex keratopathy), optic neuropathy, thyroid eye disease
Amlodipine	Chemosis (conjunctival edema)
Anticoagulants	Conjunctival, retinal, and vitreous hemorrhage
Chlorthalidone	Angle-closure glaucoma due to ciliary body swelling
Digoxin	Disturbance of color vision, photopsia, optic neuropathy
Furosemide	Angle-closure glaucoma due to ciliary body swelling
Phosphodiesterase type 5 inhibitors (eg, sildenafil, tadalafil, vardenafil)	Color vision changes, nonarteritic anterior ischemic optic neuropathy
Statins	Extraocular muscle palsy (myasthenic syndrome)
Thiazides (eg, indapamide)	Angle-closure glaucoma, nearsightedness, xanthopsia (yellow vision), band keratopathy due to hypercalcemia, macular edema
Gastrointestinal medications	
Anticholinergic agents	Angle-closure glaucoma due to mydriasis, blurring of vision due to cycloplegia, dry eyes
H_2-blockers	Retinal vascular occlusion, optic neuropathy, retrobulbar optic neuritis
Urinary tract medications	
Alpha-adrenoceptor-antagonists (eg, doxazosin, prazosin, tamsulosin, terazosin)	Intraoperative floppy iris syndrome
Phosphodiesterase type 5 inhibitors (eg, sildenafil, tadalafil, vardenafil)	Color vision changes, nonarteritic anterior ischemic optic neuropathy
Pentosan polysulfate sodium	Maculopathy
Anticholinergic agents	Angle-closure glaucoma due to mydriasis, blurring of vision due to cycloplegia, dry eyes
Finasteride	Floppy iris syndrome during intraocular surgery
CNS medications	
Amphetamines	Widening of palpebral fissure, blurring of vision due to mydriasis, elevated intraocular pressure
Anticholinergic agents including preoperative medications	Angle-closure glaucoma due to mydriasis, blurring of vision due to cycloplegia, dry eyes
Aripiprazole	Nearsightedness
Diazepam	Nystagmus
Haloperidol	Capsular cataract
Lithium carbonate	Proptosis, oculogyric crisis, nystagmus
MAO inhibitors	Nystagmus, visual hallucinations, diplopia, myasthenia gravis

(*continued*)

Table 7–3. Adverse ophthalmic effects of systemic drugs (selected list). (continued)

Medications	Possible Ophthalmic Side Effects
Morphine/opioids	Miosis, visual hallucinations, diplopia, dry eye
Neostigmine	Nystagmus, miosis
Olanzapine	Angle-closure glaucoma due to mydriasis
Phenothiazines (eg, chlorpromazine)	Pigmentary deposits in conjunctiva, cornea, lens, and retina; oculogyric crisis Chlorpromazine causes floppy iris syndrome during intraocular surgery
Phenytoin	Nystagmus
Quetiapine	Floppy iris syndrome during intraocular surgery
Retigabine	Ocular pigmentation and retinopathy
Risperidone, paliperidone	Floppy iris syndrome during intraocular surgery
SSRIs (eg, paroxetine, sertraline)	Angle-closure glaucoma, ischemic optic neuropathy, cataract
SNRIs (eg, venlafaxine)	Angle-closure glaucoma, mydriasis, dry eye
Thioridazine	Corneal and lens deposits, retinopathy, oculogyric crisis
Topiramate	Angle-closure glaucoma due to ciliary body swelling, nearsightedness, macular folds, anterior uveitis, corneal edema
Tricyclic agents (eg, imipramine)	Angle-closure glaucoma due to mydriasis, blurring of vision due to cycloplegia, dry eye
Triptans (eg, sumatriptan, zolmitriptan)	Angle-closure glaucoma due to ciliary body swelling, nearsightedness
Vigabatrin	Visual field constriction, cone dystrophy
Zonisamide	Angle-closure glaucoma due to ciliary body swelling, nearsightedness
Obstetric drugs	
Sympathomimetic tocolytics	Angle-closure glaucoma due to mydriasis
Hormonal agents	
Aromatase inhibitors (eg, anastrozole)	Dry eye, vitreo-retinal traction, retinal hemorrhages
Cabergoline	Angle-closure glaucoma
Female sex hormones	Retinal artery occlusion, retinal vein occlusion, papilledema, cranial nerve palsies, ischemic optic neuropathy
Tamoxifen	Crystalline retinal and corneal deposits, altered color perception, cataract, optic neuropathy, macular edema, retinal pigmentary change
Immunomodulators	
Alpha-interferon	Retinopathy, keratoconjunctivitis, dry eyes, optic neuropathy
Corticosteroids	Cataract (posterior subcapsular); susceptibility to viral (herpes simplex), bacterial, and fungal infections; steroid-induced glaucoma; idiopathic intracranial hypertension; central serous retinopathy
NSAIDs	Corneal opacity, vortex keratopathy, periorbital edema, dry eye
Cyclosporine	Posterior reversible leukoencephalopathy
Fingolimod	Macular edema, retinal vein occlusion
Tacrolimus	Optic neuropathy, posterior reversible leukoencephalopathy
Antibiotics	
Chloramphenicol	Optic neuropathy
Clofazimine	Crystalline deposits (conjunctiva, cornea, iris)
Ethambutol	Optic neuropathy
Fluoroquinolones	Diplopia, retinal detachment
Isoniazid	Optic neuropathy
Linezolid	Optic neuropathy

(continued)

Table 7–3. Adverse ophthalmic effects of systemic drugs (selected list). (continued)

Medications	Possible Ophthalmic Side Effects
Rifabutin	Uveitis
Streptomycin	Optic neuropathy, epidermal necrolysis
Sulfonamides	Nearsightedness, angle-closure glaucoma due to ciliary body swelling
Tetracycline, doxycycline, minocycline	Papilledema
Antivirals	
Cidofovir	Uveitis
Antimalarial agents	
Chloroquine, hydroxychloroquine	Retinal degeneration principally involving the macula, vortex keratopathy
Quinine	Retinal toxicity, pupillary abnormalities
Amebicides	
Diiodohydroxyquinolone	Optic neuropathy
Chemotherapeutic agents	
Bortezomib	Chalazia
Chlorambucil	Optic neuropathy
Cisplatin	Optic neuropathy
Docetaxel	Lacrimal (canalicular) obstruction
Fluorouracil	Lacrimal (canalicular) obstruction
MEK inhibitors: trametinib, selumetinib, cobimetinib, pimasertib	Multifocal serous retinal detachment, retinal vein occlusion, cystoid macular edema
Vincristine	Optic neuropathy
Chelating agents	
Deferoxamine, deferasirox	Retinopathy, optic neuropathy, lens opacity
Penicillamine	Ocular pemphigoid, optic neuropathy, extraocular muscle palsy (myasthenic syndrome)
Oral hypoglycemic agents	
Chlorpropamide	Refractive error, epidermal necrolysis, optic neuropathy
Thiazolidinediones (glitazones)	Increase in diabetic macular edema
Vitamins	
Vitamin A	Papilledema
Vitamin D	Band-shaped keratopathy
Rheumatologic agents	
Chloroquine, hydroxychloroquine	Retinal degeneration principally involving the macula, vortex keratopathy
Gold salts	Deposits in the cornea, conjunctiva, and lens
NSAIDs (eg, ibuprofen, naproxen, indomethacin)	Vortex keratopathy (ibuprofen, naproxen), corneal deposits (indomethacin), retinal degeneration principally involving the macula (indomethacin)
Penicillamine	Ocular pemphigoid, optic neuropathy, extraocular muscle palsy (myasthenic syndrome)
Salicylates	Subconjunctival and retinal hemorrhages, nystagmus
Dermatologic agents	
Retinoids (eg, isotretinoin, tretinoin, acitretin, and etretinate)	Papilledema, blepharoconjunctivitis, corneal opacities, decreased contact lens tolerance, decreased dark adaptation, teratogenic ocular abnormalities, idiopathic intracranial hypertension, optic neuritis
Dupilumab	Conjunctivitis
Bisphosphonates	
Alendronate, pamidronate	Scleritis, episcleritis, uveitis

cystoid macular edema, and retinal vein occlusion. Patients receiving MEK inhibitors should have a complete eye examination at baseline before the initiation of these medications and should be referred for an eye examination if blurred or reduced vision develops while taking MEK inhibitors.

Arora S et al. Retinal toxicities of systemic anticancer drugs. Surv Ophthalmol. 2022;67:97. [PMID: 34048859]

Campbell RJ et al. Evolution in the risk of cataract surgical complications among patients exposed to tamsulosin: a population-based study. Ophthalmology. 2019;126:490. [PMID: 30648549]

Jain N et al; Macula Society Pentosan Polysulfate Maculopathy Study Group. Expanded clinical spectrum of pentosan polysulfate maculopathy: a Macula Society collaborative study. Ophthalmol Retina. 2022;6:219. [PMID: 34298229]

Syed MF et al. Ocular side effects of common systemic medications and systemic side effects of ocular medications. Med Clin North Am. 2021;105:425. [PMID: 33926639]

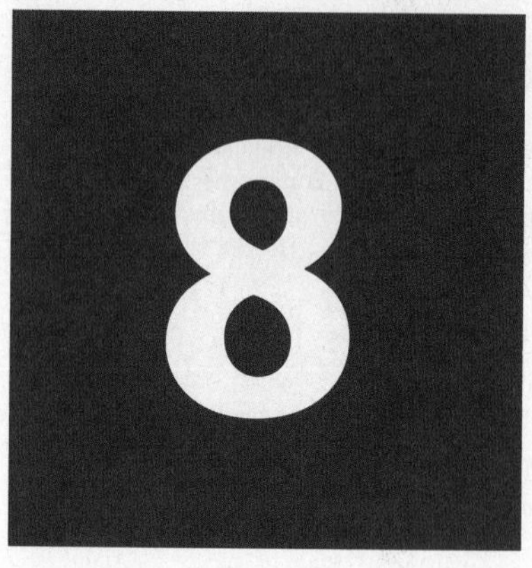

8 Otolaryngology Disorders

Elliott D. Kozin, MD
Lawrence R. Lustig, MD

DISEASES OF THE EAR

HEARING LOSS

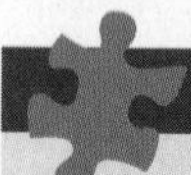

ESSENTIALS OF DIAGNOSIS

- Hearing loss is generally categorized as either conductive or sensorineural.
- Hearing loss is most commonly due to cerumen impaction, transient eustachian tube dysfunction, or age-related hearing loss.

Classification & Epidemiology

Table 8–1 categorizes hearing loss as normal, mild, moderate, severe, or profound and outlines the vocal equivalent as well as the decibel range.

A. Conductive Hearing Loss

Conductive hearing loss results from a mechanical disruption of the external auditory canal or middle ear. Several mechanisms may result in impairment of the passage of sound vibrations to the inner ear, such as obstruction (eg, cerumen impaction), mass loading (eg, middle ear effusion), stiffness (eg, otosclerosis), and discontinuity (eg, ossicular disruption). Conductive losses in adults are most commonly due to cerumen impaction or transient eustachian tube dysfunction from upper respiratory tract infection. Persistent conductive losses usually result from chronic ear infection, trauma, or otosclerosis. Perforations of the tympanic membrane may also result in a conductive hearing loss. Conductive hearing loss is often correctable with medical (eg, use of a hearing aid) or surgical (eg, repair of tympanic membrane and ossicular chain) therapy, or both. CT of the temporal bone may be used as an adjunct to physical examination to determine the potential cause of conductive hearing loss.

B. Sensorineural Hearing Loss

Sensorineural hearing losses are common in adults and generally result from deficits of the inner ear or central (brain) auditory pathway. Sensory hearing loss results from deterioration of the cochlea, usually due to loss of sensory hair cells within the organ of Corti. The most common form of sensorineural hearing loss is **age-related hearing loss** that manifests as a gradually progressive, predominantly high-frequency hearing loss. Other causes of sensorineural hearing loss include excessive noise exposure; head trauma; ototoxic medications, such as cisplatin-based chemotherapy; and systemic diseases.

Sudden sensorineural hearing loss, often called idiopathic sudden sensorineural hearing loss, is considered an otologic emergency and may be treatable with oral or intratympanic corticosteroids if delivered within several weeks of onset. Long-term severe to profound sensorineural hearing loss due to deficits at the level of the inner ear may be correctable with surgery, such as cochlear implantation. Sensorineural hearing loss may also be due to deficits at the level of the central auditory pathway, including lesions involve the eighth cranial nerve, auditory nuclei, ascending tracts, or auditory cortex. Examples of central causes of hearing loss include acoustic neuroma, multiple sclerosis, and auditory neuropathy. Treatment of hearing loss due to central causes are usually aimed at addressing the underlying pathology.

Michels TC et al. Hearing loss in adults: differential diagnosis and treatment. Am Fam Physician. 2019;100:98. [PMID: 31305044]

US Preventive Services Task Force; Krist AH et al. Screening for hearing loss in older adults: US Preventive Services Task Force recommendation statement. JAMA. 2021;325:1196. [PMID: 33755083]

Evaluation of Hearing (Audiology)

In a quiet room, the hearing level may be estimated by having the patient repeat aloud words presented in a soft whisper, a normal spoken voice, or a shout. Normal spoken voice is about 60 decibels. A 512-Hz tuning fork is useful in differentiating conductive from sensorineural hearing loss. In the **Weber test,** the tuning fork is placed directly on the

Table 8–1. Hearing loss classification.

Classification	Vocal Equivalent	Decibel (dB) Range
Normal	Soft whisper	0–20 dB
Mild	Soft spoken voice	20–40 dB
Moderate	Normal spoken voice	40–60 dB
Severe	Loud spoken voice	60–80 dB
Profound	Shout	> 80 dB

forehead or front teeth. In conductive losses, the sound is heard as louder in the ear with *poorer hearing;* however, in sensorineural losses, the sound radiates to the ear that *hears better* than the other ear. In the **Rinne test,** the tuning fork is placed alternately on the mastoid bone (bone conduction) and in front of the ear canal (air conduction). In conductive losses greater than 25 dB, bone conduction sounds louder than air conduction.

Formal audiometric studies are performed in a soundproofed room. Pure-tone thresholds in decibels (dB) are obtained over the range of 250–8000 Hz. Conductive losses create a "gap" between the air and bone thresholds, whereas in sensorineural losses, both air and bone thresholds are equally diminished. Speech discrimination measures the clarity of hearing, reported as percentage correct (90–100% is normal). Auditory brainstem-evoked response screening method is most commonly used in newborn screening and may determine the approximate location of the lesion (eg, cochlea or brain). MRI scanning is the most sensitive and specific test to determine the possible location of a defect resulting in sensorineural hearing loss.

Every patient who complains of a hearing loss should be referred for audiologic evaluation unless the cause is easily remediable (eg, cerumen impaction, otitis media). Immediate audiometric referral is indicated for patients with idiopathic sudden sensorineural hearing loss because it requires treatment (corticosteroids) within a limited several-week time period.

Feltner C et al. Screening for hearing loss in older adults: updated evidence report and systematic review for the US Preventive Services Task Force. JAMA. 2021;325:1202. [PMID: 33755082]

Powell DS et al. Hearing impairment and cognition in an aging world. J Assoc Res Otolaryngol. 2021;22:387. [PMID: 34008037]

Sharma RK et al. Age-related hearing loss and the development of cognitive impairment and late-life depression: a scoping overview. Semin Hear. 2021;42:10. [PMID: 33883788]

Hearing Amplification

Patients with hearing loss not correctable by medical therapy may benefit from hearing amplification. Contemporary hearing aids are comparatively free of distortion and have been miniaturized to the point where they often may be contained entirely within the ear canal or lie inconspicuously behind the ear.

For patients with conductive loss or unilateral profound sensorineural loss, bone-conducting hearing aids directly stimulate the ipsilateral cochlea (for conductive losses) or contralateral ear (profound unilateral sensorineural loss). In most adults with severe to profound sensory hearing loss, the **cochlear implant**—an electronic device that is surgically implanted into the cochlea to stimulate the auditory nerve—offers socially beneficial auditory rehabilitation.

Buchman CA et al. Unilateral cochlear implants for severe, profound, or moderate sloping to profound bilateral sensorineural hearing loss: a systematic review and consensus statements. JAMA Otolaryngol Head Neck Surg. 2020;146:942. [PMID: 32857157]

Dixon PR et al. Health-related quality of life changes associated with hearing loss. JAMA Otolaryngol Head Neck Surg. 2020;146:630. [PMID: 32407468]

DISEASES OF THE AURICLE

Disorders of the auricle include skin cancers due to sun exposure. Traumatic auricular hematoma must be drained to prevent significant cosmetic deformity "cauliflower ear" or canal blockage resulting from dissolution of supporting cartilage. Similarly, cellulitis of the auricle must be treated promptly to prevent perichondritis and resultant deformity. **Relapsing polychondritis** is characterized by recurrent, frequently bilateral, painful episodes of auricular erythema and edema and sometimes progressive involvement of the cartilaginous tracheobronchial tree. Treatment with corticosteroids may help forestall cartilage dissolution. Polychondritis and perichondritis may be differentiated from cellulitis by sparing of involvement of the lobule, which does not contain cartilage.

Dalal PJ et al. Risk factors for auricular hematoma and recurrence after drainage. Laryngoscope. 2020;130:628. [PMID: 31621925]

Fousekis FS et al. Ear involvement in inflammatory bowel disease: A review of the literature. J Clin Med Res. 2018;10:609. [PMID: 29977417]

DISEASES OF THE EAR CANAL

1. Cerumen Impaction

Cerumen is a protective secretion produced by the outer portion of the ear canal. *In most persons, the ear canal is self-cleansing and no hygiene measures are recommended.* Cerumen impaction is most often self-induced through ill-advised cleansing attempts by entering the canal itself, eg, digital trauma or use of a cotton-tip applicator. It may be relieved by the patient using detergent ear drops (eg, 3% hydrogen peroxide; 6.5% carbamide peroxide) and irrigation, or by the clinician using mechanical removal, suction, or irrigation. Irrigation is performed with water at body temperature to avoid a vestibular caloric response. The stream should be directed at the posterior ear canal wall adjacent to the cerumen plug. Irrigation should be performed only when the tympanic membrane is known to be intact.

Use of jet irrigators (eg, WaterPik) should be avoided since they may result in tympanic membrane perforations. Following irrigation, the ear canal should be thoroughly dried (eg, by the patient using a hair blow-dryer on low-power setting or by the clinician instilling isopropyl alcohol) to reduce the likelihood of otitis externa. Specialty referral is indicated if impaction is frequently recurrent, if it has not responded to routine measures, or if there is tympanic membrane perforation or chronic otitis media.

Horton GA et al. Cerumen management: an updated clinical review and evidence-based approach for primary care physicians. J Prim Care Community Health. 2020;11:2150132720904181. [PMID: 31994443]

2. Foreign Bodies

Foreign bodies in the ear canal are more frequent in children than in adults. Firm materials may be removed with a loop or a hook, taking care not to displace the object medially toward the tympanic membrane; microscopic guidance is helpful. Aqueous irrigation should not be performed for organic foreign bodies (eg, beans, insects), because water may cause them to swell. Living insects are best immobilized before removal by filling the ear canal with lidocaine or mineral oil. Lidocaine should *never* be used in a patient with a possible tympanic membrane perforation as this may result in a profound vestibular response.

Kim KH et al. Clinical characteristics of external auditory canal foreign bodies in children and adolescents. Ear Nose Throat J. 2020;99:648. [PMID: 31814447]

3. Otitis Externa

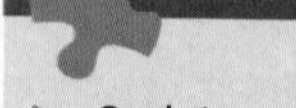

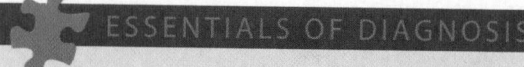

ESSENTIALS OF DIAGNOSIS

- Otalgia.
- Erythema, edema, and purulence of the external auditory canal skin.
- Diabetic or immunocompromised patients are at risk for "malignant" otitis externa (osteomyelitis of the skull base).

General Considerations

Otitis externa, often called "swimmer's ear," presents with otalgia with associated external auditory canal edema and purulent discharge. There is often a history of recent water exposure or mechanical trauma (eg, scratching, cotton applicators). Otitis externa is usually caused by gram-negative rods (eg, *Pseudomonas, Proteus*) or fungi (eg, *Aspergillus*), which grow in the presence of excessive moisture. In diabetic or immunocompromised patients, persistent otitis externa may evolve into osteomyelitis of the skull base (so-called **malignant otitis externa**). Usually caused by *Pseudomonas aeruginosa*, osteomyelitis begins in the floor of the ear canal and may extend into the middle fossa floor, the clivus, and even the contralateral skull base.

Clinical Findings

Examination reveals erythema and edema of the ear canal skin, often with a purulent exudate (Figure 8–1), as well as surrounding periauricular cellulitis. Manipulation of the auricle elicits pain. The lateral surface of the tympanic membrane is often erythematous. When the canal skin is very edematous, it may be impossible to visualize the tympanic membrane. In immunocompromised patients, such as those with diabetes, malignant otitis externa typically presents with persistent otorrhea; granulation tissue in the ear canal; deep otalgia; and in advanced cases, progressive palsies of cranial nerves, such as cranial nerve VI, VII, IX, X, XI, or XII. Diagnosis of malignant otitis externa is confirmed by the demonstration of osseous erosion on CT scanning and laboratory testing showing high inflammatory markers, such as ESR and CRP. MRI scanning is often important to rule out abscesses that may result from malignant otitis externa.

Treatment

Treatment of otitis externa involves protection of the ear from additional moisture and avoidance of further

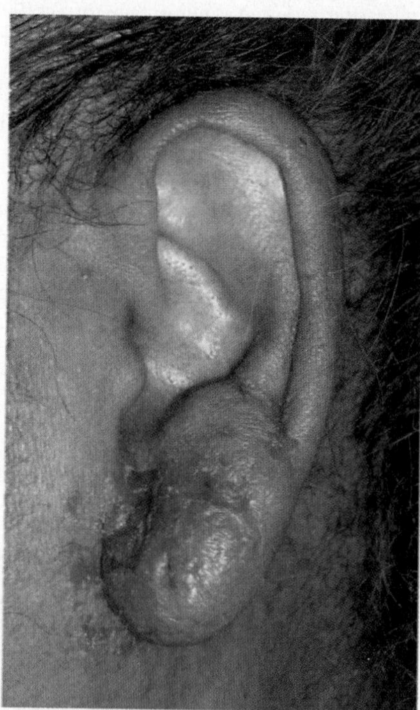

Figure 8–1. Malignant otitis externa in a 40-year-old woman with diabetes mellitus, with typical swelling and honey-colored crusting of the pinna. Both the external auditory canal and temporal bone were involved in the pseudomonal infection. (Used, with permission, from E.J. Mayeaux Jr, MD, in Usatine RP, Smith MA, Mayeaux EJ Jr, Chumley H. *The Color Atlas of Family Medicine*, 2nd ed. McGraw-Hill, 2013.)

mechanical injury by scratching. In cases of moisture in the ear (eg, swimmer's ear), acidification with a drying agent (ie, a 50/50 mixture of isopropyl alcohol/white vinegar) is often helpful. When infected, an otic antibiotic solution or suspension of an aminoglycoside (eg, neomycin/polymyxin B) or fluoroquinolone (eg, ciprofloxacin), with or without a corticosteroid (eg, hydrocortisone), is usually effective. Purulent debris filling the ear canal should be gently removed to permit entry of the topical medication. Drops should be used abundantly (five or more drops three or four times a day) to penetrate the depths of the canal. When substantial edema of the canal wall prevents entry of drops into the ear canal, a wick is placed to facilitate their entry. In recalcitrant cases—particularly when cellulitis of the periauricular tissue has developed—oral fluoroquinolones (eg, ciprofloxacin, 500 mg twice daily for 1 week) are used because of their effectiveness against *Pseudomonas*. Newer medications that are ciprofloxacin suspensions may hold promise to improve otitis externa outcomes. Any case of persistent otitis externa in an immunocompromised or diabetic individual must be referred for specialty evaluation.

Treatment of malignant otitis externa requires prolonged antipseudomonal antibiotic administration, often for several months. Although intravenous therapy is often required initially (eg, ciprofloxacin 200–400 mg every 12 hours), selected patients may be graduated to oral ciprofloxacin (500–1000 mg twice daily). To avoid relapse, antibiotic therapy should be continued, even in the asymptomatic patient, until gallium scanning indicates marked reduction or resolution of the inflammation. Surgical debridement of infected bone is reserved for cases of deterioration despite medical therapy.

Smith ME et al; INTEGRATE (The UK ENT Trainee Research Network). Acute otitis externa: consensus definition, diagnostic criteria and core outcome set development. PLoS One. 2021;16:e0251395. [PMID: 33989313]

4. Pruritus

Pruritus of the external auditory canal, particularly at the meatus, is common. While it may be associated with otitis externa or with seborrheic dermatitis or psoriasis, most cases are self-induced from excoriation or overly zealous ear cleaning. To permit regeneration of the protective cerumen blanket, patients should be instructed to avoid use of soap and water or cotton swabs in the ear canal and avoid any scratching. Patients with excessively dry canal skin may benefit from application of mineral oil, which helps counteract dryness and repel moisture. When an inflammatory component is present, topical application of a corticosteroid (eg, 0.1% triamcinolone) may be beneficial.

5. Exostoses & Osteomas

Bony overgrowths of the ear canal are a frequent incidental finding and rarely have clinical significance. They present as skin-covered bony mounds in the medial ear canal obscuring the tympanic membrane to a variable degree. Solitary osteomas are of no significance as long as they do not cause obstruction or infection. Multiple exostoses, which are generally acquired from repeated exposure to cold water (eg, "surfer's ear"), may progress and require surgical removal if completely occluding the external auditory canal or resulting in frequent infections.

Simas V et al. Lifetime prevalence of exostoses in New Zealand surfers. J Prim Health Care. 2019;11:47. [PMID: 31039989]

6. Neoplasia

The most common neoplasm of the ear canal is squamous cell carcinoma. When an apparent otitis externa does not resolve on therapy, a malignancy should be suspected and biopsy performed. This disease carries a very high 5-year mortality rate because the tumor tends to invade the lymphatics of the cranial base and must be treated with wide surgical resection and radiation therapy. Adenomatous tumors, originating from the ceruminous glands, generally follow a more indolent course.

Komune N et al. Prognostic impact of tumor extension in patients with advanced temporal bone squamous cell carcinoma. Front Oncol. 2020;10:1229. [PMID: 32850367]

Piras G et al. Management of squamous cell carcinoma of the temporal bone: long-term results and factors influencing outcomes. Eur Arch Otorhinolaryngol. 2021;278:3193. [PMID: 32979119]

Seligman KL et al. Temporal bone carcinoma: treatment patterns and survival. Laryngoscope. 2020;130:E11. [PMID: 30874314]

DISEASES OF THE EUSTACHIAN TUBE

1. Eustachian Tube Dysfunction

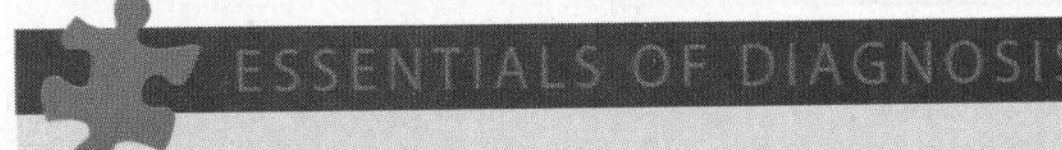

- Aural fullness.
- Discomfort with barometric pressure change.
- Retracted eardrum.

The tube that connects the middle ear to the nasopharynx—the eustachian tube—provides ventilation and drainage for the middle ear. It is normally closed, opening only during swallowing or yawning. When eustachian tube function is compromised, air trapped within the middle ear becomes absorbed and negative pressure results. The most common causes of eustachian tube dysfunction are diseases associated with edema of the tubal lining, such as viral upper respiratory tract infections and seasonal allergies. The patient usually reports a sense of fullness in the ear and mild to moderate impairment of hearing. When the tube is only partially blocked, swallowing or yawning may elicit a popping or crackling sound. Examination may reveal retraction of the tympanic membrane and decreased mobility on pneumatic otoscopy. Following a viral illness, this disorder is usually transient, lasting days to weeks. Treatment with systemic and intranasal decongestants (eg, pseudoephedrine, 60 mg orally every 4–6 hours; oxymetazoline, 0.05% spray every 8–12 hours), combined with **autoinsufflation** by forced exhalation against closed nostrils, may hasten relief. Autoinsufflation should not be recommended to patients with active intranasal infection, since this maneuver may precipitate middle ear infection. Allergic patients may also benefit from intranasal corticosteroids (eg, beclomethasone dipropionate, two sprays in each nostril twice daily for 2–6 weeks). Air travel, rapid altitudinal change, and underwater diving should be avoided until resolution.

An overly patent eustachian tube ("patulous eustachian tube") is a relatively uncommon, though quite distressing problem. Typical complaints include fullness in the ear and autophony (an exaggerated ability to hear oneself breathe and speak). A patulous eustachian tube may develop during rapid weight loss, such as following pregnancy, or it may be idiopathic. In contrast to eustachian tube dysfunction, the aural pressure is often made worse by exertion and may diminish during an upper respiratory tract infection. Although physical examination is usually normal, respiratory excursions of the tympanic membrane may occasionally be detected during vigorous breathing. Treatment includes avoidance of decongestant products and rarely surgery on the eustachian tube itself.

Froehlich MH et al. Eustachian tube balloon dilation: a systematic review and meta-analysis of treatment outcomes. Otolaryngol Head Neck Surg. 2020;163:870. [PMID: 32482125]

Tucci DL et al. Clinical consensus statement: balloon dilation of the eustachian tube. Otolaryngol Head Neck Surg. 2019;161:6. [PMID: 31161864]

2. Serous Otitis Media

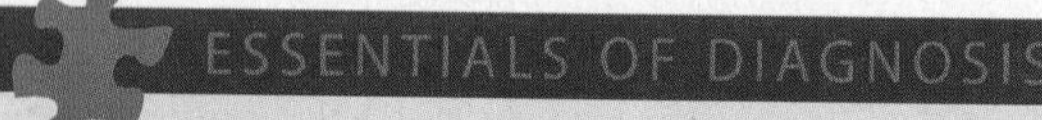

- Eustachian tube obstruction is the underlying cause.
- Resultant negative pressure causes transudation of fluid into the middle ear and stasis.

Prolonged eustachian tube dysfunction with resultant negative middle ear pressure may cause a transudation of fluid. In adults, serous otitis media usually occurs with an upper respiratory tract infection, with barotrauma, or with chronic allergic rhinitis, but when persistent and unilateral, nasopharyngeal carcinoma must be excluded. The tympanic membrane is dull and hypomobile, occasionally accompanied by air bubbles in the middle ear and conductive hearing loss. The treatment of serous otitis media is similar to that for eustachian tube dysfunction. When medication fails to bring relief after several months, a ventilating tube placed through the tympanic membrane may restore hearing and alleviate the sense of aural fullness.

Vanneste P et al. Otitis media with effusion in children: pathophysiology, diagnosis, and treatment. A review. J Otol. 2019; 14:33. [PMID: 31223299]

3. Barotrauma

Persons with poor eustachian tube function (eg, congenital narrowness or acquired mucosal edema) may be unable to equalize the barometric stress exerted on the middle ear by air travel, rapid altitudinal change, or underwater diving. The problem is generally most acute during airplane descent, since the negative middle ear pressure tends to collapse and block the eustachian tube, causing pain. Several measures are useful to enhance eustachian tube function and avoid otic barotrauma. The patient should be advised to swallow, yawn, and autoinsufflate frequently during descent. Oral decongestants (eg, pseudoephedrine, 60–120 mg) should be taken several hours before anticipated arrival time so that they will be maximally effective during descent. Topical decongestants, such as 1% phenylephrine or oxymetazoline nasal spray, should be administered 1 hour before arrival.

For acute negative middle ear pressure that persists on the ground, treatment includes decongestants and attempts at autoinsufflation. Myringotomy provides immediate relief and is appropriate in the setting of severe otalgia and hearing loss.

Underwater diving may represent an even greater barometric stress to the ear than flying. Patients should be warned to avoid diving when they have an upper respiratory infection or episode of nasal allergy. During the descent phase of the dive, if inflation of the middle ear via the eustachian tube has not occurred, pain will develop within the first 15 feet; the dive must be aborted. In all cases, divers must descend slowly and equilibrate in stages to avoid the development of severely negative pressures in the tympanum that may result in hemorrhage (hemotympanum) or in perilymphatic fistula. In the latter, the oval or round window ruptures, resulting in sensory hearing loss and acute vertigo. During the ascent phase of a saturation dive, sensory hearing loss or vertigo may develop as the first (or only) symptom of decompression sickness. Immediate recompression will return intravascular gas bubbles to solution and restore the inner ear microcirculation.

Tympanic membrane perforation is an absolute contraindication to diving, as the patient will experience an unbalanced thermal stimulus to the semicircular canals and may experience vertigo, disorientation, and even emesis.

Millan SB et al. Prevention of middle ear barotrauma with oxymetazoline/fluticasone treatment. Undersea Hyperb Med. 2021; 48:149. [PMID: 33975404]

Scarpa A et al. Inner ear disorders in SCUBA divers: a review. J Int Adv Otol. 2021;17:260. [PMID: 34100753]

DISEASES OF THE MIDDLE EAR

1. Acute Otitis Media

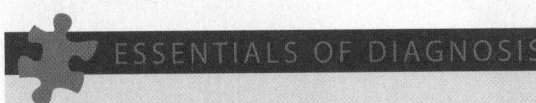

- Otalgia.
- Purulent fluid of the middle ear.
- Erythema and hypomobility of tympanic membrane.

General Considerations

Acute otitis media is a bacterial infection of the mucosally lined, air-containing spaces of the middle ear. Purulent material may extend to pneumatized mastoid air cells and petrous apex of the lateral skull base. Acute otitis media is usually precipitated by a viral upper respiratory tract infection that causes eustachian tube obstruction. This results in accumulation of fluid and mucus, which becomes secondarily infected by bacteria. The most common pathogens are *Streptococcus pneumoniae, Haemophilus influenzae,* and *Streptococcus pyogenes.*

Clinical Findings

Acute otitis media may occur at any age. Presenting symptoms and signs include otalgia, aural pressure, decreased hearing, and often fever. The typical physical findings are erythema and decreased mobility of the tympanic membrane (Figure 8–2). Occasionally, bullae will appear on the tympanic membrane.

Rarely, when middle ear empyema is severe, the tympanic membrane bulges outward. In such cases, tympanic membrane rupture is imminent. Rupture is accompanied by a sudden decrease in pain, followed by the onset of otorrhea. With appropriate therapy, spontaneous healing of the tympanic membrane occurs in most cases. Acute mastoiditis results from an infection extending from the middle ear to the mastoid air cells. It is diagnosed by pain, postauricular erythema, and occasionally proptosis of the auricle. Frank swelling over the mastoid bone or the association of cranial neuropathies or central findings indicates severe disease requiring urgent care. Evaluation includes imaging, such as CT, to determine presence of "coalescence" of air cells and associated soft-tissue abscess.

Treatment

The treatment of acute otitis media is specific antibiotic therapy, often combined with nasal decongestants. The first-choice antibiotic is amoxicillin 1 g orally every 8 hours for 5–7 days. Alternatives (useful in resistant cases) are amoxicillin-clavulanate 875/125 mg or 2 g/125 mg ER every 12 hours for 5–10 days; or cefuroxime 500 mg or cefpodoxime 200 mg orally every 12 hours for 5–7 days. Recurrent acute otitis media may be managed with long-term antibiotic prophylaxis. Single daily oral doses of sulfamethoxazole (500 mg) or amoxicillin (250 or 500 mg) are given over a period of 1–3 months. Failure of this regimen to control infection is an indication for insertion of ventilating tubes.

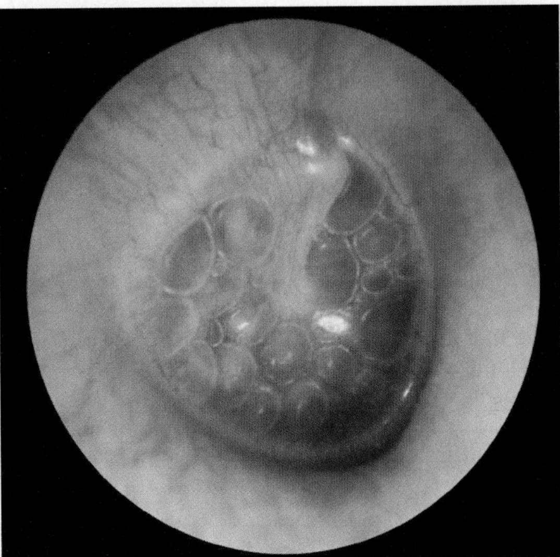

▲ Figure 8–2. Acute otitis media with effusion of right ear, with multiple air-fluid levels visible through a translucent, slightly retracted, nonerythematous tympanic membrane. (Used, with permission, from Frank Miller, MD, in Usatine RP, Smith MA, Mayeaux EJ Jr, Chumley H. *The Color Atlas of Family Medicine*, 2nd ed. McGraw-Hill, 2013.)

Surgical drainage of the middle ear (myringotomy), debridement of the mastoid (mastoidectomy), or both are reserved for patients with severe otalgia or when complications of otitis (eg, mastoiditis, meningitis) have occurred.

Hoberman A et al. Tympanostomy tubes or medical management for recurrent acute otitis media. N Engl J Med. 2021; 384:1789. [PMID: 33979487]

Szmuilowicz J et al. Infections of the ear. Emerg Med Clin North Am. 2019;37:1. [PMID: 30454772]

2. Chronic Otitis Media

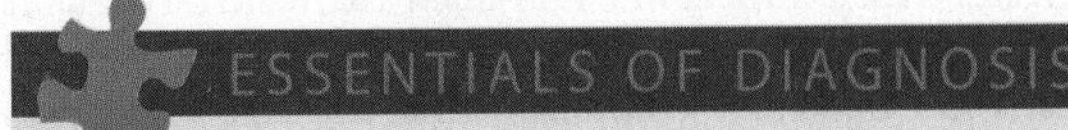

- Chronic otorrhea with or without otalgia.
- Tympanic membrane perforation with conductive hearing loss.
- Often amenable to surgical correction.

General Considerations

Chronic infection of the middle ear and mastoid generally develops as a consequence of recurrent acute otitis media, although it may follow other diseases and trauma. Perforation or retraction of the tympanic membrane may be present. The bacteriology of chronic otitis media differs from that of acute otitis media. Common organisms include *P aeruginosa, Proteus* species, *Staphylococcus aureus,* and mixed anaerobic infections.

Clinical Findings

The clinical hallmark of chronic otitis media is purulent aural discharge. Drainage may be continuous or intermittent, with increased severity during upper respiratory tract infection or following water exposure. Pain is uncommon except during acute exacerbations. Conductive hearing loss results from destruction of the tympanic membrane or ossicular chain, or both.

Treatment

The medical treatment of chronic otitis media includes regular removal of infected debris, use of earplugs to protect against water exposure, and topical antibiotic drops (ofloxacin 0.3% or ciprofloxacin with dexamethasone) for exacerbations. Oral ciprofloxacin, active against *Pseudomonas*, 500 mg twice a day for 1–6 weeks, may help dry a chronically discharging ear.

In most cases, surgery is the definitive management of tympanic membrane perforations with or without association of ossicular disruption. Successful reconstruction of the tympanic membrane may be achieved with autologous tissue, such as temporalis fascia, in about 90% of cases, often with improvement in conductive hearing.

Head K et al. Antibiotics versus topical antiseptics for chronic suppurative otitis media. Cochrane Database Syst Rev. 2020;1:CD013056. [PMID: 31902139]

Complications of Otitis Media

A. Cholesteatoma

Cholesteatoma is a special variety of chronic otitis media (Figure 8–3). The most common cause is prolonged eustachian tube dysfunction, with inward migration of the upper flaccid portion of the tympanic membrane. This creates a squamous epithelium-lined sac, which—when its neck becomes obstructed—may fill with desquamated keratin and become chronically infected. Cholesteatomas typically erode bone, including the ossicular chain with extension into the mastoid. Over time, cholesteatoma may erode into the inner ear, involve the facial nerve and, on rare occasions, spread intracranially. Otoscopic examination may reveal a retraction pocket of the tympanic membrane or a marginal tympanic membrane perforation that exudes keratin debris or granulation tissue. The treatment of cholesteatoma is surgical, including marsupialization of the sac or its complete removal. This may require the creation of a "mastoid bowl" in which the ear canal and mastoid are joined into a large common cavity that must be periodically cleaned.

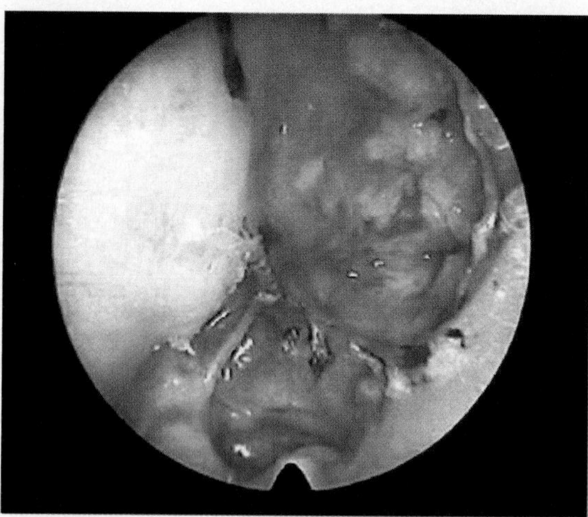

Figure 8–3. Cholesteatoma. (Used, with permission, from Vladimir Zlinsky, MD, in Roy F. Sullivan, PhD: Audiology Forum: Video Otoscopy, www.RCSullivan.com; from Usatine RP, Smith MA, Mayeaux EJ Jr, Chumley H. *The Color Atlas of Family Medicine*, 2nd ed. McGraw-Hill, 2013.)

Basonbul RA et al. Systematic review of endoscopic ear surgery outcomes for pediatric cholesteatoma. Otol Neurotol. 2021;42:108. [PMID: 33165162]

Luu K et al. Updates in pediatric cholesteatoma: minimizing intervention while maximizing outcomes. Otolaryngol Clin North Am. 2019;52:813. [PMID: 31280890]

B. Mastoiditis

Acute suppurative mastoiditis usually evolves following several weeks of inadequately treated acute otitis media. It is characterized by pain and postauricular cellulitis accompanied by a spiking fever. CT scan reveals coalescence of the mastoid air cells due to destruction of their bony septa. Initial treatment consists of intravenous antibiotics (eg, cefazolin 0.5–1.5 g every 6–8 hours) directed against the most common offending organisms (*S pneumoniae, H influenzae,* and *S pyogenes),* and myringotomy for culture and drainage. Failure of medical therapy indicates the need for surgical drainage, such as a mastoidectomy.

C. Petrous Apicitis

The medial portion of the petrous bone between the inner ear and clivus may become a site of persistent infection when the drainage of its pneumatic cell tracts becomes blocked. This may cause foul discharge, deep ear and retro-orbital pain, and sixth nerve palsy (Gradenigo syndrome); meningitis may be a complication. Treatment is with prolonged antibiotic therapy (based on culture results) or surgical drainage via petrous apicectomy or both.

Isaac H et al. Transmastoid and transtemporal drainage of petrous apicitis with otitis media. Ann Otol Rhinol Laryngol. 2021;130:314. [PMID: 32772562]

D. Facial Paralysis

Facial palsy may be associated with either acute or chronic otitis media. In the acute setting, it results from inflammation of the seventh nerve in its middle ear segment. Treatment consists of myringotomy for drainage and culture, followed by intravenous antibiotics (based on culture results). The use of corticosteroids is controversial. The prognosis is excellent, with complete recovery in most cases.

Facial palsy associated with chronic otitis media usually evolves slowly due to chronic pressure on the seventh nerve in the middle ear or mastoid by cholesteatoma. Treatment requires surgical correction of the underlying disease. The prognosis is less favorable than for facial palsy associated with acute otitis media.

Mohan S et al. Considerations in management of acute otitis media in the COVID-19 era. Ann Otol Rhinol Laryngol. 2021;130:520. [PMID: 32911957]

E. Sigmoid Sinus Thrombosis

Trapped infection within the mastoid air cells adjacent to the sigmoid sinus may cause septic thrombophlebitis. This is heralded by signs of systemic sepsis (spiking fevers, chills), at times accompanied by signs of increased intracranial pressure (headache, lethargy, nausea and vomiting, papilledema). Diagnosis can be made noninvasively by magnetic resonance venography (MRV). Primary treatment is with intravenous antibiotics (based on culture results). Additional treatment, such as anticoagulation, surgical drainage, ligation of the internal jugular vein, or some combination thereof, may be indicated when embolization is suspected.

Ziv O et al. Post-operative clinical course in children undergoing mastoidectomy due to complicated acute mastoiditis. Eur Arch Otorhinolaryngol. 2021 Oct 29. [Epub ahead of print] [PMID: 34714371]

F. Central Nervous System Infection

Otogenic meningitis is the most common intracranial complication of ear infection. In the setting of acute suppurative otitis media, it arises from hematogenous spread of bacteria, most commonly *H influenzae* and *S pneumoniae*. In chronic otitis media, it results either from passage of infection along preformed pathways, such as the petrosquamous suture line, or from direct extension of disease through the dural plates of the petrous pyramid.

Epidural abscesses arise from direct extension of disease in the setting of chronic infection. They are usually asymptomatic but may present with deep local pain, headache, and low-grade fever. They are often discovered as an incidental finding at surgery. Brain abscess may arise in the temporal lobe or cerebellum as a result of septic thrombophlebitis adjacent to an epidural abscess. The predominant causative organisms are *S aureus*, *S pyogenes*, and *S pneumoniae*. Rupture into the subarachnoid space results in meningitis and often death. (See Chapter 30.)

Botti C et al. Pneumolabyrinth: a systematic review. Eur Arch Otorhinolaryngol. 2021;278:4619. [PMID: 33881577]

3. Otosclerosis

Otosclerosis is a progressive disease with a marked familial tendency that affects the bony otic capsule. Lesions involving the footplate of the stapes result in increased impedance to the passage of sound through the ossicular chain, producing conductive hearing loss. This may be treated either through the use of a hearing aid or surgical replacement of the stapes with a prosthesis (stapedectomy). When otosclerotic lesions involve the cochlea ("cochlear otosclerosis"), permanent sensory hearing loss may occur.

Gillard DM et al. Cost-effectiveness of stapedectomy vs hearing aids in the treatment of otosclerosis. JAMA Otolaryngol Head Neck Surg. 2020;146:42. [PMID: 31697352]
Yeh CF et al. Predictors of hearing outcomes after stapes surgery in otosclerosis. Acta Otolaryngol. 2019;139:1058. [PMID: 31617779]

4. Trauma to the Middle Ear

Tympanic membrane perforation may result from impact injury or explosive acoustic trauma (Figure 8–4). Spontaneous healing occurs in most cases. Persistent perforation may result from secondary infection brought on by exposure to water. During the healing period, patients should be advised to wear earplugs while swimming or bathing. Hemorrhage behind an intact tympanic membrane (hemotympanum) may follow blunt trauma or extreme barotrauma. Spontaneous resolution over several weeks is the usual course. When a conductive hearing loss greater than 30 dB persists for more than 3 months following trauma, disruption of the ossicular chain should be suspected. Middle ear exploration with reconstruction of the ossicular chain, combined with repair of the tympanic membrane when required, will usually restore hearing.

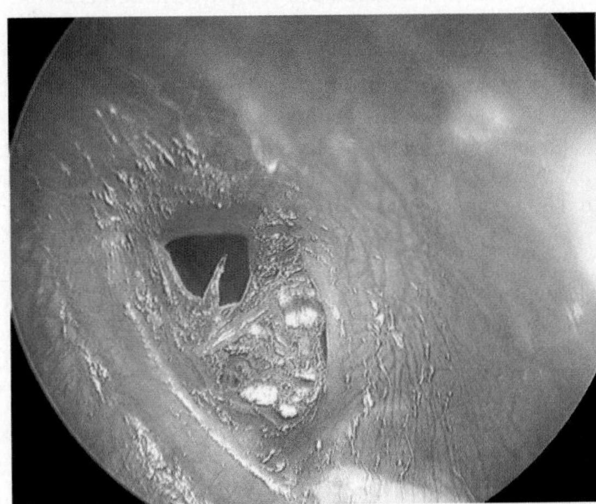

▲ **Figure 8–4.** **Traumatic perforation of the left tympanic membrane.** (Used, with permission, from William Clark, MD, in Usatine RP, Smith MA, Mayeaux EJ Jr, Chumley H. *The Color Atlas of Family Medicine*, 2nd ed. McGraw-Hill, 2013.)

Straughan AJ et al. Feel the burn! Fireworks-related otolaryngologic trauma. Ann Otol Rhinol Laryngol. 2021;130:1369. [PMID: 33834893]

5. Middle Ear Neoplasia

Primary middle ear tumors are rare. **Glomus tumors** arise either in the middle ear (glomus tympanicum) or in the jugular bulb with upward erosion into the hypotympanum (glomus jugulare). They present clinically with pulsatile tinnitus and hearing loss. A vascular mass may be visible behind an intact tympanic membrane. Large glomus jugulare tumors are often associated with multiple cranial neuropathies, especially involving nerves VII, IX, X, XI, and XII. Treatment usually requires surgery, radiotherapy, or both. **Pulsatile tinnitus thus warrants magnetic resonance angiography (MRA) and MRV to rule out a vascular mass.**

Yildiz E et al. Long-term outcome and comparison of treatment modalities of temporal bone paragangliomas. Cancers (Basel). 2021;13:5083. [PMID: 34680232]

EARACHE

Earache can be caused by a variety of otologic problems, but otitis externa and acute otitis media are the most common. Otitis externa and acute otitis media may be differentiated using history and physical examination, including pneumatic otoscopy. Pain out of proportion to the physical findings may be due to herpes zoster oticus, especially when vesicles appear in the ear canal or concha. Persistent pain and discharge from the ear suggest osteomyelitis of the skull base or cancer, and patients with these complaints should be referred for specialty evaluation.

Nonotologic causes of otalgia are numerous. The sensory innervation of the ear is derived from the trigeminal, facial, glossopharyngeal, vagal, and upper cervical nerves. Because of this rich innervation, referred otalgia is quite frequent. Temporomandibular joint dysfunction is a common cause of referred ear pain. Pain is exacerbated by chewing or psychogenic grinding of the teeth (bruxism) and may be associated with dental malocclusion. Repeated episodes of severe lancinating otalgia may occur in glossopharyngeal neuralgia. Infections and neoplasia that involve the oropharynx, hypopharynx, and larynx frequently cause otalgia. Persistent earache demands specialty referral to exclude cancer of the upper aerodigestive tract.

Norris CD et al. Secondary otalgia: referred pain pathways and pathologies. AJNR Am J Neuroradiol. 2020;41:2188. [PMID: 33093134]

DISEASES OF THE INNER EAR

1. Sensorineural Hearing Loss

Diseases of the cochlea and central auditory pathway result in hearing loss, a condition that is usually irreversible. The primary goals in the management of sensory hearing loss are prevention of further losses and functional improvement with auditory rehabilitation, such as with a hearing aid or cochlear implant.

A. Presbycusis

Presbycusis, or age-related hearing loss, is the most frequent cause of sensory hearing loss and is progressive, predominantly high-frequency, and symmetrical. Various etiologic factors (eg, prior noise trauma, drug exposure, genetic predisposition) may contribute to presbycusis. Most patients notice a loss of speech discrimination that is especially pronounced in noisy environments. About 25% of people between the ages of 65 and 75 years and almost 50% of those over 75 experience hearing difficulties. There is emerging evidence that conventional audiometry may not fully capture hearing loss (known as "hidden hearing loss"). Many patients may have subclinical hearing loss. New testing modalities are being devised to detect hearing loss in the setting of normal audiograms.

Choi JY et al. The impact of hearing loss on clinical dementia and preclinical cognitive impairment in later life. J Alzheimers Dis. 2021;81:963. [PMID: 33867361]
Drennan WR. Identifying subclinical hearing loss: extended audiometry and word recognition in noise. Audiol Neurootol. 2021 Nov 2. [Epub ahead of print] [PMID: 34727540]

B. Noise Trauma

Noise trauma is the second most common cause of sensorineural hearing loss. Sounds exceeding 85 dB for 8 hours or more are potentially injurious to the cochlea. The loss typically begins in the high frequencies (especially 4000 Hz) and, with continuing exposure, progresses to involve the speech frequencies. Among the more common sources of injurious noise are industrial machinery, weapons, and excessively loud music. Monitoring noise levels in the workplace by regulatory agencies has led to preventive programs that have reduced the frequency of occupational losses. Individuals of all ages, especially those with existing hearing losses, should wear earplugs when exposed to moderately loud noises and specially designed earmuffs when exposed to explosive noises.

Le Prell CG et al. Noise-induced hearing loss and its prevention: current issues in mammalian hearing. Curr Opin Physiol. 2020;18:32. [PMID: 32984667]
Neitzel RL et al. Risk of noise-induced hearing loss due to recreational sound: review and recommendations. J Acoust Soc Am. 2019;146:3911. [PMID: 31795675]

C. Physical Trauma

Concussive head trauma has effects on the inner ear similar to those of severe acoustic trauma. Some degree of sensory hearing loss may occur following concussion and is frequent after lateral skull base fracture.

Mizutari K. Update on treatment options for blast-induced hearing loss. Curr Opin Otolaryngol Head Neck Surg. 2019;27:376. [PMID: 31348022]

D. Ototoxicity

Ototoxic substances may affect both the auditory and vestibular systems. The most commonly used ototoxic medications are aminoglycosides; loop diuretics; and several antineoplastic agents, notably cisplatin. These medications may cause irreversible hearing loss even when administered in therapeutic doses. When using these medications, it is important to identify high-risk patients, such as those with preexisting hearing losses or kidney disease. Patients simultaneously receiving multiple ototoxic agents are at particular risk owing to ototoxic synergy. Useful measures to reduce the risk of ototoxic injury include serial audiometry, monitoring of serum peak and trough levels, and substitution of equivalent nonototoxic medications whenever possible.

It is possible for topical agents that enter the middle ear to be absorbed into the inner ear via the round window. When the tympanic membrane is perforated, use of potentially ototoxic ear drops (eg, neomycin, gentamicin) is best avoided.

Laurell G. Pharmacological intervention in the field of ototoxicity. HNO. 2019;67:434. [PMID: 30993373]

Rybak LP et al. Local drug delivery for prevention of hearing loss. Front Cell Neurosci. 2019;13:300. [PMID: 31338024]

E. Idiopathic Sudden Sensory Hearing Loss

Idiopathic sudden loss of hearing in one ear may occur at any age, but typically it occurs in persons over age 20 years. In the setting a normal otologic physical examination, symptoms may include hearing loss, aural fullness, tinnitus, and dizziness. The cause is unknown; however, idiopathic sudden hearing loss may result from a viral infection or a sudden vascular occlusion of the internal auditory artery. Obtaining an MRI is essential after the diagnosis to rule out retrocochlear pathology (eg, tumors); however, this should not delay treatment. Prompt treatment with corticosteroids has been shown to improve the odds of recovery. Intratympanic administration of corticosteroids alone or in association with oral corticosteroids has been associated with an equal or more favorable prognosis. Because treatment appears to be most effective as close to the onset of the loss as possible, and appears not to be effective after 6 weeks, a prompt audiogram should be obtained in all patients who present with sudden hearing loss without obvious middle ear pathology. Prognosis is mixed, with many patients suffering permanent deafness in the involved ear, while others have complete recovery.

Ahmadzai N et al. A systematic review and network meta-analysis of existing pharmacologic therapies in patients with idiopathic sudden sensorineural hearing loss. PLoS One. 2019;14:e0221713. [PMID: 31498809]

Chandrasekhar SS et al. Clinical practice guideline: sudden hearing loss (Update). Otolaryngol Head Neck Surg. 2019;161:S1. [PMID: 31369359]

F. Autoimmune Hearing Loss

Sensorineural hearing loss that occurs in both ears simultaneously may be associated with a wide array of systemic autoimmune disorders, such as SLE, granulomatosis with polyangiitis, and Cogan syndrome (hearing loss, keratitis, aortitis). The loss is most often progressive. The hearing level often fluctuates, with periods of deterioration alternating with partial or even complete remission. Usually, there is the gradual evolution of permanent hearing loss, which often stabilizes with some remaining auditory function but occasionally proceeds to complete deafness. Vestibular dysfunction, particularly dysequilibrium and postural instability, may accompany the auditory symptoms.

In many cases, the autoimmune pattern of audiovestibular dysfunction presents in the absence of recognized systemic autoimmune disease. Responsiveness to oral corticosteroid treatment is helpful in making the diagnosis and constitutes first-line therapy. If stabilization of hearing becomes dependent on long-term corticosteroid use, steroid-sparing immunosuppressive regimens may become necessary.

Yuen E et al. Hearing loss in patients with systemic lupus erythematosus: a systematic review and meta-analysis. Lupus. 2021;30:937. [PMID: 33645314]

2. Tinnitus

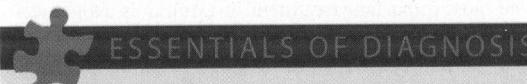

- Phantom noise or sounds.
- Persistent tinnitus often, though not always, indicates the presence of hearing loss.
- Intermittent periods of mild, high-pitched tinnitus lasting seconds to minutes are common in normal-hearing persons.

General Considerations

Tinnitus is defined as the sensation of sound in the absence of an exogenous sound source. Tinnitus can accompany any form of hearing loss, and its presence provides no diagnostic value in determining the cause of a hearing loss. Approximately 15% of the general population experiences some type of tinnitus, with prevalence beyond 20% in aging populations.

Clinical Findings

A. Symptoms and Signs

Though tinnitus is commonly associated with hearing loss, tinnitus severity correlates poorly with the degree of hearing loss. About one in seven tinnitus sufferers experiences severe annoyance, and 4% are severely disabled. When severe and persistent, tinnitus may interfere with sleep and ability to concentrate, resulting in considerable psychological distress.

Pulsatile tinnitus—often described by the patient as listening to one's own heartbeat—should be distinguished from tonal tinnitus. Although often ascribed to conductive hearing loss, pulsatile tinnitus may be far more serious and may indicate a vascular abnormality, such as glomus tumor, venous sinus stenosis, carotid vaso-occlusive disease, arteriovenous malformation, or aneurysm.

A staccato "clicking" tinnitus may result from middle ear muscle spasm (middle ear myoclonus) or sometimes palatal myoclonus. The patient typically perceives a rapid series of popping noises, lasting seconds to a few minutes, accompanied by a fluttering feeling in the ear. Specialized forms of tympanometry may formally diagnose this condition, and it is typically treated surgically.

B. Diagnostic Testing

For routine, nonpulsatile tinnitus, audiometry should be ordered to rule out an associated hearing loss. For unilateral tinnitus, particularly associated with hearing loss in the absence of an obvious causative factor (ie, noise trauma), an MRI should be obtained to rule out a retrocochlear lesion, such as vestibular schwannoma. MRA and MRV and temporal bone CT should be considered for patients who have pulsatile tinnitus to exclude a causative vascular lesion or sigmoid sinus abnormality.

Treatment

The most important treatment of tinnitus is avoidance of exposure to excessive noise, ototoxic agents, and other factors that may cause cochlear damage. Masking the tinnitus with music or through amplification of normal sounds with a hearing aid may also bring some relief. In addition to masking techniques, habituation techniques, such as tinnitus retraining therapy and cognitive behavioral therapy, may prove beneficial in those with refractory symptoms. Among patients who have emotional distress due to tinnitus, numerous antidepressant and antipsychotic medications have been tried. Unfortunately, these medications do not treat the tinnitus directly but may allow the patient to cope with it better.

Conlon B et al. Bimodal neuromodulation combining sound and tongue stimulation reduces tinnitus symptoms in a large randomized clinical study. Sci Transl Med. 2020;12:eabb2830. [PMID: 33028707]

3. Hyperacusis

Excessive sensitivity to sound may occur following hearing loss, such as that due to noise trauma, in patients susceptible to migraines, or for psychological reasons. Patients with cochlear dysfunction commonly experience "recruitment," an abnormal sensitivity to loud sounds despite a reduced sensitivity to softer ones. Fitting hearing aids and other amplification devices to patients with recruitment requires use of compression circuitry to avoid uncomfortable overamplification.

Pienkowski M. Loud music and leisure noise is a common cause of chronic hearing loss, tinnitus and hyperacusis. Int J Environ Res Public Health. 2021;18:4236. [PMID: 33923580]

Ren J et al. Prevalence of hyperacusis in the general and special populations: a scoping review. Front Neurol. 2021;12:706555. [PMID: 34539554]

4. Vertigo

ESSENTIALS OF DIAGNOSIS

- Either a sensation of motion when there is no motion or an exaggerated sense of motion in response to movement.
- Duration of vertigo episodes with associated hearing loss or other neurologic issues are the keys to diagnosis.
- Evaluation includes audiogram, electronystagmography (ENG) or videonystagmography (VNG), and head MRI.

General Considerations

Vertigo can be caused by either a peripheral or central etiology, or both (Table 8–2).

Clinical Findings

A. Symptoms and Signs

Vertigo is the cardinal symptom of vestibular disease. Vertigo is typically experienced as a distinct "spinning" sensation or a sense of tumbling or of falling forward or backward. It should be distinguished from imbalance, light-headedness, and syncope, all of which are nonvestibular in origin (Table 8–3).

1. Peripheral vestibular disease—Peripheral vestibulopathy may cause vertigo of sudden onset, may be so severe that the patient is unable to walk or stand, and is frequently accompanied by nausea and vomiting. Tinnitus and hearing loss may be associated and provide strong support for a peripheral (ie, otologic) origin.

Critical elements of the history include the duration of the discrete vertiginous episodes (seconds, minutes to hours, or days), and associated symptoms (hearing loss). Triggers should be sought, including diet (eg, increased salt intake in the case of Ménière disease), stress, fatigue, and bright lights (eg, migraine-associated dizziness).

The physical examination of the patient with vertigo includes evaluation of the ears, observation of eye motion and nystagmus in response to head turning, cranial nerve examination, and Romberg testing. In acute peripheral lesions, nystagmus is usually horizontal with a rotatory component; the fast phase usually beats away from the diseased side. Visual fixation tends to inhibit nystagmus except in very acute peripheral lesions or with CNS disease. In benign paroxysmal positioning vertigo, **Dix-Hallpike testing** (quickly lowering the patient to the supine position with the head extending over the edge and placed 30 degrees lower than the body, turned either to the left or

Table 8–2. Causes of vertigo (listed in alphabetical order within categories).

Peripheral causes
Benign paroxysmal positioning vertigo
Ethanol intoxication
Inner ear barotraumas
Ménière disease
Semicircular canal dehiscence
Vestibular neuritis/labyrinthitis
Central causes
Cerebellar ataxia syndromes
Chiari malformation
Multiple sclerosis
Seizure
Wernicke encephalopathy
Mixed central and peripheral causes
Cerebellopontine angle tumors
Vestibular schwannoma
Meningioma
Endocrinopathies
Hypothyroidism
Pendred syndrome
Hyperviscosity syndromes
Waldenström macroglobulinemia
Infections
Lyme disease
Syphilis
Migraine
Stroke and vascular insufficiency
Anterior inferior cerebellar artery stroke
Posterior inferior cerebellar artery stroke
Vasculitides
Behçet disease
Cogan syndrome
Granulomatosis with polyangiitis
Susac syndrome
Vertebral artery insufficiency
Vascular compression

right) will elicit a delayed-onset (~10 seconds) fatigable nystagmus. Nonfatigable nystagmus in this position indicates CNS disease.

Since visual fixation often suppresses observed nystagmus, many of these maneuvers are performed with Frenzel goggles, which prevent visual fixation, and often bring out subtle forms of nystagmus. The **Fukuda test** can demonstrate vestibular asymmetry when the patient steps in place with eyes closed and consistently rotates in one direction.

Table 8–3. Common vestibular disorders: differential diagnosis based on classic presentations.

Duration of Typical Vertiginous Episodes	Auditory Symptoms Present	Auditory Symptoms Absent
Seconds	Perilymphatic fistula	Benign paroxysmal positioning vertigo (cupulolithiasis), vertebrobasilar insufficiency, migraine-associated vertigo
Hours	Ménière disease, syphilis	Migraine-associated vertigo
Days	Labyrinthitis, autoimmune inner ear disease, cerebellopontine angle tumor, ototoxicity	Vestibular neuronitis, migraine-associated vertigo, multiple sclerosis, cerebellar degeneration

2. Central disease—Vertigo arising from CNS disease (Table 8–2) tends to develop gradually and then becomes progressively more severe and debilitating. Nystagmus is not always present but can occur in any direction, may be dissociated in the two eyes, and is often non-fatigable, vertical rather than horizontal in orientation, without latency, and unsuppressed by visual fixation. ENG is useful in documenting these characteristics. Evaluation of audiovestibular dysfunction requires MRI of the brain.

Episodic vertigo can occur in patients with diplopia from external ophthalmoplegia and is maximal when the patient looks in the direction where the separation of images is greatest. Cerebral lesions involving the temporal cortex may also produce vertigo; it is sometimes the initial symptom of a seizure. Finally, vertigo may be a feature of a number of systemic disorders and can occur as a side effect of certain anticonvulsant, antibiotic, hypnotic, analgesic, and tranquilizer medications or of alcohol.

Welgampola MS et al. Dizziness demystified. Pract Neurol. 2019;19:492. [PMID: 31326945]

B. Vestibular Testing

Vestibular investigations, such as audiologic evaluation, caloric stimulation, electro- or videonystagmography (ENG or VNG), vestibular-evoked myogenic potentials (VEMPs), and MRI, are indicated in patients with persistent vertigo or when CNS disease is suspected. These studies help distinguish between central and peripheral lesions and identify causes requiring specific therapy. ENG consists of objective recording of the nystagmus induced by head and body movements, gaze, and caloric stimulation. It is helpful in quantifying the degree of vestibular hypofunction.

Zuniga SA et al. Efficient use of vestibular testing. Otolaryngol Clin North Am. 2021;54:875. [PMID: 34294436]

Vertigo Syndromes Due to Peripheral Lesions

A. Ménière Disease

The cause of Ménière disease is unknown. The classic syndrome consists of episodic vertigo, with discrete vertigo spells lasting 20 minutes to several hours in association with fluctuating, often low-frequency, sensorineural hearing loss, tinnitus (usually low-tone and "blowing" in quality), and a sensation of unilateral aural pressure (Table 8–3). These symptoms in presence of headaches or migraines may suggest migraine-associated dizziness. Primary treatment is aimed at decreasing dizzy episodes. There are no treatments for reduction in hearing loss. Treatment of Ménière disease typically involves preventive measures, including low-salt diet and daily diuretics (eg, acetazolamide). For symptomatic relief of acute vertigo attacks, lorazepam (0.5–1 mg) or diazepam (2–5 mg) can be used. Nausea may be treated with oral meclizine (25 mg). In refractory cases, patients may undergo intratympanic corticosteroid or gentamicin injections, endolymphatic sac decompression, or surgical or vestibular nerve section.

Gibson WPR. Meniere's disease. Adv Otorhinolaryngol. 2019; 82:77. [PMID: 30947172]

B. Labyrinthitis

Patients with labyrinthitis suffer from acute onset of continuous, usually severe vertigo lasting several days, accompanied by hearing loss and tinnitus. During a recovery period that lasts for several weeks, the vertigo gradually improves. Hearing may return to normal or remain permanently impaired in the involved ear. The cause of labyrinthitis is unknown. Treatment consists of antibiotics, if the patient is febrile or has symptoms of a bacterial infection, oral corticosteroids, and supportive care. Vestibular suppressants are useful during the acute phase of the attack (eg, diazepam) but should be discontinued as soon as feasible to avoid long-term dysequilibrium from inadequate compensation.

Welgampola MS et al. Dizziness demystified. Pract Neurol. 2019;19:492. [PMID: 31326945]

C. Benign Paroxysmal Positioning Vertigo

Patients suffering from recurrent spells of vertigo, lasting a few (10–15) seconds per spell, associated with changes in head position (often provoked by rolling over in bed), usually have benign paroxysmal positioning vertigo (BPPV). The term "positioning vertigo" is more accurate than "positional vertigo" because it is provoked by changes in head position rather than by the maintenance of a particular posture.

The typical symptoms of BPPV occur in clusters that persist for several days. There is a brief (10–15 seconds) latency period following a head movement before symptoms develop, and the acute vertigo subsides within 10–60 seconds, though the patient may remain imbalanced for several hours. Dizziness that lasts for more than a few seconds (that is several minutes or hours) is *not* BPPV. Constant repetition of the positional change leads to habituation. Since some CNS disorders can mimic BPPV (eg, vertebrobasilar insufficiency), recurrent cases warrant head MRI/MRA. In central lesions, there is no latent period, fatigability, or habituation of the symptoms and signs. Treatment of BPPV involves physical therapy protocols (eg, the **Epley maneuver** or **Brandt-Daroff exercises**), based on the theory that it results from cupulolithiasis (free-floating statoconia, also known as otoconia) within a semicircular canal.

Argaet EC et al. Benign positional vertigo, its diagnosis, treatment and mimics. Clin Neurophysiol Pract. 2019;4:97. [PMID: 31193795]
Instrum RS et al. Benign paroxysmal positional vertigo. Adv Otorhinolaryngol. 2019;82:67. [PMID: 30947198]

D. Vestibular Neuronitis

In vestibular neuronitis, a paroxysmal, usually single attack of vertigo occurs without accompanying impairment of auditory function and will persist for several days before gradually abating. During the acute phase, examination reveals nystagmus and absent responses to caloric stimulation on one or both sides. The cause of the disorder is unclear though presumed to be viral. Treatment consists of supportive care; vestibular suppressants, such as diazepam 2–5 mg every 6–12 hours during the acute phases of the vertigo only; oral corticosteroids may potentially be used; and antiemetics, such as ondansetron and meclizine, followed by vestibular therapy if the patient does not completely compensate.

Bronstein AM et al. Long-term clinical outcome in vestibular neuritis. Curr Opin Neurol. 2019;32:174. [PMID: 30566414]
Lee JY et al. Clinical characteristics of acute vestibular neuritis according to involvement site. Otol Neurotol. 2020;41:143. [PMID: 31789808]

E. Traumatic Vertigo

Labyrinthine concussion is the most common cause of vertigo following head injury. Symptoms generally diminish within several days but may linger for a month or more. Basilar skull fractures that traverse the inner ear usually result in severe vertigo lasting several days to a week and deafness in the involved ear. Chronic posttraumatic vertigo may result from cupulolithiasis. This occurs when traumatically detached statoconia (otoconia) settle on the ampulla of the posterior semicircular canal and cause an excessive degree of cupular deflection in response to head motion. Clinically, this presents as episodic positioning vertigo. Treatment consists of supportive care and vestibular suppressant medication (diazepam) during the acute phase of the attack and vestibular therapy.

Marcus HJ et al. Vestibular dysfunction in acute traumatic brain injury. J Neurol. 2019;266:2430. [PMID: 31201499]

F. Perilymphatic Fistula

Leakage of perilymphatic fluid from the inner ear into the tympanic cavity via the round or oval window is a very rare cause of vertigo and sensory hearing loss. Most cases result from physical injury (eg, blunt head trauma, hand slap to ear); extreme barotrauma during airflight, scuba diving, etc; or vigorous Valsalva maneuvers (eg, during weight lifting). Treatment may require middle ear exploration and window sealing with a tissue graft.

Sarna B et al. Perilymphatic fistula: a review of classification, etiology, diagnosis, and treatment. Front Neurol. 2020;11:1046. [PMID: 33041986]

G. Cervicogenic Vertigo

Position receptors located in the facets of the cervical spine are important physiologically in the coordination of head and eye movements. Cervical proprioceptive dysfunction is a common cause of vertigo triggered by neck movements. This disturbance often commences after neck injury, particularly hyperextension; it is also associated with degenerative cervical spine disease. Although symptoms vary, vertigo may be triggered by assuming a particular head position as opposed to moving to a new head position (the latter typical of labyrinthine dysfunction). Cervical vertigo may often be confused with migraine-associated vertigo, which is also associated with head movement. Management consists of neck movement exercises to the extent permitted by orthopedic considerations.

Cherchi M et al. The enduring controversy of cervicogenic vertigo, and its place among positional vertigo syndromes. Audiol Res. 2021;11:491. [PMID: 34698085]
Ranalli P. An overview of central vertigo disorders. Adv Otorhinolaryngol. 2019;82:127. [PMID: 30947212]

H. Migrainous Vertigo

Episodic vertigo is frequently associated with migraine headache. Head trauma may also be a precipitating feature. The vertigo may be temporally related to the headache and last up to several hours, or it may also occur in the absence of any headache. Migrainous vertigo may resemble Ménière disease but without associated hearing loss or tinnitus. Accompanying symptoms may include head pressure; visual, motion, or auditory sensitivity and photosensitivity. Symptoms typically worsen with lack of sleep and anxiety or stress. Food triggers include caffeine, chocolate, and alcohol, among others. There is often a history of motion intolerance (easily carsick as a child). Migrainous vertigo may be familial. Treatment includes dietary and lifestyle changes (improved sleep pattern, avoidance of stress) and antimigraine prophylactic medication.

Hain T et al. Migraine associated vertigo. Adv Otorhinolaryngol. 2019;82:119. [PMID: 30947176]

I. Superior Semicircular Canal Dehiscence

Deficiency in the bony covering of the superior semicircular canal may be associated with vertigo triggered by loud noise exposure, straining, and an apparent conductive hearing loss. Autophony is also a common feature. Diagnosis is with coronal high-resolution CT scan and VEMP testing. Surgically resurfacing or plugging the dehiscent canal can improve symptoms.

Eberhard KE et al. Current trends, controversies, and future directions in the evaluation and management of superior canal dehiscence syndrome. Front Neurol. 2021;12:638574. [PMID: 33889125]

Vertigo Syndromes Due to Central Lesions

CNS causes of vertigo include brainstem vascular disease, arteriovenous malformations, tumors of the brainstem and cerebellum, multiple sclerosis, and vertebrobasilar migraine (Table 8–2). Vertigo of central origin often becomes unremitting and disabling. The associated nystagmus is often nonfatigable, vertical rather than horizontal in orientation, without latency, and unsuppressed by visual fixation. ENG is useful in documenting these characteristics. There are commonly other signs of brainstem dysfunction (eg, cranial nerve palsies; motor, sensory, or cerebellar deficits in the limbs) or of increased intracranial pressure. Auditory function is generally spared. The underlying cause should be treated.

Chari DA et al. The efficient dizziness history and exam. Otolaryngol Clin North Am. 2021;54:863. [PMID: 34294439]
Ranalli P. An overview of central vertigo disorders. Adv Otorhinolaryngol. 2019;82:127. [PMID: 30947212]

DISEASES OF THE CENTRAL AUDITORY & VESTIBULAR SYSTEMS

Lesions of the eighth cranial nerve and central audiovestibular pathways may produce hearing loss and dizziness (Table 8–3). One characteristic of neural hearing loss is deterioration of speech discrimination out of proportion to the decrease in pure tone thresholds. Another is auditory adaptation, wherein a steady tone appears to the listener to decay and eventually disappear. Auditory evoked responses are useful in distinguishing cochlear from neural losses and may give insight into the site of lesion within the central pathways.

The evaluation of central audiovestibular disorders usually requires imaging of the internal auditory canal, cerebellopontine angle, and brain with enhanced MRI.

1. Vestibular Schwannoma (Acoustic Neuroma)

Eighth cranial nerve schwannomas are among the most common intracranial tumors. Most are unilateral, but about 5% are associated with the hereditary syndrome neurofibromatosis type 2, in which bilateral eighth nerve tumors may be accompanied by meningiomas and other intracranial and spinal tumors. These benign lesions arise within the internal auditory canal and gradually grow to involve the cerebellopontine angle, eventually compressing the pons and resulting in hydrocephalus. Their typical auditory symptoms are unilateral hearing loss with a deterioration of speech discrimination exceeding that predicted by the degree of pure tone loss. Nonclassic presentations, such as sudden unilateral hearing loss, are fairly common. **Any individual with a unilateral**

or asymmetric sensorineural hearing loss should be evaluated for an intracranial mass lesion. Vestibular dysfunction more often takes the form of continuous dysequilibrium than episodic vertigo. Diagnosis is made by enhanced MRI. Treatment consists of observation, microsurgical excision, or stereotactic radiotherapy, depending on such factors as patient age, underlying health, and size of the tumor.

Kalogeridi MA et al. Stereotactic radiosurgery and radiotherapy for acoustic neuromas. Neurosurg Rev. 2020;43:941. [PMID: 30982152]

Leon J et al. Observation or stereotactic radiosurgery for newly diagnosed vestibular schwannomas: a systematic review and meta-analysis. J Radiosurg SBRT. 2019;6:91. [PMID: 31641546]

2. Vascular Compromise

Vertebrobasilar insufficiency is a common cause of vertigo in the elderly. It is often triggered by changes in posture or extension of the neck. Reduced flow in the vertebrobasilar system may be demonstrated noninvasively through MRA. Empiric treatment is with vasodilators and aspirin.

Cornelius JF et al. Compression syndromes of the vertebral artery at the craniocervical junction. Acta Neurochir Suppl. 2019;125:151. [PMID: 30610316]

3. Multiple Sclerosis

Patients with multiple sclerosis may suffer from episodic vertigo and chronic imbalance. Hearing loss in this disease is most commonly unilateral and of rapid onset. Spontaneous recovery may occur.

Kattah JC et al. Eye movements in demyelinating, autoimmune and metabolic disorders. Curr Opin Neurol. 2020;33:111. [PMID: 31770124]

OTOLOGIC MANIFESTATIONS OF AIDS

AIDS may result in many otologic signs and symptoms. The pinna and external auditory canal may be affected by Kaposi sarcoma and by persistent and potentially invasive fungal infections (particularly *Aspergillus fumigatus*). Serous otitis media due to eustachian tube dysfunction may arise from adenoidal hypertrophy (HIV lymphadenopathy), recurrent mucosal viral infections, or an obstructing nasopharyngeal tumor (eg, lymphoma). Unfortunately, ventilating tubes are seldom helpful and may trigger profuse watery otorrhea. Acute otitis media is usually caused by typical bacterial organisms, including *Proteus, Staphylococcus,* and *Pseudomonas,* and rarely, by *Pneumocystis jirovecii.* Sensorineural hearing loss is common and, in some cases, results from viral CNS infection. In cases of progressive hearing loss, cryptococcal meningitis and syphilis must be excluded. Acute facial paralysis due to herpes zoster infection (**Ramsay Hunt syndrome**) occurs commonly and follows a clinical course similar to that in nonimmunocompromised patients. Treatment is with high-dose acyclovir (see Chapter 32). Corticosteroids may also be effective as an adjunct.

Dawood G et al. Nature and extent of hearing loss in HIV-infected children: a scoping review. Int J Pediatr Otorhinolaryngol. 2020;134:110036. [PMID: 32335463]

Iacovou E et al. Diagnosis and treatment of HIV-associated manifestations in otolaryngology. Infect Dis Rep. 2012;4:e9. [PMID: 24470939]

DISEASES OF THE NOSE & PARANASAL SINUSES

INFECTIONS OF THE NOSE & PARANASAL SINUSES

Rhinosinusitis may be classified by duration of symptoms. Rhinosinusitis is called acute rhinosinusitis if less than 4 weeks' duration or as chronic rhinosinusitis if lasting more than 12 weeks, with or without acute exacerbations. Acute rhinosinusitis may also be classified by presumed etiology, such as viral rhinosinusitis or acute bacterial rhinosinusitis.

1. Viral Rhinosinusitis (Common Cold)

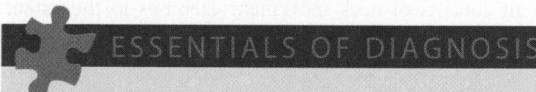

- Associated malaise, headache, and cough.
- Nasal congestion, facial pressure, rhinorrhea, and hyposmia.
- Erythematous, engorged nasal mucosa without intranasal purulence.
- Symptoms are self-limited, lasting typically < 10 days.

Clinical Findings

Due to the numerous serologic types of rhinoviruses, adenoviruses, and other viruses, patients remain susceptible to the common cold throughout life. These infections, while generally quite benign and self-limited, have been implicated in the development or exacerbation of more serious conditions, such as acute bacterial sinusitis and acute otitis media, asthma, cystic fibrosis, and bronchitis. Nasal congestion, decreased sense of smell, rhinorrhea, and sneezing accompanied by general malaise, throat discomfort and, occasionally, headache, are typical in viral infections. Nasal examination usually shows erythematous, edematous mucosa and a watery discharge. The presence of purulent nasal discharge suggests bacterial rhinosinusitis.

Najafloo R et al. Mechanism of anosmia caused by symptoms of COVID-19 and emerging treatments. ACS Chem Neurosci. 2021;12:3795. [PMID: 34609841]

Vance H et al. Addressing post-COVID symptoms: a guide for primary care physicians. J Am Board Fam Med. 2021;34:1229. [PMID: 34772779]

Treatment

The main treatment for viral rhinitis is supportive care, including rest, hydration, and use of over-the-counter analgesics and decongestants. There are no effective antiviral therapies for either the prevention or treatment of most viral rhinitis despite a common *misperception* among patients that antibiotics are helpful. Buffered hypertonic saline (3–5%) nasal irrigation has been shown to improve symptoms and reduce the need for NSAIDs. Other supportive measures, such as oral decongestants (pseudoephedrine, 30–60 mg every 4–6 hours or 120 mg twice daily), may provide some relief of rhinorrhea and nasal obstruction.

Nasal sprays, such as oxymetazoline or phenylephrine, are rapidly effective but should *not* be used for more than a few days to prevent rebound congestion. Withdrawal of the medication after prolonged use leads to **rhinitis medicamentosa,** an almost addictive need for continuous usage. Treatment of rhinitis medicamentosa requires mandatory cessation of the sprays, and this is often extremely frustrating for patients. Topical intranasal corticosteroids (eg, flunisolide, 2 sprays in each nostril twice daily), intranasal anticholinergic (ipratropium 0.06% nasal spray, 2–3 sprays every 8 hours as needed), or a short tapering course of oral prednisone may help during the withdrawal process.

Complications

Other than mild eustachian tube dysfunction or transient middle ear effusion, complications of viral rhinitis are unusual. Secondary acute bacterial rhinosinusitis is a well-accepted complication of acute viral rhinitis and is suggested by persistence of symptoms beyond 10 days with purulent green or yellow nasal secretions and unilateral facial or dental pain.

Dhama K et al. Coronavirus disease 2019-COVID-19. Clin Microbiol Rev. 2020;33:e00028. [PMID: 32580969]

2. Acute Rhinosinusitis (Rhinosinusitis)

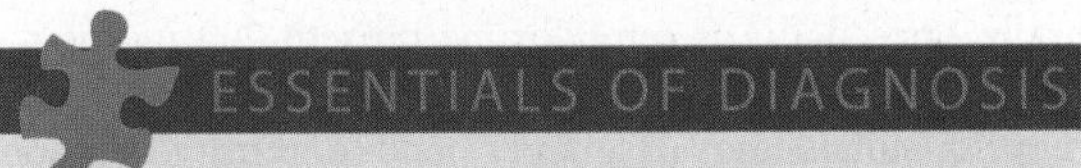

- Acute onset of symptoms.
- Purulent yellow-green nasal discharge or expectoration.
- Facial pain or pressure over the affected sinus or sinuses.
- Nasal obstruction.
- Associated cough, malaise, fever, and headache.

General Considerations

Compared with viral rhinitis, acute bacterial rhinosinusitis infections are uncommon, but they still affect nearly 20 million Americans annually and account for over 2 billion dollars in health care expenditures. Acute bacterial rhinosinusitis is believed to be the result of impaired mucociliary clearance, inflammation of the nasal cavity mucosa, and obstruction of the ostiomeatal complex. Edematous mucosa causes obstruction of the complex, resulting in the accumulation of mucus in the sinus cavity that becomes secondarily infected by bacteria. The largest of these ostiomeatal complexes is deep to the middle turbinate in the middle meatus. This complex is actually a confluence of complexes draining the maxillary, ethmoid, and frontal sinuses. The sphenoid drains from a separate complex between the septum and superior turbinate.

The typical pathogens of bacterial rhinosinusitis are *S pneumoniae*, other streptococci, *H influenzae,* and less commonly, *S aureus* and *Moraxella catarrhalis.* Pathogens vary regionally in both prevalence and drug resistance; about 25% of healthy asymptomatic individuals may, if sinus aspirates are cultured, harbor such bacteria as well.

Clinical Findings

A. Symptoms and Signs

There are no agreed-upon criteria for the diagnosis of acute bacterial rhinosinusitis in adults. Major symptoms include purulent nasal drainage, nasal obstruction or congestion, facial pain/pressure, altered smell, cough, and fever. Minor symptoms include headache, otalgia, halitosis, dental pain, and fatigue. Many of the more specific symptoms and signs relate to the affected sinus(es). Bacterial rhinosinusitis can be distinguished from viral rhinitis by persistence of symptoms for more than 10 days after onset or worsening of symptoms within 10 days after initial improvement. Acute rhinosinusitis is defined as lasting less than 4 weeks, and subacute rhinosinusitis, as lasting 4–12 weeks.

Acute maxillary sinusitis is the most common form of acute bacterial rhinosinusitis because the maxillary is the largest sinus with a single drainage pathway that is easily obstructed. Unilateral facial fullness, pressure, and tenderness over the cheek are common symptoms, but may not always be present. Pain may refer to the upper incisor and canine teeth via branches of the trigeminal nerve, which traverse the floor of the sinus. Purulent nasal drainage should be noted with nasal airway obstruction or facial pain (pressure). Maxillary sinusitis may result from dental infection, and teeth that are tender should be carefully examined for signs of abscess. Drainage of the periapical abscess or removal of the diseased tooth typically resolves the sinus infection.

Acute ethmoiditis in adults is often accompanied by maxillary sinusitis, and symptoms are similar to those described above. Localized ethmoid sinusitis may present with pain and pressure over the high lateral wall of the nose between the eyes that may radiate to the orbit.

Sphenoid sinusitis is usually seen in the setting of pansinusitis or infection of all the paranasal sinuses on at least one side. The patient may complain of a headache "in the middle of the head" and often points to the vertex.

Acute frontal sinusitis may cause pain and tenderness of the forehead. This is most easily elicited by palpation of the orbital roof just below the medial end of the eyebrow.

Hospital-associated sinusitis is a form of acute bacterial rhinosinusitis that may present without the usual symptoms. Instead, it may be a cause of fever in critically ill patients. It is often associated with prolonged presence of a nasogastric or, rarely, nasotracheal tube causing nasal mucosal inflammation and ostiomeatal complex obstruction. Pansinusitis on the side of the tube is common on imaging studies.

B. Imaging

The diagnosis of acute bacterial rhinosinusitis can usually be made on clinical grounds alone. Although more sensitive than clinical examination, routine radiographs are not cost-effective and are *not* recommended by the Agency for Health Care Policy and Research or American Association of Otolaryngology Guidelines. Consensus guidelines recommend imaging when clinical criteria are difficult to evaluate, when the patient does not respond to appropriate therapy or has been treated repeatedly with antibiotics, when intracranial involvement or cerebrospinal fluid rhinorrhea is suspected, when complicated dental infection is suspected, or when symptoms of more serious infection are noted.

When necessary, noncontrast screening coronal CT scans are more cost-effective and provide more information than conventional sinus films. CT provides a rapid and effective means to assess all of the paranasal sinuses, identify areas of greater concern (such as bony dehiscence, periosteal elevation, or maxillary tooth root exposure within the sinus), and speed appropriate therapy.

CT scans are reasonably sensitive but are not specific. Swollen soft tissue and fluid may be difficult to distinguish when opacification of the sinus is due to other conditions, such as chronic rhinosinusitis, nasal polyposis, or mucus retention cysts. Sinus abnormalities can be seen in most patients with an upper respiratory infection, while bacterial rhinosinusitis develops in only 2%.

If malignancy, intracranial extension, or opportunistic infection is suspected, MRI with gadolinium should be ordered instead of, or in addition to, CT. MRI will distinguish tumor from fluid, inflammation, and inspissated mucus far better than CT, and will better delineate tumor extent (eg, involvement of adjacent structures, such as the orbit, skull base, and palate). Bone destruction can be demonstrated as well by MRI as by CT.

Treatment

All patients with acute bacterial rhinosinusitis should have careful evaluation of pain. For symptom reduction in viral rhinitis and bacterial rhinosinusitis without complication, the European Position Paper on Rhinosinusitis and Nasal Polyps (EPOS) 2012 recommends NSAIDs, saline nasal sprays, and nasal decongestants (pseudoephedrine, 30–60 mg every 6 hours, up to 240 mg/day; nasal oxymetazoline, 0.05% or oxymetazoline, 0.05–0.1%, one or two sprays in each nostril every 6–8 hours for up to 3 days). In cases of suspected bacterial rhinosinusitis, intranasal corticosteroids (eg, high-dose mometasone furoate 200 mcg each nostril twice daily for 21 days) have demonstrated efficacy in reducing nasal symptoms and are recommended. Other medications, such as mucolytics, vitamin C, probiotics, and antihistamines, have not demonstrated efficacy in the management of acute rhinosinusitis.

Antibiotic therapy should be reserved for complicated or protracted acute bacterial rhinosinusitis. Between 40% and 69% of patients with acute bacterial rhinosinusitis improve symptomatically within 2 weeks without antibiotic therapy. Antibiotic treatment is controversial in uncomplicated cases of clinically diagnosed acute bacterial rhinosinusitis because only 5% of patients will note a shorter duration of illness with treatment, and antibiotic treatment is associated with nearly twice the number of adverse events compared with placebo. Antibiotics may be considered when symptoms last more than 10 days or when symptoms (including fever, facial pain, and swelling of the face) are severe or when cases are complicated (such as immunodeficiency). In these patients, administration of antibiotics does reduce the incidence of clinical failure by 50% and represents the most cost-effective treatment strategy.

Selection of antibiotics is usually empiric and based on a number of factors, including regional patterns of antibiotic resistance, antibiotic allergy, cost, and patient tolerance. For adults younger than 65 years with mild to moderate acute bacterial rhinosinusitis, the recommended first-line therapy is amoxicillin-clavulanate (500 mg/125 mg orally three times daily or 875 mg/125 mg orally twice daily for 5–7 days), or in those with severe sinusitis, high-dose amoxicillin-clavulanate (2000 mg/125 mg extended-release orally twice daily for 7–10 days). In patients with a high risk for penicillin-resistant *S pneumoniae* (age over 65 years, hospitalization in the prior 5 days, antibiotic use in the prior month, immunocompromised status, multiple comorbidities, or severe sinus infection), the recommended first-line therapy is the high-dose amoxicillin-clavulanate option (2000 mg/125 mg extended-release orally twice daily for 7–10 days). For those with penicillin allergy or hepatic impairment, doxycycline (100 mg orally twice daily or 200 mg orally once daily for 5–7 days) or clindamycin (150–300 mg every 6 hours) plus a cephalosporin (cefixime 400 mg orally once daily or cefpodoxime proxetil 200 mg orally twice daily) for 10 days are options. Macrolides, trimethoprim-sulfamethoxazole, and second- or third-generation cephalosporins are not recommended for empiric therapy. Dupilumab, a monoclonal antibody with inhibition of IL-4 and IL-13, is approved for patients with chronic sinusitis with nasal polyposis.

Hospital-associated infections in critically ill patients are treated differently from community-acquired infections. Removal of a nasogastric tube and improved nasal hygiene (nasal saline sprays, humidification of supplemental nasal oxygen, and nasal decongestants) are critical interventions and often curative in mild cases without aggressive antibiotic use. Endoscopic or transantral cultures may help direct medical therapy in complicated cases. In addition, broad-spectrum antibiotic coverage directed at *P aeruginosa, S aureus* (including methicillin-resistant strains), and anaerobes may be required.

Complications

Local complications of acute bacterial rhinosinusitis include orbital cellulitis and abscess, osteomyelitis, cavernous sinus thrombosis, and intracranial extension.

Orbital complications typically occur by extension of ethmoid sinusitis through the lamina papyracea, a thin layer of bone that comprises the medial orbital wall. Any change in the ocular examination necessitates immediate CT imaging. Extension in this area may cause orbital cellulitis leading to proptosis, gaze restriction, and orbital pain. Select cases are responsive to intravenous antibiotics, with or without corticosteroids, and should be managed in close conjunction with an ophthalmologist or otolaryngologist, or both. Extension through the lamina papyracea can also lead to subperiosteal abscess formation (orbital abscess). Such abscesses cause marked proptosis, ophthalmoplegia, and pain with medial gaze. While some cases respond to antibiotics, such findings should prompt an immediate referral to a specialist for consideration of decompression and evacuation. Failure to intervene quickly may lead to permanent visual impairment and a "frozen globe."

Osteomyelitis requires prolonged antibiotics as well as removal of necrotic bone. The frontal sinus is most commonly affected, with bone involvement suggested by a tender swelling of the forehead (**Pott puffy tumor**). Following treatment, secondary cosmetic reconstructive procedures may be necessary.

Intracranial complications of sinusitis can occur either through hematogenous spread, as in cavernous sinus thrombosis and meningitis, or by direct extension, as in epidural and intraparenchymal brain abscesses. Fortunately, they are rare today. Cavernous sinus thrombosis is heralded by ophthalmoplegia, chemosis, and visual loss; the diagnosis is most commonly confirmed by MRI. When identified early, cavernous sinus thrombosis typically responds to intravenous antibiotics. Frontal epidural and intracranial abscesses are often clinically silent, but may present with altered mental status, persistent fever, or severe headache.

When to Refer

Failure of acute bacterial rhinosinusitis to resolve after an adequate course of oral antibiotics necessitates referral to an otolaryngologist for evaluation. Endoscopic cultures may direct further treatment choices. Nasal endoscopy and CT scan are indicated when symptoms persist longer than 4–12 weeks. Any patients with suspected extension of disease outside the sinuses should be evaluated urgently by an otolaryngologist and imaging should be obtained.

When to Admit

- Facial swelling and erythema indicative of facial cellulitis.
- Proptosis.
- Vision change or gaze abnormality indicative of orbital cellulitis.
- Abscess or cavernous sinus involvement.
- Mental status changes suggestive of intracranial extension.
- Failure to respond to appropriate first-line treatment or symptoms persisting longer than 4 weeks.

Hoy SM. Dupilumab: a review in chronic rhinosinusitis with nasal polyps. Drugs. 2020;80:711. [PMID: 32240527]

3. Nasal Vestibulitis & *S aureus* Nasal Colonization

Inflammation of the nasal vestibule may result from folliculitis of the hairs that line this orifice and is usually the result of nasal manipulation or hair trimming. Systemic antibiotics effective against *S aureus* (such as dicloxacillin, 250 mg orally four times daily for 7–10 days) are indicated. Topical mupirocin 2% nasal ointment (applied two or three times daily) also may be a helpful addition and may prevent future occurrences. If recurrent, the addition of rifampin (10 mg/kg orally twice daily for the last 4 days of dicloxacillin treatment) may eliminate the *S aureus* carrier state. If a furuncle exists, it should be incised and drained, preferably intranasally. Adequate treatment of these infections is important to prevent retrograde spread of infection through valveless veins into the cavernous sinus and intracranial structures.

S aureus is the leading nosocomial pathogen, and nasal carriage is a well-defined risk factor in the development and spread of nosocomial infections. Nasal and extranasal methicillin-resistant *S aureus* (MRSA) colonizations are associated with a 30% risk of developing an invasive MRSA infection during hospital stays. While the vast majority have no vestibulitis symptoms, screening by nasal swabs and PCR-based assays has demonstrated a 30% rate of *S aureus* colonization in hospital patients and an 11% rate of MRSA colonization in ICU patients. Elimination of the carrier state is challenging, but studies of mupirocin 2% nasal ointment application with chlorhexidine facial washing (40 mg/mL) twice daily for 5 days have demonstrated decolonization in 39% of patients.

Septimus EJ. Nasal decolonization: what antimicrobials are most effective prior to surgery? Am J Infect Control. 2019;47S:A53. [PMID: 31146851]

4. Invasive Fungal Sinusitis

Invasive fungal sinusitis is rare and includes both rhinocerebral mucormycosis (*Mucor, Absidia,* and *Rhizopus* spp.) and other invasive fungal infections, such as *Aspergillus*. The fungus spreads rapidly through vascular channels and may be lethal if not detected early. Patients with mucormycosis almost invariably have some degree of immunocompromise, such as diabetes mellitus, long-term corticosteroid therapy, neutropenia associated with chemotherapy for hematologic malignancy, or end-stage renal disease. Occasional cases of sinonasal infection with *Aspergillus* spp. have been reported in patients with untreated HIV/AIDS. The initial symptoms may be similar to those of acute bacterial rhinosinusitis, although facial pain is often more severe.

Nasal drainage is typically clear or straw-colored, rather than purulent, and visual symptoms may be noted at presentation in the absence of significant nasal findings. On examination, the classic finding of mucormycosis is a black eschar on the middle turbinate, but this finding is not universal and may not be apparent if the infection is deep or high within the nasal bones. Often the mucosa appears normal or simply pale and dry. This may be noted on the hard palate as well. Early diagnosis requires suspicion of the disease and nasal biopsy with silver stains, revealing broad nonseptate hyphae within tissues and necrosis with vascular occlusion. Imaging, such as CT or MRI, may initially show only soft tissue changes. Consequently, biopsy and ultimate debridement should be based on the clinical setting rather than radiographic demonstration of bony destruction or intracranial changes.

Invasive fungal sinusitis represents a medical and surgical emergency. Once recognized, voriconazole may be started by intravenous infusion, and prompt wide surgical debridement is indicated for patients with reversible immune deficiency (eg, poorly controlled hyperglycemia in diabetes). Other antifungals, including amphotericin or the less nephrotoxic lipid-based amphotericin B (Ambisome) and caspofungin, are alternatives to voriconazole and may be added to voriconazole depending on the fungus. Surgical management, while necessary for any possibility of cure, often results in tremendous disfigurement and functional deficits (eg, often resulting in the loss of at least one eye). Even with early diagnosis and immediate appropriate intervention, the prognosis is guarded. In persons with diabetes, the mortality rate is about 20%. If kidney disease is present or develops, mortality is over 50%; in the setting of AIDS or hematologic malignancy with neutropenia, mortality approaches 100%. Whether to undertake aggressive surgical management should be considered carefully because many patients are gravely ill at the time of diagnosis, and overall disease-specific survival is only about 57%.

Craig JR. Updates in management of acute invasive fungal rhinosinusitis. Curr Opin Otolaryngol Head Neck Surg. 2019;27:29. [PMID: 30585877]

Kashkouli MB et al. Outcomes and factors affecting them in patients with rhino-orbito-cerebral mucormycosis. Br J Ophthalmol. 2019;103:1460. [PMID: 30514712]

ALLERGIC RHINITIS

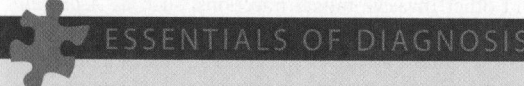

- Clear rhinorrhea, sneezing, tearing, eye irritation, and pruritus.
- Associated symptoms include cough, bronchospasm, and eczematous dermatitis.
- Environmental allergen exposure in the presence of allergen-specific IgE.

General Considerations

Allergic rhinitis is very common in the United States with population studies reporting a prevalence of 20–30% of adults and up to 40% of children. Allergic rhinitis adversely affects school and work performance, costing about $6 billion annually in the United States through direct costs of therapy as well as the indirect costs of sleep deprivation, fatigue and reduced productivity, or absenteeism. Seasonal allergic rhinitis is most commonly caused by pollens and spores. Flowering shrub and tree pollens are most common in the spring, flowering plants and grasses in the summer, and ragweed and molds in the fall. Interestingly, climate change may have an impact on the occurrence of allergic rhinitis since increased temperature and carbon dioxide exposure cause increased pollen production in ragweed plants and since the extended duration of summer correlates with longer periods of pollen production in these and other flowering weeds. Dust, household mites, air pollution, and pet dander may produce year-round symptoms, termed "perennial rhinitis."

Clinical Findings

The symptoms of "hay fever" are similar to those of viral rhinitis but are usually persistent and may show seasonal variation. Nasal symptoms are often accompanied by eye irritation, pruritus, conjunctival erythema, and excessive tearing. Many patients have a strong family history of atopy or allergy.

The clinician should be careful to distinguish allergic rhinitis from other types of nonallergic rhinitis. **Vasomotor rhinitis** (sometimes called **senile rhinitis**) is caused by increased sensitivity of the vidian nerve and is a common cause of clear rhinorrhea in elderly persons. Often patients will report that they have troubling rhinorrhea in response to numerous nasal stimuli, including warm or cold air, odors or scents, light, or particulate matter. Other types of rhinitis, including gustatory, atrophic, and drug-induced rhinorrhea, have also been described.

On physical examination, the mucosa of the turbinates is usually pale or violaceous because of venous engorgement. This is in contrast to the erythema of viral rhinitis. Nasal polyps, which are yellowish boggy masses of hypertrophic mucosa, are associated with long-standing allergic rhinitis.

Treatment

A. Intranasal Corticosteroids

Intranasal corticosteroid sprays remain the mainstay of treatment of allergic rhinitis. They are more effective—and frequently less expensive—than nonsedating antihistamines, though patients should be reminded that there may be a delay in onset of relief of 2 or more weeks. Corticosteroid sprays may also shrink hypertrophic nasal mucosa and nasal polyps, thereby providing an improved nasal airway and ostiomeatal complex drainage. Because of this effect, intranasal corticosteroids are critical in treating allergy in patients prone to recurrent acute bacterial rhinosinusitis or chronic rhinosinusitis. Available preparations include beclomethasone (42 mcg/spray twice daily per nostril), flunisolide (25 mcg/spray twice daily per nostril), mometasone furoate (200 mcg once daily per nostril), budesonide (100 mcg twice daily per nostril), and fluticasone propionate (200 mcg once daily per nostril). All are considered equally effective. Probably the most critical factors are compliance with regular use and proper introduction into the nasal cavity. In order to deliver medication to the region of the middle meatus, proper application involves holding the bottle straight up with the head tilted forward and pointing the bottle toward the ipsilateral ear when spraying. Side effects are limited, the most annoying being epistaxis (perhaps related to incorrect delivery of the drug toward the nasal septum).

B. Antihistamines

Antihistamines offer temporary, but immediate, control of many of the most troubling symptoms of allergic rhinitis. Effective oral antihistamines include nonsedating loratadine (10 mg once daily), desloratadine (5 mg once daily), and fexofenadine (60 mg twice daily or 120 mg once daily), and minimally sedating cetirizine (10 mg once daily). Brompheniramine or chlorpheniramine (4 mg orally every 6–8 hours, or 8–12 mg orally every 8–12 hours as a sustained-release tablet) and clemastine (1.34–2.68 mg orally twice daily) may be less expensive but are usually associated with some drowsiness. The safety and efficacy of the newer, less-sedating antihistamines is so compelling that one of them, the H_1-receptor antagonist nasal spray azelastine (1–2 sprays per nostril daily), is now included in the treatment guidelines of many consensus statements; however, some patients object to its bitter taste. Other side effects of oral antihistamines besides sedation include xerostomia and antihistamine tolerance (with eventual return of allergy symptoms despite initial benefit after several months of use). In such patients, typically those with perennial allergy, alternating effective antihistamines periodically can control symptoms over the long term. The FDA has approved a nasal spray containing the corticosteroid mometasone (25 mcg) and the H_1-inhibitor olopatidine hydrochloride (665 mcg) (Ryaltris) for seasonal allergic rhinitis. The dosage is 2 sprays in each nostril daily. The long-term efficacy of this medication is not yet known.

C. Adjunctive Treatment Measures

Antileukotriene medications, such as montelukast (10 mg/day orally), alone or with cetirizine (10 mg/day orally) or loratadine (10 mg/day orally), may improve nasal rhinorrhea, sneezing, and congestion. Cromolyn sodium and sodium nedocromil may be useful adjunct agents for allergic rhinitis. They work by stabilizing mast cells and preventing proinflammatory mediator release. As topical agents, they have very few side effects, but they must be initiated *well before* allergen exposure (up to 4 weeks before). The most useful form of cromolyn is probably the ophthalmologic preparation placed dropwise into the nasal cavity. Intranasal cromolyn is cleared rapidly and must be administered four times daily for continued symptom relief. In practice, it is not nearly as effective as inhaled corticosteroid.

Intranasal anticholinergic agents, such as ipratropium bromide 0.03% or 0.06% sprays (42–84 mcg per nostril three times daily), may be helpful adjuncts when rhinorrhea is a major symptom. They are not as effective for treating allergic rhinitis but are more useful for treating vasomotor rhinitis.

Avoiding or reducing exposure to airborne allergens is the most effective means of alleviating symptoms of allergic rhinitis. Depending on the allergen, this can be extremely difficult. Maintaining an allergen-free environment by covering pillows and mattresses with plastic covers, substituting synthetic materials (foam mattress, acrylics) for animal products (wool, horsehair), and removing dust-collecting household fixtures (carpets, drapes, bedspreads, wicker) is worth the attempt to help more troubled patients. Air purifiers and dust filters may also aid in maintaining an allergen-free environment. Nasal saline irrigations are a useful adjunct in the treatment of allergic rhinitis to mechanically flush the allergens from the nasal cavity. When symptoms are extremely bothersome, a search for offending allergens may prove helpful. This can either be done by serum radioallergosorbent test (RAST) testing or skin testing by an allergist.

In some cases, allergic rhinitis symptoms are inadequately relieved by medication and avoidance measures. Often, such patients have a strong family history of atopy and may also have lower respiratory manifestations, such as allergic asthma. Referral to an otolaryngologist or allergist for immunotherapy may be appropriate. Such treatment involves proper identification of offending allergens, progressively increasing doses of allergen(s), and eventual maintenance dose administration over a period of 3–5 years. Immunotherapy has been proven to reduce circulating IgE levels in patients with allergic rhinitis and reduce the need for allergy medications. Both subcutaneous and topical immunotherapy have been shown to be effective in the long-term treatment of refractory allergic rhinitis.

Fein MN et al. CSACI position statement: newer generation H_1-antihistamines are safer than first-generation H_1-antihistamines and should be the first-line antihistamines for the treatment of allergic rhinitis and urticaria. Allergy Asthma Clin Immunol. 2019;15:61. [PMID: 3158299]

Meltzer EO et al. Meta-analyses of the efficacy of pharmacotherapies and sublingual allergy immunotherapy tablets for allergic rhinitis in adults and children. Rhinology. 2021;59:422. [PMID: 34463311]

OLFACTORY DYSFUNCTION

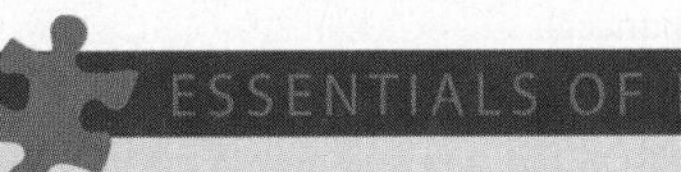

- Subjective diminished smell or taste sensation.
- Lack of objective nasal obstruction.
- Objective decrease in olfaction demonstrated by testing.

General Considerations

Anatomic blockage of the nasal cavity with subsequent airflow disruption is the most common cause of olfactory dysfunction (hyposmia or anosmia). Polyps, septal deformities, and nasal tumors may be the cause. Due to localized inflammation, transient olfactory dysfunction often accompanies the common cold, nasal allergies, and perennial rhinitis through changes in the nasal and olfactory epithelium. About 20% of olfactory dysfunction is idiopathic, although it often follows a viral illness.

CNS neoplasms, especially those that involve the olfactory groove or temporal lobe, also may affect olfaction and should be considered in patients with no other explanation for their hyposmia. Head trauma is also a rare but severe cause of olfactory dysfunction due to shearing of the olfactory sensory cells. Head trauma accounts for less than 5% of cases of hyposmia but is more commonly associated with anosmia than with hyposmia. Absent, diminished, or distorted smell has been reported in a wide variety of endocrine, nutritional, and nervous disorders.

Clinical Findings

Evaluation of olfactory dysfunction should include a thorough history of systemic illnesses and medication use as well as a physical examination focusing on the nose and nervous system. Nasal obstruction (from polyps, trauma, foreign bodies, or nasal masses) can cause functional hyposmia. Most clinical offices are not set up to test olfaction, but such tests may at times be worthwhile if only to assess whether a patient possesses any sense of smell at all. The University of Pennsylvania Smell Identification Test (UPSIT) is available commercially and is a simple, self-administered "scratch-and-sniff" test that is useful in differentiating hyposmia, anosmia, and malingering.

Treatment

Olfactory dysfunction secondary to nasal polyposis, obstruction, and chronic rhinosinusitis may respond to surgically removing the anatomic blockage, as with endoscopic sinus surgery. Unfortunately, there is no specific treatment for primary disruption of olfaction; some disturbances spontaneously resolve. The degree of olfactory dysfunction is the greatest predictor of recovery, with less severe olfactory dysfunction recovering at a much higher rate. In permanent olfactory dysfunction, counseling should be offered about seasoning foods (such as using pepper that stimulates the trigeminal as well as olfactory chemoreceptors, rather than table salt) and safety issues (such as installing home smoke alarms and using electric rather than gas appliances).

Kasiri H et al. Mometasone furoate nasal spray in the treatment of patients with COVID-19 olfactory dysfunction: a randomized, double blind clinical trial. Int Immunopharmacol. 2021;98:107871. [PMID: 34147912]

Roh D et al. The association between olfactory dysfunction and cardiovascular disease and its risk factors in middle-aged and older adults. Sci Rep. 2021;11:1248. [PMID: 33441955]

EPISTAXIS

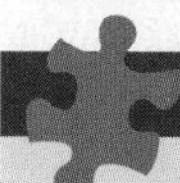

ESSENTIALS OF DIAGNOSIS

- Bleeding from a unilateral anterior nasal cavity along the septum is most common.
- Most cases may be successfully treated by direct pressure on the bleeding site for 15 minutes. When this is inadequate, topical sympathomimetics and various nasal tamponade methods are usually effective.
- Posterior, bilateral, or large-volume epistaxis should be triaged immediately to a specialist in a critical care setting.

General Considerations

Epistaxis is an extremely common problem in the primary care setting. Bleeding is most common in the anterior septum where a confluence of veins creates a superficial venous plexus (Kiesselbach plexus). Predisposing factors include nasal trauma (nose picking, foreign bodies, forceful nose blowing), rhinitis, nasal mucosal drying from low humidity or supplemental nasal oxygen, deviation of the nasal septum, atherosclerotic disease, hereditary hemorrhagic telangiectasia (Osler-Weber-Rendu syndrome), inhaled nasal cocaine (or other drugs), and alcohol abuse. Poorly controlled hypertension is associated with epistaxis. Anticoagulation or antiplatelet medications may be associated with a higher incidence, more frequent recurrence, and greater difficulty in control of epistaxis, but they do not cause it.

Clinical Findings

Laboratory assessment of bleeding parameters may be indicated, especially in recurrent epistaxis. Once the acute episode has passed, careful examination of the nose and paranasal sinuses is indicated to rule out neoplasia and hereditary hemorrhagic telangiectasia. Repeated evaluation for diagnosis and treatment of clinically significant hypertension should be performed following control of epistaxis and removal of any packing.

Treatment

Most cases of anterior epistaxis may be successfully treated by direct pressure on the site by compression of the nares continuously for 15 minutes. Venous pressure is reduced in the sitting position, and slight leaning forward. Positioning the head backwards is not recommended because this may result in blood going toward the airway, resulting in possible aspiration. Similarly, pinching the bridge of the nose is generally ineffective as the origin of bleeding typically occurs at the tip. Short-acting topical nasal decongestants (eg, phenylephrine, 0.125–1% solution, one or two sprays or oxymetazoline), which act as vasoconstrictors, may also help. When the bleeding does not readily subside, the nose should be examined, using good illumination and suction, in an attempt to locate the bleeding site. When directly visible, the bleeding site may be cauterized with silver nitrate, diathermy, or electrocautery. A supplemental patch of Surgicel or Gelfoam may be helpful with a moisture barrier, such as petroleum-based ointment, to prevent drying and crusting.

Occasionally, a site of bleeding may be inaccessible to direct control, or attempts at direct control may be unsuccessful. In such cases, there are a number of alternatives. When the site of bleeding is anterior, a hemostatic sealant, pneumatic or other nasal tamponade, or anterior packing may suffice as the latter may be accomplished with several feet of lubricated iodoform packing systematically placed in the floor of the nose and then the vault of the nose.

About 5% of nasal bleeding originates in the posterior nasal cavity, commonly associated with atherosclerotic disease and hypertension. In such cases, it may be necessary to consult an otolaryngologist for a pack to occlude the choana before placing a pack anteriorly. In emergency settings, double balloon packs (Epistat) may facilitate rapid control of bleeding with little or no mucosal trauma. Because such packing is uncomfortable, bleeding may persist, and vasovagal syncope is possible, hospitalization for monitoring and stabilization is indicated. Posterior nasal packing is quite uncomfortable and may require an opioid analgesic for pain control.

Surgical management of epistaxis, through ligation of the nasal arterial supply (internal maxillary artery and ethmoid arteries) is indicated when direct pressure and nasal packing fail. The most common approach to surgical treatment is endoscopic sphenopalatine artery ligation. This method has a reported efficacy of 73–100% in studies; however, it may miss bleeds caused by the ethmoid arterial supply. Alternatively, endovascular epistaxis control is highly effective (75–92%) and can address all sources of intranasal bleeding except those from the anterior ethmoid artery. Its use may be reserved for when a surgical approach fails because it is associated with a 1.1–1.5% risk of stroke.

After control of epistaxis, the patient is advised to avoid straining and vigorous exercise for several days. Nasal saline should be applied to the packing frequently to keep the packing moist. Avoidance of hot or spicy foods and tobacco is also advisable, since these may cause nasal vasodilation. Avoiding nasal trauma, including nose picking, is an obvious necessity. Lubrication with petroleum jelly or bacitracin ointment and increased home humidity may also be useful ancillary measures. Finally, antistaphylococcal antibiotics (eg, cephalexin, 500 mg orally four times daily, or clindamycin, 150 mg orally four times daily) generally are indicated to reduce the risk of toxic shock syndrome developing while the packing remains in place (at least 5 days).

When to Refer

- Patients with recurrent epistaxis, large-volume epistaxis, and episodic epistaxis with associated nasal obstruction should be referred to an otolaryngologist for endoscopic evaluation and possible imaging.
- Those with ongoing bleeding beyond 15 minutes should be taken to a local emergency department if the clinician is not prepared to manage acute epistaxis.

D'Aguanno V et al. Clinical recommendations for epistaxis management during the COVID-19 pandemic. Otolaryngol Head Neck Surg. 2020;163:75. [PMID: 32366173]

Tran QK et al. Prophylactic antibiotics for anterior nasal packing in emergency department: a systematic review and meta-analysis of clinically-significant infections. Am J Emerg Med. 2020;38:983. [PMID: 31839514]

Tunkel DE et al. Clinical practice guideline: nosebleed (epistaxis) executive summary. Otolaryngol Head Neck Surg. 2020;162:8. [PMID: 31910122]

NASAL TRAUMA

The nasal pyramid is the most frequently fractured bone in the body. Fracture is suggested by crepitance or palpably mobile bony segments. Epistaxis and pain are common, as are soft-tissue hematomas ("black eye"). It is important to make certain that there is no palpable step-off of the infraorbital rim, which would indicate the presence of a zygomatic complex fracture. Radiologic confirmation may at times be helpful but is not necessary in uncomplicated nasal fractures. It is also important to assess for possible concomitant additional facial, spine, pulmonary, or intracranial injuries when the circumstances of injury are suggestive, as in the case of automobile and motorcycle accidents.

Treatment is aimed at maintaining long-term nasal airway patency and cosmesis. Closed reduction can be performed under local or general anesthesia; closed reduction under general anesthesia appears to afford better patient satisfaction and decreased need for subsequent revision septoplasty or rhinoplasty.

Intranasal examination should be performed in all cases to rule out septal hematoma, which appears as a widening of the anterior septum, visible just posterior to the columella. The septal cartilage receives its only nutrition from its closely adherent mucoperichondrium. An untreated subperichondrial hematoma will result in loss of the nasal cartilage with resultant saddle nose deformity, septal perforation, or both. Septal hematomas may become infected, with *S aureus* most commonly, and should be drained with an incision in the inferior mucoperichondrium on both sides. The drained fluid should be sent for culture.

Packing for 2–5 days is often helpful to help prevent re-formation of the hematoma. Antibiotics with antistaphylococcal efficacy (eg, cephalexin, 500 mg four times daily, or clindamycin, 150 mg four times daily) should be given for 3–5 days or the duration of the packing to reduce the risk of toxic shock syndrome.

TUMORS & GRANULOMATOUS DISEASE

1. Benign Nasal Tumors

A. Nasal Polyps

Nasal polyps are pale, edematous, mucosally covered masses commonly seen in patients with allergic rhinitis. They may result in chronic nasal obstruction and a diminished sense of smell. In patients with nasal polyps and a history of asthma, aspirin should be avoided because it may precipitate a severe episode of bronchospasm, known as **triad asthma** (Samter triad). Such patients may have an immunologic salicylate sensitivity.

Use of topical intranasal corticosteroids improves the quality of life in patients with nasal polyposis and chronic rhinosinusitis. Initial treatment with topical nasal corticosteroids (see Allergic Rhinitis section for specific medications) for 1–3 months is usually successful for small polyps and may reduce the need for operation. A short course of oral corticosteroids (eg, prednisone, 6-day course using 21 [5-mg] tablets: 6 tablets [30 mg] on day 1 and tapering by 1 tablet [5 mg] each day) may also be of benefit, but when polyps are massive or medical management is unsuccessful obstructing polyps may be removed surgically. Polyps may readily be removed using endoscopic sinus surgery techniques. It may be necessary to remove polyps from the ethmoid, sphenoid, and maxillary sinuses to provide longer-lasting relief and open the affected sinuses. Intranasal corticosteroids should be continued following polyp removal to prevent recurrence, and the clinician should consider allergen testing to determine the offending allergen and avoidance measures.

Brescia G. Role of blood inflammatory cells in chronic rhinosinusitis with nasal polyps. Acta Otolaryngol. 2019;139:48. [PMID: 30686139]

Song WJ et al. Chronic rhinosinusitis with nasal polyps in older adults: clinical presentation, pathophysiology, and comorbidity. Curr Allergy Asthma Rep. 2019;19:46. [PMID: 31486905]

B. Inverted Papillomas

Inverted papillomas are benign tumors caused by HPV that usually arise on the lateral nasal wall. They present with unilateral nasal obstruction and occasionally hemorrhage. They are often easily seen on anterior rhinoscopy as cauliflower-like growths in or around the middle meatus. Because squamous cell carcinoma is seen in about 10% of inverted or schneiderian papillomas, complete excision is strongly recommended. This usually requires an endoscopic medial maxillectomy. While rare, very extensive disease may require an open inferior or total maxillectomy for complete removal. Because recurrence rates for inverted papillomas are reported to be as high as 20%, subsequent clinical and radiologic follow-up is imperative. All excised tissue (not just a portion) should be carefully reviewed by the pathologist to be sure no carcinoma is present.

Peng R et al. Outcomes of sinonasal inverted papilloma resection by surgical approach: an updated systematic review and meta-analysis. Int Forum Allergy Rhinol. 2019;9:573. [PMID: 30748098]

2. Malignant Nasopharyngeal & Paranasal Sinus Tumors

Though rare, malignant tumors of the nose, nasopharynx, and paranasal sinuses are quite problematic because they tend to remain asymptomatic until late in their course. Squamous cell carcinoma is the most common cancer found in the sinuses and nasopharynx. It is especially common in the nasopharynx, where it obstructs the eustachian tube and results in serous otitis media. Nasopharyngeal carcinoma (nonkeratinizing squamous cell carcinoma or lymphoepithelioma) is usually associated with elevated IgA antibody to the viral capsid antigen of the Epstein-Barr virus (EBV). It is particularly common in patients of southern Chinese descent and has a weaker association with tobacco exposure than other head and neck squamous cell carcinomas. Adenocarcinomas, mucosal melanomas, sarcomas, and non-Hodgkin lymphomas are less commonly encountered neoplasms of this area.

Early symptoms are nonspecific, mimicking those of rhinitis or sinusitis. Unilateral nasal obstruction, otitis media, and discharge are common, with pain and recurrent hemorrhage often clues to the diagnosis of cancer. **All adults with persistent unilateral nasal symptoms or new otitis media should be thoroughly evaluated with nasal endoscopy and nasopharyngoscopy.** A high index of suspicion remains a key to early diagnosis of these tumors. Patients often present with advanced symptoms, such as proptosis, expansion of a cheek, or ill-fitting maxillary dentures. Malar hypesthesia, due to involvement of the infraorbital nerve, is common in maxillary sinus tumors. Biopsy is necessary for definitive diagnosis, and MRI is the best imaging study to delineate the extent of disease and plan appropriate surgery and radiation.

Treatment depends on the tumor type and the extent of disease. Early stage disease may be treated with radiation therapy alone, but advanced nasopharyngeal carcinoma is best treated with concurrent radiation and chemotherapy. Chemoradiation therapy significantly decreases local, nodal, and distant failures and increases progression-free and overall survival in advanced disease. Locally recurrent nasopharyngeal carcinoma in selected cases may be treated with repeat irradiation protocols or surgery with moderate success and a high degree of concern about local wound healing. Other squamous cell carcinomas are best treated—when resectable—with a combination of surgery and irradiation. Cranial base surgery, which can be done endoscopically using image navigation, appears to be an effective modality in improving the overall prognosis in paranasal sinus malignancies eroding the ethmoid roof. Although the prognosis is poor for advanced tumors, the results of treating resectable tumors of paranasal sinus origin have improved with the wider use of skull base resections and intensity-modulated radiation therapy. Cure rates are often 45–60%.

Masarwy R et al. Neoadjuvant PD-1/PD-L1 inhibitors for resectable head and neck cancer: a systematic review and meta-analysis. JAMA Otolaryngol Head Neck Surg. 2021;147:871. [PMID: 34473219]

3. Sinonasal Inflammatory Disease (Granulomatosis with Polyangiitis & Sarcoidosis)

The nose and paranasal sinuses are involved in over 90% of cases of **granulomatosis with polyangiitis**. It is often not realized that involvement at these sites is more common than involvement of lungs or kidneys. Examination shows bloodstained crusts and friable mucosa. Biopsy, when positive, shows necrotizing granulomas and vasculitis. Other recognized sites of granulomatosis with polyangiitis in the head and neck include the subglottis and the middle ear. For treatment of granulomatosis with polyangiitis, see Chapter 20.

Sarcoidosis commonly involves the paranasal sinuses and is clinically similar to other chronic sinonasal inflammatory processes. Sinonasal symptoms, including rhinorrhea, nasal obstruction, and hyposmia or anosmia, may precede diagnosis of sarcoidosis in other organ systems. Clinically, the turbinates appear engorged with small white granulomas. Biopsy shows classic noncaseating granulomas. Notably, patients with sinonasal involvement generally have more trouble managing sarcoidosis in other organ systems.

Polymorphic reticulosis (midline malignant reticulosis, idiopathic midline destructive disease, lethal midline granuloma)—as the multitude of apt descriptive terms suggests—is not well understood but appears to be a nasal T-cell or NK-cell lymphoma. In contrast to granulomatosis with polyangiitis, involvement is limited to the mid-face, and there may be extensive bone destruction. Many destructive lesions of the mucosa and nasal structures labeled as polymorphic reticulosis are in fact non-Hodgkin lymphoma of either NK-cell or T-cell origin. Immunophenotyping, especially for CD56 expression, is essential in the histologic evaluation. Even when apparently localized, these lymphomas have a poor prognosis, with progression and death within a year the rule.

Guzman-Soto MI et al. From head to toe: granulomatosis with polyangiitis. Radiographics. 2021;41:1973. [PMID: 34652975]

DISEASES OF THE ORAL CAVITY & PHARYNX

LEUKOPLAKIA, ERYTHROPLAKIA, LICHEN PLANUS, & AND OROPHARYNGEAL CANCER

ESSENTIALS OF DIAGNOSIS

- **Leukoplakia:** A white lesion that cannot be removed by rubbing the mucosal surface.
- **Erythroplakia:** Similar to leukoplakia except that it has a definite erythematous component.
- **Oral Lichen Planus:** Most commonly presents as lacy leukoplakia but may be erosive; definitive diagnosis requires biopsy.
- **Oral Cancer:** Early lesions appear as leukoplakia or erythroplakia; more advanced lesions will be larger, with invasion into the tongue such that a mass lesion is palpable. Ulceration may be present.
- **Oropharyngeal Cancer:** Unilateral throat masses, such as emanating from the tonsils or base of tongue, typically presenting with painful swallowing and weight loss.

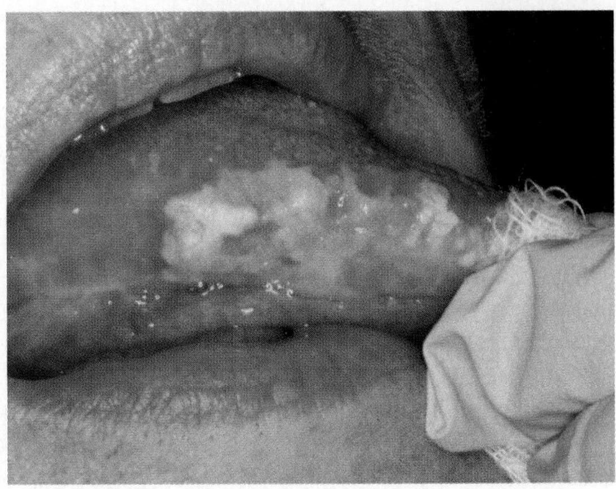

Figure 8–5. Leukoplakia with moderate dysplasia on the lateral border of the tongue. (Used, with permission, from Ellen Eisenberg, DMD, in Usatine RP, Smith MA, Mayeaux EJ Jr, Chumley H. *The Color Atlas of Family Medicine*, 2nd ed. McGraw-Hill, 2013.)

Leukoplakic regions range from small to several centimeters in diameter (Figure 8–5). Histologically, they are often hyperkeratoses occurring in response to chronic irritation (eg, from dentures, tobacco, lichen planus); about 2–6%, however, represent either dysplasia or early invasive squamous cell carcinoma. Distinguishing between **leukoplakia** and **erythroplakia** is important because about 90% of cases of erythroplakia are either dysplasia or carcinoma. **Squamous cell carcinoma** accounts for 90% of oral cancer. Alcohol and tobacco use are the major epidemiologic risk factors.

The differential diagnosis may include oral candidiasis, necrotizing sialometaplasia, pseudoepitheliomatous hyperplasia, median rhomboid glossitis, and vesiculoerosive inflammatory disease, such as erosive lichen planus. This should not be confused with the brown-black gingival melanin pigmentation—diffuse or speckled—common in non-Whites, blue-black embedded fragments of dental amalgam, or other systemic disorders associated with general pigmentation (neurofibromatosis, familial polyposis, Addison disease). Intraoral melanoma is extremely rare and carries a dismal prognosis.

Any area of erythroplakia, enlarging area of leukoplakia, or a lesion that has submucosal depth on palpation should have an incisional biopsy or an exfoliative cytologic examination. Ulcerative lesions are particularly suspicious and worrisome. Specialty referral should be sought early both for diagnosis and treatment. A systematic intraoral examination—including the lateral tongue, floor of the mouth, gingiva, buccal area, palate, and tonsillar fossae—and palpation of the neck for enlarged lymph nodes should be part of any general physical examination, especially in patients over the age of 45 who smoke tobacco or drink immoderately. Indirect or fiberoptic examination of the nasopharynx, oropharynx, hypopharynx, and larynx by an otolaryngologist, head and neck surgeon, or radiation oncologist should also be considered for such patients when there is unexplained or persistent throat or ear pain, oral or nasal bleeding, or oral erythroplakia. Fine-needle aspiration (FNA) biopsy may expedite the diagnosis if an enlarged lymph node is found.

To date, there remain no approved therapies for reversing or stabilizing leukoplakia or erythroplakia. Clinical trials have suggested a role for beta-carotene, celecoxib, vitamin E, and retinoids in producing regression of leukoplakia and reducing the incidence of recurrent squamous cell carcinomas. None have demonstrated benefit in large studies and these agents are not in general use today. The mainstays of management are surveillance following elimination of carcinogenic irritants (eg, smoking tobacco, chewing tobacco or betel nut, drinking alcohol) along with serial biopsies and excisions.

Oral lichen planus is a relatively common (0.5–2% of the population) chronic inflammatory autoimmune disease that may be difficult to diagnose clinically because of its numerous distinct phenotypic subtypes. For example, the reticular pattern may mimic candidiasis or hyperkeratosis, while the erosive pattern may mimic squamous cell carcinoma. Management begins with distinguishing it from other oral lesions. Exfoliative cytology or a small incisional or excisional biopsy is indicated, especially if squamous cell carcinoma is suspected. Therapy of lichen planus is aimed at managing pain and discomfort. Daily topical corticosteroid remains the most effective treatment for symptomatic lichen planus, but cyclosporines, retinoids, and tacrolimus have also been used. Many experts think there is a low rate (1%) of squamous cell carcinoma arising within lichen planus (in addition to the possibility of clinical misdiagnosis) and prevention of malignant transformation remains a goal of treatment.

Hairy leukoplakia occurs on the lateral border of the tongue and is a common early finding in HIV infection (see Chapter 31). It often develops quickly and appears as slightly raised leukoplakic areas with a corrugated or "hairy" surface (Figure 8–6). While much more prevalent in HIV-positive patients, hairy leukoplakia can occur following solid organ transplantation and is associated with Epstein-Barr virus infection and long-term systemic corticosteroid use. Hairy leukoplakia waxes and wanes over time with generally modest irritative symptoms. Acyclovir, valacyclovir, and famciclovir have all been used for treatment but produce only temporary resolution of the condition. It does not appear to predispose to malignant transformation.

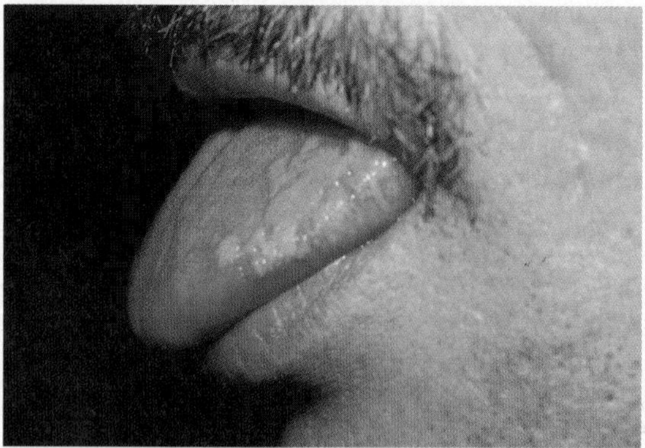

▲ **Figure 8–6.** Oral hairy leukoplakia on the side of the tongue in AIDS. (Reproduced with permission from Richard P. Usatine, MD, in Usatine RP, Smith MA, Mayeaux EJ Jr, Chumley H. *The Color Atlas of Family Medicine*, 2nd ed. McGraw-Hill, 2013.)

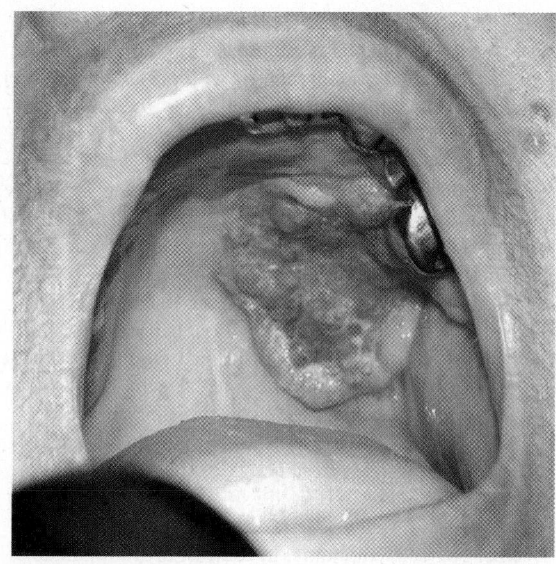

▲ **Figure 8–7.** Squamous cell carcinoma of the palate. (Used, with permission, from Frank Miller, MD, in Usatine RP, Smith MA, Mayeaux EJ Jr, Chumley H. *The Color Atlas of Family Medicine*, 2nd ed. McGraw-Hill, 2013.)

Oral cavity squamous cell carcinoma can be hard to distinguish from other oral lesions, but early detection is the key to successful management (Figure 8–7). Raised, firm, white lesions with ulcers at the base are highly suspicious and generally quite painful on even gentle palpation. Lesions less than 4 mm in depth have a low propensity to metastasize. Most patients in whom the tumor is detected before it is 2 cm in diameter are cured by local resection. Radiation is reserved for patients with positive margins or metastatic disease. Large tumors are usually treated with a combination of resection, neck dissection, and external beam radiation. Reconstruction, if required, is done at the time of resection and can involve the use of myocutaneous flaps or vascularized free flaps with or without bone. Novel fluorescence-guided surgeries are being developed to improve detection of margins and decrease recurrence.

Oropharyngeal squamous cell carcinoma generally presents later than oral cavity squamous cell carcinoma. The lesions tend to be larger and are often buried within the lymphoid tissue of the palatine or lingual tonsils. Most patients note only unilateral odynophagia and weight loss, but ipsilateral cervical lymphadenopathy is often identified by the careful clinician. While these tumors are typically associated with known carcinogens such as tobacco and alcohol, their epidemiology has changed dramatically over the past 20 years. Despite demonstrated reductions in tobacco and alcohol use within developed nations, the incidence of oropharyngeal squamous cell carcinoma has not declined over this period. Known as a possible cause of head and neck cancer since 1983, **HPV—most commonly,**

type 16—is believed to be the cause of up to 70% of all oropharyngeal squamous cell carcinoma. HPV-positive tumors are readily distinguished by immunostaining of primary tumor or FNA biopsy specimens for the p16 protein, a tumor suppressor protein that is highly correlated with the presence of HPV. These tumors often present in advanced stages of the disease with regional cervical lymph node metastases (stages III and IV), but have a better prognosis than similarly staged lesions in tobacco and alcohol users. This difference in disease control is so apparent in multicenter studies that, based on the presence or absence of the p16 protein, two distinct staging systems for oropharyngeal squamous cell carcinoma were introduced in 2018.

Machiels JP et al. Pembrolizumab given concomitantly with chemoradiation and as maintenance therapy for locally advanced head and neck squamous cell carcinoma: KEYNOTE-412. Future Oncol. 2020;16:1235. [PMID: 32490686]

ORAL CANDIDIASIS

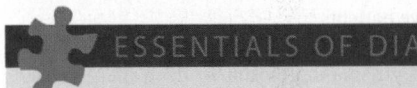

ESSENTIALS OF DIAGNOSIS

- Fluctuating throat or mouth discomfort.
- Associated with systemic or local immunosuppression, such as recent corticosteroid, chemotherapy, or antibiotic use.
- Erythema of the oral cavity or oropharynx with creamy-white, curd-like patches.
- Rapid resolution of symptoms with appropriate treatment.

Clinical Findings

A. Symptoms and Signs

Oral candidiasis (thrush) is usually painful and looks like creamy-white curd-like patches overlying erythematous mucosa (see Figure 6–11). Because these white areas are easily rubbed off (eg, by a tongue depressor)—unlike leukoplakia or lichen planus—only the underlying irregular erythema may be seen. Oral candidiasis is commonly associated with the following risk factors: (1) use of dentures, (2) debilitated state with poor oral hygiene, (3) diabetes mellitus, (4) anemia, (5) chemotherapy or local irradiation, (6) corticosteroid use (oral or systemic), or (7) broad-spectrum antibiotics. Another manifestation of candidiasis is angular cheilitis (also seen in nutritional deficiencies) (Figure 8–8).

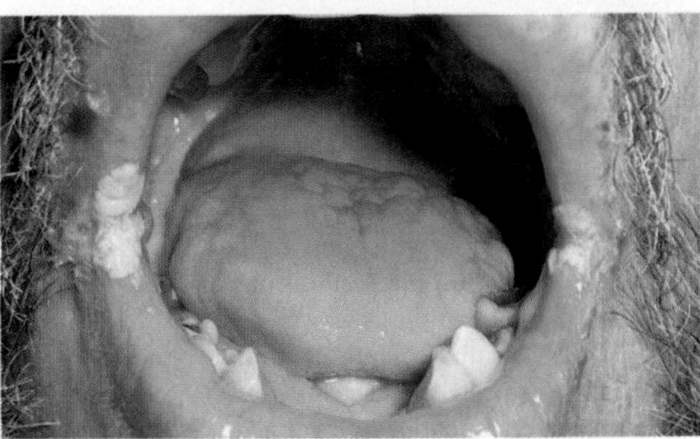

Figure 8–8. Severe angular cheilitis in HIV-positive man with oral thrush. (Reproduced with permission from Richard P. Usatine, MD, in Usatine RP, Smith MA, Mayeaux EJ Jr, Chumley H. *The Color Atlas of Family Medicine*, 2nd ed. McGraw-Hill, 2013.)

B. Diagnostic Studies

The diagnosis is made clinically. A wet preparation using potassium hydroxide will reveal spores and may show nonseptate mycelia. Biopsy will show intraepithelial pseudomycelia of *Candida albicans.*

Candidiasis is often the first manifestation of HIV infection, and HIV testing should be considered in patients with no known predisposing cause for *Candida* overgrowth (see also Chapter 31). The US Department of Health Services Clinical Practice Guideline for Evaluation and Management of Early HIV Infection recommends examination of the oral mucosa with each clinician visit as well as at a dental examination every 6 months for individuals living with HIV.

Treatment

Effective antifungal therapy may be achieved with any of the following: fluconazole (100 mg orally daily for 7 days), ketoconazole (200–400 mg orally with breakfast [requires acidic gastric environment for absorption] for 7–14 days), clotrimazole troches (10 mg dissolved orally five times daily), or nystatin mouth rinses (500,000 units [5 mL of 100,000 units/mL] held in the mouth before swallowing three times daily). In patients with HIV infection, however, longer courses of therapy with fluconazole may be needed, and oral itraconazole (200 mg/day) may be indicated in fluconazole-refractory cases. Many of the *Candida* species in these patients are resistant to first-line azoles and may require newer medications, such as voriconazole. In addition, 0.12% chlorhexidine or half-strength hydrogen peroxide mouth rinses may provide local relief. Nystatin powder (100,000 units/g) applied to dentures three or four times daily and rinsed off for several weeks may help denture wearers.

Fang J et al. Efficacy of antifungal drugs in the treatment of oral candidiasis: a Bayesian network meta-analysis. J Prosthet Dent. 2020:S0022-3913(20)30076. [PMID: 32165010]
Vila T et al. Oral candidiasis: a disease of opportunity. J Fungi (Basel). 2020;16;6:15. [PMID: 31963180]

GLOSSITIS, GLOSSODYNIA, & BURNING MOUTH SYNDROME

Inflammation of the tongue with loss of filiform papillae leads to a red, smooth-surfaced tongue (**glossitis**). Rarely painful, it may be secondary to nutritional deficiencies (eg, niacin, riboflavin, iron, or vitamin E), drug reactions, dehydration, irritants, or foods and liquids, and possibly to autoimmune reactions or psoriasis. If the primary cause cannot be identified and corrected, empiric nutritional replacement therapy may be of value.

Glossodynia is burning and pain of the tongue, which may occur with or without glossitis. In the absence of any clinical findings, it has been termed "burning mouth syndrome." Glossodynia with glossitis has been associated with diabetes mellitus, medications (eg, diuretics), tobacco, xerostomia, and candidiasis as well as the listed causes of glossitis. The burning mouth syndrome typically has no identifiable associated risk factors and seems to be most common in postmenopausal women. Treating possible underlying causes, changing long-term medications to alternative ones, and smoking cessation may resolve symptoms of glossitis. Effective treatments for the burning mouth syndrome include alpha-lipoic acid and clonazepam. Clonazepam is most effective as a rapid-dissolving tablet placed on the tongue in doses from 0.25 mg to 0.5 mg every 8–12 hours. Both glossodynia and the burning mouth syndrome are benign, and reassurance that there is no infection or tumor is likely to be appreciated. Unilateral symptoms, symptoms that cannot be related to a specific medication, and symptoms and signs involving regions supplied by other cranial nerves all may suggest neuropathology, and imaging of the brain, brainstem, and skull base with MRI should be considered.

Adamo D et al. Vortioxetine versus other antidepressants in the treatment of burning mouth syndrome: an open-label randomized trial. Oral Dis. 2021;27:1022. [PMID: 32790904]

INTRAORAL ULCERATIVE LESIONS

1. Necrotizing Ulcerative Gingivitis (Trench Mouth, Vincent Angina)

Necrotizing ulcerative gingivitis, often caused by an infection with both spirochetes and fusiform bacilli, is common in young adults under stress (classically in students at examination time). Underlying systemic diseases may also predispose to this disorder. Clinically, there is painful acute gingival inflammation and necrosis, often with bleeding, halitosis, fever, and cervical lymphadenopathy. Warm half-strength peroxide rinses and oral penicillin (250 mg three times daily for 10 days) may help. Dental gingival curettage may prove necessary.

Reddy R et al. Seventeen new cases of chronic ulcerative stomatitis with literature review. Head Neck Pathol. 2019;13:386. [PMID: 30374883]

2. Aphthous Ulcer (Canker Sore, Ulcerative Stomatitis)

Aphthous ulcers are very common and easy to recognize. Their cause remains uncertain, although an association with human herpesvirus 6 has been suggested. Found on freely moving, nonkeratinized mucosa (eg, buccal and labial mucosa and not attached gingiva or palate), they may be single or multiple, are usually recurrent, and appear as painful small round ulcerations with yellow-gray fibrinoid centers surrounded by red halos. Minor aphthous ulcers are less than 1 cm in diameter and generally heal in 10–14 days. Major aphthous ulcers are greater than 1 cm in diameter and can be disabling due to the degree of associated oral pain. Stress seems to be a major predisposing factor to the eruptions of aphthous ulcers.

Treatment is challenging because no single systemic treatment has proven effective. Avoiding local irritants, such as certain toothpastes, may decrease symptoms and episodes. Topical corticosteroids (triamcinolone acetonide, 0.1%, or fluocinonide ointment, 0.05%) in an adhesive base (Orabase Plain) do appear to provide symptomatic relief in many patients. Other topical therapies shown to be effective in controlled studies include diclofenac 3% in hyaluronan 2.5%, doxymycine-cyanoacrylate, mouthwashes containing the enzymes amyloglucosidase and glucose oxidase, and amlexanox 5% oral paste. A 1-week tapering course of prednisone (40–60 mg/day) has also been used successfully. Cimetidine maintenance therapy may be useful in patients with recurrent aphthous ulcers. Thalidomide has been used selectively in recurrent aphthous ulcerations in HIV-positive patients.

Large or persistent areas of ulcerative stomatitis may be secondary to erythema multiforme or drug allergies, acute herpes simplex, pemphigus, pemphigoid, epidermolysis bullosa acquisita, bullous lichen planus, Behçet disease, or IBD. Squamous cell carcinoma may occasionally present in this fashion. When the diagnosis is not clear, incisional biopsy is indicated.

Chaitanya N et al. Efficacy of improvised topical zinc (1%) orabase on oral mucositis during cancer chemo-radiation—a randomized study. J Nutr Sci Vitaminol (Tokyo). 2020;66:93. [PMID: 32350185]

3. Herpes Stomatitis

Herpes gingivostomatitis is common, mild, and short-lived. Clinically, there is initial burning, followed by typical small vesicles that rupture and form scabs. Lesions are most commonly found on the attached gingiva and mucocutaneous junction of the lip, but lesions can also form on the tongue, buccal mucosa, and soft palate. In most adults, it requires no intervention. In immunocompromised persons, however, reactivation of herpes simplex virus infection is frequent and may be severe. Acyclovir (200–800 mg orally five times daily for 7–10 days) or valacyclovir (1000 mg orally twice daily for 7–10 days) may shorten the course and reduce postherpetic pain. These treatments may be effective only when started within 24–48 hours of the onset of initial symptoms (pain, itching, burning) and are not effective once vesicles have erupted. Differential diagnosis includes aphthous stomatitis, erythema multiforme, syphilitic chancre, and carcinoma.

Mazzarello V et al. Do sunscreens prevent recurrent herpes labialis in summer? J Dermatolog Treat. 2019;30:179. [PMID: 29804485]

Petti S et al. The controversial natural history of oral herpes simplex virus type 1 infection. Oral Dis. 2019;25:1850. [PMID: 31733122]

PHARYNGITIS & TONSILLITIS

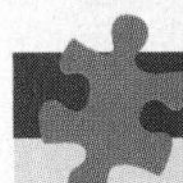

ESSENTIALS OF DIAGNOSIS

- Centor criteria for streptococcal pharyngitis: exudate or swelling on tonsils, anterior cervical adenopathy, fever, lack of cough.
- Goal is to treat group A beta-hemolytic streptococcal infection to prevent subsequent rheumatic fever (rash, arthralgias, myocardtis) and other sequelae (glomerulonephritis, posterior pharyngeal abscess).

General Considerations

Pharyngitis and tonsillitis account for over 10% of all office visits to primary care clinicians and 50% of outpatient antibiotic use. The main concern is determining who is likely to have a group A beta-hemolytic streptococcal (GABHS) infection, since this can lead to subsequent complications, such as rheumatic fever and glomerulonephritis. A second public health policy concern is reducing the extraordinary cost (both in dollars and in the development of antibiotic-resistant *S pneumoniae*) in the United States associated with unnecessary antibiotic use. Numerous well-done studies and experience with rapid laboratory tests for detection of streptococci (eliminating the delay caused by culturing) have informed a consensus recommendation.

Clinical Findings

A. Symptoms and Signs

The clinical features most suggestive of GABHS pharyngitis include fever over 38°C, tender anterior cervical adenopathy, lack of a cough, and pharyngotonsillar exudate (Figure 8–9). These four features (**the Centor criteria**), when present, strongly suggest GABHS. When two or three of the four are present, there is an intermediate likelihood of GABHS. When only one criterion is present, GABHS is unlikely. Sore throat may be severe, with odynophagia, tender adenopathy, and a scarlatiniform rash. An elevated white count and left shift are also possible. Hoarseness, cough, and coryza are not suggestive of this disease. It is also rare to have GABHS in individuals younger than 3 years old.

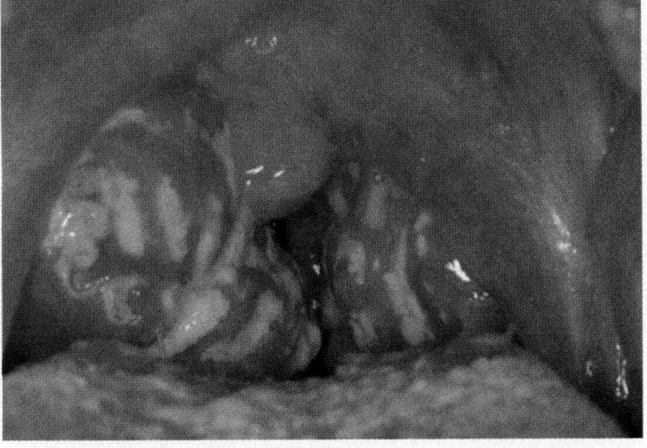

Figure 8–9. Marked exudative pharyngitis and tonsillitis due to group A beta-hemolytic streptococci. (Used, with permission, from Lawrence B. Stack, MD, in Knoop KJ, Stack LB, Storrow AB, Thurman RJ. *The Atlas of Emergency Medicine*, 5th ed. McGraw Hill, 2021.)

Marked lymphadenopathy and a shaggy, white-purple tonsillar exudate, often extending into the nasopharynx, suggest mononucleosis, especially if present in a young adult. With about 90% sensitivity, lymphocyte-to-white-blood-cell ratios of greater than 35% suggest EBV infection and not tonsillitis. Hepatosplenomegaly and a positive heterophile agglutination test or elevated anti-EBV titer are corroborative. However, about one-third of patients with infectious mononucleosis have secondary streptococcal tonsillitis, requiring treatment. Ampicillin should routinely be avoided if mononucleosis is suspected because it induces a rash that might be misinterpreted by the patient as a penicillin allergy. Diphtheria (extremely rare but described in persons with alcohol use disorder) presents with low-grade fever and an ill patient with a gray tonsillar pseudomembrane.

The most common pathogens other than GABHS in the differential diagnosis of "sore throat" are viruses, *Neisseria gonorrhoeae*, *Mycoplasma*, and *Chlamydia trachomatis*. Rhinorrhea and lack of exudate would suggest a virus, but in practice it is not possible to confidently distinguish viral upper respiratory infection from GABHS on clinical grounds alone. Infections with *Corynebacterium diphtheria*, anaerobic streptococci, and *Corynebacterium haemolyticum* (which responds better to erythromycin than penicillin) may also mimic pharyngitis due to GABHS.

B. Laboratory Findings

A single-swab throat culture is 90–95% sensitive and the rapid antigen detection testing (RADT) is 90–99% sensitive for GABHS. Results from the RADT are available in about 15 minutes.

Treatment

The Infectious Diseases Society of America recommends laboratory confirmation of the clinical diagnosis by means of either throat culture or RADT of the throat swab. The American College of Physicians–American Society of Internal Medicine (ACP-ASIM), in collaboration with the CDC, advocates use of a clinical algorithm alone—in lieu of microbiologic testing—for confirmation of the diagnosis in adults for whom the suspicion of streptococcal infection is high. Others examine the assumptions of the ACP-ASIM guideline for using a clinical algorithm alone and question whether those recommendations will achieve the stated objective of dramatically decreasing excess antibiotic use. A reasonable strategy to follow is that patients with zero or one Centor criteria are at very low risk for GABHS and therefore do not need throat cultures or RADT of the throat swab and should not receive antibiotics. Patients with two or three Centor criteria need throat cultures or RADT of the throat swab, since positive results would warrant antibiotic treatment. Patients who have all four Centor criteria are likely to have GABHS and can receive empiric therapy without throat culture or RADT.

Oral antibiotics are the preferred first-line therapy. Penicillin V potassium (250 mg orally three times daily or 500 mg twice daily for 10 days) or cefuroxime axetil (250 mg orally twice daily for 5–10 days) are both effective. The efficacy of a 5-day regimen of penicillin V potassium appears to be similar to that of a 10-day course, with a 94% clinical response rate and an 84% streptococcal eradication rate. Erythromycin (also active against *Mycoplasma* and *Chlamydia*) is a reasonable alternative to penicillin in allergic patients. Cephalosporins are somewhat more effective than penicillin in producing bacteriologic cures; 5-day courses of cefpodoxime and cefuroxime have been successful. The macrolide antibiotics have also been reported to be successful in shorter-duration regimens. Azithromycin (500 mg once daily), because of its long half-life, needs to be taken for only 3 days. For patients in whom medication compliance is in question, or those unable to take oral medication, a single intramuscular injection of benzathine penicillin or procaine penicillin, 1.2 million units is an effective alternative.

Adequate antibiotic treatment usually avoids the streptococcal complications of scarlet fever, rheumatic myocarditis, glomerulonephritis, and local abscess formation.

Antibiotics for treatment failures are also somewhat controversial. Surprisingly, penicillin-tolerant strains are not isolated more frequently in those who fail treatment than in those treated successfully with penicillin. The reasons for failure appear to be complex, and a second course of treatment with the same medication is reasonable. Alternatives to penicillin include cefuroxime and other cephalosporins, dicloxacillin (which is beta-lactamase–resistant), and amoxicillin with clavulanate. When there is a history of penicillin allergy, alternatives should be used, such as erythromycin. Erythromycin resistance—with failure rates of about 25%—is an increasing problem in many areas. In cases of severe penicillin allergy, cephalosporins should be avoided since cross-reaction occurs in greater than 8% of cases.

Ancillary treatment of pharyngitis includes analgesics and anti-inflammatory agents, such as aspirin, acetaminophen, and corticosteroids. In meta-analysis, corticosteroids increased the likelihood of complete pain resolution at 24 hours by threefold without an increase in recurrence or adverse events. Some patients find that salt water gargling is soothing. In severe cases, anesthetic gargles and lozenges (eg, benzocaine) may provide additional symptomatic relief. Occasionally, odynophagia is so intense that hospitalization for intravenous hydration and antibiotics is necessary. (See Chapter 33.)

Patients who have had rheumatic fever should be treated with a continuous course of antimicrobial prophylaxis (penicillin G, 500 mg once daily orally, or erythromycin, 250 mg twice daily orally) for at least 5 years.

Cohen JF et al. Efficacy and safety of rapid tests to guide antibiotic prescriptions for sore throat. Cochrane Database Syst Rev. 2020;6:CD012431. [PMID: 32497279]

Klein MR. Infections of the oropharynx. Emerg Med Clin North Am. 2019;37:69. [PMID: 30454781]

Sykes EA et al. Pharyngitis: approach to diagnosis and treatment. Can Fam Physician. 2020;66:251. [PMID: 32273409]

PERITONSILLAR ABSCESS & CELLULITIS

When infection penetrates the tonsillar capsule and involves the surrounding tissues, peritonsillar cellulitis results. Following therapy, peritonsillar cellulitis usually either resolves over several days or evolves into peritonsillar abscess. Peritonsillar abscess (**quinsy**) and cellulitis present with severe sore throat, odynophagia, trismus, medial deviation of the soft palate and peritonsillar fold, and an abnormal muffled ("hot potato") voice. CT may be a useful adjunct to clinical suspicion, but imaging is not required for the diagnosis. The existence of an abscess may be confirmed by aspirating pus from the peritonsillar fold just superior and medial to the upper pole of the tonsil. A 19-gauge or 21-gauge needle should be passed medial to the molar and no deeper than 1 cm, because the internal carotid artery may lie more medially than its usual location and pass posterior and deep to the tonsillar fossa. Most commonly, patients with peritonsillar abscess present to the emergency department and receive a dose of parenteral amoxicillin (1 g), amoxicillin-sulbactam (3 g), or clindamycin (600–900 mg). Less severe cases and patients who are able to tolerate oral intake may be treated for 7–10 days with oral antibiotics, including amoxicillin, 500 mg three times a day; amoxicillin-clavulanate, 875 mg twice a day; or clindamycin, 300 mg four times daily.

Although antibiotic treatment is generally undisputed, there is controversy regarding the surgical management of peritonsillar abscess. Methods include needle aspiration, incision and drainage, and tonsillectomy. Some clinicians incise and drain the area and continue with parenteral antibiotics, whereas others aspirate only and monitor as an outpatient. The data are largely equivocal for all three approaches. In patients with more severe or recurrent peritonsillar abscesses, it may be appropriate to consider immediate tonsillectomy (quinsy tonsillectomy) in the acutely infected setting, although practitioners have moved away from this approach because of the potential for complications.

About 10% of patients with peritonsillar abscess exhibit relative indications for tonsillectomy after the infection as resolved. All three approaches are effective. Regardless of the method used, one must be sure the abscess is adequately treated, since complications such as extension to the retropharyngeal, deep neck, and posterior mediastinal spaces are possible. Bacteria may also be aspirated into the lungs, resulting in pneumonia. There is controversy about whether a single abscess is a sufficient indication for tonsillectomy; about 30% of patients aged 17–30 who do not undergo early planned tonsillectomy following peritonsillar abscess ultimately undergo surgery, and only about 13% of those over 30 have their tonsils removed. Recurrent or atypical peritonsillar abscesses in older adults should also be evaluated for an underlying head and neck malignancy.

Klug TE et al. Complications of peritonsillar abscess. Ann Clin Microbiol Antimicrob. 2020;19:32. [PMID: 32731900]

Luo MS et al. Needle aspiration versus incision and drainage under local anaesthesia for the treatment of peritonsillar abscess. Eur Arch Otorhinolaryngol. 2020;277:645. [PMID: 31555918]

DEEP NECK INFECTIONS

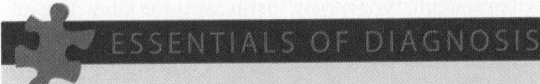

ESSENTIALS OF DIAGNOSIS

- Marked acute neck pain and swelling.
- Abscesses are emergencies because rapid airway compromise may occur.
- May spread to the mediastinum or cause sepsis.

General Considerations

Deep neck abscesses most commonly originate from odontogenic infections. Other causes include suppurative lymphadenitis; direct spread of pharyngeal infection; penetrating trauma; pharyngoesophageal foreign bodies; cervical osteomyelitis; and intravenous injection of the internal jugular vein, especially in people with substance use disorders. **Ludwig angina** is the most commonly encountered neck space infection. It is a cellulitis of the sublingual and submaxillary spaces, often arising from infection of the mandibular dentition. **Ludwig angina is an emergency** as it may cause rapid upper airway compromise and necessitate creation of a surgical airway. Recurrent deep neck infection may suggest an underlying congenital lesion, such as a branchial cleft cyst. Suppurative lymphadenopathy in middle-aged persons who smoke cigarettes and drink alcohol regularly should be considered a manifestation of malignancy (typically metastatic squamous cell carcinoma) until proven otherwise.

Clinical Findings

Patients with Ludwig angina have edema and erythema of the upper neck under the chin and often of the floor of the mouth. The tongue may be displaced upward and backward by the posterior spread of cellulitis, and coalescence of pus is often present in the floor of mouth. This may lead to occlusion of the airway. Microbiologic isolates include streptococci, staphylococci, *Bacteroides*, and *Fusobacterium*. Patients with diabetes may have different flora, including *Klebsiella*, and a more aggressive clinical course.

Patients with deep neck abscesses usually present with marked neck pain and swelling. Fever is common but not always present. **Deep neck abscesses are emergencies because they may rapidly compromise the airway.** Untreated or inadequately treated, they may spread to the mediastinum or cause sepsis.

Contrast-enhanced CT usually augments the clinical examination in defining the extent of the infection. It often will distinguish inflammation and phlegmon (requiring antibiotics) from abscess (requiring drainage) and define for the surgeon the extent of an abscess. CT with MRI may also identify thrombophlebitis of the internal jugular vein secondary to oropharyngeal inflammation. This condition, known as **Lemierre syndrome**, is rare and usually associated with severe headache. The presence of pulmonary infiltrates consistent with septic emboli in the setting of a neck abscess should lead one to suspect Lemierre syndrome or injection drug use, or both.

Treatment

Usual doses of penicillin plus metronidazole, ampicillin-sulbactam, clindamycin, or selective cephalosporins are good initial choices for treatment of Ludwig angina. Culture and sensitivity data are then used to refine the choice. Dental consultation is advisable to address the offending tooth or teeth. External drainage via bilateral submental incisions is required if the airway is threatened or when medical therapy has not reversed the process.

Treatment of deep neck abscesses includes securing the airway, intravenous antibiotics, and incision and drainage. When the infection involves the floor of the mouth, base of the tongue, or the supraglottic or paraglottic space, the airway may be secured either by intubation or tracheotomy. Tracheotomy is preferable in the patients with substantial pharyngeal edema, since attempts at intubation may precipitate acute airway obstruction. Bleeding in association with a deep neck abscess is very rare but suggests carotid artery or internal jugular vein involvement and requires prompt neck exploration both for drainage of pus and for vascular control.

Patients with Lemierre syndrome require prompt institution of antibiotics appropriate for *Fusobacterium necrophorum* as well as the more usual upper airway pathogens. The use of anticoagulation in treatment is of no proven benefit.

Fiorella ML et al. New laboratory predictive tools in deep neck space infections. Acta Otorhinolaryngol Ital. 2020;40:332. [PMID: 3329922]

Lee WS et al. Lemierre's syndrome: a forgotten and re-emerging infection. J Microbiol Immunol Infect. 2020;53:513. [PMID: 32303484]

Li RM et al. Infections of the neck. Emerg Med Clin North Am. 2019;37:95. [PMID: 30454783]

Velhonoja J et al. Deep neck space infections: an upward trend and changing characteristics. Eur Arch Otorhinolaryngol. 2020;277:863. [PMID: 31797041]

SNORING

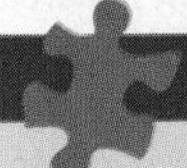

ESSENTIALS OF DIAGNOSIS

- Noise produced on inspiration due to upper aerodigestive tract blockage during sleep.
- Snoring is associated with obstructive sleep apnea (OSA) but may not alone disrupt sleep quality.

General Considerations

Ventilation disorders during sleep are extremely common. While OSA occurs in 5–10% of Americans, clinically relevant snoring may occur in as many as 59%. In general, sleep-disordered breathing problems are attributed to narrowing of the upper aerodigestive tract during sleep due to changes in position, muscle tone, and soft tissue hypertrophy or laxity. The most common sites of obstruction are the oropharynx and the base of the tongue. The spectrum of the problem ranges from simple snoring without cessation of airflow to OSA with long periods of apnea and life-threatening physiologic sequelae. OSA is discussed in Chapter 9. In contrast to OSA, snoring is almost exclusively a social problem, and despite its prevalence and association with OSA, there is comparatively little known about the management of this problem.

Clinical Findings

A. Symptoms and Signs

All patients who complain of snoring should be evaluated for OSA as discussed in Chapter 9. Symptoms of OSA (including snoring, excessive daytime somnolence, daytime headaches, and weight gain) may be present in as many as 30% of patients without demonstrable apnea or hypopnea on formal testing. Clinical examination should include examination of the nasal cavity, nasopharynx, oropharynx, and larynx to help exclude other causes of dynamic airway obstruction. In many cases of isolated snoring, the palate and uvula appear enlarged and elongated with excessive mucosa hanging below the muscular portion of the soft palate.

B. Imaging and Diagnostic Testing

Sleep examination with polysomnography is strongly advised in the evaluation of a patient with complaints of snoring. Radiographic imaging of the head or neck is generally not necessary. Additional testing may include sleep endoscopy.

Treatment

Expeditious and inexpensive management solutions of snoring are sought, often with little or no benefit. Diet modification and physical exercise can lead to improvement in snoring through the weight loss and improvement in pharyngeal tone that accompanies overall physical conditioning. Position change during sleep can be effective, and time-honored treatments, such as placing a golf or tennis ball into a pocket sewn on the back of the pajama top worn during sleep, may satisfactorily eliminate symptoms by ensuring recumbency on one side. Although numerous pharmacologic therapies have been endorsed, none demonstrate any significant utility when scrutinized.

Anatomic management of snoring can be challenging. As with OSA, snoring can come from a number of sites in the upper aerodigestive tract. While medical or surgical correction of nasal obstruction may help alleviate snoring problems, most interventions aim to improve airflow through the nasopharynx and oropharynx. Nonsurgical options include mandibular advancement appliances designed to pull the base of the tongue forward and continuous positive airway pressure via face or nasal mask. Compliance with both of these treatment options is problematic because snorers without OSA do not notice the physiologic benefits of these devices noted by patients with sleep apnea.

Surgical correction of snoring is most commonly directed at the soft palate. Historical approaches involved resection of redundant mucosa and the uvula similar to uvulopalatopharyngoplasty that is used for OSA. Regardless of how limited the procedure or what technique was used, the postoperative pain, expense of general anesthesia, and high recurrence rates limit the utility of these procedures. Office-based approaches are more widely used because of these limitations. Most of these procedures aim to stiffen the palate to prevent vibration rather than remove it. A series of procedures, including injection snoreplasty, radiofrequency thermal fibrosis, and an implantable palatal device, have been used with variable success and patient tolerance. The techniques can be technically challenging. Persistent symptoms may occur following initial treatment necessitating costly (and sometimes painful) repeat procedures. The durability of these procedures in alleviating symptoms is also poorly understood, and late failures can lead to patient and clinician frustration.

Suzuki M et al. Effect of position therapy and oral devices on sleep parameters in patients with obstructive sleep apnea. Eur Arch Otorhinolaryngol. 2021;278:4545. [PMID: 33864481]

DISEASES OF THE SALIVARY GLANDS

ACUTE INFLAMMATORY SALIVARY GLAND DISORDERS

1. Sialadenitis

Acute bacterial sialadenitis most commonly affects either the parotid or submandibular gland. It typically presents with acute swelling of the gland, increased pain and swelling with meals, and tenderness and erythema of the duct opening. Pus often can be massaged from the duct. Sialadenitis often occurs in the setting of dehydration or in association with chronic illness. Underlying Sjögren syndrome and chronic periodontitis may contribute. Ductal obstruction, often by an inspissated mucous plug, is followed by salivary stasis and secondary infection. The most common organism recovered from purulent draining saliva is *S aureus*. Treatment consists of intravenous antibiotics, such as nafcillin (1 g intravenously every 4–6 hours), and measures to increase salivary flow, including hydration, warm compresses, sialagogues (eg, lemon drops), and massage of the gland. Treatment can usually then be switched to an oral agent based on clinical improvement and microbiologic results to complete a 10-day treatment course. Less severe cases can often be treated with oral antibiotics with similar spectrum. Complete resolution of parotid swelling and pain can take 2–3 weeks. Failure of the process to improve and ultimately resolve on this regimen suggests abscess formation, ductal stricture, stone, or tumor causing obstruction. Ultrasound or CT scan may be helpful in establishing the diagnosis. In the setting of acute illness, a severe and potentially life-threatening form of sialadenitis, sometimes called suppurative sialadenitis, may develop. The causative organism is usually *S aureus*, but often no pus will drain from Stensen papilla. These patients often do not respond to rehydration and intravenous antibiotics and thus may require operative incision and drainage to resolve the infection. In patients with bilateral parotid sialadenitis, mumps should be considered.

2. Sialolithiasis

Calculus formation is more common in the Wharton duct (draining the submandibular glands) than in the Stensen duct (draining the parotid glands). Clinically, a patient may note postprandial pain and local swelling, often with a history of recurrent acute sialadenitis. Stones in the Wharton duct are usually large and radiopaque, whereas those in the Stensen duct are usually radiolucent and smaller. Those very close to the orifice of the Wharton duct may be palpated manually in the anterior floor of the mouth and removed intraorally by dilating or incising the distal duct. Those more than 1.5–2 cm from the duct are too close to the lingual nerve to be removed safely in this manner. Similarly, dilation of the Stensen duct, located on the buccal surface opposite the second maxillary molar, may relieve distal stricture or allow a small stone to pass. Sialoendoscopy for the management of chronic sialolithiasis is superior to extracorporeal shock-wave lithotripsy and fluoroscopically guided basket retrieval. Repeated episodes of sialadenitis are usually associated with stricture and chronic infection. If the obstruction cannot be safely removed or dilated, excision of the gland may be necessary to relieve recurrent symptoms.

Ferneini EM. Managing sialolithiasis. J Oral Maxillofac Surg. 2021;79:1581. [PMID: 34215413]

CHRONIC INFLAMMATORY & INFILTRATIVE DISORDERS OF THE SALIVARY GLANDS

Numerous infiltrative disorders may cause unilateral or bilateral parotid gland enlargement. Sjögren syndrome and sarcoidosis are examples of lymphoepithelial and granulomatous diseases that may affect the salivary glands. Metabolic disorders, including alcoholism, diabetes mellitus, and vitamin deficiencies, may also cause diffuse enlargement. Several medications have been associated with parotid enlargement, including thioureas, iodine, and medications with cholinergic effects (eg, phenothiazines), which stimulate salivary flow and cause more viscous saliva.

SALIVARY GLAND TUMORS

A general rule of thumb is that the smaller the size of the salivary gland with a present mass, the more likely the possibility of malignancy. Approximately 80% of salivary gland tumors occur in the parotid gland. In adults, about 80% of these are benign. In the submandibular triangle, it is sometimes difficult to distinguish a primary submandibular gland tumor from a metastatic submandibular space node. Only 50–60% of primary submandibular tumors are benign. Tumors of the minor salivary glands are most likely to be malignant, with adenoid cystic carcinoma predominating, and may be found throughout the oral cavity or oropharynx.

Most parotid tumors present as an asymptomatic mass in the superficial part of the gland. Their presence may have been noted by the patient for months or years. Facial nerve involvement correlates strongly with malignancy. Tumors may extend deep to the plane of the facial nerve or may originate in the parapharyngeal space. In such cases, medial deviation of the soft palate is visible on intraoral examination. MRI and CT scans have largely replaced sialography in defining the extent of tumor. At least one study demonstrates the potential benefit of enhanced MRI imaging in distinguishing among Warthin tumors and pleomorphic adenomas and malignant salivary gland tumors.

When the clinician encounters a patient with an otherwise asymptomatic salivary gland mass where tumor is the most likely diagnosis, the choice is whether to simply excise the mass via a parotidectomy with facial nerve dissection or submandibular gland excision or to first obtain an FNA biopsy. Although the accuracy of FNA biopsy for malignancy has been reported to be quite high, results vary among institutions. If a negative FNA biopsy would lead to a decision not to proceed to surgery, then it should be considered. Poor overall health of the patient and the possibility of inflammatory disease as the cause of the mass are situations where FNA biopsy might be helpful. In otherwise straightforward nonrecurrent cases, excision generally is indicated. In benign and small, low-grade malignant tumors, no additional treatment is needed. Postoperative irradiation is indicated for larger and high-grade cancers.

Benchetrit L et al. Major salivary gland cancer with distant metastasis upon presentation: patterns, outcomes, and imaging implications. Otolaryngol Head Neck Surg. 2021 Nov 16. [Epub ahead of print] [PMID: 34784258]

DISEASES OF THE LARYNX

HOARSENESS & STRIDOR

The primary symptoms of laryngeal disease are hoarseness and stridor. Hoarseness is caused by an abnormal vibration of the vocal folds. The voice is breathy when too much air passes incompletely apposed vocal folds, as in unilateral vocal fold paralysis or vocal fold mass. The voice is harsh when the vocal folds are stiff and vibrate irregularly, as is the case in laryngitis or malignancy. Heavy, edematous vocal folds produce a rough, low-pitched vocal quality. Stridor (a high-pitched, typically inspiratory, sound) is the result of turbulent airflow from a narrowed upper airway. Airway narrowing at or above the vocal folds produces inspiratory stridor. Airway narrowing below the vocal fold level produces either expiratory or biphasic stridor. The timing and rapidity of onset of stridor are critically important in determining the seriousness of the airway problem. **All cases of stridor should be evaluated by a specialist and rapid-onset stridor should be evaluated emergently.**

Evaluation of an abnormal voice begins with obtaining a history of the circumstances preceding its onset and an examination of the airway. **All patients with hoarseness that has persisted beyond 2 weeks should be evaluated by an otolaryngologist with laryngoscopy.** Especially when the patient has a history of tobacco use, laryngeal cancer or lung cancer (leading to paralysis of a recurrent laryngeal nerve), or concerns for cough and aspiration, must be strongly considered. In addition to structural causes of dysphonia, laryngoscopy can help identify functional problems with the voice, including vocal fold paralysis, muscle tension dysphonia, and spasmodic dysphonia.

Ross J et al. Utility of audiometry in the evaluation of patients presenting with dysphonia. Ann Otol Rhinol Laryngol. 2020;129:333. [PMID: 31731878]

COMMON LARYNGEAL DISORDERS

1. Acute Laryngitis

Acute laryngitis is probably the most common cause of hoarseness, which may persist for a week or so after other symptoms of an upper respiratory infection have cleared. Supportive care includes resting the voice, drinking enough fluid to stay hydrated, and breathing humidified air. The patient should be warned to avoid vigorous use of the voice (singing, shouting) until their voice returns to normal, since persistent use may lead to the formation of traumatic vocal fold hemorrhage, polyps, and cysts. Although thought to be usually viral in origin, both *M catarrhalis* and *H influenzae* may be isolated from the nasopharynx at higher than expected frequencies. Despite this finding, a meta-analysis has failed to demonstrate any convincing evidence that antibiotics significantly alter the natural resolution of acute laryngitis. Erythromycin may speed improvement of hoarseness at 1 week and cough at 2 weeks when measured subjectively. Oral or intramuscular corticosteroids may be used in highly selected cases of professional vocalists to speed recovery and allow scheduled performances. Examination of the vocal folds and assessment of vocal technique are mandatory prior to corticosteroid initiation, since inflamed vocal folds are at greater risk for hemorrhage and the subsequent development of traumatic vocal fold pathology.

Huang T et al. Efficacy of inhaled budesonide on serum inflammatory factors and quality of life among children with acute infectious laryngitis. Am J Otolaryngol. 2021;42:102820. [PMID: 33188988]

2. Laryngopharyngeal Reflux

ESSENTIALS OF DIAGNOSIS

- Commonly associated with hoarseness, throat irritation, heartburn, foreign body sensation, and chronic cough.
- Symptoms typically occur when upright, and many patients do not experience classic heartburn.
- Laryngoscopy is critical to exclude other causes of hoarseness.
- Diagnosis is often made based on response to PPI therapy.
- Treatment failure with PPIs is common and suggests other etiologies.

Gastroesophageal reflux into the larynx (laryngopharyngeal reflux) is considered a cause of chronic hoarseness when other causes of abnormal vocal fold vibration (such as tumor or nodules) have been excluded by laryngoscopy. GERD has also been suggested as a contributing factor to other symptoms, such as throat clearing, throat discomfort, chronic cough, a sensation of postnasal drip, esophageal spasm, and some cases of asthma. Since less than half of patients with laryngeal acid exposure have typical symptoms of heartburn and regurgitation, the lack of such symptoms should not be construed as eliminating this cause. Indeed, **most patients with symptomatic laryngopharyngeal reflux, as it is now called, do not meet criteria for GERD by pH probe testing** and these entities must be considered separately. The prevalence of this condition is hotly debated in the literature, and laryngopharyngeal reflux may not be as common as once thought.

Evaluation should initially exclude other causes of dysphonia through laryngoscopy; consultation with an otolaryngologist is advisable. Many clinicians opt for an empiric trial of a PPI since no gold standard exists for diagnosing this condition. Such an empiric trial should not precede visualization of the vocal folds to exclude other causes of hoarseness. When used, the American Academy of Otolaryngology–Head and Neck Surgery recommends twice-daily therapy with full-strength PPI (eg, omeprazole 40 mg orally twice daily or equivalent) for a minimum of 3 months. Patients may note improvement in symptoms after 3 months, but the changes in the larynx often take 6 months to resolve. If symptoms improve and cessation of therapy leads to symptoms again, then a PPI is resumed at the lowest dose effective for remission, usually daily but at times on a demand basis. Although H_2-receptor antagonists are an alternative to PPIs, they are generally both less clinically effective and less cost-effective. Nonresponders should undergo pH testing and manometry. Twenty-four-hour pH monitoring of the pharynx should best document laryngopharyngeal reflux and is advocated by some as the initial management step, but it is costly, more difficult, and less available than lower esophageal monitoring alone. Double pH probe (proximal and distal esophageal probes) testing is the best option for evaluation, since lower esophageal pH monitoring alone does not correlate well with laryngopharyngeal reflux symptoms. Oropharyngeal pH probe testing is available, but its ability to predict response to reflux treatment in patients with laryngopharyngeal reflux is not known.

Chae M et al. A prospective randomized clinical trial of combination therapy with proton pump inhibitors and mucolytics in patients with laryngopharyngeal reflux. Ann Otol Rhinol Laryngol. 2020;129:781. [PMID: 32186395]
Lechien JR et al. Laryngopharyngeal reflux: a state-of-the-art algorithm management for primary care physicians. J Clin Med. 2020;9:3618. [PMID: 33182684]

3. Recurrent Respiratory Papillomatosis

Papillomas are common lesions of the larynx and other sites where ciliated and squamous epithelia meet. Unlike oral papillomas, recurrent respiratory papillomatosis typically becomes symptomatic, with hoarseness that occasionally progresses over weeks to months. These papillomas are almost always due to HPV types 6 and 11. Repeated laser vaporizations or cold knife resections via operative laryngoscopy are the mainstay of treatment. Severe cases can cause airway compromise in adults and may require treatment as often as every 6 weeks to maintain airway patency. Extension can occur into the trachea and lungs. Tracheotomy should be avoided, if possible, since it introduces an additional squamociliary junction for which papillomas appear to have an affinity. Interferon treatment has been under investigation for many years but is only indicated in severe cases with pulmonary involvement. Rarely, cases of malignant transformation have been reported (often in smokers), but recurrent respiratory papillomatosis should generally be thought of as a benign condition. Cidofovir (a cytosine nucleotide analog in use to treat cytomegalovirus retinitis) has been used with success as intralesional therapy for recurrent respiratory papillomatosis. Because cidofovir causes adenocarcinomas in laboratory animals, its potential for carcinogenesis is being monitored. The quadrivalent and new 9 serotype recombinant human HPV vaccines (Gardasil and Gardasil 9) offer hope for the eventual prevention of this benign, but terribly morbid, disease.

Allen CT. Biologics for the treatment of recurrent respiratory papillomatosis. Otolaryngol Clin North Am. 2021;54:769. [PMID: 34099306]

4. Epiglottitis

Epiglottitis (or, more correctly, supraglottitis) should be suspected when a patient presents with a rapidly developing sore throat or when odynophagia (pain on swallowing) is out of proportion to apparently minimal oropharyngeal findings on examination. It is more common in diabetic patients and may be viral or bacterial in origin. Rarely in the era of *H influenzae* type b vaccine is this bacterium isolated in adults. Unlike in children, indirect laryngoscopy is generally safe and may demonstrate a swollen, erythematous epiglottis. Lateral plain radiographs may demonstrate an enlarged epiglottis (the epiglottis "thumb sign"). Initial treatment is hospitalization for intravenous antibiotics—eg, ceftizoxime, 1–2 g intravenously every 8–12 hours; or cefuroxime, 750–1500 mg intravenously every 8 hours; and dexamethasone, usually 4–10 mg as initial bolus, then 4 mg intravenously every 6 hours—and observation of the airway. Corticosteroids may be tapered as symptoms and signs resolve. Similarly, substitution of oral antibiotics may be appropriate to complete a 10-day course. Less than 10% of adults require intubation. Indications for intubation are dyspnea, rapid pace of sore throat (where progression to airway compromise may occur before the effects of corticosteroids and antibiotics), and endolaryngeal abscess noted on CT imaging. If the patient is not intubated, prudence suggests monitoring oxygen saturation with continuous pulse oximetry and initial admission to a monitored unit.

Gottlieb M et al. Ultrasound for airway management: an evidence-based review for the emergency clinician. Am J Emerg Med. 2020;38:1007. [PMID: 31843325]
Sideris A et al. A systematic review and meta-analysis of predictors of airway intervention in adult epiglottitis. Laryngoscope. 2020;130:465. [PMID: 31173373]

MASSES OF THE LARYNX

1. Traumatic Lesions of the Vocal Folds

Vocal fold nodules are smooth, paired lesions that form at the junction of the anterior one-third and posterior two-thirds of the vocal folds. They are a common cause of hoarseness resulting from vocal abuse. In adults, they are referred to as "singer's nodules" and in children as "screamer's nodules." Treatment requires modification of voice habits, and referral to a speech therapist is indicated. While nearly all true nodules will resolve with behavior modification, recalcitrant nodules may require surgical excision. Often, additional pathology, such as a polyp or cyst, may be encountered.

Vocal fold polyps are unilateral masses that form within the superficial lamina propria of the vocal fold. They are related to vocal trauma and seem to follow resolution of vocal fold hemorrhage. Small, sessile polyps may resolve with conservative measures, such as voice rest and corticosteroids, but larger polyps are often irreversible and require operative removal to restore normal voice.

Vocal fold cysts are also considered traumatic lesions of the vocal folds and are either true cysts with an epithelial lining or pseudocysts. They typically form from mucus-secreting glands on the inferior aspect of the vocal folds. Cysts may fluctuate in size from week to week and cause a variable degree of hoarseness. They rarely, if ever, resolve completely and may leave behind a sulcus, or vocal fold scar, if they decompress or are marsupialized. Such scarring can be a frustrating cause of permanent dysphonia.

Polypoid corditis is different from vocal fold polyps and may form from loss of elastin fibers and loosening of the intracellular junctions within the lamina propria. This loss allows swelling of the gelatinous matrix of the superficial lamina propria (called **Reinke edema**). These changes in the vocal folds are strongly associated with smoking, but also with vocal abuse, chemical industrial irritants, and hypothyroidism. While this problem is common in both male and female smokers, women seem more troubled by the characteristic decline in modal pitch caused by the increased mass of the vocal folds. If the patient stops smoking or the lesions cause stridor and airway obstruction, surgical resection of the hyperplastic vocal fold mucosa may be indicated to improve the voice or airway, or both.

A common but often unrecognized cause of hoarseness and odynophonia are **contact ulcers** or their close relatives, **granulomas**. Both lesions form on the vocal processes of the arytenoid cartilages, and patients often can correctly inform the clinician which side is affected. The cause of these ulcers and granulomas is disputed, but they are clearly related to trauma and may be related to exposure of the underlying perichondrium. They are common following intubation and generally resolve quite quickly. Chronic ulceration or granuloma formation has been associated with gastroesophageal reflux but is also common in patients with muscle tension dysphonia. Treatment is often multimodal, and an inhaled corticosteroid (eg, fluticasone 440 mcg twice daily) may be the most effective pharmacologic therapy. Adjunctive treatment measures include PPI therapy (omeprazole 40 mg orally twice daily, or equivalent) and voice therapy with special attention to vocal hygiene. Rare cases can be quite stubborn and persistent without efficacious therapy. Surgical removal is rarely, if ever, required for nonobstructive lesions.

Alegria R et al. Effectiveness of voice therapy in patients with vocal fold nodules: a systematic search and narrative review. Eur Arch Otorhinolaryngol. 2020;277:2951. [PMID: 32444967]

2. Laryngeal Leukoplakia

Leukoplakia of the vocal folds is commonly found in association with hoarseness in smokers. Direct laryngoscopy with biopsy is advised in almost all cases. Histologic examination usually demonstrates mild, moderate, or severe dysplasia. In some cases, invasive squamous cell carcinoma is present in the initial biopsy specimen. Cessation of smoking may reverse or stabilize mild or moderate dysplasia. Some patients—estimated to be less than 5% of those with mild dysplasia and about 35–60% of those with severe dysplasia—will subsequently develop squamous cell carcinoma. Treatment options include PPI therapy, close follow-up with laryngovideostroboscopy, serial resection, and external beam radiation therapy.

Sezen Goktas S et al. A new approach to vocal cord leukoplakia and evaluation of proton pump inhibitor treatment. Eur Arch Otorhinolaryngol. 2019;276:467. [PMID: 30607560]

3. Squamous Cell Carcinoma of the Larynx

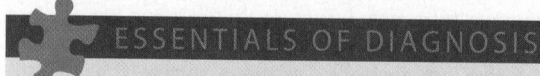

- New and persistent (> 2 weeks' duration) voice changes and hoarseness, especially in a smoker.
- Persistent throat pain, especially with swallowing; weight loss; neck mass; hemoptysis.
- Stridor or other symptoms of a compromised airway.

General Considerations

Squamous cell carcinoma of the larynx, the most common malignancy of the larynx, occurs almost exclusively in patients with a history of significant tobacco use. Based on a 2020 study, the incidence, prevalence, and mortality of laryngeal cancer are estimated at 2.76 cases/year per 100,000 individuals, 14.33 cases/year per 100,000 individuals and 1.66 deaths/year per 100,000 individuals, respectively. The incidence and prevalence have increased by 12% and 24%, respectively, during the past three decades. Mortality has declined by approximately 5%. Squamous cell carcinoma is usually seen in men aged 50–70 years. There may be an association between laryngeal cancer and HPV type 16 or 18 infection, but this association is much less strong than that between HPV 16 or 18 and oropharyngeal cancer. In both cancer types, the association with HPV seems to be strongest in nonsmokers. Laryngeal cancer is very treatable and early detection is the key to maximizing posttreatment voice, swallowing, and breathing function.

Clinical Findings

A. Symptoms and Signs

A change in voice quality is most often the presenting complaint, although throat or ear pain, hemoptysis, dysphagia, weight loss, and airway compromise may occur. Because of their early impact on vocal quality, glottic cancers are among the smallest detectable human malignancies and treatment success is very high with early lesions. Neck metastases are not common in early glottic (true vocal fold) cancer in which the vocal folds are mobile, but a third of patients in whom there is impaired fold mobility will also have involved lymph nodes at neck dissection. Supraglottic carcinoma (false vocal folds, aryepiglottic folds, epiglottis), on the other hand, often metastasizes to both sides of the neck early in the disease. Complete head and neck examination, including laryngoscopy, is mandatory for any person with the concerning symptoms listed under Essentials of Diagnosis.

B. Imaging and Laboratory Studies

Radiologic evaluation by CT or MRI is helpful in assessing tumor extent. Imaging evaluates neck nodes, tumor volume, and cartilage sclerosis or destruction. A chest CT scan is indicated if there are level VI enlarged nodes (around the trachea and the thyroid gland) or level IV enlarged nodes (inferior to the cricoid cartilage along the internal jugular vein), or if a chest film is concerning for a second primary lesion or metastases. Laboratory evaluation includes CBC and liver biochemical tests. Formal cardiopulmonary evaluation may be indicated, especially if partial laryngeal surgery is being considered. All partial laryngectomy candidates should have good to excellent lung function and exercise tolerance because chronic microaspiration may be expected following the procedure. A PET scan or CT-PET scan may be indicated to assess for distant metastases when there appears to be advanced local or regional disease.

C. Biopsy

Diagnosis is made by biopsy at the time of laryngoscopy when true fold mobility and arytenoid fixation, as well as surface tumor extent, can be evaluated. Most otolaryngologists recommend esophagoscopy and bronchoscopy at the same time to exclude synchronous primary tumor. Although an FNA biopsy of an enlarged neck node may have already been done, it is generally acceptable to assume radiographically enlarged neck nodes (greater than 1–1.5 cm) or nodes with necrotic centers are neck metastases. Open biopsies of nodal metastases should be discouraged because they may lead to higher rates of tumor treatment failure.

D. Tumor Staging

The American Joint Committee on Cancer (AJCC) staging of laryngeal cancers uses the TNM system to describe tumor extent and can be used for prognosis. Early laryngeal cancers, T1 and T2 (stage I and II) lesions, involve 1–2 laryngeal subsites locally and have no nodal metastases or profound functional abnormalities. T3 and T4 lesions may involve multiple laryngeal subsites with limitation of laryngeal mobility. These locally advanced lesions are stage III or IV cancers, and any size tumor with regional nodal metastases is at least a stage III tumor. Stage I and II lesions are generally treated with single-modality therapy (surgery or radiation), while multimodality therapy, usually including chemotherapy with radiation therapy, is reserved for more advanced stage III and IV lesions.

Treatment

Treatment of laryngeal carcinoma has four goals: cure, preservation of safe and effective swallowing, preservation of useful voice, and avoidance of a permanent tracheostoma. For early glottic and supraglottic cancers, radiation therapy is the standard of care since cure rates are greater than 95% and 80%, respectively. That said, radiation therapy carries substantial morbidity, and many early tumors (T1 and T2 lesions, without involved nodes) and selected advanced tumors (T3 and T4) may be treated with partial laryngectomy if at least one cricoarytenoid unit can be preserved. Five-year locoregional cure rates exceed 80–90% with surgery, and patient-reported satisfaction is excellent. In supraglottic tumors, even when clinically N0, elective limited neck dissection is indicated following surgical resection because of the high risk of neck node involvement.

Advanced stage III and IV tumors represent a challenging and ever-changing treatment dilemma. Twenty-five years ago, total laryngectomy was often recommended for such patients. However, the 1994 VA study (with induction cisplatin and 5-fluorouracil followed by irradiation alone in responders) demonstrated that two-thirds of patients could preserve their larynx. Subsequent studies have further defined multimodal therapy. Cisplatin-based chemotherapy concomitant with radiation therapy has been shown to be superior to either irradiation alone or induction chemotherapy followed by radiation. The same benefits have been demonstrated with the epidermal growth factor receptor blocker cetuximab with lower overall systemic toxicity and better patient tolerance. However, chemoradiation using either cetuximab or cisplatin is associated with prolonged gastrostomy-dependent dysphagia.

The high rate of dysphagia and morbidity associated with severe laryngeal stenosis following chemoradiation has prompted a reevaluation of the role of extended, but less-than-total, laryngeal resection for selected advanced laryngeal carcinoma in which at least one cricoarytenoid unit is intact (**organ preservation surgery**). In addition to the late complications, clinicians have noted that the overall success in the treatment of larynx cancer has declined in parallel with the increase in organ preservation chemoradiation therapy over the past 20 years. Some experts have proposed that this decline is the direct result of the shift in management of advanced laryngeal cancer away from surgery. Organ preservation surgery should be considered and discussed as an alternative to chemoradiation but may require referral to an appropriate regional center where such techniques are offered. After thorough evaluation of candidacy and discussion of the treatment options, patient choice plays a critical role in the ultimate decision to pursue surgery or chemoradiation as a definitive treatment modality. The patient and treating clinicians must carefully consider different early and late side effects and complications associated with different treatment modalities.

The presence of malignant adenopathy in the neck affects the prognosis greatly. Supraglottic tumors metastasize early and bilaterally to the neck, and this must be included in the treatment plans even when the neck is apparently uninvolved. Glottic tumors in which the true vocal folds are mobile (T1 or T2) have less than a 5% rate of nodal involvement; when a fold is immobile, the rate of ipsilateral nodal involvement climbs to about 30%. An involved neck is treated by surgery or chemoradiation, or both. This decision will depend on the treatment chosen for the larynx and the extent of neck involvement.

Total laryngectomy is largely reserved for patients with advanced resectable tumors with extralaryngeal spread or cartilage involvement, for those with persistent tumor following chemoradiation, and for patients with recurrent or second primary tumor following previous radiation therapy. Voice rehabilitation via a primary (or at times secondary) tracheoesophageal puncture produces intelligible and serviceable speech in about 75–85% of patients. Indwelling prostheses that are changed every 3–6 months are a common alternative to patient-inserted prostheses, which need changing more frequently.

Long-term follow-up is critical in head and neck cancer patients. In addition to the 3–4% annual rate of second tumors and monitoring for recurrence, psychosocial aspects of treatment are common. Dysphagia, impaired communication, and altered appearance may result in patient difficulties adapting to the workplace and to social interactions. In addition, smoking cessation and alcohol abatement are common challenges. Nevertheless, about 65% of patients with larynx cancer are cured, most have useful speech, and many resume their prior livelihoods with adaptations.

When to Refer

- Specialty referral should be sought early for diagnosis and treatment.
- Indirect or fiberoptic examination of the nasopharynx, oropharynx, hypopharynx, and larynx by an otolaryngologist–head and neck surgeon should be considered for patients with oral erythroplakia, unexplained throat or ear pain, unexplained oral or nasal bleeding, firm neck mass, or visible oral cavity or oropharyngeal mass.

When to Admit

- Airway compromise, hemorrhage, dehydration, significant weight loss.
- To determine an effective pain management regimen for severe pain.

Hrelec C. Management of laryngeal dysplasia and early invasive cancer. Curr Treat Options Oncol. 2021;22:90. [PMID: 34424405]

VOCAL FOLD PARALYSIS

Vocal fold paralysis can result from a lesion or damage to either the vagus or recurrent laryngeal nerve. It may result in breathy dysphonia, effortful voicing, aspiration, and rarely airway compromise. Common causes of **unilateral recurrent laryngeal nerve** involvement include thyroid surgery (and occasionally thyroid cancer), other neck surgery (anterior discectomy and carotid endarterectomy), and mediastinal or apical involvement by lung cancer. Skull base tumors often involve or abut upon lower cranial nerves and may affect the vagus nerve directly, or the vagus nerve may be damaged during surgical management of the lesion. While iatrogenic injury is the most common cause of unilateral vocal fold paralysis, the second most common cause is idiopathic. However, before deciding whether the paralysis is due to iatrogenic injury or is idiopathic, the clinician must exclude other causes, such as malignancy. In the absence of other cranial neuropathies, a CT scan with contrast from the skull base to the aorto-pulmonary window (the span of the recurrent laryngeal nerve) should be performed. If other cranial nerve deficits or high vagal weakness with palate paralysis is noted, an MRI scan of the brain and brainstem is warranted.

Unilateral vocal fold paralysis is occasionally temporary and may take over a year to resolve spontaneously. Surgical management of persistent or irrecoverable symptomatic unilateral vocal fold paralysis has evolved over the last several decades. The primary goal is medialization of the paralyzed fold in order to create a stable platform for vocal fold vibration. Additional goals include advancing diet and improving pulmonary toilet by facilitating cough. Success has been reported for years with injection laryngoplasty using Teflon, Gelfoam, fat, and collagen. Once the paralysis is determined to be permanent, formal medialization thyroplasty may be performed by creating a small window in the thyroid cartilage and placing an implant between the thyroarytenoid muscle and inner table of the thyroid cartilage. This procedure moves the vocal fold medially and creates a stable platform for bilateral, symmetric mucosal vibration.

Unlike unilateral fold paralysis, **bilateral fold paralysis** usually causes inspiratory stridor with deep inspiration and may cause rapid airway compromise. If the onset of bilateral fold paralysis is insidious, it may be asymptomatic at rest, and the patient may have a normal voice. However, the acute onset of bilateral vocal fold paralysis with inspiratory stridor at rest should be managed by a specialist immediately in a critical care environment. Causes of bilateral fold paralysis include thyroid surgery, esophageal cancer, and ventricular shunt malfunction. Unilateral or bilateral fold immobility may also be seen in trauma, cricoarytenoid arthritis secondary to advanced rheumatoid arthritis, intubation injuries, glottic and subglottic stenosis, and laryngeal cancer. The goal of intervention is the creation of a safe airway with minimal reduction in voice quality and airway protection from aspiration. A number of fold lateralization procedures for bilateral paralysis have been advocated as a means of removing the tracheotomy tube.

van Lith-Bijl JT et al. Laryngeal reinnervation: the history and where we stand now. Adv Otorhinolaryngol. 2020;85:98. [PMID: 33166981]

CRICOTHYROTOMY & TRACHEOSTOMY

The three main approaches to secure an airway include endotracheal intubation, cricothyrotomy, and tracheostomy. In an acute airway emergency where the airway above the trachea is blocked (ie, due to trauma, mass, or bleeding), cricothyrotomy secures an airway more rapidly than tracheotomy, with fewer potential immediate complications (eg, pneumothorax and hemorrhage). Depending on the airway emergency, a cricothyrotomy may need to be converted to a tracheostomy after the airway has been secured.

There are two primary indications for tracheotomy: airway obstruction at or above the level of the larynx and respiratory failure requiring prolonged mechanical ventilation. Tracheotomies may be performed via an open or percutaneous approach. In experienced hands, the various methods of percutaneous tracheotomy have been documented to be safe for carefully selected patients. Simultaneous videobronchoscopy can reduce the incidence of major complications. The major cost reduction comes from avoiding the operating room. Bedside tracheotomy (in the ICU) achieves similar cost reduction and is advocated by some experts as slightly less costly than the percutaneous procedures.

The most common indication for elective tracheotomy is the need for prolonged mechanical ventilation. There is no firm rule about how many days a patient must be intubated before conversion to tracheotomy should be advised. The incidence of serious complications, such as subglottic stenosis, increases with extended endotracheal intubation. **As soon as it is apparent that the patient will require protracted ventilatory support, tracheotomy should replace the endotracheal tube.** Less frequent indications for tracheostomy are life-threatening aspiration pneumonia, the need to improve pulmonary toilet to correct problems related to insufficient clearing of tracheobronchial secretions, and obstructive sleep apnea.

Posttracheotomy care requires humidified air to prevent secretions from crusting and occluding the inner cannula of the tracheotomy tube. The tracheotomy tube should be cleaned several times daily. The most frequent early complication of tracheotomy is dislodgment of the tracheotomy tube. Surgical creation of an inferiorly based tracheal flap sutured to the inferior neck skin may make reinsertion of a dislodged tube easier. It should be recalled that the act of swallowing requires elevation of the larynx, which is limited by tracheotomy. Therefore, frequent tracheal and bronchial suctioning is often required to clear the aspirated saliva as well as the increased tracheobronchial secretions. Care of the skin around the tracheostoma is important to prevent maceration and secondary infection.

McGrath BA et al. Tracheostomy in the COVID-19 era: global and multidisciplinary guidance. Lancet Respir Med. 2020;8: 717. [PMID: 32422180]

Pandian V et al. Critical care guidance for tracheostomy care during the COVID-19 pandemic: a global, multidisciplinary approach. Am J Crit Care. 2020;29:e116. [PMID: 32929453]

FOREIGN BODIES IN THE UPPER AERODIGESTIVE TRACT

FOREIGN BODIES IN THE TRACHEA & BRONCHI

Aspiration of foreign bodies occurs much less frequently in adults than in children. Older adults and denture wearers appear to be at greatest risk. Wider familiarity with the Heimlich maneuver has reduced deaths. If the maneuver is unsuccessful, cricothyrotomy may be necessary in the acute setting.

If there is no airway compromise, plain chest radiographs may reveal a radiopaque foreign body. Detection of radiolucent foreign bodies may be aided by CT or inspiration-expiration films that demonstrate air trapping distal to the obstructed segment. Atelectasis and pneumonia may occur later. Tracheal and bronchial foreign bodies should be removed under general anesthesia with rigid or flexible bronchoscopy by a skilled endoscopist working with an experienced anesthesiologist.

FOREIGN BODIES IN THE ESOPHAGUS

Foreign bodies in the esophagus create are typically not life-threatening situations. However, the acuity may rise depending on the type of foreign body (eg, a button battery) or if the airway is compromised. **Button battery ingestion is a surgical emergency.** If there is no concern for caustic ingestion or airway compromise, there is typically time to consult an otolaryngologist for management. It is a useful diagnostic sign of complete obstruction if the patient is drooling or cannot handle secretions. Patients may often point to the exact level of the obstruction. Indirect laryngoscopy often shows pooling of saliva at the esophageal inlet. Plain films may detect radiopaque foreign bodies, such as chicken bones. Coins tend to align in the coronal plane in the esophagus and in the sagittal direction in the trachea. If a foreign body is suspected, a CT or barium swallow may also help make the diagnosis.

The treatment of an esophageal foreign body depends on identification of its cause. In children, swallowed nonfood objects are common. In adults, however, food foreign bodies are more common, and there is the greater possibility of underlying esophageal pathology. If there is nothing sharp, such as a bone, some clinicians advocate a hospitalized 24-hour observation period prior to esophagoscopy, noting that spontaneous passage of the foreign body will occur in 50% of adult patients. In the management of meat obstruction, the use of papain (meat tenderizer) should be discouraged because it can damage the esophageal mucosa and lead to stenosis or perforation. Esophageal foreign bodies that do not pass need to be removed surgically. Endoscopic removal and examination are usually best via flexible esophagoscopy or rigid laryngoscopy and esophagoscopy. Complications of penetrating or erosive esophageal foreign bodies may include mediastinitis or erosion in the trachea with associated tracheitis.

Chirica M et al. Esophageal emergencies: WSES guidelines. World J Emerg Surg. 2019;14:26. [PMID: 31164915]

DISEASES PRESENTING AS NECK MASSES

The differential diagnosis of neck masses is heavily dependent on the location in the neck, the age of the patient, and the presence of associated disease processes. Rapid growth and tenderness suggest an inflammatory process, while firm, painless, and slowly enlarging masses are often neoplastic. In young adults, most neck masses are benign (branchial cleft cyst, thyroglossal duct cyst, reactive lymphadenitis), although malignancy should always be considered (lymphoma, metastatic thyroid carcinoma). Lymphadenopathy is common in HIV-positive persons, but a growing or dominant mass may well represent lymphoma. **In adults over age 40, cancer is the most common cause of persistent neck mass and should be definitively ruled out.** A metastasis from squamous cell carcinoma arising within the mouth, pharynx, larynx, or upper esophagus should be suspected. Risk factors for squamous cell carcinoma include smoking and HPV exposure. Especially among patients younger than 30 or older than 70, lymphoma also should be considered. In all cases, a comprehensive otolaryngologic examination is needed. Imaging and pathologic evaluation of the neck mass via FNA biopsy is likely to be the next step if a primary tumor is not obvious on physical examination.

CONGENITAL LESIONS PRESENTING AS NECK MASSES IN ADULTS

1. Branchial Cleft Cysts

Branchial cleft cysts usually present as a soft cystic mass along the anterior border of the sternocleidomastoid muscle. These lesions are usually recognized in the second or third decades of life, often when they suddenly swell or become infected. To prevent recurrent infection and possible carcinoma, they should be completely excised, along with their fistulous tracts.

First branchial cleft cysts present high in the neck, sometimes just below the ear. A fistulous connection with the floor of the external auditory canal may be present. Second branchial cleft cysts, which are far more common, may communicate with the tonsillar fossa. Third branchial cleft cysts, which may communicate with the piriform sinus, are rare and present low in the neck.

2. Thyroglossal Duct Cysts

Thyroglossal duct cysts occur along the embryologic course of the thyroid's descent from the tuberculum impar of the tongue base to its usual position in the low neck. Although they may occur at any age, they are most common before age 20. They present as a midline neck mass, often just below the hyoid bone, which moves with swallowing. Surgical excision is recommended to prevent recurrent infection and rare malignancy. This requires removal of the entire fistulous tract along with the middle portion of the hyoid bone through which many of the fistulas pass. CT or ultrasound or both are often obtained preoperatively to understand associated neck anatomy, including position of the thyroid.

INFECTIOUS & INFLAMMATORY NECK MASSES

1. Reactive Cervical Lymphadenopathy

Normal lymph nodes in the neck are usually less than 1 cm in length. Infections involving the pharynx, salivary glands, and scalp often cause tender enlargement of neck nodes. Enlarged nodes are common in HIV-infected persons. Except for the occasional node that suppurates and requires incision and drainage, treatment is directed against the underlying infection. An enlarged node (larger than 1.5 cm) or node with a necrotic center that is not associated with an obvious infection should be further evaluated, especially if the patient has a history of smoking, alcohol use, or prior cancer. Other common indications for FNA biopsy of a node include its persistence or continued enlargement. Common causes of cervical adenopathy include cancer (eg, squamous cell carcinoma, lymphoma, occasional metastases from non-head and neck sites) and infection (eg, reactive nodes, mycobacteria, and cat-scratch disease). Rare causes of adenopathy include Kikuchi disease (histiocytic necrotizing lymphadenitis) and autoimmune adenopathy.

2. Tuberculous & Nontuberculous Mycobacterial Lymphadenitis

Granulomatous neck masses are uncommon in the United States unless there are specific risk factors for particular infectious exposures or granulomatous hereditary or autoimmune illness. The differential diagnosis includes mycobacterial adenitis, sarcoidosis, and cat-scratch disease due to *Bartonella henselae*. The incidence of mycobacterial lymphadenitis is on the rise both in immunocompromised and immunocompetent individuals. The usual presentation of granulomatous disease in the neck is simply single or matted nodes. Although mycobacterial adenitis can extend to the skin and drain externally (as described for atypical mycobacteria and referred to as scrofula), this late presentation is no longer common.

FNA biopsy is usually the best initial diagnostic approach: cytology, smear for acid-fast bacilli, mycobacterial culture, and a sensitivity test can all be done. PCR from FNA (or from excised tissue) is the most sensitive test and is particularly useful when conventional methods have not been diagnostic but clinical impression remains consistent for tuberculous infection. While FNA has a high sensitivity (about 88%), its specificity is low (49%); thus, an excisional biopsy is often required to confirm the diagnosis.

See Tables 9–14 and 9–15 for current recommended treatment of tuberculosis infection, which includes infection of the lymph nodes (tuberculous lymphadenopathy). For atypical (nontuberculous) infection of the lymph nodes, treatment depends on the sensitivity results of culture, but antibiotics likely to be useful include 6 months of isoniazid and rifampin and, for at least the first 2 months, ethambutol—all in standard dosages. Some would totally excise the involved nodes prior to chemotherapy, depending on location and other factors, but this can lead to chronic draining fistulas.

3. Lyme Disease

Lyme disease, caused by the spirochete *Borrelia burgdorferi* and transmitted by ticks of the *Ixodes* genus, may have protean manifestations, but over 75% of patients have symptoms involving the head and neck. Facial paralysis, hearing loss, dysesthesias, dysgeusia, or other cranial neuropathies are most common. Headache, pain, and cervical lymphadenopathy may occur. It is essential to ask patients with cranial neuropathies about risk factors for Lyme disease. See Chapter 34 for a more detailed discussion.

Zhou G et al. Antibiotic prophylaxis for prevention against Lyme disease following tick bite: an updated systematic review and meta-analysis. BMC Infect Dis. 2021;21:1141. [PMID: 34749665]

CANCER METASTASES

In older adults, 80% of firm, persistent, and enlarging neck masses are metastatic in origin. The majority of these arise from squamous cell carcinoma of the upper aerodigestive tract, such as nasopharynx, tonsils, tongue base, and larynx. A complete head and neck examination may reveal the cancer of origin, but often imaging and examination under anesthesia are necessary to detect the primary lesion. Detecting the primary lesion is essential since it may directly impact oncologic treatment modalities. Initial radiologic screening exams typically include a CT, MRI, or PET. After imaging, many patients require direct laryngoscopy, esophagoscopy, and tracheobronchoscopy to further elucidate the primary lesion. At this time, biopsies may be taken for suspicious lesions. Fine-needle aspiration of neck masses are also routine and may help determine the diagnosis while evaluation of the primary malignancy is ongoing. Open neck biopsy should only be performed by head and neck surgeons experienced in the management of head and neck cancer since complications from open biopsy may make subsequent formal neck dissections more challenging if cancer is detected. With the exception of papillary thyroid carcinoma, non–squamous cell metastases to the neck are infrequent. While cancers that are not primary in the head or neck seldom metastasize to the cervical lymph nodes, the supraclavicular lymph nodes are quite often involved by lung, gastroesophageal, and breast cancers. Infradiaphragmatic cancers, with the exception of renal cell carcinoma and testicular cancer, rarely metastasize to the neck.

Pellini R et al. Narrow band imaging in head and neck unknown primary carcinoma: a systematic review and meta-analysis. Laryngoscope. 2020;130:1692. [PMID: 31714611]

LYMPHOMA

About 10% of lymphomas present in the head and neck. Multiple rubbery nodes, especially in young adults or in patients who have AIDS, are suggestive of lymphoma. A thorough physical examination may demonstrate other sites of nodal or organ involvement. FNA biopsy may be diagnostic, but open biopsy is often required to determine architecture and an appropriate treatment course.

Cabeçadas J et al. Lymphomas of the head and neck region: an update. Virchows Arch. 2019;474:649. [PMID: 30778677]

Payabvash S et al. Differentiation of lymphomatous, metastatic, and non-malignant lymphadenopathy in the neck with quantitative diffusion-weighted imaging: systematic review and meta-analysis. Neuroradiology. 2019;61:897. [PMID: 31175398]

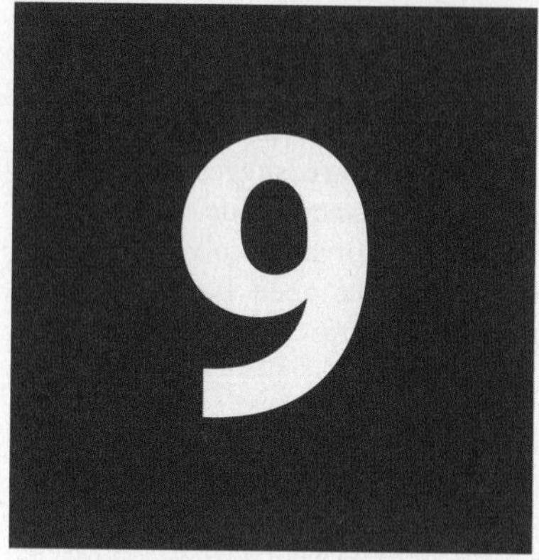

9 Pulmonary Disorders

Meghan E. Fitzpatrick, MD
Niall T. Prendergast, MD
Belinda Rivera-Lebron, MD, MS, FCCP

DISORDERS OF THE AIRWAYS

Disorders of the airways can be classified as those that involve the upper airways—loosely defined as those above and including the vocal folds—and those that involve the lower airways.

DISORDERS OF THE UPPER AIRWAYS

Acute obstruction of the upper airway can be immediately life-threatening and must be relieved promptly to avoid asphyxia. Causes of acute upper airway obstruction include trauma to the larynx or pharynx, foreign body aspiration, laryngospasm, laryngeal edema from thermal injury or angioedema, infections (acute epiglottitis, Ludwig angina, pharyngeal or retropharyngeal abscess), and acute allergic laryngitis.

Chronic obstruction of the upper airway may be caused by goiter, carcinoma of the pharynx or larynx, laryngeal or subglottic stenosis, laryngeal granulomas or webs, or bilateral vocal fold paralysis. Laryngeal or subglottic stenosis may become evident weeks or months after endotracheal intubation. Laryngomalacia refers to the collapse of the supraglottic structures during inspiration. It is the most common congenital anomaly of the larynx, manifests in infancy, and is usually resolved by 12–18 months. Inspiratory stridor, intercostal retractions on inspiration, a palpable inspiratory thrill over the larynx, and wheezing localized to the neck or trachea on auscultation are characteristic findings. Flow-volume loops may show characteristic flow limitations. Soft-tissue radiographs of the neck may show supraglottic or infraglottic narrowing. CT and MRI scans can reveal exact sites of obstruction. Flexible endoscopy may be diagnostic, but caution is necessary to avoid exacerbating upper airway edema and precipitating critical airway narrowing.

Vocal fold dysfunction syndrome, a type of inducible laryngeal obstruction, is characterized by paradoxical vocal fold adduction causing acute or chronic upper airway obstruction, or both. It presents as dyspnea and wheezing that may mimic asthma but may be distinguished from asthma or exercise-induced asthma by the lack of response to bronchodilator therapy, normal spirometry immediately after an attack, spirometric evidence of upper airway obstruction in a flow-volume loop, and a negative bronchial provocation test. However, vocal fold dysfunction may coexist with asthma, be induced by exercise, inhalational irritant exposures, laryngopharyngeal reflux of gastric contents, or psychological stress. Definitive diagnosis requires direct visualization of adduction of the vocal folds on inspiration. Treatment consists of addressing underlying precipitants (including psychogenic contributors), and speech therapy.

Eskander A et al. Acute upper airway obstruction. N Engl J Med. 2019;381:1940. [PMID: 31722154]

Petrov AA. Vocal cord dysfunction: the spectrum across the ages. Immunol Allergy Clin North Am. 2019;39:547. [PMID: 31563188]

DISORDERS OF THE LOWER AIRWAYS

Tracheal obstruction may be intrathoracic (below the suprasternal notch) or extrathoracic. Fixed tracheal obstruction may be caused by acquired or congenital tracheal stenosis, primary or secondary tracheal neoplasms, extrinsic compression (tumors of the lung, thymus, or thyroid; lymphadenopathy; congenital vascular rings; aneurysms; etc), foreign body aspiration, tracheal granulomas and papillomas, tracheal trauma, or idiopathic subglottic stenosis. Variable or dynamic tracheal obstruction may be caused by tracheomalacia, foreign body aspiration, and retained secretions.

Acquired **tracheal stenosis** is usually secondary to previous tracheotomy or endotracheal intubation. Dyspnea, cough, and inability to clear pulmonary secretions occur weeks to months after tracheal decannulation or extubation. Physical findings may be absent until tracheal diameter is reduced 50% or more, when wheezing, a palpable tracheal thrill, and harsh breath sounds may be detected. The diagnosis is usually confirmed by plain films or CT of the trachea. Complications include recurring pulmonary infection and life-threatening respiratory failure. Management is directed toward ensuring adequate ventilation and oxygenation and avoiding manipulative procedures that may increase edema of the tracheal mucosa. Surgical reconstruction, endotracheal stent placement, or laser photoresection may be required.

Bronchial obstruction may be caused by retained pulmonary secretions, aspiration, foreign bodies, bronchomalacia, bronchogenic carcinoma, compression by extrinsic masses, and tumors metastatic to the airway. Clinical and radiographic findings vary depending on the location of the obstruction and the degree of airway narrowing. Symptoms include dyspnea, cough, wheezing, and, if infection is present, fever and chills. A history of recurrent pneumonia in the same lobe or segment or slow resolution (more than 3 months) of pneumonia on successive radiographs suggests the possibility of bronchial obstruction and the need for bronchoscopy.

Radiographic findings include atelectasis (local parenchymal collapse), postobstructive infiltrates, and air trapping caused by unidirectional expiratory obstruction. CT scanning may demonstrate the nature and exact location of obstruction. Bronchoscopy is the definitive diagnostic study, particularly if tumor or foreign body aspiration is suspected. Management includes the use of bronchoscopic electrocautery, argon plasma coagulation, and laser and radiofrequency ablation.

Halvorsen T et al. Conundrums of exercise-related breathing problems. Epiglottic, laryngeal, or bronchial obstruction? Am J Respir Crit Care Med. 2020;202:e142. [PMID: 32783778]

Mahajan AK et al. Electrosurgical and laser therapy tools for the treatment of malignant central airway obstructions. Chest. 2020;157:446. [PMID: 31472155]

ASTHMA

ESSENTIALS OF DIAGNOSIS

- Episodic or chronic symptoms of wheezing, dyspnea, or cough.
- Symptoms frequently worse at night or in the early morning.
- Prolonged expiration and diffuse wheezes on physical examination.
- Limitation of airflow on pulmonary function testing (PFT) or positive bronchoprovocation challenge.
- Reversibility of airflow obstruction, either spontaneously or following bronchodilator therapy.

General Considerations

Asthma is a common disease, affecting approximately 8–10% of the population. It is slightly more common in male children (younger than 14 years) and in female adults. There is a genetic predisposition to asthma. Prevalence, hospitalizations, and fatal asthma have all increased in the United States over the past 20 years. Each year, approximately 10 million office visits, 1.8 million emergency department visits, and more than 3500 deaths in the United States are attributed to asthma. Hospitalization rates are highest among Black persons and children, and death rates are consistently highest among Black persons aged 15–24 years. The 2020 Global Initiative for Asthma (GINA) Report entitled *Global Strategy for Asthma Management and Prevention* is a comprehensive and practical resource that addresses asthma diagnosis, assessment, management, and exacerbations.

Definition & Pathogenesis

Asthma is a chronic disorder of the airways characterized by variable airway obstruction, airway hyperresponsiveness, and airway inflammation. No single histopathologic feature is pathognomonic but common findings include airway inflammatory cell infiltration with eosinophils, neutrophils, and lymphocytes (especially T cells); goblet cell hyperplasia; plugging of small airways with mucus; collagen deposition beneath the basement membrane; bronchial smooth muscle hypertrophy; airway edema; mast cell activation; and denudation of airway epithelium. The pathophysiology of asthma is heterogeneous, but a division into T2-high and T2-low endotypes (marked by high and low levels, respectively, of classic Th2 cytokines such as interleukin [IL]-4, IL-5, and IL-13) has been shown to be important regarding the selection of therapies.

Many clinical phenotypes of asthma have been identified. The most common is **allergic asthma,** which usually begins in childhood and is associated with other allergic diseases such as eczema, allergic rhinitis, or food allergy. Exposure of sensitive patients to inhaled allergens may cause symptoms immediately (immediate asthmatic response) or 4–6 hours after allergen exposure (late asthmatic response). Common allergens include house dust mites (often found in pillows, mattresses, upholstered furniture, carpets, and drapes), cockroaches, cat dander, and seasonal pollens. **Allergic asthma** falls into the T2-high endotype, as do **late-onset** T2-high asthma and **aspirin/NSAID-associated respiratory disease.** T2-low asthma phenotypes include **nonallergic asthma**, which tends to occur in adults and be marked by neutrophilic inflammation and variable response to standard therapies. **Asthma with persistent airflow limitation** is thought to be due to airway remodeling. **Asthma with obesity** refers to prominent respiratory symptoms in obese patients with little airway inflammation.

Nonspecific precipitants of asthma include upper respiratory tract infections, rhinosinusitis, postnasal drip, aspiration, gastroesophageal reflux, changes in the weather, stress, and exercise. Exposure to **products of combustion** (eg, from tobacco, methamphetamines, diesel fuel, and other agents) increases asthma symptoms and the need for medications and reduces lung function. **Air pollution** (increased air levels of respirable particles, ozone, SO_2, and NO_2) precipitates asthma symptoms and increases emergency department visits and hospitalizations. Selected individuals may experience asthma symptoms after exposure to aspirin (aspirin-exacerbated respiratory disease), NSAIDs, or tartrazine dyes. Other **medications** may precipitate asthma symptoms (see Table 9–23). **Occupational asthma** is triggered by various agents in the workplace and may occur weeks to years after initial exposure and sensitization. Women may experience **catamenial asthma** at predictable times during the menstrual cycle. **Exercise-induced bronchoconstriction** begins during exercise or within 3 minutes after its end, peaks within 10–15 minutes, and then resolves by 60 minutes. This phenomenon is thought to be a consequence of the airways' warming and humidifying an increased volume of expired air during exercise. **Cough-variant asthma** has cough instead of wheezing as the predominant symptom of bronchial hyperreactivity. Other diseases may mimic asthma; **"cardiac asthma"** is wheezing precipitated by pulmonary edema in the setting of decompensated heart failure, while **upper airway obstruction** and **paradoxical vocal fold motion** may also present with wheezing and dyspnea.

Clinical Findings

Symptoms and signs vary widely among patients as well as within individuals over time. General clinical findings in stable asthma patients and findings seen during asthma exacerbations are listed in Table 9–1.

A. Symptoms and Signs

Asthma is characterized by episodic wheezing, shortness of breath, chest tightness, and cough. Symptoms vary over time and in intensity and are often worse at night or in the early morning. Asthma symptoms may occur spontaneously or be precipitated or exacerbated by many different triggers, as discussed above. The following features decrease the likelihood that respiratory symptoms are due to asthma: isolated cough with no other symptoms, chronic sputum production, chest pain, and shortness of breath with paresthesias.

Some physical examination findings increase the probability of asthma. Nasal mucosal swelling, increased secretions, and polyps are often seen in patients with allergic asthma. Eczema, atopic dermatitis, or other allergic skin disorders may also be present. Wheezing or a prolonged expiratory phase during normal breathing correlates well with the presence of airflow obstruction; wheezing during forced expiration does not. Chest examination may be normal between exacerbations in patients with mild asthma. During severe asthma exacerbations, airflow may be too limited to produce wheezing, and the only diagnostic clue on auscultation may be globally reduced breath sounds with prolonged expiration. Hunched shoulders and use of accessory muscles of respiration suggest an increased work of breathing.

B. Laboratory Findings

Arterial blood gas (ABG) measurements may be normal during a mild asthma exacerbation, but respiratory alkalosis and an increase in the alveolar-arterial oxygen difference (A–a–Do_2) are common. During severe exacerbations, hypoxemia develops and the $Paco_2$ returns to normal. The combination of an increased $Paco_2$ and respiratory acidosis may indicate impending respiratory failure and the need for mechanical ventilation.

C. Pulmonary Function Testing

Clinicians correctly identify airflow obstruction on examination but have limited ability to gauge its severity or to predict whether it is reversible. The evaluation for asthma should therefore include **spirometry** (forced expiratory volume in 1 second [FEV_1], forced vital capacity [FVC], and FEV_1/FVC) before and after the administration of a short-acting bronchodilator. These measurements help determine the presence and extent of airflow obstruction and whether it is immediately reversible. Airflow obstruction is indicated by a reduced FEV_1/FVC ratio, generally below 0.7. Significant reversibility of airflow obstruction is defined by an increase of 12% or more and 200 mL in FEV_1 or FVC after inhaling a short-acting bronchodilator. A positive bronchodilator response supports the diagnosis of asthma, but a lack of responsiveness in the pulmonary function laboratory does not preclude success in a clinical trial of bronchodilator therapy. Severe airflow obstruction results in significant air trapping, with an increase in residual volume and consequent reduction in FVC, resulting in a pattern that may mimic a restrictive ventilatory defect.

Table 9–1. Assessing asthma control.

Components of Asthma Control	Classification of Asthma Control		
	Well Controlled	Partly Controlled	Not Controlled
Daytime asthma symptoms > 2 ×/week Nighttime awakenings due to asthma Interference with normal activity due to asthma Reliever medication needed for asthma symptoms > 2 ×/week	None of these components within past 4 weeks	1 or 2 of these components within past 4 weeks	3 or 4 of these components within past 4 weeks

Adapted from National Asthma Education and Prevention Program. Expert Panel Report 3: Guidelines for the Diagnosis and Management of Asthma. National Institutes of Health Pub. No. 08-4051. Bethesda, MD, 2007, and Global Initiative for Asthma. Global Strategy for Asthma Management and Prevention, 2019. (Available from: www.ginasthma.org.)

Bronchoprovocation testing with inhaled histamine or methacholine may be useful when asthma is suspected but spirometry is nondiagnostic. Bronchial provocation is not recommended if the FEV_1 is less than 65% of predicted. A positive methacholine test is defined as a fall in the FEV_1 of 20% or more at exposure to a methacholine concentration of less than or equal to 8 mg/mL. A negative methacholine test has a negative predictive value for asthma of 95%. Exercise challenge testing may be useful in patients with symptoms of exercise-induced bronchospasm.

Peak expiratory flow (PEF) meters are handheld devices designed as personal monitoring tools. PEF monitoring can establish peak flow variability, quantify asthma severity, and provide both patient and clinician with objective measurements on which to base treatment decisions. There are conflicting data about whether measuring PEF improves asthma outcomes but doing so is recommended to help confirm the diagnosis of asthma, to improve asthma control in patients with poor perception of airflow obstruction, and to identify environmental and occupational causes of symptoms. Predicted values for PEF vary with age, height, and sex but are poorly standardized. Comparison with reference values is less helpful than comparison with the patient's own baseline. PEF shows diurnal variation; it is generally lowest on first awakening and highest several hours before the midpoint of the waking day. PEF should be measured in the morning before the administration of a bronchodilator and in the afternoon after taking a bronchodilator. A 20% change in PEF values from morning to afternoon or from day to day suggests inadequately controlled asthma. PEF values less than 200 L/minute indicate severe airflow obstruction.

D. Additional Testing

Routine chest radiographs in patients with asthma are usually normal or show only hyperinflation. Other findings may include bronchial wall thickening and diminished peripheral lung vascular markings. Chest imaging is indicated when pneumonia, another disorder mimicking asthma, or a complication of asthma such as pneumothorax is suspected.

Skin or in vitro testing, including total serum IgE and allergen-specific IgE, to assess sensitivity to environmental allergens can identify atopy in patients with persistent asthma who may benefit from therapies directed at their allergic diathesis. Evaluations for paranasal sinus disease or gastroesophageal reflux should be considered in patients with persistent, severe, or refractory asthma symptoms. An absolute eosinophil count can identify patients eligible for anti–IL-5 therapy to manage eosinophilic airway disease.

Complications

Complications of asthma include exhaustion, dehydration, airway infection, and tussive syncope. Pneumothorax occurs but is rare. Acute hypercapnic and hypoxemic respiratory failure occurs in severe disease.

Differential Diagnosis

Patients who have atypical symptoms or poor response to therapy may have one of several conditions that mimic asthma. These disorders typically fall into upper airway disorders, lower airway disorders, systemic vasculitides, cardiac disorders, and psychiatric disorders. **Upper airway disorders** that mimic asthma include vocal fold paralysis, vocal fold dysfunction syndrome, narrowing of the supraglottic airway, and laryngeal masses or dysfunction. **Lower airway disorders** include foreign body aspiration, tracheal masses or narrowing, tracheobronchomalacia, airway edema (eg, angioedema or inhalation injury), nonasthmatic COPD (chronic bronchitis or emphysema), bronchiectasis, allergic bronchopulmonary aspergillosis (mycosis), cystic fibrosis, eosinophilic pneumonia, hypersensitivity pneumonitis, sarcoidosis, and bronchiolitis obliterans. A **systemic vasculitis** with pulmonary involvement may have an asthmatic component, such as eosinophilic granulomatosis with polyangiitis. **Cardiac disorders** include heart failure and pulmonary hypertension. **Psychiatric causes** include conversion disorders ("functional" asthma), emotional laryngeal wheezing, or episodic laryngeal dyskinesis. Rarely, Münchausen syndrome or malingering may explain a patient's complaints.

Approach to Management

The 2020 GINA Report *Global Strategy for Asthma Management and Prevention* provides guidelines for the management of asthma and identifies five important aspects of chronic asthma management: (1) assessing asthma control and severity, (2) distinguishing between severe asthma and uncontrolled asthma, (3) personalized pharmacologic therapy for asthma, (4) treatment of modifiable risk factors and control of environmental factors, and (5) guided self-management education and skills training.

1. Assessing asthma control and severity—Asthma control is assessed by evaluating symptoms, activity limitations, and risk of future exacerbations. Asthma symptoms are assessed by asking patients about their past 4 weeks including frequency of symptoms (days per week), awakening from sleep, and frequency of short-acting beta-agonist (SABA) use for relief of symptoms (Table 9–1). Future risk of exacerbations is increased by poor symptom control as well as several other risk factors: more than one exacerbation in the previous year, poor asthma medication adherence, incorrect inhaler technique, chronic sinusitis, and smoking. **Asthma severity** is evaluated retrospectively from the level of treatment needed to control symptoms and exacerbations. For example, a patient who requires Step 3 treatment to achieve control has moderate disease. Figure 9–1 describes the step therapy in a personalized asthma management plan. Typically, mild asthma responds to Step 1 or 2 treatments, moderate asthma to Step 3 treatment, and severe asthma to Step 4 or 5 treatments.

2. Uncontrolled vs severe asthma—It is important to distinguish between uncontrolled and severe asthma in patients who are using Step 4 or Step 5 treatments. The clinician must assess inhaler technique, medication adherence, comorbidities such as obstructive sleep apnea or GERD, and ongoing exposure to allergens as causes of poor

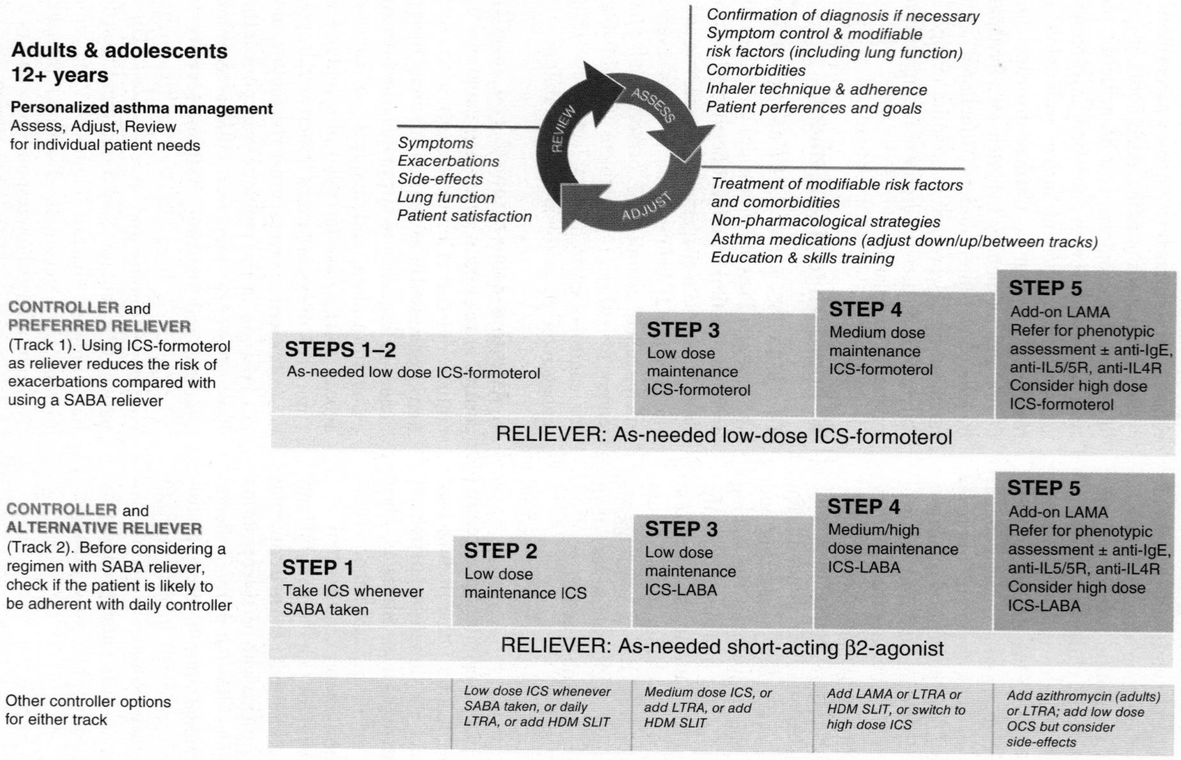

Adults & adolescents 12+ years

Personalized asthma management
Assess, Adjust, Review
for individual patient needs

REVIEW: Symptoms; Exacerbations; Side-effects; Lung function; Patient satisfaction

ASSESS: Confirmation of diagnosis if necessary; Symptom control & modifiable risk factors (including lung function); Comorbidities; Inhaler technique & adherence; Patient perferences and goals

ADJUST: Treatment of modifiable risk factors and comorbidities; Non-pharmacological strategies; Asthma medications (adjust down/up/between tracks); Education & skills training

CONTROLLER and **PREFERRED RELIEVER** (Track 1). Using ICS-formoterol as reliever reduces the risk of exacerbations compared with using a SABA reliever	**STEPS 1–2** As-needed low dose ICS-formoterol		**STEP 3** Low dose maintenance ICS-formoterol	**STEP 4** Medium dose maintenance ICS-formoterol	**STEP 5** Add-on LAMA; Refer for phenotypic assessment ± anti-IgE, anti-IL5/5R, anti-IL4R; Consider high dose ICS-formoterol
	RELIEVER: As-needed low-dose ICS-formoterol				
CONTROLLER and **ALTERNATIVE RELIEVER** (Track 2). Before considering a regimen with SABA reliever, check if the patient is likely to be adherent with daily controller	**STEP 1** Take ICS whenever SABA taken	**STEP 2** Low dose maintenance ICS	**STEP 3** Low dose maintenance ICS-LABA	**STEP 4** Medium/high dose maintenance ICS-LABA	**STEP 5** Add-on LAMA; Refer for phenotypic assessment ± anti-IgE, anti-IL5/5R, anti-IL4R; Consider high dose ICS-LABA
	RELIEVER: As-needed short-acting β2-agonist				
Other controller options for either track		*Low dose ICS whenever SABA taken, or daily LTRA, or add HDM SLIT*	*Medium dose ICS, or add LTRA, or add HDM SLIT*	*Add LAMA or LTRA or HDM SLIT, or switch to high dose ICS*	*Add azithromycin (adults) or LTRA; add low dose OCS but consider side-effects*

HDM: house dust mite; ICS: inhaled corticosteroid; LABA: long-acting beta$_2$-agonist; LAMA: long-acting muscarinic antagonist; LTRA: leukotriene receptor antagonist; OCS: oral corticosteroids; SABA: short-acting beta$_2$-agonist; SLIT: sublingual immunotherapy.

▲ **Figure 9–1. Personalized management for adults and adolescents to control symptoms and minimize future risk.** (Reproduced with permission from Global Strategy for Asthma Management and Prevention (updated 2019). Global Initiative for Asthma-GINA, 2019.)

asthma control ("uncontrolled" asthma). If the patient still requires Step 4 or 5 therapy after these issues have been addressed, then the patient has "severe" asthma and should be referred to a pulmonary or asthma specialist.

3. Pharmacotherapy for asthma—The goals of pharmacologic therapy are to minimize chronic symptoms that interfere with normal activity (including exercise), to prevent recurrent exacerbations, to reduce or eliminate the need for emergency department visits or hospitalizations, and to maintain normal or near-normal pulmonary function. Personalized asthma management is a continuous cycle that involves assessment, treatment, and review with the goals of symptom control and minimizing future risk. These goals should be met while providing therapeutic agents with the fewest adverse effects and while satisfying patients' expectations of asthma care. Management should include stepping up therapy if asthma remains uncontrolled despite adherence and good inhaler technique and stepping down to find the minimum effective therapeutic dose.

4. Treat modifiable risk factors and control environmental factors—Significant reduction in exposure to nonspecific airway irritants in all patients or to inhaled allergens in atopic patients may reduce symptoms and medication needs. Comorbid conditions that impair asthma management, such as smoking, rhinosinusitis, GERD, obesity, and obstructive sleep apnea, should be identified and treated. Nonpharmacologic interventions include increasing physical activity and breathing exercises.

5. Guided asthma self-management education and skills training—Self-management includes self-monitoring of symptoms or peak flow, a written action plan, and regular review of asthma control, treatment, and skills with a health care professional.

Treatment

A. Pharmacologic Agents

Asthma medications can be divided into three categories: (1) **long-term controller** medications (Table 9–2) used long-term to reduce airway inflammation, symptoms, and risk of future exacerbations, (2) **reliever** medications (Table 9–3) used on an as-needed basis to relieve breakthrough symptoms, and (3) **add-on therapies** for severe asthma. Figure 9–1 shows a personalized management plan for asthma to control symptoms and minimize future risk.

Most asthma medications are administered by inhalation or by oral dosing. Inhalation of an appropriate agent results in a more rapid onset of pulmonary effects as well as fewer systemic effects compared with the oral dose required to achieve the same effect on the airways. Proper inhaler technique and the use of an inhalation chamber (a "spacer") with metered-dose inhalers (MDIs) decrease oropharyngeal drug deposition and improve drug delivery to the lung. Nebulizer therapy is reserved for patients who are acutely ill and those who cannot use inhalers because of difficulties with coordination, understanding, or cooperation.

1. Inhaled corticosteroids—Inhaled corticosteroids are essential controller medications (Tables 9–3 and 9–4). Once the diagnosis of asthma is made, early initiation of inhaled corticosteroid therapy leads to a greater improvement in lung function than delayed therapy. Prescribing as-needed or daily controller inhaled corticosteroids at the start of asthma therapy conveys a message to patients that both symptom control and risk reduction are the mainstays of asthma treatment. The most important determinants of medication choice, device and dose are a patient's symptoms and risk factors, along with practical issues (such as cost and delivery mechanism). Inhaled corticosteroid dosages are classified as low-, medium-, and high-dose strengths in various published sources including GINA, but low-dose inhaled corticosteroid provides clinical benefit and is sufficient for most patients with asthma. Dosages for inhaled corticosteroids vary depending on the specific agent and delivery device (Table 9–4). For patients who require high-dose inhaled corticosteroids to achieve adequate symptom control, after 3 months of good control, the dose of inhaled corticosteroid should be decreased to the lowest dose that preserves symptom control and minimizes exacerbation risk.

Concomitant use of an MDI and an inhalation chamber coupled with mouth washing after inhaled corticosteroid use decreases systemic absorption and local side effects (cough, dysphonia, oropharyngeal candidiasis). Dry powder inhalers (DPIs) are not used with an inhalation chamber. Systemic effects (adrenal suppression, osteoporosis, skin thinning, easy bruising, and cataracts) may occur with high-dose inhaled corticosteroid therapy. Combination inhalers with an inhaled corticosteroid and a long-acting beta-2-agonist (LABA) offer convenient treatment of asthma. The GINA report recommends low-dose inhaled corticosteroid/formoterol as its preferred agent due to clinical evidence but notes that its cost and availability in different countries must be taken into consideration. Budesonide/formoterol is listed as a World Health Organization (WHO) essential medication.

2. Beta-adrenergic agonists—Beta-agonists are divided into SABAs and LABAs. SABAs (Table 9–3), including agents such as albuterol, levalbuterol, bitolterol, pirbuterol, and terbutaline, are mainstays of reliever or rescue therapy for asthma patients. There is no convincing evidence to support the use of one agent over another. All asthmatics should have immediate access to a SABA because they are the most effective bronchodilators during exacerbations and provide immediate relief of symptoms. Administration before exercise effectively prevents exercise-induced bronchoconstriction.

Inhaled SABA therapy is as effective as oral or parenteral beta-agonist therapy in relaxing airway smooth muscle and improving acute asthma and offers the advantages of rapid onset of action (less than 5 minutes) with fewer systemic side effects. Repetitive administration produces incremental bronchodilation. One or two inhalations of a

Table 9–2. Long-term controller medications for asthma.

Medication	Dosage Form	Adult Dose	Comments
Inhaled Corticosteroids (ICS)			(See Table 9–4)
Systemic Corticosteroids			(Applies to all three corticosteroids)
Methylprednisolone	2-, 4-, 6-, 8-, 16-, 32-mg tablets	40–60 mg	• Administer single dose in AM either daily or on alternate days (alternate-day therapy may produce less adrenal suppression) as needed for control. • Short courses or "bursts" as single or two divided doses for 3–10 days are effective for establishing control when initiating therapy or during a period of gradual deterioration. • There is no evidence that tapering the dose following improvement in symptom control and pulmonary function prevents relapse.
Prednisolone	5-mg tablets; 5 mg/5 mL, 15 mg/5 mL oral solution	40–60 mg	
Prednisone	1-, 2.5-, 5-, 10-, 20-, 50-mg tablets; 5 mg/mL oral solution	7.5–60 mg	
Inhaled LABA			Should not be used for symptom relief or exacerbations. Use with inhaled corticosteroids.
Formoterol	Inhalation: 20 mcg/2 mL nebulizer (DPI discontinued by FDA in United States)	20 mcg every 12 hours	• Additional doses should not be administered for at least 12 hours. • Agents should be used only with their specific inhaler and should not be taken orally. • Decreased duration of protection against EIB may occur with regular use.
Salmeterol	DPI: 50 mcg/actuation	1 blister every 12 hours	
Combined Medication			
Budesonide/formoterol	HFA MDI: 80 mcg/4.5 mcg 160 mcg/4.5 mcg	2 inhalations twice daily; dose depends on severity of asthma	• 80/4.5 mcg for asthma not controlled on low- to medium-dose ICS. • 160/4.5 mcg for asthma not controlled on medium- to high-dose ICS.
Fluticasone/salmeterol	DPI: 100 mcg/50 mcg 250 mcg/50 mcg 500 mcg/50 mcg HFA: 45 mcg/21 mcg 115 mcg/21 mcg 230 mcg/21 mcg	1 inhalation twice daily; dose depends on severity of asthma	• 100/50 mcg DPI or 45/21 mcg HFA for asthma not controlled on low- to medium-dose ICS. • 250/50 mcg DPI or 115/21 mcg HFA for asthma not controlled on medium- to high-dose ICS.
Fluticasone furoate/vilanterol	DPI: 100 mcg/25 mcg or 200 mcg/25 mcg per blister	1 puff inhaled daily	• Once-daily asthma maintenance.
Mometasone/formoterol	100 mcg/5 mcg/spray 200 mcg/5 mcg/spray	2 inhalations twice daily	
Cromolyn and Nedocromil			
Cromolyn	MDI: 0.8 mg/puff Nebulizer: 20 mg/ampule	2 puffs four times daily 1 ampule four times daily	• 4- to 6-week trial may be needed to determine maximum benefit. • Dose by MDI may be inadequate to affect hyperresponsiveness. • One dose before exercise or allergen exposure provides effective prophylaxis for 1–2 hours. Not as effective for EIB as SABA. • Once control is achieved, the frequency of dosing may be reduced.
Nedocromil	MDI: 1.75 mg/puff	2 puffs four times daily	
Inhaled Long-Acting Anticholinergic			Should not be used for symptom relief or exacerbations. Use with ICS.
Tiotropium	DPI: 18 mcg/blister	1 blister daily	

(*continued*)

Table 9–2. Long-term controller medications for asthma. (continued)

Medication	Dosage Form	Adult Dose	Comments
Leukotriene Modifiers			
Leukotriene Receptor Antagonists			
Montelukast	4- or 5-mg chewable tablet; 10-mg tablet	10 mg daily at bedtime	• Exhibits a flat dose-response curve. Doses > 10 mg will not produce a greater response in adults.
Zafirlukast	10- or 20-mg tablet	20-mg tablet twice daily	• Administration with meals decreases bioavailability; take at least 1 hour before or 2 hours after meals. • Monitor for symptoms and signs of hepatic dysfunction.
5-Lipoxygenase Inhibitor			
Zileuton	600-mg tablet	600 mg four times daily	• Monitor hepatic enzyme (ALT).
Methylxanthines			
Theophylline	Liquids, sustained-release tablets, and capsules	Starting dose: 10 mg/kg/day up to 300 mg maximum Usual maximum dose: 800 mg/day	• Adjust dose to achieve serum concentration of 5–15 mcg/mL after at least 48 hours on same dose. • Due to wide interpatient variability in theophylline metabolic clearance, routine serum theophylline level monitoring is important.
Monoclonal Antibodies			
Omalizumab	Subcutaneous injection	Dependent on pretreatment IgE level; up to 375 mg every 2 weeks	• Binds to IgE; prevents interaction with IgE receptor on mast cells and basophils. • Carries black-box warning of anaphylaxis. • Suggested IgE level 30–1500 IU/mL.
Mepolizumab	Subcutaneous injection	100 mg every 4 weeks	• Binds to IL-5; prevents interaction with receptor. • Suggested AEC ≥ 150–300/mcL (0.15–0.3 × 10^9/L).
Reslizumab	Intravenous injection	3 mg/kg every 4 weeks	• Binds to IL-5; prevents interaction with receptor. • Carries black-box warning of anaphylaxis. • Suggested AEC ≥ 400/mcL (0.4 × 10^9/L).
Benralizumab	Subcutaneous injection	30 mg every 4 weeks for 3 doses, then every 8 weeks	• Binds to IL-5 receptor; blocks receptor-ligand interaction and also causes apoptosis of basophils and eosinophils. • Suggested AEC ≥ 300/mcL (0.3 × 10^9/L).
Dupilumab	Subcutaneous injection	200 or 300 mg every 2 weeks	• Binds to IL-4Ralpha; blocks IL-4 and IL-13 signaling. • Suggested AEC ≥ 150/mcL (0.15 × 10^9/L) and/or FENO ≥ 25 ppb.

AEC, absolute eosinophil count; DPI, dry powder inhaler; EIB, exercise-induced bronchospasm; FENO, fractional exhaled nitric oxide; HFA, hydrofluoroalkane; LABA, long-acting beta-2-agonist; MDI, metered-dose inhaler; SABA, short-acting beta-2-agonist.

SABA from an MDI are usually sufficient for mild to moderate symptoms. Severe exacerbations frequently require higher doses: 6–12 puffs every 30–60 minutes of albuterol by MDI with an inhalation chamber or 2.5 mg by nebulizer provide equivalent bronchodilation. Administration by nebulization does not offer more effective delivery than MDIs used correctly but does provide higher doses. With most SABAs, the recommended dose by nebulizer for acute asthma (albuterol, 2.5 mg) is 25–30 times that delivered by a single activation of the MDI (albuterol, 0.09 mg). This difference suggests that standard dosing of inhalations from an MDI may be insufficient in the setting of an acute exacerbation. Independent of dose, nebulizer therapy may be more effective in patients who are unable to coordinate inhalation of medication from an MDI because of age, agitation, or severity of the exacerbation.

Table 9–3. Reliever medications for asthma.

Medication	Dosage Form	Adult Dose	Comments
Inhaled Short-Acting Beta-2-Agonists (SABA)			
Albuterol CFC Albuterol HFA Pirbuterol CFC Levalbuterol HFA	MDI: 90 mcg/puff, 200 puffs/canister MDI: 90 mcg/puff, 200 puffs/canister MDI: 200 mcg/puff, 400 puffs/canister MDI: 45 mcg/puff, 200 puffs/canister	2 puffs 5 minutes before exercise 2 puffs every 4–6 hours as needed 2 puffs 5 minutes before exercise 2 puffs every 4–6 hours as needed 2 puffs 5 minutes before exercise 2 puffs every 4–6 hours as needed 2 puffs 5 minutes before exercise 2 puffs every 4–6 hours as needed	• An increasing use or lack of expected effect indicates diminished control of asthma. • Not recommended for long-term daily treatment. Regular use exceeding 2 days/week for symptom control (not prevention of EIB) indicates the need to step up therapy. • Differences in potency exist, but all products are essentially comparable on a per-puff basis. • May double usual dose for mild exacerbations. • Prime the inhaler by releasing four actuations prior to use. • Periodically clean HFA activator, as drug may block/plug orifice.
Albuterol	Nebulizer solution: 0.63 mg/3 mL 1.25 mg/3 mL 2.5 mg/3 mL 5 mg/mL (0.5%)	1.25–5 mg in 3 mL of saline every 4–8 hours as needed	• May mix with budesonide inhalant suspension, cromolyn, or ipratropium nebulizer solutions. • May double dose for severe exacerbations.
Levalbuterol (R-albuterol)	Nebulizer solution: 0.31 mg/3 mL 0.63 mg/3 mL 1.25 mg/0.5 mL 1.25 mg/3 mL	0.63–1.25 mg every 8 hours as needed	• Compatible with budesonide inhalant suspension. The product is a sterile-filled, preservative-free, unit dose vial.
Anticholinergics			
Ipratropium HFA	MDI: 17 mcg/puff, 200 puffs/canister	2–3 puffs every 6 hours	• Evidence is lacking for anticholinergics producing added benefit to beta-2-agonists in long-term asthma control therapy.
	Nebulizer solution: 0.25 mg/mL (0.025%)	0.25 mg every 6 hours	
Ipratropium with albuterol	MDI: 18 mcg/puff of ipratropium bromide and 90 mcg/puff of albuterol, 200 puffs/canister	2–3 puffs every 6 hours	
	Nebulizer solution: 0.5 mg/3 mL ipratropium bromide and 2.5 mg/3 mL albuterol	3 mL every 4–6 hours	• Contains EDTA to prevent discolorations of the solution. This additive does not induce bronchospasm.
Systemic Corticosteroids			
Methylprednisolone	2-, 4-, 6-, 8-, 16-, 32-mg tablets	40–60 mg/day as single or 2 divided doses	• Short courses or "bursts" are effective for establishing control when initiating therapy or during a period of gradual deterioration. • The burst should be continued until symptoms resolve and the PEF is at least 80% of personal best. This usually requires 3–10 days but may require longer. There is no evidence that tapering the dose following improvements prevents relapse.
Prednisolone	5-mg tablets; 5 mg/5 mL, 15 mg/5 mL oral solution	40–60 mg/day as single or 2 divided doses	

(*continued*)

Table 9–3. Reliever medications for asthma. (continued)

Medication	Dosage Form	Adult Dose	Comments
Prednisone	1-, 2.5-, 5-, 10-, 20-, 50-mg tablets; 5 mg/mL oral solution	40–60 mg/day as single or 2 divided doses	
Methylprednisolone acetate	Repository injection: 40 mg/mL 80 mg/mL	240 mg intramuscularly once	• May be used in place of a short burst of oral corticosteroids in patients who are vomiting or if adherence is a problem.

CFC, chlorofluorocarbon; EIB, exercise-induced bronchospasm; HFA, hydrofluoroalkane; MDI, metered-dose inhaler; PEF, peak expiratory flow.
Adapted from National Asthma Education and Prevention Program. Expert Panel Report 3: Guidelines for the Diagnosis and Management of Asthma. National Institutes of Health Pub. No. 08-4051. Bethesda, MD, 2007.

GINA does not recommend SABA-only treatment of asthma in adults or adolescents and does not recommend scheduled daily use of SABAs. Although SABA is effective as a quick relief medication, patients who are treated with SABA alone are at increased risk for asthma-related death and urgent health care even if their symptoms are controlled. Increased use (more than one canister a month) or lack of expected effect indicates diminished asthma control and the need for additional long-term controller therapy.

LABAs provide bronchodilation for up to 12 hours after a single dose. Salmeterol and formoterol are LABAs available for asthma in the United States. In combination with an inhaled corticosteroid they are indicated for long-term prevention of asthma symptoms (including nocturnal symptoms) and for prevention of exercise-induced bronchospasm. LABAs should not be used as monotherapy because they have no anti-inflammatory effect and because monotherapy has been associated with a small but

Table 9–4. Estimated clinically comparable daily dosages for inhaled corticosteroids for adults with asthma.

Medication	Low Daily Dose	Medium Daily Dose	High Daily Dose
Beclomethasone dipropionate HFA 40 or 80 mcg/puff	80–240 mcg	> 240–480 mcg	> 480 mcg
Budesonide dipropionate DPI 90, 180, or 200 mcg/inhalation	180–400 mcg	> 400–800 mcg	> 800 mcg
Flunisolide 250 mcg/puff	500–1000 mcg	> 1000–2000 mcg	> 2000 mcg
Flunisolide HFA 80 mcg/puff	320 mcg	> 320–640 mcg	> 640 mcg
Fluticasone propionate **HFA/MDI:** 44, 110, or 220 mcg/puff **DPI:** 50, 100, or 250 mcg/inhalation	88–264 mcg 100–300 mcg	> 264–440 mcg > 300–500 mcg	> 440 mcg > 500 mcg
Mometasone furoate DPI 200 mcg/puff	200 mcg	400 mcg	> 400 mcg
Triamcinolone acetonide 75 mcg/puff	300–750 mcg	> 750–1500 mcg	> 1500 mcg

DPI, dry powder inhaler; HFA, hydrofluoroalkane; MDI, metered-dose inhaler.
Notes:
- The most important determinant of appropriate dosing is the clinician's judgment of the patient's response to therapy. Most of clinical benefit from inhaled corticosteroid therapy is seen at low doses; responsiveness varies among patients.
- Potential drug interactions: Several inhaled corticosteroids, including fluticasone, budesonide, and mometasone, are metabolized in the GI tract and liver by CYP 3A4 isoenzymes. Potent inhibitors of CYP 3A4, such as ritonavir and ketoconazole, have the potential for increasing systemic concentrations of these inhaled corticosteroids by increasing oral availability and decreasing systemic clearance. Some cases of clinically significant Cushing syndrome and secondary adrenal insufficiency have been reported.

Adapted from National Asthma Education and Prevention Program. Expert Panel Report 3: Guidelines for the Diagnosis and Management of Asthma. National Institutes of Health Pub. No. 08-4051. Bethesda, MD, 2007, and Global Initiative for Asthma. Global Strategy for Asthma Management and Prevention, 2019. (Available from: www.ginasthma.org.)

statistically significant increased risk of severe or fatal asthma attacks in two large studies. Combination inhalers containing formoterol and low-dose budesonide are the preferred option because of a large study in mild asthma that showed a 64% reduction in severe exacerbations compared with SABA-only treatment, and two large studies in mild asthma that showed noninferiority for severe exacerbations compared to low-dose inhaled corticosteroid alone.

3. Systemic corticosteroids—Systemic corticosteroids (oral prednisone or prednisolone or parenteral methylprednisolone) are most effective in achieving prompt control of asthma during acute exacerbations. Systemic corticosteroids are effective as primary treatments for patients with moderate to severe asthma exacerbations and for patients with exacerbations that do not respond promptly and completely to inhaled SABA therapy. These medications speed the resolution of airflow obstruction and reduce the rate of relapse. Delays in administering corticosteroids may result in progressive impairment. Therefore, patients with moderate to severe asthma should be prescribed oral corticosteroids so they are available for early, at-home administration. The minimal effective dose of systemic corticosteroids for asthma patients has not been identified. Outpatient prednisone "burst" therapy is 0.5–1 mg/kg/day (typically 40–60 mg) in 1–2 doses for 3–7 days. Severe exacerbations requiring hospitalization typically require 1 mg/kg of prednisone or methylprednisolone every 6–12 hours for 48 hours or until the FEV_1 (or PEF rate) returns to 50% of predicted (or 50% of baseline). The dose is then decreased to 0.5 mg/kg/day until the PEF reaches 70% of predicted or personal best. No clear advantage has been found for higher doses of corticosteroids. It may be prudent to administer corticosteroids intravenously to critically ill patients to avoid concerns about altered GI absorption.

In patients with refractory, poorly controlled asthma, systemic corticosteroids may be required for the long-term suppression of symptoms. Repeated efforts should be made to reduce the dose to the minimum needed to control symptoms. Concurrent treatment with calcium supplements and vitamin D should be initiated to prevent corticosteroid-induced bone mineral loss with long-term administration. Bone mineral density testing after 3 or more months of cumulative systemic corticosteroid exposure can guide the use of bisphosphonates for treatment of steroid-induced osteoporosis. Rapid discontinuation of systemic corticosteroids after long-term use may precipitate adrenal insufficiency.

4. Anticholinergics—Anticholinergic agents reverse vagally mediated bronchospasm but not allergen- or exercise-induced bronchospasm. They may decrease mucous gland hypersecretion. Both **short-acting muscarinic antagonists** (SAMAs) and **long-acting muscarinic antagonists** (LAMAs) are available. Ipratropium bromide, a SAMA, is less effective than SABA for relief of acute bronchospasm, but it is the inhaled drug of choice for patients with intolerance to SABA or with bronchospasm due to beta-blocker medications. Ipratropium bromide reduces the rate of hospital admissions when added to inhaled SABAs in patients with moderate to severe asthma exacerbations. Studies have shown that the addition of tiotropium to medium-dose inhaled corticosteroid and salmeterol improves lung function and reduces the frequency of asthma exacerbations.

5. Leukotriene modifiers—Leukotrienes are potent mediators that contribute to airway obstruction and asthma symptoms by contracting airway smooth muscle, increasing vascular permeability and mucous secretion, and attracting and activating airway inflammatory cells. **Zileuton** is a 5-lipoxygenase inhibitor that decreases leukotriene production, and **zafirlukast** and **montelukast** are cysteinyl leukotriene receptor antagonists. In randomized controlled trials (RCTs), these agents caused modest improvements in lung function and reductions in asthma symptoms and lessened the need for SABA rescue therapy. These agents are less effective than inhaled corticosteroid for exacerbation reduction but may be considered as alternatives in patients with asthma who are unable to take inhaled corticosteroid or who experience undesirable corticosteroid side effects.

6. Monoclonal antibody agents—Asthmatic patients who require monoclonal antibody therapies should be evaluated by either a pulmonologist or allergist experienced in their use. **Omalizumab** is a recombinant antibody that binds IgE without activating mast cells. Clinical trials in patients with moderate to severe asthma and elevated serum IgE levels have found that omalizumab, when administered subcutaneously every 2–4 weeks, reduced the need for corticosteroids. Three other IL-5 antagonist monoclonal antibodies (anti IL-5/5R) are approved for the treatment of severe asthma with peripheral blood eosinophilia that has not responded to standard treatments: **reslizumab** (administered intravenously every 4 weeks), **mepolizumab** (administered subcutaneously every 4 weeks), and **benralizumab** (administered subcutaneously every 4–8 weeks). **Dupilumab** is a monoclonal antibody (anti-IL-4Rα) that, when administered subcutaneously every 2 weeks, inhibits overactive signaling of IL-4 and IL-13.

7. Phosphodiesterase inhibitor—**Theophylline** provides mild bronchodilation in asthmatic patients. It also has anti-inflammatory and immunomodulatory properties, enhances mucociliary clearance, and strengthens diaphragmatic contractility. Sustained-release theophylline preparations are effective in controlling nocturnal symptoms and as added therapy in patients with moderate or severe persistent asthma whose symptoms are inadequately controlled by inhaled corticosteroids. Low-dose sustained-release theophylline is included as a less effective option in Step 3 treatment. Neither theophylline nor aminophylline is recommended for therapy of acute asthma exacerbations.

8. Mediator inhibitors—Cromolyn sodium and nedocromil are long-term control medications that prevent asthma symptoms and improve airway function in patients with mild persistent or exercise-induced asthma.

B. Desensitization

Immunotherapy for specific allergens may be considered in selected asthma patients who have exacerbations when exposed to allergens to which they are sensitive and when unresponsive to environmental control measures or other therapies. Studies show a reduction in asthma symptoms in patients treated with single-allergen immunotherapy. Because of the risk of immunotherapy-induced bronchoconstriction, it should be administered only in a setting where such complications can be immediately treated.

C. Vaccination

Adult patients aged 19–64 with asthma should receive the 23-valent pneumococcal polysaccharide vaccine (Pneumovax 23) and annual influenza vaccinations as well as COVID-19 vaccination. Inactive vaccines (Pneumovax) are associated with few side effects. However, the use of the intranasal live attenuated influenza vaccine may be associated with asthma exacerbations in young children.

Treatment of Asthma Exacerbations

GINA asthma treatment algorithms begin with an assessment of the severity of a patient's baseline asthma. Adjustments to that algorithm follow a stepwise approach based on a careful assessment of asthma control. Educating patients to recognize symptoms of an exacerbation and to use their action plan are important aspects of asthma management. Symptoms of exacerbations include progressive breathlessness, increasing chest tightness, decreased peak flow, and lack of improvement after SABA therapy (Table 9–5). Most instances of uncontrolled asthma are mild and can be managed successfully by patients at home with self-management plans. More severe exacerbations require evaluation and management in a primary care office (Figure 9–2) or emergency department setting (Figure 9–3).

A. Mild to Moderate Exacerbations

Mild asthma exacerbations are characterized by only minor changes in airway function (PEF greater than 60% of best) with minimal symptoms and signs of airway dysfunction. Many such patients respond quickly and fully to an inhaled SABA alone. However, an inhaled SABA may need to be continued at increased doses, eg, every 3–4 hours for 24–48 hours. Patients may also require a short-term increase in inhaled corticosteroid to four times the usual dose. In patients not improving after 48 hours, a 5- to 7-day course

Table 9–5. Evaluation and classification of severity of asthma exacerbations.

	Mild	Moderate	Severe	Respiratory Arrest Imminent
Symptoms				
Breathlessness	While walking	At rest, limits activity	At rest, interferes with conversation	While at rest, mute
Talks in	Sentences	Phrases	Words	Silent
Alertness	May be agitated	Usually agitated	Usually agitated	Drowsy or confused
Signs				
Respiratory rate	Increased	Increased	Often > 30/minute	> 30/minute
Body position	Can lie down	Prefers sitting	Sits upright	Unable to recline
Use of accessory muscles, suprasternal retractions	Usually not	Commonly	Usually	Paradoxical thoracoabdominal movement
Wheezing	Moderate, often only end expiratory	Loud; throughout exhalation	Usually loud; throughout inhalation and exhalation	Absent
Pulse/minute	< 100	100–120	> 120	Bradycardia
Pulsus paradoxus	Absent < 10 mm Hg	May be present 10–25 mm Hg	Often present > 25 mm Hg	Absence suggests respiratory muscle fatigue
Functional Assessment				
PEF or FEV_1 % predicted or % personal best	≥ 70%	40–69%	< 40%	< 25%
Pao_2 (on air, mm Hg)	Normal[1]	≥ 60[1]	< 60: possible cyanosis	< 60: possible cyanosis
Pco_2 (mm Hg)	< 42[1]	< 42[1]	≥ 42[1]	≥ 42[1]
Sao_2 (on air)	> 95%[1]	90–95%[1]	< 90%[1]	< 90%[1]

[1]Test not usually necessary.
FEV_1, forced expiratory volume in 1 second; PEF, peak expiratory flow; Sao_2, oxygen saturation.
Adapted from National Asthma Education and Prevention Program. Expert Panel Report 3: Guidelines for the Diagnosis and Management of Asthma. National Institutes of Health Pub. No. 08-4051. Bethesda, MD, 2007.

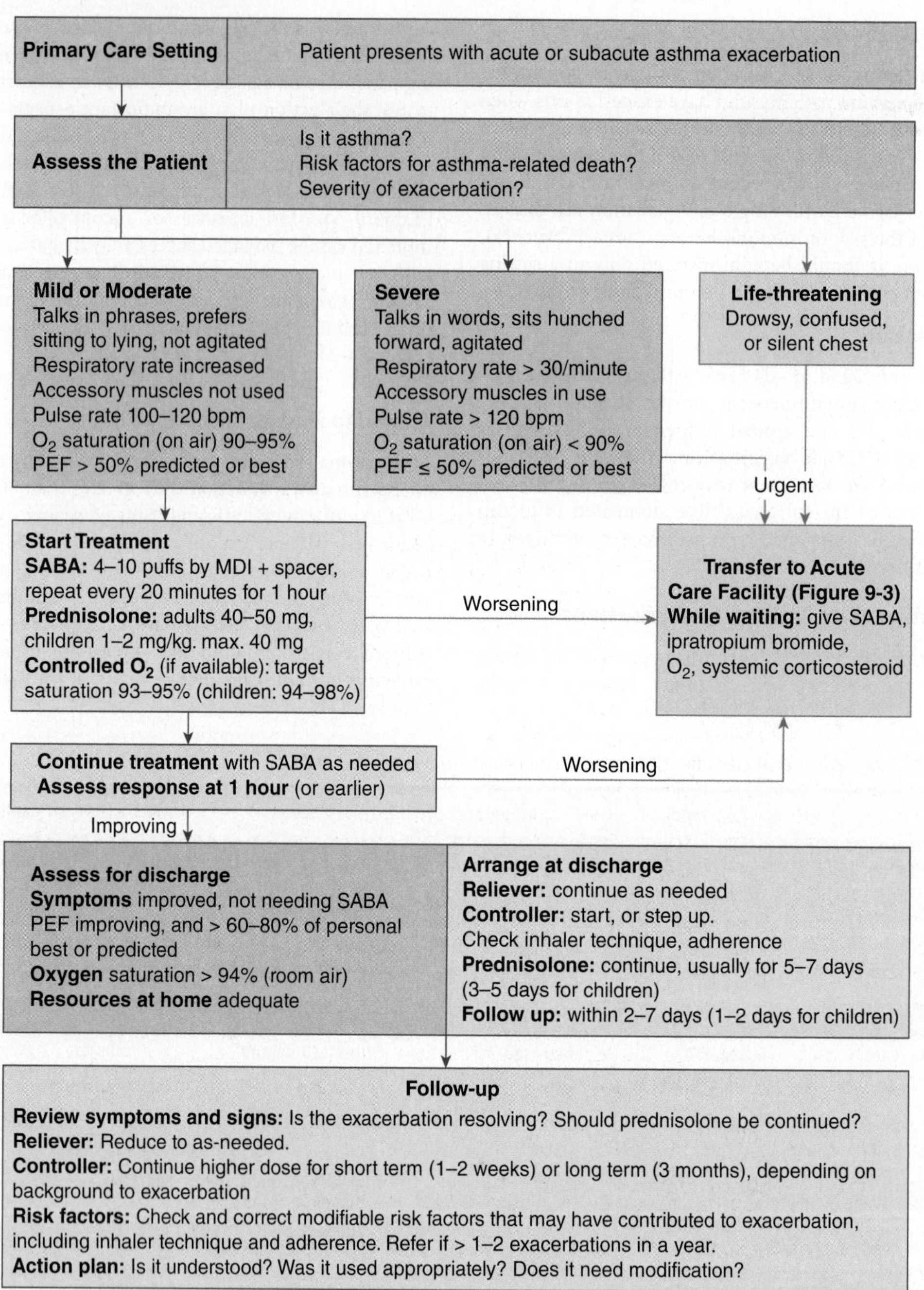

▲ **Figure 9–2.** Management of asthma exacerbations in primary care. O_2, oxygen; PEF, peak expiratory flow; SABA, short-acting beta-2-agonist (doses are for salbutamol). (Reproduced with permission from Global Strategy for Asthma Management and Prevention (updated 2019). Global Initiative for Asthma-GINA, 2019.)

of oral corticosteroids (eg, prednisone 0.5–1.0 mg/kg/day) may be necessary.

The principal goals for treating moderate asthma exacerbations are correcting hypoxemia, reversing airflow obstruction, and reducing the likelihood of obstruction recurrence. Early intervention may lessen the severity and shorten the duration of an exacerbation. Airflow obstruction is treated with continuous administration of an **inhaled SABA** and the early administration of **systemic corticosteroids.** Systemic corticosteroids should be given to patients who have a peak flow less than 70% of baseline or who do not respond to several treatments of SABA. Serial measurements of lung function to quantify the severity of airflow obstruction and its response to treatment are useful. The improvement in FEV_1 after 30–60 minutes of treatment correlates significantly with the severity of the

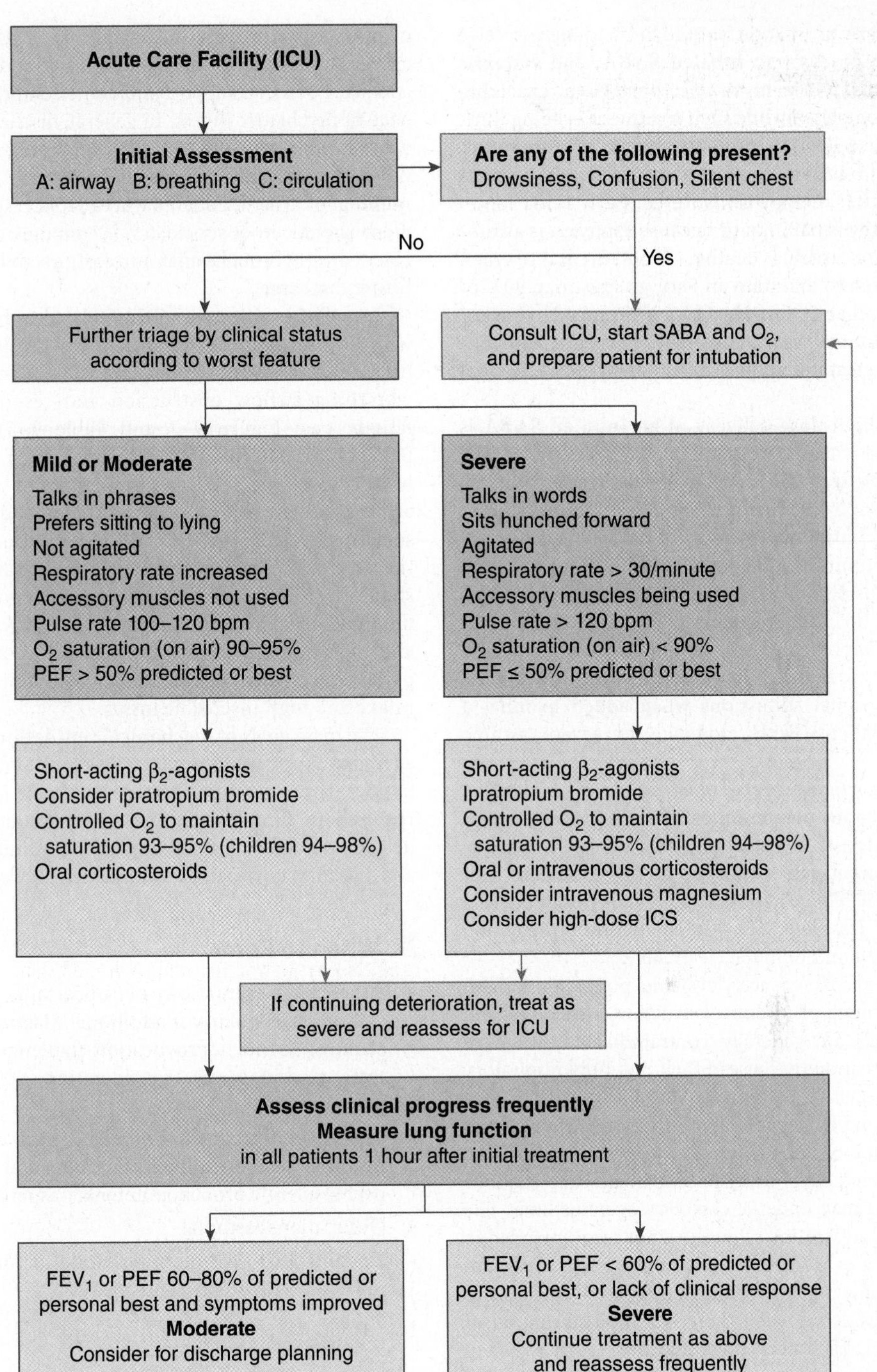

▲ **Figure 9–3.** Management of asthma exacerbations in acute care facility (eg, emergency department). FEV_1, forced expiratory volume in 1 second; ICS, inhaled corticosteroids; O_2, oxygen; PEF, peak expiratory flow; SABA, short-acting beta-2-agonist. (Reproduced with permission from Global Strategy for Asthma Management and Prevention (updated 2019). Global Initiative for Asthma-GINA, 2019.)

asthma exacerbation. Serial measurement of airflow in the emergency department may reduce the rate of hospital admissions for asthma exacerbations. Post-exacerbation care planning is important. All patients, regardless of severity, should be provided with (1) necessary medications and how to use them, (2) instruction in self-assessment, (3) a follow-up appointment, and (4) an action plan for managing recurrence.

B. Severe Exacerbations

Severe exacerbations of asthma can be life-threatening, so treatment should be started immediately. All patients with a severe exacerbation should immediately receive **oxygen,** high doses of an **inhaled SABA,** and **systemic corticosteroids.** A brief history pertinent to the exacerbation can be completed while such treatment is being initiated. More detailed assessments, including laboratory studies, usually add little early on and so should be postponed until after therapy is instituted. Early initiation of **oxygen therapy** is paramount because asphyxia is a common cause of asthma deaths. Supplemental oxygen should be given to maintain an Sao_2 greater than 90% or a Pao_2 greater than 60 mm Hg. Oxygen-induced hypoventilation is extremely rare in asthmatic patients, and concern for hypercapnia should never delay correction of hypoxemia.

Frequent high-dose delivery of an **inhaled SABA** is indicated and usually well tolerated in severe airway obstruction. At least three MDI or nebulizer treatments should be given in the first hour of therapy. Some studies suggest that continuous therapy is more effective than intermittent administration of these agents, but there is no clear consensus as long as similar doses are administered. After the first hour, the frequency of administration varies according to improvements in airflow and symptoms and occurrence of side effects. **Ipratropium bromide** reduces the rate of hospital admissions when added to inhaled SABAs in patients with moderate to severe asthma exacerbations.

Systemic corticosteroids are administered as detailed above. **Intravenous magnesium sulfate** (2 g intravenously over 20 minutes) is not recommended for routine use in asthma exacerbations. However, a 2 g infusion over 20 minutes may reduce hospitalization rates in acute severe asthma (FEV_1 less than 25% of predicted on presentation or failure to respond to initial treatment).

Mucolytic agents (eg, acetylcysteine, potassium iodide) may worsen cough or airflow obstruction. Anxiolytic and hypnotic drugs are generally contraindicated in severe asthma exacerbations because of their potential respiratory depressant effects.

Multiple studies suggest that infections with viruses (rhinovirus) and bacteria (*Mycoplasma pneumoniae, Chlamydophila pneumoniae*) predispose to acute exacerbations of asthma and may underlie chronic, severe asthma. The use of empiric antibiotics is, however, not recommended in routine asthma exacerbations since there is no consistent evidence to show improved clinical outcomes. **Antibiotics** should be considered when there is a high likelihood of acute bacterial respiratory tract infection, such as when patients have fever or purulent sputum and evidence of pneumonia or bacterial sinusitis.

In the **emergency department setting,** repeat assessment of patients with severe exacerbations should be done after the initial dose of an inhaled SABA and again after 3 doses of an inhaled SABA (60–90 minutes after initiating treatment). The response to initial treatment is a better predictor of the need for hospitalization than is the severity of the exacerbation on presentation. The decision to hospitalize a patient should be based on the duration and severity of symptoms, severity of airflow obstruction, ABG results (if available), course and severity of prior exacerbations, medication use at the time of the exacerbation, access to medical care and medications, adequacy of social support and home conditions, and presence of psychiatric illness. In general, discharge to home is appropriate if the PEF or FEV_1 has returned to 60% or more of predicted or personal best and if symptoms are minimal or absent. Patients with a rapid response to treatment should be observed for 30 minutes after the most recent dose of bronchodilator to ensure stability of response before discharge.

In the **intensive care setting,** a small subset of patients will not respond to treatment and will progress to impending respiratory failure due to a combination of worsening airflow obstruction and respiratory muscle fatigue (see Figure 9–3 and Table 9–5). Since such patients can deteriorate rapidly, they must be monitored in a critical care setting. Intubation of an acutely ill asthma patient is technically difficult and is best done semi-electively before the crisis of a respiratory arrest. At the time of intubation, the patient's intravascular volume should be closely monitored because hypotension commonly follows the administration of sedative medications and the initiation of positive-pressure ventilation; these patients are often dehydrated due to poor recent oral intake and high insensible losses.

The main goals of **mechanical ventilation** are to ensure adequate oxygenation and to avoid barotrauma. Controlled hypoventilation with permissive hypercapnia is often required to limit airway pressures. Frequent high-dose delivery of inhaled SABAs should be continued along with anti-inflammatory agents as discussed above.

When to Refer

- Atypical presentation or uncertain diagnosis of asthma, particularly if additional diagnostic testing is required (bronchoprovocation challenge, allergy skin testing, rhinoscopy, consideration of occupational exposure).
- Complicating comorbid problems, such as rhinosinusitis, tobacco use, multiple environmental allergies, suspected allergic bronchopulmonary aspergillosis.
- Occupational asthma.
- Uncontrolled symptoms despite a moderate-dose inhaled corticosteroid and a LABA.
- Patient not meeting goals of asthma therapy after 3–6 months of treatment.
- Frequent asthma-related health care utilization.
- More than two courses of oral corticosteroid therapy in the past 12 months.
- Any life-threatening asthma exacerbation or exacerbation requiring hospitalization in the past 12 months.
- Presence of social or psychological issues interfering with asthma management.

Agache I et al. EAACI Biologicals Guidelines—recommendations for severe asthma. Allergy. 2021;76:14. [PMID: 32484954]

Bleecker ER et al. Systematic literature review of systemic corticosteroid use for asthma management. Am J Respir Crit Care Med. 2020;201:276. [PMID: 31525297]

Global Initiative for Asthma. Global Strategy for Asthma Management and Prevention, 2021. https://ginasthma.org/

Menzies-Gow A et al. Difficult-to-control asthma management in adults. J Allergy Clin Immunol Pract. 22022;10:378. [PMID: 34954122]

CHRONIC OBSTRUCTIVE PULMONARY DISEASE

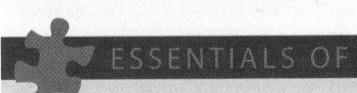

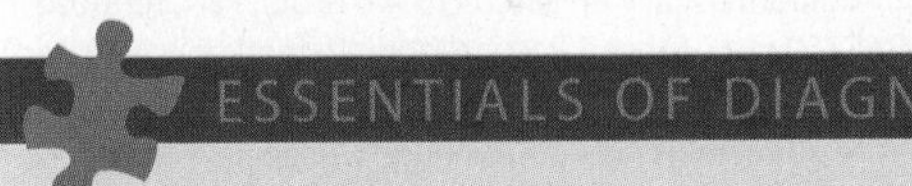

- History of cigarette smoking or other chronic inhalational exposure.
- Chronic cough, dyspnea, and sputum production.
- Rhonchi, decreased intensity of breath sounds, and prolonged expiration on physical examination.
- Airflow limitation on PFT that is not fully reversible and is most often progressive.

General Considerations

The Global Initiative for Chronic Obstructive Lung Disease (GOLD) defines COPD as a common, preventable, and treatable disease state characterized by persistent respiratory symptoms and airflow limitation due to airway and alveolar abnormalities usually caused by significant exposure to noxious particles or gases. The term "COPD" has evolved from an umbrella term for chronic bronchitis and emphysema to one that refers to a clinical syndrome of chronic respiratory symptoms, structural pulmonary abnormalities (airways or alveoli), and impaired lung function arising from multiple causes that result in airflow limitation that is not fully reversible. Symptoms include cough, dyspnea, and sputum production. COPD is a major cause of chronic morbidity and is the third leading cause of death worldwide.

The most important causes of COPD are cigarette smoking in the developed world and biomass fuel cooking in the developing world. Most smokers suffer an accelerated decline in lung function that is dose- and duration-dependent. One major study of active smokers reported yearly decreases in FEV_1 of 66 mL per year in men and 54 mL per year in women compared to 30 mL per year in men and 22 mL per year in women who sustained smoking cessation. Fifteen percent of smokers develop progressively disabling symptoms in their 40s and 50s. Approximately two-thirds of patients seen for COPD have significant exposure to tobacco smoke. The remaining one-third may have a combination of exposures to environmental tobacco smoke, occupational dusts and chemicals, and indoor air pollution from biomass fuel used for cooking and heating in poorly ventilated buildings. Outdoor air pollution, airway infection, environmental factors, and allergy have also been implicated, along with hereditary factors (most notably, deficiency of alpha-1-antitrypsin [alpha-1-antiprotease]). Atopy and bronchoconstriction in response to nonspecific airway stimuli may be important risk factors. There is evidence that lung exposures to pollution and allergens early in life can lead to poor lung growth in childhood and expiratory airflow limitation, resulting in lower than predicted spirometric values in midlife.

Clinical Findings

A. Symptoms and Signs

Patients with COPD characteristically present in the fifth or sixth decade of life complaining of excessive cough, sputum production, or shortness of breath, or a combination thereof. Symptoms have often been present for 10 years or more, yet if diagnosed early, smoking cessation can reduce the decline in lung function. Dyspnea is noted initially only on heavy exertion, but as the condition progresses it occurs with mild activity. In severe disease, dyspnea occurs at rest. As the disease progresses, two symptom patterns tend to emerge, historically referred to as "pink puffers" and "blue bloaters" (Table 9–6). Most COPD patients have features of both disorders, and their clinical course and severity may involve other factors, such as central control of ventilation and concomitant sleep-disordered breathing.

A hallmark of COPD is the acute exacerbation of symptoms beyond normal day-to-day variation, often including increased dyspnea, an increased frequency or severity of cough, and increased sputum volume or change in sputum character. These exacerbations are commonly precipitated by infection (more often viral than bacterial) or environmental factors. Pneumonia, pulmonary hypertension, right-sided heart failure, and chronic respiratory failure characterize the late stage of COPD.

B. Laboratory Findings

Spirometry provides objective information about pulmonary function and assesses the response to therapy. PFTs early in the course of COPD may reveal only abnormal closing volume and reduced mid-expiratory flow rates. Reductions in FEV_1 and in the ratio of FEV_1 to vital capacity (FEV_1% or FEV_1/FVC ratio) establish the presence of airflow obstruction. In severe disease, the FVC is markedly reduced. Lung volume measurements reveal an increase in residual volume (RV) and in total lung capacity (TLC), and an elevation of the RV/TLC ratio, indicative of air trapping, particularly common in patients with emphysema. In the setting of airflow obstruction, a reduction in the single-breath diffusing capacity for carbon monoxide (DLCO) predicts emphysema. A severely reduced DLCO predicts exertional oxyhemoglobin desaturation and is associated with coexisting pulmonary hypertension. A 6-minute walking distance of less than 350 m is associated with increased mortality.

ABG measurement characteristically shows no abnormalities early in COPD other than an increased A–a–DO_2.

Table 9–6. Patterns of disease in advanced COPD.

	Type A: Pink Puffer (Emphysema Predominant)	Type B: Blue Bloater (Bronchitis Predominant)
History and physical examination	Major complaint is dyspnea, often severe, usually presenting after age 50. Cough is rare, with scant clear, mucoid sputum. Patients are thin, with recent weight loss common. They appear uncomfortable, with evident use of accessory muscles of respiration. Chest is very quiet without adventitious sounds. No peripheral edema.	Major complaint is chronic cough, productive of mucopurulent sputum, with frequent exacerbations due to chest infections. Often presents in late 30s and 40s. Dyspnea usually mild, though patients may note limitations to exercise. Patients frequently overweight and cyanotic but seem comfortable at rest. Peripheral edema is common. Chest is noisy, with rhonchi invariably present; wheezes are common.
Laboratory studies	Hemoglobin usually normal (12–15 g/dL). Pao_2 normal to slightly reduced (65–75 mm Hg) but Sao_2 normal at rest. $Paco_2$ normal to slightly reduced (35–40 mm Hg). Chest radiograph shows hyperinflation with flattened diaphragms. Vascular markings are diminished, particularly at the apices.	Hemoglobin usually elevated (15–18 g/dL). Pao_2 reduced (45–60 mm Hg) and $Paco_2$ slightly to markedly elevated (50–60 mm Hg). Chest radiograph shows increased interstitial markings ("dirty lungs"), especially at bases. Diaphragms are not flattened.
Pulmonary function tests	Airflow obstruction ubiquitous. TLC increased, sometimes markedly so. DLCO reduced. Static lung compliance increased.	Airflow obstruction ubiquitous. TLC generally normal but may be slightly increased. DLCO normal. Static lung compliance normal.
Special Evaluations		
Ventilation-perfusion testing	Increased ventilation to high $\dot{V}/\dot{Q}$ areas, ie, high dead space ventilation.	Increased perfusion to low $\dot{V}/\dot{Q}$ areas.
Hemodynamics	Cardiac output normal to slightly low. Pulmonary artery pressures mildly elevated and increase with exercise.	Cardiac output normal. Pulmonary artery pressures elevated, sometimes markedly so, and worsen with exercise.
Nocturnal ventilation	Mild to moderate degree of oxygen desaturation not usually associated with obstructive sleep apnea.	Severe oxygen desaturation, frequently associated with obstructive sleep apnea.
Exercise ventilation	Increased minute ventilation for level of oxygen consumption; Pao_2 tends to fall; $Paco_2$ rises slightly.	Decreased minute ventilation for level of oxygen consumption. Pao_2 may rise; $Paco_2$ may rise significantly.

DLCO, single-breath diffusing capacity for carbon monoxide; TLC, total lung capacity; $\dot{V}/\dot{Q}$, ventilation-perfusion.

Indeed, ABG measurement is unnecessary unless (1) hypoxemia or hypercapnia is suspected, (2) the FEV_1 or DLCO is less than 40% of predicted, or (3) there are clinical signs of right heart failure. Hypoxemia occurs in advanced disease, particularly when chronic bronchitis predominates. Compensated respiratory acidosis occurs in patients with chronic respiratory failure, particularly in chronic bronchitis, with worsening of acidemia during acute exacerbations.

Positive sputum cultures are poorly correlated with acute exacerbations, and research techniques demonstrate evidence of preceding viral infection in most patients with exacerbations. The ECG may show sinus tachycardia, and in advanced disease, chronic pulmonary hypertension may produce electrocardiographic abnormalities typical of right-sided heart failure. Supraventricular arrhythmias (multifocal atrial tachycardia, atrial flutter, and atrial fibrillation) and ventricular irritability also occur.

C. Imaging

Radiographs of patients with chronic bronchitis typically show only nonspecific peribronchial and perivascular markings. Plain radiographs are insensitive for the diagnosis of emphysema; they show hyperinflation with flattening of the diaphragm or peripheral arterial deficiency in about half of cases. CT of the chest identifies and can quantify the emphysema phenotype associated with loss of tissue. Chest CT also detects airway narrowing and wall thickening characteristic of the bronchitic phenotype. In advanced disease, pulmonary hypertension may be suggested by enlargement of central pulmonary arteries on chest radiographs or chest CTs, and Doppler echocardiography provides an estimate of pulmonary artery pressure.

Differential Diagnosis

Clinical, imaging, and laboratory findings should enable the clinician to distinguish COPD from other obstructive pulmonary disorders, such as asthma, bronchiectasis, cystic fibrosis, bronchopulmonary aspergillosis, and central airflow obstruction. Asthma is characterized by complete or near-complete reversibility of airflow obstruction. Bronchiectasis is distinguished from COPD by recurrent pneumonia and hemoptysis, digital clubbing, and characteristic imaging abnormalities. Cystic fibrosis occurs in children, adolescents, and young adults and has characteristic imaging as well as endocrine and hepatic abnormalities. Bronchopulmonary aspergillosis is characterized by eosinophilia; elevated levels of immunoglobulin E; and episodic worsening marked by fever, malaise, productive cough, and radiographic infiltrates. Mechanical obstruction of the central airways can be distinguished from COPD by flow-volume loops.

Complications

Acute bronchitis, pneumonia, pulmonary thromboembolism, atrial dysrhythmias (such as atrial fibrillation, atrial flutter, and multifocal atrial tachycardia), and concomitant LV failure may worsen otherwise stable COPD. Pulmonary hypertension, right-sided heart failure, and chronic respiratory failure are common in advanced COPD. Spontaneous pneumothorax occurs in a small fraction of patients with emphysema. Hemoptysis may result from chronic bronchitis or may signal bronchogenic carcinoma.

Prevention

COPD is largely preventable by eliminating long-term exposure to tobacco smoke, products of biomass fuels combustion, or other inhaled toxins. Smokers with early evidence of airflow limitation can significantly alter the course of their disease by smoking cessation. Influenza vaccination reduces the frequency and severity of influenza-like illness as well as the number of COPD exacerbations. Pneumococcal vaccination appears to reduce both the frequency of community-acquired pneumonia and the number of COPD exacerbations. COVID-19 vaccination reduces mortality.

Treatment

The treatment of COPD is guided by the severity of symptoms or the presence of an exacerbation of stable symptoms. Standards for the management of patients with stable COPD and COPD exacerbations from the American Thoracic Society and GOLD, a joint expert committee of the National Heart, Lung, and Blood Institute and the WHO, are incorporated in the recommendations below. There are three commonly used ways to identify high-risk COPD patients who may require more intense treatment: (1) FEV_1 less than 50% predicted, (2) more than two exacerbations in the previous year, and (3) one or more hospitalizations for COPD exacerbation in the previous year.

A. Ambulatory Patients

1. Smoking cessation—The single most important intervention in smokers with COPD is to facilitate smoking cessation (see Chapter 1). Simply telling a patient to quit succeeds 5% of the time. Behavioral approaches, ranging from clinician advice to intensive group programs, may improve cessation rates. Pharmacologic therapy includes bupropion, nicotine replacement (transdermal patch, gum, lozenge, inhaler, or nasal spray), and varenicline (a partial agonist of nicotinic acetylcholine receptors). Combined pharmacotherapies (two forms of nicotine replacement, or nicotine replacement and bupropion), with or without behavioral approaches, have been recommended. Varenicline is effective but use has been limited by concerns about neuropsychiatric side effects. Electronic cigarettes are not recommended as a smoking cessation aid, due in part to concern for e-cigarette and vaping-associated lung injury (EVALI) (see below).

2. Oxygen therapy—Supplemental oxygen for patients with resting hypoxemia (Pao_2 < 56 mm Hg) is the only therapy with evidence of improvement in the natural history of COPD. Proven benefits of home oxygen therapy in hypoxemic patients include longer survival, reduced hospitalizations, and better quality of life. Survival in hypoxemic patients with COPD treated with supplemental oxygen therapy is directly proportional to the number of hours per day oxygen is administered: in hypoxemic COPD patients treated with continuous oxygen for 24 hours daily, the survival after 36 months is about 65%—significantly better than the survival rate of about 45% in those treated with only nocturnal oxygen. Oxygen by nasal prongs must be given for at least 15 hours a day unless therapy is specifically intended only for exercise or sleep. However, several studies of supplemental oxygen therapy showed no survival benefit in COPD patients with borderline low-normal resting oxygen levels (Pao_2 56–69 mm Hg). In a study of patients with stable COPD and resting or exercise-induced moderate desaturation, the prescription of long-term supplemental oxygen did not result in a longer time to first hospitalization or death than no long-term supplemental oxygen, nor did it provide sustained benefit in any other measured outcomes. Requirements for US Medicare coverage for a patient's home use of oxygen and oxygen equipment are listed in Table 9–7. ABG analysis is preferred over oximetry to guide initial oxygen therapy. Hypoxemic patients with pulmonary hypertension, chronic right-sided heart failure, erythrocytosis, impaired cognitive function, exercise intolerance, nocturnal restlessness, or morning headache are particularly likely to benefit from home oxygen therapy.

Table 9–7. Home oxygen therapy: requirements for Medicare coverage.[1]

Group I (any of the following):

1. $Pao_2 \leq 55$ mm Hg or $Sao_2 \leq 88\%$ taken while awake, at rest, breathing room air.
2. During sleep (prescription for nocturnal oxygen use only): $Pao_2 \leq 55$ mm Hg or $Sao_2 \leq 88\%$ for a patient whose awake, resting, room air Pao_2 is ≥ 56 mm Hg or $Sao_2 \geq 89\%$, *or* Decrease in Pao_2 > 10 mm Hg or decrease in Sao_2 > 5% associated with symptoms or signs reasonably attributed to hypoxemia (eg, impaired cognitive processes, nocturnal restlessness, insomnia).
3. During exercise (prescription for oxygen use only during exercise): $Pao_2 \leq 55$ mg Hg or $Sao_2 \leq 88\%$ taken during exercise for a patient whose awake, resting, room air Pao_2 is ≥ 56 mm Hg or $Sao_2 \geq 89\%$, *and* there is evidence that the use of supplemental oxygen during exercise improves the hypoxemia that was demonstrated during exercise while breathing room air.

Group II[2]:

Pao_2 = 56–59 mm Hg or Sao_2 = 89% if there is evidence of any of the following:

1. Dependent edema suggesting heart failure.
2. P pulmonale on ECG (P wave > 3 mm in standard leads II, III, or aVF).
3. Hematocrit > 56%.

[1]Centers for Medicare & Medicaid Services, 2003.
[2]Patients in this group must have a second oxygen test 3 months after the initial oxygen setup.

Home oxygen may be supplied by liquid oxygen systems, compressed gas cylinders, or oxygen concentrators. Most patients benefit from having both stationary and portable systems. For most patients, a flow rate of 1–3 L/minute achieves a Pao_2 greater than 55 mm Hg. Reservoir nasal cannulas or "pendants" and demand (pulse) oxygen delivery systems are available to conserve oxygen.

3. Inhaled bronchodilators—Bronchodilators do not alter the inexorable decline in lung function that is a hallmark of COPD, but they improve symptoms, exercise tolerance, FEV_1, and overall health status. Aggressiveness of bronchodilator therapy should be matched to the severity of the patient's disease. In patients who experience no symptomatic improvement, bronchodilators should be discontinued.

The most commonly prescribed short-acting bronchodilators are the SAMA **ipratropium bromide** and the SABAs (eg, albuterol/salbutamol), delivered by MDI or as an inhalation solution by nebulizer. Some clinicians prefer ipratropium as a first-line agent because of its longer duration of action and absence of sympathomimetic side effects. Some studies have suggested that ipratropium achieves superior bronchodilation in COPD patients. Typical doses are 2–4 puffs (36–72 mcg) every 6 hours. Other clinicians prefer SABAs because they are less expensive and have a more rapid onset of action, commonly leading to greater patient satisfaction. At maximal doses, beta-2-agonists have bronchodilator action equivalent to that of ipratropium but may cause tachycardia, tremor, or hypokalemia. There does not appear to be any advantage of scheduled use of SABAs compared with as-needed administration. There has been no consistent difference in efficacy demonstrated between SABAs and SAMAs. Using the SABAs and the SAMAs at submaximal doses leads to improved bronchodilation compared with either agent alone but does not improve dyspnea.

LAMAs (eg, **tiotropium, aclidinium, umeclidinium, glycopyrrolate**) and LABAs (eg, **formoterol, salmeterol, indacaterol, arformoterol, vilanterol, olodaterol**) appear to achieve bronchodilation that is equivalent or superior to what is experienced with ipratropium, in addition to similar improvements in health status. Although more expensive than short-acting agents, long-acting bronchodilators may have superior clinical efficacy in persons with advanced disease. One RCT of long-term administration of **tiotropium** added to standard therapy reported fewer exacerbations or hospitalizations and improved dyspnea scores—but no long-term effect on lung function—in the tiotropium group. Another RCT comparing the effects of tiotropium with those of salmeterol-fluticasone over 2 years reported no difference in the risk of COPD exacerbation. The incidence of pneumonia was higher in the salmeterol-fluticasone group, yet dyspnea scores were lower and there was a mortality benefit compared with tiotropium. The combination of tiotropium and formoterol (LAMA/LABA) has been shown to improve FEV_1 and FVC more than the inhaled corticosteroid/LABA combination salmeterol and fluticasone in patients with a baseline FEV_1 of less than 55% predicted. The initial drug of choice for patients with mild disease and no exacerbations is a LAMA. If the patient has more severe dyspnea and airflow obstruction, LAMA/LABA can be initiated.

The symptomatic benefits of long-acting bronchodilators are firmly established. Increased exacerbations and mortality reported in some asthmatic patients treated with salmeterol have not been observed in COPD patients, and several studies report a trend toward lower mortality in patients treated with salmeterol alone, compared with placebo. In addition, a 4-year tiotropium trial reported fewer cardiovascular events in the intervention group. Subsequent meta-analyses that include the 4-year tiotropium trial did not find an increase in cardiovascular events in treated patients. Most practitioners believe that the documented benefits of anticholinergic therapy outweigh any potential risks.

4. Corticosteroids—Multiple large clinical trials have reported a reduction in the frequency of COPD exacerbations and an increase in self-reported functional status in COPD patients treated with inhaled corticosteroids. These same trials demonstrate no effect of inhaled corticosteroids on mortality or the characteristic decline in lung function experienced by COPD patients. Thus, inhaled corticosteroids alone should not be considered first-line therapy in stable COPD patients.

Three large clinical trials of combination therapy with an inhaled corticosteroid added to a LABA demonstrated a reduced frequency of exacerbations and modest improvements in lung function. The benefits of inhaled corticosteroids must be weighed against the increased risk of bacterial pneumonia, however (relative risk was increased 1.57-fold in one study). Withdrawal of inhaled corticosteroids should be considered when patients have been stable for 2 years.

Apart from acute exacerbations, COPD is not generally responsive to oral corticosteroid therapy. Given the risks of adverse side effects, oral corticosteroids are not recommended for long-term treatment of COPD.

5. Theophylline—Oral theophylline is a fourth-line agent for treating COPD patients who do not achieve adequate symptom control with inhaled anticholinergic, beta-2-agonist, and corticosteroid therapies. Theophylline improves dyspnea ratings, exercise performance, and pulmonary function in many patients with stable COPD. Its benefits result from bronchodilation; anti-inflammatory properties; and extrapulmonary effects on diaphragm strength, myocardial contractility, and kidney function. Theophylline toxicity is a significant concern due to the medication's narrow therapeutic window, and long-term administration requires careful monitoring of serum levels. GOLD guidelines recommend theophylline only as a last resort if other bronchodilators are unavailable or unaffordable.

6. Antibiotics—Antibiotics are commonly prescribed to outpatients with COPD for the following indications: (1) to treat an acute exacerbation, (2) to treat acute bronchitis, and (3) to prevent acute exacerbations of chronic bronchitis (prophylactic antibiotics). In patients with COPD, antibiotics appear to improve outcomes slightly in all three situations. Patients with a COPD exacerbation associated with increased sputum purulence accompanied by dyspnea or an increase in the quantity of sputum are thought to benefit the most from antibiotic therapy. The choice of antibiotic depends on local bacterial resistance patterns and individual risk of *Pseudomonas aeruginosa* infection (history of *Pseudomonas* isolation, FEV_1 less than 50% of predicted, recent hospitalization [2 or more days in the past 3 months], more than three courses of antibiotics within the past year, use of systemic corticosteroids). Oral antibiotic options include doxycycline (100 mg every 12 hours), trimethoprim-sulfamethoxazole (160/800 mg every 12 hours), a cephalosporin (eg, cefpodoxime 200 mg every 12 hours or cefprozil 500 mg every 12 hours), a macrolide (eg, azithromycin 500 mg followed by 250 mg daily for 5 days), a fluoroquinolone (eg, ciprofloxacin 500 mg every 12 hours), and amoxicillin-clavulanate (875/125 mg every 12 hours). Suggested duration of therapy is 3–5 days and depends on response to therapy. There are few controlled trials of antibiotics in severe COPD exacerbations, but prompt administration is appropriate, particularly in persons with risk factors for poor outcomes (age older than 65 years, FEV_1 less than 50% of predicted, three or more exacerbations in the past year, antibiotic therapy within the past 3 months, comorbid conditions, such as cardiac disease). In COPD patients subject to frequent exacerbations despite optimal medical therapy, azithromycin (daily or three times weekly) and moxifloxacin (a 5-day course 1 week in 8 over 48 weeks) were modestly effective in clinical trials at reducing the frequency of exacerbations; monitoring for hearing loss and QT prolongation is essential.

7. Pulmonary rehabilitation—Graded aerobic physical exercise programs (eg, walking 20 minutes three times weekly or bicycling) are helpful to prevent deterioration of physical condition and to improve patients' ability to carry out daily activities. Training of inspiratory muscles by inspiring against progressively larger resistive loads reduces dyspnea and improves exercise tolerance, health status, and respiratory muscle strength in some but not all patients. Pursed-lip breathing to slow the rate of breathing and abdominal breathing exercises to relieve fatigue of accessory muscles of respiration may reduce dyspnea in some patients. Many patients undergo these exercise and educational interventions in a structured rehabilitation program. Pulmonary rehabilitation has been shown in multiple studies to improve exercise capacity, decrease hospitalizations, and enhance quality of life. Referral to a comprehensive rehabilitation program is recommended in patients who have severe dyspnea, reduced quality of life, or frequent hospitalizations despite optimal medical therapy.

8. Phosphodiesterase type 4 inhibitor—Roflumilast has been shown to reduce exacerbation frequency in patients who have moderate or severe (FEV_1 less than 50% of predicted) COPD and chronic bronchitis, with frequent exacerbations, and who are taking LABA/inhaled corticosteroid with or without a LAMA.

9. Other measures—In patients with chronic bronchitis, increased mobilization of secretions may be accomplished through adequate systemic hydration, effective cough training methods, or the use of a handheld flutter device and postural drainage, sometimes with chest percussion or vibration. Postural drainage and chest percussion should be used only in selected patients with excessive amounts of retained secretions that cannot be cleared by coughing and other methods; these measures are of no benefit in pure emphysema. Expectorant-mucolytic therapy has generally been regarded as unhelpful in patients with chronic bronchitis. Cough suppressants and sedatives should be avoided.

Human alpha-1-antitrypsin is available for replacement therapy in emphysema due to congenital deficiency (PiZZ or null genotype) of alpha-1-antitrypsin (alpha-1-antiprotease). Patients over 18 years of age with airflow obstruction by spirometry and serum levels less than 11 mmol/L (~50 mg/dL) are potential candidates for replacement therapy. Alpha-1-antitrypsin is administered intravenously in a dose of 60 mg/kg body weight once weekly.

Severe dyspnea despite optimal medical management may warrant a clinical trial of an **opioid** (eg, morphine 5–10 mg orally every 3–4 hours, oxycodone 5–10 mg orally every 4–6 hours, sustained-release morphine 10 mg orally once daily). Sedative-hypnotic drugs (eg, diazepam, 5 mg three times daily) marginally improve intractable dyspnea but cause significant drowsiness; they may benefit very anxious patients. Transnasal positive-pressure ventilation at home to rest the respiratory muscles is an approach to improve respiratory muscle function and reduce dyspnea in patients with severe COPD.

See Chapter 37 for a discussion of air travel in patients with lung disease.

B. Hospitalized Patients

Management of the hospitalized patient with an acute exacerbation of COPD includes (1) supplemental oxygen (titrated to maintain Sao_2 between 90% and 94% or Pao_2 between 60 mm Hg and 70 mm Hg); (2) inhaled beta-2-agonists (eg, albuterol 2.5 mg diluted with saline to a total of 3 mL by nebulizer, or MDI, 90 mcg per puff, four to eight puffs via spacer, every 1–4 hours as needed) with or without inhaled ipratropium bromide (500 mcg by nebulizer, or 36 mcg by MDI with spacer, every 4 hours as needed); (3) corticosteroids (prednisone 0.5 mg/kg/day orally for 7–10 days is usually sufficient, and even 5 days may be adequate); (4) broad-spectrum antibiotics; and (5) in selected cases, chest physiotherapy.

For patients without risk factors for *Pseudomonas*, management options include a fluoroquinolone (eg, levofloxacin 750 mg orally or intravenously per day, or moxifloxacin 400 mg orally or intravenously every 24 hours) or a third-generation cephalosporin (eg, ceftriaxone 1 g intravenously per day, or cefotaxime 1 g intravenously every 8 hours).

For patients with risk factors for *Pseudomonas*, therapeutic options include piperacillin-tazobactam (4.5 g intravenously every 6 hours), ceftazidime (1 g intravenously every 8 hours), cefepime (1 g intravenously every 12 hours), or levofloxacin (750 mg orally or intravenously per day for 3–7 days).

Oxygen therapy should *not* be withheld for fear of worsening respiratory acidemia; hypoxemia is more detrimental than hypercapnia. Right-sided heart failure usually responds to measures that reduce pulmonary artery pressure, such as supplemental oxygen and correction of acidemia; bed rest, salt restriction, and diuretics may add some benefit. Cardiac dysrhythmias, particularly multifocal atrial tachycardia, usually respond to aggressive treatment of COPD itself. Atrial fibrillation and flutter may require DC cardioversion after initiation of the above therapy. Theophylline should not be initiated in the acute setting, but patients taking theophylline prior to acute hospitalization should have their theophylline serum levels measured and maintained in the therapeutic range. If progressive respiratory failure ensues, tracheal intubation and mechanical ventilation are necessary. In clinical trials of COPD patients with hypercapnic acute respiratory failure, **noninvasive positive-pressure ventilation (NIPPV)** delivered via face mask reduced the need for intubation and shortened lengths of stay in the ICU. Other studies have suggested a lower risk of nosocomial infections and less use of antibiotics in COPD patients treated with NIPPV.

C. Procedures for COPD

1. Lung transplantation—Requirements for lung transplantation are severe lung disease, limited activities of daily living, exhaustion of medical therapy, ambulatory status, potential for pulmonary rehabilitation, limited life expectancy without transplantation, adequate function of other organ systems, and a good social support system. Two-year survival rate after lung transplantation for COPD is 75%. Complications include acute rejection, opportunistic infection, and obliterative bronchiolitis. Substantial improvements in pulmonary function and exercise performance have been noted after transplantation.

2. Lung volume reduction surgery—Lung volume reduction surgery, or reduction pneumoplasty, is a surgical approach to relieve dyspnea and improve exercise tolerance in patients with advanced diffuse emphysema and lung hyperinflation. Bilateral resection of 20–30% of lung volume in selected patients results in modest improvements in pulmonary function, exercise performance, and dyspnea. The duration of improvement as well as any mortality benefit remains uncertain. Prolonged air leaks occur in up to 50% of patients postoperatively. Mortality rates in centers with the largest experience with lung volume reduction surgery range from 4% to 10%.

The National Emphysema Treatment Trial compared lung volume reduction surgery with medical treatment in a randomized, multicenter clinical trial of 1218 patients with severe emphysema. Overall, surgery improved exercise capacity but not mortality when compared with medical therapy. The persistence of this benefit remains to be defined. Subgroup analysis suggested that patients with upper lobe–predominant emphysema and low exercise capacity might have improved survival, while other groups suffered excess mortality when randomized to surgery.

3. Bullectomy—Bullectomy is an older surgical procedure for palliation of dyspnea in patients with severe bullous emphysema. Bullectomy is most commonly pursued when a single bulla occupies at least 30–50% of the hemithorax.

Prognosis

The outlook for patients with clinically significant COPD is poor. The degree of pulmonary dysfunction at the time the patient is first seen is an important predictor of survival: median survival of patients with FEV_1 = 1 L or less is about 4 years. A multidimensional index (the BODE index), which includes **B**MI, airway **O**bstruction (FEV_1), **D**yspnea (modified Medical Research Council dyspnea score), and **E**xercise capacity, is a tool that predicts death and hospitalization better than FEV_1 alone. Comprehensive care programs, cessation of smoking, and supplemental oxygen may reduce the rate of decline of pulmonary function, but therapy with bronchodilators and other approaches probably have little, if any, impact on the natural course of COPD.

Dyspnea at the end of life can be extremely uncomfortable and distressing to the patient and family. As patients near the end of life, meticulous attention to palliative care is essential to effectively manage dyspnea (see Chapter 5).

When to Refer

- COPD onset occurs before the age of 40.
- Frequent exacerbations (two or more a year) despite optimal treatment.
- Severe or rapidly progressive COPD.
- Symptoms disproportionate to the severity of airflow obstruction.
- Need for long-term oxygen therapy.
- Onset of comorbid illnesses (eg, bronchiectasis, heart failure, or lung cancer).

When to Admit

- Severe symptoms or acute worsening that fails to respond to outpatient management.
- Acute or worsening hypoxemia, hypercapnia, peripheral edema, or change in mental status.
- Inadequate home care, or inability to sleep or maintain nutrition/hydration due to symptoms.
- The presence of high-risk comorbid conditions.

Agustí A et al. Update on the pathogenesis of chronic obstructive pulmonary disease. N Engl J Med. 2019;381:1248. [PMID: 31553836]

Barnes PJ. Endo-phenotyping of COPD patients. Expert Rev Respir Med. 2021;15:27. [PMID: 32730716]

Celli BR et al. Update on clinical aspects of chronic obstructive pulmonary disease. N Engl J Med. 2019;381:1257. [PMID: 31553837]

Global Initiative for Chronic Obstructive Lung Disease (GOLD). 2022 Global strategy for the prevention, diagnosis, and management of chronic obstructive lung disease. https://goldcopd.org/2022-gold-reports-2/

Lacasse Y et al; INOX Trial Group. Randomized trial of nocturnal oxygen in chronic obstructive pulmonary disease. N Engl J Med. 2020;383:1129. [PMID: 32937046]

BRONCHIECTASIS

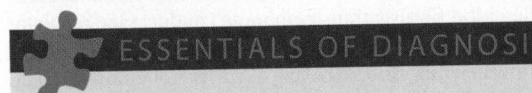

- Chronic productive cough with dyspnea and wheezing.
- Radiographic findings of dilated, thickened airways and scattered, irregular opacities.

General Considerations

Bronchiectasis is a congenital or acquired disorder of the large bronchi characterized by permanent, abnormal dilation and destruction of bronchial walls. It may be caused by recurrent inflammation or infection of the airways and may be localized or diffuse. Cystic fibrosis causes about half of all cases of bronchiectasis. Other causes include lung infections (tuberculosis and nontuberculous mycobacteria, fungal infections, lung abscess, pneumonia), immunodeficiencies (congenital or acquired hypogammaglobulinemia; common variable immunodeficiency; selective IgA, IgM, and IgG subclass deficiencies; AIDS; lymphoma; plasma cell myeloma; leukemia), alpha-1-antitrypsin deficiency, primary ciliary dyskinesia, rheumatic diseases (rheumatoid arthritis, Sjögren syndrome); allergic bronchopulmonary aspergillosis (ABPA); and localized airway obstruction (foreign body, tumor, mucoid impaction).

Clinical Findings

A. Symptoms and Signs

Symptoms of bronchiectasis include chronic cough with production of copious amounts of purulent sputum, hemoptysis, pleuritic chest pain, dyspnea, and weight loss. Physical findings may include crackles at the lung bases and wheezing.

B. Laboratory Findings and Imaging

Laboratory tests include CBC with differential, immunoglobulin quantification; testing for cystic fibrosis with sweat chloride level; and sputum culture, including for nontuberculous mycobacteria. Additional testing, if appropriate, may include aspergillus antibodies, alpha-1-antitrypsin level, ciliary testing, autoimmune serologies, and swallow assessment. Obstructive pulmonary dysfunction with hypoxemia is seen in moderate or severe disease. High-resolution CT is the diagnostic study of choice. Radiographic abnormalities include dilated and thickened bronchi that may appear as "tram tracks" or as ring-like markings; scattered irregular opacities, atelectasis, and focal consolidation may be present.

C. Microbiology

Haemophilus influenzae is the most common organism recovered from non–cystic fibrosis patients with bronchiectasis. *P aeruginosa, Streptococcus pneumoniae*, and *Staphylococcus aureus* are commonly identified. Nontuberculous mycobacteria are seen less commonly. Patients with *Pseudomonas* infection experience an accelerated course, with more frequent exacerbations and more rapid decline in lung function.

Treatment

Treatment of acute exacerbations consists of antibiotics, daily chest physiotherapy with postural drainage and chest percussion, and inhaled bronchodilators. Handheld flutter valve devices may be as effective as chest physiotherapy in clearing secretions. Antibiotic therapy should be guided by sputum smears and prior cultures. If a specific bacterial pathogen cannot be isolated, then empiric oral antibiotic therapy for 10–14 days is appropriate. Common medications include amoxicillin or amoxicillin-clavulanate, ampicillin, a second- or third-generation cephalosporin, doxycycline, or a fluoroquinolone. For recurrent exacerbations, preventive macrolide therapy for 6–12 months has been found to decrease the frequency of exacerbations. Alternatively, inhaled antibiotics have been shown to reduce exacerbations. Alternating cycles of oral antibiotics may also be considered, although data are inconclusive.

Complications of bronchiectasis include hemoptysis, right-sided heart failure, amyloidosis, and secondary visceral abscesses at distant sites (eg, brain). Bronchoscopy is sometimes necessary to evaluate hemoptysis, remove retained secretions, and rule out obstructing airway lesions. Massive hemoptysis may require embolization of bronchial arteries or surgical resection.

Chalmers JD et al. Long-term macrolide antibiotics for the treatment of bronchiectasis in adults: an individual participant data meta-analysis. Lancet Respir Med. 2019;7:845. [PMID: 31405828]

Gruffydd-Jones K et al. Primary care implications of the British Thoracic Society Guidelines for bronchiectasis in adults 2019. NPJ Prim Care Respir Med. 2019;29:24. [PMID: 31249313]

Lesan A et al. Short review on the diagnosis and treatment of bronchiectasis. Med Pharm Rep. 2019;92:111. [PMID: 31086836]

McShane PJ et al. Bronchiectasis. Chest. 2019;155:825. [PMID: 30403962]

Tejada S et al. Inhaled antibiotics for treatment of adults with non-cystic fibrosis bronchiectasis: a systematic review and meta-analysis. Eur J Intern Med. 2021;90:77. [PMID: 33947626]

ALLERGIC BRONCHOPULMONARY ASPERGILLOSIS

ABPA is a pulmonary hypersensitivity disorder caused by allergy to fungal antigens that colonize the tracheobronchial tree. It usually occurs in atopic asthmatic individuals who are 20–40 years of age or those with cystic fibrosis, in response to antigens of *Aspergillus* species. Primary criteria for the diagnosis of ABPA include (1) a clinical history of asthma or cystic fibrosis; (2) elevated serum total IgE levels (greater than 1000 IU/mL); (3) immediate cutaneous hypersensitivity to *Aspergillus* antigens or elevated serum IgE levels specific to *Aspergillus fumigatus;* and (4) at least two of the following: (a) precipitating serum antibodies to *Aspergillus* antigen or elevated serum *Aspergillus* IgG by immunoassay, (b) pulmonary radiographic abnormalities consistent with ABPA, or (c) peripheral blood eosinophil count greater than 500 cells/mcL (greater than 0.5×10^9/L). Radiographic abnormalities include transient opacities, mucoid impaction, and proximal or central bronchiectasis. High-dose corticosteroids (eg, prednisone 0.5–1 mg/kg orally per day) for at least 2 weeks with gradual taper is the treatment of choice. Patients with corticosteroid-dependent disease may benefit from itraconazole or voriconazole. Relapses are frequent. For those with frequent exacerbations, the use of biologic agents, such as anti-IgE (omalizumab), anti-IL-5 (mepolizumab, benralizumab), or anti-IL4 receptor (dupilumab), has been shown to improve outcomes. Bronchodilators (see Table 9–3) may also be helpful. Complications include hemoptysis, severe bronchiectasis, and pulmonary fibrosis.

Koutsokera A et al. Omalizumab for asthma and allergic bronchopulmonary aspergillosis in adults with cystic fibrosis. J Cyst Fibros. 2020;19:119. [PMID: 31405730]

Moldoveanu B et al. Pulmonary aspergillosis: spectrum of disease. Am J Med Sci. 2021;361:411. [PMID: 33563417]

Muthu V et al. Diagnostic cutoffs and clinical utility of recombinant *Aspergillus fumigatus* antigens in the diagnosis of allergic bronchopulmonary aspergillosis. J Allergy Clin Immunol Pract. 2020;8:579. [PMID: 31520840]

CYSTIC FIBROSIS

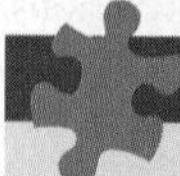

ESSENTIALS OF DIAGNOSIS

- Autosomal recessive disorder.
- Pulmonary disease: chronic or recurrent productive cough, dyspnea, and wheezing; recurrent airway infections or chronic colonization of the airways with *H influenzae, P aeruginosa, S aureus*, or *Burkholderia cenocepacia*; bronchiectasis and scarring on chest radiographs; airflow obstruction on spirometry.
- Extrapulmonary disease: sinus disease (chronic sinusitis and nasal polyposis); GI disease (pancreatic insufficiency, recurrent pancreatitis, hepatobiliary disease, meconium ileus, and distal intestinal obstruction); genitourinary problems (absent vas deferens and male infertility).
- Diagnosis: sweat chloride concentration > 60 mEq/L on two occasions; or presence of two disease-causing mutations in the cystic fibrosis transmembrane conductance regulator (*CFTR*) gene; or sweat chloride concentration 30–59 mEq/L plus one disease-causing mutation in *CFTR* gene.

General Considerations

Cystic fibrosis is the most common cause of severe chronic lung disease in young adults and the most common fatal hereditary disorder of White persons in the United States. It is an autosomal-recessive disorder affecting about 1 in 3000 White persons; 1 in 25 is a carrier. Cystic fibrosis is caused by abnormalities in a membrane chloride channel (the cystic fibrosis transmembrane conductance regulator [CFTR] protein) that results in altered chloride transport and water flux across the apical surface of epithelial cells. Over 2000 different mutations of the *CFTR* gene have been identified with potential to cause disease. The most common mutation is ΔF508.

Clinical Findings

A. Symptoms and Signs

Cystic fibrosis should be suspected in an adult with a history of chronic lung disease (especially bronchiectasis), pancreatitis, or infertility. Cough, sputum production, decreased exercise tolerance, and recurrent hemoptysis are typical complaints. Patients also often complain of chronic rhinosinusitis symptoms, steatorrhea, diarrhea, and abdominal pain. Patients with cystic fibrosis are often malnourished with low BMI. Digital clubbing (Figure 6–42), increased anteroposterior chest diameter, hyperresonance to percussion, and apical crackles are noted on physical examination. Sinus tenderness, purulent nasal secretions, and nasal polyps may also be seen. Nearly all men with cystic fibrosis have congenital bilateral absence of the vas deferens with azoospermia. Biliary cirrhosis and gallstones may occur.

B. Laboratory Findings

ABG studies often reveal hypoxemia and, in advanced disease, a chronic, compensated respiratory acidosis. PFTs show a mixed obstructive and restrictive pattern. There is a reduction in FVC, airflow rates, and TLC. Air trapping (high ratio of RV to TLC) and reduction in pulmonary diffusing capacity are common.

C. Imaging

Hyperinflation is seen early in the disease process. Peribronchial cuffing, mucus plugging, bronchiectasis (ring shadows and cysts), increased interstitial markings, small rounded peripheral opacities, and focal atelectasis are common findings. Pneumothorax can also be seen. Thin-section CT scanning often confirms the presence of bronchiectasis.

D. Diagnosis

The **quantitative sweat test** reveals elevated sodium and chloride levels (greater than 60 mEq/L) in the sweat of patients with cystic fibrosis. Two tests on different days performed in experienced laboratories are required for accurate diagnosis. A normal sweat chloride test does not exclude the diagnosis, in which case *CFTR* genotyping or other alternative diagnostic studies (such as measurement of nasal membrane potential difference, semen analysis, or assessment of pancreatic function) should be pursued, especially if there is a high clinical suspicion of cystic fibrosis. Additionally, all patients with cystic fibrosis should undergo *CFTR* genotyping to determine whether they are eligible for CFTR modulator therapy.

Treatment

Early recognition and comprehensive multidisciplinary therapy improve symptom control and survival. Referral to a regional cystic fibrosis center is strongly recommended. Treatment programs focus on the following areas: CFTR modulator medications, clearance and reduction of lower airway secretions, reversal of bronchoconstriction, treatment of respiratory tract infections and airway bacterial burden, pancreatic enzyme replacement, and nutritional and psychosocial support (including genetic and occupational counseling).

CFTR modulators include medications that alter CFTR trafficking, folding, or function. These medications are only available for patients with specific *CFTR* mutations. Examples are **ivacaftor,** a potentiator of the CFTR channel that works by increasing the time the channel remains open after being activated; and **lumacaftor, tezacaftor,** and **elexacaftor**, which work by improving CFTR protein folding and cell-surface trafficking.

Airway clearance can be promoted by postural drainage, chest percussion or vibration techniques, positive expiratory pressure or flutter valve breathing devices, directed cough, and other breathing techniques. Inhaled **recombinant human deoxyribonuclease** (rhDNase, dornase alpha) cleaves extracellular DNA in sputum, decreasing sputum viscosity; when administered long-term at a daily nebulized dose of 2.5 mg, this therapy leads to improved FEV_1 and reduces the risk of cystic fibrosis–related respiratory exacerbations as well as the need for intravenous antibiotics. Inhalation of hypertonic (7%) saline improves clearance of mucus from the airway and has been associated with small improvements in pulmonary function and fewer pulmonary exacerbations.

Short-term antibiotics are used to treat active airway infections based on results of culture and susceptibility testing of sputum. *S aureus* (including methicillin-resistant strains) and a mucoid variant of *P aeruginosa* are commonly present. *H influenzae, Stenotrophomonas maltophilia,* and *B cenocepacia* (a highly drug-resistant organism) are occasionally isolated. **Long-term antibiotic therapy,** such as azithromycin (which has immunomodulatory properties) and various inhaled antibiotics (eg, tobramycin, aztreonam, colistin, and levofloxacin) taken two to three times a day, helps slow disease progression and reduce exacerbations in patients with sputum cultures positive for *P aeruginosa*. The length of therapy depends on the persistent presence of *P aeruginosa* in the sputum. The incidence of atypical mycobacterial colonization is higher in cystic fibrosis patients, and directed antibiotic treatment is recommended for frequent exacerbations, progressive decline in lung function, or failure to thrive.

Inhaled bronchodilators (eg, albuterol) should be considered in patients who demonstrate an increase of at least 12% in FEV_1 after an inhaled bronchodilator. An **inhaled corticosteroid** should be added to the treatment regimen for patients who have cystic fibrosis with persistent asthma or ABPA.

Lung transplantation is the only definitive treatment for advanced cystic fibrosis.

Vaccination against pneumococcal and coronavirus infections and annual influenza vaccination are advised. **Screening** of family members and genetic counseling are suggested.

Prognosis

The longevity of patients with cystic fibrosis is increasing. Death occurs from pulmonary complications (eg, pneumonia, pneumothorax, or hemoptysis) or as a result of terminal chronic respiratory failure and right-sided heart failure.

Barry PJ et al; VX18-445-104 Study Group. Triple therapy for cystic fibrosis *Phe508del*-gating and -residual function genotypes. N Engl J Med. 2021;385:815. [PMID: 34437784]

Bienvenu T et al. Current and future diagnosis of cystic fibrosis: performance and limitations. Arch Pediatr. 2020;27:eS19. [PMID: 32172931]

Bierlaagh MC et al. A new era for people with cystic fibrosis. Eur J Pediatr. 2021;180:2731. [PMID: 34213646]

Lopes-Pacheco M. CFTR modulators: the changing face of cystic fibrosis in the era of precision medicine. Front Pharmacol. 2020;10:1662. [PMID: 32153386]

Turcios NL. Cystic fibrosis lung disease: an overview. Respir Care. 2020;65:233. [PMID: 31772069]

BRONCHIOLITIS

ESSENTIALS OF DIAGNOSIS

- Insidious onset of cough and dyspnea.
- Irreversible airflow obstruction and air trapping on PFTs.
- Minimal findings on chest radiograph, heterogeneous airflow obstruction, and air trapping on chest CT scan.
- Relevant exposure or risk factors: toxic fumes, viral infections, organ transplantation, connective tissue disease.

General Considerations

Bronchiolitis is a generic term applied to varied inflammatory processes that affect the bronchioles, which are small conducting airways less than 2 mm in diameter. Bronchiolitis is less common in adults than in children, but it is encountered in multiple clinical settings, such as postinfectious, inhalational injury (such as vaping), organ transplantation, connective tissue diseases, and hypersensitivity pneumonitis.

The clinical approach to bronchiolitis divides patients into groups based on etiology, but different clinical syndromes may have identical histopathologic findings. As a result, no single classification scheme has been widely accepted, and there is an overlapping array of terms to describe these disorders from the viewpoints of the clinician, the pathologist, and the radiologist.

Clinical Findings

Acute bronchiolitis can be seen following viral infections.

Constrictive bronchiolitis (also referred to as obliterative bronchiolitis or bronchiolitis obliterans) is relatively infrequent, although it is the most common finding following inhalation injury (ammonia, welding fumes, and heavy metals). It may also be seen in rheumatoid arthritis; medication reactions (busulfan, gold, and penicillamine); and chronic rejection following heart-lung, lung, or hematopoietic stem cell transplantation (bronchiolitis obliterans syndrome). Patients with constrictive bronchiolitis have airflow obstruction and air trapping on spirometry; unremarkable plain chest radiographs but heterogeneous airflow obstruction and air trapping on chest CT scans; and a progressive, deteriorating clinical course.

Proliferative bronchiolitis (organizing pneumonia) is associated with diverse pulmonary disorders, including infection, aspiration, acute respiratory distress syndrome (ARDS), hypersensitivity pneumonitis, connective tissue diseases, and organ transplantation. Compared with constrictive bronchiolitis, proliferative bronchiolitis is more likely to have an abnormal chest radiograph. Chest CT scan may show patchy consolidation, ground-glass opacities, or peripheral nodular appearance. PFTs typically reveal a restrictive ventilatory defect and impaired oxygenation.

Follicular bronchiolitis is most commonly associated with connective tissue disease, especially rheumatoid arthritis and Sjögren syndrome, and with immunodeficiency states, such as HIV or common variable immunodeficiency. Chest CT scan may show centrilobular and peribronchial nodules. It may be seen in lymphoid interstitial pneumonia.

Respiratory bronchiolitis is the most common form of bronchiolitis in adults and is usually related to cigarette smoking. It usually occurs without symptoms or physiologic evidence of lung impairment. It may be seen in respiratory bronchiolitis–associated interstitial lung disease (RB-ILD). Chest CT may show centrilobular nodules, patchy ground-glass opacities, air trapping, and "tree-in-bud" opacities.

Diffuse panbronchiolitis is most frequently diagnosed in Japan. Men are affected about twice as often as women, two-thirds are nonsmokers, and most patients have a history of chronic pansinusitis. Patients complain of dyspnea, cough, and sputum production, and chest examination shows crackles and rhonchi. PFTs reveal obstructive abnormalities, and the chest radiograph shows a distinct pattern of diffuse, small, nodular shadows with hyperinflation.

Treatment

Constrictive bronchiolitis is relatively unresponsive to corticosteroids and is frequently progressive. Corticosteroids are usually effective in **proliferative bronchiolitis** and improvement can be prompt. Therapy is initiated with prednisone at 1 mg/kg/day orally for 1–3 months. The dose is then tapered slowly to 20–40 mg/day, depending on the response, and weaned over the subsequent 3–6 months as tolerated. Relapses are common if corticosteroids are stopped prematurely or tapered too quickly. Azithromycin may be used to effectively treat **diffuse panbronchiolitis** and, additionally, it may slow down the progression of bronchiolitis obliterans syndrome in lung transplant recipients.

Gan CT et al. Long-term effect of azithromycin in bronchiolitis obliterans syndrome. BMJ Open Respir Res. 2019;6:e000465. [PMID: 31673366]

Nett RJ et al. Occupational bronchiolitis: an update. Clin Chest Med. 2020;41:661. [PMID: 33153686]

Ryu JH et al. Recent advances in the understanding of bronchiolitis in adults. F1000Res. 2020;9:F1000 Faculty Rev-568. [PMID: 32551095]

PULMONARY INFECTIONS

PNEUMONIA

Pneumonia has classically been considered in terms of the infecting organism (Table 9–8). This approach facilitates discussion of characteristic clinical presentations but is a limited guide to patient management since specific microbiologic information is usually not available at initial presentation. Current classification schemes emphasize epidemiologic factors that predict etiology and guide initial therapy. Pneumonia may be classified as **community-acquired pneumonia (CAP)** or **nosocomial pneumonia** and, within the latter, as **hospital-acquired pneumonia (HAP)** or **ventilator-associated pneumonia (VAP).** These categories are based on differing settings and infectious agents and require different diagnostic and therapeutic interventions. **Anaerobic pneumonia** and **lung abscess** can occur in both hospital and community settings.

This section sets forth the evaluation and management of pulmonary infiltrates in immunocompetent persons separately from the approach to immunocompromised persons—defined as those with HIV disease, absolute neutrophil counts less than 1000/mcL (1.0×10^9/L), or current or recent exposure to myelosuppressive or immunosuppressive medications.

1. Community-Acquired Pneumonia

ESSENTIALS OF DIAGNOSIS

- Fever or hypothermia, tachypnea, cough with or without sputum, dyspnea, chest discomfort, sweats or rigors (or both).
- Bronchial breath sounds, rhonchi, or inspiratory crackles on chest auscultation.
- Parenchymal opacity on chest radiograph (occasionally not evident at presentation).
- Occurs outside of the hospital or within 48 hours of hospital admission.

General Considerations

Community-acquired pneumonia (CAP) is a common disorder, with approximately 4–5 million cases diagnosed

Table 9–8. Characteristics of selected pneumonias.

Organism; Appearance on Smear of Sputum	Clinical Setting	Complications
Streptococcus pneumoniae (pneumococcus). Gram-positive diplococci.	Chronic cardiopulmonary disease; follows upper respiratory tract infection	Bacteremia, meningitis, endocarditis, pericarditis, empyema
Haemophilus influenzae. Pleomorphic gram-negative coccobacilli.	Chronic cardiopulmonary disease; follows upper respiratory tract infection	Empyema, endocarditis
Staphylococcus aureus. Plump gram-positive cocci in clumps.	Residence in long-term care facility, hospital-associated, influenza epidemics, cystic fibrosis, bronchiectasis, injection drug use	Empyema, cavitation
Klebsiella pneumoniae. Plump gram-negative encapsulated rods.	Alcohol abuse, diabetes mellitus; hospital-associated	Cavitation, empyema
Escherichia coli. Gram-negative rods.	Hospital-associated; rarely, community-acquired	Empyema
Pseudomonas aeruginosa. Gram-negative rods.	Hospital-associated; cystic fibrosis, bronchiectasis	Cavitation
Anaerobes. Mixed flora.	Aspiration, poor dental hygiene	Necrotizing pneumonia, abscess, empyema
Mycoplasma pneumoniae. PMNs and monocytes; no bacteria.	Young adults; summer and fall	Skin rashes, bullous myringitis; hemolytic anemia
Legionella species. Few PMNs; no bacteria.	Summer and fall; exposure to contaminated construction site, water source, air conditioner; community-acquired or hospital-associated	Empyema, cavitation, endocarditis, pericarditis
Chlamydophila pneumoniae. Nonspecific.	Clinically similar to *M pneumoniae*, but prodromal symptoms last longer (up to 2 weeks); sore throat with hoarseness common; mild pneumonia in teenagers and young adults	Reinfection in older adults with underlying COPD or heart failure may be severe or even fatal
Moraxella catarrhalis. Gram-negative diplococci.	Preexisting lung disease; elderly patients; corticosteroid or immunosuppressive therapy	Rarely, pleural effusions and bacteremia
Pneumocystis jirovecii. Nonspecific.	AIDS, immunosuppressive or cytotoxic drug therapy, cancer	Pneumothorax, respiratory failure, ARDS, death
SARS-CoV-2. Nonspecific.	Pandemic. Milder pneumonia (teenagers, young adults); more severe pneumonia (elderly, immunocompromised, multiple comorbidly ill adults)	Respiratory failure, ARDS, death

ARDS, acute respiratory distress syndrome; PMN, polymorphonuclear leukocyte; SARS-CoV-2, severe acute respiratory syndrome due to coronavirus-2 (see COVID-19 discussion, Chapter 32, and consult https://www.coronavirus.gov for the latest from the CDC).

each year in the United States, at least 25% of which require hospitalization. It is the deadliest infectious disease in the United States and is routinely among the top 10 causes of death. Mortality in milder cases treated as outpatients is less than 1%. Among patients hospitalized for CAP, in-hospital mortality is approximately 10–12% and 1-year mortality (in those over age 65) is greater than 40%. Risk factors for the development of CAP include older age; tobacco use; excessive alcohol use; comorbid medical conditions, especially COPD or other chronic lung disease; immunosuppression; and recent viral upper respiratory tract infection.

The patient's history, physical examination, and imaging studies are essential to establishing a diagnosis of CAP. None of these efforts identifies a specific microbiologic cause, however. Sputum examination may be helpful in selected patients but 40% of patients cannot produce an evaluable sputum sample; additionally, test characteristics of sputum Gram stain and culture vary by organism and lack sensitivity for some of the most common causes of pneumonia. Since patient outcomes improve when the initial antibiotic choice is appropriate for the infecting organism, the American Thoracic Society and the Infectious Diseases Society of America recommend empiric treatment based on epidemiologic data (Table 9–9). Such treatment improves initial antibiotic coverage, reduces unnecessary hospitalization, and appears to improve 30-day survival.

Definition & Pathogenesis

CAP is diagnosed outside of the hospital setting or within the first 48 hours of hospital admission. Pulmonary defense mechanisms (cough reflex, mucociliary clearance system, immune responses) normally prevent the development of lower respiratory tract infections following aspiration of oropharyngeal secretions containing bacteria or inhalation of infected aerosols. CAP occurs when there is a defect in one or more of these normal defense mechanisms or when a large infectious inoculum or a virulent pathogen overwhelms the immune response.

Prospective studies fail to identify the cause of CAP in 30–60% of cases; two or more causes are identified in up to one-third of cases. The most common bacterial pathogen identified in most studies of CAP is *S pneumoniae*, accounting for approximately two-thirds of bacterial isolates. Other common bacterial pathogens include *H influenzae, M pneumoniae, C pneumoniae, S aureus, Moraxella catarrhalis, Klebsiella pneumoniae*, other gram-negative rods, and *Legionella* species. Common viral causes of CAP include coronaviruses (SARS-CoV-2, MERS), influenza virus, respiratory syncytial virus, adenovirus, and parainfluenza virus. A detailed assessment of epidemiologic risk factors may aid in diagnosing pneumonias due to the following uncommon causes: *Chlamydophila psittaci* (psittacosis); *Coxiella burnetii* (Q fever); *Francisella tularensis* (tularemia); *Blastomyces, Coccidioides, Histoplasma* (endemic fungi); and Sin Nombre virus (hantavirus pulmonary syndrome).

Clinical Findings

A. Symptoms and Signs

Most patients with CAP experience an acute or subacute onset of fever, cough with or without sputum production, and dyspnea. Other common symptoms include sweats, chills, rigors, chest discomfort, pleurisy, hemoptysis, fatigue, myalgias, anorexia, headache, and abdominal pain. Persons over age 80, however, may have an atypical presentation, including falls, delirium, lethargy, and anorexia.

Common physical findings include fever or hypothermia, tachypnea, tachycardia, and arterial oxygen desaturation. Many patients appear acutely ill. Chest examination often reveals inspiratory crackles, rhonchi, and bronchial breath sounds. Dullness to percussion may be observed if lobar consolidation or a parapneumonic pleural effusion is present. The clinical evaluation is less than 50% sensitive compared to chest imaging for the diagnosis of CAP (see Imaging section below). In most patients, therefore, a chest radiograph is essential to the evaluation of suspected CAP.

B. Diagnostic Testing

Diagnostic testing for a specific infectious cause of CAP is not generally indicated in ambulatory patients treated as outpatients because empiric antibiotic therapy is almost always effective in this population. In ambulatory outpatients whose presentation (travel history, exposure) suggests an etiology not covered by standard therapy (eg, *Coccidioides*) or public health concerns (eg, SARS-CoV-2, *Mycobacterium tuberculosis*, influenza), diagnostic testing is appropriate. Diagnostic testing is recommended in hospitalized CAP patients for multiple reasons: the likelihood of an infectious cause unresponsive to standard therapy is higher in more severe illness, the inpatient setting allows narrowing of antibiotic coverage as specific diagnostic information is available, and the yield of testing is improved in more acutely ill patients.

Diagnostic tests are used to adjust empirically chosen therapy and to facilitate epidemiologic analysis. Three widely available diagnostic tests may guide therapy: the sputum Gram stain and culture, urinary antigen tests for *S pneumoniae* and *Legionella* species, and tests for viruses such as influenza and SARS-CoV-2 (see COVID-19 discussion, Chapter 32). The usefulness of a sputum Gram stain lies in broadening initial coverage in patients to be hospitalized for CAP, most commonly to cover *S aureus* (including community-acquired methicillin-resistant *S aureus* [CA-MRSA] strains) or gram-negative rods (including *P aeruginosa* and Enterobacteriaceae). Urinary antigen assays for *Legionella pneumophila* and *S pneumoniae* are at least as sensitive and specific as sputum Gram stain and culture. Results of antigen testing are not affected by initiation of antibiotic therapy, and positive tests may allow narrowing of initial antibiotic coverage. Urinary antigen assay for *S pneumoniae* should be ordered for patients with leukopenia or asplenia or those with severe disease. Urinary antigen assay for *L pneumophila* should be ordered for patients in an area with an outbreak, with recent travel, with severe disease, or in whom a high clinical index of suspicion exists. Rapid influenza and SARS-CoV-2 testing has intermediate sensitivity but high specificity, with sensitivity depending on the method of detection (nucleic acid or PCR-based tests have higher sensitivity than antigen-based detection). Positive tests for viruses may reduce direct isolation of hospitalized patients but do not necessarily reduce the need for antibacterial therapy, since coinfection with a bacterial pathogen is common.

Rapid turnaround multiplex-PCR amplification from lower respiratory tract samples is increasingly available. Different commercial products can identify multiple strains of bacteria and viruses, in addition to genes that encode for antibiotic resistance. Early experience with multiplex-PCR shows improved overall diagnostic yield, particularly for viral infections, and a higher incidence of bacterial/viral coinfection than previously recognized. Limitations of multiplex-PCR include cost and availability, in addition to the challenge of interpreting potentially false-positive results from a highly sensitive test, since either viral or bacterial pathogens may colonize the airways.

Additional microbiologic testing including pre-antibiotic sputum and blood cultures (at least two sets with needle sticks at separate sites) has been standard practice for patients with CAP who require hospitalization. The yield of blood and sputum cultures is low, however; false-positive results are common, and the impact of culture results on patient outcomes is small. As a result, targeted testing is recommended for patients with severe disease and for those treated empirically for MRSA or *P aeruginosa* infection. The role of culture is to allow narrowing of initial empiric antibiotic coverage, adjustment of coverage based on specific antibiotic resistance patterns, to identify unsuspected pathogens not covered by initial therapy, and to provide information for epidemiologic analysis.

Apart from microbiologic testing, hospitalized patients should undergo CBC with differential and a chemistry panel (including serum glucose, electrolytes, BUN, creatinine, bilirubin, and liver enzymes). Hypoxemic patients should have ABGs sampled. Test results help assess severity of illness and guide evaluation and management. HIV testing should be considered in all adult patients and performed in those with risk factors.

C. Imaging

A pulmonary opacity on chest radiography or CT scan is required to establish a diagnosis of CAP. Chest CT scan is more sensitive and specific than chest radiography and may be indicated in selected cases. Radiographic findings range from patchy airspace opacities to lobar consolidation with air bronchograms to diffuse alveolar or interstitial opacities. Additional findings can include pleural effusions and cavitation. Chest imaging cannot identify a specific microbiologic cause of CAP; no pattern of radiographic abnormalities is pathognomonic of any infectious cause.

Chest imaging may help assess severity and response to therapy over time. Progression of pulmonary opacities during antibiotic therapy or lack of radiographic improvement over time are poor prognostic signs and raise concerns about secondary or alternative pulmonary processes. Clearing of pulmonary opacities in patients with CAP can take 6 weeks or longer. Clearance is usually quickest in younger patients, nonsmokers, and those with only single-lobe involvement. Routine follow-up chest imaging is not indicated for most patients with CAP.

D. Special Examinations

Patients with CAP who have significant pleural fluid collections may require diagnostic thoracentesis (with pleural fluid sent for glucose, LD, and total protein levels; leukocyte count with differential; pH determination; and Gram stain and culture). Positive pleural cultures indicate the need for tube thoracostomy drainage.

Patients with cavitary opacities should have sputum fungal and mycobacterial cultures.

Sputum induction or fiberoptic bronchoscopy to obtain samples of lower respiratory secretions are indicated in patients with a worsening clinical course who cannot provide expectorated sputum samples or who may have pneumonia caused by *M tuberculosis* infection or certain opportunistic infections, including *Pneumocystis jirovecii*.

Differential Diagnosis

The differential diagnosis of lower respiratory tract infection is extensive and includes upper respiratory tract infections, reactive airway diseases, heart failure, interstitial pneumonias, lung cancer, pulmonary vasculitis, pulmonary thromboembolic disease, and atelectasis.

Treatment

Two general principles guide antibiotic therapy once the diagnosis of CAP is established: **prompt** initiation of a medication to which the etiologic pathogen is **susceptible.**

In patients who require specific diagnostic evaluation, sputum and blood culture specimens should be obtained prior to initiation of antibiotics. Since early administration of antibiotics to acutely ill patients is associated with improved outcomes, obtaining other diagnostic specimens or test results should not delay the initial dose of antibiotics.

Optimal antibiotic therapy would be pathogen directed, but a definitive microbiologic diagnosis is not typically available on presentation. A syndromic approach to therapy, based on clinical presentation and chest imaging, does not reliably predict the microbiology of CAP. Therefore, initial antibiotic choices are empiric, based on acuity (treatment as an outpatient, inpatient, or in the ICU), patient risk factors for specific pathogens, and local antibiotic resistance patterns (Table 9–9).

Since *S pneumoniae* remains a common cause of CAP in all patient groups, local prevalence of drug-resistant *S pneumoniae* significantly affects initial antibiotic choice. Prior treatment with one antibiotic in a pharmacologic class (eg, beta-lactam, macrolide, fluoroquinolone) predisposes to the emergence of drug-resistant *S pneumoniae*, with resistance developing against that class of antibiotics to which the pathogen was previously exposed. Definitions of resistance have shifted based on observations of continued clinical efficacy at achievable serum levels. In CAP, for parenteral penicillin G or oral amoxicillin, susceptible strains have a minimum inhibitory concentration (MIC) of 2 mcg/mL or less; intermediate resistance is defined as an MIC between 2 mcg/mL and 4 mcg/mL because treatment failures are uncommon with MIC of 4 mcg/mL or less. Macrolide resistance has increased; approximately one-third of *S pneumoniae* isolates now show in vitro resistance to macrolides. Treatment failures have been reported but remain rare compared to the number of patients treated. Current in vivo efficacy appears to justify maintaining macrolides as first-line therapy except in areas where there is a high prevalence of resistant strains. *S pneumoniae* resistance to fluoroquinolones is rare in the United States but is increasing.

CA-MRSA is genetically and phenotypically different from hospital-acquired MRSA strains. CA-MRSA is a rare cause of necrotizing pneumonia, empyema, respiratory failure, and shock; it appears to be associated with prior influenza infection. Linezolid may be preferred to vancomycin in treatment of CA-MRSA pulmonary infection. Daptomycin should **not** be used in any MRSA pneumonia because it does not achieve adequate concentration in the lung. For expanded discussions of specific antibiotics, see Chapters 30 and e1.

A. Treatment of Outpatients

See Table 9–9 for specific medication dosages. The most common etiologies of CAP in outpatients who do not require hospitalization are *S pneumoniae*; *M pneumoniae*; *C pneumoniae*; and respiratory viruses, including influenza. For previously healthy patients with no recent (90 days) use of antibiotics, the recommended treatment is a macrolide (clarithromycin or azithromycin), doxycycline, or amoxicillin. In areas with a high incidence of macrolide-resistant *S pneumoniae*, initial therapy in patients with no comorbidities may include the combination of a beta-lactam *plus* a macrolide, or a respiratory fluoroquinolone.

Table 9–9. Recommended empiric antibiotics for community-acquired bacterial pneumonia.

Outpatient management

1. For previously healthy patients with no risk factors for MRSA or *Pseudomonas*:
   a. Amoxicillin, 1 g orally three times daily, *or*
   b. Doxycycline, 100 mg orally twice a day, *or*
   c. In regions with a low rate (< 25%) of infection with high level (MIC ≥ 16 mcg/mL) macrolide-resistant *Streptococcus pneumoniae*, then a macrolide (clarithromycin, 500 mg orally twice a day; or azithromycin, 500 mg orally as a first dose and then 250 mg orally daily for 4 days, or 500 mg orally daily for 3 days).
2. For patients with comorbid medical conditions such as chronic heart, lung, liver, or kidney disease; diabetes mellitus; alcohol use disorder; malignancy; asplenia; immunosuppressant conditions or use of immunosuppressive drugs; or use of antibiotics within the previous 3 months (in which case an agent from a different antibiotic class should be selected):
   a. A macrolide *or* doxycycline (as above) *plus* an oral beta-lactam (amoxicillin/clavulanate 500 mg/125 mg three times daily, amoxicillin/clavulanate 875 mg/125 mg twice daily, amoxicillin/clavulanate 2 g/125 mg twice daily; cefpodoxime, 200 mg twice daily; cefuroxime, 500 mg twice daily).
   b. Monotherapy with an oral fluoroquinolone (moxifloxacin, 400 mg daily; gemifloxacin, 320 mg daily; levofloxacin, 750 mg daily).

Inpatient management of nonsevere pneumonia (typically not requiring intensive care)

1. A respiratory fluoroquinolone. Oral and intravenous doses equivalent: moxifloxacin, 400 mg daily or levofloxacin, 500–750 mg daily *or*
2. A macrolide (see above for oral therapy) *plus* a beta-lactam (see above for oral beta-lactam therapy). For intravenous therapy: ampicillin/sulbactam, 1.5–3 g every 6 hours; cefotaxime, 1–2 g every 8 hours; ceftriaxone, 1–2 g every 12–24 hours; ceftaroline, 600 mg every 12 hours.
3. For patients with prior respiratory isolation of MRSA, strongly consider adding coverage for MRSA and obtain cultures or nasal PCR to confirm infection or to allow de-escalation of therapy: vancomycin, typically starting at 15 mg/kg intravenously every 12 hours with interval dosing based on kidney function to achieve serum trough concentration 15–20 mcg/mL *or* linezolid, 600 mg orally or intravenously every 12 hours.
4. For patients with prior respiratory isolation of *Pseudomonas aeruginosa*, strongly consider adding coverage for *P aeruginosa* and obtain cultures to confirm infection or to allow de-escalation of therapy. Intravenous therapy only: piperacillin-tazobactam, 3.375–4.5 g every 6 hours; cefepime, 1–2 g every 8 hours; imipenem, 0.5–1 g every 6 hours; meropenem, 1 g every 8 hours; or aztreonam 2 g every 8 hours.

Inpatient management of severe pneumonia (typically requiring intensive care). All agents administered intravenously, except as noted.

1. Azithromycin (500 mg orally as a first dose and then 250 mg orally daily for 4 days, or 500 mg orally daily for 3 days) *or* a respiratory fluoroquinolone (as above) plus an intravenous anti-pneumococcal beta-lactam (as above).
2. For patients allergic to beta-lactam antibiotics, a fluoroquinolone *plus* aztreonam (2 g every 8 hours).
3. For patients at risk for *P aeruginosa*, add coverage for *P aeruginosa* and obtain cultures to confirm infection or to allow de-escalation of therapy: piperacillin-tazobactam, 3.375–4.5 g every 6 hours; cefepime, 1–2 g every 8 hours; imipenem, 0.5–1 g every 6 hours; meropenem, 1 g every 8 hours; or aztreonam 2 g every 8 hours.
4. For patients at risk for *Pseudomonas* infection AND who are critically ill, at increased risk for drug resistance, or if local incidence of monotherapy-resistant *Pseudomonas* is > 10%, consider adding either
   a. An anti-pseudomonal fluoroquinolone (ciprofloxacin 400 mg every 8–12 hours or levofloxacin 750 mg daily) *or*
   b. An aminoglycoside (gentamicin, tobramycin, amikacin, all weight-based dosing administered daily adjusted to appropriate trough levels).
5. For patients at risk for MRSA infection, add coverage for MRSA and obtain cultures and/or nasal PCR to confirm infection or to allow de-escalation of therapy: vancomycin, typically starting at 15 mg/kg intravenously every 12 hours with interval dosing based on kidney function to achieve serum trough concentration 15–20 mcg/mL or linezolid, 600 mg every 12 hours.

MIC, minimum inhibitory concentration; MRSA, methicillin-resistant *Staphylococcus aureus*.
Recommendations assembled from Metlay JP et al; Diagnosis and treatment of adults with community-acquired pneumonia. An official clinical practice guideline of the American Thoracic Society and Infectious Diseases Society of America. Am J Respir Crit Care Med. 2019;200(7):e45–e67.

In outpatients with chronic heart, lung, liver, or kidney disease; diabetes mellitus; alcoholism; malignancy; or asplenia or who received antibiotic therapy within the past 90 days, the recommended treatment is a macrolide or doxycycline plus a beta-lactam (high-dose amoxicillin and amoxicillin-clavulanate are preferred to cefpodoxime and cefuroxime) or monotherapy with a respiratory fluoroquinolone (moxifloxacin, gemifloxacin, or levofloxacin).

The default duration of antibiotic therapy for CAP should be 5 days; factors that may affect therapy duration are clinical stability, etiology (MRSA and *P aeruginosa* require 7 days of therapy, for example), severity of illness, complications, and comorbid medical problems.

B. Treatment of Hospitalized and ICU Patients

1. Antibiotics—The most common etiologies of CAP in patients who require hospitalization but not intensive care are *S pneumoniae*, *M pneumoniae*, *C pneumoniae*, *H influenzae*, *Legionella* species, and respiratory viruses. Some patients have aspiration as an immediate precipitant to the CAP without a specific bacterial etiology. First-line therapy in hospitalized patients is the combination of a macrolide (clarithromycin or azithromycin) plus a beta-lactam (cefotaxime, ceftriaxone, ceftaroline, or ampicillin-sulbactam) or monotherapy with a respiratory fluoroquinolone (eg, moxifloxacin, gemifloxacin, or levofloxacin) (see Table 9–9).

Almost all patients admitted to a hospital for treatment of CAP receive intravenous antibiotics. However, no studies in hospitalized patients demonstrated superior outcomes with intravenous antibiotics compared with oral antibiotics, provided patients were able to tolerate oral therapy and the medication was well absorbed. Duration of inpatient antibiotic treatment is the same as for outpatients.

The most common etiologies of CAP in patients who require admission to intensive care are *S pneumoniae*, *Legionella* species, *H influenzae*, Enterobacteriaceae species, *S aureus*, *Pseudomonas* species, and respiratory viruses. First-line antibacterial therapy in ICU patients with CAP is an anti-pneumococcal beta-lactam (cefotaxime, ceftriaxone, ceftaroline, or ampicillin-sulbactam) *plus* either azithromycin or a respiratory fluoroquinolone (moxifloxacin, gemifloxacin, or levofloxacin).

Risk factors for *Pseudomonas*, Enterobacteriaceae, or MRSA infection must be considered when choosing empiric antibiotic therapy for inpatients with CAP. Specific risk factors for these organisms include (1) prior isolation of the pathogen, (2) inpatient hospitalization within the last 90 days, or (3) exposure to intravenous antibiotics within the last 90 days. In patients with specific risk factors for *Pseudomonas* infection, combine an anti-pneumococcal, anti-pseudomonal beta-lactam (piperacillin-tazobactam, cefepime, imipenem, meropenem) with either azithromycin or a respiratory fluoroquinolone (moxifloxacin, gemifloxacin, or levofloxacin). In critically ill patients, in those at increased risk for drug resistance, or if the unit incidence of monotherapy-resistant *Pseudomonas* is greater than 10%, consider use of two agents with anti-pseudomonal efficacy: either ciprofloxacin or levofloxacin plus the above anti-pneumococcal, anti-pseudomonal beta-lactam **or** an anti-pneumococcal, anti-pseudomonal beta-lactam plus an aminoglycoside (gentamicin, tobramycin, amikacin) plus either azithromycin or a respiratory fluoroquinolone. Patients with specific risk factors for MRSA should be treated with vancomycin or linezolid. Patients with very severe disease (respiratory failure requiring mechanical ventilation or septic shock) should also be strongly considered for MRSA therapy. Provided the patient is clinically improving, negative sputum and blood cultures obtained prior to initiation of antibiotics can support de-escalation of antibiotic therapy. Additionally, all patients prescribed vancomycin or linezolid should have swabs of the nasal passages for MRSA; if the swab results are negative, MRSA coverage can be safely de-escalated, even when adequate sputum samples have not been obtained.

Patients with CAP in whom influenza is detected should be treated with the antiviral oseltamavir, whether influenza is identified as a single pathogen or as a coinfection along with a bacterial pathogen. Oseltamavir treatment is most effective when begun within 2 days but may still be beneficial within several days after symptom onset, particularly in severe cases of CAP.

2. Adjunctive treatment—Conflicting data have emerged from RCTs regarding adjunctive treatment with corticosteroids in CAP. Meta-analyses of large studies have failed to find a mortality benefit in association with corticosteroid use in mild or moderate CAP, though there may be benefit in severe disease. Based on limited data and because of the potential for complications (eg, hyperglycemia), the 2019 Infectious Diseases Society of America/American Thoracic Society (IDSA/ATS) guidelines recommend against corticosteroids in the treatment CAP of any severity. Corticosteroid treatment of influenza pneumonia may be associated with higher mortality and should be avoided. Corticosteroid treatment is recommended for SARS-CoV-2 pneumonia when oxygen is required; see Chapter 32 for further discussion. Corticosteroids are recommended to be started or continued in patients with CAP who may also have severe septic shock, acute exacerbation of asthma or COPD, or adrenal insufficiency.

Prevention

Pneumococcal vaccines prevent or lessen the severity of pneumococcal infections in immunocompetent patients. Two pneumococcal vaccines for adults are available and approved for use in the United States: one containing capsular polysaccharide antigens of 23 common strains of *S pneumoniae* (Pneumovax 23) and a conjugate vaccine containing 13 common strains (Prevnar-13). Current recommendations are for sequential administration of the two vaccines in those aged 65 years or older and in immunocompromised persons, starting with Prevnar-13. Adults with chronic illness that increases the risk of CAP (see Chapter 30) should receive the 23-valent vaccine regardless of age. Immunocompromised patients and those at highest risk for fatal pneumococcal infections should receive a single revaccination of the 23-valent vaccine 5 years after the first vaccination regardless of age. Immunocompetent persons 65 years of age or older should receive a second dose of the 23-valent vaccine if the patient first received the vaccine 6 or more years previously and was under 65 years old at the time of first vaccination.

The seasonal influenza vaccine is effective in preventing severe disease due to influenza virus with a resulting positive impact on both primary influenza pneumonia and secondary bacterial pneumonias. The seasonal influenza vaccine is recommended annually for all persons older than 6 months without contraindications, with priority given to persons at risk for complications of influenza infection (persons aged 50 years or older, immunocompromised persons, residents of long-term care facilities, patients with pulmonary or cardiovascular disorders, pregnant women) as well as health care workers and others who may transmit influenza to high-risk patients.

Vaccinations against SARS-CoV-2 are recommended for all adults without contraindications. Vaccinations (including boosters) reduce the likelihood of infection, pneumonia, hospitalization, and mortality (see COVID-19 discussion, Chapter 32).

Hospitalized patients who would benefit from pneumococcal and influenza vaccines should be vaccinated during hospitalization. The two vaccines may be administered simultaneously as soon as the patient has stabilized.

When to Admit

Once a diagnosis of CAP is made, the first management decision is to determine the site of care: Is it safe to treat the patient at home or does he or she require hospital or intensive care admission? There are two widely used clinical prediction rules available to guide admission and triage decisions, the **Pneumonia Severity Index (PSI)** and the **CURB-65.**

A. Hospital Admission Decision

The PSI is a validated prediction model that uses 20 items from demographics, medical history, physical examination, laboratory results, and imaging to stratify patients into five risk groups. The PSI is weighted toward discrimination at low predicted mortality. In conjunction with clinical judgment, it facilitates safe decisions to treat CAP in the outpatient setting. An online PSI risk calculator is available at https://www.thecalculator.co/health/Pneumonia-Severity-Index-(PSI)-Calculator-977.html. The CURB-65 assesses five simple, independent predictors of increased mortality (**C**onfusion, **U**remia, **R**espiratory rate, **B**lood pressure, and age greater than **65**) to calculate a 30-day predicted mortality (https://www.mdcalc.com/curb-65-score-pneumonia-severity). Compared with the PSI, the simpler CURB-65 is less discriminating at low mortality but excellent at identifying patients with high mortality who may benefit from ICU-level care. A modified version (CRB-65) dispenses with BUN and eliminates the need for laboratory testing. Both have the advantage of simplicity: patients with zero CRB-65 predictors have a low predicted mortality (less than 1%) and usually do not need hospitalization; hospitalization should be considered for those with one or two predictors, since they have an increased risk of death; and urgent hospitalization (with consideration of ICU admission) is required for those with three or four predictors.

Hospital admission decision should also include circumstances of care independent of pneumonia severity, including comorbidities and the patient's ability to care for themselves effectively at home.

B. ICU Admission Decision

Expert opinion has defined major and minor criteria to identify patients at high risk for death. Major criteria are septic shock with need for vasopressor support and respiratory failure with need for mechanical ventilation. Minor criteria are respiratory rate = 30 breaths or more per minute, hypoxemia (defined as Pao_2/Fio_2 = 250 or less), hypothermia (core temperature less than 36.0°C), hypotension requiring aggressive fluid resuscitation, confusion/disorientation, multilobar pulmonary opacities, leukopenia due to infection with WBC less than 4000/mcL (less than 4.0×10^9/L), thrombocytopenia with platelet count less than 100,000/mcL (less than 100×10^9/L), uremia with BUN = 20 mg/dL or more (7.1 mmol/L or more), metabolic acidosis, or elevated serum lactate level. Either one major criterion or three or more minor criteria of illness severity generally require ICU-level care.

Ebell MH et al. Accuracy of biomarkers for the diagnosis of adult community-acquired pneumonia: a meta-analysis. Acad Emerg Med. 2020;27:195. [PMID: 32100377]

López-Alcalde J et al. Short-course versus long-course therapy of the same antibiotic for community-acquired pneumonia in adolescent and adult outpatients. Cochrane Database Syst Rev. 2018;9:CD009070. [PMID: 30188565]

Metlay JP et al. Diagnosis and treatment of adults with community-acquired pneumonia. An Official Clinical Practice Guideline of the American Thoracic Society and Infectious Diseases Society of America. Am J Respir Crit Care Med. 2019;200:e45. [PMID: 31573350]

Ramirez JA et al. Treatment of community-acquired pneumonia in immunocompromised adults: a consensus statement regarding initial strategies. Chest. 2020;158:1896. [PMID: 32561442]

Torres A et al. Challenges in severe community-acquired pneumonia: a point-of-view review. Intensive Care Med. 2019;45: 159. [PMID: 30706119]

2. Nosocomial Pneumonia (Hospital-Acquired & Ventilator-Associated)

ESSENTIALS OF DIAGNOSIS

- **Hospital-acquired pneumonia (HAP)** is diagnosed in patients with clinical features and imaging consistent with pneumonia, occurring > 48 hours after admission to the hospital and excluding any infections present at the time of admission.
- **Ventilator-associated pneumonia (VAP)** requires clinical features concerning for new pneumonia with positive respiratory samples developing > 48 hours following endotracheal intubation and mechanical ventilation.

General Considerations

Hospitalized patients carry different flora with different resistance patterns than healthy patients in the community, and their health status may place them at higher risk for more severe infection. The diagnostic approach and antibiotic treatment of patients with HAP is, therefore, different from patients with CAP. Similarly, management of patients in whom VAP develops following endotracheal intubation and mechanical ventilation should address issues specific to this group of patients.

Considered together, these nosocomial pneumonias (HAP or VAP) represent an important cause of morbidity and mortality despite widespread use of preventive measures, advances in diagnostic testing, and potent new antimicrobial agents. HAP is one of the most common causes of infection among hospital inpatients and carries the highest burden of morbidity and mortality. Patients in ICUs and those who are being mechanically ventilated are at the highest risk for HAP (and VAP) and experience higher morbidity and mortality from them than other inpatients. Definitive identification of the infectious cause of a lower respiratory infection is rarely available on presentation;

initial antibiotic treatment is therefore empiric and informed by epidemiologic and patient data rather than pathogen directed.

Definition & Pathogenesis

HAP develops more than 48 hours after admission to the hospital and VAP develops in a mechanically ventilated patient more than 48 hours after endotracheal intubation. Three factors distinguish nosocomial pneumonia from CAP: (1) different infectious causes; (2) different antibiotic susceptibility patterns, specifically, a higher incidence of drug resistance; and (3) poorer underlying health status of patients putting them at risk for more severe infections. Since access to the lower respiratory tract occurs primarily through microaspiration, nosocomial pneumonia starts with a change in upper respiratory tract flora. Colonization of the pharynx and possibly the stomach with bacteria is the most important step in the pathogenesis of nosocomial pneumonia. Pharyngeal colonization is promoted by exogenous factors (eg, instrumentation of the upper airway with nasogastric and endotracheal tubes; contact with personnel, equipment, and contaminated aerosols; treatment with broad-spectrum antibiotics that promote the emergence of drug-resistant organisms); and patient factors (eg, malnutrition, advanced age, altered consciousness, swallowing disorders, and underlying pulmonary and systemic diseases). Impaired cellular and mechanical defense mechanisms in the lungs of hospitalized patients raise the risk of infection after aspiration has occurred.

Gastric acid may play a role in protection against nosocomial pneumonias. Observational studies have suggested that elevation of gastric pH due to antacids, H_2-receptor antagonists, PPIs, or enteral feeding is associated with gastric microbial overgrowth, tracheobronchial colonization, and HAP/VAP. Moreover, a 2018 meta-analysis of randomized controlled trials suggested an increased risk of HAP among enterally fed patients receiving stress ulcer prophylaxis. The IDSA and other professional organizations recommend that acid-suppressive medications (H_2-receptor antagonists and PPIs) be given only to patients at high risk for stress gastritis.

The microbiology of the nosocomial pneumonias differs from CAP but is substantially the same among HAP and VAP. The most common organisms responsible for HAP and VAP include *S aureus* (both methicillin-sensitive *S aureus* and MRSA), *P aeruginosa*, gram-negative rods, including extended spectrum beta-lactamase (ESBL)–producing organisms (*Enterobacter* species, *K pneumoniae*, and *Escherichia coli*) and non-ESBL-producing organisms. VAP patients may be infected with *Acinetobacter* species and *S maltophilia*. Anaerobic organisms (*Bacteroides*, anaerobic streptococci, *Fusobacterium*) may also cause pneumonia in the hospitalized patient; when these organisms are isolated, they are commonly part of a polymicrobial flora. VAP occurring before hospital day 4 in a previous healthy person with no antibiotic exposure is more likely to involve oral flora with minimal resistance profiles than multidrug-resistant pathogens. However, multidrug-resistant pathogens may complicate early-onset VAP in patients with antibiotic exposure in preceding 90 days, recent hospitalization, or prior colonization with multidrug-resistant pathogens.

Clinical Findings

A. Symptoms and Signs

The symptoms and signs associated with nosocomial pneumonias are nonspecific. However, two or more clinical findings (fever, leukocytosis, purulent sputum, worsening respiratory status) along with one or more new or progressive pulmonary opacities on chest imaging are characteristic features of nosocomial pneumonia. Other findings include those listed above for CAP.

The differential diagnosis of new lower respiratory tract symptoms and signs in hospitalized patients includes heart failure, atelectasis, aspiration, ARDS, pulmonary thromboembolism, pulmonary hemorrhage, and medication reactions.

B. Laboratory Findings

Diagnostic evaluation for suspected nosocomial pneumonia includes blood cultures from two different sites. Blood cultures can identify the pathogen in 15–20% of patients with nosocomial pneumonias; positivity is associated with increased risk of complications and other sites of infection. Blood counts and clinical chemistry tests do not establish a specific diagnosis; however, they help define the severity of illness and identify complications. Serum procalcitonin levels are not sufficiently sensitive to rule out HAP or VAP but may allow discontinuation of antibiotic therapy. Thoracentesis for pleural fluid analysis should be considered in patients with pleural effusions.

Examination of lower respiratory tract secretions is attended by the same disadvantages as in CAP. Gram stains and cultures of sputum are neither sensitive nor specific in the diagnosis of nosocomial pneumonias; sensitivity of sputum results further decreases following antibiotic therapy, particularly after 72 hours of antibiotics. The identification of a bacterial organism by culture of lower respiratory tract secretions does not prove that the organism is a lower respiratory tract pathogen; however, it can be used to help identify bacterial antibiotic sensitivity patterns and as a guide to adjusting empiric therapy. Nasal swab for PCR detection of MRSA is recommended to guide de-escalation of broad-spectrum antibiotic therapy in patients with HAP and VAP.

C. Imaging

Radiographic findings in HAP/VAP are nonspecific and often confounded by other processes that led initially to hospitalization or ICU admission. (See CAP above.) Imaging may demonstrate complicating features including effusion, cavitation, or barotrauma.

D. Special Examinations

When HAP is suspected in a patient who subsequently requires mechanical ventilation, secretions may be obtained by spontaneous expectoration, sputum induction, nasotracheal suctioning, and endotracheal aspiration (qualitative or semiquantitative samples), or more invasively via bronchoscopic sampling of the lower airways secretions (quantitative samples). The best approach remains a matter of debate, since qualitative or semiquantitative samples are more likely to return nonpathogenic organisms and are, thus, associated with higher antibiotic exposure (without improvement in mortality), while invasive quantitative sampling increases cost and patient risk. Invasive qualitative sampling is universally recommended when the patient does not improve during initial therapy directed at expected or isolated pathogens, or in immunocompromised persons in whom an opportunistic pathogen is suspected. Bronchoscopic sampling may also increase the diagnostic yield and identification of bacterial coinfection in patients intubated for SARS-CoV-2 pneumonia.

▶ Treatment

The initial treatment of HAP and VAP is based on risk factors for MRSA and multiple drug-resistant pathogens (Table 9–10) as well as local antibiograms and mortality risk and is thus empiric (Table 9–11). The predictive capability of sets of risk factors for drug-resistant organisms in nosocomial pneumonia vary locally; strongest predictive factors include prior isolation of drug-resistant organisms, a high local prevalence of drug-resistant organisms, and antibiotic exposure within prior 90 days. Each hospital should generate antibiograms to guide the optimal choice of antibiotics with the goals of reducing exposure to unnecessary antibiotics and the development of antibiotic resistance, thus minimizing patient harm. Because of the high mortality rate, therapy should be started as soon as HAP or VAP is suspected. After results of cultures are available, it may be possible to narrow initially broad therapy to more specific agents. Endotracheal aspiration cultures have significant negative predictive value but limited positive predictive value in the diagnosis of specific infectious causes of HAP/VAP. If an invasive diagnostic approach to suspected VAP using quantitative culture of bronchoalveolar lavage (BAL), protected specimen brush (PSB), or blind bronchial sampling (BBS) is used, antibiotics can be withheld when results are below a diagnostic threshold (BAL less than 10^4 CFU/mL, PSB or BBS less than 10^3 CFU/mL). Duration of antibiotic therapy is 7 days, consistent with clinical response, but should be individualized based on the pathogen, severity of illness, response to therapy, and comorbid conditions.

For expanded discussions of specific antibiotics, see Chapter 30.

Table 9–10. Risk factors for multidrug-resistant (MDR) pathogens, methicillin-resistant *Staphylococcus aureus* (MRSA), and *Pseudomonas* and other gram-negative bacilli in patients with hospital-acquired pneumonia (HAP) and ventilator-associated pneumonia (VAP).

Risk factors for MDR pathogens
Antibiotic therapy in the preceding 90 days
Septic shock
Acute respiratory distress syndrome preceding VAP
≥ 5 days in hospital prior to occurrence of HAP/VAP
Acute renal replacement therapy prior to HAP/VAP onset
Treatment in a unit where > 10% of gram-negative isolates are resistant to an agent being considered for monotherapy
Treatment in a unit where local antibiotic susceptibility rates are not known
Risk factors for MRSA
Antibiotic therapy in the preceding 90 days
Renal replacement therapy in the preceding 30 days
Use of gastric acid suppressive agents
Positive culture or prior MRSA colonization, especially in the preceding 90 days
Hospitalization in a unit where > 20% of *S aureus* isolates are MRSA
Hospitalization in a unit where prevalence of MRSA is not known
Risk factors for *Pseudomonas aeruginosa* and other gram-negative bacilli
Antibiotic therapy in the preceding 90 days
Structural lung disease (COPD, especially with recurrent exacerbations; bronchiectasis; or cystic fibrosis)
Recent hospitalizations, especially with manipulation of the aerodigestive tract (nasoenteric nutrition, intubation)
High-quality Gram stain of respiratory secretions with numerous and predominant gram-negative bacilli
Positive culture for *P aeruginosa* in the past year

Data from Kalil AC et al. Management of adults with hospital-acquired and ventilator-associated pneumonia: 2016 Clinical Practice Guidelines by the Infectious Diseases Society of America and the American Thoracic Society. Clin Infect Dis. 2016;63:e61.

Carr C et al. Ventilator-associated pneumonia: how do the different criteria for diagnosis match up? Am Surg. 2019;85:992. [PMID: 31638512]

Kalil AC et al. Management of adults with hospital-acquired and ventilator-associated pneumonia: 2016 Clinical Practice Guidelines by the Infectious Diseases Society of America and the American Thoracic Society. Clin Infect Dis. 2016;63:e61. [PMID: 27418577]

Lanks CW et al. Community-acquired pneumonia and hospital-acquired pneumonia. Med Clin North Am. 2019;103:487. [PMID: 30955516]

Papazian L et al. Ventilator-associated pneumonia in adults: a narrative review. Intensive Care Med. 2020;46:888. [PMID: 32157357]

Ranzani OT et al. Invasive and non-invasive diagnostic approaches for microbiological diagnosis of hospital-acquired pneumonia. Crit Care. 2019;23:51. [PMID: 30777114]

3. Anaerobic Pneumonia & Lung Abscess

ESSENTIALS OF DIAGNOSIS

- History of or predisposition to aspiration.
- Indolent symptoms, including fever, weight loss, and malaise.
- Poor dentition.
- Foul-smelling purulent sputum (in many patients).
- Infiltrate in dependent lung zone, with single or multiple areas of cavitation or pleural effusion.

Table 9–11. Recommended initial empiric antibiotics for hospital-acquired pneumonia (HAP) and ventilator-associated pneumonia (VAP).

HAP not at high risk for mortality, or VAP with no risk factors for MRSA, MDR, or *Pseudomonas* and other gram-negative bacilli

- USE **one** of the following:
  - Piperacillin-tazobactam, 4.5 g intravenously every 6 hours[1]
  - Cefepime, 2 g intravenously every 8 hours[1]
  - Levofloxacin, 750 mg intravenously daily
  - Imipenem, 500 mg intravenously every 6 hours[1]
  - Meropenem, 1 g intravenously every 8 hours[1]

HAP or VAP with risk factors for MRSA but no risk factors for MDR, *Pseudomonas*, and other gram-negative bacilli

- USE **one** of the following:
  - Piperacillin-tazobactam, 4.5 g intravenously every 6 hours[1]
  - Cefepime, 2 g intravenously every 8 hours[1]
  - Ceftazidime, 2 g intravenously every 8 hours
  - Levofloxacin, 750 mg intravenously daily
  - Ciprofloxacin, 400 mg intravenously every 8 hours
  - Imipenem, 500 mg intravenously every 6 hours[1]
  - Meropenem, 1 g intravenously every 8 hours[1]
  - Aztreonam, 2 g intravenously every 8 hours
- PLUS **one** of the following:
  - Vancomycin, 15 mg/kg intravenously every 8–12 hours with goal to target trough level = 15–20 mg/mL (consider a loading dose of 25–30 mg/kg once for severe illness)[2]
  - Linezolid, 600 mg intravenously every 12 hours

HAP with risk factors for *Pseudomonas* and other gram-negative bacilli, but no risk factors for MRSA and not at high risk for mortality

- USE **one** of the following:
  - Piperacillin-tazobactam, 4.5 g intravenously every 6 hours[1]
  - Cefepime, 2 g intravenously every 8 hours[1]
  - Ceftazidime, 2 g intravenously every 8 hours
  - Imipenem, 500 mg intravenously every 6 hours[1]
  - Meropenem, 1 g intravenously every 8 hours[1]
  - Aztreonam, 2 g intravenously every 8 hours
- PLUS **one** of the following:
  - Levofloxacin, 750 mg intravenously daily
  - Ciprofloxacin, 400 mg intravenously every 8 hours
  - Gentamicin, 5–7 mg/kg intravenously daily[2]
  - Tobramycin, 5–7 mg/kg intravenously daily[2]
  - Aztreonam, 2 g intravenously every 8 hours

HAP at high risk for mortality or VAP with risk factors for MRSA *and* risk factors for MDR, *Pseudomonas*, and other gram-negative bacilli

- USE **one** of the following:
  - Piperacillin-tazobactam, 4.5 g intravenously every 6 hours[1]
  - Cefepime, 2 g intravenously every 8 hours[1]
  - Ceftazidime, 2 g intravenously every 8 hours
  - Imipenem, 500 mg intravenously every 6 hours[1]
  - Meropenem, 1 g intravenously every 8 hours[1]
  - Aztreonam, 2 g intravenously every 8 hours
- PLUS **one** of the following:
  - Levofloxacin, 750 mg intravenously daily
  - Ciprofloxacin, 400 mg intravenously every 8 hours
  - Amikacin, 15–20 mg/kg intravenously daily[2]
  - Gentamicin, 5–7 mg/kg intravenously daily[2]
  - Tobramycin, 5–7 mg/kg intravenously daily[2]
  - Meropenem, 1 g intravenously every 8 hours[1]
  - Polymyxin B, 2.5–3.0 mg/kg per day divided in 2 daily intravenous doses
  - Colistin: consult clinical pharmacist for assistance with dosing
- PLUS **one** of the following:
  - Vancomycin, 15 mg/kg intravenously every 8–12 hours with goal to target trough level = 15–20 mg/mL (consider a loading dose of 25–30 mg/kg once for severe illness)[2]
  - Linezolid, 600 mg intravenously every 12 hours

CrCl, creatinine clearance; MDR, multidrug resistant; MRSA, methicillin-resistant *Staphylococcus aureus*.

[1]Extended infusions may be appropriate.

[2]Drug level monitoring and adjustment of dosing are required.

Data from Kalil AC et al. Management of adults with hospital-acquired and ventilator-associated pneumonia: 2016 Clinical Practice Guidelines by the Infectious Diseases Society of America and the American Thoracic Society. Clin Infect Dis. 2016;63:e61.

General Considerations

Aspiration of small amounts of oropharyngeal secretions occurs during sleep in normal individuals but rarely causes disease. Sequelae of aspiration of larger amounts of material include nocturnal asthma, chemical pneumonitis, mechanical obstruction of airways by particulate matter, bronchiectasis, and pleuropulmonary infection. Individuals predisposed to disease induced by aspiration include those with depressed levels of consciousness due to drug or alcohol use, seizures, general anesthesia, or CNS disease; those with impaired deglutition due to esophageal disease or neurologic disorders; and those with tracheal or nasogastric tubes, which disrupt the mechanical defenses of the airways.

Periodontal disease and poor dental hygiene, which increase the number of anaerobic bacteria in aspirated material, are associated with a greater likelihood of anaerobic pleuropulmonary infection. Aspiration of infected oropharyngeal contents initially leads to pneumonia in dependent lung zones, such as the posterior segments of the upper lobes and superior and basilar segments of the lower lobes. Body position at the time of aspiration determines which lung zones are dependent. The onset of symptoms is insidious. By the time the patient seeks medical attention, necrotizing pneumonia, lung abscess, or empyema may be apparent.

In most cases of aspiration and necrotizing pneumonia, lung abscess, and empyema, multiple species of anaerobic bacteria are causing the infection. Most of the remaining cases are caused by infection with both anaerobic and aerobic bacteria. *Prevotella melaninogenica*, *Peptostreptococcus*, *Fusobacterium nucleatum*, and *Bacteroides* species are commonly isolated anaerobic bacteria.

Clinical Findings

A. Symptoms and Signs

Patients with anaerobic pleuropulmonary infection usually present with constitutional symptoms, such as fever, weight loss, and malaise. Cough with expectoration of foul-smelling purulent sputum suggests anaerobic infection, though the absence of productive cough does not rule out such an infection. Dentition is often poor. Patients are rarely edentulous; if so, an obstructing bronchial lesion may be present.

B. Laboratory Findings

Expectorated sputum cultures may be difficult to interpret due to contaminating upper respiratory tract flora, but high colony count of a particular microorganism on Gram stain or in culture likely represents a true pathogen. Anaerobes and facultative anaerobes are difficult to recover on any culture, particularly following initiation of antibiotics; pleural fluid from empyema may be revealing.

C. Imaging

The different types of anaerobic pleuropulmonary infection are distinguished by their radiographic appearance. **Lung abscess** appears as a thick-walled solitary cavity surrounded by consolidation. An air-fluid level is usually present. Other causes of cavitary lung disease (tuberculosis, mycosis, cancer, infarction, necrobiotic nodules in rheumatoid arthritis, and pulmonary vasculitides) should be excluded. **Necrotizing pneumonia** is distinguished by multiple areas of cavitation within an area of consolidation. **Empyema** is characterized by the presence of purulent pleural fluid and may accompany either of the other two radiographic findings. Ultrasonography is of value in locating fluid and may also reveal pleural loculations.

Treatment

Medications of choice are directed at anaerobic organisms or facultative anaerobic streptococci and include a beta-lactam/lactamase inhibitor combination, carbapenem, or clindamycin. Second-line therapy includes a combination of penicillin and metronidazole. Duration of antibiotic therapy for anaerobic pneumonia is controversial, but it is usually given for a minimum of 3 weeks, with some experts recommending treatment until the abscess cavity has resolved on imaging.

Peripheral lung abscess must be carefully distinguished from empyema because empyema requires tube thoracostomy; if tube thoracostomy is placed inadvertently into an abscess cavity, complications, such as a bronchopleural fistula, may result. Thoracic surgery consultation is recommended for large or nonresolving abscesses or for abscesses that rupture into the pleural space. Rarely, a large abscess requires surgical intervention (percutaneous drainage, segmentectomy, lobectomy, or pneumonectomy).

Makhnevich A et al. Aspiration pneumonia in older adults. J Hosp Med. 2019;14:429. [PMID: 30794136]

Rolston KVI et al. Post-obstructive pneumonia in patients with cancer: a review. Infect Dis Ther. 2018;7:29. [PMID: 29392577]

PULMONARY INFILTRATES IN IMMUNOCOMPROMISED PATIENTS

Pulmonary infiltrates in immunocompromised patients (patients with HIV disease, absolute neutrophil counts less than 1000/mcL [less than 1.0×10^9/L], current or recent exposure to myelosuppressive or immunosuppressive medications, or those taking more than 20 mg/day of prednisone or equivalent for more than 4 weeks) may arise from infectious or noninfectious causes. Infection may be due to bacterial, mycobacterial, fungal, protozoal, helminthic, or viral pathogens. Noninfectious processes, such as pulmonary edema, alveolar hemorrhage, medication reactions, pulmonary thromboembolic disease, malignancy, and radiation pneumonitis, may mimic infection.

Although almost any pathogen can cause pneumonia in an immunocompromised patient, two clinical tools help the clinician narrow the differential diagnosis. The first is knowledge of the underlying immunologic defect. Specific immunologic defects are associated with particular infections. Defects in humoral immunity predispose to bacterial infections; defects in cellular immunity lead to infections with viruses, fungi, mycobacteria, and protozoa. Neutropenia and impaired granulocyte function predispose to infections from *S aureus*, *Aspergillus*, gram-negative bacilli, and *Candida*. Second, the time course of infection also provides clues to the etiology of pneumonia in immunocompromised patients. A fulminant pneumonia is often caused by bacterial infection, whereas an insidious pneumonia is more apt to be caused by viral, fungal, protozoal, or mycobacterial infection. Pneumonia occurring within 2–4 weeks after organ transplantation is usually bacterial, whereas several months or more after transplantation, *P jirovecii*, viruses (eg, cytomegalovirus) and fungi (eg, *Aspergillus*) are encountered more often.

Clinical Findings

Chest radiography is rarely helpful in narrowing the differential diagnosis. Examination of expectorated sputum for bacteria, fungi, mycobacteria, *Legionella*, and *P jirovecii* is important and may preclude the need for expensive, invasive diagnostic procedures. Sputum induction is often necessary for diagnosis. The sensitivity of induced sputum for detection of *P jirovecii* depends on institutional expertise, number of specimens analyzed, and detection methods.

Routine evaluation frequently fails to identify a causative organism. The clinician may begin empiric antimicrobial therapy before proceeding to invasive procedures, such as bronchoscopy, transthoracic needle aspiration, or open lung biopsy. The approach to management must be based on the severity of the pulmonary infection, the underlying disease, the risks of empiric therapy, and local expertise and experience with diagnostic procedures. BAL using flexible bronchoscopy is a safe and effective method for obtaining representative pulmonary secretions for microbiologic studies. It involves less risk of bleeding and other complications than transbronchial biopsy. BAL is especially suitable for the diagnosis of *P jirovecii* pneumonia in patients with HIV/AIDS when induced sputum analysis is negative. Surgical lung biopsy, now often performed by video-assisted thoracoscopy, provides the definitive option for diagnosis of pulmonary infiltrates in immunocompromised patients; however, a specific diagnosis is obtained in only about two-thirds of cases, and the information obtained may not affect the outcome.

Cillóniz C et al. *Pneumocystis* pneumonia in the twenty-first century: HIV-infected versus HIV-uninfected patients. Expert Rev Anti Infect Ther. 2019;17:787. [PMID: 31550942]

Del Corpo O et al. Diagnostic accuracy of serum (1-3)-β-D-glucan for *Pneumocystis jirovecii* pneumonia: a systematic review and meta-analysis. Clin Microbiol Infect. 2020;26:1137. [PMID: 32479781]

Ghembaza A et al. Risk factors and prevention of *Pneumocystis jirovecii* pneumonia in patients with autoimmune and inflammatory diseases. Chest. 2020;158:2323. [PMID: 32502592]

Haydour Q et al. Diagnosis of fungal infections: a systematic review and meta-analysis supporting American Thoracic Society Practice Guideline. Ann Am Thorac Soc. 2019;16:1179. [PMID: 3121934]

Kato H et al. Diagnosis and treatment of *Pneumocystis jirovecii* pneumonia in HIV-infected or non-HIV-infected patients-difficulties in diagnosis and adverse effects of trimethoprim-sulfamethoxazole. J Infect Chemother. 2019;25:920. [PMID: 31300379]

PULMONARY TUBERCULOSIS

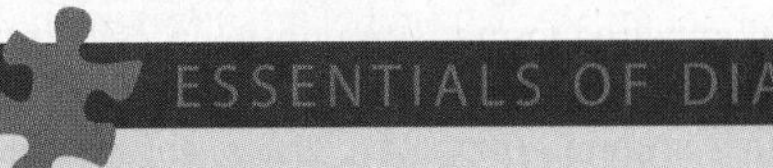

- Fatigue, weight loss, fever, night sweats, and productive cough.
- Risk factors for acquisition of infection: household exposure, incarceration, drug use, travel to or residence in endemic area.
- Chest radiograph: pulmonary opacities, including nodular or cavitating.
- Acid-fast bacilli on smear of sputum, rapid molecular testing positive, or sputum culture positive for *M tuberculosis*.

General Considerations

Tuberculosis is one of the world's most widespread and deadly illnesses. *M tuberculosis*, the organism that causes tuberculosis infection and disease, infects one-quarter of the world's population, nearly 2 billion people. Based on WHO data, there were 10 million new cases of tuberculosis worldwide in 2020 with 1.5 million people dying of the disease, a provisional increase in mortality for the first time since 2005, with a global increase in case-fatality rate to 15%. Reporting data suggest considerable disruption to tuberculosis diagnosis and treatment due to the COVID-19 pandemic. While most incident cases occur in low- and middle-income countries, tuberculosis is present in all regions of the world. In the United States, per the CDC, an estimated 13 million people are infected with *M tuberculosis*, and in 2020, there were 7174 reported active cases. Tuberculosis occurs disproportionately among disadvantaged populations, such as the malnourished, homeless, and those living in overcrowded and substandard housing. There is an increased occurrence of tuberculosis among HIV-positive individuals.

Infection with *M tuberculosis* begins when a susceptible person inhales airborne droplet nuclei containing viable organisms. Tubercle bacilli that reach the alveoli are ingested by alveolar macrophages. Infection follows if the inoculum escapes alveolar macrophage microbicidal activity. Once infection is established, lymphatic and hematogenous dissemination of tuberculosis typically occurs before the development of an effective immune response. This stage of infection, **primary tuberculosis,** is usually clinically and radiographically silent. In most persons with intact cell-mediated immunity, T-cells and macrophages surround the organisms in granulomas that limit their multiplication and spread. The infection is contained but not eradicated, since viable organisms may lie dormant within granulomas for years to decades.

Individuals with **latent tuberculosis infection** do not have active disease and cannot transmit the organism to others. However, reactivation of disease may occur if the patient's immune defenses are impaired. **Active tuberculosis** will develop in 5–15% of individuals with latent tuberculosis infection who are not given preventive therapy; half of these cases occur in the 2 years following primary infection. Diverse conditions such as gastrectomy, silicosis, diabetes mellitus, and an impaired immune response (eg, HIV infection; therapy with corticosteroids, tumor necrosis factor inhibitors or other immunosuppressive drugs) are associated with an increased risk of reactivation.

In approximately 5% of cases, the immune response is inadequate to contain the primary infection and **progressive primary tuberculosis** develops, accompanied by both pulmonary and constitutional symptoms. The clinical presentation does not definitively distinguish primary disease from reactivation of latent tuberculosis infection. Standard teaching has held that 90% of tuberculosis in adults represents activation of latent disease. However, DNA fingerprinting of the bacillus suggests that as many as one-third of new cases of tuberculosis in urban populations are primary infections resulting from person-to-person transmission.

The prevalence of drug-resistant strains is increasing worldwide, though in resourced countries including the United States, the rate of multidrug-resistant isolates has fallen to less than 1%. Risk factors for drug resistance include immigration from countries with a high prevalence of drug-resistant tuberculosis, close and prolonged contact with individuals with drug-resistant tuberculosis, unsuccessful previous therapy, and nonadherence to treatment. Drug resistance may be single or multiple. **Drug-resistant tuberculosis** is resistant to one first-line antituberculous drug, either isoniazid or rifampin. **Multidrug-resistant tuberculosis** is resistant to isoniazid and rifampin, and possibly additional agents. **Extensively drug-resistant tuberculosis** is resistant to isoniazid, rifampin, fluoroquinolones, and either aminoglycosides or capreomycin or both. Outcomes of drug-resistant tuberculosis treatment are worse than when the isolate is drug-sensitive, and outcomes appear to vary with HIV status. In a review of extensively drug-resistant tuberculosis cases in the United States, mortality was 10% in HIV-negative patients and 68% in HIV-positive patients.

Clinical Findings

A. Symptoms and Signs

The patient with pulmonary tuberculosis typically presents with slowly progressive constitutional symptoms of malaise, anorexia, weight loss, fever, and night sweats. Chronic cough is the most common pulmonary symptom. It may be dry at first but typically becomes productive of purulent sputum as the disease progresses. Blood-streaked sputum is common, but significant hemoptysis is rarely a presenting symptom; life-threatening hemoptysis may occur in advanced disease. Dyspnea is unusual unless there is extensive disease. On physical examination, the patient appears chronically ill and malnourished. On chest examination, there are no physical findings specific for tuberculosis infection. The examination may be normal or may reveal classic findings such as posttussive apical rales.

B. Laboratory Findings

Definitive diagnosis depends on recovery of *M tuberculosis* from cultures or identification of the organism by DNA or RNA amplification techniques (in concert with appropriate clinical context). At least three consecutive morning sputum specimens are advised, and samples should be collected 8 hours apart. Acid-fast staining of a sputum smear is performed initially as a screening method, with sensitivity and negative predictive values that are low (50–80%) with a single smear but may improve to 90% with serial sampling. Smear sensitivity is lower in HIV-coinfected patients. Demonstration of acid-fast bacilli on sputum smear does not establish a diagnosis of *M tuberculosis* since nontuberculous mycobacteria may colonize the airways and are increasingly recognized to cause clinical illness in patients with underlying structural lung disease.

In patients thought to have tuberculosis who cannot produce satisfactory specimens or when the smear of the spontaneously expectorated sputum is negative for acid-fast bacilli, sputum induction with 3% hypertonic saline should be performed. Flexible bronchoscopy with bronchial washings has similar diagnostic yield to induced sputum; transbronchial lung biopsies do not significantly increase the diagnostic yield but may lead to earlier diagnosis by identifying tissue granulomas. Post-bronchoscopy expectorated sputum specimens should be collected. Positive blood cultures for *M tuberculosis* are uncommon in patients with normal CD4 cell counts, but the organism may be cultured from blood in up to 50% of HIV-seropositive patients with tuberculosis whose CD4 cell counts are less than 100/mcL (less than 0.1×10^9/L); mycobacterial blood cultures should be obtained in such patients.

The slow rate of mycobacterial growth; the urgency to provide early, appropriate treatment to patients to improve their outcomes and limit community spread; and concerns about potential drug toxicities in patients treated empirically who do not have tuberculosis infection have fostered the use of rapid diagnostic techniques (Table 9–12). Molecular diagnostics offer multiple options and many advantages, though at increased expense. Nucleic acid amplification testing not only detects *M tuberculosis* (NAAT-TB) but also identifies resistance markers (NAAT-R). NAAT-TB can identify *M tuberculosis* within hours of sputum processing, allowing early isolation and treatment, though the negative predictive value is lower in smear-negative patients. NAAT-R allows rapid identification of primary drug resistance and has previously been indicated in the following patients: (1) those treated previously for tuberculosis, (2) those born (or who lived for more than 1 year) in a country with moderate tuberculosis incidence or a high incidence of multiple drug-resistant isolates, (3) contacts of patients with multidrug-resistant tuberculosis, or (4) those who are HIV seropositive. In view of the rapidity of result in concert with rifampin resistance identification, the WHO issued continued guidance in 2020 that rapid molecular testing is the ideal initial test for diagnosis and resistance profiling in persons in whom pulmonary or extrapulmonary tuberculosis is suspected.

Needle biopsy of the pleura reveals granulomatous inflammation in approximately 60% of patients with pleural effusions caused by *M tuberculosis*. Pleural fluid cultures are positive for *M tuberculosis* in 23–58% of cases of pleural tuberculosis. Culture of three pleural biopsy

Table 9–12. Essential laboratory tests for the detection of *Mycobacterium tuberculosis*.[1]

Test	Time to Result	Test Characteristics
Acid-fast bacilli light microscopy	1 day	Three morning specimens recommended. Combined sensitivity of 70% (54% for the first specimen, 11% for the second specimen, and 5% for the third specimen). First morning specimen increased yield by 12% compared to spot specimen.
Nucleic acid amplification test, detection (NAAT-TB)	1 day	Sensitivity/specificity high for smear-positive specimens, 85–97% for both; sensitivity falls in smear-negative specimens to ~66%. A positive NAAT in smear-negative patients with intermediate to high (> 30%) pretest probability of *M tuberculosis* infection is helpful while a negative NAAT is not. Should not be ordered in patients with low pretest probability of *M tuberculosis* infection.
Nucleic acid amplification test, resistance markers (NAAT-R)	1–2 days	Multiple assays for rifampin and isoniazid are available. Specificity uniformly high, > 98%. Sensitivity varies from about 84% to 96%, increases with multiple specimens. See text for indications for testing.
Mycobacterial growth detection Liquid (broth based) medium Solid (agar or egg based) medium	Up to 6–8 weeks Avg 10–14 days Avg 3–4 weeks	Liquid culture methods are more sensitive than solid culture methods (~90% and 76%, respectively) with shorter time to detection but higher contamination with bacterial growth. Specificity exceeds 99% for all methods.
Identification of *M tuberculosis* complex by DNA probe or high-performance liquid chromatography	1 day[1]	May be useful in areas of low *M tuberculosis* incidence where nontuberculous mycobacteria are commonly isolated.
First-line drug susceptibility testing (liquid medium)	1–2 weeks[1]	Gold standard. Should be performed routinely on the initial isolate.
Second-line and novel compound drug susceptibility testing Liquid (broth based) medium Solid (agar or egg based) medium	 1–2 weeks[1] 3–4 weeks[1]	

[1]Following detection of mycobacterial growth.
Adapted from Diagnostic Standards and Classification of Tuberculosis in Adults and Children. This official statement of the American Thoracic Society and the Centers for Disease Control and Prevention was adopted by the ATS Board of Directors, July 1999. This statement was endorsed by the Council of the Infectious Disease Society of America, September 1999. Am J Respir Crit Care Med. 2000;161:1376.

specimens combined with microscopic examination of a pleural biopsy yields a diagnosis in up to 90% of patients with pleural tuberculosis. Tests for pleural fluid adenosine deaminase (approximately 90% sensitivity and specificity for pleural tuberculosis at levels greater than 70 U/L) and interferon-gamma (89% sensitivity, 97% specificity in a recent meta-analysis) can be extremely helpful diagnostic aids, particularly in making decisions to pursue invasive testing in complex cases.

C. Imaging

Contrary to traditional teaching, molecular analysis demonstrates that radiographic abnormalities in pulmonary tuberculosis do not distinguish primary disease from reactivation of latent tuberculosis (Figure 9–4). The only independent predictor of an atypical pattern on chest radiograph—that is, not associated with upper lobe or cavitary disease—is an impaired patient immune response. The chest imaging pattern traditionally associated with primary disease includes small unilateral infiltrates, hilar and paratracheal lymph node enlargement, and segmental atelectasis. Pleural effusion is present in 30–40% of patients, sometimes as the sole radiographic abnormality. Reactivation tuberculosis traditionally has been associated with fibrocavitary apical disease, discrete nodules, and pneumonic infiltrates, usually in the apical or posterior segments of the upper lobes or in the superior segments of the lower lobes. Radiographic evidence of disease in other locations may be present in up to 30% of patients.

In elderly patients, lower lobe infiltrates with or without pleural effusion are frequently encountered. A "miliary" pattern (diffuse small nodular densities) can be seen with hematologic or lymphatic dissemination of the organism. Immunocompromised patients—particularly those with late-stage HIV infection—often display lower lung zone, diffuse, or miliary infiltrates; pleural effusions; and involvement of hilar and, in particular, mediastinal lymph nodes.

Resolution of active tuberculosis leaves characteristic radiographic findings. Dense nodules in the pulmonary hila, with or without obvious calcification, upper lobe fibronodular scarring, and bronchiectasis with volume loss are common findings. Ghon (calcified primary focus) and Ranke (calcified primary focus and calcified hilar lymph node) complexes are seen in a minority of patients.

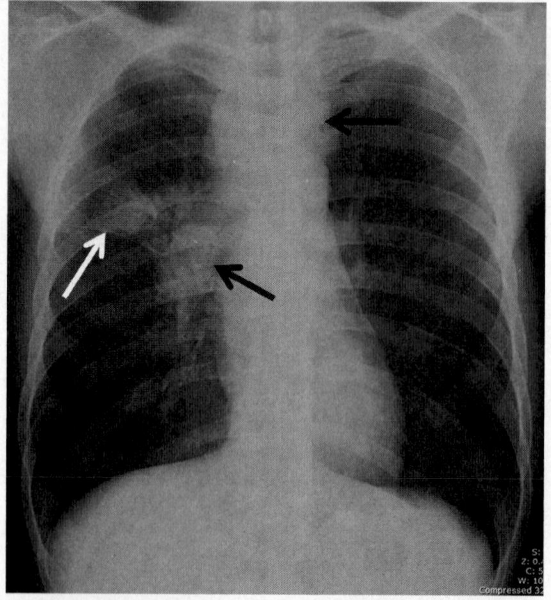

A

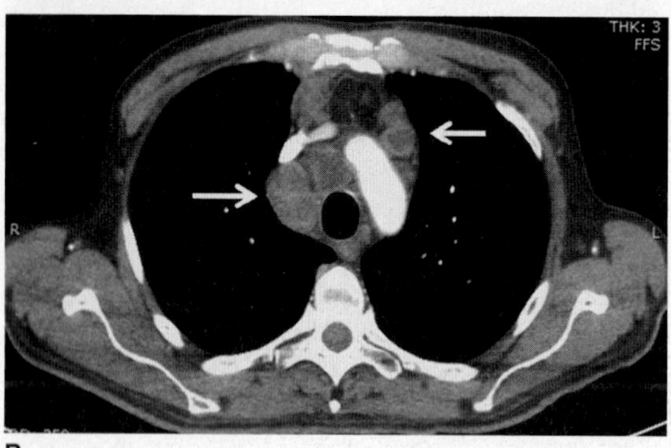

B

▲ **Figure 9–4.** Pulmonary tuberculosis. Primary pulmonary tuberculosis in a 20-year-old man with chest radiograph **(A)** showing right upper lobe consolidation (white arrow) and right hilar and mediastinal lymphadenopathy (black arrows) and contrast-enhanced CT scan **(B)** showing mediastinal lymphadenopathy (arrows). (Used, with permission, from Carlos Santiago Restrepo, MD, in Usatine RP, Smith MA, Mayeaux EJ Jr, Chumley H. *The Color Atlas of Family Medicine*, 2nd ed. McGraw-Hill, 2013.)

D. Special Examinations

Testing for latent tuberculosis infection is used to evaluate an asymptomatic person in whom *M tuberculosis* infection is suspected (eg, following contact exposure) or to establish the prevalence of tuberculosis infection in a population. Testing may be used in a person with symptoms of active tuberculosis, but a positive test does not distinguish between active and latent infection, and a negative test does not rule out active disease. Routine testing of individuals at low risk for tuberculosis is not recommended. Empiric treatment of latent tuberculosis without testing is considered appropriate in HIV-infected persons or in young (less than 5 years old) household contacts of persons with active tuberculosis in endemic areas.

The traditional approach to testing for latent tuberculosis infection is the **tuberculin skin test.** The Mantoux test is the preferred method: 0.1 mL of purified protein derivative (PPD) containing 5 tuberculin units is injected intradermally on the volar surface of the forearm using a 27-gauge needle on a tuberculin syringe. The **transverse width in millimeters of induration** at the skin test site is measured after 48–72 hours. To optimize test performance, criteria for determining a positive reaction vary depending on the likelihood of infection. Table 9–13 summarizes the criteria established by the CDC for interpretation of the Mantoux tuberculin skin test. Sensitivity and specificity of the tuberculin skin test are high: 77% and 97%, respectively. Specificity falls to 59% in populations previously vaccinated with bacillus Calmette-Guérin (BCG, an attenuated form of *Mycobacterium bovis*). False-negative tuberculin skin test reactions may result from improper testing technique; concurrent infections, including fulminant tuberculosis; malnutrition; advanced age; immunologic disorders; malignancy; corticosteroid therapy; CKD; and HIV infection. Some individuals with latent tuberculosis infection may have a negative tuberculin skin test when tested many years after exposure. Anergy testing is not recommended for routine use to distinguish a true-negative result from anergy. Poor anergy test standardization and lack of outcome data limit the evaluation of its effectiveness. Interpretation of the tuberculin skin test in persons who have previously received BCG vaccination is the same as in those who have not had BCG.

Interferon gamma release assays (including the QuantiFERON and T-SPOT tests) are in vitro assays of CD4+ T-cell–mediated interferon gamma release in response to stimulation by specific *M tuberculosis* antigens. The antigens are absent from all BCG strains and most nontuberculous mycobacteria; therefore, in whole blood, the specificity of interferon gamma release assays is superior to the tuberculin skin test in BCG-vaccinated individuals. Sensitivity is comparable to the tuberculin skin test: 60–90% depending on the specific assay and study population. Sensitivity is reduced by HIV infection, particularly in patients with low CD4 counts. Specificity is high, greater than 95%. Potential advantages of interferon gamma release assay testing include fewer false-positive results from prior BCG vaccination, better discrimination of positive responses due to nontuberculous mycobacteria, and the requirement for only one patient contact (ie, no need for the patient to return to have the tuberculin skin test read 48–72 hours later). Disadvantages include the need for specialized laboratory equipment and personnel and the substantially increased cost compared to the tuberculin skin test.

In endemic areas, interferon gamma release assays are no more sensitive than the tuberculin skin test in active tuberculosis (20–40% false-negative rate) and cannot distinguish active from latent disease. Interferon gamma release assays should not be used to exclude active tuberculosis.

Table 9–13. Classification of positive tuberculin skin test reactions.[1]

Induration Size	Group
≥ 5 mm	1. HIV-positive persons. 2. Recent contacts of a person with infectious tuberculosis. 3. Persons with fibrotic changes on chest radiographs suggestive of prior tuberculosis. 4. Patients with organ transplants and other immunosuppressed patients (receiving the equivalent of > 15 mg/day of prednisone for 1 month or more, or those taking TNF-alpha antagonists).
≥ 10 mm	1. Recent immigrants (< 5 years) from countries with a high prevalence of tuberculosis (eg, Asia, Africa, Latin America). 2. HIV-negative injection drug users. 3. Mycobacteriology laboratory personnel. 4. Residents of and employees in high-risk congregate settings: correctional institutions; long-term care facilities; hospitals and other health care facilities; residential facilities for HIV/AIDS patients; and homeless shelters. 5. Persons with medical conditions that increase the risk of progression to tuberculosis disease: gastrectomy, weight loss to ≥ 10% below ideal body weight, jejunoileal bypass, diabetes mellitus, silicosis, advanced CKD, some hematologic disorders (eg, leukemias, lymphomas), and other specific malignancies (eg, carcinoma of the head or neck and lung). 6. Children younger than 4 years or infants, children, and adolescents exposed to adults at high risk.
≥ 15 mm	1. Persons with no known risk factors for tuberculosis.

[1]A tuberculin skin test reaction is considered positive if the transverse diameter of the *indurated* area reaches the size required for the specific group. All other reactions are considered negative.
Data from https://www.cdc.gov/tb/publications/factsheets/testing/skintesting.htm.

Guidelines established by the CDC allow interferon gamma release assays to be used interchangeably with the tuberculin skin testing in the diagnosis of latent tuberculosis infection. Interferon gamma release assays are preferred in patients with prior BCG vaccination; the tuberculin skin test is preferred in children under 5 years old. Routine use of both tests is not recommended. In individuals with a positive tuberculin skin test but a low prior probability of latent tuberculosis infection and low-risk for progression to active disease, the interferon gamma release assay may be helpful as a confirmatory test to exclude a false-positive tuberculin skin test.

Treatment

A. General Measures

The goals of therapy are to cure the individual patient, minimize risk of morbidity and mortality related to treatment, reduce transmission of *M tuberculosis* to other persons, and prevent the emergence of clinically significant drug resistance in tubercle bacilli. The basic principles of antituberculous treatment are (1) to administer multiple medications to which the organisms are susceptible; (2) to provide the safest, most effective therapy for the shortest period of time; (3) to ensure adherence to therapy; and (4) to add at least two new antituberculous agents to a regimen when treatment failure is suspected.

All suspected and confirmed cases of tuberculosis should be reported promptly to local and state public health authorities. Patients with tuberculosis should be treated by clinicians who are skilled in the management of this infection. Clinical expertise is especially important in cases of drug-resistant tuberculosis.

Nonadherence to antituberculous treatment is a major cause of treatment failure, continued transmission of tuberculosis, and development of medication resistance. Adherence to treatment can be improved by providing detailed patient education about tuberculosis and its treatment in addition to a case manager who oversees all aspects of an individual patient's care. **Directly observed therapy (DOT),** which requires that a health care worker physically observe the patient ingest antituberculous medications in the home, clinic, hospital, or elsewhere, also improves adherence to treatment. The importance of direct observation of therapy cannot be overemphasized. The CDC recommends DOT for all patients with drug-resistant tuberculosis and for those receiving intermittent (twice- or thrice-weekly) therapy. Electronic DOT ("eDOT") is promising as a more efficient care model in selected populations.

Hospitalization for initial therapy of tuberculosis is not necessary for most patients. It should be considered if a patient is incapable of self-care or is likely to expose new, susceptible individuals to tuberculosis. Hospitalized patients with active disease require a private room with appropriate environmental controls, including negative-pressure ventilation where available, until tubercle bacilli are no longer found in their sputum ("smear-negative") on three consecutive smears taken on separate days.

Characteristics of antituberculous drugs are provided in Table 9–14. Additional treatment considerations can be found in Chapter 33. More complete information can be obtained from the CDC's Division of Tuberculosis Elimination website at https://www.cdc.gov/tb/topic/treatment/default.htm or the WHO tuberculosis website at https://www.who.int/health-topics/tuberculosis/.

B. Treatment of Tuberculosis in HIV-Negative Persons

Most patients with previously untreated pulmonary tuberculosis can be effectively treated with either a 6-month or a

Table 9–14. Characteristics of antituberculous medications.

Medication	Most Common Side Effects	Tests for Side Effects	Drug Interactions	Remarks
Isoniazid	Peripheral neuropathy, hepatitis, rash, mild CNS effects.	AST and ALT; neurologic examination.	Phenytoin (synergistic); disulfiram.	Bactericidal to both extracellular and intracellular organisms. Pyridoxine, 25–50 mg orally daily, is given as prophylaxis for neuropathy; 50–100 mg orally daily as treatment for it.
Rifampin	Hepatitis, fever, rash, flu-like illness, GI upset, bleeding problems, kidney failure.	CBC, platelets, AST and ALT.	Rifampin inhibits the effect of oral contraceptives, quinidine, corticosteroids, warfarin, methadone, digoxin, oral hypoglycemics; aminosalicylic acid may interfere with absorption of rifampin. Significant interactions with protease inhibitors and nonnucleoside reverse transcriptase inhibitors.	Bactericidal to all populations of organisms. Colors urine and other body secretions orange. May discolor contact lenses.
Rifapentine	Bone marrow suppression, hematuria/pyuria, hepatitis, GI upset, flu-like illness.	CBC, platelets, AST and ALT.	Strong cytochrome P450 inducer with multiple drug interactions. Use in HIV patients receiving antiretroviral therapy should be limited to experts in antiretroviral therapy.	Bactericidal to both extracellular and intracellular organisms. Colors urine and other body secretions orange. Long half-life, can be administered weekly in LTBI prophylaxis. Not for use in induction phase of therapy.
Pyrazinamide	Hyperuricemia, hepatotoxicity, rash, GI upset, joint aches.	Uric acid, AST, ALT.	Rare.	Bactericidal to intracellular organisms.
Ethambutol	Optic neuritis (reversible with discontinuance of drug; rare at 15 mg/kg); rash.	Red-green color discrimination and visual acuity.	Rare.	Bacteriostatic to both intracellular and extracellular organisms. Mainly used to inhibit development of resistant mutants. Use with caution in kidney disease or when ophthalmologic testing is not feasible.
Streptomycin	Eighth nerve damage, nephrotoxicity.	Vestibular function (audiograms); BUN and creatinine.	Neuromuscular blocking agents may be potentiated and cause prolonged paralysis.	Bactericidal to extracellular organisms. Use with caution in older patients or those with kidney disease.

LTBI, latent tuberculosis infection.

9-month regimen, though the 6-month regimen is preferred. The initial phase of a 6-month regimen consists of 2 months of daily isoniazid, rifampin, pyrazinamide, and ethambutol. Once the isolate is determined to be isoniazid-sensitive, ethambutol may be discontinued. If the *M tuberculosis* isolate is susceptible to isoniazid and rifampin, the second phase of therapy consists of isoniazid and rifampin for a minimum of 4 additional months, with treatment to extend at least 3 months beyond documentation of conversion of sputum cultures to negative for *M tuberculosis*. If DOT is used, medications may be given intermittently using one of three regimens: (1) Daily isoniazid, rifampin, pyrazinamide, and ethambutol for 2 months, followed by isoniazid and rifampin two or three times each week for 4 months if susceptibility to isoniazid and rifampin is demonstrated. (2) Daily isoniazid, rifampin, pyrazinamide, and ethambutol for 2 weeks, then administration of the same agents twice a week for 6 weeks followed by administration of isoniazid and rifampin twice each week for 4 months if susceptibility to isoniazid and rifampin is demonstrated. (3) Isoniazid, rifampin, pyrazinamide, and ethambutol three times a week for 6 months.

Patients who cannot or should not (eg, pregnant women) take pyrazinamide should receive daily isoniazid and rifampin along with ethambutol for 4–8 weeks. If susceptibility to isoniazid and rifampin is demonstrated or drug resistance is unlikely, ethambutol can be discontinued, and isoniazid and rifampin may be given for a total of 9 months of therapy. If drug resistance is a concern, patients should receive isoniazid, rifampin, and ethambutol for 9 months. Patients with smear- and culture-negative disease (eg, pulmonary tuberculosis diagnosed on clinical grounds) and patients for whom drug susceptibility testing is not available can be treated with 6 months of

Table 9–15. Recommended dosages for the initial treatment of tuberculosis.[1]

Medication	Daily[2]	Cost[3]/Day	Twice a Week[2]	Cost[3]/Wk	Three Times a Week[2]	Cost[3]/Wk
Isoniazid	5 mg/kg Max: 300 mg/dose	$0.31/300 mg	15 mg/kg Max: 900 mg/dose	$1.86	15 mg/kg Max: 900 mg/dose	$2.79
Rifampin	10 mg/kg Max: 600 mg/dose	$2.66/600 mg	10 mg/kg Max: 600 mg/dose	$5.32	10 mg/kg Max: 600 mg/dose	$7.98
Pyrazinamide	18.2–26.3 mg/kg Max: 2 g/dose	$24.33/2 g	Weight-based dosing: see references below[1]	—	Weight-based dosing: see references below[1]	—
Ethambutol	14.5–21.1 mg/kg Max: 1.6 g/dose	$3.74/1.6 g	Weight-based dosing: see references below[1]	—	Weight-based dosing: see references below[1]	—

[1]Data from Nahid P et al. Official American Thoracic Society/Centers for Disease Control and Prevention/Infectious Diseases Society of America Clinical Practice Guidelines: Treatment of drug-susceptible tuberculosis. Clin Infect Dis. 2016;63:e147.
[2]All dosing regimens should be used with directly observed therapy.
[3]IBM Micromedex Red Book (electronic version). IBM Watson Health, Greenwood Village, Colorado, USA. Available at: https://www-micromedexsolutions-com.proxy.hsl.ucdenver.edu/, accessed March 15, 2022.

isoniazid and rifampin combined with pyrazinamide for the first 2 months. This regimen assumes low prevalence of drug resistance. Previous guidelines have used streptomycin interchangeably with ethambutol. Increasing worldwide streptomycin resistance has made this medication less useful as empiric therapy.

When a twice-weekly or thrice-weekly regimen is used instead of a daily regimen, the dosages of isoniazid, pyrazinamide, and ethambutol or streptomycin must be increased. Recommended dosages for the initial treatment of tuberculosis are listed in Table 9–15. Fixed-dose combinations of isoniazid and rifampin (Rifamate) and of isoniazid, rifampin, and pyrazinamide (Rifater) are available to simplify treatment. Single tablets improve compliance but are more expensive than the individual medications purchased separately.

C. Treatment of Tuberculosis in HIV-Positive Persons

Management of tuberculosis is complex in patients with concomitant HIV disease. Experts in the management of both tuberculosis and HIV disease should be involved in the care of such patients. The CDC has published detailed recommendations for the treatment of tuberculosis in HIV-positive patients (https://www.cdc.gov/tb/topic/treatment/tbhiv.htm).

The basic approach to HIV-positive patients with tuberculosis is similar to that detailed above for patients without HIV disease. Additional considerations in HIV-positive patients include (1) longer duration of therapy and (2) drug interactions between rifamycin derivatives such as rifampin and rifabutin used to treat tuberculosis and some of the protease inhibitors and nonnucleoside reverse transcriptase inhibitors (NNRTIs) used to treat HIV. DOT is recommended for all HIV-positive tuberculosis patients. Pyridoxine (vitamin B_6), 25–50 mg orally each day, should be administered to all HIV-positive patients being treated with isoniazid to reduce central and peripheral nervous system side effects.

D. Treatment of Drug-Resistant Tuberculosis

Patients with drug-resistant *M tuberculosis* infection require careful supervision and management. Clinicians who are unfamiliar with the treatment of drug-resistant tuberculosis should seek expert advice. Tuberculosis resistant only to isoniazid can be successfully treated with a 6-month regimen of rifampin, pyrazinamide, and ethambutol or streptomycin or a 12-month regimen of rifampin and ethambutol. When isoniazid resistance is documented during a 9-month regimen without pyrazinamide, isoniazid should be discontinued. If ethambutol was part of the initial regimen, rifampin and ethambutol should be continued for a minimum of 12 months. If ethambutol was not part of the initial regimen, susceptibility tests should be repeated and two other medications to which the organism is susceptible should be added. Treatment of *M tuberculosis* isolates resistant to agents other than isoniazid and treatment of drug resistance in HIV-infected patients require expert consultation.

Multidrug-resistant tuberculosis and extensively drug-resistant tuberculosis call for an individualized daily DOT plan under the supervision of an experienced clinician. Treatment regimens are based on the patient's overall status and the results of susceptibility studies. Most drug-resistant isolates are resistant to at least isoniazid and rifampin and require a minimum of three drugs to which the organism is susceptible; expert recommendation is often for an intensive five-drug phase of treatment, followed by a two- or three-drug continuation phase of treatment for at least another 12 months. Some experts recommend at least 18–24 months of therapy.

E. Treatment of Extrapulmonary Tuberculosis

In most cases, regimens that are effective for treating pulmonary tuberculosis are also effective for treating extrapulmonary disease. However, many experts recommend

9–12 months of therapy when miliary, meningeal, or bone and joint disease is present. Treatment of skeletal tuberculosis is enhanced by early surgical drainage and debridement of necrotic bone. Corticosteroid therapy has been shown to help prevent constrictive pericarditis from tuberculous pericarditis and to reduce neurologic complications from tuberculous meningitis (Chapter 33).

F. Treatment of Pregnant or Lactating Women

Tuberculosis in pregnancy is usually treated with isoniazid, rifampin, and ethambutol for 2 months, followed by isoniazid and rifampin for an additional 7 months. Ethambutol can be stopped after the first month if isoniazid and rifampin susceptibility is confirmed. Since the risk of teratogenicity with pyrazinamide has not been clearly defined, pyrazinamide should be used only if resistance to other drugs is documented and susceptibility to pyrazinamide is likely. Streptomycin is contraindicated in pregnancy because it may cause congenital deafness. Pregnant women taking isoniazid should receive pyridoxine (vitamin B_6), 10–25 mg orally once a day, to prevent peripheral neuropathy.

Small concentrations of antituberculous drugs are present in breast milk. First-line therapy is not known to be harmful to nursing newborns at these concentrations. Therefore, breastfeeding is not contraindicated while receiving first-line antituberculous therapy. Lactating women receiving other agents should consult a tuberculosis expert.

G. Treatment Monitoring

Adults should have measurements of a CBC (including platelets) and serum bilirubin, hepatic enzymes, BUN, and creatinine before starting therapy for tuberculosis. Visual acuity and red-green color vision tests are recommended before initiation of ethambutol, and serum uric acid is recommended before starting pyrazinamide. Audiometry should be performed if streptomycin therapy is initiated.

Routine monitoring of laboratory tests for evidence of medication toxicity during therapy is not recommended unless baseline results are abnormal or liver disease is suspected. Monthly questioning for symptoms of medication toxicity is advised. Patients should be educated about common side effects of antituberculous medications and instructed to seek medical attention should these symptoms occur. Monthly follow-up of outpatients is recommended, including sputum smear and culture for *M tuberculosis*, until cultures convert to negative. Patients with negative sputum cultures after 2 months of treatment should have at least one additional sputum smear and culture performed at the end of therapy. Patients with drug-resistant isolates should have sputum cultures performed monthly during the entire course of treatment. A chest radiograph at the end of therapy provides a useful baseline for any future comparison.

Patients whose cultures do not become negative or whose symptoms do not resolve despite 3 months of therapy should be evaluated for nonadherence to the regimen and for drug-resistant organisms. DOT is recommended for the remainder of the treatment regimen, and the addition of at least two drugs not previously given should be considered pending repeat drug susceptibility testing. The clinician should seek expert assistance if drug resistance is newly found, if the patient remains symptomatic, or if smears or cultures remain positive.

Patients with only a clinical diagnosis of pulmonary tuberculosis (smears and cultures negative for *M tuberculosis*) whose symptoms and radiographic abnormalities are unchanged after 3 months of treatment usually either have another process or have had tuberculosis in the past.

H. Treatment of Latent Tuberculosis

Treatment of latent tuberculous infection is essential to controlling and eliminating tuberculosis and substantially reduces the risk that infection will progress to active disease. Targeted testing with the tuberculin skin test or interferon gamma release assays is used to identify persons who are at high risk for tuberculosis and who stand to benefit from treatment of latent infection. Table 9–13 gives the tuberculin skin test criteria for treatment of latent tuberculous infection. In general, patients with a positive tuberculin skin test or interferon gamma release assay who are at increased risk for exposure or disease are treated. It is essential that each person who meets the criteria for treatment of latent tuberculous infection undergo a careful assessment to exclude active disease. A history of past treatment for tuberculosis and contraindications to treatment should be sought. All patients at risk for HIV infection should have an HIV test. Patients suspected of having tuberculosis should receive one of the recommended multidrug regimens for active disease until the diagnosis is confirmed or excluded.

Some close contacts of persons with active tuberculosis should be evaluated for treatment of latent tuberculous infection despite a negative tuberculin skin test reaction (less than 5 mm of induration). These include immunosuppressed persons and those in whom disease may develop quickly after tuberculous infection. Close contacts who have a negative tuberculin skin test reaction on initial testing should be retested 10–12 weeks later.

Several treatment regimens for both HIV-negative and HIV-positive persons are available for the treatment of latent tuberculous infection: (1) **Isoniazid:** A 9-month oral regimen (minimum of 270 doses administered within 12 months) is preferable to 6 months of therapy. Dosing options include a daily dose of 300 mg or twice-weekly doses of 15 mg/kg. Persons at risk for developing isoniazid-associated peripheral neuropathy (those with diabetes mellitus, uremia, malnutrition, alcoholism, HIV infection, pregnancy, or seizure disorder) may be given supplemental pyridoxine (vitamin B_6), 10–50 mg/day. (2) **Isoniazid and rifampin:** A 3-month oral regimen of daily isoniazid (300 mg) and rifampin (600 mg). (3) **Isoniazid and rifapentine:** A 3-month oral regimen of once weekly isoniazid at 15 mg/kg and rifapentine at 15–30 mg/kg. (4) **Rifampin:** Patients who cannot tolerate isoniazid can be considered for a 4-month oral regimen of rifampin at 600 mg daily. HIV-positive patients receiving protease inhibitors or NNRTIs who are given rifampin or rifapentine require management by experts in both tuberculosis and HIV disease (see Treatment of Tuberculosis in HIV-Positive Persons, above).

Contacts of persons with isoniazid-resistant, rifampin-sensitive tuberculosis should receive a 2-month regimen of rifampin and pyrazinamide or a 4-month regimen of daily rifampin alone. Contacts of persons with drug-resistant tuberculosis should receive two drugs to which the infecting organism has demonstrated susceptibility. Contacts in whom the tuberculin skin test or interferon gamma release assay is negative and contacts who are HIV seronegative may be observed without treatment or treated for 6 months. HIV-positive contacts should be treated for 12 months. All contacts of persons with multidrug-resistant tuberculosis or extensively drug-resistant tuberculosis should have 2 years of follow-up regardless of type of treatment.

Persons with a positive tuberculin skin test (5 mm or more of induration) and fibrotic lesions suggestive of old tuberculosis on chest radiographs who have no evidence of active disease and no history of treatment for tuberculosis should receive 9 months of isoniazid or 4 months of rifampin (with or without isoniazid). Pregnant or breastfeeding women with latent tuberculosis should receive either daily or twice-weekly isoniazid with pyridoxine (vitamin B_6).

Baseline laboratory testing is indicated for patients at risk for liver disease, patients with HIV infection, women who are pregnant or within 3 months of delivery, and persons who use alcohol regularly. Patients receiving treatment for latent tuberculous infection should be evaluated once a month to assess for symptoms and signs of active tuberculosis and hepatitis and for adherence to their treatment regimen. Routine laboratory testing during treatment is indicated for those with abnormal baseline laboratory tests and for those at risk for developing liver disease.

BCG vaccine is an antimycobacterial vaccine developed from an attenuated strain of *M bovis*. Millions of individuals worldwide have been vaccinated with BCG. The vaccine is not generally recommended in the United States because of the low prevalence of tuberculous infection, the vaccine's interference with the ability to determine latent tuberculous infection using tuberculin skin test reactivity, and its variable effectiveness in prophylaxis of pulmonary tuberculosis. BCG vaccination in the United States should be undertaken only after consultation with local health officials and tuberculosis experts. Vaccination of health care workers should be considered on an individual basis in settings in which a high percentage of tuberculosis patients are infected with strains resistant to both isoniazid and rifampin, in which transmission of such drug-resistant *M tuberculosis* and subsequent infection are likely, and in which comprehensive tuberculous infection-control precautions have been implemented but have not been successful. The BCG vaccine is contraindicated in persons with impaired immune responses due to disease or medications.

Prognosis

Almost all properly treated immunocompetent patients with tuberculosis can be cured. Relapse rates are less than 5% with current regimens. The main cause of treatment failure is nonadherence to therapy.

Acharya B et al. Advances in diagnosis of tuberculosis: an update into molecular diagnosis of *Mycobacterium tuberculosis*. Mol Biol Rep. 2020;47:4065. [PMID: 32248381]

Ignatius EH et al. New drugs for the treatment of tuberculosis. Clin Chest Med. 2019;40:811. [PMID: 31731986]

Nahid P et al. Treatment of drug-resistant tuberculosis: an official ATS/CDC/ERS/IDSA practice guideline. AJRCCM. 2019;200:e93. [PMID: 31729908]

Shaw JA et al. Tuberculous pleural effusion. Respirology. 2019;24:962. [PMID: 31418985]

Singh R et al. Recent updates on drug resistance in *Mycobacterium tuberculosis*. J Appl Microbiol. 2020;128:1547. [PMID: 31595643]

Tiberi S et al. Multidrug and extensively drug-resistant tuberculosis: epidemiology, clinical features, management and treatment. Infect Dis Clin North Am. 2019;33:1063. [PMID: 31668191]

Zha BS et al. Treatment of drug-susceptible tuberculosis. Clin Chest Med. 2019;40:763. [PMID: 31731983]

Zhang M et al. The diagnostic utility of pleural markers for tuberculosis pleural effusion. Ann Transl Med. 2020;8:607. [PMID: 32566633]

PULMONARY DISEASE CAUSED BY NONTUBERCULOUS MYCOBACTERIA

ESSENTIALS OF DIAGNOSIS

- Chronic cough, sputum production, and fatigue; less commonly: malaise, dyspnea, fever, hemoptysis, and weight loss.
- Parenchymal opacities on chest radiograph, most often thin-walled cavities or multiple small nodules associated with bronchiectasis.
- Isolation of nontuberculous mycobacteria in a sputum culture.

General Considerations

Mycobacteria other than *M tuberculosis*—nontuberculous mycobacteria (NTM), sometimes referred to as "atypical" mycobacteria—are ubiquitous in water and soil and have been isolated from tap water. Marked geographic variability exists, both in the NTM species responsible for disease and in the prevalence of disease. These organisms are not considered communicable from person to person, have distinct laboratory characteristics, and are often resistant to most antituberculous medications (Chapter 33). Long-term epidemiologic data suggest that NTM disease has been increasing in the United States.

Definition & Pathogenesis

The diagnosis of lung disease caused by NTM is based on a combination of clinical, radiographic, and bacteriologic criteria and the exclusion of other diseases that can resemble the condition. Specific diagnostic criteria are discussed below. Complementary data are important for diagnosis because NTM organisms can reside in or colonize the airways without causing clinical disease.

Mycobacterium avium complex (MAC) is the most frequent cause of NTM pulmonary disease in humans in the United States. *Mycobacterium kansasii* is the next most frequent pulmonary pathogen. Other NTM causes of pulmonary disease include *Mycobacterium abscessus, Mycobacterium xenopi*, and *Mycobacterium malmoense;* the list of more unusual etiologic NTM species is long. Most NTM cause a chronic pulmonary infection that resembles tuberculosis but tends to progress more slowly. Disseminated disease is rare in immunocompetent persons; however, disseminated MAC disease is common in patients with AIDS.

Clinical Findings

A. Symptoms and Signs

NTM infection among immunocompetent persons frequently presents in one of three prototypical patterns: cavitary, upper lobe lesions in older male smokers that may mimic *M tuberculosis*; nodular bronchiectasis affecting the mid lung zones in middle-aged women with chronic cough; and hypersensitivity pneumonitis following environmental exposure. Most patients with NTM infection experience a chronic cough, sputum production, and fatigue. Less common symptoms include malaise, dyspnea, fever, hemoptysis, and weight loss. Symptoms from coexisting lung disease (COPD, bronchiectasis, previous mycobacterial disease, cystic fibrosis, and pneumoconiosis) may confound the evaluation. In patients with bronchiectasis, coinfection with NTM and *Aspergillus* is a negative prognostic factor. New or worsening infiltrates as well as adenopathy or pleural effusion (or both) are described in HIV-positive patients with NTM infection as part of the immune reconstitution inflammatory syndrome following institution of antiretroviral therapy.

B. Laboratory Findings

The diagnosis of NTM infection rests on recovery of the pathogen from cultures. Sputum cultures positive for atypical mycobacteria do not prove infection because NTM may exist as saprophytes colonizing the airways or may be environmental contaminants. Bronchial washings are considered to be more sensitive than expectorated sputum samples; however, their specificity for clinical disease is not known.

Bacteriologic criteria have been proposed based on studies of patients with cavitary disease with MAC or *M kansasii.* Diagnostic criteria in immunocompetent persons include the following: positive culture results from at least two separate expectorated sputum samples; or positive culture from at least one bronchial wash; or a positive culture from pleural fluid or any other normally sterile site. The diagnosis can also be established by demonstrating NTM cultured from a lung biopsy, bronchial wash, or sputum plus histopathologic changes, such as granulomatous inflammation in a lung biopsy. Rapid species identification of some NTM is possible using DNA probes or high-pressure liquid chromatography.

Diagnostic criteria are less stringent for patients with severe immunosuppression. HIV-infected patients may show significant MAC growth on culture of bronchial washings without clinical infection; therefore, HIV patients being evaluated for MAC infection must be considered individually.

Medication susceptibility testing on cultures of NTM is recommended for the following NTM: (1) *Mycobacterium avium intracellulare* to macrolides only (clarithromycin and azithromycin); (2) *M kansasii* to rifampin; and (3) rapid growers (such as *Mycobacterium fortuitum, Mycobacterium chelonae, and M abscessus*) to amikacin, doxycycline, imipenem, fluoroquinolones, clarithromycin, cefoxitin, and sulfonamides.

C. Imaging

Chest radiographic findings include infiltrates that are progressive or persist for at least 2 months, cavitary lesions, and multiple nodular densities. The cavities are often thin-walled and have less surrounding parenchymal infiltrate than is commonly seen with MTB infections. Evidence of contiguous spread and pleural involvement is often present. High-resolution CT of the chest may show multiple small nodules with or without multifocal bronchiectasis. Progression of pulmonary infiltrates during therapy or lack of radiographic improvement over time are poor prognostic signs and also raise concerns about secondary or alternative pulmonary processes. Clearing of pulmonary infiltrates due to NTM is slow.

Treatment

Establishing NTM infection does not mandate treatment in all cases, for two reasons. First, clinical disease may never develop in some patients, particularly asymptomatic patients with few organisms isolated from single specimens. Second, the spectrum of clinical disease severity is very wide; in patients with mild or slowly progressive symptoms, traditional chemotherapeutic regimens using a combination of agents may lead to drug-induced side effects worse than the disease itself. These features at least partly explain variability of adherence to treatment guidelines in practice.

Specific treatment regimens and responses to therapy vary with the species of NTM. HIV-seronegative patients with MAC pulmonary disease usually receive a combination of daily clarithromycin or azithromycin, rifampin or rifabutin, and ethambutol (Table 9–15). For patients with severe fibrocavitary disease, streptomycin or amikacin is added for the first 2 months. The optimal duration of treatment is unknown, but therapy should be continued for 12 months after sputum conversion. Medical treatment is initially successful in about two-thirds of cases, but relapses after treatment are common; long-term benefit is demonstrated in about half of all patients. Those who do not respond favorably generally have active but stable disease. Surgical resection is an alternative for the patient with progressive disease that responds poorly to chemotherapy. Disease caused by *M kansasii* responds well to drug therapy. A daily regimen of rifampin, isoniazid, and ethambutol for at least 18 months with a minimum of 12 months of negative cultures is usually successful. Rapidly growing mycobacteria (*M abscessus, M fortuitum, M chelonae*) are generally resistant to standard antituberculous therapy.

When to Refer

Patients with rapidly growing mycobacteria infection should be referred for expert management.

Abate G et al. Variability in the management of adults with pulmonary nontuberculous mycobacterial disease. Clin Infect Dis. 2021;72:1127. [PMID: 32198521]

Daley CL et al. Treatment of nontuberculous mycobacterial pulmonary disease: official ATS/ERS/ESCMID/IDSA clinical practice guideline. Eur Respir J. 2020;56:2000535. [PMID: 32636299]

Kwon YS et al. Treatment of *Mycobacterium avium* complex pulmonary disease. Tuberc Respir Dis (Seoul). 2019;82:15. [PMID: 30574687]

Mitchell JD. Surgical treatment of pulmonary nontuberculous mycobacterial infections. Thorac Surg Clin. 2019;29:77. [PMID: 30454924]

Wi YM. Treatment of extrapulmonary nontuberculous mycobacterial diseases. Infect Chemother. 2019;51:245. [PMID: 31583858]

PULMONARY NEOPLASMS

See Chapter 39 for discussions of Lung Cancer, Secondary Lung Cancer, and Mesothelioma.

SCREENING FOR LUNG CANCER

Lung cancer remains the leading cause of cancer-related mortality, in large part secondary to advanced stage at diagnosis (Chapter 39). Two large RCTs reported findings in 2011 regarding the utility of lung cancer screening. The Prostate, Lung, Colorectal and Ovarian Randomized Trial (PLCO) randomized 154,901 adults (52% current or former smokers) between the ages of 55 and 74 years to receive either no screening or annual posterior-anterior chest radiographs for 4 consecutive years. The investigators monitored the participants after screening for an average of 12 years. Results showed no mortality benefit from four annual chest radiographs either in the whole cohort or in a subset of heavy smokers who met the entry criteria for the other major trial, the National Lung Screening Trial (NLST). The NLST enrolled 53,454 current or former smokers (minimum 30-pack year exposure history) between the ages of 55 and 74 years who were randomly assigned to one of two screening modalities: three annual posterior-anterior chest radiographs or three annual low-dose chest CT scans. They were monitored for an additional 6.5 years after screening. Compared with chest radiography, low-dose chest CT detected more early-stage lung cancers and fewer advanced-stage lung cancers, indicating that CT screening systematically shifted the time of diagnosis to earlier stages, thereby providing more persons the opportunity for effective treatment. Furthermore, compared with chest radiographs, the cohort that received three annual CT scans had a statistically significant mortality benefit, with reductions in both lung cancer deaths (20.0%) and all-cause mortality (6.7%). This was the first evidence from an RCT demonstrating that lung cancer screening reduced all-cause mortality.

Additional information from PLCO, the NLST, and multiple other ongoing randomized trials is available. Trials in the Netherlands and Belgium (NELSON), Germany (LUSI), Denmark (DLCST), the United Kingdom (UKLS), and Italy (MILD, DANTE, ITALUNG) have been completed. These have revealed variable findings depending on the risk profile of the included patients, but the broad results indicate that screening is most likely to be effective, with reduction in lung cancer-specific mortality, if performed at short intervals in a high-risk population, as was done in NLST. Some studies indicate that the mortality benefit may be higher among women than among men. Issues that remain of concern regarding lung cancer screening include the following: **(1) Generalizability to practice:** NLST-participating institutions demonstrated a high level of expertise in imaging interpretation and diagnostic evaluation. Ninety-six percent of findings on CT were false positives but the vast majority of patients were monitored with serial imaging. Invasive diagnostic evaluations were uncommon and were associated with a low complication rate (1.4%). **(2) Duration of screening:** The rate of detection of new lung cancers did not fall with each subsequent annual screening over 3 years. Since new lung cancers become detectable during each year-long screening interval, the optimal number of annual CT scans is unknown as is the optimal screening interval. **(3) Overdiagnosis:** After 6.4 years of post-screening observation, there were more lung cancers in the NLST CT cohort than the chest radiography cohort (1089 and 969, respectively). Since the groups were randomized and well matched, lung cancer incidence should have been identical. Therefore, 18.5% of the lung cancers detected by CT remained clinically silent and invisible on chest radiograph for 6.4 years. Many, perhaps most, of these lung cancers would never cause clinical disease and represent overdiagnosis. **(4) Cost effectiveness:** Studies in the United States, Canada, and Europe suggest screening for lung cancer is cost effective; however, whether it is cost effective in all countries has not been determined.

In 2021, the USPSTF updated its recommendation for low-dose CT screening. Annual low-dose CT screening for lung cancer is recommended for those at high risk. High-risk criteria include age 50–80 years, at least a 20 pack-year smoking history, and either current smoking or quit date within past 15 years. Screening should be stopped once 15 years have elapsed since quitting smoking, or if a comorbid condition renders the benefits of screening null. Simulation models developed for the purposes of informing this recommendation found yearly screening using these parameters to be the most efficient in reducing lung cancer–related deaths, though more false-positive test results are expected compared to the original recommendation.

All patients participating in a screening program who still smoke should receive smoking cessation interventions.

Becker N et al. Lung cancer mortality reduction by LDCT screening–results from the randomized German LUSI trial. Int J Cancer. 2020;146:1503. [PMID: 31162856] de Koning HJ et al. Reduced lung-cancer mortality with volume CT screening in a randomized trial. N Engl J Med. 2020;382:503. [PMID: 31995683]

Iaccarino JM et al. Patient-level trajectories and outcomes after low-dose CT screening in the National Lung Screening Trial. Chest. 2019;156:965. [PMID: 31283920]

Krist AH et al. Screening for lung cancer: US Preventive Services Task Force Recommendation Statement. JAMA. 2021;325:962. [PMID: 33687470]

Pastorino U et al. Ten-year results of the Multicentric Italian Lung Detection trial demonstrate the safety and efficacy of biennial lung cancer screening. Eur J Cancer. 2019;118:142. [PMID: 31336289]

SOLITARY PULMONARY NODULE

A solitary pulmonary nodule, sometimes referred to as a "coin lesion," is a less-than-3-cm isolated, rounded opacity on chest imaging outlined by normal lung and not associated with infiltrate, atelectasis, or adenopathy. Most are asymptomatic and represent an incidental finding on chest radiography or CT scanning. The finding is important because it carries a significant risk of malignancy. The frequency of malignancy in surgical series ranges from 10% to 68% depending on patient population. Benign neoplasms, such as hamartomas, account for less than 5% of solitary nodules. Most benign nodules are infectious granulomas.

The goals of evaluation are to identify and resect malignant tumors in patients who will benefit from resection while avoiding invasive procedures in benign disease. The task is to identify nodules with a sufficiently high probability of malignancy to warrant biopsy or resection or a sufficiently low probability of malignancy to justify observation.

Symptoms alone rarely establish the cause, but clinical and imaging data can be used to assess the probability of malignancy. Malignant nodules are rare in persons under age 30. Above age 30, the likelihood of malignancy increases with age. Smokers are at increased risk, and the likelihood of malignancy increases with the number of cigarettes smoked daily. Patients with a prior malignancy have a higher likelihood of having a malignant solitary nodule.

The first step in the imaging evaluation is to review old imaging studies. Comparison with prior studies allows estimation of doubling time, which is an important marker for malignancy. Rapid progression (doubling time less than 30 days) suggests infection, while long-term stability (doubling time greater than 465 days) suggests benignity. Certain radiographic features help in estimating the probability of malignancy. Size is correlated with malignancy. A study of solitary nodules identified by CT scan showed a 1% malignancy rate in those measuring 2–5 mm, 24% in 6–10 mm, 33% in 11–20 mm, and 80% in 21–45 mm nodules. The appearance of a smooth, well-defined edge is characteristic of a benign process. Ill-defined margins or a lobular appearance suggest malignancy. A high-resolution CT finding of spiculated margins and a peripheral halo are both highly associated with malignancy. Calcification and its pattern are also helpful clues. Benign lesions tend to have dense calcification in a central or laminated pattern. Malignant lesions are associated with sparser calcification that is typically stippled or eccentric. Cavitary lesions with thick (greater than 16 mm) walls are much more likely to be malignant. High-resolution CT offers better resolution of these characteristics than chest radiography and is more likely to detect lymphadenopathy or the presence of multiple lesions. Chest CT is indicated for any suspicious solitary pulmonary nodule.

Treatment

Based on clinical and radiologic data, the clinician should assign a specific probability of malignancy to the lesion. The decision whether to recommend a biopsy or surgical excision depends on the interpretation of this probability in light of the patient's unique clinical situation. Quantitative prediction models (Brock model, VA Cooperative model) are available to assess risk of malignancy. The probabilities in parentheses below represent guidelines only and should not be interpreted as definitive.

In the case of solitary pulmonary nodules, a continuous probability function may be grouped into three categories. In patients with a **low probability (less than 5%) of malignancy** (eg, age under 30, lesions stable for more than 2 years, characteristic pattern of benign calcification), watchful waiting is appropriate. Management consists of serial imaging studies at intervals that could identify growth suggestive of malignancy. Three-dimensional reconstruction of high-resolution CT images provides a more sensitive test for growth.

Patients with a **high probability (greater than 60%) of malignancy** should proceed directly to resection following staging, provided the surgical risk is acceptable. Biopsies rarely yield a specific benign diagnosis and are not indicated.

Optimal management of patients with an **intermediate probability of malignancy (5–60%)** remains controversial. The traditional approach is to obtain a diagnostic biopsy, either through bronchoscopy or transthoracic needle aspiration (TTNA). Bronchoscopy yields a diagnosis in 10–80% of procedures depending on the size of the nodule and its location. In general, the bronchoscopic yield for nodules that are less than 2 cm and peripheral is low, although complications are generally rare. Newer bronchoscopic modalities, such as electromagnetic navigation and ultrathin bronchoscopy are being studied, although their impact upon diagnostic yield remains uncertain. TTNA has a higher diagnostic yield, reported to be between 50% and 97%. The yield is strongly operator-dependent, however, and is affected by the location and size of the lesion. Complications are higher than bronchoscopy, with pneumothorax occurring in up to 30% of patients, with up to one-third of these patients requiring placement of a chest tube.

Disappointing diagnostic yields and a high false-negative rate (up to 20–30% in TTNA) have prompted alternative approaches. **PET** detects increased glucose metabolism within malignant lesions with high sensitivity (85–97%) and specificity (70–85%). Many diagnostic algorithms have incorporated PET into the assessment of patients with inconclusive high-resolution CT findings. A positive PET increases the likelihood of malignancy, and a negative PET excludes most cancers. False-negative PET scans can occur with tumors with low metabolic activity (most notably, carcinoid tumors and adenocarcinomas, particularly minimally invasive or in situ adenocarcinomas), so follow-up CT imaging is typically performed at discrete intervals to ensure absence of growth. PET has several other drawbacks: resolution below 1 cm is poor, the test is expensive, and availability remains limited.

Sputum cytology is highly specific but lacks sensitivity. It is used in central lesions and in patients who are poor candidates for invasive diagnostic procedures.

Some centers recommend **video-assisted thoracoscopic surgery (VATS)** resection of all solitary pulmonary nodules with intermediate probability of malignancy. In some cases, the surgeon will remove the nodule and evaluate it in the operating room with frozen section. If the nodule is malignant, he or she will proceed to lobectomy and lymph node sampling, either thoracoscopically or through conversion to standard thoracotomy. This approach is less common when preoperative PET scanning is available.

All patients should be provided with an estimate of the likelihood of malignancy, and their preferences should be used to help guide diagnostic and therapeutic decisions. A strategy that recommends observation may not be preferred by a patient who desires a definitive diagnosis. Similarly, a surgical approach may not be agreeable to all patients unless the presence of cancer is definitive. Patient preferences should be elicited, and patients should be well informed regarding the specific risks and benefits associated with the recommended approach as well as the alternative strategies.

Cruickshank A et al. Evaluation of the solitary pulmonary nodule. Intern Med J. 2019;49:306. [PMID: 30897667]
Khan T et al. Diagnosis and management of peripheral lung nodule. Ann Transl Med. 2019;7:348. [PMID: 31516894]
Marcus MW et al. Probability of cancer in lung nodules using sequential volumetric screening up to 12 months: the UKLS trial. Thorax. 2019;74:761. [PMID: 31028232]
Nasim F et al. Management of the solitary pulmonary nodule. Curr Opin Pulm Med. 2019;25:344. [PMID: 30973358]
Tang K et al. The value of 18F-FDG PET/CT in the diagnosis of different size of solitary pulmonary nodules. Medicine (Baltimore). 2019;98:e14813. [PMID: 30882661]

RIGHT MIDDLE LOBE SYNDROME

Right middle lobe syndrome is recurrent or persistent atelectasis of the right middle lobe. This collapse is related to the relatively long length and narrow diameter of the right middle lobe bronchus and the oval ("fish mouth") opening to the lobe, in the setting of impaired collateral ventilation. Fiberoptic bronchoscopy or CT scan is often necessary to rule out obstructing tumor. Foreign body or other benign causes are common.

BRONCHIAL CARCINOID TUMORS

Bronchial carcinoid tumors are malignant low- and intermediate-grade neuroendocrine tumors of the lung, with a favorable prognosis compared to high-grade neuroendocrine tumors such as small cell lung cancer. Bronchial carcinoids typically occur as pedunculated or sessile growths in central bronchi. Common symptoms of bronchial carcinoid tumors are hemoptysis, cough, focal wheezing, and recurrent postobstructive pneumonia. Peripherally located bronchial carcinoid tumors are rare and present as asymptomatic solitary pulmonary nodules. **Carcinoid syndrome** (flushing, diarrhea, wheezing, hypotension) and paraneoplastic Cushing syndrome are rare. Fiberoptic bronchoscopy may reveal a pink or purple tumor in a central airway. These lesions have a well-vascularized stroma, and biopsy may be complicated by significant bleeding. CT scanning is helpful to localize the lesion and to follow its growth over time. Octreotide scintigraphy is also available for localization of these tumors.

Bronchial carcinoid tumors grow slowly; the aggressiveness is determined by the cell histology, with "typical carcinoid," a low-grade tumor, demonstrating a more indolent and favorable course than "atypical carcinoid," an intermediate-grade tumor. Bronchial carcinoid tumor staging follows the same TNM classification as other lung cancers. Surgical excision, including lymph node dissection and resection, is recommended for localized disease, and the prognosis is generally favorable. Most bronchial carcinoid tumors respond poorly to radiation and chemotherapy (see Chapter 39).

Adenomas, carcinomas, and other malignancies may rarely metastasize to the bronchi and present with endobronchial lesions. Hamartomas, myxomas, and amyloid are other rarer entities in the differential diagnosis of endobronchial mass lesions.

Girelli L et al. Results of surgical resection of locally advanced pulmonary neuroendocrine tumors. Ann Thorac Surg. 2021; 112:405. [PMID: 33130114]
Petrella F et al. The role of endobronchial treatment for bronchial carcinoid: considerations from the thoracic surgeon's point of view. Respiration. 2018;96:204. [PMID: 29953990]
Rahouma M et al. Role of wedge resection in bronchial carcinoid (BC) tumors: SEER database analysis. J Thorac Dis. 2019; 11:1355. [PMID: 31179077]
Reuling EM et al. Endobronchial treatment for bronchial carcinoid: patient selection and predictors of outcome. Respiration. 2018;95:220. [PMID: 29433123]
Singh S et al. Commonwealth Neuroendocrine Tumour Research Collaboration and the North American Neuroendocrine Tumor Society Guidelines for the Diagnosis and Management of Patients with Lung Neuroendocrine Tumors: an international collaborative endorsement and update of the 2015 European Neuroendocrine Tumor Society Expert Consensus Guidelines. J Thorac Oncol. 2020;15:1577. [PMID: 32663527]

MEDIASTINAL MASSES

Various developmental, neoplastic, infectious, traumatic, and cardiovascular disorders may cause masses that appear in the mediastinum on chest radiograph. A useful convention arbitrarily divides the mediastinum into three compartments—anterior, middle, and posterior—in order to classify mediastinal masses and assist in differential diagnosis based on contents of these anatomic regions. The anterior compartment is bounded by the sternum anteriorly and the surface of the great vessels and pericardium posteriorly. The middle compartment extends from the anterior pericardium to the anterior surface of the thoracic spine. The posterior compartment is paravertebral.

Specific mediastinal masses have a predilection for one or more of these compartments; most are located in the anterior or middle compartment.

The differential diagnosis of an **anterior mediastinal mass** includes thymoma, teratoma, thyroid lesions, lymphoma, and mesenchymal tumors (lipoma, fibroma). The differential diagnosis of a **middle mediastinal mass** includes lymphadenopathy, pulmonary artery enlargement, aneurysm of the aorta or innominate artery, developmental cyst (bronchogenic, enteric, pleuropericardial), dilated azygous or hemiazygous vein, and foramen of Morgagni hernia. The differential diagnosis of a **posterior mediastinal mass** includes hiatal hernia, neurogenic tumor, meningocele, esophageal tumor, foramen of Bochdalek hernia, thoracic spine disease, and extramedullary hematopoiesis. The neurogenic tumor group includes neurilemmoma, neurofibroma, neurosarcoma, ganglioneuroma, and pheochromocytoma.

Symptoms and signs of mediastinal masses are nonspecific and are usually caused by the effects of the mass on surrounding structures. Insidious onset of retrosternal chest pain, dysphagia, or dyspnea is often an important clue to the presence of a mediastinal mass. In about half of cases, symptoms are absent, and the mass is detected on routine chest radiograph. Physical findings vary depending on the nature and location of the mass.

CT scanning is helpful in management; additional radiographic studies of benefit include barium swallow if esophageal disease is suspected, Doppler sonography or venography of brachiocephalic veins and the superior vena cava, and angiography. MRI is useful; its advantages include better delineation of hilar structures and distinction between vessels and masses. Tissue diagnosis via either needle or excisional biopsy is generally necessary when a neoplastic process is considered. Treatment and prognosis depend on the underlying cause of the mediastinal mass.

Gentili F et al. Update in diagnostic imaging of the thymus and anterior mediastinal masses. Gland Surg. 2019;8:S188. [PMID: 31559186]

Lee HN et al. Diagnostic outcome and safety of CT-guided core needle biopsy for mediastinal masses: a systematic review and meta-analysis. Eur Radiol. 2020;30:588. [PMID: 31418086]

Miyazawa R et al. Incidental mediastinal masses detected at low-dose CT screening: prevalence and radiological characteristics. Jpn J Radiol. 2020;38:1150. [PMID: 32638279]

Sakka D et al. Mediastinal masses: clinical, radiological and pathological analysis. Eur Respir J. 2018;52:PA2579. https://erj.ersjournals.com/content/52/suppl_62/PA2579

INTERSTITIAL LUNG DISEASE (Diffuse Parenchymal Lung Disease)

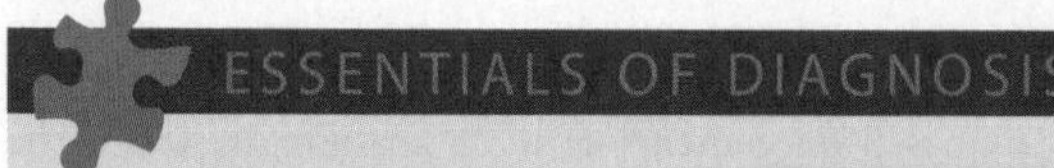

- Insidious onset of progressive dyspnea and nonproductive chronic cough.
- Tachypnea, bibasilar dry rales; digital clubbing and right heart failure with advanced disease.
- Chest radiographs with patchy distribution of ground glass, reticular, nodular, reticulonodular, or cystic opacities.
- Reduced lung volumes, pulmonary diffusing capacity, and 6-minute walk distance; hypoxemia with exercise.

Interstitial lung disease, or diffuse parenchymal lung disease, comprises a heterogeneous group of disorders that share common presentations (dyspnea), physical findings (late inspiratory crackles), and chest radiographs (septal thickening and reticulonodular changes).

The term "interstitial" is misleading since the pathologic process usually begins with injury to the alveolar epithelial or capillary endothelial cells (alveolitis). Persistent alveolitis may lead to obliteration of alveolar capillaries and reorganization of the lung parenchyma, accompanied by irreversible fibrosis. The process does not affect the airways proximal to the respiratory bronchioles. Table 9–16 outlines a selected list of differential diagnoses of interstitial lung disease. In most patients, no specific cause can be identified. In the remainder, the principal causes are medications, a variety of organic and inorganic dusts, and connective tissue diseases. The history—particularly the occupational and medication history—may provide evidence of a specific cause. The presence of diffuse parenchymal lung disease in the setting of an established connective tissue disease, such as rheumatoid arthritis, SLE, systemic sclerosis (scleroderma), polymyositis-dermatomyositis, Sjögren syndrome, and other overlap conditions, is suggestive of the cause. In some cases, lung disease precedes the more typical manifestations of the underlying connective tissue disease by months or years.

Known causes of interstitial lung disease are dealt with in their specific sections. The important idiopathic forms are discussed below.

DIFFUSE INTERSTITIAL PNEUMONIAS

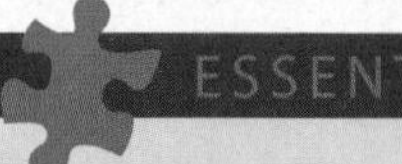
ESSENTIALS OF DIAGNOSIS

- Important to identify specific fibrosing disorders.
- Idiopathic disease may require biopsy for diagnosis.
- Accurate diagnosis identifies patients most likely to benefit from therapy.

General Considerations

The most common diagnosis among patients with diffuse interstitial lung disease is one of the interstitial pneumonias, including all the entities described in Table 9–17. Historically, a diagnosis of interstitial lung disease was based on clinical and radiographic criteria with only a small number of patients undergoing surgical lung biopsy. When biopsies were obtained, the common element of

Table 9–16. Differential diagnosis of interstitial lung disease (listed alphabetically within category).

Medication-related
Antiarrhythmic agents (amiodarone)
Antibacterial agents (nitrofurantoin, sulfonamides)
Antineoplastic agents (bleomycin, cyclophosphamide, methotrexate, nitrosoureas)
Antirheumatic agents (gold salts, penicillamine)
Phenytoin
Environmental and occupational (inhalation exposures)
Dust, inorganic (asbestos, beryllium, hard metals, silica)
Dust, organic (thermophilic actinomycetes, avian antigens, *Aspergillus* species)
Gases, fumes, and vapors (chlorine, isocyanates, paraquat, sulfur dioxide)
Ionizing radiation
Talc (injection drug users)
Infections
Fungus, disseminated (*Blastomyces dermatitidis, Coccidioides immitis, Histoplasma capsulatum*)
Mycobacteria, disseminated
Pneumocystis jirovecii
Viruses
Primary pulmonary disorders
Cryptogenic organizing pneumonia
Idiopathic interstitial pneumonia: acute interstitial pneumonia, desquamative interstitial pneumonia, nonspecific interstitial pneumonia, usual interstitial pneumonia, respiratory bronchiolitis–associated interstitial lung disease
Pulmonary alveolar proteinosis
Systemic disorders
Acute respiratory distress syndrome
Amyloidosis
Ankylosing spondylitis
Autoimmune disease: dermatomyositis, polymyositis, rheumatoid arthritis, SLE, systemic sclerosis (scleroderma)
Chronic eosinophilic pneumonia
Goodpasture syndrome
Granulomatosis polyangiitis
IBD
Idiopathic pulmonary hemosiderosis
Langerhans cell histiocytosis (eosinophilic granuloma)
Lymphangitic spread of cancer (lymphangitic carcinomatosis)
Lymphangioleiomyomatosis
Pulmonary edema
Pulmonary venous hypertension, chronic
Sarcoidosis

fibrosis led to the grouping together of several histologic patterns under the category of interstitial pneumonia or idiopathic pulmonary fibrosis (IPF). Distinct histopathologic features are now understood to represent different natural histories and responses to therapy (Table 9–17). Therefore, in the evaluation of patients with diffuse interstitial lung disease, clinicians should attempt to identify specific disorders.

Patients with diffuse interstitial pneumonia may have any of the histologic patterns described in Table 9–17. The first step in evaluation is to identify patients whose disease is truly idiopathic. As indicated in Table 9–16, most identifiable causes of diffuse interstitial pneumonia are medication-related, environmental, occupational agent exposure, or infectious. Interstitial lung diseases associated with other systemic disorders (pulmonary renal syndromes, autoimmune disease) may be identified through a careful medical history. Chest radiographs and high-resolution CT scans are diagnostic in some patients. Ultimately, many patients with apparently idiopathic disease require surgical lung biopsy to make a definitive diagnosis. The importance of accurate diagnosis is twofold. First, it allows the clinician to provide accurate information about the cause and natural history of the illness. Second, accurate diagnosis helps distinguish patients most likely to benefit from therapy.

Clinical Findings

A. Symptoms, Signs, and Imaging

The most common of the diffuse interstitial pneumonias is pulmonary fibrosis associated with the histopathologic pattern of **usual interstitial pneumonia (UIP).** When no associated cause is evident, this is **IPF.** A diagnosis of IPF/UIP can be made in patients who have (1) idiopathic disease by history and inspiratory crackles on physical examination, (2) restrictive physiology on PFTs, and (3) characteristic UIP pattern on high-resolution chest CT (peripheral, basilar predominant opacities associated with honeycombing and traction bronchiectasis) (Figure 9–5). Such patients do not need surgical lung biopsy. Assessment of pulmonary hypertension is recommended in advanced disease.

Table 9–17. Idiopathic interstitial pneumonias.

Name and Clinical Presentation	Histopathology	Radiographic Pattern	Response to Therapy and Prognosis
Usual interstitial pneumonia (UIP) Age 55–60, slight male predominance. Insidious dry cough and dyspnea lasting months to years. Clubbing present at diagnosis in 25–50%. Diffuse fine late inspiratory crackles on lung auscultation. Restrictive ventilatory defect and reduced diffusing capacity on PFTs. ANA and RF positive in ~25% in the absence of documented collagen-vascular disease.	Patchy, temporally and geographically nonuniform distribution of fibrosis, honeycomb change, and normal lung. Type I pneumocytes are lost, and there is proliferation of alveolar type II cells. "Fibroblast foci" of actively proliferating fibroblasts and myofibroblasts. Inflammation is generally mild and consists of small lymphocytes. Intra-alveolar macrophage accumulation is present but is not a prominent feature.	Diminished lung volume. High-resolution CT scanning shows increased linear or reticular bibasilar and subpleural opacities, with associated honeycombing. Unilateral disease is rare. Minimal ground-glass. Areas of normal lung may be adjacent to areas of advanced fibrosis.	No randomized study has demonstrated improved survival compared with untreated patients. Inexorably progressive. Median survival ~3 years, depending on stage at presentation. Nintedanib and pirfenidone reduce rate of decline in lung function. Refer early for lung transplantation evaluation.
Respiratory bronchiolitis–associated interstitial lung disease (RB-ILD)[1] Age 40–45. Presentation like that of UIP though in younger patients. Similar results on PFTs, but less severe abnormalities. Patients with respiratory bronchiolitis are invariably heavy smokers.	Increased numbers of macrophages evenly dispersed within the alveolar spaces. Rare fibroblast foci, little fibrosis, minimal honeycomb change. In RB-ILD the accumulation of macrophages is localized within the peribronchiolar air spaces; in DIP[1], it is diffuse. Alveolar architecture is preserved.	High-resolution CT shows nodular or reticulonodular pattern, more likely to reveal diffuse ground-glass opacities. Honeycombing is rare. May also show upper lobe emphysema.	Spontaneous remission occurs in up to 20% of patients, so natural history unclear. Smoking cessation is essential. Prognosis clearly better than that of UIP: median survival > 10 years. Corticosteroids thought to be effective, but there are no randomized clinical trials to support this view.
Acute interstitial pneumonia (AIP) Clinically known as Hamman-Rich syndrome. Wide age range, many young patients. Acute onset of dyspnea followed by rapid development of respiratory failure. Half of patients report a viral syndrome preceding lung disease. Clinical course indistinguishable from that of idiopathic ARDS.	Pathologic changes reflect acute response to injury within days to weeks. Resembles organizing phase of diffuse alveolar damage. Fibrosis and minimal collagen deposition. May appear like UIP but more homogeneous and there is no honeycomb change—though this may appear if the process persists for more than a month in a patient on mechanical ventilation.	Diffuse bilateral airspace consolidation with areas of ground-glass attenuation on high-resolution CT scan.	Supportive care (mechanical ventilation) critical but effect of specific therapies unclear. High initial mortality: 50–90% die within 2 months after diagnosis. Not progressive if patient survives. Lung function may return to normal or may be permanently impaired.
Nonspecific interstitial pneumonia (NSIP) Age 45–55. Slight female predominance. Like UIP but onset of cough and dyspnea over months, not years.	Nonspecific in that histopathology does not fit into better-established categories. Varying degrees of inflammation and fibrosis, patchy in distribution but uniform in time, suggesting response to single injury. Most have lymphocytic and plasma cell inflammation without fibrosis. Honeycombing present but scant. Some have advocated division into cellular and fibrotic subtypes.	May be indistinguishable from UIP. Most typical picture is bilateral areas of ground-glass attenuation and fibrosis on high-resolution CT. Honeycombing is rare.	Treatment with corticosteroids thought to be effective, but no prospective clinical studies have been published. Overall prognosis good but depends on the extent of fibrosis at diagnosis. Median survival > 10 years.
Cryptogenic organizing pneumonia (COP) Typically age 50–60 but wide variation. Abrupt onset, frequently weeks to a few months following a flu-like illness. Dyspnea and dry cough prominent, but constitutional symptoms are common: fatigue, fever, and weight loss. PFTs usually show restriction, but up to 25% show concomitant obstruction.	Included in the idiopathic interstitial pneumonias on clinical grounds. Buds of loose connective tissue (Masson bodies) and inflammatory cells fill alveoli and distal bronchioles.	Lung volumes normal. Chest radiograph typically shows interstitial and parenchymal disease with discrete, peripheral alveolar and ground-glass infiltrates. Nodular opacities common. High-resolution CT shows subpleural consolidation and bronchial wall thickening and dilation.	Rapid response to corticosteroids in two-thirds of patients. Long-term prognosis generally good for those who respond. Relapses are common.

[1]Includes desquamative interstitial pneumonia (DIP).
ANA, antinuclear antibody; ARDS, acute respiratory distress syndrome; PFTs, pulmonary function tests; RF, rheumatoid factor; UIP, usual interstitial pneumonia.

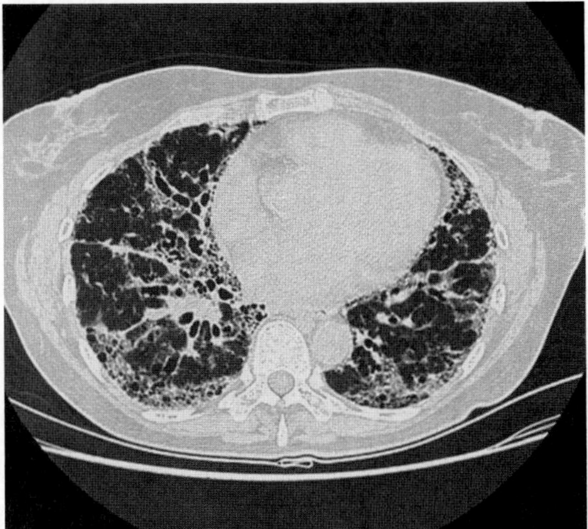

▲ **Figure 9–5.** Idiopathic pulmonary fibrosis. CT scan of the lungs showing the typical radiographic pattern of idiopathic pulmonary fibrosis, with a predominantly basilar, peripheral pattern of traction bronchiectasis, reticulation, and early honeycombing.

B. Special Studies

Three diagnostic techniques are in common use: BAL, transbronchial biopsy, and surgical lung biopsy, either through an open procedure or using VATS.

BAL may provide a specific diagnosis in cases of infection, particularly with *P jirovecii* or mycobacteria, or when cytologic examination reveals the presence of malignant cells. Additionally, BAL may be diagnostic of eosinophilic pneumonia, Langerhans cell histiocytosis, or alveolar proteinosis.

Transbronchial biopsy through the flexible bronchoscope is easily performed in most patients. The risks of pneumothorax (5%) and hemorrhage (1–10%) are low. However, the tissue specimens recovered are small, sampling error is common, and crush artifact may complicate diagnosis. Transbronchial biopsy can make a definitive diagnosis of sarcoidosis, lymphangitic spread of carcinoma, pulmonary alveolar proteinosis, miliary tuberculosis, and Langerhans cell histiocytosis. However, in IPF, transbronchial biopsy cannot confirm the diagnosis since the histologic diagnosis requires a pattern of changes rather than a single pathognomonic finding. IPF patients generally require surgical lung biopsy.

Surgical lung biopsy is the standard for diagnosis of diffuse interstitial lung disease. Two or three biopsies taken from multiple sites in the same lung, including apparently normal tissue, may yield a specific diagnosis as well as prognostic information regarding the extent of fibrosis versus active inflammation. Patients under age 60 without a specific diagnosis generally should undergo surgical lung biopsy. In older and sicker patients, the risks and benefits must be weighed carefully for three reasons: (1) the morbidity of the procedure can be significant; (2) a definitive diagnosis may not be possible even with surgical lung biopsy; and (3) when a specific diagnosis is made, there may be no effective treatment. Empiric therapy or no treatment may be preferable to surgical lung biopsy in some patients.

▶ Treatment

Patients with diffuse interstitial pneumonia should be treated by a pulmonologist. Clinical experience suggests that patients with RB-ILD, nonspecific interstitial pneumonia (NSIP), or COP (Table 9–17) frequently respond to corticosteroids and should be given a trial of therapy—typically prednisone, 1–2 mg/kg/day for a minimum of 2 months. Corticosteroid therapy is ineffective in patients with IPF and is not recommended. Nintedanib and pirfenidone are approved for the treatment of IPF based on clinical trials in highly selected patients showing a significant reduction in their rate of decline in lung function, but neither agent improved survival or quality of life. The only definitive treatment for IPF is lung transplantation, with a 5-year survival rate estimated at 50%.

▶ When to Refer

- Patients with diffuse interstitial pneumonia should be referred early to a pulmonologist for expert diagnosis and management.
- Patients with IPF should be referred early to a lung transplant program for evaluation.

Gibson CD et al. Comparison of clinical measures among interstitial lung disease (ILD) patients with usual interstitial pneumonia (UIP) patterns on high-resolution computed tomography. Lung. 2020;198:811. [PMID: 32889595]

SARCOIDOSIS

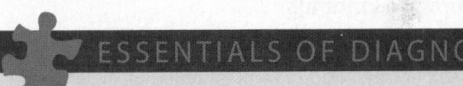

ESSENTIALS OF DIAGNOSIS

- Symptoms related to the lung, skin, eyes, peripheral nerves, liver, kidney, heart.
- Demonstration of noncaseating granulomas in a biopsy specimen.

▶ General Considerations

Sarcoidosis is a systemic disease of unknown etiology characterized in about 90% of patients by granulomatous inflammation of the lung. The incidence is highest in North American Black persons and northern European White persons. Among Black persons, women are more frequently affected than men. Onset of disease is usually in the third or fourth decade.

▶ Clinical Findings

A. Symptoms and Signs

Patients may have malaise, fever, and dyspnea of insidious onset. Symptoms caused by skin involvement (erythema nodosum, lupus pernio [Figure 9–6]), iritis, peripheral

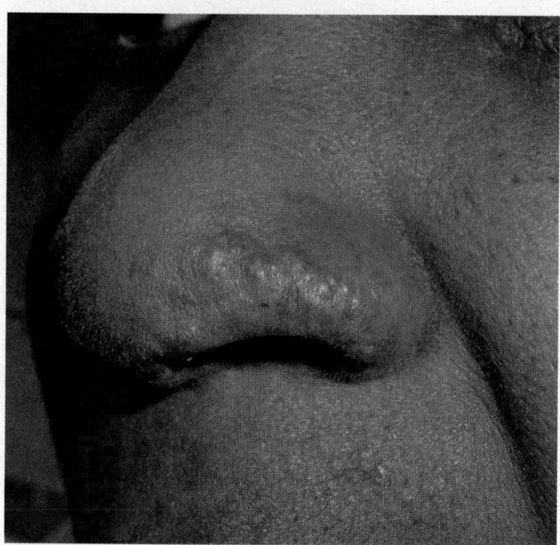

▲ **Figure 9–6. Skin involvement in sarcoidosis (lupus pernio), here involving the nasal rim.** (Reproduced with permission from Richard P. Usatine, MD, in Usatine RP, Smith MA, Mayeaux EJ Jr, Chumley HS. *The Color Atlas and Synopsis of Family Medicine*, 3rd ed. McGraw-Hill, 2019.)

neuropathy, arthritis (Chapter 20), or cardiomyopathy may also prompt the patient to seek care. Some individuals are asymptomatic and come to medical attention after abnormal findings on chest radiographs (typically bilateral hilar and paratracheal lymphadenopathy). Physical findings of interstitial lung disease with crackles are uncommon. Other symptoms and findings may include parotid gland enlargement, hepatosplenomegaly, and lymphadenopathy.

B. Laboratory Findings

Laboratory tests may show leukopenia, an elevated ESR, and hypercalcemia (about 5% of patients) or hypercalciuria (20%). ACE levels are elevated in 40–80% of patients with active disease, though this finding is neither sensitive nor specific. Physiologic testing may reveal evidence of airflow obstruction or restriction with decreased lung volumes and diffusing capacity, or both. ECG may show heart block and dysrhythmias.

C. Imaging

Radiographic findings are variable and include bilateral hilar adenopathy alone (radiographic stage I), hilar adenopathy and parenchymal involvement (radiographic stage II), parenchymal involvement alone (radiographic stage III), or advanced fibrotic changes principally in the upper lobes (radiographic stage IV). Parenchymal involvement is usually manifested radiographically by diffuse reticular infiltrates, but focal infiltrates, acinar shadows, nodules, and, rarely, cavitation may be seen. Pleural effusion is noted in less than 10% of patients.

D. Special Examinations

The diagnosis of sarcoidosis generally requires histologic demonstration of noncaseating granulomas in biopsies from a patient with other typical associated manifestations. Other granulomatous diseases (eg, berylliosis, tuberculosis, fungal infections) and lymphoma must be excluded. Biopsy of easily accessible sites (eg, palpable lymph nodes, skin lesions, or salivary glands) may be an initial step. Transbronchial lung biopsy has a high yield (75–90%) as well, especially in patients with radiographic evidence of parenchymal involvement. Some clinicians believe that tissue biopsy is not necessary when stage I radiographic findings are detected in a clinical situation that strongly favors the diagnosis of sarcoidosis (eg, a young Black woman with erythema nodosum). Biopsy is essential whenever clinical and radiographic findings suggest the possibility of an alternative diagnosis, such as lymphoma. BAL fluid in sarcoidosis is usually characterized by an increase in lymphocytes and a high CD4/CD8 cell ratio, but it does not establish a diagnosis. Patients require a yearly ophthalmologic evaluation, liver and renal function testing, PFTs, and an ECG. Cardiac MRI is favored over PET scan for patients with suspected cardiac involvement. Assessment of pulmonary hypertension is recommended in advanced disease.

▶ Treatment

Treatment is not recommended for asymptomatic disease. Oral corticosteroids (prednisone, 0.5–1.0 mg/kg/day) are indicated for patients with disabling constitutional symptoms, hypercalcemia, iritis, uveitis, arthritis, CNS involvement, cardiac involvement, granulomatous hepatitis, cutaneous lesions other than erythema nodosum, and progressive pulmonary lesions. Long-term therapy is usually required over months to years. Immunosuppressive medications, most commonly methotrexate, azathioprine, or infliximab, are used in patients who are intolerant of corticosteroids or who have corticosteroid-refractory disease. A favorable response is defined by a decrease in symptoms, reduction of radiographic abnormalities, and improvement in PFTs.

▶ Prognosis

The outlook is best for patients with hilar adenopathy alone; radiographic involvement of the lung parenchyma is associated with a worse prognosis. Erythema nodosum portends a good outcome. About 20% of patients with lung involvement suffer irreversible lung impairment, characterized by progressive fibrosis, bronchiectasis, and cavitation. Pneumothorax, hemoptysis, mycetoma formation in lung cavities, pulmonary hypertension, and respiratory failure may often complicate this advanced stage. Myocardial sarcoidosis occurs in about 5% of patients, sometimes leading to restrictive cardiomyopathy, cardiac dysrhythmias, and conduction disturbances. Death from respiratory insufficiency occurs in about 5% of patients. Patients require long-term follow-up.

Crouser ED et al. Diagnosis and detection of sarcoidosis. An Official American Thoracic Society Clinical Practice Guideline. Am J Respir Crit Care Med. 2020;201:e26. [PMID: 32293205]

Grunewald J et al. Sarcoidosis. Nat Rev Dis Primers. 2019;5:45. [PMID: 31273209]

Llanos O et al. Sarcoidosis. Med Clin North Am. 2019;103:527. [PMID: 30955519]
Ungprasert P et al. Clinical manifestations, diagnosis, and treatment of sarcoidosis. Mayo Clin Proc Innov Qual Outcomes. 2019;3:358. [PMID: 31485575]

PULMONARY ALVEOLAR PROTEINOSIS

Pulmonary alveolar proteinosis is a rare disease characterized by accumulation of lipoproteinaceous material within alveolar spaces. The condition may be primary (idiopathic) or secondary (occurring in immunodeficiency; hematologic malignancies; inhalation of mineral dusts; or following lung infections, including tuberculosis and viral infections). Progressive dyspnea is the usual presenting symptom. Chest radiograph shows bilateral alveolar infiltrates, and chest CT features a characteristic "crazy-paving" that refers to ground-glass opacities with superimposed interlobular and intralobular septal thickening. The diagnosis is based on demonstration of characteristic findings on BAL (milky appearance and periodic acid-Schiff [PAS]-positive lipoproteinaceous material) in association with clinical and radiographic features. In secondary disease, an elevated anti-GM-CSF (anti-granulocyte-macrophage colony-stimulating factor) titer in serum or BAL fluid is highly sensitive and specific.

The course of the disease varies. Some patients experience spontaneous remission; others develop progressive respiratory insufficiency. Therapy for alveolar proteinosis consists of periodic whole-lung lavage. Patients who cannot tolerate whole lung lavage or who fail to respond may benefit from inhalational or subcutaneous GM-CSF. Pulmonary infection with *Nocardia* or fungi may occur.

Salvaterra E et al. Pulmonary alveolar proteinosis: from classification to therapy. Breathe (Sheff). 2020;16:200018. [PMID: 32684997]
Trapnell BC et al. Pulmonary alveolar proteinosis. Nat Rev Dis Primers. 2019;5:16. [PMID: 30846703]
Trapnell BC et al; IMPALA Trial Investigators. Inhaled molgramostim therapy in autoimmune pulmonary alveolar proteinosis. N Engl J Med. 2020;383:1635. [PMID: 32897035]

EOSINOPHILIC PULMONARY SYNDROMES

Eosinophilic pulmonary syndromes are a diverse group of disorders typically characterized by peripheral blood eosinophilia (typically > 500 cells/mcL [0.5×10^9/L]), eosinophilic pulmonary infiltrates, dyspnea, and cough. Many patients have constitutional symptoms, including fever. Common causes include exposure to medications (nitrofurantoin, phenytoin, ampicillin, acetaminophen) or infection with helminths (eg, *Ascaris*, hookworms, *Strongyloides*) or filariae (eg, *Wuchereria bancrofti, Brugia malayi*, tropical pulmonary eosinophilia). **Löffler syndrome** refers to acute eosinophilic pulmonary infiltrates in response to transpulmonary passage of helminth larvae. Pulmonary eosinophilia can also be a feature of other illnesses, including ABPA, eosinophilic granulomatosis with polyangiitis, systemic hypereosinophilic syndromes, eosinophilic granuloma of the lung (properly referred to as pulmonary Langerhans cell histiocytosis), neoplasms, and numerous interstitial lung diseases. If an extrinsic cause is identified, therapy consists of removal of the offending medication or treatment of the underlying parasitic infection.

One-third of cases are idiopathic, and there are two common syndromes. **Acute eosinophilic pneumonia** is an acute, febrile illness characterized by cough and dyspnea, sometimes rapidly progressing to respiratory failure. The chest radiograph is abnormal but nonspecific. BAL fluid frequently shows eosinophilia, but peripheral blood eosinophilia is rare at the onset of symptoms. The response to corticosteroids is usually dramatic. **Chronic eosinophilic pneumonia** has a subacute-chronic presentation, characterized by fever, night sweats, weight loss, and dyspnea. Asthma or atopy is present in half of cases. Chest radiographs often show peripheral infiltrates, the "photographic negative" of pulmonary edema. BAL typically has a marked eosinophilia, and peripheral blood eosinophilia is present in greater than 80%. Therapy with oral prednisone (1 mg/kg/day for 1–2 weeks, followed by a gradual taper over months) usually results in dramatic improvement; however, most patients require at least 10–15 mg of prednisone every other day for a year or more (sometimes indefinitely) to prevent relapses.

Rosenberg CE et al. Approach to eosinophilia presenting with pulmonary symptoms. Chest. 2021;159:507. [PMID: 33002503]
Suzuki Y et al. Eosinophilic pneumonia: a review of the previous literature, causes, diagnosis, and management. Allergol Int. 2019;68:413. [PMID: 31253537]

DISORDERS OF THE PULMONARY CIRCULATION

PULMONARY VENOUS THROMBOEMBOLISM

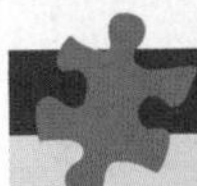

ESSENTIALS OF DIAGNOSIS

- Third most common cardiovascular cause of death in the United States.
- May present with one or more of the following: dyspnea, pleuritic chest pain, hemoptysis, syncope.
- Tachypnea, tachycardia, hypoxia may be present (alone or in any combination).
- Risk stratification with clinical scores, cardiac biomarkers, and right ventricular imaging is key for management.

General Considerations

Pulmonary venous thromboembolism (VTE), often referred to as PE, is a common, serious, and potentially fatal result of thrombus formation within the deep venous circulation that then migrates to the pulmonary circulation. PE is the third leading cause of death among hospitalized patients. Management demands a vigilant systematic approach to diagnosis and an understanding of risk factors so that appropriate therapy can be initiated.

Many substances can embolize to the pulmonary circulation, including air (during neurosurgery, from central venous catheters), amniotic fluid (during active labor), fat (long bone fractures), foreign bodies (talc in injection drug users), parasite eggs (schistosomiasis), septic emboli (acute infective endocarditis), and tumor cells (renal cell carcinoma). The most common embolus is thrombus, which may arise anywhere in the venous circulation or right heart but most often originates in the deep veins of the lower extremities. Pulmonary emboli will develop in 50–60% of patients with proximal DVT; half of these embolic events will be asymptomatic. Approximately 50–70% of patients who have symptomatic pulmonary emboli will have lower extremity DVT when evaluated.

Risk factors for PE include venous stasis, injury to the vessel wall, and hypercoagulability (Virchow triad). Venous stasis increases with immobility (obesity, stroke, bed rest—especially postoperative), hyperviscosity (polycythemia), and increased central venous pressures (low cardiac output states, pregnancy). Vessels may be damaged by prior episodes of thrombosis, orthopedic surgery, or trauma. Hypercoagulability can be caused by medications (oral contraceptives, hormonal replacement therapy) or disease (malignancy, surgery) or may be the result of inherited gene defects (factor V Leiden, prothrombin mutation) or acquired thrombophilias (protein C and protein S deficiency, antithrombin deficiency, antiphospholipid antibodies).

PE has multiple physiologic effects. Thrombus occlusion of greater than 20–25% of vascular bed causes right ventricular dilation or dysfunction and increased pulmonary vascular resistance. Vascular obstruction increases physiologic dead space (wasted ventilation) and leads to hypoxemia through right-to-left shunting, decreased cardiac output, and surfactant depletion causing atelectasis.

Clinical Findings

A. Symptoms and Signs

The clinical diagnosis of PE is notoriously challenging because the clinical symptoms and signs are similar to those of other cardiopulmonary conditions. Dyspnea and chest pain on inspiration are common. Diagnosis primarily relies on clinical prediction scores to calculate the pretest probability of PE. Wells score is most commonly used and quantifies clinical risk assessment, allowing separation of patients into low, intermediate, or high probability groups, or PE-likely versus PE-unlikely groups (Table 9–18).

B. Laboratory Findings

The **ECG** is abnormal in 70% of patients with PE. However, the most common abnormalities are sinus tachycardia and nonspecific ST and T wave changes, each seen in approximately 40% of patients. Five percent or less of patients in the PIOPED I study had P pulmonale, right ventricular hypertrophy, right axis deviation, and right bundle branch block.

ABGs usually reveal acute respiratory alkalosis due to hyperventilation and may show hypoxemia.

Table 9–18. Clinical prediction rule for PE.

Variable	Points
Clinical symptoms and signs of DVT (leg swelling and pain with palpation of deep veins)	3.0
Alternative diagnosis less likely than PE	3.0
Heart rate > 100 beats/minute	1.5
Immobilization for > 3 days or surgery in previous 4 weeks	1.5
Previous PE or DVT	1.5
Hemoptysis	1.0
Cancer (with treatment within past 6 months or palliative care)	1.0
Add **Points** *to determine* **Score**, *then refer to* **probability assessments** *below*:	
Three-tiered clinical probability assessment (Wells criteria)	**Score**
High	> 6.0
Moderate	2.0 to 6.0
Low	< 2.0
Dichotomous clinical probability assessment (Modified Wells criteria)	**Score**
PE likely	> 4.0
PE unlikely	< or = 4.0

Data from Wells PS et al. Derivation of a simple clinical model to categorize patients' probability of pulmonary embolism: increasing the models' utility with the SimpliRED D-dimer. Thromb Haemost. 2000;83:416.

Plasma levels of **D-dimer,** a degradation product of cross-linked fibrin, are elevated in the presence of thrombus. A D-dimer of less than 500 ng/mL may be used to exclude the diagnosis of PE in those patients who have low pretest probability of PE or are PE-unlikely on Wells score. Additionally, an age-adjusted D-dimer value has increased specificity than the usually specified cutoff. Due to much higher false-positive rates, D-dimer is not useful for hospital inpatients.

Serum troponin I, troponin T, and plasma BNP levels are elevated in approximately 25% of patients with PE and are useful in the risk stratification of PE because they correlate with adverse outcomes, including mechanical ventilation, prolonged hospitalization, and death.

C. Imaging and Special Examinations

1. Chest radiography—The chest radiograph is necessary to exclude other common lung diseases, but it does not establish the diagnosis of PE by itself. The chest radiograph may be normal or may show atelectasis, parenchymal infiltrates, and pleural effusions. A prominent central pulmonary artery with local oligemia (Westermark sign) or pleural-based areas of increased opacity that represent intraparenchymal hemorrhage (Hampton hump) are uncommon. Profound hypoxia with a normal chest radiograph is highly suspicious for PE.

2. Pulmonary CT-angiography—Helical CT-PA is the gold standard diagnostic study in North America for suspected PE due to its high sensitivity and specificity as well as wide availability across hospitals. CT-PA requires administration of intravenous radiocontrast dye but is otherwise noninvasive. Patients with intermediate- or high-pretest probability of PE (or PE-likely) or those with an elevated D-dimer should undergo a CT-PA.

3. Ventilation-perfusion ($\dot{V}/\dot{Q}$) lung scanning—$\dot{V}/\dot{Q}$ scanning may be used as an alternative to CT-PA in patients in whom contrast is contraindicated, such as severe contrast-induced anaphylaxis or kidney dysfunction. $\dot{V}/\dot{Q}$ scanning is performed by injecting radiolabeled microaggregated albumin into the venous system, allowing the particles to embolize to the pulmonary capillary bed (perfusion); the patient breathes a radioactive gas or aerosol while the distribution of radioactivity in the lungs is recorded (ventilation). A defect in perfusion without a corresponding defect in ventilation may indicate a PE but is not specific for the diagnosis. A normal $\dot{V}/\dot{Q}$ scan excludes the diagnosis of clinically significant PE (negative predictive value of 91% in the PIOPED I study).

4. Venous thrombosis studies—Venous ultrasonography is the test of choice to detect proximal DVT. Inability to compress the common femoral or popliteal veins in symptomatic patients is diagnostic (positive predictive value of 97%); full compressibility of both sites excludes proximal DVT (negative predictive value of 98%).

Contrast venography may be used to diagnose intraluminal filling defects, though the test is very infrequently used except in complex situations when there is discrepancy between clinical suspicion and venous ultrasound results.

5. Pulmonary angiography—Pulmonary angiography is the historical reference standard for the diagnosis of PE. At present, pulmonary angiography is only used during catheter-directed therapy (for administration of a thrombolytic or for mechanical thrombectomy) in the treatment of acute PE or to confirm the diagnosis of chronic PE in chronic thromboembolic pulmonary hypertension.

Integrated Approach to Diagnosis of Pulmonary Embolism

The diagnosis of PE uses the clinical likelihood derived from clinical prediction rules, such as Wells score (Table 9–18) along with the results of diagnostic tests, such as D-dimer, to establish a pretest probability of PE. The ideal diagnostic approach is a cost-effective, stepwise sequence to come to these decision points at minimal risk to the patient.

In patients with low pretest probability, a normal D-dimer rules out presence of PE. The Pulmonary Embolism Rule-out Criteria (PERC) may be used to identify patients for whom no testing is indicated (Table 9–19). Imaging is recommended for patients with low or intermediate pretest probability (or PE-unlikely) but a positive D-dimer or those with high pretest probability (or PE-likely).

Table 9–19. Pulmonary embolism rule-out criteria (PERC) for low-risk patients.

For patients with a Modified Wells Score ≤ 4[1] who meet ALL of the following criteria, PE is excluded, monitor off anticoagulation, and search for alternative diagnoses.

- Age < 50 years
- Heart rate < 100 bpm
- Oxyhemoglobin saturation on room air ≥ 95%
- No prior history of venous thromboembolism
- No recent (within 4 weeks) trauma or surgery requiring hospitalization
- No presenting hemoptysis
- No estrogen therapy
- No unilateral leg swelling

[1]See Table 9–18.
Data from Kline JA et al. Impact of a rapid rule-out protocol for pulmonary embolism on the rate of screening, missed cases, and pulmonary vascular imaging in an urban US emergency room. Ann Emerg Med. 2004;44:490.

Risk Stratification of Pulmonary Embolism

After a PE diagnosis is made, the next step is risk stratification since this will guide management. There are three categories based on mortality data: high-risk PE, intermediate-risk PE, and low-risk PE. Patients with high-risk PE, also known as massive PE, have hemodynamic compromise, defined as systolic blood pressure less than 90 mm Hg or a systolic blood pressure drop by 40 mm Hg or more for longer than 15 minutes, requiring a vasopressor, or causing a cardiac arrest. Patients with an intermediate-risk PE, also known as submassive PE, are hemodynamically stable but do have signs of right ventricular strain or dysfunction, either by imaging (CT-PA or echocardiogram) or cardiac biomarkers (troponin or BNP). Patients with low-risk PE have normotension without signs of right ventricular dysfunction.

PE severity scores, such as PE Severity Score Index (PESI) or the simplified PESI, compile useful patient characteristics that predict patient outcome. Such scores may also be used to decide which patients may be appropriate for outpatient PE treatment. Imaging of the right ventricle, usually using CT-PA or echocardiogram and cardiac biomarkers (troponin and/or BNP) are other useful tools that may help predict adverse outcomes.

Prevention

Discussion of strategies for the prevention of VTE can be found in Chapter 14.

Treatment

A. Anticoagulation

Anticoagulation is the mainstay therapy for VTE. It impedes additional thrombus formation, allowing endogenous fibrinolytic mechanisms to lyse existing clot, thereby decreasing mortality and recurrence of PE. Initiation of anticoagulation should be considered even prior to a confirmed diagnosis when there is high clinical suspicion and low risk of bleeding.

Unfractionated heparin binds to and accelerates the ability of antithrombin to inactivate thrombin, factor Xa, and factor IXa. Compared to unfractionated heparin, low-molecular-weight heparins (LMWHs) are as effective but have faster therapeutic activity in the treatment of VTE. Direct-acting oral anticoagulants (DOACs) offer predictable pharmacokinetics and pharmacodynamics with fixed dosing, few drug interactions, and relatively short half-life. DOACs are recommended as first-line anticoagulation for most patients.

The optimal duration of anticoagulation therapy for venous thromboembolism depends on the risk factors for VTE recurrence. Extended anticoagulation should be considered for patients with no identifiable risk factor for the index PE event, those with a persistent risk factor, those with recurrent VTE, or those with a minor risk factor (such as immobility due to prolonged car or air travel, obesity, pregnancy, or increased age). However, those with major transient/reversible risk factors (such as fracture of lower limb; hip or knee surgery; or hospitalization for heart failure, atrial fibrillation, or MI) may be considered for discontinuation of anticoagulation after 3 months. Additionally, duration of therapy needs to take into consideration the patient's age, likelihood and potential consequences of hemorrhage, and preferences for continued therapy. The D-dimer level measured a month after stopping anticoagulant therapy as well as the patient's sex may influence whether to remain off or to restart treatment. In patients who continue taking extended anticoagulation, an annual risk-benefit assessment of continuing anticoagulation therapy should be done.

The major complication of anticoagulation is hemorrhage. Risk factors for hemorrhage include the intensity of the anticoagulation; duration of therapy; concomitant administration of medications, such as aspirin, that interfere with platelet function; and patient characteristics, particularly increased age, previous GI hemorrhage, and coexistent kidney or liver disease.

B. Thrombolytic Therapy

Streptokinase, urokinase, and recombinant tissue plasminogen activator (rt-PA; alteplase) increase plasmin levels and thereby directly lyse intravascular thrombi accelerating resolution of emboli. Guidelines support systemic thrombolysis for high-risk or massive PE (hemodynamically unstable) with low risk of bleeding. Intermediate-risk or submassive PE patients (hemodynamically stable with evidence of right heart strain) do not have a mortality benefit with thrombolytic therapy but do have a significant decrease in incidence of hemodynamic collapse; however, they also have an increase in major hemorrhagic complications, including intracranial hemorrhage. Absolute contraindications to thrombolytic therapy include active bleeding and stroke within the past 3 months. Relative contraindications include uncontrolled hypertension and surgery or trauma within the past 4 weeks.

Catheter-directed thrombolysis delivers a low-dose of the thrombolytic agent directly into the PE, thereby reversing right ventricular dilation faster than anticoagulation alone. This procedure may be considered for patients with high-risk PE (though with higher risks of bleeding) and for those with intermediate-risk PE at increased risk of hemodynamic collapse.

C. Additional Measures

Mechanical pulmonary embolectomy or surgical embolectomy may be considered for selected patients with contraindications to thrombolysis or failure of thrombolysis.

Inferior vena cava filters should be inserted in patients with contraindications to anticoagulation and those with recurrent PE despite adequate anticoagulation. Consideration should be given for those with acute PE and presence of free-floating proximal end DVT, since it carries an increased risk of embolization. Once placed, it must be assessed for removal at the earliest opportunity.

Prognosis

PE is estimated to cause more than 50,000–100,000 deaths annually in the United States. The outlook for most patients is generally good. However, mortality for intermediate-risk (submassive) PE or high-risk (massive) PE may be as high as 20% and 50%, respectively. Therefore, early diagnosis and risk stratification are key. Survivors may have long-term sequelae of PE, such as exercise intolerance, chronic thromboembolic disease, and chronic thromboembolic pulmonary hypertension. Therefore, follow-up care to assess whether patients have persistent or recurrent symptoms is very important.

When to Admit

Most patients with acute PE require hospitalization. The decision to admit patients with acute PE requires assessment of factors placing them at high risk, including their severity of illness (eg, severe hypoxemia), comorbidities (eg, DVT, cardiac dysfunction), educational needs (eg, lack of knowledge about PE and its management), and/or problematic social situations (eg, prior noncompliance with follow-up care). Carefully selected patients with low-risk PE can be safely and effectively managed as outpatients with the aid of integrated clinical decision support systems.

Konstantinides SV et al. 2019 ESC Guidelines for the diagnosis and management of acute pulmonary embolism developed in collaboration with the European Respiratory Society (ERS). Eur Heart J. 2020;41:543. [PMID: 31473594]

Rivera-Lebron BN et al. Diagnosis, treatment and follow up of acute pulmonary embolism: consensus statement from the PERT Consortium. Clin Appl Hemost. 2019;25: 1076029619853037. [PMID: 31185730]

Stevens SM et al. Antithrombotic therapy for VTE disease: second update of the CHEST Guideline and Expert Panel Report. Chest. 2021;160:e545. [PMID: 34352278]

PULMONARY HYPERTENSION

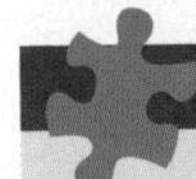

ESSENTIALS OF DIAGNOSIS

- Dyspnea, fatigue, chest pain, and syncope on exertion.
- Narrow splitting of second heart sound with loud pulmonary component; findings of right ventricular hypertrophy and heart failure in advanced disease.
- Electrocardiographic evidence of right ventricular strain or hypertrophy and right atrial enlargement.
- Enlarged central pulmonary arteries on chest radiograph.
- Elevated right ventricular systolic pressure, right ventricular dilation or dysfunction on two-dimensional echocardiography with Doppler flow studies.

General Considerations

Pulmonary hypertension is a complex problem characterized by pathologic elevation in pulmonary arterial pressure. Normal pulmonary artery systolic pressure at rest is 15–30 mm Hg, with a mean pressure less than 20 mm Hg. The pulmonary circulation is a low-pressure, low-resistance system due to its large cross-sectional area, and it can accommodate significant increase in blood flow during exercise. The primary pathologic mechanism in pulmonary hypertension is an increase in pulmonary vascular resistance that leads to an increase in the pulmonary systolic pressure. Pulmonary hypertension is defined by a mean pulmonary arterial pressure of 20 mm Hg or more on a resting cardiac catheterization.

The WHO/New York Heart Association (NYHA) functional class currently classifies pulmonary hypertension based on similarities in pathologic mechanisms and includes the following five groups.

Group 1 (pulmonary arterial hypertension [PAH]): This group gathers diseases that localize directly to the pulmonary arteries leading to structural changes, smooth muscle hypertrophy, and endothelial dysfunction. This group includes idiopathic (formerly primary) PAH; heritable PAH; drug- and toxin-induced PAH; PAH associated with HIV infection, portal hypertension, connective tissue disorders (most commonly scleroderma), congenital heart disease, and schistosomiasis; and PAH with features of veno-occlusive disease and pulmonary capillary hemangiomatosis. PAH is defined on a resting cardiac catheterization by a mean pulmonary arterial pressure of 20 mm Hg or more with a pulmonary capillary wedge pressure of 15 mm Hg or less and a pulmonary vascular resistance of 3 Wood units or more.

Group 2 (pulmonary venous hypertension due to left heart disease): This group includes LV systolic or diastolic dysfunction and valvular heart disease.

Group 3 (pulmonary hypertension due to lung disease or hypoxemia): This group is caused by advanced obstructive and restrictive lung disease, including COPD, interstitial lung disease, pulmonary fibrosis as well as other causes of chronic hypoxemia, such as sleep-disordered breathing, alveolar hypoventilation syndromes, and high-altitude exposure.

Group 4 (pulmonary hypertension due to pulmonary obstruction): This group primarily includes chronic thromboembolic pulmonary hypertension but also includes other causes of pulmonary obstructions, such as sarcoma, metastatic malignancies, and congenital pulmonary artery stenosis.

Group 5 (pulmonary hypertension secondary to unclear or multifactorial mechanisms): These patients have pulmonary hypertension secondary to hematologic disorders (eg, chronic hemolytic anemia, sickle cell anemia, myeloproliferative disorders, splenectomy), systemic disorders (eg, sarcoidosis, vasculitis, pulmonary Langerhans cell histiocytosis, neurofibromatosis type 1), metabolic disorders (eg, glycogen storage disease, Gaucher disease, thyroid disease), and miscellaneous causes (eg, ESKD with or without hemodialysis, fibrosing mediastinitis).

The clinical severity of pulmonary hypertension is classified according to the NYHA classification system, which was originally developed for heart failure but subsequently modified by the WHO; it is based primarily on symptoms and functional status.

Class I: No limitation of physical activity; no dyspnea, fatigue, chest pain, or near syncope is present with exertion.

Class II: Slight limitation of physical activity; no symptoms at rest, but ordinary physical activity causes dyspnea, fatigue, chest pain, or near syncope.

Class III: Marked limitation of physical activity; no symptoms at rest, but less than ordinary activity causes dyspnea, fatigue, chest pain, or near syncope.

Class IV: Inability to perform any physical activity without symptoms; dyspnea and fatigue are present at rest and symptoms worsen with any activity.

Clinical Findings

A. Symptoms and Signs

There are no specific symptoms or signs of pulmonary hypertension, which may delay its diagnosis and significantly affect its mortality. Typical symptoms include dyspnea with exertion and with advanced disease, at rest. Patients may have chest pain, nonproductive cough, and fatigue. Syncope may occur with exertion when there is insufficient cardiac output or if there is an arrhythmia.

Findings on physical examination can include jugular venous distention, accentuated pulmonary valve component of the second heart sound, right-sided third heart sound, tricuspid regurgitation murmur, hepatomegaly, and lower extremity edema.

B. Laboratory Findings

Routine blood work is often normal. BNP or pro-BNP may be elevated. All patients should be evaluated for HIV, liver dysfunction, and connective tissue disorders.

The ECG is typically normal except in advanced disease, where right ventricular hypertrophy (right axis deviation, incomplete right bundle branch block) and right atrial enlargement (peaked P wave in the inferior and right-sided leads) can be noted.

C. Imaging and Special Examinations

Radiographs and CT scans of the chest are useful in diagnosis. Enlargement of the right and left main pulmonary arteries is common; right ventricular and right atrial enlargement is seen in advanced disease. Chest CT scanning and PFTs are also useful in determining the cause of pulmonary hypertension for patients in Group 3 (pulmonary hypertension due to lung disease). On PFTs, the combination of normal FVC on spirometry, normal TLC on lung volume measurement, and significantly decreased diffusing capacity may be suggestive of PAH (Group 1). However, FVC and TLC may be also reduced in pulmonary hypertension due to lung disease (Group 3).

Echocardiography is the best screening study. Right ventricular assessment is made by measuring right ventricular size and function as well as right ventricular systolic pressure, which is estimated based on tricuspid jet velocity and right atrial pressure. Additionally, the echocardiogram is useful for assessing underlying cardiac disease (eg, pulmonary hypertension due to left heart disease).

Right-sided cardiac catheterization remains the gold standard for the diagnosis and quantification of pulmonary hypertension and should be performed prior to initiation of advanced therapies. Estimated pressures on echocardiogram correlate with right heart catheterization measurement but can vary by at least 10 mm Hg in more than 50% of cases so should not be used to direct therapy. Cardiac catheterization is particularly helpful in differentiating PAH from pulmonary venous hypertension by assessment of the drop in pressure across the pulmonary circulation, also known as the transpulmonary gradient. A vasodilator challenge can be performed during right heart catheterization and a significant acute vasodilator response consists of a drop in mean pulmonary pressure of greater than 10 mm Hg (or 20%) to less than 40 mm Hg.

In all patients, especially those with a history of PE or risk factors for thromboembolic disease, chronic thromboembolic pulmonary hypertension (Group 4) should be excluded prior to diagnosing idiopathic pulmonary hypertension with $\dot{V}/\dot{Q}$ lung scanning. If abnormal, CT-PA or pulmonary angiography is the next step in confirming the diagnosis and establishing the distribution and extent of disease.

Treatment

Advanced therapies, such as pulmonary vasodilators, are available to treat pulmonary hypertension. Such therapies are chosen based on the patient's functional status according to the NYHA/WHO classification. The mechanisms of action for pulmonary vasodilators follow three main pathways: (1) the nitric oxide pathway: phosphodiesterase inhibitors (sildenafil, tadalafil) and soluble guanylate cyclase stimulators (riociguat); (2) the endothelin pathway: endothelin receptor antagonists (bosentan, ambrisentan, macitentan); and (3) the prostacyclin pathway: prostacyclin analogs (intravenous epoprostenol; intravenous, subcutaneous, inhaled, or oral treprostinil; inhaled iloprost) and prostacyclin receptor agonist (selexipag). These vasodilators are only FDA approved for patients with Group 1 PAH based on their improvement in symptoms, 6-minute walk distance, WHO functional status, and hemodynamic measurements. More recently, a major RCT showed reduction in a composite outcome (death, hospitalization, progression, or unsatisfactory response) for combination therapy (using tadalafil and ambrisentan) compared to monotherapy. As a result, most patients with WHO/NYHA functional class II and III, should receive a combination of endothelin receptor antagonists and phosphodiesterase inhibitors as first-line therapy. For patients in WHO/NYHA functional class IV, a more aggressive approach is recommended with continuous prostacyclin infusion. Oral calcium channel blockers may be used in patients with a significant vasodilator response during cardiac catheterization. Anticoagulation was commonly used in the past but has fallen out of favor due to lack of efficacy.

Treatment of patients with Group 2 pulmonary hypertension (due to left heart failure) is discussed in Chapter 10. The main goal is to decrease pulmonary venous pressure by treating heart failure and volume overload, primarily with the use of diuretics.

Patients with Group 3 pulmonary hypertension (due to lung disease) should be assessed for hypoxemia at rest or with physical activity and, if present, should receive supplemental oxygen. Patients with COPD, interstitial lung disease, or obstructive sleep apnea should receive treatment for underlying disease. Inhaled treprostinil is the first therapy to be approved for patients with pulmonary hypertension due to interstitial lung disease since it improved exercise capacity based on 6-minute walk assessment.

For patients with Group 4 pulmonary hypertension (due to chronic thromboembolic disease), long-term anticoagulation is recommended. Additionally, patients with surgically accessible lesions and acceptable perioperative risk should undergo pulmonary thromboendarterectomy. For patients unable to undergo surgery or those with residual pulmonary hypertension postoperatively, medical therapy with riociguat or pulmonary artery balloon angioplasty should be considered.

Lung transplantation is a treatment option for selected patients with pulmonary hypertension when medical therapy is no longer effective. Double-lung transplant is the preferred method; in some cases, transplantation of the heart and both lungs is needed.

Prognosis

The prognosis of pulmonary hypertension varies by group. The prognosis of Group 1 patients has improved with the advent of pulmonary hypertension–specific therapy. Factors associated with poor prognosis include age older than 50 years, male sex, WHO/NYHA functional class III or IV, failure to improve to a lower functional class with therapy, and right ventricular dysfunction.

When to Refer

Patients in whom pulmonary hypertension is suspected or has been diagnosed should be referred early to a specialized pulmonary hypertension center for expert management.

When to Admit

- Patients with pulmonary hypertension, severe symptoms, and evidence of decompensated right heart failure with volume overload should be admitted to the hospital for aggressive diuresis.
- Patients with Group 1 pulmonary hypertension and functional class IV symptoms should be admitted to a specialized center for initiation of advanced therapies, such as intravenous prostacyclins.

Galiè N et al. An overview of the 6th World Symposium on Pulmonary Hypertension. Eur Respir J. 2019;53:1802148. [PMID: 30552088]

Mayeux JD et al. Management of pulmonary arterial hypertension. Curr Cardiovasc Risk Rep. 2021;15:2. [PMID: 33224405]

Sommer N et al. Current and future treatments of pulmonary arterial hypertension. Br J Pharmacol. 2021;178:6. [PMID: 32034759]

Waxman A et al. Inhaled treprostinil in pulmonary hypertension due to interstitial lung disease. N Engl J Med. 2021;384:325. [PMID: 33440084]

PULMONARY VASCULITIS

Antineutrophil cytoplasmic autoantibody (ANCA)–associated vasculitides include granulomatosis with polyangiitis, microscopic polyangiitis, and eosinophilic granulomatosis with polyangiitis. All are associated with ANCA and similar features of glomerulonephritis.

Granulomatosis with polyangiitis is a small vessel vasculitis manifested in the upper and lower respiratory tracts. Chronic sinusitis, arthralgias, fever, skin rash, and weight loss are frequent presenting symptoms. Specific pulmonary complaints occur less often. The most common sign of lung disease is nodular pulmonary infiltrates, often with cavitation, seen on chest radiography. Tracheal stenosis and endobronchial disease are sometimes seen. The diagnosis is most often based on serologic testing and biopsy of lung, sinus tissue, or kidney with demonstration of necrotizing granulomatous vasculitis (Chapter 20).

Eosinophilic granulomatosis with polyangiitis (formerly Churg-Strauss syndrome) is an idiopathic multisystem vasculitis of small and medium-sized arteries that occurs in patients with asthma. The skin and lungs are most often involved, but other organs, including the paranasal sinuses, the heart, GI tract, liver, and peripheral nerves, may also be affected. Peripheral eosinophilia greater than 1500 cells/mcL (greater than 1.5×10^9/L) or greater than 10% of peripheral WBCs is the rule. Abnormalities on chest radiographs range from transient opacities to multiple nodules. This illness may be part of a spectrum that includes polyarteritis nodosa. The diagnosis requires demonstration of histologic features, including fibrinoid necrotizing epithelioid granulomas and eosinophilic granulomas.

Anti-glomerular basement membrane (anti-GBM) antibody disease (also called Goodpasture syndrome) is a small-vessel vasculitis resulting from circulating antibodies against an antigen component of the basement membrane of the glomerulus and alveoli. It is rare, seen in young adults, and has a slight male predominance. It causes diffuse alveolar hemorrhage, rapidly progressive glomerulonephritis, and kidney failure.

Treatment

Treatment of patients with pulmonary vasculitis requires immunosuppressive therapy. Combination therapy with corticosteroids and either rituximab or cyclophosphamide is recommended for induction. Then patients should be transitioned to maintenance therapy with rituximab, methotrexate, azathioprine, or mycophenolate. For anti-GBM antibody disease, the use of plasmapheresis during induction has been shown to improve outcomes.

Prognosis

Five-year survival rates in patients with these vasculitis syndromes have been improved by combination therapy. Complete remission can be achieved in over 90% of patients with granulomatosis with polyangiitis.

Chung SA et al. 2021 American College of Rheumatology/Vasculitis Foundation guideline for the management of antineutrophil cytoplasmic antibody-associated vasculitis. Arthritis Rheumatol. 2021;73:1366. [PMID: 34235894]

Moiseev S et al; European EGPA Study Group. International consensus on ANCA testing in eosinophilic granulomatosis with polyangiitis. Am J Respir Crit Care Med. 2020;202:1360. [PMID: 32584187]

Prendecki M et al. Plasma exchange in anti-glomerular basement membrane disease. Presse Med. 2019;48:328. [PMID: 31703956]

Sacoto G et al. Lung involvement in ANCA-associated vasculitis. Presse Med. 2020;49:104039. [PMID: 32650042]

Vega Villanueva KL et al. Eosinophilic vasculitis. Curr Rheumatol Rep. 2020;22:5. [PMID: 31927633]

ALVEOLAR HEMORRHAGE SYNDROMES

Diffuse alveolar hemorrhage may occur in a variety of immune and nonimmune disorders. Alveolar infiltrates on chest radiograph, dyspnea, anemia, hemoptysis and, occasionally, fever are characteristic. Rapid clearing of diffuse lung infiltrates within 2 days is a clue to the diagnosis of diffuse alveolar hemorrhage. Pulmonary hemorrhage can be associated with an increased DLCO, although this test is infrequently obtained. Sequential BAL on bronchoscopy is the preferred method for diagnosis with lavage aliquots becoming progressively more hemorrhagic.

Causes of diffuse **immune alveolar hemorrhage** include anti-basement membrane antibody disease (Goodpasture syndrome), granulomatosis with polyangiitis, systemic necrotizing vasculitis, pulmonary capillaritis associated with idiopathic rapidly progressive glomerulonephritis, SLE, and other vasculitic and collagen vascular diseases. **Nonimmune causes** of diffuse hemorrhage include coagulopathy, mitral stenosis, necrotizing pulmonary infection, drugs (penicillamine), toxins (trimellitic anhydride), and idiopathic pulmonary hemosiderosis.

Idiopathic pulmonary hemosiderosis is a disease of children or young adults characterized by recurrent pulmonary hemorrhage; iron deficiency is typical. It is frequently associated with celiac disease. Treatment of acute episodes of hemorrhage with corticosteroids may be useful. Recurrent episodes of pulmonary hemorrhage may result in interstitial fibrosis and pulmonary failure.

Nasser M et al. Alveolar hemorrhage in vasculitis (primary and secondary). Semin Respir Crit Care Med. 2018;39:482. [PMID: 30404115]

Reisman S et al. A review of clinical and imaging features of diffuse pulmonary hemorrhage. AJR Am J Roentgenol. 2021;216:1500. [PMID: 33826359]

ENVIRONMENTAL & OCCUPATIONAL LUNG DISORDERS

SMOKE INHALATION

The inhalation of products of combustion may cause serious respiratory complications. As many as one-third of patients admitted to burn-treatment units have pulmonary injury from smoke inhalation. Morbidity and mortality due to smoke inhalation may exceed those attributed to the burns themselves. The death rate of patients with both severe burns and smoke inhalation exceeds 50%.

All patients in whom significant smoke inhalation is suspected must be assessed for three consequences of smoke inhalation: impaired tissue oxygenation, thermal injury to the upper airway, and injury to the lower airways and lung parenchyma. Impaired tissue oxygenation may result from inhalation of a hypoxic gas mixture, carbon monoxide or cyanide, or from alterations in $\dot{V}/\dot{Q}$ matching, and is an immediate threat to life. Immediate treatment with 100% oxygen is essential. The management of patients with carbon monoxide and cyanide poisoning is discussed in Chapter 38. The clinician must recognize that patients with carbon monoxide poisoning display a normal partial pressure of oxygen in arterial blood (Pao_2), but have a low *measured* (ie, not oximetric) hemoglobin saturation (Sao_2). Treatment with 100% oxygen should be continued until the measured carboxyhemoglobin level falls to less than 10% and concomitant metabolic acidosis has resolved.

Thermal injury to the mucosal surfaces of the upper airway occurs from inhalation of super-heated gases. Complications, including mucosal edema, upper airway obstruction, and impaired ability to clear oral secretions, usually become evident by 18–24 hours and produce inspiratory stridor. Respiratory failure occurs in severe cases. Early management (Chapter 37) includes the use of a high-humidity face mask with supplemental oxygen, gentle suctioning to evacuate oral secretions, elevation of the head 30 degrees to promote clearing of secretions, and topical epinephrine to reduce edema of the oropharyngeal mucous membrane. Helium-oxygen gas mixtures (Heliox) may reduce labored breathing due to critical upper airway narrowing. Close monitoring with ABGs and later with oximetry is important. Examination of the upper airway with a fiberoptic laryngoscope or bronchoscope is superior to routine physical examination. Endotracheal intubation is often necessary to maintain airway patency and is likely to be necessary in patients with deep facial burns or oropharyngeal or laryngeal edema. Tracheotomy should be avoided, if possible, because of an increased risk of pneumonia and death from sepsis.

Injury to the lower airways and lung parenchyma results from inhalation of toxic gases and products of combustion, including aldehydes and organic acids. The site of lung injury depends on the solubility of the gases inhaled, the duration of exposure, and the size of inhaled particles that transport noxious gases to distal lung units. Bronchorrhea and bronchospasm occur early after exposure along with dyspnea, tachypnea, and tachycardia. Labored breathing and cyanosis may follow. Physical examination at this stage reveals diffuse wheezing and rhonchi. Bronchiolar and alveolar edema (eg, ARDS) may develop within 1–2 days after exposure. Sloughing of the bronchiolar mucosa may occur within 2–3 days, leading to airway obstruction, atelectasis, and worsening hypoxemia. Bacterial colonization and pneumonia are common by 5–7 days after the exposure.

Treatment of smoke inhalation consists of supplemental oxygen, bronchodilators, suctioning of mucosal debris and mucopurulent secretions via an indwelling endotracheal tube, chest physical therapy to aid clearance of secretions, and adequate humidification of inspired gases. Positive end-expiratory pressure (PEEP) has been advocated to treat bronchiolar edema. Judicious fluid management and close monitoring for secondary bacterial infection round out the management protocol.

The routine use of corticosteroids for lung injury from smoke inhalation has been shown to be ineffective and may even be harmful. Routine or prophylactic use of antibiotics is not recommended.

Patients who survive should be watched for the late development of bronchiolitis obliterans.

Chao KY et al. Respiratory management in smoke inhalation injury. J Burn Care Res. 2019;40:507. [PMID: 30893426]

Galeiras R et al. Prevalence and prognostic impact of inhalation injury among burn patients: a systematic review and meta-analysis. J Trauma Acute Care Surg. 2020;88:330. [PMID: 31688831]

E-CIGARETTE- OR VAPING PRODUCT–ASSOCIATED LUNG INJURY

General Considerations

An outbreak of e-cigarette- or vaping product–associated lung injury (EVALI) began in the United States in 2019. Approximately 66% of patients have been male and 80% are under age 35. Over 95% of reported cases required hospitalization: 47% were admitted to intensive care, 22% were intubated, and many died. Based on the characteristics of these patients, the diagnosis of EVALI requires reported use of e-cigarette or vaping products within 3 months of symptom onset, compatible chest imaging findings, and an evaluation that excludes infectious etiologies.

No single causative agent has been identified. Most cases involved vaping products containing tetrahydrocannabinol (THC) or nicotine or both. Postulated factors contributing to the development of EVALI include e-cigarette flavorings, exposure to diacetyl (a popcorn flavoring that has been associated with lung injury), THC, adulteration of THC, adulteration of delivery devices, and vitamin E acetate (used as a thickening agent).

Clinical Findings

A. Symptoms and Signs

Patients with EVALI have respiratory symptoms (95%), including cough, shortness of breath, and chest pain; GI symptoms (77%), including nausea, vomiting, and diarrhea; and constitutional symptoms (85%), including fever, chills, and weight loss. The illness is usually acute to subacute with patients having symptoms for days to weeks before seeking health care.

Tachycardia and tachypnea are present in 55% and 45% of patients, respectively. Of note, 57% of cases have a recorded room air oxygen saturation of less than 95%. Given the nonspecific nature of the presentation especially during influenza season and the COVID-19 pandemic, providers must have a high degree of clinical suspicion and ask patients specifically about vaping.

B. Laboratory Findings

There are no laboratory findings specific for the diagnosis of EVALI. There may be leukocytosis, elevated CRP, and elevated ESR.

C. Imaging

Case series of chest imaging findings in EVALI show various patterns of lung injury. Chest radiographs typically show bilateral pulmonary opacities. Chest CT scans are nonspecific and may show patterns seen in other disorders, such as hypersensitivity pneumonitis, ARDS, diffuse alveolar hemorrhage, acute eosinophilic pneumonia, lipoid pneumonia, giant cell interstitial pneumonia, and organizing pneumonia.

Differential Diagnosis

The EVALI case definition requires a negative work-up for infectious causes. Other diagnoses to consider include acute eosinophilic pneumonia, ARDS, hypersensitivity pneumonitis, lipoid pneumonia, and organizing pneumonia. Influenza testing should be done in season, and SARS-CoV-2 testing, as indicated.

Treatment

In published reports of hospitalized patients with EVALI who have received corticosteroids, rapid improvement has been described. Symptoms of fatigue, dyspnea, decreased exercise capacity, and cough may persist for months.

Henry TS et al. Imaging findings of vaping-associated lung injury. AJR Am J Roentgenol. 2020;214:498. [PMID: 31593518]

Jatlaoui TC et al; Lung Injury Response Clinical Working Group. Update: interim guidance for health care providers for managing patients with suspected e-cigarette, or vaping, product use-associated lung injury—United States, November 2019. MMWR Morb Mortal Wkly Rep. 2019;68:1081. [PMID: 31751322]

Jonas AM et al. Vaping-related acute parenchymal lung injury: a systematic review. Chest. 2020;158:155. [PMID: 32442559]

Traboulsi H et al. Inhalation toxicology of vaping products and implications for pulmonary health. Int J Mol Sci. 2020;21:3495. [PMID: 32429092]

Triantafyllou GA et al. Long-term outcomes of EVALI: a 1-year retrospective study. Lancet Respir Med. 2021;9:e112. [PMID: 34710356]

PULMONARY ASPIRATION SYNDROMES

1. Acute Aspiration of Gastric Contents (Mendelson Syndrome)

Acute aspiration of gastric contents may be catastrophic. The pulmonary response depends on the characteristics and amount of gastric contents aspirated. The more acidic the material, the greater the degree of chemical pneumonitis. Aspiration of pure gastric acid (pH < 2.5) causes extensive desquamation of the bronchial epithelium, bronchiolitis, hemorrhage, and pulmonary edema. Acute gastric aspiration is one of the most common causes of ARDS. The clinical picture is one of abrupt onset of respiratory distress, with cough, wheezing, fever, and tachypnea. Crackles may be audible at the bases of the lungs. Hypoxemia may be noted immediately after aspiration occurs. Radiographic abnormalities, consisting of patchy alveolar opacities in dependent lung zones, appear within a few hours. If particulate food matter has been aspirated along with gastric acid, radiographic features of bronchial obstruction may be observed. Fever and leukocytosis are common even in the absence of infection.

Treatment of acute aspiration of gastric contents consists of supplemental oxygen, measures to maintain the airway, and the usual measures for treatment of acute respiratory failure. There is no evidence to support the routine use of prophylactic antibiotics or corticosteroids. Secondary pulmonary infection, which occurs in about one-fourth of patients, typically appears 2–3 days after aspiration. Management of infection depends on the observed flora from the tracheobronchial tree. Hypotension or shock secondary to alveolar capillary membrane injury and intravascular volume depletion is common and is managed with the judicious administration of intravenous fluids or vasopressors or both.

2. Chronic Aspiration of Gastric Contents

Chronic aspiration of gastric contents may result from primary disorders of the larynx or the esophagus, such as achalasia, esophageal stricture, systemic sclerosis (scleroderma), esophageal carcinoma, esophagitis, and GERD. In GERD, relaxation of the tone of the lower esophageal sphincter allows reflux of gastric contents into the esophagus and predisposes to chronic pulmonary aspiration, especially when supine. Cigarette smoking, consumption of alcohol or caffeine, and theophylline use are all known to relax the lower esophageal sphincter. Pulmonary disorders linked to GERD and chronic aspiration include asthma, chronic cough, bronchiectasis, and pulmonary fibrosis. Even in the absence of aspiration, acid in the esophagus may trigger bronchospasm or bronchial hyperreactivity through reflex mechanisms.

The diagnosis and management of GERD and chronic aspiration are challenging. A discussion of strategies for the evaluation, prevention, and management of extraesophageal reflux manifestations can be found in Chapter 15.

3. "Café Coronary"

Acute obstruction of the upper airway by food is associated with difficulty swallowing, old age, dental problems that impair chewing, and use of alcohol and sedative drugs. The Heimlich procedure is lifesaving in many cases.

4. Retention of an Aspirated Foreign Body

Retention of an aspirated foreign body in the tracheobronchial tree may produce both acute and chronic conditions, including atelectasis, postobstructive hyperinflation, both acute and recurrent pneumonia, bronchiectasis, and lung abscess. Occasionally, a misdiagnosis of asthma, COPD, or lung cancer is made in adult patients who have aspirated a foreign body. The plain chest radiograph usually suggests the site of the foreign body. In some cases, an expiratory film, demonstrating regional hyperinflation due to a check-valve effect, is helpful. Bronchoscopy is usually necessary to establish the diagnosis and attempt removal of the foreign body.

Hasegawa S et al. Ceftriaxone versus ampicillin/sulbactam for the treatment of aspiration-associated pneumonia in adults. J Comp Eff Res. 2019;8:1275. [PMID: 31736321]

Rodriguez AE et al. New perspectives in aspiration community acquired pneumonia. Expert Rev Clin Pharmacol. 2019; 12:991. [PMID: 31516051]

Santos JMLG et al. Interventions to prevent aspiration pneumonia in older adults: an updated systematic review. J Speech Lang Hear Res. 2021;64:464. [PMID: 33405973]

OCCUPATIONAL PULMONARY DISEASES

Many acute and chronic pulmonary diseases are directly related to inhalation of noxious substances encountered in the workplace. Disorders that are linked to occupational exposures may be classified as follows: (1) pneumoconioses, (2) hypersensitivity pneumonitis, (3) obstructive airway disorders, (4) toxic lung injury, (5) lung cancer, (6) pleural diseases, and (7) other occupational pulmonary diseases.

1. Pneumoconioses

Pneumoconioses are chronic fibrotic lung diseases caused by the inhalation of inert inorganic dusts. Pneumoconioses range from asymptomatic disorders with diffuse nodular opacities on chest radiograph to severe, symptomatic, life-shortening disorders. Clinically important pneumoconioses include coal worker's pneumoconiosis, silicosis, and asbestosis (Table 9–20). Treatment for each is supportive; pulmonary rehabilitation may be considered.

A. Coal Worker's Pneumoconiosis

In coal worker's pneumoconiosis, ingestion of inhaled coal dust by alveolar macrophages leads to the formation of coal macules, usually 2–5 mm in diameter, that appear on chest radiograph as diffuse small opacities that are especially prominent in the upper lung. Simple coal worker's pneumoconiosis is usually asymptomatic; abnormalities of PFTs are unimpressive. In complicated coal worker's pneumoconiosis (**"progressive massive fibrosis"**), conglomeration and contraction in the upper lung zones occur, with radiographic features resembling complicated silicosis. **Caplan syndrome** is a rare condition characterized by the presence of necrobiotic rheumatoid nodules (1–5 cm in diameter) in the periphery of the lung in coal workers with rheumatoid arthritis.

B. Silicosis

In silicosis, extensive or prolonged inhalation of free silica (silicon dioxide) particles (sandblasters, foundry, granite

Table 9–20. Selected pneumoconioses.

Disease	Agent	Occupations
Asbestosis	Asbestos	Mining, insulation, construction, shipbuilding
Baritosis	Barium salts	Glass and insecticide manufacturing
Coal worker's pneumoconiosis	Coal dust	Coal mining
Kaolin pneumoconiosis	Sand, mica, aluminum silicate	Mining of china clay; pottery and cement work
Shaver disease	Aluminum powder	Manufacture of corundum
Siderosis	Metallic iron or iron oxide	Mining, welding, foundry work
Silicosis	Free silica (silicon dioxide)	Rock mining, quarrying, stone cutting, tunneling, sandblasting, pottery, diatomaceous earth
Stannosis	Tin, tin oxide	Mining, tin-working, smelting
Talcosis	Magnesium silicate	Mining, insulation, construction, shipbuilding

and stone cutting, molding, ceramics) in the respirable range (0.3–5 mcm) causes the formation of small rounded opacities (silicotic nodules) throughout the lung. Calcification of the periphery of hilar lymph nodes ("eggshell" calcification) is an unusual radiographic finding that strongly suggests silicosis. Simple silicosis is usually asymptomatic and has no effect on routine PFTs; in complicated silicosis, large conglomerate densities appear in the upper lung and are accompanied by dyspnea and obstructive and restrictive pulmonary dysfunction. The incidence of pulmonary tuberculosis is increased in patients with silicosis. All patients with silicosis should have a tuberculin skin test and a chest radiograph to rule out tuberculosis.

C. Asbestosis

Asbestosis is a nodular interstitial fibrosis occurring in workers exposed to asbestos fibers (shipyard and construction workers, pipe fitters, insulators) over many years (typically 10–20 years). Patients with asbestosis usually first seek medical attention at least 15 years after exposure with the following symptoms and signs: progressive dyspnea, inspiratory crackles, and in some cases, clubbing and cyanosis. The radiographic features of asbestosis include linear streaking at the lung bases, opacities of various shapes and sizes, and honeycomb changes in advanced cases. The presence of pleural calcifications may be a clue to diagnosis. High-resolution CT scanning is the best imaging method for asbestosis because of its ability to detect parenchymal fibrosis and define the presence of coexisting pleural plaques. Cigarette smoking in asbestos workers increases the prevalence of radiographic pleural and parenchymal changes and markedly increases the incidence of lung carcinoma. It may also interfere with the clearance of short asbestos fibers from the lung. PFTs show restrictive dysfunction and reduced diffusing capacity. There is no specific treatment.

Leonard R et al. Coal mining and lung disease in the 21st century. Curr Opin Pulm Med. 2020;26:135. [PMID: 31815751]

Reynolds C et al. Occupational contributions to interstitial lung disease. Clin Chest Med. 2020;41:697. [PMID: 33153688]

Walkoff L et al. Chest imaging in the diagnosis of occupational lung diseases. Clin Chest Med. 2020;41:581. [PMID: 33153681]

Zhao H et al. Pulmonary rehabilitation can improve the functional capacity and quality of life for pneumoconiosis patients: a systematic review and meta-analysis. Biomed Res Int. 2020;2020:6174936. [PMID: 32802860]

2. Hypersensitivity Pneumonitis

Hypersensitivity pneumonitis (also called extrinsic allergic alveolitis) is a nonatopic, nonasthmatic inflammatory pulmonary disease. It is manifested mainly as an occupational disease (Table 9–21), in which exposure to inhaled organic antigens leads to an acute illness. Prompt diagnosis is essential since symptoms are usually reversible if the offending antigen is removed from the patient's environment early in the course of illness. Continued exposure may lead to progressive disease. The histopathology of acute hypersensitivity pneumonitis is characterized by

Table 9–21. Selected causes of hypersensitivity pneumonitis.

Disease	Antigen	Source
Farmer's lung	*Saccharopolyspora rectivirgula* (formerly, *Micropolyspora faeni*), *Thermoactinomyces vulgaris*	Moldy hay
"Humidifier" lung	Thermophilic actinomycetes	Contaminated humidifiers, heating systems, or air conditioners
Bird fancier's lung	Avian proteins	Bird serum and excreta
Bagassosis	*Thermoactinomyces sacchari* and *T vulgaris*	Moldy sugar cane fiber (bagasse)
Sequoiosis	*Graphium, Aureobasidium*, and other fungi	Moldy redwood sawdust
Maple bark stripper's disease	*Cryptostroma (Coniosporium) corticale*	Rotting maple tree logs or bark
Mushroom picker's disease	Same as farmer's lung	Moldy compost
Suberosis	*Penicillium frequentans*	Moldy cork dust
Detergent worker's lung	*Bacillus subtilis* enzyme	Enzyme additives

interstitial infiltrates of lymphocytes and plasma cells, with noncaseating granulomas in the interstitium and air spaces.

Clinical Findings

A. Acute Illness

The symptoms are characterized by sudden onset of malaise, chills, fever, cough, dyspnea, and nausea 4–8 hours after exposure to the offending antigen. Bibasilar crackles, tachypnea, tachycardia, and (occasionally) cyanosis are noted. Small nodular densities sparing the apices and bases of the lungs are noted on chest radiograph. Laboratory studies reveal an increase in the WBC count with a shift to the left, hypoxemia, and the presence of precipitating antibodies to the offending agent in serum. Hypersensitivity pneumonitis antibody panels against common offending antigens are available; positive results, while supportive, do not establish a definitive diagnosis. PFTs reveal restrictive dysfunction and reduced diffusing capacity.

B. Subacute and Chronic Illness

A subacute hypersensitivity pneumonitis syndrome (15% of cases) is characterized by the insidious onset of chronic cough and slowly progressive dyspnea, anorexia, and weight loss. Chronic exposure leads to progressive respiratory insufficiency and the appearance of pulmonary fibrosis on chest imaging. Surgical lung biopsy may be necessary for the diagnosis of subacute and chronic hypersensitivity pneumonitis. Even with surgical lung biopsy, however, chronic hypersensitivity pneumonitis may be difficult to diagnose because histopathologic patterns overlap with several idiopathic interstitial pneumonias.

Treatment

Treatment of acute hypersensitivity pneumonitis consists of identification of the offending agent and avoidance of further exposure. In severe acute or protracted cases, oral corticosteroids (prednisone, 0.5 mg/kg daily as a single morning dose for 2 weeks, tapered to nil over 4–6 weeks) may be given. Change in occupation is often unavoidable.

Barnes H et al. Management of fibrotic hypersensitivity pneumonitis. Clin Chest Med. 2021;42:311. [PMID: 34024406]
Creamer AW et al. Prognostic factors in chronic hypersensitivity pneumonitis. Eur Respir Rev. 2020;29:190167. [PMID: 32414744]
Nogueira R et al. Hypersensitivity pneumonitis: antigen diversity and disease implications. Pulmonology. 2019;25:97. [PMID: 30126802]

3. Other Occupational Pulmonary Diseases

Occupational diseases of the pleura may result from exposure to asbestos or talc. Inhalation of talc causes pleural plaques that are like those caused by asbestos. Benign asbestos pleural effusion occurs in some asbestos workers and may cause chronic blunting of the costophrenic angle on chest radiograph.

Occupational agents are also responsible for other pulmonary disorders, with a range of pathologies including occupational asthma, occupational COPD, interstitial lung diseases, and lung cancer. For this reason, it is important to obtain a thorough occupational history in any patient presenting with pulmonary symptoms.

Specific examples of inorganic agents associated with interstitial lung disease include anthracite coal dust (coal workers' pneumoconiosis), crystalline and nonfibrous silicates (silicosis), asbestos (asbestosis, pleural plaques, benign pleural effusion, adenoma, malignant mesothelioma), beryllium (berylliosis, which is very similar to sarcoidosis), and cobalt (hard metal lung disease). Organic dust from farm work, animal or bird exposure, or vegetable stores may cause extrinsic allergic alveolitis or hypersensitivity pneumonitis.

Unusual outbreaks (including "popcorn-worker's lung" and other diacetyl flavoring exposure causing bronchiolitis obliterans, "flock worker's lung" following synthetic fiber exposure) are occasionally reported.

Morimoto Y et al. Lung disorders induced by respirable organic chemicals. J Occup Health. 2021;63:e12240. [PMID: 34128301]
Perlman DM et al. Occupational lung disease. Med Clin North Am. 2019;103:535. [PMID: 30955520]
Wyman AE et al. Update on metal-induced occupational lung disease. Curr Opin Allergy Clin Immunol. 2018;18:73. [PMID: 29337701]

MEDICATION-INDUCED LUNG DISEASE

Typical patterns of pulmonary response to medications implicated in medication-induced respiratory disease are summarized in Table 9–22. Pulmonary injury due to medications occurs because of allergic reactions, idiosyncratic reactions, overdose, or undesirable side effects. In most patients, the mechanism of pulmonary injury is unknown.

Precise diagnosis of medication-induced pulmonary disease is often difficult because results of routine laboratory studies are not helpful and radiographic findings are not specific. A high index of suspicion and a thorough history of medication usage are critical to establishing the diagnosis of medication-induced lung disease. The clinical response to cessation of the suspected offending agent is also helpful. Acute episodes of medication-induced pulmonary disease may disappear 24–48 hours after the medication has been discontinued, but chronic syndromes may

Table 9–22. Pulmonary manifestations of selected medication toxicities.

Asthma	**Pulmonary edema**
Beta-blockers	Noncardiogenic
Aspirin	Aspirin
NSAIDs	Chlordiazepoxide
Histamine	Cocaine
Methacholine	Ethchlorvynol
Acetylcysteine	Heroin/opiates
Aerosolized pentamidine	Cardiogenic
Any nebulized medication	Beta-blockers
Chronic cough	**Pleural effusion**
ACE inhibitors	Bromocriptine
Pulmonary infiltration	Nitrofurantoin
Without eosinophilia	Any drug inducing SLE
Amitriptyline	Methysergide
Azathioprine	Chemotherapeutic agents
Amiodarone	(eg, carmustine, cyclo-
With eosinophilia	phosphamide, dasatinib,
Sulfonamides	docetaxel, GM-CSF,
L-Tryptophan	methotrexate)
Nitrofurantoin	Tyrosine kinase inhibitors
Penicillin	**Mediastinal widening**
Methotrexate	Phenytoin
Crack cocaine	Corticosteroids
Drug-induced SLE	Methotrexate
Hydralazine	**Respiratory failure**
Procainamide	Neuromuscular blockade
Isoniazid	Aminoglycosides
Chlorpromazine	Paralytic agents
Phenytoin	**CNS depression**
Interstitial pneumonitis/ fibrosis	Sedatives
Nitrofurantoin	Hypnotics
Bleomycin	Opioids
Busulfan	Alcohol
Cyclophosphamide	Tricyclic antidepressants
Immune checkpoint inhibitors	
Methysergide	
Phenytoin	

GM-CSF, granulocyte-macrophage colony-stimulating factor.

take longer to resolve. Challenge tests to confirm the diagnosis are risky and rarely performed.

Treatment of medication-induced lung disease consists of discontinuing the offending agent immediately, managing the pulmonary symptoms appropriately, and treating with corticosteroids if pulmonary toxicity is rapidly progressive. Randomized data supporting the use of corticosteroids in medication-associated pneumonitis is lacking, but observational data supports use in severe cases. Immune checkpoint inhibitors, now commonly used treatments for a variety of malignant and nonmalignant conditions, are associated with at least a 5% risk of pneumonitis, which carries mortality of up to 20% when severe. Observational data support concurrent corticosteroid treatment in these cases.

Inhalation of crack cocaine may cause a spectrum of acute pulmonary syndromes, including pulmonary infiltration with eosinophilia, pneumothorax and pneumomediastinum, bronchiolitis obliterans, and acute respiratory failure associated with diffuse alveolar damage and alveolar hemorrhage. Corticosteroids have been used with variable success to treat alveolar hemorrhage.

Long K et al. Pulmonary toxicity of systemic lung cancer therapy. Respirology. 2020;25:72. [PMID: 32729207]
Suresh K. Immune checkpoint immunotherapy for non-small cell lung cancer: benefits and pulmonary toxicities. Chest. 2018;154:1416. [PMID: 301891190]

RADIATION LUNG INJURY

The lung is an exquisitely radiosensitive organ that can be damaged by external beam radiation therapy. The degree of pulmonary injury is determined by the volume of lung irradiated, the dose and rate of exposure, and potentiating factors (eg, concurrent chemotherapy, previous radiation therapy in the same area, and simultaneous withdrawal of corticosteroid therapy). Symptomatic radiation lung injury occurs in about 10% of patients treated for carcinoma of the breast, 5–15% of patients treated for carcinoma of the lung, and 5–35% of patients treated for lymphoma. Two phases of the pulmonary response to radiation are apparent: an acute phase (radiation pneumonitis) and a chronic phase (radiation fibrosis).

1. Radiation Pneumonitis

Acute radiation pneumonitis usually occurs 2–3 months (range 1–6 months) after completion of radiotherapy and is characterized by insidious onset of dyspnea, intractable dry cough, chest fullness or pain, weakness, and fever. Late radiation pneumonitis may develop 6–12 months after completion of radiation. Occasionally, patients who are months to years removed from radiation therapy will experience "radiation recall" with an inflammatory reaction in the radiated region after treatment with a new round of chemotherapy; this phenomenon has also been reported with immune checkpoint inhibitors. The dominant histopathologic findings are a lymphocytic interstitial pneumonitis progressing to an exudative alveolitis. Inspiratory crackles may be heard in the involved area. In severe disease, respiratory distress and cyanosis occur that are characteristic of ARDS. An increased WBC count and elevated ESR are common. PFTs reveal reduced lung volumes, reduced lung compliance, hypoxemia, reduced diffusing capacity, and reduced maximum voluntary ventilation. Chest radiography, which correlates poorly with the presence of symptoms, usually demonstrates alveolar or nodular opacities limited to the irradiated area. Air bronchograms are often observed. Sharp borders of an opacity may help distinguish radiation pneumonitis from other conditions, such as infectious pneumonia, lymphangitic spread of carcinoma, and recurrent tumor; however, the opacity may extend beyond the radiation field.

No specific therapy is proved to be effective in radiation pneumonitis, but prednisone (1 mg/kg/day orally) is commonly given immediately for about 1 week; higher doses may be given in patients who are critically ill. The dose is reduced and maintained at 20–40 mg/day for several weeks, then slowly tapered. Radiation pneumonitis may improve in 2–3 weeks following onset of symptoms as the exudative phase resolves. Acute respiratory failure, if present, is treated supportively. Death from ARDS is unusual in radiation pneumonitis.

Giuranno L et al. Radiation-induced lung injury (RILI). Front Oncol. 2019;9:877. [PMID: 31555602]
Hanania AN et al. Radiation-induced lung injury: assessment and management. Chest. 2019;156:150. [PMID: 30998908]
Kasmann L et al. Radiation-induced lung toxicity—cellular and molecular mechanisms of pathogenesis, management, and literature review. Radiat Oncol. 2020;15:214. [PMID: 32912295]
Lu L et al. Radiation-induced lung injury: latest molecular developments, therapeutic approaches, and clinical guidance. Clin Exp Med. 2019;19:417. [PMID: 31313081]
Teng F et al. Radiation recall pneumonitis induced by PD-1/PD-L1 blockades: mechanisms and therapeutic implications. BMC Med. 2020;18:275. [PMID: 32943072]

2. Pulmonary Radiation Fibrosis

Radiation fibrosis may occur with or without antecedent radiation pneumonitis. Radiographic findings include obliteration of normal lung markings, dense interstitial and pleural fibrosis, reduced lung volumes, tenting of the diaphragm, and sharp delineation of the irradiated area. No specific therapy is proven effective, and corticosteroids have no value. Pulmonary fibrosis may develop after an intervening period (6–12 months) of well-being in patients who experience radiation pneumonitis. Pulmonary radiation fibrosis occurs in most patients who receive a full course of radiation therapy for cancer of the lung or breast. Most patients are asymptomatic, although slowly progressive dyspnea may occur.

Giuranno L et al. Radiation-induced lung injury (RILI). Front Oncol. 2019;9:877. [PMID: 31555602]

PLEURAL DISEASES

PLEURITIS

Pleuritic pain due to inflammation of the parietal pleura is generally localized, sharp, and fleeting; it is made worse by coughing, sneezing, deep breathing, or movement.

When the central portion of the diaphragmatic parietal pleura is irritated, pain may be referred to the ipsilateral shoulder. There are numerous causes of pleuritis. The setting in which pleuritic pain develops helps narrow the differential diagnosis. In young, otherwise healthy individuals, pleuritis is usually caused by viral respiratory infections or pneumonia (including tuberculosis in endemic regions), while PE, inflammatory disorders (serositis), malignancy, and drug reactions may also be considered in the proper context. The presence of pleural effusion, pleural thickening, or air in the pleural space requires further diagnostic and therapeutic measures.

Treatment of pleuritis consists of treating the underlying condition. Anti-inflammatory analgesic medications are often helpful for pain relief. Opioids may be used if NSAIDs are ineffective or are contraindicated, provided retention of airway secretions is not a concern.

Shaw JA et al. Pleural tuberculosis: a concise clinical review. Clin Respir J. 2018;12:1779. [PMID: 29660258]

PLEURAL EFFUSION

ESSENTIALS OF DIAGNOSIS

- May be asymptomatic; chest pain frequently seen in the setting of pleuritis, trauma, or infection; dyspnea is common with large effusions.
- Dullness to percussion and decreased breath sounds over the effusion.
- Radiographic evidence of pleural effusion.
- Diagnostic findings on thoracentesis.

General Considerations

There is constant movement of fluid from parietal pleural capillaries into the pleural space at a rate of 0.01 mL/kg body weight/h. Absorption of pleural fluid occurs through parietal pleural lymphatics. The resultant homeostasis leaves 5–15 mL of fluid in the normal pleural space. A pleural effusion is an abnormal accumulation of fluid in the pleural space. Pleural effusions may be classified by differential diagnosis (Table 9–23) or by underlying pathophysiology. Five pathophysiologic processes account for most pleural effusions: increased production of fluid in the setting of normal capillaries due to increased hydrostatic or decreased oncotic pressures **(transudates)**; increased production of fluid due to abnormal capillary permeability **(exudates)**; decreased lymphatic clearance of fluid from the pleural space **(exudates)**; infection in the pleural space **(empyema)**; and bleeding into the pleural space **(hemothorax)**.

Diagnostic thoracentesis should be performed whenever there is a new pleural effusion and no clinically apparent cause. Observation is appropriate in some situations (eg, symmetric bilateral pleural effusions in the setting of heart failure), but an atypical presentation or failure of an effusion to resolve as expected warrants thoracentesis to identify the underlying process.

Table 9–23. Causes of pleural fluid transudates and exudates.

Transudates	Exudates
Heart failure	Pneumonia (parapneumonic effusion, including empyema)
Cirrhosis with ascites	Cancer
Nephrotic syndrome	PE
Peritoneal dialysis	Bacterial infection (including empyema)
Myxedema	Tuberculosis
Atelectasis (acute)	Connective tissue disease
Constrictive pericarditis	Viral infection
Superior vena cava obstruction	Fungal infection
PE	Rickettsial infection
	Parasitic infection
	Asbestos
	Meigs syndrome
	Pancreatic disease
	Uremia
	Chronic atelectasis
	Trapped lung
	Chylothorax
	Sarcoidosis
	Drug reaction
	Post–myocardial injury syndrome

Clinical Findings

A. Symptoms and Signs

Patients with pleural effusions most often report dyspnea, cough, or respirophasic chest pain. Symptoms are more common in patients with existing cardiopulmonary disease. Small pleural effusions are less likely to be symptomatic than larger effusions. Physical findings are usually absent in small effusions. Larger effusions may present with dullness to percussion and diminished or absent breath sounds over the effusion. Compressive atelectasis may cause bronchial breath sounds and egophony just above the effusion. A massive effusion with increased intrapleural pressure may cause contralateral shift of the trachea and bulging of the intercostal spaces. A pleural friction rub indicates pulmonary infarction or pleuritis.

B. Laboratory Findings

The gross appearance of pleural fluid helps identify several types of pleural effusion. Grossly purulent fluid signifies empyema. Milky white pleural fluid should be centrifuged. A clear supernatant above a pellet of white cells indicates empyema, whereas a persistently turbid supernatant suggests a **chylous effusion;** analysis of this supernatant reveals chylomicrons and a high triglyceride level (greater than 100 mg/dL [1 mmol/L]), often from disruption of the thoracic duct. **Hemorrhagic pleural effusion** is a mixture of blood and pleural fluid. Ten thousand red cells per microliter create blood-tinged pleural fluid; 100,000 red cells/mcL (100×10^9/L) create grossly bloody pleural fluid. **Hemothorax** is the presence of gross blood in the pleural space, usually following chest trauma or instrumentation. It is defined as a ratio of pleural fluid hematocrit to peripheral blood hematocrit greater than 0.5.

Pleural fluid samples should be sent for measurement of protein, glucose, and LD in addition to total and differential WBC counts. Chemistry determinations are used to classify effusions as transudates or exudates. This classification is important because the differential diagnosis and subsequent evaluation for each entity varies (Table 9–23). A **pleural exudate** is an effusion that has one or more of the following laboratory features: (1) ratio of pleural fluid protein to serum protein greater than 0.5; (2) ratio of pleural fluid LD to serum LD greater than 0.6; (3) pleural fluid LD greater than two-thirds the upper limit of normal serum LD. Alternative diagnostic criteria that do not require the simultaneous sampling of serum but that perform similarly include the "two-test" (pleural fluid cholesterol greater than 45 mg/dL, pleural fluid LD greater than 0.45 times upper limit of normal serum LD) and the "three-test" (which adds pleural fluid protein greater than 2.9 g/dL). **Pleural transudates** occur in the setting of normal capillary integrity and demonstrate none of the laboratory features of exudates. A transudate suggests the absence of local pleural disease; characteristic laboratory findings include a glucose near to serum glucose, pH between 7.40 and 7.55 (if properly measured), and fewer than 1000 WBCs/mcL (1.0×10^9/L) with a predominance of mononuclear cells. It is worthwhile to note that discrimination of exudate from transudate is less reliable near the cutoff values for any of the criteria, and that effective diuresis may increase the protein or LD concentration in the pleural fluid as water is reabsorbed, thus creating a borderline "pseudoexudative" chemistry in transudative states such as heart failure.

Heart failure accounts for most transudates. Bacterial pneumonia, cancer, and tuberculosis (in endemic regions) are the most common causes of exudative effusion. Other causes of exudates with characteristic laboratory findings are summarized in Table 9–24.

Table 9–24. Characteristics of important exudative pleural effusions.

Etiology or Type of Effusion	Gross Appearance	WBC Count (cells/mcL)	RBC Count (cells/mcL)	Glucose	Comments
Malignancy	Turbid to bloody; occasionally serous	1000–100,000 (1.0–100 × 10^9/L) M	100 (0.1 × 10^9/L) to several hundred thousand	Equal to serum levels; < 60 mg/dL in 15% of cases	Eosinophilia uncommon; positive results on cytologic examination
Uncomplicated parapneumonic	Clear to turbid	5000–25,000 (5.0–25 × 10^9/L) P	< 5000 (5.0 × 10^9/L)	Equal to serum levels	Tube thoracostomy unnecessary
Empyema	Turbid to purulent	25,000–100,000 (25–100 × 10^9/L) P	< 5000 (5.0 × 10^9/L)	Less than serum levels; often very low	Drainage necessary; putrid odor suggests anaerobic infection
Tuberculosis	Serous to serosanguineous	5000–10,000 (5.0–10 × 10^9/L) M	< 10,000 (10 × 10^9/L)	Equal to serum levels; occasionally < 60 mg/dL	Protein > 4.0 g/dL (may exceed 5 g/dL); frequently lymphocyte predominant (> 50%); eosinophils (> 10%) or mesothelial cells (> 5%) make diagnosis unlikely; see text for additional diagnostic tests
Rheumatoid	Turbid; greenish yellow	1000–20,000 (1.0–20 × 10^9/L) M or P	< 1000 (1.0 × 10^9/L)	< 40 mg/dL	Secondary empyema common; high LD, low complement, high rheumatoid factor, cholesterol crystals are characteristic
Pulmonary infarction	Serous to grossly bloody	1000–50,000 (1.0–50 × 10^9/L) M or P	100 (0.1 × 10^9/L) to > 100,000 (100 × 10^9/L)	Equal to serum levels	Variable findings; no pathognomonic features
Esophageal rupture	Turbid to purulent; red-brown	< 5000 (5.0 × 10^9/L) to > 50,000 (50 × 10^9/L) P	1000–10,000 (1.0–10 × 10^9/L)	Usually low	High amylase level (salivary origin); pneumothorax in 25% of cases; effusion usually on left side; pH < 6.0 strongly suggests diagnosis
Pancreatitis	Turbid to serosanguineous	1000–50,000 (1.0–50 × 10^9/L) P	1000–10,000 (1.0–10 × 10^9/L)	Equal to serum levels	Usually left-sided; high amylase level

M, mononuclear cell predominance; P, polymorphonuclear leukocyte predominance.

Pleural fluid pH (normal = 7.60) is useful in the assessment of parapneumonic effusions, if it can be reliably measured, and is more useful than glucose measurement in determining need for drainage. A pH less than 7.20 suggests the need for drainage of the pleural space. An elevated amylase level in pleural fluid suggests pancreatitis, pancreatic pseudocyst, adenocarcinoma of the lung or pancreas, or esophageal rupture.

Suspected tuberculous pleural effusion should be evaluated by thoracentesis with culture, although pleural fluid culture positivity for *M tuberculosis* is low. Tests for pleural fluid adenosine deaminase (approximately 90% sensitivity and specificity for pleural tuberculosis at levels greater than 60 U/L, tuberculosis rare if level is less than 40 U/L) and interferon-gamma (89% sensitivity, 97% specificity in a meta-analysis) can be helpful diagnostic aids, particularly in making decisions to pursue invasive testing in complex patients. Closed pleural biopsy is more sensitive than pleural fluid culture for diagnosis, revealing granulomatous inflammation in approximately 60% of patients, and culture of three pleural biopsy specimens combined with histologic examination of a pleural biopsy for granulomas yields a diagnosis in up to 90% of patients.

Between 40% and 80% of exudative pleural effusions are malignant, while over 90% of malignant pleural effusions are exudative. Almost any form of cancer may cause effusions, but the most common causes are lung cancer (one-third of cases) and breast cancer. In 5–10% of malignant pleural effusions, no primary tumor is identified.

Pleural fluid specimens should be sent for cytologic examination in all cases of exudative effusions in patients suspected of harboring an underlying malignancy. The diagnostic yield depends on the nature and extent of the underlying malignancy. Sensitivity is between 50% and 65% and increases with serial sampling. In a patient with a high prior probability of malignancy, a negative cytologic examination should be followed by one repeat thoracentesis. If that examination is negative, thoracoscopy is preferred to closed pleural biopsy. The sensitivity of thoracoscopy is 92–96%.

The term **paramalignant** pleural effusion refers to an effusion in a patient with cancer when repeated attempts to identify tumor cells in the pleura or pleural fluid are nondiagnostic but when there is a presumptive relation to the underlying malignancy. For example, superior vena cava syndrome with elevated systemic venous pressures causing a transudative effusion would be "paramalignant."

C. Imaging

The lung is less dense than water and floats on pleural fluid that accumulates in dependent regions. Subpulmonic fluid may appear as lateral displacement of the apex of the diaphragm with an abrupt slope to the costophrenic sulcus or a greater than 2-cm separation between the gastric air bubble and the lung. On a standard upright chest radiograph (Figure 9–7), approximately 75–100 mL of pleural fluid must accumulate in the posterior costophrenic sulcus to be visible on the lateral view, and 175–200 mL must be present in the lateral costophrenic sulcus to be visible on the frontal view. Chest CT scans may identify as little as 10 mL

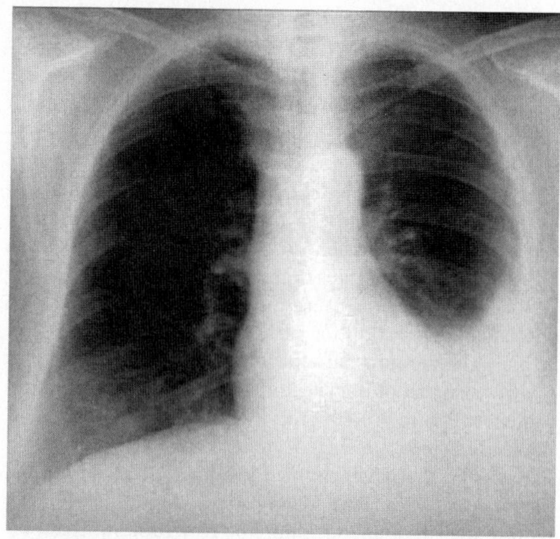

▲ **Figure 9–7. Left pleural effusion. Frontal chest radiograph showing a meniscus-shaped density at the left costophrenic angle sulcus indicative of a moderate-sized pleural effusion.** (Reproduced, with permission, from Lechner AJ, Matuschak GM, Brink DS. *Respiratory: An Integrated Approach to Disease*. McGraw-Hill, 2012.)

of fluid. At least 1 cm of fluid on the decubitus view is necessary to permit blind thoracentesis. Ultrasonography increases the safety of thoracentesis and should be incorporated routinely by trained users.

Pleural fluid may become trapped (loculated) by pleural adhesions, thereby forming unusual collections along the lateral chest wall or within lung fissures. Round or oval fluid collections in fissures that resemble intraparenchymal masses are called pseudotumors.

Treatment

A. Transudative Pleural Effusion

Transudative pleural effusions characteristically occur in the absence of pleural disease. Therefore, treatment is directed at the underlying condition. Therapeutic thoracentesis for severe dyspnea typically offers only transient benefit. Pleurodesis or indwelling pleural catheters are rarely indicated but are appropriate for management of symptoms in selected patients whose symptoms respond to drainage and whose effusions are refractory to maximal medical therapy.

B. Malignant Pleural Effusion

Chemotherapy, radiation therapy, or both offer temporary control in some malignant effusions but are generally ineffective in lung cancer in the pleural space except for small-cell lung cancer. Asymptomatic malignant effusions usually do not require specific treatment. Symptomatic patients should be offered pleural drainage, either via initial therapeutic thoracentesis to determine symptomatic response to drainage, following which an indwelling pleural catheter can be placed, or via immediate placement of an indwelling pleural catheter. Indwelling pleural catheter placement is associated with shorter hospital stays than pleurodesis. Indwelling pleural catheters often effect a pleurodesis over time, at which point the catheter can be removed.

C. Parapneumonic Pleural Effusion

Parapneumonic pleural effusions are divided into three categories, the classification of which can only be determined by sampling the fluid: uncomplicated (simple), complicated, and empyema. **Uncomplicated (simple) parapneumonic effusions** are free-flowing sterile exudates of modest size that resolve quickly with antibiotic treatment of pneumonia. They do not need drainage.

Complicated parapneumonic effusions present the most difficult management decisions. They tend to be larger than simple parapneumonic effusions and to show more evidence of inflammatory stimuli, such as low glucose level, low pH, or evidence of loculation. Inflammation probably reflects ongoing bacterial invasion of the pleural space despite rare positive bacterial cultures. Tube thoracostomy is indicated when pleural fluid glucose is less than 60 mg/dL (less than 3.3 mmol/L), or the pH is less than 7.2. These thresholds have not been prospectively validated and should not be interpreted strictly. The clinician should consider drainage of a complicated effusion if the pleural fluid pH is between 7.2 and 7.3 or the LD is greater than 1000 units/L (greater than 20 mckat/L). Pleural fluid cell count and protein have little diagnostic value in this setting.

Empyema is gross infection of the pleural space indicated by positive Gram stain or culture. Empyema should be drained, and the patient referred to a thoracic specialist to determine whether tube thoracostomy versus decortication is needed to facilitate clearance of infection and to reduce the probability of permanent fibrous encasement of the lung.

Tube thoracostomy drainage of empyema or complicated parapneumonic effusions is frequently complicated by loculation that prevents adequate drainage. Intrapleural instillation of fibrinolytic agents alone has not been shown in controlled trials to improve drainage. The combination of intrapleural tissue plasminogen activator and deoxyribonuclease (DNase), an enzyme that catalyzes extracellular DNA and degrades biofilm formation within the pleural cavity, has been found to improve clinical outcome (increased drainage, decreased length of stay, and decreased surgical referral) compared with placebo or either agent alone, and should be considered when fever, leukocytosis, or anorexia persist despite antibiotics and tube thoracostomy, or when the lung fails to reexpand.

D. Hemothorax

A small-volume hemothorax that is stable or improving on chest radiographs may be managed by close observation. In all other cases, hemothorax is treated by immediate insertion of a thoracostomy tube to (1) drain existing blood and clot, (2) quantify the amount of bleeding, (3) reduce the risk of fibrothorax, and (4) permit apposition of the pleural surfaces to reduce hemorrhage. Thoracic surgery consultation is indicated. Thoracotomy may be required to control hemorrhage, remove clot, and treat complications.

Aboudara M et al. Update in the management of pleural effusions. Med Clin North Am. 2019;103:475. [PMID: 30955515]

Bhatnagar R et al. Outpatient talc administration by indwelling pleural catheter for malignant effusion. N Engl J Med. 2018;378:1313. [PMID: 29617585]

Bramley K et al. Indwelling pleural catheter placement for nonmalignant pleural effusions. Semin Respir Crit Care Med. 2018;39:713. [PMID: 30641589]

Feller-Kopman D et al. Pleural disease. N Engl J Med. 2018;378:740. [PMID: 29466146]

Thomas R et al. Management of malignant pleural effusions—what is new. Semin Respir Crit Care Med. 2019;40:323. [PMID: 31525808]

PNEUMOTHORAX

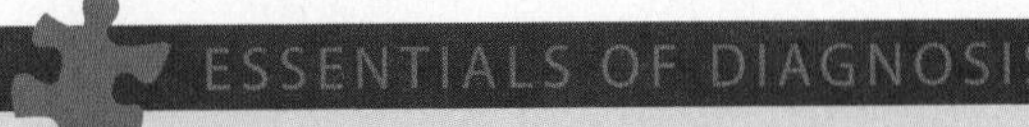

ESSENTIALS OF DIAGNOSIS

- Acute onset of unilateral chest pain and dyspnea.
- Minimal physical findings in mild cases; unilateral chest expansion, decreased tactile fremitus, hyperresonance, diminished breath sounds, mediastinal shift, cyanosis, and hypotension in tension pneumothorax.
- Presence of pleural air on chest radiograph.

General Considerations

Pneumothorax, or accumulation of air in the pleural space, is classified as spontaneous (primary or secondary), traumatic, or iatrogenic. **Primary spontaneous pneumothorax** occurs in the absence of an underlying lung disease, whereas **secondary spontaneous pneumothorax** is a complication of preexisting pulmonary disease. **Traumatic pneumothorax** results from penetrating or blunt trauma and includes **iatrogenic pneumothorax** following procedures, such as thoracentesis, pleural biopsy, subclavian or internal jugular vein catheter placement, percutaneous lung biopsy, bronchoscopy with transbronchial biopsy, and positive-pressure mechanical ventilation. **Tension pneumothorax** usually occurs in the setting of penetrating trauma, lung infection, CPR, or positive-pressure mechanical ventilation. In tension pneumothorax, the pressure of air in the pleural space exceeds alveolar and venous pressures throughout the respiratory cycle, resulting in compression of lung and reduction of venous return to the hemithorax; a check-valve mechanism may allow air to enter the pleural space on inspiration and to prevent egress of air on expiration.

Primary spontaneous pneumothorax is more likely among tall, thin individuals, more common in men, typically occurring at a young age (less than 45 years). It is thought to occur from rupture of subpleural apical blebs in response to high negative intrapleural pressures. Cigarette smoking is correlated with occurrence of primary spontaneous pneumothorax, as are connective tissue disorders such as Marfan and Ehlers-Danlos syndromes.

Secondary pneumothorax occurs as a complication of COPD, interstitial lung disease, asthma, cystic fibrosis, tuberculosis, *Pneumocystis* pneumonia, necrotizing bacterial pneumonia, menstruation (catamenial pneumothorax), and a wide variety of cystic lung diseases, including lymphangioleiomyomatosis, tuberous sclerosis, Langerhans cell histiocytosis, and Birt-Hogg-Dube syndrome (a hereditary condition with multiple benign skin tumors, lung cysts, and increased risk of both benign and malignant kidney tumors). Secondary pneumothorax, particularly in patients with underlying symptomatic lung disease, is more poorly tolerated due to the decreased respiratory reserve in this group.

Clinical Findings

A. Symptoms and Signs

Chest pain ranging from minimal to severe on the affected side and dyspnea occur in nearly all patients, and cough is commonly reported. Pneumothorax may present with life-threatening respiratory failure if underlying lung disease is present or if tension pneumothorax physiology ensues.

If pneumothorax is small (less than 15% of a hemithorax), physical findings, other than mild tachycardia, are normal. If pneumothorax is large, diminished breath sounds, decreased tactile fremitus, decreased movement of the chest, and hyperresonant percussion note are often found. Tension pneumothorax should be suspected in the presence of marked tachycardia, hypotension, and mediastinal or tracheal shift.

B. Laboratory Findings

ABG analysis is often unnecessary but reveals hypoxemia and acute respiratory alkalosis in most patients. Left-sided primary pneumothorax may produce QRS axis and precordial T-wave changes on the ECG that may be misinterpreted as acute MI.

C. Imaging

Demonstration on chest radiograph of lucency without lung markings between the chest wall and lung, and visualization of the visceral pleura (a "pleural line") is diagnostic. A few patients have secondary pleural effusion that demonstrates a characteristic air-fluid level on chest radiography. In supine patients, pneumothorax on a conventional chest radiograph may appear as an abnormally radiolucent costophrenic sulcus (the "deep sulcus" sign). In patients with tension pneumothorax, chest radiographs show a large amount of air in the affected hemithorax and contralateral shift of the mediastinum.

Chest ultrasonography, performed at the bedside by experienced clinicians or technicians, demonstrates characteristic findings in the region of the pneumothorax. These findings include absent "lung sliding," or absent "lung pulse," or presence of a "lung point," all of which demonstrate a region of lung where the parietal and visceral pleural are not in normal apposition. Ultrasound may be more sensitive than supine chest radiograph (supine positioning necessitated by clinical circumstance) for detecting pneumothorax in trauma patients, and is frequently used in critical care, though comparisons of ultrasound to chest radiograph or to CT scan report variable test characteristics.

High-resolution CT may be considered with the first spontaneous pneumothorax to evaluate for underlying cystic lung disease.

Differential Diagnosis

If the patient is young with typical clinical characteristics, the diagnosis of primary spontaneous pneumothorax is usually obvious and can be confirmed by chest radiograph. Occasionally, pneumothorax may mimic MI, PE, or pneumonia.

Complications

Tension pneumothorax may be life-threatening. Pneumomediastinum and subcutaneous emphysema may occur as complications of spontaneous pneumothorax. If pneumomediastinum is detected, rupture of the esophagus or a bronchus should be considered in the differential diagnosis.

Treatment

Treatment depends on the severity of the pneumothorax and the nature of the underlying disease. In a reliable patient with a stable, spontaneous primary pneumothorax, observation alone may be appropriate; many cases resolve spontaneously as air is absorbed from the pleural space. In fact, a 2020 US study demonstrated that even moderate to large pneumothoraces in a stable patient (no oxygen requirement, no limitation to ambulation, and no increase in size of pneumothorax over 4 hours of monitoring) can be managed without intervention provided the patient is reliable. Simple aspiration drainage of pleural air with a small-bore catheter (eg, 16-gauge angiocatheter or larger drainage catheter) can be performed for spontaneous primary pneumothoraxes that are large or progressive. Placement of a small-bore chest tube (7F to 14F) attached to a one-way Heimlich valve provides protection against development of tension pneumothorax and may permit observation from home. The patient should be treated symptomatically for cough and chest pain and monitored with serial chest radiographs every 24 hours. Similarly, a 2021 observational report of pneumothorax following percutaneous lung biopsy found monitoring and noninvasive management to be sufficient in most patients.

Patients with secondary pneumothorax, tension pneumothorax, or severe symptoms or those who have a pneumothorax on mechanical ventilation should undergo chest tube placement (tube thoracostomy). The chest tube is placed under water-seal drainage, and suction is applied until the lung expands. The chest tube can be removed after the air leak subsides.

All patients who smoke should be advised to discontinue smoking and warned that the risk of recurrence is higher if cigarette smoking is continued.

Indications for surgical management (video-assisted thoracoscopic surgery) include recurrences of spontaneous pneumothorax, any occurrence of bilateral pneumothorax, and failure of tube thoracostomy for the first episode (failure of lung to reexpand or persistent air leak). Surgical intervention is also generally recommended for any patient with a secondary pneumothorax (presence of underlying lung disease) because the risk of recurrence is high, and the consequences of recurrences are greater. Surgery permits resection or repair of blebs or bullae responsible for the pneumothorax as well as mechanical or chemical pleurodesis. Patients who are not acceptable surgical candidates can be treated with chemical pleurodesis via a chest tube.

Prognosis

An average of 30% of patients with spontaneous pneumothorax experience recurrence of the disorder after either observation or tube thoracostomy for the first episode. Recurrence after surgical therapy is less frequent. Following successful therapy, there are no long-term complications. Secondary pneumothorax has up to a 50% likelihood of recurrence following the first event if surgical intervention is not undertaken.

Brown SGA et al; PSP Investigators. Conservative versus interventional treatment for spontaneous pneumothorax. N Engl J Med. 2020;382:405. [PMID: 31995686]

Calderon Novoa F et al. Pneumothorax after percutaneous transthoracic lung biopsy. Non-invasive management in order to avoid unnecessary hospitalizations. Rev Fac Cien Med Univ Nac Cordoba. 2021;78:37. [PMID: 33787024]

Chan KK et al. Chest ultrasonography versus supine chest radiography for diagnosis of pneumothorax in trauma patients in the emergency department. Cochrane Database Syst Rev. 2020;7:CD013031. [PMID: 32702777]

Hallifax RJ et al. Ambulatory management of primary spontaneous pneumothorax: an open-label, randomised controlled trial. Lancet. 2020;396:39. [PMID: 32622394]

Plojoux J et al. New insights and improved strategies for the management of primary spontaneous pneumothorax. Clin Respir J. 2019;13:195. [PMID: 30615303]

DISORDERS OF CONTROL OF VENTILATION

The principal influences on ventilatory control are arterial P_{CO_2}, pH, P_{O_2}, and brainstem tissue pH. These variables are monitored by peripheral and central chemoreceptors. Under normal conditions, the ventilatory control system maintains arterial pH and P_{CO_2} within narrow limits; arterial P_{O_2} is more loosely controlled.

Abnormal control of ventilation can be seen with a variety of conditions ranging from rare disorders, such as primary alveolar hypoventilation, neuromuscular disorders, myxedema, starvation, and carotid body resection, to more common disorders, such as asthma, COPD, obesity, heart failure, and sleep-related breathing disorders. A few of these disorders will be discussed in this section.

HYPERVENTILATION SYNDROMES

Hyperventilation is an increase in alveolar minute ventilation that leads to hypocapnia. It may be caused by a variety of conditions, such as pregnancy, hypoxemia, obstructive and infiltrative lung diseases, sepsis, liver dysfunction, fever, and pain. Functional hyperventilation may be acute or chronic. **Acute hyperventilation** presents with hyperpnea, anxiety, paresthesias, carpopedal spasm, and tetany. **Chronic hyperventilation** may present with various nonspecific symptoms, including fatigue, dyspnea, anxiety, palpitations, and dizziness. The diagnosis of chronic hyperventilation syndrome is established if symptoms are reproduced during voluntary hyperventilation. Once organic causes of hyperventilation have been excluded, treatment of acute hyperventilation consists of breathing through pursed lips or through the nose with one nostril pinched or rebreathing expired gas from a paper bag held over the face to decrease respiratory alkalemia and its associated symptoms. Anxiolytic drugs may also be useful.

Vidotto LS et al. Dysfunctional breathing: what do we know? J Bras Pneumol. 2019;45:e20170347. [PMID: 30758427]

Zhang Z et al. Hyperventilation in neurological patients: from physiology to outcome evidence. Curr Opin Anaesthesiol. 2019;32:568. [PMID: 31211719]

OBESITY-HYPOVENTILATION SYNDROME (Pickwickian Syndrome)

In obesity-hypoventilation syndrome, awake alveolar hypoventilation appears to result from a combination of blunted ventilatory drive and increased mechanical load imposed upon the chest by obesity. Voluntary hyperventilation returns the P_{CO_2} and the P_{O_2} toward normal values, a correction not seen in lung diseases causing chronic respiratory failure, such as COPD. Diagnostic criteria include a BMI greater than 30, an arterial partial pressure of carbon dioxide greater than 45 mm Hg, and exclusion of other causes of alveolar hypoventilation. Most patients with obesity-hypoventilation syndrome also suffer from obstructive sleep apnea, which must be treated aggressively if identified as a comorbid disorder. Therapy of obesity-hypoventilation syndrome consists mainly of weight loss, which improves hypercapnia and hypoxemia as well as the ventilatory responses to hypoxia and hypercapnia. Avoidance of sedative-hypnotics, opioids, and alcohol is also recommended. NIPPV is helpful in many patients. Patients with obesity-hypoventilation syndrome have a higher risk of complications in the perioperative period, including respiratory failure, intubation, and heart failure. Recognition of these patients in the perioperative period is an important safety measure.

Kaw R et al. Obesity and obesity hypoventilation, sleep hypoventilation, and postoperative respiratory failure. Anesth Analg. 2021;132:1265. [PMID: 33857968]

Masa JF et al. Obesity hypoventilation syndrome. Eur Respir Rev. 2019;28:180097. [PMID: 30872398]

Mokhlesi B et al. Evaluation and management of obesity hypoventilation syndrome. An Official American Thoracic Society Clinical Practice Guideline. Am J Respir Crit Care Med. 2019;200:e6. [PMID: 31368798]
Ramírez Molina VR et al. Effectiveness of different treatments in obesity hypoventilation syndrome. Pulmonology. 2020;26:370. [PMID: 32553827]

SLEEP-RELATED BREATHING DISORDERS

Abnormal ventilation during sleep is manifested by apnea (breath cessation for at least 10 seconds) or hypopnea (decrement in airflow with drop in hemoglobin saturation of at least 4%). Episodes of apnea are **central** if ventilatory effort is absent for the duration of the apneic episode, **obstructive** if ventilatory effort persists throughout the apneic episode but no airflow occurs because of transient obstruction of the upper airway, or **mixed** if absent ventilatory effort precedes upper airway obstruction during the apneic episode. Pure central sleep apnea is uncommon; it may be an isolated finding or may occur in patients with primary alveolar hypoventilation or with lesions of the brainstem. Obstructive and mixed sleep apneas are more common and may be associated with life-threatening cardiac arrhythmias, severe hypoxemia during sleep, daytime somnolence, pulmonary hypertension, right-sided heart failure, systemic hypertension, and secondary erythrocytosis.

Folmer RL et al. Prevalence and management of sleep disorders in the Veterans Health Administration. Sleep Med Rev. 2020; 54:101358. [PMID: 32791487]
Gandhi KD et al. Excessive daytime sleepiness: a clinical review. Mayo Clin Proc. 2021;96:1288. [PMID: 33840518]
McNicholas WT et al. Sleep in chronic respiratory disease: COPD and hypoventilation disorders. Eur Respir Rev. 2019; 28:190064. [PMID: 31554703]

OBSTRUCTIVE SLEEP APNEA

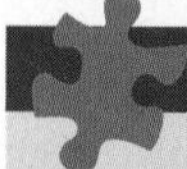

ESSENTIALS OF DIAGNOSIS

- Daytime somnolence or fatigue.
- A history of loud snoring with witnessed apneic events.
- Overnight polysomnography demonstrating apneic episodes with hypoxemia.

General Considerations

Upper airway obstruction during sleep occurs when loss of normal pharyngeal muscle tone allows the pharynx to collapse passively during inspiration. Patients with anatomically narrowed upper airways (eg, micrognathia, macroglossia, obesity, tonsillar hypertrophy) are predisposed to the development of obstructive sleep apnea. Ingestion of alcohol or sedatives before sleeping or nasal obstruction of any type, including the common cold, may precipitate or worsen the condition. Hypothyroidism and cigarette smoking are additional risk factors for obstructive sleep apnea. Before making the diagnosis of obstructive sleep apnea, a drug history should be obtained and a seizure disorder, narcolepsy, and depression should be excluded.

Clinical Findings

A. Symptoms and Signs

Most patients with obstructive or mixed sleep apnea are obese, middle-aged men. Arterial hypertension is common. Patients may complain of excessive daytime somnolence, morning sluggishness and headaches, daytime fatigue, cognitive impairment, recent weight gain, and impotence. Bed partners usually report loud cyclical snoring, breath cessation, witnessed apneas, restlessness, and thrashing movements of the extremities during sleep. Personality changes, poor judgment, work-related problems, depression, and intellectual deterioration (memory impairment, inability to concentrate) may also be observed. The USPSTF does not recommend screening asymptomatic adults for sleep apnea.

Physical examination may be normal or may reveal systemic and pulmonary hypertension with right-sided heart failure. The patient may appear sleepy or even fall asleep during the evaluation. The oropharynx is frequently found to be narrowed by excessive soft tissue folds, large tonsils, elongated uvula, or prominent tongue. Nasal obstruction by a deviated nasal septum, poor nasal airflow, and a nasal twang to the speech may be observed. A "bull neck" appearance is common.

B. Laboratory Findings

Erythrocytosis is common. Thyroid function tests (serum TSH, FT_4) should be obtained to exclude hypothyroidism.

C. Other Studies

Observation of the sleeping patient may reveal loud snoring interrupted by episodes of increasingly strong ventilatory effort that fail to produce airflow. A loud snort often accompanies the first breath following an apneic episode. Definitive diagnostic evaluation for suspected sleep apnea includes otorhinolaryngologic examination and overnight polysomnography (the monitoring of multiple physiologic factors during sleep). A complete **polysomnography** examination includes electroencephalography, electro-oculography, electromyography, ECG, pulse oximetry, and measurement of respiratory effort and airflow. Polysomnography reveals apneic episodes lasting as long as 60 seconds. Oxygen saturation falls, often to very low levels. Bradydysrhythmias, such as sinus bradycardia, sinus arrest, or atrioventricular block, may occur. Tachydysrhythmias, including paroxysmal supraventricular tachycardia, atrial fibrillation, and ventricular tachycardia, may be seen once airflow is reestablished. Home sleep studies can be done for the person without comorbidities and a moderate to high pretest probability of obstructive sleep apnea. While home studies cannot quantify the stages of sleep, they can provide a reliable index of respiratory and desaturation events.

Treatment

Weight loss and strict avoidance of alcohol and hypnotic medications are the first steps in management. Weight loss may be curative, but most patients are unable to lose the 10–20% of body weight required. **Continuous positive airway pressure (CPAP)** at night is curative in many patients. Auto-titrating CPAP machines allow a range of pressures to be prescribed (5–15 cm H_2O). Polysomnography is frequently necessary to optimize the level of CPAP necessary to abolish obstructive apneas and manage hypoxemia. Unfortunately, only about 75% of patients continue to use nasal CPAP after 1 year. Supplemental oxygen may lessen the severity of nocturnal desaturation but may also lengthen apneas; it should not be routinely prescribed without polysomnography to assess the effects of oxygen therapy. Mechanical devices inserted into the mouth at bedtime to hold the jaw forward and prevent pharyngeal occlusion have modest effectiveness in relieving apnea. However, patient compliance with these devices is suboptimal.

Uvulopalatopharyngoplasty (UPPP), a procedure consisting of resection of pharyngeal soft tissue and amputation of approximately 15 mm of the free edge of the soft palate and uvula, is helpful in approximately 50% of selected patients. It is more effective in eliminating snoring than apneic episodes. UPPP may be performed on an outpatient basis with a laser. **Nasal septoplasty** is performed if gross anatomic nasal septal deformity is present. **Tracheostomy** relieves upper airway obstruction and its physiologic consequences and represents the definitive treatment for obstructive sleep apnea. However, it has numerous adverse effects, including granuloma formation, difficulty with speech, and stoma and airway infection. Furthermore, the long-term care of the tracheostomy, especially in obese patients, can be difficult. Tracheostomy and other maxillofacial surgery approaches are reserved for patients with life-threatening arrhythmias or severe disability who have not responded to conservative therapy. **Hypoglossal nerve stimulation** can be an option for select patients who do not respond to CPAP and have certain anatomic features, including nonconcentric airway collapse; a 5-year follow-up study showed improvement in sleepiness, quality of life, and respiratory outcomes in the treatment cohort. For patients who are unable or unwilling to use CPAP, and who may not be surgical candidates, the H_3-receptor antagonist/inverse agonist pitolisant has been shown to improve sleepiness and fatigue. Full normalization of breathing patterns is not necessarily the therapeutic goal. A randomized trial of adaptive servo-ventilation in sleep apnea patients with predominant central apnea and impaired LVEF (less than 45%) reported increased cardiovascular and all-cause mortality in the treatment group.

Edwards BA et al. More than the sum of the respiratory events: personalized medicine approaches for obstructive sleep apnea. Am J Respir Crit Care Med. 2019;200:691. [PMID: 31022356]

Gottlieb DJ et al. Diagnosis and management of obstructive sleep apnea: a review. JAMA. 2020;323:1389. [PMID: 32286648]

Suurna MV et al. Obstructive sleep apnea: non-positive airway pressure treatments. Clin Geriatr Med. 2021;37:429. [PMID: 34210448]

ACUTE RESPIRATORY FAILURE

Respiratory failure is defined as respiratory dysfunction resulting in abnormalities of oxygenation or ventilation (CO_2 elimination) severe enough to threaten the function of vital organs. ABG criteria for respiratory failure are not absolute but may be arbitrarily established as a Po_2 under 60 mm Hg (7.8 kPa) or a Pco_2 over 50 mm Hg (6.5 kPa). Acute respiratory failure may occur in a variety of pulmonary and nonpulmonary disorders (Table 9–25). Only a few selected general principles of management will be reviewed here.

Clinical Findings

Symptoms and signs of acute respiratory failure are those of the underlying disease combined with those of hypoxemia or hypercapnia. The chief symptom of hypoxemia is dyspnea, though profound hypoxemia may exist in the absence of complaints. Signs of hypoxemia include cyanosis, restlessness, confusion, anxiety, delirium, tachypnea, bradycardia or tachycardia, hypotension or hypertension, cardiac dysrhythmias, and tremor. Dyspnea and headache are the cardinal symptoms of hypercapnia. Signs of hypercapnia include peripheral and conjunctival hyperemia, hypertension, tachycardia, tachypnea, impaired consciousness, papilledema, myoclonus, and asterixis. The symptoms and signs of acute respiratory failure are both insensitive and nonspecific; therefore, the clinician must maintain a high index of suspicion and obtain ABG analysis if respiratory failure is suspected.

Treatment

Treatment of the patient with acute respiratory failure consists of (1) specific therapy directed toward the underlying disease, (2) respiratory supportive care directed toward the maintenance of adequate gas exchange, and (3) general supportive care. Only the last two aspects are discussed below.

A. Respiratory Support

Respiratory support has both nonventilatory and ventilatory aspects.

1. Nonventilatory aspects—The main therapeutic goal in acute hypoxemic respiratory failure is to ensure adequate oxygenation of vital organs. Inspired oxygen concentration should be the lowest value that results in an arterial hemoglobin saturation of 88% (Po_2 55 mm Hg or 7.3 kPa) or more. Higher arterial oxygen tensions are of no proven benefit and may be deleterious. Restoration of normoxemia may rarely cause hypoventilation in patients with chronic hypercapnia; however, oxygen therapy should not be withheld for that concern. Hypoxemia in patients with obstructive airway disease is usually easily corrected by administering low-flow oxygen by nasal cannula (1–3 L/minute) or Venturi mask (24–40%). Higher concentrations of oxygen are necessary to correct hypoxemia in patients with ARDS, pneumonia, and other parenchymal lung diseases. Humidified, high-flow nasal cannulae provide

Table 9–25. Selected causes of acute respiratory failure in adults.

Airway disorders Asthma Acute exacerbation of chronic bronchitis or emphysema Obstruction of pharynx, larynx, trachea, mainstem bronchus, or lobar bronchus by edema, mucus, mass, or foreign body **Pulmonary edema** Increased hydrostatic pressure LV dysfunction (eg, myocardial ischemia, heart failure) Mitral regurgitation Left atrial outflow obstruction (eg, mitral stenosis) Volume overload states Increased pulmonary capillary permeability Acute respiratory distress syndrome Acute lung injury Unclear etiology Neurogenic Negative pressure (inspiratory airway obstruction) Re-expansion Tocolytic-associated **Parenchymal lung disorders** Pneumonia Interstitial lung diseases Diffuse alveolar hemorrhage syndromes Aspiration Lung contusion **Pulmonary vascular disorders** Thromboembolism Air embolism Amniotic fluid embolism **Chest wall, diaphragm, and pleural disorders** Rib fracture Flail chest Pneumothorax Pleural effusion Massive ascites Abdominal distention and abdominal compartment syndrome	**Neuromuscular and related disorders** Primary neuromuscular diseases Guillain-Barré syndrome Myasthenia gravis Poliomyelitis Polymyositis Drug- or toxin-induced Botulism Organophosphates Neuromuscular blocking agents Aminoglycosides Spinal cord injury Phrenic nerve injury or dysfunction Electrolyte disturbances Hypokalemia Hypophosphatemia Myxedema **CNS disorders** Drugs: sedatives, hypnotics, opioids, anesthetics Brainstem respiratory center disorders: trauma, tumor, vascular disorders, hypothyroidism Intracranial hypertension CNS infections **Increased CO_2 production** Fever Infection Hyperalimentation with excess caloric and carbohydrate intake Hyperthyroidism Seizures Rigors Drugs

adjustable oxygen delivery and flow-dependent clearance of carbon dioxide from the upper airway, resulting in reduced work of breathing and better matching of respiratory demand during respiratory distress. In hypoxemia due to acute respiratory failure, oxygenation with use of humidified, high-flow nasal cannulae has been shown to be similar and, in some cases, superior to conventional low-flow oxygen supplementation and to NIPPV.

2. Ventilatory aspects—Ventilatory support consists of maintaining patency of the airway and ensuring adequate alveolar ventilation. Mechanical ventilation may be provided via mask (noninvasive) or through tracheal intubation.

A. NONINVASIVE POSITIVE-PRESSURE VENTILATION—NIPPV delivered via a full-face mask or nasal mask is first-line therapy in COPD patients with hypercapnic respiratory failure who can protect and maintain the patency of their airway, handle their own secretions, and tolerate the mask apparatus. Several studies have demonstrated the effectiveness of this therapy in reducing intubation rates and ICU stays in patients with ventilatory failure. A bilevel positive-pressure ventilation mode is preferred for most patients. Patients with acute lung injury or ARDS or those who suffer from severely impaired oxygenation are less likely to benefit and should be intubated if they require mechanical ventilation.

B. TRACHEAL INTUBATION—Indications for tracheal intubation include (1) hypoxemia despite supplemental oxygen; (2) upper airway obstruction; (3) impaired airway protection; (4) inability to clear secretions; (5) respiratory acidosis; (6) progressive general fatigue, tachypnea, use of accessory respiratory muscles, or mental status deterioration; and (7) apnea. Patients in respiratory failure who undergo a trial of NIPPV and do not improve within 30–90 minutes should be intubated. Of note, this practice changed somewhat during the COVID-19 pandemic—periods of high-level support, whether via humidified high-flow nasal cannula or NIPPV, are tolerated for longer in part due to resource limitations (lack of ventilators) and in part due to the frequency of patient self-induced lung injury while intubated. In general, orotracheal intubation is preferred to nasotracheal intubation in urgent or emergency situations because it is easier, faster, and less traumatic. The tip of the endotracheal tube should be positioned 2–4 cm above the carina and be verified by chest radiograph immediately following intubation. Only tracheal tubes with high-volume, low-pressure air-filled cuffs should be used. Cuff inflation pressure should be kept below 20 mm Hg, if possible, to minimize tracheal mucosal injury.

C. MECHANICAL VENTILATION—Indications for mechanical ventilation include (1) apnea, (2) acute hypercapnia that is not quickly reversed by appropriate specific therapy, (3) severe hypoxemia, and (4) progressive patient fatigue despite appropriate treatment.

Several modes of positive-pressure ventilation are available. Controlled mechanical ventilation (CMV; also known as assist-control [A-C]) and synchronized intermittent mandatory ventilation (SIMV) are ventilatory modes in which the ventilator delivers a minimum number of breaths of a specified pattern (either a set volume or a set pressure) each minute. In both CMV and SIMV, the patient may trigger the ventilator to deliver additional breaths. In CMV, the ventilator responds to breaths initiated by the patient above the set rate by delivering additional full-support breaths. In SIMV, additional breaths are not supported by the ventilator unless the pressure support mode is added. Numerous alternative modes of mechanical ventilation now exist, the most popular being pressure support ventilation (PSV), proportional-assist ventilation, and CPAP.

Positive end-expiratory pressure (PEEP) is useful in improving oxygenation in patients with diffuse parenchymal lung disease, such as ARDS. It should be used cautiously in patients with localized parenchymal disease, emphysema, hyperinflation, or very high airway pressure requirements during mechanical ventilation.

D. Complications of Mechanical Ventilation—Potential complications of mechanical ventilation are numerous. Migration of the tip of the endotracheal tube into a main bronchus can cause atelectasis of the contralateral lung and overdistention of the intubated lung. Barotrauma refers to rupture and loss of integrity of the alveolar space secondary to high transmural pressures applied during positive-pressure ventilation. Barotrauma is manifested by subcutaneous emphysema, pneumomediastinum, subpleural air cysts, pneumothorax, or systemic gas embolism. Volutrauma is sometimes used to refer to subtle parenchymal injury due to overdistention of alveoli from excessive tidal volumes without alveolar rupture, mediated through inflammatory rather than physical mechanisms. The principal strategy to avoid volutrauma is the use of low tidal volume ventilation (a tidal volume of 6 mL/kg of ideal body weight is supported by the ARDS literature).

Acute respiratory alkalosis caused by overventilation is common. Hypotension induced by elevated intrathoracic pressure that results in decreased return of systemic venous blood to the heart may occur in patients treated with PEEP, particularly those with intravascular volume depletion, and in patients with severe airflow obstruction at high respiratory rates that promote dynamic hyperinflation ("breath stacking"). Ventilator-associated pneumonia is another serious complication of mechanical ventilation.

B. General Supportive Care

Hypokalemia and hypophosphatemia may worsen hypoventilation due to respiratory muscle weakness. Sedative-hypnotics and opioid analgesics should be titrated carefully to avoid oversedation, leading to prolongation of intubation. Temporary paralysis with a nondepolarizing neuromuscular blocking agent is used to facilitate mechanical ventilation and to lower oxygen consumption. Prolonged muscle weakness due to an acute myopathy is a potential complication of these agents. Myopathy is more common in patients with kidney injury and in those given concomitant corticosteroids.

Psychological and emotional support of the patient and family, skin care to avoid pressure injuries, and meticulous avoidance of health care–associated infection and complications of endotracheal tubes are vital aspects of comprehensive care for patients with acute respiratory failure.

Attention must also be paid to preventing complications associated with serious illness. Stress gastritis and ulcers may be avoided by administering sucralfate, histamine H_2-receptor antagonists, or PPIs. Meta-analyses have demonstrated that PPIs are most effective. The risk of DVT and PE may be reduced by subcutaneous administration of heparin or low-molecular-weight heparin (LMWH) (see Table 14–14), or placement of sequential compression devices on the lower extremities.

Course & Prognosis

The course and prognosis of acute respiratory failure vary and depend on the underlying disease. The prognosis of acute respiratory failure caused by uncomplicated sedative or opioid overdose is excellent. Acute respiratory failure in patients with COPD who do not require intubation and mechanical ventilation has a good immediate prognosis. On the other hand, ARDS and respiratory failure associated with sepsis have a poor prognosis.

David-João PG et al. Noninvasive ventilation in acute hypoxemic respiratory failure: a systematic review and meta-analysis. J Crit Care. 2019;49:84. [PMID: 30388493]

Grieco DL et al. Physiological comparison of high-flow nasal cannula and helmet noninvasive ventilation in acute hypoxemic respiratory failure. Am J Respir Crit Care Med. 2020; 201:303. [PMID: 31687831]

Richards H et al. Clinical benefits of prone positioning in the treatment of non-intubated patients with acute hypoxic respiratory failure: a rapid systematic review. Emerg Med J. 2021; 38:594. [PMID: 34162630]

Rochwerg B et al. High flow nasal cannula compared with conventional oxygen therapy for acute hypoxemic respiratory failure: a systematic review and meta-analysis. Intensive Care Med. 2019;45:563. [PMID: 30888444]

Schjørring OL et al; HOT-ICU Investigators. Lower or higher oxygenation targets for acute hypoxemic respiratory failure. N Engl J Med. 2021;384:1301. [PMID: 33471452]

ACUTE RESPIRATORY DISTRESS SYNDROME

ESSENTIALS OF DIAGNOSIS

- Onset of respiratory distress, often progressing to respiratory failure, within 7 days of a known clinical insult.
- New, bilateral radiographic pulmonary opacities not explained by pleural effusion, atelectasis, or nodules.
- Respiratory failure not fully explained by heart failure or volume overload.
- Impaired oxygenation, with ratio of partial pressure of oxygen in arterial blood (Pa_{O_2}) to fractional concentration of inspired oxygen (F_{IO_2}) < 300 mm Hg, with PEEP ≥ 5 cm H_2O.

General Considerations

Acute respiratory distress syndrome (ARDS) as a clinical syndrome is based on three inclusion criteria plus one

Table 9–26. Selected disorders associated with ARDS.

Systemic Insults	Pulmonary Insults
Trauma Sepsis Pancreatitis Shock Multiple transfusions Disseminated intravascular coagulation Burns Drugs and drug overdose Opioids Aspirin Phenothiazines Tricyclic antidepressants Amiodarone Chemotherapeutic agents Nitrofurantoin Protamine Thrombotic thrombocytopenic purpura Cardiopulmonary bypass Head injury Paraquat	Aspiration of gastric contents Embolism of thrombus, fat, air, or amniotic fluid Miliary tuberculosis Diffuse pneumonia (eg, SARS, COVID-19) Acute eosinophilic pneumonia Cryptogenic organizing pneumonitis Upper airway obstruction Free-base cocaine smoking Near-drowning Toxic gas inhalation Nitrogen dioxide Chlorine Sulfur dioxide Ammonia Smoke Oxygen toxicity Lung contusion Radiation exposure High-altitude exposure Lung reexpansion or reperfusion

ARDS, acute respiratory distress syndrome; SARS, severe acute respiratory syndrome.

exclusion criterion, as detailed above. The severity of ARDS is based on the level of oxygenation impairment: **mild,** Pao_2/Fio_2 ratio between 200 mm Hg and 300 mm Hg; **moderate,** Pao_2/Fio_2 ratio between 100 mm Hg and 200 mm Hg; and **severe,** Pao_2/Fio_2 ratio less than 100 mm Hg.

ARDS may follow a wide variety of clinical events (Table 9–26). Common risk factors for ARDS include sepsis, aspiration of gastric contents, shock, infection, lung contusion, nonthoracic trauma, toxic inhalation, near-drowning, and multiple blood transfusions. About one-third of ARDS patients initially have sepsis syndrome. Damage to capillary endothelial cells and alveolar epithelial cells is common to ARDS regardless of cause or mechanism of lung injury and results in increased vascular permeability and decreased production and activity of surfactant. These abnormalities in turn lead to interstitial and alveolar pulmonary edema, alveolar collapse, and hypoxemia.

Clinical Findings

ARDS is marked by the rapid onset of profound dyspnea that usually occurs 12–48 hours after the initiating event. Labored breathing, tachypnea, intercostal retractions, and crackles are noted on physical examination. Chest radiography shows diffuse or patchy bilateral infiltrates that rapidly become confluent; these characteristically spare the costophrenic angles. Air bronchograms occur in about 80% of cases. Heart size is usually normal, and pleural effusions are small or nonexistent. Marked hypoxemia occurs that is refractory to treatment with supplemental oxygen. Many patients with ARDS demonstrate multiple organ failure, particularly involving the kidneys, liver, gut, CNS, and cardiovascular system.

Differential Diagnosis

Since ARDS is a physiologic and radiographic syndrome rather than a specific disease, the concept of differential diagnosis does not strictly apply. Normal-permeability ("cardiogenic" or hydrostatic) pulmonary edema must be excluded, however, because specific therapy is available for that disorder. Emergent echocardiogram or measurement of pulmonary capillary wedge pressure by means of a flow-directed pulmonary artery catheter may be required in selected patients with suspected cardiac dysfunction; routine use in ARDS is discouraged.

Prevention

No measures that effectively prevent ARDS have been identified. Specifically, neither PEEP nor aspirin when used prophylactically has been shown to be effective in patients at risk for ARDS. Intravenous methylprednisolone does not prevent ARDS when given early to patients with sepsis syndrome or septic shock.

Treatment

The first principle in management is to identify and treat the primary condition that has led to ARDS. Meticulous supportive care must then be provided to compensate for the severe dysfunction of the respiratory system associated with ARDS and to prevent complications.

Treatment of the hypoxemia seen in ARDS usually requires tracheal intubation and positive-pressure mechanical ventilation. The lowest levels of PEEP (used to recruit atelectatic alveoli) and supplemental oxygen required to maintain the Pao_2 above 55 mm Hg (7.13 kPa) or the Sao_2 above 88% should be used. Efforts should be made to decrease Fio_2 as soon as possible to avoid oxygen toxicity. PEEP can be increased as needed if cardiac output and oxygen delivery do not decrease and airway pressures do not increase excessively (ie, plateau pressures remain below 30 cm H_2O). Prone positioning frequently improves oxygenation by helping recruit atelectatic alveoli and has been shown in some (although not all) trials to provide a mortality benefit in severe ARDS. Routine use of neuromuscular blockade is controversial; one major trial showed improved mortality and more ventilator-free days in patients with Pao_2/Fio_2 ratio less than 120 mm Hg but a subsequent trial (intended to be confirmatory) did not demonstrate a mortality benefit.

A variety of mechanical ventilation strategies are available. The most significant advance in the treatment of ARDS over the past 20 years has been the recognition of the potential for excessive alveolar stretch to cause lung injury, and the widespread adoption of low tidal volume ventilation. A multicenter study of 800 patients demonstrated that a protocol using volume-control ventilation with low tidal volumes (6 mL/kg of ideal body weight) resulted in an 8.8% absolute mortality reduction over therapy with standard tidal volumes (defined as 12 mL/kg of ideal body weight). Varying ventilator modes have been used; conventional modes of ventilation are essentially equivalent, while high-frequency oscillatory ventilation should not be used an as initial mode.

Approaches to hemodynamic monitoring and fluid management in patients with acute lung injury have been carefully studied. A prospective RCT comparing hemodynamic management guided either by a pulmonary artery catheter or a central venous catheter using an explicit management protocol demonstrated that a pulmonary artery catheter should not be routinely used for the management of acute lung injury. A subsequent randomized, prospective clinical study of restrictive fluid intake and diuresis as needed to maintain central venous pressure less than 4 mm Hg or pulmonary artery occlusion pressure less than 8 mm Hg (conservative strategy group) versus a fluid management protocol to target a central venous pressure of 10–14 mm Hg or a pulmonary artery occlusion pressure 14–18 mm Hg (liberal strategy group) showed that patients in the conservative strategy group experienced faster improvement in lung function and spent significantly fewer days on mechanical ventilation and in the ICU without an improvement in death by 60 days or worsening nonpulmonary organ failure at 28 days. Oxygen delivery can be increased in anemic patients by ensuring that the hemoglobin concentration is at least 7 g/dL (70 g/L); patients are not likely to benefit from higher levels. Increasing oxygen delivery to supranormal levels by using inotropes and high hemoglobin concentrations is not clinically useful and may be harmful. Strategies to decrease oxygen consumption include the appropriate use of sedatives, analgesics, and antipyretics.

Numerous innovative therapeutic interventions to improve outcomes in ARDS patients have been or are being investigated. Unfortunately, to date, none has consistently shown benefit in clinical trials. Systemic corticosteroids have been studied extensively with variable and inconsistent results. While a few small studies suggest some specific improved outcomes when given within the first 2 weeks after the onset of ARDS, mortality appears increased when corticosteroids are started more than 2 weeks after the onset of ARDS. Therefore, routine use of corticosteroids is not recommended.

Another therapeutic intervention is extracorporeal membrane oxygenation (ECMO). The technique has been in use since the 1970s but has been gaining wider acceptance. A 2018 trial compared the early use of ECMO in very severe ARDS with conventional strategies built on low-tidal-volume ventilation. Results failed to show a difference in 60-day mortality; however, 28% of the control group crossed over to receive ECMO. As a result, ECMO seems unlikely to become a standard first-line therapy but is likely to remain a salvage option for patients with very severe ARDS.

Course & Prognosis

Overall, ARDS mortality with low tidal volume ventilation is around 30% in large multicenter studies. The major causes of death are the primary illness and secondary complications, such as multiple organ system failure or sepsis. Many patients who die of ARDS and its complications die after withdrawal of mechanical ventilation (see Chapter 5). One troubling aspect of ARDS care is that the actual mortality of ARDS in community hospitals continues to be higher than at academic hospitals. This may reflect the fact that a significant number of community hospital–based clinicians have not adopted low tidal volume ventilation.

Different clinical syndromes that lead to ARDS carry different prognoses. For example, patients with trauma-associated ARDS have better prognosis, with a mortality rate close to 20%, whereas those with end-stage liver disease have an 80% mortality rate. This likely reflects both the effects of significant comorbidities (trauma patients tend to be younger and healthier) as well as phenotypic differences within ARDS associated with different precipitants. Post-hoc analyses of data from several major trials have shown that a hyperinflammatory phenotype associated with high levels of IL-6 and soluble tumor necrosis factor receptor in ARDS patients precipitated by sepsis is associated with more multiorgan dysfunction and higher mortality. This may have implications for precision-medicine treatment of ARDS.

Failure to improve in the first week of treatment is a poor prognostic sign, although this may not be true of ARDS from certain etiologies, including COVID-19. Survivors tend to be young and pulmonary function generally recovers over 6–12 months, although residual abnormalities often remain, including restrictive or obstructive defects, low diffusion capacity, and impaired gas exchange with exercise. Survivors of ARDS also have diminished health-related and pulmonary disease–specific quality of life as well as systemic effects, such as muscle wasting, weakness, and fatigue.

Combes A et al; EOLIA Trial Group, REVA, and ECMONet. Extracorporeal membrane oxygenation for severe acute respiratory distress syndrome. N Engl J Med. 2018;378:1965. [PMID: 29791822]

Matthay MA et al. Acute respiratory distress syndrome. Nat Rev Dis Primers. 2019;5:18. [PMID: 30872586]

Meyer NJ et al. Acute respiratory distress syndrome. Lancet. 2021;398:622. [PMID: 34217425]

National Heart, Lung, and Blood Institute PETAL Clinical Trials Network; Moss M et al. Early neuromuscular blockade in the acute respiratory distress syndrome. N Engl J Med. 2019; 380:1997. [PMID: 31112383]

Papazian L et al. Formal guidelines: management of acute respiratory distress syndrome. Ann Intensive Care. 2019;9:69. [PMID: 31197492]

Pfortmueller CA et al. COVID-19-associated acute respiratory distress syndrome (CARDS): current knowledge on pathophysiology and ICU treatment—a narrative review. Best Pract Res Clin Anaesthesiol. 2021;35:351. [PMID: 34511224]

LUNG TRANSPLANTATION

Introduction

Lung transplantation is a therapeutic option for patients with end-stage lung disease who have not responded to other therapies. The full topic is beyond the scope of this text, therefore only issues related to candidate selection and post-transplant care will be discussed.

Candidate Selection

Patients should be considered for lung transplantation if they have advanced, progressive lung disease despite appropriate medical therapy. The most common indications are interstitial lung disease, COPD, cystic fibrosis, and pulmonary arterial hypertension. The International Society of Heart and Lung Transplantation has produced guidelines for candidate selection; broadly speaking, the ideal candidate has a high (greater than 50%) risk of dying within 2 years without lung transplantation, has minimal other comorbidities, is very likely to survive transplantation, and has good social support. Contraindications are numerous and include obesity (generally BMI greater than 30 is a relative, and greater than 35 a nearly absolute, contraindication), active smoking or substance abuse, uncontrolled infection, active malignancy, significant organ dysfunction (eg, cirrhosis, CKD, heart failure, unrevascularizable coronary disease), and medical noncompliance. Each transplant center has a slightly different selection process, however common practice includes a detailed multidisciplinary evaluation. Patients should ideally be referred to transplant centers before the need for transplantation is emergent.

Care After Transplantation

As with other solid organ transplantation, care of the post–lung transplant patient is particularly concerned with immunosuppression and prophylaxis against infection, as well as with management of the side effects of immunosuppression. Most patients are immunosuppressed with a combination of a calcineurin inhibitor (eg, tacrolimus), a cell-cycle inhibitor (eg, mycophenolate mofetil), and glucocorticoids. Most centers screen for rejection with regular PFTs as well as bronchoscopies and biopsies, particularly in the first 1–2 years after transplantation.

Common complications include acute cellular rejection (treated with intensified immunosuppression), infection, chronic rejection (for which few effective treatments exist), and sequelae of immunosuppression. These include hypertension, dyslipidemia, diabetes mellitus, CKD, osteopenia/osteoporosis, and increased risk of malignancy, especially skin cancers. Post-transplant care thus necessitates close cooperation between the patient's transplant team and his or her other physicians.

Outcomes After Transplantation

While lung transplantation can be transformative for those suffering from advanced lung disease, long-term survival remains limited to those receiving kidney or liver transplants. As of the 2021 International Society of Heart and Lung Transplantation Report, median survival after lung transplantation was approximately 7 years. Survival is affected by many variables; two consistent findings have been that survival is improved in double (versus single) lung transplant patients, and in those transplanted for cystic fibrosis (versus other indications).

Bos S et al. Survival in adult lung transplantation: where are we in 2020? Curr Opin Organ Transplant. 2020;25:268. [PMID: 32332197]

Chambers DC et al. The International Thoracic Organ Transplant Registry of the International Society for Heart and Lung Transplantation: Thirty-Eighth Adult Lung Transplantation Report—2021; Focus on recipient characteristics. J Heart Lung Transplant. 2021;40:1060. [PMID: 34446355]

Gutierrez-Arias R et al. Exercise training for adult lung transplant recipients. Cochrane Database Syst Rev. 2021;7:CD012307. [PMID: 34282853]

van der Mark SC et al. Developments in lung transplantation over the past decade. Eur Respir Rev. 2020;29:190132. [PMID: 32699023]

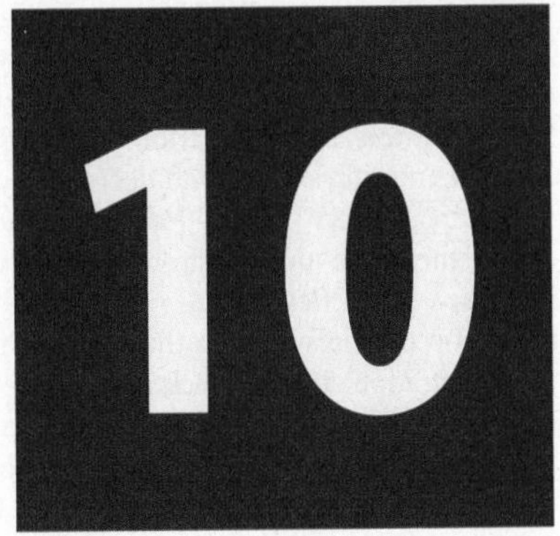

Heart Disease

Todd Kiefer, MD
Christopher B. Granger, MD
Kevin P. Jackson, MD

ADULT CONGENITAL HEART DISEASE

In the United States, there are many more adults with congenital heart disease than children, with an estimated 2 million adults in the United States surviving with congenital heart disease. In 2018, the American College of Cardiology (ACC) and American Heart Association (AHA) released updated guidelines for the assessment and treatment of patients with adult congenital heart disease. The European Society of Cardiology (ESC) completed their update on the same topic in 2020. As the number of patients with adult congenital heart disease has grown, there has been an increased appreciation of the need for more training and guidelines. A specific subspecialty board and training program has been established. The AHA also issued a scientific statement in 2015 reviewing common issues for adults with underlying congenital heart disease, another statement in 2017 for pregnant patients with congenital heart disease, and a statement in 2017 regarding noncardiac issues in these patients.

Baumgartner H et al. 2020 ESC Guidelines for the management of adult congenital heart disease. Eur Heart J. 2021;42:563. [PMID: 32860028]
Stout KK et al. 2018 AHA/ACC guideline for the management of adults with congenital heart disease: a report of the American College of Cardiology/American Heart Association Task Force on Clinical Practice Guidelines. J Am Coll Cardiol. 2019;73:e81. [PMID: 30121239]

PULMONARY VALVE STENOSIS

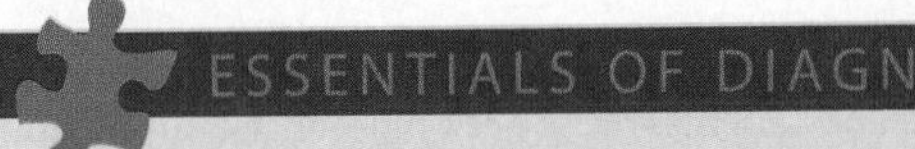

ESSENTIALS OF DIAGNOSIS

- Severe cases may present with right-sided heart failure.
- P_2 delayed and soft or absent.
- Pulmonary ejection click often present and decreases with inspiration—the only right heart sound that *decreases* with inspiration; all other right heart sounds increase.
- Echocardiography/Doppler is diagnostic.
- Patients with peak pulmonic valve gradient greater than 64 mm Hg or a mean of 35 mm Hg by echocardiography/Doppler should undergo intervention regardless of symptoms. Otherwise, operate for symptoms or evidence for right ventricular (RV) dysfunction.

General Considerations

Stenosis of the pulmonary valve or RV infundibulum increases the resistance to RV outflow, raises the RV pressure, and limits pulmonary blood flow. Pulmonic stenosis is often congenital and associated with other cardiac lesions. Pulmonary blood flow preferentially goes to the left lung in valvular pulmonic stenosis. In the absence of associated shunts, arterial saturation is normal. Peripheral pulmonic stenosis can accompany valvular pulmonic stenosis and may be part of a variety of clinical syndromes, including the congenital rubella syndrome. Patients who have had the **Ross procedure** for aortic valve disease (transfer of the pulmonary valve to the aortic position with a homograft pulmonary valve placed in the pulmonary position) may experience noncongenital postoperative pulmonic valvular or main pulmonary artery (PA) stenosis due to an immune response in the homograft. RV outflow obstructions can also occur when there is a conduit from the RV to the pulmonary artery that becomes stenotic from degenerative changes over time or when there is degeneration of a bioprosthetic replacement pulmonary valve.

Clinical Findings

A. Symptoms and Signs

Mild cases of pulmonic stenosis are asymptomatic; moderate to severe pulmonic stenosis may cause symptoms of dyspnea on exertion, syncope, chest pain, and eventually RV failure.

On examination, there is often a palpable parasternal lift due to right ventricular hypertrophy (RVH) and the pulmonary outflow tract may be palpable if the PA is enlarged. A loud, harsh systolic murmur and occasionally a prominent thrill are present in the left second and third interspaces parasternally. The murmur radiates toward the left shoulder due to the flow pattern within the main PA and increases with inspiration. In mild to moderate pulmonic stenosis, a loud ejection click can be heard to precede the murmur; this sound decreases with inspiration as the increased RV filling from inspiration prematurely opens the valve during atrial systole when inspiratory increased blood flow to the right heart occurs. The valve excursion during systole is thus less with inspiration than with expiration, and the click is therefore less audible with inspiration. *This is the only right-sided auscultatory event that decreases with inspiration.* All of the other auscultatory events increase with the increased right heart output that occurs with inspiration. In severe pulmonic stenosis, the second sound is obscured by the murmur and the pulmonary component of S_2 may be diminished, delayed, or absent. A right-sided S_4 and a prominent *a* wave in the venous pulse are present when there is RV diastolic dysfunction or a *c-v* wave may be observed in the jugular venous pressure if tricuspid regurgitation is present. Pulmonary valve regurgitation is relatively uncommon in primary pulmonic stenosis and may be very difficult to hear, as the gradient between the reduced PA diastolic pressure and the elevated RV diastolic pressure may be quite small (low-pressure pulmonary valve regurgitation).

B. ECG and Chest Radiography

Right axis deviation or RVH is noted; peaked P waves provide evidence of right atrial (RA) overload. Heart size may be normal on radiographs, or there may be a prominent RV and RA or gross cardiac enlargement, depending on the severity. There is often poststenotic dilation of the main and left pulmonary arteries. Pulmonary vascularity is usually normal, although there tends to be preferential flow to the left lung.

C. Diagnostic Studies

Echocardiography/Doppler is the diagnostic tool of choice, can provide evidence for a doming valve versus a dysplastic valve, can determine the gradient across the valve, and can provide information regarding subvalvular obstruction and the presence or absence of tricuspid or pulmonic valvular regurgitation. Mild pulmonic stenosis is present if the peak gradient by echocardiography/Doppler is less than 36 mm Hg, moderate pulmonic stenosis is present if the peak gradient is between 36 mm Hg and 64 mm Hg, and severe pulmonic stenosis is present if the peak gradient is greater than 64 mm Hg or the mean gradient is greater than 35 mm Hg. A lower gradient may be significant if there is RV dysfunction. Catheterization is usually unnecessary for the diagnosis; it should be used only if the data are unclear or in preparation for either percutaneous intervention or surgery.

Prognosis & Treatment

Patients with mild pulmonic stenosis have a normal life span with no intervention. Moderate stenosis may be asymptomatic in childhood and adolescence, but symptoms often appear as patients grow older. The degree of stenosis does worsen with time in a few patients, so serial follow-up is important. Severe stenosis is rarely associated with sudden death but can cause right heart failure in patients as early as in their 20s and 30s. Pregnancy and exercise tend to be well tolerated except in severe stenosis.

The AHA/ACC guidelines and the ESC guidelines generally agree, though the ESC suggests severe pulmonic stenosis should be considered if the RV systolic pressure is greater than 80 mm Hg. Class I (definitive) indications for intervention include all symptomatic patients and all those with a resting peak-to-peak gradient greater than 64 mm Hg or a mean greater than 35 mm Hg, regardless of symptoms. Symptoms can include cyanosis due to right-to-left shunting via a patent foramen ovale (PFO) or atrial septal defect (ASD). Percutaneous balloon valvuloplasty is highly successful in domed valve patients and is the treatment of choice. Surgical commissurotomy can also be done, or pulmonary valve replacement (with either a bioprosthetic valve or homograft) when pulmonary valve regurgitation is too severe or the valve is dysplastic. Pulmonary outflow tract obstruction due to RV to PA conduit obstruction or to homograft pulmonary valve stenosis can often be relieved with a percutaneously implanted pulmonary valve (both the Medtronic Melody valve and the Edwards Sapien XT valve are FDA approved). Frequently the seating of these valves is facilitated by placing a stent within the pulmonary artery first, then the transcatheter device within this stent. Because the new catheter valve may result in compression of the coronary artery, it is a class I requirement to assess the effect of the device on the coronary by use of a temporary balloon inflation prior to delivery of the device. Percutaneous pulmonary valve replacement is also FDA approved for those with conduit stenosis or following the Ross procedure. Percutaneous valve replacements have also been performed off-label for patients with native pulmonary valve disease, including those who have had tetralogy of Fallot repair (assuming the PA root size is small enough to seat a percutaneous valve).

Endocarditis prophylaxis is unnecessary for native valves even after valvuloplasty unless there has been prior pulmonary valve endocarditis (an unusual occurrence) (see Table 33–3). It should be used if surgical or percutaneous valve replacement has occurred. There appears to be more pulmonary valve endocarditis following percutaneous pulmonary valve replacement with the Melody valve than expected, and this is being closely monitored by the FDA.

When to Refer

All symptomatic patients (regardless of gradient) and all asymptomatic patients whose peak pulmonary valve gradient is greater than 64 mm Hg or whose mean gradient is greater than 35 mm Hg should be referred to a cardiologist with expertise in adult congenital heart disease. Patients also require intervention if cyanosis occurs due to a PFO or ASD or if there is exercise intolerance.

Hansen RL et al. Long-term outcomes up to 25 years following balloon pulmonary valvuloplasty: a multicenter study. Congenit Heart Dis. 2019;14:1037. [PMID: 31250555]

COARCTATION OF THE AORTA

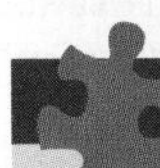

ESSENTIALS OF DIAGNOSIS

- Usual presentation is systemic hypertension.
- Echocardiography/Doppler is diagnostic; a peak gradient of > 20 mm Hg may be significant due to collaterals around the coarctation reducing gradient despite severe obstruction.
- Associated bicuspid aortic valve in 50–80% of patients.
- Delayed pulse in femoral artery compared to brachial artery.
- Systolic pressure is higher in upper extremities than in lower extremities; diastolic pressures are similar.

General Considerations

Coarctation of the aorta consists of localized narrowing of the aortic arch just distal to the origin of the left subclavian artery. If the stenosis is severe, collateral circulation develops around the coarctation site through the intercostal arteries and the branches of the subclavian arteries and can result in a lower trans-coarctation gradient by enabling blood flow to bypass the obstruction. **Coarctation is a cause of secondary hypertension and should be considered in young patients with elevated blood pressure (BP).** The renin-angiotensin system is often abnormal, however, and contributes to the hypertension occasionally seen even after coarctation repair. A bicuspid valve is seen in approximately 50–80% of the cases, and there is an increased incidence of cerebral berry aneurysms. Significant native or recurrent aortic coarctation has been defined as follows: upper extremity/lower extremity resting peak-to-peak gradient greater than 20 mm Hg or mean Doppler systolic gradient greater than 20 mm Hg; upper extremity/lower extremity gradient greater than 10 mm Hg or mean Doppler gradient greater than 10 mm Hg when there is either decreased LV systolic function or aortic regurgitation (AR); or upper extremity/lower extremity gradient greater than 10 mm Hg or mean Doppler gradient greater than 10 mm Hg when there is evidence for collateral flow around the coarctation. This should be coupled with anatomic evidence for coarctation of the aorta, typically defined by advanced imaging (cardiac magnetic resonance, CT angiography). The ESC guidelines have expanded the severity criteria and suggest stenting is appropriate if the patient is normotensive but has a peak gradient of greater than 20 mm Hg (class IIa) or if the stenosis by angiography is more than 50% (class IIb).

Clinical Findings

A. Symptoms and Signs

If cardiac failure does not occur in infancy, there are usually no symptoms until the hypertension produces LV failure. Cerebral hemorrhage, though rare, may occur. Approximately 10% of patients with coarctation of the aorta have intracranial aneurysms identified on magnetic resonance angiography or CT angiography. Increasing age has been identified as a risk factor. Strong arterial pulsations are seen in the neck and suprasternal notch. Hypertension is present in the arms, but the pressure is normal or low in the legs. This difference is exaggerated by exercise. Femoral pulsations are weak and are delayed in comparison with the brachial or radial pulse. A continuous murmur heard superiorly and midline in the back or over the left anterior chest may be present when large collaterals are present and is a clue that the coarctation is severe. The coarctation itself may result in systolic ejection murmurs heard in the left upper lung field anteriorly and near the spine on the left side posteriorly. There may be an aortic regurgitation or stenosis murmur due to an associated bicuspid aortic valve. Coarctation is associated with Turner syndrome (a sex chromosomal abnormality [XO]); a webbed neck may be present in these patients.

B. ECG and Chest Radiography

The ECG usually shows LVH. Radiography may show scalloping of the inferior portion of the ribs (**rib notching**) due to enlarged collateral intercostal arteries. Dilation of the left subclavian artery and poststenotic aortic dilation along with LV enlargement may be present. The coarctation region and the poststenotic dilation of the descending aorta may result in a **"3" sign** along the aortic shadow on the PA chest radiograph (the notch in the "3" representing the area of coarctation).

C. Diagnostic Studies

Echocardiography/Doppler is usually diagnostic and may provide additional evidence for a bicuspid aortic valve. Both MRI and CT can provide excellent images of the coarctation anatomy, and one or the other should always be done to define the coarctation anatomic structure. MRI and echocardiography/Doppler can also provide estimates of the gradient across the lesion. Cardiac catheterization provides definitive gradient information and is obviously necessary if percutaneous stenting is to be considered.

Prognosis & Treatment

Cardiac failure is common in infancy and in older untreated patients when the coarctation is severe. Patients with a demonstrated peak gradient of greater than 20 mm Hg should be considered for intervention, especially if there is evidence of collateral blood vessels. As noted above, the ESC guidelines incorporate the stenosis severity (greater than 50%) as defining severe coarctation as well. Many untreated patients with severe coarctation die of hypertension, rupture of the aorta, infective endarteritis, or cerebral hemorrhage before the age of 50. Aortic dissection also occurs with increased frequency. Coarctation of any significance may be poorly tolerated in pregnancy because of the inability to support the placental flow.

Resection of the coarctation site has a surgical mortality rate of 1–4% and includes risk of spinal cord injury.

The percutaneous interventional procedure of choice is endovascular stenting; when anatomically feasible, self-expanding and balloon-expandable covered stents have been shown to be advantageous over bare metal stents. These covered stents are FDA approved. Most coarctation repair in adults is percutaneous. Otherwise, surgical resection (usually with end-to-end anastomosis) should be performed. About 25–50% of surgically corrected patients continue to be hypertensive years after surgery because of permanent changes in the renin-angiotensin system, endothelial dysfunction, aortic stiffness, altered arch morphology, and increased ventricular stiffness. Whether the repair was by balloon dilatation, stenting, or surgical resection may make a difference in the development of hypertension. Recurrence of the coarctation stenosis following intervention requires long-term follow-up.

When to Refer

All patients with aortic coarctation and any detectable gradient should be referred to a cardiologist with expertise in adult congenital heart disease.

Fedchenko M et al. Cardiovascular risk factors in adults with coarctation of the aorta. Congenit Heart Dis. 2019;14:549. [PMID: 31099471]

Lee MGY et al. Long-term mortality and cardiovascular burden for adult survivors of coarctation of the aorta. Heart. 2019;105:1190. [PMID: 30923175]

ATRIAL SEPTAL DEFECT & PATENT FORAMEN OVALE

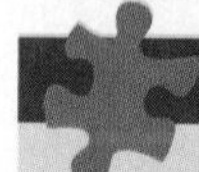

ESSENTIALS OF DIAGNOSIS

- Often asymptomatic and discovered on routine physical examination.
- With an ASD and left-to-right shunt: RV lift; S2 widely split and fixed.
- Echocardiography/Doppler is diagnostic.
- ASDs should be closed if there is evidence of an RV volume overload regardless of symptoms.
- A PFO, present in 25% of the population, rarely can lead to paradoxical emboli.

General Considerations

The most common form of ASD (80% of cases) is persistence of the ostium secundum in the mid-septum. A less common abnormality is persistence of the ostium primum (low in the septum). In most patients with an ostium primum defect, there are mitral or tricuspid valve "clefts" as well as a ventricular septal defect (VSD) as part of the atrioventricular (AV) septal defect. A sinus venosus defect is a hole, usually at the upper (or rarely the lower) part of the atrial septum, due to failure of the embryonic superior vena cava or the inferior vena cava to merge with the atria properly. The superior vena cava sinus venosus defect is usually associated with an anomalous connection of the right upper pulmonary vein into the superior vena cava. The coronary sinus ASD is rare and is basically an unroofed coronary sinus that results in shunting from the left atrium (LA) to the coronary sinus and then to the RA.

In all cases, normally oxygenated blood from the higher-pressure LA shunts into the RA, increasing RV output and pulmonary blood flow. In children, the degree of shunting across these defects may be quite large (pulmonary to systemic blood flow ratios of 3:1 or so). As the RV compliance worsens from the chronic volume overload, the RA pressure may rise and the degree of left-to-right shunting may decrease over time. Eventually, if the RA pressure exceeds the LA, the shunt may reverse and be primarily right-to-left. When this happens, systemic cyanosis appears. The major factor in the direction of shunt flow is thus the compliance of the respective atrial chambers.

The pulmonary pressures are modestly elevated in most patients with an ASD due to the high pulmonary blood flow, but severe pulmonary hypertension with cyanosis (**Eisenmenger physiology**) is actually unusual, occurring in only about 15% of the patients with an ASD alone. Increased pulmonary vascular resistance (PVR) and pulmonary hypertension secondary to pulmonary vascular disease rarely occur in childhood or young adult life in secundum defects and are more common in primum defects, especially if there is an associated VSD. Eventual RV failure may occur with any atrial shunt of significant size, and most shunts should be corrected unless they are quite small (less than 1.5:1 left-to-right shunt). In adults, a large left-to-right shunt may have begun to reverse, so the absolute left-to-right shunt measurement (Qp/Qs, where Qp = pulmonary flow and Qs = systemic flow) at the time the patient is studied may underestimate the original shunt size. In addition, in most people the LV and LA compliance normally declines more over time than the RV and RA compliance; for this reason, the natural history of small atrial septal shunts is to increase the left-to-right shunting as the patient ages. There is generally only trivial shunting with a PFO compared to a true ASD. ASDs predispose to atrial fibrillation due to RA enlargement, and paradoxical right-to-left emboli do occur. If pulmonary hypertension does occur, the 2018 guidelines recommend that the shunt should still be closed as long as the left-to-right shunt is still greater than 1.5:1 and the systolic PA pressure is less than one-half the systemic arterial pressure and the PVR calculation is less than one-third systemic vascular resistance.

Interestingly, paradoxical emboli may be more common in patients with a PFO than a true ASD, especially when there is an atrial septal aneurysm. An aneurysm of the atrial septum is not a true aneurysm but rather simply a redundancy of the atrial septum that causes it to swing back and forth (greater than 10 mm). When present with a PFO, the back-and-forth swinging tends to pull open the PFO, encouraging shunting. This may help explain why more right-to-left shunting occurs in patients with an atrial septal aneurysm and PFO than in those with a PFO alone. This creates the anatomic substrate for the occurrence of paradoxical emboli. Other factors may distort the atrial septum (such as an enlarged aorta) and result in an increased shunting in patients with a PFO. Right-to-left PFO shunting may be more prominent upright than supine, creating orthostatic hypoxemia **(platypnea orthodeoxia).** There may also be increased shunting in patients with a PFO and sleep apnea as the RA compliance may worsen during apneic spells when pulmonary pressures increase.

Clinical Findings

A. Symptoms and Signs

Patients with a small or moderate ASD or with a PFO are asymptomatic unless a complication occurs. There is only trivial shunting in a PFO unless the RA pressure increases for some other reason or the atrial septum is distorted. With larger ASD shunts, exertional dyspnea or heart failure may develop, most commonly in the fourth decade of life or later. Prominent RV and PA pulsations are then readily visible and palpable. A moderately loud systolic ejection murmur can be heard in the second and third interspaces parasternally as a result of increased flow through the pulmonary valve. S_2 is widely split and does not vary with respiration. The left-to-right shunt across the defect decreases with inspiration (as the RA pressure increases) and then increases with expiration (as the RA pressure decreases), thus keeping the RV stroke volume relatively constant in inspiration and expiration. A **"fixed" splitting** of the second sound results. In very large left-to-right shunts, a tricuspid rumble may be heard due to the high flow across the tricuspid valve in diastole.

B. ECG and Chest Radiography

Right axis deviation or RVH may be present depending on the size of the RV volume overload. Incomplete or complete right bundle branch block is present in nearly all cases of ASD, and superior axis deviation (left anterior fascicular block) is noted in the complete AV septal defect, where complete heart block is often seen as well. With sinus venosus defects, the P axis is leftward of +15° due to abnormal atrial activation with loss of the upper RA tissue from around the sinus node. This creates the negative P waves in the inferior leads. The chest radiograph shows large pulmonary arteries, increased pulmonary vascularity, and an enlarged RA and RV as with all pre-tricuspid valve cardiac left-to-right shunts. The LA is not traditionally enlarged due to an ASD shunt because the chamber is being decompressed.

C. Diagnostic Studies

Echocardiography demonstrates evidence of RA and RV volume overload. The atrial defect is usually observed by echocardiography, although sinus venosus defects may be elusive since they are high in the atrial septum. Many patients with a PFO also have an atrial septal aneurysm (defined as greater than 10-mm excursion of the septum from the static position). Echocardiography with saline injection **(bubble contrast)** can demonstrate the right-to-left component of the shunt, and both pulsed and color flow Doppler flow studies can demonstrate shunting in either direction. In platypnea orthodeoxia, the shunt may primarily result from inferior vena cava blood, and a femoral vein saline injection may be required to demonstrate the shunt. Transesophageal echocardiography (TEE) is helpful when transthoracic echocardiography quality is not optimal because it improves the sensitivity for detection of small shunts and provides a better assessment of PFO or ASD anatomy. Both CT and MRI can elucidate the atrial septal anatomy, better detect multiple fenestrations, and demonstrate associated lesions such as anomalous pulmonary venous connections. Atrial septal anatomy can be complex, and either MRI, TEE, or CT can reveal whether there is an adequate rim around the defect to allow for safe positioning of an atrial septal occluder device. These studies can also help identify any anomalous pulmonary venous connections. Cardiac catheterization can define the size and location of the shunt and determine the pulmonary pressure and PVR.

Prognosis & Treatment

Patients with small atrial shunts live a normal life span with no intervention. Large shunts usually cause disability by age 40 years. Because left-to-right shunts and RV overload tend to increase with normal age-related reduction in LV (and subsequently LA) compliance, both AHA/ACC and the ESC guidelines suggest that closure of all left-to-right shunts greater than 1.5:1 should be accomplished either by a percutaneous device or by surgery if any right heart structures are enlarged at all. If the pulmonary systolic pressure is more than two-thirds the systemic systolic pressure, then pulmonary hypertension may preclude ASD closure. The ESC guidelines add the pulmonary vascular resistance to the criteria and consider it a class IIa indication if the PVR is between 3 and 5 Wood units, and the guidelines preclude the use of closure if the PVR is greater than or equal to 5 Wood units. Testing with transient balloon occlusion of the shunt, with pulmonary vasodilators, or with both may be required in the presence of pulmonary hypertension. Preservation of the cardiac output after transient balloon occlusion and evidence for preserved pulmonary vasoreactivity with pulmonary vasodilator testing all favor closure when pulmonary hypertension and at least a 1.5:1 left-to-right shunt are present. ESC guidelines favor bringing the patient back to the catheterization laboratory for retesting on pulmonary vasodilators, rather than using acute testing, to see if the PVR can be reduced below 5 Wood units. The ESC guidelines also suggest considering fenestrated closure in the face of pulmonary hypertension. The use of bosentan or sildenafil is recommended if the PVR is over 5 Wood units and there is a right-to-left shunt. After age 40 years, cardiac arrhythmias (especially atrial fibrillation) and heart failure occur with increased frequency due to the chronic right heart volume overload. Paradoxical systemic arterial embolization also becomes more of a concern as RV compliance is lost and the left-to-right shunt begins to reverse.

PFOs are usually *not* associated with significant shunting, and therefore, the patients are hemodynamically asymptomatic and the heart size is normal. However, PFOs can be responsible for paradoxical emboli and are a possible cause of **cryptogenic strokes** in patients under age 55 years. Some shunting may occur with exercise if the right heart is enlarged or stiff. *Interestingly, the risk of recurrent paradoxical emboli is low regardless of whether the PFO is closed or not, and that observation has reduced the value of closing these defects in cryptogenic stroke.* Further confounding the advantage of PFO closure for cryptogenic stroke or transient ischemic attack (TIA) has been the discovery of frequent bouts of paroxysmal atrial fibrillation using 30-day monitoring in these patients, suggesting atrial fibrillation is actually the real stroke/TIA risk factor in some patients.

Occasionally, a PFO that has not been pathologic may become responsible for cyanosis, especially if the RA pressure is elevated from pulmonary or RV hypertension or from severe tricuspid regurgitation.

Surgery involves stitching or patching of the foramen. For ostium secundum ASDs, percutaneous closure by use of a variety of devices is preferred over surgery when the anatomy is appropriate (usually this means there must be an adequate atrial septal rim around the defect to secure the occluder device).

Patients who have hypoxemia (especially upon standing or with exercise) should have the PFO closed if no other cause for hypoxemia is evident and there is right-to-left shunting demonstrated through the PFO. For patients with cryptogenic stroke or TIA, it remains uncertain whether closure of the PFO, either by open surgical or percutaneous techniques, has any advantage over anticoagulation with either warfarin, a DOAC, or aspirin.

From a practical standpoint, **patients younger than 55 years with cryptogenic stroke/TIA and no other identifiable cause except for the presence of a PFO should still be considered for PFO closure**. A 2020 update from the guideline subcommittee of the American Academy of Neurology reaffirms no change in this overall policy. The presence of an atrial septal aneurysm (with the septum appearing "floppy" on echocardiogram) has been associated with a higher risk of recurrent stroke/TIA in patients with cryptogenic stroke/TIA. A workup for any causes for hypercoagulability and a 30-day monitor should be part of the clinical assessment to exclude other potential causes for cryptogenic stroke/TIA. In meta-analysis of data in patients with cryptogenic stroke/TIA and PFO who have their PFO closed, ischemic stroke recurrence is less frequent compared with patients receiving medical treatment. Atrial fibrillation is more frequent but mostly transient in patients who have device closure. There is no difference in TIA, all-cause mortality, or MI between those treated with medicine versus a closure device. In a large, multicenter trial in France among patients who had had a recent cryptogenic stroke attributed to PFO with an associated atrial septal aneurysm or large interatrial shunt, the rate of stroke recurrence was lower among those assigned to PFO closure combined with antiplatelet therapy than among those assigned to antiplatelet therapy alone. PFO closure was associated with an increased risk of atrial fibrillation. Residual shunting after device closure is also present in up to 25% of patients. A report from Massachusetts General Hospital found a medium to large residual shunt increased the risk of a recurrent stroke or TIA threefold.

When to Refer

- All patients with an ASD should be evaluated by a cardiologist with expertise in adult congenital disease to ensure no other structural disease is present and to investigate whether the RV is enlarged.
- If the RA and RV sizes remain normal, serial echocardiography should be performed every 3–5 years.
- If the RA and RV volumes are increased, then referral to a cardiologist who performs percutaneous closure is warranted.
- Patients younger than 55 years with cryptogenic stroke when no other source is identified except for a PFO with right-to-left shunting should be considered for PFO closure or medical therapy. An associated atrial septal aneurysm or evidence for hypercoagulability increases risk. Aspirin alone appears not to be effective. DOACs with or without device closure of the PFO may have a role in preventing recurrent stroke.
- Patients with cyanosis and a PFO with evidence of a right-to-left shunt by agitated saline bubble contrast on echocardiography, especially if the cyanosis is worsened upon assuming the upright posture.

Deng W et al. Residual shunt after PFO closure and long-term stroke recurrence. Ann Intern Med. 2020;172:717. [PMID: 33253619]

Messé SR et al. Practice advisory update summary: patent foramen ovale and secondary stroke prevention: report of the Guideline Subcommittee of the American Academy of Neurology. Neurology. 2020;94:876. [PMID: 32350058]

Oster M et al. Interventional therapy versus medical therapy for secundum atrial septal defect: a systematic review (part 2) for the 2018 AHA/ACC Guideline for the Management of Adults With Congenital Heart Disease: a report of the American College of Cardiology/American Heart Association Task Force on Clinical Practice Guidelines. Circulation. 2019;139:e814. [PMID: 30586769]

Turc G et al. Atrial septal aneurysm, shunt size and recurrent stroke risk in patients with a PFO. J Am Coll Cardiol. 2020;75:2312. [PMID: 32381162]

Wang TKM et al. Patent foramen ovale closure versus medical therapy for cryptogenic stroke: meta-analysis of randomized trials. Heart Lung Circ. 2019;28:623. [PMID: 29602754]

VENTRICULAR SEPTAL DEFECT

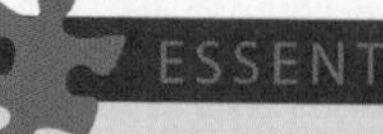

ESSENTIALS OF DIAGNOSIS

- A restrictive VSD is small and makes a louder murmur than an unrestricted one, often with an accompanying thrill. The higher the gradient across the septum, the smaller the left-to-right shunt.
- Small defects may be asymptomatic.
- Larger defects result in pulmonary hypertension (Eisenmenger physiology) if not repaired or if the pulmonary circuit is not protected by RV outflow tract obstruction.
- Echocardiography/Doppler is diagnostic.

General Considerations

Congenital VSDs occur in various parts of the ventricular septum. Membranous and muscular septal defects may spontaneously close in childhood as the septum grows and hypertrophies. A left-to-right shunt is present, with the degree depending on associated systolic RV pressure. The smaller the defect, the greater is the gradient from the LV to the RV and the louder the murmur. The presentation in adults depends on the size of the shunt and whether there is associated pulmonic or subpulmonic stenosis that has protected the lung from the systemic pressure and volume. Unprotected lungs with large shunts invariably lead to pulmonary vascular disease and severe pulmonary hypertension (Eisenmenger physiology). VSD sizes are defined by comparison to the aortic root size; a small or restrictive VSD diameter is less than 25% of the aortic root diameter, a moderately restrictive VSD diameter is 25–75% of the aorta, and an unrestricted VSD size is greater than 75% of the aortic diameter. The size can also be quantitated based on the Qp/Qs (left-to-right shunt), with a restrictive lesion being less than 1.5:1, moderately restrictive VSD being 1.5–2.2:1, and an unrestricted lesion being greater than 2.2:1.

Clinical Findings

A. Symptoms and Signs

The clinical features depend on the size of the defect and the presence or absence of RV outflow obstruction or increased PVR. Small shunts are associated with loud, harsh holosystolic murmurs in the left third and fourth interspaces along the sternum. A systolic thrill is common. Larger shunts may create both LV and RV volume and pressure overload. If pulmonary hypertension occurs, high-pressure pulmonary valve regurgitation may result. Right heart failure may gradually become evident late in the course, and the shunt will begin to balance or reverse as RV and LV systolic pressures equalize with the advent of pulmonary hypertension. Cyanosis from a developing right-to-left shunt may then occur. Cyanosis with pulmonary hypertension and an intracardiac shunt define the **Eisenmenger syndrome.**

B. ECG and Chest Radiography

The ECG may be normal or may show right, left, or biventricular hypertrophy, depending on the size of the defect and the PVR. With large shunts, the LV, the LA, and the pulmonary arteries are enlarged and pulmonary vascularity is increased on chest radiographs. The RV is often normal until late in the process. If an increased PVR (pulmonary hypertension) evolves, an enlarged PA with pruning of the distal pulmonary vascular bed is seen. In rare cases of a VSD high in the ventricular septum, an aortic cusp (right coronary cusp) may prolapse into the VSD and reduce the VSD shunt but result in acute aortic regurgitation and acute heart failure.

C. Diagnostic Studies

Echocardiography can demonstrate the size of the overloaded chambers and can usually define the defect anatomy. Doppler can qualitatively assess the magnitude of shunting by noting the gradient from LV to RV and, if some tricuspid regurgitation is present, the RV systolic pressure can be estimated. The septal leaflet of the tricuspid valve may be part of the VSD anatomy and the complex appears as a ventricular septal "aneurysm." These membranous septal aneurysms resemble a "windsock" and may fenestrate and result in a VSD shunt being present or they may remain intact. Color flow Doppler helps delineate the shunt severity and the presence of valvular regurgitation. MRI and cardiac CT can often visualize the defect and describe any other anatomic abnormalities. MRI can provide quantitative shunt data as well.

Cardiac catheterization is usually reserved for those with at least moderate shunting, to quantitate the PVR and the degree of pulmonary hypertension. The 2018 adult congenital heart disease guidelines suggest that if there is still at least a 1.5:1 left-to-right shunt and if the PVR is less than one-third that of the systemic vascular resistance, and the PA systolic pressure is more than one-half of the aortic systolic pressure, then the risk of VSD closure despite some pulmonary hypertension is acceptable and it should be done. If the PVR/systemic vascular resistance ratio or the systolic PA pressure/systolic aortic pressure ratio is greater than two-thirds or there is a net right-to-left shunt, then closure is contraindicated.

The vasoreactivity of the pulmonary circuit may be tested at catheterization using agents such as inhaled nitric oxide. The AHA/ACC guidelines suggest that if the pulmonary pressures can be lowered enough and the above ratios fall below the two-thirds value, then repair is reasonable as long as the left-to-right VSD shunt is greater than 1.5:1. The 2020 ESC guidelines focus not on the pulmonary to systemic systolic BP ratio, but on the pulmonary pressure and the PVR. A PVR of greater than or equal to 5 Wood units is considered inoperable unless pulmonary vasodilators can reduce the PVR to below that value. Bosentan, an endothelial receptor blocker that reduces pulmonary pressure in Eisenmenger syndrome, has been given a class I indication in these patients in both guidelines.

Prognosis & Treatment

Patients with a small VSD have a normal life expectancy except for the small risk of infective endocarditis. Antibiotic prophylaxis after dental work is recommended only when the VSD is residual from a prior patch closure or when there is associated pulmonary hypertension and cyanosis (see Tables 33–3, 33–4, and 33–5). With large VSD shunts, heart failure may develop early in life, and survival beyond age 40 years is unusual without intervention.

Small shunts (pulmonary-to-systemic flow ratio less than 1.5) in asymptomatic patients do not require surgery or other intervention. The presence of RV infundibular stenosis or pulmonary valve stenosis may protect the pulmonary circuit such that some patients, even with a large VSD, may still be surgical candidates as adults if there is no pulmonary hypertension.

Surgical repair of a VSD is generally a low-risk procedure unless there is significant Eisenmenger physiology. Devices for nonsurgical closure of muscular VSDs are approved and those for membranous VSDs are being implanted with promising results; however, conduction disturbance is a major complication. The percutaneous devices are also approved for closure of a VSD related to acute MI, although the results in this very high-risk patient population have not been encouraging. In the acute MI setting, the devices have also been put across the ventricular septum at surgery to help provide a firm base on which to sew a pericardial patch, given the VSD in acute MI is often associated with widespread necrosis and multiple, serpiginous pathways. A percutaneous method, wherein the two sides of the device are sewn together using a subxiphoid approach, has been described. The medications used to treat pulmonary hypertension secondary to a VSD are similar to those used to treat idiopathic ("primary") pulmonary hypertension and at times can be quite effective in relieving symptoms and reducing the degree of cyanosis. **All patients who have a right-to-left shunt present should have filters placed on any intravenous lines to avoid any contamination or air bubbles from becoming systemic.**

When to Refer

All patients with a VSD should be referred to a cardiologist with expertise in adult congenital disease to decide if long-term follow-up or further studies are warranted.

Hong ZN et al. A meta-analysis of perventricular device closure of perimembranous ventricular septal defect. J Cardiothorac Surg. 2019;14:119. [PMID: 31248430]

Kamioka N et al. Postinfarction ventricular septal defect closure. The BASSINET concept. Circ Cardiovasc Interv. 2019;12: e007788. [PMID: 31088121]

TETRALOGY OF FALLOT

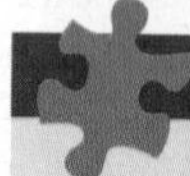

ESSENTIALS OF DIAGNOSIS

- Five features are characteristic:
  - VSD.
  - Concentric RVH.
  - RV outflow obstruction due to infundibular stenosis.
  - Septal overriding of the aorta in half the patients.
  - A right-sided aortic arch in 25%.
- Most adult patients with tetralogy of Fallot have been operated on, usually with an RV outflow patch and VSD closure. If patch overrides the pulmonary valve annulus, pulmonary regurgitation is common.
- Physical examination may be deceptive after classic tetralogy repair, with severe pulmonary valve regurgitation difficult to detect.
- Echocardiography/Doppler may underestimate significant pulmonary valve regurgitation. Be wary if the RV is enlarged or enlarging.
- Arrhythmias are common; periodic ambulatory monitoring is recommended.
- Serious arrhythmias and sudden death may occur if the QRS is wide or the RV becomes quite large, or both.

General Considerations

Patients with tetralogy of Fallot have a VSD, RV infundibular stenosis, RVH, and a dilated aorta (in about half of patients it overrides the septum). If there is an associated ASD, the complex is referred to as pentalogy of Fallot. The basic lesion is a large VSD with migration of the septum above the VSD and under the pulmonary valve. There may be pulmonary valve stenosis as well, usually due to either a bicuspid pulmonary valve or RV outflow hypoplasia. The aorta can be quite enlarged and aortic regurgitation may occur. If more than 50% of the aorta overrides the ventricular septum, it is called **double outlet RV**. Two vascular abnormalities are common: a right-sided aortic arch (in 25%) and an anomalous left anterior descending coronary artery from the right cusp (7–9%). The latter is important in that surgical correction must avoid injuring the coronary artery when repairing the RV outflow obstruction. Pulmonary branch stenosis may also be present.

Most adult patients have undergone prior surgery. If significant RV outflow obstruction is present in the neonatal period, a systemic arterial to pulmonary artery shunt may be the initial surgical procedure to improve pulmonary blood flow, though many infants undergo repair without this first step. Most adults will have had this initial palliative repair, however. The palliative procedure enables blood to reach the underperfused lung either by directly attaching one of the subclavian arteries to a main PA branch (**classic Blalock shunt**) or, more likely, by creating a conduit between the two (**modified Blalock shunt**). Total repair of the tetralogy of Fallot generally includes a VSD patch and usually an enlarging RV outflow tract patch, as well as a take-down of any prior arterial-pulmonary artery shunt. If the RV outflow tract patch extends through the pulmonary valve into the PA (transannular patch), varying degrees of pulmonary valve regurgitation develop. Most surgeons approach the inside of the RV via the right atrium and through the tricuspid valve and try to avoid a transannular patch if possible. Over the years, the volume overload from residual severe pulmonary valve regurgitation becomes the major hemodynamic problem to deal with in adults. A large RV outflow patch contributes to a relative RV volume load. Ventricular arrhythmias can originate from the edge of either the VSD or outflow tract patch and tend to increase in frequency as the size of the RV increases.

Clinical Findings

Most adult patients in whom tetralogy of Fallot has been repaired are relatively asymptomatic unless right heart failure occurs or arrhythmias become an issue. Patients can be active and generally require no specific therapy.

A. Symptoms and Signs

Physical examination should include checking both arms for any loss of pulse from a prior shunt procedure in infancy. The jugular venous pulsations (JVP) may reveal an increased *a* wave from poor RV compliance or rarely a *c-v* wave due to tricuspid regurgitation. The right-sided arch has no consequence. The precordium may be active, often with a persistent pulmonary outflow murmur. P_2 may or may not be audible. A right-sided gallop may be heard. A residual VSD or an aortic regurgitation murmur may be present.

B. ECG and Chest Radiography

The ECG reveals RVH and right axis deviation; in repaired tetralogy, there is often a right bundle branch block pattern. The chest radiograph shows a classic boot-shaped heart with prominence of the RV and a concavity in the RV outflow tract. This may be less impressive following repair. The aorta may be enlarged and right sided. **Importantly, the width of the QRS should be examined yearly because a QRS width of more than 180 msec is one of the risks for sudden death, although newer data suggest that this cutoff is not as specific as once thought.** Most experts recommend ambulatory monitoring periodically as well, especially if the patient experiences palpitations. Other identified risk factors for ventricular arrhythmias include having multiple prior cardiac surgeries, an elevated LV end-diastolic pressure (LVEDP), and older age at time of repair. In fact, it appears that the more the left side of the heart is involved, the higher the risk of sudden death.

C. Diagnostic Studies

Echocardiography/Doppler usually establishes the diagnosis by noting the unrestricted (large) VSD, the RV infundibular stenosis, and the enlarged aorta. In patients who have had tetralogy of Fallot repaired, echocardiography/Doppler also provides data regarding the amount of residual pulmonary valve regurgitation if a transannular patch is present, RV and LV function, and the presence of aortic regurgitation. Elevated N-terminal pro B-type natriuretic peptide (NT-proBNP) blood levels have also been correlated with increasing RV enlargement.

Cardiac MRI and CT can quantitate both the pulmonary regurgitation and the RV volumes. In addition, cardiac MRI and CT can identify whether there is either a native pulmonary arterial branch stenosis or a stenosis at the distal site of a prior arterial-to-PA shunt or other anomalies, such as an ASD. The ability of cardiac MRI to accurately quantitate the pulmonary regurgitation severity and provide more accurate RV volume measurements gives it an advantage over other imaging studies. Cardiac catheterization may be required to document the degree of pulmonary valve regurgitation because noninvasive studies depend on velocity gradients. Pulmonary angiography demonstrates the degree of pulmonary valve regurgitation, and RV angiography helps assess any postoperative outflow tract aneurysm.

The need for electrophysiologic studies with ventricular stimulation and potential ventricular tachycardia ablation has been suggested by some experts for patients who have had evidence for ventricular tachycardia, unexplained syncope, a wide QRS, are older, or who are about to undergo pulmonary valve replacement.

Prognosis & Treatment

A few patients with "just the right amount" of subpulmonic stenosis enter adulthood without having had surgical correction. However, most adult patients have had surgical repair, including VSD closure, resection of infundibular muscle, and insertion of an outflow tract patch to relieve the subpulmonic obstruction. Patients with pulmonary valve regurgitation should be monitored to ensure the RV volume does not progressively increase. In patients with tetralogy of Fallot, transthoracic echocardiogram monitoring of pulmonary valve regurgitation is recommended every 12–24 months based on the degree of regurgitation. Low-pressure pulmonary valve regurgitation is difficult to diagnose due to the fact that the RV diastolic pressures tend to be high and the pulmonary arterial diastolic pressure low. This means there is little gradient between the PA and the RV in diastole, so that there may be little murmur or evidence of turbulence on color flow Doppler. If the RV begins to enlarge, it must be assumed that this is due to pulmonary valve regurgitation until proven otherwise. Early surgical pulmonary valve replacement is increasingly being favored. The RV volumes from cardiac MRI are important in deciding when to intervene if the patient is not very symptomatic; an RV end-diastolic volume index of greater than 160 mm/m^2 or an RV end-systolic volume index of greater than 80 mm/m^2 is recommended as the cutoff. There are also a number of other triggers for intervention, details of which can be found in the AHA/ACC and ESC guidelines. A percutaneous approach to pulmonary valve regurgitation remains limited as the available percutaneous valve diameters are frequently too small for the size of the pulmonary annulus. The Melody valve is a bovine jugular vein prosthesis with the largest size being 22 mm in diameter. Percutaneous stented valves, particularly the Edwards SAPIEN XT, have been used successfully and can be used in patients with larger pulmonary root sizes. Often, a regular stent is placed within the PA first, with the stented valve then placed within this first stent. The expansion of the PA must not impede flow down any coronary artery; this is tested by a trial balloon expansion while imaging the coronary artery at the same time (class I requirement). There has been an increase in stented valve endocarditis noted after the placement of the Melody valve; this is being closely monitored.

If an anomalous coronary artery is present, then an extracardiac conduit around it from the RV to the PA may be necessary as part of the tetralogy repair. By 20-year follow-up, reoperation of the common tetralogy repair is needed in about 10–15%, not only for severe pulmonary valve regurgitation but also for residual infundibular stenosis. Usually the pulmonary valve is replaced with a pulmonary homograft, although a porcine bioprosthetic valve is also suitable. Percutaneous valve-in-valve stented bioprosthetic valves have successfully been used when there is surgical bioprosthetic valve dysfunction. Cryoablation of the tissue giving rise to arrhythmias is sometimes performed at the time of reoperation. Branch pulmonary stenosis may be percutaneously opened by stenting. If a conduit has been used already for repair of the RV outflow obstruction, a percutaneous approach with a stented pulmonary valve may be possible. All patients require endocarditis prophylaxis (see Tables 33–3, 33–4, and 33–5). Most adults with stable hemodynamics can be quite active, and most women can carry a pregnancy adequately if RV function is preserved.

Atrial fibrillation, reentrant atrial arrhythmias, and ventricular ectopy are common, especially after the age of 45. Left heart disease appears to cause arrhythmias more often than right heart disease. Biventricular dysfunction is not an uncommon consequence as the patient ages. The cause of associated LV dysfunction is often multifactorial and frequently unclear. Similarly, the aorta may enlarge with accompanying aortic regurgitation, and these lesions can become severe enough to warrant surgical intervention. Patients with RV or LV dysfunction or with dysfunction of both ventricles may require a prophylactic defibrillator.

When to Refer

All patients with tetralogy of Fallot should be referred to a cardiologist with expertise in adult congenital heart disease.

He F et al. Whether pulmonary valve replacement in asymptomatic patients with moderate or severe regurgitation after tetralogy of Fallot repair is appropriate: a case-control study. J Am Heart Assoc. 2019;8:e010689. [PMID: 30587056]

Ros D et al. Infectious endocarditis after percutaneous pulmonary valve implantation with a stent mounted bovine jugular vein valve. Clinical experience and the evaluation of the modified Duke criteria. Int J Cardiol. 2021;323;40. [PMID: 32860844]

Smith CA et al. Long-term outcome of tetralogy of Fallot: a study from the Pediatric Cardiac Care Consortium. JAMA Cardiol. 2019;4:34. [PMID: 30566184]

VALVULAR HEART DISEASE

The typical findings of each native valve lesion are described in Table 10–1. Table 10–2 outlines bedside maneuvers to distinguish among the various systolic murmurs.

The 2017 ACC/AHA valvular heart disease guidelines suggest all lesions may be best classified clinically into one of six categories based on anatomy and symptoms.

Stage A: Patients at risk for valvular heart disease.

Stage B: Patients with progressive valvular heart disease (mild to moderate severity) and asymptomatic.

Stage C: Asymptomatic patients who have reached criteria for severe valvular heart disease.

- **C1:** Severe valve lesion. Asymptomatic. Normal LV function.
- **C2:** Severe valve lesion. Asymptomatic. Abnormal LV function.

Stage D: Symptomatic patients as a result of valvular heart disease.

In 2020, the ACC/AHA guideline for the management of patients with valvular heart disease was published and this chapter will highlight the changes and additions from the prior guidelines, first published in 2014 and then updated in 2017.

Nishimura RA et al. 2017 AHA/ACC focused update of the 2014 AHA/ACC guideline for the management of patients with valvular heart disease: a report of the American College of Cardiology/American Heart Association Task Force on Practice Guidelines. Circulation. 2017;135:e1159. [PMID: 28298458]

Otto CM et al. 2020 ACC/AHA guideline for the management of patients with valvular heart disease. J Am Coll Cardiol. 2021; 77:450. [PMID: 33342587]

MITRAL STENOSIS

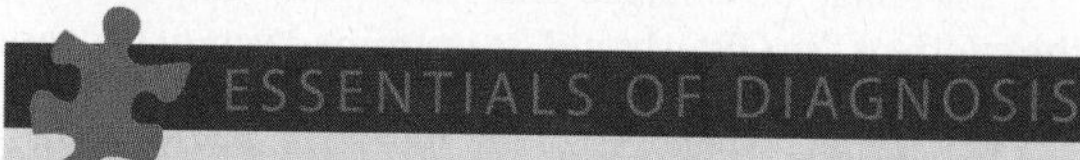

- Fatigue, exertional dyspnea, and orthopnea when the stenosis becomes severe.
- Symptoms often precipitated by onset of atrial fibrillation or pregnancy.
- Intervention indicated for symptoms, atrial fibrillation, or evidence of pulmonary hypertension. Most symptomatic patients have a mitral valve area of < 1.5 cm^2.

General Considerations

Most patients with native valve mitral stenosis are presumed to have had rheumatic heart disease, although a history of rheumatic fever is noted in only about one-third. (Also see section on Rheumatic Fever.) Rheumatic mitral stenosis results in thickening of the leaflets, fusion of the mitral commissures, retraction, thickening and fusion of the chordae, and calcium deposition in the valve. Mitral stenosis can also occur due to congenital disease with chordal fusion or papillary muscle malposition. The papillary muscles may be abnormally close together, sometimes so close that they merge into a single papillary muscle (the **"parachute mitral valve"**). In these patients, the chordae or valvular tissue (or both) may also be fused. In older patients and in those undergoing dialysis, mitral annular calcification may stiffen the mitral valve and reduce its motion to the point where a mitral gradient is present. Calcium in the mitral annulus virtually invades the mitral leaflet from the annulus inward as opposed to the calcium buildup in the leaflets and commissures as seen in rheumatic heart disease. Mitral valve obstruction may also develop in patients who have had mitral valve repair with a mitral annular ring that is too small, or in patients who have had a surgical valve replacement (prosthetic valve-patient mismatch or degeneration of the prosthetic valve over time).

Table 10–1. Differential diagnosis of valvular heart disease.

	Mitral Stenosis	Mitral Regurgitation	Aortic Stenosis	Aortic Regurgitation	Tricuspid Stenosis	Tricuspid Regurgitation
Inspection	Malar flush, precordial bulge, and diffuse pulsation in young patients.	Usually prominent and hyperdynamic apical impulse to left of MCL.	Sustained PMI, prominent atrial filling wave.	Hyperdynamic PMI to left of MCL and downward. Visible carotid pulsations. Pulsating nailbeds (Quincke sign), head bob (deMusset sign).	Giant *a* wave in jugular pulse with sinus rhythm. Peripheral edema or ascites, or both.	Large *v* wave in jugular pulse; time with carotid pulsation. Peripheral edema or ascites, or both.
Palpation	"Tapping" sensation over area of expected PMI. Right ventricular pulsation in left third to fifth ICS parasternally when pulmonary hypertension is present. P_2 may be palpable.	Forceful, brisk PMI; systolic thrill over PMI. Pulse normal, small, or slightly collapsing.	Powerful, heaving PMI to left and slightly below MCL. Systolic thrill over aortic area, sternal notch, or carotid arteries in severe disease. Small and slowly rising carotid pulse. If bicuspid AS, check for delay at femoral artery to exclude coarctation.	Apical impulse forceful and displaced significantly to left and downward. Prominent carotid pulses. Rapidly rising and collapsing pulses (Corrigan pulse).	Pulsating, enlarged liver in ventricular systole.	Right ventricular pulsation. Systolic pulsation of liver.
Heart sounds, rhythm, and blood pressure	S_1 loud if valve mobile. Opening snap following S_2. The worse the disease, the closer the S_2-opening snap interval.	S_1 normal or buried in early part of murmur (exception in mitral prolapse where murmur may be late). Prominent third heart sound when severe MR. Atrial fibrillation common. Blood pressure normal. Midsystolic clicks may be present and may be multiple.	A_2 normal, soft, or absent. Prominent S_4. Blood pressure normal, or systolic pressure normal with high diastolic pressure.	S_1 normal or reduced, A_2 loud. Wide pulse pressure with diastolic pressure < 60 mm Hg. When severe, gentle compression of femoral artery with diaphragm of stethoscope may reveal diastolic flow (Duroziez) and pressure in leg on palpation > 40 mm Hg than in arm (Hill).	S_1 often loud.	Atrial fibrillation may be present.
Murmurs						
Location and transmission	Localized at or near apex. Diastolic rumble best heard in left lateral position; may be accentuated by having patient do sit-ups. Rarely, short diastolic murmur along lower left sternal border (Graham Steell) in severe pulmonary hypertension.	Loudest over PMI; posteriorly directed jets (ie, anterior mitral prolapse) transmitted to left axilla, left infrascapular area; anteriorly directed jets (ie, posterior mitral prolapse) heard over anterior precordium. Murmur unchanged after premature beat.	Right second ICS parasternally or at apex, heard in carotid arteries and occasionally in upper interscapular area. May sound like MR at apex (Gallaverdin phenomenon), but murmur occurs after S_1 and stops before S_2.	Diastolic: louder along left sternal border in third to fourth interspace. Heard over aortic area and apex. May be associated with low-pitched mid-diastolic murmur at apex (Austin Flint) due to functional mitral stenosis. If due to an enlarged aorta, murmur may radiate to right sternal border.	Third to fifth ICS along left sternal border out to apex. Murmur increases with inspiration.	Third to fifth ICS along left sternal border. Murmur hard to hear but increases with inspiration. Sit-ups can increase cardiac output and accentuate murmur.

(*continued*)

Table 10–1. Differential diagnosis of valvular heart disease. (continued)

	Mitral Stenosis	Mitral Regurgitation	Aortic Stenosis	Aortic Regurgitation	Tricuspid Stenosis	Tricuspid Regurgitation
Timing	Relation of opening snap to A_2 important. The higher the LA pressure, the earlier the opening snap. Presystolic accentuation before S_1 if in sinus rhythm. Graham Steell begins with P_2 (early diastole) if associated pulmonary hypertension.	Pansystolic: begins with S_1 and ends at or after A_2. May be late systolic in mitral valve prolapse.	Begins after S_1, ends before A_2. The more severe the stenosis, the later the murmur peaks.	Begins immediately after aortic second sound and ends before first sound (blurring both); helps distinguish from MR.	Rumble often follows audible opening snap.	At times, hard to hear. Begins with S_1 and fills systole. Increases with inspiration.
Character	Low-pitched, rumbling; presystolic murmur merges with loud S_1.	Blowing, high-pitched; occasionally harsh or musical.	Harsh, rough.	Blowing, often faint.	As for mitral stenosis.	Blowing, coarse, or musical.
Optimum auscultatory conditions	After exercise, left lateral recumbency. Use stethoscope bell, lightly applied.	After exercise; use stethoscope diaphragm. In prolapse, findings may be more evident while standing.	Use stethoscope diaphragm. Patient resting, leaning forward, breath held in full expiration.	Use stethoscope diaphragm. Patient leaning forward, breath held in expiration.	Use stethoscope bell. Murmur usually louder and at peak during inspiration. Patient recumbent.	Use stethoscope diaphragm. Murmur usually becomes louder during inspiration.
Radiography	Straight left heart border from enlarged LA appendage. Elevation of left mainstem bronchus. Large right ventricle and pulmonary artery if pulmonary hypertension is present. Calcification in mitral valve in rheumatic mitral stenosis or in annulus in calcific mitral stenosis.	Enlarged LV and LA.	Concentric LVH. Prominent ascending aorta. Calcified aortic valve common.	Moderate to severe LV enlargement. Aortic root often dilated.	Enlarged right atrium with prominent SVC and azygous shadow.	Enlarged right atrium and right ventricle.
ECG	Broad P waves in standard leads; broad negative phase of diphasic P in V_1. If pulmonary hypertension is present, tall peaked P waves, right axis deviation, or right ventricular hypertrophy appears.	Left axis deviation or frank LVH. P waves broad, tall, or notched in standard leads. Broad negative phase of diphasic P in V_1.	LVH.	LVH.	Tall, peaked P waves. Possible right ventricular hypertrophy.	Right axis usual.

Echocardiography						
Two-dimensional echocardiography	Thickened, immobile mitral valve with anterior and posterior leaflets moving together. "Hockey stick" shape to opened anterior leaflet in rheumatic mitral stenosis. Annular calcium with thin leaflets in calcific mitral stenosis. LA enlargement, normal to small LV. Orifice can be traced to approximate mitral valve orifice area.	Thickened mitral valve in rheumatic disease; mitral valve prolapse; flail leaflet or vegetations may be seen. Dilated LV in volume overload. Operate for LV end-systolic dimension < 4.5 cm.	Dense persistent echoes from the aortic valve with poor leaflet excursion. LVH late in the disease. Bicuspid valve in younger patients.	Abnormal aortic valve or dilated aortic root. Diastolic vibrations of the anterior leaflet of the mitral valve and septum. In acute aortic regurgitation, premature closure of the mitral valve before the QRS. When severe, dilated LV with normal or decreased contractility. Operate when LV end-systolic dimension > 5.0 cm.	In rheumatic disease, tricuspid valve thickening, decreased early diastolic filling slope of the tricuspid valve. In carcinoid, leaflets fixed, but no significant thickening.	Enlarged right ventricle with paradoxical septal motion. Tricuspid valve often pulled open by displaced chordae.
Continuous and color flow Doppler and TEE	Prolonged pressure half-time across mitral valve allows estimation of gradient. MVA estimated from pressure half-time. Indirect evidence of pulmonary hypertension by noting elevated right ventricular systolic pressure measured from the tricuspid regurgitation jet.	Regurgitant flow mapped into LA. Use of PISA helps assess MR severity. TEE important in prosthetic mitral valve regurgitation.	Increased transvalvular flow velocity; severe AS when peak jet > 4 m/seconds (64 mm Hg). Valve area estimate using continuity equation is poorly reproducible.	Demonstrates regurgitation and qualitatively estimates severity based on percentage of LV outflow filled with jet and distance jet penetrates into LV. TEE important in aortic valve endocarditis to exclude abscess. Mitral inflow pattern describes diastolic dysfunction.	Prolonged pressure half-time across tricuspid valve can be used to estimate mean gradient. Severe tricuspid stenosis present when mean gradient > 5 mm Hg.	Regurgitant flow mapped into right atrium and venae cavae. Right ventricular systolic pressure estimated by tricuspid regurgitation jet velocity.

A_2, aortic second sound; AS, aortic stenosis; ICS, intercostal space; LA, left atrial; MCL, midclavicular line; MR, mitral regurgitation; MVA, measured valve area; P_2, pulmonary second sound; PISA, proximal isovelocity surface area; PMI, point of maximal impulse; S_1, first heart sound; S_2, second heart sound; S_4, fourth heart sound; SVC, superior vena cava; TEE, transesophageal echocardiography; V_1, chest ECG lead 1.

Table 10–2. Effect of various interventions on systolic murmurs.

Intervention	Hypertrophic Cardiomyopathy	Aortic Stenosis	Mitral Regurgitation	Mitral Prolapse
Valsalva	↑	↓	↓ or ×	↑ or ↓
Standing	↑	↑ or ×	↓ or ×	↑
Handgrip or squatting	↓	↓ or ×	↑	↓
Supine position with legs elevated	↓	↑ or ×	×	↓
Exercise	↑	↑ or ×	↓	↑

↑, increased; ↓, decreased; ×, unchanged.
Reproduced with permission from Paraskos JA. *Combined valvular disease. In: Dalen JE, Alpert JS, Rahimtoola SH (ed).* Valvular Heart Disease, 3e. Philadelphia: Lippincott Williams & Wilkins, 2000.

Clinical Findings

A. Symptoms and Signs

Two clinical syndromes classically occur in patients with mitral stenosis. In mild to moderate mitral stenosis, LA pressure and cardiac output may be essentially normal, and the patient is either asymptomatic or symptomatic only with extreme exertion. The measured valve area is usually between 1.5 cm^2 and 1.0 cm^2. In severe mitral stenosis (valve area less than 1.0 cm^2), severe pulmonary hypertension develops due to a "secondary stenosis" of the pulmonary vascular bed. In this condition, pulmonary edema is uncommon, but symptoms of low cardiac output and right heart failure predominate. Any measured valve area less than 1.5 cm^2 should be considered significant.

A characteristic finding of rheumatic mitral stenosis is an **opening snap** following A_2 due to the stiff mitral valve. The interval between the opening snap and aortic closure sound is long when the LA pressure is low but shortens as the LA pressure rises and approaches the aortic diastolic pressure. As mitral stenosis worsens, there is a localized low-pitched diastolic murmur whose duration increases with the severity of the stenosis as the mitral gradient continues throughout more of diastole. The diastolic murmur is best heard at the apex with the patient in the left lateral position (Table 10–1). Mitral regurgitation may be present as well.

Paroxysmal or chronic atrial fibrillation eventually develops in 50–80% of patients. Any increase in the heart rate reduces diastolic filling time and increases the mitral gradient. A sudden increase in heart rate may precipitate pulmonary edema. Therefore, heart rate control is important, with slow heart rates allowing for more diastolic filling of the LV.

B. Diagnostic Studies

Echocardiography is the most valuable technique for assessing mitral stenosis (Table 10–1). LA size can also be determined by echocardiography; increased size denotes an increased likelihood of atrial fibrillation and thrombus formation.

Because echocardiography and careful symptom evaluation provide most of the needed information, cardiac catheterization is used primarily to detect associated coronary or myocardial disease—usually after the decision to intervene has been made.

Treatment & Prognosis

In most cases, there is a long asymptomatic phase after the initial rheumatic infection, followed by subtle limitation of activity. Pregnancy and its associated increase in stroke volume and heart rate result in an increased transmitral pressure gradient and may precipitate symptoms. In particular, toward the end of pregnancy, the cardiac output continues to be maintained by an increase in heart rate, increasing the mitral gradient by shortening diastolic time. Patients with moderate to severe mitral stenosis should have the condition corrected prior to becoming pregnant if possible (when the measured valve area is about 2.0 cm^2). Pregnant patients who become symptomatic can undergo successful surgery, preferably in the third trimester, although balloon valvuloplasty is the treatment of choice if the echocardiography valve score is low enough.

The onset of atrial fibrillation often precipitates symptoms, which improve with control of the ventricular rate or restoration of sinus rhythm. Conversion to and subsequent maintenance of sinus rhythm are most commonly successful when the duration of atrial fibrillation is brief (less than 6–12 months) and the LA is not severely dilated (diameter less than 4.5 cm). Once atrial fibrillation occurs, the patient should receive warfarin even if sinus rhythm is restored, since atrial fibrillation often recurs even with antiarrhythmic therapy and 20–30% of these patients will have systemic embolization if untreated. Systemic embolization in the presence of only mild to moderate disease is not an indication for surgery but should be treated with warfarin. DOACs (dabigatran, apixaban, rivaroxaban, edoxaban) are *not* recommended by the most recent guidelines, since patients with atrial fibrillation were excluded from the approval trials.

Indications for intervention focus on symptoms such as an episode of pulmonary edema, a decline in exercise capacity, or any evidence of pulmonary hypertension (peak systolic pulmonary pressure greater than 50 mm Hg). Some experts believe that the presence of atrial fibrillation should also be a consideration for an intervention. Most

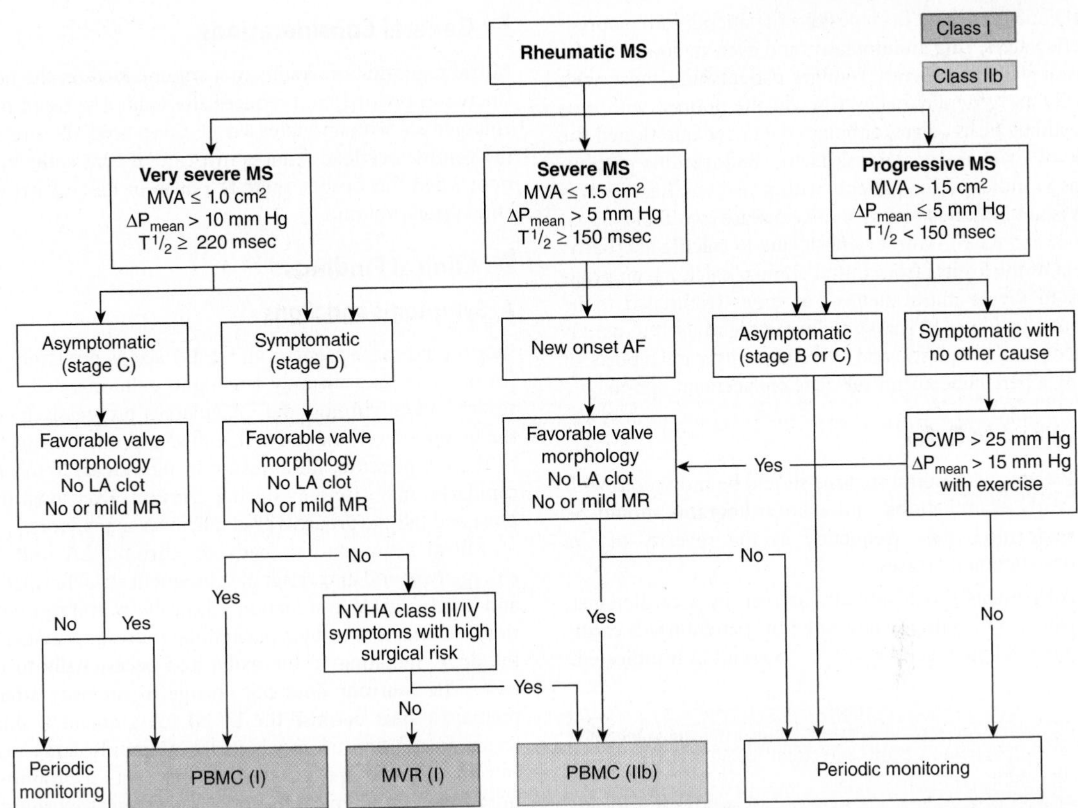

▲ **Figure 10–1.** The AHA/ACC guidelines for intervention in mitral stenosis. AF, atrial fibrillation; LA, left atrial; MR, mitral regurgitation; MS, mitral stenosis; MVA, mitral valve area; MVR, mitral valve replacement; NYHA, New York Heart Association; PBMC, percutaneous balloon mitral commissurotomy; PCWP, pulmonary capillary wedge pressure; ΔP_{mean}, mean pressure gradient; T½, half-life. (Reprinted with permission Circulation. 2014;129:e521–e643 ©2014 American Heart Association, Inc.)

interventions are not pursued until the patient is symptomatic (stage D) (Figure 10–1). In some patients, symptoms develop with calculated mitral valve areas between 1.5 cm^2 and 1.0 cm^2. Symptoms or evidence of pulmonary hypertension should drive the decision to intervene in these patients, not the estimated valve area.

Open mitral commissurotomy is now rarely performed and has been replaced by percutaneous balloon valvuloplasty. Ten-year follow-up data comparing surgery to balloon valvuloplasty suggest no real difference in outcome between the two modalities. Replacement of the valve is indicated when combined stenosis and regurgitation are present or when the mitral valve echo score is much greater than 8–10. To determine the valve score, numbers 1 to 4 are assigned to four valve characteristics: mobility, calcification, thickening, and submitral scar. Thus, a maximum score is 16. Percutaneous balloon valvuloplasty has a very low mortality rate (less than 0.5%) and a low morbidity rate (3–5%). Operative mortality rates are also low: 1–3% in most institutions. Repeat balloon valvuloplasty can be done if the morphology of the valve remains suitable. At surgery, a **Maze procedure** may be done at the same time to reduce recurrent atrial arrhythmias. It involves a number of endocardial incisions across the right and left atria to disrupt the electrical activity that sustains atrial arrhythmias. In many institutions, the LA appendage is sewn closed to help remove a potential future source for thrombosis.

Mechanical mitral prosthetic valves are more prone to thrombosis than mechanical aortic prosthetic valves. **The recommended INR range is thus higher (INR 2.5–3.5 or average of 3.0). Low-dose aspirin should be used in conjunction with warfarin if the bleeding risk is low.** DOACs are *not* recommended as an anticoagulant. It is a class IIa recommendation that warfarin be used for up to 6 months after implantation of a bioprosthetic mitral valve. Bioprosthetic valves tend to degenerate after about 10–15 years. Percutaneous balloon valvuloplasty is not effective when bioprosthetic valve stenosis occurs, but stented valve-in-valve procedures have been successful. However, valve-in-valve procedures are still uncommon due to the need for the technically challenging transseptal approach. Reported early outcomes have been positive in patients with bioprosthetic valves, ring annuloplasty, and even in some calcific mitral stenosis patients. Younger patients and those with ESKD are generally believed to do the poorest with bioprosthetic heart valves, although data have questioned the role of CKD as a major risk factor. Endocarditis prophylaxis is indicated for patients with prosthetic heart valves but is not indicated in native valve disease (see Tables 33–3, 33–4, and 33–5). Mitral stenosis due to calcific encroachment of the leaflets from mitral annular calcium can progress to severe mitral stenosis at times (estimated to be about 1 in 6 over 10 years). It does not lend itself to percutaneous valvuloplasty, and there are only case reports of using a percutaneous mitral valve replacement option.

When to Refer

- Patients with mitral stenosis should be monitored with yearly examinations, and echocardiograms should be performed more frequently as the severity of the obstruction increases.
- All patients should initially be seen by a cardiologist, who can then decide how often the patient needs cardiology follow-up and whether intervention is indicated.

Kim JY et al. Outcomes of direct oral anticoagulants in patients with mitral stenosis. J Am Coll Cardiol. 2019;73:1123. [PMID: 30871695]

Tsutsui RS et al. Natural history of mitral stenosis in patients with mitral annular calcium. JACC Cardiovasc Imaging. 2019;12:1105. [PMID: 30765312]

MITRAL REGURGITATION

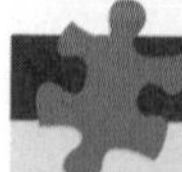

ESSENTIALS OF DIAGNOSIS

- May be asymptomatic for years (or for life).
- Severe mitral regurgitation may cause left-sided heart failure and lead to pulmonary hypertension and right-sided heart failure.
- For chronic primary mitral regurgitation, surgery is indicated for symptoms or when the LVEF is < 60% or the echocardiographic LV end-systolic dimension is > 4.0 cm. Surgery also indicated in patients who have a progressive increase in LV size or decline in LVEF.
- In patients with mitral prolapse and severe mitral regurgitation, earlier surgery is indicated if mitral repair can be performed successfully with a high degree of certainty.
- Transcatheter edge-to-edge repair, if possible, can be done in symptomatic patients at higher surgical risk regardless of whether the mitral regurgitation is primary or secondary.
- Patients with functional chronic mitral regurgitation may improve with biventricular pacing and guideline-directed management and therapy.

General Considerations

Mitral regurgitation results in a volume load on the heart (increases preload) and reduces afterload. The result is an enlarged LV with an increased EF. Over time, the stress of the volume overload reduces myocardial contractile function; when this occurs, there is a drop in EF and a rise in end-systolic volume.

Clinical Findings

A. Symptoms and Signs

In acute mitral regurgitation, the LA size is not large, and LA pressure rises abruptly, leading to pulmonary edema if severe. When chronic, the LA enlarges progressively and the increased volume can be handled without a major rise in the LA pressure; the pressure in pulmonary veins and capillaries may rise only during exertion. Exertional dyspnea and fatigue progress gradually over many years.

Mitral regurgitation leads to chronic LA and LV enlargement and may result in subsequent atrial fibrillation and eventually LV dysfunction. Clinically, mitral regurgitation is characterized by a pansystolic murmur maximal at the apex, radiating to the axilla and occasionally to the base. The murmur does not change in intensity after a premature beat because the LV to LA gradient is unaffected. In addition, a hyperdynamic LV impulse and a brisk carotid upstroke may be present along with a prominent third heart sound due to the increased volume returning to the LV in early diastole (Tables 10–1 and 10–2). In acute mitral regurgitation, the murmur intensity may be modest due to little difference between the LA and LV systolic pressures during ventricular systole. The mitral regurgitation murmur due to mitral valve prolapse tends to radiate anteriorly in the presence of posterior leaflet prolapse and posteriorly when the prolapse is primarily of the anterior leaflet. Mitral regurgitation may not be pansystolic in these patients but occur only after the mitral click (until late in the disease process when it then becomes progressively more holosystolic).

B. Diagnostic Studies

Echocardiographic information demonstrating the underlying pathologic process (rheumatic, calcific, prolapse, flail leaflet, endocarditis, cardiomyopathy), LV size and function, LA size, PA pressure, and RV function can be invaluable in planning treatment as well as in recognizing associated lesions. The valvular heart disease guidelines provide details of the classification and measures of severity for primary and secondary mitral valve regurgitation. Doppler techniques provide qualitative and semiquantitative estimates of the severity of mitral regurgitation. TEE may help reveal the cause of regurgitation and is especially useful in patients who have had mitral valve replacement, in suspected endocarditis, and in identifying candidates for valvular repair. Echocardiographic dimensions and measures of systolic function are critical in deciding the timing of surgery. Asymptomatic patients with severe mitral regurgitation (stage C1) but preserved LV dimensions should undergo at least yearly echocardiography. Exercise hemodynamics with either Doppler echocardiography or cardiac catheterization may be useful when the symptoms do not fit the anatomic severity of mitral regurgitation. BNP or NT-proBNP is useful in the early identification of LV dysfunction in the presence of mitral regurgitation and asymptomatic patients, and values that trend upward over time appear to have prognostic importance.

Cardiac MRI is occasionally useful, especially if specific myocardial causes are being sought (such as amyloid or myocarditis) or if myocardial viability assessment is needed prior to deciding whether to add coronary artery bypass grafting to mitral valve surgery.

Cardiac catheterization provides a further assessment of regurgitation and its hemodynamic impact along with LV function, resting cardiac output, and PA pressure. **The guidelines recommend coronary angiography to determine the presence of incidental CAD prior to valve surgery in all men over age 40 years and in menopausal women with coronary risk factors.** In younger patients, no coronary angiography is needed unless there is a clinical suspicion of coronary disease. Cardiac multidetector coronary CT may be adequate to screen patients with valvular heart disease for asymptomatic CAD. A normal CT coronary angiogram has a high predictive value for patients with normal or insignificant disease.

Treatment & Prognosis

A. Primary Mitral Regurgitation

The degree of LV enlargement reflects the severity and chronicity of regurgitation. LV volume overload may ultimately lead to LV failure and reduced cardiac output. LA enlargement may be considerable in **chronic mitral regurgitation** and a large amount of mitral regurgitation regurgitant volume may be tolerated. Patients with chronic lesions may thus remain asymptomatic for many years. Surgery is necessary when symptoms develop or when there is evidence for LV dysfunction, since progressive and irreversible deterioration of LV function can occur prior to the onset of symptoms. Early surgery is indicated even in asymptomatic patients with a reduced EF (less than 60%) or marked LV dilation with reduced contractility (end-systolic dimension greater than 4.0 cm) (Figure 10–2).

It is a class IIa indication for mitral valve surgery when the LVEF is greater than 60% and the LV end-systolic dimension is still less than 4.0 cm but serial imaging reveals a progressive increase in the LV end-systolic dimension or a serial decrease in the EF. Pulmonary hypertension development suggests the mitral regurgitation is severe and should prompt intervention.

Acute mitral regurgitation may develop abruptly, as with papillary muscle dysfunction following MI, valve perforation in infective endocarditis, in patients with hypertrophic cardiomyopathy (HCM), or when there are ruptured chordae tendineae in patients with mitral valve prolapse. Emergency surgery may be required.

Some patients may become hemodynamically unstable and require treatment with vasodilators or intra-aortic balloon counterpulsation that reduce the amount of retrograde regurgitant flow by lowering systemic vascular resistance and improving forward stroke volume. There is controversy regarding the role of afterload reduction in chronic mitral regurgitation, since the lesion inherently results in a reduction in afterload, and there are no data that chronic afterload reduction is effective in avoiding LV dysfunction or surgical intervention. A heightened sympathetic state has led some experts to suggest that beta-blockade be considered routinely, though this also remains speculative. The mitral regurgitation in patients with tachycardia-related cardiomyopathy may improve with normalization of the heart rate.

B. Myocardial Disease and Mitral Regurgitation (Secondary Mitral Regurgitation)

When mitral regurgitation is due to cardiac dysfunction, it may subside as the infarction heals or LV dilation diminishes. The cause of the regurgitation in most of these situations is displacement of the papillary muscles and an enlarged mitral annulus rather than papillary muscle ischemia. The fundamental problem is the lack of leaflet coaptation during systole (due to either leaflet prolapse or retraction). In acute MI, rupture of the papillary muscle may occur with catastrophic results. Transient—but sometimes severe—mitral regurgitation may occur during episodes of myocardial ischemia and contribute to flash pulmonary edema. Patients with dilated cardiomyopathies of any origin may have **secondary mitral regurgitation** due to the papillary muscle displacement or dilation of the mitral annulus, or both. If mitral valve replacement is performed, preservation of the chordae to the native valve helps prevent further ventricular dilation following surgery. Initially, several groups reported good results with mitral valve repair in patients with LVEF less than 30% and secondary mitral regurgitation. Current guidelines advise that mitral valve repair/replacement can be attempted in severe mitral regurgitation patients with an EF less than 30% or an LV end-systolic dimension greater than 5.5 cm, or both, as long as repair and preservation of the chordae are possible. Figure 10–3 outlines the recommendations for intervention in secondary mitral regurgitation.

Mitral valve replacement with chordal preservation is preferred over mitral valve repair in patients with chronic ischemic cardiomyopathy. There may also be a role for cardiac resynchronization therapy with biventricular pacemaker insertion, which has been found to reduce mitral regurgitation related to cardiomyopathy in many patients. Guidelines recommend biventricular pacing prior to surgical repair in symptomatic patients who have functional mitral regurgitation as long as other criteria (eg, a QRS of greater than 150 msec or left bundle branch block or both) are present.

There are several ongoing trials of percutaneous approaches to reducing mitral regurgitation. These approaches include the use of a **mitral clip** (MitraClip) device to create a double orifice mitral valve, various coronary catheter devices to reduce the mitral annular area, and devices to reduce the septal-lateral ventricular size and consequent mitral orifice size. Of these devices, the most success has been noted with the edge-to-edge MitraClip. Two major trials have addressed the potential advantage of

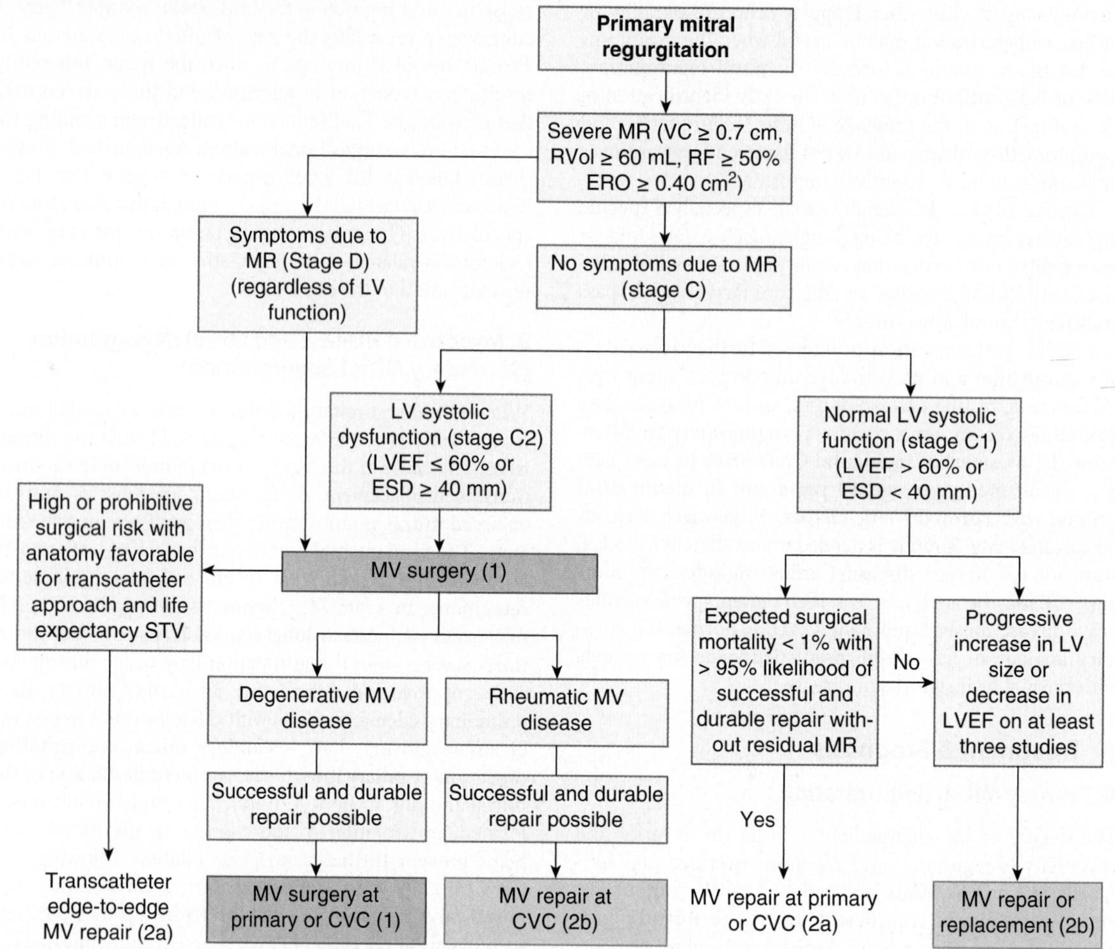

▲ **Figure 10–2. Algorithm for intervention in primary mitral regurgitation. CVC, Comprehensive valve center; ERO, effective regurgitant orifice; ESD, end-systolic dimension; MR, mitral regurgitation; MV, mitral valve; MVR, mitral valve replacement; RF, regurgitant fraction; RVol, regurgitant volume; VC, vena contracta.** (Reprinted from Journal of the American College of Cardiology,77, Otto CM et al. 2020 ACC/AHA Guideline for the Management of Patients With Valvular Heart Disease A Report of the American College of Cardiology/American Heart Association Joint Committee on Clinical Practice Guidelines, e25–e197, 2021, with permission from Elsevier.)

the percutaneous MitraClip. In the COAPT (Clinical Outcomes Assessment of MitraClip) trial among patients with heart failure and moderate-to-severe or severe secondary mitral regurgitation who remained symptomatic despite the use of maximum doses of guideline-directed medical therapy, transcatheter mitral valve repair resulted in a lower rate of hospitalization for heart failure and lower all-cause mortality within 24 months of follow-up than medical therapy alone. The absolute risk reduction in all-cause mortality in patients receiving the MitraClip in the COAPT trial was 17%, which translated to a number needed to treat (NNT) of 6 to prevent 1 death over 2 years. This rather remarkably positive result, however, was tempered by another MitraClip randomized trial in a similar population that had a rather neutral result, the MITRA-FR (Percutaneous Repair with MitraClip Device for Severe Functional/Secondary Mitral Regurgitation) study, in which the MitraClip therapy failed to show any survival benefit over medical therapy during the 1-year follow-up period. One suggestion to reconcile the differences in outcome has been suggested wherein the MitraClip is *ineffective* if the echocardiographic regurgitant orifice size is consistent with the size of the dilated LV, but the device is *effective* if the regurgitant orifice size is large compared to the size of the LV. This seemed to be verified by the results of the two trials. Current guidelines have accepted the use of the MitraClip in patients with secondary mitral regurgitation and high surgical risk. In addition, vascular plugging and occluder devices are being used in selected patients to occlude perivalvular leaks around prosthetic mitral valves. A transcatheter stented valve, which is used as a **transcatheter aortic valve replacement (TAVR)** device, can be used to open a degenerated mitral bioprosthetic valve in any position (aortic, mitral, tricuspid, or pulmonary). Transcatheter

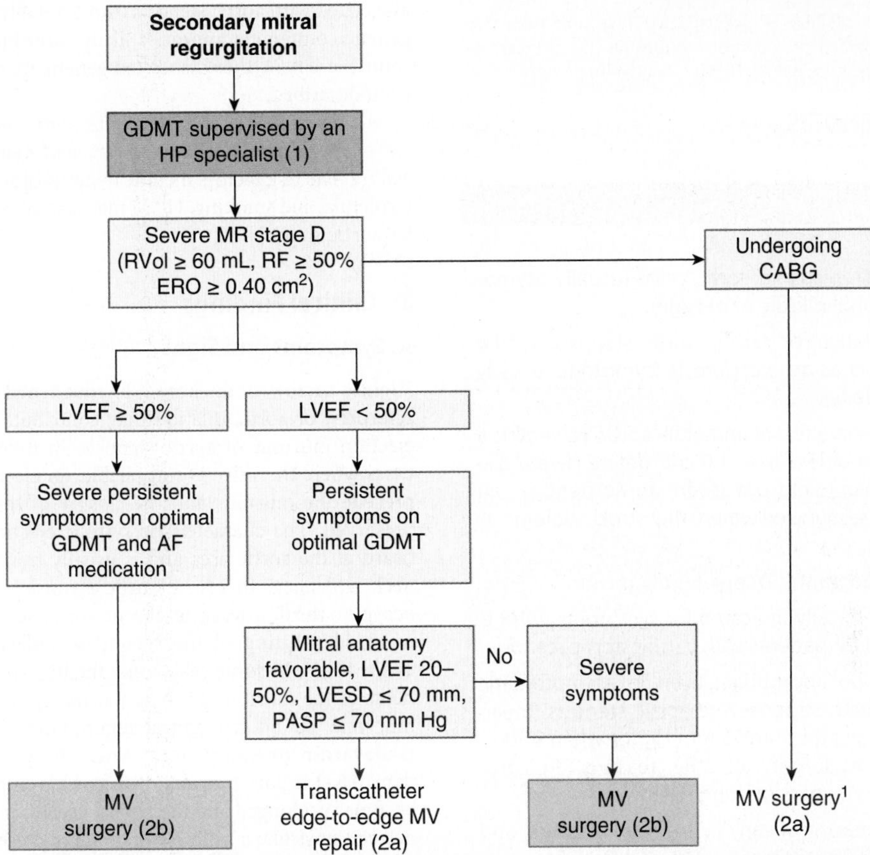

▲ **Figure 10–3. Algorithm for intervention in secondary mitral regurgitation. AF, atrial fibrillation; CABG, coronary artery bypass graft; ERO, effective regurgitant orifice; GDMT, guideline-directed management and therapy; HF, heart failure; LVESD, LV end-systolic dimension; MR, mitral regurgitation; MV, mitral valve; PASP, pulmonary artery systolic pressure; RF, regurgitant fraction; RVol, regurgitant volume.** (Reprinted from Journal of the American College of Cardiology,77, Otto CM et al. 2020 ACC/AHA Guideline for the Management of Patients With Valvular Heart Disease A Report of the American College of Cardiology/American Heart Association Joint Committee on Clinical Practice Guidelines, e25–e197, 2021, with permission from Elsevier.)

valve replacement has also been attempted in small series to repair mitral regurgitation following mitral valve repair with mixed results. Finally, the first cases of a stented mitral valve prosthesis to replace the entire mitral valve have been reported. Abbott has initiated the SUMMIT trial, a US-based pivotal trial utilizing the Tendyne percutaneous mitral valve replacement device. The mitral valve and aortic valve share a common "annulus" and some of the early attempts at percutaneous valve replacement have failed due to obstruction of the aortic outflow.

▶ When to Refer

- All patients with more than mild mitral regurgitation should be referred to a cardiologist for an evaluation.
- Serial examinations and echocardiograms should be obtained and surgical referral made if there is an increase in the LV end-systolic dimensions, a fall in the LVEF to less than 60%, symptoms, evidence for pulmonary hypertension, or the new onset of atrial fibrillation.
- There is evidence that mitral valve repair should be done early in the course of the disease to improve mortality and morbidity.
- Treatment in severe mitral regurgitation in a patient with a dilated cardiomyopathy may be of benefit.

Ailawadi G et al; EVEREST II Investigators. One-year outcomes after MitraClip for functional mitral regurgitation. Circulation. 2019;139:37. [PMID: 30586701]

Grayburn PA et al. Proportionate and disproportionate functional mitral regurgitation: a new conceptual framework that reconciles the results of the MITRA-FR and COAPT trials. JACC Cardiovasc Imaging. 2019;12:353. [PMID: 30553663]

Otto CM et al. 2020 ACC/AHA guideline for the management of patients with valvular heart disease. J Am Coll Cardiol. 2021; 77:450. [PMID: 33342587]

Pibarot P et al. MITRA-FR versus COAPT: lessons from two trials with diametrically opposed results. Eur Heart J Cardiovasc Imaging. 2019;20:620. [PMID: 31115470]

AORTIC STENOSIS

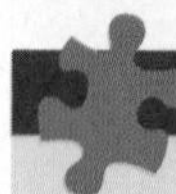

ESSENTIALS OF DIAGNOSIS

- Congenital bicuspid aortic valve (usually asymptomatic until middle or old age).
- "Degenerative" or calcific aortic stenosis; similar risk factors as atherosclerosis (symptoms usually in the elderly).
- Visual observation of immobile aortic valve plus a valve area of less than 1.0 cm^2 define severe disease; low-gradient but severe aortic stenosis can thus be recognized when the stroke volume is reduced.
- Echocardiography/Doppler is diagnostic.
- Surgery typically indicated for symptoms. TAVR is approved for patients with calcific aortic stenosis.
- Intervention appropriate even in asymptomatic patients with super-severe aortic stenosis (mean gradient greater than 55 mm Hg) or when undergoing heart surgery for other reasons (eg, coronary artery bypass grafting [CABG]).
- BNP is a marker of early LV myocardial failure, and high levels (three times normal) suggest poor prognosis and can be an indication for intervention.

General Considerations

There are two common clinical scenarios in which aortic stenosis is prevalent. The first is due to a congenitally abnormal **unicuspid** or **bicuspid valve,** rather than tricuspid. Symptoms can occur in young or adolescent individuals if the stenosis is severe, but more often emerge at age 50–65 years when calcification and degeneration of the valve become manifest. A dilated ascending aorta, due to an intrinsic defect in the aortic root media and the hemodynamic effects of the eccentric aortic jet, may accompany the bicuspid valve in about half of these patients. Coarctation of the aorta is also seen in a number of patients with congenital aortic stenosis. Offspring of patients with a bicuspid valve have a much higher incidence of the disease in either the valve, the aorta, or both (up to 30% in some series).

A second, more common pathologic process, **degenerative** or **calcific aortic stenosis**, is thought to be related to calcium deposition due to processes similar to those that occur in atherosclerotic vascular disease. Approximately 25% of patients over age 65 years and 35% of those over age 70 years have echocardiographic evidence of aortic valve thickening (sclerosis). About 10–20% of these will progress to hemodynamically significant aortic stenosis over a period of 10–15 years. Certain genetic markers are associated with aortic stenosis (most notably Notch 1), so a genetic component appears a likely contributor, at least in some patients. Other associated genetic markers have also been described.

Aortic stenosis has become the most common surgical valve lesion in developed countries, and many patients are elderly. The risk factors include hypertension, hypercholesterolemia, and smoking. HCM may also coexist with valvular aortic stenosis.

Clinical Findings

A. Symptoms and Signs

Slightly narrowed, thickened, or roughened valves **(aortic sclerosis)** or aortic dilation may contribute to the typical ejection murmur of aortic stenosis. In mild or moderate cases where the valve is still pliable, an ejection click may precede the murmur and the closure of the valve (S_2) is preserved. The characteristic systolic ejection murmur is heard at the aortic area and is usually transmitted to the neck and apex. In severe aortic stenosis, a palpable LV heave or thrill, a weak to absent aortic second sound, or reversed splitting of the second sound is present (see Table 10–1). In some cases, only the high-pitched components of the murmur are heard at the apex, and the murmur may sound like mitral regurgitation (the so-called **Gallavardin phenomenon**). When the valve area is less than 0.8–1.0 cm^2 (normal, 3–4 cm^2), ventricular systole becomes prolonged and the typical carotid pulse pattern of delayed upstroke and low amplitude is present. A delayed upstroke, though, is an unreliable finding in older patients with extensive arteriosclerotic vascular disease and a stiff, noncompliant aorta. LVH increases progressively due to the pressure overload, eventually resulting in elevation of ventricular end-diastolic pressure. Cardiac output is maintained until the stenosis is severe. LV failure, angina pectoris, or syncope may be presenting symptoms of significant aortic stenosis; importantly, all symptoms tend to first occur with exertion.

B. Redefining Severe Aortic Stenosis

There are four different anatomic syndromes that occur in patients with severe aortic stenosis. The common underlying measure of **severe aortic stenosis** is an aortic valve area of less than 1.0 cm^2 and echocardiographic evidence of an immobile aortic valve. In patients with a normal LVEF and normal cardiac output, the threshold for intervention is a peak aortic gradient of greater than 64 mm Hg and mean aortic gradient of greater than 40 mm Hg. In the same situation, **super-severe aortic stenosis** is defined as a mean gradient of greater than 55 mm Hg or peak aortic velocity greater than 5 m/seconds by Doppler.

In some patients with an aortic valve area of less than 1.0 cm^2 with a low cardiac output and stroke volume, the mean gradient may be less than 40 mm Hg. This can occur when the LV systolic function is poor (**low-gradient severe aortic stenosis with low LVEF**) or when the LV systolic function is normal **(paradoxical low-flow severe aortic stenosis with a normal LVEF).** Low flow (low output) in these situations is defined by an echocardiographic stroke volume index of less than 35 mL/minute/m^2. Prognosis in patients with low gradient, low valve area, low output, and a normal LVEF aortic stenosis may actually be worse than in patients with the traditional high gradient, low valve area, normal output, and normal LVEF aortic stenosis. If low-flow severe aortic stenosis is present in the face of a low LVEF, provocative testing with dobutamine or nitroprusside is sometimes warranted to increase the stroke volume to discover if a mean aortic valve gradient of at least 40 mm Hg can be demonstrated without increasing the aortic valve area. If the aortic valve area can be made to increase and a mean gradient of greater than 40 mm Hg cannot be demonstrated by inotropic challenge, the presumption is that the low gradient is due to an associated cardiomyopathy and not the aortic valve stenosis. In this latter situation intervention is not indicated. The guidelines acknowledge these four situations (Table 10–3). Intervention is indicated in super-severe aortic stenosis even without demonstrable symptoms (grade C) and in any of the other situations when symptoms are present: D1 defines the symptomatic high-gradient patient; D2 the symptomatic low-flow, low-gradient patient with low LVEF; and D3 the symptomatic low-flow, low-gradient patient with normal LVEF.

Symptoms of LV failure may be sudden in onset or may progress gradually. Angina pectoris frequently occurs in aortic stenosis due to underperfusion of the endocardium. Of patients with calcific aortic stenosis and angina, half have significant associated CAD. Syncope, a late finding, occurs with exertion as the LV pressure rises, stimulating the LV baroreceptors to cause peripheral vasodilation. This vasodilation results in the need for an increase in stroke volume, which increases the LV systolic pressure again, creating a cycle of vasodilation and stimulation of the baroreceptors that eventually results in a drop in systemic BP, as the stenotic valve prevents further increase in stroke volume. Less commonly, syncope may be due to arrhythmias (usually ventricular tachycardia but sometimes AV block as calcific invasion of the conduction system from the aortic valve may occur).

Table 10–3. Summary of AHA/ACC guideline definitions of symptomatic severe aortic stenosis.

Category of Severe Aortic Stenosis[1]	Properties
High Gradient	
High gradient	> 4.0 m/seconds Doppler jet velocity > 40 mm Hg mean gradient
Super-severe	> 5.0 m/seconds Doppler jet velocity > 55 mm Hg mean gradient
Low Gradient	
Low flow	Reduced LVEF (< 50%)
Low flow	Paradoxical with normal LVEF (> 50%)

[1]All categories of severe aortic stenosis have abnormal systolic opening of the aortic valve and an aortic valve area < 1.0 cm^2.

C. Diagnostic Studies

The ECG reveals LVH or secondary repolarization changes in most patients but can be normal in up to 10%. The chest radiograph may show (1) a normal or enlarged cardiac silhouette, (2) calcification of the aortic valve, and (3) dilation or calcification (or both) of the ascending aorta. The echocardiogram provides useful data about aortic valve calcification and leaflet opening, the severity of LV wall thickness, and overall ventricular function, while Doppler can provide an excellent estimate of the aortic valve gradient. Valve area estimation by echocardiography is a critical component of the diagnosis of aortic stenosis due to issues such as paradoxical low-flow aortic stenosis (low-gradient, low-flow, normal LVEF patients). Likewise, the echocardiography/Doppler can estimate the stroke volume index used to define the low-flow state when the valve area is small but the gradient is less than 40 mm Hg. Cardiac catheterization mostly provides an assessment of the hemodynamic consequence of the aortic stenosis, and the anatomy of the coronary arteries. Catheterization data can be important when there is a discrepancy between symptoms and the echocardiography/Doppler information of aortic stenosis severity. In younger patients and in patients with high aortic gradients, the aortic valve need not be crossed at catheterization. Aortic regurgitation can be semiquantified by aortic root angiography. Either BNP or NT-proBNP may provide additional prognostic data in the setting of poor LV function and aortic stenosis. A BNP greater than 550 pg/mL has been associated with a poor outcome in these patients regardless of the results of dobutamine testing. Current guidelines suggest intervention when the NT-proBNP is three times normal (class IIa indication). Stress testing can be done cautiously in patients in whom the aortic stenosis severity does not match the reported symptoms in order to confirm the reported clinical status. It should *not* be done in patients with super-severe aortic stenosis.

Prognosis & Treatment

Valve intervention is warranted in all patients who have symptomatic severe aortic stenosis (Figure 10–4). There are also times when asymptomatic aortic stenosis should undergo intervention. Asymptomatic patients with severe aortic stenosis (aortic valve area less than 1.0 cm^2) should generally undergo intervention according to the following guidelines: (1) they are undergoing other cardiac surgery (ie, CABG), (2) there is evidence for a reduced LVEF (less than 50%), (3) when the mean gradient exceeds 55 mm Hg (peak velocity greater than 5 m/seconds), (4) when there is exercise intolerance or when the BP falls more than 10 mm Hg with exercise, (5) when there is severe valvular calcium, (6) when there is evidence of a rapid increase in the peak aortic gradient (more than 0.3 m/seconds/year), (7) when there has been a progressive decrease in the LVEF, or (8) when the NT-proBNP is three times normal. Following the onset of heart failure, angina, or syncope, the prognosis without surgery is poor (50% 3-year mortality rate). Medical treatment may stabilize patients in heart failure, but intervention is indicated for all symptomatic patients with evidence of significant aortic stenosis.

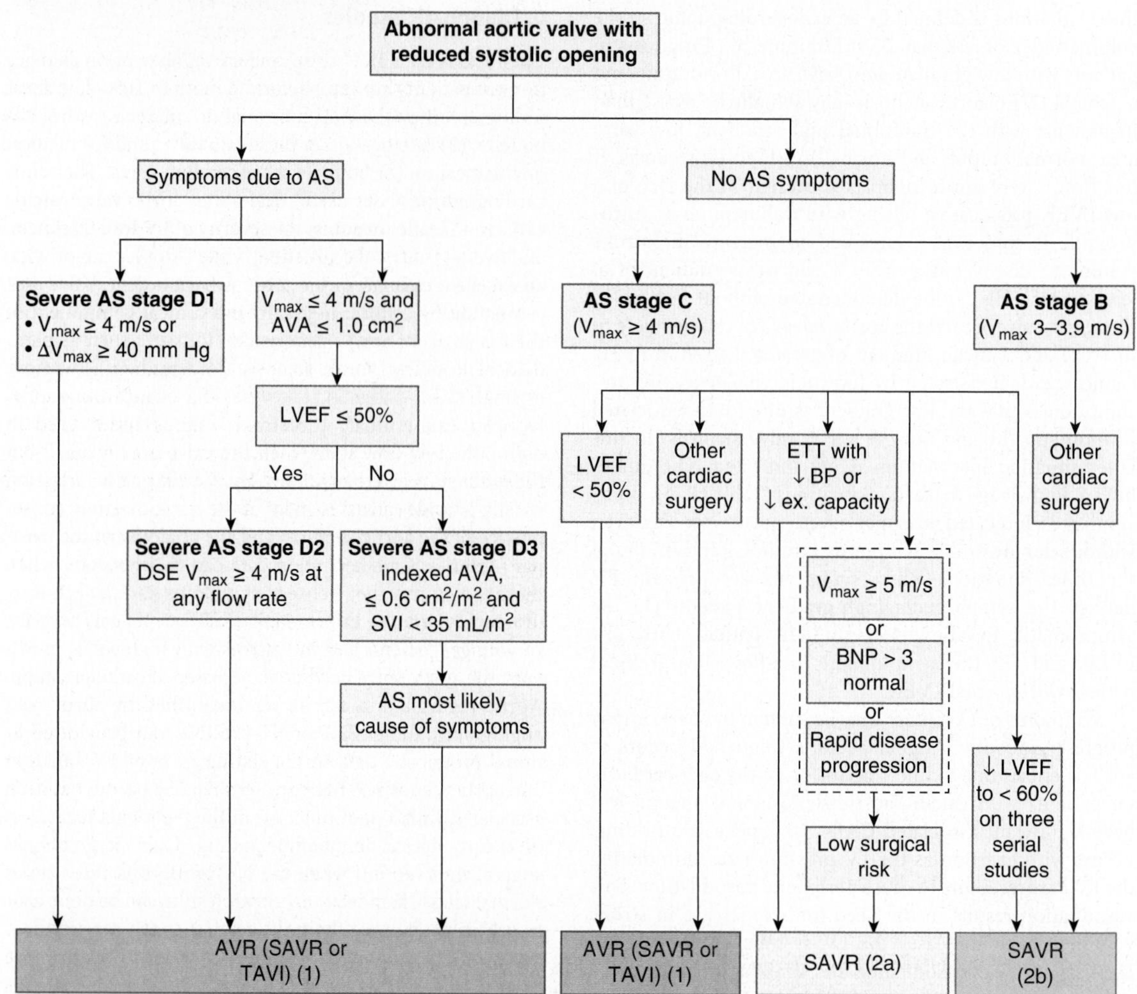

▲ **Figure 10–4.** Algorithm for the timing of intervention in aortic valve stenosis. AS, aortic stenosis; AVA, aortic valve area; AVAi, aortic valve area index; AVR, aortic valve replacement; BP, blood pressure; DSE, dobutamine stress echocardiography; ETT, exercise treadmill test; ΔP_{mean}, mean systolic pressure gradient between LV and aorta; SAVR, surgical aortic valve replacement; SVI, stroke volume index; TAVI, transcatheter aortic valve implantation; TAVR, transcatheter aortic valve replacement; V_{max}, maximum velocity. (Reprinted from Journal of the American College of Cardiology,77, Otto CM et al. 2020 ACC/AHA Guideline for the Management of Patients With Valvular Heart Disease A Report of the American College of Cardiology/American Heart Association Joint Committee on Clinical Practice Guidelines, e25–e197, 2021, with permission from Elsevier.)

The surgical mortality rate for valve replacement is low, even in older adults, and ranges from 2% to 5%. This low risk is due to the dramatic hemodynamic improvement that occurs with relief of the increased afterload. Mortality rates are substantially higher when there is an associated ischemic cardiomyopathy. Severe coronary lesions are usually bypassed at the same time as aortic valve replacement (AVR), although there are few data to suggest this practice affects outcome. In some cases, a staged procedure with stenting of the coronaries prior to surgery may be considered, especially if a percutaneous AVR approach is being considered. Around one-third to one-half of all patients with aortic stenosis have significant CAD, so this is a common concern. With the success of **transcatheter aortic valve replacement (TAVR)** or **transcatheter aortic valve implantation (TAVI),** the treatment options have greatly expanded for many patients with severe aortic stenosis. For this reason, a **Heart Valve Team** approach bringing together invasive and noninvasive cardiologists, radiologists, anesthesiologists, and cardiac surgeons is mandatory; clinical factors (such as frailty) and anatomic features (such as a calcified aorta, vascular access, etc) can affect the decision making.

Medical therapy to reduce the progression of disease has *not* been effective to date. Statins have been assessed in four major clinical trials. None revealed any benefit on the progression of aortic stenosis or on clinical outcomes despite the association of aortic stenosis with atherosclerosis. If patients with aortic stenosis have concomitant CAD, the guidelines for the use of statins should be followed. Efforts to reduce stenosis progression by blockage of the renin-angiotensin system have also been ineffective, though they are currently recommended for patients who have undergone TAVR. Control of systemic hypertension is an important adjunct, and inadequate systemic BP control is all too common due to unreasonable concerns about providing too much afterload reduction in patients with aortic stenosis. Normal systemic BP is important to maintain as the LV is affected by the total afterload (systemic BP plus the aortic valve gradient).

The interventional options in patients with aortic valve stenosis has expanded with the use of TAVR and depend on the patient's lifestyle and age. The algorithm to decide when an AVR is appropriate in various situations is outlined in Figure 10–5.

TAVR has been shown to be equivalent to surgical AVR (SAVR) in all the randomized trials of symptomatic patients, including those at low risk for surgery (less than 4%). Surgery is recommended for patients younger than 65 years or with a life expectancy of more than 20 years. TAVR is recommended for all patients older than 80 years. Either SAVR or TAVR can be considered for all patients between 65 and 80 years. The decision about whether to perform SAVR or TAVR should be made by the Heart Team; anatomic issues (such as an enlarged aorta, a coronary that might be trapped by a leaflet when the valve is inserted, an annulus too large or too small, extensive LV outflow tract calcium, etc) are often the deciding factors for whether TAVR can be done.

In young and adolescent patients, percutaneous balloon valvuloplasty still has a very small role. Balloon valvuloplasty is associated with early restenosis in the elderly population and, thus, is rarely used except as a temporizing measure prior to a more permanent SAVR or TAVR. Data suggest aortic balloon valvuloplasty in elderly people has an advantage only in those with preserved LV function, and such patients are usually excellent candidates for SAVR or TAVR.

The **Ross procedure** is generally still considered a viable option in younger patients with a bicuspid valve, and it is performed by moving the patient's own pulmonary valve and a portion of its root to the aortic position and replacing the pulmonary valve with a homograft (or rarely a bioprosthetic valve). The coronaries require reimplantation. However, dilation of the pulmonary valve autograft and consequent aortic regurgitation, plus early stenosis of the pulmonary homograft in the pulmonary position, has reduced the enthusiasm for this approach in most institutions. Current guidelines suggest the Ross procedure should only be considered in those younger than 50 years. Middle-aged and younger adults generally can tolerate the anticoagulation therapy necessary for the use of mechanical aortic valves, so patients younger than 50 years generally undergo AVR with a bileaflet mechanical valve. If the aortic root is severely dilated as well (greater than 4.5 cm), then the valve may be housed in a Dacron sheath (**Bentall procedure**) and the root replaced along with the aortic valve. Alternatively, a human homograft root and valve replacement can be used. In patients older than 50 years, bioprosthetic (either porcine or bovine pericardial) valves with a life expectancy of about 10–15 years are routinely used instead of mechanical valves to avoid need for anticoagulation. Data favor the bovine pericardial valve over the porcine aortic valve. Bioprosthetic valve degeneration in the larger valves can be potentially repaired by percutaneous valve-in-valve TAVR. If the aortic annulus is small, a bioprosthetic valve with a short sheath can be sewn to the aortic wall (the stentless AVR) rather than sewing the prosthetic annulus to the aortic annulus. (Annulus is a relative term when speaking of the aortic valve, since there is no true annulus.) Another popular surgical option when the aorta is enlarged is the use of the **Wheat procedure;** it involves aortic root replacement above the coronary arteries and replacement of the aortic valve below the coronary arteries. The coronary arteries thus remain attached to the native aorta between the new graft and prosthetic valve rather than being reimplanted onto an artificial sheath or homograft. Newer aortic valve replacements can be placed quickly through a small incision and often require only three stitches to anchor (ie, the Perceval or Intuity valve replacements). These can shorten pump times at surgery.

In patients with a bicuspid aortic valve, there is an associated ascending aortic aneurysm in about half. If the maximal dimension of the aortic root is greater than 5.5 cm, it is recommended to proceed with root replacement regardless of the severity of the aortic valve disease. It is also appropriate to intervene when the maximal aortic root size is greater than 5.0 cm in diameter if there is a family history of aortic dissection or the aortic root size increases by more than 0.5 cm in 1 year. The aortic valve may be replaced at the same time if at least moderate aortic stenosis is present or may be either left alone or repaired (valve sparing operation). If there is an indication for AVR and the root is greater than 4.5 cm in diameter, root replacement is also recommended at the time of SAVR.

The use of mechanical versus bioprosthetic AVR has changed over time. A bioprosthetic valve is acceptable for patients at any age for whom anticoagulant therapy is contraindicated, not desired, or cannot be managed, and is preferred in patients over the age of 65. An aortic mechanical valve should be used in patients younger than 50 years of age who can take warfarin. **Anticoagulation** with warfarin is required with the use of mechanical aortic valves, and the international normalized ratio (INR) should be maintained between 2.0 and 3.0 for bileaflet valves. In general, mechanical aortic valves are less subject to thrombosis than mechanical mitral valves and do not require bridging with enoxaparin unless there are other thromboembolic risk factors or it is an older generation AVR. Low-dose aspirin (eg, 81 mg daily) is recommended if there is a low bleeding risk. Some newer bileaflet mechanical valves (On-X) allow for a lower INR range from 1.5 to 2.0. Clopidogrel is recommended for the first 6 months after TAVR in combination with lifelong low-dose aspirin therapy (dual antiplatelet therapy). DOACs are *not* recommended for any mechanical valves but may be used in patients with

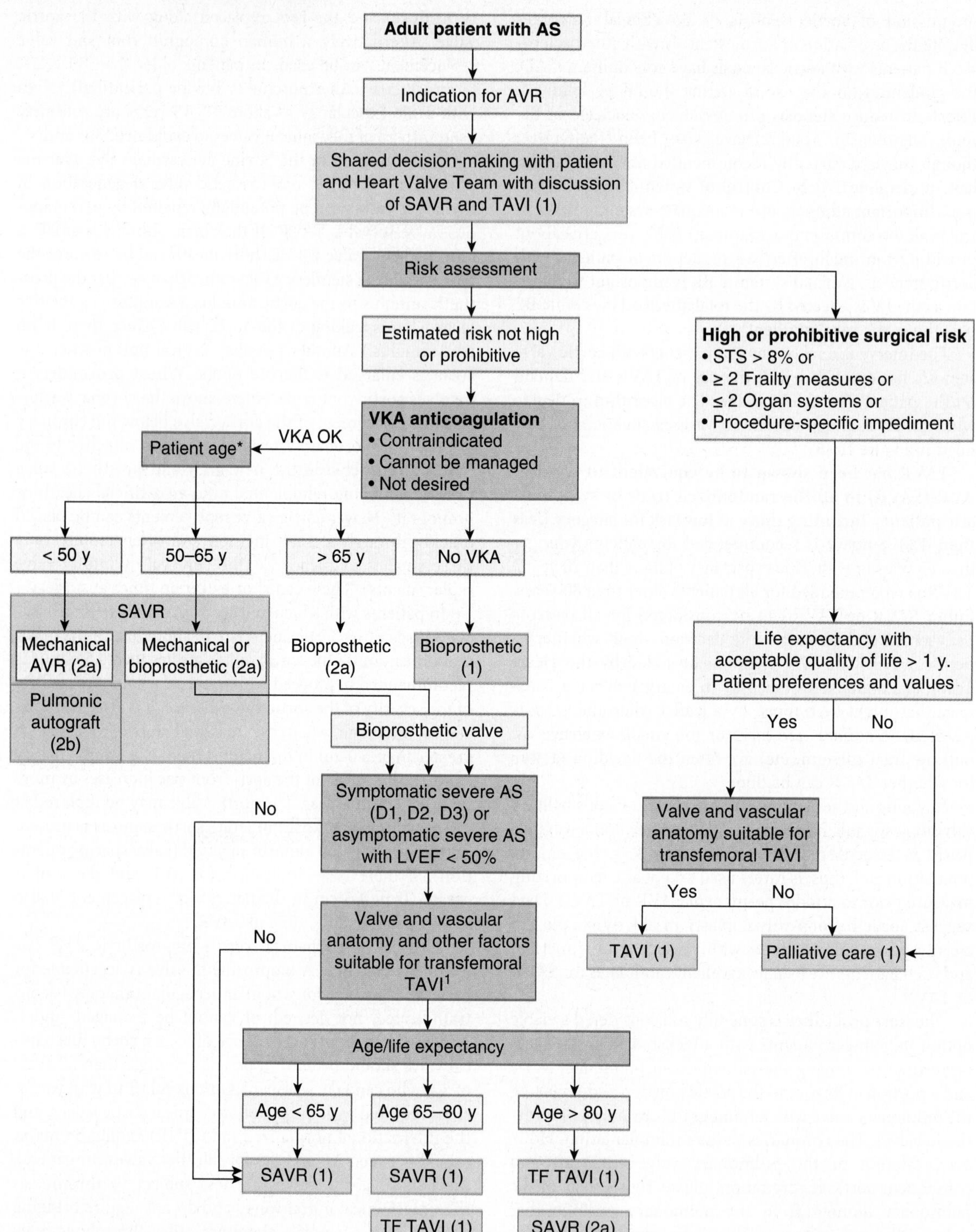

▲ **Figure 10–5. Algorithm for the type of valvular intervention in aortic valve stenosis. AS, aortic stenosis; AVR, aortic valve replacement; SAVR, surgical aortic valve replacement; STS, Society of Thoracic Surgeons; TAVI, transcatheter aortic valve implantation; TF, transfemoral; VKA, vitamin K antagonist.** (Reprinted from Journal of the American College of Cardiology,77, Otto CM et al. 2020 ACC/AHA Guideline for the Management of Patients With Valvular Heart Disease A Report of the American College of Cardiology/American Heart Association Joint Committee on Clinical Practice Guidelines, e25–e197, 2021, with permission from Elsevier.)

a bioprosthetic AVR if treating atrial fibrillation or venous thrombosis.

The use of TAVR has grown dramatically. The Edwards SAPIEN valve is a balloon-expandable valvular stent, while the CoreValve is a valvular stent that self-expands when pushed out of the catheter sheath. Cost remains a major issue. The cost of TAVR is similar to SAVR, mostly due to the cost of the valve itself. All of the professional societies stress the importance of a Heart Valve Team when considering aortic stenosis intervention.

TAVR is also being used more frequently in "valve-in-valve" procedures to reduce the gradient in patients with prosthetic valve dysfunction (regardless of whether in the aortic, mitral, tricuspid, or pulmonary position). While the results of TAVR in patients with bicuspid aortic valves (as opposed to tricuspid) have been less impressive, newer modifications have improved the success rates in these anatomic situations as well. This is supported by data from the TVT registry showing similar procedural and 1-year outcomes for patients with bicuspid or tricuspid aortic valve stenosis.

When to Refer

- All patients with echocardiographic evidence for mild-to-moderate aortic stenosis (estimated peak valve gradient greater than 30 mm Hg by echocardiography/Doppler) should be referred to a cardiologist for evaluation and to determine the frequency of follow-up.
- Any patients with symptoms suggestive of aortic stenosis (ie, exertional symptoms of chest pressure, shortness of breath, or presyncope) should be seen by a cardiologist.

Halim SA et al. Outcomes of transcatheter aortic valve replacement in patients with bicuspid aortic valve disease: a report from the Society of Thoracic Surgeons/American College of Cardiology Transcatheter Valve Therapy Registry. Circulation. 2020;141:1071. [PMID: 32098500]

Mack MJ et al; PARTNER 3 Investigators. Transcatheter aortic-valve replacement with a balloon-expandable valve in low-risk patients. N Engl J Med. 2019;380:1695. [PMID: 30883058]

Otto CM et al. 2020 ACC/AHA guideline for the management of patients with valvular heart disease. J Am Coll Cardiol. 2021; 77:450. [PMID: 33342587]

Popma JJ et al; Evolut Low Risk Trial Investigators. Transcatheter aortic-valve replacement with a self-expanding valve in low-risk patients. N Engl J Med. 2019;380:1706. [PMID: 30883053]

AORTIC REGURGITATION

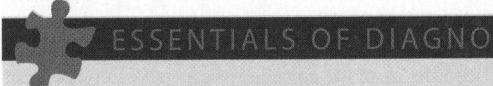

ESSENTIALS OF DIAGNOSIS

- Usually asymptomatic until middle age; presents with left-sided failure or rarely chest pain.
- Echocardiography/Doppler is diagnostic.
- Surgery for symptoms, EF < 50%, LV end-systolic dimension > 50 mm, or LV end-diastolic dimension > 65 mm.

General Considerations

Of all patients with isolated aortic valve disease, about 13% have predominately aortic regurgitation. Rheumatic aortic regurgitation has become much less common than in the preantibiotic era, and nonrheumatic causes now predominate. These include congenitally bicuspid valves, infective endocarditis, and hypertension. Many patients also have aortic regurgitation secondary to aortic root diseases, such as that associated with Marfan syndrome or aortic dissection. Rarely, inflammatory diseases, such as ankylosing spondylitis, may be implicated.

Clinical Findings

A. Symptoms and Signs

The clinical presentation is determined by the rapidity with which regurgitation develops. In **chronic aortic regurgitation,** the only sign for many years may be a soft aortic diastolic murmur. As the severity of the aortic regurgitation increases, diastolic BP falls, and the LV progressively enlarges. Most patients remain asymptomatic for long periods even at this point. LV failure is a late event and may be sudden in onset. Exertional dyspnea and fatigue are the most frequent symptoms, but paroxysmal nocturnal dyspnea and pulmonary edema may also occur. Angina pectoris or atypical chest pain may occasionally be present. Associated CAD and presyncope or syncope are less common than in aortic stenosis.

Hemodynamically, because of compensatory LV dilation, patients eject a large stroke volume, which is adequate to maintain forward cardiac output until late in the course of the disease. LV diastolic pressure may rise when heart failure occurs. Abnormal LV systolic function as manifested by reduced EF (less than 50%) and increasing end-systolic LV volume (greater than 5.0 cm) are signs that surgical intervention is warranted.

The major physical findings in chronic aortic regurgitation relate to the high stroke volume being ejected into the systemic vascular system with rapid runoff as the regurgitation takes place (see Table 10–1). This results in a **wide arterial pulse pressure.** The pulse has a rapid rise and fall (**water-hammer pulse** or **Corrigan pulse**), with an elevated systolic and low diastolic pressure. The large stroke volume and flow back into the heart are also responsible for characteristic findings, such as **Quincke pulses** (nailbed capillary pulsations), **Duroziez sign** (to-and-fro murmur over a partially compressed femoral peripheral artery), and **Musset sign** (head bob with each pulse). In younger patients, the increased stroke volume may summate with the pressure wave reflected from the periphery and create a higher than expected systolic pressure in the lower extremities compared with the central aorta. Since the peripheral bed is much larger in the leg than the arm, the BP in the leg may be over 40 mm Hg higher than in the arm (**Hill sign**) in severe aortic regurgitation. The apical impulse is prominent, laterally displaced, usually hyperdynamic, and may be sustained. A systolic flow murmur is usually present and may be quite soft and localized; the aortic diastolic murmur is usually high-pitched and decrescendo. A mid or late diastolic low-pitched mitral murmur (**Austin Flint murmur**) may be heard in advanced aortic regurgitation, owing to relative obstruction of mitral inflow produced by partial closure of the mitral valve by the rapidly rising LV diastolic pressure due to the aortic regurgitation.

In **acute aortic regurgitation** (usually from aortic dissection or infective endocarditis), LV failure is manifested primarily as pulmonary edema and may develop rapidly; surgery is urgently required in such cases. Patients with acute aortic regurgitation do not have the dilated LV of chronic aortic regurgitation and the extra LV volume is handled poorly. For the same reason, the diastolic murmur is shorter, may be minimal in intensity, and the pulse pressure may not be widened—making clinical diagnosis difficult. The mitral valve may close prematurely even before LV systole has been initiated (**preclosure**) due to the rapid rise in the LV diastolic pressure, and the first heart sound is thus diminished or inaudible. Preclosure of the mitral valve can be readily detected on echocardiography and is considered an indication for urgent surgical intervention.

B. Diagnostic Studies

The ECG usually shows moderate to severe LVH. Radiographs show cardiomegaly with LV prominence and sometimes a dilated aorta.

Echocardiography demonstrates the major diagnostic features, including whether the lesion includes the proximal aortic root and what valvular pathology is present. **Annual assessments of LV size and function are critical in determining the timing for valve replacement when the aortic regurgitation is severe.** The 2020 ACC/AHA valvular guideline provides criteria for assessing the severity of aortic regurgitation. Cardiac MRI and CT can estimate aortic root size, particularly when there is concern for an ascending aneurysm. MRI can provide a regurgitant fraction to help confirm severity. Cardiac catheterization may be unnecessary in younger patients, particularly those with acute aortic regurgitation, but can help define hemodynamics, aortic root abnormalities, and associated CAD preoperatively in older patients. Increasing data are emerging that serum BNP or NT-proBNP may be an early sign of LV dysfunction, and it is possible that these data will be added to recommendations for surgical intervention in the future.

Treatment & Prognosis

Aortic regurgitation that appears or worsens during or after an episode of infective endocarditis or aortic dissection may lead to acute severe LV failure or subacute progression over weeks or months. The former usually presents as pulmonary edema; surgical replacement of the valve is indicated even during active infection. These patients may be transiently improved or stabilized by vasodilators.

Chronic aortic regurgitation may be tolerated for many years, but the prognosis without surgery becomes poor when symptoms occur. Since aortic regurgitation places both a preload (volume) and afterload increase on the LV, medications that decrease afterload can reduce regurgitation severity, although there are no convincing data that afterload reduction alters mortality. **Recommendations advocate afterload reduction in aortic regurgitation only when there is associated systolic hypertension (systolic BP greater than 140 mm Hg).** Afterload reduction in normotensive patients does not appear warranted. ARBs, rather than beta-blockers, are the preferred additions to the medical therapy in patients with an enlarged aorta, such as in Marfan syndrome, because of the theoretical ability of an ARB to reduce aortic stiffness (by blocking TGF-beta) and to slow the rate of aortic dilation. However, clinical trials evaluating the efficacy of ARBs to reduce aortic stiffness and slow the rate of aortic dilation have not yielded a positive outcome to support their use.

Surgery is indicated once symptoms emerge or for any evidence of LV dysfunction (as exhibited by a reduction in the LVEF to less than 55% or increase in the LV end-systolic diameter to greater than 50 mm by echocardiography). In addition, it is suggested that surgery should be considered even when the LV becomes excessively enlarged (LV end-diastolic diameter greater than 65 mm). Guidelines also suggest it be considered (class IIb) if serial imaging reveals a progressive increase in the size of the LV (Figure 10–6).

The issues with AVR covered in the above section concerning aortic stenosis pertain here. Early trials of TAVR had a high incidence of postprocedural residual aortic regurgitation (18.8% in one trial). Newer TAVR valves have greatly reduced residual aortic regurgitation when used in patients with pure native aortic regurgitation (4.2%). In multivariable analysis, postprocedural at least moderate aortic regurgitation was independently associated with 1-year all-cause mortality. Compared with the early-generation devices, TAVR using the new-generation devices was associated with improved procedural outcomes in treating patients with pure native aortic regurgitation. In patients with pure native aortic regurgitation, significant postprocedural aortic regurgitation was independently associated with increased mortality.

Aortic regurgitation due to a paravalvular prosthetic valve defect can occasionally be occluded with percutaneous occluder devices. The choice of prosthetic valve for AVR depends on the patient's age and compatibility with warfarin anticoagulation similar to the choices for AVR in aortic stenosis.

The operative mortality for AVR is usually in the 3–5% range. Aortic regurgitation due to aortic root disease requires repair or replacement of the root as well as surgical treatment of the aortic valve. Though valve-sparing operations have improved recently, most patients with root replacement undergo valve replacement at the same time. Root replacement in association with valve replacement may require anastomosis of the coronary arteries, and thus the procedure is more complex than valve replacement alone. The Wheat procedure replaces the aortic root but spares the area where the coronaries attach to avoid the necessity for their reimplantation. Following any aortic valve surgery, LV size usually decreases and LV function generally improves even when the baseline EF is depressed.

Repair of the aortic root in patients with a bicuspid valve should be done once the root diameter exceeds 5.5 cm

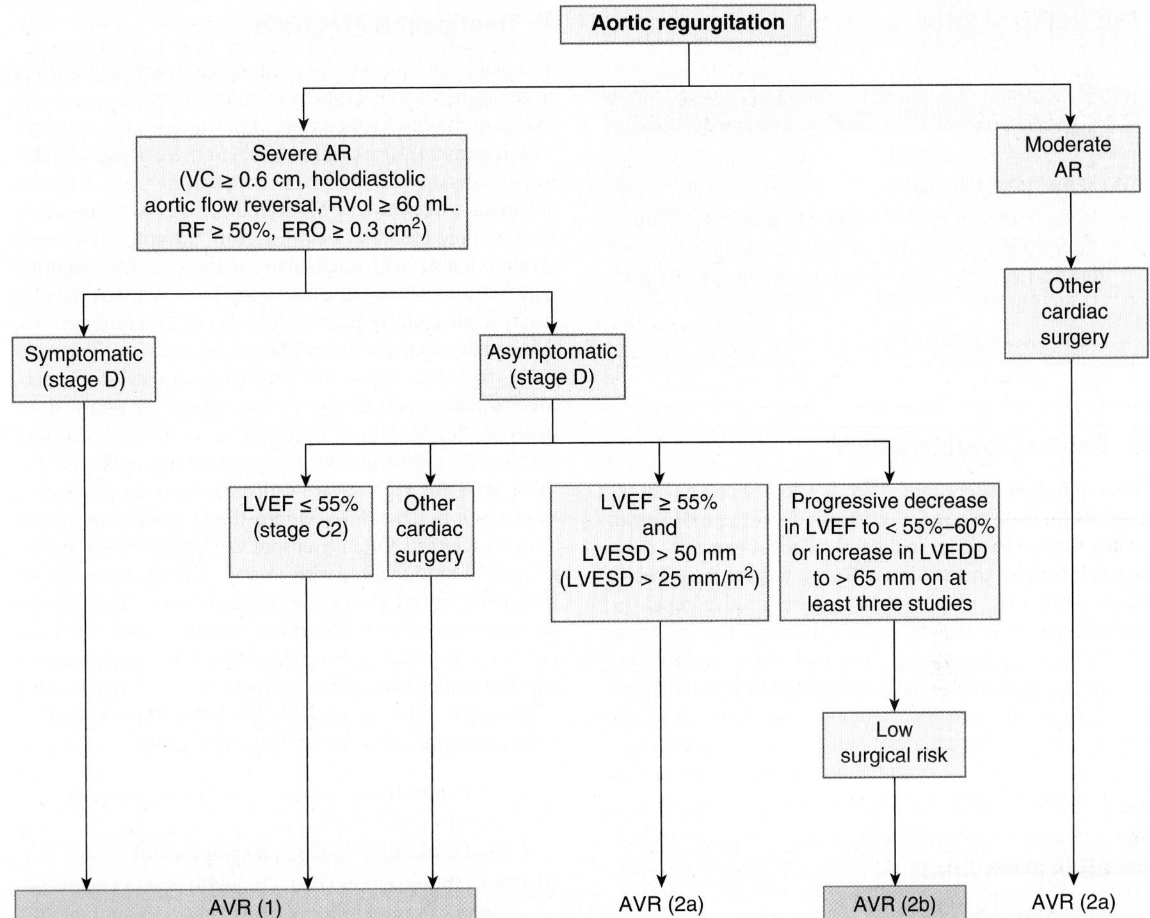

▲ **Figure 10–6.** Algorithm for intervention in aortic regurgitation. AR, aortic regurgitation; AVR, aortic valve replacement; EDD, end-diastolic dimension; ERO, effective regurgitant orifice; LVESD, LV end-systolic dimension; RF, regurgitant fraction; RVol, regurgitant volume; VC, vena contracta. (Reprinted from Journal of the American College of Cardiology,77, Otto CM et al. 2020 ACC/AHA Guideline for the Management of Patients With Valvular Heart Disease A Report of the American College of Cardiology/American Heart Association Joint Committee on Clinical Practice Guidelines, e25-e197, 2021, with permission from Elsevier.)

regardless of aortic valve disease severity. There are data that dissection is much more prevalent when the aortic root diameter exceeds 6.0 cm, and the general sense is not to let it approach that size. Patients with risk factors (family history of dissection or an increase in the diameter of the root greater than 0.5 cm in 1 year) should have the aorta repaired when the maximal dimension exceeds 5.0 cm. The following classifications summarize when to operate on the aortic root in patients with a bicuspid aortic valve based on the guidelines:

Class I indication (LOE C): aortic root diameter at sinuses or ascending aorta greater than 5.5 cm (regardless of need for AVR).

Class IIa indication (LOE C): aortic root diameter at sinuses or ascending aorta greater than 5.0 cm when there are associated risk factors (family history of dissection or increase in size more than 0.5 cm in 1 year).

Class IIa indication (LOE C): aortic root diameter greater than 4.5 cm if patient undergoing AVR for valvular reasons.

When to Refer

- Patients with audible aortic regurgitation should be seen, at least initially, by a cardiologist who can determine whether the patient needs follow-up.
- Patients with a dilated aortic root should be monitored by a cardiologist, since imaging studies other than the chest radiograph or echocardiogram may be required to decide surgical timing.

O'Gara PT et al. Timing of valve interventions in patients with chronic aortic regurgitation: are we waiting too long? J Am Coll Cardiol. 2019;73:1753. [PMID: 30846337]

Otto CM et al. 2020 ACC/AHA guideline for the management of patients with valvular heart disease. J Am Coll Cardiol. 2021;77:450. [PMID: 33342587]

TRICUSPID STENOSIS

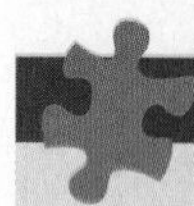

ESSENTIALS OF DIAGNOSIS

- Female predominance.
- History of rheumatic heart disease most likely. Carcinoid disease and prosthetic valve degeneration are the most common etiologies in the United States.
- Echocardiography/Doppler is diagnostic.

General Considerations

Tricuspid stenosis is rare, affecting less than 1% of the population in developed countries and less than 3% worldwide. Native valve tricuspid valve stenosis is usually rheumatic in origin. In the United States, tricuspid stenosis is more commonly due to prior tricuspid valve repair or replacement or to the carcinoid syndrome. The incidence of tricuspid stenosis after tricuspid valve replacement increases considerably after 8 years post surgery. Tricuspid regurgitation frequently accompanies the lesion. It should be suspected when right heart failure appears in the course of mitral valve disease or in the postoperative period after tricuspid valve repair or replacement.

Clinical Findings

A. Symptoms and Signs

Tricuspid stenosis is characterized by right heart failure with hepatomegaly, ascites, and dependent edema. In sinus rhythm, a giant *a* wave is seen in the JVP, which is also elevated (see Table 10–1). The typical **diastolic rumble** along the lower left sternal border mimics mitral stenosis, though in tricuspid stenosis the rumble *increases with inspiration.* In sinus rhythm, a presystolic liver pulsation may be found. It should be considered when patients exhibit signs of carcinoid syndrome.

B. Diagnostic Studies

In the absence of atrial fibrillation, the ECG reveals RA enlargement. The chest radiograph may show marked cardiomegaly with a normal PA size. A dilated superior vena cava and azygous vein may be evident.

The normal valve area of the tricuspid valve is 10 cm^2, so significant stenosis must be present to produce a gradient. Hemodynamically, a mean diastolic pressure gradient greater than 5 mm Hg is considered significant, although even a 2 mm Hg gradient can be considered abnormal. This can be demonstrated by echocardiography or cardiac catheterization. The 2017 update of the 2014 AHA/ACC guidelines suggests a tricuspid valve area of less than 1.0 cm^2 and a pressure half-time longer than 190 msec should be defined as significant because the gradient may vary depending on the heart rate.

Treatment & Prognosis

Tricuspid stenosis may be progressive, eventually causing severe right-sided heart failure. Initial therapy is directed at reducing the fluid congestion, with diuretics the mainstay (see Treatment, Heart Failure). When there is considerable bowel edema, torsemide or bumetanide may have an advantage over other loop diuretics, such as furosemide, because they are better absorbed from the gut. Aldosterone inhibitors also help, particularly if there is liver engorgement or ascites. Neither surgical nor percutaneous valvuloplasty is particularly effective for relief of tricuspid stenosis, as residual tricuspid regurgitation is common. Tricuspid valve replacement is the preferred surgical approach. Mechanical tricuspid valve replacement is rarely done because the low flow predisposes to thrombosis and because the mechanical valve cannot be crossed should the need arise for right heart catheterization or pacemaker implantation. Therefore, bioprosthetic valves are almost always preferred. Often tricuspid valve replacement is performed in conjunction with mitral valve replacement for rheumatic mitral stenosis or regurgitation. Percutaneous transcatheter valve replacement (stented valve) has been used in degenerative tricuspid prosthetic valve stenosis and a percutaneous tricuspid valve replacement device is being investigated. The indications for valve replacement in severe tricuspid stenosis are straightforward:

Class I indication (LOE C): at time of operation for left-sided valve disease.

Class I indication (LOE C): if symptomatic.

Class IIb indication (LOE C): rarely percutaneous balloon commissurotomy for isolated tricuspid stenosis in high-risk patients with no significant tricuspid regurgitation.

When to Refer

All patients with any evidence for tricuspid stenosis on an echocardiogram should be seen and monitored by a cardiologist to assess when intervention may be required.

Hirata K et al. Bioprosthetic tricuspid valve stenosis: a case series. Eur Heart J Case Rep. 2019;3:ytz110. [PMID: 31367735]

TRICUSPID REGURGITATION

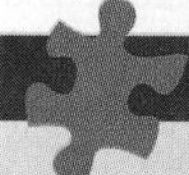

ESSENTIALS OF DIAGNOSIS

- Frequently occurs in patients with pulmonary or cardiac disease with pressure or volume overload on the right ventricle.
- Tricuspid valve regurgitation from pacemaker lead placement is becoming more common.
- Echocardiography useful in determining cause (low- or high-pressure tricuspid regurgitation).

General Considerations

Tricuspid valvular regurgitation often occurs whenever there is RV dilation from any cause. As tricuspid regurgitation increases, the RV size increases further pulling the valve open due to chordal and papillary muscle displacement. This, in turn, worsens the severity of the tricuspid regurgitation. In addition, the tricuspid annulus is shaped like a horse's saddle. With RV failure, the annulus flattens and becomes elliptical, further distorting the relationship between the leaflets and chordal attachments. In most cases, the cause of the tricuspid regurgitation is the RV geometry (functional) and not primary tricuspid valve disease. An enlarged, dilated RV may be present if there is RV systolic hypertension from valvular or subvalvular pulmonary valve stenosis, pulmonary hypertension for any reason, in severe pulmonary valve regurgitation, or in cardiomyopathy. The RV may also be injured from an MI or may be inherently dilated due to infiltrative diseases (RV dysplasia or sarcoidosis). RV dilation often occurs secondary to left heart failure. Inherent abnormalities of the tricuspid valve include **Ebstein anomaly** (displacement of the septal and posterior, but not the anterior, leaflets into the RV), tricuspid valve prolapse, carcinoid plaque formation, collagen disease inflammation, valvular tumors, or tricuspid endocarditis. In addition, pacemaker lead valvular injury is an increasingly frequent iatrogenic cause.

Clinical Findings

A. Symptoms and Signs

The symptoms and signs of tricuspid regurgitation are identical to those resulting from RV failure due to any cause. As a generality, the diagnosis can be made by careful inspection of the JVP. The JVP waveform should decline during ventricular systole (the *x* descent). The timing of this decline can be observed by palpating the opposite carotid artery. As tricuspid regurgitation worsens, more and more of this *x* descent valley in the JVP is filled with the regurgitant wave until all of the *x* descent is obliterated and a positive systolic waveform will be noted in the JVP. An associated tricuspid regurgitation murmur may or may not be audible and can be distinguished from mitral regurgitation by the left parasternal location and an increase with inspiration (**Carvallo sign**). An S_3 may accompany the murmur and is related to the high flow returning to the RV from the RA. Cyanosis may be present if the increased RA pressure stretches the atrial septum and opens a PFO or there is a true ASD (eg, in about 50% of patients with Ebstein anomaly). Severe tricuspid regurgitation results in hepatomegaly, edema, and ascites.

B. Diagnostic Studies

The ECG is usually nonspecific, though atrial flutter or atrial fibrillation is common. The chest radiograph may reveal evidence of an enlarged RA or dilated azygous vein and pleural effusion. The echocardiogram helps assess severity of tricuspid regurgitation (criteria available in the 2014 AHA/ACC valvular heart disease guidelines). In addition, echocardiography/Doppler provides RV systolic pressure as well as RV size and function. A paradoxically moving interventricular septum may be present due to the volume overload on the RV. Catheterization confirms the presence of the regurgitant wave in the RA and elevated RA pressures. If the PA or RV systolic pressure is less than 40 mm Hg, primary valvular tricuspid regurgitation should be suspected. In addition, in patients with severe tricuspid regurgitation and ascites, a hepatic wedge pressure can be performed at the time of the right heart catheterization. If there is a high gradient between the mean RA pressure and mean hepatic wedge, then cirrhosis is likely present. Normally, the gradient across the liver is less than 5 mm Hg. Mild cirrhosis is suspected if gradient is 5–10 mm Hg, moderate disease if 10–15 mm Hg, and significant cirrhosis if greater than 15 mm Hg.

Treatment & Prognosis

Mild tricuspid regurgitation is common and generally can be well managed with diuretics. When severe tricuspid regurgitation is present, bowel edema may reduce the effectiveness of diuretics, such as furosemide, and intravenous diuretics should be used initially. Torsemide or bumetanide is better absorbed in this situation when oral diuretics are added. Aldosterone antagonists have a role as well, particularly if ascites is present. At times, the efficacy of loop diuretics can be enhanced by adding a thiazide diuretic (see Treatment, Heart Failure).

Since most tricuspid regurgitation is secondary, definitive treatment usually requires elimination of the cause of the RV dysfunction. Surgical valve replacement in secondary (functional) tricuspid regurgitation is rarely if ever indicated until the cause of the RV dysfunction is resolved. If the problem is left heart disease, then treatment of the left heart issues may lower pulmonary pressures, reduce RV size, and resolve the tricuspid regurgitation. Treatment for primary and secondary causes of pulmonary hypertension will generally reduce the tricuspid regurgitation. Guidelines suggest that tricuspid valve surgery may be considered when the tricuspid annular dilation at end-diastole exceeds 4.0 cm and the patient is symptomatic. It is a class I recommendation that tricuspid annuloplasty be performed when significant tricuspid regurgitation is present and mitral valve replacement or repair is being performed for mitral regurgitation. Annuloplasty without insertion of a prosthetic ring (**DeVega annuloplasty**) may also be effective in reducing the tricuspid annular dilation. The valve leaflet itself can occasionally be primarily repaired in tricuspid valve endocarditis. If there is an inherent defect in the tricuspid valve apparatus that cannot be repaired, then replacement of the tricuspid valve is warranted. A bioprosthetic valve rather than a mechanical valve, is almost always used because the risk of mechanical valve thrombosis is increased if the INR is not stable. Anticoagulation is *not* required for bioprosthetic valves unless there is associated atrial fibrillation or flutter. Tricuspid regurgitation due to bioprosthetic degeneration has been shown to respond to transcatheter valve replacement. There are early reports of percutaneous tricuspid valve replacement for native valve tricuspid regurgitation being successful.

When to Refer

- Anyone with moderate or severe tricuspid regurgitation should be seen at least once by a cardiologist to determine whether studies and intervention are needed.
- Severe tricuspid regurgitation requires regular follow-up by a cardiologist.

Axtell AL et al. Surgery does not improve survival in patients with isolated severe tricuspid regurgitation. J Am Coll Cardiol. 2019;74:715. [PMID: 31071413]

Hahn RT et al. Anatomic relationship of the complex tricuspid valve, right ventricle, and pulmonary vasculature: a review. JAMA Cardiol. 2019;4:478. [PMID: 30994879]

PULMONARY VALVE REGURGITATION

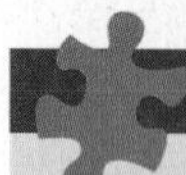

ESSENTIALS OF DIAGNOSIS

- Most cases are due to pulmonary hypertension resulting in high-pressure pulmonary valve regurgitation.
- Echocardiogram is definitive in high-pressure but may be less definitive in low-pressure pulmonary valve regurgitation.
- Low-pressure pulmonary valve regurgitation is well tolerated.

General Considerations

Pulmonary valve regurgitation can be divided into **high-pressure causes** (due to pulmonary hypertension) and **low-pressure causes** (usually due to a dilated pulmonary annulus, a congenitally abnormal [bicuspid or dysplastic] pulmonary valve, plaque from carcinoid disease, surgical pulmonary valve replacement, or the residual physiology following a surgical transannular patch used to reduce the outflow gradient in tetralogy of Fallot). Because the RV tolerates a volume load better than a pressure load, it tends to tolerate low-pressure pulmonary valve regurgitation for long periods of time without dysfunction.

Clinical Findings

Most patients are asymptomatic. Those with marked pulmonary valve regurgitation may exhibit symptoms of right heart volume overload. On examination, a hyperdynamic RV can usually be palpated (RV lift). If the PA is enlarged, it also may be palpated along the left sternal border. P_2 will be palpable in pulmonary hypertension and both systolic and diastolic thrills are occasionally noted. On auscultation, the second heart sound may be widely split due to prolonged RV systole or an associated right bundle branch block. A pulmonary valve systolic click may be noted as well as a right-sided gallop. If pulmonic stenosis is also present, the ejection click may decline with inspiration, while any associated systolic pulmonary murmur will increase. In high-pressure pulmonary valve regurgitation, the pulmonary diastolic (**Graham Steell**) murmur is readily audible. It is often contributed to by a dilated pulmonary annulus. The murmur increases with inspiration and diminishes with the Valsalva maneuver. In low-pressure pulmonary valve regurgitation, the PA diastolic pressure may be only a few mm Hg higher than the RV diastolic pressure, and there is little diastolic gradient to produce a murmur or characteristic echocardiography/Doppler findings. At times, only contrast angiography or MRI of the main PA will show the free-flowing pulmonary valve regurgitation in low-pressure pulmonary valve regurgitation. This situation is common in patients following repair of tetralogy of Fallot where, despite little murmur, there may effectively be no pulmonary valve present. This can be suspected by noting an enlarging right ventricle.

The ECG is generally of little value, although right bundle branch block is common, and there may be ECG criteria for RVH. The chest radiograph may show only the enlarged RV and PA. Echocardiography may demonstrate evidence of RV volume overload (paradoxical septal motion and an enlarged RV), and Doppler can determine peak systolic RV pressure and reveal any associated tricuspid regurgitation. The interventricular septum may appear flattened if there is pulmonary hypertension. The size of the main PA can be determined and color flow Doppler can demonstrate the pulmonary valve regurgitation, particularly in the high-pressure situation. Cardiac MRI and CT can be useful for assessing the size of the PA, for estimating regurgitant flow, for excluding other causes of pulmonary hypertension (eg, thromboembolic disease, peripheral PA stenosis), and for evaluating RV function. Cardiac catheterization is confirmatory only.

Treatment & Prognosis

Pulmonary valve regurgitation rarely needs specific therapy other than treatment of the primary cause. In low-pressure pulmonary valve regurgitation due to surgical transannular patch repair of tetralogy of Fallot, pulmonary valve replacement may be indicated if RV enlargement or dysfunction is present. In tetralogy of Fallot, the QRS will widen as RV function declines (a QRS greater than 180 msec, among other features, suggests a higher risk for sudden death) and increasing RV volumes should trigger an evaluation for potential severe pulmonary valve regurgitation. In carcinoid heart disease, pulmonary valve replacement with a porcine bioprosthesis may be undertaken, though the plaque from this disorder eventually coats the prosthetic pulmonary valve, limiting the life span of these valves. In high-pressure pulmonary valve regurgitation, treatment to control the cause of the pulmonary hypertension is key. High-pressure pulmonary valve regurgitation is poorly tolerated and is a serious condition that needs a thorough evaluation for cause and choice of therapy. Pulmonary valve replacement requires a bioprosthetic valve in most cases. Pulmonary valve regurgitation due to an RV to PA conduit or due to a pulmonary autograft replacement as part of the Ross procedure can be repaired with a percutaneous pulmonary valve (Melody valve). Bioprosthetic pulmonary valve regurgitation has also been treated using a percutaneous valve (Edwards Sapien). When the pulmonary valve is replaced percutaneously, the PA is often stented open to provide a platform for the percutaneous valve.

When to Refer

- Patients with pulmonary valve regurgitation that results in RV enlargement should be referred to a cardiologist regardless of the estimated pulmonary pressures.

MANAGEMENT OF ANTICOAGULATION FOR PATIENTS WITH PROSTHETIC HEART VALVES

The risk of thromboembolism is much lower with bioprosthetic valves than mechanical prosthetic valves. Mechanical mitral valve prostheses also pose a greater risk for thrombosis than mechanical aortic valves. For that reason, **the INR should be kept between 2.5 and 3.5 for mechanical mitral prosthetic valves but can be kept between 2.0 and 2.5 for most mechanical aortic prosthetic valves.** If there are additional risk factors in patients with a mechanical AVR (atrial fibrillation, previous thromboembolism, LV dysfunction, hypercoagulable state, or presence of older valve such as a ball-in-cage), then the INR for a mechanical AVR should be similar to a mechanical mitral valve replacement. Guidelines currently suggest the following as well: (1) a recommendation (class IIa) to expand the use of vitamin K antagonists (VKAs), such as warfarin, for up to 6 months after initial bioprosthetic valve replacement; (2) a lower target INR of 1.5–2.0 for a mechanical AVR using the On-X valve (class IIb); and (3) a consideration of VKA use with an INR of 2.5 for at least 3 months after TAVR (class IIa). Data from 2018 suggest that antiplatelet medications are inferior to warfarin for the prevention of thrombus in patients with the On-X mechanical valve. Concern regarding thrombus formation on bioprosthetic valves (including TAVR valves) also led to a class I recommendation to use multimodality imaging to identify such thrombus (class I). The DOAC rivaroxaban has *not* been found to prevent stroke related to emboli from TAVR and it should not be used. It is acceptable, though, to use DOACs for the treatment of atrial fibrillation in patients with bioprosthetic valves. For patients with a TAVR valve, it is reasonable to use dual antiplatelet therapy (clopidogrel and aspirin) for 3–6 months after the procedure. After that, lifelong low-dose aspirin should be used. As noted earlier, using warfarin for at least 3 months after TAVR is reasonable (class IIb), although that practice is widely variable. Randomized trials have not shown a benefit with DOACs after TAVR.

The European Registry of Pregnancy and Cardiac Disease (ROPAC) reported on a registry that compared pregnant women who had undergone mechanical and bioprosthetic valve replacement to pregnant women who had not. Maternal mortality was similar between the mechanical and bioprosthetic valve patients (1.5% and 1.4%, respectively) but was much higher than those without an artificial valve (0.2%). When patients with either mechanical or bioprosthetic valves were further assessed, it was found that pregnant women with mechanical valves were more likely to suffer adverse events than women with bioprosthetic valves. Hemorrhagic events occurred in 23.1% versus 9.2%, miscarriage on warfarin occurred in 28.6% versus 9.2%, and late fetal death was noted in 7.1% versus 0.7%, respectively. These data suggest **a high risk for mortality and morbidity for pregnant patients with mechanical heart valves,** and in the WHO Classification of Maternal Cardiac Risk, the presence of a mechanical valve is considered a class III (out of IV) risk for pregnancy complications.

Stoppage of warfarin for noncardiac surgery is likewise dependent on which mechanical valve is involved, the patient-specific risk factors, and the procedure contemplated. The risk of thromboembolism is highest in the first few months after valve replacement. While the interruption of warfarin therapy is generally safe, most cases of valve thrombosis occur during periods of inadequate anticoagulation, so the time interval without coverage should be kept as short as possible. High-risk features include atrial fibrillation, a prior history of thromboembolism, heart failure or low LVEF, a hypercoagulable state, a mechanical valve in the mitral position, a known high-risk valve (ball-in-cage), or concomitant hypercoagulable state (such as with an associated cancer). The use of bridging VKAs, unfractionated heparin, low-molecular-weight heparin (LMWH), and antifibrinolytics in various clinical situations in patients with valvular heart disease is summarized in Table 10–4. In general, low-risk procedures (eg, pacemaker implantation, cataract removal, and routine dental work) require no stoppage of VKAs, while in other situations the warfarin can be stopped 3 days ahead of the procedure and resumed the night after the procedure (ie, in patients with bileaflet aortic valves) without any bridging unfractionated heparin or LMWH. It is reasonable to consider bridging based on the CHA2DS2-VASc score in patients with bioprosthetic heart valves or annuloplasty rings who take anticoagulants for atrial fibrillation. In high-risk patients, principally just those with a mechanical mitral valve, the warfarin should be stopped and *bridging with either unfractionated heparin or LMWH* begun once the INR falls below therapeutic levels. Fresh frozen plasma or prothrombin complex concentrate is reasonable in an emergency situation for acute reversal if serious bleeding occurs. Most patients with a mechanical valve should not have the warfarin reversed with vitamin K, if it can be avoided, because this can result in a transient hypercoagulable state, and it may take many days to reach a therapeutic INR again.

Warfarin causes fetal skeletal abnormalities in up to 2% of women who become pregnant while taking the medication, so every effort is made to defer mechanical valve replacement in women until after childbearing age. However, if a woman with a mechanical valve becomes pregnant while taking warfarin, the risk of stopping warfarin may be higher for the mother than the risk of continuing warfarin for the fetus. The risk of warfarin to the fetal skeleton is greatest during the first trimester and, remarkably, is more related to dose than to the INR level. Guidelines suggest it is reasonable to continue warfarin for the first trimester if the dose is 5 mg/day or less. If the dose is more than 5 mg/day, it is appropriate to consider either LMWH (as long as the anti-Xa is being monitored [range: 0.8 units/mL

Table 10–4. Recommendations for administering vitamin K antagonist (VKA) therapy in patients undergoing procedures or patients with certain clinical conditions.

Procedures	Recommendations
General	Stop VKA 5 days prior and resume 12–24 hours after procedure
Bridging for mechanical heart valves	Required only for those at high risk for thromboembolism (generally only those with a mechanical mitral [not aortic] valve) Bridge with UFH or LMWH and stop UFH 4–6 hours before procedure or stop LMWH 24 hours before procedure Resume 48–72 hours after the procedure
Clinical Situations	**Recommendations**
Atrial fibrillation and moderate or severe mitral stenosis	VKA (target INR 2.0–3.0) If patient refuses, aspirin (50–100 mg) plus clopidogrel (75 mg)
Sinus rhythm and mitral stenosis	If left atrial size > 5.5 cm, then consider VKA (target 2.0–3.0)
Intermittent atrial fibrillation or history of systemic embolus and mitral stenosis	VKA (target INR 2.0–3.0)
Endocarditis	
Native valve or bioprosthetic valve endocarditis	No anticoagulation recommended
Mechanical valve endocarditis	Hold VKA until "safe to resume" (generally when mycotic aneurysm is ruled out or there is no need for urgent surgery)
Aspirin use in patients with a bioprosthetic valve	
Bioprosthetic aortic or mitral valve replacement	Aspirin (50–100 mg) indefinitely
Transcatheter valve replacement	Aspirin (50–100 mg) indefinitely plus clopidogrel (75 mg) for first 6 months. Reasonable to consider VKA to achieve INR 2.5 for first 3 months
Mitral or aortic repair	Aspirin (50–100 mg) indefinitely
Long-term anticoagulation after valve replacement	
Bioprosthetic valve in normal sinus rhythm	Aspirin (50–100 mg). Anticoagulation with a VKA to achieve an INR of 2.5 is reasonable for at least 3 months and up to 6 months after surgical MVR or AVR in patients at low risk for bleeding
Mechanical valve replacement	VKA (target INR 2.0–3.0 for mechanical aortic valve, target INR 1.5–2.5 for On-X aortic valve, target INR 2.5–3.5 for mechanical mitral valve) plus aspirin (50–100 mg)
Prosthetic valve thrombosis	
Right-sided valve	Slow infusion fibrinolytic therapy or intravenous heparin
Left-sided valve	Early surgery if thrombus large (> 0.8 cm^2), symptomatic from valvular obstruction, high surgical risk, or LA thrombus. Thrombolysis with heparin or slow-infusion fibrinolytic therapy may be tried initially if patient is stable If thrombus evident on bioprosthetic valve creating increased gradient, use of VKA reasonable to assess whether obstructive gradient can be improved
Pregnancy and a mechanical heart valve	Add aspirin (50–100 mg) for high risk VKA may be used during first trimester and throughout pregnancy if dose of warfarin is ≤ 5 mg/day If VKA dosage normally > 5 mg/day, then adjusted dose LMWH twice daily throughout pregnancy (follow anti-Xa 4 hours after dose, with target of 0.8 units/mL to 1.2 units/mL) or LMWH may be used only during the first trimester, then resume VKA during second and third trimesters ***or*** Adjusted dose UFH every 12 hours throughout pregnancy (aPTT > 2 times control) or UFH may be used only during the first trimester, then resume VKA during second and third trimester Discontinuation of VKA with initiation of UFH (2 times normal PTT) recommended before planned vaginal delivery

aPTT, activated partial thromboplastin time; AVR, aortic valve replacement; INR, international normalized ratio; LMWH, low-molecular-weight heparin; MVR, mitral valve replacement; PTT, partial thromboplastin time. UFH, unfractionated heparin.

Adapted from Nishimura RA et al. 2014 AHA/ACC guidelines for the management of patients with valvular heart disease: executive summary. Circulation. 2014;129:2440–92; and Nishimura RA et al. 2017 AHA/ACC focused update of the 2014 AHA/ACC guideline for the management of patients with valvular heart disease. J Am Coll Cardiol. 2017;70:252–289.

to 1.2 units/mL 4–6 hours post-dose]) or continuous intravenous unfractionated heparin (if the activated partial thromboplastin time [aPTT] can be monitored and is at least two times control). Guidelines suggest warfarin and low-dose aspirin are safe during the second and third trimester, and then should be stopped upon anticipation of delivery. At time of vaginal delivery, unfractionated intravenous heparin with aPTT at least two times control is desirable. DOACs (antithrombin or Xa inhibitors) should *not* be used in place of warfarin for mechanical prosthetic valves since there are no data that they are safe during pregnancy or safe for mechanical valves in general.

Management of suspected mechanical valve thrombosis depends on whether a left-sided or right-sided valve is involved, the size of the thrombus, and the patient's clinical condition. Simple fluoroscopy can help assess mechanical valve motion, although a TEE is indicated to assess thrombus size. **Therapeutic unfractionated heparin should be given to all patients with a thrombosed valve,** and this alone is generally effective. Fibrinolytic therapy is indicated if heparin therapy is ineffective and the clinical onset has been less than 2 weeks, the thrombus is smaller than 0.8 cm^2, New York Heart Association (NYHA) class symptoms are mild (functional class I or II), or the valve is right-sided. Surgery is rarely indicated; it is reserved for those with left-sided mechanical valves in NYHA functional class III or IV heart failure or in whom TEE demonstrates a mobile thrombus larger than 0.8 cm^2. The use of urgent initial therapy for a thrombosed mechanical valve should include low-dose, slow-infusion fibrinolytic therapy or urgent surgery if the patient is symptomatic.

Arya R. Pregnancy outcomes in women with mechanical prosthetic heart valves. Thromb Res. 2019;181:S37. [PMID: 31477226]

CORONARY HEART DISEASE (Atherosclerotic CAD, Ischemic Heart Disease)

CHD, or atherosclerotic CAD, is the number one cause of death in the United States and worldwide. Every minute in the United States, a person dies of CHD. About 37% of people who experience an acute coronary event, either angina or MI, will die of it in the same year. Death rates of CHD have declined every year since 1968, with about half of the decline from 1980 to 2000 due to treatments and half due to improved risk factors. CHD is still responsible for 1 in 4 of all deaths in the United States, totaling over 659,000 deaths annually. Each year, 805,000 individuals have a heart attack in the United States. CHD afflicts nearly 18.2 million Americans, and the prevalence rises steadily with age; thus, the aging of the US population promises to increase the overall burden of CHD.

Risk Factors for CAD

Most patients with CHD have some identifiable risk factor. These include a **positive family history** (the younger the onset in a first-degree relative, the greater the risk), **male sex, blood lipid abnormalities, diabetes mellitus, hypertension, physical inactivity, abdominal obesity, cigarette smoking, psychosocial factors,** and consumption of **too few fruits and vegetables** and **too much alcohol**. Many of these risk factors are modifiable. **Smoking remains the number one preventable cause of death and illness in the United States.** Although cigarette smoking rates have declined in the United States in recent decades, 12% of women and 15.6% of men still smoke. According to the World Health Organization, 1 year after quitting, the risk of CHD decreases by 50%. Various interventions have been shown to increase the likelihood of successful smoking cessation (see Chapter 1).

Hypercholesterolemia is an important modifiable risk factor for CHD. Risk increases progressively with higher levels of LDL cholesterol and declines with higher levels of HDL cholesterol. Composite risk scores, such as the Framingham score and the 10-year atherosclerotic CVD risk calculator (http://my.americanheart.org/cvriskcalculator), provide estimates of the 10-year probability of development of CHD that can guide primary prevention strategies. The 2018 ACC/AHA Guideline on the Treatment of Blood Cholesterol to Reduce Atherosclerotic Cardiovascular Risk in Adults suggests statin therapy in four populations: patients with (1) clinical atherosclerotic disease, (2) LDL cholesterol 190 mg/dL or higher, (3) diabetes who are aged 40–75 years, and (4) an estimated 10-year atherosclerotic risk of 7.5% or more aged 40–75 years (Figure 10–7). Importantly, *the guidelines do not recommend treating to a target LDL cholesterol.* Patients in these categories should be treated with a moderate- or high-intensity statin, with high-intensity statin for the higher-risk populations (Table 10–5). The ACC/AHA atherosclerotic CVD estimator allows clinicians to determine the 10-year CHD risk to determine treatment decisions (http://tools.acc.org/ascvd-risk-estimator-plus/).

The **metabolic syndrome** is defined as a constellation of three or more of the following: abdominal obesity, triglycerides 150 mg/dL or higher, HDL cholesterol less than 40 mg/dL for men or less than 50 mg/dL for women, fasting glucose 110 mg/dL or higher, and hypertension. This syndrome is increasing in prevalence at an alarming rate. Related to the metabolic syndrome, the epidemic of **obesity** in the United States is likewise a major factor contributing to CHD risk.

Myocardial Hibernation & Stunning

Areas of myocardium that are persistently underperfused but still viable may develop sustained contractile dysfunction. This phenomenon, which is termed **myocardial hibernation,** appears to represent an adaptive response that may be associated with depressed LV function. It is important to recognize this phenomenon, since this form of dysfunction is reversible following coronary revascularization. Hibernating myocardium can be identified by radionuclide testing, PET, contrast-enhanced MRI, or its retained response to inotropic stimulation with dobutamine. A related phenomenon, termed **myocardial stunning,** is the occurrence of persistent contractile dysfunction following prolonged or repetitive episodes of myocardial

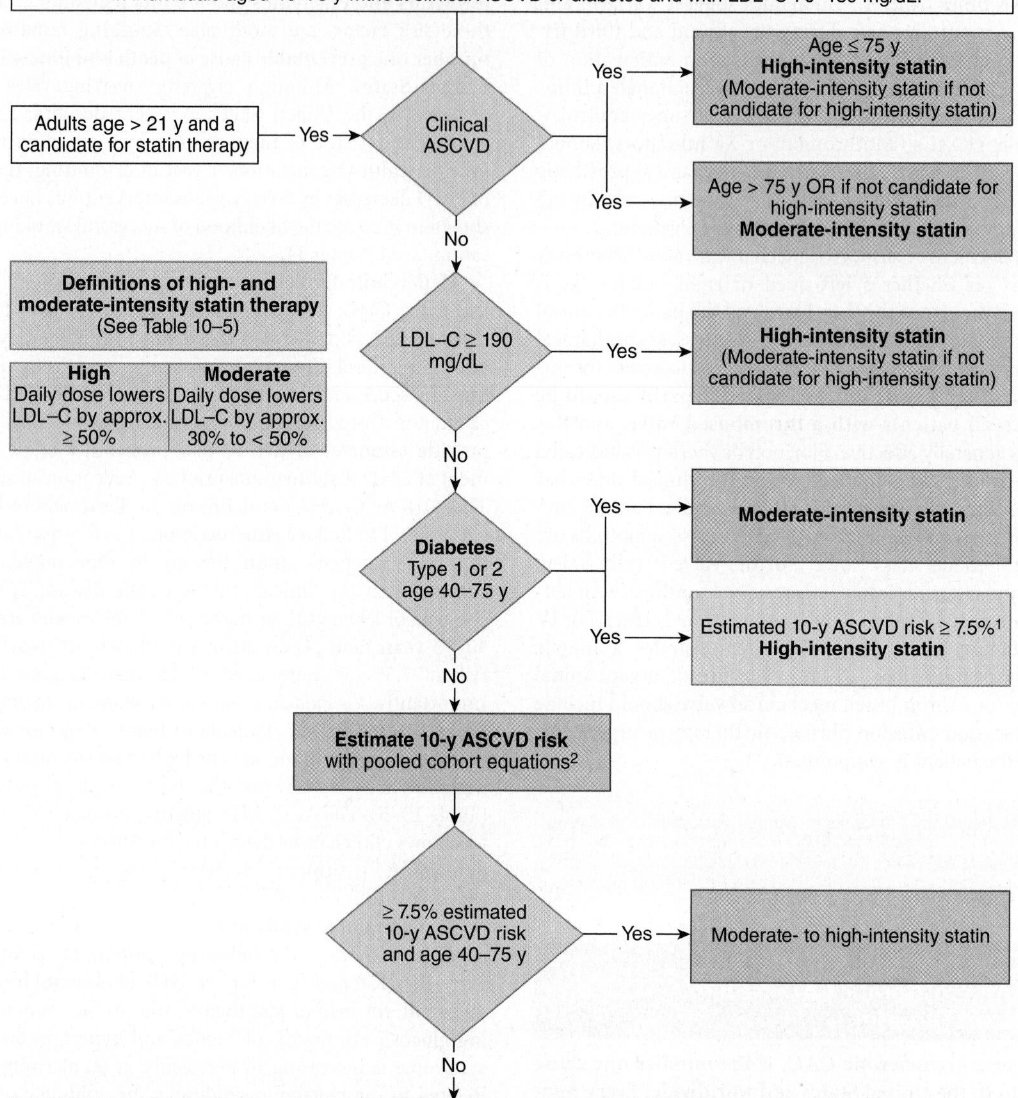
ASCVD statin benefit groups
Heart healthy lifestyle habits are the foundation of ASCVD prevention.
In individuals not receiving cholesterol-lowering drug therapy, recalculate estimated 10-y ASCVD risk every 4–6 y in individuals aged 40–75 y without clinical ASCVD or diabetes and with LDL–C 70–189 mg/dL.
Adults age > 21 y and a candidate for statin therapy
Yes
Clinical ASCVD
Yes
Age ≤ 75 y
High-intensity statin
(Moderate-intensity statin if not candidate for high-intensity statin)
Yes
Age > 75 y OR if not candidate for high-intensity statin
Moderate-intensity statin
No
Definitions of high- and moderate-intensity statin therapy
(See Table 10–5)
High
Daily dose lowers LDL–C by approx. ≥ 50%
Moderate
Daily dose lowers LDL–C by approx. 30% to < 50%
LDL–C ≥ 190 mg/dL
Yes
High-intensity statin
(Moderate-intensity statin if not candidate for high-intensity statin)
No
Diabetes
Type 1 or 2
age 40–75 y
Yes
Moderate-intensity statin
Yes
Estimated 10-y ASCVD risk ≥ 7.5%1
High-intensity statin
No
Estimate 10-y ASCVD risk
with pooled cohort equations2
≥ 7.5% estimated 10-y ASCVD risk and age 40–75 y
Yes
Moderate- to high-intensity statin
No
ASCVD prevention benefit of statin therapy may be less clear in other groups.
In selected individuals, consider additional factors influencing ASCVD risk3 and potential ASCVD risk benefits and adverse effects, drug-drug interactions, and patient preferences for statin treatment.

[1]Percent reduction in LDL–C can be used as an indication of response and adherence to therapy but is not in itself a treatment goal.

[2]The Pooled Cohort Equations can be used to estimate 10-year ASCVD risk in individuals with and without diabetes. A downloadable spreadsheet enabling estimation of 10-year and lifetime risk for ASCVD and a web-based calculator are available at http://my.americanheart.org/cvriskcalculator and http://www.cardiosource.org/science-and-quality/practice-guidelines-and-quality-standards/2013-prevention-guideline-tools.aspx.

[3]Primary LDL–C ≥ 160 mg/dL or other evidence of genetic hyperlipidemias, family history of premature ASCVD with onset < 55 years of age in a first-degree male relative or < 65 years of age in a first-degree female relative, high-sensitivity C-reactive protein > 2 mg/L, CAC score ≥ 300 Agatston units or ≥ 75 percentile for age, sex, and ethnicity, ankle-brachial index < 0.9, or elevated lifetime risk of ASCVD.

▲ **Figure 10–7. Major recommendations for statin therapy for atherosclerotic CVD prevention. ASCVD, atherosclerotic CVD; CAC, coronary artery calcium; LDL–C, LDL cholesterol.** (Adapted from Stone NJ et al. 2013 ACC/AHA guideline on the treatment of blood cholesterol to reduce atherosclerotic cardiovascular risk in adults: a report of the American College of Cardiology/American Heart Association Task Force on Practice Guidelines. Circulation. 2014;129:S1.)

Table 10–5. High-, moderate-, and low-intensity statin therapy.[1,2,3]

High-Intensity Statin Therapy	Moderate-Intensity Statin Therapy	Low-Intensity Statin Therapy
LDL–C lowering[4] ≥ 50%	LDL–C lowering[4] 30% to 49%	LDL-C lowering[4] < 30%
Atorvastatin (40 mg[5]) 80 mg **Rosuvastatin 20 mg (40 mg)**	**Atorvastatin 10 mg** (*20 mg*) **Rosuvastatin** (*5 mg*) **10 mg** **Simvastatin 20–40 mg[6]** **Pravastatin 40 mg** (*80 mg*) **Lovastatin 40 mg** (*80 mg*) *Fluvastatin XL 80 mg* **Fluvastatin 40 mg twice daily** *Pitavastatin 1–4 mg*	*Simvastatin 10 mg* **Pravastatin 10–20 mg** **Lovastatin 20 mg** *Fluvastatin 20–40 mg*

[1]Percent LDL-C reductions with the primary statin medications used in clinical practice (atorvastatin, rosuvastatin, simvastatin) were estimated using the median reduction in LDL-C from the VOYAGER database.S3.2.1-2 Reductions in LDL-C for other statin medications (fluvastatin, lovastatin, pitavastatin, pravastatin) were identified according to FDA-approved product labeling in adults with hyperlipidemia, primary hypercholesterolemia, and mixed dyslipidemia.
[2]**Boldface type** indicates specific statins and doses that were evaluated in RCTs, and the Cholesterol Treatment Trialists' 2010 meta-analysis. All these RCTs demonstrated a reduction in major cardiovascular events.
[3]Percent reductions are estimates from data across large populations. Individual responses to statin therapy varied in the RCTs and should be expected to vary in clinical practice.
[4]LDL-C lowering that should occur with the dosage listed below.
[5]Evidence from one RCT only: down-titration if unable to tolerate atorvastatin 80 mg in IDEAL study.
[6]Although simvastatin 80 mg was evaluated in RCTs, initiation of simvastatin 80 mg or titration to 80 mg is not recommended by the FDA due to the increased risk of myopathy, including rhabdomyolysis.
IDEAL, Incremental Decrease through Aggressive Lipid Lowering study; LDL–C, low-density lipoprotein cholesterol; RCTs, randomized controlled trials.

ischemia. Clinically, myocardial stunning is often seen after reperfusion of acute MI and is defined with improvement following revascularization.

Creamer MR et al. Tobacco product use and cessation indicators among adults—United States, 2018. MMWR Morb Mortal Wkly Rep. 2019;68:1013. [PMID: 31725711]
Virani SS et al; American Heart Association Council on Epidemiology and Prevention Statistics Committee and Stroke Statistics Subcommittee. Heart disease and stroke statistics—2021 update: a report from the American Heart Association. Circulation. 2021;143:e254. [PMID: 33501848]

Primary & Secondary Prevention of CHD

Although many risk factors for CHD are not modifiable, it is now clear that interventions, such as smoking cessation, treatment of dyslipidemia, and lowering of BP can both prevent coronary disease and delay its progression and complications after it is manifest.

Lowering LDL levels delays the progression of atherosclerosis and in some cases may produce regression. Even in the absence of regression, fewer new lesions develop, endothelial function may be restored, and coronary event rates are markedly reduced in patients with clinical evidence of vascular disease.

A series of clinical trials has demonstrated the efficacy of hydroxymethylglutaryl coenzyme A (HMG-CoA) reductase inhibitors (statins) in preventing death, coronary events, and strokes. Beneficial results have been found in patients who have already experienced coronary events (secondary prevention), those at particularly high risk for events (patients with diabetes and patients with peripheral artery disease), those with elevated cholesterol without multiple risk factors, and those without vascular disease or diabetes with elevated high-sensitivity CRP (hsCRP) with normal LDL levels. The benefits of statin therapy at moderate and high doses (Table 10–5) are recommended by the cholesterol treatment guidelines. The IMPROVE-IT study showed that ezetimibe, 10 mg daily, combined with simvastatin was modestly better than simvastatin alone in reducing the risk of MI and ischemic stroke, but not mortality, in stabilized patients following an acute coronary syndrome. This was associated with a reduction of LDL to 53.7 mg/dL compared to 69.7 mg/dL. With this data, ezetimibe can be used in combination with statin therapy in patients who are not at target cholesterol level for secondary prevention (for individuals at high risk for cardiovascular events with an LDL > 70 on maximal intensity statin therapy [IIa recommendation]) or cannot tolerate high-dose statin therapy.

Benefits occurred regardless of age, race, baseline cholesterol levels, or the presence of hypertension. It is clear that for patients with vascular disease, statins provide benefit for those with normal cholesterol levels, and that more aggressive statin use is associated with greater benefits. **All patients at significant risk for vascular events should**

receive a statin regardless of their cholesterol levels, and many experts recommend that with those who have prior cardiovascular events should have their LDL lowered below 70 mg/dL.

Monoclonal antibodies that inhibit proprotein convertase subtilisin/kexin type 9 (PCSK9) reduce LDL cholesterol levels significantly beyond levels associated with traditional statin therapy. These therapies have been studied in randomized trials of patients with maximally tolerated statin therapy (and for patients with statin intolerance) and have lowered LDL with signals of improved cardiovascular outcomes. The FOURIER trial showed that the PCSK9 inhibitor evolocumab, on top of statin, reduced the composite of atherothrombotic outcomes by 20% but did not reduce mortality. The ODYSSEY Outcomes trial demonstrated alirocumab reduced cardiovascular events in patients with acute coronary syndromes. Alirocumab and evolocumab have been approved by the FDA for patients on maximally tolerated statin therapy with familial hypercholesterolemia and atherosclerotic vascular disease, or both, and who require additional lowering of LDL. These medications cost several thousand dollars per year in the United States. Alirocumab has also been approved by the FDA for secondary prevention of cardiovascular events. Inclisiran (a small interfering RNA that goes to the liver and prevents the production of PCSK9) has been studied as a twice yearly injection showing reduction in LDL. The therapy was approved by the FDA in early 2022.

While fish oil supplements have *not* been shown to provide benefit for reducing risk, icosapent ethyl, a concentrated eicosapentaenoic acid at a high dose, was shown to be beneficial in the REDUCE-IT trial. Patients with established CVD or with diabetes and other risk factors, with fasting triglyceride level of 135–499 mg/dL, who were on statins were randomized to 2 g of icosapent ethyl twice daily or placebo. There was a 26% relative risk reduction in cardiovascular death, MI, and stroke, as well as a 20% relative risk reduction in cardiovascular death. Icosapent ethyl is approved by the FDA as an adjunct to maximally tolerated statin therapy to reduce the risk of MI, stroke, coronary revascularization, or unstable angina requiring hospitalization in patients with triglycerides of 150 mg/dL or more and either established CVD or diabetes mellitus and two or more additional risk factors. The role of high-dose omega-3 fatty acids was studied compared to corn oil and not shown to reduce cardiovascular events, leading to increased interest in comparative studies.

Treatment to raise HDL levels has failed to show benefit. The AIM High trial found no benefit from the addition of niacin in patients with vascular disease and a serum LDL near 70 mg/dL who were receiving statin therapy. The HPS2-THRIVE trial found no benefit but rather substantial harm of extended-release niacin (2 g) plus laropiprant (an antiflushing agent) for preventing vascular events in a population of over 25,000 patients with vascular disease who were taking simvastatin.

For *primary* prevention, aspirin has little overall benefit, including for patients with established diabetes, and is not recommended for most patients. In October 2021, the USPSTF issued guidance on the use of aspirin for primary prevention of cardiovascular events. The document recommended that patient ages 40–49 should have a shared-decision making conversation regarding the potential risk and benefits of initiating aspirin therapy for primary prevention. In addition, the document recommended that patients 60 years of age and older should not initiate aspirin for primary prevention of CVD.

Antiplatelet therapy is a very effective measure for *secondary* prevention and patients with established vascular disease should be treated with aspirin. The exact dose of aspirin in chronic CAD (81 mg vs 325 mg) was evaluated in a large pragmatic trial (ADAPTABLE). The unique pragmatic clinical trial design demonstrated that 81 mg aspirin was associated with a favorable cardiovascular event risk and bleeding risk compared with 325 mg daily.

While clopidogrel was found to be effective at preventing vascular events for 9–12 months after acute coronary syndromes, and there are some benefits in prolonging dual antiplatelet therapy after coronary stenting, clopidogrel was *not* found to be effective at preventing vascular events in combination with aspirin with longer-term treatment in the CHARISMA trial. This trial included patients with clinically evident stable atherothrombosis or with multiple risk factors; all were treated with aspirin and observed for a median of 28 months.

In the COMPASS trial, rivaroxaban, a direct factor Xa inhibitor, at a dose of 2.5 mg twice daily in addition to 100 mg of aspirin, was shown to reduce cardiovascular death, MI, and stroke by a relative risk reduction of 24% compared to 100 mg aspirin monotherapy in stable patients with CAD and peripheral artery disease. Bleeding was modestly increased. All-cause mortality was also reduced by 18%. This regimen is approved by the FDA and is used for long-term management of patients with CAD and peripheral artery disease and should be considered in this group at high risk for adverse cardiac events with a low bleeding risk profile.

The HOPE and the EUROPA trials demonstrated that ACE inhibitors (ramipril 10 mg/day and perindopril 8 mg/day, respectively) reduced fatal and nonfatal vascular events (cardiovascular deaths, nonfatal MIs, and nonfatal strokes) by 20–25% in patients at high risk, including patients with diabetes with additional risk factors or patients with clinical coronary, cerebral, or peripheral arterial atherosclerotic disease. An overview of these trials has demonstrated that while low-risk patients may *not* derive substantial benefits from ACE inhibitors, **most patients with vascular disease, even in the absence of heart failure or LV dysfunction, should be treated with an ACE inhibitor.**

Over one-third of patients with vascular disease have type 2 diabetes. In addition to controlling risk factors, using high-intensity statins and ACE inhibitors or ARBs, **there is proven benefit to reduce cardiovascular events by using oral sodium–glucose cotransporter 2 (SGLT2) inhibitors (specifically, empagliflozin, dapagliflozin, or canagliflozin) or injectable GLP1-receptor agonists (liraglutide, semaglutide, dulaglutide).** The cardiovascular benefits appear to be independent from the modest glucose lowering effects, and SGLT2 inhibitors have benefits for patients with heart failure regardless of whether they have diabetes (see Heart Failure section). In addition, newer data demonstrate the cardiovascular outcome benefits in patients with both heart failure with reduced EF and heart failure with preserved EF.

Anker SD et al; EMPEROR-Preserved Trial Investigators. Empagliflozin in heart failure with a preserved ejection fraction. N Engl J Med. 2021;385:1451. [PMID: 34449189]

Arnett DK et al. 2019 ACC/AHA guideline on the primary prevention of cardiovascular disease: part 1, lifestyle and behavioral factors. JAMA Cardiol. 2019;4:1043. [PMID: 31365022]

Bhatt DL et al; REDUCE-IT Investigators. Cardiovascular risk reduction with icosapent ethyl for hypertriglyceridemia. N Engl J Med. 2019;380:11. [PMID: 30415628]

Jones WS et al; ADAPTABLE Team. Comparative effectiveness of aspirin dosing in cardiovascular disease. N Engl J Med. 2021;384:1981. [PMID: 33999548]

Nicholls SJ et al. Effect of high-dose omega-3 fatty acids vs corn oil on major adverse cardiovascular events in patients at high cardiovascular risk: the STRENGTH randomized clinical trial. JAMA. 2020;324:2268. [PMID: 33190147]

US Preventive Services Task Force. USPSTF Bulletin: Task Force Issues Draft Recommendation Statement on Aspirin Use to Prevent Cardiovascular Disease. 2021 Oct 21. https://www.uspreventiveservicestaskforce.org/uspstf/sites/default/files/file/supporting_documents/aspirin-cvd-prevention-final-rec-bulletin.pdf

Zheng SL et al. Association of aspirin use for primary prevention with cardiovascular events and bleeding events: a systematic review and meta-analysis. JAMA. 2019;321:277. [PMID: 30667501]

CHRONIC STABLE ANGINA PECTORIS (Chronic Coronary Syndromes)

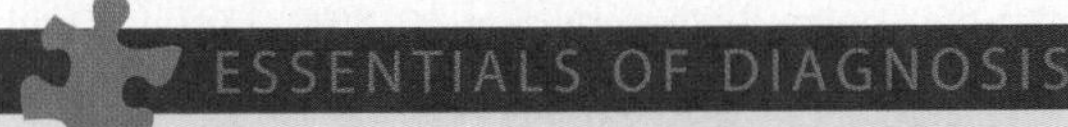

- Precordial chest pain, usually precipitated by stress or exertion, relieved rapidly by rest or nitrates.
- ECG or scintigraphic evidence of ischemia during pain or stress testing.
- Angiographic demonstration of significant obstruction of major coronary vessels.

General Considerations

Angina pectoris is the manifestation of stable CAD or chronic coronary syndromes, and it is usually due to atherosclerotic heart disease. Coronary vasospasm may occur at the site of a lesion or, less frequently, in apparently normal vessels. Other unusual causes of coronary artery obstruction, such as congenital anomalies, emboli, arteritis, or dissection may cause ischemia or infarction. Angina may also occur in the absence of coronary artery obstruction as a result of severe myocardial hypertrophy, severe aortic stenosis or regurgitation, or in response to increased metabolic demands, as in hyperthyroidism, marked anemia, or paroxysmal tachycardias with rapid ventricular rates.

Clinical Findings

A. Symptoms

The diagnosis of angina pectoris principally depends on the history, which should specifically include the following information: circumstances that precipitate and relieve angina, characteristics of the discomfort, location and radiation, duration of attacks, and effect of nitroglycerin.

1. Circumstances that precipitate and relieve angina— Angina occurs most commonly during activity and is relieved by resting. Patients may prefer to remain upright rather than lie down, as increased preload in recumbency increases myocardial work. The amount of activity required to produce angina may be relatively consistent under comparable physical and emotional circumstances or may vary from day to day. The threshold for angina is usually lower after meals, during excitement, or on exposure to cold. It is often lower in the morning or after strong emotion; the latter can provoke attacks in the absence of exertion. In addition, discomfort may occur during sexual activity, at rest, or at night as a result of coronary spasm.

2. Characteristics of the discomfort—Patients often do not refer to angina as "pain" but as a sensation of tightness, squeezing, burning, pressing, choking, aching, bursting, "gas," indigestion, or an ill-characterized discomfort. It is often characterized by clenching a fist over the mid chest. The distress of angina is rarely sharply localized and is not spasmodic.

3. Location and radiation—The distribution of the distress may vary widely in different patients but is usually the same for each patient unless unstable angina or MI supervenes. In most cases, the discomfort is felt behind or slightly to the left of the mid sternum. When it begins farther to the left or, uncommonly, on the right, it characteristically moves centrally substernally. Although angina may radiate to any dermatome from C8 to T4, it radiates most often to the left shoulder and upper arm, frequently moving down the inner volar aspect of the arm to the elbow, forearm, wrist, or fourth and fifth fingers. It may also radiate to the right shoulder or arm, the lower jaw, the neck, or even the back.

4. Duration of attacks—Angina is generally of short duration and subsides completely without residual discomfort. If the attack is precipitated by exertion and the patient promptly stops to rest, it usually lasts under 3 minutes. Attacks following a heavy meal or brought on by anger often last 15–20 minutes. Attacks lasting more than 30 minutes are unusual and suggest the development of an acute coronary syndrome with unstable angina, MI, or an alternative diagnosis.

5. Effect of nitroglycerin—The diagnosis of angina pectoris is supported if sublingual nitroglycerin promptly and invariably shortens an attack and if prophylactic nitrates permit greater exertion or prevent angina entirely.

B. Signs

Examination during angina frequently reveals a significant elevation in systolic and diastolic BP, although hypotension may also occur, and may reflect more severe ischemia or inferior ischemia (especially with bradycardia) due to a **Bezold-Jarisch reflex**. Occasionally, a gallop rhythm and an apical systolic murmur due to transient mitral regurgitation from papillary muscle dysfunction are present during pain only. Supraventricular or ventricular arrhythmias may be present, either as the precipitating factor or as a result of ischemia.

It is important to detect signs of diseases that may contribute to or accompany atherosclerotic heart disease, eg, diabetes mellitus (retinopathy or neuropathy), xanthelasma tendinous xanthomas, hypertension, thyrotoxicosis, myxedema, or peripheral artery disease. Aortic stenosis or regurgitation, HCM, and mitral valve prolapse should be sought, since they may produce angina or other forms of chest pain.

C. Laboratory Findings

Other than standard laboratory tests to evaluate for acute coronary syndrome (troponin and CK-MB) and factors contributing to ischemia (such as anemia) and to screen for risk factors that may increase the probability of true CHD (such as hyperlipidemia and diabetes mellitus), blood tests are not helpful to diagnose chronic angina.

D. ECG

The resting ECG is often normal in patients with angina. In the remainder, abnormalities include old MI, nonspecific ST–T changes, and changes of LVH. During anginal episodes, as well as during asymptomatic ischemia, *the characteristic ECG change is horizontal or downsloping ST-segment depression that reverses after the ischemia disappears.* T wave flattening or inversion may also occur. Less frequently, transient ST-segment elevation is observed; this finding suggests severe (transmural) ischemia from coronary occlusion, and it can occur with coronary spasm.

E. Pretest Probability

The history as detailed above, the physical examination findings, and laboratory and ECG findings are used to develop a pretest probability of CAD as the cause of the clinical symptoms. Other important factors to include in calculating the pretest probability of CAD are patient age, sex, and clinical symptoms. Patients with low to intermediate pretest probability for CAD should undergo noninvasive stress testing whereas patients with high pretest probability are generally referred for cardiac catheterization. National review of diagnostic cardiac catheterization findings in patients without known CAD undergoing angiography has shown that between 38% and 40% of patients do not have obstructive disease.

F. Exercise ECG

Exercise ECG testing is the most commonly used noninvasive procedure for evaluating for inducible ischemia in the patient with angina. Exercise ECG testing is often combined with imaging studies (nuclear or echocardiography), but in low-risk patients without baseline ST-segment abnormalities or in whom anatomic localization is not necessary, the exercise ECG remains the recommended initial procedure because of considerations of cost, convenience, and longstanding prognostic data.

Exercise testing can be done on a motorized treadmill or with a bicycle ergometer. A variety of exercise protocols are utilized, the most common being the **Bruce protocol,** which increases the treadmill speed and elevation every 3 minutes until limited by symptoms. At least two ECG leads should be monitored continuously.

1. Precautions and risks—The risk of exercise testing is about one infarction or death per 1000 tests, but individuals who have pain at rest or minimal activity are at higher risk and should not be tested. **Many of the traditional exclusions, such as recent MI or heart failure, are no longer used if the patient is stable and ambulatory, but symptomatic aortic stenosis remains a relative contraindication.**

2. Indications—Exercise testing is used (1) to confirm the diagnosis of angina; (2) to determine the severity of limitation of activity due to angina; (3) to assess prognosis in patients with known coronary disease, including those recovering from MI, by detecting groups at high or low risk; and (4) to evaluate responses to therapy. Because false-positive tests often exceed true positives, leading to much patient anxiety and self-imposed or mandated disability, exercise testing of asymptomatic individuals should be done only for those whose occupations place them or others at special risk (eg, airline pilots).

3. Interpretation—The usual ECG criterion for a positive test is 1-mm (0.1-mV) horizontal or downsloping ST-segment depression (beyond baseline) measured 80 msec after the J point. By this criterion, 60–80% of patients with anatomically significant coronary disease will have a positive test, but 10–30% of those without significant disease will also be positive. False positives are uncommon when a 2-mm depression is present. Additional information is inferred from the time of onset and duration of the ECG changes, their magnitude and configuration, BP and heart rate changes, the duration of exercise, and the presence of associated symptoms. In general, patients exhibiting more severe ST-segment depression (more than 2 mm) at low workloads (less than 6 minutes on the Bruce protocol) or heart rates (less than 70% of age-predicted maximum)—especially when the duration of exercise and rise in BP are limited or when hypotension occurs during the test—have more severe disease and a poorer prognosis. Depending on symptom status, age, and other factors, such patients should be referred for coronary arteriography and possible revascularization. On the other hand, less impressive positive tests in asymptomatic patients are often "false positives." Therefore, exercise testing results that do not conform to the clinical suspicion should be confirmed by stress imaging.

G. Myocardial Stress Imaging

Myocardial stress imaging (scintigraphy, echocardiography, or MRI) is indicated (1) when the resting ECG makes an exercise ECG difficult to interpret (eg, left bundle branch block, baseline ST–T changes, low voltage); (2) for confirmation of the results of the exercise ECG when they are contrary to the clinical impression (eg, a positive test in an asymptomatic patient); (3) to localize the region of ischemia; (4) to distinguish ischemic from infarcted myocardium; (5) to assess the completeness of revascularization following bypass surgery or coronary angioplasty; or (6) as a prognostic indicator in patients with known coronary disease. Published criteria summarize these indications for stress testing.

1. Myocardial perfusion scintigraphy—This test, also known as **radionuclide imaging,** provides images in which radionuclide uptake is proportionate to blood flow at the time of injection.

Stress imaging is positive in about 75–90% of patients with anatomically significant coronary disease and in 20–30% of those without it. Occasionally, other conditions, including infiltrative diseases (sarcoidosis, amyloidosis), left bundle branch block, and dilated cardiomyopathy, may produce resting or persistent perfusion defects. False-positive radionuclide tests may occur as a result of diaphragmatic attenuation or, in women, attenuation through breast tissue. Tomographic imaging (single-photon emission computed tomography [SPECT]) can reduce the severity of artifacts.

2. Radionuclide angiography—This procedure, also known as **multi-gated acquisition scan,** or **MUGA scan,** uses radionuclide tracers to image the LV and measures its EF and wall motion. In coronary disease, resting abnormalities usually represent infarction, and those that occur only with exercise usually indicate stress-induced ischemia. Exercise radionuclide angiography has approximately the same sensitivity as myocardial perfusion scintigraphy, but it is less specific in older individuals and those with other forms of heart disease. In addition, because of the precision around LVEF, the test is also used for monitoring patients exposed to cardiotoxic therapies (such as chemotherapeutic agents).

3. Stress echocardiography—Echocardiograms performed during supine exercise or immediately following upright exercise may demonstrate exercise-induced *segmental wall motion abnormalities* as an indicator of ischemia. In experienced laboratories, the test accuracy is comparable to that obtained with scintigraphy—though a higher proportion of tests is technically inadequate. While exercise is the preferred stress because of other information derived, pharmacologic stress with high-dose dobutamine (20–40 mcg/kg/minute) can be used as an alternative to exercise.

H. Other Imaging

1. Positron emission tomography—PET and SPECT scanning can accurately distinguish transiently dysfunctional ("stunned") myocardium from scar tissue.

2. CT and MRI scanning—CT scanning can image the heart and, with contrast medium and multislice technology, the coronary arteries. **Multislice CT angiography may be useful in evaluating patients with low likelihood of significant CAD to rule out disease.** Its use has been associated with lower 5-year mortality compared to standard care in patients with stable chest pain. With lower radiation exposure than radionuclide SPECT imaging, CT angiography may also be useful for evaluating chest pain and suspected acute coronary syndrome. In the large randomized comparative effectiveness PROMISE trial, patients with stable chest pain undergoing anatomic imaging with CT angiography had similar outcomes to patients undergoing functional testing (stress ECG, stress radionuclide, or stress echocardiography). CT angiography with noninvasive functional assessment of coronary stenosis (fractional flow reserve), termed **CT-FFR,** has also been evaluated in patients with low-intermediate likelihood of CAD. CT-FFR has been shown to reduce the number of patients without coronary disease requiring invasive angiography. CT-FFR has been approved for clinical use and is being used in clinical practice in the United States and Europe. The use of CT-FFR has been endorsed with a level IIa recommendation for intermediate risk patients with chest pain and no prior history of CAD with a 40–90% stenosis on CT imaging to guide need for revascularization in the 2021 ACC/AHA Guideline for the Evaluation and Diagnosis of Chest Pain.

Electron beam CT (EBCT) (Coronary Calcium Score) can quantify coronary artery calcification, which is highly correlated with atheromatous plaque and has high sensitivity, but low specificity, for obstructive coronary disease. This test has not traditionally been used in symptomatic patients. According to the AHA, persons who are at low risk (less than 10% 10-year risk) or at high risk (greater than 20% 10-year risk) for obstructive coronary disease do not benefit from coronary calcium assessment (class III, level of evidence: B). However, in clinically selected, intermediate-risk patients (5–7.5% atherosclerotic CVD), it may be reasonable to determine the atherosclerosis burden using EBCT in order to refine clinical risk prediction and to select patients for more aggressive target values for lipid-lowering therapies (class IIb, level of evidence: B).

Cardiac MRI using gadolinium provides high-resolution images of the heart and great vessels without radiation exposure or use of iodinated contrast media. Gadolinium has been associated with a rare but fatal complication in patients with severe kidney disease, called **necrotizing systemic fibrosis.** Gadolinium can demonstrate perfusion using dobutamine or adenosine to produce pharmacologic stress. Advances have been made in imaging the proximal coronary arteries. Perhaps the most clinically used indication of cardiac MRI is for identification of **myocardial fibrosis,** either from MI or infiltration, done with gadolinium contrast. This allows high-resolution imaging of myocardial viability and infiltrative cardiomyopathies.

I. Ambulatory ECG Monitoring

Ambulatory ECG recorders can monitor for ischemic ST-segment depression, but this modality is rarely used for ischemia detection. In patients with CAD, these episodes usually signify ischemia, even when asymptomatic ("silent").

J. Coronary Angiography

Selective coronary arteriography is the definitive diagnostic procedure for CAD. It can be performed with low mortality (about 0.1%) and morbidity (1–5%), but due to the invasive nature and cost, it is recommended only in patients with a high pretest probability of CAD.

Coronary arteriography should be performed in the following circumstances if percutaneous transluminal coronary angioplasty or bypass surgery is a consideration:

1. Life-limiting stable angina despite an adequate medical regimen.
2. Clinical presentation (unstable angina, postinfarction angina, etc) or noninvasive testing suggests high-risk disease (see Indications for Revascularization).
3. Concomitant aortic valve disease and angina pectoris, to determine whether the angina is due to accompanying coronary disease.
4. Asymptomatic older patients undergoing valve surgery so that concomitant bypass may be done if the anatomy is propitious.
5. Recurrence of symptoms after coronary revascularization to determine whether bypass grafts or native vessels are occluded.
6. Cardiac failure where a surgically correctable lesion, such as LV aneurysm, mitral regurgitation, or reversible ischemic dysfunction, is suspected.
7. Survivors of sudden death, symptomatic, or life-threatening arrhythmias when CAD may be a correctable cause.
8. Chest pain of uncertain cause or cardiomyopathy of unknown cause.
9. Emergently performed cardiac catheterization with intention to perform primary PCI in patients with suspected acute MI.

A narrowing of more than 50% of the luminal diameter is considered hemodynamically (and clinically) significant, although most lesions producing ischemia are associated with narrowing in excess of 70%. In those with strongly positive exercise ECGs or scintigraphic studies, three-vessel or left main disease may be present in 75–95% depending on the criteria used. **Intravascular ultrasound (IVUS)** is useful as an adjunct for assessing the results of angioplasty or stenting. In addition, IVUS is the invasive diagnostic method of choice for ostial left main lesions and coronary dissections. In **fractional flow reserve (FFR),** a pressure wire is used to measure the relative change in pressure across a coronary lesion after adenosine-induced hyperemia. Revascularization based on abnormal FFR improves clinical outcomes compared to revascularization of all angiographically stenotic lesions. FFR is an important invasive tool to aid with ischemia-driven revascularization and has become the standard tool to evaluate borderline lesions in cases in which the clinical team is evaluating the clinical and hemodynamic significance of a coronary stenosis. Additionally, pressures distally/pressures proximally during a wave-free period in diastole have been shown to demonstrate similar clinical outcomes to FFR, without the use of adenosine.

LV angiography is usually performed at the same time as coronary arteriography. Global and regional LV function are visualized, as well as mitral regurgitation if present. LV function is a major determinant of prognosis in CHD.

Differential Diagnosis

When atypical features are present—such as prolonged duration (hours or days) or darting, or knifelike pains at the apex or over the precordium—ischemia is less likely.

Anterior chest wall syndrome is characterized by a sharply localized tenderness of the intercostal muscles. Inflammation of the chondrocostal junctions may result in diffuse chest pain that is also reproduced by local pressure **(Tietze syndrome).** Intercostal neuritis (due to herpes zoster or diabetes mellitus, for example) also mimics angina.

Cervical or thoracic spine disease involving the dorsal roots produces sudden sharp, severe chest pain suggesting angina in location and "radiation" but related to specific movements of the neck or spine, recumbency, and straining or lifting. Pain due to cervical or thoracic disk disease involves the outer or dorsal aspect of the arm and the thumb and index fingers rather than the ring and little fingers.

Reflux esophagitis, peptic ulcer, chronic cholecystitis, esophageal spasm, and functional GI disease may produce pain suggestive of angina pectoris. The picture may be especially confusing because ischemic pain may also be associated with upper GI symptoms, and esophageal motility disorders may be improved by nitrates and calcium channel blockers. Assessment of esophageal motility may be helpful.

Degenerative and inflammatory lesions of the left shoulder and thoracic outlet syndromes may cause chest pain due to nerve irritation or muscular compression; the symptoms are usually precipitated by movement of the arm and shoulder and are associated with paresthesias.

Pneumonia, PE, and spontaneous pneumothorax may cause chest pain as well as dyspnea. Dissection of the thoracic aorta can cause severe chest pain that is commonly felt in the back; it is sudden in onset, reaches maximum intensity immediately, and may be associated with changes in pulses. Other cardiac disorders, such as mitral valve prolapse, HCM, myocarditis, pericarditis, aortic valve disease, or RVH, may cause atypical chest pain or even myocardial ischemia.

Treatment

Sublingual nitroglycerin is the medication of choice for acute management; it acts in about 1–2 minutes. As soon as the attack begins, one fresh tablet is placed under the tongue. This may be repeated at 3- to 5-minute intervals, but if pain is not relieved or improving after 5 minutes, the patient should call 9-1-1; pain not responding to three tablets or lasting more than 20 minutes may represent evolving infarction. The dosage (0.3, 0.4, or 0.6 mg) and the number of tablets to be used before seeking further medical attention must be individualized. Nitroglycerin buccal spray is also available as a metered (0.4 mg) delivery system. It has the advantage of being more convenient for patients who have difficulty handling the pills and of being more stable.

Prevention of Further Attacks

A. Aggravating Factors

Angina may be aggravated by hypertension, LV failure, arrhythmia (usually tachycardias), strenuous activity, cold temperatures, and emotional states. These factors should be identified and treated when possible.

B. Nitroglycerin

Nitroglycerin, 0.3–0.6 mg sublingually or 0.4–0.8 mg translingually by spray, should be taken 5 minutes before any activity likely to precipitate angina. Sublingual isosorbide dinitrate (2.5–5 mg) is only slightly longer-acting than sublingual nitroglycerin.

C. Long-Acting Nitrates

Longer-acting nitrate preparations include isosorbide dinitrate, 10–40 mg orally three times daily; isosorbide mononitrate, 10–40 mg orally twice daily or 60–120 mg once daily in a sustained-release preparation; oral sustained-release nitroglycerin preparations, 6.25–12.5 mg two to four times daily; nitroglycerin ointment, 2% ointment, 0.5–2 inches (7.5–30 mg in the morning and 6 hours later); and transdermal nitroglycerin patches that deliver nitroglycerin at rates of 0.2, 0.4, and 0.6 mg/hour rate (0.1–0.8 mg/hour), and should be taken off after 12–14 hours of use for a 10–12 hour patch-free interval daily. The main limitation to long-term nitrate therapy is *tolerance*, which can be limited by using a regimen that includes a minimum 8- to 10-hour period per day without nitrates. Isosorbide dinitrate can be given three times daily, with the last dose after dinner, or longer-acting isosorbide mononitrate once daily. Transdermal nitrate preparations should be removed overnight in most patients.

Nitrate therapy is often limited by headache. Other side effects include nausea, light-headedness, and hypotension. Importantly, phosphodiesterase inhibitors used commonly for erectile dysfunction should not be taken within 24 hours of nitrate use.

D. Beta-Blockers

Beta-blockers are the only antianginal agents that have been demonstrated to prolong life in patients with coronary disease (post-MI). **Beta-blockers should be considered for first-line therapy in most patients with chronic angina** and are recommended as such by the stable ischemic heart disease guidelines (Figure 10–8).

Beta-blockers with intrinsic sympathomimetic activity, such as pindolol, are less desirable because they may exacerbate angina in some individuals and have not been effective in secondary prevention trials. The pharmacology and side effects of the beta-blockers are discussed in Chapter 11 (see Table 11–9). The dosages of all these medications when given for angina are similar. The major contraindications are severe bronchospastic disease, bradyarrhythmias, and decompensated heart failure.

E. Ranolazine

Ranolazine is indicated for chronic angina. Ranolazine has no effect on heart rate and BP, and it has been shown in clinical trials to prolong exercise duration and time to angina, both as monotherapy and when administered with conventional antianginal therapy. It is safe to use with erectile dysfunction medications. The usual dose is 500 mg orally twice a day. Because it can cause QT prolongation, it is contraindicated in patients with existing QT prolongation; in patients taking QT prolonging medications, such as class I or III antiarrhythmics (eg, quinidine, dofetilide, sotalol); and in those taking potent and moderate CYP450 3A inhibitors (eg, clarithromycin and rifampin). Of interest, in spite of the QT prolongation, there is a significantly lower rate of ventricular arrhythmias with its use following acute coronary syndromes, as shown in the MERLIN trial.

F. Calcium Channel Blocking Agents

Unlike the beta-blockers, calcium channel blockers have *not* been shown to reduce mortality postinfarction and in some cases have increased ischemia and mortality rates. This appears to be the case with some dihydropyridines (eg, nifedipine) and with diltiazem and verapamil in patients with clinical heart failure or moderate to severe LV dysfunction. Meta-analyses have suggested that short-acting nifedipine in moderate to high doses causes an *increase* in mortality. It is uncertain whether these findings are relevant to longer-acting dihydropyridines. Nevertheless, considering the uncertainties and the lack of demonstrated favorable effect on outcomes, calcium channel blockers should be considered third-line anti-ischemic medications in the postinfarction patient. Similarly, these agents, with the exception of amlodipine (which proved safe in patients with heart failure in the PRAISE-2 trial), should be avoided in patients with heart failure or low EFs.

The pharmacologic effects and side effects of the calcium channel blockers are discussed in Chapter 11 and summarized in Table 11–7. Diltiazem, amlodipine, and verapamil are preferable because they produce less reflex tachycardia and because the former, at least, may cause fewer side effects. Nifedipine, nicardipine, and amlodipine are also approved agents for angina. Isradipine, felodipine, and nisoldipine are not approved for angina but probably are as effective as the other dihydropyridines.

G. Ivabradine

Ivabradine selectively blocks the I_f current and specifically lowers heart rate. It has been shown to reduce angina in patients with chronic stable angina and is approved in Europe. However, the SIGNIFY trial found no overall difference in clinical outcomes in patients without heart failure and angina and that there may have been harm for patients with significant angina with regard to outcomes of cardiovascular death and MI.

H. Alternative and Combination Therapies

Patients who do not respond to one class of antianginal medication often respond to another. It may, therefore, be

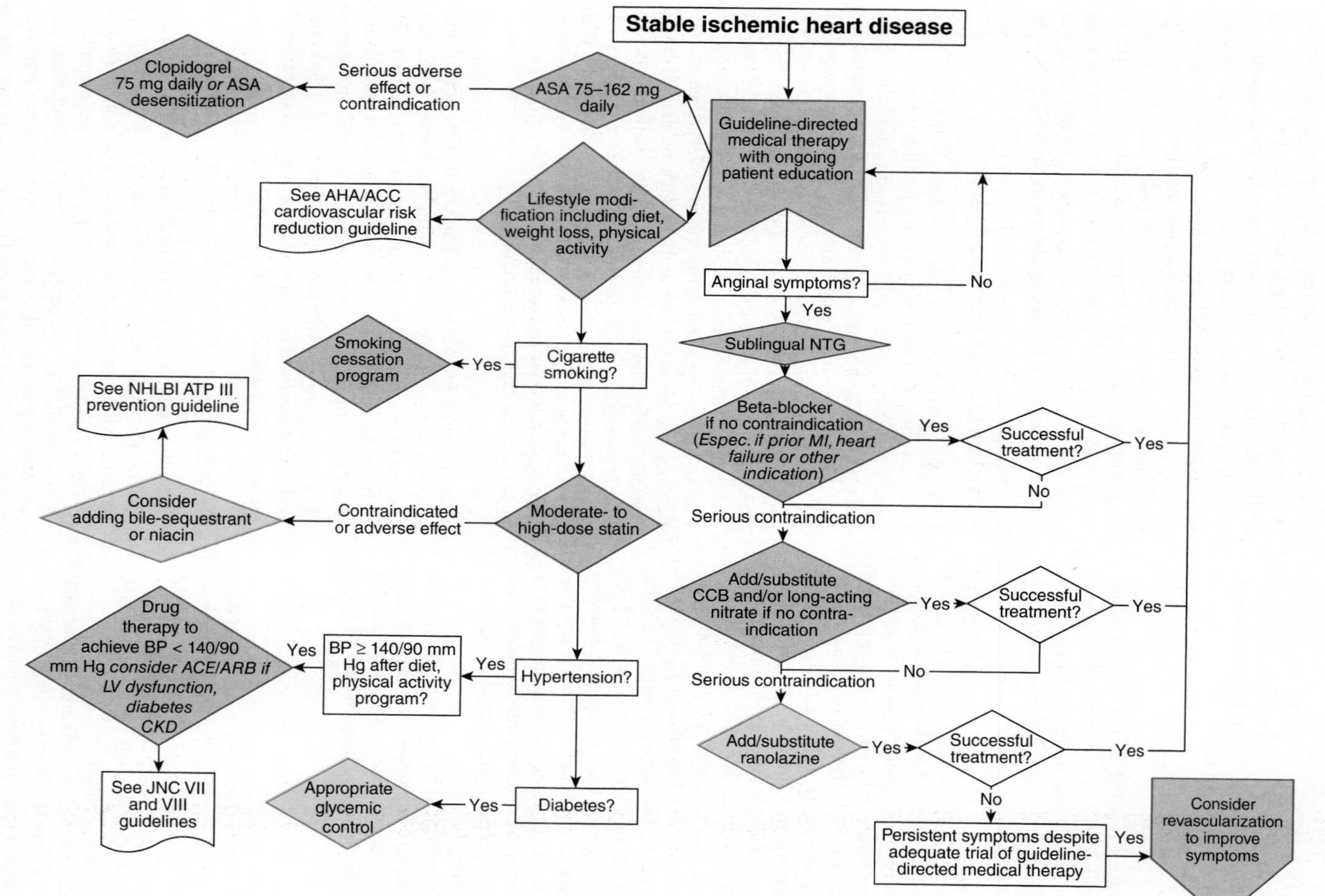

▲ **Figure 10–8.** Algorithm for guideline-directed medical therapy for patients with stable ischemic heart disease. The use of bile acid sequestrant is relatively contraindicated when triglycerides are 200 mg/dL or higher and contraindicated when triglycerides are 500 mg/dL or higher. Dietary supplement niacin must not be used as a substitute for prescription niacin. AHA/ACC, American Heart Association/American College of Cardiology; ASA, aspirin; BP, blood pressure; CCB, calcium channel blocker; NTG, nitroglycerin. (Reprinted with permission Circulation. 2012;126:e354–e471 ©2012 American Heart Association, Inc.)

worthwhile to use an alternative agent before progressing to combinations. **The stable ischemic heart disease guidelines recommend starting with a beta-blocker as initial therapy, followed by calcium channel blockers, long-acting nitrates, or ranolazine.** A few patients will have further response to a regimen including all four agents.

I. Platelet-Inhibiting Agents

Several studies have demonstrated the benefit of antiplatelet medications for patients with stable and unstable vascular disease. Therefore, **unless contraindicated, aspirin (81 mg orally daily) should be prescribed for all patients with angina.** A $P2Y_{12}$ inhibitor **clopidogrel,** 75 mg orally daily, reduces vascular events in patients with stable vascular disease (as an alternative to aspirin) and in patients with acute coronary syndromes (in addition to aspirin). Thus, it is also a good alternative in aspirin-intolerant patients. Clopidogrel in addition to aspirin did not reduce MI, stroke, or cardiovascular death in the CHARISMA trial of patients with CVD or multiple risk factors, with about a 50% increase in bleeding. However, it might be reasonable to use combination clopidogrel and aspirin for certain high-risk patients with established coronary disease, as tested in the Dual Antiplatelet Therapy (DAPT) trial. Specifically, **prolonged use of dual antiplatelet therapy with aspirin and clopidogrel may be beneficial in patients post–percutaneous stenting with drug-eluting stents who have a low bleeding risk.**

Ticagrelor, a $P2Y_{12}$ inhibitor, has been shown to reduce cardiovascular events in patients with acute coronary syndromes. Additionally, in patients with prior MI, long-term treatment with ticagrelor plus aspirin reduced cardiovascular events compared to aspirin alone. In patients with peripheral artery disease, ticagrelor monotherapy did not reduce cardiovascular events compared to clopidogrel.

Vorapaxar is an inhibitor of the protease-activated receptor-1. It was shown to reduce cardiovascular events for patients with stable atherosclerosis with a history of MI or peripheral artery disease in the TRA 2P trial. It is contraindicated for patients with a history of stroke or TIA due to increased risk of intracranial hemorrhage.

Rivaroxaban, a direct factor Xa inhibitor, when used at a dose of 2.5 mg twice daily in addition to low-dose aspirin, was found to reduce cardiovascular events including cardiovascular death, MI, or stroke when compared to aspirin monotherapy in patients with known CAD or peripheral artery disease. This agent is approved and provides another option for patients.

Current guidelines recommend **dual antiplatelet therapy (aspirin and $P2Y_{12}$ therapy) in patients with recent MI (within 1 year) or recent stenting (within 6 months) and for prolonged therapy (more than 1 year) in patients at high ischemic risk (multivessel coronary disease or polyvascular disease) and low bleeding risk.**

J. Risk Reduction

Patients with coronary disease should undergo aggressive **risk factor modification.** This approach, with a particular focus on statin treatment, treating hypertension, stopping smoking, and exercise and weight control (especially for patients with metabolic syndrome or at risk for diabetes), may markedly improve outcomes. For patients with diabetes and CVD, there is uncertainty about the optimal target blood sugar control. The ADVANCE trial suggested some benefit for tight blood sugar control with target HbA_{1C} of 6.5% or less, but the ACCORD trial found that routine aggressive targeting for blood sugar control to HbA_{1C} to less than 6.0% in patients with diabetes and coronary disease was associated with *increased* mortality. Therefore, tight blood sugar control should be avoided particularly in patients with a history of severe hypoglycemia, long-standing diabetes, and advanced vascular disease. Aggressive BP control (target systolic BP less than 120 mm Hg) in the ACCORD trial was *not* associated with reduction in CHD events despite reducing stroke. In contrast, the SPRINT trial, which did not include diabetic patients, demonstrated a reduction in cardiovascular events in patients with a reduction in death from any cause and reduction in MI with a goal systolic BP of less than 120 mm Hg versus of goal of less than 140 mm Hg. Some increase in adverse events was noted. Based on this and the totality of results, **the AHA has recommended defining hypertension at the 130 mm Hg level.**

K. Revascularization

1. Indications—There is general agreement that otherwise healthy patients in the following groups should undergo revascularization: (1) patients with unacceptable symptoms despite medical therapy to its tolerable limits; (2) patients with left main coronary artery stenosis greater than 50% with or without symptoms; (3) patients with three-vessel disease with LV dysfunction (EF less than 50% or previous transmural infarction); (4) patients with unstable angina who after symptom control by medical therapy continue to exhibit ischemia on exercise testing or monitoring; and (5) post-MI patients with continuing angina or severe ischemia on noninvasive testing. The use of revascularization for patients with acute coronary syndromes and acute ST-segment elevation MI (STEMI) is discussed below.

Data from the COURAGE trial have shown that for patients with chronic angina and disease suitable for PCI, PCI in addition to stringent guideline-directed medical therapy aimed at both risk reduction and anti-anginal care offers no mortality benefit beyond excellent medical therapy alone, and relatively moderate long-term symptomatic improvement. Therefore, **for patients with mild to moderate CAD and limited symptoms, revascularization may not provide significant functional status quality-of-life benefit.** For patients with moderate to significant coronary stenosis, such as those who have two-vessel disease associated with underlying LV dysfunction, anatomically critical lesions (greater than 90% proximal stenoses, especially of the proximal left anterior descending artery), or physiologic evidence of severe ischemia (early positive exercise tests, large exercise-induced thallium scintigraphic defects, or frequent episodes of ischemia on ambulatory monitoring), a heart team consisting of revascularization physicians (interventional cardiologists and surgeons) may be required to review and provide patients with the best revascularization options.

The ISCHEMIA trial found that for patients with moderate to severe ischemia on stress testing, coronary angiography and revascularization did not reduce the risk of cardiovascular death, MI, hospitalization for unstable angina, heart failure, or resuscitated cardiac arrest. Thus, in the context of optimal medical therapy to prevent cardiovascular events, a higher threshold for whom to evaluate with stress tests and coronary angiography may be reasonable.

2. Type of procedure—

A. Percutaneous coronary intervention including stenting—PCI, including balloon angioplasty and coronary stenting, can effectively open stenotic coronary arteries. Coronary stenting, with either bare metal stents or drug-eluting stents, has substantially reduced restenosis. Stenting can also be used selectively for left main coronary stenosis, particularly when CABG is contraindicated or deemed high risk.

PCI is possible but often less successful in bypass graft stenoses. Experienced operators are able to successfully dilate more than 90% of lesions attempted. The major early complication is intimal dissection with vessel occlusion, although this is rare with coronary stenting. The use of intravenous platelet glycoprotein IIb/IIIa inhibitors (abciximab, eptifibatide, tirofiban) substantially reduces the rate of periprocedural MI, and placement of intracoronary stents markedly improves initial and long-term angiographic results, especially with complex and long lesions. After percutaneous coronary intervention, all patients should have CK-MB and troponin measured. The definition of a periprocedural infarction has been debated, with many experts advocating for a clinical definition that incorporates different enzyme cutpoints, angiographic findings, and electrocardiographic evidence. Acute thrombosis after stent placement can largely be prevented by aggressive antithrombotic therapy (long-term aspirin, 81–325 mg, plus clopidogrel, 300–600 mg loading dose followed by 75 mg daily, for between 30 days and 1 year, and with acute use of platelet glycoprotein IIb/IIIa inhibitors).

A major limitation with PCI has been **restenosis,** which occurs in the first 6 months in less than 10% of vessels treated with drug-eluting stents, 15–30% of vessels treated with bare metal stents, and 30–40% of vessels without stenting. Factors associated with higher restenosis rates include diabetes, small luminal diameter, longer and more complex lesions, and lesions at coronary ostia or in the left anterior descending coronary artery. Drug-eluting stents that elute antiproliferative agents, such as sirolimus, everolimus, zotarolimus, or paclitaxel, have substantially reduced restenosis. In-stent restenosis is often treated with restenting with drug-eluting stents, and rarely with brachytherapy. The nearly 2 million PCIs performed worldwide per year far exceed the number of CABG operations, but the rationale for many of the procedures performed in patients with stable angina should be for angina symptom reduction. Moreover, data published in 2021 reported that 706,263 PCIs were performed in the United States from 2018 to 2019.

The COURAGE trial and the ORBITA sham-controlled trial have confirmed earlier studies in showing that, even for patients with moderate anginal symptoms and positive stress tests, PCI provides no benefit over medical therapy with respect to death or MI. PCI was more effective at relieving angina, although most patients in the medical group had improvement in symptoms. PCI was also not more effective than optimal medical therapy for exercise time in patients with one vessel coronary disease. Thus, **in patients with mild or moderate stable symptoms, aggressive lipid-lowering and antianginal therapy may be a preferable initial strategy, reserving PCI for patients with significant and refractory symptoms or for those who are unable to take the prescribed medicines.**

Several studies of PCI, including those with drug-eluting stents, versus CABG in patients with multivessel disease have been reported. The SYNTAX trial as well as previously performed trials with drug-eluting stent use in PCI patients show comparable mortality and infarction rates over follow-up periods of 1–3 years but a high rate (approximately 40%) of repeat procedures following PCI. Stroke rates are higher with CABG. As a result, the choice of revascularization procedure may depend on details of coronary anatomy and is often a matter of patient preference. However, it should be noted that less than 20% of patients with multivessel disease meet the entry criteria for the clinical trials, so these results cannot be generalized to all multivessel disease patients. Outcomes with percutaneous revascularization in patients with diabetes have generally been inferior to those with CABG. The FREEDOM trial demonstrated that **CABG surgery was superior to PCI with regard to death, MI, and stroke for patients with diabetes and multivessel coronary disease** at 5 years across all subgroups of SYNTAX score anatomy.

B. Coronary artery bypass grafting—CABG can be accomplished with a very low mortality rate (1–3%) in otherwise healthy patients with preserved cardiac function. However, the mortality rate of this procedure rises to 4–8% in older individuals and in patients who have had a prior CABG.

Grafts using one or both internal mammary arteries (usually to the left anterior descending artery or its branches) provide the best long-term results in terms of patency and flow. Segments of the saphenous vein (or, less optimally, other veins) or the radial artery interposed between the aorta and the coronary arteries distal to the obstructions are also used. One to five distal anastomoses are commonly performed.

Minimally invasive surgical techniques may involve a limited sternotomy, lateral thoracotomy (MIDCAB), or thoracoscopy (port-access). They are more technically demanding, usually not suitable for more than two grafts, and do not have established durability. Bypass surgery can be performed both on circulatory support (on-pump) and without direct circulatory support (off-pump). Randomized trial data have not shown a benefit with off-pump bypass surgery, but minimally invasive surgical techniques allow earlier postoperative mobilization and discharge.

The operative mortality rate is increased in patients with poor LV function (LVEF less than 35%) or those requiring additional procedures (valve replacement or ventricular aneurysmectomy). Patients over 70 years of age, patients undergoing repeat procedures, or those with important noncardiac disease (especially CKD and diabetes) or poor general health also have higher operative mortality and morbidity rates, and full recovery is slow. Thus, CABG should be reserved for more severely symptomatic patients in this group. Early (1–6 months) graft patency rates average 85–90% (higher for internal mammary grafts), and subsequent graft closure rates are about 4% annually. Early graft failure is common in vessels with poor distal flow, while late closure is more frequent in patients who continue smoking and those with untreated hyperlipidemia. Antiplatelet therapy with aspirin improves graft patency rates. Smoking cessation and vigorous treatment of blood lipid abnormalities (particularly with statins) are necessary. Repeat revascularization may be necessary because of recurrent symptoms due to progressive native vessel disease and graft occlusions. Reoperation is technically demanding and less often fully successful than the initial operation. In addition, in patients with ischemic mitral regurgitation, mitral repair at the time of a CABG does not offer any clinical benefit.

L. Mechanical Extracorporeal Counterpulsation

Extracorporeal counterpulsation entails repetitive inflation of a high-pressure chamber surrounding the lower half of the body during the diastolic phase of the cardiac cycle for daily 1-hour sessions over a period of 7 weeks. Randomized trials have shown that extracorporeal counterpulsation reduces angina, thus it may be considered for relief of refractory angina in patients with stable coronary disease.

M. Neuromodulation

Spinal cord stimulation can be used to relieve chronic refractory angina. Spinal cord stimulators are subcutaneously implantable via a minimally invasive procedure under local anesthesia.

Prognosis

The prognosis of angina pectoris has improved with development of therapies aimed at secondary prevention. Mortality rates vary depending on the number of vessels diseased, the severity of obstruction, the status of LV function, and the presence of complex arrhythmias. Mortality rates are progressively higher in patients with one-, two-, and three-vessel disease and those with left main coronary artery obstruction (ranging from 1% per year to 25% per year). The outlook in individual patients is unpredictable, and nearly half of the deaths are sudden. Therefore, risk stratification is attempted. Patients with accelerating symptoms have a poorer outlook. Among stable patients, those whose exercise tolerance is severely limited by ischemia (less than 6 minutes on the Bruce treadmill protocol) and those with extensive ischemia by exercise ECG or scintigraphy have more severe anatomic disease and a poorer prognosis. The **Duke Treadmill Score,** based on a standard Bruce protocol exercise treadmill test, provides an estimate of risk of death at 1 year. The score uses time on the treadmill, amount of ST-segment depression, and presence of angina (Table 10–6).

Table 10–6. Duke Treadmill Score: calculation and interpretation.

Time in minutes on Bruce protocol		= ________
−5 × amount of depression (in mm)		= ________
−4 × angina index 0 = no angina on test 1 = angina, not limiting 2 = limiting angina		= ________
Total Summed Score	**Risk Group**	**Annual Mortality**
≥ 5	Low	0.25%
−10 to 4	Intermediate	1.25%
≤ −11	High	5.25%

When to Refer

All patients with new or worsening symptoms believed to represent progressive angina or a positive stress test for myocardial ischemia with continued angina despite medical therapy (or both) should be referred to a cardiologist.

When to Admit

- Patients with elevated cardiac biomarkers, ischemic ECG findings, or hemodynamic instability.
- Patients with new or worsened symptoms, possibly thought to be ischemic, but who lack high-risk features can be observed with serial ECGs and biomarkers and discharged if stress testing shows low-risk findings.

Castro-Dominguez YS et al. Predicting in-hospital mortality in patients undergoing percutaneous coronary intervention. J Am Coll Cardiol. 2021;78:216. [PMID: 33957239]

Knuuti J et al. 2019 ESC Guidelines for the diagnosis and management of chronic coronary syndromes. Eur Heart J. 2020;41:407. [PMID: 31504439]

Writing Committee Members; Gulati M et al. 2021 AHA/ACC/ASE/CHEST/SAEM/SCCT/SCMR guideline for the evaluation and diagnosis of chest pain: a report of the American College of Cardiology/American Heart Association Joint Committee on Clinical Practice Guidelines. J Am Coll Cardiol. 2021;78:e187. [PMID: 34756653]

CORONARY VASOSPASM & ANGINA OR MI WITH NORMAL CORONARY ARTERIOGRAMS

ESSENTIALS OF DIAGNOSIS

- Precordial chest pain, often occurring at rest during stress or without known precipitant, relieved rapidly by nitrates.
- ECG evidence of ischemia during pain, sometimes with ST-segment elevation.
- Angiographic demonstration of:
  - No significant obstruction of major coronary vessels.
  - Coronary spasm that responds to intracoronary nitroglycerin or calcium channel blockers.

General Considerations

Although most symptoms of myocardial ischemia result from fixed stenosis of the coronary arteries, intraplaque hemorrhage, or thrombosis at the site of lesions, some ischemic events may be precipitated or exacerbated by coronary vasoconstriction.

Spasm of the large coronary arteries with resulting decreased coronary blood flow may occur spontaneously or may be induced by exposure to cold, emotional stress, or vasoconstricting medications, such as ergot-derivative medications. Spasm may occur both in normal and in stenosed coronary arteries. Even MI may occur as a result of spasm in the absence of visible obstructive CHD, although most instances of such coronary spasm occur in the presence of coronary stenosis.

Cocaine can induce myocardial ischemia and infarction by causing coronary artery vasoconstriction or by increasing myocardial energy requirements. It also may contribute to accelerated atherosclerosis and thrombosis. The ischemia in **Prinzmetal (variant) angina** usually results from coronary vasoconstriction. It tends to involve the right coronary artery and there may be no fixed stenoses. Myocardial ischemia may also occur in patients with normal coronary arteries as a result of disease of the coronary microcirculation or abnormal vascular reactivity. MI without obstructive coronary disease is more frequent in women and has been shown to be due to atherosclerosis or ruptured plaques in 80% of cases. The 2020 ESC guidelines recommend cardiac MRI to aid in determining the cause of MI without obstructive coronary disease.

Clinical Findings

Ischemia may be silent or result in angina pectoris.

Prinzmetal (variant) angina is a clinical syndrome in which chest pain occurs without the usual precipitating factors and is associated with ST-segment elevation rather than depression. It often affects women under 50 years of age. It characteristically occurs in the early morning, awakening patients from sleep, and is apt to be associated with arrhythmias or conduction defects. It may be diagnosed by challenge with ergonovine (a vasoconstrictor), although the results of such provocation are not specific and it entails risk.

Treatment

Patients with chest pain associated with ST-segment elevation should undergo coronary arteriography to determine whether fixed stenotic lesions are present. If they are, aggressive medical therapy or revascularization is indicated, since the presence of these lesions may represent an unstable phase of the disease. If significant lesions are not seen, there may still be endothelial disruption and plaque rupture. If spasm is suspected, avoidance of precipitants, such as cigarette smoking and cocaine, is the top priority. Episodes of coronary spasm generally respond well to nitrates, and both nitrates and calcium channel blockers (including long-acting nifedipine, diltiazem, or amlodipine [see Table 11–7]) are effective prophylactically. By allowing unopposed alpha-1-mediated vasoconstriction, beta-blockers have exacerbated coronary vasospasm, but they may have a role in management of patients in whom spasm is associated with fixed stenoses.

When to Refer

All patients with persistent symptoms of chest pain that may represent spasm should be referred to a cardiologist.

ACUTE CORONARY SYNDROMES WITHOUT ST-SEGMENT ELEVATION

ESSENTIALS OF DIAGNOSIS

- Distinction in acute coronary syndrome between patients with and without ST-segment elevation at presentation is essential to determine need for reperfusion therapy.
- Fibrinolytic therapy is harmful in acute coronary syndrome without ST-segment elevation, unlike with ST-segment elevation, where acute reperfusion saves lives.
- Antiplatelet and anticoagulation therapies and coronary intervention are mainstays of treatment.

General Considerations

Acute coronary syndromes comprise the spectrum of unstable cardiac ischemia from unstable angina to acute MI. Acute coronary syndromes are classified based on the presenting ECG as either **ST-segment elevation MI (STEMI)** or **non–ST-segment elevation MI (NSTEMI)**. This allows for immediate classification and guides determination of whether patients should be considered for acute reperfusion therapy. The evolution of cardiac biomarkers then allows determination of whether MI has occurred.

Acute coronary syndromes represent a dynamic state in which patients frequently shift from one category to another, as new ST elevation can develop after presentation and cardiac biomarkers can become abnormal with recurrent ischemic episodes.

Clinical Findings

A. Symptoms and Signs

Patients with acute coronary syndromes generally have symptoms and signs of myocardial ischemia either at rest or with minimal exertion. These symptoms and signs are similar to the chronic angina symptoms described above, consisting of substernal chest pain or discomfort that may radiate to the jaw, left shoulder or arm. Dyspnea, nausea, diaphoresis, or syncope may either accompany the chest discomfort or may be the only symptom of acute coronary syndrome. *About one-third of patients with MI have no chest pain per se*—these patients tend to be older, female, have diabetes, and be at higher risk for subsequent mortality. Patients with acute coronary syndromes have signs of heart failure in about 10% of cases, and this is also associated with higher risk of death.

Many hospitals have developed **chest pain observation units** to provide a systematic approach toward serial risk stratification to improve the triage process. In many cases, those who have not experienced new chest pain and have insignificant ECG changes and no cardiac biomarker elevation undergo treadmill exercise tests or imaging procedures to exclude ischemia at the end of an 8- to 24-hour period and are discharged directly from the emergency department if these tests are negative.

B. Laboratory Findings

Depending on the time from symptom onset to presentation, initial laboratory findings may be normal. The markers of cardiac myocyte necrosis (**myoglobin**, **CK-MB,** and **troponin I and T**) may all be used to identify acute MI, although *high-sensitivity troponin is now the recommended biomarker to diagnose acute MI* (see Laboratory Findings, Acute Myocardial Infarction with ST-Segment Elevation). In patients with STEMI, these initial markers are often within normal limits as the patient is being rushed to immediate reperfusion. In patients without ST-segment elevation, it is the presence of abnormal CK-MB or troponin values that are associated with myocyte necrosis and the diagnosis of MI. High-sensitivity troponin assays allow rapid assessment of MI in emergency departments by using 1- or 2-hour rule out algorithms. The universal definition of MI is a rise of cardiac biomarkers with at least one value above the 99th percentile of the upper reference limit together with evidence of myocardial ischemia with at least one of the following: symptoms of ischemia, ECG changes of new ischemia, new Q waves, or imaging evidence of new loss of viable myocardium or new wall motion abnormality.

Serum creatinine is an important determinant of risk, and estimated creatinine clearance is important to guide dosing of certain antithrombotics, including eptifibatide and enoxaparin.

C. ECG

Many patients with acute coronary syndromes will exhibit ECG changes during pain—either ST-segment elevation, ST-segment depression, or T-wave flattening or inversion. Dynamic ST-segment shift is the most specific for acute coronary syndrome. ST-segment elevation in lead AVR suggests left main or three-vessel disease.

Treatment

A. General Measures

Treatment of acute coronary syndromes without ST elevation should be multifaceted. Patients who are at medium or high risk should be hospitalized, maintained at bed rest or at very limited activity for the first 24 hours, monitored, and given supplemental oxygen. Sedation with a benzodiazepine agent may help if anxiety is present.

B. Specific Measures

Figure 10–9 provides an algorithm for initial management of NSTEMI.

C. Antiplatelet and Anticoagulation Therapy

Patients should receive a combination of antiplatelet and anticoagulant agents on presentation. Fibrinolytic therapy should be *avoided* in patients without ST-segment elevation since they generally do not have an acute coronary occlusion, and the risk of such therapy appears to outweigh the benefit.

1. Antiplatelet therapy—

A. ASPIRIN—Aspirin, 162–325 mg loading dose, then 81 mg daily, should be commenced immediately and continued for the first month. The 2020 ESC guidelines for longer-term aspirin treatment recommend aspirin 75–100 mg/day as preferable to higher doses with or without coronary stenting.

B. P2Y12 INHIBITORS—ACC/AHA guidelines call for either a $P2Y_{12}$ inhibitor (clopidogrel, prasugrel [at the time of PCI], or ticagrelor) as a class I recommendation. The ESC guidelines provide a stronger recommendation for a $P2Y_{12}$ inhibitor up-front, as a class IA recommendation for all patients. Both sets of guidelines recommend postponing elective CABG surgery for at least 5 days after the last dose of clopidogrel or ticagrelor and at least 7 days after the last dose of prasugrel, due to risk of bleeding.

The Clopidogrel in Unstable Angina to Prevent Recurrent Events (CURE) trial demonstrated a 20% reduction in the composite end point of cardiovascular death, MI, and stroke with the addition of clopidogrel (300-mg loading dose, 75 mg/day for 9–12 months) to aspirin in patients with non–ST-segment elevation acute coronary syndromes. The large CURRENT trial showed that "double-dose" clopidogrel (600-mg initial oral loading dose, followed by 150 mg orally daily) for 7 days reduced stent thrombosis with a modest increase in major (but not fatal) bleeding and, therefore, it is an option for patients with acute coronary syndrome undergoing PCI.

The ESC guidelines recommend ticagrelor for all patients at moderate to high risk for acute coronary syndrome (class I recommendation). Prasugrel is recommended for patients who have not yet received another $P2Y_{12}$ inhibitor, for whom a PCI is planned, and who are not at high risk for life-threatening bleeding. Clopidogrel is reserved for patients who cannot receive either ticagrelor or prasugrel. Some studies have shown an association between assays of residual platelet function and thrombotic risk during $P2Y_{12}$ inhibitor therapy, and both the European and the US guidelines do not recommend routine platelet function testing to guide therapy (class IIb recommendation).

Prasugrel is both more potent and has a faster onset of action than clopidogrel. The TRITON trial compared prasugrel with clopidogrel in patients with STEMI or NSTEMI in whom PCI was planned; prasugrel resulted in a 19% relative reduction in death from cardiovascular causes, MI,

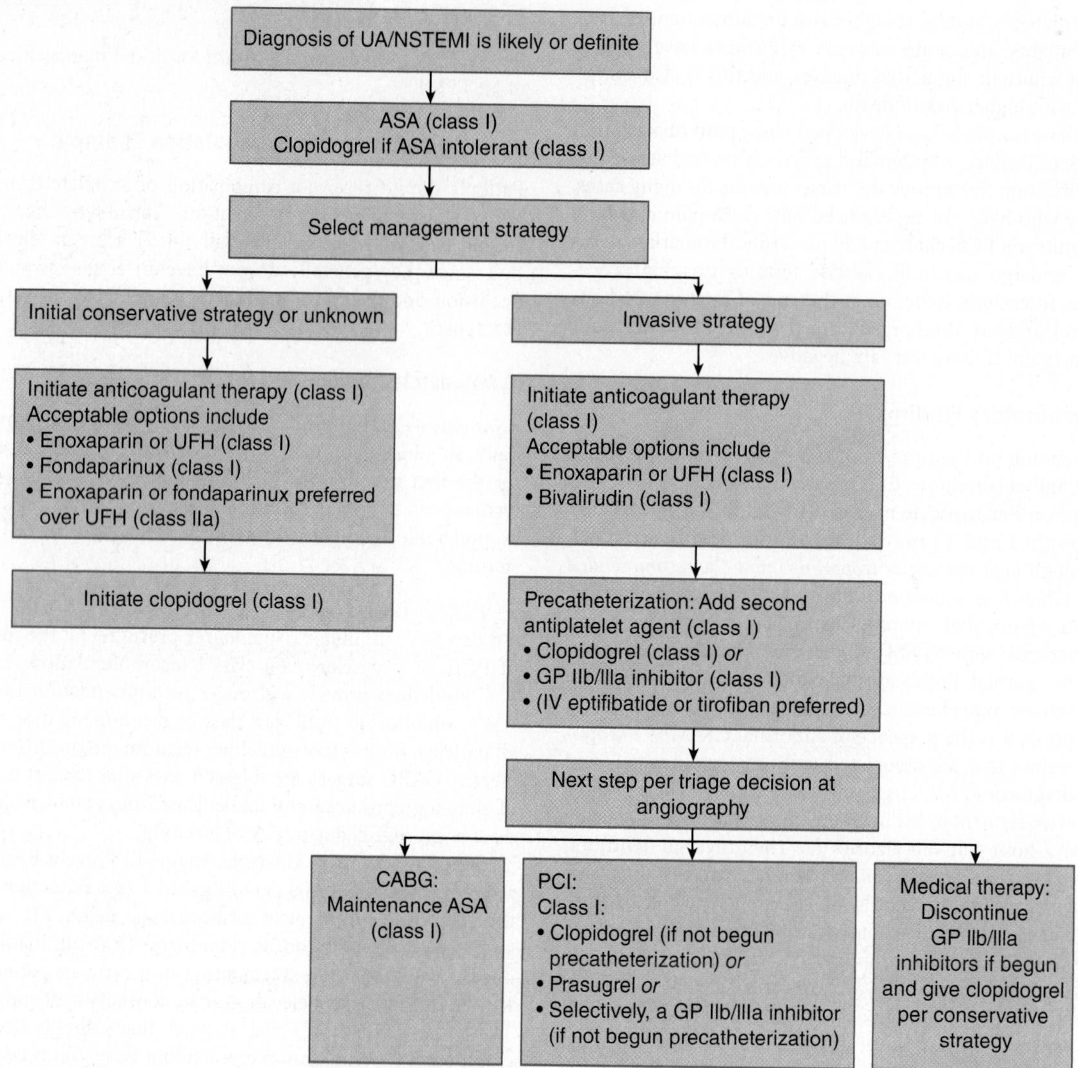

▲ **Figure 10–9.** **Flowchart for class I and class IIa recommendations for initial management of unstable angina/non–ST-segment elevation myocardial infarction (UA/NSTEMI). ASA, aspirin; CABG, coronary artery bypass grafting; GP IIb/IIIa, glycoprotein IIb/IIIa; LOE, level of evidence; UFH, unfractionated heparin.** (Reprinted with permission Circulation. 2011;123:2022–2060 ©2011 American Heart Association, Inc.)

or stroke, at the expense of an increase in serious bleeding (including fatal bleeding). Stent thrombosis was reduced by half. Because patients with prior stroke or TIA had higher risk of intracranial hemorrhage, prasugrel is contraindicated in such patients. Bleeding was also higher in patients with low body weight (less than 60 kg) and age 75 years or older, and caution should be used in these populations. For patients with STEMI treated with PCI, prasugrel appears to be especially effective (compared to clopidogrel) without a substantial increase in bleeding. For patients who will not receive revascularization, prasugrel, when compared to clopidogrel, had no overall benefit in the TRILOGY trial (the dose of prasugrel was lowered for older adults). Prasugrel appears to be at least comparable to ticagrelor for patients with STEMI regarding safety and efficacy based on the ISAR-REACT 5 trial.

Ticagrelor has a faster onset of action than clopidogrel and a more consistent and potent effect. The PLATO trial showed that when ticagrelor was started at the time of presentation in acute coronary syndrome patients (UA/NSTEMI and STEMI), it reduced cardiovascular death, MI, and stroke by 16% when compared with clopidogrel. In addition, there was a 22% relative risk reduction in mortality with ticagrelor. The overall rates of bleeding were similar between ticagrelor and clopidogrel, although non–CABG-related bleeding was modestly higher.

The finding of a lesser treatment effect in the United States may have been related to use of higher-dose aspirin, and thus when using ticagrelor, low-dose aspirin (81 mg/day) is recommended.

c. Glycoprotein IIb/IIIa inhibitors—Small-molecule inhibitors of the platelet glycoprotein IIb/IIIa receptor are useful adjuncts in high-risk patients (usually defined by fluctuating ST-segment depression or positive biomarkers) with acute coronary syndromes, particularly when they are undergoing PCI. Tirofiban, 25 mcg/kg over 3 minutes, followed by 0.15 mcg/kg/minute, and eptifibatide, 180 mcg/kg bolus followed by a continuous infusion of 2 mcg/kg/minute, have both been shown to be effective. Downward dose adjustments of the infusions are required in patients with reduced kidney function. The bolus or loading dose remains unadjusted. For example, if the estimated creatinine clearance is below 50 mL/minute, the eptifibatide infusion should be cut in half to 1 mcg/kg/minute.

2. Anticoagulant therapy—

a. Heparin—Several trials have shown that LMWH (enoxaparin 1 mg/kg subcutaneously every 12 hours) is somewhat more effective than unfractionated heparin in preventing recurrent ischemic events in the setting of acute coronary syndromes. However, the SYNERGY trial showed that unfractionated heparin and enoxaparin had similar rates of death or (re)infarction in the setting of frequent early coronary intervention.

b. Fondaparinux—Fondaparinux, a specific factor Xa inhibitor given in a dose of 2.5 mg subcutaneously once a day, was found in the OASIS-5 trial to be equally effective as enoxaparin among 20,000 patients at preventing early death, MI, and refractory ischemia, and resulted in a 50% reduction in major bleeding. This reduction in major bleeding translated into a significant reduction in mortality (and in death or MI) at 30 days. While catheter-related thrombosis was more common during coronary intervention procedures with fondaparinux, the FUTURA trial found that it can be controlled by adding unfractionated heparin (in a dose of 85 units/kg without glycoprotein IIb/IIIa inhibitors, and 60 units/kg with glycoprotein IIb/IIIa inhibitors) during the procedure. Guidelines recommend fondaparinux, describing it as especially favorable for patients who are initially treated medically and who are at high risk for bleeding, such as elderly individuals.

c. Direct thrombin inhibitors—The ACUITY trial showed that bivalirudin appears to be a reasonable alternative to heparin (unfractionated heparin or enoxaparin) plus a glycoprotein IIb/IIIa antagonist for many patients with acute coronary syndromes who are undergoing early coronary intervention. Bivalirudin (without routine glycoprotein IIb/IIIa inhibitor) is associated with substantially less bleeding than heparin plus glycoprotein IIb/IIIa inhibitor, although it may have numerically increased cardiovascular events. The ISAR REACT-4 trial showed that bivalirudin has similar efficacy compared to abciximab but better bleeding outcomes in NSTEMI patients. Bivalrudin does not currently have an FDA-approved indication for NSTEMI care.

D. Temporary Discontinuation of Antiplatelet Therapy for Procedures

Patients who have had recent coronary stents are at risk for thrombotic events, including stent thrombosis, if $P2Y_{12}$ inhibitors are discontinued for procedures (eg, dental procedures or colonoscopy). If possible, these procedures should be delayed until the end of the necessary treatment period with $P2Y_{12}$ inhibitors, which generally is at least 1 month with bare metal stents and 3–6 months with drug-eluting stents. With newer generation drug-eluting stents, elective stenting patients with bleeding risk may have $P2Y_{12}$ inhibitors stopped before 3 months. Before that time, if a procedure is necessary, risk and benefit of continuing the antiplatelet therapy through the time of the procedure should be assessed. Aspirin should generally be continued throughout the period of the procedure. Patients with polymer-free drug coated stents who are at high risk for bleeding and receiving a short course of dual antiplatelet therapy had fewer cardiovascular and bleeding events. Likewise, in the MASTER-DAPT trial, patients at high risk for bleeding treated for 1 month with DAPT had noninferior outcomes with respect to major adverse cardiac events compared with longer duration DAPT with lower rates of bleeding. A cardiologist should be consulted before temporary discontinuation of these agents.

E. Nitroglycerin

Nitrates are first-line therapy for patients with acute coronary syndromes presenting with chest pain. Nonparenteral therapy with sublingual or oral agents or nitroglycerin ointment is usually sufficient. If pain persists or recurs, intravenous nitroglycerin should be started. The usual initial dosage is 10 mcg/minute. The dosage should be titrated upward by 10–20 mcg/minute (to a maximum of 200 mcg/minute) until angina disappears or mean arterial pressure drops by 10%. Careful—usually continuous—BP monitoring is required when intravenous nitroglycerin is used. Avoid hypotension (systolic BP less than 100 mm Hg). Tolerance to continuous nitrate infusion is common.

F. Beta-Blockers

Beta-blockers are an important part of the initial treatment of unstable angina unless otherwise contraindicated. The pharmacology of these agents is discussed in Chapter 11 and summarized in Table 11–9. Use of agents with intrinsic sympathomimetic activity should be avoided in this setting. Oral medication is adequate in most patients, but intravenous treatment with metoprolol, given as three 5-mg doses 5 minutes apart as tolerated and in the absence of heart failure, achieves a more rapid effect. Oral therapy should be titrated upward as BP permits.

G. Calcium Channel Blockers

Calcium channel blockers have *not* been shown to favorably affect outcome in unstable angina, and they should be used primarily as third-line therapy in patients with continuing angina who are taking nitrates and beta-blockers or those who are not candidates for these medications. In the presence of nitrates and without accompanying beta-blockers, diltiazem or verapamil is preferred, since nifedipine and the other dihydropyridines are more likely to cause reflex tachycardia or hypotension. The initial dosage should be low, but upward titration should proceed steadily (see Table 11–7).

H. Statins

The PROVE-IT trial provides evidence for starting a statin in the days immediately following an acute coronary syndrome. In this trial, more intensive therapy with atorvastatin 80 mg/day, regardless of total or LDL cholesterol level, improved outcome compared to pravastatin 40 mg/day, with the curves of death or major cardiovascular event separating as early as 3 months after starting therapy. **High-intensity statins are recommended for all patients with acute coronary syndromes** (see Table 10–5).

Indications for Coronary Angiography

For patients with acute coronary syndrome, including NSTEMI, risk *stratification* is important for determining intensity of care. Several therapies, including glycoprotein IIb/IIIa inhibitors, LMWH heparin, and early invasive catheterization, have been shown to have the greatest benefit in higher-risk patients with acute coronary syndrome. As outlined in the ACC/AHA guidelines, patients with any high-risk feature (Table 10–7) generally warrant an early invasive strategy with catheterization and revascularization. For patients without these high-risk features, either an invasive or noninvasive approach, using exercise (or pharmacologic stress for patients unable to exercise) stress testing to identify patients who have residual ischemia and/or high risk, can be used. Moreover, based on the ICTUS trial, a strategy based on selective coronary angiography and revascularization for instability or inducible ischemia, or both, even for patients with positive troponin, is acceptable (ACC/AHA class IIb recommendation).

Two risk-stratification tools are available that can be used at the bedside, the **GRACE Risk Score** (http://www.outcomes-umassmed.org/grace) and the **TIMI Risk Score** (http://www.timi.org). The GRACE Risk Score, which applies to patients with or without ST elevation, was developed in a more generalizable registry population and has better discrimination of risk. It includes age (as a continuous variable), Killip class, BP, ST-segment deviation, cardiac arrest at presentation, serum creatinine, elevated creatine kinase (CK)-MB or troponin, and heart rate. The TIMI Risk Score includes seven variables: age 65 years or older, three or more cardiac risk factors, prior coronary stenosis of 50% or more, ST-segment deviation, two anginal events in prior 24 hours, aspirin in prior 7 days, and elevated cardiac markers.

When to Refer

- All patients with acute MI should be referred to a cardiologist.
- Patients who are taking a $P2Y_{12}$ inhibitor following coronary stenting should consult a cardiologist before discontinuing treatment for nonemergency procedures.

Table 10–7. Indications for catheterization and percutaneous coronary intervention.[1]

Acute coronary syndromes (unstable angina and non-ST elevation MI)	
Class I	Early invasive strategy for any of the following high-risk indicators:
	Recurrent angina/ischemia at rest or with low-level activity
	Elevated troponin
	ST-segment depression
	Recurrent ischemia with evidence of HF
	High-risk stress test result
	EF < 40%
	Hemodynamic instability
	Sustained ventricular tachycardia
	PCI within 6 months
	Prior CABG
	In the absence of these findings, either an early conservative or early invasive strategy
Class IIa	Early invasive strategy for patients with repeated presentations for ACS despite therapy
Class III	Extensive comorbidities in patients in whom benefits of revascularization are not likely to outweigh the risks
	Acute chest pain with low likelihood of ACS
Acute MI after fibrinolytic therapy	
Class I	Cardiogenic shock or acute severe heart failure that develops after initial presentation
	Intermediate- or high-risk findings on predischarge noninvasive ischemia testing
	Spontaneous or easily provoked myocardial ischemia
Class IIa	Failed reperfusion or reocclusion after fibrinolytic therapy
	Stable[2] patients after successful fibrinolysis, before discharge and ideally between 3 and 24 hours

[1]Class I indicates treatment is useful and effective, IIa indicates weight of evidence is in favor of usefulness/efficacy, class IIb indicates weight of evidence is less well established, and class III indicates intervention is not useful/effective and may be harmful. Level of evidence A recommendations are derived from large-scale randomized trials, and B recommendations are derived from smaller randomized trials or carefully conducted observational analyses.
[2]Although individual circumstances will vary, clinical stability is defined by the absence of low output, hypotension, persistent tachycardia, apparent shock, high-grade ventricular or symptomatic supraventricular tachyarrhythmias, and spontaneous recurrent ischemia.
ACCF/AHA, American College of Cardiology Foundation/American Heart Association; ACS, acute coronary syndrome; CABG, coronary artery bypass grafting; HF, heart failure; PCI, percutaneous coronary intervention.
Data from O'Gara PT et al. 2013 ACCF/AHA guideline for the management of ST-elevation myocardial infarction: a report of the American College of Cardiology Foundation/American Heart Association Task Force on Practice Guidelines. Circulation. 2013;127: e362–e425.

Collet JP et al. 2020 ESC Guidelines for the management of acute coronary syndromes in patients presenting without persistent ST-segment elevation. Eur Heart J. 2021;42:1289. [PMID: 32860058]

Valgimigli M et al; MASTER DAPT Investigators. Dual antiplatelet therapy after PCI in patients at high bleeding risk. N Engl J Med. 2021;385:1643. [PMID: 34449185]

ACUTE MI WITH ST-SEGMENT ELEVATION

ESSENTIALS OF DIAGNOSIS

- Sudden but not instantaneous development of prolonged (> 30 minutes) anterior chest discomfort (sometimes felt as "gas" or pressure).
- Sometimes painless, masquerading as acute heart failure, syncope, stroke, or shock.
- ECG: ST-segment elevation or left bundle branch block.
- Immediate reperfusion treatment is warranted.
- Primary PCI within 90 minutes of first medical contact is the goal and is superior to fibrinolytic therapy.
- Fibrinolytic therapy within 30 minutes of hospital presentation is the goal and reduces mortality if given within 12 hours of onset of symptoms.

General Considerations

STEMI results, in most cases, from an occlusive coronary thrombus at the site of a preexisting (though not necessarily severe) atherosclerotic plaque. More rarely, infarction may result from prolonged vasospasm, inadequate myocardial blood flow (eg, hypotension), or excessive metabolic demand. Very rarely, MI may be caused by embolic occlusion, vasculitis, aortic root or coronary artery dissection, or aortitis. Cocaine, a cause of infarction, should be considered in young individuals without risk factors. A condition that may mimic STEMI is stress cardiomyopathy (also referred to as **tako-tsubo** or **apical ballooning syndrome**). ST elevation connotes an acute coronary occlusion and warrants *immediate* reperfusion therapy with activation of emergency services.

Clinical Findings

A. Symptoms

1. Premonitory pain—There is usually a worsening in the pattern of angina preceding the onset of symptoms of MI; classically the onset of angina occurs with minimal exertion or at rest.

2. Pain of infarction—Unlike anginal episodes, most infarctions occur *at rest*, and more commonly in the early morning. The pain is similar to angina in location and radiation but it may be more severe, and it builds up rapidly or in waves to maximum intensity over a few minutes or longer. Nitroglycerin has little effect; even opioids may not relieve the pain.

3. Associated symptoms—Patients may break out in a cold sweat, feel weak and apprehensive, and move about, seeking a position of comfort. They prefer not to lie quietly. Light-headedness, syncope, dyspnea, orthopnea, cough, wheezing, nausea and vomiting, or abdominal bloating may be present singly or in any combination.

4. Painless infarction—One-third of patients with acute MI present *without* chest pain, and these patients tend to be undertreated and have poor outcomes. Older patients, women, and patients with diabetes mellitus are more likely to present without chest pain. As many as 25% of infarctions are detected on routine ECG without any recallable acute episode.

5. Sudden death and early arrhythmias—Of all deaths from MI, about half occur before the patients arrive at the hospital, with death presumably caused by ventricular fibrillation.

B. Signs

1. General—Patients may appear anxious and sometimes are sweating profusely. The heart rate may range from marked bradycardia (most commonly in inferior infarction) to tachycardia, low cardiac output, or arrhythmia. The BP may be high, especially in former hypertensive patients, or low in patients with shock. Respiratory distress usually indicates heart failure. Fever, usually low grade, may appear after 12 hours and persist for several days.

2. Chest—The **Killip classification** is the standard way to classify heart failure in patients with acute MI and has powerful prognostic value. Killip class I is absence of rales and S_3, class II is rales that do not clear with coughing over one-third or less of the lung fields or presence of an S_3, class III is rales that do not clear with coughing over more than one-third of the lung fields, and class IV is cardiogenic shock (rales, hypotension, and signs of hypoperfusion).

3. Heart—The cardiac examination may be unimpressive or very abnormal. Jugular venous distention reflects RA hypertension, and a Kussmaul sign (failure of decrease of jugular venous pressure with inspiration) is suggestive of RV infarction. Soft heart sounds may indicate LV dysfunction. Atrial gallops (S_4) are the rule, whereas ventricular gallops (S_3) are less common and indicate significant LV dysfunction. Mitral regurgitation murmurs are not uncommon and may indicate papillary muscle dysfunction or, rarely, rupture. Pericardial friction rubs are uncommon in the first 24 hours but may appear later.

4. Extremities—Edema is usually not present. Cyanosis and cold temperature indicate low output. The peripheral pulses should be noted, since later shock or emboli may alter the examination.

C. Laboratory Findings

Cardiac-specific markers of myocardial damage include quantitative determinations of CK-MB, highly sensitive and conventional troponin I, and troponin T. Each of these tests may become positive as early as 4–6 hours after the onset of an MI and should be abnormal by 8–12 hours. Troponins are more sensitive and specific than CK-MB. "Highly sensitive" or "fourth-generation" troponin assays were approved in 2017. They are the standard assays in most of Europe, with a 10- to 100-fold lower limit of detection, allowing MI to be detected earlier, using the change in value over 3 hours.

Circulating levels of troponins may remain elevated for 5–7 days or longer and therefore are generally not useful for evaluating suspected early reinfarction. Elevated CK-MB generally normalizes within 24 hours, thus being more helpful for evaluation of reinfarction. Low-level elevations of troponin in patients with severe CKD may not be related to acute coronary disease but rather a function of the physiologic washout of the marker. While many conditions including chronic heart failure are associated with elevated levels of the high-sensitivity troponin assays, these assays may be especially useful when negative to exclude MI in patients reporting chest pain.

D. ECG

The extent of the ECG abnormalities, especially the sum of the total amount of ST-segment deviation, is a good indicator of the extent of acute infarction and risk of subsequent adverse events. The classic evolution of changes is from peaked ("hyperacute") T waves, to ST-segment elevation, to Q wave development, to T wave inversion. This may occur over a few hours to several days. The evolution of new Q waves (longer than 30 msec in duration and 25% of the R wave amplitude) is diagnostic, but Q waves do not occur in 30–50% of acute infarctions (**non-Q wave infarctions**). Left bundle branch block, especially when new (or not known to be old), in a patient with symptoms of an acute MI is considered to be a **"STEMI equivalent"**; reperfusion therapy is indicated for the affected patient. Concordant ST elevation (ie, ST elevation in leads with an overall positive QRS complex) with left bundle branch block is a specific finding indicating STEMI.

E. Chest Radiography

The chest radiograph may demonstrate signs of heart failure, but these changes often lag behind the clinical findings. Signs of aortic dissection, including mediastinal widening, should be sought as a possible alternative diagnosis.

F. Echocardiography

Echocardiography provides convenient *bedside assessment* of LV global and regional function. This can help with the diagnosis and management of infarction; echocardiography has been used successfully to make judgments about admission and management of patients with suspected infarction, including in patients with ST-segment elevation or left bundle branch block of uncertain significance, since normal wall motion makes an infarction unlikely. Doppler echocardiography is generally the most convenient procedure for diagnosing postinfarction mitral regurgitation or VSD.

G. Other Noninvasive Studies

Diagnosis of MI and extent of MI can be assessed by various imaging studies in addition to echocardiography. **MRI with gadolinium contrast enhancement** is the most sensitive test to detect and quantitate extent of infarction, with the ability to detect as little as 2 g of MI. **Technetium-99m pyrophosphate scintigraphy,** when injected at least 18 hours postinfarction, complexes with calcium in necrotic myocardium to provide a "hot spot" image of the infarction. This test is insensitive to small infarctions, and false-positive studies occur, so its use is limited to patients in whom the diagnosis by ECG and enzymes is not possible—principally those who present several days after the event or have intraoperative infarctions. **Scintigraphy with thallium-201** or **technetium-based perfusion tracers** will demonstrate "cold spots" in regions of diminished perfusion, which usually represent infarction when the radiotracer is administered at rest, but abnormalities do not distinguish recent from old damage. All of these tests may be considered after the patient has had revascularization.

H. Hemodynamic Measurements

These can be helpful in managing the patient with suspected cardiogenic shock. Use of PA catheters, however, has generally not been associated with better outcomes and should be limited to patients with severe hemodynamic compromise for whom the information would be anticipated to change management.

Treatment

A. Aspirin, $P2Y_{12}$ Inhibitors (Prasugrel, Ticagrelor, and Clopidogrel)

All patients with definite or suspected acute MI should receive aspirin at a dose of 162 mg or 325 mg at once regardless of whether fibrinolytic therapy is being considered or the patient has been taking aspirin. Chewable aspirin provides more rapid blood levels. Patients with a definite aspirin allergy should be treated with a $P2Y_{12}$ inhibitor (clopidogrel, prasugrel, or ticagrelor).

$P2Y_{12}$ inhibitors, in combination with aspirin, have been shown to provide important benefits in patients with acute STEMI. Thus, guidelines call for a **$P2Y_{12}$ inhibitor to be added to aspirin for all patients with STEMI, regardless of whether reperfusion is given, and continued for at least 14 days, and generally for 1 year.** The preferred $P2Y_{12}$ inhibitors are prasugrel (60 mg orally on day 1, then 10 mg daily) or ticagrelor (180 mg orally on day 1, then 90 mg twice daily). Both of these medications demonstrated superior outcomes to clopidogrel in clinical studies of primary PCI. Clopidogrel should be administered as a loading dose of 300–600 mg orally for faster onset of action than the 75 mg maintenance dose. With fibrinolytic therapy, ticagrelor appears to be a reasonable alternative to clopidogrel, at least after an initial clopidogrel dose. Prasugrel is contraindicated in patients with a history of stroke or who are older than 75 years.

B. Reperfusion Therapy

Patients with STEMI who seek medical attention within 12 hours of the onset of symptoms should be treated with reperfusion therapy, either primary PCI or fibrinolytic therapy. Patients without ST-segment elevation (previously labeled "non-Q wave" infarctions) do not benefit, and may derive harm, from thrombolysis.

1. Primary percutaneous coronary intervention—Immediate coronary angiography and primary PCI (including stenting) of the infarct-related artery have been shown to be *superior* to thrombolysis when done by experienced operators in high-volume centers with rapid time from first medical contact to intervention ("door-to-balloon"). US and European guidelines call for first medical contact or door-to-balloon times of 90 minutes or less. Several trials have shown that if efficient transfer systems are in place, transfer of patients with acute MI from hospitals without primary PCI capability to hospitals with primary PCI capability with first door-to-device times of 120 minutes or less can improve outcome compared with fibrinolytic therapy at the presenting hospital, although this requires sophisticated systems to ensure rapid identification, transfer, and expertise in PCI. Because PCI also carries a lower risk of hemorrhagic complications, including intracranial hemorrhage, it may be the preferred strategy in many older patients and others with contraindications to fibrinolytic therapy (see Table 10–8 for factors to consider in choosing fibrinolytic therapy or primary PCI).

A. STENTING—**PCI with stenting is standard for patients with acute MI.** Although randomized trials have shown a benefit with regard to fewer repeat interventions for restenosis with the use of drug-eluting stents in STEMI patients, and current generation drug-eluting stents have similar or lower rates of stent thrombosis than bare metal stents, bare metal stents may still be used for selected patients without the ability to obtain and comply with $P2Y_{12}$ inhibitor therapy. In the subgroup of patients with cardiogenic shock, early catheterization and percutaneous or surgical revascularization are the preferred management and have been shown to reduce mortality.

"Facilitated" PCI, whereby a combination of medications (full- or reduced-dose fibrinolytic agents, with or without glycoprotein IIb/IIIa inhibitors) is given followed by immediate PCI, is *not* recommended. *Patients should be treated either with primary PCI or with fibrinolytic agents (and immediate rescue PCI for reperfusion failure), if it can be done promptly as outlined in the ACC/AHA and European guidelines.* Timely access to most appropriate reperfusion, including primary PCI, can be expanded with development of regional systems of care, including emergency medical systems and networks of hospitals. Patients treated with fibrinolytic therapy appear to have improved outcomes if transferred for routine coronary angiography and PCI within 24 hours. The AHA has a program called "Mission: Lifeline" to support the development of regional systems of care (http://www.heart.org/missionlifeline).

B. ANTIPLATELET THERAPY AFTER DRUG-ELUTING OR BARE METAL STENTS—In patients with an acute coronary syndrome, **dual antiplatelet therapy** is indicated for 1 year in all patients (including those with medical therapy and those patients undergoing revascularization irrespective of stent type). For patients undergoing elective or stable PCI, the duration of dual antiplatelet therapy is recommended for at least 1 month for patients receiving bare metal stents. For patients receiving drug-eluting stents for acute coronary syndromes, dual antiplatelet therapy is recommended for at least 1 year by the ACC/AHA and European guidelines. These recommendations are based both on the durations of therapies during the studies evaluating the stents, and the pathophysiologic understanding of the timing of endothelialization following bare metal versus drug-eluting stent implantation. The DAPT (Dual Antiplatelet Therapy) study showed fewer death, MI, and stroke events with longer (up to 30 months) dual antiplatelet therapy for patients who had received drug-eluting stents, but it also showed more bleeding and a tendency for higher mortality. Treatment with clopidogrel for longer than 1 year after drug-eluting stents, therefore, should be individualized based on thrombotic and bleeding risks.

2. Fibrinolytic therapy—

A. BENEFIT—Fibrinolytic therapy reduces mortality and limits infarct size in patients with STEMI (defined as 0.1 mV or more in two inferior or lateral leads or two contiguous precordial leads), or with left bundle branch block (not known to be old). The greatest benefit occurs if treatment is initiated within the first 3 hours after the onset of presentation, when up to a 50% reduction in mortality rate can be achieved. The magnitude of benefit declines rapidly thereafter, but a 10% relative mortality reduction can be achieved up to 12 hours after the onset of chest pain. The survival benefit is greatest in patients with large—usually anterior—infarctions. Primary PCI (including stenting) of the infarct-related artery, however, is superior to thrombolysis when done by experienced operators with rapid time from first medical contact to intervention ("door-to-balloon").

B. CONTRAINDICATIONS—Major bleeding complications occur in 0.5–5% of patients, the most serious of which is intracranial hemorrhage. The major risk factors for intracranial bleeding are age 75 years or older, hypertension at presentation (especially over 180/110 mm Hg), low body weight (less than 70 kg), and the use of fibrin-specific fibrinolytic agents (alteplase, reteplase, tenecteplase). Although patients over age 75 years have a much higher mortality rate with acute MI and therefore may derive greater benefit, the risk of severe bleeding is also higher, particularly among patients with risk factors for intracranial hemorrhage, such as severe hypertension or recent stroke. Patients presenting more than 12 hours after the onset of chest pain may also derive a small benefit, particularly if pain and ST-segment elevation persist, but rarely does this benefit outweigh the attendant risk.

Absolute contraindications to fibrinolytic therapy include previous hemorrhagic stroke, other strokes or cerebrovascular events within 1 year, known intracranial neoplasm, recent head trauma (including minor trauma), active internal bleeding (excluding menstruation), or suspected aortic dissection. Relative contraindications are BP greater than 180/110 mm Hg at presentation, other intracerebral pathology not listed above as a contraindication, known bleeding diathesis, trauma within 2–4 weeks, major surgery within 3 weeks, prolonged (more than 10 minutes) or traumatic CPR, recent (within 2–4 weeks) internal bleeding, noncompressible vascular punctures, active diabetic retinopathy, pregnancy, active peptic ulcer disease, a history of severe hypertension, current use of anticoagulants (INR greater than 2.0–3.0), and (for streptokinase) prior allergic reaction or exposure to streptokinase or anistreplase within 2 years.

C. Fibrinolytic agents—The following fibrinolytic agents are available for acute MI and are characterized in Table 10–8.

Alteplase (recombinant tissue plasminogen activator; t-PA) results in about a 50% reduction in circulating fibrinogen. In the first GUSTO trial, which compared a 90-minute dosing of t-PA (with unfractionated heparin) with streptokinase, the 30-day mortality rate with t-PA was one absolute percentage point lower (one additional life saved per 100 patients treated), though there was also a small increase in the rate of intracranial hemorrhage. An angiographic substudy confirmed a higher 90-minute patency rate and a higher rate of normal (TIMI grade 3) flow in patients.

Reteplase is a recombinant deletion mutant of t-PA that is slightly less fibrin specific. In comparative trials, it appeared to have efficacy similar to that of alteplase, but it has a longer duration of action and can be administered as two boluses 30 minutes apart.

Tenecteplase (TNK-t-PA) is a genetically engineered substitution mutant of native t-PA that has reduced plasma clearance, increased fibrin sensitivity, and increased resistance to plasminogen activator inhibitor-1. It can be given as a single weight-adjusted bolus. In the ASSENT 2 trial, this agent was equivalent to t-PA with regard to efficacy and resulted in significantly less noncerebral bleeding.

Streptokinase, commonly used outside of the United States, is somewhat less effective at opening occluded arteries and less effective at reducing mortality. It is non–fibrin-specific, causes depletion of circulating fibrinogen, and has a tendency to induce hypotension, particularly if infused rapidly. This can be managed by slowing or interrupting the infusion and administering fluids. There is controversy as to whether adjunctive heparin is beneficial in patients given streptokinase, unlike its administration with the more clot-specific agents. Allergic reactions, including anaphylaxis, occur in 1–2% of patients, and this agent should generally not be administered to patients with prior exposure.

Table 10–8. Fibrinolytic therapy for acute MI.

	Alteplase; Tissue Plasminogen Activator (t-PA)	Reteplase	Tenecteplase (TNK-t-PA)	Streptokinase
Source	Recombinant DNA	Recombinant DNA	Recombinant DNA	Group C *Streptococcus*
Half-life	5 minutes	15 minutes	20 minutes	20 minutes
Usual dose	100 mg	20 units	40 mg	1.5 million units
Administration	Initial bolus of 15 mg, followed by 50 mg infused over the next 30 minutes and 35 mg over the following 60 minutes	10 units as a bolus over 2 minutes, repeated after 30 minutes	Single weight-adjusted bolus, 0.5 mg/kg	750,000 units over 20 minutes followed by 750,000 units over 40 minutes
Anticoagulation after infusion	Aspirin, 325 mg daily; heparin, 5000 units as bolus, followed by 1000 units/hour infusion, subsequently adjusted to maintain PTT 1.5–2 times control	Aspirin, 325 mg; heparin as with t-PA	Aspirin, 325 mg daily	Aspirin, 325 mg daily; there is no evidence that adjunctive heparin improves outcome following streptokinase
Clot selectivity	High	High	High	Low
Fibrinogenolysis	+	+	+	+++
Bleeding	+	+	+	+
Hypotension	+	+	+	+++
Allergic reactions	+	+	+	++
Reocclusion	10–30%	—	5–20%	5–20%
Approximate cost[1]	$10,560.43	$5964.98	$7462.63	Not available in the United States

[1]Average wholesale price (AWP, for AB-rated generic when available) for quantity listed.
PTT, partial thromboplastin time.
Source: IBM Micromedex, Red Book (electronic version). IBM Watson Health, Greenwood Village, CO, USA. Available at https://www.micromedexsolutions.com (accessed April 8, 2020). AWP may not accurately represent the actual pharmacy cost because wide contractual variations exist among institutions.

(1) Selection of a fibrinolytic agent—In the United States, most patients are treated with alteplase, reteplase, or tenecteplase. The differences in efficacy between them are small compared with the potential benefit of treating a greater proportion of appropriate candidates in a more prompt manner. The principal objective should be to administer a thrombolytic agent within 30 minutes of presentation—or even during transport. The ability to administer tenecteplase as a single bolus is an attractive feature that may facilitate earlier treatment. The combination of a reduced-dose thrombolytic given with a platelet glycoprotein IIb/IIIa inhibitor does not reduce mortality but does cause a modest increase in bleeding complications.

(2) Postfibrinolytic management—After completion of the fibrinolytic infusion, aspirin (81–325 mg/day) and anticoagulation should be continued until revascularization or for the duration of the hospital stay (or up to 8 days). Anticoagulation with LMWH (enoxaparin or fondaparinux) is preferable to unfractionated heparin.

(A) LOW-MOLECULAR-WEIGHT HEPARIN—In the EXTRACT trial, enoxaparin significantly reduced death and MI at day 30 (compared with unfractionated heparin), at the expense of a modest increase in bleeding. In patients younger than age 75, enoxaparin was given as a 30-mg intravenous bolus and 1 mg/kg subcutaneously every 12 hours; in patients aged 75 years and older, it was given with no bolus and 0.75 mg/kg subcutaneously every 12 hours. This appeared to attenuate the risk of intracranial hemorrhage in older adults that had been seen with full-dose enoxaparin. Another antithrombotic option is fondaparinux, given at a dose of 2.5 mg subcutaneously once a day. There is no benefit of fondaparinux among patients undergoing primary PCI, and fondaparinux is not recommended as a sole anticoagulant during PCI due to risk of catheter thrombosis.

(B) UNFRACTIONATED HEPARIN—Anticoagulation with intravenous heparin (initial dose of 60 units/kg bolus to a maximum of 4000 units, followed by an infusion of 12 units/kg/hour to a maximum of 1000 units/hour, then adjusted to maintain an aPTT of 50–75 seconds beginning with an aPTT drawn 3 hours after thrombolytic) is continued for at least 48 hours after alteplase, reteplase, or tenecteplase, and with continuation of an anticoagulant until revascularization (if performed) or until hospital discharge (or day 8).

The VALIDATE trial found no benefit to bivalirudin compared to unfractionated heparin regarding the outcome of death, MI, or major bleeding.

(C) PROPHYLACTIC THERAPY AGAINST GI BLEEDING—For all patients with STEMI treated with intensive antithrombotic therapy, prophylactic treatment with PPIs, or antacids and an H_2-blocker, is advisable. However, certain PPIs, such as omeprazole and esomeprazole, may decrease the clinical effect of clopidogrel; in such cases, pantoprazole may be a better PPI option.

3. Assessment of myocardial reperfusion, recurrent ischemic pain, reinfarction—Myocardial reperfusion can be recognized clinically by the early cessation of pain and the resolution of ST-segment elevation. Although at least 50% resolution of ST-segment elevation by 90 minutes may occur without coronary reperfusion, ST resolution is a strong predictor of better outcome. Even with anticoagulation, 10–20% of reperfused vessels will reocclude during hospitalization, although reocclusion and reinfarction appear to be reduced following intervention. Reinfarction, indicated by recurrence of pain and ST-segment elevation, can be treated by readministration of a thrombolytic agent or immediate angiography and PCI.

C. General Measures

Cardiac care unit monitoring should be instituted as soon as possible. Patients without complications can be transferred to a telemetry unit after 24 hours. Activity should initially be limited to bed rest but can be advanced within 24 hours. Progressive ambulation should be started after 24–72 hours if tolerated. For patients without complications, discharge by day 4 appears to be appropriate. Low-flow oxygen therapy (2–4 L/minute) should be given if oxygen saturation is reduced, but there is no value to routine use of oxygen.

D. Analgesia

An initial attempt should be made to relieve pain with sublingual nitroglycerin. However, if no response occurs after two or three tablets, intravenous opioids provide the most rapid and effective analgesia and may also reduce pulmonary congestion. Morphine sulfate, 4–8 mg, or meperidine, 50–75 mg, should be given. Subsequent small doses can be given every 15 minutes until pain abates.

NSAIDs, other than aspirin, should be avoided during hospitalization for STEMI due to increased risk of mortality, myocardial rupture, hypertension, heart failure, and kidney injury with their use.

E. Beta-Adrenergic Blocking Agents

Trials have shown modest short-term benefit from beta-blockers started during the first 24 hours after acute MI if there are no contraindications (metoprolol 25–50 mg orally twice daily). Aggressive beta-blockade can increase shock, with overall harm in patients with heart failure. Thus, early beta-blockade should be avoided in patients with any degree of heart failure, evidence of low output state, increased risk of cardiogenic shock, or other relative contraindications to beta-blockade. Carvedilol (beginning at 6.25 mg twice a day, titrated to 25 mg twice a day) was shown to be beneficial in the CAPRICORN trial following the acute phase of large MI.

F. Nitrates

Nitroglycerin is the agent of choice for continued or recurrent ischemic pain and is useful in lowering BP or relieving pulmonary congestion. However, routine nitrate administration is not recommended, since no improvement in outcome has been observed in the ISIS-4 or GISSI-3 trials. Nitrates should be avoided in patients who received phosphodiesterase inhibitors (sildenafil, vardenafil, and tadalafil) in the prior 24 hours.

G. ACE Inhibitors

A series of trials (SAVE, AIRE, SMILE, TRACE, GISSI-III, and ISIS-4) have shown both short- and long-term improvement in survival with ACE inhibitor therapy. The benefits are greatest in patients with an EF of 40% or less, large infarctions, or clinical evidence of heart failure. Because substantial amounts of the survival benefit occur on the first day, ACE inhibitor treatment should be commenced early in patients without hypotension, especially patients with large or anterior MI. Given the benefits of ACE inhibitors for patients with vascular disease, it is reasonable to **use ACE inhibitors for *all* patients following STEMI who do not have contraindications.**

H. Angiotensin Receptor Blockers

Although there has been inconsistency in the effects of different ARBs on mortality for patients post-MI with heart failure and/or LV dysfunction, the VALIANT trial showed that valsartan 160 mg orally twice a day is *equivalent* to captopril in reducing mortality. Thus, valsartan should be used for all patients with ACE inhibitor intolerance, and is a reasonable, albeit more expensive, alternative to captopril. The combination of captopril and valsartan (at a reduced dose) was no better than either agent alone and resulted in more side effects.

I. Aldosterone Antagonists

The RALES trial showed that 25 mg of spironolactone can reduce the mortality rate of patients with advanced heart failure, and the EPHESUS trial showed a 15% relative risk reduction in mortality with eplerenone 25 mg daily for patients post-MI with LV dysfunction (LVEF of 40% or less) and either clinical heart failure or diabetes. Kidney dysfunction or hyperkalemia are contraindications, and patients must be monitored carefully for development of hyperkalemia.

J. Calcium Channel Blockers

There are no studies to support the routine use of calcium channel blockers in most patients with acute MI—and indeed, they have the potential to exacerbate ischemia and cause death from reflex tachycardia or myocardial depression. Long-acting calcium channel blockers should generally be reserved for management of hypertension or ischemia as second- or third-line medications after beta-blockers and nitrates.

K. Long-Term Antithrombotic Therapy

Discharge on aspirin, 81–325 mg/day, since it is highly effective, inexpensive, and well tolerated, is a key quality indicator of MI care. Patients who received a coronary stent should also receive a $P2Y_{12}$ inhibitor (see Antiplatelet therapy after drug-eluting or bare metal stents, above).

Patients who have received a coronary stent and who require warfarin anticoagulation present a particular challenge, since **"triple therapy"** with aspirin, clopidogrel, and warfarin has a high risk of bleeding. Triple therapy should be (1) limited to patients with a clear indication for warfarin (such as $CHADS_2$ score of 2 or more or a mechanical prosthetic valve), (2) used for the shortest period of time (such as 1 month after placement of bare metal stent; drug-eluting stents that would require longer clopidogrel duration should be avoided if possible), (3) used with low-dose aspirin and with strategies to reduce risk of bleeding (eg, PPIs for patients with a history of GI bleeding), and (4) used with consideration of a lower target anticoagulation intensity (INR 2.0–2.5, at least for the indication of atrial fibrillation) during the period of concomitant treatment with aspirin and $P2Y_{12}$ therapy. The PIONEER trial studied three treatment regimens for patients with atrial fibrillation who had coronary stent placement with a primary outcome of bleeding: (1) rivaroxaban 2.5 mg twice daily plus clopidogrel, (2) rivaroxaban 15 mg once daily plus clopidogrel, and (3) warfarin plus aspirin plus clopidogrel. There was less bleeding in the patients who received rivaroxaban plus clopidogrel than in those who received "triple therapy," although the trial was not powered to assess efficacy, and thus the low dose of rivaroxaban may be inadequate. Consensus statements recommend oral anticoagulation (with either warfarin or a DOAC) be combined with clopidogrel and with a relatively short duration of aspirin until hospital discharge up to 3 months for the typical patient with atrial fibrillation and coronary stents. Dabigatran, 110 mg and 150 mg, was also studied in patients with atrial fibrillation who underwent PCI. Dual therapy with dabigatran and clopidogrel was shown to be beneficial for bleeding compared to triple therapy, with similar rates of thrombotic cardiovascular events. However, there were too few thrombotic events to be certain about efficacy of discontinuing the aspirin, and there was a suggestion that MI and stent thrombosis occurred more often with the 110-mg dose of dabigatran than with clopidogrel alone. **Given the trial evidence to date, for a typical patient, it is reasonable to use a DOAC and clopidogrel and to discontinue aspirin at the time of hospital discharge or at 7 days after stenting.** The AUGUSTUS trial, which tested apixaban versus warfarin and aspirin versus placebo in a factorial trial, found that apixaban resulted in 31% less major and clinically relevant non major bleeding than warfarin for patients with atrial fibrillation and coronary stents or acute coronary syndromes or both. Avoiding aspirin, after an average of 6 days after the PCI, resulted in less bleeding and a nonsignificant increase in stent thrombosis. It is reasonable to stop aspirin at hospital discharge or at day 7 for patients with atrial fibrillation who are taking apixaban or warfarin at the time of discharge, although continuing aspirin for 1 month may reduce stent thrombosis.

L. Coronary Angiography

For patients who do not reperfuse based on lack of at least 50% resolution of ST elevation, **rescue angioplasty** should be performed and has been shown to reduce the composite risk of death, reinfarction, stroke, or severe heart failure. Patients treated with coronary angiography and PCI 3–24 hours after fibrinolytic therapy showed improved outcomes. Patients with recurrent ischemic pain prior to discharge should undergo catheterization and, if indicated, revascularization. PCI of a totally occluded infarct-related artery more than 24 hours after STEMI should generally not be performed in asymptomatic patients with one- or two-vessel disease without evidence of severe ischemia.

When to Refer

All patients with acute MI should be referred to a cardiologist.

Lopes RD et al; AUGUSTUS Investigators. Antithrombotic therapy after acute coronary syndrome or PCI in atrial fibrillation. N Engl J Med. 2019;380:1509. [PMID: 30883055]

Complications

A variety of complications can occur after MI even when treatment is initiated promptly.

A. Postinfarction Ischemia

In clinical trials of thrombolysis, recurrent ischemia occurred in about one-third of patients, was more common following NSTEMI than after STEMI, and had important short- and long-term prognostic implications. Vigorous medical therapy should be instituted, including nitrates and beta-blockers as well as aspirin 81–325 mg/day, anticoagulant therapy (unfractionated heparin, enoxaparin, or fondaparinux), and clopidogrel (75 mg orally daily). Most patients with postinfarction angina—and all who are refractory to medical therapy—should undergo early catheterization and revascularization by PCI or CABG.

B. Arrhythmias

Abnormalities of rhythm and conduction are common.

1. Sinus bradycardia—This is most common in inferior infarctions or may be precipitated by medications. Observation or withdrawal of the offending agent is usually sufficient. If accompanied by signs of low cardiac output, atropine intravenously is usually effective. Temporary pacing is rarely required.

2. Supraventricular tachyarrhythmias—Sinus tachycardia is common and may reflect either increased adrenergic stimulation or hemodynamic compromise due to hypovolemia or pump failure. In the latter, beta-blockade is contraindicated. Supraventricular premature beats are common and may be premonitory for atrial fibrillation. Electrolyte abnormalities and hypoxia should be corrected and causative agents (especially aminophylline) stopped. Atrial fibrillation should be rapidly controlled or converted to sinus rhythm. Intravenous beta-blockers, such as metoprolol (2.5–5 mg intravenously every 2–5 minutes, maximum 15 mg over 10-minutes) or short-acting esmolol (50–200 mcg/kg/minute), are the agents of choice if cardiac function is adequate. Intravenous diltiazem (5–15 mg/hour) may be used if beta-blockers are contraindicated or ineffective. Electrical cardioversion (commencing with 100 J) may be necessary if atrial fibrillation is complicated by hypotension, heart failure, or ischemia, but the arrhythmia often recurs. Amiodarone (150 mg intravenous bolus and then 15–30 mg/hour intravenously, or rapid oral loading dose for cardioversion of 400 mg three times daily) may be helpful to restore or maintain sinus rhythm.

3. Ventricular arrhythmias—Ventricular arrhythmias are most common in the first few hours after infarction and are a marker of high risk. Ventricular premature beats may be premonitory for ventricular tachycardia or fibrillation, but generally should *not* be treated in the absence of frequent or sustained ventricular tachycardia. Lidocaine is *not* recommended as a prophylactic measure.

Sustained ventricular tachycardia should be treated with a 1 mg/kg bolus of lidocaine if the patient is stable or by electrical cardioversion (100–200 J) if not. If the arrhythmia cannot be suppressed with lidocaine, procainamide (100 mg boluses over 1–2 minutes every 5 minutes to a cumulative dose of 750–1000 mg) or intravenous amiodarone (150 mg over 10 minutes, which may be repeated as needed, followed by 360 mg over 6 hours and then 540 mg over 18 hours) should be initiated, followed by an infusion of 0.5 mg/minute (720 mg/24 hours). Ventricular fibrillation is treated electrically (300–400 J). All patients taking antiarrhythmics should be monitored with telemetry or ECGs during initiation. Unresponsive ventricular fibrillation should be treated with additional amiodarone and repeat cardioversion while CPR is administered.

Accelerated idioventricular rhythm is a regular, wide-complex rhythm at a rate of 60–120/minute. It may occur with or without reperfusion and should not be treated with antiarrhythmics, which could cause asystole.

4. Conduction disturbances—All degrees of AV block may occur in the course of acute MI. Block at the level of the AV node is more common than infranodal block and occurs in approximately 20% of inferior MIs. First-degree block is the most common and requires no treatment. Second-degree block is usually of the Mobitz type I form (Wenckebach), is often transient, and requires treatment only if associated with a heart rate slow enough to cause symptoms. Complete AV block occurs in up to 5% of acute inferior infarctions, usually is preceded by Mobitz I second-degree block, and generally resolves spontaneously, though it may persist for hours to several weeks. The escape rhythm originates in the distal AV node or AV junction and hence has a narrow QRS complex and is reliable, albeit often slow (30–50 beats/minute). Treatment is often necessary because of resulting hypotension and low cardiac output. Intravenous atropine (1 mg) usually restores AV conduction temporarily, but if the escape complex is wide or if repeated atropine treatments are needed, temporary ventricular pacing is indicated. The prognosis for these patients is only slightly worse than for patients in whom AV block does not develop.

In anterior infarctions, the site of block is distal, below the AV node, and usually a result of extensive damage of the His-Purkinje system and bundle branches. New first-degree block (prolongation of the PR interval) is unusual in anterior infarction; Mobitz type II AV block or complete heart block may be preceded by intraventricular conduction defects or may occur abruptly. The escape rhythm, if present, is an unreliable wide-complex idioventricular rhythm. Urgent ventricular pacing is mandatory, but even with successful pacing, morbidity and mortality are high because of the extensive myocardial damage. New conduction abnormalities, such as right or left bundle branch block or fascicular blocks, may presage progression, often sudden, to second- or third-degree AV block. Temporary ventricular pacing is recommended for new-onset alternating bilateral bundle branch block, bifascicular block, or bundle branch block with worsening first-degree AV block. Patients with anterior infarction who progress to second- or third-degree block even transiently should be considered for insertion of a prophylactic permanent ventricular pacemaker before discharge.

C. Myocardial Dysfunction

Persons with hypotension not responsive to fluid resuscitation or refractory heart failure or cardiogenic shock should be considered for urgent echocardiography to assess left and right ventricular function and for mechanical complications, right heart catheterization, and continuous measurements of arterial pressure. These measurements permit the accurate assessment of volume status and may facilitate decisions about volume resuscitation, selective use of vasopressors and inotropes, and mechanical support.

1. Acute LV failure—Dyspnea, diffuse rales, and arterial hypoxemia usually indicate LV failure. General measures include supplemental oxygen to increase arterial saturation to above 95% and elevation of the trunk. Diuretics are usually the initial therapy unless RV infarction is present. Intravenous furosemide (10–40 mg) or bumetanide (0.5–1 mg) is preferred because of the reliably rapid onset and short duration of action of these medications. Higher dosages can be given if an inadequate response occurs. Morphine sulfate (4 mg intravenously followed by increments of 2 mg) is valuable in acute pulmonary edema.

Diuretics are usually effective; however, because most patients with acute infarction are not volume overloaded, the hemodynamic response may be limited and may be associated with hypotension. In mild heart failure, sublingual isosorbide dinitrate (2.5–10 mg every 2 hours) or nitroglycerin ointment (6.25–25 mg every 4 hours) may be adequate to lower pulmonary capillary wedge pressure (PCWP). In more severe failure, especially if cardiac output is reduced and BP is normal or high, sodium nitroprusside may be the preferred agent. It should be initiated only with arterial pressure monitoring; the initial dosage should be low (0.25 mcg/kg/minute) to avoid excessive hypotension, but the dosage can be increased by increments of 0.5 mcg/kg/minute every 5–10 minutes up to 5–10 mcg/kg/minute until the desired hemodynamic response is obtained. Excessive hypotension (mean BP less than 65–75 mm Hg) or tachycardia (greater than 10/minutes increase) should be avoided.

Intravenous nitroglycerin (starting at 10 mcg/minute) also may be effective but may lower PCWP with less hypotension. Oral or transdermal vasodilator therapy with nitrates or ACE inhibitors is often necessary after the initial 24–48 hours.

Inotropic agents should be avoided if possible, because they often increase heart rate and myocardial oxygen requirements and worsen clinical outcomes. Dobutamine has the best hemodynamic profile, increasing cardiac output and modestly lowering PCWP, usually without excessive tachycardia, hypotension, or arrhythmias. The initial dosage is 2.5 mcg/kg/minute, and it may be increased by similar increments up to 15–20 mcg/kg/minute at intervals of 5–10 minutes. Dopamine is more useful in the presence of hypotension, since it produces peripheral vasoconstriction, but it has a less beneficial effect on PCWP. Digoxin has not been helpful in acute infarction except to control the ventricular response in atrial fibrillation, but it may be beneficial if chronic heart failure persists.

2. Hypotension and shock—Patients with hypotension (systolic BP less than 90 mm Hg, individualized depending on prior BP) and signs of diminished perfusion (low urinary output, confusion, cold extremities) that does not respond to fluid resuscitation should be presumed to have cardiogenic shock and should be considered for urgent catheterization and revascularization. Sparing use of **intra-aortic balloon pump (IABP)** support and hemodynamic monitoring with a **PA catheter** can be considered, although these later measures have *not* been shown to improve outcome. Up to 20% will have findings indicative of intravascular hypovolemia (due to diaphoresis, vomiting, decreased venous tone, medications—such as diuretics, nitrates, morphine, beta-blockers, calcium channel blockers, and thrombolytic agents—and lack of oral intake). These should be treated with successive boluses of 100 mL of normal saline until PCWP reaches 15–18 mm Hg to determine whether cardiac output and BP respond. Pericardial tamponade due to hemorrhagic pericarditis (especially after thrombolytic therapy or CPR) or ventricular rupture should be considered and excluded by echocardiography if clinically indicated. RV infarction, characterized by a normal PCWP but elevated RA pressure, can produce hypotension. This is discussed below.

Most patients with cardiogenic shock will have moderate to severe LV systolic dysfunction, with a mean EF of 30% in the SHOCK trial. If hypotension is only modest (systolic pressure higher than 90 mm Hg) and the PCWP is elevated, diuretics should be administered. If the BP falls, inotropic support will need to be added. A large randomized trial showed *no benefit* of IABP support in cardiogenic shock.

Norepinephrine (0.1–0.5 mcg/kg/minute) is generally considered to be the most appropriate inotrope/vasopressor for cardiogenic shock based on limited randomized clinical trial evidence suggesting less arrhythmias and improved outcomes compared with dopamine. Dopamine is nonetheless also an option and can be initiated at a rate of 2–4 mcg/kg/minute and increased at 5-minute intervals to the appropriate hemodynamic end point. At dosages lower than 5 mcg/kg/minute, it improves renal blood flow; at intermediate dosages (2.5–10 mcg/kg/min), it stimulates myocardial contractility; at higher dosages (greater than 8 mcg/kg/minute), it is a potent alpha-1-adrenergic agonist. In general, BP and cardiac index rise, but PCWP does not fall. Dopamine may be combined with nitroprusside or dobutamine (see above for dosing), or the latter may be used in its place if hypotension is not severe.

Patients with cardiogenic shock not due to hypovolemia have a poor prognosis, with 30-day mortality rates of 40–80%. The IABP-SHOCK II trial found that the use of an IABP does not offer a mortality benefit at 30 days or 1 year, compared with routine care with rapid revascularization, and is likely not helpful. Surgically implanted (or percutaneous) ventricular assist devices may be used in refractory cases. Emergent cardiac catheterization and coronary angiography followed by percutaneous or surgical revascularization offer the best chance of survival. Additionally, revascularization in shock should be aimed at the culprit artery only, avoiding multivessel PCI.

D. RV Infarction

RV infarction is present in one-third of patients with inferior wall infarction but is clinically significant in less than 50% of these. It presents as hypotension with relatively preserved LV function and should be considered whenever patients with inferior infarction exhibit low BP, raised venous pressure, and clear lungs. Hypotension is often exacerbated by medications that decrease intravascular volume or produce venodilation, such as diuretics, nitrates, and opioids. RA pressure and JVP are high, while PCWP is normal or low and the lungs are clear. The diagnosis is suggested by ST-segment elevation in right-sided anterior chest leads, particularly RV_4. The diagnosis can be confirmed by echocardiography or hemodynamic measurements. Treatment consists of fluid loading beginning with 500 mL of 0.9% saline over 2 hours to improve LV filling, and inotropic agents only if necessary.

E. Mechanical Defects

Partial or complete rupture of a papillary muscle or of the interventricular septum occurs in less than 1% of acute MIs and carries a poor prognosis. These complications occur in both anterior and inferior infarctions, usually 3–7 days after the acute event. They are detected by the appearance of a new systolic murmur and clinical deterioration, often with pulmonary edema. The two lesions are distinguished by the location of the murmur (apical versus parasternal) and by Doppler echocardiography. Hemodynamic monitoring is essential for appropriate management and demonstrates an increase in oxygen saturation between the RA and PA in VSD and, often, a large *v* wave with mitral regurgitation. Treatment by nitroprusside and, preferably, **intra-aortic balloon counterpulsation (IABC)** reduces the regurgitation or shunt, but surgical correction is mandatory. In patients remaining hemodynamically unstable or requiring continuous parenteral pharmacologic treatment or counterpulsation, early surgery is recommended, though mortality rates are high (15% to nearly 100%, depending on residual ventricular function and clinical status). Patients who are stabilized medically can have delayed surgery with lower risks (10–25%), although this may be due to the death of sicker patients, some of whom may have been saved by earlier surgery.

F. Myocardial Rupture

Complete rupture of the LV free wall occurs in less than 1% of patients and usually results in immediate death. It occurs 2–7 days postinfarction, usually involves the anterior wall, and is more frequent in older women. Incomplete or gradual rupture may be sealed off by the pericardium, creating a pseudoaneurysm. This may be recognized by echocardiography, radionuclide angiography, or LV angiography, often as an incidental finding. It demonstrates a narrow-neck connection to the LV. Early surgical repair is indicated, since delayed rupture is common.

G. LV Aneurysm

An LV aneurysm, a sharply delineated area of scar that bulges paradoxically during systole, develops in 10–20% of patients surviving an acute infarction. This usually follows anterior ST-elevation infarctions. Aneurysms are recognized by persistent ST-segment elevation (beyond 4–8 weeks), and a wide neck from the LV can be demonstrated by echocardiography, scintigraphy, or contrast angiography. They rarely rupture but may be associated with arterial emboli, ventricular arrhythmias, and heart failure. Surgical resection may be performed for these indications if other measures fail. The best results (mortality rates of 10–20%) are obtained when the residual myocardium contracts well and when significant coronary lesions supplying adjacent regions are bypassed.

H. Pericarditis

The pericardium is involved in approximately 50% of infarctions, but pericarditis is often not clinically significant. Twenty percent of patients with ST-elevation infarctions will have an audible friction rub if examined repetitively. Pericardial pain occurs in approximately the same proportion after 2–7 days and is recognized by its variation with respiration and position (improved by sitting). Often, no treatment is required, but aspirin (650 mg every 4–6 hours) will usually relieve the pain. Indomethacin and corticosteroids can cause impaired infarct healing and predispose to myocardial rupture, and therefore should generally be avoided in the early post-MI period. Likewise, anticoagulation should be used cautiously, since hemorrhagic pericarditis may result.

One week to 12 weeks after infarction, **Dressler syndrome** (post-MI syndrome) occurs in less than 5% of patients. This is an autoimmune phenomenon and presents as pericarditis with associated fever, leukocytosis, and, occasionally, pericardial or pleural effusion. It may recur over months. Treatment is the same as for other forms of pericarditis. A short course of nonsteroidal agents or corticosteroids may help relieve symptoms, but the use of nonsteroidal agents in the first several weeks after MI may impair infarct healing.

I. Mural Thrombus

Mural thrombi are common in large anterior infarctions but not in infarctions at other locations. Arterial emboli occur in approximately 2% of patients with known infarction, usually within 6 weeks. Anticoagulation with heparin followed by short-term (3-month) warfarin therapy (or DOAC therapy based on limited case report experience) results in clot resolution and prevents most emboli and should be considered in all patients with large anterior infarctions and evidence of LV thrombi. Mural thrombi can be detected by echocardiography or cardiac MRI. If the thrombus is resolved at 3 months, then anticoagulation can be discontinued.

Postinfarction Management

After the first 24 hours, the focus of patient management is to prevent recurrent ischemia, improve infarct healing and prevent remodeling, and prevent recurrent vascular events. Patients with hemodynamic compromise, who are at high risk for death, need careful monitoring and management of volume status.

A. Risk Stratification

Risk stratification is important for the management of STEMI. GRACE and TIMI risk scores can be helpful tools. Patients with recurrent ischemia (spontaneous or provoked), hemodynamic instability, impaired LV function, heart failure, or serious ventricular arrhythmias should undergo cardiac catheterization (see Table 10–7). ACE inhibitor (or ARB) therapy is indicated in patients with clinical heart failure or LVEF of 40% or less. Aldosterone blockade is indicated for patients with an LVEF of 40% or less and either heart failure or diabetes mellitus.

For patients not undergoing cardiac catheterization, submaximal exercise (or pharmacologic stress testing for patients unable to exercise) before discharge or a maximal test after 3–6 weeks (the latter being more sensitive for ischemia) helps patients and clinicians plan the return to normal activity. Imaging in conjunction with stress testing adds additional sensitivity for ischemia and provides localizing information. Both exercise and pharmacologic stress imaging have successfully predicted subsequent outcome. One of these tests should be used prior to discharge in patients who have received thrombolytic therapy as a means of selecting appropriate candidates for coronary angiography.

B. Secondary Prevention

Postinfarction management should begin with identification and modification of risk factors. Treatment of hyperlipidemia and smoking cessation both prevent recurrent infarction and death. Statin therapy should be started before the patient is discharged from the hospital to reduce recurrent atherothrombotic events. BP control as well as cardiac rehabilitation and exercise are also recommended. They can be of considerable psychological benefit and appear to improve prognosis.

Beta-blockers improve survival rates, primarily by reducing the incidence of sudden death in high-risk subsets of patients, though their value may be less in patients without complications with small infarctions and normal exercise tests. While a variety of beta-blockers have been shown to be beneficial, for patients with LV dysfunction managed with contemporary treatment, carvedilol titrated to 25 mg orally twice a day has been shown to reduce mortality. Beta-blockers with intrinsic sympathomimetic activity have not proved beneficial in postinfarction patients.

Antiplatelet agents are beneficial; aspirin (75–100 mg daily, after the initial dose) and $P2Y_{12}$ inhibitor therapy for 1 year are recommended. Prasugrel provides further reduction in thrombotic outcomes compared with clopidogrel, at the cost of more bleeding, but is contraindicated for patients with prior stroke. Likewise, ticagrelor provides benefit over clopidogrel. Calcium channel blockers have *not* been shown to improve prognoses overall and should not be prescribed purely for secondary prevention. Antiarrhythmic therapy other than with beta-blockers has *not* been shown to be effective except in patients with symptomatic arrhythmias. Amiodarone has been studied in several trials of postinfarct patients with either LV dysfunction or frequent ventricular ectopy. Although survival was not improved, amiodarone was not harmful—unlike other agents in this setting. Therefore, it is the agent of choice for individuals with symptomatic postinfarction supraventricular arrhythmias. While implantable defibrillators improve survival for patients with postinfarction LV dysfunction and heart failure, the DINAMIT trial found no benefit to implantable defibrillators implanted in the 40 days following acute MI.

C. ACE Inhibitors and ARBs in Patients with LV Dysfunction

Patients who sustain substantial myocardial damage often experience subsequent progressive LV dilation and dysfunction, leading to clinical heart failure and reduced long-term survival. In patients with EFs less than 40%, long-term ACE inhibitor (or ARB) therapy prevents LV dilation and the onset of heart failure and prolongs survival. The HOPE trial, as well as an overview of trials of ACE inhibitors for secondary prevention, also demonstrated a reduction of approximately 20% in mortality rates and the occurrence of nonfatal MI and stroke with ramipril treatment of patients with coronary or peripheral vascular disease and without confirmed LV systolic dysfunction. Therefore, ACE inhibitor therapy should be strongly considered in this broader group of patients—and especially in patients with diabetes and those with even mild systolic hypertension, in whom the greatest benefit was observed (see Table 11–6).

D. Revascularization

The indications for CABG are similar to those for patients with chronic coronary syndromes, including left main stenosis and multivessel disease (particularly with type 2 diabetes or LV dysfunction, or both). For patients who have undergone primary PCI and have residual left main or multivessel disease, CABG may be appropriate, but the timing needs to take into account the high risk of stent thrombosis if $P2Y_{12}$ inhibitor therapy is interrupted. For patients with noninfarct-related CAD, stenting should generally be performed on these lesions prior to hospital discharge.

Ibanez B et al. 2017 ESC guidelines for the management of acute myocardial infarction in patients presenting with ST-segment elevation: the Task Force for the management of acute myocardial infarction in patients presenting with ST-segment elevation of the European Society of Cardiology (ESC). Eur Heart J. 2018;39:119. [PMID: 28886621]

DISORDERS OF RATE & RHYTHM

Abnormalities of cardiac rhythm and conduction can be symptomatic (syncope, near syncope, dizziness, fatigue, or palpitations) or asymptomatic. In addition, they can be lethal (sudden cardiac death) or dangerous to the extent that they reduce cardiac output, so that perfusion of the brain and myocardium is impaired. Stable supraventricular tachycardia (SVT) is generally well tolerated in patients without underlying heart disease but may lead to myocardial ischemia or heart failure in patients with coronary disease, valvular abnormalities, and systolic or diastolic myocardial dysfunction. Ventricular tachycardia, if prolonged, often results in hemodynamic compromise and may deteriorate into ventricular fibrillation if left untreated.

Whether slow heart rates produce symptoms at rest or with exertion depends on whether cerebral and peripheral perfusion can be maintained, which is generally a function of whether the patient is upright or supine and whether LV function is adequate to maintain stroke volume. If the heart rate abruptly slows, as with the onset of complete heart block or sinus arrest, syncope or convulsions (or both) may result. Unless a clear, reversible cause is found, most symptomatic patients require implantation of a permanent pacemaker.

The diagnosis of an abnormal tachyarrhythmia often can be made via cardiac monitoring, including in-hospital and ambulatory ECG monitoring, event recorders, continuous mobile cardiac telemetry, or implantable loop recorders. Additionally, optic sensors on wearable devices, such as smartwatches, utilize a passive irregular pulse notification algorithm to identify possible arrhythmia, with a positive predictive value for detection of atrial fibrillation of approximately 70%. Devices, such as certain Apple Watches and the AliveCor device, can record actual ECGs of rhythm that can be transmitted to health care providers. More invasive testing, including catheter-based electrophysiologic studies (to assess sinus node function, AV conduction, and inducibility of arrhythmias), and tests of autonomic nervous system function (tilt-table testing) can also be performed.

Treatment of tachyarrhythmias varies and can include modalities such as antiarrhythmic medications and more invasive techniques such as catheter ablation.

Antiarrhythmic Medications

Antiarrhythmic medications are frequently used to treat arrhythmias, but have variable efficacy and produce frequent side effects (Table 10–9). They are often divided into classes based on their electropharmacologic actions and many of these medications have multiple actions. The most frequently used classification scheme is the **Vaughan-Williams,** which consists of four classes.

Class I agents block membrane sodium channels. Three subclasses are further defined by the effect of the agents on the Purkinje fiber action potential. **Class Ia** medications (ie, quinidine, procainamide, disopyramide) slow the rate of rise of the action potential (V_{max}) and prolong its duration, thus slowing conduction and increasing refractoriness (moderate depression of phase 0 upstroke of the action potential). **Class Ib** agents (ie, lidocaine, mexiletine) shorten action potential duration; they do not affect conduction or refractoriness (minimal depression of phase 0 upstroke of the action potential). **Class Ic** agents (ie, flecainide, propafenone) prolong V_{max} and slow repolarization, thus slowing conduction and prolonging refractoriness, but more so than class Ia medications (maximal depression of phase 0 upstroke of the action potential).

Class II agents are the beta-blockers, which decrease automaticity, prolong AV conduction, and prolong refractoriness.

Class III agents (ie, amiodarone, dronedarone, sotalol, dofetilide, ibutilide) block potassium channels and prolong repolarization, widening the QRS and prolonging the QT interval. They decrease automaticity and conduction and prolong refractoriness.

Class IV agents are the calcium channel blockers, which decrease automaticity and AV conduction.

There are some antiarrhythmic agents that do not fall into one of these categories. The most frequently used are digoxin and adenosine. Digoxin inhibits the Na^+, K^+-ATPase pump. Digoxin prolongs AV nodal conduction and the AV nodal refractory period, but it shortens the action potential and decreases the refractoriness of the ventricular myocardium and Purkinje fibers. Adenosine can block AV nodal conduction and shortens atrial refractoriness.

Although the in vitro electrophysiologic effects of most of these agents have been defined, their use remains largely empiric. **All can exacerbate arrhythmias (proarrhythmic effect), and many depress LV function.**

The risk of antiarrhythmic agents has been highlighted by many studies, most notably the Coronary Arrhythmia Suppression Trial (CAST), in which two class Ic agents (flecainide, encainide) and a class Ia agent (moricizine) increased mortality rates in patients with asymptomatic ventricular ectopy after MI. Class Ic antiarrhythmic agents should therefore *not* be used in patients with prior MI or structural heart disease.

The use of antiarrhythmic agents for specific arrhythmias is discussed below.

Catheter Ablation for Cardiac Arrhythmias

Catheter ablation has become the primary modality of therapy for many symptomatic supraventricular arrhythmias, including AV nodal reentrant tachycardia, tachycardias involving accessory pathways, paroxysmal atrial tachycardia, and atrial flutter. Catheter ablation of atrial fibrillation is more complex and usually involves complete electrical isolation of the pulmonary veins (which are often the sites of initiation of atrial fibrillation) or placing linear lesions within the atria to prevent propagation throughout the atrial chamber. This technique is considered a reasonable therapy for symptomatic patients with medication-refractory atrial fibrillation or as an alternative to long-term antiarrhythmic medication treatment. Catheter ablation of ventricular arrhythmias has proved more difficult, but experienced centers have demonstrated reasonable success with all types of ventricular tachycardias including bundle-branch reentry, tachycardia originating in the ventricular outflow tract or papillary muscles, tachycardias originating in the specialized conduction system (fascicular

Table 10–9. Antiarrhythmic medications (listed in alphabetical order within class).

Agent	Intravenous Dosage	Oral Dosage	Therapeutic Plasma Level	Route of Elimination	Side Effects
Class Ia: Action: Sodium channel blockers: Depress phase 0 depolarization; slow conduction; prolong repolarization.					
Indications: Supraventricular tachycardia, ventricular tachycardia, symptomatic ventricular premature beats.					
Disopyramide		Immediate release: 100–200 mg every 6 hours Sustained release: 200–400 mg every 12 hours	2–8 mg/mL	Renal	Urinary retention, dry mouth, markedly ↓ LVF, QT prolongation
Procainamide	Loading: 10–17 mg/kg at 20–50 mg/minute Maintenance: 1–4 mg/minute	50 mg/kg/day in divided doses every 4 hours (short-acting)	4–10 mg/mL; NAPA (active metabolite), 10–20 mcg/mL	Renal	
Quinidine	6–10 mg/kg (intramuscularly or intravenously) over 20 minutes (rarely used parenterally)	324–648 mg every 8 hours	2–5 mg/mL	Hepatic	GI, ↓ LVF, ↑ Dig
Class Ib: Action: Shorten repolarization.					
Indications: Ventricular tachycardia, prevention of ventricular fibrillation, symptomatic ventricular premature beats.					
Lidocaine	Loading: 1 mg/kg Maintenance: 1–4 mg/minute		1–5 mg/mL	Hepatic	CNS, GI, ↓ LVF
Mexiletine		100–300 mg every 8–12 hours; maximum: 1200 mg/day	0.5–2 mg/mL	Hepatic	CNS, GI, leukopenia
Class Ic: Action: Depress phase 0 repolarization; slow conduction. (Propafenone is a weak calcium channel blocker and beta-blocker and prolongs action potential and refractoriness.)					
Indications: Ventricular tachycardia (in the absence of structural heart disease), refractory supraventricular tachycardia.					
Flecainide		50–150 mg twice daily	0.2–1 mg/mL	Hepatic	CNS, GI, AFL with 1:1 conduction, ventricular pro-arrhythmia
Propafenone		150–300 mg every 8–12 hours	Note: Active metabolites	Hepatic	CNS, GI, AFL with 1:1 conduction, ventricular pro-arrhythmia
Class II: Action: Beta-blockers, slow AV conduction.					
Indications: Supraventricular tachycardia, ventricular tachycardia, symptomatic ventricular premature beats, long QT syndrome.					
Esmolol	Loading: 500 mcg/kg over 1–2 minutes Maintenance: 50 mcg/kg/minute	Other beta-blockers may be used concomitantly	Not established	Hepatic	↓ LVF, bradycardia, AV block
Metoprolol	5 mg every 5 minutes up to 3 doses	25–200 mg daily	Not established	Hepatic	↓ LVF, bradycardia, AV block, fatigue
Propranolol	1–3 mg every 5 minute up to total of 5 mg	40–320 mg in 1–4 doses daily (depending on preparation)	Not established	Hepatic	↓ LVF, bradycardia, AV block, bronchospasm
Class III: Action: Prolong action potential.					
Indications: *Amiodarone:* refractory ventricular tachycardia, supraventricular tachycardia, prevention of ventricular tachycardia, atrial fibrillation, ventricular fibrillation; *Dofetilide:* atrial fibrillation and flutter; *Dronedarone:* atrial fibrillation (not persistent); *Ibutilide:* conversion of atrial fibrillation and flutter; *Sotalol:* ventricular tachycardia, atrial fibrillation.					
Amiodarone	150–300 mg infused rapidly, followed by 1 mg/minute infusion for 6 hours and then 0.5 mg/ minute for 18 hours	800–1600 mg/day for 7–14 days; maintain at 100–400 mg/day	1–5 mg/mL	Hepatic	Pulmonary fibrosis, hypothyroidism, hyperthyroidism, photosensitivity, corneal and skin deposits, hepatitis, ↑ Dig, neurotoxicity, GI

(*continued*)

Table 10–9. Antiarrhythmic medications (listed in alphabetical order within class). (continued)

Agent	Intravenous Dosage	Oral Dosage	Therapeutic Plasma Level	Route of Elimination	Side Effects
Dofetilide		125–500 mcg every 12 hours		Renal (dose must be reduced with kidney dysfunction)	Torsades de pointes in 3%; interaction with cytochrome P-450 inhibitors
Dronedarone		400 mg twice daily		Hepatic (contraindicated in severe impairment)	QTc prolongation, HF. Contraindicated in HF (NYHA class IV or recent decompensation), persistent AF
Ibutilide	1 mg over 10 minutes, followed by a second infusion of 0.5–1 mg over 10 minutes			Hepatic and renal	Torsades de pointes in up to 5% of patients within 3 hours after administration; patients must be monitored with defibrillator nearby
Sotalol	75 mg every 12 hours	80–160 mg every 12 hours (maximum 320 mg daily)		Renal (dosing interval should be extended if creatinine clearance is < 60 mL/minute)	Early incidence of torsades de pointes, ↓ LVF, bradycardia, fatigue (and other side effects associated with beta-blockers)
Class IV: Action: Slow calcium channel blockers.					
Indications: Supraventricular tachycardia, ventricular tachycardia (outflow tract, idiopathic).					
Diltiazem	0.25 mg/kg over 2 minutes; second 0.35-mg/kg bolus after 15 minutes if response is inadequate; infusion rate, 5–15 mg/hours	120–360 mg daily in 1–3 doses depending on preparation		Hepatic metabolism, renal excretion	Hypotension, ↓ LVF, bradycardia
Verapamil	2.5 mg bolus followed by additional boluses of 2.5–5 mg every 1–3 minutes; total 20 mg over 20 minutes; maintain at 5 mg/kg/minute	80–120 mg every 6–8 hours; 240–480 mg once daily with sustained-release preparation	0.1–0.15 mg/mL	Hepatic	Hypotension, ↓ LVF, constipation, ↑ Dig
Miscellaneous: Indications: Supraventricular tachycardia.					
Adenosine	6 mg rapidly followed by 12 mg after 1–2 minutes if needed; use half these doses if administered via central line			Adenosine receptor stimulation, metabolized in blood	Transient flushing, dyspnea, chest pain, AV block, sinus bradycardia; effect ↓ by theophylline, ↑ by dipyridamole
Digoxin	0.5 mg over 20 minutes followed by increment of 0.25 or 0.125 mg to 1–1.5 mg over 24 hours	1–1.5 mg over 24–36 hours in 3 or 4 doses; maintenance, 0.125–0.5 mg/day	0.7–2 mg/mL	Renal	AV block, arrhythmias, GI, visual changes
Ivabradine		5–7.5 mg every 12 hours		Renal and fecal	Bradycardia, phosphenes (visual brightness)

AF, atrial fibrillation; AV, atrioventricular; Dig, elevation of serum digoxin level; HF, heart failure; ↓LVF, reduced LV function; NAPA, *N*-acetylprocainamide; NYHA, New York Heart Association.

ventricular tachycardia), and ventricular tachycardias occurring in patients with ischemic or dilated cardiomyopathy. Ablation of many of these arrhythmias can be performed from the endocardial surface via endovascular catheter placement or on the epicardial surface of the heart via a percutaneous subxiphoid approach.

Catheter ablation has also been successfully performed for the treatment of ventricular fibrillation when a uniform premature ventricular contraction (PVC) can be identified. In addition, patients with symptomatic PVCs or PVCs occurring at a high enough burden to result in a cardiomyopathy (usually more than 10,000/day) may be considered for catheter ablation as well.

Catheter ablation procedures are generally safe, with an overall major complication rate ranging from 1% to 5%. Major vascular damage during catheter insertion occurs in less than 2% of patients. There is a low incidence of perforation of the myocardial wall resulting in pericardial tamponade. Sufficient damage to the AV node to require permanent cardiac pacing occurs in less than 1% of patients. When transseptal access through the interatrial septum or retrograde LV catheterization is required, additional potential complications include damage to the heart valves, damage to a coronary artery, or systemic emboli. A rare but potentially fatal complication after catheter ablation of atrial fibrillation is the development of an atrioesophageal fistula resulting from ablation on the posterior wall of the LA just overlying the esophagus, estimated to occur in less than 0.1% of procedures.

Calkins H et al. 2017 HRS/EHRA/ECAS/APHRS/SOLAECE expert consensus statement on catheter and surgical ablation of atrial fibrillation. Europace. 2018;20:e1. [PMID: 29016840]

SINUS ARRHYTHMIA, BRADYCARDIA, & TACHYCARDIA

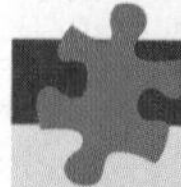

ESSENTIALS OF DIAGNOSIS

- Wide variation in sinus rate is common in young, healthy individuals and generally not pathologic.
- Symptomatic bradycardia may require permanent pacemaker implantation, especially in the elderly or patients with underlying heart disease.
- Sinus tachycardia is usually secondary to another underlying process (ie, fever, pain, anemia, alcohol withdrawal).
- Sick sinus syndrome manifests as sinus bradycardia, pauses, or inadequate heart rate response to physiologic demands (chronotropic incompetence).

General Considerations

Sinus arrhythmia is an irregularity of the normal heart rate defined as variation in the PP interval of more than 120 msec. This occurs commonly in young, healthy people due to changes in vagal influence on the sinus node during respiration (phasic) or independent of respiration (nonphasic). This is generally *not* a pathologic arrhythmia and requires no specific cardiac evaluation.

Sinus bradycardia is defined as a heart rate slower than 60 beats/minute and may be due to increased vagal influence on the normal sinoatrial pacemaker or organic disease of the sinus node. In healthy individuals, and particularly in well-trained athletes, sinus bradycardia to rates of 50 beats/minute or lower especially during sleep is a normal finding. However, in elderly patients and individuals with heart disease sinus bradycardia may be an indication of true sinus node pathology. When the sinus rate slows severely, the atrial-nodal junction or the nodal-His bundle junction may assume pacemaker activity for the heart, usually at a rate of 35–60 beats/minute.

Sinus tachycardia is defined as a heart rate faster than 100 beats/minute that is caused by rapid impulse formation from the sinoatrial node. It is a normal physiologic response to exercise or other conditions in which catecholamine release is increased. The rate infrequently exceeds 160 beats/minute but may reach 180 beats/minute in young persons. The onset and termination are usually gradual, in contrast to paroxysmal supraventricular tachycardia (PSVT) due to reentry. In rare instances, otherwise healthy individuals may present with "inappropriate" sinus tachycardia where persistently elevated basal heart rates are not in-line with physiologic demands. Long-term consequences of this disorder are few.

Sick sinus syndrome is a broad diagnosis applied to patients with sinus arrest, sinoatrial exit block (recognized by a pause equal to a multiple of the underlying PP interval or progressive shortening of the PP interval prior to a pause), or persistent sinus bradycardia. A common presentation in elderly patients is of recurrent SVTs (often atrial fibrillation) accompanied by bradyarrhythmias (**"tachy-brady syndrome"**). The long pauses that often follow the termination of tachycardia cause the associated symptoms. Sick sinus syndrome may also manifest as **chronotropic incompetence,** defined as an inappropriate heart rate response to the physiologic demands of exercise or stress, and is an under-recognized cause of poor exercise tolerance.

Clinical Findings

In most patients, sinus arrhythmia (bradycardia or tachycardia) does not cause symptoms in the absence of underlying cardiac disease or other comorbidities. When severe sinus bradycardia results in low cardiac output, however, patients may complain of weakness, confusion, or syncope if cerebral perfusion is impaired. Atrial, junctional, and ventricular ectopic rhythms are more apt to occur with slow sinus rates. Sinus bradycardia is often exacerbated by medications (digitalis, calcium channel blockers, beta-blockers, sympatholytic agents, antiarrhythmics), and non-essential agents that may be responsible should be withdrawn prior to making the diagnosis.

Sinus tachycardia is most often *a normal response* to conditions that require an increase in cardiac output, including fever, pain, anxiety, anemia, heart failure, hypovolemia, or thyrotoxicosis. Alcohol and alcohol withdrawal are common causes of sinus tachycardia and other supraventricular arrhythmias. In patients with underlying cardiac disease, sinus tachycardia may cause dyspnea or chest pain due to increased myocardial oxygen demand or reduced coronary artery blood flow.

Symptoms from sinus node dysfunction are nonspecific and may be due to other causes. It is therefore essential that symptoms be demonstrated to coincide temporally with arrhythmias. This may require prolonged ambulatory monitoring or the use of an event recorder.

Treatment

Asymptomatic patients generally do *not* require treatment. For symptomatic patients with bradycardia or sick sinus syndrome, implantation of a permanent pacemaker is usually indicated. In patients without evidence of AV nodal or bundle branch conduction abnormality, a single chamber atrial pacemaker is reasonable. Based on the results of several randomized controlled trials, *atrial-based pacing (single or dual chamber) is superior to ventricular only pacing for patients with sinus node dysfunction.* When a dual-chamber pacemaker is implanted for sinus node dysfunction with intact AV conduction, unnecessary ventricular pacing should be avoided because it may exacerbate heart failure, especially in patients with preexisting LV dysfunction. In most situations, sinus tachycardia will improve or resolve with treatment of the underlying cause. Inappropriate sinus tachycardia in the presence of symptoms (palpitations, dizziness, exertional intolerance) can be treated with a trial of beta-blockers or calcium channel blockers although treatment is often challenging. Ivabradine (5–7.5 mg twice daily), a selective inhibitor of the potassium funny channel (I_f) specific to the sinus node, may be an effective treatment option.

When to Refer

Patients with symptoms related to bradycardia or tachycardia when reversible etiologies have been excluded.

Kusumoto FM et al. 2018 ACC/AHA/HRS guideline on the evaluation and management of patients with bradycardia and cardiac conduction delay: a report of the American College of Cardiology/American Heart Association Task Force on Clinical Practice Guidelines and the Heart Rhythm Society. Heart Rhythm. 2019;16:e128. [PMID: 30412778]

AV BLOCK

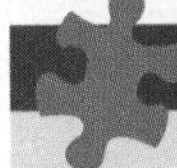

ESSENTIALS OF DIAGNOSIS

- Conduction disturbance between the atrium and ventricle that can be physiologic (due to enhanced vagal tone) or pathologic.
- Block occurs in the AV node (first-degree, second-degree Mobitz type I) or below the AV node (second-degree Mobitz type II, third-degree).
- Symptomatic AV block or block below the AV node in the absence of a reversible cause usually warrants permanent pacemaker implantation.

General Considerations

AV block can be physiologic (due to increased vagal tone) or pathologic (due to underlying heart disease such as ischemia, myocarditis, fibrosis of the conduction system, or after cardiac surgery). AV block is categorized as **first-degree** (PR interval greater than 200 msec with all atrial impulses conducted), **second-degree** (intermittent blocked beats), or **third-degree** (complete heart block, in which no atrial impulses are conducted to the ventricles). Second-degree AV block is further subclassified into **Mobitz type I (Wenckebach),** in which the AV conduction time (PR interval) progressively lengthens before the blocked beat, and **Mobitz type II,** in which there are intermittently non-conducted atrial beats not preceded by lengthening AV conduction. When only 2:1 AV block is present on the ECG, the differentiation between Mobitz type I or Mobitz type II is more difficult. If the baseline PR interval is prolonged (greater than 200 msec) or the width of the QRS complex is narrow (less than 120 msec), the block is usually nodal (Mobitz type I); if the QRS complex is wide (greater than or equal to 120 msec), the block is more likely infranodal (Mobitz type II).

AV dissociation occurs when an intrinsic ventricular pacemaker (accelerated idioventricular rhythm, ventricular premature beats, or ventricular tachycardia) is firing at a rate faster than or close to the sinus rate, such that atrial impulses arriving at the AV node when it is refractory may not be conducted. This phenomenon does not necessarily indicate AV block. No treatment is required aside from management of the causative arrhythmia.

Clinical Findings

The clinical presentation of first-degree and Mobitz type I block is typically benign and rarely produces symptoms. Normal, physiologic block of this type occurs in response to increases in parasympathetic output. This is commonly seen during sleep, with carotid sinus massage, or in well-trained athletes. It may also occur as a medication effect (calcium channel blockers, beta-blockers, digitalis, or antiarrhythmics). Pathologic causes, including myocardial ischemia or infarction (discussed earlier), inflammatory processes (ie, Lyme disease), fibrosis, calcification, or infiltration (ie, amyloidosis or sarcoidosis), should be excluded.

Mobitz type II block and complete (third-degree) heart block are almost always due to pathologic disease involving the infranodal conduction system, and symptoms including fatigue, dyspnea, presyncope or syncope are common. With complete heart block, where no atrial impulses reach the ventricle, the ventricular escape rate is usually slow (less than 50 beats/minute) and severity of symptoms may vary depending on the rate and stability of the escape rhythm. As for lesser degrees of AV block, pathologic causes should be explored.

Intraventricular conduction block is relatively common and may be transient (ie, related to increases in heart rate) or permanent. Right bundle branch block is often seen in patients with structurally normal hearts. The left bundle is composed of two components (anterior and posterior fascicles) and left bundle branch block is more often a marker of underlying cardiac disease, including ischemic heart disease, inflammatory or infiltrative disease, cardiomyopathy, and valvular heart disease. In asymptomatic patients with bifascicular block (block in two of three infranodal components—right bundle, left anterior, and left posterior fascicle), the incidence of occult complete heart block or progression to it is low (1% annually).

Treatment

Asymptomatic patients with first- or second-degree Mobitz type I AV block do not require any specific therapy. Patients should undergo treatment of any potentially reversible cause (ie, myocardial ischemia or medication effect). Symptomatic patients with any degree of heart block should be treated urgently with atropine (initial dose 0.5 mg given intravenously) or temporary pacing (transcutaneous or transvenous). The indications for permanent pacing are symptomatic bradyarrhythmias with any degree of AV block or asymptomatic high-degree AV block (second-degree Mobitz type II or third-degree heart block) not attributable to a reversible or physiologic cause. Patients with presumed cardiac syncope with normal heart rates and rhythm but bifascicular or trifascicular block on ECG should also be considered for permanent pacing.

A *standardized nomenclature for pacemaker generators* is used, usually consisting of four letters. The first letter refers to the chamber that is paced (A, atrium; V, ventricle; D, dual [for both]). The second letter refers to the chamber that is sensed (also A, V, or D). An additional option (O) indicates absence of sensing. The third letter refers to how the pacemaker responds to a sensed event (I, inhibition by a sensed impulse; T, triggering by a sensed impulse; D, dual modes of response; O, no response to sensed impulse). The fourth letter refers to the programmability or rate response capacity (R, rate modulation), a function that can increase the pacing rate in response to motion or respiratory rate when the intrinsic heart rate is inappropriately low.

A dual-chamber pacemaker that senses and paces in both chambers is the most physiologic approach to pacing patients who remain in sinus rhythm. **AV synchrony** is particularly important in patients in whom atrial contraction produces a substantial augmentation of stroke volume. For patients in permanent atrial fibrillation who require pacing for symptomatic bradycardia or pauses, catheter-based implantation of a leadless pacemaker directly to the RV endocardium may be considered. In patients with complete heart block with LV systolic dysfunction, implantation of a pacemaker capable of direct capture of the native specialized conduction system (His bundle or left bundle) or simultaneous left and right ventricular pacing (CRT-P) may be indicated. Complications from pacemaker implantation include infection, hematoma, cardiac perforation, pneumothorax, and lead dislodgement.

When to Refer

Patients with symptomatic AV block (any degree) or asymptomatic high-degree (second-degree Mobitz type II or third-degree) AV block after reversible causes have been excluded.

Upadhyay GA et al; His-SYNC Investigators. His corrective pacing or biventricular pacing for cardiac resynchronization in heart failure. J Am Coll Cardiol. 2019;74:157. [PMID: 31078637]

PAROXYSMAL SUPRAVENTRICULAR TACHYCARDIA

ESSENTIALS OF DIAGNOSIS

- Rapid, regular tachycardia most commonly seen in young adults and characterized by abrupt onset and offset.
- QRS duration narrow (< 120 msec) except in the presence of bundle branch block or accessory pathway.
- Often responsive to vagal maneuvers, AV nodal blockers, or adenosine. Cardioversion rarely required.

General Considerations

PSVT is an intermittent arrhythmia that is characterized by a sudden onset and offset and a regular ventricular response. Episodes may last from a few seconds to several hours or longer. PSVT often occurs in patients without structural heart disease. The most common mechanism for PSVT is *reentry*, which may be initiated or terminated by a fortuitously timed atrial or ventricular premature beat. The reentrant circuit usually involves dual pathways (a slow and a fast pathway) within the AV node; this is referred to as **AV nodal reentrant tachycardia (AVNRT)** and accounts for 60% of cases of PSVT. Less commonly (30% of cases), reentry is due to an *accessory pathway* between the atria and ventricles, referred to as **atrioventricular reciprocating tachycardia (AVRT)**. The pathophysiology and management of arrhythmias due to accessory pathways differ in important ways and are discussed separately below.

Clinical Findings

A. Symptoms and Signs

Symptoms of PSVT can be quite variable depending on the degree of heart rate elevation, resultant hypotension, or presence of other comorbidities. Symptoms may include palpitations, diaphoresis, dyspnea, dizziness, and mild chest pain (even in the absence of associated CHD). Syncope is rare.

B. ECG

Obtaining a 12-lead ECG when feasible is important to help determine the tachycardia mechanism. The QRS duration will be narrow (less than 120 ms) except in cases of PSVT with aberrant conduction (left bundle branch block, right bundle branch block, or antegrade conducting accessory pathway). The heart rate is regular and is usually 160–220 beats/minute but may be greater than 250 beats/minute. The P wave usually differs in contour from sinus beats and is often simultaneous with or just after the QRS complex.

Treatment

In the absence of structural heart disease, serious effects are rare, and most episodes resolve spontaneously. Particular effort should be made to terminate the episode quickly if cardiac failure, syncope, or anginal pain develops or if there is underlying cardiac or (particularly) coronary disease. Because reentry is the most common mechanism for PSVT, effective therapy requires that conduction be interrupted at some point in the reentry circuit and the vast majority of these circuits involve the AV node.

A. Mechanical Measures

A variety of maneuvers have been used to interrupt episodes, and patients may learn to perform these themselves. These maneuvers result in an acute increase in vagal tone and include the Valsalva maneuver, lowering the head between the knees, coughing, splashing cold water on the face, and breath holding. The **Valsalva maneuver** is performed with the patient semirecumbent (45 degrees), exerting around 40 mm Hg of intrathoracic pressure (by blowing through a 10 mL syringe) for at least 15 seconds. Moving the patient supine immediately following the strain maneuver and passively raising their legs for an additional 15 seconds may increase effectiveness of the maneuver. **Carotid sinus massage** is an additional technique often performed by clinicians but should be avoided if the patient has a carotid bruit. Firm but gentle pressure and massage are applied first over the right carotid sinus for 10–20 seconds and, if unsuccessful, then over the left carotid sinus. Pressure should not be exerted on both sides at the same time. **Facial contact with cold water** may cause transient bradycardia and termination of PSVT, a phenomenon known as the diving reflex. When performed properly, these maneuvers result in abrupt termination of the arrhythmia in 20–50% of cases.

B. Medication Therapy

If mechanical measures fail to terminate the arrhythmia, pharmacologic agents should be tried. **Intravenous adenosine** is recommended as the first-line agent due to its brief duration of action and minimal negative inotropic activity (Table 10–9). Because the half-life of adenosine is less than 10 seconds, the medication is given rapidly (in 1–2 seconds) as a 6 mg bolus followed by 20 mL of fluid. If this regimen is unsuccessful at terminating the arrhythmia, a second higher dose (12 mg) may be given. Adenosine causes block of electrical conduction through the AV node and results in termination of PSVT in approximately 90% of cases. Minor side effects are common and include transient flushing, chest discomfort, nausea, and headache. Adenosine may excite both atrial and ventricular tissue causing atrial fibrillation (in up to 12% of patients) or rarely ventricular arrhythmias and therefore administration should be performed with continuous cardiac monitoring and availability of an external defibrillator. Adenosine must also be used with caution in patients with reactive airways disease because it can promote bronchospasm.

When adenosine fails to terminate the arrhythmia or if a contraindication to its use is present, **intravenous calcium channel blockers**, including verapamil and diltiazem, may be used (Table 10–9). Verapamil in particular has been shown to be as effective at terminating PSVT in the acute setting (approximately 90%) as adenosine. Calcium channel blockers should be used with caution in patients with heart failure due to their negative inotropic effects. Their longer half-life compared to adenosine may result in prolonged hypotension despite restoration of normal rhythm. Etripamil, a short-acting calcium-channel blocker that is self-administered intranasally, results in rapid conversion of PSVT in preliminary studies and phase 3 trials are ongoing.

Intravenous beta-blockers include esmolol (a very short-acting beta-blocker), propranolol, and metoprolol. While beta-blockers cause less myocardial depression than calcium channel blockers, the evidence of their effectiveness to terminate PSVT is limited. Although **intravenous amiodarone** is safe, it is usually not required and often ineffective for treatment of these arrhythmias.

C. Cardioversion

If the patient is hemodynamically unstable or if adenosine, beta-blockers, and calcium channel blockers are contraindicated or ineffective, synchronized electrical cardioversion (beginning at 100 J) should be performed.

Prevention

A. Catheter Ablation

Because of concerns about the safety and the intolerability of antiarrhythmic medications, **radiofrequency ablation is the preferred approach to patients with recurrent symptomatic reentrant PSVT,** whether it is due to dual pathways within the AV node or to accessory pathways.

B. Medications

AV nodal blocking agents are the medications of choice as first-line medical therapy (Table 10–9). Beta-blockers or nondihydropyridine calcium channel blockers, such as diltiazem and verapamil, are typically used first. Patients who do not respond to agents that increase refractoriness of the AV node may be treated with antiarrhythmics. The class Ic agents (flecainide, propafenone) can be used in patients without underlying structural heart disease. In patients with evidence of structural heart disease, class III agents, such as sotalol or amiodarone, should be used because of the lower incidence of ventricular proarrhythmia during long-term therapy.

When to Refer

All patients with sustained or symptomatic PSVT should be referred to a cardiologist or cardiac electrophysiologist for long-term treatment options (including observation, pharmacotherapy, or ablation).

Page RL et al. 2015 ACC/AHA/HRS guideline for the management of adult patients with supraventricular tachycardia: a report of the American College of Cardiology/American Heart Association Task Force on Clinical Practice Guidelines and the Heart Rhythm Society. J Am Coll Cardiol. 2016;67:e27. [PMID: 26409259]

PSVT DUE TO ACCESSORY AV PATHWAYS (Preexcitation Syndromes)

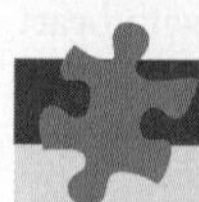

ESSENTIALS OF DIAGNOSIS

- Two classic features of Wolff-Parkinson-White (WPW) pattern on ECG are short PR interval and wide, slurred QRS complex due to manifest preexcitation (delta wave).
- Most patients with WPW pattern do not have clinical history of arrhythmia but have a higher risk of sudden cardiac death due to rapidly conducted atrial fibrillation through the accessory pathway.
- Risk factors include age younger than 20, history of tachycardia, and rapid conduction properties at electrophysiologic testing.

General Considerations

Accessory pathways or bypass tracts between the atrium and the ventricle bypass the compact AV node and can predispose to reentrant arrhythmias, such as AVRT and atrial fibrillation. When direct AV connections conduct antegrade (manifest preexcitation) they produce a classic **WPW pattern** on the baseline ECG consisting of a short PR interval and a wide, slurred QRS complex **(delta wave)** owing to early ventricular depolarization of the region adjacent to the pathway. Although the morphology and polarity of the delta wave can suggest the location of the pathway, mapping by intracardiac recordings is required for precise anatomic localization.

Accessory pathways occur in 0.1–0.3% of the population and facilitate reentrant arrhythmias owing to the disparity in refractory periods of the AV node and accessory pathway. **WPW syndrome** refers to a patient with baseline WPW pattern on ECG with associated SVT. Whether the tachycardia is associated with a narrow or wide QRS complex is frequently determined by whether antegrade conduction is through the node (narrow) or the bypass tract (wide). Some bypass tracts only conduct in a retrograde direction. In these cases, the bypass tract is termed "concealed" because it is not readily apparent on a baseline (sinus) ECG. **Orthodromic reentrant tachycardia** accounts for approximately 90% of AVRT episodes and is characterized by conduction antegrade down the AV node and retrograde up the accessory pathway, resulting in a narrow QRS complex (unless an underlying bundle branch block or interventricular conduction delay is present). **Antidromic reentrant tachycardia** conducts antegrade down the accessory pathway and retrograde through the AV node, resulting in a wide and often bizarre-appearing QRS complex that may be mistaken for ventricular tachycardia. Accessory pathways often have shorter refractory periods than specialized conduction tissue and thus tachycardias involving accessory pathways have the potential to be more rapid.

Clinical Findings

Patients with WPW in whom arrhythmia develops often have palpitations, dizziness, or mild chest pain. Most patients that have a delta wave found incidentally on ECG (WPW pattern) do not have a clinical history of arrhythmia and are therefore asymptomatic. However, these patients are still at higher risk for sudden cardiac death than the general population. Atrial fibrillation with antegrade conduction down the accessory pathway and a rapid ventricular response will develop in up to 30% of patients with WPW. If this conduction is very rapid, it can potentially degenerate to ventricular fibrillation. The 10-year risk of sudden cardiac death in patients with WPW syndrome ranges from 0.15% to 0.24%. Risk factors include age younger than 20, a history of symptomatic tachycardia, and multiple accessory pathways.

Multiple risk stratification strategies have been proposed to identify asymptomatic patients with WPW pattern ECG who may be at higher risk for lethal cardiac arrhythmias. A sudden loss of preexcitation during ambulatory monitoring or exercise testing likely indicates an accessory pathway with poor conduction properties and therefore low risk for rapid anterograde conduction. In the absence of this finding, patients may be referred for invasive electrophysiology testing. During the study, patients found to have the shortest preexcited R-R interval during atrial fibrillation of 250 msec or less or inducible SVT are at increased risk for sudden cardiac death and should undergo catheter ablation.

Treatment

A. Pharmacotherapy

Initial treatment of narrow-complex reentrant rhythms involving a bypass tract (orthodromic AVRT) is similar to other forms of PSVT and includes vagal maneuvers, intravenous adenosine, or verapamil. Treatment of wide-complex tachycardia in the presence of an accessory pathway, be it reentrant-type (antidromic AVRT) or atrial fibrillation with antegrade conduction down the bypass tract, must be managed differently. Agents such as calcium channel blockers and beta-blockers may increase the refractoriness of the AV node with minimal or no effect on the accessory pathway, often leading to faster ventricular rates and increasing the risk of ventricular fibrillation. Therefore, these agents should be avoided. Intravenous class Ia (procainamide) and class III (ibutilide) antiarrhythmic agents will increase the refractoriness of the bypass tract and are the medications of choice for wide-complex tachycardias involving accessory pathways. If hemodynamic compromise is present, electrical cardioversion is warranted.

B. Catheter Ablation

For long-term management, catheter ablation is the procedure of choice in patients with accessory pathways and recurrent symptoms or asymptomatic patients with WPW pattern on ECG and high-risk features at baseline or during electrophysiology study. Success rates for ablation of accessory pathways with radiofrequency catheters exceed 95% in appropriate patients. Major complications from catheter ablation are rare but include AV block, cardiac tamponade, and thromboembolic events. Minor complications, including hematoma at the catheter access site, occur in 1–2% of procedures. For patients not a candidate for catheter ablation, class Ic or class III antiarrhythmic medication may be considered.

When to Refer

- Asymptomatic patients with an incidental finding of WPW pattern on ECG with high-risk features.
- Patients with recurrent or prolonged tachycardia episodes despite treatment with AV nodal blocking agents.
- Patients with preexcitation and a history of atrial fibrillation or syncope.

Al-Khatib SM et al. Risk stratification for arrhythmic events in patients with asymptomatic pre-excitation: a systematic review for the 2015 ACC/AHA/HRS guideline for the management of adult patients with supraventricular tachycardia. Circulation. 2016;133:e575. [PMID: 26399661]

ATRIAL FIBRILLATION

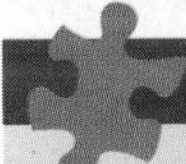

ESSENTIALS OF DIAGNOSIS

- Presents as an irregularly irregular heart rhythm on examination and ECG.
- Prevention of stroke should be considered in all patients with risk factors for stroke (those with heart failure, hypertension, age 65 or older, diabetes mellitus, prior history of stroke or TIA, or vascular disease).
- Heart rate control with beta-blocker or calcium channel blockers generally required. Restoration of sinus rhythm with cardioversion, antiarrhythmic medications, or catheter ablation in symptomatic patients.

General Considerations

Atrial fibrillation is the most common chronic arrhythmia, with an incidence and prevalence that rise with age, so that it affects approximately 9% of individuals over age 65 years. It occurs in rheumatic and other forms of valvular heart disease, dilated cardiomyopathy, ASD, hypertension, and CHD as well as in patients with no apparent cardiac disease; it may be the initial presenting sign in thyrotoxicosis, and this condition should be excluded with the initial episode. Atrial fibrillation often appears in a **paroxysmal** fashion before becoming the established rhythm. Pericarditis, chest trauma, thoracic or cardiac surgery, thyroid disorders, obstructive sleep apnea, or pulmonary disease (pneumonia, PE) as well as medications (beta-adrenergic agonists, inotropes, bisphosphonates, and certain chemotherapeutics) may cause attacks in patients with normal hearts. Acute alcohol excess and alcohol withdrawal (termed **holiday heart**) may precipitate atrial fibrillation. For regular, moderate drinkers, abstinence from alcohol reduces recurrences of atrial fibrillation by about 50%.

Atrial fibrillation, particularly when the ventricular rate is uncontrolled, can lead to LV dysfunction, heart failure, or myocardial ischemia (when underlying CAD is present). Perhaps the most serious consequence of atrial fibrillation is the propensity for thrombus formation due to stasis in the atria (particularly the left atrial appendage) and consequent embolization, most devastatingly to the cerebral circulation. ***Untreated, the rate of stroke is approximately 5% per year.*** However, patients with significant obstructive valvular disease, chronic heart failure or LV dysfunction, diabetes mellitus, hypertension, or age over 75 years and those with a history of prior stroke or other embolic events are at substantially higher risk (up to nearly 20% per year in patients with multiple risk factors). A substantial portion of the aging population with hypertension has **asymptomatic** or **"subclinical"** atrial fibrillation, which can be detected with monitoring devices and is also associated with increased risk of stroke, particularly if it lasts for 24 hours or longer. It is not clear whether, and for whom, oral anticoagulation should be used for subclinical atrial fibrillation, a question that is being addressed in ongoing clinical trials.

Clinical Findings

A. Symptoms and Signs

Atrial fibrillation itself is rarely life-threatening; however, it can have serious consequences if the ventricular rate is sufficiently rapid to precipitate hypotension, myocardial ischemia, or tachycardia-induced myocardial dysfunction. Moreover, particularly in patients with risk factors, atrial fibrillation is a major preventable cause of stroke. Although some patients—particularly older or inactive individuals—have relatively few symptoms if the rate is controlled, many patients are aware of the irregular rhythm. Most patients will complain of fatigue whether they experience other symptoms or not. The heart rate may range from quite slow to extremely rapid, but is uniformly irregular unless underlying complete heart block with junctional escape rhythm or a permanent ventricular pacemaker is in place. **Atrial fibrillation is the only common arrhythmia in which the ventricular rate is rapid and the rhythm very irregular.**

B. ECG

The surface ECG typically demonstrates erratic, disorganized atrial activity between discrete QRS complexes occurring in an irregular pattern. The atrial activity may be very fine and difficult to detect on the ECG, or quite coarse and often mistaken for atrial flutter.

C. Echocardiography

Echocardiography provides assessment of chamber volumes, LV size and function, or the presence of concomitant valvular heart disease and should be performed in all patients with a new diagnosis of atrial fibrillation. TEE is the most sensitive imaging modality to identify thrombi in the left atrium or left atrial appendage prior to any attempt at chemical or electrical cardioversion.

Treatment

A. Newly Diagnosed Atrial Fibrillation

1. Initial management—

A. HEMODYNAMICALLY UNSTABLE PATIENT—If the patient is hemodynamically unstable, usually as a result of a rapid ventricular rate or associated cardiac or noncardiac conditions, hospitalization and immediate treatment of atrial fibrillation are required. Intravenous beta-blockers (esmolol, propranolol, and metoprolol) or calcium channel blockers (diltiazem and verapamil) are usually effective at rate control in the acute setting. Urgent electrical cardioversion is only indicated in patients with shock or severe hypotension, pulmonary edema, or ongoing MI or ischemia. There is a potential risk of thromboembolism in patients undergoing cardioversion who have not received anticoagulation therapy if atrial fibrillation has been *present for more than 48 hours or is of unknown duration*; however, in hemodynamically unstable patients the need for immediate rate control outweighs that risk. An initial shock with 100–200 J is administered in synchrony with the R wave. If sinus rhythm is not restored, an additional attempt with 360 J is indicated. If this fails, cardioversion may be successful after loading with intravenous ibutilide (1 mg over 10 minutes, repeated in 10 minutes if necessary).

B. HEMODYNAMICALLY STABLE PATIENT—If the patient has no symptoms, hemodynamic instability, or evidence of important precipitating conditions (such as silent MI or ischemia, decompensated heart failure, PE, or hemodynamically significant valvular disease), hospitalization is usually not necessary. In most of these cases, atrial fibrillation is an unrecognized chronic or paroxysmal condition and should be managed accordingly (see Subsequent Management, below). For new-onset atrial fibrillation, thyroid function tests and echocardiography to assess for occult valvular or myocardial disease should be performed.

In stable patients with atrial fibrillation, a strategy of rate control and anticoagulation is appropriate. This is true whether the conditions that precipitated atrial fibrillation are likely to persist (such as following cardiac or noncardiac surgery, with respiratory failure, or with pericarditis) or might resolve spontaneously over a period of hours to days (such as atrial fibrillation due to excessive alcohol intake or electrolyte imbalance). The choice of agent is guided by the hemodynamic status of the patient, associated conditions, and the urgency of achieving rate control. In the stable patient with atrial fibrillation, a beta-blocker or calcium channel blocker (orally or intravenously) is usually the first-line agent for ventricular rate control. In the setting of MI or ischemia, beta-blockers are the preferred agent. The most frequently used agents are either metoprolol (administered as a 5 mg intravenous bolus, repeated twice at intervals of 5 minutes and then given as needed by repeat boluses or orally at total daily doses of 25–200 mg) or, in unstable patients, esmolol (0.5 mg/kg intravenously, repeated once if necessary, followed by a titrated infusion of 0.05–0.2 mg/kg/minute). If beta-blockers are contraindicated, calcium channel blockers are rapidly effective. Diltiazem (10–20 mg bolus, repeated after 15 minutes if necessary, followed by a maintenance infusion of 5–15 mg/hour) is the preferred calcium blocker if hypotension or LV dysfunction is present. Otherwise, verapamil (5–10 mg intravenously over 2–3 minutes, repeated after 30 minutes if necessary) may be used. Rate control using digoxin is slow (onset of action more than 1 hour with peak effect at 6 hours) and may be inadequate and is rarely indicated for use in the acute setting. Similarly, amiodarone, even when administered intravenously, has a relatively slow onset and is most useful as an adjunct when rate control with the previously cited agents is incomplete or contraindicated or when cardioversion is planned in the near future. Care should be taken in patients with hypotension or heart failure because the rapid intravenous administration of amiodarone may worsen hemodynamics.

Up to two-thirds of patients experiencing acute onset (shorter than 36 hours) of atrial fibrillation will spontaneously revert to sinus rhythm without the need for cardioversion. If atrial fibrillation has been present for more than a week, spontaneous conversion is unlikely and cardioversion may be considered for symptomatic patients. Importantly, **if the onset of atrial fibrillation was more than 48 hours prior to presentation (or unknown), a transesophageal echocardiogram should be performed prior to cardioversion to exclude left atrial thrombus.** If thrombus is present, the cardioversion is delayed until after a 3-week period of therapeutic anticoagulation. In either case, because atrial contractile activity may not recover for several weeks after restoration of sinus rhythm in patients who have been in atrial fibrillation for more than 48 hours, cardioversion should be followed by anticoagulation *for at least 1 month* unless there is a strong contraindication. Younger patients without heart failure, diabetes, hypertension, or other risk factors for stroke may not require long-term anticoagulation.

2. Subsequent management—If immediate cardioversion is not performed, adequate rate control can usually be achieved with beta-blockers or nondihydropyridine calcium channel blockers. Choice of the initial rate control medication is best based on the presence of accompanying conditions: Hypertensive patients can be given beta-blockers or calcium blockers (see Tables 11–9 and 11–7). Patients with CHD or heart failure should receive a beta-blocker preferentially, whereas beta-blockers should be avoided in patients with severe COPD or asthma. Long-term use of digoxin is associated with an *increase* in mortality in patients with chronic atrial fibrillation and is rarely indicated. In symptomatic patients, a resting heart rate of less than 80 beats/minute is targeted. In asymptomatic patients without LV dysfunction, a more lenient resting heart rate of up to 100–110 beats/minute is reasonable. Ambulatory monitoring to assess heart rate during exercise should be considered in all patients with a goal not to exceed maximum predicted heart rate (220 – age).

A. **Anticoagulation**—For patients with atrial fibrillation, even when it is paroxysmal or occurs rarely, the need for oral anticoagulation should be evaluated and treatment initiated for those without strong contraindication. Patients with **lone atrial fibrillation** (eg, no evidence of associated heart disease, hypertension, atherosclerotic vascular disease, diabetes mellitus, or history of stroke or TIA) under age 65 years need no antithrombotic treatment. Patients with **transient atrial fibrillation**, such as in the setting of acute MI or pneumonia, but no prior history of arrhythmia, are at high risk for future development of atrial fibrillation and appropriate anticoagulation should be initiated based on risk factors. If the cause is reversible, such as after coronary artery bypass surgery or associated with hyperthyroidism, then long-term anticoagulation is not necessary.

In addition to the traditional five risk factors that comprise the **$CHADS_2$ score** (heart failure, hypertension, age 75 years or older, diabetes mellitus, and [2 points for] history of stroke or TIA), the European and American guidelines recommend that three additional factors included in the **CHA_2DS_2-VASc** score be considered: age 65–74 years, female sex, and presence of vascular disease (Table 10–10). *The CHA_2DS_2-VASc score is especially relevant for patients who have a $CHADS_2$ score of 0 or 1;* if the CHA_2DS_2-VASc score is greater than or equal to 2, oral anticoagulation is recommended, and if CHA_2DS_2-VASc score is 1, oral anticoagulation should be considered, taking into account risk, benefit, and patient preferences. Female sex is a relatively weak factor, however, and the European guidelines have removed it from their risk assessment, so that oral anticoagulation is indicated for men who are CHA_2DS_2-VASc of 2 and women who are CHA_2DS_2-VASc of 3. (The use of warfarin is discussed in the section on Selecting Appropriate Anticoagulant Therapy in Chapter 14.) Unfortunately, studies show that *only about half* of patients with atrial fibrillation and an indication for oral anticoagulation are receiving it, and even when treated with warfarin, they are out of the target INR range nearly half the time. *One reason for undertreatment is the misperception that aspirin is useful for prevention of stroke due to atrial fibrillation.* In the European guidelines, aspirin is given a class III A recommendation, indicating that it should *not* be used because of harm (and with no good evidence of benefit). Cardioversion, if planned, should be performed after at least 3–4 weeks of anticoagulation at a therapeutic level (or after exclusion of left atrial appendage thrombus by transesophageal echocardiogram as discussed above). **Anticoagulation clinics** with systematic management of warfarin dosing and adjustment have been shown to result in better maintenance of target anticoagulation.

Four DOACs—dabigatran, rivaroxaban, apixaban, and edoxaban—have been shown to be at least as effective as warfarin for stroke prevention in patients with atrial fibrillation and have been approved by the FDA for this indication (Table 10–11). These medications have *not* been studied in patients with moderate or severe mitral stenosis, and they should *not* be used for patients with mechanical prosthetic valves. The term "nonvalvular atrial fibrillation" is no longer used in the American or European guidelines since most patients with other types of valvular heart disease have been included in trials of DOACs, which are equally effective in these patients.

Dabigatran (studied in the RE-LY trial) is superior to warfarin at preventing stroke at the 150 mg twice daily dose, and it is noninferior at the 110 mg twice daily dose, although this dose is not approved for treatment of atrial

Table 10–10. CHA_2DS_2-VASc Risk Score for assessing risk of stroke and for selecting antithrombotic therapy for patients with atrial fibrillation.

CHA_2DS_2-VASc Risk Score	
Heart failure or LVEF ≤ 40%	1
Hypertension	1
Age ≥ 75 years	2
Diabetes mellitus	1
Stroke, transient ischemic attack, or thromboembolism	2
Vascular disease (previous MI, peripheral artery disease, or aortic plaque)	1
Age 65–74 years	1
Female sex (but not a risk factor if female sex is the only factor)	1
Maximum score	9

Adjusted stroke rate according to CHA_2DS_2-VASc score

CHA_2DS_2-VASc Score	Patients (n = 7329)	Adjusted stroke rate (%/year)
0	1	0%
1	422	1.3%
2	1230	2.2%
3	1730	3.2%
4	1718	4.0%
5	1159	6.7%
6	679	9.8%
7	294	9.6%
8	82	6.7 %
9	14	15.2%

CHA_2DS_2-VASc score = 0: recommend no antithrombotic therapy

CHA_2DS_2-VASc score = 1: recommend antithrombotic therapy with oral anticoagulation or antiplatelet therapy but preferably oral anticoagulation

CHA_2DS_2-VASc score = 2: recommend oral anticoagulation

CHA_2DS_2-VASc, Cardiac failure, Hypertension, Age ≥ 75 years (doubled), Diabetes, Stroke (doubled), Vascular disease, Age 65–74, and Sex category (female).

Data from Camm AJ et al. 2012 focused update of the ESC Guidelines for the management of atrial fibrillation: an update of the 2010 ESC Guidelines for the management of atrial fibrillation. Developed with the special contribution of the European Heart Rhythm Association. Eur Heart J. 2012;33(21):2719–2747.

Table 10–11. DOACs for stroke prevention in patients with nonvalvular atrial fibrillation.

	Dabigatran	Rivaroxaban	Apixaban	Edoxaban
Class	Antithrombin	Factor Xa inhibitor	Factor Xa inhibitor	Factor Xa inhibitor
Bleeding risk compared to warfarin	Less intracranial bleeding Higher incidence of GI bleeding	Less intracranial bleeding Higher incidence of GI bleeding	Substantially lower risk of major bleeding Less intracranial bleeding	Lower risk of major bleeding Less intracranial bleeding
Dosage	110 mg twice daily 150 mg twice daily	20 mg once daily (give with food)	5 mg twice daily	60 mg once daily
Dosage adjustments	75 mg twice daily for creatinine clearance[1] 15–30 mL/minute (approved in the United States but not tested in clinical trials)	15 mg once daily for creatinine clearance[1] < 50 mL/minute	2.5 mg twice daily for patients with at least two of three risk factors: 1. Age ≥ 80 years 2. Body weight ≤ 60 kg 3. Serum creatinine ≥ 1.5 mg/dL	30 mg once daily for creatinine clearance[1] ≤ 50 mL/minute FDA recommends not to use if creatinine clearance[1] > 95 mL/minute

[1]Creatinine clearance calculated by Cockcroft-Gault equation.
Data from Nishimura RA et al. 2014 AHA/ACC guideline for the management of patients with valvular heart disease: a report of the American College of Cardiology/American Heart Association Task Force on Practice Guidelines. Circulation. 2014;129(23):e521–643.

fibrillation in the United States. Both doses result in *less* intracranial hemorrhage than warfarin but also in *more* GI bleeding than warfarin. Neither dabigatran nor any of the DOACs should be used in patients with mechanical prosthetic heart valves where the medications are less effective and riskier.

Rivaroxaban is noninferior to warfarin for stroke prevention in atrial fibrillation (in the ROCKET-AF trial). Rivaroxaban is dosed at 20 mg once daily, with a reduced dose (15 mg/day) for patients with creatinine clearances between 15 and 50 mL/minute. It should be administered *with food,* since that results in a 40% higher drug absorption. Similar to dabigatran, there is substantially less intracranial hemorrhage with rivaroxaban than warfarin.

Apixaban is more effective than warfarin at stroke prevention while having a substantially lower risk of major bleeding (in the ARISTOTLE trial) and a lower risk of all-cause mortality. The apixaban dosage is 5 mg twice daily or 2.5 mg twice daily for patients with two of three high-risk criteria (age 80 years or older, body weight 60 kg or less, and serum creatinine of 1.5 mg/dL or more). Apixaban is associated with less intracranial hemorrhage and is well tolerated. Apixaban was also shown to be superior to aspirin (and better tolerated, with comparable rates of bleeding) in the AVERROES trial of patients deemed not suitable for warfarin. Apixaban has been studied in a small trial of patients receiving hemodialysis, in which the plasma concentrations were in an acceptable range using standard dosing criteria.

Edoxaban, 60 mg once a day, is noninferior to warfarin for stroke prevention with lower rates of major bleeding and lower rates of hemorrhagic stroke (studied in the ENGAGE-AF trial). Edoxaban carries a boxed warning in FDA labelleling that it should *not* be used in patients whose creatinine clearance is more than 95 mL/minute because it is less effective in this population. The dose is decreased to 30 mg/day for patients whose creatinine clearance is less than or equal to 50 mL/minute.

These four DOACs have important advantages over warfarin, and therefore, they are recommended preferentially over VKAs. In practice, these medications are often underdosed. They should be used at the doses shown to be effective in the clinical trials as shown in Table 10–11. Even though labeled for "nonvalvular" atrial fibrillation, the DOACs are safe and effective for patients with moderate or severe valvular abnormalities, with the exception of moderate or severe mitral stenosis. In part because of lower rates of intracerebral hemorrhage, *DOACs have particular advantage over warfarin in the elderly and the frail,* including patients with history of falls. For patients who fall, oral anticoagulation should generally be used, except for patients who are suffering head trauma with falls.

There are some patients with atrial fibrillation, however, who *should* be treated with VKAs. These patients include those who have mechanical prosthetic valves, advanced kidney disease (creatinine clearance less than 25 mL/minute), or moderate or severe mitral stenosis, and those who cannot afford the newer medications. Apixaban may be a reasonable option for patients with creatinine clearance less than 25 mL/minute, with one small randomized trial of patients receiving hemodialysis suggesting that it may be reasonable. Patients who have been stable while receiving warfarin for a long time, with a high time in target INR range, and who are at lower risk for intracranial hemorrhage will have relatively less benefit with a switch to a newer medication. It is important to note, however, that most patients who have intracranial hemorrhage while taking warfarin have had a recent INR below 3.0, so that good INR control does not ensure avoidance of intracranial bleeding. One way to reduce bleeding for patients taking oral anticoagulants is to avoid concurrent aspirin, unless the patient has a clear indication, like recent MI or coronary stent. Even then, use of oral anticoagulant plus clopidogrel without aspirin, or with only a brief period of "triple" therapy and then discontinuation of aspirin, may be a reasonable approach, as has been shown in clinical trials comparing rivaroxaban and dabigatran with warfarin.

There are some important practical issues with using the DOACs. It is important to monitor kidney function at baseline and at least once a year, or more often for those with impaired kidney function. Each of the medications interacts with other medications affecting the P-glycoprotein pathway, like oral ketoconazole, verapamil, dronederone, and phenytoin. To transition patients from warfarin to a DOAC, wait until the INR decreases to about 2.0. Each of the medications has a half-life of about 10–12 hours for patients with normal kidney function. For elective procedures, stop the medications two to three half-lives (usually 24–48 hours) before procedures with low to moderate bleeding risk (ie, colonoscopy, dental extraction, cardiac catheterization), and five half-lives before procedures like major surgery. Discontinuation times should be extended in patients with impaired renal function, particularly with dabigatran. There are no practical tests to immediately measure the effect of the medications, although a normal aPTT suggests little effect with dabigatran, and a normal prothrombin suggests little effect with rivaroxaban. For rivaroxaban and apixaban, chromogenic Xa assays will measure the effect, but may not be readily available. For bleeding, standard measures (eg, diagnosing and controlling the source, stopping antithrombotic agents, and replacing blood products) should be taken. If the direct-acting medication was taken in the prior 2–4 hours, use activated oral charcoal to reduce absorption. If the patient is taking aspirin, consider platelet transfusion. Antidotes should be considered for life-threatening bleeding or for patients with need for immediate surgery, or both. For cardioversion, the DOACs appear to have similar rates of subsequent stroke as warfarin, as long as patients have been taking the medications and adherent for at least several weeks. Like with warfarin, there appears to be a 1.5- to 2-fold increased rate of bleeding associated with the use of aspirin in combination with the DOACs. Even patients with atrial fibrillation and stable coronary disease taking a DOAC at least 1 year from most recent coronary stent or coronary bypass surgery appear to have substantially greater risk than benefit from the use of aspirin. Therefore, **aspirin should *not* be used with the DOACs unless there is a clear indication, such as coronary stents or acute coronary syndrome within the prior year.**

A patient with severe bleeding while taking dabigatran may be treated with the reversal agent **idarucizumab,** which is a humanized monoclonal antibody approved by the FDA for rapid reversal of the anticoagulation effects, for use in the event of severe bleeding or the need for an urgent procedure. This treatment is widely available in the United States. **Andexanet alfa,** an intravenous factor Xa decoy, is approved for reversal of factor Xa inhibitors. Four-factor prothrombin complex concentrate may partially reverse the effects of these agents. Due to the short half-life of the DOACs (10–12 hours with normal kidney function), supportive measures (local control, packed RBCs, platelets) may suffice until the medication has cleared.

Each of the DOACs appears to be safe and effective around the time of electrical cardioversion. In each of these trials, and in one modest-sized prospective randomized trial of rivaroxaban that specifically addressed cardioversion, the rates of stroke were low (and similar to warfarin) with the DOACs when given for at least 3–4 weeks prior to cardioversion. An advantage of the DOACs is that when stable anticoagulation is desired before elective cardioversion, it is achieved faster than with warfarin.

In patients who are unsuitable for long-term anticoagulation due to excessive bleeding risk, left atrial appendage occluders (including the Watchman and Amulet devices) have been shown to protect against stroke, although they are not as effective as warfarin in preventing ischemic stroke. Occlusion of the left atrial appendage during cardiac surgery provides further protection against ischemic stroke over and above ongoing oral anticoagulant use.

B. Rate control or rhythm control—After assessing stroke risk and initiating anticoagulation where appropriate, two main treatment strategies for long-term management of atrial fibrillation exist: rate control or rhythm control, although they are not mutually exclusive. Rate control should be considered background treatment in nearly all patients with atrial fibrillation, regardless of whether rhythm restoration is eventually pursued, and may be considered the primary treatment in patients with minimal to no symptoms related to long-standing atrial fibrillation. In patients with recent-onset atrial fibrillation (less than 1 year), the EAST-AFNET 4 trial found that rhythm control with antiarrhythmic medication or catheter ablation is associated with a lower risk of death from cardiovascular causes, stroke, or hospitalization for heart failure.

The decision to pursue rhythm control is often individualized, based on symptoms, the type of atrial fibrillation (paroxysmal or persistent), comorbidities (such as heart failure), as well as general health status. As first treatment, elective cardioversion following an appropriate period of anticoagulation (minimum of 3 weeks) or exclusion of left atrial thrombus by TEE is generally recommended in patients in whom atrial fibrillation is thought to be of recent onset or when there is an identifiable precipitating factor. Similarly, cardioversion is appropriate in patients who remain symptomatic from the rhythm despite efforts to achieve rate control.

In cases in which elective cardioversion is required, it may be accomplished pharmacologically or electrically. Pharmacologic cardioversion with intravenous **ibutilide** (1 mg over 10 minutes, repeated in 10 minutes if necessary) or **procainamide** (15 mg/kg over 30 minutes) may be used in a setting in which the patient can undergo continuous ECG monitoring for at least 4–6 hours following administration. Pretreatment with intravenous magnesium (1–2 g) may prevent rare episodes of torsades de pointes associated with ibutilide administration. In patients in whom a decision has been made to continue antiarrhythmic therapy to maintain sinus rhythm (see next paragraph), cardioversion can be attempted with an agent that is being considered for long-term use. For instance, after therapeutic anticoagulation has been established, **amiodarone** can be initiated on an outpatient basis (400 mg twice daily for 2 weeks, followed by 200 mg twice daily for at least 2–4 weeks and then a maintenance dose of 200 mg daily). Because amiodarone increases the prothrombin time in patients taking warfarin and increases digoxin levels, careful monitoring of anticoagulation and medication levels is required.

Other antiarrhythmic medications that can be used for long-term maintenance therapy include propafenone, flecainide, dronedarone, dofetilide, and sotalol. **Dofetilide** (125–500 mcg twice daily orally) must be initiated in hospital due to the potential risk of torsades de pointes and the downward dose adjustment that is required for patients with renal impairment. **Propafenone** (150–300 mg orally every 8 hours) and **flecainide** (50–150 mg orally twice daily) should be avoided in patients with structural heart disease (CAD, systolic dysfunction, or significant LVH) and should be used in conjunction with an AV nodal blocking medication, especially if there is a history of atrial flutter. **Sotalol** (80–160 mg orally twice daily) should be initiated in the hospital in patients with structural heart disease due to a risk of torsades de pointes; it is not very effective for converting atrial fibrillation but can be used to maintain sinus rhythm following cardioversion. **Dronedarone** should not be used in patients with recent decompensated heart failure or when atrial fibrillation has become persistent.

In patients treated long-term with an antiarrhythmic agent, sinus rhythm will persist in 30–50%. Given this high rate of arrhythmia recurrence, the decision to maintain long-term anticoagulation should be based on risk factors (CHA_2DS_2-VASc score, Table 10–10) and not on the perceived presence or absence of atrial fibrillation, since future episodes may be asymptomatic.

B. Recurrent and Refractory Atrial Fibrillation

1. Recurrent paroxysmal atrial fibrillation—For select patients with symptomatic but rare (a few times a year) episodes of atrial fibrillation, an effective treatment strategy is on-demand pharmacologic cardioversion, termed **pill-in-the-pocket treatment**. Patients without coronary or structural heart disease may be given flecainide (200–300 mg) or propafenone (450–600 mg) in addition to a beta-blocker or nondihydropyridine calcium channel blocker as a single dose at the onset of symptoms. It is recommended that the first such treatment take place in a monitored setting (eg, the emergency department or hospital) to evaluate safety and effectiveness. For more frequent, symptomatic arrhythmic episodes, daily antiarrhythmic agents are first-line therapy; however, they are not often successful in preventing all paroxysmal atrial fibrillation episodes and long-term tolerability is poor.

2. Refractory atrial fibrillation—Atrial fibrillation should be considered refractory if it causes persistent symptoms or limits activity despite attempts at rate or rhythm control. If antiarrhythmic or rate control medications fail to improve symptoms, catheter ablation around the pulmonary veins to isolate the triggers that initiate and maintain atrial fibrillation may be considered. It is a reasonable therapy for individuals with symptomatic paroxysmal or persistent atrial fibrillation that is refractory to pharmacologic therapy and for select patients (younger than 65 years or with concurrent heart failure) as first-line therapy. The primary benefit of catheter ablation is an improvement in quality of life. In the CABANA trial, there was no difference in the primary endpoint of death, disabling stroke, serious bleeding, or cardiac arrest in patients randomized to catheter ablation versus medical therapy as first treatment for symptomatic atrial fibrillation. Ablation is successful about 50–70% of the time but repeat ablation may be required in up to 20% of patients. The procedure is routinely performed in the electrophysiology laboratory using a catheter-based approach and adverse event rates are low when performed by experienced operators. Surgical ablation can also be performed via a subxiphoid approach thoracoscopically, via thoracotomy, or via median sternotomy in the operating room as a stand-alone or adjunct procedure. Finally, in symptomatic patients with poor rate control and deemed inappropriate for pulmonary vein isolation, radiofrequency ablation of the AV node and permanent pacing ensure rate control and may facilitate a more physiologic rate response to activity, but this is usually performed only after other therapies have failed.

When to Refer

- Symptomatic atrial fibrillation with or without adequate rate control.
- Asymptomatic atrial fibrillation with poor rate control despite AV nodal blockers.
- Patients at risk for stroke who have not tolerated oral anticoagulants.

Kirchhof P et al; EAST-AFNET 4 Trial Investigators. Early rhythm-control therapy in patients with atrial fibrillation. N Engl J Med. 2020;383:1305. [PMID: 32865375]

Packer DL et al. Effect of catheter ablation vs antiarrhythmic drug therapy on mortality, stroke, bleeding, and cardiac arrest among patients with atrial fibrillation: the CABANA randomized clinical trial. JAMA. 2019;321:1261. [PMID: 30874766]

Whitlock RP et al. Left atrial appendage occlusion during cardiac surgery to prevent stroke. N Engl J Med. 2021;384:2081. [PMID: 33999547]

ATRIAL FLUTTER

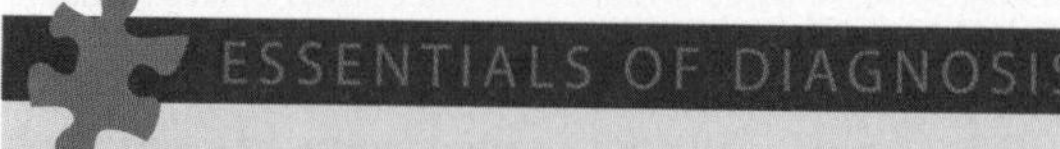

- Rapid, regular tachycardia presenting classically with 2 to 1 block in the AV node and ventricular heart rate of 150 beats/minute. ECG shows "sawtooth" pattern of atrial activity (rate 300 beats/minute).
- Stroke risk should be considered equivalent to that with atrial fibrillation.
- Catheter ablation is highly successful and is considered the definitive treatment for typical atrial flutter.

General Considerations

Atrial flutter is less common than fibrillation. It may occur in patients with structurally normal hearts but is more commonly seen in patients with COPD, valvular or structural heart disease, ASD, or surgically repaired congenital heart disease.

Clinical Findings

Patients typically present with complaints of palpitations, fatigue, or mild dizziness. In situations where the arrhythmia is unrecognized for a prolonged period of time, patients may present with symptoms and signs of heart failure (dyspnea, exertional intolerance, edema) due to tachycardia-induced cardiomyopathy. The ECG typically demonstrates a **"sawtooth"** pattern of atrial activity in the inferior leads (II, III, and AVF). The reentrant circuit generates atrial rates of 250–350 beats/minute, usually with transmission of every second, third, or fourth impulse through the AV node to the ventricles.

Treatment

Ventricular rate control is accomplished using the same agents used in atrial fibrillation, but it is generally more difficult. Conversion of atrial flutter to sinus rhythm with class I antiarrhythmic agents is also difficult to achieve, and administration of these medications has been associated with slowing of the atrial flutter rate to the point at which 1:1 AV conduction can occur at rates in excess of 200 beats/minute, with subsequent hemodynamic collapse. The intravenous class III antiarrhythmic agent ibutilide has been significantly more successful in converting atrial flutter (see Table 10–9). About 50–70% of patients return to sinus rhythm within 60–90 minutes following the infusion of 1–2 mg of this agent. Electrical cardioversion is also very effective for atrial flutter, with approximately 90% of patients converting following synchronized shocks of as little as 25–50 J.

Although the organization of atrial contractile function in this arrhythmia may provide some protection against thrombus formation, **the risk of thromboembolism should be considered equivalent to that with atrial fibrillation** due to the common coexistence of these arrhythmias. Precardioversion anticoagulation is not necessary for atrial flutter of less than 48 hours duration except in the setting of mitral valve disease. As with atrial fibrillation, anticoagulation should be continued for at least 4 weeks after electrical or chemical cardioversion and chronically in patients with risk factors for thromboembolism.

Catheter ablation is the treatment of choice for long-term management of atrial flutter owing to the high success rate and safety of the procedure. The anatomy of the typical circuit is well defined and catheter ablation within the right atrium results in immediate and permanent elimination of atrial flutter in more than 90% of patients. Due to the frequent coexistence of atrial flutter with atrial fibrillation, however, some patients may require catheter ablation of both arrhythmias. If pharmacologic therapy is chosen, class III antiarrhythmics (amiodarone or dofetilide) are generally preferred (see Table 10–9).

When to Refer

All patients with atrial flutter should be referred to a cardiologist or cardiac electrophysiologist for consideration of definitive treatment with catheter ablation.

ATRIAL TACHYCARDIA

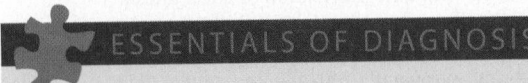

- Characterized by bursts of rapid, regular tachycardia.
- Multifocal atrial tachycardia commonly seen with severe COPD and presents with three or more distinct P wave morphologies on ECG, often confused for atrial fibrillation. Treatment of the underlying lung disease is most effective therapy.

General Considerations

Atrial tachycardia is an uncommon form of SVT characterized by paroxysms or bursts of rapid, regular arrhythmia due to focal atrial impulses originating outside of the normal sinus node. Common sites include the tricuspid annulus, the crista terminalis of the right atrium and the coronary sinus. **Multifocal atrial tachycardia** is a particular subtype seen in patients with severe COPD and characterized by varying P wave morphology (by definition, three or more foci) and markedly irregular PP intervals. The rate is usually between 100 beats/minute and 140 beats/minute, and it is often confused for atrial fibrillation. **Solitary atrial premature beats** are benign and generally not associated with underlying cardiac disease. They occur when an ectopic focus in the atria fires before the next sinus node impulse. The contour of the P wave usually differs from the patient's normal complex, unless the ectopic focus is near the sinus node. Acceleration of the heart rate by any means usually abolishes most premature beats.

Clinical Findings

Focal atrial tachycardias are usually intermittent and self-limiting although incessant forms do exist and may present with signs and symptoms of heart failure due to tachycardia-induced cardiomyopathy. Most patients report palpitations with an abrupt onset, similar to other forms of PSVT. Patients with underlying cardiac pathology (eg, CHD) can present with dyspnea or angina. Close inspection of the P wave on 12-lead ECG suggests a focus away from the sinus node, although certain locations (eg, high right atrial crista terminalis) may mimic sinus tachycardia. In this situation, the abrupt onset and offset of the arrhythmia is helpful in distinguishing atrial from sinus tachycardia, although electrophysiologic study is sometimes necessary.

Treatment

Initial management of atrial tachycardia is similar to other types of PSVT; however, vagal maneuvers and intravenous adenosine are generally less effective. Intravenous beta-blockers or calcium channel blockers can be given in the hemodynamically stable patient with a transition to oral formulations for long-term management. Antiarrhythmic medications or catheter ablation should be considered in patients who continue to have symptomatic episodes. Long-term anticoagulation is not indicated in the absence of coexistent atrial fibrillation or atrial flutter.

For patients with multifocal atrial tachycardia, treatment of the underlying condition (eg, COPD) is paramount; verapamil, 240–480 mg orally daily in divided doses, may be effective in some patients.

When to Refer

All patients with atrial tachycardia in whom initial medical management fails should be referred to a cardiologist or cardiac electrophysiologist.

VENTRICULAR PREMATURE BEATS (Ventricular Extrasystoles)

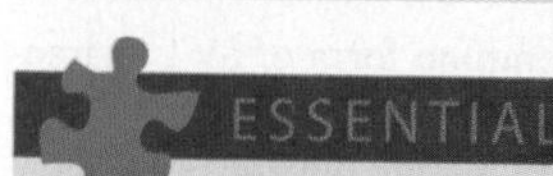

ESSENTIALS OF DIAGNOSIS

- Common but rarely symptomatic.
- Ambulatory ECG monitoring to quantify daily burden of PVCs. Asymptomatic patients with > 10% PVC burden should have periodic echocardiogram to exclude development of LV dysfunction.

General Considerations

Ventricular premature beats, or **PVCs,** are isolated beats typically originating from the outflow tract or His-Purkinje regions of ventricular tissue. In most patients, the presence of PVCs is a benign finding; however, they rarely may trigger ventricular tachycardia or ventricular fibrillation, especially in patients with underlying heart disease.

Clinical Findings

Patients may be asymptomatic or experience palpitations, dizziness, or vague chest pain. Some patients feel the irregular beat; however, symptoms can often be secondary to post-PVC augmentation of contractility or a post-PVC compensatory pause. Exercise generally abolishes premature beats in normal hearts, and the rhythm becomes regular. PVCs are characterized by wide QRS complexes that differ in morphology from the patient's normal beats. They are usually not preceded by a P wave, although retrograde ventriculoatrial conduction may occur. **Bigeminy** and **trigeminy** are arrhythmias in which every second or third beat is premature. Ambulatory ECG monitoring may reveal more frequent and complex PVCs than occur in a single routine ECG. An increased frequency of PVCs during exercise is associated with a higher risk of cardiovascular mortality and should be investigated further.

Treatment

If no associated cardiac disease is present and if the ectopic beats are asymptomatic, no therapy is indicated. Mild symptoms or anxiety from palpitations may be allayed with reassurance to the patient of the benign nature of this arrhythmia. If PVCs are frequent (bigeminal or trigeminal pattern) or multifocal, electrolyte abnormalities (ie, hypo- or hyperkalemia and hypomagnesemia) and occult cardiac disease (ie, ischemic heart disease or LV dysfunction) should be excluded. In addition, an echocardiogram should be performed in patients in whom a burden of PVCs of greater than 10,000 per day has been documented by ambulatory ECG monitoring. Pharmacologic treatment is indicated only for patients who are symptomatic or who develop cardiomyopathy thought to be due to a high burden of PVCs (generally greater than 10% of daily heart beats). Beta-blockers or nondihydropyridine calcium channel blockers are appropriate as first-line therapy. The class I and III antiarrhythmic agents (see Table 10–9) may be effective in reducing PVCs but are often poorly tolerated and can be proarrhythmic in up to 5% of patients. Catheter ablation is a well-established therapy for symptomatic individuals who do not respond to medication or for those patients whose burden of ectopic beats has resulted in a cardiomyopathy.

When to Refer

Patients with symptomatic PVCs who do not respond to initial medical management or asymptomatic patients with daily PVC burden greater than 10% on ambulatory ECG monitoring should be referred to a cardiologist or cardiac electrophysiologist.

VENTRICULAR TACHYCARDIA

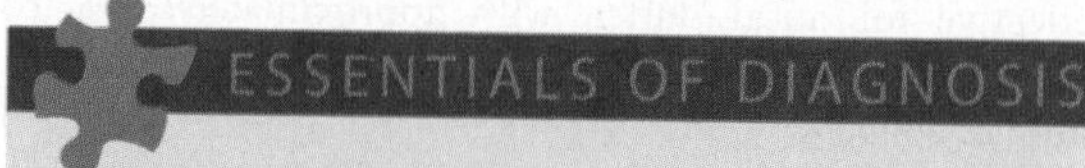

ESSENTIALS OF DIAGNOSIS

- Fast, wide QRS complex on ECG.
- Associated with ischemic heart disease, particularly in older patients.
- In the absence of reversible cause, implantable cardioverter defibrillator (ICD) is recommended if meaningful life expectancy is > 1 year.

General Considerations

Ventricular tachycardia is defined as three or more consecutive ventricular premature beats. It is classified as either **nonsustained** (lasting less than 30 seconds and terminating spontaneously) or **sustained** with a heart rate greater than 100 beats/minute. In individuals without heart disease, nonsustained ventricular tachycardia is generally associated with a benign prognosis. In patients with structural heart disease, nonsustained ventricular tachycardia is associated with an increased risk of subsequent symptomatic ventricular tachycardia and sudden death, especially when seen more than 48 hours after MI.

Ventricular tachycardia is a frequent complication of acute MI and dilated cardiomyopathy but may occur in chronic coronary disease, HCM, myocarditis, and in most other forms of myocardial disease. It can also be a consequence of atypical forms of cardiomyopathies, such as arrhythmogenic RV cardiomyopathy. However, idiopathic ventricular tachycardia can also occur in patients with structurally normal hearts. **Accelerated idioventricular rhythm** is a regular wide complex rhythm with a rate of 60–120 beats/minute, usually with a gradual onset. It occurs commonly in acute infarction and following reperfusion with thrombolytic medications. Treatment is not indicated unless there is hemodynamic compromise or more serious arrhythmias. **Torsades de pointes,** a form of ventricular tachycardia in which QRS morphology twists around the baseline, may occur in the setting of severe hypokalemia, hypomagnesemia, or after administration of a medication that prolongs the QT interval.

Clinical Findings

A. Symptoms and Signs

Patients commonly experience palpitations, dyspnea, or lightheadedness, but on rare occasion may be asymptomatic. Syncope or cardiac arrest can be presenting symptoms in patients with underlying cardiac disease or other severe comorbidities. Episodes may be triggered by exercise or emotional stress.

B. Diagnostic Studies

Comprehensive blood laboratory work should be performed because ventricular tachycardia can occur in the setting of hypokalemia and hypomagnesemia. Cardiac markers may be elevated when ventricular tachycardia presents in the setting of acute MI or as a consequence of underlying CAD and demand ischemia. In patients with sustained, hemodynamically tolerated ventricular tachycardia, a 12-lead ECG during tachycardia should be obtained. Cardiac evaluation with echocardiography or cardiac MRI, ambulatory ECG monitoring, and exercise testing may be warranted depending on the clinical situation. Survivors of cardiac arrest or life-threatening ventricular arrhythmia should be evaluated for ischemic heart disease (CT or invasive coronary angiography) and undergo revascularization when appropriate.

There is generally no role for invasive electrophysiologic study in patients with sustained ventricular tachycardia who otherwise meet criteria for ICD. In patients with structural heart disease and syncope of unknown cause, or in situations in which the mechanism of wide-complex tachycardia is uncertain, electrophysiologic study may provide important information.

C. Differentiation of Aberrantly Conducted Supraventricular Beats From Ventricular Beats

The distinction on 12-lead ECG of ventricular tachycardia from SVT with aberrant conduction may be difficult in patients with a wide-complex tachycardia; it is important because of the differing prognostic and therapeutic implications of each type. Findings favoring a **ventricular origin** include: (1) AV dissociation; (2) a QRS duration exceeding 0.14 second; (3) capture or fusion beats (infrequent); (4) left axis deviation with right bundle branch block morphology; (5) monophasic (R) or biphasic (qR, QR, or RS) complexes in V_1; and (6) a qR or QS complex in V_6. **Supraventricular origin** is favored by: (1) a triphasic QRS complex, especially if there was initial negativity in leads I and V_6; (2) ventricular rates exceeding 170 beats/minute; (3) QRS duration longer than 0.12 second but not longer than 0.14 second; and (4) the presence of preexcitation syndrome. Patients with a wide-complex tachycardia, especially those with known cardiac disease, should be presumed to have ventricular tachycardia if the diagnosis is unclear.

Treatment

A. Initial Management

The treatment of acute ventricular tachycardia is determined by the degree of hemodynamic compromise and the duration of the arrhythmia. In patients with structurally normal hearts, the prognosis is generally benign and syncope is uncommon. The etiology is often triggered activity from the right or LV outflow tract and immediate treatment with a short-acting intravenous beta-blocker or verapamil may terminate the episode.

In the presence of known or suspected structural heart disease, assessment of hemodynamic stability determines the need for urgent direct current cardioversion. When ventricular tachycardia causes hypotension, heart failure, or myocardial ischemia, immediate synchronized direct current cardioversion with 100–360 J should be performed. If ventricular tachycardia recurs, intravenous amiodarone (150-mg bolus followed by 1 mg/minute infusion for 6 hours and then 0.5 mg/minute for 18 hours) should be administered to achieve a stable rhythm with further attempts at cardioversion as necessary. Significant hypotension can occur with rapid infusions of amiodarone. The management of ventricular tachycardia in the setting of acute MI is discussed in the Complications section of Acute Myocardial Infarction with ST-Segment Elevation.

In patients with sustained ventricular tachycardia who are hemodynamically stable, medical treatment with intravenous amiodarone, lidocaine, or procainamide can be used; however, direct current cardioversion should be performed if the ventricular tachycardia fails to terminate or symptoms worsen. Empiric magnesium replacement (1–2 g intravenously) may help, especially for polymorphic ventricular tachycardia. If polymorphic ventricular tachycardia recurs, increasing the heart rate with isoproterenol infusion (up to 20 mcg/minute) or atrial pacing with a temporary pacemaker (at 90–120 beats/minute) will effectively shorten the QT interval to prevent further episodes. In patients with polymorphic ventricular tachycardia in the setting of a normal QT interval, myocardial ischemia should be considered with prompt evaluation and coronary revascularization performed as indicated.

B. Long-Term Management

Patients with symptomatic or sustained ventricular tachycardia in the absence of a reversible precipitating cause (acute MI or ischemia, electrolyte imbalance, medication toxicity, etc) are at high risk for recurrence. In patients with structurally normal hearts and ventricular tachycardia with typical outflow tract (left bundle branch block with inferior axis) or left posterior fascicle (right bundle branch block with superior axis) appearance on ECG, suppressive treatment with beta-blocker or a nondihydropyridine calcium channel blocker may be tried. Catheter ablation has a high success rate in these patients who fail initial medical treatment. In patients with significant LV dysfunction, subsequent sudden death is common and ICD implantation is recommended if meaningful survival is expected to be longer than 1 year. Beta-blockers are the mainstay for medical treatment of ventricular tachycardia in patients with structural heart disease. Antiarrhythmic medications have not been shown to lower mortality in these patients, but may decrease subsequent episodes and reduce the number of ICD shocks. Amiodarone is generally preferred in patients with structural heart disease but sotalol may be considered as well. Catheter ablation is an important treatment option for those patients with recurrent tachycardia who do not respond to or are intolerant of medical therapy; however, recurrence rates are high.

When to Refer

Any patient with sustained ventricular tachycardia or syncope of unknown cause in the presence of underlying structural cardiac disease.

Al-Khatib SM et al. 2017 AHA/ACC/HRS guideline for management of patients with ventricular arrhythmias and the prevention of sudden cardiac death: a report of the American College of Cardiology/American Heart Association Task Force on Clinical Practice Guidelines and the Heart Rhythm Society. J Am Coll Cardiol. 2018;72:e91. [PMID: 29097296]

VENTRICULAR FIBRILLATION & SUDDEN DEATH

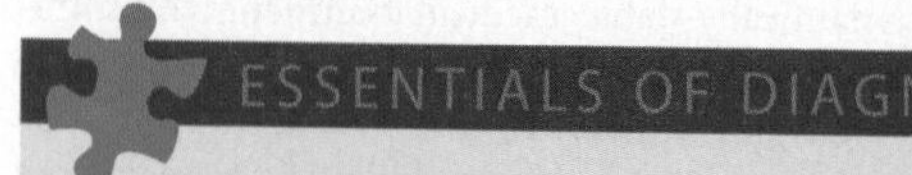

- Most patients with sudden cardiac death have underlying CHD.
- In the absence of reversible cause, ICD is recommended.

General Considerations

Sudden cardiac death is defined as unexpected nontraumatic death in clinically well or stable patients who die within 1 hour after onset of symptoms. The causative rhythm in most cases is ventricular fibrillation. **Sudden cardiac arrest** is a term reserved for the successful resuscitation of ventricular fibrillation, either spontaneously or via intervention (defibrillation).

Clinical Findings

Approximately 70% of cases of sudden cardiac death are attributable to underlying CHD; in up to 40% of patients, sudden cardiac death may be the initial manifestation of CHD. In patients younger than 35, most sudden cardiac death (SCD) is caused by inherited heart disease (long QT syndrome, catecholaminergic polymorphic ventricular tachycardia, Brugada syndrome, HCM, arrhythmogenic RV cardiomyopathy, dilated cardiomyopathy). Over the age of 35, CHD is the most common cause of SCD, although inherited causes are common up until the age of 50. Noninherited forms of heart disease can also lead to SCD, including valvular heart disease (aortic stenosis, pulmonic stenosis), congenital heart disease, and myocarditis. Prompt evaluation to exclude reversible causes of sudden cardiac arrest should begin immediately following resuscitation. Laboratory testing should be performed to exclude severe electrolyte abnormalities (particularly hypokalemia and hypomagnesemia) and acidosis and to evaluate cardiac biomarkers. Caution should be taken in attributing cardiac arrest solely to an electrolyte disturbance, however, because laboratory abnormalities may be secondary to resuscitation and not causative of the event. A 12-lead ECG should be performed to evaluate for ongoing ischemia or conduction system disease. Ventricular function should be evaluated with echocardiography. Evaluation for ischemic heart disease (CT or coronary angiography) should be performed to exclude coronary disease as the underlying cause, since revascularization may prevent recurrence. In the absence of coronary disease, contrast-enhanced cardiac MRI may be used to evaluate for the presence of myocardial scar, which is a strong predictor of recurrent ventricular tachycardia/ventricular fibrillation in patients with nonischemic cardiomyopathy.

Treatment

Unless ventricular fibrillation occurs shortly after MI, is associated with ischemia, or is seen with a correctable process (such as an electrolyte abnormality or medication toxicity), surviving patients require intervention since recurrences are frequent. Survivors of cardiac arrest appear to have improved long-term outcomes if a **targeted temperature management protocol** is rapidly initiated and continued for 24–36 hours after cardiac arrest.

Patients who survive sudden cardiac arrest have a high incidence of recurrence, so an **ICD** is generally indicated. Sudden cardiac arrest in the setting of acute ischemia or infarct should be managed with prompt coronary revascularization. However, implantation of a prophylactic ICD in patients immediately after MI is associated with a trend toward *worse* outcomes. These patients may be managed with a **wearable cardioverter defibrillator** until recovery of ventricular function can be assessed by echocardiogram at a later date (6–12 weeks following MI or coronary intervention). In patients in whom ventricular function remains low (EF less than or equal to 35%), a permanent subcutaneous ICD (when pacing is not required) or transvenous ICD should be implanted.

When to Refer

All survivors of sudden cardiac arrest should be referred to a cardiologist or cardiac electrophysiologist.

INHERITED ARRHYTHMIA SYNDROMES

ESSENTIALS OF DIAGNOSIS

- Includes long QT syndrome, Brugada syndrome, arrhythmogenic RV cardiomyopathy, and catecholaminergic polymorphic ventricular tachycardia.
- Genetic testing for patients with suspected congenital long QT syndrome based on family history, ECG or exercise testing, or severely prolonged QT interval (> 500 msec) on serial ECGs.
- Patients with long QT syndrome or catecholaminergic polymorphic ventricular tachycardia should be treated long term with an oral beta-blocker (nadolol or propranolol). ICD is indicated for patients with ventricular arrhythmia or syncope despite medical treatment.

General Considerations

Inherited arrhythmia syndromes may result in life-threatening ventricular arrhythmias due to gene mutations in cardiac channels resulting in abnormal electrolyte regulation across the cardiac cell membrane. **Congenital long QT syndrome** is an uncommon disease (1 in 2500 live births) that is characterized by a long QT interval (usually greater than 470 msec) and ventricular arrhythmia, typically polymorphic ventricular tachycardia. **Acquired long QT syndrome** is usually secondary to use of antiarrhythmic agents (sotalol, dofetilide), methadone, antidepressant medications, or certain antibiotics; electrolyte abnormalities; myocardial ischemia; or significant bradycardia. **Brugada syndrome** accounts for up to 20% of sudden cardiac death in the absence of structural heart disease and is most often due to a defect in a sodium channel gene. **Arrhythmogenic RV cardiomyopathy** is an inherited cardiomyopathy that predominantly affects the right ventricle and is characterized by areas of myocardial replacement with fibrosis and adipose tissue that frequently causes ventricular arrhythmia. **Catecholaminergic polymorphic ventricular tachycardia** is a rare but important cause of sudden cardiac death associated with exercise.

Clinical Findings

Patients with an inherited arrhythmia syndrome have a variable clinical presentation; they may be asymptomatic or have palpitations, sustained tachyarrhythmia, syncope, or sudden cardiac arrest. In young patients, syncopal episodes may be misdiagnosed as a primary seizure disorder. Personal and family history should be thoroughly reviewed in all patients. A 12-lead ECG should be performed with careful attention to any abnormality in the ST segment, T wave, and QT interval. A corrected QT interval longer than 500 msec on serial ECGs in the absence of a secondary cause (medication or electrolyte abnormality) identifies a high-risk subset of patients with long QT syndrome. Ambulatory ECG monitoring may be used to evaluate for ventricular arrhythmias as well as dynamic changes to the QT interval or T wave. Exercise ECG testing may be performed in patients with suspected long QT syndrome to assess for lack of appropriate QT interval shortening with higher heart rates. In cases where the cause of sudden cardiac arrest is suspected to be heritable, genetic testing under the guidance of a multidisciplinary genetics team is recommended to both determine the diagnosis and to facilitate the identification of first-degree family members at risk for developing the same disease.

Treatment

The management of acute polymorphic ventricular tachycardia (torsades de pointes) differs from that of other forms of ventricular tachycardia. Class Ia, Ic, or III antiarrhythmics, which prolong the QT interval, should be avoided—or withdrawn immediately if being used in patients with long QT syndrome. Intravenous beta-blockers may be effective in treating electrical storm due to long QT syndrome or catecholaminergic polymorphic ventricular tachycardia. Increasing the heart rate, whether by infusion of beta-agonist (dopamine or isoproterenol) or temporary atrial or ventricular pacing, is an effective approach that can both break and prevent the rhythm.

Long-term treatment of patients with inherited arrhythmia syndromes depends on the presence of high-risk features. Use of beta-blockers (particularly propranolol or nadolol) is the mainstay of treatment for patients with long QT syndrome or catecholaminergic polymorphic ventricular tachycardia. Surgical cervicothoracic sympathectomy should be considered for patients who do not respond to or are intolerant of beta-blockers. There is no reliable medication therapy for Brugada syndrome and prevention of arrhythmias focuses on prompt treatment of exacerbating triggers, particularly fever. Antiarrhythmic medications should be avoided in patients with inherited arrhythmia syndromes except for specific identified genetic abnormalities under the direction of a specialist. ICD implantation is generally recommended for patients with an inherited arrhythmia syndrome in whom sudden cardiac arrest is the initial presentation. An ICD should be considered in patients with recurrent sustained ventricular arrhythmias or syncope despite medical therapy.

When to Refer

Any patient with known or suspected inherited arrhythmia syndrome or with severe corrected QT interval prolongation (greater than 500 msec on serial ECGs) should be referred to a cardiologist or cardiac electrophysiologist.

Stiles MK et al. 2020 APHRS/HRS expert consensus statement on the investigation of decedents with sudden unexplained death and patients with sudden cardiac arrest, and of their families. Heart Rhythm. 2021;18:e1. [PMID: 33091602]

SYNCOPE

ESSENTIALS OF DIAGNOSIS

- Transient loss of consciousness and postural tone from vasodepressor or cardiogenic causes with prompt recovery without resuscitative measures.
- High-risk features include history of structural heart disease, abnormal ECG, and age > 60 years.

General Considerations

Syncope is a symptom defined as a transient, self-limited loss of consciousness, usually leading to a fall. Thirty percent of the adult population will experience at least one episode of syncope. It accounts for approximately 3% of emergency department visits. A specific cause of syncope is identified in about 50% of cases during the initial evaluation. The prognosis is relatively favorable except when accompanying cardiac disease is present. In many patients with recurrent syncope or near syncope, arrhythmias are not the cause. This is particularly true when the patient has no evidence of associated heart disease by history, examination, standard ECG, or noninvasive testing. The history is the most important component of the evaluation to identify the cause of syncope.

Reflex (neurally mediated) syncope may be due to excessive vagal tone or impaired reflex control of the peripheral circulation. The most frequent type is **vasovagal syncope** or the "common faint," which is often initiated by a stressful, painful, or claustrophobic experience, especially in young women. Enhanced vagal tone with resulting hypotension is the cause of syncope in **carotid sinus hypersensitivity** and **postmicturition syncope;** vagal-induced sinus bradycardia, sinus arrest, and AV block are common accompaniments and may themselves be the cause of syncope.

Orthostatic (postural) hypotension is another common cause of vasodepressor syncope, especially in elderly patients; in diabetic patients or others with autonomic neuropathy; in patients with blood loss or hypovolemia; and in patients taking vasodilators, diuretics, and adrenergic-blocking medications. In addition, a syndrome of **chronic idiopathic orthostatic hypotension** exists primarily in older men. In most of these conditions, the normal vasoconstrictive response to assuming upright posture, which compensates for the abrupt decrease in venous return, is impaired.

Cardiogenic syncope can occur on a mechanical or arrhythmic basis. There is usually no prodrome; thus, injury secondary to falling is common. Mechanical problems that can cause syncope include aortic stenosis (where syncope may occur from autonomic reflex abnormalities or ventricular tachycardia), pulmonary stenosis, HCM, congenital lesions associated with pulmonary hypertension or right-to-left shunting, and LA myxoma obstructing the mitral valve. Episodes are commonly exertional or postexertional. More commonly, cardiac syncope is due to disorders of automaticity (sick sinus syndrome), conduction disorders (AV block), or tachyarrhythmias (especially ventricular tachycardia and SVT with rapid ventricular rate).

Clinical Findings

A. Symptoms and Signs

Vasovagal syncope often has a prodrome of vasodepressor premonitory symptoms, such as nausea, diaphoresis, tachycardia, and pallor. Episodes can be aborted by lying down or removing the inciting stimulus. Cardiogenic syncope by contrast is characteristically abrupt in onset, often resulting in injury, transient (lasting for seconds to a few minutes), and followed by prompt recovery of full consciousness. In orthostatic (postural) hypotension, a greater than normal decline (20 mm Hg) in BP immediately upon arising from the supine to the standing position is observed, with or without tachycardia depending on the status of autonomic (baroreceptor) function.

B. Diagnostic Tests

The evaluation for syncope depends on findings from the history and physical examination (especially orthostatic BP evaluation, auscultation of carotid arteries, and cardiac examination).

1. ECG—A resting ECG is recommended for all patients undergoing evaluation for syncope. High-risk findings on ECG include non-sinus rhythm, complete or partial left bundle branch block, and voltage criteria indicating LV hypertrophy. Patients with a normal initial evaluation, including unremarkable history and physical, absence of cardiac disease or significant comorbidities and normal baseline ECG may not need further testing. When initial evaluation suggests a possible cardiac arrhythmia, continuous ambulatory ECG monitoring, event recorder (for infrequent episodes), or a wearable or implantable cardiac monitor can be considered. Caution is required before attributing a patient's syncopal event to rhythm or conduction abnormalities observed during monitoring without concomitant symptoms. For instance, dizziness or syncope in older patients may be unrelated to incidentally observed bradycardia, sinus node abnormalities, or ventricular ectopy.

2. Autonomic testing—**Tilt-table testing** may be useful in patients with suspected vasovagal syncope where the diagnosis is unclear after initial evaluation, especially when syncope is recurrent. The hemodynamic response to tilting determines whether there is a *cardioinhibitory*, *vasodepressor*, or *mixed* response. The overall utility of the test is improved when there is a high pretest probability of neurally mediated syncope, since the sensitivity and specificity of the test in the general population is only moderate.

3. Electrophysiologic studies—Electrophysiologic study has limited role in the evaluation of syncope, particularly in patients without structural heart disease or when there is a low suspicion for arrhythmic etiology. In patients with ischemic heart disease, LV dysfunction, known conduction disease or arrhythmia, electrophysiologic study may help elucidate the mechanism of syncope and guide treatment decisions. The diagnostic yield in patients with structural heart disease is approximately 50%.

Treatment

In patients with vasovagal syncope, treatment consists largely of education on the benign nature of the condition and counseling to avoid predisposing situations. *Counterpressure maneuvers* (squatting, leg-crossing, abdominal contraction) can be helpful in limiting or terminating episodes. Medical therapy is reserved for patients with symptoms despite these measures. Midodrine is an alpha-agonist that can increase the peripheral sympathetic neural outflow and decrease venous pooling during vasovagal episodes and has been shown to reduce the frequency of syncopal episodes in small randomized trials. Fludrocortisone and beta-blockers have also been used but generally provide minimal benefit. SSRIs have shown some benefit in select patients. There is generally no role for permanent pacemaker implantation in patients with vasovagal syncope, with the possible exception of patients older than age 40 years with prolonged (longer than 3 seconds), symptomatic episodes of asystole documented on ambulatory monitoring. Pacemaker implantation based soley upon tilt-table–induced asystolic (cardioinhibitory) response is rarely indicated.

If symptomatic bradyarrhythmias or supraventricular tachyarrhythmias are detected and felt to be the cause of syncope, therapy can usually be initiated without additional diagnostic studies. Permanent pacing is indicated in patients with cardiogenic syncope and documented severe pauses (greater than 3 seconds), bradycardia, or high-degree AV block (second-degree Mobitz type II or complete heart block) when symptoms are correlated to the arrhythmia.

An important consideration in patients who have experienced syncope, symptomatic ventricular tachycardia, or aborted sudden death is to provide recommendations concerning **automobile driving restrictions**. Patients with syncope thought to be due to temporary factors (acute MI, bradyarrhythmias subsequently treated with permanent pacing, medication effect, electrolyte imbalance) should be advised after recovery not to drive for at least 1 week. Other patients with symptomatic ventricular tachycardia or aborted sudden death, whether treated pharmacologically, with an ICD or with ablation therapy, warrant longer driving restriction (3–6 months). Significant variability in legal restrictions exist depending on region and providers should be familiar with their local driving laws and restrictions and advise patients accordingly.

When to Refer

- Patients with syncope and underlying structural heart disease, documented arrhythmia, or conduction disturbance.
- Unclear etiology of syncope with high-risk features (heart failure, abnormal ECG findings, advanced age, multiple unexplained episodes).

Brignole M et al; ESC Scientific Document Group. 2018 ESC guidelines for the diagnosis and management of syncope. Eur Heart J. 2018;39:1883. [PMID: 29562304]

HEART FAILURE

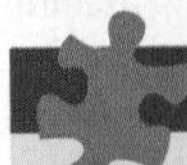

ESSENTIALS OF DIAGNOSIS

- LV failure: Either due to systolic or diastolic dysfunction. Predominant symptoms are those of low cardiac output and congestion, including dyspnea.
- RV failure: Symptoms of fluid overload predominate; usually RV failure is secondary to LV failure.
- Assessment of LV function is a crucial part of diagnosis and management.
- Optimal management of chronic heart failure includes combination medical therapies, such as ACE inhibitors, aldosterone antagonists, and beta-blockers.

General Considerations

Heart failure is a common syndrome that is increasing in incidence and prevalence. Approximately 6 million patients in the United States have heart failure, with 8 million or more patients projected to have heart failure by 2030. Each year in the United States, 809,000 patients are discharged from the hospital with a diagnosis of heart failure. It is primarily a disease of aging, with over 75% of existing and new cases occurring in individuals over 65 years of age. Seventy-five percent of heart failure patients have antecedent hypertension. The prevalence of heart failure rises from less than 1% in individuals below 60 years to nearly 10% in those over 80 years of age.

Heart failure may be right-sided or left-sided (or both). Patients with **left heart failure** may have symptoms of low cardiac output and elevated pulmonary venous pressure; dyspnea is the predominant feature. Signs of fluid retention predominate in **right heart failure**. Most patients exhibit symptoms or signs of both right- and left-sided failure, and LV dysfunction is the primary cause of RV failure. Approximately half of patients with heart failure have **preserved LV systolic function** and usually have some degree of **diastolic dysfunction.** Patients with reduced or preserved systolic function may have similar symptoms and it may be difficult to distinguish clinically between the two based on signs and symptoms. In developed countries, CAD with resulting MI and loss of functioning myocardium (**ischemic cardiomyopathy**) is the most common cause of systolic heart failure. Systemic hypertension remains an important cause of heart failure and, even more commonly in the United States, an exacerbating factor in patients with cardiac dysfunction due to other causes, such as CAD. Several processes may present with **dilated** or **congestive cardiomyopathy,** which is characterized by LV or biventricular dilation and generalized systolic dysfunction. These are discussed elsewhere in this chapter, but the most common are alcoholic cardiomyopathy, viral myocarditis (including infections by HIV; see also the COVID-19 section in Chapter 32), and dilated cardiomyopathies with no obvious underlying cause (idiopathic cardiomyopathy). Rare causes of dilated cardiomyopathy include infiltrative diseases (hemochromatosis, sarcoidosis, amyloidosis, etc), other infectious agents, metabolic disorders, cardiotoxins, and medication toxicity. Valvular heart diseases—particularly degenerative aortic stenosis and chronic aortic or mitral regurgitation—are not infrequent causes of heart failure. Persistent tachycardia, often related to atrial arrhythmias, can cause systolic dysfunction that may be reversible with controlling the rate. Diastolic cardiac dysfunction is associated with aging and related myocardial stiffening, as well as LVH, commonly resulting from hypertension. Conditions such as **hypertrophic** or **restrictive cardiomyopathy,** diabetes, and pericardial disease can produce the same clinical picture. Atrial fibrillation with or without rapid ventricular response may contribute to impaired LV filling.

Heart failure is often preventable by early detection of patients at risk and by early intervention. The importance of these approaches is emphasized by US guidelines that have incorporated a classification of heart failure that includes four stages. **Stage A** includes patients at risk for developing heart failure (such as patients with hypertension). In the majority of these patients, development of heart failure can be prevented with interventions such as the aggressive treatment of hypertension, modification of coronary risk factors, and reduction of excessive alcohol intake. **Stage B** includes patients who have structural heart disease but no current or previously recognized symptoms of heart failure. Examples include patients with previous MI, other causes of reduced systolic function, LVH, or asymptomatic valvular disease. Both ACE inhibitors and beta-blockers prevent heart failure in the first two of these conditions, and more aggressive treatment of hypertension and early surgical intervention are effective in the latter two. **Stages C** and **D** include patients with clinical heart failure and the relatively small group of patients who have become refractory to the usual therapies, respectively.

Clinical Findings

A. Symptoms

The most common symptom of patients with **left heart failure** is shortness of breath, chiefly exertional dyspnea at first and then progressing to orthopnea, paroxysmal nocturnal dyspnea, and rest dyspnea. Chronic nonproductive cough, which is often worse in the recumbent position, may occur. Nocturia due to excretion of fluid retained during the day and increased renal perfusion in the recumbent position is a common nonspecific symptom of heart failure, as is fatigue and exercise intolerance. These symptoms correlate poorly with the degree of cardiac dysfunction. Patients with **right heart failure** have predominate signs of fluid retention, with the patient exhibiting edema, hepatic congestion and, on occasion, loss of appetite and nausea due to edema of the gut or impaired GI perfusion and ascites. Surprisingly, some individuals with severe LV dysfunction will display few signs of left heart failure and appear to have isolated right heart failure. Indeed, they may be clinically indistinguishable from patients with right heart failure secondary to pulmonary disease.

Patients with acute heart failure from MI, myocarditis, and acute valvular regurgitation due to endocarditis or other conditions usually present with pulmonary edema. Patients with episodic symptoms may be having LV dysfunction due to intermittent ischemia. Patients may also present with acute exacerbations of chronic, stable heart failure. Exacerbations may be caused by alterations in therapy (or patient noncompliance), excessive salt and fluid intake, arrhythmias, excessive activity, pulmonary emboli, intercurrent infection, or progression of the underlying disease.

Patients with heart failure are often categorized by the NYHA classification as **class I** (asymptomatic), **class II** (symptomatic with moderate activity), **class III** (symptomatic with mild activity), or **class IV** (symptomatic at rest). This classification is important since some of the treatments are indicated based on NYHA classification.

B. Signs

Many patients with heart failure, including some with severe symptoms, appear comfortable at rest. Others will be dyspneic during conversation or minor activity, and those with long-standing severe heart failure may appear cachectic or cyanotic. The vital signs may be normal, but tachycardia, hypotension, and reduced pulse pressure may be present. Patients often show signs of increased sympathetic nervous system activity, including cold extremities and diaphoresis. Important peripheral signs of heart failure can be detected by examination of the neck, the lungs, the abdomen, and the extremities. RA pressure may be estimated through the height of the pulsations in the jugular venous system. With the patient at 45 degrees, measure the height of the pulsation about the sternal angle, and add 5 cm to estimate the height above the left atrium, with a pressure greater than 8 cm being abnormal. In addition to the height of the venous pressure, abnormal pulsations, such as regurgitant *v* waves, should be sought. Examination of the carotid pulse may allow estimation of pulse pressure as well as detection of aortic stenosis. Thyroid examination may reveal occult hyperthyroidism or hypothyroidism, which are readily treatable causes of heart failure. Crackles at the lung bases reflect transudation of fluid into the alveoli. Pleural effusions may cause bibasilar dullness to percussion. Expiratory wheezing and rhonchi may be signs of heart failure. Patients with severe right heart failure may have hepatic enlargement—tender or nontender—due to passive congestion. Systolic pulsations may be felt in tricuspid regurgitation. Sustained moderate pressure on the liver may increase jugular venous pressure (a positive **hepatojugular reflux** is an increase of greater than 1 cm, which correlates with elevated PCWP). Ascites may also be present. Peripheral pitting edema is a common sign in patients with right heart failure and may extend into the thighs and abdominal wall.

Cardinal cardiac examination signs are a parasternal lift, indicating pulmonary hypertension; an enlarged and sustained LV impulse, indicating LV dilation and hypertrophy; a diminished first heart sound, suggesting impaired contractility; and an S_3 gallop originating in the LV and sometimes the RV. An S_4 is usually present in diastolic heart failure. Murmurs should be sought to exclude primary valvular disease; secondary mitral regurgitation and tricuspid regurgitation murmurs are common in patients with dilated ventricles. In chronic heart failure, many of the expected signs of heart failure may be absent despite markedly abnormal cardiac function and hemodynamic measurements.

C. Laboratory Findings

A blood count may reveal anemia and a high red-cell distribution width (RDW), both of which are associated with poor prognosis in chronic heart failure through poorly understood mechanisms. Kidney function tests can determine whether cardiac failure is associated with impaired kidney function that may reflect poor kidney perfusion. CKD is another poor prognostic factor in heart failure and may limit certain treatment options. Serum electrolytes may disclose hypokalemia, which increases the risk of arrhythmias; hyperkalemia, which may limit the use of inhibitors of the renin–angiotensin system; or hyponatremia, an indicator of marked activation of the renin–angiotensin system and a poor prognostic sign. Thyroid function should be assessed to detect occult thyrotoxicosis or myxedema, and iron studies should be checked to test for hemochromatosis. In unexplained cases, appropriate biopsies may lead to a diagnosis of amyloidosis. Myocardial biopsy may exclude specific causes of dilated cardiomyopathy but rarely reveals specific reversible diagnoses.

Serum BNP is a powerful prognostic marker that adds to clinical assessment in differentiating dyspnea due to heart failure from noncardiac causes. Two markers—**BNP** and **NT-proBNP**—provide similar diagnostic and prognostic information. BNP is expressed primarily in the ventricles and is elevated when ventricular filling pressures are high. It is quite sensitive in patients with symptomatic heart failure—whether due to systolic or to diastolic dysfunction—but less specific in older patients, women, and patients with COPD. Studies have shown that BNP can help in emergency department triage in the diagnosis of acute decompensated heart failure, such that an NT-proBNP less than 300 pg/mL or BNP less than 100 pg/mL, combined with a normal ECG, makes heart failure unlikely. BNP is less sensitive and specific to diagnose heart failure in the chronic setting. BNP may be helpful in guiding the intensity of diuretic and a more consistent use of disease-modifying therapies, such as ACE inhibitors and beta-blockers, for the management of chronic heart failure. BNP, but not NT-proBNP, is increased by neprilysin inhibitors, since neprilysin degrades BNP. Thus, while NT-proBNP is still reliable, BNP should *not* be used to monitor degree of heart failure when patients are treated with sacubitril/valsartan. Worsening breathlessness or weight associated with a rising BNP (or both) might prompt increasing the dose of diuretics. However, there is no proven value in using serial natriuretic peptide measurements to guide therapy, as shown in the GUIDE-IT trial. Elevation of serum troponin, and especially of high-sensitivity troponin, is common in both chronic and acute heart failure, and it is associated with higher risk of adverse outcomes.

D. ECG and Chest Radiography

ECG may indicate an underlying or secondary arrhythmia, MI, or nonspecific changes that often include low voltage, intraventricular conduction defects, LVH, and nonspecific repolarization changes. Chest radiographs provide information about the size and shape of the cardiac silhouette. Cardiomegaly is an important finding and is a poor prognostic sign. Evidence of pulmonary venous hypertension includes relative dilation of the upper lobe veins, perivascular edema (haziness of vessel outlines), interstitial edema, and alveolar fluid. In acute heart failure, these findings correlate moderately well with pulmonary venous pressure. However, patients with chronic heart failure may show relatively normal pulmonary vasculature despite markedly elevated pressures. Pleural effusions are common and tend to be bilateral or right-sided.

E. Additional Studies

The clinical diagnosis of systolic myocardial dysfunction is often inaccurate. The primary confounding conditions are diastolic dysfunction of the heart with decreased relaxation and filling of the LV (particularly in hypertension and in hypertrophic states) and pulmonary disease.

The most useful test is the echocardiogram because it can differentiate heart failure with and without preserved LV systolic function. The echocardiogram can define the size and function of both ventricles and of the atria. LVEF is the most commonly used measurement to define systolic function. RV function is assessed by contractility and other measures, such as tricuspid annular plane systolic excursion. Echocardiography will also allow detection of pericardial effusion, valvular abnormalities, intracardiac shunts, and segmental wall motion abnormalities suggestive of old MI as opposed to more generalized forms of dilated cardiomyopathy.

Radionuclide angiography as well as cardiac MRI also measure LVEF and permit analysis of regional wall motion. These tests are especially useful when echocardiography is technically suboptimal, such as in patients with severe pulmonary disease. MRI can assess for presence of scar tissue and of infiltrative disease. When myocardial ischemia is suspected as a cause of LV dysfunction, as it should be unless there is another clear cause, stress testing or coronary angiography should be performed.

F. Cardiac Catheterization

In most patients with heart failure, clinical examination and noninvasive tests can determine LV size and function and valve function to support and refine the diagnosis. Left heart catheterization may be helpful to define the presence and extent of CAD, although CT angiography may also be appropriate, especially when the likelihood of coronary disease is low. Evaluation for coronary disease is particularly important when LV dysfunction may be partially reversible by revascularization. The combination of angina or noninvasive evidence of significant myocardial ischemia with symptomatic heart failure is often an indication for coronary angiography if the patient is a potential candidate for revascularization. Right heart catheterization may be useful to select and monitor therapy in patients refractory to standard therapy.

Treatment: Heart Failure With Reduced LVEF

The treatment of heart failure is aimed at relieving symptoms, improving functional status, and preventing death and hospitalizations. Figure 10–10 outlines the role of the major pharmacologic and device therapies for heart failure with reduced LVEF (less than or equal to 40%). **The evidence of clinical benefit, including reducing death and hospitalization, as well as reducing sudden cardiac death, of most therapies is limited to patients with heart failure with reduced LVEF (40% or less).** The SGLT2 inhibitors, which reduce heart failure hospitalization for patients with preserved EF, are one *exception* to this general finding. It is now recognized that patients with mildly reduced EF (41–49%) may derive benefit from mineralocorticoid receptor antagonist and angiotensin receptor-neprilysin inhibitor (ARNI) (sacubitril/valsartan). Treatment of heart failure with preserved LVEF is aimed at improving symptoms and treating comorbidities. Achieving target (or maximally tolerated up to target) dosing to obtain the benefits of these treatments that have been shown in clinical trials is important (Table 10–12).

A. Correction of Reversible Causes

The major reversible causes of heart failure with reduced LVEF, also called **chronic systolic heart failure,** include valvular lesions, myocardial ischemia, uncontrolled hypertension, arrhythmias (especially persistent tachycardias), alcohol- or drug-induced myocardial depression, hypothyroidism, intracardiac shunts, and high-output states. Calcium channel blockers with negative inotropy (specifically verapamil or diltiazem), antiarrhythmic medications, thiazolidinediones, and NSAIDs may be important contributors to worsening heart failure. Some metabolic and infiltrative cardiomyopathies may be partially reversible, or their progression may be slowed; these include hemochromatosis, sarcoidosis, and amyloidosis. Once possible reversible components are being addressed, the measures outlined below are appropriate.

B. Pharmacologic Treatment

See also the following section Acute Heart Failure & Pulmonary Edema.

1. Diuretic therapy—Diuretics are the most effective means of providing symptomatic relief to patients with moderate to severe heart failure with dyspnea and fluid overload, for heart failure with either reduced or preserved LVEF. Few patients with symptoms or signs of fluid retention can be optimally managed without a diuretic. However, excessive diuresis can lead to electrolyte imbalance

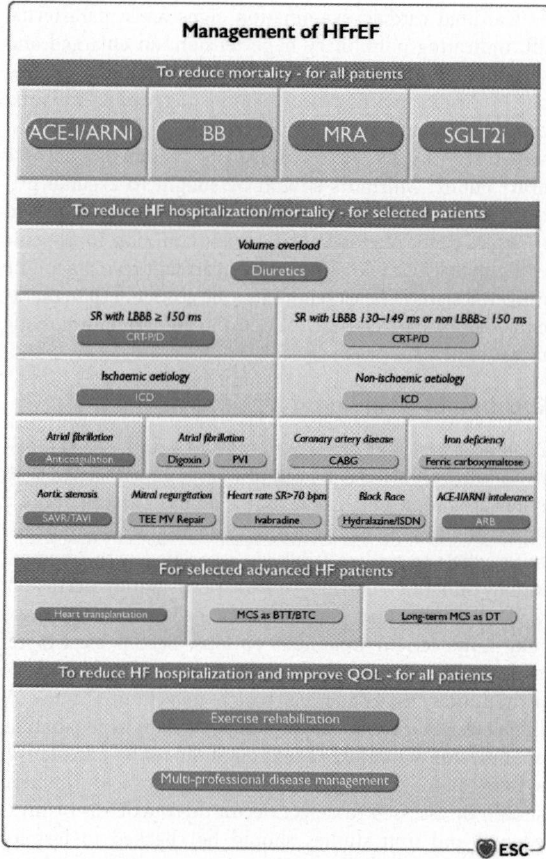

▲ **Figure 10–10.** Strategic phenotypic overview of the management of heart failure with reduced EF. ARNI, angiotensin receptor-neprilysin inhibitor; BB, beta-blocker; b.p.m., beats per minute; BTC, bridge to candidacy; BTT, bridge to transplantation; CABG, coronary artery bypass graft; CRT-D, cardiac resynchronization therapy with defibrillator; CRT-P, cardiac resynchronization therapy pacemaker; DT, destination therapy; HF, heart failure; HFrEF, heart failure with reduced EF; ICD, implantable cardioverter-defibrillator; ISDN, isosorbide dinitrate; LBBB, left bundle branch block; MCS, mechanical circulatory support; MRA, mineralocorticoid receptor antagonist; MV, mitral valve; PVI, pulmonary vein isolation; QOL, quality of life; SAVR, surgical aortic valve replacement; SGLT2i, sodium-glucose co-transporter 2 inhibitor; SR, sinus rhythm; TAVI, transcatheter aortic valve replacement; TEE, transcatheter edge to edge. Color code for classes of recommendation: green for class of recommendation I; yellow for class of recommendation IIa. The figure shows management options with class I and IIa recommendations. (McDonagh TA et al; 2021 ESC Guidelines for the diagnosis and treatment of acute and chronic heart failure. Eur Heart J. 2021;42(36):3599–3726, by permission of Oxford University Press.)

Table 10–12. Evidence-based doses of disease-modifying medications in key randomized trials in HFrEF or after MI (medications listed in alphabetical order within classes).

Medications	Starting Dose	Target Dose
ACE Inhibitors		
Captopril	6.25 mg three times daily	50 mg three times daily
Enalapril	2.5 mg twice daily	10–20 mg twice daily
Lisinopril	2.5–5.0 mg once daily	20–35 once daily
Ramipril	2.5 mg once daily	10 mg once daily
Trandolapril	0.5 mg once daily	4 mg once daily
Beta-Blockers		
Bisoprolol	1.25 mg once daily	10 mg once daily
Carvedilol	3.125 mg twice daily	25 mg twice daily
Metoprolol succinate (CR/XL)	12.5–25 mg once daily	200 mg once daily
Nebivolol	1.25 once daily	10 mg once daily
ARBs		
Candesartan	4–8 mg once daily	32 mg once daily
Losartan	50 mg once daily	150 mg once daily
Valsartan	40 mg twice daily	160 mg twice daily
Aldosterone Antagonist		
Eplerenone	25 mg once daily	50 mg once daily
Spironolactone	25 mg once daily	50 mg once daily
ARNI		
Sacubitril/valsartan	49/51 mg twice daily	97/103 mg twice daily
I_f Channel Blocker		
Ivabradine	5 mg twice daily	7.5 mg twice daily
SGLT2 Inhibitors		
Dapagliflozin	10 mg once daily	10 mg once daily
Empagliflozin	10 mg once daily	10 mg once daily

ARNI, angiotensin receptor-neprilysin inhibitor; HFrEF, heart failure with reduced EF.

and neurohormonal activation. **A combination of a diuretic and an ACE inhibitor or ARNI should be the initial treatment in most symptomatic patients with heart failure and reduced LVEF, with the early addition of a beta-blocker.**

When fluid retention is mild, **thiazide diuretics** or a similar type of agent (hydrochlorothiazide, 25–100 mg; metolazone, 2.5–5 mg; chlorthalidone, 25–50 mg; etc) may be sufficient. Thiazide or related diuretics often provide better control of hypertension than short-acting loop agents. The thiazides are generally *ineffective* when the GFR falls below 30–40 mL/minute/1.73 m^2, a not infrequent occurrence in patients with severe heart failure. Metolazone maintains its efficacy down to a GFR of approximately 20–30 mL/minute/1.73 m^2. Adverse reactions include hypokalemia and intravascular volume depletion with resulting prerenal azotemia, skin rashes, neutropenia and thrombocytopenia, hyperglycemia, hyperuricemia, and hepatic dysfunction.

Patients with more severe heart failure should be treated with one of the oral **loop diuretics.** These include furosemide (20–320 mg daily), bumetanide (1–8 mg daily), and torsemide (20–200 mg daily). These agents have a rapid onset and a relatively short duration of action. In patients with preserved kidney function, two or more daily doses are preferable to a single larger dose. In acute situations or when GI absorption is in doubt, they should be given intravenously. Torsemide may be effective when furosemide is not, related to better absorption and a longer half life. Larger doses (up to 500 mg of furosemide or equivalent) may be required with severe renal impairment. The major adverse reactions include intravascular volume depletion, prerenal azotemia, and hypotension. Hypokalemia, particularly with accompanying digitalis therapy, is a major problem. Less common side effects include skin rashes, GI distress, and ototoxicity (the latter more common with ethacrynic acid and possibly less common with bumetanide).

The **oral potassium-sparing agents** are often useful in combination with the loop diuretics and thiazides, with the first choice being the aldosterone inhibitors spironolactone (12.5–100 mg daily) or eplerenone (25–100 mg daily). Aldosterone is often increased in heart failure. These medications spare loss of potassium, they have some diuretic effect (especially at higher doses), and they also improve clinical outcomes, including survival. Their onsets of action are slower than the other potassium-sparing agents, and spironolactone's side effects include gynecomastia and hyperkalemia. Combinations of potassium supplements or ACE inhibitors and potassium-sparing medications can increase the risk of hyperkalemia but have been used with success in patients with persistent hypokalemia.

Patients with refractory edema may respond to combinations of a loop diuretic and thiazide-like agents. Metolazone, because of its maintained activity with CKD, is the most useful agent for such a combination. Extreme caution must be observed with this approach, since massive diuresis and electrolyte imbalances often occur; 2.5 mg of metolazone orally should be added to the previous dosage of loop diuretic. In many cases this is necessary only once or twice a week, but dosages up to 10 mg daily have been used in some patients.

2. Inhibitors of the renin–angiotensin–aldosterone system—Inhibition of the renin–angiotensin–aldosterone system with ACE inhibitors should be part of the initial therapy of this syndrome based on their mortality benefits.

A. ACE INHIBITORS—At least seven ACE inhibitors have been shown to be effective for the treatment of heart failure or the related indication of postinfarction LV dysfunction (see Table 11–6). ACE inhibitors reduce mortality by approximately 20% in patients with symptomatic heart failure and have also been shown to prevent hospitalizations, increase exercise tolerance, and reduce symptoms in these patients. As a result, ACE inhibitors generally should be part of first-line treatment of patients with symptomatic LV systolic dysfunction (EF less than 40%), usually in combination with a diuretic. They are also indicated for the management of patients with reduced EFs without symptoms because they prevent the progression to clinical heart failure.

Because ACE inhibitors may induce significant hypotension, particularly following the initial doses, they must be started with caution. Hypotension is most prominent in patients with already low BPs (systolic pressure less than 100 mm Hg), hypovolemia, prerenal azotemia (especially if it is diuretic induced), and hyponatremia (an indicator of activation of the renin–angiotensin system). These patients should generally be started at low dosages (captopril 6.25 mg orally three times daily, enalapril 2.5 mg orally daily, or the equivalent), but other patients may be started at twice these dosages. Within several days (for those with the markers of higher risk) or at most 2 weeks, patients should be questioned about symptoms of hypotension, and both kidney function and potassium levels should be monitored.

ACE inhibitors should be titrated to the dosages proved effective in clinical trials (captopril 50 mg three times daily, enalapril 10 mg twice daily, ramipril 10 mg daily, lisinopril 20 mg daily, or the equivalent) over a period of 1–3 months. Most patients will tolerate these doses. *Asymptomatic hypotension is not a contraindication to up-titrating or continuing ACE inhibitors.* Some patients exhibit increases in serum creatinine or potassium, but they do *not* require discontinuation if the levels stabilize—even at values as high as 3 mg/dL and 5.5 mEq/L, respectively. Kidney dysfunction is more frequent in patients with diabetes, older patients, and those with low systolic pressures, and these groups should be monitored more closely. The most common side effects of ACE inhibitors in heart failure patients are dizziness (often not related to the level of BP) and cough, though the latter is often due as much to heart failure or intercurrent pulmonary conditions as to the ACE inhibitor. ACE inhibitor–induced cough is more common in women than in men.

B. Angiotensin II receptor blockers—Another approach to inhibiting the renin–angiotensin–aldosterone system is the use of specific ARBs (see Table 11–6), which will decrease adverse effects of angiotensin II by blocking the AT_1 receptor. In addition, because there are alternative pathways of angiotensin II production in many tissues, the receptor blockers may provide more complete blockade of the AT_1 receptor.

However, these agents do *not* share the effects of ACE inhibitors on other potentially important pathways that produce increases in bradykinin, prostaglandins, and nitric oxide in the heart, blood vessels, and other tissues. ARBs, specifically candesartan or valsartan, provide important benefits as an alternative to ACE inhibitors in chronic heart failure with reduced LVEF. (A large trial of patients with chronic heart failure and preserved LVEF found no benefit from the ARB irbesartan.) **While they have the same level of recommendation in the guidelines, generally ACE inhibitors are preferred over ARBs for patients who tolerate them.**

C. Spironolactone and eplerenone—Inhibiting aldosterone has become a mainstay of management of symptomatic heart failure with reduced LVEF. The RALES trial compared spironolactone 25 mg daily with placebo in patients with advanced heart failure (current or recent class IV) already receiving ACE inhibitors and diuretics and showed a 29% reduction in mortality as well as similar decreases in other clinical end points. Based on the EMPHASIS-HF trial, the efficacy and safety of aldosterone antagonism—in the form of eplerenone, 25–50 mg orally daily—is established for patients with mild or moderate heart failure. Hyperkalemia was uncommon in severe heart failure clinical trial patients who received high doses of diuretic as maintenance therapy; however, hyperkalemia in patients taking spironolactone appears to be common in general practice. Potassium levels must be monitored closely during initiation of spironolactone (after 1 and 4 weeks of therapy) and periodically thereafter, particularly for patients with even mild degrees of kidney injury, and in patients receiving ACE inhibitors.

D. Combination sacubitril and valsartan—The most recently approved medication to improve clinical outcome in patients with heart failure and reduced LVEF is the combination of valsartan and sacubitril, called an **angiotensin receptor-neprilysin inhibitor (ARNI).** Compared to the ACE inhibitor enalapril, the ARNI was shown to reduce cardiovascular death and hospitalization for heart failure by 20% for patients with heart failure and reduced LVEF in a large randomized trial (PARADIGM-HF) of patients who had been taking an ACE inhibitor or ARB. Cardiovascular death itself was also reduced by 20%.

This evidence led to a class I recommendation by the ACC/AHA and the ESC guidelines for the use of **sacubitril/valsartan as a *replacement* for ACE inhibitors for patients with heart failure with reduced EF who remain symptomatic on an ACE inhibitor, beta-blocker, and mineralocorticoid inhibitor.** Patients with baseline systolic BP less than 100 mm Hg were not included in the PARADIGM trial, and symptomatic hypotension is more common with sacubitril/valsartan than ACE inhibitor. Sacubitril/valsartan can be safely started in the hospital for patients admitted with decompensated failure, once they are stable with systolic BP of at least 100 mm Hg and there has been a 36-hour washout period since the last dose of ACE inhibitor.

While there was some evidence of benefit, sacubitril/valsartan did not result in significant improvement in the primary outcome of total heart failure hospitalizations and cardiovascular death in the PARAGON-HF trial studying a population of patients with heart failure and preserved LVEF (45% or greater). However, the FDA has approved sacubitril/valsartan in this population, particularly for patients with EF "below normal," that is for EF less than 50% including patients with mildly reduced EF (41–49%).

3. Beta-blockers—Beta-blockers are part of the foundation of care of chronic heart failure based on their lifesaving benefits. The mechanism of this benefit remains unclear, but it is likely that chronic elevations of catecholamines and sympathetic nervous system activity cause progressive myocardial damage, leading to worsening LV function and dilation. The primary evidence for this hypothesis is that over a period of 3–6 months, beta-blockers produce consistent substantial rises in EF (averaging 10% absolute increase) and reductions in LV size and mass.

Three medications have strong evidence of reducing mortality: **carvedilol** (a nonselective beta-1- and beta-2-receptor blocker), the beta-1-selective **extended-release agent metoprolol succinate** (but not short-acting metoprolol tartrate), and **bisoprolol** (beta-1-selective agent).

There is currently a strong recommendation that **stable patients (defined as having no recent deterioration or evidence of volume overload) with mild, moderate, and even severe heart failure should be treated with a beta-blocker unless there is a noncardiac contraindication.** In the COPERNICUS trial, carvedilol was both well tolerated and highly effective in reducing both mortality and heart failure hospitalizations in a group of patients with severe (NYHA class III or IV) symptoms, but care was taken to ensure that they were free of fluid retention at the time of initiation. In this study, one death was prevented for every 13 patients treated for 1 year—as dramatic an effect as has been seen with a pharmacologic therapy in the history of cardiovascular medicine. One trial comparing carvedilol and (short-acting) metoprolol tartrate (COMET) found significant reductions in all-cause mortality and cardiovascular mortality with carvedilol. Thus, patients with chronic heart failure should be treated with extended-release metoprolol succinate, bisoprolol, or carvedilol but *not* short-acting metoprolol tartrate.

Because even apparently stable patients may deteriorate when beta-blockers are initiated, initiation must be done gradually and with great care. Carvedilol is initiated at a dosage of 3.125 mg orally twice daily and may be increased to 6.25, 12.5, and 25 mg twice daily at intervals of approximately 2 weeks. The protocols for sustained-release metoprolol use were started at 12.5 or 25 mg orally daily and doubled at intervals of 2 weeks to a target dose of 200 mg daily (using the Toprol XL sustained-release preparation). Bisoprolol was administered at a dosage of 1.25, 2.5, 3.75, 5, 7.5, and 10 mg orally daily, with increments at 1- to 4-week intervals. More gradual up-titration is often more convenient and may be better tolerated. The SENIORS trial of 2135 patients found that nebivolol was effective in elderly patients (70 years and older) with chronic heart failure, although the evidence of degree of benefit was not as strong as with the three proven beta-blockers carvedilol, metoprolol succinate, or bisoprolol.

Patients should be instructed to monitor their weight at home as an indicator of fluid retention and to report any increase or change in symptoms immediately. Before each dose increase, patients should be seen and examined to ensure that there has not been fluid retention or worsening of symptoms. If heart failure worsens, this can usually be managed by increasing diuretic doses and delaying further increases in beta-blocker doses, though downward adjustments or discontinuation is sometimes required. Carvedilol, because of its beta-blocking activity, may cause dizziness or hypotension. This can usually be managed by reducing the doses of other vasodilators and by slowing the pace of dose increases.

4. SGLT2 inhibitors—Two large clinical trials of patients with type 2 diabetes have shown that inhibitors of SGLT2 substantially reduce the risk of cardiovascular death and hospitalization for heart failure for patients with reduced LVEF, with or without diabetes. Dapagliflozin also reduced all-cause mortality. Dagliflozin and empagliflozin reduce cardiovascular death and heart failure hospitalization, and they have been approved for treating heart failure with reduced LVEF. SGLT2 inhibitors also reduced kidney disease progression, and patients with eGFR of 20 mL/minute/1.73 m^2 have been included in these trials.

5. Digitalis glycosides—The efficacy of digitalis glycosides in reducing the symptoms of heart failure has been established in at least four multicenter trials that have demonstrated that digoxin withdrawal is associated with worsening symptoms and signs of heart failure, more frequent hospitalizations for decompensation, and reduced exercise tolerance. Digoxin should be considered for patients who remain symptomatic when taking diuretics and ACE inhibitors as well as for patients with heart failure who are in atrial fibrillation and require rate control. However, there is uncertainty about the safety of digoxin in this population with atrial fibrillation, especially with higher digoxin concentrations.

Digoxin has a half-life of 24–36 hours and is eliminated almost entirely by the kidneys. The oral maintenance dose may range from 0.125 mg three times weekly to 0.5 mg daily. It is lower in patients with kidney dysfunction, in older patients, and in those with smaller lean body mass. Although an oral loading dose of 0.75–1.25 mg (depending primarily on lean body size) over 24–48 hours may be given if an early effect is desired, in most patients with chronic heart failure it is sufficient to begin with the expected maintenance dose (usually 0.125–0.25 mg daily). Amiodarone, quinidine, propafenone, and verapamil are among the medications that may increase digoxin levels up to 100%. It is prudent to measure a blood level after 7–14 days (and at least 6 hours after the last dose was administered). Optimum serum digoxin levels are 0.7–1.2 ng/mL. Digoxin may induce ventricular arrhythmias, especially when hypokalemia or myocardial ischemia is present. Digoxin toxicity is discussed in Chapter 38.

6. Nitrates and hydralazine—Although ACE inhibitors, which have vasodilating properties, improve prognosis, such a benefit is not established with the direct-acting vasodilators. The combination of hydralazine and isosorbide dinitrate has been shown to *improve outcomes in Black persons*, but the effect is less clear than the well-established benefits of ACE inhibitors. ARBs or ARNIs have largely supplanted the use of the hydralazine–isosorbide dinitrate combination in ACE-intolerant patients.

See section Acute Myocardial Infarction with ST-Segment Elevation earlier in this chapter for a discussion on the intravenous vasodilating medications and their dosages.

A. Nitrates—Intravenous vasodilators (sodium nitroprusside or nitroglycerin) are used primarily for acute or severely decompensated chronic heart failure, especially when accompanied by hypertension or myocardial ischemia. If neither of the latter is present, therapy is best initiated and adjusted based on hemodynamic measurements. The starting dosage for nitroglycerin is generally about 10 mcg/minute, which is titrated upward by 10–20 mcg/minute (to a maximum of 200 mcg/minute) until mean arterial pressure drops by 10%. Hypotension (BP less than 100 mm Hg systolic) should be avoided. For sodium nitroprusside, the starting dosage is 5–10 mcg/minute, with upward titration to a maximum dose of 400 mcg/minute.

Isosorbide dinitrate, 20–40 mg orally three times daily, and nitroglycerin ointment, 2%, 15–16 mg (1.4 inches; 1 inch = 15 mg) every 6–8 hours, appear to be equally effective, although the ointment is generally reserved for inpatient use only. The nitrates are moderately effective in relieving shortness of breath, especially in patients with mild to moderate symptoms, but less successful—probably because they have little effect on cardiac output—in advanced heart failure. Nitrate therapy is generally well tolerated, but headaches and hypotension may limit the dose of all agents. The development of tolerance to long-term nitrate therapy occurs. This is minimized by intermittent therapy, especially if a daily 8- to 12-hour nitrate-free interval is used, but probably develops to some extent in most patients receiving these agents. Transdermal nitroglycerin patches have no sustained effect in patients with heart failure and should *not* be used for this indication.

B. Hydralazine—Oral hydralazine is a potent arteriolar dilator; when used as a single agent, it has not been shown to improve symptoms or exercise tolerance during long-term treatment. The combination of nitrates and oral hydralazine produces greater hemodynamic effects as well as clinical benefits.

7. Ivabradine—Ivabradine inhibits the I_f channel in the sinus node and has the specific effect of slowing sinus rate. Ivabradine is approved by the FDA for use in stable patients with heart failure and heart rate of 70 beats/minute who are taking the maximally tolerated dose of beta-blockers or in patients in whom beta-blockers are contraindicated. It is approved by the European Medicines Agency for use in patients with a heart rate of 75 beats/minute or more. Both the US and the European guidelines give it a class IIa recommendation for patients in sinus rhythm with a heart rate of 70 beats/minute or more with an EF of 35% or less, and persisting symptoms despite treatment with an evidence-based dose of beta-blocker (or a maximum tolerated dose below that), ACE inhibitor (or ARB), and an aldosterone antagonist (or ARB). In a trial of patients with chronic angina, ivabradine did not reduce cardiovascular events, and there may have been more events with ivabradine (than placebo) in patients with symptomatic angina.

8. Vericiguat (a soluble guanylate cyclase stimulator)—In January 2021, the FDA approved vericiguat to reduce the risk of cardiovascular death and heart failure hospitalization following a hospitalization for heart failure in patients with chronic heart failure and LVEF less than 45%. The VICTORIA trial showed a modest but significant reduction in cardiovascular death and heart failure hospitalization with vericiguat, on top of other effective therapies, in this high-risk population.

9. Combination of medical therapies—Optimal management of chronic heart failure involves using combinations of proven life-saving therapies. In addition to ACE inhibitors and beta-blockers, patients who remain symptomatic should be considered for mineralocorticoid (aldosterone) receptor antagonists and for sacubitril/valsartan. This combination, titrated to full tolerated doses, with careful monitoring of kidney function and potassium, will provide the greatest pharmacologic benefit to the majority of patients with heart failure with reduced LVEF.

10. Treatments that may cause harm in heart failure with reduced LVEF—Several therapies should be *avoided,* when possible, in patients with systolic heart failure. These include thiazolidinediones (glitazones) that cause worsening heart failure, most calcium channel blockers (with the exception of amlodipine and felodipine), NSAIDs, and cyclooxygenase-2 inhibitors that cause sodium and water retention and renal impairment, and the combination of an ACE inhibitor, ARB, and aldosterone blocker that increases the risk of hyperkalemia.

11. Anticoagulation—Patients with LV failure and reduced EF are at somewhat increased risk for developing intracardiac thrombi and systemic arterial emboli. However, this risk appears to be primarily in patients who are in atrial fibrillation, who have had thromboemboli, or who have had a large recent anterior MI. In general, these patients should receive warfarin for 3 months following the MI. Other patients with heart failure have embolic rates of approximately two per 100 patient-years of follow-up, which approximates the rate of major bleeding, and routine anticoagulation is not warranted except in patients with prior embolic events or mobile LV thrombi. A clinical trial of low-dose rivaroxaban failed to show substantial benefit in patients with heart failure with reduced LVEF.

12. Antiarrhythmic therapy—Patients with moderate to severe heart failure have a high incidence of both symptomatic and asymptomatic arrhythmias. Although less than 10% of patients have syncope or presyncope resulting from ventricular tachycardia, ambulatory monitoring reveals that up to 70% of patients have asymptomatic episodes of nonsustained ventricular tachycardia. These arrhythmias indicate a poor prognosis independent of the severity of LV dysfunction, but many of the deaths are probably not arrhythmia related. Beta-blockers, because of their marked favorable effect on prognosis in general and on the incidence of sudden death specifically, should be initiated in these as well as all other patients with heart failure (see Beta-Blockers). Other evidence-based therapies for heart failure, including ACE inhibitors, ARBs, mineralocorticoid receptor antagonists, and ARNIs, have all been shown to reduce sudden cardiac death. Empiric antiarrhythmic therapy with amiodarone did not improve outcome in the SCD-HeFT trial, and most other agents are contraindicated because of their proarrhythmic effects in this population and their adverse effect on cardiac function. For patients with systolic heart failure and atrial fibrillation, a rhythm control strategy has not been shown to improve outcome compared to a rate control strategy and thus should be reserved for patients with a reversible cause of atrial fibrillation or refractory symptoms. Then, amiodarone is the medication of choice.

13. Statin therapy—Even though vascular disease is present in many patients with chronic heart failure, the role of statins has not been well defined in the heart failure population. The CORONA and the GISSI-HF trials show no benefits of statins in the chronic heart failure population.

C. Nonpharmacologic Treatment

1. Implantable cardioverter defibrillators (ICDs)—Indications for ICDs include not only patients with symptomatic or asymptomatic arrhythmias but also patients with chronic heart failure and LV systolic dysfunction who are receiving contemporary heart failure treatments, including beta-blockers. In the second Multicenter Automatic Defibrillator Implantation Trial (MADIT II), 1232 patients with prior MI and an EF less than 30%, were randomized to an ICD or a control group. Mortality was 31% lower in the ICD group, which translated into 9 lives saved for each 100 patients who received a device and were monitored for 3 years. The Centers for Medicare and Medicaid Services provides reimbursement coverage to include patients with chronic heart failure and ischemic or nonischemic cardiomyopathy with an EF of 35% or less.

2. Biventricular pacing (resynchronization)—Many patients with heart failure due to systolic dysfunction have abnormal intraventricular conduction that results in dyssynchronous and hence inefficient contractions. Several studies have evaluated the efficacy of "multisite" pacing, using leads that stimulate the RV from the apex and the LV from the lateral wall via the coronary sinus. Patients with wide QRS complexes (generally 120 msec or more), reduced EFs, and moderate to severe symptoms have been evaluated. Results from trials with up to 2 years of follow-up have shown an increase in EF, improvement in symptoms and exercise tolerance, and reduction in death and hospitalization. The best responders to cardiac resynchronization therapy are patients with wider QRS, left bundle branch block, and nonischemic cardiomyopathy, and the lowest responders are those with narrow QRS and non–left bundle branch block pattern. Thus, as recommended in the 2013 European guidelines, resynchronization therapy is indicated for patients with class II, III, and ambulatory class IV heart failure, EF of 35% or less, and left bundle branch block pattern with QRS duration of 120 msec or more. Patients with non–left bundle branch block pattern and prolonged QRS duration may be considered for treatment.

3. Case management, diet, and exercise training—Thirty to 50 percent of heart failure patients who are hospitalized will be readmitted within 3–6 months. Strategies to prevent clinical deterioration, such as case management, home monitoring of weight and clinical status, and patient adjustment of diuretics, can prevent rehospitalizations and should be part of the treatment regimen of advanced heart failure. Involvement of a multidisciplinary team (rather than a single physician) and in-person (rather than just telephonic) communication appear to be important features of successful programs.

Patients should routinely practice moderate salt restriction (2–2.5 g sodium or 5–6 g salt per day). More severe sodium restriction is usually difficult to achieve and unnecessary because of the availability of potent diuretic agents.

Exercise training improves activity tolerance in significant part by reversing the peripheral abnormalities associated with heart failure and deconditioning. In severe heart failure, restriction of activity may facilitate temporary recompensation. A large trial showed no significant benefit (nor harm) from a structured exercise training program on death or hospitalization, although functional status and symptoms were improved. Thus, *in stable patients, a prudent increase in activity or a regular exercise regimen can be encouraged.* Indeed, a gradual exercise program is associated with diminished symptoms and substantial increases in exercise capacity.

4. Coronary revascularization—Since underlying CAD is the cause of heart failure in the majority of patients, coronary revascularization has been thought to be able to both improve symptoms and prevent progression. While the STITCH trial failed to show an overall survival benefit from CABG among patients with multivessel coronary disease who were candidates for CABG, but who also had heart failure and an LVEF of 35% or less, at 5 years, there was benefit at 10 years of follow-up. Thus, revascularization does appear warranted for some patients with heart failure, including those with more severe angina or left main coronary disease (excluded from the STITCH trial).

5. Cardiac transplantation—Because of the poor prognosis of patients with advanced heart failure, cardiac transplantation is widely used. Many centers have 1-year survival rates exceeding 80–90%, and 5-year survival rates above 70%. Infections, hypertension and kidney dysfunction caused by cyclosporine, rapidly progressive coronary atherosclerosis, and immunosuppressant-related cancers have been the major complications. The high cost and limited number of donor organs require careful patient selection early in the course.

6. Other surgical treatment options—Externally powered and implantable **ventricular assist devices** can be used in patients who require ventricular support either to allow the heart to recover or as a bridge to transplantation. The latest generation devices are small enough to allow patients unrestricted mobility and even discharge from the hospital. *Continuous flow* devices appear to be more effective than *pulsatile flow* devices. However, complications are frequent, including bleeding, thromboembolism, and infection, and the cost is very high, exceeding $200,000 in the initial 1–3 months.

Although 1-year survival was improved in the REMATCH randomized trial, all 129 patients died by 26 months. Newer-generation continuous flow pump ventricular assist devices have been shown to result in better survival than the first-generation pulsatile flow device used in REMATCH.

7. Palliative care—Despite the technologic advances of recent years, it should be remembered that many patients with chronic heart failure are elderly and have multiple comorbidities. Many of them will not experience meaningful improvements in survival with aggressive therapy. The goal of management for these patients and all those with serious illness should include symptomatic improvement and palliative care as they approach the end of life (see Chapter 5).

Treatment: Heart Failure With Preserved LVEF

Although half of all heart failure occurs among patients with normal LVEF, often with diastolic dysfunction, **the only therapy shown to reduce cardiovascular death or heart failure hospitalization in this population is empagliflozin.** The mainstays of treating heart failure with preserved EF are SGLT2 inhibitors and fluid management to avoid overload with diuretic therapy and to treat comorbidities like hypertension, diabetes, and arrhythmias.

A. Correction of Reversible Causes

Hypertension, pericardial disease, and atrial tachycardias are potentially reversible factors that can contribute to heart failure with preserved LVEF. Since tachycardia is associated with shorter overall diastolic filling time, controlling accelerated heart rate may be important. With effective treatment available for familial and wild-type transthyretin amyloid cardiomyopathy, this diagnosis should be considered for patients with unexplained heart failure with preserved EF.

B. Pharmacologic Treatment

1. Diuretic therapy—Diuretics are important to control symptoms of fluid overload in patients with heart failure with preserved LVEF, similar to symptoms from systolic heart failure.

2. Inhibitors of the renin-angiotensin-aldosterone system—ACE inhibitors and ARBs have *not* been shown to improve outcome in patients with heart failure and preserved LVEF, despite being good therapies for the comorbidity of hypertension. Sacubitril/valsartan does *not* substantially improve outcome in patients with heart failure and preserved LVEF. Spironolactone has *not* been shown to improve outcome in a large trial of patients with heart failure and preserved LVEF, but there may have been some benefit in patients enrolled in the Americas who had more clearly defined heart failure. Spironolactone should remain a therapeutic option, especially for patients who also have hypertension.

C. Nonpharmacologic Treatment

Unlike in patients with heart failure and reduced LVEF, ICD and resynchronization device treatments do *not* have a role in patients with preserved LVEF. Revascularization for patients with heart failure and preserved LVEF should be guided by the same considerations as for patients with heart failure with reduced LVEF.

Prognosis

Once manifest, heart failure with reduced LVEF carries a poor prognosis. Even with appropriate treatment, the 5-year mortality is approximately 50%. Mortality rates vary from less than 5% per year in those with no or few symptoms to greater than 30% per year in those with severe and refractory symptoms. These figures emphasize the critical importance of early detection and intervention. Higher mortality is related to older age, lower LVEF, more severe symptoms, CKD, and diabetes. The prognosis of heart failure has improved in the past two decades, probably at least in part because of the more widespread use of ACE inhibitors and beta-blockers, which markedly improve survival in those with heart failure with reduced LVEF.

When to Refer

Patients with new symptoms of heart failure not explained by an obvious cause should be referred to a cardiologist. Patients with continued symptoms of heart failure and reduced LVEF (35% or less) should be referred to a cardiologist for consideration of placement of an ICD or cardiac resynchronization therapy (if QRS duration is 120 msec or more, especially with left bundle branch block pattern).

When to Admit

- Patients with unexplained new or worsened symptoms or positive cardiac biomarkers concerning for acute myocardial necrosis.
- Patients with hypoxia, gross fluid overload, or pulmonary edema not readily resolved in an outpatient setting.

Al-Khatib SM et al. 2017 AHA/ACC/HRS guideline for management of patients with ventricular arrhythmias and the prevention of sudden cardiac death: executive summary: a report of the American College of Cardiology/American Heart Association Task Force on Clinical Practice Guidelines and the Heart Rhythm Society. Circulation. 2018;138:e210. [PMID: 29084733]

Armstrong PW et al; VICTORIA Study Group. Vericiguat in patients with heart failure and reduced ejection fraction. N Engl J Med. 2020;382:1883. [PMID: 32222134]

Bozkurt B et al. Universal definition and classification of heart failure: a report of the Heart Failure Society of America, Heart Failure Association of the European Society of Cardiology, Japanese Heart Failure Society and Writing Committee of the Universal Definition of Heart Failure. J Card Fail. 2021 Mar 1. [Epub ahead of print] [PMID: 33663906]

McDonagh TA et al. 2021 ESC guidelines for the diagnosis and treatment of acute and chronic heart failure: developed by the Task Force for the diagnosis and treatment of acute and chronic heart failure of the European Society of Cardiology (ESC) with the special contribution of the Heart Failure Association (HFA) of the ESC. Eur J Heart Fail. 2022;24:4. [PMID: 35083827]

McMurray JJV et al; DAPA-HF Trial Committees and Investigators. Dapagliflozin in patients with heart failure and reduced ejection fraction. N Engl J Med. 2019;381:1995. [PMID: 31535829]

Solomon SD et al; PARAGON-HF Investigators and Committees. Angiotensin-neprilysin inhibition in heart failure with preserved ejection fraction. N Engl J Med. 2019;381:1609. [PMID: 31475794]

Velazquez EJ et al; PIONEER-HF Investigators. Angiotensin-neprilysin inhibition in acute decompensated heart failure. N Engl J Med. 2019;380:539. [PMID: 30415601]

ACUTE HEART FAILURE & PULMONARY EDEMA

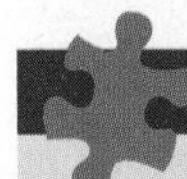

ESSENTIALS OF DIAGNOSIS

- Acute onset or worsening of dyspnea at rest.
- Tachycardia, diaphoresis, cyanosis.
- Pulmonary rales, rhonchi; expiratory wheezing.
- Radiograph shows interstitial and alveolar edema with or without cardiomegaly.
- Arterial hypoxemia.

General Considerations

Typical causes of acute cardiogenic pulmonary edema include acute MI or severe ischemia, exacerbation of chronic heart failure, acute severe hypertension, AKI, acute volume overload of the LV (valvular regurgitation), and mitral stenosis. By far the most common presentation in developed countries is one of acute or subacute deterioration of chronic heart failure, precipitated by discontinuation of medications, excessive salt intake, myocardial ischemia, tachyarrhythmias (especially rapid atrial fibrillation), or intercurrent infection. Often in the latter group, there is preceding volume overload with worsening edema and progressive shortness of breath for which earlier intervention can usually avoid the need for hospital admission.

Clinical Findings

Acute pulmonary edema presents with a characteristic clinical picture of severe dyspnea, the production of pink, frothy sputum, and diaphoresis and cyanosis. Rales are present in all lung fields, as are generalized wheezing and rhonchi. Pulmonary edema may appear acutely or subacutely in the setting of chronic heart failure or may be the first manifestation of cardiac disease, usually acute MI, which may be painful or silent. Less severe decompensations usually present with dyspnea at rest, rales, and other evidence of fluid retention but without severe hypoxia.

Noncardiac causes of pulmonary edema include intravenous opioids, increased intracerebral pressure, high altitude, sepsis, medications, inhaled toxins, transfusion reactions, shock, and disseminated intravascular coagulation. These are distinguished from cardiogenic pulmonary edema by the clinical setting, history, and physical examination. Conversely, in most patients with cardiogenic pulmonary edema, an underlying cardiac abnormality can usually be detected clinically or by ECG, chest radiograph, or echocardiogram.

The chest radiograph reveals signs of pulmonary vascular redistribution, blurriness of vascular outlines, increased interstitial markings, and, characteristically, the butterfly pattern of distribution of alveolar edema. The heart may be enlarged or normal in size depending on whether heart failure was previously present. Assessment of cardiac function by echocardiography is important, since a substantial proportion of patients has normal EFs with elevated atrial pressures due to diastolic dysfunction. In cardiogenic pulmonary edema, BNP is elevated, and the PCWP is invariably elevated, usually over 25 mm Hg. In noncardiogenic pulmonary edema, the wedge pressure may be normal or even low.

Treatment

In full-blown pulmonary edema, the patient should be placed in a sitting position with legs dangling over the side of the bed; this facilitates respiration and reduces venous return. **Oxygen** is delivered by mask to obtain an arterial Po_2 greater than 60 mm Hg. Noninvasive pressure support ventilation may improve oxygenation and prevent severe CO_2 retention while pharmacologic interventions take effect. However, if respiratory distress remains severe, endotracheal intubation and mechanical ventilation may be necessary.

Morphine is highly effective in pulmonary edema and may be helpful in less severe decompensations when the patient is uncomfortable. The initial dosage is 2–8 mg intravenously (subcutaneous administration is effective in milder cases) and may be repeated after 2–4 hours. Morphine increases venous capacitance, lowering LA pressure, and relieves anxiety, which can reduce the efficiency of ventilation. However, morphine may lead to CO_2 retention by reducing the ventilatory drive. It should be avoided in patients with opioid-induced pulmonary edema, who may improve with opioid antagonists, and in those with neurogenic pulmonary edema.

Intravenous diuretic therapy (furosemide, 40 mg, or bumetanide, 1 mg—or higher doses if the patient has been receiving long-term diuretic therapy) is usually indicated even if the patient has not exhibited prior fluid retention. These agents produce venodilation prior to the onset of diuresis. The DOSE trial has shown that, for acute decompensated heart failure, bolus doses of furosemide are of similar efficacy as continuous intravenous infusion, and that higher-dose furosemide (2.5 times the prior daily dose) resulted in more rapid fluid removal without a substantially higher risk of kidney impairment.

Nitrate therapy accelerates clinical improvement by reducing both BP and LV filling pressures. Sublingual nitroglycerin or isosorbide dinitrate, topical nitroglycerin, or intravenous nitrates will ameliorate dyspnea rapidly prior to the onset of diuresis, and these agents are particularly valuable in patients with accompanying hypertension.

Intravenous nesiritide, a recombinant form of human BNP, is a potent vasodilator that reduces ventricular filling pressures and improves cardiac output. Its hemodynamic effects resemble those of intravenous nitroglycerin with a more predictable dose–response curve and a longer duration of action. In clinical studies, nesiritide (administered as 2 mcg/kg by intravenous bolus injection followed by an infusion of 0.01 mcg/kg/minute, which may be up-titrated if needed) produced a rapid improvement in both dyspnea and hemodynamics. The primary adverse effect is hypotension, which may be symptomatic and sustained. Because most patients with acute heart failure respond well to conventional therapy, the role of nesiritide may be primarily in patients who continue to be symptomatic after initial treatment with diuretics and nitrates.

A randomized placebo-controlled trial of 950 patients evaluating intravenous milrinone in patients admitted for decompensated heart failure who had no definite indications for inotropic therapy showed no benefit in increasing survival, decreasing length of admission, or preventing readmission. In addition, rates of sustained hypotension and atrial fibrillation were significantly increased. Thus, the role of positive inotropic agents appears to be limited to patients with refractory symptoms and signs of low cardiac output, particularly if life-threatening vital organ hypoperfusion (such as deteriorating kidney function) is present. In some cases, dobutamine or milrinone may help maintain patients who are awaiting cardiac transplantation.

Bronchospasm may occur in response to pulmonary edema and may itself exacerbate hypoxemia and dyspnea. Treatment with inhaled beta-adrenergic agonists or intravenous aminophylline may be helpful, but both may also provoke tachycardia and supraventricular arrhythmias.

In most cases, pulmonary edema responds rapidly to therapy. When the patient has improved, the cause or precipitating factor should be ascertained. In patients without prior heart failure, evaluation should include echocardiography and, in many cases, cardiac catheterization and coronary angiography. Patients with acute decompensation of chronic heart failure should be treated to achieve a euvolemic state and have their medical regimen optimized. Generally, an oral diuretic and an ACE inhibitor should be initiated, with efficacy and tolerability confirmed prior to discharge. In selected patients, early but careful initiation of beta-blockers in low doses should be considered.

MYOCARDITIS & THE CARDIOMYOPATHIES

INFECTIOUS MYOCARDITIS

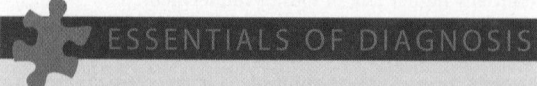

- Often follows an upper respiratory infection.
- May present with chest pain (pleuritic or nonspecific) or signs of heart failure.
- Echocardiogram documents cardiomegaly and contractile dysfunction. Initial heart size is generally normal with thickened walls.
- Myocardial biopsy, though not sensitive, may reveal a characteristic inflammatory pattern. MRI has a role in diagnosis.
- COVID-19 myocarditis impacts between 3% and 58% of people with COVID-19 based on underlying myocardial risk and imaging.

General Considerations

Cardiac dysfunction due to primary myocarditis is presumably caused by either an acute viral infection or a post viral immune response. Secondary myocarditis is the result of inflammation caused by nonviral pathogens, medications, chemicals, physical agents, or inflammatory diseases (such as SLE). The list of both infectious and noninfectious causes of myocarditis is extensive (Table 10–13).

Myopericarditis due to the coronavirus has been of particular concern during the COVID-19 pandemic. Much remains unknown. There is speculation that the SARS-CoV-2 spike protein may be able to bind to the ACE-2 membrane receptor on cardiomyocytes creating direct cellular injury and T-lymphocyte–mediated cytotoxicity augmented by a cytokine storm. This process activates more T cells and furthers a cycle of T-cell activation and further release of cytokines.

The currently accepted definition of myocarditis is biopsy dependent and includes the observation of 14 or more lymphocytes/mcL including up to 4 monocytes/mcL with the presence of 7 or more CD3-positive T lymphocytes/mcL. Injury can be **fulminant, subclinical,** or **chronic.** Both cellular and humoral inflammatory processes contribute to the progression to chronic injury, and there are subgroups that appear to benefit from immunosuppression.

Genetic predisposition is a likely factor in at least a few cases. Autoimmune myocarditis (eg, giant cell myocarditis) may occur with no identifiable viral infection. The heterogeneity of the clinical syndromes and the incomplete understanding of the immunopathology hinder a more complete understanding of the mechanisms involved.

Myocarditis following SARS-CoV-2 infection or vaccination have been reported in the medical literature. In both scenarios, younger male patients seem to be at highest risk for this overall rare event. With vaccination, the CDC reports rates of 13.3 myocarditis cases per 100,000 recipients of the Moderna vaccine and 2.7 cases per 100,000 recipients of the Pfizer-BioNTech vaccine; with natural COVID-19 infection, a rate of 150 cases of myocarditis per 100,000 people has been described. This variation in the myocarditis rates between the two vaccines is not understood and is the focus on ongoing research. With COVID-19, myocarditis appears to affect ethnic groups disproportionately with death rates highest among Black persons likely due to both an increase in comorbidities and health care disparities. In a German study of 100 patients who had recovered from COVID-19, cardiac MRI revealed some degree of abnormality in 78 patients, with inflammation noted in 60, independent of severity of the illness.

Table 10–13. Causes of myocarditis.

1. INFECTIOUS CAUSES
RNA viruses: Picornaviruses (coxsackie A and B, echovirus, poliovirus, hepatitis virus), orthomyxovirus (influenza), paramyxoviruses (respiratory syncytial virus, mumps), togaviruses (rubella), flaviviruses (dengue fever, yellow fever), SARS-CoV-2
DNA viruses: Adenovirus (A1, 2, 3, and 5), erythrovirus (Bi9V and 2), herpesviruses (human herpes virus 6 A and B, cytomegalovirus, Epstein-Barr virus, varicella-zoster), retrovirus (HIV)
Bacteria: Chlamydia (*Chlamydophila pneumoniae, C psittaci*), *Haemophilus influenzae, Legionella, Pneumophilia, Brucella, Clostridium, Francisella tularensis, Neisseria meningitis, Mycobacterium* (tuberculosis), *Salmonella, Staphylococcus, streptococcus* A, *Streptococcus pneumoniae,* tularemia, tetanus, syphilis, *Vibrio cholerae*
Spirocheta: *Borrelia recurrentis*, leptospira, *Treponema pallidum*
Rickettsia: *Coxiella burnetii, R rickettsii, R prowazekii*
Fungi: *Actinomyces, Aspergillus, Candida, Cryptococcus, Histoplasma, Nocardia*
Protozoa: *Entamoeba histolytica, Plasmodium falciparum, Trypanosoma cruzi, T burcei, T gondii, Leishmania*
Helminthic: *Ascaris, Echinococcus granulosus, Schistosoma, Trichenella spiralis, Wuchereria bancrofti*
2. NONINFECTIOUS CAUSES
Autoimmune diseases: Dermatomyositis, inflammatory bowel disease, rheumatoid arthritis, Sjögren syndrome, SLE, granulomatosis with polyangiitis, giant cell myocarditis
Medications: Aminophylline, amphetamine, anthracyclin, catecholamines, chloramphenicol, cocaine, cyclophosphamide, doxorubicin, 5-FU, mesylate, methysergide, phenytoin, trastuzumab, zidovudine
Hypersensitivity reactions due to medications: Azithromycin, benzodiazepines, clozapine, cephalosporins, dapsone, dobutamine, lithium, diuretics, thiazide, methyldopa, mexiletine, streptomycin, sulfonamides, NSAIDs, tetanus toxoid, tetracycline, tricyclic antidepressants
Hypersensitivity reactions due to venoms: Bee, wasp, black widow spider, scorpion, snake
Systemic diseases: Eosinophilic granulomatosis with polyangiitis (formerly known as Churg-Strauss syndrome), collagen diseases, sarcoidosis, Kawasaki disease, systemic sclerosis
Other: Heat stroke, hypothermia, transplant rejection, radiation injury

Schultheiss HP et al. The manage of myocarditis. Eur Heart J. 2011;32(21):2616–25, by permission of Oxford University Press and the European Society of Cardiology.

Clinical Findings

A. Symptoms and Signs

Patients may present several days to a few weeks after the onset of an acute febrile illness or a respiratory infection or they may present with heart failure without antecedent symptoms. The onset of heart failure may be gradual or may be abrupt and fulminant. In acute fulminant myocarditis, low output and shock may be present with severely depressed LV systolic function. The LV chamber size is typically not very enlarged. A pericardial friction rub may be present. In the European Study of Epidemiology and Treatment of Inflammatory Heart Disease, 72% of participants had dyspnea, 32% had chest pain, and 18% had arrhythmias. Pulmonary and systemic emboli may occur. Pleural-pericardial chest pain is common. Examination reveals tachycardia, a gallop rhythm, and other evidence of heart failure or conduction defects. At times, the presentation may mimic an acute MI with ST changes, positive cardiac markers, and regional wall motion abnormalities despite normal coronaries. Microaneurysms may also occur and may be associated with serious ventricular arrhythmias. It has been estimated that approximately 10% of all dilated cardiomyopathy patients have viral myocarditis as the cause.

B. ECG and Chest Radiography

ECG may show sinus tachycardia, other arrhythmias, nonspecific repolarization changes, and intraventricular conduction abnormalities. The presence of Q waves or left bundle branch block portends a higher rate of death or cardiac transplantation. Ventricular ectopy may be the initial and only clinical finding. The chest radiograph is nonspecific, but cardiomegaly is frequent, though not universal. Evidence for pulmonary venous hypertension is common and frank pulmonary edema may be present.

C. Diagnostic Studies

There is no specific laboratory finding that is consistently present, though the WBC count is usually elevated and the ESR and CRP usually are increased. Troponin I or T levels are elevated in about one-third of patients, but CK-MB is elevated in only 10%. Other biomarkers, such as BNP and NT-proBNP, are usually elevated. Echocardiography provides the most convenient way of evaluating cardiac function and can exclude many other processes. MRI with gadolinium enhancement reveals spotty areas of injury throughout the myocardium, but both T2- and T1-weighted images are needed to achieve optimal results; correlation with endomyocardial biopsy results is poor.

D. Endomyocardial Biopsy

Confirmation of myocarditis still requires histologic evidence. The AHA/ACC/ESC class I recommendations for biopsy are (1) in patients with heart failure, a normal-sized or dilated LV less than 2 weeks after onset of symptoms, and hemodynamic compromise; or (2) in patients with a dilated LV 2 weeks to 3 months after onset of symptoms, new ventricular arrhythmias or AV nodal block (Mobitz II or complete heart block) or who do not respond to usual care after 1–2 weeks. In some cases, the identification of inflammation without viral genomes by PCR suggests that immunosuppression might be useful. Because the cardiac involvement is often patchy, the diagnosis even with biopsy can be missed in up to one-half of cases.

Treatment & Prognosis

Patients with fulminant myocarditis may present with acute cardiogenic shock. Acute myocarditis has been implicated as a cause of sudden death in 5–22% of such cases in athletes younger than 35 years. The ventricles are usually not dilated but thickened (possibly due to myxedema). There is a high death rate. Traditionally, there has been a paradox noted, wherein patients with fulminant myocarditis were thought to more likely fully recover after the event. Several recent observations have challenged this concept. Patients with subacute disease have a dilated cardiomyopathy and generally make an incomplete recovery. Those who present with chronic disease tend to have only mild dilation of the LV and eventually present with a more restrictive cardiomyopathy. Treatment is directed toward the clinical scenario with ACE inhibitors and beta-blockers if LVEF is less than 40%. NSAIDs should be used if myopericarditis-related chest pain occurs. Colchicine has been suggested if pericarditis predominates. Arrhythmias should be suppressed.

For COVID-19–related myocarditis, treatment is generally supportive. A 2020 review noted that of the attempted therapies, such as remdesivir, glucocorticoids, IL-6 inhibitors (tocilizumab), intravenous immunoglobulin (IVIG), and colchicine, only corticosteroids appeared to have any favorable effect on outcomes. The data are still incomplete, however, as of early 2022.

Specific antimicrobial therapy is indicated when an infecting agent is identified. Exercise should be limited during the recovery phase. Some experts believe digoxin should be avoided, and it likely has little value in this setting anyway. Controlled trials of immunosuppressive therapy with corticosteroids and IVIG have not suggested a benefit, though some recommend IVIG given at 2 g/kg over 24 hours in proven cases. Uncontrolled trials suggest that interferon might have a supportive role. Similarly, antiviral medication (such as pleconaril for enteroviruses) has been tried empirically. Studies are lacking as to when to discontinue the chosen therapy if the patient improves. Patients with fulminant myocarditis require aggressive short-term support, including an IABP or an LV assist device. If severe pulmonary infiltrates accompany the fulminant myocarditis, extracorporeal membrane oxygenation (ECMO) support may be temporarily required and has had notable success.

The question of what to do with the athlete in whom evidence of COVID-19 myocarditis has developed has led to a series of national discussions, some prompted by the cardiac MRI findings in young adults with minimal symptoms. The higher troponin levels associated with poorer outcomes have generally occurred only in hospitalized patients. The findings of an abnormal cardiac MRI have not consistently proven to result in any long-term cardiac injury. Table 10–14 outlines the suggested guidelines by a Task Force from the American College of Cardiology Sports and Exercise Section.

When to Refer

Patients in whom myocarditis is suspected should be seen by a cardiologist at a tertiary care center where facilities are available for diagnosis and therapies available should a fulminant course ensue. The facility should have ventricular support devices and transplantation options available.

Table 10–14. American College of Cardiology Sports and Exercise Section Guidelines for athletes with COVID-19 myocarditis.

Myocarditis diagnosis if both of the following are present
- A clinical syndrome of < 3 months, duration
- Otherwise unexplained increase in serum troponin levels, ECG changes, arrhythmias, high-grade AV block, regional wall motion abnormalities, or pericardial effusion. MRI findings suggesting myocarditis including T1- or T2-weighted imaging or late gadolinium enhancement.

Sports eligibility after myocarditis
- Must obtain a resting echocardiogram, 24-hour ambulatory ECG monitoring, and an exercise ECG no earlier than 3–6 months after the illness (class I, LOE C)
- Can resume exercise training if ALL of the following are met (class IIa, LOE C)
  - Normal ventricular function
  - Serum markers of myocardial injury, heart failure, and inflammation have returned to normal
  - Clinically relevant arrhythmias on ambulatory ECG monitoring or exercise ECG are absent.

AV, atrioventricular, LOE, level of evidence.

Boehmer TK et al. Association between COVID-19 and myocarditis using hospital-based administrative data—United States, March 2020–January 2021. MMWR Morb Mortal Wkly Rep. 2021;70:1228. [PMID: 34473684]

Kim JH et al. Coronavirus disease 2019 and the athletic heart: emerging perspectives on pathology, risks, and return to play. JAMA Cardiol. 2021;6:219. [PMID: 33104154]

Moslehi JJ et al. Fulminant myocarditis: evolving diagnosis, evolving biology, evolving prognosis. J Am Coll Cardiol. 2019; 74:312. [PMID: 31319913]

Puntmann VO et al. Outcomes of cardiovascular magnetic resonance imaging in patients recently recovered from coronavirus disease 2019 (COVID-19). JAMA Cardiol. 2020;5:1265. [PMID: 32730619]

Sawalha K et al. Systematic review of COVID-19 related myocarditis: insights on management and outcome. Cardiovasc Revasc Med. 2021;23:107. [PMID: 32847728]

Sharma AN et al. Fulminant myocarditis: epidemiology, pathogenesis, diagnosis, and management. Am J Cardiol. 2019; 124: 1954. [PMID: 31679645]

Siripanthong B et al. Recognizing COVID-19-related myocarditis: the possible pathophysiology and proposed guideline for diagnosis and management. Heart Rhythm. 2020;17:1463. [PMID: 32387246]

Witberg G et al. Myocarditis after Covid-19 vaccination in a large health care organization. N Engl J Med. 2021;385:2132. [PMID: 34614329]

NONINFECTIOUS MYOCARDITIS

A variety of medications, illicit drugs, and toxic substances can produce acute or chronic myocardial injury; the clinical presentation varies widely. The phenothiazines, lithium, chloroquine, disopyramide, antimony-containing compounds, and arsenicals can also cause ECG changes, arrhythmias, or heart failure. Hypersensitivity reactions to sulfonamides, penicillins, and aminosalicylic acid as well as other medications can result in cardiac dysfunction.

Radiation can cause an acute inflammatory reaction as well as a chronic fibrosis of heart muscle, usually in conjunction with pericarditis.

Cardiotoxicity from cocaine may occur from coronary artery spasm, MI, arrhythmias, and myocarditis. A cocaine cardiomyopathy has also been described. Because many of these processes are believed to be mediated by cocaine's inhibitory effect on norepinephrine reuptake by sympathetic nerves, beta-blockers have been used in patients with fixed stenosis. In documented coronary spasm, calcium channel blockers and nitrates may be effective. Usual therapy for heart failure or conduction system disease is warranted when symptoms occur. Other recreational drug use has been associated with myocarditis in various case reports.

Systemic disorders are also associated with myocarditis. These include giant cell myocarditis, eosinophilic myocarditis, celiac disease, granulomatosis with polyangiitis, and sarcoidosis. A benefit from immunosuppressive therapy, especially in giant cell myocarditis has been suggested in a number of observational studies, including those directed primarily at T cells (ie, using muromonab-CD3). Treatment of eosinophilic myocarditis includes the use of high-dose corticosteroids and removal of the offending medication or underlying trigger, if known. Most studies suggest that HIV is only indirectly responsible for HIV cardiomyopathy, and other factors, gp 120 protein, adverse reaction to antiretroviral therapy, and opportunistic infections have been implicated more often. Epstein-Barr and herpes simplex viruses have been identified in some patients' myocardium.

The problem of cardiovascular side effects from cancer chemotherapy agents is an ever growing one and has spawned a new clinical area in cardiology called **cardio-oncology.** Anthracyclines (doxorubicin, daunorubicin, idarubicin, epirubicin, and mitoxantrone) remain the cornerstone of treatment of many malignancies but may result in cardiomyopathy. Heart failure can be expected in 5% of patients treated with a cumulative dose of 400–450 mg/m^2, and this rate is doubled if the patient is over age 65. While symptoms and evidence for myocardial dysfunction usually appear within 1 year of starting therapy, late onset manifestation of heart failure may appear up to a decade later. The major mechanism of cardiotoxicity is thought to be due to oxidative stress inducing both apoptosis and necrosis of myocytes. There is also disruption of the sarcomere. This pathologic understanding is the rationale behind the superoxide dismutase mimetic and iron-chelating agent, dexrazoxane, to protect from the injury. The use of trastuzumab in combination with anthracyclines increases the risk of cardiac dysfunction up to 28%; this has been an issue since combined use of these agents is particularly effective in *HER2*-positive breast cancer. Other risk factors for patients receiving anthracyclines include the use of paclitaxel, concurrent radiation, and preexisting CVD (including hypertension, peripheral vascular disease, CAD, and diabetes). A summary of cardiotoxic cancer therapeutic agents and their role may be found in the 2019 AHA statement on cardio-oncology.

In patients receiving chemotherapy, it is important to look for subtle signs of cardiovascular compromise. Serial echocardiography, cardiac MR, or both can provide concrete data regarding LV function. Echo/Doppler myocardial global strain abnormalities may be the first abnormality observed (even prior to a drop in the LVEF) and assessment of the T2 signal from cardiac MRI may also provide early detection of cardiotoxicity. Biomarkers such as BNP or NT-proBNP may be of some value when serial measures are obtained. Other biomarkers may appear early in the course of myocardial injury (especially troponin and myeloperoxidase) and may allow for early detection of cardiotoxicity before other signs become evident. There is some evidence that beta-blocker therapy may reduce the negative effects on myocardial function. There are anecdotal data from animal models that NSAIDs may be harmful in patients with myocarditis. They should be avoided along with alcohol and strenuous physical exercise.

When to Refer

Many patients with myocardial injury from toxic agents can be monitored safely if ventricular function remains relatively preserved (EF greater than 40%) and no heart failure symptoms occur. Diastolic dysfunction may be subtle.

Once heart failure or a reduced LVEF becomes evident or significant conduction system disease becomes manifest, the patient should be evaluated and monitored by a cardiologist in case myocardial dysfunction worsens and further intervention becomes warranted.

Campia U et al. Cardio-oncology: vascular and metabolic perspectives: a scientific statement from the American Heart Association. Circulation. 2019;139:e579. [PMID: 30786722]

Ye L et al. Myocardial strain imaging by echocardiography for the prediction of cardiotoxicity of chemotherapy treated patients: a meta-analysis. JACC Cardiovasc Imaging. 2020;13:881. [PMID: 31734206]

Yu AF et al. Cardiac magnetic resonance and cardio-oncology: does T(2) signal the end of anthracycline cardiotoxicity? J Am Coll Cardiol. 2019;73:792. [PMID: 30784672]

DILATED CARDIOMYOPATHY

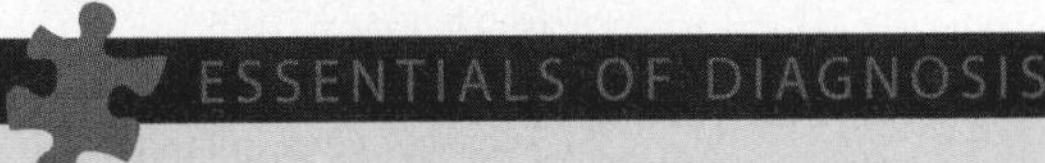

- Symptoms and signs of heart failure.
- Echocardiogram confirms LV dilation, thinning, and global dysfunction.
- Severity of RV dysfunction critical in long-term prognosis.

General Considerations

Heart failure definitions have changed over the years and patients with a dilated cardiomyopathy are generally placed into the category of heart failure with reduced EF where the LVEF is defined as less than or equal to 40%. *In about half of the patients in this category, there is LV enlargement and it is this group that defines dilated cardiomyopathy*. This is a large group of heterogeneous myocardial disorders characterized by reduced myocardial contractility in the absence of abnormal loading conditions such as with hypertension or valvular disease. The prevalence averages 36 cases/100,000 in the United States and accounts for approximately 10,000 deaths annually. Black patients are afflicted three times as often as White patients. The prognosis is poor with 50% mortality at 5 years once symptoms emerge.

The causes are multiple and diverse. Up to 20–35% have a familial etiology. It is common for hereditary causes to first present with conduction system disease prior to a reduced LVEF. A 2020 report of 2538 patients with a dilated cardiomyopathy in whom genetics were available suggested a clear association with at least 12 differing genes. Recent attention has focused particularly on the Lamin A/C genotype. While a large proportion of dilated cardiomyopathy causes are listed as idiopathic, it is likely that genetic variants may be responsible for many of these. Endocrine, inflammatory, and metabolic causes include obesity, diabetes, thyroid disease, celiac disease, SLE, acromegaly, and growth hormone deficiency. Toxic, drug-induced, and inflammatory causes are listed in the prior section. Nutritional diseases such as deficiency of thiamine, selenium, and carnitine have also been documented. Dilated cardiomyopathy may also be caused by prolonged tachycardia either from supraventricular arrhythmias, from very frequent PVCs (more than 15% of heart beats), or from frequent RV pacing. Dilated cardiomyopathy is also associated with HIV, Chagas disease, rheumatologic disorders, iron overload, sleep apnea, amyloidosis, sarcoidosis, chronic alcohol usage, ESKD, or cobalt exposure ("Quebec beer-drinkers, cardiomyopathy"). Peripartum cardiomyopathy and stress-induced disease (tako-tsubo) are discussed separately.

Clinical Findings

A. Symptoms and Signs

In most patients, symptoms of heart failure develop gradually. It is important to seek out a history of familial dilated cardiomyopathy and to identify behaviors that might predispose patients to the disease. The physical examination reveals rales, an elevated JVP, cardiomegaly, S_3 gallop rhythm, often the murmurs of functional mitral or tricuspid regurgitation, peripheral edema, or ascites. In severe heart failure, Cheyne-Stokes breathing, pulsus alternans, pallor, and cyanosis may be present.

B. ECG and Chest Radiography

The major findings are listed in Table 10–15. Sinus tachycardia is common. Other common abnormalities include

Table 10–15. Classification of the cardiomyopathies.

	Dilated	Hypertrophic	Restrictive
Frequent causes	Idiopathic, alcoholic, major catecholamine discharge, myocarditis, postpartum, chemotherapy, endocrinopathies, genetic diseases, burnt out HOCM, CAD, tachycardia-induced, cocaine	Hereditary syndrome, possibly chronic hypertension in older adults	Amyloidosis, post-radiation, post–open heart surgery, diabetes, endomyocardial fibrosis, Fabry disease, sarcoidosis
Symptoms	Left or biventricular heart failure	Dyspnea, chest pain, syncope	Dyspnea, fatigue, right heart failure > left heart failure
Physical examination	Cardiomegaly, S_3, elevated jugular venous pressure, rales	Sustained point of maximal impulse, S_4, variable systolic murmur, bisferiens carotid pulse	Elevated jugular venous pressure
ECG	ST–T changes, conduction abnormalities, ventricular ectopy	LVH, exaggerated septal Q waves	ST–T changes, conduction abnormalities, low voltage
Chest radiograph	Enlarged heart, pulmonary congestion	Mild cardiomegaly	Mild to moderate cardiomegaly
Echocardiogram, nuclear studies, MRI, PET, CT	LV dilation and dysfunction	LVH, asymmetric septal or other myocardial wall thickness > 15 mm, small LV size, normal or supranormal function, systolic anterior mitral motion, diastolic dysfunction. May be nonobstructive or apical	Small or normal LV size, normal or mildly reduced LV function. Gadolinium hyperenhancement on MRI
Cardiac catheterization	LV dilation and dysfunction, high diastolic pressures, low cardiac output. Coronary angiography important to exclude ischemic cause	Small, hypercontractile LV, dynamic outflow gradient, diastolic dysfunction	High diastolic pressure, "square root" sign, normal or mildly reduced LV function

HOCM, hypertrophic obstructive cardiomyopathy.

left bundle branch block and ventricular or atrial arrhythmias. The chest radiograph reveals cardiomegaly, evidence for left and/or right heart failure, and pleural effusions (right more frequently than left).

C. Diagnostic Studies

In the 2017 AHA/ACCF heart failure guideline focused update, patients with dyspnea should have a BNP or NT-proBNP measured to help establish prognosis and disease severity (class I, level of evidence [LOE] A).

An echocardiogram is indicated to exclude unsuspected valvular or other lesions and confirm the presence of ventricular dilatation, reduced LV systolic function and associated RV systolic dysfunction, or pulmonary hypertension. Mitral Doppler inflow patterns also help in the diagnosis of concomitant diastolic dysfunction. Color flow Doppler can reveal tricuspid or mitral regurgitation, and continuous Doppler can estimate PA pressures. Intracavitary thrombosis is occasionally seen. Exercise or pharmacologic stress myocardial perfusion imaging may uncover underlying coronary disease. Radionuclide ventriculography provides a noninvasive measure of the EF and both RV and LV wall motion, though its use has been supplanted by cardiac MRI in most institutions. Cardiac MRI is particularly helpful in inflammatory or infiltrative processes, such as sarcoidosis or hemochromatosis, and is the diagnostic study of choice for RV dysplasia. MRI can also help define an ischemic etiology by noting gadolinium hyperenhancement consistent with myocardial scar from infarction or prior myocarditis. Cardiac catheterization is seldom of specific value unless myocardial ischemia is suspected, although right heart catheterization should be considered to help guide therapy when the clinical syndrome is not clear cut (class I indication, LOE C). Myocardial biopsy is rarely useful in establishing the diagnosis, although occasionally the underlying cause (eg, sarcoidosis, hemochromatosis) can be discerned. Its use is considered a class IIa indication with LOE of C. It should not be used routinely. Biopsy is most useful in transplant rejection.

Treatment

The management of heart failure is outlined in the section on heart failure. Standard therapy includes control of BP and of contributing factors such as obesity, smoking, diabetes or potentially cardiotoxic agents. All patients with a remote history of MI or acute coronary syndrome and reduced LVEF should be given ACE inhibitors, ARBs, or sacubitril/valsartan. Beta-blockers should be included in this population as well. **All patients with dilated cardiomyopathy regardless of etiology should be treated with beta-blockers and ACE inhibitors. If still symptomatic, aldosterone antagonists should be added, and ARNI used instead of an ACE inhibitor or ARB.** The use of the combination of all three of ACE inhibition, ARB, and aldosterone antagonists can create harm, though, and is discouraged due to concerns for hyperkalemia. Calcium channel blockers should be avoided except as necessary to control ventricular response in atrial fibrillation or flutter. If congestive symptoms are present, diuretics and an aldosterone antagonist should be added. In patients with class II–IV heart failure symptoms, an aldosterone receptor antagonist should be added when the LVEF is less than 35% (unless contraindicated). Care in the use of mineralocorticoid receptor antagonists is warranted when the GFR is less than 30 mL/minute/1.73 m^2 or when the potassium is elevated. All patients with diabetes should be taking mineralocorticoid antagonists if the LVEF is less than or equal to 40%. Systemic BP control is extremely important. Use of the angiotensin receptor-neprilysin inhibitor, sacubitril/valsartan, has been approved for NYHA Heart Failure of Functional class II–IV. If the resting heart rate is greater than 70 beats per minute, the LVEF is less than 35%, and the patient has chronic stable heart failure, the use of ivabradine to slow the heart rate has also been approved. Ivabradine should not replace other beta-blockers, however. Digoxin is a second-line medication but remains favored as an adjunct by some clinicians; digoxin may be beneficial to reduce recurrent hospitalizations and to control the ventricular response in atrial fibrillation in sedentary patients. Given the question of abnormal nitric oxide utilization in Blacks, the use of hydralazine-nitrate combination therapy is recommended in this population. Sodium restriction is helpful, especially in acute heart failure. Continuous positive airway pressure can improve LV function in patients with sleep apnea.

When atrial fibrillation is present, heart rate control is important if sinus rhythm cannot be established or maintained. There are few data, however, to suggest an advantage of sinus rhythm over atrial fibrillation on long-term outcomes. Many patients may be candidates for cardiac synchronization therapy with biventricular pacing if there is significant mitral regurgitation and the QRS width is greater than 150 msec.

To help prevent sudden death, an ICD is reasonable (class IIa, LOE B) in asymptomatic ischemic cardiomyopathy patients with an LVEF of less than 30% on appropriate medical therapy (at least 3 months post-MI). Cardiac rehabilitation and exercise training have consistently been found to improve clinical status.

Few cases of cardiomyopathy are amenable to specific therapy for the underlying cause. Alcohol use should be discontinued, since there is often marked recovery of cardiac function following a period of abstinence in alcoholic cardiomyopathy. Endocrine causes (hyperthyroidism or hypothyroidism, acromegaly, and pheochromocytoma) should be treated. Immunosuppressive therapy is not indicated in chronic dilated cardiomyopathy. There are some patients who may benefit from implantable LV assist devices either as a bridge to transplantation or as a temporary measure until cardiac function returns. LV assist devices can be considered as *destination therapy* in patients who are not candidates for cardiac transplantation. Arterial and pulmonary emboli are more common in dilated cardiomyopathy than in ischemic cardiomyopathy, and suitable candidates may benefit from long-term anticoagulation. All patients with atrial fibrillation should be so treated. DOACs are preferred over warfarin unless there is associated mitral stenosis. Either warfarin or a DOAC should be considered when a mobile LV thrombus is observed on the echocardiogram.

Prognosis

The prognosis of dilated cardiomyopathy without clinical heart failure is variable, with some patients remaining stable, some deteriorating gradually, and others declining rapidly. Once heart failure is manifest, the natural history is similar to that of other causes of heart failure, with an annual mortality rate of around 11–13%. The underlying cause of heart failure has prognostic value in patients with unexplained cardiomyopathy. Patients with peripartum cardiomyopathy or stress-induced cardiomyopathy appear to have a better prognosis than those with other forms of cardiomyopathy. Patients with cardiomyopathy due to infiltrative myocardial diseases, HIV infection, or doxorubicin therapy have an especially poor prognosis.

When to Refer

Patients with new or worsening symptoms of heart failure with dilated cardiomyopathy should be referred to a cardiologist. Patients with continued symptoms of heart failure and reduced LVEF (35% or less) should be referred for consideration of placement of an ICD or cardiac resynchronization therapy (if QRS duration is 150 msec or more, especially with a left bundle branch block pattern). Patients with advanced refractory symptoms should be referred for consideration of heart transplant or LV assist device therapy.

When to Admit

Patients with hypoxia, fluid overload, or pulmonary edema not readily resolved in an outpatient setting should be admitted.

Mazzarotto F et al. Reevaluating the genetic contribution of monogenetic dilated cardiomyopathy. Circulation. 2020;141:387. [PMID: 31983221]

Rosenbaum AN et al. Genetics of dilated cardiomyopathy: practical implications for heart failure management. Nat Rev Cardiol. 2020;17:286. [PMID: 31605094]

STRESS CARDIOMYOPATHY

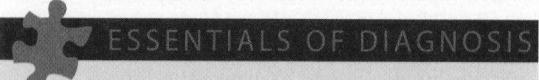

ESSENTIALS OF DIAGNOSIS

- Occurs after a major catecholamine discharge.
- Acute chest pain or shortness of breath.
- Predominately affects postmenopausal women.
- Presents as an acute anterior MI, but coronaries normal at cardiac catheterization.
- Imaging reveals apical LV ballooning due to anteroapical stunning of the myocardium.
- Most patients recover completely, although there are complications similar to MI.

General Considerations

Stress cardiomyopathy (**tako-tsubo syndrome**) generally follows a high catecholamine surge. The resulting shape of the LV acutely suggests a rounded ampulla form similar to a Japanese octopus pot (tako-tsubo pot). Mid-ventricular ballooning has also been described. The key feature is that the myocardial stunning that occurs does *not* follow the pattern suggestive of coronary ischemia (even though about 15% of patients will have coexisting CAD, and some may have concomitant plaque rupture MI). Over two-thirds of patients report a prior stressful event, either emotional or physical, including hypoglycemia, lightning strikes, earthquakes, postventricular tachycardia, during alcohol withdrawal, following surgery, during hyperthyroidism, after stroke, and following emotional stress ("broken-heart syndrome"). Virtually any event that triggers excess catecholamines has been implicated in a wide number of case reports. Pericarditis and even tamponade have been described in isolated cases. Recurrences have also been described. In Western countries it predominantly affects women (up to 90%), primarily postmenopausal. Among patients with stress cardiomyopathy, compared to patients with acute coronary syndrome, there are more neurologic and psychiatric disorders. Patients with COPD, migraines, or affective disorders who take beta-agonists may have an increased risk of a poor outcome. The prognosis was initially thought to be benign, but subsequent studies have demonstrated that *both short-term mortality and long-term mortality are higher than thought.* Indeed, mortality reported during the acute phase in hospitalized patients is approximately 4–5%, a figure comparable to that of STEMI in the era of primary percutaneous coronary interventions. Approximately 10% of patients will have cardiac and neurologic adverse outcomes over the next year.

The structures that mediate the stress response are in both the central and autonomic nervous systems. Acute stressors induce brain activation, increasing bioavailability of cortisol and catecholamine. Both circulating epinephrine and norepinephrine released from adrenal medullary chromaffin cells and norepinephrine released locally from sympathetic nerve terminals are significantly increased. This catecholamine surge leads to myocardial damage through multiple mechanisms, including, direct catecholamine toxicity, adrenoceptor-mediated damage, epicardial and microvascular coronary vasoconstriction and/or spasm, and increased cardiac workload. The relative preponderance among postmenopausal women suggests that estrogen deprivation may be facilitating, possibly via endothelial dysfunction.

Clinical Findings

A. Symptoms and Signs

The symptoms are similar to any acute coronary syndrome. Typical angina and dyspnea are usually present. Syncope is rare, although arrhythmias are not uncommon.

B. ECG and Chest Radiography

The ECG reveals ST-segment elevation as well as deep anterior T-wave inversion. The chest radiograph is either normal or reveals pulmonary congestion. The dramatic T-wave inversions gradually resolve over time.

C. Diagnostic Studies

The echocardiogram reveals LV apical dyskinesia usually not consistent with any particular coronary distribution. The urgent cardiac catheterization reveals the LV apical ballooning in association with normal coronaries. Initial cardiac enzymes are positive but often taper quickly. In almost all cases, MRI hyperenhancement studies reveal no long-term scarring.

Treatment

Immediate therapy is similar to any acute MI. Initiation of long-term therapy depends on whether LV dysfunction persists. Most patients receive aspirin, beta-blockers, and ACE inhibitors until the LV fully recovers. Despite the presumed association with high catecholamines, the use of ACE inhibitors or ARBs, but not beta-blockers, has been associated with improved long-term survival. See Treatment of Heart Failure With Reduced LVEF.

Prognosis

The rate of severe in-hospital complications, including shock and death, appear to be similar between those with an acute coronary syndrome and tako-tsubo. Overall, prognosis is good unless there is a serious complication (such as mitral regurgitation, ventricular rupture, or ventricular tachycardia). Recovery of the LVEF is expected in most cases after a period of days to weeks.

When to Refer

All patients with an acute coronary syndrome should be urgently seen by a cardiologist for further evaluation and monitored until resolution of the ventricular dysfunction.

HYPERTROPHIC CARDIOMYOPATHY

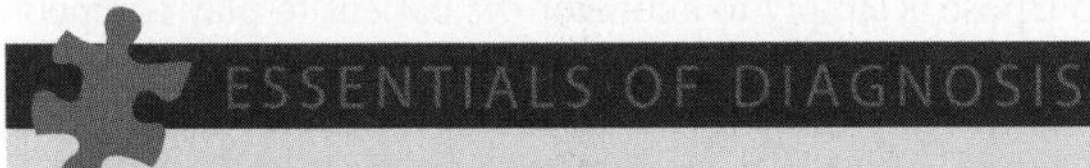

- May present with dyspnea, chest pain, syncope.
- Though LV outflow gradient is classic, symptoms are primarily related to diastolic dysfunction.
- Echocardiogram is diagnostic. Any area of LV wall thickness > 1.5 cm defines the disease.
- Increased risk of sudden death.

General Considerations

In 2020, an ACC/AHA joint committee on clinical practice guidelines issued updated guidelines for the diagnosis and treatment of HCM. The guidelines address many clinical scenarios and provide a host of clinically relevant suggestions. HCM is noted when there is LVH unrelated to any pressure or volume overload. The definition has evolved over time; while it traditionally was defined by LV outflow obstruction due to septal hypertrophy, currently it is considered present any time that *any portion of LV wall is measured at more than 1.5 cm thick on an echocardiogram.* This allows for many forms to be considered that do not create LV outflow obstruction. The increased wall thickness reduces LV systolic stress, increases the EF, and can result in an "empty ventricle" at end-systole. The interventricular septum may be disproportionately involved (**asymmetric septal hypertrophy**), but in some cases the hypertrophy is localized to the mid-ventricle or to the apex. In a normal heart, the LV apex may be paper thin; in HCM, the LV obstruction may trap blood just above the apex and the LV pressure may be very high there. This can result in the apex becoming aneurysmal. The LV outflow tract is usually narrowed during systole due to the hypertrophied septum and systolic anterior motion of the mitral valve occurs as the anterior mitral valve leaflet is pulled into the LV outflow. The obstruction is worsened by factors that increase myocardial contractility (sympathetic stimulation, digoxin, and postextrasystolic beat) or that decrease LV filling (Valsalva maneuver, peripheral vasodilators). The amount of obstruction is preload and afterload dependent and can vary from day to day. The consequence of the hypertrophy is *elevated LV diastolic pressures* rather than systolic dysfunction. Rarely, systolic dysfunction develops late in the course of the disease. The LV is usually more involved than the RV, and the atria are frequently significantly enlarged.

HCM is inherited as an autosomal-dominant trait with variable penetrance and is caused by mutations of one of a large number of genes, most of which code for myosin heavy chains or proteins regulating calcium handling. The prognosis is related to the specific gene mutation. Patients usually present in early adulthood. Elite athletes may demonstrate considerable hypertrophy that can be confused with HCM, but generally diastolic dysfunction is not present in the athlete and this finding helps separate pathologic disease from **athletic hypertrophy**. The apical variety is particularly common in those of Asian descent. A **HCM in older adults** (usually in association with hypertension) has also been defined as a distinct entity (often a sigmoid interventricular septum is noted with a knob of cardiac muscle below the aortic valve). Mitral annular calcification is often present. Mitral regurgitation is variable and often dynamic, depending on the degree of outflow tract obstruction.

Clinical Findings

A. Symptoms and Signs

The most frequent symptoms are dyspnea and chest pain. Syncope is also common and is typically postexertional, when diastolic filling diminishes due to fluid loss and tachycardia increasing LV outflow tract obstruction. Residual circulating catecholamines accentuate the changes. Arrhythmias are an important problem. Atrial fibrillation is a long-term consequence of chronically elevated LA pressures and is a poor prognostic sign. Ventricular arrhythmias are also common, and sudden death may occur, often after extraordinary exertion.

Features on physical examination include a bisferiens carotid pulse, triple apical impulse (due to the prominent atrial filling wave and early and late systolic impulses), and a loud S_4. The JVP may reveal a prominent *a* wave due to reduced RV compliance. In cases with LV outflow obstruction, a loud systolic murmur is present along the left sternal border that increases with upright posture or Valsalva maneuver and decreases with squatting. These maneuvers help differentiate the murmur of HCM from that of aortic stenosis. In HCM, reducing the LV volume *increases* the outflow obstruction and the murmur intensity; whereas in valvular aortic stenosis, reducing the stroke volume across the valve *decreases* the murmur. Mitral regurgitation is frequently present as well.

B. ECG and Chest Radiography

LVH is nearly universal in symptomatic patients, though entirely normal ECGs are present in up to 25%, usually in those with localized hypertrophy. Exaggerated septal Q waves inferolaterally may mimic MI. The chest radiograph is often unimpressive. Unlike with aortic stenosis, the ascending aorta is not dilated.

C. Diagnostic Studies

The echocardiogram is diagnostic, revealing LVH (involving the septum more commonly than the posterior walls), systolic anterior motion of the mitral valve, early closing followed by reopening of the aortic valve, a small and hypercontractile LV, and delayed relaxation and filling of the LV during diastole. The septum is usually 1.3–1.5 times the thickness of the posterior wall. Septal motion tends to be reduced. Doppler ultrasound reveals turbulent flow and a dynamic gradient in the LV outflow tract and, commonly, mitral regurgitation. Abnormalities in the diastolic filling pattern are present in 80% of patients.

Echocardiography can usually differentiate the disease from ventricular noncompaction, a congenital myocardial disease pattern with marked trabeculation that partially fills the LV cavity. Myocardial perfusion imaging may suggest septal ischemia in the presence of normal coronary arteries. Cardiac MRI confirms the hypertrophy and contrast enhancement frequently reveals evidence of scar at the junction of the RV attachment to the interventricular septum. Cardiac catheterization confirms the diagnosis and defines the presence or absence of CAD. Frequently, coronary arterial bridging (squeezing of the coronary in systole) occurs, especially in the septal arteries. Exercise studies are recommended to assess for ventricular arrhythmias and to document the BP response. Loop monitoring is recommended for determination of ventricular ectopy.

▶ Treatment

Beta-blockers should be the initial medication in symptomatic individuals, especially when dynamic outflow obstruction is noted on the echocardiogram. The resulting slower heart rates assist with diastolic filling of the stiff LV. Dyspnea, angina, and arrhythmias respond in about 50% of patients. Calcium channel blockers, especially verapamil, have also been effective in symptomatic patients. Verapamil or nondihydropyridine calcium channel blockers, such as diltiazem, are class I recommendations. Their effect is due primarily to improved diastolic function; however, their vasodilating actions can also increase outflow obstruction and cause hypotension. Verapamil should not be used if there is hypotension or a resting gradient of over 100 mm Hg. Disopyramide is also effective because of its negative inotropic effects; it is usually used as an addition to the medical regimen rather than as primary therapy or to help control atrial arrhythmias. Oral diuretics are frequently necessary due to the high LV diastolic pressure and elevated LA pressures but should be used with caution to avoid dehydration that would increase obstruction. Digoxin is relatively contraindicated, except rarely for rate control in atrial fibrillation. For acute hypotension that does not respond to fluids, phenylephrine may be considered. In HCM patients without outflow obstruction, similar treatment should be used only if symptomatic and the use of oral diuretics is safer. In a very small number of these patients, apical myomectomy may be considered.

Patients do best in sinus rhythm, and atrial fibrillation should be aggressively treated with antiarrhythmics or radiofrequency ablation. DOACs are preferred over warfarin if atrial fibrillation occurs. Patients with HCM should be treated regardless of their CHA_2DS_2-VASc score.

The 2020 AHA/ACC guidelines recommend a preventive ICD for HCM patients with documented cardiac arrest or sustained ventricular tachycardia (class I). It is a class IIa recommendation for an ICD if there are one or more of the following risk factors: (1) sudden death in one or more first-degree or close relative 50 years of age or younger, (2) any LV wall greater than or equal to 30 mm, (3) any recent syncope likely to have been arrhythmogenic, (4) LV apical aneurysm, or (5) LV systolic dysfunction (EF less than 50%). It is a class IIb recommendation for an ICD if there is significant (greater than 15%) late gadolinium enhancement on cardiac MRI. In those who receive an ICD, antitachycardia pacing should be programmed to minimize shocks. The use of an ICD is contraindicated, though, if the purpose is simply to allow for the patient to play competitive sports.

Excision of part of the outflow myocardial septum (**myotomy–myomectomy**) by experienced surgeons is successful in patients with symptoms unresponsive to medical therapy. A few surgeons advocate mitral valve replacement, since this results in resolution of the gradient and prevents associated mitral regurgitation. In some cases, myomectomy has been combined with an Alfieri stitch on the mitral valve (a stitch that binds the midportion of the anterior and posterior mitral valve leaflets together). Rare cases of progression to LV dilation or patients with intractable symptoms can be considered for cardiac transplantation. Nonsurgical septal ablation can be performed by injection of alcohol into septal branches of the left coronary artery to create a controlled myocardial infarct in the regions of greatest wall thickness. It is now considered first-line therapy, if feasible, for those with LV outflow tract obstruction greater than 50 mm Hg who do not respond to medical therapy or who are not deemed surgical candidates.

In "burnt out" HCM, the medical therapy is similar to that of dilated cardiomyopathy. In those with refractory arrhythmias or heart failure, cardiac transplantation is an option.

Pregnancy results in an increased risk in patients with symptoms or outflow tract gradients of greater than 50 mm Hg. Genetic counseling is indicated before planned conception. In pregnant patients with HCM, continuation of beta-blocker therapy is recommended. For more details on the impact of HCM on sport, activity, and occupation (such as driving commercially or piloting an aircraft), the reader is referred to the discussions in the 2020 AHA/ACC guidelines.

When to Refer

Patients should be referred to a cardiologist to establish care, consider genetic testing, review the presence of any high-risk features, and discuss medications or the need for any intervention. This is particularly important if any symptoms are present.

Ommen SR. 2020 AHA/ACC guidelines for the diagnosis and treatment of patients with hypertrophic cardiomyopathy: executive summary. Circulation. 2020;142:e533. [PMID: 33215938]

RESTRICTIVE CARDIOMYOPATHY

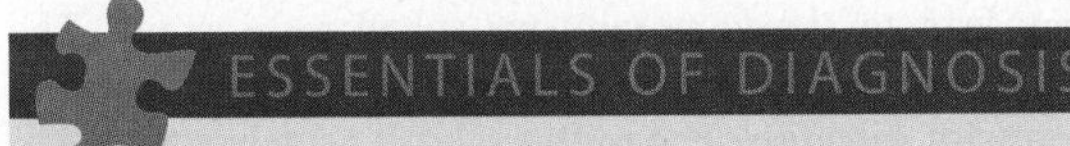

- Right heart failure tends to dominate over left heart failure.
- Pulmonary hypertension is present.
- Amyloidosis is the most common cause.
- Echocardiography is key to diagnosis.
- Radionuclide imaging or myocardial biopsy can confirm amyloid.

General Considerations

Restrictive cardiomyopathy is characterized by *impaired diastolic filling with reasonably preserved LV chamber size*. The condition is relatively uncommon, with the most frequent cause being amyloidosis. The diagnosis of **cardiac amyloidosis** has dramatically increased in the last few years since diagnostic testing has improved and there is an awareness of its prevalence. The prevalence of AL amyloid is approximately 12 cases per million, the prevalence of variant or hereditary ATTR amyloid is about 0.3 cases per million, and the prevalence of wild type ATTR amyloid is 155–191 cases per million. Many experts believe the actual prevalence of wild type ATTR is much higher. While light-chain amyloid proteins can be toxic to cardiomyocytes, they may also internalize into many cell types and this may explain some of the cardiac dysfunction observed. ATTR refers to transthyretin, a protein normally found in the liver that helps transport thyroid hormones and vitamin A. Wild type (normal) occurs more commonly in the elderly and in men, and previously was referred to as "senile systemic amyloidosis." Hereditary or variant ATTR is genetically transmitted, deposition occurs at an earlier age, and it has associated neurologic impact. TTR is a tetramer that can dissociate into four monomers and aggregate as amyloid fibrils. The differential diagnosis of a restrictive cardiomyopathy includes infiltrative disorders beside amyloidosis, such as sarcoidosis, Gaucher disease, and Hurler syndrome. Storage diseases such as hemochromatosis, Fabry disease, and glycogen storage diseases can also produce the picture. Noninfiltrative diseases, such as familial cardiomyopathy and pseudoxanthoma elasticum, can be implicated rarely, and other secondary causes include diabetes, systemic sclerosis (scleroderma), radiation, chemotherapy, CAD, and longstanding hypertension.

Clinical Findings

A. Symptoms and Signs

Restrictive cardiomyopathy must be distinguished from constrictive pericarditis (see Table 10–15). The key feature is that *ventricular interaction is accentuated with respiration in constrictive pericarditis* and that interaction is absent in restrictive cardiomyopathy. In addition, the pulmonary arterial pressure is invariably elevated in restrictive cardiomyopathy due to the high PCWP and is normal in uncomplicated constrictive pericarditis. Symptoms may include angina, syncope, stroke, and peripheral neuropathy. Periorbital purpura, a thickened tongue, and hepatomegaly are all suggestive physical findings of amyloidosis.

B. Diagnostic Studies

Conduction disturbances are frequently present. Low voltage on the ECG combined with ventricular hypertrophy on the echocardiogram is suggestive of disease. Technetium pyrophosphate imaging (bone scan imaging) can also identify amyloid deposition in the myocardium, and it has become the noninvasive imaging modality of choice for diagnosing transthyretin amyloidosis. With typical scintographic findings in patients without a monoclonal gammopathy, biopsy is no longer necessary for diagnosis. Cardiac MRI presents a distinctive pattern of diffuse hyperenhancement of the gadolinium image in amyloidosis and is a useful screening test. Late gadolinium hyperenhancement of a high degree suggests more extensive cardiac involvement. The echocardiogram reveals a small, thickened LV with bright myocardium (speckled), rapid early diastolic filling revealed by the mitral inflow Doppler, and biatrial enlargement. Characteristic longitudinal strain patterns may help identify cardiac amyloidosis. The LV chamber size is usually normal with a reduced LVEF. Atrial septal thickening may be evident and an amyloid variant that primarily affects the atria has been described. Rectal, abdominal fat, or gingival biopsies can confirm systemic involvement, but myocardial involvement may still be present if these are negative and requires endomyocardial biopsy for the confirmation that cardiac amyloid is present. Demonstration of tissue infiltration on biopsy specimens using special stains followed by immunohistochemical studies and genetic testing are essential to define which specific protein is involved. TTR gene sequencing in patients in whom the TTR wild type or TTR mutant variant is suspected and mass spectroscopy on all tissue in question are recommended highly. BNP and NT-proBNP are traditionally elevated and have been used to help distinguish constrictive pericarditis from a restrictive cardiomyopathy.

Treatment

Treatment for AL amyloidosis includes alkylator-based chemotherapy or high-dose melphalan followed by autologous stem cell transplantation. In immunoglobin light chain amyloidosis, standard- or high-dose chemotherapy with stem cell rescue is often pursued. Treatment of ATTR amyloid is undergoing an evolution. Tafamidis helps prevent the misfolding of the TTR tetramer and is now approved for treatment. Patisiran is also available, and it inhibits both variant and wild type TTR production. For the variant TTR polyneuropathy, subcutaneous inotersen is available (it binds to TTR mRNA preventing transcription).

In acute heart failure, diuretics can help, but excessive diuresis can produce worsening kidney dysfunction. As with most patients with severe right heart failure, loop diuretics, thiazides, and aldosterone antagonists are all useful. Atrial thrombi are not uncommon, although the role of anticoagulation in amyloidosis remains ill defined. Digoxin may precipitate arrhythmias and should not be used. Beta-blockers help slow heart rates and improve filling by increasing diastolic time. Verapamil presumably works by improving myocardial relaxation and increasing diastolic filling time. Slow heart rates are desired to allow for increased diastolic filling time. ACE inhibition or angiotensin II receptor blockade may improve diastolic relaxation and filling at times and can be tried with caution if the systemic BP is adequate. Corticosteroids may be helpful in sarcoidosis, but they are more effective for conduction abnormalities in this disease than in heart failure.

When to Refer

All patients with the diagnosis of a restrictive cardiomyopathy should be referred to a cardiologist to decide etiology and plan appropriate treatment. Unexplained LVH with relatively preserved LVEF and symptoms of heart failure should raise the question of cardiac amyloid, particularly now that there is effective treatment available.

Kitaoka H et al; Japanese Circulation Society Joint Working Group. JCS 2020 guideline on diagnosis and treatment of cardiac amyloidosis. Circ J. 2020;84:1610. [PMID: 32830187]

Marques N et al. Specific therapy for transthyretin cardiac amyloidosis: a systematic literature review and evidence-based recommendations. J Am Heart Assoc. 2020;9:e016614. [PMID: 32969287]

RHEUMATIC FEVER

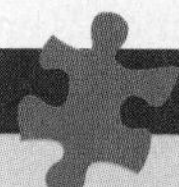

ESSENTIALS OF DIAGNOSIS

- More common in developing countries (100 cases/100,000 population) than in the United States (~2 cases/100,000 population).
- Peak incidence between ages 5 and 15 years.
- May involve mitral and other valves acutely, rarely leading to heart failure.

General Considerations

Rheumatic fever is a systemic immune process that is a sequela of a beta-hemolytic streptococcal infection of the pharynx. It is a major scourge in developing countries and responsible for 320,000 deaths in young people worldwide each year. Over 15 million people have evidence for rheumatic heart disease. Signs of **acute rheumatic fever** usually commence 2–3 weeks after infection but may appear as early as 1 week or as late as 5 weeks. The disease has become quite uncommon in the United States, except in immigrants. The peak incidence is between ages 5 and 15 years; rheumatic fever is rare before age 4 years or after age 40 years. Rheumatic carditis and valvulitis may be self-limited or may lead to slowly progressive valvular deformity. The characteristic lesion is a perivascular granulomatous reaction with valvulitis. The mitral valve is acutely attacked in 75–80% of cases, the aortic valve in 30% (but rarely as the sole valve involved), and the tricuspid and pulmonary valves in under 5% of cases.

The clinical profile of the infection includes carditis in 50–70% and arthritis in 35–66%, followed by chorea (10–30%, predominantly in girls) then subcutaneous nodules (0–10%) and erythema marginatum (in less than 6%). Echocardiography has been found to be superior to auscultation, and the 2015 guidelines introduced **subclinical carditis** to the Jones criteria to represent abnormal echocardiographic findings when auscultatory findings were either not present or not recognized.

Chronic rheumatic heart disease results from single or repeated attacks of rheumatic fever that produce rigidity and deformity of valve cusps, fusion of the commissures, or shortening and fusion of the chordae tendineae. Valvular stenosis or regurgitation results, and the two often coexist. In chronic rheumatic heart disease, the mitral valve alone is abnormal in 50–60% of cases; combined lesions of the aortic and mitral valves occur in 20%; pure aortic lesions are less common. Tricuspid involvement occurs in about 10% of cases, but only in association with mitral or aortic disease and is thought to be more common when recurrent infections have occurred. The pulmonary valve is rarely affected long term. A history of rheumatic fever is obtainable in only 60% of patients with rheumatic heart disease. While there has been progress against this disease, it remains a major cardiovascular problem in the poorest regions of the world.

Clinical Findings

The presence of two major criteria—or one major and two minor criteria—establishes the diagnosis. While India, New Zealand, and Australia have all published revised guidelines since 2001, the 2015 recommendations have revised the Jones criteria (Table 10–16) in a scientific statement from the AHA where subclinical carditis is now recognized with the advent of echocardiography. The revised criteria also recognize that a lower threshold should be used to diagnosis acute rheumatic fever in high-risk populations.

A. Major Criteria

1. Carditis—Carditis is most likely to be evident in children and adolescents. Any of the following suggests the presence of carditis: (1) pericarditis; (2) cardiomegaly, detected by physical signs, radiography, or echocardiography; (3) heart failure, right- or left-sided—the former perhaps more prominent in children, with painful liver engorgement due to tricuspid regurgitation; and (4) mitral or aortic regurgitation murmurs, indicative of dilation of a valve ring with or without associated valvulitis or morphologic findings on echocardiography of rheumatic valvulitis. The Carey–Coombs short mid-diastolic mitral murmur may be present due to inflammation of the mitral valve. It is a class I (LOE B) indication to perform echocardiography/Doppler studies on all cases of suspected or confirmed acute rheumatic fever.

2. Erythema marginatum and subcutaneous nodules—Erythema marginatum begins as rapidly enlarging macules that may be less notable on black skin and that assume the shape of rings or crescents with clear centers. They may be raised, confluent, and either transient or persistent and usually on the trunk or proximal extremities. Subcutaneous nodules are uncommon except in children. They are small (2 cm or less in diameter), firm, and nontender and are attached to fascia or tendon sheaths over bony prominences. They persist for days or weeks, are recurrent, and are indistinguishable from rheumatoid nodules. Neither the rash nor nodules ever occur as the sole manifestation of acute rheumatic fever.

3. Sydenham chorea—This is the most definitive manifestation of acute rheumatic fever. Defined as involuntary choreoathetoid movements primarily of the face, tongue, and upper extremities, Sydenham chorea may be the sole manifestation of rheumatic fever. Girls are more frequently affected than boys, and occurrence in adults is rare.

4. Polyarthritis—This is a migratory polyarthritis that involves the large joints sequentially. In adults and in certain moderate- to high-risk populations, only a single joint may be affected. The arthritis lasts 1–5 weeks and subsides without residual deformity. Prompt response of arthritis to therapeutic doses of salicylates or nonsteroidal agents is characteristic.

B. Minor Criteria

These include fever, polyarthralgia, reversible prolongation of the PR interval, and an elevated ESR or CRP. A lower threshold is set for patients at high risk (Table 10–16). The 2015 guidelines stipulate that evidence for a preceding

Table 10–16. The 2015 revised Jones criteria.[1]

Population	Criteria	
	Major	Minor
Low risk	Carditis (clinical or subclinical)	Polyarthralgia
	Arthritis (polyarthritis only)	Fever (≥ 38.5°C)
	Chorea	ESR ≥ 60 mm/hour or CRP ≥ 3.0 mg/dL (or both)
	Erythema marginatum	Prolonged PR interval (unless carditis is major criterion)
	Subcutaneous nodules	
Moderate and high risk	Carditis (clinical or subclinical)	Monoarthralgia
	Arthritis (monoarthritis, polyarthritis, polyarthralgia)	Fever (≥ 38°C)
	Chorea	ESR ≥ 30 mm/hour or CRP ≥ 3.0 mg/dL (or both)
	Erythema marginatum	Prolonged PR interval (unless carditis is a major criterion)
	Subcutaneous nodules	

[1]For all patients with evidence of preceding group A streptococcal pharyngitis: initial acute rheumatic fever can be diagnosed when 2 major criteria or 1 major plus 2 minor criteria are met. Recurrent acute rheumatic fever can be diagnosed when 2 major or 1 major plus 2 minor or 3 minor criteria are met. Reprinted with permission Circulation. 2015;131:1806–1818 ©2015 American Heart Association, Inc.

streptococcal infection can be defined by an increase or rising anti-streptolysin O titer or streptococcal antibodies (anti-DNAase B), a positive throat culture for group A beta-hemolytic streptococcal or a positive rapid group A streptococcal carbohydrate antigen test in a child with a high pretest probability of streptococcal pharyngitis.

Treatment

A. General Measures

The patient should be kept at strict bed rest until the temperature returns to normal (without the use of antipyretic medications) and the ESR, plus the resting pulse rate, and the ECG have all returned to baseline.

B. Medical Measures

1. Salicylates—The salicylates markedly reduce fever and relieve joint pain and swelling. They have no effect on the natural course of the disease. Adults may require large doses of aspirin, 0.6–0.9 g every 4 hours; children are treated with lower doses.

2. Penicillin—Penicillin (benzathine penicillin, 1.2 million units intramuscularly once, or procaine penicillin, 600,000 units intramuscularly daily for 10 days) is used to eradicate streptococcal infection if present. Erythromycin may be substituted (40 mg/kg/day).

3. Corticosteroids—There is no proof that cardiac damage is prevented or minimized by corticosteroids. A short course of corticosteroids (prednisone, 40–60 mg orally daily, with tapering over 2 weeks) usually causes rapid improvement of the joint symptoms and is indicated when response to salicylates has been inadequate.

Prevention of Recurrent Rheumatic Fever

Improvements in socioeconomic conditions and public health are critical to reducing bouts of rheumatic fever. The initial episode of rheumatic fever can usually be prevented by early treatment of streptococcal pharyngitis with penicillin (see Chapter 33). Prevention of recurrent episodes of rheumatic fever is critical. Recurrences of rheumatic fever are most common in patients who have had carditis during their initial episode and in children, 20% of whom will have a second episode within 5 years. The preferred method of prophylaxis is with benzathine penicillin G, 1.2 million units intramuscularly every 4 weeks. Oral penicillin (250 mg twice daily) is less reliable.

If the patient is allergic to penicillin, sulfadiazine (or sulfisoxazole), 1 g daily, or erythromycin, 250 mg orally twice daily, may be substituted. The macrolide azithromycin is similarly effective against group A streptococcal infection. If the patient has not had an immediate hypersensitivity (anaphylactic-type) reaction to penicillin, then cephalosporin may also be used.

Recurrences are uncommon after 5 years following the first episode and in patients over 21 years of age. Prophylaxis is usually discontinued after these times except in groups with a high risk of streptococcal infection—parents or teachers of young children, nurses, military recruits, etc. Secondary prevention of rheumatic fever depends on whether carditis has occurred. Current guidelines suggest that if there is no evidence for carditis, preventive therapy can be stopped at age 21 years. If carditis has occurred but there is no residual valvular disease, it can be stopped at 10 years after the acute rheumatic fever episode. If carditis has occurred with residual valvular involvement, it should be continued for 10 years after the last episode or until age 40 years if the patient is in a situation in which reexposure would be expected.

Prognosis

Initial episodes of rheumatic fever may last months in children and weeks in adults. The immediate mortality rate is 1–2%. Persistent rheumatic carditis with cardiomegaly, heart failure, and pericarditis implies a poor prognosis; 30% of children thus affected die within 10 years after the initial attack. After 10 years, two-thirds of patients will have detectable valvular abnormalities (usually thickened valves with limited mobility), but significant symptomatic valvular heart disease or persistent cardiomyopathy occurs in less than 10% of patients with a single episode. In developing countries, acute rheumatic fever occurs earlier in life and recurs more frequently; thus, the evolution to chronic valvular disease is both accelerated and more severe.

Dooley LM et al. Rheumatic heart disease: a review of the current status of global research activity. Autoimmun Rev. 2021;20:102740. [PMID: 33333234]

DISEASES OF THE PERICARDIUM

ACUTE INFLAMMATORY PERICARDITIS

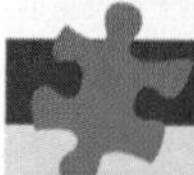

ESSENTIALS OF DIAGNOSIS

- Anterior pleuritic chest pain that is worse supine than upright.
- Pericardial rub.
- Fever common.
- ESR or inflammatory CRP usually elevated.
- ECG reveals diffuse ST-segment elevation with associated PR depression.

General Considerations

Acute (less than 2 weeks) inflammation of the pericardium may be infectious in origin or may be due to systemic diseases (autoimmune syndromes, uremia), neoplasm, radiation, drug toxicity, hemopericardium, postcardiac surgery, or contiguous inflammatory processes in the myocardium or lung. In many of these conditions, the pathologic process involves both the pericardium and the myocardium. Overall pericarditis accounts for 0.2% of hospital admissions and about 5% of patients with nonischemic chest pain seen in the emergency department. The ESC in 2015 proposed four categories of pericarditis: acute, incessant, current, and chronic. Each category has its own diagnostic criteria. In **acute pericarditis,** there are four criteria: (1) pericardial chest pain, (2) pericardial rub, (3) new widespread ST-elevation or PR depression, and (4) new or worsening pericardial effusion. To establish the diagnosis of acute pericarditis, at least two of these four criteria must be present. **Incessant pericarditis** is defined by its duration; it lasts longer than 4–6 weeks but less than 3 months without remission. **Recurrent pericarditis** can be diagnosed in a patient with one reported episode of pericarditis who has been symptom free for at least 4–6 weeks. Finally, **chronic pericarditis** is diagnosed when it persists for more than 3 months.

Viral infections (especially infections with coxsackieviruses and echoviruses but also influenza, Epstein-Barr, varicella, hepatitis, mumps, and HIV viruses) are the most common cause of acute pericarditis and probably are responsible for many cases classified as idiopathic. COVID-19 has been associated with both acute pericarditis and even cardiac tamponade. Males—usually under age 50 years—are most commonly affected. The differential diagnosis primarily requires exclusion of acute MI. **Tuberculous pericarditis** is rare in developed countries but remains common in certain areas of the world. It results from direct lymphatic or hematogenous spread; clinical pulmonary involvement may be absent or minor, although associated pleural effusions are common. **Bacterial pericarditis** is equally rare and usually results from direct extension from pulmonary infections. Pneumococci, though, can cause a primary pericardial infection. *Borrelia burgdorferi,* the organism responsible for Lyme disease, can also cause myopericarditis (and occasionally heart block). **Uremic pericarditis** is a common complication of CKD. The pathogenesis is uncertain; it occurs both with untreated uremia and in otherwise stable dialysis patients. Spread of adjacent lung cancer as well as invasion by breast cancer, renal cell carcinoma, Hodgkin disease, and lymphomas are the most common **neoplastic processes** involving the pericardium and have become the most frequent causes of pericardial tamponade in many countries. Pericarditis may occur 2–5 days after infarction due to an inflammatory reaction to transmural myocardial necrosis **(post-MI** or **postcardiotomy pericarditis [Dressler syndrome]). Radiation** can initiate a fibrinous and fibrotic process in the pericardium, presenting as subacute pericarditis or constriction. Radiation pericarditis usually follows treatments of more than 4000 cGy delivered to ports including more than 30% of the heart.

Other causes of pericarditis include **connective tissue diseases,** such as SLE and rheumatoid arthritis, **drug-induced pericarditis** (minoxidil, penicillins, clozapine), and **myxedema.** In addition, pericarditis may result from **pericardial injury** from invasive cardiac procedures (such as cardiac pacemaker and defibrillator perforation and intracardiac ablation, especially atrial fibrillation ablation), and the implantation of intracardiac devices (such as ASD occluder devices).

Pericarditis and myocarditis may coexist in 20–30% of patients. Myocarditis is often suspected when there is an elevation of serum troponins, although there are no data that suggest troponin elevations are associated with a poor prognosis.

Clinical Findings

A. Symptoms and Signs

The presentation and course of inflammatory pericarditis depend on its cause, but most syndromes have associated chest pain, which is usually pleuritic and postural (relieved by sitting). The pain is substernal but may radiate to the neck, shoulders, back, or epigastrium. Dyspnea may also be present and the patient is often febrile. A pericardial **friction rub** is characteristic, with or without evidence of fluid accumulation or constriction. The presentation of tuberculous pericarditis tends to be subacute, but nonspecific symptoms (fever, night sweats, fatigue) may be present for days to months. Pericardial involvement develops in 1–8% of patients with pulmonary tuberculosis. Symptoms and signs of bacterial pericarditis are similar to those of other types of inflammatory pericarditis, but patients appear toxic and are often critically ill. Uremic pericarditis can present with or without symptoms; fever is absent. Often neoplastic pericarditis is painless, and the presenting symptoms relate to hemodynamic compromise or the primary disease. At times the pericardial effusion is very large, consistent with its chronic nature. Post-MI or postcardiotomy pericarditis (Dressler syndrome) usually presents as a recurrence of pain with pleural-pericardial features. A rub is often audible, and repolarization changes on the ECG may be confused with ischemia. Large effusions are uncommon, and spontaneous resolution usually occurs in a few days. Dressler syndrome occurs days to weeks to several months after MI or open heart surgery, may be recurrent, and probably represents an autoimmune syndrome. Patients present with typical pain, fever, malaise, and leukocytosis. Rarely, other symptoms of an autoimmune disorder, such as joint pain and fever, may occur. Tamponade is rare with Dressler syndrome after MI but not when it occurs postoperatively. The clinical onset of radiation pericarditis is usually within the first year but may be delayed for many years; often a full decade or more may pass before constriction becomes evident.

B. Laboratory Findings and Diagnostic Studies

The diagnosis of viral pericarditis is usually clinical, and leukocytosis is often present. Rising viral titers in paired sera may be obtained for confirmation but are rarely done. Cardiac enzymes may be slightly elevated, reflecting an epicardial myocarditis component. The echocardiogram is often normal or reveals only a trivial amount of extra fluid during the acute inflammatory process. The diagnosis of tuberculous pericarditis can be inferred if acid-fast bacilli are found elsewhere. The tuberculous pericardial effusions are usually small or moderate but may be large when chronic. The yield of mycobacterial organisms by pericardiocentesis is low; pericardial biopsy has a higher yield but may also be negative, and pericardiectomy may be required. If bacterial pericarditis is suspected on clinical grounds, diagnostic pericardiocentesis can be confirmatory. In uremic patients not on dialysis, the incidence of pericarditis correlates roughly with the level of BUN and creatinine. The pericardium is characteristically "shaggy" in uremic pericarditis, and the effusion is hemorrhagic and exudative. The diagnosis of neoplastic pericarditis can occasionally be made by cytologic examination of the effusion or by pericardial biopsy, but it may be difficult to establish clinically if the patient has received mediastinal radiation within the previous year. Neoplastic pericardial effusions develop over a long period of time and may become quite huge (more than 2 L). The ESR is high in post-MI or postcardiotomy pericarditis and can help confirm the diagnosis. Large pericardial effusions and accompanying pleural effusions are frequent. Myxedema pericardial effusions due to hypothyroidism usually are characterized by the presence of cholesterol crystals within the fluid.

C. Other Studies

The ECG usually shows generalized ST and T wave changes and may manifest a characteristic progression beginning with diffuse ST elevation, followed by a return to baseline and then to T-wave inversion. Atrial injury is often present and manifested by PR depression, especially in the limb leads. The chest radiograph is frequently normal but may show cardiac enlargement (if pericardial fluid is present), as well as signs of related pulmonary disease. Mass lesions and enlarged lymph nodes may suggest a neoplastic process. About 60% of patients have a pericardial effusion (usually mild) detectable by echocardiography. MRI and CT scan can visualize neighboring tumor in neoplastic pericarditis. A screening chest CT or MRI is often recommended to ensure there are no extracardiac diseases contiguous to the pericardium. A consensus statement from the American Society of Echocardiography proposes adding an elevated CRP and late gadolinium enhancement of the pericardium to confirmatory criteria for the diagnosis of pericarditis. There are data that the degree of quantitative delayed enhancement of the pericardium is associated with a higher rate of recurrent pericarditis. PET scanning can also be used to help define pericardial inflammation.

Treatment

For acute pericarditis, experts suggest a restriction in activity until symptom resolution. For athletes, the duration of exercise restriction should be until resolution of symptoms and normalization of all laboratory tests (generally 3 months). The 2015 ESC guidelines recommend aspirin 750–1000 mg every 8 hours for 1–2 weeks with a taper by decreasing the dose 250–500 mg every 1–2 weeks or ibuprofen 600 mg every 8 hours for 1–2 weeks with a taper by decreasing the dose by 200–400 mg every 1–2 weeks. Gastroprotection should be included. Studies support initial treatment of the acute episode with colchicine to prevent recurrences. Colchicine should be added to the NSAID at 0.5–0.6 mg once (for patients less than 70 kg) or twice (for patients more than 70 kg) daily and continued for at least 3 months. Tapering of colchicine is not mandatory; however, in the last week of treatment, the dosage can be reduced every other day for patients less than 70 kg or once a day for those more than 70 kg. Aspirin and colchicine should be used instead of NSAIDs in post-MI pericarditis (Dressler syndrome), since NSAIDs and corticosteroids may have an adverse effect on myocardial healing. Aspirin in doses of 750–1000 mg three times daily for 1–2 weeks plus 3 months of colchicine is the recommended treatment for Dressler syndrome. Despite initial treatment, recurrence has been reported in about 30%.

Colchicine should be used for at least 6 months as therapy in all refractory cases and in recurrent pericarditis. At times a longer duration of therapy is required. The CRP is used to assess the effectiveness of treatment, and once it is normalized, tapering is initiated. Indomethacin in doses of 25–50 mg every 8 hours can also be considered in recurrent pericarditis in place of ibuprofen. Systemic corticosteroids can be added in patients with severe symptoms, in refractory cases, or in patients with immune-mediated etiologies, but such therapy may entail a higher risk of recurrence and may actually prolong the illness. Colchicine is recommended in addition to corticosteroids, again for at least 3 months, to help prevent recurrences. Prednisone in doses of 0.25–0.5 mg/kg/day orally is generally suggested with tapering over a 4- to 6-week period. Recent studies have confirmed the advantage of adding anakinra, an interleukin-1 receptor antagonist, for the treatment of recurrent pericarditis, especially for corticosteroid-dependent and colchicine-resistant pericarditis.

As a rule, symptoms subside in several days to weeks. The major early complication is **tamponade,** which occurs in less than 5% of patients. There may be recurrences in the first few weeks or months. Rarely, when colchicine therapy alone fails or cannot be tolerated (usually due to GI symptoms), the pericarditis may require more significant immunosuppression, such as cyclophosphamide, azathioprine, intravenous human immunoglobulins, interleukin-1 receptor antagonists (anakinra), or methotrexate. If colchicine plus more significant immunosuppression fails, surgical pericardial stripping may be considered in recurrent cases even without clinical evidence for constrictive pericarditis.

Standard antituberculous medication therapy is usually successful for tuberculous pericarditis (see Chapter 9), but constrictive pericarditis can occur. Uremic pericarditis usually resolves with the institution of—or with more aggressive—dialysis. Tamponade is fairly common, and partial pericardiectomy (**pericardial window**) may be necessary. Whereas anti-inflammatory agents may relieve the pain and fever associated with uremic pericarditis, indomethacin and systemic corticosteroids do not affect its natural history. The prognosis with neoplastic effusion is poor, with only a small minority surviving 1 year. If it is compromising the clinical comfort of the patient, the effusion is initially drained percutaneously. Attempts at balloon pericardiotomy have been abandoned because outcomes were not more effective than simple drainage. A pericardial window, either by a subxiphoid approach or via video-assisted thoracic surgery, allows for partial pericardiectomy. Installation of chemotherapeutic agents or tetracycline may be used to reduce the recurrence rate. Symptomatic therapy is the initial approach to radiation pericarditis, but recurrent effusions and constriction often require surgery.

Prognosis

There are data that patients with acute pericarditis and any of the following criteria have the poorest prognosis: fever higher than 38°C, subacute onset, large effusion with or without tamponade, lack of response to anti-inflammatory medication after 1 week, myopericarditis, traumatic pericarditis, and those on oral anticoagulation. About 15% of patients have at least one of these high-risk findings.

When to Refer

Patients who do not respond initially to conservative management, who have recurrences, or who appear to be developing constrictive pericarditis should be referred to a cardiologist for further assessment.

Imazio M et al. Anakinra for corticosteroid-dependent and colchicine-resistant pericarditis. The IRAP (International Registry of Anakinra for Pericarditis) study. Eur J Prev Cardiol 2020;27:956. [PMID: 31610707]

PERICARDIAL EFFUSION & TAMPONADE

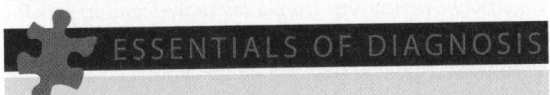

Pericardial effusion

- Clinical impact determined by the speed of accumulation.
- May or may not cause pain.

Tamponade

- Tachycardia with an elevated JVP and either hypotension or a paradoxical pulse.
- Low voltage or electrical alternans on ECG.
- Echocardiography is diagnostic.

Pericardial effusion can develop during any of the acute pericarditis processes. Because the pericardium covers the ascending aorta and arch, aortic dissection and/or rupture can lead to tamponade as well. The *speed of accumulation* determines the physiologic importance of the effusion. Because of pericardial stretch, effusions larger than 1000 mL that develop slowly may produce no hemodynamic effects. Conversely, smaller effusions that appear rapidly can cause tamponade due to the curvilinear relationship between the volume of fluid and the intrapericardial pressure. Tamponade is characterized by elevated intrapericardial pressure (greater than 15 mm Hg), which restricts venous return and ventricular filling. As a result, the stroke volume and arterial pulse pressure fall, and the heart rate and venous pressure rise. Shock and death may result.

Clinical Findings

A. Symptoms and Signs

Pericardial effusions may be associated with pain if they occur as part of an acute inflammatory process or may be painless, as is often the case with neoplastic or uremic effusion. Dyspnea and cough are common, especially with tamponade. Cardiac tamponade can be a life-threatening syndrome evidenced by tachycardia, hypotension, pulsus paradoxicus, raised JVP, muffled heart sounds, and decreased ECG voltage or electrical alternans. Other symptoms may result from the primary disease. The prognosis is a function of the cause. Large idiopathic chronic effusions (over 3 months) have a 30–35% risk of progression to cardiac tamponade.

A pericardial friction rub may be present even with large effusions. In cardiac tamponade, tachycardia, tachypnea, a narrow pulse pressure, and a relatively preserved systolic pressure are characteristic. **Pulsus paradoxus** is defined as a decline of greater than 10 mm Hg in systolic pressure during inspiration. Since the RV and LV share the same pericardium, when there is significant pericardial effusion, as the RV enlarges with inspiratory filling, septal motion toward the LV chamber reduces LV filling and results in an accentuated drop in the stroke volume and systemic BP with inspiration (the paradoxical pulse). Central venous pressure is elevated and, since the intrapericardial, and thus intracardiac, pressures are high even at the initiation of diastole, there is no evident *y* descent in the RA, RV, or LV hemodynamic tracings because the pericardial pressure prevents early ventricular filling. This differs from constriction where most of the initial filling of the RV and LV occurs during early diastole (rapid *y* descent), and it is only in mid to late diastole that the ventricles can no longer fill. In tamponade, ventricular filling is inhibited throughout diastole. Edema or ascites are rarely present in tamponade; these signs favor a more chronic process.

B. Laboratory Findings

Laboratory tests tend to reflect the underlying processes (see causes of pericarditis under General Considerations above).

C. Diagnostic Studies

Chest radiograph can suggest chronic effusion by an enlarged cardiac silhouette with a globular configuration but may appear normal in acute situations. The ECG often reveals nonspecific T wave changes and reduced QRS voltage. **Electrical alternans** is present only occasionally but is pathognomonic and is believed to be due to the heart swinging within the large effusion. Echocardiography is the primary method for demonstrating pericardial effusion and is quite sensitive. If tamponade is present, the high intrapericardial pressure may collapse lower pressure cardiac structures, such as the RA and RV. Cardiac CT and MRI also demonstrate pericardial fluid, pericardial thickening, and any associated contiguous lesions within the chest. Diagnostic pericardiocentesis or biopsy may be indicated for microbiologic and cytologic studies; a pericardial biopsy may be performed relatively simply through a small subxiphoid incision or by use of a video-assisted thoracoscopic surgical procedure. Unfortunately, the quality of the pericardial fluid itself rarely leads to a diagnosis, and any type of fluid (serous, serosanguinous, bloody, etc) can be seen in most diseases. Pericardial fluid analysis is most useful in excluding a bacterial cause and is occasionally helpful in malignancies. Effusions due to hypothyroidism or lymphatic obstruction may contain cholesterol or be chylous in nature, respectively.

Treatment

Small effusions can be followed clinically by careful observations of the JVP and by testing for a change in the paradoxical pulse. The most common cause of a paradoxical pulse is severe pulmonary disease, especially asthma, where marked changes in intrapleural pressures occur with inspiration and expiration. Serial echocardiograms are indicated if no intervention is immediately contemplated. Vasodilators and diuretics should be avoided. **When tamponade is present, urgent pericardiocentesis or cardiac surgery is required.** Because the pressure–volume relationship in the pericardial fluid is curvilinear and upsloping, removal of even a small amount of fluid often produces a dramatic fall in the intrapericardial pressure and immediate hemodynamic benefit; but complete drainage with a catheter is preferable. Continued or repeat drainage may be indicated, especially in malignant effusions. Pericardial windows via video-assisted thoracoscopy have been particularly effective in preventing recurrences when the underlying cause of the effusion continues to be present and are more effective than needle pericardiocentesis, subxiphoid surgical windows, or percutaneous balloon pericardiotomy. Effusions related to recurrent inflammatory pericarditis can be treated as noted above (see Acute Inflammatory Pericarditis). The presence of pericardial fluid in patients with pulmonary hypertension is a poor prognostic sign.

When to Refer

- Any unexplained pericardial effusion should be referred to a cardiologist.
- Trivial pericardial effusions are common, especially in heart failure, and need not be referred unless symptoms of pericarditis are evident.
- Hypotension or a paradoxical pulse suggesting the pericardial effusion is hemodynamically compromising the patient is a medical emergency and requires immediate drainage.
- Any echocardiographic signs of tamponade.

CONSTRICTIVE PERICARDITIS

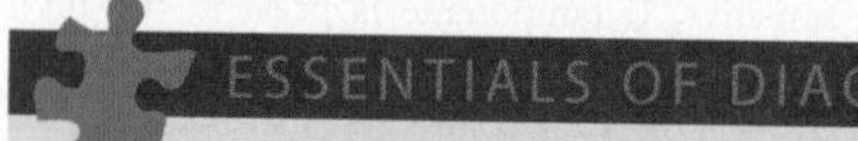

- Clinical evidence of right heart failure.
- No fall or an elevation of the JVP with inspiration (Kussmaul sign).
- Echocardiographic evidence for septal bounce and reduced mitral inflow velocities with inspiration.
- At times may be difficult to differentiate from restrictive cardiomyopathy.
- Cardiac catheterization may be necessary when clinical and echocardiographic features are equivocal.

General Considerations

Pericardial inflammation can lead to a thickened, fibrotic, adherent pericardium that restricts diastolic filling and produces chronically elevated venous pressures. In the past, tuberculosis was the most common cause of constrictive pericarditis, but while it remains so in underdeveloped countries, it is rare now in the rest of the world. Constrictive pericarditis rarely occurs following recurrent pericarditis. The risk of constrictive pericarditis due to viral or idiopathic pericarditis is less than 1%. Its occurrence increases following immune-mediated or neoplastic pericarditis (2–5%) and is highest after purulent bacterial pericarditis (20–30%). Other causes include post cardiac surgery, radiation therapy, and connective tissue disorders. A small number of cases are drug-induced or secondary to trauma, asbestosis, sarcoidosis, or uremia. At times, both pericardial tamponade and constrictive pericarditis may coexist, a condition referred to as **effusive-constrictive pericarditis**. The only definitive way to diagnose this condition is to reveal the underlying constrictive physiology once the pericardial fluid is drained. The differentiation of constrictive pericarditis from a restrictive cardiomyopathy may require cardiac catheterization and the utilization of all available noninvasive imaging methods.

Clinical Findings

A. Symptoms and Signs

The principal symptoms are slowly progressive dyspnea, fatigue, and weakness. Chronic edema, hepatic congestion, and ascites are usually present. Ascites often seems out of proportion to the degree of peripheral edema. The examination reveals these signs and a characteristically elevated jugular venous pressure with a rapid *y* descent. This can be detected at bedside by careful observation of the jugular pulse and noting an apparent increased pulse wave at the end of ventricular systole (due to the relative accentuation of the *v* wave by the rapid *y* descent). **Kussmaul sign**—a failure of the JVP to fall with inspiration—is also a frequent finding. The apex may actually retract with systole and a pericardial "knock" may be heard in early diastole. Pulsus paradoxus is unusual. Atrial fibrillation is common.

B. Diagnostic Studies

At times, constrictive pericarditis is extremely difficult to differentiate from restrictive cardiomyopathy and the two may coexist. When unclear, the use of both noninvasive testing and cardiac catheterization is required to sort out the difference.

1. Radiographic findings—The chest radiograph may show normal heart size or cardiomegaly. Pericardial calcification is best seen on the lateral view and is uncommon. It rarely involves the LV apex, and finding of calcification at the LV apex is more consistent with LV aneurysm.

2. Echocardiography—Echocardiography rarely demonstrates a thickened pericardium. A **septal "bounce"** reflecting the rapid early filling is common, though. RV/LV interaction may be demonstrated by an inspiratory reduction in the mitral inflow Doppler pattern of greater than 25%, much as in tamponade. Usually the initial mitral inflow into the LV is very rapid, and this can be demonstrated as well by the Doppler inflow (E wave) pattern. Other echocardiographic features, such as the ratio of the medial and lateral mitral annular motion (e' velocity), the respiration-related septal shift, and hepatic vein expiratory diastolic reversal ratio, also suggest constrictive physiology.

3. Cardiac CT and MRI—These imaging tests are only occasionally helpful. Pericardial thickening of more than 4 mm must be present to establish the diagnosis, but no pericardial thickening is demonstrable in 20–25% of patients with constrictive pericarditis. Some MRI techniques demonstrate the septal bounce and can provide further evidence for ventricular interaction.

4. Cardiac catheterization—This procedure is often confirmatory or can be diagnostic in difficult cases where the echocardiographic features are unclear or mixed. As a generality, the pulmonary pressure is low in constriction (as opposed to restrictive cardiomyopathy). In constrictive pericarditis, because of the need to demonstrate RV/LV interaction, cardiac catheterization should include simultaneous measurement of both the LV and RV pressure tracings with inspiration and expiration. This interaction can be demonstrated by cardiac MRI. Hemodynamically, patients with constriction have equalization of end-diastolic pressures throughout their cardiac chambers, there is rapid early filling then an abrupt increase in diastolic pressure (**"square-root" sign**), the RV end-diastolic pressure is more than one-third the systolic pressure, simultaneous measurements of RV and LV systolic pressure reveal a discordance with inspiration (the RV rises as the LV falls), and there is usually a Kussmaul sign (failure of the RA pressure to fall with inspiration). In restrictive cardiomyopathy, there is concordance of RV and LV systolic pressures with inspiration.

Treatment

Therapy should be aimed at the specific etiology initially. If there is laboratory evidence of ongoing inflammation, then anti-inflammatory medications may have a role. Once the hemodynamics are evident, the mainstay of treatment is diuresis. As in other disorders of right heart failure, the diuresis should be aggressive, using loop diuretics (oral torsemide or bumetanide if bowel edema is suspected or intravenous furosemide), thiazides, and aldosterone antagonists (especially in the presence of ascites and liver congestion). Surgical pericardiectomy should be recommended when diuretics are unable to control symptoms. Pericardiectomy removes only the pericardium between the phrenic nerve pathways, however, and most patients still require diuretics after the procedure, though symptoms are usually dramatically improved. Morbidity and mortality after pericardiectomy are high (up to 15%) and are greatest in those with the most disability prior to the procedure. Poor prognostic predictors include prior radiation, kidney dysfunction, higher pulmonary systolic pressures, abnormal LV systolic function, a lower serum sodium level, liver dysfunction, and older age. Pericardial calcium has no impact on survival.

When to Refer

If the diagnosis of constrictive pericarditis is unclear or the symptoms of fluid retention resist medical therapy, then referral to a cardiologist is warranted to both establish the diagnosis and recommend therapy.

Anasari-Gilani K et al. Multimodality approach to the diagnosis and management of constrictive pericarditis. Echocardiography. 2020;30:632. [PMID: 32240548]

Goldstein JA et al. Hemodynamics of constrictive pericarditis and restrictive cardiomyopathy. Catheter Cardiovasc Interv. 2020;95:1240. [PMID: 31904891]

PULMONARY HYPERTENSION

ESSENTIALS OF DIAGNOSIS

- Mean PA pressure ≥ 25 mm Hg.
- Dyspnea and often cyanosis.
- Enlarged pulmonary arteries on chest radiograph.
- Elevated JVP and RV heave.
- Echocardiography is often diagnostic.

General Considerations

The normal pulmonary bed offers about one-tenth as much resistance to blood flow as the systemic arterial system. Based on the 2019 Sixth World Symposium on Pulmonary Hypertension, the definition of pulmonary hypertension was changed. It was defined by a mean PA pressure of 20 mm Hg with a pulmonary vascular resistance of greater than or equal to 3 Wood units. Three categories were then defined:

1. Precapillary pulmonary hypertension: mean pulmonary artery pressure greater than 20 mm Hg, PVR greater than or equal to 3.0 Wood units, PCWP less than or equal to 15 mm Hg
2. Isolated post-capillary pulmonary hypertension: mean pulmonary artery pressure greater than 20 mm Hg, PVR less than 3.0 Wood units, PCWP greater than 15 mm Hg
3. Combined pre- and post-pulmonary hypertension: mean pulmonary artery pressure greater than 20 mm Hg, PVR greater than or equal to 3.0 Wood units, PCWP greater than 15 mm Hg

The clinical classification of pulmonary hypertension by the Sixth World Symposium on Pulmonary Hypertension is outlined in Table 10–17.

Group I includes **pulmonary arterial hypertension (PAH)** related to an underlying pulmonary vasculopathy. It includes the former "primary pulmonary hypertension" under the term "idiopathic pulmonary hypertension" and is defined as pulmonary hypertension and elevated PVR in the absence of other disease of the lungs or heart. Its cause

Table 10–17. Updated classification of pulmonary hypertension (PH).

Pulmonary arterial hypertension (PAH)
Idiopathic PAH
Heritable PAH
Drug- and toxin-induced PAH
PAH associated with connective tissue disease, HIV infection, portal hypertension, congenital heart disease, schistosomiasis
PAH long-term responders to calcium channel blockers
PAH with overt features of venous/capillaries (PVOD/PCH) involvement
Persistent PH of the newborn syndrome
PH due to left heart disease
Due to heart failure with preserved LVEF
Due to heart failure with reduced LVEF
Valvular heart disease
Congenital/acquired cardiovascular conditions leading to post-capillary pulmonary hypertension
PH due to lung diseases or hypoxia (or both)
Obstructive lung disease
Restrictive lung disease
Other lung disease with mixed obstructive/restrictive pattern
Hypoxia without lung disease
Developmental lung disorders
PH due to pulmonary artery obstructions
Chronic thromboembolic pulmonary hypertension
Other pulmonary artery obstructions
PH with unclear or multifactorial mechanisms
Hematologic disorders
Systemic and metabolic disorders
Others
Complex congenital heart disease

PVOD/PCH, pulmonary veno-occlusive disease/ pulmonary capillary hemangiomatosis.

Reproduced with permission of the © ERS 2022: European Respiratory Journal 53 (1) 1801913; DOI: 10.1183/13993003.01913-2018. Published 24 January 2019.

is unknown. About 6–10% have heritable PAH. Drug and toxic pulmonary hypertension have been described as associated with the use of anorexigenic agents that increase serotonin release and block its uptake. These include aminorex fumarate, fenfluramine, and dexfenfluramine. In some cases, there is epidemiologic linkage to ingestion of rapeseed oil or L-tryptophan and use of recreational drugs, such as amphetamines and cocaine. Pulmonary hypertension associated with connective tissue disease includes cases associated with systemic sclerosis—up to 8–12% of patients with systemic sclerosis may be affected. Pulmonary hypertension has also been associated with HIV infection, portal hypertension, congenital heart disease (Eisenmenger syndrome), schistosomiasis, and chronic hemolytic anemia (eg, sickle cell anemia). In rare instances, obstruction of the pulmonary venous circulation may occur (pulmonary veno-occlusive disease and capillary hemangiomatosis).

Group II includes all cases related to left heart disease. **Group III** includes cases due to parenchymal lung disease, impaired control of breathing, or living at high altitude. This group encompasses those with idiopathic pulmonary fibrosis and COPD. **Group IV** represents patients with chronic thromboembolic disease or other pulmonary artery obstruction. **Group V** includes multifactorial causes such as hematologic, systemic, and metabolic disorders.

Clinical Findings

A. Symptoms and Signs

Common to all is exertional dyspnea, chest pain, fatigue, and lightheadedness as early symptoms; later symptoms include syncope, abdominal distention, ascites, and peripheral edema as RV function worsens. Chronic lung disease, especially sleep apnea, often is overlooked as a cause for pulmonary hypertension as is chronic thromboembolic disease. Patients with idiopathic pulmonary hypertension are characteristically young women who have evidence of right heart failure that is usually progressive, leading to death in 2–8 years without therapy. This is a decidedly different prognosis than patients with Eisenmenger physiology due to a left-to-right shunt; 40% of patients with Eisenmenger physiology are alive 25 years after the diagnosis has been made. Patients have manifestations of low cardiac output, with weakness and fatigue, as well as edema and ascites as right heart failure advances. Peripheral cyanosis is present, and syncope on effort may occur.

B. Diagnostic Studies

The ESC and European Respiratory Society updated guidelines for the diagnosis and treatment of pulmonary hypertension in 2019. All patients with a high risk for PAH should undergo *confirmatory right heart catheterization.*

The laboratory evaluation of idiopathic pulmonary hypertension must exclude a secondary cause. A hypercoagulable state should be sought by measuring protein C and S levels, the presence of a lupus anticoagulant, the level of factor V Leiden, prothrombin gene mutations, and D-dimer. Chronic pulmonary emboli must be excluded (usually by ventilation-perfusion lung scan or contrast spiral CT); the ventilation-perfusion scan is the more sensitive test but not specific. If it is normal, then chronic thromboembolic pulmonary hypertension is very unlikely. The chest radiograph helps exclude a primary pulmonary etiology—evidence for patchy pulmonary edema may raise the suspicion of pulmonary veno-occlusive disease due to localized obstruction in pulmonary venous drainage. A sleep study may be warranted if sleep apnea is suspected. The ECG is generally consistent with RVH and RA enlargement. Echocardiography with Doppler helps exclude an intracardiac shunt and usually demonstrates an enlarged RV and RA—at times they may be huge and hypocontractile. Severe pulmonic or tricuspid valve regurgitation may be present. Interventricular septal flattening seen on the echocardiogram is consistent with pulmonary hypertension. Doppler interrogation of the tricuspid regurgitation jet provides an estimate of RV systolic pressure. Pulmonary function tests help exclude other disorders, though primary pulmonary hypertension may present with only a reduced carbon monoxide diffusing capacity of the lung (DL_{CO}) or severe desaturation (particularly if a

PFO has been stretched open and a right-to-left shunt is present). A declining DL_{CO} may precede the development of pulmonary hypertension in a patient with systemic sclerosis. Chest CT demonstrates enlarged pulmonary arteries and excludes other causes (such as emphysema or interstitial lung disease). Pulmonary angiography (or magnetic resonance angiography or CT angiography) reveals loss of the smaller acinar pulmonary vessels and tapering of the larger ones. Catheterization allows measurement of pulmonary pressures and testing for vasoreactivity using a variety of agents, but **nitric oxide** is the preferred testing agent due to its ease of use and short half-life. A positive response is defined as one that decreases the pulmonary mean pressure by greater than 10 mm Hg, with the final mean PA pressure less than 40 mm Hg. Abdominal ultrasound is recommended to exclude portal hypertension. A lung biopsy is no longer suggested as relevant for the diagnosis.

Treatment & Prognosis

The treatment of PAH continues to evolve and depends on the etiology. For group I patients with a normal PCWP, treatment is related to the response to nitric oxide challenge with those responsive being initially treated with calcium channel blockers. The vast majority of patients, unfortunately, do not respond to the acute vasoreactivity testing. Specific PAH therapy is therefore recommended in this situation. This begins with monotherapy but expands to the use of sequential medication therapy when pulmonary pressures are not improved. In critically ill hypotensive patients inotropic support may be required and eventually lung transplantation considered. Balloon atrial septostomy is considered a IIb recommendation (on the notion that increased right-to-left shunting will improve cardiac output), but it is very rarely utilized.

Medication monotherapy varies in effectiveness depending on the etiologic classification. Only those in class I who respond to nitric oxide should get calcium channel blockers. The current medication therapies include endothelin-receptor blockers (ambrisentan, bosentan, macitentan), phosphodiesterase type-5 inhibitors (sildenafil, tadalafil, and vardenafil), a guanylate cyclase stimulator (riociquat), prostanoids (epoprostenol, iloprost, teprostinil, and beraprost), and an IP-receptor agonist (selexipag). Various medication combinations have been approved and, when ineffective, sequential medication therapies may be used. Many medications interfere with HIV treatment, and this needs to be assessed if relevant. Due to inherent lung disease or left heart disease, there are no therapies that are specific to PAH. Bosentan, an endothelin receptor blocker, has received a class I indication for patients with Eisenmenger syndrome. Anticoagulation is often recommended and is required lifelong in chronic thromboembolic pulmonary hypertension. The number of patients with inoperable chronic thromboembolic pulmonary hypertension being treated with balloon pulmonary angioplasty has increased dramatically since favorable results have been reported. Riociguat remains the only approved medical therapy for chronic thromboembolic pulmonary hypertension patients in this latter group.

Counseling and patient education are also important. Aerobic exercise is recommended but no heavy physical exertion or isometric exercise. Routine immunizations are advised. Pregnancy should be strongly discouraged and preventive measures taken to ensure it does not occur. Maternal mortality in severe PAH may be up to 50%.

Warfarin anticoagulation is recommended in all patients with idiopathic PAH and no contraindication. Diuretics are useful for the management of right-sided heart failure; clinical experience suggests loop diuretics (torsemide or bumetanide, which are absorbed even if bowel edema is present) plus spironolactone are preferable. Oxygen should be used to maintain oxygen saturation greater than 90%. Acute vasodilator testing (generally with nitric oxide) should be performed in all patients with idiopathic PAH who may be potential candidates for long-term therapy with calcium channel blockers. Patients with PAH caused by conditions other than idiopathic PAH respond poorly to oral calcium channel blockers, and there is little value of acute vasodilator testing in these patients.

When to Refer

All patients with suspected pulmonary hypertension should be referred to either a cardiologist or pulmonologist who specializes in pulmonary hypertension.

Frost A et al. Diagnosis of pulmonary hypertension. Eur Respir J. 2019;53:1801904. [PMID: 30545972]

Galiè N et al. An overview of the 6th World Symposium on Pulmonary Hypertension. Eur Respir J. 2019;53:1802148. [PMID: 30552088]

Kataoka M et al. Balloon pulmonary angioplasty (percutaneous transluminal pulmonary angioplasty) for chronic thromboembolic pulmonary hypertension: a Japanese perspective. JACC Cardiovasc Interv. 2019;12:1382. [PMID: 31103538]

Simonneau G et al. Haemodynamic definitions and updated clinical classification of pulmonary hypertension. Eur Respir J. 2019;53:1801913. [PMID: 30545968]

NEOPLASTIC DISEASES OF THE HEART

PRIMARY CARDIAC TUMORS

Primary cardiac tumors are rare and constitute only a small fraction of all tumors that involve the heart or pericardium. The most common primary tumor is **atrial myxoma**; it comprises about 50% of all tumors in adult case series. It is generally attached to the atrial septum and is more likely to grow on the LA side of the septum rather than the RA. Patients with myxoma can rarely present with the characteristics of a systemic illness, with obstruction of blood flow at the mitral valve level, or with signs of peripheral embolization. The syndrome includes fever, malaise, weight loss, leukocytosis, elevated ESR, and emboli (peripheral or pulmonary, depending on the location of the tumor). This is sometimes confused with infective endocarditis, lymphoma, other cancers, or autoimmune diseases. In most cases, the tumor may grow to considerable size and produce symptoms by simply obstructing mitral inflow. Episodic pulmonary edema (classically occurring when an upright posture is assumed) and signs of low output may result. Physical examination may reveal a diastolic sound related to motion of the tumor ("tumor plop") or a diastolic murmur similar to that of mitral stenosis. Right-sided myxomas may cause symptoms of right-sided failure. Familial myxomas occur as part of the Carney complex, which consists of myxomas, pigmented skin lesions, and endocrine neoplasia.

The diagnosis of atrial myxoma is established by echocardiography or by pathologic study of embolic material. Cardiac MRI is useful as an adjunct. Contrast angiography is frequently unnecessary, although it may demonstrate a "tumor blush" when the mass is vascular. Surgical excision is usually curative, though recurrences do occur and serial echocardiographic follow-up is recommended.

The second most common primary cardiac tumors are **valvular papillary fibroelastomas** and **atrial septal lipomas.** These tend to be benign and usually require no therapy. Papillary fibroelastomas are usually on the pulmonary or aortic valves, may embolize or cause valvular dysfunction, and should be removed if large and mobile. Other primary cardiac tumors include rhabdomyomas (that often appear multiple in both the RV and LV), fibrous histiocytomas, hemangiomas, and a variety of unusual sarcomas. Some sarcomas may be of considerable size before discovery. Primary pericardial tumors, such as mesotheliomas related to asbestos exposure, may also occur. The diagnosis may be supported by an abnormal cardiac contour on radiograph. Echocardiography is usually helpful but may miss tumors infiltrating the ventricular wall. Cardiac MRI is the diagnostic procedure of choice along with gated CT imaging for all cardiac tumors.

SECONDARY CARDIAC TUMORS

Metastases from malignant tumors can also affect the heart. Most often this occurs in malignant melanoma, but other tumors that are known to metastasize to the heart include bronchogenic carcinoma; carcinoma of the breast; lymphoma; renal cell carcinoma; sarcomas; and, in patients with AIDS, Kaposi sarcoma. These are often clinically silent but may lead to pericardial tamponade, arrhythmias and conduction disturbances, heart failure, and peripheral emboli. The ECG may reveal regional Q waves. The diagnosis is often made by echocardiography, but cardiac MRI and CT scanning can often better delineate the extent of involvement. Metastatic tumors, especially lung or breast, may invade the pericardium and result in very large pericardial effusions as they result in slow accumulation of fluid. The prognosis is poor for all secondary cardiac tumors and treatment is generally palliative. On occasion, surgical resection for debulking or removal and chemotherapy may be effective in relieving symptoms.

Treatment

Many primary tumors may be resectable. Atrial myxomas should be removed surgically due to the high incidence of embolization from these friable tumors. Recurrences require lifelong monitoring with echocardiography. Papillary fibroelastomas are usually benign but they should be removed if they appear mobile and are larger than 10 mm in size or if there is evidence of embolization at the time of discovery. Large pericardial effusions from metastatic tumors may be drained for comfort, but the fluid invariably recurs. Rhabdomyomas may be surgically cured if the tumor is accessible and can be removed while still leaving enough functioning myocardium intact.

When to Refer

All patients with suspected cardiac tumors should be referred to a cardiologist or cardiac surgeon for evaluation and possible therapy.

Rahouma M et al. Cardiac tumors prevalence and mortality: a systematic review and meta-analysis. Int J Surg. 2020;76:178. [PMID: 32169566]

TRAUMATIC HEART DISEASE

Trauma is the leading cause of death in patients aged 1–44 years; cardiac and vascular trauma is second only to neurologic injury as the reason for these deaths. Penetrating wounds to the heart are often lethal unless immediately surgically repaired. In a 20-year review of penetrating trauma at a single institution, it was found that gunshot wounds were fatal 13 times more often than stab wounds and that factors such as hypotension, Glasgow Coma Score less than 8, Revised Trauma Score less than 7.84, associated injuries, and the more severe the injuries (Injury Severity Score greater than 25) all added to the mortality and morbidity risk.

Blunt trauma is a more frequent cause of cardiac injuries. This type of injury is common in motor vehicle accidents and may occur with any form of chest trauma, including CPR efforts. The most common injuries are myocardial contusions or hematomas. The RV is particularly prone to contusion as it sits directly under the sternum. Other forms of nonischemic cardiac injury include metabolic injury due to burns, electrical current, or sepsis. These may be asymptomatic (particularly in the setting of more severe injuries) or may present with chest pain of a nonspecific nature or, not uncommonly, with a pericardial component. Elevations of cardiac enzymes are frequent, and can be quite high, but the levels do not correlate with prognosis. There are some data that the presence of certain other cardiac biomarkers, such as NT-proBNP, correlate better with significant myocardial injury. Echocardiography may reveal an akinetic myocardial segment or pericardial effusion. Cardiac MRI may also suggest acute injury. Coronary CT angiography or angiography can reveal a coronary dissection or acute occlusion if that is a concern. Pericardiocentesis is warranted if tamponade is evident. As noted above, tako-tsubo transient segmental myocardial dysfunction can occur due to the accompanying stress.

Severe trauma may also cause myocardial or valvular rupture. Cardiac rupture can involve any chamber, but survival is most likely if injury is to one of the atria or the RV. Hemopericardium or pericardial tamponade is the usual clinical presentation, and surgery is almost always necessary. Mitral and aortic valve rupture may occur during severe blunt trauma—the former presumably if the impact occurs during systole and the latter if during diastole. Patients reach the hospital in shock or severe heart failure. Immediate surgical repair is essential. The same types of injuries may result in transection of the aorta, either at the level of the arch or distal to the takeoff of the left subclavian artery at the ligamentum arteriosum. Transthoracic echocardiography and TEE are the most helpful and immediately available diagnostic techniques. CT and MRI may also be required to better define the injury before surgical intervention.

Blunt trauma may also result in damage to the coronary arteries. Acute or subacute coronary thrombosis is the most common presentation. The clinical syndrome is one of acute MI with attendant ECG, enzymatic, and contractile abnormalities. Emergent revascularization is sometimes feasible, either by the percutaneous route or by coronary artery bypass surgery. LV aneurysms are common outcomes of traumatic coronary occlusions, likely due to sudden occlusion with no collateral vascular support. Coronary artery dissection or rupture may also occur in the setting of blunt cardiac trauma.

As expected, patients with severe preexisting conditions fare the least well after cardiac trauma. Data from ReCONECT, a trauma consortium, reveal that mortality is linked to volume of cases seen at various centers, preexisting coronary disease or heart failure, intubation, age, and a severity scoring index.

Qamar SR et al. State of the art imaging review of blunt and penetrating cardiac trauma. Can Assoc Radiol J. 2020;71:301. [PMID: 32066272]

Schellenberg M et al. Critical decisions in the management of thoracic trauma. Emerg Med Clin North Am. 2018;36:135. [PMID: 29132573]

HEART DISEASE & PREGNANCY

General principles to discuss with the patient include preconceptual counseling, pregnancy risk assessment, genetic risks, environmental risks, and pregnancy management. For some patients, it may also include a discussion regarding contraception, termination of a pregnancy, and a conversation about not only the delivery but what will happen post-pregnancy (including issues such as an eventual need for heart surgery or transplantation). In a review of 1315 pregnancies in patients with heart disease, 3.6% had serious cardiovascular complications and half were found to be preventable. Two-thirds of the complications occurred in the antepartum period. Adverse fetal and neonatal events, as expected, were much more common in those pregnancies with cardiovascular events.

The **Cardiac Disease in Pregnancy Investigation (CARPREG I)** scoring system for risk from cardiac events for women with heart disease noted four major risk factors: (1) NYHA FC III or IV heart failure, (2) prior cardiac events, (3) mitral or aortic obstruction, and (4) LVEF less than 40%. One point is assigned to each. Patients with no points had a 5% risk, those with 1 point had a complication rate of 27%, while for those with 2 or more points, the risk was 74%. Other reviews have suggested that the major risk for adverse outcomes or death to either the mother or fetus include pulmonary hypertension (with pulmonary pressure greater than three-quarters of systemic pressure), maternal cyanosis, systemic ventricular dysfunction, poor maternal functional class, severe left-sided valvular obstruction, aortic coarctation, significantly dilated aortic root, significant unrepaired heart defects, and warfarin therapy in patients with mechanical valves. In 2018, this group reported the results from a follow-up study (CARPREG II). Cardiac complications occurred in 16% of pregnancies and were primarily related to arrhythmias and heart failure. Although the overall rates of cardiac complications during pregnancy did not change over the years, the frequency of pulmonary edema decreased (8% from 1994 to 2001 vs. 4% from 2001 to 2014). Ten predictors of maternal cardiac complications were identified: five general predictors (prior cardiac events or arrhythmias, poor functional class or cyanosis, high-risk valve disease/LV outflow tract obstruction, systemic ventricular dysfunction, no prior cardiac interventions); four lesion-specific predictors (mechanical valves, high-risk aortopathies, pulmonary hypertension, CAD); and one delivery of care predictor (late pregnancy assessment). These 10 predictors were incorporated into a new risk index **(CARPREG II)** shown in Figure 10–11.

The World Health Organization offers guidelines for the management of pregnancy in patients with congenital heart disease. This 2011 guideline also outlines risks to the fetus. Table 10–18 summarizes the observations and recommendations. Medication usage during pregnancy is always a difficult decision since *most have not been studied*. ACE inhibitors and amiodarone are contraindicated. Beta-blockers (including labetalol, metoprolol, and sotalol), digoxin, and calcium channel blockers are generally well tolerated (especially nifedipine, amlodipine, or verapamil, although there is controversy with diltiazem). There are concerns about the use of atenolol and premature birth, and it should not be used. Labetalol has been found to be particularly useful for treating hypertension as has methyldopa (though this is rarely used). Diuretics can generally be given safely. Pregnancy is a hypercoagulable state; the use of warfarin is discussed above under valvular disease and congenital heart disease, but fundamentally the risk is dose related (not INR related) and warfarin can be used during the first trimester if the dose is 5 mg or less. For many patients, the most common potential complication is an atrial arrhythmia or systemic hypertension (systemic BP greater than 140/90 mm Hg). Patients should be hospitalized if BP exceeds 170/110 mm Hg.

Patients with adult congenital heart disease are at risk not only for cardiovascular events but also for obstetric events such as hypertension, preeclampsia, placenta previa or abruption, and early delivery.

Pfaller B et al. Preventing complications in pregnant women with cardiac disease. J Am Coll Cardiol. 2020;75:1443. [PMID: 32216913]

Schlichting LE et al. Maternal comorbidities and complications of delivery in pregnant women with congenital heart disease. J Am Coll Cardiol. 2019;73:2181. [PMID: 31047006]

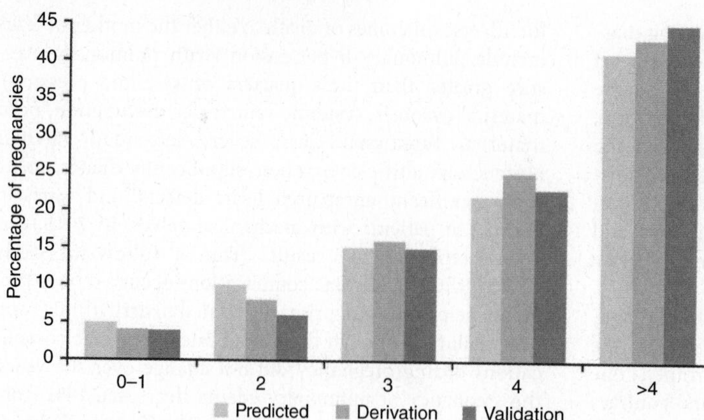

PREDICTOR	POINTS
Prior cardiac events or arrhythmias	3
Baseline NYHA III-IV or cyanosis	3
Mechanical valve	3
Ventricular dysfunction	2
High-risk left-sided valve disease/ left ventricular outflow tract obstruction	2
Pulmonary hypertension	2
Coronary artery disease	2
High-risk aortopathy	2
No prior cardiac intervention	1
Late pregnancy assessment	1

▲ **Figure 10–11.** Risk index for material cardiac complications in pregnancy (CARPREG II). The risk index is divided into five categories based on the sum of the points for a given pregnancy: 0 to 1 point; 2 points; 3 points; 4 points; and > 4 points. The predicted risks for primary cardiac events stratified according to point score were 0 to 1 point (5%), 2 points (10%), 3 points (15%), 4 points (22%), and > 4 points (41%). NYHA, New York Heart Association. (Reproduced with permission from Silversides CK, Grewal J, Mason J, et al. Pregnancy outcomes in women with heart disease: the CARPREG II Study. J Am Coll Cardiol. 2018;71(21):2419–2430.)

CARDIOVASCULAR COMPLICATIONS OF PREGNANCY

Pregnancy-related hypertension (eclampsia and preeclampsia) is discussed in Chapter 19.

1. Cardiomyopathy of Pregnancy (Peripartum Cardiomyopathy)

In approximately 1 in 3000 to 4000 live births, dilated cardiomyopathy develops in the mother in the final month of pregnancy or within 6 months after delivery. Risk factors include preeclampsia, twin pregnancies, and African ethnicity. The cause is slowly being elucidated. The vasculo-hormonal hypothesis requires two events. One is genetic, a reduction in a STAT3 transcription factor that results in cleavage of prolactin from the pituitary by cathepsin D. This results in a 16-kd fragment that increases microRNA 146a that results in myocardial apoptosis. The second is from the placenta, soluble tyrosine kinase that blocks VEGF (vascular endothelial growth factor). It appears both components may be necessary to effectively result in peripartum cardiomyopathy. The course of the disease is variable; most cases improve or resolve completely over several months, but others progress to refractory heart failure. About 60% of patients make a complete recovery. Serum BNP levels are routinely elevated in pregnancy, but serial values may be useful in predicting who may be at increased risk for a worse outcome. Beta-blockers have been administered judiciously to these patients, with at least anecdotal success. Diuretics, hydralazine, and nitrates help treat the heart failure with minimal risk to the fetus. Sotalol is acceptable for ventricular or atrial arrhythmias if other beta-blockers are ineffective. Some experts advocate anticoagulation because of an increased risk of thrombotic events, and both warfarin and heparin have their proponents. In severe cases, transient use of extracorporeal membrane oxygenation (ECMO) has been lifesaving. Recurrence in subsequent pregnancies is common, particularly if cardiac function has not completely recovered, and subsequent pregnancies are to be discouraged if the EF remains less than 55%. The risk of recurrent heart failure in a subsequent pregnancy has been estimated to be 21%. Delivery of the baby is important, though the peak incidence of the problem is in the first week after delivery and a few cases appear up to 5 weeks after delivery. Since the anti-angiogenic cleaved prolactin fragment is considered causal for peripartum cardiomyopathy, bromocriptine (a prolactin release inhibitor) has been reported to be beneficial. A multicenter trial in Europe found LVEF improved to a greater extent in patients with peripartum cardiomyopathy who were given bromocriptine than those who were not given bromocriptine. In addition, bromocriptine treatment was associated with high rate of full LV recovery and low morbidity and mortality in peripartum cardiomyopathy patients compared with other peripartum cardiomyopathy cohorts not treated with bromocriptine.

For a complete review of the current issues surrounding peripartum cardiomyopathy, the reader is referred to the state-of-art article noted below.

Davis MB et al. Peripartum cardiomyopathy: JACC State-of-the-Art Review. J Am Coll Cardiol. 2020;75:207. [PMID: 31948651]
Honigberg MC et al. Peripartum cardiomyopathy. BMJ. 2019;364:k5287. [PMID: 30700415]

2. Coronary Artery & Aortic Vascular Abnormalities During Pregnancy

An acute coronary syndrome occurs in 2.8–8.1 per 1,000,000 pregnancies. Many are women over 35 years. It is known that pregnancy predisposes to dissection of the aorta

Table 10–18. Management strategies for women with valve disease, complex congenital heart disease, pulmonary hypertension, aortopathy, and dilated cardiomyopathy.

High-Risk Heart Disease in Pregnancy
- Preconception counseling and pregnancy risk stratification for all women with high-risk heart disease of childbearing age
- In women considering pregnancy: Switch to safer cardiac medications and emphasize importance of close monitoring
- In women avoiding pregnancy: Discuss safe and effective contraception choices or termination in early pregnancy

Disease	Management Strategy		
	Pregnancy Not Advised	Pregnancy Management	Delivery
Valve disease	• Severe mitral and aortic valve disease • Mechanical prosthetic valves if effective anticoagulation not possible	• Close follow-up • Medication therapy for heart failure or arrhythmias • Balloon valvuloplasty or surgical valve replacement in refractory cases	• Vaginal delivery preferred • C-section in case of fetal or maternal instability • Early delivery for clinical and hemodynamic deterioration • Consider hemodynamic monitoring during labor and delivery
Complex congenital heart disease	• Significant ventricular dysfunction • Severe AV valve dysfunction • Falling Fontan circulation • Oxygen saturation < 85%	• Close follow-up	• Vaginal delivery preferred • C-section in case of fetal or maternal instability • Consider hemodynamic monitoring during labor and delivery
Pulmonary hypertension	• Established pulmonary arterial hypertension	• Close follow-up • Early institution of pulmonary vasodilators	• Vaginal delivery preferred • C-section in case of fetal or maternal instability • Timing of delivery depends on clinical and RV function • Early delivery advisable • Diuresis after delivery to prevent RV volume overload • Extended hospital stay after delivery
Aortopathy	*For some women—* • Marfan syndrome • Bicuspid aortic valve • Turner syndrome • Rapid growth of aortic diameter or family history of premature aortic dissection	• Treat hypertension • Beta-blockers to reduce heart rate • Frequent echocardiographic assessment • Surgery during pregnancy or after C-section if large increase in aortic diameter	• C-section in cases of significant aortic dilation – Marfan syndrome > 40 mm – Bicuspid aortic valve > 45 mm – Turner syndrome: aortic size index > 20 mm/m^2
Dilated cardiomyopathy	• LVEF < 40% • History of peripartum cardiomyopathy	• Close follow-up • Beta-blockers • Diuretic agents for volume overload • Vasodilators for hemodynamic and symptomatic improvement	• Vaginal delivery preferred • C-section in case of fetal or maternal instability • Consider hemodynamic monitoring during labor and delivery • Early delivery for clinical and hemodynamic deterioration

AV, atrioventricular; C-section, cesarean section; RV, right ventricular.
Reproduced with permission from Elkayam U et al. High-risk cardiac disease in pregnancy: Part I. J Am Coll Cardiol. 2016;68(4):396–410.

and other arteries, perhaps because of the accompanying connective tissue changes. The risks are particularly high in patients with Marfan, Ehlers-Danlos, or Loeys-Dietz syndromes. The risk is highest in the third trimester, and coronary dissection, thrombosis, and atherosclerosis have about equal prevalence. The most frequent cause in one study was coronary dissection, and it has a peak incidence in the early postpartum period. Paradoxical emboli through a PFO to the coronary arteries have been implicated in a few instances. Clinical management is essentially similar to that of other patients with acute infarction, unless there is a connective tissue disorder. If nonatherosclerotic dissection is present, coronary intervention may be risky, as further dissection can be aggravated. In most instances, conservative management is warranted. At times, extensive aortic dissection requires surgical intervention. Marfan patients are particularly susceptible to further aortic expansion during pregnancy when the aortic diameter is more than 4.5 cm (greater or equal to 27 mm/m^2), and pregnancy should be discouraged in these situations. Some data, however, suggest that there is an increased risk of dissection during pregnancy even when the elective repair is reasonable (ie, when the aortic root is greater than 4.0 cm in women with Marfan syndrome contemplating pregnancy). Acute infarction during pregnancy is associated with an 8% maternal mortality and 56% incidence of premature delivery. If PCI is required, it is now recommended that a drug-eluting stent be considered rather than a bare metal stent. Medications that appear to be safe during pregnancy include aspirin, beta-blockers, clopidogrel, heparin or enoxaparin, and nitrates. Medications that are not safe include aldosterone inhibitors, ACE inhibitors or ARBs, DOACs, and statins. If need be, fibrinolytics, GP IIb/IIIa inhibitors, bivalirudin, and calcium channel blockers can be used.

Tweet MS et al. Pregnancy-associated myocardial infarction: prevalence, causes, and interventional management. Circ Cardiovasc Interv. 2020 Aug 1. [Epub ahead of print] [PMID: 32862672]

3. Management of Labor

Although vaginal delivery is usually well tolerated, unstable patients (including patients with severe hypertension and worsening heart failure) should have planned cesarean section. Spinal anesthesia results in a large drop in the systemic vascular resistance and can worsen right-to-left shunting. An increased risk of aortic rupture has been noted during delivery in patients with coarctation of the aorta and severe aortic root dilation with Marfan syndrome, and vaginal delivery should be avoided in these patients. For most patients, even those with complex congenital heart disease, vaginal delivery is the preferred method, however. Immediately following delivery, there are numerous fluid shifts that occur with the initial blood loss, reducing preload and accompanied by the loss of afterload reduction that had been provided by the placenta. Quickly, however, venous return increases as the uterus is no longer compressing the inferior vena cava and there is an infusion of fluid into the vascular system as the uterus quickly shrinks back toward its normal size. The sudden increase in preload and loss of afterload following delivery can result in heart failure during the first 48–72 hours after the delivery and that remains the high-risk time for susceptible patients.

CARDIOVASCULAR SCREENING OF ATHLETES

The sudden death of a competitive athlete inevitably becomes an occasion for local, if not national, publicity. On each occasion, the public and the medical community ask whether such events could be prevented by more careful or complete screening. Although each event is tragic, it must be appreciated that there are approximately 5 million competitive athletes at the high school level or above in any given year in the United States. The number of cardiac deaths occurring during athletic participation is unknown but estimates at the high school level range from one in 100,000 to one in 300,000 participants. Death rates among more mature athletes increase as the prevalence of CAD rises. These numbers highlight the problem of how best to screen individual participants. Even an inexpensive test such as an ECG would generate an enormous cost if required of all athletes, and it is likely that only a few at-risk individuals would be detected. Echocardiography, either as a routine test or as a follow-up examination for abnormal ECGs, would be prohibitively expensive except for the elite professional athlete. Thus, *the most feasible approach is that of a careful medical history and cardiac examination performed by personnel aware of the conditions responsible for most sudden deaths in competitive athletes.*

It is important to point out that sudden death is much more common in the older than the younger athlete. Older athletes will generally seek advice regarding their fitness for participation. These individuals should recognize that strenuous exercise is associated with an increase in risk of sudden cardiac death and that appropriate training substantially reduces this risk. Preparticipation screening for risk of sudden death in the older athlete is a complex issue and at present is largely focused on identifying inducible ischemia due to significant coronary disease.

In a series of 158 athletic deaths in the United States between 1985 and 1995, hypertrophic cardiomyopathy (36%) and coronary anomalies (19%) were by far the most frequent underlying conditions. LVH was present in another 10%, ruptured aorta (presumably due to Marfan syndrome or cystic medial necrosis) in 6%, myocarditis or dilated cardiomyopathy in 6%, aortic stenosis in 4%, and arrhythmogenic RV dysplasia in 3%. In addition, commotio cordis, or sudden death due to direct myocardial injury, may occur. More common in children, ventricular tachycardia or ventricular fibrillation may occur even after a minor direct blow to the heart; it is thought to be due to the precipitation of a PVC just prior to the peak of the T wave on ECG.

A careful family and medical history and cardiovascular examination will identify most individuals at risk. An update in 2014 recommends that **all middle school and higher athletes undergo a medical screen questionnaire and examination.** The 12 elements in the examination are outlined in Table 10–19.

A family history of premature sudden death or CVD, or of any of these predisposing conditions should mandate further workup, including an ECG and echocardiogram. Symptoms of unexplained fatigue or dyspnea, exertional chest pain, syncope, or near syncope also warrant further evaluation. A Marfan-like appearance, significant elevation of BP, abnormalities of heart rate or rhythm, and pathologic heart murmurs or heart sounds should also be investigated before clearance for athletic participation is given. Such an evaluation is recommended before participation at the high school and college levels and every 2 years during athletic competition.

Stress-induced syncope or chest pressure may be the first clue to an anomalous origin of a coronary artery. Anatomically, this lesion occurs most often when the left anterior descending artery or left main coronary arises from

Table 10–19. 12-element AHA recommendations for preparticipation cardiovascular screening of competitive athletes.

Medical History
Personal History
1. Exertional chest pain/discomfort
2. Unexplained syncope/near-syncope
3. Excessive exertional and unexplained dyspnea/fatigue
4. Prior recognition of a heart murmur
5. Elevated systemic blood pressure
Family History
6. Premature death (sudden and unexpected, or otherwise) before age of 50 years due to heart disease in one or more relatives
7. Disability from heart disease in a close relative before age of 50 years
8. Specific knowledge of certain cardiac conditions in family members: hypertrophic cardiomyopathy, dilated cardiomyopathy, long QT syndrome or other ion channelopathies, Marfan syndrome, or other important arrhythmias
Physical Examination
9. Heart murmur
10. Diminished femoral pulse (to exclude coarctation)
11. Phenotype of Marfan syndrome
12. Brachial artery blood pressure (sitting position)

Reproduced with permission from Lawless CE, Asplund C, Asif IM, et al. Protecting the heart of the American athlete: proceedings of the American College of Cardiology Sports and Exercise Cardiology Think Tank October 18, 2012, Washington, DC. J Am Coll Cardiol. 2014;64(20):2146–2171.

the right coronary cusp and traverses between the aorta and pulmonary trunks. The "slit-like" orifice that results from the angulation at the vessel origin is thought to cause ischemia when the aorta and pulmonary arteries enlarge during vigorous exercise and tension is placed on the coronary.

The toughest distinction may be in sorting out the healthy athlete with LVH from the athlete with hypertrophic cardiomyopathy. In general, the healthy athlete's heart is *less* likely to have an unusual pattern of LVH (such as asymmetric septal hypertrophy), or to have LA enlargement, an abnormal ECG, an LV cavity less than 45 mm in diameter at end-diastole, an abnormal diastolic filling pattern, or a family history of hypertrophic cardiomyopathy. The athlete is more likely to be male than the individual with hypertrophic cardiomyopathy, where women are equally at risk. Cardiac MRI is emerging as a useful means to separate the athlete's heart from hypertrophic obstructive cardiomyopathy. Increased risk is also evident in patients with the WPW syndrome, a prolonged QTc interval, or those who demonstrate the abnormal ST changes in leads V1 and V2 consistent with the Brugada syndrome.

Selective use of routine ECG and stress testing is recommended in men above age 40 years and women above age 50 years who continue to participate in vigorous exercise and at earlier ages when there is a positive family history for premature CAD, hypertrophic cardiomyopathy, or multiple risk factors. Because at least some of the risk features (long QT, LVH, Brugada syndrome, WPW syndrome) may be evident on routine ECG screening, several cost-effectiveness studies have been done. Most suggest that preparticipation ECGs are of potential value, though what to do when the QTc is mildly increased is unclear. Many experts feel the high incidence of false-positive ECG studies makes it very ineffective as a screening tool. With the low prevalence of cardiac anomalies in the general public, it has been estimated that 200,000 individual athletes would need to be screened to identify the single individual who would die suddenly. A report from Canada reviewing 74 sudden cardiac arrests during sports activity noted that the vast majority occurred during noncompetitive sports. The incidence during competitive sports was 0.76 per 100,000 athlete-years, and there was not a clear association with structural heart disease in most. Genetic testing of all athletes who demonstrate T-wave inversions on their ECG also has been shown to be ineffective; the genetic testing contributed an additional diagnosis in only 2.5% of subjects over that obtained by routine clinical means.

The issue of routine screening, therefore, remains controversial. A report from the United Kingdom in 2018, screening adolescent soccer players from 1996 to 2016 (that included ECG and echocardiography), identified diseases associated with sudden death in only 0.38% of the 11,168 athletes screened for a total of 118,351 person-years. The incidence of sudden death was about 7 per 100,000 athletes and most were related to cardiomyopathies that had not been detected on the screening procedures.

In 2017, a position paper from a number of European societies presented arguments regarding the use of a number of preparticipation screening options. The manuscript also provided input from a number of international sports organizations. They concluded that there were data to support obtaining the clinical history, performing a physical examination, and performing a 12-lead ECG on all participants. They did not recommend echocardiography as a screening tool.

In 2017, a consensus statement from the American Medical Society for Sports Medicine was published summarizing the current recommendations for the appropriate screening options in the various clinical scenarios. Once a high-risk individual has been identified, guidelines from the Bethesda conference and the ESC can be used to help determine whether the athlete may continue to participate in sporting events. Table 10–20 summarizes these recommendations.

Screening for return to play after myocardial/pericardial involvement with COVID-19 is currently an important issue (see also Infectious Myocarditis above). An expert consensus statement from the ACC suggests the following:

1. In the athlete who has had COVID-19, the ECG and high-sensitivity troponin should be normal. If any clinical concerns remain, then a transthoracic echocardiogram should be obtained.

Table 10–20. Recommendations for competitive sports participation among athletes with potential causes of SCD.

Condition	36th Bethesda Conference	European Society of Cardiology
Structural Cardiac Abnormalities		
HCM	Exclude athletes with a probable or definitive clinical diagnosis from all competitive sports. Genotype-positive/phenotype-negative athletes may still compete.	Exclude athletes with a probable or definitive clinical diagnosis from all competitive sports. Exclude genotype-positive/phenotype-negative individuals from competitive sports.
ARVC	Exclude athletes with a probable or definitive diagnosis from competitive sports.	Exclude athletes with a probable or definitive diagnosis from competitive sports.
CCAA	Exclude from competitive sports.	Not applicable.
	Participation in all sports 3 months after successful surgery would be permitted for an athlete with ischemia, ventricular arrhythmia or tachyarrhythmia, or LV dysfunction during maximal exercise testing.	
Electrical Cardiac Abnormalities		
WPW	Athletes without structural heart disease, without a history of palpitations, or without tachycardia can participate in all competitive sports. In athletes with symptoms, electrophysiological study and ablation are recommended. Return to competitive sports is allowed after corrective ablation, provided that the ECG has normalized.	Athletes without structural heart disease, without a history of palpitations, or without tachycardia can participate in all competitive sports. In athletes with symptoms, electrophysiological study and ablation are recommended. Return to competitive sports is allowed after corrective ablation, provided that the ECG has normalized.
LQTS	Exclude any athlete with a previous cardiac arrest or syncopal episode from competitive sports. Asymptomatic patients restricted to competitive low-intensity sports. Genotype-positive/phenotype-negative athletes may still compete.	Exclude any athlete with a clinical or genotype diagnosis from competitive sports.
BrS	Exclude from all competitive sports except those of low intensity.	Exclude from all competitive sports.
CPVT	Exclude all patients with a clinical diagnosis from competitive sports. Genotype-positive/phenotype-negative patients may still compete in low-intensity sports.	Exclude all patients with a clinical diagnosis from competitive sports. Genotype-positive/phenotype-negative patients are also excluded.
Acquired Cardiac Abnormalities		
Commotio cordis	Eligibility for returning to competitive sport in survivors is a matter of individual clinical judgment. Survivors must undergo a thorough cardiovascular workup including 12-lead ECG, ambulatory ECG monitoring, and echocardiography.	Not applicable.
Myocarditis	Exclude from all competitive sports. Convalescent period of 6 months. Athletes may return to competition when test results normalize.	Exclude from all competitive sports. Convalescent period of 6 months. Athletes may return to competition when test results normalize.

ARVC, arrhythmogenic right ventricular cardiomyopathy; BrS, Brugada syndrome; CCAA, congenital coronary artery anomalies; CPVT, catecholaminergic polymorphic ventricular tachycardia; HCM, hypertrophic cardiomyopathy; LQTS, long QT syndrome; SCD, sudden cardiac death; WPW, Wolff-Parkinson-White syndrome.

Reproduced with permission from Chandra N et al. Sudden cardiac death in young athletes: practical challenges and diagnostic dilemmas. J Am Coll Cardiol. 2013;61(10):1027–1040.

2. Point-of-care echocardiography is not recommended, as the most common echocardiogram abnormalities may be missed by point-of-care echocardiography. These include RV dysfunction, diastolic LV abnormalities, and early signs of LV dysfunction (including abnormal global longitudinal strain). These are "red flags."
3. If any "red flags" from echocardiogram are present, then cardiac MRI should be obtained. MRI provides better assessment of RV function and abnormalities of myocardial edema (T2 imaging), intracellular and extracellular signaling (T1 imaging), and late gadolinium enhancement. The long-term significance of these findings is unknown.
4. Other imaging modalities can include coronary CT, chest CTA (looking for PE, given the hypercoagulable state COVID-19 creates), and rarely PET imaging.
5. Cardiopulmonary exercise testing is to be avoided during the acute phase but is valuable at 3–6 months after the illness if symptoms persist and as part of return to play guidelines.

Phelan D et al. Screening of potential cardiac involvement in competitive athletes recovering from COVID-19: an expert consensus statement. JACC Cardiovasc Imaging. 2020;13:2635. [PMID: 33303102]

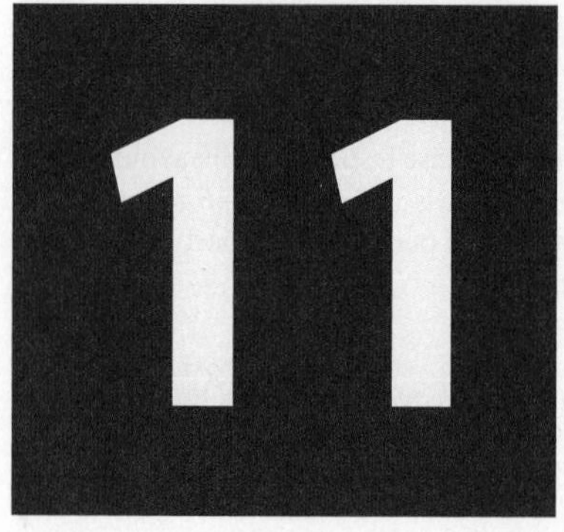

Systemic Hypertension

Michael Sutters, MD, MRCP (UK)

Based on the National Health and Nutrition Survey period 2017–2018, about 45% of adults in the United States have a blood pressure greater than 130/80 mm Hg or are being treated for hypertension. About 80% of people with hypertension are aware of the diagnosis and 75% are receiving treatment, but hypertension is controlled in only 52% of those affected. Cardiovascular morbidity and mortality increase as both systolic and diastolic blood pressures rise, but in individuals over age 50 years, the systolic pressure and pulse pressure are better predictors of complications than diastolic pressure. The prevalence of hypertension increases with age. Adequate blood pressure control reduces the incidence of acute coronary syndrome by 20–25%, stroke by 30–35%, and heart failure by 50%.

HOW IS BLOOD PRESSURE MEASURED & HYPERTENSION DIAGNOSED?

Blood pressure should be measured with a well-calibrated sphygmomanometer. The bladder width within the cuff should encircle at least 80% of the arm circumference. Readings should be taken after the patient has been resting comfortably, back supported in the sitting or supine position, for at least 5 minutes and at least 30 minutes after smoking or coffee ingestion. Blood pressure readings made in the office with devices that permit multiple automated measurements after a pre-programmed rest period produce data that are independent of digit preference bias (tendency to favor numbers that end with zero or five) and avoid the "white coat" phenomenon (where blood pressure is elevated in the clinic but normal at home). Blood pressure measurements taken outside the office environment, either by intermittent self-monitoring (home blood pressure) or with an automated device programmed to take measurements at regular intervals (ambulatory blood pressure), are more powerful predictors of outcomes and are advocated in clinical guidelines.

A single elevated blood pressure reading is not sufficient to establish the diagnosis of hypertension. The major exceptions to this rule are hypertension presenting with unequivocal evidence of life-threatening end-organ damage, as seen in hypertensive emergency, or hypertensive urgency where blood pressure is greater than 220/125 mm Hg but life-threatening end-organ damage is absent. In less severe cases, the diagnosis of hypertension depends on a series of measurements of blood pressure since readings can vary and tend to regress toward the mean with time. Patients whose initial blood pressure is in the hypertensive range exhibit the greatest fall toward the normal range between the first and second encounters. However, the concern for diagnostic precision needs to be balanced by an appreciation of the importance of establishing the diagnosis of hypertension as quickly as possible since a 3-month delay in treatment of hypertension in high-risk patients is associated with a twofold increase in cardiovascular morbidity and mortality. The 2017 guidelines from the American College of Cardiology and American Heart Association (ACC/AHA) (based on conventional office-based measurements) define **normal blood pressure** as less than 120/80 mm Hg, **elevated blood pressure** as 120–129/less than 80 mm Hg, **stage 1 hypertension** as 130–139/80–89 mm Hg, and **stage 2 hypertension** as greater than or equal to 140/90 mm Hg. As exemplified by Hypertension Canada's 2017 guidelines (Figure 11–1), automated and home blood pressure measurements have assumed greater prominence in the diagnostic algorithms published by many national hypertension workgroups. Equivalent blood pressures for these different modes of measurement are described in Table 11–1.

Blood pressure is normally lowest at night and the loss of this nocturnal dip is a dominant predictor of cardiovascular risk, particularly risk of thrombotic stroke. An accentuation of the normal morning increase in blood pressure is associated with increased likelihood of cerebral hemorrhage.

It is important to recognize that patients in whom hypertension is diagnosed do not automatically require drug treatment; this decision depends on the clinical setting and evaluation of cardiovascular risk.

White Coat, Masked, & Labile Hypertension

The term "white coat" hypertension applies to patients whose blood pressure is elevated in the office but normal at home. Cardiovascular risk in white coat hypertension is elevated but less so than in established hypertension. Masked hypertension describes the opposite situation,

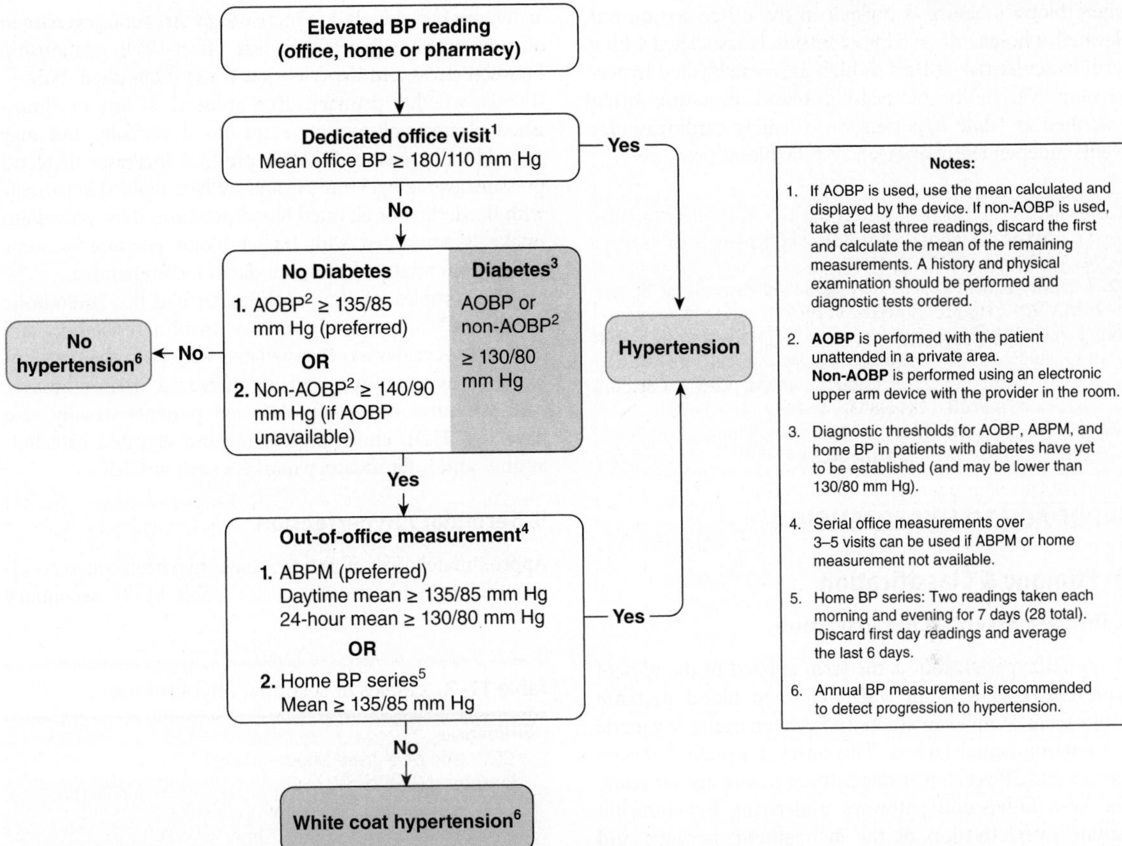

▲ **Figure 11–1. According to these recommendations, if AOBP measurements are not available, blood pressures recorded manually in the office may be substituted if taken as the mean of the last two readings of three consecutive readings. Note that the blood pressure threshold for diagnosing hypertension is higher if recorded manually in these guidelines. If home blood pressure monitoring is unavailable, office measurements recorded over three to five separate visits can be substituted. ABPM, ambulatory blood pressure measurement; AOBP, automated office blood pressure; BP, blood pressure.** (Reproduced with permission from Leung AA, Daskalopoulou SS, Dasgupta K, et al. Hypertension Canada's 2017 guidelines for diagnosis, risk assessment, prevention, and treatment of hypertension in adults. Can J Cardiol. 2017;33(5):557–576.)

Table 11–1. Corresponding blood pressure values across a range of blood pressure measurement methods.

Manual Measurement in Clinic[1]	Home Blood Pressure Measurement	Ambulatory Blood Pressure Measurement (Daytime)	Ambulatory Blood Pressure Measurement (Nighttime)	Ambulatory Blood Pressure Measurement (24-Hour)
120/80 mm Hg	120/80 mm Hg	120/80 mm Hg	100/65 mm Hg	115/75 mm Hg
130/80 mm Hg	130/80 mm Hg	130/80 mm Hg	110/65 mm Hg	125/75 mm Hg
140/90 mm Hg	135/85 mm Hg	135/85 mm Hg	120/70 mm Hg	130/80 mm Hg
160/100 mm Hg	145/90 mm Hg	145/90 mm Hg	140/85 mm Hg	145/90 mm Hg

[1]Clinic manual blood pressures are critically dependent on technique. The use of automated devices in an unattended setting typically result in systolic blood pressures 9–13 mm Hg lower than clinic manual pressures. Data abstracted from Greenland P et al. The New 2017 ACC/AHA Guidelines "up the pressure" on diagnosis and treatment of hypertension. JAMA. 2017;318:2083.

where blood pressure is normal in the office setting but elevated at home. Masked hypertension is associated with a cardiovascular risk at least as high as in established hypertension. Variability of systolic blood pressure, often described as labile hypertension, predicts cardiovascular events independently of mean systolic blood pressure.

Greenland P et al. The New 2017 ACC/AHA Guidelines "up the pressure" on diagnosis and treatment of hypertension. JAMA. 2017;318:2083. [PMID: 29159417]

Jin J. JAMA patient page. Checking blood pressure at home. JAMA. 2017;318:310. [PMID: 28719694]

Leung AA et al; Hypertension Canada. Hypertension Canada's 2017 guidelines for diagnosis, risk assessment, prevention, and treatment of hypertension in adults. Can J Cardiol. 2017;33:557. [PMID: 28449828]

Melville S et al. Out-of-office blood pressure monitoring in 2018. JAMA. 2018;320:1805. [PMID: 30398589]

APPROACH TO HYPERTENSION

Etiology & Classification

A. Primary Essential Hypertension

"Essential hypertension" is the term applied to the 95% of hypertensive patients in which elevated blood pressure results from complex interactions between multiple genetic and environmental factors. The onset is usually between ages 25 and 50 years; it is uncommon before age 20 years. The best understood pathways underlying hypertension include overactivation of the sympathetic nervous and renin-angiotensin-aldosterone systems (RAAS), blunting of the pressure-natriuresis relationship, variation in cardiovascular and renal development, and elevated intracellular sodium and calcium levels.

Exacerbating factors include obesity, sleep apnea, increased salt intake, excessive alcohol use, cigarette smoking, polycythemia, NSAID therapy, and low potassium intake. Obesity is associated with an increase in intravascular volume; elevated cardiac output; activation of the renin-angiotensin system; and, probably, increased sympathetic outflow. Lifestyle-driven weight reduction lowers blood pressure modestly, but the dramatic weight reduction following bariatric surgery results in improved blood pressure in most patients, and actual remission of hypertension in 20–40% of cases. In patients with sleep apnea, treatment with continuous positive airway pressure (CPAP) has been associated with improvements in blood pressure. Increased salt intake probably elevates blood pressure in some individuals so dietary salt restriction is recommended in patients with hypertension. Excessive use of alcohol also raises blood pressure, perhaps by increasing plasma catecholamines. Hypertension can be difficult to control in patients who consume more than 40 g of ethanol (two drinks) daily or drink in "binges." Cigarette smoking raises blood pressure by increasing plasma norepinephrine. Although the long-term effect of smoking on blood pressure is less clear, the synergistic effects of smoking and high blood pressure on cardiovascular risk are well documented. The relationship of exercise to hypertension is variable. Aerobic exercise lowers blood pressure in previously sedentary individuals, but increasingly strenuous exercise in already active subjects has less effect. The relationship between stress and hypertension is not established. Polycythemia, whether primary, drug-induced, or due to diminished plasma volume, increases blood viscosity and may raise blood pressure. NSAIDs produce increases in blood pressure averaging 5 mm Hg and are best avoided in patients with borderline or elevated blood pressures. Low potassium intake is associated with higher blood pressure in some patients; an intake of 90 mmol/day is recommended.

The complex of abnormalities termed the **"metabolic syndrome"** (upper body obesity, insulin resistance, and hypertriglyceridemia) is associated with both the development of hypertension and an increased risk of adverse cardiovascular outcomes. Affected patients usually also have low HDL cholesterol levels and elevated catecholamines and inflammatory markers such as CRP.

B. Secondary Hypertension

Approximately 5% of patients have hypertension secondary to identifiable specific causes (Table 11–2). Secondary

Table 11–2. Causes of secondary hypertension.

Endocrine
Conn syndrome (hyperaldosteronism)
Licorice
Cushing syndrome (hypercortisolism)
Thyroid disease
Pheochromocytoma
Acromegaly
Mutations in steroid gene regulatory domains
Hypercalcemia
Renal
Parenchymal kidney disease
Polycystic kidney disease
Systemic sclerosis (scleroderma)
Page kidney (subcapsular compression of the kidney)
Mutations in genes encoding ion transport proteins
Vascular
Renal artery stenosis
Coarctation
Autonomic
Stress
Neurogenic
Medications
NSAIDs
Corticosteroids
Calcineurin inhibitors
Stimulants
Decongestants
Angiogenesis inhibitors
Tyrosine kinase inhibitors
Estrogen
Erythropoietin
Alcohol, cocaine
Gemcitabine
Atypical antipsychotics
MAO inhibitors
Other
Obstructive sleep apnea
Pregnancy

hypertension should be suspected in patients in whom hypertension develops at an early age or after the age of 50 years, and in those previously well controlled who become refractory to treatment. Hypertension resistant to maximum doses of three medications is another clue, although multiple medications are usually required to control hypertension in persons with diabetes.

1. Genetic causes—Hypertension can be caused by mutations in single genes, inherited on a Mendelian basis. Although rare, these conditions provide important insight into blood pressure regulation and possibly the genetic basis of essential hypertension. Glucocorticoid remediable aldosteronism is an autosomal dominant cause of early-onset hypertension with normal or high aldosterone and low renin levels. The syndrome of hypertension exacerbated in pregnancy is inherited as an autosomal dominant trait. In these patients, a mutation in the mineralocorticoid receptor makes it abnormally responsive to progesterone and, paradoxically, to spironolactone. Liddle syndrome is an autosomal dominant condition characterized by early-onset hypertension, hypokalemic alkalosis, low renin, and low aldosterone levels. Gordon syndrome, or pseudohypoaldosteronism type II, is most often transmitted in an autosomal dominant pattern and presents with early-onset hypertension associated with hyperkalemia, metabolic acidosis, and relative suppression of aldosterone.

2. Kidney disease—Renal parenchymal disease is the most common cause of secondary hypertension, which results from increased intravascular volume and increased activity of the RAAS. Increased sympathetic nerve activity may also contribute.

3. Renal vascular hypertension—Renal artery stenosis is present in 1–2% of hypertensive patients. The most common cause is atherosclerosis, but fibromuscular dysplasia should be suspected in women under 50 years of age. Excessive renin release occurs due to reduction in renal perfusion pressure, while attenuation of pressure natriuresis contributes to hypertension in patients with a single kidney or bilateral lesions.

Renal vascular hypertension should be suspected in the following circumstances: (1) the documented onset is before age 20 or after age 50 years, (2) the hypertension is resistant to three or more drugs, (3) there are epigastric or renal artery bruits, (4) there is atherosclerotic disease of the aorta or peripheral arteries (15–25% of patients with symptomatic lower limb atherosclerotic vascular disease have renal artery stenosis), (5) there is an abrupt increase (more than 25%) in the level of serum creatinine after administration of ACE inhibitors, or (6) episodes of pulmonary edema are associated with abrupt surges in blood pressure. (See Renal Artery Stenosis, Chapter 22.)

4. Primary hyperaldosteronism—Hyperaldosteronism should be considered in people with resistant hypertension, blood pressures consistently greater than 150/100 mm Hg, hypokalemia (although this is often absent), or adrenal incidentaloma, and in those with a family history of hyperaldosteronism. Mild hypernatremia and metabolic alkalosis may also occur. Hypersecretion of aldosterone is estimated to be present in 5–10% of hypertensive patients and, besides noncompliance, is the most common cause of resistant hypertension. The initial screening step is the simultaneous measurement of aldosterone and renin in blood in a morning sample collected after 30 minutes quietly seated. Hyperaldosteronism is suggested when the plasma aldosterone concentration is elevated (normal: 1–16 ng/dL) in association with suppression of plasma renin activity (normal: 1–2.5 ng/mL/hour). However, the plasma aldosterone/renin ratio (normal less than 30) is not highly specific as a screening test. This is because renin levels may approach zero, which leads to exponential increases in the plasma aldosterone/renin ratio even when aldosterone levels are normal. Hence, an elevated plasma aldosterone/renin ratio should probably not be taken as evidence of hyperaldosteronism unless the aldosterone level is actually elevated.

During the workup for hyperaldosteronism, an initial plasma aldosterone/renin ratio can be measured while the patient continues taking usual medications. If under these circumstances the ratio proves normal or equivocal, medications that alter renin and aldosterone levels, including ACE inhibitors, ARBs, diuretics, beta-blockers, and clonidine, should be discontinued for 2 weeks before repeating the plasma aldosterone/renin ratio; spironolactone and eplerenone should be held for 4 weeks. Slow-release verapamil and alpha-blockers can be used to control blood pressure during this drug washout period. Patients with a plasma aldosterone level greater than 16 ng/dL and an aldosterone/renin ratio of 30 or more might require further evaluation for primary hyperaldosteronism.

The lesion responsible for hyperaldosteronism is an adrenal adenoma or bilateral adrenal hyperplasia.

5. Cushing syndrome—Hypertension occurs in about 80% of patients with spontaneous Cushing syndrome. Excess glucocorticoid may act through salt and water retention (via mineralocorticoid effects), increased angiotensinogen levels, or permissive effects in the regulation of vascular tone. Diagnosis and treatment of Cushing syndrome are discussed in Chapter 26.

6. Pheochromocytoma—Pheochromocytomas are uncommon; they are probably found in less than 0.1% of all patients with hypertension and in approximately two individuals per million population. Chronic vasoconstriction of the arterial and venous beds leads to a reduction in plasma volume and predisposes to postural hypotension. Glucose intolerance develops in some patients. Hypertensive crisis in pheochromocytoma may be precipitated by a variety of drugs, including tricyclic antidepressants, antidopaminergic agents, metoclopramide, and naloxone. The diagnosis and treatment of pheochromocytoma are discussed in Chapter 26.

7. Coarctation of the aorta—This uncommon cause of hypertension is discussed in Chapter 10. Evidence of radial-femoral delay should be sought in all younger patients with hypertension.

8. Hypertension associated with pregnancy—Hypertension occurring de novo or worsening during pregnancy, including preeclampsia and eclampsia, is one of the most common causes of maternal and fetal morbidity and mortality (see Chapter 19). Autoantibodies with the potential to activate the angiotensin II type 1 receptor have been causally implicated in preeclampsia, in resistant hypertension, and in progressive systemic sclerosis.

9. Estrogen use—A small increase in blood pressure occurs in most women taking oral contraceptives. A more significant increase of 8/6 mm Hg systolic/diastolic is noted in about 5% of women, mostly in obese individuals older than age 35 who have been treated for more than 5 years. This is caused by increased hepatic synthesis of angiotensinogen. The lower dose of postmenopausal estrogen does not generally cause hypertension but rather maintains endothelium-mediated vasodilation.

10. Other causes of secondary hypertension—Hypertension has been associated with hypercalcemia, acromegaly, hyperthyroidism, hypothyroidism, baroreceptor denervation (sometimes seen after treatment of head and neck cancer), compression of the rostral ventrolateral medulla, and increased intracranial pressure. Certain medications may cause or exacerbate hypertension—most importantly cyclosporine, tacrolimus, angiogenesis inhibitors, and erythrocyte-stimulating agents (such as erythropoietin). Decongestants, NSAIDs, cocaine, and alcohol should also be considered. Over-the-counter products should not be overlooked, eg, a dietary supplement marketed to enhance libido was found to contain yohimbine, an alpha-2–antagonist, which can produce severe rebound hypertension in patients taking clonidine.

When to Refer

Referral to a hypertension specialist should be considered in cases of severe, resistant, or early-/late-onset hypertension or when secondary hypertension is suggested by screening.

Byrd JB et al. Primary aldosteronism. Circulation. 2018;138:823. [PMID: 30359120]

Herrmann SM et al. Renovascular hypertension. Endocrinol Metab Clin North Am. 2019;48:765. [PMID: 31655775]

Complications of Untreated Hypertension

Many adverse outcomes in hypertension are associated with thrombosis rather than bleeding, possibly because increased vascular shear stress converts the normally anticoagulant endothelium to a prothrombotic state. The excess morbidity and mortality related to hypertension approximately doubles for each 6 mm Hg increase in diastolic blood pressure. However, target-organ damage varies markedly between individuals with similar levels of office hypertension; home and ambulatory pressures are superior to office readings in the prediction of end-organ damage (Table 11–1).

A. Hypertensive Cardiovascular Disease

Cardiac complications are the major causes of morbidity and mortality in primary (essential) hypertension. For any level of blood pressure, LVH is associated with incremental cardiovascular risk in association with heart failure (through systolic or diastolic dysfunction), ventricular arrhythmias, myocardial ischemia, and sudden death.

The occurrence of heart failure is reduced by 50% with antihypertensive therapy. Hypertensive LVH regresses with therapy and is most closely related to the degree of systolic blood pressure reduction. Diuretics have produced equal or greater reductions of LV mass when compared with other drug classes. Conventional beta-blockers are less effective in reducing LVH but play a specific role in patients with established CAD or impaired LV function.

B. Hypertensive Cerebrovascular Disease and Dementia

Hypertension is the major predisposing cause of hemorrhagic and ischemic stroke. Cerebrovascular complications are more closely correlated with systolic than diastolic blood pressure. The incidence of these complications is markedly reduced by antihypertensive therapy. Preceding hypertension is associated with a higher incidence of subsequent dementia of both vascular and Alzheimer types. Home and ambulatory blood pressure may be a better predictor of cognitive decline than office readings in older people. Effective blood pressure control reduces the risk of cognitive dysfunction developing later in life.

C. Hypertensive Kidney Disease

Chronic hypertension is associated with injury to vascular, glomerular, and tubulointerstitial compartments within the kidney, accounting for about 25% of ESKD. Nephrosclerosis is particularly prevalent in persons of sub-Saharan African ancestry, in whom susceptibility is linked to *APOL1* mutations and hypertension results from kidney disease rather than causing it.

D. Aortic Dissection

Hypertension is a contributing factor in many patients with dissection of the aorta. Its diagnosis and treatment are discussed in Chapter 12.

E. Atherosclerotic Complications

Most Americans with hypertension die of complications of atherosclerosis, but the impact of antihypertensive therapy on atherosclerotic complications is less clear than that seen in the prevention of heart failure, stroke, and kidney disease. Prevention of cardiovascular outcomes related to atherosclerosis probably requires control of multiple risk factors, of which hypertension is only one.

Supiano MA et al. New guidelines and SPRINT results: implications for geriatric hypertension. Circulation. 2019;140:976. [PMID: 31525101]

Clinical Findings

The clinical and laboratory findings arise from involvement of the target organs: heart, brain, kidneys, eyes, and peripheral arteries.

A. Symptoms

Mild to moderate primary (essential) hypertension is largely asymptomatic for many years. The most frequent symptom, headache, is also nonspecific. Accelerated hypertension is associated with somnolence, confusion, visual disturbances, and nausea and vomiting (hypertensive encephalopathy).

Hypertension in patients with pheochromocytomas that secrete predominantly norepinephrine is usually sustained but may be episodic. The typical attack lasts from minutes to hours and is associated with headache, anxiety, palpitation, profuse perspiration, pallor, tremor, and nausea and vomiting. Blood pressure is markedly elevated, and angina or acute pulmonary edema may occur. In primary aldosteronism, patients may have muscular weakness, polyuria, and nocturia due to hypokalemia; hypertensive emergency is rare. Chronic hypertension often leads to LVH and diastolic dysfunction, which can present with exertional and paroxysmal nocturnal dyspnea. Cerebral involvement causes stroke due to thrombosis or hemorrhage from microaneurysms of small penetrating intracranial arteries. Hypertensive encephalopathy is probably caused by acute capillary congestion and exudation with cerebral edema and may present as posterior reversible encephalopathy syndrome, comprising headache, visual disturbances, altered mental state, and seizures. These symptoms usually improve rapidly with control of hypertension.

B. Signs

Like symptoms, physical findings depend on the cause of hypertension, its duration and severity, and the degree of effect on target organs.

1. Blood pressure—Blood pressure is taken in both arms and, if lower extremity pulses are diminished or delayed, in the legs to exclude coarctation of the aorta. If blood pressure differs between right and left arms, the higher reading should be recorded as the actual blood pressure and subclavian stenosis suspected in the other arm. An orthostatic drop of at least 20/10 mm Hg is often present in pheochromocytoma. Older patients may have falsely elevated readings by sphygmomanometry because of noncompressible vessels. This may be suspected in the presence of Osler sign—a palpable brachial or radial artery when the cuff is inflated above systolic pressure. Occasionally, it may be necessary to make direct measurements of intra-arterial pressure, especially in patients with apparent severe hypertension who do not tolerate therapy.

2. Retinas—Narrowing of arterial diameter to less than 50% of venous diameter, copper or silver wire appearance, exudates, hemorrhages, and hypertensive retinopathy are associated with a worse prognosis. The typical changes of severe hypertensive retinopathy are shown in Figure 11–2 (see Chapter 7).

3. Heart—An LV heave indicates severe hypertrophy. Aortic regurgitation may be auscultated in up to 5% of patients, and hemodynamically insignificant aortic regurgitation

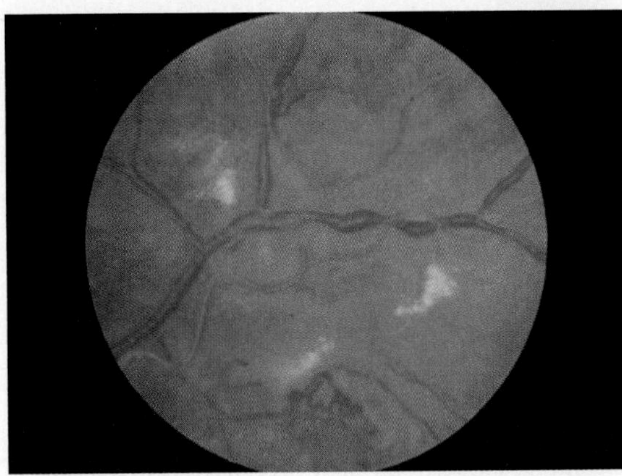

▲ **Figure 11–2. Severe, chronic hypertensive retinopathy with hard exudates, increased vessel light reflexes, and sausage-shaped veins.** (Used, with permission, from Richard E. Wyszynski, MD, in Knoop KJ, Stack LB, Storrow AB, Thurman RJ. *The Atlas of Emergency Medicine*, 4th ed. McGraw-Hill, 2016.)

can be detected by Doppler echocardiography in 10–20%. A presystolic (S_4) gallop due to decreased compliance of the LV is quite common in patients in sinus rhythm.

4. Pulses—Radial-femoral delay suggests coarctation of the aorta; loss of peripheral pulses occurs due to atherosclerosis, less commonly aortic dissection, and rarely Takayasu arteritis, all of which can involve the renal arteries.

C. Laboratory Findings

Recommended testing includes hemoglobin; serum electrolytes and serum creatinine; fasting blood sugar level (hypertension is a risk factor for the development of diabetes, and hyperglycemia can be a presenting feature of pheochromocytoma); plasma lipids (necessary to calculate cardiovascular risk and as a modifiable risk factor); serum uric acid (hyperuricemia is a relative contraindication to diuretic therapy); and UA.

D. ECG and Chest Radiographs

Electrocardiographic criteria are highly specific but not very sensitive for LVH. The "strain" pattern of ST–T wave changes is a sign of more advanced disease and is associated with a poor prognosis. A chest radiograph is not necessary in the workup of uncomplicated hypertension.

E. Echocardiography

The primary role of echocardiography should be to evaluate patients with clinical symptoms or signs of cardiac disease.

F. Diagnostic Studies

Additional diagnostic studies are indicated only if the clinical presentation or routine tests suggest secondary or complicated hypertension. These may include 24-hour urine free cortisol, urine or plasma metanephrines, and plasma aldosterone and renin concentrations to screen for endocrine causes of hypertension. Renal ultrasound will detect structural changes (such as polycystic kidneys, asymmetry, and hydronephrosis); increased echogenicity and reduced cortical volume are reliable indicators of advanced CKD. Evaluation for renal artery stenosis should be undertaken in concert with subspecialist consultation.

G. Summary

Since most hypertension is essential or primary, few studies are necessary beyond those listed above. If conventional therapy is unsuccessful or if secondary hypertension is suspected, further studies and perhaps referral to a hypertension specialist are indicated.

Nonpharmacologic Therapy

Lifestyle modification is recommended for all patients with elevated blood pressure. A diet rich in fruits, vegetables, and low-fat dairy foods and low in saturated and total fats (DASH diet) has been shown to lower blood pressure. Increased dietary fiber lowers blood pressure. For every 7 g of dietary fiber ingested, cardiovascular risk could be lowered by 9%. The effect of diet on blood pressure may be mediated by shifts in the microbial species in the gut, the intestinal microbiota. Hand squeezing exercises three times a week can lower systolic blood pressure by 6 mm Hg. The protocol comprises four repeats of 2 minutes at 30% of maximum force (using a handheld dynamometer) with 1- to 3-minute rest intervals between squeezes. The acute increase in systolic blood pressure during vigorous exercise, known as the exercise pressor response, is around 50 mm Hg in normal individuals. In hypertensive persons, the exercise pressor response is elevated to about 75 mm Hg above resting systolic blood pressure. This exaggerated response is not reduced by antihypertensive medications, even in those with otherwise controlled hypertension, and is exacerbated by increased dietary sodium intake.

Additional lifestyle changes, listed in Table 11–3, can prevent or mitigate hypertension or its cardiovascular consequences.

Fu J et al. Nonpharmacologic interventions for reducing blood pressure in adults with prehypertension to established hypertension. J Am Heart Assoc. 2020;9:e016804. [PMID: 32975166]

Smart NA et al. An evidence-based analysis of managing hypertension with isometric resistance exercise—are the guidelines current? Hypertens Res. 2020;43:249. [PMID: 31758166]

Who Should Be Treated With Medications?

Treatment should be offered to all persons in whom blood pressure reduction, irrespective of initial blood pressure levels, will reduce cardiovascular risk with an acceptably low rate of medication-associated adverse effects.

Table 11–3. The impact of lifestyle modifications.

Modification	Intervention	Resulting Decrease in Blood Pressure
Weight loss	Target BMI 18.5–24.9	5–20 mm Hg/ 10-kg loss
DASH diet	Fruit, vegetables, low fat dairy	8–14 mm Hg
Sodium intake	< 100 mmol/day (< 6 g salt)	2–8 mm Hg
Alcohol intake	Male ≤ 2 drinks/day Female ≤ 1 drink/day	4 mm Hg
Exercise	Aerobic 30 minutes/day Dynamic 90-150 minutes/ week Isometric (hand grip 4 repetitions 3 times/week)	5–10 mm Hg
Mindfulness	Meditation and breathing control	5 mm Hg

DASH, Dietary Approaches to Stop Hypertension.

The ACC/AHA, Hypertension Canada (HC), and the European Society of Hypertension and European Society of Cardiology (ESH/ESC) have developed independent guidelines for the evaluation and management of hypertension. There is broad agreement that drug treatment is necessary in those with office-based blood pressures exceeding 160/100 mm Hg, irrespective of cardiac risk. Similarly, the American, Canadian, and European guidelines agree that treatment thresholds should be lower in the presence of elevated cardiovascular risk. American guidelines stand apart in recommending initiation of antihypertensive pharmacotherapy in those with blood pressure of 140–159/90–99 mm Hg, even if cardiovascular risk is not elevated. By contrast, the Canadian guidelines suggest lifestyle modifications in this low-cardiovascular-risk group, while the European guidelines recommend initiation of pharmacotherapy only if elevated pressure in this low-risk population persists after lifestyle modification. There is no outcomes evidence that mortality or risk of cardiovascular events can be reduced by treating mild hypertension (140/90–160/100 mm Hg) in low-risk individuals. Table 11–4 compares these three sets of guidelines. Since evaluation of total cardiovascular risk (Table 11–5) is important in deciding who to treat with antihypertensive medications, risk calculators are essential clinical tools. The ACC has an online toolkit relevant to primary prevention (https://tools.acc.org/ascvd-risk-estimator-plus/#!/calculate/estimate/), and an associated app called ASCVD Risk Estimator Plus (downloadable at https://www.acc.org/ASCVDApp). The interaction between risk and age deserves careful attention. At any given level of calculated risk, treatment is likely to have a greater impact in the young than the elderly. Consequently, there is a possibility that setting absolute risk thresholds for treatment might lead to undertreatment of the young and overtreatment of the elderly.

Table 11–4. Comparison of blood pressure treatment thresholds from the 2017 ACC/AHA guidelines, the 2018 Hypertension Canada guidelines, and the 2018 ESH/ESC guidelines.

Guidelines[1]	Cardiovascular Risk	Threshold for Pharmacotherapy (mm Hg)	Target (mm Hg)
ACC/AHA	Not increased	> 140/90	< 130/80 (reasonable)
Hypertension Canada	Not increased	> 160/100	< 140/90 (< 130/80 for diabetes)
ESH/ESC	Not increased	> 140/90[2]	All < 140/90, most < 130/80, not < 120
ACC/AHA	Increased	< 130/80	< 130/80 (recommended)
Hypertension Canada	Increased	> 140 systolic[3]	< 120 systolic
ESH/ESC	Increased	> 130/80	120–130/< 80
ACC/AHA > 65 yr	Risk due to advanced age	> 130/80	< 130 systolic
Hypertension Canada (for older adults)[4]	Increased	Not specified[4]	Not specified[4]
ESH/ESC > 65 yr	Not increased	> 140/90[5]	130–140/> 80[6]

[1]In all three sets of guidelines, blood pressure values are based on nonautomated office blood pressure readings.
[2]Consider drug treatment if lifestyle changes fail to control blood pressure.
[3]Consider drug treatment at systolic blood pressure > 130 mm Hg if very high risk, eg, established cardiovascular disease, especially coronary disease. **Note:** The > 140/80 mm Hg threshold for treatment of high-risk patients in the Canadian guidelines refers to automated blood pressure readings, which are lower than nonautomated readings.
[4]Recommendations for persons > 75 years are not explicitly stated in the Hypertension Canada guidelines. They removed separate goals for the elderly but consider age > 75 years to be a risk signifier triggering an approach that many would view as overly aggressive in the extremely old.
[5]The European guidelines indicate a slightly more conservative treatment threshold of > 160/90 mm Hg for those > 80 years.
[6]This target range is also suggested in the European guidelines for patients > 80 years.
ACC, American College of Cardiology; AHA, American Heart Association; ESC, European Society of Cardiology; ESH, European Society of Hypertension.

Table 11–5. Cardiovascular risk factors.

Major risk factors
Hypertension[1]
Cigarette smoking
Obesity (BMI ≥ 30)[1]
Physical inactivity
Dyslipidemia[1]
Diabetes mellitus[1]
Microalbuminuria or estimated GFR < 60 mL/minute/1.73 m²
Age (> 55 years for men, > 65 years for women)
Family history of premature cardiovascular disease (< 55 years for men, < 65 years for women)
Target-organ damage
Heart
LVH
Angina or prior MI
Prior coronary revascularization
Heart failure
Brain
Stroke or transient ischemic attack
CKD
Peripheral arterial disease
Retinopathy

[1]Components of the metabolic syndrome.
Data from Chobanian AV et al. The Seventh Report of the Joint National Committee on Prevention, Detection, Evaluation, and Treatment of High Blood Pressure: the JNC 7 report. JAMA. 2003;289:2560.

Goals of Treatment

Traditionally, the most widely accepted goal for blood pressure management has been less than 140/90 mm Hg. However, observational studies suggest that there does not seem to be a blood pressure level below which decrements in cardiovascular risk taper off, and a number of randomized controlled trials have suggested that treatment to blood pressure targets considerably below 140 mm Hg may benefit certain patient groups.

The SPRINT study suggests that outcomes improve in nondiabetic patients with considerably elevated cardiovascular risk when treatment lowers systolic pressure to less than 120 mm Hg compared to less than 140 mm Hg. On the other hand, in the HOPE3 study of largely nondiabetic patients at somewhat lower risk than those in SPRINT, reducing blood pressure by an average of 6/3 mm Hg systolic/diastolic from a baseline of 138/82 mm Hg provided no significant outcomes benefits. Therefore, it appears that blood pressure targets should be lower in people at greater estimated cardiovascular risk. In response to the SPRINT study, the 2018 HC guidelines urge prescribers to consider a blood pressure goal of less than 120/80 mm Hg in patients considered at elevated risk for cardiovascular events. The 2017 ACC/AHA guidelines take a different approach by defining a 130/80 mm Hg goal as "reasonable" in nonelevated risk hypertensive patients, strengthening this to "recommended" in elevated risk hypertensive patients.

The 2018 ESH/ESC guidelines specify a target of less than 140 mm Hg systolic for all, and less than 130 mm Hg for most if tolerated. There is a trend toward recommending similar treatment targets in the elderly; this topic is discussed in greater detail below. Some experts note that manual office measurements of around 130/80 mm Hg are likely to approximate the lower blood pressure targets specified in the SPRINT study, which used automated office blood pressure measuring devices that have been demonstrated to read as much as 16/7 mm Hg lower than manual office readings. The 2018 Canadian guidelines acknowledge this disparity in measurement methods by specifying that automated office devices should be used in the monitoring of patients selected for the aggressive blood pressure goal of less than 120/80 mm Hg. Table 11–4 compares the treatment threshold and target recommendations laid out in the American, Canadian, and European guidelines.

Treatment to blood pressures less than 130 mm Hg systolic seems especially important in stroke prevention. The ACCORD study examined the effect of treatment of systolic pressures to below 130–135 mm Hg in patients with diabetes; the study's two by two factorial design addressed glycemic control as well as blood pressure control. In the original analysis, the lower blood pressure treatment goal significantly increased the risk of serious adverse effects (with no additional gain in terms of heart, kidney, or retinal disease). There was, however, significant additional reduction in the risk of stroke, indicating that lower blood pressure targets might be justified in diabetic patients at high risk for cerebrovascular events. Post hoc analysis of the ACCORD study after 9 years of follow-up suggested that a beneficial effect of lower blood pressure in older high-risk persons (mostly on nonfatal myocardial infarctions) could be detected in the standard glycemic control group. Similarly, in the SPS3 trial in patients who have had a lacunar stroke, treating the systolic blood pressure to less than 130 mm Hg (mean systolic blood pressure of 127 mm Hg among treated versus mean systolic blood pressure 138 mm Hg among untreated patients) probably reduced the risk of recurrent stroke (and with an acceptably low rate of adverse effects from treatment). Blood pressure management in acute stroke is discussed below.

How Low to Go?

Although observational studies indicate that the blood pressure–risk relationship holds up at levels considerably below 120 mm Hg, there has been uncertainty about whether this is true for treated blood pressure. This question was addressed in a secondary analysis of data from the ONTARGET and TRANSCEND studies in which participants with elevated cardiovascular risk but no history of stroke were treated with telmisartan (plus or minus ramipril) or placebo. The risk of the composite cardiovascular endpoint was lowest at a treated systolic blood pressure range between 120 mm Hg and 140 mm Hg. Increased risk was observed at blood pressures below and above this range. The risk of stroke was the only exception, with incremental benefit observed below a treated systolic of 120 mm Hg. With respect to diastolic blood pressure on treatment, composite risk began to increase at levels below 70 mm Hg. This suggests that the blood pressure–cardiovascular risk relationship evident in observational studies of untreated hypertension may not hold in the case of treated blood pressure and that there are grounds for a degree of caution in treating below a systolic pressure of 120 mm Hg.

In seeking to simplify decision making in the treatment of hypertension, some authors have suggested that a systolic blood pressure goal in the 120–130 mm Hg range would be safe and effective in high-risk patients, and a systolic blood pressure of around 130 mm Hg would be reasonable in lower-risk patients, irrespective of diastolic pressures. Diastolic blood pressure will track with systolic blood pressure; the main concern about diastolic blood pressure is that treatment will lower it too much in patients who have wider pulse pressures. However, it seems that a lower diastolic blood pressure as a consequence of treatment does not negate the benefits of systolic blood pressure control, even though wider pulse pressures at baseline are associated with cardiovascular mortality.

Treatment of Other Cardiovascular Risk Factors

Data from multiple studies indicate that statins should be part of the strategy to reduce overall cardiovascular risk. The HOPE3 study of persons at intermediate cardiovascular risk showed that 10 mg of rosuvastatin reduced average LDL cholesterol from 130 mg/dL to 90 mg/dL (3.36–2.33 mmol/L), and significantly reduced the risk of multiple cardiovascular events, including MI and coronary revascularization. Low-dose aspirin (81 mg/day) is no longer recommended in the primary prevention of MI or stroke. Low-dose aspirin is effective in prevention of recurrent cardiovascular events, but blood pressure should first be controlled to minimize the risk of cerebral hemorrhage.

Sheppard JP et al. Benefits and harms of antihypertensive treatment in low-risk patients with mild hypertension. JAMA Intern Med. 2018;178:1626. [PMID: 30383082]

Visseren FLJ et al; ESC Scientific Document Group. 2021 ESC Guidelines on cardiovascular disease prevention in clinical practice. Eur J Prev Cardiol. 2022;29:5. [PMID: 34558602]

DRUG THERAPY: CURRENT ANTIHYPERTENSIVE AGENTS

There are many classes of antihypertensive drugs of which six (ACE inhibitors, ARBs, renin inhibitors, calcium channel blockers, diuretics, and beta-blockers) are suitable for initial therapy based on efficacy and tolerability. The specific classes of antihypertensive medications are discussed below, and guidelines for the choice of initial medications are offered.

A. Angiotensin-Converting Enzyme Inhibitors

ACE inhibitors are commonly used as the initial medication in mild to moderate hypertension (Table 11–6). Their primary mode of action is inhibition of the RAAS, but they

Table 11–6. Antihypertensive drugs: renin and ACE inhibitors and ARBs.

Medication (Proprietary Name)	Oral Dosage	Cost of 30 Days of Treatment (Average Dosage)[1]	Adverse Effects	Comments
Renin Inhibitors				
Aliskiren (Tekturna)	*Initial:* 150 mg once daily *Range:* 150–300 mg once daily	$234.40 (150 mg)	Angioedema, hypotension, hyperkalemia. Contraindicated in pregnancy.	Probably metabolized by CYP3A4. Absorption is inhibited by high-fat meal.
Aliskiren and HCTZ (Tekturna HCT)	*Initial:* 150 mg/12.5 mg once daily *Range:* 150 mg/12.5 mg–300 mg/25 mg once daily	$293.54 (150 mg/12.5 mg)		
ACE Inhibitors				
Benazepril (Lotensin)	*Initial:* 10 mg once daily *Range:* 5–40 mg in 1 or 2 doses	$28.50 (20 mg)	Cough, hypotension, dizziness, hyperkalemia, kidney dysfunction, angioedema; taste alteration and rash (may be more frequent with captopril); rarely, proteinuria, blood dyscrasia. Contraindicated in pregnancy.	More fosinopril is excreted by the liver in patients with kidney dysfunction (dose reduction may or may not be necessary). Captopril and lisinopril are active without metabolism. Captopril, enalapril, lisinopril, and quinapril are approved for heart failure.
Benazepril and HCTZ (Lotensin HCT)	*Initial:* 5 mg/6.25 mg once daily *Range:* 5 mg/6.25 mg–20 mg/25 mg	$32.10 (any dose)		
Benazepril and amlodipine (Lotrel)	*Initial:* 10 mg/2.5 mg once daily *Range:* 10 mg/2.5 mg–40 mg/10 mg	$99.60 (20 mg/10 mg)		
Captopril (Capoten)	*Initial:* 25 mg twice daily *Range:* 50–450 mg in 2 or 3 doses	$76.20 (25 mg)		
Captopril and HCTZ (Capozide)	*Initial:* 25 mg/15 mg twice daily *Range:* 25 mg/15 mg–50 mg/25 mg	$171.00 (25 mg/15 mg)		
Enalapril (Vasotec)	*Initial:* 5 mg once daily *Range:* 5–40 mg in 1 or 2 doses	$28.50 (20 mg)		
Enalapril and HCTZ (Vaseretic)	*Initial:* 5 mg/12.5 mg once daily *Range:* 5 mg/12.5 mg–10 mg/25 mg	$35.70 (10 mg/25 mg)		
Fosinopril (Monopril)	*Initial:* 10 mg once daily *Range:* 10–80 mg in 1 or 2 doses	$15.90 (20 mg)		
Fosinopril and HCTZ (Monopril-HCT)	*Initial:* 10 mg/12.5 mg once daily *Range:* 10 mg/12.5 mg–20 mg/12.5 mg	$44.40 (any dose)		

(*continued*)

Table 11–6. Antihypertensive drugs: renin and ACE inhibitors and ARBs. (continued)

Medication (Proprietary Name)	Oral Dosage	Cost of 30 Days of Treatment (Average Dosage)[1]	Adverse Effects	Comments
Lisinopril (Prinivil, Zestril)	*Initial:* 5–10 mg once daily *Range:* 5–40 mg once daily	$2.40 (20 mg)		
Lisinopril and HCTZ (Prinzide or Zestoretic)	*Initial:* 10 mg/12.5 mg once daily *Range:* 10 mg/12.5 mg–20 mg/12.5 mg	$7.20 (20 mg/12.5 mg)		
Moexipril (Univasc)	*Initial:* 7.5 mg once daily *Range:* 7.5–30 mg in 1 or 2 doses	$41.70 (7.5 mg)		
Perindopril (Aceon)	*Initial:* 4 mg once daily *Range:* 4–16 mg in 1 or 2 doses	$84.00 (8 mg)		
Perindopril and amlodipine (Prestalia)	*Initial:* 3.5 mg/2.5 mg once daily *Range:* 3.5 mg/2.5–14 mg/10 mg once daily	$204.30 (7 mg/5 mg)		
Quinapril (Accupril)	*Initial:* 10 mg once daily *Range:* 10–80 mg in 1 or 2 doses	$36.60 (20 mg)		
Quinapril and HCTZ (Accuretic)	*Initial:* 10 mg/12.5 mg once daily *Range:* 10 mg/12.5 mg–20 mg/25 mg	$36.60 (20 mg/12.5 mg)		
Ramipril (Altace)	*Initial:* 2.5 mg once daily *Range:* 2.5–20 mg in 1 or 2 doses	$42.30 (5 mg)		
Trandolapril (Mavik)	*Initial:* 1 mg once daily *Range:* 1–8 mg once daily	$36.30 (4 mg)		
Trandolapril and verapamil (Tarka)	*Initial:* 2 mg/180 mg ER once daily *Range:* 2 mg/180 mg ER–8 mg/480 mg ER	$158.70 (any dose)		
ARBs				
Azilsartan (Edarbi)	*Initial:* 40 mg once daily *Range:* 40–80 mg once daily	$271.87 (80 mg)	Hyperkalemia, kidney dysfunction, rare angioedema. Combinations have additional side effects. Contraindicated in pregnancy.	Losartan has a flat dose-response curve. Valsartan and irbesartan have wider dose-response ranges and longer durations of action. Addition of low-dose diuretic (separately or as combination pills) increases the response.
Azilsartan and chlorthalidone (Edarbychlor)	*Initial:* 40 mg/12.5 mg once daily *Range:* 40 mg/12.5–40 mg/25 mg once daily	$256.62 (any dose)		
Candesartan cilexitil (Atacand)	*Initial:* 16 mg once daily *Range:* 8–32 mg once daily	$91.80 (16 mg)		
Candesartan cilexitil and HCTZ (Atacand HCT)	*Initial:* 16 mg/12.5 mg once daily *Range:* 32 mg/12.5 mg once daily	$141.60 (16 mg/12.5 mg)		
Eprosartan (Teveten)	*Initial:* 600 mg once daily *Range:* 400–800 mg in 1–2 doses	$102.78 (600 mg)		
Irbesartan (Avapro)	*Initial:* 150 mg once daily *Range:* 150–300 mg once daily	$13.80 (150 mg)		

Irbesartan and HCTZ (Avalide)	*Initial:* 150 mg/12.5 mg once daily *Range:* 150 mg/12.5 mg–300 mg/25 mg once daily	$20.10 (150 mg/12.5 mg)		
Losartan and HCTZ (Hyzaar)	*Initial:* 50 mg/12.5 mg once daily *Range:* 50 mg/12.5 mg–100 mg/25 mg once daily	$74.10 (50 mg/12.5 mg/)		
Olmesartan (Benicar)	*Initial:* 20 mg once daily *Range:* 20–40 mg once daily	$188.40 (20 mg)		
Olmesartan and HCTZ (Benicar HCT)	*Initial:* 20 mg/12.5 mg once daily *Range:* 20 mg/12.5 mg–40 mg/25 mg once daily	$188.40 (20 mg/12.5 mg)		
Olmesartan and amlodipine (Azor)	*Initial:* 20 mg/5 mg once daily *Range:* 20 mg/5 mg–40 mg/10 mg	$234.90 (20 mg/5 mg)		
Olmesartan and amlodipine and HCTZ (Tribenzor)	*Initial:* 20 mg/5 mg/12.5 mg once daily *Range:* 20 mg/5 mg/12.5 mg–40 mg/10 mg/25 mg once daily	$235.20 (20 mg/5 mg/12.5 mg)		
Telmisartan (Micardis)	*Initial:* 40 mg once daily *Range:* 20–80 mg once daily	$130.20 (40 mg)		
Telmisartan and HCTZ (Micardis HCT)	*Initial:* 40 mg/12.5 mg once daily *Range:* 40 mg/12.5 mg–80 mg/25 mg once daily	$144.90 (40 mg/12.5 mg)		
Telmisartan and amlodipine (Twynsta)	*Initial:* 40 mg/5 mg once daily *Range:* 40 mg/5 mg–80 mg/10 mg once daily	$171.30 (any dose)		
Valsartan (Diovan)	*Initial:* 80 mg once daily *Range:* 80 mg/12.5 mg–320 mg/25 mg once daily	$16.50 (160 mg)		
Valsartan and HCTZ (Diovan HCT)	*Initial:* 80 mg/12.5 mg once daily *Range:* 80–320 mg valsartan once daily	$128.10 (160 mg/12.5 mg)		
Valsartan and amlodipine (Exforge)	*Initial:* 160 mg/5 mg once daily *Range:* 160 mg/5 mg–320 mg/10 mg once daily	$186.00 (160 mg/10 mg)		
Other Combination Products				
Amlodipine and valsartan and HCTZ (Exforge HCT)	*Initial:* 5 mg/160 mg/12.5 mg once daily *Range:* 5 mg/160 mg/12.5 mg–10 mg/320 mg/25 mg once daily	$171.00 (160 mg valsartan)		

[1]Average wholesale price (AWP, for AB-rated generic when available) for quantity listed.
Source: IBM Micromedex Red Book (electronic version) IBM Watson Health. Greenwood Village, CO, USA. Available at https://www.micromedexsolutions.com, accessed March 16, 2022. AWP may not accurately represent the actual pharmacy cost because wide contractual variations exist among institutions.
ER, extended release; HCTZ, hydrochlorothiazide.

also inhibit bradykinin degradation, stimulate the synthesis of vasodilating prostaglandins, and can reduce sympathetic nervous system activity. ACE inhibitors appear to be more effective in younger White patients. They are relatively less effective in Black and older persons and in predominantly systolic hypertension. Although as single therapy they achieve adequate antihypertensive control in only about 40–50% of patients, the combination of an ACE inhibitor and a diuretic or calcium channel blocker is potent.

ACE inhibitors are the agents of choice in persons with type 1 diabetes with frank proteinuria or evidence of kidney dysfunction because they delay the progression to ESKD. Many authorities have expanded this indication to include persons with type 1 and type 2 diabetes mellitus with microalbuminuria who do not meet the usual criteria for antihypertensive therapy. ACE inhibitors may also delay the progression of nondiabetic kidney disease. The Heart Outcomes Prevention Evaluation (HOPE) trial demonstrated that the ACE inhibitor ramipril reduced the number of cardiovascular deaths, nonfatal myocardial infarctions, and nonfatal strokes and also reduced the incidence of new-onset heart failure, kidney dysfunction, and new-onset diabetes in a population of patients at high risk for vascular events. Although this was not specifically a hypertensive population, the benefits were associated with a modest reduction in blood pressure, and the results inferentially support the use of ACE inhibitors in similar hypertensive patients. ACE inhibitors are a drug of choice (usually in conjunction with a diuretic and a beta-blocker) in patients with heart failure with reduced ejection fraction and are indicated also in asymptomatic patients with reduced ejection fraction.

How to initiate therapy—A baseline metabolic panel should be drawn prior to starting medications that interfere with the RAAS, repeated 1–2 weeks after initiation of therapy to evaluate changes in creatinine and potassium. Minor dose adjustments of these medications rarely trigger significant shifts in these values.

Side effects—An advantage of the ACE inhibitors is their relative freedom from troublesome side effects (Table 11–6). Severe hypotension can occur in patients with bilateral renal artery stenosis; significant increases in creatinine may ensue but are usually reversible with the discontinuation of the ACE inhibitor. Hyperkalemia may develop in patients with kidney disease and type IV renal tubular acidosis (commonly seen in patients with diabetes) and in older adults. A chronic dry cough is common, seen in 10% of patients or more, and may require stopping the drug. Skin rashes are observed with any ACE inhibitor. Angioedema is an uncommon but potentially dangerous side effect of all agents of this class because of their inhibition of kininase. Exposure of the fetus to ACE inhibitors during the second and third trimesters of pregnancy has been associated with a variety of defects due to hypotension and reduced renal blood flow.

B. Angiotensin II Receptor Blockers

ARBs can improve cardiovascular outcomes in patients with hypertension as well as in patients with related conditions, such as heart failure and type 2 diabetes with nephropathy. ARBs have not been compared with ACE inhibitors in randomized controlled trials in patients with hypertension, but two trials comparing losartan with captopril in heart failure and post–MI LV dysfunction showed trends toward worse outcomes in the losartan group. By contrast, valsartan seems as effective as ACE inhibitors in these settings. Within group heterogeneity of antihypertensive potency and duration of action might explain such observations. The Losartan Intervention for Endpoints (LIFE) trial in nearly 9000 hypertensive patients with electrocardiographic evidence of LVH—comparing losartan with the beta-blocker atenolol as initial therapy—demonstrated a significant reduction in stroke with losartan. Of note is that in diabetic patients, death and MI were also reduced, and there was a lower occurrence of new-onset diabetes. In a subgroup analysis from the LIFE trial, atenolol appeared to be superior to losartan in African Americans, while the opposite was the case in non-African Americans. A similar reduced efficacy of lisinopril compared to diuretics and calcium channel blockers was observed in Black persons in the Antihypertensive and Lipid-Lowering Treatment to Prevent Heart Attach Trial (ALLHAT), suggesting that ACE inhibitors and ARBs may not be the preferred agents in Black patients (see Table 11–12). In the treatment of hypertension, combination therapy with an ACE inhibitor and an ARB is not advised because it generally offers no advantage over monotherapy at maximum dose with addition of a complementary class where necessary.

Side effects—Unlike ACE inhibitors, the ARBs rarely cause cough and are less likely to be associated with skin rashes or angioedema (Table 11–6). However, as seen with ACE inhibitors, hyperkalemia can be a problem, and patients with bilateral renal artery stenosis may exhibit hypotension and worsened kidney function. Olmesartan has been linked to a sprue-like syndrome, presenting with abdominal pain, weight loss, and nausea, which subsides upon drug discontinuation. There is evidence from an observational study suggesting that ARBs and ACE inhibitors are less likely to be associated with depression than calcium channel blockers and beta-blockers.

C. Renin Inhibitors

Since renin cleavage of angiotensinogen is the rate-limiting step in the renin-angiotensin cascade, the most efficient inactivation of this system would be expected with renin inhibition. Conventional ACE inhibitors and ARBs probably offer incomplete blockade, even in combination. Aliskiren, a renin inhibitor, binds the proteolytic site of renin, thereby preventing cleavage of angiotensinogen. Aliskiren effectively lowers blood pressure, reduces albuminuria, and limits LVH, but it has yet to be established as a first-line drug based on outcomes data. The combination of aliskiren with ACE inhibitors or ARBs in persons with type 2 diabetes mellitus offers no advantage and might even increase the risk of adverse cardiac or renal consequences.

D. Calcium Channel Blocking Agents

These agents act by causing peripheral vasodilation but with less reflex tachycardia and fluid retention than other vasodilators. They are effective as single-drug therapy in approximately 60% of patients in all demographic groups and all grades of hypertension (Table 11–7). For these reasons, they may be preferable to beta-blockers and ACE inhibitors in Black and older persons. Verapamil and diltiazem should be combined cautiously with beta-blockers because of their potential for depressing atrioventricular (AV) conduction and sinus node automaticity as well as contractility.

Calcium channel blockers are equivalent to ACE inhibitors and thiazide diuretics in prevention of CHD, major cardiovascular events, cardiovascular death, and total mortality. A protective effect against stroke with calcium channel blockers is well established, and in two trials (ALLHAT and the Systolic Hypertension in Europe trial), these agents appeared to be more effective than diuretic-based therapy.

Side effects—The most common side effects of calcium channel blockers are headache, peripheral edema, bradycardia, and constipation (especially with verapamil in older adults) (Table 11–7). The dihydropyridine agents—nifedipine, nicardipine, isradipine, felodipine, nisoldipine, and amlodipine—are more likely to produce symptoms of vasodilation, such as headache, flushing, palpitations, and peripheral edema. Edema is minimized by coadministration of an ACE inhibitor or ARB. Calcium channel blockers have negative inotropic effects and should be used cautiously in patients with cardiac dysfunction. Amlodipine is the only calcium channel blocker with established safety in patients with severe heart failure.

E. Diuretics

Thiazide diuretics (Table 11–8) are the antihypertensives that have been most extensively studied and most consistently effective in clinical trials. They lower blood pressure initially by decreasing plasma volume, but during long-term therapy, their major hemodynamic effect is reduction of peripheral vascular resistance. Most of the antihypertensive effect of these agents is achieved at lower dosages (typically, 12.5 mg of hydrochlorothiazide or equivalent), but their biochemical and metabolic effects are dose related. Chlorthalidone has the advantage of better 24-hour blood pressure control than hydrochlorothiazide in clinical trials. Thiazides may be used at higher doses if plasma potassium is above 4.5 mmol/L. The loop diuretics (such as furosemide) may lead to electrolyte and volume depletion more readily than the thiazides and have short durations of action. Because of these adverse effects, loop diuretics should be reserved for use in patients with kidney dysfunction (serum creatinine greater than 2.5 mg/dL [208.3 mcmol/L]; estimated eGFR less than 30 mL/minute/1.73 m^2) in which case they are more effective than thiazides. Relative to beta-blockers and ACE inhibitors, diuretics are more potent in Black persons, older individuals, obese persons, and other subgroups with increased plasma volume or low plasma renin activity (or both). They are relatively more effective in cigarette smokers than in nonsmokers. Long-term thiazide administration also mitigates the loss of bone mineral content in older women at risk for osteoporosis.

Overall, diuretics administered alone control blood pressure in 50% of patients with mild to moderate hypertension and can be used effectively in combination with all other agents. They are also useful for lowering isolated or predominantly systolic hypertension.

Side effects—The adverse effects of diuretics relate primarily to the metabolic changes listed in Table 11–8. Erectile dysfunction, skin rashes, and photosensitivity are less frequent. Hypokalemia has been a concern but is uncommon at the recommended dosages. The risk can be minimized by limiting dietary salt or increasing dietary potassium; potassium replacement is not usually required to maintain serum K^+ at greater than 3.5 mmol/L. Higher serum K^+ levels are prudent in patients at special risk from intracellular potassium depletion, such as those taking digoxin or with a history of ventricular arrhythmias, in which case a potassium-sparing agent could be used. Compared with ACE inhibitors and ARBs, diuretic therapy is associated with a slightly higher incidence of mild new-onset diabetes. Diuretics also increase serum uric acid and may precipitate gout. Increases in blood glucose, triglycerides, and LDL cholesterol may occur but are relatively minor during long-term low-dose therapy. The potential for worsening of diabetes is outweighed by the advantages of blood pressure control, and diuretics should not be withheld from diabetic patients.

F. Aldosterone Receptor Antagonists

Spironolactone and eplerenone are natriuretic in sodium-retaining states, such as heart failure and cirrhosis, but only very weakly so in hypertension. These drugs have reemerged in the treatment of hypertension, particularly in resistant patients and are helpful additions to most other antihypertensive medications. Consistent with the increasingly appreciated importance of aldosterone in essential hypertension, the aldosterone receptor blockers are effective at lowering blood pressure in all hypertensive patients regardless of renin level and are also effective in Black persons. Aldosterone plays a central role in target-organ damage, including the development of ventricular and vascular hypertrophy and renal fibrosis. Aldosterone receptor antagonists ameliorate these consequences of hypertension, to some extent independently of effects on blood pressure.

Side effects—Spironolactone can cause breast pain and gynecomastia in men through activity at the progesterone receptor, an effect not seen with the more specific eplerenone. Hyperkalemia is a problem with both drugs, chiefly in patients with CKD. Hyperkalemia is more likely if the pretreatment plasma potassium exceeds 4.5 mmol/L.

G. Beta-Blocking Agents

These drugs are effective in hypertension because they decrease the heart rate and cardiac output. The beta-blockers also decrease renin release and are more efficacious in populations with elevated plasma renin activity, such as younger White patients. They neutralize the reflex tachycardia caused by vasodilators and are especially useful in patients with associated conditions that benefit from the

Table 11–7. Antihypertensive drugs: calcium channel blocking agents.

Medication (Proprietary Name)	Oral Dosages	Cost of 30 Days of Treatment (Average Dosage)[1]	Special Properties			Adverse Effects	Comments
			Peripheral Vasodilation	Cardiac Automaticity and Conduction	Contractility		
Nondihydropyridine Agents							
Diltiazem							
(Cardizem SR)	*Initial:* 90 mg twice daily *Range:* 180–360 mg in 2 doses	\$283.80 (120 mg twice daily)	++	↓↓	↓↓	Edema, headache, bradycardia, bloating and constipation, dizziness, AV block, heart failure, urinary frequency.	Also approved for angina.
(Cardizem CD)	*Initial:* 180 mg ER once daily *Range:* 180–360 mg ER once daily	\$42.00 (240 mg once daily)					
(Cartia XT)	*Initial:* 180 or 240 mg ER once daily *Range:* 180–480 mg ER once daily	\$42.00 (240 mg once daily)					
Dilt-XR	*Initial:* 180 or 240 mg ER once daily *Range:* 180–540 mg ER once daily	\$42.90 (240 mg once daily)					
(Taztia XT)	*Initial:* 120 or 180 mg ER once daily *Range:* 120–540 mg ER once daily	\$53.40 (240 mg once daily)					
(Tiazac)	*Initial:* 120 or 240 mg ER once daily *Range:* 120–540 mg ER once daily	\$53.40 (240 mg once daily)					
Verapamil							
(Calan)	*Initial:* 40 mg three times daily *Range:* 120–480 mg in 3 divided doses	\$35.10 (80 mg three times daily)	++	↓↓↓	↓↓↓	Same as diltiazem but more likely to cause constipation and heart failure.	Also approved for angina and arrhythmias.
(Calan SR)	*Initial:* 120 mg ER once daily *Range:* 120–480 mg ER in 1 or 2 doses	\$49.20 (240 mg once daily)					
(Verelan)	*Initial:* 120 or 240 mg ER once daily *Range:* 240–480 mg ER once daily	\$68.70 (240 mg once daily)					
(Verelan PM)	*Initial:* 100 or 200 mg ER once daily *Range:* 100–400 mg ER once daily	\$75.90 (200 mg once daily)					

Dihydropyridines							
Amlodipine (Norvasc)	*Initial:* 2.5 mg once daily *Range:* 2.5–10 mg once daily	$3.00 (10 mg once daily)	+++	↓/0	↓/0	Edema, dizziness, palpitations, flushing, headache, hypotension, tachycardia, bloating and constipation, urinary frequency.	Amlodipine, nicardipine, and nifedipine also approved for angina.
Amlodipine and atorvastatin (Caduet)	*Initial:* 2.5 mg/10 mg once daily *Range:* 10 mg/80 mg once daily	$281.10 (10 mg/40 mg daily)	+++	↓/0	↓/0	Edema (amlodipine), myopathy and hepatotoxicity (atorvastatin).	
Felodipine (Plendil)	*Initial:* 5 mg ER once daily *Range:* 5–10 mg ER once daily	$65.40 (10 mg ER daily)	+++	↓/0	↓/0		
Isradipine (DynaCirc)	*Initial:* 2.5 mg twice daily *Range:* 2.5–5 mg twice daily	$225.60 (5 mg twice daily)	+++	↓/0	↓		
Nicardipine (Cardene)	*Initial:* 20 mg three times daily *Range:* 20–40 mg three times daily	$200.70 (20 mg three times daily)	+++	↓/0	↓		
Nifedipine (Adalat CC)	*Initial:* 30 mg ER once daily *Range:* 30–90 mg ER once daily	$68.70/60 mg daily	+++	↓	↓↓		
Nifedipine (Procardia XL)	*Initial:* 30 or 60 mg ER once daily *Range:* 30–120 mg ER once daily	$19.80/60 mg daily					
Nisoldipine (Sular)	*Initial:* 17 mg daily *Range:* 17–34 mg daily	$251.70 (34 mg once daily)	+++	↓/0	↓		

[1]Average wholesale price (AWP, for AB-rated generic when available) for quantity listed.
Source: IBM Micromedex Red Book (electronic version) IBM Watson Health. Greenwood Village, CO, USA. Available at https://www.micromedexsolutions.com, accessed March 16, 2022. AWP may not accurately represent the actual pharmacy cost because wide contractual variations exist among institutions.
AV, atrioventricular; ER, extended release.

Table 11–8. Antihypertensive drugs: diuretics (in descending order of preference).

Drugs	Proprietary Names	Oral Doses	Cost of 30 Days of Treatment[1] (Average Dosage)	Adverse Effects	Comments
Thiazides and Related Diuretics					
Hydrochlorothiazide (HCTZ)	Esidrix, Microzide	*Initial:* 12.5 or 25 mg once daily *Range:* 12.5–50 mg once daily	\$2.40 (25 mg)	↓K^+, ↓Mg^{2+}, ↑Ca^{2+}, ↓Na+, ↑uric acid, ↑glucose, ↑LDL cholesterol, ↑triglycerides; rash, erectile dysfunction.	Low dosages effective in many patients without associated metabolic abnormalities
Chlorthalidone	Thalitone	*Initial:* 12.5 or 25 mg once daily *Range:* 12.5–50 mg once daily	\$36.30 (25 mg)		Better 24-hour blood pressure control than HCTZ because of longer half-life
Metolazone	Zaroxolyn	*Initial:* 1.25 or 2.5 mg once daily *Range:* 1.25–5 mg once daily	\$70.80 (5 mg)		More effective with concurrent kidney disease
Indapamide	Lozol	*Initial:* 2.5 mg once daily *Range:* 2.5–5 mg once daily	\$30.60 (2.5 mg)		Does not alter serum lipid levels
Bendroflumethiazide	Aprinox Neo-Naclex	*Initial:* 2.5 mg once daily	—		Not available in United States
Loop Diuretics					
Furosemide	Lasix	*Initial:* 20 mg twice daily *Range:* 40–320 mg in 2 or 3 doses	\$5.40 (40 mg)	Same as thiazides, but with higher risk of excessive diuresis and electrolyte imbalance. Increases calcium excretion.	Short duration of action a disadvantage; should be reserved for patients with kidney disease or fluid retention. Poor antihypertensive.
Ethacrynic acid	Edecrin	*Initial:* 50 mg once daily *Range:* 50–100 mg once or twice daily	\$1437.00 (25 mg)		
Bumetanide	(generic)	*Initial:* 0.25 mg twice daily *Range:* 0.5–10 mg in 2 or 3 doses	\$32.40 (1 mg)		
Torsemide	Demadex	*Initial:* 5 mg once daily *Range:* 5–10 mg once daily	\$21.00 (10 mg)		Effective blood pressure medication at low dosage.
Aldosterone Receptor Blockers					
Spironolactone	Aldactone	*Initial:* 12.5 or 25 mg once daily *Range:* 12.5–100 mg once daily	\$5.70 (25 mg)	Hyperkalemia, metabolic acidosis, gynecomastia.	Can be useful add-on therapy in patients with refractory hypertension.
Amiloride	(generic)	*Initial:* 5 mg once daily *Range:* 5–10 mg once daily	\$6.90 (5 mg)		
Eplerenone	Inspra	*Initial:* 25 mg once daily *Range:* 25–100 mg once daily	\$123.00 (25 mg)		

Combination Products					
HCTZ and triamterene	Dyazide, Maxzide-25 (25/37.5 mg)	*Ilnitial:* 25 mg/37.5 mg once daily *Range*: 25 mg/37.5 mg–50 mg/75 mg once daily	$10.80	Same as thiazides plus GI disturbances, hyperkalemia rather than hypokalemia, headache; triamterene can cause kidney stones and kidney dysfunction; spironolactone causes gynecomastia. Hyperkalemia can occur if this combination is used in patients with advanced kidney disease or those taking ACE inhibitors.	Use should be limited to patients with demonstrable need for a potassium-sparing agent.
HCTZ and amiloride	(generic) (50/5 mg)	*Initial:* 25 mg/2.5 mg once daily *Range:* 50 mg/5 mg–100 mg/10 mg once daily	$34.80		
HCTZ and spironolactone	Aldactazide (25/25 mg; 50/50 mg)	*Initial:* 25 mg/25 mg once daily *Range:* 25 mg/25 mg–100 mg/100 mg once daily	$37.20 (25/25 mg)		

[1]Average wholesale price (AWP, for AB-rated generic when available) for quantity listed.
Source: IBM Micromedex Red Book (electronic version) IBM Watson Health. Greenwood Village, CO, USA. Available at https://www.micromedexsolutions.com, accessed March 16, 2022. AWP may not accurately represent the actual pharmacy cost because wide contractual variations exist among institutions.

cardioprotective effects of these agents. These include individuals with angina pectoris, previous myocardial infarction, and stable heart failure as well as those with migraine headaches and somatic manifestations of anxiety.

Although all beta-blockers appear to be similar in antihypertensive potency, they differ in a number of pharmacologic properties (these differences are summarized in Table 11–9), including specificity to the cardiac beta-1-receptors (cardioselectivity) and whether they also block the beta-2-receptors in the bronchi and vasculature; *at higher dosages, however, all agents are nonselective.* The beta-blockers also differ in their pharmacokinetics, lipid solubility—which determines whether they cross the blood-brain barrier predisposing to CNS side effects—and route of metabolism. Metoprolol reduces mortality and morbidity in patients with chronic stable heart failure with reduced ejection fraction (see Chapter 10). Carvedilol and nebivolol maintain cardiac output and are beneficial in patients with LV systolic dysfunction. Carvedilol and nebivolol may reduce peripheral vascular resistance by concomitant alpha-blockade (carvedilol) and increased nitric oxide release (nebivolol). Because of the lack of efficacy in primary prevention of MI and inferiority compared with other drugs in prevention of stroke and LVH, traditional beta-blockers should not be used as first-line agents in the treatment of hypertension without specific compelling indications (such as active CAD). Vasodilating beta-blockers may emerge as alternative first-line antihypertensives, but this possibility has yet to be rigorously tested in outcome studies.

Side effects—The side effects of beta-blockers include inducing or exacerbating bronchospasm in predisposed patients; sinus node dysfunction and AV conduction depression (resulting in bradycardia or AV block); nasal congestion; Raynaud phenomenon; and CNS symptoms with nightmares, excitement, depression, and confusion. Fatigue, lethargy, and erectile dysfunction may occur. The traditional beta-blockers (but not the vasodilator beta-blockers carvedilol and nebivolol) have an adverse effect on lipids and glucose metabolism. Beta-blockers are used cautiously in patients with type 1 diabetes since they can mask the symptoms of hypoglycemia and prolong these episodes by inhibiting gluconeogenesis. These drugs should also be used with caution in patients with advanced peripheral vascular disease associated with rest pain or nonhealing ulcers, but they are generally well tolerated in patients with mild claudication. Nebivolol can be safely used in patients with stage II claudication (claudication at 200 m).

In treatment of pheochromocytoma, beta-blockers should not be administered until alpha-blockade (eg, phentolamine) has been established. Otherwise, blockade of vasodilatory beta-2-adrenergic receptors will allow unopposed vasoconstrictor alpha-adrenergic–receptor activation with worsening of hypertension. *For the same reason, beta-blockers should not be used to treat hypertension arising from cocaine use.*

Great care should be exercised if the decision is made, in the absence of compelling indications, to remove beta-blockers from the treatment regimen because abrupt withdrawal can precipitate acute coronary events and severe increases in blood pressure.

H. Alpha-Antagonists

Prazosin, terazosin, and doxazosin (Table 11–10) block postsynaptic alpha-receptors, relax smooth muscle, and reduce blood pressure by lowering peripheral vascular resistance. These agents are effective as single-drug therapy in some individuals, but tachyphylaxis may appear during long-term therapy. Unlike beta-blockers and diuretics, alpha-blockers have no adverse effect on serum lipid levels. In fact, alpha-blockers increase HDL cholesterol while reducing total cholesterol; whether this is beneficial in the long term has not been established.

Side effects—Side effects are relatively common (Table 11–10). These include marked hypotension after the first dose which, therefore, should be small and given at bedtime. Post-dosing palpitations, headache, and nervousness may continue to occur during long-term therapy; these symptoms may be less frequent or severe with doxazosin because of its more gradual onset of action. In ALLHAT, persons receiving doxazosin as initial therapy had a significant increase in heart failure hospitalizations and a higher incidence of stroke relative to those receiving diuretics, prompting discontinuation of this arm of the study. Cataractectomy in patients exposed to alpha-blockers can be complicated by the floppy iris syndrome, even after discontinuation of the drug, so the ophthalmologist should be alerted that the patient has been taking the drug prior to surgery.

To summarize, alpha-blockers should generally not be used as initial agents to treat hypertension—except perhaps in men with symptomatic prostatism or nightmares linked to PTSD.

I. Drugs With Central Sympatholytic Action

Methyldopa, clonidine, guanabenz, and guanfacine (Table 11–10) lower blood pressure by stimulating alpha-adrenergic receptors in the CNS, thus reducing efferent peripheral sympathetic outflow. There is considerable experience with methyldopa in pregnant women, and it is still used for this population. Clonidine is available in patches, which may have particular value in noncompliant patients. All of these central sympatholytic agents are effective as single therapy in some patients, but they are usually used as second- or third-line agents because of the high frequency of drug intolerance.

Side effects—Side effects include sedation, fatigue, dry mouth, postural hypotension, and erectile dysfunction. An important concern is rebound hypertension following withdrawal. Methyldopa also causes hepatitis and hemolytic anemia and should be restricted to individuals who have already tolerated long-term therapy.

J. Peripheral Sympathetic Inhibitors

These agents are usually used only in refractory hypertension. Reserpine remains a cost-effective antihypertensive agent (Table 11–10). Its reputation for inducing mental depression and its other side effects—sedation, nasal stuffiness, sleep disturbances, and peptic ulcers—has made it unpopular, though these problems are uncommon at low dosages. Guanethidine and guanadrel inhibit catecholamine

Table 11–9. Antihypertensive drugs: beta-blocking agents.

Medication (Proprietary Name)	Oral Dosage	Cost of 30 Days of Treatment (Average Dosage)[1]	Special Properties					Comments[5]
			Beta-1 Selectivity[2]	ISA[3]	MSA[4]	Lipid Solubility	Renal vs Hepatic Elimination	
Acebutolol (Sectral)	*Initial:* 400 mg once daily *Range:* 200–1200 mg in 1 or 2 doses	$47.10 (400 mg)	+	+	+	+	H > R	Positive ANA; rare LE syndrome; also indicated for arrhythmias. Doses > 800 mg have beta-1 and beta-2 effects.
Atenolol (Tenormin)	*Initial:* 25 mg once daily *Range:* 25–100 mg once daily	$24.90 (50 mg)	+	0	0	0	R	Also indicated for angina and post-MI. Doses > 100 mg have beta-1 and beta-2 effects.
Atenolol/chlorthalidone (Tenoretic)	*Initial:* 50 mg/25 mg once daily *Range:* 50 mg/25 mg–100 mg/25 mg once daily	$56.40 (50 mg/25 mg)	+	0	0	0	R	
Betaxolol (Kerlone)	*Initial:* 10 mg once daily *Range:* 10–40 mg once daily	$36.90 (10 mg)	+	0	0	+	H > R	
Bisoprolol (Zebeta)	*Initial:* 5 mg once daily *Range:* 5–20 mg once daily	$42.00 (10 mg)	+	0	0	0	R = H	Also effective for heart failure.
Bisoprolol and HCTZ (Ziac)	*Initial:* 2.5 mg/6.25 mg once daily *Range:* 2.5 mg/6.25 mg–10 mg/6.25 mg once daily	$101.10 (2.5/6.25 mg)	+	0	0	0	R = H	Low-dose combination approved for initial therapy.
Carvedilol (Coreg)	*Initial:* 6.25 mg twice daily *Range:* 12.5–50 mg in 2 doses	$5.40 (25 mg)	0	0	0	+++	H > R	Alpha:beta blocking activity 1:9; may cause orthostatic symptoms; effective for heart failure. Nitric oxide potentiating vasodilatory activity.[6]
Carvedilol (Coreg CR)	*Initial:* 20 mg ER once daily *Range:* 20–80 mg ER once daily	$297.30 (any tablet)	0	0	0	+++	H > R	
Labetalol (Trandate)	*Initial:* 100 mg twice daily *Range:* 200–2400 mg in 2 doses	$23.40 (200 mg)	0	0/+	0	++	H	Alpha:beta blocking activity 1:3; more orthostatic hypotension, fever, hepatotoxicity.
Metoprolol (Lopressor)	*Initial:* 50 mg twice daily *Range:* 50–200 mg twice daily	$7.80 (50 mg)	+	0	+	+++	H	Also indicated for angina and post-MI. Approved for heart failure. Doses > 100 mg have beta-1 and beta-2 effects.
Metoprolol (Toprol-XL [SR preparation])	*Initial:* 25 mg once daily *Range:* 25–400 mg once daily	$6.00 (100 mg)						

(continued)

Table 11–9. Antihypertensive drugs: beta-blocking agents. (continued)

Medication (Proprietary Name)	Oral Dosage	Cost of 30 Days of Treatment (Average Dosage)[1]	Special Properties					Comments[5]
			Beta-1 Selectivity[2]	ISA[3]	MSA[4]	Lipid Solubility	Renal vs Hepatic Elimination	
Metoprolol and HCTZ (Lopressor HCT)	*Initial:* 50 mg/12.5 mg twice daily *Range:* 50 mg/25 mg–200 mg/50 mg in single or divided doses	\$131.40 (100 mg/25 mg)	+	0	+	+++	H	
Nadolol (Corgard)	*Initial:* 20 mg once daily *Range:* 20–320 mg once daily	\$7.20 (40 mg)	0	0	0	0	R	
Nebivolol (Bystolic)	*Initial:* 5 mg once daily *Range:* 40 mg once daily	\$100.80 (5 mg)	+	0	0	++	H	Nitric oxide potentiating vasodilatory activity.[6]
Pindolol (Visken)	*Initial:* 5 mg twice daily *Range:* 10–60 mg in 2 doses	\$79.20 (5 mg)	0	++	+	+	H > R	In adults, 35% renal clearance
Propranolol								
(Inderal)	*Initial:* 20 mg twice daily *Range:* 40–640 mg in 2 doses	\$18.60 (40 mg)	0	0	++	+++	H	Also indicated for angina and post-MI.
(Inderal LA)	*Initial:* 80 mg ER once daily *Range:* 120–640 mg ER once daily	\$89.40 (120 mg)						
(InnoPran XL)	*Initial:* 80 mg ER once nightly *Range:* 80–120 mg ER once nightly	\$906.00 (120 mg)						
Propranolol and HCTZ (generic)	*Initial:* 40 mg/25 mg twice daily *Range:* 40 mg/25 mg–80 mg/25 mg twice daily	\$84.60 (80 mg/25 mg)	0	0	++	+++	H	
Timolol (generic)	*Initial:* 5 mg twice daily *Range:* 10–60 mg in 2 doses	\$102.00 (10 mg)	0	0	0	++	H > R	Also indicated for post-MI; 80% hepatic clearance.

[1]Average wholesale price (AWP, for AB-rated generic when available) for quantity listed.
Source: IBM Micromedex Red Book (electronic version) IBM Watson Health. Greenwood Village, CO, USA. Available at https://www.micromedexsolutions.com, accessed March 16, 2022. AWP may not accurately represent the actual pharmacy cost because wide contractual variations exist among institutions.
[2]Agents with beta-1 selectivity are less likely to precipitate bronchospasm and decrease peripheral blood flow in low doses, but selectivity is only relative.
[3]Agents with ISA cause less resting bradycardia and lipid changes.
[4]MSA generally occurs at concentrations greater than those necessary for beta-blockade. The clinical importance of MSA by beta-blockers has not been defined.
[5]Adverse effects of all beta-blockers: bronchospasm, fatigue, sleep disturbance and nightmares, bradycardia and atrioventricular block, worsening of heart failure, cold extremities, GI disturbances, erectile dysfunction, ↑ triglycerides, ↓ HDL cholesterol, rare blood dyscrasias.
[6]Carvedilol and nebivolol stimulate release of nitric oxide by vascular endothelium, which may augment the vasodilatory effects of drugs such as hydralazine and prazosin.
ANA, antinuclear antibody; ER, extended release; HCTZ, hydrochlorothiazide; ISA, intrinsic sympathomimetic activity; LE, lupus erythematosus; MSA, membrane-stabilizing activity; SR, sustained release; 0, no effect; +, some effect; ++, moderate effect; +++, most effect.

Table 11–10. Alpha-blocking agents, sympatholytics, and vasodilators.

Medication (Proprietary Names)	Dosage	Cost of 30 Days of Treatment (Average Dosage)[1]	Adverse Effects	Comments
Alpha-Blockers				
Doxazosin (Cardura)	*Initial:* 1 mg at bedtime *Range:* 1–16 mg once daily	$8.70 (4 mg)	Syncope with first dose; postural hypotension, dizziness, palpitations, headache, weakness, drowsiness, sexual dysfunction, anticholinergic effects, urinary incontinence; first-dose effects may be less with doxazosin.	May ↑ HDL and ↓ LDL cholesterol. May provide short-term relief of obstructive prostatic symptoms. Less effective in preventing cardiovascular events than diuretics.
Doxazosin (Cardura XL)	*Initial:* 4 mg ER once daily *Range:* 4–8 mg ER once daily	$212.10 (4 mg ER)		
Prazosin (Minipress)	*Initial:* 1 mg at bedtime *Range:* 2–20 mg in 2 or 3 doses	$130.80 (5 mg)		
Terazosin (Hytrin)	*Initial:* 1 mg at bedtime *Range:* 1–20 mg in 1 or 2 doses	$48.30 (5 mg)		
Central Sympatholytics				
Clonidine (Catapres)	*Initial:* 0.1 mg twice daily *Range:* 0.2–0.6 mg in 2 doses	$3.00 (0.1 mg)	Sedation, dry mouth, sexual dysfunction, headache, bradyarrhythmias; side effects may be less with guanfacine. Contact dermatitis with clonidine patch.	"Rebound" hypertension may occur even after gradual withdrawal.
Clonidine (Catapres TTS [transdermal patch])	*Initial:* 0.1 mg/day patch weekly *Range:* 0.1–0.3 mg/day patch weekly	$223.06 (0.2 mg patch)		
Clonidine and chlorthalidone (Clorpres)	*Initial:* 0.1 mg/15 mg one to three times daily *Range:* 0.1 mg/15 mg–0.6 mg/30 mg in single or divided doses	$166.20 (0.1 mg/15 mg)		
Guanfacine (Tenex)	*Initial:* 1 mg once daily *Range:* 1–3 mg once daily	$26.10 (1 mg)		
Methyldopa (Aldochlor)	*Initial:* 250 mg twice daily *Range:* 500–2000 mg in 2 doses	$39.60 (500 mg)	Hepatitis, hemolytic anemia, fever.	Avoid in favor of safer agents.
Peripheral Neuronal Antagonists				
Reserpine (generic)	*Initial:* 0.05 mg once daily *Range:* 0.05–0.25 mg once daily	$35.70 (0.1 mg)	Depression (less likely at low dosages, ie, < 0.25 mg), night terrors, nasal stuffiness, drowsiness, peptic disease, GI disturbances, bradycardia.	
Direct Vasodilators				
Hydralazine (Apresoline)	*Initial:* 25 mg twice daily *Range:* 50–300 mg in 2–4 doses	$9.00 (25 mg)	GI disturbances, tachycardia, headache, nasal congestion, rash, LE-like syndrome.	May worsen or precipitate angina.
Minoxidil (generic)	*Initial:* 5 mg once daily *Range:* 10–40 mg once daily	$38.40 (10 mg)	Tachycardia, fluid retention, headache, hirsutism, pericardial effusion, thrombocytopenia.	Should be used in combination with beta-blocker and diuretic.

[1]Average wholesale price (AWP, for AB-rated generic when available) for quantity listed.
Source: IBM Micromedex Red Book (electronic version) IBM Watson Health. Greenwood Village, CO, USA. Available at https://www.micromedexsolutions.com, accessed March 16, 2022. AWP may not accurately represent the actual pharmacy cost because wide contractual variations exist among institutions.
ER, extended release; LE, lupus erythematosus.

release from peripheral neurons but frequently cause orthostatic hypotension (especially in the morning or after exercise), diarrhea, and fluid retention.

K. Arteriolar Dilators

Hydralazine and minoxidil (Table 11–10) relax vascular smooth muscle and produce peripheral vasodilation. When given alone, they stimulate reflex tachycardia; increase myocardial contractility; and cause headache, palpitations, and fluid retention. To counteract these effects, the agents are usually given in combination with diuretics and beta-blockers in resistant patients. Hydralazine produces frequent GI disturbances and may induce a lupus-like syndrome. Minoxidil causes hirsutism and marked fluid retention; this very potent agent is reserved for the most refractory of cases.

Antihypertensive Medications & the Risk of Cancer

A number of observational studies have examined the association between long-term exposure to antihypertensive medications and cancer. Weak associations have been suggested by some of these studies, but results have been mixed. In the absence of large-scale prospective studies with cancer as a prespecified outcome measure, the effect of antihypertensive drugs on the risk of cancer remains uncertain. By contrast, the beneficial effect of these drugs on cardiovascular outcomes has been clearly established. Concern about increased risk of cancer should not be minimized, but at present there are no compelling data to prompt a change in prescribing patterns.

Procedures That Modulate the Activity of the Autonomic Nervous System

Before the advent of antihypertensive medications, lumbar sympathectomy was used to lower blood pressure. In a more specific and less invasive approach, the renal sympathetic nerves can be ablated using radiofrequency energy applied to the luminal surface of the renal arteries. However, the Symplicity HTN-3 study of renal sympathetic denervation did not show any difference in blood pressure reduction compared to a sham procedure group. Subsequently, the SPYRAL HTN-OFF MED study, using a more intensive and closely controlled ablation strategy, demonstrated modest but clinically meaningful blood pressure reductions compared to the sham control group. This effect on blood pressure has been confirmed by several subsequent studies. Although not yet accepted in general clinical practice, it seems probable that renal sympathetic nerve ablation will emerge as an alternative or adjunctive modality in the treatment of hypertension and may have a role in the management of resistant hypertension and drug intolerance.

Developing an Antihypertensive Regimen

Historically, data from large placebo-controlled trials supported the overall conclusion that antihypertensive therapy with diuretics and beta-blockers had a major beneficial effect on a broad spectrum of cardiovascular outcomes, reducing the incidence of stroke by 30–50% and of heart failure by 40–50%, and halting progression to accelerated hypertension syndromes. The decreases in fatal and nonfatal CHD and cardiovascular and total mortality were less dramatic, ranging from 10% to 15%. Similar placebo-controlled data pertaining to the newer agents are generally lacking, except for stroke reduction with the calcium channel blocker nitrendipine in the Systolic Hypertension in Europe trial. However, there is substantial evidence that ACE inhibitors, and to a lesser extent ARBs, reduce adverse cardiovascular outcomes in other related populations (eg, patients with diabetic nephropathy, heart failure, or post-MI and individuals at high risk for cardiovascular events). Most large clinical trials that have compared outcomes in relatively unselected patients have failed to show a difference between newer agents—such as ACE inhibitors, calcium channel blockers, and ARBs—and the older diuretic-based regimens with regard to survival, myocardial infarction, and stroke. Where differences have been observed, they have mostly been attributable to subtle asymmetries in blood pressure control rather than to any inherent advantages of one agent over another. Recommendations for initial treatment identify ACE inhibitors, ARBs, and calcium channel blockers as valid choices. Because of their adverse metabolic profile, initial therapy with thiazides might best be restricted to older patients. Thiazides are acceptable as first-line therapy in Black persons because of specific efficacy in this group.

As discussed above, beta-blockers are not ideal first-line drugs in the treatment of hypertension without compelling indications for their use (such as active CAD and heart failure). Vasodilator beta-blockers (such as carvedilol and nebivolol) may produce better outcomes than traditional beta-blockers; however, this possibility remains speculative.

Theoretically, restoration of nocturnal dipping by dosing some antihypertensive medications at the end of the day seems desirable. However, the impact that nocturnal dosing of antihypertensive medications has on hypertension control and clinical outcomes remains unresolved. The HYGIA study reported significant benefits of evening compared to morning dosing. However, because of the risk of ischemic events from profound nocturnal hypotension and because clinical benefits remain uncertain, many experts have criticized this study and urged caution before general acceptance of nocturnal dosing.

Medications that interrupt the renin-angiotensin cascade are more effective in young, White persons, in whom renin tends to be higher. Calcium channel blockers and diuretics are more effective in older or Black persons, in whom renin levels are generally lower. Many patients require two or more medications and even then a substantial proportion fail to achieve the goal blood pressure. A stepped care approach to the drug treatment of hypertension is outlined in Table 11–11. In diabetic patients, three or four drugs are usually required to reduce systolic blood pressure to goal. In many patients, blood pressure cannot be adequately controlled with any combination. As a result, debating the appropriate first-line agent is less relevant than determining the most appropriate combinations of agents.

Table 11–11. A stepped care approach to the initiation and titration of antihypertension medications.[1,2]

Step 1	ACE inhibitor/ARB **or**[3] Calcium channel blocker **or** Thiazide diuretic[4]
Step 2	ACE inhibitor/ARB **plus** Calcium channel blocker **or** thiazide diuretic[5]
Step 3	ACE inhibitor/ARB **plus** calcium channel blocker **plus** thiazide diuretic
Step 4	ACE inhibitor/ARB **plus** calcium channel blocker **plus** thiazide diuretic **plus** spironolactone[6]

[1]Allow 2 weeks to reach full effect of each drug. Proceed through steps until target blood pressure is attained.
[2]Beta-blockers can be used at any stage if specifically indicated, eg, heart failure or angina.
[3]Initiation with combination therapy should be considered in patients with higher levels of blood pressure and higher cardiovascular risk.
[4]Thiazide or calcium channel blocker is more effective initial therapy in older people and Blacks.
[5]If required, add a calcium channel blocker rather than diuretic in younger patients to avoid long-term exposure to metabolic side effects of diuretics.
[6]Alternatives to spironolactone include eplerenone, amiloride, or triamterene. Watch for hyperkalemia, especially if also receiving ACE inhibitor/ARB. Avoid potassium-sparing diuretics in advanced CKD. If more than three drugs are required at maximum dose, consider specialist referral.

The mnemonic ABCD can be used to remember four classes of antihypertensive medications. These four classes can be divided into two categories: AB and CD. AB refers to drugs that block the RAAS (**A**CE/ARB and **b**eta-blockers). CD refers to those that work in other pathways (**c**alcium channel blockers and **d**iuretics). Combinations of drugs between the two categories are more potent than combinations from within a category. Many experts recommend the use of fixed-dose combination (between two categories) antihypertensive agents as first-line therapy in patients with substantially elevated systolic pressures (greater than 160/100 mm Hg) or difficult-to-control hypertension (which is often associated with diabetes or kidney dysfunction). Because of the unwanted metabolic effects of thiazides, calcium channel blockers may be the preferred second agent in the younger hypertensive patient who is already taking an ACE inhibitor or ARB. However, studies have repeatedly confirmed the effectiveness of thiazide diuretics as first-line agents in prevention of multiple clinical endpoints. Based on the results from the ACCOMPLISH trial, a combination of ACE inhibitor and calcium channel blocker may prove optimal for patients at high risk for cardiovascular events. The initial use of low-dose combinations allows faster blood pressure reduction without substantially higher intolerance rates and is likely to be better accepted by patients. Data from the ALTITUDE study (in patients with type 2 diabetes and CKD or cardiovascular disease or both) indicate that the addition of aliskiren to either ARB or ACE inhibitor was associated with worse outcomes and cannot be recommended, at least in this population. A suggested approach to treatment, tailored to patient demographics, is outlined in Table 11–12.

In sum, as a prelude to treatment, the patient should be informed of common side effects and the need for diligent compliance. In patients with blood pressure less than 160/90 mm Hg in whom pharmacotherapy is indicated, treatment should start with a single agent or two-drug combination at a low dose. Follow-up visits usually should be at 4- to 6-week intervals to allow for full medication effects to be established (especially with diuretics) before further titration or adjustment. If, after titration to usual doses, the patient has shown a discernible but incomplete response and a good tolerance of the initial drug, another medication should be added. See Goals of Treatment, above. As a rule of thumb, a blood pressure reduction of 10 mm Hg can be expected for each antihypertensive agent added to the regimen and titrated to the optimum dose. In those with more severe hypertension, or with comorbidities (such as diabetes) that are likely to render them resistant to treatment, initiation with combination therapy is advised and more frequent follow-up is indicated. Most guidelines recommend the use of home blood pressure monitors in the diagnosis of hypertension. Digital technology makes it possible to monitor the patient's self-measured response to therapy with direct transmission of blood pressure readings to the clinic. The availability of blood pressure profiles generated from multiple home-gathered data points over continuous intervals allows more precise control of the overall hypertensive burden.

Patients who are compliant with their medications and who do not respond to conventional combination regimens should usually be evaluated for secondary hypertension before proceeding to more complex regimens.

Medication Nonadherence

Adherence to antihypertensive treatment is alarmingly poor. In one European study of antihypertensive medication compliance, there was a 40% discontinuation rate at 1 year after initiation. Collaborative care, using clinicians, pharmacists, social workers, and nurses to encourage compliance, has had a variable and often rather modest effect on blood pressure control. Adherence is enhanced by patient education and by use of home blood pressure measurement. The choice of antihypertensive medication is important. Better compliance has been reported for patients whose medications could be taken once daily or as combination pills. Adherence is best with ACE inhibitors and ARBs, and worse with beta-blockers and diuretics.

Table 11–12. Choice of antihypertensive agent based on demographic considerations.[1,2]

	Black Persons, All Ages[3]	All Others, Age < 55 Years	All Others, Age > 55 Years
First-line	CCB or diuretic[4,5]	ACE inhibitor or ARB[6] or CCB or diuretic[4,5]	CCB or diuretic[4,5]
Second-line	ARB[6] or ACE inhibitor[6,7] or vasodilating beta-blocker[8]	Vasodilating beta-blocker[8]	ACE inhibitor[6] or ARB[6] or vasodilating beta-blocker[8]
Resistant hypertension	Aldosterone receptor blocker	Aldosterone receptor blocker	Aldosterone receptor blocker
Additional options	Centrally acting alpha-agonist or peripheral alpha-antagonist[9]	Centrally acting alpha-agonist or peripheral alpha-antagonist[9]	Centrally acting alpha-agonist or peripheral alpha-antagonist[9]

[1]Compelling indications may alter the selection of an antihypertensive drug.
[2]Start with full dose of one agent, or lower doses of combination therapy. In more severe hypertension (≥ 140/90 mm Hg), consider initiating therapy with a fixed-dose combination.
[3]The reasons why the responses to some medications tend to differ in Black patients are complex and poorly understood. Observations such as these should not be taken as evidence of biological differences based on racial categories.
[4]For patients with significant kidney dysfunction, use loop diuretic instead of thiazide.
[5]The adverse metabolic effects of thiazide diuretics and beta-blockers should be considered in younger patients but may be less important in the older patient.
[6]Women of childbearing age should avoid ACE inhibitors and ARBs or discontinue as soon as pregnancy is diagnosed.
[7]Despite the elevated risk of angioedema and cough in Black patients, ACE inhibitors are generally well tolerated and are a useful adjunct.
[8]There are theoretical advantages in the use of vasodilating beta-blockers such as carvedilol and nebivolol.
[9]Alpha-antagonists may precipitate or exacerbate orthostatic hypotension in older adults.
CCB, calcium channel blocker.

Sex-Specific Considerations in Hypertension

Because of the preponderance of male recruitment into large-scale clinical trials, the impact of a patient's sex on the evaluation and management of hypertension remains uncertain. The limited data that exist suggest a steeper relationship in women between 24-hour ambulatory and nighttime systolic blood pressure and the risk of cardiovascular events. There are many sex-specific effects on the mechanisms and end-organ impact of hypertension. In younger adults, men are more likely to be hypertensive than women, a relationship that reverses in later life. Regression of LVH in response to ACE inhibitors is less pronounced in women. Women are more likely to have isolated systolic hypertension, probably because they develop more active LV systolic function and greater vascular stiffness than men. Fibromuscular dysplasia of the renal artery is much more common in women than men. The side effects of many antihypertensive drugs are more pronounced in women than men, including ACE inhibitor–associated cough and hyponatremia and hypokalemia in response to diuretics. Conversely, thiazides can help preserve bone density. Dependent edema due to amlodipine is more likely in women, and women are more sensitive to beta-blockers. There are no data to support a different blood pressure target in women, but this question has not been examined in dedicated clinical trials.

Treatment of Hypertension in Diabetes

Hypertensive patients with diabetes are at particularly high risk for cardiovascular events. Data from the ACCORD study of diabetic patients demonstrated that most of the benefits of blood pressure lowering were seen with a systolic target of less than 140 mm Hg. Although there was a reduction in stroke risk at a systolic target below 120/70 mm Hg, treatment to this lower target was associated with an *increased* risk of serious adverse effects. US and Canadian guidelines recommend a blood pressure goal of less than 130/80 mm Hg in diabetic patients. Because of the beneficial effects of ACE inhibitors in diabetic nephropathy, they should be part of the initial treatment regimen. ARBs or perhaps renin inhibitors may be substituted in those intolerant of ACE inhibitors. While the ONTARGET study showed that combinations of ACE inhibitors and ARBs in persons with atherosclerosis or type 2 diabetes with end-organ damage appeared to minimize proteinuria, this strategy slightly increased the risks of progression to dialysis and of death; thus, it is not recommended. Most diabetic patients require combinations of three to five agents to achieve target blood pressure, usually including a diuretic and a calcium channel blocker or beta-blocker. Canagliflozin improves glycemic control through inhibition of the sodium-glucose co-transporter 2 (SGLT2) and, in addition, generally lowers blood pressure by 3–4 mm Hg. This drug was associated with improved renal outcomes and reduced cardiovascular risk in the CREDENCE trial of patients with diabetic nephropathy and can be considered when additional blood pressure control is needed in patients with type 2 diabetes. In addition to rigorous blood pressure control, treatment of persons with diabetes should include aggressive treatment of other risk factors.

Treatment of Hypertension in Chronic Kidney Disease

Hypertension is present in 40% of patients with a GFR of 60–90 mL/minute/1.73 m^2 and 75% of patients with a GFR less than 30 mL/minute/1.73 m^2. The rate of progression of CKD is markedly slowed by treatment of hypertension. In the SPRINT trial, the reduction in cardiovascular risk associated with lower blood pressure targets was also observed in the subgroup with a GFR of less than 60 mL/minute/1.73 m^2. However, an effect of *lower* blood pressure targets on the slowing of CKD progression appears to be restricted to those with pronounced proteinuria. In the SPRINT trial, the lower blood pressure goal was associated with increased risk of AKI, but this was generally reversible and not associated with elevated biomarkers for ischemic injury. Most experts recommend a blood pressure target of less than 130/80 mm Hg in patients with CKD, with consideration of more intensive lowering if proteinuria greater than 1 g per 24 hours is present. Medications that interrupt the renin-angiotensin cascade can slow the progression of kidney disease and are preferred for initial therapy, especially in those with albuminuria of greater than 300 mg/g creatinine. Transition from thiazide to loop diuretic is often necessary to control volume expansion as the eGFR falls below 30 mL/minute/1.73 m^2. ACE inhibitors remain protective and safe in kidney disease associated with significant proteinuria and serum creatinine as high as 5 mg/dL (380 mcmol/L). However, the use of drugs blocking the RAAS cascade in patients with advanced CKD should be supervised by a nephrologist. Kidney function and electrolytes should be measured 1 week after initiating treatment and subsequently monitored carefully in patients with kidney disease. An increase in creatinine of 20–30% is acceptable and expected; more exaggerated responses suggest the possibility of renal artery stenosis or volume contraction. Although lower blood pressure levels are associated with acute decreases in GFR, this appears not to translate into an increased risk of developing ESKD in the long term. Persistence with ACE inhibitor or ARB therapy as the serum potassium level exceeds 5.5 mEq/L is probably not warranted, since other antihypertensive medications are renoprotective as long as goal blood pressures are maintained. However, diuretics can often be helpful in controlling mild hyperkalemia, and there are novel cation exchange polymers (such as patiromer) that sequester potassium in the gut and are more effective and better tolerated than sodium polystyrene sulfonate.

Treatment of Hypertension in Black Patients

Substantial evidence indicates that African Americans are not only more likely to become hypertensive and more susceptible to the cardiovascular and renal complications of hypertension but also respond differently to many antihypertensive medications. The REGARDS study illustrates these differences. At systolic blood pressures less than 120 mm Hg, Black and White Americans between 45 and 64 years of age had equal risk of stroke. For a 10 mm Hg increase in systolic blood pressure, the risk of stroke was threefold higher in Black participants. At levels above 140–159/90–99 mm Hg, the hazard ratio for stroke in Black compared to White participants between 45 and 64 years of age was 2.35. This increased susceptibility may reflect environmental factors, such as structural racism, diet, activity, stress, or access to health care services; differences in occurrence of comorbid conditions such as diabetes or obesity; or genetic ancestry and epigenetics. More studies are needed to determine the source of these differences, and it should be noted that racial disparities are not synonymous with inherent biologic differences based on race. In all persons with hypertension, a multifaceted program of education and lifestyle modification is warranted. Early introduction of combination therapy has been advocated, but there are no clinical trial data to support a lower than usual blood pressure goal in Black patients. Because it appears that ACE inhibitors and ARBs—in the absence of concomitant diuretics—are less effective in Black than in White patients, initial therapy should generally be a diuretic or a diuretic in combination with a calcium channel blocker. However, inhibitors of the RAAS do lower blood pressure in Black patients, are useful adjuncts to the recommended diuretic and calcium channel blockers and should be used in patients with hypertension and compelling indications such as heart failure and kidney disease (especially in the presence of proteinuria) (Table 11–13). *Black patients have an elevated risk of ACE inhibitor–associated angioedema and cough, so ARBs would be the preferred choice.*

Treating Hypertension in Older Adults

Several studies in persons over 60 years of age have confirmed that antihypertensive therapy prevents fatal and

Table 11–13. Recommended antihypertensive medications for coexisting indications.

Indication	Antihypertensive Medication					
	Diuretic	Beta-Blocker	ACE Inhibitor	ARB	Calcium Channel Blocker	Aldosterone Antagonist
Heart failure	√	√	√	√		√
Following MI		√	√			√
High coronary disease risk	√	√	√		√	
Diabetes	√	√	√	√	√	
Chronic kidney disease			√	√		
Recurrent stroke prevention	√		√			

nonfatal MI and reduces overall cardiovascular mortality. The HYVET study indicated that a reasonable ultimate blood pressure goal is 150/80 mm Hg. Updated guidelines suggest that blood pressure goals should not generally be influenced by age alone. An exploratory subgroup analysis of the SPRINT study found that people older than age 75 years showed benefit at the 120 mm Hg systolic treatment target. Importantly, these benefits were also evident in patients classified as frail. This more aggressive approach was, however, associated with greater risk of falls and worsening kidney function, indicating that close monitoring is required in elderly patients treated to lower blood pressure goals. It is also important to note the exclusion criteria of the SPRINT study, which included diabetes mellitus, stroke, and orthostatic hypotension.

Blood pressure treatment goals should be individualized in the very elderly. In the SPRINT MIND study, the lower systolic blood pressure target of 120 mm Hg was associated with a 15% reduction in the incidence of mild cognitive impairment and probable all cause dementia compared to the 140 mm Hg in the target group. Based upon this data, aggressive control of hypertension in high-risk individuals would have a significant impact on the prevalence of dementia. As discussed above, it is important to note that blood pressure measurements in the SPRINT study were made by automated devices, which are known to read lower than conventional office measurements.

How to initiate antihypertensive therapy in older patients—The same medications are used in older patients but at 50% lower doses. Pressure should be reduced more gradually with a safe intermediate systolic blood pressure goal of 160 mm Hg. As treatment is initiated, older patients should be carefully monitored for orthostasis, altered cognition, and electrolyte disturbances. The elderly are especially susceptible to problems associated with polypharmacy, including drug interactions and dosing errors.

Management of Supine Hypertension in Patients With Orthostatic Hypotension

Supine hypertension is common in patients with orthostatic hypotension and is associated with increased cardiovascular risk. Treatment of orthostasis can exacerbate supine hypertension and vice versa. Life expectancy is often reduced in patients with profound autonomic nervous system dysfunction. Treatment of nocturnal hypertension might be considered with the use of shorter acting agents (eg, captopril, hydralazine, losartan, or quick-release nifedipine). In patients with supine hypertension, medications used to increase blood pressure during the day should not be given within 5 hours of bedtime.

Follow-Up of Patients Receiving Hypertension Therapy

Once blood pressure is controlled on a well-tolerated regimen, follow-up visits can be infrequent and laboratory testing limited to those appropriate for the patient and the medications used. Yearly monitoring of blood lipids is recommended, and an ECG could be repeated at 2- to 4-year intervals depending on whether initial abnormalities are present and on the presence of coronary risk factors. Patients who have had excellent blood pressure control for several years, especially if they have lost weight and initiated favorable lifestyle modifications, might be considered for a trial of reduced antihypertensive medications.

Deere BP et al. Hypertension and race/ethnicity. Curr Opin Cardiol. 2020;35:342. [PMID: 32398604]

Milani RV et al. New aspects in the management of hypertension in the digital era. Curr Opin Cardiol. 2021;36:398. [PMID: 33871402]

Suchard MA et al. Comprehensive comparative effectiveness and safety of first-line antihypertensive drug classes: a systematic, multinational, large-scale analysis. Lancet. 2019;394:1816. [PMID: 31668726]

Supiano MA et al. New guidelines and SPRINT results: implications for geriatric hypertension. Circulation. 2019;140:976. [PMID: 31525101]

Vogel B et al. The Lancet Women and Cardiovascular Disease Commission: reducing the global burden by 2030. Lancet. 2021;397:2385. [PMID: 34010613]

RESISTANT HYPERTENSION

Resistant hypertension is defined as the failure to reach blood pressure control in patients who are adherent to full doses of an appropriate three-drug regimen (including a diuretic). In the approach to resistant hypertension, the clinician should first confirm compliance and rule out "white coat hypertension," ideally using ambulatory or home-based measurement of blood pressure. Exacerbating factors should be considered (as outlined above). Finally, identifiable causes of resistant hypertension should be sought (Table 11–14). The clinician should pay particular attention to the type of diuretic being used in relation to the patient's kidney function. Aldosterone may play an important role in resistant hypertension and aldosterone receptor blockers can be very useful. If goal blood pressure cannot be achieved following completion of these steps, consultation with a hypertension specialist should be considered. Renal sympathetic nerve ablation is a consideration for these patients in the absence of other options, but further trials are needed before this procedure can be routinely integrated into clinical practice.

Wei FF et al. Diagnosis and management of resistant hypertension: state of the art. Nat Rev Nephrol. 2018;14:428. [PMID: 29700488]

HYPERTENSIVE URGENCIES & EMERGENCIES

Hypertensive urgencies are situations in which blood pressure must be reduced within a few hours. These include patients with asymptomatic severe hypertension (systolic blood pressure greater than 220 mm Hg or diastolic pressure greater than 125 mm Hg that persists after a period of observation) and those with optic disk edema, progressive target-organ complications, and severe perioperative hypertension. Elevated blood pressure levels alone—in the absence of symptoms of new or progressive

Table 11–14. Causes of resistant hypertension.

Improper blood pressure measurement
Nonadherence
Volume overload and pseudotolerance
Excess sodium intake
Volume retention from kidney disease
Inadequate diuretic therapy
Drug-induced or other causes
Inadequate doses
Inappropriate combinations
NSAIDs; cyclooxygenase-2 inhibitors
Cocaine, amphetamines, other illicit drugs
Sympathomimetics (decongestants, anorectics)
Oral contraceptives
Adrenal steroids
Cyclosporine and tacrolimus
Erythropoietin
Licorice (including some chewing tobacco)
Selected over-the-counter dietary supplements and medicines (eg, ephedra, ma huang, bitter orange)
Associated conditions
Obesity
Excess alcohol intake
Identifiable causes of hypertension (see Table 11–2)

Data from Chobanian AV et al. The Seventh Report of the Joint National Committee on Prevention, Detection, Evaluation, and Treatment of High Blood Pressure: the JNC 7 report. JAMA. 2003;289:2560.

target-organ damage—rarely require emergency therapy. Parenteral drug therapy is not usually required; partial reduction of blood pressure with relief of symptoms is the goal. Effective oral agents are clonidine, captopril, and slow-release nifedipine.

Hypertensive emergencies require substantial reduction of blood pressure within 1 hour to avoid the risk of serious morbidity or death. Although blood pressure is usually strikingly elevated (diastolic pressure greater than 130 mm Hg), the correlation between pressure and end-organ damage is often poor. *It is the presence of critical multiple end-organ injury that determines the seriousness of the emergency and the approach to treatment.* Emergencies include hypertensive encephalopathy (headache, irritability, confusion, and altered mental status due to cerebrovascular spasm), hypertensive nephropathy (hematuria, proteinuria, and AKI due to arteriolar necrosis and intimal hyperplasia of the interlobular arteries), intracranial hemorrhage, aortic dissection, preeclampsia-eclampsia, pulmonary edema, unstable angina, or myocardial infarction. Encephalopathy or nephropathy accompanying hypertensive retinopathy has historically been called malignant hypertension, but the therapeutic approach is identical to that used in other hypertensive emergencies.

Parenteral therapy is indicated in most hypertensive emergencies, especially if encephalopathy is present. The initial goal in hypertensive emergencies is to reduce the pressure by no more than 25% (within minutes to 1 or 2 hours) and then toward a level of 160/100 mm Hg within 2–6 hours. Excessive reductions in pressure may precipitate coronary, cerebral, or renal ischemia. To avoid such declines, the use of agents that have a predictable, dose-dependent, transient, and progressive antihypertensive effect is preferable (Table 11–15). *In that regard, the use of sublingual or oral fast-acting nifedipine preparations is best avoided.*

Acute ischemic stroke is often associated with marked elevation of blood pressure, which will usually fall spontaneously. In such cases, antihypertensives should only be used if the systolic blood pressure exceeds 180–200 mm Hg, and blood pressure should be reduced cautiously by 10–15% over 24 hours (Table 11–15). If thrombolytics are to be given, blood pressure should be maintained at less than 185/110 mm Hg during treatment and for 24 hours following treatment.

In **intracerebral hemorrhage,** the aim is to minimize bleeding by reducing the systolic blood pressure in most patients to 140 mm Hg within the first 6 hours. In acute subarachnoid hemorrhage, as long as the bleeding source remains uncorrected, a compromise must be struck between preventing further bleeding and maintaining cerebral perfusion in the face of cerebral vasospasm. In this situation, blood pressure goals depend on the patient's usual blood pressure. In previously normotensive patients, the target should be a systolic blood pressure of 110–120 mm Hg; in hypertensive patients, blood pressure should be reduced to 20% below baseline pressure. In the treatment of hypertensive emergencies complicated by (or precipitated by) CNS injury, labetalol and nicardipine are good choices since they are nonsedating and do not appear to cause significant increases in cerebral blood flow or intracranial pressure. Patients with subarachnoid hemorrhage should receive nimodipine for 3 weeks following presentation to minimize cerebral vasospasm. *In hypertensive emergencies arising from catecholaminergic mechanisms, such as pheochromocytoma or cocaine use, beta-blockers can worsen the hypertension because of unopposed peripheral vasoconstriction; nicardipine, clevidipine, or phentolamine is preferred.* Labetalol is useful in these patients if the heart rate must be controlled but should not be used as first-line therapy because it exhibits more beta- than alpha-blockade. Table 11–15 provides guidelines for the choice of antihypertensive agent based on the site of end-organ damage. ACE inhibitors are specifically indicated for hypertensive crisis from systemic sclerosis (scleroderma).

In acute aortic dissection, systolic blood pressure and heart rate should be reduced within 30 minutes to below 120 mm Hg and less than 60 beats per minute, using a combination of vasodilation and beta-blockade.

Pharmacologic Management

A. Parenteral Agents

Sodium nitroprusside is no longer the treatment of choice for acute hypertensive problems; in most situations, appropriate control of blood pressure is best achieved using combinations of nicardipine or clevidipine plus labetalol or esmolol. (Table 11–16 lists drugs, dosages, and adverse effects.)

1. Nicardipine—Intravenous nicardipine is the most potent and the longest acting of the parenteral calcium channel blockers. As a primarily arterial vasodilator, it has

Table 11–15. Treatment of hypertensive emergency depending on primary site of end-organ damage. *See* Table 11–16 *for dosages.*

Type of Hypertensive Emergency	Recommended Drug Options and Combinations	Drugs to Avoid
Myocardial ischemia and infarction	Nicardipine plus esmolol[1] Nitroglycerin plus labetalol Nitroglycerin plus esmolol[1]	Hydralazine, diazoxide, minoxidil, nitroprusside
Acute kidney injury	Fenoldopam Nicardipine Clevidipine	
Aortic dissection	Esmolol plus nicardipine Esmolol plus clevidipine Labetalol Esmolol plus nitroprusside	Hydralazine, diazoxide, minoxidil
Acute pulmonary edema, LV systolic dysfunction	Nicardipine plus nitroglycerin[2] plus a loop diuretic Clevidipine plus nitroglycerin[2] plus a loop diuretic	Hydralazine, diazoxide, beta-blockers
Acute pulmonary edema, diastolic dysfunction	Esmolol plus low-dose nitroglycerin plus a loop diuretic Labetalol plus low-dose nitroglycerin plus a loop diuretic	
Ischemic stroke (systolic blood pressure > 180–200 mm Hg)	Nicardipine Clevidipine Labetalol	Nitroprusside, methyldopa, clonidine, nitroglycerin
Intracerebral hemorrhage (systolic blood pressure > 140–160 mm Hg)	Nicardipine Clevidipine Labetalol	Nitroprusside, methyldopa, clonidine, nitroglycerin
Hyperadrenergic states, including cocaine use	Nicardipine plus a benzodiazepine Clevidipine plus a benzodiazepine Phentolamine Labetalol	Beta-blockers
Preeclampsia, eclampsia	Labetalol Nicardipine	Diuretics, ACE inhibitors

[1]Avoid if there is LV systolic dysfunction.
[2]Drug of choice if LV systolic dysfunction is associated with ischemia.

the potential to precipitate reflex tachycardia, and for that reason, it should not be used without a beta-blocker in patients with CAD.

2. Clevidipine—Intravenous clevidipine is an L-type calcium channel blocker with a 1-minute half-life, which facilitates swift and tight control of severe hypertension. It acts on arterial resistance vessels and is devoid of venodilatory or cardiodepressant effects.

3. Labetalol—This combined beta- and alpha-blocking agent is the most potent adrenergic blocker for rapid blood pressure reduction. Other beta-blockers are far less potent. Excessive blood pressure drops are unusual. Experience with this agent in hypertensive syndromes associated with pregnancy has been favorable.

4. Esmolol—This rapidly acting beta-blocker is approved only for treatment of supraventricular tachycardia, but is often used for lowering blood pressure. It is less potent than labetalol and should be reserved for patients in whom there is particular concern about serious adverse events related to beta-blockers.

5. Fenoldopam—Fenoldopam is a peripheral dopamine-1 (DA_1) receptor agonist that causes a dose-dependent reduction in arterial pressure without evidence of tolerance, rebound, withdrawal, or deterioration of kidney function. In higher dosage ranges, tachycardia may occur. This drug is natriuretic, which may simplify volume management in AKI.

6. Enalaprilat—This is the active form of the oral ACE inhibitor enalapril. The onset of action is usually within 15 minutes, but the peak effect may be delayed for up to 6 hours. Thus, enalaprilat is used primarily as an adjunctive agent.

7. Diuretics—Intravenous loop diuretics can be very helpful when the patient has signs of heart failure or fluid retention, but the onset of their hypotensive response is slow, making them an adjunct rather than a primary agent for hypertensive emergencies. Low dosages should be used initially (furosemide, 20 mg, or bumetanide, 0.5 mg). They facilitate the response to vasodilators, which often stimulate fluid retention.

8. Hydralazine—Hydralazine can be given intravenously or intramuscularly, but its effect is less predictable than that of other drugs in this group. It produces reflex tachycardia and should not be given without beta-blockers in patients

Table 11–16. Drugs for hypertensive emergencies and urgencies (in descending order of preference).

Agent	Action	Dosage	Onset	Duration	Adverse Effects	Comments
Hypertensive Emergencies						
Nicardipine (Cardene)	Calcium channel blocker	5 mg/hour intravenously; may increase by 1–2.5 mg/hour every 15 minutes to 15 mg/hour	1–5 minutes	3–6 hours	Hypotension, tachycardia, headache.	May precipitate myocardial ischemia.
Clevidipine (Cleviprex)	Calcium channel blocker	1–2 mg/hour intravenously initially; double rate every 90 seconds until near goal, then by smaller amounts every 5–10 minutes to a maximum of 32 mg/hour	2–4 minutes	5–15 minutes	Headache, nausea, vomiting.	Lipid emulsion: contraindicated in patients with allergy to soy or egg.
Labetalol (Trandate)	Beta- and alpha-blocker	20–40 mg intravenously every 10 minutes to 300 mg; 2 mg/minute infusion	5–10 minutes	3–6 hours	Nausea, hypotension, bronchospasm, bradycardia, heart block.	Avoid in acute LV systolic dysfunction, asthma. May be continued orally.
Esmolol (Brevibloc)	Beta-blocker	Loading dose 500 mcg/kg intravenously over 1 minute; maintenance, 25–200 mcg/kg/minute	1–2 minutes	10–30 minutes	Bradycardia, nausea.	Avoid in acute LV systolic dysfunction, asthma. Weak antihypertensive.
Fenoldopam (Corlopam)	Dopamine receptor agonist	0.1–1.6 mcg/kg/minute intravenously	4–5 minutes	< 10 minutes	Reflex tachycardia, hypotension, increased intraocular pressure.	May protect kidney function.
Enalaprilat (Vasotec)	ACE inhibitor	1.25 mg intravenously every 6 hours	15 minutes	6 hours or more	Excessive hypotension.	Additive with diuretics; may be continued orally.
Furosemide (Lasix)	Diuretic	10–80 mg orally or intravenously	15 minutes	4 hours	Hypokalemia, hypotension.	Adjunct to vasodilator.
Hydralazine (Apresoline)	Vasodilator	5–20 mg intravenously; may repeat after 20 minutes	10–30 minutes	2–6 hours	Tachycardia, headache, vomiting, diarrhea	Avoid in CAD, dissection. Rarely used except in pregnancy.
Nitroglycerin	Vasodilator	0.25–5 mcg/kg/minute intravenously	2–5 minutes	3–5 minutes	Headache, nausea, hypotension, bradycardia.	Tolerance may develop. Useful primarily with myocardial ischemia.
Nitroprusside (Nitropress)	Vasodilator	0.25–10 mcg/kg/minute intravenously	Seconds	3–5 minutes	Anxiety, increased intracranial pressure, vomiting, bowel obstruction; thiocyanate and cyanide toxicity, especially with kidney and liver dysfunction; hypotension. Coronary steal, decreased cerebral blood flow, increased intracranial pressure.	No longer the first-line agent.
Hypertensive Urgencies						
Clonidine (Catapres)	Central sympatholytic	0.1–0.2 mg orally initially; then 0.1 mg every hour to 0.8 mg orally	30–60 minutes	6–8 hours	Sedation.	Rebound may occur.
Captopril (Capoten)	ACE inhibitor	12.5–25 mg orally	15–30 minutes	4–6 hours	Excessive hypotension.	
Nifedipine (Adalat, Procardia)	Calcium channel blocker	10 mg orally initially; may be repeated after 30 minutes	15 minutes	2–6 hours	Excessive hypotension, tachycardia, headache, angina, myocardial infarction, stroke.	Response unpredictable.

with possible coronary disease or aortic dissection. Hydralazine is used primarily in pregnancy and in children, but even in these situations, it is not a first-line drug.

9. Nitroglycerin, intravenous—This agent should be reserved for patients with accompanying acute coronary ischemic syndromes.

10. Nitroprusside sodium—This agent is given by controlled intravenous infusion gradually titrated to the desired effect. It lowers the blood pressure within seconds by direct arteriolar and venous dilation. Monitoring with an intra-arterial line avoids hypotension. Nitroprusside—in combination with a beta-blocker—is useful in patients with aortic dissection.

B. Oral Agents

Patients with less severe acute hypertensive syndromes can often be treated with oral therapy. Suitable drugs will reduce the blood pressure over a period of hours. In those presenting as a consequence of noncompliance, it is usually sufficient to restore the patient's previously established oral regimen.

1. Clonidine—Clonidine, 0.2 mg orally initially, followed by 0.1 mg every hour to a total of 0.8 mg, will usually lower blood pressure over a period of several hours. Sedation is frequent, and rebound hypertension may occur if the drug is stopped.

2. Captopril—Captopril, 12.5–25 mg orally, will also lower blood pressure in 15–30 minutes. The response is variable and may be excessive. Captopril is the drug of choice in the management of systemic sclerosis hypertensive crisis.

3. Nifedipine—The effect of fast-acting nifedipine capsules is unpredictable and may be excessive, resulting in hypotension and reflex tachycardia. Because MI and stroke have been reported in this setting, the use of sublingual nifedipine is not advised. Nifedipine retard, 20 mg orally, appears to be safe and effective.

C. Subsequent Therapy

When the blood pressure has been brought under control, combinations of oral antihypertensive agents can be added as parenteral drugs are tapered off over a period of 2–3 days.

Jolly H et al. Management of hypertensive emergencies and urgencies: narrative review. Postgrad Med J. 2021 Oct 20. [Epub ahead of print] [PMID: 34670853]

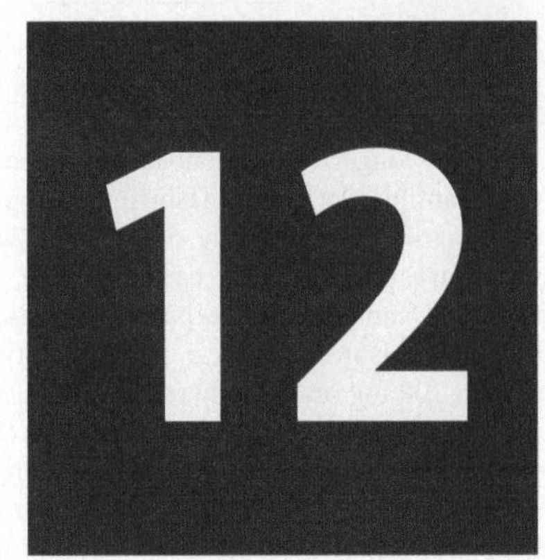

Blood Vessel & Lymphatic Disorders

Warren J. Gasper, MD
James C. Iannuzzi, MD, MPH
Meshell D. Johnson, MD

ATHEROSCLEROTIC PERIPHERAL VASCULAR DISEASE

Occlusive atherosclerotic lesions in the extremities, or peripheral artery disease (PAD), is evidence of a systemic atherosclerotic process. The prevalence of PAD is 30% in patients who are 70 years old without other risk factors, or 50 years old with risk factors such as diabetes mellitus or tobacco use. Pathologic changes of atherosclerosis may be diffuse, but flow-limiting stenoses occur segmentally. In the lower extremities, stenoses classically occur in three anatomic segments: the aortoiliac segment, femoral-popliteal segment, and the infrapopliteal or tibial segment of the arterial tree.

Approximately two-thirds of patients with PAD are either asymptomatic or do not have classic symptoms. Intermittent claudication, which is pain with ambulation that occurs from insufficient blood flow relative to demand, is typically described as severe and cramping primarily in the calf muscles.

OCCLUSIVE DISEASE: AORTA & ILIAC ARTERIES

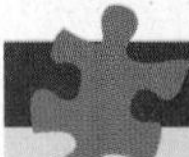

ESSENTIALS OF DIAGNOSIS

- Claudication: cramping pain or tiredness in the calf, thigh, or hip while walking.
- Diminished femoral pulses.
- Tissue loss (ulceration, gangrene) or rest pain.

General Considerations

Lesions in the distal aorta and proximal common iliac arteries classically occur in White men aged 50–60 years who smoke cigarettes. Disease progression may lead to complete occlusion of one or both common iliac arteries, which can precipitate occlusion of the entire abdominal aorta to the level of the renal arteries.

Clinical Findings

A. Symptoms and Signs

The pain from aortoiliac lesions may extend into the thigh and buttocks and erectile dysfunction may occur from bilateral common iliac disease. Rarely, patients complain only of weakness in the legs when walking, or simply extreme limb fatigue. The symptoms are relieved with rest and are reproducible when the patient walks again. Femoral pulses and distal pulses are absent or very weak. Bruits may be heard over the aorta, iliac, and femoral arteries.

B. Doppler and Vascular Findings

The ratio of systolic blood pressure detected by Doppler examination at the ankle compared with the brachial artery (referred to as the ankle-brachial index [ABI]) is reduced to below 0.9 (normal ratio is 0.9–1.2); this difference is exaggerated by exercise. Both the dorsalis pedis and the posterior tibial arteries are measured and the higher of the two artery pressures is used for calculation. Segmental waveforms or pulse volume recordings obtained by strain gauge technology through blood pressure cuffs demonstrate blunting of the arterial inflow throughout the lower extremity.

C. Imaging

CT angiography (CTA) and magnetic resonance angiography (MRA) can identify the anatomic location of disease. Due to overlying bowel, duplex ultrasound has a limited role in imaging the aortoiliac segment. Imaging is required only when symptoms necessitate intervention, since a history and physical examination with vascular testing should appropriately identify the involved levels of the arterial tree.

Treatment

A. Medical and Exercise Therapy

The cornerstones of aortoiliac disease treatment are cardiovascular risk factor reduction and a supervised or structured exercise program. Essential elements include cigarette smoking cessation, antiplatelet therapy, lipid and blood pressure management, and weight loss. Nicotine replacement therapy, bupropion, and varenicline have established benefits in cigarette smoking cessation (see Chapter 1). While no longer recommended for primary prevention of CVD, antiplatelet agents (aspirin [81 mg orally daily] or clopidogrel [75 mg orally daily]) remain important for secondary prevention of cardiovascular events in those with PAD and to reduce peripheral vascular morbidity. Low-dose rivaroxaban (2.5 mg orally twice daily) with aspirin 100 mg orally daily reduces both major cardiovascular and limb-related adverse events in symptomatic patients. All patients with PAD should receive high-dose statin (eg, atorvastatin 80 mg daily if tolerated) to treat hypercholesterolemia and arterial inflammation. A trial of cilostazol, 100 mg orally twice a day, may improve walking distance in approximately two-thirds of patients but may take 2–4 weeks to be effective and 12 weeks until full effect.

Supervised exercise programs for PAD provide significant improvements in pain, walking distance, and quality of life and may be more effective than an endovascular treatment alone. A minimum training goal is a walking session of 30–45 minutes at least 3 days per week for a minimum of 12 weeks. Structured community or home-based exercise programs as well as alternative exercises (cycling, upper-body ergometry) may also be effective. The Society for Vascular Surgery Supervised Exercise Therapy App, a patient-facing mobile app, has shown promise.

B. Endovascular Therapy

Focal atherosclerotic lesions in the aorta or iliac arteries can be effectively treated with angioplasty and stenting. This approach matches the results of surgery for single stenoses but both effectiveness and durability decrease with longer or multiple stenoses.

C. Surgical Intervention

A prosthetic aorto-femoral bypass graft that bypasses the diseased aorta or iliac artery segments is a highly effective and durable treatment for this disease. Patients may also be treated with a graft from the axillary artery to the femoral arteries (axillo-femoral bypass graft) or with a graft from the contralateral femoral artery (femoral-femoral bypass) when iliac disease is limited to one side. The operative risk of axillo-femoral and femoral-to-femoral bypass grafts is lower because the abdominal cavity is not entered and the aorta is not cross-clamped, but the grafts are less durable.

Complications

The complications of aorto-femoral bypass are those of any major abdominal surgery in a patient population with a high prevalence of CVD. Mortality is low (2–3%), but morbidity is higher and includes a 5–10% rate of MI. While endovascular approaches are safer and the complication rate is 1–3%, they are less durable with extensive disease.

Prognosis

Patients with isolated aortoiliac disease may have a further reduction in walking distance without intervention, but symptoms rarely progress to rest pain or threatened limb loss. Life expectancy is limited by attendant CVD with a mortality rate of 25–40% at 5 years.

Symptomatic relief is generally excellent with supervised exercise or after intervention. After aorto-femoral bypass, a patency rate of 90% at 5 years is reported. Endovascular patency rates and symptom relief for patients with short stenoses are also good with 80% symptom free at 3 years. Recurrence rates following endovascular treatment of extensive disease are 30–50%.

When to Refer

Patients with progressive reduction in walking distance despite risk factor modification and supervised exercise programs and those with limitations that interfere with their activities of daily living should be referred for consultation to a vascular surgeon.

When to Admit

- Patients with evidence of chronic limb-threatening ischemia, including lower extremity rest pain and tissue loss since these may quickly progress to limb-threatening conditions.
- Patients with acute limb ischemia should also be admitted with intravenous anticoagulation and surgical consultation.
- Patients with acute limb ischemia for treatment with intravenous anticoagulation and to obtain surgical consultation.

Bonaca M P et al. Rivaroxaban in peripheral artery disease after revascularization. N Engl J Med. 2020;382:1994. [PMID: 32222135]

Morcos R et al. The evolving treatment of peripheral arterial disease through guideline-directed recommendations. J Clin Med. 2018;7:9. [PMID: 29315259]

OCCLUSIVE DISEASE: FEMORAL & POPLITEAL ARTERIES

ESSENTIALS OF DIAGNOSIS

- Cramping pain or tiredness in the calf with exercise.
- Reduced popliteal and pedal pulses.
- Foot pain at rest, relieved by dependency.
- Foot gangrene or ischemic ulcers.

General Considerations

The superficial femoral artery is the peripheral artery most commonly occluded by atherosclerosis. Atherosclerosis of the femoral-popliteal segment usually occurs about a decade after the development of aortoiliac disease, has an even gender distribution, and commonly affects Black and

Latinx patients. The disease frequently occurs where the superficial femoral artery passes through the abductor magnus tendon in the distal thigh (Hunter canal). The common femoral artery and the popliteal artery are less often diseased but lesions in these vessels are debilitating, resulting in short-distance claudication.

Clinical Findings

A. Symptoms and Signs

Symptoms of intermittent claudication caused by lesions of the common femoral artery, superficial femoral artery, and popliteal artery are confined to the calf. Claudication occurs at 2–4 blocks when there is occlusion or stenosis of the superficial femoral artery at the adductor canal, provided good collateral vessels from the profunda femoris are maintained. However, with concomitant disease of the profunda femoris or the popliteal artery, much shorter distances may trigger symptoms. With short-distance claudication, dependent rubor of the foot may be present; pallor on elevation distinguishes rubor from erythema. Chronic low blood flow states will also cause atrophic changes in the lower leg and foot with loss of hair, thinning of the skin and subcutaneous tissues, and disuse atrophy of the muscles. With segmental occlusive disease of the superficial femoral artery, the common femoral pulsation is normal, but the popliteal and pedal pulses are reduced.

B. Doppler and Vascular Findings

ABI values less than 0.9 are diagnostic of PAD and levels below 0.4 suggest chronic limb-threatening ischemia (formerly critical limb ischemia). ABI readings depend on arterial compression; since vessels may be calcified in diabetes mellitus, CKD, and in older adults, ABIs can be misleading. In such patients, the toe-brachial index is usually reliable with a value less than 0.7 considered diagnostic of PAD. Pulse volume recordings with cuffs placed at the high thigh, mid-thigh, calf, and ankle will delineate the levels of obstruction with reduced pressures and blunted waveforms.

C. Imaging

Duplex ultrasonography, CTA, and MRA all adequately show the anatomic location of the obstructive lesions and are performed only if revascularization is planned. After revascularization, patients can be monitored with annual ultrasonograms.

Treatment

A. Medical and Exercise Therapy

As with aortoiliac disease, risk factor reduction, medical optimization with an antiplatelet agent, high-dose statin, and exercise treatment are the cornerstone of therapy. Dual treatment with rivaroxaban (2.5 mg orally twice daily) and aspirin (81 mg orally daily) has been shown to reduce limb-related events, major amputation, and cardiovascular events. Cilostazol, 100 mg orally twice a day, may improve intermittent claudication symptoms.

B. Surgical Intervention

Intervention is indicated if claudication is progressive, incapacitating, or interferes significantly with essential daily activities or employment. Intervention is mandatory if there is ischemic rest pain or ischemic ulcers threaten the foot.

1. Bypass surgery—The most effective and durable treatment for superficial femoral artery lesions is a femoral-popliteal bypass with autologous saphenous vein. Synthetic material, usually polytetrafluoroethylene, can be used, but these grafts do not have the durability of vein bypass.

2. Endovascular techniques—Endovascular techniques, such as angioplasty and stenting, are often used for lesions of the superficial femoral artery. These techniques have lower morbidity than bypass surgery but also have decreased durability.

Endovascular therapy is most effective in patients undergoing aggressive risk factor modification in whom lesions measure less than 10 cm long. Paclitaxel-eluting stents or paclitaxel-coated balloons offer modest improvement over bare metal stents and noncoated balloons, but the effect is not as robust as in the coronary arteries. The 1-year patency rate is 50% for balloon angioplasty, 70% for drug-coated balloons, 80% for bare metal stents, and 90% for drug-eluting stents. However, by 3 years, the patency rates are significantly worse for all four techniques and reintervention for restenosis is common. After a meta-analysis of clinical trial data showed increased mortality at 3–5 years after treatment with paclitaxel-coated devices, the US FDA recommends judicious use of the devices. However, an interim analysis of the SWEDEPAD trial demonstrated no significant difference in all-cause mortality at 2.5 years; similarly, a subgroup analysis of the VOYAGER PAD trial found no mortality difference between drug-coated devices and angioplasty.

3. Thromboendarterectomy—Removal of the atherosclerotic plaque is limited to the lesions of the common femoral and the profunda femoris arteries where bypass grafts and endovascular techniques have a more limited role.

Complications

Open surgical procedures of the lower extremities, particularly long bypasses with vein harvest, have a risk of wound infection that is higher than in other areas of the body. Wound infection or seroma can occur in as many as 10–15% of cases. MI rates after open surgery are 5–10%, with a 1–4% mortality rate. Complication rates of endovascular surgery are 1–5%, making these therapies attractive despite their lower durability.

Prognosis

The prognosis for motivated patients with isolated superficial femoral artery disease is excellent, and surgery is not recommended for mild or moderate claudication in these patients. However, when claudication significantly limits daily activity and cardiovascular health, intervention may be warranted. All interventions require close postprocedure follow-up with repeated ultrasound surveillance so that recurrent narrowing can be treated promptly with angioplasty or bypass to prevent complete occlusion. The reported patency rate of bypass grafts of the femoral artery, superficial femoral artery, and popliteal artery is 65–70% at 3 years, whereas the patency of angioplasty is less than 50% at 3 years.

Because of the extensive atherosclerotic disease, including associated coronary lesions, 5-year survival with lower extremity PAD is 70% and decreases to 50% when there is involvement of the tibial arteries. However, with aggressive risk factor modification, substantial improvement in longevity has been reported.

When to Refer

Patients with progressive symptoms, short-distance claudication, rest pain, or any ulceration should be referred to a peripheral vascular specialist.

When to Admit

Individuals presenting with chronic limb threatening ischemia (eg, ischemic rest pain, tissue loss) may warrant admission because of a high risk of progression to limb loss. If there is concern for a foot infection, particularly in patients with diabetes, admission for broad-spectrum antibiotics and emergent surgical evaluation should be considered since emergent debridement may be necessary to prevent ascending infections that could be limb- and life-threatening.

Bauersachs RM et al. Total ischemic event reduction with rivaroxaban after peripheral arterial revascularization in the VOYAGER PAD Trial. J Am Coll Cardiol. 2021;78:317. [PMID: 34010631]

Nordanstig J et al. Mortality with paclitaxel-coated devices in peripheral artery disease. N Engl J Med. 2020;383:2538. [PMID: 33296560]

OCCLUSIVE DISEASE: TIBIAL & PEDAL ARTERIES

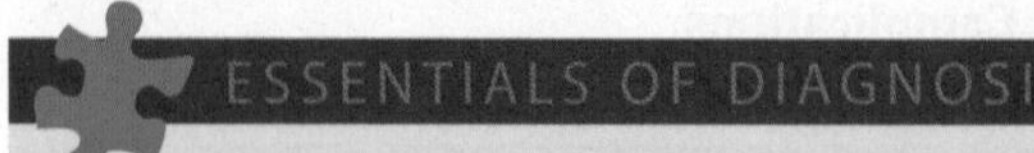

- Severe pain of the forefoot that is relieved by dependency (ischemic rest pain).
- Pain or numbness of the foot with walking.
- Ulcer or gangrene, and not claudication, is a frequent initial manifestation.
- Pallor when the foot is elevated.

General Considerations

Occlusive processes of the tibial arteries of the lower leg and pedal arteries in the foot occur primarily in patients with diabetes. There often is extensive calcification of the artery wall.

Clinical Findings

A. Symptoms and Signs

Unless there are concomitant lesions in the aortoiliac or femoral/superficial femoral artery segments, the first manifestation of leg ischemia due to tibial artery disease is frequently an ischemic ulcer or foot gangrene, rather than claudication. Chronic limb-threatening ischemia is defined as the presence of ischemic rest pain or ulcers and is associated with the highest rate of amputation. Classically, ischemic rest pain is confined to the dorsum of the foot and is relieved with dependency: the pain does not occur with standing, sitting, or dangling the leg over the edge of the bed. It is severe and burning in character, and because it is present only when recumbent, it may awaken the patient from sleep.

On examination, femoral and popliteal pulses may or may not be present depending on disease extent, but palpable pedal pulses will be absent. Dependent rubor may be prominent with pallor on elevation. The skin of the foot is generally cool, atrophic, and hairless.

B. Doppler and Vascular Findings

The ABI is often below 0.4; however, the ABI may be falsely elevated due to calcification of the arterial media layer (Mönckeberg medial calcific sclerosis) and may not be compressible. Toe-brachial indexes are preferred for assessing perfusion and predicting wound healing.

C. Imaging

Digital subtraction angiography is the gold standard method to delineate the anatomy of the tibial-popliteal segment. MRA or CTA is less helpful for detection of lesions in this location due to the small vasculature and other technical issues related to image resolution.

Differential Diagnosis

It is important to differentiate rest pain from diabetic neuropathic dysesthesia. Leg night cramps cause pain in the leg rather than the foot and should not be confused with ischemic rest pain. Dependent rubor in the presence of a toe wound can often be mistaken for cellulitis; pallor on elevation helps confirm the diagnosis of rubor.

Treatment

Good foot care may prevent ulcers, and most diabetic patients will do well with a conservative regimen. However, if ulcerations appear and there is no significant healing within 2–3 weeks, blood flow studies (ankle-brachial index/toe-brachial index) are indicated. Poor blood flow and a foot ulcer or nightly ischemic rest pain requires expeditious revascularization to avoid a major amputation.

A. Bypass and Endovascular Techniques

Bypass with vein to the distal tibial or pedal arteries is an effective therapy to treat rest pain and heal ischemic foot ulcers. Because the foot often has relative sparing of vascular disease, these bypasses have had adequate patency rates

(70% at 3 years). In nearly all series, limb preservation rates are much higher than patency rates.

Endovascular treatment of tibial or pedal artery disease with plain balloon angioplasty is effective for short segment lesions. The technical failure and reocclusion rates increase drastically with long segment disease in multiple tibial arteries. Stents and drug-coated balloons have not been successful in the tibial vessels to date.

B. Amputation

Patients with ischemic rest pain or ulcers have a 30–40% 1-year risk for major amputation that increases if revascularization cannot be done. Because of the distal nature of the tibial artery disease, diabetic patients are more likely to be asymptomatic until more severe ischemic disease with tissue loss develops, which can be exacerbated by peripheral neuropathy. Diabetic patients with PAD have a 4-fold risk of chronic limb-threatening ischemia compared with nondiabetic patients with PAD and have a risk of amputation up to 20-fold when compared to an age-matched population. Tibial artery disease is a major risk factor for amputation and is included as a factor in the Global Limb Anatomic Staging System (GLASS) vascular guidelines.

Complications

The complications of intervention are similar to those listed for superficial femoral artery disease; the overall cardiovascular risk of intervention increases with decreasing ABI. Patients with chronic limb-threatening ischemia require aggressive risk factor modification. Wound infection rates after bypass are higher if there is an open wound in the foot.

Prognosis

Patients with tibial atherosclerosis have extensive atherosclerotic burden and a high prevalence of diabetes. Their prognosis without intervention is poor and complicated by the risk of amputation.

When to Refer

Patients with diabetes and foot ulcers should be referred for a formal vascular evaluation.

When to Admit

Any diabetic patient with a foot ulcer and foot infection should be evaluated for an emergent operative incision and drainage. Broad-spectrum intravenous antibiotics should be given empirically (eg, vancomycin to cover methicillin-resistant *Staphylococcus aureus* [MRSA] plus either ertapenem or piperacillin/tazobactam to cover gram-negative and anaerobic organisms). Multidisciplinary limb preservation centers, staffed with vascular surgeons, podiatrists, plastic and orthopedic surgeons, prosthetics and orthotic specialists, and diabetes specialists, should be sought since they have improved limb salvage rates.

Conte MS et al. Global vascular guidelines on the management of chronic limb-threatening ischemia. J Vasc Surg. 2019;69:3. [PMID: 31159978]

ACUTE ARTERIAL OCCLUSION OF A LIMB

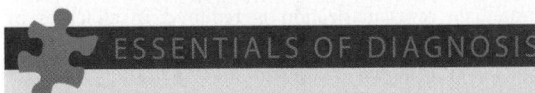

- Sudden pain in a limb with absent limb pulses.
- Usually some neurologic dysfunction with numbness, weakness, or complete paralysis.
- Loss of light touch sensation requires revascularization within 3 hours for limb viability.

General Considerations

Acute occlusion may be due to an embolus or to thrombosis of a diseased atherosclerotic segment. Emboli large enough to occlude proximal arteries in the lower extremities are almost always cardiac in origin. Atrial fibrillation is the most common cause of cardiac thrombus formation; other causes are valvular disease or thrombus formation on the ventricular surface of a large anterior myocardial infarct.

Emboli from arterial sources such as arterial ulcerations or calcified excrescences are usually small and go to the distal arterial tree (toes).

The typical patient with primary thrombosis will have a history of claudication and an abrupt worsening of symptoms. If the stenosis is chronic, collateral blood vessels will develop, and the resulting occlusion may cause only a minimal increase in symptoms.

Clinical Findings

A. Symptoms and Signs

The sudden onset of extremity pain, with loss or reduction in pulses, is diagnostic of acute arterial occlusion. This often will be accompanied by neurologic dysfunction, such as numbness or paralysis in extreme cases. With popliteal occlusion, symptoms may affect only the foot. With proximal occlusions, the whole leg may be affected. Signs of severe arterial ischemia include pallor, coolness of the extremity, and mottling. Impaired neurologic function progressing to anesthesia with paralysis indicates irreversible injury requiring amputation.

B. Doppler and Laboratory Findings

There will be little or no flow found with Doppler examination of the distal vessels. Imaging, if done, may show an abrupt cutoff of contrast with embolic occlusion. Blood work may show myoglobinemia and metabolic acidosis.

C. Imaging

Whenever possible, imaging should be done in the operating room because obtaining angiography, MRA, or CTA may delay revascularization and jeopardize the viability of the extremity. However, in cases with only modest symptoms and where light touch of the extremity is maintained, imaging may be helpful in planning the revascularization procedure.

Treatment

Immediate revascularization is required in all cases of symptomatic acute arterial thrombosis. *Evidence of neurologic injury, including loss of light touch sensation, indicates that collateral flow is inadequate to maintain limb viability and revascularization should be accomplished within 3 hours.* Longer delays carry a significant risk of irreversible tissue damage approaching 100% at 6 hours.

A. Heparin

As soon as the diagnosis is made, an initial weight-based bolus of unfractionated heparin should be infused intravenously (80 units/kg) followed by a continuous heparin infusion to maintain the activated partial thromboplastin time (aPTT) in the therapeutic range (60–85 seconds) (12–18 units/kg/hour). This helps prevent clot propagation and may also relieve associated vessel spasm. Anticoagulation may improve symptoms, but revascularization will still be required.

B. Endovascular Techniques

Pharmacomechanical thrombectomy catheters can achieve rapid revascularization and are most effective for the smaller arteries of the lower leg. Catheter-directed chemical thrombolysis into the clot with tissue plasminogen activator (TPA) may be done but often requires 24 hours or longer to fully lyse the thrombus. TPA can only be used in patients with mild ischemia, as determined by an intact neurologic examination. Patients with moderate to severe ischemia require immediate revascularization. Absolute contraindications for TPA include bleeding diathesis, GI bleeding, intracranial trauma, or neurosurgery within the past 3 months. Frequent vascular and access site examinations are required during the thrombolytic procedure to guard against the development of a hematoma.

C. Surgical Intervention

General anesthesia is usually indicated for surgical exploration of an acute arterial occlusion of a limb; local anesthesia may be used in extremely high-risk patients if the exploration is limited to the common femoral artery. In extreme cases, it may be necessary to perform thromboembolectomy from the femoral, popliteal, and even the pedal vessels to revascularize the limb. The combined use of devices that pulverize and aspirate clot and intraoperative thrombolysis with TPA improves outcomes.

Complications

Complications of revascularization of an acutely ischemic limb include severe metabolic acidosis, hyperkalemia, AKI, and cardiac arrest. When several hours have elapsed but recovery of viable tissue may still be possible, significant levels of lactic acid, potassium, and other harmful agents such as myoglobin may be released into the circulation during revascularization. Administering sodium bicarbonate (150 mEq $NaHCO_3$ in 1 L of dextrose 5% in water at a rate of 1–1.5 L in the first hour and then adjust the rate to manage acidosis) before reestablishing arterial flow is required. Surgery in the presence of thrombolytic agents and heparin carries a high risk of postoperative wound hematoma.

Prognosis

There is a 10–25% risk of amputation with an acute arterial embolic occlusion, and a 25% or higher in-hospital mortality rate. Prognosis for acute thrombotic occlusion of an atherosclerotic segment is generally better because the collateral flow can maintain extremity viability. The longer-term survival reflects the overall condition of the patient. In high-risk patients, an acute arterial occlusion is associated with a dismal prognosis.

OCCLUSIVE CEREBROVASCULAR DISEASE

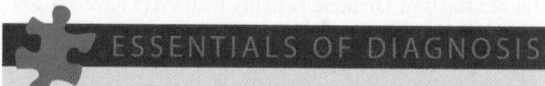

- Sudden onset of weakness and numbness of an extremity or the face, aphasia, dysarthria, or unilateral blindness (amaurosis fugax).
- Bruit heard loudest in the mid neck.

General Considerations

Unlike the other vascular territories, symptoms of ischemic cerebrovascular disease are predominantly due to emboli. When collateral flow reestablishes perfusion, ischemia reverses (transient ischemic attacks [TIAs]) but signals a high risk for additional emboli and stroke. Most ischemic strokes are due to emboli from the heart. One-quarter of all ischemic strokes may be due to emboli from an arterial source; approximately 90% of these emboli originate from the proximal internal carotid artery, an area uniquely prone to the development of atherosclerosis. The aortic arch may also be an atheroembolic source. Intracranial atherosclerotic lesions are uncommon in western populations but are the most frequent location of cerebrovascular disease in Asian populations.

Clinical Findings

A. Symptoms and Signs

Generally, the symptoms of a TIA last only a few seconds to minutes (but may continue up to 24 hours) while a stroke is defined as persistent symptoms beyond 24 hours. The most common lesions associated with carotid disease involve the anterior circulation in the cortex with both motor and sensory involvement. Emboli to the retinal artery cause unilateral blindness; transient monocular blindness is termed "amaurosis fugax." Posterior circulation symptoms referable to the brainstem, cerebellum, and visual regions of the brain may be due to atherosclerosis of the vertebral basilar systems and are much less common.

Signs of cerebrovascular disease may include carotid artery bruits. However, there is poor correlation between the degree of stenosis and the presence of the bruit.

Furthermore, the presence of a bruit does not correlate with stroke risk. Nonfocal symptoms, such as dizziness and unsteadiness, seldom are related to cerebrovascular atherosclerosis.

B. Imaging

Duplex ultrasonography is the imaging modality of choice with high specificity and sensitivity for detecting and grading the degree of stenosis at the carotid bifurcation (see Chapter 24).

Excellent depiction of the full anatomy of the cerebrovascular circulation from aortic arch to cranium can be obtained with MRA or CTA. Each of the modalities may have false-positive or false-negative findings. Since the decision to intervene in cases of carotid stenosis depends on an accurate assessment of the degree of stenosis, it is recommended that at least two modalities be used to confirm the degree of stenosis. Diagnostic cerebral angiography is reserved when carotid artery stenting is planned or other imaging modalities are contraindicated.

Treatment

See Chapter 24 for a discussion of the medical management of occlusive cerebrovascular disease.

A. Asymptomatic Patients

Large studies have shown a 5-year reduction in stroke rate from 11.5% to 5.0% with surgical treatment of asymptomatic carotid stenosis that is greater than 60%; these patients with asymptomatic carotid stenosis may benefit from carotid intervention if their risk from intervention is low and their expected survival is longer than 5 years. Aggressive risk factor modification, including high-potency statins, may be as valuable as surgical intervention in these patients; the large NIH-sponsored CREST2 study is examining this issue.

Mild to moderate disease (30–50% stenosis) indicates the need for ongoing monitoring and aggressive risk factor modification. Patients with carotid stenosis that suddenly worsens likely have an unstable plaque and are at particularly high risk for embolic stroke.

B. Symptomatic Patients

Large randomized trials have shown that patients with TIAs or strokes from which they have completely or nearly completely recovered will benefit from carotid intervention if the ipsilateral carotid artery has a stenosis of more than 70% (Figure 12–1), and they are likely to benefit if the artery has a stenosis of 50–69%. In these situations, carotid endarterectomy (CEA) and, in selected cases, carotid artery stenting, have been shown to have a durable effect in preventing further events. In symptomatic patients, intervention should ideally be planned within 2 weeks since delays increase the risk of a second event.

Complications

The most common complication from carotid intervention is cranial nerve injury, while the most dreaded complication is stroke from embolization or carotid occlusion.

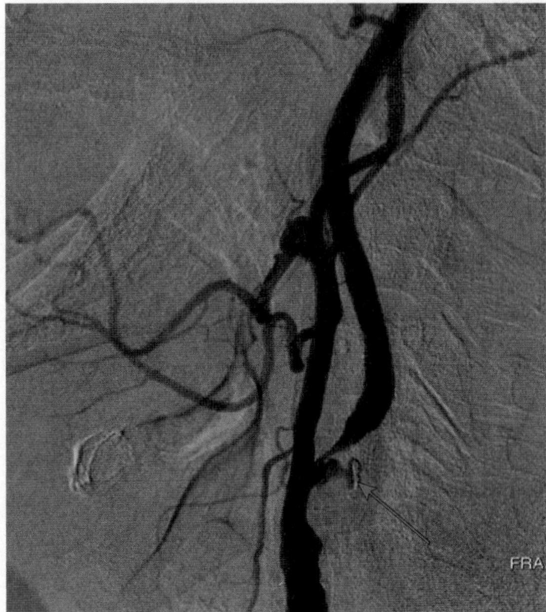

▲ **Figure 12–1. Digital subtraction angiography of a high-grade (90%) stenosis of the internal carotid artery with ulceration (arrow).** (Used, with permission, from Dean SM, Satiani B, Abraham WT. *Color Atlas and Synopsis of Vascular Diseases.* McGraw-Hill, 2014.)

The American Heart Association's recommendations for upper limits of acceptable combined morbidity and mortality for these interventions is 3% for patients with asymptomatic carotid stenosis, 5% for those with TIAs, and 7% for patients with previous stroke. Higher rates of morbidity and mortality negate the therapeutic benefit of carotid intervention.

A. Carotid Endarterectomy

In the 2010 CREST study, the stroke risk for CEA was 2.3%. CEA also carries a 1–2% risk of permanent cranial nerve injury (usually the vagus nerve). A postoperative neck hematoma can cause acute airway compromise. CAD is a comorbidity in most of these patients. MI rates after CEA are approximately 2–6%.

B. Carotid Angioplasty and Stenting

Carotid artery stenting had a stroke risk of 4.1% in the 2010 CREST study; patients over 70 years of age and women had higher stroke rates with carotid artery stenting than with CEA. However, the risk of MI was lower with carotid artery stenting compared to CEA (1.1% vs 2.3%). Carotid artery stenting is indicated for reoperative cases, prior neck radiation, and high carotid bifurcations not otherwise accessible surgically. Nonetheless, emboli are more common during transfemoral carotid artery stenting in spite of embolic protection devices, especially when the carotid artery is heavily calcified. Transcervical carotid stenting, performed through a small incision at the base of the neck, avoids the aortic arch, uses cerebral protective flow reversal, and has lower reported embolization rates than transfemoral carotid stenting.

Prognosis

Twenty-five percent of patients with carotid stenosis and a TIA or small stroke will have further brain ischemia within 18 months with most of the events occurring within the first 6 months. Historically, patients with asymptomatic carotid stenosis likely had an annual stroke rate of just over 2% which may be lower in the statin era. Prospective ultrasound screening at least annually is recommended in asymptomatic patients with known carotid stenosis to identify plaque progression, which increases stroke risk. Concomitant CAD is common and is an important factor both for perioperative risk and long-term prognosis. Aggressive risk factor modification should be prescribed for patients with cerebrovascular disease regardless of planned intervention.

When to Refer

Both asymptomatic and symptomatic patients with a carotid stenosis of 70% or greater by ultrasound criteria and patients with carotid stenosis of 50% or greater with symptoms of a TIA or stroke should be referred to a vascular specialist for consultation.

When to Admit

Individuals with a TIA or stroke should be admitted for further workup and evaluation. Further imaging is warranted in these patients and anticoagulation with heparin should be initiated after ruling out hemorrhagic stroke.

Brott TG et al; CREST Investigators. Long-term results of stenting versus endarterectomy for carotid-artery stenosis. N Engl J Med. 2016;374:1021. [PMID: 26890472]

Paraskevas KI et al. An updated systematic review and meta-analysis of results of transcervical carotid artery stenting with flow reversal. J Vasc Surg. 2020;72:1489. [PMID: 32422272]

VISCERAL ARTERY INSUFFICIENCY (Intestinal Angina)

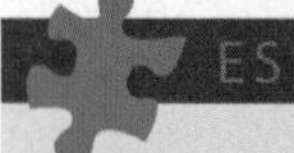

ESSENTIALS OF DIAGNOSIS

- Severe postprandial abdominal pain.
- Weight loss with a "fear of eating."
- **Acute mesenteric ischemia:** severe abdominal pain yet minimal findings on physical examination.

General Considerations

Acute mesenteric ischemia results from occlusive mesenteric arterial disease, either embolic occlusion or primary thrombosis of at least one major mesenteric artery. Ischemia can also result from **nonocclusive mesenteric ischemia,** which is generally seen in patients with low flow states, such as severe heart failure, sepsis, or hypotension. **Chronic mesenteric ischemia,** also called intestinal angina, occurs when increased flow demands during feeding are not met resulting in abdominal pain. Because of the rich collateral mesenteric network, generally at least two of the three major visceral vessels (celiac, superior mesenteric, inferior mesenteric arteries) must be affected before symptoms develop. **Ischemic colitis,** a variant of mesenteric ischemia, usually occurs in the distribution of the inferior mesenteric artery. The intestinal mucosa is the most sensitive to ischemia and will slough if underperfused.

Clinical Findings

A. Symptoms and Signs

1. Acute mesenteric ischemia—Visceral arterial embolism presents acutely with severe abdominal pain. In contrast, patients with primary visceral arterial thrombosis often have an antecedent history consistent with chronic mesenteric ischemia. The key finding with acute mesenteric ischemia is severe, steady, diffuse abdominal pain with an absence of focal tenderness or distention. This "pain out of proportion" to physical examination findings occurs because ischemia initially is mucosal and does not impact the peritoneum until transmural ischemia inflames the peritoneal lining. A high WBC count, lactic acidosis, hypotension, and abdominal distention may aid in the diagnosis.

2. Chronic mesenteric ischemia—Patients are generally over 45 years of age and may have evidence of atherosclerosis in other vasculature. Symptoms consist of epigastric or periumbilical postprandial pain lasting 1–3 hours. To avoid the pain, patients limit food intake and may develop a fear of eating. Weight loss is universal. In severe cases of intestinal angina, patients may become dehydrated, which can cause hypotension and an acute thrombosis.

3. Ischemic colitis—Characteristic symptoms are left lower quadrant pain and tenderness, abdominal cramping, and mild diarrhea (non-bloody or bloody). Rectal discharge will appear mucus-like or bloody and should prompt further evaluation.

B. Imaging and Colonoscopy

Contrast-enhanced CT is accurate at determining the presence of ischemic intestine. In acute or chronic mesenteric ischemia, a CTA or MRA can demonstrate narrowing of the proximal visceral vessels. In acute mesenteric ischemia from a nonocclusive low flow state, angiography is needed to display the typical "pruned tree" appearance of the distal visceral vascular bed. Ultrasound scanning of the mesenteric vessels may show proximal obstructing lesions.

In patients with ischemic colitis, flexible sigmoidoscopy should be performed to assess the grade of ischemia that occurs most often in watershed areas, such as the rectal sigmoid and splenic flexure.

Treatment

1. Acute mesenteric ischemia—A high suspicion of acute mesenteric ischemia dictates immediate exploration to assess bowel viability. If the bowel remains viable, arterial bypass using a prosthetic conduit can be done either from the supra-celiac aorta or common iliac artery to the celiac and the superior mesentery artery. Angioplasty and stenting of the arteries can be used but do not avoid a surgical evaluation of bowel viability.

2. Chronic mesenteric ischemia—Angioplasty and stenting of the proximal vessel may be beneficial depending on the anatomy of the stenosis. Should an endovascular solution not be available, an aorto-visceral artery bypass is the preferred management. The long-term results are highly durable.

3. Ischemic colitis—The mainstay of treatment is maintenance of blood pressure and perfusion until collateral circulation becomes well established. The patient must be monitored closely for evidence of perforation necessitating resection.

Prognosis

The combined morbidity and mortality rates are 10–15% from surgical intervention of chronic mesenteric ischemia, in part due to patients' malnutrition and frailty. The combined morbidity and mortality rates from surgical intervention of acute mesenteric ischemia is 50–69%, although only 25% of patients will survive 1 year. However, without intervention, both acute and chronic mesenteric ischemia are uniformly fatal. Adequate collateral circulation usually develops in those who have ischemic colitis, and the prognosis for this entity is better than chronic mesenteric ischemia.

When to Refer

Any patient in whom there is a suspicion of mesenteric ischemia should be urgently referred for imaging and possible intervention.

When to Admit

Indications for admission include the presence of abdominal pain out of proportion to abnormal physical findings (there are no findings of peritonitis and the abdomen is soft) or a history of worsening intestinal angina with inability to tolerate a diet.

Alahdab F et al. A systematic review and meta-analysis of endovascular versus open surgical revascularization for chronic mesenteric ischemia. J Vasc Surg. 2018;67:1598. [PMID: 29571626]

Lim S et al. Contemporary management of acute mesenteric ischemia in the endovascular era. Vasc Endovascular Surg. 2019;53:42. [PMID: 30360689]

ACUTE MESENTERIC VEIN OCCLUSION

The hallmarks of acute mesenteric vein occlusion are postprandial pain and evidence of a hypercoagulable state. Acute mesenteric vein occlusion presents similarly to the arterial occlusive syndromes but is much less common. Patients at risk include those with paroxysmal nocturnal hemoglobinuria; protein C, protein S, or antithrombin deficiencies; or the *JAK2* mutation. Thrombolysis is the mainstay of therapy. Aggressive long-term anticoagulation is required.

NONATHEROSCLEROTIC VASCULAR DISEASE

THROMBOANGIITIS OBLITERANS (Buerger Disease)

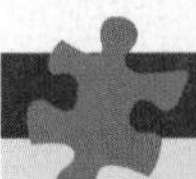

ESSENTIALS OF DIAGNOSIS

- Typically occurs in male cigarette smokers.
- Distal extremities involved with severe ischemia, progressing to tissue loss.
- Thrombosis of the superficial veins may occur.
- Smoking cessation is essential to stop disease progression.

General Considerations

Thromboangiitis obliterans (Buerger disease) is a segmental, inflammatory, and thrombotic process of the distal-most arteries and occasionally veins of the extremities. Pathologic examination reveals arteritis in the affected vessels. The cause is not known but it is rarely seen in patients who do not smoke cigarettes. Arteries most commonly affected are the plantar and digital vessels of the foot and lower leg. In advanced stages, the fingers and hands may become involved. The incidence of thromboangiitis obliterans has decreased dramatically.

Clinical Findings

A. Symptoms and Signs

Thromboangiitis obliterans may be initially difficult to differentiate from atherosclerotic peripheral vascular disease, but in most cases, the lesions are on the toes and the patient is younger than 40 years. The observation of superficial thrombophlebitis may aid the diagnosis. Because the distal vessels are usually affected, intermittent claudication is not common, but rest pain, particularly pain in the distal most extremity (ie, toes), is frequent. This pain often progresses to tissue loss and amputation unless the patient stops smoking. The progression of the disease seems to be intermittent with acute and dramatic episodes followed by some periods of remission.

B. Imaging

MRA or invasive angiography can demonstrate the obliteration of the distal arterial tree typical of thromboangiitis obliterans.

Differential Diagnosis

In atherosclerotic peripheral vascular disease, the onset of tissue ischemia tends to be less dramatic than in thromboangiitis obliterans, and symptoms of proximal arterial involvement, such as claudication, predominate.

Symptoms of Raynaud disease may be difficult to differentiate from thromboangiitis obliterans and may coexist in 40% of patients. Repetitive atheroemboli may also mimic thromboangiitis obliterans. It may be necessary to image the proximal arterial tree to rule out sources of arterial microemboli.

Treatment

Cessation of cigarette smoking is the mainstay of therapy and will halt the disease in most cases. As the distal arterial tree is occluded, revascularization is often not possible. Intra-arterial infusion of prostacyclin analogs has been reported to improve ulcer healing in select cases. Sympathectomy is rarely effective.

Prognosis

If smoking cessation can be achieved, the outlook for thromboangiitis obliterans may be better than in patients with premature peripheral vascular disease. If smoking cessation is not achieved, then the prognosis is generally poor, with amputation of both lower and upper extremities a possible outcome.

Cacione DG et al. Pharmacological treatment for Buerger's disease. Cochrane Database Syst Rev. 2020;5:CD011033. [PMID: 32364620]

ARTERIAL ANEURYSMS

ABDOMINAL AORTIC ANEURYSM

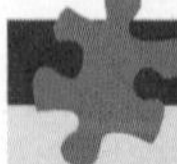

ESSENTIALS OF DIAGNOSIS

- Most aortic aneurysms are asymptomatic until rupture.
- 80% of AAAs measuring 5 cm are palpable; the usual threshold for treatment is 5.5 cm.
- Back or abdominal pain with aneurysmal tenderness may precede rupture.
- Rupture is catastrophic: excruciating abdominal pain that radiates to the back; hypotension.

General Considerations

Dilatation of the infrarenal aorta is a normal part of aging. The aorta of a healthy young man measures approximately 2 cm. An aneurysm is considered present when the aortic diameter exceeds 3 cm, but aneurysms rarely rupture until their diameter exceeds 5 cm. AAAs are found in 2% of men over 55 years of age; the male to female ratio is 4:1. Ninety percent of abdominal atherosclerotic aneurysms originate below the renal arteries. The aneurysms usually involve the aortic bifurcation and often involve the common iliac arteries.

Aortic inflammation is uncommon with atherosclerotic aneurysms and may be due to inflammation from aortic vasculitis, as in Takayasu disease or Behçet disease. Rarely, inflammatory aortitis is due to infections, including *Salmonella,* tuberculosis, and syphilis. Periaortic inflammation without vasculitis or infection (inflammatory aneurysm) is due to retroperitoneal fibrosis, either idiopathic or secondary (IgG_4-related disease).

Clinical Findings

A. Symptoms and Signs

1. Asymptomatic—Although 80% of 5-cm infrarenal aneurysms are palpable on routine physical examination, most aneurysms are discovered on ultrasound or CT imaging as part of a screening program or during the evaluation of unrelated abdominal symptoms.

2. Symptomatic—

A. PAIN—Aneurysmal expansion may be accompanied by pain that is mild to severe midabdominal discomfort often radiating to the lower back. The pain may be constant or intermittent and is exacerbated by even gentle pressure on the aneurysm sack. Pain may also accompany inflammatory aneurysms. Most aneurysms have a thick layer of thrombus lining the aneurysmal sac, but embolization to the lower extremities is rarely seen.

B. RUPTURE—The sudden escape of blood into the retroperitoneal space causes severe pain and hypotension. Free rupture into the peritoneal cavity is a lethal event.

B. Laboratory Findings

In acute cases of a contained retroperitoneal rupture, the hematocrit may be normal, since there has been no opportunity for hemodilution.

Patients with aneurysms may also have CAD, carotid disease, kidney disease, and emphysema, which are typically seen in elderly men who smoke cigarettes. Preoperative testing may indicate the presence of these comorbid conditions, which increase the risk of intervention.

C. Imaging

Abdominal ultrasonography is the diagnostic study of choice for initial screening for the presence of an aneurysm. In approximately three-quarters of patients with aneurysms, curvilinear calcifications outlining portions of the aneurysm wall may be visible on plain radiographs of the abdomen or back. CT scans provide a more reliable assessment of aneurysm diameter and should be done when the aneurysm nears the diameter threshold (5.5 cm) for treatment. Contrast-enhanced CT scans show the arteries above and below the aneurysm. CT imaging will often demonstrate mural thrombus within the aneurysm and is not an indication for anticoagulation.

Once an aneurysm is identified, routine follow-up with ultrasound will determine size and growth rate. The frequency of imaging depends on aneurysm size ranging from every 2 years for aneurysms smaller than 4 cm to every 6 months for aneurysms at or approaching 5 cm. When an aneurysm measures approximately 5 cm, a CTA with contrast should be done to more accurately assess the size of the aneurysm and define the anatomy.

Screening

Guidelines recommend abdominal ultrasound screening in men 65–75 years old with exposure to 100 or more lifetime cigarettes but conflict on whether women with the same exposure should be screened. Guidelines do not recommend repeated screening if the aorta shows no enlargement. While patients are monitored, smoking cessation and treatment of underlying hypertension, hyperlipidemia, and diabetes should be considered.

Treatment

A. Elective Repair

The risk of rupture increases with aneurysm diameter. In general, elective repair is indicated for aortic aneurysms 5.5 cm or larger in diameter or aneurysms that demonstrate rapid expansion (more than 0.5 cm in 6 months). Symptoms such as pain or tenderness may indicate impending rupture and require urgent repair regardless of the aneurysm's diameter.

B. Aneurysmal Rupture

A ruptured aneurysm is a lethal event. Approximately half the patients exsanguinate prior to reaching a hospital. In the remainder, bleeding may be temporarily contained in the retroperitoneum (contained rupture), allowing the patient to undergo emergent surgery. However, only half of those patients will survive. Endovascular repair is recommended for ruptured aneurysm treatment, with the results offering improvement over open repair for these critically ill patients.

C. Aortic Inflammation/Inflammatory Aneurysm

Aortic or periaortic inflammation requires medical treatment for the underlying cause (vasculitis, infection, or retroperitoneal fibrosis). Indications for surgical treatment are based on the size of the aneurysm (5.5 cm or larger), associated compression of retroperitoneal structures (such as the ureter), or pain upon palpation of the aneurysm. Interestingly, the inflammation that encases an inflammatory aneurysm recedes after either endovascular or open surgical aneurysm repair.

D. Assessment of Operative Risk

Aneurysms appear to be a variant of systemic atherosclerosis. Patients with aneurysms have a high rate of coronary disease, but a 2004 trial demonstrated minimal value in addressing stable CAD prior to aneurysm resection. However, in patients with significant symptoms of coronary disease, the coronary disease should be treated first. Aneurysm repair should follow shortly thereafter because there is a slightly increased risk of aneurysm rupture after the coronary procedures.

E. Open Surgical Resection Versus Endovascular Repair

In open surgical aneurysm repair, a graft is sutured to the nondilated vessels above and below the aneurysm. This involves an abdominal incision, extensive dissection, and interruption of aortic blood flow. The mortality rate is low (2–5%) in centers that have a high volume for this procedure and when it is performed in good-risk patients. Older, sicker patients may not tolerate the cardiopulmonary stresses of the operation. With endovascular aortic repair, a stent-graft is introduced through small incisions over the femoral arteries and positioned within the aorta under fluoroscopic guidance. The stent must be able to seal securely against the wall of the aorta above and below the aneurysm, thereby excluding blood from flowing into the aneurysm sac. To successfully treat an aneurysm, the anatomic requirements for endovascular repairs are more precise than for open repairs. Most studies have found that endovascular aortic repair offers patients reduced operative morbidity and mortality as well as shorter recovery periods. Long-term survival is equivalent between the two techniques. Patients who undergo endovascular repair, however, likely need additional interventions and need lifelong monitoring, since there is a 10–15% incidence of continued aneurysm growth after endovascular repair.

Complications

MI, the most common complication, occurs in up to 10% of patients who undergo open aneurysm repair. The incidence of MI is substantially lower with endovascular repair. For routine infrarenal aneurysms, renal injury is unusual; however, when it does occur, or if the baseline creatinine is elevated, it is a significant complicating factor in the postoperative period. Respiratory complications are similar to those seen in most major abdominal surgery. GI hemorrhage, even years after aortic surgeries, suggests the possibility of **graft enteric fistula,** most commonly between the aorta and the distal duodenum; the incidence of this complication is higher when the initial surgery is performed on an emergency basis.

Prognosis

The mortality rate for an open elective surgical resection is 1–5%, and the mortality rate for endovascular therapy is 0.5–2%. Of those who survive surgery, approximately 60% are alive at 5 years; MI is the leading cause of death. The long-term survival (5 years or more) after open and endovascular repairs is equivalent.

Mortality rates of untreated aneurysms vary with aneurysm diameter. The mortality rate among patients with large aneurysms has been defined as follows: 12% annual risk of rupture with an aneurysm larger than 6 cm in diameter and a 25% annual risk of rupture in aneurysms of more than 7 cm diameter. In general, a patient with an aortic aneurysm larger than 5.5 cm has a threefold greater chance of dying of a consequence of rupture of the aneurysm than of dying of the surgical resection.

At present, endovascular aneurysm repair may be less definitive than open surgical repair and requires close follow up with an imaging procedure. Device migration, component separation, and graft limb thrombosis or kinking are common reasons for repeat intervention. With complete exclusion of blood from the aneurysm sac, the pressure is lowered, which causes the aneurysm to shrink. An "endoleak" from the top or bottom seal zones (type 1) or through a graft defect (type 3) is associated with a persistent risk of rupture. Indirect leakage of blood through lumbar and inferior mesenteric branches of the aneurysm (type-2 endoleak) produces an intermediate picture with somewhat reduced pressure in the sac, slow shrinkage, and low rupture risk. However, type-2 endoleak warrants close observation as aneurysm dilatation can change aneurysm morphology leading to type-1 endoleak and rupture.

When to Refer

- Any patient with a 4.5-cm or larger aortic aneurysm should be referred to a vascular specialist for observation and assessment.
- Urgent referrals should be made if the patient complains of pain and gentle palpation of the aneurysm confirms that it is the source, regardless of the aneurysmal size.

When to Admit

- Patients with a tender aneurysm to palpation or signs of aortic rupture require emergent hospital admission.
- Evidence of infection after repair.

O'Donnell TFX et al. Abdominal aortic aneurysm screening guidelines: United States Preventive Services Task Force and Society for Vascular Surgery. J Vasc Surg. 2020;71:1457. [PMID: 32334726]

Jin J. Screening for abdominal aortic aneurysm. JAMA Patient Page. JAMA. 2019;322:2256. [PMID: 31821432]

Lederle FA et al; OVER Veterans Affairs Cooperative Study Group. Open versus endovascular repair of abdominal aortic aneurysm. N Engl J Med. 2019;380:2126. [PMID: 31141634]

Schanzer A et al. Management of abdominal aortic aneurysms. N Engl J Med. 2021;385:1690. [PMID: 34706173]

THORACIC AORTIC ANEURYSMS

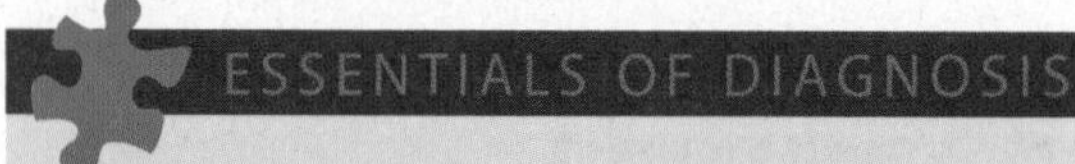

- Widened mediastinum on chest radiograph.
- With rupture, sudden onset of chest pain radiating to the back.

General Considerations

Most thoracic aortic aneurysms are due to atherosclerosis; syphilis is a rare cause. Disorders of connective tissue and Ehlers-Danlos and Marfan syndromes also are rare causes but have important therapeutic implications. Traumatic, false aneurysms, caused by partial tearing of the aortic wall with deceleration injuries, may occur just beyond the origin of the left subclavian artery. Less than 10% of aortic aneurysms occur in the thoracic aorta.

Clinical Findings

A. Symptoms and Signs

Most thoracic aneurysms are asymptomatic. When symptoms occur, they depend largely on the size and the position of the aneurysm and its rate of growth. Substernal back or neck pain may occur. Pressure on the trachea, esophagus, or superior vena cava can result in the following symptoms and signs: dyspnea, stridor or brassy cough, dysphagia, and edema in the neck and arms as well as distended neck veins. Stretching of the left recurrent laryngeal nerve causes hoarseness. With aneurysms of the ascending aorta, aortic regurgitation may be present due to dilation of the aortic valve annulus. Rupture of a thoracic aneurysm is catastrophic because bleeding is rarely contained, allowing no time for emergent repair.

B. Imaging

The aneurysm may be diagnosed on chest radiograph by the calcified outline of the dilated aorta. CT scanning with contrast enhancement is the modality of choice, but MRA can be used to demonstrate the anatomy and aneurysmal size and to exclude lesions that can mimic aneurysms, such as neoplasms or substernal goiter. There is no low-cost alternative (eg, ultrasonography) for screening or surveillance. Cardiac catheterization and echocardiography may be required to describe the relationship of the coronary vessels to an aneurysm of the ascending aorta.

Treatment

Indications for repair depend on the location of dilation, rate of growth, associated symptoms, and overall condition of the patient. Aneurysms that involve the proximal aortic arch or ascending aorta represent particularly challenging problems and may be considered for repair when they measure 5.5 cm. Open surgery is usually required, carrying substantial risk of morbidity (including stroke, diffuse neurologic injury, and intellectual impairment) because interruption of arch blood flow is required. Descending thoracic aneurysms measuring 5.5 cm or larger should be considered for repair, since there is a 5-year survival of 54% in untreated patients. Aneurysms of the descending thoracic aorta are treated routinely by endovascular grafting. Repair of aortic arch aneurysms should be undertaken only if there is a skilled surgical team with an acceptable record of outcomes for these complex procedures. The availability of thoracic aortic endograft technique using complex branched endovascular reconstructions for aneurysms involving the arch or visceral aorta (custom-made grafts with branches to the vessels involved in the aneurysm) does not change the indications for aneurysm repair.

Complications

With the exception of endovascular repair for discrete saccular aneurysms of the descending thoracic aorta, the morbidity and mortality of thoracic aneurysm repair is higher than for infra-renal AAA repair. Paraplegia remains a devastating complication. Most large series report approximately 4–10% rate of paraplegia following endovascular repair of thoracic aortic aneurysms. The spinal arterial supply is segmental through intercostal branches of the aorta with variable degrees of intersegmental connection. Therefore, the more extensive the aneurysm, the greater is the risk of paraplegia with repair. Prior infrarenal abdominal aortic surgery, subclavian or internal iliac artery occlusion, and hypotension all increase the paraplegia risk. Involvement of the aortic arch also increases the risk of stroke, even when the aneurysm does not directly affect the carotid artery.

Prognosis

Generally, degenerative aneurysms of the thoracic aorta will enlarge (on average 0.1 cm/y) and require repair to prevent death from rupture. Saccular aneurysms, particularly those distal to the left subclavian artery and the descending thoracic aorta, have good results with endovascular repair. Resection of aneurysms of the aortic arch requires a skilled surgical team and should be attempted only in low-risk patients. Branched or fenestrated endovascular grafting technology has demonstrated reduced morbidity and mortality.

When to Refer

- Ascending aortic aneurysms larger than 4.5 cm should be referred to a cardiac surgeon for observation and assessment and considered for repair at 5.5 cm.
- Descending thoracic aortic aneurysm should be referred to a vascular specialist when they reach 5 cm for observation and assessment and considered for repair at 5.5 cm.

When to Admit

- Any patient with chest or back pain with a known or suspected thoracic aorta aneurysm must be brought to the hospital and undergo urgent imaging studies to rule out the aneurysm as a cause of the pain.

Tenorio ER et al. Endovascular repair for thoracoabdominal aortic aneurysms: current status and future challenges. Ann Cardiothorac Surg. 2021;10:744. [PMID: 34926178]

Upchurch GR et al. Society for Vascular Surgery clinical practice guidelines of thoracic endovascular aortic repair for descending thoracic aortic aneurysms. J Vasc Surg. 2021;73:55S. [PMID: 32628988]

PERIPHERAL ARTERY ANEURYSMS

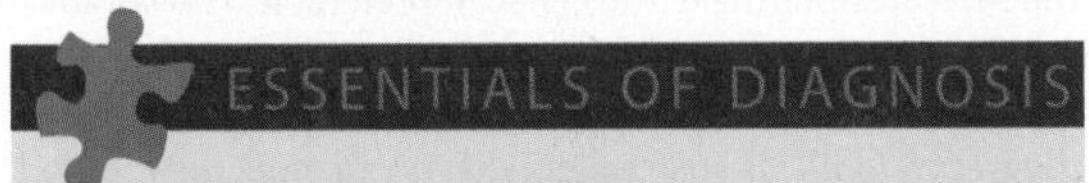

- Widened, prominent pulses.
- Acute leg or foot pain and paresthesias with loss of distal pulses.
- High association of popliteal aneurysms with AAAs.

General Considerations

Like aortic aneurysms, peripheral artery aneurysms are silent until critically symptomatic. However, unlike aortic aneurysms, the presenting manifestations are due to peripheral embolization and thrombosis. Popliteal artery aneurysms account for 70% of peripheral arterial aneurysms. Popliteal aneurysms may embolize repetitively over time and occlude distal arteries. Due to the redundant parallel arterial supply to the foot, ischemia does not occur until a final embolus occludes flow.

Primary femoral artery aneurysms are much less common. However, pseudoaneurysms of the femoral artery following arterial punctures for arteriography and cardiac catheterization occur with an incidence ranging from 0.05% to 6% of arterial punctures.

Clinical Findings

A. Symptoms and Signs

The patient may be aware of a pulsatile mass when the aneurysm is in the groin, but popliteal aneurysms are often undetected by the patient and clinician. Rarely, peripheral aneurysms may produce symptoms by compressing the local vein or nerve. The first symptom may be due to ischemia of acute arterial occlusion. The symptoms range from sudden-onset pain and paralysis to short-distance claudication that slowly lessens as collateral circulation develops. Symptoms from recurrent embolization to the leg are often transient, if they occur at all. Sudden ischemia may appear in a toe or part of the foot, followed by slow resolution, and the true diagnosis may be elusive. The onset of recurrent episodes of pain in the foot, particularly if accompanied by cyanosis, suggests embolization and requires investigation of the heart and proximal arterial tree.

Because popliteal pulses are somewhat difficult to palpate even in normal individuals, a particularly prominent or easily felt pulse is suggestive of aneurysm and should be investigated by ultrasound. Since popliteal aneurysms are bilateral in 60% of cases, the diagnosis of thrombosis of a popliteal aneurysm is often aided by the palpation of a pulsatile aneurysm in the contralateral popliteal space. Approximately 50% of patients with popliteal aneurysms have an aneurysmal abdominal aorta.

B. Imaging Studies

Duplex color ultrasound is the most efficient investigation to confirm the diagnosis of peripheral aneurysm, measure its size and configuration, and demonstrate mural thrombus. MRA or CTA is required to define the aneurysm and local arterial anatomy for reconstruction. Arteriography is not recommended because mural thrombus reduces the apparent diameter of the lumen on angiography. Patients with popliteal aneurysms should undergo abdominal ultrasonography to determine whether an AAA is also present.

Treatment

To prevent limb loss, immediate or urgent surgery is indicated when acute embolization or thrombosis has caused acute ischemia. Open surgical bypass is generally indicated. Similarly, surgery is indicated when an aneurysm is associated with any peripheral embolization, the aneurysm is larger than 2 cm, or a mural thrombus is present. Endovascular exclusion of the aneurysm can be done but has anatomic constraints and is reserved for high-risk patients. Intra-arterial thrombolysis may be done in the setting of acute ischemia, if examination (light touch) remains intact, suggesting that immediate surgery is not imperative. Acute pseudoaneurysms of the femoral artery due to arterial punctures can be successfully treated using ultrasound-guided compression or thrombin injection. Open surgery with prosthetic interposition grafting is preferred for primary aneurysms of the femoral artery.

Prognosis

Approximately one-third of untreated patients will require an amputation. The long-term patency of bypass grafts for femoral and popliteal aneurysms is generally excellent but depends on the adequacy of the outflow tract. Late graft occlusion is less common than in similar surgeries for occlusive disease.

When to Refer

- Peripheral arterial aneurysms measuring 2 cm or with ultrasound evidence of thrombus within the aneurysm should be referred to a vascular specialist.

When to Admit

Patients with symptoms of ischemia or any signs of embolization should be admitted.

AORTIC DISSECTION

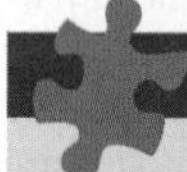

ESSENTIALS OF DIAGNOSIS

- Sudden searing chest pain with radiation to the back, abdomen, or neck in a hypertensive patient.
- Widened mediastinum on chest radiograph.
- Pulse discrepancy in the extremities.
- Acute aortic regurgitation may develop.

General Considerations

Aortic dissection occurs when a spontaneous intimal tear develops and blood dissects into the media of the aorta. The tear can result from repetitive torque applied to the ascending and proximal descending aorta during the cardiac cycle; hypertension is an important component of this disease process. Dissections are classified by the entry point and distal extent. **Type A dissection** involves the arch proximal to the left subclavian artery, and **type B dissection** occurs in the proximal descending thoracic aorta typically just beyond the left subclavian artery. Dissections may occur in the absence of hypertension but abnormalities of smooth muscle, elastic tissue, or collagen are more common in these patients. Pregnancy, bicuspid aortic valve, and coarctation also are associated with increased risk of dissection.

Blood entering the intimal tear may extend the dissection into the abdominal aorta, the lower extremities, the carotid arteries, or less commonly, the subclavian arteries. Both absolute pressure levels and the pulse pressure are important in propagation of dissection. *Aortic dissection is a true emergency and requires immediate control of blood pressure to limit the extent of the dissection.* With type A dissection, which has the worse prognosis, death may occur within hours due to rupture of the dissection into the pericardial sac or dissection into the coronary arteries, resulting in MI. Rupture into the pleural cavity is also possible. The intimal/medial flap of the aortic wall created by the dissection may occlude major aortic branches, resulting in ischemia of the brain, intestines, kidney, or extremities.

Clinical Findings

A. Symptoms and Signs

Severe persistent chest pain of sudden onset radiating down the back or possibly into the anterior chest is characteristic. Radiation of the pain into the neck may also occur. The patient is usually hypertensive. Syncope, hemiplegia, or paralysis of the lower extremities may occur. Mesenteric ischemia or kidney injury may develop. Peripheral pulses may be diminished or unequal. A diastolic murmur may develop as a result of a dissection in the ascending aorta close to the aortic valve, causing valvular regurgitation, heart failure, and cardiac tamponade.

B. Electrocardiographic Findings

LVH from long-standing hypertension is often present. Acute changes suggesting myocardial ischemia do not develop unless dissection involves the coronary artery ostium. Classically, inferior wall abnormalities predominate since dissection leads to compromise of the right rather than the left coronary artery. In some patients, the ECG may be completely normal.

C. Imaging

A multiplanar CT scan with contrast enhancement is the immediate diagnostic imaging modality of choice; clinicians should have a low threshold for obtaining a CT scan in any hypertensive patient with chest pain and equivocal findings on ECG. The CT scan should include both the chest and abdomen to fully delineate the extent of the dissected aorta. MRA is an excellent imaging modality for chronic dissections, but in the acute situation, the longer imaging time and the difficulty of monitoring patients in the MRI scanner make the CT scan preferable. Chest radiographs may reveal an abnormal aortic contour or widened superior mediastinum. Although transesophageal echocardiography (TEE) is an excellent diagnostic imaging method, it is generally not readily available in the acute setting.

Differential Diagnosis

Aortic dissection is most commonly misdiagnosed as MI or other causes of chest pain such as pulmonary embolization. Dissections may occur with minimal pain; branch vessel occlusion of the lower extremity can mimic arterial embolus.

Treatment

A. Medical

Aggressive measures to lower blood pressure should occur when an aortic dissection is suspected, even before the diagnostic studies have been completed. Treatment requires a simultaneous reduction of the systolic blood pressure to 100–120 mm Hg and heart rate to 60–70 beats/minute. Beta-blockers should be first-line therapy because they reduce the LV ejection force that weakens the arterial wall. Labetalol, both an alpha- and beta-blocker, lowers heart rate and achieves rapid blood pressure control. Give 20 mg over 2 minutes by intravenous injection. Additional doses of 40–80 mg intravenously can be given every 10 minutes (maximum dose 300 mg) until the desired blood pressure has been reached. Alternatively, 2 mg/minute may be given by intravenous infusion, titrated to desired effect. The short half-life of esmolol allows for rapid titration and for testing a patient's reaction to a beta-blocker if there are concerns about asthma or bradycardia. Give a loading dose of esmolol, 0.5 mg/kg intravenously over 1 minute, followed by an infusion of 0.0025–0.02 mg/kg/minute. Titrate the infusion to a goal heart rate of 60–70 beats/minute. For patients who cannot tolerate a beta-blocker or who need a second agent to control the hypertension, intravenous calcium channel blocker infusions, such as nicardipine, are an alternative. Start nicardipine 5 mg/hour intravenously and titrate the infusion to the desired effect. If beta-blockade alone does not control the hypertension, nitroprusside may be added as follows: 50 mg of nitroprusside in 1000 mL of 5% dextrose and water, infused at a rate of 0.5 mL/minute for a 70-kg person (0.3 mcg/kg/minute); the infusion rate is increased by 0.5 mL every 5 minutes until adequate control of the pressure has been achieved. Morphine sulfate is the appropriate drug to use for pain relief. Long-term medical care of patients should include beta-blockers in their antihypertensive regimen.

B. Surgical Intervention

1. Type A dissection—*Urgent surgical intervention is required for all type A dissections.* If a skilled cardiovascular team is not available, the patient should be transferred to an appropriate facility. The procedure involves grafting and replacing the diseased portion of the arch and brachiocephalic vessels as necessary. Replacement of the aortic valve may be required with reattachment of the coronary arteries.

2. Type B dissection with malperfusion—*Urgent surgery is required for type B dissections if there is aortic branch compromise resulting in malperfusion of the renal, visceral, or extremity vessels.* The immediate goal of surgery is to restore flow to the ischemic tissue. Endovascular stenting of the entry tear at the level of the subclavian artery may result in obliteration of the false lumen and restore flow into the branch vessel from the true lumen. The results, however, are unpredictable and should only be attempted by an experienced team.

3. Type B dissection without malperfusion—For acute type B dissections without malperfusion, blood pressure control is the primary treatment. Long-term aortic-specific survival and late aneurysm formation rates are improved with early thoracic stent graft repair, especially in healthy patients with high-risk anatomic features (aortic diameter greater than 4 cm or partial false lumen thrombosis).

Prognosis & Follow-Up

The mortality rate for untreated type A dissections is approximately 1% per hour for 72 hours and over 90% at 3 months. Mortality is also extremely high for untreated type B dissections with malperfusion or rupture. The surgical and endovascular therapies for these patients are technically demanding and require an experienced team to achieve perioperative mortalities of less than 10%. Aneurysmal enlargement of the residual false lumen may develop despite adequate antihypertensive therapy. Yearly CT scans are required to monitor for aneurysm development. Indications for late aneurysm repair are determined by aneurysm size (6 cm or larger), similar to undissected thoracic aneurysms.

When to Admit

- All patients with an acute dissection should be hospitalized for blood pressure management and observation.
- Urgent surgical repair is indicated for all type A dissections and for type B dissections with malperfusion, rupture, or persistent symptoms.

Bossone E et al. Epidemiology and management of aortic disease: aortic aneurysms and acute aortic syndromes. Nat Rev Cardiol. 2021;18:331. [PMID: 33353985]

VENOUS DISEASES

VARICOSE VEINS

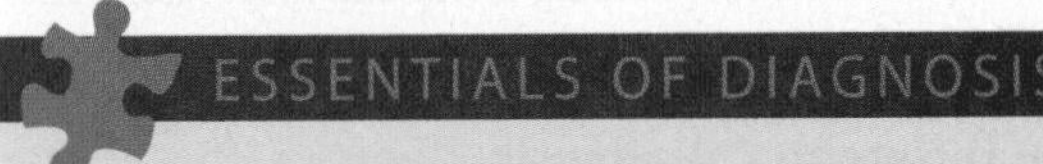

- Dilated, tortuous superficial veins in the legs.
- Asymptomatic or aching discomfort or pain.
- Often hereditary.
- Increased frequency after pregnancy.

General Considerations

Varicose veins develop in the lower extremities. Periods of high venous pressure related to prolonged standing or heavy lifting are contributing factors, but the highest incidence occurs in women after pregnancy. Varicosities develop in over 20% of all adults.

The combination of progressive venous reflux and venous hypertension is the hallmark of chronic venous disease. The superficial veins are involved, typically the great saphenous vein and its tributaries, but the short saphenous vein (posterior lower leg) may also be affected. Distention of the vein prevents the valve leaflets from coapting, creating incompetence and reflux of blood toward the foot.

Secondary varicosities can develop as a result of obstructive changes and valve damage in the deep venous system following thrombophlebitis, or rarely as a result of proximal venous occlusion due to neoplasm or fibrosis. Congenital or acquired arteriovenous fistulas or venous malformations are also associated with varicosities and should be considered in young patients with varicosities.

Clinical Findings

A. Symptoms and Signs

Symptom severity is not correlated with the number and size of the varicosities; extensive varicose veins may produce no subjective symptoms, whereas minimal varicosities may produce many symptoms. Dull, aching heaviness or a feeling of fatigue of the legs brought on by periods of standing is the most common complaint. Itching from venous eczema may occur either above the ankle or directly overlying large varicosities.

Dilated, tortuous veins of the thigh and calf are visible and palpable when the patient is standing. Longstanding varicose veins may progress to chronic venous insufficiency with associated ankle edema, brownish skin hyperpigmentation, and chronic skin induration or fibrosis. A bruit or thrill is never found with primary varicose veins and, when found, alerts the clinician to the presence of an arteriovenous fistula or malformation.

B. Imaging

The identification of the source of venous reflux that feeds the symptomatic veins is necessary for effective surgical treatment. Duplex ultrasonography by a technician experienced in the diagnosis and localization of venous reflux is the test of choice for planning therapy. In most cases, reflux will arise from the greater saphenous vein.

Differential Diagnosis

Varicose veins due to primary superficial venous reflux should be differentiated from those secondary to previous or ongoing obstruction of the deep veins (post-thrombotic syndrome). Pain or discomfort secondary to neuropathy should be distinguished from symptoms associated with coexistent varicose veins. Similarly, vein symptoms should be distinguished from pain due to intermittent claudication, which occurs after a predictable amount of exercise and resolves with rest. In adolescent patients with varicose veins, imaging of the deep venous system is obligatory to exclude a congenital malformation or atresia of the deep veins. *Surgical treatment of varicose veins in these patients is contraindicated because the varicosities may play a significant role in venous drainage of the limb.*

Complications

Superficial thrombophlebitis of varicose veins is uncommon. The typical presentation is acute localized pain with tender, firm veins. The process is usually self-limiting, resolving within several weeks. The risk of DVT or embolization is very low unless the thrombophlebitis extends into the great saphenous vein in the upper medial thigh. Predisposing conditions include pregnancy, local trauma, or prolonged periods of sitting.

In older patients, superficial varicosities may bleed with even minor trauma. The amount of bleeding can be alarming as the pressure in the varicosity is high.

Treatment

A. Nonsurgical Measures

Nonsurgical treatment is effective. Elastic graduated compression stockings (20–30 mm Hg pressure) reduce the venous pressure in the leg and may prevent the progression of disease. Good control of symptoms can be achieved when stockings are worn daily during waking hours and legs are elevated, especially at night. Compression stockings are well-suited for elderly patients or patients who do not want surgery.

B. Varicose Vein Sclerotherapy

Direct injection of a sclerosing agent induces permanent fibrosis and obliteration of the target veins. Chemical irritants (eg, glycerin) or hypertonic saline are often used for small, less-than-4-mm reticular veins or telangiectasias. Foam sclerotherapy is used to treat the great saphenous vein, varicose veins larger than 4 mm, and perforating veins. Sclerotherapy of varicose veins without treatment of underlying saphenous vein reflux is associated with varicosity recurrence rates over 50% as uncorrected reflux progressively dilates adjacent veins. Complications such as phlebitis, tissue necrosis, or infection may occur with any sclerosing agent.

C. Surgical Reflux Treatment

Treatment options for reflux arising from the great saphenous vein include surgical vein stripping (removal) or endovenous treatments using thermal devices (laser or radiofrequency catheter), cyanoacrylate glue injection, or foam sclerosant injection. Endovenous treatments can often be performed with local anesthesia alone and the early success is equal to vein stripping. Long-term success is highest with vein stripping and thermal treatments while the long-term durability of cyanoacrylate glue and foam is unknown. One major complication of thermal treatments is endothermal heat-induced thrombosis of the deep vein and may require prolonged anticoagulation. Less common sources of reflux include the small saphenous vein (for varicosities in the posterior calf) and incompetent perforator veins arising directly from the deep venous system. Correction of reflux is performed at the same time as excision of the symptomatic varicose veins. When superficial venous reflux is present, concomitant reflux in the deep venous system is often secondary to volume overload, which will resolve with correction of the superficial reflux.

Prognosis

Surgical treatment of superficial vein reflux and excision of varicose veins provide excellent results. The 5-year success rate (as defined as lack of pain and recurrent varicosities) is 85–90%. Simple excision (phlebectomy) or injection sclerotherapy without correction of reflux is associated with recurrence rates over 50%. Even after adequate treatment, secondary tissue changes may persist.

When to Refer

- Absolute indications for referral for saphenous ablation include thrombophlebitis and bleeding.
- Pain and cosmetic concerns are responsible for the majority of referrals for ablation.

Kabnick LS et al. Classification and treatment of endothermal heat-induced thrombosis: recommendations from the American Venous Forum and the Society for Vascular Surgery. J Vasc Surg Venous Lymphat Disord. 2021;9:6. [PMID: 33012690]

DePopas E et al. Varicose veins and lower extremity venous insufficiency. Semin Intervent Radiol. 2018;35:56. [PMID: 29628617]

SUPERFICIAL VENOUS THROMBOPHLEBITIS

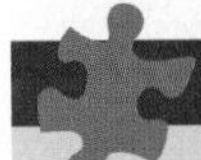

ESSENTIALS OF DIAGNOSIS

- Red, painful induration along a superficial vein, usually at the site of a recent intravenous line.
- Marked swelling of the extremity may not occur.

General Considerations

Short-term venous catheterization of superficial arm veins as well as the use of longer-term peripherally inserted central catheter (PICC) lines are the most common cause of superficial thrombophlebitis. Intravenous catheter sites should be observed daily for signs of local inflammation and should be removed if a local reaction develops in the vein. Serious thrombotic or septic complications can occur if this policy is not followed; *S aureus* is the most common pathogen. Other organisms, including fungi, may also be responsible.

Superficial thrombophlebitis may occur spontaneously, often in pregnant or postpartum women or in individuals with varicose veins, or it may be associated with trauma, as with a blow to the leg or following intravenous therapy with irritating solutions. It also may be a manifestation of systemic hypercoagulability secondary to abdominal cancer such as carcinoma of the pancreas and may be the earliest sign of these conditions. Superficial thrombophlebitis related to a PICC may be associated with occult DVT in about 20% of cases, but occult DVT is much less commonly associated with spontaneous superficial thrombophlebitis of the saphenous vein (about 5% of cases). Pulmonary emboli are exceedingly rare and occur from an associated DVT (see Chapters 9 and 14).

Clinical Findings

A. Symptoms and Signs

In spontaneous superficial thrombophlebitis, the great saphenous vein is most often involved. The patient usually experiences a dull pain in the region of the involved vein. Local findings consist of induration, redness, and tenderness along the course of a vein. The process may be localized, or it may involve most of the great saphenous vein and its tributaries. The inflammatory reaction generally subsides in 1–2 weeks; a firm cord may remain for a much longer period. Edema of the extremity is uncommon.

Localized redness and induration at the site of a recent intravenous line requires urgent attention. Proximal extension of the induration and pain with chills and high fever suggest septic phlebitis and requires urgent treatment.

B. Imaging

Duplex ultrasound of the involved extremity is the standard of care to establish the extent of superficial thrombophlebitis and detect the presence of DVT.

Differential Diagnosis

The linear rather than circular nature of the lesion and the distribution along the course of a superficial vein serve to differentiate superficial phlebitis from cellulitis, erythema nodosum, erythema induratum, panniculitis, and fibrositis. Lymphangitis and deep thrombophlebitis must also be considered.

Treatment

For focal, spontaneous thrombophlebitis not near the saphenofemoral junction, local heat and NSAIDs are usually effective in limiting the process. Prophylactic dose fondaparinux or rivaroxaban is recommended for 5 cm or longer superficial thrombophlebitis of the saphenous veins (Table 14–14) and full anticoagulation is reserved for disease that is rapidly progressing or if there is concern for extension into the deep system (Table 14–16). Active malignancy, a history of venous thromboembolism, and known thrombophilia are also indications for full dose anticoagulation. The usual course of treatment of superficial thrombophlebitis is 6 weeks. When the lower extremity superficial thrombosis is less than 5 cm but the patient has risk factors such as hospitalization, immobilization, or recent surgery, prophylactic dose anticoagulation may be deferred unless there is extension of the thrombus on repeat ultrasonography 7–10 days later. If the induration is extensive or is progressing toward the saphenofemoral junction (leg) or cephalo-axillary junction (arm) despite anticoagulation, ligation and division of the vein at the junction of the deep and superficial veins is indicated.

Septic superficial thrombophlebitis is an intravascular abscess and requires urgent treatment with heparin or fondaparinux (see Table 14–16) to limit further thrombus formation and removal of the offending catheter in catheter-related infections (see Chapter 30). Treat with antibiotics (eg, vancomycin, 15 mg/kg intravenously every 12 hours, plus ceftriaxone, 1 g intravenously every 24 hours). If cultures are positive, therapy should be continued for 7–10 days or for 4–6 weeks if complicating endocarditis cannot be excluded. Surgical excision of the involved vein may also be necessary to control the infection.

Prognosis

With spontaneous thrombophlebitis, the course is generally benign and brief. In patients with phlebitis secondary to varicose veins, recurrent episodes are likely unless correction of the underlying venous reflux and excision of varicosities is done. In contrast, the mortality from septic thrombophlebitis is 20% or higher and requires aggressive treatment. However, if the involvement is localized, the mortality is low and prognosis is excellent with early treatment.

Duffett L et al. Treatment of superficial vein thrombosis: a systematic review and meta-analysis. Thromb Haemost. 2019;119:479. [PMID: 30716777]

CHRONIC VENOUS INSUFFICIENCY

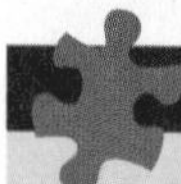

ESSENTIALS OF DIAGNOSIS

- History of prior DVT or leg injury.
- Edema, (brawny) skin hyperpigmentation, subcutaneous lipodermosclerosis in the lower leg.
- Venous ulcers: large ulcerations at or above the medial ankle.

General Considerations

Chronic venous insufficiency is a severe manifestation of venous hypertension. One of the most common etiologies is prior deep venous thrombophlebitis, although about 25% of patients do not have a known history of DVT. In these cases, there may be a history of leg trauma or surgery; obesity is often a complicating factor. Progressive superficial venous reflux is also a common cause. Other causes include congenital or neoplastic obstruction of the pelvic veins or a congenital or acquired arteriovenous fistula.

The basic pathology is caused by valve leaflets that do not coapt because they are either thickened and scarred (post-thrombotic syndrome) or in a dilated vein and are therefore functionally inadequate. With the valves unable to stop venous blood from returning to the foot (venous reflux), the leg develops venous hypertension and an abnormally high hydrostatic force is transmitted to the subcutaneous veins and tissues of the lower leg. The resulting edema results in dramatic and deleterious secondary changes. The stigmata of chronic venous insufficiency include fibrosis of the subcutaneous tissue and skin, pigmentation of skin (hemosiderin taken up by the dermal macrophages) and, later, ulceration, which is extremely slow to heal. Itching may precipitate the formation of ulceration or local wound cellulitis. Dilation of the superficial veins may occur, leading to varicosities. Although surgical treatment for venous reflux can improve symptoms, controlling edema and the secondary skin changes usually require lifelong compression therapy.

Clinical Findings

A. Symptoms and Signs

Progressive pitting edema of the leg (particularly the lower leg) is the primary presenting symptom. Secondary changes in the skin and subcutaneous tissues develop over time (Figure 12–2). The usual symptoms are itching, a dull discomfort made worse by periods of standing, and pain if an ulceration is present. The skin at the ankle is usually taut from swelling, shiny, and a brownish pigmentation (hemosiderin) often develops. If the condition is longstanding, the subcutaneous tissues become thick and fibrous. Ulcerations may occur, usually just above the ankle, on the medial or anterior aspect of the leg. Healing results in a thin scar on a fibrotic base that often breaks down with minor trauma or further bouts of leg swelling. Varicosities may appear (Figure 12–3) that are associated with incompetent perforating veins. Cellulitis, which is often difficult to distinguish from the hemosiderin pigmentation, may be diagnosed by blanching erythema with pain.

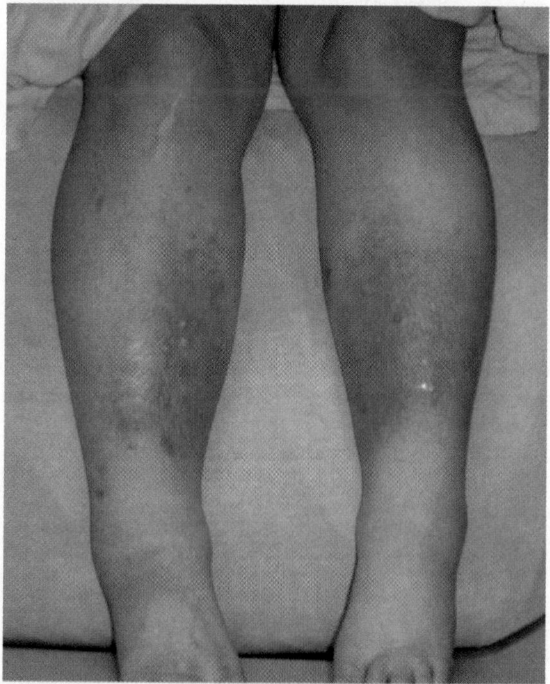

▲ **Figure 12–2. Bilateral pretibial edema and erythema consistent with stasis dermatitis (sometimes mimicking cellulitis) in chronic venous insufficiency.** (Used, with permission, from Dean SM, Satiani B, Abraham WT. *Color Atlas and Synopsis of Vascular Diseases.* McGraw-Hill, 2014.)

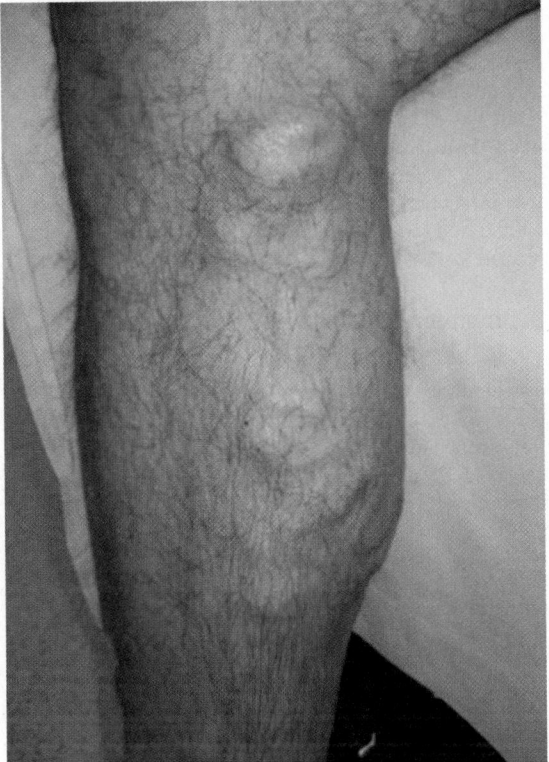

▲ **Figure 12–3.** Varicose veins, manifested as blue, subcutaneous, tortuous veins more than 3 mm in diameter. (Used, with permission, from Dean SM, Satiani B, Abraham WT. *Color Atlas and Synopsis of Vascular Diseases.* McGraw-Hill, 2014.)

B. Imaging

Patients with post-thrombotic syndrome or signs of chronic venous insufficiency should undergo duplex ultrasonography to determine whether superficial reflux is present and to evaluate the degree of deep reflux and obstruction.

Differential Diagnosis

Patients with heart failure, CKD, or decompensated liver disease may have bilateral edema of the lower extremities. Many medications can cause edema (eg, calcium channel blockers, NSAIDs, thiazolidinediones). Swelling from lymphedema involves the feet and may be unilateral, but varicosities are absent. Edema from these causes pits easily and brawny discoloration is rare. Lipedema is a disorder of adipose tissue that occurs almost exclusively in women, is bilateral and symmetric, and is characterized by stopping at a distinct line just above the ankles.

Primary varicose veins may be difficult to differentiate from the secondary varicosities of post-thrombotic syndrome or venous obstruction.

Other conditions associated with chronic ulcers of the leg include neuropathic ulcers from diabetes mellitus, arterial insufficiency (often manifests as painful lateral ankle ulcers with absent pulses; conversely, medial ankle ulcers, are usually due to venous insufficiency), autoimmune diseases (eg, Felty syndrome), sickle cell anemia, erythema induratum (bilateral and usually on the posterior aspect of the lower part of the leg), and fungal infections.

Prevention

Irreversible tissue changes and associated complications in the lower legs can be reduced through early and aggressive anticoagulation of acute DVT to minimize the valve damages and by prescribing compression stockings if chronic edema develops after the DVT has resolved. Treatment of acute iliofemoral DVT with catheter-directed thrombolysis or mechanical thrombectomy does not reduce post-thrombotic syndrome and chronic venous insufficiency.

Treatment

A. General Measures

Fitted, graduated compression stockings (20–30 mm Hg pressure or higher) worn from the foot to just below the knee during the day and evening are the mainstays of treatment and are usually sufficient. When they are not, additional measures, such as avoidance of long periods of sitting or standing, intermittent elevations of the involved leg, and sleeping with the legs kept above the level of the heart, may be necessary to control the swelling. Pneumatic compression of the leg, which can pump the fluid out of the leg, is used in refractory cases.

B. Ulceration

As the primary pathology is edema and venous hypertension, healing of the ulcer will not occur until the edema is controlled and compression is applied. Circumferential nonelastic bandages on the lower leg enhance the pumping action of the calf muscles on venous blood flow out of the calf. A lesion can often be treated on an ambulatory basis by means of a semi-rigid gauze boot made with Unna paste (Gelocast, Medicopaste) or a multi-layer compression dressing (eg, Profore). Initially, the ulcer needs to be debrided and the boot changed every 2–3 days to control ulcer drainage. As the edema and drainage subside, the boot is changed every 5–7 days until the ulcer heals. The ulcer, tendons, and bony prominences must be adequately padded. Alternatively, knee-high graduated compression stockings with an absorbent dressing may be used, if wound drainage is minimal. Home compression therapy with a pneumatic compression device is used in refractory cases, but many patients have severe pain with the "milking" action of the pump device. Some patients will require hospital admission for complete bed rest and leg elevation to achieve ulcer healing. After the ulcer has healed, daily graduated compression stocking therapy is mandatory to prevent ulcer recurrence.

C. Vein Treatment (Reflux or Obstruction)

Treatment of superficial vein reflux (see Varicose Veins, above) has been shown to decrease the recurrence rate of venous ulcers. Where there is substantial obstruction of the femoral or popliteal deep venous system, superficial varicosities supply the venous return and should not be removed.

Venous stents as treatment of chronic iliac deep vein stenosis or obstruction may improve venous ulcer healing and reduce the ulcer recurrence rate in severe cases.

Prognosis

Edema often recurs, particularly if support stockings that have at least 20–30 mm Hg compression are not worn consistently.

When to Refer

- Patients with significant saphenous reflux should be evaluated for ablation.
- Patients with ulcers should be monitored by an interdisciplinary wound care team so that these challenging wounds receive aggressive care.

Raffetto JD et al. Why venous leg ulcers have difficulty healing: overview on pathophysiology, clinical consequences, and treatment. J Clin Med. 2020;10:29. [PMID: 33374372]

SUPERIOR VENA CAVAL OBSTRUCTION

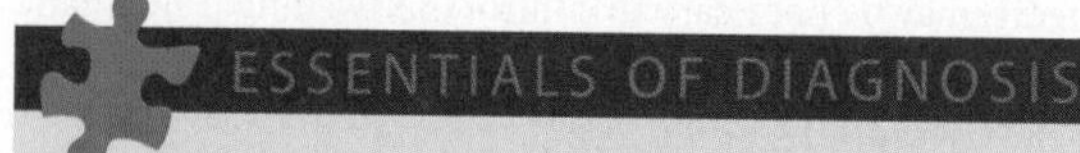

- Swelling of the neck, face, and upper extremities.
- Dilated veins over the upper chest and neck.

General Considerations

Partial or complete obstruction of the superior vena cava is a relatively rare condition that is usually secondary to neoplastic or inflammatory processes in the superior mediastinum. The most frequent causes are (1) neoplasms, such as carcinoma of the lung with direct extension (over 80%), lymphomas, or primary malignant mediastinal tumors; (2) chronic fibrotic mediastinitis, either of unknown origin or secondary to tuberculosis, histoplasmosis, pyogenic infections, or drugs (especially methysergide); (3) DVT, often by extension of the process from the axillary or subclavian vein into the innominate vein and vena cava associated with catheterization of these veins for dialysis or for hyperalimentation; (4) aneurysm of the aortic arch; and (5) constrictive pericarditis.

Clinical Findings

A. Symptoms and Signs

The onset of symptoms is acute or subacute. Symptoms include swelling of the neck and face and upper extremities. Symptoms are often perceived as congestion and present as headache, dizziness, visual disturbances, stupor, syncope, or cough. There is progressive obstruction of the venous drainage of the head, neck, and upper extremities. The cutaneous veins of the upper chest and lower neck become dilated, and flushing of the face and neck develops. Brawny edema of the face, neck, and arms occurs later, and cyanosis of these areas then appears. Cerebral and laryngeal edema ultimately result in impaired function of the brain as well as respiratory insufficiency. Bending over or lying down accentuates the symptoms; sitting quietly is generally preferred. The manifestations are more severe if the obstruction develops rapidly and if the azygos junction or the vena cava between that vein and the heart is obstructed.

B. Laboratory Findings

The venous pressure is elevated (often more than 20 cm of water) in the arm and is normal in the leg. Since lung cancer is a common cause, bronchoscopy is often performed; transbronchial biopsy, however, is relatively contraindicated because of venous hypertension and the risk of bleeding.

C. Imaging

Chest radiographs and a CT scan can define the location and often the nature of the obstructive process, and contrast venography or magnetic resonance venography (MRV) will map out the extent and degree of the venous obstruction and the collateral circulation. Brachial venography or radionuclide scanning following intravenous injection of technetium (Tc-99m) pertechnetate demonstrates a block to the flow of contrast material into the right heart and enlarged collateral veins. These techniques also allow estimation of blood flow around the occlusion as well as serial evaluation of the response to therapy.

Treatment

Conservative measures, such as elevation of the head of the bed and lifestyle modification to avoid bending over, are useful. Balloon angioplasty of the obstructed caval segment combined with stent placement provides prompt relief of symptoms and is the procedure of choice for all etiologies. Occasionally, anticoagulation is needed, while thrombolysis is rarely needed.

Urgent treatment for neoplasm consists of (1) cautious use of intravenous diuretics and (2) mediastinal irradiation, starting within 24 hours, with a treatment plan designed to give a high daily dose of radiation but a short total course of therapy to rapidly shrink the local tumor. Intensive radiation therapy combined with chemotherapy will palliate the process in up to 90% of patients. In patients with a subacute presentation, radiation therapy alone usually suffices. Chemotherapy is added if lymphoma or small-cell carcinoma is diagnosed.

Long-term outcome is complicated by risk of re-occlusion from either thrombosis or neoplasm growth. Surgical procedures to bypass the obstruction are complicated by bleeding from high venous pressure. In cases where the thrombosis is secondary to an indwelling catheter, thrombolysis may be attempted. Clinical judgment is required since a long-standing clot may be fibrotic and the risk of bleeding can outweigh the potential benefit.

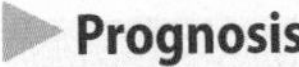

Prognosis

The prognosis depends on the nature and degree of obstruction and its speed of onset. Slowly developing forms secondary to fibrosis may be tolerated for years. A high degree of obstruction of rapid onset secondary to cancer is often fatal in a few days or weeks because of increased intracranial pressure and cerebral hemorrhage, but treatment of the tumor with radiation and chemotherapeutic drugs may result in significant palliation. Balloon angioplasty and stenting provide good relief but may require re-treatment for recurrent symptoms due to thrombosis or restenosis.

When to Refer

- Any patient with progressive head and neck swelling should be referred to rule out superior vena cava syndrome.

When to Admit

- Any patient with acute edema of the head and neck or with signs and symptoms of airway compromise, such as hoarseness or stridor, should be admitted.

Azizi AH et al. Superior vena cava syndrome. JACC Cardiovasc Interv. 2020;13:2896. [PMID: 33357528]

DISEASES OF THE LYMPHATIC CHANNELS

LYMPHANGITIS & LYMPHADENITIS

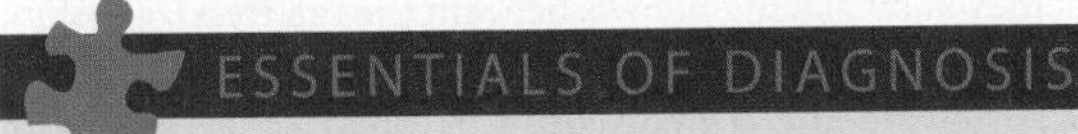

ESSENTIALS OF DIAGNOSIS

- Red streak from wound or cellulitis toward regional lymph nodes, which are usually enlarged and tender.
- Chills, fever, and malaise may be present.

General Considerations

Lymphangitis and lymphadenitis are common manifestations of a bacterial infection that is usually caused by hemolytic streptococci or *S aureus* (or by both organisms) and becomes invasive, generally from an infected wound, cellulitis, or an abscess. The wound may be very small or superficial, or an established abscess may be present, feeding bacteria into the lymphatics. The involvement of the lymphatics is often manifested by a red streak in the skin extending in the direction of the regional lymph nodes.

Clinical Findings

A. Symptoms and Signs

Throbbing pain is usually present at the site of bacterial invasion from a wound, cellulitis, or abscess. Malaise, anorexia, sweating, chills, and fever of 38–40°C develop quickly, often with a rapid pulse. The red streak, when present, may be definite or may be faint and easily missed, especially in dark-skinned patients. The involved regional lymph nodes may be significantly enlarged and are usually quite tender. The infection may progress rapidly, often in a matter of hours, and may lead to septicemia and death.

B. Laboratory Findings

Leukocytosis with a left shift is usually present. Blood cultures may be positive, most often for staphylococcal or streptococcal species. Culture and sensitivity studies of the wound exudate or pus may be helpful in treatment of the more severe or refractory infections but are often difficult to interpret because of skin contaminants.

Differential Diagnosis

The erythema and induration of superficial thrombophlebitis are localized in and around the thrombosed vein. Venous thrombosis is not associated with lymphadenitis, and an entrance wound with secondary cellulitis is generally absent.

Cat-scratch fever *(Bartonella henselae)* is a cause of lymphadenitis; the nodes, though often very large, are relatively nontender. Exposure to cats is common, but the patient may have forgotten about the scratch.

It is extremely important to differentiate cellulitis from acute streptococcal hemolytic gangrene or a necrotizing soft tissue infection. These are deeper infections that may be extensive and are potentially lethal. Patients are more seriously ill; there may be redness due to leakage of red cells, creating a non-blanching erythema; subcutaneous crepitus, a late finding, may be palpated or auscultated; and subcutaneous air may be present on radiography or CT scan. Immediate surgical consultation is needed for wide debridement of all involved deep tissues if a necrotizing infection is suspected.

Treatment

A. General Measures

Prompt treatment should include heat (hot, moist compresses or heating pad), elevation when feasible, and immobilization of the infected area. Analgesics may be prescribed for pain.

B. Specific Measures

Empiric antibiotic therapy for hemolytic streptococci or *S aureus* (or both organisms) should always be instituted. Cephalosporins or extended-spectrum penicillins are commonly used (eg, cephalexin, 0.5 g orally four times daily for 7–10 days; see Table 30–6). Trimethoprim-sulfamethoxazole (two double-strength tablets orally twice daily for 7–10 days) should be considered when there is concern that the pathogen is MRSA (see Tables 30–4 and 30–6). Vancomycin, 15 mg/kg intravenously every 12 hours, is used for patients with signs of a systemic inflammatory response.

C. Wound Care

Any wound that is the initiating site of lymphangitis should be treated aggressively. Any necrotic tissue must be debrided and loculated pus drained.

Prognosis

With proper therapy including an antibiotic effective against the invading bacteria, control of the infection can usually be achieved in a few days. Delayed or inadequate therapy can lead to overwhelming infection with septicemia.

When to Admit

- Infections causing lymphangitis should be treated in the hospital with intravenous antibiotics.
- Debridement may be required and prompt surgical consultation is prudent.

LYMPHEDEMA

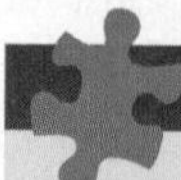

ESSENTIALS OF DIAGNOSIS

- Painless persistent edema of one or both lower extremities, primarily in young women.
- Pitting edema without ulceration, varicosities, or stasis pigmentation.
- Lymphangitis and cellulitis may occur.

General Considerations

The **primary form** of lymphedema is caused by congenital hypo- or hyperplastic proximal or distal lymphatics. The obstruction may be in the pelvic or lumbar lymph channels and nodes when the disease is extensive and progressive. The **secondary form** of lymphedema involves inflammatory or mechanical lymphatic obstruction from trauma, regional lymph node resection or irradiation, or extensive involvement of regional nodes by malignant disease or filariasis. Lymphedema may occur following surgical removal of the lymph nodes in the groin or axillae. Episodes of acute and chronic inflammation may be superimposed, with further stasis and secondary fibrosis.

Clinical Findings

Hypertrophy of the limb results, with markedly thickened and fibrotic skin and subcutaneous tissue (Figure 12–4) in very advanced cases.

T_2-weighted MRI has been used to identify lymphatics and proximal obstructing masses. Lymphangiography and radioactive isotope studies may identify focal defects in lymph flow but are of little value in planning therapy.

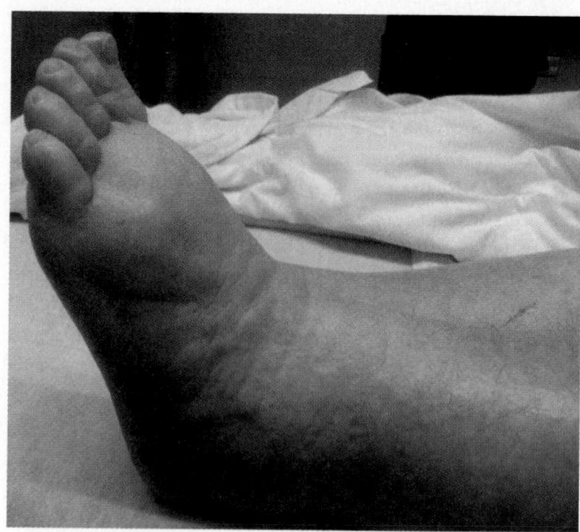

Figure 12–4. Lymphedema with a dorsal pedal hump and exaggerated skin folds near the ankle. (Used, with permission, from Dean SM, Satiani B, Abraham WT. *Color Atlas and Synopsis of Vascular Diseases.* McGraw-Hill, 2014.)

Treatment

There is no effective cure for lymphedema; treatment strategies can control the lymphedema and allow normal function. Most patients can be treated with some of the following measures: (1) Aid the flow of lymph out of the extremity through intermittent elevation, especially during the sleeping hours (foot of bed elevated 15–20 degrees, achieved by placing pillows beneath the mattress); constant use of graduated elastic compression stockings; and massage toward the trunk—either by hand or by means of pneumatic pressure devices designed to milk edema out of an extremity. Wound care centers specializing in the care of patients with lymphedema may be helpful. (2) Avoid secondary by means of good hygiene and treatment of any trichophytosis of the toes. Once an infection starts, it should be treated by periods of elevation and antibiotic therapy that covers *Staphylococcus* and *Streptococcus* organisms (see Table 30–6). Infections can be a serious and recurring problem and are often difficult to control. Prophylactic antibiotics have not been shown to be of benefit. (3) Intermittent courses of diuretic therapy, especially in those with premenstrual or seasonal exacerbations, are rarely helpful. (4) Amputation is used only for the rare complication of lymphangiosarcoma in the extremity.

Prognosis

With aggressive treatment, including pneumatic compression devices, good relief of symptoms can be achieved. The long-term outlook is dictated by the associated conditions and avoidance of recurrent cellulitis.

Chen K et al. Surgical management of postmastectomy lymphedema and review of the literature. Ann Plast Surg. 2021;86:S173. [PMID: 33346539]

SHOCK

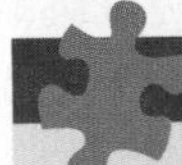

ESSENTIALS OF DIAGNOSIS

- Hypotension, tachycardia, oliguria, altered mental status.
- Peripheral hypoperfusion and impaired oxygen delivery.
- Four classifications: hypovolemic, cardiogenic, obstructive, or distributive.

General Considerations

Shock occurs when the rate of arterial blood flow is inadequate to meet tissue metabolic needs. This results in regional hypoxia and subsequent lactic acidosis from anaerobic metabolism in peripheral tissues as well as eventual end-organ damage and failure.

Classification

Table 12–1 outlines common causes and mechanisms associated with each type of shock.

A. Hypovolemic Shock

Hypovolemic shock results from decreased intravascular volume secondary to loss of blood or fluids and electrolytes. The etiology may be suggested by the clinical setting (eg, trauma) or by signs and symptoms of blood loss (eg, GI bleeding) or dehydration (eg, vomiting or diarrhea). Compensatory vasoconstriction may transiently maintain the blood pressure but unreplaced losses of over 15% of the intravascular volume can result in hypotension and progressive tissue hypoxia.

B. Cardiogenic Shock

Cardiogenic shock results from cardiac failure with the resultant inability of the heart to maintain adequate tissue perfusion. The clinical definition of cardiogenic shock is evidence of tissue hypoxia due to decreased cardiac output (cardiac index less than 2.2 L/minute/m^2) in the presence of adequate intravascular volume. This is most often caused by MI but can also be due to cardiomyopathy, myocardial contusion, valvular incompetence or stenosis, or arrhythmias. See Chapter 10.

C. Obstructive Shock

Pericardial tamponade, tension pneumothorax, and massive PE can cause an acute decrease in cardiac output resulting in shock. These are medical emergencies requiring prompt diagnosis and treatment.

D. Distributive Shock

Distributive or vasodilatory shock has many causes including sepsis, anaphylaxis, traumatic spinal cord injury, or acute adrenal insufficiency. The reduction in systemic vascular resistance results in inadequate cardiac output and tissue hypoperfusion despite normal circulatory volume.

Table 12–1. Classification of shock by mechanism and common causes.

Classification
Hypovolemic shock
Blood loss
Traumatic hemorrhage
Exsanguination
Hemothorax
Hemoperitoneum
Fracture (femur and pelvis)
Nontraumatic hemorrhage
GI bleed
AAA rupture
Ectopic pregnancy rupture
Volume loss
Burns
Skin integrity loss (toxic epidermal necrolysis)
Vomiting
Diarrhea
Hyperosmolar states (eg, hyperosmolar hyperglycemic state)
Third spacing (eg, ascites, pancreatitis)
Decreased intake
Cardiogenic shock
Dysrhythmia
Bradycardias and blocks
Tachycardias
Myocardial disease
Left or right ventricular infarction
Dilated cardiomyopathy
Mechanical
Valvular
Aortic regurgitation from dissection
Papillary muscle rupture from ischemia
Acute valvular rupture from abscess
Ventricular aneurysm rupture
Ventricular septum rupture
Ventricular free wall rupture
Obstructive shock
Tension pneumothorax
Pericardial disease
Pericardial tamponade
Constrictive pericarditis
High-risk (massive) PE
Severe pulmonary hypertension
Auto PEEP from mechanical ventilation
Distributive (vasodilatory) shock
Anaphylactic shock
Septic shock
Neurogenic shock
Drug-induced vasodilation
Adrenal insufficiency

Reproduced with permission from Stone CK, Humphries RL (editors). *Current Emergency Diagnosis & Treatment*, 7th ed. NY: McGraw-Hill, 2011.
PEEP, positive end expiratory pressure.

1. Septic shock—Sepsis is the most common cause of distributive shock and carries a mortality rate of 20–50%. The Society of Critical Care Medicine and the European Society of Intensive Care Medicine's 2016 definition for **sepsis** is life-threatening organ dysfunction caused by a dysregulated host response to infection from any organism (bacterial, viral, or fungal). **Septic shock** is clinically defined as sepsis with fluid-unresponsive hypotension (systolic blood pressure less than 100 mm Hg), serum lactate level higher than 2 mmol/L, and a need for vasopressors to keep mean arterial pressure (MAP) above 65 mm Hg. The most common cause of septic shock in hospitalized patients is infection with gram-positive or gram-negative organisms, with a growing incidence of infection from multidrug-resistant organisms. Sepsis from viral and fungal organisms is increasing but remain less than that for bacterial infections. Risk factors for septic shock include bacteremia, extremes of age, diabetes mellitus, cancer, immunosuppression, and history of a recent invasive procedure.

CLINICAL TOOLS TO IDENTIFY SEPSIS AND SEPTIC SHOCK—Multiple tools exist to screen for sepsis. The Third International Consensus Definitions for Sepsis and Septic Shock (SEPSIS-3) recommend using the Sequential Organ Failure Assessment (SOFA) score to define sepsis (https://en.wikipedia.org/wiki/SOFA_score); an increase of 2 or more SOFA score points in a patient with infection is diagnostic of sepsis with a predicted 10% mortality.

Systemic inflammatory response syndrome (SIRS) criteria is another screening tool. SIRS is defined as a systemic response to a nonspecific infectious or noninfectious insult resulting in at least two of the following findings: (1) body temperature higher than 38°C (100.4°F) or lower than 36°C (96.8°F), (2) heart rate faster than 90 beats per minute, (3) respiratory rate more than 20 breaths per minute or hyperventilation with an arterial carbon dioxide tension ($PaCO_2$) less than 32 mm Hg, or (4) abnormal WBC count (greater than 12,000/mcL or less than 4000/mcL or greater than 10% immature [band] forms). Vasodilatory shock from SIRS is often due to burns; pancreatitis; autoimmune disorders, such as vasculitis or inflammatory colitis; air or amniotic fluid embolus; ischemia; or trauma. The SEPSIS-3 group also introduced the quick SOFA (qSOFA) scoring system, but the poor sensitivity of this measurement led the Surviving Sepsis Campaign Guidelines 2021 to strongly recommend against its use as a single screening tool. Regardless of the screening tools used, performance improvement programs for sepsis screening and standardized treatment procedures are highly encouraged.

2. Neurogenic shock—Neurogenic shock is caused by traumatic spinal cord injury or effects of an epidural or spinal anesthetic. This results in loss of sympathetic tone with a reduction in systemic vascular resistance and hypotension without a compensatory tachycardia. Reflex vagal parasympathetic stimulation evoked by pain, gastric dilation, or fright may simulate neurogenic shock, producing hypotension, bradycardia, and syncope.

3. Endocrine shock—Endocrine shock can arise from hyper- or hypothyroidism or adrenal insufficiency (either primary adrenal crisis from Addison disease or secondary adrenal insufficiency [see Chapter 26]). Adrenal insufficiency most often occurs with abrupt cessation of long-term corticosteroid use, but it can also be precipitated by infection, trauma, surgery, or pituitary injury. In addition to hypotension, symptoms include weakness, nausea, abdominal pain, and confusion. Hypothyroidism can lead to myxedema coma, presenting with vasodilation and depressed cardiac output. Shock from hyperthyroidism most often produces high-output cardiac failure.

Clinical Findings

A. Symptoms and Signs

Hypotension is traditionally defined as a systolic blood pressure of 90 mm Hg or less or a MAP of less than 60–65 mm Hg but must be evaluated relative to the patient's normal blood pressure. A drop in systolic pressure of greater than 10–20 mm Hg or an increase in pulse of more than 15 beats per minute with positional change suggests depleted intravascular volume. However, blood pressure is often not the best indicator of end-organ perfusion because compensatory mechanisms, such as increased heart rate, increased cardiac contractility, and vasoconstriction can occur to prevent hypotension. Patients with hypotension often have cool or mottled extremities and weak or thready peripheral pulses. Splanchnic vasoconstriction may lead to oliguria, bowel ischemia, and liver dysfunction, which can ultimately result in multiorgan failure. Mentation may be normal or patients may become restless, agitated, confused, lethargic, or comatose as a result of inadequate perfusion of the brain.

Hypovolemic shock is evident when signs of hypoperfusion, such as oliguria, altered mental status, and cool extremities, are present. Jugular venous pressure is low, and there is a narrow pulse pressure indicative of reduced stroke volume. Rapid replacement of fluids can restore tissue perfusion. In **cardiogenic shock,** there are also signs of global hypoperfusion with oliguria, altered mental status, and cool extremities. Jugular venous pressure is elevated and there may be evidence of pulmonary edema with respiratory compromise in the setting of left-sided heart failure. *A transthoracic echocardiogram (TTE) or a transesophageal echocardiogram (TEE) is an effective diagnostic tool to differentiate hypovolemic from cardiogenic shock.* In hypovolemic shock, the LV will be small because of decreased filling, but contractility is often preserved. In cardiogenic shock, there is a decrease in LV contractility. The LV may appear dilated and full because of the inability of the LV to eject a sufficient stroke volume.

In **obstructive shock**, the central venous pressure may be elevated but the TTE or TEE may show reduced LV filling, a pericardial effusion in the case of tamponade, thickened pericardium in the case of pericarditis, or right ventricular dysfunction in the case of massive PE. Pericardiocentesis or pericardial window for pericardial tamponade, chest tube placement for tension pneumothorax, or catheter-directed thrombolytic therapy for massive PE can be life saving in cases of obstructive shock.

In **distributive shock,** signs include hyperdynamic heart sounds, warm extremities initially, and a wide pulse pressure indicative of large stroke volume. The echocardiogram may show a hyperdynamic LV. **Septic shock** is diagnosed when there is clinical evidence of infection in the setting of persistent hypotension and evidence of organ hypoperfusion, such as lactic acidosis, decreased urinary output, or altered mental status despite adequate volume resuscitation (see Clinical Tools to Identify Sepsis and Septic Shock, above). **Neurogenic shock** is diagnosed when there is evidence of CNS injury and persistent hypotension despite adequate volume resuscitation. A history of long-term corticosteroid use or thyroid disease can increase the likelihood of **endocrine shock.**

B. Laboratory Findings and Imaging

Blood tests should include CBC, electrolytes, glucose, arterial blood gas determinations, coagulation parameters, lactate levels, typing and cross-matching, and bacterial cultures. An ECG and chest radiograph should be part of the initial assessment. Point-of-care ultrasonography can rapidly assess global cardiac function, presence of pericardial effusion, and intravascular volume status via inferior vena cava inspection in cases of undifferentiated hypotension. A TTE can more formally assess right- and left-sided filling pressures and cardiac output.

Treatment

A. General Measures

Treatment depends on prompt diagnosis and an accurate appraisal of inciting conditions. Initial management consists of basic life support with an assessment of the patient's circulation, airway, and breathing. This may entail airway intubation and mechanical ventilation. Ventilatory failure should be anticipated in patients with severe metabolic acidosis due to shock. Mechanical ventilation along with sedation can decrease respiratory muscle oxygen demand and allow improved oxygen delivery to hypoperfused tissues. Intravenous access and fluid resuscitation should be instituted along with cardiac monitoring and assessment of hemodynamic parameters such as blood pressure and heart rate. Cardiac monitoring can detect myocardial ischemia or malignant arrhythmias, which can be treated by standard advanced cardiac life support (ACLS) protocols.

Unresponsive or minimally responsive patients should have their glucose checked immediately, and if their glucose levels are low, 1 ampule of 50% dextrose intravenously should be given. An arterial line should be placed for continuous blood pressure measurement, and an indwelling urinary catheter should be inserted to monitor urinary output.

B. Hemodynamic Measurements

Early consideration is given to placement of a central venous catheter (CVC) (also known as a central line) for infusion of fluids and medications and for hemodynamic pressure measurements. A CVC can provide measurements of the central venous pressure (CVP) and the central venous oxygen saturation ($ScvO_2$), both of which can be used to manage septic and cardiogenic shock. Pulmonary artery catheters (PACs) allow measurement of the pulmonary artery pressure, left-sided filling pressure or the pulmonary capillary wedge pressure (PCWP), the mixed venous oxygen saturation (SvO_2), and cardiac output. Multiple studies suggest that PACs do not increase overall mortality or length of hospital stay but are associated with higher use of inotropes and intravenous vasodilators in select groups of critically ill patients. The attendant risks associated with PACs (infection, arrhythmias, vein thrombosis, and pulmonary artery rupture) can be as high as 4–9%; thus, the routine use of PACs cannot be recommended. However, in complex situations, PACs may be useful in distinguishing between cardiogenic and septic shock, so the value of the information they might provide must be carefully weighed in each patient. TTE is a noninvasive alternative to the PAC. TTE can provide information about the pulmonary artery pressure and current cardiac function, including cardiac output. The $ScvO_2$, which is obtained through the CVC, can be used as a surrogate for the SvO_2, which is obtained through the PAC. Pulse pressure variation, as determined by arterial line waveform analysis, or stroke volume variation is much more sensitive than CVP as dynamic measures of fluid responsiveness in volume resuscitation, but these measurements have only been validated in patients who are mechanically ventilated with tidal volumes of 8 mL/kg, not triggering the ventilator, and in normal sinus rhythm. Point-of-care ultrasound measurements of the inferior vena cava (IVC) can suggest intravascular volume status and guide fluid replacement. If the patient is mechanically ventilated and the IVC dilates ~15–20% with inspiration, they are likely to respond to intravenous fluids. If the patient is spontaneously breathing, they may be fluid-responsive if their IVC is less than 2 cm in diameter and collapses by more than 50% with each inspiration.

A CVP less than 5 mm Hg suggests hypovolemia, and a CVP greater than 18 mm Hg suggests volume overload, cardiac failure, tamponade, or pulmonary hypertension. A cardiac index lower than 2 L/minute/m^2 indicates a need for inotropic support. A cardiac index higher than 4 L/minute/m^2 in a hypotensive patient is consistent with early septic shock. The systemic vascular resistance is low (less than 800 dynes · s/cm^{-5}) in sepsis and neurogenic shock and high (greater than 1500 dynes · s/cm^{-5}) in hypovolemic and cardiogenic shock. Treatment is directed at maintaining a CVP of 8–12 mm Hg, a MAP of 65 mm Hg or higher, a cardiac index of 2–4 L/minute/m^2, and a $ScvO_2$ greater than 70%.

C. Volume Replacement

Volume replacement is critical in the initial management of shock. **Hemorrhagic shock** is treated with immediate efforts to achieve hemostasis and rapid infusions of blood substitutes, such as type-specific or type O negative packed RBCs or whole blood, which provides extra volume and clotting factors. Each unit of PRBC or whole blood is expected to raise the hematocrit by 3%. **Hypovolemic shock** secondary to dehydration is managed with rapid boluses of isotonic crystalloid solutions, usually in 1-L increments. **Cardiogenic shock** in the absence of fluid overload requires smaller boluses of crystalloid fluid challenges, usually in increments of 250 mL. **Septic shock** usually requires large volumes of fluid for resuscitation (typically 30 mL/kg) as the associated capillary leak releases fluid into the extravascular space. *Caution must be used in cases of large-volume resuscitation with unwarmed fluids because this can produce hypothermia, which can lead to hypothermia-induced coagulopathy.* Warming of fluids before administration can avoid this complication.

Choice of resuscitation fluid—Crystalloid solution is the resuscitation fluid of choice in most settings. Historically, 0.9% saline was the most widely used crystalloid solution in resuscitation. Data suggest that balanced crystalloids, like lactated Ringer solution or Plasma-Lyte, are associated with less kidney injury, fewer instances of hyperchloremic metabolic acidosis, and decreased overall mortality. Comparisons of 0.9% saline and colloid (albumin) solutions in critically ill patients found no difference in outcome except in patients with traumatic brain injury, where albumin resuscitation led to higher mortality. Thus, the use of balanced crystalloid solutions for volume resuscitation in shock is favored. If the patient does not respond to fluid resuscitation, early use of vasopressors should be considered.

D. Early Goal-Directed Therapy

Compensated shock can occur in the setting of normalized hemodynamic parameters with ongoing global tissue hypoxia. Traditional endpoints of resuscitation such as blood pressure, heart rate, urinary output, mental status, and skin perfusion can therefore be misleading. Following set protocols for the treatment of septic shock by adjusting the use of fluids, vasopressors, and inotropes to meet hemodynamic targets (MAP 65 mm Hg or higher, CVP 8–12 mm Hg, $ScvO_2$ greater than 70%) is termed **early goal-directed therapy (EGDT).** Lactate clearance (a decline of lactate levels) of more than 10% can be used as a substitute for $ScvO_2$ criteria if $ScvO_2$ monitoring is not available.

The 2021 Surviving Sepsis Campaign's recommendations for patients with sepsis or septic shock are to measure lactate level; obtain blood cultures prior to administration of broad-spectrum antibiotics, *which should occur within 1 hour of sepsis diagnosis;* and administer 30 mL/kg balanced crystalloid (lactated Ringer solution or Plasma-Lyte) for hypotension or lactate greater than 4 mmol/L within the first 3 hours of presentation. Smaller resuscitation volumes may be appropriate for patients with heart failure, cirrhosis, or advanced kidney disease. Vasopressors should be administered for hypotension not responsive to initial fluid resuscitation to maintain MAP 65 mm Hg or higher. Remeasure lactate if initial level was high, and reassess volume status and tissue perfusion frequently. A meta-analysis of hemodynamic optimization trials suggests that early treatment before the development of organ failure results in improved survival, and patients who respond well to initial efforts demonstrate a survival advantage over nonresponders.

E. Medications

1. Vasoactive therapy—Vasopressors and inotropic agents are administered only after adequate fluid resuscitation. Choice of vasoactive therapy depends on the presumed etiology of shock as well as cardiac output. If there is continued hypotension with evidence of high cardiac output after adequate volume resuscitation (as in septic shock), then vasopressor support is needed to improve vasomotor tone. If there is evidence of low cardiac output with high filling pressures, inotropic support is needed to improve contractility.

A. DISTRIBUTIVE (VASODILATORY) SHOCK—When increased vasoconstriction is required to maintain an adequate perfusion pressure, alpha-adrenergic catecholamine agonists (such as norepinephrine and phenylephrine) are generally used. Although norepinephrine is both an alpha-adrenergic and beta-adrenergic agonist, it preferentially increases MAP over cardiac output. The initial dose is 1–2 mcg/minute as an intravenous infusion, titrated to maintain MAP at 65 mm Hg or higher. The usual maintenance dose is 2–4 mcg/minute intravenously (maximum dose is 30 mcg/minute). Patients with refractory shock may require dosages of 10–30 mcg/minute intravenously. Epinephrine, also with both alpha-adrenergic and beta-adrenergic effects, may be used in severe shock and during acute resuscitation. It is the vasopressor of choice for anaphylactic shock. For severe shock, give epinephrine 1 mcg/minute as a continuous intravenous infusion initially and titrate to hemodynamic response; the usual dosage range is 1–10 mcg/minute intravenously.

Dopamine has variable effects according to dosage. At low doses (2–5 mcg/kg/minute intravenously), stimulation of dopaminergic and beta-adrenergic receptors produces increased glomerular filtration, heart rate, and contractility. At doses of 5–10 mcg/kg/minute, beta-1-adrenergic effects predominate, resulting in an increase in heart rate and cardiac contractility. At higher doses (greater than 10 mcg/kg/minute), alpha-adrenergic effects predominate, resulting in peripheral vasoconstriction. The maximum dose is typically 50 mcg/kg/minute.

There is no evidence documenting a survival benefit from, or the superiority of, a particular vasopressor in septic shock. Norepinephrine is the initial vasopressor of choice in septic shock to maintain the MAP at 65 mm Hg or higher. Phenylephrine can be used for hyperdynamic septic shock if dysrhythmias or tachycardias prevent the use of agents with beta-adrenergic activity. In meta-analyses, the use of dopamine as a first-line vasopressor in septic shock resulted in an *increase* in 28-day mortality and a higher incidence of arrhythmic events. Dopamine should only be used as an alternative to norepinephrine in select patients with septic shock, including patients with significant bradycardia or low potential for tachyarrhythmias.

Vasopressin (ADH) is often used as an *adjunctive therapy* to catecholamine vasopressors in the treatment of distributive shock. Vasopressin causes peripheral vasoconstriction via V1 receptors located on smooth muscle cells. Vasopressin also potentiates the effects of catecholamines on the vasculature and stimulates cortisol production. Intravenous infusion of vasopressin at a low dose (0.01–0.04 units/minute) as a second agent to norepinephrine has been beneficial in septic patients with hypotension refractory to fluid resuscitation and conventional catecholamine vasopressors. Higher doses of vasopressin decrease cardiac output and may put patients at greater risk for splanchnic and coronary artery ischemia. Studies do not favor the use of vasopressin as first-line therapy.

Angiotensin II, a component of the renin-angiotensin-aldosterone system axis, is a potent direct vasoconstrictor that acts on the arteries and veins to increase blood pressure. Angiotensin II (Giapreza) can be considered as an *additional agent* in vasodilatory shock that is refractory to catecholamines and vasopressin. The recommended starting dose is 20 ng/kg/minute via continuous intravenous infusion through a central venous line. It can be titrated every 5 minutes by increments of up to 15 ng/kg/minute as needed to achieve MAP goals, but not to exceed 80 ng/kg/minute during the first 3 hours of use. Maintenance doses should not exceed 40 ng/kg/minute. Concurrent venous thromboembolism (VTE) prophylaxis is indicated as studies revealed a higher incidence of VTE with angiotensin II use.

B. Cardiogenic shock—Given meta-analyses documenting decreased mortality, expert opinion suggests norepinephrine be the first-line vasopressor for cardiogenic shock. Dobutamine, a predominantly beta-adrenergic agonist, increases contractility and decreases afterload. It is used for patients with low cardiac output and high PCWP but who do not have hypotension. Dobutamine can be added to a vasopressor if there is reduced myocardial function (decreased cardiac output and elevated PCWP), or if there are signs of hypoperfusion despite adequate volume resuscitation and an adequate MAP. The initial dose is 0.1–0.5 mcg/kg/minute intravenous infusion, which can be titrated every few minutes to hemodynamic effect; the usual dosage range is 2–20 mcg/kg/minute intravenously. Tachyphylaxis can occur after 48 hours secondary to the downregulation of beta-adrenergic receptors. Milrinone is a phosphodiesterase inhibitor that can be substituted for dobutamine. A 2021 study of patients with cardiogenic shock found no significant difference in mortality when comparing milrinone to dobutamine. Amrinone is another phosphodiesterase inhibitor that can be used. These phosphodiesterase inhibitor drugs increase cyclic AMP levels and increase cardiac contractility, bypassing the beta-adrenergic receptor. Vasodilation is a side effect of both amrinone and milrinone.

2. Antibiotics—Definitive therapy for septic shock includes early initiation of empiric broad-spectrum antibiotics (see Table 30–5) after appropriate cultures have been obtained and within 1 hour of recognition of septic shock. Imaging studies may prove useful to attempt localization of sources of infection. Surgical management may also be necessary if necrotic tissue or loculated infections are present in attempts to control the source of infection.

3. Corticosteroids—Corticosteroids are the treatment of choice in patients with shock secondary to adrenal insufficiency, defined as a cortisol response of 9 mcg/dL or less after one injection of 250 mcg of corticotropin. Studies supporting corticosteroid use in patients with shock from sepsis or other etiologies are mixed but meta-analyses are slightly in favor of their use. The ADRENAL study demonstrated shorter time to shock resolution (3 days vs 4 days) but no difference in 90-day mortality. The APROCCHSS study demonstrated lower 90-day all-cause mortality for patients receiving hydrocortisone plus fludrocortisone. Notably, some worse outcomes were observed from increased rates of secondary infections. Corticosteroids can be administered in refractory shock to decrease shock duration; the current recommended regimen is hydrocortisone 50 mg intravenously every 6 hours for 5–7 days.

F. Other Treatment Modalities

Cardiac failure may require use of transcutaneous or transvenous pacing or placement of an intra-arterial balloon pump or LV assist device. Emergent revascularization by percutaneous angioplasty or coronary artery bypass surgery appears to improve long-term outcome with increased survival compared with initial medical stabilization for patients with myocardial ischemia leading to cardiogenic shock (see Chapter 10). Urgent renal replacement therapy may be indicated for maintenance of fluid and electrolyte balance during AKI resulting in shock from multiple modalities. Studies do not support the use of intravenous vitamin C as treatment for sepsis.

Annane D et al; CRICS-TRIGGERSEP Network. Hydrocortisone plus fludrocortisone for adults with septic shock. N Engl J Med. 2018;378:809. [PMID: 29490185]

Evans L et al. Surviving sepsis campaign: international guidelines for management of sepsis and septic shock 2021. Intensive Care Med. 2021;47:1181. [PMID: 34599691]

Gando S et al; Japanese Association for Acute Medicine (JAAM) Sepsis Prognostication in Intensive Care Unit and Emergency Room (SPICE) (JAAM SPICE) Study Group. The SIRS criteria have better performance for predicting infection than qSOFA scores in the emergency department. Sci Rep. 2020;10:8095. [PMID: 32415144]

Khanna A et al; ATHOS-3 Investigators. Angiotensin II for the treatment of vasodilatory shock. N Engl J Med. 2017;377:419. [PMID: 28528561]

Mathew R et al. Milrinone as compared with dobutamine in the treatment of cardiogenic shock. N Engl J Med. 2021;385:516. [PMID: 34347952]

Sevransky JE et al; VICTAS Investigators. Effect of vitamin C, thiamine, and hydrocortisone on ventilator- and vasopressor-free days in patients with sepsis: the VICTAS randomized clinical trial. JAMA. 2021;325:742. [PMID: 33620405]

Venkatesh B et al; ADRENAL Trial Investigators and the Australian–New Zealand Intensive Care Society Clinical Trials Group. Adjunctive glucocorticoid therapy in patients with septic shock. N Engl J Med. 2018;378:797. [PMID: 29347874]

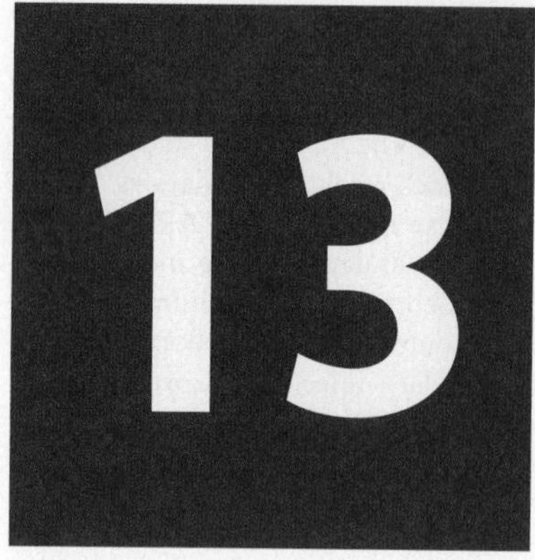

Blood Disorders

Lloyd E. Damon, MD
Charalambos Babis Andreadis, MD, MSCE

ANEMIAS

General Approach to Anemias

Anemia is present in adults if the hematocrit is below 41% (hemoglobin less than 13.6 g/dL [135 g/L]) in males or below 36% (hemoglobin less than 12 g/dL [120 g/L]) in females. Congenital anemia is suggested by the patient's personal and family history. The most common cause of anemia is iron deficiency. Poor diet may result in folic acid deficiency and contribute to iron deficiency, but bleeding is the most common cause of iron deficiency in adults. Physical examination demonstrates pallor. Attention to physical signs of primary hematologic diseases (lymphadenopathy; hepatosplenomegaly; or bone tenderness, especially in the sternum or anterior tibia) is important. Mucosal changes such as a smooth tongue suggest megaloblastic anemia.

Anemias are classified according to their pathophysiologic basis, ie, whether related to diminished production (relative or absolute reticulocytopenia) or to increased production due to accelerated loss of RBCs (reticulocytosis) (Table 13–1), and according to RBC size (Table 13–2). A reticulocytosis occurs in one of three pathophysiologic states: acute blood loss, recent replacement of a missing erythropoietic nutrient, or reduced RBC survival (ie, hemolysis). A severely microcytic anemia (mean corpuscular volume [MCV] less than 70 fL) is due either to iron deficiency or thalassemia, while a severely macrocytic anemia (MCV greater than 120 fL) is almost always due to either megaloblastic anemia or to cold agglutinins in blood analyzed at room temperature. A bone marrow biopsy is generally needed to complete the evaluation of anemia when the blood laboratory evaluation fails to reveal an etiology, when there are additional cytopenias present, or when an underlying primary or secondary bone marrow process is suspected.

IRON DEFICIENCY ANEMIA

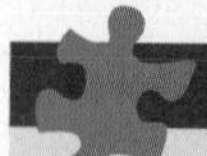

ESSENTIALS OF DIAGNOSIS

- Iron deficiency: serum ferritin is < 12 ng/mL (27 pmol/L) or < 30 ng/mL (67 pmol/L) if also anemic.
- Caused by bleeding unless proved otherwise.
- Responds to iron therapy.

General Considerations

Iron deficiency is the most common cause of anemia worldwide. The causes are listed in Table 13–3. Aside from circulating RBCs, the major location of iron in the body is the storage pool as ferritin or as hemosiderin in macrophages.

The average American diet contains 10–15 mg of iron per day. About 10% of this amount is absorbed in the stomach, duodenum, and upper jejunum under acidic conditions. Dietary iron present as heme is efficiently absorbed (10–20%) but nonheme iron less so (1–5%), largely because of interference by phosphates, tannins, and other food constituents. The major iron transporter from the diet across the intestinal lumen is ferroportin, which also facilitates the transport of iron to apotransferrin in macrophages for delivery to erythroid progenitor cells in the bone marrow prepared to synthesize hemoglobin. Hepcidin, which is increasingly produced during inflammation, negatively regulates iron transport by promoting the degradation of ferroportin. Small amounts of iron—approximately 1 mg/day—are normally lost through exfoliation of skin and GI mucosal cells.

Menstrual blood loss plays a major role in iron metabolism. The average monthly menstrual blood loss is approximately 50 mL but may be five times greater in some individuals. Women with heavy menstrual losses must absorb 3–4 mg of iron from the diet each day to maintain adequate iron stores, which is not commonly achieved. Women with menorrhagia of this degree will almost always become iron deficient without iron supplementation.

In general, iron metabolism is balanced between absorption of 1 mg/day and loss of 1 mg/day. Pregnancy and lactation upset the iron balance since requirements increase to 2–5 mg of iron per day. Normal dietary iron cannot supply these requirements, and medicinal iron is needed during pregnancy and lactation. Decreased iron absorption can also cause iron deficiency, such as in people affected by celiac disease (gluten enteropathy), and it also commonly occurs after gastric resection or jejunal bypass surgery.

Table 13–1. Classification of anemia by RBC pathophysiology.

Decreased RBC production (relative or absolute reticulocytopenia)
Hemoglobin synthesis lesion: iron deficiency, thalassemia, anemia of chronic disease, hypoerythropoietinemia
DNA synthesis lesion: megaloblastic anemia, folic acid deficiency, DNA synthesis inhibitor medications
Hematopoietic stem cell lesion: aplastic anemia, leukemia
Bone marrow infiltration: carcinoma, lymphoma, fibrosis, sarcoidosis, Gaucher disease, others
Immune-mediated inhibition: aplastic anemia, pure RBC aplasia
Increased RBC destruction or accelerated RBC loss (reticulocytosis)
Acute blood loss
Hemolysis (intrinsic)
Membrane lesion: hereditary spherocytosis, elliptocytosis
Hemoglobin lesion: sickle cell, unstable hemoglobin
Glycolysis lesion: pyruvate kinase deficiency
Oxidation lesion: glucose-6-phosphate dehydrogenase deficiency
Hemolysis (extrinsic)
Immune: warm antibody, cold antibody
Microangiopathic: disseminated intravascular coagulation, thrombotic thrombocytopenic purpura, hemolytic-uremic syndrome, mechanical cardiac valve, paravalvular leak
Infection: *Clostridium perfringens*, malaria
Hypersplenism

The most important cause of iron deficiency anemia in adults is chronic blood loss, especially menstrual and GI blood loss. Iron deficiency demands a search for a source of GI bleeding if other sites of blood loss (excess uterine bleeding, hematuria, and repeated blood donations) are excluded. Prolonged aspirin or NSAID use may cause it without a documented structural lesion. Celiac disease, even when asymptomatic, can cause iron deficiency through poor absorption in the GI tract. Zinc deficiency is another cause of poor iron absorption. Chronic hemoglobinuria may lead to iron deficiency, but this is uncommon. Traumatic hemolysis due to a prosthetic cardiac valve and other causes of intravascular hemolysis (eg, paroxysmal nocturnal hemoglobinuria) should also be considered. The cause of iron deficiency is not found in up to 5% of cases.

Table 13–2. Classification of anemia by mean RBC volume (MCV).

Microcytic
Iron deficiency
Thalassemia
Anemia of chronic disease
Lead toxicity
Zinc deficiency
Macrocytic (Megaloblastic)
Vitamin B_{12} deficiency
Folate deficiency
DNA synthesis inhibitors
Macrocytic (Nonmegaloblastic)
Aplastic anemia
Myelodysplasia
Liver disease
Reticulocytosis
Hypothyroidism
Bone marrow failure state (eg, aplastic anemia, marrow infiltrative disorder, etc)
Copper deficiency
Normocytic
Kidney disease
Non-thyroid endocrine gland failure
Copper deficiency
Mild form of most acquired microcytic or macrocytic etiologies of anemia

Table 13–3. Causes of iron deficiency.

Deficient diet
Decreased absorption
Autoimmune gastritis
Celiac disease
Helicobacter pylori gastritis
Hereditary iron-refractory iron deficiency anemia
Zinc deficiency
Increased requirements
Pregnancy
Lactation
Blood loss (chronic)
GI
Menstrual
Blood donation
Hemoglobinuria
Iron sequestration
Pulmonary hemosiderosis
Idiopathic

Pure iron deficiency might prove refractory to oral iron replacement. Refractoriness is defined as a hemoglobin increment of less than 1 g/dL (10 g/L) after 4–6 weeks of 100 mg/day of elemental oral iron. The differential diagnosis in these cases (Table 13–3) includes malabsorption from autoimmune gastritis, *Helicobacter pylori* gastric infection, celiac disease, and hereditary iron-refractory iron deficiency anemia. Iron-refractory iron deficiency anemia is a rare autosomal recessive disorder due to mutations in the transmembrane serine protease 6 (*TMPRSS6*) gene, which normally downregulates hepcidin. In iron-refractory iron deficiency anemia, hepcidin levels are normal to high and ferritin levels are low-normal despite the iron deficiency.

Clinical Findings

A. Symptoms and Signs

The primary symptoms of iron deficiency anemia are those of the anemia itself (easy fatigability, tachycardia, palpitations, and dyspnea on exertion). Severe deficiency causes skin and mucosal changes, including a smooth tongue, brittle nails, spooning of nails (koilonychia), and cheilosis. Dysphagia due to the formation of esophageal webs (Plummer-Vinson syndrome) may occur in severe iron deficiency. Pica (ie, craving for specific foods [ice chips, etc] not rich in iron) develops in many iron-deficient patients.

B. Laboratory Findings

Iron deficiency develops in stages. The first is depletion of iron stores without anemia followed by anemia with a normal RBC size (normal MCV) followed by anemia with reduced RBC size (low MCV). The reticulocyte count is low or inappropriately normal. Ferritin is a measure of total body iron stores. A ferritin value less than 12 ng/mL (27 pmol/L) (in the absence of scurvy) is a highly reliable indicator of reduced iron stores. Note that the lower limit of normal for ferritin is often below 12 ng/mL (27 pmol/L) in women due to the fact that the normal ferritin range is generated by including healthy menstruating women who are iron deficient but not anemic. However, because serum ferritin levels may rise in response to inflammation or other stimuli, a normal or elevated ferritin level does not exclude a diagnosis of iron deficiency. A ferritin level less than 30 ng/mL (67 pmol/L) almost always indicates iron deficiency in anyone who is anemic. As iron deficiency progresses, serum iron values decline to less than 30 mcg/dL (67 pmol/L) and transferrin (the iron transport protein) levels rise to compensate, leading to transferrin saturations of less than 15%. Low transferrin saturation is also seen in anemia of inflammation, so caution in the interpretation of this test is warranted. Isolated iron deficiency anemia has a low hepcidin level, not yet a clinically available test. As the MCV falls (ie, microcytosis), the blood smear shows hypochromic microcytic cells. With further progression, anisocytosis (variations in RBC size) and poikilocytosis (variation in shape of RBCs) develop. Severe iron deficiency will produce a bizarre peripheral blood smear, with severely hypochromic cells, target cells, and pencil-shaped or cigar-shaped cells. Bone marrow biopsy for evaluation of iron stores is rarely performed. If the biopsy is done, it shows the absence of iron in erythroid progenitor cells by Prussian blue staining. The platelet count is commonly increased, but it usually remains under 800,000/mcL (800×10^9/L).

Differential Diagnosis

Other causes of microcytic anemia include anemia of chronic disease (specifically, anemia of inflammation), thalassemia, lead poisoning, zinc deficiency, and congenital X-linked sideroblastic anemia. Anemia of chronic disease is characterized by normal or increased iron stores in bone marrow macrophages and a normal or elevated ferritin level; the serum iron and transferrin saturation are low, often drastically so, and the total iron-binding capacity (TIBC) (the blood's capacity for iron to bind to transferrin) and transferrin are either normal or low. Thalassemia produces a greater degree of microcytosis for any given level of hemoglobin than does iron deficiency and, unlike virtually every other cause of anemia, has a normal or elevated (rather than a low) RBC count as well as a reticulocytosis. In thalassemia, RBC morphology on the peripheral smear resembles severe iron deficiency.

Treatment

The diagnosis of iron deficiency anemia can be made either by the laboratory demonstration of an iron-deficient state or by evaluating the response to a therapeutic trial of iron replacement. Since the anemia itself is rarely life-threatening, the most important part of management is identification of the cause—especially a source of occult blood loss.

A. Oral Iron

Ferrous sulfate, 325 mg once daily or every other day on an empty stomach, is a standard approach for replenishing iron stores. As oral iron stimulates hepcidin production, once daily or every other day dosing maximizes iron absorption compared to multiple doses per day, and with fewer side effects. Nausea and constipation limit compliance with ferrous sulfate. Extended-release ferrous sulfate with mucoprotease is a well-tolerated oral preparation. Taking ferrous sulfate with food reduces side effects but also its absorption. An appropriate response to oral iron is a return of the hematocrit level halfway toward normal within 3 weeks with full return to baseline after 2 months. Iron therapy should continue for 3–6 months after restoration of normal hematologic values to replenish iron stores. Failure of response to iron therapy is usually due to noncompliance, although occasional patients may absorb iron poorly, particularly if the stomach is achlorhydric. Such patients may benefit from concomitant administration of oral ascorbic acid. Other reasons for failure to respond include incorrect diagnosis (anemia of chronic disease, thalassemia), celiac disease, and ongoing blood loss that exceeds the rate of new erythropoiesis. Treatment of *H pylori* infection, in appropriate cases, can improve oral iron absorption.

B. Parenteral Iron

The indications are intolerance of or refractoriness to oral iron (including those with iron-refractory iron deficiency anemia), GI disease (usually IBD) precluding the use of oral iron, and continued blood loss that cannot be corrected, such as chronic hemodialysis. Historical parenteral iron preparations, such as high-molecular-weight iron dextran, were problematic due to long infusion times (hours), polyarthralgia, and hypersensitivity reactions, including anaphylaxis. Current parenteral iron preparations coat the iron in protective carbohydrate shells or contain low-molecular-weight iron dextran, are safe, and can be administered over 15 minutes to 1 hour. Most iron-deficient patients need 1–1.5 g of parenteral iron; this dose corrects for the iron deficit and replenishes iron stores for the future.

Ferric pyrophosphate citrate (Triferic) is an FDA-approved additive to the dialysate designed to replace the 5–7 mg of iron that patients with CKD tend to lose during each hemodialysis treatment. Ferric pyrophosphate citrate delivers sufficient iron to the marrow to maintain hemoglobin and not increase iron stores; it may obviate the need for intravenous iron in hemodialysis patients.

When to Refer

Patients should be referred to a hematologist if the suspected diagnosis is not confirmed or if they are not responsive to oral iron therapy.

Camaschella C. Iron deficiency. Blood. 2019;133:30. [PMID: 30401704]
Cappellini MD et al. Iron deficiency anaemia revisited. J Intern Med. 2020;287:153. [PMID: 31665543]
Pasricha SR et al. Iron deficiency. Lancet. 2021;397:233. [PMID: 33285139]

ANEMIA OF CHRONIC DISEASE

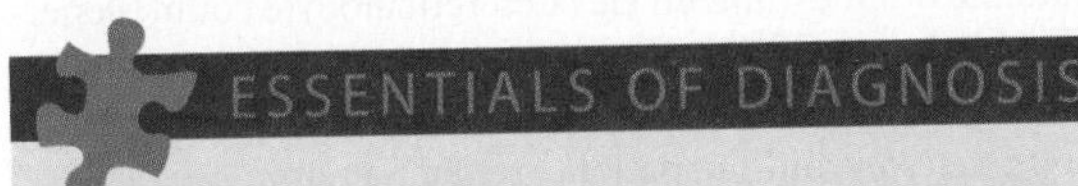

- Mild or moderate normocytic or microcytic anemia.
- Normal or increased ferritin and normal or reduced transferrin.
- Underlying chronic disease.

General Considerations

Many chronic systemic diseases are associated with mild or moderate anemia. The anemias of chronic disease are characterized according to etiology and pathophysiology. First, the **anemia of inflammation** is associated with chronic inflammatory states (such as IBD, rheumatologic disorders, chronic infections, and malignancy) and is mediated through hepcidin (a negative regulator of ferroportin) primarily via elevated IL-6, resulting in reduced iron uptake in the gut and reduced iron transfer from macrophages to erythroid progenitor cells in the bone marrow. This is referred to as iron-restricted erythropoiesis since the patient is iron replete. There is also reduced responsiveness to erythropoietin, the elaboration of hemolysins that shorten RBC survival, and the production of other inflammatory cytokines that dampen RBC production. The serum iron is low in the anemia of inflammation. Second, the **anemia of organ failure** can occur with kidney disease, liver failure, and endocrine gland failure. Erythropoietin is reduced and the RBC mass decreases in response to the diminished signal for RBC production; the serum iron is normal (except in CKD where it is low due to the reduced hepcidin clearance and subsequent enhanced degradation of ferroportin). Third, the **anemia of older adults** is present in up to 20% of individuals over age 85 years in whom a thorough evaluation for an explanation of anemia is negative. The anemia is a consequence of (1) a relative resistance to RBC production in response to erythropoietin, (2) a decrease in erythropoietin production relative to the nephron mass, (3) a negative erythropoietic influence of higher levels of chronic inflammatory cytokines in older adults, and (4) the presence of various somatic mutations in myeloid genes typically associated with myeloid neoplasms. The latter condition is now referred to as **clonal cytopenias of undetermined significance,** which has a 15–20% per year rate of transformation to a myeloid neoplasm, such as a myelodysplastic syndrome (MDS). The serum iron is normal.

Clinical Findings

A. Symptoms and Signs

The clinical features are those of the causative condition. The diagnosis should be suspected in patients with known chronic diseases. In cases of significant anemia, coexistent iron deficiency or folic acid deficiency should be suspected. Decreased dietary intake of iron or folic acid is common in chronically ill patients, many of whom will also have ongoing GI blood losses. Patients undergoing hemodialysis regularly lose both iron and folic acid during dialysis.

B. Laboratory Findings

The hematocrit rarely falls below 60% of baseline (except in kidney failure). The MCV is usually normal or slightly reduced. RBC morphology is usually normal, and the reticulocyte count is mildly decreased or normal.

1. Anemia of inflammation—In the anemia of inflammation, serum iron and transferrin values are low, and the transferrin saturation may be extremely low, leading to an erroneous diagnosis of iron deficiency. In contrast to iron deficiency, serum ferritin values should be normal or increased. A serum ferritin value less than 30 ng/mL (67 pmol/L) indicates coexistent iron deficiency. Anemia of inflammation has elevated hepcidin levels; however, no clinical test is yet available. A particular challenge is the diagnosis of iron deficiency in the setting of the anemia of inflammation, in which the serum ferritin can be as high as 200 ng/mL (450 pmol/L). The diagnosis is established by a bone marrow biopsy with iron stain. Absent iron staining indicates iron deficiency, whereas iron localized in marrow macrophages indicates pure anemia of inflammation. However, bone marrow biopsies are rarely done for this purpose. Two other tests support iron deficiency in the setting of inflammation: a reticulocyte hemoglobin concentration of less than 28 pg or a soluble serum transferrin receptor (units: mg/L) to log ferritin (units: mcg/L) ratio of 1–8 (a ratio of less than 1 is virtually diagnostic of pure anemia of chronic disease). A functional test is hemoglobin response to oral or parenteral iron in the setting of inflammation when iron deficiency is suspected. A note of caution: certain circumstances of iron-restricted erythropoiesis (such as malignancy) will partially respond to parenteral iron infusion even when the iron stores are replete due to the immediate distribution of iron to erythropoietic progenitor cells after the infusion.

2. Other anemias of chronic disease—In the anemias of organ failure and of older adults, the iron studies are generally normal. The anemia of older persons is a diagnosis of exclusion. Clonal cytopenias of undetermined significance are diagnosed by sending a blood or bone marrow sample for myeloid gene sequencing.

Treatment

In most cases, no treatment of the anemia of chronic disease is necessary and the primary management is to address the condition causing the anemia. When the anemia is severe or is adversely affecting the quality of life or functional status, then treatment involves either RBC transfusions or parenteral recombinant erythropoietin (epoetin alfa or darbepoetin). The FDA-approved indications for recombinant erythropoietin are hemoglobin less than 10 g/dL and anemia due to rheumatoid arthritis, IBD, hepatitis C, zidovudine therapy in HIV-infected patients, myelosuppressive chemotherapy of solid malignancy (treated with palliative intent only), or CKD (eGFR of less than 60 mL/minute). The dosing and schedule of recombinant erythropoietin are individualized to maintain the hemoglobin between 10 g/dL (100 g/L) and 12 g/dL (120 g/L). The use of recombinant erythropoietin is associated with an increased risk of venothromboembolism and arterial thrombotic episodes, especially if the hemoglobin rises to greater than 12 g/dL (120 g/L). There is concern that recombinant erythropoietin is associated with reduced survival in patients with malignancy. For patients with end-stage renal disease receiving recombinant erythropoietin who are on hemodialysis, the anemia of CKD can be more effectively corrected by adding soluble ferric pyrophosphate to their dialysate than by administering intravenous iron supplementation.

When to Refer

Referral to a hematologist is not usually necessary.

de Las Cuevas Allende R et al. Anaemia of chronic diseases: pathophysiology, diagnosis and treatment. Med Clin (Barc). 2021;156:235. [PMID: 33358297]

Steensma DP. The clinical challenge of idiopathic cytopenias of undetermined significance (ICUS) and clonal cytopenias of undetermined significance (CCUS). Curr Hematol Malig Rep. 2019;14:536. [PMID: 31696381]

Weiss G et al. Anemia of inflammation. Blood. 2019;133:40. [PMID: 30401705]

THE THALASSEMIAS

ESSENTIALS OF DIAGNOSIS

- Microcytosis disproportionate to the degree of anemia.
- Positive family history.
- Lifelong personal history of microcytic anemia.
- Normal or elevated RBC count.
- Abnormal RBC morphology with microcytes, hypochromia, acanthocytes, and target cells.
- In beta-thalassemia, elevated levels of hemoglobin A_2 and F.

General Considerations

The thalassemias are hereditary disorders characterized by reduction in the synthesis of globin chains (alpha or beta). Reduced globin chain synthesis causes reduced hemoglobin synthesis and a hypochromic microcytic anemia because of defective hemoglobinization of RBCs. Thalassemias can be considered among the hyperproliferative hemolytic anemias, the anemias related to abnormal hemoglobin, and the hypoproliferative anemias, since all of these factors play a role in their pathophysiology. The hallmark laboratory features are small (low MCV) and pale (low mean corpuscular hemoglobin [MCH]) RBCs, anemia, and a normal to elevated RBC count (ie, a large number of the small and pale RBCs are being produced). Although patients often exhibit an elevated reticulocyte count, generally the degree of reticulocyte output is inadequate to meet the degree of RBC destruction (hemolysis) occurring in the bone marrow and the patients remain anemic.

Normal adult hemoglobin is primarily hemoglobin A, which represents approximately 98% of circulating hemoglobin. Hemoglobin A is formed from a tetramer of two alpha-globin chains and two beta-globin chains—and is designated alpha2beta2. Two copies of the alpha-globin gene are located on each chromosome 16, and there is no substitute for alpha-globin in the formation of adult hemoglobin. One copy of the beta-globin gene resides on each chromosome 11 adjacent to genes encoding the beta-like globins delta and gamma (the so-called beta-globin gene cluster region). The tetramer of alpha2delta2 forms hemoglobin A_2, which normally composes 1–3% of adult hemoglobin. The tetramer alpha2gamma2 forms hemoglobin F, which is the major hemoglobin of fetal life and which composes less than 1% of normal adult hemoglobin.

The thalassemias are described as **thalassemia trait** when there are laboratory features without significant clinical impact, **thalassemia intermedia** when there is an occasional RBC transfusion requirement or other moderate clinical impact, and **thalassemia major** when the disorder is life-threatening and the patient is transfusion-dependent. Most patients with thalassemia major die of the consequences of iron overload from RBC transfusions.

Alpha-thalassemia is due primarily to gene deletions causing reduced alpha-globin chain synthesis (Table 13–4). Each alpha-globin gene produces one-quarter of the total alpha-globin quantity, so there is a predictable proportionate decrease in alpha-globin output with each lost alpha-globin gene. Since all adult hemoglobins are alpha

Table 13–4. Alpha-thalassemia syndromes.

Number of Alpha-Globin Genes Transcribed	Syndrome	Hematocrit	MCV
4	Normal	Normal	Normal
3	Silent carrier	Normal	Normal
2	Thalassemia minor (or trait)	28–40%	60–75 fL
1	Hemoglobin H disease	22–32%	60–70 fL
0	Hydrops fetalis[1]	< 18%	< 60 fL

[1]Die in utero.

MCV, mean corpuscular volume.

Table 13–5. Beta-thalassemia syndromes.

	Beta-Globin Genes Transcribed	Hb A	Hb A_2	Hb F	Transfusions
Normal	Homozygous beta	97–99%	1–3%	< 1%	None
Thalassemia minor	Heterozygous $beta^0$	80–95%	4–8%	1–5%	None
	Heterozygous $beta^+$	80–95%	4–8%	1–5%	None
Thalassemia intermedia	Homozygous $beta^+$ (mild)	0–30%	4–8%	6–10%	Occasional
Thalassemia major	Homozygous $beta^0$	0%	4–10%	90–96%	Dependent
	Homozygous $beta^+$ (severe)	0–10%	4–10%	90–96%	Dependent

Hb, hemoglobin; $beta^0$, no beta-globin produced; $beta^+$, some beta-globin produced.

containing, alpha-thalassemia produces no change in the proportions of hemoglobins A, A_2, and F on hemoglobin electrophoresis. In severe forms of alpha-thalassemia, excess beta chains may form a beta-4 tetramer called hemoglobin H. In the presence of reduced alpha chains, the excess beta chains are unstable and precipitate, causing damage to RBC membranes. This leads to both intramedullary (bone marrow) and peripheral blood hemolysis.

Beta-thalassemias are usually caused by point mutations rather than deletions (Table 13–5). These mutations result in premature chain termination or in problems with transcription of RNA and ultimately cause reduced or absent beta-globin chain synthesis. The molecular defects leading to beta-thalassemia are numerous and heterogeneous. Defects that result in absent beta-globin chain expression are termed $beta^0$, whereas those causing reduced but not absent synthesis are termed $beta^+$. In $beta^+$ thalassemia, the degree of reduction of beta-globin synthesis is consistent within families but is quite variable between families. The reduced beta-globin chain synthesis in beta-thalassemia results in a relative increase in the proportions of hemoglobins A_2 and F compared to hemoglobin A on hemoglobin electrophoresis, as the beta-like globins (delta and gamma) substitute for the missing beta chains. In the presence of reduced beta chains, the excess alpha chains are unstable and precipitate, causing damage to RBC membranes. This leads to both intramedullary (bone marrow) and peripheral blood hemolysis. The bone marrow demonstrates erythroid hyperplasia under the stimuli of anemia and ineffective erythropoiesis (intramedullary destruction of the developing erythroid cells). In cases of severe thalassemia, the marked expansion of the erythroid compartment in the bone marrow may cause severe bony deformities, osteopenia, and pathologic bone fractures.

Clinical Findings

A. Symptoms and Signs

The **alpha-thalassemia** syndromes are seen primarily in persons from southeast Asia and China and, less commonly, in Blacks and persons of Mediterranean origin (Table 13–4). Normally, adults have four copies of the alpha-globin chain. When three alpha-globin genes are present, the patient is hematologically normal (silent carrier). When two alpha-globin genes are present, the patient is said to have **alpha-thalassemia trait,** a form of thalassemia minor. In alpha-thalassemia-1 trait, the alpha gene deletion is heterozygous (alpha –/alpha –) and affects mainly those of Asian descent. In alpha-thalassemia-2 trait, the alpha gene deletion is homozygous (alpha alpha/– –) and affects mainly Blacks. These patients are clinically normal and have a normal life expectancy and performance status, with a mild microcytic anemia. When only one alpha globin chain is present (alpha –/– –), the patient has **hemoglobin H disease** (alpha-thalassemia-3). This is a chronic hemolytic anemia of variable severity (thalassemia minor or intermedia). Physical examination might reveal pallor and splenomegaly. Affected individuals usually do not need transfusions; however, they may be required during transient periods of hemolytic exacerbation caused by infection or other stressors or during periods of erythropoietic shutdown caused by certain viruses ("aplastic crisis"). When all four alpha-globin genes are deleted, no normal hemoglobin is produced and the affected fetus is stillborn (**hydrops fetalis**). In hydrops fetalis, the only hemoglobin species made is gamma and is called hemoglobin Bart's (gamma4).

Beta-thalassemia primarily affects persons of Mediterranean origin (Italian, Greek) and to a lesser extent Asians and Blacks (Table 13–5). Patients homozygous for beta-thalassemia ($beta^0/beta^0$ or some with $beta^+/beta^+$) have **beta-thalassemia major** (Cooley anemia). Affected children are normal at birth, but after 6 months, when hemoglobin synthesis switches from hemoglobin F to hemoglobin A, severe anemia develops that requires transfusion. Numerous clinical problems ensue, including stunted growth, bony deformities (abnormal facial structure, pathologic bone fractures), hepatosplenomegaly, jaundice (due to gallstones, hepatitis-related cirrhosis, or both), and thrombophilia. The clinical course is modified significantly by transfusion therapy, but transfusional iron overload (hemosiderosis) results in a clinical picture similar to hemochromatosis, with heart failure, cardiac arrhythmias, cirrhosis, endocrinopathies, and pseudoxanthoma elasticum (calcification and fragmentation of the elastic fibers of the skin, retina, and cardiovascular system), usually after more than 100 units of RBCs have been transfused. Iron overloading occurs because the human body has no active iron excretory mechanism. Before the application of allogeneic stem cell transplantation and the development of more effective forms of iron chelation, death from iron overload usually occurred between the ages of 20 and 30 years.

Patients homozygous for a milder form of beta-thalassemia ($beta^+/beta^+$, but allowing a higher rate of beta-globin synthesis) have **beta-thalassemia intermedia**. These patients have chronic hemolytic anemia but do not require transfusions except under periods of stress or during aplastic crises. They also may develop iron overload because of periodic transfusion. They survive into adult life but with hepatosplenomegaly and bony deformities. Patients heterozygous for beta-thalassemia ($beta/beta^0$ or $beta/beta^+$) have **beta-thalassemia minor** and a clinically insignificant microcytic anemia.

Prenatal diagnosis is available, and genetic counseling should be offered and the opportunity for prenatal diagnosis discussed.

B. Laboratory Findings

1. Alpha-thalassemia trait—These patients have mild or no anemia, with hematocrits between 28% and 40%. The MCV is strikingly low (60–75 fL) despite the modest anemia, and the red blood count is normal or increased. The peripheral blood smear shows microcytes, hypochromia, occasional target cells, and acanthocytes (cells with irregularly spaced spiked projections). The reticulocyte count and iron parameters are normal. Hemoglobin electrophoresis is normal. Alpha-thalassemia trait is thus usually diagnosed by exclusion. Genetic testing to demonstrate alpha-globin gene deletion is available.

2. Hemoglobin H disease—These patients have a more marked anemia, with hematocrits between 22% and 32%. The MCV is remarkably low (60–70 fL) and the peripheral blood smear is markedly abnormal, with hypochromia, microcytosis, target cells, and poikilocytosis. The reticulocyte count is elevated and the RBC count is normal or elevated. Hemoglobin electrophoresis will show a fast-migrating hemoglobin (hemoglobin H), which comprises 10–40% of the hemoglobin. A peripheral blood smear can be stained with supravital dyes to demonstrate the presence of hemoglobin H.

3. Beta-thalassemia minor—These patients have a modest anemia with hematocrit between 28% and 40%. The MCV ranges from 55 fL to 75 fL, and the RBC count is normal or increased. The reticulocyte count is normal or slightly elevated. The peripheral blood smear is mildly abnormal, with hypochromia, microcytosis, and target cells. In contrast to alpha-thalassemia, basophilic stippling is present. Hemoglobin electrophoresis shows an elevation of hemoglobin A_2 to 4–8% and occasional elevations of hemoglobin F to 1–5%.

4. Beta-thalassemia intermedia—These patients have a moderate anemia with hematocrit between 17% and 33%. The MCV ranges from 55 fL to 75 fL, and the RBC count is normal or increased. The reticulocyte count is elevated. The peripheral blood smear is abnormal with hypochromia, microcytosis, basophilic stippling, and target cells. Hemoglobin electrophoresis shows up to 30% hemoglobin A, an elevation of hemoglobin A_2 up to 10%, and elevation of hemoglobin F from 6% to 10%.

5. Beta-thalassemia major—These patients have severe anemia, and without transfusion the hematocrit may fall to less than 10%. The peripheral blood smear is bizarre, showing severe poikilocytosis, hypochromia, microcytosis, target cells, basophilic stippling, and nucleated RBCs. Little or no hemoglobin A is present. Variable amounts of hemoglobin A_2 are seen, and the predominant hemoglobin present is hemoglobin F.

Differential Diagnosis

Mild forms of thalassemia must be differentiated from iron deficiency. Compared to iron deficiency anemia, patients with thalassemia have a lower MCV, a normal or elevated RBC count (rather than low), a more abnormal peripheral blood smear at modest levels of anemia, and usually a reticulocytosis. Iron studies are normal, or the transferrin saturation or ferritin (or both) are elevated. Severe forms of thalassemia may be confused with other hemoglobinopathies. The diagnosis of beta-thalassemia is made by the above findings and hemoglobin electrophoresis showing elevated levels of hemoglobins A_2 and F (provided the patient is replete in iron), or beta-gene sequencing. The diagnosis of alpha-thalassemia is made by exclusion since there is no change in the proportion of the normal adult hemoglobin species or confirmed by alpha gene deletion studies. The only other microcytic anemia with a normal or elevated RBC count is iron deficiency in a patient with polycythemia vera.

Treatment

Patients with mild thalassemia (alpha-thalassemia trait or beta-thalassemia minor) require no treatment and should be identified so that they will not be subjected to repeated evaluations and mistaken treatment for iron deficiency. Patients with hemoglobin H disease should take folic acid supplementation (1 mg/day orally) and avoid medicinal iron and oxidative drugs such as sulfonamides. Patients with severe thalassemia are maintained on a regular transfusion schedule (in part to suppress endogenous erythropoiesis and therefore bone marrow expansion) and receive folic acid supplementation. Splenectomy is performed if hypersplenism causes a marked increase in the transfusion requirement or refractory symptoms. Patients with regular transfusion requirements should be treated with iron chelation (oral or parenteral) to prevent or delay life-limiting organ damage from iron overload. A new agent, **luspatercept**, has been FDA approved for transfusion-dependent beta-thalassemia. It is a TGF-beta ligand trap that promotes erythroid maturation and reduces transfusion needs.

Allogeneic stem cell transplantation is the treatment of choice for beta-thalassemia major and the only available cure. Children who have not yet experienced organ damage from iron overload do well, with long-term survival in more than 80% of cases. Autologous hematopoietic stem cell gene therapy is showing promise for thalassemia major.

When to Refer

All patients with thalassemia intermedia or major should be referred to a hematologist. Any patient with an unexplained microcytic anemia should be referred to help establish a diagnosis. Patients with thalassemia minor or intermedia should be offered genetic counseling because offspring of thalassemic couples are at risk for inheriting thalassemia major.

Cappellini MD et al. The use of luspatercept for thalassemia in adults. Blood Adv. 2021;5:326. [PMID: 33570654]

Kattamis A et al. Changing patterns in the epidemiology of β-thalassemia. Eur J Haematol. 2020;105:692. [PMID: 32886826]

Pinto VM et al. Management of iron overload in beta-thalassemia patients: clinical practice update based on case series. Int J Mol Sci. 2020;21:8771. [PMID: 33233561]

VITAMIN B_{12} DEFICIENCY

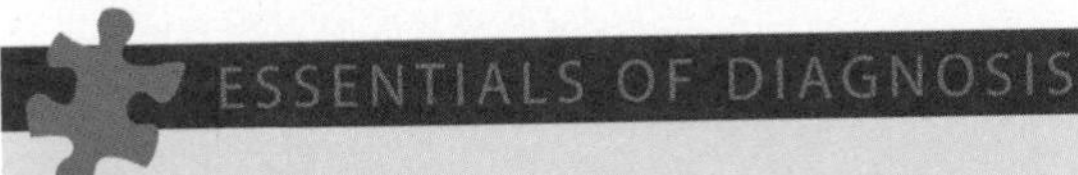

- Macrocytic anemia.
- Megaloblastic blood smear (macro-ovalocytes and hypersegmented neutrophils).
- Low serum vitamin B_{12} level.

General Considerations

Vitamin B_{12} belongs to the family of cobalamins and serves as a cofactor for two important reactions in humans. As methylcobalamin, it is a cofactor for methionine synthetase in the conversion of homocysteine to methionine, and as adenosylcobalamin for the conversion of methylmalonyl-coenzyme A (CoA) to succinyl-CoA. Vitamin B_{12} comes from the diet and is present in all foods of animal origin. The daily absorption of vitamin B_{12} is 5 mcg.

The liver contains 2–5 mg of stored vitamin B_{12}. Since daily utilization is 3–5 mcg, the body usually has sufficient stores of vitamin B_{12} so that it takes more than 3 years for vitamin B_{12} deficiency to occur if all intake or absorption immediately ceases.

Since vitamin B_{12} is present in foods of animal origin, dietary vitamin B_{12} deficiency is rare but is seen in vegans—strict vegetarians who avoid all dairy products, meat, and fish (Table 13–6). Pernicious anemia is an autoimmune illness whereby autoantibodies destroy gastric parietal cells (that produce intrinsic factor) and cause atrophic gastritis or bind to and neutralize intrinsic factor, or both. Abdominal surgery may lead to vitamin B_{12} deficiency in several ways. Gastrectomy will eliminate the site of intrinsic factor production; blind loop syndrome will cause competition for vitamin B_{12} by bacterial overgrowth in the lumen of the intestine; and surgical resection of the ileum will eliminate the site of vitamin B_{12} absorption. Rare causes of vitamin B_{12} deficiency include fish tapeworm (*Diphyllobothrium latum*) infection, in which the parasite uses luminal vitamin B_{12}; pancreatic insufficiency (with failure to inactivate competing cobalamin-binding proteins [R-factors]); severe Crohn disease, causing sufficient destruction of the ileum to impair vitamin B_{12} absorption; and perhaps prolonged use of PPIs.

Table 13–6. Causes of vitamin B_{12} deficiency.

Dietary deficiency
Decreased production or availability of intrinsic factor
Pernicious anemia (autoimmune)
Gastrectomy
Helicobacter pylori infection
Competition for vitamin B_{12} in the gut
Blind loop syndrome
Fish tapeworm (rare)
Pancreatic insufficiency
PPIs
Decreased ileal absorption of vitamin B_{12}
Surgical resection
Crohn disease
Transcobalamin II deficiency (rare)

Clinical Findings

A. Symptoms and Signs

Vitamin B_{12} deficiency causes a moderate to severe anemia of slow onset; patients may have few symptoms relative to the degree of anemia. In advanced cases, the anemia may be severe, with hematocrits as low as 10–15%, and may be accompanied by leukopenia and thrombocytopenia. The deficiency also produces changes in mucosal cells, leading to glossitis, as well as other vague GI disturbances such as anorexia and diarrhea. Vitamin B_{12} deficiency also leads to a complex neurologic syndrome. Peripheral nerves are usually affected first, and patients complain initially of paresthesias. As the posterior columns of the spinal cord become impaired, patients complain of difficulty with balance or proprioception, or both. In more advanced cases, cerebral function may be altered as well, and on occasion, dementia and other neuropsychiatric abnormalities may be present. It is critical to recognize that the nonhematologic manifestations of vitamin B_{12} deficiency can be manifest despite a completely normal CBC.

Patients are usually pale and may be mildly icteric or sallow. Typically, later in the disease course, neurologic examination may reveal decreased vibration and position sense or memory disturbance (or both).

B. Laboratory Findings

The diagnosis of vitamin B_{12} deficiency is made by finding a low serum vitamin B_{12} (cobalamin) level. Whereas the normal vitamin B_{12} level is greater than 300 pg/mL (221 pmol/L), most patients with overt vitamin B_{12} deficiency have serum levels less than 200 pg/mL (148 pmol/L), with symptomatic patients often having levels less than 100 pg/mL (74 pmol/L). The diagnosis of vitamin B_{12} deficiency in low or low-normal values (level of 200–300 pg/mL [147.6–221.3 pmol/L]) is best confirmed by finding an elevated level of serum methylmalonic acid or homocysteine. Of note, elevated levels of serum methylmalonic acid can be due to kidney disease.

The anemia of vitamin B_{12} deficiency is typically moderate to severe with the MCV quite elevated (110–140 fL). However, it is possible to have vitamin B_{12} deficiency with a normal MCV from coexistent thalassemia or iron deficiency; in other cases, the reason is obscure. Patients with neurologic symptoms and signs that suggest possible vitamin B_{12} deficiency should be evaluated for that deficiency despite a normal MCV or the absence of anemia. In typical cases, the peripheral blood smear is megaloblastic, defined as RBCs that appear as macro-ovalocytes, (although other shape changes are usually present) and neutrophils that are hypersegmented (six [or greater]-lobed neutrophils or mean neutrophil lobe counts greater than four). The reticulocyte count is reduced. Because vitamin B_{12} deficiency can affect all hematopoietic cell lines, the WBC count and the platelet count are reduced in severe cases.

Other laboratory abnormalities include elevated serum LD and a modest increase in indirect bilirubin. These two findings reflect the intramedullary destruction of developing abnormal erythroid cells.

Bone marrow morphology is characteristically abnormal. Marked erythroid hyperplasia is present as a response to defective RBC production (ineffective erythropoiesis). Megaloblastic changes in the erythroid series include abnormally large cell size and asynchronous maturation of the nucleus and cytoplasm—ie, cytoplasmic maturation continues while impaired DNA synthesis causes retarded nuclear development. In the myeloid series, giant bands and meta-myelocytes are characteristically seen.

Differential Diagnosis

Vitamin B_{12} deficiency should be differentiated from folic acid deficiency, the other common cause of megaloblastic anemia, in which RBC folic acid is low while vitamin B_{12} levels are normal. The bone marrow findings of vitamin B_{12} deficiency are sometimes mistaken for a MDS or even acute erythrocytic leukemia. The distinction between vitamin B_{12} deficiency and myelodysplasia is based on the characteristic morphology and the low vitamin B_{12} and elevated methylmalonic acid levels.

Treatment

Initially, patients with vitamin B_{12} deficiency are usually treated with parenteral therapy. Intramuscular or subcutaneous injections of 100–1000 mcg of vitamin B_{12} are adequate for each dose (with the higher dose recommended initially). Replacement is usually given daily for the first week, weekly for the next month, and then monthly for life. The vitamin deficiency will recur if patients discontinue their therapy. Oral or sublingual methylcobalamin (1 mg/day) may be used instead of parenteral therapy once initial correction of the deficiency has occurred. Oral or sublingual replacement is effective, even in pernicious anemia, since approximately 1% of the dose is absorbed in the intestine via passive diffusion in the absence of active transport. It must be continued indefinitely and serum vitamin B_{12} levels must be monitored to ensure adequate replacement. For patients with neurologic symptoms caused by vitamin B_{12} deficiency, long-term parenteral vitamin B_{12} therapy is recommended, though its superiority over oral vitamin B_{12} therapy has not been proven. Because some patients are concurrently folic acid deficient from intestinal mucosal atrophy, simultaneous folic acid replacement (1 mg daily) is advised for the first several months of vitamin B_{12} replacement.

Patients respond to therapy with an immediate improvement in their sense of well-being. Hypokalemia may complicate the first several days of therapy, particularly if the anemia is severe. A brisk reticulocytosis occurs in 5–7 days, and the hematologic picture normalizes in 2 months. CNS symptoms and signs are potentially reversible if they have been present for less than 6 months. RBC transfusions are rarely needed despite the severity of anemia, but when given, diuretics are also recommended to avoid heart failure because this anemia develops slowly and the plasma volume is increased at the time of diagnosis.

When to Refer

Referral to a hematologist is not usually necessary.

Lewis CA et al. Iron, vitamin B_{12}, folate and copper deficiency after bariatric surgery and the impact on anaemia: a systematic review. Obes Surg. 2020;30:4542. [PMID: 32785814]

Socha DS et al. Severe megaloblastic anemia: vitamin deficiency and other causes. Cleve Clin J Med. 2020;87:153. [PMID: 32127439]

Wolffenbuttel BHR et al. The many faces of cobalamin (vitamin B_{12}) deficiency. Mayo Clin Proc Innov Qual Outcomes. 2019;3:200. [PMID: 31193945]

FOLIC ACID DEFICIENCY

ESSENTIALS OF DIAGNOSIS

- Macrocytic anemia.
- Megaloblastic blood smear (macro-ovalocytes and hypersegmented neutrophils).
- Reduced folic acid levels in RBCs or serum.
- Normal serum vitamin B_{12} level.

General Considerations

"Folic acid" is the term commonly used for pteroylmonoglutamic acid. Folic acid is present in most fruits and vegetables (especially citrus fruits and green leafy vegetables). Daily dietary requirements are 50–100 mcg. Total body stores of folic acid are approximately 5 mg, enough to supply requirements for 2–3 months.

The most common cause of folic acid deficiency is inadequate dietary intake (Table 13–7). Alcoholic or anorectic patients, persons who do not eat fresh fruits and vegetables, and those who overcook their food are candidates for folic acid deficiency. Reduced folic acid absorption is rarely seen, since absorption occurs from the entire GI tract. However, medications such as phenytoin, trimethoprim-sulfamethoxazole, or sulfasalazine may interfere with its absorption. Folic acid absorption is poor in some

Table 13–7. Causes of folic acid deficiency.

Dietary deficiency
Decreased absorption
Celiac disease
Medications: phenytoin, sulfasalazine, trimethoprim-sulfamethoxazole
Concurrent vitamin B_{12} deficiency
Increased requirement
Chronic hemolytic anemia
Pregnancy
Exfoliative skin disease
Excess loss: hemodialysis
Inhibition of reduction to active form
Methotrexate

patients with vitamin B_{12} deficiency due to GI mucosal atrophy. Folic acid requirements are increased in pregnancy, hemolytic anemia, and exfoliative skin disease, and in these cases the increased requirements (5–10 times normal) may not be met by a normal diet.

Clinical Findings

A. Symptoms and Signs

The clinical features are similar to those of vitamin B_{12} deficiency. However, isolated folic acid deficiency does not result in neurologic abnormalities.

B. Laboratory Findings

Megaloblastic anemia is identical to anemia resulting from vitamin B_{12} deficiency. A RBC folic acid level below 150 ng/mL (340 nmol/L) is diagnostic of folic acid deficiency. Whether to order a serum or a RBC folate level remains unsettled since there are few, if any, data to support one test over the other. Usually the serum vitamin B_{12} level is normal, but it should always be measured when folic acid deficiency is suspected. In some instances, folic acid deficiency is a consequence of the GI mucosal atrophy from vitamin B_{12} deficiency.

Differential Diagnosis

The megaloblastic anemia of folic acid deficiency should be differentiated from vitamin B_{12} deficiency by the finding of a normal vitamin B_{12} level and a reduced RBC (or serum) folic acid level. Alcoholic patients, who often have nutritional deficiency, may also have anemia of liver disease. Pure anemia of liver disease causes a macrocytic anemia but does not produce megaloblastic morphologic changes in the peripheral blood; rather, target cells are present. Hypothyroidism is associated with mild macrocytosis and also with pernicious anemia.

Treatment

Folic acid deficiency is treated with daily oral folic acid (1 mg). The response is similar to that seen in the treatment of vitamin B_{12} deficiency, with rapid improvement and a sense of well-being, reticulocytosis in 5–7 days, and total correction of hematologic abnormalities within 2 months. Large doses of folic acid may produce hematologic responses in cases of vitamin B_{12} deficiency, but permit neurologic damage to progress; hence, obtaining a serum vitamin B_{12} level in suspected folic acid deficiency is paramount.

When to Refer

Referral to a hematologist is not usually necessary.

Lewis CA et al. Iron, vitamin B_{12}, folate and copper deficiency after bariatric surgery and the impact on anaemia: a systematic review. Obes Surg. 2020;30:4542. [PMID: 32785814]

Shulpekova Y et al. The concept of folic acid in health and disease. Molecules. 2021;26:3731. [PMID: 34207319]

Socha DS et al. Severe megaloblastic anemia: vitamin deficiency and other causes. Cleve Clin J Med. 2020;87:153. [PMID: 32127439]

HEMOLYTIC ANEMIAS

The hemolytic anemias are a group of disorders in which RBC survival is reduced, either episodically or continuously. The bone marrow has the ability to increase erythroid production up to eightfold in response to reduced RBC survival, so anemia will be present only when the ability of the bone marrow to compensate is outstripped. This will occur when RBC survival is extremely short or when the ability of the bone marrow to compensate is impaired.

Hemolytic disorders are generally classified according to whether the defect is intrinsic to the RBC or due to some external factor (Table 13–8). Intrinsic defects have been described in all components of the RBC, including the membrane, enzyme systems, and hemoglobin; most of these disorders are hereditary. Hemolytic anemias due to external factors are classified as immune,

Table 13–8. Classification of hemolytic anemias.

Intrinsic
Membrane defects: hereditary spherocytosis, hereditary elliptocytosis, paroxysmal nocturnal hemoglobinuria
Glycolytic defects: pyruvate kinase deficiency, severe hypophosphatemia
Oxidation vulnerability: glucose-6-phosphate dehydrogenase deficiency, methemoglobinemia
Hemoglobinopathies: sickle cell syndromes, thalassemia, unstable hemoglobins
Extrinsic
Immune: autoimmune, lymphoproliferative disease, drug-induced, idiopathic
Microangiopathic: thrombotic thrombocytopenic purpura, hemolytic-uremic syndrome, disseminated intravascular coagulation, valve hemolysis, metastatic adenocarcinoma, vasculitis, copper overload
Infection: *Plasmodium, Clostridium, Borrelia*
Hypersplenism
Burns

microangiopathic hemolytic anemias, drug-induced, and RBC infections.

Certain laboratory features are common to all hemolytic anemias. Haptoglobin, a normal plasma protein that binds and clears free hemoglobin released into plasma, is depressed in hemolytic disorders. However, the haptoglobin level is influenced by many factors and is not always a reliable indicator of hemolysis, particularly in end-stage liver disease (its site of synthesis). When intravascular hemolysis occurs, transient hemoglobinemia ensues. Hemoglobin is filtered through the renal glomerulus and is usually reabsorbed by tubular cells. Hemoglobinuria will be present only when the capacity for reabsorption of hemoglobin by renal tubular cells is exceeded. In the absence of hemoglobinuria, evidence for prior intravascular hemolysis is the presence of hemosiderin in shed renal tubular cells (positive urine hemosiderin). With severe intravascular hemolysis, hemoglobinemia and methemalbuminemia may be present. Hemolysis increases the indirect bilirubin, and the total bilirubin may rise to 4 mg/dL (68 mcmol/L) or more. Bilirubin levels higher than this may indicate some degree of hepatic dysfunction. Serum LD levels are strikingly elevated in cases of microangiopathic hemolysis (thrombotic thrombocytopenic purpura, hemolytic-uremic syndrome) and may be elevated in other hemolytic anemias.

PAROXYSMAL NOCTURNAL HEMOGLOBINURIA

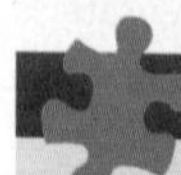

ESSENTIALS OF DIAGNOSIS

- Episodic hemoglobinuria.
- Thrombosis is common.
- Suspect in confusing cases of hemolytic anemia with or without pancytopenia.
- Flow cytometry demonstrates deficiencies of CD55 and CD59.

General Considerations

Paroxysmal nocturnal hemoglobinuria (PNH) is a rare acquired clonal hematopoietic stem cell disorder that results in abnormal sensitivity of the RBC membrane to lysis by complement and therefore hemolysis. Free hemoglobin is released into the blood that scavenges nitric oxide and promotes esophageal spasms, male erectile dysfunction, kidney damage, and thrombosis. Patients with significant PNH have shortened survival; thrombosis is the primary cause of death.

Clinical Findings

A. Symptoms and Signs

Classically, patients report episodic hemoglobinuria resulting in reddish-brown urine. Hemoglobinuria is most often noticed in the first morning urine due to the fall in blood pH while sleeping (hypoventilation) that facilitates this hemolysis. Besides anemia, these patients are prone to thrombosis, especially within mesenteric and hepatic veins, CNS veins (sagittal vein), and skin vessels (with formation of painful nodules). As this is a hematopoietic stem cell disorder, PNH may appear de novo or arise in the setting of aplastic anemia or myelodysplasia with possible progression to acute myeloid leukemia (AML). It is common that patients with idiopathic aplastic anemia have a small PNH clone (less than 2%) on blood or bone marrow analysis; this should not be considered true PNH per se, especially in the absence of a reticulocytosis or thrombosis.

B. Laboratory Findings

Anemia is of variable severity and frequency, so reticulocytosis may or may not be present at any given time. Abnormalities on the blood smear are nondiagnostic but may include macro-ovalocytes and polychromasia. Since the episodic hemolysis is mainly intravascular, urine hemosiderin is a useful test. Serum LD is characteristically quite elevated. Iron deficiency is commonly present, related to chronic iron loss from hemoglobinuria.

The WBC count and platelet count may be decreased and are always decreased in the setting of aplastic anemia. The best screening test is flow cytometry of blood erythrocytes, granulocytes, and monocytes to demonstrate deficiency of CD55 and CD59. The proportion of erythrocytes deficient in these proteins might be low due to the ongoing destruction of affected erythrocytes. The FLAER assay (fluorescein-labeled proaerolysin) by flow cytometry is more sensitive. Bone marrow morphology is variable and may show either generalized hypoplasia or erythroid hyperplasia or both. The bone marrow karyotype may be either normal or demonstrate a clonal abnormality.

Treatment

Many patients with PNH have mild disease not requiring intervention. In severe cases and in those occurring in the setting of myelodysplasia or previous aplastic anemia, allogeneic hematopoietic stem cell transplantation may prove curative. In patients with severe hemolysis (usually requiring RBC transfusions) or thrombosis (or both), treatment with eculizumab is warranted. Eculizumab is a humanized monoclonal antibody against complement protein C5 given every 2 weeks. Binding of eculizumab to C5 prevents its cleavage so the membrane attack complex cannot assemble. Eculizumab improves quality of life and reduces hemolysis, transfusion requirements, fatigue, and thrombosis risk. Eculizumab increases the risk of *Neisseria meningitidis* infections; patients receiving the antibody should undergo meningococcal vaccination (including vaccines for serogroup B) and take oral penicillin (or equivalent) meningococcal prophylaxis. Ravulizumab is a longer-acting version of eculizumab; it is given every 8 weeks and demonstrates fewer breakthrough hemolytic episodes than eculizumab. A C3 inhibitor, pegcetacoplan, is also available for PNH and blocks both intra- and extravascular hemolysis pathways. Iron replacement is indicated for treatment of iron deficiency when present, which may improve the anemia while also causing a transient increase in hemolysis. For unclear reasons, corticosteroids are effective in decreasing hemolysis.

When to Refer

Most patients with PNH should be under the care of a hematologist.

Brodsky RA. How I treat paroxysmal nocturnal hemoglobinuria. Blood. 2021;137:1304. [PMID: 33512400]

Hillmen P et al. Pegcetacoplan versus eculizumab in paroxysmal nocturnal hemoglobinuria. N Engl J Med. 2021;384:1028. [PMID: 33730455]

Patriquin CJ et al. How we treat paroxysmal nocturnal hemoglobinuria: a consensus statement of the Canadian PNH Network and review of the national registry. Eur J Haematol. 2019;102:36. [PMID: 30242915]

GLUCOSE-6-PHOSPHATE DEHYDROGENASE DEFICIENCY

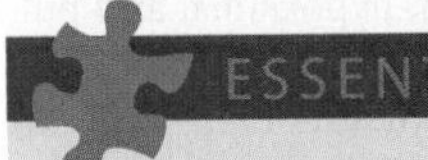

ESSENTIALS OF DIAGNOSIS

- X-linked recessive disorder seen commonly in American Black men.
- Episodic hemolysis in response to oxidant drugs or infection.
- Bite cells and blister cells on the peripheral blood smear.
- Reduced levels of glucose-6-phosphate dehydrogenase between hemolytic episodes.

General Considerations

Glucose-6-phosphate dehydrogenase (G6PD) deficiency is a hereditary enzyme defect that causes episodic hemolytic anemia because of the decreased ability of RBCs to deal with oxidative stresses. G6PD deficiency leads to excess oxidized glutathione that forces hemoglobin to denature and form precipitants called Heinz bodies. Heinz bodies cause RBC membrane damage, which leads to premature removal of these RBCs by reticuloendothelial cells within the spleen (ie, extravascular hemolysis).

Numerous G6PD isoenzymes have been described. The usual isoenzyme found in American Blacks is designated G6PD-A and that found in Whites is designated G6PD-B, both of which have normal function and stability and therefore no hemolytic anemia. Ten to 15 percent of American Blacks have the variant G6PD isoenzyme designated A–, in which there is both a reduction in normal enzyme activity and a reduction in its stability. The A– isoenzyme activity declines rapidly as the RBC ages past 40 days, a fact that explains the clinical findings in this disorder. More than 150 G6PD isoenzyme variants have been described, including some Mediterranean, Ashkenazi Jewish, and Asian variants with very low enzyme activity, episodic hemolysis, and exacerbations due to oxidizing substances including fava beans. Patients with G6PD deficiency seem to be protected from malaria parasitic infection, have less CAD, and possibly have fewer cancers and greater longevity.

Clinical Findings

G6PD deficiency is an X-linked disorder affecting 10–15% of American hemizygous Black males and rare female homozygotes. Female carriers are rarely affected—only when an unusually high percentage of cells producing the normal enzyme are X-inactivated.

A. Symptoms and Signs

Patients are usually healthy, without chronic hemolytic anemia or splenomegaly. Hemolysis occurs episodically due to oxidative stress on the RBCs, generated either by infection or exposure to certain medications. Medications initiating hemolysis that should be avoided include dapsone, methylene blue, phenazopyridine, primaquine, rasburicase, toluidine blue, nitrofurantoin, trimethoprim/sulfamethoxazole, sulfadiazine, pegloticase, and quinolones. Other medications, such as chloroquine, quinine, high-dose aspirin, and isoniazid, have been implicated but are less certain as offenders since they are often given during infections. Even with continuous use of the offending medication, the hemolytic episode is self-limited because older RBCs (with low enzyme activity) are removed and replaced with a population of young RBCs (reticulocytes) with adequate functional levels of G6PD. Severe G6PD deficiency (as in Mediterranean variants) may produce a chronic hemolytic anemia.

B. Laboratory Findings

Between hemolytic episodes, the blood is normal. During episodes of hemolysis, the hemoglobin rarely falls below 8 g/dL (80 g/L), and there is reticulocytosis and increased serum indirect bilirubin. The peripheral blood cell smear often reveals a small number of "bite" cells—cells that appear to have had a bite taken out of their periphery, or "blister" cells. This indicates pitting of precipitated membrane hemoglobin aggregates (ie, Heinz bodies) by the splenic macrophages. Heinz bodies may be demonstrated by staining a peripheral blood smear with cresyl violet; they are not visible on the usual Wright-Giemsa–stained blood smear. Specific enzyme assays for G6PD reveal a low level but may be falsely normal if they are performed during or shortly after a hemolytic episode during the period of reticulocytosis. In these cases, the enzyme assays should be repeated weeks after hemolysis has resolved. In severe cases of G6PD deficiency, enzyme levels are always low.

Treatment

No treatment is necessary except to avoid known oxidant medications.

Garcia AA et al. Treatment strategies for glucose-6-phosphate dehydrogenase deficiency: past and future perspectives. Trends Pharmacol Sci. 2021;42:829. [PMID: 34389161]

Georgakouli K et al. Exercise in glucose-6-phosphate dehydrogenase deficiency: harmful or harmless? A narrative review. Oxid Med Cell Longev. 2019;2019:8060193. [PMID: 31089417]

SICKLE CELL ANEMIA & RELATED SYNDROMES

ESSENTIALS OF DIAGNOSIS

- Recurrent pain episodes.
- Positive family history and lifelong history of hemolytic anemia.
- Irreversibly sickled cells on peripheral blood smear.
- Hemoglobin S is the major hemoglobin seen on electrophoresis.

General Considerations

Sickle cell anemia is an autosomal recessive disorder in which an abnormal hemoglobin leads to chronic hemolytic anemia with numerous clinical consequences. A single DNA base change leads to an amino acid substitution of valine for glutamate in the sixth position on the beta-globin chain. The abnormal beta chain is designated beta^{s} and the tetramer of alpha-2beta^{s}-2 is designated hemoglobin SS. Hemoglobin S is unstable and polymerizes in the setting of various stressors, including hypoxemia and acidosis, leading to the formation of sickled RBCs. Sickled cells result in hemolysis and the release of ATP, which is converted to adenosine. Adenosine binds to its receptor (A2B), resulting in the production of 2,3-biphosphoglycerate and the induction of more sickling, and to its receptor (A2A) on natural killer cells, resulting in pulmonary inflammation. The free hemoglobin from hemolysis scavenges nitric oxide causing endothelial dysfunction, vascular injury, and pulmonary hypertension.

The rate of sickling is influenced by the intracellular concentration of hemoglobin S and by the presence of other hemoglobins within the cell. Hemoglobin F cannot participate in polymer formation, and its presence markedly retards sickling. Factors that increase sickling are RBC dehydration and factors that lead to formation of deoxyhemoglobin S (eg, acidosis and hypoxemia), either systemic or local in tissues. Hemolytic crises may be related to splenic sequestration of sickled cells (primarily in childhood before the spleen has been infarcted as a result of repeated sickling) or with coexistent disorders such as G6PD deficiency.

The beta^{S} gene is carried in 8% of American Blacks, and 1 of 400 American Black children will be born with sickle cell anemia; prenatal diagnosis is available when sickle cell anemia is suspected. Genetic counseling should be made available to patients.

Clinical Findings

A. Symptoms and Signs

The disorder has its onset during the first year of life, when hemoglobin F levels fall as a signal is sent to switch from production of gamma-globin to beta-globin. Chronic hemolytic anemia produces jaundice, pigment (calcium bilirubinate) gallstones, splenomegaly (early in life), and poorly healing skin ulcers over the lower tibia. Life-threatening severe anemia can occur during hemolytic or aplastic crises, the latter generally associated with viral or other infection caused by immunoincompetence from hyposplenism or by folic acid deficiency causing reduced erythropoiesis.

Acute painful episodes due to acute vaso-occlusion from clusters of sickled RBCs may occur spontaneously or be provoked by infection, dehydration, or hypoxia. Common sites of acute painful episodes include the spine and long appendicular bones. These episodes last hours to days and may produce low-grade fever. Acute vaso-occlusion may cause strokes due to sagittal sinus venous thrombosis or to bland or hemorrhagic CNS arterial ischemia. Vaso-occlusion may also cause priapism. Vaso-occlusive episodes are not associated with increased hemolysis.

Repeated episodes of vascular occlusion especially affect the heart, lungs, and liver. The acute chest syndrome is characterized by acute chest pain, hypoxemia, and pulmonary infiltrates on a chest radiograph and must be distinguished from an infectious pneumonia. Ischemic necrosis of bones may occur, rendering the bone susceptible to osteomyelitis due to salmonellae and (somewhat less commonly) staphylococci. Infarction of the papillae of the renal medulla causes renal tubular concentrating defects and gross hematuria, more often encountered in sickle cell trait than in sickle cell anemia. Retinopathy is often present and may lead to visual impairment. Pulmonary hypertension may develop and is associated with a poor prognosis. These patients are prone to delayed puberty. An increased incidence of infection is related to hyposplenism as well as to defects in the alternate complement pathway.

On examination, patients are often chronically ill and jaundiced. There is often hepatomegaly, but the spleen is not palpable in adult life. The heart may be enlarged with a hyperdynamic precordium and systolic murmurs and, in some cases, a pronounced increase in P2. Nonhealing cutaneous ulcers of the lower leg and retinopathy may be present.

B. Laboratory Findings

Chronic hemolytic anemia is present. The hematocrit is usually 20–30%. The peripheral blood smear is characteristically abnormal, with sickled cells comprising 5–50% of RBCs. Other findings include reticulocytosis (10–25%), nucleated RBCs, and hallmarks of hyposplenism such as Howell-Jolly bodies and target cells. The WBC count is characteristically elevated to 12,000–15,000/mcL ($12–15 \times 10^9$/L), and reactive thrombocytosis may occur. Indirect bilirubin levels are high.

The diagnosis of sickle cell anemia is confirmed by hemoglobin electrophoresis (Table 13–9). Hemoglobin S will usually comprise 85–98% of hemoglobin. In homozygous S disease, no hemoglobin A will be present. Hemoglobin F levels are sometimes increased, and high hemoglobin F levels (15–20%) are associated with a more benign

Table 13–9. Hemoglobin distribution in sickle cell syndromes.

Genotype	Clinical Diagnosis	Hb A	Hb S	Hb A_2	Hb F
AA	Normal	97–99%	0%	1–2%	< 1%
AS	Sickle trait	60%	40%	1–2%	< 1%
AS, alpha-thalassemia	Sickle trait, alpha-thalassemia	70–75%	25–30%	1–2%	< 1%
SS	Sickle cell anemia	0%	86–98%	1–3%	5–15%
SS, alpha-thalassemia (3 genes)	SS alpha-thalassemia, silent	0%	90%	3%	7–9%
SS, alpha-thalassemia (2 genes)	SS alpha-thalassemia, trait	0%	80%	3%	11–21%
S, beta^0-thalassemia	Sickle beta^0-thalassemia	0%	70–80%	3–5%	10–20%
S, beta$^+$-thalassemia	Sickle beta$^+$-thalassemia	10–20%	60–75%	3–5%	10–20%

Hb, hemoglobin; beta^0, no beta-globin produced; beta$^+$, some beta-globin produced.

clinical course. Patients with S-beta$^+$-thalassemia and SS alpha-thalassemia also have a more benign clinical course than straight sickle cell anemia (SS) patients.

Treatment

When allogeneic hematopoietic stem cell transplantation is performed before the onset of significant end-organ damage, it can cure more than 80% of children with sickle cell anemia who have suitable HLA-matched donors, with a reasonably good quality of life. Transplantation remains investigational in adults. Other therapies modulate disease severity: hydroxyurea increases hemoglobin F levels epigenetically. Hydroxyurea (500–750 mg orally daily) reduces the frequency of painful crises in patients whose quality of life is disrupted by frequent vaso-occlusive pain episodes (three or more per year). Long-term follow-up of patients taking hydroxyurea demonstrates it improves overall survival and quality of life with little evidence for secondary malignancy. The use of omega-3 (n-3) fatty acid supplementation may also reduce vaso-occlusive episodes and reduce transfusion needs in patients with sickle cell anemia. L-glutamine has been shown to favorably modulate sickle pain crises and acute chest syndrome. A monoclonal antibody (crizanlizumab-tmca) reduces vaso-occlusive episodes by 50%. It blocks P-selectin on activated endothelial cells and thus disrupts the adverse interactions of platelets, RBCs, and leukocytes with the endothelial wall. Voxelotor inhibits the polymerization of deoxygenated sickle RBCs and increases the hemoglobin in SS patients age 12 years or older, and thus can reduce transfusion needs.

Supportive care is the mainstay of treatment for sickle cell anemia. Patients are maintained on folic acid supplementation (1 mg orally daily) and given transfusions for aplastic or hemolytic crises. When acute painful episodes occur, precipitating factors should be identified and infections treated if present. The patient should be kept well hydrated, given generous analgesics, and supplied oxygen if hypoxic. Pneumococcal vaccination reduces the incidence of infections with this pathogen while hydroxyurea and L-glutamine reduce hospitalizations for acute pain. ACE inhibitors are recommended in patients with microalbuminuria.

Exchange transfusions are indicated for the treatment of severe or intractable acute vaso-occlusive crises, acute chest syndrome, priapism, and stroke. Long-term transfusion therapy has been shown to be effective in reducing the risk of recurrent stroke in children. Phenotypically matched transfused RBCs are recommended to reduce the risk of RBC alloimmunization. It has been recommended that children with SS who are aged 2–16 years have annual transcranial ultrasounds and, if the Doppler velocity is abnormal (200 cm/s or greater), the clinician should strongly consider beginning transfusions to prevent stroke. Iron chelation is needed for those on chronic transfusion therapy.

Prognosis

Sickle cell anemia becomes a chronic multisystem disease, leading to organ failure that may result in early death. With improved supportive care, average life expectancy is now between 40 and 50 years of age.

When to Refer

Patients with sickle cell anemia should have their care coordinated with a hematologist and should be referred to a Comprehensive Sickle Cell Center, if available.

When to Admit

Patients should be admitted for management of acute chest syndrome, for aplastic crisis, or for painful episodes that do not respond to outpatient interventions.

DeBaun MR et al. American Society of Hematology 2020 guidelines for sickle cell disease: prevention, diagnosis, and treatment of cerebrovascular disease in children and adults. Blood Adv. 2020;4:1554. [PMID: 32298430]

Howard J et al. Voxelotor in adolescents and adults with sickle cell disease (HOPE): long-term follow-up results of an international, randomised, double-blind, placebo-controlled, phase 3 trial. Lancet Haematol. 2021;8:e323. [PMID: 33838113]

Kutlar A et al. Effect of crizanlizumab on pain crises in subgroups of patients with sickle cell disease: a SUSTAIN study analysis. Am J Hematol. 2019;94:55. [PMID: 30295335]
Pecker LH et al. Sickle cell disease. Ann Intern Med. 2021;174:ITC1. [PMID: 33428443]
Vichinsky E et al. A phase 3 randomized trial of voxelotor in sickle cell disease. N Engl J Med. 2019;381:509. [PMID: 31199090]

SICKLE CELL TRAIT

People with the heterozygous hemoglobin genotype AS have **sickle cell trait.** These persons are hematologically normal, with no anemia and normal RBCs on peripheral blood smear. Hemoglobin electrophoresis will reveal that approximately 40% of hemoglobin is hemoglobin S (Table 13–9). People with sickle cell trait experience more rhabdomyolysis during vigorous exercise but do not have increased mortality compared to the general population. They may be at increased risk for venous thromboembolism. Chronic sickling of RBCs in the acidotic renal medulla results in microscopic and gross hematuria, hyposthenuria (poor urine concentrating ability), and possibly CKD. No treatment is necessary but genetic counseling is recommended.

Liem RI. Balancing exercise risk and benefits: lessons learned from sickle cell trait and sickle cell anemia. Hematology Am Soc Hematol Educ Program. 2018;2018:418. [PMID: 30504341]
Pecker LH et al. The current state of sickle cell trait: implications for reproductive and genetic counseling. Hematology Am Soc Hematol Educ Program. 2018;2018:474. [PMID: 30504348]

SICKLE THALASSEMIA

Patients with homozygous sickle cell anemia and alpha-thalassemia have less vigorous hemolysis and run higher hemoglobins than SS patients due to reduced RBC sickling related to a lower hemoglobin concentration within the RBC and higher hemoglobin F levels (Table 13–9). The MCV is low, and the RBCs are hypochromic.

Patients who are compound heterozygotes for beta^s and beta-thalassemia are clinically affected with sickle cell syndromes. Sickle beta^0-thalassemia is clinically very similar to homozygous SS disease. Vaso-occlusive crises may be somewhat less severe, and the spleen is not always infarcted. The MCV is low, in contrast to the normal MCV of sickle cell anemia. Hemoglobin electrophoresis reveals no hemoglobin A but will show an increase in hemoglobins A_2 and F (Table 13–9).

Sickle beta$^+$-thalassemia is a milder disorder than homozygous SS disease, with fewer pain episodes but more acute chest syndrome than sickle beta^0-thalassemia. The spleen is usually palpable. The hemolytic anemia is less severe, and the hematocrit is usually 30–38%, with reticulocytes of 5–10%. Hemoglobin electrophoresis shows the presence of some hemoglobin A and elevated hemoglobins A_2 and F (Table 13–9). The MCV is low.

AUTOIMMUNE HEMOLYTIC ANEMIA

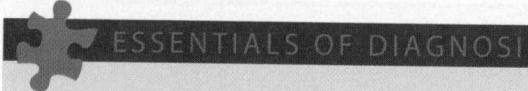

- Acquired hemolytic anemia caused by IgG autoantibody.
- Spherocytes and reticulocytosis on peripheral blood smear.
- Positive antiglobulin (Coombs) test.

General Considerations

Warm autoimmune hemolytic anemia is an acquired disorder in which an IgG autoantibody is formed that binds to a RBC membrane protein and does so most avidly at body temperature (ie, a "warm" autoantibody). The antibody is most commonly directed against a basic component of the Rh system present on RBCs. When IgG antibodies coat the RBC, the Fc portion of the antibody is recognized by macrophages present in the spleen and other portions of the reticuloendothelial system. The interaction between splenic macrophages and the antibody-coated RBC results in removal of RBC membrane and the formation of a spherocyte due to the decrease in surface-to-volume ratio of the surviving RBC. These spherocytic cells have decreased deformability and are unable to squeeze through the 2-mcm fenestrations of splenic sinusoids and become trapped in the red pulp of the spleen. When large amounts of IgG are present on RBCs, complement may be fixed. Direct complement lysis of cells is rare, but the presence of C3b on the surface of RBCs allows Kupffer cells in the liver to participate in the hemolytic process via C3b receptors. The destruction of RBCs in the spleen and liver designates this as extravascular hemolysis. The clinical distinction between extra- and intravascular hemolysis is not always straightforward.

Approximately one-half of all cases of autoimmune hemolytic anemia are idiopathic. The disorder may also be seen in association with SLE, other rheumatic disorders, chronic lymphocytic leukemia (CLL), or lymphomas. It must be distinguished from drug-induced hemolytic anemia. When penicillin (or other medications, especially cefotetan, ceftriaxone, and piperacillin) coats the RBC membrane, the autoantibody is directed against the membrane-drug complex. Fludarabine, an antineoplastic, causes autoimmune hemolytic anemia through immunoincompetence: there is defective self- versus non–self-immune surveillance permitting the escape of a B-cell clone, which produces the offending autoantibody.

Clinical Findings

A. Symptoms and Signs

Autoimmune hemolytic anemia typically produces an anemia of rapid onset that may be life-threatening. Patients complain of fatigue and dyspnea and may present with angina pectoris or heart failure. On examination, jaundice and splenomegaly are usually present.

B. Laboratory Findings

The anemia is of variable degree but may be very severe, with hematocrit of less than 10%. Reticulocytosis is present, and spherocytes are seen on the peripheral blood smear. In cases of severe hemolysis, the stressed bone marrow may also release nucleated RBCs. As with other hemolytic disorders, the serum indirect bilirubin is increased and the haptoglobin is low. Approximately 10% of patients with autoimmune hemolytic anemia have coincident immune thrombocytopenia (Evans syndrome).

The antiglobulin (Coombs) test forms the basis for diagnosis. The Coombs reagent is a rabbit IgM antibody raised against human IgG or human complement. The direct antiglobulin (Coombs) test (DAT) is performed by mixing the patient's RBCs with the Coombs reagent and looking for agglutination, which indicates the presence of IgG or both IgG and complement on the RBC surface. The indirect antiglobulin (Coombs) test is performed by mixing the patient's serum with a panel of type O RBCs. After incubation of the test serum and panel RBCs, the Coombs reagent is added. Agglutination in this system indicates the presence of free antibody (autoantibody or alloantibody) in the patient's serum.

The direct antiglobulin test is positive (for IgG or both IgG and complement) in about 90% of patients with autoimmune hemolytic anemia. A "super-Coombs" test might be positive in some of the 10% negative group. The indirect antiglobulin test may or may not be positive. A positive indirect antiglobulin test indicates the presence of a large amount of autoantibody that has saturated binding sites on the RBC and consequently appears in the serum. Because the patient's serum usually contains the autoantibody, it may be difficult to obtain a "compatible" cross-match with homologous RBCs for transfusions since the cross-match indicates the possible presence (true or false) of a RBC "alloantibody."

Treatment

Initial treatment consists of oral prednisone, 1–2 mg/kg/day. Patients with DAT-negative and DAT-positive warm autoimmune hemolysis respond equally well to corticosteroids. Transfused RBCs will survive similarly as the patient's own RBCs (ie, shortened survival). Because of difficulty in performing the cross-match, possible "incompatible" blood may need to be given. Decisions regarding transfusions should be made in consultation with a hematologist and a blood bank specialist. Death from cardiovascular collapse can occur in the setting of rapid hemolysis. In patients with rapid hemolysis, therapeutic plasmapheresis should be performed early in management to remove autoantibodies.

Patients with warm autoimmune hemolytic anemia refractory to prednisone may also be treated with a variety of agents. Treatment with rituximab, a monoclonal antibody against the B cell antigen CD20, is effective in many cases. The suggested dose is 375 mg/m^2 intravenously weekly for 4 weeks. Rituximab is used in conjunction with corticosteroids as initial therapy in some patients with severe disease. In patients with past hepatitis B virus (HBV) infection, rituximab should be used with an anti-HBV agent since HBV reactivation, fulminant hepatitis and, rarely, death can otherwise occur. Danazol, 400–800 mg/day orally, is less often effective than in immune thrombocytopenia but is well suited for long-term use because of its low toxicity profile. Immunosuppressive agents, including cyclophosphamide, vincristine, azathioprine, mycophenolate mofetil, alemtuzumab (an anti-CD52 antibody), or cyclosporine, may also be used. High-dose intravenous immune globulin (1 g/kg daily for 2 days) may be effective in controlling hemolysis, but the benefit is short-lived (1–3 weeks) and immune globulin is very expensive. If prednisone or other medical therapies are ineffective, splenectomy can be considered, which may cure the disorder. The long-term prognosis for patients with this disorder is good, especially if there is no other underlying autoimmune disorder or lymphoproliferative disorder. Treatment of an associated lymphoproliferative disorder will also treat the hemolytic anemia.

When to Refer

Patients with autoimmune hemolytic anemia should be referred to a hematologist for confirmation of the diagnosis and subsequent care.

When to Admit

Patients should be hospitalized for symptomatic anemia or rapidly falling hemoglobin levels.

Barcellini W et al. How I treat warm autoimmune hemolytic anemia. Blood. 2021;137:1283. [PMID: 33512406]

Brodsky RA. Warm autoimmune hemolytic anemia. N Engl J Med. 2019;381:647. [PMID: 31412178]

Hill QA et al. Defining autoimmune hemolytic anemia: a systematic review of the terminology used for diagnosis and treatment. Blood Adv. 2019;3:1897. [PMID: 31235526]

Jäger U et al. Diagnosis and treatment of autoimmune hemolytic anemia in adults: recommendations from the First International Consensus Meeting. Blood Rev. 2020;41:100648. [PMID: 31839434]

COLD AGGLUTININ DISEASE

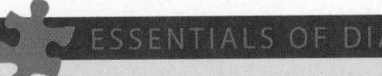

- Increased reticulocytes on peripheral blood smear.
- Antiglobulin (Coombs) test positive only for complement.
- Positive cold agglutinin titer.

General Considerations

Cold agglutinin disease is an acquired hemolytic anemia due to an IgM autoantibody (called a "cold agglutinin") usually directed against the I/i antigen on RBCs. These IgM autoantibodies characteristically will react poorly with cells at 37°C but avidly at lower temperatures, usually at 0–4°C (ie, "cold" autoantibody). Since the blood temperature (even in the most peripheral parts of the body) rarely goes lower than 20°C, only cold autoantibodies reactive at relatively higher temperatures will produce clinical effects. Hemolysis results indirectly from attachment of IgM, which in the cooler parts of the circulation (fingers, nose, ears) binds and fixes complement. When the RBC returns to a warmer temperature, the IgM antibody dissociates, leaving complement on the cell. Complement lysis of RBCs rarely occurs. Rather, C3b, present on the RBCs, is recognized by Kupffer cells (which have receptors for C3b), and RBC sequestration and destruction in the liver ensues (extravascular hemolysis). However, in some cases, the complement membrane attack complex forms, lysing the RBCs (intravascular hemolysis). The clinical distinction between extra- and intra-vascular hemolysis is not always straightforward.

Most cases of chronic cold agglutinin disease are idiopathic. Others occur in association with Waldenström macroglobulinemia, lymphoma, or CLL, in which a monoclonal IgM paraprotein is produced. Acute postinfectious cold agglutinin disease occurs following mycoplasma pneumonia or viral infection (infectious mononucleosis, measles, mumps, or cytomegalovirus [CMV] with autoantibody directed against antigen i rather than I).

Clinical Findings

A. Symptoms and Signs

In chronic cold agglutinin disease, symptoms related to RBC agglutination occur on exposure to cold, and patients may complain of mottled or numb fingers or toes, acrocyanosis, episodic low back pain, and dark-colored urine. Hemolytic anemia is occasionally severe, but episodic hemoglobinuria may occur on exposure to cold. The hemolytic anemia in acute postinfectious syndromes is rarely severe.

B. Laboratory Findings

Mild anemia is present with reticulocytosis and rarely spherocytes. The blood smear made at room temperature shows agglutinated RBCs (there is no agglutination on a blood smear made at body temperature). The direct antiglobulin (Coombs) test will be positive for complement only. Serum cold agglutinin titer will semi-quantitate the autoantibody. A monoclonal IgM is often found on serum protein electrophoresis and confirmed by serum immunoelectrophoresis. There is indirect hyperbilirubinemia and the haptoglobin is low during periods of hemolysis. Serum free hemoglobin is often elevated, and hemoglobinuria is present when intravascular hemolysis is occurring.

Treatment

Treatment is largely symptomatic, based on avoiding exposure to cold. Splenectomy and prednisone are usually ineffective (except when associated with a lymphoproliferative disorder) since hemolysis takes place in the liver and blood stream. Rituximab is the treatment of choice but in patients with past HBV infection, it must be used with anti-HBV prophylaxis. The rituximab dose is 375 mg/m^2 intravenously weekly for 4 weeks. Relapses may be effectively retreated. High-dose intravenous immunoglobulin (2 g/kg) may be temporarily effective, but it is rarely used because of the high cost and short duration of benefit. Patients with severe disease may be treated with cytotoxic agents, such as bendamustine (plus rituximab), cyclophosphamide, fludarabine, or bortezomib, or with immunosuppressive agents, such as cyclosporine. As in warm IgG-mediated autoimmune hemolysis, it may be difficult to find compatible blood for transfusion. RBCs should be transfused through an in-line blood warmer.

Berentsen S. How I treat cold agglutinin disease. Blood. 2021;137:1295. [PMID: 33512410]

Jäger U et al. Diagnosis and treatment of autoimmune hemolytic anemia in adults: recommendations from the First International Consensus Meeting. Blood Rev. 2020;41:100648. [PMID: 31839434]

APLASTIC ANEMIA

ESSENTIALS OF DIAGNOSIS

- Pancytopenia.
- No abnormal hematopoietic cells seen in blood or bone marrow.
- Hypocellular bone marrow.

General Considerations

Aplastic anemia is a condition of bone marrow failure that arises from suppression of, or injury to, the hematopoietic stem cell. The bone marrow becomes hypoplastic, fails to produce mature blood cells, and pancytopenia develops.

There are a number of causes of aplastic anemia (Table 13–10). Direct hematopoietic stem cell injury may be caused by radiation, chemotherapy, toxins, or pharmacologic agents. SLE may rarely cause suppression of the hematopoietic stem cell by an IgG autoantibody directed against it. However, the most common pathogenesis of aplastic anemia appears to be autoimmune suppression of

Table 13–10. Causes of aplastic anemia.

Autoimmune: idiopathic, SLE
Congenital: defects in telomere length maintenance or DNA repair (dyskeratosis congenita, Fanconi anemia, etc)
Chemotherapy, radiotherapy
Toxins: benzene, toluene, insecticides
Medications: chloramphenicol, gold salts, sulfonamides, phenytoin, carbamazepine, quinacrine, tolbutamide
Post-viral hepatitis (viral agent known or unknown)
Non-hepatitis viruses (EBV, parvovirus, CMV, echovirus 3, others)
Pregnancy
Paroxysmal nocturnal hemoglobinuria
Malignancy: large granular lymphocytic leukemia (T-LGL)

CMV, cytomegalovirus; EBV, Epstein-Barr virus.

hematopoiesis by a T-cell-mediated cellular mechanism, so-called idiopathic aplastic anemia. In some cases of idiopathic aplastic anemia, defects in maintenance of the hematopoietic stem cell telomere length (eg, dyskeratosis congenita) or in DNA repair pathways (eg, Fanconi anemia) have been identified and are likely linked to both the initiation of bone marrow failure and the propensity to later progress to myelodysplasia, PNH, or AML. Complex detrimental immune responses to viruses can also cause aplastic anemia.

Clinical Findings

A. Symptoms and Signs

Patients come to medical attention because of the consequences of bone marrow failure. Anemia leads to symptoms of weakness and fatigue, neutropenia causes vulnerability to bacterial or fungal infections, and thrombocytopenia results in mucosal and skin bleeding. Physical examination may reveal signs of pallor, purpura, and petechiae. Other abnormalities such as hepatosplenomegaly, lymphadenopathy, or bone tenderness should *not* be present, and their presence should lead to questioning the diagnosis.

B. Laboratory Findings

The hallmark of aplastic anemia is pancytopenia (neutropenia, anemia, and thrombocytopenia). However, early in the evolution of aplastic anemia, only one or two cell lines may be reduced.

Anemia may be severe and is always associated with reticulocytopenia. RBC morphology is unremarkable, but there may be mild macrocytosis (increased MCV). Neutrophils and platelets are reduced in number, and no immature or abnormal forms are seen on the blood smear. The bone marrow aspirate and the bone marrow biopsy appear hypocellular, with only scant amounts of morphologically normal hematopoietic progenitors. The prior dictum that the bone marrow karyotype should be normal (or germline if normal variant) has evolved and some clonal abnormalities or other genetic aberrations may be present even in the setting of idiopathic aplastic anemia.

Differential Diagnosis

Aplastic anemia must be differentiated from other causes of pancytopenia (Table 13–11). Hypocellular forms of myelodysplasia or acute leukemia may occasionally be confused with aplastic anemia. These are differentiated by the presence of cellular morphologic abnormalities, increased percentage of blasts, or abnormal karyotype in bone marrow cells typical of MDS or acute leukemia. Hairy cell leukemia has been misdiagnosed as aplastic anemia and should be recognized by the presence of splenomegaly and by abnormal "hairy" lymphoid cells in a hypocellular bone marrow biopsy. Pancytopenia with a normocellular bone marrow may be due to SLE, disseminated infection, hypersplenism, nutritional (eg, vitamin B_{12} or folate) deficiency, or myelodysplasia. Isolated thrombocytopenia may occur early as aplastic anemia develops and may be confused with immune thrombocytopenia.

Table 13–11. Causes of pancytopenia.

Bone marrow disorders
Aplastic anemia
Myelodysplasia
Acute leukemia
Chronic idiopathic myelofibrosis
Infiltrative disease: lymphoma, myeloma, carcinoma, hairy cell leukemia, etc
Non–bone marrow disorders
Hypersplenism (with or without portal hypertension)
SLE
Infection: tuberculosis, HIV, leishmaniasis, brucellosis, CMV, parvovirus B19
Nutritional deficiency (megaloblastic anemia)
Medications
Cytotoxic chemotherapy
Ionizing radiation

CMV, cytomegalovirus.

Treatment

Mild cases of idiopathic aplastic anemia may be treated with supportive care, including erythropoietic (epoetin or darbepoetin) or myeloid (filgrastim or sargramostim or biosimilars) growth factors, or both. RBC transfusions and platelet transfusions are given as necessary, and antibiotics are used to treat or prevent infections.

Severe aplastic anemia is defined by a neutrophil count of less than 500/mcL (0.5×10^9/L), platelets less than 20,000/mcL (20×10^9/L), reticulocytes less than 1%, and bone marrow cellularity less than 20%. The treatment of choice for young adults (under age 40 years) who have an HLA-matched sibling is allogeneic bone marrow transplantation. Children or young adults may also benefit from allogeneic bone marrow transplantation using an unrelated donor. Because of the increased risks associated with unrelated donor allogeneic bone marrow transplantation compared to sibling donors, this treatment is usually reserved for patients who have not responded to immunosuppressive therapy.

For adults over age 40 years or those without HLA-matched hematopoietic stem cell donors, the treatment of choice for severe idiopathic aplastic anemia is immunosuppression and hematopoietic stimulation with equine antithymocyte globulin (ATG) plus cyclosporine and eltrombopag (the thrombopoietin mimetic) (response rates approaching 90%). Equine ATG is given in the hospital in conjunction with transfusion and antibiotic support. A proven regimen is equine ATG 40 mg/kg/day intravenously for 4 days in combination with cyclosporine, 6 mg/kg orally twice daily, and eltrombopag, 150 mg orally daily. Equine ATG is superior to rabbit ATG, resulting in a higher response rate and better survival. ATG should be used in combination with corticosteroids (prednisone or methylprednisolone 1–2 mg/kg/day orally for 1 week, followed by a taper over 2 weeks) to avoid ATG infusion reactions and serum sickness. Responses usually occur in 1–3 months and are usually only partial, but the blood counts rise high enough to give patients a safe and transfusion-free life. The full benefit of immunosuppression is generally assessed at 4 months post-equine ATG. Cyclosporine and eltrombopag are maintained at full doses for 6 months and then stopped in responding patients. Androgens (such as fluoxymesterone 10–20 mg/day orally in divided doses or danazol 200 mg orally twice daily) have been widely used in the past, with a low response rate, and may be considered in mild cases.

Course & Prognosis

Patients with severe aplastic anemia have a rapidly fatal illness if left untreated. Allogeneic bone marrow transplant from an HLA-matched sibling donor produces survival rates of over 80% in recipients under 20 years old and of about 65–70% in those 20 to 50 years old. Respective survival rates drop by 10–15% when the donor is HLA-matched but unrelated. Equine ATG-cyclosporine immunosuppressive treatment leads to a response in approximately 70% of patients (including those with hepatitis virus–associated aplastic anemia) and in up to 90% of patients with the addition of eltrombopag. Up to one-third of patients will relapse with aplastic anemia after ATG-based therapy. Clonal hematologic disorders, such as PNH, AML, or myelodysplasia, may develop in one-quarter of patients treated with immunosuppressive therapy after 10 years of follow-up. Factors that predict response to ATG-cyclosporine therapy are patient's age, reticulocyte count, lymphocyte count, and age-adjusted telomere length of leukocytes at the time of diagnosis.

When to Refer

All patients should be referred to a hematologist.

When to Admit

Admission is necessary for treatment of neutropenic infection, the administration of ATG, or allogeneic bone marrow transplantation.

DeZern AE et al. Approach to the diagnosis of aplastic anemia. Blood Adv. 2021;5:2660. [PMID: 34156438]

Georges GE et al. Severe aplastic anemia: allogeneic bone marrow transplantation as first line treatment. Blood Adv. 2020;2:2020. [PMID: 30108110]

Marsh JCW et al. The case for upfront HLA-matched unrelated donor hematopoietic stem cell transplantation as a curative option for adult acquired severe aplastic anemia. Biol Blood Marrow Transplant. 2019;25:e277. [PMID: 31129354]

Zhu Y et al. Allo-HSCT compared with immunosuppressive therapy for acquired aplastic anemia: a system review and meta-analysis. BMC Immunol. 2020;2:10. [PMID: 32138642]

NEUTROPENIA

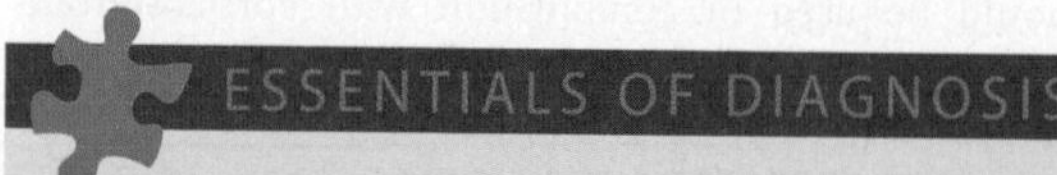

- Neutrophils < 1800/mcL (1.8×10^9/L).
- Severe if neutrophils < 500/mcL (0.5×10^9/L).

General Considerations

Neutropenia is present when the absolute neutrophil count is less than 1800/mcL (1.8×10^9/L), although Black, Asian, and other persons in specific ethnic groups may have normal neutrophil counts as low as 800–1200/mcL (1.2×10^9/L) or even less. The neutropenic patient is increasingly vulnerable to infection by gram-positive and gram-negative bacteria and by fungi. The risk of infection is related to the severity of neutropenia. The risk of serious infection rises sharply with neutrophil counts below 500/mcL (0.5×10^9/L), and a high risk of infection within days occurs with neutrophil counts below 100/mcL (0.1×10^9/L) ("profound neutropenia"). The classification of neutropenic syndromes is unsatisfactory as the pathophysiology and natural history of different syndromes overlap. Patients with "chronic benign neutropenia" are free of infection despite very low stable neutrophil counts; they respond adequately to infections and inflammatory stimuli with an appropriate neutrophil release from the bone marrow. In contrast, the neutrophil count of patients with cyclic neutropenia periodically oscillates (usually in 21-day cycles) between normal and low, with infections occurring during the nadirs. Congenital neutropenia is lifelong neutropenia punctuated with bouts of infection.

A variety of bone marrow disorders and non-marrow conditions may cause neutropenia (Table 13–12). All of the causes of aplastic anemia (Table 13–10) and pancytopenia (Table 13–11) may cause neutropenia. The new onset of an isolated neutropenia is most often due to an idiosyncratic reaction to a medication, and agranulocytosis (complete absence of neutrophils in the peripheral blood) is almost always due to a drug reaction. In these cases, examination of the bone marrow shows an almost complete absence of granulocyte precursors with other cell lines undisturbed. Neutropenia in the presence of a normal bone marrow may

Table 13–12. Causes of neutropenia.

Bone marrow disorders
Congenital
Dyskeratosis congenita
Fanconi anemia
Cyclic neutropenia
Congenital neutropenia
Hairy cell leukemia
Large granular lymphoproliferative disorder
Myelodysplasia
Non–bone marrow disorders
Medications: antiretroviral medications, cephalosporins, chlorpromazine, chlorpropamide, cimetidine, methimazole, myelosuppressive cytotoxic chemotherapy, penicillin, phenytoin, procainamide, rituximab, sulfonamides
Aplastic anemia
Benign chronic neutropenia
Pure WBC aplasia
Hypersplenism
Sepsis
Other immune
Autoimmune (idiopathic)
Felty syndrome
SLE
HIV infection

be due to immunologic peripheral destruction (autoimmune neutropenia), sepsis, or hypersplenism. The presence in the serum of antineutrophil antibodies supports the diagnosis of autoimmune neutropenia but does not prove this as the pathophysiologic reason for neutropenia. **Felty syndrome** is an immune neutropenia associated with seropositive nodular rheumatoid arthritis and splenomegaly. Severe neutropenia may be associated with clonal disorders of T lymphocytes, often with the morphology of large granular lymphocytes, referred to as CD3-positive T-cell large granular lymphoproliferative disorder. Isolated neutropenia is an uncommon presentation of hairy cell leukemia or MDS. By its nature, myelosuppressive cytotoxic chemotherapy causes neutropenia in a predictable manner.

Clinical Findings

Neutropenia results in stomatitis and in infections due to gram-positive or gram-negative aerobic bacteria or to fungi such as *Candida* or *Aspergillus*. The most common infectious syndromes are sinusitis, cellulitis, pneumonia, septicemia, and neutropenic fever of unknown origin. Fever in neutropenic patients should always be initially assumed to be of infectious origin until proven otherwise (Chapter 30).

Treatment

Treatment of neutropenia depends on its cause. Potential causative medications should be discontinued. Myeloid growth factors (filgrastim or sargramostim or biosimilar myeloid growth factors) help facilitate neutrophil recovery after offending medications are stopped. Chronic myeloid growth factor administration (daily or every other day) is effective at dampening the neutropenia seen in cyclic or congenital neutropenia. When Felty syndrome leads to repeated bacterial infections, splenectomy has been the treatment of choice, but sustained use of myeloid growth factors is effective and provides a nonsurgical alternative. Patients with autoimmune neutropenia respond briefly to immunosuppression with corticosteroids and are best managed with intermittent doses of myeloid growth factors. The neutropenia associated with large granular lymphoproliferative disorder may respond to therapy with oral methotrexate, cyclophosphamide, or cyclosporine.

Fevers during neutropenia should be considered as infectious until proven otherwise. Febrile neutropenia is a life-threatening circumstance. Enteric gram-negative bacteria are of primary concern and often empirically treated with fluoroquinolones or third- or fourth-generation cephalosporins (see Infections in the Immunocompromised Patient, Chapter 30). For protracted neutropenia, fungal infections are problematic and empiric coverage with azoles (fluconazole for yeast and voriconazole, itraconazole, posaconazole, or isavuconazole for molds) or echinocandins is recommended. The neutropenia following myelosuppressive chemotherapy is predictable and is partially ameliorated by the use of myeloid growth factors. For patients with acute leukemia undergoing intense chemotherapy or patients with solid cancer undergoing high-dose chemotherapy, the prophylactic use of antimicrobial agents and myeloid growth factors is recommended.

When to Refer

Refer to a hematologist if neutrophils are persistently and unexplainably less than 1000/mcL (1.0×10^9/L).

When to Admit

Neutropenia by itself is not an indication for hospitalization. However, many patients with severe neutropenia may have a serious underlying disease that may require inpatient treatment. Most patients with febrile neutropenia require hospitalization to treat infection.

Abdel-Azim H et al. Strategies to generate functionally normal neutrophils to reduce infection and infection-related mortality in cancer chemotherapy. Pharmacol Ther. 2019;204:107403. [PMID: 31470030]

Atallah-Yunes SA et al. Benign ethnic neutropenia. Blood Rev. 2019;37:100586. [PMID: 31255364]

Frater JL. How I investigate neutropenia. Int J Lab Hematol. 2020;42:121. [PMID: 32543073]

Singh N et al. Isolated chronic and transient neutropenia. Cureus. 2019;11:e5616. [PMID: 31720132]

LEUKEMIAS & OTHER MYELOPROLIFERATIVE NEOPLASMS

Myeloproliferative disorders are due to acquired clonal abnormalities of the hematopoietic stem cell. Since the stem cell gives rise to myeloid, erythroid, and platelet cells, qualitative and quantitative changes are seen in all of these cell lines. Classically, the myeloproliferative disorders produce characteristic syndromes with well-defined clinical and laboratory features (Tables 13–13 and 13–14). However, these disorders are grouped together because they may evolve from one into another and because hybrid disorders are commonly seen. All of the myeloproliferative disorders may progress to AML.

Table 13–13. World Health Organization classification of myeloproliferative disorders (modified).

Myeloproliferative neoplasms
Chronic myeloid leukemia, *BCR-ABL1*–positive
Chronic neutrophilic leukemia
Polycythemia vera
Primary myelofibrosis (PMF)
Essential thrombocythemia
Chronic eosinophilic leukemia, not otherwise specified (NOS)
Myeloproliferative neoplasm, unclassifiable
Mastocytosis
Myelodysplastic/myeloproliferative neoplasms (MDS/MPN)
Myelodysplastic syndromes
Acute myeloid leukemia and related neoplasms
Acute myeloid leukemia with recurrent genetic abnormalities
Acute myeloid leukemia with myelodysplasia-related changes
Therapy-related myeloid neoplasms
Acute myeloid leukemia, NOS
Myeloid sarcoma
Myeloid proliferations related to Down syndrome
Acute leukemias of ambiguous lineage
B lymphoblastic leukemia/lymphoma
T lymphoblastic leukemia/lymphoma

Table 13–14. Laboratory features of myeloproliferative neoplasms.

	White Count	Hematocrit	Platelet Count	RBC Morphology
Polycythemia vera	N or ↑	↑↑	N or ↑	N
Essential thrombocytosis	N or ↑	N	↑↑	N
Primary myelofibrosis	N or ↓ or ↑	↓	↓ or N or ↑	Abn
Chronic myeloid leukemia	↑↑	N or ↓	N or ↑ or ↓	N

Abn, abnormal; N, normal.

The Philadelphia chromosome seen in chronic myeloid leukemia (CML) was the first recurrent cytogenetic abnormality to be described in a human malignancy. Since that time, there has been tremendous progress in elucidating the genetic nature of these disorders, with identification of mutations in *JAK2, MPL, CALR, CSF3R*, and other genes.

Masarova L et al. The rationale for immunotherapy in myeloproliferative neoplasms. Curr Hematol Malig Rep. 2019;14:310. [PMID: 31228096]

Schwede M et al. Diagnosis and management of neutrophilic myeloid neoplasms. Clin Adv Hematol Oncol. 2021;19:450. [PMID: 34236344]

POLYCYTHEMIA VERA

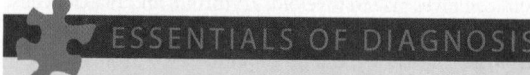

- *JAK2 (V617F)* mutation.
- Splenomegaly.
- Normal arterial oxygen saturation.
- Usually elevated white blood count and platelet count.

General Considerations

Polycythemia vera is an acquired myeloproliferative disorder that causes overproduction of all three hematopoietic cell lines, most prominently the RBCs. Erythroid production is independent of erythropoietin, and the serum erythropoietin level is low. True erythrocytosis, with an elevated RBC mass, should be distinguished from spurious erythrocytosis caused by a constricted plasma volume.

A mutation in exon 14 of *JAK2 (V617F)*, a signaling molecule, has been demonstrated in 95% of cases. Additional *JAK2* mutations have been identified (exon 12) and suggest that *JAK2* is involved in the pathogenesis of this disease and is a therapeutic target.

Clinical Findings

A. Symptoms and Signs

Headache, dizziness, tinnitus, blurred vision, and fatigue are common complaints related to expanded blood volume and increased blood viscosity. Generalized pruritus, especially following a warm shower or bath, is related to histamine release from the basophilia. Epistaxis is related to engorgement of mucosal blood vessels in combination with abnormal hemostasis. Sixty percent of patients are men, and the median age at presentation is 60 years. Polycythemia rarely occurs in persons under age 40 years.

Physical examination reveals plethora and engorged retinal veins. The spleen is palpable in 75% of cases but is nearly always enlarged when imaged. Thrombosis is the most common complication of polycythemia vera and the major cause of morbidity and death in this disorder. Thrombosis appears to be related both to increased blood viscosity and abnormal platelet function. Uncontrolled polycythemia leads to a very high incidence of thrombotic complications of surgery, and elective surgery should be deferred until the condition has been treated. Paradoxically, in addition to thrombosis, increased bleeding can occur. There is also a high incidence of peptic ulcer disease.

B. Laboratory Findings

According to the WHO 2016 criteria, the hallmark of polycythemia vera is a hematocrit (at sea level) that exceeds 49% in males or 48% in females. RBC morphology is normal (Table 13–14). The white blood count is usually elevated to 10,000–20,000/mcL ($10–20 \times 10^9$/L), and the platelet count is variably increased, sometimes to counts exceeding 1,000,000/mcL (1000×10^9/L). Platelet morphology is usually normal. WBCs are usually normal, but basophilia and eosinophilia are frequently present. Erythropoietin is suppressed and serum levels, usually low. The diagnosis should be confirmed with *JAK2* mutation screening. The absence of a mutation in either exon 14 (most common) or 12 should lead the clinician to question the diagnosis.

The bone marrow is hypercellular, with hyperplasia of all hematopoietic elements, but bone marrow examination is not necessary to establish the diagnosis. Iron stores are usually absent from the bone marrow, having been transferred to the increased circulating RBC mass. Iron deficiency may also result from chronic GI blood loss. Bleeding may lower the hematocrit to the normal range (or lower), creating diagnostic confusion, and may lead to a situation with significant microcytosis yet a normal hematocrit.

Vitamin B_{12} levels are strikingly elevated because of increased levels of transcobalamin III (secreted by WBCs). Overproduction of uric acid may lead to hyperuricemia.

Although RBC morphology is usually normal at presentation, microcytosis, hypochromia, and poikilocytosis may result from iron deficiency following treatment by phlebotomy. Progressive hypersplenism may also lead to elliptocytosis (eg, with RBCs the size and shape of those in hereditary elliptocytosis).

Differential Diagnosis

Spurious polycythemia, in which an elevated hematocrit is due to contracted plasma volume rather than increased RBC mass, may be related to diuretic use or may occur without obvious cause.

A secondary cause of polycythemia should be suspected if splenomegaly is absent and the high hematocrit is not accompanied by increases in other cell lines. Secondary causes of polycythemia include hypoxia and smoking; carboxyhemoglobin levels may be elevated in smokers (Table 13–15). A renal CT scan or sonogram may be considered to look for an erythropoietin-secreting cyst or tumor. A positive family history should lead to investigation for a congenital high-oxygen-affinity hemoglobin. An absence of a mutation in *JAK2* suggests a different diagnosis. However, *JAK2* mutations are also commonly found in other myeloproliferative disorders, essential thrombocytosis, and myelofibrosis.

Polycythemia vera should be differentiated from other myeloproliferative disorders (Table 13–14). Marked elevation of the white blood count (above 30,000/mcL [30×10^9/L]) suggests CML. Abnormal RBC morphology and nucleated RBCs in the peripheral blood are seen in myelofibrosis. Essential thrombocytosis is suggested when the platelet count is strikingly elevated.

Treatment

The treatment of choice is phlebotomy. One unit of blood (approximately 500 mL) is removed weekly until the hematocrit is less than 45%; the hematocrit is maintained at less than 45% by repeated phlebotomy as necessary. Patients for whom phlebotomy is problematic (because of poor venous access or logistical reasons) may be managed primarily with hydroxyurea. Because repeated phlebotomy intentionally produces iron deficiency, the requirement for phlebotomy should gradually decrease. It is important to avoid medicinal iron supplementation, as this can thwart the goals of a phlebotomy program. A diet low in iron is not necessary but will increase the intervals between phlebotomies. Maintaining the hematocrit at normal levels has been shown to decrease the incidence of thrombotic complications.

Occasionally, myelosuppressive therapy is indicated. Indications include a high phlebotomy requirement, thrombocytosis, and intractable pruritus. There is evidence that reduction of the platelet count to less than 600,000/mcL (600×10^9/L) will reduce the risk of thrombotic complications. Hydroxyurea is widely used when myelosuppressive therapy is indicated. The usual dose is 500–1500 mg/day orally, adjusted to keep platelets less than 500,000/mcL (500×10^9/L) without reducing the neutrophil count to less than 2000/mcL (2.0×10^9/L). Alkylating agents, such as busulfan and pipobroman, can be used for refractory cases but have been shown to increase the risk of conversion of this disease to acute leukemia and thus should be used with caution.

A randomized phase 3 trial comparing ropeginterferon alfa-2b, a novel interferon, to hydroxyurea demonstrated improved disease control rates in patients presenting without splenomegaly with 53% vs 38% of patients achieving a complete hematologic response and with improved disease burden at 3 years' follow-up. Toxicity included abnormal liver biochemical tests in the ropeginterferon alfa-2b group, and leukopenia and thrombocytopenia in the standard therapy group, with serious adverse events occurring in 2% in the former and 4% in the latter group. As a result, ropeginterferon alfa-2b was approved by the European Medicines Agency as first-line therapy for patients without symptomatic splenomegaly.

Low-dose aspirin (75–81 mg/day orally) has been shown to reduce the risk of thrombosis without excessive bleeding and should be part of therapy for all patients without contraindications to aspirin. Aspirin should be used with caution in patients with extreme thrombocytosis due to the likelihood of acquired von Willebrand disease. Allopurinol 300 mg orally daily may be indicated for hyperuricemia. Antihistamine therapy with diphenhydramine or other H_1-blockers and, rarely, SSRIs are used to manage pruritus.

Prognosis

Polycythemia is an indolent disease with median survival of over 15 years. The major cause of morbidity and mortality is arterial thrombosis. Over time, polycythemia vera may convert to myelofibrosis. In approximately 5% of cases, the disorder progresses to AML, which is usually refractory to therapy.

When to Refer

Patients with polycythemia vera should be referred to a hematologist.

When to Admit

Inpatient care is rarely required.

Barbui T et al. The 2016 revision of WHO classification of myeloproliferative neoplasms: clinical and molecular advances. Blood Rev. 2016;30:453. [PMID: 27341755]

Gangat N et al. *JAK2* unmutated erythrocytosis: current diagnostic approach and therapeutic views. Leukemia. 2021;35:2166. [PMID: 34021251]

Gisslinger H et al; PROUD-PV Study Group. Ropeginterferon alfa-2b versus standard therapy for polycythaemia vera (PROUD-PV and CONTINUATION-PV): a randomised, non-inferiority, phase 3 trial and its extension study. Lancet Haematol. 2020;7:e196. [PMID: 32014125]

Table 13–15. Causes of polycythemia.

Spurious polycythemia
Secondary polycythemia
Hypoxia: cardiac disease, pulmonary disease, high altitude
Carboxyhemoglobin: smoking
Erythropoietin-secreting tumors, eg, kidney lesions (rare)
Abnormal hemoglobins (rare)
Polycythemia vera

Ronner L et al. Improving the investigative approach to polycythaemia vera: a critical assessment of current evidence and vision for the future. Lancet Haematol. 2021;8:e605. [PMID: 34329580]

Tefferi A et al. Polycythemia vera and essential thrombocythemia: 2021 update on diagnosis, risk-stratification and management. Am J Hematol. 2020;95:1599. [PMID: 32974939]

ESSENTIAL THROMBOCYTOSIS

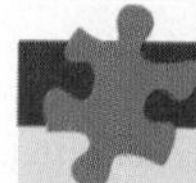

ESSENTIALS OF DIAGNOSIS

- Elevated platelet count in absence of other causes.
- Normal RBC mass.
- Absence of *bcr/abl* gene (Philadelphia chromosome).

General Considerations

Essential thrombocytosis is an uncommon myeloproliferative disorder in which marked proliferation of the megakaryocytes in the bone marrow leads to elevation of the platelet count. As with polycythemia vera, the finding of a high frequency of mutations of *JAK2* and others in these patients has advanced the understanding of this disorder.

Clinical Findings

A. Symptoms and Signs

The median age at presentation is 50–60 years, and there is a slightly increased incidence in women. The disorder is often suspected when an elevated platelet count is found. Less frequently, the first sign is thrombosis, which is the most common clinical problem. The risk of thrombosis rises with age. Venous thromboses may occur in unusual sites such as the mesenteric, hepatic, or portal vein. Some patients experience erythromelalgia, painful burning of the hands accompanied by erythema; this symptom is reliably relieved by aspirin. Bleeding, typically mucosal, is less common and is related to a concomitant qualitative platelet defect. Splenomegaly is present in at least 25% of patients.

B. Laboratory Findings

An elevated platelet count is the hallmark of this disorder and may be over 2,000,000/mcL (2000×10^9/L) (Table 13–14). The WBC count is often mildly elevated, usually not above 30,000/mcL (30×10^9/L), but with some immature myeloid forms. The hematocrit is normal. The peripheral blood smear reveals large platelets, but giant degranulated forms seen in myelofibrosis are not observed. RBC morphology is normal.

The bone marrow shows increased numbers of megakaryocytes but no other morphologic abnormalities. The peripheral blood should be tested for the *bcr/abl* fusion gene (Philadelphia chromosome) since it can differentiate CML, where it is present, from essential thrombocytosis, where it is absent.

Differential Diagnosis

Essential thrombocytosis must be distinguished from secondary causes of an elevated platelet count. In reactive thrombocytosis, the platelet count seldom exceeds 1,000,000/mcL (1000×10^9/L). Inflammatory disorders such as rheumatoid arthritis and ulcerative colitis cause significant elevations of the platelet count, as may chronic infection. The thrombocytosis of iron deficiency is observed only when anemia is significant. The platelet count is temporarily elevated after a splenectomy. *JAK2* mutations are found in over 50% of cases. *MPL* and *CALR* mutations frequently occur in patients with *JAK2*-negative essential thrombocytosis.

Regarding other myeloproliferative disorders, the lack of erythrocytosis distinguishes it from polycythemia vera. Unlike myelofibrosis, RBC morphology is normal, nucleated RBCs are absent, and giant degranulated platelets are not seen. In CML, the Philadelphia chromosome (or *bcr/abl* by molecular testing) establishes the diagnosis.

Treatment

Patients are considered at high risk for thrombosis if they are older than 60 years, have a *JAK2* mutation, and have a previous history of thrombosis. They also have a higher risk for bleeding. The risk of thrombosis can be reduced by control of the platelet count, which should be kept under 500,000/mcL (500×10^9/L). The treatment of choice is oral hydroxyurea in a dose of 500–1000 mg/day. In rare cases in which hydroxyurea is not well tolerated because of anemia, low doses of anagrelide, 1–2 mg/day orally, may be added. Higher doses of anagrelide can be complicated by headache, peripheral edema, and heart failure. Pegylated interferon alfa-2 can induce significant hematologic responses and can potentially target the malignant clone in *CALR*-mutant cases. Strict control of coexistent cardiovascular risk factors is mandatory for all patients.

Vasomotor symptoms such as erythromelalgia and paresthesias respond rapidly to aspirin. Historically, low-dose aspirin (81 mg/day orally) has been used to reduce the risk of thrombotic complications in low-risk patients, but a recent study found that once daily dosing is not as effective as an every 12-hour regimen. In the unusual event of severe bleeding, the platelet count can be lowered rapidly with plateletpheresis. In cases of marked thrombocytosis (greater than or equal to 1,000,000/mcL [1000×10^9/L]) or of any evidence of bleeding, acquired von Willebrand syndrome must be excluded before starting low-dose aspirin.

Course & Prognosis

Essential thrombocytosis is an indolent disorder that allows long-term survival. Average survival is longer than 15 years from diagnosis, and the survival of patients younger than age 50 years does not appear different from matched controls. The major source of morbidity—thrombosis—can be reduced by appropriate platelet control. Late in the disease course, the bone marrow may become fibrotic, and massive splenomegaly may occur, sometimes with splenic infarction. There is a 10–15% risk of progression to myelofibrosis after 15 years, and a 1–5% risk of transformation to acute leukemia over 20 years.

When to Refer

Patients with essential thrombocytosis should be referred to a hematologist.

Bewersdorf JP et al. Novel and combination therapies for polycythemia vera and essential thrombocythemia: the dawn of a new era. Expert Rev Hematol. 2020;13:1189. [PMID: 33076714]

Rocca B et al. A randomized double-blind trial of 3 aspirin regimens to optimize antiplatelet therapy in essential thrombocythemia. Blood. 2020;136:171. [PMID: 32266380]

PRIMARY MYELOFIBROSIS

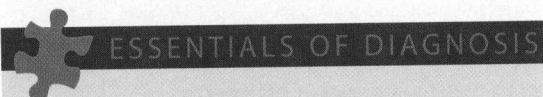

- Striking splenomegaly.
- Teardrop poikilocytosis on peripheral smear.
- Leukoerythroblastic blood picture; giant abnormal platelets.
- Initially hypercellular, then hypocellular bone marrow with reticulin or collagen fibrosis.

General Considerations

Primary myelofibrosis is a myeloproliferative disorder characterized by clonal hematopoiesis that is often but not always accompanied by *JAK2*, *CALR*, or *MPL* mutations; bone marrow fibrosis; anemia; splenomegaly; and a leukoerythroblastic peripheral blood picture with teardrop poikilocytosis. Myelofibrosis can also occur as a secondary process following the other myeloproliferative disorders (eg, polycythemia vera, essential thrombocytosis). It is believed that fibrosis occurs in response to increased secretion of platelet-derived growth factor (PDGF) and possibly other cytokines. In response to bone marrow fibrosis, extramedullary hematopoiesis takes place in the liver, spleen, and lymph nodes. In these sites, mesenchymal cells responsible for fetal hematopoiesis can be reactivated. According to the 2016 WHO classification, "prefibrotic" primary myelofibrosis is distinguished from "overtly fibrotic" primary myelofibrosis; the former might mimic essential thrombocytosis in its presentation, and it is prognostically relevant to distinguish the two.

Clinical Findings

A. Symptoms and Signs

Primary myelofibrosis develops in adults over age 50 years and is usually insidious in onset. Patients most commonly present with fatigue due to anemia or abdominal fullness related to splenomegaly. Uncommon presentations include bleeding and bone pain. On examination, splenomegaly is almost invariably present and is commonly massive. The liver is enlarged in more than 50% of cases.

Later in the course of the disease, progressive bone marrow failure takes place as it becomes increasingly more fibrotic. Progressive thrombocytopenia leads to bleeding. The spleen continues to enlarge, which leads to early satiety. Painful episodes of splenic infarction may occur. The patient becomes cachectic and may experience severe bone pain, especially in the upper legs. Hematopoiesis in the liver leads to portal hypertension with ascites and esophageal varices, and occasionally myelopoiesis in the epidural space causes transverse myelitis.

B. Laboratory Findings

Patients are almost invariably anemic at presentation. The white blood count is variable—either low, normal, or elevated—and may be increased to 50,000/mcL (50×10^9/L). The platelet count is variable. The peripheral blood smear is dramatic, with significant poikilocytosis and numerous teardrop forms in the RBC line. Nucleated RBCs are present, and the myeloid series is shifted, with immature forms including a small percentage of promyelocytes or myeloblasts. Platelet morphology may be bizarre, and giant degranulated platelet forms (megakaryocyte fragments) may be seen. The triad of teardrop poikilocytosis, leukoerythroblastic blood, and giant abnormal platelets is highly suggestive of myelofibrosis.

The bone marrow usually cannot be aspirated (dry tap), though early in the course of the disease, biopsy shows it to be hypercellular, with a marked increase in megakaryocytes. Fibrosis at this stage is detected by a silver stain demonstrating increased reticulin fibers. Later, biopsy reveals more severe fibrosis, with eventual replacement of hematopoietic precursors by collagen. There is no characteristic chromosomal abnormality. *JAK2* is mutated in ~65% of cases, and *MPL* and *CALR* are mutated in the majority of the remaining cases; 10% of cases are "triple-negative."

Differential Diagnosis

A leukoerythroblastic blood picture from other causes may be seen in response to severe infection, inflammation, or infiltrative bone marrow processes. However, teardrop poikilocytosis and giant abnormal platelet forms will not be present. Bone marrow fibrosis may be seen in metastatic carcinoma, Hodgkin lymphoma, and hairy cell leukemia. These disorders are diagnosed by characteristic morphology of involved tissues.

Of the other myeloproliferative disorders, CML is diagnosed when there is marked leukocytosis, normal RBC morphology, and the presence of the *bcr/abl* fusion gene. Polycythemia vera is characterized by an elevated hematocrit. Essential thrombocytosis shows predominant platelet count elevations.

Treatment

Observation with supportive care is a reasonable treatment strategy for asymptomatic patients with low risk or an intermediate risk, especially in the absence of high-risk mutations.

Anemic patients are supported with transfusion. Anemia can also be controlled with androgens, prednisone, thalidomide, or lenalidomide. First-line therapy for myelofibrosis-associated splenomegaly is hydroxyurea 500–1000 mg/day orally, which is effective in reducing spleen size by half in approximately 40% of patients. Both thalidomide and lenalidomide may improve splenomegaly and thrombocytopenia in some patients. Splenectomy is not routinely performed but is indicated for medication-refractory splenic enlargement causing recurrent painful episodes, severe thrombocytopenia, or an unacceptable transfusion requirement. Perioperative complications can occur in 28% of patients and include infections, abdominal vein thrombosis, and bleeding. Radiation therapy has a role for painful sites of extramedullary hematopoiesis, pulmonary hypertension, or severe bone pain. Transjugular intrahepatic portosystemic shunt might also be considered to alleviate symptoms of portal hypertension.

Certain patients with intermediate-risk and those with high- or very high-risk disease should be considered for allogeneic stem cell transplant, which is currently the only potentially curative treatment modality for primary myelofibrosis. Nontransplant candidates may be treated with JAK2 inhibitors or immunomodulatory agents for symptom control. Ruxolitinib, an FDA-approved JAK2 inhibitor, results in reduction of spleen size and improvement of constitutional symptoms but does not induce complete clinical or cytogenetic remissions or significantly affect the *JAK2/CALR/MPL* mutant allele burden. Moreover, ruxolitinib can exacerbate cytopenias. Another FDA-approved selective JAK2 inhibitor, fedratinib, can lead to sustained reduction in spleen size and improvement in disease-associated symptoms for patients with advanced- stage myelofibrosis. However, it carries a significant risk of serious and fatal encephalopathy, including Wernicke encephalopathy, and providers should regularly assess thiamine levels in all patients. The immunomodulatory medications lenalidomide and pomalidomide result in control of anemia in 25% and thrombocytopenia in ~58% of cases, without significant reduction in splenic size.

Course & Prognosis

The median survival from time of diagnosis is approximately 5 years. Therapies with biologic agents and the application of reduced-intensity allogeneic stem cell transplantation appear to offer the possibility of improving the outcome for many patients. End-stage myelofibrosis is characterized by generalized asthenia, liver failure, and bleeding from thrombocytopenia, with some cases terminating in AML. Two new prognostic systems for primary myelofibrosis have recently been introduced: GIPSS (genetically inspired prognostic scoring system) and MIPSS70+ version 2.0 (MIPSSv2; genetic variant- (formerly, mutation-) and karyotype-enhanced international prognostic scoring system). GIPSS is based exclusively on mutations and karyotype. MIPSSv2 includes, in addition to genetic and karyotypic variants, clinical risk factors. Patients with certain pathogenic variants including *ASXL1* and *SRSF2* have an adverse prognosis regardless of clinical features. By contrast, patients with type 1/like *CALR* variants, compared to their counterparts with other driver mutations, experience significantly better survival.

When to Refer

Patients in whom myelofibrosis is suspected should be referred to a hematologist.

When to Admit

Admission is not usually necessary.

Rumi E et al. The genetic basis of primary myelofibrosis and its clinical relevance. Int J Mol Sci. 2020;21:8885. [PMID: 33255170]

Talpaz M et al. Fedratinib, a newly approved treatment for patients with myeloproliferative neoplasm-associated myelofibrosis. Leukemia. 2021;35:1. [PMID: 32647323]

Tefferi A. Primary myelofibrosis: 2021 update on diagnosis, risk-stratification and management. Am J Hematol. 2021;96:145. [PMID: 33197049]

CHRONIC MYELOID LEUKEMIA

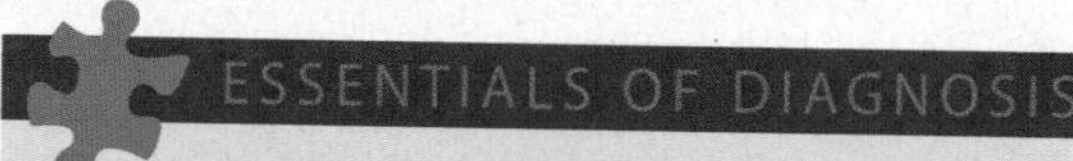

- Elevated WBC count.
- Markedly left-shifted myeloid series but with a low percentage of promyelocytes and blasts.
- Presence of *bcr/abl* gene (Philadelphia chromosome).

General Considerations

CML is a myeloproliferative disorder characterized by overproduction of myeloid cells. These myeloid cells continue to differentiate and circulate in increased numbers in the peripheral blood.

CML is characterized by a specific chromosomal abnormality and a specific molecular abnormality. The **Philadelphia chromosome** is a reciprocal translocation between the long arms of chromosomes 9 and 22. The fusion gene *bcr/abl* produces a novel protein that possesses tyrosine kinase activity. This disorder is the first recognized example of tyrosine kinase "addiction" by cancer cells.

Early CML ("chronic phase") does not behave like a malignant disease. Normal bone marrow function is retained, WBCs differentiate, and despite some qualitative abnormalities, the neutrophils combat infections normally. However, untreated CML is inherently unstable, and without treatment, the disease progresses to an "accelerated" phase and then an "acute blast" phase, which is morphologically indistinguishable from acute leukemia.

Clinical Findings

A. Symptoms and Signs

CML is a disorder of middle age (median age at presentation is 55 years). Patients usually complain of fatigue, night sweats, and low-grade fevers related to the hypermetabolic state caused by overproduction of WBCs. Patients may also complain of abdominal fullness related to splenomegaly. In some cases, an elevated white blood count is discovered incidentally. Rarely, the patient will present with a clinical syndrome related to leukostasis with blurred vision, respiratory distress, or priapism. The white blood count in these cases is usually greater than 100,000/mcL (100×10^9/L) but less than 500,000/mcL (500×10^9/L). On examination, the spleen is enlarged (often markedly so), and sternal tenderness may be present as a sign of marrow overexpansion. In cases discovered during routine laboratory monitoring, these findings are often absent. Acceleration of the disease is often associated with fever (in the absence of infection), bone pain, and splenomegaly.

B. Laboratory Findings

CML is characterized by an elevated WBC count; the median white blood count at diagnosis is 150,000/mcL (150×10^9/L), although in some cases the WBC count is only modestly increased (Table 13–14). The peripheral blood is characteristic. The myeloid series is left shifted, with mature forms dominating and with cells usually present in proportion to their degree of maturation. Blasts are usually less than 5%. Basophilia and eosinophilia may be present. At presentation, the patient is usually not anemic. RBC morphology is normal, and nucleated RBCs are rarely seen. The platelet count may be normal or elevated (sometimes to strikingly high levels). A bone marrow biopsy is essential to ensure sufficient material for a complete karyotype and for morphologic evaluation to confirm the phase of disease. The bone marrow is hypercellular, with left-shifted myelopoiesis. Myeloblasts compose less than 5% of marrow cells. The hallmark of the disease is the *bcr/abl* gene that is detected by PCR testing of the peripheral blood and bone marrow.

With progression to the accelerated and blast phases, progressive anemia and thrombocytopenia occur, and the percentage of blasts in the blood and bone marrow increases. Blast-phase CML is diagnosed when blasts comprise more than 20% of bone marrow cells.

Differential Diagnosis

Early CML must be differentiated from the reactive leukocytosis associated with infection. In such cases, the white blood count is usually less than 50,000/mcL (50×10^9/L), splenomegaly is absent, and the *bcr/abl* gene is not present.

CML must be distinguished from other myeloproliferative disease (Table 13–14). The hematocrit should not be elevated, the RBC morphology is normal, and nucleated RBCs are rare or absent. Definitive diagnosis is made by finding the *bcr/abl* gene.

Treatment

Treatment is usually not emergent even with white blood counts over 200,000/mcL (200×10^9/L), since the majority of circulating cells are mature myeloid cells that are smaller and more deformable than primitive leukemic blasts. In the rare instances in which symptoms result from extreme hyperleukocytosis (priapism, respiratory distress, visual blurring, altered mental status), emergent leukapheresis is performed in conjunction with myelosuppressive therapy.

In chronic-phase CML, the goal of therapy is normalization of the hematologic abnormalities and suppression of the malignant *bcr/abl*-expressing clone. The treatment of choice consists of a tyrosine kinase inhibitor (eg, imatinib, nilotinib, dasatinib, bosutinib) targeting the aberrantly active abl kinase. It is expected that a hematologic complete remission, with normalization of blood counts and splenomegaly will occur within 3 months of treatment initiation. Second, a reduction of *bcr/abl* transcripts to less than 10% on the international scale should be achieved, ideally within 3 months but certainly within 6 months. Finally, a major molecular response (less than or equal to 0.1% transcripts) is desired within 12 months. Patients who achieve this level of molecular response have an excellent prognosis, with overall survival approaching 100% since disease progression is uncommon. On the other hand, patients have a worse prognosis if these targets are not achieved, molecular response is subsequently lost, or new pathogenic variants or cytogenetic abnormalities develop.

Imatinib mesylate was the first tyrosine kinase inhibitor to be approved and it results in nearly universal (98%) hematologic control of chronic-phase disease at a dose of 400 mg/day. The rate of a major molecular response with imatinib in chronic-phase disease is ~30% at 1 year. The second-generation tyrosine kinase inhibitors, nilotinib, dasatinib, and bosutinib are also used as front-line therapy and can significantly increase the rate of a major molecular response compared to imatinib and result in a lower rate of progression to advanced-stage disease. However, these agents are associated with additional toxicity and have not been shown to benefit overall survival. Since they can still salvage 90% of patients who do not respond to treatment with imatinib, they may be reserved for use in that situation.

Patients taking tyrosine kinase inhibitors should be monitored with a quantitative PCR assay. Those with a consistent increase in *bcr/abl* transcript or those with a suboptimal molecular response as defined above should undergo testing for a pathogenic variant of *abl* and then be switched to an alternative tyrosine kinase inhibitor. The *T315I* variant of *abl* is specifically resistant to therapy with imatinib, dasatinib, nilotinib, and bosutinib but appears to be sensitive to the third-generation agent ponatinib. However, ponatinib is associated with a high rate of vascular thrombotic complications. For patients with the *T315I* variant as well as patients who have not responded to multiple tyrosine kinase inhibitors, including ponatinib, the allosteric inhibitor asciminib can be tried. It has shown a 54% complete hematologic response rate and a 48% sustained major molecular response in heavily pretreated patients. Dose-limiting toxic effects include asymptomatic elevations in the lipase level and clinical pancreatitis. Lastly, omacetaxine—a non–tyrosine kinase inhibitor therapy approved for patients with CML who are resistant to at least two tyrosine kinase inhibitors—can produce major cytogenetic responses in 18% of patients. Patients in whom a good molecular response to any of these agents cannot be achieved or in whom disease progresses despite therapy should be considered for allogeneic stem cell transplantation.

Patients with advanced-stage disease (accelerated phase or myeloid/lymphoid blast crisis) should be treated with a tyrosine kinase inhibitor alone or in combination with myelosuppressive chemotherapy. The doses of tyrosine kinase inhibitors in that setting are usually higher than those appropriate for chronic-phase disease. Since the duration of response to tyrosine kinase inhibitors in this setting is limited, patients who have accelerated or blast-phase disease should ultimately be considered for allogeneic stem cell transplantation.

Course & Prognosis

Patients with good molecular responses to tyrosine kinase inhibitor therapy have an excellent prognosis, with essentially 100% survival at last follow up. Studies suggest that tyrosine kinase inhibitor therapy may be safely discontinued after 2 years in patients who achieve a sustained major molecular response, with ~50% of patients remaining in molecular remission at least 1 year posttreatment. Of importance, more than 80% of recurrences occur within the first 6–8 months after stopping therapy, and loss of major molecular response is uncommon after 1 year. About 90–95% of patients who experience molecular recurrence regain their initial molecular level after restarting tyrosine kinase inhibitor therapy.

When to Refer

All patients with CML should be referred to a hematologist.

When to Admit

Hospitalization is rarely necessary and should be reserved for symptoms of leukostasis at diagnosis or for transformation to acute leukemia.

Cortes J. How to manage CML patients with comorbidities. Hematology Am Soc Hematol Educ Program. 2020;2020:237. [PMID: 33275749]

Craddock CF. We do still transplant CML, don't we? Hematology Am Soc Hematol Educ Program. 2018;2018:177. [PMID: 30504307]

Harrington P et al. Novel developments in chronic myeloid leukaemia. Curr Opin Hematol. 2021;28:122. [PMID: 33464004]

Hochhaus A et al. European LeukemiaNet 2020 recommendations for treating chronic myeloid leukemia. Leukemia. 2020;34:966. [PMID: 32127639]

Morita K et al. Current status and novel strategy of CML. Int J Hematol. 2021;113:624. [PMID: 33782818]

MYELODYSPLASTIC SYNDROMES

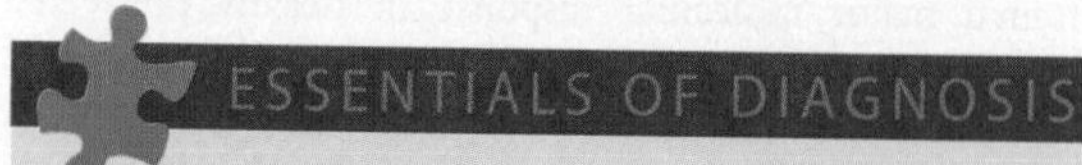

ESSENTIALS OF DIAGNOSIS

- Cytopenias with a hypercellular bone marrow.
- Morphologic abnormalities in one or more hematopoietic cell lines.

General Considerations

The MDS are a group of acquired clonal disorders of the hematopoietic stem cell. They are characterized by the constellation of cytopenias, a usually hypercellular marrow, morphologic dysplasia, and genetic abnormalities. The disorders are usually idiopathic but may be caused by prior exposure to cytotoxic chemotherapy, radiation, or both. In addition to cytogenetics, sequencing can detect genetic pathogenic variants in 80–90% of MDS patients. Importantly, acquired clonal variants identical to those seen in MDS can occur in the hematopoietic cells of ~10% of apparently healthy older individuals, defining the disorder of **clonal hematopoiesis of indeterminate potential (CHIP).**

Myelodysplasia encompasses several heterogeneous syndromes. A key distinction is whether there is an increase in bone marrow blasts (greater than 5% of marrow elements). The category of MDS with excess blasts represents a more aggressive form of the disease, often leading to AML. Those without excess blasts are characterized by the degree of dysplasia, eg, MDS with single lineage dysplasia and MDS with multilineage dysplasia. The morphologic finding of **ringed sideroblasts** is used to define a subcategory of the lower-risk MDS syndromes. Patients with **isolated 5q loss,** which is characterized by the cytogenetic finding of loss of part of the long arm of chromosome 5, comprise an important subgroup of patients with a different natural history. Lastly, a proliferative syndrome including sustained peripheral blood monocytosis more than 1000/mcL (1.0×10^9/L) is termed **chronic myelomonocytic leukemia (CMML),** a disorder that shares features of myelodysplastic and myeloproliferative disorders. An International Prognostic Scoring System (IPSS) classifies patients by risk status based on the percentage of bone marrow blasts, cytogenetics, and severity of cytopenias. The IPSS is associated with the rate of progression to AML and with overall survival, which can range from a median of 6 years for the low-risk group to 5 months for the high-risk patients.

Clinical Findings

A. Symptoms and Signs

Patients are usually over age 60 years. Many patients are asymptomatic when the diagnosis is made because of the finding of abnormal blood counts. Fatigue, infection, or bleeding related to bone marrow failure are usually the presenting symptoms and signs. The course may be indolent, and the disease may present as a wasting illness with fever, weight loss, and general debility. On examination, splenomegaly may be present in combination with pallor, bleeding, and various signs of infection. MDS can also be accompanied by a variety of paraneoplastic syndromes prior to or following this diagnosis.

B. Laboratory Findings

Anemia may be marked with the MCV normal or increased, and transfusion support may be required. On the peripheral blood smear, macro-ovalocytes may be seen. The WBC count is usually normal or reduced, and neutropenia is common.

The neutrophils may exhibit morphologic abnormalities, including deficient numbers of granules or deficient segmentation of the nucleus, even a bilobed nucleus (the so-called Pelger-Huët abnormality). The myeloid series may be left shifted, and small numbers of promyelocytes or blasts may be seen. The platelet count is normal or reduced, and hypogranular platelets may be present.

The bone marrow is characteristically hypercellular but occasionally may be hypocellular. Erythroid hyperplasia is common, and signs of abnormal erythropoiesis include megaloblastic features, nuclear budding, or multinucleated erythroid precursors. The Prussian blue stain may demonstrate ringed sideroblasts. In the marrow, too, the myeloid series is often left shifted, with variable increases in blasts. Deficient or abnormal granules may be seen. A characteristic abnormality is the presence of dwarf megakaryocytes with a unilobed nucleus. Genetic abnormalities define MDS; there are frequent cytogenetic abnormalities involving chromosomes 5 and 7. Some patients with an indolent form have an isolated partial deletion of chromosome 5 (MDS with isolated del[5q]). Aside from cytogenetic abnormalities, the most commonly genes with pathogenic variants are *SF3B1, TET2, SRSF2, ASXL1, DNMT3A, RUNX1, U2AF1, TP53,* and *EZH2.*

Differential Diagnosis

MDS should be distinguished from megaloblastic anemia, aplastic anemia, myelofibrosis, HIV-associated cytopenias, and acute or chronic drug effect. In subtle cases, cytogenetic evaluation of the bone marrow may help distinguish this clonal disorder from other causes of cytopenias. As the number of blasts increases in the bone marrow, myelodysplasia is arbitrarily separated from AML by the presence of less than 20% blasts.

Treatment

Myelodysplasia is a heterogeneous disease, and the appropriate treatment depends on a number of factors. For patients with anemia who have a low serum erythropoietin level (500 U/L or less), erythropoiesis-stimulating agents may raise the hematocrit and reduce the RBC transfusion requirement in 40%. Addition of intermittent granulocyte colony-stimulating factor (G-CSF) therapy may augment the erythroid response to epoetin. Unfortunately, the patients with the highest transfusion requirements and those with erythropoietin levels above 200 U/L are the least likely to respond. Patients who remain dependent on RBC transfusion and who can tolerate it should receive iron chelation in order to prevent serious iron overload; the dose of oral agent deferasirox is 20 mg/kg/day in divided dosing. Patients affected primarily with severe neutropenia may benefit from the use of myeloid growth factors such as filgrastim. Oral thrombopoietin analogs, such as romiplostim and eltrombopag, have shown effectiveness in raising the platelet count in myelodysplasia. Finally, occasional patients can benefit from immunosuppressive therapy including ATG. Predictors of response to ATG include age younger than 60 years, absence of 5q−, and presence of HLA DR15.

For patients who do not respond to these interventions, there are several therapeutic options available. Lenalidomide is the treatment of choice in patients with MDS with isolated del(5q) with significant responses in 70% of patients, and responses typically lasting longer than 2 years. In addition, nearly half of these patients enter a cytogenetic remission with clearing of the abnormal 5q− clone. The recommended initial dose is 10 mg/day orally. The most common side effects are neutropenia and thrombocytopenia, but venous thrombosis occurs and warrants prophylaxis with aspirin, 81 mg/day orally. A novel agent, luspatercept, has been developed to target signaling via the SMAD2–SMAD3 pathway, which is constitutively increased in the bone marrow cells of patients with MDS and ineffective erythropoiesis. In a randomized study, luspatercept induced transfusion independence in 38% of lower-risk MDS patients who had not responded to growth factor therapy compared to 13% in the placebo arm. The most common adverse events included fatigue, diarrhea, asthenia, nausea, and dizziness.

For patients with high-risk MDS, hypomethylating agents are the treatment of choice. Azacitidine can improve both symptoms and blood counts and prolong overall survival and time to conversion to acute leukemia. It is used at a dose of 75 mg/m^2 daily for 5–7 days every 28 days and up to six cycles of therapy may be required to achieve a response. Decitabine, a related hypomethylating agent, given at 20 mg/m^2 daily for 5 days every 28 days can produce similar hematologic responses but has not demonstrated a benefit in overall survival compared to supportive care alone. Unfortunately, the progress that has been made over the past decade in understanding the complex molecular mechanisms underlying MDS has not yet translated into new therapeutic options. The addition of the BCL2 inhibitor venetoclax to 5-azacytidine has recently been shown to be well tolerated and may lead to higher response rates.

Allogeneic stem cell transplantation is the only curative therapy for myelodysplasia, but its role is limited by the advanced age of many patients and the variably indolent course of the disease.

Course & Prognosis

Myelodysplasia is an ultimately fatal disease, and allogeneic transplantation is the only curative therapy, with cure rates of 30–60% depending primarily on the risk status of the disease. Patients most commonly die of infections or bleeding. Patients with MDS with isolated del(5q) have a favorable prognosis, with 5-year survival over 90%. Other patients with low-risk disease (with absence of both excess blasts and adverse cytogenetics) may also do well, with similar survival. Those with excess blasts or CMML have a higher (30–50%) risk of developing acute leukemia, and short survival (less than 2 years) without allogeneic transplantation.

When to Refer

All patients with myelodysplasia should be referred to a hematologist.

When to Admit

Hospitalization is needed only for specific complications, such as severe infection.

Angelucci E et al. Iron chelation in transfusion-dependent patients with low- to intermediate-1-risk myelodysplastic syndromes: a randomized trial. Ann Intern Med. 2020;172:513. [PMID: 32203980]

Chan O et al. Chronic myelomonocytic leukemia diagnosis and management. Leukemia. 2021;35:1552. [PMID: 33714974]

Kröger N et al. Comparison between 5-azacytidine treatment and allogeneic stem-cell transplantation in elderly patients with advanced MDS according to donor availability (VidazaAllo Study). J Clin Oncol. 2021;39:3318. [PMID: 34283629]

Park S et al. Clinical effectiveness and safety of erythropoietin-stimulating agents for the treatment of low- and intermediate-risk myelodysplastic syndrome: a systematic literature review. Br J Haematol. 2019;184:134. [PMID: 30549002]

Platzbecker U et al. Current challenges and unmet medical needs in myelodysplastic syndromes. Leukemia. 2021;35:2182. [PMID: 34045662]

Stomper J et al. Hypomethylating agents (HMA) for the treatment of acute myeloid leukemia and myelodysplastic syndromes: mechanisms of resistance and novel HMA-based therapies. Leukemia. 2021;35:1873. [PMID: 33958699]

ACUTE LEUKEMIA

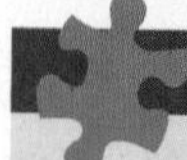

ESSENTIALS OF DIAGNOSIS

- Short duration of symptoms, including fatigue, fever, and bleeding.
- Cytopenias or pancytopenia.
- Blasts in peripheral blood in 90% of patients.
- More than 20% blasts in the bone marrow.

General Considerations

Acute leukemia is a malignancy of the hematopoietic progenitor cell. Malignant immature cells proliferate in an uncontrolled fashion and replace normal bone marrow elements. Most cases arise with no clear cause. However, radiation and some toxins (benzene) are leukemogenic. In addition, a number of chemotherapeutic agents (especially cyclophosphamide, melphalan, other alkylating agents, and etoposide) may cause leukemia. The leukemias seen after toxin or chemotherapy exposure often develop from a myelodysplastic prodrome and are often associated with abnormalities in chromosomes 5 and 7. Those related to etoposide or anthracyclines may have abnormalities in chromosome 11q23 (MLL locus).

Most of the clinical findings in acute leukemia are due to replacement of normal bone marrow elements by the malignant cells. Less common manifestations result from organ infiltration (skin, GI tract, meninges). Acute leukemia is potentially curable with combination chemotherapy.

The myeloblastic subtype, AML, is primarily an adult disease with a median age at presentation of 60 years and an increasing incidence with advanced age. Acute promyelocytic leukemia (APL) is characterized by the chromosomal translocation t(15;17), which produces the fusion gene *PML-RAR*-alpha, leading to a block in differentiation that can be overcome with pharmacologic doses of retinoic acid. The lymphoblastic subtype of acute leukemia, ALL, comprises 80% of the acute leukemias of childhood. The peak incidence is between 3 and 7 years of age. It is also seen in adults, causing approximately 20% of adult acute leukemias.

Classification of the Leukemias

A. Acute Myeloid Leukemia (AML)

AML is primarily categorized based on recurrent structural chromosomal and molecular abnormalities. The cytogenetic abnormalities can be identified on traditional karyotyping or metaphase fluorescence in situ hybridization (FISH) and the molecular abnormalities are identified by either targeted or genome-wide sequencing of tumor DNA. Favorable cytogenetics such as t(8;21) producing a chimeric RUNX1/RUNX1T1 protein and inv(16)(p13;q22) are seen in 15% of cases and are termed the "core-binding factor" leukemias. These patients have a higher chance of achieving both short- and long-term disease control. Unfavorable cytogenetics confer a very poor prognosis. These consist of chromosomal translocations [t(6;9), t(3;3) or inv (3), t(v;11q23)], isolated monosomy 5 or 7, the presence of two or more other monosomies, or three or more separate cytogenetic abnormalities and account for 25% of the cases. The majority of cases of AML are of intermediate risk by traditional cytogenetics and have either a normal karyotype or chromosomal abnormalities that do not confer strong prognostic significance. However, there are several recurrent gene pathogenic variants with prognostic significance in this subgroup. On the one hand, internal tandem duplication in the gene *FLT3* occurs in ~30% of AML and is conditionally associated with a poor prognosis in the setting of wild type *NPM1*. Other pathogenic variants conferring a poor prognosis occur in *RUNX1*, *ASXL1*, and *TP53*. On the other hand, a relatively favorable group of patients has been identified that lacks *FLT3-ITD* pathogenic variants and includes variants of nucleophosmin 1 (*NPM1*) or carries *CEBPA* biallelic variants.

B. Acute Promyelocytic Leukemia (APL)

In considering the various types of AML, APL is discussed separately because of its unique biologic features and response to non-chemotherapy treatments. APL is characterized by the cytogenetic finding of t(15;17) and the fusion gene *PML-RAR*-alpha. It is a highly curable form of leukemia (over 90%) with integration of all-trans-retinoic acid (ATRA) and arsenic trioxide (ATO) in induction, consolidation, and maintenance regimens.

C. Acute Lymphoblastic Leukemia (ALL)

ALL is most usefully classified by immunologic phenotype as follows: common, early B lineage, and T cell. Hyperdiploidy (with more than 50 chromosomes), especially of chromosomes 4, 10, and 17, and translocation t(12;21) (TEL-AML1), is associated with a better prognosis. Unfavorable cytogenetics are hypodiploidy (less than 44 chromosomes), the Philadelphia chromosome t(9;22), the t(4;11) translocation (which has fusion genes involving the *MLL* gene at 11q23), and a complex karyotype with more than five chromosomal abnormalities.

D. Mixed Phenotype Acute Leukemias

These leukemias consist of blasts that lack differentiation along the lymphoid or myeloid lineage or blasts that express both myeloid and lymphoid lineage-specific antigens. This group is considered very high risk and has a poor prognosis. The limited available data suggest that an "acute lymphoblastic leukemia–like" regimen followed by allogeneic stem cell transplant may be advisable; addition of a tyrosine kinase inhibitor in patients with t(9;22) translocation is recommended.

Clinical Findings

A. Symptoms and Signs

Most patients have been ill only for days or weeks. Bleeding (usually due to thrombocytopenia) occurs in the skin and mucosal surfaces, with gingival bleeding, epistaxis, or menorrhagia. Less commonly, widespread bleeding is seen in patients with disseminated intravascular coagulation (DIC) (in APL and monocytic leukemia). Infection is due to neutropenia, with the risk of infection rising as the neutrophil count falls below 500/mcL (0.5×10^9/L). Common presentations include cellulitis, pneumonia, and perirectal infections; death within a few hours may occur if treatment with appropriate antibiotics is delayed. Fungal infections are also commonly seen.

Patients may also seek medical attention because of gum hypertrophy and bone and joint pain. The most dramatic presentation is hyperleukocytosis, in which a markedly elevated circulating blast count (total white blood count greater than 100,000/mcL [100×10^9/L]) leads to impaired circulation, presenting as headache, confusion, and dyspnea. Such patients require emergent chemotherapy with adjunctive leukapheresis since mortality approaches 40% in the first 48 hours.

On examination, patients appear pale and have purpura and petechiae; signs of infection may not be present. Stomatitis and gum hypertrophy may be seen in patients with monocytic leukemia, as may rectal fissures. There is variable enlargement of the liver, spleen, and lymph nodes. Bone tenderness may be present, particularly in the sternum, tibia, and femur.

B. Laboratory Findings

The hallmark of acute leukemia is the combination of pancytopenia with circulating blasts. However, blasts may be absent from the peripheral smear in as many as 10% of cases ("aleukemic leukemia"). The bone marrow is usually hypercellular and dominated by blasts (greater than 20%).

Hyperuricemia may be seen. If DIC is present, the fibrinogen level will be reduced, the prothrombin time prolonged, and fibrin degradation products or fibrin D-dimers present. Patients with ALL (especially T cell) may have a mediastinal mass visible on chest radiograph. Meningeal leukemia will have blasts present in the spinal fluid, seen in approximately 5% of cases at diagnosis; it is more common in monocytic types of AML and can be seen with ALL.

The **Auer rod,** an eosinophilic needle-like inclusion in the cytoplasm, is a characteristic of AML (though sometimes seen in APL, high-grade MDS, and myeloproliferative disorders). The phenotype of leukemia cells is usually demonstrated by flow cytometry or immunohistochemistry. AML cells usually express myeloid antigens such as CD13 or CD33 and myeloperoxidase. ALL cells of B lineage will express CD19, and most cases will express CD10, formerly known as the "common ALL antigen." ALL cells of T lineage will usually not express mature T-cell markers, such as CD3, CD4, or CD8, but will express some combination of CD2, CD5, and CD7 and will not express surface immunoglobulin. Almost all cells express terminal deoxynucleotidyl transferase (TdT).

Differential Diagnosis

AML must be distinguished from other myeloproliferative disorders, CML, and MDS. Acute leukemia may also resemble a left-shifted bone marrow recovering from a previous toxic insult. If the diagnosis is in doubt, a bone marrow study should be repeated in several days to see if maturation has taken place. ALL must be separated from other lymphoproliferative disease such as CLL, lymphomas, and hairy cell leukemia. It may also be confused with the atypical lymphocytosis of mononucleosis and pertussis.

Treatment

Acute leukemia is considered a curable disease, especially among younger patients without significant comorbidities. The first step in treatment is to obtain complete remission, defined as normal peripheral blood with resolution of cytopenias, normal bone marrow with no excess blasts, and normal clinical status. The type of initial chemotherapy depends on the subtype of leukemia.

1. AML—Most patients with AML who are treated with a curative intent receive a combination of an anthracycline (daunorubicin or idarubicin) plus cytarabine, either alone or in combination with other agents (eg, gemtuzumab ozogamicin). This therapy will produce complete remissions in 80–90% of patients under age 60 years and in 50–60% of older patients (see Table 39–2). Patients with secondary AML (evolved from prior myelodysplastic or myeloproliferative disorders) or treatment-associated AML should receive the drug Vyxeos (a liposomal formulation of daunorubicin and cytarabine). Patients with a pathogenic variant of *FLT3* benefit from the addition of the FLT3 kinase inhibitor midostaurin to their regimen. Post-remission therapy options include additional chemotherapy and allogeneic stem cell transplantation. Patients with a favorable genetic profile can be treated with chemotherapy alone or with autologous transplant with cure rates of 60–80%. For intermediate-risk patients with AML, cure rates are 35–40% with chemotherapy and 40–60% with allogeneic transplantation. Patients who do not enter remission (primary induction failure) or those with high-risk genetics have cure rates of less than 10% with chemotherapy alone and are referred for allogeneic stem cell transplantation.

Patients who are not treated with initial curative intent (those older than 75 years or with significant comorbidities) can derive benefit from newer targeted agents, including the bcl2 inhibitor venetoclax added to a hypomethylating agent or low-dose cytarabine, enasidenib (targeting *IDH2* mutations), ivosidenib (targeting *IDH2* mutations), or glasdegib. Some of these patients can still benefit from a reduced-intensity allogeneic transplant if they achieve good disease control.

Once leukemia has recurred after initial chemotherapy, the prognosis is poor. For patients in second remission, allogeneic transplantation offers a 20–30% chance of cure. Targeted therapies described above are useful for selected patients and can offer long-term disease control.

2. ALL—Adults with ALL are treated with combination chemotherapy, including daunorubicin, vincristine, prednisone, and asparaginase. This treatment produces complete remissions in 90% of patients. Those patients with Philadelphia chromosome-positive ALL (or *bcr-abl*-positive ALL) should receive a tyrosine kinase inhibitor, such as dasatinib or ponatinib, added to their initial chemotherapy. Remission induction therapy for ALL is less myelosuppressive than treatment for AML and does not necessarily produce prolonged marrow aplasia. Patients should also receive CNS prophylaxis so that meningeal sequestration of leukemic cells does not develop.

After achieving complete remission, patients may be treated with either additional cycles of chemotherapy or high-dose chemotherapy and stem cell transplantation. Treatment decisions are made based on patient age and disease risk factors. Adults younger than 39 years have uniformly better outcomes when treated under pediatric protocols. For older patients, minimal residual disease testing early on can identify high-risk patients who will not be cured with chemotherapy alone and who will do better with allogeneic transplantation. For patients with relapsed disease, the bispecific antibody blinatumomab targeting CD19 and the antibody-drug conjugate inotuzumab ozogamicin targeting CD22 have shown remarkable activity and are considered superior to traditional chemotherapy options. Chimeric antigen receptor T cell therapy targeting CD19 is an additional option for patients with relapsed or refractory B-ALL but is currently used as a bridge to allogeneic transplantation.

Prognosis

Approximately 70–80% of adults with AML under age 60 years achieve complete remission and ~50% are cured using risk-adapted post-remission therapy. Older adults with AML achieve complete remission in up to 50% of instances. The cure rates for older patients with AML have been very low (approximately 10–20%) even if they achieve remission and are able to receive post-remission chemotherapy.

Patients younger than 39 years with ALL have excellent outcomes after undergoing chemotherapy followed by risk-adapted intensification and transplantation (cure rates of 60–80%). Patients with adverse cytogenetics, poor response to chemotherapy, or older age have a much lower chance of cure (cure rates of 20–40%).

When to Refer

All patients should be referred to a hematologist.

When to Admit

Most patients with acute leukemia will be admitted for treatment.

Dholaria B et al. The evolving role of allogeneic haematopoietic cell transplantation in the era of chimaeric antigen receptor T-cell therapy. Br J Haematol. 2021;193:1060. [PMID: 33928630]

DiNardo CD et al. How I treat acute myeloid leukemia in the era of new drugs. Blood. 2020;135:85. [PMID: 31765470]

McMurry H et al. IDH inhibitors in AML—promise and pitfalls. Curr Hematol Malig Rep. 2021;16:207. [PMID: 33939107]

Sekeres MA et al. American Society of Hematology 2020 guidelines for treating newly diagnosed acute myeloid leukemia in older adults. Blood Adv. 2020;4:3528. [PMID: 32761235]

Swaminathan M et al. Novel therapies for AML: a round-up for clinicians. Expert Rev Clin Pharmacol. 2020;13:1389. [PMID: 33412978]

CHRONIC LYMPHOCYTIC LEUKEMIA

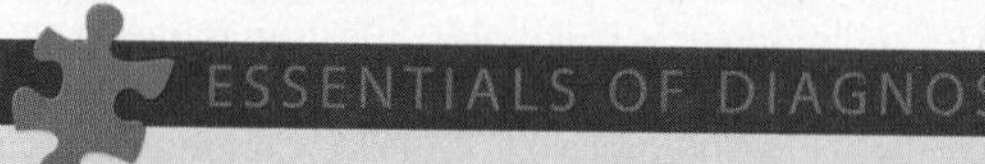

- B-cell lymphocytosis with CD19 expression > 5000/mcL (> 5.0 × 10^9/L).
- Coexpression of CD19, CD5 on lymphocytes.

General Considerations

CLL is a clonal malignancy of B lymphocytes. The disease is usually indolent, with slowly progressive accumulation of long-lived small lymphocytes. These cells are immune-incompetent and respond poorly to antigenic stimulation.

CLL is manifested clinically by immunosuppression, bone marrow failure, and organ infiltration with lymphocytes. Immunodeficiency is also related to inadequate antibody production by the abnormal B cells. With advanced disease, CLL may cause damage by direct tissue infiltration.

CLL usually pursues an indolent course, but some subtypes behave more aggressively; a variant, prolymphocytic leukemia, is more aggressive. The morphology of the latter is different, characterized by larger and more immature cells. In 5–10% of cases, CLL may be complicated by autoimmune hemolytic anemia or autoimmune thrombocytopenia. In approximately 5% of cases an aggressive large-cell lymphoma (**Richter syndrome**) can develop.

Clinical Findings

A. Symptoms and Signs

CLL is a disease of older patients, with 90% of cases occurring after age 50 years and a median age at presentation of 70 years. Many patients will be incidentally discovered to have lymphocytosis. Others present with fatigue or lymphadenopathy. On examination, 80% of patients will have diffuse lymphadenopathy and 50% will have enlargement of the liver or spleen.

The long-standing Rai classification system remains prognostically useful: stage 0, lymphocytosis only; stage I, lymphocytosis plus lymphadenopathy; stage II, organomegaly (spleen, liver); stage III, anemia; stage IV, thrombocytopenia. These stages can be collapsed into low risk (stages 0–I), intermediate risk (stage II), and high risk (stages III–IV).

B. Laboratory Findings

The hallmark of CLL is isolated lymphocytosis. The WBC count is elevated and may be markedly abnormal (elevated to several hundred thousand). Usually 75–98% of the circulating cells are lymphocytes. Lymphocytes appear small and mature, with condensed nuclear chromatin, and are morphologically indistinguishable from normal lymphocytes, but smaller numbers of larger and activated lymphocytes may be seen. The hematocrit and platelet count are usually normal at presentation. The bone marrow is variably infiltrated with small lymphocytes. The immunophenotype of CLL demonstrates coexpression of the B lymphocyte lineage marker CD19 with the T lymphocyte marker CD5; this finding is commonly observed only in CLL and mantle cell lymphoma. CLL is distinguished from mantle cell lymphoma by the expression of CD23, CD200, and LEF-1, low expression of surface immunoglobulin and CD20, and the absence of a translocation or overexpression of cyclin D1. Patients whose CLL cells have pathogenic variants of the immunoglobulin gene (IgVH somatic mutation) have a more indolent form of disease; these cells typically express low levels of the surface antigen CD38 and do not express the zeta-associated protein (ZAP-70). Conversely, patients whose cells have nonvariant IgVH genes and high levels of ZAP-70 expression do less well and require treatment sooner. The assessment of genomic changes by FISH provides important prognostic information. The finding of deletion of chromosome 17p (TP53) confers the worst prognosis, while deletion of 11q (ATM) confers an inferior prognosis to the average genotype, and isolated deletion of 13q has a more favorable outcome. Hypogammaglobulinemia is present in 50% of patients and becomes more common with advanced disease. In some, a small amount of IgM paraprotein is present in the serum.

Differential Diagnosis

Few syndromes can be confused with CLL. Viral infections producing lymphocytosis should be obvious from the presence of fever and other clinical findings; however, fever may occur in CLL from concomitant bacterial infection. Pertussis may cause a particularly high total lymphocyte count. Other lymphoproliferative diseases such as Waldenström macroglobulinemia, hairy cell leukemia, or lymphoma (especially mantle cell lymphoma or small lymphocyte lymphoma) in the leukemic phase are distinguished on the basis of the morphology and immunophenotype of circulating lymphocytes and bone marrow. Monoclonal B-cell lymphocytosis is a disorder characterized by fewer than 5000/mcL (5.0×10^9/L) B cells and is considered a precursor to B-CLL.

Treatment

The treatment of CLL is evolving as several active targeted agents are now available. Most cases of early indolent CLL require no specific therapy, and the standard of care for early-stage disease has been observation. Indications for treatment include progressive fatigue, symptomatic lymphadenopathy, anemia, or thrombocytopenia. These patients have either symptomatic and progressive Rai stage II disease or stage III/IV disease. Initial treatment for patients with CLL consists of targeted biologic therapy in most cases. Options include single agent ibrutinib or acalabrutinib (inhibitors of Bruton tyrosine kinase that target B-cell receptor signaling) or venetoclax (a bcl2 inhibitor resulting in apoptosis) in combination with anti-CD20 antibody therapy. Choice between these agents is based on toxicity as well as preference. Ibrutinib is a well-tolerated, oral agent given at 420 mg daily; it can be associated with hypertension, atrial fibrillation, rash, and increased infections. Caution should be exercised when this agent is used in conjunction with CYP3A inhibitors or inducers. In addition, there is a potential for serious bleeding when it is used in patients taking warfarin. Acalabrutinib, a more specific BTK inhibitor, administered in a dose of 100 mg orally twice daily, is another option that is associated with a lower risk of adverse cardiovascular events. Venetoclax (slowly titrated up to 400 mg daily) is usually given for a shorter course of therapy and is associated with tumor lysis syndrome and neutropenia; some patients may require hospitalization for initial therapy. Venetoclax has to be combined with a monoclonal anti-CD20 antibody, usually obinutuzumab, which can result in infusion reactions. Traditional combination chemotherapy is used only in selected cases (see Table 39–3). For older patients, chlorambucil, 0.6–1 mg/kg orally every 4 weeks, in combination with obinutuzumab is another therapy option.

Patients who relapse while taking a BTK inhibitor should undergo testing to identify recurrent BTK pathogenic variants (eg, *C481S*) that may respond to the novel agent pirtobrutinib. Alternatively, they can be treated with a combination of venetoclax and the anti-CD20 antibody obinutuzumab. For patients who relapse following venetoclax-based therapy, a BTK inhibitor is often used. Other options for relapsed disease include idelalisib and duvelisib (inhibitors of PI3 kinase delta), which are associated with higher toxicity. The dosage for idelalisib is 150 mg orally twice a day, and the dosage for duvelisib is 25 mg orally twice a day. There are risks for colitis, liver injury, and fatal infectious complications in patients treated with PI3k inhibitors. Patients should be given antimicrobial prophylaxis and monitored closely while taking these agents.

Of note, BTK and PI3k inhibitors can be initially associated with marked lymphocytosis due to release of tumor cells from the lymph nodes into the peripheral blood. This results in a significant early reduction in lymphadenopathy but a potentially misleading, more delayed clearance of lymphocytes from peripheral blood and bone marrow.

Associated autoimmune hemolytic anemia or immune thrombocytopenia may require treatment with rituximab, prednisone, or splenectomy. Fludarabine should be avoided in patients with autoimmune hemolytic anemia since it may exacerbate it. Rituximab should be used with anti-HBV agent prophylaxis in patients with past HBV infection. Patients with recurrent bacterial infections and hypogammaglobulinemia benefit from prophylactic infusions of gamma globulin (0.4 g/kg/month), but this treatment is cumbersome and expensive, justified only when these infections are severe. Patients undergoing therapy with a nucleoside analog (fludarabine, pentostatin) should receive anti-infective prophylaxis for *Pneumocystis jirovecii* pneumonia, herpes viruses, and invasive fungal infections until there is evidence of T-cell recovery.

Allogeneic transplantation offers potentially curative treatment for patients with CLL, but it should be used only in patients whose disease cannot be controlled by the available therapies. Nonmyeloablative allogeneic transplant can result in over 40% long-term disease control in CLL but with risk of moderate toxicity. Chimeric antigen receptor T-cell therapy is currently being evaluated for patients with refractory disease.

Prognosis

Targeted therapies have changed the prognosis of CLL. Patients with stage 0 or stage I disease have a median survival of 10–15 years, and these patients may be reassured that they can live a normal life. Patients with stage III or stage IV disease had a median survival of less than 2 years in the past, but with current therapies, 5-year survival is more than 70% and the long-term outlook appears to be substantially changed. For patients with high-risk and resistant forms of CLL, there is evidence that allogeneic transplantation can overcome risk factors and lead to long-term disease control.

When to Refer

All patients with CLL should be referred to a hematologist.

When to Admit

Hospitalization is rarely needed.

Ahn IE et al. Targeting bruton's tyrosine kinase in CLL. Front Immunol. 2021;12:687458. [PMID: 34248972]

Lew TE et al. How I treat chronic lymphocytic leukemia after venetoclax. Blood. 2021;138:361. [PMID: 33876212]

Patel K et al. Current and future treatment strategies in chronic lymphocytic leukemia. J Hematol Oncol. 2021;14:69. [PMID: 33902665]

HAIRY CELL LEUKEMIA

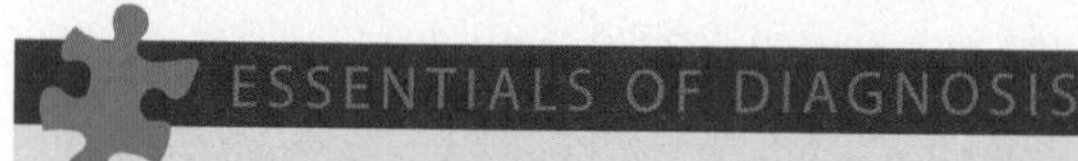

- Pancytopenia.
- Splenomegaly, often massive.
- Hairy cells present on blood smear and especially in bone marrow biopsy.

General Considerations

Hairy cell leukemia is a rare malignancy of hematopoietic stem cells differentiated as mature B lymphocytes with hairy cytoplasmic projections. The V600E pathogenic variant in the *BRAF* gene is recognized as the causal genetic event of hairy cell leukemia since it is detectable in almost all cases at diagnosis and is present at relapse.

Clinical Findings

A. Symptoms and Signs

The disease characteristically presents in middle-aged men. The median age at presentation is 55 years, and there is a striking 5:1 male predominance. Most patients present with gradual onset of fatigue, others complain of symptoms related to markedly enlarged spleen, and some come to attention because of infection.

Splenomegaly is almost invariably present and may be massive. The liver is enlarged in 50% of cases; lymphadenopathy is uncommon.

Hairy cell leukemia is usually an indolent disorder whose course is dominated by pancytopenia and recurrent infections, including mycobacterial infections.

B. Laboratory Findings

The hallmark of hairy cell leukemia is pancytopenia. Anemia is nearly universal, and 75% of patients have thrombocytopenia and neutropenia. The "hairy cells" are usually present in small numbers on the peripheral blood smear and have a characteristic appearance with numerous cytoplasmic projections. The bone marrow is usually inaspirable (dry tap), and the diagnosis is made by characteristic morphology on bone marrow biopsy. The hairy cells have a characteristic histochemical staining pattern with tartrate-resistant acid phosphatase (TRAP). On immunophenotyping, the cells coexpress the antigens CD11c, CD20, CD22, CD25, CD103, and CD123. Pathologic examination of the spleen shows marked infiltration of the red pulp with hairy cells. This is in contrast to the usual predilection of lymphomas to involve the white pulp of the spleen.

Differential Diagnosis

Hairy cell leukemia should be distinguished from other lymphoproliferative diseases that involve the bone marrow. It also may be confused with other causes of pancytopenia, including hypersplenism due to any cause, aplastic anemia, and paroxysmal nocturnal hemoglobinuria.

Treatment

Treatment is indicated for symptomatic disease, ie, splenic discomfort, recurrent infections, or significant cytopenias. The treatment of choice is a nucleoside analog, specifically pentostatin or cladribine for a single course, producing a complete remission in 70–95% of patients. Treatment is associated with infectious complications, and patients should be closely monitored. The median duration of response is over 8 years and patients who relapse a year or more after initial therapy can be treated again with one of these agents. Rituximab can be used in the relapsed setting either as a single agent or in combination with a nucleoside analog. The BRAF inhibitor vemurafenib exhibits ~100% overall response rate in patients with refractory/relapsed hairy cell leukemia, with 35–40% complete remissions. The median relapse-free survival is ~19 months in patients who achieved complete remission and 6 months in those who obtained a partial response. Based on its superior safety profile compared to nucleoside analogs, vemurafenib is currently being evaluated as an initial therapy in combination with the anti-CD20 antibody obinutuzumab. Moxetumomab pasudotox is a recombinant CD22-targeting immunotoxin approved for patients with refractory disease. It has shown a durable complete response rate of 31% in the pivotal trial. However, it can be associated with capillary leak and hemolytic-uremic syndrome attributable to the diphtheria toxin moiety.

Course & Prognosis

More than 95% of patients with hairy cell leukemia live longer than 10 years.

Bohn JP et al. The biology of classic hairy cell leukemia. Int J Mol Sci. 2021;22:7780. [PMID: 34360545]

Chihara D et al. Treatment of hairy cell leukemia. Expert Rev Hematol. 2020;13:1107. [PMID: 32893700]

Grever MR et al. Consensus guidelines for the diagnosis and management of patients with classic hairy cell leukemia. Blood. 2017;129:553. [PMID: 27903528]

Liebers N et al. BRAF inhibitor treatment in classic hairy cell leukemia: a long-term follow-up study of patients treated outside clinical trials. Leukemia. 2020;34:1454. [PMID: 31740808]

LYMPHOMAS

NON-HODGKIN LYMPHOMAS

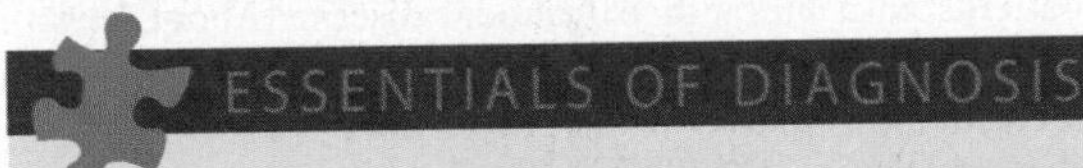

- Often present with painless lymphadenopathy.
- Diagnosis is made by tissue biopsy.

General Considerations

The non-Hodgkin lymphomas are a heterogeneous group of cancers of lymphocytes usually presenting as enlarged lymph nodes. The disorders vary in clinical presentation and course from indolent to rapidly progressive.

Molecular biology has provided clues to the pathogenesis of these disorders, often a matter of balanced chromosomal translocations whereby an oncogene becomes juxtaposed next to either an immunoglobulin gene (B-cell lymphoma) or the T-cell receptor gene or related gene (T-cell lymphoma). The net result is oncogene overexpression and development of lymphoma. The best-studied example is Burkitt lymphoma, in which a characteristic cytogenetic abnormality of translocation between the long arms of chromosomes 8 and 14 has been identified. The protooncogene c-*myc* is translocated from its normal position on chromosome 8 to the immunoglobulin heavy chain locus on chromosome 14. Overexpression of c-*myc* is related to malignant transformation through excess B-cell proliferation. In follicular lymphoma, the t(14;18) translocation is characteristic and *bcl-2* is overexpressed, resulting in protection against apoptosis, the usual mechanism of B-cell death.

Classification of the lymphomas is a dynamic area still undergoing evolution. The 2017 grouping (Table 13–16) separates diseases based on both clinical and pathologic features. Eighty-five percent of non-Hodgkin lymphomas are B-cell and 15% are T-cell or NK-cell in origin. Even though non-Hodgkin lymphomas represent a diverse group of diseases, they are historically divided in two categories based on clinical behavior and pathology: the indolent (low-grade) and the aggressive (intermediate- or high-grade).

Table 13–16. World Health Organization classification of lymphomas (modified from 2017 version).

Precursor B-cell lymphoblastic lymphoma
Mature B-cell lymphomas
Chronic lymphocytic leukemia/small lymphocytic lymphoma
Monoclonal B-cell lymphocytosis
Hairy cell leukemia
Plasma cell myeloma
Diffuse large B-cell lymphoma
Primary diffuse large B-cell lymphoma of the CNS
High-grade B-cell lymphoma, with *MYC* and *BCL2* and/or *BCL6* rearrangements
Mediastinal (thymic) large B-cell lymphoma
Follicular lymphoma
Lymphoplasmacytic lymphoma (Waldenström macroglobulinemia)
Mantle cell lymphoma
Burkitt lymphoma
Marginal zone lymphoma
MALT type
Nodal type
Splenic type
Mature T- (and NK-) cell lymphomas
Anaplastic large-cell lymphoma
Angioimmunoblastic T-cell lymphoma
Peripheral T-cell lymphoma, NOS
Cutaneous T-cell lymphoma (mycosis fungoides, Sézary syndrome)
Extranodal NK-/T-cell lymphoma, nasal type
Adult T-cell leukemia/lymphoma
T-cell large granular lymphocytic leukemia
Hodgkin lymphoma
Nodular lymphocyte predominant Hodgkin lymphoma
Classic Hodgkin lymphoma
Posttransplant lymphoproliferative disorders
Histiocytic and dendritic cell neoplasms

MALT, mucosa-associated lymphoid tissue; NOS, not otherwise specified.

Clinical Findings

A. Symptoms and Signs

Patients with non-Hodgkin lymphomas usually present with lymphadenopathy. Involved lymph nodes may be present peripherally or centrally (in the retroperitoneum, mesentery, and pelvis). The indolent lymphomas are usually disseminated at the time of diagnosis, and bone marrow involvement is frequent. Many patients with lymphoma have constitutional symptoms such as fever, drenching night sweats, and weight loss of greater than 10% of prior body weight (referred to as "B symptoms").

On examination, lymphadenopathy may be isolated or diffuse, and extranodal sites of disease (such as the skin, GI tract, liver, and bone marrow) may be found. Patients with Burkitt lymphoma are noted to have abdominal pain or abdominal fullness because of the predilection of the disease for the abdomen.

Once a pathologic diagnosis is established, staging is done using a whole-body PET/CT scan, a bone marrow biopsy, and, in patients with high-grade lymphoma or intermediate-grade lymphoma with high-risk features, a lumbar puncture.

B. Laboratory Findings

The peripheral blood is usually normal even with extensive bone marrow involvement by lymphoma. Circulating lymphoma cells in the blood are not commonly seen.

Bone marrow involvement is manifested as paratrabecular monoclonal lymphoid aggregates. In some high-grade lymphomas, the meninges are involved and malignant cells are found with cerebrospinal fluid cytology. The serum LD, a useful prognostic marker, is incorporated in risk stratification of treatment.

The diagnosis of lymphoma is made by tissue biopsy. Needle aspiration may yield evidence for non-Hodgkin lymphoma, but a lymph node biopsy (or biopsy of involved extranodal tissue) is required for accurate diagnosis and classification.

Treatment

A. Indolent Lymphomas

The most common lymphomas in this group are follicular lymphoma, marginal zone lymphomas, and small lymphocytic lymphoma (SLL). The treatment of **indolent lymphomas** depends on the stage of disease and the clinical status of the patient. A small number of patients have limited disease with only one or two contiguous abnormal lymph node groups and may be treated with localized irradiation with curative intent. However, most patients (85%) with indolent lymphoma have disseminated disease at the time of diagnosis and are not considered curable. Historically, treatment of these patients has not affected overall survival; therefore, treatment is offered only when symptoms develop or for high tumor bulk. Following each treatment response, patients will experience a relapse at traditionally shorter intervals. Some patients will have temporary spontaneous remissions (8%). There are an increasing number of reasonable treatment options for indolent lymphomas, but no consensus exists on the best strategy. Treatment with rituximab (375 mg/m^2 intravenously weekly for 4 weeks) is commonly used either alone or in combination with chemotherapy and may be the only agent to affect overall survival in these disorders. Patients should be screened for hepatitis B because rare cases of fatal fulminant hepatitis have been described with the use of anti-CD20 monoclonal therapies without anti-HBV agent prophylaxis. Rituximab is added to chemotherapy regimens including bendamustine; cyclophosphamide, vincristine, and prednisone (R-CVP); and cyclophosphamide, doxorubicin, vincristine, and prednisone (R-CHOP) (see Table 39–2). The immunomodulatory agent lenalidomide in combination with anti-CD20 therapy is an alternative option with similar outcomes to chemotherapy. The regimens mentioned above can also be used for patients with relapsed disease. Other treatment options include the PI3K delta inhibitors (idelalisib, umbralisib, and duvalisib) and the PI3K alpha inhibitor (copanlisib). Chimeric antigen receptor T-cell therapy targeting CD19 is available for patients with at least two relapses. Stem cell transplantation (either allogeneic or autologous) is also an option for these patients.

Patients with mucosa-associated lymphoid tissue (MALT) tumors of the stomach may be appropriately treated with combination antibiotics directed against *H pylori* and with acid blockade but require frequent endoscopic monitoring. Alternatively, MALT tumors confined to the stomach can also be cured with whole-stomach radiotherapy. MALT tumors of the spleen are usually associated with hepatitis C and may remit following hepatitis C eradication therapy.

B. Aggressive Lymphomas

Patients with **diffuse large B-cell lymphoma** are treated with curative intent. Most patients are treated with six cycles of immunochemotherapy such as R-CHOP (see Table 39–2). Involved nodal radiotherapy may be added for patients with bulky or extranodal disease. About 25% of patients with diffuse large B-cell lymphoma have been identified as "double-protein expressors" with overexpression of MYC and BCL2 proteins by immunohistochemistry. While the outcomes with R-CHOP are inferior, no definitive alternative treatment recommendations can be made at this time. **High-grade lymphoma** with chromosomal translocations affecting *MYC*, such as t(8;14), and translocations affecting *BCL2*, such as t(14;18), or *BCL6* (3q27), also called "double-hit lymphoma," has a very aggressive course. Patients with this disease may do better with dose-adjusted R-EPOCH as front-line therapy.

Patients with diffuse large B-cell lymphoma or high-grade lymphoma who relapse after initial chemotherapy can still be cured by autologous hematopoietic stem cell transplantation if their disease remains responsive to chemotherapy. An additional or alternative potentially curative option is chimeric antigen receptor T-cell therapy targeting CD19 therapy, which produces durable complete response rates of ~40%.

Mantle cell lymphoma is not effectively treated with standard immunochemotherapy regimens. Intensive initial immunochemotherapy including autologous hematopoietic stem cell transplantation has been shown to improve outcomes. The BTK inhibitors ibrutinib, acalabrutinib, and zanubrutinib are active in relapsed or refractory patients with mantle cell lymphoma. Chimeric antigen receptor T cell therapy targeting CD19 therapy with brexucabtagene autoleucel shows promising activity in patients whose disease progresses after treatment with BTK inhibitors. Reduced-intensity allogeneic stem cell transplantation offers curative potential for selected patients. For **primary CNS lymphoma,** repetitive cycles of high-dose intravenous methotrexate with rituximab early in the treatment course produce better results than whole-brain radiotherapy and with less cognitive impairment.

Patients with **highly aggressive lymphomas** (Burkitt or lymphoblastic) require urgent, intense, cyclic chemotherapy in the hospital similar to that given for ALL, and they also require intrathecal chemotherapy as CNS prophylaxis.

Patients with **peripheral T-cell lymphomas** usually have advanced stage nodal and extranodal disease and typically have inferior response rates to therapy compared to patients with aggressive B-cell lymphomas. Autologous stem cell transplantation is often incorporated in first-line therapy. The antibody-drug conjugate brentuximab vedotin has significant activity in patients with CD30-positive peripheral T-cell lymphomas, such as anaplastic large-cell lymphoma. The combination of brentuximab vedotin with cyclophosphamide, *adriamycin*, and prednisone is the initial treatment of choice for CD30-positive peripheral T-cell lymphomas.

Prognosis

The median survival of patients with indolent lymphomas is 10–15 years. These diseases ultimately become refractory to chemotherapy. This often occurs at the time of histologic progression of the disease to a more aggressive form of lymphoma.

The International Prognostic Index is widely used to categorize patients with aggressive lymphoma into risk groups. Factors that confer adverse prognosis are age over 60 years, elevated serum LD, stage III or stage IV disease, more than one extranodal site of disease, and poor performance status. Cure rates range from more than 80% for low-risk patients (zero risk factors) to less than 50% for high-risk patients (four or more risk factors).

For patients who relapse after initial chemotherapy, autologous hematopoietic stem cell transplantation and chimeric antigen receptor T-cell therapy offer a 40–50% chance of long-term lymphoma-free survival.

The treatment of older patients with lymphoma has been difficult because of poorer tolerance of aggressive chemotherapy. The use of reduced-intensity regimens (eg, R-miniCHOP) with myeloid growth factors and prophylactic antibiotics are preferred.

When to Refer

All patients with lymphoma should be referred to a hematologist or an oncologist.

When to Admit

Admission is necessary only for specific complications of lymphoma or its treatment and for the treatment of all high-grade lymphomas.

Ferreri AJM et al. Evolving treatments for primary central nervous system lymphoma. Am Soc Clin Oncol Educ Book. 2019;39:454. [PMID: 31099614]

Lumish M et al. How we treat mature B-cell neoplasms (indolent B-cell lymphomas). J Hematol Oncol. 2021;14:5. [PMID: 33407745]

Sehn LH et al. Diffuse large B-cell lymphoma. N Engl J Med. 2021;384:842. [PMID: 33657296]

Tavares A et al. Diffuse large B-cell lymphoma in very elderly patients: towards best tailored treatment—a systematic review. Crit Rev Oncol Hematol. 2021;160:103294. [PMID: 33675907]

Westin JR et al. Efficacy and safety of CD19-directed CAR-T cell therapies in patients with relapsed/refractory aggressive B-cell lymphomas: observations from the JULIET, ZUMA-1, and TRANSCEND trials. Am J Hematol. 2021;96:1295. [PMID: 34310745]

HODGKIN LYMPHOMA

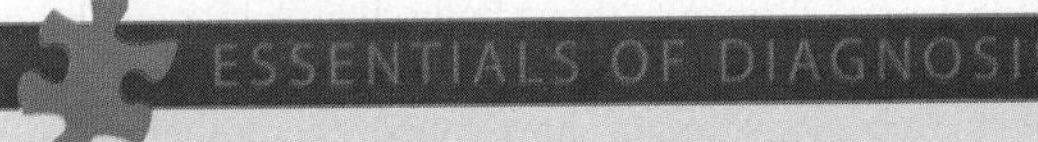

- Often painless lymphadenopathy.
- Constitutional symptoms may or may not be present.
- Pathologic diagnosis by lymph node biopsy.

General Considerations

Hodgkin lymphoma is characterized by lymph node biopsy showing Reed-Sternberg cells in an appropriate reactive cellular background. The malignant cell is derived from B lymphocytes of germinal center origin.

Clinical Findings

There is a bimodal age distribution, with one peak in the 20s and a second over age 50 years. Most patients seek medical attention because of a painless mass, commonly in the neck. Others may seek medical attention because of constitutional symptoms such as fever, weight loss, or drenching night sweats, or because of generalized pruritus. An unusual symptom of Hodgkin lymphoma is pain in an involved lymph node following alcohol ingestion.

An important feature of Hodgkin lymphoma is its tendency to arise within single lymph node areas and spread in an orderly fashion to contiguous areas of lymph nodes. Late in the course of the disease, vascular invasion leads to widespread hematogenous dissemination.

Hodgkin lymphoma is divided into two subtypes: classic Hodgkin (nodular sclerosis, mixed cellularity, lymphocyte rich, and lymphocyte depleted) and non-classic Hodgkin (nodular lymphocyte predominant). Hodgkin lymphoma should be distinguished pathologically from other malignant lymphomas and may occasionally be confused with reactive lymph nodes seen in infectious mononucleosis, cat-scratch disease, or drug reactions (eg, phenytoin).

Patients undergo a staging evaluation to determine the extent of disease, including serum chemistries, whole-body PET/CT scan, and bone marrow biopsy.

Treatment

Chemotherapy is the mainstay of treatment for Hodgkin lymphoma, and ABVD (doxorubicin, bleomycin, vinblastine, dacarbazine) remains the standard first-line regimen due to its manageable toxicity. The substitution of the antibody-drug conjugate brentuximab vedotin for bleomycin (AAVD) has demonstrated somewhat superior progression-free survival and is frequently used for patients with higher risk disease. The more intense regimen, escalated BEACOPP (bleomycin, etoposide, doxorubicin, cyclophosphamide, vincristine, procarbazine, prednisone), is associated with increased toxicity and is reserved for patients with activity on an interim PET/CT scan after starting ABVD. Low-risk patients are those with stage I or II disease without bulky lymphadenopathy or evidence of systemic inflammation. They traditionally receive a combination of short-course chemotherapy with involved nodal radiotherapy, but involved nodal radiotherapy can be eliminated for those with an early negative PET/CT scan without a significant change in outcomes (see Table 39–3). High-risk patients are those with stage III or IV disease or with stage II disease and a large mediastinal or other bulky mass or systemic inflammation. These patients are treated with a full course of chemotherapy for six cycles. Pulmonary toxicity can unfortunately occur following either chemotherapy (bleomycin) or radiation and should be treated aggressively in these patients, since it can lead to permanent fibrosis and death. A negative interim PET/CT scan after two cycles of chemotherapy can be used to identify patients with an excellent progression-free survival who can have bleomycin eliminated from their treatment. Conversely, an abnormal interim PET/CT scan is associated with a worse prognosis and should prompt early intensification of treatment to achieve a complete response (CR).

Classic Hodgkin lymphoma relapsing after initial treatment is treatable with high-dose chemotherapy and autologous hematopoietic stem cell transplantation. This offers a 35–50% chance of cure when disease is still chemotherapy responsive. Immune checkpoint inhibition by PD1 blockade with nivolumab or pembrolizumab has shown remarkable activity in patients with relapsed or refractory disease (overall response rate [ORR], 65%). These agents as well as brentuximab vedotin are increasingly incorporated in second-line regimens prior to or, for ineligible patients, in lieu of stem cell transplantation.

Prognosis

All patients should be treated with curative intent. Prognosis in advanced stage Hodgkin lymphoma is influenced by seven features: stage, age, gender, hemoglobin, albumin, WBC count, and lymphocyte count. The cure rate is 75% if zero to two risk features are present and 55% when three or more risk features are present. The prognosis of patients with stage IA or IIA disease is excellent, with 10-year survival rates in excess of 90%. Patients with advanced disease (stage III or IV) have 10-year survival rates of 50–60%. Inferior results are seen in patients who are older, those who have bulky disease, and those with lymphocyte depletion or mixed cellularity on histologic examination. Non-classic Hodgkin lymphoma (nodular lymphocyte predominant) is highly curable with radiotherapy alone for early-stage disease; however, for high-stage disease, it is characterized by long survival with repetitive relapses after chemotherapy or monoclonal anti-CD20 antibody therapy.

When to Refer

- All patients should be sent to an oncologist or hematologist.
- Secondary referral to a radiation oncologist might be appropriate.

When to Admit

Patients should be admitted for complications of the disease or its treatment.

Kuruvilla J et al; KEYNOTE-204 investigators. Pembrolizumab versus brentuximab vedotin in relapsed or refractory classical Hodgkin lymphoma (KEYNOTE-204): an interim analysis of a multicentre, randomised, open-label, phase 3 study. Lancet Oncol. 2021;22:512. [PMID: 33721562]

Longley J et al. Personalized medicine for Hodgkin lymphoma: mitigating toxicity while preserving cure. Hematol Oncol. 2021;39:39. [PMID: 34105815]

PLASMA CELL MYELOMA

ESSENTIALS OF DIAGNOSIS

- Bone pain, often in the spine, ribs, or proximal long bones.
- Monoclonal immunoglobulin (ie, paraprotein) in the serum or urine.
- Clonal plasma cells in the bone marrow or in a tissue biopsy, or both.
- Organ damage due to plasma cells (eg, bones, kidneys, hypercalcemia, anemia) or other defined criteria.

General Considerations

Plasma cell myeloma (previously called multiple myeloma) is a malignancy of hematopoietic stem cells terminally differentiated as plasma cells. It is characterized by infiltration of the bone marrow, bone destruction, and paraprotein production. The diagnosis is established when monoclonal plasma cells (either kappa or lambda light chain restricted) are found in the bone marrow (any percentage) or in a tumor (plasmacytoma). This is associated with end-organ damage (such as bone disease [lytic lesions seen on bone radiographs, MRI, or PET/CT scan], anemia [hemoglobin less than 10 g/dL {100 g/L}], hypercalcemia [calcium greater than 11 mg/dL {2.75 mmol/L}], or kidney injury [creatinine greater than 2 mg/dL {176.8 mcmol/L} or creatinine clearance less than 40 mL/minute]) with or without paraprotein elaboration. Sixty percent or more clonal plasma cells in the bone marrow, or a serum free kappa to lambda ratio of greater than 100 or less than 0.01 (both criteria regardless of end-organ damage), are also diagnostic of plasma cell myeloma. Smoldering myeloma is defined as 10–59% clonal plasma cells in the bone marrow, a serum paraprotein level of 3 g/dL (30 g/L) or higher, or both, without plasma cell–related end-organ damage.

Malignant plasma cells can form tumors (plasmacytomas) that may cause spinal cord compression or other soft-tissue–related problems. Bone disease is common and due to excessive osteoclast activation mediated largely by the interaction of the receptor activator of NF-kappa-B (RANK) with its ligand (RANKL). In plasma cell myeloma, osteoprotegerin (a decoy receptor for RANKL) is underproduced, thus promoting the binding of RANK with RANKL with consequent excessive bone resorption.

The paraproteins (monoclonal immunoglobulins) secreted by the malignant plasma cells may cause additional problems. Very high paraprotein levels (either IgG or IgA) may cause hyperviscosity, although this is more common with the IgM paraprotein as in Waldenström macroglobulinemia. The light chain component of the immunoglobulin, when produced in excess, often leads to kidney injury (frequently aggravated by hypercalcemia or hyperuricemia, or both). Light chain components may be deposited in tissues as amyloid, resulting in kidney failure with albuminuria and a vast array of other systemic syndromes (restrictive cardiomyopathy, autonomic and peripheral neuropathy, enlarged tongue, etc).

Myeloma patients are prone to recurrent infections for a number of reasons, including neutropenia, the underproduction of normal immunoglobulins (so-called immunoparesis), and the immunosuppressive effects of chemotherapy. Myeloma patients are especially prone to infections with encapsulated organisms such as *Streptococcus pneumoniae* and *Haemophilus influenzae* and should receive vaccinations against them.

Clinical Findings

A. Symptoms and Signs

Myeloma is a disease of older adults (median age 65 years). The most common presenting complaints are those related to anemia, bone pain, kidney disease, and infection. Bone pain is most common in the back, hips, or ribs or may present as a pathologic fracture, especially of the femoral neck or vertebrae. Patients may also come to medical attention because of spinal cord compression from a plasmacytoma or the hyperviscosity syndrome (mucosal bleeding, vertigo, nausea, visual disturbances, alterations in mental status, hypoxia). Many patients are diagnosed because of laboratory findings of elevated total protein, hypercalcemia, proteinuria, elevated ESR, or abnormalities on serum protein electrophoresis obtained for symptoms or in routine screening studies. A few patients come to medical attention because of organ dysfunction due to amyloidosis.

Examination may reveal pallor, bone tenderness, or soft tissue masses. Patients may have neurologic signs related to neuropathy or spinal cord compression. Fever occurs mainly with infection. Acute oliguric or nonoliguric kidney injury may be present due to hypercalcemia, hyperuricemia, light chain cast injury, or primary amyloidosis.

B. Laboratory Findings

Anemia is nearly universal. RBC morphology is normal, but rouleaux formation is common and may be marked. The absence of rouleaux formation, however, excludes neither plasma cell myeloma nor the presence of a serum paraprotein. The neutrophil and platelet counts are usually normal at presentation. Only rarely will plasma cells be visible on peripheral blood smear (plasma cell leukemia if greater than 20%).

The hallmark of myeloma is the finding of a paraprotein on serum or urine protein electrophoresis (PEP) or immunofixation electrophoresis (IFE). The majority of patients will have a monoclonal spike visible in the gamma- or beta-globulin region of the PEP. The semi-quantification of the paraprotein on the PEP is referred to as the M-protein, and IFE will reveal this to be a monoclonal immunoglobulin. Approximately 15% of patients will have no demonstrable paraprotein in the serum on PEP because their myeloma cells produce only light chains and not intact immunoglobulin (but often seen on serum IFE), and the light chains pass rapidly through the glomerulus into the urine. Urine PEP and IFE usually demonstrate the light chain paraprotein in this setting. The free light chain assay will sometimes demonstrate excess monoclonal light chains in serum and urine, and in a small proportion of patients, will be the only means to identify and quantify the paraprotein being produced. Overall, the paraprotein is IgG (60%), IgA (20%), or light chain only (15%) in plasma cell myeloma, with the remainder being rare cases of IgD, IgM, or biclonal gammopathy. In sporadic cases, no paraprotein is present ("nonsecretory myeloma"); these patients have particularly aggressive disease.

The bone marrow will be infiltrated by variable numbers of monoclonal plasma cells. The plasma cells may be morphologically abnormal often demonstrating multi-nucleation and vacuolization. The plasma cells will display marked skewing of the normal kappa-to-lambda light chain ratio, which will indicate their clonality. Many benign inflammatory processes can result in bone marrow plasmacytosis, but with the absence of clonality and morphologic atypia.

C. Imaging

Bone radiographs are important in establishing the diagnosis of myeloma. Lytic lesions are most commonly seen in the axial skeleton: skull, spine, proximal long bones, and ribs.

At other times, only generalized osteoporosis is seen. The radionuclide bone scan is not useful in detecting bone lesions in myeloma since there is little osteoblastic component. In the evaluation of patients with known or suspected plasma cell myeloma, MRI and PET/CT scans are more sensitive to detect bone disease than plain radiographs and are preferred.

Differential Diagnosis

When a patient is discovered to have a paraprotein, the distinction between plasma cell myeloma or another lymphoproliferative malignancy with a paraprotein (CLL/SLL, Waldenström macroglobulinemia, non-Hodgkin lymphoma, primary amyloid, cryoglobulinemia) or monoclonal gammopathy of undetermined significance (MGUS) must be made. Plasma cell myeloma, smoldering plasma cell myeloma, and MGUS must be distinguished from reactive (benign) polyclonal hypergammaglobulinemia (which is commonly seen in cirrhosis or chronic inflammation).

Treatment

Patients with low-risk smoldering myeloma are observed. Those with high-risk smoldering disease may be treated with lenalidomide (an immunomodulatory agent) and dexamethasone since this therapy prolongs the time to symptomatic myeloma and may prolong survival compared to no treatment though at the expense of treatment-related side effects.

Most patients with plasma cell myeloma require treatment at diagnosis because of bone pain or other symptoms and complications related to the disease. The initial treatment generally involves therapy with an immunomodulatory agent, such as lenalidomide; a proteasome inhibitor, such as bortezomib or carfilzomib; the anti-CD38 monoclonal antibody, daratumumab; and moderate- or high-dose dexamethasone. An immunomodulatory agent is sometimes replaced with an alkylating agent, cyclophosphamide, in the setting of kidney injury. The major side effects of lenalidomide are neutropenia and thrombocytopenia, skin rash, venous thromboembolism, peripheral neuropathy, and possibly birth defects. Bortezomib and carfilzomib have the advantages of producing rapid responses and of being effective in poor-prognosis myeloma. The major side effect of bortezomib is neuropathy (both peripheral and autonomic), which is largely ameliorated when given subcutaneously rather than intravenously. Carfilzomib rarely causes neuropathy but sometimes causes acute pulmonary hypertension or cardiac systolic dysfunction that is usually reversible. For patients with plasma cell myeloma, including newly diagnosed, autologous stem cell transplant–ineligible patients as well as relapsed or refractory patients, daratumumab (1800 mg) plus hyaluronidase-fihj (30,000 units) is administered subcutaneously into the abdomen over 3–5 minutes.

An oral proteasome inhibitor, ixazomib, is available for relapsed disease. Pomalidomide, an immunomodulatory agent, is effective as salvage therapy after relapse. Other salvage agents include daratumumab, elotuzumab (an anti-SLAMF7 monoclonal antibody), selinexor (causes cell cycle arrest and apoptosis), and belantamab mafodotin (an anti-BCMA antibody conjugated to a cytotoxic agent).

After initial therapy, many patients under age 80 years are consolidated with autologous hematopoietic stem cell transplantation following high-dose melphalan (an alkylating chemotherapeutic agent). Autologous stem cell transplantation prolongs both duration of remission and overall survival. Lenalidomide or thalidomide prolong remission and survival when given as posttransplant maintenance therapy but at the expense of an elevated rate of second malignancies. Proteasome inhibitors prolong remissions in high-risk patients after autologous stem cell transplantation. For patients with multi-agent refractory disease, chimeric antigen receptor T-cell therapy targeting the early plasma cell antigen BCMA has shown remarkable activity with response rates exceeding 70% and median duration of response of over 11 months.

Localized radiotherapy may be useful for palliation of bone pain or for eradicating tumor at the site of pathologic fracture. Vertebral collapse with its attendant pain and mechanical disturbance can be treated with vertebroplasty or kyphoplasty. Hypercalcemia and hyperuricemia should be treated aggressively with immobilization and hydration. The bisphosphonates (pamidronate or zoledronic acid) or the RANKL-inhibitor (denosumab) given intravenously monthly reduces pathologic fractures in patients with bone disease. These medications are important adjuncts in this subset of patients. The bisphosphonates are also used to treat myeloma-related hypercalcemia. However, long-term bisphosphonates have been associated with a risk of osteonecrosis of the jaw and other bony areas, so their use is limited to 1–2 years after definitive initial therapy in most patients. Myeloma patients with oliguric or anuric kidney disease at diagnosis due to high free light chain levels should be treated aggressively with chemotherapy and considered for therapeutic plasma exchange (to reduce the paraprotein burden) because return of kidney function can sometimes occur.

Prognosis

The outlook for patients with myeloma has been steadily improving for the past decade. The median survival of patients is more than 7 years. Patients with low-stage disease who lack high-risk genomic changes respond very well to treatment and derive significant benefit from autologous hematopoietic stem cell transplantation with survival approaching a decade. The International Staging System for myeloma relies on two factors: beta-2-microglobulin and albumin. Stage 1 patients have both beta-2-microglobulin less than 3.5 mg/L and albumin greater than 3.5 g/dL (survival more than 5 years). Stage 3 is established when beta-2-microglobulin is greater than 5.5 mg/L (survival less than 2 years). Stage 2 is established with values in between stage 1 and 3. Other adverse prognostic findings are an elevated serum LD or bone marrow genetic abnormalities established by FISH involving the immunoglobulin heavy chain locus at chromosome 14q32, multiple copies of the 1q21-23 locus, or 17p chromosome abnormalities (causing the loss or mutation of *TP53*).

When to Refer

All patients with plasma cell myeloma should be referred to a hematologist or an oncologist.

When to Admit

Hospitalization is indicated for treatment of AKI, hypercalcemia, or suspicion of spinal cord compression, for certain chemotherapy regimens, or for autologous hematopoietic stem cell transplantation.

Berbari HE et al. Initial therapeutic approaches to patients with multiple myeloma. Adv Ther. 2021;38:3694. [PMID: 34145483]

Goldschmidt H et al. Navigating the treatment landscape in multiple myeloma: which combinations to use and when? Ann Hematol. 2019;98:1. [PMID: 30470875]

Lonial S et al. Belantamab mafodotin for relapsed or refractory multiple myeloma (DREAMM-2): a two-arm, randomised, open-label, phase 2 study. Lancet Oncol. 2020;21:207. [PMID: 31859245]

Moreau P et al. Treatment of relapsed and refractory multiple myeloma: recommendations from the International Myeloma Working Group. Lancet Oncol. 2021;22:e105. [PMID: 33662288]

van de Donk NWCJ et al. CAR T-cell therapy for multiple myeloma: state of the art and prospects. Lancet Haematol. 2021;8:e446. [PMID: 34048683]

MONOCLONAL GAMMOPATHY OF UNDETERMINED SIGNIFICANCE

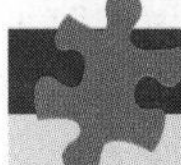

ESSENTIALS OF DIAGNOSIS

- Monoclonal immunoglobulin (ie, paraprotein) in the serum (< 3 g/dL [< 30 g/L]) or urine or both.
- Clonal plasma cells in the bone marrow < 10% (diagnostic).
- No symptoms and no organ damage from the paraprotein.

General Considerations

MGUS is present in 1% of all adults (3% of those over age 50 years and more than 5% of those over age 70 years). Among all patients with paraproteins, MGUS is far more common than plasma cell myeloma. MGUS is defined as bone marrow clonal plasma cells less than 10% in the setting of a paraprotein in the serum or urine or both (serum M-protein less than 3 g/dL [30 g/L]) and the absence of plasma cell–related end-organ damage. If an excess of serum free light chains (kappa or lambda) is established, the kappa to lambda ratio is 100 or less or 0.01 or greater (otherwise, this is diagnostic of plasma cell myeloma). In approximately one-quarter of cases, MGUS progresses to overt malignant disease in a median of one decade. The transformation of MGUS to plasma cell myeloma is approximately 1% per year. Two adverse risk factors for progression of MGUS to a plasma cell or lymphoid malignancy are an abnormal serum kappa to lambda free light chain ratio and a serum monoclonal protein (M-protein) level 1.5 g/dL or greater. Patients with MGUS have shortened survival (median 8.1 years vs 12.4 years for age- and sex-matched controls). In addition, 12% of patients with MGUS will convert to primary amyloidosis in a median of 9 years. Plasma cell myeloma, smoldering plasma cell myeloma, and MGUS must be distinguished from reactive (benign) polyclonal hypergammaglobulinemia (common in cirrhosis or chronic inflammation).

Laboratory Findings

To establish the diagnosis, serum and urine should be sent for PEP and IFE to search for a monoclonal protein; serum should be sent for free light chain analysis and quantitative immunoglobulins. Additional tests include a hemoglobin and serum albumin, calcium, and creatinine. If these additional tests are normal (or if abnormal but otherwise explained), then a bone marrow biopsy is usually deferred provided the serum M-protein is less than 3 g/dL (less than 30 g/L). In asymptomatic individuals, a skeletal survey (radiographs) is performed, but if there are some bone complaints or a question regarding bone disease, MRI or PET/CT imaging is preferred. MGUS is diagnosed if patients do not meet the criteria for smoldering plasma cell myeloma or plasma cell myeloma.

Treatment

Patients with MGUS are observed without treatment.

Ho M et al. Changing paradigms in diagnosis and treatment of monoclonal gammopathy of undetermined significance (MGUS) and smoldering multiple myeloma (SMM). Leukemia. 2020;34:3111. [PMID: 33046818]

Kyle RA et al. Long-term follow up of monoclonal gammopathy of undetermined significance. N Engl J Med. 2018;378:241. [PMID: 29342381]

Seth S et al. Monoclonal gammopathy of undetermined significance: current concepts and future prospects. Curr Hematol Malig Rep. 2020;15:45. [PMID: 32222885]

WALDENSTRÖM MACROGLOBULINEMIA

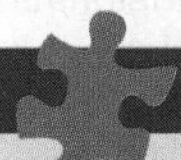

ESSENTIALS OF DIAGNOSIS

- Monoclonal IgM paraprotein.
- Infiltration of bone marrow by plasmacytic lymphocytes.
- Absence of lytic bone disease.
- *L265P* pathogenic variant in the gene *MYD88*.

General Considerations

Waldenström macroglobulinemia is a syndrome of IgM hypergammaglobulinemia that occurs in the setting of a low-grade non-Hodgkin lymphoma characterized by B cells that are morphologically a hybrid of lymphocytes and plasma cells. These cells characteristically secrete the IgM paraprotein, and many clinical manifestations of the disease are related to this macroglobulin.

Clinical Findings

A. Symptoms and Signs

This disease characteristically develops insidiously in patients in their 60s or 70s. Patients usually present with fatigue related to anemia. Hyperviscosity of serum may be manifested in a number of ways. Mucosal and GI bleeding is related to engorged blood vessels and platelet dysfunction. Other complaints include nausea, vertigo, and visual disturbances. Alterations in consciousness vary from mild lethargy to stupor and coma. The IgM paraprotein may also cause symptoms of cold agglutinin disease (hemolysis) or chronic demyelinating peripheral neuropathy.

On examination, there may be hepatosplenomegaly or lymphadenopathy. The retinal veins are engorged. Purpura may be present. There should be no bone tenderness.

B. Laboratory Findings

Anemia is nearly universal, and rouleaux formation is common, although the RBCs are agglutinated when the blood smear is prepared at room temperature. The anemia is related in part to expansion of the plasma volume by 50–100% due to the presence of the paraprotein. Other blood counts are usually normal. The abnormal plasmacytic lymphocytes may appear in small numbers on the peripheral blood smear. The bone marrow is characteristically infiltrated by the plasmacytic lymphocytes. The *L265P* pathogenic variant in *MYD88* is detectable in more than 90% of patients.

The hallmark of macroglobulinemia is the presence of a monoclonal IgM spike seen on serum PEP in the beta-globulin region. The serum viscosity is usually increased above the normal of 1.4–1.8 times that of water. Symptoms of hyperviscosity usually develop when the serum viscosity is over four times that of water, and marked symptoms usually arise when the viscosity is over six times that of water. Because paraproteins vary in their physicochemical properties, there is no strict correlation between the concentration of paraprotein and serum viscosity.

The IgM paraprotein may cause a positive antiglobulin (Coombs) test for complement and have cold agglutinin or cryoglobulin properties. If macroglobulinemia is suspected but the serum PEP shows only hypogammaglobulinemia, the test should be repeated while taking special measures to maintain the blood at 37°C, since the paraprotein may precipitate out at room temperature. Bone radiographs are normal, and there is no evidence of kidney injury.

Differential Diagnosis

Waldenström macroglobulinemia is differentiated from MGUS by the finding of bone marrow infiltration with monoclonal malignant cells. It is distinguished from CLL by bone marrow morphology, the absence of CD5 expression, and the absence of lymphocytosis, and it is distinguished from plasma cell myeloma by bone marrow morphology, the finding of the characteristic IgM paraprotein, and the absence of lytic bone disease.

Treatment

Patients with marked hyperviscosity syndrome (stupor, coma, pulmonary edema) should be treated on an emergency basis with plasmapheresis. On a chronic basis, some patients can be managed with periodic plasmapheresis alone. As with other indolent malignant lymphoid diseases, rituximab (375 mg/m^2 intravenously weekly for 4–8 weeks) has significant activity. However, a word of caution: the IgM often rises first after rituximab therapy before it falls and for patients with hyperviscosity, an additional cytotoxic agent needs to be initiated at the same time. Combination therapy is recommended for advanced disease (see Table 39–3) with addition of bendamustine showing excellent response rates. The oral BTK inhibitors ibrutinib (420 mg daily) and zanubrutinib (160 mg twice daily) have shown significant activity with a 90% response rate and a 73% major response rate that can result in durable remissions. Proteasome inhibitors (bortezomib, carfilzomib) and lenalidomide have also been shown to have activity in this disease. Autologous hematopoietic stem cell transplantation is reserved for relapsed or refractory patients.

Prognosis

Waldenström macroglobulinemia is an indolent disease with a median survival rate of 5 years, and 10% of patients are alive at 15 years.

When to Refer

All patients should be referred to a hematologist or an oncologist.

When to Admit

Patients should be admitted for treatment of hyperviscosity syndrome.

Bustoros M et al. Progression risk stratification of asymptomatic Waldenström macroglobulinemia. J Clin Oncol. 2019;37:1403. [PMID: 30990729]

Gertz MA. Waldenström macroglobulinemia: 2021 update on diagnosis, risk stratification, and management. Am J Hematol. 2021;96:258. [PMID: 33368476]

AMYLOIDOSIS

ESSENTIALS OF DIAGNOSIS

- Congo red positive amyloid protein on tissue biopsy.
- Primary amyloid protein is kappa or lambda immunoglobulin light chain.
- Serum or urine (or both) light chain paraprotein.

General Considerations

Amyloidosis is a rare condition whereby a protein abnormally deposits in tissue resulting in organ dysfunction.

The propensity of a protein to be amyloidogenic is a consequence of disturbed translational or posttranslational protein folding and lack of consequential water solubility. The input of amyloid protein into tissues far exceeds its output, so amyloid build up inexorably proceeds to organ dysfunction and ultimately organ failure and premature death.

Amyloidosis is classified according to the type of amyloid protein deposited. The six main categories are **primary** (immunoglobulin light chain [AL]), **secondary** (serum protein A, produced in inflammatory conditions [AA]), **hereditary** (mutated transthyretin [TTR]; many others), **senile** (wild-type TTR; atrial natriuretic peptide; others), **dialysis-related** (beta-2-microglobulin, not filtered out by dialysis membranes [Abeta-2M]), and **LECT2** (associated with Latinx ethnicity). Amyloidosis is further classified as **localized** (amyloid deposits only in a single tissue type or organ) or, most common, **systemic** (widespread amyloid deposition).

Clinical Findings

A. Symptoms and Signs

Patients with **localized amyloidosis** have symptoms and signs related to the affected single organ, such as hoarseness (vocal cords) or proptosis and visual disturbance (orbits). Patients with **systemic amyloidosis** have symptoms and signs of unexplained medical syndromes, including heart failure (infiltrative/restrictive cardiomyopathy), nephrotic syndrome, malabsorption and weight loss, hepatic dysfunction, autonomic insufficiency, carpal tunnel syndrome (often bilateral), and sensorimotor peripheral neuropathy. Other symptoms and signs include an enlarged tongue; waxy, rough plaques on skin; contusions (including the periorbital areas); cough or dyspnea; and disturbed deglutition. These symptoms and signs arise insidiously, and the diagnosis of amyloidosis is generally made late in the disease process.

B. Laboratory Findings

The diagnosis of amyloid protein requires a tissue biopsy that demonstrates deposition of a pink interstitial substance in the tissue with the hematoxylin and eosin stain. This protein stains red with Congo red and becomes an apple-green color when the light is polarized. Amyloid is a triple-stranded fibril composed of the amyloid protein, amyloid protein P, and glycosaminoglycan. The amyloid fibrils form beta-pleated sheets as demonstrated by electron microscopy. In primary amyloidosis, the amyloid protein is either the kappa or lambda immunoglobulin light chain.

When systemic amyloidosis is suspected, a blind aspiration of the abdominal fat pad will reveal amyloid two-thirds of the time. If the fat pad aspiration is unrevealing, then the affected organ needs biopsy. In 90% of patients with primary amyloidosis, analysis of the serum and urine will reveal a kappa or lambda light chain paraprotein by PEP, IFE, or free light chain assay; in the remainder, mass spectroscopy demonstrates light chain in the tissue biopsy. Lambda amyloid is more common than kappa amyloid, a relative proportion opposite from normal B-cell stoichiometry. Most patients with primary amyloidosis have a small excess of kappa- or lambda-restricted plasma cells in the bone marrow (but less than 10%). The bone marrow may or may not demonstrate interstitial amyloid deposition or amyloid in the blood vessels.

Patients with primary cardiac amyloidosis have an infiltrative cardiomyopathy with thick ventricular walls on echocardiogram that sometimes shows a specific speckling pattern. Paradoxically, QRS voltages are low on ECG. Cardiac MRI has a distinctive delayed enhancement of gadolinium that is virtually diagnostic. With renal amyloid, albuminuria is present, which can be in the nephrotic range. Late in renal involvement, kidney function decreases (see Chapter 22, Renal Amyloidosis).

Differential Diagnosis

Amyloidosis must be distinguished from MGUS and plasma cell myeloma or other malignant lymphoproliferative disorders with an associated paraprotein. Of note, 12% of patients with MGUS will convert to primary amyloidosis in a median of 9 years. One-fifth of patients who have primary amyloidosis will meet the diagnostic criteria for plasma cell myeloma; conversely, 5% of patients with plasma cell myeloma will have amyloid deposition of their paraprotein at diagnosis.

Treatment

The treatment approach to primary amyloidosis closely resembles that of plasma cell myeloma. Prospective, randomized trials of plasma cell myeloma chemotherapy versus colchicine have demonstrated a survival benefit to chemotherapy. The goal is reduction of light chain production and thus tissue deposition as a means to arrest progressive end-organ dysfunction. Active agents in primary amyloidosis include melphalan, cyclophosphamide, dexamethasone, lenalidomide, bortezomib and daratumumab (see Table 39–3). As in plasma cell myeloma, autologous hematopoietic stem cell transplantation after high-dose melphalan is used in patients with reasonable organ function and a good performance status. The treatment-related mortality, however, is higher in patients with primary amyloidosis than in plasma cell myeloma (6% vs 1%). Some patients will demonstrate end-organ improvement after therapy. Agents are being developed that facilitate amyloid dissolution or correct protein folding abnormalities in the amyloid protein. Treatment of AA amyloid is treatment of the underlying cause of inflammation. Treatment of familial TTR is liver transplantation and of acquired or inherited TTR is tafamidis or inotersen.

Prognosis

Untreated primary amyloidosis is associated with progressive end-organ failure and premature death. There is no known cure for primary amyloidosis. Although virtually every tissue examined at autopsy will contain amyloid, patients with primary amyloidosis usually have one or two primary failing organs that clinically drive the presentation and prognosis. The cardiac biomarkers BNP, N-terminal pro-BNP, and troponins T and I are prognostic in this disease regardless of overt clinical cardiac involvement. Historically, patients with predominantly cardiac or autonomic nerve presentations had survivals of 3–9 months, those with carpal tunnel syndrome or nephrosis had survivals of 1.5–3 years, and those with peripheral neuropathy had survivals of 5 years. These survivals are roughly doubled with plasma cell myeloma-like treatment. In those patients able to undergo autologous hematopoietic stem cell transplantation, the median survival is about 5 years (and approaches 10 years for those achieving a complete hematologic remission).

When to Refer

- All patients who have primary amyloidosis or in whom it is suspected should be referred to a hematologist or oncologist.
- Patients with hereditary amyloidosis should be referred to a hepatologist for consideration of liver transplantation.

When to Admit

- Patients with systemic amyloidosis require hospitalization to treat exacerbations of end-organ failure, including heart, liver, or kidney.
- Patients with primary amyloidosis require hospitalization to undergo autologous hematopoietic stem cell transplantation.

Brunger AF et al. Causes of AA amyloidosis: a systematic review. Amyloid. 2020;27:1. [PMID: 31766892]

Gertz MA et al. Systemic amyloidosis recognition, prognosis, and therapy: a systematic review. JAMA. 2020;324:79. [PMID: 32633805]

Kastritis E et al; ANDROMEDA Trial Investigators. Daratumumab-based treatment for immunoglobulin light-chain amyloidosis. N Engl J Med. 2021;385:46. [PMID: 34192431]

Palladini G et al. Management of AL amyloidosis in 2020. Blood. 2020;136:2620. [PMID: 33270858]

BLOOD TRANSFUSIONS

Most blood products are leukoreduced in-line during acquisition and are thus prospectively leukocyte-poor. Leukoreduced blood products reduce the incidence of leukoagglutination reactions, platelet alloimmunization, transfusion-related acute lung injury, and CMV exposure.

RBC TRANSFUSIONS

RBC transfusions are given to raise the hemoglobin levels in patients with clinically significant anemia or to replace losses after acute bleeding episodes.

Preparations of RBCs for Transfusion

Several types of preparations containing RBCs are available (whole blood, packed RBCs, frozen RBCs, or autologous non-frozen RBCs).

A. Fresh Whole Blood

The advantage of whole blood for transfusion is the simultaneous presence of RBCs, plasma, and fresh platelets. Fresh whole blood is not absolutely necessary, since all the above components are available separately. The major indications for use of whole blood are cardiac surgery with hemorrhage or massive hemorrhage when more than 10 units of blood is required in a 24-hour period.

B. Packed RBCs

Packed RBCs are the component most commonly used to raise the hemoglobin. Each unit has a volume of about 300 mL, of which approximately 200 mL consists of RBCs. One unit of packed RBCs will usually raise the hemoglobin by approximately 1 g/dL. Current guidelines recommend a transfusion “trigger” hemoglobin threshold of 7–8 g/dL (70–80 g/L) for hospitalized patients, including those who are critically ill, those undergoing cardiothoracic surgery or repair of a hip fracture, those with upper GI bleeding, and those with hematologic malignancy undergoing chemotherapy or hematopoietic cell transplant.

C. Autologous Packed RBCs

Patients scheduled for elective surgery may donate blood for autologous transfusion. These units may be stored for up to 35 days before freezing is necessary.

Compatibility Testing

Before transfusion, the recipient’s and the donor’s blood are typed and cross-matched to avoid hemolytic transfusion reactions. Although many antigen systems are present on RBCs, only the ABO and Rh systems are specifically tested prior to all transfusions. The A and B antigens are the most important because everyone who lacks one or both RBC antigens has IgM isoantibodies (called isoagglutinins) in his or her plasma against the missing antigen(s). The isoagglutinins activate complement and can cause rapid intravascular lysis of the incompatible RBCs. In emergencies, type O/Rh-negative blood can be given to any recipient, but usually packed RBCs are given to minimize transfusion of donor plasma containing anti-A and anti-B antibodies with the use of whole blood.

The other important antigen routinely tested for is the D antigen of the Rh system. Approximately 15% of the population lacks this antigen. In patients lacking the antigen, anti-D antibodies are not naturally present, but the D antigen is highly immunogenic. A recipient whose RBCs lack D and who receives D-positive blood often develop anti-D antibodies that can cause severe lysis of subsequent transfusions of D-positive RBCs or abort a D-positive fetus.

Blood typing includes a cross-match assay of recipient serum for alloantibodies directed against donor RBCs by mixing recipient serum with panels of RBCs representing commonly occurring minor RBC antigens. The screening is particularly important if the recipient has had previous transfusions or pregnancy.

Hemolytic Transfusion Reactions

The most severe hemolytic transfusion reactions are acute (temporally related to the transfusion), involving incompatible mismatches in the ABO system that are isoagglutinin-mediated. Most of these cases are due to clerical errors and mislabeled specimens. With current compatibility testing and double-check clerical systems, the risk of an acute hemolytic reaction is 1 in 76,000 transfused units of RBCs. Death from acute hemolytic reaction occurs in 1 in 1.8 million transfused units. When hemolysis occurs, it is rapid and intravascular, releasing free hemoglobin into the plasma. The severity of these reactions depends on the dose of RBCs given. The most severe reactions are those seen in surgical patients under anesthesia.

Delayed hemolytic transfusion reactions are caused by minor RBC antigen discrepancies and are typically less severe. The hemolysis usually takes place at a slower rate and is mediated by IgG alloantibodies causing extravascular RBC destruction. These transfusion reactions may be delayed for 5–10 days after transfusion. In such cases, the recipient has received RBCs containing an immunogenic antigen, and in the time since transfusion, a new alloantibody has formed. The most common antigens involved in such reactions are Duffy, Kidd, Kell, and C and E loci of the Rh system. The current risk of a delayed hemolytic transfusion reaction is 1 in 6000 transfused units of RBCs.

A. Symptoms and Signs

Major acute hemolytic transfusion reactions cause fever and chills, with backache and headache. In severe cases, there may be apprehension, dyspnea, hypotension, and cardiovascular collapse. Patients under general anesthesia will not manifest such symptoms, and the first indication may be tachycardia, generalized bleeding, or oliguria. *The transfusion must be stopped immediately.* In severe cases, acute DIC, AKI from tubular necrosis, or both can occur. Death occurs in 4% of acute hemolytic reactions due to ABO incompatibility. Delayed hemolytic transfusion reactions are usually without any or only mild symptoms or signs.

B. Laboratory Findings

When an acute hemolytic transfusion episode is suspected, the identification of the recipient and of the transfusion product bag label should be rechecked. The transfusion product bag with its pilot tube must be returned to the blood bank, and a fresh sample of the recipient's blood must accompany the bag for retyping and re–cross-matching of donor and recipient blood samples. The hemoglobin will fail to rise by the expected amount after a transfusion. Coagulation studies may reveal evidence of AKI or acute DIC. The plasma-free hemoglobin in the recipient will be elevated resulting in hemoglobinuria.

In cases of delayed hemolytic reactions, there will be an unexpected drop in hemoglobin and an increase in the total and indirect bilirubins. The new offending alloantibody is easily detected in the patient's serum.

C. Treatment

If an acute hemolytic transfusion reaction is suspected, the transfusion should be stopped at once. The patient should be vigorously hydrated to prevent ATN. Forced diuresis with mannitol may help prevent or minimize AKI.

Leukoagglutinin Reactions

Most transfusion reactions are not hemolytic but represent reactions to antigens present on transfused passenger leukocytes in patients who have been sensitized to leukocyte antigens through previous transfusions or pregnancy. Transfusion products relatively rich in leukocyte-rich plasma, especially platelets, are most likely to cause this. Moderate to severe leukoagglutinin reactions occur in 1% of RBC transfusions and 2% of platelet transfusions. The risk of a leukoagglutination reaction is minimal if the transfused blood product is leukoreduced in-line upon collection. Most commonly, fever and chills develop in patients within 12 hours after transfusion. In severe cases, cough and dyspnea may occur and the chest radiograph may show transient pulmonary infiltrates. Because no hemolysis is involved, the hemoglobin rises by the expected amount despite the reaction.

Leukoagglutinin reactions may respond to acetaminophen (500–650 mg orally) and diphenhydramine (25 mg orally or intravenously); corticosteroids, such as hydrocortisone (1 mg/kg intravenously), are also of value. Overall, leukoagglutination reactions are diminishing through the routine use of in-line leukotrapping during blood donation (ie, leukoreduced blood). Patients experiencing severe leukoagglutination episodes despite receiving leukoreduced blood transfusions should receive leukopoor or washed blood products.

Hypersensitivity Reactions

Urticaria or bronchospasm may develop during or soon after a transfusion. These reactions are almost always due to exposure to allogeneic plasma proteins rather than to leukocytes. The risk is low enough that the routine use of antihistamine premedications has been eliminated before packed RBC transfusions. However, a hypersensitivity reaction, including anaphylactic shock, may develop in patients who are IgA deficient because of antibodies to IgA in the patient's plasma directed against the IgA in the transfused blood product. Patients with such reactions may require transfusion of washed or even frozen RBCs to avoid future severe reactions.

Contaminated Blood

Blood products can be contaminated with bacteria. Platelets are especially prone to bacterial contamination because they cannot be refrigerated. Bacterial contamination occurs in 1 of every 30,000 RBC donations and 1 of every 5000 platelet donations. Receipt of a blood product contaminated with gram-positive bacteria will cause fever and bacteremia, but rarely causes a sepsis syndrome. Receipt of a blood product contaminated with gram-negative bacteria often causes septic shock, acute DIC, and AKI due to the transfused endotoxin and is usually fatal. Strategies to reduce bacterial contamination include enhanced venipuncture site skin cleansing, diverting of the first few milliliters of donated blood, use of single-donor blood products (as opposed to pooled-donor products), and point-of-care rapid bacterial screening in order to discard questionable units. Blood products infused with psoralen and then exposed to UVA light will have no living organisms in them but add cost to acquisition of the blood product. The current risk of a septic transfusion reaction from a culture-negative unit of single-donor platelets (not psoralen treated) is 1 in 60,000. In any patient who may have received contaminated blood, the recipient and the donor blood bag should both be cultured, and antibiotics should be given immediately to the recipient.

Infectious Diseases Transmitted Through Transfusion

Despite the use of only volunteer blood donors and the routine screening of blood, transfusion-associated viral diseases remain a problem. All blood products (RBCs, platelets, plasma, cryoprecipitate) can transmit viral diseases. All blood donors are screened with questionnaires designed to detect (and therefore reject) donors at high risk for transmitting infectious diseases. For example, the American Red Cross does not accept blood donation from persons with SARS-CoV-2 virus or from contacts of persons who have or are suspected to have the causal SARS-CoV-2 virus. All blood is screened for hepatitis B surface antigen, antibody to hepatitis B core antigen, antibody to syphilis, antibodies to HIV-1 and HIV-2 and NAT (nucleic acid amplification) for HIV, antibody to hepatitis C virus (HCV) and NAT for hepatitis C, antibody to human T-cell lymphotropic/leukemia virus (HTLV), and NAT for West Nile virus. Zika virus contamination is screened for by donor questionnaire, but the routine use of an FDA-approved detection test has not been uniformly adopted to screen donated blood. It is recommended that blood donors get screened once for antibodies against *Trypanosoma cruzi*, the infectious agent that causes Chagas disease (and if negative, no further screening for additional blood donations).

With improved screening, the risk of posttransfusion hepatitis has steadily decreased after the receipt of screened "negative" blood products. The risk of acquiring hepatitis B is about 1 in 200,000 transfused units in the United States. The risk of hepatitis C acquisition is 1 in 1.5 to 2 million transfused units in the United States. The risk of HIV acquisition is 1 in 2 million transfused units. Unscreened but leukoreduced blood products appear to be equivalent to CMV screened-negative blood products in terms of the risk of CMV transmission to a CMV-seronegative recipient.

Transfusion Graft-Versus-Host Disease

Allogeneic passenger lymphocytes in transfused blood products will engraft in some recipients and mount an alloimmune attack against tissues expressing discrepant HLA antigens causing graft-versus-host disease (GVHD). The symptoms and signs of transfusion-associated GVHD include fever, rash, diarrhea, hepatitis, lymphadenopathy, and severe pancytopenia. The outcome is usually fatal. Transfusion-associated GVHD occurs most often in recipients with immune defects, malignant lymphoproliferative disorders, solid tumors being treated with chemotherapy or immunotherapy, treatment with immunosuppressive medications (especially purine analogs such as fludarabine), or older patients undergoing cardiac surgery. HIV infection alone does not increase the risk. The use of leukoreduced blood products is inadequate to prevent transfusion-associated GVHD. This complication can be avoided by irradiating blood products (25 Gy or more) to prevent lymphocyte proliferation in blood products given to recipients at high risk for transfusion-associated GVHD.

Transfusion-Related Acute Lung Injury

Transfusion-related acute lung injury (TRALI) occurs in 1 in every 5000 transfused units of blood products. TRALI is clinically defined as noncardiogenic pulmonary edema after a blood product transfusion without other explanation. Transfused surgical and critically ill patients seem most susceptible. It has been associated with allogeneic antibodies in the donor plasma component that bind to recipient leukocyte antigens, including HLA antigens and other granulocyte- and monocyte-specific antigens (such as human neutrophil antigen [HNA]-1a, -1b, -2a, and -3a). In 20% of cases, no antileukocyte antibodies are identified raising the concern that bioactive lipids or other substances that accumulate while the blood product is in storage can also mediate TRALI in susceptible recipients. Ten to 20% of female blood donors and 1–5% of male blood donors have antileukocyte antibodies in their serum. The risk of TRALI is reduced through the use of male-only plasma donors, when possible. There is no specific treatment for TRALI, only supportive care.

PLATELET TRANSFUSIONS

Platelet transfusions are indicated in cases of thrombocytopenia due to decreased platelet production. They are of some use in immune thrombocytopenia when active bleeding is evident, but the clearance of transfused platelets is rapid as they are exposed to the same pathophysiologic forces experienced by the recipient's endogenous platelets. The risk of bleeding rises when the platelet count falls to less than 80,000/mcL (80×10^9/L), and the risk of life-threatening spontaneous bleeding increases when the platelet count is less than 5000/mcL (5×10^9/L). Because of this, prophylactic platelet transfusions are often given at these very low levels, usually when less than 10,000/mcL (10×10^9/L). Platelet transfusions are also given prior to invasive procedures or surgery in thrombocytopenic patients, and the goal is often to raise the platelet count to 50,000/mcL (50×10^9/L) or more.

Platelets for transfusion are most commonly derived from single-donor apheresis collections (roughly the equivalent to the platelets recovered from six donations of whole blood). A single donor unit of platelets should raise the platelet count by 50,000 to 60,000 platelets per mcL

(50–60 × 10^9/L) in a transfusion-naïve recipient without hypersplenism or ongoing platelet consumptive disorder. Transfused platelets typically last for 2 or 3 days. Platelet transfusion responses may be suboptimal with poor platelet increments and short platelet survival times. This may be due to one of several causes, including fever, sepsis, hypersplenism, DIC, large body habitus, low platelet dose in the transfusion, or platelet alloimmunization (from prior transfusions, prior pregnancy, or prior organ transplantation). Many, but not all, alloantibodies causing platelet destruction are directed at HLA antigens. Patients requiring long periods of platelet transfusion support should be monitored to document adequate responses to transfusions so that the most appropriate product can be used. If random platelet transfusions prove inadequate, then the patient should be cross-matched with potential donors who might prove better able to provide adequate platelet-transfusion increments and platelet survival. Patients requiring ongoing platelet transfusions who become alloimmunized may benefit from HLA-matched platelets derived from either volunteer donors or family members.

TRANSFUSION OF PLASMA COMPONENTS

Fresh frozen plasma (FFP) is available in units of approximately 200 mL. FFP contains normal levels of all coagulation factors (about 1 unit/mL of each factor). FFP is used to correct coagulation factor deficiencies (such as in liver disease) and to treat thrombotic thrombocytopenic purpura or other thrombotic microangiopathies. FFP is also used to correct or prevent coagulopathy in trauma patients receiving massive transfusion of packed RBC (PRBC). An FFP:PRBC ratio of 1:2 or more is associated with improved survival in trauma patients receiving massive transfusions, regardless of the presence of a coagulopathy.

Cryoprecipitate is made from fresh plasma by cooling the plasma to 4°C and collecting the precipitate. One unit of cryoprecipitate has a volume of approximately 15–20 mL and contains approximately 250 mg of fibrinogen and between 80 and 100 units of factor VIII and von Willebrand factor. Cryoprecipitate is most commonly used to supplement fibrinogen in cases of acquired hypofibrinogenemia (eg, acute DIC) or in rare instances of congenital hypofibrinogenemia. One unit of cryoprecipitate will raise the fibrinogen level by about 8 mg/dL (0.24 mcmol/L). Cryoprecipitate is sometimes used to temporarily correct the acquired qualitative platelet dysfunction associated with kidney disease.

Frank SM et al. Clinical utility of autologous salvaged blood: a review. J Gastrointest Surg. 2020;24:464. [PMID: 31468332]
Solves Alcaina P. Platelet transfusion: and update on challenges and outcomes. J Blood Med. 2020;11:19. [PMID: 32158298]
Zeeuw van der Laan EAN et al. Update on the pathophysiology of transfusion-related acute lung injury. Curr Opin Hematol. 2020;27:386. [PMID: 32868671]

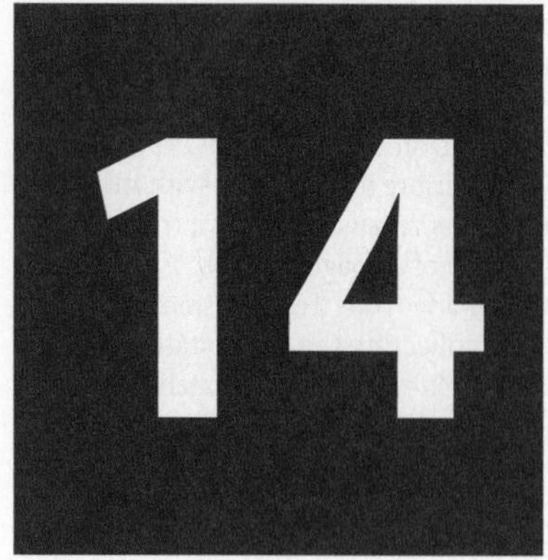

Disorders of Hemostasis, Thrombosis, & Antithrombotic Therapy

Andrew D. Leavitt, MD
Erika Leemann Price, MD, MPH

To evaluate patients for defects of hemostasis, the clinical context must be considered carefully (Table 14–1). **Heritable defects** are suggested by bleeding that begins in infancy or childhood, is recurrent, and occurs at multiple anatomic sites, although other patterns of presentation are possible. **Acquired disorders** of hemostasis typically are associated with bleeding that begins later in life and may relate to introduction of medications (eg, agents that affect platelet activity) or to onset of underlying medical conditions (such as kidney disease, liver disease, myelodysplasia, aortic stenosis, prosthetic aortic valve, myeloproliferative neoplasms, plasma cell disorders), or may be idiopathic (acquired hemophilia A, acquired von Willebrand disease). Importantly, however, a sufficient hemostatic challenge (such as major trauma) may produce excessive bleeding even in individuals with normal hemostasis. Obtaining a personal history of hemostatic challenges (eg, circumcision, trauma, injury during youth sports, tooth extractions, prior surgery, pregnancy and delivery) and a family history of bleeding are essential when evaluating someone for a possible bleeding disorder.

PLATELET DISORDERS

THROMBOCYTOPENIA

Selected causes of thrombocytopenia are shown in Table 14–2. The age of the patient and presence of comorbid conditions can help direct the diagnostic workup.

The risk of clinically relevant spontaneous bleeding (including petechial hemorrhage and bruising) does not typically increase appreciably until the platelet count falls below 10,000–20,000/mcL ($10–20 \times 10^9$/L), although patients with dysfunctional platelets or local vascular defects can bleed with higher platelet counts. Suggested platelet counts to prevent spontaneous bleeding or to provide adequate hemostasis around the time of invasive procedures are found in Table 14–3. However, most medical centers develop their own local guidelines to have a consistent approach to such complex situations.

DECREASED PLATELET PRODUCTION

1. Bone Marrow Failure

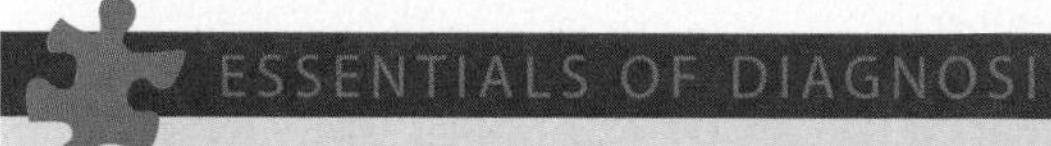

ESSENTIALS OF DIAGNOSIS

- Determine if bone marrow failure is congenital or acquired.
- Most congenital marrow failure disorders present in childhood.

General Considerations

Congenital conditions that cause thrombocytopenia include amegakaryocytic thrombocytopenia, the thrombocytopenia-absent radius syndrome, and Wiskott-Aldrich syndrome; these disorders usually feature isolated thrombocytopenia, whereas patients with Fanconi anemia and dyskeratosis congenita typically include cytopenias in other blood cell lineages. Mutations in genes (*FLI1, MYH9, GATA1, ETV6*, among others) that cause thrombocytopenia are being identified.

Acquired causes of bone marrow failure (see Chapter 13) leading to thrombocytopenia include, but are not limited to, acquired aplastic anemia, myelodysplastic syndrome (MDS), acquired amegakaryocytic thrombocytopenia (albeit a rare disorder), alcohol, and drugs. Unlike aplastic anemia, MDS is more common among older patients.

Clinical Findings

See Chapter 13 for symptoms and signs of aplastic anemia. Acquired aplastic anemia typically presents with reductions in multiple blood cell lineages, and the CBC reveals pancytopenia (anemia, thrombocytopenia, and neutropenia). A bone marrow biopsy is required for diagnosis and reveals marked hypocellularity. MDS also presents as cytopenias and can have pancytopenia, but the marrow typically demonstrates hypercellularity and dysplastic features. The presence of macrocytosis, ringed sideroblasts on iron

Table 14–1. Evaluation of the bleeding patient.

Necessary Component of Evaluation	Diagnostic Correlate
Location	
Mucocutaneous (bruises, petechiae, gingivae, nosebleeds, GI, GU)	Suggests qualitative/quantitative platelet defects; vWD
Joints, soft tissue	Suggests disorders of coagulation factors
Onset	
Infancy/childhood	Suggests heritable condition
Adulthood	Suggests milder heritable condition or acquired defect of hemostasis (eg, ITP, medication, acquired factor VIII deficiency; acquired vWD)
Clinical Context	
Postsurgical	Anatomic/surgical defect must be ruled out
Pregnancy	vWD, HELLP syndrome, ITP, acquired factor VIII inhibitor
Sepsis	May indicate DIC
Exposure to anticoagulants	Rule out excessive anticoagulation
Personal History[1]	
Absent	Suggests acquired rather than congenital defect, or anatomic/surgical defect (if applicable)
Present	Suggests established acquired defect or congenital disorder
Family History	
Absent	Suggests acquired defect or no defect of hemostasis
Present	May signify hemophilia A or B, vWD, other heritable bleeding disorders

[1]Prior spontaneous bleeding and excessive bleeding with circumcision, menses, dental extractions, trauma, minor procedures (eg, endoscopy, biopsies), and major procedures (surgery).
DIC, disseminated intravascular coagulation; GU, genitourinary; HELLP, hemolysis, elevated liver enzymes, low platelets; ITP, immune thrombocytopenia; vWD, von Willebrand disease.

staining of the bone marrow aspirate, dysplasia of hematopoietic elements, or cytogenetic abnormalities (especially monosomy 5 or 7 and trisomy 8) is more suggestive of MDS.

Differential Diagnosis

Adult patients with acquired amegakaryocytic thrombocytopenia (rare) have isolated thrombocytopenia and reduced or absent megakaryocytes in the bone marrow, which along with failure to respond to immunomodulatory regimens typically administered in immune thrombocytopenia (ITP), distinguishes them from patients with ITP.

Table 14–2. Selected causes of thrombocytopenia.

Decreased production of platelets
Congenital bone marrow failure
Amegakaryocytic thrombocytopenia, Wiskott-Aldrich syndrome, Fanconi anemia
Acquired bone marrow failure
Aplastic anemia, myelodysplastic syndrome, leukemia
Exposure to chemotherapy, irradiation, medications (https://ouhsc.edu/platelets/ditp.html)
Marrow infiltration (neoplastic, infectious)
Nutritional (deficiency of vitamin B_{12}, folate)
Other: HIV, alcohol
Other inherited thrombocytopenias
Bernard-Soulier syndrome, gray platelet syndrome, May-Hegglin anomaly, Hemansky Pudlak syndrome, MYH9 mutations, and others
Increased destruction of platelets
Immune thrombocytopenia (primary)
Immune thrombocytopenia (secondary), including drug-induced, lymphoproliferative disorders (eg, CLL) or viral infections (eg, hepatitis C virus, Epstein-Barr virus, or HIV)
Heparin-induced thrombocytopenia
Thrombotic microangiopathy/microangiopathic hemolytic anemias
Disseminated intravascular coagulation
Posttransfusion purpura
Mechanical (aortic valvular dysfunction; extracorporeal bypass)
von Willebrand disease, type 2B
Hemophagocytosis
Increased sequestration of platelets
Hypersplenism (eg, cirrhosis, myeloproliferative disorders, lymphoma)
Other conditions causing thrombocytopenia
Gestational thrombocytopenia
Pseudothrombocytopenia

CLL, chronic lymphocytic leukemia.

Treatment

A. Congenital Conditions

Treatment is varied but may include blood product support, blood cell growth factors, androgens and, in some cases, allogeneic hematopoietic stem cell transplantation.

Table 14–3. Desired platelet count ranges.

Clinical Scenario	Platelet Count /mcL (× 10^9/L)
Prevention of spontaneous mucocutaneous bleeding	> 10,000–20,000 (> 10–20)
Insertion of central venous catheters	> 20,000–50,000[1] (> 20–50)
Administration of therapeutic anticoagulation	> 30,000–50,000 (> 30–50)
Minor surgery and selected invasive procedures[2]	> 50,000–80,000 (> 50–80)
Major surgery	> 80,000–100,000 (> 80–100)

[1]A platelet target within the higher reference range is required for tunneled catheters.
[2]Such as endoscopy with biopsy.

B. Acquired Conditions

Patients with severe aplastic anemia are treated with immunosuppressive therapy or allogeneic hematopoietic stem cell transplantation (see Chapter 13).

Treatment of thrombocytopenia due to MDS, if clinically significant bleeding is present or if the risk of bleeding is high, is limited to chronic transfusion of platelets in most instances (Table 14–3). Additional treatment is discussed in Chapter 13.

Nurden AT et al. Inherited thrombocytopenias: history, advances and perspectives. Haematologica. 2020;105:2004. [PMID: 32527953]

2. Bone Marrow Infiltration

Replacement of the normal bone marrow elements by leukemic cells, plasma cell myeloma, lymphoma, or nonhematologic tumors or by infections (such as mycobacterial disease or ehrlichiosis) may cause thrombocytopenia; however, abnormalities in other blood cell lines are usually present. These entities are easily diagnosed after examining the bone marrow biopsy and aspirate or determining the infecting organism from an aspirate specimen, and they often lead to a leukoerythroblastic peripheral blood smear (left-shifted myeloid lineage cells, nucleated RBCs, and teardrop-shaped RBCs). Treatment of thrombocytopenia is directed at eradication of the underlying infiltrative disorder, but platelet transfusion may be required if clinically significant bleeding is present.

3. Chemotherapy & Irradiation

Chemotherapeutic agents and irradiation may lead to thrombocytopenia by direct toxicity to megakaryocytes, hematopoietic progenitor cells, or both. The severity and duration of chemotherapy-induced depressions in the platelet count are determined by the specific agent and regimen used, although the platelet count typically resolves more slowly following a chemotherapeutic insult than does neutropenia or anemia, especially if multiple cycles of treatment have been given. Until recovery occurs, patients may be supported with transfused platelets if bleeding is present or the risk of bleeding is high (Table 14–3). Studies suggest that that platelet growth factors, such as eltrombopag and romiplostim, may help prevent chemotherapy-induced thrombocytopenia and allow patients to receive their full chemotherapy doses on schedule. Checkpoint inhibitors can also lead to thrombocytopenia that mimics immune thrombocytopenic purpura.

Soff GA et al. Romiplostim treatment of chemotherapy-induced thrombocytopenia. J Clin Oncol. 2019;37:2892. [PMID: 31545663]

Wang Z et al. Recombinant human thrombopoietin (rh-TPO) for the prevention of severe thrombocytopenia induced by high-dose cytarabine: a prospective, randomized, self-controlled study. Leuk Lymphoma. 2018;59:2821. [PMID: 29909708]

4. Nutritional Deficiencies

Thrombocytopenia, typically in concert with anemia, may be observed with a deficiency of folate (that may accompany alcohol use disorder) or vitamin B_{12} (concomitant neurologic findings may be manifest). In addition, thrombocytopenia can occur in very severe iron deficiency, albeit rarely, whereas thrombocytosis is far more common. Replacing the deficient vitamin or mineral results in improvement in the platelet count.

5. Cyclic Thrombocytopenia

Cyclic thrombocytopenia is a rare disorder that produces cyclic oscillations of the platelet count, usually with a periodicity of 3–6 weeks. The pathophysiologic mechanism responsible for the condition is unclear. Severe thrombocytopenia and bleeding typically occur at the platelet nadir. Oral contraceptive medications, androgens, azathioprine, and thrombopoietic growth factors have been used successfully in the management of cyclic thrombocytopenia.

INCREASED PLATELET DESTRUCTION

1. Immune Thrombocytopenia

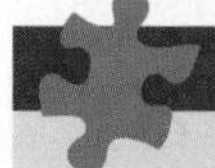

ESSENTIALS OF DIAGNOSIS

- Isolated thrombocytopenia (rule out pseudothrombocytopenia by review of peripheral smear).
- Assess for any new causative medications and HIV, hepatitis B, hepatitis C, and *Helicobacter pylori* infections.
- Immune thrombocytopenia (ITP) is a diagnosis of exclusion.

General Considerations

ITP is an autoimmune condition in which pathogenic antibodies bind platelets, accelerating their clearance from the circulation; additional pathophysiologic mechanisms include a role for T cells. Many patients with ITP also lack appropriate compensatory platelet production, thought, at least in part, to reflect the antibody's effect on megakaryocytopoiesis and thrombopoiesis. ITP is primary (idiopathic) in most adult patients, although it can be secondary (ie, associated with autoimmune disease, such as SLE; lymphoproliferative disease, such as lymphoma; medications; and infections caused by hepatitis C virus, HIV, and *H pylori*), and ITP can be exacerbated by SARS-CoV-2 vaccination. Antiplatelet antibody targets include glycoproteins IIb/IIIa and Ib/IX on the platelet membrane, although antibodies are demonstrable in only two-thirds of patients; testing for such antibodies is not standard of care given the significant false-positive and false-negative results. In addition to production of antiplatelet antibodies, HIV and hepatitis C virus may lead to thrombocytopenia through additional mechanisms (for instance, by direct suppression of platelet production [HIV] and cirrhosis-related decreased thrombopoietin [TPO] production and secondary splenomegaly [hepatitis C virus]).

Lee EJ...Leavitt AD et al. SARS-CoV-2 vaccination and immune thrombocytopenia in de novo and pre-existing ITP patients. Blood. 2022;139:1564. [PMID: 34587251]

Clinical Findings

A. Symptoms and Signs

Mucocutaneous bleeding may be present, depending on the platelet count. Clinically relevant spontaneous bruising, epistaxis, gingival bleeding, or other types of hemorrhage generally do not occur until the platelet count has fallen below 10,000–20,000/mcL (10–20 × 10^9/L). Individuals with secondary ITP (such as due to autoimmune disease, HIV or HCV infection, SLE, or lymphoproliferative malignancy) may have additional disease-specific findings.

B. Laboratory Findings

Typically, patients have isolated thrombocytopenia. If substantial bleeding has occurred, anemia may also be present. Hepatitis B and C viruses and HIV infections should be excluded by serologic testing. *H pylori* infections can sometimes cause isolated thrombocytopenia.

Bone marrow should be examined in patients with unexplained cytopenias in two or more lineages, in patients older than 40 years with isolated thrombocytopenia, or in those who do not respond to primary ITP-specific therapy. A bone marrow biopsy is not necessary in all cases to make an ITP diagnosis in younger patients. Megakaryocyte morphologic abnormalities and hypocellularity or hypercellularity are not characteristic of ITP. ITP patients often have increased numbers of bone marrow megakaryocytes. If there are clinical findings suggestive of a lymphoproliferative malignancy, a CT scan should be performed. In the absence of such findings, otherwise asymptomatic patients younger than 40 years lacking the above infections and with unexplained isolated thrombocytopenia of recent onset may be considered to have ITP.

Treatment

Individuals with platelet counts less than 25,000–30,000/mcL (25–30 × 10^9/L) or those with significant bleeding should be treated; the remainder may be monitored serially for progression, but that is a patient-specific decision. The mainstay of initial treatment of new-onset primary ITP is a short course of prednisone with or without intravenous immunoglobulin (IVIG) or anti-D (WinRho) (Figure 14–1). A short course of high-dose dexamethasone is also an option for initial treatment. Response to corticosteroids is generally seen within 3–7 days of initiating treatment, with response to IVIG typically seen in 24–36 hours. Platelet transfusions may be given concomitantly if active bleeding is present. Adding the anti-B-cell monoclonal antibody rituximab to corticosteroids as first-line treatment may improve the initial response rate, but it is associated with increased toxicity and is not regarded as standard first-line therapy in most centers.

Although over two-thirds of patients with ITP respond to initial treatment with oral corticosteroids, most relapse following reduction of the corticosteroid dose. Patients with a persistent platelet count less than 30,000/mcL (30 × 10^9/L) or clinically significant bleeding are appropriate candidates for second-line treatments (Figure 14–1). These treatments are chosen empirically, bearing in mind potential toxicities and patient preference. IVIG or anti-D (WinRho) temporarily increases platelet counts (duration, up to 3 weeks, rarely longer). Serial IVIG or anti-D treatment is an option for some adult patients while alternate safe treatment is pursued. Rituximab leads to clinical responses in about 50% of adults with corticosteroid-refractory chronic ITP, which decreases to about 20% at 5 years. The TPO-mimetics romiplostim (administered subcutaneously weekly), eltrombopag (taken orally daily), and avatrombopag (taken orally daily) are used in adult patients with chronic ITP who have not responded durably to corticosteroids or IVIG. Romiplostim, eltrombopag, or avatrombopag can be taken indefinitely to maintain the platelet response and can be used as second-line therapy, but many patients can discontinue taking these agents and maintain an adequate platelet count (above 30,000/mcL [30 × 10^9/L]). The Syk inhibitor fostamatinib treats patients with ITP who do not respond to corticosteroids, TPO-mimetics, or rituximab. Splenectomy is now used infrequently; it has a durable response rate of over 50% and may be considered for cases of severe ITP that fail to respond durably to initial treatment or are refractory to second-line agents; patients should receive pneumococcal, *Haemophilus influenzae* type b, and meningococcal vaccination at least 2 weeks before therapeutic splenectomy. If available, laparoscopic splenectomy is preferred. Additional treatments for ITP are found in Figure 14–1.

For thrombocytopenia associated with HIV or hepatitis C virus, effective treatment of either infection leads to an amelioration of thrombocytopenia in most cases; refractory thrombocytopenia may require the use of IVIG, splenectomy, TPO-mimetic, or anti-CD20 therapy. Occasionally, ITP treatment response is impaired due to *H pylori* infection, which should be ruled out in the appropriate situation.

Management goals for **pregnancy-associated ITP** are a platelet count of 10,000–30,000/mcL (10–30 × 10^9/L) in the first trimester, greater than or equal to 30,000/mcL (30 × 10^9/L) during the second or third trimester, and greater than 50,000/mcL (50 × 10^9/L) prior to cesarean section or vaginal delivery. Moderate-dose oral prednisone or intermittent IVIG infusions are standard treatment options. Splenectomy is reserved for failure to respond to these therapies and may be performed in the first or second trimester. Management requires close interaction between obstetrician and hematologist. TPO-mimetics are not approved for use during pregnancy.

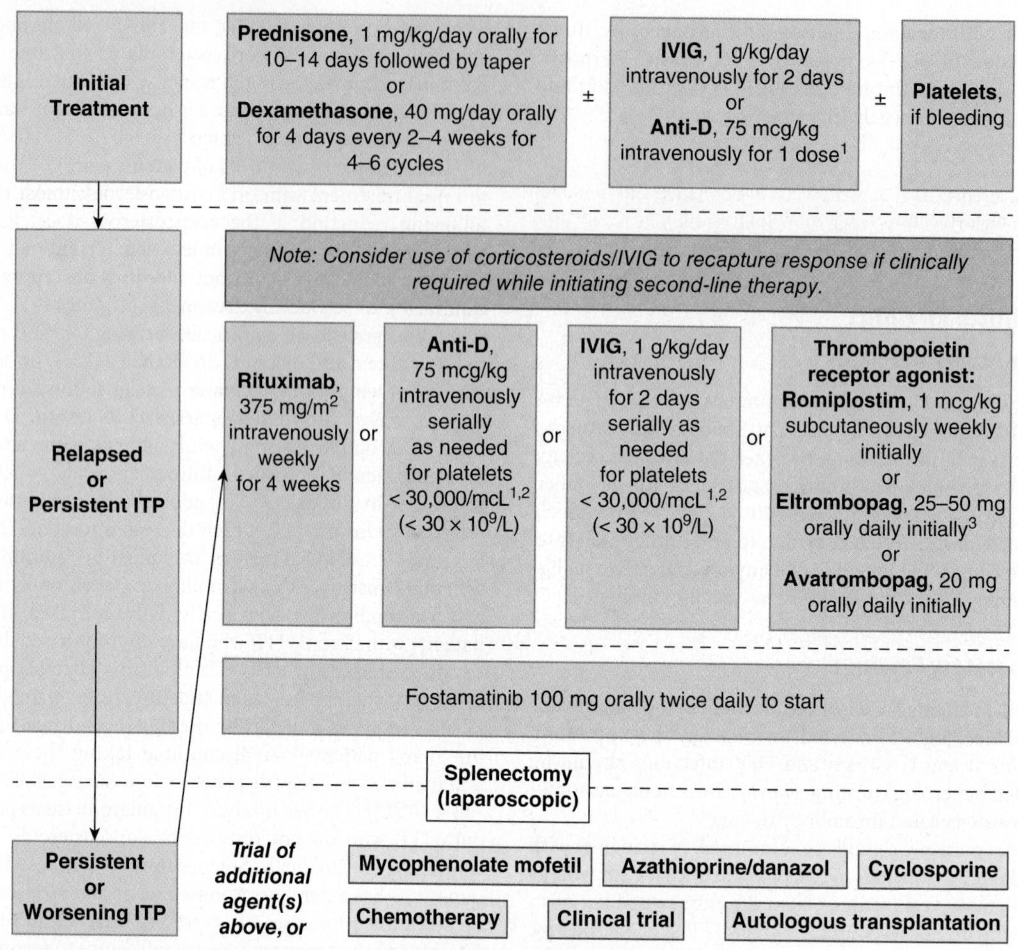

▲ **Figure 14–1.** Management of immune thrombocytopenia (ITP), a simplified overview.

When to Refer

All patients with ITP need to be managed by a hematologist because of the complexity of the decision making.

When to Admit

Patients with major hemorrhage or severe thrombocytopenia associated with bleeding should be admitted and monitored in-hospital until the platelet count has consistently risen to more than 20,000–30,000/mcL (20–30 × 10^9/L) and hemodynamic stability has been achieved.

Bussel J et al. Fostamatinib for the treatment of adult persistent and chronic immune thrombocytopenia: results of two phase 3, randomized, placebo-controlled trials. Am J Hematol. 2018;93:921. [PMID: 29696684]

Miltiadous O et al. Identifying and treating refractory ITP: difficulty in diagnosis and role of combination treatment. Blood. 2020;135:472. [PMID: 31756253]

Neunert C et al. American Society of Hematology 2019 guidelines for immune thrombocytopenia. Blood Adv. 2019;3:3829. [PMID: 31794604]

2. Thrombotic Microangiopathy

ESSENTIALS OF DIAGNOSIS

- Microangiopathic hemolytic anemia and thrombocytopenia, without another plausible explanation, are sufficient for a presumptive diagnosis of thrombotic microangiopathy (TMA).
- Fever, neurologic impairment, and kidney disease may occur but are not required for diagnosis.
- Kidney injury is more common and more severe in hemolytic-uremic syndrome (HUS).

General Considerations

The TMAs include, but are not limited to, thrombotic thrombocytopenic purpura (TTP) and HUS. These disorders are characterized by thrombocytopenia due to the incorporation of platelets into fibrin thrombi in the microvasculature, and microangiopathic hemolytic anemia, which results from shearing of erythrocytes in fibrin networks in the microcirculation.

In idiopathic TTP, autoantibodies against ADAMTS-13 (a disintegrin and metalloproteinase with thrombospondin type 1 repeat, member 13), also known as the von Willebrand factor (vWF) cleaving protease (vWFCP), lead to accumulation of ultra-large vWF multimers. The ultra-large multimers bridge and aggregate platelets in the absence of hemostatic triggers, which in turn leads to the vessel obstruction and various organ dysfunctions seen in TTP. In some cases of pregnancy-associated TMA, an antibody to ADAMTS-13 is present. In contrast, the activity of the ADAMTS-13 in congenital TTP is decreased due to a mutation in the gene encoding the molecule. Classic HUS, called Shiga toxin–mediated HUS, is thought to be secondary to toxin-mediated endothelial damage and is often contracted through the ingestion of undercooked ground beef contaminated with *Escherichia coli* (especially types O157:H7 or O145).

Complement-mediated HUS (formerly called atypical HUS) is not related to Shiga toxin. Patients with complement-mediated HUS often have genetic defects in proteins that regulate complement activity. Damage to endothelial cells, hematopoietic stem cell transplantation in the setting of cancer, or HIV infection may also lead to TMA. Certain medications (eg, cyclosporine, quinine, ticlopidine, clopidogrel, mitomycin C, and bleomycin) are associated with the development of TMA, possibly by promoting injury to endothelial cells, although inhibitory antibodies to ADAMTS-13 have been demonstrated in some cases.

Clinical Findings

A. Symptoms and Signs

Microangiopathic hemolytic anemia and thrombocytopenia are presenting signs in all patients with TTP and most patients with HUS; in a subset of patients with HUS, the platelet count remains in the normal range. Only about 25% of patients with TTP manifest all components of the original pentad of findings (microangiopathic hemolytic anemia, thrombocytopenia, fever, kidney disease, and neurologic abnormalities) (Table 14–4). Most patients (especially children) with HUS have a recent or current diarrheal illness, often bloody. Neurologic manifestations, including headache, somnolence, delirium, seizures, paresis, and coma, may result from deposition of microthrombi in the cerebral vasculature.

B. Laboratory Findings

Laboratory features of TMA include those associated with microangiopathic hemolytic anemia (anemia, elevated LD, elevated indirect bilirubin, decreased haptoglobin, schistocytes on the blood smear, elevated reticulocyte count, and a negative direct antiglobulin test); thrombocytopenia; elevated creatinine; positive stool culture for *E coli* O157:H7 or stool assays for Shiga toxin; reductions in ADAMTS-13 activity with the presence (acquired TTP) or absence (inherited TTP) of ADAMTS-13 inhibitor; and mutations of genes encoding complement proteins (complement-mediated HUS; specialized laboratory assessment). Routine coagulation studies (prothrombin time [PT], activated

Table 14–4. Presentation and management of thrombotic microangiopathies.

	TTP	Complement-Mediated HUS	Shiga Toxin–Mediated HUS
Patient population	Adults	Children (occasionally adults)	Usually children, often following bloody diarrhea
Pathogenesis	Acquired autoantibody to ADAMTS-13	Some cases: heritable deficiency in function of complement regulatory proteins	Bacterial (such as enterotoxogenic *Escherichia coli;* Shiga toxin)
Thrombocytopenia	Typically severe, except in very early clinical course	Variable	May be mild/absent in a minority of patients
Fever	Typical	Variable	Atypical
Kidney disease	Typical, but may be mild	Typical	Typical
Neurologic impairment	Variable	Less than half of cases	Less than half of cases
Laboratory investigation	Decreased activity of ADAMTS-13; inhibitor usually identified	Defects in complement regulatory proteins	Typically normal ADAMTS-13 activity Positive stool culture for *E coli* 0157:H7 or detectable antibody to Shiga toxin
Management	Immediate TPE in most cases Hemodialysis for severe kidney disease Caplacizumab (selected patients) Platelet transfusions contraindicated unless TPE underway	Immediate TPE initially in most cases Eculizumab Supportive care Hemodialysis for severe kidney disease	Hemodialysis for severe kidney disease Supportive care TPE rarely beneficial (exception: selected cases in adults)

ADAMTS-13, a disintegrin and metalloproteinase with a thrombospondin type 1 motif, member 13; HUS, hemolytic-uremic syndrome; TPE, therapeutic plasma exchange; TTP, thrombotic thrombocytopenic purpura.

partial thromboplastin time [aPTT], fibrinogen) are within the normal range in most patients with TTP or HUS.

Treatment

With the exception of children or adults with endemic diarrhea-associated HUS, who generally recover with supportive care only, plasma exchange must be initiated as soon as the diagnosis of TMA is suspected and in all cases of TTP. *Immediate administration of plasma exchange is essential in most cases of TTP because the mortality rate without treatment is over 95%.* Plasma exchange usually is administered once daily until the platelet count and LD have returned to normal for at least 2 days, after which the frequency of treatments may be tapered or stopped while the platelet count and LD are monitored for relapse. In cases of insufficient response to once-daily plasma exchange, twice-daily treatments can be considered. Fresh frozen plasma (FFP) may be administered if immediate access to plasma exchange is not available or in cases of familial TMA. *Platelet transfusions are contraindicated* in the treatment of TMA due to reports of worsening TMA, possibly due to propagation of platelet-rich microthrombi. In cases of documented life-threatening bleeding, however, platelet transfusions may be given slowly and preferably after plasma exchange is underway. RBC transfusions may be administered in cases of clinically significant anemia. Hemodialysis should be considered for patients with significant kidney injury. Caplacizumab, a bi-specific antibody that targets the A1 domain of vWF and prevents vWF interaction with the platelet glycoprotein Ib-IX-V receptor, can reduce the time to platelet count normalization and 30-day mortality. The role of caplacizumab in the treatment of TTP remains controversial given its high cost and limited benefit, despite its inclusion in 2020 guidelines.

In cases of TTP relapse following initial treatment, plasma exchange should be reinstituted. If ineffective, or in cases of primary refractoriness, second-line treatments including rituximab (which has shown efficacy when administered preemptively in selected cases of relapsing TTP), corticosteroids, IVIG, vincristine, cyclophosphamide, and splenectomy should be used. Idiopathic TTP is a relapsing autoimmune disorder (antibody inhibitor to ADAMTS-13) for most patients; careful monitoring of the ADAMTS-13 activity and inhibitor status and use of rituximab can prevent dangerous relapses.

Complement-mediated HUS may respond to plasma infusion initially; however, once this diagnosis is strongly suspected, apheresis is typically stopped and serial infusions of the anti-complement C5 antibody eculizumab are given, which have produced sustained remissions in some patients. Hemodialysis or kidney transplantation may be necessary for irreversible kidney injury.

When to Refer

Consultation by a hematologist or transfusion medicine specialist familiar with plasma exchange is required at the time of presentation. Patients with TMA and TTP require ongoing care by a hematologist.

When to Admit

All patients with newly suspected or diagnosed TMA should be hospitalized immediately.

Goshua G et al. Cost effectiveness of caplacizumab in acquired thrombotic thrombocytopenic purpura. Blood. 2021;137:969. [PMID: 33280030]

Scully M et al; HERCULES Investigators. Caplacizumab treatment for acquired thrombotic thrombocytopenic purpura. N Engl J Med. 2019;380:335. [PMID: 30625070]

Zheng XL et al. ISTH guidelines for the diagnosis of thrombotic thrombocytopenic purpura. J Thromb Haemost. 2020;18: 2486. [PMID: 32914582]

Zheng XL et al. ISTH guidelines for treatment of thrombotic thrombocytopenic purpura. J Thromb Haemost. 2020;18: 2496. [PMID: 32914526]

3. Heparin-Induced Thrombocytopenia

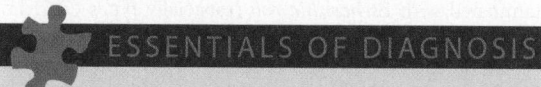

- Thrombocytopenia within 5–14 days of exposure to heparin.
- Decline in baseline platelet count of ≥ 50%.
- Thrombosis occurs in up to 50% of cases; bleeding is uncommon.

General Considerations

Heparin-induced thrombocytopenia (HIT) is an acquired disorder that affects approximately 3% of patients exposed to unfractionated heparin and ~0.3–0.6% of patients exposed to low-molecular-weight heparin (LMWH). The condition results from formation of IgG antibodies to heparin-platelet factor 4 (PF4) complexes; the antibody:heparin-PF4 complex binds to and activates platelets independent of physiologic hemostasis, which leads to thrombocytopenia and thromboses. von Willebrand factor has been postulated to play a role in the thrombotic events that take place long after heparin is cleared from the patient's system.

Clinical Findings

A. Symptoms and Signs

Patients are often asymptomatic, and due to the prothrombotic nature of HIT, bleeding usually does not occur. Thrombosis (at any venous or arterial site), however, may be detected in up to 50% of patients, up to 30 days post diagnosis. If thrombosis has not already been detected, the use of duplex Doppler ultrasound of the lower extremities should be considered to rule out subclinical DVT.

B. Laboratory Findings

A presumptive diagnosis of HIT is made when new-onset thrombocytopenia is detected in a patient (typically a hospitalized patient) within 5–14 days of initial exposure to heparin; other presentations (eg, rapid-onset HIT) are less common and reflect recent prior heparin exposure. A decline of 50% or more from the baseline platelet count is typical. The 4T score (http://www.qxmd.com/calculate-online/hematology/hit-heparin-induced-thrombocytopenia-probability) is a clinical prediction rule for assessing pretest probability for HIT. Low 4T scores have been shown to be more predictive of excluding HIT than are intermediate or high scores of predicting its presence. Once HIT is clinically suspected, the clinician must establish the diagnosis by performing a screening PF4-heparin antibody ELISA. If the PF4-heparin antibody ELISA is positive, the diagnosis must be confirmed using a functional assay (such as serotonin release assay). The magnitude of a positive ELISA result correlates with the clinical probability of HIT, but even high ELISA optical density values may be falsely positive. The confirmatory functional assay is essential.

Treatment

Treatment should be initiated as soon as the diagnosis of HIT is suspected, before laboratory test results are available.

Management of HIT (Table 14–5) involves the immediate discontinuation of all forms of heparin. Despite thrombocytopenia, platelet transfusions are rarely necessary and should be avoided. Due to the substantial frequency of thrombosis among HIT patients, an alternative anticoagulant should be administered immediately while awaiting confirmatory testing. A direct thrombin inhibitor (DTI), such as argatroban or bivalirudin, is preferred in critical illness because of the shorter duration of action. The use of the subcutaneous indirect anti-Xa inhibitor fondaparinux for initial treatment of HIT is a reasonable option in clinically stable patients. For confirmed HIT, the DTI should be continued until the platelet count has recovered to at least 100,000/mcL (100×10^9/L), at which point treatment with a vitamin K antagonist (warfarin) may be initiated. The DTI should be continued until therapeutic anticoagulation with the vitamin K antagonist warfarin has been achieved (ie, INR of 2.0–3.0); the infusion of argatroban must be temporarily discontinued before the INR is obtained so that it reflects the anticoagulant effect of warfarin alone. There is a growing use of oral anti-Xa agents instead of vitamin K antagonists in selected patients. In all patients with HIT, some form of anticoagulation (warfarin, fondaparinux, or an oral anti-Xa agent) should be continued for at least 30 days, due to a persistent risk of thrombosis even after the platelet count has recovered, but in patients in whom thrombosis has been documented, anticoagulation should continue for 3–6 months.

Subsequent exposure to heparin should be avoided in all patients with a prior history of HIT, if possible. If its use is regarded as necessary for a procedure, it should be withheld until PF4-heparin antibodies are no longer detectable by ELISA (usually as of 100 days following an episode of HIT), and exposure should be limited to the shortest time period possible. A common example is a cardiac catheterization. The heparin is gone before the antibody returns, so HIT is avoided.

Table 14–5. Management of suspected or proven HIT.

Agent	Indication	Dosing
I. Discontinue all forms of heparin. Send PF4-heparin ELISA. Send confirmatory serotonin release assay if positive ELISA.		
II. Begin treatment with direct thrombin inhibitor, or in some circumstances, fondaparinux.		
Argatroban	Prophylaxis or treatment of HIT	Continuous intravenous infusion of 0.5–1.2 mcg/kg/minute, titrate to aPTT = 1.5 to 3 × the baseline value.[1] Max infusion rate is 10 mcg/kg/minute.
Bivalirudin	Percutaneous coronary intervention[2]	Bolus of 0.75 mg/kg intravenously followed by initial continuous intravenous infusion of 1.75 mg/kg/hour. Manufacturer indicates monitoring should be by ACT.
Fondaparinux	Treatment of HIT	5–10 mg (weight based)
III. Perform Doppler ultrasound of lower extremities to rule out subclinical thrombosis (if indicated).		
IV. Follow platelet counts daily until recovery occurs.		
V. When platelet count has recovered, transition anticoagulation to warfarin, fondaparinux, or an oral anti-Xa agent; treat for 30 days (HIT) or 3–6 months (HITT).		
VI. Document heparin allergy in medical record (confirmed cases).		

[1]Liver insufficiency: initial infusion rate = 0.5 mcg/kg/minute.
[2]Not approved for HIT/HITT.
ACT, activated clotting time; aPTT, activated partial thromboplastin time; HIT, heparin-induced thrombocytopenia; HITT, heparin-induced thrombocytopenia and thrombosis; PF4, platelet factor 4.

When to Refer

Due to the tremendous thrombotic potential of the disorder and the complexity of use of the DTI, all patients with HIT should be evaluated by a hematologist.

When to Admit

Most patients with HIT are hospitalized at the time of detection of thrombocytopenia. Admission is a clinical decision for an outpatient in whom HIT is suspected and who is a candidate for subcutaneous fondaparinux or an oral anti-Xa agent. Other outpatients may need admission for intravenous DTIs. Regardless, a hematologist needs to be involved as soon as the diagnosis is suspected or treatment is indicated.

Cuker A et al. American Society of Hematology 2018 guidelines for management of venous thromboembolism: heparin-induced thrombocytopenia. Blood Adv. 2018;2:3360. [PMID: 30482768]

Johnston I et al. Recognition of PF4-VWF complexes by heparin-induced thrombocytopenia antibodies contributes to thrombus propagation. Blood. 2020;135:1270. [PMID: 32077913]

Warkentin TE. Laboratory diagnosis of heparin-induced thrombocytopenia. Int J Lab Hematol. 2019;41:15. [PMID: 31069988]

4. Disseminated Intravascular Coagulation

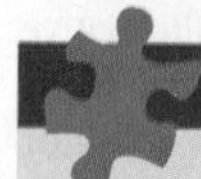

ESSENTIALS OF DIAGNOSIS

- Associated with cancer, sepsis, trauma, and obstetrical patients.
- Prolonged PT and aPTT, and low/declining fibrinogen.
- Thrombocytopenia.

General Considerations

Disseminated intravascular coagulation (DIC) is caused by uncontrolled local or systemic activation of coagulation, which leads to depletion of coagulation factors and fibrinogen, and often results in thrombocytopenia as platelets are activated and consumed.

Numerous disorders are associated with DIC, including sepsis (in which coagulation is activated by presence of lipopolysaccharide), cancer, trauma, burns, and pregnancy-associated complications (in which tissue factor is released). Aortic aneurysm and cavernous hemangiomas may promote localized intravascular coagulation, and snake bites may result in DIC due to the introduction of exogenous toxins.

Clinical Findings

A. Symptoms and Signs

Bleeding in DIC usually occurs at multiple sites, such as at intravenous catheters or incisions, and may be widespread (purpura fulminans). Malignancy-related DIC may manifest principally as thrombosis (Trousseau syndrome).

B. Laboratory Findings

In early DIC, the platelet count and fibrinogen levels often remain within the normal range, albeit reduced from baseline levels. There is progressive thrombocytopenia (rarely severe), prolongation of the PT, decrease in fibrinogen levels, and eventually elevation in the aPTT. D-dimer levels typically are elevated due to the activation of coagulation and diffuse cross-linking of fibrin followed by fibrinolysis. Schistocytes on the blood smear, due to shearing of red cells through the microvasculature, are present in 10–20% of patients. Laboratory abnormalities in the HELLP syndrome (hemolysis, elevated liver enzymes, low platelets), a severe form of DIC with a particularly high mortality rate that occurs in peripartum women, include elevated liver transaminases and kidney injury due to gross hemoglobinuria and pigment nephropathy. Malignancy-related DIC may initially feature normal platelet counts and coagulation studies, but clinicians often see a dropping platelet count and fibrinogen, with a rising INR, highlighting the importance of serial laboratory values to help make the diagnosis.

Treatment

The underlying causative disorder must be treated (eg, antimicrobials, chemotherapy, surgery, or delivery of conceptus). If clinically significant bleeding is present, hemostasis must be achieved (Table 14–6).

Blood products are administered if clinically significant hemorrhage has occurred or is thought likely to occur without intervention based on progressively increasing PT and PTT and decreasing fibrinogen and platelets levels (Table 14–6). The goal of platelet therapy for most cases is greater than 20,000/mcL (20×10^9/L) or greater than 50,000/mcL (50×10^9/L) for serious bleeding, such as intracranial bleeding. FFP is typically given only to patients with a prolonged aPTT and PT and significant bleeding. Cryoprecipitate may be given for bleeding or for fibrinogen levels less than 80–100 mg/dL. The clinician should correct the fibrinogen level with cryoprecipitate prior to giving FFP for prolonged PT and aPTT to see if the fibrinogen replacement alone corrects the PT and aPTT. The PT, aPTT, fibrinogen, and platelet count should be monitored at least every 6–8 hours in acutely ill patients with DIC.

In some cases of refractory bleeding despite replacement of blood products, administration of low doses of heparin can be considered. The clinician must remember that DIC is primarily a disorder of excessive clotting with secondary fibrinolysis, and that heparin can interfere with thrombin generation, which leads to less consumption of coagulation proteins and platelets. An infusion of 5 units/kg/hour (no bolus) may be used with appropriate clinical

Table 14–6. Management of DIC.

I. Assess for underlying cause of DIC and treat.	
II. Establish baseline platelet count, PT, aPTT, D-dimer, fibrinogen.	
III. Transfuse blood products only if ongoing bleeding or high risk of bleeding.	**Platelets:** goal > 20,000/mcL (20×10^9/L) (most patients) or > 50,000/mcL (50×10^9/L) (severe bleeding, eg, intracranial hemorrhage)
	Cryoprecipitate: goal fibrinogen level > 80–100 mg/dL
	Fresh frozen plasma: goal PT and aPTT < 1.5 × normal
	Packed RBCs: goal hemoglobin > 8 g/dL or improvement in symptomatic anemia
IV. Follow platelets, aPTT, PT, fibrinogen every 4–12 hours as clinically indicated.	
V. If persistent bleeding due to severe consumption or consumption that requires excessive blood product use, consider use of heparin[1] (initial infusion, 5 units/kg/hour) and titrate to desired clinical goals; do not administer bolus.	
VI. Follow laboratory parameters every 4–12 hours as clinically indicated until DIC resolves	

[1]Contraindicated if platelets cannot be maintained at > 50,000/mcL (50×10^9/L), in cases of GI or CNS bleeding, in conditions that may require surgical management, or placental abruption.
aPTT, activated partial thromboplastin time; DIC, disseminated intravascular coagulation; PT, prothrombin time.

judgement, up-titrated as clinically indicated. *Heparin, however, can be contraindicated if the platelet count cannot be maintained above 30,000/mcL (30 × 10^9/L) and in cases of CNS hemorrhage, GI bleeding, placental abruption, and any other condition that is likely to require imminent surgery.* Fibrinolysis inhibitors may be considered in select DIC patients with bleeding, but this can promote dangerous clotting and should be undertaken with great caution and only in consultation with a hematologist.

1. HELLP syndrome—The treatment must include evacuation of the uterus (eg, delivery of a term or near-term infant or removal of retained placental or fetal fragments).

2. Trousseau syndrome—Patients require treatment of the underlying malignancy and administration of unfractionated heparin or subcutaneous therapeutic-dose LMWH as treatment of thrombosis, since warfarin typically is less effective at secondary prevention of thromboembolism in the disorder. Typically, the heparin or LMWH treatment will gradually return the fibrinogen, PT (INR), aPTT, and platelet count back to normal, but it can take many days. Oral anti-Xa agents or oral DTIs can be considered once stabilized with parenteral heparin or LMWH, but extended LMWH is often used in this setting.

Immediate initiation of medical treatment (usually within 24 hours of diagnosis) is required for acute promyelocytic leukemia (APL)–associated DIC, along with administration of blood products as clinically indicated.

When to Refer

- Diffuse bleeding unresponsive to administration of blood products should be evaluated by a hematologist.
- All patients with DIC should be cared for by a hematologist prior to starting treatment with heparin or LMWH.

When to Admit

Most patients with DIC are hospitalized when DIC is detected.

Cuker A et al. American Society of Hematology 2018 guidelines for management of venous thromboembolism: heparin-induced thrombocytopenia. Blood Adv. 2018;2:3360. [PMID: 30482768]

Levi M et al. Disseminated intravascular coagulation: an update on pathogenesis and diagnosis. Expert Rev Hematol. 2018;11:663. [PMID: 29999440]

Levi M. Pathogenesis and diagnosis of disseminated intravascular coagulation. Int J Lab Hematol. 2018;40:15. [PMID: 29741245]

Warkentin TE et al. Direct oral anticoagulants for treatment of HIT: update of Hamilton experience and literature review. Blood. 2017;130:1104. [PMID: 28646118]

OTHER CONDITIONS CAUSING THROMBOCYTOPENIA

1. Drug-Induced Thrombocytopenia

Drug-induced thrombocytopenia is often immune-mediated but can also be due to marrow suppression. Table 14–7 lists medications associated with thrombocytopenia. The typical presentation of drug-induced, antibody-mediated thrombocytopenia is severe thrombocytopenia and mucocutaneous bleeding 5–14 days after exposure to a new drug, although a range of presentations is possible. Discontinuation of the offending agent leads to resolution of thrombocytopenia within 3–7 days in most cases, but recovery kinetics depend on rate of drug clearance, which can be affected by liver and kidney function. Patients with severe thrombocytopenia should be given platelet transfusions with or without IVIG. The University of Oklahoma Health Sciences center maintains a useful website for drug-induced thrombocytopenia (https://www.ouhsc.edu/platelets/).

Table 14–7. Selected medications causing drug-associated thrombocytopenia.[1]

Class	Examples
Chemotherapy	Most agents
Antiplatelet agents	Abciximab, eptifibatide, tirofiban Anagrelide Ticlopidine
Antimicrobial agents	Adefovir, indinavir, ritonavir Fluconazole Isoniazid Linezolid Penicillins Remdesivir Rifampin Sulfa drugs Vancomycin
Cardiovascular agents	Amiodarone Atorvastatin, simvastatin Captopril Digoxin Hydrochlorothiazide Procainamide
GI agents	Cimetidine, famotidine
Neuropsychiatric agents	Carbamazepine Haloperidol Methyldopa Phenytoin
Analgesic agents	Acetaminophen Diclofenac, ibuprofen, naproxen, sulindac
Anticoagulant agents	Heparin Low-molecular-weight heparin
Immunomodulator agents	Interferon-alpha Rituximab
Immunosuppressant agents	Mycophenolate mofetil Tacrolimus
Other agents	Immunizations Iodinated contrast dye

[1]See also https://www.ouhsc.edu/platelets/.

2. Posttransfusion Purpura

Posttransfusion purpura (PTP) is a rare disorder of sudden-onset thrombocytopenia that occurs within 1 week after transfusion of red cells, platelets, or plasma. Antibodies against the human platelet antigen PL^{A1} are detected in most individuals with PTP. Patients with PTP often are either multiparous women or persons who have received transfusions previously. Severe thrombocytopenia and bleeding are typical. Initial treatment consists of administration of IVIG (1 g/kg/day for 2 days), which should be administered as soon as the diagnosis is suspected. Platelets are not indicated unless severe bleeding is present, but if they are to be administered, HLA-matched PL^{A1}-negative platelets are preferred. A second course or IVIG, plasma exchange, corticosteroids, TPO-mimetics, or splenectomy may be required in case of refractoriness. PL^{A1}-negative or washed blood products are preferred for subsequent transfusions, but data supporting various treatment options are limited.

Vu K, Leavitt AD. Posttransfusion purpura with antibodies against human platelet antigen-4a following checkpoint inhibitor therapy: a case report and review of the literature. Transfusion. 2018;58:2265. [PMID: 30222869]

3. von Willebrand Disease Type 2B

von Willebrand disease (vWD) type 2B leads to chronic, characteristically mild to moderate thrombocytopenia due to an abnormal vWF molecule that binds platelets with increased affinity, resulting in aggregation and clearance (see von Willebrand Disease, below).

4. Platelet Sequestration

One-third of the platelet mass is typically sequestered in the spleen. Splenomegaly, due to a variety of conditions, may lead to thrombocytopenia of variable severity. When possible, treatment of the underlying disorder should be pursued, but splenectomy, splenic embolization, or splenic irradiation may be considered in selected cases.

5. Pregnancy

Gestational thrombocytopenia is thought to result from progressive expansion of the blood volume that typically occurs during pregnancy, leading to hemodilution. Cytopenias result even though blood cell production is normal or increased. Platelet counts less than 100,000/mcL (100×10^9/L), however, are observed in less than 10% of pregnant women in the third trimester; decreases to less than 70,000/mcL (70×10^9/L) should prompt consideration of pregnancy-related ITP as well as preeclampsia or a pregnancy-related thrombotic microangiopathy.

6. Infection or Sepsis

The exact mechanism underlying sepsis-related thrombocytopenia remains ill-defined. Immune-mediated destruction and enhanced clearance by the liver are possible explanations, and there may be significant overlap with concomitant DIC. Regardless, the platelet count typically improves with effective antimicrobial treatment or after the infection has resolved. Hemophagocytosis may occur in some critically ill patients; a defect in immunomodulation may lead to bone marrow macrophages (histiocytes) engulfing cellular components of the marrow. The phenomenon typically resolves with resolution of the infection, but with certain infections (Epstein-Barr virus) immunosuppression may be required. Hemophagocytosis also may occur with malignancy, in which case the disorder is usually unresponsive to treatment with immunosuppression and requires treatment of the malignancy.

7. Pseudothrombocytopenia

Pseudothrombocytopenia results from ethylenediaminetetraacetic acid (EDTA) anticoagulant-induced platelet clumping; the phenomenon typically disappears when blood is collected in a tube containing citrate anticoagulant. Pseudothrombocytopenia diagnosis requires review of the peripheral blood smear and is not associated with bleeding.

Ghimire S et al. Current understanding and future implications of sepsis-induced thrombocytopenia. Eur J Haematol. 2021;106:301. [PMID: 33191517]

Koyama K et al. Time course of immature platelet count and its relation to thrombocytopenia and mortality in patients with sepsis. PLoS One. 2018;13:e0192064. [PMID: 29381746]

QUALITATIVE PLATELET DISORDERS

CONGENITAL DISORDERS OF PLATELET FUNCTION

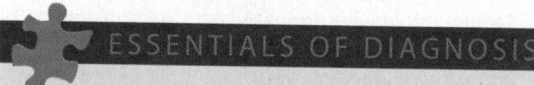

- Usually diagnosed in childhood.
- Family history usually is positive.
- May be diagnosed in adulthood when there is excessive bleeding.

General Considerations

Heritable qualitative platelet disorders are far less common than acquired platelet function disorders and lead to variably severe bleeding, often beginning in childhood. Occasionally, however, disorders of platelet function may go undetected until later in life when excessive bleeding occurs following a sufficient hemostatic challenge. Thus, the true incidence of hereditary qualitative platelet disorders is unknown.

Bernard-Soulier syndrome (BSS) is a rare, autosomal recessive bleeding disorder due to reduced or abnormal platelet membrane expression of glycoprotein Ib/IX (vWF receptor).

Glanzmann thrombasthenia results from an abnormality in the platelet glycoprotein IIb/IIIa receptor on the platelet membrane. Glycoprotein IIb/IIIa is the fibrinogen receptor critical for linking platelets during initial platelet aggregation/platelet plug formation. Inheritance is autosomal recessive.

Under normal circumstances, activated platelets release the contents of platelet granules to reinforce the aggregatory response. Storage pool disease includes a spectrum of defects in release of alpha or dense (delta) platelet granules, or both (alpha-delta storage pool disease).

Clinical Findings

A. Symptoms and Signs

Bleeding due to defective platelets is usually mucocutaneous, but it is not limited to mucocutaneous surfaces. The onset of bleeding with Glanzmann thrombasthenia is usually in infancy or childhood, but some forms are milder and present later in life. The degree of deficiency in IIb/IIIa may not correlate well with bleeding symptoms. Patients with storage pool disease are affected by variable bleeding, ranging from mild and trauma-related to spontaneous.

B. Laboratory Findings

Patients with Bernard-Soulier syndrome have abnormally large platelets (approaching the size of red cells), moderate thrombocytopenia, and a prolonged bleeding time. Platelet aggregation studies show a marked defect in response to ristocetin, whereas aggregation in response to other agonists is normal; the addition of normal platelets corrects the abnormal aggregation. The diagnosis can be confirmed by platelet flow cytometry.

In Glanzmann thrombasthenia, platelet aggregation studies show marked impairment of aggregation in response to stimulation with various agonists, which reflects the critical role of the fibrinogen receptor in platelet plug formation.

Storage pool disease includes defects in the number, content, or function of platelet alpha or dense granules, or both. The gray platelet syndrome comprises abnormalities of platelet alpha granules, thrombocytopenia, and marrow fibrosis. The blood smear shows agranular platelets, and the diagnosis is confirmed with electron microscopy.

Treatment

The mainstay of treatment (including periprocedural prophylaxis) is transfusion of normal platelets, although desmopressin acetate (DDAVP), antifibrinolytic agents, and recombinant human activated factor VII each have a role in selected clinical situations.

Orsini S et al; European Hematology Association-Scientific Working Group (EHA-SWG) on thrombocytopenias and platelet function disorders. Bleeding risk of surgery and its prevention in patients with inherited platelet disorders. Haematologica. 2017;102:1192. [PMID: 28385783]

ACQUIRED DISORDERS OF PLATELET FUNCTION

Platelet dysfunction is more commonly acquired than inherited; the widespread use of platelet-altering medications accounts for most of the cases of qualitative defects. In cases where platelet function is irreversibly altered, platelet inhibition typically recovers within 7–9 days following discontinuation of the drug, which is the time it takes to replace all of the impaired platelets with newly produced platelets. In cases where platelet function is non-irreversibly affected, platelet inhibition recovers with clearance of the drug from the system. Transfusion of platelets may be required if clinically significant bleeding is present.

Lee RH et al. Impaired hemostatic activity of healthy transfused platelets in inherited and acquired platelet disorders: mechanisms and implications. Sci Transl Med. 2019;11:eaay0203. [PMID: 31826978]

Zheng SL et al. Association of aspirin use for primary prevention with cardiovascular events and bleeding events: a systematic review and meta-analysis. JAMA. 2019;321:277. [PMID: 30667501]

DISORDERS OF COAGULATION

CONGENITAL DISORDERS OF COAGULATION

1. Hemophilia A & B

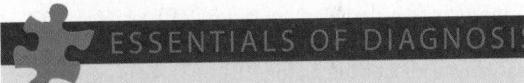

- **Hemophilia A:** congenital deficiency of coagulation factor VIII.
- **Hemophilia B:** congenital deficiency of coagulation factor IX.
- Recurrent hemarthroses and arthropathy.
- Risk of development of inhibitory antibodies to factor VIII or factor IX.
- Many older patients received blood products contaminated with HIV or hepatitis C virus.

General Considerations

Hemophilia A occurs in ~1 per 5000 live male births, whereas hemophilia B occurs in ~1 in 25,000 live male births. Inheritance is X-linked recessive for both, leading to affected males and carrier (affected) females with variable bleeding tendencies. Daughters of all affected males are obligate carriers. There is no race predilection. Factor activity testing is indicated for male infants with a hemophilic maternal pedigree who are asymptomatic or who experience excessive bleeding, for all daughters of affected males (100% chance of being affected) and carrier mothers (50% chance of being affected), and for otherwise asymptomatic adolescents or adults who experience unexpected excessive bleeding with trauma or invasive procedures.

Inhibitors to factor VIII develop in approximately 20–25% of patients with severe hemophilia A; inhibitors to factor IX develop in less than 5% of patients with severe hemophilia B. Risk of inhibitor formation exists for both plasma-derived and recombinant factor products.

A substantial proportion of older patients with hemophilia acquired infection with HIV or HCV or both in the

1980s due to exposure to contaminated factor concentrates and blood products.

Clinical Findings

A. Symptoms and Signs

Severe hemophilia (factor VIII activity less than 1%) presents in infants or in early childhood with spontaneous bleeding into joints, soft tissues, or other locations. Spontaneous bleeding is much less common in patients with mild hemophilia (factor VIII activity greater than 5%), but bleeding is common with provoked bleeding (eg, surgery, trauma). Intermediate clinical symptoms are seen in patients with moderate hemophilia (factor VIII activity 1–5%). Female carriers of hemophilia can have a wide range of factor VIII activity and therefore have variable bleeding tendencies.

Significant hemophilic arthropathy can be minimized in patients who receive long-term regular prophylaxis with factor concentrate starting in early childhood, whereas destructive joint disease is common in adults who have experienced recurrent hemarthroses. Patients tend to have one or two "target" joints into which they bleed most often.

Inhibitor development to factor VIII or factor IX is characterized by bleeding episodes that are resistant to treatment with clotting factor VIII or IX concentrate, and by new or atypical bleeding.

B. Laboratory Findings

Hemophilia A or B is diagnosed by an isolated reproducibly low factor VIII or factor IX activity level, in the absence of other conditions. If the aPTT is prolonged, it typically corrects upon mixing with normal plasma. Depending on the level of residual factor VIII or factor IX activity, and the sensitivity of the thromboplastin used in the aPTT coagulation reaction, the aPTT may or may not be prolonged, although it typically is markedly prolonged in severe hemophilia. Hemophilia is classified according to the level of factor activity in the plasma. **Mild hemophilia** has greater than 5% factor activity; **moderate hemophilia** has 1–5% factor activity; and **severe hemophilia** has less than 1% factor activity. Female carriers may become symptomatic if significant lyonization has occurred favoring the defective factor VIII or factor IX gene, leading to factor VIII or factor IX activity level markedly less than 50%. Typically, a clinical bleeding diathesis occurs once the factor activity is less than 20%, but this appears to be patient-specific, and bleeding can occur in trauma, surgery, and delivery if the factor activity is less than 50%.

In the presence of an inhibitor to factor VIII or factor IX, there is accelerated clearance of and suboptimal or absent rise in measured activity of infused factor, and the aPTT does not correct on mixing. The Bethesda assay measures the potency of the inhibitor.

Treatment

A. Factor VIII or IX Products

Plasma-derived or recombinant factor VIII or IX products are the mainstay of treatment. The optimal care for individuals with severe hemophilia is primary prophylaxis: by the age of 4 years, most children with severe hemophilia have begun twice- or thrice-weekly infusions of factor to prevent the recurrent joint bleeding that otherwise would characterize the disorder and lead to severe musculoskeletal morbidity. In selected cases of less severe hemophilia, or as an adjunct to prophylaxis in severe hemophilia, treatment with factor products is given peri-procedurally, prior to high-risk activities (such as sports), or as needed for bleeding episodes (Table 14–8). Recombinant factor VIII and factor IX molecules that are bioengineered to have an extended half-life may allow for extended dosing intervals in patients who are treated prophylactically. The decision to switch to a long-acting product is patient specific. The long-acting factor IX products have clear added value in reducing frequency of factor injections often to weekly or less. Long-acting factor VIII products have not achieved a similar degree of extended half-life. Patients with mild hemophilia A may respond to as-needed (on demand) intravenous or intranasal DDAVP. Antifibrinolytic agents may be useful in cases of mucosal bleeding and are commonly used adjunctively, such as following dental procedures.

B. Factor VIII or IX Inhibitors

Factor inhibitors (antibodies that interfere with activity or half-life) are a major clinical problem for patients with hemophilia. It may be possible to overcome low-titer inhibitors (less than 5 Bethesda units [BU]) by giving larger doses of factor, whereas treatment of bleeding in the presence of a high-titer inhibitor (more than 5 BU) requires infusion of an activated prothrombin complex concentrate (such as FEIBA [factor eight inhibitor bypassing activity]) or recombinant activated factor VII. Recombinant porcine factor VIII is also an option but is reserved for selective circumstances because of its cost. Inhibitor tolerance induction, achieved by giving large doses (50–300 units/kg intravenously of factor VIII daily) for 6–18 months, succeeds in eradicating the inhibitor in 70% of patients with hemophilia A and in 30% of patients with hemophilia B. Patients with hemophilia B who receive inhibitor tolerance induction, however, are at risk for development of nephrotic syndrome and anaphylactic reactions, making eradication of their inhibitors more problematic. Additional immunomodulation may allow for eradication in selected inhibitor tolerance induction–refractory patients. Emicizumab is a novel bi-specific antibody that brings activated factor IX and factor X together, effectively replacing the cofactor function of factor VIII in the clotting cascade, providing a major therapeutic advance for patients with inhibitors. Emicizumab has also been demonstrated to be an effective option for patients without inhibitors. It is given subcutaneously weekly, every other week, or every 4 weeks, making it easier to administer than intravenous factor products.

C. Gene Therapy

Gene therapy clinical trials for hemophilia A and B have shown great promise for patients with severe hemophilia A

Table 14–8. Treatment of bleeding in selected inherited disorders of hemostasis.

Disorder	Subtype	Treatment for Minor Bleeding	Treatment for Major Bleeding	Comment
Hemophilia A	Mild Moderate or severe	DDAVP[1] Factor VIII product	DDAVP[1] or factor VIII product Factor VIII product	Treat for 3–10 days for major bleeding or following surgery, keeping factor activity level 50–80% initially. Adjunctive EACA may be useful for mucosal bleeding or procedures
Hemophilia B	Mild, moderate, or severe	Factor IX product	Factor IX product	
von Willebrand disease	Type 1 Type 2 Type 3	DDAVP[1] DDAVP,[1] vWF product vWF product	DDAVP,[1] vWF product vWF product vWF product	
Factor XI deficiency	—	FFP or EACA	FFP	Adjunctive EACA should be used for mucosal bleeding or procedures

[1]Mild hemophilia A and type 2A or 2B vWD patients: therapeutic trial must have previously confirmed an adequate response (ie, elevation of factor VIII or vWF activity level into the normal range) and (for type 2B) no exacerbation of thrombocytopenia. DDAVP is not typically effective for type 2M vWD. A vWF-containing factor VIII concentrate is preferred for treatment of type 2N vWD.

Notes:

DDAVP dose is 0.3 mcg/kg intravenously in 50 mL saline over 20 minutes, or nasal spray 300 mcg for weight > 50 kg or 150 mcg for < 50 kg, every 24 hours, maximum of three doses in a 72-hour period. If more than two doses are used in a 48-hour period, free water restriction and monitoring for hyponatremia is essential.

EACA dose is 50 mg/kg orally four times daily for 3–5 days; maximum 24 g/day, useful for mucosal bleeding/dental procedures.

Factor VIII product dose is 50 units/kg for severe hemophilia A intravenously initially followed by 25 units/kg every 8 hours followed by lesser doses at longer intervals once hemostasis has been established.

Factor IX product dose is 100 units/kg (120 units/kg if using Benefix) intravenously initially for severe hemophilia B followed by 50 units/kg (60 units/kg if using Benefix) every 8 hours followed by lesser doses at longer intervals once hemostasis has been established.

vWF-containing factor VIII product dose is 60–80 RCoF units/kg intravenously every 12 hours initially followed by lesser doses at longer intervals once hemostasis has been established.

FFP is typically administered in 4-unit boluses and may not need to be re-bolused after the initial administration due to the long half-life of factor XI.

DDAVP, desmopressin acetate; EACA, epsilon-aminocaproic acid; FFP, fresh frozen plasma; vWF, von Willebrand factor.

and B. For most patients, gene therapy has eliminated spontaneous bleeding as well as the need for factor replacement. While phase 3 clinical trials have been restricted to patients 18 years of age and older, the results look extremely promising. It is hoped that this potentially life-changing therapy will become an approved treatment outside of clinical trials in late 2022.

D. Antiretroviral Therapy

Antiretroviral treatment should be administered to hemophilia patients with HIV infection. Patients with hepatitis C infection should be referred for treatment to eradicate the virus.

When to Refer

All patients with hemophilia should be seen regularly in a comprehensive hemophilia treatment center.

When to Admit

- Major invasive procedures because of the need for serial infusions of clotting factor concentrate.
- Bleeding that is unresponsive to outpatient treatment.

George LA et al. Hemophilia B gene therapy with a high-specific-activity factor IX variant. N Engl J Med. 2017;377:2215. [PMID: 29211678]

Mahlangu J et al. Emicizumab prophylaxis in patients who have hemophilia A without inhibitors. N Engl J Med. 2018;379:811. [PMID: 30157389]

Manco-Johnson MJ et al; Joint Outcomes Committee of the Universal Data Collection, US Hemophilia Treatment Center Network. Prophylaxis usage, bleeding rates, and joint outcomes of hemophilia, 1999 to 2010: a surveillance project. Blood. 2017;129:2368. [PMID: 28183693]

Oldenburg J et al. Emicizumab prophylaxis in hemophilia A with inhibitors. N Engl J Med. 2017;377:809. [PMID: 28691557]

Pasi KJ et al. Multiyear follow-up of AAV5-hFVIII-SQ gene therapy for hemophilia A. N Engl J Med. 2020;382:29. [PMID: 31893514]

2. von Willebrand Disease

ESSENTIALS OF DIAGNOSIS

- The most common inherited bleeding disorder.
- vWF binds platelets to subendothelial surfaces, aggregates platelets, and prolongs the half-life of factor VIII.

General Considerations

vWF is an unusually large multimeric glycoprotein that binds to subendothelial collagen and its platelet receptor, glycoprotein Ib, bridging platelets to the subendothelial matrix at the site of vascular injury and contributing to linking them together in the platelet plug. vWF also has a binding site for factor VIII, prolonging factor VIII half-life in the circulation.

Between 75% and 80% of patients with vWD have type 1, a *quantitative abnormality* of the vWF molecule that usually does not feature an identifiable causal mutation in the vWF gene.

Type 2 vWD is seen in 15–20% of patients with vWD. In type 2A or 2B vWD, a *qualitative defect* in the vWF molecule is causative. Types 2N and 2M vWD are due to defects in vWF that decrease binding to factor VIII or to platelets, respectively. Type 2M vWD features a normal multimer pattern. Importantly, type 2N vWD can clinically resemble hemophilia A because factor VIII activity levels are decreased, and vWF activity and antigen (Ag) are normal. Type 3 vWD is rare, and like type 1, is a quantitative defect, with mutational homozygosity or compound heterozygosity yielding very low levels of vWF and severe bleeding in infancy or childhood. Due to its factor VIII carrier function, a severely low vWF level leads to low factor VIII activity and prolonged aPTT.

Clinical Findings

A. Symptoms and Signs

Patients with type 1 vWD usually have mild or moderate platelet-type bleeding (mucocutaneous) that may be evident in childhood. Heavier bleeding may occur with menses, surgery, or following delivery. Patients with type 2 vWD usually have moderate to severe bleeding that presents in childhood or adolescence. Patient with type 3 vWD demonstrate a severe bleeding phenotype that typically manifests in childhood or infancy.

B. Laboratory Findings

In type 1 vWD, the vWF activity (ristocetin co-factor or VWF:GPIbM assay) and the vWF Ag are mildly depressed, whereas the vWF multimer pattern is normal (Table 14–9). Laboratory testing of type 2A or 2B vWD typically shows a ratio of vWF Ag:vWF activity of approximately 2:1 and a multimer pattern that lacks the highest molecular weight multimers. Thrombocytopenia is common in type 2B vWD due to a gain-of-function mutation of the vWF molecule, which leads to increased vWF binding to its receptor on platelets, resulting in platelet clearance; a ristocetin-induced platelet aggregation (RIPA) study shows an increase in platelet aggregation in response to low concentrations of ristocetin. Except in the more severe forms of vWD that feature a significantly decreased factor VIII activity, aPTT is most commonly normal in patients with vWD. The PT is not affected by vWD. vWD type 2N has normal vWF antigen and activity but a low factor VIII due to impaired vWF binding to factor VIII.

Treatment

The treatment of vWD is outlined in Table 14–8. DDAVP is useful in the treatment of mild bleeding in most cases of type 1 and some cases of type 2 vWD. DDAVP causes release of vWF and factor VIII from storage sites (endothelial cells), leading to a two- to sevenfold increase in vWF and factor VIII. A therapeutic DDAVP trial to document sufficient rise in vWF level is critical prior to relying on DDAVP as a treatment option. Due to tachyphylaxis and the risk of significant hyponatremia secondary to fluid retention, DDAVP treatment should be limited to one dose per 24 hours and no more than three doses over 5 days. vWF-containing factor VIII concentrates or recombinant VWF products are used in all other clinical scenarios, and when bleeding is not controlled with DDAVP. Cryoprecipitate is no longer used as a source of vWD in clinical practice. Antifibrinolytic agents (eg, aminocaproic acid or tranexamic acid) may be used adjunctively for mucosal bleeding or procedures. Pregnant patients with type 1 vWD usually do not require treatment at the time of delivery because of the physiologic increase in vWF levels (up to threefold that of baseline) that are observed by parturition. However, levels need to be confirmed in late pregnancy, and if they are low or if excessive bleeding is encountered, vWF products may be given. Moreover, patients are at risk for significant bleeding 1–2 weeks postpartum when vWF levels fall secondary to the fall in estrogen levels and related return to baseline vWF levels.

James PD et al. ASH ISTH NHF WFH 2021 guidelines on the diagnosis of von Willebrand disease. Blood Adv. 2021;5:280. [PMID: 33570651]

Table 14–9. Laboratory diagnosis of von Willebrand disease.

Type		vWF Activity	vWF Antigen	Factor VIII	RIPA	Multimer Pattern
1		↓	↓	Nl or ↓	↓	Normal pattern; uniform ↓ intensity of bands
2	A	↓↓	↓	↓	↓	Large and intermediate multimers decreased or absent
	B	↓↓	↓	↓	↑	Large multimers decreased or absent
	M	↓	↓	↓	↓	Normal pattern; uniform ↓ intensity of bands
	N	Nl	Nl	↓↓	Nl	Nl
3		↓↓↓	↓↓↓	↓↓↓	↓↓↓	Multimers absent

Nl, normal; RIPA, ristocetin-induced platelet aggregation; vWF, von Willebrand factor.

3. Factor XI Deficiency

Factor XI deficiency (also called hemophilia C) is inherited in an autosomal recessive manner, leading to heterozygous, compound heterozygous, or homozygous defects. It is most prevalent among individuals of Ashkenazi Jewish descent but is in the differential diagnosis of any unexplained prolonged aPTT. In contrast to hemophilia A and B, factor XI levels do not correlate well with bleeding symptoms. Mild bleeding is most common, and diagnosis is often made after unexpected, excessive bleeding following surgery or trauma. Importantly, factor XI deficiency that can lead to provoked excessive bleeding does not always prolong the aPTT. FFP is the mainstay of treatment when plasma-derived factor XI concentrate is not available. Adjunctive aminocaproic acid or tranexamic acid is administered for procedures or bleeding episodes involving the mucosa (Table 14–8).

Verghese L et al. Management of parturients with factor XI deficiency—10 year case series and review of literature. Eur J Obstet Gynecol Reprod Biol. 2017;215:85. [PMID: 28622635]

4. Less Common Heritable Disorders of Coagulation

Congenital deficiencies of clotting factors II, V, VII, and X are rare and typically are inherited in an autosomal recessive pattern. A prolongation in the PT (and aPTT for factor X, factor V, and factor II deficiency) that corrects upon mixing with normal plasma is typical. Definitive diagnosis requires testing for specific factor activity. The treatment of factor II deficiency is with a prothrombin complex concentrate; factor V deficiency is treated with infusions of FFP or platelets (which contain factor V in alpha granules); factor VII deficiency is treated with recombinant human activated factor VII. Factor X deficiency is treated with an FDA-approved plasma-derived factor X product (Coagadex).

Deficiency of factor XIII characteristically leads to delayed bleeding that occurs hours to days after a hemostatic challenge, such as surgery or trauma. The condition is usually life-long, and spontaneous intracranial hemorrhages as well as recurrent pregnancy loss appear to occur with increased frequency in these patients compared with other congenital deficiencies. Cryoprecipitate can be used to provide factor XIII, but if available, plasma-derived factor XIII concentrate (Corifact) is preferred to treat bleeding or for surgical prophylaxis. Regular prophylactic factor XIII replacement is indicated for patients with severe factor XIII deficiency. Factor XIII has an A and B subunit. Recombinant factor XIII A-subunit (Tretten) is an option for patients deficient in the factor XIII A subunit. Factor XIII deficiency does not cause a prolongation of the PT or aPTT.

National Hemophilia Foundation. Products Licensed in the US. https://www.hemophilia.org/healthcare-professionals/guidelines-on-care/products-licensed-in-the-us8

Peyvandi F et al. Treatment of rare factor deficiencies in 2016. Hematology Am Soc Hematol Educ Program. 2016;2016:663. [PMID: 27913544]

ACQUIRED DISORDERS OF COAGULATION

1. Acquired Antibodies to Factor II

Patients with antiphospholipid antibodies occasionally have antibody specificity to coagulation factor II (prothrombin) that accelerates factor II clearances and can lead to severe hypoprothrombinemia and bleeding. Mixing studies may or may not reveal the presence of an inhibitor, as the antibody typically binds to a non-enzymatically active portion of the molecule leading to accelerated clearance, but characteristically the PT is prolonged and levels of factor II are low. FFP should be administered to treat bleeding. Treatment is immunosuppressive.

2. Acquired Antibodies to Factor V

Products containing bovine factor V (such as topical thrombin or fibrin glue, frequently used in surgical procedures) can lead to formation of an anti–factor V antibody that cross-reacts with human factor V. Clinicopathologic manifestations range from a prolonged PT in an otherwise asymptomatic individual to severe bleeding. Mixing studies suggest the presence of an inhibitor, and the factor V activity level is low. In cases of serious or life-threatening bleeding, IVIG or platelet transfusions, or both, should be administered, and immunosuppression (as for acquired inhibitors to factor VIII) may be offered.

3. Acquired Antibodies to Factor VIII

Acquired hemophilia A due to factor VIII inhibitors is the most common acquired factor-specific bleeding disorder. Spontaneous antibodies to factor VIII can occur in adults without a prior history of hemophilia; older adults and patients with lymphoproliferative malignancy or autoimmune disease and those who are postpartum or postsurgical are at highest risk. The clinical presentation, which should be viewed as a medical emergency, typically includes extensive soft tissue ecchymoses, hematomas, and mucosal bleeding, as opposed to hemarthrosis characteristic of congenital hemophilia A. The aPTT is typically prolonged and does not correct upon mixing; factor VIII activity is low and a Bethesda assay reveals the titer of the inhibitor. Inhibitors of low titer (less than 5 BU) may often be overcome by infusion of high doses of factor VIII concentrates, whereas high-titer inhibitors (greater than 5 BU) must be treated with serial infusions of activated prothrombin complex concentrates, recombinant human activated factor VII, or recombinant porcine factor VIII. Emicizumab is also a treatment option. Along with establishment of hemostasis by one of these measures, immunosuppressive treatment with corticosteroids with or without oral cyclophosphamide or rituximab must be instituted to eradicate the autoantibody. Treatment with IVIG and plasmapheresis can be considered in refractory cases. Unlike in congenital factor VIII deficiency of hemophilia A, the patient's bleeding does not correlate well with the factor VIII activity level, so the clinician must be concerned with any elevation of aPTT secondary to acquired factor VIII inhibitor. All such patients require immediate referral to a hematologist.

Gibson CJ et al. Clinical problem-solving. A bruising loss. N Engl J Med. 2016;375:76. [PMID: 27406351]
Thomas VM et al. Off-label use of emicizumab in persons with acquired haemophilia A and von Willebrand disease: a scoping review of the literature. Haemophilia. 2022;28:4. [PMID: 34820989]

4. Vitamin K Deficiency

Vitamin K deficiency may occur as a result of deficient dietary intake of vitamin K (from green leafy vegetables, soybeans, and other sources), malabsorption, or decreased production by intestinal bacteria (due to treatment with chemotherapy or antibiotics). Vitamin K is required for normal function of vitamin K epoxide reductase that assists in posttranslational gamma-carboxylation of the coagulation factors II, VII, IX, and X, which is necessary for their activity. Thus, mild to moderate vitamin K deficiency typically features a prolonged PT (activity of the vitamin K–dependent factors is more reflected than in the aPTT; aPTT is prolonged if the deficiency is more severe) that corrects upon mixing; activity levels of individual clotting factors II, VII, IX, and X typically are low. Importantly, a concomitantly low factor V activity level is not indicative of isolated vitamin K deficiency and may indicate an underlying defect in liver synthetic function. Hospitalized patients on broad-spectrum antibiotics and with poor or no oral intake are at high risk for vitamin K deficiency.

For treatment, vitamin K_1 (phytonadione) may be administered via intravenous or oral routes; the subcutaneous route is not recommended due to erratic absorption. The oral dose is 5–10 mg/day and absorption is typically excellent; at least partial improvement in the PT should be observed within 18–24 hours of administration. Intravenous administration results in faster normalization of a prolonged PT than oral administration; due to infrequent reported serious adverse reactions, parenteral doses should be administered slowly (eg, over 30 minutes) with concomitant monitoring.

5. Coagulopathy of Liver Disease

Impaired liver function due to cirrhosis or other causes leads to decreased synthesis of clotting factors, including factors II, V, VII, IX, X, and fibrinogen; factor VIII levels, largely made in endothelial cells, may be elevated despite depressed levels of other coagulation factors. The PT (and with advanced disease, the aPTT) is typically prolonged and usually corrects on mixing with normal plasma. A normal factor V level, with decreased activity of factors II, VII, IX, and X suggests vitamin K deficiency rather than liver disease. Qualitative and quantitative deficiencies of fibrinogen also are prevalent among patients with advanced liver disease, typically leading to a prolonged PT, thrombin time, and reptilase time.

The coagulopathy of liver disease usually does not require hemostatic treatment unless bleeding occurs. Infusion of FFP may be considered if active bleeding is present and the aPTT and PT are prolonged; however, the effect is transient and concern for volume overload may limit infusions. Patients with bleeding and a fibrinogen level consistently below 80–100 mg/dL should receive cryoprecipitate. Liver transplantation, if feasible, results in production of coagulation factors at normal levels. The use of recombinant human activated factor VII in patients with bleeding varices is controversial, although some patient subgroups may experience benefit. The coagulopathy of liver disease can predispose to bleeding or thrombosis, so caution and experience are needed for optimal management.

Hunt BJ. Bleeding and coagulopathies in critical care. N Engl J Med. 2014;370:847. [PMID: 24571757]
Saner FH et al. Assessment and management of coagulopathy in critically-ill patients with liver failure. Curr Opin Crit Care. 2019;25:179. [PMID: 30855324]
Tripodi A et al. Changing concepts of cirrhotic coagulopathy. Am J Gastroenterol. 2017;112:274. [PMID: 27801884]

6. Warfarin Ingestion

See Antithrombotic Therapy section, below.

7. Disseminated Intravascular Coagulation

See above.

8. Heparin/Fondaparinux/Direct-Acting Oral Anticoagulant Use

See Classes of Anticoagulants, below.

9. Lupus Anticoagulants

Lupus anticoagulants prolong the aPTT by interfering with interactions between the clotting cascade and the phospholipid surface on which they function, but they do not lead to bleeding. Rather, they predispose to thrombosis. Lupus anticoagulants were so named because of their early identification in patients with autoimmune disease, although they also occur with increased frequency in individuals with underlying infection, inflammation, or malignancy, and they also can occur in asymptomatic individuals in the general population. A prolongation in the aPTT is observed that does not correct completely on mixing but that normalizes with excessive phospholipid. Specialized testing such as a positive hexagonal phase phospholipid neutralization assay, a prolonged dilute Russell viper venom time, and positive platelet neutralization assays can confirm the presence of a lupus anticoagulant. Rarely, the antibodies also interfere with factor II activity, and that tiny subset of lupus anticoagulant patients are at risk for bleeding.

Müller-Calleja N et al. Tissue factor pathway inhibitor primes monocytes for antiphospholipid antibody-induced thrombosis. Blood. 2019;134:1119. [PMID: 31434703]

OTHER CAUSES OF BLEEDING

Occasionally, abnormalities of the vasculature and integument may lead to bleeding despite normal hemostasis; congenital or acquired disorders may be causative. Congenital abnormalities include Ehlers-Danlos syndrome, osteogenesis imperfecta, hereditary hemorrhagic telangiectasia (Osler-Weber-Rendu disease) (see Chapter 40), and Marfan syndrome. Acquired disorders include integument thinning due to prolonged corticosteroid administration or normal aging, amyloidosis, vasculitis, and scurvy (acquired defects). The bleeding time often is prolonged. If possible, treatment of the underlying condition should be pursued, but if this is not possible or feasible (ie, congenital syndromes), globally hemostatic agents such as antifibrinolytic agents or DDAVP can be considered for treatment of bleeding.

ANTITHROMBOTIC THERAPY

The currently available anticoagulants include unfractionated heparin, LMWHs, fondaparinux, vitamin K antagonists (ie, warfarin), and DOACs (ie, dabigatran, rivaroxaban, apixaban, edoxaban). (For a discussion of injectable DTIs, see section Heparin-Induced Thrombocytopenia above.)

Classes of Anticoagulants

A. Unfractionated Heparin and LMWHs

About one-third of the molecules in a given preparation of unfractionated heparin contain the crucial pentasaccharide sequence necessary for binding of antithrombin and exerting its anticoagulant effect upon thrombin. The degree of anticoagulation with unfractionated heparin is typically monitored by aPTT or anti-Xa level in patients who are receiving the drug in therapeutic doses, although the pharmacokinetics of unfractionated heparin are poorly predictable. Only a fraction of an infused dose of heparin is metabolized by the kidneys, making it safe to use in most patients with significant kidney disease.

Due to less protein and cellular binding, pharmacokinetics of the LMWHs are much more predictable than those of unfractionated heparin, allowing for fixed weight-based dosing. All LMWHs are principally renally cleared and must be avoided or used with extreme caution in individuals with creatinine clearance less than 30 mL/minute. Compared to unfractionated heparin, LMWHs have a longer half-life, which allows once- or twice-daily subcutaneous dosing and thus greater convenience and outpatient therapy in selected cases. Most patients do not require monitoring, although monitoring using the anti-Xa activity level is appropriate for patients with moderate kidney disease, those with elevated BMI or low weight, and selected pregnant patients. LMWHs are associated with a lower frequency of HIT and thrombosis (approximately 0.6%) than unfractionated heparin (3%).

B. Fondaparinux

Fondaparinux is a synthetic molecule consisting of the highly active pentasaccharide sequence found in LMWHs. As such, it exerts almost no thrombin inhibition and works to indirectly inhibit factor Xa through binding to antithrombin. Fondaparinux, like the LMWHs, is almost exclusively metabolized by the kidneys, and should be avoided in patients with creatinine clearance less than 30 mL/minute. Predictable pharmacokinetics allow for weight-based dosing.

C. Vitamin K Antagonist (Warfarin)

The vitamin K antagonist warfarin inhibits the activity of the vitamin K–dependent carboxylase that is important for the posttranslational modification of coagulation factors II, VII, IX, and X. Although warfarin is taken orally, which is a significant advantage over the heparins and heparin derivatives, interindividual differences in nutritional status, comorbid diseases, concomitant medications, and genetic polymorphisms lead to a poorly predictable anticoagulant response. Individuals taking warfarin must undergo periodic monitoring to verify the intensity of the anticoagulant effect, reported as the INR, which corrects for differences in potency of commercially available thromboplastin used to perform the PT.[1]

D. Direct-Acting Oral Anticoagulants

Unlike warfarin, the DOACs act directly against coagulation factors. Dabigatran is a DTI; rivaroxaban, apixaban, and edoxaban are direct factor Xa inhibitors. DOACs (1) have a predictable dose effect and therefore do not require laboratory monitoring, (2) have anticoagulant activity independent of vitamin K with no need for dietary stasis, and (3) are renally metabolized to varying degrees so there are restrictions or dose reductions related to reduced kidney function (Table 14–10). While the DOACs have fewer drug interactions than warfarin, if DOACs are given with potentially interacting medications, there is no reliable way to measure the impact on anticoagulant activity of the concomitant administration. There is also no reliable way to measure adherence. The clinician must carefully consider kidney function, concomitant medications, indication for use, candidacy for lead-in parenteral therapy (as required for acute VTE treatment with edoxaban and dabigatran only) and anticipated patient adherence. Providers must be careful to dose each DOAC properly for the indication, kidney function, and weight of patient, and to check for drug interactions. (See Table 14–10 for details.) For morbidly obese patients (more than 120 kg or BMI ≥ 40), standard doses of apixaban or rivaroxaban should be chosen rather than dabigatran or edoxaban. DOACs are not recommended for VTE treatment in the acute setting following bariatric surgery due to concerns regarding absorption but can be considered for ongoing treatment after the initial 4 weeks of therapy; when available, apixaban or rivaroxaban trough levels can be checked to ensure they are within expected ranges. Reversal agents are available for the oral DTI (dabigatran) and for the factor Xa inhibitors (apixaban, rivaroxaban, edoxaban) (Table 14–11).

Routine monitoring is not recommended for patients taking DOACs. However, there are clinical scenarios where assessing anticoagulant activity may be helpful, including active bleeding, pending urgent surgery, suspected therapeutic failure, or concern for accumulation. Drug-specific anti-Xa levels are not widely available, and guidance is

[1]Importantly, because the INR is not standardized for abnormalities of factor V and fibrinogen, the INR should be used only in reference to anticoagulation in patients who are receiving warfarin.

Table 14–10. DOACs for VTE treatment and prevention.[1] Dosing for atrial fibrillation is provided in Table 10–13.

	Dabigatran	Rivaroxaban	Apixaban	Edoxaban
Mechanism	Oral direct thrombin inhibitor	Oral direct factor Xa inhibitor	Oral direct factor Xa inhibitor	Oral direct factor Xa inhibitor
Approved uses for VTE	VTE treatment and secondary prevention VTE prophylaxis post-hip replacement	VTE treatment and secondary prevention VTE prophylaxis post-hip or knee replacement VTE prophylaxis in select adult patients hospitalized for acute medical illness	VTE treatment and secondary prevention VTE prophylaxis post-hip or knee replacement	VTE treatment and secondary prevention
Frequency of dosing for VTE	Twice daily following 5-day parenteral lead-in for acute VTE	Twice daily for first 21 days of acute VTE therapy, then daily Once daily for DVT prophylaxis	Twice daily	Once daily following 5-day parenteral lead-in for acute VTE
Food	With or without food	With food (for 15- and 20-mg tablets)	With or without food	With or without food
Crushable?	No	Can crush; do not administer via J tube	Can crush and administer orally or via NG tube	No data
Renal clearance	80%	30–60%	25%	50%
Kinetics	t ½ = 12–17 hours; tmax = 2 hours	t ½ = 5–9 hours; tmax = 3 hours	t ½ = 12 hours; tmax = 3 hours	t ½ = 10–14 hours; tmax = 2 hours
Impact on INR	↑ (or →)	↑↑ (or → at low concentrations)	↑ (or →)	↑
Impact on aPTT	↑↑	↑	↑	↑
Drug interactions (list not comprehensive)	**Avoid** rifampin, St John's wort, and possibly carbamazepine **Caution** with amiodarone, clarithromycin, dronedarone, ketoconazole, quinidine, verapamil No dose adjustment if CrCl > 50 mL/minute **Reduce dose** to 75 mg orally twice daily if CrCl 30–50 mL/minute and concurrent use of dronedarone or ketoconazole	**Avoid** carbamazepine, conivaptan, indinavir/ritonavir, itraconazole, ketoconazole, lopinavir/ritonavir, phenytoin, rifampin, ritonavir, St John's wort **Caution** with the concurrent use of combined P-gp inhibitors and/or weak or moderate inhibitors of CYP3A4 (eg, amiodarone, azithromycin, diltiazem, dronedarone, erythromycin, felodipine, quinidine, ranolazine, verapamil) particularly in patients with impaired kidney function	**Avoid** carbamazepine, phenytoin, rifampin, St John's wort. If on apixaban 5 mg twice daily, decrease to 2.5 mg twice daily if starting itraconazole, ketoconazole, or ritonavir. If already on decreased dose of apixaban, avoid co-administration. **Caution** with clarithromycin	**Avoid** rifampin **Reduce dose** with certain P-gp inhibitors (eg, amiodarone, azithromycin, verapamil, ketoconazole, clarithromycin). Use has not been studied with many other P-gp inhibitors and inducers. Some experts recommend avoiding concurrent use altogether
Switching from DOAC to warfarin (per AC Forum Clinical Guidance)	Start warfarin and overlap with dabigatran; CrCl C50 mL/minute, overlap 3 days CrCl 30–50 mL/minute, overlap 2 days CrCl 15–30 mL/minute, overlap 1 day	Stop DOAC; start warfarin and LMWH at time of next scheduled DOAC dose and bridge until INR ≥ 2.0	Stop DOAC; start warfarin and LMWH at time of next scheduled DOAC dose and bridge until INR ≥ 2.0	For 60-mg dose, reduce dose to 30 mg and start warfarin concomitantly For 30-mg dose, reduce dose to 15 mg and start warfarin concomitantly Stop edoxaban when INR ≥ 2.0
Warfarin to DOAC	Start when INR < 2.0	Start when INR < 3.0	Start when INR < 2.0	Start when INR ≤ 2.5
Special considerations	Dyspepsia is common and starts within first 10 days GI bleeding risk higher with dabigatran than with warfarin	GI bleeding risk higher with rivaroxaban than with warfarin		Do not use if CrCl < 15 mL/minute

Table 14–11. Medications to consider for reversing anticoagulant effect during life-threatening bleeding.[1]

Anticoagulants	Guidance
Parenteral	
Heparins	Protamine provides total (for unfractionated heparin) or partial (for LMWHs) reversal of anticoagulant effect. • Administration: Very slow infusion • Maximum dose: 50 mg intravenously • Caution: risk of anaphylactoid reactions and true hypersensitivity reactions, especially if allergy to other protamine-containing medications (such as NPH insulin) or to fish (black box warning) • Dosing depends on dose given and time elapsed • Dosing calculator at https://clincalc.com/Protamine/
Unfractionated heparin	Protamine (100% neutralization) • 1 mg protamine neutralizes approximately 100 units of heparin sulfate • Monitor drug activity with aPTT and/or heparin anti-Xa activity
LMWH (enoxaparin, dalteparin)	Protamine (approximately 60% neutralization) • Last dose < 8 hours ago: 1 mg protamine for each 100 units of dalteparin or 1 mg enoxaparin • Last dose > 8 hours ago: 0.5 mg protamine for each 100 units of dalteparin or 1 mg enoxaparin • Degree of reversal can be assessed with LMWH anti-Xa activity
Oral	
DOACs	Guidance for all DOAC-associated major bleeding: • Supportive measures recommended for all patients • If ingested within 2 hours, administer activated charcoal • Reversal agent is recommended ONLY if bleeding is life-threatening or into a critical organ • Reversal agent is not recommended for DOAC overdose without bleeding
Dabigatran	Idarucizamab 5 g intravenously once If idarucizamab is not available: administer APCC 50 units/kg intravenously
Apixaban	Andexanet alfa: Last dose ≤ 5 mg AND within 8 hours: low dose[2] Last dose > 5 mg AND within 8 hours: high dose[3] Last dose > 8 hours ago: low dose[2] If andexanet alfa is not available: administer four-factor PCC 2000 units
Rivaroxaban	Andexanet alfa: Last dose ≤ 10 mg AND within 8 hours: low dose[2] Last dose > 10 mg AND within 8 hours: high dose[3] Last dose > 8 hours ago: low dose[2] If andexanet alfa is not available: administer four-factor PCC 2000 units
Warfarin	See Table 14–21

[1]Guidance adopted from 2019 Anticoagulation Forum and American Society of Hematology 2019 guidelines.
[2]Low-dose andexanet alfa: initial 400 mg intravenous bolus at target rate of 30 mg/minute followed by continuous infusion at 4 mg/minute for up to 120 minutes.
[3]High-dose andexanet alfa: initial 800 mg intravenous bolus at target rate of 30 mg/minute followed by continuous infusion at 8 mg/minute for up to 120 minutes. Begin infusion within 2 minutes after intravenous bolus to prevent rebound anti-Xa activity.
APCC, three-factor prothrombin complex concentrate; FFP, fresh frozen plasma; LMWH, low-molecular-weight heparin; PCC, four-factor prothrombin complex concentrate.
Data from Cuker A et al. Reversal of direct oral anticoagulants: Guidance from the Anticoagulation Forum. Am J Hematol. 2019;94(6):697–709; data from Witt DM et al. American Society of Hematology 2018 guidelines for management of venous thromboembolism: optimal management of anticoagulation therapy. Blood Adv. 2018;2(22):3257–3291.

lacking regarding clinical approach to the results. DOACs have varying effects on the PT and aPTT. In the absence of drug-specific levels, a normal dilute thrombin time excludes the presence of clinically relevant dabigatran levels; an elevated aPTT suggests clinically relevant levels of dabigatran. An elevated PT suggests clinically relevant levels of rivaroxaban. However, a normal aPTT or normal PT does not rule out clinically significant amounts of dabigatran or rivaroxaban, respectively.

Douxfils J et al. Laboratory testing in patients treated with direct oral anticoagulants: a practical guide for clinicians. J Thromb Haemost. 2018;16:209. [PMID: 29193737]

Prevention of Venous Thromboembolic Disease

The frequency of venous thromboembolic disease (VTE) among hospitalized patients ranges widely. Up to 60% of VTE cases occur during or after hospitalization, with especially high incidence among critical care patients and high-risk surgical patients.

Avoidance of fatal PE, which occurs in up to 5% of high-risk inpatients as a consequence of hospitalization or surgery, is a major goal of pharmacologic prophylaxis. Tables 14–12 and 14–13 provide risk stratification for DVT/VTE among hospitalized surgical and medical inpatients. Standard pharmacologic prophylactic regimens are listed in Table 14–14; prophylactic anticoagulation regimens differ in their recommended duration of use. Prophylactic strategies should be guided by individual risk stratification, with all moderate- and high-risk patients receiving pharmacologic prophylaxis, unless contraindicated. Contraindications to VTE prophylaxis for hospital inpatients at high risk for VTE are listed in Table 14–15. In patients at high risk for VTE with absolute contraindications to pharmacologic prophylaxis, mechanical devices such as intermittent pneumatic compression devices should be used, ideally in portable form with at least an 18-hour daily wear time.

Table 14–12. Risk stratification for DVT/VTE among surgical inpatients.

High risk[1]
- Recent major orthopedic surgery/arthroplasty/fracture
- Abdominal/pelvic cancer undergoing surgery
- Spinal cord injury[2] or major trauma within 90 days
- More than three of the intermediate risk factors (see below)

Intermediate risk
- Not ambulating independently outside of room at least twice daily
- Active infectious or inflammatory process
- Active malignancy
- Major surgery (nonorthopedic)
- History of VTE
- Stroke
- Central venous access or PICC line
- IBD
- Prior immobilization (> 72 hours) preoperatively
- Obesity (BMI > 30)
- Patient age > 50 years
- Hormone replacement or oral contraceptive therapy
- Hypercoagulable state
- Nephrotic syndrome
- Burns
- Cellulitis
- Varicose veins
- Paresis
- HF (systolic dysfunction)
- COPD exacerbation

Low risk
- Minor procedure and age < 40 years with no additional risk factors
- Ambulatory with expected length of stay of < 24 hours or minor surgery

[1]Risk is highest in first month and persists for up to 90 days.
[2]Direct spinal cord trauma is a contraindication to VTE prophylaxis in the immediate post-injury period; consult with neurosurgical experts regarding timing of initiation.
HF, heart failure; PICC, peripherally inserted central catheter; VTE, venous thromboembolism.

Table 14–13. Padua Risk Assessment Model for VTE prophylaxis in hospitalized medical patients.

Condition	Points[1]
Active cancer, history of VTE, immobility, laboratory thrombophilia	3 points each
Recent (≤ 1 mo) trauma and/or surgery	2 points each
Age ≥ 70; acute MI or ischemic stroke; acute infection or rheumatologic disorder; BMI ≥ 30; hormonal therapy	1 point each

[1]A score ≥ 4 connotes high risk of VTE in the noncritically ill medical patients and pharmacologic prophylaxis is indicated, absent absolute contraindications.
CVA, cerebrovascular accident; VTE, venous thromboembolism.

1. Primary VTE prophylaxis for medical patients—It is recommended that VTE prophylaxis be used judiciously in hospitalized medical patients who are not critically ill since a comprehensive review of evidence suggested harm from bleeding in low-risk patients given low-dose heparin, and skin necrosis from compression stockings in stroke patients. Risk assessment models like the Padua Risk Score (Table 14–13) and the IMPROVE risk score can help clinicians identify patients who may benefit from DVT prophylaxis. The IMPROVE investigators also developed a bleeding risk model that may aid in identifying acutely ill medical inpatients at increased risk for bleeding: https://www.outcomes-umassmed.org/IMPROVE/risk_score/index.html. While two of the anti-Xa oral anticoagulants (rivaroxaban) have been approved for extended duration prophylaxis after discharge for medically ill patients, how to identify those who will have clinical benefit from this practice is still unclear. For the prevention of VTE in severe COVID-19, see below.

2. Primary VTE prophylaxis for surgical patients—The Caprini score may help guide decisions in surgical patients about VTE prophylaxis (https://www.mdcalc.com/caprini-score-venous-thromboembolism-2005). In addition, certain high-risk surgical patients should be considered for extended-duration prophylaxis of up to 1 month, including those undergoing total hip replacement, hip fracture repair, and abdominal and pelvic cancer surgery. If bleeding is present, if the risk of bleeding is high, or if the risk of VTE is high for the inpatient (Table 14–12) and therefore combined prophylactic strategies are needed, some measure of thromboprophylaxis may be provided through mechanical devices such as intermittent pneumatic compression devices and graduated compression stockings.

3. Primary VTE prophylaxis for ambulatory cancer patients—Some ambulatory cancer patients undergoing chemotherapy who are at moderate to high risk of VTE (Khorana risk score ≥ 2) (https://www.mdcalc.com/khorana-risk-score-venous-thromboembolism-cancer-patients) may benefit from pharmacologic DVT prophylaxis, although bleeding risk is increased and caution should be taken, particularly in patients with GI or intracranial malignancy, and other risk factors for

Table 14–14. Pharmacologic prophylaxis of VTE in selected clinical scenarios.[1]

Anticoagulant	Dose	Frequency	Clinical Scenario	Comment
LMWH and Fondaparinux				
Enoxaparin	40 mg subcutaneously	Once daily	Medical inpatients at high risk for VTE and most critical care patients[2]	—
			Surgical patients (moderate risk for VTE)	—
			Abdominal/pelvic cancer surgery	Consider continuing for 4 weeks total duration after abdominopelvic cancer surgery.
		Twice daily	Bariatric surgery	Higher doses may be required.
	30 mg subcutaneously	Twice daily	Orthopedic surgery[3]	Give for at least 10 days. For THR, TKR, or HFS, consider continuing up to 1 month after surgery in high-risk patients.
			Major trauma	Not applicable to patients with isolated lower extremity trauma.
			Spinal cord injury[4]	—
Dalteparin	2500 units subcutaneously	Once daily	Medical inpatients at high risk for VTE[2]	—
			Abdominal surgery (moderate risk for VTE)	Give for 5–10 days.
	5000 units subcutaneously	Once daily	Orthopedic surgery[3]	First dose = 2500 units. Give for at least 10 days. For THR, TKR, or HFS, consider continuing up to 1 month after surgery in high-risk patients.
			Abdominal surgery (higher risk for VTE)	Give for 5–10 days. Consider continuing for 4 weeks total duration after abdomino-pelvic cancer surgery.
			Medical inpatients	—
Fondaparinux	2.5 mg subcutaneously	Once daily	Orthopedic surgery[3]	Give for at least 10 days. For THR, TKR, or HFS, consider continuing up to 1 month after surgery in high-risk patients.
Direct-Acting Oral Anticoagulants				
Rivaroxaban	10 mg orally	Once daily	Orthopedic surgery: THR, TKR	Give for 12 days following TKR; give for 35 days following THR.
Apixaban	2.5 mg orally	Twice daily	Following THR or TKR	Give for 12 days following TKR; give for 35 days following THR.
Dabigatran	110 mg orally first day, then 220 mg	Once daily	Following THR	For patients with CrCl > 30 mL/minute. Consider continuing up to 1 month after surgery in high-risk patients.
Unfractionated Heparin				
Unfractionated heparin	5000 units subcutaneously	Three times daily	Higher VTE risk with low bleeding risk	Includes gynecologic surgery for malignancy and urologic surgery, medical patients with multiple risk factors for VTE.
	5000 units subcutaneously	Twice daily	Hospitalized patients at intermediate risk for VTE	Includes gynecologic surgery (moderate risk).
			Patients with epidural catheters	LMWHs usually avoided due to risk of spinal hematoma.
			Patients with severe kidney disease[5]	LMWHs contraindicated.

(*continued*)

Table 14–14. Pharmacologic prophylaxis of VTE in selected clinical scenarios.[1] (continued)

Anticoagulant	Dose	Frequency	Clinical Scenario	Comment
Warfarin and Aspirin				
Warfarin	(Variable) oral	Once daily	Orthopedic surgery[3]	Titrate to goal INR = 2.5. Give for at least 10 days. For high-risk patients undergoing THR, TKR, or HFS, consider continuing up to 1 month after surgery.
Aspirin	81 mg orally	Twice daily	TKR, THR	For patients at otherwise low VTE risk following major orthopedic surgery. Give for at least 14 days.

[1]All regimens administered subcutaneously, except for warfarin. See Table 14–15 for contraindications.
[2]See Prevention of Venous Thromboembolic Disease text, above, for definition of high-risk patients.
[3]Includes TKR, THR, and HFS.
[4]Direct spinal cord trauma is a contraindication to VTE prophylaxis in the immediate post-injury period; consult with neurosurgical experts regarding timing of initiation.
[5]Defined as creatinine clearance < 30 mL/minute.
CrCl, creatine clearance; HFS, hip fracture surgery; LMWH, low-molecular-weight heparin; P-gp, P-glycoprotein; THR, total hip replacement; TKR, total knee replacement; VTE, venous thromboembolic disease.

anticoagulant-related bleeding (such as thrombocytopenia and kidney dysfunction). DOACs should be avoided when there are possible interactions with chemotherapeutic agents.

Treatment of VTE Disease

A. Anticoagulant Therapy for VTE

Treatment for VTE should be offered to patients with objectively confirmed DVT or PE, or to those in whom the clinical suspicion is high for the disorder but who have not yet undergone diagnostic testing (see Chapter 9). The management of VTE primarily involves administration of anticoagulants; the goal is to prevent recurrence, extension and embolization of thrombosis and to reduce the risk of post-thrombotic syndrome. Suggested anticoagulation regimens are found in Table 14–16.

Table 14–15. Contraindications to VTE prophylaxis for medical or surgical hospital inpatients at high risk for VTE.

Absolute contraindications
- Acute hemorrhage from wounds or drains or lesions
- Intracranial hemorrhage within prior 24 hours
- Heparin-induced thrombocytopenia (HIT): consider using fondaparinux
- Severe trauma to head or spinal cord or extremities
- Epidural anesthesia/spinal block within 12 hours of initiation of anticoagulation (concurrent use of an epidural catheter and anticoagulation other than low prophylactic doses of unfractionated heparin should require review and approval by service who performed the epidural or spinal procedure, eg, anesthesia/pain service, and in many cases, should be avoided entirely)
- Currently receiving warfarin or heparin or LMWH or direct thrombin inhibitor for other indications

Relative contraindications
- Coagulopathy (INR > 1.5)
- Intracranial lesion or neoplasm
- Severe thrombocytopenia (platelet count < 50,000/mcL [50×10^9/L])
- Intracranial hemorrhage within past 6 months
- GI or genitourinary hemorrhage within past 6 months

LMWH, low-molecular-weight heparin; VTE, venous thromboembolic disease.
Adapted from guidelines used at the Veterans Affairs Medical Center, San Francisco, CA.

B. Selecting Appropriate Initial Anticoagulant Therapy for VTE

Most patients with DVT alone may be treated as outpatients, provided that their risk of bleeding is low and they have good follow-up. Table 14–17 outlines proposed selection criteria for outpatient treatment of DVT.

Among patients with PE, risk stratification at time of diagnosis should direct treatment and triage. Patients with persistent hemodynamic instability are classified as high-risk patients (previously referred to as having "massive PE") and have an early PE-related mortality of more than 15%. These patients should be admitted to an ICU and generally receive thrombolysis and anticoagulation with intravenous heparin. Intermediate-risk patients (previously "submassive PE") have a mortality rate of up to 15% and should be admitted to a higher level of inpatient care, with consideration of thrombolysis on a case-by-case basis. Catheter-directed techniques, if available, may be an option for patients who are poor candidates for systemic thrombolysis and/or in centers with expertise. Low-risk patients have a mortality rate less than 3% and are candidates for expedited discharge or outpatient therapy.

For hemodynamically stable patients, additional assessment focusing on right ventricular dysfunction is warranted to differentiate between low-risk, low-intermediate risk, and high-intermediate risk PE. The Bova score (https://www.mdcalc.com/bova-score-pulmonary-embolism-complications) and the simplified PE severity index accurately identify patients at low risk for 30-day PE-related mortality (Table 14–18) who are potential candidates for expedited discharge or outpatient treatment.

Because the Bova score includes serum troponin and evidence of right ventricular dysfunction (by CT or echocardiography), it also identifies patients with high-intermediate risk PE who warrant close monitoring and may require escalation of therapy. An RV/LV ratio less than 1.0 on chest CT angiogram has been shown to have good negative predictive value for adverse outcome but suffers from inter observer variability. Echocardiography may provide better assessment of right ventricular dysfunction when there is concern. Serum biomarkers such as BNP and troponin are most useful for their negative predictive value, and mainly in combination with other predictors.

Selection of an initial anticoagulant should be determined by patient characteristics (kidney function, immediate bleeding risk, weight) and the clinical scenario (eg, whether thrombolysis is being considered, active cancer, thrombosis location) as described in Table 14–16.

1. Parenteral anticoagulants for VTE—

Heparins—In patients in whom parenteral anticoagulation is being considered, LMWHs are more effective than unfractionated heparin in the immediate treatment of DVT and PE; they are preferred as initial treatment because of predictable pharmacokinetics, which allow for subcutaneous, once- or twice-daily dosing with no requirement for monitoring in most patients. Accumulation of LMWH and increased rates of bleeding have been observed among patients with severe kidney disease (creatinine clearance less than 30 mL/minute), leading to a recommendation to use intravenous unfractionated heparin preferentially in these patients. *If concomitant thrombolysis is being considered, unfractionated heparin is preferred.* Patients with VTE and a perceived higher risk of bleeding (ie, post-surgery) may be better candidates for treatment with

Table 14–16. Initial anticoagulation for VTE.[1]

Anticoagulant	Dose/Frequency	Clinical Scenario: DVT, Lower Extremity	DVT, Upper Extremity	PE	VTE, With Concomitant Severe Kidney Disease[2]	VTE, Cancer-Related	Comment
Unfractionated Heparin							
Unfractionated heparin	80 units/kg intravenous bolus, then continuous intravenous infusion of 18 units/kg/hour	×	×	×	×		Bolus may be omitted if risk of bleeding is perceived to be elevated. Maximum bolus, 10,000 units. Requires aPTT or heparin anti-Xa monitoring. Most patients: begin warfarin at time of initiation of heparin.
	330 units/kg subcutaneously × 1, then 250 units/kg subcutaneously every 12 hours	×					Fixed-dose; no aPTT monitoring required
LMWH and Fondaparinux							
Enoxaparin[3]	1 mg/kg subcutaneously every 12 hours **or** 1.5 mg/kg subcutaneously daily	×	×	×			Most patients: begin warfarin at time of initiation of LMWH
Dalteparin[3]	200 units/kg subcutaneously once daily for first month, then 150 units/kg/day	×	×	×		×	Preferred LMWH for cancer patients; administer for at least 3–6 months (no transition to warfarin)
Fondaparinux	5–10 mg subcutaneously once daily; use 7.5 mg for body weight 50–100 kg; 10 mg for body weight > 100 kg	×	×	×			

(*continued*)

Table 14–16. Initial anticoagulation for VTE.[1] (continued)

Anticoagulant	Dose/Frequency	Clinical Scenario					Comment
		DVT, Lower Extremity	DVT, Upper Extremity	PE	VTE, With Concomitant Severe Kidney Disease[2]	VTE, Cancer-Related	
Direct-Acting Oral Anticoagulants (DOACs)							
Rivaroxaban	15 mg orally twice daily with food for 21 days, then 20 mg orally daily with food	×	×	×		×	Contraindicated if CrCl < 30 mL/minute Monotherapy without need for initial parenteral therapy Caution in luminal GI or genitourinary cancer
Apixaban	10 mg orally twice daily for first 7 days, then 5 mg twice daily	×	×	×		×	Contraindicated if CrCl < 25 mL/minute Monotherapy without need for initial parenteral therapy
Dabigatran	5–10 days of parenteral anticoagulation, then begin 150 mg orally twice daily	×	×	×			Contraindicated if CrCl < 15 mL/minute Initial need for parenteral therapy
Edoxaban	5–10 days of parenteral anticoagulation, then 60 mg orally once daily; 30 mg once daily recommended if CrCl is 15–50 mL/minute, if weight ≤ 60 kg, or if certain P-gp inhibitors are present	×	×	×		×	Contraindicated if CrCl < 15 mL/minute Initial need for parenteral therapy Caution in luminal GI or genitourinary cancer

[1]Obtain baseline hemoglobin, platelet count, aPTT, PT/INR, and creatinine prior to initiation of anticoagulation. *Anticoagulation is contraindicated in the setting of active bleeding.*
[2]Defined as creatinine clearance < 30 mL/minute.
[3]If body weight < 50 kg, reduce dose and monitor anti-Xa levels.
CrCl, creatinine clearance; P-gp, P-glycoprotein; VTE, venous thromboembolic disease (includes DVT and PE).
Note: An "×" denotes appropriate use of the anticoagulant.

unfractionated heparin than LMWH given its shorter half-life and reversibility. Unfractionated heparin can be effectively neutralized with protamine sulfate while protamine may only have partial reversal effect on LMWH. Use of unfractionated heparin leads to HIT and thrombosis in approximately 3% of patients, so daily CBCs are recommended during the initial 10–14 days of exposure.

Weight-based, fixed-dose daily subcutaneous fondaparinux may also be used for the initial treatment of DVT and PE, with no increase in bleeding over that observed with LMWH. Its lack of reversibility, long half-life, and renal clearance limit its use in patients with an increased risk of bleeding or kidney disease.

2. Oral anticoagulants for VTE—

A. Direct-acting oral anticoagulants—DOACs have a predictable dose effect, few drug-drug interactions, rapid onset of action, and freedom from laboratory monitoring (Table 14–10). Dabigatran, rivaroxaban, apixaban, and edoxaban are approved for treatment of acute DVT and PE. While rivaroxaban and apixaban can be used as monotherapy eliminating the need for parenteral therapy, patients treated with dabigatran or edoxaban must first receive 5–10 days of parenteral anticoagulation and then be transitioned to the oral agent per prescribing information. Unlike warfarin, DOACs do not require an overlap since these agents are immediately active; the DOAC is started when the parenteral agent is stopped. Compared to warfarin and LMWH, the DOACs are all noninferior with respect to prevention of recurrent VTE; both rivaroxaban and apixaban have a lower bleeding risk than warfarin with LMWH bridge. While DOACs are recommended as first-line therapy for acute VTE, agent selection should be individualized with consideration of kidney

Table 14–17. Patient selection for outpatient treatment of DVT.

Patients considered appropriate for outpatient treatment
- No clinical signs or symptoms of PE and pain controlled
- Confirmed ability to pay for medication (either by insurance or out-of-pocket)
- Capable and willing to comply with frequent follow-up
- Initially, patients may need to be seen daily to weekly

Potential contraindications for outpatient treatment
- DVT involving inferior vena cava, iliac, common femoral, or upper extremity vein (these patients might benefit from vascular intervention)
- Comorbid conditions requiring inpatient management
- Active peptic ulcer disease, GI bleeding in past 14 days, liver synthetic dysfunction
- Brain metastases, current or recent CNS or spinal cord injury/surgery in the last 10 days, CVA ≤ 4–6 weeks
- Familial bleeding diathesis
- Active bleeding from source other than GI
- Thrombocytopenia
- Creatinine clearance < 30 mL/minute
- Weight < 55 kg (male) or < 45 kg (female)
- Recent surgery, spinal or epidural anesthesia in the past 3 days
- History of heparin-induced thrombocytopenia
- Inability to reliably take medication at home, recognize changes in health status, or understand or follow directions

CVA, cerebrovascular accident.

function, concomitant medication use, indication, cost, and adherence. Heparins may be preferable as initial therapy when hospitalized patients have clinical instability and fluctuating renal or hepatic function; when bleeding risk is high; or when there is concern that thrombolysis may be required.

B. Warfarin—If warfarin is chosen as the oral anticoagulant it should be initiated along with the parenteral anticoagulant, which is continued until INR is in therapeutic range. Most patients require 5 mg of warfarin daily for initial treatment, but lower doses (2.5 mg daily) should be considered for patients of Asian descent, older adults, and those with hyperthyroidism, heart failure, liver disease, recent major surgery, malnutrition, certain polymorphisms for the *CYP2C9* or the *VKORC1* genes or who are receiving concurrent medications that increase sensitivity to warfarin. Conversely, individuals of African descent, those with larger BMI or hypothyroidism, and those who are receiving medications that increase warfarin metabolism (eg, rifampin) may require higher initial doses (7.5 mg daily). Daily INR results should guide dosing adjustments in the hospitalized patient while at least biweekly INR results guide dosing in the outpatient during the initial period of therapy (Table 14–19). Web-based warfarin dosing calculators incorporating clinical and genetic factors are available to help clinicians choose appropriate starting doses (eg, see www.warfarindosing.org). Because an average of 5 days is required to achieve a steady-state reduction in the activity of vitamin K–dependent coagulation factors, the parenteral anticoagulant should be continued for at least 5 days and until the INR is more than 2.0. Meticulous follow-up should be arranged for all patients taking warfarin because of the bleeding risk associated with initiation of therapy. Once stabilized, the INR should be checked at an interval no longer than every 6 weeks and warfarin dosing should be adjusted by guidelines (Table 14–20) since this strategy has been shown to improve the time patients spend in the therapeutic range and their clinical outcomes. Supratherapeutic INRs should be managed according to evidence-based guidelines (Table 14–21).

Table 14–18. Simplified Pulmonary Embolism Severity Index (PESI).

		Points
Age > 80 years old		1
Cancer		1
Chronic cardiopulmonary disease		1
Systolic blood pressure < 100 mm Hg		1
Oxygen saturation ≤ 90%		1
Severity Class	**Points**	**30-Day Mortality**
Low risk	0	1%
High risk	≥ 1	10%

Data from Jiménez D et al; RIETE Investigators. Simplification of the pulmonary embolism severity index for prognostication in patients with acute symptomatic pulmonary embolism. Arch Intern Med. 2010;170:1383.

C. Duration of Anticoagulation Therapy for VTE

The clinical scenario in which the thrombosis occurred is the strongest predictor of recurrence and, in most cases, guides duration of anticoagulation (Table 14–22). In the first year after discontinuation of anticoagulation therapy, the frequency of recurrent VTE among individuals whose thrombosis occurred in the setting of a transient, major, reversible risk factor (such as surgery) is approximately 3% after completing 3 months of anticoagulation, compared with at least 8% for individuals whose thrombosis was unprovoked, and greater than 20% in patients with cancer. Men have a greater than twofold higher risk of recurrent VTE compared to women; recurrent PE is more likely to develop in patients with clinically apparent PE than in those with DVT alone and has a case fatality rate of nearly 10%; and proximal DVT has a higher recurrence risk than distal DVT.

1. Provoked versus unprovoked VTE—Patients with provoked VTE are generally treated with a minimum of 3 months of anticoagulation, whereas unprovoked VTE should prompt consideration of indefinite anticoagulation provided the patient is not at high risk for bleeding. Merely extending duration of anticoagulation beyond 3 months for unprovoked PE will not reduce risk of recurrence once anticoagulation is stopped; if anticoagulants are stopped after 3, 6, 12, or 18 months in such a patient, the risk of recurrence after cessation of therapy is similar. Individual risk stratification may help identify patients most likely to suffer recurrent disease and thus most likely to benefit

Table 14–19. Warfarin dosing adjustment guidelines for initiation of warfarin therapy.

Measurement Day	INR	Action
For Hospitalized Patients Newly Starting Therapy		
Day 1		5 mg (2.5 or 7.5 mg in select populations[1])
Day 2	< 1.5	Continue dose
	≥ 1.5	Decrease or hold dose[2]
Day 3	≤ 1.2	Increase dose[2]
	> 1.2 and < 1.7	Continue dose
	≥ 1.7	Decrease dose[2]
Day 4 until therapeutic	Daily increase < 0.2 units	Increase dose[2]
	Daily increase 0.2–0.3 units	Continue dose
	Daily increase 0.4–0.6 units	Decrease dose[2]
	Daily increase ≥ 0.7 units	Hold dose
For Outpatients Newly Starting Therapy		
Measure PT/INR on Day 1	Baseline	Start treatment with 2–7.5 mg
Measure PT/INR on Day 3–4	< 1.5	Increase weekly dose by 5–25%
	1.5–1.9	No dosage change
	2.0–2.5	Decrease weekly dose by 25–50%
	> 2.5	Decrease weekly dose by 50% or HOLD dose
Measure PT/INR on Day 5–7	< 1.5	Increase weekly dose by 10–25%
	1.5–1.9	Increase weekly dose by 0–20%
	2.0–3.0	No dosage change
	> 3.0	Decrease weekly dose by 10–25% or HOLD dose
Measure PT/INR on Day 8–10	< 1.5	Increase weekly dose by 15–35%
	1.5–1.9	Increase weekly dose by 5–20%
	2.0–3.0	No dosage change
	> 3.0	Decrease weekly dose by 10–25% or HOLD dose
Measure PT/INR on Day 11–14	< 1.6	Increase weekly dose by 15–35%
	1.6–1.9	Increase weekly dose by 5–20%
	2.0–3.0	No dosage change
	> 3.0	Decrease weekly dose by 5–20% or HOLD dose

[1]See text.
[2]In general, dosage adjustments should not exceed 2.5 mg or 50%.
Data from Kim YK et al. J Thromb Haemost. 2010;8:101. From Center for Health Quality, Outcomes, and Economic Research, VA Medical Center, Bedford, MA.

from ongoing anticoagulation therapy (see below). Normal D-dimer levels 1 month after cessation of anticoagulation are associated with lower recurrence risk, although some would argue not low enough to consider stopping anticoagulant therapy, particularly in men.

2. Risk scoring systems to guide therapy duration—The HERDOO2 risk scoring system uses BMI, age, D-dimer, and post-phlebitic symptoms to identify women at lower risk for recurrence after unprovoked VTE (https://www.mdcalc.com/herdoo2-rule-discontinuing-anticoagulation-unprovoked-vte). The Vienna Prediction Model, a simple scoring system based on age, sex, D-dimer, and location of thrombosis, can help estimate an individual's recurrence risk to guide duration of therapy decisions.

3. Cancer-related VTE—LMWH has been the mainstay of treatment for cancer-related VTE based on lower VTE recurrence in cancer patients treated with dalteparin compared with warfarin. Studies have also shown that DOACs (edoxaban, rivaroxaban, and apixaban) are at least as effective as LMWH for VTE treatment. The use of edoxaban and rivaroxaban is associated with increased bleeding, though, particularly for patients with GI cancer.

Table 14–20. Warfarin-dosing adjustment guidelines for patients receiving long-term therapy, with target INR 2–3.

Patient INR	Weekly Dosing Change	
	Dose Change	Follow-Up INR
≤ 1.5	Increase by 10–15%	Within 1 week
1.51–1.79	If falling or low on two or more occasions, increase weekly dose by 5–10%.	7–14 days
1.80–2.29	Consider not changing the dose unless a consistent pattern has been observed.	7–14 days
2.3–3.0 (in range)	No change in dosage.	28 days (42 days if INR in range three times consecutively)
3.01–3.20	Consider not changing the dose unless a consistent pattern has been observed.	7–14 days
3.21–3.69	Do not hold warfarin. If rising or high on two or more occasions, decrease weekly dose by 5–10%.	7–14 days
3.70–4.99	Hold warfarin for 1 day and decrease weekly dose by 5–10%.	Within 1 week, sooner if clinically indicated
5.0–8.99	Hold warfarin. Clinical evaluation for bleeding. When INR is therapeutic, restart at lower dose (decrease weekly dose by 10–15%). Check INR at least weekly until stable. Consider vitamin K if bleeding risk is high (see Table 14–21).	Within 1 week, sooner if clinically indicated, then weekly until stabilized
≥ 9	See Table 14–21	

From Center for Health Quality, Outcomes, and Economic Research, VA Medical Center, Bedford, MA. Data from Kim YK et al. J Thromb Haemost. 2010;8:101. See also Van Spall HE et al. Variation in warfarin dose adjustment practice is responsible for differences in the quality of anticoagulation control between centers and countries: an analysis of patients receiving warfarin in the randomized evaluation of long-term anticoagulation therapy (RE-LY) trial. Circulation. 2012;126:2309.

The International Society for Thrombosis and Haemostasis suggests use of the oral factor Xa inhibitors apixaban, rivaroxaban, or edoxaban for cancer patients with a diagnosis of acute VTE, no drug-drug interactions, and a low risk of bleeding. However, the use of LMWH is suggested for those with a high risk of bleeding, including patients with luminal GI cancers with an intact primary tumor and those at risk for bleeding from the genitourinary or GI tract. For patients with intracranial malignancy and VTE, bleeding risk depends on tumor type (primary versus metastatic) and other characteristics; whenever possible, interdisciplinary consultation is recommended to help determine risk of initiating anticoagulation. DOACs do not appear to confer higher bleeding risk compared to LMWH in patients with brain tumors. Clinicians must be aware that chemotherapeutic agents may interact with DOACs and their use should be avoided in cases of potential interactions because there is no easily accessible and reliable way to measure the anticoagulant effect of DOACs.

4. Thrombophilia workup in determining duration— Laboratory workup for thrombophilia is not recommended routinely for determining duration of therapy because clinical presentation is a much stronger predictor of recurrence risk. The workup may be pursued in patients younger than 50 years, with a strong family history, with a clot in unusual locations, or with recurrent thromboses (Table 14–23). In addition, a workup for thrombophilia may be considered in women of childbearing age in whom results may influence fertility and pregnancy outcomes and management or in those patients in whom results will influence duration of therapy. An important hypercoagulable state to identify is antiphospholipid syndrome because these patients have a marked increase in recurrence rates, are at risk for both arterial and venous disease, in general receive bridge therapy during any interruption of anticoagulation, and should not receive DOACs as first-line antithrombotic therapy due to increased arterial events compared to warfarin. Due to effects of anticoagulants and acute thrombosis on many of the tests, the thrombophilia workup should be delayed in most cases until at least 3 months after the acute event, if indicated at all (Table 14–24). The benefit of anticoagulation must be weighed against the bleeding risks posed, and the benefit-risk ratio should be assessed at the initiation of therapy, at 3 months, and then at least annually in any patient receiving prolonged anticoagulant therapy. Bleeding risk scores, such as the Riete score (https://www.mdcalc.com/riete-score-risk-hemorrhage-pulmonary-embolism-treatment) have been developed to estimate risk of these complications. Their performance, however, may not offer any advantage over a clinician's subjective assessment, particularly in older individuals. Consideration of bleeding risk is of particular importance when identifying candidates for extended duration therapy for treatment of unprovoked VTE; defined courses should be considered for patients at high bleeding risk.

D. Secondary Prevention

Antithrombotic therapy for secondary prevention offered after the initial 3–6 months of treatment should be considered in patients with VTE that is not majorly provoked; it is most compelling for those with unprovoked VTE. For most patients who continue to take a DOAC to prevent recurrence, the dose can be reduced to prophylactic intensity after the initial 6 months of therapy. In patients deemed poor candidates for ongoing DOAC or warfarin use but who warrant some secondary prevention, low-dose (81–100 mg) aspirin may be used; however, this will

Table 14–21. American College of Chest Physicians evidence-based clinical practice guidelines for the management of supratherapeutic INR.

Clinical Situation	INR	Recommendations
No significant bleed	Above therapeutic range but < 5.0	• Lower dose or omit dose (see Table 14–20). • Monitor more frequently and resume at lower dose when INR falls within therapeutic range (if INR only slightly above range, may not be necessary to decrease dose)
	≥ 5.0 but < 9.0	• Hold next 1–2 doses • Monitor more frequently and resume therapy at lower dose (see Table 14–20) when INR falls within therapeutic range • *Patients at high risk for bleeding*[1]: Hold warfarin and consider giving vitamin K_1 1–2.5 mg orally; check INR in 24–48 hour to ensure response to therapy
	≥ 9.0	• Hold warfarin • Vitamin K_1 2.5–5 mg orally • Monitor frequently and resume therapy at lower dose when INR within therapeutic range
Serious/life-threatening bleed		• Hold warfarin and give 10 mg vitamin K by slow intravenous infusion supplemented by FFP, PCC, or recombinant factor VIIa (PCC preferred)

[1]Patients at higher risk for bleeding include elderly people, and conditions that increase the risk of bleeding include kidney disease, hypertension, falls, liver disease, and history of GI or genitourinary bleeding.
FFP, fresh frozen plasma; PCC, prothrombin complex concentrate.

provide far less reduction in risk of recurrent VTE with similar bleeding risk.

Connors JM. Thrombophilia testing and venous thrombosis. N Engl J Med. 2017;377:2298. [PMID: 29211668]
Cuker A et al. Reversal of direct oral anticoagulants: guidance from the Anticoagulation Forum. Am J Hematol. 2019;94:697. [PMID: 30916798]
Garcia D et al. Diagnosis and management of the antiphospholipid syndrome. N Engl J Med. 2018;378:2010. [PMID: 29791828]
Khorana AA et al. Role of direct oral anticoagulants in the treatment of cancer-associated venous thromboembolism: guidance from the SSC of the ISTH. J Thromb Haemost. 2018;16:1891. [PMID: 30027649]
Konstantinides SV et al. The 2019 ESC Guidelines on the diagnosis and management of acute pulmonary embolism. Eur Heart J. 2019;40:3453. [PMID: 31697840]

Table 14–22. Duration of treatment of VTE.

Scenario	Suggested Duration of Therapy	Comments
Provoked by major transient risk factor (eg, major surgery, major trauma, major hospitalization)	3 months	VTE prophylaxis upon future exposure to transient risk factor
Unprovoked	At least 3 months; consider indefinite if bleeding risk allows	May individually risk-stratify for recurrence with D-dimer, clinical risk scores, and clinical presentation Consider transition to DOAC secondary prevention dose after initial treatment period
Recurrent unprovoked	Indefinite	If recurrent despite therapeutic anticoagulation, consider hematology consultation for further evaluation and guidance
Cancer-related	≥ 3–6 months or as long as cancer is active, whichever is longer	LMWH or carefully selected DOAC recommended for initial treatment (see Table 14–16)
Underlying significant thrombophilia (eg, antiphospholipid antibody syndrome, antithrombin deficiency, protein C deficiency, protein S deficiency, ≥ two concomitant thrombophilic conditions)	Indefinite	To avoid false positives, consider delaying investigation for laboratory thrombophilia until 3 months after event

LMWH, low-molecular-weight heparin; VTE, venous thromboembolic disease.

Table 14–23. Candidates for thrombophilia workup if results will influence management.

Patients < 50 years of age
Strong family history of VTE
Clot in unusual locations
Recurrent thromboses
Women of childbearing age
Suspicion for APS (avoid DOACs if APS is strongly suspected or confirmed)

APS, antiphospholipid syndrome; VTE, venous thromboembolism.

Stevens SM et al. Antithrombotic therapy for VTE disease: second update of the CHEST Guideline and Expert Panel Report. Chest. 2021;160:e545. [PMID: 34352278]

Streiff MB et al. Update on Guidelines for the management of cancer-associated thrombosis. Oncologist. 2021;26:e24. [PMID: 33275332]

Streiff MB et al. Cancer-associated venous thromboembolic disease, version 2.2021, NCCN Clinical Practice Guidelines in Oncology. J Natl Compr Canc Netw. 2021;19:1181. [PMID: 34666313]

Witt DM et al. American Society of Hematology 2018 guidelines for management of venous thromboembolism: optimal management of anticoagulation therapy. Blood Adv. 2018;2:3257. [PMID: 30482765]

E. Thrombolytic Therapy

1. Thrombolytic therapy for high risk, massive PE— Anticoagulation alone is appropriate treatment for most patients with PE. However, patients with high-risk, massive PE (defined as PE causing sustained hypotension [systolic blood pressure greater than 90 mm Hg]) or requirement for inotropic support) have an in-hospital mortality rate that approaches 30% and, absent contraindications (Table 14–25), require immediate thrombolysis in combination with anticoagulation (Table 14–26).

2. Thrombolytic therapy for intermediate-risk, submassive PE—Systemic thrombolytic therapy has been used in carefully selected patients with intermediate-risk, submassive PE (defined as PE without hemodynamic instability but with evidence of right ventricular compromise and myocardial injury). Thrombolysis in this cohort decreases risk of hemodynamic compromise but increases the risk of major hemorrhage and stroke. A lower dose of alteplase (tPA) commonly used for PE treatment (50 mg rather than 100 mg) has been evaluated in small trials. Catheter-directed therapy for acute PE may be considered for high-risk or intermediate-risk PE when systemic thrombolysis has failed or as an alternative to systemic thrombolytic therapy.

3. Thrombolytic therapy for other indications—In patients with large proximal iliofemoral DVT, data from randomized controlled trials are limited on the benefit of catheter-directed thrombolysis in addition to treatment with anticoagulation but do show increased risk of major bleeding. Thrombolytic therapy should be reserved for patients at the highest risk for limb ischemia from extensive acute thrombosis.

Table 14–24. Laboratory evaluation of thrombophilia.

Hypercoagulable State	When to Suspect	Laboratory Workup	Influence of Anticoagulation and Acute Thrombosis
Antiphospholipid antibody syndrome	Unexplained DVT/PE CVA/TIA before age 50 years Recurrent thrombosis (despite anticoagulation) Thrombosis at an unusual site Arterial and venous thrombosis Livedo reticularis, Raynaud phenomenon, thrombocytopenia, recurrent early pregnancy loss	Anti-cardiolipin IgG and/or IgM medium or high titer (ie, > 40 GPL or MPL, or > the 99th percentile)[1] Anti-beta-2 glycoprotein I IgG and/or IgM medium or high titer (> the 99th percentile)[1] Lupus anticoagulant[1]	Lupus anticoagulant can be falsely positive or falsely negative on anticoagulation
Protein C, S, antithrombin deficiencies	Thrombosis < 50 years of age with family history of VTE	Screen with protein C activity, free protein S, antithrombin activity[2]; if free protein S is normal, check protein S activity	Acute thrombosis can result in decreased protein C, S and antithrombin activity. Warfarin can decrease protein C and S activity; heparin can decrease antithrombin activity. DOACs can increase protein C, S, and antithrombin activity
Factor V Leiden, prothrombin gene mutation	Thrombosis on OCPs, cerebral vein thrombosis, DVT/PE in White population	PCR for factor V Leiden or prothrombin gene mutation	No influence
Hyperhomocysteinemia		Fasting homocysteine	No influence

[1]Detected on two occasions not < 12 weeks apart.
[2]Nephrotic syndrome and liver disease can reduce protein C, protein S, and antithrombin; pregnancy causes decreased free protein S.
CVA/TIA, cerebrovascular accident/transient ischemic attack; OCPs, oral contraceptives; VTE, venous thromboembolism.

Table 14–25. Contraindications to thrombolytic therapy for PE.

	Contraindication		
	Absolute	Major	Relative
American Heart Association	Previous intracranial hemorrhage Structural intracranial disease Ischemic stroke within 3 months Suspected aortic dissection Active bleeding or bleeding diathesis Recent surgery encroaching on the spinal canal or brain Recent closed-head or facial trauma with radiographic evidence of bony fracture or brain injury		Age > 75 years Anticoagulant therapy Pregnancy Noncompressible vascular punctures Traumatic or prolonged CPR (> 10 minutes) Recent internal bleeding (within 2–4 weeks) Chronic, poorly controlled hypertension Systolic BP > 180 mm Hg or diastolic BP > 110 mm Hg Dementia Ischemic stroke > 3 months ago Major surgery within 3 weeks
European Society of Cardiology	Previous hemorrhagic stroke or stroke of unknown origin CNS damage or neoplasms Ischemic stroke within 6 months GI bleeding within 1 month Recent major trauma, surgery, or head injury in the preceding 3 weeks Known bleeding risk		TIA in preceding 6 months Anticoagulant therapy Pregnancy Noncompressible puncture site Traumatic resuscitation Active peptic ulcer disease Infective endocarditis Refractory hypertension (systolic BP > 180 mm Hg) Advanced liver disease
American College of Chest Physicians		Previous intracranial hemorrhage Structural intracranial disease Ischemic stroke within 3 months Active bleeding Bleeding diathesis Recent brain or spinal surgery Recent head trauma with fracture or brain injury	Age > 75 years Anticoagulant therapy Pregnancy Recent invasive procedure Traumatic CPR Recent non-intracranial bleeding Pericarditis or pericardial fluid Systolic BP > 180 mm Hg or diastolic BP > 110 mm Hg Weight < 60 kg Ischemic stroke > 3 months ago Recent surgery Diabetic retinopathy Female Black race

Reproduced with permission from Kaplovitch E, Shaw JR, Douketis J. Thrombolysis in pulmonary embolism: an evidence-based approach to treating life-threatening pulmonary emboli. Crit Care Clin. 2020;36(3):465–480.

Chiasakul T et al. Thrombolytic therapy in acute venous thromboembolism. Hematology Am Soc Hematol Educ Program. 2020;2020:612. [PMID: 33275702]

Hennemeyer C et al. Outcomes of catheter-directed therapy plus anticoagulation versus anticoagulation alone for submassive and massive pulmonary embolism. Am J Med. 2019;132:240. [PMID: 30367851]

Kiser TH et al. Half-dose versus full-dose alteplase for treatment of pulmonary embolism. Crit Care Med. 2018;46:1617. [PMID: 29979222]

Konstantinides SV et al. 2019 ESC Guidelines on the diagnosis and management of acute pulmonary embolism. Eur Heart J. 2019;40:3453. [PMID: 31697840]

Vedantham S et al; ATTRACT Trial Investigators. Pharmacomechanical catheter-directed thrombolysis for deep-vein thrombosis. N Engl J Med. 2017;377:2240. [PMID: 29211671]

F. Nonpharmacologic Therapy

1. Graduated compression stockings—Graduated compressions stockings may provide symptomatic relief to selected patients with ongoing swelling but do not reduce risk of postthrombotic syndrome at 6 months. They are contraindicated in patients with peripheral vascular disease.

2. Inferior vena caval (IVC) filters—There is a paucity of data to support the use of permanent or retrievable IVC filters for the prevention of PE in any clinical scenario. There are two randomized, controlled trials of IVC filters for prevention of PE. In the first study, patients with documented DVT received full- intensity, time-limited anticoagulation with or without placement of a permanent IVC filter. Patients with permanent IVC filters had a lower rate

Table 14–26. Thrombolytic regimens for acute PE.

Alteplase[1]		Streptokinase[1]		Urokinase[1]		Reteplase	Tenecteplase
Classical Regimen	Accelerated Regimen	Classical Regimen	Accelerated Regimen	Classical Regimen	Accelerated Regimen		
100 mg infusion over 2 hour	0.6 mg/kg (up to 50 mg) bolus over 15 minutes	250,000 IU bolus over 30 minutes, followed by 100,000 IU/hour over 12–24 hours	1.5 million IU infusion over 2 hours	4400 IU/kg bolus followed by 4400 IU/kg/hour infusion over 12–24 hours	3 million IU infusion over 2 hours	Two boluses of 10 units given 30 minutes apart	Weight-based bolus over 5 s: < 60 kg: 30 mg ≥ 60 to < 70 kg: 35 mg ≥ 70 to < 80 kg: 40 mg ≥ 80 to < 90 kg: 45 mg ≥ 90 kg: 50 mg

[1]FDA approved thrombolytic for PE.

Reproduced with permission from Kaplovitch E, Shaw JR, Douketis J. Thrombolysis in pulmonary embolism: an evidence-based approach to treating life-threatening pulmonary emboli. Crit Care Clin. 2020;36(3):465–480.

of nonfatal asymptomatic PE at 12 days but an increased rate of DVT at 2 years. In the second study, patients with symptomatic PE and residual proximal DVT plus at least one additional risk factor for severity received full intensity anticoagulation with or without a retrievable IVC filter. IVC filter use did not reduce the risk of symptomatic recurrent PE at 3 months. While IVC filters were once commonly used to prevent VTE recurrence in the setting of anticoagulation failure, many experts now recommend switching to an alternative agent or increasing the intensity of the current anticoagulant regimen instead. Most experts agree with placement of a retrievable IVC filter in patients with acute proximal DVT or PE and an absolute contraindication to anticoagulation; evidence to support this practice, however, is lacking. The remainder of the indications (submassive/intermediate-risk PE, free-floating iliofemoral DVT, perioperative risk reduction) are controversial. Whenever possible, the filter should be removed once anticoagulation has been started and has been shown to be tolerated. Rates of IVC filter retrieval are very low, often due to failure to arrange for removal. Thus, if a device is placed, removal should be arranged at the time of device placement.

Complications of IVC filters include local thrombosis, tilting, migration, fracture, and inability to retrieve the device. When considering placement of an IVC filter, it is best to consider both short- and long-term complications, since devices intended for removal may become permanent. To improve patient safety, institutions should develop systems that guide appropriate patient selection for IVC filter placement, tracking, and removal.

3. Mechanical embolectomy—Patients with high-risk VTE and very high bleeding risk may be considered for mechanical embolectomy if local expertise and resources are available.

When to Refer

- Presence of large iliofemoral VTE, unprovoked upper extremity DVT, IVC thrombosis, portal vein thrombosis, or Budd-Chiari syndrome for consideration of catheter-directed thrombolysis.
- High-risk PE for urgent embolectomy or catheter-directed therapies.
- Intermediate-risk PE if considering thrombolysis.
- History of HIT or prolonged PTT plus kidney failure for alternative anticoagulation regimens.
- Consideration of IVC filter placement.
- Clots in unusual locations (eg, renal, hepatic, or cerebral vein), or simultaneous arterial and venous thrombosis, to assess possibility of a hypercoagulable state.
- Recurrent VTE while receiving therapeutic anticoagulation.

When to Admit

- Documented or suspected intermediate- or high-risk PE, low-risk PE at high risk for bleeding, poor candidate for outpatient treatment.
- DVT with poorly controlled pain, high bleeding risk, or concerns about follow-up.
- Large iliofemoral DVT for consideration of thrombolysis.
- Acute PE/DVT and absolute contraindication to anticoagulation for IVC filter placement.
- Venous thrombosis despite therapeutic anticoagulation.
- Suspected Paget-Schroetter syndrome (spontaneous upper extremity thrombosis related to thoracic outlet syndrome).

Bikdeli B et al. Systematic review of efficacy and safety of retrievable inferior vena caval filters. Thromb Res. 2018;165:79. [PMID: 29579576]

PRIMARY VTE PREVENTION & TREATMENT IN SEVERE COVID-19

Patients hospitalized with severe COVID-19 have an increased incidence of thrombotic complications, including venous (DVT, PE) and arterial (stroke, limb occlusion) events.

Although the reasons for this hypercoagulability are not yet well understood, the profound systemic inflammatory response associated with severe COVID-19 is thought to play a role.

Clinical Findings

While the hypercoagulability in COVID-19 resembles DIC, laboratory and clinical findings are somewhat different. Laboratory findings in patients with severe COVID-19 may include markedly elevated D-dimer and modestly prolonged prothrombin time. However, patients with COVID-19 tend to have elevated fibrinogen levels; thrombocytopenia is rare and nonsevere; and bleeding complications are unusual. Thrombosis in patients with COVID-19 is associated with a poor prognosis and often occurs despite standard pharmacologic prophylaxis.

Risk Stratification & Initial Prognostication in Severe COVID-19

Given the prevalence and prognostic value of abnormal laboratory findings at presentation, patients hospitalized with COVID-19 should have PT/INR, PTT, D-dimers, and fibrinogen measured at presentation. Serial monitoring should be considered even in patients who are otherwise clinically stable. Worsening laboratory parameters during hospitalization should prompt consideration of transfer to a higher level of care and heightened clinical suspicion for thrombosis.

VTE Prophylaxis for Severe COVID-19

In the absence of strong contraindications, all patients hospitalized with COVID-19 should receive pharmacologic VTE prophylaxis. LMWH is preferred over unfractionated heparin to minimize staff exposure and the chance of HIT.

For patients with a prior history of VTE who take an oral anticoagulant for secondary prevention at the time of admission, transition to LMWH should be considered due to its shorter half-life and potential anti-inflammatory properties.

Some patients who are hospitalized in the acute care setting with COVID-19, who have very elevated D-dimer values (over 4 times the upper limit of normal) and require supplemental oxygen, and who have *low* bleeding risk, may benefit from therapeutic dosing of anticoagulation. Patients who are critically ill in ICUs have not been shown to benefit from therapeutic dosing. At this time, there is also no clear benefit from VTE prophylaxis for patients with COVID-19 who do not require hospitalization. Trials are ongoing to evaluate the benefit of pharmacologic VTE prophylaxis with DOACs for COVID-19 patients following hospital discharge.

For updated recommendations regarding pharmacologic dosing and post-discharge prophylaxis, refer to professional society guidance (links at end of this section) since guidance in this area is evolving rapidly.

Diagnosis & Management of VTE in Severe COVID-19

Logistical challenges complicate the diagnosis of thromboembolism in patients with COVID-19 due to patient instability and risks of staff exposures. D-dimers are generally elevated in hospitalized patients who have COVID-19. A substantial increase in D-dimers may suggest COVID-19–associated coagulopathy with or without thrombotic events. Clinicians should remain vigilant for signs and symptoms of thrombosis and consider obtaining surveillance laboratory testing at least every 3–4 days with low threshold for imaging. Ideally, thrombosis should be confirmed radiographically, but in situations where these studies cannot safely be obtained and clinical suspicion is very high, empiric treatment may be considered.

Guidance from the Anticoagulation Forum (https://acforum.org/web/), the International Society for Thrombosis and Haemostasis (https://academy.isth.org/isth/#!*menu=8*browseby=2*sortby=1*label=19794), and the American Society for Hematology (https://www.hematology.org/covid-19) is evolving and should be frequently consulted.

ATTACC Investigators; ACTIV-4a Investigators; REMAP-CAP Investigators; Lawler PR et al. Therapeutic anticoagulation with heparin in noncritically ill patients with Covid-19. N Engl J Med. 2021;385:790. [PMID: 34351721]

Carrier M et al; AVERT Investigators. Apixaban to prevent venous thromboembolism in patients with cancer. N Engl J Med. 2019;380:711. [PMID: 30511879]

Connors JM et al. COVID-19 and its implications for thrombosis and anticoagulation. Blood. 2020;135:2033. [PMID: 32339221]

Khorana AA et al; CASSINI Investigators. Rivaroxaban for thromboprophylaxis in high-risk ambulatory patients with cancer. N Engl J Med. 2019;380:720. [PMID: 30786186]

REMAP-CAP Investigators; ACTIV-4a Investigators; ATTACC Investigators; Goligher EC et al. Therapeutic anticoagulation with heparin in critically ill patients with Covid-19. N Engl J Med. 2021;385:777. [PMID: 34351722]

Schünemann HJ et al. American Society of Hematology 2018 guidelines for management of venous thromboembolism: prophylaxis for hospitalized and nonhospitalized medical patients. Blood Adv. 2018;2:3198. [PMID: 30482763]

Spyropoulos AC et al. Efficacy and safety of therapeutic-dose heparin vs standard prophylactic or intermediate-dose heparins for thromboprophylaxis in high-risk hospitalized patients with COVID-19: the HEP-COVID randomized clinical trial. JAMA Intern Med. 2021;181:1612. [PMID: 34617959]

Gastrointestinal Disorders

Kenneth R. McQuaid, MD

SYMPTOMS & SIGNS OF GI DISEASE

DYSPEPSIA

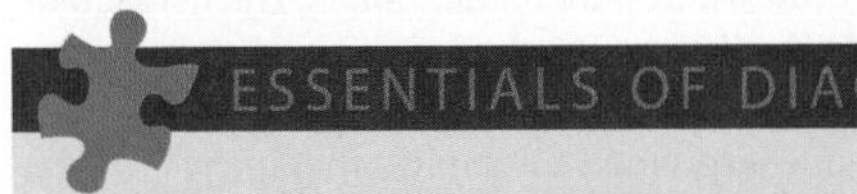

ESSENTIALS OF DIAGNOSIS

- Predominant epigastric pain or discomfort.
- May be associated with heartburn, nausea, postprandial fullness, or vomiting.
- Endoscopy is warranted in all patients age 60 years or older and selected younger patients with "alarm" features.
- In all other patients, testing for *Helicobacter pylori* is recommended; if positive, antibacterial treatment is given.
- Patients who are *H pylori* negative or do not improve after *H pylori* eradication should be prescribed a trial of empiric PPI therapy.
- Patients with persistent symptoms should be offered a trial of a tricyclic antidepressant.

General Considerations

Dyspepsia refers to acute, chronic, or recurrent pain or discomfort centered in the upper abdomen. Predominant epigastric pain that is present for at least 1 month is clinically relevant. Dyspepsia occurs in 10–20% of the adult population and accounts for 3% of general medical office visits. The epigastric pain may be associated with heartburn, nausea, postprandial fullness, or vomiting. Heartburn (retrosternal burning) should be distinguished from dyspepsia. When heartburn is the dominant complaint, gastroesophageal reflux is nearly always present.

Etiology

A. Food or Drug Intolerance

Acute, self-limited "indigestion" may be caused by overeating, eating too quickly, eating high-fat foods, eating during stressful situations, or drinking too much alcohol or coffee. Prescription and nonprescription medications should be carefully reviewed since many may cause dyspepsia.

B. Functional Dyspepsia

Functional dyspepsia refers to dyspepsia for which no organic etiology has been determined by endoscopy or other testing. This is the most common cause of *chronic* dyspepsia, accounting for up to 75% of patients. Symptoms may arise from a complex interaction of increased visceral afferent sensitivity, gastric delayed emptying or impaired accommodation to food or psychosocial stressors or symptoms may develop de novo following an enteric infection. Although benign, these chronic symptoms may be difficult to treat.

C. Luminal GI Tract Dysfunction

Peptic ulcer disease is present in 5–15% of patients with dyspepsia. GERD is present in up to 20% of patients with dyspepsia, even without significant heartburn. Gastric or esophageal cancer is identified in less than 1%; cancer is extremely rare in persons under age 60 years with uncomplicated dyspepsia. Other causes include gastroparesis (especially in diabetes mellitus) and parasitic infection (*Giardia, Strongyloides, Anisakis*).

D. *Helicobacter pylori* Infection

Chronic gastric infection with *H pylori* is an important cause of peptic ulcer disease but may cause dyspepsia in a subset of patients in the absence of peptic ulcer disease.

E. Pancreatic Disease

Pancreatic carcinoma and chronic pancreatitis may cause chronic epigastric pain, but it is more severe, sometimes radiates to the back, and usually is associated with anorexia, rapid weight loss, steatorrhea, or jaundice.

F. Biliary Tract Disease

The abrupt onset of epigastric or right upper quadrant pain due to cholelithiasis or choledocholithiasis should be readily distinguished from dyspepsia.

G. Other Conditions

Diabetes mellitus, thyroid disease, CKD, myocardial ischemia, intra-abdominal malignancy, gastric volvulus or paraesophageal hernia, chronic gastric or intestinal ischemia, and pregnancy are sometimes accompanied by acute or chronic epigastric pain or discomfort.

Clinical Findings

A. Symptoms and Signs

Given the nonspecific nature of dyspeptic symptoms, the history has limited diagnostic utility. It should clarify the chronicity, location, and quality of the epigastric pain, and its relationship to meals. The pain may be accompanied by one or more upper abdominal symptoms including postprandial fullness, heartburn, nausea, or vomiting. Concomitant weight loss, persistent vomiting, constant or severe pain, progressive dysphagia, hematemesis, or melena warrants endoscopy or abdominal CT imaging. Potentially offending medications and excessive alcohol use should be identified and discontinued if possible. The patient should be asked about a family history of upper GI cancer. The patient's reason for seeking care should be determined. Recent changes in employment, marital discord, physical and sexual abuse, anxiety, depression, and fear of serious disease may all contribute to the development and reporting of symptoms. Patients with functional dyspepsia often are younger, report a variety of abdominal and extragastrointestinal complaints, show signs of anxiety or depression, or have used psychotropic medications.

The symptom profile alone does not differentiate between functional dyspepsia and organic GI disorders. Based on the clinical history alone, primary care clinicians misdiagnose nearly half of patients with peptic ulcers or gastroesophageal reflux.

The physical examination is rarely helpful. Signs of serious organic disease such as weight loss, organomegaly, abdominal mass, or fecal occult blood must be further evaluated.

B. Laboratory Findings

In patients younger than age 60 with uncomplicated dyspepsia (in whom gastric cancer is rare), a noninvasive test for *H pylori* (urea breath test, fecal antigen test) should be performed first. Although serologic tests are inexpensive, performance characteristics are poor in low-prevalence populations, whereas breath and fecal antigen tests have 95% accuracy. If *H pylori* breath test or fecal antigen test results are negative in a patient not taking NSAIDs, peptic ulcer disease is virtually excluded. In patients older than age 60 years, initial laboratory work should include a CBC, serum electrolytes, liver enzymes, calcium, and thyroid function tests but the cost-effectiveness of such studies is uncertain.

C. Upper Endoscopy

Upper endoscopy is mainly indicated to look for upper gastric or esophageal malignancy in *all* patients over age 60 years with new-onset dyspepsia (in whom there is increased malignancy risk). In patients under age 60, the risk of malignancy is less than 1% so recent guidelines recommend against routine endoscopy for most younger patients—except those with prominent "alarm" features, such as progressive weight loss, rapidly progressive dysphagia, persistent vomiting, evidence of bleeding or iron deficiency anemia, palpable abdominal mass, or a family history of upper GI cancer. For patients born in regions in which there is a higher incidence of gastric cancer, such as Central or South America, China and Southeast Asia, or Africa, an age threshold of 45 years may be more appropriate.

Endoscopy may also be warranted when symptoms fail to respond to initial empiric management or when frequent symptom relapse occurs after discontinuation of empiric therapy.

D. Other Tests

In patients with refractory symptoms or progressive weight loss, antibodies for celiac disease or stool testing for ova and parasites or *Giardia* antigen, fat, or elastase may be considered. Abdominal imaging (ultrasonography or CT) is performed only when pancreatic, biliary tract, vascular disease, or volvulus is suspected. Gastric emptying studies may be useful in patients with recurrent nausea and vomiting who have not responded to empiric therapies.

Treatment

Initial empiric treatment is recommended for patients who are younger than age 60 years and who lack severe or worrisome "alarm" features that warrant further testing with endoscopy or abdominal imaging. Those whose symptoms do not to respond to or relapse after empiric treatment should undergo upper endoscopy with subsequent treatment directed at the specific disorder identified (eg, peptic ulcer, gastroesophageal reflux, cancer). When endoscopy is performed, gastric biopsies should be obtained to test for *H pylori* infection. If infection is present, antibacterial treatment should be given.

A. Empiric Therapy

Patients younger than age 60 should be tested for *H pylori* and, if positive, treated for 14 days with an effective regimen (see Table 15–10). *H pylori* eradication therapy proves definitive for patients with underlying peptic ulcers and may improve symptoms in a small subset (less than 10%) of infected patients with functional dyspepsia.

H pylori–negative patients and patients with persistent dyspepsia after *H pylori* eradication most likely have functional dyspepsia or atypical GERD and should be treated with a PPI for 4 weeks. Meta-analysis of six randomized controlled trials reported symptom improvement in 50% of patients treated with a PPI versus 27% of those treated with a placebo. For patients who have symptom relapse after discontinuation of the PPI, intermittent or long-term PPI therapy may be considered.

B. Treatment of Functional Dyspepsia

Patients who have no significant findings on endoscopy as well as patients under age 60 who do not respond to *H pylori* eradication or empiric PPI therapy are presumed to have functional dyspepsia. Patients with mild, intermittent symptoms may respond to reassurance and lifestyle or dietary changes. A food diary, in which patients record their food intake, symptoms, and daily events, may reveal dietary or psychosocial precipitants of pain. Herbal therapies (peppermint, caraway) may offer benefit with little risk of adverse effects.

Antisecretory drugs (PPIs or H_2-receptor antagonists) have demonstrated limited efficacy in the treatment of functional dyspepsia. A small number of patients (less than 10%) derive benefit from *H pylori* eradication therapy. Low doses of tricyclic antidepressants (eg, desipramine or nortriptyline, 25–50 mg orally at bedtime) benefit some patients, possibly by moderating visceral afferent sensitivity. Doses should be increased slowly to minimize side effects. SSRIs do not appear to be beneficial. Although some prokinetics have demonstrated modest improvement in global symptoms compared to placebo in controlled trials, the more effective agents are either not available in the United States (domperidone) or were removed from the market to due rare but serious adverse events (cisapride). Metoclopramide (5–10 mg three times daily) may improve symptoms but cannot be recommended for long-term use due to the risk of tardive dyskinesia.

Chisty A. Update on indigestion. Med Clin North Am. 2021; 105:19. [PMID: 33246519]

Ford AC et al. Systematic review and network meta-analysis: efficacy of drugs for functional dyspepsia. Aliment Pharmacol Ther. 2021;53:8. [PMID: 32936964]

Pasricha PJ et al. Functional dyspepsia and gastroparesis in tertiary care are interchangeable syndromes with common clinical and pathological features. Gastroenterology. 2021;160: 2006. [PMID: 33548234]

NAUSEA & VOMITING

Nausea is a vague, intensely disagreeable sensation of sickness or "queasiness" and is distinguished from anorexia. Vomiting often follows, as does retching (spasmodic respiratory and abdominal movements). Vomiting should be distinguished from regurgitation, the effortless reflux of liquid or food stomach contents; and from rumination, the chewing and swallowing of food that is regurgitated volitionally after meals.

The brainstem vomiting center is composed of a group of neuronal areas within the medulla that coordinate emesis. It may be stimulated by four sources of afferent input: (1) Afferent vagal fibers from the GI viscera are rich in serotonin 5-HT_3 receptors; these may be stimulated by biliary or GI distention, mucosal or peritoneal irritation, or infections. (2) Fibers of the vestibular system, which have high concentrations of histamine H_1 and muscarinic cholinergic receptors. (3) Higher CNS centers (amygdala); here, certain sights, smells, or emotional experiences may induce vomiting. (4) The chemoreceptor trigger zone, located outside the blood-brain barrier in the medulla, is rich in opioid, serotonin 5-HT_3, neurokinin 1 (NK_1), and dopamine D_2 receptors. This region may be stimulated by drugs and chemotherapeutic agents, toxins, hypoxia, uremia, acidosis, and radiation therapy. Although the causes of nausea and vomiting are many, a simplified list is provided in Table 15–1.

Clinical Findings

A. Symptoms and Signs

Acute symptoms without abdominal pain are typically caused by food poisoning, infectious gastroenteritis, drugs, or systemic illness. A 2021 prospective study of 1992 consecutive patients with COVID-19 hospitalized at 36 North American medical centers reports that 27% had nausea, 16% had vomiting, and 11% had abdominal pain. GI symptoms were mild in 74% and the initial manifestation of disease in 13%. Inquiry should be made into recent changes in medications, diet, other intestinal symptoms, or similar illnesses in family members. The acute onset of severe pain and vomiting suggests peritoneal irritation, acute gastric or intestinal obstruction, or pancreaticobiliary disease. Persistent vomiting suggests pregnancy, gastric outlet obstruction, gastroparesis, intestinal dysmotility, psychogenic disorders, and CNS or systemic disorders. Vomiting that occurs in the morning before breakfast is common with pregnancy, uremia, alcohol intake, and increased intracranial pressure. Inquiry should be made into use of cannabis products. Suspect cannabinoid hyperemesis syndrome in patients with prolonged use, especially in those who report compulsive showering or bathing. Vomiting immediately after meals strongly suggests bulimia or psychogenic causes. Vomiting of undigested food one to several hours after meals is characteristic of gastroparesis or a gastric outlet obstruction; physical examination may reveal a succussion splash. Patients with acute or chronic symptoms should be asked about neurologic symptoms (eg, headache, stiff neck, vertigo, and focal paresthesias or weakness) that suggest a CNS cause.

B. Special Examinations

With vomiting that is severe or protracted, serum electrolytes should be obtained to look for hypokalemia, azotemia, or metabolic alkalosis resulting from loss of gastric contents. Flat and upright abdominal radiographs or abdominal CT are obtained in patients with severe pain or suspicion of mechanical obstruction to look for free intraperitoneal air or dilated loops of small bowel. The cause of gastric outlet obstruction is best demonstrated by upper endoscopy, and the cause of small intestinal obstruction is best demonstrated by abdominal CT. Gastroparesis is confirmed by nuclear scintigraphic studies or ^{13}C-octanoic acid breath tests, which show delayed gastric emptying and either upper endoscopy or barium upper GI series showing no evidence of mechanical gastric outlet obstruction. Abnormal liver biochemical tests or elevated amylase or lipase suggest pancreaticobiliary disease, which may be investigated with an abdominal sonogram or CT scan. CNS causes are best evaluated with either head CT or MRI.

Table 15–1. Causes of nausea and vomiting.

Visceral afferent stimulation	**Mechanical obstruction** Gastric outlet obstruction: peptic ulcer disease, malignancy, gastric volvulus Small intestinal obstruction: adhesions, hernias, volvulus, Crohn disease, carcinomatosis **Dysmotility** Gastroparesis: diabetic, postviral, postvagotomy Small intestine: systemic sclerosis (scleroderma), amyloidosis, chronic intestinal pseudo-obstruction, familial myoneuropathies **Peritoneal irritation** Peritonitis: perforated viscus, appendicitis, spontaneous bacterial peritonitis **Infections** Viral gastroenteritis: Norwalk agent, rotavirus, COVID-19 "Food poisoning": toxins from *Bacillus cereus, Staphylococcus aureus, Clostridium perfringens* Acute systemic infections **Hepatobiliary or pancreatic disorders** Acute or chronic pancreatitis Cholecystitis or choledocholithiasis **Topical GI irritants** Alcohol, NSAIDs, oral antibiotics **Postoperative** **Other** Cardiac disease: acute MI, heart failure Urologic disease: stones, pyelonephritis Vascular: chronic mesenteric ischemia, superior mesenteric artery syndrome
Vestibular disorders	**Vestibular disorders** Labyrinthitis, Ménière syndrome, motion sickness
CNS disorders	**Increased intracranial pressure** CNS tumors, subdural or subarachnoid hemorrhage **Migraine** **Cyclical vomiting syndrome** **Infections** Meningitis, encephalitis **Psychogenic** Anticipatory vomiting, anorexia nervosa and bulimia, psychiatric disorders
Irritation of chemoreceptor trigger zone	**Antitumor chemotherapy** **Medications and drugs** Opioids Marijuana Anticonvulsants Antiparkinsonism medications Beta-blockers, antiarrhythmics, digoxin Oral contraceptives Cholinesterase inhibitors Diabetes medications (metformin, acarbose, pramlintide, exenatide) **Radiation therapy** **Systemic disorders** Diabetic ketoacidosis Uremia Adrenocortical crisis Parathyroid disease Hypothyroidism Pregnancy Paraneoplastic syndrome

Complications

Complications include dehydration, hypokalemia, metabolic alkalosis, aspiration, rupture of the esophagus (Boerhaave syndrome), and bleeding secondary to a mucosal tear at the gastroesophageal junction (Mallory-Weiss syndrome).

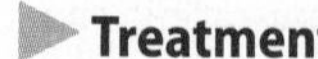

Treatment

A. General Measures

Most causes of acute vomiting are mild, self-limited, and require no specific treatment. Patients should ingest clear liquids (broths, tea, soups, carbonated beverages) and small quantities of dry foods (soda crackers). Ginger may be an effective nonpharmacologic treatment. For more severe acute vomiting, hospitalization may be required. Patients unable to eat and losing gastric fluids may become dehydrated, resulting in hypokalemia with metabolic alkalosis. Intravenous 0.45% saline solution with 20 mEq/L of potassium chloride is given in most cases to maintain hydration. A nasogastric suction tube for gastric or mechanical small bowel obstruction improves patient comfort and permits monitoring of fluid loss.

B. Antiemetic Medications

Medications may be given either to prevent or to control vomiting. Combinations of drugs from different classes may provide better control of symptoms with less toxicity in some patients. Table 15–2 outlines common antiemetic dosing regimens.

1. Serotonin 5-HT_3-receptor antagonists—Ondansetron, granisetron, and palonosetron are effective in preventing chemotherapy- and radiation-induced emesis when initiated prior to treatment; dolasetron has been discontinued in the United States. Due to its prolonged half-life and internalization of the 5-HT_3-receptor, palonosetron is superior to other 5-HT_3-receptor antagonists for the prevention of acute and delayed chemotherapy-induced emesis from moderately or highly emetogenic chemotherapeutic regimens. Although 5-HT_3-receptor antagonists are effective as single agents for the prevention of chemotherapy-induced nausea and vomiting, their efficacy is enhanced by combination therapy with a corticosteroid (dexamethasone)

Table 15–2. Common antiemetic dosing regimens.

	Dosage	Route
Serotonin 5-HT_3 Antagonists		
Ondansetron	Doses vary: 4–8 mg for postoperative nausea and vomiting	Intravenously, orally
	8 mg single dose IV or 8 mg twice daily orally for moderately or highly emetogenic chemotherapy	Intravenously, orally
Granisetron	1 mg once daily	Intravenously
	1–2 mg once daily	Orally
Palonosetron	0.25 mg once as a single dose 30 minutes before start of chemotherapy	Intravenously
	0.5 mg once as single dose	Orally
Corticosteroids		
Dexamethasone	4–12 mg once pre-induction for prevention of postoperative nausea and vomiting	Intravenously, orally
	8 mg once daily for chemotherapy	Intravenously, orally
Dopamine Receptor Antagonists		
Metoclopramide	10–20 mg or 0.5 mg/kg every 6–8 hours	Intravenously
	10–20 mg every 6–8 hours	Orally
Prochlorperazine	5–10 mg every 4–6 hours	Intravenously, intramuscularly, orally
	25 mg suppository every 12 hours	Per rectum
Promethazine	12.5–25 mg every 6–8 hours	Intravenously, orally
	25 mg every 6–8 hours	Per rectum
Trimethobenzamide	200 mg every 6–8 hours	Orally
	250–300 mg every 6–8 hours	Intravenously, orally
Olanzapine	5–10 mg once daily on days 1–4 for chemotherapy	
Neurokinin Receptor Antagonists[1]		
Aprepitant	125 mg once before chemotherapy; then 80 mg on days 1 and 2 after chemotherapy	Orally
Fosaprepitant	150 mg once 30 minutes before chemotherapy	Intravenously
Rolapitant	180 mg once before chemotherapy	Orally
Netupitant/palonosetron	Netupitant 300 mg/palonosetron 0.50 mg once before chemotherapy	Orally

[1]Neurokinin receptor antagonists are used solely for highly emetogenic chemotherapy regimens in combination with 5-HT_3 antagonists or dexamethasone or both.

and an NK_1-receptor antagonist. Serotonin antagonists increasingly are used for the prevention of postoperative nausea and vomiting because of increased restrictions on the use of other antiemetic agents (such as droperidol).

2. Corticosteroids—Corticosteroids (eg, dexamethasone) have antiemetic properties, but the basis for these effects is unknown. These agents enhance the efficacy of serotonin receptor antagonists for preventing acute and delayed nausea and vomiting in patients receiving moderately to highly emetogenic chemotherapy regimens.

3. Neurokinin receptor antagonists—Aprepitant, fosaprepitant, and rolapitant are highly selective antagonists for NK_1-receptors in the area postrema. They are used in combination with corticosteroids and serotonin antagonists for the prevention of acute and delayed nausea and vomiting with highly emetogenic chemotherapy regimens. Netupitant is another oral NK_1-receptor antagonist that is administered in a fixed-dose combination with palonosetron. Combined therapy with an NK_1 receptor antagonist prevents acute emesis in 80–90% and delayed emesis in more than 70% of patients treated with highly emetogenic regimens.

4. Dopamine antagonists—The phenothiazines, butyrophenones, and substituted benzamides (eg, prochlorperazine, promethazine) have antiemetic properties that are due to dopaminergic blockade as well as to their sedative effects. High doses of these agents are associated with antidopaminergic side effects, including extrapyramidal reactions and depression. With the advent of more effective and safer antiemetics, these agents are infrequently used, mainly in outpatients with minor, self-limited symptoms. The atypical antipsychotic agent olanzapine has potent antiemetic properties that may be mediated by blockade of both dopamine and serotonin neurotransmitters. In patients receiving highly emetic chemotherapy, the addition of olanzapine to a standard regimen (dexamethasone, serotonin-$5HT_3$ receptor antagonist, and NK_1- receptor antagonist) significantly reduces the risk of acute and delayed nausea and vomiting.

5. Antihistamines and anticholinergics—These drugs (eg, meclizine, dimenhydrinate, transdermal scopolamine) may be valuable in the prevention of vomiting arising from stimulation of the labyrinth, ie, motion sickness, vertigo, and migraines. They may induce drowsiness. A combination of oral vitamin B_6 and doxylamine is recommended by the American College of Obstetricians and Gynecologists as first-line therapy for nausea and vomiting during pregnancy.

6. Cannabinoids—Marijuana has been used widely as an appetite stimulant and antiemetic. Some states allow the use of medical marijuana with a clinician's certification. Strains of medical marijuana with different proportions of various naturally occurring cannabinoids (primarily THC and cannabidiol [CBD]) can be chosen to minimize its psychoactive effects. Excessive cannabinoid may cause nausea, vomiting, and abdominal pain (cannabinoid hyperemesis syndrome), which may be temporarily relieved with hot showers or bathing.

Hsu YC et al. Effectiveness of palonosetron versus granisetron in preventing chemotherapy-induced nausea and vomiting: a systematic review and meta-analysis. Eur J Clin Pharmacol. 2021;77:1597. [PMID: 33993343]

Laszkowska M et al. Disease course and outcomes of COVID-19 among hospitalized patients with gastrointestinal manifestations. Clin Gastroenterol Hepatol. 2021;19:1402. [PMID: 33007514]

Qayed E et al. Low incidence of severe gastrointestinal complications in COVID-19 patients admitted to the intensive care unit: a large, multicenter study. Gastroenterology. 2021;160:1403. [PMID: 33010411]

Weibel S et al. Drugs for preventing postoperative nausea and vomiting in adults after general anaesthesia: an abridged Cochrane network meta-analysis. Anaesthesia. 2021;76:962. [PMID: 33170514]

HICCUPS

Though usually a benign and self-limited annoyance, hiccups may be persistent and a sign of serious underlying illness. In patients on mechanical ventilation, hiccups can trigger a full respiratory cycle and result in respiratory alkalosis.

Causes of benign, self-limited hiccups include gastric distention (carbonated beverages, air swallowing, overeating), sudden temperature changes (hot then cold liquids, hot then cold shower), alcohol ingestion, and states of heightened emotion (excitement, stress, laughing). There are over 100 causes of recurrent or persistent hiccups due to GI, CNS, cardiovascular, and thoracic disorders. Persistent hiccups may be an atypical presentation of COVID-19.

▶ Clinical Findings

Evaluation of the patient with persistent hiccups should include a detailed neurologic examination, serum creatinine, liver chemistry tests, and a chest radiograph. When the cause remains unclear, CT; MRI of the head, chest, and abdomen; upper endoscopy; and echocardiography may help.

▶ Treatment

A number of simple remedies may be helpful in patients with acute benign hiccups. (1) Irritation of the nasopharynx by tongue traction, lifting the uvula with a spoon, catheter stimulation of the nasopharynx, or eating 1 teaspoon (tsp) (7 g) of dry granulated sugar. (2) Interruption of the respiratory cycle by breath holding, Valsalva maneuver, sneezing, gasping (fright stimulus), or rebreathing into a bag. (3) Stimulation of the vagus by carotid massage. (4) Irritation of the diaphragm by holding knees to chest or by continuous positive airway pressure during mechanical ventilation. (5) Relief of gastric distention by belching or insertion of a nasogastric tube.

A number of drugs have been promoted as being useful in the treatment of hiccups. Chlorpromazine, 25–50 mg orally or intramuscularly, is most commonly used. Other agents reported to be effective include anticonvulsants (phenytoin, carbamazepine), benzodiazepines (lorazepam, diazepam), metoclopramide, baclofen, and gabapentin. For severe, intractable hiccups, phrenic nerve block, vagal nerve stimulation and, occasionally, general anesthesia have been used with variable efficacy.

Adam E. A systematic review of the effectiveness of oral baclofen in the management of hiccups in adult palliative care patients. J Pain Palliat Care Pharmacother. 2020;34:43. [PMID: 31910072]

Prince G et al. Persistent hiccups as an atypical presenting complaint of COVID-19. Am J Emerg Med. 2020;38:1546. [PMID: 32345563]

CONSTIPATION

Constipation occurs in 15% of adults and up to one-third of older adults and is a common reason for seeking medical attention. It is more common in women. Older individuals are predisposed due to comorbid medical conditions, medications, poor eating habits, decreased mobility, and in some cases, inability to sit on a toilet (bed-bound patients). The first step in evaluating the patient is to determine what is meant by "constipation." Patients may define constipation as infrequent stools (fewer than three in a week), hard or lumpy stools, excessive straining, or a sense of incomplete evacuation. Table 15–3 summarizes the many causes of constipation, which are discussed below.

Table 15–3. Causes of constipation in adults.

Most common
Inadequate fiber or fluid intake
Poor bowel habits
Irritable bowel syndrome
Systemic disease
Endocrine: hypothyroidism, hyperparathyroidism, diabetes mellitus
Metabolic: hypokalemia, hypercalcemia, uremia, porphyria
Neurologic: Parkinson disease, multiple sclerosis, sacral nerve damage (prior pelvic surgery, tumor), paraplegia, autonomic neuropathy
Medications
Opioids
Diuretics
Calcium channel blockers
Anticholinergics
Psychotropics
Calcium and iron supplements
Clonidine
Cholestyramine
Structural abnormalities
Anorectal: rectal prolapse, rectocele, rectal intussusception, anorectal stricture, anal fissure, solitary rectal ulcer syndrome
Perineal descent
Colonic mass with obstruction: adenocarcinoma
Colonic stricture: radiation, ischemia, diverticulosis
Hirschsprung disease
Idiopathic megarectum
Slow colonic transit
Idiopathic: isolated to colon
Psychogenic
Eating disorders
Chronic intestinal pseudo-obstruction
Pelvic floor dyssynergia

Etiology

A. Primary Constipation

Most patients have constipation that cannot be attributed to any structural abnormalities or systemic disease. These patients may be further categorized as having normal colonic transit time, slow transit, or defecatory disorders (with or without slow colonic transit). Normal colonic transit time is approximately 35 hours; more than 72 hours is significantly abnormal. Slow colonic transit is commonly idiopathic (due to dysfunction of the enteric nervous system) but may be part of a generalized GI dysmotility syndrome. Normal defecation requires coordination between relaxation of the anal sphincter and pelvic floor musculature while abdominal pressure is increased. Patients with defecatory disorders (also known dyssynergic defecation)—women more often than men—have impaired relaxation or paradoxical contraction of the anal sphincter and/or pelvic floor muscles during attempted defecation that impedes the bowel movement. This problem may be acquired during childhood or adulthood. Patients may complain of excessive straining, sense of incomplete evacuation, need for digital manipulation, or adoption of a non-sitting (eg, standing) position during defecation. Patients with predominant complaints of abdominal pain or bloating with chronic idiopathic constipation are more appropriately given a diagnosis of irritable bowel syndrome (IBS) with constipation.

B. Secondary Constipation

Constipation may be caused by systemic disorders, medications, or obstructing colonic lesions. Systemic disorders that can cause constipation include neurologic gut dysfunction, myopathies, endocrine disorders, or electrolyte abnormalities (eg, hypercalcemia or hypokalemia); medication side effects are often responsible (eg, anticholinergics or opioids). Colonic lesions that obstruct fecal passage, such as neoplasms and strictures, are an uncommon cause but important in new-onset constipation. Such lesions should be excluded in patients older than age 50 years, in patients with "alarm" symptoms or signs (hematochezia, weight loss, anemia, or positive fecal occult blood tests [FOBT] or fecal immunochemical tests [FIT]), and in patients with a family history of colon cancer or inflammatory bowel disease. Defecatory difficulties also can be due to a variety of anorectal problems that impede or obstruct flow (perineal descent, rectal prolapse, rectocele), some of which may require surgery, and to Hirschsprung disease (usually suggested by lifelong constipation).

Clinical Findings

A. Symptoms and Signs

All patients should undergo a history and physical examination to distinguish primary from secondary causes of constipation. Physical examination should include digital rectal examination with assessment for anatomic abnormalities, such as anal stricture, rectocele, rectal prolapse, or perineal descent during straining as well as assessment of pelvic floor motion during simulated defecation (ie, the patient's ability to "expel the examiner's finger"). Further diagnostic tests should be performed in patients with any of the following: signs of systemic disease, recent onset of constipation without apparent cause, "alarm" symptoms (hematochezia, weight loss, anemia, positive FOBT or FIT), family history of colon cancer or IBD, and age 45–50 years or older with no prior colonoscopy screening. These tests should include laboratory studies (CBC; serum electrolytes, calcium, glucose, and TSH) and a colonoscopy or flexible sigmoidoscopy.

B. Special Examinations

Patients with refractory constipation not responding to routine medical management warrant further diagnostic studies. Anorectal manometry including a balloon expulsion test should be performed first to evaluate for defecatory disorders. Inability to expel a balloon (attached to a 16F indwelling urinary catheter) filled with 50 mL of warm water within 1–2 minutes while sitting on a toilet is strongly suggestive of pelvic floor dyssynergia. Defecography to further assess pelvic floor function may be considered in selected patients. Subsequent colon transit studies are recommended only after defecatory disorders have been excluded. Colon transit time may be assessed by radiopaque markers, scintigraphy, or wireless motility capsule.

Treatment

A. Chronic Constipation

1. Dietary and lifestyle measures—Patients should be instructed on normal defecatory function and optimal toileting habits, including regular timing, proper positioning, and abdominal pressure. Adequate dietary fluid and fiber intake should be emphasized. Sorbitol-containing fruits and dried fruits (prunes, plums, apricots, cherries, mangos) and fruit-based laxatives are well tolerated and associated with improvement in stool consistency and frequency. Increased dietary fiber may cause distention or flatulence, which often diminishes over several days. Soluble fiber supplements (eg, psyllium, methylcellulose) are a convenient, well-tolerated way to increase dietary fiber (Table 15–4). Response to fiber therapy is not immediate and increases in dosage should be made gradually over 7–10 days. Fiber is most likely to benefit patients with normal colonic transit. However, fiber may not benefit patients with symptoms of colonic inertia, defecatory disorders, opioid-induced constipation, or IBS; it may even exacerbate these symptoms. Regular exercise is associated with a decreased risk of constipation. When possible, discontinue medications that may be causing or contributing to constipation. Probiotics are widely promoted in direct advertising to patients for treatment of constipation. Meta-analysis of randomized controlled trials suggests probiotics improve stool frequency and consistency; however, more study is needed.

2. Laxatives—Laxatives may be given on an intermittent or chronic basis for constipation that does not respond to dietary and lifestyle changes (Table 15–4). In a 2020 survey of US adults with constipation symptoms (hard, lumpy, or infrequent stools or straining), 45% were taking fibers supplements or nonprescription laxatives; only 3% were taking prescription laxatives. There is no evidence that long-term use of these agents is harmful.

A. Osmotic laxatives—Treatment usually is initiated with regular (daily) use of an osmotic laxative. Nonabsorbable osmotic agents promote defecation by increased retention of water in the intestinal lumen, leading to softening of the stool and secondary stimulation of colonic peristalsis. Polyethylene glycol 3350 (MiraLax) should be the first-line agent in most situations due to its established efficacy in controlled clinical trials and low incidence of adverse events. MiraLax 17 g once daily has demonstrated superiority to placebo, lactulose, and prucalopride. Nondigestible carbohydrates (sorbitol, lactulose) are efficacious but less preferred because they may cause bloating, cramps, and flatulence. Magnesium-containing laxatives (magnesium hydroxide [milk of magnesia], magnesium oxide, magnesium sulfate) may be suitable for intermittent therapy but should not be given to patients with chronic renal insufficiency. When used in conventional doses, the onset of action of osmotic agents is generally within 24 hours. For more rapid treatment of acute constipation, purgative laxatives may be used, such as magnesium citrate (8–10 oz) or large-volume polyethylene glycol solutions (2–4 L, administered over 2–4 hours). Magnesium citrate may cause hypermagnesemia.

B. Stimulant laxatives—For patients with incomplete response to osmotic agents, stimulant laxatives may be prescribed as needed as a "rescue" agent or on a regular basis (daily or alternate days). These agents stimulate fluid secretion and colonic contraction, resulting in a bowel movement within 6–12 hours after oral ingestion or 15–60 minutes after rectal administration. Oral agents are usually administered once daily at bedtime. Common nonprescription preparations include bisacodyl and senna (Table 15–4).

C. Secretagogues—Several agents stimulate intestinal chloride secretion either through activation of chloride channels (lubiprostone) or guanylcyclase C (linaclotide and plecanatide), resulting in increased intestinal fluid and accelerated colonic transit. In multicenter controlled trials, patients treated with lubiprostone 24 mcg orally twice daily, linaclotide 145 mcg once daily, or plecanatide 3 mg once daily increased the number of bowel movements compared with patients treated with placebo. Because these agents are expensive, they should be reserved for patients who have suboptimal response or side effects with less expensive agents.

D. Serotonin 5-HT-receptor agonist—Prucalopride is a high-affinity 5-HT_4-agonist that is approved in the United States for the treatment of chronic constipation (2 mg once daily). In six clinical trials, 19–38% of patients treated with prucalopride experienced at least three spontaneous bowel movements per week, which was 5–23% more than with placebo. In contrast to prior, less-selective

Table 15–4. Pharmacologic management of constipation.

Agent	Dosage	Onset of Action	Comments
Fiber Laxatives			
Psyllium	1 tbs (3.5 g fiber) once or twice daily	Days	(Metamucil; Perdiem)
Methylcellulose	1 tbs (2 g fiber) once or twice daily	Days	(Citrucel) Less gas, flatulence
Calcium polycarbophil	1 or 2 tablets once or twice daily	12–24 hours	(FiberCon) Does not cause gas; pill form
Guargum	1 tbsp once or twice daily	Days	(Benefiber) Non-gritty, tasteless, less gas
Stool Surfactants			
Docusate sodium	100 mg once or twice daily	12–72 hours	(Colace) Marginal benefit
Mineral oil	15–45 mL once or twice daily	6–8 hours	May cause lipoid pneumonia if aspirated
Osmotic Laxatives			
Magnesium hydroxide	15–30 mL orally once or twice daily	6–24 hours	(Milk of magnesia) May cause hypermagnesemia if CKD
Lactulose or 70% sorbitol	15–60 mL orally once daily to three times daily	6–48 hours	Cramps, bloating, flatulence
Polyethylene glycol (PEG 3350)	17 g in 8 oz liquid once or twice daily	6–24 hours	(MiraLAX); More effective, less bloating than lactulose, sorbitol
Stimulant Laxatives			
Bisacodyl	5–20 mg orally as needed	6–8 hours	May cause cramps; avoid daily use if possible
Bisacodyl suppository	10 mg per rectum as needed	1 hour	
Senna	17.2–34.4 mg orally	8–12 hours	(ExLax; Senekot; SennaS) May cause cramps; avoid daily use if possible
Lubiprostone	24 mcg orally twice daily	12–48 hours	Expensive; may cause nausea. Contraindicated in pregnancy
Linaclotide	72–145 mcg orally once daily		Expensive; contraindicated in pediatric patients
Plecanatide	3–6 mg once daily		Expensive; contraindicated in pediatric patients
Enemas			
Tap water	500 mL per rectum	5–15 minutes	
Sodium phosphate enema	120 mL per rectum	5–15 minutes	Commonly used for acute constipation or to induce movement prior to medical procedures
Mineral oil enema	100–250 mL per rectum	5–15 minutes	To soften and lubricate fecal impaction
Agents used for Acute Purgative or to Clean Bowel Prior to Medical Procedures			
Polyethylene glycol (PEG 3350)	4 L orally administered over 2–4 hours	< 4 hours	(GoLYTELY; CoLYTE; NuLYTE, MoviPrep) Used to cleanse bowel before colonoscopy
Magnesium citrate	10 oz orally	3–6 hours	Lemon-flavored

5-HT_4-agonists (cisapride, tegaserod), which were removed from the market due to adverse cardiovascular events, prucalopride does not have affinity for hERG K^+ channels and does not appear to have any cardiovascular risk.

E. Opioid-receptor antagonists—Long-term use of opioids can cause constipation by increasing tonic, nonpropulsive colonic contractions that lead to increased intestinal fluid absorption and dry, hard stools. Methylnaltrexone (450 mg orally once daily), naloxegol (12.5–25 mg orally once daily), and naldemedine (0.2 mg orally once daily) are mu-opioid receptor antagonists that block peripheral opioid receptors (including in the GI tract) without affecting central analgesia. These medications are recommended for the treatment of opioid-induced constipation in patients receiving prolonged opioid therapy who have not had an adequate laxative response with an osmotic agent (usually PEG-3300) and a stimulant laxative (usually bisacodyl or senna) (see Chapter 5). A subcutaneous formulation of methylnaltrexone also is approved for treatment of patients receiving palliative care for advanced illness who have not responded to conventional laxative regimens.

B. Fecal Impaction

Severe impaction of stool in the rectal vault may result in obstruction to further fecal flow, leading to partial or complete large bowel obstruction. Predisposing factors include medications (eg, opioids), severe psychiatric disease, prolonged bed rest, neurogenic disorders of the colon, and spinal cord disorders. Clinical presentation includes decreased appetite, nausea and vomiting, and abdominal pain and distention. There may be paradoxical "diarrhea" as liquid stool leaks around the impacted feces. Firm feces are palpable on digital examination of the rectal vault. Initial treatment is directed at relieving the impaction with enemas (saline, mineral oil, or diatrizoate) or digital disruption of the impacted fecal material. Long-term care is directed at maintaining soft stools and regular bowel movements (as above).

When to Refer

- Patients with "alarm" symptoms or who are over age 45–50 should be referred for colonoscopy.
- Patients with refractory constipation should be considered for anorectal manometry, balloon expulsion test, and colonic transit study.
- Patients with defecatory disorders may benefit from biofeedback therapy.
- Rarely, surgery (subtotal colectomy) is required for patients with severe colonic inertia.

Bharucha AE et al. Mechanisms, evaluation, and management of chronic constipation. Gastroenterology. 2020;18:1232. [PMID: 31945360]
Oh SJ et al. Chronic constipation in the United States: results from a population-based survey assessing healthcare seeking and use of pharmacotherapy. Am J Gastroenterol. 2020; 115:895. [PMID: 32324606]
Rao S et al. Efficacy and safety of over-the-counter therapies for chronic constipation: an updated systematic review. Am J Gastroenterol. 2021;116:1156. [PMID: 33767108]

GASTROINTESTINAL GAS

1. Belching

Belching (eructation) is the involuntary or voluntary release of gas from the stomach or esophagus. It occurs most frequently after meals, when gastric distention results in transient lower esophageal sphincter (LES) relaxation. Belching is a normal reflex and does not itself denote GI dysfunction. Virtually all stomach gas comes from swallowed air. With each swallow, 2–5 mL of air is ingested, and excessive amounts may result in distention, flatulence, and abdominal pain. This may occur with rapid eating, gum chewing, smoking, and the ingestion of carbonated beverages. Evaluation should be restricted to patients with other complaints such as dysphagia, heartburn, early satiety, or vomiting.

Chronic excessive belching is almost always caused by supragastric belching (voluntary diaphragmatic contraction, followed by upper esophageal relaxation with air inflow to the esophagus) or true air swallowing (aerophagia), both of which are behavioral disorders that are more common in patients with anxiety or psychiatric disorders. These patients may benefit from referral to a behavioral or speech therapist.

Zad M et al. Chronic burping and belching. Curr Treat Options Gastroenterol. 2020;18:33. [PMID: 31974815]

2. Bloating & Flatus

Bloating is a complaint of increased abdominal pressure that may or may not be accompanied by visible distention. Organic causes of acute bloating with distention, vomiting, and/or pain include ascites, GI obstruction (gastric fundoplication, gastric outlet obstruction, small intestine or colon obstruction, and constipation). Complaints of chronic abdominal distention or bloating are common. Some patients swallow excess air (aerophagia, poorly fitting dentures, sleep apnea, and rapid eating) or produce excess gas (excessive FODMAP [fermentable oligosaccharides, disaccharides, monosaccharides, and polyols] ingestion and malabsorption). Others have impaired gas propulsion or expulsion, increased bowel wall tension, enhanced visceral sensitivity, or altered viscerosomatic reflexes leading to abdominal protrusion. Many of these patients have an underlying functional GI disorder such as IBS or functional dyspepsia. Constipation should be treated, and exercise (which accelerates gas propulsion) is recommended. Medications that inhibit GI motility should be avoided (opioids and calcium channel blockers).

Healthy adults pass **flatus** up to 20 times daily and excrete up to 750 mL. Flatus is derived from two sources: swallowed air (primarily nitrogen) and bacterial fermentation of undigested carbohydrate (which produces H_2, CO_2, and methane). A number of short-chain carbohydrates (FODMAPs) are incompletely absorbed in the small intestine and pass into the colon. These include lactose (dairy products); fructose (fruits, corn syrups, and some sweeteners); polyols (stone-fruits, mushrooms, and some sweeteners); and oligosaccharides (legumes, lentils, cruciferous vegetables, garlic, onion, pasta, and whole grains). Abnormal gas production may be caused by increased ingestion of these carbohydrates or, less commonly, by disorders of malabsorption. Foul odor may be caused by garlic, onion, eggplant, mushrooms, and certain herbs and spices.

Determining abnormal from normal amounts of flatus is difficult. Patients who report excess flatus may also complain of bloating, cramping, and altered stool habits (diarrhea or constipation). Patients with a long-standing history of flatulence and no other symptoms or signs of malabsorption disorders can be treated conservatively. Gum chewing and carbonated beverages should be avoided to reduce air swallowing. Lactose intolerance may be assessed by a 2-week trial of a lactose-free diet or by a hydrogen breath test. A list of foods containing FODMAPs should be provided and high FODMAP foods eliminated for 2–4 weeks. If symptoms improve, FODMAP groups may be sequentially introduced to identify triggers. Multiple low-FODMAP dietary guides are available; however, referral to a knowledgeable dietician may be helpful.

The nonprescription agent Beano (alpha-d-galactosidase enzyme) reduces gas caused by foods containing galacto-oligosaccharides (legumes, chickpeas, lentils) but not other FODMAPs. Activated charcoal may afford relief. Simethicone has no proven benefit.

Many patients report reduced flatus production with use of probiotics, although there has been limited controlled study of these agents for this purpose.

Lacy BE et al. Management of chronic abdominal distention and bloating. Clin Gastroenterol Hepatol. 2021;19:219. [PMID: 32246999]

Scarlata K. Low FODMAP diet: what your patients need to know. Am J Gastroenterol. 2019;114:189. [PMID: 30356177]

DIARRHEA

Diarrhea can range in severity from an acute self-limited episode to a severe, life-threatening illness. To properly evaluate the complaint, the clinician must determine the patient's normal bowel pattern and the nature of the current symptoms.

Approximately 10 L/day of fluid enter the duodenum of which all but 1.5 L/day are absorbed by the small intestine. The colon absorbs most of the remaining fluid, with less than 200 mL/day lost in the stool. Although diarrhea sometimes is defined as a stool weight of more than 200–300 g/24 hours, quantification of stool weight is necessary only in some patients with chronic diarrhea. In most cases, the physician's working definition of diarrhea is increased stool frequency (more than three bowel movements per day) or liquidity of feces.

The causes of diarrhea are myriad. In clinical practice, it is helpful to distinguish acute from chronic diarrhea, as the evaluation and treatment are entirely different (Tables 15–5 and 15–6).

1. Acute Diarrhea

ESSENTIALS OF DIAGNOSIS

- Diarrhea of < 2 weeks' duration is most commonly caused by invasive or noninvasive pathogens and their enterotoxins.

Acute noninflammatory diarrhea

- Watery, nonbloody.
- Usually mild, self-limited.
- Caused by a virus or noninvasive, toxin-producing bacterium.
- Diagnostic evaluation is limited to patients with diarrhea that is severe or persists beyond 7 days.

Acute inflammatory diarrhea

- Blood or pus, fever.
- Usually caused by an invasive or toxin-producing bacterium.
- Diagnostic evaluation requires routine stool bacterial testing (including *E coli* O157:H5 and O157:H7) in all patients and testing as clinically indicated in others for *Clostridioides difficile* and parasites.

Table 15–5. Causes of acute infectious diarrhea.

Noninflammatory Diarrhea	Inflammatory Diarrhea
Viral Noroviruses, astrovirus, adenovirus, rotavirus, sapovirus, SARS-CoV-2	**Viral** Cytomegalovirus
Protozoal *Giardia lamblia* *Cryptosporidium* *Cyclospora*	**Protozoal** *Entamoeba histolytica*
Bacterial 1. Preformed enterotoxin production *Staphylococcus aureus* *Bacillus cereus* *Clostridium perfringens* 2. Enterotoxin production Enterotoxigenic *Escherichia coli* (ETEC) *Vibrio cholerae, Vibrio vulnificus*	**Bacterial** 1. Cytotoxin production Enterohemorrhagic *E coli* O157:H5 and O157:H7 (EHEC) *Vibrio parahaemolyticus* *Clostridioides difficile* 2. Mucosal invasion *Shigella* *Campylobacter jejuni* *Salmonella* Enteroinvasive *E coli* (EIEC) *Listeria monocytogenes* *Aeromonas* *Yersinia enterocolitica* 3. Infectious proctitis *Chlamydia* *Neisseria gonorrhoeae*

Etiology & Clinical Findings

Diarrhea acute in onset and persisting for less than 2 weeks is most commonly caused by infectious agents, bacterial toxins (either preformed or produced in the gut), or medications. Community outbreaks (including norovirus and SARS-CoV-2 in nursing homes, schools, cruise ships) suggest a viral etiology or a common food source. Similar recent illnesses in family members suggest an infectious origin. Among patients with COVID-19 infection, watery diarrhea (usually mild) occurs in one-third and may be the presenting symptom in 3–16%. Ingestion of improperly stored or prepared food implicates "food poisoning" due to bacterial toxins that are either present in the ingested food (preformed) or produced within the GI tract after ingestion. Pregnant women have an increased risk of developing listeriosis. Day care attendance or exposure to unpurified water (camping, swimming) may result in infection with *Giardia* or *Cryptosporidium*. Large *Cyclospora* outbreaks have been traced to contaminated produce. Recent travel abroad suggests "traveler's diarrhea" (see Chapter 30). Antibiotic administration within the preceding several

Table 15–6. Causes of chronic diarrhea.

Osmotic diarrhea CLUES: Stool volume decreases with fasting; increased stool osmotic gap 1. Medications: antacids, lactulose, sorbitol 2. Disaccharidase deficiency: lactose intolerance 3. Factitious diarrhea: magnesium (antacids, laxatives) **Secretory diarrhea** CLUES: Large volume (> 1 L/day); little change with fasting; normal stool osmotic gap 1. Hormonally mediated: VIPoma, carcinoid, medullary carcinoma of thyroid (calcitonin), Zollinger-Ellison syndrome (gastrin) 2. Factitious diarrhea (laxative abuse); phenolphthalein, senna 3. Villous adenoma 4. Bile salt malabsorption (idiopathic, ileal resection; Crohn ileitis; postcholecystectomy) 5. Medications **Inflammatory conditions** CLUES: Fever, hematochezia, abdominal pain 1. Ulcerative colitis 2. Crohn disease 3. Microscopic colitis 4. Malignancy: lymphoma, adenocarcinoma (with obstruction and pseudodiarrhea) 5. Radiation enteritis **Medications** Common offenders: SSRIs, cholinesterase inhibitors, NSAIDs, PPIs, angiotensin II receptor blockers, metformin, allopurinol	**Malabsorption syndromes** CLUES: Weight loss, abnormal laboratory values; fecal fat > 10 g/24 hours 1. Small bowel mucosal disorders: celiac disease, tropical sprue, Whipple disease, eosinophilic gastroenteritis, small bowel resection (short bowel syndrome), Crohn disease 2. Lymphatic obstruction: lymphoma, carcinoid, infectious (tuberculosis, MAI), Kaposi sarcoma, sarcoidosis, retroperitoneal fibrosis 3. Pancreatic disease: chronic pancreatitis, pancreatic carcinoma 4. Bacterial overgrowth: motility disorders (diabetes, vagotomy), systemic sclerosis (scleroderma), fistulas, small intestinal diverticula **Motility disorders** CLUES: Prior abdominal surgery or systemic disease 1. Postsurgical: vagotomy, partial gastrectomy, blind loop with bacterial overgrowth 2. Systemic disorders: systemic sclerosis (scleroderma), diabetes mellitus, hyperthyroidism 3. Irritable bowel syndrome **Chronic infections** 1. Parasites: *Giardia lamblia, Entamoeba histolytica, Strongyloides stercoralis, Capillaria philippinensis* 2. AIDS-related: viral: cytomegalovirus; bacterial: *Clostridioides difficile,* MAI; protozoal: microsporidia (*Enterocytozoon bieneusi*), *Cryptosporidium, Cystoisospora belli* (formerly *Isospora belli*) **Factitious** See Osmotic and Secretory diarrhea above

MAI, *Mycobacterium avium-intracellulare.*

weeks increases the likelihood of *C difficile* colitis. Finally, risk factors for HIV infection or sexually transmitted diseases should be determined. (AIDS-associated diarrhea is discussed in Chapter 31; infectious proctitis is discussed later in this chapter under Anorectal Infections.) Persons engaging in anal intercourse or oral-anal sexual activities are at risk for a variety of infections that cause proctitis, including gonorrhea, syphilis, lymphogranuloma venereum, and herpes simplex.

The nature of the diarrhea helps distinguish among different infectious causes (Table 15–5 and Chapter 30, Table 30–3).

A. Noninflammatory Diarrhea

Watery, nonbloody diarrhea associated with periumbilical cramps, bloating, nausea, or vomiting suggests a small bowel source caused by either a virus (rotavirus, norovirus, adenovirus, astrovirus, coronavirus), a toxin-producing bacterium (enterotoxigenic *E coli* [ETEC], *Staphylococcus aureus, Bacillus cereus, Clostridium perfringens*), or another agent (*Giardia*) that disrupts normal absorption and secretory process in the small intestine. Prominent vomiting suggests viral enteritis or food poisoning due to a preformed toxin *(S aureus, B cereus)*. Although typically mild, the diarrhea (which originates in the small intestine) can be voluminous and result in dehydration with hypokalemia and metabolic acidosis (eg, cholera). Because tissue invasion does not occur, fecal leukocytes are not present.

B. Inflammatory Diarrhea

The presence of fever and bloody diarrhea (dysentery) indicates colonic tissue damage caused by invasion (shigellosis, salmonellosis, *Campylobacter* or *Yersinia* infection, amebiasis) or a toxin (*C difficile*, Shiga-toxin–producing *E coli* [STEC; also known as enterohemorrhagic *E coli*]). Because these organisms predominantly involve the colon, the diarrhea is small in volume (less than 1 L/day) and associated with left lower quadrant cramps, urgency, and tenesmus. Fecal leukocytes or lactoferrin usually are present in infections with invasive organisms. *E coli* O157:H7 is a Shiga-toxin–producing noninvasive organism most commonly acquired from contaminated meat that has resulted in several outbreaks of an acute, often severe hemorrhagic colitis. A major complication of STEC is hemolytic-uremic syndrome, which develops in 6–22% of cases. In immunocompromised and HIV-infected patients, cytomegalovirus (CMV) can cause intestinal ulceration with watery or bloody diarrhea. *Listeria monocytogenes* has been implicated in several outbreaks of foodborne gastroenteritis, which have been characterized by fever (60–100%), watery diarrhea, and nausea or vomiting.

Infectious dysentery must be distinguished from acute ulcerative colitis, which may also present acutely with fever, abdominal pain, and bloody diarrhea. Immune checkpoint inhibitor therapy for malignancies may cause GI side effects in 8–27% of patients that range from mild diarrhea to severe enterocolitis characterized by abdominal pain and inflammatory diarrhea with mucus, blood, elevated lactoferrin or calprotectin, and colitis at endoscopy. Diarrhea that persists for more than 14 days is not attributable to bacterial pathogens (except for *C difficile*) and should be evaluated as chronic diarrhea.

Evaluation

In over 90% of patients with acute noninflammatory diarrhea, the illness is mild and self-limited, responding within 5 days to simple rehydration therapy or antidiarrheal agents. The isolation rate of bacterial pathogens from stool cultures in patients with acute noninflammatory diarrhea is under 3%; therefore, diagnostic investigation is unnecessary except in suspected outbreaks or in patients at high risk for spreading infection to others.

The goal of initial evaluation of acute diarrhea is to distinguish patients with mild disease from those with more serious illness. Prompt medical evaluation is indicated in the following situations (Figure 15–1): (1) signs of inflammatory diarrhea manifested by any of the following: fever (higher than 38.5°C), WBC 15,000/mcL (15×10^9/L) or more, bloody diarrhea, or severe abdominal pain; (2) the passage of six or more unformed stools in 24 hours; (3) profuse watery diarrhea and dehydration; (4) frail older patients or nursing home residents; (5) immunocompromised patients (AIDS, posttransplantation); (6) exposure to antibiotics; (7) hospital-acquired diarrhea (onset following at least 3 days of hospitalization); or (8) systemic illness.

Physical examination pays note to the patient's level of hydration, mental status, and the presence of abdominal tenderness or peritonitis. Peritoneal findings may be present in infection with *C difficile* or STEC. Hospitalization is required in patients with severe dehydration, organ failure, marked abdominal pain, or altered mental status.

Stool should be sent for microbial assessment when patients have dysentery (bloody stools), severe illness, or persistent diarrhea beyond 7 days. Until recently, stool specimens were sent for microscopy (to assess for fecal white cells and protozoa) and bacterial cultures. These traditional methods provided a positive diagnosis in 60–75% of patients with dysenteric diarrhea but required 48–72 hours. Currently, many centers perform microbial assessment using multiplex molecular techniques with nucleic acid amplification (eg, PCR assays) that screen for

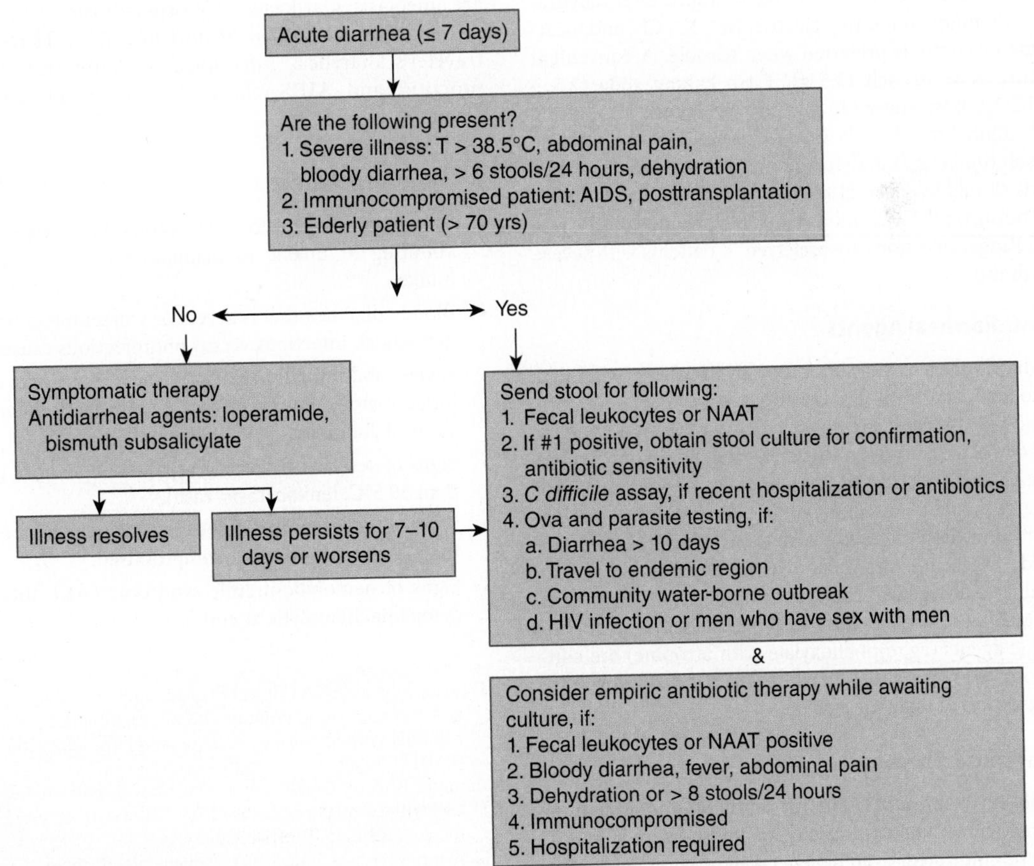

Figure 15–1. Evaluation of acute diarrhea. NAAT, nucleic acid amplification test.

a panel of pathogens, including viruses, protozoa, and bacteria, within 1–5 hours. If the PCR assay detects a bacterial pathogen, stool culture is recommended for confirmation and antibiotic sensitivity testing. In patients who are hospitalized or who have a history of antibiotic exposure, a stool sample should be tested for *C difficile*. Patients with severe diarrhea or dysentery and a known history of inflammatory bowel disease or prior immune checkpoint inhibitor therapy require expedited evaluation with stool studies and possible sigmoidoscopy or colonoscopy with biopsy to exclude infection (*C difficile*, other bacteria, CMV) prior to therapy with intravenous corticosteroids.

Treatment

A. Diet

Most mild diarrhea will not lead to dehydration provided the patient takes adequate oral fluids containing carbohydrates and electrolytes. Patients find it more comfortable to rest the bowel by avoiding high-fiber foods, fats, milk products, caffeine, and alcohol. Drinking tea and "flat" carbonated beverages and eating soft, easily digested foods (eg, soups, crackers, bananas, applesauce, rice, toast) are encouraged.

B. Rehydration

In more severe diarrhea, dehydration can occur quickly, especially in children and frail older adults. Oral rehydration with fluids containing glucose, Na^+, K^+, Cl^-, and bicarbonate or citrate is preferred when feasible. A convenient mixture is ½ tsp salt (3.5 g), 1 tsp baking soda (2.5 g $NaHCO_3$), 8 tsp sugar (40 g), and 8 oz orange juice (1.5 g KCl), diluted to 1 L with water. Alternatively, oral electrolyte solutions (eg, Pedialyte, Gatorade) are readily available. Fluids should be given at rates of 50–100 mL/kg/24 hours depending on the hydration status. Intravenous fluids (lactated Ringer injection) are preferred in patients with severe dehydration.

C. Antidiarrheal Agents

Antidiarrheal agents may be used safely in patients with mild to moderate diarrheal illnesses to improve patient comfort. Opioid agents help decrease the stool number and liquidity and control fecal urgency. However, they should not be used in patients with bloody diarrhea, high fever, or systemic toxicity and should be discontinued in patients whose diarrhea is worsening despite therapy. With these provisos, such drugs provide excellent symptomatic relief. Loperamide is preferred, in a dosage of 4 mg orally initially, followed by 2 mg after each loose stool (maximum: 8 mg/24 hours). Anticholinergic agents (eg, diphenoxylate with atropine) are contraindicated in acute diarrhea because of the rare precipitation of toxic megacolon.

D. Antibiotic Therapy

1. Empiric treatment—Empiric antibiotic treatment of patients with acute, community-acquired diarrhea generally is not indicated. Even patients with inflammatory diarrhea caused by invasive pathogens usually have symptoms that will resolve within several days without antimicrobials. In centers in which stool microbial testing with rapid molecular assays is not available, empiric treatment may be considered while the stool bacterial culture is incubating, particularly in patients with non–hospital-acquired diarrhea who have moderate to severe fever, tenesmus, or bloody stools and no suspicion of infection with STEC. It should also be considered in patients who are immunocompromised or who have significant dehydration. The oral medications of choice for empiric treatment are the fluoroquinolones (eg, ciprofloxacin 500 mg twice daily, ofloxacin 400 mg, or levofloxacin 500 mg once daily for 1–3 days) or azithromycin (eg, 1 g single dose or 500 mg daily for 3 days). Empiric treatment of noninflammatory traveler's diarrhea is discussed in Chapter 30.

2. Specific antimicrobial treatment—Antibiotics are not recommended in patients with nontyphoid *Salmonella*, *Campylobacter*, or *Yersinia*, except in severe disease, because they do not hasten recovery or reduce the period of fecal bacterial excretion. STEC infection should not be treated with antibiotics due to an increased risk of hemolytic-uremic syndrome, especially in children. The infectious bacterial diarrheas for which treatment is recommended are shigellosis, cholera, extraintestinal salmonellosis, listeriosis, and *C difficile*. The parasitic infections for which treatment is indicated are amebiasis, giardiasis, cryptosporidiosis, cyclosporiasis, and *Enterocytozoon bienusi* infection. Therapy for traveler's diarrhea, infectious (sexually transmitted) proctitis, and AIDS-related diarrhea is presented in Chapters 30 and 31.

When to Admit

- Severe dehydration for intravenous fluids, especially if vomiting or unable to maintain sufficient oral fluid intake.
- Bloody diarrhea that is severe or worsening in order to distinguish infectious versus noninfectious cause.
- Severe abdominal pain, worrisome for toxic colitis, inflammatory bowel disease, intestinal ischemia, or surgical abdomen.
- Signs of severe infection or sepsis (temperature higher than 39.5°C, leukocytosis, rash).
- Severe or worsening diarrhea in patients who are older than 70 years or immunocompromised.
- Signs of hemolytic-uremic syndrome (AKI, thrombocytopenia, hemolytic anemia).

Dougan M et al. AGA Clinical Practice update on the diagnosis and management of immune checkpoint inhibitor colitis and hepatitis: expert review. Gastroenterology. 2021;160:1384. [PMID: 33080231]

Elmuner BJ et al. Digestive manifestations in patients hospitalized with coronavirus disease 2019. Clin Gastroenterol Hepatol. 2021;19:1355. [PMID: 33010411]

Siciliano V et al. Clinical management of infectious diarrhea. Rev Recent Clin Trials. 2020;15:298. [PMID: 32598272]

2. Chronic Diarrhea

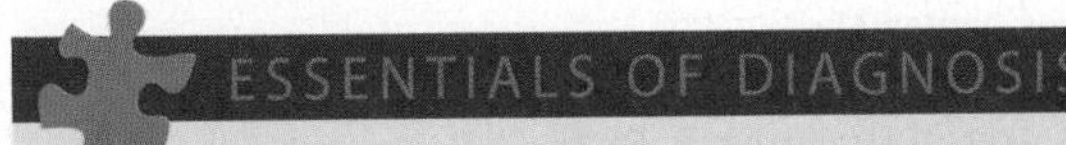

- Diarrhea present for > 4 weeks.
- Before embarking on extensive workup, common causes should be excluded, including medications, chronic infections, and IBS.

Etiology

The causes of chronic diarrhea may be grouped into the following major pathophysiologic categories: medications, osmotic diarrheas, secretory conditions, inflammatory conditions, malabsorptive conditions, motility disorders, chronic infections, and systemic disorders (Table 15–6).

A. Medications

Numerous medications can cause diarrhea. All medications should be carefully reviewed, and discontinuation of potential culprits should be considered.

B. Osmotic Diarrheas

As stool leaves the colon, fecal osmolality is equal to the serum osmolality, ie, approximately 290 mOsm/kg. Under normal circumstances, the major osmoles are Na^+, K^+, Cl^-, and HCO_3^-. The stool osmolality may be estimated by multiplying the stool ($Na^+ + K^+$) × 2. The **osmotic gap** is the difference between the *measured* osmolality of the stool (or serum) and the *estimated* stool osmolality and is normally less than 50 mOsm/kg. An increased osmotic gap (greater than 75 mOsm/kg) implies that the diarrhea is caused by ingestion or malabsorption of an osmotically active substance. The most common causes are carbohydrate malabsorption (lactose, fructose, sorbitol), laxative abuse, and malabsorption syndromes. Osmotic diarrheas resolve during fasting. Those caused by malabsorbed carbohydrates are characterized by abdominal distention, bloating, and flatulence due to increased colonic gas production.

Carbohydrate malabsorption is common and should be considered in all patients with chronic, postprandial diarrhea. Patients should be asked about their intake of dairy products (lactose), fruits and artificial sweeteners (fructose and sorbitol), processed foods and soft drinks (high-fructose corn syrup), and alcohol. The diagnosis of carbohydrate malabsorption may be established by an elimination trial for 2–3 weeks or by hydrogen breath tests.

Ingestion of magnesium- or phosphate-containing compounds (laxatives, antacids) should be considered in enigmatic chronic diarrhea. The fat substitute olestra also causes diarrhea and cramps in occasional patients.

C. Secretory Conditions

Increased intestinal secretion or decreased absorption results in a high-volume watery diarrhea with a normal osmotic gap. There is little change in stool output during the fasting state, and dehydration and electrolyte imbalance may develop. Causes include endocrine tumors (stimulating intestinal or pancreatic secretion), bile salt malabsorption (stimulating colonic secretion), and microscopic colitis. Microscopic colitis is a common cause of chronic watery diarrhea in older adults (see Inflammatory Bowel Disease, below).

D. Inflammatory Conditions

Diarrhea is present in most patients with inflammatory bowel disease (ulcerative colitis, Crohn disease). A variety of other symptoms may be present, including abdominal pain, fever, weight loss, and hematochezia.

E. Malabsorptive Conditions

The major causes of malabsorption are small intestinal mucosal diseases, intestinal resections, lymphatic obstruction, small intestinal bacterial overgrowth, and pancreatic insufficiency. Its characteristics are weight loss, osmotic diarrhea, steatorrhea, and nutritional deficiencies. Significant diarrhea in the absence of weight loss is not likely to be due to malabsorption. The physical and laboratory abnormalities related to deficiencies of vitamins or minerals are discussed in Chapter 29.

F. Motility Disorders (Including IBS)

IBS is the most common cause of chronic diarrhea in young adults (see Irritable Bowel Syndrome, below). It should be considered in patients with lower abdominal pain and altered bowel habits who have no other evidence of serious organic disease (weight loss, nocturnal diarrhea, anemia, or GI bleeding). Abnormal intestinal motility secondary to systemic disorders, radiation enteritis, or surgery may result in diarrhea due to rapid transit or to stasis of intestinal contents with bacterial overgrowth, resulting in malabsorption.

G. Chronic Infections

Chronic parasitic infections may cause diarrhea through a number of mechanisms. Pathogens most commonly associated with diarrhea include the protozoans *Giardia*, *Entamoeba histolytica*, and *Cyclospora* as well as the intestinal nematodes. Strongyloidiasis and capillariasis should be excluded in patients from endemic regions, especially in the presence of eosinophilia. Bacterial infections with *C difficile* and, uncommonly, *Aeromonas* and *Plesiomonas* may cause chronic diarrhea.

Immunocompromised patients are susceptible to infectious organisms that can cause acute or chronic diarrhea (see Chapter 31), including microsporidia, *Cryptosporidium*, CMV, *Cystoisospora belli* (formerly *Isospora belli*), *Cyclospora*, and *Mycobacterium avium* complex.

H. Systemic Conditions

Chronic systemic conditions, such as thyroid disease, diabetes, and collagen vascular disorders, may cause diarrhea through alterations in motility or intestinal absorption.

Clinical Findings

The history and physical examination commonly suggest the underlying pathophysiology that guides the subsequent diagnostic workup (Figure 15–2). The clinician should establish whether the diarrhea is continuous or intermittent, whether it has a relationship to meals, and whether it occurs at night or during fasting. The stool appearance may suggest a malabsorption disorder (greasy or malodorous), inflammatory disorder (containing blood or pus), or a secretory process (watery). The presence of abdominal pain suggests IBS or inflammatory bowel disease. Medications, diet, and recent psychosocial stressors should be reviewed. Physical examination should assess for signs of malnutrition, dehydration, and inflammatory bowel disease.

Because chronic diarrhea is caused by so many conditions, the subsequent diagnostic approach is guided by the relative suspicion for the underlying cause, and no specific algorithm can be followed in all patients. Prior to embarking on an extensive evaluation, the most common causes of chronic diarrhea should be considered, including medications, IBS, and lactose intolerance. The presence of nocturnal diarrhea, weight loss, anemia, or positive results on FOBT are inconsistent with these disorders and warrant further evaluation. AIDS-associated diarrhea is discussed in Chapter 31.

A. Initial Diagnostic Tests

1. Routine laboratory tests—CBC, serum electrolytes, liver chemistries, calcium, phosphorus, albumin, TSH, vitamin A and D levels, prothrombin time with INR, ESR, and CRP should be obtained in most patients. Serologic testing for celiac disease with an IgA tissue transglutaminase (IgA anti-tTG) test is recommended in the evaluation of most patients with chronic diarrhea even in the absence of signs of malabsorption. Anemia occurs in malabsorption syndromes (folate, iron, or vitamin B_{12} deficiency) as well as in inflammatory conditions. Hypoalbuminemia is present in malabsorption, protein-losing enteropathies, and inflammatory diseases. Hyponatremia and nonanion gap metabolic acidosis occur in secretory diarrheas. Increased ESR or CRP suggests inflammatory bowel disease. Elevated fasting levels (greater than 48 ng/mL) of the bile acid precursor 7αC4 are strongly predictive of bile acid diarrhea.

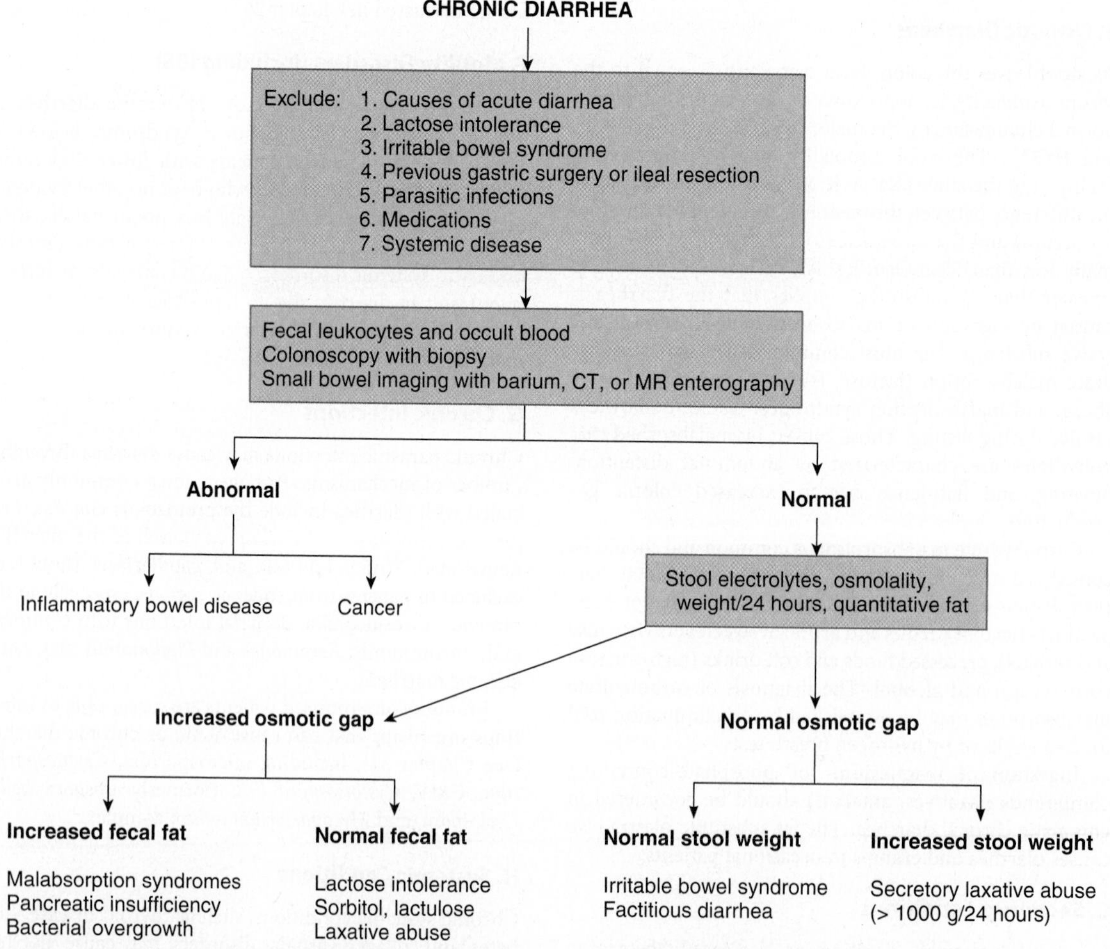

▲ **Figure 15–2.** Decision diagram for diagnosis of causes of chronic diarrhea.

2. Routine stool studies—Stool samples should be analyzed for ova and parasites, electrolytes (to calculate osmotic gap), qualitative staining for fat (Sudan stain), occult blood, and either leukocytes or fecal calprotectin or lactoferrin. Parasitic infections (*Giardia*, *E histolytica*, *Cryptosporidia*, and *Cyclospora*) may be diagnosed with stool multiplex PCR assays that test for a panel of pathogens within 1–5 hours, or, where PCR is unavailable, by microscopy with special stains. As discussed previously, an increased osmotic gap suggests an osmotic diarrhea or disorder of malabsorption. A positive fecal fat stain suggests a disorder of malabsorption. In patients with positive fecal fat or suspicion for chronic pancreatitis, a stool sample should be sent for measurement of pancreatic elastase, which is low with pancreatic insufficiency. The presence of fecal leukocytes or elevated calprotectin or lactoferrin may suggest inflammatory bowel disease.

3. Endoscopic examination and mucosal biopsy—Most patients with chronic persistent diarrhea undergo colonoscopy with mucosal biopsy to exclude inflammatory bowel disease (including Crohn disease and ulcerative colitis), microscopic colitis, and colonic neoplasia. Upper endoscopy with small bowel biopsy is performed when a small intestinal malabsorptive disorder is suspected (celiac disease, Whipple disease) from abnormal laboratory studies or a positive fecal fat stain. It may also be done in patients with advanced AIDS to document *Cryptosporidium*, microsporidia, and *M avium-intracellulare* infection.

B. Further Studies

If the cause of diarrhea is still not apparent, further studies may be warranted.

1. 24-hour stool collection quantification of total weight and fat—A stool weight of less than 200–300 g/24 hours excludes diarrhea and suggests a functional disorder such as IBS. A weight greater than 1000–1500 g suggests a significant secretory process, including neuroendocrine tumors. A fecal fat determination in excess of 10 g/24 hours confirms a malabsorptive disorder. Fecal elastase less than 100 mcg/g may be caused by pancreatic insufficiency. (See Celiac Disease and specific tests for malabsorption, below.)

2. Other imaging studies—Calcification on a plain abdominal radiograph confirms a diagnosis of chronic pancreatitis, although abdominal CT and endoscopic ultrasonography are more sensitive for the diagnosis of chronic pancreatitis as well as pancreatic cancer. Small intestinal imaging with CT or MRI enterography is helpful in the diagnosis of Crohn disease, small bowel lymphoma, carcinoid, and jejunal diverticula. Neuroendocrine tumors may be localized using CT, and metastases may be detected using somatostatin receptor PET scanning. Retention of less than 11% at 7 days of intravenous 75Se-homotaurocholate on scintigraphy suggests bile salt malabsorption; however, this test is unavailable in the United States.

3. Laboratory tests—

A. Serologic tests for neuroendocrine tumors—Secretory diarrheas due to neuroendocrine tumors are rare but should be considered in patients with chronic, high-volume watery diarrhea (greater than 1 L/day) with a normal osmotic gap that persists during fasting. Measurements of the secretagogues of various neuroendocrine tumors may be assayed, including serum chromogranin A (pancreatic neuroendocrine tumors), vasoactive intestinal peptide (VIP) (VIPoma), calcitonin (medullary thyroid carcinoma), gastrin (Zollinger-Ellison syndrome), and urinary 5-hydroxyindoleacetic acid (5-HIAA) (carcinoid).

B. Breath test—The diagnosis of small bowel bacterial overgrowth is suggested by a noninvasive breath test (glucose or lactulose); however, a high rate of false-positive test results limits the utility of these tests. A definitive diagnosis of bacterial overgrowth is determined by aspirate of small intestinal contents for quantitative aerobic and anaerobic bacterial culture; however, this procedure is not available at most centers.

Treatment

A number of antidiarrheal agents may be used in certain patients with chronic diarrheal conditions and are listed below. Opioids are safe in most patients with chronic, stable symptoms.

Loperamide: 4 mg orally initially, then 2 mg after each loose stool (maximum: 16 mg/day).

Diphenoxylate with atropine: One tablet orally three or four times daily as needed.

Codeine and **deodorized tincture of opium:** Because of potential habituation, these drugs are avoided except in cases of chronic, intractable diarrhea. Codeine may be given in a dosage of 15–60 mg orally every 4 hours; tincture of opium, 0.3–1.2 mL orally every 6 hours as needed.

Clonidine: Alpha-2-adrenergic agonists inhibit intestinal electrolyte secretion. Clonidine, 0.1–0.3 mg orally twice daily, or a clonidine patch, 0.1–0.2 mg/day, may help in some patients with secretory diarrheas, diabetic diarrhea, or cryptosporidiosis.

Octreotide: This somatostatin analog stimulates intestinal fluid and electrolyte absorption and inhibits intestinal fluid secretion and the release of GI peptides. It is given for secretory diarrheas due to neuroendocrine tumors (VIPomas, carcinoid). Effective doses range from 50 mcg to 250 mcg subcutaneously three times daily.

Bile salt binders: Cholestyramine 2–4 g or colestipol (1–2 g once to three times daily) or colesevelam (625 mg, 1–3 tablets once or twice daily) may be useful in patients with bile salt-induced diarrhea, which may be idiopathic or secondary to intestinal resection or ileal disease.

Borup C et al. Biochemical diagnosis of bile acid diarrhea: prospective comparison with the ^{75}Seleno-taurohomocholic acid test. Am J Gastroenterol. 2020;115:2086. [PMID: 32740083]

Burgers K et al. Chronic diarrhea in adults: evaluation and differential diagnosis. Am Fam Physician. 2020;15:472. [PMID: 32293842]

Howe JR et al. North American Neuroendocrine Tumor Society consensus paper on the surgical management of pancreatic neuroendocrine tumors. Pancreas. 2020;49:1. [PMID: 31856076]

Sadowski DC et al. Canadian Association of Gastroenterology clinical practice guideline on the management of bile acid diarrhea. Clin Gastroenterol Hepatol. 2020;18:24. [PMID: 31526844]

GI BLEEDING

1. Acute Upper GI Bleeding

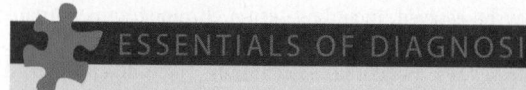

- Hematemesis (bright red blood or "coffee grounds").
- Melena in most cases; hematochezia in massive upper GI bleeds.
- Volume status to determine severity of blood loss; hematocrit is a poor early indicator of blood loss.
- Endoscopy diagnostic and may be therapeutic.

General Considerations

There are over 250,000 hospitalizations a year in the United States for acute upper GI bleeding. In the United States, the mortality rate for nonvariceal upper GI bleeding has declined steadily over the past 20 years to 2.1%. Mortality is higher in patients who are older than age 60 years and in patients in whom bleeding develops during hospitalization. Patients seldom die of exsanguination but rather of complications from an underlying disease.

The most common presentation of upper GI bleeding is hematemesis or melena. Hematemesis may be either bright red blood or brown "coffee grounds" material. Melena develops after as little as 50–100 mL of blood loss in the upper GI tract, whereas hematochezia requires a loss of more than 1000 mL. Although hematochezia generally suggests a lower bleeding source (eg, colonic), severe upper GI bleeding may present with hematochezia in 10% of cases.

Upper GI bleeding is self-limited in 80% of patients; urgent medical therapy and endoscopic evaluation are obligatory in the rest. Patients with bleeding more than 48 hours prior to presentation have a low risk of recurrent bleeding.

Etiology

Peptic ulcers account for 40% of major upper GI bleeding with an overall mortality rate of less than 5%. In North America, the incidence of bleeding from ulcers is declining due to eradication of *H pylori* and prophylaxis with PPIs in high-risk patients.

Portal hypertension accounts for 10–20% of upper GI bleeding. Bleeding usually arises from esophageal varices and less commonly gastric or duodenal varices or portal hypertensive gastropathy. Approximately 25% of patients with cirrhosis have medium to large esophageal varices, of whom 30% experience acute variceal bleeding within a 2-year period. Due to improved care, the hospital mortality rate has declined over the past 20 years from 40% to 15%. Nevertheless, a mortality rate of 60–80% is expected at 1–4 years due to recurrent bleeding or other complications of chronic liver disease.

Lacerations of the gastroesophageal junction cause 5–10% of cases of upper GI bleeding. Many patients report a history of heavy alcohol use or retching. Less than 10% have continued or recurrent bleeding.

Vascular anomalies are found throughout the GI tract and may be the source of chronic or acute GI bleeding. They account for 7% of cases of acute upper tract bleeding. The most common are **angioectasias** (angiodysplasias), which are 1–10 mm distorted, aberrant submucosal vessels caused by chronic, intermittent obstruction of submucosal veins. They have a bright red stellate appearance and occur throughout the GI tract but most commonly in the right colon. **Telangiectasias** are small, cherry red lesions caused by dilation of venules that may be part of systemic conditions (hereditary hemorrhagic telangiectasia, CREST syndrome) or occur sporadically. The **Dieulafoy lesion** is an aberrant, large-caliber submucosal artery, most commonly in the proximal stomach that causes recurrent, intermittent bleeding.

Gastric neoplasms cause about 1% of upper GI hemorrhages.

Erosive gastritis is superficial, so it is a relatively unusual cause of severe GI bleeding (less than 5% of cases) and more commonly results in chronic blood loss. Gastric mucosal erosions are due to NSAIDs, alcohol, or severe medical or surgical illness (stress-related mucosal disease).

Severe erosive esophagitis due to chronic gastroesophageal reflux may rarely cause significant upper GI bleeding, especially in patients who are bedbound long-term.

An aortoenteric fistula complicates 2% of abdominal aortic grafts or, rarely, can occur as the initial presentation of a previously untreated aneurysm. Unusual causes of upper GI bleeding include hemobilia (from hepatic tumor, angioma, penetrating trauma), and pancreatic malignancy and pseudoaneurysm (hemosuccus pancreaticus).

Initial Evaluation & Treatment

A. Stabilization

The initial step is assessment of the hemodynamic status. A systolic blood pressure lower than 100 mm Hg identifies a high-risk patient with severe acute bleeding. A heart rate over 100 beats/minute with a systolic blood pressure over 100 mm Hg signifies moderate acute blood loss. A normal systolic blood pressure and heart rate suggest relatively minor hemorrhage. Postural hypotension and tachycardia are useful when present but may be due to causes other than blood loss. Because the hematocrit may take 24–72 hours to equilibrate with the extravascular fluid, it is not a reliable indicator of the severity of acute bleeding.

In patients with significant bleeding, two 18-gauge or larger intravenous lines should be started prior to further diagnostic tests. Blood is sent for CBC, prothrombin time with INR, serum creatinine, liver enzymes, and blood typing and screening (in anticipation of the possible need for transfusion). In patients without hemodynamic compromise or overt active bleeding, aggressive fluid repletion can be delayed until the extent of the bleeding is further clarified. Patients with evidence of hemodynamic compromise are given 0.9% saline or lactated Ringer infusion and cross-matched for 2–4 U of packed RBCs. It is rarely necessary to administer type-specific or O-negative blood.

Central venous pressure monitoring is desirable in some cases, but line placement should not interfere with rapid volume resuscitation.

Placement of a nasogastric tube is not routinely recommended in clinical guidelines but may be helpful in the initial assessment and triage of selected patients with suspected active upper tract bleeding. The aspiration of red blood or "coffee grounds" confirms an upper GI source of bleeding, though up to 18% of patients with confirmed upper tract sources of bleeding have nonbloody aspirates—especially when bleeding originates in the duodenum. Erythromycin (250 mg) administered intravenously 30 minutes prior to upper endoscopy promotes gastric emptying and may improve the quality of endoscopic evaluation when substantial amounts of blood or clot in the stomach is suspected. Efforts to stop or slow bleeding by gastric lavage with large volumes of fluid are of no benefit and expose the patient to an increased risk of aspiration.

B. Blood Replacement

The amount of fluid and blood products required is based on assessment of vital signs, evidence of active bleeding from nasogastric aspirate, and laboratory tests. In patients who are hemodynamically stable, a restrictive policy for RBC transfusion is recommended utilizing a threshold of less than 7 g/dL in most patients but less than 8 g/dL in patients with known CVD. In the absence of continued bleeding, the hemoglobin should rise approximately 1 g/dL for each unit of transfused packed RBCs. Sufficient packed RBCs should be given to maintain a hemoglobin of 7–9 g/dL. In patients with severe GI bleeding, it is desirable to transfuse blood before the hemoglobin reaches 7 g/dL to prevent decreases below that level occurring from hemodilution with fluid resuscitation. Transfusion of blood should not be withheld from patients with massive active bleeding regardless of the hemoglobin value. In actively bleeding patients, platelets are transfused if the platelet count is under 50,000/mcL (50×10^9/L) and considered if there is impaired platelet function due to aspirin or clopidogrel use (regardless of the platelet count). Uremic patients (who also have dysfunctional platelets) with active bleeding are given three doses of desmopressin (DDAVP), 0.3 mcg/kg intravenously, at 12-hour intervals. In patients with active bleeding who have been taking anticoagulation therapy, the benefits of reversal of anticoagulation (reduced bleeding and reduced need for blood products) must be weighed against the risks (thromboembolism, ischemia). In general, endoscopy may be performed safely and effective hemostasis treatment applied if the INR is less than 2.5. In patients taking warfarin, anticoagulation with active bleeding and INR greater than 2.5, either fresh frozen plasma or four factor prothrombin complex (Kcentra®) may be administered. In the face of massive bleeding, administration of four factor prothrombin complex concentrates is preferred (rather than fresh frozen plasma) because it is more rapid and effective at correcting the INR and requires a smaller volume. In patients receiving anticoagulation therapy with the direct thrombin inhibitor (dabigatran) or factor Xa inhibitors (rivaroxaban, apixaban, edoxaban), restoration of normal anticoagulation usually requires 24–48 hours (presuming normal kidney and liver function). Therefore, reversal should only be considered in patients with life-threatening bleeding. Idarucizumab (an intravenous monoclonal antibody) is approved for the reversal of dabigatran, and andexanet alfa (a modified factor Xa decoy protein) is approved for the reversal of apixaban and rivaroxaban. For management of coagulation abnormalities in patients with cirrhosis and upper GI bleeding, see Esophageal Varices.

C. Initial Triage

A preliminary assessment of risk based on several clinical factors aids in the resuscitation as well as the rational triage of the patient. Clinical predictors of increased risk of further bleeding and death include liver disease, heart failure, syncope, systolic blood pressure less than 110 mm Hg, pulse greater than 100 beats/minute, bright red blood in the nasogastric aspirate or on rectal examination, and initial hemoglobin less than 13 g/dL (in men) or less than 12 g/dL (in women).

1. High risk—Patients with active bleeding manifested by hematemesis or bright red blood on nasogastric aspirate, shock, persistent hemodynamic derangement despite fluid resuscitation, serious comorbid medical illness, or evidence of advanced liver disease require admission to an ICU. Endoscopy should be performed within 12–24 hours in most patients, but only after adequate hemodynamic resuscitation and management of other active comorbidities (eg, acute coronary syndrome). In a large randomized controlled trial of patients with acute upper GI bleeding deemed at high risk for recurrent bleeding or death, there was no difference in 30-day mortality among patients in whom endoscopy was performed within 6 hours versus within 6–24 hours.

2. Low to moderate risk—All other patients are admitted to an observation unit, medical ward, or step-down unit after appropriate stabilization for further evaluation and treatment. Patients without evidence of active bleeding undergo nonemergent endoscopy, usually within 24 hours.

Subsequent Evaluation & Treatment

Specific treatment of the various causes of upper GI bleeding is discussed elsewhere in this chapter. The following general comments apply to most patients with bleeding.

The clinician's impression of the bleeding source is correct in only 40% of cases. Signs of chronic liver disease implicate bleeding due to portal hypertension, but a different lesion is identified in 25% of patients with cirrhosis. A history of dyspepsia, NSAID use, or peptic ulcer disease suggests peptic ulcer. Acute bleeding preceded by heavy alcohol ingestion or retching suggests a Mallory-Weiss tear, though most patients with Mallory-Weiss tears have neither.

A. Upper Endoscopy

Virtually all patients with upper tract bleeding should undergo upper endoscopy within 24 hours of arriving in the emergency department. The benefits of endoscopy in this setting are threefold.

1. To identify the source of bleeding—The appropriate acute and long-term medical therapy is determined by the cause of bleeding. Patients with portal hypertension will be treated differently from those with ulcer disease. If surgery or radiologic interventional therapy is required for uncontrolled bleeding, the source of bleeding identified at endoscopy will determine the approach.

2. To determine the risk of rebleeding and guide triage—Patients with a nonbleeding Mallory-Weiss tear, esophagitis, gastritis, and ulcers that have a clean, white base have a very low risk (less than 5%) of rebleeding. Patients with one of these findings who are younger than 60 years, without hemodynamic instability or transfusion requirement, without serious coexisting illness, and who have stable social support may be discharged from the emergency department or medical ward after endoscopy with outpatient follow-up. All others with one of these low-risk lesions should be observed on a medical ward for 24–48 hours. Patients with ulcers that are actively bleeding or have a visible vessel or adherent clot, or who have variceal bleeding usually require at least a 3-day hospitalization with closer initial observation in an ICU or step-down unit.

3. To render endoscopic therapy—Hemostasis can be achieved in actively bleeding lesions with endoscopic modalities such as cautery, injection, or endoclips. About 90% of bleeding or nonbleeding varices can be effectively treated immediately with application of rubber bands to the varices. Similarly, 90% of bleeding ulcers, angiomas, or Mallory-Weiss tears can be controlled with either endoscopic injection of epinephrine, direct cauterization of the vessel by a heater probe or multipolar electrocautery probe, clips, or application of a hemostatic powder spray (TC-325). Certain nonbleeding lesions, such as ulcers with visible blood vessels, and angioectasias are also treated with these therapies. Specific endoscopic therapy of varices, peptic ulcers, and Mallory-Weiss tears is dealt with elsewhere in this chapter.

B. Acute Pharmacologic Therapies

1. Acid inhibitory therapy—**Intravenous PPIs** (esomeprazole or pantoprazole, 80 mg bolus, followed by 8 mg/hours continuous infusion for 72 hours) reduce the risk of rebleeding in patients with peptic ulcers with high-risk features (active bleeding, visible vessel, or adherent clot) after endoscopic treatment. **Oral PPIs** (omeprazole, esomeprazole, or pantoprazole 40 mg; lansoprazole or dexlansoprazole 30–60 mg) once or twice daily are sufficient for lesions at low-risk for rebleeding (eg, esophagitis, gastritis, clean-based ulcers, and Mallory-Weiss tears).

Administration of continuous intravenous PPI *before* endoscopy results in a decreased number of ulcers with lesions that require endoscopic therapy. It therefore is standard clinical practice at many institutions to administer either an intravenous or a high-dose oral PPI prior to endoscopy in patients with significant upper GI bleeding. Based on the findings during endoscopy, the intravenous PPI may be continued or discontinued.

2. Octreotide—Continuous intravenous infusion of octreotide (100 mcg bolus, followed by 50–100 mcg/hour) reduces splanchnic blood flow and portal blood pressures and is effective in the initial control of bleeding related to portal hypertension. It is administered promptly to all patients with active upper GI bleeding and evidence of liver disease or portal hypertension until the source of bleeding can be determined by endoscopy. In countries where it is available, terlipressin may be preferred to octreotide for the treatment of bleeding related to portal hypertension because of its sustained reduction of portal and variceal pressures and its proven reduction in mortality.

C. Other Treatment

1. Intra-arterial embolization—Angiographic treatment is used in patients with persistent bleeding from ulcers, angiomas, or Mallory-Weiss tears who have failed endoscopic therapy and are poor operative risks. Compared with surgical intervention for recurrent or refractory bleeding, embolization achieves equivalent clinical success rates with lower mortality.

2. Transvenous intrahepatic portosystemic shunts (TIPS)—Placement of a wire stent from the hepatic vein through the liver to the portal vein provides effective decompression of the portal venous system and control of acute variceal bleeding. It is indicated in patients in whom endoscopic modalities have failed to control acute variceal bleeding.

Laine L et al. ACG Clinical Guideline: upper gastrointestinal and ulcer bleeding. Am J Gastroenterol. 2021;116:899. [PMID: 33929377]

Lau JY et al. Timing of endoscopy for acute upper gastrointestinal bleeding. N Engl J Med. 2020;382:1299. [PMID: 32242355]

Mullady DK et al. AGA Clinical Practice Update on endoscopic therapies for non-variceal upper gastrointestinal bleeding: expert review. Gastroenterology. 2020;159:1120. [PMID: 32574620]

2. Acute Lower GI Bleeding

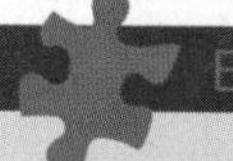

ESSENTIALS OF DIAGNOSIS

- Hematochezia usually present.
- Ten percent of cases of hematochezia due to upper GI source.
- Evaluation with colonoscopy in stable patients.
- Massive active bleeding calls for evaluation with CT angiography, followed by upper endoscopy, or angiography.

General Considerations

Lower GI bleeding is defined as that arising below the ligament of Treitz, ie, the small intestine or colon; however, up to 95% of cases arise from the colon. The severity of lower GI bleeding ranges from mild anorectal bleeding to massive, large-volume hematochezia. Bright red blood that drips into the bowl after a bowel movement or is mixed with solid brown stool signifies mild bleeding, usually from an anorectosigmoid source, and can be evaluated in the outpatient setting. In patients hospitalized with GI bleeding, lower tract bleeding is one-third as common as upper GI hemorrhage and tends to have a more benign course. Patients hospitalized with lower GI tract bleeding are less likely to present with shock or orthostasis (less than 5%) or to require transfusions (less than 40%). Spontaneous cessation of bleeding occurs in over 75% of cases, and hospital mortality is approximately 1%.

Etiology

The cause of these lesions depends on both the age of the patient and the severity of the bleeding. In patients under 50 years of age, the most common causes are infectious colitis, anorectal disease, and inflammatory bowel disease. In older patients, significant hematochezia is most often seen with diverticulosis, angioectasias, malignancy, or ischemia. There is an increased risk of lower GI bleeding in patients taking aspirin, nonaspirin antiplatelet agents, NSAIDs, and anticoagulants.

A. Diverticulosis

Hemorrhage occurs in 3–5% of all patients with diverticulosis and is the most common cause of major lower tract bleeding, accounting for over 50% of cases. Diverticular bleeding usually presents as acute, painless, large-volume maroon or bright red hematochezia in patients over age 50 years. More than 95% of cases require less than 4 units of blood transfusion. Bleeding subsides spontaneously in 80% but may recur in up to 25% of patients.

B. Angioectasias

Angioectasias (angiodysplasias) occur throughout the upper and lower intestinal tracts and cause painless bleeding ranging from melena or hematochezia to occult blood loss. They are responsible for 5% of cases of lower GI bleeding, where they are most often seen in the cecum and ascending colon. They are flat, red lesions (2–10 mm) with ectatic peripheral vessels radiating from a central vessel and are most common in patients over age 70 years and in those with CKD. Bleeding in younger patients more commonly arises from the small intestine.

Ectasias can be identified in up to 6% of persons over age 60 years, so the mere presence of ectasias does not prove that the lesion is the source of bleeding, since active bleeding is seldom seen.

C. Neoplasms

Benign polyps and malignant carcinomas are associated with chronic occult blood loss or intermittent anorectal hematochezia. They may cause up to 7% of acute lower GI hemorrhage.

After endoscopic removal of colonic polyps, important bleeding may occur up to 2 weeks later in 0.1–1% of patients overall but in 3–10% following mucosal resection of large (greater than 2 cm) polyps. In up to one-half of cases, colonoscopy is required to treat postpolypectomy hemorrhage and minimize the need for transfusions.

D. Inflammatory Bowel Disease

Patients with inflammatory bowel disease (especially ulcerative colitis) often have diarrhea with variable amounts of hematochezia. Bleeding varies from occult blood loss to recurrent hematochezia mixed with stool. Symptoms of abdominal pain, tenesmus, and urgency are often present.

E. Anorectal Disease

Anorectal disease (hemorrhoids, fissures) usually results in small amounts of bright red blood noted on the toilet paper, streaking of the stool, or dripping into the toilet bowl; clinically significant blood loss can sometimes occur. Hemorrhoids are the source in 10% of patients admitted with lower bleeding. Rectal ulcers may account for up to 8% of lower bleeding, usually in older adults or debilitated patients with constipation.

F. Ischemic Colitis

This condition is seen commonly in older patients, most of whom have atherosclerotic disease. Most cases occur spontaneously due to transient episodes of nonocclusive ischemia. Ischemic colitis may also occur in 5% of patients after surgery for ileoaortic aneurysm or an AAA. In younger patients, colonic ischemia may develop due to vasculitis, coagulation disorders, estrogen therapy, and long-distance running. Ischemic colitis results in hematochezia or bloody diarrhea associated with mild cramps. In most patients, the bleeding is mild and self-limited.

G. Others

Chronic radiation-induced changes in the rectum may cause anorectal bleeding that develops months to years after pelvic radiation of urologic, gynecologic, or anorectal malignancies. Endoscopy reveals multiple rectal vascular ectasias ("radiation proctopathy"). Acute infectious colitis (see Acute Diarrhea, above) commonly causes bloody diarrhea. Rare causes of lower tract bleeding include vasculitic ischemia, solitary rectal ulcer, NSAID-induced ulcers in the small bowel or right colon, small bowel diverticula, and colonic varices.

Clinical Findings

A. Symptoms and Signs

The color of the stool helps distinguish upper from lower GI bleeding, especially when observed by the clinician. Brown stools mixed or streaked with blood predict a source in the rectosigmoid or anus. Large volumes of bright red blood suggest a colonic source; maroon stools imply a lesion in the right colon or small intestine; and black stools (melena) predict a source proximal to the ligament of Treitz. Although 10% of patients admitted with self-reported hematochezia have an upper GI source of bleeding (eg, peptic ulcer), this almost always occurs in the setting of massive hemorrhage with hemodynamic instability. Painless large-volume bleeding usually suggests diverticular bleeding. Bloody diarrhea associated with cramping abdominal pain, urgency, or tenesmus is characteristic of inflammatory bowel disease, infectious colitis, or ischemic colitis.

B. Diagnostic Tests

Important considerations in management include exclusion of an upper tract source, anoscopy and sigmoidoscopy, colonoscopy, CT angiography and angiography, and small intestine push enteroscopy or capsule imaging. The studies selected depend on the severity of bleeding at presentation and the presence of hemodynamic instability with suspected ongoing, active bleeding.

1. Anoscopy and sigmoidoscopy—In otherwise healthy patients without anemia under age 45 years with small-volume bleeding, anoscopy and sigmoidoscopy are performed to look for evidence of anorectal disease, inflammatory bowel disease, or infectious colitis. If a lesion is found, no further evaluation is needed immediately unless the bleeding persists or is recurrent. In patients over age 45 years with small-volume hematochezia, the entire colon must be evaluated with colonoscopy to exclude tumor.

2. Colonoscopy—In patients with acute, large-volume bleeding requiring hospitalization, colonoscopy is the preferred initial study in most cases. A meta-analysis of four randomized trials comparing colonoscopy within 24 hours versus elective colonoscopy found that colonoscopy within 24 hours did not reduce length of stay, rebleeding, or mortality. Thus, for patients with stable vital signs and whose lower GI bleeding appears to have stopped (more than 75% of patients), colonoscopy can be performed electively during the hospital stay after appropriate resuscitation and bowel cleansing. For patients who are resuscitated and hemodynamically stable but have signs of continued active bleeding (less than 25% of patients), earlier colonoscopy (within 12–24 hours) can be considered after oral administration of colonic lavage solution (4–8 L of GoLytely, CoLYTE, or NuLyte) over 2–5 hours to clear the bowel of clots. The probable site of bleeding can be identified in 70–85% of patients, and a high-risk lesion can be identified and treated in up to 25%.

3. CT angiography—In patients with massive lower GI bleeding, hemodynamic instability, and suspected active bleeding, urgent radiographic imaging is warranted. Multidetector CT angiography is preferred to technetium-labeled RBC scanning to detect active arterial bleeding and to help localize bleeding to the stomach, upper GI tract, small intestine, right colon, or left colon. In patients with active bleeding demonstrated at CT angiography or in those not effectively treated at colonoscopy, urgent angiography is performed in an attempt to facilitate selective transcatheter embolization therapy.

4. Exclusion of an upper tract source—A nasogastric tube with aspiration should be considered, especially in patients with hemodynamic compromise. Aspiration of red blood or dark brown ("coffee grounds") guaiac-positive material strongly implicates an upper GI source of bleeding. Upper endoscopy should be performed in most patients presenting with hematochezia and hemodynamic instability to exclude an upper GI source, unless prior CT angiography has demonstrated a bleeding site in the lower GI tract.

Treatment

Initial stabilization, blood replacement, and triage are managed in the same manner as described above in Acute Upper GI Bleeding. In patients with ongoing bleeding, consideration should be given to temporary discontinuation of antiplatelet agents for up to 5 days and anticoagulants for 7 days. Compared to persons who do not take long-term low-dose aspirin, the incidence of recurrent lower GI bleeding within 5 years was higher in those who resumed low-dose aspirin postdischarge (18.9% vs 6.9%); however, these patients had a lower risk of serious cardiovascular events (22.8% vs 36.5%) and death (8.2% vs 26.7%).

A. Therapeutic Colonoscopy

High-risk lesions (eg, angioectasia or diverticulum, rectal ulcer with active bleeding, or a visible vessel) may be treated endoscopically with epinephrine injection, cautery (bipolar or heater probe), application of metallic endoclips or bands, or application of a hemostatic powder (TC-325). Radiation-associated vascular ectasias are effectively treated with cautery, preferably with an argon plasma coagulator or with radiofrequency wave ablation or with endorectal instillation of formalin.

B. Intra-arterial Embolization

When a bleeding lesion is identified, angiography with selective embolization achieves immediate hemostasis in more than 95% of patients. Major complications occur in 5% (mainly ischemic colitis) and rebleeding occurs in up to 25%.

C. Surgical Treatment

Emergency surgery is rarely required with acute lower GI bleeding due to the efficacy of colonoscopic and angiographic therapies.

Surgery may be considered in patients with recurrent diverticular hemorrhage depending on the severity of bleeding and the patient's other comorbid conditions.

Expert Panel on Interventional Radiology; Karuppasamy K et al. ACR Appropriateness Criteria®. Radiologic management of lower gastrointestinal bleeding: 2021 update. J Am Coll Radiol. 2021;18:S139. [PMID: 33958109]

Furtado FS et al. Endorectal instillation or argon plasma coagulation for hemorrhagic radiation proctopathy therapy: a prospective and randomized clinical trial. Gastrointest Endosc. 2021;93:1393. [PMID: 33220297]

Niikura R et al. Efficacy and safety of early vs elective colonoscopy for acute lower gastrointestinal bleeding. Gastroenterology. 2020;158:168. [PMID: 31563627]
Triantafyllou K et al. Diagnosis and management of acute lower gastrointestinal bleeding: European Society of Gastrointestinal Endoscopy (ESGE) guideline. Endoscopy. 2021;53:850. [PMID: 34062566]
Tsay C et al. Early colonoscopy does not improve outcomes of patients with lower gastrointestinal bleeding: systematic review of randomized trials. Clin Gastroenterol Hepatol. 2020;18:1696. [PMID: 31843595]

3. Suspected Small Bowel Bleeding

Bleeding from the small intestine can be overt or occult. *Overt* small bowel bleeding manifests as melena, maroon stools, or bright red blood per rectum. Up to 5–10% of patients admitted to hospitals with clinically overt GI bleeding do not have a cause identified on upper endoscopy or colonoscopy and may be suspected to have a small bowel source. In up to one-fourth of cases, however, a source of bleeding has been overlooked in the upper or lower tract on prior endoscopic studies. *Occult* small bowel bleeding refers to bleeding that is manifested by recurrent positive FOBTs or FITs or recurrent iron deficiency anemia, or both in the absence of visible blood loss.

Evaluation of Suspected Overt Small Bowel Bleeding

The likely etiology of overt small bowel bleeding depends on the age of the patient. The most common causes of small intestinal bleeding in patients younger than 40 years are neoplasms (stromal tumors, lymphomas, adenocarcinomas, carcinoids), Crohn disease, celiac disease, and Meckel diverticulum. These disorders also occur in patients over age 40; however, angioectasias and NSAID-induced ulcers are far more common.

The evaluation of suspected overt small bowel bleeding depends on the age and overall health status of the patient, associated symptoms, and severity of the bleeding. Before pursuing evaluation of the small intestine, upper endoscopy and colonoscopy are often repeated to ascertain that a lesion in these regions has not been overlooked. Repeat upper endoscopy should be performed with a longer instrument (usually a colonoscope) to evaluate the distal duodenum. If these studies are unrevealing and the patient is hemodynamically stable, capsule endoscopy should be performed to evaluate the small intestine. Further management depends on the capsule endoscopic findings, most commonly, angioectasias (25%), ulcers (10–25%), and neoplasms (1–10%). Multiphasic CT enterography may be considered if capsule endoscopy is unrevealing, since it is more sensitive for the detection of small bowel neoplasms and can exclude hepatic or pancreatic sources of bleeding. Laparotomy is warranted if a small bowel tumor is identified by capsule endoscopy or radiographic studies. Most other lesions identified by capsule imaging can be further evaluated with enteroscopes that use overtubes with balloons to advance the scope through most of the small intestine in a forward and retrograde direction (balloon-assisted enteroscopy). Neoplasms can be biopsied or resected, and angioectasias may be cauterized.

For active, hemodynamically significant acute bleeding, multiphasic CT angiography may be useful to identify and localize active small bowel bleeding and guide subsequent urgent angiography with embolization. A nuclear scan for Meckel diverticulum should be obtained in patients under age 30. With the advent of capsule imaging and advanced endoscopic technologies for evaluating and treating bleeding lesions in the small intestine, intraoperative enteroscopy of the small bowel is seldom required.

4. Occult GI Bleeding

Occult GI bleeding refers to bleeding that is not apparent to the patient. Chronic GI blood loss of less than 100 mL/day may cause no appreciable change in stool appearance. Thus, occult bleeding in an adult is identified by a positive FOBT, FIT, or by iron deficiency anemia in the absence of visible blood loss. FOBT or FIT may be performed in patients with GI symptoms or as a screening test for colorectal neoplasia (see Chapter 39). From 2% to 6% of patients in screening programs have a positive FOBT or FIT.

In the United States, 2% of men and 5% of women have iron deficiency anemia (serum ferritin less than 30–45 mcg/L). In premenopausal women, iron deficiency anemia is most commonly attributable to menstrual and pregnancy-associated iron loss; however, a GI source of chronic blood loss is present in 10%. Occult blood loss may arise from anywhere in the GI tract. Among men and postmenopausal women, a potential GI cause of blood loss can be identified in the colon in 15–30% and in the upper GI tract in 35–55%; a malignancy is present in the lower GI tract in 8.9% and upper tract in 2.0%. Iron deficiency on rare occasions is caused by malabsorption (especially celiac disease) or malnutrition. The most common causes of occult bleeding with iron deficiency are (1) neoplasms; (2) vascular abnormalities (angioectasias); (3) acid-peptic lesions (esophagitis, peptic ulcer disease, erosions in hiatal hernia); (4) infections (nematodes, especially hookworm; tuberculosis); (5) medications (especially NSAIDs or aspirin); and (6) other causes such as inflammatory bowel disease.

Evaluation of Occult Bleeding

Asymptomatic adults with positive FOBTs or FITs that are performed for routine colorectal cancer screening should undergo colonoscopy (see Chapter 39). All symptomatic adults with positive FOBTs or FITs or iron deficiency anemia should undergo evaluation of the lower and upper GI tract with colonoscopy and upper endoscopy, unless the anemia can be definitively ascribed to a nongastrointestinal source (eg, menstruation, blood donation, or recent surgery). Patients with iron deficiency anemia should be evaluated for possible celiac disease with either IgA anti-tTG or duodenal biopsy. After evaluation of the upper and lower GI tract with upper endoscopy and colonoscopy, the origin of occult bleeding remains unexplained in 30–50% of patients. In some of these patients, a source for occult bleeding from a small intestine source is suspected.

For patients with iron deficiency anemia who have no significant findings on upper endoscopy or colonoscopy and who are without symptoms of small intestinal disease, a 2020 AGA guideline recommends an initial trial of empiric iron therapy. Once daily administration of oral formulations containing 150 mg of elemental iron are commonly recommended, but lower daily doses (60–100 mg) or alternate day dosing may be equally efficacious and better tolerated. A sustained rise in ferritin and hemoglobin with 1–2 months of iron therapy may obviate the need for further studies.

Further investigation of the small intestine is recommended in patients who have anemia that responds poorly to empiric iron supplementation, who have signs of ongoing bleeding (fecal occult blood), or who have worrisome symptoms (abdominal pain, weight loss). Capsule endoscopy is recommended as the initial study in most patients to look for vascular ectasias and to exclude a small intestinal neoplasia or inflammatory bowel disease. If a small intestine source is identified, push enteroscopy, balloon-assisted enteroscopy, abdominal CT, angiography, or laparotomy is pursued, as indicated. When possible, antiplatelet agents (aspirin, NSAIDs, clopidogrel) should be discontinued. Patients with occult bleeding without a bleeding source identified after upper endoscopy, colonoscopy, and capsule endoscopy have a low risk of recurrent bleeding and usually can be managed with close observation.

Ko CW et al. AGA clinical practice guidelines on the gastrointestinal evaluation of iron deficiency anemia. Gastroenterology. 2020;159:1085. [PMID: 32810434]

Kuo JR et al. The clinician's guide to suspected small bowel bleeding. Am J Gastroenterol. 2019;114:591. [PMID: 30747768]

Ohmiya N et al. Development of a comorbidity index to identify patients with small bowel bleeding at risk for rebleeding and small bowel vascular diseases. Clin Gastroenterol Hepatol. 2019;17:896. [PMID: 30130626]

DISEASES OF THE PERITONEUM

ASSESSMENT OF THE PATIENT WITH ASCITES

Etiology of Ascites

The term "ascites" denotes the pathologic accumulation of fluid in the peritoneal cavity. Healthy men have little or no intraperitoneal fluid, but women normally may have up to 20 mL depending on the phase of the menstrual cycle. The causes of ascites may be classified into two broad pathophysiologic categories: that which is associated with a normal peritoneum and that which occurs due to a diseased peritoneum (Table 15–7). The most common cause of ascites is portal hypertension secondary to chronic liver disease, which accounts for over 80% of patients with ascites. The management of portal hypertensive ascites is discussed in Chapter 16. The most common causes of nonportal hypertensive ascites include infections (tuberculous peritonitis), intra-abdominal malignancy, inflammatory disorders of the peritoneum, and ductal disruptions (chylous, pancreatic, biliary).

Table 15–7. Causes of ascites.

Normal Peritoneum
Portal hypertension (SAAG ≥ 1.1 g/dL)
1. Hepatic congestion[1]
Heart failure
Constrictive pericarditis
Tricuspid insufficiency
Budd-Chiari syndrome
Veno-occlusive disease
2. Liver disease[2]
Cirrhosis
Alcoholic hepatitis
Fulminant hepatic failure
Massive hepatic metastases
Hepatic fibrosis
Acute fatty liver of pregnancy
3. Portal vein occlusion
4. Miscellaneous
Myxedema
Hypoalbuminemia (SAAG < 1.1 g/dL)
Nephrotic syndrome
Protein-losing enteropathy
Severe malnutrition with anasarca
Miscellaneous conditions (SAAG < 1.1 g/dL)
Chylous ascites
Pancreatic ascites
Bile ascites
Nephrogenic ascites
Urine ascites
Ovarian disease
Diseased peritoneum (SAAG < 1.1 g/dL)[2]
Infections
Bacterial peritonitis
Tuberculous peritonitis
Fungal peritonitis
HIV-associated peritonitis
Malignant conditions
Peritoneal carcinomatosis
Primary mesothelioma
Pseudomyxoma peritonei
Massive hepatic metastases
Hepatocellular carcinoma
Other conditions
Familial Mediterranean fever
Vasculitis
Granulomatous peritonitis
Eosinophilic peritonitis

[1]Hepatic congestion is usually associated with SAAG ≥ 1.1 g/dL and ascitic fluid total protein > 2.5 g/dL.

[2]There may be cases of "mixed ascites" in which portal hypertensive ascites is complicated by a secondary process such as infection. In these cases, the SAAG is ≥ 1.1 g/dL.

SAAG, serum-ascites albumin gradient = serum albumin minus ascitic fluid albumin.

Clinical Findings

A. Symptoms and Signs

The history usually is one of increasing abdominal girth, with the presence of abdominal pain depending on the cause. Because most ascites is secondary to chronic liver disease with portal hypertension, patients should be asked about risk factors for liver disease, especially alcohol consumption, transfusions, tattoos, injection drug use, a history of viral hepatitis or jaundice, and birth in an area endemic for hepatitis. A history of cancer or marked weight loss arouses suspicion of malignant ascites. Fevers may suggest infected peritoneal fluid, including bacterial peritonitis (spontaneous or secondary). Patients with chronic liver disease and ascites are at greatest risk for developing spontaneous bacterial peritonitis. In immigrants, immunocompromised hosts, or severely malnourished alcoholics, tuberculous peritonitis should be considered.

Physical examination should look for signs of portal hypertension and chronic liver disease. Elevated jugular venous pressure may suggest right-sided heart failure or constrictive pericarditis. A large tender liver is characteristic of acute alcoholic hepatitis or Budd-Chiari syndrome (thrombosis of the hepatic veins). Large abdominal wall veins with cephalad flow suggest portal hypertension; inferiorly directed flow implies hepatic vein obstruction. Signs of chronic liver disease include palmar erythema, cutaneous spider angiomas, gynecomastia, muscle wasting and asterixis from hepatic encephalopathy. Anasarca results from heart failure or nephrotic syndrome with hypoalbuminemia. Finally, firm lymph nodes in the left supraclavicular region or umbilicus suggest intra-abdominal malignancy.

The physical examination is relatively insensitive for detecting ascitic fluid. In general, patients must have at least 1500 mL of fluid to be detected reliably by this method. Even the experienced clinician may find it difficult to distinguish between obesity and small-volume ascites. Abdominal ultrasound establishes the presence of fluid.

B. Laboratory Testing

1. Abdominal paracentesis—Abdominal paracentesis is performed as part of the diagnostic evaluation in all patients with new onset of ascites to help determine the cause. It also is recommended for patients admitted to the hospital with cirrhosis and ascites (in whom the prevalence of bacterial peritonitis is 10–20%) and when patients with known ascites deteriorate clinically (with fever, abdominal pain, worsened hepatic encephalopathy or worsened kidney function) to exclude bacterial peritonitis.

A. INSPECTION—Cloudy ascitic fluid is seen with infection. Milky fluid indicates chylous ascites (due to hypertriglyceridemia). Bloody fluid suggests either a traumatic paracentesis or malignant ascites (in up to 20% of cases).

B. ROUTINE STUDIES—

(1) Cell count—An ascitic WBC count with differential is the most important test. Normal ascitic fluid contains less than 500 leukocytes/mcL (0.5×10^9/L) and less than 250 polymorphonuclear neutrophils (PMNs)/mcL. Any inflammatory condition can cause an elevated ascitic WBC count. A PMN count of greater than 250/mcL (0.25×10^9/L) (neutrocytic ascites) with a PMN percentage of more than 75% of all white cells is highly suggestive of bacterial peritonitis, either spontaneous primary peritonitis or secondary peritonitis (due to an intra-abdominal source of infection, eg, a perforated viscus or appendicitis). An elevated WBC with a predominance of lymphocytes arouses suspicion of tuberculosis or peritoneal carcinomatosis.

(2) Albumin and total protein—The serum-ascites albumin gradient (SAAG) is the best single test for the classification of ascites into portal hypertensive and nonportal hypertensive causes (Table 15–7). Calculated by subtracting the ascitic fluid albumin from the serum albumin, the gradient correlates directly with the portal pressure. An SAAG of 1.1 g/dL or more suggests underlying portal hypertension, while gradients less than 1.1 g/dL implicate nonportal hypertensive causes.

The accuracy of the SAAG exceeds 95% in classifying ascites. It should be recognized, however, that approximately 4% of patients have "mixed ascites," ie, underlying cirrhosis with portal hypertension complicated by a second cause for ascites formation (such as malignancy or tuberculosis). Thus, a high SAAG is indicative of portal hypertension but does not exclude concomitant malignancy.

The ascitic fluid total protein provides some additional clues to the cause. An elevated SAAG and a high protein level (greater than 2.5 g/dL) are seen in most cases of hepatic congestion secondary to cardiac disease or Budd-Chiari syndrome. However, a high ascitic fluid protein is also found in up to 20% of cases of uncomplicated cirrhosis and in two-thirds of patients with malignant ascites.

(3) Culture and Gram stain—The best technique consists of the inoculation of aerobic and anaerobic blood culture bottles with 5–10 mL of ascitic fluid at the patient's bedside, which increases the sensitivity for detecting bacterial peritonitis to over 85% in patients with neutrocytic ascites (greater than 250 PMNs/mcL [0.25×10^9/L]), compared with approximately 50% sensitivity by conventional agar plate or broth cultures.

C. OPTIONAL STUDIES—Other ascitic fluid laboratory tests of utility include glucose and LD (helpful in distinguishing spontaneous from secondary bacterial peritonitis); amylase (elevation suggests pancreatic ascites or perforation of the GI tract with leakage of pancreatic secretions); and creatinine (suggests leakage of urine from the bladder or ureters). An ascitic bilirubin concentration that is greater than the serum bilirubin suggests perforation of the biliary tree. Ascitic fluid cytologic examination is ordered if peritoneal carcinomatosis is suspected. Adenosine deaminase may be useful for the diagnosis of tuberculous peritonitis.

C. Imaging

Abdominal ultrasound is useful in confirming presence of ascites and in guiding paracentesis. Both ultrasound and CT imaging are useful in distinguishing between causes of portal and nonportal hypertensive ascites. Doppler ultrasound and CT can detect Budd-Chiari syndrome. In patients with nonportal hypertensive ascites, these studies are useful in detecting lymphadenopathy and masses in the mesentery, liver, ovaries, and pancreas. Furthermore, they permit directed percutaneous needle biopsies of these lesions. However, ultrasound and CT are not useful for detecting peritoneal carcinomatosis; the role of PET imaging is unclear.

D. Laparoscopy

In evaluating some patients with nonportal hypertensive ascites (low SAAG) or mixed ascites, laparoscopy permits direct visualization and biopsy of the peritoneum, liver, and some intra-abdominal lymph nodes. Cases of suspected peritoneal tuberculosis or suspected malignancy with nondiagnostic CT imaging and ascitic fluid cytology are best evaluated by laparoscopy.

Aithal GP et al. Guidelines on the management of ascites in cirrhosis. Gut. 2021;70:9. [PMID: 33067334]

SPONTANEOUS BACTERIAL PERITONITIS

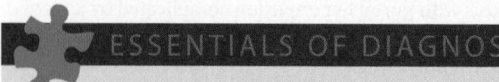

- A history of chronic liver disease and ascites.
- Fever and abdominal pain.
- Peritoneal signs uncommonly encountered on examination.
- Ascitic fluid neutrophil count > 250 WBCs/mcL (0.25×10^9/L).

General Considerations

"Spontaneous" bacterial infection of ascitic fluid occurs in the absence of an apparent intra-abdominal source of infection. It is seen with few exceptions in patients with ascites caused by chronic liver disease. Translocation of enteric bacteria across the gut wall or mesenteric lymphatics leads to seeding of the ascitic fluid, as may bacteremia from other sites. Approximately 20–30% of cirrhotic patients with ascites develop spontaneous peritonitis; however, the incidence is greater than 40% in patients with ascitic fluid total protein less than 1 g/dL, probably due to decreased ascitic fluid opsonic activity.

Virtually all cases of spontaneous bacterial peritonitis are caused by a monomicrobial infection. The most common pathogens are enteric gram-negative bacteria (*E coli, Klebsiella pneumoniae*) or gram-positive bacteria (*Streptococcus pneumoniae*, viridans streptococci, *Enterococcus* species). Anaerobic bacteria are not associated with spontaneous bacterial peritonitis.

Clinical Findings

A. Symptoms and Signs

Spontaneous bacterial peritonitis is symptomatic in 80–90% of patients; fever and abdominal pain are the most common symptoms (present in two-thirds). In many cases, however, the presentation is subtle (eg, a change in mental status due to precipitation or exacerbation of hepatic encephalopathy or a sudden worsening of kidney function).

Physical examination typically demonstrates signs of chronic liver disease with ascites. Abdominal tenderness is present in less than 50% of patients, and its presence suggests other processes. Spontaneous bacterial peritonitis may be present in 10–20% of patients hospitalized with chronic liver disease, sometimes in the absence of any suggestive symptoms or signs.

B. Laboratory Findings

The most important diagnostic test is abdominal paracentesis. Ascitic fluid should be sent for cell count with differential, and blood culture bottles should be inoculated at the bedside; Gram stain and reagent strips are insensitive.

In the proper clinical setting, an ascitic fluid PMN count of greater than 250 cells/mcL (neutrocytic ascites) is presumptive evidence of bacterial peritonitis. The percentage of PMNs is greater than 50–70% of the ascitic fluid WBCs and commonly approximates 100%. Patients with neutrocytic ascites are presumed to be infected and should be started—regardless of symptoms—on antibiotics. Although 10–30% of patients with neutrocytic ascites have negative ascitic bacterial cultures ("culture-negative neutrocytic ascites"), it is presumed that these patients nonetheless have bacterial peritonitis and should be treated empirically. Occasionally, a positive blood culture identifies the organism when ascitic fluid culture is negative.

Differential Diagnosis

Spontaneous bacterial peritonitis must be distinguished from secondary bacterial peritonitis, in which ascitic fluid has become secondarily infected by an intra-abdominal infection. Secondary bacterial infection accounts for 3% of cases of infected ascitic fluid. Causes include appendicitis, diverticulitis, perforated peptic ulcer, and perforated gallbladder. Even in the presence of perforation, clinical symptoms and signs of peritonitis may be lacking owing to the separation of the visceral and parietal peritoneum by the ascitic fluid.

Ascitic fluid total protein, LD, and glucose are useful in distinguishing spontaneous bacterial peritonitis from secondary infection. Up to two-thirds of patients with secondary bacterial peritonitis have at least two of the following: decreased glucose level (less than 50 mg/dL), elevated LD level (greater than serum), and elevated total protein (greater than 1 g/dL). Ascitic neutrophil counts greater than 10,000/mcL (10×10^9/L) also are suspicious; however, most patients with secondary peritonitis have neutrophil counts within the range of spontaneous peritonitis. The presence of multiple organisms on ascitic fluid Gram stain or culture is diagnostic of secondary peritonitis.

If secondary bacterial peritonitis is suspected, abdominal CT imaging of the upper and lower GI tracts should be obtained to look for evidence of an intra-abdominal source of infection. If these studies are negative and secondary peritonitis still is suspected, repeat paracentesis should be performed after 48 hours of antibiotic therapy to see if the PMN count is decreasing. In secondary bacterial peritonitis, the PMN count is not below the pretreatment value at 48 hours.

Neutrocytic ascites may also be seen in some patients with peritoneal carcinomatosis, pancreatic ascites, or tuberculous ascites. In these circumstances, however, PMNs account for less than 50% of the ascitic WBCs.

Prevention

Up to 70% of patients who survive an episode of spontaneous bacterial peritonitis will have another episode within 1 year. Oral once-daily prophylactic therapy with ciprofloxacin, 500 mg, or trimethoprim-sulfamethoxazole, one double-strength tablet, has been shown to reduce the rate of recurrent infections to less than 20%. Prophylaxis should be considered also in patients who have not had prior bacterial peritonitis but are at increased risk for infection due to low-protein ascites (total ascitic protein less than 1.5 g/dL) with impaired kidney function (serum creatinine 1.2 g/dL or higher) or decompensated cirrhosis (Child-Pugh class C). When used in appropriately selected high-risk patients, prophylactic antibiotics are associated with a lower risk of spontaneous bacterial peritonitis, hepatorenal syndrome, and mortality.

Treatment

Empiric therapy for spontaneous bacterial peritonitis should be initiated with a third-generation cephalosporin (such as cefotaxime, 2 g intravenously every 8–12 hours, or ceftriaxone, 1–2 g intravenously every 24 hours) or a combination beta-lactam/beta-lactamase agent (such as ampicillin/sulbactam, 2 g/1 g intravenously every 6 hours). Because of a high risk of nephrotoxicity in patients with chronic liver disease, aminoglycosides should not be used. Although the optimal duration of therapy is unknown, an empiric course of 5–10 days is recommended, or treatment until the ascites fluid PMN count decreases to less than 250 cells/mcL. For most infections, 5 days is sufficient; however, infections caused by more serious, virulent pathogens (*S aureus*, viridans streptococci, *Pseudomonas*, or Enterobacteriaceae) warrant 10 days of treatment. Patients without significant clinical improvement after 5 days should undergo repeat paracentesis to assess treatment efficacy. If the ascitic neutrophil count has not decreased by 25%, antibiotic coverage should be adjusted (guided by culture and sensitivity results, if available) and secondary causes of peritonitis excluded. If the ascitic PMN count has decreased but remains more than 250 cells/mcL, antibiotics should be continued for an additional 2–3 days before paracentesis is repeated. Patients with suspected secondary bacterial peritonitis should be given broad-spectrum coverage for enteric aerobic and anaerobic flora with a third-generation cephalosporin and metronidazole, pending identification and definitive (usually surgical) treatment of the cause.

Kidney injury develops in up to 40% of patients and is a major cause of death. Intravenous albumin increases effective arterial circulating volume and renal perfusion, decreasing both kidney injury and mortality. Intravenous albumin, 1.5 g/kg on day 1 and 1 g/kg on day 3, should be administered to patients at high risk for hepatorenal failure (ie, patients with baseline creatinine greater than 1 mg/dL, BUN greater than 30 mg/dL, or bilirubin greater than 4 mg/dL). Nonselective beta-blockers increase the risk of hepatorenal syndrome in patients with bacterial peritonitis. They should be discontinued permanently due to their adverse impact on cardiac output, renal perfusion, and long-term survival in advanced cirrhosis.

Prognosis

The mortality rate of spontaneous bacterial peritonitis is 25%, but if the disease is recognized and treated early, it is less than 10%. Since the majority of patients have underlying severe liver disease, many may die of liver failure, hepatorenal syndrome, or bleeding complications of portal hypertension. The most effective treatment for recurrent spontaneous bacterial peritonitis is liver transplantation.

Biggin S et al. Diagnosis, evaluation, and management of ascites, spontaneous bacterial peritonitis and hepatorenal syndrome: 2021 Practice Guidance by the American Association for the Study of Liver Disease. Hepatology. 2021;74:1014. [PMID: 33942342]

Fernandez J et al. Efficacy of albumin treatment for patients with cirrhosis and infections unrelated to spontaneous bacterial peritonitis. Clin Gastroenterol Hepatol. 2020;18:963. [PMID: 31394283]

Komolafe O et al. Antibiotic prophylaxis to prevent spontaneous bacterial peritonitis in people with liver cirrhosis: a network meta-analysis. Cochrane Database Syst Rev. 2020;1: CD013125. [PMID: 31978256]

MALIGNANT ASCITES

Two-thirds of cases of malignant ascites are caused by peritoneal carcinomatosis. The most common causes are primary adenocarcinomas of the ovary, uterus, pancreas, stomach, colon, lung, or breast. The remaining one-third is due to lymphatic obstruction or portal hypertension due to hepatocellular carcinoma or diffuse hepatic metastases. Patients present with nonspecific abdominal discomfort and weight loss associated with increased abdominal girth. Nausea or vomiting may be caused by partial or complete intestinal obstruction. Abdominal CT may be useful to demonstrate the primary malignancy or hepatic metastases but seldom confirms the diagnosis of peritoneal carcinomatosis. In patients with carcinomatosis, paracentesis demonstrates a low serum ascites-albumin gradient (less than 1.1 mg/dL), an increased total protein (greater than 2.5 g/dL), and an elevated WBC (often both neutrophils and mononuclear cells) but with a lymphocyte predominance. Cytology is positive in over 95%, but laparoscopy may be required in patients with negative cytology to confirm the diagnosis and to exclude tuberculous peritonitis, with which it may be confused. Malignant ascites attributable to portal hypertension usually is associated with an increased serum ascites-albumin gradient (greater than 1.1 g/dL), a variable total protein, and negative ascitic cytology. Ascites caused by peritoneal carcinomatosis does not respond to diuretics.

Patients may be treated with periodic large-volume paracentesis for symptomatic relief. Indwelling catheters can be left in place for patients approaching the end of life who require periodic paracentesis for symptomatic relief. Intraperitoneal chemotherapy is sometimes used to shrink the tumor, but the overall prognosis is extremely poor, with only 10% survival at 6 months. Ovarian cancers represent an exception to this rule. With newer treatments consisting of surgical debulking and intraperitoneal chemotherapy, long-term survival from ovarian cancer is possible.

Ba M et al. Cytoreductive surgery and HIPEC for malignant ascites from colorectal cancer—a randomized study. Medicine (Baltimore). 2020;99:e21546. [PMID: 32872001]

Bleicher J et al. A palliative approach to management of peritoneal carcinomatosis and malignant ascites. Surg Oncol Clin N Am. 2021;30:475. [PMID: 34053663]

Hodge C et al. Palliation of malignant ascites. J Surg Oncol. 2019;120:67. [PMID: 30903617]

FAMILIAL MEDITERRANEAN FEVER

This is a rare autosomal recessive disorder of unknown pathogenesis that almost exclusively affects people of Mediterranean ancestry, especially Sephardic Jews, Armenians, Turks, and Arabs. Patients lack a protease in serosal fluids that normally inactivates interleukin-8 and the chemotactic complement factor 5A. Symptoms present in most patients before the age of 20 years. It is characterized by episodic bouts of acute peritonitis that may be associated with serositis involving the joints and pleura. Peritoneal attacks are marked by the sudden onset of fever, severe abdominal pain, and abdominal tenderness with guarding or rebound tenderness. If left untreated, attacks resolve within 24–48 hours. Because symptoms resemble those of surgical peritonitis, patients may undergo unnecessary exploratory laparotomy. Colchicine, 0.6 mg orally two or three times daily, has been shown to decrease the frequency and severity of attacks.

Accetturo M. Improvement of *MEFV* gene variants classification to aid treatment decision making in familial Mediterranean fever. Rheumatology. 2020;59:754. [PMID: 31411330]

Bodur H et al. Familial Mediterranean fever: assessment of clinical manifestations, pregnancy, genetic mutational analyses, and disease severity in a national cohort. Rheumatol Int. 2020;40:29. [PMID: 31522233]

MESOTHELIOMA

(**See** Chapter 39.)

DISEASES OF THE ESOPHAGUS

(**See** Chapter 39 **for Esophageal Cancer.**)

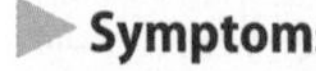

Symptoms

Heartburn, dysphagia, and odynophagia almost always indicate a primary esophageal disorder.

A. Heartburn

Heartburn (pyrosis) is the feeling of substernal burning, often radiating to the neck. Most commonly caused by the reflux of acidic (or, rarely, alkaline) material into the esophagus, heartburn is highly suggestive of GERD.

B. Dysphagia

Dysphagia is defined as difficulty swallowing food or liquid due to the sensation of it sticking in the throat or chest, with a discomfort, or a choking sensation. In a 2020 survey of US adults, 15% of adults reported recent dysphagia that required compensatory maneuvers (avoiding certain foods or cutting into smaller pieces; eating more slowly; drinking liquids). Up to one-half of these adults previously had sought evaluation for their symptoms. Difficulties in swallowing may arise from problems in transferring the food bolus from the oropharynx to the upper esophagus (oropharyngeal dysphagia) or from impaired transport of the bolus through the body of the esophagus (esophageal dysphagia). The history usually suggests the correct diagnosis.

1. Oropharyngeal dysphagia—The oropharyngeal phase of swallowing is a complex process requiring elevation of the tongue, closure of the nasopharynx, relaxation of the upper esophageal sphincter, closure of the airway, and pharyngeal peristalsis. A variety of mechanical and neuromuscular conditions can disrupt this process (Table 15–8). Problems with the oral phase of swallowing cause drooling or spillage of food from the mouth, inability to chew or initiate swallowing, or dry mouth. Pharyngeal dysphagia is characterized by an immediate sense of the bolus catching in the neck, the need to swallow repeatedly to clear food from the pharynx, or coughing or choking during meals. There may be associated dysphonia, dysarthria, or other neurologic symptoms.

Table 15–8. Causes of oropharyngeal dysphagia.

Neurologic disorders
Brainstem cerebrovascular accident, mass lesion
Amyotrophic lateral sclerosis, multiple sclerosis, pseudobulbar palsy, post-polio syndrome, Guillain-Barré syndrome
Parkinson disease, Huntington disease, dementia
Tardive dyskinesia
Muscular and rheumatologic disorders
Myopathies, polymyositis
Oculopharyngeal dystrophy
Sjögren syndrome
Metabolic disorders
Thyrotoxicosis, amyloidosis, Cushing disease, Wilson disease
Medication side effects: anticholinergics, phenothiazines
Infectious diseases
Polio, diphtheria, botulism, Lyme disease, syphilis, mucositis (*Candida*, herpes)
Structural disorders
Zenker diverticulum
Cervical osteophytes, cricopharyngeal bar, proximal esophageal webs
Oropharyngeal tumors
Postsurgical or radiation changes
Pill-induced injury
Motility disorders
Upper esophageal sphincter dysfunction

Table 15–9. Causes of esophageal dysphagia.

Cause	Clues
Mechanical obstruction	**Solid foods worse than liquids**
Schatzki ring	Intermittent dysphagia; not progressive
Peptic stricture	Chronic heartburn; progressive dysphagia
Esophageal cancer	Progressive dysphagia; age over 50 years
Eosinophilic esophagitis	Young adults; small-caliber lumen, proximal stricture, corrugated rings, or white papules
Motility disorder	**Solid and liquid foods**
Achalasia	Progressive dysphagia
Spastic esophageal disorders	Intermittent; not progressive; may have chest pain
Systemic sclerosis (scleroderma)	Chronic heartburn; Raynaud phenomenon
Ineffective esophageal motility	Intermittent; not progressive; commonly associated with GERD

2. Esophageal dysphagia—Esophageal dysphagia may be caused by **mechanical obstructions** of the esophagus or by **motility disorders** (Table 15–9). Patients with **mechanical obstruction** experience dysphagia, primarily for solids. This is recurrent, predictable, and, if the lesion progresses, will worsen as the lumen narrows. Patients with **motility disorders** have dysphagia for both solids and liquids. It is episodic, unpredictable, and can be progressive.

C. Odynophagia

Odynophagia is sharp substernal pain on swallowing that may limit oral intake. It usually reflects severe erosive disease. It is most commonly associated with infectious esophagitis due to *Candida*, herpesviruses, or CMV, especially in immunocompromised patients. It may also be caused by corrosive injury due to caustic ingestions and by pill-induced ulcers.

Diagnostic Studies

A. Upper Endoscopy

Endoscopy is the study of choice for evaluating persistent heartburn, dysphagia, odynophagia, and structural abnormalities detected on barium esophagography. In addition to direct visualization, it allows biopsy of mucosal abnormalities and of normal mucosa (to evaluate for eosinophilic esophagitis) as well as dilation of strictures.

B. Videoesophagography

Oropharyngeal dysphagia is best evaluated with rapid-sequence videoesophagography.

C. Barium Esophagography

Patients with esophageal dysphagia often are evaluated first with a barium esophagography to differentiate between mechanical lesions and motility disorders, providing important information about the latter in particular. In patients in whom there is a high suspicion of a mechanical lesion, many clinicians will proceed first to endoscopic evaluation because it better identifies mucosal lesions (eg, erosions) and permits mucosal biopsy and dilation. However, barium study is more sensitive for detecting subtle esophageal narrowing due to rings, achalasia, and proximal esophageal lesions.

D. Esophageal Manometry

Esophageal motility may be best assessed using high-resolution manometry with multiple, closely spaced sensors. Manometry is indicated (1) to determine the location of the LES to allow precise placement of a conventional electrode pH probe; (2) to establish the etiology of dysphagia in patients in whom a mechanical obstruction cannot be found, especially if a diagnosis of achalasia is suspected by endoscopy or barium study; and (3) for the preoperative assessment of patients being considered for antireflux surgery to exclude an alternative diagnosis (eg, achalasia) or possibly to assess peristaltic function in the esophageal body.

E. Esophageal pH Recording and Impedance Testing

The pH within the esophageal lumen may be monitored continuously for 24–48 hours. There are two kinds of systems in use: catheter-based and wireless. Catheter-based systems use a long transnasal catheter that is connected directly to the recording device. With wireless systems, a capsule is attached directly to the esophageal mucosa under endoscopic visualization and data are transmitted by radiotelemetry to the recording device. The recording provides information about the amount of esophageal acid reflux and the temporal correlations between symptoms and reflux.

Esophageal pH monitoring devices provide information about the amount of esophageal acid reflux but not nonacid reflux. Techniques using combined pH and multichannel intraluminal impedance allow assessment of acid and nonacid liquid reflux. They may be useful in evaluation of patients with atypical reflux symptoms or persistent symptoms despite therapy with PPIs to diagnose hypersensitivity, functional symptoms, and symptoms caused by nonacid reflux.

Adkins C et al. Prevalence and characteristics of dysphagia based on population-based survey. Clin Gastroenterol Hepatol. 2020;18:1970. [PMID: 31669055]

Gyawali CP et al. ACG Clinical Guidelines: clinical use of esophageal physiologic testing. Am J Gastroenterol. 2020;115:1412. [PMID: 32769426]

Yadlapati R et al. Esophageal motility disorders on high-resolution manometry: Chicago Classification version 4.0. Neurogastroenterol Motil. 2021;33:e14058. [PMID: 33373111]

GASTROESOPHAGEAL REFLUX DISEASE

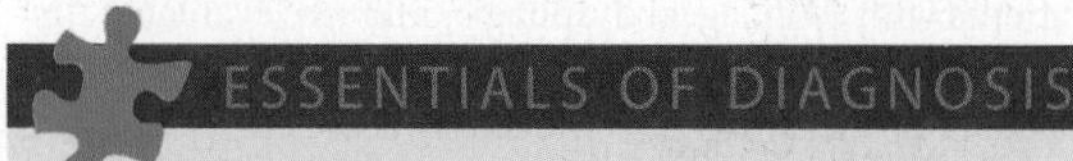

- Heartburn; may be exacerbated by meals, bending, or recumbency.
- Typical uncomplicated cases do not require diagnostic studies.
- Endoscopy demonstrates abnormalities in one-third of patients.

General Considerations

GERD is a condition that develops when the reflux of stomach contents causes troublesome symptoms or complications. In a 2020 survey of US adults, 31% reported GERD symptoms within the prior week. The two most common symptoms are heartburn and regurgitation. However, other symptoms of GERD include dyspepsia, dysphagia, belching, chest pain, cough, and hoarseness. Although most patients have mild disease, esophageal mucosal damage (reflux esophagitis) develops in up to one-third and more serious complications develop in a few others. Several factors may contribute to GERD.

A. Dysfunction of the Gastroesophageal Junction

The antireflux barrier at the gastroesophageal junction depends on LES pressure, the intra-abdominal location of the sphincter (resulting in a "flap valve" caused by angulation of the esophageal-gastric junction), and the extrinsic compression of the sphincter by the crural diaphragm. In most patients with GERD, baseline LES pressures are normal (10–35 mm Hg). Most reflux episodes occur during transient relaxations of the LES that are triggered by gastric distention by a vagovagal reflex. A subset of patients with GERD have an incompetent (less than 10 mm Hg) LES that results in increased acid reflux, especially when supine or when intra-abdominal pressures are increased by lifting or bending. A hypotensive sphincter is present in up to 50% of patients with severe erosive GERD.

Hiatal hernias are found in one-fourth of patients with nonerosive GERD, three-fourths of patients with severe erosive esophagitis, and over 90% of patients with Barrett esophagus. They are caused by movement of the LES above the diaphragm, resulting in dysfunction of the gastroesophageal junction reflux barrier. Hiatal hernias are common and may cause no symptoms; however, in patients with gastroesophageal reflux, they are associated with higher amounts of acid reflux and delayed esophageal acid clearance, leading to more severe esophagitis and Barrett esophagus. Increased reflux episodes occur during normal swallowing-induced relaxation, transient LES relaxations, and straining due to reflux of acid from the hiatal hernia sac into the esophagus.

Truncal obesity may contribute to GERD, presumably due to an increased intra-abdominal pressure, which contributes to dysfunction of the gastroesophageal junction and increased likelihood of hiatal hernia.

B. Irritant Effects of Refluxate

Esophageal mucosal damage is related to the potency of the refluxate and the amount of time it is in contact with the mucosa. Acidic gastric fluid (pH less than 4.0) is extremely caustic to the esophageal mucosa and is the major injurious agent in the majority of cases. In some patients, reflux of bile or alkaline pancreatic secretions may be contributory.

C. Abnormal Esophageal Clearance

Acid refluxate normally is cleared and neutralized by esophageal peristalsis and salivary bicarbonate. Patients with severe GERD may have diminished clearance due to hypotensive peristaltic contractions (less than 30 mm Hg) or intermittent failed peristalsis after swallowing. Certain medical conditions such as systemic sclerosis (scleroderma) are associated with diminished peristalsis. Sjögren syndrome, anticholinergic medications, and oral radiation therapy may exacerbate GERD due to impaired salivation.

D. Delayed Gastric Emptying

Impaired gastric emptying due to gastroparesis or partial gastric outlet obstruction potentiates GERD.

Clinical Findings

A. Symptoms and Signs

The typical symptom is heartburn. This most often occurs 30–60 minutes after meals and upon reclining. Patients often report relief from taking antacids or baking soda. When this symptom is dominant, the diagnosis is established with a high degree of reliability. Many patients, however, have less specific dyspeptic symptoms with or without heartburn. Overall, a clinical diagnosis of gastroesophageal reflux has a sensitivity and specificity of only 65%. Severity is not correlated with the degree of tissue damage. In fact, some patients with severe esophagitis are only mildly symptomatic. Patients may complain of regurgitation—the spontaneous reflux of sour or bitter gastric contents into the mouth. Dysphagia occurs in one-third of patients and may be due to erosive esophagitis, abnormal esophageal peristalsis, or the development of an esophageal stricture.

"Atypical" or "extraesophageal" manifestations of gastroesophageal disease may occur, including asthma, chronic cough, chronic laryngitis, sore throat, noncardiac chest pain, and sleep disturbances. In the absence of heartburn or regurgitation, atypical symptoms are unlikely to be related to gastroesophageal reflux.

Physical examination and laboratory data are normal in uncomplicated disease.

B. Special Examinations

Initial diagnostic studies are not warranted for patients with typical GERD symptoms suggesting uncomplicated reflux disease. Patients with typical symptoms of heartburn and regurgitation should be treated empirically with a twice-daily H_2-receptor antagonist or a once-daily PPI for 4–8 weeks. Further investigation is required in patients with symptoms that persist despite empiric acid inhibitory therapy to identify complications of reflux disease and to diagnose other conditions, particularly in patients with "alarm features" (troublesome dysphagia, odynophagia, weight loss, iron deficiency anemia).

1. Upper endoscopy—Upper endoscopy is excellent for documenting the type and extent of tissue damage in gastroesophageal reflux; for detecting other gastroesophageal lesions that may mimic GERD; and for detecting GERD complications, including esophageal stricture, Barrett metaplasia, and esophageal adenocarcinoma. In the absence of prior antisecretory therapy, up to one-third of patients with GERD have visible mucosal damage (known as reflux esophagitis), characterized by single or multiple erosions or ulcers in the distal esophagus at the squamocolumnar junction. In patients treated with a PPI prior to endoscopy, preexisting reflux esophagitis may be partially or completely healed. The Los Angeles (LA) classification grades reflux esophagitis on a scale of A (one or more isolated mucosal breaks 5 mm or less that do not extend between the tops of two mucosal folds) to D (one or more mucosal breaks that involve at least 75% of the esophageal circumference).

2. Barium esophagography—This study should not be performed to diagnose GERD. In patients with severe dysphagia, it is sometimes obtained prior to endoscopy to identify a stricture.

3. Esophageal pH or combined esophageal pH-impedance testing—Esophageal pH monitoring measures the amount of esophageal acid reflux, whereas combined pH-impedance testing measures both acidic and nonacidic reflux. Both tests may also be useful to establish whether there is a temporal relationship between reflux events and symptoms. They are the most accurate studies for documenting gastroesophageal reflux but are unnecessary in most patients who have typical symptoms and satisfactory response to empiric antisecretory therapy. They are indicated in patients with typical symptoms who have unsatisfactory response to empiric therapy, patients with atypical or extraesophageal symptoms, and patients who are being considered for antireflux surgery.

Differential Diagnosis

Symptoms of GERD may be similar to those of other diseases such as angina pectoris, eosinophilic esophagitis, esophageal motility disorders, dyspepsia, peptic ulcer, or functional disorders. Reflux erosive esophagitis may be confused with pill-induced damage, eosinophilic esophagitis, or infections (CMV, herpes, *Candida*).

Complications

A. Barrett Esophagus

This is a condition in which the squamous epithelium of the esophagus is replaced by metaplastic columnar epithelium containing goblet and columnar cells (specialized intestinal metaplasia). Present in 1.5% of the general population and 7–10% of patients with chronic reflux, Barrett esophagus is believed to arise from chronic reflux-induced injury to the esophageal squamous epithelium; however, it is also increased in patients with truncal obesity independent of GERD. Barrett esophagus is suspected at endoscopy from the presence of orange, gastric type epithelium that extends upward more than 1 cm from the gastroesophageal junction into the distal tubular esophagus in a tongue-like or circumferential fashion. Biopsies obtained at endoscopy confirm the diagnosis. Three types of columnar epithelium may be identified: gastric cardiac, gastric fundic, and specialized intestinal metaplasia. There is agreement that the latter carries an increased risk of dysplasia; however, some authorities believe that gastric cardiac mucosa also raises risk.

Barrett esophagus should be treated with long-term PPIs once or twice daily to control reflux symptoms. Although these medications do not appear to cause regression of Barrett esophagus, they may reduce the risk of cancer. Paradoxically, one-third of patients report minimal or no symptoms of GERD, suggesting decreased acid sensitivity of Barrett epithelium. Indeed, over 90% of individuals with Barrett esophagus in the general population do not seek medical attention.

The most serious complication of Barrett esophagus is esophageal adenocarcinoma. It is believed that most adenocarcinomas of the esophagus and many such tumors of the gastric cardia arise from dysplastic epithelium in Barrett esophagus. The incidence of adenocarcinoma in patients with Barrett esophagus is estimated at 0.2–0.5% per year. Although this still is an 11-fold increased risk compared with patients without Barrett esophagus, adenocarcinoma of the esophagus remains a relatively uncommon malignancy in the United States (9000 cases/year). Given the large number of adults with chronic GERD relative to the small number in whom adenocarcinoma develops and the costs and risks of upper endoscopy, a 2019 clinical guideline recommended against endoscopic screening for Barrett esophagus in adults with GERD except in those with one or more risk factors for adenocarcinoma (aged older than 50 years, truncal obesity, current or prior history of smoking, or male gender) or in adults with a family history of Barrett esophagus or esophageal adenocarcinoma.

In patients known to have nondysplastic Barrett esophagus, surveillance endoscopy every 3–5 years is recommended to look for low- or high-grade dysplasia or adenocarcinoma. During endoscopy, biopsies are obtained from nodular or irregular mucosa (which have an increased risk of high-grade dysplasia or cancer) as well as randomly from the esophagus every 1–2 cm. In a 2021 population-based study, initial surveillance endoscopy detected low-grade dysplasia in 10.6%, high-grade dysplasia in 3.1%, and esophageal cancer in 1.8%. In patients with nondysplastic Barrett esophagus, the risk of progression to high-grade dysplasia or cancer is related to the length of Barrett epithelium. This risk is 0.29%/year for those with columnar epithelium lengths of 1–3 cm (short-segment) and 0.91%/year in those with lengths greater than 3 cm (long-segment).

The finding of dysplasia should be confirmed by a second, expert pathologist. The detection of dysplasia is increased with use of the WATS (wide-area trans-epithelial sampling) technique in which a brush is deployed through the endoscope to obtain deep epithelial samples that are analyzed by a central laboratory computer.

Endoscopic therapy now is the standard of care for patients who have Barrett esophagus with dysplasia (low-grade, high-grade) or well-differentiated mucosal adenocarcinoma (Tis or T1a). Therapy should be performed by endoscopists with expertise in advanced resection and ablation techniques. All nodules should be removed with mucosal snare resection or dissection techniques to assess for the presence and depth of cancer. Following resection, ablation of any remaining Barrett mucosa—including flat (nonnodular) high-grade dysplasia—is performed with radiofrequency wave electrocautery or cryotherapy. Current guidelines also recommend that patients with flat *low-grade* dysplasia (confirmed by a second expert pathologist) also be considered for ablation, reserving annual endoscopic surveillance to patients with increased comorbidities and reduced life-expectancy. The efficacy of endoscopic ablation therapies in patients with Barrett dysplasia is supported by several studies. When high-dose PPIs are administered to normalize intraesophageal pH, radiofrequency wave ablation electrocautery eradication of Barrett columnar epithelium is followed by complete healing with normal squamous epithelium in greater than 78% of patients and elimination of dysplasia in 91%.

Endoscopic ablation techniques have a risk of complications (bleeding, perforation, strictures). Therefore, endoscopic eradication therapy currently is not recommended for patients with nondysplastic Barrett esophagus for whom the risk of developing esophageal cancer is low and treatment does not appear to be cost-effective.

B. Peptic Stricture

Stricture formation occurs in about 5% of patients with esophagitis. It is manifested by the gradual development of solid food dysphagia progressive over months to years. Most strictures are located at the gastroesophageal junction. Endoscopy with biopsy is mandatory in all cases to differentiate peptic stricture from stricture by esophageal carcinoma. Active erosive esophagitis is often present. Up to 90% of symptomatic patients are effectively treated by dilation with graduated polyvinyl catheters passed over a wire placed at the time of endoscopy or fluoroscopically, or by balloons passed fluoroscopically or through an endoscope. Dilation is continued over one to several sessions. A luminal diameter of 15–18 mm is usually sufficient to relieve dysphagia. Long-term therapy with a PPI is required to decrease the likelihood of stricture recurrence.

▶ Treatment

A. Medical Treatment

The goal of treatment is to provide symptomatic relief, to heal esophagitis (if present), and to prevent complications. In the majority of patients with uncomplicated disease, empiric treatment is initiated based on a compatible history without the need for further confirmatory studies. Patients not responding and those with suspected complications undergo further evaluation with upper endoscopy or esophageal manometry and pH recording.

1. Mild, intermittent symptoms—Patients with mild or intermittent symptoms that do not impact adversely on quality of life may benefit from lifestyle modifications with medical interventions taken as needed. Patients may find that eating smaller meals and elimination of acidic foods (citrus, tomatoes, coffee, spicy foods), foods that precipitate reflux (fatty foods, chocolate, peppermint, alcohol), and cigarettes may reduce symptoms. Weight loss should be recommended for patients who are overweight or have had recent weight gain. All patients should be advised to avoid lying down within 3 hours after meals (the period of greatest reflux). Patients with nocturnal symptoms should also elevate the head of the bed on 6-inch blocks or a foam wedge to reduce reflux and enhance esophageal clearance.

Patients with infrequent heartburn (less than once weekly) may be treated on demand with antacids or oral H_2-receptor antagonists. Antacids provide rapid relief of heartburn; however, their duration of action is less than 2 hours. Many are available over the counter. Those containing magnesium should not be used for patients with kidney disease, and patients with acute or chronic kidney disease should be cautioned appropriately.

The oral H_2-receptor antagonists come in a variety of strengths: cimetidine 200 mg; famotidine 10 mg and 20 mg; and nizatidine 75 mg and 150 mg. Most of these drug strengths are now available over the counter without need for a prescription. When taken for active heartburn, these agents have a delay in onset of at least 30 minutes. However, once these agents take effect, they provide heartburn relief for up to 8 hours.

2. Troublesome symptoms—

A. INITIAL THERAPY—Patients with troublesome reflux symptoms and patients with known complications of GERD (erosive esophagitis, Barrett esophagus, stricture) should be treated with a once-daily oral PPI (omeprazole or rabeprazole, 20 mg; omeprazole, 40 mg with sodium bicarbonate; lansoprazole, 30 mg; dexlansoprazole, 60 mg; esomeprazole or pantoprazole, 40 mg) taken 30 minutes before breakfast for 4–8 weeks. Because there appears to be little difference between these agents in efficacy or side effect profiles, the choice of agent is determined by cost. Oral omeprazole, 20 mg, and lansoprazole, 15 mg, are available as over-the-counter formulations. Once-daily PPIs achieve adequate control of heartburn in 70–80% of patients, complete heartburn resolution in over 50%, and healing of erosive esophagitis (when present) in 75–85%. In contrast, PPIs are less effective in reducing bothersome regurgitation. Because of their superior efficacy and ease of use, PPIs are preferred to H_2-receptor antagonists for the initial treatment of acute and chronic GERD.

B. LONG-TERM THERAPY—In those who achieve good symptomatic relief with a course of empiric once-daily PPI, therapy may be discontinued after 8–12 weeks. Most patients (over 80%) will experience relapse of GERD symptoms, usually within 3 months. Patients whose symptoms relapse may be treated with either continuous PPI therapy, intermittent 2- to 4-week courses, or "on demand" therapy (ie, drug taken until symptoms abate) depending on symptom frequency and patient preference. Alternatively, twice-daily H_2-receptor antagonists may be used to control symptoms in patients without erosive esophagitis. Patients who require twice-daily PPI therapy for initial symptom control and patients with complications of GERD, including severe erosive esophagitis, Barrett esophagus, or peptic stricture, should be maintained on long-term therapy with a once- or twice-daily PPI titrated to the lowest effective dose to achieve satisfactory symptom control.

PPIs are considered to be extremely safe. Although a number of safety concerns have been raised in retrospective observational studies, it is difficult to determine whether the modest associations identified are due to a causal relationship. Long-term use of PPIs likely does have a small increased risk of infectious gastroenteritis (including *C difficile*), small intestinal bacterial overgrowth, and micronutrient deficiencies (iron, vitamin B_{12}, magnesium). A large prospective study of over 17,000 patients taking PPIs for a median of 3 years did not find an increased risk of other previously reported adverse events, including pneumonia, bone fractures, kidney disease (due to interstitial nephritis), dementia, or MI. Long-term PPI therapy should be prescribed to patients with appropriate indications and at the lowest effective dose.

3. Unresponsive disease—Up to one-third of patients report inadequate relief of heartburn or regurgitation with once-daily PPI therapy. Approximately 25% respond to an increase in PPI therapy to twice daily (30–45 minutes before breakfast and dinner). Patients unresponsive to twice-daily therapy should undergo endoscopy for detection of severe, inadequately treated reflux esophagitis and for other gastroesophageal conditions (including eosinophilic esophagitis and achalasia) that may mimic GERD. Truly refractory esophagitis may be caused by medical noncompliance, resistance to PPIs, gastrinoma with gastric acid hypersecretion (Zollinger-Ellison syndrome), or pill-induced esophagitis. Patients without endoscopically visible esophagitis should undergo ambulatory esophageal pH monitoring with impedance monitoring to determine whether the symptoms are correlated with reflux (both acid and nonacid reflux) episodes. The study generally is performed on twice-daily PPI therapy to determine the number of reflux episodes (acid and nonacid) and symptom association with reflux episodes. Refractory GERD is diagnosed in patients with confirmed reflux (increased acid reflux or significant correlation of symptoms with acid or nonacid reflux episodes) despite PPI therapy. These patients may be candidates for surgical or endoscopic therapy. Approximately 30% of patients with unresponsive symptoms do not have increased reflux or a significant symptom correlation with reflux episodes and are diagnosed with "functional heartburn," a functional disorder. Treatment with a low-dose tricyclic antidepressant (eg, imipramine or nortriptyline 25 mg orally at bedtime) may be beneficial.

4. Extraesophageal reflux manifestations—Establishing a causal relationship between gastroesophageal reflux and extraesophageal symptoms (eg, asthma, hoarseness, cough, sleep disturbances) is difficult. Gastroesophageal reflux seldom is the sole cause of extraesophageal disorders but may be a contributory factor. Although ambulatory esophageal pH testing can document the presence of increased acid esophageal reflux, it does not prove a causative connection. Current guidelines recommend that a trial of a twice-daily PPI be administered for 2–3 months in patients with suspected extraesophageal GERD syndromes who also have typical GERD symptoms. Improvement of extraesophageal symptoms suggests but does not prove that acid reflux is the causative factor. Esophageal impedance-pH testing may be performed in patients whose extraesophageal symptoms persist after 3 months of PPI therapy and may be considered before PPI therapy in patients without typical GERD symptoms in whom other causes of extraesophageal symptoms have been excluded.

B. Surgical Treatment

Surgical fundoplication affords good to excellent relief of symptoms and healing of esophagitis in over 85% of properly selected patients and can be performed laparoscopically with low complication rates in most instances. Although patient satisfaction is high, typical reflux symptoms recur in 10–30% of patients. Furthermore, new symptoms of dysphagia, bloating, increased flatulence, dyspepsia, or diarrhea develop in over 30% of patients. In a 2019 randomized controlled trial of patients with refractory heartburn and confirmed reflux (acid or nonacid) despite twice-daily PPI therapy, fundoplication resulted in 67% adequate symptom relief at 1 year compared with 12–28% with continued medical therapy.

A minimally invasive magnetic artificial sphincter is FDA approved for the treatment of GERD in patients with hiatal hernias less than 3 cm in size. The device is made up of a flexible, elastic string of titanium beads (wrapped around a magnetic core) that is placed laparoscopically below the diaphragm at the gastroesophageal junction. The magnets are designed to open with pressures generated during swallowing but remain closed during gastroesophageal reflux events, which generate lower pressure than swallowing. In prospective clinical trials with up to 5 years of follow up, magnetic sphincter augmentation has demonstrated GERD symptom relief equivalent to laparoscopic fundoplication but far fewer side effects (long-term dysphagia 4–10%, bloating 8%, diarrhea 2%, nausea/vomiting 2%). In 2020, results were reported comparing magnetic sphincter augmentation with twice-daily PPI therapy in patients with GERD and moderate to severe regurgitation. After 1 year, sphincter augmentation led to significant improvement of regurgitation in 96% of patients and of GERD symptoms in 81% of patients compared with 19% and 8% of patients, respectively, treated with twice-daily PPIs. Given the excellent safety and efficacy data demonstrated with this device to date, it should be considered as an alternative to fundoplication surgery for patients with GERD, especially those with troublesome regurgitation, and hiatal hernias less than 3 cm in size.

Surgical treatment is not recommended for patients who are well controlled with medical therapies but should be considered for those with severe reflux disease who are unwilling to accept lifelong medical therapy due to its expense, inconvenience, or theoretical risks as well as for patients with proven refractory GERD symptoms or bothersome regurgitation despite PPI therapy. Gastric bypass (rather than fundoplication) should be considered for obese patients with GERD.

Several endoscopic procedures have been developed to treat GERD; however, none have found wide acceptance, largely due to limited long-term efficacy.

When to Refer

- Patients with typical GERD whose symptoms do not resolve with empiric management with a twice-daily PPI.
- Patients with suspected extraesophageal GERD symptoms that do not resolve with 3 months of twice-daily PPI therapy.
- Patients with significant dysphagia or other "alarm" symptoms for upper endoscopy.
- Patients with Barrett esophagus for endoscopic surveillance.
- Patients who have Barrett esophagus with dysplasia or early mucosal cancer.
- Surgical therapy is considered.

Bell R et al. Magnetic sphincter augmentation superior to proton pump inhibitors for regurgitation in a 1-year randomized trial. Clin Gastroenterol Hepatol. 2020;18:1736. [PMID: 31518717]

Desai M et al. Management of peptic strictures. Am J Gastroenterol. 2020;115:967. [PMID: 32618639]

Dhaliwal L et al. Neoplasia detection rate in Barrett's esophagus and its impact on missed dysplasia: results from a large population-based study. Clin Gastroenterol Hepatol. 2021;19:922. [PMID: 32707339]

Dunn CP et al. Understanding the GERD barrier. J Clin Gastroenterol. 2021;55:459. [PMID: 33883513]

Yanes M et al. Mortality, reoperation, and hospital stay within 90 days of primary and secondary antireflux surgery in a population-based multinational study. Gastroenterology. 2021;160:2283. [PMID: 33587926]

INFECTIOUS ESOPHAGITIS

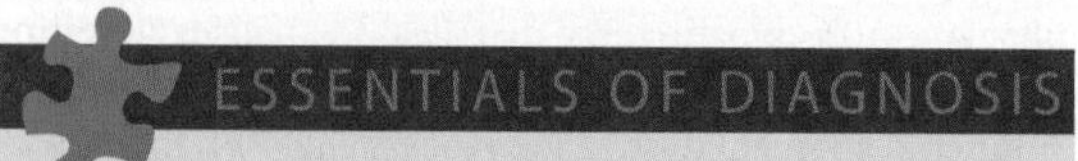

- Immunosuppressed patient.
- Odynophagia, dysphagia, and chest pain.
- Endoscopy with biopsy establishes diagnosis.

General Considerations

Infectious esophagitis occurs most commonly in immunosuppressed patients. Patients with AIDS, solid organ transplants, leukemia, lymphoma, and those receiving immunosuppressive drugs are at particular risk for opportunistic infections. *Candida albicans*, herpes simplex, and CMV are the most common pathogens. *Candida* infection may occur also in patients who have uncontrolled diabetes and those being treated with systemic corticosteroids, radiation therapy, or systemic antibiotic therapy. Herpes simplex can affect normal hosts, in which case the infection is generally self-limited.

Clinical Findings

A. Symptoms and Signs

The most common symptoms are odynophagia and dysphagia. Substernal chest pain occurs in some patients. Patients with candidal esophagitis are sometimes asymptomatic. Oral thrush is present in only 75% of patients with candidal esophagitis but also occurs in 25–50% of patients with viral esophagitis and is therefore an unreliable indicator of the cause of esophageal infection. Patients with esophageal CMV infection may have infection at other sites such as the colon and retina. Oral ulcers (herpes labialis) are often associated with herpes simplex esophagitis.

B. Special Examinations

Treatment may be empiric. For diagnostic certainty, endoscopy with biopsy and brushings (for microbiologic and histopathologic analysis) is preferred because of its high diagnostic accuracy. The endoscopic signs of candidal esophagitis are diffuse, linear, yellow-white plaques adherent to the mucosa. CMV esophagitis is characterized by one to several large, shallow, superficial ulcerations. Herpes esophagitis results in multiple small, deep ulcerations.

Treatment

A. Candidal Esophagitis

Systemic therapy is required for esophageal candidiasis. An empiric trial of antifungal therapy is often administered without performing diagnostic endoscopy. Initial therapy is generally with fluconazole, 400 mg on day 1, then 200–400 mg/day orally for 14–21 days. Patients not responding to empiric therapy within 3–5 days should undergo endoscopy with brushings, biopsy, and culture to distinguish resistant fungal infection from other infections (eg, CMV, herpes). Esophageal candidiasis not responding to fluconazole therapy may be treated with itraconazole suspension (not capsules), 200 mg/day orally, or voriconazole, 200 mg orally twice daily. Refractory infection may be treated intravenously with caspofungin, 50 mg daily.

B. Cytomegalovirus Esophagitis

In patients with HIV infection, immune restoration with antiretroviral therapy is the most effective means of controlling CMV disease. Initial therapy is with ganciclovir, 5 mg/kg intravenously every 12 hours for 3–6 weeks. Neutropenia is a frequent dose-limiting side effect. Once resolution of symptoms occurs, it may be possible to complete the course of therapy with oral valganciclovir, 900 mg once daily.

Patients who either do not respond to or cannot tolerate ganciclovir are treated acutely with foscarnet, 90 mg/kg intravenously every 12 hours for 3–6 weeks. The principal toxicities are AKI, hypocalcemia, and hypomagnesemia.

C. Herpetic Esophagitis

Immunocompetent patients may be treated symptomatically and generally do not require specific antiviral therapy. Immunosuppressed patients may be treated with oral acyclovir, 400 mg orally five times daily, or 250 mg/m^2 intravenously every 8–12 hours, usually for 14–21 days. Oral famciclovir, 500 mg orally three times daily, or valacyclovir, 1 g twice daily, are also effective but more expensive than generic acyclovir. Nonresponders require therapy with foscarnet, 40 mg/kg intravenously every 8 hours for 21 days.

Prognosis

Most patients with infectious esophagitis can be effectively treated with complete symptom resolution. Depending on the patient's underlying immunodeficiency, relapse of symptoms off therapy can raise difficulties. Long-term suppressive therapy is sometimes required.

Hoversten P et al. Risk factors, endoscopic features, and clinical outcomes of cytomegalovirus esophagitis based on a 10-year analysis at a single center. Clin Gastroenterol. 2020;18:736. [PMID: 31077832]

Narasimhalu T et al. Educational case: infectious esophagitis. Acad Pathol. 2020;7:2374289520903438. [PMID: 32083170]

PILL-INDUCED ESOPHAGITIS

A number of different medications may injure the esophagus, presumably through direct, prolonged mucosal contact or mechanisms that disrupt mucosal integrity. The most commonly implicated are the NSAIDs, potassium chloride pills, quinidine, zalcitabine, zidovudine, alendronate and risedronate, emepronium bromide, iron, vitamin C, and antibiotics (doxycycline, tetracycline, clindamycin, trimethoprim-sulfamethoxazole). Because injury is most likely to occur if pills are swallowed without water or while supine, hospitalized or bed-bound patients are at greater risk. Symptoms include severe retrosternal chest pain, odynophagia, and dysphagia, often beginning several hours after taking a pill. These may occur suddenly and persist for days. Some patients (especially older patients) have relatively little pain, presenting with dysphagia. Endoscopy may reveal one to several discrete ulcers that may be shallow or deep. Chronic injury may result in severe esophagitis with stricture, hemorrhage, or perforation. Healing occurs rapidly when the offending agent is eliminated. To prevent pill-induced damage, patients should take pills with 4 oz of water and remain upright for 30 minutes after ingestion. Known offending agents should not be given to patients with esophageal dysmotility, dysphagia, or strictures.

Syed M. Pill-induced oesophagitis. Postgrad Med J. 2021;97:349. [PMID: 32423921]

BENIGN ESOPHAGEAL LESIONS

1. Mallory-Weiss Syndrome (Mucosal Laceration of Gastroesophageal Junction)

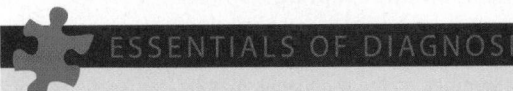

- Hematemesis; usually self-limited.
- Prior history of vomiting, retching in 50%.
- Endoscopy establishes diagnosis.

General Considerations

Mallory-Weiss syndrome is characterized by a nonpenetrating mucosal tear at the gastroesophageal junction that is hypothesized to arise from events that suddenly raise transabdominal pressure, such as lifting, retching, or vomiting. Alcoholism is a strong predisposing factor. Mallory-Weiss tears are responsible for approximately 5% of cases of upper GI bleeding.

Clinical Findings

A. Symptoms and Signs

Patients usually present with hematemesis with or without melena. A history of retching, vomiting, or straining is obtained in about 50% of cases.

B. Special Examinations

As with other causes of upper GI hemorrhage, upper endoscopy should be performed after the patient has been appropriately resuscitated. The diagnosis is established by identification of a 0.5- to 4-cm linear mucosal tear usually located either at the gastroesophageal junction or, more commonly, just below the junction in the gastric mucosa.

Differential Diagnosis

At endoscopy, other potential causes of upper GI hemorrhage are found in over 35% of patients with Mallory-Weiss tears, including peptic ulcer disease, erosive gastritis, arteriovenous malformations, and esophageal varices. Patients with underlying portal hypertension are at higher risk for continued or recurrent bleeding.

Treatment

Patients are initially treated as needed with fluid resuscitation and blood transfusions. Most patients stop bleeding spontaneously and require no therapy. Endoscopic hemostatic therapy is employed in patients who have continuing active bleeding. Injection with epinephrine (1:10,000), cautery with a bipolar or heater probe coagulation device, or mechanical compression of the artery by application of an endoclip or band is effective in 90–95% of cases. Angiographic arterial embolization or operative intervention is required in patients who fail endoscopic therapy.

He L et al. The prediction value of scoring systems in Mallory-Weiss syndrome patients. Medicine (Baltimore). 2019;98:e15751. [PMID: 31145291]

2. Eosinophilic Esophagitis

General Considerations

Eosinophilia of the esophagus may be caused by eosinophilic esophagitis and GERD (and, rarely, celiac disease, Crohn disease, and pemphigus).

Eosinophilic esophagitis is a disorder in which food or environmental antigens are thought to stimulate an inflammatory response. Initially recognized in children, it is increasingly identified in young or middle-aged adults (estimated prevalence 43/100,000). A history of allergies or atopic conditions (asthma, eczema, hay fever) is present in over half of patients.

Clinical Findings

Most adults have a long history of dysphagia for solid-foods or an episode of food impaction. Heartburn or chest pain may be present. Children may have abdominal pain, vomiting, or failure to thrive. On laboratory tests, a few have eosinophilia or elevated IgE levels. Barium swallow studies may demonstrate a small-caliber esophagus; focal or long, tapered strictures; or multiple concentric rings. However, endoscopy with esophageal biopsy and histologic evaluation is required to establish the diagnosis. Endoscopic appearances include **E**dema, concentric **R**ings ("trachealization"), **E**xudates (white plaques), **F**urrows (vertical lines), and **S**trictures (EREFS); however, the esophagus is grossly normal in up to 5% of patients. Multiple biopsies (4–8) from the proximal and distal esophagus should be obtained to demonstrate multiple (greater than 15/high-powered field) eosinophils in the mucosa. Consideration should be given to the disorders that may cause increased esophageal eosinophils, including hypereosinophilic syndrome, eosinophilic gastroenteritis, achalasia, connective tissue disorders, drug hypersensitivity, and Crohn disease. Skin testing for food allergies may be helpful to identify causative factors.

Treatment

The goals of therapy are improvement of symptoms, reduction of inflammation, and prevention and treatment of esophageal strictures. Treatment options include PPIs, topical corticosteroids, food elimination diets, and esophageal dilation. First-line therapy for most adults is a PPI orally twice daily for 2 months followed by repeat endoscopy and mucosal biopsy. Up to one-third of symptomatic patients with increased esophageal eosinophils have clinical and histologic improvement with PPI treatment. It is hypothesized that esophageal acid exposure may contribute to antigen-mediated eosinophilic inflammation. PPI therapy should be discontinued in patients with persistent symptoms and inflammation.

In patients with continued symptoms, optimal treatment is uncertain. Referral to an allergist for evaluation of coexisting atopic disorders and for testing for food and environmental allergens may be considered, but studies suggest limited predictive value in adults. Empiric elimination of suspected dietary allergens leads to clinical, endoscopic and histologic improvement in 50–70% of adults. The most common allergenic foods are dairy, eggs, wheat, and soy followed by peanuts and shellfish. With progressive reintroduction of each food group, the trigger food group may be identified in up to 85% of patients. Topical corticosteroids lead to symptom resolution in 70% of adults. Either budesonide in sucralose suspension, 1 mg, or powdered fluticasone, 880 mcg (from foil-lined inhaler diskus), is administered twice daily for 6–8 weeks with similar efficacy. Symptomatic relapse is common after discontinuation of therapy and may require maintenance topical corticosteroid therapy. Budesonide orodispersible tablets 0.5 or 1.0 mg twice daily are approved in Europe for initial and maintenance therapy of eosinophilic esophagitis but are not yet available in the United States. In a 2011 phase 3 randomized controlled trial of patients who achieved clinical and histologic remission after 6 weeks of budesonide orodispersible tablet 1.0 mg twice daily, 75% of participants who continued budesonide 0.5 mg or 1.0 mg twice daily for 48 weeks remained in remission compared with only 4.4% of patients given placebo. Esophageal candidiasis occurred in 13–18% of treated patients. Graduated dilation of strictures should be conducted in patients with dysphagia and strictures or narrow-caliber esophagus but should be performed cautiously because there is an increased risk of perforation and postprocedural chest pain.

Hirano I et al. AGA Institute and the Joint Task Force on Allergy-Immunology Practice Parameters clinical guidelines for the management of eosinophilic esophagitis. Gastroenterology. 2020;158:1776. [PMID: 32359562]
Muir A et al. Eosinophilic esophagitis: a review. JAMA. 2021;326:1310. [PMID:34609446]
Rank MA et al. Technical review on the management of eosinophilic esophagitis: a report of the AGA Institute and the Joint Task Force on Allergy-Immunology Practice Parameters. Gastroenterology. 2020;158:1789. [PMID: 32359563]
Straumann A et al. Budesonide orodispersible tablets maintain remission in a randomized, placebo-controlled trial of patients with eosinophilic esophagitis. Gastroenterology. 2020;159:1672. [PMID: 32721437]

3. Esophageal Webs & Rings

Esophageal webs are thin, diaphragm-like membranes of squamous mucosa that typically occur in the mid or upper esophagus and may be multiple. They may be congenital but also occur with eosinophilic esophagitis, graft-versus-host disease, pemphigoid, epidermolysis bullosa, pemphigus vulgaris, and, rarely, in association with iron deficiency anemia (Plummer-Vinson syndrome). Esophageal "Schatzki" rings are smooth, circumferential, thin (less than 4 mm in thickness) mucosal structures located in the distal esophagus at the squamocolumnar junction. Their pathogenesis is controversial. They are associated in nearly all cases with a hiatal hernia, and reflux symptoms are common, suggesting that acid gastroesophageal reflux may be contributory in many cases. Most webs and rings are over 20 mm in diameter and are asymptomatic. Solid food dysphagia most often occurs with rings less than 13 mm in diameter. Characteristically, dysphagia is intermittent and not progressive. Large poorly chewed food boluses such as beefsteak are most likely to cause symptoms. Obstructing boluses may pass by drinking extra liquids or after regurgitation. In some cases, an impacted bolus must be extracted endoscopically. Esophageal webs and rings are best visualized using a barium esophagogram with full esophageal distention. Endoscopy is less sensitive than barium esophagography.

The majority of symptomatic patients with a single ring or web can be effectively treated with the passage of bougie or endoscopic balloon dilators to disrupt the lesion or endoscopic electrosurgical incision of the ring. A minimum lumen diameter of 15–18 mm achieves symptom remission in most patients. A single dilation may suffice, but repeat dilations are required in many patients. Patients who have heartburn or who require repeated dilation should receive long-term acid suppressive therapy with a PPI.

Vermeulen BD et al. Risk factors and clinical outcomes of endoscopic dilation in benign esophageal strictures: a long-term follow-up study. Gastrointest Endosc. 2020;91:1058. [PMID: 31917167]

4. Zenker Diverticulum

Zenker diverticulum is a protrusion of pharyngeal mucosa that develops at the pharyngoesophageal junction between the inferior pharyngeal constrictor and the cricopharyngeus. The cause is believed to be loss of elasticity of the upper esophageal sphincter, resulting in restricted opening during swallowing. Symptoms of dysphagia and regurgitation tend to develop insidiously over years in older, predominantly male patients. Initial symptoms include vague oropharyngeal dysphagia with coughing or throat discomfort. As the diverticulum enlarges and retains food, patients may note halitosis, spontaneous regurgitation of undigested food, nocturnal choking, gurgling in the throat, or a protrusion in the neck. Complications include aspiration pneumonia, bronchiectasis, and lung abscess. The diagnosis is best established by a videoesophagography.

Symptomatic patients require cricopharyngeal myotomy with incision of the septum between the diverticulum and esophagus. Minimally invasive intraluminal approaches that use flexible endoscopes or rigid esophagoscopes are preferred. Significant improvement occurs in over 90% of patients with a recurrence rate of 11%. Giant diverticula require surgical transcervical myotomy with diverticulectomy. Small asymptomatic diverticula may be observed.

Brewer Gutierrez OI et al. Zenker's diverticulum per-oral endoscopic myotomy techniques: changing paradigms. Gastroenterology. 2019;156:2134. [PMID: 30851303]

Jirapinyo P et al. Devices and techniques for flexible endoscopic management of Zenker's diverticulum (with videos). Gastrointest Endosc. 2021;94:3. [PMID: 33926711]

Wagh MS et al. How to approach a patient with Zenker's diverticulum. Gastroenterology. 2021;160:10. [PMID: 33220254]

5. Esophageal Varices

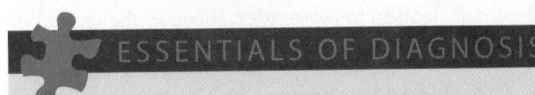

ESSENTIALS OF DIAGNOSIS

- Develop secondary to portal hypertension.
- Found in 50% of patients with cirrhosis.
- One-third of patients with varices develop upper GI bleeding.
- Diagnosis established by upper endoscopy.

General Considerations

Esophageal varices are dilated submucosal veins that develop in patients with underlying portal hypertension and that may result in serious upper GI bleeding. The causes of portal hypertension are discussed in Chapter 16. Under normal circumstances, there is a 2–6 mm Hg pressure gradient between the portal vein and the inferior vena cava. When the gradient exceeds 10–12 mm Hg, significant portal hypertension exists. Esophageal varices are the most common cause of important GI bleeding due to portal hypertension, though gastric varices and, rarely, intestinal varices may also bleed. Bleeding from esophageal varices most commonly occurs in the distal 5 cm of the esophagus.

The most common cause of portal hypertension is cirrhosis. Approximately 50% of patients with cirrhosis have esophageal varices. Bleeding from varices occurs in 30% of patients with esophageal varices. In the absence of any treatment, variceal bleeding spontaneously stops in about 50% of patients. Patients surviving this bleeding episode have a 60% chance of recurrent variceal bleeding, usually within the first 6 weeks. With current therapies, the in-hospital mortality rate associated with bleeding esophageal varices is 15%.

A number of factors have been identified that may portend an increased risk of bleeding from esophageal varices. The most important are (1) the size of the varices; (2) the presence at endoscopy of red wale markings (longitudinal dilated venules on the varix surface); (3) the severity of liver disease (as assessed by Child scoring); and (4) active alcohol abuse—patients with cirrhosis who continue to drink have an extremely high risk of variceal bleeding.

Clinical Findings

A. Symptoms and Signs

Patients with bleeding esophageal varices present with symptoms and signs of acute GI hemorrhage. (See Acute Upper GI Bleeding, above.) In some cases, there may be preceding retching or dyspepsia attributable to alcoholic gastritis or withdrawal. Varices per se do not cause symptoms of dyspepsia, dysphagia, or retching. Variceal bleeding usually is severe, resulting in hypovolemia manifested by postural vital signs or shock. But 20% of patients with chronic liver disease in whom bleeding develops have a nonvariceal source of bleeding.

B. Laboratory Findings

These are identical to those listed above in the section on Acute Upper GI Bleeding.

Initial Management

A. Acute Resuscitation

The initial management of patients with acute upper GI bleeding is also discussed in the section on Acute Upper GI Bleeding. Variceal hemorrhage is life-threatening; rapid assessment and resuscitation with fluids or blood products are essential. Overtransfusion should be avoided because it leads to increased central and portal venous pressures, increasing the risk of rebleeding. Most patients with bleeding esophageal varices have advanced liver disease with coagulopathy due to thrombocytopenia; deficiencies of liver-derived clotting factors I (fibrinogen), II, VII, IX, and X; and accelerated intravascular fibrinolysis. The INR does not provide an accurate reflection of coagulopathy in advanced liver disease. Fresh frozen plasma should not be administered routinely in stable patients with an elevated INR because it has no proven benefit but does have potential harms, including increased portal pressures and risk of portal vein or deep venous thrombosis. In patients with decompensated cirrhosis and active severe upper GI bleeding, platelet transfusion is recommended for platelet counts below 50,000/mcL (50×10^9/L) and fresh frozen plasma may be considered for INRs greater than 1.8. Recombinant factor VIIa has not demonstrated efficacy in controlled studies and is not recommended. The role of prothrombin complex concentrates requires further study. Patients with advanced liver disease are at high risk for poor outcome regardless of the bleeding source and should be in an ICU.

B. Pharmacologic Therapy

1. Antibiotic prophylaxis—Cirrhotic patients admitted with upper GI bleeding have a greater than 50% chance of developing a severe bacterial infection during hospitalization—such as bacterial peritonitis, pneumonia, or UTI. Most infections are caused by gram-negative organisms of gut origin. Prophylactic administration of intravenous third-generation cephalosporins (eg, ceftriaxone, 1 g/day) for 5–7 days reduces the risk of serious infection to 10–20% as well as hospital mortality, especially in patients with Child-Pugh class C cirrhosis.

2. Vasoactive drugs—Octreotide and somatostatin infusions reduce portal pressures in ways that are poorly understood. Octreotide (50 mcg intravenous bolus followed by 50 mcg/hour) or somatostatin (250 mcg/hour)—not available in the United States—reduces splanchnic and hepatic blood flow and portal pressures in cirrhotic patients. Both agents appear to provide acute control of variceal bleeding in up to 80% of patients although neither has been shown to reduce mortality. Combined treatment with octreotide or somatostatin infusion and endoscopic therapy with band ligation (or sclerotherapy) is superior to either modality alone in controlling acute bleeding and early rebleeding, and it may improve survival. In patients with advanced liver disease and upper GI hemorrhage, it is reasonable to initiate therapy with octreotide or somatostatin on admission and continue for 3–5 days if varices are confirmed by endoscopy. If bleeding is determined by endoscopy not to be secondary to portal hypertension, the infusion can be discontinued.

Terlipressin, 1–2 mg intravenously every 4 hours (not available in the United States), is a synthetic vasopressin analog that causes a significant and sustained reduction in portal and variceal pressures while preserving renal perfusion. Where available, terlipressin may be preferred to somatostatin or octreotide. Terlipressin is contraindicated in patients with significant coronary, cerebral, or peripheral vascular disease.

3. Vitamin K—In cirrhotic patients with an abnormal prothrombin time, vitamin K (10 mg intravenously) should be administered.

4. Lactulose—Encephalopathy may complicate an episode of GI bleeding in patients with severe liver disease. In patients with encephalopathy, lactulose should be administered in a dosage of 30 mL orally every 1–2 hours until evacuation occurs then reduced to 15–45 mL/hour every 8–12 hours as needed to promote two or three bowel movements daily. (See Chapter 16.)

C. Emergent Endoscopy

Emergent endoscopy is performed after the patient's hemodynamic status has been appropriately stabilized (usually within 12–24 hours). In patients with active bleeding, endotracheal intubation is commonly performed to protect against aspiration during endoscopy. An endoscopic examination is performed to exclude other or associated causes of upper GI bleeding such as Mallory-Weiss tears, peptic ulcer disease, and portal hypertensive gastropathy. In many patients, variceal bleeding has stopped spontaneously by the time of endoscopy, and the diagnosis of variceal bleeding is made presumptively. Immediate endoscopic treatment of the varices generally is performed with banding. In clinical practice, sclerotherapy is now seldom used. These techniques arrest active bleeding in 80–90% of patients and reduce the chance of in-hospital recurrent bleeding to about 20%.

If banding is undertaken, repeat sessions are scheduled at intervals of 2–4 weeks until the varices are obliterated or reduced to a small size. For patients with platelet counts less than 50,000/mcL (50×10^9/L), consideration should be given to preprocedure administration of avatrombopag, an FDA-approved oral thrombopoietin receptor agonist. In phase 3 clinical trials at a dose of 40–60 mg/day for 5 consecutive days beginning 10–13 days prior to endoscopy, 68% of patients with baseline platelet counts less than 40,000/mcL (40×10^9/L) and 88% with baseline counts 40,000–50,000/mcL achieved platelet counts greater than 50,000/mcL (50×10^9/L) and avoided periprocedural platelet transfusions.

D. Balloon Tube Tamponade

In patients with massive variceal GI bleeding, mechanical tamponade with specially designed nasogastric tubes containing large gastric and esophageal balloons (Minnesota or Sengstaken-Blakemore tubes) may provide initial control of hemorrhage in 60–90% of patients. Balloon tamponade is used as a temporizing measure only in patients with bleeding that cannot be controlled with pharmacologic or endoscopic techniques until more definitive decompressive therapy (eg, TIPS) can be provided.

E. Portal Decompressive Procedures

In the 10–20% of patients with variceal bleeding that cannot be controlled with pharmacologic or endoscopic therapy, emergency portal decompression may be considered.

1. Transvenous intrahepatic portosystemic shunts (TIPS)—Over a wire that is passed through a catheter inserted in the jugular vein, an expandable wire mesh stent (8–12 mm in diameter) is passed through the liver parenchyma, creating a portosystemic shunt from the portal vein to the hepatic vein. TIPS can control acute hemorrhage in over 90% of patients actively bleeding from gastric or esophageal varices. However, when TIPS is performed in the actively bleeding patient, the mortality approaches 40%, especially in patients requiring ventilatory support or blood pressure support and patients with renal insufficiency, bilirubin greater than 3 mg/dL, or encephalopathy. Therefore, TIPS should be considered in the 10–20% of patients with acute variceal bleeding that cannot be controlled with pharmacologic and endoscopic therapy, but it may not be warranted in patients with a particularly poor prognosis.

2. Emergency portosystemic shunt surgery—Emergency portosystemic shunt surgery is associated with a 40–60% mortality rate. At centers where TIPS is available, emergency portosystemic shunts are no longer performed.

Prevention of Rebleeding

Once the initial bleeding episode has been controlled, therapy is warranted to reduce the high risk (60%) of rebleeding.

A. Combination Beta-Blockers and Variceal Band Ligation

Nonselective beta-adrenergic blockers (propranolol, nadolol) reduce the risk of rebleeding from esophageal varices to about 40%. Likewise, long-term treatment with band ligation reduces the incidence of rebleeding to about 30%. In most patients, two to six treatment sessions (performed at 2- to 4-week intervals) are needed to eradicate the varices.

Meta-analyses of randomized controlled trials suggest that a *combination* of band ligation plus beta-blockers is superior to either variceal band ligation alone (RR 0.68) or beta-blockers alone (RR 0.71). Therefore, combination therapy is recommended for patients without contraindications to beta-blockers. Recommended starting doses of beta-blockers are propranolol (20 mg orally twice daily), long-acting propranolol (60 mg orally once daily), or nadolol (20–40 mg orally once daily), with gradual increases in the dosage every 1–2 weeks until the heart rate falls by 25% or reaches 55–60 beats/minute, provided the systolic blood pressure remains above 90 mm Hg and the patient has no side effects. The average dosage of long-acting propranolol is 120 mg once daily and for nadolol, 80 mg once daily. One-third of patients with cirrhosis are intolerant of beta-blockers, experiencing fatigue or hypotension. Drug administration at bedtime may reduce the frequency and severity of side effects.

B. Transvenous Intrahepatic Portosystemic Shunt

TIPS has resulted in a significant reduction in recurrent bleeding compared with endoscopic sclerotherapy or band ligation—either alone or in combination with beta-blocker therapy. At 1 year, rebleeding rates in patients treated with TIPS versus various endoscopic therapies average 20% and 40%, respectively. However, TIPS was also associated with a higher incidence of encephalopathy (35% vs 15%) and did not result in a decrease in mortality. Another limitation of TIPS is that stenosis and thrombosis of the stents occur in the majority of patients over time with a consequent risk of rebleeding. Given these problems, TIPS should be reserved for patients who have recurrent (two or more) episodes of variceal bleeding that have failed endoscopic or pharmacologic therapies. TIPS is also useful in patients with recurrent bleeding from gastric varices or portal hypertensive gastropathy (for which endoscopic therapies cannot be used). TIPS is likewise considered in patients who are noncompliant with other therapies or who live in remote locations (without access to emergency care).

C. Surgical Portosystemic Shunts

Shunt surgery has a significantly lower rate of rebleeding compared with endoscopic therapy but also a higher incidence of encephalopathy. With the advent and widespread adoption of TIPS, surgical shunts are seldom performed.

D. Liver Transplantation

Candidacy for orthotopic liver transplantation should be assessed in all patients with chronic liver disease and bleeding due to portal hypertension. Transplant candidates should be treated with band ligation or TIPS to control bleeding pretransplant.

Prevention of First Episodes of Variceal Bleeding

Among patients with varices that have not previously bled, bleeding occurs in 12% of patients each year, with a lifetime risk of 30%. Because of the high mortality rate associated with variceal hemorrhage, prevention of the initial bleeding episode is desirable. Therefore, it is recommended that patients with chronic liver disease with compensated cirrhosis or suspected cirrhosis should undergo diagnostic endoscopy or capsule endoscopy to determine whether varices are present. Transient elastography (FibroScan) is a noninvasive method for assessing liver stiffness and fibrosis that may be used to stratify patients at high risk for varices (who may benefit from endoscopy) versus those at low risk (in whom endoscopy is not needed). Varices are present in 40% of patients with Child-Pugh class A cirrhosis and in 85% with Child-Pugh class C cirrhosis. In patients without varices on screening endoscopy, a repeat endoscopy is recommended in 3 years, since varices develop in 8% of patients per year. Patients with varices have a higher risk of bleeding if they have varices larger than 5 mm, varices with red wale markings, or Child-Pugh class B or C cirrhosis. The risk of bleeding in patients with varices smaller than 5 mm is 5% per year and with large varices is 15–20% per year. Patients with small varices without red wale marks and compensated (Child-Pugh class A) cirrhosis have a low risk of bleeding; hence, prophylaxis is unnecessary, but endoscopy should be repeated in 1–2 years to reassess size.

Nonselective beta-adrenergic blockers are recommended to reduce the risk of first variceal hemorrhage in patients with medium/large varices and patients with small varices who either have variceal red wale marks or advanced cirrhosis (Child-Pugh class B or C). (See Combination Beta-Blockers and Variceal Band Ligation, above.) Band ligation is not recommended for small varices due to technical difficulties in band application. Prophylactic band ligation may be preferred over beta-blockers for patients at higher risk for bleeding, especially patients with medium/large varices with red wale markings or with advanced cirrhosis (Child-Pugh class B or C) as well as patients with contraindications to or intolerance of beta-blockers.

When to Refer

- All patients with upper GI bleeding and suspected varices should be evaluated by a physician skilled in therapeutic endoscopy.
- Patients being considered for TIPS procedures or liver transplantation.
- Patients with cirrhosis for endoscopic evaluation for varices.

When to Admit

All patients with acute upper GI bleeding and suspected cirrhosis should be admitted to an ICU.

Baiges A et al. Treatment of acute variceal bleeding in 2021—when to use transjugular intrahepatic portosystemic shunts? Clin Liver Dis. 2021;25:345. [PMID: 33838854]

Nicoară-Farcău O et al; Preemptive TIPS Individual Data Metanalysis, International Variceal Bleeding Study and Baveno Cooperation Study groups. Effects of early placement of transjugular portosystemic shunts in patients with high-risk acute variceal bleeding: a meta-analysis of individual patient data. Gastroenterology. 2021;160:193. [PMID: 32980344]

Pfisterer N et al. Clinical algorithms for the prevention of variceal bleeding and rebleeding in patients with liver cirrhosis. World J Hepatol. 2021;13:731. [PMID: 34367495]

Plaz Torres MC et al. Secondary prevention of variceal bleeding in adults with previous oesophageal variceal bleeding due to decompensated liver cirrhosis: a network meta-analysis. Cochrane Database Syst Rev. 2021;3:CD013122. [PMID: 33784794]

Roccarina D et al. Primary prevention of variceal bleeding in people with oesophageal varices due to liver cirrhosis: a network meta-analysis. Cochrane Database Syst Rev. 2021;4:CD013121. [PMID: 33822357]

Zanetto A et al. Recent advances in the management of acute variceal hemorrhage. J Clin Med. 2021;10:3818. [PMID: 34501265]

ESOPHAGEAL MOTILITY DISORDERS

1. Achalasia

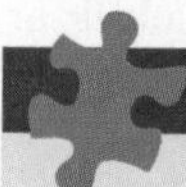

ESSENTIALS OF DIAGNOSIS

- Gradual, progressive dysphagia for solids and liquids.
- Regurgitation of undigested food.
- Barium esophagogram with "bird's beak" distal esophagus.
- Esophageal manometry confirms diagnosis.

General Considerations

Achalasia is an idiopathic motility disorder characterized by loss of peristalsis in the distal two-thirds (smooth muscle) of the esophagus and impaired relaxation of the LES. There appears to be denervation of the esophagus resulting primarily from loss of nitric oxide–producing inhibitory neurons in the myenteric plexus. The cause of the neuronal degeneration is unknown.

Clinical Findings

A. Symptoms and Signs

There is a steady increase in the incidence of achalasia with age; however, it can be seen in individuals as young as 25 years. Patients complain of the gradual onset of dysphagia for solid foods and, in the majority, for liquids also. Symptoms at presentation may have persisted for months to years. Substernal discomfort or fullness may be noted after eating. Many patients eat more slowly and adopt specific maneuvers such as lifting the neck or throwing the shoulders back to enhance esophageal emptying. Regurgitation of undigested food is common and may occur during meals or up to several hours later. Nocturnal regurgitation can provoke coughing or aspiration. Up to 50% of patients report substernal chest pain that is unrelated to meals or exercise and may last up to hours. Weight loss is common. Physical examination is unhelpful.

B. Imaging

Chest radiographs may show an air-fluid level in the enlarged, fluid-filled esophagus. Barium esophagography discloses characteristic findings, including esophageal dilation, loss of esophageal peristalsis, poor esophageal emptying, and a smooth, symmetric "bird's beak" tapering of the distal esophagus. Five minutes after ingestion of 8 oz of barium, a column height of more than 2 cm has a sensitivity and specificity of greater than 85% in differentiating achalasia from other causes of dysphagia. Without treatment, the esophagus may become markedly dilated ("sigmoid esophagus").

C. Special Examinations

After esophagography, endoscopy is always performed to evaluate the distal esophagus and gastroesophageal junction to exclude a distal stricture or a submucosal infiltrating carcinoma. The diagnosis is confirmed by high-resolution esophageal manometry demonstrating absence of normal peristalsis and impaired esophagogastric junction relaxation after swallowing. An integrated post-swallow relaxation pressure greater than 15 mm Hg has a diagnostic sensitivity of 97%. Three achalasia subtypes are recognized based on esophageal contractility and pressure patterns: types I and II (both with 100% failed peristalsis) and type III (failed peristalsis with 20% or more distal premature "spastic" contractions).

Differential Diagnosis

Chagas disease is associated with esophageal dysfunction that is indistinguishable from idiopathic achalasia and should be considered in patients from endemic regions (Central and South America); it is becoming more common in the southern United States. Primary or metastatic tumors can invade the gastroesophageal junction, resulting in a picture resembling that of achalasia, called "pseudoachalasia." Endoscopic ultrasonography and chest CT may be required to examine the distal esophagus in suspicious cases.

Treatment

Several effective treatment options are available, all of which promote improved esophageal emptying by lowering distal esophageal pressure either through endoscopic injection with botulinum toxin or disruption of the LES by pneumatic balloon dilation or cardioesophageal myotomy (surgical or endoscopic).

A. Botulinum Toxin Injection

Endoscopically guided injection of botulinum toxin directly into the LES results in a marked reduction in LES pressure with initial improvement in symptoms in 65–85% of patients. However, symptom relapse occurs in over 50% of patients within 6–9 months and in all patients within 2 years. Because it is inferior to pneumatic dilation therapy and surgery in producing sustained symptomatic relief, this therapy is most appropriate for patients with comorbidities who are poor candidates for more invasive procedures.

B. Pneumatic Dilation

Over 80% of patients derive good to excellent relief of dysphagia after one to three sessions of pneumatic dilation of the LES. Dilation is less effective in patients who are younger than age 45, have the type III variant, or have a dilated esophagus. Perforations occur in less than 3% of dilations but infrequently require operative repair. In a 2021 network meta-analysis of nine randomized controlled trials, laparoscopic Heller myotomy and POEM were not significantly different in treatment success but both were superior to pneumatic dilation. Patients who do not respond to initial treatment with pneumatic dilation may be treated with cardiomyotomy (Heller or POEM).

C. Surgical Heller Cardiomyotomy

A modified Heller cardiomyotomy of the LES and cardia (usually performed with a laparoscopic approach) results in symptomatic improvement in approximately 90% of patients. Because gastroesophageal reflux develops in up to 20% of patients after myotomy, most surgeons also perform an antireflux procedure (fundoplication), and most patients are prescribed a once-daily PPI. Symptoms recur in greater than 5–15% of cases within 10 years but usually respond to pneumatic dilation. A 2017 systematic review of five randomized comparative cardiomyotomy trials detected a higher clinical success rate after 1 year with laparoscopic myotomy than Heller myotomy (RR 1.14) but no significant differences after 2–5 years.

D. Per Oral Endoscopic Myotomy (POEM)

POEM is a less invasive endoscopic procedure in which the endoscope dissects through the submucosal space to the lower esophageal sphincter, where the circular muscle fibers of the cardia and distal esophagus are incised. Because a fundoplication is not performed, long-term antisecretory therapy for gastroesophageal reflux with a PPI is required in most patients. POEM may be the preferred treatment modality for type III achalasia (where a longer myotomy of the distal esophagus is indicated). A randomized controlled trial of 221 patients with achalasia showed that satisfactory symptom improvement was equivalent both in patients treated with POEM (83%) and in those treated with surgical myotomy (81.7%) 2 years after treatment. Serious adverse events occurred in 2.7% of patients treated with POEM and 7.3% with surgical myotomy, but postoperative reflux esophagitis was higher with POEM (44%) than with surgical myotomy (29%).

In summary, optimal treatment of achalasia depends on the patient's age, achalasia subtype, provider's expertise, and patient's preferences or concerns regarding surgery or posttreatment gastroesophageal reflux.

Management of Refractory Achalasia

Complete esophagectomy or percutaneous gastrostomy is required in the 1% of patients in whom massive dilation of the esophagus (megaesophagus) develops despite dilation or myotomy. In megaesophagus, dysphagia, food retention, and regurgitation may decrease nutrition and quality of life and increase risk of aspiration.

Carlson DA et al. Personalized approach to the management of achalasia: how we do it. Am J Gastroenterol. 2020;115:1556. [PMID: 32558688]

Khashab M et al. ASGE guideline on the management of achalasia. Gastrointest Endosc. 2020;91:213. [PMID: 31839408]

Mundre P et al. Efficacy of surgical or endoscopic treatment of idiopathic achalasia: a systematic review and network meta-analysis. Lancet Gastroenterol Hepatol. 2021;6:30. [PMID: 33035470]

Vaezi MF et al. ACG Clinical Guideline: diagnosis and management of achalasia. Am J Gastroenterol. 2020;115:1393. [PMID: 32773454]

2. Other Primary Esophageal Motility Disorders

Clinical Findings

A. Symptoms and Signs

Abnormalities in esophageal motility may cause dysphagia or chest pain. Dysphagia for liquids as well as solids tends to be intermittent and nonprogressive. Periods of normal swallowing may alternate with periods of dysphagia, which usually is mild though bothersome—rarely severe enough to result in significant alterations in lifestyle or weight loss. Dysphagia may be provoked by stress, large boluses of food, or hot or cold liquids. Some patients may experience anterior chest pain that may be confused with angina pectoris but usually is nonexertional. The pain generally is unrelated to eating. (See Chest Pain of Undetermined Origin, below.)

B. Diagnostic Tests

The evaluation of suspected esophageal motility disorders includes barium esophagography, upper endoscopy, and, in some cases, esophageal manometry. Barium esophagography is useful to exclude mechanical obstruction and to evaluate esophageal motility. The presence of simultaneous contractions (spasm), disordered or failed peristalsis, or delayed emptying supports a diagnosis of esophageal dysmotility. Upper endoscopy also is performed to exclude a mechanical obstruction (as a cause of dysphagia) and to look for evidence of erosive reflux esophagitis (a common cause of chest pain) or eosinophilic esophagitis (confirmed by esophageal biopsy). Manometry is not routinely used for mild to moderate symptoms because the findings seldom influence further medical management, but it may be useful in patients with persistent, disabling dysphagia to exclude achalasia and to look for other disorders of esophageal motility. These include esophagogastric junction outflow obstruction, spastic esophageal disorders (distal esophageal spasm and hypercontractile ["jackhammer"] esophagus), and esophageal hypomotility (ineffective or failed peristalsis). The further evaluation of noncardiac chest pain is discussed below.

Treatment

For patients with mild symptoms of dysphagia, therapy is directed at symptom reduction and reassurance. Patients should be instructed to chew carefully, eat more slowly, and take smaller bites of food with liquids. Because unrecognized gastroesophageal reflux may cause dysphagia, a trial of a PPI (esomeprazole 40 mg, lansoprazole 30 mg) orally twice daily should be administered for 4–8 weeks. Opioids may exacerbate esophageal dysmotility and should be discontinued, if possible. No medications have been shown to improve symptoms in patients with esophageal hypomotility. Treatment of patients with severe dysphagia or chest pain attributed to spastic disorders is empiric. Uncontrolled studies report benefit with (1) smooth muscle relaxants (isosorbide [10–20 mg four times daily] or nitroglycerin [0.4 mg sublingually as needed]); (2) calcium channel blockers (nifedipine [10 mg] or diltiazem [60–90 mg] 30–45 minutes before meals); (3) phosphodiesterase type 5 inhibitors (eg, sildenafil); (4) botulinum toxin injection into the lower esophagus; (5) esophageal dilation; or (6) POEM.

De Bortoli N et al. Hypercontractile esophagus from pathophysiology to management: proceedings from the Pisa symposium. Am J Gastroenterol. 2021;116:263. [PMID: 33273259]

DeLay K et al. Clinical updates in esophageal motility disorders beyond achalasia. Clin Gastroenterol Hepatol. 2021;19:1789. [PMID: 34405804]

Mittal R et al. Esophageal motility disorders and gastroesophageal reflux disease. N Engl J Med. 2020;383:1961. [PMID: 33176086]

Yadlapati R et al. Esophageal motility disorders on high-resolution manometry: Chicago Classification version 4.0. Neurogastroenterol Motil. 2021;33:e14058. [PMID: 33373111]

DISEASES OF THE STOMACH & DUODENUM

(See Chapter 39 for Gastric Cancers.)

GASTRITIS & GASTROPATHY

The term "gastropathy" should be used to denote conditions in which there is epithelial or endothelial damage without inflammation, and "gastritis" should be used to denote conditions in which there is histologic evidence of inflammation. In clinical practice, the term "gastritis" is commonly applied to three categories: (1) erosive and hemorrhagic "gastritis" (gastropathy); (2) nonerosive, nonspecific (histologic) gastritis; and (3) specific types of gastritis, characterized by distinctive histologic and endoscopic features diagnostic of specific disorders.

1. Erosive & Hemorrhagic "Gastritis" (Gastropathy)

ESSENTIALS OF DIAGNOSIS

- Most commonly seen in alcoholic or critically ill patients, or patients taking NSAIDs.
- Often asymptomatic; may cause epigastric pain, nausea, and vomiting.
- May cause hematemesis; usually insignificant bleeding.

General Considerations

The most common causes of erosive gastropathy are medications (especially NSAIDs), alcohol, stress due to severe medical or surgical illness, and portal hypertension ("portal gastropathy"). Major risk factors for stress gastritis include mechanical ventilation, coagulopathy, trauma, burns, shock, sepsis, CNS injury, liver failure, kidney disease, and multiorgan failure. The use of enteral nutrition reduces the risk of stress-related bleeding. Uncommon causes of erosive gastropathy include ischemia, caustic ingestion, and radiation. Erosive and hemorrhagic gastropathy typically are diagnosed at endoscopy, often being performed because of dyspepsia or upper GI bleeding. Endoscopic findings include subepithelial hemorrhages, petechiae, and erosions. These lesions are superficial, vary in size and number, and may be focal or diffuse. There usually is no significant inflammation on histologic examination.

Clinical Findings

A. Symptoms and Signs

Erosive gastropathy is usually asymptomatic. Symptoms, when they occur, include anorexia, epigastric pain, nausea, and vomiting. There is poor correlation between symptoms and the number or severity of endoscopic abnormalities. The most common clinical manifestation of erosive gastritis is upper GI bleeding, which presents as hematemesis, "coffee grounds" emesis, or bloody aspirate in a patient receiving nasogastric suction, or as melena. Because erosive gastritis is superficial, hemodynamically significant bleeding is rare.

B. Laboratory Findings

The laboratory findings are nonspecific. The hematocrit is low if significant bleeding has occurred; iron deficiency may be found.

C. Special Examinations

Upper endoscopy is the most sensitive method of diagnosis. Although bleeding from gastritis is usually insignificant, it cannot be distinguished on clinical grounds from more serious lesions such as peptic ulcers or esophageal varices. Hence, endoscopy is generally performed within 24 hours in patients with upper GI bleeding to identify the source.

Differential Diagnosis

Epigastric pain may be due to peptic ulcer, gastroesophageal reflux, gastric cancer, biliary tract disease, food poisoning, viral gastroenteritis, and functional dyspepsia. With severe pain, one should consider a perforated or penetrating ulcer, pancreatic disease, esophageal rupture, ruptured aortic aneurysm, gastric volvulus, GI ischemia, and myocardial ischemia. Causes of upper GI bleeding include peptic ulcer disease, esophageal varices, Mallory-Weiss tear, and angioectasias.

Specific Causes & Treatment

A. Stress Gastritis

1. Prophylaxis—Stress-related mucosal erosions and subepithelial hemorrhages may develop within 72 hours in critically ill patients. Clinically overt bleeding occurs in 6% of ICU patients, but clinically important bleeding in less than 1.5%. Bleeding is associated with a higher mortality rate but is seldom the cause of death. Two of the most important risk factors for bleeding are coagulopathy (platelets less than 50,000/mcL [50×10^9/L] or INR greater than 1.5) and respiratory failure with the need for mechanical ventilation for over 48 hours. When these two risk factors are absent, the risk of significant bleeding is only 0.1%. Other risk factors include traumatic brain injury, severe burns, sepsis, shock, liver disease, and prior history of peptic ulcer disease and GI bleeding. Early enteral tube feeding may decrease the risk of significant bleeding.

Prophylaxis should be routinely administered to critically ill patients with risk factors for significant bleeding upon admission. Prophylactic suppression of gastric acid with H_2-receptor antagonists (intravenous) or PPIs (oral or intravenous) have both been shown to reduce the incidence of clinically overt and significant bleeding. A meta-analysis of 57 randomized controlled trials suggested that PPIs were more effective than H_2-receptor antagonists in reducing clinically significant bleeding (OR 0.38) but may increase the risk of pneumonia (OR 1.27). A 2020 randomized clinical trial of 26,828 patients in 50 ICUs requiring mechanical ventilation reported a lower incidence of clinically significant bleeding in patients given prophylactic PPIs (1.3%) than in those given H_2-antagonists (1.8%) but a nonsignificant higher mortality (HR, 1.05; 95% CI, 1.00–1.10).

The optimal, cost-effective prophylactic regimen remains uncertain; hence, clinical practices vary. For patients with nasoenteric tubes, immediate-release omeprazole (40 mg at 1 and 6 hours on day 1; then 40 mg once daily beginning on day 2) may be preferred because of lower cost and ease of administration. For patients requiring intravenous administration, continuous intravenous infusions of H_2-receptor antagonists provide adequate control of intragastric pH in most patients in the following doses over 24 hours: cimetidine (900–1200 mg) or famotidine (20 mg). Alternatively, intravenous PPIs, although more expensive, may be preferred due to superior efficacy. The optimal dosing of intravenous PPIs is uncertain; however, in clinical trials pantoprazole doses ranging from 40 mg to 80 mg and administered every 8–24 hours appear equally effective.

2. Treatment—Once bleeding occurs, patients should receive continuous infusions of a PPI (esomeprazole or pantoprazole, 80 mg intravenous bolus, followed by 8 mg/hour continuous infusion) as well as sucralfate suspension, 1 g orally every 4 to 6 hours. Endoscopy should be performed in patients with clinically significant bleeding to look for treatable causes, especially stress-related peptic ulcers with active bleeding or visible vessels. When bleeding arises from diffuse gastritis, endoscopic hemostasis techniques are not helpful.

B. NSAID Gastritis

Of patients receiving NSAIDs in clinical trials, 25–50% have gastritis and 10–20% have ulcers at endoscopy; however, symptoms of significant dyspepsia develop in about 5%. NSAIDs that are more selective for the cyclooxygenase (COX)-2 enzyme ("coxibs"), such as celecoxib, etodolac, and meloxicam, decrease the incidence of endoscopically visible ulcers by approximately 75% and significant ulcer complications by up to 50% compared with nonselective NSAIDs (nsNSAIDs). COX-2 selective NSAIDs are associated with increased risk of cardiovascular complications and therefore should be used with caution in patients with cardiovascular risk factors (see Peptic Ulcer Disease – NSAID-Induced Ulcers).

Dyspepsia is increased 1.5- to 2-fold with both nsNSAID and coxib use. However, dyspeptic symptoms correlate poorly with mucosal abnormalities (erosions or ulcers) or the development of adverse clinical events (ulcer bleeding or perforation). Given the frequency of dyspeptic symptoms in patients taking NSAIDs, it is neither feasible nor desirable to investigate all such cases. Patients with "alarm" symptoms or signs, such as severe pain, weight loss, vomiting, GI bleeding, or anemia, should undergo diagnostic upper endoscopy. For other patients, symptoms may improve with discontinuation of the agent, reduction to the lowest effective dose, or administration with meals. PPIs have demonstrated efficacy in controlled trials for the treatment of NSAID-related dyspepsia and superiority to H_2-receptor antagonists for healing of NSAID-related ulcers even in the setting of continued NSAID use. Therefore, an empiric 2- to 4-week trial of an oral PPI (omeprazole, rabeprazole, or esomeprazole, 20–40 mg/day; lansoprazole or dexlansoprazole, 30 mg/day; pantoprazole, 40 mg/day) is recommended for patients with NSAID-related dyspepsia, especially those in whom continued NSAID treatment is required. If symptoms do not improve, diagnostic upper endoscopy should be conducted.

C. Alcoholic Gastritis

Excessive alcohol consumption may lead to dyspepsia, nausea, emesis, and minor hematemesis—a condition sometimes labeled "alcoholic gastritis." However, it is not proven that alcohol alone actually causes significant erosive gastritis. Therapy with H_2-receptor antagonists, PPIs, or sucralfate for 2–4 weeks often is empirically prescribed.

D. Portal Hypertensive Gastropathy

Portal hypertension commonly results in gastric mucosal and submucosal congestion of capillaries and venules, which is correlated with the severity of the portal hypertension and underlying liver disease. Usually asymptomatic, it may cause chronic GI bleeding in 10% of patients and, less commonly, clinically significant bleeding with hematemesis. Treatment with propranolol or nadolol reduces the incidence of recurrent acute bleeding by lowering portal pressures. Patients who fail propranolol therapy may be successfully treated with portal decompressive procedures (see section above on treatment of esophageal varices).

PEPTIC Investigators for the Australian and New Zealand Intensive Care Society Clinical Trials Group, Alberta Health Services Critical Care Strategic Clinical Network, and the Irish Critical Care Trials Group; Young PJ et al. Effect of stress ulcer prophylaxis with PPIs vs histamine-2 receptor blockers on in-hospital mortality among ICU patients receiving invasive mechanical ventilation: the PEPTIC randomized clinical trial. JAMA. 2020;323:616. [PMID: 31950977]

Rice TW et al. PPIs vs histamine-2 receptor blockers for stress ulcer prophylaxis in critically ill patients: issues of interpretability in pragmatic trials. JAMA. 2020;323:611. [PMID: 31950973]

Wang Y et al. Efficacy and safety of gastrointestinal bleeding prophylaxis in critically ill patients: a systematic review and network meta-analysis. BMJ. 2020;368:16744. [PMID: 31907166]

2. Nonerosive, Nonspecific Gastritis & Intestinal Metaplasia

Nonerosive gastritis is characterized by histologic inflammation. The main types of nonerosive gastritis are those due to *H pylori* infection, those associated with pernicious anemia, and eosinophilic gastritis, and possibly other genetic and environmental factors (see Specific Types of Gastritis below). The diagnosis of nonerosive gastritis is based on histologic assessment of mucosal biopsies. Endoscopic findings are normal in many cases and do not reliably predict the presence of histologic inflammation. While clinically silent in most patients, ongoing inflammation and glandular destruction may lead to patchy or diffuse atrophy of the normal cardia, fundic or antral mucosa with subsequent development of gastric intestinal metaplasia, diagnosed histologically by the presence of goblet cells and Paneth cells. Gastric intestinal metaplasia is believed to an important precursor to the development of gastric cancer. The prevalence of gastric metaplasia varies dramatically worldwide, ranging from 3% to 5% in the United States and Northern European countries to over 20% in East Asia and South America. In the United States, the prevalence is higher among Latinx, Black, and American Indian persons. The estimated risk of developing gastric cancer with intestinal metaplasia is 1.6% within 10 years. Population-based screening for intestinal metaplasia and early gastric cancer is not endorsed by professional guidelines in regions with low gastric cancer incidence but is practiced in high-incidence regions.

In patients undergoing endoscopy for other indications in whom gastric biopsies are obtained, gastric intestinal metaplasia may be identified incidentally. Testing for *H pylori* is recommended, and if present, followed by eradication, which is associated with a 46% reduction in risk of gastric cancer. Routine surveillance in patients with gastric dysplasia for cancer is not recommended by professional guidelines but may be considered in higher risk individuals (eg, family history of gastric cancer).

Altayar O et al. AGA technical review on gastric intestinal metaplasia—epidemiology and risk factors. Gastroenterology. 2020;158:732. [PMID: 31816301]

Gawron AJ et al. AGA technical review on gastric intestinal metaplasia—natural history and clinical outcomes. Gastroenterology. 2020;158:705. [PMID: 31816300]

Shah SC et al. Surveillance of gastric intestinal metaplasia. Am J Gastroenterol. 2020;115:641. [PMID: 32058339]

A. *Helicobacter pylori* Gastritis

H pylori is a spiral gram-negative rod that resides beneath the gastric mucous layer adjacent to gastric epithelial cells. Although not invasive, it causes gastric mucosal inflammation with PMNs and lymphocytes.

In developed countries, the prevalence of *H pylori* is rapidly declining. In the United States, the prevalence rises from less than 10% in non-immigrants under age 30 years to over 50% in those over age 60 years. The prevalence is higher in non-Whites and immigrants from developing countries and is correlated inversely with socioeconomic status. Transmission is from person to person, mainly during infancy and childhood; however, the mode of transmission is unknown.

Acute infection with *H pylori* may cause a transient clinical illness characterized by nausea and abdominal pain that may last for several days and is associated with acute histologic gastritis with PMNs. After these symptoms resolve, the majority progress to chronic infection with chronic, diffuse mucosal inflammation (gastritis) characterized by PMNs and lymphocytes. Most persons are asymptomatic and suffer no sequelae. Many patients have inflammation that predominates in the gastric antrum but spares the gastric body (where acid is secreted). People with this phenotype tend to have increased gastrin; increased acid production; and increased risk of developing peptic ulcers, especially duodenal ulcers. Over time, inflammation may become more diffuse, involving the gastric body. In some patients, this may lead to destruction of acid-secreting glands with resultant mucosal atrophy, decreased acid secretion, and intestinal metaplasia. This phenotype is associated with an increased risk of gastric ulcers and gastric cancer. Chronic *H pylori* gastritis leads to the development of duodenal or gastric ulcers in up to 10%, gastric cancer in 0.1–3%, and low-grade B cell gastric lymphoma (mucosa-associated lymphoid tissue lymphoma; MALToma) in less than 0.01%. *H pylori* is estimated to account for 80–89% of non-cardia gastric cancers.

Eradication of *H pylori* may be achieved with antibiotics in over 85% of patients and leads to resolution of the chronic gastritis (see Table 15–10). Testing for *H pylori* is indicated for patients with either active or a past history of documented peptic ulcer disease, gastric metaplasia (see above), gastric MALToma, or a personal or family history of gastric carcinoma. Testing and empiric treatment are cost-effective in young patients (less than 60 years of age) with uncomplicated dyspepsia prior to further medical evaluation. Testing for and treating *H pylori* in patients with functional dyspepsia is generally recommended (see Dyspepsia, above). In addition, to reduce the risk of ulcer-related bleeding, testing for (and, if positive, treating) *H pylori* infection is recommended in patients taking low-dose aspirin or NSAIDs long-term. Some groups recommend population-based screening of all asymptomatic persons in regions in which there is a high prevalence of *H pylori* and gastric cancer (such as Japan, Korea, and China) to reduce the incidence of gastric cancer. Population-based screening of asymptomatic individuals is not recommended in western countries, in which the incidence of gastric cancer is low, but should be considered in immigrants from high-prevalence regions.

1. Noninvasive testing for *H pylori*—Although serologic tests are easily obtained and widely available, clinical guidelines no longer endorse their use for testing for *H pylori* infection. Laboratory-based quantitative serologic ELISA tests have an overall accuracy of only 80%. By contrast, the fecal antigen immunoassay and [^{13}C] urea breath test have excellent sensitivity and specificity (greater than 90–95%). Although more expensive and cumbersome to perform, these tests of active infection are more cost-effective in most clinical settings because they reduce unnecessary treatment for patients without active infection.

Recent PPIs or antibiotics significantly reduce the sensitivity of urea breath tests and fecal antigen assays. Prior to testing, PPIs should be discontinued for 14 days and antibiotics for at least 28 days.

2. Endoscopic testing for *H pylori*—When upper endoscopy is performed in patients with symptoms suggestive of upper GI disease (dyspepsia, dysphagia, vomiting, weight loss, GI bleeding), gastric biopsy specimens can be obtained for histology and detection of *H pylori* with a sensitivity and specificity of greater than 95%. Molecular-based testing of biopsy specimens for antibiotic susceptibility is commercially available but not yet in widespread clinical use.

Graham DY. Molecular-based *Helicobacter pylori* susceptibility testing is almost ready for prime time. Gastroenterology. 2021;160:1936. [PMID: 33647279]

Gupta S et al. AGA clinical practice guidelines on management of gastric intestinal metaplasia. Gastroenterology. 2020;158:693. [PMID: 31816298]

B. Pernicious Anemia Gastritis

Pernicious anemia gastritis is a rare autoimmune disorder involving the fundic glands with resultant achlorhydria, decreased intrinsic factor secretion, and vitamin B_{12} malabsorption. Of patients with B_{12} deficiency, a small number have pernicious anemia. Most patients have malabsorption secondary to chronic *H pylori* infection that results in atrophic gastritis, small intestine bacterial overgrowth, or dietary insufficiency. Fundic histology in pernicious anemia is characterized by severe gland atrophy and intestinal metaplasia caused by autoimmune destruction of the gastric fundic mucosa. Anti-intrinsic factor antibodies are present in 70% of patients. Achlorhydria leads to pronounced hypergastrinemia (greater than 1000 pg/mL) due to loss of acid inhibition of gastrin G cells. Hypergastrinemia may induce hyperplasia of gastric enterochromaffin-like cells that may lead to the development of small, multicentric carcinoid tumors in 5% of patients. Metastatic spread is uncommon in lesions smaller than 2 cm. The risk of gastric adenocarcinoma is increased threefold, with a prevalence of 1–3%. Endoscopy with biopsy is indicated in patients with pernicious anemia at the time of diagnosis. Endoscopic surveillance for dysplasia or cancer is not recommended. Pernicious anemia is discussed in detail in Chapter 13.

Annibale E et al. A current clinical overview of atrophic gastritis. Expert Rev Gastroenterol Hepatol. 2020;14:93. [PMID: 31951768]

Massironi S et al. The changing face of chronic autoimmune atrophic gastritis: an updated comprehensive perspective. Autoimmun Rev. 2019;18:215. [PMID: 30639639]

Table 15–10. Treatment options for peptic ulcer disease.

Active *Helicobacter pylori*–associated ulcer

1. Treat with anti–*H pylori* regimen for 14 days. Best empiric treatment options:

   Standard Bismuth Quadruple Therapy
   - PPI orally twice daily[1,2]
   - Bismuth subsalicylate 262 mg two tablets orally four times daily or bismuth subcitrate 120–400 mg orally four times daily
   - Tetracycline 500 mg orally four times daily
   - Metronidazole 500 mg three times daily

   OR
   - PPI orally twice daily[1]
   - Bismuth subcitrate potassium 140 mg/metronidazole 125 mg/tetracycline 125 mg (Pylera) three capsules orally four times daily[3]

   Rifabutin-Based Triple Therapy (Talicia)—four capsules, each capsule contains omeprazole 10 mg/rifabutin 12.5 mg/amoxicillin 250 mg, orally every 8 hours, thus total dosages are
   - Omeprazole 40 mg orally every 8 hours
   - Rifabutin 50 mg orally every 8 hours
   - Amoxicillin 1000 mg orally every 8 hours

   Standard Triple Therapy (No longer recommended except in locales where clarithromycin resistance is < 15%)
   - PPI orally twice daily
   - Clarithromycin 500 mg orally twice daily
   - Amoxicillin 1 g orally twice daily (or, if penicillin allergic, metronidazole 500 mg orally twice daily)
2. After completion of course of *H pylori* eradication therapy, continue treatment with PPI[1] once daily for 4–6 weeks if ulcer is large (> 1 cm) or complicated.
3. Confirm successful eradication of *H pylori* with urea breath test, fecal antigen test, or endoscopy with biopsy at least 4 weeks after completion of antibiotic treatment and 2 weeks after completion of PPI treatment.

Active ulcer not attributable to *H pylori*

Consider other causes: NSAIDs, Zollinger-Ellison syndrome, gastric malignancy. Treatment options:
- PPIs[1]:
  Uncomplicated duodenal ulcer: treat for 4 weeks
  Uncomplicated gastric ulcer: treat for 8 weeks
- H_2-receptor antagonists:
  Uncomplicated duodenal ulcer: cimetidine 800 mg, nizatidine 300 mg, famotidine 40 mg, orally once daily at bedtime for 6 weeks
  Uncomplicated gastric ulcer: cimetidine 400 mg, nizatidine 150 mg, famotidine 20 mg, orally twice daily for 8 weeks
  Complicated ulcers: PPIs[1] are the preferred drugs

Prevention of ulcer relapse

1. NSAID-induced ulcer: prophylactic therapy for high-risk patients (prior ulcer disease or ulcer complications, use of corticosteroids or anticoagulants, age > 60 years, serious comorbid illnesses). Treatment options:
   - PPI once daily
   - Celecoxib (contraindicated in patients with increased risk of CVD)
   - Misoprostol 200 mcg orally 4 times daily
2. Long-term "maintenance" therapy indicated in patients with recurrent ulcers who either are *H pylori*–negative or who have failed attempts at eradication therapy: once-daily oral PPI[1]

[1]Oral PPIs: omeprazole 40 mg, rabeprazole 20 mg, lansoprazole 30 mg, dexlansoprazole 30–60 mg, pantoprazole 40 mg, esomeprazole 40 mg. PPIs are administered 30 minutes before meals.
[2]Preferred regimen in regions with high clarithromycin resistance or in patients who have previously received a macrolide antibiotic or are penicillin allergic. Effective against metronidazole-resistant organisms.
[3]Pylera is an FDA-approved formulation containing bismuth subcitrate 140 mg/tetracycline 125 mg/metronidazole 125 mg per capsule. Packaged for 10-day course; however, 14-day treatment recommended.
[4]Talicia is an FDA approved combination formulation, with each capsule containing omeprazole 10 mg/rifabutin 12.5 mg/amoxicillin 250 mg. Talicia is administered as four capsules orally every 8 hours, thus the dosage is omeprazole 40 mg/rifabutin 50 mg/amoxicillin 1000 mg orally every 8 hours for 14 days.

3. Specific Types of Gastritis

Infections

Acute bacterial infection of the gastric submucosa and muscularis with a variety of aerobic or anaerobic organisms produces a rare, rapidly progressive, life-threatening condition known as phlegmonous or necrotizing gastritis, which requires broad-spectrum antibiotic therapy and, in many cases, emergency gastric resection. Viral infection with CMV is seen in patients with AIDS and after bone marrow or solid organ transplantation. Endoscopic findings include thickened gastric folds and ulcerations. Fungal infection with mucormycosis and *Candida* may occur in immunocompromised and diabetic patients. Larvae of *Anisakis marina* ingested in raw fish or sushi may become embedded in the gastric mucosa, producing severe abdominal pain. Pain persists for several days until the larvae die. Endoscopic removal of the larvae provides rapid symptomatic relief.

PEPTIC ULCER DISEASE

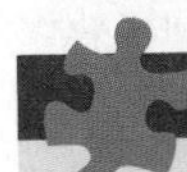

ESSENTIALS OF DIAGNOSIS

- History of dyspepsia present in 80–90% of patients with variable relationship to meals.
- Ulcer symptoms characterized by rhythmicity and periodicity.
- Ulcer complications present without antecedent symptoms in 10–20% of patients.
- Most NSAID-induced ulcers are asymptomatic.
- Upper endoscopy with gastric biopsy for *H pylori* is the diagnostic procedure of choice in most patients.
- Gastric ulcer biopsy or documentation of complete healing necessary to exclude gastric malignancy.

General Considerations

Peptic ulcer is a break in the gastric or duodenal mucosa that arises when the normal mucosal defensive factors are impaired or are overwhelmed by aggressive luminal factors such as acid and pepsin. In the United States, there are about 500,000 new cases per year of peptic ulcer and 4 million ulcer recurrences; the lifetime prevalence of ulcers in the adult population is approximately 10%. Ulcers occur either in the duodenum, where over 95% are in the bulb or pyloric channel, or in the stomach, where benign ulcers are located most commonly in the antrum (60%) or at the junction of the antrum and body on the lesser curvature (25%).

Although ulcers can occur in any age group, duodenal ulcers most commonly occur in patients between the ages of 30 and 55 years, whereas gastric ulcers are more common in patients between the ages of 55 and 70 years. The incidence of duodenal ulcer disease has been declining dramatically for the past 30 years (due to the eradication of *H pylori*), but the incidence of gastric ulcers has not been declining (due to the widespread use of NSAIDs and low-dose aspirin).

Etiology

There are two major causes of peptic ulcer disease: NSAIDs and chronic *H pylori* infection. Evidence of *H pylori* infection or NSAID ingestion should be sought in all patients with peptic ulcer. Alcohol, dietary factors, and stress do not appear to cause ulcer disease. Less than 5–10% of ulcers are caused by other conditions, including acid hypersecretory states (such as Zollinger-Ellison syndrome or systemic mastocytosis), CMV (especially in transplant recipients), Crohn disease, lymphoma, medications (eg, alendronate), or chronic medical illness (cirrhosis or CKD), or are idiopathic.

A. *H pylori*–Associated Ulcers

H pylori infection with associated gastritis appears to be a necessary cofactor for the majority of duodenal and gastric ulcers not associated with NSAIDs. Ulcer disease will develop in an estimated 10% of infected patients. The prevalence of *H pylori* infection in duodenal ulcer patients is 70–90%. The association with gastric ulcers is lower, but *H pylori* is found in most patients in whom NSAIDs cannot be implicated.

The natural history of *H pylori*–associated peptic ulcer disease is well defined. In the absence of specific antibiotic treatment to eradicate the organism, 85% of patients will have an endoscopically visible recurrence within 1 year. Half of these will be symptomatic. After successful eradication of *H pylori* with antibiotics, ulcer recurrence rates are reduced dramatically to 5–20% at 1 year. Most of these ulcer recurrences are due to NSAID use or, rarely, reinfection with *H pylori*.

B. NSAID-Induced Ulcers

There is a 10–20% prevalence of gastric ulcers and a 2–5% prevalence of duodenal ulcers in long-term NSAID users. Approximately 2–5%/year of long-term NSAID users will have an ulcer that causes clinically significant dyspepsia or a serious complication. The incidence of serious GI complications (hospitalization, bleeding, perforation) is 0.2–1.9%/year. Meta-analyses of clinical trials detected an increased risk of upper GI bleeding in patients taking low-dose aspirin (1 of 1000), coxibs (2 of 1000), and nsNSAIDs (4–6 of 1000). The risk of NSAID complications is greater within the first 3 months of therapy and in patients who are older than 60 years; who have a prior history of ulcer disease; or who take NSAIDs in combination with aspirin, corticosteroids, or anticoagulants.

Traditional nsNSAIDs inhibit prostaglandins through reversible inhibition of both COX-1 and COX-2 enzymes. Aspirin causes irreversible inhibition of COX-1 and COX-2 as well as of platelet aggregation. Coxibs (or selective NSAIDs) preferentially inhibit COX-2—the principal enzyme involved in prostaglandin production at sites of inflammation—while providing relative sparing of COX-1, the principal enzyme involved with mucosal cytoprotection in the stomach and duodenum. Celecoxib is the only coxib currently available in the United States, although other older NSAIDs (etodolac, meloxicam) may have similar COX-2/COX-1 selectivity.

Coxibs decrease the incidence of endoscopically visible ulcers by approximately 75% compared with nsNSAIDs. Of greater clinical importance, the risk of significant clinical events (obstruction, perforation, bleeding) is reduced by up to 50% in patients taking coxibs versus nsNSAIDs. However, a twofold increase in the incidence in cardiovascular complications (MI, cerebrovascular infarction, and death) has been detected in patients taking coxibs compared with placebo, prompting the voluntary withdrawal of two highly selective coxibs (rofecoxib and valdecoxib) from the market by the manufacturers. A review by an FDA panel suggested that all NSAIDs (other than aspirin and, possibly, naproxen) may be associated with an increased risk of cardiovascular complications, but concluded that celecoxib, which has less COX-2 selectivity than rofecoxib and valdecoxib, does not have higher risk than other nsNSAIDs when used in currently recommended doses (200 mg/day). In 2016, a large, randomized, noninferiority trial comparing ibuprofen, naproxen, and celecoxib in arthritis patients with increased cardiovascular risk found no difference in cardiovascular safety between the three drugs over 3 years. However, celecoxib was associated with significantly fewer serious GI events than both naproxen (hazard ratio 0.71) and ibuprofen (hazard ratio 0.65).

Use of even low-dose aspirin (81–325 mg/day) leads to a twofold increased risk of GI bleeding complications. In population studies, GI bleeding occurs in 1.2% of patients each year. Patients with a prior history of peptic ulcers or GI bleeding have a markedly increased risk of complications on low-dose aspirin. It should be noted that low-dose aspirin in combination with NSAIDs or coxibs increases the risk of ulcer complications by up to tenfold compared with NSAIDs or low-dose aspirin alone. Dual antiplatelet therapy with aspirin and a thienopyridine (eg, clopidogrel) incurs a twofold to threefold increased risk of bleeding compared with aspirin alone.

H pylori infection increases the risk of ulcer disease and complications over threefold in patients taking NSAIDs or low-dose aspirin. It is hypothesized that NSAID initiation may potentiate or aggravate ulcer disease in susceptible infected individuals.

Clinical Findings

A. Symptoms and Signs

Epigastric pain (dyspepsia), the hallmark of peptic ulcer disease, is present in 80–90% of patients. However, this complaint is not sensitive or specific enough to serve as a reliable diagnostic criterion for peptic ulcer disease. The clinical history cannot accurately distinguish duodenal from gastric ulcers. Less than 25% of patients with dyspepsia have ulcer disease at endoscopy. Twenty percent of patients with ulcer complications such as bleeding have no antecedent symptoms ("silent ulcers"). Nearly 60% of patients with NSAID-related ulcer complications do not have prior symptoms.

Pain is typically well localized to the epigastrium and not severe. It is described as gnawing, dull, aching, or "hunger-like." Approximately 50% of patients report relief of pain with food or antacids (especially those with duodenal ulcers) and a recurrence of pain 2–4 hours later. However, many patients deny any relationship to meals or report worsening of pain. Two-thirds of duodenal ulcers and one-third of gastric ulcers cause nocturnal pain that awakens the patient. A change from a patient's typical rhythmic discomfort to constant or radiating pain may reflect ulcer penetration or perforation. Most patients have symptomatic periods lasting up to several weeks with intervals of months to years in which they are pain free (periodicity).

Nausea and anorexia may occur with gastric ulcers. Significant vomiting and weight loss are unusual with uncomplicated ulcer disease and suggest gastric outlet obstruction or gastric malignancy.

The physical examination is often normal in uncomplicated peptic ulcer disease. Mild, localized epigastric tenderness to deep palpation may be present. FOBT or FIT is positive in one-third of patients.

B. Laboratory Findings

Laboratory tests are normal in uncomplicated peptic ulcer disease but are ordered to exclude ulcer complications or confounding disease entities. Anemia may occur with acute blood loss from a bleeding ulcer or less commonly from chronic blood loss. Leukocytosis suggests ulcer penetration or perforation. An elevated serum amylase in a patient with severe epigastric pain suggests ulcer penetration into the pancreas. A fasting serum gastrin level to screen for Zollinger-Ellison syndrome is obtained in some patients.

C. Endoscopy

Upper endoscopy is the procedure of choice for the diagnosis of duodenal and gastric ulcers. Duodenal ulcers are virtually never malignant and do not require biopsy. Three to 5 percent of benign-appearing gastric ulcers prove to be malignant. Hence, biopsies of the ulcer margin are almost always performed. Provided that the gastric ulcer appears benign to the endoscopist and adequate biopsy specimens reveal no evidence of cancer, dysplasia, or atypia, the patient may be monitored without further endoscopy. If these conditions are not fulfilled, follow-up endoscopy should be performed 12 weeks after the start of therapy to document complete healing; nonhealing ulcers are suspicious for malignancy.

D. Imaging

Abdominal CT imaging is obtained in patients with suspected complications of peptic ulcer disease (perforation, penetration, or obstruction). Barium upper GI series is no longer recommended.

E. Testing for *H pylori*

In patients in whom an ulcer is diagnosed by endoscopy, gastric mucosal biopsies should be obtained for histologic evaluation. Noninvasive assessment for *H pylori* with fecal antigen assay or urea breath testing may be done in patients with a history of peptic ulcer disease to diagnose active infection or in patients following its treatment to confirm successful eradication. Both tests have a sensitivity and specificity of 92–95%. PPIs may cause false-negative urea breath tests and fecal antigen tests and should be withheld for at least 14 days before testing. Because of its lower sensitivity (85%) and specificity (79%), serologic testing should not be performed unless fecal antigen testing or urea breath testing is unavailable.

Differential Diagnosis

Peptic ulcer disease must be distinguished from other causes of epigastric distress (dyspepsia). Over 50% of patients with dyspepsia have no obvious organic explanation for their symptoms and are classified as having functional dyspepsia (see sections above on Dyspepsia and Functional Dyspepsia). Atypical gastroesophageal reflux may be manifested by epigastric symptoms. Biliary tract disease is characterized by discrete, intermittent episodes of pain that should not be confused with other causes of dyspepsia. Severe epigastric pain is atypical for peptic ulcer disease unless complicated by a perforation or penetration. Other causes include acute pancreatitis, acute cholecystitis or choledocholithiasis, esophageal rupture, gastric volvulus, gastric or intestinal ischemia, and ruptured aortic aneurysm.

Pharmacologic Agents

Agents that enhance the healing of peptic ulcers may be divided into three categories: (1) acid-antisecretory agents, (2) mucosal protective agents, and (3) agents that promote healing through eradication of *H pylori*.

A. Acid-Antisecretory Agents

1. PPIs—PPIs covalently bind the acid-secreting enzyme H^+-K^+-ATPase, or "proton pump," permanently inactivating it.

There are six oral PPIs currently available: omeprazole, rabeprazole, esomeprazole, lansoprazole, dexlansoprazole, and pantoprazole. Despite minor differences in their pharmacology, they are equally efficacious in the treatment of peptic ulcer disease. Treatment with oral PPIs results in over 90% healing of duodenal ulcers after 4 weeks and 90% of gastric ulcers after 8 weeks when given once daily (30 minutes before breakfast) at the following recommended doses: omeprazole, 20–40 mg; esomeprazole, 40 mg; rabeprazole, 20 mg; lansoprazole, 30 mg; dexlansoprazole, 30–60 mg; and pantoprazole, 40 mg. Compared with H_2-receptor antagonists, PPIs provide faster pain relief and more rapid ulcer healing.

The PPIs are remarkably safe for short-term therapy. (For potential long-term risks, see Gastroesophageal Reflux Disease.) Long-term use may lead to increased risk of enteric infections (including *C difficile*) and micronutrient deficiencies (vitamin B_{12}, iron, magnesium, and possibly calcium). Observational studies report an association with a number of adverse events, including interstitial nephritis, pneumonia, bone fracture, MI, and dementia, but these have not been confirmed in large prospective studies. Nonetheless, long-term PPI therapy should be prescribed only for patients with appropriate indications. Serum gastrin levels rise significantly in 3% of patients receiving long-term therapy but return to normal limits within 2 weeks after discontinuation.

2. H_2-receptor antagonists—Although H_2-receptor antagonists are effective in the treatment of peptic ulcer disease, PPIs are now the preferred agents because of their ease of use and superior efficacy. Three H_2-receptor antagonists are available: cimetidine, famotidine, and nizatidine. For uncomplicated peptic ulcers, H_2-receptor antagonists may be administered once daily at bedtime as follows: nizatidine 300 mg, famotidine 40 mg, and cimetidine 800 mg. Duodenal and gastric ulcer healing rates of 85–90% are obtained within 6 weeks and 8 weeks, respectively. NOTE: Ranitidine has now been withdrawn from the US market by the FDA after an ongoing investigation showed that, when stored at higher-than-normal temperatures, it could contain an increased and unsafe quantity of N-nitrosodimethylamine (NDMA), a probable human carcinogen.

B. Agents Enhancing Mucosal Defenses

Bismuth sucralfate, misoprostol, and antacids all have been shown to promote ulcer healing through the enhancement of mucosal defensive mechanisms. Given the greater efficacy and safety of antisecretory agents and better compliance of patients, these agents are no longer used as first-line therapy for active ulcers in most clinical settings.

C. *H pylori* Eradication Therapy

Eradication of *H pylori* has proved difficult. Combination regimens that use two or three antibiotics with a PPI or bismuth are required to achieve adequate rates of eradication and to reduce the number of failures due to antibiotic resistance. In the United States, up to 50% of strains are resistant to metronidazole and 10–20% are resistant to clarithromycin. Recommended regimens are listed in Table 15–10. Ideally, the optimal regimen would be determined by antibiotic susceptibility testing; however, this requires endoscopic biopsy. In most clinical settings, therapy is chosen empirically. Commercial laboratories now offer culture-based and molecular-based susceptibility testing, which may be helpful for patients who have not responded to an initial empiric course of treatment.

Until recently, in the United States a 14-day course of so-called triple therapy with a PPI, clarithromycin, and either amoxicillin (or metronidazole, if penicillin allergic) was recommended as first-line therapy. However, updated guidelines recommend that triple therapy no longer be used (due to increasing clarithromycin resistance) except in areas with known low-level clarithromycin resistance (less than 15%) or when susceptibility has been confirmed by molecular- or culture-based tests. In most settings, empiric treatment for 14-days is recommended with either a bismuth-based quadruple therapy regimen or a rifabutin-based triple therapy regimen. Both achieve a greater than 85% eradication rate. The bismuth-based quadruple therapy regimen consists of bismuth, tetracycline, a PPI, and metronidazole or tinidazole (Table 15–10). It is effective even for metronidazole-resistant strains. The rifabutin-based regimen contains omeprazole, rifabutin, and amoxicillin (Talicia). Four capsules are taken orally every 8 hours. Rifabutin-resistant strains are rare.

Medical Treatment

Patients should be encouraged to eat balanced meals at regular intervals. There is no justification for bland or restrictive diets. Moderate alcohol intake is not harmful. Smoking retards the rate of ulcer healing and increases the frequency of recurrences and should be prohibited.

A. Treatment of *H pylori*–Associated Ulcers

1. Treatment of active ulcer—The goals of treatment of active *H pylori*–associated ulcers are to relieve dyspeptic symptoms, to promote ulcer healing, and to eradicate *H pylori* infection. Uncomplicated *H pylori*–associated ulcers should be treated for 14 days with one of the PPI-based *H pylori* eradication regimens listed in Table 15–10. At that point, no further antisecretory therapy is needed, provided the ulcer was small (less than 1 cm) and dyspeptic symptoms have resolved. For patients with large or complicated ulcers, an antisecretory agent should be continued for an additional 2–4 weeks (duodenal ulcer) or 4–6 weeks (gastric ulcer) after completion of the antibiotic regimen to ensure complete ulcer healing. A once-daily oral PPI (as listed in Table 15–10) is recommended. Confirmation of *H pylori* eradication is recommended for all patients more than 4 weeks after completion of antibiotic therapy and more than 2 weeks after discontinuation of the PPI either with noninvasive tests (urea breath test, fecal antigen test) or endoscopy with biopsy for histology.

2. Therapy to prevent recurrence—Successful eradication reduces ulcer recurrences to less than 20% after 1–2 years. The most common cause of recurrence after antibiotic therapy is failure to achieve successful eradication. Once cure has been achieved, reinfection rates are less than 0.5% per year. Although *H pylori* eradication has reduced the need for long-term maintenance antisecretory therapy to prevent ulcer recurrences, there remains a subset of patients who require long-term therapy with a PPI once daily. This subset includes patients with *H pylori*–positive ulcers who have not responded to repeated attempts at eradication therapy, patients with a history of *H pylori*–positive ulcers who have recurrent ulcers despite successful eradication, and patients with idiopathic ulcers (ie, *H pylori*–negative and not taking NSAIDs). In all patients with recurrent ulcers, NSAID usage (unintentional or surreptitious) and hypersecretory states (including gastrinoma) should be excluded.

B. Treatment of NSAID-Induced Ulcers

1. Treatment of active ulcers—In patients with NSAID-induced ulcers, the offending agent should be discontinued whenever possible. Both gastric and duodenal ulcers respond rapidly to therapy with H_2-receptor antagonists or PPIs (Table 15–10) once NSAIDs are eliminated. All patients with NSAID-associated ulcers should undergo testing for *H pylori* infection. Antibiotic eradication therapy should be given if *H pylori* tests are positive.

2. Prevention of NSAID-induced ulcers—Clinicians should carefully weigh the benefits of NSAID therapy with the risks of cardiovascular and GI complications. Ulcer complications occur in up to 2% of all nsNSAID-treated patients per year, but in up to 10–20% per year of patients with multiple risk factors. These include age over 60 years, history of ulcer disease or complications, concurrent use of antiplatelet therapy (low-dose aspirin or clopidogrel, or both), concurrent therapy with anticoagulants or corticosteroids, and serious underlying medical illness. After considering the patient's risk of cardiovascular and GI complications due to NSAID use, the clinician can decide what type of NSAID (nsNSAID vs coxib) is appropriate and what strategies should be used to reduce the risk of such complications. To minimize cardiovascular and GI risks, all NSAIDs should be used at the lowest effective dose and for the shortest time necessary.

A. Test for and treat *H pylori* infection—All patients with a known history of peptic ulcer disease who are treated with NSAIDs or antiplatelet agents (aspirin, clopidogrel) should be tested for *H pylori* infection and treated, if positive. Although *H pylori* eradication may decrease the risk of NSAID-related complications, cotherapy with a PPI is still required in high-risk patients.

B. PPI—Treatment with an oral PPI given once daily (rabeprazole 20 mg, omeprazole 20–40 mg, lansoprazole 30 mg, dexlansoprazole 30–60 mg, or pantoprazole or esomeprazole 40 mg) is effective in the prevention of NSAID-induced gastric and duodenal ulcers and is approved by the FDA for this indication. Among high-risk patients taking nsNSAIDs or coxibs, the incidence of endoscopically visible gastric and duodenal ulcers after 6 months of therapy in patients treated with esomeprazole 20–40 mg/day was 5%, compared with 17% who were given placebo. Nonetheless, PPIs are not fully protective in high-risk patients in preventing NSAID-related complications. In prospective, controlled trials of patients with a prior history of NSAID-related ulcer complications, the incidence of recurrent bleeding was almost 5% after 6 months in patients taking nsNSAIDs and a PPI. In prospective, controlled trials of patients with a prior history of ulcer complications related to low-dose aspirin, the incidence of recurrent ulcer bleeding in patients taking low-dose aspirin alone was approximately 15% per year compared with 0–2% per year in patients taking low-dose aspirin and PPI and 9–14% per year in patients taking clopidogrel. Thus, PPIs are highly effective in preventing complications related to low-dose aspirin, even in high-risk patients. Enteric coating of aspirin may reduce direct topical damage to the stomach but does not reduce its other complications.

C. Recommendations to reduce risk of ulcer complications from nsNSAIDs and coxibs—For patients with a low risk of CVD who have no risk factors for GI complications, an nsNSAID alone may be given. For patients with one or two GI risk factors, a coxib alone or an nsNSAID should be given with a PPI once daily to reduce the risk of GI complications. NSAIDs should be avoided, if possible, in patients with multiple risk factors; if required, however, combination therapy of celecoxib or a partially COX-2 selective nsNSAID (etodolac, meloxicam) with a PPI once daily is recommended.

For patients with an increased risk of cardiovascular complications, it is preferable to avoid NSAIDs, if possible. Almost all patients with increased cardiovascular risk also will be taking antiplatelet therapy with low-dose aspirin or clopidogrel, or both. Because combination therapy with an nsNSAID and antiplatelet therapy increases the risks of GI complications, these patients should all receive cotherapy with a PPI once daily or misoprostol.

D. Recommendations to reduce risk of ulcer complications with use of antiplatelet agents—The risk of significant GI complications in persons taking low-dose aspirin (81–325 mg/day) or clopidogrel, or both, for cardiovascular prophylaxis is 0.5%/year. Aspirin, 81 mg/day, is recommended in most patients because it has a lower risk of GI complications but equivalent cardiovascular protection compared with higher aspirin doses. Complications are increased with combinations of aspirin and clopidogrel or aspirin and anticoagulants. Clopidogrel does not cause GI ulcers or erosions. However, its antiplatelet activity may promote bleeding from erosions or ulcers caused by low-dose aspirin or *H pylori*. Patients with dyspepsia or prior ulcer disease should be tested for *H pylori* infection and treated, if positive. Patients younger than 60–70 years who have no other risk factors for GI complications may be treated with low-dose aspirin or dual antiplatelet therapy without a PPI. Virtually all other patients who require low-dose aspirin or aspirin plus anticoagulant therapy should receive a PPI once daily.

At the present time, the optimal management of patients who require dual antiplatelet therapy with clopidogrel and aspirin is uncertain. Clopidogrel is a prodrug that is activated by the cytochrome P450 CYP2C19 enzyme. All PPIs inhibit CYP2C19 to varying degrees, with omeprazole having the highest and pantoprazole the least level of inhibition. In vitro and in vivo platelet aggregation studies demonstrate that PPIs (especially omeprazole) may attenuate the antiplatelet effects of clopidogrel, although the clinical importance of this interaction is uncertain. The FDA has issued a warning that patients should avoid using clopidogrel with omeprazole and esomeprazole. A 2010 expert consensus panel concluded that once daily treatment with an oral PPI (pantoprazole 40 mg; rabeprazole 20 mg; lansoprazole or dexlansoprazole 30 mg) may be recommended for patients who have an increased risk of upper GI bleeding (prior history of peptic ulcer disease or GI bleeding; concomitant NSAIDs). For patients with a lower risk of GI bleeding, the risks and benefits of PPIs must be weighed. Pending further recommendations, an acceptable alternative is to treat with an oral H_2-receptor antagonist (famotidine 20 mg, nizatidine 150 mg) twice daily; however, PPIs are more effective in preventing upper GI bleeding. Cimetidine is a CYP2C19 inhibitor and should not be used. An alternative strategy is ticagrelor, an antiplatelet agent approved for use with low-dose aspirin in the treatment of acute coronary syndrome. Like clopidogrel, ticagrelor blocks the platelet ADP p2y12 receptor; however, it does not require hepatic activation, it does not interact with the CYP2C19 enzyme, and its efficacy is not diminished by PPIs.

C. Refractory Ulcers

Ulcers that are truly refractory to medical therapy are now uncommon. Less than 5% of ulcers are unhealed after 8 weeks of once daily therapy with PPIs, and almost all benign ulcers heal with twice-daily therapy. Thus, noncompliance is the most common cause of ulcer nonhealing. NSAID and aspirin use, sometimes surreptitious, are commonly implicated in refractory ulcers and must be stopped. Single or multiple linear gastric ulcers may occur in large hiatal hernias where the stomach slides back and forth through the diaphragmatic hiatus ("Cameron lesions"); this may be a cause of iron deficiency anemia. Other causes of nonhealing ulcers include acid hypersecretion (Zollinger-Ellison syndrome), unrecognized malignancy (adenocarcinoma or lymphoma), medications causing GI ulceration (eg, iron or bisphosphonates), Crohn disease, and unusual infections (*H heilmanii*, CMV, mucormycosis). Fasting serum gastrin levels should be obtained to exclude gastrinoma with acid hypersecretion (Zollinger-Ellison syndrome). Repeat ulcer biopsies are mandatory after 2–3 months of therapy in all nonhealed ulcers to look for malignancy or infection. Patients with persistent nonhealing ulcers are referred for surgical therapy after exclusion of NSAID use and persistent *H pylori* infection.

Guevara B et al. *Helicobacter pylori*: a review of current diagnostic and management strategies. Dig Dis Sci. 2020;65:1917. [PMID: 32170476]

Howden CW et al. Recent developments pertaining to *H pylori* infection. Am J Gastroenterol. 2021;116:1. [PMID: 33378314]

Hulten KG et al. National and regional US antibiotic resistance to *Helicobacter pylori*: lessons from a clinical trial. Gastroenterology. 2021;161:342. [PMID: 33798524]

Kurlander JE et al. Trials of dual antiplatelet therapy after percutaneous coronary intervention lack strategies to ensure appropriate gastroprotection. Am J Gastroenterol. 2021;116:821. [PMID: 33982954]

COMPLICATIONS OF PEPTIC ULCER DISEASE

1. GI Hemorrhage

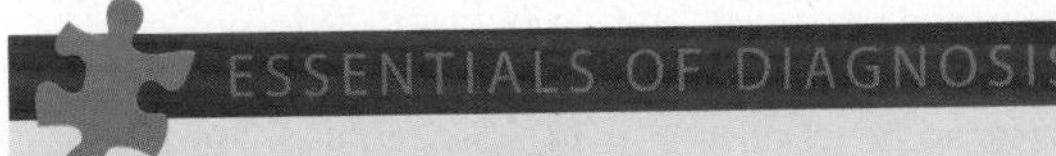

- "Coffee grounds" emesis, hematemesis, melena, or hematochezia.
- Emergent upper endoscopy is diagnostic and therapeutic.

General Considerations

Approximately 50% of all episodes of upper GI bleeding are due to peptic ulcer. Clinically significant bleeding occurs in 10% of ulcer patients. About 80% of patients stop bleeding spontaneously and generally have an uneventful recovery; the remaining 20% have more severe bleeding. The overall mortality rate for ulcer bleeding is 7%, but it is higher in older patients, in patients with comorbid medical problems, and in patients with hospital-associated bleeding. Mortality is also higher in patients who present with persistent hypotension or shock, bright red blood in the vomitus or nasogastric lavage fluid, or severe coagulopathy.

Clinical Findings

A. Symptoms and Signs

Up to 20% of patients have no antecedent symptoms of pain; this is particularly true of patients receiving NSAIDs. Common presenting signs include melena and hematemesis. Massive upper GI bleeding or rapid GI transit may result in hematochezia rather than melena; this may be misinterpreted as signifying a lower tract bleeding source. Nasogastric lavage that demonstrates "coffee grounds" or bright red blood confirms an upper tract source. Recovered nasogastric lavage fluid that is negative for blood does not exclude active bleeding from a duodenal ulcer.

B. Laboratory Findings

The hematocrit may fall as a result of bleeding or expansion of the intravascular volume with intravenous fluids. The BUN may rise as a result of absorption of blood nitrogen from the small intestine and prerenal azotemia.

Treatment

A. Medical Therapy

1. Antisecretory agents—Intravenous PPIs should be administered for 3 days in patients with ulcers whose endoscopic appearance suggests a high risk of rebleeding after endoscopic therapy. Intravenous PPIs have been associated with a reduction in rebleeding, transfusions, need for further endoscopic therapy, and surgery in the subset of patients with high-risk ulcers, ie, an ulcer with active bleeding, visible vessel, or adherent clot. After initial successful endoscopic treatment of ulcer hemorrhage, intravenous esomeprazole, pantoprazole, or omeprazole (80 mg bolus injection, followed by 8 mg/hour continuous infusion for 72 hours) reduces the rebleeding rate from approximately 20% to less than 10%; however, intravenous omeprazole is not available in the United States.

High-dose oral PPIs (omeprazole 40 mg twice daily) also appear to be effective in reducing rebleeding but have not been compared with the intravenous regimen. Intravenous H_2-receptor antagonists have not been demonstrated to be of any benefit in the treatment of acute ulcer bleeding.

2. Long-term prevention of rebleeding—Recurrent ulcer bleeding develops within 3 years in one-third of patients if no specific therapy is given. In patients with bleeding ulcers who are *H pylori*–positive, successful eradication effectively prevents recurrent ulcer bleeding in almost all cases. It is therefore recommended that all patients with bleeding ulcers be tested for *H pylori* infection and treated if positive. Four weeks after completion of antibiotic therapy, a urea breath or fecal antigen test for *H pylori* should be administered or endoscopy performed with biopsy and histology for confirmation of successful eradication. In patients in whom *H pylori* persists or the small subset of patients whose ulcers are not associated with NSAIDs or *H pylori*, long-term acid suppression with a once-daily PPI should be prescribed to reduce the likelihood of recurrence of bleeding.

B. Endoscopy

Endoscopy is the preferred diagnostic procedure in almost all cases of upper GI bleeding because of its high diagnostic accuracy, its ability to predict the likelihood of recurrent bleeding, and its availability for therapeutic intervention in high-risk lesions. Endoscopy should be performed within 24 hours in most cases. In cases of severe active bleeding, endoscopy should be performed after patients have been appropriately resuscitated and are hemodynamically stable.

On the basis of clinical and endoscopic criteria, it is possible to predict which patients are at a higher risk of rebleeding and therefore to make more rational use of hospital resources. Nonbleeding ulcers under 2 cm in size with a base that is clean have a less than 5% chance of rebleeding. Most young (under age 60 years), otherwise healthy patients with clean-based ulcers may be safely discharged from the emergency department or hospital after endoscopy. Ulcers that have a flat red or black spot have a less than 10% chance of significant rebleeding. Patients who are hemodynamically stable with these findings should be admitted to a hospital ward for 24–72 hours and may begin immediate oral feedings and antiulcer (or anti–*H pylori*) medication.

By contrast, the risk of rebleeding or continued bleeding in ulcers with a nonbleeding visible vessel is 50%, and with active bleeding, it is 80–90%. Endoscopic therapy with thermocoagulation (bipolar or heater probes) or application of endoscopic clips (akin to a staple) is the standard of care for such lesions because it reduces the risk of rebleeding, the number of transfusions, and the need for subsequent surgery. The optimal treatment of ulcers with a dense clot that adheres despite vigorous washing is controversial; removal of the clot followed by endoscopic treatment of an underlying vessel may be considered in selected high-risk patients. For actively bleeding ulcers, a combination of epinephrine injection followed by thermocoagulation or clip application commonly is used. These techniques achieve successful hemostasis of actively bleeding lesions in 90% of patients. Endoscopic application of a topical hemostatic powder (Hemospray) may provide temporary hemostasis for up to 24 hours in patients with massive bleeding that interferes with effective application of thermocoagulation or endoclip placement. After endoscopic therapy followed by an intravenous PPI, significant rebleeding occurs in less than 10% of cases, of which over 70% can be managed successfully with repeat endoscopic treatment. After endoscopic treatment, patients should remain hospitalized for at least 72 hours, when the risk of rebleeding falls to below 3%.

C. Recurrent Bleeding

Less than 5% of patients have persistent or recurrent bleeding that cannot be controlled with endoscopic techniques. The availability of newer, larger over-the-scope clips has further reduced the risk of persistent bleeding requiring other more aggressive interventions. In a randomized prospective study of patients with recurrent ulcer bleeding after conventional medical and endoscopic therapy, persistent bleeding occurred in 6% of patients treated with over-the-scope clips versus 42.4% treated with further conventional endoscopic modalities. For patients in whom endoscopic therapy is unsuccessful, percutaneous radiologic embolization or surgery should be considered. Overall surgical mortality for emergency ulcer bleeding is less than 6%. The prognosis is poorer for patients over age 60 years, those with serious underlying medical illnesses or CKD, and those who require more than 10 units of blood transfusion.

2. Ulcer Perforation

Perforations develop in less than 5% of ulcer patients, usually from ulcers on the anterior wall of the stomach or duodenum. Perforation results in a chemical peritonitis that causes sudden, severe generalized abdominal pain that prompts most patients to seek immediate attention. Older adults or debilitated patients and those receiving long-term corticosteroid therapy may experience minimal initial symptoms, presenting late with bacterial peritonitis, sepsis, and shock. On physical examination, patients appear ill, with a rigid, quiet abdomen and rebound tenderness. Hypotension develops later after bacterial peritonitis has developed. If hypotension is present early with the onset of pain, other abdominal emergencies should be considered such as a ruptured aortic aneurysm, mesenteric infarction, or acute pancreatitis. Leukocytosis is almost always present. A mildly elevated serum amylase (less than twice normal) is sometimes seen with ulcer perforation. Abdominal CT usually establishes the diagnosis without need for further studies. The absence of free air may lead to a misdiagnosis of pancreatitis, cholecystitis, or appendicitis.

Laparoscopic closure of perforations can be performed in many centers, significantly reducing operative morbidity compared with open laparotomy.

3. Gastric Outlet Obstruction

Gastric outlet obstruction occurs in less than 2% of patients with ulcer disease and is due to edema or cicatricial narrowing of the pylorus or duodenal bulb. With the advent of potent antisecretory therapy with PPIs and the eradication of *H pylori*, obstruction now is less commonly caused by peptic ulcers than by gastric neoplasms or extrinsic duodenal obstruction by intra-abdominal neoplasms. The most common symptoms are early satiety, vomiting, and weight loss. Later, vomiting may develop that typically occurs one to several hours after eating and consists of partially digested food contents. Patients may develop dehydration, metabolic alkalosis, and hypokalemia. On physical examination, a succussion splash may be heard in the epigastrium. In most cases, nasogastric aspiration will result in evacuation of a large amount (greater than 200 mL) of foul-smelling fluid, which establishes the diagnosis. Patients are treated initially with intravenous isotonic saline and KCl to correct fluid and electrolyte disorders, an intravenous PPI, and nasogastric decompression of the stomach. Upper endoscopy is performed after 24–72 hours to define the nature of the obstruction and to exclude gastric neoplasm.

Hussein M et al. Hemostatic spray powder (TC-325) in the primary endoscopic treatment of peptic-ulcer bleeding: a multicenter international registry. Endoscopy. 2021;53:36. [PMID: 32459010]

Laine L et al. ACG Clinical Guideline: upper gastrointestinal and ulcer bleeding. Am J Gastroenterol. 2021;116:899. [PMID: 33929377]

Mullady DK et al. AGA Clinical Practice Update on endoscopic therapies for non-variceal upper gastrointestinal bleeding: expert review. Gastroenterology. 2021;159:1120. [PMID: 32574620]

ZOLLINGER-ELLISON SYNDROME (Gastrinoma)

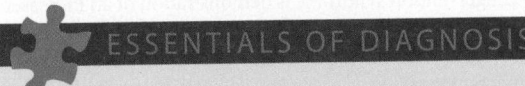

- Peptic ulcer disease; may be severe and atypical.
- Gastric acid hypersecretion.
- Diarrhea common, relieved by nasogastric suction.
- Most cases are sporadic; 25% occur with multiple endocrine neoplasia type 1 (MEN 1).

General Considerations

Zollinger-Ellison syndrome is caused by gastrin-secreting gut neuroendocrine tumors (gastrinomas), which result in hypergastrinemia and acid hypersecretion. Less than 1% of peptic ulcer disease is caused by gastrinomas. Primary gastrinomas may arise in the pancreas (25%), duodenal wall (45%), or lymph nodes (5–15%), and in other locations including unknown primary sites (20%). Approximately 80% arise within the "gastrinoma triangle" bounded by the porta hepatis, the neck of the pancreas, and the third portion of the duodenum. Most gastrinomas are solitary or multifocal nodules that are potentially resectable. Approximately 25% of patients have small multicentric gastrinomas associated with MEN 1 that are more difficult to resect. Over two-thirds of gastrinomas are malignant, and one-third have already metastasized to the liver at initial presentation.

Clinical Findings

A. Symptoms and Signs

Over 90% of patients with Zollinger-Ellison syndrome develop peptic ulcers. In most cases, the symptoms are indistinguishable from other causes of peptic ulcer disease, and therefore, the syndrome may go undetected for years. Ulcers usually are solitary and located in the duodenal bulb, but they may be multiple or occur more distally in the duodenum. Isolated gastric ulcers do not occur. Gastroesophageal reflux symptoms occur often. Diarrhea occurs in one-third of patients, in some cases in the absence of peptic symptoms. Gastric acid hypersecretion can cause direct intestinal mucosal injury and pancreatic enzyme inactivation, resulting in diarrhea, steatorrhea, and weight loss; nasogastric aspiration of stomach acid stops the diarrhea. Screening for Zollinger-Ellison syndrome with fasting gastrin levels should be done in patients with ulcers that are refractory to standard therapies, giant ulcers (larger than 2 cm), ulcers located distal to the duodenal bulb, multiple duodenal ulcers, frequent ulcer recurrences, ulcers associated with diarrhea, ulcers occurring after ulcer surgery, and ulcers with complications. Ulcer patients with hypercalcemia or family histories of ulcers (suggesting MEN 1) should also be screened. Finally, patients with peptic ulcers who are *H pylori* negative and who are not taking NSAIDs should be screened.

B. Laboratory Findings

The most sensitive and specific method for identifying Zollinger-Ellison syndrome is demonstration of an increased fasting serum gastrin concentration (greater than 150 pg/mL [150 ng/L]). If possible, levels should be obtained with patients not taking H_2-receptor antagonists for 24 hours or PPIs for 6 days; however, withdrawal of the PPI may result in marked gastric hypersecretion with serious consequences and patients should be closely monitored. The median gastrin level is 500–700 pg/mL (500–700 ng/L), and 60% of patients have levels less than 1000 pg/mL (1000 ng/L). Hypochlorhydria with increased gastric pH is a much more common cause of hypergastrinemia than is gastrinoma. Therefore, a measurement of gastric pH (and, where available, a gastric secretory study) is performed in patients with fasting hypergastrinemia. Most patients have a basal acid output of over 15 mEq/hour. A gastric pH of greater than 3.0 implies hypochlorhydria and excludes gastrinoma. In a patient with a serum gastrin level of greater than 1000 pg/mL (1000 ng/L) and gastric pH < 2, the diagnosis of Zollinger-Ellison syndrome is established. With lower gastrin levels (150–1000 pg/mL [150–1000 ng/L]) and acid secretion, a secretin stimulation test may be performed to distinguish Zollinger-Ellison syndrome from other causes of hypergastrinemia. Intravenous secretin (2 U/kg) produces a rise in serum gastrin of over 200 pg/mL (200 ng/L) within 2–30 minutes in 85% of patients with gastrinoma. An elevated serum calcium suggests hyperparathyroidism and MEN 1 syndrome. In all patients with Zollinger-Ellison syndrome, serum parathyroid hormone (PTH), prolactin, LH-FSH, and growth hormone (GH) levels should be obtained to exclude MEN 1.

C. Imaging

Imaging studies are obtained in an attempt to determine whether there is metastatic disease and, if not, to identify the site of the primary tumor. CT and MRI scans are commonly obtained first to look for large hepatic metastases and primary lesions, but they have low sensitivity for small lesions. Gastrinomas express somatostatin receptors that bind radiolabeled octreotide and Gallium-68 dotatate. Full body ^{68}Ga-PET scans (preferably combined with CT) have a sensitivity of greater than 90% for detection of primary tumor in the pancreas, duodenum, and lymph nodes as well as for detection of metastatic disease in liver and bone. Where available, ^{68}Ga-PET/CT has supplanted somatostatin receptor scintigraphy with single PET. In patients with negative ^{68}Ga-PET/CT or somatostatin receptor scintigraphy, endoscopic ultrasonography may be useful to detect small gastrinomas in the duodenal wall, pancreas, or peripancreatic lymph nodes.

Differential Diagnosis

Gastrinomas are one of several gut neuroendocrine tumors that have similar histopathologic features and arise either from the gut or pancreas. These include carcinoid, insulinoma, VIPoma, glucagonoma, and somatostatinoma. These tumors usually are differentiated by the gut peptides that they secrete; however, poorly differentiated neuroendocrine tumors may not secrete any hormones. Patients may present with symptoms caused by tumor metastases (jaundice, hepatomegaly) rather than functional symptoms. Once a diagnosis of a neuroendocrine tumor is established from the liver biopsy, the specific type of tumor can subsequently be determined. Both carcinoid and gastrinoma tumors may be detected incidentally during endoscopy after biopsy of a submucosal nodule and must be distinguished by subsequent studies.

Hypergastrinemia due to gastrinoma must be distinguished from other causes of hypergastrinemia. Atrophic gastritis with decreased acid secretion is detected by gastric secretory analysis. Other conditions associated with hypergastrinemia (eg, gastric outlet obstruction, vagotomy, CKD) are associated with a negative secretin stimulation test.

Treatment

A. Metastatic Disease

The most important predictor of survival is the presence of metastases (liver or bone). In patients with multiple metastases, initial therapy should be directed at controlling hypersecretion. Oral PPIs (omeprazole, esomeprazole, rabeprazole, pantoprazole, lansoprazole, dexlansoprazole) are given at a dose of 40–120 mg/day, titrated to achieve a basal acid output of less than 10 mEq/hour. At this level, there is complete symptomatic relief and ulcer healing. Systemic therapies include long-acting somatostatin analogs (Octreotide LAR, lanreotide), tyrosine kinase inhibitors, and peptide receptor radionucleotide therapy. Owing to the slow growth of these tumors, 30% of patients with hepatic metastases have a survival of 10 years.

B. Localized Disease

Cure can be achieved only if the gastrinoma can be resected before hepatic metastatic spread has occurred. Lymph node metastases do not adversely affect prognosis. Laparotomy should be considered in all patients in whom preoperative studies fail to demonstrate hepatic or other distant metastases. A combination of preoperative studies, duodenotomy with careful duodenal inspection, and intraoperative palpation and sonography allows successful localization and resection in the majority of cases. The 15-year survival of patients who do not have liver metastases at initial presentation is over 95%. Surgery usually is not recommended in patients with MEN 1 due to the presence of multifocal tumors and long-term survival in the absence of surgery in most patients.

Rossi RE et al. Gastrinoma and Zollinger Ellison syndrome: a roadmap for the management between new and old therapies. World J Gastroenterol. 2021;27:5890. [PMID: 34629807]

DISEASES OF THE SMALL INTESTINE

MALABSORPTION

The term “malabsorption” denotes disorders in which there is a disruption of digestion and nutrient absorption. The clinical and laboratory manifestations of malabsorption are summarized in Table 15–11.

Table 15–11. Clinical manifestations and laboratory findings in malabsorption of various nutrients.

Manifestations	Laboratory Findings	Malabsorbed Nutrients
Steatorrhea (bulky, light-colored stools)	Increased fecal fat; decreased serum cholesterol; decreased serum carotene, vitamin A, vitamin D	Triglycerides, fatty acids, phospholipids, cholesterol. Fat-soluble vitamins: A, D, E, K
Diarrhea (increased fecal water)	Increased stool volume and weight; increased fecal fat; increased stool osmolality gap	Fats, carbohydrates
Weight loss; muscle wasting	Increased fecal fat; decreased carbohydrate (D-xylose) absorption	Fat, protein, carbohydrates
Microcytic anemia	Low serum iron	Iron
Macrocytic anemia	Decreased serum vitamin B_{12} or RBC folate	Vitamin B_{12} or folic acid
Paresthesia; tetany; positive Trousseau and Chvostek signs	Decreased serum calcium or magnesium	Calcium, vitamin D, magnesium
Bone pain; pathologic fractures; skeletal deformities	Osteopenia on radiograph; osteoporosis (adults); osteomalacia (children)	Calcium, vitamin D
Bleeding tendency (ecchymoses, epistaxis)	Prolonged prothrombin time or INR	Vitamin K
Edema	Decreased serum total protein and albumin; increased fecal loss of alpha-1-antitrypsin	Protein
Milk intolerance (cramps, bloating, diarrhea)	Abnormal lactose tolerance test	Lactose

1. Celiac Disease

ESSENTIALS OF DIAGNOSIS

- *Typical symptoms*: weight loss, chronic diarrhea, abdominal distention, growth retardation.
- *Atypical symptoms*: dermatitis herpetiformis, iron deficiency anemia, osteoporosis.
- Abnormal serologic test results.
- Abnormal small bowel biopsy.
- Clinical improvement on gluten-free diet.

General Considerations

Celiac disease (also called sprue, celiac sprue, and gluten enteropathy) is a permanent dietary disorder caused by an immunologic response to gluten, a storage protein found in certain grains, that results in diffuse damage to the proximal small intestinal mucosa with malabsorption of nutrients. Although symptoms may manifest between 6 months and 24 months of age after the introduction of weaning foods, most cases present in childhood or adulthood. Population screening with serologic tests suggests that the global prevalence of this disease is 1.4%. In North America, the prevalence of biopsy-confirmed disease is 0.5%. Although the precise pathogenesis is unclear, celiac disease arises in a small subset of genetically susceptible (-DQ2 or -DQ8) individuals when dietary gluten stimulates an inappropriate immunologic response.

Clinical Findings

The most important step in diagnosing celiac disease is to consider the diagnosis. Because of its protean manifestations, celiac disease is underdiagnosed in the adult population.

A. Symptoms and Signs

The GI symptoms and signs of celiac disease depend on the length of small intestine involved and the patient's age when the disease presents. "Classic" symptoms of malabsorption, including diarrhea, steatorrhea, weight loss, abdominal distention, weakness, muscle wasting, or growth retardation, more commonly present in infants (younger than 2 years). Older children and adults are less likely to manifest signs of serious malabsorption. They may report chronic diarrhea, dyspepsia, or flatulence due to colonic bacterial digestion of malabsorbed nutrients, but the severity of weight loss is variable. Many adults have minimal or no GI symptoms but present with extraintestinal "atypical" manifestations, including fatigue, depression, iron deficiency anemia, osteoporosis, short stature, delayed puberty, amenorrhea, or reduced fertility. Approximately 40% of patients with positive serologic tests consistent with disease have no symptoms of disease; the natural history of these patients with "silent" disease is unclear.

Physical examination may be normal in mild cases or may reveal signs of malabsorption such as loss of muscle mass or subcutaneous fat, pallor due to anemia, easy bruising due to vitamin K deficiency, hyperkeratosis due to vitamin A deficiency, bone pain due to osteomalacia, or neurologic signs (peripheral neuropathy, ataxia) due to vitamin B_{12} or vitamin E deficiency (Table 15–11). Abdominal examination may reveal distention with hyperactive bowel sounds.

Dermatitis herpetiformis is regarded as a cutaneous variant of celiac disease. It is a characteristic skin rash consisting of pruritic papulovesicles over the extensor surfaces of the extremities and over the trunk, scalp, and neck.

Dermatitis herpetiformis occurs in less than 10% of patients with celiac disease; however, almost all patients who present with dermatitis herpetiformis have evidence of celiac disease on intestinal mucosal biopsy, though it may not be clinically evident.

B. Laboratory Findings

1. Routine laboratory tests—Depending on the severity of illness and the extent of intestinal involvement, nonspecific laboratory abnormalities may be present that may raise the suspicion of malabsorption and celiac disease (Table 15–11). Limited proximal involvement may result only in microcytic anemia due to iron deficiency. Up to 3% of adults with iron deficiency not due to GI blood loss have undiagnosed celiac disease. Megaloblastic anemia may be due to folate or vitamin B_{12} deficiency (due to terminal ileal involvement or associated autoimmune gastritis). Low serum calcium or elevated alkaline phosphatase may reflect impaired calcium or vitamin D absorption with osteomalacia or osteoporosis. Dual-energy x-ray densitometry scanning is recommended for all patients with celiac disease to screen for osteoporosis. Elevations of prothrombin time, or decreased vitamin A or D levels reflect impaired fat-soluble vitamin absorption. A low serum albumin may reflect small intestine protein loss or poor nutrition. Other deficiencies may include zinc and vitamin B_6. Mild elevations of aminotransferases are found in up to 40%.

2. Serologic tests—Serologic tests should be performed in all patients in whom there is a suspicion of celiac disease. Patient self-elimination of gluten before serologic testing may result in false-negative test results. The recommended test is the IgA tissue transglutaminase-2 antibody (IgA anti-tTG2), which has a 98% sensitivity and 98% specificity for the diagnosis of celiac disease. Antigliadin antibodies are not recommended because of their lower sensitivity and specificity. An IgA level should be obtained in patients with a negative IgA TG antibody when celiac disease is strongly suspected because up to 3% of patients with celiac disease have IgA deficiency. In patients with IgA deficiency, tests that measures IgG antibodies to tissue transglutaminase (IgG tTG) or to deamidated gliadin peptides (anti-DGP) have excellent sensitivity and specificity. Levels of all antibodies become undetectable after 3–24 months of dietary gluten withdrawal and may be used to monitor dietary compliance, especially in patients whose symptoms fail to resolve after institution of a gluten-free diet.

C. Mucosal Biopsy

Endoscopic mucosal biopsy of the proximal duodenum (bulb) and distal duodenum is the standard method for confirmation of the diagnosis in patients with a positive serologic test for celiac disease. At endoscopy, atrophy or scalloping of the duodenal folds may be observed. Histology reveals abnormalities ranging from intraepithelial lymphocytosis alone to extensive infiltration of the lamina propria with lymphocytes and plasma cells, hypertrophy of the intestinal crypts, and blunting or complete loss of intestinal villi. In patients in whom celiac disease is first suspected on intestinal biopsies, celiac serologic tests should be obtained to confirm the diagnosis. Partial or complete reversion of these abnormalities occurs within 3–24 months after a patient is placed on a gluten-free diet, but symptom resolution remains incomplete in 30% of patients. If a patient with a compatible biopsy demonstrates prompt clinical improvement on a gluten-free diet and a decrease in serologic markers, a repeat biopsy is unnecessary.

Differential Diagnosis

Many patients with chronic diarrhea or flatulence are erroneously diagnosed as having IBS. Celiac disease must be distinguished from other causes of malabsorption, as outlined above. Severe panmalabsorption of multiple nutrients is almost always caused by mucosal disease. The histologic appearance of celiac disease may resemble other mucosal diseases such as tropical sprue, bacterial overgrowth, cow's milk intolerance, viral gastroenteritis, eosinophilic gastroenteritis, and mucosal damage caused by acid hypersecretion associated with gastrinoma. Documentation of clinical response to gluten withdrawal therefore is essential to the diagnosis.

Over the past decade, there has been a growing proportion (now 10%) of the population reporting symptoms after gluten ingestion who do not have serologic or histologic evidence of celiac disease. This has led to increases in gluten-free offerings from the restaurant and food industry. Foods with gluten often contain a number of other FODMAPs. Blinded clinical trials suggest that self-reported wheat sensitivity is not due to gluten intolerance and that the symptom improvement reported by patients with gluten restriction is due to broader FODMAP elimination.

Treatment

Removal of all gluten (wheat, rye, and barley) from the diet is essential to therapy but strict adherence can be difficult to achieve. Even among patients who report adherence to the gluten-free diet, gluten peptides can be detected in almost 40% of stool and urine specimens over a 4-week period. Although oats appear to be safe for many patients, commercial products may be contaminated with wheat or barley during processing. Because of the pervasive use of gluten products in manufactured foods and additives, in medications, and by restaurants, it is imperative that patients and their families confer with a knowledgeable dietitian to comply satisfactorily with this lifelong diet. Several excellent dietary guides and patient support groups are available. Most patients with celiac disease also have lactose intolerance either temporarily or permanently and should avoid dairy products until the intestinal symptoms have improved on the gluten-free diet. Dietary supplements (folate, iron, zinc, calcium, and vitamins A, B_6, B_{12}, D, and E) should be provided in the initial stages of therapy but usually are not required long-term with a gluten-free diet. Patients with confirmed osteoporosis may require long-term calcium, vitamin D, and bisphosphonate therapy.

Improvement in symptoms should be evident within a few weeks on the gluten-free diet. The most common reason for treatment failure is incomplete removal of gluten. Intentional or unintentional rechallenge with gluten may trigger acute severe diarrhea with dehydration and electrolyte imbalance and may require TPN and intravenous or oral corticosteroids (prednisone 40 mg or budesonide 9 mg) for 2 or more weeks while a gluten-free diet is reinitiated.

Prognosis & Complications

If appropriately diagnosed and treated, patients with celiac disease have an excellent prognosis. Celiac disease may be associated with other autoimmune disorders, including Addison disease, Graves disease, type 1 diabetes mellitus, myasthenia gravis, systemic sclerosis, Sjögren syndrome, atrophic gastritis, and pancreatic insufficiency. In some patients, celiac disease may evolve and become refractory to the gluten-free diet. The most common cause is intentional or unintentional dietary noncompliance, which may be suggested by positive serologic tests. Celiac disease that is truly refractory to gluten withdrawal occurs in 0.5–1.5% and generally carries a poor prognosis. There are two types of refractory disease, which are distinguished by their intraepithelial lymphocyte phenotype. This diagnosis should be considered in patients previously responsive to the gluten-free diet in whom new weight loss, abdominal pain, and malabsorption develop.

Celiac Disease Foundation, 20350 Ventura Blvd, Suite #240, Woodland Hills, CA 91364. https://celiac.org

Lebwohl B et al. Epidemiology, presentation, and diagnosis of celiac disease. Gastroenterology. 2021;160:63. [PMID: 32950520]

Rubin JE et al. Celiac disease. Ann Intern Med. 2020;172:ITC1. [PMID: 31905394]

Silvester JA et al. Celiac disease: fallacies and facts. Am J Gastroenterol. 2021;116:1148. [PMID: 33767109]

Stefanolo JP et al. Real-world gluten exposure in patients with celiac disease on gluten-free diets, determined from gliadin immunogenic peptides in urine and fecal specimens. Clin Gastroenterol Hepatol. 2021;19:484. [PMID: 32217152]

2. Whipple Disease

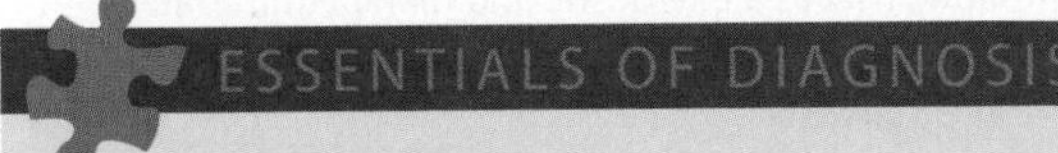

- Multisystem disease.
- Fever, lymphadenopathy, arthralgias.
- Weight loss, malabsorption, chronic diarrhea.
- Duodenal biopsy with periodic acid-Schiff (PAS)-positive macrophages with characteristic bacillus.

General Considerations

Whipple disease is a rare multisystem illness with an estimated prevalence of 1 per 100,000 caused by infection with the bacillus *Tropheryma whipplei*. It may occur at any age but most commonly affects White men in the fourth to sixth decades. The source of infection is unknown, but no cases of human-to-human spread have been documented.

Clinical Findings

A. Symptoms and Signs

The clinical manifestations are protean; however, the most common are arthralgias, diarrhea, abdominal pain, and weight loss. Arthralgias or a migratory, nondeforming arthritis occurs in 80% and is typically the first symptom experienced. GI symptoms occur in approximately 75% of cases. They include abdominal pain, diarrhea, and some degree of malabsorption with distention, flatulence, and steatorrhea. Weight loss is the most common presenting symptom—seen in almost all patients. Loss of protein due to intestinal or lymphatic involvement may result in protein-losing enteropathy with hypoalbuminemia and edema. In the absence of GI symptoms, the diagnosis often is delayed for several years. Intermittent low-grade fever occurs in over 50% of cases.

Physical examination may reveal hypotension (a late finding), low-grade fever, and evidence of malabsorption (see Table 15–11). Lymphadenopathy is present in 50%. Heart murmurs due to valvular involvement may be evident. Peripheral joints may be enlarged or warm, and peripheral edema may be present. Neurologic findings are protean, and include ophthalmoplegia, dementia (confusion, memory loss), cerebellar ataxia, chronic meningitis, myelopathy, and seizures. Hyperpigmentation on sun-exposed areas is evident in up to 40%.

B. Laboratory Findings

If significant malabsorption is present, patients may have laboratory abnormalities as outlined in Table 15–11. There may be steatorrhea.

C. Histologic Evaluation

The diagnosis of Whipple disease is established in 90% of cases by endoscopic biopsy of the duodenum with histologic evaluation, which demonstrates infiltration of the lamina propria with PAS-positive macrophages that contain gram-positive bacilli (which are not acid-fast) and dilation of the lacteals. The remainder of cases are diagnosed by *T whipplei*–specific PCR or immunohistochemistry of duodenal biopsies or extraintestinal fluids (cerebrospinal, synovial) or tissue (lymph nodes, synovium, endocardium). The sensitivity of PCR is 97% and the specificity 100%. Because asymptomatic CNS infection occurs in 40% of patients, examination of the cerebrospinal fluid by PCR for *T whipplei* should be performed routinely.

Differential Diagnosis

Whipple disease should be considered in patients who present with signs of malabsorption, fever of unknown origin, lymphadenopathy, seronegative arthritis, culture-negative endocarditis, or multisystem disease. Small bowel biopsy readily distinguishes Whipple disease from other mucosal malabsorptive disorders, such as celiac disease.

Treatment

Antibiotic therapy results in a dramatic clinical improvement within several weeks, even in some patients with neurologic involvement. The optimal regimen is unknown.

Complete clinical response usually is evident within 1–3 months; however, relapse may occur in up to one-third of patients after discontinuation of treatment. Therefore, prolonged treatment for at least 1 year is required. Drugs that cross the blood-brain barrier are preferred. A randomized controlled trial in 40 patients with 3–10 years' follow-up demonstrated 100% remission with either ceftriaxone 1 g intravenously twice daily or meropenem 1 g intravenously three times daily for 2 weeks, followed by trimethoprim-sulfamethoxazole 160/800 mg twice daily for 12 months. After treatment, repeat duodenal biopsies for histologic analysis and cerebrospinal fluid PCR should be obtained every 6 months for at least 1 year. The absence of PAS-positive material predicts a low likelihood of clinical relapse.

Prognosis

If untreated, the disease is fatal. Because some neurologic signs may be permanent, the goal of treatment is to prevent this progression. Patients must be followed closely after treatment for signs of symptom recurrence.

Elchert JA et al. Epidemiology of Whipple's disease in the USA between 2012 and 2017: a population-based national study. Dig Dis Sci. 2019;64:1305. [PMID: 30488239]

Ferrieres L et al. Whipple's disease; diagnosis and predictive factor of relapse. Eur J Gastroenterol Hepatol. 2020;32:325. [PMID: 31764405]

Hujoel IA et al. *Tropheryma whipplei* infection (Whipple disease) in the USA. Dig Dis Sci. 2019;64:213. [PMID: 29572616]

3. Bacterial Overgrowth

ESSENTIALS OF DIAGNOSIS

- Symptoms of diarrhea, bloating, and flatulence.
- Advanced cases associated with weight loss, steatorrhea, and deficiencies of iron or vitamins A, D, and B_{12}.
- Diagnosis suggested by breath tests using glucose or lactulose as substrates.
- Diagnosis confirmed by jejunal aspiration with quantitative bacterial cultures.

General Considerations

The small intestine normally contains a small number of bacteria. Bacterial overgrowth in the small intestine of whatever cause may result in malabsorption via several mechanisms. Passage of malabsorbed bile acids and carbohydrates into the colon leads to an osmotic and secretory diarrhea and increased flatulence.

Causes of bacterial overgrowth include (1) gastric achlorhydria (including PPI therapy); (2) anatomic abnormalities of the small intestine with stagnation (afferent limb of Billroth II gastrojejunostomy, resection of ileocecal valve, small intestine diverticula, obstruction, blind loop); (3) small intestine motility disorders (vagotomy, systemic sclerosis, diabetic enteropathy, chronic intestinal pseudo-obstruction); (4) gastrocolic or coloenteric fistula (Crohn disease, malignancy, surgical resection); and (5) miscellaneous disorders. Bacterial overgrowth is an important cause of diarrhea in older patients, perhaps because of decreased gastric acidity or impaired intestinal motility. It may also be present in a subset of patients with IBS.

Clinical Findings

Many patients with bacterial overgrowth are asymptomatic. Symptoms are nonspecific and include diarrhea, bloating, flatulence, and sometimes steatorrhea with weight loss. Bacterial overgrowth should be considered in any patient with these symptoms, especially patients with a predisposing cause (such as prior GI surgery) and older adults with unexplained diarrhea and weight loss. Bacterial synthesis of folic acid and consumption of cobalamin may cause elevated serum folate and decreased vitamin B_{12} levels. Severe cases may result in clinically significant vitamin and mineral deficiencies, including fat-soluble vitamins A or D, and low serum albumin (Table 15–11). A specific diagnosis can be established firmly only by an aspirate and culture of distal duodenal secretion that demonstrates over 10^3 organisms/mL. However, this is an invasive and laborious test that requires careful collection and culturing techniques and therefore is not available in most clinical settings. Noninvasive breath hydrogen and methane tests with glucose or lactulose as substrates are generally preferred because of their ease of use. Following ingestion of glucose 75 g or lactulose 10 g, a rise in exhaled breath hydrogen of 20 ppm or methane of 10 ppm or more within 90 minutes is suggestive of bacterial overgrowth and has 65% diagnostic agreement with small bowel cultures. A small bowel study (CT or MR enterography, barium radiography) may be obtained to look for mechanical factors predisposing to intestinal stasis.

A 2020 American College of Gastroenterology guideline suggests breath testing when bacterial overgrowth is suspected. However, many clinicians prefer to use an empiric antibiotic trial as a diagnostic and therapeutic strategy.

Treatment

Where possible, the anatomic defect that has potentiated bacterial overgrowth should be corrected. Otherwise, treatment for 7–10 days with oral broad-spectrum antibiotics improves symptoms in up to 90% of patients for weeks to months. Recommended regimens include ciprofloxacin, 250 mg twice daily; amoxicillin clavulanate, 875 mg twice daily; trimethoprim-sulfamethoxazole (one double-strength tablet) twice daily; rifaximin, 400–550 mg three times daily; or a combination of neomycin, 500 mg twice daily, plus metronidazole, 250 mg three times daily.

Within 6 months of completing antibiotic therapy, symptoms recur in over 25% of patients. In patients with more frequent symptomatic relapse, cyclic antibiotic therapy (eg, 1 week out of 4) may be sufficient. Continuous antibiotics should be avoided, if possible, to avoid development of bacterial antibiotic resistance.

Pimental M et al. ACG Clinical Guideline: small intestinal bacterial overgrowth. Am J Gastroenterol. 2020;115:165. [PMID: 32023228]

Quigley EM et al. AGA Clinical Practice Update on small intestinal bacterial overgrowth: expert review. Gastroenterology. 2020;159:1526. [PMID: 32679220]

4. Short Bowel Syndrome

Short bowel syndrome is the malabsorptive condition that arises secondary to removal of significant segments of the small intestine. The most common causes in adults are Crohn disease, mesenteric infarction, radiation enteritis, volvulus, tumor resection, and trauma. The type and degree of malabsorption depend on the length and site of the resection and the degree of adaptation of the remaining bowel.

Terminal Ileal Resection

Resection of the terminal ileum results in malabsorption of bile salts and vitamin B_{12}, which are normally absorbed in this region. Patients with low serum vitamin B_{12} levels or resection of over 50 cm of ileum require monthly subcutaneous or intramuscular vitamin B_{12} injections. In patients with less than 100 cm of ileal resection, bile salt malabsorption stimulates fluid secretion from the colon, resulting in watery diarrhea. This may be treated with administration of bile salt-binding resins one to three times daily with meals (cholestyramine, 2–4 g/day orally, colestipol tablets, 2 g orally, or colesevelam, 625 mg orally). Resection of over 100 cm of ileum leads to a reduction in the bile salt pool that results in steatorrhea and malabsorption of fat-soluble vitamins. Treatment is with a low-fat diet and vitamins supplemented with medium-chain triglycerides, which do not require micellar solubilization. Unabsorbed fatty acids bind with calcium, reducing its absorption and enhancing the absorption of oxalate. Oxalate kidney stones may develop. Calcium supplements should be administered to bind oxalate and increase serum calcium. Cholesterol gallstones due to decreased bile salts are common also. In patients with resection of the ileocolonic valve, bacterial overgrowth may occur in the small intestine, further complicating malabsorption.

Extensive Small Bowel Resection

Resection of up to 40–50% of the total length of small intestine usually is well tolerated. A more massive resection may result in "short bowel syndrome," characterized by weight loss and diarrhea due to nutrient, water, and electrolyte malabsorption. If the colon is preserved, 100 cm of proximal jejunum may be sufficient to maintain adequate oral nutrition with a low-fat, high–complex carbohydrate diet, though fluid and electrolyte losses may still be significant. In patients in whom the colon has been removed, at least 200 cm of proximal jejunum is typically required to maintain oral nutrition. Antidiarrheal agents (loperamide, 2–4 mg orally three times daily) slow transit and reduce diarrheal volume. Octreotide reduces intestinal transit time and fluid and electrolyte secretion. Gastric hypersecretion initially complicates intestinal resection and should be treated with PPIs.

Patients with less than 100–200 cm of proximal jejunum remaining almost always require parenteral nutrition. Teduglutide (recombinant) is a glucagon-like peptide-2 analogue that stimulates small bowel growth and absorption and is FDA approved for the treatment of short bowel syndrome. In clinical trials, it resulted in a reduced need for parenteral nutrition. Small intestine transplantation has a reported 5-year graft survival rate of 40%. Currently, it is performed chiefly in patients in whom serious problems develop due to parenteral nutrition.

Da Roach HM et al. Treating short bowel syndrome with pharmacotherapy. Expert Opin Pharmacother. 2020;21:709. [PMID: 32057270]

Harpain F et al. Teduglutide in short bowel syndrome patients: a way back to normal life? JPEN J Parenter Enteral Nutr. 2022;46:300. [PMID: 34614239]

Massironi S et al. Understanding short bowel syndrome: current status and future perspectives. Dig Liver Dis. 2020;52:253. [PMID: 31892505]

Pironi L. Translation of evidence into practice with teduglutide in the management of adults with intestinal failure due to short-bowel syndrome: a review of recent literature. JPEN J Parenter Enteral Nutr. 2020;44:968. [PMID: 31802516]

Sadowski DC et al. Canadian Association of Gastroenterology clinical practice guideline on the management of bile acid diarrhea. Clin Gastroenterol Hepatol. 2020;18:24. [PMID: 31526844]

5. Lactase Deficiency

ESSENTIALS OF DIAGNOSIS

- Diarrhea, bloating, flatulence, and abdominal pain after ingestion of milk-containing products.
- Diagnosis supported by symptomatic improvement on lactose-free diet.
- Diagnosis confirmed by hydrogen breath test.

General Considerations

Lactase is a brush border enzyme that hydrolyzes the disaccharide lactose into glucose and galactose. The concentration of lactase enzyme levels is high at birth but declines steadily in most people of non-European ancestry during childhood and adolescence and into adulthood. As many as 90% of Asian Americans, 70% of African Americans, 95% of Native Americans, 50% of Mexican Americans, and 60% of Jewish Americans are lactose intolerant compared with less than 25% of White adults. Lactase deficiency may also arise secondary to other GI disorders that affect the proximal small intestinal mucosa. These include Crohn disease, celiac disease, viral gastroenteritis, giardiasis, short bowel syndrome, and malnutrition. Malabsorbed lactose is fermented by intestinal bacteria, producing gas and organic acids. The nonmetabolized lactose and organic acids result in an increased stool osmotic load with an obligatory fluid loss.

Clinical Findings

A. Symptoms and Signs

Patients have great variability in clinical symptoms, depending both on the severity of lactase deficiency and the amount of lactose ingested. Because of the nonspecific nature of these symptoms, there is a tendency for both lactose-intolerant and lactose-tolerant individuals to mistakenly attribute a variety of abdominal symptoms to lactose intolerance. Most patients with lactose intolerance can drink at least one 8-oz serving of milk daily (12 g of lactose) without symptoms, though rare patients have almost complete intolerance. With mild to moderate amounts of lactose malabsorption, patients may experience bloating, abdominal cramps, and flatulence. With higher lactose ingestions, an osmotic diarrhea will result. Isolated lactase deficiency does not result in other signs of malabsorption or weight loss. If these findings are present, other GI disorders should be pursued.

B. Laboratory Findings

The most widely available test for the diagnosis of lactase deficiency is the hydrogen breath test. After ingestion of 50 g of lactose, a rise in breath hydrogen of more than 20 ppm within 90 minutes is a positive test, indicative of bacterial carbohydrate metabolism. In clinical practice, many clinicians prescribe an empiric trial of a lactose-free diet for 2 weeks. Resolution of symptoms (bloating, flatulence, diarrhea) is suggestive of lactase deficiency (though a placebo response cannot be excluded) and may be confirmed, if necessary, with a hydrogen breath test.

Differential Diagnosis

The symptoms of late-onset lactose intolerance are nonspecific and may mimic several GI disorders, such as inflammatory bowel disease, mucosal malabsorptive disorders, IBS, and pancreatic insufficiency. Furthermore, lactase deficiency frequently develops secondary to other GI disorders (as listed above).

Treatment

The goal of treatment in patients with isolated lactase deficiency is achieving patient comfort. Patients usually find their "threshold" of intake at which symptoms will occur. Foods that are high in lactose include milk (12 g/cup), ice cream (9 g/cup), and cottage cheese (8 g/cup). Aged cheeses have a lower lactose content (0.5 g/oz). Unpasteurized yogurt contains bacteria that produce lactase and is generally well tolerated.

By spreading dairy product intake throughout the day in quantities of less than 12 g of lactose (one cup of milk), most patients can take dairy products without symptoms and do not require lactase supplements. Most food markets provide milk that has been pretreated with lactase, rendering it 100% lactose free (Fairlife). Lactase enzyme replacement is commercially available as nonprescription formulations (Lactaid, Lactrase, Dairy Ease). Caplets or drops of lactase may be taken with milk products, improving lactose absorption and eliminating symptoms. The number of caplets ingested depends on the degree of lactose intolerance. Patients who choose to restrict or eliminate milk products should consider calcium supplementation (calcium citrate 650 mg 2 tablets orally two times daily) to meet calcium intake needs and reduce risk of osteoporosis.

Catanzaro R et al. Lactose intolerance: an update on its pathogenesis, diagnosis, and treatment. Nutr Res. 2021;89:23. [PMID: 33887513]

INTESTINAL MOTILITY DISORDERS

1. Acute Paralytic Ileus

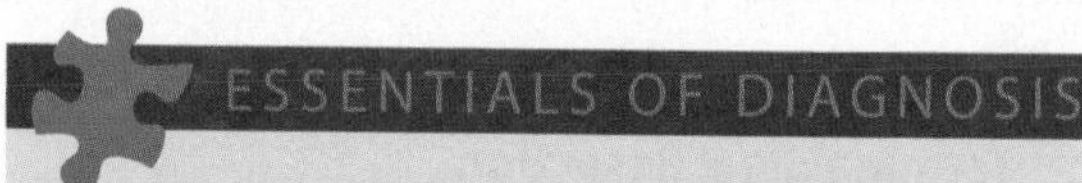

- Precipitating factors: surgery, peritonitis, electrolyte abnormalities, medications, severe medical illness.
- Nausea, vomiting, obstipation, distention.
- Minimal abdominal tenderness; decreased bowel sounds.
- Plain abdominal radiography with gas and fluid distention in small and large bowel.

General Considerations

Ileus is a condition in which there is neurogenic failure or loss of peristalsis in the intestine in the absence of any mechanical obstruction. It is commonly seen in hospitalized patients as a result of (1) intra-abdominal processes such as recent GI or abdominal surgery or peritoneal irritation (peritonitis, pancreatitis, ruptured viscus, hemorrhage); (2) severe medical illness such as pneumonia, respiratory failure requiring intubation, sepsis or severe infections, uremia, diabetic ketoacidosis, and electrolyte abnormalities (hypokalemia, hypercalcemia, hypomagnesemia, hypophosphatemia); and (3) medications that affect intestinal motility (opioids, anticholinergics, phenothiazines). Following surgery, small intestinal motility usually normalizes first (often within hours), followed by the stomach (24–48 hours), and the colon (48–72 hours). Postoperative ileus is reduced with minimally invasive (eg, laparoscopic) surgery, by the use of patient-controlled or epidural analgesia, and by avoidance of intravenous opioids as well as early ambulation, gum chewing, and initiation of a clear liquid diet.

Clinical Findings

A. Symptoms and Signs

Patients who are conscious report mild diffuse, continuous abdominal discomfort with nausea and vomiting. Generalized abdominal distention is present with minimal abdominal tenderness but no signs of peritoneal irritation (unless due to the primary disease). Bowel sounds are diminished to absent.

B. Laboratory Findings

The laboratory abnormalities are attributable to the underlying condition. Serum electrolytes (sodium, potassium), magnesium, phosphorus, and calcium, should be obtained to exclude abnormalities as contributing factors.

C. Imaging

Plain film radiography of the abdomen demonstrates distended gas-filled loops of the small and large intestine. Air-fluid levels may be seen. Under some circumstances, it may be difficult to distinguish ileus from partial small bowel obstruction. A CT scan may be useful in such instances to exclude mechanical obstruction, especially in postoperative patients.

Differential Diagnosis

Ileus must be distinguished from mechanical obstruction of the small bowel or proximal colon. Pain from small bowel mechanical obstruction is usually intermittent, cramping, and associated initially with profuse vomiting. Acute gastroenteritis, acute appendicitis, and acute pancreatitis may all present with ileus.

Treatment

The primary medical or surgical illness that has precipitated adynamic ileus should be treated. Most cases of ileus respond to restriction of oral intake with gradual liberalization of diet as bowel function returns. Severe or prolonged ileus requires nasogastric suction and parenteral administration of fluids and electrolytes. Alvimopan is a peripherally acting mu-opioid receptor antagonist with limited absorption or systemic activity that reverses opioid-induced inhibition of intestinal motility.

Wells CI et al. Post-operative ileus: definitions, mechanisms and controversies. ANZ J Surg. 2022;92:62. [PMID: 34676664]

2. Acute Colonic Pseudo-Obstruction (Ogilvie Syndrome)

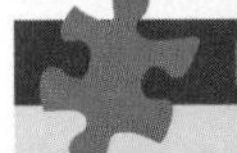

ESSENTIALS OF DIAGNOSIS

- Severe abdominal distention.
- Arises in postoperative state or with severe medical illness.
- May be precipitated by electrolyte imbalances, medications.
- Absent to mild abdominal pain; minimal tenderness.
- Massive dilation of cecum or right colon.

General Considerations

Spontaneous massive dilation of the cecum and proximal colon may occur in many different settings in hospitalized patients. Progressive cecal dilation may lead to ischemia and spontaneous perforation with dire consequences. The risk of perforation increases with duration of distention beyond 6 days but correlates poorly with absolute cecal size. Early detection and management are important to reduce morbidity and mortality. Colonic pseudo-obstruction is most commonly detected in postsurgical patients (mean 3–5 days), after trauma, and in medical patients with respiratory failure, metabolic imbalance, malignancy, MI, heart failure, pancreatitis, or a recent neurologic event (stroke, subarachnoid hemorrhage, trauma). Liberal use of opioids or anticholinergic agents may precipitate colonic pseudo-obstruction in susceptible patients.

Clinical Findings

A. Symptoms and Signs

Many patients are on ventilatory support or are unable to report symptoms due to altered mental status. Abdominal distention is frequently noted by the clinician as the first sign, often leading to a plain film radiograph that demonstrates colonic dilation. Some patients are asymptomatic, although most report constant but mild abdominal pain. Nausea and vomiting may be present. Bowel movements may be absent, but up to 40% of patients continue to pass flatus or stool. Abdominal tenderness with some degree of guarding or rebound tenderness may be detected; however, signs of peritonitis are absent unless perforation has occurred. Bowel sounds may be normal or decreased.

B. Laboratory Findings

Laboratory findings reflect the underlying medical or surgical problems. Serum sodium, potassium, magnesium, phosphorus, and calcium should be obtained to exclude abnormalities as contributing factors. Significant fever or leukocytosis raises concern for colonic ischemia or perforation.

C. Imaging

Radiographs demonstrate colonic dilation, usually confined to the cecum and proximal colon. The upper limit of normal for cecal size is 9 cm. A cecal diameter greater than 10–12 cm is associated with an increased risk of colonic perforation. Varying amounts of small intestinal dilation and air-fluid levels due to adynamic ileus may be seen. Generally, a CT scan should be obtained to exclude a distal colonic mechanical obstruction due to malignancy, volvulus, or fecal impaction.

Differential Diagnosis

Colonic pseudo-obstruction should be distinguished from distal colonic mechanical obstruction (as above) and toxic megacolon, which is acute dilation of the colon due to inflammation (inflammatory bowel disease) or infection (*C difficile*–associated colitis, CMV). Patients with toxic megacolon manifest fever; dehydration; significant abdominal pain; leukocytosis; and diarrhea, which is often bloody.

Treatment

Conservative treatment is the appropriate first step for patients with no or minimal abdominal tenderness, no fever, no leukocytosis, and a cecal diameter smaller than 12 cm. The underlying illness is treated appropriately. A nasogastric tube and a rectal tube should be placed. Patients should be ambulated or periodically rolled from side to side and to the knee-chest position in an effort to promote expulsion of colonic gas. All drugs that reduce intestinal motility, such as opioids, anticholinergics, and calcium channel blockers, should be discontinued if possible. Enemas may be administered judiciously if large amounts of stool are evident on radiography. Oral laxatives are not helpful and may cause perforation, pain, or electrolyte abnormalities.

Conservative treatment is successful in over 80% of cases within 1–2 days. Patients must be watched for signs of worsening distention or abdominal tenderness. Cecal size should be assessed by abdominal radiographs every 12 hours. Intervention should be considered in patients with any of the following: (1) no improvement or clinical deterioration after 24–48 hours of conservative therapy; (2) cecal dilation greater than 10 cm for a prolonged period (more than 3–4 days); or (3) patients with cecal dilation greater than 12 cm. Neostigmine injection should be given unless contraindicated. A single dose (2 mg intravenously) results in rapid (within 30 minutes) colonic decompression in 75–90% of patients. Cardiac monitoring during neostigmine infusion is indicated for possible bradycardia that may require atropine administration. Colonoscopic decompression is indicated in patients who fail to respond to neostigmine. Colonic decompression with aspiration of air or placement of a decompression tube is successful in 70% of patients. However, the procedure is technically difficult in an unprepared bowel and has been associated with perforations in the distended colon. Dilation recurs in up to 50% of patients. In patients in whom colonoscopy is unsuccessful, a tube cecostomy can be created through a small laparotomy or with percutaneous radiologically guided placement.

Prognosis

In most cases, the prognosis is related to the underlying illness. The risk of perforation or ischemia is increased with cecal diameter more than 12 cm and when distention has been present for more than 6 days. With aggressive therapy, the development of perforation is unusual.

Jeong SJ et al. Endoscopic management of benign colonic obstruction and pseudo-obstruction. Clin Endosc. 2020;53:18. [PMID: 31645090]

Naveed M et al. American Society for Gastrointestinal Endoscopy guideline on the role of endoscopy in the management of acute colonic pseudo-obstruction and colonic volvulus. Gastrointest Endosc. 2020;91:228. [PMID: 31791596]

3. Chronic Intestinal Pseudo-Obstruction & Gastroparesis

Gastroparesis and chronic intestinal pseudo-obstruction are chronic conditions characterized by intermittent, waxing and waning symptoms and signs of gastric or intestinal obstruction in the absence of any mechanical lesions to account for the findings. They are caused by a heterogeneous group of endocrine disorders (diabetes mellitus, hypothyroidism, cortisol deficiency), postsurgical conditions (vagotomy, partial gastric resection, fundoplication, gastric bypass, Whipple procedure), neurologic conditions (Parkinson disease, muscular and myotonic dystrophy, autonomic dysfunction, multiple sclerosis, postpolio syndrome, porphyria), rheumatologic syndromes (progressive systemic sclerosis), infections (postviral, Chagas disease), amyloidosis, paraneoplastic syndromes, medications, and eating disorders (anorexia); a cause may not always be identified.

Clinical Findings

A. Symptoms and Signs

Gastric involvement leads to chronic or intermittent symptoms of gastroparesis with early satiety, nausea, vomiting (1–3 hours after meals) and epigastric pain. Upper abdominal symptoms correlate poorly with the severity of gastric emptying. Patients with predominantly small bowel involvement may have abdominal distention, vomiting, diarrhea, and varying degrees of malnutrition. Abdominal pain is not common and should prompt investigation for structural causes of obstruction. Bacterial overgrowth in the stagnant intestine may result in malabsorption. Colonic involvement may result in constipation or alternating diarrhea and constipation.

B. Imaging

Plain film radiography may demonstrate dilation of the esophagus, stomach, small intestine, or colon resembling ileus or mechanical obstruction. Mechanical obstruction of the stomach, small intestine, or colon is much more common than gastroparesis or intestinal pseudo-obstruction and must be excluded with endoscopy or CT enterography, especially in patients with prior surgery, recent onset of symptoms, or abdominal pain. In cases of unclear origin, studies based on the clinical picture are obtained to exclude underlying systemic disease. Gastric scintigraphy with a low-fat solid meal remains the preferred method for assessing gastric emptying. Gastric retention of 60% after 2 hours or more than 10% after 4 hours is abnormal. A wireless motility capsule and a nonradioactive or 13-C labeled breath test using blue-green algae (*Spirulina platensis*) also are available. Small bowel manometry is useful for distinguishing visceral from myopathic disorders and for excluding cases of mechanical obstruction that are otherwise difficult to diagnose by endoscopy or radiographic studies.

Treatment

There is no specific therapy for gastroparesis or pseudo-obstruction. Acute exacerbations are treated with

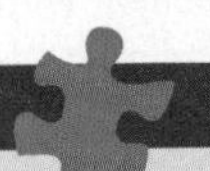

nasogastric suction and intravenous fluids. Long-term treatment is directed at maintaining nutrition. Patients should eat small, frequent meals that are low in fiber, milk, gas-forming foods, and fat. Foods that are well tolerated include tea, ginger ale, soup, white rice, potatoes and sweet potatoes, fish, gluten-free foods, and applesauce. Some patients may require liquid enteral supplements. Agents that reduce GI motility (opioids, anticholinergics) should be avoided. In diabetic patients, glucose levels should be maintained below 200 mg/dL since hyperglycemia may slow gastric emptying even in the absence of diabetic neuropathy, and amylin and GLP-1 analogs (exenatide or pramlintide) should be discontinued.

Currently available prokinetic agents have shown limited improvement of gastric emptying or upper GI symptoms in patients with gastroparesis. Metoclopramide (5–20 mg orally or 5–10 mg intravenously or subcutaneously four times daily) may enhance gastric emptying but not small bowel dysmotility. Since the use of metoclopramide for more than 3 months is associated with a less than 1% risk of tardive dyskinesia, patients are advised to discontinue the medication if neuromuscular side effects, particularly involuntary movements, develop. Older patients are at greatest risk. In 2019, a small, blinded, crossover trial involving 34 patients with confirmed gastroparesis showed that prucalopride, a serotonin 5-HT_4-receptor agonist (currently FDA approved for treatment of chronic constipation), significantly improved gastric emptying and symptoms after 2 weeks of therapy (2 mg daily orally) compared with placebo. Several uncontrolled studies report symptom improvement with endoscopic modalities that reduce intrapyloric pressure, including botulinum toxin injection, dilation, and myotomy (G-POEM). In a systematic review of 10 studies involving 292 patients, endoscopic pyloromyotomy led to symptomatic improvement in 84%. Bacterial overgrowth should be treated with intermittent antibiotics. Patients with predominant small bowel distention may require a venting gastrostomy to relieve distress. Some patients may require placement of a jejunostomy for long-term enteral nutrition. Patients unable to maintain adequate enteral nutrition require TPN or small bowel transplantation. Difficult cases should be referred to centers with expertise in this area.

Abdelfatah MM et al. Long-term outcome of gastric per-oral endoscopic pyloromyotomy in treatment of gastroparesis. Clin Gastroenterol Hepatol. 2021;19:816. [PMID: 32450364]

Carlin JL et al. Efficacy and safety of tradipitant in patients with diabetic and idiopathic gastroparesis in a randomized, placebo-controlled trial. Gastroenterology. 2021;160:76. [PMID: 32693185]

Lacy BE et al. Controversies in gastroparesis: discussing the sticky points. Am J Gastroenterol. 2021;116:1572. [PMID: 33767098]

Parsi MA et al. Techniques and devices for the endoscopic treatment of gastroparesis (with video). Gastrointest Endosc. 2020;92:483. [PMID: 32684298]

Vijayvargiya P et al. Effects of promotility agents on gastric emptying and symptoms: a systematic review and meta-analysis. Gastroenterology. 2019;156:1650. [PMID: 30711628]

APPENDICITIS

ESSENTIALS OF DIAGNOSIS

- *Early:* periumbilical pain; *later:* right lower quadrant pain and tenderness.
- Anorexia, nausea and vomiting, obstipation.
- Tenderness or localized rigidity at McBurney point.
- Low-grade fever and leukocytosis.

General Considerations

Appendicitis is the most common abdominal surgical emergency, affecting approximately 10% of the population. It occurs most commonly between the ages of 10 and 30 years. It is initiated by obstruction of the appendix by a fecalith, inflammation, foreign body, or neoplasm. Obstruction leads to increased intraluminal pressure, venous congestion, infection, and thrombosis of intramural vessels. If untreated, gangrene and perforation develop within 36 hours.

Clinical Findings

A. Symptoms and Signs

Appendicitis usually begins with vague, often colicky periumbilical or epigastric pain. Within 12 hours the pain shifts to the right lower quadrant, manifested as a steady ache that is worsened by walking or coughing. Almost all patients have nausea with one or two episodes of vomiting. Protracted vomiting or vomiting that begins before the onset of pain suggests another diagnosis. A sense of constipation is typical, and some patients administer cathartics in an effort to relieve their symptoms—though some report diarrhea. Low-grade fever (below 38°C) is typical; high fever or rigors suggest another diagnosis or appendiceal perforation.

On physical examination, localized tenderness with guarding in the right lower quadrant can be elicited with gentle palpation with one finger. When asked to cough, patients may be able to precisely localize the painful area, a sign of peritoneal irritation. Light percussion may also elicit pain. Although rebound tenderness is also present, it is unnecessary to elicit this finding if the above signs are present. The psoas sign (pain on passive extension of the right hip) and the obturator sign (pain with passive flexion and internal rotation of the right hip) are indicative of adjacent inflammation and strongly suggestive of appendicitis.

B. Atypical Presentations of Appendicitis

Owing to the variable location of the appendix, there are a number of "atypical" presentations. Because the retrocecal appendix does not touch the anterior abdominal wall, the pain remains less intense and poorly localized; abdominal tenderness is minimal and may be elicited in the right flank.

The psoas sign may be positive. With pelvic appendicitis, there is pain in the lower abdomen, often on the left, with an urge to urinate or defecate. Abdominal tenderness is absent, but tenderness is evident on pelvic or rectal examination; the obturator sign may be present. In older adult patients, the diagnosis of appendicitis is often delayed because patients present with minimal, vague symptoms and mild abdominal tenderness.

C. Laboratory Findings

Moderate leukocytosis (10,000–20,000/mcL [$10–20 \times 10^9$/L]) with neutrophilia is common. Microscopic hematuria and pyuria are present in 25% of patients.

D. Imaging

Both abdominal ultrasound and CT are useful in diagnosing appendicitis as well as excluding other diseases presenting with similar symptoms, including adnexal disease in younger women. However, CT appears to be more accurate (sensitivity 94%, specificity 95%, positive likelihood ratio 13.3, negative likelihood ratio 0.09). Abdominal CT is also useful in cases of suspected appendiceal perforation to diagnose a periappendiceal abscess. In patients in whom there is a clinically high suspicion of appendicitis, some surgeons feel that preoperative diagnostic imaging is unnecessary. However, studies suggest that even in this group, imaging studies suggest an alternative diagnosis in up to 15%.

Differential Diagnosis

Given its frequency and myriad presentations, appendicitis should be considered in the differential diagnosis of all patients with abdominal pain. A several-hour period of close observation with reassessment usually clarifies the diagnosis. In a 2020 retrospective review of 123,711 adults with appendicitis, the diagnosis was more commonly missed in women, patients with comorbidities, and patients who experienced abdominal pain with constipation. Absence of classic migration of pain (from epigastrium to right lower abdomen); right lower quadrant pain; fever; or guarding each makes appendicitis less likely. Widespread use of ultrasonography and CT has reduced the number of incorrect diagnoses to less than 2%. Still, in some cases, diagnostic laparotomy or laparoscopy is required.

The most common causes of diagnostic confusion are gastroenteritis and gynecologic disorders. Viral gastroenteritis presents with nausea, vomiting, low-grade fever, and diarrhea and can be difficult to distinguish from appendicitis. The onset of vomiting before pain makes appendicitis less likely. As a rule, the pain of gastroenteritis is more generalized and the tenderness less well localized. Acute salpingitis or tubo-ovarian abscess should be considered in young, sexually active women with fever and bilateral abdominal or pelvic tenderness. A twisted ovarian cyst may also cause sudden severe pain. The sudden onset of lower abdominal pain in the middle of the menstrual cycle suggests mittelschmerz. Sudden severe abdominal pain with diffuse pelvic tenderness and shock suggests a ruptured ectopic pregnancy. A positive pregnancy test and pelvic ultrasonography are diagnostic. Retrocecal or retroileal appendicitis (often associated with pyuria or hematuria) may be confused with ureteral colic or pyelonephritis. Other conditions that may resemble appendicitis are diverticulitis, carcinoid of the appendix, perforated colonic cancer, Crohn ileitis, perforated peptic ulcer, cholecystitis, and mesenteric adenitis. It is virtually impossible to distinguish appendicitis from Meckel diverticulitis, but both require surgical treatment.

Complications

Perforation occurs in 20% of patients and should be suspected in patients with pain persisting for over 36 hours, high fever, diffuse abdominal tenderness or peritoneal findings, a palpable abdominal mass, or marked leukocytosis. Localized perforation results in a contained abscess, usually in the pelvis. A free perforation leads to suppurative peritonitis with toxicity. Septic thrombophlebitis (pylephlebitis) of the portal venous system is rare and suggested by high fever, chills, bacteremia, and jaundice.

Treatment

The treatment of early, uncomplicated appendicitis is surgical appendectomy in most patients. When possible, a laparoscopic approach is preferred to open laparotomy. Prior to surgery, patients should be given broad-spectrum antibiotics with gram-negative and anaerobic coverage to reduce the incidence of postoperative infections. Recommended preoperative intravenous regimens include cefoxitin or cefotetan 1–2 g every 8 hours; ampicillin-sulbactam 3 g every 6 hours; or ertapenem 1 g as a single dose. Up to 80–90% of patients with uncomplicated appendicitis treated with antibiotics alone for 7 days have resolution of symptoms and signs. Therefore, conservative management with antibiotics alone may be considered in patients with a nonperforated appendicitis with surgical contraindications or with a strong preference to avoid surgery; however, appendectomy generally still is recommended in most patients to prevent recurrent appendicitis (20–35% within 1 year).

Emergency appendectomy is required in patients with perforated appendicitis with generalized peritonitis. The optimal treatment of stable patients with perforated appendicitis and a contained abscess is controversial. Surgery in this setting can be difficult. Many recommend percutaneous CT-guided drainage of the abscess with intravenous fluids and antibiotics to allow the inflammation to subside. An interval appendectomy may be performed after 6 weeks to prevent recurrent appendicitis.

Prognosis

The mortality rate from uncomplicated appendicitis is extremely low. Even with perforated appendicitis, the mortality rate in most groups is only 0.2%, though it approaches 15% in older adults.

Di Saverio S et al. Diagnosis and treatment of acute appendicitis: 2020 update of the WSES Jerusalem guidelines. World J Emerg Surg. 2020;15:27. [PMID: 32295644]

Flum DR et al. A randomized trial comparing antibiotics with appendectomy for appendicitis. N Engl J Med. 2020;383:1907. [PMID: 33017106]
Mahajan P et al. Factors associated with potentially missed diagnosis of appendicitis in the emergency department. JAMA Netw Open. 2020;3:e200612. [PMID: 32150270]
Sippola S et al. Effect of oral moxifloxacin versus intravenous ertapenem plus oral levofloxacin for treatment of uncomplicated acute appendicitis: the APPAC II randomized clinical trial. JAMA. 2021;325:353. [PMID: 33427870]

INTESTINAL TUBERCULOSIS

Intestinal tuberculosis is common in underdeveloped countries but rare in the United States except in immigrant groups or in patients with untreated AIDS. It is caused by both *Mycobacterium tuberculosis* and *M bovis*. Active pulmonary disease is present in less than 50% of patients. The most frequent site of involvement is the ileocecal region; however, any region of the GI tract may be involved. Patients may be without symptoms or complain of chronic abdominal pain, obstructive symptoms, weight loss, and diarrhea. An abdominal mass may be palpable. Complications include intestinal obstruction, hemorrhage, and fistula formation. The purified protein derivative (PPD) skin test may be negative, especially in patients with weight loss or AIDS. Abdominal CT may show thickening of the cecum and ileocecal valve and massive lymphadenopathy. Colonoscopy may demonstrate an ulcerated mass, multiple ulcers with steep edges and adjacent small sessile polyps, small ulcers or erosions, or small diverticula, most commonly in the ileocecal region. The differential diagnosis includes Crohn disease, carcinoma, lymphoma, and intestinal amebiasis. The diagnosis is established by either endoscopic or surgical biopsy revealing acid-fast bacilli, caseating granuloma, or positive cultures for the organism. Detection of tubercle bacilli in biopsy specimens by PCR is now the most sensitive means of diagnosis.

Treatment with standard antituberculous regimens (Tables 9–14 and 9–15) is effective.

Lu S et al. Clinical diagnosis and endoscopic analysis of 10 cases of intestinal tuberculosis. Medicine (Baltimore). 2020;99: e21175. [PMID: 32664157]

PROTEIN-LOSING ENTEROPATHY

Protein-losing enteropathy comprises a number of conditions that result in excessive loss of serum proteins into the GI tract.

Hypoalbuminemia is the sine qua non of protein-losing enteropathy. However, other serum proteins such as alpha-1-antitrypsin also are lost from the gut epithelium. In protein-losing enteropathy caused by lymphatic obstruction, loss of lymphatic fluid commonly results in lymphocytopenia (less than 1000/mcL), hypoglobulinemia, and hypocholesterolemia.

In most cases, protein-losing enteropathy is recognized as a sequela of a known GI disorder. In patients in whom the cause is unclear, evaluation is indicated and is guided by the clinical suspicion. Protein-losing enteropathy must be distinguished from other causes of hypoalbuminemia, which include liver disease and nephrotic syndrome, and from heart failure. Protein-losing enteropathy is confirmed by determining the gut alpha-1-antitrypsin clearance (24-hour volume of feces × stool concentration of alpha-1-antitrypsin ÷ serum alpha-1-antitrypsin concentration). A clearance of more than 27 mL/24 hours is abnormal.

Laboratory evaluation of protein-losing enteropathy includes serum protein electrophoresis, lymphocyte count, and serum cholesterol to look for evidence of lymphatic obstruction. Serum ANA and C3 levels are useful to screen for autoimmune disorders. Stool samples should be examined for ova and parasites. Evidence of malabsorption is evaluated by means of a stool qualitative fecal fat determination. Intestinal imaging is performed with small bowel enteroscopy, CT enterography, or wireless capsule endoscopy of the small intestine. Colonic diseases are excluded with colonoscopy. CT of the abdomen is performed to look for evidence of neoplasms or lymphatic obstruction. Rarely, lymphangiography is helpful. In some situations, laparotomy with full-thickness intestinal biopsy is required to establish a diagnosis.

Treatment is directed at the underlying cause.

Elli L et al. Protein-losing enteropathy. Curr Opin Gastroenterol. 2020;36:238. [PMID: 32073507]
Tseng YJ et al. Protein-losing enteropathy and primary intestinal lymphangiectasia. QJM. 2020;113:224. [PMID: 31309229]

DISEASES OF THE COLON & RECTUM

(See Chapter 39 **for Colorectal Cancer.)**

IRRITABLE BOWEL SYNDROME

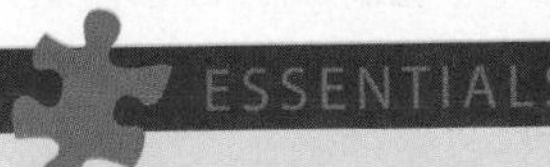

ESSENTIALS OF DIAGNOSIS

- Chronic functional disorder characterized by abdominal pain with alterations in bowel habits.
- Symptoms usually begin in late teens to early twenties.
- Limited evaluation to exclude organic causes of symptoms.

General Considerations

IBS can be defined as an idiopathic clinical entity characterized by chronic (more than 3 months) abdominal pain that occurs in association with altered bowel habits. These symptoms may be continuous or intermittent. The 2016 Rome IV consensus definition of IBS is recurrent abdominal pain that occurs an average of at least 1 day/week and is associated with two or more of the following three features: (1) related to defecation (relief or worsening), (2) associated with a change in frequency of stool, or (3) associated with a change in form (appearance) of stool. Other symptoms supporting the diagnosis include abnormal stool frequency; abnormal stool form (lumpy or hard; loose or watery); abnormal stool passage (straining, urgency, or feeling of incomplete evacuation); and abdominal bloating or a feeling of abdominal distention.

Patients may have other somatic or psychological complaints such as dyspepsia, heartburn, chest pain, headaches, fatigue, myalgias, urologic dysfunction, gynecologic symptoms, anxiety, or depression.

The disorder is a common problem presenting to both gastroenterologists and primary care physicians. Up to 5% of adults have symptoms compatible with the diagnosis, but most never seek medical attention. Approximately two-thirds of patients with IBS are women.

Pathogenesis

A. Abnormal Motility

A variety of abnormal myoelectrical and motor abnormalities have been identified in the colon and small intestine. In some cases, these are temporally correlated with episodes of abdominal pain or emotional stress. Differences between patients with constipation-predominant (slow intestinal transit or pelvic floor dyssynergia) and diarrhea-predominant (rapid intestinal transit, bile acid malabsorption) syndromes are reported.

B. Visceral Hypersensitivity

Patients often have a lower visceral pain threshold, reporting abdominal pain at lower volumes of colonic gas insufflation or colonic balloon inflation than controls. Many patients complain of bloating and distention, which may be due to several different factors including increased visceral sensitivity, increased gas production, impaired gas transit through the intestine, or impaired rectal expulsion. Many patients also report rectal urgency despite small rectal volumes of stool.

C. Intestinal Inflammation

It is postulated that dietary factors, medications (antibiotics), or infections may increase intestinal permeability, leading to intestinal inflammation that may contribute to alterations in intestinal motility or visceral hypersensitivity.

Symptoms compatible with IBS develop within 1 year in over 10% of patients after an episode of bacterial gastroenteritis compared with less than 2% of controls. Women and patients with antibiotic exposure or psychological stress at the onset of gastroenteritis appear to be at increased risk for developing "postinfectious" IBS.

Alterations in the intestinal microbiome composition may cause increased postprandial gas as well as bloating and distention due to degradation of undigested, fermentable carbohydrates in the small intestine or colon. A subset of patients with IBS appear to have small intestinal bacterial overgrowth. However, estimates of the proportions of patients affected vary widely in part due to the different methods used to diagnose bacterial overgrowth. In a 2020 meta-analysis of 25 studies of IBS patients who underwent testing for bacterial overgrowth, an increase in breath hydrogen or methane excretion was reported in 62% following lactulose ingestion but in 21% following glucose ingestion, and only 14% using the "gold standard" of jejunal aspirates and bacterial cultures.

D. Psychosocial Abnormalities

More than 50% of patients with irritable bowel who seek medical attention have underlying depression, anxiety, or somatization. Psychological abnormalities may influence how the patient perceives or reacts to illness and minor visceral sensations. Chronic stress may alter intestinal motility or modulate pathways that affect central and spinal processing of visceral afferent sensation.

Clinical Findings

A. Symptoms and Signs

Irritable bowel is a chronic condition. Symptoms usually begin in the late teens to twenties. The diagnosis is established in the presence of compatible symptoms and the judicious use of tests to exclude organic disease.

Abdominal pain usually is intermittent, crampy, and in the lower abdominal region. Pain is typically associated with a change in stool frequency or form and may be improved or worsened by defecation. It does not usually occur at night or interfere with sleep. Patients with IBS may be classified into one of four categories based on the predominant stool habits and stool form: IBS with diarrhea, IBS with constipation, IBS with mixed constipation and diarrhea, or IBS that is not subtyped. It is important to clarify what the patient means by these complaints. Patients with irritable bowel and constipation report infrequent bowel movements (less than three per week), hard or lumpy stools, or straining. Patients with IBS with diarrhea refer to loose or watery stools, frequent stools (more than three per day), urgency, or fecal incontinence. Many patients report that they have a firm stool in the morning followed by progressively looser movements. Complaints of visible distention and bloating are common, though these are not always clinically evident.

The patient should be asked about "alarm" symptoms that suggest a diagnosis other than IBS and warrant further investigation. The acute onset of symptoms raises the likelihood of organic disease, especially in patients older than 45 years. Nocturnal diarrhea, severe constipation or diarrhea, hematochezia, weight loss, and fever are incompatible with a diagnosis of IBS and warrant investigation for underlying disease. Patients who have a family history of cancer, IBD, or celiac disease should undergo additional evaluation. Eating habits and nutrient intake should be evaluated to screen for eating disorders.

A physical examination should be performed to look for evidence of organic disease and to allay the patient's anxieties. The physical examination usually is normal. Abdominal tenderness, especially in the lower abdomen, is common but not pronounced. A digital rectal examination should be performed in patients with constipation to screen for paradoxical anal squeezing during attempted straining that may suggest pelvic floor dyssynergia. A pelvic examination is recommended for postmenopausal women with recent onset constipation and lower abdominal pain to screen for gynecologic malignancy.

B. Laboratory Findings and Special Examinations

Although the vague nature of symptoms and patient anxiety may prompt clinicians to consider a variety of diagnostic studies, overtesting should be avoided, since the likelihood of serious organic disease is low. Nonetheless, AGA and ACG practice guidelines recommend selected laboratory tests in patients with chronic diarrhea to exclude other diagnoses. A CBC should be obtained to screen for iron deficiency anemia. A fecal calprotectin level is recommended to screen for inflammatory bowel disease; a value of greater than 50 mcg/g may warrant further endoscopic evaluation. Serologic testing for celiac disease (TG IgA) should be performed. Stool specimen examinations should be obtained in patients with increased likelihood of parasitic infection (eg, day care workers, campers, foreign travelers) for *Giardia* antigen or for multiple organisms (*Giardia, Cryptosporidium, Cyclospora, Entamoeba histolytica*) using nucleic acid amplification (PCR) tests. If these tests are negative, further testing is not necessary in most patients and education, reassurance, and initial empiric treatment is recommended. Routine sigmoidoscopy or colonoscopy is not recommended in patients younger than 45 years with symptoms of IBS without "alarm" symptoms but should be considered along with further laboratory testing in patients who do not improve with conservative management. In all patients aged 45 years or older who have not had a previous evaluation, colonoscopy should be obtained to exclude malignancy. When colonoscopy is performed, random mucosal biopsies should be obtained to look for evidence of microscopic colitis (which may have similar symptoms). Patients with symptoms or signs of pelvic floor disorder (dyssynergic defecation) should be referred for anorectal physiology testing (manometry and balloon expulsion test). Routine testing for bacterial overgrowth with hydrogen breath tests is not recommended.

Differential Diagnosis

A number of disorders may present with similar symptoms. Examples include colonic neoplasia, inflammatory bowel disease (ulcerative colitis, Crohn disease, microscopic colitis), bile-acid diarrhea, hyper- or hypothyroidism, parasites, malabsorption (especially celiac disease, bacterial overgrowth, lactase deficiency), causes of chronic secretory diarrhea (carcinoid), and gynecologic disorders (endometriosis, ovarian cancer). Psychiatric disorders such as depression, panic disorder, and anxiety must be considered as well. Women with refractory symptoms have an increased incidence of prior sexual and physical abuse. These diagnoses should be excluded in patients with presumed IBS who do not improve within 2–4 weeks of empiric treatment or in whom subsequent "alarm" symptoms develop.

Treatment

A. General Measures

As with other functional disorders, the most important interventions the clinician can offer are reassurance, education, and support. This includes identifying and responding to the patient's concerns, careful explanation of the pathophysiology and natural history of the disorder, setting realistic treatment goals, and involving the patient in the treatment process. Because irritable bowel symptoms are chronic, the patient's reasons for seeking consultation at this time should be determined. These may include major life events or recent psychosocial stressors, dietary or medication changes, concerns about serious underlying disease, or reduced quality of life and impairment of daily activities. In discussing with the patient the importance of the mind-gut interaction, it may be helpful to explain that alterations in visceral motility and sensitivity may be exacerbated by environmental, social, or psychological factors such as foods, medications, hormones, and stress. Symptoms such as pain, bloating, and altered bowel habits may lead to anxiety and distress, which in turn may further exacerbate bowel disturbances due to disordered communication between the gut and the CNS. Fears that the symptoms will progress, require surgery, or degenerate into serious illness should be allayed. The patient should understand that IBS is a chronic disorder characterized by periods of exacerbation and quiescence. The emphasis should be shifted from finding the cause of the symptoms to finding a way to cope with them. Moderate exercise is beneficial. Clinicians must resist the temptation to chase chronic complaints with new or repeated diagnostic studies.

B. Dietary Therapy

Patients commonly report dietary intolerances. Proposed mechanisms for dietary intolerance include food allergy, hypersensitivity, effects of gut hormones, changes in bacterial flora, increased bacterial gas production (arising in the small or large intestine), and direct chemical irritation. Fatty foods, alcohol, caffeine, spicy foods, and grains are poorly tolerated by many patients with IBS. In patients with diarrhea, bloating, and flatulence, lactose intolerance should be excluded with a hydrogen breath test or a trial of a lactose-free diet. A host of poorly absorbed, fermentable, monosaccharides and short-chain carbohydrates (FODMAPs) may exacerbate bloating, flatulence, and diarrhea in some patients. These include six food groups: fructose (corn syrups, apples, pears, honey, watermelon, raisins), lactose, fructans (garlic, onions, leeks, asparagus, artichokes), wheat-based products (breads, pasta, cereals, cakes), sorbitol (stone fruits), and raffinose (legumes, lentils, brussel sprouts, soybeans, cabbage). Dietary restriction of these fermentable carbohydrates for 2–4 weeks may improve symptoms (especially abdominal pain and bloating) in 50–65% of patients. Responders should gradually reintroduce different FODMAPs to identify food triggers. Ingestion of alpha-galactosidase supplement ("Beano") with meals containing foods with high galactoside content (eg, beans, peas, lentils, soy) may improve bowel symptoms. Gluten has not been demonstrated to increase bowel symptoms independent of other FODMAPs, and a gluten-free diet is not recommended.

Poorly fermentable soluble fiber (psyllium, oatmeal) improves global symptoms in many patients and is recommended by the 2021 American College of Gastroenterology guideline. Fermentable or insoluble fiber (bran, whole grains) may increase gas and bloating.

C. Pharmacologic Measures

More than two-thirds of patients with IBS have mild symptoms that respond readily to education, reassurance, and dietary interventions. Drug therapy should be reserved for patients with moderate to severe symptoms that do not respond to conservative measures. These agents should be viewed as being adjunctive rather than curative. Given the wide spectrum of symptoms, no single agent is expected to provide relief in all or even most patients. Nevertheless, therapy targeted at the specific dominant symptom (pain, constipation, or diarrhea) may be beneficial.

1. Antispasmodic agents—Over-the-counter, enteric-coated peppermint oil formulations (thought to relax smooth intestine) are widely available. In a 2020 randomized controlled trial, a formulation that is released in the small intestine improved abdominal pain in a higher proportion of treated patients (47%) compared with patients given placebo (34%). Based on these results and a meta-analysis of seven other randomized, controlled trials that suggested benefit, the 2021 ACG guideline has suggested that peppermint oil may be useful to relieve global IBS symptoms and abdominal pain.

Anticholinergic agents are not recommended by current guidelines due to a lack of well-designed trials demonstrating efficacy, although some practitioners continue to prescribe these agents to treat acute pain or bloating. Available agents include hyoscyamine, 0.125 mg orally (or sublingually as needed) or sustained-release, 0.037 mg or 0.75 mg orally twice daily; dicyclomine, 10–20 mg orally; or methscopolamine, 2.5–5 mg orally before meals and at bedtime. Anticholinergic side effects are common, including urinary retention, constipation, tachycardia, and dry mouth. Hence, these agents should be used with caution in older patients and in patients with constipation.

2. Antidiarrheal agents—Loperamide (2 mg orally three or four times daily) is effective for the treatment of patients with diarrhea, reducing stool frequency, liquidity, and urgency although it does not improve abdominal pain. It may best be used "prophylactically" in situations in which diarrhea is anticipated (such as stressful situations) or would be inconvenient (social engagements). Increased intracolonic bile acids due to alterations in enterohepatic circulation may contribute to diarrhea in a subset of patients with diarrhea. An empiric trial of bile salt–binding agents (cholestyramine, 2–4 g one to three times daily with meals; colesevelam, 625 mg, 1–3 tablets twice daily) may be considered. Eluxadoline (75–100 mg twice daily) is an opioid antagonist that is approved for treatment of IBS with diarrhea. In phase 3 trials, it decreased abdominal pain and improved stool consistency in approximately 25% of patients versus 16–19% with placebo; however, sphincter of Oddi dysfunction and pancreatitis developed in a small percentage (0.5%) of patients. Given its minimal efficacy, adverse side effect profile, and unproven benefit versus loperamide, further study is needed before its use can be recommended.

3. Anticonstipation agents—Treatment with oral osmotic laxatives such as polyethylene glycol 3350 (MiraLAX, 17–34 g/day) may increase stool frequency, improve stool consistency, and reduce straining but do not improve abdominal pain. Lactulose and sorbitol produce increased flatus and distention and should be avoided in patients with IBS. The secretagogues lubiprostone (8 mcg orally twice daily), linaclotide (290 mcg orally once daily), and plecanatide (3 mg orally once daily) are FDA approved for treatment of IBS with constipation based on modest demonstrated efficacy and are recommended in the 2021 ACG guideline. Through different mechanisms, these agents stimulate increased intestinal chloride and fluid secretion, resulting in accelerated colonic transit. In clinical trials, lubiprostone led to global symptom improvement in 18% of patients compared with 10% of patients who received placebo (a therapeutic gain of 8%). Using different FDA-approved endpoints for significant clinical response (30% reduction in abdominal pain and more than three spontaneous bowel movements per week), phase 3 trials of linaclotide and plecanatide have demonstrated similar therapeutic gains: linaclotide 12.5% versus placebo 4% and plecanatide 26% versus placebo 16%. Tegaserod is a 5-HT_4-receptor agonist that stimulates peristalsis. After original approval in 2002, it was voluntarily withdrawn from the market in 2007 because of cardiovascular safety concerns. Tegaserod (6 mg orally twice daily) was reapproved by the FDA in 2019 for women under age 65 with IBS and constipation after evaluation of clinical and safety data from 29 placebo-controlled trials and newer treatment outcome data. It may be considered for treatment of women age younger than 65 years with one or fewer cardiovascular risk factors whose IBS with constipation has not improved with secretagogue therapy. Patients with intractable constipation should undergo further assessment for slow colonic transit and pelvic floor dysfunction (see Constipation, above).

4. Psychotropic agents—Patients with predominant symptoms of pain or bloating may benefit from low doses of tricyclic antidepressants, which are believed to have effects on motility, visceral sensitivity, and central pain perception that are independent of their psychotropic effects. Because of their anticholinergic effects, these agents may be more useful in patients with diarrhea-predominant than constipation-predominant symptoms. Oral nortriptyline, desipramine, or imipramine may be started at a low dosage of 10 mg at bedtime and increased gradually to 50–150 mg as tolerated. Response rates do not correlate with dosage, and many patients respond to doses of 50 mg or less daily. Side effects are common, and lack of efficacy with one agent does not preclude benefit from another. Agents with higher anticholinergic activity may improve diarrhea but worsen constipation. Improvement should be evident within 4 weeks. The oral SSRIs (sertraline, 25–100 mg daily; citalopram, 10–20 mg; paroxetine, 20–50 mg daily; or fluoxetine, 10–40 mg daily) may be used to treat irritable bowel symptoms as well as treat mood disorders. SSRIs may accelerate GI transit and improve constipation. Anxiolytics should not be used chronically in IBS because of their habituation potential. Patients with major depression or anxiety disorders should be identified and treated with therapeutic doses of appropriate agents.

5. Serotonin receptor antagonists—Alosetron is a 5-HT_3 antagonist that is FDA approved for the treatment of women with severe IBS with predominant diarrhea. Unfortunately, due to cases of severe constipation and a small (1:1000) but significant risk of ischemic colitis, alosetron is restricted to women with severe IBS with diarrhea who have not responded to conventional therapies and who have been educated about the relative risks and benefits of the agent. A randomized crossover trial of another 5-HT_3 antagonist, ondansetron 4–8 mg three times daily, showed overall superior symptom improvement, including stool frequency, consistency, and urgency. At this time, 5-HT_3 antagonists may be considered after careful discussion of the risks and benefits in carefully selected patients with severe diarrhea-predominant IBS.

6. Nonabsorbable antibiotics—Rifaximin (550 mg, three times daily for 14 days) may be considered in patients with refractory symptoms, especially bloating. A 2012 meta-analysis identified a 9.9% greater improvement in bloating with rifaximin compared with placebo, a modest gain that is similar to other less expensive therapies. Symptom improvement may be attributable to suppression of bacteria in either the small intestine or colon, resulting in decreased bacterial carbohydrate fermentation, diarrhea, and bloating.

7. Probiotics—Meta-analyses of small controlled clinical trials of probiotics report improved symptoms of pain, bloating, and flatulence in some patients; however, there is no proven benefit. Probiotics are not recommended for IBS treatment in the 2020 AGA and 2021 ACG guidelines.

D. Psychological Therapies

Cognitive-behavioral therapies, relaxation techniques, yoga, and hypnotherapy appear to be beneficial in some patients. Patients with underlying psychological abnormalities may benefit from evaluation by a psychiatrist or psychologist. Patients with severe disability should be referred to a pain management center.

Prognosis

Most patients with IBS learn to cope with their symptoms and lead productive lives.

Black DJ et al. Efficacy of pharmacological therapies in patients with IBS with diarrhoea or mixed stool pattern: systematic review and network meta-analysis. Gut. 2020;69:74. [PMID: 30996042]

Camilleri M. Diagnosis and treatment of irritable bowel syndrome: a review. JAMA. 2021;325:865. [PMID: 33651094]

Lacy BE et al. ACG clinical guideline: management of irritable bowel syndrome. Am J Gastroenterol. 2021;116:17. [PMID: 33315591]

Shah A et al. Small intestinal bacterial overgrowth in irritable bowel syndrome: a systematic review and meta-analysis of case-control studies. Am J Gastroenterol. 2020;115:190. [PMID: 31913194]

Weerts ZZ et al. Efficacy and safety of peppermint oil in a randomized, double-blind trial of patients with irritable bowel syndrome. Gastroenterology. 2020;158:123. [PMID: 31470006]

ANTIBIOTIC-ASSOCIATED COLITIS

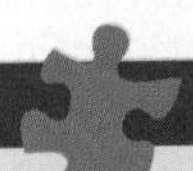

ESSENTIALS OF DIAGNOSIS

- Most cases of antibiotic-associated diarrhea are not attributable to *C difficile* and are usually mild and self-limited.
- Symptoms of antibiotic-associated colitis vary from mild to fulminant; almost all colitis is attributable to *C difficile*.
- Diagnosis in most cases established by stool assay.

General Considerations

Antibiotic-associated diarrhea is a common clinical occurrence. Characteristically, the diarrhea occurs during the period of antibiotic exposure, is dose related, and resolves spontaneously after discontinuation of the antibiotic. In most cases, this diarrhea is mild, self-limited, and does not require any specific laboratory evaluation or treatment. Stool examination usually reveals no fecal leukocytes, and stool cultures reveal no pathogens. Although *C difficile* is identified in the stool of 15–25% of cases of antibiotic-associated diarrhea, it is also identified in 5–10% of patients treated with antibiotics who do not have diarrhea. Most cases of antibiotic-associated diarrhea are due to changes in colonic bacterial fermentation of carbohydrates and are not due to *C difficile*.

Antibiotic-associated colitis is a significant clinical problem almost always caused by *C difficile* infection that colonizes the colon and releases two toxins: TcdA and TcdB. Found throughout hospitals in patient rooms and bathrooms, *C difficile* is readily transmitted from patient to patient by hospital personnel. Fastidious hand washing and use of disposable gloves are helpful in minimizing transmission and reducing infections in hospitalized patients. In hospitalized patients, *C difficile* colitis occurs in approximately 20% of those who are colonized at admission and 3.5% of those not colonized. In both hospital-associated and community infections, most episodes of colitis occur in people who have received antibiotics that disrupt the normal bowel flora and thus allow the bacteria to flourish. Although almost all antibiotics have been implicated, colitis most commonly develops after use of ampicillin, clindamycin, third-generation cephalosporins, and fluoroquinolones. Symptoms usually begin during or shortly after antibiotic therapy but may be delayed for up to 8 weeks. All patients with acute diarrhea should be asked about recent antibiotic exposure. Patients who are older; debilitated; immunocompromised; receiving multiple antibiotics or prolonged (more than 10 days) antibiotic therapy; receiving enteral tube feedings, PPIs, or chemotherapy; or who have IBD have a higher risk of acquiring *C difficile* and developing *C difficile*–associated diarrhea.

Pathogenic strains of *C difficile* produce two toxins: toxin TcdA is an enterotoxin and toxin TcdB is a cytotoxin. A more virulent strain of *C difficile* (NAP1) that contains an 18-base pair deletion of the TcdC inhibitory gene results in higher toxin A and B production. This hypervirulent strain is more prevalent among hospital-associated infections and associated with outbreaks of severe disease but now appears to be declining in incidence.

Clinical Findings

A. Symptoms and Signs

Most patients report mild to moderate greenish, foul-smelling watery diarrhea 3–15 times per day with lower abdominal cramps. Physical examination is normal or reveals mild left lower quadrant tenderness. The stools may have mucus but seldom gross blood. Over half of hospitalized patients diagnosed with *C difficile* colitis have severe disease as defined by a white blood count greater than 15,000/mcL (15×10^9/L) or serum creatinine greater than 1.5 g/dL. Fever is uncommon.

Fulminant disease occurs in up to 10% of patients. It is characterized by hypotension or shock, ileus, or megacolon. Most patients have abdominal pain or tenderness, distention, and profuse diarrhea; however, diarrhea may be absent or appear to be improving in patients with ileus. Laboratory data suggestive of severe disease include a WBC greater than 30,000/mcL (30×10^9/L), serum albumin less than 2.5 g/dL (due to protein-losing enteropathy), elevated serum lactate, and rising serum creatinine.

B. Special Examinations

1. Stool studies—Stool testing for *C difficile* is recommended in hospitalized patients with dysentery or three or more liquid stools within 24 hours or outpatients with diarrhea persisting longer than 1 week. Three types of diagnostic tests are in common use: (1) an immunoassay for glutamate dehydrogenase (GDH) protein has high sensitivity and negative predictive value (95%) for the detection of toxigenic and nontoxigenic *C difficile,* though it does not distinguish active infection with toxin secretion from colonization; (2) PCR tests amplify the *C difficile* toxin gene (usually *TcdB*); they have extremely high sensitivity (97–99%) for detection of *C difficile* as well as the ability to detect the hypervirulent NAP1 strain but like the GDH assay cannot distinguish active infection from colonization; (3) rapid enzyme immunoassays (EIAs) detect the presence of *C difficile*–toxins TcdA and TcdB with 75–95% sensitivity, confirming active toxin-secreting infection. As the initial diagnostic test, most laboratories screen for *C difficile* with either the PCR toxin gene test or the GDH protein assay. A negative PCR or GDH assay effectively excludes infection. Treatment based on PCR or GDH testing alone may result in unnecessary treatment of patients with *C difficile* colonization. Therefore, laboratories may perform secondary testing with toxin EIA to distinguish colonization from active toxin-producing infection.

2. Flexible sigmoidoscopy—Flexible sigmoidoscopy is not needed in patients who have typical symptoms and a positive stool test. It may clarify the diagnosis in patients with positive *C difficile* toxin assays who have atypical symptoms or who have persistent diarrhea despite appropriate therapy. In patients with mild to moderate symptoms, there may be no abnormalities or only patchy or diffuse, nonspecific colitis indistinguishable from other causes. In patients with severe illness, true **pseudomembranous colitis** is seen.

3. Imaging studies—Abdominal radiographs or noncontrast abdominal CTs are obtained in patients with severe or fulminant symptoms to look for evidence of colonic dilation and wall thickening. Abdominal CT also is useful in the evaluation of hospitalized patients with abdominal pain or ileus without significant diarrhea, in whom the presence of colonic wall thickening suggests unsuspected *C difficile* colitis. CT is also useful in the detection of possible perforation.

Differential Diagnosis

In the hospitalized patient in whom acute diarrhea develops after admission, the differential diagnosis includes simple antibiotic-associated diarrhea (not related to *C difficile*), enteral feedings, medications, and ischemic colitis. Other infectious causes are unusual in hospitalized patients in whom diarrhea develops more than 72 hours after admission, and it is not cost-effective to obtain stool cultures unless tests for *C difficile* are negative. *Klebsiella oxytoca* may cause a distinct form of antibiotic-associated hemorrhagic colitis that is segmental (usually in the right or transverse colon); spares the rectum; and is more common in younger, healthier outpatients.

Complications

Severe colitis may progress quickly to fulminant disease, resulting in hemodynamic instability, respiratory failure, metabolic acidosis, megacolon (more than 7-cm diameter), perforation, and death. Chronic untreated colitis may result in weight loss and protein-losing enteropathy.

Treatment

A. Initial Treatment

To reduce transmission within health care facilities, patients with suspected or proven *C difficile* infection should be placed on strict contact precautions and health care workers should apply careful handwashing before and after contact. If possible, therapy with the inciting antibiotic should be discontinued as soon as possible. The treatment of an initial episode of *C difficile* colitis is determined by the severity of disease. For patients with nonsevere disease, oral fidaxomicin (200 mg orally two times daily) and vancomycin (125 mg orally four times daily) are equally effective for initial treatment, but recurrence rates are lower with fidaxomicin than vancomycin (15% vs 25%). Fidaxomicin may be preferred as first-line treatment for patients believed to be at higher risk for recurrent disease. Recommended treatment duration is 10 days in most situations but is extended in patients requiring prolonged antibiotic therapy for other infections. Metronidazole (500 mg orally three times daily) is no longer recommended for initial therapy except in mild disease when vancomycin or fidaxomicin is unavailable. Symptomatic improvement occurs in most patients within 72 hours. Following treatment, stool assays may remain positive for several weeks after symptom resolution.

For patients with fulminant disease, vancomycin 500 mg orally four times daily along with metronidazole 500 mg intravenously every 8 hours are recommended. In patients with ileus, vancomycin may be administered by nasoenteric tube and by rectal enema (500 mg in 100 mL normal saline by enema every 6 hours). The efficacy of fidaxomicin for severe or fulminant disease requires further investigation. Early surgical consultation is recommended for all patients with severe or fulminant disease. Total abdominal colectomy or loop ileostomy with colonic lavage may be required in patients with toxic megacolon, perforation, sepsis, or hemorrhage. Poor surgical candidates should be considered for **fecal microbiota transplantation (FMT)** administered by colonoscopy at 3- to 5-day intervals (see below).

B. Treatment of Relapse

Up to 20% of patients have a relapse of diarrhea from *C difficile* within 8 weeks after stopping initial therapy. This may be due to reinfection or failure to eradicate the organism. Guidelines recommend that the first recurrence be treated with fidaxomicin 200 mg orally twice daily for 10 days or with a prolonged tapering regimen of vancomycin 125 mg orally four times daily for 14 days; twice daily for 7 days; once daily for 7 days; then every other 2 or 3 days for 2–8 weeks. Second recurrence should be treated with an additional vancomycin tapering regimen, as above.

For patients with two or more relapses, guidelines recommend consideration of FMT, in which a suspension of fecal bacteria from a healthy donor is given to the patient with infection. Fecal specimens that have been screened for infectious agents are commercially available. The fecal microbiota usually is instilled into the patient by one of two methods: infusion through a colonoscope into the terminal ileum and colon or ingestion of multiple freeze-dried capsules. Meta-analysis of 34 studies of FMT for recurrent or refractory *C difficile* suggests that efficacy is somewhat higher following colonoscopic administration (92–94%) than oral administration (74–96%); however, the oral capsule method may be preferred for non-hospitalized patients due to relative ease of administration. Randomized studies have demonstrated significantly higher resolution of *C difficile* diarrhea with FMT (92–94%) than with vancomycin (19–31%) or fidaxomicin (42%). FMT carries the potential risk of transmission of serious, even sometimes fatal, infection. However, with proper screening and stool testing of donors, the risk of such infection appears to be low.

Cheng YW et al. Fecal microbiota transplant decreases mortality in patients with refractory severe or fulminant *Clostridioides difficile* infection. Clin Gastroenterol Hepatol. 2020;18:2234. [PMID: 31923639]

Kelly CR et al. ACG Clinical Guidelines: prevention, diagnosis, and treatment of *Clostridioides difficile* infections. Am J Gastroenterol. 2021;116:1124. [PMID: 34003176]

Rao K et al. Diagnosis and treatment of *Clostridioides (Clostridium) difficile* infection in adults in 2020. JAMA. 2020;323:1403. [PMID: 32150234]

Saha S et al. Long-term safety of fecal microbiota transplantation for recurrent *Clostridioides difficile* infection. Gastroenterology. 2021;160:1961. [PMID: 33444573]

INFLAMMATORY BOWEL DISEASE

The term "inflammatory bowel disease" includes ulcerative colitis and Crohn disease. The diagnosis and management of each will be reviewed in the sections below. In the United States, there are approximately 1.6 million people with IBD with adjusted annual incidences of 12.2 cases/100,000 person-years for ulcerative colitis and 10.7 cases/100,000 person-years for Crohn disease. These diseases can occur at any age but most commonly begin in adolescents and adults under age 40 years. The natural history of both varies from mild, often intermittent disease symptoms to severe disease characterized by elevated inflammatory markers and mucosal ulcerations that may lead to intestinal complications (bleeding, strictures, fistulas, surgery), nutritional deficiencies, and impaired quality of life. Both diseases may be associated with several extraintestinal manifestations, including oral ulcers, oligoarticular or polyarticular nondeforming peripheral arthritis, spondylitis or sacroiliitis, episcleritis or uveitis, erythema nodosum, pyoderma gangrenosum, hepatitis and sclerosing cholangitis, and thromboembolic events.

Pharmacologic Therapy

Although ulcerative colitis and Crohn disease appear to be distinct entities, several pharmacologic agents are used to treat both. Despite extensive research, there are still no specific therapies for these diseases. The mainstays of therapy are 5-aminosalicylic acid derivatives, corticosteroids, immunomodulating drugs (such as mercaptopurine or azathioprine and methotrexate) and other small-molecule agents, and biologic therapies.

A. 5-Aminosalicylic Acid (5-ASA)

5-ASA is a topically active agent that has a variety of anti-inflammatory effects. It is readily absorbed from the small intestine but demonstrates minimal colonic absorption. Several oral and topical compounds have been designed to target delivery of 5-ASA to the colon or distal small intestine.

1. Oral formulations—Mesalamine compounds are oral 5-ASA formulations that are either coated in various pH-sensitive resins (Asacol, Apriso, and Lialda) that release 5-ASA throughout the colon or packaged in timed-release capsules (Pentasa) that release 5-ASA in the small intestine and colon. Side effects of these compounds are uncommon but include nausea, rash, diarrhea, pancreatitis, and acute interstitial nephritis. Sulfasalazine and balsalazide are two oral formulations that contain 5-ASA linked by an azo bond to another agent (sulfapyridine or an inert peptide, respectively) in order to prevent small intestine absorption. Following cleavage of the azo bond by colonic bacteria, 5-ASA is released in the colon. The sulfapyridine group is absorbed and may cause side effects in 15–30% of patients, including nausea, oligospermia, leukopenia, agranulocytosis, impaired folate metabolism, and hypersensitivity (fever, rash, hemolytic anemia, pneumonitis). Because of its side effects, sulfasalazine is used less frequently than balsalazide and other 5-ASA agents.

2. Topical mesalamine—5-ASA is provided in the form of suppositories (Canasa; 1000 mg) and enemas (Rowasa; 4 g/60 mL). These formulations can deliver much higher concentrations of 5-ASA to the distal colon than oral compounds. Side effects are uncommon.

B. Corticosteroids

A variety of intravenous, oral, and topical corticosteroid formulations have been used in inflammatory bowel disease. They have utility in the short-term treatment of moderate to severe disease. However, long-term use is associated with serious, potentially irreversible side effects and is to be avoided. The agents, route of administration, duration of use, and tapering regimens used are based more on personal bias and experience than on data from rigorous clinical trials. In hospitalized adult patients with severe disease, current guidelines recommend intravenous methylprednisolone 40–60 mg/day, which may be given in single or divided doses. Oral formulations are prednisone or methylprednisolone. Budesonide is an oral corticosteroid with high topical anti-inflammatory activity but low systemic activity due to high first-pass hepatic metabolism. An enteric-coated formulation is available (Entocort) that targets delivery to the terminal ileum and proximal colon. An enteric coated, multi-matrix, delayed-release formulation (budesonide Multi Matrix [MMX] formulation [Uceris]) is available that releases budesonide throughout the colon. Topical preparations are provided as hydrocortisone suppositories (25 mg and 30 mg), foam (10%, 80 mg), and enemas (100 mg) and as budesonide foam (2 mg).

C. Immunomodulating Drugs and Other Small Molecules

1. Thiopurines (mercaptopurine and azathioprine)—In current clinical practice, these drugs are mainly used in combination with anti-TNF agents (see section D.1. below) in patients with moderate to severe Crohn disease and ulcerative colitis to reduce antibody formation against the biologic agent and to increase the likelihood of clinical remission through increased anti-TNF drug levels and possible synergistic effects. In some settings, they continue to be used as monotherapy to maintain remission in patients with quiescent disease. Side effects of mercaptopurine and azathioprine, including allergic reactions (fever, rash, or arthralgias) and nonallergic reactions (nausea, vomiting, pancreatitis, hepatotoxicity, bone marrow suppression, infections), occur in 15% of patients. Thiopurines are associated with up to a 2.5-fold increased risk of non-Hodgkin lymphomas (0.5/1000 patient-years). The risk rises after 1–2 years of exposure and is higher in men younger than age 30 years and patients older than age 50 years. Thiopurines also are associated with a risk of human papillomavirus (HPV)–related cervical dysplasia and with an increased risk of non-melanoma skin cancer. Younger patients also are at risk for severe primary Epstein-Barr virus (EBV) infection, if not previously exposed.

About 1 person in 300 has a homozygous mutation of one of the enzymes that metabolizes thiopurine methyltransferase (TPMT), placing them at risk for profound immunosuppression; 1 person in 9 is heterozygous for TPMT, resulting in intermediate enzyme activity. Measurement of TPMT functional activity is recommended prior to initiation of therapy. Treatment should be withheld in patients with absent TPMT activity. The most effective dose of mercaptopurine is 1–1.5 mg/kg and for azathioprine, is 2–3 mg/kg daily. For patients with normal TPMT activity, both drugs may be initiated at the weight-calculated dose. A CBC should be obtained weekly for 4 weeks, biweekly for 4 weeks, and then every 1–3 months for the duration of therapy. Liver biochemical tests should be measured periodically. Some clinicians prefer gradual dose escalation, especially for patients with intermediate TPMT activity or for whom TPMT measurement is not available; both drugs may be started at 25 mg/day and increased by 25 mg every 1–2 weeks while monitoring for myelosuppression until the target dose is reached. If the white blood count falls below 4000/mcL (4.0×10^9/L) or the platelet count falls below 100,000/mcL (100×10^9/L), the medication should be held for at least 1 week before reducing the daily dose by 25–50 mg. Measurement of thiopurine metabolites (6-TG and 6-MMP) is of unproved value in most patients but is recommended in patients who have not responded to standard, weight-based dosing or in whom adverse effects develop.

2. Methotrexate—Low-dose oral methotrexate (12.5 mg once weekly) is used in combination with anti-TNF agents to prevent immunogenicity. Methotrexate is an analog of dihydrofolic acid. Side effects of methotrexate include nausea, vomiting, stomatitis, infections, bone marrow suppression, hepatic fibrosis, and life-threatening pneumonitis. A CBC and liver chemistries should be monitored every 3 months. Folate supplementation (1 mg/day) should be administered. Because methotrexate is teratogenic, it should be discontinued in men and women at least 6 months before conception and during pregnancy.

3. Janus kinase inhibitors—Tofacitinib is a nonbiologic small-molecule inhibitor of Janus kinase (JAK 1/3), which is involved through the JAK-STAT pathway in modulation of multiple interleukins. It is currently approved by the FDA as second-line therapy for the treatment of moderate to severe ulcerative colitis (not Crohn disease) that has not responded to anti-TNF therapy. It has rapid oral absorption and lacks immunogenicity. The FDA has issued a black box warning about an increased risk of blood clots and deaths in rheumatoid arthritis patients taking tofacitinib 10 mg orally twice daily compared with patients taking 5 mg orally twice daily of anti-TNF agents. Tofacitinib should not be prescribed to patients deemed at higher risk for thrombosis. It has a low risk of adverse events, including infections, with the exception of herpes zoster (it occurs in up to 5% of patients). Prior to initiating treatment, patients without a history of varicella vaccination should undergo testing for varicella antibodies and receive varicella vaccination if antibody negative. Vaccination with inactivated (not live) recombinant zoster (Shingrix) is recommended in all patients without confirmed varicella vaccination or prior varicella infection.

4. Sphingosine 1-phosphate receptor modulators—Ozanimod is an oral agent that binds to lymphocyte sphingosine 1-phosphate receptors (types 1 and 5), thereby blocking their ability to leave lymph nodes. It is currently approved for the treatment of moderate to severe ulcerative colitis. It leads to a mean 45% reduction of peripheral lymphocyte count that may last for up to 2 weeks after drug discontinuation. Liver chemistries and CBC should be obtained 3–6 months after drug initiation. Severe lymphopenia less than 200×10^9/L (less than 0.2×10^9/L) should prompt drug dosage reduction or discontinuation. The risk of serious adverse events from ozanimod is low but includes hypertension, bradyarrhythmia, liver transaminase elevation, and macular edema. Herpes simplex reactivation (1.3%) or herpes zoster (2.2%) may occur. Prior to initiation of therapy, patients without a history of varicella vaccination should undergo testing for varicella antibodies and, if antibody negative, be given inactivated recombinant zoster (Shingrix) vaccine (see Immunizations below).

D. Biologic Therapies

A number of biologic therapies are available or in clinical testing that target various components of the immune system. Biologic agents are highly effective for patients with moderate to severe disease and when administered early in the disease course may improve the natural history of disease. The potential benefits of these agents must be weighed with their high cost and risk of rare but serious and potentially life-threatening side effects.

1. Anti-TNF therapies—Four monoclonal antibodies to TNF currently are available for the treatment of inflammatory bowel disease: infliximab, adalimumab, golimumab, and certolizumab. All four agents bind and neutralize soluble as well as membrane-bound TNF on macrophages and activated T lymphocytes, thereby preventing TNF stimulation of effector cells.

Infliximab is a chimeric (75% human/25% mouse) IgG_1 antibody that is administered by intravenous infusion. A three-dose regimen of 5 mg/kg administered at 0, 2, and 6 weeks is recommended for acute induction, followed by infusions every 8 weeks for maintenance therapy. Acute infusion reactions occur in 5–10% of infusions but are uncommon in patients receiving regularly scheduled infusions or concomitant immunomodulators (ie, azathioprine or methotrexate). Most reactions are mild and can be treated by slowing the infusion rate and administering acetaminophen and diphenhydramine. Severe reactions (hypotension, severe shortness of breath, rigors, severe chest discomfort) occur in less than 1% and may require oxygen, diphenhydramine, hydrocortisone, and epinephrine. With repeated, intermittent intravenous injections, antibodies to infliximab develop in up to 40% of patients, which are associated with a shortened duration or loss of response and increased risk of acute or delayed infusion reactions. Giving infliximab in a regularly scheduled maintenance therapy (eg, every 8 weeks) or in combination with other immunomodulating agents (azathioprine, mercaptopurine, or methotrexate) significantly reduces the development of antibodies to less than 10%.

Adalimumab and golimumab are fully human IgG_1 antibodies that are administered by subcutaneous injection. For adalimumab, a dose of 160 mg at week 0 and 80 mg at week 2 is recommended for acute induction, followed by maintenance therapy with 40 mg subcutaneously every other week. For golimumab, a dose of 200 mg at week 0 and 100 mg at week 2 is recommended for acute induction, followed by maintenance therapy with 100 mg subcutaneously every 4 weeks.

Certolizumab is a fusion compound in which the Fab1 portion of a chimeric (95% human/5% mouse) TNF-antibody is bound to polyethylene glycol in order to prolong the drug half-life. However, certolizumab is infrequently used due to lower clinical efficacy.

Hypersensitivity reactions are rare with subcutaneous anti-TNF therapies. Antibodies to adalimumab or golimumab develop in 5% of patients and to certolizumab in 10%, which may lead to shortened duration or loss of response to the drug.

Serious infections with anti-TNF therapies may occur in 2–5% of patients, including sepsis, pneumonia, abscess, and cellulitis; however, controlled studies suggest the increased risk may be attributable to increased severity of disease and concomitant use of corticosteroids or immunomodulators. Patients treated with anti-TNF therapies are at increased risk for the development of opportunistic infections with intracellular bacterial pathogens including tuberculosis, mycoses (candidiasis, histoplasmosis, coccidioidomycosis, nocardiosis), and listeriosis, and with reactivation of viral infections, including hepatitis B, herpes simplex, varicella zoster, and EBV. Prior to use of these agents, patients should be screened for latent tuberculosis with PPD testing and a chest radiograph. Antinuclear and anti-DNA antibodies occur in a large percentage of patients; however, the development of drug-induced lupus is rare. All agents may cause severe hepatic reactions leading to acute hepatic failure; liver biochemical tests should be monitored routinely during therapy. Anti-TNF therapies may increase the risk of skin cancer, hence annual dermatologic examinations are recommended. There may be a small risk of non-Hodgkin lymphoma in patients taking anti-TNF monotherapy; however, the risk is much higher in patients receiving a combination of anti-TNF and a thiopurine (6.1-fold increase; 0.95/1000 person-years). Rare cases of optic neuritis and demyelinating diseases, including multiple sclerosis have been reported. Anti-TNF therapies may worsen heart failure in patients with cardiac disease.

In patients with active inflammatory bowel disease, monitoring of anti-TNF trough levels and any anti-drug antibodies is useful to optimize drug levels and guide therapy. Therapeutic drug monitoring is indicated in patients who have poor clinical response or who have lost clinical response. Patients with high titers of anti-drug antibodies should be switched to a different anti-TNF agent. Anti-TNF therapy is considered to have failed when patients have a poor response despite adequate anti-TNF trough concentrations; another class of drugs should be tried. Increasingly, experts recommend proactive measurement of drug and antibody concentrations in all patients to optimize clinical response and minimize drug antibody formation (more common at low drug levels). At present, recommended trough concentrations during maintenance therapy are greater than 7 mcg/mL for infliximab, greater than 7–10 mcg/mL for adalimumab, and greater than 1 mcg/mL for golimumab.

2. Anti-integrins—Anti-integrins decrease the trafficking of circulating leukocytes through the vasculature, reducing chronic inflammation. Vedolizumab is FDA approved for patients with moderately active ulcerative colitis or Crohn disease who have an inadequate response to or intolerance of corticosteroids, immunomodulators, or anti-TNF agents. Induction therapy is given as a 300-mg intravenous dose at weeks 0, 2, and 6. This is followed by maintenance therapy of 300 mg intravenously every 4–8 weeks based on clinical response or serum trough concentrations. Thus far, vedolizumab does not appear to be associated with an increased risk of serious infections or malignancy. Infusion reactions are uncommon. Antibodies develop in 3.7% but may not interfere with drug efficacy. Combination therapy with immunomodulators does not appear to increase rates of clinical response or remission. Therapeutic drug monitoring is of uncertain utility.

3. Anti-IL-12/23 antibody—Ustekinumab is a human IgG_1 monoclonal antibody that binds the p40 subunit of IL-12 and IL-23, interfering with their receptor binding on T cells, NK cells, and antigen presenting cells. Ustekinumab is FDA approved for the treatment of patients with moderate to severe Crohn disease and for those with moderate to severe ulcerative colitis. Induction therapy is given as a single, weight-based intravenous dose (approximately 5–7 mg/kg), followed by 90 mg every 8 weeks by subcutaneous injection. There has been no demonstrated increase in severe infections or malignancy, and other serious events are rare. Antibodies to ustekinumab develop in less than 2.3% of patients and their impact on treatment efficacy is uncertain. Combination therapy with immunomodulators does not appear to increase rates of clinical response or remission. Therapeutic drug monitoring is of uncertain utility.

Beaugerie L et al. Predicting, preventing, and managing treatment-related complications in patients with inflammatory bowel diseases. Clin Gastroenterol Hepatol. 2020;18:1324. [PMID: 32059920]

Buchner AM et al. Biosimilars in inflammatory bowel disease. Am J Gastroenterol. 2021;116:45. [PMID: 33110013]

Hu A et al. Combination therapy does not improve rate of clinical or endoscopic remission in patients with inflammatory bowel diseases treated with vedolizumab or ustekinumab. Clin Gastroenterol Hepatol. 2021;19:1366. [PMID: 32668338]

Shukla R et al. Therapeutic drug monitoring of non-anti-tumor necrosis factor biologics. Clin Gastroenterol Hepatol. 2021; 19:1108. [PMID:335563]

Singh S et al. Comparative risk of serious infections with biologic and/or immunosuppressive therapy in patients with inflammatory bowel diseases: a systematic review and meta-analysis. Clin Gastroenterol Hepatol. 2020;18:69. [PMID: 30876964]

Immunizations

Due to increased risk of vaccine-preventable infections, vaccination status should be confirmed in ***all*** patients with IBD. Inactivated vaccines—hepatitis A and B, recombinant herpes zoster (Shingrix), influenza, and DTaP (tetanus, diphtheria, pertussis) vaccines—may be safely administered in patients receiving immunosuppressive agents; however, efficacy may be attenuated. Pneumococcal vaccine is recommended for patients who are over age 65 or who are receiving immunosuppressive agents. Live virus vaccines (varicella; measles, mumps, rubella) should considered ***before*** initiating immunosuppressives for previously unvaccinated patients who lack serologic evidence of prior infection. Live virus vaccines should ***not*** be administered to patients taking immunosuppressive agents.

Benchimol EI et al. Canadian Association for Gastroenterology clinical practice guideline for immunizations in patients with inflammatory bowel disease—Part 1: live vaccines. Gastroenterology. 2021;161:669. [PMID: 33617891]

Jones JL et al. Canadian Association of Gastroenterology clinical practice guideline for immunizations in patients with inflammatory bowel disease—Part 2: inactivated vaccines. Gastroenterology. 2021;161:681. [PMID: 34476339]

Lifestyle & Social Support for Patients

IBD is a lifelong illness that can have profound physical, psychological, and social impacts on the individual and their family. A therapeutic relationship between the patient and clinician that involves trust, open communication, and shared decision-making is critical to achieving optimal outcomes. Adherence to a healthy lifestyle is associated with improved outcomes, including reduced mortality. Patients may be encouraged to stop or avoid smoking, maintain light alcohol consumption, and engage in moderate to vigorous physical activity. Diets that are low in saturated fats and red meats and high in fruits, vegetables (including the Mediterranean diet) may be encouraged in patients without intestinal strictures. Patients should be screened for anxiety and depression, and psychological support (including cognitive behavioral therapy) offered when appropriate. Patients should be encouraged to become involved in the Crohn's and Colitis Foundation of America (CCFA) for patient-centered educational materials and local support groups (https://www.crohnscolitisfoundation.org/).

Levine A et al. Dietary guidance from the International Organization for Study of Inflammatory Bowel Diseases. Clin Gastroenterol Hepatol. 2020;18:1381. [PMID: 32068150]

Lewis JD et al. A randomized trial comparing the specific carbohydrate diet to a Mediterranean diet in adults with Crohn's disease. Gastroenterology. 2021;161:837. [PMID: 34052278]

Lo CH et al. Healthy lifestyle is associated with reduced mortality in patients with inflammatory bowel disease. Clin Gastroenterol Hepatol. 2021;19:87. [PMID: 32142939]

1. Crohn Disease

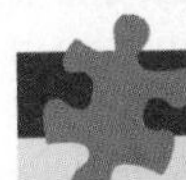

ESSENTIALS OF DIAGNOSIS

- Insidious onset.
- Intermittent bouts of low-grade fever, diarrhea, and right lower quadrant pain.
- Right lower quadrant mass and tenderness.
- Perianal disease with abscess, fistulas.
- Radiographic or endoscopic evidence of ulceration, stricturing, or fistulas of the small intestine or colon.

General Considerations

One-third of cases of Crohn disease involve the small bowel only, most commonly the terminal ileum (ileitis). Half of all cases involve the small bowel and colon, most often the terminal ileum and adjacent proximal ascending colon (ileocolitis). In 20% of cases, the colon alone is affected. One-third of patients have associated perianal disease (fistulas, fissures, abscesses). Less than 5% of patients have symptomatic involvement of the upper intestinal tract. Unlike ulcerative colitis, Crohn disease is a *transmural* process that may involve *any* segment of the GI tract. It results in mucosal inflammation and ulceration, stricturing, fistula development, and abscess formation. Cigarette smoking is strongly associated with the development of Crohn disease, resistance to medical therapy, and early disease relapse.

Clinical Findings

A. Symptoms and Signs

Because of the variable location of involvement and severity of inflammation, Crohn disease may present with a variety of symptoms and signs. In eliciting the history, the clinician should take particular note of fevers, weight loss, abdominal pain, number of liquid bowel movements per day, general sense of well-being, and prior surgical resections. Physical examination should focus on the patient's temperature, weight, and nutritional status, abdominal tenderness or mass, rectal examination, and extraintestinal manifestations. Approximately 20–30% of patients have an indolent, nonprogressive course. The majority will require specific therapies (often biologic agents) to reduce inflammation, improve quality of life, and reduce the risk of surgery and hospitalization. Most commonly, there is one or a combination of the following clinical constellations.

1. Luminal inflammatory disease—This is the most common presentation at diagnosis (60–80%). Patients report malaise, weight loss, and loss of energy. In patients with ileitis or ileocolitis, there may be diarrhea, usually nonbloody and often intermittent. In patients with colitis involving the rectum or left colon, there may be bloody diarrhea and fecal urgency, mimicking the symptoms of ulcerative colitis. Cramping or steady right lower quadrant or periumbilical pain is common. Physical examination reveals focal tenderness, usually in the right lower quadrant. A palpable, tender mass that represents thickened or matted loops of inflamed intestine may be present in the lower abdomen.

2. Intestinal stricturing—Narrowing of the small bowel may occur as a result of inflammation or fibrotic stenosis. Patients report postprandial bloating, cramping pains, and loud borborygmi. This may occur in patients with active inflammatory symptoms or later in the disease from chronic fibrosis without other systemic symptoms or signs of inflammation.

3. Penetrating disease and fistulae—Sinus tracts that penetrate through the bowel, where they may be contained or form fistulas to adjacent structures, develop in a subset of patients. Penetration through the bowel can result in an intra-abdominal or retroperitoneal phlegmon or abscess manifested by fevers, chills, a tender abdominal mass, and leukocytosis. Fistulas between the small intestine and colon commonly are asymptomatic, but can result in diarrhea, weight loss, bacterial overgrowth, and malnutrition. Fistulas to the bladder produce recurrent infections. Fistulas to the vagina result in malodorous drainage and problems with personal hygiene. Fistulas to the skin usually occur at the site of surgical scars.

4. Perianal disease—One-third of patients with either large or small bowel involvement develop perianal disease manifested by large painful skin tags, anal fissures, perianal abscesses, and fistulas.

5. Extraintestinal manifestations—Extraintestinal manifestations may include arthralgias, arthritis, iritis or uveitis, pyoderma gangrenosum, or erythema nodosum. Oral aphthous lesions are common.

B. Laboratory Findings

Laboratory values may reflect inflammatory activity or nutritional complications of disease. A CBC and serum albumin should be obtained in all patients. Anemia may reflect chronic inflammation, mucosal blood loss, iron deficiency, or vitamin B_{12} malabsorption secondary to terminal ileal inflammation or resection. Leukocytosis may reflect inflammation or abscess formation or may be secondary to corticosteroid therapy. Hypoalbuminemia may be due to intestinal protein loss, malabsorption, bacterial overgrowth, or chronic inflammation. The ESR or CRP level is elevated in many patients during active inflammation; however, one-third have a normal CRP level. Fecal calprotectin is an excellent noninvasive test. Elevated levels are correlated with active inflammation as demonstrated by ileocolonoscopy or radiologic CT or MR enterography. Stool specimens are sent for examination for routine pathogens and *C difficile* toxin by microscopy, culture, and toxin assay or by rapid multiplex PCR diagnostic assessment.

C. Special Diagnostic Studies

In most patients, the initial diagnosis of Crohn disease is based on a compatible clinical picture with supporting endoscopic, pathologic, and radiographic findings. Colonoscopy usually is performed first to evaluate the colon and terminal ileum and to obtain mucosal biopsies. Typical endoscopic findings include aphthoid, linear or stellate ulcers, strictures, and segmental involvement with areas of normal-appearing mucosa adjacent to inflamed mucosa. Large or deep mucosal ulcers portend a higher risk for progressive disease. In 10% of cases, it may be difficult to distinguish ulcerative colitis from Crohn disease. Granulomas on biopsy are present in less than 25% of patients but are highly suggestive of Crohn disease. CT or MR enterography is obtained in patients with suspected small bowel involvement. Suggestive findings include ulcerations, strictures, and fistulas; in addition, CT or MR enterography may identify bowel wall thickening and vascularity, mucosal enhancement, and fat stranding. MR enterography, where available, may be preferred due its lack of radiation exposure. Capsule imaging may help establish a diagnosis when clinical suspicion for small bowel involvement is high but radiographs are normal or nondiagnostic. Barium upper GI series with small bowel follow through should no longer be performed.

Complications

A. Abscess

The presence of a tender abdominal mass with fever and leukocytosis suggests an abscess. Emergent CT or MR of the abdomen is necessary to confirm the diagnosis. Patients should be given broad-spectrum antibiotics. Smaller abscesses (less than 3 cm) respond to antibiotic therapy but larger abscesses usually require percutaneous or surgical drainage.

B. Obstruction

Small bowel obstruction may develop secondary to active inflammation or chronic fibrotic stricturing and is often acutely precipitated by dietary indiscretion. Patients should be given intravenous fluids with nasogastric suction. Systemic corticosteroids are indicated in patients with symptoms or signs of active inflammation but are unhelpful in patients with inactive, fixed disease. Patients unimproved on medical management require surgical resection of the stenotic area or stricturoplasty.

C. Abdominal and Rectovaginal Fistulas

Many fistulas are asymptomatic and require no specific therapy. For symptomatic fistulas, medical therapy is effective in a subset of patients and is usually tried first in outpatients who otherwise are stable. Anti-TNF agents may promote closure in up to 60% within 10 weeks; however, relapse occurs in over one-half of patients within 1 year despite continued therapy. Surgical therapy is required for symptomatic fistulas that do not respond to medical therapy. Fistulas that arise above (proximal to) areas of intestinal stricturing commonly require surgical treatment.

D. Perianal Disease

Patients with fissures, fistulas, and skin tags commonly have perianal discomfort. Successful treatment of active intestinal disease also may improve perianal disease. Specific treatment of perianal disease can be difficult and is best approached jointly with a surgeon with an expertise in colorectal disorders. Pelvic MRI is the best noninvasive study for evaluating perianal fistulas. Patients should be instructed on proper perianal skin care, including gentle wiping with a premoistened pad (baby wipes) followed by drying with a cool hair dryer, daily cleansing with sitz baths or a water wash, and use of perianal cotton balls or pads to absorb drainage. Oral antibiotics (metronidazole, 250 mg three times daily, or ciprofloxacin, 500 mg twice daily) may promote symptom improvement or healing in patients with fissures or uncomplicated fistulas; however, recurrent symptoms are common. Immunomodulators or anti-TNF agents or both promote short-term symptomatic improvement from anal fistulas in two-thirds of patients and complete closure in up to one-half of patients; however, less than one-third maintain symptomatic remission during long-term maintenance treatment.

Anorectal abscesses should be suspected in patients with severe, constant perianal pain, or perianal pain in association with fever. Superficial abscesses are evident on perianal examination, but deep perirectal abscesses may require digital examination or pelvic CT or MR scan. Depending on the abscess location, surgical drainage may be achieved by incision, or catheter or seton placement. Surgery should be considered for patients with severe, refractory symptoms but is best approached after medical therapy of the Crohn disease has been optimized.

E. Carcinoma

Patients with colonic Crohn disease are at increased risk for developing colon carcinoma; hence, annual screening colonoscopy to detect dysplasia or cancer is recommended for patients with a history of 8 or more years of Crohn colitis. Patients with Crohn disease also have an increased risk of lymphoma and small bowel adenocarcinoma; however, both are rare.

F. Hemorrhage

Unlike ulcerative colitis, severe hemorrhage is unusual in Crohn disease.

G. Malabsorption

Malabsorption may arise after extensive surgical resections of the small intestine and from bacterial overgrowth in patients with enterocolonic fistulas, strictures, and stasis. Serum levels of vitamins A, D, and B_{12} should be obtained at diagnosis and monitored periodically in patients with ileal inflammation or resection.

Differential Diagnosis

Chronic cramping abdominal pain and diarrhea are typical of both IBS and Crohn disease, but radiographic examinations are normal in the former. Celiac disease may cause diarrhea with malabsorption. Acute fever and right lower quadrant pain may resemble appendicitis or *Yersinia enterocolitica* enteritis. Intestinal lymphoma causes fever, pain, weight loss, and abnormal small bowel radiographs that may mimic Crohn disease. Patients with undiagnosed AIDS may present with fever and diarrhea. Segmental colitis may be caused by tuberculosis, *E histolytica, Chlamydia*, or ischemic colitis. *C difficile* or CMV infection may develop in patients with inflammatory bowel disease, mimicking disease recurrence. In patients from tuberculosis-endemic countries, it can be extremely difficult to distinguish active intestinal tuberculosis from Crohn disease, even with biopsies and PCR analyses. Diverticulitis or appendicitis with abscess formation may be difficult to distinguish acutely from Crohn disease. NSAIDs may exacerbate inflammatory bowel disease and may also cause NSAID-induced colitis characterized by small bowel or colonic ulcers, erosions, or strictures, often most severe in the terminal ileum and right colon.

Treatment of Active Disease

Crohn disease is a chronic lifelong illness characterized by exacerbations and remissions. Although no specific therapy exists, early treatment that successfully achieves endoscopic and histologic remission is associated with a reduced risk of disease complications, including fistulas, abscesses, and surgeries. Risk stratification is therefore appropriate to guide selection of the optimal treatment. Risk factors for an aggressive disease course include (1) young age at disease onset; (2) early need for corticosteroids; (3) perianal disease, fistulizing or stricturing disease, or upper GI involvement; (4) laboratory markers of severe inflammation, including low albumin or hemoglobin, elevated CRP, or elevated fecal calprotectin; or (5) endoscopic findings of deep ulcerations. Approximately, 20–30% of patients have mild, intermittent disease with a nonprogressive course. Most patients have moderate to severe disease for which early use of biologic therapies is warranted to control inflammation and to slow or arrest disease progression.

A. Mild/Low-Risk Disease

Patients may be characterized as having mild disease with a low risk of disease progression if they have mild symptoms, no significant weight loss, normal or only mildly elevated inflammatory markers (CRP, fecal calprotectin, serum albumin), absence of intestinal complications (stricturing, abscess, fistula, perianal disease), and limited intestinal involvement with superficial mucosal ulcers.

1. Nutrition—Patients should eat a well-balanced diet with as few restrictions as possible. Eating smaller but more frequent meals may be helpful. Patients with diarrhea should be encouraged to drink fluids to avoid dehydration. Many patients report that certain foods worsen symptoms, especially fried or greasy foods. Because lactose intolerance is common, a trial off dairy products is warranted if flatulence or diarrhea is a prominent complaint. Probiotics have not proven beneficial for Crohn disease.

2. Symptomatic therapy—Loperamide (2–4 mg) may be given for diarrhea as needed up to four times daily.

3. Drug therapy—It is recommended that therapy for mild, low-risk Crohn disease begin with medications that are less potent but have a lower risk of adverse effects. Recommended drug treatment depends on the location of disease involvement.

A. TERMINAL ILEUM OR ASCENDING COLON DISEASE—For patients with mild disease involving the terminal ileum or ascending colon, initial treatment is recommended with extended-release budesonide (Entocort), 9 mg once daily for 8 weeks, which induces remission in 50–70% of patients. If disease remission is achieved, budesonide is tapered over 2–4 weeks in 3 mg increments and the patient observed. For treatment of mild ileocolonic Crohn disease, 5-ASA agents remain in widespread clinical use despite an absence of clinical trial data supporting their efficacy. Formulations that release mesalamine in the distal small intestine (Asacol 2.4–4.8 g/day or Pentasa 2–4 g/day) are most often prescribed.

B. LEFT-SIDED OR DIFFUSE COLITIS—For patients with mild colitis that is diffuse or involves only the left side of the colon, oral corticosteroids (prednisone or prednisolone) are recommended. The initial dose of either agent is 40 mg once daily for 1–2 weeks, followed in those who respond by gradual tapering of 5–10 mg/week over 4–8 weeks. Sulfasalazine (1.5–3 g orally twice daily) appears effective in improving symptoms and inducing remission in patients with mild Crohn disease involving the colon (not small intestine) and is recommended in current treatment guidelines. Sulfasalazine is associated with potentially severe side effects in up to 30% of patients (see Inflammatory Bowel Disease: Pharmacologic Therapy). For patients who respond, sulfasalazine 2–4 g/day may be continued as long-term maintenance. Because of sulfasalazine's side effects, many clinicians prescribe other oral 5-ASA agents for mild Crohn colitis despite an absence of clinical data supporting efficacy. Such agents include those that release 5-ASA throughout the colon: delayed-release mesalamine (Lialda or Asacol 2.4–4.8 g/day; Apriso 2.25–4.5 g/day) and balsalazide 2.25 g three times daily.

C. LONG-TERM FOLLOW-UP—In patients with mild Crohn disease who respond to initial therapy with budesonide or prednisone, treatment should be discontinued and the patient monitored periodically for disease recurrence (symptoms, CRP, fecal calprotectin, or endoscopy every 1–2 years). Patients who respond to treatment with sulfasalazine or other 5-ASA formulations should continue long-term maintenance therapy. Patients with mild disease who either do not respond to initial therapy or those who experience symptom relapse more than once every 1–2 years following tapering of corticosteroids should be reclassified as moderate to high risk for disease progression and "stepped up" to more potent therapies (oral corticosteroids, immunomodulators, or biologic agents).

B. Moderate to Severe/High-Risk Crohn Disease

Moderate to severe disease may be characterized by frequent diarrhea, weight loss, daily abdominal pain, abdominal tenderness, and perianal disease. Evidence of significant inflammation includes elevated CRP (greater than 5 mg/dL); anemia; low serum albumin; elevated fecal calprotectin (greater than 150–200 mcg/g); or the findings of deep ulceration, stricture, or penetrating disease on endoscopy or radiologic imaging. Patients characterized as having moderate to severe Crohn disease warrant early treatment with biologic agents (with or without immunomodulators) to promote sustained clinical remission and intestinal mucosal healing ("endoscopic remission"). The choice of therapies depends on patient age and comorbidities, patient preference, the presence of extraintestinal manifestations, and "tiering" of agents by third-party payors. Sustained clinical remission with intestinal mucosal healing should be the therapeutic goal in most patients; however, this cannot always be achieved.

1. Nutrition—Patients with obstructive symptoms should be placed on a low-roughage diet, ie, no raw fruits or vegetables, popcorn, nuts, etc. TPN sometimes is used short term in patients with active disease and progressive weight loss, especially those awaiting surgery who have malnutrition but cannot tolerate enteral feedings because of high-grade obstruction, high-output fistulas, severe diarrhea, or abdominal pain. Parenteral vitamin B_{12} (1000 mcg subcutaneously per month) and oral vitamin D supplementation commonly are needed for patients with previous ileal resection or extensive terminal ileal disease.

2. Symptomatic therapy—Involvement of the terminal ileum with Crohn disease or prior ileal resection may lead to reduced absorption of bile acids that may induce secretory diarrhea from the colon. Secretory diarrhea responds to agents that bind the malabsorbed bile salts: cholestyramine 2–4 g or colestipol 1–2 g one to three times daily with meals; or colesevelam, 625 mg, one to three tablets twice daily. Patients with extensive ileal disease (requiring more than 100 cm of ileal resection) have severe bile salt malabsorption causing steatorrhea. Such patients may benefit from a low-fat diet; bile salt–binding agents exacerbate the diarrhea and should not be given. Patients with Crohn disease are at risk for the development of small intestinal bacterial overgrowth due to enteral fistulas, ileal resection, and impaired motility and may benefit from a course of broad-spectrum antibiotics (see Bacterial Overgrowth, above). Other causes of diarrhea include lactase deficiency and short bowel syndrome. Use of oral antidiarrheal agents may provide benefit in some patients.

3. Drug therapy—The goal of drug treatment for moderate to severe, high-risk Crohn disease is to induce and maintain clinical disease remission, including mucosal healing, whenever possible.

A. CORTICOSTEROIDS—Corticosteroids dramatically suppress the acute clinical symptoms and signs in most patients with both small and large bowel disease; however, they do not alter the natural history of the underlying disease. Because of their rapidity of onset, corticosteroids commonly are used in patients with moderate to severe disease to promote early symptomatic improvement while other disease-modifying agents with slower onset of action are initiated. Hospitalization is warranted in some patients with symptoms or signs of severe disease, especially those with high fever, persistent vomiting, evidence of intestinal obstruction, severe weight loss, severe abdominal tenderness, or suspicion of an abscess. In patients with a tender, palpable inflammatory abdominal mass, CT of the abdomen should be obtained prior to administering corticosteroids to rule out an abscess. If no abscess is identified, parenteral corticosteroids (methylprednisolone 40–60 mg daily) should be administered. Outpatients with moderate to severe disease may be treated with oral prednisone or methylprednisolone, 40 mg/day for 1–2 weeks followed by slow tapering of 5–10 mg/week over 4–8 weeks. Remission or significant improvement occurs in greater than 80% of patients after 8–16 weeks of therapy. It is recommended in most patients that a biologic agent be initiated as the corticosteroid is tapered and withdrawn. Use of long-term low corticosteroid doses should be avoided because of associated complications. If a decision is made not to initiate a biologic agent, long-term treatment with an immunomodulator (azathioprine, mercaptopurine, or methotrexate) is recommended to attempt to provide a steroid-free disease maintenance. However, approximately 20% of patients cannot be completely withdrawn from corticosteroids without experiencing a symptomatic flare-up.

B. BIOLOGIC THERAPIES—Induction therapy with a biologic agent is recommended for almost all patients with moderate to severe Crohn disease; those with a favorable clinical response to induction treatment should be maintained on long-term therapy with a goal of achieving clinical and endoscopic remission. Current treatment options include anti-TNF monoclonal antibodies (infliximab, adalimumab, certolizumab), anti-integrin monoclonal antibody (vedolizumab), and anti-IL-12/23 monoclonal antibody (ustekinumab) (see Inflammatory Bowel Disease: Pharmacology, above). In the absence of head-to-head comparative trials of these agents, relative differences in efficacy and safety are suggested by network meta-analyses. The choice of biologic agent depends on the disease severity, patient age and comorbidities, patient preference, and drug cost/pharmacy tiering.

(1) Anti-TNF therapies—For most patients with moderate to severe Crohn disease, two anti-TNF therapies (infliximab or adalimumab) are recommended as the preferred first-line agents to induce remission either as monotherapy or in combination with immunomodulating agents (azathioprine, mercaptopurine, or methotrexate). Up to two-thirds of patients have significant clinical improvement during acute induction therapy (see Inflammatory Bowel Disease: Pharmacology above for dosing). Although direct comparisons of these anti-TNF agents are unavailable, indirect evidence suggests that intravenous, weight-based infliximab infusion may be preferred to subcutaneous, fixed-dose adalimumab for patients with severe disease, extraintestinal manifestations, perianal disease, or obesity. Certolizumab appears inferior to other anti-TNF agents. Compared with anti-TNF monotherapy, clinical trials suggest that combination of an anti-TNF agent (infliximab or adalimumab) with an immunomodulator (azathioprine, mercaptopurine, or methotrexate) achieves higher rates of clinical and mucosal healing. This benefit is ascribed to increased anti-TNF serum drug levels, reduced development of neutralizing anti-TNF antibodies, and synergistic

anti-inflammatory effects. Despite these benefits, the role of combination therapy versus monotherapy is controversial due to an increased risk of adverse events, including myelosuppression, infections, and malignancies (lymphoma, skin cancer). Due to the complexity and higher risks of combination therapy, many clinicians prefer monotherapy with drug monitoring to optimize anti-TNF trough levels and reduce the risk of developing anti-drug antibodies. Retrospective clinical trial data suggest that remission rates are similar between combination therapy and anti-TNF monotherapy when adjusted for trough levels. Combination therapy is favored for patients at higher risk for disease progression or who previously developed antibodies to a biologic agent.

After initial clinical response, symptom relapse occurs in more than 80% of patients within 1 year in the absence of further maintenance therapy. Therefore, scheduled maintenance therapy is usually recommended (eg, infliximab, 5 mg/kg infusion every 8 weeks; or adalimumab, 40 mg subcutaneous injection every 1–2 weeks). With long-term maintenance therapy, approximately two-thirds of patients have continued clinical response and up to one-half have complete symptom remission. Serum anti-TNF trough levels and drug antibody levels may guide therapy in patients who have lost response. Patients with low serum anti-TNF trough levels and absent drug antibodies should receive increased anti-TNF dosing (infliximab 10 mg/kg; adalimumab 80 mg) or decreased dosing intervals (infliximab every 6 weeks; adalimumab every week). Patients with high antibodies to the anti-TNF agent and low anti-TNF trough levels should be switched to another anti-TNF agent. Patients with inadequate response despite adequate anti-TNF trough levels should be changed to an alternative biologic agent, such as vedolizumab or ustekinumab. In patients receiving combination therapy, consideration should be given to stopping or reducing the dose of the immunomodulating agent after 6–12 months for patients in remission, most especially men younger than age 30 years who have a higher risk of hepatosplenic T-cell lymphoma and for adults older than age 50–60 years in whom there is a higher risk of lymphoma and of infectious complications.

(2) Anti-IL-12/IL-23 antibody—Ustekinumab is also appropriate as first-line induction therapy for patients with moderate to severe Crohn disease and is preferred in those deemed to be at increased risk for complications of anti-TNF therapy. It is also recommended in patients who did not respond to or lost response to prior anti-TNF therapy. In a phase 3 trial involving 741 patients with Crohn disease in whom anti-TNF therapy failed, clinical response was seen in 34% of patients 6 weeks after a single dose of intravenous ustekinumab compared to 21.5% with placebo. In a second phase 3 trial composed of patients in whom conventional therapy with immunomodulators or corticosteroids (but not anti-TNF) had failed, clinical improvement occurred in 55% compared to 28.7% with placebo. Among patients from both induction trials who were enrolled in a chronic maintenance trial (ustekinumab versus placebo subcutaneously every 8 weeks), 53% of those given ustekinumab were in clinical remission at week 44 versus 36% given the placebo.

(3) Anti-integrins—Vedolizumab may be chosen as a first-line agent for induction therapy in patients with moderate Crohn disease who are deemed at increased risk for complications from anti-TNF therapy due to advanced age, multiple comorbidities, or prior malignancy. Vedolizumab may also be used as a second- or third-line agent in patients who have not responded or lost response to anti-TNF agents or ustekinumab. For both first-line therapy in patients not previously treated with biologic agents and second-line therapy in patients who did not respond to anti-TNF therapy, a 2021 AGA guideline provides a "conditional" recommendation for vedolizumab versus a "strong" recommendation for ustekinumab due to low certainty of evidence. In a phase 3 trial, among patients demonstrating initial clinical improvement with vedolizumab induction therapy, 39% of patients treated with long-term vedolizumab (300 mg intravenously every 8 weeks) were in remission at 1 year compared with 21.6% of patients given placebo. Vedolizumab may be less effective than anti-TNF or ustekinumab in the treatment of extraintestinal manifestations and fistulous disease.

Indications for Surgery

Over 50% of patients will require at least one surgical procedure. The main indications for surgery are intractability to medical therapy, intra-abdominal abscess, massive bleeding, symptomatic refractory internal or perianal fistulas, and intestinal obstruction. Patients with chronic obstructive symptoms due to a short segment of ileal stenosis are best treated with resection or stricturoplasty (rather than long-term medical therapy), which promotes rapid return of well-being and elimination of corticosteroids. After surgery, endoscopic evidence of recurrence occurs in 60% within 1 year. Endoscopic recurrence precedes clinical recurrence by months to years; clinical recurrence occurs in 20% of patients within 1 year and 80% within 10–15 years. In a controlled trial of 297 patients undergoing ileocolonic resection, endoscopic recurrence occurred in 30% of patients treated with infliximab every 8 weeks compared with 60% treated with placebo. It may be reasonable to initiate empiric infliximab postoperatively for patients at high risk for disease recurrence and to perform endoscopy in low-risk patients 6 months after surgery in order to identify patients with early endoscopic recurrence who may benefit from biologic therapy.

Prognosis

With proper medical and surgical treatment, the majority of patients are able to cope with this chronic disease and its complications and lead productive lives. Few patients die as a direct consequence of the disease.

When to Refer

- For expertise in endoscopic procedures or capsule endoscopy.
- For follow-up of any patient requiring hospitalization.
- Patients with moderate to severe disease for whom therapy with immunomodulators or biologic agents is being considered.
- When surgery may be necessary.

When to Admit

- An intestinal obstruction is suspected.
- An intra-abdominal or perirectal abscess is suspected.
- A serious infectious complication is suspected, especially in patients who are immunocompromised due to concomitant use of corticosteroids, immunomodulators, or anti-TNF agents.
- Patients with severe symptoms of diarrhea, dehydration, weight loss, or abdominal pain.
- Patients with severe or persisting symptoms despite treatment with corticosteroids.

Agrawal M et al. Approach to the management of recently diagnosed inflammatory bowel disease patients: a user's guide for adult and pediatric gastroenterologists. Gastroenterology. 2021;161:47. [PMID: 33940007]

Barnes EL et al. Perioperative and postoperative management of patients with Crohn's disease and ulcerative colitis. Clin Gastroenterol Hepatol. 2020;18:1356. [PMID: 31589972]

Feuerstein JD et al. AGA Clinical practice guidelines on the medical management of moderate to severe luminal and perianal fistulizing Crohn's disease. Gastroenterology. 2021;160:2496. [PMID: 34051983]

Nguyen NH et al. Positioning therapies in the management of Crohn's disease. Clin Gastroenterol Hepatol. 2020;18:1268. [PMID: 31676360]

Siegel CA et al. Identifying patients with inflammatory bowel diseases at high vs low risk of complications. Clin Gastroenterol Hepatol. 2020;18:1261. [PMID: 31778805]

Tilg H et al. How to manage Crohn's disease after ileocolonic resection? Gastroenterology. 2020;159:816. [PMID: 32739244]

Ungaro RC et al. Deep remission at 1 year prevents progression of early Crohn's disease. Gastroenterology. 2020;159:130. [PMID: 32224129]

2. Ulcerative Colitis

ESSENTIALS OF DIAGNOSIS

- Bloody diarrhea.
- Lower abdominal cramps and fecal urgency.
- Anemia, low serum albumin.
- Negative stool studies for pathogens.
- Sigmoidoscopy is the key to diagnosis.

General Considerations

Ulcerative colitis is a chronic, recurrent disease involving only the colon. It is characterized by diffuse mucosal inflammation that results in friability, erosions, and ulcers with bleeding. Ulcerative colitis invariably involves the rectum and may extend proximally in a continuous fashion to involve part or all of the colon. Approximately one-fourth of patients have disease confined to the rectosigmoid region (proctosigmoiditis); one-half have disease that extends to the splenic flexure (left-sided colitis); and one-fourth have disease that extends more proximally (extensive colitis). In patients with distal colitis, the disease progresses with time to more extensive involvement in 25%. There is some correlation between disease extent and symptom severity. In most patients, the disease is characterized by periods of symptomatic flare-ups and periods of mild activity or remission. Approximately 15% of patients may have an aggressive course with increased risk of hospitalization or surgery. Of patients hospitalized with severe colitis, colectomy is required in up to 30% for unresponsive or "fulminant" disease. Ulcerative colitis is more common in nonsmokers and former smokers. Disease severity may be lower in active smokers and may worsen in patients who stop smoking. Appendectomy before the age of 20 years for acute appendicitis is associated with a reduced risk of developing ulcerative colitis.

Clinical Findings

A. Symptoms and Signs

The clinical profile in ulcerative colitis is highly variable. Bloody diarrhea is the hallmark. Several clinical and laboratory parameters help classify patients as having mild, moderate, or severe disease (Table 15–12). Patients should be asked about stool frequency, the presence and amount of rectal bleeding, cramps, abdominal pain, fecal urgency, tenesmus, and extraintestinal symptoms. Physical examination should focus on the patient's volume status as determined by orthostatic blood pressure and pulse measurements and by nutritional status. On abdominal examination, the clinician should look for tenderness and evidence of peritoneal inflammation. Red blood may be present on digital rectal examination.

1. Mild to moderate disease—Patients with mild to moderate disease have fewer than four to six bowel movements per day, mild to moderate rectal bleeding, and no constitutional symptoms. Stools may be formed or loose in consistency. Because of rectal inflammation, there is fecal urgency and tenesmus. Left lower quadrant cramps relieved by defecation are common, but there is no significant abdominal pain or tenderness. There may be mild anemia and hypoalbuminemia.

2. Severe disease—Patients with severe disease have more than six bloody bowel movements per day, resulting in

Table 15–12. Ulcerative colitis: assessment of disease activity.

	Mild	Moderate	Severe
Stool frequency (per day)	< 4	4–6	> 6–10
Blood in stools	Intermittent	Frequent	Continuous
Hematocrit (%)	Normal	30–40	< 30
CRP	Normal or elevated	Elevated	Elevated
ESR (mm/h)	< 30	> 30	> 30
Endoscopy Mayo Subscore	1	2–3	3

severe anemia, hypovolemia, and impaired nutrition with hypoalbuminemia. Abdominal pain and tenderness are present. "Fulminant colitis" is a subset of severe disease characterized by rapidly worsening symptoms with signs of toxicity.

B. Laboratory Findings

The degree of abnormality of the hematocrit, serum albumin, and inflammatory markers (ESR and CRP) reflects disease severity (Table 15–12).

C. Endoscopy

In acute colitis, the diagnosis is readily established by sigmoidoscopy. The mucosal appearance is characterized by edema, friability, mucopus, and erosions. The "Mayo" endoscopic scoring system is commonly used in clinical practice and therapeutic trials. A score of 0 indicates normal or inactive colitis; 1 indicates erythema, decreased vascularity; 2 indicates friability, marked erythema, erosions; and 3 indicates ulcerations, severe friability, spontaneous bleeding. Mayo endoscopic scores 1–2 are consistent with mild to moderate disease clinical activity, and Mayo scores 2–3 are usually seen in patients with moderate to severe clinical activity. Colonoscopy should not be performed in patients with fulminant disease because of the risk of perforation. After patients have demonstrated improvement on therapy, colonoscopy is performed to determine the extent of disease.

D. Imaging

Abdominal imaging with plain radiographs or CT is obtained in patients with severe colitis to look for significant colonic dilation. Barium enemas are of little utility and may precipitate toxic megacolon.

Differential Diagnosis

The initial presentation of ulcerative colitis is indistinguishable from other causes of colitis, clinically as well as endoscopically. Thus, the diagnosis of idiopathic ulcerative colitis is reached after excluding other known causes of colitis. Infectious colitis should be excluded by sending stool specimens for routine testing to exclude *Salmonella, Shigella, Campylobacter, E coli* O157, *C difficile*, and amebiasis. Where available, microbial assessment using multiplex molecular techniques provides results within 1–4 hours with excellent sensitivity and is preferred to conventional labor-intensive stool microscopy, culture, and toxin testing. CMV colitis occurs in immunocompromised patients, including patients receiving prolonged corticosteroid therapy, and is diagnosed on mucosal biopsy. Gonorrhea, chlamydial infection, herpes, and syphilis are considerations in sexually active patients with proctitis. In older adult patients with CVD, ischemic colitis may involve the rectosigmoid. A history of radiation to the pelvic region can result in proctitis months to years later. Crohn disease involving the colon but not the small intestine may be confused with ulcerative colitis. In 10% of patients, a distinction between Crohn disease and ulcerative colitis may not be possible.

Treatment

There are three main treatment objectives: (1) to terminate the acute, symptomatic attack; (2) to achieve complete remission of clinical and endoscopic disease activity; and (3) to prevent recurrence of attacks. The treatment of acute ulcerative colitis depends on the extent of colonic involvement and the severity of illness. Patients with systemic signs of inflammation (ie, anemia, low serum albumin, elevated CRP or ESR levels) and ulcerations with extensive disease on colonoscopy are at increased risk for hospitalization or surgery, and early aggressive therapy with biologic agents is warranted.

A. Mild to Moderate Distal Colitis

Patients with disease confined to the rectum or rectosigmoid region generally have mild to moderate but distressing symptoms. Patients may be treated with topical mesalamine, topical corticosteroids, or oral aminosalicylates (5-ASA) according to patient preference and cost considerations. Topical mesalamine is the drug of choice and is superior to topical corticosteroids and oral 5-ASA. Mesalamine is administered as a suppository, 1000 mg once daily at bedtime for proctitis, and as an enema, 4 g at bedtime for proctosigmoiditis, for 4–8 weeks, with 75% of patients improving. Patients who either decline or are unable to manage topical therapy may be treated with oral 5-ASA, as discussed below. Although topical corticosteroids are a less expensive alternative to mesalamine, they are also less effective. Hydrocortisone enema or foam (80–100 mg) or budesonide foam are prescribed for proctitis or proctosigmoiditis. Systemic effects from short-term use are very slight. For patients with distal disease who do not improve with topical or oral mesalamine therapy within 6 weeks, the following options may be considered: (1) a combination of a topical agent with an oral 5-ASA agent; (2) topical corticosteroid; or (3) addition of oral prednisone (as described below) or budesonide MMX 9 mg/day for 4–8 weeks to rectal and oral 5-ASA.

Most patients with proctitis or proctosigmoiditis who achieve complete remission with oral or rectal 5-ASA should continue indefinitely on the same therapy to reduce the likelihood of symptomatic relapse. Maintenance treatment with 5-ASA reduces the 12-month relapse rate from 75% to less than 40%. Some patients, however, may prefer intermittent therapy for symptomatic relapse. Topical corticosteroids are ineffective for maintaining remission of distal colitis.

B. Mild to Moderate Colitis

1. 5-ASA agents—Disease extending above the sigmoid colon is best treated with both an oral and rectal 5-ASA agent. For induction of remission, the optimal dose of oral 5-ASA (mesalamine) is 2–3 g once daily in combination with mesalamine 1 g suppository or 4 g enema at bedtime. Most patients improve within 4–8 weeks. Some patients may prefer to initiate therapy with an oral agent, adding topical therapy if initial response is inadequate. These agents achieve clinical improvement in 75% of patients and remission in 20–30%. Oral sulfasalazine (1.5–2 g twice daily) is uncommonly used due to its side effects.

2. Corticosteroids—Patients with mild to moderate colitis who do not improve within 4–8 weeks of 5-ASA therapy should have an oral corticosteroid therapy added with budesonide MMX or prednisone. Budesonide MMX (Uceris) 9 mg/day orally for 4–8 weeks may be preferred in mild to moderate colitis due to its low incidence of corticosteroid-associated side effects, especially in those for whom other systemic corticosteroids are deemed high risk. For patients who require more than one course of corticosteroid therapy every 1–2 years for symptomatic relapse, treatment should be "stepped up" to include a thiopurine (azathioprine or mercaptopurine) or a biologic agent, as described below for Moderate to Severe Colitis.

C. Moderate to Severe Colitis

1. Corticosteroids—An oral corticosteroid (prednisone or methylprednisolone) is commonly prescribed as the first-line agent for nonhospitalized patients with moderate to severe colitis or as second-line therapy in patients in whom initial 5-ASA therapy was ineffective. The initial oral dose of prednisone is 40 mg daily. Rapid improvement is observed in most cases within 2 weeks. Thereafter, tapering of prednisone should proceed by 5–10 mg/wk. After tapering to 20 mg/day, slower tapering (2.5 mg/wk) is sometimes required. Complete tapering of prednisone without symptomatic flare-ups is possible in the majority of patients. Corticosteroids should not be continued long-term to control symptoms because of an unacceptable risk of adverse side effects. Patients achieving remission should be maintained on oral mesalamine (2–4 g/day). Up to 30% of patients either do not respond to prednisone or have symptomatic flares during tapering that prevent its complete withdrawal. The addition of a thiopurine (azathioprine or mercaptopurine) is sometimes used to promote complete steroid withdrawal and maintain long-term remission. Biologic agents or small molecules (tofacitinib, ozanimod) are recommended for patients in whom corticosteroids cannot be completely withdrawn or who require more than one course of corticosteroids every 1–2 years.

2. Biologic agents and small molecules—Anti-TNF antibodies (infliximab, adalimumab, golimumab), vedolizumab (integrin antibody), ustekinumab (IL-12/23 antibody), tofacitinib (Janus kinase inhibitor), and ozanimod (sphingosine 1-phoshate receptor modulator) have demonstrated efficacy for treatment of moderate to severe colitis. The preferred agent depends on several considerations: prior exposure and response to biologic agents; disease severity; patient comorbidities; preferred mode of administration (intravenous, subcutaneous, oral); and pharmacy/insurance company tiering.

A. Treatment of patients naïve to prior biologic therapy—A 2020 AGA guideline recommends either infliximab or vedolizumab as first-line therapies for moderate to severe colitis based on their efficacy and safety profiles. These two agents had the highest rankings of all biologic agents for induction of clinical remission in a 2020 network meta-analysis. Although infliximab may be the more effective agent (especially for severe disease), vedolizumab may be the preferred first-line therapy in older adult patient who have increased medical comorbidities due to its significantly lower incidence of infectious complications.

An induction regimen of infliximab (5 mg/kg intravenously administered at 0, 2, and 6 weeks) results in clinical response in 65% of patients. During long-term maintenance treatment with infliximab (5–10 mg/kg every 4–8 weeks), clinical improvement or remission is achieved in approximately 50% of patients. Network meta-analyses suggest superiority of infliximab (weight-based, intravenous infusion) over the other anti-TNF agents adalimumab and golimumab (fixed-dose, subcutaneous injection). Treatment with adalimumab or golimumab may nonetheless be selected in patients with moderate (not severe) disease who prefer the convenience of subcutaneous, self-injection.

Vedolizumab induction (300 mg intravenously at 0, 2, and 6 weeks) led to clinical improvement in 47.1% of patients compared with 25.5% who were given placebo. Among patients who demonstrated initial clinical improvement, 41.8% of those given long-term maintenance treatment with vedolizumab (300 mg intravenously every 8 weeks) were in clinical remission at 1 year compared with 15.9% of those given placebo. The 2019 VARSITY trial randomized patients with moderate to severe ulcerative colitis to induction and maintenance therapy with vedolizumab versus adalimumab. At 1 year, clinical remission (31.3% vs 22.5%) and endoscopic improvement (39.7% vs 27.7%) were seen in significantly more patients treated with vedolizumab than adalimumab. This was the first controlled trial in ulcerative colitis comparing agents from different biologic classes. Due to its efficacy and superior safety profile, vedolizumab may become the preferred first-line biologic agent for the treatment of moderate ulcerative colitis.

When initiating induction therapy with anti-TNF agents, many clinicians add an immunomodulator (azathioprine, mercaptopurine, or methotrexate) for the first year to increase the likelihood of disease remission and to reduce the development of antibodies that may result in secondary loss of response to anti-TNF therapies. If monotherapy is preferred, proactive drug monitoring of serum trough levels and anti-drug antibody titers should be obtained during induction and maintenance therapy in order to optimize drug dosing. Vedolizumab and ustekinumab have a lower incidence of anti-drug antibodies; hence, immunomodulator cotherapy is not generally prescribed.

Ozanimod is a once daily oral small molecule that was approved by the FDA in 2021 for the treatment of moderate to severe ulcerative colitis. During the first week of therapy, ozanimod dosage is titrated upward (days 1–4: 0.23 mg orally once daily; days 5–7: 0.46 mg orally once daily). On day 8 and thereafter, the dosage is 0.92 mg orally once daily. In phase 3 trials of patients with moderate to severe ulcerative colitis who had not previously received biologic therapy, ozanimod treatment resulted in higher clinical response than placebo after 10 weeks (52.5% versus 29.1%) and higher clinical remission after 52 weeks (41% versus 22%). Among patients who had previously not responded to treatment with an anti-TNF agent, ozanimod treatment achieved clinical response after 10 weeks in 36.9% versus 18.5% with placebo. Clinical experience with this novel agent is limited, but it should be considered in non-hospitalized, biologically naive patients who prefer the convenience of oral therapy.

B. Second-line treatment for patients who have not responded to infliximab—In patients with moderate to severe colitis who have not responded to or lost response to infliximab, the 2020 AGA treatment guideline recommends ustekinumab or tofacitinib rather than vedolizumab or adalimumab as second-line therapy based on network meta-analyses. In phase 3 trials, the clinical response rates at 8 weeks following intravenous administration of ustekinumab 6 mg/kg vs placebo were 62% vs 31%, respectively. Among responders who entered long-term maintenance treatment with ustekinumab 90 mg or placebo subcutaneous injection every 8 weeks, clinical remission was significantly higher with ustekinumab (44%) than with placebo (24%).

Tofacitinib, an oral, small-molecule JAK 1/3 inhibitor, was approved by the FDA in 2018 for the treatment of moderate to severe ulcerative colitis. However, in 2019 the FDA issued a black box warning about an increased risk of thrombosis and death in rheumatoid arthritis patients treated with tofacitinib 10 mg orally twice daily for prolonged periods. Therefore, the 2020 AGA treatment guideline recommends that tofacitinib currently be restricted to second-line therapy in patients who have not responded or who have lost response to anti-TNF therapy. A network meta-analysis of controlled trials found that tofacitinib ranked highest among therapies for induction of remission in patients who have received anti-TNF therapy.

3. Probiotics—Probiotics have not demonstrated significant benefit versus placebo in the treatment of mild to moderate ulcerative colitis in randomized, controlled trials.

D. Severe and Fulminant Colitis

About 15% of patients with ulcerative colitis have a more severe course. Of these, a small subset has a fulminant course with rapid progression of symptoms over 1–2 weeks and signs of severe toxicity. These patients appear quite ill, with fever, prominent hypovolemia, hemorrhage requiring transfusion, and abdominal distention with tenderness. Toxic megacolon develops in less than 2% of cases of ulcerative colitis. It is characterized by colonic dilation of more than 6 cm on plain films with signs of toxicity.

1. General measures—Discontinue all oral intake for 24–48 hours or until the patient demonstrates clinical improvement. TPN is indicated only in patients with poor nutritional status or if feedings cannot be reinstituted within 7–10 days. All opioid or anticholinergic agents should be discontinued. Restore circulating volume with fluids, correct electrolyte abnormalities, and consider transfusion for significant anemia (hematocrit less than 25–28%). A plain abdominal radiograph or CT scan should be ordered on admission to look for evidence of colonic dilation. Send stools for assessment of bacterial pathogens, *C difficile* and parasites, either by conventional bacterial culture, *C difficile* toxin assay, and ova and parasite examinations or by rapid, multiplex PCR assay. CMV superinfection should be considered in patients receiving long-term immunosuppressive therapy who are unresponsive to corticosteroid therapy. Due to a high risk of venous thromboembolic (VTE) disease, VTE prophylaxis should be administered to all hospitalized patients with inflammatory bowel disease. Surgical consultation should be sought for all patients with severe disease.

Patients with fulminant disease are at higher risk for toxic megacolon or perforation and must be monitored closely. Abdominal examinations should be repeated to look for evidence of worsening distention or pain. A 2020 AGA guideline does not recommend the use of empiric broad-spectrum antibiotics in the absence of confirmed infection. In addition to the therapies outlined above, nasogastric suction should be initiated. Patients with toxic megacolon should be instructed to roll from side to side and onto the abdomen in an effort to decompress the distended colon. Serial abdominal plain films should be obtained to look for worsening dilation or signs of ischemia. Patients with fulminant disease or toxic megacolon who worsen or do not improve within 48–72 hours should undergo surgery to prevent perforation. If the operation is performed before perforation, the mortality rate should be low.

2. Corticosteroid therapy—Methylprednisolone, 40–60 mg, is administered intravenously. There appears to be no difference in efficacy between single-dose, divided dose, or continuous infusion regimens. Higher or "pulse" doses are of no benefit. Hydrocortisone enemas (100 mg) may also be administered twice daily for treatment of urgency or tenesmus. Clinical improvement with systemic corticosteroids should be evident within 3–5 days in 50–75% of patients. Once symptomatic improvement has occurred, oral fluids are reinstituted. If these fluids are well tolerated, intravenous corticosteroids are discontinued and the patient is started on oral prednisone (as described for moderate disease). Patients without significant improvement within 3–5 days of intravenous corticosteroid therapy should be referred for surgery or considered for anti-TNF therapies or cyclosporine.

3. Anti-TNF therapies—Intravenous infusion of infliximab, 5–10 mg/kg, has been shown in uncontrolled and controlled studies to be effective in treating severe colitis in patients who did not improve within 4–7 days of intravenous corticosteroid therapy. In a controlled study of patients hospitalized for ulcerative colitis, colectomy was required within 3 months in 69% who received placebo therapy, compared with 47% who received infliximab. Thus, infliximab therapy should be considered in patients with severe ulcerative colitis who have not improved with intravenous corticosteroid therapy. Recent studies have demonstrated more rapid clearance of infliximab in patients with severe ulcerative colitis. Uncontrolled trials have found lower colectomy rates in patients administered higher doses of infliximab (three infusions of 5–10 mg/kg within 2–3 weeks) than with conventional dosing (5 mg/kg at 0, 2, and 6 weeks).

4. Cyclosporine—Intravenous cyclosporine (2–4 mg/kg/day as a continuous infusion) benefits 60–75% of patients with severe colitis who have not improved after 7–10 days of corticosteroids, but it is associated with significant toxicity (nephrotoxicity, seizures, infection, hypertension). Up to two-thirds of responders may be maintained in remission with a combination of oral cyclosporine for 3 months and long-term therapy with mercaptopurine or azathioprine. A 2011 randomized study of patients with severe colitis refractory to intravenous corticosteroids found similar response rates (85%) with cyclosporine and infliximab therapy.

5. Surgical therapy—Patients with severe disease who do not improve after corticosteroid, infliximab, or cyclosporine therapy are unlikely to respond to further medical therapy, and surgery is recommended.

Risk of Colon Cancer

In patients with ulcerative colitis with disease proximal to the rectum and in patients with Crohn colitis, there is an increased risk of developing colon carcinoma. Although older meta-analyses from referral centers reported a high risk (8% after 20 years), more recent systematic reviews of population-based studies report a 2.4-fold increased risk (1.4% after a mean of 14 years of follow-up). Colonoscopies are recommended beginning 8 years after disease diagnosis. The use of high-definition colonoscopes with electronic enhancement or spray application of dilute blue dye (chromoendoscopy) enhances the detection of subtle mucosal lesions, thereby significantly increasing the detection of dysplasia compared with standard colonoscopy. At colonoscopy, all polypoid and nonpolypoid lesions should be resected, when possible, and biopsies obtained of endoscopically unresectable lesions. Subsequent surveillance colonoscopies are performed every 1–5 years, depending on ulcerative colitis extent and activity, and presence of colonic scarring, pseudopolyps, or dysplasia.

Surgery in Ulcerative Colitis

Surgery is required in 25% of patients. Severe hemorrhage, perforation, and documented carcinoma are absolute indications for surgery. Surgery is indicated also in patients with fulminant colitis or toxic megacolon that does not improve within 48–72 hours, in patients with invisible flat dysplasia or non-endoscopically resectable dysplastic lesions on surveillance colonoscopy, and in patients with refractory disease requiring long-term corticosteroids to control symptoms.

Although total proctocolectomy (with placement of an ileostomy) provides complete cure of the disease, most patients seek to avoid it out of concern for the impact it may have on their bowel function, their self-image, and their social interactions. After complete colectomy, patients may have a standard ileostomy with an external appliance, a continent ileostomy, or an internal ileal pouch that is anastomosed to the anal canal (ileal pouch–anal anastomosis). The latter maintains intestinal continuity, thereby obviating an ostomy. Under optimal circumstances, patients have five to seven loose bowel movements per day without incontinence. Endoscopic or histologic inflammation in the ileal pouch ("pouchitis") develops in over 40% of patients within 1 year and in up to 80% over the long term, resulting in increased stool frequency, fecal urgency, cramping, and bleeding, but usually resolves with a 2-week course of oral metronidazole (250–500 mg three times daily) or ciprofloxacin (500 mg twice daily). Patients with frequently relapsing pouchitis may need continuous antibiotics. Probiotics do not appear to be of benefit.

Prognosis

Ulcerative colitis is a lifelong disease characterized by exacerbations and remissions. For most patients, the disease is readily controlled by medical therapy without need for surgery. The majority never require hospitalization. A subset of patients with more severe disease will require surgery, which results in complete cure of the disease. Properly managed, most patients with ulcerative colitis lead close to normal productive lives.

When to Refer

- Colonoscopy: for evaluation of activity and extent of active disease and for surveillance for neoplasia in patients with quiescent disease for more than 8 years.
- For follow-up of any patient requiring hospitalization.

When to Admit

- Patients with severe disease manifested by frequent bloody stools, anemia, weight loss, and fever.
- Patients with fulminant disease manifested by rapid progression of symptoms, worsening abdominal pain, distention, high fever, and tachycardia.
- Patients with moderate to severe symptoms that do not respond to oral corticosteroids and require a trial of bowel rest and intravenous corticosteroids.
- Patients in whom surgical colectomy is indicated.

Danese S et al. Positioning therapies in ulcerative colitis. Clin Gastroenterol Hepatol. 2020;18:1280. [PMID: 31982609]

Deepak P et al. Safety of tofacitinib in a real-world cohort of patients with ulcerative colitis. Clin Gastroenterol Hepatol. 2021;19:1592. [PMID: 32629130]

Feuerstein JD et al. AGA clinical practice guidelines on the management of moderate to severe ulcerative colitis. Gastroenterology. 2020;158:1450. [PMID: 30576644]

Murthy S et al. AGA clinical practice update on endoscopic surveillance and management of colorectal dysplasia in inflammatory bowel disease: expert review. Gastroenterology. 2021;161:1042. [PMID: 34416977]

Rubin DT et al. ACG clinical guideline: ulcerative colitis in adults. Am J Gastroenterol. 2019;114:384. [PMID: 30840605]

Sandborn WJ et al. Ozanimod as induction and maintenance therapy for ulcerative colitis. N Engl J Med. 2021;385:1280. [PMID: 34587385]

Singh S et al. First- and second-line pharmacotherapies for patients with moderate to severe active ulcerative colitis: an updated network meta-analysis. Clin Gastroenterol Hepatol. 2020;18:2179. [PMID: 31945470]

3. Microscopic Colitis

Microscopic colitis is an idiopathic condition that is found in up to 15% of patients who have chronic or intermittent watery diarrhea with normal-appearing mucosa at endoscopy. There are two major subtypes—collagenous colitis and lymphocytic colitis. In both, histologic evaluation of mucosal biopsies reveals chronic inflammation (lymphocytes, plasma cells) in the lamina propria and increased intraepithelial lymphocytes. **Collagenous colitis** is further characterized by the presence of a thickened band (greater than 10 mcm) of subepithelial collagen. Both forms occur more commonly in women, especially in the fifth to sixth decades. Symptoms tend to be chronic or recurrent but may remit in most patients after several years. A more severe illness characterized by abdominal pain, fatigue, dehydration, and weight loss may develop in a subset of patients. The cause of **microscopic colitis** usually is unknown. Several medications have been implicated as etiologic agents, including NSAIDs, PPIs, low-dose aspirin, SSRIs, ACE inhibitors, beta-blockers, and menopausal estrogen hormonal therapy. Diarrhea usually abates within 30 days of stopping the offending medication. Celiac disease may be present in 2–9% of patients and should be excluded with serologic testing (IgA anti-tTG). Treatment is largely empiric since there are few well-designed, controlled treatment trials. Antidiarrheal therapy with loperamide is the first-line treatment for mild symptoms, providing symptom improvement in up to 70%. The next option is delayed-release budesonide (Entocort), 9 mg/day for 6–8 weeks. Budesonide induces clinical remission in greater than 80% of patients; however, relapse occurs in most patients after stopping therapy. Remission is maintained in 75% of patients treated long-term with low doses of budesonide. In clinical practice, budesonide is tapered to the lowest effective dose for suppressing symptoms (3 mg every other day to 6 mg daily). For patients who do not respond to budesonide, uncontrolled studies report that treatment with bile-salt binding agents (cholestyramine, colestipol) or 5-ASAs (sulfasalazine, mesalamine) may be effective in some patients. Less than 3% of patients have refractory or severe symptoms, which may be treated with immunosuppressive agents (azathioprine or methotrexate) or anti-TNF agents (infliximab, adalimumab).

Miehlke S et al. European guidelines on microscopic colitis: United European Gastroenterology and European Microscopic Colitis group statement and recommendations. United European Gastroenterol J. 2021;9:13. [PMID: 33619914]

Zylberberg HM et al. Medication use and microscopic colitis: a multicentre retrospective cohort study. Aliment Pharmacol Ther. 2021;54:526. [PMID: 33852749]

DIVERTICULAR DISEASE OF THE COLON

Colonic diverticulosis increases with age, ranging from a prevalence of 5% in those under age 40 to over 50% by age 60 years in Western societies. Most are asymptomatic, discovered incidentally at endoscopy or on barium enema. Complications occur in less than 5%, including GI bleeding and diverticulitis.

Colonic diverticula may vary in size from a few millimeters to several centimeters and in number from one to several dozen. Almost all patients with diverticulosis have involvement in the sigmoid and descending colon; however, only 15% have proximal colonic disease.

For over 40 years, it has been believed that diverticulosis arises after many years of a diet deficient in fiber. Recent epidemiologic studies challenge this theory, finding no association between the prevalence of asymptomatic diverticulosis and low dietary fiber intake or constipation. Thus, the etiology of diverticulosis is uncertain. The extent to which abnormal motility and hereditary factors contribute to diverticular disease is unknown. Patients with abnormal connective tissue are also disposed to development of diverticulosis, including Ehlers-Danlos syndrome, Marfan syndrome, and systemic sclerosis.

1. Uncomplicated Diverticulosis

More than 90% of patients with diverticulosis have uncomplicated disease and no specific symptoms. In most, diverticulosis is an incidental finding detected during colonoscopy. Some patients have nonspecific complaints of chronic constipation, abdominal pain, or fluctuating bowel habits. Physical examination is usually normal but may reveal mild left lower quadrant tenderness with a thickened, palpable sigmoid and descending colon. Screening laboratory studies should be normal in uncomplicated diverticulosis.

There is no reason to perform imaging studies for the purpose of diagnosing asymptomatic, uncomplicated disease. Diverticula are well seen on colonoscopy and CT. Involved segments of colon may also be narrowed and deformed.

Patients in whom diverticulosis is discovered should be encouraged to increase dietary fiber either through diet (fruits, vegetables, whole grains) or fiber supplements (psyllium, methylcellulose), which is associated with a lower risk of diverticulitis in prospective cohort studies. Studies suggest that the risk of diverticulitis may be further reduced with exercise and avoidance of red meats and NSAIDs.

Ma W et al. Intake of dietary fiber, fruits, and vegetables and risk of diverticulitis. Am J Gastroenterol. 2019;114:1531. [PMID: 31397679]

Strate LL et al. Epidemiology, pathophysiology, and treatment of diverticulitis. Gastroenterology. 2019;156:1282. [PMID: 30660732]

2. Diverticulitis

ESSENTIALS OF DIAGNOSIS

- Acute abdominal pain and fever.
- Left lower abdominal tenderness and mass.
- Leukocytosis.

Clinical Findings

A. Symptoms and Signs

Diverticulitis is defined as macroscopic inflammation of a diverticulum that may reflect a spectrum from inflammation alone, to microperforation with localized paracolic inflammation, to macroperforation with either abscess or generalized peritonitis. Thus, there is a range from mild to severe disease. Most patients with localized inflammation or infection report mild to moderate aching abdominal pain, usually in the left lower quadrant. Constipation or loose stools may be present. Nausea and vomiting are frequent. In many cases, symptoms are so mild that the patient may not seek medical attention until several days after onset. Physical findings include a low-grade fever, left lower quadrant tenderness, and a palpable mass. Stool occult blood is common, but hematochezia is rare. Leukocytosis is mild to moderate. Patients with free perforation present with a more dramatic picture of generalized abdominal pain and peritoneal signs.

B. Imaging

In those presenting for the first time with mild symptoms, an abdominal CT is obtained to look for evidence of diverticulitis (colonic diverticula, wall thickening, pericolic fat infiltration) and to exclude other causes of abdominal pain. An abdominal CT is also indicated in patients with fever, leukocytosis, and sepsis or peritonitis or in those who are immunocompromised to look for evidence of complicated disease (abscess, phlegmon, perforation, fistula). Patients who respond to acute medical management should undergo complete colonic evaluation with colonoscopy or CT colonography 6–8 weeks after resolution of clinical symptoms to exclude colorectal cancer (which may mimic diverticulitis). Cancer is identified in 1.3% and 7.9% of patients following a diagnosis of uncomplicated or complicated diverticulitis, respectively. Endoscopy and colonography are contraindicated during the initial stages of an acute attack because of the risk of free perforation.

Differential Diagnosis

Diverticulitis must be distinguished from other causes of lower abdominal pain, including perforated colonic carcinoma, Crohn disease, appendicitis, ischemic colitis, *C difficile*–associated colitis, and gynecologic disorders (ectopic pregnancy, ovarian cyst or torsion), by abdominal CT scan, pelvic ultrasonography, or radiographic studies of the distal colon that use water-soluble contrast enemas.

Complications

Complications, such as phlegmon, abscess, perforation, peritonitis, or sepsis, develop in approximately 12% of patients with acute diverticulitis. Chronic inflammation or an untreated abscess may lead to smoldering disease (ongoing pain, leukocytosis); formation of fistulas to the bladder, ureter, vagina, uterus, bowel, and abdominal wall; or stricturing of the colon with partial or complete obstruction.

Treatment

A. Medical Management

Most patients with uncomplicated disease can be managed with conservative measures. Patients with mild symptoms and no peritoneal signs may be managed initially as outpatients on a clear liquid diet for 2–3 days. Although broad-spectrum oral antibiotics with anaerobic activity commonly are prescribed, large clinical trials confirm that antibiotics are not beneficial in uncomplicated disease. A 2021 AGA guideline suggests that antibiotics should be used selectively for uncomplicated disease, including patients who are immunocompromised, have significant comorbid disease, or have small pericolonic abscesses (less than 3–4 cm). Reasonable regimens include amoxicillin and clavulanate potassium (875 mg/125 mg) twice daily; or metronidazole, 500 mg three times daily plus either ciprofloxacin, 500 mg twice daily, or trimethoprim-sulfamethoxazole, 160/800 mg twice daily orally, for 7–10 days or until the patient is afebrile for 3–5 days. Symptomatic improvement usually occurs within 3 days, at which time the diet may be advanced. Once the acute episode has resolved, a high-fiber diet is recommended.

Patients with increasing pain, fever, or inability to tolerate oral fluids require hospitalization. Hospitalization is required in patients who are immunocompromised, have significant comorbid illness, have abscesses greater than 3–4 cm, or have signs of severe diverticulitis (high fevers, leukocytosis, or peritoneal signs). Patients should be given nothing by mouth and should receive intravenous fluids. If ileus is present, a nasogastric tube should be placed. Intravenous antibiotics should be given to cover anaerobic and gram-negative bacteria. Single-agent therapy with either a second-generation cephalosporin (eg, cefoxitin), piperacillin-tazobactam, or ticarcillin clavulanate appears to be as effective as combination therapy (eg, metronidazole or clindamycin plus an aminoglycoside or third-generation cephalosporin [eg, ceftazidime, cefotaxime]). Symptomatic improvement should be evident within 2–3 days. Intravenous antibiotics should be continued for 5–7 days, before changing to oral antibiotics.

B. Surgical Management

Surgical consultation and repeat abdominal CT should be obtained on all patients with severe disease or those who do not improve after 72 hours of medical management. Patients with a localized abdominal abscess 4 cm in size or larger are usually treated urgently with a percutaneous catheter drain placed by an interventional radiologist. This permits control of the infection and resolution of the immediate infectious inflammatory process. Indications for emergent surgical management include generalized peritonitis, large undrainable abscesses, and clinical deterioration despite medical management and percutaneous drainage. Following recovery from complicated diverticulitis, a subsequent elective one-stage surgical resection has generally been recommended to reduce recurrent episodes of complicated disease; however, a conservative approach may be selected for some patients. Patients with chronic disease resulting in fistulas or colonic obstruction will require elective surgical resection.

Prognosis

Diverticulitis recurs in 15–20% of patients treated with medical management over 10–20 years. However, less than

5% have more than two recurrences. Among patients who have an episode of uncomplicated diverticulitis, less than 5% later develop complicated disease. Therefore, elective surgical resection is no longer routinely recommended in patients with recurrent bouts of uncomplicated disease but is individualized based on patient preference, age, comorbid disease, and frequency and severity of attacks. Diverticulosis is not associated with an increased risk of colorectal cancer.

When to Refer

- Failure to improve within 72 hours of medical management.
- Presence of significant peridiverticular abscesses (4 cm or larger) requiring possible percutaneous or surgical drainage.
- Generalized peritonitis or sepsis.
- Recurrent attacks.
- Chronic complications, including colonic strictures or fistulas.

When to Admit

- Severe pain or inability to tolerate oral intake.
- Signs of sepsis or peritonitis.
- CT showing signs of complicated disease (abscess, perforation, obstruction).
- Failure to improve with outpatient management.
- Immunocompromised or frail, older patient.

Hall J et al. The American Society of Colon and Rectal Surgeons clinical practice guidelines for the treatment of left-sided colonic diverticulitis. Dis Colon Rectum. 2020;63:728. [PMID: 32384404]

Jaung R et al. Antibiotics do not reduce length of hospital stay for uncomplicated diverticulitis in a pragmatic double-blind randomized trial. Clin Gastroenterol Hepatol. 2021;19:503. [PMID: 32240832]

Peery AF et al. AGA clinical practice update on medical management of colonic diverticulitis: expert review. Gastroenterology. 2021;160:906. [PMID: 33279517]

Tehranian S et al. Prevalence of colorectal cancer and advanced adenoma in patients with acute diverticulitis: implications for follow up colonoscopy. Gastrointest Endosc. 2020;91:634. [PMID: 31521778]

3. Diverticular Bleeding

Half of all cases of acute lower GI bleeding are attributable to diverticulosis (see Acute Lower GI Bleeding, above).

POLYPS OF THE COLON

Polyps are discrete mass lesions that protrude into the intestinal lumen. Although most commonly sporadic, they may be inherited as part of a familial polyposis syndrome. Polyps may be divided into four major pathologic groups: mucosal adenomatous polyps (tubular, tubulovillous, and villous), mucosal serrated polyps (hyperplastic, sessile serrated polyps, and traditional serrated adenoma), mucosal nonneoplastic polyps (juvenile polyps, hamartomas, inflammatory polyps), and submucosal lesions (lipomas, lymphoid aggregates, carcinoids, pneumatosis cystoides intestinalis). Of polyps removed at colonoscopy, over 70% are adenomatous; most of the remainder are serrated.

NONFAMILIAL ADENOMATOUS & SERRATED POLYPS

Adenomas and serrated polyps may be non-polypoid (flat, slightly elevated, or depressed), sessile, or pedunculated (containing a stalk). Their significance is that over 95% of cases of adenocarcinoma of the colon are believed to arise from these lesions. Early detection and removal of these precancerous lesions through screening programs has resulted in a 34% reduction in deaths from colorectal cancer since 2000. It is proposed that there is a polyp → carcinoma sequence whereby nonfamilial colorectal cancer develops through a continuous process from normal mucosa to adenomatous or serrated polyp and later to carcinoma. An estimated 75% of cancers arise in adenomas after inactivation of the *APC* gene leads to chromosomal instability and inactivation or loss of other tumor suppressor genes. The remaining 25% of cancers arise through the serrated pathway in which hyperplastic polyps develop *Kras* mutations (forming traditional serrated adenomas) or *BRAF* oncogene activation (forming sessile serrated lesions) with widespread methylation of CpG-rich promoter regions that leads to inactivation of tumor suppressor genes or mismatch repair genes (*MLH1*) with microsatellite instability.

A. Adenomas

Adenomas are present in more than 30% of men and 20% of women over the age of 50. Most adenomas are smaller than 5 mm and have a low risk of becoming malignant. Adenomas are classified as "advanced" if they are 1 cm or larger or contain villous features or high-grade dysplasia. In the general population, the prevalence of advanced adenomas is 6%. Advanced lesions are believed to have a higher risk of harboring or progressing to malignancy. It has been estimated from longitudinal studies that it takes an average of 5 years for a medium-sized polyp to develop from normal-appearing mucosa and 10 years for a gross cancer to arise.

B. Serrated Polyps

There are three types of serrated polyps: hyperplastic polyps, sessile serrated lesions, and traditional serrated adenomas. It is believed that sessile serrated lesions (prevalence 5–12%) and traditional serrated adenomas (prevalence less than 1%) entail an increased risk of colorectal cancer similar or greater to that of adenomas and account for up to 20–30% of colorectal cancers. Many pathologists cannot reliably distinguish between hyperplastic polyps and sessile serrated lesions. Diminutive hyperplastic polyps (less than 5 mm) are extremely common (prevalence 20–30%), especially in the rectum, and believed to be without significant risk.

Clinical Findings

A. Symptoms and Signs

Most patients with adenomatous and serrated polyps are completely asymptomatic. Chronic occult blood loss may lead to iron deficiency anemia. Large polyps may ulcerate, resulting in intermittent hematochezia.

B. Fecal Occult Blood or Multitarget DNA Tests

FOBT, FIT, and fecal DNA tests are available as part of colorectal cancer screening programs (see Chapter 39). FIT is a fecal immunochemical test for hemoglobin with a single specimen having a sensitivity of approximately 80% for colorectal cancer and 20–30% for advanced adenomas but a much lower sensitivity for serrated lesions. FIT is more sensitive than guaiac-based tests for the detection of colorectal cancer and advanced adenomas. In 2014, a test combining a fecal DNA test with a fecal immunochemical test for stool hemoglobin (under the proprietary name "Cologuard") was approved by the FDA. In a prospective comparative trial conducted in persons at average risk for colorectal cancer undergoing colonoscopy, the sensitivity for colorectal cancer for Cologuard was 92.3% compared to 73.8% for FIT and the sensitivity for large (greater than 1 cm) adenomas or serrated polyps for Cologuard was 42.4% compared to 23.8% for FIT.

C. Radiologic Tests

CT colonography ("virtual colonoscopy") uses data from helical CT with computer-enabled luminal image reconstruction to generate two-dimensional and three-dimensional images of the colon. Using optimal imaging software with multidetector helical CT scanners, several studies report a sensitivity of 90% or more for the detection of polyps larger than 10 mm in size. However, the accuracy for detection of polyps 5–9 mm in size is significantly lower (sensitivity 50%). A small proportion of these diminutive polyps harbor advanced histology (up to 1.2%) or carcinoma (less than 1%). Abdominal CT also results in a radiation exposure that may lead to a small risk of cancer.

D. Endoscopic Tests

Colonoscopy allows evaluation of the entire colon and is the best means of detecting and removing adenomatous and serrated polyps. It should be performed in all patients who have positive FOBT, FIT, or fecal DNA tests or iron deficiency anemia (see Occult GI Bleeding above) since the prevalence of colonic neoplasms is increased in these patients. Colonoscopy should also be performed in patients with polyps detected on CT colonography or adenomas detected on flexible sigmoidoscopy to remove these polyps and to fully evaluate the entire colon. The newest generation of capsule endoscopy of the colon has an 86% sensitivity and 88% specificity for detection of adenomas greater than 6 mm compared with colonoscopy, but only 29% sensitivity and 33% specificity for sessile serrated polyps. Capsule endoscopy may be considered in patients who are unsuitable or unwilling to undergo colonoscopy or who have an incomplete colonoscopy.

Treatment

A. Colonoscopic Polypectomy

Most adenomatous and serrated polyps are less than 2 cm in size and are readily amenable to colonoscopic removal; this can be done with biopsy forceps (for those less than 3 mm), with cold snare excision (for those less than 10 mm), or with cold snare or hot snare cautery (for those 10–20 mm). Sessile polyps larger than 2 cm may be removed by appropriately trained physicians using a variety of endoscopic techniques (eg, saline-lift mucosal resection or dissection) or infrequently may require surgical resection. Patients with large sessile polyps removed in piecemeal fashion should undergo repeated colonoscopy in 6 months to verify complete polyp removal. Complications after colonoscopic polypectomy include perforation in 0.2% and clinically significant bleeding in 0.3–1.0% of all patients, but in 4–8% following mucosal resection of large lesions.

B. Postpolypectomy Surveillance

Adenomas and serrated polyps can be found in 30–40% of patients when another colonoscopy is performed within 3–5 years after the initial examination and polyp removal. Periodic colonoscopic surveillance is therefore recommended to detect these "metachronous" lesions, which either may be new or may have been overlooked during the initial examination. Most of these polyps are small, without high-risk features, and of little immediate clinical significance. The probability of detecting advanced neoplasms at surveillance colonoscopy depends on the number, size, and histologic features of the polyps removed on initial (index) colonoscopy. The US Multi-Society Task Force Guideline provides the following recommendations for repeat colonoscopy that depend on the findings at baseline colonoscopy: (1) **10 years:** normal colonoscopy or fewer than 20 hyperplastic polyps less than 10 mm in the distal colon or rectum; (2) **7–10 years:** 1–2 adenomas less than 10 mm; (3) **5–10 years**: 1–2 sessile serrated polyps less than 10 mm; (4): **3–5 years:** 3–4 adenomas or sessile serrated polyps less than 10 mm; (5) **3 years:** 5–10 adenomas *or* sessile serrated polyps less than 10 mm; *or* 1 or more adenomas or sessile serrated polyp 10 mm or larger *or* an adenoma containing villous features or high-grade dysplasia *or* a sessile serrated polyp with dysplasia. Patients with more than 10 adenomas should have a repeat colonoscopy at 1 year and may be considered for evaluation for a familial polyposis syndrome.

Gupta S et al. Recommendations for follow-up after colonoscopy and polypectomy: a consensus updated by the US Multi-Society Task Force on Colorectal Cancer. Gastroenterology. 2020;158:1131. [PMID: 32039982]

Kaltenbach T et al. Endoscopic removal of colorectal lesions—recommendations of the US Multi-Society Task Force on Colorectal Cancer. Gastroenterology. 2020;158:1095. [PMID: 32058340]

Meester RG et al. Prevalence and clinical features of sessile serrated polyps: a systematic review. Gastroenterology. 2020;159: 105. [PMID: 32199884]

HEREDITARY COLORECTAL CANCER & POLYPOSIS SYNDROMES

Up to 4% of all colorectal cancers are caused by germline genetic mutations that impose on carriers a high lifetime risk of developing colorectal cancer (see Chapter 39). Because the diagnosis of these disorders has important implications for treatment of affected patients and for screening of family members, it is important to consider these disorders in patients with a family history of colorectal cancer that has affected more than one family member, those with a personal or family history of colorectal cancer developing at an early age (50 years or younger), those with a personal or family history of multiple polyps (more than 10), and those with a personal or family history of multiple extracolonic malignancies.

1. Familial Adenomatous Polyposis

ESSENTIALS OF DIAGNOSIS

- Inherited condition characterized by early development of hundreds to thousands of colonic adenomatous polyps.
- Variety of extracolonic manifestations (eg, duodenal adenomas, desmoid tumors, and osteomas) and extracolonic cancers (stomach, duodenum, thyroid).
- Attenuated variant with < 100 (average 25) colonic adenomas.
- Genetic testing confirms mutation of *APC* gene (90%) or *MUTYH* gene (8%).
- Prophylactic colectomy recommended to prevent otherwise inevitable colorectal cancer (adenocarcinoma).

General Considerations

Familial adenomatous polyposis (FAP) is a syndrome affecting 1:10,000 people and accounts for approximately 0.5% of colorectal cancers. The classic form of FAP is characterized by the development of hundreds to thousands of colonic adenomatous polyps and a variety of extracolonic manifestations. Of patients with classic FAP, approximately 90% have a mutation in the *APC* gene that is inherited in an autosomal dominant fashion and 8% have mutations in the *MUTYH* gene that are inherited in an autosomal recessive fashion. FAP arises de novo in 25% of patients in the absence of genetic mutations in the parents. An attenuated variant of FAP also has been recognized in which an average of only 25 polyps (range of 1–100) develop.

Clinical Findings

A. Symptoms and Signs

In classic FAP, colorectal polyps develop by a mean age of 15 years and cancer often by age 40 years. Unless prophylactic colectomy is performed, colorectal cancer is inevitable by age 50 years. In attenuated FAP, the mean age for development of cancer is about 56 years.

Adenomatous polyps of the duodenum and periampullary area develop in over 90% of patients, resulting in a 5–8% lifetime risk of adenocarcinoma. Adenomas occur less frequently in the gastric antrum and small bowel and, in those locations, have a lower risk of malignant transformation. Gastric fundus gland polyps occur in over 50% but have an extremely low (0.6%) malignant potential.

A variety of other benign extraintestinal manifestations, including soft tissue tumors of the skin, desmoid tumors, osteomas, and congenital hypertrophy of the retinal pigment, develop in some patients with FAP. These extraintestinal manifestations vary among families, depending in part on the type or site of mutation in the *APC* gene. Desmoid tumors are locally invasive fibromas, most commonly intra-abdominal, that may cause bowel obstruction, ischemia, or hemorrhage. They occur in 15% of patients and are the second leading cause of death in FAP. Malignancies of the CNS (Turcot syndrome) and tumors of the thyroid and liver (hepatoblastomas) may also develop in patients with FAP.

B. Genetic Testing

Genetic counseling and testing should be offered to patients found to have multiple adenomatous polyps at endoscopy and to first-degree family members of patients with FAP. Most centers now perform genetic testing using a multigene panel of 14–67 hereditary cancer genes, including *APC* and *MUTYH*. *APC* gene mutations are identified in 80% of patients with more than 1000, and 56% with 100–1000 polyps (ie, the classic phenotype of FAP). Current guidelines recommend that genetic testing be considered in individuals with as few as 10 adenomas to exclude a diagnosis of attenuated disease, most especially in patients less than age 50–60 years.

Treatment

Once the diagnosis has been established, complete proctocolectomy with ileoanal anastomosis or colectomy with ileorectal anastomosis is recommended in most patients, usually before age 20 years. Colonoscopy every 1–2 years with polypectomy may be considered for patients with attenuated FAP and a low number of polyps. Upper endoscopic evaluation of the stomach, duodenum, and periampullary area should be performed every 1–3 years to look for adenomas or carcinoma with resection of duodenal or ampullary polyps greater than 10 mm, increasing in size, or suspicious for high-grade dysplasia or cancer. Sulindac and celecoxib have been shown to decrease the number and size of polyps in the rectal stump but not the duodenum.

Kupfer SS et al. Patients in whom to consider genetic evaluation and testing for hereditary colorectal cancer syndromes. Am J Gastroenterol. 2020;115:1. [PMID: 31634263]

Yang J et al. American Society for Gastrointestinal Endoscopy guideline on the role of endoscopy in familial adenomatous polyposis syndromes. Gastrointest Endosc. 2020;91:963. [PMID: 32169282]

2. Hamartomatous Polyposis Syndromes

Hamartomatous polyposis syndromes are rare and account for less than 0.1% of colorectal cancers. They include Peutz-Jeghers syndrome, familial juvenile polyposis, and Cowden disease.

Tacheci I et al. Peutz-Jeghers syndrome. Curr Opin Gastroenterol. 2021;37:245. [PMID: 33591027]

Wagner A et al. The management of Peutz-Jeghers syndrome: European Hereditary Tumour Group (EHTG) guideline. J Clin Med. 2021;10:473. [PMID: 33513864]

3. Lynch Syndrome

ESSENTIALS OF DIAGNOSIS

- Autosomal dominant inherited condition.
- Caused by pathogenic variants in a gene that detects and repairs DNA base-pair mismatches, resulting in DNA microsatellite instability and inactivation of tumor suppressor genes.
- Increased lifetime risk of colorectal cancer (22–75%), endometrial cancer (30–60%), and other cancers; they may develop at young ages.
- Evaluation warranted in patients with personal history of early-onset colorectal cancer or family history of colorectal, endometrial, or other Lynch syndrome–related cancers at young age or in multiple family members.
- Diagnosis suspected by tumor tissue immunohistochemical staining for mismatch repair proteins or by testing for microsatellite instability.
- Diagnosis confirmed by genetic testing.

General Considerations

Lynch syndrome (also known as hereditary nonpolyposis colon cancer [HNPCC]) is an autosomal dominant condition in which there is a markedly increased risk of developing colorectal cancer as well as a host of other cancers, including endometrial, ovarian, kidney, bladder, hepatobiliary, gastric, and small intestinal cancers. It is estimated to account for up to 3% of all colorectal cancers. Affected individuals have a 22–75% lifetime risk of developing colorectal carcinoma and a 30–60% lifetime risk of endometrial cancer, depending on the variant gene. Unlike individuals with familial adenomatous polyposis, patients with Lynch syndrome develop only a few adenomas, which may be flat and more often contain villous features or high-grade dysplasia. In contrast to the traditional polyp → cancer progression (which may take over 10 years), these polyps are believed to undergo rapid transformation over 1–2 years from normal tissue → adenoma → cancer. Colon and endometrial cancer tend to develop at an earlier age (mean age 45–50 years) than sporadic, nonhereditary cancers. A germline pathogenic variant is identified in 20% of patients in whom colon cancer was diagnosed before age 50. Compared to patients with sporadic tumors of similar pathologic stage, those with Lynch syndrome tumors have improved survival. However, synchronous or metachronous cancers occur within 10 years in up to 45% of patients.

Lynch syndrome is caused by a defect in one of several genes that are important in the detection and repair of DNA base-pair mismatches: *MLH1, MSH2, MSH6,* and *PMS2* or EPCAM, a promoter for *MSH2*. Germline pathogenic variants in *MLH1* and *MSH2* account for almost 90% of the known variants in families with Lynch syndrome. Variants in any of these mismatch repair genes result in a characteristic phenotypic DNA abnormality known as microsatellite instability.

Clinical Findings

A thorough family cancer history is essential to identify families that may be affected by the Lynch syndrome so that appropriate genetic and colonoscopic screening can be offered. The National Colorectal Cancer Roundtable recommends a simple three-question tool for identifying increased risk and meriting more detailed assessment: (1) Have you had colorectal cancer or polyps diagnosed before age 50? (2) Do you have three or more relatives with colorectal cancer? and (3) Do you have a first-degree relative with colorectal cancer or another Lynch syndrome–related cancer diagnosed before age 50? The PREMM5 probability model is available for calculating the likelihood of Lynch syndrome based on family and personal history (https://premm.dfci.harvard.edu/). Genetic evaluation is recommended for those with a personal or family history of colorectal cancer under age 50, a history of multiple family members with cancer, or a greater than 5% PREMM5 model-predicted chance of Lynch syndrome. Genetic testing can be performed with multigene panels that test for germline cancer genes (ie, Lynch, familial adenomatous polyposis, and hamartomatous syndromes) as well as others of uncertain significance for approximately $250. Referral to a genetic counselor is recommended.

Personal and family history alone are insufficient to identify a significant proportion of patients with Lynch syndrome. For this reason, the National Comprehensive Cancer Network recommend that *all* colorectal cancers should undergo testing for Lynch syndrome with either immunohistochemistry or microsatellite instability. Universal testing has the greatest sensitivity for the diagnosis of Lynch syndrome and is cost-effective. Individuals whose tumors have normal immunohistochemical staining or do not have microsatellite instability are unlikely to have germline pathogenic variants in mismatch repair genes, do not require further genetic testing, and do not require intensive cancer surveillance. Up to 15% of sporadic (noninherited) tumors have microsatellite instability or absent *MLH1* staining due to somatic (noninherited) methylation of the *MLH1* gene promoter and somatic *BRAF* mutations, which must be excluded before further genetic testing is considered. Germline testing for gene mutations is positive in more than 90% of individuals whose tumors show absent histochemical staining of one of the mismatch repair genes or high level of microsatellite instability without a *BRAF* mutation.

Screening & Treatment

If a pathogenic variant is detected in a patient with cancer in one of the known mismatch genes, genetic testing of other first-degree family members is indicated. If genetic testing documents a Lynch syndrome gene variant, affected relatives should be screened with colonoscopy every 1–2 years beginning at age 25 (or at age 5 years younger than the age at diagnosis of the youngest affected family member). If cancer is found, subtotal colectomy with ileorectal anastomosis (followed by annual surveillance of the rectal stump) should be performed. Women should undergo screening for endometrial and ovarian cancer beginning at age 30–35 years with pelvic examination, transvaginal ultrasound, and endometrial sampling. Prophylactic hysterectomy and oophorectomy are recommended to women at age 40 or once they have finished childbearing. Screening for gastric cancer with upper endoscopy should be considered every 2–3 years beginning at age 30–35 years.

Biller LH et al. Familial burden and other clinical factors associated with various types of cancer in individuals with Lynch syndrome. Gastroenterology. 2021;161:143. [PMID: 33794268]

Ladabaum U. What is Lynch-like syndrome and how should we manage it? Clin Gastroenterol Hepatol. 2020;18:294. [PMID: 31408703]

Xi L et al. Recent advances in Lynch syndrome. Exp Hematol Oncol. 2021;10:37. [PMID: 34118983]

ANORECTAL DISEASES

(See Chapter 39 for Carcinoma of the Anus.)

HEMORRHOIDS

ESSENTIALS OF DIAGNOSIS

- Bright red blood per rectum.
- Protrusion, discomfort.
- Characteristic findings on external anal inspection and anoscopic examination.

General Considerations

Internal hemorrhoids are subepithelial vascular cushions consisting of connective tissue, smooth muscle fibers, and arteriovenous communications between terminal branches of the superior rectal artery and rectal veins. They are a normal anatomic entity, occurring in all adults, that contribute to normal anal pressures and ensure a water-tight closure of the anal canal. They commonly occur in three primary locations—right anterior, right posterior, and left lateral. External hemorrhoids arise from the inferior hemorrhoidal veins located below the dentate line and are covered with squamous epithelium of the anal canal or perianal region.

Hemorrhoids may become symptomatic as a result of activities that increase venous pressure, resulting in distention and engorgement. Straining at stool, diarrhea, constipation, prolonged sitting, pregnancy, obesity, and low-fiber diets all may contribute. With time, redundancy and enlargement of the venous cushions may develop and result in bleeding or protrusion.

Clinical Findings

A. Symptoms and Signs

Patients often attribute a variety of perianal complaints to "hemorrhoids." However, the principal problems attributable to internal hemorrhoids are bleeding, prolapse, and mucoid discharge. Bleeding is manifested by bright red blood that may range from streaks of blood visible on toilet paper or stool to bright red blood that drips into the toilet bowl after a bowel movement. Uncommonly, bleeding is severe and prolonged enough to result in anemia. Initially, internal hemorrhoids are confined to the anal canal (stage I). Over time, the internal hemorrhoids may gradually enlarge and protrude from the anal opening. At first, this mucosal prolapse occurs during straining and reduces spontaneously (stage II). With progression over time, the prolapsed hemorrhoids may require manual reduction after bowel movements (stage III) or may remain chronically protruding (stage IV). Chronically prolapsed hemorrhoids may result in a sense of fullness or discomfort and mucoid discharge, resulting in irritation of perianal skin and soiling of underclothes. Pain is unusual with internal hemorrhoids, occurring only when there is extensive inflammation and thrombosis of irreducible tissue or with thrombosis of an external hemorrhoid.

B. Examination

External hemorrhoids are readily visible on perianal inspection. Nonprolapsed internal hemorrhoids are not visible but may protrude through the anus with gentle straining while the clinician spreads the buttocks. Prolapsed hemorrhoids are visible as protuberant purple nodules covered by mucosa. The perianal region should also be examined for other signs of disease such as fistulas, fissures, skin tags, condyloma, anal cancer, or dermatitis. On digital examination, uncomplicated internal hemorrhoids are neither palpable nor painful. Anoscopic evaluation, best performed in the prone jackknife position, provides optimal visualization of internal hemorrhoids.

Differential Diagnosis

Small volume rectal bleeding may be caused by an anal fissure or fistula, neoplasms of the distal colon or rectum, ulcerative colitis or Crohn colitis, infectious proctitis, or rectal ulcers. Rectal prolapse, in which a full thickness of rectum protrudes concentrically from the anus, is readily distinguished from mucosal hemorrhoidal prolapse. Proctosigmoidoscopy or colonoscopy should be performed in all patients with hematochezia to exclude disease in the rectum or sigmoid colon that could be misinterpreted in the presence of hemorrhoidal bleeding.

Treatment

A. Conservative Measures

Most patients with early (stage I and stage II) disease can be managed with conservative treatment. To decrease straining with defecation, patients should be given instructions for a high-fiber diet and told to increase fluid intake with meals, avoid straining, and limit sitting time on the toilet to less than 5 minutes. Dietary fiber may be supplemented with bran powder (1–2 tbsp twice daily added to food or in 8 oz of liquid) or with commercial bulk laxatives (eg, Benefiber, Metamucil, Citrucel). Suppositories and rectal ointments have no demonstrated utility in the management of mild disease. Mucoid discharge may be treated effectively by the local application of a cotton ball tucked next to the anal opening after bowel movements.

B. Medical Treatment

Patients with stage I, stage II, and stage III hemorrhoids and recurrent bleeding despite conservative measures may be treated without anesthesia with rubber band ligation, injection sclerotherapy, or application of electrocoagulation (bipolar cautery or infrared photocoagulation). The choice of therapy is dictated by operator preference, but rubber band ligation is preferred due to its ease of use and high rate of efficacy. Major complications occur in less than 2%, including pelvic sepsis, pelvic abscess, urinary retention, and bleeding. Recurrence is common unless patients alter their dietary habits. Edematous, prolapsed (stage IV) internal hemorrhoids, may be treated acutely with topical creams, foams, or suppositories containing various combinations of emollients, topical anesthetics, (eg, pramoxine, dibucaine), vasoconstrictors (eg, phenylephrine), astringents (witch hazel), and corticosteroids. Common preparations include Preparation H (several formulations), Anusol HC, Proctofoam, Nupercainal, Tucks, and Doloproct (not available in the United States).

C. Surgical Treatment

Surgical excision (traditional hemorrhoidectomy or stapled hemorrhoidopexy) is reserved for less than 5–10% of patients with chronic severe bleeding due to stage III or stage IV hemorrhoids or patients with acute thrombosed stage IV hemorrhoids with necrosis. Complications of surgical hemorrhoidectomy include postoperative pain (which may persist for 2–4 weeks) and impaired continence.

Thrombosed External Hemorrhoid

Thrombosis of the external hemorrhoidal plexus results in a perianal hematoma. It most commonly occurs in otherwise healthy young adults and may be precipitated by coughing, heavy lifting, or straining at stool. The condition is characterized by the relatively acute onset of an exquisitely painful, tense and bluish perianal nodule covered with skin that may be up to several centimeters in size. Pain is most severe within the first few hours but gradually eases over 2–3 days as edema subsides. Symptoms may be relieved with warm sitz baths, analgesics, and ointments. With symptom resolution, a perianal skin tag may persist, which can be a source of irritation. If the patient is evaluated in the first 24–48 hours, removal of the clot may hasten symptomatic relief. With the patient in the lateral position, the skin around and over the lump is injected subcutaneously with 1% lidocaine using a tuberculin syringe with a 30-gauge needle. An ellipse of skin is then excised and the clot evacuated. A dry gauze dressing is applied for 12–24 hours, and daily sitz baths are then begun.

When to Refer

- Stage I, II, or III: When conservative measures fail and expertise in medical procedures is needed (injection, banding, thermocoagulation).
- Stage IV: When surgical therapy is required.

Gardner IH et al. Benign anorectal disease: hemorrhoids, fissures, and fistulas. Ann Gastroenterol. 2020;33:9. [PMID: 31892792]

Muldoon R. Review of American Society of Colon and Rectal Surgeons clinical practice guidelines for the management of hemorrhoids. JAMA Surg. 2020;155:773. [PMID: 32584937]

Wald A et al. ACG Clinical guideline: management of benign anorectal disorders. Am J Gastroenterol. 2021;116:1987. [PMID: 34618700]

ANORECTAL INFECTIONS

A number of organisms can cause inflammation of the anal and rectal mucosa. Proctitis is characterized by anorectal discomfort, tenesmus, constipation, and mucus or bloody discharge. Most cases of proctitis are sexually transmitted, especially by anal-receptive intercourse. Infectious proctitis must be distinguished from noninfectious causes of anorectal symptoms, including anal fissures or fistulae, perirectal abscesses, anorectal carcinomas, and inflammatory bowel disease (ulcerative colitis or Crohn disease).

Etiology & Management

Several organisms may cause infectious proctitis.

A. *Neisseria gonorrhoeae*

Gonorrhea may cause itching, burning, tenesmus, and a mucopurulent discharge, although many anorectal infections are asymptomatic. Nucleic acid amplification testing for gonorrhea and chlamydia has excellent sensitivity and specificity and is preferred in most clinical settings due to ease of transport and laboratory processing. Rectal swab specimens should be taken during anoscopy. Swabs should also be taken from the pharynx and urethra in men and from the pharynx and cervix in women. Culture with sensitivity testing may be required in patients with suspected infection recurrence. Complications of untreated infections include strictures, fissures, fistulas, and perirectal abscesses. (For treatment, see Chapter 33.)

B. *Treponema pallidum*

Anal syphilis may be asymptomatic or may lead to perianal pain and discharge. With primary syphilis, the chancre may be at the anal margin or within the anal canal and may mimic a fissure, fistula, or ulcer. Proctitis or inguinal lymphadenopathy may be present. With secondary syphilis, condylomata lata (pale-brown, flat verrucous lesions) may be seen, with secretion of foul-smelling mucus. Although the diagnosis may be established with dark-field microscopy or fluorescent antibody testing of scrapings from the chancre or condylomas, this requires proper equipment and trained personnel. The VDRL or RPR test is positive in 75% of primary cases and in 99% of secondary cases. (For treatment, see Chapter 34.)

C. *Chlamydia trachomatis*

Chlamydial infection may cause proctitis similar to gonorrheal proctitis; however, some infections are asymptomatic. It also may cause lymphogranuloma venereum, characterized by proctocolitis with fever and bloody diarrhea, painful perianal ulcerations, anorectal strictures and fistulas, and inguinal adenopathy (buboes). Previously rare in developed countries, an increasing number of cases have been identified among men who have sex with men. The diagnosis is established by PCR-based testing of rectal discharge or rectal biopsy. Recommended treatment is doxycycline 100 mg orally twice daily for 21 days.

D. Herpes Simplex Type 2

Herpes simplex type 2 virus is a common cause of anorectal infection. Symptoms occur 4–21 days after exposure and include severe pain, itching, constipation, tenesmus, urinary retention, and radicular pain from involvement of lumbar or sacral nerve roots. Small vesicles or ulcers may be seen in the perianal area or anal canal. Sigmoidoscopy is not usually necessary but may reveal vesicular or ulcerative lesions in the distal rectum. Diagnosis is established by viral culture, PCR, or antigen detection assays of vesicular fluid. Symptoms resolve within 2 weeks, but viral shedding may continue for several weeks. Patients may remain asymptomatic with or without viral shedding or may have recurrent mild relapses. Treatment of acute infection for 7–10 days with acyclovir, 400 mg, or famciclovir, 250 mg orally three times daily, or valacyclovir, 1 g twice daily, has been shown to reduce the duration of symptoms and viral shedding. Patients with AIDS and recurrent relapses may benefit from long-term suppressive therapy (see Chapter 31).

E. Condylomata Acuminata

Condylomata acuminata (warts) are a significant cause of anorectal symptoms. Caused by the HPV, they may occur on the perianal area, in the anal canal, or on the genitals. Perianal or anal warts are seen in up to 25% of men who have sex with men. HIV-positive individuals with condylomas have a higher relapse rate after therapy and a higher rate of progression to high-grade dysplasia or anal cancer. The warts are located on the perianal skin and extend within the anal canal up to 2 cm above the dentate line. Patients may have no symptoms or may report itching, bleeding, and pain. The warts may be small and flat or verrucous, or may form a confluent mass that may obscure the anal opening. Warts must be distinguished from condyloma lata (secondary syphilis) or anal cancer. Biopsies should be obtained from large or suspicious lesions. Treatment can be difficult. Sexual partners should also be examined and treated. The treatment of anogenital warts is discussed in Chapter 30. The HPV vaccine, Gardasil-9 valent, has demonstrated efficacy in preventing anogenital warts and is now recommended for all persons aged 9–14 (two or three doses) and persons aged 15–45 (three doses), as well as all men of any age who have sex with men (see Chapters 1 and 30). HIV-positive individuals with condylomas who have detectable serum HIV RNA levels should have anoscopic surveillance for anal cancer every 3–6 months.

Blanco JL et al. Effective treatment of lymphogranuloma venereum proctitis with azithromycin. Clin Infect Dis. 2021;73:614. [PMID: 33462582]

Davidson KW et al. Screening for chlamydia and gonorrhea: US Preventive Services Task Force recommendations statement. JAMA. 2021;326:949. [PMID: 34519796]

Workowski KA et al. Sexually transmitted infection treatment guidelines, 2021. MMWR Recomm Rep. 2021;70:1. [PMID: 34292926]

FECAL INCONTINENCE

In a 2018 survey, 4.7% of US adults reported fecal incontinence within the prior 30 days. There are five general requirements for bowel continence: (1) solid or semisolid stool (even healthy young adults have difficulty maintaining continence with liquid rectal contents); (2) a distensible rectal reservoir (as sigmoid contents empty into the rectum, the vault must expand to accommodate); (3) a sensation of rectal fullness (if the patient cannot sense this, overflow may occur before the patient can take appropriate action); (4) intact pelvic nerves and muscles; and (5) the ability to reach a toilet in a timely fashion.

Minor Incontinence

Many patients complain of inability to control flatus or slight soilage of undergarments that tends to occur after bowel movements or with straining or coughing. This may be due to local anal problems such as prolapsed hemorrhoids that make it difficult to form a tight anal seal or isolated weakness of the internal anal sphincter, especially if stools are somewhat loose. Patients should be treated with fiber supplements to provide greater stool bulk. Coffee and other caffeinated beverages should be eliminated. The perianal skin should be cleansed with moist, lanolin-coated tissue (baby wipes) to reduce excoriation and infection. After wiping, loose application of a cotton ball near the anal opening may absorb small amounts of fecal leakage. Prolapsing hemorrhoids may be treated with band ligation or surgical hemorrhoidectomy. Control of flatus and seepage may be improved by Kegel perineal exercises. Conditions such as ulcerative proctitis that cause tenesmus and urgency, chronic diarrheal conditions, and IBS may result in difficulty in maintaining complete continence, especially if a toilet is not readily available.

Loperamide may be helpful to reduce urge incontinence in patients with loose stools and may be taken in anticipation of situations in which a toilet may not be readily available. Older patients may require more time or assistance to reach a toilet, which may lead to incontinence. Scheduled toileting and the availability of a bedside commode are helpful. Older adult patients with chronic constipation may develop stool impaction leading to "overflow" incontinence.

Major Incontinence

Complete uncontrolled loss of stool reflects a significant problem with central perception or neuromuscular function. Incontinence that occurs without awareness suggests a loss of central awareness (eg, dementia, cerebrovascular accident, multiple sclerosis) or peripheral nerve injury (eg, spinal cord injury, cauda equina syndrome, pudendal nerve damage due to obstetric trauma or pelvic floor prolapse, aging, or diabetes mellitus). Incontinence that occurs despite awareness and active efforts to retain stool suggests sphincteric damage, which may be caused by traumatic childbirth (especially forceps delivery), episiotomy, prolapse, prior anal surgery, and physical trauma.

Physical examination should include careful inspection of the perianal area for hemorrhoids, rectal prolapse, fissures, fistulas, and either gaping or a keyhole defect of the anal sphincter (indicating severe sphincteric injury or neurologic disorder). The perianal skin should be stimulated to confirm an intact anocutaneous reflex. Digital examination during relaxation gives valuable information about resting tone (due mainly to the internal sphincter) and contraction of the external sphincter and pelvic floor during squeezing. It also excludes fecal impaction. Anoscopy is required to evaluate for hemorrhoids, fissures, and fistulas. Proctosigmoidoscopy is useful to exclude rectal carcinoma or proctitis. Anal ultrasonography or pelvic MRI is the most reliable test for definition of anatomic defects in the external and internal anal sphincters. Anal manometry may also be useful to define the severity of weakness, to assess sensation, and to predict response to biofeedback training.

Patients who are incontinent only of loose or liquid stools are treated with bulking agents and antidiarrheal drugs (eg, loperamide, 2 mg before meals and prophylactically before social engagements, shopping trips, etc). Patients with incontinence of solid stool benefit from scheduled toilet use after glycerin suppositories or tap water enemas. Biofeedback training with pelvic floor strengthening (Kegel) exercises (alternating 5-second squeeze and 10-second rest for 10 minutes twice daily) may be helpful in motivated patients to lower the threshold for awareness of rectal filling, strengthen the pelvic floor, and improve continence. In a 2019 randomized controlled trial, global incontinence symptom improvement occurred in 38% of patients instructed on daily pelvic floor contraction exercises (three sets of 10 contractions sustained for up to 10 seconds and two sets of 3 contractions sustained for up to 30 seconds) compared with 18% who did not perform these exercises. Operative management is seldom needed but should be considered in patients with major incontinence due to prior injury to the anal sphincter who have not responded to medical therapy.

When to Refer

- Conservative measures fail.
- Anorectal tests are deemed necessary (manometry, ultrasonography, electromyography).
- A surgically correctable lesion is suspected.

Mazor Y et al. Factors associated with response to anorectal biofeedback therapy in patients with fecal incontinence. Clin Gastroenterol Hepatol. 2021;19:492. [PMID: 32251788]

Pasricha T et al. Fecal incontinence in the elderly. Clin Geriatr Med. 2021;37:71. [PMID: 33213775]

Sbeit W et al. Diagnostic approach to faecal incontinence: what test and when to perform? World J Gastroenterol. 2021;27:1553. [PMID: 33958842]

Whitehead WE et al. Fecal incontinence diagnosed by Rome IV criteria in the United States, Canada, and the United Kingdom. Clin Gastroenterol Hepatol. 2020;18:385. [PMID: 31154029]

OTHER ANAL CONDITIONS

Anal Fissures

Anal fissures are linear or rocket-shaped ulcers that are usually less than 5 mm in length. Most fissures are believed to arise from trauma to the anal canal during defecation, perhaps caused by straining, constipation, or high internal sphincter tone. They occur most commonly in the posterior midline, but 10% occur anteriorly. Fissures that occur off the midline should raise suspicion for Crohn disease, HIV/AIDS, tuberculosis, syphilis, or anal carcinoma. Patients complain of severe, tearing pain during defecation followed by throbbing discomfort that may lead to constipation due to fear of recurrent pain. There may be mild associated hematochezia, with blood on the stool or toilet paper. Anal fissures are confirmed by visual inspection of the anal verge while gently separating the buttocks. Acute fissures look like cracks in the epithelium. Chronic fissures result in fibrosis and the development of a skin tag at the outermost edge (sentinel pile). Digital and anoscopic examinations may cause severe pain and may not be possible. Medical management is directed at promoting effortless, painless bowel movements. Fiber supplements and sitz baths should be prescribed. Topical anesthetics (5% lidocaine; 2.5% lidocaine plus 2.5% prilocaine) may provide temporary relief. Healing occurs within 2 months in up to 45% of patients with conservative management. Chronic fissures may be treated with topical 0.125–0.4% nitroglycerin, diltiazem 2% ointment, or nifedipine 0.5% (1 cm of ointment) applied 2–3 times daily just inside the anus with the tip of a finger for 4–8 weeks, or injection of botulinum toxin (20 units) into the internal anal sphincter. All these treatments result in healing in 60–90% of patients with chronic anal fissure, but headaches occur in up to 40% of patients treated with nitroglycerin. Botulinum toxin may cause transient anal incontinence. Fissures recur in up to

40% of patients after treatment. Chronic or recurrent fissures benefit from lateral internal sphincterotomy; however, minor incontinence may complicate this procedure.

Kyriakakis R et al. What predicts successful nonoperative management with botulinum toxin for anal fissure? Am J Surg. 2020;219:442. [PMID: 31679653]
Lu Y et al. Diagnosis and treatment of anal fissures in 2021. JAMA. 2021;325:688. [PMID: 33591336]
Wald A et al. ACG clinical guidelines: management of benign anorectal disorders. Am J Gastroenterol. 2021;116:1987. [PMID: 34618700]

Perianal Abscess & Fistula

The anal glands located at the base of the anal crypts at the dentate line may become infected, leading to abscess formation. Other causes of abscess include anal fissure and Crohn disease. Abscesses may extend upward or downward through the intersphincteric plane. Symptoms of perianal abscess are throbbing, continuous perianal pain. Erythema, fluctuance, and swelling may be found in the perianal region on external examination or in the ischiorectal fossa on digital rectal examination. Perianal abscesses are treated with local incision and drainage, while ischiorectal abscesses require drainage in the operating room. After drainage of an abscess, most patients are found to have a fistula in ano.

Fistula in ano most often arises in an anal crypt and is usually preceded by an anal abscess. In patients with fistulas that connect to the rectum, other disorders such as Crohn disease, lymphogranuloma venereum, rectal tuberculosis, and cancer should be considered. Fistulas are associated with purulent discharge that may lead to itching, tenderness, and pain. The treatment of Crohn-related fistula is discussed elsewhere in this chapter. Treatment of simple idiopathic fistula in ano is by surgical incision or excision under anesthesia. Care must be taken to preserve the anal sphincters. Surgical fistulotomy for treatment of complex (high, transphincteric) anal fissures carries a high risk of incontinence. Techniques for healing the fistula while preserving the sphincter include an endoanal advancement flap over the internal opening and insertion of a bioprosthetic plug into the fistula opening.

Amato A et al. Evaluation and management of perianal abscess and anal fistula: SICCR position statement. Tech Coloproctol. 2020;24:127. [PMID: 31974827]
Cooper CR et al. Perianal fistulas. Dis Colon Rectum. 2020; 63:129. [PMID: 31914108]
Wasmann KA et al. Treatment of perianal fistulas in Crohn's disease, seton versus anti-TNF versus surgical closure following anti-TNF [PISA]: a randomised controlled trial. J Crohns Colitis. 2020;14:1049. [PMID: 31919501]

Perianal Pruritus

Perianal pruritus is characterized by perianal itching and discomfort. It may be caused by poor anal hygiene associated with fistulas, fissures, prolapsed hemorrhoids, skin tags, and minor incontinence. Conversely, overzealous cleansing with soaps may contribute to local irritation or contact dermatitis. Contact dermatitis, atopic dermatitis, bacterial infections (*Staphylococcus* or *Streptococcus*), parasites (pinworms, scabies), candidal infection (especially in diabetics), sexually transmitted disease (condylomata acuminata, herpes, syphilis, molluscum contagiosum), and other skin conditions (psoriasis, Paget disease, lichen sclerosis) must be excluded. In patients with idiopathic perianal pruritus, examination may reveal erythema, excoriations, or lichenified, eczematous skin. Education is vital to successful therapy. Spicy foods, coffee, chocolate, and tomatoes may cause irritation and should be eliminated. After bowel movements, the perianal area should be cleansed with nonscented wipes premoistened with lanolin followed by gentle drying. A piece of cotton ball should be tucked next to the anal opening to absorb perspiration or fecal seepage. Anal ointments and lotions may exacerbate the condition and should be avoided. A short course of high-potency topical corticosteroid may be tried, although efficacy has not been demonstrated. Diluted capsaicin cream (0.006%) led to symptomatic relief in 75% of patients in a double-blind crossover study.

Cohee MW et al. Benign anorectal conditions: evaluation and management. Am Fam Physician. 2020;101:24. [PMID: 31894930]
Ortega AE et al. Idiopathic pruritus ani and acute perianal dermatitis. Clin Colon Rectal Surg. 2019;32:327. [PMID: 31507341]

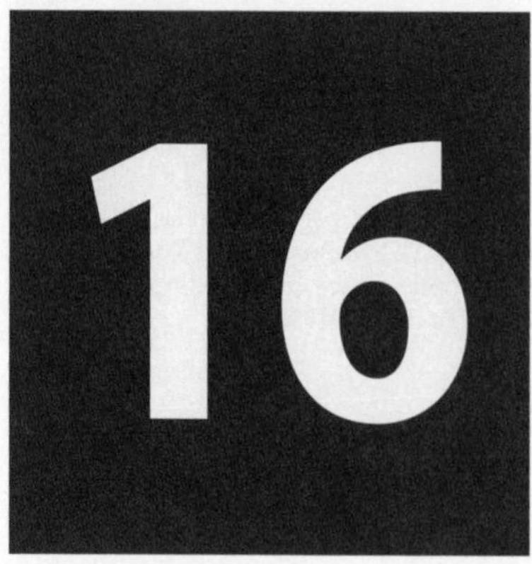

Liver, Biliary Tract, & Pancreas Disorders

Lawrence S. Friedman, MD

JAUNDICE & EVALUATION OF ABNORMAL LIVER BIOCHEMICAL TESTS

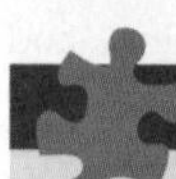

ESSENTIALS OF DIAGNOSIS

- Jaundice results from accumulation of bilirubin in body tissues; the cause may be hepatic or nonhepatic.
- Hyperbilirubinemia may be due to abnormalities in the formation, transport, metabolism, or excretion of bilirubin.
- Persistent mild elevations of the aminotransferase levels are common in clinical practice and caused most often by nonalcoholic fatty liver disease (NAFLD).
- Evaluation of obstructive jaundice begins with ultrasonography and is usually followed by cholangiography.

General Considerations

Jaundice (icterus) results from the accumulation of bilirubin—a product of heme metabolism—in body tissues. Hyperbilirubinemia may be due to abnormalities in the formation, transport, metabolism, or excretion of bilirubin. Total serum bilirubin is normally 0.2–1.2 mg/dL (3.42–20.52 mcmol/L). Mean levels are higher in men than women, higher in White persons and Latinx persons than Black persons and correlate with an increased risk of symptomatic gallstone disease and inversely with the risk of stroke, respiratory disease, CVD, and mortality. Jaundice may not be recognizable until serum bilirubin levels are about 3 mg/dL (51.3 mcmol/L).

Jaundice may be caused by predominantly unconjugated or conjugated bilirubin in the serum (Table 16–1). Unconjugated hyperbilirubinemia may result from overproduction of bilirubin because of hemolysis; impaired hepatic uptake of bilirubin due to certain drugs; or impaired conjugation of bilirubin by glucuronide, as in Gilbert syndrome due to mild decreases in uridine diphosphate (UDP) glucuronyl transferase, or Crigler-Najjar syndrome caused by moderate decreases (type II) or absence (type I) of UDP glucuronyl transferase. Hemolysis alone rarely elevates the serum bilirubin level to more than 7 mg/dL (119.7 mcmol/L). Predominantly conjugated hyperbilirubinemia may result from impaired excretion of bilirubin from the liver due to hepatocellular disease, drugs, sepsis, or hereditary hepatocanalicular transport defects (such as Dubin-Johnson syndrome, progressive familial intrahepatic cholestasis syndromes, and intrahepatic cholestasis of pregnancy) or from extrahepatic biliary obstruction. Features of some hyperbilirubinemic syndromes are summarized in Table 16–2.

Clinical Findings

A. Unconjugated Hyperbilirubinemia

Stool and urine color are normal, and there is mild jaundice and indirect (unconjugated) hyperbilirubinemia with no bilirubin in the urine. Splenomegaly occurs in all hemolytic disorders except in sickle cell disease.

B. Conjugated Hyperbilirubinemia

Conjugated hyperbilirubinemia is often accompanied by pruritus, light-colored stools, and jaundice, although the patient may be asymptomatic. Malaise, anorexia, low-grade fever, and right upper quadrant discomfort are frequent with hepatocellular disease. Dark urine, jaundice, and, in women, amenorrhea occur. An enlarged tender liver, spider telangiectasias, palmar erythema, ascites, gynecomastia, sparse body hair, fetor hepaticus, and asterixis may be present, depending on the cause, severity, and chronicity of liver dysfunction.

C. Biliary Obstruction

There may be right upper quadrant pain, weight loss (suggesting carcinoma), jaundice, pruritus, dark urine, and light-colored stools. Symptoms and signs may be intermittent if caused by a stone, carcinoma of the ampulla, or cholangiocarcinoma. Pain may be absent early in pancreatic cancer. Occult blood in the stools suggests cancer of the ampulla. A palpable gallbladder (Courvoisier sign) is

Table 16–1. Classification of jaundice.

Type of Hyperbilirubinemia	Location and Cause
Unconjugated hyperbilirubinemia (predominantly indirect bilirubin)	Increased bilirubin production (eg, hemolytic anemias, hemolytic reactions, hematoma, pulmonary infarction) Impaired bilirubin uptake and storage (eg, posthepatitis hyperbilirubinemia, Gilbert syndrome, Crigler-Najjar syndrome, drug reactions)
Conjugated hyperbilirubinemia (predominantly direct bilirubin)	**Hereditary Cholestatic Syndromes** (see also Table 16–2)
	Faulty excretion of bilirubin conjugates (eg, Dubin-Johnson syndrome, Rotor syndrome) or pathogenic variant in genes coding for bile salt transport proteins (eg, progressive familial intrahepatic cholestasis syndromes, benign recurrent intrahepatic cholestasis, and some cases of intrahepatic cholestasis of pregnancy)
	Hepatocellular Dysfunction
	Biliary epithelial and hepatocyte damage (eg, hepatitis, hepatic cirrhosis) Intrahepatic cholestasis (eg, certain drugs, biliary cirrhosis, sepsis, postoperative jaundice) Hepatocellular damage or intrahepatic cholestasis resulting from miscellaneous causes (eg, spirochetal infections, infectious mononucleosis, cholangitis, sarcoidosis, lymphomas, hyperthyroidism, industrial toxins)
	Biliary Obstruction
	Choledocholithiasis, biliary atresia, carcinoma of biliary duct, sclerosing cholangitis, IgG_4-related cholangitis, ischemic cholangiopathy, COVID cholangiopathy, choledochal cyst, external pressure on bile duct, pancreatitis, pancreatic neoplasms

Ig, immunoglobulin.

characteristic, but neither specific nor sensitive, of a pancreatic head tumor. Fever and chills are more common in benign obstruction with associated cholangitis.

Diagnostic Studies

(See Tables 16–3 and 16–4.)

A. Laboratory Findings

Elevated serum alanine and AST (ALT and AST) levels reflect hepatocellular injury. Normal reference values for ALT and AST are lower than generally reported when persons with risk factors for fatty liver are excluded. The upper limit of normal for ALT is 29–33 U/L in men and 19–25 U/L in women. Levels decrease with age and correlate with BMI and mortality from liver disease and inversely with caffeine consumption and physical activity. Levels are mildly elevated in more than 25% of persons with untreated celiac disease and in type 1 diabetic patients with so-called glycogenic hepatopathy and often rise transiently in healthy persons who begin taking 4 g of acetaminophen per day or experience rapid weight gain on a fast-food diet. Levels may rise strikingly but transiently in patients with acute biliary obstruction from choledocholithiasis. NAFLD is by far the most common cause of persistent mildly to moderately elevated aminotransferase levels. Elevated ALT and AST levels, often greater than 1000 U/L (20 mckat/L), are the hallmark of hepatocellular necrosis or inflammation. Modest elevations are frequent in systemic infections, including COVID-19. The differential diagnosis of any liver test elevation always includes toxicity caused by drugs, herbal and dietary supplements, and toxins.

Elevated alkaline phosphatase levels are seen in cholestasis or infiltrative liver disease (such as tumor, granulomatous disease, or amyloidosis). Isolated alkaline phosphatase elevations of hepatic rather than bone, intestinal, or placental origin are confirmed by concomitant elevation of gamma-glutamyl transpeptidase or 5′-nucleotidase levels.

B. Imaging

Demonstration of dilated bile ducts by ultrasonography or CT indicates biliary obstruction (90–95% sensitivity). Ultrasonography, CT, and MRI may also demonstrate hepatomegaly, intrahepatic tumors, and portal hypertension. MRI is the most accurate technique for identifying isolated liver lesions such as hemangiomas, focal nodular hyperplasia, or focal fatty infiltration and for detecting hepatic iron overload. The most sensitive techniques for detection of individual small hepatic metastases in patients eligible for resection are multiphasic helical or multislice CT; MRI with use of gadolinium or ferumoxides as contrast agents; CT arterial portography, in which imaging follows intravenous contrast infusion via a catheter placed in the superior mesenteric artery; and intraoperative ultrasonography. Because of its much lower cost, ultrasonography is preferable to CT (~six times more expensive) or MRI (~seven times more expensive) as a screening test for hepatocellular carcinoma in persons with cirrhosis. PET can be used to detect small pancreatic tumors and metastases. Ultrasonography can detect gallstones with a sensitivity of 95%.

Magnetic resonance cholangiopancreatography (MRCP) is a sensitive, noninvasive method of detecting bile duct stones, strictures, and dilatation; however, it is less reliable than endoscopic retrograde cholangiopancreatography (ERCP) for distinguishing malignant from benign strictures. ERCP requires a skilled endoscopist and may be used to demonstrate pancreatic or ampullary causes of jaundice, carry out sphincterotomy and stone extraction, insert a stent

Table 16–2. Hyperbilirubinemic disorders.

	Nature of Defect	Type of Hyperbilirubinemia	Clinical and Pathologic Characteristics
Gilbert syndrome[1]	Reduced activity of uridine diphosphate glucuronyl transferase	Unconjugated (indirect) bilirubin	Benign, asymptomatic hereditary jaundice. Hyperbilirubinemia increased by 24- to 36-hour fast. No treatment required. Associated with reduced mortality from CVD.
Dubin-Johnson syndrome[2]	Reduced excretory function of hepatocytes	Conjugated (direct) bilirubin	Benign, asymptomatic hereditary jaundice. Gallbladder does not visualize on oral cholecystography. Liver darkly pigmented on gross examination. Biopsy shows centrilobular brown pigment. Prognosis excellent.
Rotor syndrome[3]	Reduced hepatic reuptake of bilirubin conjugates	Conjugated (direct) bilirubin	Similar to Dubin-Johnson syndrome, but the liver is not pigmented, and the gallbladder is visualized on oral cholecystography. Prognosis excellent.
Recurrent or progressive intrahepatic cholestasis[4]	Cholestasis, often on a familial basis	Predominantly conjugated (direct) bilirubin	Episodic attacks of or progressive jaundice, itching, and malaise. Onset in early life and may persist for a lifetime. Alkaline phosphatase increased. Cholestasis found on liver biopsy. (Biopsy may be normal during remission.) Prognosis is generally excellent for "benign" recurrent intrahepatic cholestasis but may not be for familial forms.
Intrahepatic cholestasis of pregnancy[5]	Cholestasis	Predominantly conjugated (direct) bilirubin	Benign cholestatic jaundice, usually occurring in the third trimester of pregnancy. Itching, GI symptoms, abnormal liver excretory function tests, and elevated serum bile acid levels (> 10 mcmol/L). Cholestasis noted on liver biopsy. Prognosis excellent, but recurrence with subsequent pregnancies or use of oral contraceptives is characteristic.

[1]Gilbert syndrome generally results from the addition of extra dinucleotide(s) TA sequences to the TATA promoter of the conjugating enzyme *UGT1A1*.
[2]Dubin-Johnson syndrome is caused by a pathogenic variant in the *ABCC2* gene coding for organic anion transporter multidrug resistance protein 2 in bile canaliculi on chromosome 10q24.
[3]Rotor syndrome is caused by pathogenic variants in the genes coding for organic anion transporting polypeptides OATP1B1 and OATP1B3 on chromosome 12p.
[4]Pathogenic variants in genes that control hepatocellular transport systems that are involved in the formation of bile and inherited as autosomal recessive traits are on chromosomes 18q21–22, 2q24, 7q21, and others in families with progressive familial intrahepatic cholestasis. Pathogenic variants of genes on chromosome 18q21–22 alter a P-type ATPase expressed in the small intestine and liver and those on chromosome 2q24 alter the bile acid export pump and also cause benign recurrent intrahepatic cholestasis. Pathogenic variants in the *ABCB4* gene on chromosome 7 that encodes multidrug resistance protein 3 account for progressive familial intrahepatic cholestasis type 3. Less common causes of progressive familial intrahepatic cholestasis are pathogenic variants in genes that encode TJP2, FXR, MY05B, and others.
[5]Pathogenic variants in genes (especially *ABCB4* and *ABCB11*) that encode biliary canalicular transporters account for many cases of intrahepatic cholestasis of pregnancy.

Table 16–3. Liver biochemical tests: normal values and changes in hepatocellular and obstructive jaundice.

Tests	Normal Values	Hepatocellular Jaundice	Obstructive Jaundice
Bilirubin[1]			
Direct	0.1–0.3 mg/dL (1.71–5.13 mcmol/L)	Increased	Increased
Indirect	0.2–0.7 mg/dL (3.42–11.97 mcmol/L)	Increased	Increased
Urine bilirubin	None	Increased	Increased
Serum albumin	3.5–5.5 g/dL (35–55 g/L)	Decreased	Generally unchanged
Alkaline phosphatase	30–115 U/L (0.6–2.3 mkat/L)	Mildly increased (+)	Markedly increased (++++)
Prothrombin time	INR of 1.0–1.4. After vitamin K, 10% decrease in 24 hours	Prolonged if damage is severe; does not respond to parenteral vitamin K	Prolonged if obstruction is marked; generally responds to parenteral vitamin K
ALT, AST	ALT, ≤ 30 U/L (0.6 mkat/L) (men), ≤ 19 U/L (0.38 mkat/L) (women); AST, 5–40 U/L (0.1–0.8 mkat/L)	Increased, as in viral hepatitis	Minimally increased

[1]Measured by the van den Bergh reaction, which overestimates direct bilirubin in normal persons.

Table 16–4. Causes of serum aminotransferase elevations.[1]

Mild Elevations (< 5 × normal)	Severe Elevations (> 15 × normal)
Hepatic: ALT-predominant	Acute viral hepatitis (A–E, herpes)
Chronic hepatitis B, C, and D	Medications/toxins
Acute viral hepatitis (A-E, EBV, CMV, others)	Ischemic hepatitis
Steatosis/steatohepatitis	Autoimmune hepatitis
Hemochromatosis	Wilson disease
Medications/toxins	Acute bile duct obstruction
Autoimmune hepatitis	Acute Budd-Chiari syndrome
Alpha-1-antitrypsin (alpha-1-antiprotease) deficiency	Hepatic artery ligation
Wilson disease	
Celiac disease	
Glycogenic hepatopathy	
Hepatic: AST-predominant	
Alcohol-related liver injury (AST:ALT > 2:1)	
Cirrhosis	
COVID-19	
Nonhepatic	
Strenuous exercise	
Hemolysis	
Myopathy	
Thyroid disease	
Macro-AST	

[1]Almost any liver disease can cause moderate aminotransferase elevations (5–15 × normal).

CMV, cytomegalovirus; EBV, Epstein-Barr virus.

Reproduced with permission from Green RM et al. AGA technical review on the evaluation of liver chemistry tests. *Gastroenterology.* 2002;123(4):1367–1384.

through an obstructing lesion, or facilitate direct cholangiopancreatoscopy. Complications of ERCP include pancreatitis (5% or less) and, less commonly, cholangitis, bleeding, or duodenal perforation after sphincterotomy. Percutaneous transhepatic cholangiography is an alternative approach to evaluating the anatomy of the biliary tract. Serious complications of PTC occur in 3% and include fever, bacteremia, bile peritonitis, and intraperitoneal hemorrhage. Endoscopic ultrasonography (EUS) is the most sensitive test for detecting small lesions of the ampulla or pancreatic head and for detecting portal vein invasion by pancreatic cancer. It is also accurate for detecting or excluding bile duct stones.

C. Liver Biopsy

Percutaneous liver biopsy is considered the definitive study for determining the cause and histologic severity of hepatocellular dysfunction or infiltrative liver disease, although it is subject to sampling error. It is generally performed under ultrasound or, in some patients with suspected metastatic disease or a hepatic mass, CT guidance. A transjugular route can be used in patients with coagulopathy or ascites, and in selected cases endoscopic ultrasound-guided liver biopsy has proved advantageous. The risk of bleeding after a percutaneous liver biopsy is approximately 0.6% and is increased in persons with a platelet count of 50,000/mcL (50×10^9/L) or less. The risk of death is less than 0.1%. Panels of blood tests (eg, FibroSure, NAFLD fibrosis score, enhanced liver fibrosis score) and, more accurately, ultrasound (vibration-controlled transient elastography, a point-of-care technique), point-shear wave, or bidimensional shear wave (integrated in ultrasound devices), or magnetic resonance elastography to measure liver stiffness are used for estimating the stage of liver fibrosis and degree of portal hypertension without the need for liver biopsy; they are most useful for excluding advanced fibrosis.

When to Refer

Patients with jaundice should be referred for diagnostic procedures.

When to Admit

Patients with liver failure should be hospitalized.

European Association for the Study of the Liver. EASL Clinical Practice Guidelines on non-invasive tests for evaluation of liver disease severity and prognosis—2021 update. J Hepatol. 2021;75:659. [PMID: 34166721]

Khalifa A et al. The utility of liver biopsy in the evaluation of liver disease and abnormal liver function tests. Am J Clin Pathol. 2021;156:259. [PMID: 33693456]

Neuberger J et al. Guidelines on the use of liver biopsy in clinical practice from the British Society of Gastroenterology, the Royal College of Radiologists and the Royal College of Pathology. Gut. 2020;69:1382. [PMID: 32467090]

Roediger R et al. Intrahepatic cholestasis of pregnancy: natural history and current management. Semin Liver Dis. 2021;41:103. [PMID: 33764488]

Tran AN et al. Care of the patient with abnormal liver test results. Ann Intern Med. 2021;174:ITC129. [PMID: 34516271]

DISEASES OF THE LIVER

See Chapter 39 for Hepatocellular Carcinoma.

ACUTE HEPATITIS A

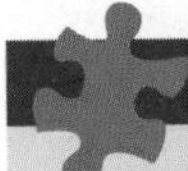

ESSENTIALS OF DIAGNOSIS

- Prodrome of anorexia, nausea, vomiting, malaise, aversion to smoking.
- Fever, enlarged and tender liver, jaundice.
- Normal to low white cell count; markedly elevated aminotransferases.

General Considerations

Hepatitis can be caused by viruses, including the five hepatotropic viruses—A, B, C, D, and E—and many drugs and toxic agents; the clinical manifestations may be similar regardless of cause. Hepatitis A virus (HAV) is a 27-nm RNA hepatovirus (in the picornavirus family) that causes epidemics or sporadic cases of hepatitis. HAV infection is hyperendemic in developing countries. Globally, over 1.5 million people are infected with HAV annually. The virus is transmitted by the fecal-oral route by either person-to-person contact or ingestion of contaminated food or water, and its spread is favored by crowding and poor sanitation. Since introduction of the HAV vaccine in the United States in 1995, the incidence rate of HAV infection has declined from as much as 14 to 0.4 per 100,000 population, with a corresponding decline in the mortality rate from 0.1 to 0.02 death per 100,000 population and an increase in the mean age of infection and death. Nevertheless, over 80% of persons aged 20–60 years in the United States are still susceptible to HAV, and vulnerable populations are especially at risk. The highest incidence rate (2.1 per 100,000) is in adults aged 30–39. Common source outbreaks resulting from contaminated food, including inadequately cooked shellfish, or untreated ground water from wells continue to occur, although no drinking water–associated outbreaks have occurred in the United States since 2009. In 2017, an outbreak beginning in California and extending to at least 33 other states affected a large number of homeless persons and resulted in many deaths. Outbreaks also occur among people who inject drugs or unvaccinated residents in institutions and among men who have sex with men and international adoptees and their contacts. In the United States, international travel emerged as an important risk factor, accounting for over 40% of cases in the early 2000s but a lower percentage in the 2010s. Overall, however, reports of HAV infection increased by nearly 300% during 2016–2018 compared to 2013–2015.

The incubation period averages 30 days. HAV is excreted in feces for up to 2 weeks before clinical illness but rarely after the first week of illness. The mortality rate for hepatitis A is low, and acute liver failure due to hepatitis A is uncommon except for rare instances in which it occurs in a patient with concomitant chronic hepatitis C. There is no chronic carrier state. In the United States, about 30% of the population have serologic evidence of previous HAV infection.

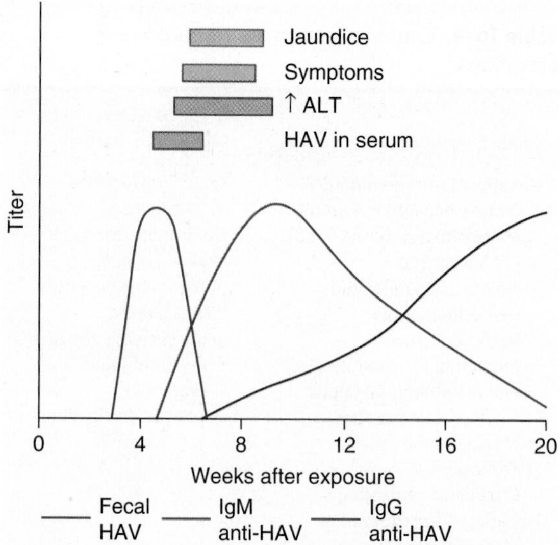

▲ **Figure 16–1. The typical course of acute type A hepatitis. (Anti-HAV, antibody to hepatitis A virus; HAV, hepatitis A virus.)** (Reproduced with permission from Koff RS. Acute viral hepatitis. In: Friedman LS, Keeffe EB. *Handbook of Liver Disease*, 4th ed. Philadelphia: Saunders Elsevier, 2018.)

Clinical Findings

A. Symptoms and Signs

Figure 16–1 shows the typical course of acute hepatitis A. Clinical illness is more severe in adults than in children, in whom it is usually asymptomatic. The onset may be abrupt or insidious, with malaise, myalgia, arthralgia, easy fatigability, upper respiratory symptoms, and anorexia. A distaste for smoking, paralleling anorexia, may occur early. Nausea and vomiting are frequent, and diarrhea or constipation may occur. Fever is generally present but is low-grade except in occasional cases in which systemic toxicity may occur. Defervescence and a fall in pulse rate often coincide with the onset of jaundice.

Abdominal pain is usually mild and constant in the right upper quadrant or epigastrium, often aggravated by jarring or exertion, and rarely may be severe enough to simulate cholecystitis. Jaundice occurs after 5–10 days but may appear at the same time as the initial symptoms. In many patients, jaundice never develops. With the onset of jaundice, prodromal symptoms often worsen, followed by progressive clinical improvement. Stools may be acholic during this phase. Hepatomegaly—rarely marked—is present in over half of cases. Liver tenderness is usually present. Splenomegaly is reported in 15% of patients, and soft, enlarged lymph nodes—especially in the cervical or epitrochlear areas—may be noted.

The acute illness usually subsides over 2–3 weeks with complete clinical and laboratory recovery by 9 weeks. In some cases, clinical, biochemical, and serologic recovery may be followed by one or two relapses, but recovery is the rule. Acute cholecystitis occasionally complicates the course of acute hepatitis A. Other occasional extrahepatic complications include AKI, arthritis, vasculitis, acute pancreatitis, aplastic anemia, and a variety of neurologic manifestations.

B. Laboratory Findings

The WBC count is normal to low, especially in the preicteric phase. Large atypical lymphocytes may occasionally be seen. Mild proteinuria is common, and bilirubinuria often precedes the appearance of jaundice. Strikingly elevated ALT or AST levels occur early, followed by elevations of bilirubin and alkaline phosphatase; in a minority of patients, the latter persist after aminotransferase levels have normalized. Cholestasis is occasionally marked. Antibody to hepatitis A (anti-HAV) appears early in the course of the illness (Figure 16–1). Both IgM and IgG anti-HAV are detectable in serum soon after the onset. Peak titers of IgM anti-HAV occur during the first week of clinical disease and usually disappear within 3–6 months. Detection of IgM anti-HAV is an excellent test for diagnosing acute hepatitis A. Titers of IgG anti-HAV rise after 1 month of the disease and may persist for years. IgG anti-HAV (in the absence of IgM anti-HAV) indicates previous exposure to HAV, noninfectivity, and immunity.

Differential Diagnosis

The differential diagnosis includes other viruses that cause hepatitis, particularly hepatitis B (HBV) and C (HCV) viruses, and diseases such as infectious mononucleosis, cytomegalovirus infection, herpes simplex virus infection, Middle East respiratory syndrome, and infections caused by many other viruses, including influenza, Ebola virus, and SARS-CoV-2; spirochetal diseases such as leptospirosis and secondary syphilis; brucellosis; rickettsial diseases such as Q fever; drug-induced liver injury; and ischemic hepatitis (shock liver). Occasionally, autoimmune hepatitis may have an acute onset mimicking acute viral hepatitis. Rarely, metastatic cancer of the liver, lymphoma, or leukemia may present as a hepatitis-like picture.

The prodromal phase of viral hepatitis must be distinguished from other infectious disease such as influenza and COVID-19, upper respiratory infections, and the prodromal stages of the exanthematous diseases. Cholestasis may mimic obstructive jaundice.

Prevention

Strict isolation of patients is not necessary, but hand washing after bowel movements is required. Unvaccinated persons who are exposed to HAV are advised to receive postexposure prophylaxis with a single dose of HAV vaccine or immune globulin (0.01 mL/kg), or both, within 2 weeks of exposure. The vaccine is preferred in healthy persons aged 1 year to 40 years, whereas immune globulin plus the vaccine is preferred in those who are younger than 1 year or older than 40 years, are immunocompromised, or have chronic liver disease.

Vaccination with one of two effective inactivated hepatitis A vaccines available in the United States provides long-term immunity and is recommended for persons living in or traveling to endemic areas (including military personnel), persons over age 40, patients with chronic liver disease upon diagnosis after prescreening for immunity, men who have sex with men, persons with HIV infection, animal handlers, persons who use injection or noninjection drugs, persons experiencing homelessness, persons who are incarcerated, close personal contacts of international adoptees, persons living in group settings for those with developmental disabilities, and persons who request protection against HAV. For healthy travelers, a single dose of vaccine at any time before departure can provide adequate protection. Routine vaccination is advised by the Advisory Committee on Immunization Practices of the CDC for all children aged 12–23 months in the United States, with catch-up vaccination for children and adolescents aged 2–18 years who have not previously received the HAV vaccine. HAV vaccine is also effective in the prevention of secondary spread to household contacts of primary cases. The recommended dose for adults is 1 mL (1440 ELISA units) of Havrix (GlaxoSmithKline) or 1 mL (50 units) of Vaqta (Merck) intramuscularly, followed by a booster dose at 6–18 months. A combined hepatitis A and B vaccine (Twinrix, GlaxoSmithKline) is available.

Treatment

Bed rest is recommended only if symptoms are marked. If nausea and vomiting are pronounced or if oral intake is substantially decreased, intravenous 10% glucose is indicated.

Dietary management consists of palatable meals as tolerated, without overfeeding; breakfast is usually tolerated best. Strenuous physical exertion, alcohol, and hepatotoxic agents should be avoided. Small doses of oxazepam are safe because metabolism is not hepatic; morphine sulfate should be avoided. Corticosteroids have no benefit in patients with viral hepatitis, including those with acute liver failure.

Prognosis

In most patients, clinical recovery is generally complete within 3 months. Laboratory evidence of liver dysfunction may persist for a longer period, but most patients recover completely. Hepatitis A does not cause chronic liver disease, although it may persist for up to 1 year, and clinical and biochemical relapses may occur before full recovery. The mortality rate is less than 1.0%, with a higher rate in older adults than in younger persons.

When to Admit

- Encephalopathy is present.
- INR greater than 1.6.
- The patient is unable to maintain hydration.

Desai AN et al. Management of hepatitis A in 2020–2021. JAMA. 2020;324:383. [PMID: 32628251]

Freedman M et al. Recommended adult immunization schedule, United States, 2020. Ann Intern Med. 2020;172:337. [PMID: 32016359]

Hofmeister MG et al. Factors associated with hepatitis A mortality during person-to-person outbreaks: a matched case-control study—United States, 2016–2019. Hepatology. 2021;74:28. [PMID: 33217769]

Nelson NP et al. Prevention of hepatitis A virus infection in the United States: recommendations of the Advisory Committee on Immunization Practices, 2020. MMWR Recomm Rep. 2020;69:1. [PMID: 32614811]

Saviano A et al. Liver disease and coronavirus disease 2019: from pathogenesis to clinical care. Hepatology. 2021;74:1088. [PMID: 33332624]

ACUTE HEPATITIS B

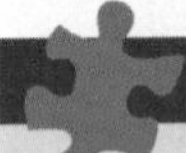

ESSENTIALS OF DIAGNOSIS

- Prodrome of anorexia, nausea, vomiting, malaise, aversion to smoking.
- Fever, enlarged and tender liver, jaundice.
- Normal to low WBC count; markedly elevated aminotransferases early in the course.
- Liver biopsy shows hepatocellular necrosis and mononuclear infiltrate but is rarely indicated.

General Considerations

Hepatitis B virus (HBV) is a 42-nm hepadnavirus with a partially double-stranded DNA genome, inner core protein (hepatitis B core antigen, HBcAg), and outer surface coat (hepatitis B surface antigen, HBsAg). There are 10 different genotypes (A–J). HBV is usually transmitted by inoculation of infected blood or blood products or by sexual contact, and it is present in saliva, semen, and vaginal secretions. HBsAg-positive mothers may transmit HBV at delivery.

Since 1990, the incidence of HBV infection in the United States has decreased from 8.5 to 1.5 cases per 100,000 population. The prevalence is 0.27% in persons aged 6 or older. Because of universal vaccination since 1992, exposure to HBV is low among persons aged 18 or younger. HBV is prevalent in men who have sex with men and in people who inject drugs (about 7% of HIV-infected persons are coinfected with HBV), but the greatest number of cases result from heterosexual transmission. Other groups at risk include patients and staff at hemodialysis centers, physicians, dentists, nurses, and personnel working in clinical and pathology laboratories and blood banks. Half of all patients with acute hepatitis B in the United States have previously been incarcerated or treated for a sexually transmitted disease. The risk of HBV infection from a blood transfusion in the United States is no higher than 1 in 350,000 units transfused. Screening for HBV infection is recommended for high-risk groups by the USPSTF.

The incubation period of hepatitis B is 6 weeks to 6 months (average 12–14 weeks). The onset of hepatitis B is more insidious, and the aminotransferase levels are higher on average, than in HAV infection. Acute liver failure occurs in less than 1%, with a mortality rate of up to 60%. Following acute hepatitis B, HBV infection persists in 1–2% of immunocompetent adults, but in a higher percentage of children and immunocompromised adults. There are an estimated 2.4 million persons (including an estimated 1.47 million foreign-born persons from endemic areas) with chronic hepatitis B in the United States and 248 million worldwide. Compared with the general population, the prevalence of chronic HBV infection is increased two- to threefold in non-Latinx Black persons and tenfold in Asian persons. Persons with chronic hepatitis B, particularly when HBV infection is acquired early in life and viral replication persists, are at substantial risk for cirrhosis and hepatocellular carcinoma (up to 25–40%); men are at greater risk than women.

Clinical Findings

A. Symptoms and Signs

The clinical picture of viral hepatitis is extremely variable, ranging from asymptomatic infection without jaundice to acute liver failure and death in a few days to weeks. Figure 16–2 shows the typical course of acute HBV infection. The onset may be abrupt or insidious, and the clinical features are similar to those for acute hepatitis A. Serum sickness may be seen early in acute hepatitis B. Fever is generally present and is low-grade. Defervescence and a fall in pulse rate often coincide with the onset of jaundice. Infection caused by HBV may be associated with glomerulonephritis and polyarteritis nodosa.

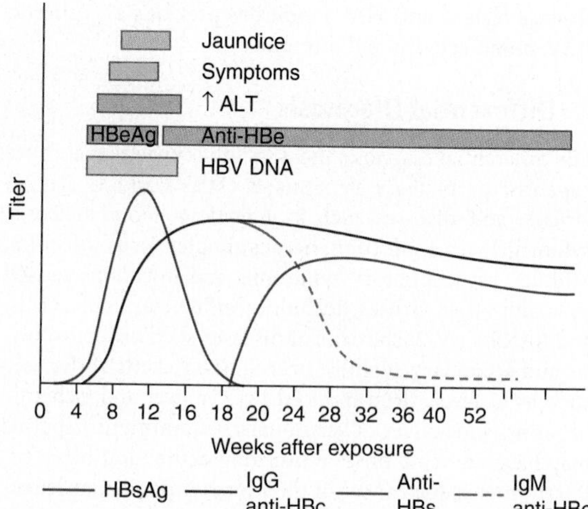

Figure 16–2. The typical course of acute type B hepatitis. Anti-HBe, antibody to HBeAg; anti-HBc, antibody to hepatitis B core antigen; anti-HBs, antibody to HBsAg; HBeAg, hepatitis Be antigen; HBsAg, hepatitis B surface antigen. (Reproduced with permission from Koff RS. Acute viral hepatitis. In: Friedman LS, Keeffe EB. *Handbook of Liver Disease*, 3rd ed. Philadelphia: Saunders Elsevier, 2012.)

The acute illness usually subsides over 2–3 weeks with complete clinical and laboratory recovery by 16 weeks. In 5–10% of cases, the course may be more protracted, but less than 1% will develop acute liver failure. Hepatitis B may become chronic.

B. Laboratory Findings

The laboratory features are similar to those for acute hepatitis A, although serum aminotransferase levels are higher on average in acute hepatitis B, and marked cholestasis is not a feature. Marked prolongation of the prothrombin time in severe hepatitis correlates with increased mortality.

There are several antigens and antibodies as well as HBV DNA that relate to HBV infection and that are useful in diagnosis. Interpretation of common serologic patterns is shown in Table 16–5.

1. HBsAg—The appearance of HBsAg in serum is the first evidence of infection, appearing before biochemical evidence of liver disease, and persisting throughout the clinical illness. Persistence of HBsAg more than 6 months after the acute illness signifies chronic hepatitis B.

2. Anti-HBs—Specific antibody to HBsAg (anti-HBs) appears in most individuals after clearance of HBsAg and after successful vaccination against hepatitis B. Disappearance of HBsAg and the appearance of anti-HBs signal recovery from HBV infection, noninfectivity, and immunity.

Table 16–5. Common serologic patterns in hepatitis B virus (HBV) infection and their interpretation.

HBsAg	Anti-HBs	Anti-HBc	HBeAg	Anti-HBe	Interpretation
+	–	IgM	+	–	Acute hepatitis B
+	–	IgG[1]	+	–	Chronic hepatitis B with active viral replication
+	–	IgG	–	+	Inactive HBV carrier state (low HBV DNA level) or HBeAg-negative chronic hepatitis B with active viral replication (high HBV DNA level)
+	+	IgG	+ or –	+ or –	Chronic hepatitis B with heterotypic anti-HBs (about 10% of cases)
–	–	IgM	+ or –	–	Acute hepatitis B
–	+	IgG	–	+ or –	Recovery from hepatitis B (immunity)
–	+	–	–	–	Vaccination (immunity)
–	–	IgG	–	–	False-positive; less commonly, infection in remote past

[1]Low levels of IgM anti-HBc may also be detected.

3. Anti-HBc—IgM anti-HBc appears shortly after HBsAg is detected. In the setting of acute hepatitis, IgM anti-HBc indicates a diagnosis of acute hepatitis B, and it fills the serologic gap in rare patients who have cleared HBsAg but do not yet have detectable anti-HBs. IgM anti-HBc can persist for 3–6 months, and sometimes longer. IgM anti-HBc may also reappear during flares of previously inactive chronic hepatitis B. IgG anti-HBc also appears during acute hepatitis B but persists indefinitely, whether the patient recovers (with the appearance of anti-HBs in serum) or chronic hepatitis B develops (with persistence of HBsAg). In asymptomatic persons such as blood donors, an isolated anti-HBc with no other positive HBV serologic results may represent a falsely positive result or latent infection in which HBV DNA is detectable in serum only by PCR testing.

4. HBeAg—HBeAg is a secretory form of HBcAg that appears in serum during the incubation period shortly after the detection of HBsAg. HBeAg indicates viral replication and infectivity. Persistence of HBeAg beyond 3 months indicates an increased likelihood of chronic hepatitis B. Its disappearance is often followed by the appearance of anti-HBe, generally signifying diminished viral replication and decreased infectivity.

5. HBV DNA—The presence of HBV DNA in serum generally parallels the presence of HBeAg, although HBV DNA is a more sensitive and precise marker of viral replication and infectivity. In some patients with chronic hepatitis B, HBV DNA is present at high levels without HBeAg in serum because of development of a pathogenic variant in the core promoter or pre-core region of the gene that codes HBcAg; these variants prevent synthesis of HBeAg in infected hepatocytes. When additional variants in the core gene are also present, the severity of HBV infection is enhanced and the risk of cirrhosis is increased.

Differential Diagnosis

The differential diagnosis includes hepatitis A and the same disorders listed for the differential diagnosis of acute hepatitis A. In addition, coinfection with hepatitis D virus (HDV) must be considered.

Prevention

Strict isolation of patients is not necessary. Thorough hand washing by medical staff who may contact contaminated utensils, bedding, or clothing is essential. Medical staff should handle disposable needles carefully and not recap them. Screening of donated blood for HBsAg, anti-HBc, and anti-HCV has reduced the risk of transfusion-associated hepatitis markedly. All pregnant women should undergo testing for HBsAg. HBV-infected persons should practice safe sex. Immunoprophylaxis of the neonate reduces the risk of perinatal transmission of HBV infection; when the mother's serum HBV DNA level is 200,000 IU/mL or higher (or the mother's serum HBsAg level is above 4–4.5 $\log_{10}$ IU/mL), antiviral treatment of the mother should also be initiated in the third trimester (see Chronic Hepatitis B & Chronic Hepatitis D). HBV-infected health care workers are not precluded from practicing medicine or dentistry if they follow CDC guidelines.

Hepatitis B immune globulin (HBIG) may be protective—or may attenuate the severity of illness—if given within 7 days after exposure (adult dose is 0.06 mL/kg body weight) followed by initiation of the HBV vaccine series. This approach is recommended for unvaccinated persons exposed to HBsAg-contaminated material via mucous membranes or through breaks in the skin and for individuals who have had sexual contact with a person with HBV infection (irrespective of the presence or absence of HBeAg in the source). HBIG is also indicated for newborn infants of HBsAg-positive mothers, with initiation of the vaccine series at the same time, both within 12 hours of birth (administered at different injection sites).

The CDC recommends HBV vaccination of all infants and children in the United States and all adults who are at risk for hepatitis B (including persons under age 60 with diabetes mellitus) or who request vaccination. Over 90% of recipients of the vaccine mount protective antibody to hepatitis B; immunocompromised persons, including patients receiving dialysis (especially those with diabetes mellitus), respond poorly (see Table 30–7). The standard regimen for adults is 10–20 mcg (depending on the formulation) repeated again at 1 and 6 months, but alternative schedules have been approved, including accelerated schedules of 0, 1, 2, and 12 months and of 0, 7, and 21 days plus 12 months. For greatest reliability of absorption, the deltoid muscle is the preferred site of inoculation. A newer vaccine, Heplisav-B, which uses a novel immune system–stimulating ingredient, was approved by the FDA for adults in 2017. Immunization requires only two injections, and Heplisav-B appears to be more effective than previous HBV vaccines. When documentation of seroconversion is considered desirable, postimmunization anti-HBs titers may be checked. Protection appears to be excellent even if the titer wanes—persisting for at least 20 years—and booster reimmunization is not routinely recommended but is advised for immunocompromised persons in whom anti-HBs titers fall below 10 mIU/mL. For vaccine nonresponders, three additional vaccine doses may elicit seroprotective anti-HBs levels in 30–50% of persons. Doubling of the standard dose or use of Heplisav-B may also be effective. Universal vaccination of neonates in countries endemic for HBV has reduced the incidence of hepatocellular carcinoma. Incomplete immunization is the most important predictor of liver disease among vaccinees. Unfortunately, approximately 64 million high-risk adults in the United States remain susceptible to HBV.

Treatment

Treatment of acute hepatitis B is the same as that for acute hepatitis A. Encephalopathy or severe coagulopathy indicates acute liver failure, and hospitalization at a liver transplant center is mandatory. Antiviral therapy is generally unnecessary in patients with acute hepatitis B but is usually prescribed in cases of acute liver failure caused by HBV as well as in spontaneous reactivation of chronic hepatitis B presenting as acute-on-chronic liver failure (see Acute Liver Failure).

Prognosis

In most patients, clinical recovery is complete in 3–6 months. Laboratory evidence of liver dysfunction may persist for a longer period, but most patients recover completely. The mortality rate for acute hepatitis B is 0.1–1% but is higher with superimposed hepatitis D.

Chronic hepatitis, characterized by elevated aminotransferase levels for more than 3–6 months, develops in 1–2% of immunocompetent adults with acute hepatitis B, but in as many as 90% of infected neonates and infants and a substantial proportion of immunocompromised adults. Ultimately, cirrhosis develops in up to 40% of those with chronic hepatitis B; the risk of cirrhosis is even higher in HBV-infected patients coinfected with HCV or HIV. Patients with cirrhosis are at risk for hepatocellular carcinoma at a rate of 3–5% per year. Even in the absence of cirrhosis, patients with chronic hepatitis B—particularly those with active viral replication—are at increased risk for hepatocellular carcinoma.

When to Refer

Refer patients with acute hepatitis who require liver biopsy for diagnosis.

When to Admit

- Encephalopathy is present.
- INR greater than 1.6.
- The patient is unable to maintain hydration.

Hwang JP et al. USPSTF 2020 Hepatitis B Screening Recommendation: evidence to broaden screening and strengthen linkage to care. JAMA. 2020;324:2380. [PMID: 33320206]

Sfeir MM et al. Serologic testing for hepatitis B. JAMA. 2021;326:2423. [PMID: 34797375]

US Preventive Services Task Force; Krist AH et al. Screening for hepatitis B virus infection in adolescents and adults: US Preventive Services Task Force Recommendation Statement. JAMA. 2020;324:2415. [PMID: 33320230]

Wong RJ et al. An updated assessment of chronic hepatitis B prevalence among foreign-born persons living in the United States. Hepatology. 2021;74:607. [PMID: 33655536]

ACUTE HEPATITIS C & OTHER CAUSES OF ACUTE VIRAL HEPATITIS

Viruses other than HAV and HBV that can cause hepatitis are hepatitis C virus (HCV), HDV, and hepatitis E virus (HEV) (an enterically transmitted hepatitis seen in epidemic form in Asia, the Middle East, and North Africa and sporadically in Western countries). Human pegivirus (formerly hepatitis G virus [HGV]) rarely, if ever, causes frank hepatitis. In immunocompromised and rare immunocompetent persons, cytomegalovirus, Epstein-Barr virus, and herpes simplex virus should be considered in the differential diagnosis of hepatitis. Middle East respiratory syndrome (MERS), severe acute respiratory syndrome (SARS), SARS coronavirus infection (SARS-CoV-2), Ebola virus infection, and influenza may be associated with elevated serum aminotransferase levels (occasionally marked). Unidentified pathogens account for a small percentage of cases of acute viral hepatitis.

1. Hepatitis C

HCV is a single-stranded RNA virus (hepacivirus) with properties similar to those of flaviviruses. Seven major genotypes of HCV have been identified. In the past, HCV was responsible for over 90% of cases of posttransfusion hepatitis, yet only 4% of cases of hepatitis C were attributable to blood transfusions. Over 60% of cases are transmitted by injection drug use, and both reinfection and superinfection of HCV are common in people who actively inject drugs. Body piercing, tattoos, and hemodialysis are risk factors. The risk of sexual and maternal–neonatal transmission is low and may be greatest in a subset of patients with high circulating levels of HCV RNA. Having multiple sexual partners may increase the risk of HCV infection, and HIV coinfection, unprotected receptive anal intercourse with ejaculation, and sex while high on methamphetamine increase the risk of HCV transmission in men who have sex with men. Transmission via breastfeeding has not been documented. An outbreak of hepatitis C in patients with immune deficiencies has occurred in some recipients of intravenous immune globulin. Hospital- and outpatient facility–acquired transmission has occurred via multidose vials of saline used to flush Portacaths; through reuse of disposable syringes; through drug "diversion" and tampering with injectable opioids by an infected health care worker; through contamination of shared saline, radiopharmaceutical, and sclerosant vials; via inadequately disinfected endoscopy equipment; and between hospitalized patients on a liver unit. In the developing world, unsafe medical practices lead to a substantial number of cases of HCV infection. Incarceration in prison is a risk factor, with a seroprevalence of 26% in the United States and rates as high as 90% in some states. In many patients, the source of infection is unknown. Coinfection with HCV is found in at least 30% of HIV-infected persons. HIV infection leads to an increased risk of acute liver failure and more rapid progression of chronic hepatitis C to cirrhosis; in addition, HCV increases the hepatotoxicity of antiretroviral therapy. The number of cases of chronic HCV infections in the United States is reported to have decreased from 3.2 million in 2001 to 2.3 million in 2013 with a small increase to 2.4 million between 2013 and 2016, although estimates of at least 4.6 million exposed and 3.5 million infected have also been reported. The incidence of new cases of acute, symptomatic hepatitis C declined from 1992 to 2005, but after 2002 an increase was observed in persons aged 15 to 24, because of injection drug use, and since 2010 there has been a 3.8-fold increase in its overall incidence. An increase has also been observed in women of reproductive age. Worldwide, 71 million people are infected with HCV, with the highest rates in central and east Asia, north Africa, and the Middle East.

Clinical Findings

A. Symptoms and Signs

Figure 16–3 shows the typical course of HCV infection. The incubation period for hepatitis C averages 6–7 weeks, and clinical illness is often mild, usually asymptomatic, and

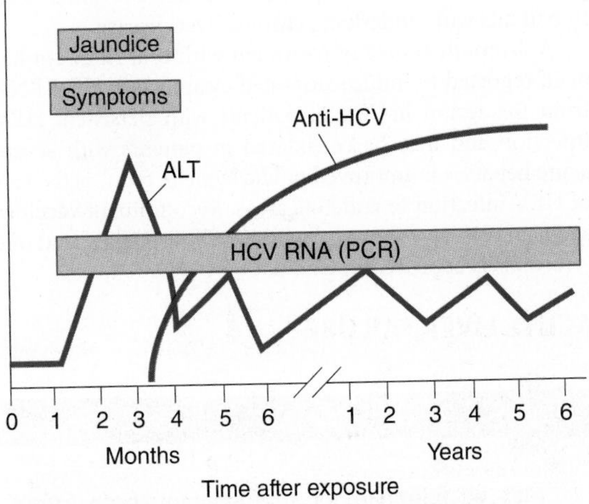

▲ **Figure 16–3.** The typical course of acute and chronic hepatitis C. Anti-HCV, antibody to hepatitis C virus by enzyme immunoassay; HCV RNA PCR, hepatitis C viral RNA by PCR.

characterized by waxing and waning aminotransferase elevations and a high rate (greater than 80%) of chronic hepatitis. In pregnant patients with chronic hepatitis C, serum aminotransferase levels frequently normalize despite persistence of viremia, only to increase again after delivery.

B. Laboratory Findings

Diagnosis of hepatitis C is based on an enzyme immunoassay (EIA) that detects antibodies to HCV. Anti-HCV is not protective, and in patients with acute or chronic hepatitis, its presence in serum generally signifies that HCV is the cause. A diagnosis of hepatitis C may be confirmed by using an assay for HCV RNA. Occasional persons are found to have anti-HCV without HCV RNA in the serum, suggesting recovery from HCV infection in the past.

Complications

HCV is a pathogenic factor in mixed cryoglobulinemia and membranoproliferative glomerulonephritis and may be related to lichen planus, autoimmune thyroiditis, lymphocytic sialadenitis, idiopathic pulmonary fibrosis, sporadic porphyria cutanea tarda, monoclonal gammopathies, CVD, and type 2 diabetes mellitus. HCV infection confers a 20–30% or more increased risk of B-cell non-Hodgkin (predominantly marginal zone) lymphoma, and chronic HCV infection (especially genotype 1) is associated with an increased risk of end-stage renal disease. Hepatic steatosis is a particular feature of infection with HCV genotype 3 and may also occur in patients infected with other HCV genotypes who have risk factors for fatty liver. HCV infection during pregnancy is associated with preterm birth and intrahepatic cholestasis of pregnancy.

Prevention

Testing donated blood for HCV has helped reduce the risk of transfusion-associated hepatitis C from 10% in 1990 to about one case per two million units in 2011. The USPSTF recommends that asymptomatic adults aged 18–79 be screened for HCV infection. The CDC recommends HCV screening for all persons over age 18 at least once in a lifetime and all pregnant women (in both cases except in settings where the prevalence of HCV infection is less than 0.1% [very rare]). HCV-infected persons should practice safe sex, but there is little evidence that HCV is spread easily by sexual contact or perinatally, and no specific preventive measures are recommended for infected persons in a monogamous relationship or for infected pregnant women. Because most cases of HCV infection are acquired by injection drug use, public health officials have recommended avoidance of shared needles and creation of needle exchange programs for injection drug users. As yet, there is no vaccine for HCV. Vaccination against HAV (after prescreening for prior immunity) and HBV is recommended for patients with chronic hepatitis C.

Treatment

A 6-week course of ledipasvir and sofosbuvir has been shown to prevent chronic hepatitis in patients with acute genotype-1 hepatitis C and lack of spontaneous clearance after 3 months (see Chronic Viral Hepatitis). Treatment of acute hepatitis C may be cost effective and is particularly recommended in people who inject drugs.

Prognosis

In most patients, clinical recovery is complete in 3–6 months. Laboratory evidence of liver dysfunction may persist for a longer period. The overall mortality rate is less than 1%, but the rate is reportedly higher in older people and has declined since 2013. Acute liver failure due to HCV is rare in the United States.

Chronic hepatitis, which progresses slowly in many cases, develops in as many as 85% of all persons with acute hepatitis C. Ultimately, cirrhosis develops in up to 30% of those with chronic hepatitis C; the risk of cirrhosis and hepatic decompensation is higher in patients coinfected with both HCV and HBV or HIV. Patients with cirrhosis are at risk for hepatocellular carcinoma at a rate of 3–5% per year. Long-term morbidity and mortality in patients with chronic hepatitis C is lower in Black than in White patients and lowest in those infected with HCV genotype 2 and highest in those with HCV genotype 3.

Cacoub P et al. Extrahepatic manifestations of chronic HCV infection. N Engl J Med. 2021;384:1038. [PMID: 33730456]

Jin F et al. Prevalence and incidence of hepatitis C virus infection in men who have sex with men: a systematic review and meta-analysis. Lancet Gastroenterol Hepatol. 2021;6:39. [PMID: 33217341]

Kushner T et al. Changing epidemiology, implications, and recommendations for hepatitis C in women of childbearing age and during pregnancy. J Hepatol. 2021;74:734. [PMID: 33248169]

Schillie S et al. CDC recommendations for hepatitis C screening among adults—United States, 2020. MMWR Recomm Rep. 2020;69:1. [PMID: 32271723]

2. Hepatitis D

HDV is a defective RNA virus that causes hepatitis only in association with HBV infection and specifically only in the presence of HBsAg; it is cleared when the latter is cleared.

HDV may coinfect with HBV or may superinfect a person with chronic hepatitis B, usually by percutaneous exposure. When acute hepatitis D is coincident with acute HBV infection, the infection is generally similar in severity to acute hepatitis B alone. In chronic hepatitis B, superinfection by HDV appears to carry a worse short-term prognosis, often resulting in acute liver failure or severe chronic hepatitis that progresses rapidly to cirrhosis.

New cases of hepatitis D are infrequent in the United States primarily because of the control of HBV infection, and cases seen today are usually from cohorts infected years ago who survived the initial impact of hepatitis D and now have cirrhosis. These patients are at risk for decompensation and have a threefold increased risk of hepatocellular carcinoma. HDV is estimated to cause 18% of cases of cirrhosis and 20% of cases of hepatocellular carcinoma associated with HBV infection. New cases are seen primarily in immigrants from endemic areas, including Africa, central Asia, Eastern Europe, and the Amazon region of Brazil. As many as 13% of HBV carriers are infected with HDV worldwide; principal risk factors are injecting drug use, high-risk sexual behavior, and HIV and HCV coinfections. The diagnosis of hepatitis D is made by detection of antibody to hepatitis D antigen (anti-HDV) and, where available, hepatitis D antigen (HDAg) or HDV RNA in serum.

Rizzetto M et al. The changing context of hepatitis D. J Hepatol. 2021;74:1200. [PMID: 33484770]

3. Hepatitis E

HEV is a 27- to 34-nm RNA hepevirus (in the Hepeviridae family) that is a major cause of acute hepatitis throughout Central and Southeast Asia (about 16% of the population there have antibodies to the virus), and it should be considered in patients with acute hepatitis after a trip to an endemic area. In rare cases, hepatitis E can be mistaken for drug-induced liver injury. In industrialized countries, it may be spread by swine, and having a pet in the home and consuming undercooked organ meats or infected cow's milk are risk factors. The risk appears to be increased in patients undergoing hemodialysis.

Illness generally is self-limited (no carrier state), but instances of chronic hepatitis with rapid progression to cirrhosis attributed to HEV genotype 3 have been reported in transplant recipients (particularly when tacrolimus rather than cyclosporine is used as the main immunosuppressant) and, rarely, in persons with HIV infection, preexisting liver disease, or cancer undergoing chemotherapy. The diagnosis of acute hepatitis E is made most readily by testing for IgM anti-HEV in serum, although available tests may not be reliable.

Reported extrahepatic manifestations include arthritis; pancreatitis; thyroiditis; myocarditis; glomerulonephritis; monoclonal gammopathy; thrombocytopenia; aplastic anemia; a variety of neurologic complications, including Guillain-Barré syndrome and neuralgic amyotrophy (which involves the brachial plexuses bilaterally); and hemophagocytic lymphohistiocytosis. In endemic regions, the mortality rate is high (15–25%) in pregnant women. The risk of hepatic decompensation and death is increased in patients with underlying chronic liver disease.

A 3-month course of treatment with oral ribavirin has been reported to induce sustained clearance of HEV RNA from the serum in 78% of patients with persistent HEV infection and may be considered in patients with severe acute hepatitis E. Improved public hygiene reduces the risk of HEV infection in endemic areas. Recombinant vaccines against HEV have shown promise in clinical trials, and one (Hecolin) is approved in China.

ACUTE LIVER FAILURE

ESSENTIALS OF DIAGNOSIS

- May be fulminant or subfulminant; both forms carry a poor prognosis.
- Acetaminophen and idiosyncratic drug reactions are the most common causes.

General Considerations

Acute liver failure may be fulminant or subfulminant. Fulminant hepatic failure is characterized by the development of hepatic encephalopathy within 8 weeks after the onset of acute liver injury. Coagulopathy (INR 1.5 or higher) is invariably present. Subfulminant hepatic failure occurs when these findings appear between 8 weeks and 6 months after the onset of acute liver injury and carries an equally poor prognosis. Acute-on-chronic liver failure refers to acute deterioration in liver function (often caused by infection) and associated failure of other organs in a person with preexisting chronic liver disease.

An estimated 1600 cases of acute liver failure occur each year in the United States. Toxicity caused by acetaminophen (a direct hepatotoxin) is the most common cause, accounting for at least 45% of cases. Suicide attempts account for 44% of cases of acetaminophen-induced hepatic failure, and unintentional overdoses ("therapeutic misadventures"), which are often a result of a decrease in the threshold toxic dose because of chronic alcohol use or fasting and have been reported after weight loss surgery, account for at least 48%. Other causes include idiosyncratic (in some cases, immune-mediated) drug reactions (the second most common cause, with antibiotics, antituberculosis drugs, and antiepileptics implicated most commonly), viral hepatitis, poisonous mushrooms (*Amanita phalloides*), shock, heat stroke, Budd-Chiari syndrome, malignancy (most commonly lymphomas), Wilson disease, Reye syndrome, fatty liver of pregnancy and other disorders of fatty acid oxidation, autoimmune hepatitis, parvovirus B19 infection, and rarely grand mal seizures. The cause is indeterminate in approximately 5.5% of cases. The risk of acute liver failure is increased in patients with diabetes mellitus, and outcome is worsened by obesity. Herbal and dietary supplements are thought to be contributory to acute liver failure in a substantial portion of cases, regardless of cause, and may be associated with lower rates of transplant-free survival. Acute-on-chronic liver failure is often precipitated by a bacterial infection or an alcohol binge and alcohol-associated hepatitis.

Viral hepatitis accounts for only 12% of all cases of acute liver failure. The decline of viral hepatitis as the principal cause of acute liver failure is due in part to universal vaccination of infants and children against hepatitis B and the availability of the hepatitis A vaccine. Acute liver failure may occur after reactivation of hepatitis B in carriers who receive immunosuppressive therapy. In endemic areas, hepatitis E is an important cause of acute liver failure, particularly in pregnant women. Hepatitis C is a rare cause of acute liver failure in the United States, but acute hepatitis A or B superimposed on chronic hepatitis C may cause acute liver failure.

Clinical Findings

GI symptoms, systemic inflammatory response, and kidney dysfunction are common. Clinically significant bleeding is uncommon and reflects severe systemic inflammation rather than coagulopathy. Adrenal insufficiency and subclinical myocardial injury (manifesting as an elevated serum troponin I level) often complicate acute liver failure. Jaundice may be absent or minimal early in the course, but laboratory tests show severe hepatocellular damage. In acetaminophen toxicity, serum aminotransferase elevations are often towering (greater than 5000 U/L), and acetaminophen is undetectable in plasma in 50% of cases. In acute liver failure due to microvesicular steatosis (eg, fatty liver of pregnancy), serum aminotransferase elevations may be modest (less than 300 U/L). Over 10% of patients have an elevated serum amylase level at least three times the upper limit of normal, often because of renal dysfunction. The blood ammonia level is typically elevated and correlates (along with the Model for End-Stage Liver Disease [MELD] score) with the development of encephalopathy and intracranial hypertension. Intracranial hypertension rarely develops when the blood ammonia level is less than 75 mcmol/L and is invariable when it is greater than 200 mcmol/L. The severity of extrahepatic organ dysfunction (as assessed by the Sequential Organ Failure Assessment [SOFA]) also correlates with the likelihood of intracranial hypertension. AKI frequently complicates acute-on-chronic liver failure.

Treatment

The treatment of acute liver failure is directed toward achieving metabolic and hemodynamic stability. Intravascular volume should be preserved, but large-volume infusions of hypotonic fluids should be avoided. Norepinephrine is the preferred vasopressor; vasopressin may be added for persistent hypotension. Hypoglycemia should be prevented. Intermittent renal replacement therapy may be required. To preserve muscle mass and immune function, enteral administration of protein, 1–1.5 g/kg/day, is advised, with careful monitoring of the ammonia level.

Cerebral edema and sepsis are the leading causes of death. Prophylactic antibiotic therapy decreases the risk of infection, observed in up to 90%, but has no effect on survival and is not routinely recommended. Microbiological screening cultures should be obtained for patients admitted to hospital. For suspected sepsis, broad coverage is indicated. Despite a high rate of adrenal insufficiency, corticosteroids do not reduce mortality and may lower overall survival in patients with a high MELD score, although they may reduce vasopressor requirements. Stress gastropathy prophylaxis with an H_2-receptor blocker or PPI is recommended. Administration of acetylcysteine (140 mg/kg orally followed by 70 mg/kg orally every 4 hours for an additional 17 doses or 150 mg/kg in 5% dextrose intravenously over 15 minutes followed by 50 mg/kg over 4 hours and then 100 mg/kg over 16 hours) prevents acetaminophen toxicity if administered within 12 hours of ingestion and may be beneficial when given up to 72 hours after ingestion. For massive acetaminophen overdoses, treatment with intravenous acetylcysteine may need to be extended in duration until the serum aminotransferase levels are declining and serum acetaminophen levels are undetectable. Treatment with acetylcysteine improves cerebral blood flow and oxygenation as well as transplant-free survival in patients with stage 1 or 2 encephalopathy due to acute liver failure of any cause. Penicillin G (300,000 to 1 million U/kg/day) or silibinin (silymarin or milk thistle), which is not licensed in the United States, is administered to patients with mushroom poisoning. Nucleoside analogs are recommended for patients with acute liver failure caused by HBV (see Chronic Viral Hepatitis), and intravenous acyclovir has shown benefit in those with herpes simplex virus hepatitis. Plasmapheresis combined with D-penicillamine has been used in acute liver failure due to Wilson disease. Subclinical seizure activity is common in patients with acute liver failure, but the value of prophylactic phenytoin is uncertain.

Early transfer to a liver transplantation center is essential. The head of the patient's bed should be elevated to 30 degrees, and patients with stage 3 or 4 encephalopathy should be intubated. In some centers, extradural sensors are placed in patients at high risk for intracranial hypertension to monitor intracranial pressure for impending cerebral edema with the goal of maintaining the intracranial pressure below 20 mm Hg and the cerebral perfusion pressure above 70 mm Hg but may be associated with complications. Lactulose is of uncertain value. Mannitol, 0.5 g/kg, or 100–200 mL of a 20% solution by intravenous infusion over 10 minutes, may decrease cerebral edema but should be used with caution in patients with advanced CKD. Intravenously administered hypertonic saline to induce hypernatremia (serum sodium concentration of 145–155 mEq/L [145–155 mmol/L]) also may reduce intracranial hypertension. Hypothermia to a temperature of 32–34°C may reduce intracranial pressure when other measures have failed and may improve survival long enough to permit liver transplantation, although a controlled trial showed no benefit, and some authorities recommend a target core temperature of 35–36°C. The value of hyperventilation is uncertain. A short-acting barbiturate, propofol, or intravenous boluses of indomethacin, 25 mg, are considered for refractory intracranial hypertension. Hemodialysis raises intracranial pressure and should be avoided, but continuous renal replacement therapy may be used, if necessary, in patients with AKI.

Prognosis

With earlier recognition of acute liver failure, the frequency of cerebral edema has declined, and overall survival has improved steadily since the 1970s and is now as high as 75%. However, the survival rate in acute liver failure with severe encephalopathy is as low as 20%. The cause of liver injury is the most important determinant of transplant-free survival. In acetaminophen hepatotoxicity, the transplant-free survival is 75%, and no more than 8% of patients undergo liver transplantation. Survival rates are also favorable for hepatitis A, ischemic hepatitis, and pregnancy-related liver disease. For patients with acute liver failure not due to acetaminophen, the outlook is poor in patients younger than 10 and older than 40 years of age and in those with an idiosyncratic drug reaction but appears to be improved when acetylcysteine is administered to patients with stage 1 or 2 encephalopathy. Other adverse prognostic factors are a serum bilirubin level greater than 18 mg/dL (307.8 mcmol/L), INR higher than 6.5, onset of encephalopathy more than 7 days after the onset of jaundice, and a low factor V level (less than 20% of normal in patients younger than 30 years and 30% or less in those 30 years of age or older). For acetaminophen-induced acute liver failure, indicators of a poor outcome are acidosis (pH < 7.3), INR greater than 6.5, and azotemia (serum creatinine 3.4 mg/dL [283.22 mcmol/L] or higher), whereas a rising serum alpha-fetoprotein level predicts a favorable outcome. Other predictors of poor survival in patients with acute liver failure are an elevated blood lactate level (greater than 3.5 mEq/L [3.5 mmol/L]), elevated blood ammonia level (greater than 211 mcg/dL [124 mcmol/L]), and possibly hyperphosphatemia (greater than 3.7 mg/dL [1.2 mmol/L]). The development of thrombocytopenia in the first week is associated with the development of multiorgan system failure and a poor outcome. A number of prognostic indices have been proposed: the "BiLE" score, based on the serum bilirubin, serum lactate, and etiology; the Acute Liver Failure Early Dynamic (ALFED) model, based on the arterial ammonia level, serum bilirubin, INR, and hepatic encephalopathy; and the Acute Liver Failure Study Group (ALFSG) index, based on coma grade, INR, serum bilirubin and phosphorous levels, and serum levels of M30, a cleavage product of cytokeratin-18 caspase. The likelihood of transplant-free survival on admission has been reported to be predicted by a regression model that incorporates the grade of hepatic encephalopathy, etiology, vasopressor use, and log transformations of the serum bilirubin and INR. For acetaminophen-induced acute liver failure, a model that incorporates hepatic encephalopathy grade equal to or greater than 3, Glasgow coma score, cardiovascular failure, mean arterial pressure, INR, serum bilirubin, serum AST, serum creatinine, arterial pH, and arterial lactate has shown good discrimination. In general, emergency liver transplantation is considered for patients with stage 2 to stage 3 encephalopathy or a MELD score of 30.5 or higher (see Cirrhosis) and is associated with a 70% survival rate at 5 years. For mushroom poisoning, liver transplantation should be considered when the interval between ingestion and the onset of diarrhea is less than 8 hours or the INR is 6.0 or higher, even in the absence of encephalopathy. Acute-on-chronic liver failure has a poor prognosis, particularly when associated with kidney dysfunction; some patients may be candidates for liver transplantation.

When to Admit

All patients with acute liver failure should be hospitalized.

Stravitz RT et al. Acute liver failure. Lancet. 2019;394:869. [PMID: 31498101]

CHRONIC VIRAL HEPATITIS

ESSENTIALS OF DIAGNOSIS

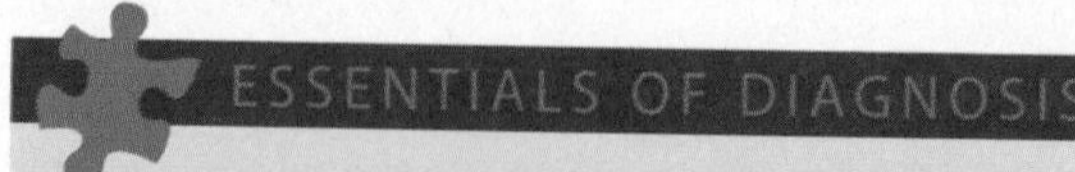

- Defined by chronic infection (HBV, HCV, HDV) for longer than 3–6 months.
- Diagnosis is usually made by antibody tests and viral nucleic acid in serum.

General Considerations

Chronic hepatitis is defined as chronic necroinflammation of the liver of more than 3–6 months' duration, demonstrated by persistently elevated serum aminotransferase levels or characteristic histologic findings, often in the absence of symptoms. In many cases, the diagnosis of chronic hepatitis may be made on initial presentation. The causes of chronic hepatitis include HBV, HCV, and HDV as well as autoimmune hepatitis; alcohol-associated and nonalcoholic steatohepatitis; certain medications, such as isoniazid and nitrofurantoin; Wilson disease; alpha-1-antitrypsin (antiprotease) deficiency; and, rarely, celiac disease. Mortality from chronic HBV and HCV infection has been rising in the United States, and HCV has surpassed HIV as a cause of death. Chronic hepatitis is categorized based on etiology; grade of portal, periportal, and lobular inflammation (minimal, mild, moderate, or severe); and stage of fibrosis (none, mild, moderate, severe, cirrhosis). In the absence of advanced cirrhosis, patients are often asymptomatic or have mild nonspecific symptoms. The World Health Organization has outlined a strategy for eliminating chronic viral hepatitis by 2030 (by vaccinating against hepatitis B, ensuring blood safety and injection safety, timely birth dosing of hepatitis B vaccine, harm reduction from injecting drug use, and testing and treating persons coinfected with hepatitis viruses and HIV).

1. Chronic Hepatitis B & Chronic Hepatitis D

Clinical Findings & Diagnosis

Chronic hepatitis B afflicts 248 million people worldwide (2 billion overall have been infected; endemic areas include Asia and sub-Saharan Africa) and an estimated 2.4 million (predominantly males) in the United States. It may be noted as a continuum of acute hepatitis B or diagnosed because of repeated detection of HBsAg in serum, often with elevated aminotransferase levels.

Five phases of chronic HBV infection are recognized: immune tolerant phase, immune active (or immune clearance) phase, inactive HBsAg carrier state, reactivated chronic hepatitis B phase, and the HBsAg-negative phase. In the immune tolerant phase **(HBeAg-positive chronic HBV infection)**, HBeAg and HBV DNA are present in serum and are indicative of active viral replication, and serum aminotransferase levels are normal, with little necroinflammation in the liver. This phase is common in infants and young children whose immature immune system fails to mount an immune response to HBV.

Persons in the immune tolerant phase and those who acquire HBV infection later in life may enter an immune active phase **(HBeAg-positive chronic hepatitis B)**, in which aminotransferase and HBV DNA levels are elevated and necroinflammation is present in the liver, with a risk of progression to cirrhosis (at a rate of 2–5.5% per year) and of hepatocellular carcinoma (at a rate of more than 2% per year in those with cirrhosis); low-level IgM anti-HBc is present in serum in about 70%.

Patients enter the inactive HBsAg carrier state **(HBeAg-negative chronic HBV infection)** when biochemical improvement follows immune clearance. This improvement coincides with disappearance of HBeAg and reduced HBV DNA levels (less than 10^5 copies/mL, or less than 20,000 IU/mL) in serum, appearance of anti-HBe, and integration of the HBV genome into the host genome in infected hepatocytes. Patients in this phase are at a low risk for cirrhosis (if it has not already developed) and for hepatocellular carcinoma, and those with persistently normal serum aminotransferase levels infrequently have histologically significant liver disease, especially if the HBsAg level is low.

The reactivated chronic hepatitis B phase **(HBeAg-negative chronic hepatitis B)** may result from infection by a pre-core mutant of HBV or from spontaneous mutation of the pre-core or core promoter region of the HBV genome during the course of chronic hepatitis caused by wild-type HBV. HBeAg-negative chronic hepatitis B accounts for less than 10% of cases of chronic hepatitis B in the United States, up to 50% in southeast Asia, and up to 90% in Mediterranean countries, reflecting in part differences in the frequencies of HBV genotypes. In reactivated chronic hepatitis B, there is a rise in serum HBV DNA levels and possible progression to cirrhosis (at a rate of 8–10% per year), particularly when additional pathogenic variants in the core gene of HBV are present. Risk factors for reactivation include male sex and HBV genotype C as well as immunosuppression. Treatment of HCV infection with direct-acting antiviral agents has been reported to lead to instances of HBV reactivation.

In patients with either HBeAg-positive or HBeAg-negative chronic hepatitis B, the risk of cirrhosis and of hepatocellular carcinoma correlates with the serum HBV DNA level. Other risk factors include advanced age, male sex, alcohol use, cigarette smoking, HBV genotype C, and coinfection with HCV or HDV. HIV coinfection is also associated with an increased frequency of cirrhosis when the CD4 count is low.

Only 1% of treated and untreated patients per year reach the **HBsAg-negative phase,** in which anti-HBe may remain detectable, serum ALT levels are normal, and HBV DNA is undetectable in serum but remains present in the liver. This phase is also referred to as a "functional cure." In some cases, anti-HBs appears in serum.

Acute **hepatitis D** infection superimposed on chronic HBV infection may result in severe chronic hepatitis, which may progress rapidly to cirrhosis and may be fatal. Patients with long-standing chronic hepatitis D and B often have inactive cirrhosis and are at risk for decompensation and hepatocellular carcinoma. The diagnosis is confirmed by detection of anti-HDV or HDAg (or HDV RNA) in serum.

Treatment

Patients with active viral replication (HBeAg and HBV DNA [10^5 copies/mL or more, or 20,000 IU/mL or more] in serum and elevated aminotransferase levels) may be treated with a nucleoside or nucleotide analog or with pegylated interferon. Nucleoside and nucleotide analogs are preferred because they are better tolerated and can be taken orally. For patients who are HBeAg-negative, the threshold for treatment is a serum HBV DNA level of 10^4 copies/mL, or 2000 IU/mL. If the threshold HBV DNA level for treatment is met but the serum ALT level is normal, treatment may still be considered in patients over age 35–40 if liver biopsy or a noninvasive assessment of liver fibrosis demonstrates a fibrosis stage of 2 of 4 (moderate) or higher. Therapy is aimed at reducing and maintaining the serum HBV DNA level to the lowest possible levels, thereby leading to normalization of the ALT level and histologic improvement. An additional goal in HBeAg-positive patients is seroconversion to anti-HBe, and some responders eventually clear HBsAg. Although nucleoside and nucleotide analogs generally have been discontinued 6–12 months after HBeAg-to-anti-HBe seroconversion, some patients (especially Asian patients) serorevert to HBeAg after discontinuation, have a rise in HBV DNA levels and recurrence of hepatitis activity, and require long-term therapy, which also is required when seroconversion does not occur and in patients with cirrhosis (at least until HBsAg clears and possibly indefinitely). HBeAg-negative patients with chronic hepatitis B also generally require long-term therapy because relapse is frequent when therapy is stopped. The goal of therapy is "functional cure," characterized by loss of HBsAg, with or without appearance of anti-HBs, and undetectable HBV DNA in serum, associated with improved patient outcomes.

The available nucleoside and nucleotide analogs—entecavir, tenofovir, lamivudine, adefovir, and telbivudine—differ in efficacy and rates of resistance; however, in HBeAg-positive patients, they all achieve an HBeAg-to-anti-HBe seroconversion rate of about 20% at 1 year, with higher rates after more prolonged therapy. The preferred first-line oral agents are entecavir and tenofovir. Entecavir is rarely associated with resistance unless a patient is already resistant to lamivudine. The daily dose is 0.5 mg orally for patients not resistant to lamivudine and 1 mg for patients who previously became resistant to lamivudine. Suppression of HBV DNA in serum occurs in nearly all treated patients, and histologic improvement is observed in 70% of patients. Entecavir has been reported to cause lactic acidosis when used in patients with decompensated cirrhosis. Tenofovir disoproxil fumarate, 300 mg orally daily, is equally effective and is used as a first-line agent or when resistance to a nucleoside analog has developed. Like entecavir, tenofovir has a low rate of resistance when used as initial therapy. Long-term use may lead to an elevated serum creatinine level and reduced serum phosphate level (Fanconi-like syndrome) that is reversible with discontinuation of the drug. Tenofovir alafenamide, 25 mg orally daily, is an alternative formulation of tenofovir that is associated with a lower rate of renal and bone toxicity than tenofovir disoproxil fumarate.

Nucleoside and nucleotide analogs are well tolerated even in patients with decompensated cirrhosis (for whom the treatment threshold may be an HBV DNA level less than 10^4 copies/mL and therapy should be continued indefinitely) and may be effective in patients with rapidly progressive hepatitis B ("fibrosing cholestatic hepatitis") following organ transplantation.

Nucleoside analogs are also recommended to prevent reactivation in both inactive HBV carriers and those positive only for anti-HBc prior to the initiation of immunosuppressive therapy (especially B-cell–depleting agents, such as rituximab, and anti-tumor necrosis factor antibody or moderate- or high-dose corticosteroid therapy) or cancer chemotherapy. In patients infected with both HBV and HIV, antiretroviral therapy, including two drugs active against both viruses (eg, tenofovir plus lamivudine or emtricitabine), has been recommended when treatment of HIV infection is indicated. Tenofovir, telbivudine, and lamivudine have been shown to be safe in pregnant women. Antiviral therapy has been recommended, beginning in the third trimester, when the mother's serum HBV DNA level is 200,000 IU/mL or higher to reduce levels at the time of delivery.

Peginterferon alfa-2a is still an alternative to the oral agents in selected cases. A dose of 180 mcg subcutaneously once weekly for 48 weeks leads to sustained normalization of aminotransferase levels, disappearance of HBeAg and HBV DNA from serum, and appearance of anti-HBe in up to 40% of treated patients and results in improved survival. A response is most likely in patients with a low baseline HBV DNA level and high aminotransferase levels and is more likely in those who are infected with HBV genotype A than with other genotypes (especially genotype D). Moreover, many complete responders eventually clear HBsAg and develop anti-HBs in serum. Relapses are uncommon in complete responders who seroconvert from HBeAg to anti-HBe. Peginterferon may be considered to avoid long-term therapy with an oral agent, as in young women who may want to become pregnant in the future. Patients with HBeAg-negative chronic hepatitis B have a response rate of 60% after 48 weeks of therapy with peginterferon, but the response may not be durable once peginterferon is stopped. The response to peginterferon is poor in patients with HIV coinfection.

In **chronic hepatitis D**, peginterferon alfa-2b (1.5 mcg/kg/wk for 48 weeks) may lead to normalization of serum aminotransferase levels, histologic improvement, and elimination of HDV RNA from serum in 20–50% of patients, but relapse may occur, and tolerance is poor. Nucleoside and nucleotide analogs are generally not effective in treating chronic hepatitis D.

Prognosis

The sequelae of chronic hepatitis secondary to hepatitis B include cirrhosis, liver failure, and hepatocellular carcinoma. The 5-year mortality rate is 0–2% in those without cirrhosis, 14–20% in those with compensated cirrhosis, and 70–86% following decompensation. The risk of cirrhosis and hepatocellular carcinoma correlates with serum HBV DNA levels, and a focus of therapy is to suppress HBV DNA levels below 300 copies/mL (60 IU/mL). In patients with cirrhosis, even low levels of HBV DNA in serum increase the risk of hepatocellular carcinoma compared with undetectable levels. HBV genotype C is associated with a higher risk of cirrhosis and hepatocellular carcinoma than other genotypes. Antiviral treatment improves the prognosis in responders, prevents (or leads to regression of) cirrhosis, and decreases the frequency of liver-related complications (although the risk of hepatocellular carcinoma does not become as low as that in inactive HBV carriers and hepatocellular carcinoma may even occur after clearance of HBsAg). A risk score (PAGE-B) based on a patient's age, sex, and platelet count has been reported to predict the 5-year risk of hepatocellular carcinoma in White patients taking entecavir or tenofovir.

Anderson RT et al. Association between seroclearance of hepatitis B surface antigen and long-term clinical outcomes of patients with chronic hepatitis B virus infection: systematic review and meta-analysis. Clin Gastroenterol Hepatol. 2021;19:463. [PMID: 32473348]

Shiffman ML (guest editor). Challenging issues in the management of chronic hepatitis B virus. Clin Liver Dis. 2021;25:673. [Full issue]

Wang Y et al. Hepatitis B reactivation: a review of clinical guidelines. J Clin Gastroenterol. 2021;55:393. [PMID: 33828065]

2. Chronic Hepatitis C

Clinical Findings & Diagnosis

Chronic hepatitis C develops in up to 85% of patients with acute hepatitis C. It is clinically indistinguishable from chronic hepatitis due to other causes and may be the most common. Worldwide, 71 million people are infected with HCV, with 1.8% of the US population infected. Peak prevalence in the United States (about 4%) is in persons born between 1945 and 1964. In approximately 40% of cases, serum aminotransferase levels are persistently normal. The diagnosis is confirmed by detection of anti-HCV by EIA. In rare cases of suspected chronic hepatitis C but a negative EIA, HCV RNA is detected by PCR testing. Progression to cirrhosis occurs in 20% of affected patients after 20 years, with an increased risk in men, those who drink more than 50 g of alcohol daily, and those who acquire HCV infection after age 40 years. The rate of fibrosis progression accelerates after age 50. Black persons have a higher rate of chronic hepatitis C but lower rates of fibrosis progression and response to therapy than White persons. Immunosuppressed persons—including patients with hypogammaglobulinemia or HIV infection with a low CD4 count or those receiving immunosuppressants—appear to progress more rapidly to cirrhosis than immunocompetent persons with chronic hepatitis C. Tobacco and cannabis smoking and hepatic steatosis also appear to promote progression of fibrosis, whereas coffee consumption appears to slow progression. Persons with chronic hepatitis C and persistently normal serum aminotransferase levels usually have mild chronic hepatitis with slow or absent progression to cirrhosis; however, cirrhosis is present in 10% of these patients. Serum fibrosis testing (eg, FibroSure) or elastography may be used to identify the absence of fibrosis or presence of cirrhosis.

Treatment

The introduction of direct-acting antiviral agents has rapidly expanded the therapeutic armamentarium against HCV (Table 16–6). With the introduction of all-oral regimens, the criterion for a sustained virologic response was shortened from 24 weeks to 12 weeks following the completion of treatment. The definition of clearance of HCV RNA requires use of a sensitive real-time reverse transcriptase-PCR assay to monitor HCV RNA during treatment (the lower limit of quantification should be 25 IU/mL or less, and the limit of detection should be 10–15 IU/mL).

Several types of direct-acting antiviral agents have been developed (Tables 16–6 and 16–7). HCV protease inhibitors ("...previrs") generally have high antiviral potency but differ with respect to the development of resistance (although resistance-associated substitutions in the HCV genome tend not to persist after therapy with these agents is stopped). Examples include glecaprevir and voxilaprevir. Medications in this class are contraindicated in patients with decompensated cirrhosis.

NS5A inhibitors ("...asvirs"), such as ledipasvir and velpatasvir, are characterized by high antiviral potency at picomolar doses. The cross-genotype efficacy of these agents varies.

HCV polymerase inhibitors ("...buvirs") are categorized as nucleoside or nucleotide analog and non-nucleoside polymerase inhibitors. Nucleos(t)ide analogs are active against all HCV genotypes and have a high barrier to resistance. Sofosbuvir has been the sole available agent in this category. Non-nucleos(t)ide polymerase inhibitors, such as dasabuvir, are the weakest class of compounds against HCV because of a low barrier to resistance. Drugs in this class are generally more active against HCV genotype 1b than HCV genotype 1a. They have been developed to be used only in combination with the other direct-acting antiviral agents, mainly protease inhibitors and NS5A inhibitors.

In late 2019, the American Association for the Study of Liver Diseases and the Infectious Diseases Society of America recommended two preferred and highly effective combination regimens: glecaprevir plus pibrentasvir for 8 weeks for genotypes 1–6 and sofosbuvir plus velpatasvir for 12 weeks for genotypes 1, 2, 4, 5, or 6; subsequently sofosbuvir and velpatasvir was approved for genotype 3 (see Table 16–7). The combination of glecaprevir and pibrentasvir is approved for 8 weeks in treatment-naïve, noncirrhotic or compensated cirrhotic and treatment-experienced noncirrhotic patients, including those coinfected with HIV, and for 12 weeks in treatment-experienced, compensated cirrhotic patients. Sofosbuvir and velpatasvir should also be administered for 12 weeks in treatment-experienced compensated cirrhotic patients. Additional modifications may be required in patients with genotype-3 treatment-experienced compensated or decompensated cirrhosis. The combination of glecaprevir and pibrentasvir is also a pangenotypic option for patients with CKD, including those receiving dialysis. The combination of sofosbuvir, velpatasvir, and voxilaprevir is occasionally recommended as "rescue" therapy in patients with nonresponse or relapse following treatment with an NS5A-containing regimen. Where available, testing for resistance-associated substitutions may be helpful in some cases before re-treatment. Use of any regimen containing a protease inhibitor is contraindicated in patients with decompensated cirrhosis.

Table 16–6. Direct-acting antiviral agents for HCV infection (in alphabetical order within class).[1]

Agent	Genotype(s)	Dose[2]	Comment
NS3/4A Protease Inhibitors			
Glecaprevir	1–6	300 mg orally once daily	Used in combination with pibrentasvir[3] with or without ribavirin
Grazoprevir	1 and 4	100 mg orally once daily	Used in combination with elbasvir[4]
Paritaprevir	1 and 4	150 mg orally once daily	Used in combination with ombitasvir and dasabuvir; ritonavir (100 mg) boosted[5]; for genotype 1b with cirrhosis and genotype 1a, used with ribavirin. Used in combination with ombitasvir, ritonavir boosting, and ribavirin for genotype 4[6]
Simeprevir	1 and 4	150 mg orally once daily	Used in combination with sofosbuvir
Voxilaprevir	1–6	100 mg orally once daily	Used in combination with sofosbuvir and velpatasvir[7]
NS5A Inhibitors			
Daclatasvir[8]	1–6	60 mg orally once daily	Used in combination with sofosbuvir (genotypes 1–6, with or without ribavirin depending on presence of cirrhosis) or with asunaprevir (not available in the United States)
Elbasvir	1 and 4	50 mg orally once daily	Used in combination with grazoprevir (see above)
Ledipasvir	1, 4–6	90 mg orally once daily	Used in combination with sofosbuvir[9]
Ombitasvir	1 and 4	25 mg orally once daily	Used in combination with paritaprevir (ritonavir boosted) with or without dasabuvir and with or without ribavirin as per paritaprevir above
Pibrentasvir	1–6	120 mg orally once daily	Used in combination with glecaprevir with or without ribavirin
Velpatasvir	1–6	100 mg orally once daily	Used in combination with sofosbuvir,[10] may be used with sofosbuvir and voxilaprevir
NS5B Nucleos(t)ide Polymerase Inhibitor			
Sofosbuvir	1–6	400 mg orally once daily	Used in combination with ribavirin (genotypes 2 and 3) or with simeprevir (genotypes 1 and 4) or with daclatasvir (all genotypes) or with ledipasvir (genotypes 1, 3, and 4) or with velpatasvir (all genotypes) or with velpatasvir and voxilaprevir (all genotypes)
NS5B Non-Nucleos(t)ide Polymerase Inhibitor			
Dasabuvir	1 and 4	250 mg orally twice daily	Used in combination with paritaprevir (ritonavir boosted) and ombitasvir with or without ribavirin as per paritaprevir above

[1]Regimens approved by the FDA as of early 2022.
[2]The preferred regimen and duration of treatment may vary depending on HCV genotype, presence or absence of cirrhosis or CKD, or nonresponse to prior therapy for HCV infection. In selected cases, testing for resistance-associated substitutions may be considered.
[3]Marketed as Mavyret (AbbVie).
[4]Marketed as Zepatier (Merck) for HCV genotypes 1 and 4 infection.
[5]Marketed as Viekira Pak and Viekira XR (AbbVie).
[6]Marketed as Technivie (AbbVie).
[7]Marketed as Vosevi (Gilead Sciences).
[8]Approved by the FDA for use with sofosbuvir in HCV genotypes 1 and 3 infection but taken off the market in the United States in 2019.
[9]Marketed as Harvoni (Gilead Sciences).
[10]Marketed as Epclusa (Gilead Sciences).

Overall treatment rates are still less than 20% and lowest among Latinx persons and persons with Medicaid or indigent care insurance. The cost of direct-acting antiviral agents has been high (although declining), and lack of insurance coverage has often been a barrier to their use. Additional factors to consider in the selection of a regimen are the presence of cirrhosis or kidney dysfunction, prior treatment, potential drug interactions (of which there are many), and the likelihood that a patient may require liver transplantation in the future. Certain cytochrome P450/P-glycoprotein inducing medications, such as carbamazepine, phenytoin, and phenobarbital, contraindicate the use of all HCV direct-acting antiviral regimens. HCV infection is easy to cure with oral direct-acting agents, with expected sustained virologic response rates well above 90%. Treatment failure is infrequent and most likely in patients infected with HCV genotype 1a or 3, particularly in association with cirrhosis.

Antiviral therapy has been shown to be beneficial in the treatment of cryoglobulinemia associated with chronic hepatitis C; an acute flare of cryoglobulinemia may first require treatment with rituximab, cyclophosphamide plus methylprednisolone, or plasma exchange. As noted above, patients with HCV and HIV coinfection

Table 16–7. Preferred FDA-approved oral direct-acting antiviral (DAA) treatment regimens for HCV infection.[1]

Regimen	Indication	Duration of Treatment in Noncirrhotic Treatment-Naïve Patients (weeks)
Glecaprevir and pibrentasvir	Genotypes 1–6 and DAA-experienced genotype 1	8
Sofosbuvir and velpatasvir	Genotypes 1–6, and DAA-experienced genotypes 1b and 2	12
Sofosbuvir, velpatasvir, and voxilaprevir	DAA-experienced genotypes 1–6	–

[1]Based on the American Association for the Study of Liver Diseases/Infectious Diseases Society of America 2018 Guidance. In late 2019, two preferred regimens were proposed: glecaprevir and pibrentasvir for 8 weeks (genotypes 1–6) and sofosbuvir and velpatasvir for 12 weeks (genotypes 1, 2, 4, 5, 6). See HCV Guidance: Recommendation for testing, managing, and treating hepatitis C. http://www.hcvguidelines.org, accessed December 17, 2021.

have been shown to respond well to treatment of HCV infection. Moreover, in persons coinfected with HCV and HIV, long-term liver disease–related mortality increases as HIV infection–related mortality is reduced by antiretroviral therapy. Occasional instances of reactivation of HBV infection, as well as herpesvirus, have occurred with direct-acting antiviral agents for HCV infection, and all candidates should be prescreened for HBV infection, with the initiation of antiviral prophylactic therapy in those who are HbsAg positive before treatment of HCV infection is begun.

Prognosis

Chronic hepatitis C is an indolent, often subclinical disease that may lead to cirrhosis and hepatocellular carcinoma after decades. The overall mortality rate in patients with transfusion-associated hepatitis C may be no different from that of an age-matched control population. Nevertheless, mortality or transplantation rates clearly rise to 5% per year once cirrhosis develops. A risk score combining age, sex, platelet count, and AST-to-ALT ratio has been proposed. There is some evidence that HCV genotype 1b is associated with a higher risk of hepatocellular carcinoma than other genotypes. Antiviral therapy has a beneficial effect on mortality, cardiovascular events, type 2 diabetes mellitus, and quality of life, is cost effective, appears to retard and even reverse fibrosis, and reduces (but does not eliminate) the risk of decompensated cirrhosis and hepatocellular carcinoma in responders with advanced fibrosis. Even patients who achieve a sustained virologic response remain at an increased risk for mortality compared with the general population. An increased risk of death from extrahepatic cancers has been described in this group, as well as in patients who achieve suppression of HBV infection. Although mortality from cirrhosis and hepatocellular carcinoma due to hepatitis C is still substantial, the need for liver transplantation for chronic hepatitis C has declined, and survival after transplantation has improved. The risk of mortality from drug addiction is higher than that for liver disease in patients with chronic hepatitis C. HCV infection appears to be associated with increased cardiovascular mortality, especially in persons with diabetes mellitus and hypertension. Statin use has been reported to be associated with improved virologic response to antiviral therapy and decreased progression of liver fibrosis and frequency of hepatocellular carcinoma.

When to Refer

- For liver biopsy.
- For antiviral therapy.

When to Admit

For complications of decompensated cirrhosis.

European Association for the Study of the Liver. EASL recommendations on treatment of hepatitis C: final update of the series. J Hepatol. 2020;73:1170. [PMID: 32956768]

Ioannou GN. HCC surveillance after SVR in patients with F3/F4 fibrosis. J Hepatol. 2021;74:458. [PMID: 33303216]

Negro F. Residual risk of liver disease after hepatitis C virus eradication. J Hepatol. 2021;74:952. [PMID: 33276027]

Sarrazin C. Treatment failure with DAA therapy: importance of resistance. J Hepatol. 2021;74:1472. [PMID: 33716089]

AUTOIMMUNE HEPATITIS

ESSENTIALS OF DIAGNOSIS

- Usually young to middle-aged women.
- Chronic hepatitis with high serum globulins and characteristic liver histology.
- Positive antinuclear antibody (ANA) or smooth muscle antibody, or both, in most cases in the United States.
- Responds to corticosteroids.

General Considerations

Autoimmune hepatitis is usually seen in young women but can occur in either sex at any age. The incidence, which has been rising, and prevalence are estimated to be approximately 2 and 31 per 100,000 population, respectively.

The risk of autoimmune hepatitis is increased in first-degree relatives of affected patients.

Clinical Findings

A. Symptoms and Signs

The onset is usually insidious. About 25% of cases present with acute severe hepatitis (and occasionally acute liver failure), and some cases follow a viral illness (such as hepatitis A, Epstein-Barr infection, or measles) or exposure to a drug or toxin (such as nitrofurantoin, minocycline, hydralazine, methyldopa, infliximab, or an immune checkpoint inhibitor). Exacerbations may occur postpartum. Amenorrhea may be a presenting feature, and the frequency of depression appears to be increased. Thirty-four percent of patients, and particularly older patients, are asymptomatic. Examination may reveal a healthy-appearing young woman with multiple spider telangiectasias, cutaneous striae, acne, hirsutism, and hepatomegaly. Extrahepatic features include arthritis, Sjögren syndrome, thyroiditis, nephritis, ulcerative colitis, and Coombs-positive hemolytic anemia. Patients, especially older patients, with autoimmune hepatitis are at increased risk for cirrhosis, which, in turn, increases the risk of hepatocellular carcinoma (at a rate of about 1% per year).

B. Laboratory Findings

Serum aminotransferase levels may be greater than 1000 U/L, and the total bilirubin is usually increased. Autoimmune hepatitis has been classified as type I or type II, although the clinical features and response to treatment are similar between the two types. In type I (classic) autoimmune hepatitis, ANA or smooth muscle antibodies (either or both) are usually detected in serum. Serum gamma-globulin levels are typically elevated (up to 5–6 g/dL [0.05–0.06 g/L]). In acute severe autoimmune hepatitis, ANA are absent and serum IgG is normal, each in up to 39% of cases. Antibodies to soluble liver antigen (anti-SLA) characterize a variant of type I that is marked by severe disease, a high relapse rate after treatment, and absence of the usual antibodies (ANA and smooth muscle antibodies). Type II, seen more often in girls under age 14 in Europe, is characterized by circulating antibodies to liver-kidney microsome type 1 (anti-LKM1) without smooth muscle antibodies or ANA. In some cases, antibodies to liver cytosol type 1, are detected. Type II autoimmune hepatitis can be seen in patients with autoimmune polyglandular syndrome type 1. Concurrent primary biliary cholangitis (PBC) or primary sclerosing cholangitis ("overlap syndrome") has been recognized in 7–13% and 6–11% of patients with autoimmune hepatitis, respectively. Liver biopsy is indicated to help establish the diagnosis (interface hepatitis is the hallmark), evaluate disease severity and stage of fibrosis, and determine the need for treatment. Histologic features of NAFLD are found in 17–30% of patients with autoimmune hepatitis. Cirrhosis is present in 28–33% of adults at presentation.

Simplified diagnostic criteria based on the detection of autoantibodies (1 point for a titer of greater than 1:40 or 2 points for a titer of greater than 1:80), elevated IgG levels (1 point for IgG level greater than or equal to upper limit of normal or 2 points for level greater than or equal to 1.1 times upper limit of normal), characteristic histologic features (1 or 2 points depending on how typical the features are), and exclusion of viral hepatitis (2 points) can be useful for diagnosis; a total score of 6 indicates probable and a score of 7 indicates definite autoimmune hepatitis with a high degree of specificity but moderate sensitivity. Diagnostic criteria for an overlap of autoimmune hepatitis and PBC ("Paris criteria") have been proposed.

Treatment

Prednisone with or without azathioprine (often started 2 weeks after prednisone) improves symptoms; decreases the serum bilirubin, aminotransferase, and gamma-globulin levels; and reduces hepatic inflammation. Symptomatic patients with aminotransferase levels elevated tenfold (or fivefold if the serum globulins are elevated at least twofold) are optimal candidates for therapy, and asymptomatic patients with modest enzyme elevations may be considered for therapy depending on the clinical circumstances and histologic severity; however, asymptomatic patients usually remain asymptomatic, have either mild hepatitis or inactive cirrhosis on liver biopsy specimens, and have a good long-term prognosis without therapy.

Prednisone is given initially in a dose of 30 mg orally daily with azathioprine, 50 mg orally daily, which is generally well tolerated and permits the use of lower corticosteroid doses than a regimen beginning with prednisone 60 mg orally daily alone. A decrease in serum AST levels by 80% after 8 weeks predicts normalization of AST levels at 1 year. Intravenous corticosteroids or prednisone, 60 mg orally daily, is recommended for patients with acute severe autoimmune hepatitis; azathioprine is often started 2 weeks later. In patients with noncirrhotic autoimmune hepatitis, budesonide, 3 mg orally two or three times daily, may be at least as effective as prednisone as first-line treatment and associated with fewer side effects. Whether patients should undergo testing for the genotype of thiopurine methyltransferase prior to treatment with azathioprine to predict toxicity is debated. Adjusting the dose of azathioprine based on metabolite levels, as in IBD, has been suggested. Blood counts are monitored weekly for the first 2 months of therapy and monthly thereafter because of the small risk of bone marrow suppression. The dosage of prednisone is lowered from 30 mg/day after 1 week to 20 mg/day and again after 2 or 3 weeks to 15 mg/day. Treatment is response-guided, and ultimately, a maintenance dosage of 10 mg/day should be achieved. While symptomatic improvement is often prompt, biochemical improvement is more gradual, with normalization of serum aminotransferase levels after an average of 22 months. Histologic resolution of inflammation lags biochemical remission by 3–6 months and repeat liver biopsy should be considered in persons with at least 2 years of biochemical remission. Failure of aminotransferase levels to return to normal invariably predicts lack of histologic resolution.

The response rate to therapy with prednisone and azathioprine is 80%, with remission in 65% by 3 years. Older patients are more likely to respond than younger patients and those with, hyperbilirubinemia or a high MELD score (12 or higher, see Cirrhosis). Fibrosis may reverse with therapy and rarely progresses after apparent biochemical and histologic remission. Once complete remission is achieved, therapy may be withdrawn, but the subsequent relapse rate is 90% by 3 years. Relapses may again be treated in the same manner as the initial episode, with the same remission rate. After successful treatment of a relapse, the patient may continue taking azathioprine (up to 2 mg/kg) or the lowest dose of prednisone with or without azathioprine (50 mg/day) needed to maintain aminotransferase levels as close to normal as possible; another attempt at withdrawing therapy may be considered in patients remaining in remission long term (eg, 4 years or longer). During pregnancy, flares can be treated with prednisone, and maintenance azathioprine does not have to be discontinued.

Nonresponders to corticosteroids and azathioprine (failure of serum aminotransferase levels to decrease by 50% after 6 months) may be considered for a trial of cyclosporine, tacrolimus, sirolimus, everolimus, methotrexate, rituximab, or infliximab. Mycophenolate mofetil, 500 mg increased to 1 g twice daily, is an effective alternative to azathioprine in patients who cannot tolerate it but is less effective in nonresponders to azathioprine and is a known teratogen that must be withdrawn prior to conception. It may be effective in up to 60% of patients refractory to or intolerant of corticosteroids. Occasionally, 6-mercaptopurine may be tolerated in patients who do not tolerate azathioprine. Bone density should be monitored—particularly in patients receiving maintenance corticosteroid therapy—and measures undertaken to prevent or treat osteoporosis (see Chapter 26). Liver transplantation may be required for treatment failures and patients with a severe acute presentation (immediately in those with acute liver failure and after 2 weeks in those with acute severe autoimmune hepatitis and a lack of improvement with corticosteroids), but the outcome may be worse than that for PBC because of an increased rate of infectious complications. As immunosuppression is reduced, the disease has been recognized to recur in up to 70% of transplanted livers at 5 years (and rarely to develop de novo); sirolimus can be effective in such cases.

Prognosis

Overall long-term mortality of patients with autoimmune hepatitis and cirrhosis appears to be twofold higher than that of the general population despite response to immunosuppressive therapy. Factors that predict the need for liver transplantation or that predict liver-related death include the following: (1) age 20 years or younger or age 60 years or older at presentation, (2) low serum albumin level at diagnosis, (3) cirrhosis at diagnosis, (4) the presence of anti-SLA, and (5) incomplete normalization of the serum ALT level after 6 months of treatment. The disease appears to be more aggressive in Black patients than in White patients.

When to Refer

- For liver biopsy.
- For immunosuppressive therapy.

When to Admit

- Hepatic encephalopathy.
- INR greater than 1.6.

Ben Merabet Y et al. Sustained remission after treatment withdrawal in autoimmune hepatitis: a multicenter retrospective study. Dig Dis Sci. 2021;66:2107. [PMID: 32607807]

Mack CL et al. Diagnosis and management of autoimmune hepatitis in adults and children: 2019 practice guidance and guidelines from the American Association for the Study of Liver Diseases. Hepatology. 2020;72:671. [PMID: 31863477]

McNally BB et al. Azathioprine monotherapy is equivalent to dual therapy in maintaining remission in autoimmune hepatitis. Dig Dis Sci. 2021;66:1715. [PMID: 32436124]

ALCOHOL-ASSOCIATED LIVER DISEASE

ESSENTIALS OF DIAGNOSIS

- Chronic alcohol intake usually exceeds 80 g/day in men and 30–40 g/day in women with alcohol-associated hepatitis or cirrhosis.
- Fatty liver is often asymptomatic.
- Fever, right upper quadrant pain, tender hepatomegaly, and jaundice characterize alcohol-associated hepatitis, but the patient may be asymptomatic.
- AST is usually elevated but infrequently > 300 U/L (6 mckat/L); AST is > ALT, often by a factor of two or more.
- Alcohol-associated hepatitis is often reversible, but it is the most common precursor of cirrhosis in the United States.

General Considerations

Excessive alcohol intake can lead to fatty liver, hepatitis, and cirrhosis. Validated tools, such as the Alcohol Use Disorders Inventory Test (AUDIT), can be used to identify persons with alcohol abuse and dependence (see Table 1–7). Alcohol-associated hepatitis is characterized by acute or chronic inflammation and parenchymal necrosis of the liver induced by alcohol and is often a reversible disease, but it is the most common precursor of cirrhosis in the United States. It is associated with four to five times the number of hospitalizations and deaths as hepatitis C. Mortality from alcohol-associated liver disease has been increasing since 1999.

The frequency of alcohol-associated cirrhosis is estimated to be 10–15% among persons who consume over 50 g of alcohol (4 oz of 100-proof whiskey, 15 oz of wine, or four 12-oz cans of beer) daily for over 10 years (although the risk of cirrhosis may be lower for wine than for a comparable intake of beer or spirits). The risk of cirrhosis is lower (5%) in the absence of other cofactors such as chronic viral hepatitis and obesity. Genetic factors may also account for differences in susceptibility to and severity of liver disease. Women appear to be more susceptible than men, in part because of lower gastric mucosal alcohol dehydrogenase levels, but young men who drink excessively are at increased risk for liver disease later in life when they are no longer drinking as much.

Clinical Findings

A. Symptoms and Signs

The clinical presentation of alcohol-associated liver disease can vary from asymptomatic hepatomegaly to a rapidly fatal acute illness (acute-on-chronic liver failure) or end-stage cirrhosis. A recent period of heavy drinking, complaints of anorexia and nausea, and the demonstration of hepatomegaly and jaundice strongly suggest the diagnosis. Abdominal pain and tenderness, splenomegaly, ascites, fever, and encephalopathy may be present. Infection, including invasive aspergillosis, is common in patients with severe alcohol-associated hepatitis.

B. Laboratory Findings

In patients with steatosis, mild liver enzyme elevations may be the only laboratory abnormality. Anemia (usually macrocytic) may be present. Leukocytosis with a shift to the left is common in patients with severe alcohol-associated hepatitis. Leukopenia is occasionally seen and resolves after cessation of drinking. About 10% of patients have thrombocytopenia related to a direct toxic effect of alcohol on megakaryocyte production or to hypersplenism.

AST is usually elevated but infrequently above 400 U/L (6 mckat/L). AST is greater than ALT, usually by a factor of two or more. Serum alkaline phosphatase is generally elevated, but seldom more than three times the normal value. Serum bilirubin is increased in 60–90% of patients with alcohol-associated hepatitis.

Serum bilirubin levels greater than 10 mg/dL (171 mcmol/L) and marked prolongation of the prothrombin time (6 seconds or more above control) indicate severe alcohol-associated hepatitis with a mortality rate above 30%. The serum albumin is depressed, and the gamma-globulin level (especially IgA) is elevated in 50–75% of individuals, even in the absence of cirrhosis. Increased transferrin saturation, hepatic iron stores, and sideroblastic anemia are found in many alcoholic patients. Folic acid deficiency may coexist.

C. Imaging

Imaging studies can detect moderate to severe hepatic steatosis reliably but not inflammation or fibrosis. Ultrasonography helps exclude biliary obstruction and identifies subclinical ascites. CT with intravenous contrast or MRI may be indicated in selected cases to evaluate patients for collateral vessels, space-occupying lesions of the liver, or concomitant disease of the pancreas.

D. Liver Biopsy

Liver biopsy, if done, demonstrates macrovesicular fat and, in patients with alcohol-associated hepatitis, polymorphonuclear infiltration with hepatic necrosis, Mallory (or Mallory-Denk) bodies (alcoholic hyaline), and perivenular and perisinusoidal fibrosis. Micronodular cirrhosis may be present as well. The findings are similar to those of nonalcoholic steatohepatitis.

Differential Diagnosis

Alcohol-associated hepatitis may be closely mimicked by cholecystitis and cholelithiasis and by drug toxicity. Other causes of hepatitis or chronic liver disease may be excluded by serologic or biochemical testing, imaging studies, or liver biopsy. A formula based on the AST/ALT ratio, BMI, mean corpuscular volume, and sex has been reported to reliably distinguish alcohol-associated liver disease from NAFLD.

Treatment

A. General Measures

Abstinence from alcohol is essential. Hospitalized patients should be monitored for alcohol withdrawal; the Clinical Institute Withdrawal Assessment for Alcohol-Revised (CIWA-Ar) is often used in practice (see Figure 25–3). Acamprosate, naltrexone, or baclofen may be considered in combination with counseling to reduce the likelihood of recidivism. Baclofen appears to be safe in persons with advanced alcohol-associated liver disease but can worsen hepatic encephalopathy. Fatty liver is quickly reversible with abstinence. Every effort should be made to provide sufficient amounts of carbohydrates and calories in anorectic patients to reduce endogenous protein catabolism, promote gluconeogenesis, and prevent hypoglycemia. Nutritional support (30–40 [and no less than 21.5] kcal/kg with 1.0–1.5 g/kg as protein) improves liver disease, but not necessarily survival, in patients with malnutrition. Intensive enteral nutrition is difficult to implement, however. The administration of micronutrients, particularly folic acid, thiamine, and zinc, is indicated, especially when deficiencies are noted; glucose administration increases the thiamine requirement and can precipitate Wernicke-Korsakoff syndrome if thiamine is not coadministered. Nephrotoxic drugs should be avoided in patients with severe alcohol-associated hepatitis.

B. Pharmacologic Measures

Methylprednisolone, 32 mg/day orally, or the equivalent, for 1 month, may reduce short-term (1-month but not 6-month) mortality in patients with alcohol-associated hepatitis and encephalopathy, a modified Maddrey discriminant function index (defined by the patient's prothrombin time minus the control prothrombin time times 4.6 plus the total bilirubin in mg/dL) of 32 or more, or a MELD score of 20 or more, particularly those with a MELD score between 25 and 39 (see Cirrhosis). Concomitant GI bleeding or infection may not preclude treatment with corticosteroids if otherwise indicated, but treatment with prednisolone increases the risk of serious infections during and after treatment is completed. The combination of corticosteroids and N-acetylcysteine has been reported to further improve 1-month but not 6-month survival and reduce the risk of hepatorenal syndrome and infections; the combination may be superior to corticosteroids alone, but more data are needed.

Pentoxifylline, 400 mg orally three times daily for 4 weeks, decreases the risk of hepatorenal syndrome. It does not appear to reduce short-term mortality. Its use is not recommended in some guidelines, but it has been used when corticosteroids are contraindicated. The addition of pentoxifylline to prednisolone does not appear to improve survival but may reduce the frequency of hepatorenal syndrome compared with prednisolone alone.

Prognosis

A. Short-Term

The overall mortality rate for alcohol-associated hepatitis is 34% (20% within 1 month) without corticosteroid therapy. Individuals in whom the prothrombin time prohibits liver biopsy have a 42% mortality rate at 1 year. Other unfavorable prognostic factors are older age, a serum bilirubin greater than 10 mg/dL (171 mcmol/L), hepatic encephalopathy, coagulopathy, azotemia, leukocytosis, sepsis and other infections, systematic inflammatory response syndrome (which is associated with multiorgan failure), lack of response to corticosteroid therapy, a low serum transferrin level, and possibly a paucity of steatosis on a liver biopsy specimen and reversal of portal blood flow by Doppler ultrasonography. Concomitant GI bleeding does not appear to worsen survival. Failure of the serum bilirubin level to decline after 7 (and probably 4) days of treatment with corticosteroids predicts nonresponse and poor long-term survival, as does the Lille model (which includes age, serum creatinine, serum albumin, prothrombin time [or INR], serum bilirubin on admission, and serum bilirubin on day 7). The MELD score used for cirrhosis and the Glasgow alcohol-associated hepatitis score (based on age, WBC count, BUN, prothrombin time ratio, and bilirubin level) also correlate with mortality from alcohol-associated hepatitis and have higher specificities than the discriminant function and Lille score. A scoring system based on age, serum bilirubin, INR, and serum creatinine (ABIC) has been proposed, and at least one study has shown that the development of AKI is the most accurate predictor of 90-day mortality. Another scoring system based on hepatic encephalopathy, systemic inflammatory response syndrome, and MELD score has also been reported to predict AKI and mortality. The combination of the MELD score and Lille model has been reported to be the best predictor of short-term mortality among the scoring systems. Histologic features associated with 90-day mortality include the degree of fibrosis and neutrophil infiltration, presence of megamitochondria, and bilirubinostasis.

B. Long-Term

The 3-year mortality rate of persons who recover from acute alcohol-associated hepatitis is 10 times greater than that of control individuals of comparable age; the 5-year mortality rate is as high as 85%. Histologically severe disease is associated with continued excessive mortality rates after 3 years, whereas the death rate is not increased after the same period in those whose liver biopsy specimens show only mild alcohol-associated hepatitis. Complications of portal hypertension (ascites, variceal bleeding, hepatorenal syndrome), coagulopathy, and severe jaundice following recovery from acute alcohol-associated hepatitis also suggest a poor long-term prognosis.

The most important long-term prognostic factor is continued excessive drinking. The overall 10-year survival among all persons with alcohol-associated liver disease is 88% among those who are abstinent compared with 73% in those who experience a relapse in drinking. There is no safe level of drinking in persons with alcohol-associated liver disease or other liver diseases. The risk of alcohol-associated cirrhosis is greater in women than in men and associated with obesity, cigarette smoking, chronic hepatitis C, and low vitamin D levels; the risk is inversely associated with coffee drinking. Alcohol-associated cirrhosis is a risk factor for hepatocellular carcinoma, and the risk is highest in carriers of the *C282Y* pathogenic variant for hemochromatosis or those with increased hepatic iron. A 6-month period of abstinence is generally required before liver transplantation is considered, although this requirement has been questioned and early liver transplantation has been performed in selected patients with alcohol-associated hepatitis, with good outcomes. Optimal candidates have adequate social support, do not smoke, have no psychosis or personality disorder, are adherent to therapy, and have regular appointments with a psychiatrist or psychologist who specializes in addiction treatment. Patients with alcohol-associated liver disease are at higher risk for posttransplant malignancy than those with other types of liver disease because of alcohol and tobacco use.

When to Refer

Refer patients with alcohol-associated hepatitis who require liver biopsy for diagnosis.

When to Admit

- Hepatic encephalopathy.
- INR greater than 1.6.
- Total bilirubin 10 mg/dL or more.
- Inability to maintain hydration.

Arab JP et al. Identification of optimal therapeutic window for steroid use in severe alcohol-associated hepatitis: a worldwide study. J Hepatol. 2021;75:1026. [PMID: 34166722]

Avila MA et al. Recent advances in alcohol-related liver disease (ALD): summary of a Gut round table meeting. Gut. 2020;69:764. [PMID: 3187928]

Crabb DW et al. Diagnosis and treatment of alcohol-associated liver diseases: 2019 practice guidance from the American Association for the Study of Liver Diseases. Hepatology. 2020;71:306. [PMID: 31314133]

Kwo PY (editor). Alcoholic hepatitis. Clin Liver Dis. 2021;25:483. [Full issue]

Singal AK et al. Diagnosis and treatment of alcohol-associated liver disease: a review. JAMA. 2021;326:165. [PMID: 34255003]

DRUG- & TOXIN-INDUCED LIVER INJURY

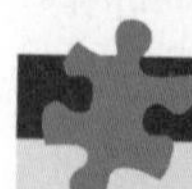

ESSENTIALS OF DIAGNOSIS

- Drug-induced liver injury can mimic viral hepatitis, biliary tract obstruction, or other types of liver disease.
- Clinicians must inquire about the use of many widely used therapeutic agents, including over-the-counter "natural" and herbal and dietary supplements, in any patient with liver disease.

General Considerations

Many therapeutic agents may cause drug-induced liver injury, with jaundice occurring in 30% of cases and up to 10% of patients with drug-induced liver injury dying or undergoing liver transplantation within 6 months of onset. In any patient with liver disease, the clinician must inquire carefully about the use of potentially hepatotoxic drugs or exposure to hepatotoxins, including over-the-counter herbal and dietary supplements. The medications most commonly implicated are antibiotics because of their widespread use. In some cases, coadministration of a second agent may increase the toxicity of the first (eg, isoniazid and rifampin, acetaminophen and alcohol, combinations of immune checkpoint inhibitors). The diagnosis often depends on exclusion of other causes of liver disease. A relationship between increased serum ALT levels in premarketing clinical trials and postmarketing reports of hepatotoxicity has been identified. Except for drugs used to treat tuberculosis and HIV infection, obeticholic acid, and possibly azithromycin, the risk of hepatotoxicity is not increased in patients with preexisting cirrhosis, but hepatotoxicity may be more severe and the outcome worse when it does occur. Older persons may be at higher risk for hepatotoxicity from certain agents, such as amoxicillin-clavulanic acid, isoniazid, and nitrofurantoin, and more likely to have persistent and cholestatic, rather than hepatocellular, injury compared with younger persons. Drug toxicity may be categorized based on pathogenesis or predominant histologic appearance. Drug-induced liver injury can mimic viral hepatitis, biliary tract obstruction, vanishing bile duct syndrome, or other types of liver disease (and vice versa). The development of jaundice in a patient with serum aminotransferase levels at least three times the upper limit of normal predicts a mortality rate of at least 10% ("Hy's Law"). A model based on the presence of comorbidities, the MELD score, and serum albumin has been reported to predict 6-month mortality.

Categorization by Pathogenesis

A. Direct Hepatotoxicity

Liver toxicity caused by this group of drugs is characterized by dose-related severity, a latent period following exposure, and susceptibility in all individuals. One example is acetaminophen (the toxicity of which is enhanced by fasting because of depletion of glutathione and by long-term alcohol use both because of depletion of glutathione and because of induction of cytochrome P450 2E1; and the toxicity of which is possibly reduced by statins, fibrates, and NSAIDs and acetylcysteine treatment). Other examples include alcohol, *Amanita phalloides* mushrooms, carbon tetrachloride, chloroform, heavy metals, mercaptopurine, niacin, obeticholic acid, plant alkaloids, phosphorus, pyrazinamide, tetracyclines, tipranavir, valproic acid, and vitamin A.

B. Idiosyncratic Reactions

Except for acetaminophen, most severe hepatotoxicity is idiosyncratic. Reactions of this type are (1) sporadic, (2) not related to dose above a general threshold of 100 mg/day, and (3) occasionally associated with features suggesting an allergic reaction, such as fever and eosinophilia (including drug rash with eosinophilia and systemic symptoms [DRESS] syndrome), which may be associated with a favorable outcome. In many instances, the drug is lipophilic, and toxicity results directly from a reactive metabolite that is produced only in certain individuals on a genetic basis. Illness tends to be more severe in Black persons than in White persons. Drug-induced liver injury may be observed only during postmarketing surveillance and not during preclinical trials. Examples include abacavir, abeparvovec, alemtuzumab, atabecestat, amiodarone, aspirin, carbamazepine, chloramphenicol, dapsone, diclofenac, disulfiram, duloxetine, ezetimibe, flavocoxid (a "medical food"), fluoroquinolones (levofloxacin and moxifloxacin, in particular), flutamide, halothane, isoniazid, ketoconazole, lamotrigine, methyldopa, natalizumab, nevirapine, oxacillin, phenytoin, pyrazinamide, quinidine, remdesivir, rivaroxaban, streptomycin, temozolomide, thiazolidinediones, tolvaptan, and perhaps tacrine. Statins, like all cholesterol-lowering agents, may cause serum aminotransferase elevations but rarely cause true hepatitis, and even more rarely cause acute liver failure, and are no longer considered contraindicated in patients with liver disease. Most acute idiosyncratic drug-induced liver injury is reversible with discontinuation of the offending agent. Risk factors for chronicity (longer than 1 year) are older age, dyslipidemia, and severe acute injury.

C. Indirect Hepatotoxicity

Indirect hepatotoxicity refers to liver injury that results when use of a drug leads to exacerbation of preexisting liver disease. An example is a flare of HBV infection in the setting of immunosuppressive therapy for a nonhepatic autoimmune disease.

Categorization by Histopathology

A. Cholestatic Injury

1. Noninflammatory—Drug-induced cholestasis results from inhibition or genetic deficiency of various hepatobiliary transporter systems. The following drugs cause cholestasis: anabolic steroids containing an alkyl or ethinyl group at carbon 17, azathioprine, cetirizine, cyclosporine, diclofenac, estrogens, febuxostat, indinavir (increased risk of indirect hyperbilirubinemia in patients with Gilbert syndrome), mercaptopurine, methyltestosterone, tamoxifen, temozolomide, and ticlopidine.

2. Inflammatory—The following drugs cause inflammation of portal areas with bile duct injury (cholangitis [and, in some cases, bile duct loss]), often with allergic features such as eosinophilia: amoxicillin-clavulanic acid (among the most common causes of drug-induced liver injury), azathioprine, azithromycin, captopril, celecoxib, cephalosporins, chlorothiazide, chlorpromazine, chlorpropamide, erythromycin, mercaptopurine, pazopanib, penicillamine, prochlorperazine, semisynthetic penicillins (eg, cloxacillin), sulfadiazine, and temozolomide. Ketamine abuse may cause secondary biliary cirrhosis. Cholestatic and mixed cholestatic-hepatocellular toxicity is more likely than pure hepatocellular toxicity to lead to chronic liver disease.

B. Hepatocellular Injury

Medications that may result in acute or chronic hepatitis that is histologically and, in some cases, clinically similar to autoimmune hepatitis include minocycline and nitrofurantoin, most commonly, as well as aspirin, isoniazid (increased risk in HBV and HCV carriers), methyldopa, NSAIDs, propylthiouracil, terbinafine, tumor necrosis factor inhibitors, and varenicline. Histologic features that favor a drug cause include portal tract neutrophils and hepatocellular cholestasis. Hepatitis also can occur in patients taking cocaine, diclofenac, dimethyl fumarate, efavirenz, imatinib mesylate, ipilimumab, nivolumab, and other checkpoint inhibitors, which may also cause cholangitis, methylenedioxymethamphetamine (MDMA; ecstasy), nefazodone (has a black box warning for a potential to cause liver failure), nevirapine (like other HIV protease inhibitors, increased risk in HBV and HCV carriers), pioglitazone, ritonavir (greater rate than other HIV protease inhibitors), rosiglitazone, saquinavir, sulfonamides, telithromycin, tocilizumab, and zafirlukast, as well as a variety of alternative remedies (eg, black cohosh, chaparral, garcinia cambogia, germander, green tea extract, Herbalife products, Hydroxycut, jin bu huan, kava, saw palmetto, skullcap, usnic acid, and other traditional Chinese herbal preparations), in addition to dietary supplements (eg, 1,3-dimethylamylamine in OxyELITE Pro, a weight loss supplement withdrawn from the US market).

C. Other Reactions

1. Fatty liver—

A. MACROVESICULAR—This type of liver injury may be produced by alcohol, amiodarone, corticosteroids, haloperidol, irinotecan, lomitapide, methotrexate, mipomersen, tamoxifen, vinyl chloride (in exposed workers), zalcitabine, and possibly oxaliplatin.

B. MICROVESICULAR—Often resulting from mitochondrial injury, microvesicular steatosis is associated with aspirin (Reye syndrome), didanosine, linezolid, stavudine, tetracyclines, valproic acid, and zidovudine.

2. Granulomas—Allopurinol, hydralazine, pembrolizumab and other immune checkpoint inhibitors, phenytoin, pyrazinamide, quinidine, quinine, sulfasalazine, and vemurafenib can lead to granulomas and, in some cases, granulomatous hepatitis.

3. Fibrosis and cirrhosis—Methotrexate and vitamin A are associated with fibrosis and cirrhosis.

4. Sinusoidal obstruction syndrome (veno-occlusive disease)—This disorder may result from treatment with antineoplastic agents (eg, pre–bone marrow transplant, busulfan, gemtuzumab ozogamicin, inotuzumab ozogamicin, oxaliplatin), mycophenolate mofetil, and pyrrolizidine alkaloids (eg, comfrey).

5. Peliosis hepatis (blood-filled cavities)—Peliosis hepatis may be caused by anabolic steroids and oral contraceptive steroids as well as azathioprine and mercaptopurine, which may also cause nodular regenerative hyperplasia and other forms of liver injury.

6. Nodular regenerative hyperplasia—Nodular regenerative hyperplasia may be caused by azathioprine, 5-fluorouracil, oxaliplatin, and thioguanine.

7. Neoplasms—Neoplasms may result from therapy with oral contraceptive steroids, including estrogens (hepatic adenoma but not focal nodular hyperplasia) and vinyl chloride (angiosarcoma).

When to Refer

Refer patients with drug- and toxin-induced hepatitis who require liver biopsy for diagnosis.

When to Admit

Patients with liver failure should be hospitalized.

Chalasani NP et al. ACG Clinical Guideline: diagnosis and management of idiosyncratic drug-induced liver injury. Am J Gastroenterol. 2021;116:878. [PMID: 33929376]

Dougan M et al. AGA Clinical Practice Update on diagnosis and management of immune checkpoint inhibitor colitis and hepatitis: expert review. Gastroenterology. 2021;160:1384. [PMID: 33080231]

Gholam PM (editor). Drug hepatotoxicity. Clin Liver Dis 2020;24:1. [Full issue]

Hoofnagle JH et al. Drug-induced liver injury—types and phenotypes. N Engl J Med. 2019;381:264. [PMID: 31314970]

National Institute of Diabetes and Digestive and Kidney Diseases. LiverTox. 2021 Dec 21. https://livertox.nih.gov

NONALCOHOLIC FATTY LIVER DISEASE

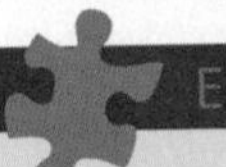

ESSENTIALS OF DIAGNOSIS

- Often asymptomatic.
- Elevated aminotransferase levels, hepatomegaly, or steatosis on ultrasonography.
- Predominantly macrovesicular steatosis with or without inflammation and fibrosis on liver biopsy.

General Considerations

NAFLD is estimated to affect 37% of the US adult population and has increased in incidence at least fivefold since the late 1990s. Even adolescents and young adults may be affected. The principal causes of NAFLD are obesity (present in 40% or more of affected patients), diabetes mellitus (in 20% or more), and hypertriglyceridemia (in 20% or more) in association with insulin resistance as part of the metabolic syndrome. In fact, the alternative designation "metabolic-associated (or metabolic dysfunction-associated) fatty liver disease" (MAFLD) has been proposed. The risk of NAFLD in persons with metabolic syndrome is 4 to 11 times higher than that of persons without insulin resistance. Nonobese persons (more frequently Asians) account for 10–20% of persons with NAFLD and have metabolic profiles characteristic of insulin resistance. Other causes of fatty liver include corticosteroids, amiodarone, diltiazem, methotrexate, tamoxifen, irinotecan, oxaliplatin, antiretroviral therapy, toxins (vinyl chloride, carbon tetrachloride, yellow phosphorus), endocrinopathies such as Cushing syndrome and hypopituitarism, polycystic ovary syndrome, hypothyroidism, hypobetalipoproteinemia and other metabolic disorders, obstructive sleep apnea (with chronic intermittent hypoxia), excessive dietary fructose consumption, malnutrition, starvation and refeeding syndrome, and total parenteral nutrition. NAFLD may be a predisposing factor in liver injury caused by some drugs. The risk of NAFLD is increased in persons with psoriasis and appears to correlate with the activity of psoriasis. Soft drink consumption and cholecystectomy have been reported to be associated with NAFLD. Physical activity protects against the development of NAFLD.

In addition to macrovesicular steatosis, histologic features may include focal infiltration by polymorphonuclear neutrophils and Mallory hyalin, a picture indistinguishable from that of alcohol-associated hepatitis and referred to as nonalcoholic steatohepatitis (NASH), which affects 3–6% of the US population and leads to cirrhosis in approximately 20% of affected persons. In patients with NAFLD, older age, obesity, and diabetes mellitus are risk factors for advanced hepatic fibrosis and cirrhosis, whereas coffee consumption reduces the risk. The frequency and severity of NAFLD is greater in men than in women during reproductive age, but after menopause the frequency is higher in women than men, suggesting that estrogen is protective. However, in women, synthetic hormone use (oral contraceptives and hormone replacement therapy) increases the histologic severity of NASH. Cirrhosis caused by NASH appears to be uncommon in Black persons. Persons with NAFLD are at increased risk for CVD, CKD, and colorectal cancer.

Microvesicular steatosis is seen with Reye syndrome, with toxicity caused by didanosine, stavudine, linezolid, valproic acid, or high-dose tetracycline, and with acute fatty liver of pregnancy and may result in acute liver failure.

Clinical Findings

A. Symptoms and Signs

Most patients with NAFLD are asymptomatic or have mild right upper quadrant discomfort. Hepatomegaly is present in up to 75% of patients, but stigmata of chronic liver disease are uncommon. Signs of portal hypertension generally signify advanced liver fibrosis or cirrhosis, but occasionally occur in patients with mild or no fibrosis and severe steatosis.

B. Laboratory Findings

Laboratory studies may show mildly elevated aminotransferase and alkaline phosphatase levels; however, laboratory values may be normal in up to 80% of persons with hepatic steatosis. In contrast to alcohol-associated liver disease, the ratio of ALT to AST is almost always greater than 1.0 in NAFLD, but it decreases, often to less than 1.0, as advanced fibrosis and cirrhosis develop. Antinuclear or smooth muscle antibodies and an elevated serum ferritin level may each be detected in 30% of patients with NASH. Iron deficiency is also common and associated with female sex, obesity, increased waist circumference, diabetes mellitus, and persons who are Black or Native Americans.

C. Imaging

Macrovascular steatosis may be demonstrated on ultrasonography, CT, or MRI. However, imaging does not distinguish steatosis from steatohepatitis or detect fibrosis. Where available, MRI-proton density fat fraction or magnetic resonance spectroscopy allows hepatic fat content to be quantitated and appears to correlate with the risk of fibrosis progression; ultrasound or magnetic resonance elastography to assess liver stiffness can be used to estimate hepatic fibrosis.

D. Liver Biopsy and Risk Scores

Percutaneous liver biopsy is diagnostic and has been the standard approach to assessing the degree of inflammation and fibrosis. The risks of the procedure must be balanced against the impact of the added information on management decisions and assessment of prognosis. Liver biopsy is generally not recommended in asymptomatic persons with unsuspected hepatic steatosis detected on imaging but normal liver biochemistry test results. The histologic spectrum of NAFLD includes fatty liver, isolated portal fibrosis, steatohepatitis, and cirrhosis. Noninvasive approaches to the assessment of fibrosis are now preferred, with liver biopsy reserved when results of noninvasive testing are inconclusive. The FIB-4 score is often used particularly to exclude advanced fibrosis because of its simplicity. It is based on age, platelet count, and serum AST and ALT levels. A risk score for predicting advanced fibrosis, known as BARD, is based on BMI more than 28, AST/ALT ratio 0.8 or more, and diabetes mellitus; it has a high negative predictive value (ie, a low score reliably excludes advanced fibrosis). Another risk score for advanced fibrosis, the NAFLD Fibrosis Score (http://nafldscore.com) based on age, hyperglycemia, BMI, platelet count, albumin, and AST/ALT ratio, has a positive predictive value of over 80% and identifies patients at increased risk for liver-related complications and death. A clinical scoring system to predict the likelihood of NASH in morbidly obese persons includes six predictive factors: hypertension, type 2 diabetes mellitus, sleep apnea, AST greater than 27 U/L

(0.54 mckat/L), ALT greater than 27 U/L (0.54 mckat/L), and persons who are not Black. The role of liver stiffness measurement by elastography to assess the fibrosis stage continues to evolve; in general, results are less accurate in obese than in nonobese persons.

Treatment

Treatment consists of lifestyle changes to remove or modify the offending factors often in the context of a multidisciplinary clinic. Weight loss, dietary fructose restriction, increased dietary fiber, and moderate exercise (through reduction of abdominal obesity) often lead to improvement in liver biochemical tests and steatosis in obese patients with NAFLD. A Mediterranean diet can reduce liver fat without weight loss and is often recommended. Loss of 5% of body weight appears necessary to improve steatosis, loss of greater than or equal to 7% improves steatohepatitis, and loss of greater than or equal to 10% improves fibrosis. Exercise may reduce liver fat with minimal or no weight loss and no reduction in ALT levels. Resistance training and aerobic exercise are equally effective in reducing hepatic fat content in patients with NAFLD and type 2 diabetes mellitus. Although avoidance of alcohol is recommended, modest wine consumption may not be detrimental in nonsmokers. Various drugs for the treatment of NASH are under study. Vitamin E 800 IU/day (to reduce oxidative stress) appears to be of benefit in patients with NASH who do not have diabetes mellitus. There is controversy as to whether vitamin E increases the risk of prostate cancer in men and hemorrhagic stroke; moreover, the benefit is often not sustained. Thiazolidinediones reverse insulin resistance and, in most relevant studies, have improved both serum aminotransferase levels and histologic features of steatohepatitis but lead to weight gain. Metformin, which reduces insulin resistance, improves abnormal liver chemistries but may not reliably improve liver histology. Pentoxifylline improves liver biochemical test levels but is associated with a high rate of side effects, particularly nausea. Ursodeoxycholic acid, 12–15 mg/kg/day, has not consistently resulted in biochemical and histologic improvement in patients with NASH but may be effective when given in combination with vitamin E. Hepatic steatosis due to total parenteral nutrition may be ameliorated—and perhaps prevented—with supplemental choline. Obeticholic acid, a farnesoid X receptor agonist that has been approved for the treatment of PBC, has been shown to improve liver fibrosis in patients with NASH. Statins are not contraindicated in persons with NAFLD and may protect against histologic progression in some patients. Bariatric surgery may be considered in patients with a BMI greater than 35 and leads to histologic regression of NASH in most patients (but worsening in a few). Liver transplantation is indicated in appropriate candidates with advanced cirrhosis caused by NASH, the third most common (and most rapidly increasing) indication for liver transplantation in the United States. Liver transplantation for NASH with advanced cirrhosis may be associated with increased mortality from CVD and sepsis compared with liver transplantation for other indications.

Prognosis

Fatty liver often has a benign course and is readily reversible with discontinuation of alcohol (or no more than one glass of wine per day, which has been reported in some, but not other, studies to reduce the frequency of NASH in persons with NAFLD), or treatment of other underlying conditions; if untreated, fibrosis progresses at an average rate of one stage every 14 years, with 20% of patients progressing more rapidly. In patients with NAFLD, the likelihood of NASH is increased by the following factors: obesity, older age, ethnicity other than Black, female sex, diabetes mellitus, hypertension, higher ALT or AST level, higher AST/ALT ratio, low platelet count, elevated fasting C-peptide level, and a high ultrasound steatosis score. NASH may be associated with hepatic fibrosis in 40% of cases with progression at a rate of one stage every 7 years; cirrhosis develops in 9–25%; and decompensated cirrhosis occurs in 30–50% of cirrhotic patients over 10 years. The course may be more aggressive in diabetic persons than in nondiabetic persons. In the United States, NAFLD is associated with 8% of all-cause mortality and more than one-third of deaths associated with liver disease and with diabetes mellitus. Risk factors for fibrosis in patients with fatty liver without NASH are severe steatosis and the I148M variant of the *PNPLA3* gene. Heterozygous alpha-1-antitrypsin deficiency also appears to be a risk factor for fibrosis in patients with NASH. Mortality is increased in patients with NAFLD, correlates with fibrosis stage, and is the result of CVD and malignancy (including hepatocellular carcinoma, colorectal cancer, and breast cancer) as well as liver disease. Risk factors for mortality are older age, male sex, White race, the I148M variant of the *PNPLA3* gene, smoking, higher BMI, hypertension, diabetes mellitus, and advanced fibrosis stage. In the general population, in fact, both excess adiposity and reduced activity are significant predictors of liver-related mortality. Steatosis is a cofactor for the progression of fibrosis in patients with other causes of chronic liver disease, such as hepatitis C, and NAFLD appears to be a risk factor for CKD. Hepatocellular carcinoma is a complication of cirrhosis caused by NASH, as it is for other causes of cirrhosis, and has been reported even in the absence of cirrhosis. NASH accounts for a substantial percentage of cases labeled as cryptogenic cirrhosis and can recur following liver transplantation. Central obesity is an independent risk factor for death from cirrhosis of any cause.

When to Refer

Refer patients with NAFLD who require liver biopsy for diagnosis and those with evidence of advanced fibrosis for management.

Kim D et al. Physical activity, measured objectively, is associated with lower mortality in patients with nonalcoholic fatty liver disease. Clin Gastroenterol Hepatol. 2021;19:1240. [PMID: 32683103]

Liebe R et al. Diagnosis and management of secondary causes of steatohepatitis. J Hepatol. 2021;74:1455. [PMID: 33577920]

Powell EE et al. Non-alcoholic fatty liver disease. Lancet. 2021;397:2212. [PMID: 33894145]

Younossi ZM et al. AGA Clinical Practice Update on lifestyle modification using diet and exercise to achieve weight loss in the management of nonalcoholic fatty liver disease: expert review. Gastroenterology. 2021;160:912. [PMID: 33307021]

Younossi ZM et al. Role of noninvasive tests in clinical gastroenterology practices to identify patients with nonalcoholic steatohepatitis at high risk of adverse outcomes: expert panel recommendations. Am J Gastroenterol. 2021;116:254. [PMID: 33284184]

CIRRHOSIS

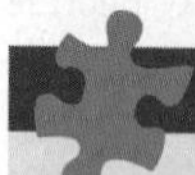

ESSENTIALS OF DIAGNOSIS

- Result of injury that leads to both fibrosis and regenerative nodules.
- May be reversible if cause is removed.
- The clinical features result from hepatic cell dysfunction, portosystemic shunting, and portal hypertension.

General Considerations

Cirrhosis is the result of hepatocellular injury with inflammation that leads to both fibrosis and regenerative nodules throughout the liver. The prevalence rate is 0.27%, with an estimated 1.5 billion persons having chronic liver disease and 2.14 million liver-related deaths worldwide. Hospitalization rates for cirrhosis and portal hypertension are rising in the United States, and patients with chronic liver disease have longer hospital stays, more readmissions, and less access to post-acute care than patients with other chronic diseases. Causes include chronic viral hepatitis; alcohol; drug toxicity; autoimmune and metabolic liver diseases, including NAFLD; and miscellaneous disorders. Celiac disease appears to be associated with an increased risk of cirrhosis. Many patients have more than one risk factor (eg, chronic hepatitis and alcohol use) and likely genetic predisposition. Mexican American and Black persons have a higher frequency of cirrhosis than White persons because of a higher rate of risk factors. In persons at increased risk for liver injury (eg, heavy alcohol use, obesity, iron overload), higher coffee and tea consumption and statin use reduce the risk of cirrhosis.

Clinically, cirrhosis is considered to progress through three stages that correlate with the thickness of fibrous septa: compensated, compensated with varices, and decompensated (ascites, variceal bleeding, encephalopathy, or jaundice).

A diagnosis of acute-on-chronic liver failure should be made in a patient with cirrhosis and acute decompensation (new or worsening ascites, GI hemorrhage, overt encephalopathy, worsening nonobstructive jaundice, or bacterial infection associated with other organ failure). Precipitating factors include infections, hemodynamic instability, heavy alcohol use, and drug hepatotoxicity.

Clinical Findings

A. Symptoms and Signs

The clinical features of cirrhosis result from hepatocyte dysfunction, portosystemic shunting, and portal hypertension. Patients may have no symptoms for long periods. The onset of symptoms may be insidious or, less often, abrupt. Fatigue, disturbed sleep, muscle cramps, and weight loss are common. In advanced cirrhosis, anorexia is usually present and may be extreme, with associated nausea and occasional vomiting, as well as reduced muscle strength and exercise capacity. Abdominal pain may be present and is related either to hepatic enlargement and stretching of Glisson capsule or to the presence of ascites. Abdominal wall hernias occur in 20% of persons with cirrhosis. Menstrual abnormalities (usually amenorrhea), erectile dysfunction, loss of libido, sterility, and gynecomastia may occur. Hematemesis is the presenting symptom in 15–25%. The risk of falls is increased in patients with cirrhosis and the falls are associated with mortality.

Skin manifestations consist of spider telangiectasias (invariably on the upper half of the body), palmar erythema (mottled redness of the thenar and hypothenar eminences), Dupuytren contractures, and Terry nails. Evidence of vitamin deficiencies (glossitis and cheilosis) is common. Weight loss, wasting (due to sarcopenia), and the appearance of chronic illness are present in advanced cirrhosis. Jaundice—usually not an initial sign—is mild at first, increasing in severity during the later stages of the disease. In 70% of cases, the liver is enlarged, palpable, and firm if not hard and has a sharp or nodular edge; the left lobe may predominate. Splenomegaly is present in 35–50% of cases and is associated with an increased risk of complications of portal hypertension. The superficial veins of the abdomen and thorax are dilated, reflecting the intrahepatic obstruction to portal blood flow, as do rectal varices. The abdominal wall veins fill from below when compressed. Ascites, pleural effusions, peripheral edema, and ecchymoses are late findings. Ascites is classified as grade 1, or mild, when it is detectable only by ultrasound; grade 2, or moderate, when associated with symmetrical abdominal distention; and grade 3, or gross, when associated with marked abdominal distention. Encephalopathy, characterized by day-night reversal, asterixis, tremor, dysarthria, delirium, drowsiness, and, ultimately, coma, also occurs late in the course except when precipitated by an acute hepatocellular insult or an episode of GI bleeding or infection. Fever is present in up to 35% of patients and usually reflects associated alcohol-associated hepatitis, spontaneous bacterial peritonitis, or another intercurrent infection.

B. Laboratory Findings

Laboratory abnormalities are either absent or minimal in early or compensated cirrhosis. Anemia, a frequent finding, is often macrocytic; causes include suppression of erythropoiesis by alcohol as well as folate deficiency, hemolysis, hypersplenism, and occult or overt blood loss from the GI tract. The WBC count may be low, reflecting hypersplenism, or high, suggesting infection. Thrombocytopenia, the most common cytopenia in cirrhotic patients, is secondary to alcohol-induced marrow suppression, sepsis, folate deficiency, or splenic sequestration. Prolongation of the prothrombin time may result from reduced levels of clotting factors (except factor VIII). However, bleeding risk correlates poorly with the prothrombin time because of concomitant abnormalities of fibrinolysis, and among hospitalized patients under age 45, cirrhosis is associated with an increased risk of venous thromboembolism.

Blood chemistries reflect hepatocellular injury and dysfunction, manifested by modest elevations of AST and alkaline phosphatase and progressive elevation of the bilirubin. Serum albumin decreases as the disease progresses; gamma-globulin levels are increased and may be as high as in autoimmune hepatitis. The risk of diabetes mellitus is increased in patients with cirrhosis, particularly when associated with HCV infection, alcoholism, hemochromatosis, or NAFLD. Vitamin D deficiency has been reported in as many as 91% of patients with cirrhosis. In cirrhosis of all causes, the following are common: (1) blunted cardiac inotropic and chronotropic responses to exercise, stress, and drugs, (2) prolongation of the QT interval in the setting of a hyperkinetic circulation, and (3) systolic and diastolic ventricular dysfunction in the absence of other known causes of cardiac disease ("cirrhotic cardiomyopathy"). Relative adrenal insufficiency appears to be common in patients with advanced cirrhosis, even in the absence of sepsis, and in those with acute-on-chronic liver failure.

C. Imaging

Ultrasonography is helpful for assessing liver size and detecting ascites or hepatic nodules, including small hepatocellular carcinomas. Together with a Doppler study, it may establish patency of the splenic, portal, and hepatic veins. Hepatic nodules are characterized further by contrast-enhanced CT or MRI. Nodules indeterminant for malignancy may be biopsied under ultrasound or CT guidance.

D. Liver Biopsy

Liver biopsy may show inactive cirrhosis (fibrosis with regenerative nodules) with no specific features to suggest the underlying cause. Alternatively, there may be additional features of alcohol-associated liver disease, chronic hepatitis, NASH, or other specific causes of cirrhosis. Liver biopsy may be performed by laparoscopy or, in patients with coagulopathy and ascites, by a transjugular or endoscopic ultrasonographic approach. Combinations of routine blood tests (eg, AST, platelet count), including the FibroSure test, serum markers of hepatic fibrosis (eg, hyaluronic acid, amino-terminal propeptide of type III collagen, tissue inhibitor of matrix metalloproteinase 1), and ultrasound or magnetic resonance elastography are potential alternatives to liver biopsy for the diagnosis or exclusion of cirrhosis. In persons with chronic hepatitis C, for example, a low FibroSure or elastography score reliably excludes advanced fibrosis, a high score reliably predicts advanced fibrosis, and intermediate scores are inconclusive. The combination of increased liver stiffness and a platelet count below 150,000/mcL (150×10^9/L) is an indicator of clinically significant portal hypertension.

E. Other Tests

Esophagogastroduodenoscopy confirms the presence of varices and detects specific causes of bleeding in the esophagus, stomach, and proximal duodenum. In selected cases, wedged hepatic vein pressure measurement may establish the presence and cause of portal hypertension.

Differential Diagnosis

The most common causes of cirrhosis are alcohol, chronic hepatitis C infection, NAFLD, and hepatitis B infection. Hemochromatosis is the most commonly identified genetic disorder that causes cirrhosis. Other diseases associated with cirrhosis include Wilson disease, alpha-1-antitrypsin (alpha-1-antiprotease) deficiency, and celiac disease. PBC occurs more frequently in women than men. Secondary biliary cirrhosis may result from chronic biliary obstruction due to a stone, stricture, or neoplasm. Heart failure and constrictive pericarditis may lead to hepatic fibrosis ("cardiac cirrhosis") complicated by ascites. Hereditary hemorrhagic telangiectasia can lead to portal hypertension because of portosystemic shunting and nodular transformation of the liver as well as high-output heart failure. Many cases of cirrhosis are "cryptogenic," in which unrecognized NAFLD may play a role.

Complications

Upper GI tract bleeding may occur from varices, portal hypertensive gastropathy, or gastroduodenal ulcer (see Chapter 15). Varices may also result from portal vein thrombosis, which may complicate cirrhosis. Liver failure may be precipitated by alcoholism, surgery, and infection. Hepatic Kupffer cell (reticuloendothelial) dysfunction and decreased opsonic activity lead to an increased risk of systemic infection (which may be increased further by the use of PPIs, which increase mortality fourfold). These infections include nosocomial infections, which may be classified as spontaneous bloodstream infections, UTIs, pulmonary infections, spontaneous bacterial peritonitis, *Clostridioides difficile* infection, and intervention-related infections. These nosocomial infections are increasingly caused by multidrug-resistant bacteria. Osteoporosis occurs in 12–55% of patients with cirrhosis. The risk of hepatocellular carcinoma is increased greatly in persons with cirrhosis (see Chapter 39). Varices, ascites, and encephalopathy may arise when there is clinically significant portal hypertension (hepatic venous pressure gradient greater than 10 mm Hg).

Treatment

A. General Measures

Most important is abstinence from alcohol. The diet should be palatable, with adequate calories (20–40 kcal/kg body weight per day depending on the patient's BMI and the presence or absence of malnutrition) and protein (1.2–1.5 g/kg/day depending on the presence or absence of malnutrition) and, if there is fluid retention, sodium restriction. In the presence of hepatic encephalopathy, protein intake should be reduced to no less than 60–80 g/day.

Vitamin supplementation is desirable. Muscle cramps may be helped by L-carnitine, 300 mg orally four times a day, calcium, quinidine, baclofen, muscle relaxants, or intravenous albumin. In patients with clinically significant portal hypertension, carvedilol, a nonselective beta receptor antagonist with alpha-1 blocking activity, appears to reduce the frequency of decompensating events, although it may lead to hypotension particularly in patients with decompensated cirrhosis. Patients with cirrhosis should receive the HAV, HBV, pneumococcal, and COVID-19 vaccines and a yearly influenza vaccine. Liver transplantation in appropriate candidates is curative. Care coordination and palliative care, when appropriate, have been shown to improve outcomes and reduce readmission rates.

B. Treatment of Complications

1. Ascites and edema—Diagnostic paracentesis is indicated for patients who have new ascites or who have been hospitalized for a complication of cirrhosis; it reduces mortality, especially if performed within 12 hours of admission. Serious complications of paracentesis, including bleeding, infection, or bowel perforation, occur in 1.6% of procedures and are associated with therapeutic (vs diagnostic) paracentesis and possibly with Child-Pugh class C, a platelet count less than 50,000/mcL (50×10^9/L), and alcohol-associated cirrhosis. In patients with coagulopathy, however, pre-paracentesis prophylactic transfusions are not necessary. In addition to a cell count and culture, the ascitic albumin level should be determined: a serum-ascites albumin gradient (serum albumin minus ascitic fluid albumin) greater than or equal to 1.1 suggests portal hypertension. An elevated ascitic adenosine deaminase level is suggestive of tuberculous peritonitis, but the sensitivity of the test is reduced in patients with portal hypertension. Occasionally, cirrhotic ascites is chylous (rich in triglycerides); other causes of chylous ascites are malignancy, tuberculosis, and recent abdominal surgery or trauma.

In individuals with ascites, the urinary sodium concentration is often less than 10 mEq/L (10 mmol/L). Free water excretion is also impaired in cirrhosis, and hyponatremia may develop.

In all patients with cirrhotic ascites, dietary sodium intake may initially be restricted to 2000 mg/day; the intake of sodium may be liberalized slightly after diuresis ensues. NSAIDs are contraindicated, and aminoglycosides, ACE inhibitors, and angiotensin II antagonists should be avoided. In some patients, ascites diminishes promptly with bed rest and dietary sodium restriction alone. Fluid intake is often restricted (to 800–1000 mL/day) in patients with hyponatremia. Treatment of severe hyponatremia (serum sodium less than 120 mEq/L [120 mmol/L]) with vasopressin receptor antagonists (eg, intravenous conivaptan, 20 mg daily) can be considered, but such treatment is expensive, causes thirst, and does not improve survival; oral tolvaptan is contraindicated in patients with liver disease because of potential hepatotoxicity. Long-term intravenous administration of albumin has been reported to improve 18-month survival in patients with cirrhotic ascites.

A. Diuretics—Spironolactone, generally in combination with furosemide, should be used in patients who do not respond to salt restriction alone. The dose of spironolactone is initially 100 mg orally daily and may be increased by 100 mg every 3–5 days (up to a maximal conventional daily dose of 400 mg/day, although higher doses have been used) until diuresis is achieved, typically preceded by a rise in the urinary sodium concentration. A "spot" urine sodium concentration that exceeds the potassium concentration correlates with a 24-hour sodium excretion greater than 78 mmol/day, which predicts diuresis in patients adherent to a salt-restricted diet. Monitoring for hyperkalemia is important. In patients who cannot tolerate spironolactone because of side effects, such as painful gynecomastia, amiloride (another potassium-sparing diuretic) may be used in a starting dose of 5–10 mg orally daily. Diuresis is augmented by the addition of a loop diuretic such as furosemide. This potent diuretic, however, will maintain its effect even with a falling GFR, with resulting prerenal azotemia. The dose of oral furosemide is increased in concert with spironolactone and ranges from 40 mg/day to 160 mg/day, and blood pressure, urinary output, mental status, and serum electrolytes (especially potassium) should be monitored in patients taking the drug. The goal of weight loss in the ascitic patient without associated peripheral edema should be no more than 1–1.5 lb/day (0.5–0.7 kg/day).

B. Large-volume paracentesis—In patients with massive ascites and respiratory compromise, ascites which is refractory to diuretics ("diuretic resistant"), or which produces intolerable diuretic side effects ("diuretic intractable") (affecting 5–10% of patients with cirrhosis and ascites), large-volume paracentesis (more than 5 L) is effective. Intravenous albumin concomitantly at a dosage of 6–8 g/L of ascites fluid removed protects the intravascular volume and may prevent post-paracentesis circulatory dysfunction, although the usefulness of this practice is debated and albumin is expensive. Large-volume paracentesis can be repeated daily until ascites is largely resolved and may decrease the need for hospitalization. If possible, diuretics should be continued in the hope of preventing recurrent ascites.

C. Transjugular intrahepatic portosystemic shunt (TIPS)—TIPS is an effective treatment of variceal bleeding refractory to standard therapy (eg, endoscopic band ligation) and has shown benefit in the treatment of severe refractory ascites, specifically in patients on maximum diuretic therapy who require at least three large-volume paracenteses per year. The technique involves insertion of an expandable metal stent between a branch of the hepatic vein and the portal vein over a catheter inserted via the internal jugular vein. Increased renal sodium excretion and control of ascites refractory to diuretics can be achieved in about 75% of selected cases. The success rate is lower in patients with underlying CKD. TIPS may be considered for refractory hepatic hydrothorax (translocation of ascites across the diaphragm to the pleural space); video-assisted thoracoscopy with pleurodesis using talc may be effective when TIPS is contraindicated. Complications of

TIPS include hepatic encephalopathy in 20–30% of cases, infection, shunt stenosis in up to 60% of cases, and shunt occlusion in up to 30% of cases when bare stents are used; polytetrafluoroethylene-covered stents are associated with long-term patency rates of 80–90%. Long-term patency often requires periodic shunt revisions. In most cases, patency can be maintained by balloon dilation, local thrombolysis, or placement of an additional stent. TIPS is particularly useful in patients who require short-term control of variceal bleeding or ascites until liver transplantation can be performed. In patients with refractory ascites, TIPS results in lower rates of ascites recurrence and hepatorenal syndrome but a higher rate of hepatic encephalopathy (the frequency of which is reduced with prophylactic rifaximin) than occurs with repeated large-volume paracentesis; benefits to sarcopenia and to survival have been demonstrated. CKD, diastolic cardiac dysfunction, refractory encephalopathy, and hyperbilirubinemia (greater than 5 mg/dL [85.5 mcmol/L]) are associated with mortality after TIPS, and patients with a serum bilirubin greater than 3 mg/dL (50 mcmol/L), platelets less than 75,000/mcL (75×10^9/L), preexisting encephalopathy, active infection, severe heart failure, or severe pulmonary hypertension may not benefit from TIPS.

2. Spontaneous bacterial peritonitis—Spontaneous bacterial peritonitis is heralded by abdominal pain, increasing ascites, fever, and progressive encephalopathy in a patient with cirrhotic ascites; symptoms are typically mild. (Analogously, spontaneous bacterial empyema may complicate hepatic hydrothorax and is managed similarly.) Risk factors in cirrhotic patients with ascites include gastroesophageal variceal bleeding and possibly use of a PPI. Paracentesis reveals an ascitic fluid with, most commonly, a total white cell count of up to 500 cells/mcL (0.5×10^9/L) with a high polymorphonuclear (PMN) cell count (250/mcL [0.25×10^9/L] or more) and a protein concentration of 1 g/dL (10 g/L) or less. Cultures of ascites give the highest yield—80–90% positive—when specialized culture bottles are inoculated at the bedside. Common isolates are *Escherichia coli* and *Streptococcus* spp. Gram-positive cocci are the most common isolates in patients who have undergone an invasive procedure such as central venous line placement, and the frequency of enterococcal isolates is increasing. Anaerobes are uncommon. Pending culture results, if there are 250 or more PMNs/mcL or symptoms or signs of infection, intravenous antibiotic therapy should be initiated with cefotaxime, 2 g every 8–12 hours for at least 5 days. Alternative choices include ceftriaxone, amoxicillin-clavulanic acid, and levofloxacin (in patients not receiving fluoroquinolone prophylaxis). Oral ofloxacin, 400 mg twice daily for 7 days, or, in a patient not already taking a fluoroquinolone for prophylaxis against bacterial peritonitis, a 2-day course of intravenous ciprofloxacin, 200 mg twice daily, followed by oral ciprofloxacin, 500 mg twice daily for 5 days, may be effective alternative regimens in selected patients. Piperacillin-tazobactam is recommended for patients with risk factors for multidrug-resistant organisms, including hospital-acquired spontaneous bacterial peritonitis, and specific therapy should be guided by local resistance patterns. Vancomycin should be added in patients with prior bacterial peritonitis or a positive surveillance swab for methicillin-resistant *Staphylococcus aureus*. Daptomycin should be added in patients with a positive surveillance swab for vancomycin-resistant enterococcus. Meropenem can be used in patients with current or recent exposure to piperacillin-tazobactam. In patients with spontaneous bacterial peritonitis in the setting of acute-on-chronic liver failure, treatment with meropenem and daptomycin is recommended. Supplemental administration of intravenous albumin, 1.5 g/kg at diagnosis and 1 g/kg on day 3 (which may have anti-inflammatory effects in addition to expanding plasma volume), prevents further renal impairment and reduces mortality, particularly in patients with a serum creatinine greater than 1 mg/dL (83.3 mcmol/L), BUN greater than 30 mg/dL (10.8 mmol/L), or total bilirubin greater than 4 mg/dL (68.4 mcmol/L). Nonselective beta-blockers should be held in patients who develop hypotension (mean arterial pressure less than 65 mm Hg) or AKI. Given the increasing failure of initial empiric antibiotic therapy, response to therapy should be documented by a decrease in the PMN count of at least 25% on repeat paracentesis 48 hours after initiation of therapy. The overall mortality rate is high—up to 30% during hospitalization and up to 70% by 1 year. Mortality may be predicted by the 22/11 model: MELD score greater than 22 and peripheral WBC count higher than 11,000/mcL (11×10^9/L). Another model predictive of mortality includes the BUN, WBC count, Child-Pugh score, and mean arterial pressure. Patients with cirrhosis and septic shock have a high frequency of relative adrenal insufficiency, which if present requires administration of hydrocortisone.

In survivors of bacterial peritonitis, the risk of recurrent peritonitis may be decreased by long-term ciprofloxacin (eg, 500 mg orally once per day), norfloxacin (400 mg orally daily; no longer available in the United States), or trimethoprim-sulfamethoxazole (eg, one double-strength tablet once per day). In cases of recurrent peritonitis, the causative organism is often resistant to fluoroquinolones and may become multidrug resistant in some cases. In high-risk cirrhotic patients without prior peritonitis (eg, those with an ascitic protein less than 1.5 g/dL and serum bilirubin greater than 3 mg/dL (51.3 mcmol/L), serum creatinine greater than 1.2 mg/dL (99.96 mcmol/L), BUN 25 mg/dL (9 mmol/L) or more, sodium 130 mEq/L (130 mmol/L) or less, or Child-Pugh score of 9 or more, the risk of peritonitis, hepatorenal syndrome, and mortality for at least 1 year may be reduced by prophylactic trimethoprim-sulfamethoxazole, one double-strength tablet once per day, ciprofloxacin, 500 mg once per day, or norfloxacin, 400 mg orally once a day (though not in the United States). In patients hospitalized for acute variceal bleeding, intravenous ceftriaxone (1 g per day), followed by oral trimethoprim-sulfamethoxazole (one double-strength tablet once per day) or ciprofloxacin (500 mg every 12 hours), for a total of 7 days, reduces the risk of bacterial peritonitis.

3. Hepatorenal syndrome—Hepatorenal syndrome occurs in up to 10% of patients with advanced cirrhosis and ascites. It is characterized by azotemia (increase in serum creatinine level of greater than 0.3 mg/dL [26.5 mcmol/L]) within 48 hours or increase by 50% or more from baseline within the previous 7 days or a urine volume less than 0.5 mL/kg/hour for 6 hours or longer in the absence of (1) current or recent nephrotoxic drug use, (2) macroscopic signs of structural kidney injury, or (3) shock and failure of kidney function to improve following 2 days of diuretic withdrawal and volume expansion with albumin, 1 g/kg up to a maximum of 100 g/day. Oliguria, hyponatremia, and a low urinary sodium concentration are typical features. Hepatorenal syndrome is diagnosed only when other causes of acute kidney injury (including prerenal azotemia and ATN) have been excluded. AKI-hepatorenal syndrome (formerly type 1 hepatorenal syndrome) is typically associated with at least doubling of the serum creatinine to a level greater than 2.5 mg/dL (208.25 mcmol/L) or by halving of the creatinine clearance to less than 20 mL/minute (0.34 mL/s/1.73 m^2 BSA) in less than 2 weeks. CKD (or non-AKI)-hepatorenal syndrome (formerly type 2 hepatorenal syndrome) is more slowly progressive and chronic. An acute decrease in cardiac output is often the precipitant.

In addition to discontinuation of diuretics, clinical improvement and an increase in short-term survival may follow one of the following regimens for 7–14 days: (1) intravenous terlipressin (not yet approved by the US FDA, though elsewhere it remains the preferred agent where available) or (2) intravenous norepinephrine plus intravenous albumin 1 g/kg on day 1 followed by 40–50 g/day for the duration of therapy. (3) Oral midodrine plus octreotide, subcutaneously or intravenously, is less effective than terlipressin. Oral midodrine, 7.5 mg three times daily, added to diuretics, increases the blood pressure and has been reported to convert refractory ascites to diuretic-sensitive ascites. (4) Prolongation of survival has been associated with use of MARS (Molecular Adsorbent Recirculating System), a modified dialysis method that selectively removes albumin-bound substances. (5) Improvement in kidney function may follow placement of a TIPS, although data are limited; survival after 1 year is reported to be predicted by the combination of a serum bilirubin level less than 3 mg/dL (50 mcmol/L) and a platelet count greater than 75,000/mcL (75×10^9/L).

Continuous venovenous hemofiltration and hemodialysis are of uncertain value in hepatorenal syndrome. Liver transplantation is the ultimate treatment of choice, but many patients die before a donor liver can be obtained. Mortality correlates with the MELD score and presence of a systemic inflammatory response. AKI-hepatorenal syndrome is often irreversible in patients with a systemic infection. The 3-month probability of survival in cirrhotic patients with hepatorenal syndrome (15%) is lower than that for renal failure associated with infections (31%), hypovolemia (46%), and parenchymal kidney disease (73%).

4. Hepatic encephalopathy—Hepatic encephalopathy is a state of disordered CNS function resulting from failure of the liver to detoxify noxious agents of gut origin because of hepatocellular dysfunction and portosystemic shunting. The clinical spectrum ranges from day-night reversal and mild intellectual impairment to coma. Patients with covert (formerly minimal) hepatic encephalopathy have no recognizable clinical symptoms but demonstrate mild cognitive, psychomotor, and attention deficits on standardized psychometric tests and an increased rate of traffic accidents. The stages of overt encephalopathy are (1) mild confusion, (2) drowsiness, (3) stupor, and (4) coma. A revised staging system known as SONIC (**S**pectrum **O**f **N**eurocognitive **I**mpairment in **C**irrhosis) encompasses absent, covert, and stages 2 to 4 encephalopathy. Ammonia is the most readily identified and measurable toxin but is not solely responsible for the disturbed mental status. Bleeding into the intestinal tract may significantly increase the amount of protein in the bowel and precipitate encephalopathy. Other precipitants include constipation, alkalosis, and potassium deficiency induced by diuretics, opioids, hypnotics, and sedatives; medications containing ammonium or amino compounds; paracentesis with consequent hypovolemia; hepatic or systemic infection; and portosystemic shunts (including TIPS). In one study, risk factors for hepatic encephalopathy in patients with cirrhosis included a higher serum bilirubin level and use of a nonselective beta-blocker, whereas a higher serum albumin level and use of a statin were protective. The diagnosis is based primarily on detection of characteristic symptoms and signs, including asterixis. A smartphone app called EncephalApp using the "Stroop test" (asking the patient to name the color of a written word rather than the word itself, even when the word is the name of a different color) has proved useful for detecting covert hepatic encephalopathy.

Oral protein intake is withheld during acute episodes if the patient cannot eat. When the patient resumes oral intake, protein intake should be 60–80 g/day as tolerated; vegetable protein is better tolerated than meat protein. GI bleeding should be controlled and blood purged from the GI tract. This can be accomplished with 120 mL of magnesium citrate by mouth or nasogastric tube every 3–4 hours until the stool is free of gross blood or by administration of lactulose. The value of treating patients with covert hepatic encephalopathy is uncertain; probiotic agents may have some benefit.

Lactulose, a nonabsorbable synthetic disaccharide syrup, is digested by bacteria in the colon to short-chain fatty acids, resulting in acidification of colon contents. This acidification favors the formation of ammonium ion in the $NH_4^+ \leftrightarrow NH_3 + H^+$ equation; NH_4^+ is not absorbable, whereas NH_3 is absorbable and thought to be neurotoxic. Lactulose also leads to a change in bowel flora so that fewer ammonia-forming organisms are present. When given orally, the initial dose of lactulose for acute hepatic encephalopathy is 30 mL three or four times daily. The dose should then be titrated so that the patient produces 2–3 soft stools per day. When given rectally because the patient is unable to take medicines orally, the dose is 200 g/300 mL given as a solution of lactulose in saline or sorbitol in a retention enema for 30–60 minutes; it may be repeated every 4–6 hours. Bowel cleansing with a polyethylene glycol colonoscopy preparation is also effective in patients with acute overt hepatic encephalopathy and may be preferable. Continued use of lactulose after an episode of acute encephalopathy reduces the frequency of recurrences.

The ammonia-producing intestinal flora may also be controlled with an oral antibiotic. The nonabsorbable agent rifaximin, 550 mg orally twice daily, is preferred and has been shown as well to maintain remission of and reduce the risk of rehospitalization for hepatic encephalopathy over a 24-month period, with or without the concomitant use of lactulose. Metronidazole, 250 mg orally three times daily, has also shown benefit. Patients who do not respond to lactulose alone may improve with an antibiotic added to treatment with lactulose.

Sodium benzoate, 5 g orally twice daily, ornithine aspartate, 9 g orally three times daily, and L-acyl-carnitine (an essential factor in the mitochondrial transport of long-chain fatty acids), 4 g orally daily, may lower blood ammonia levels, but there is less experience with these drugs than with lactulose. Flumazenil is effective in about 30% of patients with severe hepatic encephalopathy, but the drug is short-acting and intravenous administration is required. Use of special dietary supplements enriched with branched-chain amino acids is usually unnecessary except in occasional patients who are intolerant of standard protein supplements. Opioids and sedatives metabolized or excreted by the liver should be avoided. If agitation is marked, oxazepam, 10–30 mg, which is not metabolized by the liver, may be given cautiously by mouth or by nasogastric tube. Zinc deficiency should be corrected, if present, with oral zinc sulfate, 600 mg/day in divided doses.

5. Coagulopathy—Hypoprothrombinemia caused by malnutrition and vitamin K deficiency may be treated with vitamin K (eg, phytonadione, 5 mg orally or intravenously daily); however, this treatment is ineffective when synthesis of coagulation factors is impaired because of hepatic disease. In such cases, correcting the prolonged prothrombin time would require large volumes of fresh frozen plasma (see Chapter 14). Because the effect is transient, the value of plasma infusions, even for active bleeding or before an invasive procedure, has been questioned because of concomitant alterations in anti-hemostatic factors and because bleeding risk does not correlate with the INR. Recombinant activated factor VIIa may be an alternative but is expensive and poses a 1–2% risk of thrombotic complications. Bleeding risk in critically ill patients with cirrhosis has been shown to correlate with bleeding on hospital admission, a platelet count less than 30,000/mcL (30×10^9/L), a fibrinogen level less than 60 mg/dL (1.764 mcmol/L), and an activated partial thromboplastin time greater than 100 seconds. In patients with active bleeding or undergoing an invasive procedure, goals for management according to some guidelines include a hematocrit value greater than 25%, platelet count greater than 50,000/mcL (50×10^9/L), and fibrinogen level greater than 120 mg/dL (3.528 mcmol/L). A thrombopoietin analog, eg, avatrombopag or lusutrombopag, reduces the need for platelet transfusions in patients with cirrhosis and a platelet count less than 50,000/mcL (50×10^9/L) who undergo invasive procedures but must be administered for at least 3–5 days for the platelet count to start to rise.

6. Hemorrhage from esophageal varices—See Chapter 15.

7. Hepatopulmonary syndrome and portopulmonary hypertension—Shortness of breath in patients with cirrhosis may result from pulmonary restriction and atelectasis caused by massive ascites or hepatic hydrothorax. The hepatopulmonary syndrome—the triad of chronic liver disease, an increased alveolar-arterial gradient while the patient is breathing room air, and intrapulmonary vascular dilatations or arteriovenous communications that result in a right-to-left intrapulmonary shunt—occurs in 5–32% of patients with cirrhosis. Patients often have greater dyspnea (platypnea) and arterial deoxygenation (orthodeoxia) in the upright than in the recumbent position. The diagnosis should be suspected in a cirrhotic patient with a pulse oximetry level of 96% or lower.

Contrast-enhanced echocardiography is a sensitive screening test for detecting pulmonary vascular dilatations, whereas macroaggregated albumin lung perfusion scanning is more specific and may be used to confirm the diagnosis. High-resolution CT may be useful for detecting dilated pulmonary vessels that may be amenable to embolization in patients with severe hypoxemia (PO_2 less than 60 mm Hg [7.8 kPa]) who respond poorly to supplemental oxygen.

Medical therapy has been disappointing. Long-term oxygen therapy is recommended for severely hypoxemic patients. The syndrome may reverse with liver transplantation, although postoperative morbidity and mortality from severe hypoxemic respiratory failure are increased in patients with a preoperative arterial PO_2 less than 44 mm Hg (5.9 kPa) or with substantial intrapulmonary shunting. TIPS may provide palliation in patients with hepatopulmonary syndrome awaiting transplantation.

Portopulmonary hypertension occurs in 0.7% of patients with cirrhosis. Female sex, autoimmune hepatitis, and genetic variation in aromatase have been reported to be risk factors, and large spontaneous portosystemic shunts are present in many affected patients and are associated with a lack of response to treatment. In cases confirmed by right-sided heart catheterization, treatment with the prostaglandins epoprostenol, iloprost, or treprostinil (the latter two are easier to administer); the endothelin-receptor antagonists ambrisentan and macitentan or bosentan (no longer used because of potential hepatotoxicity); the phosphodiesterase-5 inhibitors sildenafil, tadalafil, or vardenafil; the oral prostacyclin receptor agonist selexipag; or the direct cyclic GMP analog riociguat may reduce pulmonary hypertension and thereby facilitate liver transplantation. Beta-blockers worsen exercise capacity and are contraindicated, and calcium channel blockers should be used with caution because they may worsen portal hypertension. Liver transplantation is contraindicated in patients with moderate to severe pulmonary hypertension (mean pulmonary pressure greater than 35 mm Hg).

C. Liver Transplantation

Liver transplantation is indicated in selected cases of irreversible, progressive chronic liver disease, acute-on-chronic liver failure, acute liver failure, and certain metabolic diseases in which the metabolic defect is in the liver. Absolute contraindications include malignancy (except relatively small hepatocellular carcinomas in a cirrhotic liver—see Chapter 39), advanced cardiopulmonary disease (except hepatopulmonary syndrome), and sepsis. Relative contraindications include age over 70 years, morbid obesity, portal and mesenteric vein thrombosis, active alcohol or drug abuse, severe malnutrition, and lack of patient understanding. With the emergence of effective antiretroviral therapy for HIV disease, a major cause of mortality in these patients has shifted to liver disease caused by HCV and HBV infection; experience to date suggests that the outcome of liver transplantation is comparable to that for non–HIV-infected liver transplant recipients. Patients with alcoholism should generally be abstinent for 6 months. Liver transplantation should be considered in patients with worsening functional status, rising bilirubin, decreasing albumin, worsening coagulopathy, refractory ascites, recurrent variceal bleeding, or worsening encephalopathy; prioritization is based on the MELD (or MELD-Na) score. Treatment of HCV infection should be deferred until after transplantation in patients in whom the MELD score is 21 or higher. Combined liver-kidney transplantation is indicated in patients with associated kidney failure presumed to be irreversible. The major impediment to more widespread use of liver transplantation is a shortage of donor organs. Adult living donor liver transplantation is an option for some patients and extended-criteria donors are used. Five-year survival rates over 80% are now reported. Hepatocellular carcinoma, hepatitis B and C, Budd-Chiari syndrome, and autoimmune liver disease may recur in the transplanted liver. The incidence of recurrence of hepatitis B can be reduced by preoperative and postoperative treatment with a nucleoside or nucleotide analog and perioperative administration of HBIG, and hepatitis C can be treated with direct-acting antiviral agents. Immunosuppression is achieved with combinations of cyclosporine, tacrolimus, sirolimus, corticosteroids, azathioprine, and mycophenolate mofetil and may be complicated by infections, advanced CKD, neurologic disorders, and drug toxicity, as well as graft rejection, vascular occlusion, or bile leaks. Patients taking these drugs are at risk for obesity, diabetes mellitus, and hyperlipidemia and may develop recurrent or de novo NAFLD following transplantation.

Prognosis

The risk of death from compensated cirrhosis is 4.7 times that of the risk in the general population, and the risk from decompensated cirrhosis is 9.7 times higher. Use of statins appears to decrease the risk of decompensation in patients with compensated cirrhosis, in whom the risk of decompensation can be predicted with a scoring system that includes serum albumin, serum bilirubin, age, serum AST and ALT, and platelet count. Prognostic scoring systems for cirrhosis include the Child-Pugh score and MELD score (Table 16–8). The MELD-Na score, which incorporates the serum bilirubin, creatinine, and sodium levels and the INR, is also a measure of mortality risk in patients with

Table 16–8. Child-Pugh and Model for End-Stage Liver Disease (MELD) scoring systems for staging cirrhosis.

Child-Pugh Scoring System			
	Numerical Score		
Parameter	1	2	3
Ascites	None	Slight	Moderate to severe
Encephalopathy	None	Slight to moderate	Moderate to severe
Bilirubin, mg/dL (mcmol/L)	< 2.0 (34.2)	2–3 (34.2–51.3)	> 3.0 (51.3)
Albumin, g/dL (g/L)	> 3.5 (35)	2.8–3.5 (28–35)	< 2.8 (28)
Prothrombin time (seconds increased)	1–3	4–6	> 6.0
	Total Numerical Score and Corresponding Child-Pugh Class		
	Score	Class	
	5–6	A	
	7–9	B	
	10–15	C	

MELD Scoring Systems

Original MELD score = 11.2 $\log_e$ (INR) + 3.78 $\log_e$ (bilirubin [mg/dL]) + 9.57 $\log_e$ (creatinine [mg/dL]) + 6.43. (Range 6–40.)
MELD-Na score = MELD + (140 – Na) × (1 – 0.025 × MELD).

end-stage liver disease and is particularly useful for predicting short- and intermediate-term survival and complications of cirrhosis (eg, bacterial peritonitis) as well as determining allocation priorities for donor livers. Additional (MELD-exception) points are given for patients with conditions such as hepatopulmonary syndrome and hepatocellular carcinoma that may benefit from liver transplantation. A MELD score of 17 or more is required for liver transplant listing. In patients with a relatively low MELD score (less than 21) and a low priority for liver transplantation, an elevated hepatic venous pressure gradient, persistent ascites, hepatic encephalopathy, and a low health-related quality of life are additional independent predictors of mortality, and further modifications of the MELD score are under consideration. Only 50% of patients with severe hepatic dysfunction (serum albumin less than 3 g/dL [30 g/L], bilirubin greater than 3 mg/dL [51.3 mcmol/L], ascites, encephalopathy, cachexia, and upper GI bleeding) survive 6 months without transplantation. The risk of death in this subgroup of patients with advanced cirrhosis is associated with muscle wasting, age 65 years or older, mean arterial pressure 82 mm Hg or less, severe kidney dysfunction, cognitive dysfunction, ventilatory insufficiency, prothrombin time 16 seconds or longer, delayed and suboptimal treatment of sepsis, and second infections. For cirrhotic patients admitted to an intensive care unit, the Royal Free Hospital score, consisting of the serum bilirubin, INR, serum lactate, alveolar-arterial oxygen gradient, and BUN, has been reported to predict mortality. The combination of the MELD score and serum lactate at the time of hospitalization has been reported to predict inpatient mortality better than the MELD score alone. Severe kidney dysfunction increases mortality up to sevenfold in patients with cirrhosis, and at least 25% of patients who survive an episode of AKI develop CKD. The ratio of neutrophils to lymphocytes in peripheral blood has been reported to correlate with mortality 1 year after a nonelective hospitalization in patients with cirrhosis. Obesity and diabetes mellitus appear to be risk factors for clinical deterioration and cirrhosis-related mortality, as is continued alcohol use in patients with alcohol-associated cirrhosis. The use of beta-blockers for portal hypertension is beneficial early in the course. However, beta-blockers may become ineffective and may be associated with reduced survival in patients with refractory ascites, spontaneous bacterial peritonitis, sepsis, or severe alcohol-associated hepatitis because of their negative effect on cardiac compensatory reserve. In general, beta-blockers should be discontinued when the systolic blood pressure is less than 90 mm Hg, the serum sodium level is less than 130 mEq/L, or AKI has developed, although results of some studies have challenged these guidelines. Patients with cirrhosis are at risk for the development of hepatocellular carcinoma, with rates of 3–5% per year for alcohol-associated and viral hepatitis–related cirrhosis. Liver transplantation has markedly improved the outlook for patients with cirrhosis who are candidates and are referred for evaluation early in the course. Patients with compensated cirrhosis are given additional priority for liver transplantation if they are found to have a lesion larger than 2 cm in diameter consistent with hepatocellular carcinoma. In-hospital mortality from cirrhosis declined from 9.1% in 2002 to 5.4% in 2010 and that from variceal bleeding in patients with cirrhosis declined from over 40% in 1980 to 15% in 2000. Rates and costs of hospital admissions increased substantially between 2005 and 2015, primarily because of increases in the rates of cirrhosis caused by NAFLD. Patients hospitalized with cirrhosis and an infection are at high risk for subsequent infections, particularly if they are older, taking a PPI, or receiving antibiotic prophylaxis for spontaneous bacterial peritonitis.

When to Refer

- For liver biopsy.
- When the MELD score is 14 or higher.
- For upper endoscopy to screen for gastroesophageal varices.

When to Admit

- GI bleeding.
- Stage 3–4 hepatic encephalopathy.
- Worsening kidney function.
- Severe hyponatremia.
- Serious infection.
- Profound hypoxia.

Biggins SW et al. Diagnosis, evaluation, and management of ascites, spontaneous bacterial peritonitis and hepatorenal syndrome: 2021 practice guidance by the American Association for the Study of Liver Diseases. Hepatology. 2021;74:1014. [PMID: 33942342]

Cardenas A et al (editors). Complication of cirrhosis. Clin Liver Dis. 2021;25:253. [Full issue]

Ginès P et al. Liver cirrhosis. Lancet. 2021;398:1359. [PMID: 34543610]

Tandon P et al. AGA Clinical Practice Update on palliative care management in cirrhosis: expert review. Clin Gastroenterol Hepatol. 2021;19:646. [PMID: 33221550]

Wong F et al. Terlipressin plus albumin for the treatment of type 1 hepatorenal syndrome. N Engl J Med. 2021;384:818. [PMID: 33657294]

PRIMARY BILIARY CHOLANGITIS

ESSENTIALS OF DIAGNOSIS

- Occurs in middle-aged women.
- Often asymptomatic.
- Elevation of alkaline phosphatase, positive antimitochondrial antibodies, elevated IgM, increased cholesterol.
- Characteristic liver biopsy.
- In later stages, can present with fatigue, jaundice, features of cirrhosis, xanthelasmas, xanthomas, steatorrhea.

General Considerations

PBC is a chronic disease of the liver characterized by autoimmune destruction of small intrahepatic bile ducts and cholestasis. The designation “primary biliary cholangitis” has replaced “primary biliary cirrhosis” because many patients do not have cirrhosis. The disease is insidious in onset, occurs usually in women aged 40–60 years, and is often detected by the chance finding of elevated alkaline phosphatase levels. Estimated incidence and prevalence rates in the United States are 4.5 and 65.4 per 100,000, respectively, in women, and 0.7 and 12.1 per 100,000, respectively, in men. These rates may be increasing. The frequency of the disease among first-degree relatives of affected persons is 1.3–6%, the risk is increased in second- and third-degree relatives, and the concordance rate in identical twins is high. PBC is associated with HLA *DRB1*08* and *DQB1*. The disease may be associated with Sjögren syndrome, autoimmune thyroid disease, Raynaud syndrome, systemic sclerosis (scleroderma), hypothyroidism, and celiac disease; all patients with PBC should be screened for these conditions. Infection with *Novosphingobium aromaticivorans* or *Chlamydophila pneumoniae* may trigger or cause PBC. A history of UTIs (caused by *E coli* or *Lactobacillus delbrueckii*) and smoking, and possibly use of hormone replacement therapy and hair dye, are risk factors, and clustering of cases in time and space argues for a causative role of environmental agents.

Clinical Findings

A. Symptoms and Signs

Many patients are asymptomatic for years. The onset of clinical illness is insidious and is heralded by fatigue (excessive daytime somnolence) and pruritus. With progression, physical examination reveals hepatosplenomegaly. Xanthomatous lesions may occur in the skin and tendons and around the eyelids. Jaundice, steatorrhea, and signs of portal hypertension are late findings, although occasional patients have esophageal varices despite an early histologic stage. Autonomic dysfunction, including orthostatic hypotension and associated fatigue and cognitive dysfunction, appear to be common. The risk of low bone density, osteoporosis, and fractures is increased in patients with PBC (who tend to be older women) possibly due in part to polymorphisms of the vitamin D receptor.

B. Laboratory Findings

Blood counts are normal early in the disease. Liver biochemical tests reflect cholestasis with elevation of alkaline phosphatase, cholesterol (especially high-density lipoproteins and lipoprotein X), and, in later stages, bilirubin. Antimitochondrial antibodies are present in 95% of patients, and serum IgM levels are elevated.

Diagnosis

The diagnosis of PBC is based on the detection of cholestatic liver chemistries (often initially an isolated elevation of the alkaline phosphatase) and antimitochondrial antibodies in a titer greater than 1:40 in serum. Baseline ultrasonography should be obtained. Liver biopsy is not necessary for diagnosis unless antimitochondrial antibodies are absent but permits histologic staging: I, portal inflammation with granulomas; II, bile duct proliferation, periportal inflammation; III, interlobular fibrous septa; and IV, cirrhosis. Estimations of histologic stage by an "enhanced liver fibrosis (ELF) assay," which incorporates serum levels of hyaluronic acid, tissue inhibitor of metalloproteinase-1, and procollagen III aminopeptide, and by elastography have shown promise.

Differential Diagnosis

The disease must be differentiated from chronic biliary tract obstruction (stone or stricture), carcinoma of the bile ducts, primary sclerosing cholangitis, sarcoidosis, cholestatic drug toxicity (eg, chlorpromazine), and (in some cases) chronic hepatitis. Patients with a clinical and histologic picture of PBC but no antimitochondrial antibodies are said to have antimitochondrial antibody-negative PBC (previously termed "autoimmune cholangitis"), which has been associated with lower serum IgM levels and a greater frequency of smooth muscle antibodies and ANA. Many such patients are found to have antimitochondrial antibodies by immunoblot against recombinant proteins (rather than standard immunofluorescence). Some patients have overlapping features of PBC and autoimmune hepatitis.

Treatment

Cholestyramine (4 g) in water or juice three times daily may be beneficial for pruritus; colestipol and colesevelam may be better tolerated but have not been shown to reduce pruritus. Rifampin, 150–300 mg orally twice daily, is inconsistently beneficial. Opioid antagonists (eg, naloxone, 0.2 mcg/kg/minute by intravenous infusion, or naltrexone, starting at 12.5 mg/day by mouth) show promise in the treatment of pruritus but may cause opioid withdrawal symptoms. The 5-hydroxytryptamine (5-HT_3) serotonin receptor antagonist ondansetron, 4 mg orally three times a day as needed, and the SSRI sertraline, 75–100 mg/day orally, may also provide some benefit. For refractory pruritus, plasmapheresis or extracorporeal albumin dialysis may be needed. Modafinil, 100–200 mg/day orally, may improve daytime somnolence but is poorly tolerated. Deficiencies of vitamins A, D, and K may occur if steatorrhea is present and are aggravated when cholestyramine is administered.

Ursodeoxycholic acid (13–15 mg/kg/day in one or two doses) is the preferred medical treatment for PBC. It has been shown to slow the progression of disease (particularly in early-stage disease), stabilize histology, improve long-term survival, reduce the risk of developing esophageal varices, and delay (and possibly prevent) the need for liver transplantation, even in the absence of liver biochemical improvement. Complete normalization of liver biochemical tests occurs in 20% of treated patients within 2 years and 40% within 5 years, and survival is similar to that of healthy controls when the drug is given to patients with stage 1 or 2 PBC. The rate of improvement in the alkaline phosphatase to normal or near-normal levels has been reported to be lower in men than women (72% vs 80%) and higher in women whose disease is diagnosed after age 70 than before age 30 (90% vs 50%). Ursodeoxycholic acid has also been reported to reduce the risk of recurrent colorectal adenomas in patients with PBC. Side effects include weight gain and rarely loose stools. The drug can be continued during pregnancy.

Obeticholic acid, a farnesoid X receptor agonist, may be added in patients with an incomplete response or intolerance to ursodeoxycholic acid. Obeticholic acid is begun in a dose of 5 mg orally daily and increased to 10 mg daily at 6 months if tolerated, based on the decline in serum alkaline phosphatase and bilirubin levels. In patients with Child-Pugh class B or C cirrhosis, the recommended initial dose was 5 mg weekly; however, the drug can cause serious liver injury in patients with advanced cirrhosis, and its use in these patients has been restricted by the FDA. Treatment with obeticholic acid has been shown to stabilize or reverse hepatic fibrosis. The principal side effect is pruritus. Given the expense of the drug, the cost-effectiveness of obeticholic acid has been questioned.

Bezafibrate (not available in the United States) and fenofibrate, which activate peroxisome proliferator–activated receptors (PPARs) and inhibit bile acid synthesis, have shown promise as second-line agents and improve symptoms (including pruritus), liver biochemical test levels, and fibrosis. Colchicine (0.6 mg orally twice daily) and methotrexate (15 mg/wk orally) have had some reported benefit in improving symptoms and serum levels of alkaline phosphatase and bilirubin. Methotrexate may also improve liver histology in some patients, but overall response rates have been disappointing. For patients with advanced disease, liver transplantation is the treatment of choice.

Prognosis

Without liver transplantation, survival averages 7–10 years once symptoms develop but has improved for younger women since the introduction of ursodeoxycholic acid. Progression to liver failure and portal hypertension may be accelerated by smoking; outcomes are worse in men than in women. Patients with early-stage disease in whom the alkaline phosphatase and AST are less than 1.5 times normal and bilirubin is 1 mg/dL (17.1 mcmol/L) or less after 1 year of therapy with ursodeoxycholic acid (Paris II criteria) are at low long-term risk for cirrhosis and have a life expectancy similar to that of the healthy population. Attainment of a serum bilirubin level less than 0.6 times the upper limit of normal or a normal alkaline phosphatase level is associated with the lowest risk for liver transplantation or death. Pregnancy is well tolerated in younger patients. In advanced disease, an adverse prognosis is indicated by a high Mayo risk score that includes older age, high serum bilirubin, edema, low serum albumin, and prolonged prothrombin time as well as by variceal hemorrhage. Other prognostic models include the Globe index, which is based on age, serum bilirubin, serum albumin, serum alkaline phosphatase, and platelet count and, in treated patients, the UK-PBC score, which is based on the baseline serum albumin and platelet count and the serum bilirubin, aminotransferases, and alkaline phosphatase after 12 months of ursodeoxycholic acid. An increase in liver stiffness of more than 2.1 kPa per year indicates an adverse prognosis. A prediction tool for varices has been proposed based on the serum albumin, serum alkaline phosphatase, platelet count, and splenomegaly. Fatigue is associated with an increased risk of cardiac mortality and may not be reversed by liver transplantation. Among asymptomatic patients, a decline in liver function is observed in up to 50% by 5 years, and at least one-third will become symptomatic within 15 years. The risk of hepatocellular carcinoma appears to be increased in patients with PBC; risk factors include older age, male sex, prior blood transfusions, advanced histologic stage, signs of cirrhosis or portal hypertension, and a biochemical nonresponse to ursodeoxycholic acid. Liver transplantation should be considered when the MELD-Na score is at least 15, total serum bilirubin at least 6, or Mayo risk score at least 7.8. Liver transplantation for advanced PBC is associated with a 1-year survival rate of 85–90%. The disease recurs in the graft in 20% of patients by 3 years and 37% by 10 years. A reduced risk of recurrence, graft loss, and death is associated with preventive treatment with ursodeoxycholic acid in combination with cyclosporine (rather than tacrolimus).

When to Refer

- For liver biopsy.
- For liver transplant evaluation.

When to Admit

- GI bleeding.
- Stage 3–4 hepatic encephalopathy.
- Worsening kidney function.
- Severe hyponatremia.
- Profound hypoxia.

Goet JC et al; GLOBAL PBC Study Group. A comparison of prognostic scores (Mayo, UK-PBC, and GLOBE) in primary biliary cholangitis. Am J Gastroenterol. 2021;116:1514. [PMID: 33941746]

John BV et al. Male sex is associated with higher rates of liver-related mortality in primary biliary cholangitis and cirrhosis. Hepatology. 2021;74:879. [PMID: 33636012]

Lleo A et al. Primary biliary cholangitis. Lancet. 2020;396:1915. [PMID: 33308474]

Murillo Perez CF et al. Goals of treatment for improved survival in primary biliary cholangitis: treatment target should be bilirubin within the normal range and normalization of alkaline phosphatase. Am J Gastroenterol. 2020;115:1066. [PMID: 32618657]

Tanaka A et al. Association of bezafibrate with transplant-free survival in patients with primary biliary cholangitis. J Hepatol. 2021;75:565. [PMID: 33882268]

HEMOCHROMATOSIS

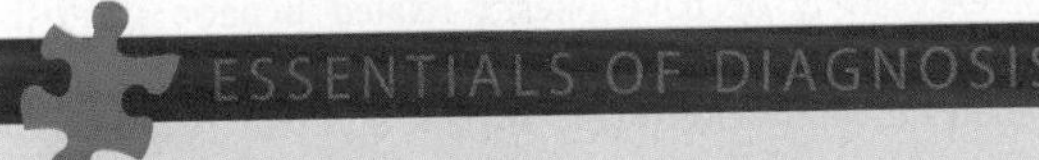

- Usually suspected because of a family history or an elevated iron saturation or serum ferritin.
- Most patients are asymptomatic; the disease is rarely recognized clinically before the fifth decade.
- Hepatic abnormalities and cirrhosis, heart failure, hypogonadism, and arthritis.
- *HFE* gene mutation (usually C282Y/C282Y) is found in most cases.

General Considerations

Hemochromatosis is an autosomal recessive disease caused in most cases by a pathogenic variant in the *HFE* gene on chromosome 6. The HFE protein is thought to play an important role in the process by which duodenal crypt cells sense body iron stores, and the variant gene leads to increased iron absorption from the duodenum. A decrease in the synthesis or expression of hepcidin, the principal iron regulatory hormone, is thought to be a key pathogenic factor in all forms of hemochromatosis. About 85% of persons with well-established hemochromatosis are homozygous for the C282Y variant (type 1a hemochromatosis). The frequency of the C282Y variant averages 7% in Northern European and North American White populations, resulting in a 0.5% frequency of homozygotes (of whom 38–50% will develop biochemical evidence of iron overload but only 28% of men and 1% of women will develop clinical symptoms). The C282Y gene variant and hemochromatosis are uncommon in Black and Asian American populations. A second genetic variant (H63D) may contribute to the development of iron overload in a small percentage (1.5%) of persons who are compound heterozygotes for C282Y and H63D (type 1b); iron overload–related disease develops in only a few patients (particularly those who have a comorbidity such as diabetes mellitus and fatty liver). A third gene variant (S65C) may lead to increased serum iron and ferritin levels without clinical significance (type 1c). High serum ferritin levels are seen in hyperferritinemia cataract syndrome associated with pathogenic variants in the *FTL* (ferritin L-chain) gene. An uncommon juvenile-onset variant that is characterized by severe iron overload, cardiac dysfunction, hypogonadotropic hypogonadism, and a high mortality rate is usually linked to a variant gene on chromosome 1q designated *HJV* that produces a protein called hemojuvelin (type 2a) or, rarely, to a variant of the *HAMP* gene on chromosome 19 that encodes hepcidin (type 2b). Rare instances of hemochromatosis result from pathogenic variants in the genes that encode transferrin receptor 2 (*TFR2*) (type 3) and ferroportin (*SLC40A1*) (type 4a). Type 4b hemochromatosis is characterized by resistance of ferroportin to hepcidin.

Hemochromatosis is characterized by increased accumulation of iron as hemosiderin in the liver, pancreas, heart, adrenals, testes, pituitary, and kidneys. Cirrhosis is more likely to develop in affected persons who drink alcohol excessively or have obesity-related hepatic steatosis than in those who do not; other risk factors include age and diabetes mellitus. Eventually, hepatic and pancreatic insufficiency, heart failure, and hypogonadism may develop. Heterozygotes do not develop cirrhosis in the absence of associated disorders such as viral hepatitis or NAFLD.

Clinical Findings

A. Symptoms and Signs

The onset of clinical disease is usually after age 50 years—earlier in men than in women; however, because of widespread liver biochemical testing and iron screening, the diagnosis is usually made long before symptoms develop. Early symptoms are nonspecific (eg, fatigue, arthralgia). Later clinical manifestations include a symmetric arthropathy that is similar to osteoarthritis and calcium pyrophosphate deposition disease (and ultimately the need for joint replacement surgery in some cases), hepatomegaly and evidence of hepatic dysfunction, skin pigmentation (combination of slate-gray due to iron and brown due to melanin, sometimes resulting in a bronze color), cardiac enlargement with or without heart failure or conduction defects, diabetes mellitus with its complications, and erectile dysfunction in men. Interestingly, population studies have shown an increased prevalence of liver disease but not of diabetes mellitus, arthritis, or heart disease in C282Y homozygotes. In patients in whom cirrhosis develops, bleeding from esophageal varices may occur, and there is a 15–20% frequency of hepatocellular carcinoma; the risk of intrahepatic cholangiocarcinoma is also increased. Affected patients are at increased risk of infection with *Vibrio vulnificus, Listeria monocytogenes, Yersinia enterocolitica*, and other siderophilic organisms. The risk of porphyria cutanea tarda is increased in persons with the C282Y or H63D variants, and C282Y homozygotes have twice the risk of colorectal and breast cancer than persons without the C282Y variant.

B. Laboratory Findings

Laboratory findings include mildly abnormal liver tests (AST, alkaline phosphatase), an elevated plasma iron with greater than 45% transferrin saturation, a low unsaturated iron-binding capacity, and an elevated serum ferritin (although a normal iron saturation or a normal ferritin does not exclude the diagnosis). Affected men are more likely than affected women to have an elevated ferritin level. Testing for *HFE* variants is indicated in any patient with evidence of iron overload. Interestingly, in persons with an elevated serum ferritin, the likelihood of detecting C282Y homozygosity decreases with increasing ALT and AST levels, which likely reflect hepatic inflammation and secondary iron overload. In contrast to secondary iron overload, the serum ALT level is often normal.

C. Imaging

MRI and CT may show changes consistent with iron overload of the liver, and MRI-based techniques (eg, T2 spin echo and T2* gradient-recalled echo MRI) can quantitate hepatic iron stores and help assess the degree of hepatic fibrosis.

D. Liver Biopsy

In patients who are homozygous for C282Y, liver biopsy is often indicated to determine whether cirrhosis is present. Biopsy can be deferred, however, in patients in whom the serum ferritin level is less than 1000 mcg/L, serum AST level is normal, and hepatomegaly is absent; the likelihood of cirrhosis is low in these persons. Serum biomarkers of fibrosis may be an alternative to liver biopsy for identifying advanced fibrosis. Risk factors for advanced fibrosis include male sex, excess alcohol consumption, and diabetes mellitus. Liver biopsy also may be indicated when iron overload is suspected even though the patient is neither homozygous for C282Y nor a C282Y/H63D compound heterozygote. In patients with hemochromatosis, the liver biopsy characteristically shows extensive iron deposition in hepatocytes and in bile ducts, and the hepatic iron index—hepatic iron content per gram of liver converted to micromoles and divided by the patient's age—is generally higher than 1.9 (though no longer used for diagnosis). Only 5% of patients with hereditary hemochromatosis identified by screening in a primary care setting have cirrhosis.

Screening

Iron studies and *HFE* testing are recommended for all first-degree family members of a proband; children of an affected person (C282Y homozygote) need to be screened only if the patient's spouse carries the C282Y or H63D mutation. General population screening for hemochromatosis is not recommended because the clinical penetrance of C282Y homozygosity and morbidity and mortality from hemochromatosis are low. Patients with otherwise unexplained chronic liver disease, chondrocalcinosis, erectile dysfunction, and type 1 diabetes mellitus (especially late-onset) should be screened for iron overload.

Treatment

Affected persons are advised to avoid foods rich in iron (such as red meat), alcohol, vitamin C, raw shellfish, and supplemental iron, although dietary restrictions may not be necessary in those undergoing phlebotomy. Weekly phlebotomies of 1 or 2 units (250–500 mL) of blood (each containing about 250 mg of iron) are indicated in all symptomatic patients, and those with a serum ferritin level of at least 300 mcg/L (men) or 200 mcg/L (women) with an increased fasting iron saturation (greater than or equal to 45%); these phlebotomies should be continued for up to 2–3 years to achieve depletion of iron stores. The hematocrit and serum iron values should be monitored. When iron store depletion is achieved (iron saturation less than 50% and serum ferritin level 50–100 mcg/L), phlebotomies (every 2–4 months) to maintain serum ferritin levels between 50 mcg/L and 100 mcg/L are continued, although compliance has been reported to decrease with time. Administration of a PPI, which reduces intestinal iron absorption, decreases the maintenance phlebotomy volume requirement. In C282Y homozygous women, a BMI greater than 28 is associated with a lower phlebotomy requirement, possibly because hepcidin levels are increased by overweight. Complications of hemochromatosis—arthropathy, diabetes mellitus, heart disease, portal hypertension, and hypopituitarism—also require treatment.

The chelating agent deferoxamine is indicated for patients with hemochromatosis and anemia or in those with secondary iron overload due to thalassemia who cannot tolerate phlebotomies. The drug is administered intravenously or subcutaneously in a dosage of 20–40 mg/kg/day infused over 24 hours and can mobilize 30 mg of iron per day; however, treatment is painful and time-consuming. Two oral chelators, deferasirox, 20 mg/kg once daily, and deferiprone, 25 mg/kg three times daily, have been approved for treatment of iron overload due to blood transfusions and may be appropriate in persons with hemochromatosis who cannot tolerate phlebotomy; however, these agents have a number of side effects and drug-drug interactions.

The course of hemochromatosis appears to be favorably altered by phlebotomy therapy, although the evidence for a benefit is surprisingly sparse. With phlebotomy therapy, hepatic fibrosis may regress, and in precirrhotic patients, cirrhosis may be prevented. Cardiac conduction defects may improve with treatment. Joint disease, diabetes mellitus, and hypogonadism may not reverse with treatment of hemochromatosis. More severe joint symptoms are associated with persistent increases in the transferrin saturation, even if the serum ferritin level is maintained below 50 mcg/L. In patients with cirrhosis, varices may reverse, the risk of variceal bleeding declines, and the risk of hepatocellular carcinoma may be reduced. In those with an initial serum ferritin level greater than 1000 mcg/L (2247 pmol/L), the risk of death is fivefold greater than in those with a serum ferritin of 1000 mcg/L (2247 pmol/L) or less. In treated patients, only those with a serum ferritin greater than 2000 mcg/L (4494 pmol/L) are reported to have increased mortality, mainly related to liver disease. Since 1997, posttransplant survival rates have been excellent. Following liver transplantation, serum iron studies and hepcidin levels are normal, and phlebotomy is not required.

When to Refer

- For liver biopsy.
- For initiation of therapy.

Chin J et al. Utility of serum biomarker indices for staging of hepatic fibrosis before and after venesection in patients with hemochromatosis caused by variants in HFE. Clin Gastroenterol Hepatol. 2021;19:1459. [PMID: 32745684]

Kowdley KV et al. ACG Clinical Guideline: hereditary hemochromatosis. Am J Gastroenterol. 2019;114:1202. [PMID: 31335359]

Moore AB et al. Case 25-2021: a 48-year-old man with fatigue and leg swelling. N Engl J Med. 2021;385:745. [PMID: 34407347]

WILSON DISEASE

ESSENTIALS OF DIAGNOSIS

- Rare autosomal recessive disorder that usually occurs in persons under age 40.
- Excessive deposition of copper in the liver and brain.
- Serum ceruloplasmin, the plasma copper-carrying protein, is low.
- Urinary excretion of copper and hepatic copper concentration are high.

General Considerations

Wilson disease (hepatolenticular degeneration) is a rare autosomal recessive disorder that usually occurs in persons between 3 and 55 years of age. The worldwide prevalence is generally stated to be about 30 per million population, but the frequency of the allele appears to be greater than implied by this estimate. The condition is characterized by excessive deposition of copper in the liver and brain. The genetic defect, localized to chromosome 13 (*ATP7B*), has been shown to affect a copper-transporting adenosine triphosphatase in the liver and leads to copper accumulation in the liver and oxidative damage of hepatic mitochondria. Most patients are compound heterozygotes (ie, carry two different pathogenic variants). Over 600 variants in the Wilson disease gene have been identified. The H1069Q variant accounts for

37–63% of disease alleles in populations of Northern European descent. The major physiologic aberration in Wilson disease is excessive absorption of copper from the small intestine and decreased excretion of copper by the liver, resulting in increased tissue deposition, especially in the liver, brain, cornea, and kidney.

Clinical Findings

Wilson disease tends to present as liver disease in adolescents (more common in females) and neuropsychiatric disease in young adults (more common in males), but there is great variability, and onset of symptoms after age 40 is more common than previously thought. The diagnosis should always be considered in any child or young adult with hepatitis, splenomegaly with hypersplenism, Coombs-negative hemolytic anemia, portal hypertension, and neurologic or psychiatric abnormalities. Wilson disease should also be considered in persons under 40 years of age with chronic hepatitis or acute liver failure.

Hepatic involvement may range from elevated liver biochemical tests (although the alkaline phosphatase may be low, particularly in patients with acute severe liver disease) to cirrhosis and portal hypertension. In patients with acute liver failure (seen more often in women than in men), the diagnosis of Wilson disease is suggested by an alkaline phosphatase (in U/L)-to-total bilirubin (in mg/dL) ratio less than 4 and an AST-to-ALT ratio greater than 2.2. The neurologic manifestations of Wilson disease are related to basal ganglia dysfunction and include an akinetic-rigid syndrome similar to parkinsonism, pseudosclerosis with tremor, ataxia, and a dystonic syndrome. Dysarthria, dysphagia, incoordination, and spasticity are common. Migraines, insomnia, and seizures have been reported. Psychiatric features include behavioral and personality changes and emotional lability and may precede characteristic neurologic features. The risk of depression is increased. The pathognomonic sign of the condition is the brownish or gray-green Kayser-Fleischer ring, which represents fine pigmented granular deposits in Descemet membrane in the cornea (Figure 16–4). The ring is usually most marked at the superior and inferior poles of the cornea. It is sometimes seen with the naked eye and is readily detected by slit-lamp examination. It may be absent in patients with hepatic manifestations only but is usually present in those with neuropsychiatric disease. Renal calculi, aminoaciduria, renal tubular acidosis, hypoparathyroidism, infertility, hemolytic anemia, and subcutaneous lipomas may occur.

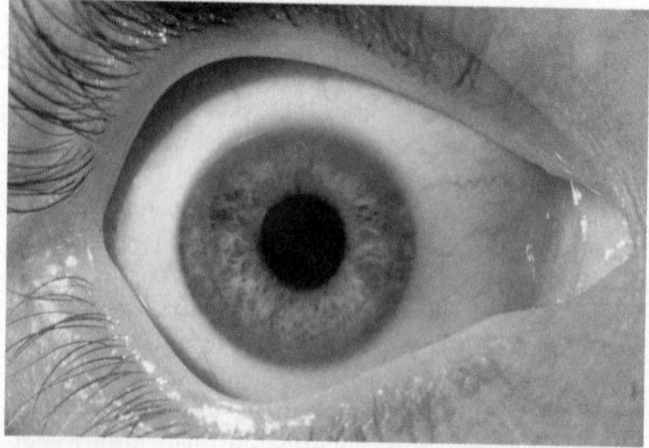

Figure 16–4. Brownish Kayser-Fleischer ring at the rim of the cornea in a patient with Wilson disease. (Used, with permission, from Mediscan/Alamy Stock Photo.)

Diagnosis

The diagnosis can be challenging, even with the use of scoring systems (eg, the Leipzig criteria), and is generally based on demonstration of increased urinary copper excretion (greater than 40 mcg/24 hours and usually greater than 100 mcg/24 hours) or low serum ceruloplasmin levels (less than 14 mg/dL [140 mg/L]; less than 10 mg/dL [100 mg/L] strongly suggests the diagnosis), and elevated hepatic copper concentration (greater than 250 mcg/g of dry liver) as well as Kayser-Fleischer rings, neurologic symptoms, and Coombs-negative hemolytic anemia. However, increased urinary copper (on three separate 24-hour collections) and a low serum ceruloplasmin level (by a standard immunologic assay), while useful, are neither completely sensitive nor specific for Wilson disease, although an enzymatic assay for ceruloplasmin appears to be more accurate and more sensitive for screening than urinary copper excretion; lipemia can interfere with the measurement of ceruloplasmin by the standard assay. The ratio of exchangeable copper to total copper in serum has been reported to be a reliable test for the diagnosis of Wilson disease. Liver biopsy may show acute or chronic hepatitis or cirrhosis. MRI of the brain may show evidence of increased basal ganglia, brainstem, and cerebellar copper even early in the course of the disease. If available, molecular analysis of *ATP7B* pathogenic variants can be diagnostic.

Treatment

Early treatment to remove excess copper before it can produce hepatic or neurologic damage is essential. Initially, restriction of dietary copper (shellfish, organ foods, nuts, mushrooms, and chocolate) may be of value. Oral D-penicillamine (0.75–2 g/day in divided doses taken 1 hour before or 2 hours after food) has traditionally been the drug of choice and enhances urinary excretion of chelated copper. Oral pyridoxine, 50 mg per week, is added because D-penicillamine is an antimetabolite of this vitamin. If D-penicillamine treatment cannot be tolerated because of GI intolerance, hypersensitivity, autoimmune reactions, nephrotoxicity, or bone marrow toxicity, trientine hydrochloride, 250–500 mg three times a day, a chelating agent as effective as D-penicillamine but with a lower rate of adverse effects, is used and is increasingly prescribed as a first-line agent, although its cost has become exorbitant. Oral zinc acetate or zinc gluconate, 50 mg of elemental zinc three times a day taken 30 minutes before or 2 hours after a meal, interferes with intestinal absorption of copper, promotes fecal copper excretion, and has been used as first-line therapy in asymptomatic or pregnant patients and those with neurologic disease, in combination with a chelating agent, or as maintenance therapy after decoppering with a chelating agent, but adverse GI effects often lead to discontinuation and its long-term efficacy and safety (including a risk of hepatotoxicity) have been questioned; it can lead to copper deficiency in normal persons.

Treatment should continue indefinitely. The doses of penicillamine and trientine should be reduced during pregnancy. Supplemental vitamin E, an antioxidant, has been recommended but not rigorously studied. Once the serum nonceruloplasmin copper level is within the normal range (50–150 mcg/L), the dose of chelating agent can be reduced to the minimum necessary for maintaining that level. The prognosis is good in patients who are effectively treated before liver or brain damage has occurred, but long-term survival is reduced in patients with cirrhosis at diagnosis (84% after 20 years). Liver transplantation is indicated for acute liver failure (often after plasma exchange or dialysis with MARS as a stabilizing measure) and decompensated cirrhosis (with excellent outcomes). Liver transplantation is generally not recommended for intractable isolated neuropsychiatric disease. All first-degree relatives, especially siblings, require screening with serum ceruloplasmin, liver biochemical tests, and slit-lamp examination or, if the causative pathogenic gene variant is known, with variant analysis.

When to Refer

All patients with Wilson disease should be referred for diagnosis and treatment.

When to Admit

- Acute liver failure.
- GI bleeding.
- Stage 3–4 hepatic encephalopathy.
- Worsening kidney function.
- Severe hyponatremia.
- Profound hypoxia.

Collins CJ et al. Direct measurement of ATP7B peptides is highly effective in the diagnosis of Wilson disease. Gastroenterology. 2021;160:2367. [PMID: 33640437]

Dong Y et al. Role for biochemical assays and Kayser-Fleischer rings in diagnosis of Wilson's disease. Clin Gastroenterol Hepatol. 2021;19:590. [PMID: 32485301]

Shribman S et al. Clinical presentations of Wilson disease. Ann Transl Med. 2019;7:S60. [PMID: 31179297]

HEPATIC VENOUS OUTFLOW OBSTRUCTION (Budd-Chiari Syndrome)

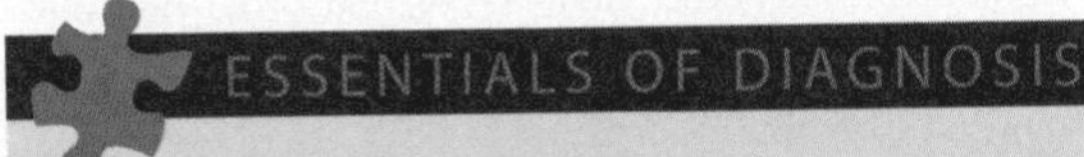

ESSENTIALS OF DIAGNOSIS

- Right upper quadrant pain and tenderness.
- Ascites.
- Imaging studies show occlusion/absence of flow in the hepatic vein(s) or inferior vena cava.
- Clinical picture is similar in sinusoidal obstruction syndrome, but major hepatic veins are patent.

General Considerations

Factors that predispose patients to hepatic venous outflow obstruction, or Budd-Chiari syndrome, including hereditary and acquired hypercoagulable states, can be identified in up to 85% of affected patients; multiple disorders are found in up to 45%. Up to 50% of cases are associated with polycythemia vera or other myeloproliferative neoplasms (which entail a 1% risk of Budd-Chiari syndrome). These cases are often associated with a specific pathogenic variant (*V617F*) in the gene that codes for JAK2 tyrosine kinase and may otherwise be subclinical. Other predispositions to thrombosis (eg, activated protein C resistance [factor V Leiden mutation] [25% of cases], protein C or S or antithrombin deficiency [23%], antiphospholipid antibodies [20%], hyperprothrombinemia [factor II *G20210A* pathogenic variant] [rarely], the methylenetetrahydrofolate reductase *TT677* variant) may be identified in other cases. Hepatic vein obstruction may be associated with caval webs, right-sided heart failure or constrictive pericarditis, neoplasms that cause hepatic vein occlusion, paroxysmal nocturnal hemoglobinuria, hyperhomocysteinemia, Behçet syndrome, vasculitis, sarcoidosis, IBD, celiac disease, blunt abdominal trauma, use of oral contraceptives, and pregnancy. In India, China, and South Africa, Budd-Chiari syndrome is associated with a poor standard of living and often the result of occlusion of the hepatic portion of the inferior vena cava, presumably due to prior thrombosis. The clinical presentation is mild, but the course is frequently complicated by hepatocellular carcinoma.

Some cytotoxic agents and pyrrolizidine alkaloids (comfrey or "bush teas") may cause **sinusoidal obstruction syndrome** (previously known as veno-occlusive disease because the terminal venules are often occluded), which mimics Budd-Chiari syndrome clinically. Sinusoidal obstruction syndrome may occur in patients who have undergone hematopoietic stem cell transplantation, particularly those with pretransplant serum aminotransferase elevations or fever during cytoreductive therapy with cyclophosphamide, azathioprine, carmustine, busulfan, etoposide, or gemtuzumab ozogamicin or those receiving high-dose cytoreductive therapy or high-dose total body irradiation.

Clinical Findings

A. Symptoms and Signs

The presentation is most commonly subacute but may be fulminant, acute, or chronic; it may present as acute-on-chronic liver failure (see Cirrhosis). Clinical manifestations generally include ascites, painful hepatic enlargement, jaundice, splenomegaly, and AKI. With chronic disease, bleeding varices and hepatic encephalopathy may be evident; hepatopulmonary syndrome may occur.

B. Imaging

Hepatic imaging studies may show a prominent caudate lobe since its venous drainage may be occluded. The screening test of choice is contrast-enhanced, color, or pulsed-Doppler ultrasonography, which has a sensitivity of 85% for detecting evidence of hepatic venous or inferior vena caval thrombosis. MRI with spin-echo and gradient-echo sequences and intravenous gadolinium injection allows visualization of the obstructed veins and collateral vessels. Direct venography can delineate caval webs and occluded hepatic veins ("spider-web" pattern) most precisely but is rarely required. Concomitant splanchnic vein thrombosis may be found in 4–21% of cases.

C. Liver Biopsy

Percutaneous or transjugular liver biopsy in Budd-Chiari syndrome may be considered when the results of noninvasive imaging are inconclusive and frequently shows characteristic centrilobular congestion and fibrosis and often multiple large regenerative nodules. Liver biopsy is rarely required, however, and is often contraindicated in sinusoidal obstruction syndrome because of thrombocytopenia, and the diagnosis is based on clinical findings.

Treatment

Ascites should be treated with salt restriction and diuretics. Treatable causes of Budd-Chiari syndrome should be sought. Prompt recognition and treatment of an underlying hematologic disorder may avoid the need for surgery; however, the optimal anticoagulation regimen is uncertain, and anticoagulation is associated with a high risk of bleeding, particularly in patients with portal hypertension and those undergoing invasive procedures. Low-molecular-weight heparins are preferred over unfractionated heparin because of a high rate of heparin-induced thrombocytopenia with the latter. Warfarin is also an acceptable treatment, and direct-acting oral anticoagulants seem to have comparable efficacy but lack a reversal agent. Infusion of a thrombolytic agent into recently occluded veins has been attempted with success. Defibrotide, an adenosine receptor agonist that increases endogenous tissue plasminogen activator levels, has been approved by the FDA for the prevention and treatment of the sinusoidal obstruction syndrome. The drug is given as an intravenous infusion every 6 hours for a minimum of 21 days. Serious adverse effects include hypotension and hemorrhage; the drug is expensive and has no benefit in severe sinusoidal obstruction syndrome.

Balloon angioplasty, often with placement of an intravascular metallic stent, is preferred in patients with an inferior vena caval web and is being performed commonly in patients with hepatic vein thrombosis. TIPS placement may be attempted in patients with Budd-Chiari syndrome and persistent hepatic congestion or failed thrombolytic therapy and possibly in those with sinusoidal obstruction syndrome. Late TIPS dysfunction is less frequent with the use of polytetrafluoroethylene-covered stents than uncovered stents. TIPS is preferred over surgical decompression (side-to-side portacaval, mesocaval, or mesoatrial shunt), which, in contrast to TIPS, has generally not been proven to improve long-term survival. Older age, a higher serum bilirubin level, and a greater INR predict a poor outcome with TIPS. When TIPS is technically not feasible because of complete hepatic vein obstruction, ultrasound-guided direct intrahepatic portosystemic shunt is an alternative approach. Liver transplantation can be considered in patients with acute liver failure, cirrhosis with hepatocellular dysfunction, and failure of a portosystemic shunt, and outcomes have improved with the advent of patient selection based on the MELD score. Patients with Budd-Chiari syndrome often require lifelong anticoagulation and treatment of the underlying myeloproliferative disease; antiplatelet therapy with aspirin and hydroxyurea has been suggested as an alternative to warfarin in patients with a myeloproliferative disorder. For all patients with Budd-Chiari syndrome, a poor outcome has been reported to correlate with Child-Pugh class C and a lack of response to interventional therapy of any kind.

Prognosis

The overall 5-year survival rate is 50–90% with treatment (but less than 10% without intervention). Adverse prognostic factors in patients with Budd-Chiari syndrome are older age, high Child-Pugh score, ascites, encephalopathy, sepsis, elevated total bilirubin, prolonged prothrombin time, elevated serum creatinine, acute respiratory failure, concomitant portal vein thrombosis, cancer, and histologic features of acute liver disease superimposed on chronic liver injury. The 3-month mortality may be predicted by the Rotterdam score, which is based on encephalopathy, ascites, prothrombin time, and bilirubin. A serum ALT level at least fivefold above the upper limit of normal on presentation indicates hepatic ischemia and predicts a poor outcome, particularly when the ALT level decreases slowly. The risk of hepatocellular carcinoma is increased, and patients with chronic Budd-Chiari syndrome should undergo surveillance with abdominal ultrasonography and serum alpha-fetoprotein levels every 6 months; risk factors include cirrhosis, combined hepatic vein and inferior vena cava obstruction, and a long-segment inferior vena cava block.

When to Admit

All patients with hepatic vein obstruction should be hospitalized.

Alukal JJ et al. A nationwide analysis of Budd-Chiari syndrome in the United States. J Clin Exp Hepatol. 2021;11:181. [PMID: 33746442]

Sharma A et al. An update on the management of Budd-Chiari syndrome. Dig Dis Sci. 2021;66:1780. [PMID: 32691382]

Simonetto DA et al. ACG Clinical Guideline: disorders of the hepatic and mesenteric circulation. Am J Gastroenterol. 2020;115:18. [PMID: 31895720]

Thuluvath PJ et al. A scoring model to predict in-hospital mortality in patients with Budd-Chiari syndrome. Am J Gastroenterol. 2021;116:1905. [PMID: 33900212]

THE LIVER IN HEART FAILURE

Ischemic hepatitis, also called **ischemic hepatopathy, hypoxic hepatitis, shock liver**, or **acute cardiogenic liver injury**, may affect 2.5 of every 100 patients admitted to an ICU and results from an acute fall in cardiac output due to acute MI, arrhythmia, or septic or hemorrhagic shock, usually in a patient with passive congestion of the liver. Rare cases have occurred in patients with COVID-19. Clinical hypotension may be absent (or unwitnessed). In some cases, the precipitating event is arterial hypoxemia due to respiratory failure, sleep apnea, severe anemia, heat stroke, carbon monoxide poisoning, cocaine use, or bacterial endocarditis. More than one precipitant is common. Statin therapy prior to admission may protect against ischemic hepatitis.

The hallmark of ischemic hepatitis is a rapid and striking elevation of serum aminotransferase levels (often greater than 5000 U/L); an early rapid rise in the serum LD level (with an ALT-to-LD ratio less than 1.5) is also typical. Elevations of serum alkaline phosphatase and bilirubin are usually mild, but jaundice is associated with worse outcomes. The prothrombin time may be prolonged, and encephalopathy or hepatopulmonary syndrome may develop. The mortality rate due to the underlying disease is high (particularly in patients receiving vasopressor therapy or with septic shock, acute kidney disease, or coagulopathy), but in patients who recover, the aminotransferase levels return to normal quickly, usually within 1 week—in contrast to viral hepatitis.

In patients with **passive congestion of the liver** ("nutmeg liver") due to right-sided heart failure, the serum bilirubin level may be elevated, occasionally as high as 40 mg/dL (684 mcmol/L), due in part to hypoxia of perivenular hepatocytes, and its level is a predictor of mortality and morbidity. Serum alkaline phosphatase levels are normal or slightly elevated, and, in the absence of superimposed ischemia, aminotransferase levels are only mildly elevated. Hepatojugular reflux is present, and with tricuspid regurgitation the liver may be pulsatile. Ascites may be out of proportion to peripheral edema, with a high serum ascites-albumin gradient (greater than or equal to 1.1) and an ascitic fluid protein level of more than 2.5 g/dL (25 g/L). A markedly elevated serum N-terminal-proBNP or BNP level (greater than 364 pg/mL [364 ng/L]) has been reported to distinguish ascites due to heart failure from ascites due to cirrhosis in the absence of renal insufficiency. In severe cases, signs of encephalopathy may develop. Liver stiffness measurement by elastography is increased even in the absence of fibrosis. Mortality is generally attributable to the underlying heart disease but has also been reported to correlate with a noninvasive measure of liver stiffness. The MELD score excluding the INR (MELD-XI) predicts the clinical outcome.

Breu AC et al. A multicenter study into causes of severe acute liver injury. Clin Gastroenterol Hepatol. 2019;17:1201. [PMID: 30103039]

Fortea JI et al. Congestive hepatopathy. Int J Mol Sci. 2020;21:9420. [PMID: 33321947]

Horvatits T et al. Liver injury and failure in critical illness. Hepatology. 2019;70:2204. [PMID: 31215660]

NONCIRRHOTIC PORTAL HYPERTENSION

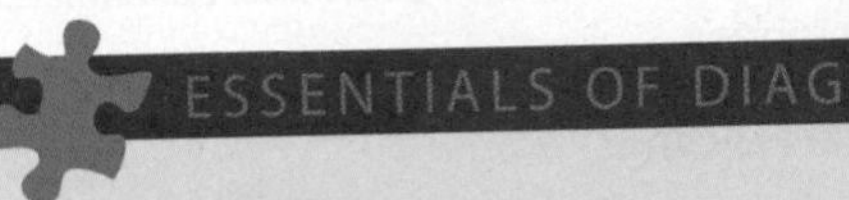

ESSENTIALS OF DIAGNOSIS

- Splenomegaly or upper GI bleeding from esophageal or gastric varices in patients without liver disease.
- Portal vein thrombosis complicating cirrhosis.

General Considerations

Causes of noncirrhotic portal hypertension include extrahepatic portal vein obstruction (portal vein thrombosis often with cavernous transformation [portal cavernoma]), splenic vein obstruction (presenting as gastric varices without esophageal varices), schistosomiasis, nodular regenerative hyperplasia, and arterial-portal vein fistula. Idiopathic noncirrhotic portal hypertension is common in India and has been attributed to chronic infections, exposure to medications or toxins, prothrombotic disorders, immunologic disorders, and genetic disorders that result in obliterative vascular lesions in the liver. It is rare in Western countries, where increased mortality is attributable to associated disorders and older age; the term portosinusoidal vascular disease has been proposed.

Portal vein thrombosis may occur in 10–25% of patients with cirrhosis, is associated with the severity of the liver disease and related in part to acquired protein C deficiency and splenorenal shunts (resulting in stagnant portal venous blood flow), and may be associated with hepatocellular carcinoma and possibly clinical deterioration but not with increased mortality. Other risk factors for portal vein thrombosis are oral contraceptive use, pregnancy, chronic inflammatory diseases (including pancreatitis), injury to the portal venous system (including surgery), other malignancies, and treatment of thrombocytopenia with eltrombopag. Portal vein thrombosis may be classified as type 1, involving the main portal vein; type 2, involving one (2a) or both (2b) branches of the portal vein; or type 3, involving the trunk and branches of the portal vein. Additional descriptors are occlusive or nonocclusive, recent or chronic, and extension (into the mesenteric vein) as well as the nature of any underlying liver disease. Splenic vein thrombosis may complicate pancreatitis or pancreatic cancer. Pylephlebitis (septic thrombophlebitis of the portal vein) may complicate intra-abdominal inflammatory disorders such as appendicitis or diverticulitis, particularly when anaerobic organisms (especially *Bacteroides* species) are involved. Nodular regenerative hyperplasia results from altered hepatic perfusion and can be associated with collagen vascular diseases; myeloproliferative disorders; and drugs, including azathioprine, 5-fluorouracil, oxaliplatin, and thioguanine. In patients infected with HIV, long-term use of didanosine and use of a combination of didanosine and stavudine have been reported to account for some cases of noncirrhotic portal hypertension often due to nodular regenerative hyperplasia; genetic factors may play a role. The term "obliterative portal venopathy" is used to describe primary occlusion of intrahepatic portal veins in the absence of cirrhosis, inflammation, or hepatic neoplasia.

Clinical Findings

A. Symptoms and Signs

Acute portal vein thrombosis usually causes abdominal pain. Aside from splenomegaly, the physical findings are not remarkable, although hepatic decompensation can follow severe GI bleeding, and intestinal infarction may occur when portal vein thrombosis is associated with mesenteric venous thrombosis. Ascites may occur in 25% of persons with noncirrhotic portal hypertension. Covert hepatic encephalopathy is reported to be common in patients with noncirrhotic portal vein thrombosis.

B. Laboratory Findings

Liver biochemical test levels are usually normal, but there may be findings of hypersplenism. An underlying hypercoagulable state is found in many noncirrhotic patients with portal vein thrombosis in the absence of an obvious provoking factor; this includes myeloproliferative neoplasms (often associated with a specific pathogenic variant [*V617F*] in the gene coding for JAK2 tyrosine kinase, which is found in 24% of cases of portal vein thrombosis), pathogeni variant *G20210A* of prothrombin, factor V Leiden variant, protein C and S deficiency, antiphospholipid syndrome, pathogenic variant *TT677* of methylenetetrahydrofolate reductase, elevated factor VIII levels, hyperhomocysteinemia, and a variant of the gene that codes for thrombin-activatable fibrinolysis inhibitor. It is possible, however, that in many cases evidence of hypercoagulability is a secondary phenomenon due to portosystemic shunting and reduced hepatic blood flow.

C. Imaging

Color Doppler ultrasonography is usually the initial diagnostic test for portal vein thrombosis. Contrast-enhanced CT or magnetic resonance angiography (MRA) of the portal system is generally confirmatory and can assess extension of thrombus into the mesenteric veins and exclude tumor thrombus in patients with cirrhosis. EUS may be helpful in some cases. In patients with jaundice, magnetic resonance cholangiography may demonstrate compression of the bile duct by a large portal cavernoma (portal biliopathy), a finding that may be more common in patients with an underlying hypercoagulable state than in those without one. In patients with pylephlebitis, CT may demonstrate an intra-abdominal source of infection, thrombosis or gas in the portal venous system, or a hepatic abscess.

D. Other Studies

Endoscopy shows esophageal or gastric varices. Needle biopsy of the liver may be indicated to diagnose schistosomiasis, nodular regenerative hyperplasia, and noncirrhotic portal fibrosis and may demonstrate sinusoidal dilatation. A low liver stiffness measurement by elastography may help distinguish noncirrhotic portal hypertension from cirrhosis.

Treatment

If splenic vein thrombosis is the cause of variceal bleeding, splenectomy is curative. For other causes of noncirrhotic portal hypertension, band ligation followed by beta-blockers to reduce portal pressure is initiated for variceal bleeding, with portosystemic shunting (including TIPS) reserved for failures of endoscopic therapy; rarely, progressive liver dysfunction requires liver transplantation. Anticoagulation, particularly with low-molecular-weight or unfractionated heparin, or thrombolytic therapy may be indicated for isolated acute portal vein thrombosis (and leads to at least partial recanalization in up to 75% of cases when started within 6 months of thrombosis) and possibly for acute splenic vein thrombosis; an oral anticoagulant is continued long-term if a hypercoagulable disorder is identified or if an acute portal vein thrombosis extends into the mesenteric veins. The decision to prescribe an anticoagulant for a patient with cirrhosis and portal vein thrombosis depends on the presence of ascites, the patient's fall risk, the extent and progression of the clot, and the patient's candidacy for liver transplantation. Partial portal vein thrombosis may resolve in 30–50% of cases. There is a paucity of data on the use of direct-acting oral anticoagulants in patients with cirrhosis and portal vein thrombosis. The use of enoxaparin to prevent portal vein thrombosis and hepatic decompensation in patients with cirrhosis has shown promise.

When to Refer

All patients with noncirrhotic portal hypertension should be referred.

Northup PG et al. Vascular liver disorders, portal vein thrombosis, and procedural bleeding in patients with liver disease: 2020 practice guidance by the American Association for the Study of Liver Diseases. Hepatology. 2021;73:366. [PMID: 33219529]

Senzolo M et al. Current knowledge and management of portal vein thrombosis in cirrhosis. J Hepatol. 2021;75:442. [PMID: 33930474]

Simonetto DA et al. ACG Clinical Guideline: disorders of the hepatic and mesenteric circulation. Am J Gastroenterol. 2020;115:18. [PMID: 31895720]

PYOGENIC HEPATIC ABSCESS

ESSENTIALS OF DIAGNOSIS

- Fever, right upper quadrant pain, jaundice.
- Often occur in setting of biliary disease, but up to 40% are "cryptogenic" in origin.
- Detected by imaging studies.

General Considerations

The incidence of liver abscess is 3.6 per 100,000 population in the United States and has increased since the 1990s. The liver can be invaded by bacteria via (1) the bile duct (acute "suppurative" [formerly ascending] cholangitis); (2) the portal vein (pylephlebitis); (3) the hepatic artery, secondary to bacteremia; (4) direct extension from an infectious process; and (5) traumatic implantation of bacteria through the abdominal wall or GI tract (eg, a fish or chicken bone). Risk factors for liver abscess include older age and male sex. Predisposing conditions and factors include presence of malignancy, diabetes mellitus, IBD, and cirrhosis; necessity for liver transplantation; endoscopic sphincterotomy; and use of a PPI. Statin use may reduce the risk of pyogenic liver abscess. Pyogenic liver abscess has been observed to be associated with a subsequent increased risk of GI malignancy and hepatocellular carcinoma.

Acute cholangitis resulting from biliary obstruction due to a stone, stricture, or neoplasm is the most common identifiable cause of hepatic abscess in the United States. In 10% of cases, liver abscess is secondary to appendicitis or diverticulitis. At least 40% of abscesses have no demonstrable cause and are classified as cryptogenic; a dental source is identified in some cases. The most frequently encountered organisms are *E coli, Klebsiella pneumoniae, Proteus vulgaris, Enterobacter aerogenes*, and multiple microaerophilic and anaerobic species (eg, *Streptococcus anginosus* [also known as *S milleri*]). Liver abscess caused by virulent strains of *K pneumoniae* may be associated with thrombophlebitis of the portal or hepatic veins and hematogenously spread septic ocular or CNS complications; the abscess may be gas-forming, associated with diabetes mellitus, and result in a high mortality rate. *Staphylococcus aureus* is usually the causative organism in patients with chronic granulomatous disease. Uncommon causative organisms include *Salmonella, Haemophilus, Yersinia*, and *Listeria*. Hepatic candidiasis, tuberculosis, and actinomycosis are seen in immunocompromised patients and those with hematologic malignancies. Rarely, hepatocellular carcinoma can present as a pyogenic abscess because of tumor necrosis, biliary obstruction, and superimposed bacterial infection (see Chapter 39); even more rarely, liver abscess may be the result of a necrotic liver metastasis. The possibility of an amoebic liver abscess must always be considered (see Chapter 35).

Clinical Findings

A. Symptoms and Signs

The presentation is often insidious. Fever (either steady or spiking fever) is almost always present and may antedate other symptoms or signs. Pain may be a prominent complaint and is localized to the right upper quadrant or epigastric area. Jaundice and tenderness in the right upper abdomen are the chief physical findings. The risk of AKI is increased.

B. Laboratory Findings

Laboratory examination reveals leukocytosis with a shift to the left. Liver biochemical tests are nonspecifically abnormal. Blood cultures are positive in 50–100% of cases.

C. Imaging

Chest films usually reveal elevation of the diaphragm if the abscess is in the right lobe of the liver. Ultrasonography, CT, or MRI may reveal the presence of intrahepatic lesions. On MRI, characteristic findings include high signal intensity on T2-weighted images and rim enhancement. The characteristic CT appearance of hepatic candidiasis, usually seen in the setting of systemic candidiasis, is that of multiple "bull's-eyes," but imaging studies may be negative in neutropenic patients.

Treatment

Treatment should consist of antimicrobial agents (generally a third-generation cephalosporin such as ceftriaxone 2 g intravenously every 24 hours and metronidazole 500 mg intravenously every 6 hours) that are effective against coliform organisms and anaerobes. Antibiotics are administered for 2–3 weeks, and sometimes for up to 6 weeks. If the abscess is at least 5 cm in diameter or the response to antibiotic therapy is not rapid, intermittent needle aspiration, percutaneous or EUS-guided catheter drainage or stent placement or, if necessary, surgical (eg, laparoscopic) drainage should be done. Other suggested indications for abscess drainage are patient age of at least 55 years, symptom duration of at least 7 days, and involvement of two lobes of the liver. The underlying source (eg, biliary disease, dental infection) should be identified and treated. The mortality rate is still substantial (at least 5% in most studies) and is highest in patients with underlying biliary malignancy or severe multiorgan dysfunction. Other risk factors for mortality include older age, cirrhosis, CKD, and other cancers. Hepatic candidiasis often responds to intravenous amphotericin B (total dose of 2–9 g). Fungal abscesses are associated with mortality rates of up to 50% and are treated with intravenous amphotericin B and drainage.

When to Admit

Nearly all patients with pyogenic hepatic abscess should be hospitalized.

Mukthinuthalapati VVPK et al. Risk factors, management, and outcomes of pyogenic liver abscess in a US safety net hospital. Dig Dis Sci. 2020;65:1529. [PMID: 31559551]

BENIGN LIVER NEOPLASMS

Benign neoplasms of the liver must be distinguished from hepatocellular carcinoma, intrahepatic cholangiocarcinoma, and metastases (see Chapter 39). The most common benign neoplasm of the liver is the **cavernous hemangioma,** often an incidental finding on ultrasonography or CT. This lesion may enlarge in women who take hormonal therapy and must be differentiated from other space-occupying intrahepatic lesions, usually by contrast-enhanced MRI, CT, or ultrasonography. Rarely, fine-needle biopsy is necessary to differentiate these lesions and does not appear to carry an increased risk of bleeding. Surgical resection of cavernous hemangiomas is infrequently necessary but may be required for abdominal pain or rapid enlargement, to exclude malignancy, or to treat Kasabach-Merritt syndrome (consumptive coagulopathy complicating a hemangioendothelioma or rapidly growing hemangioma, usually in infants).

In addition to rare instances of sinusoidal dilatation and peliosis hepatis, two distinct benign lesions with characteristic clinical, radiologic, and histopathologic features are focal nodular hyperplasia and hepatocellular adenoma. **Focal nodular hyperplasia** occurs at all ages and in both sexes and is probably not caused by oral contraceptives. It is often asymptomatic and appears as a hypervascular mass, often with a central hypodense "stellate" scar on contrast-enhanced ultrasonography, CT, or MRI. Focal nodular hyperplasia may also occur in patients with cirrhosis, with exposure to certain drugs such as azathioprine, and with antiphospholipid syndrome. The prevalence of hepatic hemangiomas is increased in patients with focal nodular hyperplasia.

Hepatocellular adenoma occurs most commonly in women in the third and fourth decades of life and is usually caused by oral contraceptives; acute abdominal pain may occur if the tumor undergoes necrosis or hemorrhage. The tumor may be associated with pathogenic variants in a variety of genes, some of which are associated with an increased risk of malignant transformation. Rare instances of multiple hepatocellular adenomas in association with maturity-onset diabetes of the young occur in families with a germline pathogenic variant in *HNF1alpha*. Hepatocellular adenomas also occur in patients with glycogen storage disease and familial adenomatous polyposis. The tumor is hypovascular.

Cystic neoplasms of the liver, such as cystadenoma and cystadenocarcinoma, must be distinguished from simple and echinococcal cysts, Von Meyenburg complexes (hamartomas), and polycystic liver disease.

Clinical Findings

The only physical finding in focal nodular hyperplasia or hepatocellular adenoma is a palpable abdominal mass in a minority of cases. Liver function is usually normal. Contrast-enhanced ultrasonography, arterial phase helical CT, and especially multiphase dynamic MRI with contrast can distinguish an adenoma from focal nodular hyperplasia without the need for biopsy in 80–90% of cases and may suggest a specific subtype of adenoma (eg, homogeneous fat pattern in *HNF1alpha*-variant adenomas and marked and persistent arterial enhancement in inflammatory adenomas).

Treatment

Oral contraceptives should not necessarily be discontinued in women who have focal nodular hyperplasia, although affected women who continue taking oral contraceptives should have annual ultrasonography for 2–3 years to ensure that the lesion is not enlarging. The prognosis is excellent.

Hepatocellular adenoma may undergo bleeding, necrosis, and rupture, often after hormone therapy; in the third trimester of pregnancy; or in men, in whom the rate of malignant transformation is high. A lesion less than 5 cm in diameter, however, poses little risk of complications to a pregnant woman, who should undergo ultrasonography during each trimester and 12 weeks postpartum. Resection is advised in all affected men and in women in whom the tumor causes symptoms or is 5 cm or greater in diameter, even in the absence of symptoms. If an adenoma is less than 5 cm in size, resection is also recommended if a beta-catenin gene pathogenic variant is present in a biopsy sample. In selected cases, laparoscopic resection or percutaneous radiofrequency ablation may be feasible. Rarely, liver transplantation is required. Regression of benign hepatic tumors may follow cessation of oral contraceptives. Transarterial embolization is the initial treatment for adenomas complicated by hemorrhage or rupture.

When to Refer

- Diagnostic uncertainty.
- For surgery.

When to Admit

- Severe pain.
- Rupture.

Herman P et al. Guidelines for the treatment of hepatocellular adenoma in the era of molecular biology: an experience-based surgeons' perspective. J Gastrointest Surg. 2021;25:1494. [PMID: 32666496]

Klompenhouwer AJ et al. New insights in the management of hepatocellular adenoma. Liver Int. 2020;40:1529. [PMID: 32464711]

Myers L et al. Focal nodular hyperplasia and hepatic adenoma: evaluation and management. Clin Liver Dis. 2020;24:389. [PMID: 32620279]

Yataco ML et al. Management of the incidental liver lesion. Am J Gastroenterol. 2021;116:855. [PMID: 33298700]

DISEASES OF THE BILIARY TRACT

See Chapter 39 for Carcinoma of the Biliary Tract.

CHOLELITHIASIS (Gallstones)

ESSENTIALS OF DIAGNOSIS

- Often asymptomatic.
- Classic biliary pain ("episodic gallbladder pain") characterized by infrequent episodes of steady severe pain in epigastrium or right upper quadrant with radiation to right scapula.
- Gallstones detected on ultrasonography.

General Considerations

Gallstones are more common in women than in men and increase in incidence in both sexes and all races with age. In the United States, the prevalence of gallstones is 8.6% in women and 5.5% in men. The highest rates are in persons over age 60, and rates are higher in Mexican American persons than in White and Black persons who are not of Latinx descent. Although cholesterol gallstones are less common in Black persons, cholelithiasis attributable to hemolysis occurs in over a third of individuals with sickle cell disease. Persons who are native to either the northern or southern hemisphere have a high rate of cholesterol cholelithiasis. As many as 75% of Pima and other American Indian women over 25 years of age have cholelithiasis. Obesity is a risk factor for gallstones, especially in women. Rapid weight loss, as occurs after bariatric surgery, also increases the risk of symptomatic gallstone formation. Diabetes mellitus, glucose intolerance, and insulin resistance are risk factors for gallstones, and a high intake of carbohydrate and high dietary glycemic load increase the risk of cholecystectomy in women. Hypertriglyceridemia may promote gallstone formation by impairing gallbladder motility. The prevalence of gallbladder disease is increased in men (but not women) with cirrhosis and HCV infection. Moreover, cholecystectomy has been reported to be associated with an increased risk of NAFLD and cirrhosis, possibly because gallstones and liver disease share risk factors. Gallstone disease is associated with increased overall, cardiovascular, and cancer mortality.

The incidence of gallstones is high in individuals with Crohn disease; approximately one-third of those with inflammatory involvement of the terminal ileum have gallstones due to disruption of bile salt resorption that results in decreased solubility of the bile. Drugs such as clofibrate, octreotide, and ceftriaxone can cause gallstones. Prolonged fasting (over 5–10 days) can lead to formation of biliary "sludge" (microlithiasis), which usually resolves with refeeding but can lead to gallstones or biliary symptoms. Pregnancy, particularly in obese women and those with insulin resistance, is associated with an increased risk of gallstones and of symptomatic gallbladder disease. Hormone replacement therapy appears to increase the risk of gallbladder disease and need for cholecystectomy; the risk is lower with transdermal than oral therapy. Gallstones detected by population screening have been reported to be associated with an increased risk of right-sided colon cancers. A low-carbohydrate diet and a Mediterranean diet as well as physical activity and cardiorespiratory fitness may help prevent gallstones. Consumption of caffeinated coffee appears to protect against gallstones in women, and a high intake of magnesium and of polyunsaturated and monounsaturated fats reduces the risk of gallstones in men. A diet high in fiber and rich in fruits and vegetables and statin use reduce the risk of cholecystectomy, particularly in women. Aspirin and other NSAIDs may protect against gallstones.

Gallstones are classified according to their predominant chemical composition as cholesterol or calcium bilirubinate stones. The latter comprise less than 20% of the gallstones found in patients in the United States or Europe but 30–40% of gallstones found in patients in Japan.

Clinical Findings

Table 16–9 lists the clinical and laboratory features of several diseases of the biliary tract as well as their treatment. Cholelithiasis is frequently asymptomatic and is discovered during a routine imaging study, surgery, or autopsy. Symptoms (biliary [or "episodic gallbladder"] pain) develop in 10–25% of patients (1–4% annually), and acute cholecystitis develops in 20% of these symptomatic persons over time. Risk factors for the development of symptoms or complications include female sex; young age; awareness of having gallstones; and large, multiple, and older stones. Occasionally, small intestinal obstruction due to "gallstone ileus" (or Bouveret syndrome when the obstructing stone is in the pylorus or duodenum) presents as the initial manifestation of cholelithiasis.

Treatment

NSAIDs (eg, diclofenac 50–75 mg intramuscularly) can be used to relieve biliary pain. Laparoscopic cholecystectomy is the treatment of choice for symptomatic gallbladder disease. Pain relief after cholecystectomy is most likely in patients with episodic pain (generally once a month or less), pain lasting 30 minutes to 24 hours, pain in the evening or at night, and the onset of symptoms 1 year or less before presentation. Patients may go home within 1 day of the procedure and return to work within days (instead of weeks for those undergoing open cholecystectomy). The procedure is often performed on an outpatient basis and is suitable for most patients, including those with acute cholecystitis. Conversion to a conventional open cholecystectomy may be necessary in 2–8% of cases (higher for acute cholecystitis than for uncomplicated cholelithiasis). Bile duct injuries occur in 0.1% of cases done by experienced surgeons, and the overall complication rate is 11% and correlates with the patient's comorbidities, duration of surgery, and emergency admissions for gallbladder disease prior to cholecystectomy. There is generally no need for prophylactic cholecystectomy in an asymptomatic person unless the gallbladder is calcified, gallstones are 3 cm or greater in diameter, or the patient is a Native American or a candidate for bariatric surgery or cardiac transplantation. Cholecystectomy may increase the risk of esophageal, proximal small intestinal, and colonic adenocarcinomas as well as hepatocellular carcinoma because of increased duodenogastric reflux and changes in intestinal exposure to bile. In pregnant patients, a conservative approach to biliary pain is advised, but for patients with repeated attacks of biliary pain or acute cholecystitis, cholecystectomy can be performed—even by the laparoscopic route—preferably in the second trimester. Enterolithotomy alone is considered adequate treatment in most patients with gallstone ileus.

Ursodeoxycholic acid is a bile salt that when given orally for up to 2 years dissolves some cholesterol stones and may be considered in occasional, selected patients who refuse cholecystectomy. The dose is 8–10 mg/kg in two or three divided doses daily. It is most effective in patients with a functioning gallbladder, as determined by gallbladder visualization on oral cholecystography, and multiple small "floating" gallstones (representing not more than 15% of patients with gallstones). In half of patients, gallstones recur within 5 years after treatment is stopped.

Table 16–9. Diseases of the biliary tract.

	Clinical Features	Laboratory Features	Diagnosis	Treatment
Asymptomatic gallstones	Asymptomatic	Normal	Ultrasonography	None
Symptomatic gallstones	Biliary pain	Normal	Ultrasonography	Laparoscopic cholecystectomy
Cholesterolosis of gallbladder	Usually asymptomatic	Normal	Oral cholecystography	None
Adenomyomatosis	May cause biliary pain	Normal	Oral cholecystography	Laparoscopic cholecystectomy if symptomatic
Porcelain gallbladder	Usually asymptomatic, high risk of gallbladder cancer	Normal	Radiograph or CT	Laparoscopic cholecystectomy
Acute cholecystitis	Epigastric or right upper quadrant pain, nausea, vomiting, fever, Murphy sign	Leukocytosis	Ultrasonography, HIDA scan	Antibiotics, laparoscopic cholecystectomy
Chronic cholecystitis	Biliary pain, constant epigastric or right upper quadrant pain, nausea	Normal	Ultrasonography (stones), oral cholecystography (nonfunctioning gallbladder)	Laparoscopic cholecystectomy
Choledocholithiasis	Asymptomatic or biliary pain, jaundice, fever; gallstone pancreatitis	Cholestatic liver biochemical tests; leukocytosis and positive blood cultures in cholangitis; elevated amylase and lipase in pancreatitis	Ultrasonography (dilated ducts), EUS, MRCP, ERCP	Endoscopic sphincterotomy and stone extraction; antibiotics for cholangitis

ERCP, endoscopic retrograde cholangiopancreatography; EUS, endoscopic ultrasonography; HIDA, hepatic iminodiacetic acid; MRCP, magnetic resonance cholangiopancreatography.

Ursodeoxycholic acid, 500–600 mg daily, and diets higher in fat reduce the risk of gallstone formation with rapid weight loss. Lithotripsy in combination with bile salt therapy for single radiolucent stones smaller than 20 mm in diameter was an option in the past but is no longer generally used in the United States.

When to Refer

Patients should be referred when they require surgery.

Gutt C et al. The treatment of gallstone disease. Dtsch Arztebl Int. 2020;117:148. [PMID: 32234195]

Sutherland JM et al. A cost-utility study of laparoscopic cholecystectomy for the treatment of symptomatic gallstones. J Gastrointest Surg. 2020;24:1314. [PMID: 31144191]

ACUTE CHOLECYSTITIS

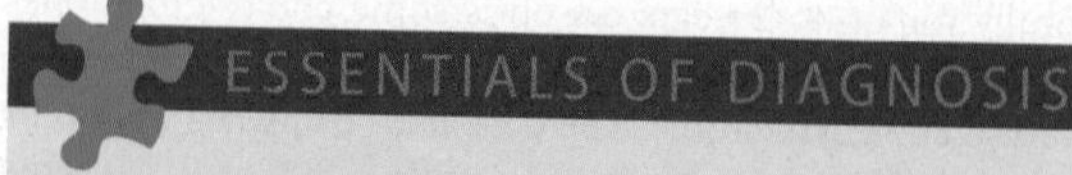

- Steady, severe pain and tenderness in the right hypochondrium or epigastrium.
- Nausea and vomiting.
- Fever and leukocytosis.

General Considerations

Cholecystitis is associated with gallstones in over 90% of cases. It occurs when a stone becomes impacted in the cystic duct and inflammation develops behind the obstruction. Acalculous cholecystitis should be considered when unexplained fever or right upper quadrant pain occurs within 2–4 weeks of major surgery or in a critically ill patient who has had no oral intake for a prolonged period; multiorgan failure is often present. Acute cholecystitis may be caused by infectious agents (eg, cytomegalovirus, cryptosporidiosis, microsporidiosis) in patients with AIDS or by vasculitis (eg, polyarteritis nodosa, Henoch-Schönlein purpura).

Clinical Findings

A. Symptoms and Signs

The acute attack is often precipitated by a large or fatty meal and is characterized by the sudden appearance of steady pain localized to the epigastrium or right hypochondrium, which may gradually subside over a period of 12–18 hours. Vomiting occurs in about 75% of patients and in half of instances affords variable relief. Fever is typical. Right upper quadrant abdominal tenderness (often with a Murphy sign, or inhibition of inspiration by pain on palpation of the right upper quadrant) is almost always present and is usually associated with muscle guarding and rebound tenderness (Table 16–9). A palpable gallbladder is present in about 15% of cases. Jaundice is present in about 25% of cases and, when persistent or severe, suggests the possibility of choledocholithiasis.

B. Laboratory Findings

The WBC count is usually high (12,000–15,000/mcL [12–15 × 10^9/L]). Total serum bilirubin values of 1–4 mg/dL (17.1–68.4 mcmol/L) may be seen even in the absence of bile duct obstruction. Serum aminotransferase and alkaline phosphatase levels are often elevated—the former as high as 300 U/mL, and even higher when associated with acute cholangitis. Serum amylase may also be moderately elevated.

C. Imaging

Plain films of the abdomen may show radiopaque gallstones in 15% of cases. Right upper quadrant abdominal ultrasonography, which is often performed first, may show gallstones but is not as sensitive for acute cholecystitis (sensitivity 67%, specificity 82%); findings suggestive of acute cholecystitis are gallbladder wall thickening, pericholecystic fluid, and a sonographic Murphy sign. ^{99m}Tc hepatobiliary imaging (using iminodiacetic acid compounds), also known as the hepatic iminodiacetic acid (HIDA) scan, is useful in demonstrating an obstructed cystic duct, which is the cause of acute cholecystitis in most patients. This test is reliable if the bilirubin is under 5 mg/dL (85.5 mcmol/L) (98% sensitivity and 81% specificity for acute cholecystitis). False-positive results can occur with prolonged fasting, liver disease, and chronic cholecystitis, and the specificity can be improved by intravenous administration of morphine, which induces spasm of the sphincter of Oddi. CT may show complications of acute cholecystitis, such as perforation or gangrene.

Differential Diagnosis

The disorders most likely to be confused with acute cholecystitis are perforated peptic ulcer, acute pancreatitis, appendicitis in a high-lying appendix, perforated colonic carcinoma or diverticulum of the hepatic flexure, liver abscess, hepatitis, pneumonia with pleurisy on the right side, and myocardial ischemia. Definite localization of pain and tenderness in the right upper quadrant, with radiation of pain around to the infrascapular area, strongly favors the diagnosis of acute cholecystitis. True cholecystitis without stones suggests acalculous cholecystitis.

Complications

A. Gangrene of the Gallbladder

Continuation or progression of right upper quadrant abdominal pain, tenderness, muscle guarding, fever, and leukocytosis after 24–48 hours suggests severe inflammation and possible gangrene of the gallbladder, resulting from ischemia due to splanchnic vasoconstriction and intravascular coagulation. Necrosis may occasionally develop without specific signs in persons who are obese, diabetic, older, or immunosuppressed. Gangrene may lead to gallbladder perforation, usually with formation of a pericholecystic abscess, and rarely to generalized peritonitis. Other serious acute complications include emphysematous cholecystitis (secondary infection with a gas-forming organism) and empyema.

B. Chronic Cholecystitis and Other Complications

Chronic cholecystitis results from repeated episodes of acute cholecystitis or chronic irritation of the gallbladder wall by stones and is characterized pathologically by varying degrees of chronic inflammation of the gallbladder. Calculi are usually present. In about 4–5% of cases, the villi of the gallbladder undergo polypoid enlargement due to deposition of cholesterol that may be visible to the naked eye ("strawberry gallbladder," cholesterolosis). In other instances, hyperplasia of all or part of the gallbladder wall may be so marked as to give the appearance of a myoma (adenomyomatosis). Hydrops of the gallbladder results when acute cholecystitis subsides but cystic duct obstruction persists, producing distention of the gallbladder with a clear mucoid fluid. Occasionally, a stone in the neck of the gallbladder may compress the common hepatic duct and cause jaundice (Mirizzi syndrome). Xanthogranulomatous cholecystitis is a rare, aggressive variant of chronic cholecystitis characterized by grayish-yellow nodules or streaks, representing lipid-laden macrophages, in the wall of the gallbladder and often presents with acute jaundice.

Cholelithiasis with chronic cholecystitis may be associated with acute exacerbations of gallbladder inflammation, bile duct stones, fistulization to the bowel, pancreatitis and, rarely, carcinoma of the gallbladder. Calcified (porcelain) gallbladder is associated with gallbladder carcinoma and is generally an indication for cholecystectomy; the risk of gallbladder cancer may be higher when calcification is mucosal rather than intramural.

Treatment

Acute cholecystitis usually subsides on a conservative regimen, including withholding oral feedings, intravenous fluids, analgesics, and intravenous antibiotics (generally a second- or third-generation cephalosporin such as ceftriaxone 1 g intravenously every 24 hours, with the addition of metronidazole, 500 mg intravenously every 6 hours), although the need for antibiotics has been questioned in patients undergoing immediate cholecystectomy. In severe cases, a fluoroquinolone such as ciprofloxacin, 400 mg intravenously every 12 hours, plus metronidazole, may be given. Morphine or meperidine may be administered for pain. Because of the high risk of recurrent attacks (up to 10% by 1 month and over 20% by 1 year), cholecystectomy—generally laparoscopically—should be performed within 24 hours of admission to the hospital for acute cholecystitis. Compared with delayed surgery, surgery within 24 hours is associated with a shorter length of stay, lower costs, and greater patient satisfaction. If nonsurgical treatment has been elected, the patient (especially if diabetic or older) must be watched carefully for recurrent symptoms, evidence of gangrene of the gallbladder, or cholangitis.

In high-risk patients, ultrasound-guided aspiration of the gallbladder, if feasible, percutaneous or EUS-guided cholecystostomy, or endoscopic insertion of a stent or nasobiliary drain into the gallbladder may postpone or even avoid the need for surgery. ERCP with transpapillary gallbladder drainage may be preferable in patients with coagulopathy or ascites. Immediate cholecystectomy is mandatory when there is evidence of gangrene or perforation. Surgical treatment of chronic cholecystitis is the same as for acute cholecystitis. If indicated, cholangiography can be performed during laparoscopic cholecystectomy. Choledocholithiasis can also be excluded by either preoperative or postoperative MRCP or ERCP.

Prognosis

The overall mortality rate of cholecystectomy is less than 0.2%, but hepatobiliary tract surgery is a more formidable procedure in older patients, in whom mortality rates are higher, as they are in persons with diabetes mellitus and cirrhosis. A technically successful surgical procedure in an appropriately selected patient is generally followed by complete resolution of symptoms.

When to Admit

All patients with acute cholecystitis should be hospitalized.

Podboy A et al. Comparison of EUS-guided endoscopic transpapillary and percutaneous gallbladder drainage for acute cholecystitis: a systematic review with network meta-analysis. Gastrointest Endosc. 2021;93:797. [PMID: 32987004]

Saumoy M et al. Endoscopic therapies for gallbladder drainage. Gastrointest Endosc. 2021;94:671. [PMID: 34344541]

Sobani ZA et al. Endoscopic transpapillary gallbladder drainage for acute cholecystitis. Dig Dis Sci. 2021;66:1425. [PMID: 32588249]

Sobani ZA et al. Endoscopic ultrasound-guided gallbladder drainage. Dig Dis Sci. 2021;66:2154. [PMID: 32749635]

Teoh AYB et al. EUS-guided gallbladder drainage versus laparoscopic cholecystectomy for acute cholecystitis: a propensity score analysis with 1-year follow-up data. Gastrointest Endosc. 2021;93:577. [PMID: 32615177]

PRE- & POSTCHOLECYSTECTOMY SYNDROMES

1. Precholecystectomy

In a small group of patients (mostly women) with biliary pain, conventional radiographic studies of the upper GI tract and gallbladder—including cholangiography—are unremarkable. Emptying of the gallbladder may be markedly reduced on gallbladder scintigraphy following injection of cholecystokinin; cholecystectomy may be curative in such cases. Histologic examination of the resected gallbladder may show chronic cholecystitis or microlithiasis. An additional diagnostic consideration is sphincter of Oddi dysfunction.

2. Postcholecystectomy

Following cholecystectomy, some patients complain of continuing symptoms, ie, right upper quadrant pain, flatulence, and fatty food intolerance. The persistence of symptoms in this group of patients suggests the possibility of an incorrect diagnosis prior to cholecystectomy, eg, esophagitis, pancreatitis, radiculopathy, or functional bowel disease. Choledocholithiasis or bile duct stricture should be ruled out. Pain may also be associated with dilatation of the cystic duct remnant, neuroma formation in the ductal wall, foreign body granuloma, anterior cutaneous nerve entrapment syndrome, or traction on the bile duct by a long cystic duct.

The clinical presentation of right upper quadrant pain, chills, fever, or jaundice suggests biliary tract disease. EUS is recommended to demonstrate or exclude a stone or stricture. Biliary pain associated with elevated liver biochemical tests or a dilated bile duct in the absence of an obstructing lesion suggests sphincter of Oddi dysfunction. Biliary manometry may be useful for documenting elevated baseline sphincter of Oddi pressures typical of sphincter dysfunction when biliary pain is associated with elevated liver biochemical tests (twofold) or a dilated bile duct (greater than 10 mm) ("sphincter disorder," formerly type II sphincter of Oddi dysfunction), but is not necessary when both are present ("sphincter stenosis," formerly type I sphincter of Oddi dysfunction) and is associated with a high risk of pancreatitis. In the absence of either elevated liver biochemical tests or a dilated bile duct ("functional pain," formerly type III sphincter of Oddi dysfunction), a nonbiliary source of symptoms should be suspected; biliary sphincterotomy does not benefit this group. (Analogous criteria have been developed for pancreatic sphincter dysfunction.) Biliary scintigraphy after intravenous administration of morphine and MRCP following intravenous administration of secretin have been studied as screening tests for sphincter dysfunction. Endoscopic sphincterotomy is most likely to relieve symptoms in patients with a sphincter disorder or stenosis, although many patients continue to have some pain. In some cases, treatment with a calcium channel blocker, long-acting nitrate, phosphodiesterase inhibitor (eg, vardenafil), duloxetine, or tricyclic antidepressant or possibly injection of the sphincter with botulinum toxin may be beneficial. The rate of psychosocial comorbidity with sphincter of Oddi dysfunction does not appear to differ from that of the general population. In refractory cases, surgical sphincteroplasty or removal of the cystic duct remnant may be considered.

When to Refer

Patients with sphincter of Oddi dysfunction should be referred for diagnostic procedures.

Miyatani H et al. Clinical course of biliary-type sphincter of Oddi dysfunction: endoscopic sphincterotomy and functional dyspepsia as affecting factors. Ther Adv Gastrointest Endosc. 2019;12:2631774519867184. [PMID: 31448369]

Smith ZL et al. The next EPISOD: trends in utilization of endoscopic sphincterotomy for sphincter of Oddi dysfunction from 2010–2019. Clin Gastroenterol Hepatol. 2022;20:e600. [PMID: 33161159]

CHOLEDOCHOLITHIASIS & CHOLANGITIS

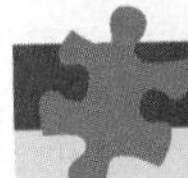

ESSENTIALS OF DIAGNOSIS

- Often a history of biliary pain, which may be accompanied by jaundice.
- Occasional patients present with painless jaundice.
- Nausea and vomiting.
- Cholangitis should be suspected with fever followed by hypothermia and gram-negative shock, jaundice, and leukocytosis.
- Stones in bile duct most reliably detected by ERCP or EUS.

General Considerations

About 15% of patients with gallstones in the gallbladder have choledocholithiasis (bile duct stones). The percentage rises with age, and the frequency in older adults with gallstones may be as high as 50%. Bile duct stones usually originate in the gallbladder but may also form spontaneously in the bile duct after cholecystectomy. The risk is increased twofold in persons with a juxtapapillary duodenal diverticulum. Symptoms and possible cholangitis result if there is obstruction.

Clinical Findings

A. Symptoms and Signs

A history of biliary pain or jaundice may be obtained. Biliary pain results from rapid increases in bile duct pressure due to obstructed bile flow. The features that suggest the presence of a bile duct stone are (1) frequently recurring attacks of right upper abdominal pain that is severe and persists for hours, (2) chills and fever associated with severe pain, and (3) a history of jaundice associated with episodes of abdominal pain (Table 16–9). The combination of right upper quadrant pain, fever (and chills), and jaundice represents **Charcot triad** and denotes the classic picture of acute cholangitis. The addition of altered mental status and hypotension (**Reynolds pentad**) signifies acute suppurative cholangitis and is an endoscopic emergency. According to the Tokyo guidelines (revised in 2018), the diagnosis of acute cholangitis is established by an elevated WBC signifying systemic inflammation and elevated cholestatic liver biochemical test levels or imaging evidence of biliary dilatation, or both.

Hepatomegaly may be present in calculous biliary obstruction, and tenderness is usually present in the right upper quadrant and epigastrium. Bile duct obstruction lasting more than 30 days results in liver damage leading to cirrhosis. Hepatic failure with portal hypertension occurs in untreated cases. In a population-based study from Denmark, acute cholangitis was reported to be a marker of occult GI cancer.

B. Laboratory Findings

Acute obstruction of the bile duct typically produces a transient albeit striking increase in serum aminotransferase levels (often greater than 1000 U/L [20 mckat/L]). Bilirubinuria and elevation of the serum bilirubin are present if the bile duct remains obstructed; levels commonly fluctuate. Serum alkaline phosphatase levels rise more slowly. Not uncommonly, serum amylase elevations are present because of secondary pancreatitis. When extrahepatic obstruction persists for more than a few weeks, differentiation of obstruction from chronic cholestatic liver disease becomes more difficult. Leukocytosis is present in patients with acute cholangitis. Prolongation of the prothrombin time can result from the obstructed flow of bile to the intestine. In contrast to hepatocellular dysfunction, hypoprothrombinemia due to obstructive jaundice will respond to intravenous vitamin K, 10 mg, or water-soluble oral vitamin K (phytonadione), 5 mg, within 24–36 hours. In patients with acute calculous cholecystitis, predictors of concomitant choledocholithiasis are serum aminotransferase levels over three times the upper limit of normal, an alkaline phosphatase level above normal, a serum lipase over three times the upper limit of normal, a bilirubin of 1.8 mg/dL or more, and a bile duct diameter above 6 mm.

C. Imaging

Ultrasonography and CT may demonstrate dilated bile ducts, and radionuclide imaging may show impaired bile flow. EUS, helical CT, and magnetic resonance cholangiography are accurate in demonstrating bile duct stones and may be used in patients thought to be at intermediate risk for choledocholithiasis (age older than 55 years, cholecystitis, bile duct diameter greater than 6 mm on ultrasonography, serum bilirubin 1.8–4 mg/dL [30.78–68.4 mcmol/L], elevated serum liver enzymes, or pancreatitis). A decision analysis has suggested that magnetic resonance cholangiography is preferable when the risk of bile duct stones is low (less than 40%), and EUS is preferable when the risk is intermediate (40–91%). ERCP (occasionally with intraductal ultrasonography) or percutaneous transhepatic cholangiography provides the most direct and accurate means of determining the cause, location, and extent of obstruction, but in patients at intermediate risk of choledocholithiasis, initial cholecystectomy with intraoperative cholangiography results in a shorter length of hospital stay, fewer bile duct investigations, and no increase in morbidity. If the likelihood that obstruction is caused by a stone is high (bile duct stone seen on ultrasonography, serum bilirubin greater than 4 mg/dL [68.4 mcmol/L], or acute cholangitis), ERCP with sphincterotomy and stone extraction or stent placement is the procedure of choice; meticulous technique is required to avoid causing acute cholangitis. Because the sensitivity of these criteria for choledocholithiasis is only 80%, it is not unreasonable for magnetic resonance cholangiography or EUS to be done before ERCP.

Differential Diagnosis

The most common cause of obstructive jaundice is a bile duct stone. Next in frequency are neoplasms of the pancreas, ampulla of Vater, or bile duct or an obstructed stent placed previously for decompression of an obstructing tumor. Extrinsic compression of the bile duct may result from metastatic carcinoma (usually from the GI tract or breast) involving porta hepatis lymph nodes or, rarely, from a large duodenal diverticulum. Gallbladder cancer extending into the bile duct often presents as obstructive jaundice. Chronic cholestatic liver diseases (PBC, sclerosing cholangitis, drug-induced) must be considered. Hepatocellular jaundice can usually be differentiated by the history, clinical findings, and liver biochemical tests, but liver biopsy is necessary on occasion. Recurrent pyogenic cholangitis should be considered in persons from Asia (and occasionally elsewhere) with intrahepatic biliary stones (particularly in the left ductal system) and recurrent cholangitis.

Treatment

In general, bile duct stones, even small ones, should be removed, even in an asymptomatic patient. A bile duct stone in a patient with cholelithiasis or cholecystitis is usually treated by endoscopic sphincterotomy and stone extraction followed by laparoscopic cholecystectomy within 72 hours in patients with cholecystitis and within 2 weeks in those without cholecystitis. In selected cases, laparoscopic cholecystectomy and ERCP can be performed in a single session. An alternative approach, which is also associated with a shorter duration of hospitalization in patients at intermediate risk for choledocholithiasis, is laparoscopic cholecystectomy and bile duct exploration.

For patients older than 70 years or poor-risk patients with cholelithiasis and choledocholithiasis, cholecystectomy may be deferred after endoscopic sphincterotomy because the risk of subsequent cholecystitis is low (although the risk of subsequent complications is lower when cholecystectomy is performed). ERCP with sphincterotomy, biliary drainage, and stone removal or stent placement generally within 48 hours, should be performed before cholecystectomy in patients with gallstones and cholangitis, jaundice (serum total bilirubin greater than 4 mg/dL [68.4 mcmol/L]), a dilated bile duct (greater than 6 mm), or stones in the bile duct seen on ultrasonography or CT. (Stones may ultimately recur in up to 12% of patients, particularly in older patients, when the bile duct diameter is 15 mm or greater or when brown pigment stones are found at the time of the initial sphincterotomy.) For bile duct stones 1 cm or more in diameter, endoscopic sphincterotomy followed by large balloon dilation has been recommended. Endoscopic balloon dilation of the sphincter of Oddi is otherwise considered in patients with coagulopathy because the risk of bleeding is lower with balloon dilation than with sphincterotomy. Balloon dilation is not associated with a higher rate of pancreatitis than endoscopic sphincterotomy if adequate dilation for more than 1 minute is carried out, and it may be associated with a lower rate of stone recurrence. An alternative approach is placement of a short fully covered metal stent to mitigate bleeding risk. EUS-guided biliary drainage and PTC with drainage are second-line approaches if ERCP fails or is not possible. In patients with biliary pancreatitis that resolves rapidly, the stone usually passes into the intestine, and ERCP prior to cholecystectomy is not necessary if intraoperative cholangiography is planned.

Choledocholithiasis discovered at laparoscopic cholecystectomy may be managed via laparoscopic or, if necessary, open bile duct exploration or by postoperative endoscopic sphincterotomy. Operative findings of choledocholithiasis are palpable stones in the bile duct, dilatation or thickening of the wall of the bile duct, or stones in the gallbladder small enough to pass through the cystic duct. Laparoscopic intraoperative cholangiography (or intraoperative ultrasonography) should be done at the time of cholecystectomy in patients with liver enzyme elevations but a bile duct diameter of less than 5 mm; if a ductal stone is found, the duct should be explored. In the post-cholecystectomy patient with choledocholithiasis, endoscopic sphincterotomy with stone extraction is preferable to transabdominal surgery. Lithotripsy (endoscopic or external), peroral cholangioscopy (choledoscopy), or biliary stenting may be a therapeutic consideration for large stones. For the patient with a T tube and bile duct stone, the stone may be extracted via the T tube.

Postoperative antibiotics are not administered routinely after biliary tract surgery. Cultures of the bile are always taken at operation. If biliary tract infection was present preoperatively or is apparent at operation, ampicillin-sulbactam (3 g intravenously every 6 hours) or piperacillin-tazobactam (3.375 or 4.5 g intravenously every 6 hours) or a third-generation cephalosporin (eg, ceftriaxone, 1 g intravenously every 24 hours) is administered postoperatively and adjusted when the results of sensitivity tests on culture specimens are available. A T-tube cholangiogram should be done before the tube is removed, usually about 3 weeks after surgery.

Urgent ERCP with sphincterotomy and stone extraction (within 24–48 hours) is generally indicated for choledocholithiasis complicated by acute cholangitis and is preferred to surgery. Before ERCP, liver function should be evaluated thoroughly. The prothrombin time may be restored to normal by intravenous administration of vitamin K. For mild-to-moderately severe community-acquired acute cholangitis, ciprofloxacin (400 mg intravenously every 12 hours) penetrates well into bile and is effective treatment, with metronidazole (500 mg intravenously every 6–8 hours) for anaerobic coverage. An alternative regimen is ampicillin-sulbactam (3 g intravenously every 6 hours). Regimens for patients with severe or hospital-acquired acute cholangitis, and those potentially infected with an antibiotic-resistant pathogen, include intravenous piperacillin-tazobactam (3.375 or 4 g every 6 hours) or a carbapenem such as meropenem (1 g intravenously every 8 hours). Aminoglycosides (eg, gentamicin 5–7 mg/kg intravenously every 24 hours) may be added in cases of severe sepsis or septic shock but should not be given for more than a few days because the risk of aminoglycoside nephrotoxicity is increased in patients with cholestasis. Regimens that include drugs active against anaerobes are required when a biliary-enteric communication is present.

Emergent decompression of the bile duct, generally by ERCP, is required for patients who are septic or fail to improve on antibiotics within 12–24 hours. Medical therapy alone is most likely to fail in patients with tachycardia, a serum albumin less than 3 g/dL (30 g/L), marked hyperbilirubinemia, a high serum ALT level, a high WBC count, and a prothrombin time greater than 14 seconds on admission. If sphincterotomy cannot be performed, the bile duct can be decompressed by a biliary stent or nasobiliary catheter. Once decompression is achieved, antibiotics are generally continued for at least another 3 days. Cholecystectomy can be undertaken after resolution of cholangitis unless the patient remains unfit for surgery. Mortality from acute cholangitis has been reported to correlate with a high total bilirubin level, prolonged partial thromboplastin time, malnutrition, presence of a liver abscess, and unsuccessful ERCP.

When to Refer

All symptomatic patients with choledocholithiasis should be referred.

When to Admit

All patients with acute cholangitis should be hospitalized.

Alsayid M et al. The impact of laparoscopic cholecystectomy on 30-day readmission rate for acute cholangitis patients: a single-center study. Dig Dis Sci. 2021;66:861. [PMID: 32248392]

An Z et al. Acute cholangitis: causes, diagnosis, and management. Gastroenterol Clin North Am. 2021;50:403. [PMID: 34024448]

Buxbaum JL et al. ASGE guideline on the management of cholangitis. Gastrointest Endosc. 2021;94:207. [PMID: 34023065]

Buxbaum J et al. Toward an evidence-based approach for cholangitis diagnosis. Gastrointest Endosc. 2021;94:297. [PMID: 33905719]

Iqbal U et al. Emergent versus urgent ERCP in acute cholangitis: a systematic review and meta-analysis. Gastrointest Endosc. 2020;91:753. [PMID: 31628955]

BILIARY STRICTURE

Benign biliary strictures are the result of surgical (including liver transplantation) anastomosis or injury in about 95% of cases. The remainder of cases are caused by blunt external injury to the abdomen, pancreatitis, IgG_4-related disease, erosion of the duct by a gallstone, or prior endoscopic sphincterotomy.

Signs of injury to the duct may or may not be recognized in the immediate postoperative period. If complete occlusion has occurred, jaundice will develop rapidly; more often, however, a tear has been made accidentally in the duct, and the earliest manifestation of injury may be excessive or prolonged loss of bile from the surgical drains. Bile leakage resulting in a bile collection (biloma) may predispose to localized infection, which in turn accentuates scar formation and the ultimate development of a fibrous stricture.

Cholangitis is the most common complication of stricture. Typically, the patient experiences episodes of pain, fever, chills, and jaundice within a few weeks to months after cholecystectomy. Physical findings may include jaundice during an acute attack of cholangitis and right upper quadrant abdominal tenderness. Serum alkaline phosphatase is usually elevated. Hyperbilirubinemia is variable, fluctuating during exacerbations and usually remaining in the range of 5–10 mg/dL (85.5–171 mcmol/L). Blood cultures may be positive during an acute episode of cholangitis. Secondary biliary cirrhosis will inevitably develop if a stricture is not treated.

MRCP or multidetector CT is valuable in demonstrating the stricture and outlining the anatomy. ERCP is the first-line interventional approach and permits biopsy and cytologic specimens to exclude malignancy (in conjunction with EUS-guided fine-needle aspiration, an even more sensitive test for distal bile duct malignancy), sphincterotomy to allow a bile leak to close, and dilation (often repeated) and stent placement, thereby avoiding surgical repair in some cases. When ERCP is unsuccessful, dilation of a stricture may be accomplished by PTC or under EUS guidance. Placement of multiple plastic stents appears to be more effective than placement of a single stent. The use of fully covered self-expanding metal stents, which are more easily removed endoscopically than uncovered metal stents, as well as bioabsorbable stents, is an alternative to use of plastic stents and requires fewer ERCPs to achieve stricture resolution; stent migration may occur in 10% of cases. Uncovered metal stents, which often cannot be removed endoscopically, are generally avoided in benign strictures unless life expectancy is less than 2 years. Strictures related to chronic pancreatitis are more difficult than postsurgical strictures to treat endoscopically and may be best managed with a temporary covered metal stent. Following liver transplantation, endoscopic management is more successful for anastomotic than for nonanastomotic strictures. Results for nonanastomotic strictures may be improved with repeated dilations or the use of multiple plastic stents. Biliary strictures after live liver donor liver transplantation, particularly in patients with a late-onset (after 24 weeks) stricture or with intrahepatic biliary dilatation, are also challenging and require aggressive endoscopic therapy; in addition, the risk of post-ERCP pancreatitis appears to be increased.

When malignancy cannot be excluded with certainty, additional diagnostic approaches may be considered—if available—including intraductal ultrasonography, peroral cholangioscopy, confocal laser endomicroscopy, optical coherence tomography, fluorescence in situ hybridization, and, most recently, next-generation genetic sequencing. Differentiation from cholangiocarcinoma may ultimately require surgical exploration in 20% of cases. Operative treatment of a stricture frequently necessitates performance of an end-to-end ductal repair, choledochojejunostomy, or hepaticojejunostomy to reestablish bile flow into the intestine.

When to Refer

All patients with biliary stricture should be referred.

When to Admit

Patients with acute cholangitis should be hospitalized.

Han S et al. Combination of ERCP-based modalities increases diagnostic yield for biliary strictures. Dig Dis Sci. 2021;66:1276. [PMID: 32430658]

Ramchandani M et al. Fully covered self-expanding metal stent vs multiple plastic stents to treat benign biliary strictures secondary to chronic pancreatitis: a multicenter randomized trial. Gastroenterology. 2021;161:185. [PMID: 33741314]

PRIMARY SCLEROSING CHOLANGITIS

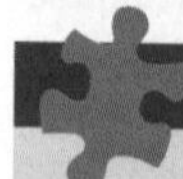

ESSENTIALS OF DIAGNOSIS

- Most common in men aged 20–50 years.
- Often associated with ulcerative colitis.
- Progressive jaundice, itching, and other features of cholestasis.
- Diagnosis based on characteristic cholangiographic findings.
- At least 10% risk of cholangiocarcinoma.

General Considerations

Primary sclerosing cholangitis is an uncommon disease thought to result from an increased immune response to intestinal endotoxins and characterized by diffuse inflammation of the biliary tract leading to fibrosis and strictures of the biliary system. From 60% to 70% of affected persons are male, usually 20–50 years of age (median age 41). The incidence is nearly 3.3 per 100,000 in Asian Americans, 2.8 per 100,000 in Latinx Americans, and 2.1 per 100,000 in Black persons, with an intermediate (and increasing) incidence in White persons and a prevalence of 16.2 per 100,000 population (21 per 100,000 men and 6 per 100,000 women) in the United States.

Primary sclerosing cholangitis is closely associated with IBD (more commonly ulcerative colitis than Crohn colitis), which is present in approximately two-thirds of patients with primary sclerosing cholangitis; however, clinically significant sclerosing cholangitis develops in only 1–4% of patients with ulcerative colitis. Smoking is associated with a decreased risk of primary sclerosing cholangitis in patients who also have IBD. Coffee consumption is also associated with a decreased risk of primary sclerosing cholangitis, and statin use is associated with improved outcomes in patients with primary sclerosing cholangitis. Women with primary sclerosing cholangitis may be more likely to have recurrent UTIs and less likely to use hormone replacement therapy than healthy controls. Associations with CVD and diabetes mellitus have been reported. Primary sclerosing cholangitis is associated with the histocompatibility antigens HLA-B8 and -DR3 or -DR4, and first-degree relatives of patients with primary sclerosing cholangitis have a fourfold increased risk of primary sclerosing cholangitis and a threefold increased risk of ulcerative colitis. A subset of patients with primary sclerosing cholangitis have increased serum IgG_4 levels and distinct HLA associations (with a poorer prognosis) but do not meet criteria for IgG_4-related sclerosing cholangitis. The diagnosis of primary sclerosing cholangitis may be difficult to make after biliary surgery.

Clinical Findings

A. Symptoms and Signs

Primary sclerosing cholangitis presents as progressive obstructive jaundice, frequently associated with fatigue, pruritus, anorexia, and indigestion. A patient's disease may be diagnosed in the presymptomatic phase because of an elevated alkaline phosphatase level or a subclinical phase based on abnormalities on magnetic resonance cholangiography despite normal liver enzyme levels. Complications of chronic cholestasis, such as osteoporosis, malabsorption of fat-soluble vitamins, and malnutrition, may occur late in the course. Risk factors for osteoporosis include older age, lower BMI, and longer duration of IBD. Esophageal varices on initial endoscopy are most likely in patients with a higher Mayo risk score based on age, bilirubin, albumin, and AST and a higher AST/ALT ratio, and new varices are likely to develop in those with a lower platelet count and higher bilirubin at 2 years. In patients with primary sclerosing cholangitis, ulcerative colitis is frequently characterized by rectal sparing and backwash ileitis.

B. Diagnostic Findings

The diagnosis of primary sclerosing cholangitis is generally made by MRCP, the sensitivity of which approaches that of ERCP. Characteristic cholangiographic findings are segmental fibrosis of bile ducts with saccular dilatations between strictures. Biliary obstruction by a stone or tumor should be excluded. Liver biopsy is not necessary for diagnosis when cholangiographic findings are characteristic. The disease may be confined to small intrahepatic bile ducts in about 15% of cases, in which case MRCP and ERCP are normal, and the diagnosis is suggested by liver biopsy findings. These patients have a longer survival than patients with involvement of the large ducts and do not appear to be at increased risk for cholangiocarcinoma unless large-duct sclerosing cholangitis develops (which occurs in about 20% over 7–10 years). Liver biopsy may show characteristic periductal fibrosis ("onion-skinning") and allows staging, which is based on the degree of fibrosis and which correlates with liver stiffness as measured by elastography. Perinuclear ANCA as well as antinuclear, anticardiolipin, antithyroperoxidase, and anti-*Saccharomyces cerevisiae* antibodies and rheumatoid factor are frequently detected in serum.

Occasional patients have clinical and histologic features of both sclerosing cholangitis and autoimmune hepatitis. Cholangitis in IgG_4-related disease is sometimes difficult to distinguish from primary sclerosing cholangitis (and even cholangiocarcinoma), is associated with autoimmune pancreatitis (see Chronic Pancreatitis), and is responsive to corticosteroids. A serum IgG_4 level more than four times the upper limit of normal or an IgG_4:IgG_1 ratio of more than 0.24 strongly suggests IgG_4-related sclerosing cholangitis, but in up to one-third of cases, the serum IgG_4 level is normal. Primary sclerosing cholangitis must also be distinguished from idiopathic adulthood ductopenia (a rare disorder that affects young to middle-aged adults who manifest cholestasis resulting from loss of interlobular and septal bile ducts yet who have a normal cholangiogram. Primary sclerosing cholangitis must also be distinguished from other cholangiopathies (including PBC; cystic fibrosis; eosinophilic cholangitis; AIDS cholangiopathy; histiocytosis X; allograft rejection; graft-versus-host disease; ischemic cholangiopathy [often with biliary "casts," a rapid progression to cirrhosis, and a poor outcome] caused by hepatic artery thrombosis, shock, respiratory failure, or drugs, intra-arterial chemotherapy, sarcoidosis, and post-COVID cholangiopathy).

Complications

Cholangiocarcinoma may complicate the course of primary sclerosing cholangitis in up to 20% of cases (1.2% per year) and may be difficult to diagnose by cytologic examination or biopsy because of false-negative results. A serum CA 19-9 level above 100 U/mL is suggestive but not diagnostic of cholangiocarcinoma. Annual MRI with MRCP or right upper quadrant ultrasonography (MRCP is more sensitive than ultrasonography) and, by some guidelines but not others, serum CA 19-9 testing (a level of 20 is the threshold for further investigation) are recommended for surveillance, with ERCP and biliary cytology if the results are suggestive of malignancy. PET, peroral cholangioscopy, and confocal laser endomicroscopy may play roles in the early detection of cholangiocarcinoma. Patients with ulcerative colitis and primary sclerosing cholangitis are at high risk (tenfold higher than ulcerative colitis patients without primary sclerosing cholangitis) for colorectal neoplasia. The risks of gallstones, cholecystitis, gallbladder polyps, and gallbladder carcinoma appear to be increased in patients with primary sclerosing cholangitis.

Treatment

Episodes of acute bacterial cholangitis may be treated with ciprofloxacin (750 mg twice daily orally or intravenously). Ursodeoxycholic acid in standard doses (10–15 mg/kg/day orally) may improve liver biochemical test results but does not appear to alter the natural history. However, withdrawal of ursodeoxycholic acid may result in worsening of liver biochemical test levels and increased pruritus, and ursodeoxycholic acid in intermediate doses (17–23 mg/kg/day) has been reported to be beneficial.

Careful endoscopic evaluation of the biliary tract may permit balloon dilation of localized strictures, and repeated dilation of a dominant stricture may improve survival, although such patients have reduced survival compared with patients who do not have a dominant stricture. Short-term (2–3 weeks) placement of a stent in a major stricture also may relieve symptoms and improve biochemical abnormalities, with sustained improvement after the stent is removed, but may not be superior to balloon dilation alone; long-term stenting may increase the rate of complications such as cholangitis and is not recommended.

Cholecystectomy is indicated in patients with primary sclerosing cholangitis and a gallbladder polyp greater than 8 mm in diameter. In patients without cirrhosis, surgical resection of a dominant bile duct stricture may lead to longer survival than endoscopic therapy by decreasing the subsequent risk of cholangiocarcinoma. When feasible, extensive surgical resection of cholangiocarcinoma complicating primary sclerosing cholangitis may result in 5-year survival rates of greater than 50%. In patients with ulcerative colitis, primary sclerosing cholangitis is an independent risk factor for the development of colorectal dysplasia and cancer (especially in the right colon), and strict adherence to a colonoscopic surveillance program (yearly for those with ulcerative colitis and every 5 years for those without ulcerative colitis) is recommended. Whether treatment with ursodeoxycholic acid reduces the risk of colorectal dysplasia and carcinoma in patients with ulcerative colitis and primary sclerosing cholangitis is still uncertain. For patients with cirrhosis and clinical decompensation, liver transplantation is the treatment of choice; primary sclerosing cholangitis recurs in the graft in 30% of cases, with a possible reduction in the risk of recurrence when colectomy has been performed for ulcerative colitis before transplantation.

Prognosis

Survival of patients with primary sclerosing cholangitis averages 9–17 years, and up to 21 years in population-based studies. Adverse prognostic markers are older age, hepatosplenomegaly, higher serum bilirubin and AST levels, lower albumin levels, a history of variceal bleeding, a dominant bile duct stricture, and extrahepatic duct changes. Variceal bleeding is also a risk factor for cholangiocarcinoma. Patients in whom serum alkaline phosphatase levels decline by 40% or more (spontaneously, with ursodeoxycholic acid therapy, or after treatment of a dominant stricture) have longer transplant-free survival times than those in whom the alkaline phosphatase does not decline. Moreover, improvement in the serum alkaline phosphatase to less than 1.5 times the upper limit of normal is associated with a reduced risk of cholangiocarcinoma. Risk of progression can be predicted by three findings on MRI and MRCP: a cirrhotic appearance to the liver, portal hypertension, and enlarged perihepatic lymph nodes.

The Amsterdam-Oxford model has been proposed to predict transplant-free survival and is based on disease subtype (large- versus small-duct involvement), age at diagnosis, serum albumin, platelet count, serum AST, serum alkaline phosphatase, and serum bilirubin. Another promising scoring system is the UK-PSC risk score based on age, serum bilirubin, serum alkaline phosphatase, albumin, platelet count, presence of extrahepatic disease, and variceal hemorrhage. The PSC risk estimate tool (PREsTo) based on nine variables (bilirubin, albumin, alkaline phosphatase, platelets, AST, hemoglobin, sodium, patient age, and number of years since the diagnosis of primary sclerosing cholangitis) has been reported to accurately predict hepatic decompensation. Transplant-free survival can also be predicted by serum levels of markers of liver fibrosis—hyaluronic acid, tissue inhibitor of metalloproteinase-1, and propeptide of type III procollagen. Reduced quality of life is associated with older age, large-duct disease, and systemic symptoms. Maternal primary sclerosing cholangitis is associated with preterm birth and cesarean section delivery; risk of congenital malformations is not increased. Interestingly, patients with milder ulcerative colitis tend to have more severe primary cholangitis and a higher rate of liver transplantation. Actuarial survival rates with liver transplantation are as high as 72% at 5 years, but rates are much lower once cholangiocarcinoma has developed. Following transplantation, patients have an increased risk of nonanastomotic biliary strictures and—in those with ulcerative colitis—colon cancer, and the disease recurs in 30%. The retransplantation rate is higher than that for PBC. Patients who are unable to undergo liver transplantation will ultimately require high-quality palliative care (see Chapter 5).

Eaton JE et al. Early cholangiocarcinoma detection with magnetic resonance imaging versus ultrasound in primary sclerosing cholangitis. Hepatology. 2021;73:1868. [PMID: 32974892]

Eaton JE et al. Primary sclerosing cholangitis risk estimate tool (PREsTo) predicts outcomes of the disease: a derivation and validation study using machine learning. Hepatology. 2020;71:214. [PMID: 29742811]

Nicoletti A et al. Guideline review: British Society of Gastroenterology/UK-PSC guidelines for the diagnosis and management of primary sclerosing cholangitis. Frontline Gastroenterol. 2020;12:62. [PMID: 33456743]

Trivedi PJ et al. Effects of primary sclerosing cholangitis on risks of cancer and death in people with inflammatory bowel disease, based on sex, race, and age. Gastroenterology. 2020;159:915. [PMID: 32445859]

DISEASES OF THE PANCREAS

See Chapter 39 for Carcinoma of the Pancreas and Periampullary Area.

ACUTE PANCREATITIS

ESSENTIALS OF DIAGNOSIS

- Abrupt onset of deep epigastric pain, often with radiation to the back.
- History of previous episodes, often related to alcohol intake.
- Nausea, vomiting, sweating, weakness.
- Abdominal tenderness and distention and fever.
- Leukocytosis, elevated serum amylase, elevated serum lipase.

General Considerations

The annual incidence of acute pancreatitis ranges from 110 to 140 per 100,000 population and has increased since 1990. Most cases of acute pancreatitis are related to biliary tract disease (45%) (a passed gallstone, usually 5 mm or less in diameter) or heavy alcohol intake (20%), with worldwide variations. The exact pathogenesis is not known but may include edema or obstruction of the ampulla of Vater, reflux of bile into pancreatic ducts, and direct injury of pancreatic acinar cells by prematurely activated pancreatic enzymes. Among the numerous other causes or associations are (1) hyperlipidemias (chylomicronemia, hypertriglyceridemia, or both); (2) hypercalcemia; (3) abdominal trauma (including surgery); (4) medications (including azathioprine, mercaptopurine, asparaginase, pentamidine, didanosine, valproic acid, tetracyclines, dapsone, isoniazid, metronidazole, estrogen and tamoxifen [by raising serum triglycerides], sulfonamides, mesalamine, celecoxib, sulindac, leflunomide, thiazides, simvastatin, fenofibrate, enalapril, methyldopa, procainamide, sitagliptin, exenatide, possibly corticosteroids, and others); (5) vasculitis; (6) infections (eg, hepatitis viruses, mumps, cytomegalovirus, *M avium intracellulare* complex, SARS-CoV-2); (7) peritoneal dialysis; (8) cardiopulmonary bypass, single- or double-balloon enteroscopy; (9) ERCP; and (10) a scorpion bite (rare). Medication-induced acute pancreatitis is generally dose-related and associated with worse outcomes than that due to other causes. In patients with pancreas divisum, a congenital anomaly in which the dorsal and ventral pancreatic ducts fail to fuse, acute pancreatitis may result from stenosis of the minor papilla with obstruction to flow from the accessory pancreatic duct, although concomitant gene variants, particularly in the cystic fibrosis transmembrane conductance regulator (*CFTR*) gene, may account for acute pancreatitis in these patients. Acute pancreatitis may also result from an anomalous junction of the pancreaticobiliary duct (pancreaticobiliary malunion). Rarely, acute pancreatitis may be the presenting manifestation of a pancreatic or ampullary neoplasm or pancreatic cyst. Celiac disease appears to be associated with an increased risk of acute and chronic pancreatitis. Apparently "idiopathic" acute pancreatitis is often caused by occult biliary microlithiasis but unlikely to be caused by sphincter of Oddi dysfunction involving the pancreatic duct. Between 15% and 25% of cases are truly idiopathic. Smoking, high dietary glycemic load, and abdominal adiposity increase the risk of pancreatitis, and older age and obesity increase the risk of a severe course; vegetable consumption, dietary fiber, and use of statins may reduce the risk of pancreatitis, and coffee drinking may reduce the risk of nonbiliary pancreatitis.

Clinical Findings

A. Symptoms and Signs

Epigastric abdominal pain, generally abrupt in onset, is steady, boring, and severe and often made worse by walking and lying supine and better by sitting and leaning forward. The pain usually radiates into the back but may radiate to the right or left. Nausea and vomiting are usually present. Weakness, sweating, and anxiety are noted in severe attacks. There may be a history of alcohol intake or a heavy meal immediately preceding the attack or a history of milder similar episodes or biliary pain in the past.

The upper abdomen is tender, most often without guarding, rebound, or rigidity. The abdomen may be distended, and bowel sounds may be absent with associated ileus. Fever of 38.4–39°C, tachycardia, hypotension (even shock), pallor, and cool clammy skin are present in severe cases. Mild jaundice may be seen. Occasionally, an upper abdominal mass due to the inflamed pancreas or a pseudocyst may be palpated. AKI (usually prerenal azotemia) may occur early in the course of acute pancreatitis.

B. Laboratory Findings

Serum lipase and amylase are elevated—usually more than three times the upper limit of normal—within 24 hours in 90% of cases; their return to normal is variable depending on the severity of disease. Lipase remains elevated longer than amylase and is slightly more accurate for the diagnosis of acute pancreatitis. Leukocytosis (10,000–30,000/mcL [10–30 × 10^9/L]), proteinuria, granular casts, glycosuria (10–20% of cases), hyperglycemia, and elevated serum bilirubin may be present. BUN and serum alkaline phosphatase may be elevated and coagulation tests abnormal. An elevated serum creatinine level (greater than 1.8 mg/dL [149.94 mcmol/L]) at 48 hours is associated with the development of pancreatic necrosis. In patients with clear evidence of acute pancreatitis, a serum ALT level of more than 150 U/L (3 mkat/L) suggests biliary pancreatitis. A decrease in serum calcium may reflect saponification and correlates with severity of the disease. Levels lower than 7 mg/dL (1.75 mmol/L) (when serum albumin is normal) are associated with tetany and an unfavorable prognosis. Patients with acute pancreatitis caused by hypertriglyceridemia generally have fasting triglyceride levels above 1000 mg/dL (10 mmol/L) and often have other risk factors for pancreatitis; in some cases, the serum amylase is not elevated substantially because of an inhibitor in the serum of patients with marked hypertriglyceridemia that interferes with measurement of serum amylase. An early rise in the hematocrit value above 44% suggests hemoconcentration and predicts pancreatic necrosis. An elevated CRP concentration (greater than 150 mg/L [1500 mg/L]) at 48 hours suggests severe disease.

Other diagnostic tests that offer the possibility of simplicity, rapidity, ease of use, and low cost—including urinary trypsinogen-2, trypsinogen activation peptide, and carboxypeptidase B—are not widely available. In patients in whom ascites or a left pleural effusion develops, fluid amylase content is high. Electrocardiography may show ST–T wave changes.

C. Assessment of Severity

In addition to the individual laboratory parameters noted above, the severity of acute alcohol-associated pancreatitis can be assessed using several scoring systems (none of which has been shown to have high prognostic accuracy), including the **Ranson criteria** (Table 16–10). The **Sequential Organ Failure Assessment (SOFA)** score or **modified Marshall scoring system** can be used to assess injury to other organs, and the **Acute Physiology and Chronic Health Evaluation (APACHE II)** score is another tool for assessing severity. The severity of acute pancreatitis can also be predicted by the **Pancreatitis Activity Scoring System (PASS)** based on organ failure, intolerance to a solid diet, systemic inflammatory response syndrome, abdominal pain, and dose of intravenous morphine (or its equivalent) required to control pain. Another simple 5-point clinical scoring system (the **Bedside Index for Severity in Acute Pancreatitis,** or **BISAP**) based on **B**UN above 25 mg/dL (9 mmol/L), **I**mpaired mental status, **S**ystemic inflammatory response syndrome, **A**ge older than 60 years, and **P**leural effusion during the first 24 hours (before the onset of organ failure) identifies patients at increased risk for mortality. More simply, the presence of a systemic inflammatory response alone and an elevated BUN level on admission as well as a rise in BUN within the first 24 hours of hospitalization are independently associated with increased mortality; the greater the rise in BUN after admission, the greater the mortality rate. A model based on the change in serum amylase in the first 2 days after admission and the BMI has been proposed. The absence of rebound abdominal tenderness or guarding, a normal hematocrit value, and a normal serum creatinine level (the "**harmless acute pancreatitis score**," or **HAPS**) predict a nonsevere course with 98% accuracy. The **revised Atlanta classification** of the severity of acute pancreatitis uses the following three categories: (1) **mild** disease is the absence of organ failure and local ([peri] pancreatic necrosis or fluid collections) or systemic complications; (2) **moderate** disease is the presence of transient (under 48 hours) organ failure or local or systemic complications, or both; and (3) **severe** disease is the presence of persistent (48 hours or more) organ failure. A similar **"determinant-based" classification** also includes a

Table 16–10. Ranson criteria for assessing the severity of acute pancreatitis.

Three or more of the following predict a severe course complicated by pancreatic necrosis with a sensitivity of 60–80%

- Age over 55 years
- WBC count > 16 × 10^3/mcL (> 16 × 10^9/L)
- Blood glucose > 200 mg/dL (> 11 mmol/L)
- Serum LD > 350 U/L (> 7 mkat/L)
- AST > 250 U/L (> 5 mkat/L)

Development of the following in the first 48 hours indicates a worsening prognosis

- Hematocrit drop of more than 10 percentage points
- BUN rise > 5 mg/dL (> 1.8 mmol/L)
- Arterial Po_2 of < 60 mm Hg (< 7.8 kPa)
- Serum calcium of < 8 mg/dL (< 0.2 mmol/L)
- Base deficit over 4 mEq/L
- Estimated fluid sequestration of > 6 L

Mortality rates correlate with the number of criteria present

Number of Criteria	Mortality Rate
0–2	1%
3–4	16%
5–6	40%
7–8	100%

category of **critical** acute pancreatitis characterized by both persistent organ failure and infected peripancreatic necrosis.

D. Imaging

Plain radiographs of the abdomen may show gallstones (if calcified), a "sentinel loop" (a segment of air-filled small intestine most commonly in the left upper quadrant), the "colon cutoff sign"—a gas-filled segment of transverse colon abruptly ending at the area of pancreatic inflammation—or focal linear atelectasis of the lower lobes of the lungs with or without pleural effusions. Ultrasonography is often not helpful in diagnosing acute pancreatitis because of intervening bowel gas but may identify gallstones in the gallbladder. Unenhanced CT is useful for demonstrating an enlarged pancreas when the diagnosis of pancreatitis is uncertain, differentiating pancreatitis from other possible intra-abdominal catastrophes, and providing an initial assessment of prognosis but is often unnecessary early in the course (Table 16–11). Rapid-bolus intravenous contrast-enhanced CT following aggressive volume resuscitation is of particular value after the first 3 days of severe acute pancreatitis for identifying areas of necrotizing pancreatitis and assessing the degree of necrosis (although the use of intravenous contrast may increase the risk of complications of pancreatitis and of AKI and should be avoided when the serum creatinine level is above 1.5 mg/dL [124.95 mcmol/L]). MRI appears to be a suitable alternative to CT. Perfusion CT on day 3 demonstrating areas of ischemia in the pancreas has been reported to predict the development of pancreatic necrosis. The presence of a fluid collection in the pancreas correlates with an increased mortality rate. CT-guided needle aspiration of areas of necrotizing pancreatitis after the third day may disclose infection, usually by enteric organisms, which typically requires debridement; however, the false-negative rate is 25%. The presence of gas bubbles on CT implies infection by gas-forming organisms. EUS is useful in identifying occult biliary disease (eg, small stones, sludge, microlithiasis), which is present in many patients with apparently idiopathic acute pancreatitis and is indicated in persons over age 40 to exclude malignancy. ERCP is generally not indicated after a first attack of acute pancreatitis unless there is associated cholangitis or jaundice or a bile duct stone is known to be present, but EUS or MRCP should be considered, especially after repeated attacks of idiopathic acute pancreatitis. Following a single attack of idiopathic acute pancreatitis, a negative EUS examination predicts a low risk of relapse.

Differential Diagnosis

Acute pancreatitis must be differentiated from an acutely perforated duodenal ulcer, acute cholecystitis, acute intestinal obstruction, leaking aortic aneurysm, renal colic, and acute mesenteric ischemia. Serum amylase may also be elevated in proximal intestinal obstruction, gastroenteritis, mumps not involving the pancreas (salivary amylase), and ectopic pregnancy and after administration of opioids and abdominal surgery. Serum lipase may also be elevated in many of these conditions.

Complications

Intravascular volume depletion secondary to leakage of fluids into the pancreatic bed and to ileus with fluid-filled loops of bowel may result in prerenal azotemia and even ATN without overt shock. This sequence usually occurs within 24 hours of the onset of acute pancreatitis and lasts 8–9 days. Some patients require renal replacement therapy.

According to the revised Atlanta classification, fluid collections and necrosis may be acute (within the first 4 weeks) or chronic (after 4 weeks) and sterile or infected. Chronic collections, including pseudocysts and walled-off necrosis, are characterized by encapsulation. Sterile or infected necrotizing pancreatitis may complicate the course in 5–10% of cases and accounts for most of the deaths. The risk of infection does not correlate with the extent of necrosis. Pancreatic necrosis is often associated with fever, leukocytosis, and, in some cases, shock and is associated with organ failure (eg, GI bleeding, respiratory failure, AKI) in 50% of cases. It may lead to complete transection of the pancreatic duct (disconnected pancreatic duct syndrome), which may result in recurrent fluid collections or persistent fistulae months or years after necrosis has resolved. Because infected pancreatic necrosis is often an indication for

Table 16–11. Estimated mortality rates of pancreatitis based on severity.

Point Value for Appearance of Pancreas Based on CT scan		Additional Points for Percentage of Pancreatic Necrosis		Estimated Mortality Rate Based on Total Points Sum	
Condition of Pancreas	Points	Percentage of Necrosis	Points	Total Points	Estimated Mortality Rate
Normal pancreas	0	0%	0	0	0%
Enlargement of pancreas	1 point	0%	0	1	0%
Inflammation of the pancreas or peripancreatic fat or both	2 points	< 30%	2 points	4	< 3%
Single new peripancreatic fluid collection	3 points	30–50%	4 points	7	> 6%
Two or more new peripancreatic fluid collections or retroperitoneal air	4 points	> 50%	6 points	10	~17%

debridement, fine-needle aspiration of necrotic tissue under CT guidance should be performed (if necessary, repeatedly) for Gram stain and culture.

A serious complication of acute pancreatitis is acute respiratory distress syndrome (ARDS); cardiac dysfunction may be superimposed. It usually occurs 3–7 days after the onset of pancreatitis in patients who have required large volumes of fluid and colloid to maintain blood pressure and urinary output. Most patients with ARDS require intubation, mechanical ventilation, and supplemental oxygen.

Pancreatic abscess (also referred to as infected or suppurative pseudocyst) is a suppurative process characterized by rising fever, leukocytosis, and localized tenderness and an epigastric mass usually 6 or more weeks into the course of acute pancreatitis. The abscess may be associated with a left-sided pleural effusion or an enlarging spleen secondary to splenic vein thrombosis. In contrast to infected necrosis, the mortality rate is low following drainage.

Pseudocysts, encapsulated fluid collections with high amylase content, commonly appear in pancreatitis when CT is used to monitor the evolution of an acute attack. Pseudocysts that are smaller than 6 cm in diameter often resolve spontaneously. They most commonly are within or adjacent to the pancreas but can present almost anywhere (eg, mediastinal, retrorectal) by extension along anatomic planes. Multiple pseudocysts are seen in 14% of cases. Pseudocysts may become secondarily infected, necessitating drainage as for an abscess. Pancreatic ascites may present after recovery from acute pancreatitis as a gradual increase in abdominal girth and persistent elevation of the serum amylase level in the absence of frank abdominal pain. Marked elevations in ascitic protein (greater than 3 g/dL) and amylase (greater than 1000 U/L [20 mkat/L]) concentrations are typical. The condition results from disruption of the pancreatic duct or drainage of a pseudocyst into the peritoneal cavity.

Rare complications of acute pancreatitis include hemorrhage caused by erosion of a blood vessel to form a pseudoaneurysm and by colonic necrosis. Portosplenomesenteric venous thrombosis frequently develops in patients with necrotizing acute pancreatitis but rarely leads to complications. Other local complications include abdominal compartment syndrome, intestinal ischemia, and gastric outlet obstruction. Chronic pancreatitis develops in about 10% of cases of acute pancreatitis. Diabetes mellitus and exocrine pancreatic insufficiency may develop after acute pancreatitis.

Treatment

A. Treatment of Acute Disease

1. Mild disease—In most patients, acute pancreatitis is a mild disease ("nonsevere acute pancreatitis") that subsides spontaneously within several days. The pancreas is "rested" by a regimen of withholding food and liquids by mouth, bed rest, and, in patients with moderately severe pain or ileus and abdominal distention or vomiting, nasogastric suction. Goal-directed therapy with early aggressive fluid resuscitation (one-third of the total 72-hour fluid volume administered within 24 hours of presentation, 250–500 mL/hour initially) may reduce the frequency of systemic inflammatory response syndrome and organ failure in this group of patients and appears to have the greatest benefit in patients with acute pancreatitis predicted to be mild in severity when started within 4 hours of the patient's arrival at the hospital. Lactated Ringer solution may be preferable to normal saline; however, overly aggressive fluid resuscitation may lead to morbidity as well.

Pain is controlled with meperidine, up to 100–150 mg intramuscularly every 3–4 hours as necessary. In those with severe liver or kidney dysfunction, the dose may need to be reduced. Morphine had been thought to cause sphincter of Oddi spasm but is now considered an acceptable alternative and, given the potential side effects of meperidine, may even be preferable. Oral intake of fluid and foods can be resumed when the patient is largely free of pain and has bowel sounds (even if the serum amylase is still elevated). Clear liquids are given first (this step may be skipped in patients with mild acute pancreatitis), followed by gradual advancement to a low-fat diet, guided by the patient's tolerance and by the absence of pain. Pain may recur on refeeding in 20% of patients.

Following recovery from acute biliary pancreatitis, laparoscopic cholecystectomy is generally performed, preferably during the same hospital admission, and is associated with a reduced rate of recurrent gallstone-related complications compared with delayed cholecystectomy. In selected cases endoscopic sphincterotomy alone may be done. In patients with recurrent pancreatitis associated with pancreas divisum, insertion of a stent in the minor papilla (or minor papilla sphincterotomy) may reduce the frequency of subsequent attacks, although complications of such therapy are frequent. In patients with recurrent acute pancreatitis attributed to pancreatic sphincter of Oddi dysfunction, biliary sphincterotomy alone is as effective as combined biliary and pancreatic sphincterotomy in reducing the frequency of recurrent acute pancreatitis, but chronic pancreatitis may still develop in treated patients. Hypertriglyceridemia with acute pancreatitis has been treated with combinations of insulin, heparin, apheresis, and hemofiltration, but the benefit of these approaches has not been proven.

2. Severe disease—In more severe pancreatitis—particularly necrotizing pancreatitis—there may be considerable leakage of fluids, necessitating large amounts of intravenous fluids (eg, 500–1000 mL/hour for several hours, then 250–300 mL/hour) to maintain intravascular volume. Risk factors for high levels of fluid sequestration include younger age, alcohol etiology, higher hematocrit value, higher serum glucose, and systemic inflammatory response syndrome in the first 48 hours of hospital admission. Hemodynamic monitoring in an ICU is required, and the importance of aggressive goal-directed intravenous hydration targeted to result in adequate urinary output, stabilization of blood pressure and heart rate, restoration of central venous pressure, and a modest decrease in hematocrit value cannot be overemphasized. Calcium gluconate must be given intravenously if there is evidence of hypocalcemia with tetany. Infusions of fresh frozen plasma or serum albumin may be necessary in patients with coagulopathy or hypoalbuminemia. With colloid solutions, the risk of ARDS may be increased. If shock persists after adequate volume replacement (including packed red cells), vasopressors may be required. For the patient requiring a large volume of parenteral fluids, central venous pressure and blood gases should be monitored at regular intervals.

Enteral nutrition via a nasojejunal or possibly nasogastric feeding tube is preferable to parenteral nutrition in patients who will otherwise be without oral nutrition for at least 7–10 days and it reduces the risk of multiorgan failure and mortality when started within 48 hours of admission. However, it is not tolerated in some patients (eg, those with an ileus) and may not reduce the rates of infection and death compared with resumption of oral feeding after 72 hours. Parenteral nutrition (including lipids) should be considered in patients who have severe pancreatitis and ileus; glutamine supplementation appears to reduce the risk of infectious complications and mortality.

The routine use of antibiotics to prevent conversion of sterile necrotizing pancreatitis to infected necrosis is of no benefit and generally is not indicated in patients with less than 30% pancreatic necrosis. Imipenem (500 mg intravenously every 6 hours) or possibly cefuroxime (1.5 g intravenously three times daily, then 250 mg orally twice daily) administered for no more than 14 days to patients with sterile necrotizing pancreatitis has been reported in some studies to reduce the risk of pancreatic infection and mortality, but in general, prophylactic antibiotics are not recommended; meropenem and the combination of ciprofloxacin and metronidazole do not appear to reduce the frequency of infected necrosis, multiorgan failure, or mortality. When infected necrotizing pancreatitis is confirmed, imipenem or meropenem should be continued. Drug-resistant organisms are increasingly prevalent. In occasional cases, a fungal infection is found, and appropriate antifungal therapy should be prescribed.

NSAIDs (eg, indomethacin administered rectally) and aggressive hydration with lactated Ringer solution have been reported to reduce the frequency and severity of post-ERCP pancreatitis in persons at high risk, and rectal indomethacin is widely used, but studies of the benefit of indomethacin in unselected patients have yielded conflicting results. Placement of a stent across the pancreatic duct or orifice has been shown to reduce the risk of post-ERCP pancreatitis by 60–80% and is a common practice.

B. Treatment of Complications and Follow-Up

A surgeon should be consulted in all cases of severe acute pancreatitis. If the diagnosis is in doubt and investigation indicates a strong possibility of a serious surgically correctable lesion (eg, perforated peptic ulcer), exploratory laparotomy is indicated. When acute pancreatitis is found unexpectedly, it is usually wise to close without intervention. If the pancreatitis appears mild and cholelithiasis or microlithiasis is present, cholecystectomy or cholecystostomy may be justified. When severe pancreatitis results from choledocholithiasis and jaundice (serum total bilirubin above 5 mg/dL [85.5 mcmol/L]) or cholangitis is present, ERCP with endoscopic sphincterotomy and stone extraction is indicated. MRCP may be useful in selecting patients for therapeutic ERCP. Endoscopic sphincterotomy does not appear to improve the outcome of severe pancreatitis in the absence of cholangitis or jaundice.

Necrosectomy may improve survival in patients with necrotizing pancreatitis and clinical deterioration with multiorgan failure or lack of resolution by 4 weeks and is often indicated for infected necrosis, although a select group of relatively stable patients with infected pancreatic necrosis may be managed with antibiotics alone. The goal is to debride necrotic pancreas and surrounding tissue and establish adequate drainage. Outcomes are best if necrosectomy is delayed until the necrosis has organized, usually about 4 weeks after disease onset. A "step-up" approach in which nonsurgical endoscopic transluminal (transgastric or transduodenal) or percutaneous catheter drainage of walled-off pancreatic necrosis under radiologic guidance, with subsequent endoscopic and, if necessary, open surgical necrosectomy has been shown to reduce mortality and resource utilization in selected patients with necrotizing pancreatitis and confirmed or suspected secondary infection. In some cases, laparoscopic guidance (video-assisted retroperitoneal debridement) is an additional option, depending on local expertise. Lumen-apposing metal stents (LAMS) or double-pigtail plastic stents are used for endoscopic transluminal drainage, with removal of LAMS after 4 weeks to minimize the risk of complications. Treatment is labor intensive, and multiple procedures are often required, although costs and complication rates are lower than those for surgery. Endoscopic or surgical interventions may be required for chronic disconnected pancreatic duct syndrome.

The development of a pancreatic abscess is an indication for prompt percutaneous or surgical drainage. Chronic pseudocysts require endoscopic, percutaneous catheter, or surgical drainage when infected or associated with persisting pain, pancreatitis, or bile duct obstruction. For pancreatic infections, imipenem, 500 mg every 8 hours intravenously, is a good choice of antibiotic because it achieves bactericidal levels in pancreatic tissue for most causative organisms. Pancreatic duct leaks and fistulas may require endoscopic or surgical therapy.

Prognosis

Mortality rates for acute pancreatitis have declined from at least 10% to around 5% since the 1980s, but the mortality rate for severe acute pancreatitis (more than three Ranson criteria; see Table 16–10) remains at least 20%, with rates of 10% and 25% in those with sterile and infected necrosis, respectively. Severe acute pancreatitis is predicted by features of the systemic inflammatory response on admission; a persistent systemic inflammatory response is associated with a mortality rate of 25% and a transient response with a mortality rate of 8%. Half of the deaths, usually from multiorgan failure, occur within the first 2 weeks. Multiorgan failure is associated with a mortality rate of at least 30%, and if it persists beyond the first 48 hours, a mortality rate of over 50%. Later deaths occur because of complications of infected necrosis. The risk of death doubles when both organ failure and infected necrosis are present. Moreover, hospital-acquired infections increase the mortality of acute pancreatitis, independent of severity. Readmission to the hospital for acute pancreatitis within 30 days may be predicted by a scoring system based on five factors during the index admission: eating less than a solid diet at discharge; nausea, vomiting, or diarrhea at discharge; pancreatic necrosis; use of antibiotics at discharge; and pain at discharge. Male sex, an alcohol etiology, and severe acute disease are risk factors. Recurrences are common (24%) in alcohol-associated pancreatitis, particularly in patients who smoke (40%), but can be reduced by repeated, regularly scheduled interventions to eliminate alcohol consumption and smoking after discharge from the hospital. A severe initial attack also increases the risk of recurrence and of subsequent exocrine pancreatic insufficiency. The risk of chronic pancreatitis following an episode of acute alcohol-associated pancreatitis is 8% in 5 years, 13% in 10 years, and 16% in 20 years, and the risk of diabetes mellitus is increased more than twofold over 5 years. Overall, chronic pancreatitis develops in 36% of patients with recurrent acute pancreatitis; alcohol use and smoking are principal risk factors. An association between a diagnosis of acute pancreatitis and long-term risk of pancreatic cancer has been reported.

When to Admit

Nearly all patients with acute pancreatitis should be hospitalized.

Baron TH et al. American Gastroenterological Association Clinical Practice Update: management of pancreatic necrosis. Gastroenterology. 2020;158:67. [PMID: 31479658]

Boxhoorn L et al. Acute pancreatitis. Lancet. 2020;396:726. [PMID: 32891214]

Lee A et al. Lactated Ringers vs normal saline resuscitation for mild acute pancreatitis: a randomized trial. Gastroenterology. 2021;160:955. [PMID: 33159924]

Mederos MA et al. Acute pancreatitis: a review. JAMA. 2021;325:382. [PMID: 33496779]

CHRONIC PANCREATITIS

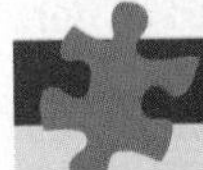

ESSENTIALS OF DIAGNOSIS

- Chronic or intermittent epigastric pain, steatorrhea, weight loss, abnormal pancreatic imaging.
- A mnemonic for the predisposing factors of chronic pancreatitis is TIGAR-O: toxic-metabolic, idiopathic, genetic, autoimmune, recurrent and severe acute pancreatitis, or obstructive.

General Considerations

The prevalence of chronic pancreatitis in the United States is 25–99 per 100,000 population with a peak in persons aged 46–55 years. Chronic pancreatitis occurs most often in patients with alcoholism (45–80% of all cases). The risk of chronic pancreatitis increases with the duration and amount of alcohol consumed, but pancreatitis develops in only 5–10% of heavy drinkers. Tobacco smoking is a risk factor for idiopathic chronic pancreatitis and has been reported to accelerate progression of alcohol-associated chronic pancreatitis. About 2% of patients with hyperparathyroidism develop pancreatitis. In tropical Africa and Asia, tropical pancreatitis, related in part to malnutrition, is the most common cause of chronic pancreatitis. By contrast, in Western societies, obesity can lead to pancreatic steatosis, which may lead ultimately to pancreatic exocrine and endocrine insufficiency and an increased risk of pancreatic cancer. A stricture, stone, or tumor obstructing the pancreas can lead to obstructive chronic pancreatitis. Autoimmune pancreatitis is associated with hypergammaglobulinemia (IgG_4 in particular), often with autoantibodies and other autoimmune diseases, and is responsive to corticosteroids. Affected persons are at increased risk for various cancers. Type 1 autoimmune pancreatitis (lymphoplasmacytic sclerosing pancreatitis, or simply autoimmune pancreatitis) is a multisystem disease, typically in a patient over age 60, characterized by lymphoplasmacytic infiltration and fibrosis on biopsy, associated bile duct strictures, retroperitoneal fibrosis, renal and salivary gland lesions, and a high rate of relapse after treatment. It is the pancreatic manifestation of IgG_4-related disease. Type 2 ("idiopathic duct-centric chronic pancreatitis") affects the pancreas alone, typically in a patient aged 40–50 years, and is characterized by intense duct-centric lymphoplasmacytic infiltration on biopsy, lack of systemic IgG_4 involvement, an association with IBD in 25% of cases, often a tumor-like mass, and a low rate of relapse after treatment. Between 10% and 30% of cases of chronic pancreatitis are idiopathic, with either early onset (median age 20) or late onset (median age 58). Genetic factors may predispose to chronic pancreatitis in nearly half of the early-onset cases and a quarter of the late-onset cases and include pathogenic variants of the *CFTR* gene, the pancreatic secretory trypsin inhibitory gene (*PSTI*, also known as the serine protease inhibitor, *SPINK1*), the chymotrypsin-C (*CTRC*) gene, and the genes for carboxypeptidase A1 (*CPA1*) and possibly uridine 5′-diphosphate glucuronosyltransferase (*UGT1A7*). A variant of the cationic trypsinogen gene on chromosome 7 (serine protease 1, *PRSS1*) is associated with hereditary pancreatitis, transmitted as an autosomal dominant trait with variable penetrance. A useful mnemonic for the predisposing factors to chronic pancreatitis is **TIGAR-O:** **T**oxic-metabolic, **I**diopathic, **G**enetic, **A**utoimmune, **R**ecurrent and severe acute pancreatitis, or **O**bstructive.

The pathogenesis of chronic pancreatitis may be explained by the SAPE (**S**entinel **A**cute **P**ancreatitis **E**vent) hypothesis by which the first (sentinel) acute pancreatitis event initiates an inflammatory process that results in injury and later fibrosis ("necrosis-fibrosis"). In many cases, chronic pancreatitis is a self-perpetuating disease characterized by chronic pain or recurrent episodes of acute pancreatitis and ultimately by pancreatic exocrine or endocrine insufficiency (sooner in alcohol-associated pancreatitis than in other types). After many years, chronic pain may resolve spontaneously or following surgery tailored to the cause of pain. Over 80% of adults develop diabetes mellitus within 25 years after the clinical onset of chronic pancreatitis.

Clinical Findings

A. Symptoms and Signs

Persistent or recurrent episodes of epigastric and left upper quadrant pain are typical. Anorexia, nausea, vomiting, constipation, flatulence, and weight loss are common. During attacks, tenderness over the pancreas, mild muscle guarding, and ileus may be noted. Attacks may last for only a few hours or for as long as 2 weeks; pain may eventually be almost continuous. Steatorrhea (as indicated by bulky, foul, fatty stools) may occur late in the course.

B. Laboratory Findings

Serum amylase and lipase may be elevated during acute attacks; however, normal values do not exclude the diagnosis. Serum alkaline phosphatase and bilirubin may be elevated owing to compression of the bile duct. Glycosuria may be present. Excess fecal fat may be demonstrated on chemical analysis of the stool. Exocrine pancreatic insufficiency generally is confirmed by response to therapy with pancreatic enzyme supplements; the secretin stimulation test can be used if available (and has a high negative predictive value for ruling out early acute chronic pancreatitis), as can detection of decreased fecal chymotrypsin or elastase levels, although the latter tests lack sensitivity and specificity. Vitamin B_{12} malabsorption is detectable in about 40% of patients, but clinical deficiency of vitamin B_{12} and fat-soluble vitamins is rare. Accurate diagnostic tests are available for the major trypsinogen gene pathogenic variants, but because of uncertainty about the mechanisms linking heterozygous *CFTR* and *PSTI* variants with pancreatitis, genetic testing for mutations in these two genes is recommended primarily in younger patients in whom the etiology of chronic pancreatitis is unclear. Elevated IgG_4 levels, ANA, antibodies to lactoferrin and carbonic anhydrase II, and other autoantibodies are often found in patients with autoimmune pancreatitis (especially type 1). Pancreatic biopsy, if necessary, shows a lymphoplasmacytic inflammatory infiltrate with characteristic IgG_4 immunostaining, which is also found in biopsy specimens of the major papilla, bile duct, and salivary glands, in type 1 autoimmune pancreatitis.

C. Imaging

CT or MRI is recommended as initial testing for diagnosis of chronic pancreatitis, although plain films show calcifications due to pancreaticolithiasis in 30% of affected patients. CT may show calcifications not seen on plain films as well as ductal dilatation and heterogeneity or atrophy of the gland. Occasionally, the findings raise suspicion of pancreatic cancer ("tumefactive chronic pancreatitis"). Secretin-enhanced MRCP may be considered in selected cases. When CT or MRI is inconclusive, EUS (with pancreatic tissue sampling) may be needed. Endoscopic ultrasonographic ("Rosemont") criteria for the diagnosis of chronic pancreatitis include hyperechoic foci with shadowing indicative of calculi in the main pancreatic duct and lobularity with honeycombing of the pancreatic parenchyma. ERCP is the most sensitive imaging study for chronic pancreatitis and may show dilated ducts, intraductal stones, strictures, or pseudocyst but is infrequently used for diagnosis alone; moreover, the results may be normal in patients with so-called minimal change pancreatitis. Histology is the gold standard for diagnosis when clinical suspicion is strong but imaging studies are inconclusive.

Characteristic imaging features of autoimmune pancreatitis include diffuse enlargement of the pancreas, a peripheral rim of hypoattenuation, and irregular narrowing of the main pancreatic duct. In the United States, the diagnosis of autoimmune pancreatitis is based on the **HISORt** criteria: **H**istology, **I**maging, **S**erology, other **O**rgan involvement, and **R**esponse to corticosteroid **T**herapy.

Complications

Opioid addiction is common. Other frequent complications include often brittle diabetes mellitus, pancreatic pseudocyst or abscess, cholestatic liver enzymes with or without jaundice, bile duct stricture, exocrine pancreatic insufficiency, malnutrition, osteoporosis, and peptic ulcer. Pancreatic cancer develops in 5% of patients after 20 years; the risk may relate to tobacco and alcohol use. In patients with hereditary pancreatitis, the risk of pancreatic cancer rises after 50 years of age and reaches 19% by age 70 (see Chapter 39).

Treatment

A. Medical Measures

A low-fat diet should be prescribed. Alcohol is forbidden because it frequently precipitates attacks. Opioids should be avoided if possible. Preferred agents for pain are acetaminophen, NSAIDs, and, if an opioid is necessary, tramadol, along with pain-modifying agents such as tricyclic antidepressants, SSRIs, and gabapentin or pregabalin. Exocrine pancreatic insufficiency is treated with pancreatic enzyme replacement therapy selected based on high lipase activity (Table 16–12). A total dose of at least 40,000 units of lipase in capsules is given with each meal. Doses of 90,000 units or more of lipase per meal may be required in some cases. The tablets should be taken at the start of, during, and at the end of a meal. Concurrent administration of an H_2-receptor antagonist (eg, famotidine, 20 mg orally twice daily), a PPI (eg, omeprazole, 20–60 mg orally daily), or sodium bicarbonate (650 mg orally before and after meals) decreases the inactivation of lipase by acid and may thereby further decrease steatorrhea. In selected cases of alcohol-associated pancreatitis and in cystic fibrosis, enteric-coated microencapsulated preparations may offer an advantage; however, in patients with cystic fibrosis, high-dose pancreatic enzyme replacement therapy has been associated with strictures of the ascending colon. Pain secondary to idiopathic chronic pancreatitis may be alleviated in some cases by pancreatic enzyme replacement therapy (not enteric-coated preparations) or by octreotide, 200 mcg subcutaneously three times daily, although some guidelines recommend against such therapy. Associated diabetes mellitus should be treated (see Chapter 27). Autoimmune pancreatitis is treated with prednisone 40 mg/day orally for 1–2 months, followed by a taper of 5 mg every

Table 16–12. FDA-approved pancreatic enzyme (pancrelipase) preparations.

Product	Enzyme Content/Unit Dose, USP Units		
	Protease	Lipase	Amylase
Immediate-Release Capsules			
Nonenteric-coated			
Viokace 10,440	10,440	39,150	39,150
Viokace 20,880	20,880	78,300	78,300
Delayed-Release Capsules			
Enteric-coated minimicrospheres			
Creon 3000	3000	15,000	9500
Creon 6000	6000	30,000	19,000
Creon 12,000	12,000	60,000	38,000
Creon 24,000	24,000	120,000	76,000
Creon 36,000	36,000	180,000	114,000
Enteric-coated minitablets			
Ultresa 13,800	13,800	27,600	27,600
Ultresa 20,700	20,700	46,000	41,400
Ultresa 23,000	23,000	46,000	41,400
Enteric-coated beads			
Zenpep 3000	3000	16,000	10,000
Zenpep 5000	5000	27,000	17,000
Zenpep 10,000	10,000	55,000	34,000
Zenpep 15,000	15,000	82,000	51,000
Zenpep 20,000	20,000	109,000	68,000
Zenpep 25,000	25,000	136,000	85,000
Enteric-coated microtablets			
Pancreaze 4200	4200	17,500	10,000
Pancreaze 10,500	10,500	43,750	25,000
Pancreaze 16,800	16,800	70,000	40,000
Pancreaze 21,000	21,000	61,000	37,000
Bicarbonate-buffered enteric-coated microspheres			
Pertzye 8000	8000	30,250	28,750
Pertzye + 16,000	16,000	60,500	57,500

USP, US Pharmacopeia.

2–4 weeks. Nonresponse or relapse occurs in 45% of type 1 cases (particularly in those with concomitant IgG_4-associated cholangitis); rituximab is an effective induction and maintenance agent, and azathioprine or long-term low-dose corticosteroid use appears to reduce the risk of relapse.

B. Endoscopic and Surgical Treatment

Endoscopic therapy or surgery may be indicated in chronic pancreatitis to treat underlying biliary tract disease, ensure free flow of bile into the duodenum, drain persistent pseudocysts, treat other complications, eliminate obstruction of the pancreatic duct, attempt to relieve pain, or exclude pancreatic cancer. Liver fibrosis may regress after biliary drainage. Distal bile duct obstruction may be relieved by endoscopic placement of multiple plastic stents or a fully covered self-expandable metal stent in the bile duct. When obstruction of the duodenal end of the pancreatic duct can be demonstrated by ERCP, dilation of or placement of such stents in the duct and pancreatic duct stone lithotripsy or surgical resection of the tail of the pancreas with implantation of the distal end of the duct by pancreaticojejunostomy may be performed. Endoscopic therapy is successful in about 50% of cases. In patients who do not respond to endoscopic therapy, surgery is successful in about 50%. When the pancreatic duct is diffusely dilated, anastomosis between the duct after it is split longitudinally and a defunctionalized limb of jejunum (modified Puestow procedure), in some cases combined with resection of the head of the pancreas (Beger or Frey procedure), is associated with relief of pain in 80% of cases. In advanced cases, subtotal or total pancreatectomy with islet autotransplantation may be considered as a last resort but has variable efficacy and causes pancreatic insufficiency and diabetes mellitus. Endoscopic or surgical (including laparoscopic) drainage is indicated for symptomatic pseudocysts and, in many cases, those over 6 cm in diameter. EUS may facilitate selection of an optimal site for endoscopic drainage. Pancreatic ascites or pancreaticopleural fistulas due to a disrupted pancreatic duct can be managed by endoscopic placement of a stent across the disrupted duct. Pancreatic sphincterotomy or fragmentation of stones in the pancreatic duct by lithotripsy and endoscopic removal of stones from the duct may relieve pain in selected patients. For patients with chronic pain and nondilated ducts, a percutaneous celiac plexus nerve block may be considered under either CT or EUS guidance, with pain relief (albeit often short-lived) in approximately 50% of patients (see Chapter 5). A single session of radiation therapy to the pancreas has been reported to relieve otherwise refractory pain.

Prognosis

Chronic pancreatitis often leads to disability and reduced life expectancy; pancreatic cancer is the main cause of death. The prognosis is best in patients with recurrent acute pancreatitis caused by a remediable condition, such as cholelithiasis, choledocholithiasis, stenosis of the sphincter of Oddi, or hyperparathyroidism, and in those with autoimmune pancreatitis. Medical management of hyperlipidemia, if present, may also prevent recurrent attacks of pancreatitis. The Chronic Pancreatitis Diagnosis Score based on pain, hemoglobin A_{1c} level, C-reactive protein level, BMI, and platelet count has been shown to correlate with hospital admissions and number of hospital days. In alcohol-associated pancreatitis, pain relief is most likely when a dilated pancreatic duct can be decompressed. In patients with disease not amenable to decompressive surgery, addiction to opioids is a frequent outcome of treatment. A poorer quality of life is associated with constant rather than intermittent pain, pain-related disability or unemployment, current smoking, and comorbidities.

When to Refer

All patients with chronic pancreatitis should be referred for diagnostic and therapeutic procedures.

When to Admit

- Severe pain.
- New jaundice.
- New fever.

Beyer G et al. Chronic pancreatitis. Lancet. 2020;396:499. [PMID: 32798493]

Gardner TB et al. ACG Clinical Guideline: chronic pancreatitis. Am J Gastroenterol. 2020;115:322. [PMID: 32022720]

Issa Y et al; Dutch Pancreatitis Study Group. Effect of early surgery vs endoscopy-first approach on pain in patients with chronic pancreatitis: the ESCAPE randomized clinical trial. JAMA. 2020;323:237. [PMID: 31961419]

Kempeneers MA et al. Pain patterns in chronic pancreatitis: a nationwide longitudinal cohort study. Gut. 2021;70:1724. [PMID: 33158979]

Lewis MD et al. Differences in age at onset of symptoms, and effects of genetic variants, in patients with early vs late-onset idiopathic chronic pancreatitis in a North American cohort. Clin Gastroenterol Hepatol. 2021;19:349. [PMID: 32240833]

Breast Disorders

Armando E. Giuliano, MD, FACS, FRCSEd
Sara A. Hurvitz, MD, FACP

BENIGN BREAST DISORDERS

FIBROCYSTIC CONDITION

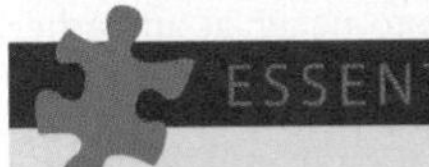

ESSENTIALS OF DIAGNOSIS

- Painful breast masses; often multiple and bilateral.
- Rapid fluctuation in mass size is common.
- Pain often worsens during premenstrual phase of cycle.
- Most common age is 30–50 years. Rare in postmenopausal women not receiving hormonal replacement.

General Considerations

Fibrocystic condition is the most frequent lesion of the breast. Although commonly referred to as "fibrocystic disease," it does not, in fact, represent a pathologic or anatomic disorder. It is common in women 30–50 years of age but rare in postmenopausal women who are not taking hormonal replacement. Estrogen is considered a causative factor. There may be an increased risk in women who drink alcohol, especially women between 18 and 22 years of age. Fibrocystic condition encompasses a wide variety of benign histologic changes in the breast epithelium, some of which are found so commonly in normal breasts that they are probably variants of normal but have nonetheless been termed a "condition" or "disease."

The microscopic findings of fibrocystic condition include cysts (gross and microscopic), papillomatosis, adenosis, fibrosis, and ductal epithelial hyperplasia. Although it has been thought that a fibrocystic condition increases the risk of breast cancer, *only the variants with a component of epithelial proliferation (especially with atypia), papillomatosis, or increased breast density on mammogram represent true risk factors.*

Clinical Findings

A. Symptoms and Signs

Fibrocystic condition may produce an asymptomatic mass in the breast that is discovered by accident, but pain or tenderness often calls attention to it. Discomfort often occurs or worsens during the premenstrual phase of the cycle, at which time the cysts tend to enlarge. Fluctuations in size and rapid appearance or disappearance of a breast mass are common, as are multiple or bilateral masses and serous nipple discharge. Patients will give a history of a transient lump in the breast or cyclic breast pain.

B. Diagnostic Tests

Mammography and ultrasonography should be used to evaluate a mass in a patient with fibrocystic condition. Ultrasonography alone may be used in women under 30 years of age; mammography may be helpful, but the breast tissue in young women is usually too radiodense to permit a worthwhile study. Ultrasonography is useful in differentiating a cystic mass from a solid mass, especially in women with dense breasts. Simple cysts are not worrisome and require no treatment or follow-up unless they are symptomatic and causing pain, in which case they may be aspirated. Ultrasonography can reliably distinguish fibroadenoma from carcinoma but not from a phyllodes tumor. Because a mass due to fibrocystic condition may nonetheless be difficult to distinguish from carcinoma on the basis of clinical findings and imaging studies, *suspicious lesions should be biopsied.* Core needle biopsy, rather than fine-needle aspiration (FNA), is the preferable technique. If the lesion is cystic, needle aspiration will suffice. Excisional biopsy is rarely necessary but should be done for lesions with atypia or where imaging and biopsy results are discordant. Surgery should be conservative since the primary objective is to exclude cancer. Simple mastectomy or extensive removal of breast tissue is rarely, if ever, indicated for fibrocystic condition.

Differential Diagnosis

Pain, fluctuation in size, and multiplicity of lesions are the features consistent with fibrocystic condition and most helpful in differentiating it from carcinoma. If a dominant mass is present, the diagnosis of cancer should be assumed until disproven by imaging or biopsy. Final diagnosis depends on analysis of a biopsy specimen.

Treatment

When the diagnosis of fibrocystic condition has been established by previous biopsy or is likely because the history is classic, aspiration of a discrete mass suggestive of a cyst is indicated to alleviate pain and, more importantly, to confirm the cystic nature of the mass. The patient is reexamined at intervals thereafter. If no fluid is obtained by aspiration, if fluid is bloody, if a mass persists after aspiration, or if at any time during follow-up a persistent or recurrent mass is noted, biopsy should be performed.

Breast pain associated with generalized fibrocystic condition is best treated by avoiding trauma and by wearing a good supportive brassiere during the night and day. Most hormone therapy is not advisable because it does not cure the condition and has undesirable side effects; danazol (100–200 mg orally twice daily), a synthetic androgen, is the only treatment approved by the US FDA for patients with severe pain. This treatment suppresses pituitary gonadotropins, but androgenic effects (acne, edema, hirsutism) usually make this treatment intolerable; in practice, it is rarely used. Similarly, tamoxifen reduces some symptoms of fibrocystic condition, but because of its side effects, it is not useful for young women unless it is given to reduce the risk of cancer. Postmenopausal women receiving hormone replacement therapy may stop or change doses of hormones to reduce pain. Oil of evening primrose, a natural form of gamolenic acid, has been shown to decrease pain in 44–58% of users. The dosage of gamolenic acid is six capsules of 500 mg orally twice daily. Studies have also demonstrated a low-fat diet or decreasing dietary fat intake may reduce the painful symptoms associated with fibrocystic condition. Topical treatments such as NSAIDs are rarely of value.

The role of caffeine consumption in the development and treatment of fibrocystic condition is controversial. Some studies suggest that eliminating caffeine from the diet is associated with improvement while other studies refute the benefit. Many patients report relief of symptoms after giving up coffee, tea, and chocolate. Similarly, many women find vitamin E (400 IU daily) helpful; however, these observations remain anecdotal.

Prognosis

Exacerbations of pain, tenderness, and cyst formation may occur at any time until menopause, when symptoms usually subside, except in patients receiving hormonal replacement. The patient should be advised to examine her own breasts regularly just after menstruation and to inform her clinician if a mass appears. The risk of breast cancer developing in women with fibrocystic condition with a proliferative or atypical epithelial hyperplasia or papillomatosis is higher than that of the general population. These women should be monitored carefully with physical examinations and imaging studies.

Balci FL et al. Clinical factors affecting the therapeutic efficacy of evening primrose oil on mastalgia. Ann Surg Oncol. 2020;27:4844. [PMID: 32748152]

Chetlen AL et al. Mastalgia: imaging work-up appropriateness. Acad Radiol. 2017;24:345. [PMID: 27916596]

Osouli Tabrizi S et al. The effect of the herbal medicine on severity of cyclic mastalgia: a systematic review and meta-analysis. J Complement Integr Med. 2021 May 20. [Epub ahead of print] [PMID: 34107571]

Qu P et al. Detection rate is not higher for women with BBD history in breast cancer screening. J Public Health (Oxf). 2021;43:333. [PMID: 31774529]

FIBROADENOMA OF THE BREAST

This common benign neoplasm occurs most frequently in young women, usually within 20 years after puberty. It is somewhat more frequent and tends to occur at an earlier age in Black women. Multiple tumors are found in 10–15% of patients.

The typical **fibroadenoma** is a round or ovoid, rubbery, discrete, relatively movable, nontender mass 1–5 cm in diameter. Clinical diagnosis in young patients is generally not difficult. In women over 30 years, fibrocystic condition of the breast and carcinoma of the breast must be considered. Cysts can be identified by aspiration or ultrasonography. Fibroadenoma does not normally occur after menopause but may occasionally develop after administration of hormones.

No treatment is usually necessary if the diagnosis can be made by core needle biopsy. Excision with pathologic examination of the specimen is performed if the diagnosis is uncertain or the lesion grows significantly. Cryoablation, or freezing of the fibroadenoma, appears to be a safe procedure if the lesion is a biopsy-proven fibroadenoma prior to ablation. Cryoablation is not appropriate for all fibroadenomas because some are too large to freeze or the diagnosis may not be certain. There is no clinical advantage to cryoablation of a histologically proven fibroadenoma beyond the relief that some patients experience when the mass is gone. However, at times a mass of scar or fat necrosis replaces the mass of the fibroadenoma. Reassurance seems preferable to treatment. Distinguishing a large fibroadenoma from a phyllodes tumor based on needle biopsy results or imaging alone is usually not possible; histologic examination after excision is usually required. Presumed fibroadenomas larger than 3–4 cm should be excised to rule out phyllodes tumors.

Phyllodes tumor is a fibroadenoma-like tumor with cellular stroma that grows rapidly. It may reach a large size and, if inadequately excised, will recur locally. The lesion can be benign or malignant. If benign, phyllodes tumor is treated by local excision. The treatment of malignant phyllodes tumor is more controversial, but complete removal of the tumor with a margin of normal tissue avoids recurrence. Because these tumors may be large, total mastectomy is sometimes necessary. Lymph node dissection is not performed, since the sarcomatous portion of the tumor metastasizes to the lungs and not the lymph nodes.

Erickson LA et al. Fibroadenoma of the breast. Mayo Clin Proc. 2020;95:2573. [PMID: 33153651]
Rayzah M. Phyllodes tumors of the breast: a literature review. Cureus. 2020;12:e10288. [PMID: 32923300]
Tummidi S et al. Fibroadenoma versus phyllodes tumor: a vexing problem revisited! BMC Cancer. 2020;20:648. [PMID: 32660435]

NIPPLE DISCHARGE

In order of decreasing frequency, the following are the most common causes of nipple discharge in the nonlactating breast: duct ectasia, intraductal papilloma, and carcinoma. The important characteristics of the discharge and other factors to be evaluated are listed in Table 17–1.

1. Discharge from a single duct—Spontaneous, unilateral, serous or serosanguineous discharge from a single duct is usually caused by an ectatic duct or an intraductal papilloma or, rarely, by an intraductal cancer. A mass may not be palpable. The involved duct may be identified by pressure at different sites around the nipple at the margin of the areola. Bloody discharge is suggestive of cancer but is more often caused by a benign papilloma in the duct. Cytologic examination may identify malignant cells, but negative findings do not rule out cancer, which is more likely in older women. In any case, the involved bloody duct—and a mass if present—should be excised. A ductogram (a mammogram of a duct after radiopaque dye has been injected), like cytology, is of limited value since excision of the suspicious ductal system is indicated regardless of findings. Ductoscopy, evaluation of the ductal system with a small scope inserted through the nipple, has been attempted but is not effective management.

Table 17–1. Characteristics of nipple discharge in the nonpregnant, nonlactating woman.

Finding	Significance
Serous	Most likely benign FCC, ie, duct ectasia
Bloody	More likely neoplastic–papilloma, carcinoma
Associated mass	More likely neoplastic
Unilateral	Either neoplastic or non-neoplastic
Bilateral	Most likely non-neoplastic
Single duct	More likely neoplastic
Multiple ducts	More likely FCC
Milky	Endocrine disorders, medications
Spontaneous	Either neoplastic or non-neoplastic
Produced by pressure at single site	Either neoplastic or non-neoplastic
Persistent	Either neoplastic or non-neoplastic
Intermittent	Either neoplastic or non-neoplastic
Related to menses	More likely FCC
Premenopausal	More likely FCC
Taking hormones	More likely FCC

FCC, fibrocystic condition.

2. Discharge from multiple ducts—In premenopausal women, spontaneous multiple duct discharge, unilateral or bilateral, most noticeable just before menstruation, is often due to fibrocystic condition. Discharge may be green or brownish. Papillomatosis and ductal ectasia are usually detected only by biopsy. If a mass is present, it should be removed.

A milky discharge from multiple ducts in the nonlactating breast may occur from hyperprolactinemia. Serum prolactin levels should be obtained to search for a pituitary tumor. TSH helps exclude causative hypothyroidism. Numerous antipsychotic medications and other medications may also cause a milky discharge that ceases on discontinuance of the medication.

Oral contraceptive agents or estrogen replacement therapy may cause clear, serous, or milky discharge from a single duct, but multiple duct discharge is more common. In the premenopausal woman, the discharge is more evident just before menstruation and disappears on stopping the medication. If it does not stop, is from a single duct, and is copious, exploration should be performed since this may be a sign of cancer.

A purulent discharge may originate in a subareolar abscess and require removal of the abscess and the related lactiferous sinus.

When localization of the discharge is not possible, no mass is palpable, and the discharge is nonbloody, the patient should be reexamined every 3 or 4 months for a year, and a mammogram and an ultrasound should be performed. Although most discharge is from a benign process, patients may find it annoying or disconcerting. To eliminate the discharge, proximal duct excision can be performed both for treatment and diagnosis.

Çetin K et al. Evaluation and management of pathological nipple discharges without using intraductal imaging methods. Ir J Med Sci. 2020;189:451. [PMID: 31631245]
Gupta D et al. Nipple discharge: current clinical and imaging evaluation. AJR Am J Roentgenol. 2021;216:330. [PMID: 33295815]
Zacharioudakis K et al. Can we see what is invisible? The role of MRI in the evaluation and management of patients with pathological nipple discharge. Breast Cancer Res Treat. 2019;178:115. [PMID: 31352554]

FAT NECROSIS

Fat necrosis is a rare lesion of the breast but is of clinical importance because it produces a mass (often accompanied by skin or nipple retraction) that is usually indistinguishable from carcinoma even with imaging studies. Fat necrosis can occur after trauma; after fat injections to augment breast size or fill defects after breast surgery; and after segmental resection, radiation therapy, or flap reconstruction following mastectomy.

The resultant mass may be confused with cancer. If untreated, the mass gradually disappears. If imaging is not typical of fat necrosis, the safest course is to obtain a biopsy. Core needle biopsy is usually adequate.

Lee J et al. Natural course of fat necrosis after breast reconstruction: a 10-year follow-up study. BMC Cancer. 2021;21:166. [PMID: 33593330]

BREAST ABSCESS

During nursing, an area of redness, tenderness, and induration may develop in the breast. The organism most commonly found in these abscesses is *Staphylococcus aureus* (see Puerperal Mastitis, Chapter 19).

Infection in the nonlactating breast is rare. A subareolar abscess may develop in young or middle-aged women who are not lactating. Often needle or catheter drainage is adequate to treat an abscess, but surgical incision and drainage may be necessary; these infections tend to recur after incision and drainage unless the area is explored during a quiescent interval, with excision of the involved lactiferous duct or ducts at the base of the nipple. In the nonlactating breast, inflammatory carcinoma must always be considered. Thus, incision and biopsy of any indurated tissue with a small piece of erythematous skin is indicated when suspected abscess or cellulitis in the nonlactating breast does not resolve promptly with antibiotics.

Luo J et al. Abscess drainage with or without antibiotics in lactational breast abscess: study protocol for a randomized controlled trial. Infect Drug Resist. 2020;13:183. [PMID: 32021332]

Sugawara C et al. Factors associated with surgical treatment in postpartum women with mastitis or breast abscess: a retrospective cohort study. Breastfeed Med. 2022;17:233. [PMID: 34936486]

DISORDERS OF THE AUGMENTED BREAST

At least 4 million American women have had breast implants. Breast augmentation is performed by placing implants under the pectoralis muscle or, less desirably, in the subcutaneous tissue of the breast. Most implants are made of an outer silicone shell filled with a silicone gel, saline, or some combination of the two. Capsule contraction or scarring around the implant develops in about 15–25% of patients, leading to a firmness and distortion of the breast that can be painful. Some require removal of the implant and surrounding capsule.

Implant rupture may occur in as many as 5–10% of women, and bleeding of gel through the capsule is noted even more commonly. Although silicone gel may be an immunologic stimulant, there is *no increase* in autoimmune disorders in patients with such implants. The FDA has advised symptomatic women with ruptured silicone implants to discuss possible surgical removal with their clinicians. However, women who are asymptomatic and have no evidence of rupture of a silicone gel prosthesis do not require removal of the implant. Women with symptoms of autoimmune illnesses often undergo removal, but no benefit has been shown.

Studies have failed to show any association between implants and an increased incidence of breast cancer. However, breast cancer may develop in a patient with an augmentation prosthesis, as it does in women without them. Detection in patients with implants may be more difficult because mammography is less able to detect early lesions. Mammography is better if the implant is subpectoral rather than subcutaneous. Local recurrence is usually cutaneous or subcutaneous and is easily detected by palpation. Rarely, lymphoma of the breast with silicone implants has been reported.

If a cancer develops in a patient with implants, it should be treated in the same manner as in women without implants. Such women should be offered the option of mastectomy or breast-conserving therapy, which may require removal or replacement of the implant. Radiotherapy of the augmented breast often results in marked capsular contracture. Adjuvant treatments should be given for the same indications as for women who have no implants.

Coroneos CJ et al. US FDA breast implant postapproval studies: long-term outcomes in 99,993 patients. Ann Surg. 2019;269:30. [PMID: 30222598]

Montemurro P et al. Controllable factors to reduce the rate of complications in primary breast augmentation: a review of the literature. Aesthetic Plast Surg. 2021;45:498. [PMID: 32358668]

CARCINOMA OF THE FEMALE BREAST

ESSENTIALS OF DIAGNOSIS

- Risk factors: Age, nulliparity, childbirth after age 30, family history of breast cancer or deleterious mutations (*BRCA1*, *BRCA2,* or others), and personal history of breast cancer or some types of proliferative conditions.
- Early findings: Mammographic abnormalities and no palpable mass, or single, nontender, firm to hard mass with ill-defined margins.
- Later findings: Skin or nipple retraction; axillary lymphadenopathy; breast enlargement, erythema, edema, pain; fixation of mass to skin or chest wall.

Incidence & Risk Factors

Breast cancer will develop in *one of eight* American women. Next to skin cancer, breast cancer is the most common cancer in women; it is second only to lung cancer as a cause of death. In 2021 there were approximately 281,550 new cases and 43,600 deaths from breast cancer in the United States. Worldwide, breast cancer is diagnosed in approximately 2.3 million women, and about 685,000 die of breast cancer each year.

The most significant risk factor for the development of breast cancer is age. A woman's risk of breast cancer rises rapidly until her early 60s, peaks in her 70s, and then declines. A significant family history of breast or ovarian cancer imparts a high risk of developing breast cancer. Germline mutations in the *BRCA* family of tumor suppressor genes or other breast cancer susceptibility genes accounts for approximately 5–10% of breast cancer diagnoses and tend to cluster in certain ethnic groups, including women of Ashkenazi Jewish descent. Women with a mutation in the *BRCA1* gene, located on chromosome 17, have an estimated 85% chance of developing breast cancer in their lifetime. Other genes associated with an increased risk of breast and other cancers include *BRCA2* (associated with a gene on chromosome 13); ataxia-telangiectasia mutation (*ATM*), *BARD1, CHEK2, PALB2, RAD51D*; and mutation of the tumor suppressor gene *p53*. Primary care clinicians should assess a woman's personal and family history for breast, ovarian, tubal, or peritoneal cancer (as family history of ovarian and peritoneal cancers increases a woman's risk of breast cancer) using a familial risk assessment tool (eg, https://bcrisktool.cancer.gov/calculator.html). Those with a positive result should receive genetic counseling in order to decide whether genetic testing is indicated.

Even when genetic testing fails to reveal a predisposing genetic mutation, women with a strong family history of breast cancer are at higher risk for development of breast cancer. Compared with a woman with no affected family members, a woman who has one first-degree relative with breast cancer has double the risk of developing breast cancer and a woman with two first-degree relatives with breast cancer has triple the risk of developing breast cancer. The risk is further increased for a woman whose affected family member was premenopausal at the time of diagnosis or had bilateral breast cancer. Lifestyle and reproductive factors also contribute to risk of breast cancer. Nulliparous women and women whose first full-term pregnancy occurred after the age of 30 have an elevated risk. Early menarche (under age 12) and late natural menopause (after age 55) are associated with an increase in risk, especially for hormone receptor–positive (estrogen receptor [ER]-positive or progesterone receptor [PR]-positive or both) breast cancer. Combined oral contraceptive pills also appear to increase the risk of breast cancer, with longer use associated with higher risk. Several studies show that concomitant administration of progesterone and estrogen to postmenopausal women may increase the incidence of breast cancer, compared with the use of estrogen alone or with no hormone replacement treatment. A prior history of chest wall radiation increases the risk of breast cancer years later. Alcohol consumption, high dietary intake of fat, and lack of exercise may also increase the risk of breast cancer. Fibrocystic breast condition is also associated with an increased incidence of cancer only when it is accompanied by proliferative changes, papillomatosis, atypical epithelial hyperplasia, or increased breast density on mammogram. A woman who had cancer in one breast is at increased risk for cancer developing in the other breast. In these women, a contralateral cancer develops at rate of approximately 1% per year. Women with cancer of the uterine corpus have a risk of breast cancer significantly higher than that of the general population, and women with breast cancer have a comparably increased risk of endometrial cancer. Breast cancer tends to be diagnosed more frequently in women of higher socioeconomic status.

Table 17–2. Factors associated with increased risk of breast cancer (listed in alphabetical order).

Age	Older
Family history	Breast cancer in parent, sibling, or child (especially bilateral or premenopausal)
Genetics	*BRCA1, BRCA2*, or other unknown mutations
Menstrual history	Early menarche (under age 12) Late menopause (after age 55)
Previous medical history	Endometrial cancer Proliferative forms of fibrocystic disease Cancer in other breast
Race	White
Reproductive history	Nulliparous or late first pregnancy

Women at greater than average risk for developing breast cancer (Table 17–2) should be identified by their clinicians and monitored carefully. Several risk assessment models have been validated to estimate a woman's risk of developing cancer. Women with genetic mutations in whom breast cancer develops may be treated in the same way as women who do not have mutations (ie, lumpectomy), though there is an increased risk of ipsilateral and contralateral breast cancer after lumpectomy for these women.

Bahl M. Management of high-risk breast lesions. Radiol Clin North Am. 2021;59:29. [PMID: 33222998]

Breast Cancer Association Consortium; Dorling L et al. Breast cancer risk genes—association analysis in more than 113,000 women. N Engl J Med. 2021;384:428. [PMID: 33471991]

Daly AA et al. A review of modifiable risk factors in young women for the prevention of breast cancer. Breast Cancer (Dove Med Press). 2021;13:241 [PMID: 33883932]

Jin J. JAMA patient page. Should I be tested for *BRCA* mutations? JAMA. 2019;322:702. [PMID: 31429898]

Kanadys W et al. Use of oral contraceptives as a potential risk factor for breast cancer: a systematic review and meta-analysis of case-control studies up to 2010. Int J Environ Res Public Health. 2021;18:4638. [PMID: 33925599]

Kim G et al. Assessing risk of breast cancer: a review of risk prediction models. J Breast Imaging. 2021;3:144. [PMID: 33778488]

Minami CA et al. Menopausal hormone therapy and long-term breast cancer risk: further data from the Women's Health Initiative Trials. JAMA. 2020;324:347. [PMID: 32720989]

Palmer JR et al. A validated risk prediction model for breast cancer in US Black women. J Clin Oncol. 2021;39:3866. [PMID: 34623926]

Siegel RL et al. Cancer statistics, 2021. CA Cancer J Clin. 2021; 71:7. [PMID: 33433946]

Smith SG et al. The impact of body mass index on breast cancer incidence among women at increased risk: an observational study from the International Breast Intervention Studies. Breast Cancer Res Treat. 2021;188:215. [PMID: 33656637]

Tung NM et al. Management of hereditary breast cancer: American Society of Clinical Oncology, American Society for Radiation Oncology, and Society of Surgical Oncology Guideline. J Clin Oncol. 2020;38:2080. [PMID: 32243226]

US Preventive Services Task Force; Owens DK et al. Risk assessment, genetic counseling, and genetic testing for *BRCA*-related cancer: US Preventive Services Task Force Recommendation Statement. JAMA. 2019;322:652. [PMID: 31429903]

Prevention

Multiple clinical trials have evaluated the use of selective ER modulators (SERMs), including tamoxifen and raloxifene, or aromatase inhibitors for prevention of breast cancer in women with no personal history of breast cancer but at high risk for developing the disease. A network meta-analysis of six of these studies including 50,927 women demonstrated a 32% reduction in breast cancer incidence with the use of tamoxifen compared to placebo and a 47% reduction in risk of breast cancer with the use of an aromatase inhibitor compared with placebo. An increased risk of endometrial cancer, cataracts, and venous thromboembolic events has been associated with tamoxifen and a higher rate of fractures and musculoskeletal side effects are associated with aromatase inhibitors. While preventive agents have been shown to be effective at reducing the risk of breast cancer and saving costs, the use of this intervention by women has been relatively low, possibly due to the perceived risks and side effects of therapy.

Some women at high risk may consider prophylactic mastectomy or oophorectomy.

Chlebowski RT et al. Breast cancer prevention: time for a change. JCO Oncol Pract. 2021;17:709. [PMID: 34319769]

Cuzick J et al. Use of anastrozole for breast cancer prevention (IBIS-II): long-term results of a randomised controlled trial. Lancet. 2020;395:117. [PMID: 31839281]

Graham D et al. Breast cancer risk-reducing medications. JAMA. 2020;324:310. [PMID: 32692388]

Shieh Y et al. Medications for primary prevention of breast cancer. JAMA. 2020;324:291. [PMID: 32692377]

US Preventive Services Task Force; Owens DK et al. Medication use to reduce risk of breast cancer: US Preventive Services Task Force Recommendation Statement. JAMA. 2019;322:857. [PMID: 31479144]

Early Detection of Breast Cancer

A. Screening Programs

Screening detects breast cancer before it has spread to the lymph nodes in about 80% of the women evaluated. This increases the chance of survival to greater than 85% at 5 years.

Substantial evidence supports the use of **routine screening mammography;** however, recommendations relating to timing and frequency vary by different agencies and countries. About one-third of the abnormalities detected on screening mammograms will be found to be malignant when biopsy is performed. The probability of cancer on a screening mammogram is directly related to the Breast Imaging Reporting and Data System (BIRADS) assessment, and workup should be performed based on this classification. The sensitivity of mammography varies from approximately 60% to 90%. This sensitivity depends on several factors, including patient age, breast density, tumor size, tumor histology (lobular versus ductal), location, and mammographic appearance. In young women with dense breasts, mammography is less sensitive than in older women with fatty breasts, in whom mammography can detect at least 90% of malignancies. Smaller tumors, particularly those without calcifications, are more difficult to detect, especially in dense breasts. The lack of sensitivity and the low incidence of breast cancer in young women have led to questions concerning the value of mammography for screening in women 40–50 years of age. The specificity of mammography in women under 50 years varies from about 30% to 40% for nonpalpable mammographic abnormalities to 85% to 90% for clinically evident malignancies. Guidelines from at least six separate organizations exist in the United States and each differs slightly, making it somewhat complex for clinicians and patients to navigate. While the American College of Radiology, American Medical Association, and National Comprehensive Cancer Network (NCCN) recommend starting mammography screening at age 40, the USPSTF recommends starting screening at age 50. Most guidelines recommend annual screening; however, the American Cancer Society recommends decreasing the frequency of screening to every 1–2 years starting at age 55 years and the USPSTF recommends routine mammography be done no more than every 2 years beginning at age 50 years. It is generally agreed that mammography should continue until life expectancy is shorter than 7–10 years, although the USPSTF recommends stopping screening after age 74 years regardless of life expectancy. Thus, clinicians should have an informed discussion with patients about screening mammography regarding its potential risks (eg, false positives, overdiagnosis, radiation exposure) and benefits (eg, early diagnosis), taking into consideration a patient's individual risk factors.

B. Imaging

1. Mammography—Mammography is the most reliable means of detecting breast cancer before a mass can be palpated. Most slowly growing cancers can be identified by mammography at least 2 years before reaching a size detectable by palpation.

Indications for mammography are as follows: (1) screening at regular intervals asymptomatic women at risk for developing breast cancer; (2) evaluating each breast when a diagnosis of potentially curable breast cancer has been made, and at regular intervals thereafter; (3) evaluating a questionable or ill-defined breast mass or other suspicious change in the breast; (4) searching for an occult breast cancer in women with metastatic disease in axillary nodes or elsewhere from an unknown primary; (5) screening women prior to cosmetic operations or prior to biopsy of a mass, to examine for an unsuspected cancer; (6) monitoring women with breast cancer who have been treated with breast-conserving surgery and radiation; and (7) monitoring the contralateral breast in women with breast cancer treated with mastectomy.

Calcifications are the most easily recognized mammographic abnormality. The most common findings associated with carcinoma of the breast are clustered pleomorphic microcalcifications. Such calcifications are usually at least five to eight in number, aggregated in one part of the breast and differing from each other in size and shape, often including branched or V- or Y-shaped configurations. There may be an associated mammographic mass density or, at times, only a mass density with no calcifications. Such a density usually has irregular or ill-defined borders and may lead to architectural distortion within the breast, but may be subtle and difficult to detect.

Patients with a dominant or suspicious mass on examination must undergo biopsy despite mammographic findings. The mammogram should be obtained prior to biopsy so that other suspicious areas can be noted and the contralateral breast can be evaluated. *Mammography is never a substitute for biopsy* because it may not reveal clinical cancer, especially in a very dense breast.

Communication and documentation among the patient, the referring clinician, and the interpreting physician are critical for high-quality screening and diagnostic mammography. The patient should be told about *how* she will receive timely results of her mammogram; that mammography does not "rule out" cancer; and that she may receive a correlative examination such as ultrasound at the mammography facility if referred for a suspicious lesion. She should also be aware of the technique and need for breast compression and that this may be uncomfortable. The mammography facility should be informed in writing by the clinician of abnormal physical examination findings. The Agency for Health Care Policy and Research Clinical Practice Guidelines strongly recommend that all mammography reports be communicated in writing to the patient and referring clinician. Legislation has been passed in a number of US states that requires imaging facilities to report to patients the density of their breasts. This may prompt women with dense breasts to discuss with their clinician whether or not additional screening options would be appropriate in addition to mammogram.

2. Other imaging—MRI and ultrasound may be useful screening modalities in women who are at high risk for breast cancer but not for the general population. The *sensitivity* of MRI is much higher than mammography; however, the *specificity* is significantly lower and this results in multiple unnecessary biopsies. The increased sensitivity despite decreased specificity may be considered a reasonable trade-off for those at increased risk for developing breast cancer but not for normal-risk population. The NCCN guidelines recommend MRI in addition to screening mammography for high-risk women, including those with deleterious mutations, those who have a lifetime risk of breast cancer of at least 20%, and those with a personal history of lobular carcinoma in situ (LCIS).

Women who received radiation therapy to the chest in their teens or twenties are also known to be at high risk for developing breast cancer and screening MRI may be considered in addition to mammography. A Netherlands study (Dense Tissue and Early Breast Neoplasm Screening "DENSE") involving over 40,000 women with extremely dense breast tissue demonstrated that the addition of annual MRI to screening mammography was associated with a lower rate of cancers being diagnosed in 2 years.

Houser M et al. Current and future directions of breast MRI. J Clin Med. 2021;10:5668. [PMID: 34884370]

C. Clinical Breast Examination and Self-Examination

Breast self-examination has *not* been shown to improve survival. Because of the lack of strong evidence demonstrating value, the American Cancer Society no longer recommends monthly breast self-examination. Nonetheless, patients should recognize and report any breast changes to their clinicians as it remains an important facet of proactive care.

Destounis SV et al. Update on breast density, risk estimation, and supplemental screening. AJR Am J Roentgenol. 2020;214:296. [PMID: 31743049]

García-Albéniz X et al. Continuation of annual screening mammography and breast cancer mortality in women older than 70 years. Ann Intern Med. 2020;172:381. [PMID: 32092767]

Harkness EF et al. Risk-based breast cancer screening strategies in women. Best Pract Res Clin Obstet Gynaecol. 2020;65:3. [PMID: 31848103]

Hong S et al. Effect of digital mammography for breast cancer screening: a comparative study of more than 8 million Korean women. Radiology. 2020;294:247. [PMID: 31793847]

Clinical Findings Associated with Early Detection of Breast Cancer

A. Symptoms and Signs

The presenting complaint in about 70% of patients with breast cancer is a lump (usually painless) in the breast. About 90% of these breast masses are discovered by the patient. Less frequent symptoms are breast pain; nipple discharge; erosion, retraction, enlargement, or itching of the nipple; and redness, generalized hardness, enlargement, or shrinking of the breast. Rarely, an axillary mass or swelling of the arm may be the first symptom. Back or bone pain, jaundice, or weight loss may be the result of systemic metastases, but these symptoms are rarely seen on initial presentation.

The relative frequency of carcinoma in various anatomic sites in the breast is shown in Figure 17–1.

Inspection of the breast is the first step in physical examination and should be carried out with the patient sitting, arms at her sides and then overhead. Abnormal variations in breast size and contour, minimal nipple retraction, and slight edema, redness, or retraction of the skin can be identified (Figure 17–2). Asymmetry of the breasts and retraction or dimpling of the skin can often be accentuated by having the patient raise her arms overhead or press her hands on her hips to contract the pectoralis muscles. Axillary and supraclavicular areas should be thoroughly palpated for enlarged nodes with the patient sitting. Palpation of the breast for masses or other changes should be performed with the patient both seated and supine with the arm abducted. Palpation with a rotary motion of the

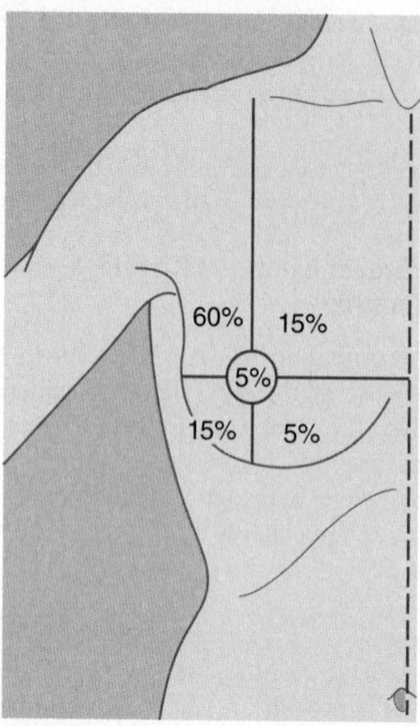

▲ **Figure 17–1.** Frequency of breast carcinoma at various anatomic sites.

examiner's fingers as well as a horizontal stripping motion has been recommended.

Breast cancer usually consists of a nontender, firm or hard mass with poorly delineated margins (caused by local infiltration). Small (1–2 mm) erosions of the nipple epithelium may be the only manifestation of Paget disease of the breast (Figure 17–3). Watery, serous, or bloody discharge from the nipple is an occasional early sign but is more often associated with benign disease.

A lesion smaller than 1 cm in diameter may be difficult or impossible for the examiner to feel but may be discovered by the patient. The patient should always be asked to demonstrate the location of the mass. If the clinician fails to confirm the patient's suspicions and imaging studies are normal, the examination should be repeated in 2–3 months, preferably 1–2 weeks after the onset of menses. During the premenstrual phase of the cycle, increased innocuous nodularity may suggest neoplasm or may obscure an

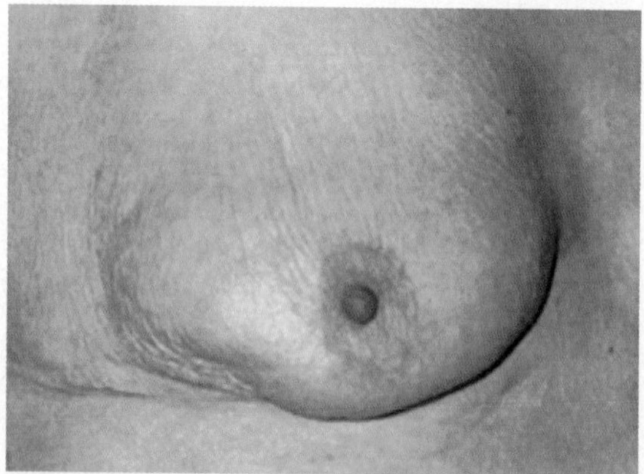

▲ **Figure 17–2.** Skin dimpling. (Used, with permission, from Armando E. Giuliano, MD.)

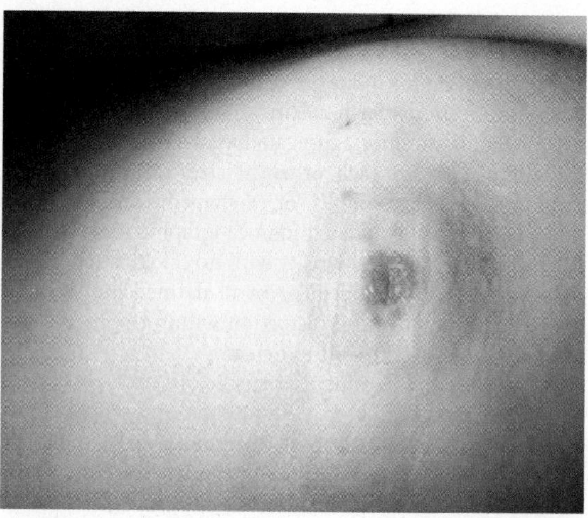

▲ **Figure 17–3.** Paget disease. (Used, with permission, from Armando E. Giuliano, MD.)

underlying lesion. If there is any question regarding the nature of an abnormality under these circumstances, the patient should be asked to return after her menses.

Metastases tend to first involve regional lymph nodes, which may be palpable. One or two movable, nontender, not particularly firm axillary lymph nodes 5 mm or less in diameter are frequently present and are generally not significant. Firm or hard nodes larger than 1 cm are typical of metastases. Axillary nodes that are matted or fixed to skin or deep structures indicate advanced disease (at least stage III). If the examiner thinks that the axillary nodes are involved, that impression will be borne out by histologic section in about 85% of cases. The incidence of positive axillary nodes increases with the size of the primary tumor. Noninvasive cancers (in situ) do not metastasize. Metastases in node(s) are present in about 30% of patients with clinically negative nodes.

In most cases, no nodes are palpable in the supraclavicular fossa. Firm or hard nodes of any size in this location or just beneath the clavicle should be biopsied. Ipsilateral supraclavicular or infraclavicular nodes containing cancer indicate that the tumor is in an advanced stage (stage III or IV). Edema of the ipsilateral breast or arm, commonly caused by metastatic infiltration of regional lymphatics, is also a sign of advanced cancer.

B. Laboratory Findings

Liver or bone metastases may be associated with elevation of serum alkaline phosphatase. Hypercalcemia is an occasional important finding in advanced cancer of the breast. Serum tumor markers such as carcinoembryonic antigen and CA 15-3 or CA 27-29 are *not* recommended for diagnosis of early lesions or for routine surveillance for recurrence after a breast cancer diagnosis.

C. Imaging

1. For lesions felt only by the patient—Ultrasonography is often valuable and mammography essential when an area is felt by the patient to be abnormal but the clinician feels no mass. MRI should not be used to rule out cancer because MRI has a false-negative rate of about 3–5%. Although lower than mammography, this false-negative rate cannot permit safe elimination of the possibility of cancer. False-negative results with imaging are more likely seen in infiltrating lobular carcinomas and ductal carcinoma in situ (DCIS) than invasive ductal carcinoma.

2. For metastatic lesions—For patients with suspicious symptoms or signs (bone pain, abdominal symptoms, elevated liver biochemical tests) or locally advanced disease (clinically abnormal lymph nodes or large primary tumors), staging scans are indicated prior to surgery or systemic therapy. Chest imaging with CT or radiographs may be done to evaluate for pulmonary metastases. Abdominal imaging with CT or ultrasound may be obtained to evaluate for liver metastases. Bone scans using ^{99m}Tc-labeled phosphates or phosphonates are more sensitive than skeletal radiographs in detecting metastatic breast cancer. Bone scanning has not proved to be of clinical value as a routine preoperative test in the absence of symptoms, physical findings, or abnormal alkaline phosphatase or calcium levels. The frequency of abnormal findings on bone scan parallels the status of the axillary lymph nodes on pathologic examination. PET scanning alone or combined with CT (PET-CT) may also be used for detecting soft tissue or visceral metastases in patients with locally advanced disease or with symptoms or signs of metastatic disease.

D. Diagnostic Tests

1. Aspiration—If a tumor is palpable and feels like a cyst, an 18-gauge needle can be used to aspirate the fluid and make the diagnosis of cyst. If a cyst is aspirated and the fluid is nonbloody, it does not have to be examined cytologically. If the mass does not recur, no further diagnostic test is necessary.

2. Biopsy—The diagnosis of breast cancer depends ultimately on examination of tissue or cells removed by biopsy. Treatment should never be undertaken without an unequivocal histologic or cytologic diagnosis of cancer. About 60% of lesions clinically thought to be cancer prove on biopsy to be benign, while about 30% of clinically benign lesions are found to be malignant. These findings demonstrate the fallibility of clinical judgment and the necessity for biopsy. *The safest course is biopsy examination of all suspicious lesions found on physical examination or imaging, or both.*

There is only one probable exception to the need for a histologic diagnosis of a breast mass: a nonsuspicious, presumably fibrocystic mass, in a premenopausal woman. Rather, these masses can be observed through one or two menstrual cycles. However, the mass must be biopsied if it does not completely resolve during this time and ultrasonographic findings show that it is not cystic or benign appearing (like a fibroadenoma or intramammary lymph node). Figures 17–4 and 17–5 present algorithms for management of breast masses in premenopausal and postmenopausal patients.

The simplest biopsy method is needle biopsy, either by aspiration of tumor cells (FNA cytology) or by obtaining a small core of tissue with a hollow needle (core needle biopsy).

Core (large) needle biopsy removes a core of tissue with a large cutting needle for histologic examination and *is the diagnostic procedure of choice* for both palpable and image-detected abnormalities. Handheld biopsy devices make large-core needle (14-gauge) biopsy of a palpable mass easy and cost effective in the office with local anesthesia. As in the case of any needle biopsy, the main problem is sampling error due to improper positioning of the needle, giving rise to a false-negative test result. This is extremely unusual with image-guided biopsies. Core needle biopsy allows the tumor to be tested for the expression of biological markers, such as ER, PR, and *HER2*.

FNA cytology is a technique whereby cells are aspirated with a small needle and examined cytologically. This technique can be performed easily with virtually no morbidity and is much less expensive than excisional or open biopsy. The main disadvantages are that it requires a pathologist skilled in the cytologic diagnosis of breast cancer and it is subject to sampling problems. Furthermore, noninvasive cancers usually cannot be distinguished from invasive cancers. The incidence of false-positive diagnoses is extremely low, perhaps 1–2%. The false-negative rate is as high as 10%. Most experienced clinicians would not leave a suspicious dominant mass in the breast even when FNA cytology is negative unless the clinical diagnosis, breast imaging studies, and cytologic studies were all in agreement, such as for a fibrocystic lesion or fibroadenoma. Given the stated limitations, *core needle biopsy, rather than FNA, is the modality of choice for sampling an abnormal breast mass.* FNA can be useful for biopsy of suspicious lymph nodes near the axillary vein.

Open biopsy under local anesthesia as a separate procedure prior to deciding upon definitive treatment has become less common with the increased use of core needle biopsy. Core needle biopsy, when positive, offers a more rapid approach with less expense and morbidity, but when nondiagnostic it must be followed by open biopsy. It generally consists of an **excisional biopsy,** which is done through an incision with the intent to remove the entire abnormality, not simply a sample. Intraoperative frozen section examination of a breast biopsy has generally been abandoned unless there is a high clinical suspicion of malignancy in a patient well prepared for the diagnosis of cancer and its treatment options.

3. Biopsy with ultrasound guidance—Ultrasonography may show signs suggestive of carcinoma, such as an irregular mass or a mass within a cyst in the rare case of intracystic carcinoma. Nonpalpable mammographic densities that appear benign should be investigated with ultrasound to determine whether the lesions are cystic or solid or have features suggestive of a malignancy. These may even be needle biopsied with ultrasound guidance.

4. Biopsy with mammographic guidance—When a suspicious abnormality is identified by mammography alone and cannot be palpated by the clinician, the lesion should

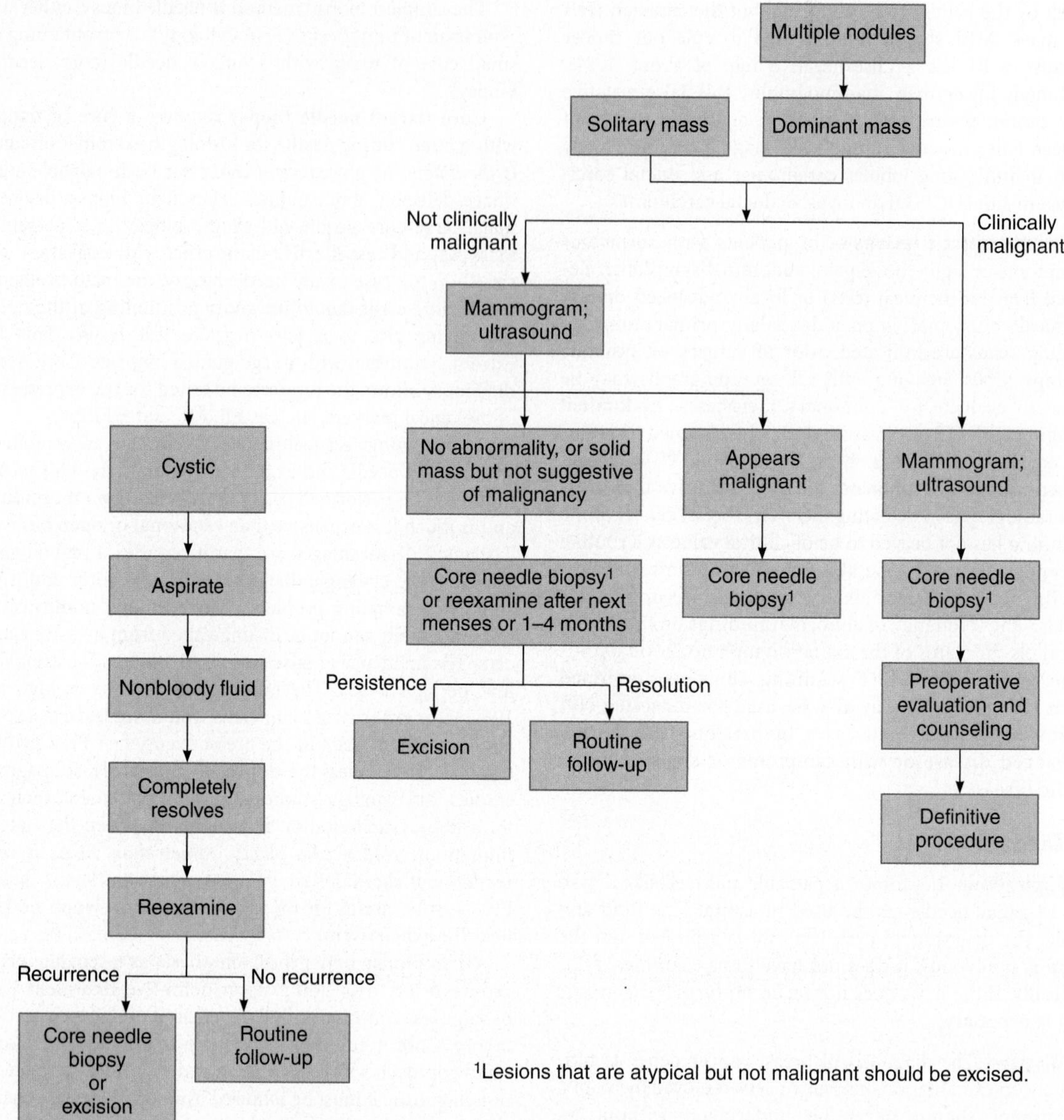

▲ **Figure 17–4. Evaluation of breast masses in premenopausal women.** (Reproduced with permission from Giuliano AE, Srour MK. Breast disease. In: Berek JS, Hacker NF. Berek & Hacker's [editors], *Gynecologic Oncology*. 7th ed. Philadelphia: Wolters Kluwer, 2021.)

be biopsied under mammographic guidance. Mammographic guidance can be used for core needle biopsies or excisional biopsies.

A metal clip should be placed after any image-guided core biopsy to facilitate finding the site of the lesion if subsequent treatment is necessary. Some atypical lesions such as atypical ductal hyperplasia or papilloma may require excision because they are associated with a malignancy in 15–25% of cases.

5. Other imaging modalities—Other modalities of breast imaging have been investigated for diagnostic purposes. Automated breast ultrasonography is useful in distinguishing cystic from solid lesions but should be used only as a supplement to physical examination and mammography. MRI is highly sensitive but not specific and should not be used for screening except in highly selective cases. For example, MRI is useful in differentiating scar from recurrence post-lumpectomy and is valuable to screen high-risk women (eg, women with deleterious mutations). It may also be of value to examine for multicentricity when there is a known primary cancer; to examine the contralateral breast in women with cancer; to examine the extent of cancer, especially lobular carcinomas; or to determine the response to neoadjuvant chemotherapy. Moreover, MRI-detected suspicious findings that are not seen on mammogram or ultrasound may be biopsied under MRI guidance.

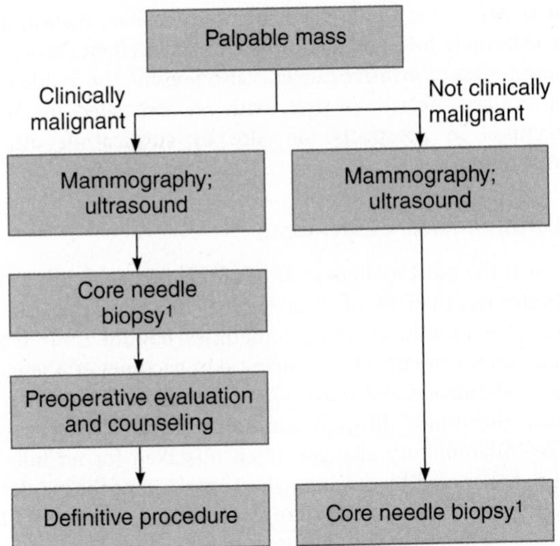

▲ **Figure 17–5. Evaluation of breast masses in post-menopausal women.** (Reproduced with permission from Giuliano AE, Srour MK. Breast disease. In: Berek JS, Hacker NF. Berek & Hacker's [editors], *Gynecologic Oncology*. 7th ed. Philadelphia: Wolters Kluwer, 2021.)

PET scanning does not appear useful in evaluating the breast itself but is useful to examine for distant metastases.

6. Cytology—Cytologic examination of nipple discharge or cyst fluid may be helpful on rare occasions. As a rule, mammography (or ductography) and breast biopsy are required when nipple discharge or cyst fluid is bloody or cytologically questionable.

Sutton EJ et al. Accuracy of magnetic resonance imaging-guided biopsy to verify breast cancer pathologic complete response after neoadjuvant chemotherapy: a nonrandomized controlled trial. JAMA Netw Open. 2021;4:e2034045. [PMID: 33449096]

Differential Diagnosis

The most common lesions in the differential diagnosis of breast cancer are the following, in descending order of frequency: fibrocystic condition of the breast, fibroadenoma, intraductal papilloma, lipoma, and fat necrosis.

Staging

The American Joint Committee on Cancer and the International Union Against Cancer have a joint TNM (tumor, regional lymph nodes, distant metastases) staging system for breast cancer (Table 17–3). All patients are assigned an anatomic stage based on TNM. The eighth edition is a landmark change because it adds biologic markers (ER, PR, HER2, histologic grade, and 21-gene Recurrence Score) to modify the anatomic staging. Thus, each patient is assigned not only an anatomic stage but also a prognostic stage, incorporating these biological factors. The *clinical* prognostic stage, in which T, N, M, grade, and HER2 and hormone receptor status are incorporated, is assigned to all breast cancer patients and is the only prognostic staging classification appropriate for patients who receive neoadjuvant (presurgical) systemic therapy or who do not undergo surgery. The *pathologic* prognostic stage is assigned to those patients who undergo surgery as their initial breast cancer treatment. This is based on T, N, M,

Table 17–3. American Joint Commission on Cancer TNM anatomic stage groups.[1]

When T Is...	And N Is...	And M Is...	Then the Stage Group Is[2]...
Tis	N0	M0	0
T1	N0	M0	IA
T0	N1mi	M0	IB
T1	N1mi	M0	IB
T0	N1	M0	IIA
T1	N1	M0	IIA
T2	N0	M0	IIA
T2	N1	M0	IIB
T3	N0	M0	IIB
T1	N2	M0	IIIA
T2	N2	M0	IIIA
T3	N1	M0	IIIA
T3	N2	M0	IIIA
T4	N0	M0	IIIB
T4	N1	M0	IIIB
T4	N2	M0	IIIB
Any T	N3	M0	IIIC
Any T	Any N	M1	IV

[1]The Anatomic Stage Group table should only be used in global regions where biomarker tests are not routinely available. Cancer registries in the United States must use the prognostic stage group table for case reporting.

[2]T1 includes micrometastases (T1mi). T0 and T1 tumors with lymph node micrometastases only are excluded from stage IIA and are classified as stage IB. M0 includes M0 with isolated tumor cells (i+). The designation pM0 is not valid; any M0 is clinical. If a patient presents with M1 disease before neoadjuvant systemic therapy, then the stage is stage IV and remains stage IV regardless of response to neoadjuvant therapy. Stage designation may be changed if postsurgical imaging studies reveal the presence of distant metastases, provided the studies are performed within 4 months of diagnosis in the absence of disease progression and provided the patient has not received neoadjuvant therapy. Staging after neoadjuvant therapy is denoted with a "yc" or "yp" prefix to the T and N classification. No stage group is assigned if there is a complete pathological response (pCR) to neoadjuvant therapy: for example, ypT0ypN0cM0.

Reproduced with permission from Giuliano AE et al. Breast cancer – major changes in the American Joint Committee on Cancer eighth edition cancer staging manual. *CA Cancer J Clin.* 2017;67(4):290–303.

Table 17–4. Histologic types of breast cancer.

Type	Frequency of Occurrence
Infiltrating ductal (not otherwise specified)	80–90%
Medullary	5–8%
Colloid (mucinous)	2–4%
Tubular	1–2%
Papillary	1–2%
Invasive lobular	6–8%
Noninvasive	4–6%
Intraductal	2–3%
Lobular in situ	2–3%
Rare cancers	< 1%
Juvenile (secretory)	
Adenoid cystic	
Epidermoid	
Sudoriferous	

grade, HER2, hormone receptor status, and in some patients with small ER-positive, HER2-negative, node-negative tumors, 21-gene recurrence score.

Pathologic Types

Numerous pathologic subtypes of breast cancer can be identified histologically (Table 17–4).

Except for the in situ cancers, the histologic subtypes have only a slight bearing on prognosis when outcomes are compared after accurate staging. The noninvasive cancers by definition are confined by the basement membrane of the ducts and lack the ability to spread. Histologic parameters for invasive cancers, including lymphovascular invasion and tumor grade, have been shown to be of prognostic value. Immunohistochemical analysis for expression of hormone receptors and for overexpression of HER2 in the primary tumor offers prognostic and therapeutic information.

Special Clinical Forms of Breast Cancer

A. Paget Carcinoma

Paget carcinoma is uncommon (about 1% of all breast cancers). Over 85% of cases are associated with an underlying invasive or noninvasive cancer, usually a well-differentiated infiltrating ductal carcinoma or a DCIS. Gross nipple changes are often minimal, and a tumor mass may not be palpable.

Because the nipple changes appear innocuous, the diagnosis is frequently missed. The first symptom is often itching or burning of the nipple, with superficial erosion or ulceration. These are often diagnosed and treated as dermatitis or bacterial infection, leading to delay or failure in detection. The diagnosis is established by biopsy of the area of erosion. When the lesion consists of nipple changes only or an associated DCIS, the incidence of axillary metastases is extremely low, and the prognosis is excellent. When a breast mass or invasive cancer is also present, the incidence of axillary metastases rises, with an associated marked decrease in prospects for cure by surgical or other treatment.

B. Inflammatory Carcinoma

This is the most malignant form of breast cancer and constitutes less than 3% of all cases. The clinical findings consist of a rapidly growing, sometimes painful mass that enlarges the breast. The overlying skin becomes erythematous, edematous, and warm. Often there is no distinct mass since the tumor diffusely infiltrates the involved breast. The inflammatory changes, often mistaken for an infection, are caused by carcinomatous invasion of the subdermal lymphatics, with resulting edema and hyperemia. If the clinician suspects infection but the lesion does not respond to antibiotics within 1–2 weeks, biopsy should be performed. Metastases tend to occur early and widely; while rarely deemed curable in the past, anti-HER2 therapy (if HER2 overexpressing or amplified), surgery, and chemotherapy have resulted in some long-term cures for patients with inflammatory carcinoma. Mastectomy is indicated when chemotherapy and radiation have resulted in clinical remission with no evidence of distant metastases. In these cases, residual disease in the breast may be eradicated. Sentinel node biopsy is not indicated due to the high false-negative rate.

Breast Cancer Occurring During Pregnancy or Lactation

Breast cancer complicates up to one in 3000 pregnancies. Its incidence is increasing as women are having children at an older age. The diagnosis is frequently delayed because physiologic changes in the breast may obscure the lesion and screening mammography is not done in young or pregnant women. Termination of pregnancy has not been shown to improve maternal prognosis. The decision whether to terminate the pregnancy must be made on an individual basis, taking into account the patient's wishes, the clinical stage of the cancer and overall prognosis, the gestational age of the fetus, and the potential for premature ovarian failure in the future with systemic therapy.

It is important for primary care and reproductive specialists to aggressively work up any breast abnormality discovered in a pregnant woman. Pregnancy (or lactation) is not a contraindication to operation or treatment, and therapy should be based on the stage of the disease as in the nonpregnant (or nonlactating) woman. Women with early-stage gestational breast cancer who choose to continue their pregnancy should undergo surgery to remove the tumor and systemic therapy if indicated. Often neoadjuvant systemic therapy may be given during pregnancy and the operation and radiation therapy delayed. Retrospective reviews of patients treated with anthracycline-containing regimens for gestational cancers (including leukemia and lymphomas) have established the relative safety of these regimens during pregnancy for both the patient and the fetus.

Taxane-based and trastuzumab-based regimens have not been evaluated extensively, however. Radiation therapy should be delayed until after delivery.

Bilateral Breast Cancer

Bilateral breast cancer occurs in less than 5% of cases, but there is as high as a 20–25% incidence of later occurrence of cancer in the second breast. Bilaterality occurs more often in familial breast cancer, in women under age 50 years, and when there is a deleterious mutation. The incidence of second breast cancers increases directly with the length of time the patient is alive after her first cancer—about 1–2% per year. Tamoxifen or aromatase inhibitors decrease the risk of a contralateral hormone receptor–positive cancer.

In patients with breast cancer, mammography should be performed before primary treatment and at regular intervals thereafter to search for occult cancer in the opposite breast or conserved ipsilateral breast.

LCIS and Noninvasive Cancer

Noninvasive cancer can occur within the ducts (DCIS) or lobules (LCIS). DCIS tends to be unilateral and is believed to progress to invasive cancer if untreated. Invasive cancer will develop in the same breast in approximately 40–60% of women who have unresected DCIS. In the eighth edition of the American Joint Committee on Cancer (AJCC) Cancer Staging Manual, LCIS is no longer considered a cancer. LCIS is generally agreed to be a marker of an increased risk of breast cancer rather than a direct precursor of breast cancer itself. The probability of breast cancer (DCIS or invasive cancer in either breast) in a woman in whom LCIS has been diagnosed is estimated to be 1% per year. If LCIS is detected on core needle biopsy, an excisional biopsy without lymph node sampling may be performed to rule out DCIS or invasive cancer, but NCCN guidelines suggest observation alone is satisfactory. The incidence of LCIS is rising, likely due to increased use of screening mammography. In addition, the rate of mastectomy after the diagnosis of LCIS is increasing in spite of the fact that mastectomy is only recommended in those patients who otherwise have an increased risk of breast cancer through family history, genetic mutation, or past exposure to thoracic radiation. Pleomorphic LCIS may behave more like DCIS and may be associated with invasive carcinoma. For this reason, pleomorphic LCIS should be surgically removed with clear margins.

The treatment of intraductal lesions is controversial. DCIS can be treated by wide excision with or without radiation therapy or with total mastectomy. Conservative management is advised in patients with small lesions amenable to lumpectomy. Patients in whom LCIS is diagnosed or who have received lumpectomy for DCIS may discuss chemoprevention (with hormonal blockade therapy) with their clinician, which is effective in reducing the risk of invasive breast cancer. Axillary metastases from in situ cancers should not occur unless there is an occult invasive cancer. Because a sentinel lymph node biopsy after mastectomy cannot be performed, it should be performed in a patient undergoing mastectomy for DCIS in case an invasive component is discovered.

Giuliano AE et al. Eighth edition of the AJCC Cancer Staging Manual: breast cancer. Ann Surg Oncol. 2018;25:1783. [PMID: 29671136]

Hester RH et al. Inflammatory breast cancer: early recognition and diagnosis is critical. Am J Obstet Gynecol. 2021;225:392. [PMID: 33845027]

Paris I et al. Pregnancy-associated breast cancer: a multidisciplinary approach. Clin Breast Cancer. 2021;21:e120. [PMID: 32778512]

Sisti A et al. Paget disease of the breast: a national retrospective analysis of the US population. Breast Dis. 2020;39:119. [PMID: 32390594]

Tumor Biomarkers & Gene Expression Profiling

Hormone receptor–positive tumors are ER-positive or PR-positive, or both. Treatment with a hormonally targeted agent (anti-estrogen or anti-ER) is an essential therapy for hormone receptor–positive breast cancer. Hormone receptor–negative cancers do not respond to endocrine treatments. Patients whose tumors are hormone receptor–positive tend to have a more indolent disease course than those whose tumors are hormone receptor–negative.

The *HER2* (*human epidermal growth factor receptor 2*) gene is an oncogene; breast cancer cells that overproduce the *HER2* gene (HER2-amplified or "HER2-positive" cancers) overproduce the growth-promoting protein HER2. HER2-positive breast cancer is generally more aggressive than breast cancer with normal HER2 expression (HER2-negative breast cancer). Targeted therapies that block HER2 have been shown to significantly improve outcomes for patients with HER2-positive disease.

Determining the ER, PR, and HER2 status of the tumor at the time early breast cancer is diagnosed and, if possible, at the time of recurrence is critical, both to gauge a patient's prognosis and to determine the best treatment regimen. In addition to ER, PR, and HER2 status, other important prognostic factors include the rate at which tumor divides (assessed by an immunohistochemical stain for Ki67) and the grade and differentiation of the cells. These markers may be obtained on core biopsy or surgical specimens, but not reliably on FNA cytology. Individually these biomarkers are predictive and thus provide insight to guide appropriate therapy. Moreover, when combined, they provide useful information regarding risk of recurrence and prognosis in the curative setting.

In general, tumors that lack expression of HER2, ER, and PR ("**triple-negative**") have a higher risk of early recurrence and metastases and are associated with a worse survival compared with other types. Neither endocrine therapy nor HER2-targeted agents are useful for this type of breast cancer. Chemotherapy has been the primary treatment option for triple-negative breast cancer. In contrast, patients with early-stage, hormone receptor–positive breast cancer may not benefit from the addition of chemotherapy to hormonally targeted treatments. Several molecular tests have been developed to assess risk of recurrence and to predict which patients are most likely to benefit from chemotherapy for early-stage disease. Oncotype DX (Genomic Health/Exact Sciences) evaluates the expression of 21 genes relating to ER, HER2, and proliferation in a tumor specimen and categorizes a patient's risk of recurrence (recurrence score) as high, intermediate, or low risk. Patients in low- or intermediate-risk categories do not benefit from chemotherapy, especially when age 50 or over. This test is primarily indicated for ER-positive, lymph node–negative tumors, but results from the RxPONDER trial suggest that postmenopausal women with 1–3 positive lymph nodes with a recurrence score of less than 25 may not benefit from the use of chemotherapy.

MammaPrint (Agendia) is an FDA-approved 70-gene signature assay that is available for evaluating prognosis. This test classifies patients into good and poor prognostic groups to predict clinical outcome and may be used on patients with hormone receptor–positive or hormone receptor–negative breast cancer. ASCO guidelines indicate this assay may be best used to help determine whether chemotherapy may be safely withheld in patients with hormone receptor–positive, HER2-negative, node-positive breast cancer at high clinical risk. ASCO does not recommend using this assay in hormone receptor–negative or HER2-positive breast cancer. The eighth edition of the AJCC staging system incorporates genomic assays to provide a prognostic stage. Patients with low-risk genomic assays may be downstaged from their TNM stage.

Kalinsky K et al. 21-gene assay to inform chemotherapy benefit in node-positive breast cancer. N Engl J Med. 2021;16:2336. [PMID: 34914339]

Liveringhouse CL et al. Genomically guided breast radiation therapy: a review of the current data and future directions. Adv Radiat Oncol. 2021;6:100731. [PMID: 34409215]

Press MF et al. Assessment of ERBB2/HER2 status in HER2-equivocal breast cancers by FISH and 2013/2014 ASCO-CAP guidelines. JAMA Oncol. 2019;5:366. [PMID: 30520947]

Wolff AC et al. Human epidermal growth factor receptor 2 testing in breast cancer: American Society of Clinical Oncology/College of American Pathologists Clinical Practice Guideline Focused Update. Arch Pathol Lab Med. 2018;142:1364. [PMID: 29846104]

Curative Treatment

Most patients with early breast cancer can be cured. Treatment with a curative intent is advised for clinical stage I, II, and III disease (see Table 39–2). Patients with locally advanced (T3, T4) and even inflammatory tumors may be cured with multimodality therapy. When distant metastatic disease (outside the breast or regional lymph nodes) is diagnosed, palliation becomes the goal of therapy. Treatment with palliative intent is appropriate for all patients with stage IV disease and for patients with unresectable local cancers.

A. Choice and Timing of Primary Therapy

The extent of disease and its biologic aggressiveness are the principal determinants of the outcome of primary therapy. Clinical and pathologic staging help in assessing extent of disease (see Table 17–3), but each is imprecise. Other factors such as tumor grade, hormone receptor assays, *HER2* amplification, and genomic assays are of prognostic and predictive value for benefits from systemic therapy but are not as relevant in determining the type of local therapy. In contrast, the presence of a germline deleterious mutation in *BRCA1* or *BRCA2* may have implications for both local and systemic therapy options; thus, genetic testing of patients with newly diagnosed breast cancer should be considered.

Controversy has surrounded the choice of primary therapy of stage I, II, and III breast carcinoma. Traditionally, the standard of care for stage I, stage II, and most stage III cancer has been surgical resection followed by adjuvant (postoperative) radiation or systemic therapy, or both, when indicated. Administering chemotherapy before surgery (in the neoadjuvant setting) may shrink large tumors, making some patients who require mastectomy candidates for lumpectomy. In addition, the response to neoadjuvant therapy may determine the need for additional postoperative systemic therapy, which may result in improved survival for some tumor types. It is important for patients to understand all the surgical options, including reconstructive options, prior to having surgery. Patients with large primary tumors, inflammatory cancer, or palpably enlarged lymph nodes should have staging scans performed to rule out distant metastatic disease prior to definitive surgery. In general, adjuvant systemic therapy is started when the breast has adequately healed, ideally within 4–8 weeks after surgery. While no prospective studies have defined the appropriate timing of adjuvant chemotherapy, a single-institution study of over 6800 patients suggests that *systemic therapy should be started within 60 days of surgery,* especially in women with stage II or III breast cancer, triple-negative breast cancer, or HER2-positive disease.

B. Surgical Resection

1. Breast-conserving therapy—Multiple, large, randomized studies including the Milan and NSABP trials show that disease-free and overall survival rates are similar for patients with stage I and stage II breast cancer treated with partial mastectomy (breast-conserving lumpectomy or "breast conservation") plus axillary dissection followed by radiation therapy and for those treated by modified radical mastectomy (total mastectomy plus axillary dissection).

Tumor size is a major consideration in determining the feasibility of breast conservation. The NSABP lumpectomy trial randomized patients with tumors as large as 4 cm. To achieve an acceptable cosmetic result, the patient must have a breast of sufficient size to enable excision of a 4-cm tumor without considerable deformity. Therefore, large tumor size is only a relative contraindication. Subareolar tumors, also difficult to excise without deformity, are not contraindications to breast conservation. Oncoplastic techniques combining principles of plastic and reconstructive surgery with surgical oncologic principles are enabling resection of large tumors with excellent cosmetic results. Clinically detectable multifocality is a relative contraindication to breast-conserving surgery, as is fixation to the chest wall or skin or involvement of the nipple or overlying skin.

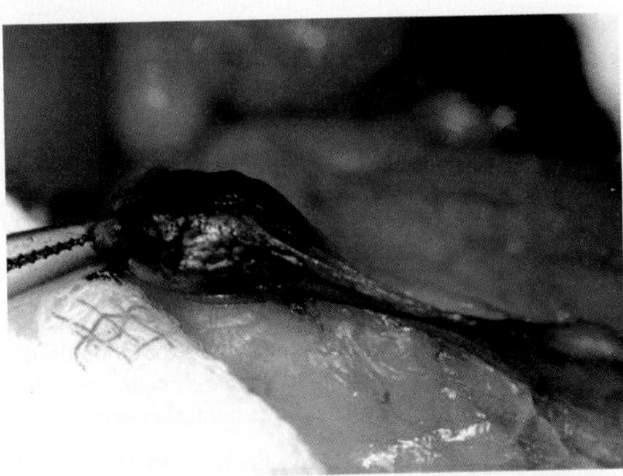

▲ **Figure 17–6.** Sentinel node. (Used, with permission, from Armando E. Giuliano, MD.)

The patient—not the surgeon—should be the judge of what is cosmetically acceptable. Given the relatively high risk of poor outcome after radiation, concomitant systemic sclerosis (scleroderma) is a contraindication to breast-conserving surgery. A history of prior therapeutic radiation to the ipsilateral breast or chest wall (or both) is also generally a contraindication for breast conservation, although accelerated partial breast irradiation may permit a second breast irradiation.

Axillary dissection is primarily used to properly stage cancer and plan radiation and systemic therapy. Intraoperative lymphatic mapping and sentinel node biopsy identify lymph nodes most likely to harbor metastases if present (Figure 17–6). **Sentinel node biopsy** is a proven alternative to axillary dissection in patients without clinical evidence of axillary lymph node metastases. If sentinel node biopsy reveals no evidence of axillary metastases, it is highly likely that the remaining lymph nodes are free of disease and axillary dissection may be omitted. An important study from the American College of Surgeons Oncology Group randomized women with sentinel node metastases to undergo completion of axillary dissection or to receive no further axillary-specific treatment after lumpectomy; no difference in 10-year survival was found. *Omission of axillary dissection is acceptable for women with tumor-free sentinel nodes or those with involvement of one or two sentinel nodes who are treated with lumpectomy, whole breast irradiation, and adjuvant systemic therapy.*

Breast-conserving surgery with sentinel node biopsy and radiation is the preferred form of treatment for patients with early-stage breast cancer. Despite the numerous randomized trials showing no survival benefit of mastectomy over breast-conserving partial mastectomy with irradiation or of axillary dissection over sentinel node biopsy, these conservative procedures still appear to be underutilized.

2. Mastectomy—Modified radical mastectomy was previously the standard therapy for most patients with early-stage breast cancer. This operation removes the entire breast, overlying skin, nipple, and areolar complex usually with underlying pectoralis fascia with the axillary lymph nodes in continuity. The major advantage of modified radical mastectomy is that radiation therapy may not be necessary, although radiation may be used when lymph nodes are involved with cancer or when the primary tumor is 5 cm or larger. The disadvantage of mastectomy is the cosmetic and psychological impact associated with breast loss. Radical mastectomy, which removes the underlying pectoralis muscle, should be performed rarely, if at all. Axillary node dissection is not indicated for noninvasive cancers because nodal metastases are rarely present. Skin-sparing mastectomies, including those with preservation of the nipple-areolar complex, provide excellent cosmetic and oncologic results; skin-sparing and nipple-sparing mastectomy, however, is not appropriate for all patients. Breast reconstruction, immediate or delayed, should be discussed with patients who choose or require mastectomy. Patients should have an interview with a reconstructive plastic surgeon to discuss options prior to making a decision regarding reconstruction. Time is well spent preoperatively in educating the patient and family about these matters.

C. Radiotherapy

Radiotherapy after breast-conserving surgery consists of 5–7 weeks of radiation for a total dose of 5000–6000 cGy. Most radiation oncologists use a boost dose to the cancer location. Shorter fractionation schedules may be reasonable for women with low-risk, early-stage breast cancer. Guidelines by the American Society of Radiation Oncology and the European Society for Radiotherapy indicate that it is appropriate to discuss partial breast radiation for women over the age of 50 with node-negative, hormone receptor–positive, small (T1) tumors with surgical margins of at least 2 mm. Moreover, in women over the age of 70 with small (less than 2 cm), lymph node–negative, hormone receptor–positive cancers, radiation therapy may be avoided. The recurrence rates after intraoperative radiation, while low, appear significantly higher than postoperative whole breast radiation therapy. However, in all these situations, a balanced discussion with a radiation oncologist to weigh the risks and benefits of each approach is warranted.

Studies suggest that radiotherapy after mastectomy may improve recurrence rates and survival in younger patients and those with tumors 5 cm or larger or positive lymph nodes.

Giuliano AE et al. Locoregional recurrence after sentinel lymph node dissection with or without axillary dissection in patients with sentinel lymph node metastases: long-term follow-up from the American College of Surgeons Oncology Group (Alliance) ACOSOG Z0011 Randomized Trial. Ann Surg. 2016;264:413. [PMID: 27513155]

Giuliano AE. The evolution of sentinel node biopsy for breast cancer: personal experience. Breast J. 2020;26:17. [PMID: 31876042]

Korde LA et al. Neoadjuvant chemotherapy, endocrine therapy and targeted therapy for breast cancer: ASCO Guideline. J Clin Oncol. 2021;39:1485. [PMID: 33507815]

Murphy BM et al. Surgical management of axilla following neoadjuvant endocrine therapy. Ann Surg Oncol. 2021;28:8729. [PMID: 34275042]

Vicini FA et al. Long-term primary results of accelerated partial breast irradiation after breast-conserving surgery for early-stage breast cancer: a randomised, phase 3, equivalence trial. Lancet. 2019;394:2155. [PMID: 31813636]

D. Adjuvant Systemic Therapy

Systemic therapy improves survival and is advocated for most patients with curable breast cancer. In practice, most medical oncologists use chemotherapy for patients with either node-positive or higher-risk (eg, hormone receptor–negative or HER2-positive) node-negative breast cancer and use endocrine therapy for all hormone receptor–positive invasive breast cancer unless contraindicated. Prognostic factors other than nodal status that are used to determine the patient's risks of recurrence are tumor size, ER and PR status, nuclear grade, histologic type, proliferative rate (Ki-67), oncogene expression (Table 17–5), and patient's age and menopausal status. In general, systemic chemotherapy decreases the chance of recurrence by about 30%, hormonal modulation decreases the relative risk of recurrence by 40–50% (for hormone receptor–positive cancer), HER2-targeted therapy decreases the relative risk of recurrence by approximately 40% (for HER2-positive cancer). Systemic chemotherapy is usually given sequentially, rather than concurrently, with radiation. In terms of sequencing, typically chemotherapy is given before radiation and endocrine therapy is started concurrent with or after radiation therapy. Three additional agents became available in 2021 for use in the curative setting for patients with high-risk breast cancer: olaparib, a poly(adenosine diphosphate-ribose) polymerase inhibitor that was shown to reduce the relative risk of an invasive recurrency for *BRCA1/2* carriers with high-risk disease by just over 40%; abemaciclib, a cyclin dependent kinase 4/6 inhibitor shown to improve the invasive disease-free survival for those with high-risk HR-positive disease by approximately 30%; and pembrolizumab, an immune checkpoint inhibitor shown to improve the event-free survival for patients with stage II or greater triple-negative breast cancer by over 35%.

The long-term advantage of systemic therapy is well established. All patients with invasive hormone receptor–positive tumors should consider the use of hormone-modulating therapy. Almost all patients with HER2-positive tumors should receive trastuzumab-containing chemotherapy regimens. In general, adjuvant systemic chemotherapy should not be given to women who have small node-negative breast cancers with favorable histologic findings and tumor biomarkers. The ability to predict more accurately which patients with HER2-negative, hormone receptor–positive, lymph node–negative tumors should receive chemotherapy has improved with the advent of prognostic tools, such as Oncotype DX and MammaPrint (see Biomarkers and Gene Expression Profiling above). These validated tools enable clinicians to better select patients who can safely omit chemotherapy.

Table 17–5. Prognostic factors for recurrence in node-negative breast cancer.

Prognostic Factors	Increased Recurrence	Decreased Recurrence
Size[1]	T3, T2	T1, T0
Hormone receptors (ER, PR)	Negative	Positive
Histologic grade	High	Low
S phase fraction	> 5%	< 5%
Lymphatic or vascular invasion	Present	Absent
HER2 oncogene amplification	High	Low
Epidermal growth factor receptor	High	Low
High Oncotype DX Recurrence Score or other genomic prognostic assays	High score	Low score

ER, estrogen receptor; PR, progesterone receptor.
[1]See Table 17–3 for TNM staging for breast cancer.

1. Chemotherapy—The Early Breast Cancer Trialists' Collaborative Group (EBCTCG) meta-analysis involving over 28,000 women enrolled in 60 trials of adjuvant polychemotherapy versus no chemotherapy demonstrated a significant beneficial impact of chemotherapy on clinical outcome in non–stage IV breast cancer. This study showed that *adjuvant chemotherapy reduces the risk of recurrence and breast cancer–specific mortality in all women and women under the age of 50 derived the greatest benefit.*

A. ANTHRACYCLINE- AND CYCLOPHOSPHAMIDE-CONTAINING REGIMENS—On the basis of the superiority of anthracycline-containing regimens in metastatic breast cancer, both doxorubicin and epirubicin have been studied extensively in the adjuvant setting. Studies comparing Adriamycin (doxorubicin) and cyclophosphamide (AC) or epirubicin and cyclophosphamide (EC) to cyclophosphamide-methotrexate-5-fluorouracil (CMF) have shown that treatments with anthracycline-containing regimens are at least as effective as treatment with CMF. Retrospective analyses of several studies suggest that anthracyclines may be primarily effective in tumors with HER2 overexpression or alteration in the expression of topoisomerase IIa (the target of anthracyclines and close to the *HER2* gene). Given this, for HER2-negative, node-negative breast cancer, four cycles of AC or six cycles of CMF are probably equally effective.

B. TAXANES—Multiple trials of taxanes (paclitaxel and docetaxel) have been conducted to evaluate their use in combination with anthracycline-based regimens. The majority of these trials showed an improvement in disease-free survival and at least one showed an improvement in overall survival with the taxane-based regimen. A meta-analysis of taxane versus non-taxane anthracycline-based regimen trials showed an improvement in disease-free and overall survival for the taxane-based regimens. Several regimens have been reported including AC followed by paclitaxel (AC-P) or docetaxel (Taxotere) (AC-T), docetaxel concurrent with AC (TAC), 5-fluorouracil-epirubicin-cyclophosphamide (FEC)-docetaxel, and FEC-paclitaxel.

While it is generally agreed that *taxanes should be used for most patients receiving chemotherapy for early breast cancer, data are mounting against the routine use of anthracyclines for HR-positive or HER2-positive disease.* A balanced discussion regarding the potential risks versus benefits of the addition of anthracyclines is warranted, especially in hormone receptor–positive or HER2-positive disease.

C. Duration and dose of chemotherapy—The ideal duration of adjuvant chemotherapy remains uncertain. However, based on the meta-analysis performed in the Oxford Overview (EBCTCG), the current recommendation is for 3–6 months of the commonly used regimens. Data suggest that the timing and sequencing of anthracycline-taxane–based chemotherapy may be important. Multiple trials beginning in the 1980s sought to demonstrate whether dose-intensification of adjuvant chemotherapy by shortening the intervals between cycles ("dose-dense"), or by giving chemotherapy at full dose sequentially rather than concurrently at reduced doses is associated with better outcomes. The EBCTCG meta-analysis included 37,298 patients treated on 26 trials and showed a significant 3.4% absolute decrease and 14% relative risk reduction in breast cancer recurrences with dose-intensification. Moreover, the absolute 10-year breast cancer mortality was improved by 2.4%. While impressive, the benefit of dose-intensification appeared to be strongest in node-positive disease. Its benefit, if any, in HER2-positive disease in the era of HER2-targeted therapy has not been validated. Additionally, the use of dose-intensification in (non-anthracycline) taxane-based regimens has not been evaluated.

D. Chemotherapy side effects—Chemotherapy side effects, which are discussed in Chapter 39, are generally well controlled.

2. Targeted therapy—Targeted therapy refers to agents that are directed specifically against a protein or molecule expressed uniquely on tumor cells or in the tumor microenvironment.

A. HER2 targeted therapy—Approximately 20% of breast cancers are characterized by amplification of the *HER2* oncogene leading to overexpression of the HER2 oncoprotein. The poor prognosis associated with HER2 overexpression has been drastically improved with the development of HER2-targeted therapy. Trastuzumab (Herceptin [H]), a monoclonal antibody that binds to HER2, is effective in combination with chemotherapy (AC-TH or TCH [docetaxel, carboplatin, trastuzumab]) in patients with HER2-overexpressing early breast cancer. Both AC-TH and TCH are FDA-approved for nonmetastatic, HER2-positive breast cancer. In these regimens, trastuzumab is given with chemotherapy and then continued beyond the course of chemotherapy with a goal, in general, to complete a full year. Neoadjuvant chemotherapy plus dual *HER2*-targeted therapy with trastuzumab and pertuzumab (also a HER2-targeted monoclonal antibody that prevents dimerization of HER2 with HER3 and has been shown to be synergistic in combination with trastuzumab) is a standard of care option available to patients with stage II/III HER2-positive breast cancer (see Neoadjuvant Therapy). Adjuvant trastuzumab with pertuzumab is primarily restricted to patients with high-risk, node-positive disease. Neratinib, an orally bioavailable dual HER1 (EGFR), HER2 tyrosine kinase inhibitor, is FDA-approved as extended adjuvant therapy (to be given after completion of 1 year of trastuzumab). The phase 3 placebo-controlled EXTENET study demonstrated that neratinib improves invasive disease-free survival when given for 1 year after completion of a year of standard adjuvant trastuzumab-based therapy (median follow-up 5.2 years, stratified HR 0.73, $P = 0.0083$). The benefit of neratinib appears to be restricted to those with tumor co-expression of ER, PR, or both. Neratinib is associated with GI toxicity, most notably moderate to severe diarrhea in approximately 40% of patients who did not use antidiarrheal prophylaxis. Measures such as starting at a lower dose of neratinib and escalating as tolerated or using prophylactic colestipol or budesonide have been shown to mitigate this side effect.

Patients who undergo neoadjuvant trastuzumab-based chemotherapy and have residual disease remaining at the time of surgery have a comparatively poor outcome compared to those who achieve a pathologic complete response. In the phase 3 randomized KATHERINE trial, 1486 patients with residual disease after standard neoadjuvant trastuzumab/taxane-based therapy (18% of whom also received neoadjuvant pertuzumab) were randomized to receive the antibody-drug conjugate trastuzumab emtansine or standard trastuzumab for 14 cycles after surgery. Patients treated with trastuzumab emtansine had a statistically significantly improved 3-year invasive disease-free survival (88% vs 77%), associated with a 50% relative risk reduction. Adjuvant trastuzumab emtansine is FDA-approved for patients with residual disease after standard trastuzumab-containing neoadjuvant therapy.

Retrospective studies have shown that even small (stage T1a,b) *HER2*-positive tumors have a worse prognosis compared with same-sized *HER2*-negative tumors and may thus be appropriate for trastuzumab-based regimens.

Cardiomyopathy develops in a small but significant percentage (0.4–4%) of patients who receive trastuzumab-based regimens. For this reason, anthracyclines and trastuzumab should not be given concurrently and cardiac function is monitored periodically throughout HER2-targeted therapy.

B. Endocrine therapy—Adjuvant hormone modulation therapy is highly effective in decreasing relative risk of recurrence by 40–50% and mortality by 25% in women with hormone receptor–positive tumors regardless of menopausal status.

(1) Tamoxifen—The traditional 5-year regimen of adjuvant estrogen-receptor antagonist/agonist tamoxifen was compared to a 10-year regimen in the Adjuvant Tamoxifen Longer Against Shorter (ATLAS) trial. Disease-free and overall survival were significantly improved in women who received 10 years of tamoxifen, particularly after year 10. Though these results are impressive, the clinical application of long-term tamoxifen use must be discussed with patients individually, taking into consideration risks of tamoxifen (such as secondary uterine cancers, venous thromboembolic events, and side effects that impact quality of life). Ovarian suppression in addition to tamoxifen has been shown to significantly improve 8-year disease-free survival (83.2% vs 78.9%) and 8-year overall survival (93.3% vs 91.5%) compared to tamoxifen alone in the randomized Suppression of Ovarian Function Trial (SOFT) study, though the benefits appeared to be seen primarily in chemotherapy-treated patients with higher risk disease.

(2) Aromatase inhibitors for postmenopausal women—AIs, including anastrozole, letrozole, and exemestane, reduce estrogen production and are also effective in the adjuvant setting for postmenopausal women. At least seven large randomized trials enrolling more than 24,000 postmenopausal patients with hormone receptor–positive nonmetastatic breast cancer have compared the use of AIs with tamoxifen or placebo as adjuvant therapy. All these studies have shown small but statistically significant improvements in disease-free survival (absolute benefits of 2–6%) with the use of AIs. In addition, AIs have been shown to reduce the risk of contralateral breast cancers and to have fewer associated serious side effects (such as endometrial cancers and thromboembolic events) than tamoxifen. However, they are associated with accelerated bone loss and an increased risk of fractures as well as a musculoskeletal syndrome characterized by arthralgias or myalgias (or both) in the majority of patients. The ASCO and the NCCN have recommended that *postmenopausal women with hormone receptor–positive breast cancer be offered an AI either initially or after tamoxifen therapy.* HER2 status should not affect the use or choice of hormone therapy. In general, AIs are given for 5 years. However, a number of studies are evaluating extended adjuvant therapy for 7–10 years total. The use of extended adjuvant AIs is reserved for high-risk patients after a balanced discussion regarding potential risks versus benefits.

(3) Aromatase inhibitors for premenopausal women—*AIs should not be used in a patient with functioning (premenopausal) ovaries since they do not block ovarian production of estrogen.* However, a combined analysis of the SOFT and Tamoxifen and Exemestane Trial (TEXT) studies showed for the first time that exemestane plus ovarian suppression with triptorelin was associated with a reduced risk of relapse compared to tamoxifen, making this a viable adjuvant therapy option for *premenopausal* women with high-risk ER-positive breast cancers.

C. Bisphosphonates and other bone-modifying agents—Multiple randomized studies have evaluated the use of adjuvant bisphosphonates in addition to standard local and systemic therapy for early-stage breast cancer and have shown, in addition to improvement in bone density, a consistent reduction in the risk of metastatic recurrence in postmenopausal patients. A meta-analysis evaluating more than 18,000 women with early-stage breast cancer treated with bisphosphonates or placebo showed that bisphosphonates reduce the risk of cancer recurrence (especially in bone) and improve breast cancer–specific survival primarily in postmenopausal women. Side effects associated with bisphosphonate therapy include bone pain, fever, osteonecrosis of the jaw (rare, less than 1%), esophagitis or ulcers (for oral bisphosphonates), and kidney injury. The jointly published guidelines of the Cancer Care Ontario and ASCO recommend that bisphosphonate use (zoledronic acid or clodronate) be considered in the adjuvant therapy plan for postmenopausal breast cancer patients. In addition, denosumab, an antibody directed against receptor activator of nuclear factor kappa B ligand (RANK-L), blocks osteoclastic activity. It was evaluated in two phase 3 adjuvant trials with discordant results: The "D-CARE" study randomized patients with early-stage breast cancer (all biologic subtypes) to receive denosumab or placebo and failed to demonstrate a reduction in breast cancer recurrences or deaths. It is speculated that one possible reason for this negative result may be due to the fact that premenopausal patients (who do not have a demonstrated metastatic recurrence benefit from bisphosphonates) were included in the study. In contrast, the ABCSG-18 trial restricted enrollment to postmenopausal women and did show an improvement in disease-free survival with denosumab.

D. Cyclin dependent kinase 4/6 inhibitors—Hormonally driven breast cancer may be particularly sensitive to inhibition of cell cycle regulatory proteins, called cyclin dependent kinases 4 and 6 (CDK 4/6). Three oral CDK4/6 inhibitors are palbociclib, ribociclib, and abemaciclib. In 2021, the FDA approved adjuvant abemaciclib for patients with HR-positive, HER2-negative, node-positive, high-risk breast cancer with a Ki-67 score of at least 20%. Patients who may be candidates for adjuvant abemaciclib thus need their tumor tested for Ki-67 by an FDA-approved immunohistochemical assay.

E. PARP inhibitors—*BRCA*-mutation–associated cancers are deficient in double-strand DNA repair mechanisms and become reliant on an alternative enzyme, poly (adenosine diphosphate-ribose) polymerase (PARP), for DNA repair and survival. Thus, targeting PARP selectively kills breast cancer cells in patients who carry a germline mutation in *BRCA1* or *BRCA2*. Two PARP inhibitors (olaparib and talazoparib) are FDA-approved for the treatment of *BRCA*-associated metastatic breast cancer. The NCCN guidelines include adjuvant olaparib for select patients and recommend germline genetic testing for any patient who may be a candidate for adjuvant olaparib.

While olaparib should be given in combination with standard adjuvant endocrine therapy for HR-positive disease, the use of olaparib in combination with abemaciclib (see above) has not been studied and is not recommended. Thus, if a patient is a candidate for both agents, decisions regarding which agent to use must be made on a case-by-case basis in discussion with the patient. The use of olaparib has also not been studied in combination with capecitabine (see CREATE-X trial below), thus, there are no data to guide selection between these agents in triple-negative *BRCA*-mutation–associated breast cancer with residual disease after neoadjuvant chemotherapy.

3. Adjuvant therapy in older women—Data relating to the optimal use of adjuvant systemic treatment for women over the age of 65 are limited. Results from the EBCTCG overview indicate that while adjuvant chemotherapy yields a smaller benefit for older women compared with younger women, it still improves clinical outcomes. Moreover, individual studies do show that older women with higher risk disease derive benefits from chemotherapy. One study compared the use of oral chemotherapy (capecitabine) to standard chemotherapy in older women and concluded that standard chemotherapy is preferred. Another study (USO TC vs AC) showed that women over the age of 65 derive similar benefits from the taxane-based regimen as women who are younger. The benefits of endocrine therapy for hormone receptor–positive disease appear to be independent of age. In general, decisions relating to the use of systemic therapy should take into account a patient's comorbidities and physiological age, more so than chronologic age.

E. Neoadjuvant Therapy

The use of systemic therapy prior to resection of the primary tumor (neoadjuvant) is a standard option that should be considered and discussed with patients. This enables the assessment of sensitivity of the tumor to the selected systemic therapy. Patients with hormone receptor–negative, triple-negative, or HER2-positive breast cancer are more likely to have a pathologic complete response (meaning no residual invasive cancer in the breast and sampled nodes at the time of surgery) to neoadjuvant chemotherapy than those with hormone receptor–positive breast cancer. A pathologic complete response at the time of surgery, especially in hormone receptor–negative tumors, is associated with improvement in event-free and overall survival. Neoadjuvant chemotherapy also increases the chance of breast conservation by shrinking the primary tumor in women who would otherwise need mastectomy for local control. Survival after neoadjuvant chemotherapy is similar to that seen with postoperative adjuvant chemotherapy.

1. HER2-positive breast cancer—Dual targeting of HER2 with two monoclonal antibodies, trastuzumab and pertuzumab, showed positive results in two phase 2 clinical trials in the neoadjuvant setting, the TRYPHAENA and the NEOSPHERE studies.

Based on these clinical trials, three regimens are FDA-approved in the HER2-positive neoadjuvant setting: docetaxel (T), cyclophosphamide I, trastuzumab (H), and pertuzumab (P) (TCHP) for six cycles; FEC for three cycles followed by THP for three cycles; or THP for four cycles (followed by three cycles of postoperative FEC). The randomized TRAIN-2 trial compared nine cycles of non-anthracycline, TCHP-type therapy versus FEC-TCHP and demonstrated no improvement in pathologic complete response or event-free survival with the use of anthracycline, thus providing further support for the use of a non-anthracycline regimen for HER2-positive disease. After completing surgery, patients should resume HER2-targeted therapy. If there is residual disease, the standard of care is to give 14 cycles of trastuzumab emtansine based on the KATHERINE trial that showed a significantly improved invasive disease-free survival for patients who received trastuzumab emtansine if they had a non-pathologic complete response to neoadjuvant treatment. In the case of pathologic complete response, trastuzumab with (ie, if node-positive) or without pertuzumab is given to complete 1 year of total therapy with consideration for the use of neratinib as extended adjuvant therapy for high-risk (lymph node–positive, hormone receptor–positive) disease.

2. Hormone receptor–positive, HER2-negative breast cancer—Patients with hormone receptor–positive breast cancer have a lower chance of achieving a pathologic complete response with neoadjuvant therapy than those patients with triple-negative or HER2-positive breast cancers. Studies indicate similar clinical response rates with neoadjuvant endocrine therapy compared to neoadjuvant chemotherapy. Typically, responses are not appreciated unless 4–6 or more months of therapy are given. Outside of the clinical trial setting, the use of neoadjuvant hormonal therapy is generally restricted to postmenopausal patients who are unable or unwilling to tolerate chemotherapy.

3. Triple-negative breast cancer—Recent studies have showed that targeted therapy demonstrated meaningful improvements in long-term outcomes for patients with curable breast cancer that is lacking in *HER2* amplification or hormone receptor expression. A meta-analysis of nine randomized trials including over 2100 patients and a median follow-up of 47–67 months demonstrated not only an improved pathologic complete response rate with the addition of platinum to chemotherapy but also a significantly improved event-free survival and a trend toward improved overall survival.

The anti-PD-1 immune checkpoint inhibitor pembrolizumab was FDA-approved in 2021 for treatment of triple-negative breast cancer in the neoadjuvant setting in combination with chemotherapy, followed by adjuvant pembrolizumab to complete a year. Patients treated with neoadjuvant or adjuvant pembrolizumab should receive it in combination with the taxane, platinum, anthracycline–based regimen. It is not clear whether use of pembrolizumab solely in the adjuvant setting (without use in neoadjuvant setting) benefits patients; thus, it is not recommended.

Questions remain regarding optimal adjuvant treatment of patients with residual disease after neoadjuvant therapy. A standard option based on the CREATE-X study is to use eight cycles of adjuvant capecitabine after neoadjuvant therapy. It is not known whether adding capecitabine to adjuvant pembrolizumab benefits patients who have received neoadjuvant pembrolizumab plus chemotherapy and have residual disease at the time of definitive breast surgery; the combined use of these two agents is not the standard of care. For patients with a *BRCA1* or *BRCA2* mutation and residual triple-negative breast cancer at the time of definitive breast surgery, the use of adjuvant olaparib is an option. However, the combination or sequencing of olaparib and pembrolizumab is untested in this setting.

4. Timing of sentinel lymph node biopsy in neoadjuvant setting—There is considerable concern about the timing of sentinel lymph node biopsy, since the chemotherapy may affect cancer present in the lymph nodes. Several studies have shown that sentinel node biopsy can be done after neoadjuvant therapy. However, a large multicenter study, ACOSOG 1071, demonstrated a false-negative rate of 10.7% when the sentinel lymph node biopsy was performed after neoadjuvant therapy, while the false-negative rate before neoadjuvant therapy is less than 1–5%. The SENTINA trial showed similarly poor results for sentinel node biopsy after neoadjuvant therapy. The false-negative rate falls to an acceptable level if three nodes are removed and isotope and dye are used. Some physicians recommend performing sentinel lymph node biopsy before administering the chemotherapy in order to avoid a false-negative result and to aid in planning subsequent radiation therapy. Others prefer to perform sentinel lymph node biopsy after neoadjuvant therapy to avoid a second operation and assess post-chemotherapy nodal status. An effective approach for sentinel node biopsy for patients who had involved nodes pre-chemotherapy is to place a clip in the positive node and be sure to excise it at the time of sentinel node biopsy. Important questions remain to be answered involving the use of neoadjuvant therapy, including which neoadjuvant agents to use, duration of treatment, and additional postoperative therapy.

Burstein HJ et al. Adjuvant endocrine therapy for women with hormone receptor-positive breast cancer: ASCO Clinical Practice Guideline Focused Update. J Clin Oncol. 2019;37:423. [PMID: 30452337]

Denduluri N et al. Selection of optimal adjuvant chemotherapy and targeted therapy for early breast cancer: ASCO guideline update. J Clin Oncol. 2021;39:685. [PMID: 33079579]

Gnant M et al. Adjuvant palbociclib for early breast cancer: the PALLAS trial results (ABCSG-42/AFT-05/BIG-14-03). J Clin Oncol. 2022;40:282. [PMID: 34874182]

Gnant M et al; Austrian Breast and Colorectal Cancer Study Group. Duration of adjuvant aromatase-inhibitor therapy in postmenopausal breast cancer. N Engl J Med. 2021;385:495. [PMID: 34320285]

Hurvitz SA et al. Anthracycline use in *ERBB2*-positive breast cancer: it is time to re-TRAIN. JAMA Oncol. 2021;7:975. [PMID: 34014297]

Hurvitz SA et al. A careful reassessment of anthracycline use in curable breast cancer. NPJ Breast Cancer. 2021;7:134. [PMID: 34625570]

Poggio F et al. Adding a platinum agent to neoadjuvant chemotherapy for triple negative breast cancer: the end of the debate. Ann Oncol. 2022;33:347. [PMID: 34861375]

Schmid P et al; KEYNOTE-522 Investigators. Pembrolizumab for early triple-negative breast cancer. N Engl J Med. 2020; 382:810. [PMID: 32101663]

Tutt ANJ et al; OlympiA Clinical Trial Steering Committee and Investigators. Adjuvant olaparib for patients with *BRCA1*- or *BRCA2*-mutated breast cancer. N Engl J Med. 2021;384:2394. [PMID: 34081848]

Van der Voort A et al. Three-year follow up of neoadjuvant chemotherapy with or without anthracyclines in the presence of dual *ERBB2* blockade in patients with *ERBB2*-positive breast cancer: a secondary analysis of the TRAIN-2 randomized, phase 3 trial. JAMA Oncol. 2021;7:978. [PMID: 34014249]

von Minckwitz G et al; KATHERINE Investigators. Trastuzumab emtansine for residual invasive HER2-positive breast cancer. N Engl J Med. 2019;380:617. [PMID: 30516102]

Palliative Treatment

Palliative treatments are aimed to manage symptoms, improve quality of life, and even prolong survival, without the expectation of achieving cure. Even when cure of the disease is not expected, palliative treatments are appropriate for breast cancer metastatic to distant sites. In the United States, it is uncommon to have distant metastases at the time of diagnosis (de novo metastases). However, most patients who have a breast cancer recurrence after initial local and adjuvant therapy have metastatic rather than local (in breast) disease. Breast cancer most commonly metastasizes to the liver, lungs, and bone, causing symptoms such as fatigue, change in appetite, abdominal pain, cough, dyspnea, or bone pain. Headaches, imbalance, vision changes, vertigo, and other neurologic symptoms may be signs of brain metastases. Triple-negative (ER-, PR-, HER2-negative) and HER2-positive tumors have a higher rate of brain metastases than hormone receptor–positive, HER2-negative tumors.

A. Radiotherapy and Bisphosphonates

Palliative radiotherapy may be advised for primary treatment of locally advanced cancers with distant metastases to control ulceration, pain, and other manifestations in the breast and regional nodes. Irradiation of the breast and chest wall and the axillary, internal mammary, and supraclavicular nodes should be undertaken in an attempt to cure locally advanced and inoperable lesions when there is no evidence of distant metastases. A small number of patients in this group are cured in spite of extensive breast and regional node involvement.

Palliative irradiation is of value also in the treatment of certain bone or soft tissue metastases to control pain or avoid fracture. Radiotherapy is especially useful in the treatment of isolated bony metastases, chest wall recurrences, and brain metastases and, sometimes, in lieu of the preferred option of orthopedic surgery for acute spinal cord compression.

In addition to radiotherapy, bisphosphonate therapy has shown excellent results in delaying and reducing skeletal events in women with bony metastases. Pamidronate and zoledronic acid are FDA-approved intravenous bisphosphonates given for bone metastases or hypercalcemia of malignancy from breast cancer. Denosumab is FDA-approved for the treatment of bone metastases from breast cancer, with data showing that it reduced the time to first skeletal-related event (eg, pathologic fracture) compared to zoledronic acid.

Caution should be exercised when combining radiation therapy with chemotherapy because toxicity of either or both may be augmented by their concurrent administration. In general, *only one type of therapy should be given at a time* unless it is necessary to irradiate a destructive lesion of weight-bearing bone while the patient is receiving chemotherapy. Systemic therapy should be changed only if the disease is clearly progressing or if intolerable side effects have developed. This is especially difficult to determine for patients with destructive bone metastases, since changes in the status of these lesions are difficult to determine radiographically.

B. Targeted Therapy

1. Hormonally based therapy for metastatic disease— The following therapies have all been shown to be effective in hormone receptor–positive metastatic breast cancer: administration of medications that block or downregulate ERs (such as tamoxifen or fulvestrant, respectively) or medications that block the synthesis of hormones (such as AIs); ablation of the ovaries, adrenal, or pituitary glands; and the administration of hormones (eg, estrogens, androgens, progestins); see Table 17–6. Because only 5–10% of

Table 17–6. Hormonally targeted agents commonly used for management of metastatic breast cancer (listed in alphabetical order).

Medications	Action	Dose, Route, Frequency	Major Side Effects
Anastrozole (Arimidex)	AI	1 mg orally daily	Hot flushes, skin rashes, nausea and vomiting, bone loss
Exemestane (Aromasin)	AI	25 mg orally daily	Hot flushes, increased arthralgia/arthritis, myalgia, bone loss
Fulvestrant (Faslodex)	Steroidal estrogen receptor antagonist	500 mg intramuscularly days 1, 15, 29 and then monthly	GI upset, headache, back pain, hot flushes, pharyngitis, injection site pain
Goserelin (Zoladex)	Synthetic LH-releasing analog	3.6 mg subcutaneously monthly	Arthralgias, blood pressure changes, hot flushes, headaches, vaginal dryness, bone loss
Letrozole (Femara)	AI	2.5 mg orally daily	Hot flushes, arthralgia/arthritis, myalgia, bone loss
Leuprolid (Lupron)	Synthetic LH-releasing analog	3.75 or 7.5 mg subcutaneously monthly	Arthralgias, blood pressure changes, hot flushes, headaches, vaginal dryness, bone loss
Megestrol acetate (Megace)	Progestin	40 mg orally four times daily	Fluid retention, venous thromboembolic events; rarely used except in late stage, treatment-refractory disease
Tamoxifen citrate (Nolvadex)	SERM	20 mg orally daily	Hot flushes, uterine bleeding, thrombophlebitis, rash
Toremifene citrate (Fareston)	SERM	60 mg orally daily	Hot flushes, sweating, nausea, vaginal discharge, dry eyes, dizziness

AI, aromatase inhibitor; SERM, selective estrogen receptor modulator.

women with ER-negative tumors respond, they should not receive endocrine therapy. Women within 1 year of their last menstrual period are arbitrarily considered to be premenopausal and should have surgical (bilateral oophorectomy) or chemical ovarian ablation (using a gonadotropin-releasing hormone [GnRH] analog such as leuprolide [Lupron], goserelin [Zoladex], or triptorelin). Premenopausal women who have had chemical or surgical ovarian ablation are then eligible to receive the same hormonally targeted therapies that are available to postmenopausal women. Guidelines indicate that sequential hormonal therapy (Table 17–6) is the preferred treatment for hormone receptor–positive metastatic breast cancer except in the rare case when disease is immediately threatening visceral organs.

A. First-line treatment options—

(1) Hormonally targeted agents—Single-agent hormonally targeted therapy options include the pure ER degrader/antagonist fulvestrant (500 mg intramuscularly days 1 and 15, then every month), tamoxifen (20 mg orally daily), or an AI (anastrozole, letrozole, or exemestane; all oral daily). The average time to disease progression associated with single-agent first-line tamoxifen is 5–8 months and with AI is approximately 8–12 months. The side effect profile of AIs differs from tamoxifen. The main side effects of tamoxifen are nausea, skin rash, and hot flushes. Rarely, tamoxifen induces hypercalcemia in patients with bony metastases. Tamoxifen also increases the risk of venous thromboembolic events and uterine hyperplasia and cancer. The main side effects of AIs include hot flushes, vaginal dryness, and joint stiffness; however, osteoporosis and bone fractures are significantly higher than with tamoxifen. Results from the phase 3 FALCON study (comparing first-line treatment with fulvestrant to anastrozole) showed that the use of first-line fulvestrant significantly improves progression-free survival by almost 3 months with the largest treatment effect observed in patients without visceral disease.

(2) Hormonally targeted therapy plus cyclin dependent kinase inhibition—Hormonally driven breast cancer is particularly sensitive to inhibition of cell cycle regulatory proteins, called cyclin dependent kinases 4 and 6 (CDK 4/6). Studies of three CDK4/6 inhibitors (palbociclib 125 mg daily, ribociclib 600 mg daily, and abemaciclib 150 mg twice daily) combined with an endocrine agent (AI or fulvestrant) all demonstrated a median progression-free survival of over 2 years; the longest median progression-free survival reported in metastatic ER-positive breast cancer to date. Similar progression-free survival benefits were achieved with ribociclib in younger women in the phase 3 randomized trial (MONALEESA-7) that exclusively enrolled premenopausal women (treated with goserelin to suppress ovarian function in combination with endocrine therapy). **Collectively, clinical trials support the use of a CDK4/6 inhibitor plus an AI as the gold standard treatment in the first-line setting of hormone-receptor–positive metastatic breast cancer**. Importantly, these therapies yield objective response rates as good as or better than that seen with chemotherapy. All three CDK inhibitors are FDA-approved in the first-line setting in combination with endocrine therapy. Thus far, ribociclib is the only CDK4/6 inhibitor to report an overall survival benefit (in MONALEESA-2, MONALEESA-3, and MONALEESA-7) when added to endocrine therapy in patients

who previously have not received endocrine therapy for metastatic disease (first-line setting). In general, CDK4/6 inhibitors are well tolerated, though monitoring patients for neutropenia (especially with ribociclib and palbociclib) and management of diarrhea (especially with abemaciclib) are necessary. Febrile neutropenia and infections are rare, and use of growth factors is not required; however, palbociclib and ribociclib are given for 3 consecutive weeks, stopping for 1 week to allow white cell count to recover. Abemaciclib is given twice daily continuously (28-day cycles).

B. Treatment options when disease progresses after hormonal-based therapy—

(1) Fulvestrant plus CDK4/6 inhibitor—Palbociclib, ribociclib, and abemaciclib have been evaluated in phase 3 trials (PALOMA-3, MONALEESA-3, MONARCH-2, respectively) in patients whose disease has progressed on prior endocrine therapy. All three have shown a significant improvement in median progression-free survival; ribociclib and abemaciclib have shown a significant improvement in overall survival when added to fulvestrant. Palbociclib, ribociclib, and abemaciclib are FDA-approved in combination with fulvestrant for this indication and are **the gold standard second-line regimen in patients who have not received a CDK4/6 inhibitor in the first-line setting.** Abemaciclib is also FDA-approved as a single agent (200 mg orally twice daily) for patients with advanced ER-positive breast cancer who have received prior endocrine therapy and chemotherapy. At this time, use of any CDK4/6 inhibitor after disease progression on a CDK4/6 inhibitor is not appropriate outside of a clinical trial.

(2) Secondary or tertiary hormonal therapy—Patients who have disease progression following first-line endocrine-based therapy may be offered a different form of endocrine therapy. For example, if a patient has been treated with an AI as first-line therapy, fulvestrant or tamoxifen should be considered at the time of disease progression as second-line therapy.

(3) Everolimus plus endocrine therapy—Everolimus (Afinitor) is an oral inhibitor of the mammalian target of rapamycin (MTOR)—a protein whose activation has been associated with the development of endocrine resistance. A phase 3, placebo-controlled trial (BOLERO-2) evaluated the AI exemestane with or without everolimus in 724 patients with AI-resistant, hormone receptor–positive metastatic breast cancer and found that patients treated with everolimus had a significantly improved progression-free survival (7.8 months vs 3.2 months) but no significant difference in overall survival. Everolimus has also been evaluated in combination with fulvestrant and shown to have similar improvements in progression-free survival compared to single-agent fulvestrant. The main side effect of everolimus is stomatitis (mouth sores). This can be avoided, almost completely, by the prophylactic use of oral steroid mouthwash starting with cycle 1.

(4) Phosphatidylinositol-3-kinase (PI3K) inhibitors plus endocrine therapy—Approximately 40% of hormone receptor–positive breast cancers have activation of the PI3K-AKT-mTOR pathway, most commonly due to an activating mutation of PI3K on the *PIK3CA* gene. Alpelisib is an oral alpha-isoform selective inhibitor of PI3K with clinical activity in *PIK3CA*-mutated breast cancer. Alpelisib is FDA-approved for *PIK3CA*-mutated hormone receptor–positive breast cancer. Side effects of alpelisib include hyperglycemia, diarrhea, rash, and transaminitis.

2. HER2-targeted agents—For patients with HER2-positive tumors, trastuzumab plus chemotherapy significantly improves clinical outcomes, including survival compared to chemotherapy alone. Pertuzumab is an FDA-approved monoclonal antibody that targets the extracellular domain of *HER2* at a different epitope than targeted by trastuzumab and inhibits receptor dimerization. Treatment with the combination of pertuzumab, trastuzumab, and docetaxel imparts a significantly longer progression-free and overall survival compared with treatment with docetaxel and trastuzumab **and is the first-line gold standard for HER2-positive metastatic breast cancer.** Trastuzumab emtansine had been the second-line gold standard for HER2-positive metastatic breast cancer. In 2021, the FDA-approved antibody-drug conjugate, trastuzumab deruxtecan (T-DXd), replaced T-DM1 as the second-line gold standard (after trastuzumab and taxane-based therapy).

In addition to pertuzumab, trastuzumab, trastuzumab emtansine, and trastuzumab deruxtecan, four other HER2-targeted therapies are FDA-approved for patients who have received two or more prior lines of therapy for advanced-stage disease. A novel HER2-selective oral tyrosine kinase inhibitor, tucatinib, penetrates the blood-brain barrier, potentially improving outcomes for those with brain metastases from breast cancer. A large, randomized trial (HER2CLIMB) compared capecitabine plus trastuzumab plus either tucatinib or placebo in patients with pretreated, HER2-positive advanced disease and demonstrated an improved progression-free survival in the overall population, improved progression-free survival in those with CNS metastases, and importantly, a significantly improved overall survival. Other agents are neratinib (in combination with capecitabine), lapatinib (in combination with capecitabine or trastuzumab), and margetuximab, a monoclonal antibody similar to trastuzumab that is designed to improve the antibody-dependent cellular cytotoxicity mechanism of action when used with chemotherapy.

3. Targeting triple-negative breast cancer—Breast cancers lacking expression of the hormone receptors ER and PR and without overexpression of HER2 behave more aggressively and have traditionally been amenable only to therapy with cytotoxic chemotherapy. However, data supporting the use of immune modulation in the treatment of breast cancer have been practice-changing. PD-L1 is a protein on cancer cell surfaces (as well as other cells) that couples with T cells. This coupling, or immune checkpoint, protects the cancer cells from being destroyed by T cells. Checkpoint inhibitor drugs prevent the PD-1/PD-L1 coupling from taking place, thus allowing the T cells to attack the tumor. A PD-1-targeted immune checkpoint inhibitor, pembrolizumab, is FDA-approved for patients with PD-L1-positive disease in combination with chemotherapy (taxane or gemcitabine/carboplatin) based on results from the KEYNOTE 355 trial. Another FDA-approved therapy for triple-negative disease is sacituzumab govitecan, an antibody-drug conjugate that delivers SN-38 (active metabolite of the chemotherapy irinotecan) to Trop-2 overexpressing breast cancer cells.

4. Targeting PARP in *BRCA1/2* mutation–associated breast cancer—Poly (adenosine diphosphate-ribose) polymerase (PARP) is an enzyme important in single-strand DNA repair. Patients who carry germline mutations in *BRCA1* or *BRCA2* have tumors with deficient double-strand DNA repair mechanisms. Experts have theorized that inhibiting PARP selectively kills *BRCA1/2*-mutated cancers. A phase 3 clinical trial (OlympiAD) that compared olaparib (an oral PARP inhibitor) to treatment of physician's choice (single-agent chemotherapy) demonstrated a significantly improved progression-free survival (7.0 months vs 4.2 months), an improved response rate, and a lower rate of adverse events than standard therapy. Talazoparib, a second PARP inhibitor, has also been shown to improve outcomes similarly in the phase 3 EMBRACA study. Both olaparib and talazoparib are FDA-approved for *BRCA*-mutated metastatic breast cancer as single agents.

C. Palliative Chemotherapy

Cytotoxic medications should be considered for the treatment of metastatic breast cancer (1) if life- or organ-threatening visceral metastases are present (especially brain, liver, or lymphangitic pulmonary), (2) if hormonal treatment is unsuccessful or the disease has progressed after an initial response to hormonal manipulation (for hormone receptor–positive breast cancer), or (3) if the tumor is ER-negative or HER2-positive. Prior adjuvant chemotherapy does not seem to alter response rates in patients who relapse. A number of chemotherapy medications (including vinorelbine, paclitaxel, docetaxel, gemcitabine, ixabepilone, carboplatin, cisplatin, capecitabine, albumin-bound paclitaxel, eribulin, and liposomal doxorubicin) may be used as single agents with first-line objective response rates ranging from 30% to 50%.

Combination chemotherapy yields statistically significantly higher response rates and progression-free survival rates compared with sequential single-agent therapy but has not been conclusively shown to improve overall survival rates. Combinations that have been tested in phase 3 studies and have proven efficacy compared with single-agent therapy include capecitabine/docetaxel, gemcitabine/paclitaxel, and capecitabine/ixabepilone (see Tables 39–3 and 39–13). It is generally appropriate to treat willing patients with multiple sequential lines of therapy as long as they tolerate the treatment and as long as their performance status is good (eg, at least ambulatory and able to care for self, up out of bed more than 50% of waking hours).

Bardia A…Hurvitz SA et al. Sacituzumab govitecan in metastatic triple-negative breast cancer. N Engl J Med. 2021. 2021;384:1529. [PMID: 33882206]

Bardia A et al. Elacestrant, an oral selective estrogen receptor degrader (SERD), vs investigator's choice of endocrine monotherapy for ER+/HER2- advanced/metastatic breast cancer (mBC) following progression on prior endocrine and CDK4/6 inhibitor therapy: results of EMERALD phase 3 trial. San Antonio Breast Cancer Symposium 2021. GS2-02.

Burstein HJ. Systemic therapy for estrogen receptor-positive, HER2-negative breast cancer. N Engl J Med. 2020;383:2557. [PMID: 33369357]

Cortes J...Hurvitz SA. Trastuzumab deruxtecan versus trastuzumab emtansine for breast cancer. N Engl J Med. 2022; 386:1143. [PMID: 35320644]

Cortes J et al. Pembrolizumab plus chemotherapy versus placebo plus chemotherapy for previously untreated locally recurrent inoperable or metastatic triple-negative breast cancer (KEYNOTE-355): a randomised, placebo-controlled, double-blind, phase 3 clinical trial. Lancet. 2020;396:1817. [PMID: 33278935]

Diéras V et al. Veliparib with carboplatin and paclitaxel in BRCA-mutated advanced breast cancer (BROCADE3): a randomised, double-blind, placebo-controlled, phase 3 trial. Lancet Oncol. 2020;21:1269. [PMID: 32861273]

Modi S...Hurvitz SA et al. Trastuzumab deruxtecan in previously treated HER2-positive breast cancer. N Engl J Med. 2020; 382:610. [PMID: 31825192]

Murthy RK...Hurvitz SA et al. Tucatinib, trastuzumab, and capecitabine for HER2-positive metastatic breast cancer. N Engl J Med. 2020;382:597. [PMID: 31825569]

National Comprehensive Cancer Network. NCCN Guidelines: Breast Cancer. https://www.nccn.org/guidelines/guidelines-detail?category=1&id=1419

Rugo HS et al; SOPHIA Study Group. Efficacy of margetuximab vs trastuzumab in patients with pretreated ERBB2-positive advanced breast cancer: a phase 3 randomized clinical trial. JAMA Oncol. 2021;7:573. [PMID: 33480963]

Saura C...Hurvitz SA et al. Neratinib plus capecitabine versus lapatinib plus capecitabine in HER2-positive metastatic breast cancer previously treated with ≥2 HER2-directed regimens: phase III NALA trial. J Clin Oncol. 2020;38:3138. [PMID: 32678716]

Slamon DJ et al. Overall survival with ribociclib plus fulvestrant in advanced breast cancer. N Engl J Med. 2020;382:514. [PMID: 31826360]

Swain S et al. Pertuzumab, trastuzumab, and docetaxel for HER2-positive metastatic breast cancer (CLEOPATRA): end-of-study results from a double-blind, randomised, placebo-controlled, phase 3 study. Lancet Oncol. 2020;21:519. [PMID: 32171426]

Prognosis

Stage of breast cancer is the most reliable indicator of prognosis (Tables 17-3 and 17–7). Axillary lymph node status is the best-analyzed prognostic factor and correlates with survival at all tumor sizes. When cancer is localized to the breast

Table 17–7. Approximate survival of patients with breast cancer by TNM stage.

TNM Stage	5 Years	10 Years
0	95%	90%
I	85%	70%
IIA	70%	50%
IIB	60%	40%
IIIA	55%	30%
IIIB	30%	20%
IV	5–10%	2%
All	65%	30%

with no evidence of regional spread after pathologic examination, the clinical cure rate with most accepted methods of therapy is 75% to more than 90%. In fact, patients with small mammographically detected biologically favorable tumors and no evidence of axillary spread have a 5-year survival rate greater than 95%. When the axillary lymph nodes are involved with tumor, the survival rate drops to 50–70% at 5 years and probably around 25–40% at 10 years. The use of biologic markers, such as ER, PR, grade, and HER2, helps identify high-risk tumor types as well as direct treatment used (see Biomarkers & Gene Expression Profiling). Gene analysis studies can predict disease-free survival for some subsets of patients. The eighth edition of the AJCC Staging Manual has incorporated these factors into staging, resulting in incorporation of biologic factors to predict outcome.

Five-year statistics do not accurately reflect the final outcome of therapy. The mortality rate of breast cancer patients exceeds that of age-matched normal controls for nearly 20 years. Thereafter, the mortality rates are equal, though deaths that occur among breast cancer patients are often directly the result of tumor.

In general, breast cancer appears to be somewhat more aggressive and associated with worse outcomes in younger than in older women, and this may be related to the fact that fewer younger women have ER-positive tumors. Disparities in treatment outcome for different racial and ethnic backgrounds have been reported by several studies. These differences appear to be not only due to different socioeconomic factors (and a resulting difference in access to health care) but also due to differences in the subtype of breast cancer diagnosed.

For those patients whose disease progresses despite treatment, some studies suggest supportive group therapy may improve survival. Especially as they approach the end of life, such patients will require meticulous palliative care (see Chapter 5).

DeSantis CE et al. Cancer statistics for African Americans, 2019. CA Cancer J Clin. 2019;69:211. [PMID: 30762872]

Giuliano AE et al. Eighth edition of the AJCC Cancer Staging Manual: Breast Cancer. Ann Surg Oncol. 2018;25:1783. [PMID: 29671136]

Jemal A et al. Factors that contributed to black-white disparities in survival among nonelderly women with breast cancer between 2004 and 2013. J Clin Oncol. 2018;36:14. [PMID: 29035645]

Miller KD et al. Cancer statistics for hispanics/latinos, 2018. CA Cancer J Clin. 2018;68:425. [PMID: 30285281]

Follow-Up Care

After primary therapy, patients with breast cancer should be monitored long term in order to detect recurrences and to observe the opposite breast for a second primary carcinoma. Local and distant recurrences occur most frequently within the first 2–5 years, especially for hormone receptor–negative tumors. During the first 2 years, most patients should be examined every 6 months, then annually thereafter. Special attention is paid to the contralateral breast because a new primary breast malignancy will develop in 20–25% of patients. In some cases, especially in hormone receptor–positive breast cancer, metastases are dormant for long periods and may appear 20 years or longer after removal of the primary tumor. Although studies have failed to show an adverse effect of hormonal replacement in disease-free patients, it is rarely used after breast cancer treatment, particularly if the tumor was hormone receptor–positive. Even pregnancy has not been associated with shortened survival of patients rendered disease free—yet many oncologists are reluctant to advise a young patient with breast cancer that it is safe to become pregnant. The use of estrogen replacement for conditions such as osteoporosis, vaginal dryness, and hot flushes may be considered for a woman with a history of breast cancer after discussion of the benefits and risks; however, it is not routinely recommended, especially given the availability of nonhormonal agents for these conditions (such as bisphosphonates and denosumab for osteoporosis).

A. Local Recurrence

The incidence of local recurrence correlates with tumor size, the presence and number of involved axillary nodes, the histologic type of tumor, the presence of skin edema or skin and fascia fixation with the primary tumor, and the type of definitive surgery and local irradiation. Local recurrence on the chest wall after total mastectomy and axillary dissection develops in as many as 8% of patients. When the axillary nodes are not involved, the local recurrence rate is less than 5%, but the rate is as high as 25% when they are heavily involved. A similar difference in local recurrence rate is noted between small and large tumors. Factors such as multifocal cancer, in situ tumors, lymphovascular invasion, positive resection margins, chemotherapy, and radiotherapy have an effect on local recurrence in patients treated with breast-conserving surgery. Adjuvant systemic therapy greatly decreases the rate of local recurrence. Genomic analysis with identification of high mutation scores also predicts local recurrence.

Chest wall recurrences usually appear within the first several years but may occur as late as 15 or more years after mastectomy. All suspicious nodules and skin lesions should be biopsied. Local excision or localized radiotherapy may be feasible if an isolated nodule is present. If lesions are multiple or accompanied by evidence of regional involvement in the internal mammary or supraclavicular nodes, the disease is best managed by radiation treatment of the entire chest wall including the parasternal, supraclavicular, and axillary areas as well as systemic therapy.

Local recurrence after mastectomy usually signals the presence of widespread disease and is an indication for tests to search for metastases. Distant metastases will develop within a few years in most patients with locally recurrent tumor after mastectomy. When there is no evidence of metastases beyond the chest wall and regional nodes, irradiation for cure after complete local excision should be attempted. After partial mastectomy, local recurrence does not have as serious a prognostic significance as after mastectomy. However, those patients in whom a recurrence develops have a worse prognosis than those who do not. It is speculated that the ability of a cancer to recur locally after radiotherapy is a sign of aggressiveness and resistance to therapy. Completion of the mastectomy should be done for local recurrence after partial mastectomy; some of these patients will survive for prolonged periods, especially if the breast recurrence is DCIS or occurs more than 5 years after initial treatment. Systemic chemotherapy or hormonal treatment should be used for women in whom disseminated disease develops or those in whom local recurrence occurs. In rare cases, re-irradiation with accelerated partial breast techniques may be effective.

B. Breast Cancer Survivorship Issues

Given that most women with nonmetastatic breast cancer will be cured, a significant number of women face survivorship issues stemming from either the diagnosis or the treatment of the breast cancer, or both. These challenges include psychological struggles, cognitive dysfunction (also called "chemo brain"), upper extremity lymphedema, weight management problems, cardiovascular issues, bone loss, postmenopausal side effects, and fatigue. One randomized study reported that survivors who received psychological intervention from the time of diagnosis had a lower risk of recurrence and breast cancer–related mortality. A randomized study in older, overweight cancer survivors showed that diet and exercise reduced the rate of self-reported functional decline compared with no intervention.

1. Edema of the arm—Significant edema of the arm occurs in about 10–30% of patients after axillary dissection with or without mastectomy. It occurs more commonly in obese women, in women who had radiotherapy, and in women who had postoperative infection. Partial mastectomy with radiation to the axillary lymph nodes is followed by chronic edema of the arm in 10–20% of patients. Sentinel lymph node dissection has proved to be an accurate form of axillary staging without the side effects of edema or infection. Judicious use of radiotherapy, with treatment fields carefully planned to spare the axilla as much as possible, can greatly diminish the incidence of edema, which will occur in only 5% of patients if no radiotherapy is given to the axilla after a partial mastectomy and lymph node dissection.

Late or secondary edema of the arm may develop years after treatment as a result of axillary recurrence or infection in the hand or arm, with obliteration of lymphatic channels. When edema develops, a careful examination of the axilla for recurrence or infection is performed. Infection in the arm or hand on the dissected side should be treated with antibiotics, rest, and elevation. If there is no sign of recurrence or infection, the swollen extremity should be treated with rest and elevation. A mild diuretic may be helpful. If there is no improvement, a compressor pump or manual compression decreases the swelling, and the patient is then fitted with an elastic glove or sleeve. Most patients are not bothered enough by mild edema to wear an uncomfortable glove or sleeve and will treat themselves with elevation or manual compression alone. Rarely, edema may be severe enough to interfere with use of the limb. A prospective randomized study has shown that twice weekly progressive weight lifting improves lymphedema symptoms and exacerbations and improves extremity strength.

2. Breast reconstruction—Breast reconstruction is usually feasible after total or modified radical mastectomy. Reconstruction should be discussed with patients prior to mastectomy, because it offers an important psychological focal point for recovery. Reconstruction is not an obstacle to the diagnosis of recurrent cancer. The most common breast reconstruction has been implantation of a silicone gel or saline prosthesis in the subpectoral plane between the pectoralis minor and pectoralis major muscles. Alternatively, autologous tissue can be used for reconstruction.

Autologous tissue flaps have the advantage of not feeling like a foreign body to the patient. The most popular autologous technique is reconstruction using abdominal tissue flaps. This includes the deep inferior epigastric perforator (DIEP) flap and the more traditional transrectus abdominis muscle (TRAM) flap. A latissimus dorsi flap can be swung from the back but offers less volume than the TRAM flap and thus often requires supplementation with an implant. Reconstruction may be performed immediately (at the time of initial mastectomy) or may be delayed until later, usually when the patient has completed adjuvant therapy. When considering reconstructive options, concomitant illnesses should be considered, since the ability of an autologous flap to survive depends on medical comorbidities. In addition, the need for radiotherapy may affect the choice of reconstruction as radiation may increase fibrosis around an implant or decrease the volume of a flap. Skin-sparing and nipple-sparing mastectomies with immediate reconstruction, when feasible, may afford superior cosmetic outcomes.

3. Risks of pregnancy—Clinicians are often asked to advise patients regarding the potential risk of future pregnancy after definitive treatment for early-stage breast cancer. *To date, no adverse effect of pregnancy on survival of women who have had breast cancer has been demonstrated.* When counseling patients, oncologists must take into consideration the patients' overall prognosis, age, comorbidities, and life goals.

In patients with inoperable or metastatic cancer (stage IV disease), induced abortion may be advisable because of the possible adverse effects of hormonal treatment, radiotherapy, or chemotherapy upon the fetus in addition to the expectant mother's poor prognosis.

Lambertini M et al. Pregnancy after breast cancer: a systematic review and meta-analysis. J Clin Oncol 2021;39:3293. [PMID: 34197218]

Ma KK et al. Obstetric outcomes in young women with breast cancer: prior, postpartum, and subsequent pregnancies. Am J Perinatol. 2020;37:370. [PMID: 30726999]

Marsden J et al. The risks and benefits of hormone replacement therapy before and after a breast cancer diagnosis. Post Reprod Health. 2020;26:126. [PMID: 32997592]

McLaughlin SA et al. Breast cancer-related lymphedema: risk factors, screening, management, and the impact of locoregional treatment. J Clin Oncol. 2020;38:2341. [PMID: 32442064]

Naoum GE et al. Quantifying the impact of axillary surgery and nodal irradiation on breast cancer-related lymphedema and local tumor control: long-term results from a prospective screening trial. J Clin Oncol. 2020;38:3430. [PMID: 32730184]

Tevaawerk A et al. Survivorship, version 1.2021. J Natl Compr Canc Netw. 2021;19:676. [PMID: 34214969]

Van Dyk K et al. The cognitive effects of endocrine therapy in survivors of breast cancer: a prospective longitudinal study up to 6 years after treatment. Cancer. 2019;125:681. [PMID: 30485399]

Wagner LI et al. Patient-reported cognitive impairment among women with early breast cancer randomly assigned to endocrine therapy alone versus chemoendocrine therapy: results from TAILORx. J Clin Oncol. 2020;38:1875. [PMID: 32271671]

CARCINOMA OF THE MALE BREAST

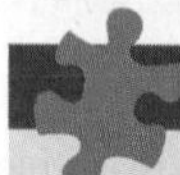

ESSENTIALS OF DIAGNOSIS

- A painless lump beneath the areola in a man usually over 50 years of age.
- Nipple discharge, retraction, or ulceration may be present.
- Generally poorer prognosis than in women.

General Considerations

Breast cancer in men is a rare disease; the incidence is only about 1% of all breast cancer diagnoses. The average age at occurrence is about 70 years, and there may be an increased incidence of breast cancer in men with prostate cancer. As in women, hormonal influences are probably related to the development of male breast cancer. There is a high incidence of both breast cancer and gynecomastia in Bantu men, theoretically owing to failure of estrogen inactivation by associated liver disease. It is important to note that first-degree relatives of men with breast cancer are considered to be at high risk. This risk should be taken into account when discussing options with the patient and family. In addition, *BRCA2* mutations are common in men with breast cancer. Men with breast cancer, especially with a history of prostate cancer, should receive genetic counseling.

Clinical Findings

A painless lump, occasionally associated with nipple discharge, retraction, erosion, or ulceration, is the primary complaint. Examination usually shows a hard, ill-defined, nontender mass beneath the nipple or areola. Gynecomastia not uncommonly precedes or accompanies breast cancer in men and may itself be a risk factor. Nipple discharge is an uncommon presentation for breast cancer in men but is an ominous finding associated with carcinoma in nearly 75% of cases.

Breast cancer staging is the same in men as in women. Gynecomastia and metastatic cancer from another site (eg, prostate) must be considered in the differential diagnosis. Benign tumors are rare, and biopsy should be performed on all males with a defined breast mass.

Treatment

Treatment consists of modified radical mastectomy in operable patients, who should be chosen by the same criteria as women with the disease. Breast-conserving therapy remains underutilized. Irradiation is the first step in treating localized metastases in the skin, lymph nodes, or skeleton that are causing symptoms. Examination of the cancer for hormone receptors and *HER2* overexpression is of value in determining adjuvant therapy. Over 95% of men have ER-positive tumors and less than 10% have overexpression of *HER2*. Androgen receptor is also commonly overexpressed in male breast cancer, though this does not impact systemic therapy decisions. Adjuvant systemic therapy and radiation are used for the same indications as in breast cancer in women.

Because breast cancer in men is frequently hormone receptor–positive, diagnosed late, and is a disseminated disease, endocrine therapy is of considerable importance in its management. Tamoxifen is the main medication for management of advanced breast cancer in men. Tamoxifen (20 mg orally daily) should be the initial treatment. There are few data regarding the use of AIs in men, but they are used frequently. Castration in advanced breast cancer is a successful measure and more beneficial than the same procedure in women but is rarely used. Objective evidence of regression may be seen in 60–70% of men with endocrine therapy for metastatic disease—approximately twice the proportion in women. Bone is the most frequent site of metastases from breast cancer in men (as in women), and endocrine therapy relieves bone pain in most patients so treated. The longer the interval between mastectomy and recurrence, the longer is the remission following treatment.

Chemotherapy should be administered for the same indications and using the same dosage schedules as for women with metastatic disease or for adjuvant treatment.

Prognosis

A large population-based, international breast cancer study reported that after adjustment for prognostic features (age, stage, treatment), men have a similar relative survival stage for stage compared to women. For node-positive disease, 5-year survival is approximately 69%, and for node-negative disease, it is about 88%.

For those patients whose disease progresses despite treatment, meticulous efforts at palliative care are essential (see Chapter 5).

Giordano SH. Breast cancer in men. N Engl J Med. 2018;378:2311. [PMID: 29897847]

Hassett MJ et al. Management of male breast cancer: ASCO guideline. J Clin Oncol. 2020;38:1849. [PMID: 32058842]

Leone J et al. Tumor subtypes and survival in male breast cancer. Breast Cancer Res Treat. 2021;188:695. [PMID: 33770314]

Pizatto M et al. Trends in male breast cancer mortality: a global overview. Eur J Cancer Prev. 2021;30:472. [PMID: 33470692]

Gynecologic Disorders

Jill Brown, MD, MPH, MHS, FACOG[1]
Katerina Shvartsman, MD, FACOG[1]

ABNORMAL UTERINE BLEEDING IN WOMEN OF REPRODUCTIVE AGE

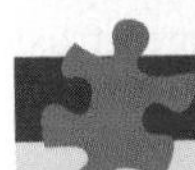

ESSENTIALS OF DIAGNOSIS

- Accurate diagnosis of abnormal uterine bleeding (AUB) depends on appropriate categorization and diagnostic tests.
- Evaluating AUB depends on the age and risk factors of the patient.
- Pregnancy should always be ruled out as a cause of AUB in reproductive age women.

General Considerations

Normal menstrual frequency varies from 24 to 38 days with bleeding lasting an average of 5 days (range, 2–8 days) and a mean blood loss of 40 mL per cycle. AUB refers to menstrual bleeding of abnormal quantity, duration, or schedule. The International Federation of Gynecology and Obstetrics (FIGO) introduced the classification system for AUB in 2011, which was then endorsed by the American College of Obstetrics and Gynecology. This classification system pairs AUB with descriptive terms denoting the bleeding pattern (ie, **heavy**, **light** and **menstrual**, **intermenstrual**) and etiology (the acronym **PALM-COEIN** standing for **P**olyp, **A**denomyosis, **L**eiomyoma, **M**alignancy and hyperplasia, **C**oagulopathy, **O**vulatory dysfunction, **E**ndometrial, **I**atrogenic, and **N**ot yet classified). In adolescents, AUB often occurs because of persistent **anovulation** due to the immaturity of the hypothalamic-pituitary-ovarian axis. Once regular menses have been established during adolescence, **ovulatory dysfunction** AUB (AUB-O) accounts for most cases. AUB in women aged 19–39 years is often a result of pregnancy, structural lesions, anovulatory cycles, use of hormonal contraception, or endometrial hyperplasia.

Clinical Findings

A. Symptoms and Signs

The diagnosis depends on the following: (1) confirming uterine source of the bleeding; (2) excluding pregnancy and confirming patient is premenopausal; (3) ascertaining whether the bleeding pattern suggests regular ovulatory bleeding or anovulatory bleeding; (4) determining contribution of structural abnormalities (PALM), including risk for malignancy/hyperplasia; (5) identifying risk of medical conditions that may impact bleeding (eg, inherited bleeding disorders, endocrine disease, risk of infection); and (6) assessing contribution of medications, including contraceptives, anticoagulants, and natural product supplements that may affect bleeding.

B. Laboratory Studies

A CBC, pregnancy test, and thyroid tests should be done. For adolescents with heavy menstrual bleeding and adults with a positive screening history for bleeding disorders, coagulation studies should be considered, since up to 18% of women with severe heavy menstrual bleeding have an underlying coagulopathy. Vaginal or urine samples should be obtained for testing to rule out infectious causes. If indicated, cervical cytology should also be obtained.

C. Imaging

Transvaginal ultrasound is useful to assess for presence of fibroids, suspicion of adenomyosis, and to evaluate endometrial thickness. Sonohysterography or hysteroscopy may help to diagnose endometrial polyps or subserous myomas. MRI is not a primary imaging modality for AUB but can more definitively diagnose submucous myomas and adenomyosis.

D. Endometrial Sampling

The purpose of endometrial sampling is to determine if hyperplasia or carcinoma is present. Sampling methods

---

[1]Dr. Brown and Dr. Shvartsman are employees of the Uniformed Services University (USU). The opinions and assertions expressed in this chapter are Dr. Brown's and Dr. Shvartsman's and do not reflect the official policy or position of the USU or the Department of Defense.

Table 18–1. Common gynecologic diagnostic procedures.

Colposcopy
Visualization of cervical, vaginal, or vulvar epithelium under 5–50 × magnification with and without dilute acetic acid to identify abnormal areas requiring biopsy. An office procedure.

Dilation & curettage (D&C)
Dilation of the cervix and curettage of the entire endometrial cavity, using a metal curette or suction cannula and often using forceps for the removal of endometrial polyps. Can usually be done in the office under local anesthesia or in the operating room under sedation or general anesthesia. D&C is often combined with hysteroscopy for improved sensitivity.

Endometrial biopsy
Blind sampling of the endometrium by means of a curette or small aspiration device without cervical dilation. Diagnostic accuracy similar to D&C. An office procedure performed with or without local anesthesia.

Endocervical curettage
Removal of endocervical epithelium with a small curette for diagnosis of cervical dysplasia and cancer. An office procedure performed with or without local anesthesia.

Hysterosalpingography
Injection of radiopaque dye through the cervix to visualize the uterine cavity and oviducts. Mainly used in investigation of infertility or to identify a space-occupying lesion.

Hysteroscopy
Visual examination of the uterine cavity with a small fiberoptic endoscope passed through the cervix. Curettage, endometrial ablation, biopsies of lesions, and excision of myomas or polyps can be performed concurrently. Can be done in the office under local anesthesia or in the operating room under sedation or general anesthesia. Greater sensitivity for diagnosis of uterine pathology than D&C.

Laparoscopy
Visualization of the abdominal and pelvic cavity through a small fiberoptic endoscope passed through a subumbilical incision. Permits diagnosis, tubal sterilization, and treatment of many conditions previously requiring laparotomy. General anesthesia is used.

Saline infusion sonohysterography
Introduction of saline solution into endometrial cavity with a catheter to visualize submucous myomas or endometrial polyps by transvaginal ultrasound. May be performed in the office with oral or local analgesia, or both.

and other gynecologic diagnostic procedures are described in Table 18–1. Polyps, endometrial hyperplasia and, occasionally, submucous myomas are identified on endometrial biopsy. Endometrial sampling should be performed in patients with AUB who are 45 years or older, or in younger patients with a history of unopposed estrogen exposure (including obesity or chronic ovulatory dysfunction) or failed medical management and persistent AUB.

Treatment

Treatment for premenopausal patients with AUB depends on the etiology of the bleeding, determined by history, physical examination, laboratory findings, imaging, and endometrial sampling. Patients with AUB due to structural abnormalities (eg, submucosal myomas, endometrial polyps, or pelvic [endometrial] neoplasms) or bleeding diathesis (thrombophilias) may require targeted therapy. A large proportion of premenopausal patients, however, have ovulatory dysfunction AUB (AUB-O).

Treatment for AUB-O should include consideration of potentially contributing medical conditions, such as thyroid dysfunction. Often AUB-O can be treated hormonally. For women amenable to using contraceptives, estrogen-progestin contraceptives and the 52-mg levonorgestrel-releasing intrauterine device (IUD) are both effective treatments. The choice between the two depends on whether any contraindications to these treatments exist and on patient preference. Oral or injectable progestin-only medications are also generally effective, but there is little consensus on optimal regimens, and they appear to be less effective than other medical therapies like the hormonal IUD and tranexamic acid. Nonhormonal options include NSAIDs, such as naproxen or mefenamic acid, in the usual anti-inflammatory doses taken during menses, and tranexamic acid 1300 mg three times per day orally for up to 5 days. Both have been shown to decrease menstrual blood loss by about 40%, with tranexamic acid superior to NSAIDs in direct comparative studies.

Women who are experiencing heavier bleeding can be given a taper of any of the combination oral contraceptives (with 30–35 mcg of ethinyl estradiol) to control the bleeding. There are several commonly used contraceptive dosing regimens, including one pill three times daily (every 8 hours) for 1 or 2 days followed by one pill twice daily through day 5 and then one pill daily through day 20; after withdrawal bleeding occurs, pills are taken in the usual dosage for three cycles. In cases of heavy bleeding requiring hospitalization, intravenous conjugated estrogens, 25 mg every 4 hours for three or four doses, can stop acute bleeding. This can be followed by oral conjugated estrogens, 2.5 mg daily, or ethinyl estradiol, 20 mcg orally daily, for 3 weeks, with the addition of medroxyprogesterone acetate, 10 mg orally daily for the last 10 days of treatment, or a combination oral contraceptive daily for 3 weeks. This will stabilize the endometrium and control the bleeding.

For women with ineffective results from medical management or who do not desire medical management, surgical options can be considered. Heavy menstrual bleeding due to structural lesions (eg, fibroids, adenomyosis, polyps) is the most common indication for surgery. Minimally invasive procedural options for fibroids include uterine artery embolization and focused ultrasound ablation. Surgical options include myomectomy or hysterectomy. For adenomyosis, the definitive treatment is hysterectomy. Polyps can often be excised hysteroscopically. For women without structural abnormalities, endometrial ablation has similar results compared to the hormonal IUD in reducing menstrual blood loss. Hysteroscopic surgical approaches include endometrial ablation with laser photocoagulation or electrocautery. Nonhysteroscopic techniques include balloon thermal ablation, cryoablation, free-fluid thermal ablation, impedance bipolar radiofrequency ablation, and microwave ablation. The latter methods are well-adapted to outpatient therapy under local anesthesia. While hysterectomy was used commonly in the past for bleeding unresponsive to medical therapy, the low risk of complications and the good short-term results of both endometrial ablation and hormonal IUD make them attractive alternatives to hysterectomy.

When to Refer

- If bleeding is not controlled with first-line therapy.
- If expertise is needed for a surgical procedure.

When to Admit

If bleeding is uncontrollable with first-line therapy or the patient is not hemodynamically stable.

Belcaro C et al. Comparison between different diagnostic strategies in low-risk reproductive age and pre-menopausal women presenting abnormal uterine bleeding. Diagnostics (Basel). 2020;10:884. [PMID: 33142970]

Bofill Rodriguez M et al. Cyclical progestogens for heavy menstrual bleeding. Cochrane Database Syst Rev. 2019;8: CD001016. [PMID: 31425626]

Bryant-Smith AC et al. Antifibrinolytics for heavy menstrual bleeding. Cochrane Database Syst Rev. 2018;4:CD000249. [PMID: 29656433]

Wouk N et al. Abnormal uterine bleeding in premenopausal women. Am Fam Physician. 2019;99:435. [PMID: 30932448]

POSTMENOPAUSAL UTERINE BLEEDING

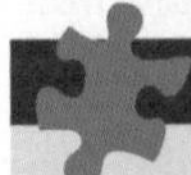

ESSENTIALS OF DIAGNOSIS

- Any uterine bleeding in a postmenopausal woman (12 months or more following cessation of menstrual cycles) is abnormal and should be evaluated.
- Transvaginal ultrasound measurement of the endometrium is an important tool in evaluating the cause of postmenopausal bleeding.

General Considerations

Menopause is defined as 1 year without menstrual bleeding. The most common causes of postmenopausal bleeding are endometrial atrophy, endometrial proliferation or hyperplasia, endometrial or cervical cancer, and administration of estrogens without or with added progestin. Other causes include atrophic vaginitis, trauma, endometrial polyps, abrasion of the cervix associated with prolapse of the uterus, and blood dyscrasias.

Diagnosis

The vulva and vagina should be inspected for areas of bleeding, ulcers, or neoplasms. Cervical cytology should be obtained, if indicated. Transvaginal sonography should be used to measure endometrial thickness. An endometrial stripe measurement of 4 mm or less indicates a low likelihood of hyperplasia or endometrial cancer. If the endometrial thickness is greater than 4 mm, endometrial sampling is indicated. If there is focal thickening of the endometrium on ultrasound or persistent bleeding despite negative results on endometrial biopsy, guided sampling with hysteroscopy is more appropriate than random endometrial sampling.

Treatment

Management options for endometrial hyperplasia without atypia include surveillance, oral contraceptives, or progestin therapy. Surveillance may be used if the risk of occult cancer or progression to cancer is low and the inciting factor (eg, anovulation) has been eliminated. Therapy may include taking cyclic or continuous progestin therapy (medroxyprogesterone acetate, 10–20 mg/day orally, or norethindrone acetate, 15 mg/day orally) or using a hormonal IUD. Repeat sampling should be performed if symptoms recur. Hysterectomy is the preferred treatment for endometrial hyperplasia with atypia (also called endometrial intraepithelial neoplasia) or carcinoma of the endometrium. In some patients with endometrial hyperplasia with atypia, progestin therapy with scheduled repeat endometrial sampling may be an alternative to hysterectomy. Patients who elect this approach include those who desire future childbearing or those who are not candidates for surgery.

When to Refer

- Expertise in performing ultrasonography is required.
- Endometrial hyperplasia with atypia is present.
- Hysteroscopy is indicated.

Khafaga A et al. Abnormal uterine bleeding. Obstet Gynecol Clin North Am. 2019;46:595. [PMID: 31677744]

Saccardi C et al. Endometrial cancer risk prediction according to indication of diagnostic hysteroscopy in post-menopausal women. Diagnostics (Basel). 2020;10:257. [PMID: 32349386]

LEIOMYOMA OF THE UTERUS (Fibroid Tumor)

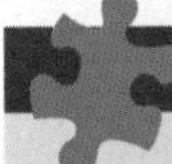

ESSENTIALS OF DIAGNOSIS

- Irregular enlargement of the uterus (may be asymptomatic).
- Heavy or irregular uterine bleeding.
- Pelvic pain, dysmenorrhea, and pressure.

General Considerations

Uterine leiomyomas are the most common benign neoplasm of the female genital tract. They are discrete, round, firm, often multiple, uterine tumors composed of smooth muscle and connective tissue. The most commonly used classification is by anatomic location: (1) intramural,

(2) submucous, (3) subserous, and (4) cervical. Submucous myomas may become pedunculated and descend through the cervix into the vagina.

Clinical Findings

A. Symptoms and Signs

In nonpregnant women, myomas are frequently asymptomatic. The two most common symptoms of uterine leiomyomas for which women seek treatment are AUB and pelvic pain or pressure. Occasionally, degeneration occurs, causing intense pain. Myomas that significantly distort the uterine cavity may affect pregnancy by interfering with implantation, rapidly distending in early pregnancy, or impairing uterine contractility postpartum. Torsion of subserosal pedunculated fibroids may lead to necrosis and pain.

B. Laboratory Findings

Iron deficiency anemia may result from blood loss.

C. Imaging

Ultrasonography will confirm the presence of uterine myomas and can be used sequentially to monitor growth. MRI can delineate intramural and submucous myomas accurately and is typically used before uterine artery embolization to determine fibroid size and location in relation to uterine blood supply. Hysterography or hysteroscopy can also confirm cervical or submucous myomas.

Differential Diagnosis

Irregular myomatous enlargement of the uterus must be differentiated from the similar, but symmetric enlargement that may occur with pregnancy or adenomyosis. Subserous myomas must be distinguished from ovarian tumors. Leiomyosarcoma is an unusual tumor occurring in 0.5% of women operated on for symptomatic myomas. It is rare under the age of 40 but increases in incidence thereafter.

Treatment

A. Nonsurgical Measures

Women who have small asymptomatic myomas can be managed expectantly and evaluated annually. In patients wishing to defer surgical management, nonhormonal therapies (such as NSAIDs and tranexamic acid) have been shown to decrease menstrual blood loss. Women with heavy bleeding related to fibroids may respond to estrogen-progestin oral contraceptives or the hormonal IUD, although an IUD cannot be used with a distorted cavity or cavity length greater than 10 cm. Hormonal therapies, such as GnRH agonists, GnRH antagonists, and selective progesterone receptor modulators (eg, low-dose mifepristone and ulipristal acetate), have been shown to reduce myoma volume, uterine size, and menstrual blood loss. The FDA has also approved the combination of relugolix 40 mg, estradiol 1 mg, and norethindrone acetate 0.5 mg (Myfembree) as the first once-daily treatment for the management of heavy menstrual bleeding associated with uterine fibroids in premenopausal women with a treatment duration of up to 24 months.

However, ulipristal acetate was withdrawn from the market in the European Union and Canada as of September 2020 due to rare reports of serious drug-induced liver injury. And selective progesterone receptor modulators are not approved for fibroid treatment in the United States.

B. Surgical Measures

Surgical intervention is based on the patient's symptoms, desire for future fertility or uterine preservation, and long-term treatment goals. A variety of surgical measures are available for the treatment of myomas: myomectomy (hysteroscopic, laparoscopic, or abdominal) and hysterectomy (vaginal, laparoscopy-assisted vaginal, laparoscopic, abdominal, or robotic). Submucous myomas may be amenable to hysteroscopic resection. Myomectomy is the surgical treatment of choice for women who wish to preserve fertility.

Because the risk of surgical complications increases with the increasing size of the myoma, preoperative reduction of myoma size is sometimes desirable before hysterectomy. GnRH analogs, such as depot leuprolide, 3.75 mg intramuscularly monthly, can be used preoperatively for 3- to 4-month periods to temporarily reduce the size of myomas and surrounding vascularity. GnRH analogs also can be a bridge to surgery in patients who are anemic. By stopping menses, patients may increase their hemoglobin level, perhaps decreasing their need for blood transfusion perioperatively.

Uterine artery embolization is a minimally invasive treatment for uterine fibroids. In uterine artery embolization, the goal is to block the blood vessels supplying the fibroids, causing them to shrink. Magnetic resonance–guided high-intensity focused ultrasound, myolysis/radiofrequency ablation, and laparoscopic or vaginal occlusion of uterine vessels are newer interventions used to treat fibroids with a smaller body of evidence to support their use.

Prognosis

In women desiring future fertility, myomectomy may be offered. Patients should be counseled that recurrence may occur by 40 months in 25% of cases, postoperative pelvic adhesions may impact fertility, and cesarean delivery may be necessary secondary to disruption of the myometrium. Approximately 80% of women have long-term improvement in symptoms following uterine artery embolization. However, direct comparison of women with symptomatic fibroids who underwent myomectomy or uterine artery embolization showed that fibroid-related quality of life at 2 years post-procedure was higher among women who underwent myomectomy. Definitive surgical therapy (ie, hysterectomy) is curative.

When to Refer

Refer to a gynecologist for treatment of symptomatic leiomyomata.

When to Admit

For acute abdomen associated with an infarcted leiomyoma or for hemorrhage not controlled by outpatient measures.

Al-Hendy A et al. Treatment of uterine fibroid symptoms with relugolix combination therapy. N Engl J Med. 2021;384:630. [PMID: 33596357]
Ali M et al. An evaluation of relugolix/estradiol/norethindrone acetate for the treatment of heavy menstrual bleeding associated with uterine fibroids in premenopausal women. Expert Opin Pharmacother. 2022;23:421. [PMID: 35068291]
Chudnoff S et al. Ultrasound-guided transcervical ablation of uterine leiomyomas. Obstet Gynecol 2019;133:13. [PMID: 30531573]
Donnez J et al. The current place of medical therapy in uterine fibroid management. Best Pract Res Clin Obstet Gynaecol. 2018;46:57. [PMID: 29169896]
Manyonda I et al; FEMME Collaborative Group. Uterine-artery embolization or myomectomy for uterine fibroids. N Engl J Med. 2020;383:440. [PMID: 32726530]
Osuga Y et al. Oral gonadotropin-releasing hormone antagonist relugolix compared with leuprorelin injections for uterine leiomyomas: a randomized clinical trial. Obstet Gynecol. 2019;133:423. [PMID: 30741797]

CERVICAL POLYPS

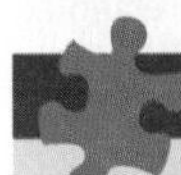
ESSENTIALS OF DIAGNOSIS

- Irregular or postcoital bleeding.
- Polyps visible in the cervical os on speculum examination.

Clinical Findings

Cervical polyps commonly occur during the reproductive years, particularly after age 40, and are occasionally noted in postmenopausal women. The cause is not known, but inflammation may play an etiologic role. The principal symptoms are discharge and abnormal vaginal bleeding. However, abnormal bleeding should not be ascribed to a cervical polyp without sampling the endocervix and endometrium. The polyps are visible in the cervical os on speculum examination.

Cervical polyps must be differentiated from polypoid neoplastic disease of the endometrium, small submucous pedunculated myomas, large nabothian cysts, and endometrial polyps. Cervical polyps rarely contain foci of dysplasia (0.5%) or of malignancy (0.5%). Asymptomatic polyps in women under age 45 may be left untreated.

Treatment

Cervical polyps can generally be removed in the office by avulsion with uterine packing forceps or ring forceps.

When to Refer

- Polyp with a wide base.
- Inability to differentiate endocervical from endometrial polyp.

Budak A et al. Role of endometrial sampling in cases with asymptomatic cervical polyps. J Gynecol Obstet Hum Reprod. 2019;48:207. [PMID: 30660657]

PELVIC PAIN

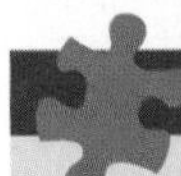
ESSENTIALS OF DIAGNOSIS

- Determine if pain is acute or chronic.
- Categorize if pain is cyclic or continuous.
- Consider nongynecologic causes.

1. Primary Dysmenorrhea

Primary dysmenorrhea is menstrual pain associated with menstrual cycles in the absence of pathologic findings. Primary dysmenorrhea usually begins within 1–2 years after menarche and may become progressively more severe. The frequency of cases increases up to age 20 and then decreases with both increasing age and parity. Half to three-quarters of women are affected by dysmenorrhea at some time, and 5–6% have incapacitating pain.

Clinical Findings

Primary dysmenorrhea is low, midline, wave-like, cramping pelvic pain often radiating to the back or inner thighs. Cramps may last for 1 or more days and may be associated with nausea, diarrhea, headache, and flushing. The pain is produced by uterine vasoconstriction, anoxia, and sustained contractions mediated by prostaglandins. The pelvic examination is normal between menses; examination during menses may produce discomfort, but there are no pathologic findings.

Treatment

NSAIDs (ibuprofen, ketoprofen, mefenamic acid, naproxen) and the cyclooxygenase (COX)-2 inhibitor (celecoxib) are generally helpful. The medication should be started 1–2 days before expected menses. Symptoms can be suppressed with use of combined hormonal contraceptives, depo-medroxyprogesterone acetate (DMPA), etonogestrel subdermal implant (Nexplanon), or the hormonal IUD. Oral contraceptives taken continuously can suppress menstruation completely and prevent dysmenorrhea. Other therapies that have shown some benefit include local heat, thiamine 100 mg/day orally, vitamin E 200 units/day orally, and high-frequency transcutaneous electrical nerve stimulation around the time of menses. These options may be offered to patients who desire nonhormonal therapy, although they have less supporting evidence.

2. Endometriosis

General Considerations

Endometriosis is an aberrant growth of endometrium outside of the uterus, particularly in the dependent parts of the pelvis and in the ovaries. Its principal manifestations are chronic pain and infertility. While retrograde menstruation is the most widely accepted cause, its pathogenesis and natural course are not fully understood. The overall prevalence in the United States is 6–10%.

Clinical Findings

The clinical manifestations of endometriosis are variable and unpredictable in both presentation and course. Dysmenorrhea, chronic pelvic pain, and dyspareunia are among the well-recognized symptoms. Many women with endometriosis, however, remain asymptomatic, and most women with endometriosis have a normal pelvic examination. However, in some women, pelvic examination can disclose tender nodules in the cul-de-sac or rectovaginal septum, uterine retroversion with decreased uterine mobility, uterine tenderness, or adnexal mass or tenderness.

Endometriosis must be distinguished from pelvic inflammatory disease, ovarian neoplasms, and uterine myomas. Bowel invasion by endometrial tissue may produce blood in the stool that must be distinguished from that produced by bowel neoplasm.

Imaging is useful mainly in the presence of a pelvic or adnexal mass. Transvaginal ultrasonography is the imaging modality of choice to detect the presence of deeply penetrating endometriosis of the rectum or rectovaginal septum; MRI should be reserved for equivocal cases of rectovaginal or bladder endometriosis. A definitive diagnosis of endometriosis is made only by histology of lesions removed at surgery.

Treatment

A. Medical Treatment

Although there is no conclusive evidence that NSAIDs improve the pain associated with endometriosis, these agents are a reasonable option in appropriately selected patients. Medical treatment, using a variety of hormonal therapies, is effective in the amelioration of pain associated with endometriosis. Most of these regimens are designed to inhibit ovulation and to lower hormone levels, thus preventing cyclic stimulation of endometriotic implants and inducing atrophy. The optimum duration of hormonal therapies is not clear, and their relative merits in terms of side effects and long-term risks and benefits show insignificant differences when compared with one another and even, in mild cases, with placebo. Commonly used medical regimens include the following:

1. Combined hormonal (estrogen-progestin) contraceptives are first-line treatment because they suppress ovulation, which may inhibit stimulation of endometriosis. Any of the combination oral contraceptives, the contraceptive patch, or the vaginal ring may be used continuously, which is preferred for treatment of endometriosis. Breakthrough bleeding can be treated with conjugated estrogens, 1.25 mg orally daily for 1 week, or estradiol, 2 mg daily orally for 1 week. Alternatively, a short hormone-free interval to allow a withdrawal bleed can be used whenever bothersome breakthrough bleeding occurs.
2. Progestins, specifically oral norethindrone acetate and subcutaneous DMPA, have been approved by the US FDA for treatment of endometriosis-associated pain. The etonogestrel implant has also been shown to decrease endometriosis-related pain.
3. Intrauterine progestin, using the hormonal IUD, has been shown to be effective in reducing endometriosis-associated pelvic pain and may be considered before surgery.
4. GnRH agonists are highly effective in reducing pain associated with endometriosis; however, they are not superior to other methods such as combined hormonal contraceptives. The GnRH analog (such as long-acting injectable leuprolide acetate, 3.75 mg intramuscularly monthly, used for 6 months) suppresses ovulation. Side effects of vasomotor symptoms and bone demineralization may be relieved by "add-back" therapy, such as conjugated equine estrogen, 0.625 mg orally daily, or norethindrone, 5 mg orally daily.
5. GnRH antagonists suppress pituitary gonadotropin production and create a hypoestrogenic state, like GnRH agonists, but they are effective immediately rather than requiring 7–14 days for GnRH suppression. Injectable and oral forms (eg, cetrorelix and elagolix, respectively) are available.
6. Danazol is an androgenic medication used to treat endometriosis-associated pain. It may be used for 4–6 months in the lowest dose necessary to suppress menstruation, usually 200–400 mg orally twice daily. However, danazol has a high incidence of androgenic side effects, including decreased breast size, weight gain, acne, and hirsutism, that are more severe than with other medications available.
7. Aromatase inhibitors (such as anastrozole or letrozole) in combination with conventional therapy have been evaluated with positive results in premenopausal women with endometriosis-associated pain and pain recurrence.

B. Surgical Measures

Surgical treatment of endometriosis—particularly extensive disease—is effective both in reducing pain and in promoting fertility. Laparoscopic ablation of endometrial implants significantly reduces pain. Ablation of implants and, if necessary, removal of ovarian endometriomas enhance fertility, although subsequent pregnancy rates are inversely related to the severity of disease. Women with disabling pain for whom childbearing is not a consideration can be treated definitively with hysterectomy plus bilateral salpingo-oophorectomy. In premenopausal women, hormone replacement may then relieve vasomotor symptoms.

Prognosis

There is little systematic research regarding either the progression of the disease or the prediction of clinical outcomes. The prognosis for reproductive function in early or moderately advanced endometriosis appears to be good with conservative therapy. Hysterectomy, with bilateral salpingo-oophorectomy, often is regarded as definitive treatment of endometriosis associated with intractable pelvic pain, adnexal masses, or multiple previous ineffective conservative surgical procedures. However, symptoms may recur even after hysterectomy and oophorectomy.

When to Refer

Refer to a gynecologist for laparoscopic diagnosis or surgical treatment.

When to Admit

Rarely necessary except for acute abdomen associated with ruptured or bleeding endometrioma.

3. Other Etiologies of Pelvic Pain

Additional causes of pelvic pain may include adenomyosis, fibroids, PID, malpositioned IUD, or other abnormalities of the pelvic organs, including the bowel or bladder.

Clinical Findings

The history may be suggestive of the causes mentioned above. Physical examination may be useful to narrow the differential diagnosis.

Diagnosis

Targeted physical examination may help identify the anatomic source of pelvic pain. PID should be considered in sexually active women with pelvic pain and examination findings of cervical motion tenderness, uterine tenderness, or adnexal tenderness without another explanation for the pain. Pelvic imaging is useful for diagnosing uterine fibroids or other anomalies. Adenomyosis (the presence of endometrial glands and stroma within the myometrium) may be detected with ultrasound or MRI. Laparoscopy may help diagnose endometriosis or other pelvic abnormalities not visualized by imaging.

Treatment

Treatment should be directed at the underlying cause. For example, PID should be treated with antibiotics as described below. If pain symptoms are marked or prolonged or unresponsive to medical management, diagnostic laparoscopy may be warranted. Definitive surgery depends on the intraoperative findings and the underlying etiology. For example, adenomyosis or endometriosis may respond to hormonal approaches, but if those are unsuccessful, hysterectomy remains the definitive treatment of choice for women for whom childbearing is not a consideration.

When to Refer

- Standard therapy fails to relieve pain.
- Suspicion of pelvic pathology, such as endometriosis, leiomyomas, adenomyosis, or PID.

American College of Obstetricians and Gynecologists' Committee on Practice Bulletins—Gynecology. Chronic pelvic pain: ACOG Practice Bulletin, Number 218. Obstet Gynecol. 2020;135:e98. [PMID: 32080051]

Brown J et al. Oral contraceptives for pain associated with endometriosis. Cochrane Database Syst Rev. 2018;5:CD001019. [PMID: 29786828]

Carey ET al. Updates in the approach to chronic pelvic pain: what the treating gynecologist should know. Clin Obstet Gynecol. 2019;62:666. [PMID: 31524660]

Samy A et al. Medical therapy options for endometriosis related pain, which is better? A systematic review and network meta-analysis of randomized controlled trials. J Gynecol Obstet Hum Reprod. 2021;50:101798. [PMID: 32479894]

Singh SS et al. Surgical outcomes in patients with endometriosis: a systematic review. J Obstet Gynaecol Can. 2020;42:881. [PMID: 31718952]

Vilasagar S et al. A practical guide to the clinical evaluation of endometriosis-associated pelvic pain. J Minim Invasive Gynecol. 2020;27:270. [PMID: 31669551]

PELVIC ORGAN PROLAPSE

General Considerations

Pelvic organ prolapse, including cystocele, rectocele, and enterocele, are vaginal hernias commonly seen in multiparous women. **Cystocele** is a hernia of the bladder wall into the vagina, causing a soft anterior fullness. Cystocele may be accompanied by **urethrocele,** which is not a hernia but a sagging of the urethra following its detachment from the pubic symphysis usually during childbirth. **Rectocele** is a herniation of the terminal rectum into the posterior vagina, causing a collapsible pouch-like fullness. **Enterocele** is a vaginal vault hernia containing small intestine, usually in the posterior vagina and resulting from a deepening of the pouch of Douglas. Two or all three types of hernia may occur in combination. The cause of pelvic organ prolapse is multifactorial. Risk factors include vaginal birth, genetic predisposition, advancing age, prior pelvic surgery, connective tissue disorders, and increased intra-abdominal pressure associated with obesity or straining associated with chronic constipation or coughing.

Clinical Findings

Symptoms of pelvic organ prolapse may include a sensation of a bulge or protrusion in the vagina, urinary or fecal incontinence, constipation, sense of incomplete bladder or bowel emptying, and dyspareunia.

Treatment

Treatment depends on the extent of prolapse; associated symptoms; impact on the patient's quality of life; the patient's age; and her desire to retain her uterus and ability for coitus.

A. General Measures

Supportive measures include a high-fiber diet and laxatives to improve constipation. Weight reduction in obese patients and limitation of straining and lifting are helpful. Pelvic muscle training (Kegel exercises) is a simple, noninvasive intervention that may improve pelvic function; it has demonstrated clear benefit for women with urinary or fecal symptoms, especially incontinence. Pessaries may reduce a cystocele, rectocele, or enterocele and are helpful in women who do not wish to undergo surgery or who are poor surgical candidates.

B. Surgical Measures

The most common surgical procedure is vaginal or abdominal hysterectomy with additional attention to restoring apical support with a suspension procedure, such as vaginal uterosacral suspension, sacrospinous fixation, or by abdominal sacral colpopexy. Since stress urinary incontinence and urinary retention may coexist with apical prolapse, women should be evaluated for these conditions before surgery. An anti-incontinence procedure may be done in conjunction with prolapse surgery if indicated. Surgical mesh placed transvaginally for pelvic organ prolapse repair was introduced into clinical practice in 2002; however, in 2011 the US FDA issued warnings about concerns for serious complications associated with this practice (including mesh erosion and pain). Use of these methods subsequently declined significantly. In April 2019, the US FDA withdrew its approval of surgical mesh for the indication of transvaginal repair of pelvic organ prolapse. Patients planning to have surgical repair of pelvic organ prolapse should discuss all treatment options with their clinician. Women who have received transvaginal mesh for the surgical repair of pelvic organ prolapse and have no associated symptoms or complications should continue with their annual check-ups and other routine follow-up care. They should let their clinician know that they have a surgical mesh implant, especially if they plan to have another pelvic surgery or related medical procedure. In addition, they should notify their clinician if they develop symptoms such as persistent vaginal bleeding or discharge, pelvic or groin pain, or dyspareunia.

Generally, surgical repair of pelvic organ prolapse is reserved until after completion of childbearing. If a woman with symptomatic prolapse desires pregnancy, the same procedures for vaginal suspension can be performed without hysterectomy, though limited data on pregnancy outcomes or prolapse outcomes are available. For older women who do not desire coitus, colpocleisis, the partial obliteration of the vagina, is an effective and straightforward procedure. Uterine suspension with sacrospinous cervicocolpopexy may be an effective approach in older women who wish to avoid hysterectomy but preserve coital function.

When to Refer

- Refer to urogynecologist or gynecologist for incontinence evaluation.
- Refer if nonsurgical therapy is ineffective.
- Refer for removal of mesh if symptoms develop.

American College of Obstetricians and Gynecologists. Practice Bulletin No. 214: pelvic organ prolapse. Obstet Gynecol. 2019;134:e126. [PMID: 31651832]

Carter P et al. Management of mesh complications following surgery for stress urinary incontinence or pelvic organ prolapse: a systematic review. BJOG. 2020;127:28. [PMID: 31541614]

Gluck O et al. Laparoscopic sacrocolpopexy: a comprehensive literature review on current practice. Eur J Obstet Gynecol Reprod Biol. 2020;245:94. [PMID: 31891897]

Hemming C et al. Surgical interventions for uterine prolapse and for vault prolapse: the two VUE RCTs. Health Technol Assess. 2020;24:1. [PMID: 32138809]

Ko KJ et al. Current surgical management of pelvic organ prolapse: strategies for the improvement of surgical outcomes. Investig Clin Urol. 2019;60:413. [PMID: 31692921]

PREMENSTRUAL SYNDROME

General Considerations

The **premenstrual syndrome (PMS)** is a recurrent, variable cluster of troublesome physical and emotional symptoms that develop during the 5 days before the onset of menses and subside within 4 days after menstruation begins. PMS intermittently affects about 40% of all premenopausal women, primarily those 25–40 years of age. In about 5–8% of affected women, the syndrome may be severe. Although not every woman experiences all the symptoms or signs at one time, many describe bloating, breast pain, headache, swelling, irritability, aggressiveness, depression, inability to concentrate, libido change, lethargy, and food cravings. When emotional or mood symptoms predominate, along with physical symptoms, and there is a clear functional impairment with work or personal relationships, the term **"premenstrual dysphoric disorder" (PMDD)** may be applied. The pathogenesis of PMS/PMDD is still uncertain, and treatment methods are mainly empiric. The clinician should provide support for both the patient's emotional and physical distress, including the following:

1. Careful evaluation of the patient, with understanding, explanation, and reassurance.
2. Advice to keep a daily diary of all symptoms for 2–3 months, such as the Daily Record of Severity of Problems, to evaluate the timing and characteristics of symptoms. If symptoms occur throughout the month rather than in the 2 weeks before menses, the patient may have depression or other mental health diagnosis instead of or in addition to PMS.

Treatment

For mild to moderate symptoms, a program of aerobic exercise; reduction of caffeine, salt, and alcohol intake; and use of alternative therapies, such as acupuncture and herbal treatments may be helpful, although these interventions remain unproven.

Medications that prevent ovulation, such as hormonal contraceptives, may lessen physical symptoms. These include continuous combined hormonal contraceptive methods (pill, patch, or vaginal ring) or GnRH agonist with "add-back" therapy (eg, conjugated equine estrogen, 0.625 mg orally daily, with medroxyprogesterone acetate, 2.5–5 mg orally daily).

When mood disorders predominate, several serotonin reuptake inhibitors have been shown to be effective in relieving tension, irritability, and dysphoria with few side effects. First-line medication therapy includes serotonergic antidepressants (citalopram, escitalopram, fluoxetine, sertraline, venlafaxine) either daily or only on symptom days. There are limited data to support the use of calcium, vitamin D, and vitamin B_6 supplementation. There is insufficient evidence to support cognitive behavioral therapy.

Yonkers KA et al. Premenstrual disorders. Am J Obstet Gynecol. 2018;218:68. [PMID: 28571724]

MENOPAUSAL SYNDROME

See Chapter 26, Endocrine Disorders.

POLYCYSTIC OVARY SYNDROME

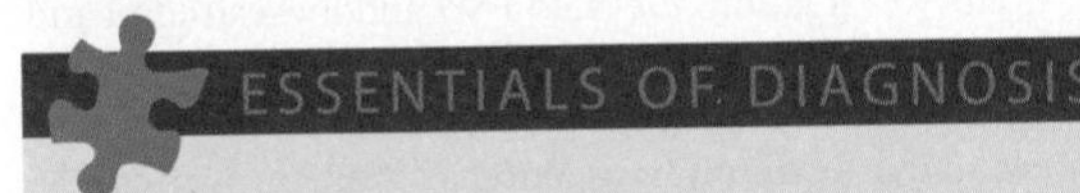

- Clinical or biochemical evidence of hyperandrogenism.
- Oligoovulation or anovulation.
- Polycystic ovaries on ultrasonography.

General Considerations

Polycystic ovary syndrome (PCOS) is a common endocrine disorder of unknown etiology affecting 5–10% of reproductive age women. The Rotterdam Criteria, endorsed by the National Institutes of Health, identify **hyperandrogenism, ovulatory dysfunction,** and **polycystic ovaries** as the key diagnostic features of the disorder in adult women; at least two of these features must be present for diagnosis.

Clinical Findings

PCOS often presents as a menstrual disorder (ranging from amenorrhea to heavy menstrual bleeding) and infertility. Skin disorders due to peripheral androgen excess, including hirsutism and acne, are common. Patients may also show signs of insulin resistance and hyperinsulinemia, and these women are at increased risk for early-onset type 2 diabetes mellitus and metabolic syndrome. Unrecognized or untreated PCOS is a risk factor for CVD. Patients who do become pregnant are at increased risk for perinatal complications, such as gestational diabetes and preeclampsia. In addition, they have an increased long-term risk of endometrial cancer secondary to chronic exposure to unopposed estrogen.

Differential Diagnosis

Anovulation in the reproductive years may also be due to (1) premature ovarian failure (high FSH, low estradiol); (2) functional hypothalamic amenorrhea, often associated with rapid weight loss or extreme physical exertion (low to normal FSH for age); (3) discontinuation of hormonal contraceptives (return to ovulation typically occurs within 90 days); (4) pituitary adenoma with elevated prolactin (galactorrhea may or may not be present); and (5) hyperthyroidism or hypothyroidism. To rule out other etiologies in women with suspected PCOS, serum FSH, estradiol, prolactin, and TSH should be evaluated. Because of the high risk of insulin resistance and dyslipidemia, all women with suspected PCOS should have a hemoglobin A_{1C} and fasting glucose along with a lipid profile. Women with clinical evidence of androgen excess should have total testosterone, free (bioavailable) testosterone, and 17-hydroxyprogesterone measured. Women with stigmata of Cushing syndrome should have a 24-hour urinary free cortisol or a low-dose dexamethasone suppression test. Congenital adrenal hyperplasia and androgen-secreting adrenal tumors also tend to have high circulating androgen levels and anovulation with polycystic ovaries; these disorders must also be ruled out in women with presumed PCOS and high serum androgens.

Treatment

In obese patients with PCOS, weight reduction and exercise are often effective in reversing the metabolic effects and in inducing ovulation. For women who do not respond to weight loss and exercise and do not desire pregnancy, combined hormonal contraceptives are first-line treatment to manage hyperandrogenism and menstrual irregularities. Intermittent or continuous progestin therapy or a hormonal IUD may be used for endometrial protection in women who cannot or choose not to use combined hormonal contraceptives. Metformin therapy may be used as a second-line therapy to improve menstrual function. Metformin has little or no benefit in the treatment of hirsutism, acne, or infertility. Contraceptive counseling should be offered to prevent unplanned pregnancy in case of a return of ovulatory cycles. For women who are seeking pregnancy and remain anovulatory, clomiphene, letrozole, or other medications can be used for ovarian stimulation (see section on Infertility below). Women with PCOS are at greater risk than normal women for twin gestation with ovarian stimulation.

If hirsutism does not improve after 6 months of treatment with combined hormonal contraceptives, an antiandrogen, such as spironolactone, may be added. Topical eflornithine cream applied to affected facial areas twice daily for 6 months may be helpful in most women. Hirsutism may also be managed with depilatory creams, electrolysis, and laser therapy. The combination of laser therapy and topical eflornithine may be particularly effective.

Weight loss, exercise, and treatment of unresolved metabolic derangements are important in preventing CVD. Women with PCOS should be managed aggressively and should have regular monitoring of lipid profiles and glucose.

When to Refer

- If expertise in diagnosis is needed.
- If patient is infertile.

American College of Obstetricians and Gynecologists. Practice Bulletin No. 194: polycystic ovary syndrome. Obstet Gynecol. 2018;131:e157. [PMID: 29794677]

Gadalla MA et al. Medical and surgical treatment of reproductive outcomes in polycystic ovary syndrome: an overview of systematic reviews. Int J Fertil Steril. 2020;13:257. [PMID: 31710185]

Huddleston HG et al. Diagnosis and treatment of polycystic ovary syndrome. JAMA. 2022;327:274. [PMID: 35040896]

Shi S et al. Letrozole and human menopausal gonadotropin for ovulation induction in clomiphene resistance polycystic ovary syndrome patients: a randomized controlled study. Medicine (Baltimore). 2020;99:e18383. [PMID: 31977842]

INFERTILITY

A couple is said to be infertile if pregnancy does not result after 1 year of normal sexual activity without contraception. Up to 20% of couples experience infertility in their reproductive lives; the incidence of infertility increases with age, with a decline in fertility beginning in the early 30s and accelerating in the late 30s. The male partner contributes to about 40% of cases of infertility, and a combination of factors is common. CDC National Survey of Family Growth data from 2011–2015 noted that 12% of women in the United States aged 15–44 report impaired fecundity.

A. Initial Testing

During the initial interview, the clinician can present an overview of infertility and discuss an evaluation and management plan. Private consultations with each partner separately are then conducted. Pertinent details (eg, sexually transmitted infection history or prior pregnancies) must be obtained. The ill effects of cigarettes, alcohol, and other recreational drugs on male fertility should be discussed. Prescription medications that impair male potency and factors that may lead to scrotal hyperthermia, such as tight underwear or frequent use of saunas or hot tubs, should be discussed. The gynecologic history should include the menstrual pattern, the use and types of contraceptives, frequency and success of coitus, and correlation of intercourse with time of ovulation. The American Society for Reproductive Medicine provides patient information on the infertility evaluation and treatment (https://www.asrm.org/topics/topics-index/infertility/).

General physical and genital examinations are performed on the female partner. Basic laboratory studies include assessment of **ovarian reserve** (eg, antimüllerian hormone, and day 3 FSH and estradiol) and thyroid function tests. If the woman has regular menses with moliminal symptoms, the likelihood of ovulatory cycles is very high. A luteal phase serum progesterone above 3 ng/mL establishes ovulation. Couples should be advised that coitus resulting in conception occurs during the 6-day window before the day of ovulation. Ovulation predictor kits have largely replaced basal body temperatures for predicting ovulation, but temperature charting may be used to identify most fertile days. Basal body temperature charts cannot predict ovulation; they can only retrospectively confirm that ovulation occurred.

A semen analysis should be completed to rule out a male factor for infertility (see Chapter 29).

B. Further Testing

1. Gross deficiencies of sperm (number, motility, or appearance) require a repeat confirmatory analysis.
2. A screening pelvic ultrasound and hysterosalpingography to identify uterine cavity or tubal anomalies should be performed. Hysterosalpingography is performed within 3 days following the menstrual period if structural abnormalities are suspected. This radiographic study will demonstrate uterine abnormalities (septa, polyps, submucous myomas) and tubal obstruction. Women who have had prior pelvic inflammatory disease or abnormal tubes seen on hysterosalpingography or laparoscopy should receive doxycycline, 100 mg orally twice daily for 5 days.
3. Absent or infrequent ovulation requires additional laboratory evaluation. Elevated FSH and low estradiol and antimüllerian hormone levels indicate ovarian insufficiency. Patients with elevated prolactin levels should be evaluated for pituitary adenoma. Women over age 35 may require further assessment of **ovarian reserve.** A markedly elevated FSH (greater than 15–20 IU/L) on day 3 of the menstrual cycle suggests inadequate ovarian reserve. Although less widely performed, a clomiphene citrate challenge test, with measurement of FSH on day 10 after administration of clomiphene from days 5–9, can help confirm a diagnosis of diminished ovarian reserve. The number of antral follicles during the early follicular phase of the cycle can provide useful information about ovarian reserve and can confirm serum testing. An antimüllerian hormone level can be measured at any time during the menstrual cycle and is less likely to be affected by hormones.
4. If all the above testing is normal, **unexplained infertility** is diagnosed. In approximately 25% of women whose basic evaluation is normal, the first-line therapy is usually controlled ovarian hyperstimulation (commonly with clomiphene citrate) and intrauterine insemination. IVF may be recommended as second-line therapy.

Treatment

A. Medical Measures

Fertility may be restored by treatment of endocrine abnormalities, particularly hypothyroidism or hyperthyroidism. Women who are anovulatory because of low body weight or exercise may become ovulatory when they gain weight or decrease their exercise levels; conversely, obese women who are anovulatory may become ovulatory with loss of even 5–10% of body weight.

B. Surgical Measures

Excision of ovarian tumors or ovarian foci of endometriosis can improve fertility. Microsurgical relief of tubal obstruction due to salpingitis or tubal ligation will reestablish fertility in many cases, although with severe disease or proximal obstruction, IVF is preferable. Peritubal adhesions or endometriotic implants often can be treated via laparoscopy.

In a male with a varicocele, sperm characteristics may be improved following surgical treatment. For men who have sperm production but obstructive azoospermia, trans-epidermal sperm aspiration or microsurgical epidermal sperm aspiration has been successful.

C. Induction of Ovulation

1. Clomiphene citrate—Clomiphene citrate stimulates gonadotropin release, especially FSH. It acts as a selective estrogen receptor modulator, similar to tamoxifen and raloxifene, and binds to the estrogen receptor. A low level of estrogen decreases the negative feedback on the hypothalamus, thereby increasing the release of FSH and LH. When FSH and LH are present in the appropriate amounts and timing, ovulation occurs.

After a normal menstrual period or induction of withdrawal bleeding with progestin, clomiphene 50 mg orally should be given daily for 5 days, typically on days 3–7 of the cycle. If ovulation does not occur, the clomiphene dosage is increased to 100 mg orally daily for 5 days. While doses of 150 mg may be used, doses greater than 100 mg do not appear to improve clinical pregnancy rates. The rate of ovulation following clomiphene treatment is approximately 80% in the absence of other infertility factors. The pregnancy rate is 30–40%, and twinning occurs in 5% of these pregnancies. Three or more fetuses are rare (less than 0.5% of cases). Pregnancy is most likely to occur within the first three ovulatory cycles and unlikely to occur after cycle 6. In addition, several studies have suggested a twofold to threefold increased risk of ovarian cancer with the use of clomiphene for more than 1 year, so treatment with clomiphene is usually limited to a maximum of six cycles.

2. Letrozole—The aromatase inhibitor letrozole appears to be at least as effective as clomiphene for induction of ovulation in women with PCOS. There is a reduced risk of multiple pregnancy, a lack of antiestrogenic effects, and a reduced need for ultrasound monitoring. The dose of letrozole is 2.5–7.5 mg daily, starting on day 3 of the menstrual cycle. In women who have a history of estrogen-dependent tumors, such as breast cancer, letrozole is preferred over other agents because the estrogen levels with this medication are much lower.

3. Human menopausal gonadotropins (hMG) or recombinant FSH—hMG or recombinant FSH is indicated in cases of hypogonadotropism and most other types of anovulation resistant to clomiphene treatment. Because of the complexities, laboratory tests, and expense associated with this treatment, these patients should be referred to an infertility specialist.

D. Artificial Insemination in Azoospermia

If azoospermia is present, artificial insemination by a donor usually results in pregnancy, assuming female function is normal. Using frozen sperm provides the opportunity for screening for sexually transmitted infections, including HIV infection.

E. Assisted Reproductive Technology (ART)

Couples who have not responded to traditional infertility treatments and those with occlusive tubal disease, severe endometriosis, oligospermia, and immunologic or unexplained infertility, may benefit from ART. All ART procedures involve ovarian stimulation to produce multiple oocytes, oocyte retrieval by transvaginal sonography–guided needle aspiration, and handling of the oocytes outside the body. With IVF, the eggs are fertilized in vitro and the embryos transferred to the uterus. Intracytoplasmic sperm injection allows fertilization with a single sperm. While originally intended for couples with male factor infertility, it is now used in two-thirds of all IVF procedures in the United States.

The chance of a multiple gestation pregnancy (ie, twins, triplets) is increased in all assisted reproductive procedures, increasing the risk of preterm delivery and other pregnancy complications. To minimize this risk, most infertility specialists recommend transferring only one embryo in appropriately selected patients with a favorable prognosis.

Prognosis

The prognosis for conception and normal pregnancy is good if minor (even multiple) disorders can be identified and treated; it is poor if the causes of infertility are severe, untreatable, or of prolonged duration (over 3 years).

In the absence of identifiable causes of infertility, 60% of couples will achieve a spontaneous pregnancy within 3 years. Couples in which the woman is younger than 35 years who do not achieve pregnancy within 1 year of trying may be candidates for infertility treatment, and within 6 months for women age 35 years and older. Also, offering appropriately timed information about adoption is considered part of a complete infertility regimen.

When to Refer

Refer to reproductive endocrinologist if ART is indicated, or surgery is required.

American College of Obstetricians and Gynecologists. Committee Opinion No. 781: infertility workup for the women's health specialist. Obstet Gynecol. 2019;133:e377. [PMID: 31135764]

Hodgson RM et al. Interventions for endometriosis-related infertility: a systematic review and network meta-analysis. Fertil Steril. 2020;113:374. [PMID: 32106991]

Merritt BA et al. Imaging of infertility, Part 1: hysterosalpingograms to magnetic resonance imaging. Radiol Clin North Am. 2020;58:215. [PMID: 32044003]

Merritt BA et al. Imaging of infertility, Part 2: hysterosalpingograms to magnetic resonance imaging. Radiol Clin North Am. 2020;58:227. [PMID: 32044004]

Shi S et al. Letrozole and human menopausal gonadotropin for ovulation induction in clomiphene resistance polycystic ovary syndrome patients: a randomized controlled study. Medicine (Baltimore). 2020;99:e18383. [PMID: 31977842]

CONTRACEPTION & FAMILY PLANNING

Unintended pregnancies are a worldwide problem but disproportionately impact developing countries. There were 121 million unintended pregnancies annually from 2015 to 2019, corresponding to a global rate of 64 per 1000 women aged 15–49; 61% of these cases resulted in an abortion. In middle- and high-income countries, the unintended pregnancy rate fell by 21% from 1990–1994 to 2015–2019, whereas it fell by 18% in low-income countries over this time frame. It is important for primary care providers to educate their patients about the benefits of contraception and to provide options that are appropriate and desirable for the patient.

1. Oral Contraceptives

A. Combined Oral Contraceptives

1. Efficacy and methods of use—Combined oral contraceptives have a perfect use failure rate of 0.3% and a typical use failure rate of 8%. Their primary mode of action is suppression of ovulation. The pills can be started on the first day of the menstrual cycle, the first Sunday after the onset of the cycle, or on any day of the cycle. If started more than 5 days after the first day of the cycle, a backup method should be used for the first 7 days. If an active pill is missed at any time, and no intercourse occurred in the past 5 days, two pills should be taken immediately, and a backup method should be used for 7 days. If intercourse occurred in the previous 5 days, emergency contraception should be offered. A backup method should be used for 7 days.

2. Benefits of oral contraceptives—Noncontraceptive benefits of oral contraceptives include lighter menses and improvement of dysmenorrhea, decreased risk of ovarian and endometrial cancer, and improvement in acne. Functional ovarian cysts are less likely with oral contraceptive use. There is also a beneficial effect on bone mass.

3. Selection of an oral contraceptive—Any of the combination oral contraceptives containing 35 mcg or less of ethinyl estradiol or 3 mg of estradiol valerate are suitable for most women. There is some variation in potency of the various progestins in the pills, but there are essentially no clinically significant differences for most women among the progestins in the low-dose pills. There is insufficient evidence that triphasic oral contraceptives provide any benefit compared to monophasic oral contraceptives in terms of effectiveness, bleeding patterns, or discontinuation rates. Therefore, monophasic pills are recommended as a first choice for women starting oral contraceptive use. Women who have acne or hirsutism may benefit from treatment with desogestrel, drospirenone, or norgestimate, since they are the least androgenic. Pills are typically packaged in 21- or 28-day cyclic regimens but may be taken continuously to allow the user to decide if and when she has a withdrawal bleed. Studies have shown no significant risk from long-term amenorrhea in patients taking continuous oral contraceptives. The low-dose oral contraceptives commonly used in the United States are listed in Table 18–2.

4. Drug interactions—Several medications interact with oral contraceptives potentially decreasing their efficacy, typically by inducing microsomal enzymes in the liver. Some commonly prescribed medications in this category are phenytoin, phenobarbital (and other barbiturates), primidone, topiramate, carbamazepine, rifampin, and St. John's wort. Women taking these medications should use another means of contraception for maximum safety.

Antiretroviral medications, specifically ritonavir-boosted protease inhibitors, may significantly decrease the efficacy of combined oral contraceptives. Other antiretrovirals, such as nonnucleoside reverse transcriptase inhibitors, have smaller effects on oral contraceptive efficacy.

5. Contraindications and adverse effects—Oral contraceptives have been associated with many adverse effects; they are contraindicated with some conditions and should be used with caution in others (Table 18–3).

A. MYOCARDIAL INFARCTION—The risk of MI is higher with use of oral contraceptives in certain populations, but the risk attributable to oral contraceptives is low in reproductive age women. Cigarette smoking, obesity, hypertension, diabetes mellitus, or hypercholesterolemia increases the risk. Smokers over age 35 and women with other cardiovascular risk factors should use other non-estrogen–containing methods of birth control.

B. THROMBOEMBOLIC DISEASE—A three- to fivefold increased rate of venous thromboembolism is found in oral contraceptive users, but the absolute risk is low (5–6 per 100,000 woman-years compared to a rate of 50–300 per 100,000 pregnancies). Several studies have reported a two-fold increased risk in women using oral contraceptives containing the progestins, gestodene (not available in the United States), drospirenone, or desogestrel, compared with women using oral contraceptives with levonorgestrel and norethindrone. Women in whom thromboembolism develops should stop using oral contraceptives, as should those at increased risk for thromboembolism associated with surgery, fracture, serious injury, hypercoagulable condition, or immobilization. Women with a known thrombophilia should not use estrogen-containing contraceptives.

C. CEREBROVASCULAR DISEASE—Overall, a small increased risk of hemorrhagic stroke and subarachnoid hemorrhage and a somewhat greater increased risk of thrombotic stroke have been found; smoking, hypertension, and age over 35 years are associated with increased risk. Women should stop using estrogen-containing contraceptives if such warning symptoms as severe headache, blurred or lost vision, or other transient neurologic disorders develop.

D. CARCINOMA—There is no increased risk of breast cancer in women aged 35–64 who are current or former users of oral contraceptives. Women with a family history of breast cancer or women who started oral contraceptive use at a young age are not at increased risk. Combination oral contraceptives reduce the risk of endometrial carcinoma by 40% after 2 years of use and 60% after 4 or more years of use. The risk of ovarian cancer is reduced by 30% with pill use for less than 4 years, by 60% with pill use for 5–11 years, and by 80% with use for 12 or more years. Oral contraceptives have been associated with developing benign hepatocellular adenomas and peliosis hepatis (blood-filled cavities) (but not focal nodular hyperplasia or hepatocellular carcinoma); hepatocellular adenomas may rarely cause rupture of the liver, hemorrhage, and death. The risk of hepatocellular adenoma increases with higher dosage, longer duration of use, and older age.

E. HYPERTENSION—Oral contraceptives may cause hypertension in some women; the risk is increased with longer duration of use and older age. Women in whom hypertension develops while using oral contraceptives should use other non-estrogen–containing contraceptive methods. However, with regular blood pressure monitoring, nonsmoking women with well-controlled mild hypertension may use oral contraceptives.

Table 18–2. Commonly used low-dose oral contraceptives (listed within each group in order of increasing estrogen dose).

Name	Progestin	Estrogen (Ethinyl Estradiol)	Cost per Month[1]
Combination			
Alesse[2,3]	0.1 mg levonorgestrel	20 mcg	$35.20
Loestrin 1/20[2]	1 mg norethindrone acetate	20 mcg	$38.22
Mircette[2]	0.15 mg desogestrel	20 mcg	$59.98
Yaz[2]	3 mg drospirenone	20 mcg	$22.68
Loestrin 21 1.5/30[2]	1.5 mg norethindrone acetate	30 mcg	$34.44
Low Ogestrel[2]	0.3 mg norgestrel	30 mcg	$30.52
Levora[2]	0.15 mg levonorgestrel	30 mcg	$30.92
Desogen[2]	0.15 mg desogestrel	30 mcg	$35.55
Yasmin[2]	3 mg drospirenone	30 mcg	$22.12
Brevicon[2], Modicon[2]	0.5 mg norethindrone	35 mcg	$32.17
Demulen 1/35[2]	1 mg ethynodiol diacetate	35 mcg	$29.88
Ortho-Novum 1/35[2]	1 mg norethindrone	35 mcg	$10.33
Ortho-Cyclen[2]	0.25 mg norgestimate	35 mcg	$32.23
Gildagia[2]	0.4 mg norethindrone	35 mcg	$44.84
Combination: Extended-Cycle			
LoSeasonique (91-day cycle)[2]	0.10 mg levonorgestrel (days 1–84)/0 mg levonorgestrel (days 85–91)	20 mcg (84 days)/10 mcg (7 days)	$82.63
Amethyst (28-day pack)	90 mcg levonorgestrel	20 mcg	$59.40
Seasonique (91-day cycle)[2]	0.15 mg levonorgestrel (days 1–84)/0 mg levonorgestrel (days 85–91)	30 mcg (84 days)/10 mcg (7 days)	$67.70
Triphasic			
Estrostep[2]	1 mg norethindrone acetate (days 1–5) 1 mg norethindrone acetate (days 6–12) 1 mg norethindrone acetate (days 13–21)	20 mcg 30 mcg 35 mcg	$203.28
Cyclessa[2]	0.1 mg desogestrel (days 1–7) 0.125 mg desogestrel (days 8–14) 0.15 mg desogestrel (days 15–21)	25 mcg	$62.22
Tri-Lo-Estarylla	0.18 mg norgestimate (days 1–7) 0.215 mg norgestimate (days 8–14) 0.25 mg norgestimate (days 15–21)	25 mcg	$61.56
Trivora[2,3]	0.05 mg levonorgestrel (days 1–6) 0.075 mg levonorgestrel (days 7–11) 0.125 mg levonorgestrel (days 12–21)	30 mcg 40 mcg 30 mcg	$27.48
Ortho-Novum 7/7/7[2,3]	0.5 mg norethindrone (days 1–7) 0.75 mg norethindrone (days 8–14) 1 mg norethindrone (days 15–21)	35 mcg	$32.17
Tri Estarylla[2,3]	0.18 mg norgestimate (days 1–7) 0.215 mg norgestimate (days 8–14) 0.25 mg norgestimate (days 15–21)	35 mcg	$39.32
Tri-Norinyl[2,3]	0.5 mg norethindrone (days 1–7) 1 mg norethindrone (days 8–16) 0.5 mg norethindrone (days 17–21)	35 mcg	$73.11
Progestin-Only Pill			
Ortho Micronor[2,3]	0.35 mg norethindrone to be taken continuously	None	$36.90
Slynd	4 mg drospirenone (days 1–24)	None	$194.00

[1]Average wholesale price (AWP, for AB-rated generic when available) for quantity listed. Source: IBM Micromedex® Red Book (electronic version. IBM Watson Health, Greenwood Village, Colorado, USA. Available at: https://www-micromedexsolutions-com.proxy.hsl.ucdenver.edu/ (cited March 27, 2022).
[2]Generic equivalent available.
[3]Multiple other brands available.

Table 18–3. Contraindications to use of combined hormonal contraceptives.

Absolute contraindications
Pregnancy
Thrombophlebitis or thromboembolic disorders (past or present)
Stroke or CAD (past or present)
Cancer of the breast (known or suspected)
Undiagnosed abnormal vaginal bleeding
Estrogen-dependent cancer (known or suspected)
Hepatocellular adenoma (past or present)
Uncontrolled hypertension
Diabetes mellitus with vascular disease
Age ≥ 35 and smoking ≥ 15 cigarettes daily
Known thrombophilia
Migraine with aura
Active hepatitis
Surgery or orthopedic injury requiring prolonged immobilization
Relative contraindications
Migraine without aura
Hypertension
Heart or kidney disease
Diabetes mellitus
Gallbladder disease
Cholestasis during pregnancy
Sickle cell disease (S/S or S/C type)
Lactation

F. Headache—Migraine or other vascular headaches may occur or worsen with pill use. If severe or frequent headaches develop while using this method, it should be discontinued. Women with migraine headaches *with aura* should not use oral contraceptives due to the increased risk of stroke.

G. Lactation—Combined oral contraceptives can impair the quantity and quality of breast milk. While it is preferable to avoid the use of combination oral contraceptives during lactation, the effects on milk quality are small and are not associated with developmental abnormalities in infants. Combination oral contraceptives should not be started earlier than 4 weeks postpartum to allow for establishment of lactation and to avoid compounding the increased risk of postpartum thromboembolic disease. Progestin-only pills, levonorgestrel implants, and DMPA are alternatives with no adverse effects on milk supply.

H. Obesity—Obese and overweight women have generally been excluded from oral contraceptive trials until recently. Obesity is an independent risk factor for thromboembolic complications. However, obese women should not be denied effective contraception because of concerns about oral contraceptive complications or efficacy. Evidence suggests that efficacy is similar for overweight and obese women as for normal-weight individuals.

I. Other disorders—Depression may occur or be worsened with oral contraceptive use. Fluid retention may occur. Patients who had cholestatic jaundice during pregnancy may develop it while taking birth control pills.

6. Minor side effects—Nausea and dizziness may occur in the first few months of pill use. Spotting or breakthrough bleeding between menstrual periods may occur; this may be helped by switching to a pill of slightly greater estrogen potency. Missed menstrual periods may occur, especially with low-dose pills. A pregnancy test should be performed if pills have been skipped or an expected menstrual period is missed. Fatigue and decreased libido can occur. Chloasma may occur, as in pregnancy, and is increased by exposure to sunlight.

B. Progestin Minipill

1. Efficacy and methods of use—A formulation containing 0.35 mg of norethindrone alone is available in the United States. The efficacy is similar to that of combined oral contraceptives but depends highly on consistent use (eg, taking the pill within the same 3-hour window every day). A progestin-only pill containing drospirenone was approved by the US FDA in 2019, and a desogestrel-only pill is available in several countries outside the United States. The minipill is believed to prevent conception by causing thickening of the cervical mucus to make it hostile to sperm, by altering ovum transport (which may account for the slightly higher rate of ectopic pregnancy with these pills), and by inhibiting implantation. Ovulation is inhibited inconsistently with this method. The minipill is begun on the first day of a menstrual cycle and then taken continuously for as long as contraception is desired; there is no "placebo week."

2. Advantages—The low dose of progestin and absence of estrogen make the minipill safe for women with contraindications to estrogen therapy. Because estrogen may decrease initial milk production during lactation, the progestin minipill is an ideal choice for breastfeeding women. It also is often tried by women who want minimal doses of hormones and by patients who are over age 35. The minipill lacks the cardiovascular side effects of combination pills.

3. Complications and contraindications—There are few contraindications to the minipill (ie, current breast cancer). The minipill typically should be avoided in women with malabsorptive disease, current or past ischemic heart disease, and history of stroke. Minipill users often have bleeding irregularities (eg, prolonged flow, spotting, or amenorrhea); such patients may need regular pregnancy tests if there is a concern about contraceptive effectiveness. Many of the absolute contraindications and relative contraindications listed in Table 18–3 apply to the minipill; however, the contraceptive benefit of the minipill may outweigh the risks for patients who smoke, who are over age 35, or who have conditions such as superficial or deep venous thrombosis or known thromboembolic disorders or diabetes mellitus with vascular disease. Minor side effects of combination oral contraceptives such as mild headache may also occur with the minipill.

Bastianelli C et al. Pharmacodynamics of combined estrogen-progestin oral contraceptives: 4. Effects on uterine and cervical epithelia. Expert Rev Clin Pharmacol. 2020;13:163. [PMID: 31975619]

Bearak J et al. Global, regional, and subregional trends in unintended pregnancy and its outcomes from 1990 to 2014: estimates from a Bayesian hierarchical model. Lancet Glob Health. 2018;6:e380. [PMID: 29519649]

Bearak J et al. Unintended pregnancy and abortion by income, region, and the legal status of abortion: estimates from a comprehensive model for 1990-2019. Lancet Glob Health. 2020;8:E1152. [PMID: 32710833]

Serfaty D. Update on contraceptive contraindications. J Gynecol Obstet Hum Reprod. 2019;48:297. [PMID: 30796985]

Shufelt C et al. Hormonal contraception in women with hypertension. JAMA. 2020;324:1451. [PMID: 32955577]

Teal S et al. Contraception selection, effectiveness, and adverse effects: a review. JAMA. 2021;326:2507. [PMID: 34962522]

2. Contraceptive Injections & Implants (Long-Acting Progestins)

The injectable progestin depot medroxyprogesterone acetate (**DMPA**) is approved for contraceptive use in the United States. There has been extensive worldwide experience with this method over the past 3 decades. The medication is given as a deep intramuscular injection of 150 mg every 3 months and has a typical use failure rate of 4%. A subcutaneous preparation, containing 104 mg of DMPA is also available in the United States. Common side effects include irregular bleeding, amenorrhea, weight gain, and headache. It is associated with bone mineral loss that is reversible after discontinuation of the method. Users commonly have irregular bleeding initially and subsequently develop amenorrhea. Ovulation may be delayed after its discontinuation. Contraindications are similar to those for the minipill.

A single-rod, subdermal progestin implant, etonogestrel (**Nexplanon**), is approved for use in the United States. Nexplanon is a 40-mm by 2-mm rod containing 68 mg of the progestin etonogestrel that is inserted in the inner aspect of the nondominant arm. It is approved for use for 3 years, but data suggest it maintains effectiveness through 5 years. Hormone levels drop rapidly after removal, and there is no delay in the return of fertility. In clinical trials, the pregnancy rate was 0.0% with 3 years of use. Typical use failure is 0.1%. The side-effect profile is similar to that of the minipill and DMPA. Irregular bleeding has been the most common reason for discontinuation.

American College of Obstetricians and Gynecologists. Practice Bulletin No. 206: use of hormonal contraception in women with coexisting medical conditions. 2019;133:e128. [PMID: 30681544]

Bahamondes L et al. Long-acting reversible contraceptive (LARCs) methods. Best Pract Res Clin Obstet Gynaecol. 2020;66:28. [PMID: 32014434]

Dianat S et al. Side effects and health benefits of depot medroxyprogesterone acetate: a systematic review. Obstet Gynecol. 2019;133:332. [PMID: 30633132]

Espey E et al. Barriers and solutions to improve adolescent intrauterine device access. J Pediatr Adolesc Gynecol. 2019;32:S7. [PMID: 31585618]

Horvath S et al. From uptake to access: a decade of learning from ACOG LARC program. Am J Obstet Gynecol. 2020;222:S866. [PMID: 31794720]

Teal S et al. Contraception selection, effectiveness, and adverse effects: a review. JAMA. 2021;326:2507. [PMID: 34962522]

3. Other Combined Hormonal Contraceptives

A **transdermal contraceptive patch** is available that delivers a daily dose of norelgestromin (150 mcg) and ethinyl estradiol (35 mcg) and measures 20 cm^2. The patch is applied to the lower abdomen, upper torso, or buttock once a week for 3 consecutive weeks, followed by 1 week without the patch. It appears that the average steady-state concentration of ethinyl estradiol with the patch is approximately 60% higher than with a 35-mcg pill. However, there is no evidence for an increased incidence of estrogen-related side effects. The mechanism of action, side effects, and efficacy are similar to those associated with oral contraceptives, although compliance may be better. However, discontinuation due to side effects is more frequent.

A **contraceptive vaginal ring** that releases 120 mcg of etonogestrel and 15 mcg of ethinyl estradiol daily (Nuvaring) is available. The ring is soft and flexible and is placed in the upper vagina for 3 weeks, removed, and replaced 1 week later, or can be removed and immediately replaced after 4 weeks for continuous cycling, similar to oral contraceptives. The 1-year reusable segesterone acetate/ethinyl estradiol vaginal ring (Annovera) was approved by the US FDA in 2018. The ring is worn for 3 weeks and removed for 1 week, and that pattern is repeated for a total of 13 cycles. The efficacy, mechanism of action, and systemic side effects of combined hormonal vaginal rings are similar to those associated with oral contraceptives. Ring users may experience increased vaginal discharge.

4. Intrauterine Devices

In the United States, the following IUDs are available: the hormone (levonorgestrel)-releasing **Mirena, Liletta, Kyleena,** and **Skyla** IUDs and the copper-bearing **TCu380A (Paragard).** The mechanism of action of the copper IUD is thought to involve either spermicidal or inhibitory effects on sperm capacitation and transport. The hormonal IUDs also cause thickening of cervical mucus, prevent endometrial thickening, and can inhibit ovulation. IUDs are not abortifacients.

Skyla is FDA-approved for use for 3 years, Kyleena for 5 years, Liletta for 6 years, Mirena for 7 years, and the TCu380A for 10 years. The hormonal IUDs have the advantage of reducing cramping and menstrual flow. Mirena also is FDA-approved for the treatment of heavy menstrual bleeding.

The IUD is an excellent contraceptive method for most women. The devices are highly effective, with failure rates similar to those achieved with surgical sterilization. IUDs may be used in nulliparous women and adolescents. Women who are not in mutually monogamous relationships should also use condoms for protection from sexually transmitted infections. Hormonal IUDs may have a protective effect against upper tract infection similar to that of oral contraceptives.

A. Insertion

Insertion can be performed at any time during the menstrual cycle if pregnancy can be reasonably excluded. IUDs can be safely inserted in the immediate postabortal and postpartum periods. Both types of IUDs (hormonal and copper-bearing) may be inserted up to 48 hours after vaginal delivery, or prior to closure of the uterus at the time of cesarean section. Insertion immediately following abortion

Table 18–4. Contraindications to IUD use.

Absolute contraindications
Pregnancy
Acute or subacute pelvic inflammatory disease or purulent cervicitis
Significant anatomic abnormality of uterus
Unexplained uterine bleeding
Wilson disease or copper allergy (copper IUD)
Breast cancer (hormonal IUD)
Cervical, endometrial, or gestational trophoblastic neoplasia
Relative contraindications
Active liver disease (hormonal IUD)
Menorrhagia or severe dysmenorrhea (copper IUD)

IUD, intrauterine device.

is acceptable if there is no sepsis and if follow-up insertion a month later will not be possible; otherwise, it is wise to wait until 4 weeks postabortion. NSAIDs given as premedication may be helpful.

B. Contraindications and Complications

Contraindications to use of IUDs are outlined in Table 18–4.

1. Pregnancy—The copper-containing or levonorgestrel 52-mg IUD can be inserted within 5 days following a single episode of unprotected midcycle coitus as a **postcoital contraceptive**. An IUD should not be inserted into a pregnant uterus. If pregnancy occurs as an IUD failure, there is a greater chance of spontaneous abortion if the IUD is left in situ (50%) than if it is removed (25%). Women using an IUD who become pregnant should have the IUD removed if the string is visible. It can be removed at the time of abortion if that is desired. If the string is not visible and the patient wants to continue the pregnancy, she should be informed of the increased risk of miscarriage, infection, preterm birth, and abruption. She should be informed that any flu-like symptoms such as fever, myalgia, headache, or nausea warrant immediate medical attention for possible septic abortion.

Since the risk of ectopic pregnancy is increased in IUD users who become pregnant with an IUD in situ, clinicians should search for adnexal masses in early pregnancy and should always check the products of conception for placental tissue following abortion.

2. Pelvic infection—There is an increased risk of pelvic infection during the first month following insertion; however, prophylactic antibiotics are not recommended at the time of insertion since they do not appear to decrease this risk. The subsequent risk of pelvic infection appears to be primarily related to the risk of acquiring sexually transmitted infections. Infertility rates do not appear to be increased among women who have previously used the currently available IUDs. At the time of insertion, women with an increased risk of sexually transmitted infections should be screened for gonorrhea and chlamydia. Women with a history of recent or recurrent pelvic infection are not good candidates for an IUD.

3. Heavy menstrual bleeding or severe dysmenorrhea—The copper IUD can cause heavier menstrual periods, bleeding between periods, and more cramping, so it is generally not suitable for women who already suffer from these problems. Alternatively, the hormonal IUD Mirena has been approved by the US FDA to treat heavy menstrual bleeding. NSAIDs are also helpful in decreasing bleeding and pain in IUD users.

4. Complete or partial expulsion—Spontaneous expulsion of the IUD occurs in up to 10% of women during the first year of use. Any IUD should be removed if the body of the device can be seen or felt in the cervical os.

5. Missing IUD strings—If the transcervical tail cannot be seen, this may signify unnoticed expulsion, perforation of the uterus with abdominal migration of the IUD, or simply retraction of the string into the cervical canal or uterus. Once pregnancy is ruled out, the clinician may probe for the IUD with sterile sound or forceps designed for IUD removal. If the IUD cannot be detected, pelvic ultrasound will demonstrate if the IUD is intrauterine. Alternatively, obtain anteroposterior and lateral radiographs of the pelvis to evaluate for an extrauterine IUD. If the IUD is in the abdominal cavity, it should generally be removed by laparoscopy or laparotomy. Perforations of the uterus are less likely if insertion is performed slowly, with meticulous care taken to follow directions applicable to each type of IUD.

Averbach SH et al. Expulsion of intrauterine devices after postpartum placement by timing of placement, delivery type, and intrauterine device type: a systematic review and meta-analysis. Am J Obstet Gynecol. 2020;223:177. [PMID: 32142826]

De Nadai MN et al. Intracervical block for levonorgestrel-releasing intrauterine system placement among nulligravid women: a randomized double-blind controlled trial. Am J Obstet Gynecol. 2020;222:245. [PMID: 31541635]

Mazza D et al. Increasing long-acting reversible contraceptives: the Australian Contraceptive ChOice pRoject (ACCORd) cluster randomized trial. Am J Obstet Gynecol. 2020;222:S921. [PMID: 31837291]

Teal S et al. Contraception selection, effectiveness, and adverse effects: a review. JAMA. 2021;326:2507. [PMID: 34962522]

Turok DK et al. Levonorgestrel vs. copper intrauterine devices for emergency contraception. N Engl J Med. 2021;384:335. [PMID: 33503342]

5. Diaphragm & Cervical Cap

The **diaphragm (with contraceptive jelly)** is a safe and effective contraceptive method with features that make it acceptable to some women and not others. Typical use failure is 17%. The advantages of this method are that it has no systemic side effects and gives significant protection against pelvic infection and cervical dysplasia as well as pregnancy. The disadvantages are that it must be inserted near the time of coitus and that pressure from the rim predisposes some women to cystitis after intercourse.

The **cervical cap (with contraceptive jelly)** is similar to the diaphragm but fits snugly over the cervix only (the diaphragm stretches from behind the cervix to behind the pubic symphysis). The cervical cap is more difficult to insert and remove than the diaphragm. The main advantages are that it can be used by women who cannot be fitted for a diaphragm because of a relaxed anterior vaginal wall or by women who have discomfort with or in whom repeated bladder infections develop with the diaphragm. However, reported typical use failure rates are 14% in nulliparous women and 29% in parous women.

Because of the small risk of toxic shock syndrome, a cervical cap or diaphragm should not be left in the vagina for over 24 hours, nor should these devices be used during the menstrual period.

6. Contraceptive Foam, Cream, Film, Sponge, Jelly, & Suppository

These products are available without prescription, are easy to use, and have typical failure rates of 10–22%. All contain the spermicide nonoxynol-9, which also has some viricidal and bactericidal activity. Nonoxynol-9 does not appear to adversely affect the vaginal colonization of hydrogen peroxide–producing lactobacilli. The US FDA requires products containing nonoxynol-9 to include a warning that the products do not protect against HIV or other sexually transmitted infections and that use of these products can irritate the vagina and rectum and may increase the risk of HIV acquisition from an infected partner. A different on-demand vaginal contraceptive, a vaginal pH regulator gel containing lactic acid–citric acid–potassium bitartrate (commercial name Phexxi), was FDA-approved for use in the United States in 2020. The supporting clinical trial estimated 27.5 pregnancies per 100 woman-years.

Phexxi—a nonhormonal contraceptive gel. Med Lett Drugs Ther. 2020;62:129. [PMID: 32970042]

7. Condom

The male condom of latex, polyurethane or animal membrane affords protection against pregnancy—equivalent to that of a diaphragm and spermicidal jelly; latex and polyurethane (but not animal membrane) condoms also offer protection against many sexually transmitted infections, including HIV. When a spermicide, such as vaginal foam, is used with the condom, perfect use failure rate is approximately 2% and typical use, 13%. The disadvantages of condoms are dulling of sensation and spillage of semen due to tearing, slipping, or leakage with detumescence of the penis. Latex condoms should not be used with oil-based lubricants since these can degrade the condom and make it less effective.

Two female condoms, one made of polyurethane and the other of synthetic nitrile, are available in the United States. The reported failure rates range from 5% to 21%; the efficacy is comparable to that of the diaphragm. These are the only female-controlled method that offers significant protection against both pregnancy and sexually transmitted infections.

Beksinska M et al. Male and female condoms: their key role in pregnancy and STI/HIV prevention. Best Pract Res Clin Obstet Gynaecol. 2020;66:55. [PMID: 32007451]

8. Contraception Based on Awareness of Fertile Periods

These methods are most effective when the couple restricts intercourse to the post-ovular phase of the cycle or uses a barrier method at other times. Well-instructed, motivated couples may achieve low pregnancy rates with fertility awareness methods. Examples of some of these include monitoring cervical mucus changes, basal body temperature fluctuations, and menstrual cycle calculations to avoid having intercourse on fertile days. However, comparative efficacy trials of these methods against other contraceptive methods do not exist.

9. Emergency Contraception

Emergency contraception can decrease the risk of pregnancy after intercourse but before the establishment of pregnancy. These methods should be started as soon as possible and within 120 hours after unprotected coitus: (1) Levonorgestrel, 1.5 mg orally as a single dose (available in the United States prepackaged as Plan B and available over-the-counter for women aged 17 years and older), has a 1–2% failure rate when taken within 72 hours. It remains efficacious up to 120 hours after intercourse, though less so compared with earlier use. (2) If the levonorgestrel regimen is not available, a combination oral contraceptive containing ethinyl estradiol and levonorgestrel 1.5 mg given twice in 12 hours may be used. Used within 72 hours, the failure rate of these regimens is approximately 3%, but antinausea medication is often necessary. (3) Ulipristal acetate, a selective progesterone receptor modulator, taken orally as a single 30 mg dose, has been shown to be more effective than levonorgestrel, especially when used between 72 and 120 hours, particularly among overweight and obese women. Patients should wait 5 days after taking ulipristal to start or restart a hormonal contraceptive method. (4) Copper or levonorgestrel 52-mg IUD insertion within 5 days after one episode of unprotected midcycle coitus will also prevent pregnancy. Copper IUD use for emergency contraception is the most effective available method, with first cycle pregnancy rates of 0.1%. All victims of sexual violence should be offered emergency contraception.

Goldstuck ND et al. The efficacy of intrauterine devices for emergency contraception and beyond: a systemic review update. Int J Womens Health. 2019;11:471. [PMID: 31686919]

Shen J et al. Interventions for emergency contraception. Cochrane Database Syst Rev. 2019;1:CD001324. [PMID: 30661244]

Upadhya KK; Committee on Adolescence. Emergency contraception. Pediatrics. 2019;144:e20193149. [PMID: 31740497]

10. Sterilization

In the United States, sterilization is the most popular method of birth control for couples who want no more children. Although sterilization is reversible in some instances, reversal surgery for both women and men is costly, complicated, and not always successful. Therefore, patients should be counseled carefully before sterilization and should view the procedure as permanent.

Female sterilization procedures include laparoscopic bipolar electrocoagulation, salpingectomy, plastic ring application on the uterine tubes, or minilaparotomy with tubal resection. Salpingectomy may be preferred for the added benefit of decreasing ovarian cancer risk. The advantages of laparoscopy are minimal postoperative pain, small incisions, and rapid recovery. The advantages of minilaparotomy are that it can be performed with standard surgical instruments under local or general anesthesia. However, there is more postoperative pain and a longer recovery period. The cumulative 10-year failure rate for all methods combined is 1.85%, varying from 0.75% for postpartum partial salpingectomy and laparoscopic unipolar coagulation to 3.65% for spring clips; this fact should be discussed with women preoperatively. Some studies have found an increased risk of menstrual irregularities as a long-term complication of tubal ligation, but findings in different studies have been inconsistent. A method of transcervical sterilization, Essure, involving placement of an expanding nickel-titanium microcoil into the proximal uterine tube under hysteroscopic guidance, was approved by the US FDA in 2002. However, as of 2018, Essure was no longer marketed due to concerns related to complications and side effects reported by users.

Male sterilization by vasectomy is a safe, simple procedure in which the vas deferens is severed and sealed through a scrotal incision under local anesthesia. Long-term follow-up studies on vasectomized men show no excess risk of CVD. Despite past controversy, there is no definite association of vasectomy with prostate cancer.

When to Refer

Refer to experienced clinicians for etonogestrel subdermal (Nexplanon) insertion, IUD insertion, tubal occlusion or ligation, or vasectomy.

ACOG Practice Bulletin No. 208 Summary: benefits and risks of sterilization. Obstet Gynecol. 2019;133:592. [PMID: 30801465]

Mercier RJ et al. Expedited scheduling of interval tubal ligation: a randomized controlled trial. Obstet Gynecol. 2019;134:1178. [PMID: 31764727]

Zamorano AS et al. Postpartum salpingectomy: a procedure whose time has come. Am J Obstet Gynecol. 2019;220:8. [PMID: 30591122]

11. Abortion

Since the legalization of abortion in the United States in 1973, the related maternal mortality rate has fallen markedly because illegal and self-induced abortions have been replaced by safer procedures. Abortions in the first trimester of pregnancy are performed by vacuum aspiration under local anesthesia or with medical regimens. Dilation and evacuation, a variation of vacuum aspiration is generally used in the second trimester. Techniques utilizing intra-amniotic instillation of hypertonic saline solution or various prostaglandins regimens, along with medical or osmotic dilators are occasionally used after 18 weeks. Several medical abortion regimens using mifepristone and multiple doses of misoprostol have been reported as being effective in the second trimester. Overall, legal abortion in the United States has a mortality rate of less than 1:100,000. Rates of morbidity and mortality rise with length of gestation. In the United States, more than 60% of abortions are performed before 9 weeks, and more than 90% are performed before 13 weeks' gestation; only 1.2% are performed after 20 weeks. If abortion is chosen, every effort should be made to encourage the patient to seek an early procedure. In the United States, while numerous state laws limiting access to abortion and a federal law banning a rarely used variation of dilation and evacuation have been enacted, abortion remains legal and available until fetal viability (definition varies by state), under *Roe v. Wade*.

Complications resulting from abortion include retained products of conception (often associated with infection and heavy bleeding), uterine perforation, and unrecognized ectopic pregnancy. Immediate analysis of the removed tissue for placenta can exclude or corroborate the diagnosis of ectopic pregnancy. Women who have fever, bleeding, or abdominal pain after abortion should be examined; use of broad-spectrum antibiotics and reaspiration of the uterus are frequently necessary. Hospitalization is advisable if postabortal endometritis requires administration of intravenous antibiotics. Complications following illegal abortion often need emergency care for hemorrhage, septic shock, or uterine perforation.

Prophylactic antibiotics are recommended before surgical abortion; for example, a single dose of doxycycline 200 mg orally can be given 1 hour before the procedure. Rh immune globulin should be given to all Rh-negative women following abortion. Contraception should be thoroughly discussed, and contraception provided at the time of abortion. There is growing evidence to support the safety and efficacy of immediate postabortal insertion of IUDs.

Mifepristone (RU 486) is approved by the US FDA as an oral abortifacient at a dose of 200 mg orally on day 1, followed by misoprostol 800 mcg buccally 24–48 hours later. The WHO recommended regimen includes mifepristone orally followed by misoprostol vaginally, sublingually, or buccally. These combinations are 93% successful in terminating pregnancies of up to 70 days' gestation with few complications. There is a 5–10% risk of incomplete abortion requiring curettage and approximately 1% risk of requiring intervention for excessive bleeding. Overall, the risk of uterine infection is lower with medical than with surgical abortion.

Baiju N et al. Effectiveness, safety and acceptability of self-assessment of the outcome of first-trimester medical abortion: a systematic review and meta-analysis. BJOG. 2019;126:1536. [PMID: 31471989]

Mark KS et al. Risk of complication during surgical abortion in obese women. Am J Obstet Gynecol. 2018;218:238. [PMID: 29074080]

Schmidt-Hansen M et al. Follow-up strategies to confirm the success of medical abortion of pregnancies up to 10 weeks' gestation: a systematic review with meta-analyses. Am J Obstet Gynecol. 2020;222:551. [PMID: 31715147]

FEMALE SEXUAL DYSFUNCTION

General Considerations

Female sexual dysfunction is a common problem. Depending on the questions asked, surveys have shown that from 35% to 98% of women report sexual concerns. Questions related to sexual functioning should be asked as part of the routine medical history. Three helpful questions to broach the topic are "Are you currently involved in a sexual relationship?," "With men, women, or both?," and "Do you have any sexual concerns or any pain with sex?" If the woman is not involved in a sexual relationship, she should be asked if there are any concerns that are contributing to a lack of sexual behavior. If a history of sexual dysfunction is elicited, a complete history of factors that may affect sexual function should be taken. These factors include her reproductive history (including pregnancies and mode of delivery) as well as history of infertility, sexually transmitted infection, rape or sexual violence, gynecologic or urologic disorders, endocrine abnormalities (such as diabetes mellitus or thyroid disease), neurologic problems, CVD, psychiatric disease, and current prescription and over-the-counter medication use. A detailed history of the specific sexual dysfunction should be elicited, and a gynecologic examination should focus on findings that may contribute to sexual complaints.

Etiology

A. Disorders of Sexual Desire

Sexual desire in women is a complex and poorly understood phenomenon. Emotion is a key factor. Relationship conflict, fear or anxiety related to previous sexual encounters, or history of sexual abuse or violence may contribute to a lack of desire. Physical factors such as chronic illness, fatigue, depression, and specific medical disorders (such as diabetes mellitus, thyroid disease, or adrenal insufficiency) may also contribute. Menopause and attitudes toward aging may play a role. In addition, sexual desire may be influenced by other sexual dysfunction, such as arousal disorders, dyspareunia, or anorgasmia.

B. Sexual Arousal Disorders

Sexual arousal disorders may be both subjective and objective. Sexual stimulation normally leads to genital vasocongestion and lubrication. Some women may have a physiologic response to sexual stimuli but may not subjectively feel aroused because of factors such as distractions; negative expectations; anxiety; fatigue; depression; or medications, such as SSRIs or oral contraceptives. Other women with vaginal atrophy may lack both a subjective and physiologic response to sexual stimuli.

C. Orgasmic Disorders

Despite subjective and physiologic arousal, women may experience a marked delay in orgasm, diminished sensation of an orgasm, or anorgasmia. The etiology of orgasmic disorders is complex and typically multifactorial, but the cause of a particular patient's orgasmic disorder is usually amenable to treatment.

D. Sexual Pain Disorders

Dyspareunia (female sexual pain) is defined as recurrent or persistent genital pain that is provoked by sexual contact. **Vulvodynia** is a frequent cause of dyspareunia in premenopausal women. It is defined as vulvar pain of at least 3 months' duration without an identifiable cause. The discomfort may be experienced as either constant or intermittent, focal or diffuse, and spontaneous or provoked. There are generally no physical findings, except a subset of patients may have vulvar erythema.

Vaginismus is defined as recurrent or persistent involuntary spasm of the musculature of the lower third of the vagina that interferes with sexual intercourse, resulting from fear, pain, sexual violence, or a negative attitude toward sex, and causing marked distress or interpersonal difficulty. Other medical causes of sexual pain may include vulvovaginitis; vulvar disease, including lichen planus, lichen sclerosus, and lichen simplex chronicus; and pelvic disease, such as endometriosis or chronic PID; or vaginal atrophy.

Treatment

A. Disorders of Sexual Desire

In the absence of specific medical disorders, arousal or orgasmic disorders or dyspareunia, the focus of therapy is psychological. Cognitive behavioral therapy, sexual therapy, and couples therapy may all play a role. Success with pharmacologic therapy, particularly the use of dopamine agonists or testosterone with estrogen, has been reported. For premenopausal women with hypoactive sexual desire, bremelanotide 1.75 mg subcutaneously given at least 45 minutes before sexual activity can be effective therapy.

B. Sexual Arousal Disorders

As with disorders of sexual desire, arousal disorders may respond to psychological therapy. The phosphodiesterase inhibitors used in men do not appear to benefit most women with sexual arousal disorders. However, there is evidence to suggest a role for sildenafil in women with sexual dysfunction due to multiple sclerosis, type 1 diabetes mellitus, and spinal cord injury, and a role for antidepressant medications if other approaches fail.

Flibanserin (Addyi), an antidepressant, was approved by the US FDA in August 2015 as an effective treatment of hypoactive sexual desire disorder in premenopausal women; however, to be effective, it must be used long term and it has significant risks that require specific certifications of providers and pharmacies for dispensation to patients in the United States. While this medication remains available, it is rarely prescribed.

C. Orgasmic Disorders

For many women, counseling or sex therapy may be adequate treatment. There is an FDA-cleared vacuum device that increases clitoral blood flow; it may improve the likelihood of orgasm.

D. Sexual Pain Disorders

Specific painful disorders, such as endometriosis, vulvovaginitis, vulvar dermatoses, or vaginal atrophy, should be treated as outlined in other sections of this chapter.

Vaginismus may be treated initially with sexual counseling, education about anatomy and sexual function, and pelvic floor physical therapy by a specialized provider. The patient can be instructed in self-dilation, using a lubricated finger or dilators of graduated sizes. Before coitus (with adequate lubrication) is attempted, the patient—and then her partner—should be able to easily and painlessly introduce two fingers into the vagina. Penetration should never be forced, and the woman should always be the one to control the depth of insertion during dilation or intercourse. Injection of botulinum toxin has been used successfully in refractory cases.

Since the cause of vulvodynia is unknown, management is difficult. Few treatment approaches have been subjected to methodologically rigorous trials. A variety of topical agents have been tried, although only topical anesthetics (eg, estrogen cream and a compounded mixture of topical amitriptyline 2% and baclofen 2% in a water washable base) have been useful in relieving vulvodynia. Useful oral medications include amitriptyline in gradually increasing doses from 10 mg/day to 75–100 mg/day; gabapentin, starting at 300 mg three times daily and increasing to 1200 mg three times daily; and various SSRIs. Biofeedback and physical therapy, with a therapist experienced with the treatment of vulvar pain, have been shown to be helpful. Surgery—usually consisting of vestibulectomy—has been useful for women with introital dyspareunia. See also Chapter e6.

When to Refer

- When symptoms or concerns persist despite first-line therapy.
- For expertise in surgical procedures.

Clayton AH et al. Female sexual dysfunction. Med Clin North Am. 2019;103:681. [PMID: 31078200]

Kingsberg SA et al. Bremelanotide for the treatment of hypoactive sexual desire disorder: two randomized phase 3 trials. Obstet Gynecol. 2019;134:899. [PMID: 31599840]

Rogers RG et al. An International Urogynecological Association (IUGA)/International Continence Society (ICS) joint report on the terminology for the assessment of sexual health of women with pelvic floor dysfunction. Int Urogynecol J. 2018;29:647. [PMID: 29577166]

SEXUAL VIOLENCE

ESSENTIALS OF DIAGNOSIS

- The legal definition of rape varies by state and geographic location. The term "sexual violence" is used by the CDC and will be used in this discussion. It can be committed by a stranger, but more commonly the assailant is known to the victim, including a current or former partner or spouse (a form of intimate partner violence [IPV]).
- All victims of sexual violence should be offered emergency contraception.
- The many individuals affected, the enormous health care costs, and the need for a multidisciplinary approach make sexual violence and IPV important health care issues.
- Knowledge of state laws and collection of evidence requirements are essential for clinicians evaluating possible victims of sexual violence, including IPV.

General Considerations

Rape, or sexual assault, is legally defined in different ways in various jurisdictions. Clinicians and emergency department personnel who deal with victims of sexual violence should be familiar with the laws pertaining to sexual assault in their own state. From a medical and psychological viewpoint, it is essential that persons treating victims of sexual violence recognize the nonconsensual and violent nature of the crime. About 95% of people who report sexual violence are women. Each year in the United States, 4.8 million incidents of physical or sexual assault are reported by women. Penetration may be vaginal, anal, or oral and may be by the penis, hand, or a foreign object. The assailant may be unknown to the victim or, more frequently, may be an acquaintance or even the spouse.

"Unlawful sexual intercourse," or statutory rape, is intercourse with a female before the age of majority even with her consent.

Health care providers can have a significant impact in increasing the reporting of sexual violence and in identifying resources for the victims. The International Rescue Committee has developed a multimedia training tool to encourage competent, compassionate, and confidential clinical care for sexual violence survivors in low-resource settings. They have studied this intervention in over 100 health care providers and found that knowledge increased from 49% to 62% ($P < 0.001$) and confidence from 58% to 73% ($P < 0.001$) in clinical care for sexual violence survivors following training. There was also a documented increase in eligible survivors receiving emergency contraception from 50% to 82% ($P < 0.01$), HIV postexposure prophylaxis from 42% to 92% ($P < 0.001$), and sexually transmitted infection prophylaxis and treatment from 45% to 96% ($P < 0.01$). This training encourages providers to offer care in the areas of pregnancy and sexually transmitted infection prevention as well as assistance for psychological trauma.

Because sexual violence is a personal crisis, each patient will react differently, but anxiety disorders and PTSD are common sequelae. The **rape trauma syndrome** comprises two principal phases: (1) Immediate or acute: shaking, sobbing, and restless activity may last from a few days to a few weeks. The patient may experience anger, guilt, or shame or may repress these emotions. Reactions vary depending on the victim's personality and the circumstances of the attack. (2) Late or chronic: problems related to the attack may develop weeks or months later. Sexual violence survivors are at increased risk for developing several psychological and behavioral adverse effects, including PTSD, sleep disturbances, anxiety, depression, suicide attempt, and medication misuse.

Clinicians and emergency department personnel who deal with victims of sexual violence should work with community rape crisis centers or other sources of ongoing psychological support and counseling.

Examination

The clinician who first sees the alleged victim of sexual violence should be empathetic and prepared with appropriate evidence collection and treatment materials. Standardized information and training, such as the program created by the International Rescue Committee, can be a helpful resource to the providers caring for these patients. Many emergency departments have a protocol for sexual violence victims and personnel who are trained in interviewing and examining victims of sexual violence.

Treatment

1. Give analgesics or sedatives if indicated. Administer tetanus toxoid if deep lacerations contain soil or dirt particles.
2. Give ceftriaxone, 250 mg intramuscularly, plus azithromycin, 1 g orally, to prevent gonorrhea and chlamydia. In addition, give metronidazole, 2 g orally, as a single dose to treat trichomoniasis. Incubating syphilis will probably be prevented by these medications, but the VDRL test should be repeated 6 weeks after the assault.
3. Prevent pregnancy by using one of the methods discussed under Emergency Contraception.
4. Vaccinate against hepatitis B.
5. Offer HIV prophylaxis (see Chapter 31).
6. Because women who are sexually assaulted are at increased risk for long-term psychological sequelae, such as PTSD and anxiety disorders, it is critical that the patient and her family and friends have a source of ongoing counseling and psychological support.

When to Refer

All women who seek care for sexual assault should be referred to a facility that has expertise in the management of victims of sexual violence and is qualified to perform expert forensic examination, if requested.

Adams JA et al. Interpretation of medical findings in suspected child sexual abuse: an update for 2018. J Pediatr Adolesc Gynecol. 2018;31:225. [PMID: 29294380]

American College of Obstetricians and Gynecologists. ACOG Committee Opinion No. 777: sexual assault. Obstet Gynecol. 2019;133:e296. [PMID: 30913202]

Pastor-Moreno G et al. Intimate partner violence during pregnancy and risk of fetal and neonatal death: a meta-analysis with socioeconomic context indicators. Am J Obstet Gynecol. 2020;222:123. [PMID: 31394067]

BARTHOLIN DUCT CYSTS & ABSCESSES

Trauma or infection may involve the Bartholin duct, causing obstruction of the gland. Drainage of secretions is obstructed, leading to pain, swelling, and abscess formation (Figure 18–1).

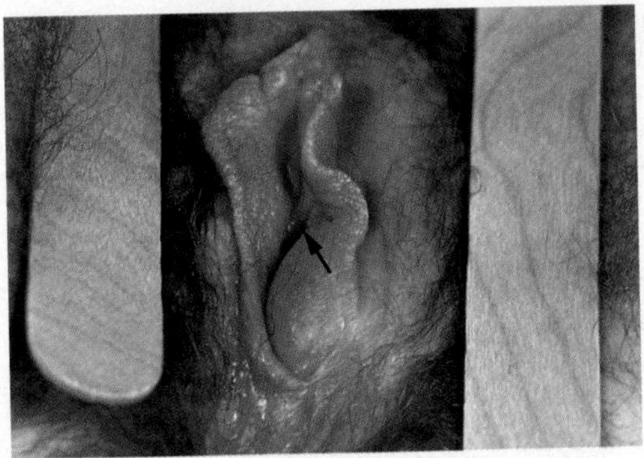

▲ **Figure 18–1.** Bartholin cyst (abscess). The Bartholin gland is located in the lower two-thirds of the introitus. (From Susan Lindsley, Public Health Image Library, CDC.)

The principal symptoms are periodic painful swelling on either side of the introitus and dyspareunia. A fluctuant swelling, usually 1–4 cm in diameter lateral to either labium minus, is a sign of occlusion of a Bartholin duct. Tenderness is suggestive of active infection.

Purulent drainage or secretions from the gland should be tested for *Neisseria gonorrhoeae*, *Chlamydia trachomatis*, and other pathogens, and treated accordingly (see Chapter 33); frequent warm sitz baths may be helpful. Abscesses or cysts that are symptomatic should undergo incision and drainage with additional efforts to keep the drainage tract open (eg, Word catheter or marsupialization). Marsupialization should be considered for recurrence. Antibiotics are unnecessary unless cellulitis is present. In women under 40, asymptomatic cysts do not require therapy; in women over age 40, biopsy or removal should be considered to rule out vulvar carcinoma.

When to Refer

When surgical therapy (marsupialization) is indicated.

Dole DM et al. Management of Bartholin duct cysts and gland abscesses. J Midwifery Womens Health. 2019;64:337. [PMID: 30734519]

Omole F et al. Bartholin duct cyst and gland abscess: office management. Am Fam Physician. 2019;99:760. [PMID: 31194482]

VAGINITIS

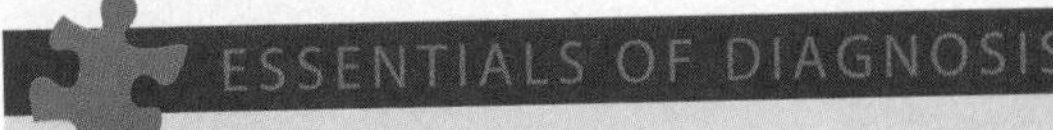

ESSENTIALS OF DIAGNOSIS

- Vaginal irritation.
- Pruritus.
- Abnormal or malodorous discharge.

General Considerations

Inflammation and infection of the vagina are common gynecologic complaints, resulting from a variety of pathogens, allergic reactions to vaginal contraceptives or other products, vaginal atrophy, or friction during coitus. The normal vaginal pH is 4.5 or less, and *Lactobacillus* is the predominant organism. Normal secretions during the middle of the cycle, or during pregnancy, can be confused with vaginitis.

Clinical Findings

When the patient complains of vaginal irritation, pain, pruritus or unusual or malodorous discharge, a history should be taken, noting the onset, location, duration, and characterization of symptoms including triggers and alleviating factors. Additional history should include the LMP; recent sexual activity; use of contraceptives, tampons, or douches; and recent changes in medications or use of antibiotics. The physical examination should include careful inspection of the vulva and speculum examination of the vagina and cervix. A vaginal, cervical, or urine sample can be obtained for detection of gonococcus and chlamydia, if clinically indicated. Evaluation for yeast, bacterial vaginosis, and trichomonas should be performed. The vaginal pH should be tested; it is frequently greater than 4.5 in infections due to trichomonads and bacterial vaginosis. A bimanual examination to look for evidence of pelvic infection, namely cervical motion, uterine, or adnexal tenderness, should follow. Point-of-care testing is available for all three main organisms that cause vaginitis and can be used if microscopy is not available or for confirmatory testing of microscopy.

A. Vulvovaginal Candidiasis

Pregnancy, diabetes mellitus, and use of broad-spectrum antibiotics or corticosteroids predispose patients to *Candida* infections. Heat, moisture, and occlusive clothing also contribute to the risk. Pruritus, vulvovaginal erythema, and a white curd-like discharge that is not malodorous are found (Figure 18–2). Microscopic examination with 10% potassium hydroxide reveals hyphae and spores. A swab for cultures or for PCR testing may be performed if *Candida* is suspected but not demonstrated.

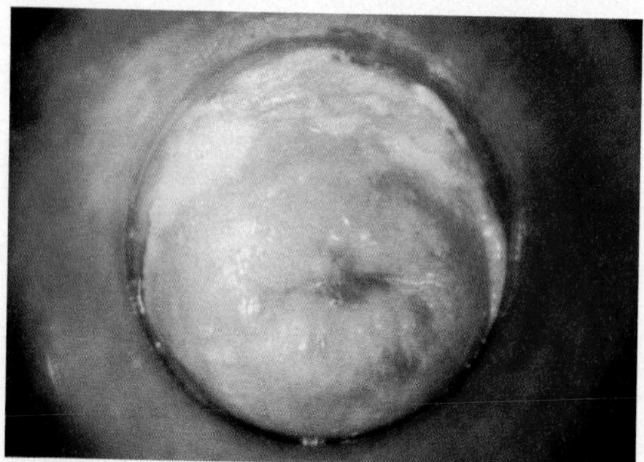

▲ **Figure 18–2.** Cervical candidiasis. (Public Health Image Library, CDC.)

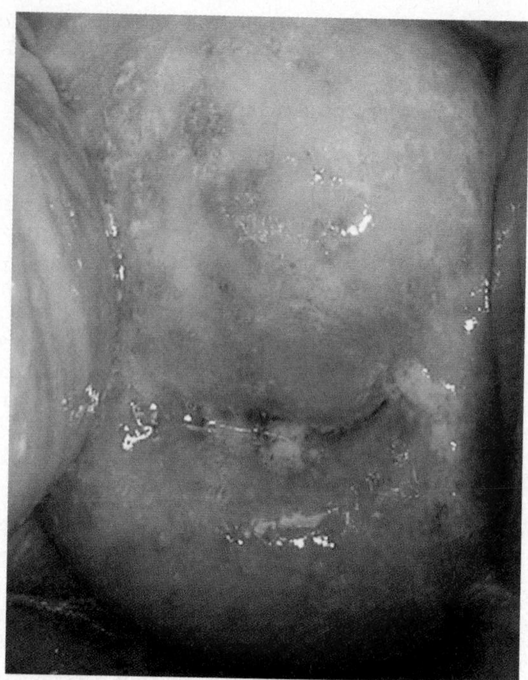

▲ **Figure 18–3.** Strawberry cervix in *Trichomonas vaginalis* infection, with inflammation and punctate hemorrhages. (Reproduced with permission from Richard P. Usatine, MD, in Usatine RP, Smith MA, Mayeaux EJ Jr, Chumley H, Tysinger J. *The Color Atlas of Family Medicine*. McGraw-Hill, 2009.)

B. *Trichomonas vaginalis* Vaginitis

This sexually transmitted protozoal flagellate infects the vagina, Skene ducts, and lower urinary tract in women and the lower genitourinary tract in men. Pruritus and a malodorous frothy, yellow-green discharge occur, along with diffuse vaginal erythema and red macular lesions on the cervix in severe cases ("**strawberry cervix**," Figure 18–3). Motile organisms with flagella seen by microscopic examination of a wet mount with saline solution is confirmatory but are identified in only 60–70% of cases. Nucleic acid amplification tests are highly sensitive and specific to identify *T vaginalis*. Other rapid diagnostic tests with improved sensitivity compared to wet mount (eg, Affirm VP III and OSOM *Trichomonas* Rapid Test) are commercially available.

C. Bacterial Vaginosis

Bacterial vaginosis is a polymicrobial disease that is *not* considered a sexually transmitted infection, but sexual activity is a risk factor. An overgrowth of *Gardnerella* and other anaerobes is often associated with increased malodorous discharge without obvious vulvitis or vaginitis. The discharge is grayish and sometimes frothy, with a pH of 5.0–5.5. An amine-like ("fishy") odor is present if a drop of discharge is alkalinized with 10% potassium hydroxide. On wet mount in saline, epithelial cells are covered with bacteria to such an extent that cell borders are obscured

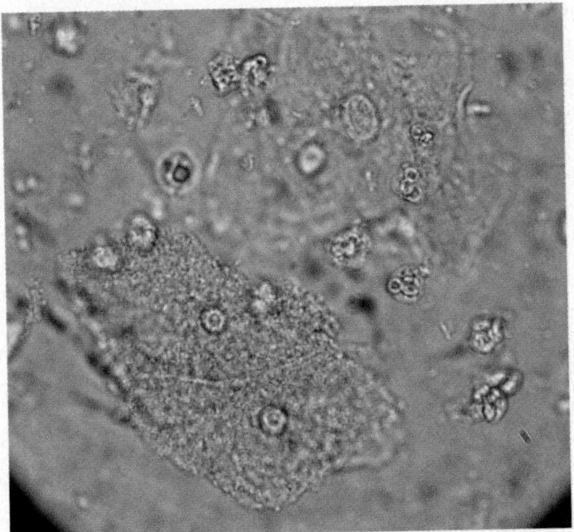

▲ **Figure 18–4.** Clue cells seen in bacterial vaginosis due to *Gardnerella vaginalis.* (Reproduced with permission from Richard P. Usatine, MD, in Usatine RP, Smith MA, Mayeaux EJ Jr, Chumley H, Tysinger J. *The Color Atlas of Family Medicine*. McGraw-Hill, 2009.)

(**clue cells**, Figure 18–4). Vaginal cultures are generally not useful in diagnosis; however, molecular testing is available.

Treatment

A. Vulvovaginal Candidiasis

A variety of topical and oral regimens are available to treat vulvovaginal candidiasis. Women with uncomplicated vulvovaginal candidiasis will usually respond to a 1- to 3-day regimen of a topical azole or a one-time dose of oral fluconazole 150 mg. Women with complicated infection (including four or more episodes in 1 year [*recurrent* vulvovaginal candidiasis], severe symptoms and signs, non-albicans species, uncontrolled diabetes mellitus, HIV infection, corticosteroid treatment, or pregnancy) should receive 7–14 days of a topical regimen or two doses of oral fluconazole 3 days apart. In recurrent non-albicans infections, boric acid 600 mg in a gelatin capsule intravaginally once daily for 2 weeks is approximately 70% effective. If recurrence occurs, referral to a gynecologist or an infectious disease specialist is indicated.

1. Single-dose regimens—Effective single-dose regimens include miconazole (1200-mg vaginal suppository), tioconazole (6.5% cream, 5 g vaginally), sustained-release butoconazole (2% cream, 5 g vaginally), or fluconazole (150-mg oral tablet).

2. Three-day regimens—Effective 3-day regimens include butoconazole (2% cream, 5 g vaginally once daily), clotrimazole (2% cream, 5 g vaginally once daily), terconazole (0.8% cream, 5 g, or 80-mg vaginal suppository once daily), or miconazole (200-mg vaginal suppository once daily).

3. Seven-day regimens—The following regimens are given once daily: clotrimazole (1% cream), miconazole (2% cream, 5 g, or 100-mg vaginal suppository), or terconazole (0.4% cream, 5 g).

4. Recurrent vulvovaginal candidiasis (maintenance therapy)—Clotrimazole (500-mg vaginal suppository once weekly or 200 mg cream twice weekly) or fluconazole (100, 150, or 200 mg orally once weekly) is an effective regimen for maintenance therapy for up to 6 months.

B. *Trichomonas vaginalis* Vaginitis

Treatment of both partners simultaneously is recommended; metronidazole 500 mg orally twice a day for 7 days or tinidazole, 2 g orally as a single dose is usually used.

In the case of treatment failure with metronidazole in the absence of reexposure, the patient should be re-treated with metronidazole or tinidazole, 2 g orally once daily for 7 days. If this is not effective in eradicating the organisms, metronidazole and tinidazole susceptibility testing can be arranged with the CDC at 404-718-4141 or at https://www.cdc.gov/std. Women infected with *T vaginalis* are at increased risk for concurrent infection with other sexually transmitted diseases (STDs) and should be offered comprehensive STD testing.

C. Bacterial Vaginosis

The recommended regimens are metronidazole (500 mg orally, twice daily for 7 days), clindamycin vaginal cream (2%, 5 g, once daily for 7 days), or metronidazole gel (0.75%, 5 g, twice daily for 5 days). Alternative regimens include clindamycin (300 mg orally twice daily for 7 days), clindamycin ovules (100 g intravaginally at bedtime for 3 days), tinidazole (2 g orally once daily for 2 days), tinidazole (1 g orally once daily for 5 days) or secnidazole (2 g oral granules in single dose). The National STD Curriculum offers a helpful training module to clinicians to review current recommendations for treatment of vaginitis (https://www.std.uw.edu/custom/self-study/vaginitis).

American College of Obstetricians and Gynecologists. ACOG Practice Bulletin No. 215: vaginitis in nonpregnant patient. Obstet Gynecol. 2020;135:e1. [PMID: 31856123]

Giovanini AF et al. Bacterial vaginosis and desquamative inflammatory vaginitis. N Engl J Med. 2019;380:1088. [PMID: 30865815]

Neal CM et al. Noncandidal vaginitis: a comprehensive approach to diagnosis and management. Am J Obstet Gynecol. 2020; 222:114. [PMID: 31513780]

PELVIC INFLAMMATORY DISEASE (Salpingitis, Endometritis)

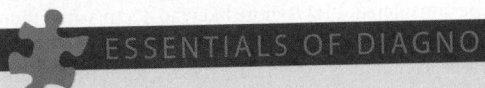

- Lower abdominal or pelvic pain.
- Uterine, adnexal, or cervical motion tenderness.
- Absence of a competing diagnosis.

General Considerations

Pelvic inflammatory disease is a polymicrobial infection of the upper genital tract associated with the sexually transmitted organisms *N gonorrhoeae* and *C trachomatis* as well as endogenous organisms, including anaerobes, *Haemophilus influenzae*, enteric gram-negative rods, and streptococci. It is most common in young, nulliparous, sexually active women with multiple partners and is a leading cause of infertility and ectopic pregnancy. The use of barrier methods of contraception may provide significant protection.

Clinical Findings

A. Symptoms and Signs

Patients with PID most commonly present with lower abdominal pain. Additional complaints may include AUB and abnormal vaginal discharge. Systemic features such as fever typically indicate more severe disease, including pelvic abscess. Right upper quadrant pain may indicate an associated perihepatitis **(Fitz-Hugh-Curtis syndrome).** Diagnosis of PID is complicated by the fact that women may have subtle or mild symptoms that are not readily recognized as PID, such as postcoital bleeding, urinary frequency, or low back pain.

B. Minimum Diagnostic Criteria

PID is diagnosed clinically. Women with cervical motion, uterine, or adnexal tenderness meet diagnostic criteria for PID and should be treated with antibiotics unless there is a competing diagnosis, such as ectopic pregnancy or appendicitis.

C. Additional Criteria

No single historical, physical, or laboratory finding is definitive for acute PID. The following criteria may be used to enhance the specificity of the diagnosis: (1) oral temperature higher than 38.3°C, (2) abnormal cervical or vaginal discharge with white cells on saline microscopy (greater than 1 leukocyte per epithelial cell), (3) elevated ESR, (4) elevated CRP, and (5) laboratory documentation of cervical infection with *N gonorrhoeae* or *C trachomatis*. Testing for gonorrhea and chlamydia should be performed. Treatment should not be delayed while awaiting results.

Differential Diagnosis

Appendicitis, ectopic pregnancy, septic abortion, hemorrhagic or ruptured ovarian cysts or tumors, torsion of an ovarian cyst, degeneration of a myoma, and acute enteritis must be considered. PID is more likely to occur when there is a prior history of PID, recent sexual contact, recent onset of menses, recent insertion of an IUD, or recent intercourse with a partner who has a sexually transmitted infection. Acute PID is highly unlikely when recent (within 60 days) intercourse has not taken place. A sensitive serum pregnancy test should be obtained to rule out ectopic pregnancy. Pelvic ultrasonography is helpful to rule out tubo-ovarian abscess. Laparoscopy should be considered when imaging is not informative, and the patient has not responded to outpatient treatment for PID or has not improved after 72 hours of inpatient treatment; it should also be considered when an acutely ill patient has a high suspicion of a competing diagnosis requiring surgical intervention (eg, appendicitis). The appendix should be visualized at laparoscopy to rule out appendicitis. Cultures should be obtained at laparoscopy.

Treatment

A. Antibiotics

Early treatment with appropriate antibiotics effective against *N gonorrhoeae*, *C trachomatis*, and the endogenous organisms listed above is essential to prevent long-term sequelae. The sexual partner should be treated appropriately. Most women with mild to moderate disease can be treated successfully as an outpatient. The recommended outpatient regimen is ceftriaxone (500 mg intramuscularly; 1 g for persons who weigh 150 kg or greater) plus doxycycline (100 mg orally twice a day for 14 days) with metronidazole 500 mg orally twice a day **or** a single dose of cefoxitin (2 g intramuscularly) with probenecid (1 g orally) plus doxycycline (100 mg orally twice daily for 14 days) and metronidazole 500 mg orally twice daily for 14 days. For patients with severe disease or those who meet criteria for hospitalization, there are two recommended regimens. One regimen includes either cefotetan, 2 g intravenously every 12 hours, or cefoxitin, 2 g intravenously every 6 hours or ceftriaxone, 1 g intravenously every 24 hours, plus doxycycline, 100 mg orally or intravenously every 12 hours. The other recommended regimen is clindamycin, 900 mg intravenously every 8 hours, plus gentamicin, a loading dose of 2 mg/kg intravenously or intramuscularly followed by a maintenance dose of 1.5 mg/kg every 8 hours (or as a single daily dose, 3–5 mg/kg). These regimens should be continued for at least 24 hours after the patient shows significant clinical improvement. Then, an oral regimen should be given for a total course of antibiotics of 14 days with doxycycline, 100 mg orally twice a day and metronidazole, 500 mg orally twice a day.

B. Surgical Measures

Surgery is reserved for cases of suspected tubo-ovarian abscess rupture or cases with a poor response to antibiotics. Unless rupture is suspected, the clinician should institute high-dose antibiotic therapy in the hospital, and monitor therapy with ultrasound. In 70% of cases, antibiotics are effective, but in 30%, there is inadequate response in 48–72 hours and surgical intervention is required. Unilateral adnexectomy is acceptable for unilateral abscess. Hysterectomy and bilateral salpingo-oophorectomy may be necessary for overwhelming infection or in cases of chronic disease with intractable pelvic pain.

Prognosis

Despite treatment, long-term sequelae, including repeated episodes of infection, chronic pelvic pain, dyspareunia, ectopic pregnancy, or infertility, develop in one-fourth of women with acute disease. The risk of infertility increases with repeated episodes of salpingitis: it is estimated at 10% after the first episode, 25% after a second episode, and 50% after a third episode.

When to Admit

The following patients with acute PID should be admitted for intravenous antibiotic therapy:

- The patient has a tubo-ovarian abscess (direct inpatient observation for at least 24 hours before switching to outpatient parenteral therapy).
- The patient is pregnant.
- The patient cannot follow or tolerate an outpatient regimen.
- The patient has not responded clinically to outpatient therapy within 72 hours.
- The patient has severe illness, nausea and vomiting, or high fever.
- Another surgical emergency, such as appendicitis, cannot be ruled out.

Curry A et al. Pelvic inflammatory disease: diagnosis, management and prevention. Am Fam Physician. 2019;100:357. [PMID: 31524362]

Ross J et al. 2017 European guideline for the management of pelvic inflammatory disease. Int J STD AIDS. 2018;29:108. [PMID: 29198181]

US Preventive Services Task Force; Krist AH et al. Behavioral counseling interventions to prevent sexually transmitted infections: US Preventive Services Task Force Recommendation Statement. JAMA. 2020;324:674. [PMID: 32809008]

Workowski KA et al. Sexually transmitted infections treatment guidelines, 2021. MMWR Recomm Rep. 2021;70:1. [PMID: 34292926]

CONDYLOMA ACUMINATA

Warty growths on the vulva, perianal area, vaginal walls, or cervix are caused by various types of HPV. Pregnancy and immunosuppression favor growth. Ninety percent of genital warts are caused by HPV 6 and 11. With increasing use of the HPV vaccine in the United States, the prevalence of HPV types 6, 11, 16 and 18 decreased from 11.5% in 2003–2006 to 4.3% in 2009–2012 among girls aged 14–19 years, and from 18.5% to 12.1% in women aged 20–24 years. Vulvar lesions may be obviously wart-like or may be diagnosed only after application of 4% acetic acid (vinegar) and colposcopy, when they appear whitish, with prominent papillae. Vaginal lesions may show diffuse hypertrophy or a cobblestone appearance.

Recommended treatments for vulvar warts include podophyllum resin 10–25% in tincture of benzoin (do not use during pregnancy or on bleeding lesions) or 80–90% trichloroacetic or bichloroacetic acid, carefully applied to avoid the surrounding skin. The pain of bichloroacetic or trichloroacetic acid application can be lessened by a sodium bicarbonate paste applied immediately after treatment. Podophyllum resin must be washed off after 2–4 hours. Freezing with liquid nitrogen or a cryoprobe and electrocautery are also effective. Patient-applied regimens, useful when the entire lesion is accessible to the patient, include podofilox 0.5% solution or gel, imiquimod 5% cream, or sinecatechins 15% ointment. Vaginal warts may be treated with cryotherapy with liquid nitrogen or trichloroacetic acid. Extensive warts may require treatment with CO_2 laser, electrocautery, or excision under local or general anesthesia.

Grennan D. JAMA patient page. Genital warts. JAMA. 2019;321:520. [PMID: 30721297]

Meites E et al. Human papillomavirus vaccination for adults: updated recommendations of the Advisory Committee on Immunization Practices. MMWR Morb Mortal Wkly Rep. 2019;68:698. [PMID: 31415491]

CERVICAL INTRAEPITHELIAL NEOPLASIA (CIN) (Dysplasia of the Cervix)

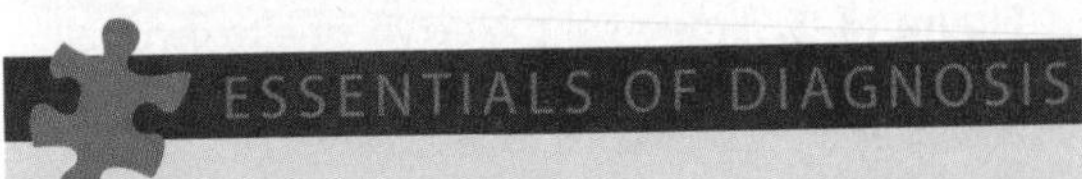

- The presumptive diagnosis is made by an abnormal Papanicolaou smear.
- Diagnose by colposcopically directed biopsy.

General Considerations

The squamocolumnar junction of the cervix is an area of active squamous cell proliferation. In childhood, this junction is located on the exposed vaginal portion of the cervix. At puberty, because of hormonal influence and possibly because of changes in the vaginal pH, the squamous margin begins to encroach on the single-layered, mucus-secreting epithelium, creating an area of metaplasia (**transformation zone**). Infection with HPV (see Prevention, below) may lead to cellular abnormalities, which over time may develop into squamous cell dysplasia or cancer. There are varying degrees of dysplasia (Table 18–5), defined by the degree of cellular atypia; all atypia must be observed and treated if persistent or worsening.

Table 18–5. Classification systems for Papanicolaou smears.

Dysplasia	CIN	Bethesda System
Benign	Benign	Normal
Benign with inflammation	Benign with inflammation	Normal, ASC-US
Mild dysplasia	CIN I	Low-grade SIL
Moderate dysplasia	CIN II	High-grade SIL
Severe dysplasia	CIN III	High-grade SIL
Carcinoma in situ	—	—
Invasive cancer	Invasive cancer	Invasive cancer

ASC-US, atypical squamous cells of undetermined significance; CIN, cervical intraepithelial neoplasia; SIL, squamous intraepithelial lesion.

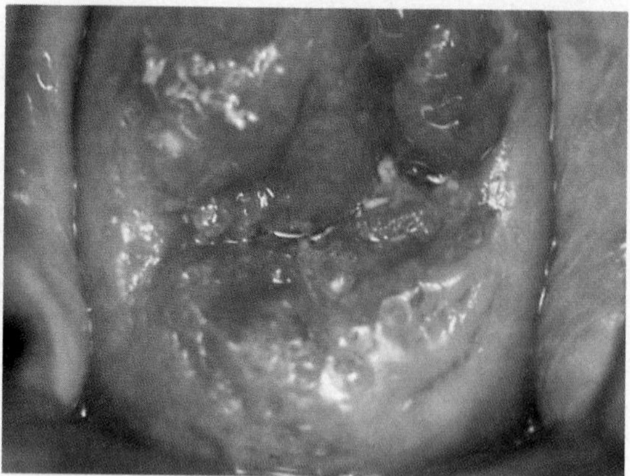

▲ **Figure 18–5.** Erosion of the cervix due to cervical intraepithelial neoplasia (CIN), a precursor lesion to cervical cancer. (Public Health Image Library, CDC.)

Clinical Findings

There are no specific symptoms or signs of CIN. The presumptive diagnosis is made by cytologic screening of an asymptomatic population with no grossly visible cervical changes. All visible abnormal cervical lesions should be biopsied (Figure 18–5).

Screening & Diagnosis

A. Cytologic Examination (Papanicolaou Smear)

In immunocompetent women, cervical cancer screening should begin at age 21. The recommendation to start screening at age 21 years regardless of the age of onset of sexual intercourse is based on the very low incidence of cancer in younger women and the potential for adverse effects associated with treatment of young women with abnormal cytology screening results. In contrast to the high rate of infection with HPV in sexually active adolescents, invasive cervical cancer is very rare in women younger than age 21 years. The USPSTF 2018 statement recommends screening for cervical cancer in women aged 21–65 years as follows: for women aged 21–29 years, screening with cytology (conventional [Papanicolaou smear] or liquid-based) alone every 3 years; and for women aged 30–65 years, screening with cytology alone every 3 years, with high-risk HPV testing alone every 5 years, or with a combination of cytology and high-risk HPV testing (co-testing) every 5 years. These recommendations apply to women who have a cervix, regardless of their sexual history or HPV vaccination status. They do not apply to women who have a previous diagnosis of cervical cancer or a high-grade precancerous cervical lesion (ie, CIN grade II or III), women with immune compromise (eg, living with HIV), or women with in utero exposure to diethylstilbestrol; such women may require more frequent screening.

The USPSTF recommends against screening for cervical cancer for women younger than age 21 years, for women older than age 65 years who have had adequate prior screening and are not otherwise at high risk for cervical cancer, and for women who have had a hysterectomy with removal of the cervix and who have no history of cervical cancer or a high-grade precancerous lesion.

The goal of screening is to identify high-grade precancerous cervical lesions to prevent their progression to cervical cancer. These high-grade cervical lesions may be treated with excisional and ablative therapies. Screening and management guidelines are continually undergoing evaluation and change frequently.

Cytologic reports from the laboratory may describe findings in one of several ways (see Table 18–5). The Bethesda System uses the terminology "atypical squamous cells of unknown significance" (**ASC-US**) and "squamous intraepithelial lesions," either low-grade (**LSIL**) or high-grade (**HSIL**). HPV DNA testing can be used adjunctively as a triage test to stratify risk in women age 21 years and older with a cytologic diagnosis of ASC-US and in postmenopausal women with a cytologic diagnosis of ASC-US or LSIL.

Women with ASC-US and a negative HPV screening may be followed up in 1 year with a repeat Papanicolaou smear and HPV co-testing. If the HPV screen is positive, colposcopy is indicated. If HPV screening is unavailable, repeat cytology may be done at 12 months. Women aged 21–24 with low-grade squamous intraepithelial lesion (LSIL) should have repeat Papanicolaou smear in 1 year. Women aged 25 or older with squamous intraepithelial lesion (SIL) or atypical glandular cells should undergo colposcopy. For the most current guidelines, please consult these sources: https://www.uspreventiveservicestaskforce.org/uspstf/document/RecommendationStatementFinal/cervical-cancer-screening (August 2018) and https://www.asccp.org/guidelines (April 2019).

Chor J et al. Cervical cancer screening guideline for individuals at average risk. JAMA. 2021;326:2193. [PMID: 34766970]

B. Colposcopy

Women who have positive HPV screening or women aged 25 or older with squamous intraepithelial lesion or atypical glandular cells should be referred for colposcopy. Viewing the cervix with 10–20 × magnification allows for assessment of the size and margins of an abnormal transformation zone and determination of extension into the endocervical canal. The application of 3–5% acetic acid (vinegar) dissolves mucus, and the acid's desiccating action sharpens the contrast between normal and actively proliferating squamous epithelium. Abnormal changes include white patches and vascular atypia, which indicate areas of greatest cellular activity.

C. Biopsy

Colposcopically directed biopsy and endocervical curettage are office procedures. Data from both cervical biopsy and endocervical curettage are important in deciding on treatment.

Prevention

Virtually all cervical dysplasias and cancers are associated with cervical infection with HPV. There are over 100 recognized HPV subtypes. Types 6 and 11 tend to cause genital warts and mild dysplasia and rarely progress to cervical cancer; types 16, 18, 31, and others cause higher-grade dysplasia. The HPV 9-valent (Gardasil-9) recombinant vaccine (9vHPV) is indicated for the prevention of cervical, vaginal, and vulvar cancers (in women) and anal cancers (in women and men) caused by HPV types 16, 18, 31, 33, 45, 52, and 58; genital warts (in women and men) caused by HPV types 6 and 11; and precancerous/dysplastic lesions of cervix, vagina, vulva (in women), and anus (in women and men) caused by HPV types 6, 11, 16, 18, 31, 33, 45, 52, and 58. Gardasil-9 is recommended for vaccination of females and males aged 9–45 years old. The earlier HPV 4-valent vaccine known as Gardasil that was indicated for prevention of diseases related to HPV types 6, 11, 16, and 18 has been discontinued in the United States. The use of HPV vaccination in the United States continues to increase; however, the HPV vaccination continues to lag far behind other vaccines recommended for adolescents. In 2018, 51% of adolescents were up to date with the three-dose HPV vaccine series compared with 48% in 2017.

Because complete coverage of all carcinogenic HPV types is not provided by either vaccine, all women need to have regular cervical cancer screening as outlined above. In addition to vaccination, preventive measures include limiting the number of sexual partners and thus exposure to HPV, using a condom for coitus, smoking cessation, and avoiding exposure to secondhand smoke.

Treatment

Treatment varies depending on the degree and extent of CIN. Biopsies should precede treatment, except in cases of high-grade squamous intraepithelial lesion (HSIL) where it may be appropriate to proceed directly to a LEEP.

A. Cryosurgery

The use of freezing (cryosurgery) is effective for noninvasive small lesions visible on the cervix without endocervical extension.

B. CO_2 Laser

This well-controlled method minimizes tissue destruction. It is colposcopically directed and requires special training. It may be used with large visible lesions and involves vaporization of the transformation zone on the cervix and the distal 5–7 mm of endocervical canal.

C. Loop Excision

When the CIN is clearly visible in its entirety, a wire loop can be used for excisional biopsy. This office procedure, called **LEEP (loop electrosurgical excision procedure)**, done with local anesthesia is quick and straightforward. Cutting and hemostasis are achieved with a low-voltage electrosurgical machine.

D. Conization of the Cervix

Conization is surgical removal of the entire transformation zone and endocervical canal. It typically is reserved for cases of severe dysplasia (CIN III) or carcinoma in situ, particularly those with endocervical extension. It can be performed with scalpel, CO_2 laser, needle electrode, or large-loop excision.

Follow-Up

Because recurrence is possible—especially in the first 2 years after treatment—and because the false-negative rate of a single cervical cytologic test is 20%, close follow-up after colposcopy and biopsy is imperative. Following excisional or ablative procedure, HPV-based testing should be performed at 6 months and then annually for 3 years followed by HPV-based testing every 3 years for at least 25 years. Colposcopy and endocervical sampling should be performed for any abnormality.

The American Society for Colposcopy and Cervical Pathology Guidelines for cervical cancer screening and management of abnormal Papanicolaou smears are available online (https://www.asccp.org/guidelines).

When to Refer

- Patients with CIN II/III should be referred to an experienced colposcopist.
- Patients requiring conization biopsy should be referred to a gynecologist.

Chor J et al. Cervical cancer screening guideline for individuals at average risk. JAMA. 2021;326:2193. [PMID: 34766970]
Kalliala I et al. Incidence and mortality from cervical cancer and other malignancies after treatment of cervical intraepithelial neoplasia: a systematic review and meta-analysis of the literature. Ann Oncol. 2020;31:213. [PMID: 31959338]
Oshman LD et al. Human papillomavirus vaccination for adults: updated recommendations of the Advisory Committee on Immunization Practices (ACIP). JAMA. 2020;323:468. [PMID: 31930397]
Perkins RB et al. 2019 ASCCP risk-based management consensus guidelines for abnormal cervical cancer screening tests and cancer precursors. J Low Genit Tract Dis. 2020;24:102. [PMID: 32243307]
US Preventive Services Task Force; Curry SJ et al. Screening for cervical cancer: US Preventive Services Task Force Recommendation Statement. JAMA. 2018;320:674. [PMID: 30140884]

CARCINOMA OF THE CERVIX

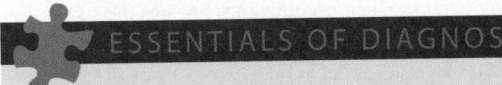

- Increased risk in women who smoke and those with HIV or high-risk HPV types.
- Gross lesions should be evaluated by colposcopically directed biopsies and not cytology alone.

General Considerations

Cervical cancer is the third most common cancer in the world and the leading cause of cancer death among women in developing countries. It is considered a sexually transmitted infection as both squamous cell and adenocarcinoma of the cervix are secondary to infection with HPV, primarily types 16 and 18. Women infected with HIV and with other forms of immunosuppression are at an increased risk for high-risk HPV infection and CIN. Smoking appears to be a cofactor for squamous cell carcinoma (SCC). SCC accounts for approximately 80% of cervical cancers, while adenocarcinoma accounts for 15%, and adenosquamous carcinoma for 3–5%; neuroendocrine or small cell carcinomas are rare.

SCC appears first in the intraepithelial layers (the preinvasive stage, or carcinoma in situ). Preinvasive cancer (CIN III) is most commonly diagnosed in women 25–35 years of age. Two to 10 years are required for carcinoma to penetrate the basement membrane and become invasive. While cervical cancer mortality has declined steadily in the United States due to high rates of screening and improved treatment, the rate of decline has slowed in recent years. In general, Black women experienced much higher incidence and mortality than White women. The 5-year survival rate ranges from 73% for stage II cervical cancer to less than 20% for stage IV.

Clinical Findings

A. Symptoms and Signs

Early cervical cancer is often asymptomatic. The most common signs are irregular or heavy bleeding and postcoital spotting. Bladder and rectal dysfunction or fistulas and pain are late sequelae.

B. Cervical Biopsy and Endocervical Curettage or Conization

These procedures are necessary steps after a positive Papanicolaou smear to determine the extent and depth of invasion of the cancer. Even if the smear is positive, definitive diagnosis must be established through biopsy before additional treatment is given.

C. "Staging" or Estimate of Gross Spread of Cancer of the Cervix

Staging of invasive cervical cancer is achieved by clinical evaluation, usually conducted under anesthesia. Further examinations, such as ultrasonography, CT, MRI, lymphangiography, laparoscopy, and fine-needle aspiration, are valuable for treatment planning.

Complications

Metastases to regional lymph nodes occur with increasing frequency from stage I to stage IV. Paracervical extension occurs in all directions from the cervix. The ureters may become obstructed lateral to the cervix, causing hydroureter and hydronephrosis and consequently impaired kidney function. Almost two-thirds of patients with untreated carcinoma of the cervix die of uremia when ureteral obstruction is bilateral. Pain in the back, in the distribution of the lumbosacral plexus, is often indicative of neurologic involvement. Gross edema of the legs may be indicative of vascular and lymphatic stasis due to tumor. Vaginal fistulas to the rectum and urinary tract are severe late complications. Hemorrhage causes death in 10–20% of patients with extensive invasive carcinoma.

Prevention

Vaccination with the recombinant 9-valent HPV vaccine (Gardasil-9) can prevent cervical cancer by targeting the HPV types that pose the greatest risk and protect against low-grade and precancerous lesions caused by other HPV types (see Cervical Intraepithelial Neoplasia).

Treatment

A. Emergency Measures

Vaginal hemorrhage originates from gross ulceration and cavitation in later stage cervical carcinoma. Ligation and suturing of the cervix are usually not feasible, but emergent vaginal packing, cautery, tranexamic acid, and irradiation are helpful to stop bleeding temporarily. Ligation, resection, or embolization of the uterine or hypogastric arteries may be lifesaving when other measures fail.

B. Specific Measures

1. Carcinoma in situ (stage 0)—In women for whom childbearing is not a consideration, total hysterectomy is the definitive treatment. In women who wish to retain the uterus, acceptable alternatives include cryosurgery, laser surgery, LEEP, or cervical conization. HPV-based testing should be repeated at 6 months and then annually for 3 years followed by HPV-based testing every 3 years for at least 25 years.

2. Invasive carcinoma—Microinvasive carcinoma (stage IA1) is treated with simple, extrafascial hysterectomy. Stages IA2 and IB1 cancers are typically treated with modified radical hysterectomy and pelvic lymphadenectomy. Women with stage IB1 may be candidates for fertility-sparing surgery, which includes radical trachelectomy and lymph node dissection with preservation of the uterus and ovaries. Women with IB2 cancers typically undergo radical hysterectomy and pelvic lymphadenectomy. Adjuvant chemotherapy or radiation may be used for women with risk factors for recurrence. Women with locally advanced disease (stage IB3 to IVA) usually are treated with primary chemoradiation. Metastatic disease (stage IVB) typically is treated with chemotherapy.

Prognosis

The overall 5-year relative survival rate for carcinoma of the cervix is 68% in White women and 55% in Black women in the United States. Survival rates are inversely proportionate to the stage of cancer: stage 0, 99–100%; stage IA, more than 94%; stage IB–IIA, 73–90%; stage IIB, 65%; stage III, 40%; and stage IV, less than 20%.

When to Refer

All patients with invasive cervical carcinoma (stage IA or higher) should be referred to a gynecologic oncologist.

American Cancer Society. Survival rates for cervical cancer, by stage, January 3, 2020. https://www.cancer.org/cancer/cervical-cancer/detection-diagnosis-staging/survival.html
Benson R et al. Locally advanced cervical cancer—neoadjuvant chemotherapy followed by concurrent chemoradiation and targeted therapy as maintenance: a phase II study. J Cancer Res Ther. 2019;15:1359. [PMID: 31898673]
Johnson CA et al. Cervical cancer: an overview of pathophysiology and management. Semin Oncol Nurs. 2019;35:166. [PMID: 30878194]
Stolnicu S et al. Recent advances in invasive adenocarcinoma of the cervix. Virchows Arch. 2019;475:537. [PMID: 31209635]
US Preventive Services Task Force; Curry SJ et al. Screening for cervical cancer: US Preventive Services Task Force Recommendation Statement. JAMA. 2018;320:674. [PMID: 30140884]

CARCINOMA OF THE ENDOMETRIUM

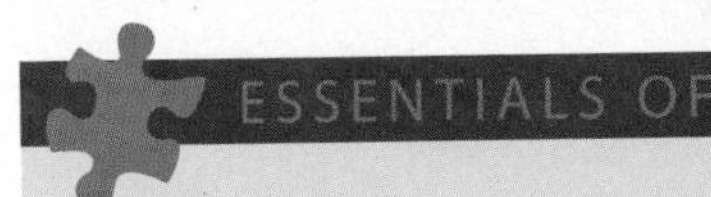

- AUB is the presenting sign in 90% of cases.
- After a negative pregnancy test, endometrial tissue is required to confirm the diagnosis.

General Considerations

Adenocarcinoma of the endometrium is the most common cancer of the female genital tract in developed countries. It occurs most often in women 50–70 years of age. Obesity, nulliparity, diabetes mellitus, polycystic ovaries with prolonged anovulation, unopposed estrogen therapy, and the extended use of tamoxifen for the treatment of breast cancer are risk factors. Women with a family history of colon cancer (hereditary nonpolyposis colorectal cancer, Lynch syndrome) are at significantly increased risk, with a lifetime incidence as high as 30%.

Abnormal bleeding is the presenting sign in 90% of cases. Any postmenopausal bleeding requires investigation. Pain generally occurs late in the disease, with metastases or infection.

Papanicolaou smear of the cervix occasionally shows atypical endometrial cells but is an insensitive diagnostic tool. Endocervical and endometrial sampling is the only reliable means of diagnosis and is important to differentiate endometrial cancer from hyperplasia, which often can be treated hormonally. Simultaneous hysteroscopy can be a valuable addition to localize polyps or other lesions within the uterine cavity. Pelvic ultrasonography may determine the thickness of the endometrium as an indication of hypertrophy and possible neoplastic change. The finding of a thin endometrial lining on ultrasound (4 mm or less) in a postmenopausal woman is clinically reassuring in cases where very little tissue is obtainable through endometrial biopsy.

Prevention

Prompt endometrial sampling for patients who report abnormal menstrual bleeding or postmenopausal uterine bleeding will reveal many incipient and clinical cases of endometrial cancer. Younger women with chronic anovulation are at risk for endometrial hyperplasia and subsequent endometrial cancer; they can significantly reduce the risk of hyperplasia with the use of oral contraceptives, cyclic progestin therapy, or a hormonal IUD.

Staging

Staging and prognosis are based on surgical and pathologic evaluation only. Examination under anesthesia, endometrial and endocervical sampling, chest radiography, intravenous urography, cystoscopy, sigmoidoscopy, transvaginal sonography, and MRI will help determine the extent of the disease and its appropriate treatment.

Treatment

Treatment consists of total hysterectomy and bilateral salpingo-oophorectomy. Peritoneal washings for cytologic examination are routinely taken and lymph node sampling may be done. Women with high-risk endometrial cancer (serous adenocarcinoma, clear cell carcinoma, grade 3 deeply invasive endometrioid carcinoma, and stages III/IV disease) are generally treated with surgery followed by chemotherapy and/or radiation therapy.

Prognosis

With early diagnosis and treatment, the overall 5-year survival for stage I disease is 80–90%. With stage I disease, the depth of myometrial invasion is the strongest predictor of survival, with a 90% 5-year survival with less than 50% depth of invasion and 80% survival with 50% or more invasion. Survival rates decrease with increasing stage of disease.

When to Refer

All patients with endometrial carcinoma should be referred to a gynecologic oncologist.

Chargari C et al. Brachytherapy: an overview for clinicians. CA Cancer J Clin. 2019;69:386. [PMID: 31361333]
Cusimano MC et al. Laparoscopic and robotic hysterectomy in endometrial cancer patients with obesity: a systematic review and meta-analysis of conversions and complications. Am J Obstet Gynecol. 2019;221:410. [PMID: 31082383]
Passarello K et al. Endometrial cancer: an overview of pathophysiology, management and care. Semin Oncol Nurs. 2019; 35:157. [PMID: 30867105]

CARCINOMA OF THE VULVA

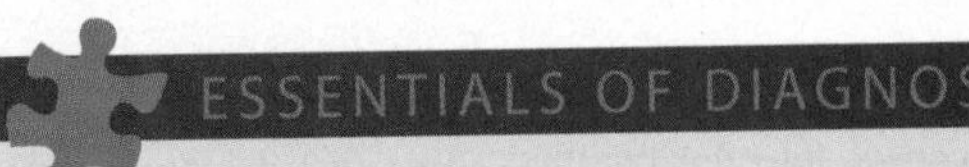

- Two independent pathways for development: HPV or chronic inflammation.
- History of prolonged vulvar irritation, with pruritus, local discomfort, or slight bloody discharge.
- Early lesions may suggest or include non-neoplastic epithelial disorders.

- Late lesions appear as a mass, an exophytic growth, or a firm, ulcerated area in the vulva.
- Biopsy is necessary for diagnosis.

General Considerations

Most cancers of the vulva are squamous lesions that classically occur in women over 50. Vulvar low-grade squamous intraepithelial lesions (LSIL) are benign and do not require intervention. Vulvar high-grade squamous intraepithelial lesions (HSIL) and differentiated vulvar intraepithelial neoplasia (dVIN) are premalignant conditions. Vulvar HSIL (VIN usual type) is associated with HPV, while dVIN is associated with vulvar dermatoses, eg, lichens sclerosus. About 70–90% of premalignant lesions are vulvar HSIL, but HSIL is the precursor for only 20% of vulvar cancers, while dVIN is the precursor for approximately 80% of vulvar cancers. Given that high percentages of HSIL and vulvar cancers are HPV-related, immunization with the HPV vaccine is beneficial to reduce the risk of HPV-related vulvar disease.

Differential Diagnosis

Other vulvar lesions must be considered. Vulvar intraepithelial neoplasia may resemble vulvar cancer and must be distinguished by histology. Benign vulvar disorders that must be excluded in the diagnosis of carcinoma of the vulva include inflammatory vulvar dermatoses (psoriasis, lichen sclerosus, lichen planus), chronic granulomatous lesions (eg, lymphogranuloma venereum, syphilis), condylomas, epidermal inclusion cysts, hidradenomas, or neurofibromas. Lichen sclerosus and other associated leukoplakic changes in the skin should be biopsied. The likelihood that a superimposed vulvar cancer will develop in a woman with a non-neoplastic epithelial disorder is low (1–5%).

Diagnosis

Biopsy is essential for the diagnosis of VIN and vulvar cancer and should be performed with any localized atypical vulvar lesion, including white patches and hyperpigmented lesions. Multiple skin-punch specimens can be taken in the office under local anesthesia, with care to include tissue from the edges of each lesion sampled. Colposcopy of vulva, vagina, and cervix can help in identifying areas for biopsy and in planning further treatment.

Staging

Vulvar cancer generally spreads by direct extension into the vagina, urethra, perineum, and anus, with discontinuous spread into the inguinal and femoral lymph nodes. Staging is based on a combined clinical and surgical/pathologic system.

Treatment

Invasive carcinoma confined to the vulva without evidence of spread to adjacent organs or to the regional lymph nodes is treated with wide local excision and inguinal lymphadenectomy or wide local excision alone if invasion is less than 1 mm. To avoid the morbidity of inguinal lymphadenectomy, some guidelines recommend sentinel lymph node sampling for women with early-stage vulvar cancer. Patients with more advanced disease may receive preoperative radiation, chemotherapy, or both.

Prognosis

Vulvar squamous cell carcinomas seldom metastasize. With adequate excision, the prognosis is excellent. Patients with invasive vulvar SCC 2 cm in diameter or less, without inguinal lymph node metastases, have an 85–90% 5-year survival rate. If the lesion is larger than 2 cm and lymph node involvement is present, the likelihood of 5-year survival is approximately 40%.

When to Refer

All patients with invasive vulvar carcinoma should be referred to a gynecologic oncologist.

Gadducci A et al. Locally advanced squamous cell carcinoma of the vulva: a challenging question for gynecologic oncologists. Gynecol Oncol. 2020;158:208. [PMID: 32460996]

Morrison J et al. British Gynaecological Cancer Society (BGCS) vulval cancer guidelines: recommendations for practice. Eur J Obstet Gynecol Reprod Biol. 2020;252:502. [PMID: 32620514]

Singh N et al. Vulval squamous cell carcinoma and its precursors. Histopathology. 2020;76:128. [PMID: 31846523]

Tan A et al. Diagnosis and management of vulvar cancer: a review. J Am Acad Dermatol. 2019;81:1387. [PMID: 31349045]

OVARIAN TUMORS & OVARIAN CANCER

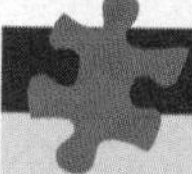

ESSENTIALS OF DIAGNOSIS

- Symptoms include vague GI discomfort, pelvic pressure, or pain.
- Many cases of early-stage cancer are asymptomatic.
- Pelvic examination and ultrasound are mainstays of diagnosis.

General Considerations

Ovarian tumors are common. Most are benign, but malignant ovarian tumors are the leading cause of death from gynecologic cancer. The wide range of types and patterns of ovarian tumors is due to the complexity of ovarian embryology and differences in tissues of origin.

In women with no family history of ovarian cancer, the lifetime risk in the United States is 1.3%, whereas a woman with one affected first-degree relative has a 5% lifetime risk. Worldwide, the risk of ovarian cancer is 2.7%. Ultrasound or tumor marker screening for women with one or no affected first-degree relatives has not been shown to reduce mortality from ovarian cancer, and the risks associated with unnecessary prophylactic surgical procedures outweigh the benefits in low-risk women. With two or more affected first-degree relatives, the risk is 7%. Approximately 3% of women with two or more affected first-degree relatives will have a **hereditary ovarian cancer syndrome** with a lifetime ovarian cancer risk of 40%. Women with a *BRCA1* gene pathogenic variant have a 45% lifetime risk of ovarian cancer and those with a *BRCA2* pathogenic variant, a 25% risk. Consideration should be given to screening with transvaginal sonography and serum CA 125 testing, starting at age 30–35 years for women with *BRCA1* pathogenic variant or age 35–40 for women with *BRCA2* pathogenic variant or 5–10 years earlier than the earliest age that ovarian cancer was first diagnosed in any family member. Of note, this screening regimen has not been shown to reduce mortality; thus, prophylactic oophorectomy should be considered at conclusion of childbearing.

Clinical Findings

A. Symptoms and Signs

Most women with both benign and malignant ovarian neoplasms are either asymptomatic or experience only mild nonspecific GI symptoms or pelvic pressure. Women with advanced malignant disease may experience abdominal pain and bloating, and a palpable abdominal mass with ascites is often present.

B. Laboratory Findings

Serum CA 125 is elevated in 80% of women with epithelial ovarian cancer overall but in only 50% of women with early disease. However, CA 125 may be elevated in premenopausal women with benign disease (such as endometriosis), minimizing its usefulness in ovarian cancer screening. In premenopausal women with ovarian masses, other tumor markers (such as human chorionic gonadotropin [hCG], LD, or alpha-fetoprotein) may be indicators of the tumor type.

C. Imaging

Transvaginal sonography is useful for screening high-risk women but has inadequate sensitivity for screening low-risk women. Ultrasound is helpful in differentiating ovarian masses that are benign and likely to resolve spontaneously from those with malignant potential. Color Doppler imaging may further enhance the specificity of ultrasound diagnosis.

Differential Diagnosis

Once an ovarian mass has been detected, it must be categorized as functional, benign neoplastic, or potentially malignant. Predictive factors include age, size of the mass, ultrasound configuration, serum CA 125 level, the presence of symptoms, and whether the mass is unilateral or bilateral. Simple cysts up to 10 cm in diameter are almost universally benign in both premenopausal and postmenopausal patients. Most will resolve spontaneously and may be monitored without intervention. If the mass is larger or unchanged on repeat transvaginal sonography, or if symptomatic, surgical evaluation is warranted.

Treatment

If a malignant ovarian mass is suspected, surgical evaluation should be performed by a gynecologic oncologist. For benign neoplasms, tumor excision or unilateral oophorectomy is usually performed. For ovarian cancer in an early stage, the standard therapy is complete surgical staging including hysterectomy and bilateral salpingo-oophorectomy with omentectomy and selective lymphadenectomy. With more advanced disease, aggressive removal of all visible tumor improves survival. Except for women with low-grade ovarian cancer in an early stage, postoperative chemotherapy is indicated (see Table 39–3). Several chemotherapy regimens are effective, such as the combination of cisplatin or carboplatin with paclitaxel, with clinical response rates of up to 60–70%.

Prognosis

Advanced disease is diagnosed in approximately 75% of women with ovarian cancer. The overall 5-year survival is approximately 17% with distant metastases but is 89% with early-stage disease.

When to Refer

If a malignant mass is suspected, surgical evaluation should be performed by a gynecologic oncologist.

Centers for Disease Control and Prevention (CDC). Ovarian cancer screening. 2021. https://www.cdc.gov/cancer/ovarian/basic_info/screening.htm

Fujiwara K et al. Landscape of systemic therapy for ovarian cancer in 2019: primary therapy. Cancer. 2019;125:4582. [PMID: 31967679]

González-Martín A et al. Immunotherapy with checkpoint inhibitors in patients with ovarian cancer: still promising? Cancer. 2019;125:4616. [PMID: 31967676]

Lee JM et al. New strategies in ovarian cancer treatment. Cancer. 2019;125:4623. [PMID: 31967682]

Momenimovahed Z et al. Ovarian cancer in the world: epidemiology and risk factors. Int J Womens Health. 2019;11:287. [PMID: 31118829]

Pignata S et al. Treatment of recurrent epithelial ovarian cancer. Cancer. 2019;125:4609. [PMID: 31967680]

US Preventive Services Task Force; Grossman DC et al. Screening for ovarian cancer: US Preventive Services Task Force Recommendation Statement. JAMA. 2018;319:588. [PMID: 29450531]

Obstetrics & Obstetric Disorders

Vanessa L. Rogers, MD
Scott W. Roberts, MD

DIAGNOSIS OF PREGNANCY

It is advantageous to diagnose pregnancy as promptly as possible. Prenatal care can begin early for a desired pregnancy, and potentially harmful medications and activities such as drug and alcohol use, smoking, and occupational chemical exposure can be eliminated. If an unwanted pregnancy occurs, counseling about options can be provided at an early stage.

Pregnancy Tests

All urine or blood pregnancy tests rely on the detection of human chorionic gonadotropin (hCG) produced by the placenta. Levels increase shortly after implantation, approximately double every 48 hours (this rise can range from 30% to 100% in normal pregnancies), reach a peak at 50–75 days, and fall to lower levels in the second and third trimesters. Pregnancy tests are performed on serum or urine and are accurate at the time of the missed period or shortly after it.

Compared with intrauterine pregnancies, **ectopic pregnancies** may show lower levels of hCG that plateau or fall in serial determinations. Quantitative assays of hCG repeated at 48-hour intervals are used in the diagnosis of ectopic pregnancy as well as in cases of molar pregnancy and early pregnancy loss. Comparison of hCG levels between laboratories may be misleading in a given patient because different international standards may produce results that vary by as much as twofold. Consistent follow-up is necessary to make the correct diagnosis and management plan. **Pregnancy of unknown location** is a term used to describe a situation where a woman has a positive pregnancy test, but the location and viability of the pregnancy are not known because it is not seen on transvaginal ultrasound.

Manifestations of Pregnancy

The following symptoms and signs are usually due to pregnancy, but none are diagnostic. A record of the time of coitus or insemination is helpful for diagnosing and dating a pregnancy.

A. Symptoms

Amenorrhea, nausea and vomiting, breast tenderness and tingling, urinary frequency and urgency, "quickening" (perception of first movement noted at about the 18th week), weight gain.

B. Signs (in Weeks From Last Menstrual Period)

Breast changes (enlargement, vascular engorgement, colostrum) begin early in pregnancy and continue until the postpartum period. Cyanosis of the vagina and cervical portio and softening of the cervix occur in about the 7th week. Softening of the cervicouterine junction takes place in the 8th week, and generalized enlargement and diffuse softening of the corpus occurs after the 8th week. When a woman's abdomen will start to enlarge depends on her body habitus but typically starts in the 16th week.

The uterine fundus is palpable above the pubic symphysis by 12–15 weeks from the last menstrual period and reaches the umbilicus by 20–22 weeks. Fetal heart tones can be heard by Doppler at 10–12 weeks' gestation.

Differential Diagnosis

The nonpregnant uterus enlarged by myomas can be confused with the gravid uterus, but it is usually firm and irregular. An ovarian tumor may be found midline, displacing the nonpregnant uterus to the side or posteriorly. Ultrasonography and a pregnancy test will provide accurate diagnosis in these circumstances.

ESSENTIALS OF PRENATAL CARE

Prenatal visits should begin as early as possible after the diagnosis of pregnancy. The initial visit should include a history, physical examination, advice to the patient, and appropriate tests and procedures (see *CMDT Online* at AccessMedicine.com for a discussion of routine prenatal care).

A. Medications

Only medications prescribed or authorized by the obstetric provider should be taken since certain medications are contraindicated during pregnancy (Table 19–1).

Table 19–1. Common drugs that are teratogenic or fetotoxic.[1]

ACE inhibitors	Lithium
Alcohol	Methotrexate
Androgens	Misoprostol
Angiotensin-II receptor blockers	NSAIDs (third trimester)
Antiepileptics (phenytoin, valproic acid, carbamazepine)	Opioids (prolonged use)
	Radioiodine (antithyroid)
Benzodiazepines	Reserpine
Cyclophosphamide	Ribavirin
Diazoxide	Sulfonamides (second and third trimesters)
Diethylstilbestrol	
Disulfiram	Tetracycline (third trimester)
Ergotamine	Thalidomide
Estrogens	Tobacco smoking
Griseofulvin	Warfarin and other coumarin anticoagulants
Isotretinoin	

[1]Many other drugs are also contraindicated during pregnancy. Evaluate any drug for its need versus its potential adverse effects. Further information can be obtained from the manufacturer or from any of several teratogenic registries around the country. Go to https://www.fda.gov/ScienceResearch/SpecialTopics/WomensHealthResearch/ucm134848.htm for more information.

B. Alcohol and Other Drugs

Pregnant women should be encouraged to abstain from alcohol, tobacco, and all recreational ("street") drugs. No safe level of alcohol intake has been established for pregnancy. Fetal effects are manifest in the **fetal alcohol syndrome,** which includes growth restriction; facial, skeletal, and cardiac abnormalities; and serious CNS dysfunction.

Cigarette smoking results in fetal exposure to carbon monoxide and nicotine, which may eventuate to adverse pregnancy outcomes. An increased risk of placental abruption (abruptio placentae), placenta previa, and premature rupture of the membranes is documented among women who smoke. Preterm delivery, low birth weight, and ectopic pregnancy are also more likely among cigarette smokers. Women who smoke should quit smoking or at least reduce the number of cigarettes smoked per day to as few as possible. Complete cessation is preferred over reduction with the best outcomes seen in women who stop smoking prior to 15 weeks' gestation. Clinicians should ask all pregnant women about their smoking history and offer smoking cessation counseling during pregnancy, since women are more motivated to change at this time. Pregnant women should also avoid exposure to environmental smoke ("passive smoking"), smokeless tobacco, and e-cigarettes. Pharmacotherapy for smoking cessation has been used with mixed results. Studies of bupropion and nicotine replacement systems are inadequate to properly weigh risks and benefits.

Sometimes compounding the above effects on pregnancy outcome are the independent adverse effects of illicit drugs. Cocaine use in pregnancy is associated with an increased risk of premature rupture of membranes, preterm delivery, placental abruption, intrauterine growth restriction, neurobehavioral deficits, and sudden infant death syndrome. Similar adverse effects on pregnancy are associated with amphetamine use, perhaps reflecting the vasoconstrictive properties of both amphetamines and cocaine. Adverse effects associated with opioid use include intrauterine growth restriction, prematurity, and fetal death. For pregnant women with opioid use disorder, opioid agonist therapy is the standard of care (see Chapter 5).

C. Radiographs and Noxious Exposures

Radiographs should be avoided unless essential and approved by a clinician. Abdominal shielding should be used whenever possible. The patient should be told to inform her other health care providers that she is pregnant. Chemical or radiation hazards should be avoided as should excessive heat in hot tubs or saunas. Patients should be told to avoid handling cat feces or cat litter and to wear gloves when gardening to avoid infection with toxoplasmosis.

LACTATION

Drugs taken by a nursing mother may accumulate in milk and be transmitted to the infant (Table 19–2). The amount of drug entering the milk depends on the drug's lipid solubility, mechanism of transport, and degree of ionization.

Sattari M et al. Maternal implications of breastfeeding: a review for the internist. Am J Med. 2019;132:912. [PMID: 30853481]

TRAVEL & IMMUNIZATIONS DURING PREGNANCY

During an otherwise normal low-risk pregnancy, travel can be planned most safely up to the 32nd week. Commercial flying in pressurized cabins does not pose a threat to the fetus. An aisle seat will allow frequent walks. Adequate fluids should be taken during the flight. Travel can also increase women's chances of exposure to SARS-CoV-2, the virus that causes COVID-19. Pregnant women infected with SARS-CoV-2 are believed to be at increased risk for preterm birth and for serious illness compared with women who are not pregnant. Pregnant women should limit their exposure to people outside their household, wear a mask while outside the home, practice frequent hand washing, and social distance.

Vaccination against COVID-19 is recommended for women who are pregnant, trying to get pregnant, or may become pregnant, and who are breastfeeding. The CDC has determined that the benefits of vaccination outweigh any risks. There is no evidence that vaccination causes problems with fertility in men or women. Pregnant women who have been vaccinated may receive the COVID-19 booster shot. There have been rare reports of thrombosis with thrombocytopenia syndrome in women younger than 50 years old who received the Johnson and Johnson's Janssen vaccine. This risk has not been found with the Pfizer-BioNTech and Moderna vaccines; women younger than 50 years old with access to multiple vaccines may want to factor this into their decision-making process.

Traveling to endemic areas of yellow fever (Africa or Latin America) or of Zika virus (Latin America) is not advisable; since Zika virus can be sexually transmitted,

Table 19–2. Drugs and substances that require a careful assessment of risk before they are prescribed for breastfeeding women.[1]

Drugs	Concern
Atenolol	Hypotension and bradycardia in the infant. Metoprolol and propranolol are preferred.
Ciprofloxacin	Adverse effects on fetal cartilage and bone. Must weigh risks versus benefits.
Codeine, oxycodone	CNS depression. Unpredictable metabolism.
Cyclophosphamide	Neonatal neutropenia. No breastfeeding.
Diphenhydramine	Present in small quantities in milk; sources are conflicting regarding its safety.
Fluoxetine	Present in breast milk in higher levels than other SSRIs. Watch for adverse effects like an infant's fussiness and crying.
Lisinopril	Unknown effects. Captopril or enalapril is preferred if an ACE inhibitor is needed.
Lithium	Circulating levels in the neonate are variable. Follow infant's serum creatinine and BUN levels and thyroid function tests.
Tetracyclines	Adverse effects on fetal bone growth and dental staining.
Valproic acid	Long-term effects are unknown. Although levels in milk are low, it is teratogenic, so it should be avoided if possible.

[1]The above list is not all-inclusive. For additional information, see the reference from which this information is adapted: Rowe H et al. Maternal medication, drug use, and breastfeeding. Pediatr Clin North Am. 2013;60:275, or the online drug and lactation database, Lactmed, at https://www.ncbi.nlm.nih.gov/books/NBK501922/.

partner travel should also be discussed (see Chapter 32). Similarly, it is inadvisable to travel to areas of Africa or Asia where chloroquine-resistant falciparum malaria is a hazard, since complications of malaria are more common in pregnancy.

Ideally, all immunizations should precede pregnancy. *Live virus products are contraindicated during pregnancy (measles, rubella, yellow fever, and smallpox).* Inactivated polio vaccine should be given subcutaneously instead of the oral live-attenuated vaccine. The varicella vaccine should be given 1–3 months before becoming pregnant. It is not recommended in pregnancy. Vaccines against pneumococcal pneumonia, meningococcal meningitis, and hepatitis A can be used as indicated. Pregnant women who are high risk for hepatitis B and who have not been previously vaccinated should be vaccinated during pregnancy. The HPV vaccine is not recommended for pregnant women. However, adverse outcomes have not been described when used during pregnancy. If a woman who has started the vaccine series is pregnant, the remaining doses should be administered when she is no longer pregnant.

The CDC lists pregnant women as a high-risk group for influenza. Annual influenza vaccination is indicated in all women who are pregnant or will be pregnant during the "flu season." It can be given in the first trimester. The CDC also recommends that every pregnant woman receive a dose of Tdap during each pregnancy irrespective of her prior vaccination history. The optimal timing for such Tdap administration is between 27 and 36 weeks' gestation, to maximize the antibody response of the pregnant woman against pertussis and the passive antibody transfer to the infant. For any woman who was not previously vaccinated with Tdap and for whom the vaccine was not given during her pregnancy, Tdap should be administered immediately postpartum. Further, any teenagers or adults not previously vaccinated who will have close contact with the infant should also receive it, ideally 2 weeks before exposure to the child. This vaccination strategy is called "cocooning," and its purpose is to protect the infant aged younger than 12 months who is at particularly high risk for lethal pertussis.

Hepatitis A vaccine contains formalin-inactivated virus and can be given in pregnancy when needed. Pooled immune globulin to prevent hepatitis A is safe and does not carry risk of HIV transmission. Chloroquine can be used for malaria prophylaxis in pregnancy, and proguanil is also safe.

Water should be purified by boiling in settings where there is potential for microbial contamination, since iodine purification may provide more iodine than is safe during pregnancy.

Prophylactic antibiotics or bismuth subsalicylate should not be used during pregnancy to prevent diarrhea. Oral rehydration and treatment of bacterial diarrhea with erythromycin or ampicillin if necessary is preferred.

Centers for Disease Control and Prevention. COVID-19 Vaccines While Pregnant or Breastfeeding. 2021 Dec 6. https://www.cdc.gov/coronavirus/2019-ncov/vaccines/recommendations/pregnancy.html

OBSTETRIC COMPLICATIONS OF THE FIRST & SECOND TRIMESTERS

VOMITING OF PREGNANCY & HYPEREMESIS GRAVIDARUM

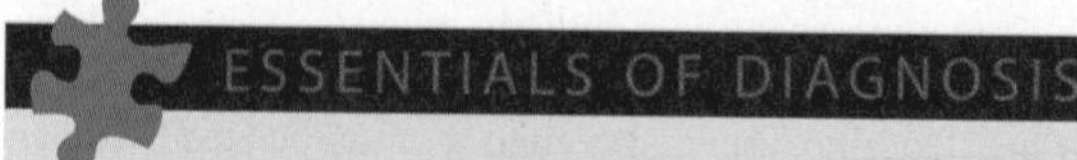

- **Hyperemesis gravidarum**
  - Persistent, severe vomiting.
  - Weight loss, dehydration, hypochloremic alkalosis, hypokalemia.

- May have transient elevation of liver enzymes.
- Appears related to high or rising serum hCG.
- More common with multifetal pregnancies or hydatidiform mole.

General Considerations

Nausea and vomiting begin soon after the first missed period and cease by the fifth month of gestation. Up to three-fourths of women complain of nausea and vomiting during early pregnancy, with the vast majority noting nausea throughout the day. This problem exerts no adverse effects on the pregnancy and does not presage other complications.

Persistent, severe vomiting during pregnancy—hyperemesis gravidarum—can be disabling and require hospitalization. Hyperthyroidism can be associated with hyperemesis gravidarum, so it is advisable to determine TSH and free thyroxine (FT_4) values in these patients.

Treatment

A. Mild Nausea and Vomiting of Pregnancy

In most instances, only reassurance and dietary advice are required. Because of possible teratogenicity, drugs used during the first half of pregnancy should be restricted to those of major importance to life and health. Pyridoxine (vitamin B_6), 50–100 mg/day orally, is nontoxic and may be helpful in some patients. Pyridoxine alone or in combination with doxylamine (10 mg doxylamine succinate and 10 mg pyridoxine hydrochloride, two tablets at bedtime) is first-line pharmacotherapy. Antiemetics, antihistamines, and antispasmodics are generally unnecessary.

B. Hyperemesis Gravidarum

With more severe nausea and vomiting, it may become necessary to hospitalize the patient. In this case, a private room with limited activity is preferred. It is recommended to give nothing by mouth until the patient is improving, and maintain hydration and electrolyte balance by giving appropriate parenteral fluids and vitamin supplements as indicated. Antiemetics such as promethazine (12.5–25 mg orally, rectally, or intravenously every 4–6 hours), metoclopramide (5–10 mg orally or intravenously every 6 hours), or ondansetron (4–8 mg orally or intravenously every 8 hours) should be started. Ondansetron has been associated in some studies with congenital anomalies. Data are limited, but the risks and benefits of treatment should be addressed with the patient. If there is an increased risk, it is probably low. Antiemetics will likely need to be given intravenously initially. Rarely, total parenteral nutrition may become necessary but only if enteral feedings cannot be done. As soon as possible, the patient should be placed on a dry diet consisting of six small feedings daily. Antiemetics may be continued orally as needed. After inpatient stabilization, the patient can be maintained at home even if she requires intravenous fluids in addition to her oral intake. There are conflicting studies regarding the use of corticosteroids for the control of hyperemesis gravidarum, and it has also been associated with fetal anomalies, specifically oral clefts. The increase in risk is likely small. However, this treatment should be withheld before 10 weeks' gestation and until more accepted treatments have been exhausted.

When to Refer

- Patient does not respond to first-line outpatient management.
- There is concern for other pathology (ie, hydatidiform mole).

When to Admit

- Patient cannot tolerate any food or water.
- Patient cannot ingest necessary medications.
- Weight loss.
- Presence of a hydatidiform mole.

American College of Obstetricians and Gynecologists. ACOG Practice Bulletin No. 189: nausea and vomiting of pregnancy. Obstet Gynecol. 2018;131:e15. [Reaffirmed 2019] [PMID: 29266076]

SPONTANEOUS PREGNANCY LOSS

ESSENTIALS OF DIAGNOSIS

- Intrauterine pregnancy at less than 20 weeks' gestation.
- Low or falling levels of hCG.
- Bleeding, midline cramping pain.
- Open cervical os.
- Complete or partial expulsion of products of conception.

General Considerations

About three-fourths of spontaneous pregnancy losses (spontaneous abortions) occur before the 16th week; of these, three-fourths occur before the 8th week. Almost 20% of all clinically recognized pregnancies result in a spontaneous loss.

More than 60% of spontaneous losses result from chromosomal defects due to maternal or paternal factors; about 15% appear to be associated with maternal trauma, infections, dietary deficiencies, diabetes mellitus, hypothyroidism, antiphospholipid antibody syndrome, or anatomic malformations. There is no reliable evidence that spontaneous pregnancy loss may be induced by psychic stimuli such as severe fright, grief, anger, or anxiety. In about one-fourth of cases, the cause cannot be determined. There is no evidence that video display terminals or associated electromagnetic fields are related to an increased risk of spontaneous pregnancy loss.

It is important to distinguish women with a history of incompetent cervix from those with early pregnancy loss which typically occur in the first trimester. Factors that predispose to incompetent cervix, a problem of the second trimester, are a history of incompetent cervix with a previous pregnancy, cervical conization or surgery, cervical injury, diethylstilbestrol (DES) exposure, and anatomic abnormalities of the cervix. Before pregnancy or during the first trimester, there are no methods for determining whether the cervix will eventually be incompetent. After 14–16 weeks, ultrasound may be used to evaluate the internal anatomy of the lower uterine segment and cervix for the funneling and shortening abnormalities consistent with cervical incompetence.

Clinical Findings

A. Symptoms and Signs

1. Incompetent cervix—Characteristically, incompetent cervix presents as "silent" cervical dilation (ie, with minimal uterine contractions) in the second trimester. When the cervix reaches 4 cm or more, active uterine contractions or rupture of the membranes may occur secondary to the degree of cervical dilation. This does not change the primary diagnosis.

2. Threatened spontaneous abortion—Bleeding or cramping occurs, but the pregnancy continues. The cervix is not dilated.

3. Inevitable spontaneous abortion—The cervix is dilated and the membranes may be ruptured, but passage of the products of conception has not yet occurred. Bleeding and cramping persist, and passage of the products of conception is considered inevitable.

4. Complete abortion—Products of conception are completely expelled. Pain ceases, but spotting may persist. Cervical os is closed.

5. Incomplete abortion—The cervix is dilated. Some portion of the products of conception remains in the uterus. Only mild cramps are reported, but bleeding is persistent and often excessive.

6. Missed abortion—The pregnancy has ceased to develop, but the conceptus has not been expelled. Missed abortion may also be referred to as early pregnancy loss. Symptoms of pregnancy disappear. There may be a brownish vaginal discharge but no active bleeding. Pain does not develop. The cervix is semifirm and slightly patulous; the uterus becomes smaller and irregularly softened; the adnexa are normal.

B. Laboratory Findings

Pregnancy tests show low or falling levels of hCG. A CBC should be obtained if bleeding is heavy. Determine Rh type and give Rh_0(D) immune globulin if Rh-negative. All tissue recovered should be assessed by a pathologist and may be sent for genetic analysis in selected cases.

C. Ultrasonographic Findings

Transvaginal ultrasound can detect the gestational sac 5–6 weeks from the last menstruation, a fetal pole at 6 weeks, and fetal cardiac activity at 6–7 weeks. Serial observations are often required to evaluate changes in size of the embryo. Diagnostic criteria of early pregnancy loss are a crown-rump length of 7 mm or more and no heartbeat or a mean sac diameter of 25 mm or more and no embryo.

Differential Diagnosis

The bleeding that occurs in abortion of a uterine pregnancy must be differentiated from the abnormal bleeding of an ectopic pregnancy and anovulatory bleeding in a nonpregnant woman. The passage of hydropic villi in the bloody discharge is diagnostic of hydatidiform mole.

Treatment

A. General Measures

1. Threatened spontaneous abortion—Studies have failed to demonstrate benefit of bedrest for 1–2 days followed by gradual resumption of usual activities. Abstinence from sexual activity has also been suggested without proven benefit. Data are lacking to support the administration of progestins to all women with a threatened abortion. If during the patient's evaluation, an infection is diagnosed (ie, UTI), it should be treated.

2. Missed abortion—This calls for counseling regarding the fate of the pregnancy and planning for its elective termination at a time chosen by the patient and clinician. Management can be medical or surgical. Each has risks and benefits. Medically induced first-trimester termination with prostaglandins (ie, misoprostol given vaginally or orally in a dose of 200–800 mcg) is safe, effective, less invasive, and more private than surgical intervention; however, if it is unsuccessful or if there is excessive bleeding, a surgical procedure (dilation and curettage) may still be needed. Patients must be counseled about the different therapeutic options.

B. Surgical Measures

1. Inevitable or incomplete spontaneous abortion—Prompt removal of any products of conception remaining within the uterus is required to stop bleeding and prevent infection. Analgesia and a paracervical block are useful, followed by uterine exploration with ovum forceps or uterine aspiration. Regional anesthesia may be required.

2. Cerclage and restriction of activities—A cerclage is the treatment of choice for incompetent cervix, but a viable intrauterine pregnancy should be confirmed before placement of the cerclage.

Cerclage should be undertaken with caution when there is advanced cervical dilation or when the membranes are prolapsed into the vagina. *Rupture of the membranes and infection are specific contraindications to cerclage.* Testing for *N gonorrhoeae, C trachomatis*, and group B streptococci should be obtained before elective placement of a cerclage. *N gonorrhoeae* and *C trachomatis* should be treated before placement.

When to Refer

- Patient with history of a second-trimester loss.
- Vaginal bleeding in a pregnant patient that resembles menstruation.

- Patient with an open cervical os.
- No signs of uterine growth in serial examinations of a pregnant patient.
- Leakage of amniotic fluid.

When to Admit

- Open cervical os.
- Heavy vaginal bleeding.
- Leakage of amniotic fluid.

American College of Obstetricians and Gynecologists. ACOG Practice Bulletin No. 200: early pregnancy loss. Obstet Gynecol. 2018;132:e197. [PMID: 30157093]

RECURRENT PREGNANCY LOSS

According to the American Society of Reproductive Medicine, recurrent pregnancy loss is defined as the loss of two or more previable (less than 24 weeks' gestation or 500 g) pregnancies in succession. Recurrent pregnancy loss affects about 1–5% of couples. Abnormalities related to recurrent abortion can be identified in approximately 50% of these couples. If a woman has lost three previous pregnancies without identifiable cause, she still has at least a 55% chance of carrying a fetus to viability.

Recurrent pregnancy loss is a clinical rather than pathologic diagnosis. The clinical findings are similar to those observed in other types of pregnancy loss. It is appropriate to begin a medical evaluation in a woman who has had two first-trimester losses.

Treatment

A. Preconception Therapy

Preconception therapy is aimed at detection of maternal or paternal defects that may contribute to pregnancy loss. A thorough history and examination is essential. A random blood glucose test and thyroid function studies (including thyroid antibodies) can be done if history indicates a possible predisposition to diabetes mellitus or thyroid disease. Detection of lupus anticoagulant and other hemostatic abnormalities (proteins S and C and antithrombin deficiency, hyperhomocysteinemia, anticardiolipin antibody, factor V Leiden mutations) and an antinuclear antibody test may be indicated. Hysteroscopy, saline infusion sonogram, or hysterography can be used to exclude submucosal myomas and congenital anomalies of the uterus. In women with recurrent pregnancy losses, resection of a uterine septum, if present, has been recommended. Chromosomal (karyotype) analysis of both partners can be done to rule out balanced translocations (found in 3–4% of infertile couples), but karyotyping is expensive and may not be helpful.

Many therapies have been tried to prevent recurrent abortion from immunologic causes. Low-molecular-weight heparin (LMWH), aspirin, intravenous immunoglobulin, and corticosteroids have all been used but the definitive treatment has not yet been determined (see Antiphospholipid Syndrome, below). Prophylactic low-dose heparin and low-dose aspirin have been recommended for women with antiphospholipid antibodies and recurrent pregnancy loss.

B. Postconception Therapy

The patient should be provided early prenatal care and scheduled frequent office visits. Empiric sex steroid hormone therapy is complicated and should be done by an expert if undertaken.

Prognosis

The prognosis is excellent if the cause of pregnancy losses can be corrected or treated.

ECTOPIC PREGNANCY

ESSENTIALS OF DIAGNOSIS

- Amenorrhea or irregular bleeding and spotting.
- Pelvic pain, usually adnexal.
- Adnexal mass by clinical examination or ultrasound.
- Failure of serum beta-hCG to double every 48 hours.
- No intrauterine pregnancy on transvaginal ultrasound with serum beta-hCG > 2000 milli-units/mL.

General Considerations

Ectopic implantation occurs in approximately 2% of first trimester pregnancies. About 98% of ectopic pregnancies are tubal. Other sites of ectopic implantation are the peritoneum or abdominal viscera, the ovary, and the cervix. Any condition that prevents or inhibits migration of the fertilized ovum to the uterus can predispose to an ectopic pregnancy, including a history of infertility, pelvic inflammatory disease, ruptured appendix, and prior tubal surgery. Combined intrauterine and extrauterine pregnancy of two embryos (heterotopic) may occur rarely. In the United States, undiagnosed or undetected ectopic pregnancy is one of the most common causes of maternal death during the first trimester.

Clinical Findings

A. Symptoms and Signs

Severe lower quadrant pain occurs in almost every case. It is sudden in onset, stabbing, intermittent, and does not radiate. Backache may be present during attacks. Shock occurs in about 10%, often after pelvic examination. At least two-thirds of patients give a history of abnormal menstruation; many have been infertile.

Blood may leak from the tubal ampulla over a period of days, and considerable blood may accumulate in the peritoneum. Slight but persistent vaginal spotting is usually reported, and a pelvic mass may be palpated. Abdominal distention and mild paralytic ileus are often present.

B. Laboratory Findings

The CBC may show anemia and slight leukocytosis. Quantitative serum pregnancy tests will show levels generally lower than expected for normal pregnancies of the same duration. If beta-hCG levels are followed over a few days, there may be a slow rise or a plateau rather than the near doubling every 2 days associated with normal early intrauterine pregnancy or the falling levels that occur with spontaneous abortion.

C. Imaging

Ultrasonography can reliably demonstrate a gestational sac 5–6 weeks from the last menstruation and a fetal pole at 6 weeks if located in the uterus. An empty uterine cavity raises a strong suspicion of extrauterine pregnancy, which can occasionally be revealed by transvaginal ultrasound. Specified levels of serum beta-hCG have been reliably correlated with ultrasound findings of an intrauterine pregnancy; a beta-hCG level of 6500 milli-units/mL with an empty uterine cavity by transabdominal ultrasound is highly suspicious for an ectopic pregnancy. Similarly, a beta-hCG value of 2000 milli-units/mL or more can be indicative of an ectopic pregnancy if no products of conception are detected within the uterine cavity by transvaginal ultrasound. Serum beta-hCG values can vary by laboratory, so clinical decisions should not be made based solely on beta-hCG levels.

D. Special Examinations

Laparoscopy is the surgical procedure of choice both to confirm an ectopic pregnancy and in most cases to permit removal of the ectopic pregnancy without the need for exploratory laparotomy.

Ectopic pregnancy should be suspected when postabortal tissue examination fails to reveal chorionic villi. Steps must be taken for immediate diagnosis, including prompt microscopic tissue examination, ultrasonography, and serial beta-hCG titers every 48 hours.

Differential Diagnosis

Clinical and laboratory findings suggestive or diagnostic of pregnancy will distinguish ectopic pregnancy from many acute abdominal illnesses such as acute appendicitis, acute pelvic inflammatory disease, ruptured corpus luteum cyst or ovarian follicle, and urinary calculi. Uterine enlargement with clinical findings similar to those found in ectopic pregnancy is also characteristic of an aborting uterine pregnancy or hydatidiform mole.

Treatment

Patients must be warned about the complications of an ectopic pregnancy and monitored closely. In a stable patient with normal liver and renal function tests, methotrexate (50 mg/m^2) intramuscularly—given as single or multiple doses—is acceptable medical therapy for early ectopic pregnancy. Favorable criteria are that the pregnancy should be less than 3.5 cm in largest dimension and unruptured, with no active bleeding and no fetal heart tones. Several small studies have not found an increased risk of fetal malformations or pregnancy losses in women who conceive within 6 months of methotrexate therapy.

When a patient with an ectopic pregnancy is unstable or when surgical therapy is planned, the patient is hospitalized. Blood is typed and cross-matched. The goal is to diagnose and operate before there is frank rupture of the tube and intra-abdominal hemorrhage. *The use of methotrexate in an unstable patient is absolutely contraindicated.*

Surgical treatment is definitive. In most patients, diagnostic laparoscopy is the initial surgical procedure performed. Depending on the size of the ectopic pregnancy and whether or not it has ruptured, salpingostomy with removal of the ectopic pregnancy or a partial or complete salpingectomy can usually be performed. Clinical conditions permitting, patency of the contralateral tube can be established by injection of indigo carmine into the uterine cavity and flow through the contralateral tube confirmed visually by the surgeon; iron therapy for anemia may be necessary during convalescence. Rh_0(D) immune globulin (300 mcg) should be given to Rh-negative patients.

Prognosis

Repeat tubal pregnancy occurs in about 10% of cases. This should not be regarded as a contraindication to future pregnancy, but the patient requires careful observation and early ultrasound confirmation of an intrauterine pregnancy.

When to Refer

- Severe abdominal pain.
- Palpation of an adnexal mass on pelvic examination.
- Abdominal pain and vaginal bleeding in a pregnant patient.

When to Admit

Presence of symptoms or signs of a ruptured ectopic pregnancy.

Carusi D. Pregnancy of unknown location: evaluation and management. Semin Perinatol. 2019;43:95. [PMID: 30606496]

GESTATIONAL TROPHOBLASTIC DISEASE (Hydatidiform Mole & Choriocarcinoma)

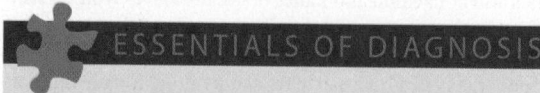

Hydatidiform mole

- Amenorrhea.
- Irregular uterine bleeding.
- Serum beta-hCG > 40,000 milli-units/mL.
- Passage of grapelike clusters of enlarged edematous villi per vagina.

- ▶ Uterine ultrasound shows characteristic heterogeneous echogenic image and no fetus or placenta.
- ▶ Cytogenetic composition is 46,XX (85%), of paternal origin.

Choriocarcinoma

- ▶ Persistence of detectable beta-hCG after mole evacuation.

General Considerations

Gestational trophoblastic disease is a spectrum of disorders that includes hydatidiform mole (partial and complete), invasive mole (local extension into the uterus or vagina), choriocarcinoma (malignancy often complicated by distant metastases), and placental site trophoblastic tumor. Complete moles show no evidence of a fetus on ultrasonography. The majority are 46,XX, with all chromosomes of paternal origin. Partial moles generally show evidence of an embryo or gestational sac; are triploid, slower-growing, and less symptomatic; and often present clinically as a missed abortion. Partial moles tend to follow a benign course, while complete moles have a greater tendency to become choriocarcinoma.

In North America, the frequency of gestational trophoblastic disease is 1:1500 pregnancies. The highest rates occur in Asian persons. Risk factors include prior spontaneous abortion, a history of mole, and age younger than 21 or older than 35. Approximately 10% of women require further treatment after evacuation of the mole; choriocarcinoma develops in 2–3% of women.

Clinical Findings

A. Symptoms and Signs

Uterine bleeding, beginning at 6–16 weeks, is observed in most instances. In some cases, the uterus is larger than would be expected in a normal pregnancy of the same duration. Excessive nausea and vomiting may occur. Bilaterally enlarged cystic ovaries are sometimes palpable. They result from ovarian hyperstimulation due to excess beta-hCG.

Preeclampsia-eclampsia may develop during the second trimester of an untreated molar pregnancy, but this is unusual because most are diagnosed early.

Choriocarcinoma may be manifested by continued or recurrent uterine bleeding after evacuation of a mole or following delivery, abortion, or ectopic pregnancy. An ulcerative vaginal tumor, pelvic mass, or distant metastases may be the presenting manifestation.

B. Laboratory Findings

Hydatidiform moles are generally characterized by high serum beta-hCG values, which can range from high normal to the millions. Levels are higher with complete moles than with partial moles. Serum beta-hCG values, if extremely high, can assist in making the diagnosis, but they are more helpful in managing response to treatment. Hemoglobin/hematocrit, creatinine, blood type, liver biochemical tests, and thyroid function tests should also be measured. High beta-hCG levels can cause the release of thyroid hormone, and rarely, symptoms of hyperthyroidism. Patients with hyperthyroidism may require beta-blocker therapy until the mole has been evacuated.

C. Imaging

The preoperative diagnosis of hydatidiform mole is confirmed by ultrasound. Placental vesicles can be easily seen on transvaginal ultrasound. A preoperative chest film is indicated to rule out pulmonary metastases of the trophoblast.

Treatment

A. Specific (Surgical) Measures

The uterus should be emptied as soon as the diagnosis of hydatidiform mole is established, preferably by suction curettage. The products of conception removed from the uterus should be sent to a pathologist for review. Ovarian cysts should not be resected nor ovaries removed; spontaneous regression of theca lutein cysts will occur with elimination of the mole. In patients who have completed their childbearing, hysterectomy is an acceptable alternative. Hysterectomy does not preclude the need for follow-up of beta-hCG levels.

B. Follow-Up Measures

Weekly quantitative beta-hCG level measurements are initially required. Following successful surgical evacuation, moles show a progressive decline in beta-hCG. After three negative weekly tests (less than 5 milli-units/mL), the interval may be increased to every 1 month for an additional 6 months. The purpose of this follow-up is to identify persistent nonmetastatic and metastatic disease, including choriocarcinoma, which is more likely to occur if the initial beta-hCG is high and the uterus is large. If levels plateau or begin to rise, the patient should be evaluated by repeat laboratory tests, chest film, and dilatation and curettage (D&C) before the initiation of chemotherapy. Effective contraception (preferably birth control pills) should be prescribed to avoid the hazard and confusion of elevated beta-hCG from a new pregnancy. The beta-hCG levels should be negative for 6 months before pregnancy is attempted again. Because the risk of recurrence of a molar pregnancy is 1–2%, an ultrasound should be performed in the first trimester of the pregnancy following a mole to ensure that the pregnancy is normal. In addition, a beta-hCG level should then be checked 6 weeks postpartum (after the subsequent normal pregnancy) to ensure there is no persistent trophoblastic tissue, and the placenta should be examined by a pathologist.

C. Antitumor Chemotherapy

If malignant tissue is discovered at surgery or during the follow-up examination, chemotherapy is indicated. For low-risk patients with a good prognosis, methotrexate is considered first-line therapy followed by dactinomycin (see Table 39–3). Patients with high-risk disease should be referred to a cancer center, where multiple-agent chemotherapy probably will be given.

Prognosis

Five-year survival after courses of chemotherapy, even when metastases have been demonstrated, can be expected in at least 85% of cases of choriocarcinoma.

When to Refer

- Uterine size exceeds that anticipated for gestational age.
- Vaginal bleeding similar to menstruation.
- Pregnant patient with a history of a molar pregnancy.

When to Admit

- Confirmed molar pregnancy by ultrasound and laboratory studies.
- Heavy vaginal bleeding in a pregnant patient under evaluation.

Elias KM et al. State-of-the-art workup and initial management of newly diagnosed molar pregnancy and postmolar gestational trophoblastic neoplasia. J Natl Compr Canc Netw. 2019;17:1396. [PMID: 31693988]

OBSTETRICAL COMPLICATIONS OF THE SECOND & THIRD TRIMESTERS

PREECLAMPSIA-ECLAMPSIA

ESSENTIALS OF DIAGNOSIS

Gestational hypertension

- Blood pressure of ≥ 140/90 mm Hg systolic or > 90 mm Hg diastolic after 20 weeks' gestation.

Preeclampsia

- Blood pressure of ≥ 140 mm Hg systolic or ≥ 90 mm Hg diastolic after 20 weeks' gestation.
- Proteinuria of ≥ 0.3 g in 24 hours.

Preeclampsia with severe features

- Blood pressure of ≥ 160 mm Hg systolic or ≥ 110 mm Hg diastolic.
- Progressive kidney injury.
- Thrombocytopenia.
- Hemolysis, elevated liver enzymes, low platelets (HELLP).
- Pulmonary edema.
- Vision changes or headache.
- When hypertension is present with severe features of preeclampsia, seizure prophylaxis could be beneficial.

Eclampsia

- Seizures in a patient with evidence of preeclampsia.

General Considerations

Preeclampsia is defined as the presence of newly elevated blood pressure and proteinuria during pregnancy. Eclampsia is diagnosed when seizures develop in a patient with evidence of preeclampsia. Historically, three elements were required for the diagnosis of preeclampsia: hypertension, proteinuria, and edema. Edema was difficult to objectively quantify and is no longer a required element. In addition, proteinuria may not always be present in preeclampsia with severe features.

Preeclampsia-eclampsia most commonly occurs in the third trimester but can occur any time after 20 weeks' gestation and up to 6 weeks postpartum.

Risk factors for early preeclampsia-eclampsia are maternal comorbid conditions, such as hypertension, kidney disease, and SLE.

Preeclampsia-eclampsia is a disease unique to pregnancy, with the only cure being delivery of the fetus and placenta. Preeclampsia develops in approximately 7% of pregnant women in the United States; of those, eclampsia will develop in 5% (0.04% of pregnant women). Primiparas are most frequently affected; however, the incidence of preeclampsia-eclampsia is increased with multifetal gestations, preeclampsia in a previous pregnancy, and comorbid diseases such as chronic hypertension, pregestational diabetes, gestational diabetes, thrombophilia, kidney disease, SLE, prepregnancy BMI above 30, antiphospholipid antibody syndrome, maternal age 35 years or older, assisted reproductive technology, and obstructive sleep apnea. Eclampsia is a significant cause of maternal death.

Clinical Findings

The severity of preeclampsia-eclampsia is based on its effect on six major target areas: the CNS, the kidneys, the liver, the hematologic system, the vascular system, and the fetal-placental unit. By evaluating each of these areas for the presence of mild to severe preeclampsia, the degree of involvement can be assessed, and an appropriate management plan can be formulated that balances the severity of disease and gestational age (Table 19–3).

A. Preeclampsia

1. Without severe features—Patients usually have few complaints, and the diastolic blood pressure is less than 110 mm Hg. Edema may be present. The platelet count is over 100,000/mcL ($100 \times 10^9/L$), antepartum fetal testing is reassuring, CNS irritability is minimal, epigastric pain is not present, and liver enzymes are not elevated. Proteinuria is present with urine protein greater than or equal to 0.3/24 hours. Gestational hypertension may be present in the absence of proteinuria.

2. With severe features—Symptoms are more dramatic and persistent. Patients may complain of headache and changes in vision. The blood pressure is often above 160/110 mm Hg. Thrombocytopenia (platelet count less than 100,000/mcL [$100 \times 10^9/L$]) may be present and progress to disseminated intravascular coagulation. Severe epigastric pain may be present from hepatic subcapsular

Table 19–3. Indicators of mild and severe preeclampsia-eclampsia and gestational hypertension with severe features.

Site	Indicator	Mild	Severe
CNS	Symptoms and signs	Hyperreflexia	Seizures, blurred vision, scotomas, headache, clonus, irritability
Kidney	Proteinuria Urinary output	> 0.3 g/24 hours > 30 mL/hour	> 0.3 g/24 hours < 30 mL/hour
Liver	AST, ALT, LD	Normal liver enzymes	Elevated liver enzymes, epigastric pain, ruptured liver
Hematologic	Platelets Hemoglobin	Normal Normal	< 100,000/mcL (100 × 10^9/L) Low, normal, or elevated
Vascular	Blood pressure Retina	< 160/110 mm Hg Arteriolar spasm	> 160/110 mm Hg Retinal hemorrhages
Fetal-placental unit	Growth restriction Oligohydramnios Fetal distress	Absent Absent Absent	Present Present Present

hemorrhage with significant stretch or rupture of the liver capsule. HELLP syndrome (hemolysis, elevated liver enzymes, low platelets) is an advanced form of severe preeclampsia.

B. Eclampsia

The occurrence of seizures defines eclampsia. It is a manifestation of severe CNS involvement. Other findings of preeclampsia are observed.

Differential Diagnosis

Other diseases that can mimic preeclampsia-eclampsia include chronic hypertension, CKD, primary seizure disorders, gallbladder and pancreatic disease, immune thrombocytopenia, thrombotic thrombocytopenic purpura, and hemolytic-uremic syndrome.

Treatment

The American College of Obstetricians and Gynecologists (ACOG) supports considering the use of low-dose aspirin (81 mg orally daily) initiated between 12 weeks' and 28 weeks' gestation for women at increased risk for preeclampsia; risk factors include a history of preeclampsia, multifetal gestation, chronic hypertension, diabetes mellitus, kidney disease, or autoimmune diseases (such as SLE or antiphospholipid syndrome). Clinicians may also consider low-dose aspirin (81 mg orally daily) if more than one of the following moderate risk factors are present: nulliparity, obesity, family history of preeclampsia, Black race, age greater than 35 years, low socioeconomic status, and personal history factors (eg, mother having a previous baby with low birth weight). In clinical studies, diuretics, dietary restriction or enhancement, sodium restriction, and vitamin-mineral supplements (eg, calcium or vitamin C and E) have not been confirmed to be useful. The only cure is delivery of the fetus at a time as favorable as possible for its survival.

A. Preeclampsia

Early recognition is the key to treatment. This requires careful attention to the details of prenatal care—especially subtle changes in blood pressure and weight. The objectives are to prolong pregnancy, if possible, to allow fetal lung maturity while preventing progression to severe disease and eclampsia. The critical factors are the gestational age of the fetus, fetal pulmonary maturity, and the severity of maternal disease. Preeclampsia-eclampsia without severe features and gestational hypertension at term is managed by delivery. Before term, severe preeclampsia-eclampsia requires delivery with very few exceptions. Epigastric pain, seizures, severe range blood pressures, thrombocytopenia, and visual disturbances are strong indications for delivery of the fetus. Marked proteinuria alone can be managed more conservatively.

1. Home management—Home management may be attempted for patients with gestational hypertension and preeclampsia without severe features and a stable home situation. This requires assistance at home, rapid access to the hospital, a reliable patient, and the ability to obtain frequent blood pressure readings. A home health nurse can often provide frequent home visits and assessments.

2. Hospital care—Hospitalization is required for women with preeclampsia with severe features or those with unpredictable home situations. Regular assessments of blood pressure, urine protein, and fetal heart tones and activity are required. A CBC with platelet count, electrolyte panel, and liver enzymes should be checked regularly, with frequency dependent on severity. A 24-hour urine collection for total protein and creatinine clearance should be obtained on admission and repeated as indicated. Magnesium sulfate is not used until the diagnosis of severe preeclampsia is made and delivery planned (see Eclampsia, below).

Fetal evaluation should be obtained as part of the workup. If the patient is being admitted to the hospital, fetal testing should be performed on the same day to assess fetal well-being. This may be done by fetal heart rate testing with nonstress testing or by biophysical profile. A regular schedule of fetal surveillance must then be followed. Daily fetal kick counts can be recorded by the patient herself. If the fetus is less than 34 weeks' gestation, corticosteroids (betamethasone 12 mg intramuscularly every 24 hours for two doses, or dexamethasone 6 mg intramuscularly every 12 hours for four doses) can be administered to the mother. *However, when a woman clearly has unstable severe preeclampsia, delivery should not be delayed for fetal lung maturation or administration of corticosteroids.* In women with gestational hypertension or preeclampsia without severe features at or beyond 37 weeks' gestation, delivery rather than expectant management (eg, watchful waiting or close monitoring) upon diagnosis is recommended.

The method of delivery is determined by the maternal and fetal status. A vaginal delivery is preferred because it has less blood loss than a cesarean section and requires less coagulation factors. Cesarean section is reserved for the usual fetal indications. For mild preeclampsia, delivery should take place at term.

B. Eclampsia

1. Emergency care—If the patient is convulsing, she is turned on her side to prevent aspiration and to improve blood flow to the placenta. The seizure may be stopped by giving an intravenous bolus of magnesium sulfate (the preferred agent), 4–6 g over 4 minutes or until the seizure stops. A continuous intravenous infusion of magnesium sulfate is then started at a rate of 2–3 g/hour unless the patient has reduced kidney function (serum creatinine 1.0–1.5 mg/dL). Reducing maintenance dosing to 1 g/hour or temporarily stopping infusion may be necessary to address instances of kidney dysfunction and magnesium toxicity. Magnesium blood levels may be checked every 4–6 hours and ideally the infusion rate adjusted to maintain a therapeutic blood level (4–7 mEq/L). Urinary output is checked hourly, and the patient assessed for signs of possible magnesium toxicity such as loss of deep tendon reflexes or decrease in respiratory rate and depth, which can be reversed with calcium gluconate, 1 g intravenously over 2 minutes. If seizures continue, an additional dose of magnesium sulfate, 2 g intravenously, may be infused. Alternative agents should be used only if magnesium sulfate is unavailable.

2. General care—In patients who have preeclampsia with severe features, magnesium sulfate should be given intravenously, 4- to 6-g load over 15–20 minutes followed by 2–3 g/hour maintenance, for seizure prophylaxis. Eclampsia necessitates delivery once the patient is stabilized. It is important, however, that assessment of the status of the patient and fetus take place first. Continuous fetal monitoring must be performed and maternal blood typed and cross-matched quickly. A urinary catheter is inserted to monitor urinary output, and a CBC with platelets, electrolytes, creatinine, and liver enzymes are obtained. If hypertension is present with systolic values of 160 mm Hg or higher or diastolic values 110 mm Hg or higher, antihypertensive medications should be administered to reduce the blood pressure to 140–150/90–100 mm Hg. Lower blood pressures than this may induce placental insufficiency through reduced perfusion. Hydralazine, given in 5- to 10-mg increments intravenously every 20 minutes, is frequently used to lower blood pressure. Labetalol, 10–20 mg intravenously, every 20 minutes as needed, can also be used. Immediate-release oral nifedipine 10–20 mg may be administered and then repeated in 20 minutes, followed by 10–20 mg every 4–6 hours for a maximum daily dosage of 180 mg. This medication is helpful if the patient does not have intravenous access.

3. Delivery—Delivery is mandated once eclampsia has occurred. Vaginal delivery is preferred. Subsequent prolonged fetal heart rate decelerations are frequent after an eclamptic seizure. However, delivery should proceed only after there is maternal hemodynamic stabilization. Furthermore, maternal resuscitation is usually followed by normalization of the fetal tracing. The rapidity with which delivery must be achieved depends on the fetal and maternal status following the seizure and the availability of laboratory data on the patient. Oxytocin, given intravenously and titrated to a dose that results in adequate contractions, may be used to induce or augment labor. Oxytocin should only be administered by a clinician specifically trained in its use. Regional analgesia or general anesthesia is acceptable. Cesarean section is used for the usual obstetric indications.

4. Postpartum—Magnesium sulfate infusion (2–3 g/hour with noted exceptions, see above) should be continued for 24 hours postpartum. Late-onset preeclampsia-eclampsia can occur during the postpartum period. It is usually manifested by either hypertension or seizures. Treatment is the same as before delivery—ie, with hydralazine and magnesium sulfate.

When to Refer

- New onset of hypertension and proteinuria in a pregnant patient more than 20 weeks' gestation.
- New onset of seizure activity in a pregnant patient.

When to Admit

- Symptoms of preeclampsia with severe features in a pregnant patient with elevated blood pressure above baseline.
- Evaluation for preeclampsia when severe features of the disease are suspected.
- Evaluation for preeclampsia in a patient with an unstable home environment.
- Evidence of eclampsia.

American College of Obstetricians and Gynecologists. Practice Bulletin No. 222: gestational hypertension and preeclampsia. Obstet Gynecol. 2020;135:e237. [PMID: 32443079]

PRETERM LABOR

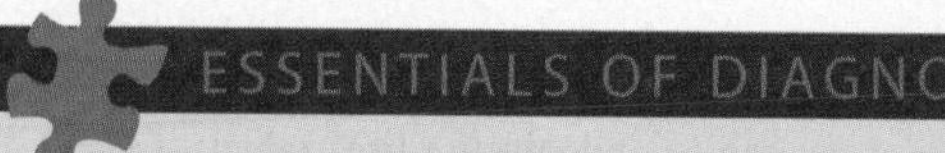

- Preterm regular uterine contractions approximately 5 minutes apart.
- Cervical dilatation, effacement, or both.

General Considerations

Preterm birth is defined as birth between 20 0/7 and 36 6/7 weeks' gestation, and spontaneous preterm labor with or without premature rupture of the fetal membranes causes at least two-thirds of all preterm births. Prematurity is the largest single contributor to infant mortality, and survivors are at risk for a myriad of short- and long-term complications. It also the most common reason for antepartum hospitalization. Rates of infant death and long-term neurologic impairment are inversely related to gestational age at birth. The cusp of viability in contemporary practice is 23–25 weeks' gestation, and infants born before 23 weeks rarely survive. About two-thirds of the preterm births occur between 34 weeks and 36 weeks and 6 days (termed "late preterm birth"), and good outcomes are expected at these gestational ages. Importantly, however, even these late preterm infants are at significantly increased risk for both morbidity and mortality when compared to those infants born at term.

Major risk factors for spontaneous preterm labor include a past history of preterm birth and a short cervical length as measured by transvaginal ultrasound. Other known risk factors include Black race, multifetal pregnancies, intrauterine infection, substance abuse, smoking, periodontal disease, and socioeconomic deprivation. Numerous preterm births are preceded by ruptured membranes.

Clinical Findings

In women with regular uterine contractions and cervical change, the diagnosis of preterm labor is straightforward. However, symptoms such as pelvic pressure, cramping, or vaginal discharge may be the first complaints in high-risk patients who later develop preterm labor. Because these complaints may be vague and irregular uterine contractions are common, distinguishing which patients merit further evaluation can be problematic. In some cases, this distinction can be facilitated by the use of fetal fibronectin measurement in cervicovaginal specimens. This test is most useful when it is negative (less than 50 ng/mL), since the negative predictive value for delivery within 7–14 days is 93–97%. A negative test, therefore, usually means the patient can be reassured and discharged home. Because of its low sensitivity, however, fetal fibronectin is not recommended as a screening test in asymptomatic women.

Treatment

A. General Measures

Patients must be educated to identify symptoms associated with preterm labor to avoid unnecessary delay in their evaluation. In patients who are believed to be at increased risk for preterm delivery, randomized trials have failed to demonstrate improved outcomes in women placed on activity restriction. Paradoxically, such recommendations may place a woman at an *increased* risk to deliver preterm. Women with preterm labor at the threshold of viability present unique ethical and obstetric challenges and are best managed in consultation with maternal-fetal medicine and neonatology specialists. The families in such situations should be actively and continually engaged about decisions regarding the aggressiveness of resuscitative efforts.

B. Corticosteroids

In pregnancies between 23 weeks' and 34 weeks' gestation where preterm birth is anticipated, a single short course of corticosteroids should be administered to promote fetal lung maturity. Such therapy has been demonstrated to reduce the frequency of respiratory distress syndrome, intracranial hemorrhage, and even death in preterm infants. Betamethasone, 12 mg intramuscularly repeated once 24 hours later, and dexamethasone, 6 mg intramuscularly repeated every 12 hours for four doses, both cross the placenta and are the preferred treatments in this setting. A single repeat course of antenatal corticosteroids should be considered in women who are at risk for preterm delivery within the next 7 days, and whose prior dose of antenatal corticosteroids was administered more than 14 days previously. Rescue course corticosteroids could be provided as early as 7 days from the prior dose, if indicated by the clinical scenario. Administration of betamethasone may be considered in pregnant women between 34 0/7 and 36 6/7 weeks' gestation at imminent risk for preterm birth within 7 days, and who have not received a previous course of antenatal corticosteroids.

C. Antibiotics

Despite the finding that preterm labor is associated with intrauterine infection in certain cases, there is no evidence that antibiotics forestall delivery in women with preterm labor and intact membranes. However, women in preterm labor should receive antimicrobial prophylaxis against group B *streptococcus* unless a single standard culture of the distal vagina and anorectum has been negative for the organism in the preceding 5 weeks. Notably, there is usually not enough time in this clinical setting to culture and test isolates. The recommended regimen for antimicrobial prophylaxis against group B *Streptococcus* is penicillin G, 5 million units intravenously as a loading dose and then 2.5–3 million units intravenously every 4 hours until delivery. In penicillin-allergic patients not at high risk for anaphylaxis, 2 g of cefazolin can be given intravenously as an initial dose and then 1 g intravenously every 8 hours until delivery. In patients at high risk for anaphylaxis, vancomycin, 20 mg/kg intravenously every 8 hours until delivery, can be used. Clindamycin, 900 mg intravenously every 8 hours until delivery, can also be used after a group B streptococcal isolate has been confirmed to be susceptible to clindamycin.

D. Tocolytic Agents

Evidence supports the use of first-line tocolytic treatment to forestall delivery with beta-adrenergic receptor agonists, calcium channel blockers, or indomethacin for short-term prolongation of pregnancy (up to 48 hours) to allow for the administration of antenatal corticosteroids, and (if appropriate), transport the patient to a facility better equipped to care for premature infants. Maintenance therapy (continuation of treatment beyond 48 hours) is not effective at preventing preterm birth and is not recommended.

Beta-adrenergic drugs, such as terbutaline, can be given every 30 minutes as an intravenous infusion starting at 2.5 mcg/minute or as a subcutaneous injection starting at 250 mcg. Oral terbutaline is not recommended because of the lack of proven efficacy and concerns about maternal safety. Serious maternal side effects have been reported with the use of terbutaline and include tachycardia, pulmonary edema, arrhythmias, metabolic derangements (such as hyperglycemia and hypokalemia), and even death. Pulmonary edema occurs with increased frequency with concomitant administration of corticosteroids, large-volume intravenous fluid infusion, maternal sepsis, or prolonged tocolysis. Because of these safety concerns, the US FDA warns that terbutaline be administered exclusively in a hospital setting and discontinued after 48–72 hours of treatment.

Nifedipine, 20 mg orally every 6 hours, and **indomethacin**, 50 mg orally once then 25 mg orally every 6 hours up to 48 hours, have been used with limited success.

Magnesium sulfate is commonly used (but no longer recommended as a first-line agent) for tocolysis, and there is evidence that it may also be protective against cerebral palsy in infants from 24 weeks' to 32 weeks' gestation when given at time of birth. Magnesium sulfate is given intravenously as a 4- to 6-g bolus followed by a continuous infusion of 2 g/hour. Magnesium levels are not typically checked but should be monitored if there is any concern for toxicity. Magnesium sulfate is entirely cleared by the kidney and must, therefore, be used with caution in women with any degree of kidney disease.

Before attempts are made to prevent preterm delivery with tocolytic agents, the patient should be assessed for conditions in which delivery would be indicated. Severe preeclampsia, lethal fetal anomalies, placental abruption, and intrauterine infection are all examples of indications for preterm delivery. In such cases, attempts to forestall delivery would be inappropriate.

Preterm Birth Prevention

Strategies aimed at preventing preterm birth in high-risk women—principally those with a history of preterm birth or a shortened cervix (or both)—have focused on the administration of progesterone or progesterone compounds and the use of cervical cerclage. Prospective randomized controlled trials have demonstrated reductions in rates of preterm birth in high-risk women with singleton pregnancies who received progesterone supplementation, although the optimal preparation, dose, and route of administration (intramuscular injection versus vaginal suppository) are unclear. Although the issue has not been settled, there is some evidence that progesterone therapy may decrease rates of preterm birth in nulliparous women who have a shortened cervix as measured by transvaginal ultrasound. The ACOG does not recommend universal transvaginal cervical length screening but acknowledges that this strategy may be considered.

There is also evidence that women with a previous spontaneous preterm birth and a shortened cervix (less than 25 mm before 24 weeks' gestation) may benefit from placement of a cervical cerclage. Incidentally detected short cervical length in the second trimester in the absence of a prior singleton preterm birth is not diagnostic of cervical insufficiency, and cerclage is not indicated in this setting. In twin and triplet gestations, however, neither progesterone administration nor cervical cerclage placement has been effective at prolonging pregnancy, and these therapies are not recommended in women with multifetal pregnancies.

When to Refer

- Symptoms of increased pelvic pressure or cramping in high-risk patients.
- Regular uterine contractions.
- Rupture of membranes.
- Vaginal bleeding.

When to Admit

- Cervical dilation of 2 cm or more before 34 weeks' gestation.
- Contractions that cause cervical change.
- Rupture of membranes.

American College of Obstetricians and Gynecologists. ACOG Practice Bulletin, No 234: prediction and prevention of spontaneous preterm birth. Obstet Gynecol. 2021;138:945. [PMID: 34794160]

American College of Obstetricians and Gynecologists. Practice Advisory: use of antenatal corticosteroids at 22 weeks of gestation. 2021 Sep. https://www.acog.org/clinical/clinical-guidance/practice-advisory/articles/2021/09/use-of-antenatal-corticosteroids-at-22-weeks-of-gestation

American College of Obstetricians and Gynecologists. Practice Bulletin No. 217: prelabor rupture of membranes. Obstet Gynecol. 2020;135:e80. [PMID: 32080050]

THIRD-TRIMESTER BLEEDING

Five to 10 percent of women have vaginal bleeding in late pregnancy. The clinician must distinguish between placental causes (placenta previa, placental abruption, vasa previa) and nonplacental causes (labor, infection, disorders of the lower genital tract, systemic disease. The approach to bleeding in late pregnancy depends on the underlying cause, the gestational age at presentation, the degree of blood loss, and the overall status of the mother and her fetus. The cause of antepartum bleeding after mid-pregnancy is unknown in one-third of cases.

Treatment

A. General Measures

The patient should initially be observed closely with continuous fetal monitoring to assess for fetal distress. A CBC with platelets and a prothrombin time (INR) should be obtained and repeated serially if the bleeding continues. If hemorrhage is significant or if there is evidence of acute hypovolemia, the need for transfusion should be anticipated and an appropriate volume of red cells prepared with cross-matching. Ultrasound examination should be performed to determine placental location. Digital pelvic examinations are done only after ultrasound examination has ruled out placenta previa. Administration of anti-D immune globulin may be required for women who are Rh negative.

B. Placenta Previa

Placenta previa occurs when the placenta implants over the internal cervical os. Risk factors for this condition include previous cesarean delivery, increasing maternal age, multiparity, and cigarette smoking. If the diagnosis is initially made in the first or second trimester, the ultrasound should be repeated in the third trimester. Persistence of placenta previa at this point is an indication for cesarean as the route of delivery. Painless vaginal bleeding is the characteristic symptom in placenta previa and can range from light spotting to profuse hemorrhage. Hospitalization for extended evaluation is the appropriate initial management approach. For pregnancies that have reached 37 weeks' gestation or beyond with continued bleeding, cesarean delivery is generally indicated. Pregnancies at 36 weeks or earlier are candidates for expectant management provided the bleeding is not prodigious, and a subset of these women can be discharged if the bleeding and contractions completely subside.

C. Morbidly Adherent Placenta

Morbidly adherent placenta is a general term describing an abnormally adherent placenta that has invaded into the uterus. The condition can be further classified depending on whether the depth of invasion is limited to the endometrium (*accreta*), extends into the myometrium (*increta*), or invades beyond the uterine serosa (*percreta*). The most important risk factor for a morbidly adherent placenta is a prior uterine scar—typically from one or more prior cesarean deliveries. The focus of invasion usually involves the scar itself, and *placenta previa* is commonly associated with morbid adherence. Obstetric care providers are concerned with the incidence of these syndromes has increased dramatically over the last 50 years commensurate with the increasing cesarean delivery rate.

After delivery of the infant, almost always in a repeat cesarean section, the morbidly adherent placenta does not separate normally, and the bleeding that results can be torrential. Emergency hysterectomy is usually required to stop the hemorrhage, and transfusion requirements are often massive. Because of the considerable increase in both maternal morbidity and mortality associated with this condition, careful preoperative planning is imperative when the diagnosis is suspected antenatally. Ultrasound findings such as intraplacental lacunae, bridging vessels into the bladder, and loss of the retroplacental clear space suggest placental invasion in women who have placenta previa. *Importantly, however, even if ultrasound findings are subtle, an abnormally adherent placenta should be suspected in any patient with one or more prior cesarean deliveries and an anterior placenta previa.* Ideally, delivery planning should involve a multidisciplinary team, and the surgery should take place at an institution with appropriate personnel and a blood bank equipped to handle patients requiring massive transfusion. It has been demonstrated that a systematic approach to management with a multidisciplinary team improves patient outcomes. Evidence-based recommendations regarding delivery timing are lacking, but the goal is to have a planned, late-preterm cesarean delivery. As such, delivery at 34–36 weeks in a stable patient seems a reasonable approach.

D. Placental Abruption

Placental abruption is the premature separation of the placenta from its implantation site before delivery. Risk factors for abruption include hypertension, multiparity, cocaine use, cigarette smoking, previous abruption, and thrombophilias. Classic symptoms are vaginal bleeding, uterine tenderness, and frequent contractions, but the clinical presentation is highly variable. There is often concealed hemorrhage when the placenta abrupts, which causes increased pressure in the intervillous space. Excess amounts of thromboplastin escape into the maternal circulation and defibrination occurs. Profound coagulopathy and acute hypovolemia from blood loss can occur and are more likely with an abruption severe enough to kill the fetus. Ultrasound may be helpful to exclude placenta previa, but failure to identify a retroplacental clot does not exclude abruption. In most cases, abruption is an indication for immediate cesarean delivery because of the high risk of fetal death.

American College of Obstetricians and Gynecologists. Obstetric Care Consensus No. 7: placenta accreta spectrum. Obstet Gynecol. 2018;132:e259. [PMID: 30461695]

American College of Obstetricians and Gynecologists. Practice Bulletin No. 183: postpartum hemorrhage. Obstet Gynecol. 2017;130:e168. [Reaffirmed 2019] [PMID: 28937571]

OBSTETRIC COMPLICATIONS OF THE PERIPARTUM PERIOD

PUERPERAL MASTITIS

Postpartum mastitis occurs sporadically in nursing mothers, usually with symptom onset after discharge from the hospital. *Staphylococcus aureus* is usually the causative agent. Women nursing for the first time and those with difficulty breastfeeding appear to be at greatest risk. Rarely, inflammatory carcinoma of the breast can be mistaken for puerperal mastitis (see also Chapter 17). Unfortunately, strategies aimed at preventing mastitis in breastfeeding women have been unsuccessful.

Mastitis frequently begins within 3 months after delivery and may start with an engorged breast and a sore or fissured nipple. Cellulitis is typically unilateral with the affected area of breast being red, tender, and warm. Fever and chills are common complaints as well. Treatment consists of antibiotics effective against penicillin-resistant staphylococci (dicloxacillin 500 mg orally every 6 hours or a cephalosporin for 10–14 days) and regular emptying of the breast by nursing or by using a mechanical suction device. Although nursing from the infected breast is safe for the infant, local inflammation of the nipple may complicate latching. Failure to respond to usual antibiotics within 3 days may represent an organizing abscess or infection with a resistant organism. The risk for abscess formation is increased when the causative organism is methicillin-resistant *S aureus* (MRSA), compared with infection from nonresistant staphylococcal species. If an abscess is suspected, ultrasound of the breast can help confirm the diagnosis. In these cases, aspiration or surgical evacuation is usually required. Changing antibiotics based on culture sensitivity (to vancomycin or trimethoprim-sulfamethoxazole, for example) is useful, especially if the clinical course is not improving appropriately.

CHORIOAMNIONITIS & METRITIS

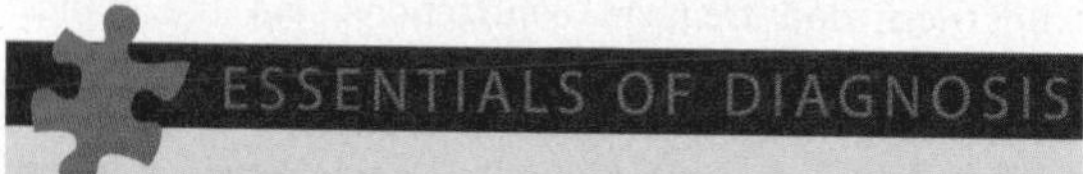

- Fever not attributable to another source.
- Uterine tenderness.
- Tachycardia in the mother, fetus, or both.

General Considerations

Pelvic infections are relatively common problems encountered during the peripartum period. Chorioamnionitis is an infection of the amnion and chorion (fetal parts), usually occurring during labor. Uterine infection after delivery is often called endometritis or endomyometritis, but the term "metritis" is probably most accurate to emphasize that the infection extends throughout the uterine tissue. These infections are polymicrobial and are most commonly attributed to urogenital pathogens. The single most important risk factor for puerperal infection is cesarean delivery, which increases the risk from 5- to 20-fold. Other recognized risk factors include prolonged labor, use of internal monitors, nulliparity, multiple pelvic examinations, prolonged rupture of membranes, and lower genital tract infections. Although maternal complications such as dysfunctional labor and postpartum hemorrhage are increased with clinical chorioamnionitis, the principal reason to initiate treatment is to prevent morbidity in the offspring. Neonatal complications such as sepsis, pneumonia, intraventricular hemorrhage, and cerebral palsy are increased in the setting of chorioamnionitis. Intrapartum initiation of antibiotics, however, significantly reduces neonatal morbidity.

Clinical Findings

Puerperal infections are diagnosed principally by the presence of fever (38°C or higher) in the absence of any other source and one or more of the following signs: maternal or fetal tachycardia (or both), and uterine tenderness. Foul-smelling lochia may be present but is an insensitive marker of infection as many women without infection may experience an unpleasant odor. Likewise, some life-threatening infections such as necrotizing fasciitis are typically odorless. Cultures are typically not done because of the polymicrobial nature of the infection.

Treatment

Treatment is empiric with broad-spectrum antibiotics that will cover gram-positive and gram-negative organisms if still pregnant and gram-negative organisms and anaerobes if postpartum. A common regimen for chorioamnionitis is ampicillin, 2 g intravenously every 6 hours, and gentamicin, 2 mg/kg intravenous load then 1.5 mg/kg intravenously every 8 hours. A common regimen for metritis is gentamicin, 2 mg/kg intravenous load then 1.5 mg/kg intravenously every 8 hours, and clindamycin, 900 mg intravenously every 8 hours. Antibiotics are stopped in the mother when she has been afebrile and asymptomatic for 24 hours. No oral antibiotics are subsequently needed. Patients with metritis who do not respond in the first 24–48 hours may have an enterococcal component of metritis and require additional gram-positive coverage (such as ampicillin) to the regimen.

MEDICAL CONDITIONS COMPLICATING PREGNANCY

ANEMIA

Normal pregnancy is characterized by an increase in maternal plasma volume of about 50% and an increase in red cell volume of about 25%. Because of these changes, the mean hemoglobin and hematocrit values are lower than in the nonpregnant state. Anemia in pregnancy is considered when the hemoglobin measurement is below 11 g/dL in the first trimester, 10.5 g/dL in the second trimester, and 11 g/dL in the third trimester. By far, the most common causes are iron deficiency and acute blood loss anemia, the latter usually occurring in the peripartum period. Symptoms such as fatigue and dyspnea that would otherwise suggest the presence of anemia in nonpregnant women are common in pregnant women; therefore, periodic measurement of hematocrits in pregnancy is essential so that anemia can be identified and treated. In addition to its impact on maternal health, untoward pregnancy outcomes such as low birthweight and preterm delivery have been associated with second- and third-trimester anemia.

A. Iron Deficiency Anemia

The increased requirement for iron over the course of pregnancy is appreciable to support fetal growth and expansion of maternal blood volume. Dietary intake of iron generally cannot meet this demand, and all pregnant women should receive about 30 mg of elemental iron per day in the second and third trimesters. Oral iron therapy is commonly associated with GI side effects, such as nausea and constipation, and these symptoms often contribute to noncompliance. If supplementation is inadequate, however, anemia often becomes evident by the third trimester of pregnancy. Because iron deficiency is by far the most common cause of anemia in pregnancy, treatment is usually empiric and consists of 60–100 mg of elemental iron per day and a diet containing iron-rich foods. Iron studies can confirm the diagnosis, if necessary (see Chapter 13), and further evaluation should be considered in patients who do not respond to oral iron. Intermittent iron supplementation (eg, every other day) has been associated with fewer side effects and may be reasonable for women who cannot tolerate daily therapy.

B. Folic Acid Deficiency Anemia

Megaloblastic anemia in pregnancy is almost always caused by folic acid deficiency, since vitamin B_{12} deficiency is uncommon in the childbearing years. Folate deficiency is usually caused by inadequate dietary intake of fresh leafy vegetables, legumes, and animal proteins.

The diagnosis is made by finding macrocytic red cells and hypersegmented neutrophils on a blood smear (see Chapter 13). However, blood smears in pregnancy may be difficult to interpret since they frequently show iron deficiency changes as well. With established folate deficiency, a supplemental dose of 1 mg/day and a diet with increased folic acid will generally correct the anemia.

C. Sickle Cell Anemia

Women with sickle cell anemia are subject to serious complications in pregnancy. The anemia becomes more severe, and acute pain crises often occur more frequently. When compared with women who do not have hemoglobinopathies, women with hemoglobin SS are at increased risk for infections (especially pulmonary and urinary tract), thromboembolic events, pregnancy-related hypertension, transfusion, cesarean delivery, preterm birth, and fetal growth restriction. There also continues to be an increased rate of maternal mortality, despite an increased recognition of the high-risk nature of these pregnancies. Intensive medical treatment may improve the outcomes for both mother and fetus. Prophylactically transfusing packed red cells to lower the level of hemoglobin S and elevate the level of hemoglobin A is a controversial practice without clear benefit. Most women with sickle cell disease will not require iron supplementation, but folate requirements can be appreciable due to red cell turnover from hemolysis.

D. Other Anemias

Although many of the inherited or acquired causes of anemia are relatively rare in women of childbearing age, they can be encountered in pregnancy. The implications for the mother and her offspring vary widely depending on the etiology of anemia. For example, mild microcytic anemia may be caused by iron deficiency, but it could also represent anemia of chronic disease because of previously undiagnosed malignancy. As such, women who have anemia caused by a disorder besides a nutritional deficiency are best managed in conjunction with a maternal-fetal medicine specialist and a hematologist. Additionally, women who have an inherited form of anemia (hemoglobinopathies and thalassemia syndromes, for example) should be offered genetic counseling; prenatal diagnosis, if available, should be discussed if the parents wish to know whether the fetus is affected.

American College of Obstetricians and Gynecologists. ACOG Practice Bulletin No. 233: anemia in pregnancy. Obstet Gynecol. 2021;138:e55. [PMID: 34293770]

American College of Obstetricians and Gynecologists. ACOG Practice Bulletin No. 78: hemoglobinopathies in pregnancy. Obstet Gynecol 2007;109:229. [Reaffirmed 2019] [PMID: 17197616]

ANTIPHOSPHOLIPID SYNDROME

The antiphospholipid syndrome (APS) is characterized by autoantibodies, notably in association with arterial and venous thrombosis and adverse pregnancy outcomes (see Chapter 20).

THYROID DISEASE

Thyroid disease is relatively common in pregnancy, and in their overt states, both hypothyroidism and hyperthyroidism have been consistently associated with adverse pregnancy outcomes. There are gestational age-specific effects that pregnancy has on thyroid function tests; failure to recognize these physiologic alterations can cause misclassification or misdiagnosis. Women who have a history of a thyroid disorder or symptoms that suggest thyroid dysfunction should be screened with thyroid function tests. Screening asymptomatic pregnant women, however, is of unproven benefit and is not currently recommended.

Overt hypothyroidism is defined by an elevated serum TSH level with a depressed FT_4 level. During pregnancy, several factors occur that affect maternal thyroid hormones: (1) Rising estrogen levels increase thyroxine binding globulin (TBG) serum concentrations, reducing FT_4 levels. (2) Placental deiodinase promotes the turnover of T_4. (3) Supplemental iron and prenatal multivitamins containing iron can bind to oral T_4 and reduce its intestinal absorption.

The most common etiology of hypothyroidism during pregnancy is Hashimoto (autoimmune) thyroiditis. Many of the symptoms of hypothyroidism mimic those of normal pregnancy, making its clinical identification difficult. Maternal hypothyroidism has consistently been associated with an increase in complications such as spontaneous abortion, preterm birth, preeclampsia, placental abruption, and impaired neuropsychological development in the offspring; the fetus is at least partially dependent on maternal T_4 for its CNS development—particularly in the second trimester. *Therefore, for women who need levothyroxine, it is prudent to increase the dosages by approximately 20–30% as soon as pregnancy is confirmed. Pregnant women with overt hypothyroidism or myxedema should be treated immediately with levothyroxine at full replacement doses of 1.6 mcg/kg/day (about 100–150 mcg daily).* For titration, the levothyroxine dosage may be increased according to clinical response and serum TSH, measuring serum TSH every 4–6 weeks and trying to keep the serum TSH level in a trimester-specific gestational reference range. An increase in the dose of levothyroxine may be required in the second and third trimesters. By mid-pregnancy, women require an average of 47% increase in their levothyroxine dosage.

Subclinical hypothyroidism is defined as an increased serum TSH with a normal FT_4 level. Although some studies have found associations with untoward pregnancy outcomes such as miscarriage, preterm birth, and preeclampsia, others have failed to confirm these findings. There is no evidence that treatment of subclinical hypothyroidism will prevent any of these outcomes. The ACOG and the American Association of Clinical Endocrinologists recommend against universal screening for thyroid disease in pregnancy.

Overt hyperthyroidism, defined as excessive production of thyroxine with a depressed (usually undetectable) serum TSH level, is also associated with increased risks in pregnancy. Spontaneous pregnancy loss, preterm birth, preeclampsia, and maternal heart failure occur with increased frequency with untreated thyrotoxicosis. Thyroid storm, although rare, can be a life-threatening complication. Medical treatment of thyrotoxicosis is usually accomplished with the antithyroid drugs propylthiouracil or methimazole. Although teratogenicity has not been clearly established, in utero exposure to methimazole has been associated with aplasia cutis and choanal and esophageal atresia in the offspring of pregnancies so treated. Propylthiouracil is not believed to be teratogenic, but it has been associated with the rare complications of hepatotoxicity and agranulocytosis. Recommendations by the American Thyroid Association are to treat with propylthiouracil in the first trimester and convert to methimazole for the remainder of the pregnancy. The therapeutic target for the FT_4 level is the upper limit of the normal reference range. The TSH levels generally stay suppressed even with adequate treatment. A beta-blocker can be used for such symptoms as palpitations or tremors. Fetal hypothyroidism or hyperthyroidism is uncommon but can occur with maternal Graves disease, which is the most common cause of hyperthyroidism in pregnancy. *Radioiodine ablation is absolutely contraindicated in pregnancy because it may destroy the fetal thyroid as well.*

Postpartum thyroiditis is discussed in Chapter 26; see Thyroiditis.

American College of Obstetricians and Gynecologists. Practice Bulletin No. 223: thyroid disease in pregnancy. Obstet Gynecol. 2020;135:e261 [PMID: 32443080]

DIABETES MELLITUS

Normal pregnancy can be characterized as a state of increased insulin resistance that helps ensure a steady stream of glucose delivery to the developing fetus. Thus, both mild fasting hypoglycemia and postprandial hyperglycemia are physiologic. These metabolic changes are felt to be hormonally mediated with likely contributions from human placental lactogen, estrogen, and progesterone.

A. Gestational Diabetes Mellitus

Gestational diabetes mellitus is abnormal glucose tolerance in pregnancy and is generally believed to exaggerate the pregnancy-induced physiologic changes in carbohydrate metabolism. Alternatively, pregnancy may unmask an underlying propensity for glucose intolerance, which will be evident in the nonpregnant state at some future time if not in the immediate postpartum period. Indeed, at least 50% of women with gestational diabetes will have an overt diabetes diagnosis at some point in their lifetime. During the pregnancy, the principal concern in women identified to have gestational diabetes is excessive fetal growth, which can cause increased maternal and perinatal morbidity. Shoulder dystocia occurs more frequently in infants of mothers with diabetes because of fetal overgrowth and increased fat deposition on the shoulders. Cesarean delivery and preeclampsia are also significantly increased in women with diabetes, both gestational and overt.

All asymptomatic pregnant women should undergo laboratory screening for gestational diabetes after 24 weeks' gestation. The diagnostic thresholds for glucose tolerance tests in pregnancy are not universally agreed upon, and importantly, adverse pregnancy outcomes appear to occur along a continuum of glucose intolerance even if the diagnosis of gestational diabetes is not formally assigned. A two-stage testing strategy is recommended by the ACOG, starting with a 50-g screening test offered to all pregnant women at 24–28 weeks' gestation. If this test is abnormal, the diagnostic test is a 100-g oral glucose tolerance test (Table 19–4).

Women in whom gestational diabetes is diagnosed should undergo nutrition counseling, and medications are typically initiated for those with persistent fasting hyperglycemia. Insulin has historically been considered the standard medication used to achieve glycemic control. Oral hypoglycemic agents, principally glyburide and metformin, have been evaluated in short-term clinical trials and appear to achieve similar degrees of glycemic control to insulin without increasing maternal or neonatal morbidity. These medications, however, have not been approved by the US FDA for this indication; the long-term safety of oral agents has not been adequately studied in the women

Table 19–4. Screening and diagnostic criteria for gestational diabetes mellitus.

Screening for gestational diabetes mellitus

1. 50-g oral glucose load, administered between 24 and 28 weeks, without regard to time of day or time of last meal.
2. Venous plasma glucose measured 1 hour later.
3. Value of 140 mg/dL (7.8 mmol/L) or above in venous plasma indicates the need for a diagnostic glucose tolerance test.

Diagnosis of gestational diabetes mellitus

1. 100-g oral glucose load, administered in the morning after overnight fast lasting at least 8 hours but not more than 14 hours, and following at least 3 days of unrestricted diet (> 150 g carbohydrate) and physical activity.
2. Venous plasma glucose is measured fasting and at 1, 2, and 3 hours. Patient should remain seated and should not smoke throughout the test.
3. The diagnosis of gestational diabetes is made when two or more of the following venous plasma concentrations are met or exceeded: fasting, 95 mg/dL (5.3 mmol/L); 1 hour, 180 mg/dL (10 mmol/L); 2 hours, 155 mg/dL (8.6 mmol/L); 3 hours, 140 mg/dL (7.8 mmol/L).

or in their offspring, and study quality of these agents has been poor. The current standard of care is insulin, unless circumstances preclude its use. In those cases, metformin is a reasonable choice. Insulin regimens commonly include multiple daily injections of a split-dose mix of intermediate-acting and short-acting agents. Regular and NPH insulins, as well as insulin lispro and aspart, do not cross the placenta. Once therapy is initiated, blood glucose surveillance is important to assess for adequacy of glycemic control. Capillary blood glucose levels should be checked four times per day, once fasting and three times after meals. Euglycemia is considered to be 60–90 mg/dL (3.3–5.0 mmol/L) while fasting and less than 120 mg/dL (6.7 mmol/L) 2 hours postprandially. Intensive therapy with dietary modifications or insulin therapy, or both, has been demonstrated to decrease rates of macrosomia, shoulder dystocia, and preeclampsia. Because of the increased prevalence of overt diabetes in women identified to have gestational diabetes, they should be screened at 6–12 weeks' postpartum with a fasting plasma glucose test or a 2-hour oral glucose tolerance test (75-g glucose load).

B. Overt Diabetes Mellitus

Overt diabetes is diabetes mellitus that antedates the pregnancy. There is an inverse relationship between glycemic control and fetal malformations, and women whose periconceptional glycosylated hemoglobin levels are at or near normal levels have rates of malformations that approach baseline. In gestational diabetes, fetal overgrowth from inadequately controlled hyperglycemia remains a significant concern because of the increased maternal and perinatal morbidity that accompany macrosomia. Women with overt diabetes are subject to several other complications as well. Spontaneous pregnancy loss and third-trimester stillbirths occur with increased frequency in these women. There is also at least a twofold to threefold increased risk for fetal malformations (risk in in normal pregnancies is 2–3%), as hyperglycemia during organogenesis is teratogenic. The most common malformations in offspring of diabetic women are cardiac, skeletal, and neural tube defects. For the mother, the likelihood of infections and pregnancy-related hypertension is increased.

Preconception counseling and evaluation in a diabetic woman is ideal to maximize the pregnancy outcomes. This provides an opportunity to optimize glycemic control and evaluate for evidence of end-organ damage. The initial evaluation of diabetic women should include a complete chemistry panel, HbA_{1c} determination, 24-hour urine collection for total protein and creatinine clearance, funduscopic examination, and an ECG. Hypertension is common and may require treatment. Optimally, euglycemia should be established before conception and maintained during pregnancy with daily home glucose monitoring by the patient. A well-planned dietary program is a key component, with an intake of 1800–2200 kcal/day divided into three meals and three snacks. Insulin is given subcutaneously in a split-dose regimen as described above for women with gestational diabetes. The use of continuous insulin pump therapy may be helpful for some patients (see Chapter 27).

Throughout the pregnancy, diabetic women should be seen every 2–3 weeks and more frequently depending on the clinical condition. Adjustments in the insulin regimen may be necessary as the pregnancy progresses to maintain optimal glycemic control. A specialized ultrasound is often performed around 20 weeks to screen for fetal malformations. Symptoms and signs of infections should be evaluated and promptly treated. In the third trimester, fetal surveillance is indicated, and women with diabetes should receive serial antenatal testing (usually in the form of a nonstress test or biophysical profile). The timing of delivery is dictated by the quality of diabetic control, the presence or absence of medical complications, and fetal status. The goal is to reach 39 weeks (38 completed weeks) and then proceed with delivery. Confirmation of lung maturity may be appropriate if preterm delivery is contemplated.

American College of Obstetricians and Gynecologists. Practice Bulletin No. 201: pregestational diabetes mellitus. Obstet Gynecol. 2018;132:e228. [PMID: 30461693]

American College of Obstetricians and Gynecologists. Practice Bulletin No. 190: gestational diabetes mellitus. Obstet Gynecol. 2018;131:e49. [PMID: 29370047]

CHRONIC HYPERTENSION

Chronic hypertension is estimated to complicate up to 5% of pregnancies. To establish this diagnosis, hypertension should antedate the pregnancy or be evident before 20 weeks' gestation to differentiate it from pregnancy-related hypertension. This distinction can be problematic when the initial presentation is after 20 weeks, but chronic hypertension is confirmed if the blood pressure remains elevated beyond 12 weeks postpartum. Risk factors for chronic hypertension include older maternal age, Black race, and obesity.

Women with chronic hypertension are at increased risk for adverse maternal and perinatal outcomes. Superimposed preeclampsia develops in up to 20% of women with mild hypertension, but the risk increases up to 50% when there is severe baseline hypertension (160/110 mm Hg or higher) and may be even higher when there is evidence of end-organ damage. When preeclampsia is superimposed on chronic hypertension, there is a tendency for it to occur at an earlier gestational age, be more severe, and impair fetal growth. Women with chronic hypertension are also at increased risk for placental abruption, cesarean delivery, preterm birth, and perinatal mortality.

Ideally, women with chronic hypertension should undergo a preconceptional evaluation to detect end-organ damage, assess the need for antihypertensive therapy, and discontinue teratogenic medications. The specific tests ordered may vary depending on the severity of the hypertensive disorder, but an evaluation of liver, kidney, and cardiac function (eg, 24-hour urine protein and maternal echocardiogram if mother takes medications) is appropriate.

If the woman is not known to have chronic hypertension, then initiation of antihypertensive therapy in pregnant women is indicated only if the blood pressure is sustained at or above 160/110 mm Hg or if there is evidence of end-organ damage. Treatment of hypertension has not been demonstrated to improve pregnancy outcomes, but it is indicated in women with significant hypertension for long-term maternal cardiovascular health. Although methyldopa (Table 11–10) has the longest record of safety in pregnancy, nifedipine (Table 11–7) and labetalol (Table 11–9) are also acceptable, and these three agents are recommended above all others when initiating therapy in pregnancy. Care must be taken not to excessively reduce the blood pressure, as this may decrease uteroplacental perfusion. The goal is a modest reduction in blood pressure and avoidance of severe hypertension.

If a woman with mild chronic hypertension is stable on a medical regimen when she becomes pregnant, it is usually appropriate to continue this therapy, although the benefits of doing so are not well established. *ACE inhibitors and ARBs, however, are contraindicated in all trimesters of pregnancy.* These medications are teratogenic in the first trimester and cause fetal hypocalvaria and AKI in the second and third trimesters.

When there is sustained severe hypertension despite multiple medications or significant end-organ damage from hypertensive disease, pregnancy is not likely to be tolerated well. In these situations, therapeutic abortion may be appropriate. If the pregnancy is continued, the woman must be counseled that the maternal and perinatal risks are appreciable, and complications such as superimposed preeclampsia and fetal growth restriction should be anticipated.

American College of Obstetricians and Gynecologists. Practice Bulletin No. 203: chronic hypertension in pregnancy. Obstet Gynecol. 2019;133:e26. [PMID: 30575676]

HEART DISEASE

Normal pregnancy physiology is characterized by cardiovascular adaptations in the mother. Cardiac output increases markedly because of both augmented stroke volume and an increase in the resting heart rate, and the maternal blood volume expands by up to 50%. These changes may not be tolerated well in women with functional or structural abnormalities of the heart. Thus, although only a small number of pregnancies are complicated by cardiac disease, these contribute disproportionately to overall rates of maternal morbidity and mortality. Most cardiac disease in women of childbearing age in the United States is caused by congenital heart disease and not rheumatic heart disease. Ischemic heart disease, however, is being seen more commonly in pregnant women due to increasing rates of comorbid conditions, such as diabetes mellitus, hypertension, and obesity.

For practical purposes, the best single measurement of cardiopulmonary status is defined by the New York Heart Association Functional Classification. Most pregnant women with cardiac disease have class I or II functional disability, and although good outcomes are generally anticipated in this group, complications such as preeclampsia, preterm birth, and low birth weight appear to occur with increased frequency. Women with more severe disability (class III or IV) are rare in contemporary obstetrics; however, the maternal mortality is markedly increased in this setting and is usually the result of heart failure. Because of these risks, therapeutic abortion for maternal health should be considered in women who are severely disabled from cardiac disease. Specific conditions that have been associated with a high risk for maternal death include Eisenmenger syndrome, primary pulmonary hypertension, Marfan syndrome with aortic root dilatation, and severe aortic or mitral stenosis. In general, these conditions should be considered contraindications to pregnancy.

The importance of preconceptional counseling for women with heart disease cannot be overstated. A thorough evaluation before pregnancy provides an opportunity for comprehensive risk assessment and detailed planning. Once pregnant, women with cardiac disease are best treated by a team of practitioners with experience in caring for such patients. Heart failure and arrhythmias are the most common cardiovascular complications associated with heart disease in pregnancy, and adverse maternal and fetal outcomes are increased when they occur. Symptoms of volume overload should therefore be evaluated and treated promptly. Labor management depends on the underlying cardiac lesion and the degree of disability. Women with a history of arrhythmia should have continuous cardiac monitoring throughout labor, delivery, and the immediate postpartum period. Cesarean delivery is generally reserved for obstetric indications but may be appropriate for women in whom Valsalva maneuvers are contraindicated. The early postpartum period is a critical time for fluid management. Patients who are predisposed to heart failure should be monitored closely during the puerperium.

Infective endocarditis prophylaxis is not recommended for a vaginal or cesarean delivery in the absence of infection, except in the small subset of patients at highest risk for adverse outcomes from endocarditis. The women at highest risk include those with cyanotic heart disease, prosthetic valves, or both. Prophylactic antibiotics for endocarditis, if required, should be given intravenously (see Table 33–5). If infection is present, such as chorioamnionitis, the underlying infection should be treated with the usual regimen and additional agents are not needed specifically for endocarditis prophylaxis.

American College of Obstetricians and Gynecologists. Practice Bulletin No. 199: use of prophylactic antibiotics in labor and delivery. Obstet Gynecol. 2018;132:e103. [PMID: 30134425]

Canobbio MM et al. Management of pregnancy in patients with complex congenital heart disease: a scientific statement for healthcare professionals from the American Heart Association. Circulation. 2017;135:e50. [PMID: 28082385]

ASTHMA

(**See also** Chapter 9.)

Asthma is one of the most common medical conditions encountered in pregnancy. Women with mild to moderate asthma can generally expect excellent pregnancy outcomes, but severe or poorly controlled asthma has been associated with several pregnancy complications, including preterm birth, small-for-gestational-age infants, and preeclampsia. The effects of pregnancy on asthma are likely minimal as asthma severity in the pregnancy has been reported to be similar to its severity during the year preceding the pregnancy. Strategies for treatment are similar to those in nonpregnant women. Patients should be educated about symptom management and avoidance of asthma triggers. Baseline pulmonary function tests can objectively assess lung function and may help the patient with self-monitoring of her asthma severity using a peak flow meter. As in nonpregnant women, treatment algorithms generally follow a stepwise approach, and commonly used medications, particularly those for mild to moderate asthma symptoms, are generally considered safe in pregnancy. Concerns about teratogenicity and medication effects on the fetus should be thoroughly discussed with the patient to decrease noncompliance rates. Inhaled beta-2-agonists are indicated for all asthma patients, and low to moderate dose inhaled corticosteroids are added for persistent symptoms when a rescue inhaler alone is inadequate. Systemic corticosteroid administration is reserved for severe exacerbations but should not be withheld, if indicated, irrespective of gestational age. Cromolyn, leukotriene receptor antagonists, and theophylline are appropriate alternative therapies if first-line management is ineffective. The primary goals of management in pregnancy include minimizing symptoms and avoiding hypoxic episodes to the fetus. Prostaglandin F2a and ergonovine—medications frequently used to treat postpartum uterine atony—should be avoided because they can precipitate bronchospasm in women with asthma.

American College of Obstetricians and Gynecologists. Practice Bulletin No. 90: asthma in pregnancy. Obstet Gynecol. 2008;111:457. [Reaffirmed 2019] [PMID: 18238988]

SEIZURE DISORDERS

Epilepsy is one of the most common serious neurologic disorders in pregnant women. Many of the commonly used antiepileptic drugs are known human teratogens. Therefore, the principal objectives in managing pregnancy in epileptic women are achieving adequate control of seizures while minimizing exposure to medications that can cause congenital malformations. Certain women who are contemplating pregnancy and have been seizure-free for 2–5 years may be considered candidates for discontinuation of antiseizure medication before pregnancy. For those who continue to require treatment, however, therapy with one medication is preferred. Selecting a regimen should be based on the type of seizure disorder and the risks associated with each medication. Valproic acid should not be considered first-line therapy because it has consistently been associated with higher rates of fetal malformations than most other commonly used antiepileptic drugs, and it may be associated with impaired neurocognitive development in the offspring. Phenytoin and carbamazepine both have established patterns of associated fetal malformations. Concerns about teratogenicity have prompted increasing use of the newer antiepileptic drugs such as lamotrigine, topiramate, oxcarbazepine, and levetiracetam. Although the safety of these medications in pregnancy continues to be evaluated, experiences from ongoing registries and large, population-based studies suggest that in utero exposure to the newer antiepileptic drugs in the first trimester of pregnancy carries a lower risk of major malformations than older medications. Lamotrigine and levetiracetam are considered the least teratogenic. One birth registry, however, found an increase in oral clefts among women taking lamotrigine. Several small studies have found an association between levetiracetam and low birth weight. Some studies suggest that topiramate is associated with a slightly increased risk of oral clefts. Although it is recommended that pregnant women with epilepsy be given supplemental folic acid, it is unclear if supplemental folate decreases rates of fetal malformations in women taking anticonvulsant therapy. Antiepileptic medications may be affected by volume of distribution changes in pregnancy, and serum levels should be followed when appropriate.

American College of Obstetricians and Gynecologists. Clinical Updates in Women's Health Care: Seizures. 2021 Jan 1. https://www.acog.org/clinical/journals-and-publications/clinical-updates/2021/01/seizures

Harden C et al. Epilepsy in pregnancy. Neurol Clin. 2019;37:53. [PMID: 30470275]

INFECTIOUS CONDITIONS COMPLICATING PREGNANCY

URINARY TRACT INFECTION

The urinary tract is especially vulnerable to infections during pregnancy because the altered secretions of steroid sex hormones and the pressure exerted by the gravid uterus on the ureters and bladder cause hypotonia and congestion and predispose to urinary stasis. Labor and delivery and urinary retention postpartum also may initiate or aggravate infection. *Escherichia coli* is the offending organism in over two-thirds of cases.

From 2% to 15% of pregnant women have asymptomatic bacteriuria, which some believe to be associated with an increased risk of preterm birth. It is estimated that pyelonephritis will develop in 20–40% of these women if untreated.

An evaluation for asymptomatic bacteriuria at the first prenatal visit is recommended for all pregnant women. If a urine culture is positive, treatment should be initiated. Nitrofurantoin (100 mg orally twice daily), ampicillin (250 mg orally four times daily), and cephalexin (250 mg orally four times daily) are acceptable medications for 4–7 days. Sulfonamides should be avoided in the third trimester because they may interfere with bilirubin binding and thus impose a risk of neonatal hyperbilirubinemia and kernicterus. Fluoroquinolones are also contraindicated because of their potential teratogenic effects on fetal cartilage and bone. Patients with recurrent bacteriuria should receive suppressive medication (once daily dosing of an appropriate antibiotic) for the remainder of the pregnancy. Acute pyelonephritis requires hospitalization for intravenous administration of antibiotics and crystalloids until the patient is afebrile; this is followed by a full course of oral antibiotics.

Kalinderi K et al. Urinary tract infection during pregnancy: current concepts on a common multifaceted problem. J Obstet Gynaecol. 2018;38:448. [PMID: 29402148]

GROUP B STREPTOCOCCAL INFECTION

Group B streptococci frequently colonize the lower female genital tract, with an asymptomatic carriage rate in pregnancy of 10–30%. This rate depends on maternal age, gravidity, and geographic variation. Vaginal carriage is asymptomatic and intermittent, with spontaneous clearing in approximately 30% and recolonization in about 10% of women. Adverse perinatal outcomes associated with group B streptococcal colonization include UTI, intrauterine infection, premature rupture of membranes, preterm delivery, and postpartum metritis.

Women with postpartum metritis due to infection with group B streptococci, especially after cesarean section, develop fever, tachycardia, and abdominal pain, usually within 24 hours after delivery. Approximately 35% of these women are bacteremic.

Group B streptococcal infection is a common cause of neonatal sepsis. Transmission rates are high, yet the rate of neonatal sepsis is surprisingly low at less than 1:1000 live births. Unfortunately, the mortality rate associated with early-onset disease can be as high as 20–30% in premature infants. In contrast, it is approximately 2–3% in those at term. Moreover, these infections can contribute markedly to chronic morbidity, including developmental delays and neurologic disabilities. Late-onset disease develops through contact with hospital nursery personnel. Up to 45% of these health care workers can carry the bacteria on their skin and transmit the infection to newborns.

The 2019 ACOG recommendations for screening and prophylaxis for group B streptococcal colonization are available at https://www.acog.org/clinical/clinical-guidance/committee-opinion/articles/2020/02/prevention-of-group-b-streptococcal-early-onset-disease-in-newborns.

VARICELLA

Commonly known as chickenpox, varicella-zoster virus (VZV) infection has a fairly benign course when incurred during childhood but may cause serious illness in adults, particularly during pregnancy. Infection results in lifelong immunity. Approximately 95% of women born in the United States have VZV antibodies by the time they reach reproductive age. The incidence of VZV infection during pregnancy has been reported as up to 7:10,000. *The vaccine is contraindicated in pregnancy because the effects of the vaccine on the fetus are unknown.* Nonpregnant women who are vaccinated should avoid pregnancy for 1 month after injection. Inadvertent vaccination in early pregnancy or within a month of pregnancy is not an indication for termination, although women should be counseled about theoretical risks.

Clinical Findings

A. Symptoms and Signs

The incubation period for this infection is 10–20 days. A primary infection follows and is characterized by a flu-like syndrome with malaise, fever, and development of a pruritic maculopapular rash on the trunk, which becomes vesicular and then crusts. Pregnant women are prone to the development of VZV pneumonia, often a fulminant infection sometimes requiring respiratory support. After primary infection, the virus becomes latent, ascending to dorsal root ganglia. Subsequent reactivation can occur as zoster, often under circumstances of immunocompromise, although this is rare during pregnancy.

Two types of fetal infection have been documented. The first is congenital VZV syndrome, which typically occurs in 0.4–2% of fetuses exposed to primary VZV infection during the first trimester. Anomalies include limb and digit abnormalities, microphthalmos, and microcephaly.

Infection during the second and third trimesters is less threatening. Maternal IgG crosses the placenta, protecting the fetus. The only infants at risk for severe infection are those born after maternal viremia but before development of maternal protective antibody. Maternal infection manifesting 5 days before or up to 2 days after delivery is the time period believed to be most hazardous for transmission to the fetus.

B. Laboratory Findings

Diagnosis is commonly made on clinical grounds. Laboratory verification is made by ELISA, fluorescent antibody, and hemagglutination inhibition antibody techniques. Vesicular fluid can be sent for qualitative varicella PCR assay.

Treatment

Varicella-zoster immune globulin (VZIG) has been shown to prevent or modify the symptoms of infection in exposed persons. Treatment success depends on identification of susceptible women at or just following exposure. Exposed women with a questionable or negative history of chickenpox should be checked for antibody, since the overwhelming majority will have been previously exposed. If the antibody is negative, VZIG (625 units intramuscularly) should ideally be given within 96 hours of exposure for greatest efficacy, but the CDC reports it can be given for up to 10 days. There are no known adverse effects of VZIG administration during pregnancy, although the incubation period for disease can be lengthened. Infants born to women in whom symptoms develop in the period from 5 days before delivery to 2 days after delivery should also receive VZIG (125 units).

Pregnant women with varicella may benefit from treatment with oral acyclovir, 800 mg orally four times daily for 5 days, if started within 24 hours of rash onset. Treatment has been shown to improve maternal symptoms but does not prevent congenital varicella. Infected pregnant women should be closely observed and hospitalized at the earliest signs of pulmonary involvement. Intravenous acyclovir (10 mg/kg intravenously every 8 hours) is recommended in the treatment of VZV pneumonia.

American College of Obstetricians and Gynecologists. ACOG Practice Bulletin No. 151: cytomegalovirus, parvovirus B19, varicella zoster, and toxoplasmosis in pregnancy. Obstet Gynecol. 2015;125:1510. [Reaffirmed 2019] [PMID: 26000539]

TUBERCULOSIS

The diagnosis of tuberculosis in pregnancy is made by history taking, physical examination, and testing, with special attention to women in high-risk groups. Women at high risk include those from endemic areas, those infected with HIV, drug users, health care workers, and close contacts of people with tuberculosis. Screening chest radiographs should only be obtained in pregnant patients who have a positive test or with suggestive findings in the history and physical examination. Abdominal shielding must be used if a chest radiograph is obtained. Both tuberculin skin testing and interferon gamma release assays are acceptable tests in pregnancy.

Decisions on treatment depend on whether the patient has active disease or is at high risk for progression to active disease. Pregnant women with active disease or who are high risk for progression should be treated during pregnancy as the risks of complications from tuberculosis outweigh the risks of treatment. Pregnant women with latent disease not at high risk for disease progression can receive treatment postpartum, which does not preclude breastfeeding. The concentration of medication in breast milk is neither toxic nor adequate for treatment of the newborn. Isoniazid, ethambutol, and rifampin are used to treat tuberculosis (see Chapters 9 and 33). Because isoniazid therapy may cause vitamin B_6 deficiency, a supplement of 50 mg/day of vitamin B_6 should be given simultaneously. There is concern that isoniazid, particularly in pregnant women, can cause hepatitis. Liver biochemical tests should be performed monthly in pregnant women who receive treatment. Streptomycin, ethionamide, and most other antituberculous drugs should be avoided in pregnancy. If adequately treated, tuberculosis in pregnancy has an excellent prognosis.

Miele K et al. Tuberculosis in pregnancy. Obstet Gynecol. 2020; 135:1444. [PMID: 32459437]

HIV/AIDS DURING PREGNANCY

Asymptomatic HIV infection is associated with a normal pregnancy rate and no increased risk of adverse pregnancy outcomes. There is no evidence that pregnancy causes AIDS progression.

Previously, two-thirds of HIV-positive neonates acquired their infection close to, or during, the time of delivery. Routine HIV screening in pregnancy, including the use of rapid HIV tests in Labor and Delivery units, and using antiretroviral drugs has markedly reduced this transmission risk to approximately 1%. In an HIV-positive pregnant woman, a CD4 count, plasma RNA level, and resistance testing (if virus is detectable, and the patient has not already had this) should be obtained at the first prenatal visit. Treatment should not be delayed while waiting for the results of resistance testing. Prior or current antiretroviral use should be reviewed. The patient should be tested for HLA-B*5701 if abacavir may be prescribed; HLA-B*5701 positivity puts the patient at risk for a serious hypersensitivity reaction and its use is contraindicated.

A woman already taking and tolerating an acceptable antiretroviral regimen need not discontinue it in the first trimester. Patients should also be tested for hepatitis A, hepatitis C, tuberculosis, toxoplasmosis, and cytomegalovirus.

Women not taking medication should be offered combination antiretroviral therapy (commonly a dual nucleoside reverse transcriptase inhibitor combination and either a ritonavir-boosted protease inhibitor or an integrase strand transfer inhibitor) after counseling regarding the potential impact of therapy on both mother and fetus (see Chapter 31). Antiretroviral therapy should be offered regardless of viral load and CD4 count. Whether to start in the first or second trimester should be determined on a case-by-case basis, but it should be started as early as reasonably possible. It can be started in the first trimester after explanation of risks and benefits, provided the mother is not experiencing nausea and vomiting. Most medications used to treat HIV/AIDS have thus far proven to be safe in pregnancy with an acceptable risk/benefit ratio. The physiologic changes that occur during pregnancy may alter the effect of some medications. Before starting any regimen, the safety and efficacy of the medications selected should be reviewed. Standard of care also includes administration of intravenous zidovudine (2 mg/kg intravenously over 1 hour followed by 1 mg/kg/hour intravenously) begun 3 hours before cesarean delivery and continued through the surgery until cord clamping in women whose viral load near delivery (after 34–36 weeks' gestation or within 4–6 weeks of delivery) is more than 1000 copies/mL or unknown. Antiretroviral therapy on the patient's usual schedule should be continued in labor. Intravenous zidovudine is not required for antiretroviral therapy–compliant women whose viral load is less than or equal to 50 copies/mL near delivery; data are limited in cases where the viral load is between 50 copies/mL and 1000 copies/mL.

The use of prophylactic elective cesarean section at 38 weeks' gestation (before the onset of labor or rupture of the membranes) to prevent vertical transmission of HIV infection from mother to fetus has been shown to further reduce the transmission rate. In patients with a viral load of less than 1000 copies/mL near delivery, there may be no additional benefit of cesarean delivery, and those women can be offered a vaginal delivery. Amniotomy should not be performed in the setting of viremia unless there is a clear obstetric indication. Amniotomy, however, has not been associated with an increased risk of perinatal transmission when the mother is receiving antiretroviral therapy and virologically suppressed. Internal monitors, particularly the fetal scalp electrode, should be avoided as should operative deliveries (forceps-assisted and vacuum-assisted vaginal deliveries). Methergine (used for postpartum hemorrhage) should be avoided, if possible, in patients receiving regimens that include cytochrome P450 (CYP) 3A4 inhibitors and CYP3A4 enzyme inducers. HIV-infected women should be advised not to breastfeed their infants.

The Public Health Task Force provides guidelines for the management of HIV/AIDS in pregnancy (https://hivinfo.nih.gov). In addition, there is the National Perinatal HIV Hotline, which provides free consultation regarding perinatal HIV care (1-888-448-8765).

Panel on Treatment of Pregnant Women with HIV Infection and Prevention of Perinatal Transmission. Recommendations for the use of antiretroviral drugs in pregnant women with HIV infection and interventions to reduce perinatal HIV transmission in the United States. 2021 Dec 30. https://clinicalinfo.hiv.gov/sites/default/files/guidelines/documents/Perinatal_GL.pdf

MATERNAL HEPATITIS B & C CARRIER STATE

A. Hepatitis B Virus

There are an estimated 350 million chronic carriers of hepatitis B virus worldwide. In the United States, 1.4 million people are infected, with the highest rate among Asian American persons. All pregnant women should be screened for HBsAg. Transmission of the virus to the baby after delivery is likely if both surface antigen and e antigen are positive. Vertical transmission can be blocked by the immediate postdelivery administration to the newborn of hepatitis B immunoglobulin and hepatitis B vaccine intramuscularly. The vaccine dose is repeated at 1 and 6 months of age. Third trimester administration of tenofovir disoproxil fumarate, 300 mg orally once per day starting at 28–32 weeks and continuing through delivery (first line), lamivudine, or telbivudine to women with a viral load of greater than 10^6–10^8 copies/mL has been shown to reduce vertical transmission particularly if the viral load is less than 10^6 copies/mL at delivery. This therapy appears safe in pregnancy although long-term follow-up data are lacking. Pregnant women with chronic hepatitis B should have liver biochemical tests and viral load testing during the pregnancy. Hepatitis B infection is not a contraindication to breastfeeding, and antiviral therapy if given need not be continued postpartum.

B. Hepatitis C Virus

This infection is the most common chronic blood-borne infection in the United States. Because risk-based screening misses approximately 50% of cases and postpartum treatment is highly effective, universal screening in pregnancy is recommended. The average rate of hepatitis C virus (HCV) infection among infants born to HCV-positive, HIV-negative women is 5–6%. However, the average infection rate increases to 10–11% when mothers are coinfected with HCV and HIV. The principal factor associated with transmission is HCV RNA in the mother at the time of birth. Treatment is not recommended in pregnancy. Interferon and ribavirin have been considered contraindicated. Ledipasvir/sofosbuvir (Harvoni) has been shown to be safe in animal studies. Direct-acting antiviral regimens should only be initiated during pregnancy if in the setting of a clinical trial. Cesarean section is not recommended solely for a maternal history of hepatitis C. During labor, early rupture of membranes and placement of a fetal scalp electrode should be avoided if safe to do so because of the unknown risk of increased vertical transmission. Breastfeeding is not contraindicated.

Dotters-Katz SK et al. Society for Maternal-Fetal Medicine Consult Series No. 56: hepatitis C in pregnancy-updated guidelines: replaces Consult No. 43. Am J Obstet Gynecol. 2021;225:B8. [PMID: 34116035]
Jin J. JAMA patient page. Screening for hepatitis B in pregnant women. JAMA. 2019;322:376. [PMID: 31334796]

HERPES GENITALIS

Infection of the lower genital tract by herpes simplex virus type 2 (HSV-2) (see also Chapter 6) is a common STD with potentially serious consequences to pregnant women and their newborn infants. Although up to 25% of pregnant women may have antibodies to HSV-2, a history of the infection is unreliable, and the incidence of neonatal infection is not known. There are estimated to be 1200–1500 cases of neonatal infection annually in the United States. Many infected neonates are born to women with no history, symptoms, or signs of infection.

Women who have had *primary* herpes infection late in pregnancy are at high risk for shedding virus at delivery; however, it can be difficult to differentiate primary from nonprimary infection. Women with a primary infection or nonprimary first outbreak and women with a clinical history of genital herpes should be offered prophylactic acyclovir, 400 mg orally three times daily, starting at 36 weeks' gestation, to decrease the likelihood of active lesions at the time of labor and delivery. For treatment, see Chapter 32.

Women with a history of *recurrent* genital herpes have a lower neonatal attack rate than women infected during the pregnancy, but they should still be monitored with clinical observation and culture of any suspicious lesions. Since asymptomatic viral shedding is not predictable by antepartum cultures, recommendations do not include routine cultures in individuals with a history of herpes without active disease. However, when labor begins, vulvar and cervical inspection should be performed. Cesarean delivery is indicated at the time of labor if there are prodromal symptoms or active genital lesions.

American College of Obstetricians and Gynecologists. ACOG Practice Bulletin No. 220: management of genital herpes in pregnancy. Obstet Gynecol. 2020;135:e193. [PMID: 32332414]

SYPHILIS, GONORRHEA, & *CHLAMYDIA TRACHOMATIS* INFECTION

These STDs have significant consequences for mother and child (see also Chapters 33 and 34). Untreated syphilis in pregnancy can cause late abortion, stillbirth, transplacental infection, and congenital syphilis. Gonorrhea can produce large-joint arthritis by hematogenous spread as well as ophthalmia neonatorum. Maternal chlamydial infections are largely asymptomatic but are manifested in the newborn by inclusion conjunctivitis and, at age 2–4 months, by pneumonia. The diagnosis of each can be reliably made by appropriate laboratory tests. All women should be tested for syphilis as part of their routine prenatal care. Pregnant women younger than 25 years and those at increased risk for *C trachomatis* should be screened for chlamydia at their first prenatal visit. Repeat testing depends on risk factors, prevalence, and state laws. A pregnant woman treated for *C trachomatis* should be tested for cure 4 weeks later and then retested 3 months later because of high reinfection rates. Women who remain at high risk should be tested in the third trimester. Women younger than 25 years and those at increased risk should be tested for gonorrhea at their first prenatal appointment. Women with positive tests for gonorrhea should be treated and then retested 3 months later. Women who remain at high risk should be tested in the third trimester. The sexual partners of women with STDs should be identified and treated if possible; the local health department can assist with this process.

Workowski KA et al. Sexually transmitted infections treatment guidelines, 2021. MMWR Recomm Rep. 2021:70:1. [PMID: 34292926]

GASTROINTESTINAL, HEPATIC, & BILIARY DISORDERS OF PREGNANCY

Complications involving the GI tract, liver, and gallbladder are common in pregnancy. Nausea and vomiting in the first trimester affect most pregnant women to some degree (see Obstetric Complications of the First & Second Trimesters). *Nausea and vomiting in the last half of pregnancy, however, are never normal;* a thorough evaluation of such complaints is mandatory. Some of these conditions are incidental to pregnancy (eg, appendicitis), while others are related to the gravid state and tend to resolve with delivery (eg, acute fatty liver of pregnancy). Importantly, the myriad anatomic and physiologic changes associated with normal pregnancy must be considered when assessing for a disease state. Likewise, interpretation of laboratory studies must consider the pregnancy-associated changes in hepatic protein production.

For conditions in which surgery is clinically indicated, operative intervention should never be withheld based solely on a woman being pregnant. While purely elective surgery is avoided during pregnancy, women who undergo surgical procedures for an urgent or emergent indication during pregnancy do not appear to be at increased risk for adverse outcomes. Obstetric complications, when they occur, are more likely to be associated with the underlying maternal illness. Recommendations have held that the optimal time for semi-elective surgery is the second trimester to avoid exposure to anesthesia in the first trimester and the enlarged uterus in the third. Importantly, however, there is no convincing evidence that general anesthesia induces malformations or increases the risk for abortion.

CHOLELITHIASIS & CHOLECYSTITIS

Cholelithiasis is common in pregnancy as physiologic changes such as increased cholesterol production and incomplete gallbladder emptying predispose to gallstone formation. The diagnosis is usually suspected based on classic symptoms of nausea, vomiting, and right upper quadrant pain, usually after meals, and is confirmed with right upper quadrant ultrasound. Symptomatic cholelithiasis without cholecystitis is usually managed conservatively, but recurrent symptoms are common. Cholecystitis results from obstruction of the cystic duct and often is accompanied by bacterial infection. Medical management with antibiotics is reasonable in selected cases, but definitive treatment with cholecystectomy will help prevent complications such as gallbladder perforation and pancreatitis. Cholecystectomy has successfully been performed in all trimesters of pregnancy and should not be withheld based on the stage of pregnancy if clinically indicated. Laparoscopy is preferred in the first half of pregnancy but becomes more technically challenging in the last trimester due to the enlarged uterus and cephalad displacement of abdominal contents.

Obstruction of the common bile duct, which can lead to cholangitis, is an indication for surgical removal of gallstones and establishment of biliary drainage. Endoscopic retrograde cholangiopancreatography (ERCP) with or without sphincterotomy is a nonsurgical alternative. ERCP should only be undertaken when there is therapeutic intent. Pregnant women can safely undergo ERCP provided that precautions are taken to minimize fetal exposure to radiation. There does, however, appear to be a slightly higher rate of post-procedure pancreatitis in pregnant women who undergo ERCP. Magnetic resonance cholangiopancreatography (MRCP) can also be of use in patients with suspected common bile duct obstruction. This study is useful for those women in whom the etiology of common duct dilatation is unclear on ultrasound. MRCP can provide detailed evaluation of the entire biliary system and the pancreas while avoiding ionizing radiation.

The most common cause of acute pancreatitis in pregnancy is gallstone disease. The diagnosis can be confirmed with an appropriate history and an elevated serum amylase or lipase. Although pregnancy is associated with a rise in serum amylase, a value of at least two times the upper limit of normal suggests pancreatitis with the appropriate clinical scenario. Management is conservative, including bowel rest, intravenous fluids, supplemental nutrition if necessary, and analgesics. CT imaging should be avoided unless severe complications such as necrosis, abscess, or hemorrhage are suspected.

Abushamma S et al. A guide to upper gastrointestinal tract, biliary, and pancreatic disorders: clinical updates in women's health care primary and preventive care review. Obstet Gynecol. 2021;137:1152. [PMID: 34011887]

ACUTE FATTY LIVER OF PREGNANCY

Acute fatty liver of pregnancy, a disorder limited to the gravid state, occurs in the third trimester of pregnancy and causes acute hepatic failure. With improved recognition and immediate delivery, the maternal mortality rate in contemporary reports is about 4%. The disorder is usually seen after the 35th week of gestation and is more common in primigravidas and those with twins. The incidence is about 1:10,000 deliveries.

The etiology of acute fatty liver of pregnancy is likely poor placental mitochondrial function. Many cases may be due to a homozygous fetal deficiency of long-chain acyl coenzyme A dehydrogenase (LCHAD).

Clinical Findings

Clinical onset is gradual, with nausea and vomiting being the most common presenting symptoms. Varying degrees of flu-like symptoms are also typical. Eventually, symptoms progress to those of fulminant hepatic failure: jaundice, encephalopathy, disseminated intravascular coagulation, and death. On examination, the patient shows signs of hepatic failure.

Laboratory findings include marked elevation of alkaline phosphatase but only moderate elevations of ALT and AST. Hypocholesterolemia and hypofibrinogenemia are typical, and hypoglycemia can be extreme. Coagulopathy is also frequently seen with depressed procoagulant protein production. Kidney function should be assessed for hepatorenal syndrome. The WBC count is elevated, and the platelet count is depressed.

Differential Diagnosis

The differential diagnosis is that of fulminant hepatitis. Liver aminotransferases for fulminant hepatitis are higher (greater than 1000 U/mL) than those for acute fatty liver of pregnancy (usually 500–1000 U/mL). Preeclampsia may involve the liver but rarely causes jaundice; the elevations in liver biochemical tests in patients with preeclampsia rarely reach the levels seen in patients with acute fatty liver of pregnancy.

Treatment

Diagnosis of acute fatty liver of pregnancy mandates immediate delivery. Intensive supportive care with ICU-level observation is essential and typically includes administration of blood products and glucose and correction of acidemia. Vaginal delivery is preferred. Resolution of encephalopathy and laboratory derangements occurs over days with supportive care, and recovery is usually complete. Rare cases of liver transplantation have been reported.

Nelson DB et al. Acute fatty liver of pregnancy. Clin Obstet Gynecol. 2020;63:152. [PMID: 31725416]

INTRAHEPATIC CHOLESTASIS OF PREGNANCY

Intrahepatic cholestasis of pregnancy is characterized by incomplete clearance of bile acids in genetically susceptible women. The principal symptom is pruritus, which can be generalized but tends to have a predilection for the palms and soles. Presentation is typically in the third trimester, and women with multifetal pregnancies are at increased risk. The finding of an elevated serum bile acid level, ideally performed in the fasting state, confirms the diagnosis. Associated laboratory derangements include modest elevations in hepatic transaminase levels and mild hyperbilirubinemia. Although rare, the bilirubin level may be sufficiently elevated to result in clinical jaundice. The symptoms and laboratory abnormalities resolve quickly after delivery but can recur in subsequent pregnancies or with exposure to combination oral contraceptives.

Adverse fetal outcomes, particularly preterm birth, nonreassuring fetal status, meconium-stained amniotic fluid, and stillbirth, have consistently been reported in women with cholestasis of pregnancy. The risk for adverse perinatal outcomes appears to correlate with disease severity as measured by the degree of bile acid elevation, and women with fasting bile acids greater than 40 mcmol/L have been reported to be at greatest risk. Because of the risks associated with cholestasis of pregnancy, many clinicians recommend antenatal testing in the third trimester, and if cholestasis is present, elective early delivery to reduce the risk of stillbirth. The diagnosis of cholestasis of pregnancy is made when the level of bile salts is 10 mcmol/L or more (not necessarily fasting) with maternal symptoms. The Society for Maternal-Fetal Medicine (SMFM) 2021 recommends early delivery (36 weeks' gestation) when the patient's bile acid level is greater than 100 mcmol/L and other fetal tests are normal; in the symptomatic patient whose bile acid level is below 100 mcmol/L, the SMFM suggests delivery between 36 and 39 weeks' gestation. The ACOG endorses ursodeoxycholic acid as the first-line agent for the treatment of maternal symptoms of intrahepatic cholestasis of pregnancy. A 2019 randomized controlled trial did not find that ursodeoxycholic acid improved perinatal outcomes.

Lee RH et al. Society for Maternal-Fetal Medicine Consult Series No. 53: intrahepatic cholestasis of pregnancy: replaces Consult No. 13. Am J Obstet Gynecol. 2021;224:B2. [PMID: 33197417]

APPENDICITIS

Appendicitis occurs in about 1 of 1500 pregnancies. The diagnosis is more difficult to make clinically in pregnant women where the appendix is displaced cephalad from McBurney point. Furthermore, nausea, vomiting, and mild leukocytosis occur in normal pregnancy, so with or without these findings, any complaint of right-sided pain should raise suspicion. Imaging can help confirm the diagnosis if clinical findings are equivocal. Abdominal sonography is a reasonable initial imaging choice, but nonvisualization of the appendix is common in pregnancy. CT scanning is more sensitive than ultrasound, and with proper shielding, the radiation exposure to the fetus is minimized. MRI is also used to evaluate for appendicitis in pregnant women and is a reasonable alternative to CT scanning.

An operative approach to appendicitis, rather than a conservative nonoperative approach, is indicated for pregnant patients. Conservative management is associated with increases in maternal morbidity, including septic shock, peritonitis, and venous thromboembolism.

Unfortunately, the diagnosis of appendicitis is not made until the appendix has ruptured in at least 20% of obstetric patients. Peritonitis in these cases can lead to preterm labor or abortion. With early diagnosis and appendectomy, the prognosis is good for mother and baby.

Weinstein MS et al. Appendicitis and cholecystitis in pregnancy. Clin Obstet Gynecol. 2020;63:405. [PMID: 32187083]

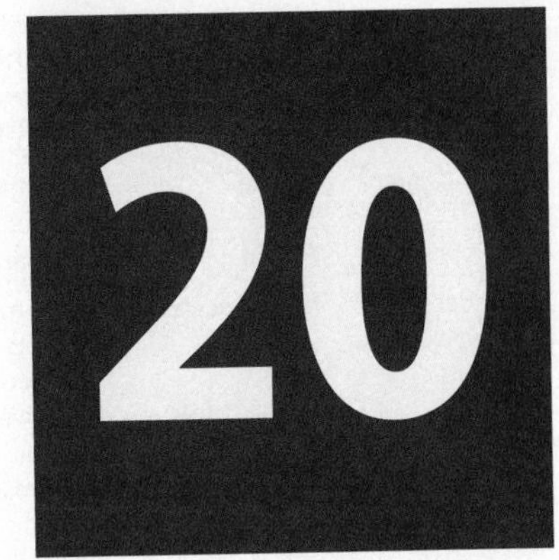

Rheumatologic, Immunologic, & Allergic Disorders

Rebecca L. Manno, MD, MHS
Jinoos Yazdany, MD, MPH
Teresa K. Tarrant, MD
Mildred Kwan, MD, PhD

RHEUMATOLOGIC DISORDERS

Diagnosis & Evaluation

A. Examination of the Patient

Two helpful clinical clues for diagnosing arthritis are the joint pattern and the presence or absence of extra-articular manifestations. The joint pattern is defined by the answers to three questions: (1) Is inflammation present? (2) How many joints are involved? and (3) What joints are affected? Joint inflammation manifests as warmth, swelling, and morning stiffness of at least 30 minutes' duration. Overlying erythema occurs with the intense inflammation of crystal-induced and septic arthritis. Both the number of affected joints and the specific sites of involvement affect the differential diagnosis (Table 20–1). Some diseases—gout, for example—are characteristically monoarticular, whereas other diseases, such as rheumatoid arthritis, are usually polyarticular. The location of joint involvement can also be distinctive. Only two diseases frequently cause prominent involvement of the distal interphalangeal (DIP) joint: osteoarthritis and psoriatic arthritis. Extra-articular manifestations such as fever (eg, gout, Still disease, endocarditis, vasculitis, SLE), rash (eg, SLE, psoriatic arthritis, inflammatory myositis), nodules (eg, rheumatoid arthritis, gout), or neuropathy (eg, vasculitis) narrow the differential diagnosis further.

B. Arthrocentesis and Examination of Joint Fluid

If the diagnosis is uncertain, synovial fluid should be examined whenever possible (Table 20–2). Most large joints are easily aspirated, and contraindications to arthrocentesis are few. The aspirating needle should never be passed through an overlying cellulitis or psoriatic plaque because of the risk of introducing infection. For patients who are receiving DOACs or long-term anticoagulation therapy with warfarin, joints can be aspirated with a small-gauge needle (eg, 22F); the INR should be less than 3.0 for patients taking warfarin.

1. Types of studies—

A. GROSS EXAMINATION—Clarity is an approximate guide to the degree of inflammation. Noninflammatory fluid is transparent, mild inflammation produces translucent fluid, and purulent effusions are opaque. Traumatic taps, trauma, and bleeding disorders are the most common causes of bloody effusions.

B. CELL COUNT—Normal synovial fluid contains less than 200 white cells/mcL (0.2×10^9/L). Higher synovial fluid white cell counts can discriminate between noninflammatory (less than 2000 white cells/mcL [2.0×10^9/L]), inflammatory (2000–75,000 white cells/mcL [$2.0–75 \times 10^9$/L]), and purulent (greater than 100,000 white cells/mcL [100×10^9/L]) joint effusions. Synovial fluid glucose and protein levels add little information and should not be ordered.

C. MICROSCOPIC EXAMINATION—Compensated polarized light microscopy identifies and distinguishes monosodium urate (gout, negatively birefringent) and calcium pyrophosphate (pseudogout, positive birefringent) crystals. Gram stain has specificity but limited sensitivity (50%) for septic arthritis.

D. CULTURE—Bacterial cultures and special studies for gonococci, tubercle bacilli, or fungi are ordered as appropriate.

2. Interpretation—Synovial fluid analysis is diagnostic in infectious or microcrystalline arthritis. Although the severity of inflammation in synovial fluid can overlap among various conditions, the synovial fluid white cell count is a helpful guide to diagnosis (Table 20–3).

DEGENERATIVE & CRYSTAL-INDUCED ARTHRITIS

DEGENERATIVE JOINT DISEASE (Osteoarthritis)

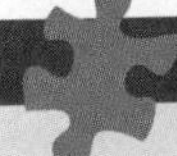

ESSENTIALS OF DIAGNOSIS

- A degenerative disorder with minimal articular inflammation.
- No systemic symptoms.
- Pain relieved by rest; morning stiffness brief.
- Radiographic findings: narrowed joint space, osteophytes, increased subchondral bone density, bony cysts.

Table 20–1. Diagnostic value of the joint pattern.

Characteristic	Status	Representative Disease
Inflammation	Present	Rheumatoid arthritis, SLE, gout
	Absent	Osteoarthritis
Number of involved joints	Monoarticular	Gout, trauma, septic arthritis, Lyme disease, osteoarthritis
	Oligoarticular (2–4 joints)	Reactive arthritis, psoriatic arthritis, IBD
	Polyarticular (≥ 5 joints)	Rheumatoid arthritis, SLE
Site of joint involvement	Distal interphalangeal	Osteoarthritis, psoriatic arthritis (not rheumatoid arthritis)
	Metacarpophalangeal, wrists	Rheumatoid arthritis, SLE, calcium pyrophosphate deposition disease (not osteoarthritis)
	First metatarsal phalangeal	Gout, osteoarthritis

General Considerations

Osteoarthritis, the most common form of joint disease, is chiefly a disease of aging. Ninety percent of all people have radiographic features of osteoarthritis in weight-bearing joints by age 40. Symptomatic disease increases with age. Sex is also a risk factor; osteoarthritis develops in women more frequently than in men.

This arthropathy is characterized by degeneration of cartilage and by hypertrophy of bone at the articular margins. Inflammation is usually minimal. Hereditary and mechanical factors may be involved in the pathogenesis.

Obesity is a risk factor for osteoarthritis of the knee, hand, and probably of the hip. Recreational running does not increase the incidence of osteoarthritis, but participation in competitive contact sports (eg, football) does. Jobs requiring frequent bending and carrying increase the risk of knee osteoarthritis (see Chapter 41).

Clinical Findings

A. Symptoms and Signs

Degenerative joint disease is divided into two types: (1) primary, which most commonly affects some or all of the following: the DIP and the proximal interphalangeal (PIP) joints of the fingers, the carpometacarpal joint of the thumb, the hip, the knee, the metatarsophalangeal (MTP) joint of the big toe, and the cervical and lumbar spine; and (2) secondary, which may occur in any joint as a sequela to articular injury. The injury may be acute, as in a fracture; or chronic, as from occupational overuse of a joint or metabolic disease (eg, hyperparathyroidism, hemochromatosis, ochronosis) or joint inflammation (eg, rheumatoid arthritis).

The onset is insidious. Initially, there is articular stiffness, seldom lasting more than 15 minutes; this develops later into pain on motion of the affected joint and is made worse by activity or weight bearing and relieved by rest. Flexion contracture or varus deformity of the knee is not unusual, and bony enlargements of the DIP (Heberden nodes) and PIP (Bouchard nodes) are occasionally prominent (Figure 20–1). There is no ankylosis, but limitation of motion of the affected joint or joints is common. Crepitus may often be felt over the knee. Joint effusion and other articular signs of inflammation are mild. However, in some cases a one-way valve effect between the knee joint and gastrocnemius-semimembranosus bursa can lead to accumulation of synovial fluid, called a popliteal (Baker) cyst. There are no systemic manifestations.

B. Laboratory Findings

Osteoarthritis does not cause elevation of the ESR or other laboratory signs of inflammation. Synovial fluid is noninflammatory.

C. Imaging

Radiographs may reveal narrowing of the joint space; osteophyte formation and lipping of marginal bone; and thickened, dense subchondral bone. Bone cysts may also be present.

Table 20–2. Examination of joint fluid.

Measure	(Normal)	Group I (Noninflammatory)	Group II (Inflammatory)	Group III (Purulent)
Volume (mL) (knee)	< 3.5	Often > 3.5	Often > 3.5	Often > 3.5
Clarity	Transparent	Transparent	Translucent to opaque	Opaque
Color	Clear	Yellow	Yellow to opalescent	Yellow to green
WBC per mcL	< 200 (0.2×10^9/L)	< 2000 (2.0×10^9/L)	2000–75,000[1] ($2.0–75.0 \times 10^9$/L)	> 100,000[2] (100×10^9/L)
Polymorphonuclear leukocytes	< 25%	< 25%	50% or more	75% or more
Culture	Negative	Negative	Negative	Usually positive[2]

[1]Gout, rheumatoid arthritis, and other inflammatory conditions occasionally have synovial fluid WBC counts > 75,000/mcL (75×10^9/L) but rarely > 100,000/mcL (100×10^9/L).

[2]Most purulent effusions are due to septic arthritis. Septic arthritis, however, can present with group II synovial fluid, particularly if infection is caused by organisms of low virulence (eg, *Neisseria gonorrhoeae*) or if antibiotic therapy has been started.

Table 20–3. Differential diagnosis by joint fluid groups.

Noninflammatory (< 2000 white cells/mcL [< 2 × 10⁹/L])	Inflammatory (2000–75,000 white cells/mcL [2.0–75.0 × 10⁹/L])	Purulent (> 100,000 white cells/mcL [> 100 × 10⁹/L])	Hemorrhagic
Osteoarthritis Traumatic arthritis Osteonecrosis Charcot arthropathy	Rheumatoid arthritis SLE Polymyositis or dermatomyositis Systemic sclerosis Systemic necrotizing vasculitides Polychondritis Gout Calcium pyrophosphate deposition disease Hydroxyapatite deposition disease Juvenile rheumatoid arthritis Ankylosing spondylitis Psoriatic arthritis Reactive arthritis IBD arthritis Hypogammaglobulinemia Sarcoidosis Rheumatic fever Indolent/low virulence infections (viral, mycobacterial, fungal, Whipple disease, Lyme disease)	Septic arthritis (bacterial)	Trauma Pigmented villonodular synovitis Tuberculosis Neoplasia Coagulopathy Charcot arthropathy

Reprinted by permission from Springer Nature: Springer, Primer on the Rheumatic Diseases 13th ed by Klippel JH et al (eds) © 2008.

Differential Diagnosis

Because articular inflammation is minimal and systemic manifestations are absent, degenerative joint disease should seldom be confused with other arthritides. The distribution of joint involvement in the hands also helps distinguish osteoarthritis from rheumatoid arthritis. Osteoarthritis chiefly affects the DIP and PIP joints and spares the wrist and metacarpophalangeal (MCP) joints; rheumatoid arthritis involves the wrists and MCP joints and spares the DIP joints. Furthermore, the joint enlargement is bony-hard and cool in osteoarthritis but spongy and warm in rheumatoid arthritis. Skeletal symptoms due to degenerative changes in joints—especially in the spine—may cause coexistent metastatic neoplasia, osteoporosis, plasma cell myeloma, or other bone disease to be overlooked.

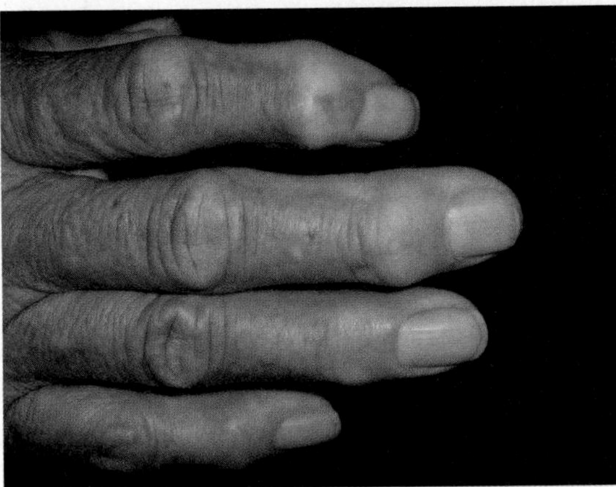

▲ **Figure 20–1.** Osteoarthritis in an older woman with Heberden nodes at the distal interphalangeal joints. There is some swelling beginning at the proximal interphalangeal joints creating Bouchard nodes. (Reproduced with permission from Richard P. Usatine, MD, in Usatine RP, Smith MA, Mayeaux EJ Jr, Chumley H. *The Color Atlas of Family Medicine,* 2nd ed. McGraw-Hill, 2013.)

Prevention

Weight reduction reduces the risk of developing symptomatic knee, hip and hand osteoarthritis. Correcting leg length discrepancy of greater than 1 cm with shoe modification may prevent knee osteoarthritis from developing in the shorter leg.

Treatment

A. General Measures

Patients with osteoarthritis of the hand may benefit from assistive devices and instruction on techniques for joint protection; splinting is beneficial for those with symptomatic osteoarthritis of the first carpometacarpal joint. Patients with mild to moderate osteoarthritis of the knee or hip should participate in a regular exercise program (eg, a supervised walking program, hydrotherapy classes) and, if overweight, should lose weight. A randomized, controlled trial of 156 individuals with knee osteoarthritis found that physical therapy was more effective at reducing pain and disability at 1 year than intra-articular glucocorticoid injections. Reduction in pain with weight loss can be significant; one study showed that loss of 10% or more of body weight resulted in a 50% reduction in pain scores of knee osteoarthritis. Using assistive devices (eg, a cane on the contralateral side) can improve functional status.

B. Medical Management

1. Oral NSAIDs—NSAIDs (see Table 5–5) are more effective than acetaminophen for osteoarthritis but have greater toxicity. NSAIDs inhibit cyclooxygenase (COX), the enzyme that converts arachidonic acid to prostaglandins. COX exists in two isomers—COX-1, which is expressed continuously in many cells and is responsible for the homeostatic effects of prostaglandins, and COX-2, which is induced by cytokines and expressed in inflammatory tissues. Most NSAIDs inhibit both isomers. Celecoxib is the only selective COX-2 inhibitor available in the United States.

GI toxicity, such as gastric ulceration, perforation, and GI hemorrhage, are the most common serious side effects of NSAIDs. The overall rate of bleeding with NSAID use in the general population is low (1:6000 users or less) but is increased by the risk factors of long-term use, higher NSAID dose, concomitant corticosteroids or anticoagulants, SSRIs, the presence of rheumatoid arthritis, history of peptic ulcer disease or alcoholism, and age over 70. *PPIs (eg, esomeprazole 20–40 mg orally daily) reduce the incidence of serious GI toxicity and should be used for patients with risk factors for NSAID-induced GI toxicity.* Patients who have recently recovered from an NSAID-induced bleeding gastric ulcer appear to be at high risk for rebleeding (about 5% in 6 months) when an NSAID is reintroduced, even if prophylactic measures (such as PPIs) are used. Compared with nonselective NSAIDs, celecoxib is less likely to cause upper GI tract adverse events, including bleeding.

All of the NSAIDs, including aspirin and celecoxib, can produce renal toxicity, including interstitial nephritis, nephrotic syndrome, prerenal azotemia, and aggravation of hypertension. Hyperkalemia due to hyporeninemic hypoaldosteronism is seen rarely. Renal toxicity is uncommon but is increased by the following risk factors: CKD, volume depletion from diuretic use or GI loss, HF, cirrhosis, or use of ACE inhibitors or ARBs.

All NSAIDs, except the nonacetylated salicylates and celecoxib, interfere with platelet function and prolong bleeding time. Aspirin irreversibly inhibits platelet function, so the bleeding time effect resolves only as new platelets are made. In contrast, the effect of nonselective NSAIDs on platelet function is reversible and resolves as the drug is cleared. Concomitant administration of a nonselective NSAID can interfere with the ability of aspirin to acetylate platelets and thus may interfere with the cardioprotective effects of low-dose aspirin. *All NSAIDs are associated with a small increase in the absolute risk of MI and stroke in patients with or without risk factors for heart disease or known heart disease.* While the cardiovascular risk is related to the dose and duration of treatment, stroke and MI can occur within the first week of treatment. Cardiovascular risks associated with naproxen, ibuprofen, and moderate dose celecoxib (200 mg orally daily) are comparable.

2. Topical therapies—Topical NSAIDs (eg, 4 g of diclofenac gel 1% applied to the affected joint four times daily) appear more effective than placebo for knee and hand osteoarthritis. Because they have lower rates of systemic side effects than with oral NSAIDs, topical NSAIDs are preferable for patients with risk factors for NSAID-induced GI toxicity. Topical NSAIDs are preferred for patients 75 years of age or older. Topical capsaicin may be of benefit for osteoarthritis of the hand or the knee.

3. Acetaminophen, opioids, chondroitin, and glucosamine—Acetaminophen is not recommended given that its impact on pain is frequently negligible and hepatotoxicity can occur from high doses. Opioids are generally not appropriate for the long-term management of pain due to osteoarthritis. Chondroitin sulfate and glucosamine, alone or in combination, are no better than placebo in reducing the pain of knee or hip osteoarthritis.

4. Intra-articular injections—Intra-articular injections of corticosteroids, hyaluronate, or platelet-rich plasma have not convincingly produced long-term benefits in reducing pain or preserving function in osteoarthritis. A 2-year controlled trial demonstrated that injecting the knee with triamcinolone every 12 weeks was no more effective than injecting saline in reducing knee pain and resulted in more cartilage volume loss. Similarly, platelet-rich plasma injections were no better than saline injections in improving knee pain or slowing disease progression in a randomized, controlled trial of patients with knee osteoarthritis.

5. Duloxetine—For patients with osteoarthritis in multiple joints who either have not responded to or cannot use NSAIDs, the selective serotonin and norepinephrine reuptake inhibitor duloxetine, 30–60 mg orally daily, can reduce pain. Nausea occurs in 6–15% of patients.

6. Physical therapy—Physical therapy is beneficial for knee osteoarthritis. A randomized, controlled trial of 156 patients with knee osteoarthritis compared intra-articular glucocorticoid injections to physical therapy; those receiving physical therapy had less pain and functional disability after 1 year compared to those receiving injections.

C. Surgical Measures

Total hip and knee replacements provide excellent symptomatic and functional improvement when involvement of that joint severely restricts walking or causes pain at rest, particularly at night. Arthroscopic surgery for knee osteoarthritis is ineffective. Severe first carpometacarpal osteoarthritis can be treated surgically when other treatments are inadequate.

Prognosis

Symptoms may be severe and limit activity considerably (especially with involvement of the hips, knees, and cervical spine).

When to Refer

Refer patients to an orthopedic surgeon when recalcitrant symptoms or functional impairment, or both, warrant consideration of joint replacement surgery of the hip, knee, or thumb.

Deyle GD et al. Physical therapy versus glucocorticoid injection for osteoarthritis of the knee. N Engl J Med. 2020;382:1420. [PMID: 32268027]

Kolasinski SL et al. 2019 American College of Rheumatology/Arthritis Foundation guideline for the management of osteoarthritis of the hand, hip, and knee. Arthritis Rheumatol. 2020;72:220. [PMID: 31908163]

CRYSTAL DEPOSITION ARTHRITIS

1. Gouty Arthritis

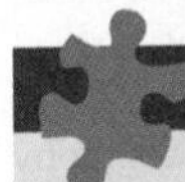

ESSENTIALS OF DIAGNOSIS

- Acute, monoarticular arthritis, often of the first MTP joint; recurrence is common.
- Polyarticular involvement more common in patients with longstanding disease.
- Identification of urate crystals in joint fluid or tophi is diagnostic.
- Dramatic therapeutic response to NSAIDs.
- With chronicity, urate deposits in subcutaneous tissue, bone, cartilage, joints, and other tissues.

General Considerations

Gout is a metabolic disease of a heterogeneous nature, often familial, associated with abnormal deposits of urate in tissues and characterized initially by a recurring acute arthritis, usually monoarticular, and later by chronic deforming arthritis. Urate deposition occurs when serum uric acid is supersaturated (ie, at levels greater than 6.8 mg/dL [404.5 mcmol/L]). Hyperuricemia is due to overproduction or underexcretion of uric acid—sometimes both. The disease is especially common in Pacific islanders, eg, Filipinos and Samoans. Primary gout has a heritable component, and genome-wide surveys have linked risk of gout to several genes whose products regulate urate handling by the kidney. Secondary gout, which also may have a heritable component, is related to acquired causes of hyperuricemia, eg, medication use (especially diuretics, low-dose aspirin, cyclosporine, and niacin), myeloproliferative disorders, plasma cell myeloma, hemoglobinopathies, CKD, hypothyroidism, psoriasis, sarcoidosis, and lead poisoning (Table 20–4). Alcohol ingestion promotes hyperuricemia by increasing urate production and decreasing the renal excretion of uric acid. Finally, hospitalized patients frequently suffer attacks of gout because of changes in diet, fluid intake, or medications that lead either to rapid reductions or increases in the serum urate level.

About 90% of patients with primary gout are men, usually over 30 years of age. In women, the onset is typically postmenopausal. The characteristic lesion is the tophus, a nodular deposit of monosodium urate monohydrate crystals with an associated foreign body reaction. Tophi are found in cartilage, subcutaneous and periarticular tissues, tendon, bone, the kidneys, and elsewhere. Urates have been demonstrated in the synovial tissues (and fluid) during acute arthritis; the acute inflammation of gout is believed to be initiated by the ingestion of uncoated urate crystals by monocytes and synoviocytes. The precise relationship of hyperuricemia to gouty arthritis is still obscure, since chronic hyperuricemia is found in people who never develop gout or uric acid stones. Rapid fluctuations in serum urate levels, either increasing or decreasing, are important factors in precipitating acute gout. The mechanism of the late, chronic stage of gouty arthritis is better understood. This is characterized pathologically by tophaceous invasion of the articular and periarticular tissues, with structural derangement and secondary degeneration (osteoarthritis).

Table 20–4. Origin of hyperuricemia.

Primary hyperuricemia
Increased production of purine
Idiopathic
Specific enzyme defects (eg, Lesch-Nyhan syndrome, glycogen storage diseases)
Decreased renal clearance of uric acid (idiopathic)
Secondary hyperuricemia
Increased catabolism and turnover of purine
Myeloproliferative disorders
Carcinoma and sarcoma (disseminated)
Chronic hemolytic anemias
Cytotoxic drugs
Psoriasis
Down syndrome
Decreased renal clearance of uric acid
CKD
Drug-induced (eg, thiazides, low-dose aspirin, cyclosporine, niacin)
Ketoacidemia (eg, diabetic ketoacidosis, starvation)
Hypothyroidism
Preeclampsia
Functional impairment of tubular transport
Hyperlacticacidemia
Diabetes insipidus (vasopressin-resistant)
Bartter syndrome
Sarcoidosis
Lead poisoning

From Rodnan GP. Gout and other crystalline forms of arthritis. *Postgrad Med.* 1975;58(5):6–14. Reprinted by permission of the publisher (Taylor & Francis Ltd, http://www.tandfonline.com).

Uric acid kidney stones are present in 5–10% of patients with gouty arthritis. Hyperuricemia correlates highly with the likelihood of developing stones, with the risk of stone formation reaching 50% in patients with a serum urate level greater than 13 mg/dL. Chronic urate nephropathy is caused by the deposition of monosodium urate crystals in the renal medulla and pyramids. Although progressive CKD occurs in a substantial percentage of patients with chronic gout, the role of hyperuricemia in causing this outcome is controversial, because many patients with gout have numerous confounding risk factors for CKD (eg, hypertension, NSAID use, alcohol use, lead exposure, and other risk factors for vascular disease). In a 2020 randomized, controlled trial in patients with CKD and a high risk of its progression, urate-lowering treatment with allopurinol did not slow the decline in eGFR compared with placebo.

Clinical Findings

A. Symptoms and Signs

Acute gouty arthritis is sudden in onset and frequently nocturnal. It may develop without apparent precipitating cause or may follow rapid increases or decreases in serum urate levels. Common precipitants are alcohol excess (particularly beer), changes in medications that affect urate metabolism, and, in the hospitalized patient, fasting before medical procedures. The MTP joint of the great toe is the most susceptible joint ("podagra"), although others, especially those of the feet, ankles, and knees, are commonly affected (Figure 20–2). Gouty attacks may develop in periarticular soft tissues such as the arch of the foot. Hips and shoulders are rarely affected. More than one joint may occasionally be affected during the same attack; in such cases, the distribution of the arthritis is usually asymmetric. As the attack progresses, the pain becomes intense. The involved joints are swollen and exquisitely tender and the overlying skin tense, warm, and dusky red. Fever is common and may reach 39°C. Tophi may be found in the pinna of the ears, feet, olecranon and prepatellar bursae, and hands. They usually develop years after the initial attack of gout.

Asymptomatic periods of months or years commonly follow the initial acute attack. After years of recurrent severe monoarthritis attacks of the lower extremities and untreated hyperuricemia, gout can evolve into a chronic, deforming polyarthritis of upper and lower extremities that mimics rheumatoid arthritis.

Chronic lead intoxication may cause attacks of gouty arthritis (saturnine gout).

B. Laboratory Findings

Although serial measurements of the serum uric acid detect hyperuricemia in 95% of patients, a single uric acid determination during an acute flare of gout is normal in up to 25% of cases. A normal serum uric acid level, therefore, does not exclude gout, especially in patients taking urate-lowering drugs. During an acute attack, the peripheral blood white cell count (neutrophilia) is frequently elevated. Identification of sodium urate crystals in joint fluid or material aspirated from a tophus establishes the diagnosis. The crystals, which may be extracellular or found within neutrophils, are needle-like and negatively birefringent when examined by polarized light microscopy.

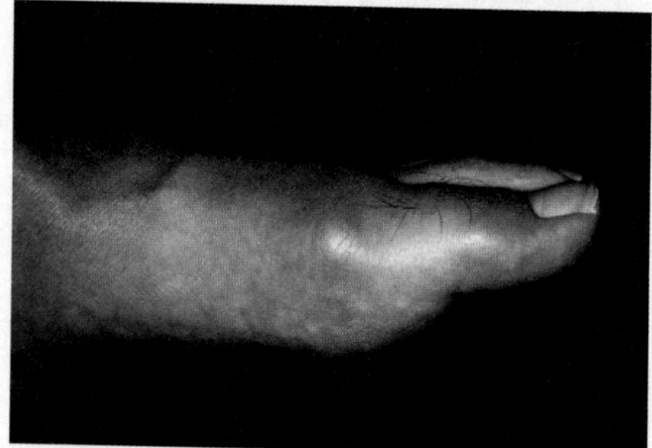

▲ **Figure 20–2.** Typical inflammatory changes of gout at first metatarsophalangeal joint (podagra). (Reproduced with permission from Richard P. Usatine, MD, in Usatine RP, Smith MA, Mayeaux EJ Jr, Chumley H. *The Color Atlas of Family Medicine*, 2nd ed. McGraw-Hill, 2013.)

C. Imaging

Early in the disease, radiographs show no changes. Later, punched-out erosions with an overhanging rim of cortical bone ("rat bite") develop. When these are adjacent to a soft tissue tophus, they are diagnostic of gout. Ultrasonography and dual-energy CT can be used to confirm the diagnosis of gout; tophi that are too small to appreciate on physical examination and smaller deposits of urate crystals can frequently be detected by these imaging modalities.

Differential Diagnosis

Acute gout is often confused with cellulitis. Bacteriologic studies usually exclude acute pyogenic arthritis but rarely, acute gout and pyogenic arthritis can coexist. Pseudogout is distinguished by the identification of calcium pyrophosphate crystals (positive birefringence) in the joint fluid, usually normal serum uric acid, and the radiographic appearance of chondrocalcinosis.

Chronic tophaceous arthritis may resemble chronic rheumatoid arthritis; gout is suggested by an earlier history of monoarthritis and is established by the demonstration of urate crystals in a suspected tophus. Likewise, hips and shoulders are generally spared in tophaceous gout. Biopsy may be necessary to distinguish tophi from rheumatoid nodules.

Treatment

A. Asymptomatic Hyperuricemia

As a general rule, uric acid–lowering drugs should not be instituted until acute gout, renal calculi, or tophi become apparent.

B. Acute Attack

Treatment of the acute attack focuses on reducing inflammation, not lowering serum uric acid.

1. NSAIDs—Oral NSAIDs in full dose (eg, naproxen 500 mg twice daily or indomethacin 25–50 mg every 8 hours; see Table 5–5) are effective treatment for acute gout and should be continued until the symptoms have resolved (usually 5–10 days). Contraindications include active peptic ulcer disease, impaired kidney function, and a history of allergic reaction to NSAIDs.

2. Colchicine—Oral colchicine is an appropriate treatment option for acute gout, provided the duration of the attack is less than 36 hours. For acute gout, colchicine should be administered orally as follows: a loading dose of 1.2 mg followed by a dose of 0.6 mg 1 hour later for a total dose of

1.8 mg the first day; thereafter 0.6 mg twice per day is used until resolution. Patients who are already taking prophylactic doses of colchicine and have an acute flare of gout may receive the full loading dose (1.2 mg) followed by 0.6 mg 1 hour later (before resuming the usual 0.6 mg once or twice daily) provided they have not received this regimen within the preceding 14 days (in which case, NSAIDs or corticosteroids should be used). Colchicine dose should be reduced or avoided altogether if there is significant kidney or liver impairment. Using oral colchicine during the intercritical period to prevent gout attacks is discussed below.

3. Corticosteroids—Corticosteroids often give dramatic symptomatic relief in acute episodes of gout and will control most attacks. They are especially useful in patients with contraindications to NSAIDs. Corticosteroids may be given intravenously (eg, methylprednisolone, 40 mg/day) or orally (eg, prednisone, 40–60 mg/day). Corticosteroids can be given at the suggested dose for 5–10 days and then simply discontinued or given at the suggested initial dose for 2–5 days and then tapered over 7–10 days. If the patient's gout is monoarticular or oligoarticular, intra-articular administration of the corticosteroid (eg, triamcinolone, 10–40 mg depending on the size of the joint) is very effective. Because gouty and septic arthritis can coexist, albeit rarely, joint aspiration and Gram stain with culture of synovial fluid should be performed when intra-articular corticosteroids are given.

4. Interleukin-1 inhibitors—Anakinra (an interleukin-1 receptor antagonist) and canakinumab (a monoclonal antibody against interleukin-1 beta) have efficacy for the management of acute gout, but these drugs have not been approved by the FDA for this indication. Anakinra can be used in hospitalized patients with acute gout in whom comorbidities prevent the use of NSAIDs, colchicine, or glucocorticoids.

C. Management Between Attacks

Treatment during symptom-free periods is intended to minimize urate deposition in tissues and to reduce the frequency and severity of recurrences. Potentially reversible causes of hyperuricemia are a high-purine diet, obesity, alcohol consumption, and use of certain medications (Table 20–4). Patients with a single episode of gout who have normal kidney function and are able to lose weight and stop drinking alcohol are at low risk for another attack and may not require long-term medical therapy. In contrast, patients with mild CKD or a history of multiple attacks of gout will likely benefit from pharmacologic treatment. In general, the higher the uric acid level and the more frequent the attacks, the more likely that long-term medical therapy will be beneficial. All patients with tophaceous gout should receive urate-lowering therapy.

1. Diet—Excessive alcohol consumption can precipitate attacks and should be avoided. Beer consumption appears to confer a higher risk of gout than does whiskey or wine. Although dietary purines usually contribute only 1 mg/dL to the serum uric acid level, moderation in eating foods with high purine content is advisable. Patients should avoid organ meats and beverages sweetened with high fructose corn syrup. A high liquid intake and, more importantly, a daily urinary output of 2 L or more will aid urate excretion and minimize urate precipitation in the kidney.

2. Avoidance of hyperuricemic medications—Thiazide and loop diuretics inhibit renal excretion of uric acid and, if possible, should be avoided in patients with gout. Similarly, niacin can raise serum uric acid levels and should be discontinued if there are therapeutic alternatives. Low doses of aspirin also aggravate hyperuricemia.

3. Colchicine prophylaxis—Colchicine can be used when urate-lowering therapy is started to suppress attacks precipitated by abrupt changes in the serum uric acid level. The usual dose is 0.6 mg orally either once or twice a day. Colchicine is renally cleared. Patients who have coexisting moderate CKD should take colchicine only once a day or once every other day to avoid peripheral neuromyopathy and other complications of colchicine toxicity. In patients with concomitant CAD, chronic colchicine use can reduce major cardiovascular events.

4. Reduction of serum uric acid—Indications for urate-lowering therapy in a person with gout include frequent acute arthritis (two or more episodes per year), tophaceous deposits, or CKD (stage 2 or worse). The American College of Rheumatology guidelines recommend a treat-to-target approach for urate-lowering therapy. In some cases, particularly in patients with tophi or frequent attacks, control of gout may require lowering serum uric acid to less than 5 mg/dL or 297.4 mcmol/L. Lowering serum uric acid levels does not benefit an acute gout flare.

Three classes of agents may lower the serum uric acid—xanthine oxidase inhibitors (allopurinol or febuxostat), uricosuric agents, and uricase (pegloticase).

A. Xanthine oxidase inhibitors—Allopurinol and febuxostat are the preferred first-line agents for lowering urate and have similar efficacy. They reduce plasma uric acid levels by blocking the final enzymatic steps in the production of uric acid. Allopurinol and febuxostat should not be used together, but they can be tried sequentially if the initial agent fails to lower serum uric acid to the target level or if it is not tolerated. The most frequent adverse effect with either medication is the precipitation of an acute gouty attack; thus, patients generally should be receiving prophylactic doses of colchicine.

Hypersensitivity to allopurinol occurs in 2% of cases, usually within the first few months of therapy, and it can be life-threatening. The most common initial sign of hypersensitivity is a pruritic rash that may progress to toxic epidermal necrolysis, particularly if allopurinol is continued; vasculitis and hepatitis are other manifestations. *Patients should be instructed to stop allopurinol immediately if a rash develops.* CKD and concomitant thiazide therapy are risk factors. There is a strong association between allopurinol hypersensitivity and HLA-B*58:01, which is a prevalent allele in certain populations. It is recommended to screen for HLA-B*58:01 before initiating allopurinol in all persons of Chinese, Thai, and Korean descent, as well as in African-American persons.

The initial daily dose of allopurinol is 100 mg/day orally (50 mg/day for those with stage 4 or worse CKD); the dose of allopurinol should be titrated upward every 2–5 weeks to achieve the target serum uric acid level. A typical dose of allopurinol is 300 mg, but most patients require greater than 300 mg daily to achieve the target uric acid level. The maximum daily dose is 800 mg.

Allopurinol interacts with other drugs. The combined use of allopurinol and ampicillin causes a drug rash in 20% of patients. Allopurinol can increase the half-life of probenecid, while probenecid increases the excretion of allopurinol. Thus, a patient taking both drugs may need to use slightly higher than usual doses of allopurinol and lower doses of probenecid.

Febuxostat can also rarely cause hypersensitivity reactions, and those with previous hypersensitivity to allopurinol appear to have slightly higher risk. It can be given without dose adjustment to patients with mild to moderate kidney disease. However, abnormal liver tests may develop in 2–3% of patients taking febuxostat. Despite initial concern that febuxostat was associated with more cardiovascular events than allopurinol, a large, randomized, controlled trial in 2020 showed that the two drugs have similar cardiovascular safety. The initial dose of febuxostat is 40 mg/day orally. If the target serum uric acid is not reached in 4 weeks, the dose of febuxostat can be increased to 80 mg/day and then to the maximum dose of 120 mg/day.

B. Uricosuric drugs—Uricosuric drugs lower serum uric acid levels by blocking the tubular reabsorption of filtered urate, thereby increasing uric acid excretion by the kidney. Probenecid (0.5 g/day orally) is the uricosuric available in the United States; lesinurad (200 mg/day orally) is also available in some countries. These drugs are typically reserved for patients who cannot achieve a serum uric acid of less than or equal to 6.0 mg/dL with allopurinol or febuxostat alone. Probenecid should not be used in patients with a creatinine clearance of less than 50 mL/minute due to limited efficacy; contraindications include a history of nephrolithiasis (uric acid or calcium stones) and evidence of high uric acid excretion (ie, greater than 800 mg of uric acid in a 24-hour urine collection). To reduce the development of uric acid stones (which occur in up to 11%), patients should be advised to increase their fluid intake and clinicians should consider prescribing an alkalinizing agent (eg, potassium citrate, 30–80 mEq/day orally) to maintain a urinary pH > 6.0.

C. Uricase—Pegloticase, a recombinant uricase that must be administered intravenously (8 mg every 2 weeks), is indicated for the rare patient with refractory chronic tophaceous gout. Pegloticase carries an FDA black box warning, which advises administering the drug only in health care settings and by health care professionals prepared to manage anaphylactic and other serious infusion reactions.

D. Chronic Tophaceous Arthritis

With rigorous drug adherence, allopurinol, febuxostat, and pegloticase shrink tophi and in time can lead to their disappearance. Resorption of extensive tophi requires maintaining a serum uric acid below 6 mg/dL. Surgical excision of large tophi offers mechanical improvement in selected deformities.

E. Gout in the Transplant Patient

Hyperuricemia and gout commonly develop in many transplant patients because they have decreased kidney function and require drugs that inhibit uric acid excretion (especially cyclosporine and diuretics). Treating acute gout in these patients is challenging. Often the best approach for monoarticular gout—after excluding infection—is injecting corticosteroids into the joint. For polyarticular gout, increasing the dose of systemic corticosteroid may be the only alternative. Since transplant patients often have multiple attacks of gout, long-term relief requires lowering the serum uric acid with allopurinol or febuxostat. (Kidney dysfunction seen in many transplant patients makes uricosuric agents ineffective.) Both allopurinol and febuxostat inhibit the metabolism of azathioprine and should be avoided in patients who take azathioprine.

Prognosis

Without treatment, the acute attack may last from a few days to several weeks. The intervals between acute attacks vary up to years, but the asymptomatic periods often become shorter if the disease progresses. Chronic gouty arthritis occurs after repeated attacks of acute gout, but only after inadequate treatment. The younger the patient at the onset of disease, the greater the tendency to a progressive course. Destructive arthropathy is rarely seen in patients whose first attack is after age 50.

Badve SV et al; CKD-FIX Study Investigators. Effects of allopurinol on the progression of chronic kidney disease. N Engl J Med. 2020;382:2504. [PMID: 32579811]

Mackenzie IS et al; FAST Study Group. Long-term cardiovascular safety of febuxostat compared with allopurinol in patients with gout (FAST): a multicentre, prospective, randomised, open-label, non-inferiority trial. Lancet. 2020;396:1745. [PMID: 33181081]

2. Calcium Pyrophosphate Deposition

Calcium pyrophosphate deposition (CPPD) in fibrocartilage and hyaline cartilage (chondrocalcinosis) can cause an acute crystal-induced arthritis ("pseudogout"), a degenerative arthropathy, and a chronic inflammatory polyarthritis ("pseudorheumatoid arthritis"). CPPD also can be an asymptomatic condition detected as incidental chondrocalcinosis on radiographs. The prevalence of CPPD increases with age. Hyperparathyroidism, familial hypocalciuric hypercalcemia, hemochromatosis, and hypomagnesemia confer risk of CPPD, but most cases have no associated condition.

Pseudogout is most often seen in persons aged 60 or older, is characterized by acute, recurrent and rarely chronic arthritis involving large joints (most commonly the knees and the wrists) and is almost always accompanied by radiographic chondrocalcinosis of the affected joints. The crowned dens syndrome, caused by pseudogout of the atlantoaxial junction associated with "crown-like" calcifications around the dens, manifests with severe neck pain, rigidity, and high fever that can mimic meningitis or polymyalgia rheumatica. Pseudogout, like gout, frequently develops 24–48 hours after major surgery. Identification of weakly positively birefringent calcium pyrophosphate crystals in joint aspirates is diagnostic. NSAIDs are helpful in the treatment of acute episodes. Colchicine, 0.6 mg orally once or twice daily, is more effective for prophylaxis than for acute attacks. Aspiration of the inflamed joint and intra-articular injection of triamcinolone, 10–40 mg, depending on the size of the joint, are also of value in resistant cases. In patients with contraindications to other therapies, the use of anakinra, an IL-1 inhibitor, is an option.

The degenerative arthropathy associated with CPPD can involve joints not usually affected by osteoarthritis (eg, glenohumeral joint, wrist, patellofemoral compartment of the knee). The "pseudorheumatoid arthritis" of CPPD affects the metacarpophalangeal joints and wrists. In both conditions, radiographs demonstrate chondrocalcinosis and degenerative changes such as asymmetric joint space narrowing and osteophyte formation.

Cipolletta E et al. Biologics in the treatment of calcium pyrophosphate deposition disease: a systematic literature review. Clin Exp Rheumatol. 2020;38:1001. [PMID: 32359034]

Parperis K et al. Management of calcium pyrophosphate crystal deposition disease: a systematic review. Semin Arthritis Rheum. 2021;51:84. [PMID: 33360232]

AUTOIMMUNE DISEASES

RHEUMATOID ARTHRITIS

ESSENTIALS OF DIAGNOSIS

- Usually insidious onset with morning stiffness and joint pain.
- Symmetric polyarthritis with predilection for small joints of the hands and feet; deformities common with progressive disease.
- Radiographic findings: juxta-articular osteoporosis, joint erosions, and joint space narrowing.
- Rheumatoid factor and antibodies to cyclic citrullinated peptides (anti-CCP) are present in 70–80%.
- Extra-articular disease: subcutaneous nodules, interstitial lung disease, pleural effusion, pericarditis, splenomegaly, scleritis, and vasculitis.

General Considerations

Rheumatoid arthritis is a chronic systemic inflammatory disease whose major manifestation is synovitis of multiple joints. It has a prevalence of 1% and is more common in women than men (female:male ratio of 3:1). Rheumatoid arthritis can begin at any age, but the peak onset is in the fourth or fifth decade for women and the sixth to eighth decades for men. The cause is not known. Susceptibility to rheumatoid arthritis is genetically determined with multiple genes contributing. Inheritance of HLA-DRB1 alleles encoding a distinctive five-amino-acid sequence known as the "shared epitope" is the best characterized genetic risk factor. Untreated, rheumatoid arthritis causes joint destruction with consequent disability and shortens life expectancy. Early, aggressive treatment is the standard of care.

The pathologic findings in the joint include chronic synovitis with formation of a pannus, which erodes cartilage, bone, ligaments, and tendons. Effusion and other manifestations of inflammation are common.

Clinical Findings

A. Symptoms and Signs

1. Joint symptoms—The clinical manifestations of rheumatoid arthritis are highly variable, but joint symptoms usually predominate. Although acute presentations may occur, the onset of articular signs of inflammation is usually insidious, with prodromal symptoms of vague periarticular pain or stiffness. Symmetric swelling of multiple joints with tenderness and pain is characteristic. Monoarticular disease is occasionally seen initially. Stiffness persisting for longer than 30 minutes (and usually many hours) is prominent in the morning. Stiffness may recur after daytime inactivity and be much more severe after strenuous activity. Although any diarthrodial joint may be affected, PIP joints of the fingers, MCP joints (Figure 20–3), wrists, knees, ankles, and MTP joints are most often involved. Synovial cysts and rupture of tendons may occur. Entrapment syndromes are common—particularly of the median nerve at the carpal

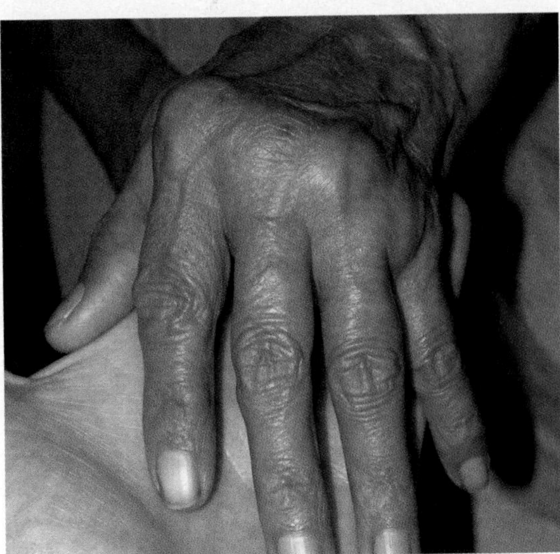

▲ **Figure 20–3.** Rheumatoid arthritis with ulnar deviation at the metacarpophalangeal joints. (Reproduced with permission from Richard P. Usatine, MD, in Usatine RP, Smith MA, Mayeaux EJ Jr, Chumley H, Tysinger J. *The Color Atlas of Family Medicine*. McGraw-Hill, 2009.)

tunnel of the wrist. Rheumatoid arthritis can affect the neck but spares the other components of the spine and does not involve the sacroiliac joints. In advanced disease, atlantoaxial (C1–C2) subluxation can lead to myelopathy.

2. Rheumatoid nodules—Twenty percent of patients have subcutaneous rheumatoid nodules, most commonly situated over bony prominences but also observed in the bursae and tendon sheaths (Figure 20–4). Nodules are occasionally seen in the lungs, the sclerae, and other tissues. Nodules correlate with the presence of rheumatoid factor in serum ("seropositivity"), as do most other extra-articular manifestations.

3. Ocular symptoms—Dryness of the eyes, mouth, and other mucous membranes is found especially in advanced disease (see Sjögren syndrome). Other ocular manifestations include episcleritis, scleritis, scleromalacia due to scleral nodules, and peripheral ulcerative keratitis.

4. Other symptoms—Interstitial lung disease is not uncommon (estimates of prevalence vary widely according to method of detection) and manifests clinically as cough and progressive dyspnea. Pericarditis and pleural disease are usually silent clinically, but symptomatic effusions can occur. Occasionally, a small-vessel vasculitis develops and manifests as tiny hemorrhagic infarcts in the nail folds or finger pulps. Necrotizing arteritis is well reported but rare. A small subset of patients with rheumatoid arthritis has Felty syndrome, the occurrence of splenomegaly and neutropenia, usually in the setting of severe, destructive arthritis. Felty syndrome must be distinguished from large granular lymphoproliferative disorder, with which it shares many features.

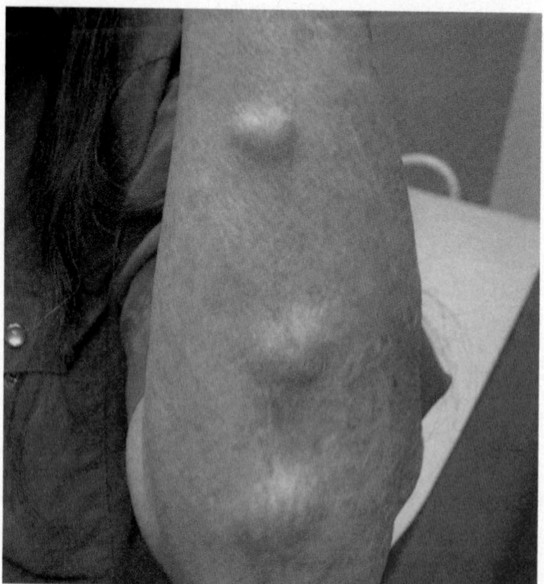

▲ **Figure 20–4.** Rheumatoid nodules over the extensor surface of the forearm. (Reproduced with permission from Richard P. Usatine, MD, in Usatine RP, Smith MA, Mayeaux EJ Jr, Chumley H. *The Color Atlas of Family Medicine*, 2nd ed. McGraw-Hill, 2013.)

B. Laboratory Findings

Anti-CCP antibodies and rheumatoid factor, an IgM antibody directed against the Fc region of IgG, are present in 70–80% of patients with established rheumatoid arthritis. Rheumatoid factor has a sensitivity of only 50% in early disease. Anti-CCP antibodies are the most specific blood test for rheumatoid arthritis (specificity ~95%). Rheumatoid factor can occur in other autoimmune diseases and in chronic infections, including hepatitis C, syphilis, subacute bacterial endocarditis, and tuberculosis. The prevalence of rheumatoid factor positivity also rises with age in healthy individuals. Approximately 20% of rheumatoid arthritis patients have antinuclear antibodies.

The ESR and levels of CRP are typically elevated in proportion to disease activity. Anemia of chronic disease is common. The platelet count is often elevated, roughly in proportion to the severity of overall joint inflammation. Initial joint fluid examination confirms the inflammatory nature of the arthritis (see Table 20–2).

Arthrocentesis is needed to diagnose superimposed septic arthritis, which is a common complication of rheumatoid arthritis and should be considered whenever a patient with rheumatoid arthritis has one joint inflamed out of proportion to the rest.

C. Imaging

Of all the laboratory tests, radiographic changes are the most specific for rheumatoid arthritis. Radiographs obtained during the first 6 months of symptoms, however, are usually normal. The earliest changes occur in the hands or feet and consist of soft tissue swelling and juxta-articular demineralization. Later, diagnostic changes of uniform joint space narrowing and erosions develop. The erosions are often first evident at the ulnar styloid and at the juxta-articular margin, where the bony surface is not protected by cartilage. Characteristic changes also occur in the cervical spine, with C1–2 subluxation, but these changes usually take many years to develop. Although both MRI and ultrasonography are more sensitive than radiographs in detecting bony and soft tissue changes in rheumatoid arthritis, their value in early diagnosis relative to that of plain radiographs has not been established.

Differential Diagnosis

The differentiation of rheumatoid arthritis from other joint conditions and immune-mediated disorders can be difficult. In contrast to rheumatoid arthritis, osteoarthritis spares the wrists and the MCP joints. Osteoarthritis is not associated with constitutional manifestations, and the joint pain is characteristically relieved by rest, unlike the morning stiffness of rheumatoid arthritis. Signs of articular inflammation, prominent in rheumatoid arthritis, are usually minimal in degenerative joint disease. CPPD disease can cause a degenerative arthropathy of the MCPs and wrists; radiographs are usually diagnostic. Although gouty arthritis is almost always intermittent and monoarticular in the early years, it may evolve with time into a chronic polyarticular process that mimics rheumatoid arthritis. Gouty tophi can resemble rheumatoid nodules but are not associated with rheumatoid factor, whose sensitivity for rheumatoid nodules approaches 100%. The early history of intermittent monoarthritis and the presence of synovial urate crystals are distinctive features of gout.

Spondyloarthropathies, particularly earlier in their course, can be a source of diagnostic uncertainty; predilection for lower extremities and involvement of the spine and sacroiliac joints point to the correct diagnosis. Chronic Lyme arthritis typically involves only one joint, most commonly the knee, and is associated with positive serologic tests (see Chapter 34). Acute viral infections, most notably with Chikungunya virus and parvovirus B19, can cause a polyarthritis that mimics early-onset rheumatoid arthritis. However, fever is common, the arthritis usually resolves within weeks, and serologic studies confirm recent infection. Chronic infection with hepatitis C can cause a chronic nonerosive polyarthritis associated with rheumatoid factor; tests for anti-CCP antibodies are negative.

Malar rash, photosensitivity, discoid skin lesions, alopecia, high titer antibodies to double-stranded DNA or Smith, glomerulonephritis, and CNS abnormalities point to the diagnosis of SLE. Polymyalgia rheumatica occasionally causes polyarthralgias in patients over age 50, but these patients remain rheumatoid factor–negative and have chiefly proximal muscle pain and stiffness, centered on the shoulder and hip girdles. Joint pain that can be confused with rheumatoid arthritis presents in a substantial minority of patients with granulomatosis with polyangiitis. This diagnostic error can be avoided by recognizing that, in contrast to rheumatoid arthritis, the arthritis of granulomatosis with polyangiitis preferentially involves larger joints (eg, hips, ankles, wrists) and usually spares the small joints of the hand. Rheumatic fever is characterized by the migratory nature of the arthritis, an elevated antistreptolysin titer, and a more dramatic and prompt response to aspirin; carditis and erythema marginatum may occur in adults, but chorea and subcutaneous nodules occur only in children. Finally, a variety of cancers produce paraneoplastic syndromes, including polyarthritis. One form is hypertrophic pulmonary osteoarthropathy most often produced by lung and GI carcinomas, characterized by a rheumatoid-like arthritis associated with clubbing, periosteal new bone formation, and a negative rheumatoid factor. Diffuse swelling of the hands with palmar fasciitis occurs in a variety of cancers, especially ovarian carcinoma.

Treatment

The primary objectives in treating rheumatoid arthritis are reduction of inflammation and pain, preservation of function, and prevention of deformity. Disease-modifying antirheumatic drugs (DMARDs) should be started as soon as the diagnosis of rheumatoid disease is certain and then adjusted with the aim of suppressing disease activity. NSAIDs provide some symptomatic relief in rheumatoid arthritis but do not prevent erosions or alter disease progression. They are not appropriate for monotherapy and should only be used in conjunction with DMARDs, if at all. The American College of Rheumatology recommends using standardized assessments, such as the Disease Activity Score 28 Joints or the Clinical Disease Activity Index, to gauge therapeutic responses, with the target of low disease activity or remission by these measures.

A. Corticosteroids

Low-dose corticosteroids (eg, oral prednisone 5–10 mg daily) produce a prompt anti-inflammatory effect and slow the rate of articular erosion. These are often used as a "bridge" to reduce disease activity until the slower acting DMARDs take effect or as adjunctive therapy for active disease that persists despite treatment with DMARDs. No more than 10 mg of prednisone or equivalent per day is appropriate for articular disease. Higher doses are used to manage serious extra-articular manifestations (eg, pericarditis, necrotizing scleritis). When corticosteroids are to be discontinued, they should be tapered gradually on a planned schedule appropriate to the duration of treatment. All patients receiving long-term corticosteroid therapy should take measures to prevent osteoporosis (Table 26–17).

Intra-articular corticosteroids may be helpful for symptom control if one or two joints are the chief source of difficulty. Intra-articular triamcinolone, 10–40 mg depending on the size of the joint to be injected, may be given but not more than four times a year.

B. DMARDs

1. Synthetic DMARDs—

A. Methotrexate—Methotrexate is the initial synthetic DMARD of choice for patients with rheumatoid arthritis. It is generally well tolerated and often produces a beneficial effect in 2–6 weeks. The usual initial dose is 7.5 or 10 mg of methotrexate orally once weekly. If the patient has tolerated methotrexate but has not responded in 1 month, the dose can be increased to 15 mg orally weekly. The maximal oral dose is usually 20 mg weekly. The most frequent side effects are gastric irritation and stomatitis. Cytopenia, most commonly leukopenia or thrombocytopenia but rarely pancytopenia due to bone marrow suppression, is another important potential problem of methotrexate therapy. The risk of developing pancytopenia is much higher in patients whose serum creatinine is greater than 2 mg/dL (176.8 mcmol/L). Hepatotoxicity with fibrosis and cirrhosis is an important toxic effect that correlates with cumulative dose and is uncommon with appropriate monitoring of liver biochemical tests. Methotrexate is contraindicated in a patient with any form of chronic hepatitis, in pregnant women, and in any patient with significant kidney dysfunction (estimated GFR less than 30 mL/minute/1.73 m^2). Heavy alcohol use increases hepatotoxicity, so patients should be advised to drink alcohol in extreme moderation, if at all. Diabetes mellitus, obesity, and kidney disease also increase the risk of hepatotoxicity. Liver biochemical tests should be monitored at least every 12 weeks, along with a CBC. The dose of methotrexate should be reduced if aminotransferase levels are elevated, and the drug should be discontinued if abnormalities persist despite dosage reduction. All patients should be prescribed either daily folate (1 mg orally) or weekly leucovorin calcium

(2.5–5 mg taken orally 24 hours after the dose of methotrexate) to reduce gastric irritation, stomatitis, cytopenias, and hepatotoxicity. Hypersensitivity to methotrexate can cause an acute or subacute interstitial pneumonitis that can be life-threatening but which usually responds to cessation of the drug and institution of corticosteroids. Because methotrexate is teratogenic, women of childbearing age must use effective contraception while taking the medication. Methotrexate is associated with an increased risk of B-cell lymphomas, some of which resolve following the discontinuation of the medication as well as all types of skin cancer. The combination of methotrexate and other folate antagonists, such as trimethoprim-sulfamethoxazole, should be used cautiously since pancytopenia can result. Amoxicillin can decrease renal clearance of methotrexate, leading to toxicity. Probenecid also increases methotrexate drug levels and toxicity and should be avoided.

B. Sulfasalazine—This drug is a second-line agent for rheumatoid arthritis. It is usually introduced at a dosage of 500 mg orally twice daily and then increased each week by 500 mg until the patient improves or the daily dose reaches 3000 mg. Side effects, particularly neutropenia and thrombocytopenia, occur in 10–25% and are serious in 2–5%. Sulfasalazine also causes hemolysis in patients with glucose-6-phosphate dehydrogenase (G6PD) deficiency, so a G6PD level should be checked before initiation. Patients with aspirin sensitivity should not be given sulfasalazine. Patients taking sulfasalazine should have CBC monitored every 2–4 weeks for the first 3 months, then every 3 months.

C. Leflunomide—Leflunomide, a pyrimidine synthesis inhibitor, is administered orally as a single daily dose of 20 mg. The most frequent side effects are diarrhea, rash, reversible alopecia, and hepatotoxicity. Some patients experience dramatic unexplained weight loss. The drug is teratogenic and has a half-life of 2 weeks, but active metabolites can be detected for up to 2 years. Thus, it is contraindicated in premenopausal women who wish to bear children.

D. Antimalarials—Hydroxychloroquine sulfate is the antimalarial agent most often used in rheumatoid arthritis. Monotherapy with hydroxychloroquine should be reserved for patients with very mild disease because only a small percentage will respond and often only after 3–6 months of therapy. Hydroxychloroquine is often used in combination with other conventional DMARDs, particularly methotrexate and sulfasalazine (so-called "triple therapy"). The advantage of hydroxychloroquine is its comparatively low toxicity, especially at a dosage of 200–400 mg/day orally (not to exceed 5 mg/kg/day). The prevalence of the most important adverse effect, retinal toxicity that can lead to visual loss, is a function of duration of therapy, occurring in less than 2% of patients (dosed properly) during the first 10 years of use but rising to 20% after 20 years of treatment. Ophthalmologic examinations every 12 months are required. Rare reactions include neuropathies and myopathies of both skeletal and cardiac muscle, which usually improve when the drug is withdrawn.

E. Janus kinase inhibitors—Tofacitinib, baricitinib, and upadacitinib, inhibitors of Janus kinase, are used to manage severe rheumatoid arthritis that is refractory to methotrexate or other agents. Janus kinase inhibitors are oral agents that can be used either as monotherapy or in combination with methotrexate. Tofacitinib is administered in a dose of 5 mg twice daily; baricitinib is 2 mg or 4 mg daily, and upadacitinib is 15 mg daily. Janus kinase inhibitors can increase the risk of infections. Patients should be screened and treated for latent tuberculosis prior to receiving these drugs. Vaccination against varicella is also recommended. There is an FDA black box warning for Janus kinase inhibitors about slightly higher risks of serious heart-related events, cancer, blood clots, and death based on data from a large, randomized, controlled trial comparing tofacitinib with tumor necrosis factor (TNF) inhibitors in patients taking methotrexate.

2. Biologic DMARDs—

A. Tumor necrosis factor inhibitors—Inhibitors of TNF—a proinflammatory cytokine—are frequently added to the treatment of patients who have not responded adequately to methotrexate and can be used as initial therapy in combination with methotrexate for patients with poor prognostic factors.

Five TNF inhibitors are in use: etanercept, infliximab, adalimumab, golimumab, and certolizumab pegol. Etanercept, a soluble recombinant TNF receptor:Fc fusion protein, is usually administered at a dosage of 50 mg subcutaneously once per week. Infliximab, a chimeric monoclonal antibody, is administered at a dosage of 3–10 mg/kg intravenously; infusions are repeated after 2, 6, 10, and 14 weeks and then are administered every 8 weeks. Adalimumab, a human monoclonal antibody that binds to TNF, is given at a dosage of 40 mg subcutaneously every other week. The dose for golimumab, a human anti-TNF monoclonal antibody, is 50 mg subcutaneously once monthly. Certolizumab pegol is a PEGylated Fab fragment of an anti-TNF monoclonal antibody; the dose is 200–400 mg subcutaneously every 2 to 4 weeks. Each drug produces substantial improvement in more than 60% of patients and is usually well tolerated. Minor irritation at injection sites is the most common side effect of etanercept and adalimumab. Rarely, nonrecurrent leukopenia develops in patients. TNF inhibitors have been associated with a several-fold increased risk of serious bacterial infections and a striking increase in granulomatous infections, particularly reactivation of tuberculosis. Screening for latent tuberculosis (see Chapter 9) is mandatory before initiating TNF blockers. It is prudent to suspend TNF blockers when a fever or other manifestations of a clinically important infection develops. Demyelinating neurologic complications that resemble multiple sclerosis have been reported rarely in patients taking TNF inhibitors, but the true magnitude of this risk—likely small—has not been determined with precision. Most observational studies have not found a higher risk of malignancy with TNF inhibitors, but the FDA has issued a safety alert about case reports of malignancies, including leukemias. Infliximab was associated with increased morbidity in a heart failure trial; therefore, TNF inhibitors should be used with extreme caution in patients with heart failure. Infliximab can rarely cause anaphylaxis and induce anti-DNA antibodies (but rarely clinically evident SLE).

B. ABATACEPT—Abatacept, a recombinant protein made by fusing a fragment of the Fc domain of human IgG with the extracellular domain of a T-cell inhibitory receptor (CTLA4), blocks T-cell costimulation and produces clinically meaningful responses in approximately 50% of individuals whose disease does not respond to the combination of methotrexate and a TNF inhibitor.

C. RITUXIMAB—Rituximab, a humanized mouse monoclonal antibody that depletes B cells, can be used in combination with methotrexate or leflunomide for patients whose disease has been refractory to treatment with a TNF inhibitor. Because rituximab reduces the humoral immune response, it should be used with caution during the COVID-19 pandemic as multiple studies suggest a higher risk of mortality from COVID-19 in patients using this drug.

D. TOCILIZUMAB AND SARILUMAB—Tocilizumab and sarilumab are monoclonal antibodies that block the receptor for IL-6, an inflammatory cytokine involved in the pathogenesis of rheumatoid arthritis. They are used most often in combination with methotrexate for patients whose disease has been refractory to treatment with a TNF inhibitor. These drugs have been associated with GI perforations, although this adverse event is rare.

3. Combination DMARDs—As a general rule, DMARDs have greater efficacy when administered in combination than when used individually. The most commonly used combination is methotrexate with a TNF inhibitor. Still, most patients who require DMARD therapy are given methotrexate monotherapy initially because this regimen is effective in up to one-third of patients and is less expensive and less toxic than combination therapy. The combination of methotrexate, sulfasalazine, and hydroxychloroquine ("triple therapy") is economical, effective, and not inferior to the combination of methotrexate plus etanercept for those who have not responded to methotrexate monotherapy. The choice of a second-line biologic agent for patients who have not responded to TNF inhibitors is often based on patient and provider preference and insurance coverage since comparative effectiveness data are sparse. *Biologic DMARDs should not be combined.*

Course & Prognosis

After months or years, deformities may occur; the most common are ulnar deviation of the fingers (Figure 20–3), boutonniére deformity (hyperextension of the DIP joint with flexion of the PIP joint), "swan-neck" deformity (flexion of the DIP joint with extension of the PIP joint), valgus deformity of the knee, and volar subluxation of the MTP joints. The excess mortality associated with rheumatoid arthritis is largely due to CVD that is unexplained by traditional risk factors and that appears to result from deleterious effects of chronic systemic inflammation on the vascular system.

When to Refer

Early referral to a rheumatologist is essential for diagnosis and the timely introduction of effective therapy.

Fraenkel L et al. 2021 American College of Rheumatology guideline for the treatment of rheumatoid arthritis. Arthritis Care Res (Hoboken). 2021;73:924. [PMID: 34101387]

Smolen JS et al. EULAR recommendations for the management of rheumatoid arthritis with synthetic and biological disease-modifying antirheumatic drugs: 2019 update. Ann Rheum Dis. 2020;79:685. [PMID: 31969328]

Solomon DH et al. Adverse effects of low-dose methotrexate: a randomized trial. Ann Intern Med. 2020;172:369. [PMID: 32066146]

ADULT STILL DISEASE

Still disease is a systemic form of juvenile chronic arthritis in which high spiking fevers are much more prominent, especially at the outset, than arthritis. This rare syndrome also occurs in adults. Most adults are in their 20s or 30s; onset after age 60 is rare. The fever is dramatic, often with daily spikes to 40°C, associated with sweats and chills, and then plunging to normal or several degrees below normal in the absence of antipyretics. Many patients initially complain of sore throat. An evanescent salmon-colored nonpruritic rash, chiefly on the chest and abdomen, is a characteristic feature. The rash can easily be missed since it often appears only with the fever spike. Many patients also have lymphadenopathy and pericardial effusions. Joint symptoms are mild or absent initially, but a destructive arthritis, especially of the wrists, may develop months later. Anemia and leukocytosis, with white blood counts sometimes exceeding 40,000/mcL (40×10^9/L), are the rule. Serum ferritin levels are often strikingly elevated (greater than 3000 mg/mL or 6741 pmol/L). (Other conditions, including viral infections, malignancy, and multiple blood transfusions, can also cause extreme elevations in ferritin levels.) The diagnosis of adult Still disease is suggested by the quotidian fever pattern, sore throat, and the classic rash but requires exclusion of other causes of fever. About half of the patients respond to NSAIDs, and half require prednisone, sometimes in doses greater than 60 mg/day orally. Targeting IL-1 with anakinra or canakinumab or IL-6 with tocilizumab can be effective for patients with refractory disease. The course of adult Still disease can be monophasic, intermittent, or chronic. Macrophage activation syndrome is a life-threatening complication of adult Still disease and manifests as fever; splenomegaly; cytopenias; hypertriglyceridemia; hypofibrinogenemia; marked elevation of serum ferritin; elevated soluble CD25; depressed natural killer cell activity; and hemophagocytosis in bone marrow, spleen, and lymph nodes.

Kedor C et al. Canakinumab for Treatment of Adult-Onset Still's Disease to Achieve Reduction of Arthritic Manifestation (CONSIDER): phase II, randomised, double-blind, placebo-controlled, multicentre, investigator-initiated trial. Ann Rheum Dis. 2020;79:1090. [PMID: 32404342]

SYSTEMIC LUPUS ERYTHEMATOSUS

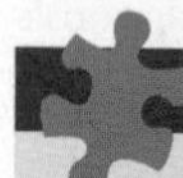

ESSENTIALS OF DIAGNOSIS

- Occurs mainly in young women.
- Rash over areas exposed to sunlight.
- Joint symptoms in 90% of patients.
- Anemia, leukopenia, thrombocytopenia.
- Glomerulonephritis, CNS disease, and complications of antiphospholipid antibodies are major sources of disease morbidity.
- Serologic findings: antinuclear antibodies (100%), anti–double-stranded DNA antibodies (approximately two-thirds), and low serum complement levels (particularly during disease flares).

General Considerations

SLE is an inflammatory autoimmune disorder characterized by autoantibodies to nuclear antigens. It can affect multiple organ systems. Many of its clinical manifestations are secondary to the trapping of antigen-antibody complexes in capillaries of visceral structures or to autoantibody-mediated destruction of host cells (eg, thrombocytopenia). The clinical course is marked by spontaneous remission and relapses. The severity may vary from a mild episodic disorder to a rapidly fulminant, life-threatening illness.

The incidence of SLE is influenced by many factors, including sex, environmental exposures, and genetic inheritance. About 85% of patients are women and most cases develop after menarche and before menopause. Among older individuals, the sex distribution is more equal. Race is also a factor, as SLE occurs in 1:250 Black women but in 1:1000 White women. Familial occurrence of SLE has been repeatedly documented, and the disorder is concordant in 25–70% of identical twins. If a mother has SLE, her daughters' risks of developing the disease are 1:40 and her sons' risks are 1:250. Serologic abnormalities (positive antinuclear antibody) are seen in asymptomatic family members, and the prevalence of other rheumatic diseases is increased among close relatives of patients.

The diagnosis of SLE should be suspected in patients having a multisystem disease with a positive test for antinuclear antibodies. It is imperative to ascertain that the condition has not been induced by a drug (see Drug-Induced Lupus below).

The traditional criteria of diagnosing SLE if at least 4 of 11 criteria in Table 20–5 were met were updated in 2019 to require an antinuclear antibody (ANA) titer of 80 or more (Table 20–6), highlighting that SLE should almost never be diagnosed in the absence of an elevated ANA titer. Criteria are developed as guidelines for the inclusion of patients in research studies and do not supplant clinical judgment in the diagnosis of SLE.

Table 20–5. Criteria for the classification of SLE. (A patient is classified as having SLE if any 4 or more of 11 criteria are met.)

1. Malar rash
2. Discoid rash
3. Photosensitivity
4. Oral ulcers
5. Arthritis
6. Serositis
7. Kidney disease
   a. > 0.5 g/day proteinuria, or
   b. ≥ 3+ dipstick proteinuria, or
   c. Cellular casts
8. Neurologic disease
   a. Seizures, or
   b. Psychosis (without other cause)
9. Hematologic disorders
   a. Hemolytic anemia, or
   b. Leukopenia (< 4000/mcL [4.0×10^9/L]), or lymphopenia (< 1500/mcL [1.5×10^9/L]), or
   c. Thrombocytopenia (< 100,000/mcL [100×10^9/L])
10. Immunologic abnormalities
    a. Antibody to native DNA, or
    b. Antibody to Sm, or
    c. Antibodies to antiphospholipid antibodies based on (1) IgG or IgM anti-cardiolipin antibodies, (2) lupus anticoagulant, or (3) false-positive serologic test for syphilis
11. Positive ANA

ANA, antinuclear antibody.
Reproduced with permission from Tan EM et al. The 1982 revised criteria for the classification of systemic lupus erythematosus. *Arthritis Rheum.* 1982;25(11):1271–127, and data from Hochberg MC. Updating the American College of Rheumatology revised criteria for the classification of systemic lupus erythematosus. *Arthritis Rheum.* 1997;40(9):1725.

Clinical Findings

A. Symptoms and Signs

The systemic features include fever, anorexia, malaise, and weight loss. Most patients have skin lesions at some time; the characteristic "butterfly" (malar) rash affects less than half of patients. Other cutaneous manifestations are panniculitis (lupus profundus), discoid lupus and typical fingertip lesions (periungual erythema, nail fold infarcts, and splinter hemorrhages). Alopecia is common. Mucous membrane lesions tend to occur during periods of exacerbation. Raynaud phenomenon, present in about 20% of patients, often antedates other features of the disease.

Joint symptoms, with or without active synovitis, occur in over 90% of patients and are often the earliest manifestation. The arthritis can lead to reversible swan-neck deformities, but radiographic erosions and subcutaneous nodules are rare.

Ocular manifestations include keratoconjunctivitis sicca and retinal vasculopathy (cotton-wool spots, episcleritis, scleritis, and optic neuropathy). Pleurisy and pleural effusion are common. Pneumonitis, interstitial lung disease, and pulmonary hypertension can rarely occur. Alveolar hemorrhage is uncommon but life-threatening.

Table 20–6. 2019 European League Against Rheumatism/American College of Rheumatology classification criteria for SLE.

Criteria	Definition
ANA	ANA at a titer of ≥ 1:80 at least once. Testing by immunofluorescence on HEp-2 cells or a solid-phase ANA screening immunoassay with at least equivalent performance is highly recommended
Fever	Temperature > 38.3°C
Leukopenia	WBC count < 4000/mcL (4.0×10^9/L)
Thrombocytopenia	Platelet count < 100,000/mcL (100×10^9/L)
Autoimmune hemolysis	Evidence of hemolysis, such as reticulocytosis, low haptoglobin, elevated indirect bilirubin, elevated LD, and positive direct antiglobulin (Coombs) test
Delirium	Characterized by: (1) change in consciousness or level of arousal with reduced ability to focus; (2) symptom development over hours to < 2 days; (3) symptom fluctuation throughout the day; (4) either acute/subacute change in cognition (eg, memory deficit or disorientation) or change in behavior, mood, or affect (eg, restlessness, reversal of sleep/wake cycle)
Psychosis	Characterized by delusions or hallucinations or both without insight and absence of delirium
Seizure	Primary generalized seizure or partial/focal seizure
Nonscarring alopecia	Nonscarring alopecia observed by a clinician[1]
Oral ulcers	Oral ulcers observed by a clinician[1]
Subacute cutaneous or discoid lupus	Subacute cutaneous lupus erythematosus observed by a clinician[1]: Annular or papulosquamous (psoriasiform) cutaneous eruption, usually photodistributed If skin biopsy is performed, typical changes must be present (interface vacuolar dermatitis consisting of a perivascular lymphohistiocytic infiltrate, often with dermal mucin noted). **or** Discoid lupus erythematosus observed by a clinician[1]: Erythematous-violaceous cutaneous lesions with secondary changes of atrophic scarring, dyspigmentation, often follicular hyperkeratosis/plugging (scalp), leading to scarring alopecia on the scalp If skin biopsy is performed, typical changes must be present (interface vacuolar dermatitis consisting of a perivascular and/or periappendageal lymphohistiocytic infiltrate. In the scalp, follicular keratin plugs may be seen. In longstanding lesions, mucin deposition may be noted)
Acute cutaneous lupus	Malar rash or generalized maculopapular rash observed by a clinician[1] If skin biopsy is performed, typical changes must be present (interface vacuolar dermatitis consisting of a perivascular lymphohistiocytic infiltrate, often with dermal mucin noted. Perivascular neutrophilic infiltrate may be present early in the course)
Pleural or pericardial effusion	Imaging evidence (such as ultrasonography, radiography, CT scan, MRI) of pleural or pericardial effusion, or both
Acute pericarditis	Presence of two or more of the following: 1. Pericardial chest pain (typically sharp, worse with inspiration, improved by leaning forward) 2. Pericardial rub 3. ECG with new widespread ST elevation or PR depression 4. New or worsened pericardial effusion on imaging (such as ultrasonography, radiography, CT scan, MRI)
Joint involvement	Presence of either synovitis involving > 2 joints characterized by swelling or effusion or tenderness in > 2 joints and at least 30 minutes of morning stiffness
Proteinuria	> 0.5 g/24 hours by 24-hour urine or equivalent spot urine protein-to-creatinine ratio
Class II or V lupus nephritis on renal biopsy according to ISN/RPS 2003 classification	*Class II:* Mesangial proliferative lupus nephritis: purely mesangial hypercellularity of any degree or mesangial matrix expansion by light microscopy, with mesangial immune deposit. A few isolated subepithelial or subendothelial deposits may be visible by immunofluorescence or electron microscopy but not by light microscopy *Class V:* Membranous lupus nephritis: global or segmental subepithelial immune deposits or their morphologic sequelae by light microscopy and by immunofluorescence or electron microscopy, with or without mesangial alterations

(*continued*)

Table 20–6. 2019 European League Against Rheumatism/American College of Rheumatology classification criteria for SLE. (continued)

Criteria	Definition
Class III or IV lupus nephritis on renal biopsy according to ISN/RPS 2003 classification	*Class III:* Focal lupus nephritis: active or inactive focal, segmental, or global endocapillary, or extracapillary glomerulonephritis involving < 50% of all glomeruli, typically with focal subendothelial immune deposits, with or without mesangial alterations *Class IV:* Diffuse lupus nephritis: active or inactive diffuse, segmental, or global endocapillary or extracapillary glomerulonephritis involving ≥ 50% of all glomeruli, typically with diffuse subendothelial immune deposits, with or without mesangial alterations. This class includes cases with diffuse wire loop deposits but with little or no glomerular proliferation
Positive antiphospholipid antibodies	Anti-cardiolipin antibodies (IgA, IgG, or IgM) at medium or high titer (> 40 APL, GPL, or MPL, or > 99th percentile) or positive anti-beta-2GPI antibodies (IgA, IgG, or IgM) or positive lupus anticoagulant
Low C3 OR low C4	C3 OR C4 below the lower limit of normal
Low C3 AND low C4	Both C3 AND C4 below the lower limits of normal
Anti-dsDNA antibodies *or* anti-Sm antibodies	Anti-dsDNA antibodies in an immunoassay with demonstrated ≥ 90% specificity for SLE against relevant disease controls *or* anti-Sm antibodies

[1]This may include physical examination or review of a photograph.

anti-beta-2GPI, anti–beta-2-glycoprotein 1; anti-dsDNA, anti–double-stranded DNA; ANA, antinuclear antibodies; Ig, immunoglobulin; ISN, International Society of Nephrology; RPS, Renal Pathology Society.

Reproduced with permission from Aringer M et al. 2019 European League Against Rheumatism/ American College of Rheumatology classification criteria for systemic lupus erythematosus. *Arthritis Rheumatol*. 2019;71(9):1400–1412.

The pericardium is affected in the majority of patients. Heart failure may result from myocarditis and hypertension. Cardiac arrhythmias are common. Atypical verrucous endocarditis of Libman-Sacks is usually clinically silent but occasionally can produce acute or chronic valvular regurgitation—most commonly mitral regurgitation, which can be a source of systemic emboli.

Neurologic complications of SLE include psychosis, cognitive impairment, seizures, peripheral and cranial neuropathies, transverse myelitis, and strokes. Severe depression and psychosis are sometimes exacerbated by the administration of large doses of corticosteroids.

Several forms of glomerulonephritis may occur, including mesangial, focal proliferative, diffuse proliferative, and membranous (see Chapter 22). Some patients may also have interstitial nephritis. With appropriate therapy, the survival rate even for patients with serious kidney disease (proliferative glomerulonephritis) is favorable, albeit a substantial portion of patients with severe lupus nephritis develop ESKD.

Hematologic manifestations include leukopenia, autoimmune hemolytic anemia, immune thrombocytopenia, and thrombotic thrombocytopenic purpura.

B. Laboratory Findings

SLE is characterized by the production of many different autoantibodies (Tables 20–7 and 20–8). Antinuclear antibody tests based on immunofluorescence assays using HEp-2 cells (a human cell line) as a source of nuclei are nearly 100% sensitive for SLE but not specific—ie, they are positive in low titer in up to 20% of healthy adults and also in many patients with other immune-mediated conditions such as rheumatoid arthritis, thyroid disease, systemic sclerosis (scleroderma), and Sjögren syndrome. False-negative results can occur with tests for antinuclear antibodies based on multiplex assays that use specific nuclear antigens rather than cell lines. Antibodies to double-stranded DNA and to Sm are specific for SLE but not sensitive, since they are present in only 60% and 30% of patients, respectively. Depressed serum complement—a finding suggestive of disease activity—often returns toward normal in remission. Anti–double-stranded DNA antibody levels also correlate with disease activity in some patients; anti-Sm levels do not. Other autoantibodies commonly seen in SLE include antibodies to SS-A/Ro, SS-B/La, ribonucleoprotein (RNP), and phospholipid. Antibodies to SS-A/Ro are associated with subacute cutaneous lupus; during pregnancy these autoantibodies can cross the placenta and damage the developing fetal conduction system, producing congenital heart block.

During disease flares, elevations in the ESR are common, but the serum CRP is usually normal unless there is serositis or arthritis. An elevated CRP in the absence of these manifestations should increase clinical suspicion for infection. Abnormality of urinary sediment, including hematuria with or without casts, and proteinuria (varying from mild to nephrotic range) can indicate active lupus nephritis.

Differential Diagnosis

The differential diagnosis is broad, including drug-induced lupus, rheumatoid arthritis, systemic vasculitis, systemic sclerosis, primary antiphospholipid syndrome, inflammatory myopathies, viral hepatitis, sarcoidosis, acute drug

Table 20–7. Frequency (%) of autoantibodies in rheumatic diseases.[1]

	ANA	Anti-DNA	Rheumatoid Factor	Anti-Sm	Anti-SS-A	Anti-SS-B	Anti-SCL-70	Anti-Centromere	Anti-Jo-1	ANCA	Anti-CCP
Rheumatoid arthritis	30–60	0–5	70	0	0–5	0–2	0	0	0	0	70–80
SLE	95–100	50	20	20	15–20	5–20	0	0	0	0–1	10–15
Sjögren syndrome	95	0	75	0	65	65	0	0	0	0	0
Diffuse systemic sclerosis	> 95	0	30	0	0	0	33	3	0	0	10
Limited systemic sclerosis	> 95	0	30	0	0	0	20	50	0	0	10
Polymyositis/ dermatomyositis	80	0	33	0	0	0	0	0	20–30	0	3
Granulomatosis with polyangiitis	0–15	0	50	0	0	0	0	0	0	93–96[1]	0

[1]Frequency for generalized, active disease.
ANA, antinuclear antibodies; Anti-Sm, anti-Smith antibody; Anti-SCL-70, anti-scleroderma antibody; ANCA, antineutrophil cytoplasmic antibody; anti-CCP, anti-cyclic citrullinated peptides.

reactions, and infections or malignancies with multisystem involvement.

Treatment

Since the various manifestations of SLE affect prognosis differently and since SLE activity often waxes and wanes, drug therapy—both the choice of agents and the intensity of their use—must be tailored to match disease severity.

Table 20–8. Frequency (%) of laboratory abnormalities in SLE.

Anemia	60%
Leukopenia	45%
Thrombocytopenia	30%
Antiphospholipid antibodies	
Anti-cardiolipin antibody	25%
Lupus anticoagulant	7%
Anti–beta-2-glycoprotein 1	25%
Direct Coombs-positive	30%
Proteinuria	30%
Hematuria	30%
Hypocomplementemia	60%
ANA	95–100%
Anti-double-stranded DNA	50%
Anti-Sm	20%

ANA, antinuclear antibody; Anti-Sm, anti-Smith antibody.
Reproduced with permission from Hochberg MC, Boyd RE, Ahearn JM, et al. Systemic lupus erythematosus: a review of clinico-laboratory features and immunogenetic markers in 150 patients with emphasis on demographic subsets. *Medicine (Baltimore)*. 1985;64(5):285–295.

Patients should be cautioned against sun exposure and should apply broad-spectrum UVA/UVB sunscreen while outdoors. Milder skin lesions often respond to the topical administration of corticosteroids. Minor joint symptoms can usually be alleviated by NSAIDs.

Antimalarials (hydroxychloroquine) may be helpful in treating lupus rashes or joint symptoms. They also reduce the incidence of disease flares and prolong survival in SLE. The dose of hydroxychloroquine is 200 or 400 mg/day orally and should not exceed 5 mg/kg/day; annual monitoring for retinal toxicity is recommended. Neuropathy and myopathy are rare adverse effects of hydroxychloroquine and may be erroneously ascribed to the underlying disease.

Corticosteroids are required for the control of certain complications. (Systemic corticosteroids rarely are given for minor skin rashes, leukopenia, or the anemia associated with chronic disease.) Glomerulonephritis, hemolytic anemia, myocarditis, alveolar hemorrhage, CNS involvement, and severe thrombocytopenia all require corticosteroid treatment and often other interventions. For serious manifestations, either methylprednisolone 250–1000 mg given intravenously over 30 minutes daily for 3 days or prednisone 40–60 mg orally is needed initially; however, the lowest dose of corticosteroid that controls the condition should be used over time (Table 26–17). Immunosuppressive agents (such as cyclophosphamide, mycophenolate mofetil, azathioprine, methotrexate, or tacrolimus) are used for long-term control of disease. Belimumab, a monoclonal antibody that inhibits the activity of a B-cell growth factor, is FDA-approved for treating antibody-positive SLE patients with active non-renal lupus that has not responded to standard therapies (eg, antimalarials or immunosuppressive therapies). Belimumab is also approved for the treatment of active lupus nephritis. Anifrolumab, a type 1 interferon receptor antagonist, is approved to treat non-renal lupus that has not responded to standard therapies.

Voclosporin, a novel calcineurin inhibitor, is approved to treat active lupus nephritis when used in combination with mycophenolate mofetil.

Treatment of lupus nephritis includes an induction phase and a maintenance phase. Mycophenolate mofetil (1000 mg or 1500 mg orally twice daily) and cyclophosphamide are first-line induction treatments for lupus nephritis and are generally given with corticosteroids to achieve disease control. Cyclophosphamide is usually administered using the Euro-Lupus regimen (500 mg intravenously every 2 weeks for six doses) but can also be administered according to the National Institutes of Health regimen (3–6 monthly intravenous pulses [0.5–1 g/m^2]) for induction. Evidence increasingly suggests that renal response can be enhanced with combination immunosuppressive therapy. For example, belimumab can improve renal response when added to cyclophosphamide or mycophenolate mofetil. Similarly, voclosporin can improve renal response when added to mycophenolate; voclosporin can be helpful in nephrotic syndrome as the drug stabilizes renal podocytes and can quickly reduce proteinuria. Mycophenolate mofetil or azathioprine is typically used for maintenance therapy for lupus nephritis; patients who were induced with combination therapy using belimumab or voclosporin should generally continue these therapies for at least 1–2 years during the maintenance phase of treatment. Close follow-up is needed to watch for potential side effects when immunosuppressants are given; these agents should be administered by clinicians experienced in their use. When higher doses of cyclophosphamide are required, gonadotropin-releasing hormone analogs can be given to protect a woman against the risk of premature ovarian failure. Rituximab is usually reserved for life-threatening or organ-threatening manifestations that have failed conventional therapies.

Course & Prognosis

Ten-year survival rates exceeding 85% are routine. In most patients, the illness pursues a relapsing and remitting course. Prednisone, often needed in doses of 40 mg/day orally or more during severe flares, can usually be tapered to low doses (5–10 mg/day) or be discontinued when the disease is inactive. However, there are some in whom the disease pursues a virulent course, leading to serious impairment of vital structures such as lungs, heart, brain, or kidneys, and the disease may lead to death. Mortality in SLE shows a bimodal pattern. In the early years after diagnosis, infections—especially with opportunistic organisms—are the leading cause of death, followed by active SLE, chiefly due to kidney or CNS disease. In later years, accelerated atherosclerosis, linked to chronic inflammation, becomes a major cause of death. Indeed, the incidence of MI is five times higher in persons with SLE than in the general population. Therefore, SLE patients should avoid cigarette smoking and minimize other conventional risk factors for atherosclerosis (eg, hypercholesterolemia, hypertension, obesity, and inactivity).

Fertility is normal in SLE. Women are advised to pursue pregnancy under close supervision and when SLE is well-controlled and no teratogenic medications are being used. With more patients living longer, avascular necrosis of bone, affecting most commonly the hips and knees, is responsible for substantial morbidity. Nonetheless, the outlook for most patients with SLE is increasingly favorable.

When to Refer

- Appropriate diagnosis and management of SLE requires the active participation of a rheumatologist.
- The severity of organ involvement dictates referral to other subspecialists, such as nephrologists and pulmonologists.

When to Admit

- Rapidly progressive glomerulonephritis, pulmonary hemorrhage, transverse myelitis, and other severe organ-threatening manifestations of lupus usually require in-patient assessment and management.
- Severe infections, particularly in the setting of immunosuppressant therapy, should prompt admission.

Furie R et al. Two-year, randomized, controlled trial of belimumab in lupus nephritis. N Engl J Med. 2020;383:1117. [PMID: 32937045]

Morand EF et al; TULIP-2 Trial Investigators. Trial of anifrolumab in active systemic lupus erythematosus. N Engl J Med. 2020;382:211. [PMID: 31851795]

Rovin BH et al. Efficacy and safety of voclosporin versus placebo for lupus nephritis (AURORA 1): a double-blind, randomised, multicentre, placebo-controlled, phase 3 trial. Lancet. 2021; 397:2070. [PMID: 33971155]

DRUG-INDUCED LUPUS

ESSENTIALS OF DIAGNOSIS

- Symptomatic during exposure to offending drug; symptoms resolve when drug is stopped.
- Unlike in SLE, kidney involvement is unlikely.
- Elevated ANA but unlikely to have anti-DNA antibodies unless secondary to TNF inhibitors.

Drug-induced lupus shares several clinical and serologic features with SLE but is due to ongoing exposure to a drug and resolves when the offending drug is discontinued. In contrast to SLE, the sex ratio is nearly equal. As a general rule, drug-induced lupus presents with fever, arthralgia, myalgia, and serositis but not kidney involvement, neurologic symptoms, or other features of SLE. Serologic testing reveals elevated titers of antinuclear antibodies in all patients, but antibodies to DNA, Sm, RNP, SS-A, and SS-B are rare. Antibodies to histones occur in up to 95% of patients but also are seen in SLE and thus do not distinguish drug-induced lupus from SLE; the absence of antihistone antibodies, however, make either diagnosis unlikely. Complement levels are usually normal. The list of drugs implicated as possible causes of drug-induced lupus in observational studies and case reports is extensive. There are definite associations between the development of drug-induced lupus and the use of hydralazine, isoniazid, and minocycline as well as several less commonly prescribed drugs (procainamide, methyldopa, chlorpromazine). The incidence of drug-induced lupus in patients taking hydralazine for a year or longer is as high as 5–8%; for most other medications, the risk is considerably lower (less than 1%). TNF inhibitors can induce antibodies to DNA but usually not anti-histone antibodies; the incidence of lupus-like syndromes resulting from these medications is low (0.5–1%). Drug-induced lupus generally resolves within weeks to months after discontinuing the offending agent.

Arnaud L et al. Drug-induced systemic lupus: revisiting the ever-changing spectrum of the disease using the WHO pharmacovigilance database. Ann Rheum Dis. 2019;78:504. [PMID: 30793701]

Kawka L et al. Characterization of drug-induced cutaneous lupus: analysis of 1994 cases using the WHO pharmacovigilance database. Autoimmun Rev. 2021;20:102705. [PMID: 33188917]

ANTIPHOSPHOLIPID SYNDROME

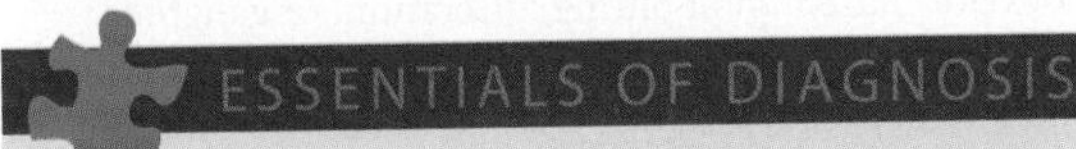

- Hypercoagulability; recurrent arterial or venous thromboses.
- Thrombocytopenia is common.
- Recurrent fetal loss.
- Recurrent events are frequent; lifetime anticoagulation with warfarin is recommended.

General Considerations

The clinical features of primary antiphospholipid syndrome (APS) are venous or arterial occlusions or certain pregnancy complications. Laboratory criteria include the identification of at least one of the following three antiphospholipid antibodies: IgG or IgM anti-cardiolipin, IgG or IgM antibodies to beta-2-glycoprotein 1, and lupus anticoagulant. In less than 1% of patients with antiphospholipid antibodies, a potentially devastating syndrome known as the "**catastrophic antiphospholipid syndrome**" occurs, leading to diffuse thromboses, thrombotic microangiopathy, and multiorgan system failure. Catastrophic APS has a mortality rate approaching 50%.

Clinical Findings

A. Symptoms and Signs

Patients are often asymptomatic until suffering a thrombotic complication of this syndrome or a pregnancy loss. Thrombotic events may occur in either the arterial or venous circulations. Thus, deep venous thromboses, pulmonary emboli, and cerebrovascular accidents are typical clinical events. Budd-Chiari syndrome, cerebral sinus vein thrombosis, myocardial or digital infarctions, hemorrhagic infarction of the adrenal glands (due to adrenal vein thrombosis), and other thrombotic events also occur. Other symptoms and signs of APS include thrombocytopenia, mental status changes, livedo reticularis, skin ulcers, microangiopathic nephropathy, and cardiac valvular thickening or vegetations. Pregnancy losses include unexplained fetal death after 10 weeks' gestation; one or more premature births before 34 weeks because of eclampsia, preeclampsia, or placental insufficiency; or three or more unexplained miscarriages before 10 weeks' gestation.

B. Laboratory Findings

Thrombocytopenia occurs in 22–42% of patients and is usually moderate (platelet counts above 50,000/mcL [50×10^9/L]). The presence of thrombocytopenia does not reduce the risk of thrombosis.

Three types of antiphospholipid antibodies are associated with this syndrome: (1) anti-cardiolipin antibodies, (2) antibodies to beta-2-glycoprotein, and (3) a "lupus anticoagulant" that prolongs certain phospholipid-dependent coagulation tests (see below). Anti-cardiolipin antibodies can produce a biologic false-positive test for syphilis (ie, a positive rapid plasma reagin but negative specific anti-treponemal assay). In general, IgG anti-cardiolipin antibodies are believed to be more pathologic than IgM. In case-control studies, 3.1% of patients in the general population who experienced a venous thrombotic event (in the absence of cancer) tested positive for the lupus anticoagulant (versus 0.9% of controls, yielding an odds ratio of 3.6). For women younger than 50 years in whom a thrombotic stroke developed, the odds ratio for having the lupus anticoagulant is 43.1. Presence of the lupus anticoagulant is a stronger risk factor for thrombosis or pregnancy loss than is the presence of antibodies to either beta-2-glycoprotein 1 or anti-cardiolipin. A clue to the presence of a lupus anticoagulant, which may occur in individuals who do not have SLE, may be detected by a prolongation of the partial thromboplastin time (which, paradoxically, is associated with a thrombotic tendency rather than a bleeding risk). Testing for the lupus anticoagulant involves phospholipid-dependent functional assays of coagulation, such as the Russell viper venom time (RVVT).

Differential Diagnosis

The exclusion of other autoimmune disorders, particularly those in the SLE spectrum, is essential because such disorders may be associated with manifestations requiring alternative treatments. Other genetic or acquired conditions associated with hypercoagulability such as protein C, protein S, or antithrombin deficiency and factor V Leiden should be excluded. Catastrophic APS has a broad differential, including sepsis, pulmonary-renal syndromes, systemic vasculitis, disseminated intravascular coagulation, and thrombotic thrombocytopenic purpura.

Treatment

Patients should be given warfarin to maintain an INR of 2.0–3.0; DOACs are less effective than warfarin. Patients who have recurrent thrombotic events while taking warfarin may require higher INRs (greater than 3.0), but the bleeding risk increases substantially with this degree of anticoagulation.

For pregnancy-associated APS, the combination of prophylactic doses of low-molecular-weight heparin (Table 14–14) and low-dose aspirin (81 mg) is the usual approach to prevent pregnancy complications. In pregnant women with a history of thrombotic events outside of pregnancy, full-dose low-molecular-weight heparin is administered (Table 14–16). Anticoagulation is typically continued through pregnancy and the early postpartum period for thromboprophylaxis. The benefit of using corticosteroids and intravenous immunoglobulin in these patients is unclear; neither treatment is recommended.

However, in patients with catastrophic APS, either intravenous immunoglobulin or plasmapheresis plus intravenous heparin and high doses of corticosteroids are administered. Resistant disease may require biologic therapy with monoclonal antibodies against CD20 on B cells (rituximab) or against complement component C5 (eculizimab), although data to support these therapies are limited to case series.

Tektonidou MG et al. EULAR recommendations for the management of antiphospholipid syndrome in adults. Ann Rheum Dis. 2019;78:1296. [PMID: 31092409]

RAYNAUD PHENOMENON

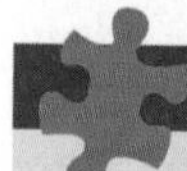

ESSENTIALS OF DIAGNOSIS

- Paroxysmal bilateral digital pallor and cyanosis followed by rubor.
- Precipitated by cold or emotional stress; relieved by warmth.
- **Primary form:** benign course; usually affects young women.
- **Secondary form:** more severe, sometimes causing digital ulceration or gangrene.

General Considerations

Raynaud phenomenon (RP) is a syndrome of paroxysmal digital ischemia, most commonly caused by an exaggerated response of digital arterioles to cold or emotional stress. The initial phase of RP, mediated by excessive vasoconstriction, consists of well-demarcated digital pallor or cyanosis; the subsequent (recovery) phase of RP, caused by vasodilation, leads to intense hyperemia and rubor. Although RP chiefly affects fingers, it can also affect toes and other acral areas such as the nose and ears. RP is classified as primary (idiopathic or Raynaud disease) or secondary. Nearly one-third of the population reports being "sensitive to the cold" but does not experience the paroxysms of digital pallor, cyanosis, and erythema characteristic of RP. Primary RP occurs in 2–6% of adults, is especially common in young women, and poses more of a nuisance than a threat to good health. In contrast, secondary RP is less common, is chiefly associated with rheumatic diseases (especially systemic sclerosis) and can be severe enough to cause digital ulceration or gangrene.

Clinical Findings

In early attacks of RP, only one or two fingertips may be affected; as it progresses, all fingers down to the distal palm may be involved. The thumbs are rarely affected. During recovery there may be intense rubor, throbbing, paresthesia, pain, and slight swelling. Attacks usually terminate spontaneously or upon returning to a warm room or putting the extremity in warm water. The patient is usually asymptomatic between attacks. Sensory changes that often accompany vasomotor manifestations include numbness, tingling, diminished sensation, and aching pain.

Primary RP appears more commonly in women between ages 15 and 30, symmetrically involving the fingers of both hands, unlike secondary RP (which may be unilateral and may involve only one or two fingers). It tends to be mildly progressive. Spasm becomes more frequent and prolonged. Unlike secondary RP, primary RP does not cause digital pitting, ulceration, or gangrene.

Nailfold capillary abnormalities are among the earliest clues of secondary rather than primary RP. The nailfold capillary pattern can be visualized by placing a drop of grade B immersion oil at the patient's cuticle and then viewing the area with an ophthalmoscope set to 40 diopters. Dropout of capillaries and dilation of the remaining capillary loops indicate a secondary form of RP, most commonly systemic sclerosis (Figure 20–5) (Table 20–9). While highly specific for secondary RP, nailfold capillary changes have a low sensitivity. Digital pitting or ulceration or other abnormal physical findings (eg, skin tightening, loss of extremity pulse, rash, swollen joints) provides evidence of secondary RP.

Primary RP must be differentiated from the numerous causes of secondary RP (Table 20–9). The history and examination may suggest the diagnosis of systemic sclerosis, SLE, or mixed connective tissue disease; RP is often the first manifestation of limited systemic sclerosis (CREST syndrome). The diagnosis of many of these rheumatic diseases is supported with specific serologic tests.

RP may occur in patients with the thoracic outlet syndromes. In these disorders, involvement is generally unilateral, and symptoms referable to brachial plexus compression tend to dominate the clinical picture. Carpal tunnel syndrome should also be considered, and nerve conduction tests are appropriate in selected cases.

Differential Diagnosis

The differentiation from Buerger disease (thromboangiitis obliterans) is usually not difficult, since thromboangiitis obliterans is generally a disease of men, particularly cigarette smokers; peripheral pulses are often diminished or absent; and, when RP occurs in association with thromboangiitis obliterans, it is usually in only one or two digits.

In acrocyanosis, cyanosis of the hands is permanent and diffuse; the sharp and paroxysmal line of demarcation with pallor does not occur with acrocyanosis. Frostbite may lead to chronic RP.

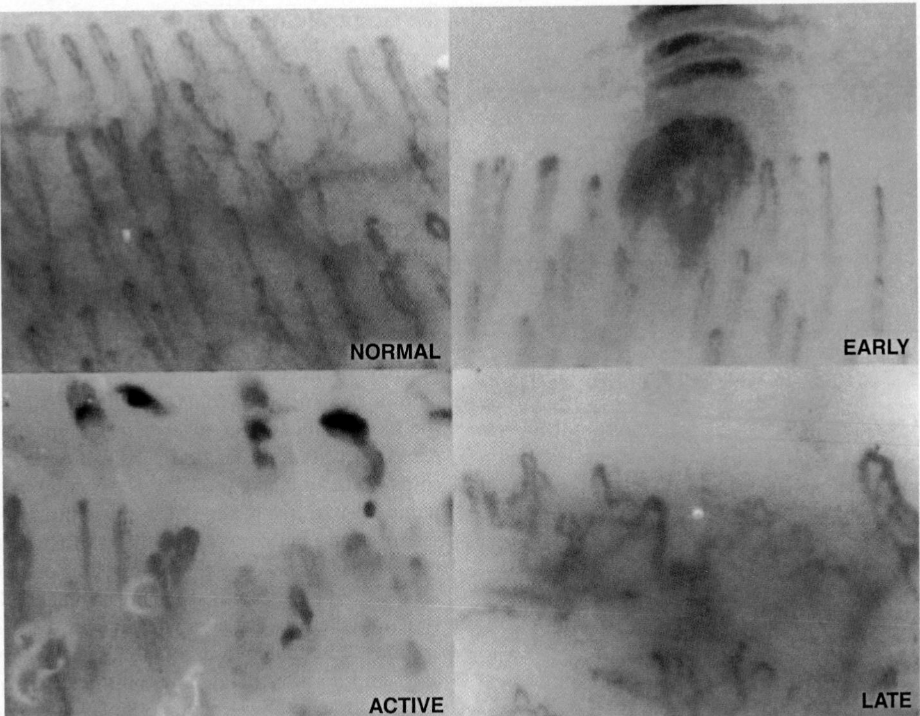

▲ **Figure 20–5.** The systemic sclerosis (scleroderma) pattern: early, active, and late nailfold videocapillaroscopy patterns versus normal. (Reproduced with permission from Cutolo M, Pizzorni C, Secchi ME, Sulli A. Capillaroscopy. *Best Pract Res Clin Rheumatol*. 2008;22(6):1093–1108.)

Treatment

A. General Measures

Patients should wear gloves or mittens whenever in temperatures that precipitate attacks. Keeping the body warm is also a cornerstone of initial therapy. Wearing warm shirts, coats, and hats will help prevent the exaggerated vasospasm that causes RP and that is not prevented by warming only the hands. The hands should be protected from injury at all times; wounds heal slowly, and infections are consequently hard to control. Softening and lubricating lotion to control fissured dry skin should be applied to the hands frequently. Cigarette smoking should be stopped and sympathomimetic drugs (eg, decongestants, diet pills, and amphetamines) should be avoided. For most patients with primary RP, general measures alone are sufficient to control symptoms. Medical or surgical therapy should be considered in patients who have severe symptoms or are experiencing tissue injury from digital ischemia.

B. Medications

Calcium channel blockers are first-line therapy for RP. Calcium channel blockers produce a modest benefit and are more effective in primary RP than secondary RP. Slow-release nifedipine (30–120 mg/day orally), amlodipine (5–20 mg/day orally), felodipine, isradipine, and nisoldipine are more effective than verapamil, nicardipine, and diltiazem. Other medications that may be effective include angiotensin II receptor blockers, topical nitrates, phosphodiesterase inhibitors (eg, sildenafil, tadalafil, and vardenafil), or SSRIs (fluoxetine). Severe or refractory episodes of RP in which there is a threat of digital loss may require treatment with intravenous infusions of prostacyclin or prostacyclin analogs (eg, epoprostenol, iloprost, treprostinil).

C. Surgical Measures

Sympathectomy may be indicated when attacks have become frequent and severe, when they interfere with work and well-being, and particularly when trophic changes have developed and medical measures have failed. Digital sympathectomy may improve secondary RP.

Prognosis

Primary RP is benign and largely a nuisance for affected individuals who are exposed to cold winters or excessive air conditioning. The prognosis of secondary RP depends on the underlying disease; unfortunately, severe pain from ulceration and gangrene is not rare with systemic sclerosis.

When to Refer

Appropriate management of patients with secondary RP often requires consultation with a rheumatologist.

When to Admit

Patients with critical digital ischemia as evidenced by severe pain and demarcation should be admitted for intensive therapy.

Table 20–9. Causes of secondary Raynaud phenomenon.

Rheumatic diseases
Systemic sclerosis
SLE
Mixed connective tissue disease
Dermatomyositis/polymyositis
Sjögren syndrome
Vasculitis (polyarteritis nodosa, Takayasu disease, Buerger disease)
Neurovascular compression and occupational trauma
Carpal tunnel syndrome
Thoracic outlet obstruction
Vibration injury
Drugs and substances
Beta-blockers
Serotonin agonists (sumatriptan)
Sympathomimetic drugs (decongestants)
Chemotherapy (bleomycin, vinblastine)
Ergotamine
Caffeine
Nicotine
Cocaine
Epoxy resins
Hematologic disorders
Cryoglobulinemia
Polycythemia vera
Paraproteinemia
Cold agglutinins
Endocrine disorders
Hypothyroidism
Pheochromocytoma
Miscellaneous
Atherosclerosis
Embolic disease
Migraine
Sequela of frostbite

Hughes M et al. Raynaud phenomenon and digital ulcers in systemic sclerosis. Nat Rev Rheumatol. 2020;16:208. [PMID: 32099191]

SYSTEMIC SCLEROSIS (Scleroderma)

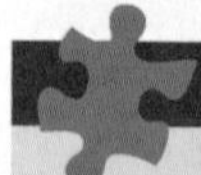

ESSENTIALS OF DIAGNOSIS

- **Limited disease** (CREST syndrome): skin thickening confined to face, neck, and distal extremities.
- **Diffuse disease** (20%): widespread thickening of skin, including truncal involvement, with areas of increased pigmentation and depigmentation.
- Raynaud phenomenon and antinuclear antibodies are present in virtually all patients.
- **Systemic features:** gastroesophageal reflux, GI hypomotility, pulmonary fibrosis, pulmonary hypertension, renal involvement.

General Consideration

Systemic sclerosis (scleroderma) is a rare chronic disorder characterized by diffuse fibrosis of the skin and internal organs. Symptoms usually appear in the third to fifth decades, and women are affected two to three times as frequently as men.

Two forms of systemic sclerosis are generally recognized: limited (80% of patients) and diffuse (20%). In limited systemic sclerosis, which often has one or more features of the CREST syndrome (calcinosis cutis, Raynaud phenomenon, esophageal motility disorder, sclerodactyly, and telangiectasia), the hardening of the skin (scleroderma) is limited to the face, neck, and skin distal to the elbows and knees. In contrast, diffuse systemic sclerosis, the skin changes also involve the trunk and proximal extremities. Tendon friction rubs over the forearms and shins occur uniquely (but not universally) in diffuse systemic sclerosis. In general, patients with limited systemic sclerosis have better outcomes than those with diffuse disease, largely because life-threatening lung or kidney disease is rare. Cardiac disease is also more characteristic of diffuse systemic sclerosis. Patients with limited disease, however, are more susceptible to digital ischemia, leading to finger loss, and to life-threatening pulmonary hypertension. Small and large bowel hypomotility, which may occur in either form of systemic sclerosis, can cause constipation alternating with diarrhea, malabsorption due to bacterial overgrowth, pseudoobstruction, and severe bowel distention with rupture.

Clinical Findings

A. Symptoms and Signs

Raynaud phenomenon is usually the initial manifestation and can precede other signs and symptoms by years in cases of limited systemic sclerosis. Polyarthralgia, weight loss, and malaise are common early features of diffuse systemic sclerosis but are infrequent in limited disease. Cutaneous disease usually, but not always, develops before visceral involvement and can manifest initially as nonpitting subcutaneous edema associated with pruritus. With time the skin becomes thickened and hidebound, with loss of normal folds. Telangiectasia, pigmentation, and depigmentation are characteristic. Ulceration of the fingertips and subcutaneous calcification are seen. Dysphagia and symptoms of reflux due to esophageal dysfunction are common and result from abnormalities in motility and later from fibrosis. Fibrosis and atrophy of the GI tract cause hypomotility. Large-mouthed diverticuli occur in the jejunum, ileum, and colon. Diffuse pulmonary fibrosis and pulmonary vascular disease are reflected in restrictive lung physiology and low diffusing capacities. Cardiac abnormalities include pericardial effusions, heart block, myocardial fibrosis, and right heart failure secondary to pulmonary hypertension. Systemic sclerosis–associated renal crisis, resulting from intimal proliferation of smaller renal arteries and usually associated with hypertension, is a life-threatening emergency. Many cases can be treated effectively with ACE inhibitors.

B. Laboratory Findings

Mild anemia is often present. In renal crisis, the peripheral blood smear shows findings consistent with a microangiopathic hemolytic anemia (due to mechanical damage to red cells from diseased small vessels). Elevation of the ESR is unusual. Mild proteinuria with few cells or casts can occur. Antinuclear antibody tests are nearly always positive, frequently in high titers (Table 20–7). The scleroderma antibody (anti-SCL-70), directed against topoisomerase III, is found in one-third of patients with diffuse systemic sclerosis and in 20% of those with limited disease. Anti-SCL-70 antibodies may portend a poor prognosis, with a high likelihood of serious internal organ involvement (eg, interstitial lung disease). Anticentromere antibodies are seen in 50% of those with limited systemic sclerosis and in 3% of individuals with diffuse disease (Table 20–7). Anticentromere antibodies are highly specific for limited systemic sclerosis, but they also occur occasionally in overlap syndromes. Anti-RNA polymerase III antibodies develop in 10–20% of systemic sclerosis patients overall and are associated with rapidly progressive skin disease, renal crisis, and a higher risk of concomitant solid cancers, especially breast cancer.

Differential Diagnosis

Early in its course, systemic sclerosis can cause diagnostic confusion with other causes of Raynaud phenomenon, particularly SLE, mixed connective tissue disease, and the inflammatory myopathies. Eosinophilic fasciitis is a rare disorder presenting with skin hardening that resembles diffuse systemic sclerosis. The inflammatory abnormalities, however, are limited to the fascia rather than the dermis and epidermis. Moreover, patients with eosinophilic fasciitis are distinguished from those with systemic sclerosis by the presence of peripheral blood eosinophilia, the absence of Raynaud phenomenon, a good response to prednisone, and an association (in some cases) with paraproteinemias. Diffuse skin thickening and visceral involvement are features of scleromyxedema; the presence of a paraprotein, the absence of Raynaud phenomenon, and distinct skin histology point to scleromyxedema. Diabetic cheiropathy typically develops in longstanding, poorly controlled diabetes mellitus and can mimic sclerodactyly. Morphea and linear scleroderma cause sclerodermatous changes limited to circumscribed areas of the skin and usually have excellent outcomes.

Treatment

Treatment of systemic sclerosis focuses on the organ systems involved. Although there is no effective therapy for the underlying disease process, interventions for management of specific organ manifestations have improved substantially. Treatment for Raynaud phenomenon is discussed above. The hypertensive crises in scleroderma renal crisis must be treated early and aggressively (in the hospital) with ACE inhibitors, eg, captopril, initiated at 25 mg orally every 6 hours and titrated up as tolerated to a maximum of 100 mg every 6 hours. Patients with severe esophageal disease should take medications in liquid or crushed form. Esophageal reflux can be reduced and the risk of scarring diminished by avoiding late-night meals and using PPIs (eg, omeprazole, 20–40 mg/day orally), which achieve near-complete inhibition of gastric acid production and are effective for refractory esophagitis. Patients with delayed gastric emptying maintain their weight better if they eat small, frequent meals and remain upright for at least 2 hours after eating. Oral prokinetic agents such as metoclopramide (10 mg four times daily) or cisapride (10–20 mg four times daily) can improve dysphagia caused by esophageal hypomotility. Erythromycin (250 mg three times daily) can be used if prokinetic agents fail. Since erythromycin impairs the metabolism of cisapride, combined use of these two agents is contraindicated. Long-term octreotide (0.1 mg subcutaneously twice daily), a somatostatin analog, helps some patients with bacterial overgrowth and pseudoobstruction. Malabsorption due to bacterial overgrowth responds to antibiotics, eg, rifaximin, 550 mg three times orally daily, often prescribed cyclically. Apart from the patient with myositis, prednisone has little or no role in the treatment of systemic sclerosis; doses higher than 15 mg/day have been associated with scleroderma renal crisis. In patients with early diffuse systemic sclerosis (scleroderma), methotrexate can be used in the treatment of skin disease, arthritis, and myositis. The usual initial dose is 7.5 mg of methotrexate orally once weekly. If the patient has tolerated methotrexate but has not responded in 1 month, the dose can be increased to 15 mg orally once per week. The maximal dose is usually 20 mg/week.

For patients who require treatment for interstitial lung disease, mycophenolate mofetil (1000–1500 mg orally twice daily) can improve dyspnea and pulmonary function tests modestly. Cyclophosphamide has similar efficacy but greater toxicity; this drug should only be administered by physicians familiar with its use. The IL-6 inhibitor tocilizumab, 162 mg subcutaneously once weekly, slows the rate of decline in pulmonary function and may be used as an alternative for patients who cannot tolerate mycophenolate mofetil. Azathioprine is an additional option for treatment of systemic sclerosis–associated lung disease. In patients who do not respond to or cannot take the agents above, nintedanib (an inhibitor of multiple tyrosine kinases) can slow the progression of systemic sclerosis–associated lung disease and is FDA-approved for this indication.

Treatment of pulmonary hypertension in systemic sclerosis is largely extrapolated from general trials of pulmonary hypertension. Therapies include phosphodiesterase type 5 inhibitors (sildenafil, tadalafil, vardenafil), a guanylate cyclase stimulant (riociguat), endothelin-1 receptor antagonists (bosentan, ambrisentan, macitentan), and an endothelin-A receptor antagonist (ambrisentan). Refractory pulmonary hypertension may require prostacyclin pathway agonists (epoprostenol, treprostinil, iloprost, selexipag). For patients with severe, diffuse systemic sclerosis, myeloablation followed by autologous stem cell transplantation is superior to immunosuppression with cyclophosphamide but has greater toxicity.

The 9-year survival rate in systemic sclerosis averages approximately 40%. The prognosis tends to be worse in those with diffuse disease, in Black patients, men, and older patients. Lung disease—in the form of pulmonary fibrosis or pulmonary arterial hypertension—is the leading cause of mortality. Those persons in whom severe internal organ involvement does not develop in the first 3 years have a substantially better prognosis, with 72% surviving at least 9 years. Studies conducted in a small number of patients with simultaneous onset of cancer and systemic sclerosis have demonstrated that the disease developed due to an immune response directed at the cancer.

When to Refer

- Appropriate management of systemic sclerosis requires frequent consultations with a rheumatologist.
- Severity of organ involvement dictates referral to cardiologists, pulmonologists, gastroenterologists, or nephrologists.

Distler O et al; SENSCIS Trial Investigators. Nintedanib for systemic sclerosis-associated interstitial lung disease. N Engl J Med. 2019;380:2518. [PMID: 31112379]

Khanna D et al; focuSSced investigators. Tocilizumab in systemic sclerosis: a randomised, double-blind, placebo-controlled, phase 3 trial. Lancet Respir Med. 2020;8:963. Erratum in: Lancet Respir Med. 2020;8:e75. [PMID: 32866440]

IMMUNE-MEDIATED INFLAMMATORY MYOPATHIES

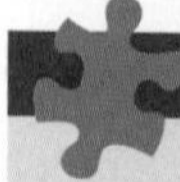

ESSENTIALS OF DIAGNOSIS

- Progressive muscle weakness.
- **Dermatomyositis:** characteristic cutaneous manifestations (Gottron papules, heliotrope rash); increased risk of malignancy.
- Elevated creatine kinase, myositis-specific antibodies, diagnostic muscle biopsy.
- Mimics include infectious, metabolic, or drug-induced myopathies.

General Considerations

Immune-mediated inflammatory myopathies include polymyositis, dermatomyositis, myositis resulting from a rheumatic disease or overlap syndrome, inclusion body myositis (IBM), and immune-mediated necrotizing myopathy. These disorders are characterized by progressive muscle weakness, and all but IBM demonstrate an inflammatory infiltrate in muscle tissue.

Polymyositis and dermatomyositis are systemic disorders of unknown cause whose principal manifestation is muscle weakness. Although their clinical presentations (aside from the presence of certain skin findings in dermatomyositis, some of which are pathognomonic) and treatments are similar, the two diseases are pathologically distinct. They affect persons of any age group, but the peak incidence is in the fifth and sixth decades of life and women are affected twice as commonly as men. There is an increased risk of malignancy, especially in dermatomyositis. Indeed, up to one patient in four with dermatomyositis has an occult malignancy. Malignancies may be evident at the time of presentation with the muscle disease but may not be detected until months afterward in some cases. The malignancies most commonly associated with dermatomyositis are lung, ovarian, breast, colorectal, cervical, bladder, nasopharyngeal, esophageal, pancreatic, and renal cancer. Patients may have skin disease without overt muscle involvement, a condition termed dermatomyositis sine myositis; these patients can have aggressive interstitial lung disease. Myositis may also overlap with other connective tissue diseases, especially systemic sclerosis, SLE, mixed connective tissue disease, and Sjögren syndrome.

IBM affects older men and is characterized by more distal weakness in the upper extremities and is generally less symmetric. Immune-mediated necrotizing myopathies include those associated with the signal recognition particle or with anti-3-hydroxy-3-methylglutaryl coenzyme A reductase (anti-HMGCR) autoantibodies in the setting of statin use. This latter entity is distinct from the more common statin-induced myopathy, which occurs in about 1% of statin users. Unlike anti-HMGCR necrotizing myopathy, statin-induced myopathy generally resolves within 6 months of drug discontinuation.

Clinical Findings

A. Symptoms and Signs

Polymyositis may begin abruptly, but the usual presentation is one of progressive muscle weakness over weeks to months. The weakness chiefly involves proximal muscle groups of the upper and lower extremities and the neck. Leg weakness (eg, difficulty in rising from a chair or climbing stairs) typically precedes arm symptoms. In contrast to myasthenia gravis, polymyositis and dermatomyositis do not cause facial or ocular muscle weakness. In contrast to polymyalgia rheumatica (PMR), pain and tenderness of affected muscles occur in only one-fourth of cases, and these are rarely the chief complaints. About one-fourth of patients have dysphagia. In contrast to systemic sclerosis, which affects the smooth muscle of the lower esophagus and can cause a "sticking" sensation below the sternum, polymyositis or dermatomyositis involves the striated muscles of the upper pharynx and can make initiation of swallowing difficult. Clinically significant myocarditis is uncommon even though there is often creatine kinase-MB elevation. Respiratory muscle weakness can be severe enough to cause CO_2 retention and respiratory failure.

Dermatomyositis has a characteristic rash that is dusky red and may appear in a malar distribution, mimicking the classic rash of SLE. Facial erythema beyond the malar distribution is also characteristic of dermatomyositis. Erythema also occurs over other areas of the face, neck, shoulders, and upper chest and back ("shawl sign"). Periorbital edema and a purplish (heliotrope) suffusion over the eyelids are typical signs (Figure 20–6). Coloration of the heliotrope and other rashes of dermatomyositis can be affected by skin tone. In Black persons, the rashes may

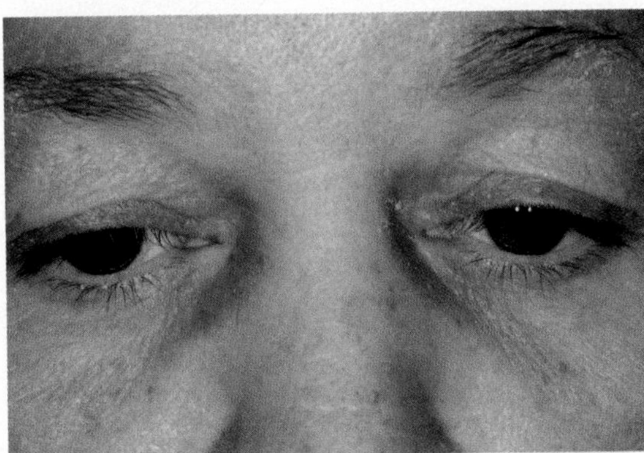

▲ **Figure 20–6.** Bilateral heliotrope rash, which is a pathognomonic sign of dermatomyositis. (Reproduced with permission from Richard P. Usatine, MD, in Usatine RP, Smith MA, Mayeaux EJ Jr, Chumley H. *The Color Atlas of Family Medicine*, 2nd ed. McGraw-Hill, 2013.)

appear more hyperpigmented than erythematous or violaceous. Periungual erythema, dilations of nailfold capillaries, Gottron papules (raised violaceous lesions overlying the dorsa of DIP, PIP, and MCP joints), and Gottron sign (erythematous rash on the extensors surfaces of the fingers, elbows, and knees) are highly suggestive. Infrequently, the cutaneous findings of this disease precede the muscle inflammation by weeks or months. Diagnosing polymyositis in patients over age 70 years can be difficult because weakness may be overlooked or attributed erroneously to idiopathic frailty. A subset of patients with polymyositis and dermatomyositis have the **"antisynthetase syndrome,"** a group of findings including inflammatory nonerosive arthritis, fever, Raynaud phenomenon, "mechanic's hands" (hyperkeratosis along the radial and palmar aspects of the fingers), interstitial lung disease, and often severe muscle disease associated with certain autoantibodies (eg, anti-Jo-1 antibodies).

IBM, because of its tendency to mimic polymyositis, is a common cause of "treatment-resistant polymyositis." The typical patient with IBM is a man over the age of 50 years. The onset of IBM is more insidious than that of polymyositis or dermatomyositis (eg, occurring over years rather than months), and the distal motor weakness is commonly asymmetric. Creatine kinase levels are often minimally elevated and are normal in 25%. Electromyography may show a mixed picture of myopathic and neurogenic abnormalities. The disease is associated with antibodies to cytoplasmic 5'-nucleotidase 1A (cN1A). IBM is less likely to respond to therapy.

Immune-mediated necrotizing myopathy, although similar to polymyositis, is distinct because of the presence of muscle necrosis. Autoantibodies aid in diagnosis; anti-SRP antibodies are associated with severe muscle weakness, pain, and cardiac involvement. Anti-HMGCR antibodies occur in the setting of statin use and are associated with proximal muscle weakness and marked creatine kinase elevations. Many patients have a severe and unrelenting disease course with persistent weakness, unlike other statin-induced myopathies, which are generally self-limited after drug discontinuation.

B. Laboratory Findings

Measurement of serum levels of muscle enzymes, especially creatine kinase and aldolase, is most useful in diagnosis and in assessment of disease activity. Inflammatory myositis can be misdiagnosed as hepatitis because of elevations in serum levels of muscle-derived ALT and AST levels. Anemia is uncommon. The ESR and CRP are often normal and are not reliable indicators of disease activity. Rheumatoid factor is found in a minority of patients. Antinuclear antibodies can be present, especially when there is an associated connective tissue disease. A number of autoantibodies are seen exclusively in patients with myositis and are associated with distinctive clinical features (Table 20–10). Examples of myositis-specific antibodies include (1) anti-Jo-1 antibody (antisynthetase syndrome), (2) anti-Mi-2 (dermatomyositis), (3) anti-155/140 (dermatomyositis with malignancy), (4) anti-MDA5 (melanocyte differentiation-associated protein 5, linked to dermatomyositis with cutaneous ulcerations and rapidly progressive interstitial lung disease), and (5) anti-signal recognition particle (immune-mediated necrotizing myopathy). Chest radiographs are usually normal unless there is associated interstitial lung disease. Electromyographic abnormalities can point toward a myopathic, rather than a neurogenic, cause of weakness. MRI can detect early and patchy muscle involvement, can guide

Table 20–10. Myositis-specific antibodies.

Antibody	Clinical Association
Anti-Jo-1, PL-7, PL-12	Polymyositis or dermatomyositis with interstitial lung disease, arthritis, mechanic's hands, Raynaud phenomenon (antisynthetase syndrome). No increased malignancy risk.
Anti-Mi-2	Dermatomyositis with rash more than myositis, good prognosis
Anti-MDA5 (anti-CADM 140)	Dermatomyositis with rapidly progressive lung disease, cutaneous ulcers
Anti-TIF-1 (p155/140)	Severe skin manifestations, cancer-associated dermatomyositis
Anti-NXP-2	Juvenile dermatomyositis
Anti-SAE	Cancer-associated dermatomyositis, dermatomyositis with pulmonary arterial hypertension
Anti-SRP	Severe, acute necrotizing myopathy with more cardiac involvement
Anti-HMG CoA reductase	Necrotizing myopathy related to statin use
PM-Scl, Ro, Ku, U 1-3 RNP	Polymyositis/dermatomyositis overlap syndromes
Anti-cN1A	Inclusion body myositis

Reproduced with permission from Imboden JB, Hellmann DB, Stone JH (editors): *Current Diagnosis & Treatment Rheumatology*, 3rd ed. McGraw-Hill, 2013.

biopsies, and often is more useful than electromyography. The search for an occult malignancy should begin with a history and physical examination, supplemented with a CBC, comprehensive biochemical panel, and UA and should include age- and risk-appropriate cancer screening tests. Given the especially strong association of ovarian carcinoma and dermatomyositis, transvaginal ultrasonography, CT scanning, and CA-125 levels may be useful in women. No matter how extensive the initial screening, some malignancies will not become evident for months after the initial presentation of the myopathy.

C. Muscle Biopsy

Biopsy of clinically involved muscle is often required. The pathology findings in polymyositis and dermatomyositis are distinct. In dermatomyositis, the cellular infiltrate is mostly perifascicular and perivascular, while in polymyositis, the inflammatory infiltrate involves the fascicle itself. The presence of prominent necrosis with a paucity of inflammatory cells suggests an immune-mediated necrotizing myopathy. Muscle biopsy in IBM shows characteristic intracellular vacuoles by light microscopy and either tubular or filamentous inclusions in the nucleus or cytoplasm by electron microscopy. False-negative biopsies sometimes occur in these disorders because of the sometimes patchy distribution of pathologic abnormalities.

Differential Diagnosis

Muscle inflammation may occur as a component of SLE, systemic sclerosis, Sjögren syndrome, and overlap syndromes. In those cases, associated findings usually permit the precise diagnosis of the primary condition.

Hypothyroidism is a common cause of proximal muscle weakness associated with elevations of serum creatine kinase. Hyperthyroidism and Cushing disease may both be associated with proximal muscle weakness with normal levels of creatine kinase. Patients with polymyalgia rheumatica are over the age of 50 and—in contrast to patients with polymyositis—have pain but no objective weakness; creatine kinase levels are normal. Disorders of the peripheral nervous system and CNS (eg, chronic inflammatory polyneuropathy, multiple sclerosis, myasthenia gravis, Lambert-Eaton disease, and amyotrophic lateral sclerosis) can produce weakness but are distinguished by characteristic symptoms and neurologic signs and often by distinctive electromyographic abnormalities. A number of systemic vasculitides (polyarteritis nodosa, microscopic polyangiitis, eosinophilic granulomatosis with polyangiitis, granulomatosis with polyangiitis, and mixed cryoglobulinemia) can produce profound weakness through vasculitic neuropathy. The muscle weakness associated with these disorders, however, is typically distal and asymmetric, at least in the early stages.

Limb-girdle muscular dystrophy can present in early adulthood with a clinical picture that mimics polymyositis: proximal muscle weakness, elevations in serum creatine kinase, and inflammatory cells on muscle biopsy. Failure to respond to treatment for polymyositis or the presence of atypical clinical features such as scapular winging or weakness of ankle plantar flexors should prompt genetic testing for limb-girdle muscular dystrophy.

Many drugs, including corticosteroids, alcohol, clofibrate, penicillamine, tryptophan, and hydroxychloroquine, can produce proximal muscle weakness. Long-term use of colchicine at doses as low as 0.6 mg twice a day in patients with moderate CKD can produce a mixed neuropathy-myopathy that mimics polymyositis. The weakness and muscle enzyme elevation reverse with cessation of the drug. HIV is associated with a myopathy indistinguishable from polymyositis.

Statins can cause myopathy and rhabdomyolysis, in addition to the anti-HMGCR myopathy described above. Although only about 0.1% of patients taking a statin drug alone develop myopathy, concomitant administration of other drugs (especially gemfibrozil, cyclosporine, niacin, macrolide antibiotics, azole antifungals, and protease inhibitors) increases the risk.

The use of immune checkpoint inhibitors to treat cancer can cause rheumatic and musculoskeletal symptoms, including myalgia and myositis.

Treatment

Most patients respond to corticosteroids. Initially, prednisone, 40–60 mg or more orally daily is often required. The dose is then adjusted downward while monitoring muscle strength and serum levels of muscle enzymes. Long-term use of corticosteroids is often needed, and the disease may recur when they are withdrawn. Patients with an associated neoplasm have a poor prognosis, although remission may follow treatment of the tumor; corticosteroids may or may not be effective in these patients. Immunosuppressive drugs like methotrexate (15–25 mg orally weekly), azathioprine (1.5 mg/kg orally once daily) or mycophenolate mofetil (1–1.5 g orally twice daily) are often started to reduce cumulative corticosteroid exposure. Intravenous immunoglobulin is effective for dermatomyositis resistant to prednisone and anti-HMGCR myopathy. Intravenous immunoglobulin is FDA-approved for the treatment of dermatomyositis. Rituximab is effective in some patients with inflammatory myositis unresponsive to prednisone. Since the rash of dermatomyositis is often photosensitive, patients should limit sun exposure. Hydroxychloroquine (200–400 mg/day orally not to exceed 5 mg/kg) can help ameliorate the skin disease.

When to Refer

- All patients with myositis should be referred to a rheumatologist or neurologist.
- Severe lung disease may require consultation with a pulmonologist.

When to Admit

- Signs of rhabdomyolysis.
- New onset of dysphagia.
- Respiratory insufficiency with hypoxia or carbon dioxide retention.

Aggarwal R et al. Prospective, double-blind, randomized, placebo-controlled phase III study evaluating efficacy and safety of octagam 10% in patients with dermatomyositis ("ProDERM Study"). Medicine (Baltimore). 2021;100:e23677. [PMID: 33429735]

Allenbach Y et al. Immune-mediated necrotizing myopathy: clinical features and pathogenesis. Nat Rev Rheumatol. 2020; 16:689. [PMID: 33093664]

Lundberg IE et al. Idiopathic inflammatory myopathies. Nat Rev Dis Primers. 2021;7:86. [PMID: 34857798]

MIXED CONNECTIVE TISSUE DISEASE, OVERLAP, & UNDIFFERENTIATED SYNDROMES

Many patients with symptoms and signs of a connective tissue disease have features of more than one type of rheumatic disease. Special attention has been drawn to a subset of antinuclear antibody–positive patients who have high titers of RNP autoantibodies and overlapping features of SLE, systemic sclerosis, rheumatoid arthritis, and inflammatory myositis. Swollen or puffy hands are a common early feature of this disease, referred to as mixed connective tissue disease. Raynaud phenomenon, arthralgias, and myalgias are common. Unlike patients with SLE, renal or CNS disease is uncommon. A key reason to identify this subset of patients is that pulmonary hypertension and interstitial lung disease are major causes of mortality, and regular screening for these manifestations is required. Some patients have features of more than one connective tissue disease (eg, rheumatoid arthritis and SLE, SLE and systemic sclerosis) in the absence of high-titer anti-RNP antibodies and are called having an "overlap syndrome;" others have only a few features of autoimmunity and cannot yet be classified ("undifferentiated connective tissue disease"). Treatments are guided more by the distribution and severity of patients' organ system involvement than by therapies specific to these overlap syndromes.

Reiseter S et al. Progression and mortality of interstitial lung disease in mixed connective tissue disease: a long-term observational nationwide cohort study. Rheumatology (Oxford). 2018;57:255. [PMID: 28379478]

Sciascia S et al. Differentiating between UCTD and early-stage SLE: from definitions to clinical approach. Nat Rev Rheumatol. 2022;18:9. [PMID: 34764455]

SJÖGREN SYNDROME

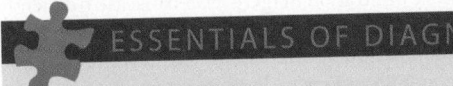

- Women (average age 50 years) comprise 90% of patients.
- Dryness of eyes and dry mouth (sicca components) are the most common features; they occur alone or with rheumatoid arthritis or other connective tissue disease.
- Rheumatoid factor and antinuclear antibodies are common.
- Increased incidence of lymphoma.

General Considerations

Sjögren syndrome is a systemic autoimmune disorder whose clinical presentation is usually dominated by dryness of the eyes and mouth due to immune-mediated dysfunction of the lacrimal and salivary glands. The disorder is predominantly seen in women, with a ratio of 9:1; most cases develop between the ages of 40 and 60 years. Sjögren syndrome can occur in isolation ("primary" Sjögren syndrome) or in association with another rheumatic disease. Sjögren syndrome is most frequently associated with rheumatoid arthritis but also occurs with SLE, primary biliary cholangitis, systemic sclerosis, polymyositis, Hashimoto thyroiditis, polyarteritis, and interstitial pulmonary fibrosis.

Clinical Findings

A. Symptoms and Signs

Keratoconjunctivitis sicca results from inadequate tear production caused by lymphocyte and plasma cell infiltration of the lacrimal glands. Ocular symptoms are usually mild. Burning, itching, and the sensation of having a foreign body or a grain of sand in the eye occur commonly. For some patients, the initial manifestation is the inability to tolerate wearing contact lenses. Many patients with more severe ocular dryness notice ropy secretions across their eyes, especially in the morning. For most patients, symptoms of dryness of the mouth (xerostomia) dominate those of dry eyes. Patients frequently complain of a "cotton mouth" sensation and difficulty swallowing foods, especially dry foods like crackers, unless they are washed down with liquids. The persistent oral dryness causes most patients to carry water bottles or other liquid dispensers from which they sip constantly. A few patients have such severe xerostomia that they have difficulty speaking. Persistent xerostomia results in rampant dental caries; caries at the gum line strongly suggest Sjögren syndrome. Some patients are most troubled by loss of taste and smell. Parotid enlargement, which may be chronic or relapsing, develops in one-third of patients. Dryness may involve the nose, throat, larynx, bronchi, vagina, and skin.

Systemic manifestations include dysphagia, small-vessel vasculitis, pleuritis, obstructive airways disease and interstitial lung disease (in the absence of cigarette smoking), neuropsychiatric dysfunction (most commonly peripheral neuropathies), and pancreatitis; they may be related to the associated diseases noted above. Renal tubular acidosis (type I, distal) occurs in 20% of patients. Chronic interstitial nephritis, which may cause impaired kidney function, may be seen.

B. Laboratory Findings

Laboratory findings include mild anemia, leukopenia, and eosinophilia. Polyclonal hypergammaglobulinemia, rheumatoid factor positivity (70%), and antinuclear antibodies (95%) are all common findings. Antibodies against SS-A and SS-B are often present in primary Sjögren syndrome and tend to correlate with the presence of extraglandular manifestations (Table 20–7).

Useful ocular diagnostic tests include the Schirmer test, which measures the quantity of tears secreted. Lip biopsy, a simple procedure, reveals characteristic lymphoid foci in accessory salivary glands. Biopsy of the parotid gland should be reserved for patients with atypical presentations such as unilateral gland enlargement that suggest a neoplastic process.

Differential Diagnosis

Isolated complaints of dry mouth are most commonly due to medication side effects. Chronic hepatitis C can cause sicca symptoms and rheumatoid factor positivity; minor salivary gland biopsies reveal lymphocytic infiltrates but not to the extent of Sjögren syndrome, and tests for anti-SS-A and anti-SS-B are negative. Diffuse infiltration of CD8 T cells producing parotid gland enlargement can develop in HIV-infected individuals. Involvement of the lacrimal or salivary glands, or both, in sarcoidosis can mimic Sjögren syndrome; biopsies reveal noncaseating granulomas. IgG_4-related systemic disease can cause lacrimal and salivary gland enlargement that mimics Sjögren syndrome.

Treatment & Prognosis

Treatment of sicca symptoms is symptomatic and supportive. Artificial tears applied frequently will relieve ocular symptoms and avert further desiccation. Topical ocular 0.05% cyclosporine also improves ocular symptoms and signs of dryness. The mouth should be kept well lubricated. Sipping water frequently or using sugar-free gums and hard candies usually relieves dry mouth symptoms. Pilocarpine (5 mg orally four times daily) and the acetylcholine derivative cevimeline (30 mg orally three times daily) may improve xerostomia symptoms. Atropinic (anticholingeric) drugs and decongestants decrease salivary secretions and should be avoided. A program of oral hygiene, including fluoride treatment, is essential to preserve dentition. If there is an associated rheumatic disease, its systemic treatment is not altered by the presence of Sjögren syndrome. Extraglandular disease, including arthritis, vasculitis, or pulmonary manifestations, is treated with similar immunosuppressive medications as SLE or rheumatoid arthritis.

Although Sjögren syndrome may compromise patients' quality of life significantly, the disease is usually associated with a normal life span. Poor prognoses are influenced mainly by the presence of systemic features associated with underlying disorders, the development in some patients of lymphocytic vasculitis, the occurrence of a painful peripheral neuropathy, and the complication (in a minority of patients) of lymphoma. Severe systemic inflammatory manifestations are treated with prednisone or various immunosuppressive medications. The patients at greatest risk for developing lymphoma are those with severe exocrine dysfunction, marked parotid gland enlargement, splenomegaly, vasculitis, peripheral neuropathy, anemia, and mixed monoclonal cryoglobulinemia (3–10% of the total Sjögren population).

When to Refer

- Presence of systemic symptoms or signs.
- Ocular dryness not responsive to artificial tears.

When to Admit

Presence of severe systemic signs such as vasculitis unresponsive to outpatient management.

Ramos-Casals M et al. EULAR recommendations for the management of Sjögren's syndrome with topical and systemic therapies. Ann Rheum Dis. 2020;79:3. [PMID: 31672775]

Seror R et al. Current and future therapies for primary Sjögren syndrome. Nat Rev Rheumatol. 2021;17:475. [PMID: 34188206]

IgG_4-RELATED DISEASE

ESSENTIALS OF DIAGNOSIS

- Mainly affects men older than 50 years.
- Lymphoplasmacytic infiltrates causing tumors or fibrosis in any organ or tissue.
- Subacute onset; constitutional symptoms rare.
- Diagnostic histopathology.

General Considerations

IgG_4-related disease is a systemic disorder of unknown cause marked by highly characteristic fibroinflammation that contains IgG_4 plasma cells and can infiltrate virtually any organ. The disorder chiefly affects men (75% of patients) over the age of 50 years.

Clinical Findings

A. Symptoms and Signs

IgG_4-related disease can affect any organ of the body, can be localized or generalized, demonstrates the same distinctive histopathology at all sites of involvement, produces protean manifestations depending on location and extent of involvement, and causes disease that ranges in severity from asymptomatic to organ- or life-threatening. The inflammatory infiltration in IgG_4-related disease frequently produces tumefactive masses that can be found during physical examination or on imaging. Some of the common presenting manifestations include enlargement of submandibular glands, proptosis from periorbital infiltration, retroperitoneal fibrosis, mediastinal fibrosis, inflammatory aortic aneurysm, and pancreatic mass with autoimmune pancreatitis. IgG_4-related disease can also affect the thyroid (formerly Riedel thyroiditis), kidney, meninges, pituitary, sinuses, lung, prostate, breast, and bone. Most symptomatic patients with IgG_4-related disease present subacutely; fever and constitutional symptoms are usually absent. Nearly half of the patients with IgG_4-related disease also have allergic disorders such as sinusitis or asthma.

B. Laboratory Findings

Serum IgG_4 levels are usually, but not invariably, elevated so this finding cannot be used as the sole diagnostic criterion. The infiltrating lesions in IgG_4-related disease often produce tumors or fibrotic changes that are evident on CT or MRI imaging. However, the cornerstone of diagnosis is histopathology. The key pathological findings are a dense lymphoplasmacytic infiltrate rich in IgG_4 plasma cells, storiform (matted and irregularly whorled) fibrosis, and obliterative phlebitis.

Differential Diagnosis

IgG_4-related disease can mimic many disorders including sarcoidosis, Sjögren syndrome (lacrimal gland enlargement), pancreatic cancer (pancreatic mass), chronic infections (eg, HIV, hepatitis C), and granulomatosis with polyangiitis (proptosis). Lymphoma can mimic some of the histopathologic features of IgG_4-related disease.

Treatment & Prognosis

Patients who are asymptomatic and have no organ-threatening disease can be monitored carefully. Spontaneous resolution can occur. Initial therapy is usually oral prednisone 0.6 mg/kg/day, tapered over weeks or months depending on response. Given that corticosteroid monotherapy may fail to control the disease and can cause significant long-term toxicity, immunosuppressants, especially rituximab, are often used. The degree of fibrosis in affected organs determines the patient's responsiveness to treatment.

When to Refer

- Presence of systemic symptoms or signs.
- Symptoms or signs not responsive to prednisone.

When to Admit

Presence of severe systemic signs unresponsive to outpatient management.

Wallace ZS et al. The 2019 American College of Rheumatology/European League Against Rheumatism classification criteria for IgG_4-related disease. Arthritis Rheumatol. 2020;72:7. [PMID: 31793250]

Zhang W et al. Management of IgG_4-related disease. Lancet Rheumatol. 2019;1:e55. https://doi.org/10.1016/S2665-9913(19)30017.

VASCULITIS SYNDROMES

Vasculitis is a heterogeneous group of disorders characterized by inflammation within the walls of affected blood vessels. The major forms of primary systemic vasculitis are listed in Table 20–11. The first consideration in classifying cases of vasculitis is the size of the major vessels involved: large, medium, or small. The presence of the clinical signs and symptoms shown in Table 20–12 helps distinguish among these three groups. After determining the size of the major vessels involved, other issues that contribute to the classification include the following:

Table 20–11. Classification scheme of primary vasculitides according to size of predominant blood vessels involved.

Predominantly large-vessel vasculitides
Takayasu arteritis
Giant cell arteritis (temporal arteritis)
Behçet disease[1]
Predominantly medium-vessel vasculitides
Polyarteritis nodosa
Buerger disease
Primary angiitis of the CNS
Predominantly small-vessel vasculitides
Cutaneous leukocytoclastic angiitis ("hypersensitivity vasculitis")
Immune-complex–mediated
IgA vasculitis (Henoch-Schönlein purpura)
Hypocomplementemic urticarial vasculitis (anti-C1q vasculitis)
Essential cryoglobulinemia[2]
"ANCA-associated" vasculitis[3]
Granulomatosis with polyangiitis[2]
Microscopic polyangiitis[2]
Eosinophilic granulomatosis with polyangiitis[2]

[1]May involve small-, medium-, and large-sized blood vessels.
[2]Frequent overlap of small- and medium-sized blood vessel involvement.
[3]Not all forms of these disorders are always associated with ANCA.
ANCA, antineutrophil cytoplasmic antibodies.

- Does the process involve arteries, veins, or both?
- What are the patient's demographic characteristics (age, sex, ethnicity, cigarette smoking status)?
- Which organs are involved?
- Is there hypocomplementemia or other evidence of immune complex deposition?
- Is there granulomatous inflammation on tissue biopsy?
- Are antineutrophil cytoplasmic antibodies (ANCA) present?

Table 20–12. Typical clinical manifestations of large-, medium-, and small-vessel vasculitis.

Large Vessel	Medium vessel	Small vessel
Fever, weight loss, malaise, arthralgias/arthritis	Fever, weight loss, malaise, arthralgias/arthritis	Fever, weight loss, malaise, arthralgias/arthritis
Limb claudication	Cutaneous nodules	Purpura
Asymmetric blood pressures	Ulcers	Vesiculobullous lesions
Absence of pulses	Livedo reticularis	Urticaria
Bruits	Digital gangrene	Glomerulonephritis
Aortic dilation	Mononeuritis multiplex	Alveolar hemorrhage
	Microaneurysms	Cutaneous extravascular necrotizing granulomas
		Splinter hemorrhages
		Uveitis
		Episcleritis
		Scleritis

In addition to the disorders considered to be primary vasculitides, there are also multiple forms of vasculitis that are associated with other known underlying conditions. These "secondary" forms of vasculitis occur in the setting of chronic infections (eg, hepatitis B or C, subacute bacterial endocarditis), connective tissue disorders, IBD, malignancies, and reactions to medications. Only the major primary forms of vasculitis are discussed here.

Felicetti M et al. One year in review 2020: vasculitis. Clin Exp Rheumatol. 2020;38:3. [PMID: 32359039]

POLYMYALGIA RHEUMATICA & GIANT CELL ARTERITIS

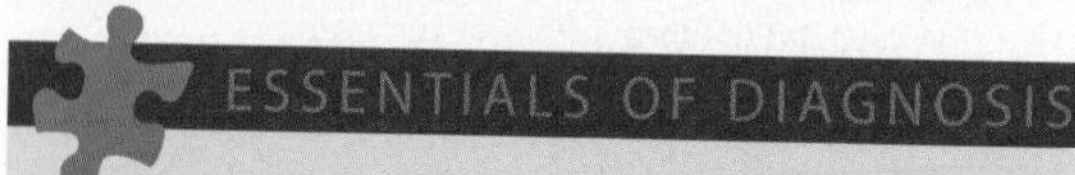

- Age over 50 years.
- Markedly elevated ESR and CRP.
- **Polymyalgia rheumatica:** pain and stiffness in shoulders and hips lasting for several weeks without other explanation.
- **Giant cell arteritis:** headache, jaw claudication, polymyalgia rheumatica; without treatment, permanent blindness may occur.

General Considerations

Polymyalgia rheumatica and giant cell arteritis probably represent a spectrum of one disease. Both affect the same population (patients over the age of 50), and the incidence of the disease increases with each decade of life. Both show preference for the same HLA haplotypes and show similar patterns of cytokines in blood and arteries. Giant cell arteritis is a systemic panarteritis affecting medium-sized and large vessels. Giant cell arteritis was previously called temporal arteritis because the temporal artery is frequently involved, as are other extracranial branches of the carotid artery. However, the aorta and its major branches may be also involved in giant cell arteritis. Polymyalgia rheumatica and giant cell arteritis frequently coexist. The important differences between the two conditions are that polymyalgia rheumatica alone is not a systemic vasculitis, does not cause blindness, and responds to low-dose (10–20 mg/day orally) prednisone; giant cell arteritis can cause blindness, aortitis, and large artery complications that require high-dose (40–60 mg/day) prednisone.

Clinical Findings

A. Polymyalgia Rheumatica

Polymyalgia rheumatica is a clinical diagnosis based on pain and stiffness of the shoulder and pelvic girdle areas, frequently in association with fever, malaise, and weight loss. In approximately two-thirds of cases, polymyalgia occurs in the absence of giant cell arteritis. Because of the stiffness and pain in the shoulders, hips, and lower back, patients have trouble combing their hair, putting on a coat, or rising from a chair. In contrast to polymyositis and polyarteritis nodosa, polymyalgia rheumatica does not cause muscular weakness either through primary muscle inflammation or secondary to nerve infarction.

B. Giant Cell Arteritis

The mean age at onset is approximately 79 years. About 50% of patients with giant cell arteritis also have polymyalgia rheumatica. The classic symptoms suggesting that a patient has arteritis are headache, scalp tenderness, visual symptoms (particularly amaurosis fugax or diplopia), jaw claudication, or throat pain. Of these symptoms, jaw claudication has the highest positive predictive value. The temporal artery can be normal on physical examination but may be nodular, enlarged, tender, or pulseless. Blindness usually results from anterior ischemic optic neuropathy, caused by occlusive arteritis of the posterior ciliary branch of the ophthalmic artery. The ischemic optic neuropathy of giant cell arteritis may produce no funduscopic findings for the first 24–48 hours after the onset of blindness.

Asymmetry of pulses in the arms, a murmur of aortic regurgitation, or bruits near the clavicle resulting from subclavian artery stenoses identify patients in whom giant cell arteritis has affected the aorta or its major branches. Clinically evident large vessel involvement—characterized chiefly by aneurysm of the thoracic aorta or stenosis of the subclavian, vertebral, carotid, and basilar arteries—occurs in approximately 25% of patients with giant cell arteritis, sometimes years after the diagnosis. Subclinical large artery disease is the rule: PET scans reveal inflammation in the aorta and its major branches in nearly 85% of untreated patients. Forty percent of patients with giant cell arteritis have nonclassical symptoms at presentation, including large artery involvement causing chiefly aortic regurgitation or arm claudication, respiratory tract problems (most frequently dry cough), mononeuritis multiplex (most frequently with painful paralysis of a shoulder), or fever of unknown origin. Giant cell arteritis accounts for 15% of all cases of fever of unknown origin in patients over the age of 65. The fever can be as high as 40°C and is frequently associated with rigors and sweats. Thus, in an older patient with fever of unknown origin and marked elevations of acute-phase reactants in the absence of an infectious source, giant cell arteritis must be considered even in the absence of specific features such as headache or jaw claudication. In some cases, instead of having the well-known symptom of jaw claudication, patients complain of vague pain affecting other locations, including the tongue, nose, or ears. Indeed, unexplained head or neck pain in an older patient may signal the presence of giant cell arteritis.

C. Laboratory Findings

1. Polymyalgia rheumatica—Acute-phase reactants (generally ESR higher than 30 mm/hour and CRP more than 0.5 mg/dL) are universally present.

2. Giant cell arteritis—Nearly 90% of patients with giant cell arteritis have ESRs higher than 50 mm/hour. The ESR in this disorder is often more than 100 mm/hour, but cases in which the ESR is lower or even normal do occur. In one series, 5% of patients with biopsy-proven giant cell arteritis had ESRs below 40 mm/hour. Although the CRP is slightly more sensitive, patients with biopsy-proven giant cell arteritis with normal CRP have also been described. Most patients also have a mild normochromic, normocytic anemia and thrombocytosis. The alkaline phosphatase (liver source) is elevated in 20% of patients with giant cell arteritis.

Differential Diagnosis

The differential diagnosis of malaise, anemia, and striking acute-phase reactant elevations includes rheumatic diseases (such as rheumatoid arthritis or systemic vasculitides), plasma cell myeloma, other malignant disorders, and chronic infections (such as bacterial endocarditis and osteomyelitis).

Treatment

A. Polymyalgia Rheumatica

Patients with isolated polymyalgia rheumatica (ie, those not having "above the neck" symptoms of headache, jaw claudication, scalp tenderness, or visual symptoms) are treated with prednisone, 10–20 mg/day orally. If the patient does not experience a dramatic improvement within 72 hours, the diagnosis should be revisited. Usually after 2–4 weeks of treatment, slow tapering of prednisone can be attempted. Most patients require some dose of prednisone for a minimum of approximately 1 year; 6 months is too short in most cases. Care must be taken to prevent corticosteroid side effects (Table 26–17). Disease flares are common (50% or more) as prednisone is tapered, which may necessitate increasing prednisone. Tapering of prednisone should be based on symptoms and not solely on laboratory values because the ESR can fluctuate, and it is not specific for polymyalgia rheumatica disease activity. Adding weekly methotrexate may increase the chance of successfully tapering prednisone in some patients.

B. Giant Cell Arteritis

The urgency of early diagnosis and treatment in giant cell arteritis relates to the prevention of blindness. Once blindness develops, it is usually permanent. Therefore, when a patient has symptoms and findings suggestive of cranial involvement from giant cell arteritis, therapy with prednisone (1 mg/kg/daily or max 80 mg/day orally) should be initiated immediately, and a temporal artery biopsy performed promptly thereafter. For patients who seek medical attention for visual loss, intravenous pulse methylprednisolone (eg, 1 g daily for 3 days) should be started; unfortunately, few patients recover vision no matter what the initial treatment. Although it is prudent to obtain a temporal artery biopsy as soon as possible after instituting treatment, diagnostic findings of giant cell arteritis may still be present 2 weeks (or longer) after starting corticosteroids. An adequate biopsy specimen is essential (at least 2 cm in length), because the disease may be segmental. Obtaining a unilateral biopsy is recommended in 2021 guidelines (positive in approximately 80–85% of patients) since bilateral biopsies only increase the yield by less than 15%. The presence of a "halo sign" on temporal artery ultrasonography may obviate the need for temporal artery biopsy, although biopsy remains the gold standard for giant cell arteritis diagnosis. Temporal artery biopsy is abnormal in only 50% of patients with *large artery* giant cell arteritis. In these patients, magnetic resonance angiography or CT angiography will establish the diagnosis by demonstrating long stretches of narrowing, thickening, or aneurysmal dilation of the aorta and the subclavian and axillary arteries, or both. Thoracic aortic aneurysms occur 17 times more frequently in patients with giant cell arteritis than in normal individuals and can cause aortic regurgitation, dissection, or rupture. The aneurysms can develop at any time but typically occur 7 years after the diagnosis of giant cell arteritis is made; hence, routine screening for this complication in cranial and large vessel giant cell arteritis is recommended.

Prednisone should be continued at a high dose orally for about 1 month before tapering. After 1 month of high-dose prednisone, most patients will have a normal ESR. When tapering and adjusting the dosage of prednisone, the ESR (or CRP) is a useful, but not absolute, guide to disease activity. A common error is treating the ESR rather than the patient. The ESR often rises slightly as the prednisone is tapered, even as the disease remains quiescent. Because older individuals often have baseline ESRs that are above the normal range, mild ESR elevations should not be an occasion for renewed treatment with prednisone in patients who are asymptomatic. Tocilizumab, an inhibitor of the IL-6 receptor, is FDA-approved for giant cell arteritis and can reduce the prolonged use of prednisone and decrease the risk of disease flare.

Hellmich B et al. 2018 update of the EULAR recommendations for the management of large vessel vasculitis. Ann Rheum Dis. 2020;79:19. [PMID: 31270110]

Maz M et al. 2021 American College of Rheumatology/Vasculitis Foundation guideline for the management of giant cell arteritis and Takayasu arteritis. Arthritis Rheumatol. 2021;73:1349. [PMID: 34235884]

TAKAYASU ARTERITIS

Takayasu arteritis is a granulomatous vasculitis of the aorta and its major branches. Rare in North America but more prevalent in the Far East, it primarily affects women and typically has its onset in early adulthood. Takayasu arteritis can present with nonspecific constitutional symptoms of malaise, fever, and weight loss or with manifestations of vascular inflammation and damage: diminished pulses, unequal blood pressures in the arms, carotidynia (tenderness over the carotid arteries), bruits over carotid and subclavian arteries, retinopathy, limb claudication, and hypertension. There are no specific laboratory abnormalities; the ESR and the CRP level are elevated in most cases. The diagnosis is established by imaging studies, usually MRI, which can detect inflammatory thickening of the walls of affected vessels, or CT angiography, which can provide images of the stenoses, occlusions, and dilations characteristic of arteritis. High-dose corticosteroids (eg, oral prednisone, 1 mg/kg) are recommended for newly diagnosed or severely relapsing Takayasu arteritis. The addition of methotrexate, azathioprine, mycophenolate mofetil, or TNF inhibitors is recommended for refractory disease and as steroid-sparing agents; TNF inhibitors are first-line additions. There are limited data for other biologic therapies, such as anti-IL6 therapy (tocilizumab) and tofacitinib. Takayasu arteritis has a chronic relapsing and remitting course that requires ongoing monitoring and adjustment of therapy.

Gribbons KB et al. Patterns of arterial disease in Takayasu arteritis and giant cell arteritis. Arthritis Care Res (Hoboken). 2020;72:1615. [PMID: 31444857]
Michailidou D et al. Clinical symptoms and associated vascular imaging findings in Takayasu's arteritis compared to giant cell arteritis. Ann Rheum Dis. 2020;79:262. [PMID: 31649025]

POLYARTERITIS NODOSA

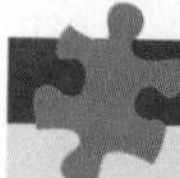

ESSENTIALS OF DIAGNOSIS

- Medium-sized arteries are affected.
- Clinical findings depend on the arteries involved; lungs are spared.
- Common features include fever, abdominal pain, extremity pain, livedo reticularis, mononeuritis multiplex.
- Kidney involvement causes renin-mediated hypertension.
- Associated with hepatitis B (10% of cases).

General Considerations

Polyarteritis nodosa is a necrotizing arteritis of medium-sized vessels that has a predilection for involving the skin, peripheral nerves, mesenteric vessels (including renal arteries), heart, and brain but spares the lungs. Polyarteritis nodosa is rare, with a prevalence of 30 per 1 million people. Approximately 10% of cases of polyarteritis nodosa are caused by hepatitis B. Most cases of hepatitis B–associated disease occur within 6 months of hepatitis B infection. Mutations in the gene for adenosine deaminase 2 have been identified in early-onset familial polyarteritis.

Clinical Findings

A. Symptoms and Signs

The clinical onset is usually insidious, with fever, malaise, weight loss, and other symptoms developing over weeks to months. Pain in the extremities is often a prominent early feature caused by arthralgia, myalgia (particularly affecting the calves), or neuropathy. The combination of mononeuritis multiplex (with the most common finding being footdrop) and features of a systemic illness is one of the earliest specific clues to the presence of an underlying vasculitis.

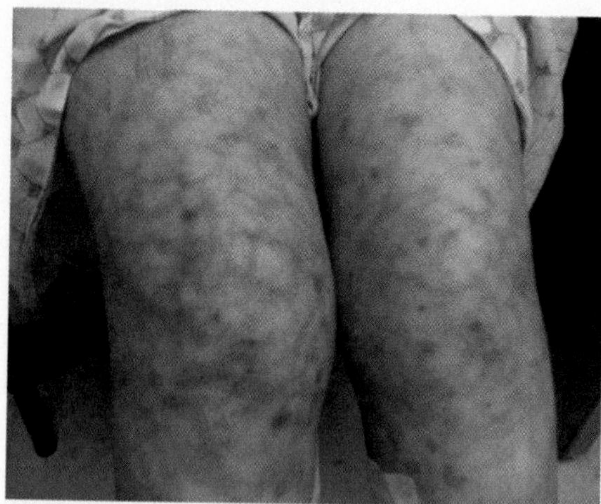

Figure 20–7. Livedo reticularis as a manifestation of antiphospholipid antibody syndrome. (Used, with permission, from Imboden JB et al. *Current Diagnosis & Treatment: Rheumatology*, 3rd ed. McGraw-Hill, 2013.)

Polyarteritis nodosa is among the forms of vasculitis most commonly associated with vasculitic neuropathy.

In polyarteritis nodosa, the typical skin findings—livedo reticularis (Figure 20–7), subcutaneous nodules, and skin ulcers—reflect the involvement of deeper, medium-sized blood vessels. Digital gangrene is common. The most common cutaneous presentation is lower extremity ulcerations, usually occurring near the malleoli. Involvement of the renal arteries leads to a renin-mediated hypertension (much less characteristic of vasculitides involving smaller blood vessels). For unclear reasons, classic polyarteritis nodosa seldom (if ever) involves the lung, with the occasional exception of the bronchial arteries.

Abdominal pain—particularly diffuse periumbilical pain precipitated by eating—is common but often difficult to attribute to mesenteric vasculitis in the early stages. Nausea and vomiting are frequent symptoms. Infarction compromises the function of major viscera and may lead to acalculous cholecystitis or appendicitis. Some patients present dramatically with an acute abdomen caused by mesenteric vasculitis and gut perforation or with hypotension resulting from rupture of a microaneurysm in the liver, kidney, or bowel.

Newly acquired hypertension from renin-mediated kidney disease frequently occurs. Subclinical cardiac involvement is common in polyarteritis nodosa, and overt cardiac dysfunction may occur (eg, MI secondary to coronary vasculitis, or myocarditis).

B. Laboratory Findings

Most patients with polyarteritis nodosa have anemia, and leukocytosis is common. Acute-phase reactants are often (but not always) strikingly elevated. A major challenge in making the diagnosis of polyarteritis nodosa, however, is the absence of a disease-specific serologic test (eg, an autoantibody). Patients with classic polyarteritis nodosa are ANCA-negative but may have low titers of rheumatoid factor or antinuclear antibodies, both of which are nonspecific findings. Tests for active hepatitis B infection (HBsAg, HBeAg, hepatitis B viral load) should be performed. Patients with childhood onset of polyarteritis nodosa should undergo genetic evaluation for mutations in the genes for adenosine deaminase 2.

C. Biopsy and Angiography

The diagnosis of polyarteritis nodosa requires confirmation with either a tissue biopsy or vascular imaging. Biopsies of symptomatic sites such as skin and nerve and muscle (or both), are essential for diagnosis. A deep biopsy, not a punch biopsy, of skin ulcers or nodules should be made to ensure a medium-size vessel is included in the sample. Current guidelines recommend a biopsy of the nerve and muscle (instead of the nerve alone) in patients with neuropathic symptoms. Patients in whom polyarteritis nodosa is suspected—eg, based on mesenteric ischemia or new-onset hypertension occurring in the setting of a systemic illness—may be diagnosed by the angiographic finding of aneurysmal dilations in the renal, mesenteric, or hepatic arteries.

Differential Diagnosis

Genetic collagen vascular disorders (such as Ehlers-Danlos and Loey-Dietz syndromes), fibromuscular dysplasia, and segmental arterial mediolysis should be considered when imaging findings suggest polyarteritis nodosa in the absence of other clinical features of the disorder.

Treatment

High-dose pulse methylprednisolone (eg, 1 g intravenously daily for 3 days) is recommended as the initial treatment for severe polyarteritis nodosa. Adding cyclophosphamide lowers the risk of disease-related death and morbidity among patients who have severe disease. Methotrexate or azathioprine are used to maintain remissions induced by cyclophosphamide. For patients with polyarteritis nodosa associated with hepatitis B, the preferred treatment regimen is a short course of prednisone accompanied by anti-HBV therapy and plasmapheresis (three times a week for up to 6 weeks). Inhibitors of TNF are first-line therapy for the polyarteritis associated with deficiency of adenosine deaminase 2.

Prognosis

Without treatment, the 5-year survival rate in this disorder is about 10%. With appropriate therapy, remissions are possible in many cases and the 5-year survival rate has improved to 60–90%. Poor prognostic factors are CKD with serum creatinine greater than 1.6 mg/dL (141 mcmol/L), proteinuria greater than 1 g/day, GI ischemia, CNS disease, and cardiac involvement. In the absence of any of these five factors, 5-year survival is nearly 90%. Survival at 5 years drops to 75% with one poor prognostic factor present and to about 50% with two or more factors. Substantial morbidity and death may result from adverse effects of cyclophosphamide and corticosteroids (Table 26–17). These therapies require careful monitoring and expert management. In contrast to many other forms of systemic vasculitis, disease relapses in polyarteritis following the successful induction of remission occur in only about 20% of cases.

Chung SA et al. 2021 American College of Rheumatology/Vasculitis Foundation Guideline for the management of polyarteritis nodosa. Arthritis Rheumatol. 2021;73:1384. [PMID: 34235883]

Hočevar A et al. Clinical approach to diagnosis and therapy of polyarteritis nodosa. Curr Rheumatol Rep. 2021;23:14. [PMID: 33569653]

GRANULOMATOSIS WITH POLYANGIITIS

ESSENTIALS OF DIAGNOSIS

- Classic triad of upper and lower respiratory tract disease and glomerulonephritis.
- Suspect if upper respiratory tract symptoms (eg, nasal congestion, sinusitis) are refractory to usual treatment.
- Kidney disease is often rapidly progressive.
- Venous thromboembolism commonly occurs.
- ANCAs (90% of patients), usually directed against proteinase-3 (but may be directed against myeloperoxidase).
- Tissue biopsy usually necessary for diagnosis.

General Considerations

Granulomatosis with polyangiitis (formerly Wegener granulomatosis), which has an estimated incidence of approximately 12 cases per million individuals per year, is one of three vasculitides associated with ANCA. The other "ANCA-associated vasculitides" include microscopic polyangiitis and eosinophilic granulomatosis with polyangiitis. Granulomatosis with polyangiitis is characterized by vasculitis of small arteries, arterioles, and capillaries, necrotizing granulomatous lesions of both upper and lower respiratory tract, glomerulonephritis, and other vasculitic organ manifestations. Without treatment, generalized disease is invariably fatal, with most patients surviving less than 1 year after diagnosis. It occurs most commonly in the fourth and fifth decades of life and affects men and women with equal frequency.

Clinical Findings

A. Symptoms and Signs

The disorder usually develops over 4–12 months. Upper respiratory tract symptoms develop in 90% of patients and lower respiratory tract symptoms develop in 60% of patients; some patients may have both upper and lower respiratory tract symptoms. Upper respiratory tract symptoms can include nasal congestion, sinusitis, otitis media, mastoiditis, inflammation of the gums, or stridor due to

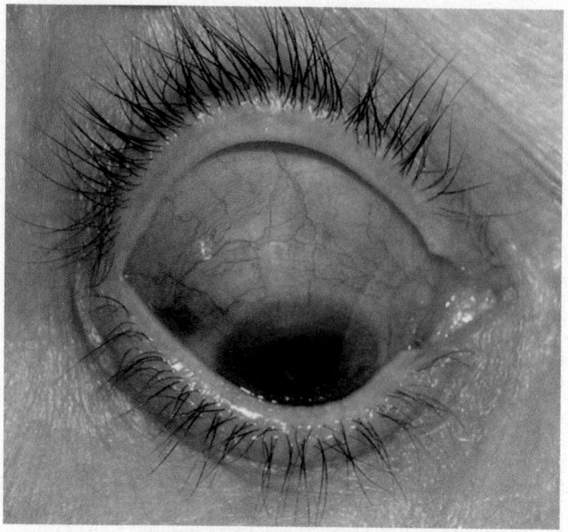

▲ **Figure 20–8.** Scleritis in a patient with granulomatosis with polyangiitis. (Used, with permission, from Everett Allen, MD, in Usatine RP, Smith MA, Mayeaux EJ Jr, Chumley H. *The Color Atlas of Family Medicine*, 2nd ed. McGraw-Hill, 2013.)

subglottic stenosis. Since many of these symptoms are common, the underlying disease is not often suspected until the patient develops systemic symptoms, or the original problem is refractory to treatment. The lungs are affected initially in 40% and eventually in 80%, with symptoms including cough, dyspnea, and hemoptysis. Other early symptoms can include a migratory oligoarthritis with a predilection for large joints; a variety of symptoms related to ocular disease (unilateral proptosis from orbital pseudotumor; red eye from scleritis [Figure 20–8], episcleritis, anterior uveitis, or peripheral ulcerative keratitis); purpura or other skin lesions; and dysesthesia due to neuropathy. Renal involvement, which develops in three-fourths of the cases, may be subclinical until kidney disease is advanced. Fever, malaise, and weight loss are common.

Physical examination can be remarkable for congestion, crusting, ulceration, bleeding, and even perforation of the nasal septum. Destruction of the nasal cartilage with "saddle nose" deformity occurs late. Otitis media, proptosis, scleritis, episcleritis, and conjunctivitis are other common findings. Newly acquired hypertension, a frequent feature of polyarteritis nodosa, is rarely a symptom of granulomatosis with polyangiitis. Venous thrombotic events (eg, DVT and PE) are a common occurrence in granulomatosis with polyangiitis. Although limited forms of granulomatosis with polyangiitis have been described in which the kidney is spared initially, kidney disease will develop in most untreated patients.

B. Laboratory Findings

1. Serum tests and UA—Most patients have anemia, mild leukocytosis, and elevated acute-phase reactants. If there is kidney involvement, proteinuria occurs and the urinary sediment contains red cells, often with red cell casts.

Serum tests for ANCA help in the diagnosis of granulomatosis with polyangiitis (Table 20–7). The two key ANCA subtypes relevant to systemic vasculitis are those directed against proteinase-3 (PR3) and myeloperoxidase (MPO). Antibodies to these two antigens are termed "PR3-ANCA" and "MPO-ANCA," respectively. The cytoplasmic pattern of immunofluorescence (c-ANCA) caused by PR3-ANCA has a high specificity (more than 90%) for granulomatosis with polyangiitis but may less commonly be seen in the other forms of ANCA-associated vasculitis). A substantial percentage of patients with "limited" granulomatosis with polyangiitis, disease that does not pose an immediate threat to life and is often confined to the sinus and upper respiratory tract, are ANCA-negative. ANCA levels correlate erratically with disease activity, and changes in titer should not dictate changes in therapy in the absence of supporting clinical data. The perinuclear (p-ANCA) pattern, caused by MPO-ANCA, is more likely to occur in microscopic polyangiitis or eosinophilic granulomatosis with polyangiitis but may be found in granulomatosis with polyangiitis. Approximately 10–25% of patients with classic granulomatosis with polyangiitis have MPO-ANCA. All positive immunofluorescence assays for ANCA should be confirmed by enzyme immunoassays for the specific autoantibodies directed against PR3 or MPO.

2. Histologic findings—Although ANCA testing is helpful, there remains the need in most cases for diagnostic confirmation by tissue biopsy. Histologic features of granulomatosis with polyangiitis include vasculitis, granulomatous inflammation, geographic necrosis, and acute and chronic inflammation. The full range of pathologic changes is usually evident only on thoracoscopic lung biopsy; granulomas, observed only rarely in kidney biopsy specimens, are found much more commonly on lung biopsy specimens. Nasal biopsies often do not show vasculitis but may show chronic inflammation and other changes that rule out nasopharyngeal cancer or infection. Kidney biopsy discloses a segmental necrotizing glomerulonephritis with multiple crescents; this is characteristic but not diagnostic. Pathologists characterize the kidney lesion of granulomatosis with polyangiitis (and other forms of "ANCA-associated vasculitis") as a pauci-immune glomerulonephritis because of the relative absence (compared with immune complex–mediated disorders) of IgG, IgM, IgA, and complement proteins within glomeruli.

C. Imaging

Chest CT is more sensitive than chest radiography; lesions include infiltrates, nodules, masses, and cavities. Pleural effusions are uncommon. Often the radiographs prompt concern about lung cancer. Hilar adenopathy large enough to be evident on chest film is unusual in granulomatosis with polyangiitis; if present, sarcoidosis, tumor, or infection is more likely. Other common radiographic abnormalities include extensive sinusitis and even bony sinus erosions.

▶ Differential Diagnosis

Due to refractory and severe sinusitis, granulomatosis with polyangiitis may be misdiagnosed as chronic infectious sinonasal disease and treated with antibiotics alone. Initial complaints of joint pain can lead to a misdiagnosis of rheumatoid arthritis. Lung cancer may be the first diagnostic consideration for some middle-aged patients with cough, hemoptysis, and lung masses. Granulomatosis with polyangiitis shares with SLE, anti–glomerular basement membrane disease, and microscopic polyangiitis the ability to cause an acute pulmonary-renal syndrome. Although both granulomatosis with polyangiitis and microscopic polyangiitis may have MPO-ANCA positivity, microscopic polyangiitis does not involve the sinuses or upper respiratory tract and does not have granulomatous inflammation on histopathology. Cocaine use can destroy midline tissues—the nose and palate—that mimics granulomatosis with polyangiitis. Patients using cocaine may have a drug-induced positive result for PR-3-ANCA, and lesional biopsies may demonstrate vasculitis from exposure to the toxin. COPA syndrome, a rare genetic autoinflammatory interferonopathy condition, has many features of a systemic vasculitis such as diffuse alveolar hemorrhage, glomerulonephritis, and inflammatory arthritis. Multiple autoantibodies may be simultaneously present in COPA syndrome including ANA, PR3-ANCA, MPO-ANCA, and rheumatoid factor, which is a clue that their presence lacks specificity. COPA syndrome should be considered when children (younger than 20 years of age) present with multiorgan inflammatory symptoms (especially lung) that mimic granulomatosis with polyangiitis.

Treatment

Early treatment is crucial to preventing the devastating end-organ and catastrophic complications of this disease. Current practice divides treatment into two phases: induction of remission and maintenance of remission. Plasma exchange does not reduce the incidence of ESKD or death in severe ANCA-associated vasculitis.

A. Induction of Remission

Choice of induction therapy is dictated by whether the patient has mild disease (ie, no significant kidney dysfunction) or severe disease (ie, life- or organ-threatening disease such as rapidly progressive glomerulonephritis or pulmonary hemorrhage). American College of Rheumatology/Vasculitis Foundation recommendations for the treatment of granulomatosis with polyangiitis favor rituximab as first-line induction therapy. Cyclophosphamide may also be used for induction therapy. Avacopan, an oral C5a receptor inhibitor, is FDA-approved as add-on treatment for severe ANCA-associated vasculitis induction therapy in combination with rituximab or cyclophosphamide plus corticosteroids. Although the standard induction regimen of corticosteroids in ANCA-associated vasculitis is 1 mg/kg orally daily, faster corticosteroid dose reductions have demonstrated equal efficacy with fewer corticosteroid-related complications, such as infections.

1. Rituximab plus prednisone (plus avacopan)—Rituximab, a B-cell–depleting antibody, is FDA-approved in combination with corticosteroids (prednisone 1 mg/kg orally daily) for the treatment of granulomatosis with polyangiitis and microscopic polyangiitis. Studies demonstrate that rituximab is as effective as cyclophosphamide for remission induction in these conditions.

2. Cyclophosphamide plus prednisone (plus avacopan)—Remissions can be induced in more than 90% of patients treated with prednisone (1 mg/kg daily) plus cyclophosphamide (2 mg/kg/day orally or 15 mg/kg intravenously every 2 weeks for 3 doses, then every 3 weeks for at least 3 doses with adjustments required for acute or CKD and patients over age 70). To minimize toxicity, patients are treated with cyclophosphamide for only 3–6 months; once remission is achieved, the patient is switched to a non-cyclophosphamide maintenance regimen.

Both rituximab and cyclophosphamide increase the risk of developing life-threatening opportunistic infections (including progressive multifocal leukoencephalopathy [PML]). *Whenever cyclophosphamide or rituximab is used,* Pneumocystis jirovecii *prophylaxis with one single-strength oral trimethoprim-sulfamethoxazole daily is essential.*

3. Methotrexate plus prednisone—For nonsevere disease without life- or organ-threatening manifestations, methotrexate up to 25 mg oral or subcutaneous weekly, plus corticosteroids may be effective induction therapy.

B. Maintenance of Remission

Options for maintaining remission in patients with normal or near normal kidney function after rituximab or cyclophosphamide induction include azathioprine (up to 2 mg/kg/day orally), methotrexate (20–25 mg/week either orally or subcutaneously), mycophenolate mofetil, or rituximab. Per treatment guidelines, rituximab, dosed at a fixed interval of 1 g every 6 months or 500 mg every 4 months, is favored as first-line maintenance treatment.

Charles P et al. Long-term rituximab use to maintain remission of antineutrophil cytoplasmic antibody-associated vasculitis: a randomized trial. Ann Intern Med. 2020;173:179. [PMID: 32479166]

Chung SA et al. 2021 American College of Rheumatology/Vasculitis Foundation guideline for the management of antineutrophil cytoplasmic antibody-associated vasculitis. Arthritis Rheumatol. 2021;73:1366. [PMID: 34235894]

Jayne DRW et al; ADVOCATE Study Group. Avacopan for the treatment of ANCA-associated vasculitis. N Engl J Med. 2021;384:599. [PMID: 33596356]

MICROSCOPIC POLYANGIITIS

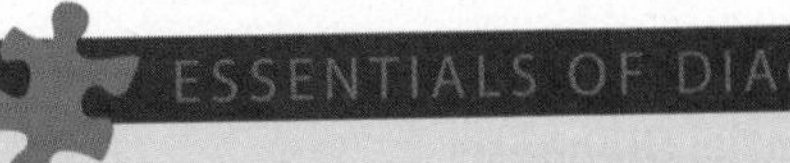

- Necrotizing vasculitis of small- and medium-sized arteries and veins.
- Most common cause of pulmonary-renal syndrome (diffuse alveolar hemorrhage and glomerulonephritis).
- ANCA in 75% of cases.

General Considerations

Microscopic polyangiitis is a pauci-immune nongranulomatous necrotizing vasculitis that (1) affects small blood vessels (capillaries, venules, or arterioles), (2) often causes glomerulonephritis and pulmonary capillaritis, and (3) is often associated with ANCA on immunofluorescence testing (directed against MPO, a constituent of neutrophil granules). Because microscopic polyangiitis may involve medium-sized as well as small blood vessels and because it tends to affect capillaries within the lungs and kidneys, its spectrum overlaps those of both polyarteritis nodosa and granulomatosis with polyangiitis.

In rare instances, medications, particularly propylthiouracil, hydralazine, allopurinol, penicillamine, minocycline, and sulfasalazine, induce a systemic vasculitis associated with high titers of p-ANCA and features of microscopic polyangiitis.

Clinical Findings

A. Symptoms and Signs

A wide variety of findings suggesting vasculitis of small blood vessels may develop in microscopic polyangiitis. These include "palpable" (or "raised") purpura and other signs of cutaneous vasculitis (ulcers, splinter hemorrhages, vesiculobullous lesions).

Microscopic polyangiitis is the most common cause of pulmonary-renal syndromes, being several times more common than anti–glomerular basement membrane disease. Pulmonary hemorrhage may occur with pathologic findings typically of capillaritis. Interstitial lung fibrosis that mimics usual interstitial pneumonitis may be part of the presenting condition and conveys a poor prognosis.

Vasculitic neuropathy (mononeuritis multiplex) is also common in microscopic polyangiitis.

B. Laboratory Findings

Three-fourths of patients with microscopic polyangiitis are ANCA-positive, usually with anti-myeloperoxidase antibodies (MPO-ANCA) that cause a p-ANCA pattern on immunofluorescence testing. ANCA directed against proteinase-3 (PR3-ANCA) can also be observed.

Elevated acute-phase reactants are typical of active disease. Microscopic hematuria, proteinuria, and RBC casts in the urine may occur. The kidney lesion is a segmental, necrotizing glomerulonephritis, often with localized intravascular coagulation and the observation of intraglomerular thrombi upon renal biopsy.

Differential Diagnosis

Distinguishing this disease from granulomatosis with polyangiitis may be challenging. Microscopic polyangiitis is not associated with the chronic destructive upper respiratory tract disease often found in granulomatosis with polyangiitis. As noted, a critical difference between the two diseases is the absence of granulomatous inflammation in microscopic polyangiitis. Because their treatments may differ, microscopic polyangiitis must also be differentiated from polyarteritis nodosa.

Treatment

Microscopic polyangiitis is usually treated in the same way as granulomatosis with polyangiitis: patients with severe disease, typically involving pulmonary hemorrhage and glomerulonephritis, require urgent induction treatment with corticosteroids and either cyclophosphamide or rituximab. Following successful induction of remission, maintenance treatment should be continued with rituximab, as first line, or azathioprine, methotrexate, or mycophenolate (all second-line maintenance therapy). In cases of drug-induced MPO-ANCA–associated vasculitis, the offending medication should be discontinued; significant organ involvement (eg, pulmonary hemorrhage, glomerulonephritis) requires immunosuppressive therapy.

Prognosis

The key to effecting good outcomes is early diagnosis. Compared with patients who have granulomatosis with polyangiitis, those who have microscopic polyangiitis are more likely to have significant fibrosis on renal biopsy because of later diagnosis.

Merkel PA et al. Long-term safety of rituximab in granulomatosis with polyangiitis and in microscopic polyangiitis. Arthritis Care Res (Hoboken). 2021;73:1372. [PMID: 32475029]

Nguyen Y et al. Microscopic polyangiitis: clinical characteristics and long-term outcomes of 378 patients from the French Vasculitis Study Group Registry. J Autoimmun. 2020;112:102467. [PMID: 32340774]

EOSINOPHILIC GRANULOMATOSIS WITH POLYANGIITIS

Eosinophilic granulomatosis with polyangiitis (previously called Churg-Strauss syndrome) is an ANCA-associated vasculitis (along with granulomatosis with polyangiitis and microscopic polyangiitis), although the presence of ANCA occurs in less than 50% of patients (usually anti-MPO). It is characterized by peripheral eosinophilia, sinusitis with polyposis, asthma, lung infiltrates, vasculitic skin involvement, glomerulonephritis, and vasculitic neuropathy. Myocarditis can lead to arrhythmias and heart failure if untreated. Eosinophilic granulomatosis with polyangiitis should be considered in patients with an unexplained peripheral eosinophilia and vasculitis. Laboratory workup for unexplained eosinophilia should include ANCA testing, serum tryptase levels, peripheral flow cytometry for PDGF receptor abnormalities (which can be seen in eosinophilic leukemia) and testing for helminthic infections. Eosinophilic infiltrates on tissue samples strongly suggest the diagnosis of eosinophilic granulomatosis with polyangiitis, especially if accompanied by vasculitis (purpura, glomerulonephritis, vasculitic ulcers, mononeuritis multiplex). Corticosteroids remain first-line treatment with azathioprine and methotrexate demonstrating efficacy for mild to moderate disease. Mepolizumab, an IL-5 inhibitor, is FDA-approved for the treatment of eosinophilic granulomatosis with polyangiitis, although it has not been studied for severe life- or organ-threatening vasculitic disease manifestations (which generally require cyclophosphamide).

Canzian A et al. Use of biologics to treat relapsing and/or refractory eosinophilic granulomatosis with polyangiitis: data from a European collaborative study. Arthritis Rheumatol. 2021;73:498. [PMID: 33001543]

LEVAMISOLE-ASSOCIATED PURPURA

Exposure to levamisole, a prevalent adulterant of illicit cocaine in North America, can induce a distinctive clinical syndrome of retiform purpura and cutaneous necrosis affecting the extremities, ears, and skin overlying the zygomatic arch. The syndrome has been linked to neutropenia, agranulocytosis, and pauci-immune glomerulonephritis. It is associated with the lupus anticoagulant, IgM antibodies to cardiolipin, and very high titers of p-ANCAs (due to autoantibodies to elastase, lactoferrin, cathepsin-G, and other neutrophil components rather than to myeloperoxidase alone). Biopsies reveal widespread thrombosis of small cutaneous vessels with varying degrees of vasculitis. There is no consensus on treatment of levamisole-induced purpura, but early lesions can resolve with abstinence. There may be long-term sequelae of levamisole exposure, such as deforming cutaneous lesions, arthralgias, and arthritis.

Emil NS et al. Atypical chronic inflammatory ANCA-positive deforming arthritis after cocaine-levamisole exposure. J Clin Rheumatol. 2020;26:24. [PMID: 30273264]

CRYOGLOBULINEMIA

Cryoglobulinemia can be associated with an immune-complex–mediated, small-vessel vasculitis. Chronic infection with hepatitis C is the most common underlying condition; cryoglobulinemic vasculitis also can occur with other chronic infections (such as subacute bacterial endocarditis, osteomyelitis, HIV, and hepatitis B), with connective tissue diseases (especially Sjögren syndrome), and with lymphoproliferative disorders. The cryoglobulins associated with vasculitis are cold-precipitable immune complexes consisting of rheumatoid factor and IgG (rheumatoid factor is an autoantibody to the constant region of IgG). The rheumatoid factor component can be monoclonal (type II cryoglobulins) or polyclonal (type III cryoglobulins). Type I cryoglobulins are cryoprecipitable monoclonal proteins that lack rheumatoid factor activity; these cause cold-induced hyperviscosity syndromes, not vasculitis, and are associated with B-cell lymphoproliferative diseases.

▶ Clinical Findings

Cryoglobulinemic vasculitis typically manifests as recurrent palpable purpura (predominantly on the lower extremities) and peripheral neuropathy. A proliferative glomerulonephritis may develop and can manifest as rapidly progressive glomerulonephritis. Abnormal liver biochemical tests, abdominal pain, digital gangrene, and pulmonary disease may also occur. The diagnosis is based on a compatible clinical picture and a positive serum test for cryoglobulins. The presence of a disproportionately low C4 level or rheumatoid factor or both can be diagnostic clues to the presence of cryoglobulinemia.

▶ Treatment

Antiviral regimens are first-line therapy for hepatitis C–associated cryoglobulinemic vasculitis that is neither life- nor organ-threatening. Interferon-free direct-acting antiviral agents are preferred because of the excellent long-term response in clinical trials. Patients with severe cryoglobulinemic vasculitis (eg, extensive digital gangrene, extensive neuropathy, and rapidly progressive glomerulonephritis) and hepatitis C should receive immunosuppressive therapy with corticosteroids and either rituximab or cyclophosphamide plus antiviral treatment. Plasma exchange may provide additional benefit in selected cases. Relapse of vasculitis with cryoglobulinemia following clearing of hepatitis C infection has been reported in a small percentage of patients.

Boleto G et al. Cryoglobulinemia after the era of chronic hepatitis C infection. Semin Arthritis Rheum. 2020;50:695. [PMID: 32521323]

Kolopp-Sarda MN et al. Cryoglobulinemic vasculitis: pathophysiological mechanisms and diagnosis. Curr Opin Rheumatol. 2021;33:1. [PMID: 33186245]

IgA VASCULITIS (Henoch-Schönlein Purpura)

IgA vasculitis (Henoch-Schönlein purpura), the most common systemic vasculitis in children, occurs in adults as well. Typical clinical features are palpable purpura, arthritis, and hematuria. Abdominal pain occurs less frequently in adults than in children. Pathologic features on skin biopsy include leukocytoclastic vasculitis with IgA deposition. Biopsy of the kidney reveals segmental glomerulonephritis with crescents and mesangial deposition of IgA. The cause is not known.

The purpuric skin lesions are typically located on the lower extremities but may also be seen on the hands, arms, trunk, and buttocks. Joint symptoms are present in the majority of patients, with the knees and ankles being most commonly involved. Abdominal pain secondary to vasculitis of the intestinal tract is often associated with GI bleeding. Hematuria signals the presence of a renal lesion that is usually reversible, although it occasionally may progress to CKD (see Henoch-Schönlein purpura, Chapter 22). Children tend to have more frequent and more serious GI vasculitis, whereas adults more often suffer from glomerulonephritis. Chronic courses with persistent or intermittent skin disease are more likely to occur in adults than in children.

The value of corticosteroids has been controversial. In children, prednisone (1–2 mg/kg/day orally) does not decrease the frequency of proteinuria 1 year after onset of disease. Severe disease is often treated with aggressive immunosuppressive agents, but there is no consensus regarding the efficacy of this approach or the optimal therapeutic regimen.

Audemard-Verger A et al. Impact of aging on phenotype and prognosis in IgA vasculitis. Rheumatology (Oxford). 2021; 60:4245. [PMID: 33410479]

Ozen S et al. European consensus-based recommendations for diagnosis and treatment of immunoglobulin A vasculitis—the SHARE initiative. Rheumatology (Oxford). 2019;58:1607. [PMID: 30879080]

RELAPSING POLYCHONDRITIS

This disease is characterized by inflammatory destructive lesions of cartilaginous structures, principally the ears, nose, trachea, and larynx. Nearly 40% of cases are associated with another disease, especially other immunologic disorders (ANCA vasculitis, SLE, rheumatoid arthritis, or Hashimoto thyroiditis), cancers (plasma cell myeloma), or hematologic disorders (myelodysplastic syndrome). Relapsing polychondritis is episodic and affects men and women equally. The cartilage is painful, swollen, and tender during an attack and subsequently becomes atrophic, resulting in permanent deformity. Biopsy of the involved cartilage shows inflammation and chondrolysis. Laryngotracheal and bronchial chondritis can lead to life-threatening airway narrowing and collapse. Noncartilaginous manifestations of the disease include fever, episcleritis, uveitis, deafness, aortic regurgitation, inflammatory arthritis, and rarely, glomerulonephritis. Large vessel vasculitis is a frequently overlooked but potentially catastrophic complication. Diagnosing this uncommon disease is especially difficult since the signs of cartilage inflammation (such as red ears or nasal pain) may be more subtle than the fever, arthritis, rash, or other systemic manifestations and there are no serologic markers for the disease.

Prednisone, 0.5–1 mg/kg/day orally, is often effective. Dapsone (100–200 mg/day orally) or methotrexate (7.5–20 mg orally per week) may also have efficacy, sparing the need for long-term high-dose corticosteroid treatment. Involvement of the tracheobronchial tree may respond to inhibitors of TNF.

A newly described genetic syndrome, VEXAS (vacuoles, E1 enzyme, X-linked, autoinflammatory, somatic), is caused by somatic mutations in *UBA1* in hematopoietic progenitor cells. Clinical features include hematologic manifestations (cytopenias, bone marrow failure) and a spectrum of inflammatory features such as chondritis, vasculitis, fever, and arthritis. This rare syndrome (predominately in males because it is X-linked) should be considered in the differential diagnosis of chondritis especially in the presence of an unexplained macrocytosis and evidence of systemic inflammation (ie, high ESR/CRP).

Ferrada MA et al. Somatic mutations in *UBA1* define a distinct subset of relapsing polychondritis patients with VEXAS. Arthritis Rheumatol. 2021;73:1886. [PMID: 33779074]

Tomelleri A et al. Large-vessel vasculitis affecting the aorta and its branches in relapsing polychondritis: case series and systematic review of the literature. J Rheumatol. 2020;47:1780. [PMID: 31839593]

BEHÇET DISEASE

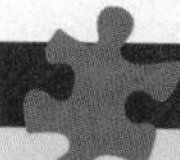

ESSENTIALS OF DIAGNOSIS

- Recurrent, painful oral and genital aphthous ulcers.
- Erythema nodosum–like lesions; follicular rash; pathergy phenomenon.
- Anterior or posterior uveitis. Posterior uveitis may be asymptomatic until significant damage to the retina has occurred.
- Neurologic lesions can mimic multiple sclerosis.

General Considerations

Named after the Turkish dermatologist who first described it, Behçet disease is of unknown cause and most commonly occurs in persons of Asian, Turkish, or Middle Eastern background. The protean manifestations are believed to result from vasculitis that may involve all types of blood vessels: small, medium, and large, on both the arterial and venous side of the circulation.

Clinical Findings

A. Symptoms and Signs

The hallmark of Behçet disease is painful aphthous ulcerations in the mouth. These lesions, which usually are multiple, may be found on the tongue, gums, and inner surfaces of the oral cavity. Genital lesions, similar in appearance, are also common but do not occur in all patients. Other cutaneous lesions of Behçet disease include tender, erythematous, papular lesions that resemble erythema nodosum. On biopsy, however, many of these lesions are shown to be secondary to vasculitis rather than septal panniculitis. These erythema nodosum–like lesions tend to ulcerate, which is a major difference between the lesions of Behçet disease and the erythema nodosum seen in sarcoidosis and IBD. An erythematous follicular rash that occurs frequently on the upper extremities may be a subtle feature of the disease. The **pathergy phenomenon** is frequently underappreciated (unless the patient is asked); in this phenomenon, sterile pustules develop at sites where needles have been inserted into the skin (eg, for phlebotomy).

A nonerosive arthritis occurs in about two-thirds of patients, most commonly affecting the knees and ankles. Eye involvement may be one of the most devastating complications of Behçet disease. Posterior uveitis, in essence a retinal venulitis, may lead to the insidious destruction of large areas of the retina before the patient becomes aware of visual problems. Anterior uveitis, associated with the triad of photophobia, blurred vision, and a red eye, is intensely symptomatic. This complication may lead to a hypopyon, the accumulation of pus in the anterior chamber. If not treated properly, anterior uveitis may lead to synechial formation between the iris and lens, resulting in permanent pupillary distortion.

CNS involvement can cause major morbidity in Bechet disease. Findings include sterile meningitis (recurrent meningeal headaches associated with a lymphocytic pleocytosis), cranial nerve palsies, seizures, encephalitis, mental disturbances, and spinal cord lesions. The CNS lesions may mimic multiple sclerosis radiologically. Aphthous ulcerations of the ileum and cecum and other forms of GI involvement develop in approximately a quarter of patients. Large vessel vasculitis can lead to pulmonary artery aneurysms and life-threatening pulmonary hemorrhage. Finally, patients have a hypercoagulable tendency that may lead to complicated venous thrombotic events, particularly deep venous thromboses, pulmonary emboli, cerebral sinus thrombosis, and other problems associated with clotting.

The clinical course may be chronic but is often characterized by remissions and exacerbations.

B. Laboratory Findings

There are no pathognomonic laboratory features of Behçet disease. Although acute-phase reactants are often elevated, there is no autoantibody or other assay that is distinctive. No markers of hypercoagulability specific to Behçet have been identified. Behçet disease has a genetic risk factor (HLA B51), but this gene is neither necessary nor sufficient to cause the disease.

Treatment

Both colchicine (0.6 mg once to three times daily orally) and topical corticosteroids (oral dexamethasone suspension 1 mg twice daily swish and spit of 0.5 mg/5 mL) may ameliorate the mucocutaneous ulcerative symptoms. Apremilast, a selective phosphodiesterase-4 inhibitor, is FDA-approved for the treatment of oral ulcers in Behçet disease. Corticosteroids (1 mg/kg/day of oral prednisone) are a mainstay of initial therapy for severe disease manifestations. Azathioprine (2 mg/kg/day orally) may be an effective steroid-sparing agent. Infliximab, cyclosporine, or cyclophosphamide is indicated for severe ocular and CNS complications of Behçet disease.

Hatemi G et al. One year in review 2021: Behçet's syndrome. Clin Exp Rheumatol. 2021;39:3. [PMID: 34524077]

Posarelli C et al. Behcet's syndrome and ocular involvement: changes over time. Clin Exp Rheumatol. 2020;38:86. [PMID: 33253088]

PRIMARY ANGIITIS OF THE CENTRAL NERVOUS SYSTEM

Primary angiitis of the CNS is a syndrome with several possible causes that produces small- and medium-sized vasculitis limited to the brain and spinal cord. Biopsy-proved cases have predominated in men who have a history of weeks to months of headaches, encephalopathy, and multifocal strokes. Systemic symptoms and signs are absent, and routine laboratory tests, including ESR and CRP, may be normal. MRI of the brain is almost always abnormal, and the spinal fluid often reveals a mild lymphocytosis and a modest increase in protein level. Angiograms classically reveal a "string of beads" pattern produced by alternating segments of arterial narrowing and dilation. However, neither the MRI nor the angiogram appearance is specific for vasculitis. Indeed, in one study, none of the patients who had biopsy-proved CNS vasculitis had an angiogram showing "the string of beads," and none of the patients with the classic angiographic findings had a positive brain biopsy for vasculitis. Review of many studies suggests that the sensitivity of angiography varies greatly (from 40% to 90%) and the specificity is only approximately 30%. Several conditions, including vasospasm, can produce the same angiographic pattern as vasculitis. Definitive diagnosis requires a compatible clinical picture with exclusion of infection (including subacute bacterial endocarditis), neoplasm (especially intravascular lymphoma), or drug exposure (eg, cocaine) that can mimic primary angiitis of the CNS *and* a positive brain biopsy. In contrast to biopsy-proved cases, patients with angiographically defined CNS vasculopathy are chiefly women who have had an abrupt onset of headaches and stroke (often in the absence of encephalopathy) with normal spinal fluid findings. Many patients who fit this clinical profile may have reversible cerebral vasoconstriction rather than true vasculitis. Such cases are best treated with calcium channel blockers (such as nimodipine or verapamil) and possibly a short course of corticosteroids. Biopsy-proved cases usually improve with prednisone therapy and often require cyclophosphamide. Treatment response correlates with the size of arteries involved: vasculitis of small cortical and leptomeningeal vessels is associated with a better response and outcome than vasculitis of larger arteries. Cases of CNS vasculitis associated with cerebral amyloid angiopathy often respond well to corticosteroids, albeit the long-term natural history remains poorly defined.

Krawezyk M et al. Primary CNS vasculitis: a systematic review on clinical characteristics associated with abnormal biopsy and angiograph. Autoimmun Rev. 2021;20:102714. [PMID: 33197577]

Salvarani C et al. Long-term remission, relapses and maintenance therapy in adult primary central nervous system vasculitis: A single-center 35-year experience. Autoimmun Rev. 2020;19:102497. [PMID: 32062032]

LIVEDO RETICULARIS & LIVEDO RACEMOSA

Livedo reticularis produces a mottled, purplish discoloration of the skin with reticulated cyanotic areas surrounding paler central cores (Figure 20–7). This distinctive "fishnet" pattern is caused by spasm or obstruction of perpendicular arterioles, combined with pooling of blood in surrounding venous plexuses. Idiopathic livedo reticularis is a benign condition that worsens with cold exposure, improves with warming, and primarily affects the extremities. Apart from cosmetic concerns, it is usually asymptomatic. The presence of systemic symptoms or the development of cutaneous ulcerations points to the presence of an underlying disease.

Secondary livedo reticularis, called livedo racemosa, occurs in association with diseases that cause vascular obstruction or inflammation. Livedo racemosa resembles idiopathic livedo reticularis but has a wider skin distribution, including trunk, buttocks, and extremities. Its lesions are more irregular, broken, and circular. Of particular importance is the link with antiphospholipid antibody syndrome. Livedo racemosa is the presenting manifestation in 25% of patients with antiphospholipid antibody syndrome and is strongly associated with the subgroup that has arterial thromboses, including those with antiphospholipid antibody–positive Sneddon syndrome (livedo reticularis and cerebrovascular events). Other underlying causes of livedo racemosa include the vasculitides (particularly polyarteritis nodosa), cholesterol emboli syndrome, thrombocythemia, cryoglobulinemia, cold agglutinin disease, primary hyperoxaluria (due to vascular deposits of calcium oxalate), and disseminated intravascular coagulation.

Weishaupt C et al. Characteristics, risk factors and treatment reality in livedoid vasculopathy—a multicentre analysis. J Eur Acad Dermatol Venereol. 2019;33:1784. [PMID: 31009111]

SERONEGATIVE SPONDYLOARTHROPATHIES

The seronegative spondyloarthropathies are ankylosing spondylitis, psoriatic arthritis, reactive arthritis, the arthritis associated with IBD, and undifferentiated spondyloarthropathy. These disorders are noted for male predominance, onset usually before age 40, inflammatory arthritis of the spine and sacroiliac joints, asymmetric oligoarthritis of large peripheral joints, enthesopathy (inflammation of where ligaments, tendons, and joint capsule insert into bone), ocular inflammation, the absence of autoantibodies, and a striking association with HLA-B27. HLA-B27 is positive in up to 90% of patients with ankylosing spondylitis and 75% with reactive arthritis. HLA-B27 also occurs in 50% of the psoriatic and IBD patients who have sacroiliitis. Patients with only peripheral arthritis in these latter two syndromes do not show an increase in HLA-B27.

AXIAL SPONDYLOARTHRITIS (Ankylosing Spondylitis)

ESSENTIALS OF DIAGNOSIS

- Chronic low backache and stiffness in young adults, worst in the morning.
- Progressive limitation of back motion and chest expansion.
- Transient (50%) or persistent (25%) peripheral arthritis.
- Anterior uveitis in 20–25%.
- Diagnostic radiographic changes in sacroiliac joints.
- Negative serologic tests for rheumatoid factor and anti-CCP antibodies.
- HLA-B27 testing is most helpful when there is an intermediate probability of disease.

General Considerations

Axial spondyloarthritis (SpA) is a general term for inflammatory arthritides that affect the spine and the sacroiliac joints. Axial SpA can be radiographic (changes present on plain radiographs) or nonradiographic. Ankylosing spondylitis, the prototypic radiographic axial SpA, is a chronic inflammatory disease of the joints of the axial skeleton, manifested clinically by pain and progressive fusion of the spine. The age at onset is usually in the late teens or early 20s. The incidence is greater in males than in females.

Clinical Findings

A. Symptoms and Signs

The onset is usually gradual, with intermittent bouts of back pain that may radiate into the buttocks. The back pain is worse in the morning and associated with stiffness that lasts hours. Pain and stiffness improve with activity, in contrast to back pain due to mechanical causes, which improves with rest and worsens with activity. As the disease advances, symptoms progress in a cephalad direction and back motion becomes limited, with the normal lumbar curve flattened and the thoracic curvature exaggerated. Chest expansion is often limited due to costovertebral joint involvement. In advanced cases, the entire spine becomes fused, allowing no motion in any direction. Transient acute arthritis of the peripheral joints occurs in about 50% of cases, and permanent changes in the peripheral joints—most commonly the hips, shoulders, and knees—are seen in about 25%. Enthesopathy, a hallmark of the spondyloarthropathies, can manifest as swelling of the Achilles tendon at its insertion, plantar fasciitis (producing heel pain), or dactylitis, which is fusiform "sausage" swelling of a finger or toe.

Anterior uveitis is associated in up to 25% of cases and may be a presenting feature of ankylosing spondylitis. Cardiac involvement, characterized by atrioventricular conduction defects, aortic regurgitation, or aortic root widening, occurs in 3–5% of patients with longstanding severe disease. Pulmonary fibrosis of the upper lobes, with progression to cavitation and bronchiectasis mimicking tuberculosis, may rarely occur, characteristically long after the onset of skeletal symptoms.

B. Laboratory Findings

The ESR is elevated in 85% of cases, but rheumatoid factor and anti-CCP antibodies, which are usually positive in rheumatoid arthritis, are negative. The presence of elevated ESR or CRP conveys increased risk of disease progression and accumulation of damage. Anemia of chronic disease may be present but is often mild. HLA-B27 is found in 90% of White patients and 50% of Black patients with ankylosing spondylitis. Because this antigen occurs in 8% of the healthy White persons and 2% of healthy Black persons, it is not a specific diagnostic test but is most useful when there is intermediate probability of disease.

C. Imaging

The earliest radiographic changes are usually in the sacroiliac joints. In the first 2 years of the disease, sacroiliac changes may be detectable only by MRI. Indeed, patients who have symptoms and findings of ankylosing spondylitis and sacroiliitis evident by MRI but not by conventional radiographs are classified as having nonradiographic axial spondyloarthritis. With disease progression, erosion and sclerosis of the sacroiliac joints become evident on plain radiographs. The sacroiliitis of ankylosing spondylitis is bilateral and symmetric. Inflammation where the annulus fibrosus attaches to the vertebral bodies initially causes sclerosis ("the shiny corner sign") and then characteristic squaring of the vertebral bodies. The term "bamboo spine" describes the late radiographic appearance of the spinal column in which the vertebral bodies are fused by vertically oriented, bridging syndesmophytes formed by the ossification of the annulus fibrosus and calcification of the anterior and lateral spinal ligaments.

Differential Diagnosis

Low back pain due to mechanical causes, disk disease, and degenerative arthritis is very common. Onset of back pain before age 30 and an "inflammatory" quality of the back pain (ie, profound morning stiffness and pain that improve with activity) should raise the possibility of ankylosing spondylitis. In contrast to ankylosing spondylitis, rheumatoid arthritis predominantly affects multiple, small, peripheral joints of the hands and feet. Rheumatoid arthritis spares the sacroiliac joints and only affects the cervical component of the spine. Bilateral sacroiliitis indistinguishable from ankylosing spondylitis is seen with the spondylitis associated with IBD. Sacroiliitis associated with reactive arthritis and psoriasis, on the other hand, is often asymmetric or even unilateral. Osteitis condensans ilii (sclerosis on the iliac side of the sacroiliac joint) is an asymptomatic, postpartum radiographic finding that is occasionally mistaken for sacroiliitis. Diffuse idiopathic skeletal hyperostosis (DISH) causes exuberant osteophytes ("enthesophytes") of the spine that may be difficult to distinguish from the syndesmophytes of ankylosing spondylitis. The enthesophytes of DISH are thicker and more anterior than the syndesmophytes of ankylosing spondylitis, and sacroiliac joints are normal in DISH.

Treatment

NSAIDs remain first-line treatment of ankylosing spondylitis. TNF inhibitors have established efficacy for NSAID-resistant axial disease; responses are often substantial and durable. TNF inhibitors may also have disease-modifying effects and slow radiographic progression. Secukinumab and ixekizumab inhibit the proinflammatory cytokine IL-17A; these agents are highly effective and FDA-approved for the treatment of ankylosing spondylitis. Corticosteroids have minimal impact on the arthritis—particularly the spondylitis—of ankylosing spondylitis and can worsen osteopenia. All patients should be referred to a physical therapist for instruction in postural exercises and a safe exercise program.

Prognosis

Most patients have persistent symptoms over decades; rare individuals experience long-term remissions. The severity of disease varies greatly, with about 10% of patients having work disability after 10 years. Developing hip disease within the first 2 years of disease onset presages a worse prognosis. Biologic agents provide symptomatic relief, improve quality of life, and may slow disease progression for many patients with ankylosing spondylitis.

Koo BS et al. Tumour necrosis factor inhibitors slow radiographic progression in patients with ankylosing spondylitis: 18-year real-world evidence. Ann Rheum Dis. 2020;79:1327. [PMID: 32660979]

Sari I et al. Factors predictive of radiographic progression in ankylosing spondylitis. Arthritis Care Res (Hoboken). 2021;73:275. [PMID: 31675169]

PSORIATIC ARTHRITIS

ESSENTIALS OF DIAGNOSIS

- Psoriasis precedes arthritis in 80% of cases.
- **Arthritis:** usually asymmetric, with "sausage" appearance of fingers and toes (dactylitis); polyarthritis that may resemble rheumatoid arthritis.
- Sacroiliac joint involvement common.
- **Radiographic findings:** osteolysis; pencil-in-cup deformity; relative lack of osteoporosis; bony ankylosis; asymmetric sacroiliitis and atypical syndesmophytes.

General Considerations

Although psoriasis usually precedes the onset of arthritis, arthritis may precede skin disease by up to 2 years or occur simultaneously in approximately 20% of cases.

Clinical Findings

A. Symptoms and Signs

The patterns or subsets of joint involvement in psoriatic arthritis include the following:

1. A symmetric polyarthritis that resembles rheumatoid arthritis. Usually, fewer joints are involved than in rheumatoid arthritis.
2. An oligoarthritis that may lead to considerable destruction of the affected joints.
3. A pattern of disease in which the DIP joints are primarily affected. Early, this may be monoarticular, and often the joint involvement is asymmetric. Nail pitting and onycholysis frequently accompany DIP involvement.
4. A severe deforming arthritis (arthritis mutilans) with osteolysis.
5. A spondylitic form in which sacroiliitis and spinal involvement predominate; 50% of these patients are HLA-B27 positive.

Arthritis is at least five times more common in patients with severe psoriatic skin disease than in those with only mild skin findings. Occasionally, however, patients may have a single patch of psoriasis (typically hidden in the scalp, gluteal cleft, or umbilicus) and are unaware of its presence. Thus, a detailed search for cutaneous lesions is essential in patients with arthritis of new onset. Also, the psoriatic lesions may have cleared when arthritis appears—in such cases, the history is most useful in diagnosing previously unexplained cases of monoarthritis or oligoarthritis. Nail pitting is sometimes a clue. "Sausage" swelling, or dactylitis, of one or more digits is a common manifestation of enthesopathy in psoriatic arthritis.

B. Laboratory Findings

The ESR is elevated in approximately 50% of patients with psoriatic arthritis; normal values do not rule out the diagnosis. Rheumatoid factor and anti-CCP antibodies are not present. Uric acid levels may be high, reflecting the active turnover of skin affected by psoriasis.

C. Imaging

Radiographic findings are most helpful in distinguishing the disease from other forms of arthritis. There are marginal erosions of bone and irregular destruction of joint and bone, which, in the phalanx, may give the appearance of a sharpened pencil. Fluffy periosteal new bone may be marked, especially at the insertion of muscles and ligaments into bone. Such changes will also be seen along the shafts of metacarpals, metatarsals, and phalanges. Psoriatic spondylitis causes asymmetric sacroiliitis and syndesmophytes. In psoriatic arthritis as in ankylosing spondylitis, MRI is more sensitive in detecting axial abnormalities than conventional radiographs, especially in the first few years of disease onset. Ultrasonography and MRI are more sensitive than conventional radiographs in detecting peripheral arthritis, enthesitis, and dactylitis.

Treatment

In patients with active psoriatic arthritis, a TNF inhibitor biologic agent is recommended as first-line agent. If a TNF inhibitor is contraindicated or not tolerated, methotrexate (or non-biologic agents, such as leflunomide, sulfasalazine, cyclosporine, or apremilast) may be effective.

Patients who do not respond to TNF inhibitors or oral small molecule agents can be treated with ustekinumab, a monoclonal antibody that inhibits IL-12 and IL-23; r an IL-17 inhibitor, secukinumab, or ixekizumab or IL-23 inhibitor, guselkumab. Tofacitinib (JAK-STAT inhibitor) and abatacept (CTLA4 inhibitor) may be options with failure of the above therapies. Corticosteroids are less effective in psoriatic arthritis than in other forms of inflammatory arthritis and may precipitate pustular psoriasis during tapers.

McInnes IB et al. Efficacy and safety of guselkumab, an interleukin-23p19-specific monoclonal antibody, through one year in biologic-naive patients with psoriatic arthritis. Arthritis Rheumatol. 2021;73:604. [PMID: 33043600]

REACTIVE ARTHRITIS

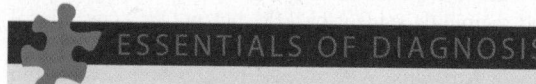

- Oligoarthritis, conjunctivitis, urethritis, keratoderma blennorrhagicum, and mouth ulcers.
- Usually follows dysentery or a sexually transmitted infection.
- HLA-B27–positive in 50–80% of patients.

General Considerations

Reactive arthritis is precipitated by antecedent GI or genitourinary infections. and manifests as an asymmetric sterile oligoarthritis, typically of the lower extremities. It is frequently associated with enthesitis. Extra-articular manifestations are common and include urethritis, conjunctivitis, uveitis, keratoderma blennorrhagicum, and mucocutaneous lesions. Reactive arthritis occurs most commonly in young men and is associated with HLA-B27 in 80% of White patients and 50–60% of Black patients.

Clinical Findings

A. Symptoms and Signs

Most cases of reactive arthritis develop within 1–4 weeks after either a GI infection (usually with *Shigella, Salmonella, Yersinia, or Campylobacter*) or a sexually transmitted infection (with *Chlamydia trachomatis* or perhaps *Ureaplasma urealyticum*). Whether the inciting infection is sexually transmitted or dysenteric does not affect the subsequent manifestations but does influence the gender ratio. The spectrum of pathogens known to cause reactive arthritis is broadening to include *Mycobacterium, Staphylococcus*, and SARS-CoV-2. Synovial fluid from affected joints is culture-negative. A clinically indistinguishable syndrome can occur without an apparent antecedent infection, suggesting that subclinical infection can precipitate reactive arthritis or that there are other, as yet unrecognized, triggers.

The arthritis is most commonly asymmetric and frequently involves the large weight-bearing joints (knee and ankle); sacroiliitis or ankylosing spondylitis is observed in at least 20% of patients, especially after frequent recurrences. Systemic symptoms including fever and weight loss are common at the onset of disease. The mucocutaneous lesions may include balanitis (Figure 20–9), stomatitis, and keratoderma blennorrhagicum, indistinguishable from pustular psoriasis. Involvement of the fingernails in reactive arthritis mimics psoriatic changes. When present, conjunctivitis is mild and occurs early in the disease course. Anterior uveitis, which can develop at any time in HLA-B27–positive patients, is a more clinically significant ocular complication. Carditis and aortic regurgitation may occur. While most signs of the disease disappear within days or weeks, the arthritis may persist for several months or become chronic. Recurrences involving any combination of the clinical manifestations are common and are

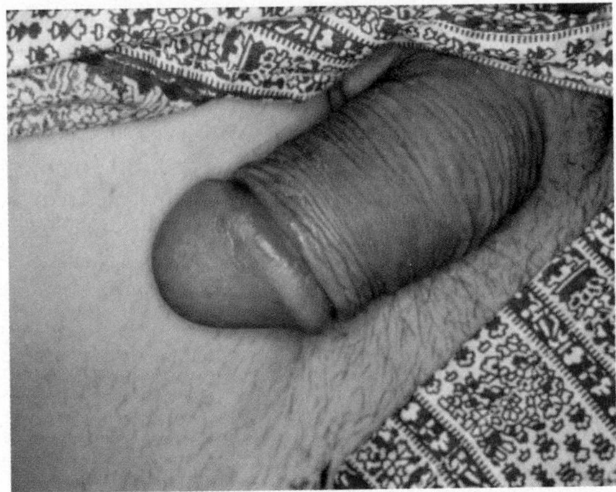

▲ **Figure 20–9.** Circinate balanitis due to reactive arthritis. (From Susan Lindsley, Dr. M. F. Rein, Public Health Image Library, CDC.)

sometimes followed by permanent sequelae, especially in the joints (eg, articular destruction).

B. Imaging

Radiographic signs of permanent or progressive joint disease may be seen in the sacroiliac and peripheral joints.

Differential Diagnosis

Gonococcal arthritis can initially mimic reactive arthritis, but the marked improvement after 24–48 hours of antibiotic administration in gonococcal arthritis and the culture results distinguish the two disorders. Rheumatoid arthritis, ankylosing spondylitis, and psoriatic arthritis must also be considered. By causing similar oral, ocular, and joint lesions, Behçet disease may mimic reactive arthritis. The oral lesions of reactive arthritis, however, are typically painless, in contrast to those of Behçet disease.

Treatment

NSAIDs have been the mainstay of therapy. Antibiotics given at the time of a nongonococcal sexually transmitted infection reduce the chance that the individual will develop this disorder. For chronic reactive arthritis associated with chlamydial infection, a randomized trial demonstrated that 6 months of rifampin (300 mg orally twice daily) in combination with either doxycycline (100 mg orally twice daily) or azithromycin (500 mg orally daily for 5 days then twice weekly) was more effective than placebo. Patients who do not respond to NSAIDs may respond to sulfasalazine or methotrexate. For those patients with recent-onset disease that is refractory to NSAIDs and these DMARDs, anti-TNF agents, which are effective in the other spondyloarthropathies, may be effective.

Taniguchi Y et al. Expanding the spectrum of reactive arthritis (ReA): classic ReA and infection-related arthritis including poststreptococcal ReA, Poncet's disease, and iBCG-induced ReA. Rheumatol Int. 2021;41:1387. [PMID: 33939015]

INFLAMMATORY BOWEL DISEASE–ASSOCIATED SPONDYLOARTHRITIS

One-fifth of patients with IBD have arthritis, which complicates Crohn disease somewhat more frequently than it does ulcerative colitis. In both diseases, two distinct forms of arthritis occur. The first is peripheral arthritis—usually a nondeforming asymmetric oligoarthritis of large joints—in which the activity of the joint disease parallels that of the bowel disease. The arthritis usually begins months to years after the bowel disease, but occasionally the joint symptoms develop earlier and may be prominent enough to cause the patient to overlook intestinal symptoms. The second form of arthritis is a spondylitis that is indistinguishable by symptoms or radiographs from ankylosing spondylitis and follows a course independent of the bowel disease. About 50% of these patients are HLA-B27 positive.

Controlling the intestinal inflammation usually eliminates the peripheral arthritis. NSAIDs can be effective when the arthritis is mild but must be used cautiously since they can exacerbate IBD. TNF inhibitors are useful therapies because they are effective both for the bowel and joints.

Levine I et al. Prevalence, predictors, and disease activity of sacroiliitis among patients with Crohn's disease. Inflamm Bowel Dis. 2021;27:809. [PMID: 32793977]

INFECTIOUS ARTHRITIS

NONGONOCOCCAL ACUTE BACTERIAL (Septic) ARTHRITIS

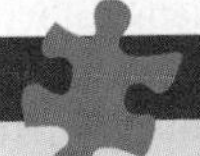

ESSENTIALS OF DIAGNOSIS

- Acute onset of inflammatory monoarticular arthritis, most often in large weight-bearing joints and wrists.
- Common risk factors include previous joint damage and injection drug use.
- Infection with causative organism commonly found elsewhere in body.
- Joint effusions are usually large; synovial fluid WBC counts > 50,000/mcL (50×10^9/L) are common.

General Considerations

Lyme disease is discussed in Chapter 34.

Nongonococcal acute bacterial arthritis is most often due to hematogenous seeding of the joint; direct inoculation from penetrating trauma is rare. The key risk factors are bacteremia (eg, injection drug use, endocarditis, infection at other sites), damaged joints (eg, rheumatoid arthritis), prosthetic joints, compromised immunity (eg, advanced age, diabetes mellitus, advanced CKD, alcohol use disorder, cirrhosis, or immunosuppressive therapy), and loss of skin integrity (eg, cutaneous ulcer or psoriasis). *Staphylococcus aureus* is the most common cause of nongonococcal septic arthritis, accounting for about 50% of all cases. Methicillin-resistant *S aureus* (MRSA) and group B *Streptococcus* are frequent and important causes of septic arthritis. Gram-negative septic arthritis causes about 10% of cases and is especially common in injection drug users and immunocompromised persons; *Escherichia coli* and *Pseudomonas aeruginosa* are the most common pathogens. Pathologic changes include varying degrees of acute inflammation, with synovitis, effusion, abscess formation in synovial or subchondral tissues, and, if treatment is not adequate, articular destruction.

Clinical Findings

A. Symptoms and Signs

The onset is acute, with pain, swelling, and heat of the affected joint worsening over hours. The knee is most frequently involved; other commonly affected sites are the hip, wrist, shoulder, and ankle. Unusual sites, such as the sternoclavicular or sacroiliac joint, can be involved in injection drug users. Chills and fever are common but are absent in up to 20% of patients. Infection of the hip usually does not produce apparent swelling but results in groin pain aggravated by walking. More than one joint is involved in 15% of cases of septic arthritis; risk factors for multiple joint involvement include rheumatoid arthritis, associated endocarditis, and infection with group B streptococci.

B. Laboratory Findings

Synovial fluid analysis is critical for diagnosis. The leukocyte count of the synovial fluid is always inflammatory (greater than 2000/mcL [2×10^9/L]), usually exceeds 50,000/mcL (50×10^9/L), and often is more than 100,000/mcL (100×10^9/L), with 90% or more polymorphonuclear cells (Table 20–2). Synovial fluid cell count in septic arthritis may be lower in immunocompromised patients, especially those on biologic therapies such as TNF inhibitors. Gram stain of the synovial fluid is positive in 75% of staphylococcal infections and in 50% of gram-negative infections. Synovial fluid cultures are positive in 70–90% of cases; administration of antibiotics prior to arthrocentesis reduces the likelihood of a positive culture result. Blood cultures are positive in approximately 50% of patients.

C. Imaging

Imaging tests generally add little to the diagnosis of septic arthritis. Other than demonstrating joint effusion, radiographs are usually normal early in the disease; however, evidence of demineralization may develop within days of onset. MRI and CT are more sensitive in detecting fluid in joints that are not accessible to physical examination (eg, the hip). Bony erosions and narrowing of the joint space followed by osteomyelitis and periostitis may be seen within 2 weeks.

D. Prosthetic Joint Infection

The clinical and laboratory manifestations of prosthetic joint infection are influenced by whether the infection is early (less than 3 months after surgery), delayed (3–12 months after surgery), or late (more than 12 months after surgery). Early infections present with acute redness and swelling and are usually caused by *S aureus* and gram-negative organisms. Delayed infections often present with subtle manifestations: pain is common but only 50% of patients will have fever. Less virulent organisms, such as coagulase-negative *Staphylococcus*, *Propionibacterium acnes*, and enterococci, are common causes of delayed infections. Late infections present with acute pain, swelling, and fever and are often caused by hematogenous seeding of *S aureus*, gram-negative bacilli, and hemolytic streptococci.

Differential Diagnosis

Gout and pseudogout can cause acute, very inflammatory monoarticular arthritis and fever; failure to find crystals on synovial fluid analysis excludes these diagnoses. The most common articular manifestation of chronic Lyme disease is inflammatory monoarthritis of the knee, which yields synovial fluid that is Gram stain and culture negative. Acute rheumatic fever commonly involves an inflammatory migratory oligoarthritis. Pyogenic arthritis may be superimposed on other types of joint disease, notably rheumatoid arthritis. Septic arthritis must be excluded by joint fluid examination in any patient with rheumatoid arthritis who has a joint strikingly more inflamed than the other joints, especially if the patient is receiving biologic DMARD therapy.

Prevention

The American Academy of Orthopedic Surgeons advocates prescribing antibiotic prophylaxis for any patient with a prosthetic joint replacement who undergoes a procedure that can cause bacteremia. However, the topic remains controversial.

Treatment

The effective treatment of septic arthritis requires appropriate antibiotic therapy together with drainage of the infected joint. Hospitalization is always necessary. If the likely causative organism cannot be determined clinically or from the synovial fluid Gram stain, treatment should be started with broad-spectrum antibiotic coverage effective against staphylococci, streptococci, and gram-negative organisms. The recommended initial treatment is to vancomycin (1 g intravenously every 12 hours, adjusted for age, weight, and renal function) plus a third-generation cephalosporin: ceftriaxone, 1–2 g intravenously daily (or every 12 hours if concomitant meningitis or endocarditis is suspected); or cefotaxime, 1–2 g intravenously every 8 hours. Antibiotic therapy should be adjusted when culture results become available; the duration of antibiotic therapy is usually 4–6 weeks.

Early orthopedic consultation is essential. Effective drainage is usually achieved through early arthroscopic lavage and debridement. Options for treating prosthetic joint infections depend, in part, on the timing of the infection and include chronic suppression, debridement without removal of the prosthesis, or one- or two-stage exchange of the prosthesis.

Prognosis

The outcome of septic arthritis depends largely on the antecedent health of the patient, the causative organism (eg, *S aureus* bacterial arthritis is associated with a poor functional outcome in about 40% of cases), and the promptness of treatment. The mortality rate is 30% for patients with polyarticular sepsis. Bony ankylosis and articular destruction commonly occur if treatment is delayed or inadequate.

Goff DS et al. Review of guidelines for dental antibiotic prophylaxis for prevention of endocarditis and prosthetic joint infections and need for dental stewardship. Clin Infect Dis. 2020;71:455. [PMID: 31728507]

Mabille C et al. Medical versus surgical treatment in native hip and knee septic arthritis. Infect Dis Now. 2021;51:164. [PMID: 32387296]

GONOCOCCAL ARTHRITIS

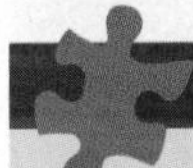

ESSENTIALS OF DIAGNOSIS

- Prodromal migratory polyarthralgias.
- Tenosynovitis is the most common sign.
- Purulent monoarthritis in 50%.
- Characteristic skin lesions.
- Most common in young women during menses or pregnancy.
- Symptoms of urethritis frequently absent.
- Dramatic response to antibiotics.

General Considerations

In contrast to nongonococcal bacterial arthritis, gonococcal arthritis usually occurs in otherwise healthy individuals. Host factors, however, influence the expression of the disease: gonococcal arthritis is two to three times more common in women than in men, is especially common during menses and pregnancy, and is rare after age 40. Gonococcal arthritis is also common in men who have sex with men, whose high incidence of asymptomatic gonococcal pharyngitis and proctitis predisposes them to disseminated gonococcal infection. Recurrent disseminated gonococcal infection should prompt testing of the patient's CH50 level to evaluate for a congenital deficiency of a terminal complement component (C5, C6, C7, or C8).

Clinical Findings

A. Symptoms and Signs

One to 4 days of migratory polyarthralgias involving the wrist, knee, ankle, or elbow are common at the outset. Thereafter, two patterns emerge. The first pattern is characterized by tenosynovitis that most often affects the wrists, fingers, ankles, or toes and is seen in 60% of patients. The second pattern is purulent monoarthritis that most frequently involves the knee, wrist, ankle, or elbow and is seen in 40% of patients. Less than half of patients have fever, and less than one-fourth have any genitourinary symptoms. Most patients will have asymptomatic, but highly characteristic, skin lesions that usually consist of 2 to 10 small necrotic pustules distributed over the extremities, especially the palms and soles.

B. Laboratory Findings

The peripheral blood leukocyte count averages about 10,000 cells/mcL (10×10^9/L) and is elevated in less than one-third of patients. The synovial fluid WBC count usually ranges from 30,000 to 60,000 cells/mcL ($30–60 \times 10^9$/L). The synovial fluid Gram stain is positive in one-fourth of cases and culture in less than half. Positive blood cultures are uncommon. Urethral, throat, cervical, and rectal cultures should be done in all patients, and are often positive in the absence of local symptoms. Urinary nucleic acid amplification tests have excellent sensitivity and specificity for the detection of *Neisseria gonorrhoeae* in genitourinary sites.

C. Imaging

Radiographs are usually normal or show only soft tissue swelling.

Differential Diagnosis

Reactive arthritis can produce acute monoarthritis, urethritis, and fever in a young person but is distinguished by negative cultures and failure to respond to antibiotics. Lyme disease involving the knee is less acute, does not show positive cultures, and may be preceded by known tick exposure and characteristic rash. The synovial fluid analysis will exclude gout, pseudogout, and nongonococcal bacterial arthritis. Rheumatic fever and sarcoidosis can produce migratory tenosynovitis. Infective endocarditis with septic arthritis can mimic disseminated gonococcal infection. Meningococcemia occasionally presents with a clinical picture that resembles disseminated gonococcal infection; blood cultures establish the correct diagnosis. Rocky mountain spotted fever and dengue can produce arthritis and skin findings. Early hepatitis B infection is associated with circulating immune complexes that can cause an urticarial rash and polyarthralgias.

Treatment

The treatment of disseminated gonorrhea (arthritis-dermatitis syndrome) per CDC guidelines is ceftriaxone (1 g daily intravenously or intramuscularly). Once susceptibility testing has been obtained, 24–48 hours after clinical improvement, the antibiotic regimen can be changed to an oral agent to complete a 7-day course.

Prognosis

Generally, gonococcal arthritis responds dramatically in 24–48 hours after initiation of antibiotics, and drainage of the infected joint(s) is rarely needed. Complete recovery is the rule.

Centers for Disease Control and Prevention (CDC). Sexually Transmitted Infections Treatment Guidelines, 2021: gonococcal infections among adolescents and adults. https://www.cdc.gov/std/treatment-guidelines/gonorrhea-adults.htm

RHEUMATIC MANIFESTATIONS OF HIV INFECTION

Infection with HIV has been associated with various rheumatic symptoms and may coexist with autoimmune rheumatic diseases, such as rheumatoid arthritis, psoriatic arthritis, or spondyloarthritis. Acute new HIV infection (viremia) causes severe arthralgias in an oligoarticular, asymmetric pattern that resolve within 24 hours; the joint examination is normal. HIV-associated arthritis is an asymmetric oligoarticular process with objective findings of arthritis and a self-limited course that ranges from weeks to months. Along with antiretroviral therapies, immunosuppressive medications can be used if necessary in HIV-infected patients, though with caution. Muscle weakness associated with an elevated creatine kinase can be due to nucleoside reverse transcriptase inhibitor–associated myopathy or HIV-associated myopathy; the clinical presentations of each resemble idiopathic polymyositis but the muscle biopsies show minimal inflammation. Less commonly, an inflammatory myositis indistinguishable from idiopathic polymyositis occurs. Other rheumatic manifestations of HIV include diffuse infiltrative lymphocytosis syndrome (with parotid gland enlargement) and various forms of vasculitis.

VIRAL ARTHRITIS

Arthralgias occur frequently in the course of acute infections with many viruses, but frank arthritis is uncommon with the notable exceptions of acute parvovirus B19 infection and Chikungunya fever. Parvovirus B19 causes an acute polyarthritis in 50–60% of adult cases (infected children develop the febrile exanthem known as "slapped cheek fever"). The arthritis can mimic rheumatoid arthritis but is almost always self-limited and resolves within several weeks. The diagnosis is established by the presence of IgM antibodies specific for parvovirus B19. Chikungunya fever is an arthropod-borne viral infection that is endemic to West Africa but has spread to multiple locations including the Indian Ocean islands, the Caribbean and Central and Latin America. Clinical manifestations include high fever, rash, and incapacitating bone pain. Acute polyarthralgia and polyarthritis are common and can persist for months or years. For Chikungunya-associated chronic arthritis, treatment with methotrexate or other DMARD agents may be an option.

Self-limited polyarthritis is common in acute hepatitis B infection and typically occurs before the onset of jaundice. Urticaria or other types of skin rash may be present. The clinical picture resembles that of serum sickness. Serum transaminase levels are elevated, and tests for hepatitis B surface antigen are positive. Serum complement levels are often low during active arthritis and become normal after remission of arthritis. The incidence of hepatitis B–associated polyarthritis has fallen substantially with the introduction of hepatitis B vaccination.

Chronic infection with hepatitis C is associated with chronic polyarthralgia (up to 20% of cases) and with chronic polyarthritis (3–5%). This can mimic rheumatoid arthritis; the presence of rheumatoid factor in most hepatitis C infections leads to further diagnostic confusion. Distinguishing hepatitis C–associated arthritis/arthralgias from the co-occurrence of hepatitis C and rheumatoid arthritis can be difficult. Rheumatoid arthritis always causes objective arthritis (not just arthralgias) and can be erosive (hepatitis C–associated arthritis is nonerosive). The presence of anti-CCP antibodies helps to diagnose rheumatoid arthritis.

Adarsh MB et al. Methotrexate in early Chikungunya arthritis: a 6 month randomized controlled open-label trial. Curr Rheumatol Rev. 2020;16:319. [PMID: 31858912]

TUBERCULOSIS OF BONES & JOINTS

SPINAL TUBERCULOSIS (Pott Disease)

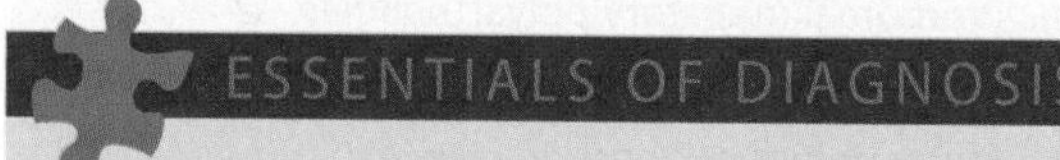

- Seen primarily in individuals from developing countries or immunocompromised patients.
- Back pain and gibbus deformity with radiographic evidence of vertebral involvement.
- Less than 20% have active pulmonary tuberculosis.
- Evidence of *Mycobacterium tuberculosis* in aspirate or biopsies of spinal lesions.

General Considerations

In the developing world, children primarily bear the burden of musculoskeletal tuberculosis. In the United States, however, musculoskeletal infection is more often seen in adults who have immigrated from countries where tuberculosis is prevalent, or it develops in the setting of immunosuppression (eg, HIV infection, therapy with biologic agent). Spinal tuberculosis (Pott disease) accounts for about 50% of musculoskeletal infection due to *M tuberculosis* (see Chapter 9). Seeding of the vertebrae may occur through hematogenous spread from the respiratory tract at the time of primary infection, with clinical disease developing years later due to reactivation, or through lymphatics from infected foci in the pleura or kidneys. The thoracic and lumbar vertebrae are the most common sites of spinal involvement; vertebral infection is associated with paravertebral cold abscesses in 75% of cases.

Clinical Findings

A. Symptoms and Signs

Patients have back pain, often present for months and sometimes associated with radicular pain and lower extremity weakness. Constitutional symptoms are usually absent, and less than 20% have active pulmonary disease. Destruction of the vertebral body anteriorly can produce the characteristic wedge-shaped gibbus deformity.

B. Laboratory Findings

Most patients have a positive reaction to purified protein derivative (PPD) or a positive interferon-gamma release assay. Cultures of paravertebral abscesses and biopsies of vertebral lesions are positive in up to 70–90%. Biopsies reveal characteristic caseating granulomas in most cases. Isolation of *M tuberculosis* from an extraspinal site is sufficient to establish the diagnosis in the proper clinical setting.

C. Imaging

Radiographs can reveal lytic and sclerotic lesions and bony destruction of vertebrae but are normal early in the disease course. CT scanning can demonstrate paraspinal soft tissue extensions of the infection; MRI is the imaging technique of choice to detect compression of the spinal cord or cauda equina.

Differential Diagnosis

Spinal tuberculosis must be differentiated from subacute and chronic spinal infections due to pyogenic organisms, *Brucella*, fungi, and malignancy.

Complications

Paraplegia due to compression of the spinal cord or cauda equina is the most serious complication of spinal tuberculosis.

Treatment

Antimicrobial therapy should be administered for 6–9 months, usually in the form of isoniazid, rifampin, pyrazinamide, and ethambutol for 2 months followed by isoniazid and rifampin for an additional 4–7 months (see also Chapter 9). Medical management alone is often sufficient. Surgical intervention, however, may be indicated when there is neurologic compromise or severe spinal instability.

Guillouzouic A et al. Treatment of bone and joint tuberculosis in France: a multicentre retrospective study. J Clin Med. 2020;9:2529. [PMID: 32764500]

Kim JH et al. Prognostic factors for unfavourable outcomes of patients with spinal tuberculosis in a country with an intermediate tuberculosis burden: a multicentre cohort study. Bone Joint J. 2019;101:1542. [PMID: 31786996]

TUBERCULOUS ARTHRITIS

Infection of peripheral joints by *M tuberculosis* usually presents as a monoarticular arthritis lasting for weeks to months (or longer), but less often, it can have an acute presentation that mimics septic arthritis. Any joint can be involved; the hip and knee are most commonly affected. Constitutional symptoms and fever are present in only a small number of cases. Tuberculosis also can cause a chronic tenosynovitis of the hand and wrist. Joint destruction occurs far more slowly than in septic arthritis due to pyogenic organisms. Synovial fluid is inflammatory but not to the degree seen in pyogenic infections, with synovial white cell counts in the range of 10,000–20,000 cells/mcL ($10–20 \times 10^9$/L). Smears of synovial fluid are positive for acid-fast bacilli in a minority of cases; synovial fluid cultures, however, are positive in 80% of cases. Because culture results may take weeks, the diagnostic procedure of choice usually is synovial biopsy, which yields characteristic pathologic findings and positive cultures in greater than 90%. Antimicrobial therapy is the mainstay of treatment. Rarely, a reactive, sterile polyarthritis associated with erythema nodosum (Poncet disease) develops in patients with active pulmonary or extrapulmonary tuberculosis.

McGuire E et al. Extraspinal articular tuberculosis: an 11-year retrospective study of demographic features and clinical outcomes in East London. J Infect. 2020;81:383. [PMID: 32579987]

MISCELLANEOUS RHEUMATOLOGIC DISORDERS

FIBROMYALGIA

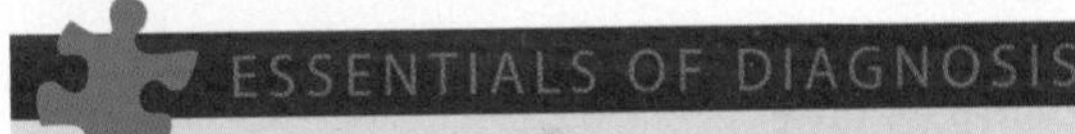

- Most frequent in women aged 20–50.
- Chronic widespread musculoskeletal pain syndrome with multiple tender points.
- Fatigue, headaches, numbness common.
- Objective signs of inflammation absent; laboratory studies normal.

General Considerations

Fibromyalgia is a common syndrome, affecting 3–10% of the general population. It shares many features with myalgic encephalomyelitis/chronic fatigue syndrome, namely, an increased frequency among women aged 20–50, absence of objective findings, and absence of diagnostic laboratory test results. While many of the clinical features of the two conditions overlap, musculoskeletal pain predominates in fibromyalgia, whereas lassitude dominates myalgic encephalomyelitis/chronic fatigue syndrome.

The cause is unknown, but aberrant perception of painful stimuli, sleep disorders, depression, and viral infections have all been proposed. Fibromyalgia may coexist with other rheumatic and medical conditions, such as SLE, hypothyroidism, rheumatoid arthritis, or sleep apnea.

Clinical Findings

The patient complains of chronic aching pain and stiffness, frequently involving the entire body but with prominence of pain around the neck, shoulders, low back, and hips. Fatigue, sleep disorders, subjective numbness with paresthesias, chronic headaches, and irritable bowel symptoms are common. Even minor exertion aggravates pain and increases fatigue. Physical examination is normal except for "trigger points" of pain produced by palpation of various areas such as the trapezius, the medial fat pad of the knee, and the lateral epicondyle of the elbow.

Differential Diagnosis

Fibromyalgia is a diagnosis of exclusion. A detailed history and repeated physical examination can obviate the need for extensive laboratory testing. Rheumatoid arthritis and SLE present with objective physical findings and laboratory abnormalities. Thyroid function tests are useful since hypothyroidism can produce a fibromyalgia-like syndrome. The idiopathic inflammatory myopathies produce demonstrable weakness. Polymyalgia rheumatica produces shoulder and pelvic girdle pain, is associated with anemia and elevated ESR, and occurs after age 50. The diagnosis of fibromyalgia should be made hesitantly in a patient over age 50 and should never be invoked to explain fever, weight loss, or any other objective signs. Hypophosphatemic states, such as oncogenic osteomalacia, can cause musculoskeletal pain unassociated with physical findings but pain is limited to a few areas and labs reveal a low serum phosphate level.

Treatment

A multidisciplinary approach is most effective. Patient education is essential. Patients can be comforted that they have a diagnosable syndrome treatable by specific although imperfect therapies, and that the course is not progressive. Cognitive behavioral therapy, including programs that emphasize mindfulness meditation, is often helpful. Exercise programs are also beneficial, particularly tai chi and yoga. These medications have shown modest efficacy: amitriptyline, fluoxetine, duloxetine, milnacipran, cyclobenzaprine, pregabalin, gabapentin, or low-dose naltrexone. Tramadol and acetaminophen combinations have ameliorated symptoms modestly in short-term trials. NSAIDs are generally ineffective. Cannabinoids may have a role in the treatment of fibromyalgia; however, dose, formulation, and frequency are unknown. Opioids and corticosteroids are ineffective and should not be used. Depression and anxiety are extremely common among patients with fibromyalgia; concurrent treatment of these comorbid conditions is highly recommended.

Prognosis

All patients have chronic symptoms. With treatment, however, many do eventually resume increased activities. Progressive or objective findings do not develop.

Kleykamp BA et al. The prevalence of psychiatric and chronic pain comorbidities in fibromyalgia: an ACTTION systematic review. Semin Arthritis Rheum. 2021;51:166. [PMID: 33383293]

Kurlyandchik I et al. Safety and efficacy of medicinal cannabis in the treatment of fibromyalgia: a systematic review. J Altern Complement Med. 2021;27:198. [PMID: 33337931]

THORACIC OUTLET SYNDROMES

Thoracic outlet syndromes result from compression of the neurovascular structures supplying the upper extremity. Symptoms and signs arise from intermittent or continuous pressure on elements of the brachial plexus (more than 90% of cases) or the subclavian or axillary vessels (veins or arteries) by a variety of anatomic structures of the shoulder girdle region. The neurovascular bundle can be compressed between the anterior or middle scalene muscles and a normal first thoracic rib or a cervical rib. Most commonly thoracic outlet syndromes are caused by scarred scalene neck muscle secondary to neck trauma or sagging of the shoulder girdle resulting from aging, obesity, or pendulous breasts. Faulty posture, occupation, or thoracic muscle hypertrophy from physical activity (eg, weightlifting, baseball pitching) may be other predisposing factors.

Thoracic outlet syndromes present in most patients with some combination of four symptoms involving the upper extremity: pain, numbness, weakness, and swelling. The predominant symptoms depend on whether the compression chiefly affects neural or vascular structures. The onset of symptoms is usually gradual but can be sudden. Some patients spontaneously notice aggravation of symptoms with specific positioning of the arm. Pain radiates from the point of compression to the base of the neck, the axilla, the shoulder girdle region, arm, forearm, and hand. Paresthesias are common and distributed to the volar aspect of the fourth and fifth digits. Sensory symptoms may be aggravated at night or by prolonged use of the extremities. Weakness and muscle atrophy are the principal motor abnormalities. Vascular symptoms consist of arterial ischemia characterized by pallor of the fingers on elevation of the extremity, sensitivity to cold and, rarely, gangrene of the digits or venous obstruction marked by edema, cyanosis, and engorgement.

Symptoms can be provoked within 60 seconds over 90% of the time by having a patient elevate the arms in a "stick-em-up" position (ie, abducted 90 degrees in external rotation). Reflexes are usually not altered. Obliteration of the radial pulse with certain maneuvers of the arm or neck, once considered a highly sensitive sign of thoracic outlet obstruction, does not occur in most cases.

Chest radiography will identify patients with cervical ribs (although most patients with cervical ribs are asymptomatic). MRI with the arms held in different positions is useful in identifying sites of impaired blood flow. Intra-arterial or venous obstruction is confirmed by angiography. Determination of conduction velocities of the ulnar and other peripheral nerves of the upper extremity may help localize the site of their compression.

Thoracic outlet syndrome must be differentiated from osteoarthritis of the cervical spine, tumors of the superior pulmonary sulcus, cervical spinal cord, or nerve roots, and periarthritis of the shoulder.

Treatment is directed toward relief of compression of the neurovascular bundle. Greater than 95% of patients can be treated successfully with conservative therapy consisting of physical therapy and avoiding postures or activities that compress the neurovascular bundle. Operative treatment, required by less than 5% of patients, is more likely to relieve the neurologic rather than the vascular component that causes symptoms.

COMPLEX REGIONAL PAIN SYNDROME

Complex regional pain syndrome (formerly called reflex sympathetic dystrophy) is a rare disorder of the extremities characterized by autonomic and vasomotor instability. The cardinal symptoms and signs are pain localized to an arm or leg, swelling of the involved extremity, disturbances of color and temperature in the affected limb, dystrophic changes in the overlying skin and nails, and limited range of motion. Strikingly, the findings are not limited to the distribution of a single peripheral nerve. Most cases are preceded by surgery or direct physical trauma, often of a relatively minor nature, to the soft tissues, bone, or nerve. Early mobilization after injury or surgery reduces the likelihood of developing the syndrome. Any extremity can be involved, but the syndrome most commonly occurs in the hand and is associated with ipsilateral restriction of shoulder motion ("shoulder-hand" syndrome). This syndrome proceeds through phases: pain, swelling, and skin color and temperature changes develop early and, if untreated, lead to atrophy and dystrophy. The swelling in complex regional pain syndrome is diffuse ("catcher's mitt hand") and not restricted to joints. Pain is often burning in quality, intense, and often greatly worsened by minimal stimuli such as light touch. The shoulder-hand variant of this disorder sometimes complicates MI or injuries to the neck or shoulder. Complex regional pain syndrome may occur after a knee injury or after arthroscopic knee surgery. There are no systemic symptoms. In the early phases of the syndrome, bone scans are sensitive, showing diffuse increased uptake in the affected extremity; radiographs eventually reveal severe generalized osteopenia. This syndrome should be differentiated from other rheumatoid arthritis, thoracic outlet obstruction, and mononeuritis multiplex, among others.

Early treatment offers the best prognosis for recovery. For mild cases, NSAIDs (eg, naproxen 250–500 mg twice daily orally) can be effective. For more severe cases associated with edema, prednisone, 30–60 mg/day orally for 2 weeks and then tapered over 2 weeks, can be effective. Pain management is important and allows for effective physical therapy, which is critical to restore function. Some patients may benefit from antidepressant agents (eg, nortriptyline initiated at a dosage of 10 mg orally at bedtime and gradually increased to 40–75 mg at bedtime) or anticonvulsants (eg, gabapentin 300 mg three times daily orally). Bisphosphonates, calcitonin, regional nerve blocks, and dorsal-column stimulation have also been reported to be helpful. Vitamin C supplementation (1 g orally daily) may have a role in preventing the development of complex regional pain syndrome following surgical procedures known to be a risk factor (eg, total knee replacement, foot or ankle surgery). The prognosis partly depends on the stage in which the lesions are encountered and the extent and severity of associated organic disease.

Jacques H et al. Prospective randomized study of the vitamin C effect on pain and complex pain regional syndrome after total knee arthroplasty. Int Orthop. 2021;45:1155. [PMID: 33438072]

RHEUMATOLOGIC MANIFESTATIONS OF CANCER

Rheumatologic syndromes may be the presenting manifestations for a variety of cancers. Dermatomyositis in adults is often associated with cancer. Hypertrophic pulmonary osteoarthropathy, which is characterized by the triad of polyarthritis, clubbing, and periosteal new bone formation, is associated with both malignant diseases (eg, lung and intrathoracic cancers) and nonmalignant ones (eg, cyanotic heart disease, cirrhosis, and lung abscess). Cancer-associated polyarthritis is rare, has both oligoarticular and polyarticular forms, and should be considered when "seronegative rheumatoid arthritis" develops abruptly in an older patient. Palmar fasciitis manifests as bilateral palmar swelling with finger contractures and may be the first indication of cancer, particularly ovarian carcinoma. Remitting seronegative synovitis with non-pitting edema ("RS3PE") presents with a symmetric small-joint polyarthritis associated with non-pitting edema of the hands; it can be idiopathic or associated with malignancy. Palpable purpura due to leukocytoclastic vasculitis may be the presenting complaint in myeloproliferative disorders. Hairy cell leukemia can be associated with medium-sized vessel vasculitis such as polyarteritis nodosa. Acute leukemia can produce severe joint and bone pain without florid synovitis. Rheumatic manifestations of myelodysplastic syndromes include cutaneous vasculitis, lupus-like syndromes, neuropathy, and episodic intense arthritis. Erythromelalgia, a painful warmth and redness of the extremities that (unlike Raynaud) improves with cold exposure or with elevation of the extremity, is often associated with myeloproliferative diseases, particularly essential thrombocythemia.

Immune-related adverse events from immune checkpoint inhibitors used to treat a variety of malignancies include pneumonitis, colitis, and inflammatory arthritis. These events are common and often can be managed with corticosteroids alone and adjustment of immunotherapy. However, the persistence of some autoimmune conditions despite cessation of cancer treatment, namely inflammatory arthritis, may require long-term immunosuppression.

NEUROGENIC ARTHROPATHY (Charcot Joint)

Neurogenic arthropathy is joint destruction resulting from loss or diminution of proprioception, pain, and temperature perception. Although initially described in the knees of patients with tabes dorsalis, it is more frequently seen in association with diabetic neuropathy (foot and ankle) or syringomyelia (shoulder). As normal muscle tone and protective reflexes are lost, secondary degenerative joint disease ensues, resulting in an enlarged, boggy, relatively painless joint with extensive cartilage erosion, osteophyte formation, and multiple loose joint bodies. Radiographs can reveal striking osteolysis that mimics osteomyelitis or dramatic destruction of the joint with subluxation, fragmentation of bone, and bony sclerosis.

Treatment is directed toward the primary disease; mechanical devices are used to assist in weight bearing and prevention of further trauma. Surgical strategies, including arthrodesis, with or without orthobiologics, can be considered if nonsurgical management fails. Pharmacotherapy has not demonstrated efficacy for this condition.

PALINDROMIC RHEUMATISM

Palindromic rheumatism is a disease of unknown cause characterized by frequent recurring attacks (at irregular intervals) of acutely inflamed joints. Periarticular pain with swelling and transient subcutaneous nodules may also occur. The attacks cease within several hours to several days. The knee and finger joints are most commonly affected, but any peripheral joint may be involved. Although hundreds of attacks may take place over a period of years, there is no permanent articular damage. Laboratory findings are usually normal. Palindromic rheumatism must be distinguished from acute gouty arthritis and an atypical acute onset of rheumatoid arthritis. In some patients, palindromic rheumatism is a prodrome of rheumatoid arthritis.

Symptomatic treatment with NSAIDs is usually all that is required during the attacks. Hydroxychloroquine may be of value in preventing recurrences.

OSTEONECROSIS (Avascular Necrosis of Bone)

Osteonecrosis is a complication of corticosteroid use, alcohol use, trauma, SLE, pancreatitis, gout, sickle cell disease, dysbaric syndromes (eg, "the bends"), and infiltrative diseases (eg, Gaucher disease). The most commonly affected sites are the proximal and distal femoral heads, leading to hip or knee pain. Other commonly affected sites include the ankle, shoulder, and elbow. Osteonecrosis of the jaw is associated with the dose-related use of bisphosphonates, usually when high-dose intravenous bisphosphonate therapy is used for treating metastatic cancer or plasma cell myeloma rather than osteoporosis. Initially, radiographs are normal; MRI, CT scan, and bone scan are more sensitive techniques. Treatment involves avoidance of weight bearing on the affected joint for at least several weeks. The value of surgical core decompression is controversial. For osteonecrosis of the hip, a variety of procedures designed to preserve the femoral head have been developed for early disease, including vascularized and nonvascularized bone grafting procedures. These procedures are most effective in avoiding or forestalling the need for total hip arthroplasty in young patients who do not have advanced disease. Without intervention, the natural history of avascular necrosis is progression of the bony infarction to cortical collapse, resulting in significant joint dysfunction. Total hip replacement is the usual outcome for all patients who are candidates.

ALLERGIC & IMMUNOLOGIC DISORDERS

Teresa K. Tarrant, MD
Mildred Kwan, MD, PhD

IMMEDIATE HYPERSENSITIVITY

1. Food Allergy

Immediate hypersensitivity IgE-mediated allergic reactions to foods commonly occur within 2 hours of ingestion and are much less common in adults as a de novo food allergy than in children. Typical reactions include a combination of emesis, diarrhea, urticaria with or without angioedema, bronchial hypersensitivity, and hypotension. A serum tryptase may be elevated during anaphylactic reactions within a few hours after the exposure. The most common systemic food allergies are caused by milk, egg, wheat, soy, fish, shellfish, peanuts, and tree nut allergens. Shellfish, peanuts, and tree nuts are the most common causes of food anaphylaxis in adults; milk and egg allergies are more common in children but often resolve by adulthood. Diagnosis of food allergy is based on a correlative history, skin tests, and serum specific IgE tests. There is no role for specific IgG or IgA testing for evaluating food immediate hypersensitivity. Because of frequent false-positive IgE tests the use of indiscriminate screening of IgE panels to foods is not recommended; oral food challenge with a reproducible immediate hypersensitivity reaction remains the gold standard for diagnosis. Food challenge, however, should only be conducted by an experienced provider in a setting equipped to treat anaphylaxis. Management of food allergy involves strict avoidance of the food and guaranteed access to epinephrine autoinjectors. The use of oral immunotherapy to treat food allergy in children and adolescents, should only be performed by an experienced allergist immunologist.

Other IgE-mediated food reactions include oral allergy syndrome and hypersensitivity to alpha-gal (galactose-alpha-1,3-galactose). Oral allergy syndrome and pollen-associated food allergy syndrome result from cross-reactivity between certain food and pollen proteins. Affected individuals have known seasonal pollen allergies (most commonly tree pollens) and experience itching of the oral mucosa upon ingestion of cross-reactive raw fruits and vegetables. In contrast to systemic food allergy, symptoms are mostly limited to the oropharynx.

Barshow SM et al. Mechanisms of oral immunotherapy. Clin Exp Allergy. 2021;51:527. [PMID: 33417257]

2. Venom Allergy

Most systemic allergic reactions to insect stings are caused by honeybees, vespids (yellow jackets, hornets, wasps, honeybee), and fire ants. Systemic anaphylactic reactions can occur after stinging events at any age. Patients at highest risk for anaphylaxis from subsequent stings are those who have had a history of recent or severe reactions, or both;

thus, the risk of a systemic reaction declines over elapsed time since the last sting. If a systemic allergy is suspected because symptoms include generalized urticaria, anaphylaxis, angioedema, wheezing, or diarrhea, refer the patient to an allergist for confirmative venom allergy testing; initiation of venom immunotherapy is commonly recommended. In the interim, patients should be given self-administrated epinephrine for those with continuing exposure.

Golden DB et al. Stinging insect hypersensitivity: a practice parameter update 2016. Ann Allergy Asthma Immunol. 2017; 118:28. [PMID: 28007086]

3. Anaphylaxis

General Considerations

Anaphylaxis is the most serious and potentially life-threatening manifestation of mast cell and basophil mediator release. The National Institute of Allergy and Infectious Diseases/Food Allergy and Anaphylaxis Network definition of anaphylaxis and criteria for diagnosis are shown in Table 20–13. Anaphylaxis is defined under these circumstances: (1) an allergen exposure followed by the acute onset of illness involving skin or mucosal tissue and either respiratory compromise or hypotension (systolic blood pressure less than 90 mm Hg or 30% less than known baseline); (2) a likely allergen exposure followed by the acute onset of two or more of these conditions: skin or mucosal tissue involvement, respiratory compromise, hypotension, and persistent GI symptoms; or (3) a known allergen exposure followed by hypotension.

IgE-dependent anaphylaxis is an acute syndrome initiated by a new allergen exposure after a prior exposure has sensitized the patient with anti-allergen IgE antibodies; IgE-mediated anaphylaxis cannot occur on first-time exposure to allergens like medications, insect venoms, latex, and foods. Conversely, other anaphylactic reactions (sometimes called "anaphylactoid"), such as radiocontrast media, certain medications (most NSAIDs, opioids, and vancomycin), and COVID mRNA vaccine reactions, are due to different immunologic mechanisms and can occur with first-time exposure.

Clinical Findings

A. Symptoms and Signs

Symptoms and signs typically start to occur within 30 minutes of initial exposure but may rarely appear up to several hours later. These include: (1) skin manifestations (typically urticaria, flushing, blotchy rashes, and pruritus); (2) respiratory distress (wheezing, stridor, bronchospasm, and airway angioedema); (3) GI symptoms (cramping, emesis, and diarrhea [especially in food allergy]); and (4) hypotension. Anaphylaxis is potentially fatal, especially if untreated.

B. Laboratory Findings

Laboratory evaluation obtained shortly after onset of symptoms can support a diagnosis of anaphylaxis but should not take the place of expedient treatment. Elevated serum tryptase within 4–6 hours following onset of anaphylaxis is most useful because it is a specific biomarker of mast cell degranulation. Plasma histamine generally peaks 30 minutes after onset of symptoms, making it difficult to obtain during peak levels. Referral to an allergist is necessary because of concern for future reactions and need for appropriate education and intervention. Specific serum IgE

Table 20–13. NIAID/FAAN consensus criteria for anaphylaxis. Anaphylaxis is likely when any one of the three criteria is fulfilled.

Presentation	Time to Onset of Symptoms	Clinical Manifestations
Criterion 1: Acute onset of illness	Minutes to 2–3 hours	One of the following combinations of symptoms: Skin or mucosa, or both[1] *with* Respiratory compromise[2] *or* ↓ blood pressure or end-organ dysfunction[3]
Criterion 2: After exposure to **likely** allergens	Minutes to 2–3 hours	Involvement of two or more of the following systems: Skin or mucosa, or both[1] Respiratory compromise[2] ↓ blood pressure or end-organ dysfunction[3] Persistent GI symptoms[4]
Criterion 3: After exposure to **known** allergens	Minutes to 2–3 hours	Involvement of the cardiovascular system: ↓ blood pressure

[1]Indicates presence of pruritus, flushing, hives, or angioedema.
[2]Indicates presence of dyspnea, wheeze-bronchospasm, decreased peak expiratory flow, stridor, or hypoxemia.
[3]Indicates decreased blood pressure; end-organ dysfunction includes collapse, syncope, or incontinence.
[4]Indicates presence of vomiting, crampy abdominal pain, or diarrhea.
Reproduced with permission from Renae Boerneke and Mildred Kwan, University of North Carolina. And this article was published in The Journal of Allergy and Clinical Immunology, Volume 117, Sampson HA, Muñoz-Furlong A, Campbell RL, et al. Second symposium on the definition and management of anaphylaxis: summary report–Second National Institute of Allergy and Infectious Disease/Food Allergy and Anaphylaxis Network symposium, 391–397, © Elsevier 2006.

or skin testing to suspected allergens may be performed optimally 4–6 weeks after a severe reaction; this delayed testing is to avoid falsely negative testing during a post-reaction "refractory" period where IgE consumed during anaphylaxis has not yet been regenerated. The positive predictive value of these tests depends highly on a suggestive temporal relationship to suspected allergen exposure.

Treatment

Administration of intramuscular epinephrine (0.01 mg/kg of a 1:1000 [1 mg/mL] solution, maximum 0.5 mg in adults) at the onset of suspected anaphylaxis is the cornerstone of therapy and should not be delayed. There is no absolute contraindication to administering intramuscular epinephrine in the setting of anaphylaxis. Supportive measures, such as oxygen, intravenous fluids and, if required, airway management are also appropriate. Adjunctive therapies may include antihistamines, bronchodilators, and corticosteroids. Self-administered epinephrine at the earliest signs of recurrence can be life-sparing, whereas antihistamines and corticosteroids have limited value in reversing anaphylaxis.

When to Refer

Patients with new or unexplained onset of anaphylaxis should be evaluated by an allergist.

Shaker MS et al. Anaphylaxis—a 2020 practice parameter update, systematic review, and Grading of Recommendations, Assessment, Development and Evaluation (GRADE) analysis. J Allergy Clin Immunol. 2020;145:1082. [PMID: 32001253]

Cutaneous or skin prick allergen testing produces a localized pruritic wheal (induration) and flare (erythema) that is maximal at 15–20 minutes. Such testing is used most commonly to diagnose allergic respiratory disease (rhinitis and asthma) and IgE-mediated allergy to food, drugs (penicillins), and hymenoptera venom. Allergen extracts are available for pollens, fungi, animal danders, and dust mites and are appropriately selected for the patient's geographic area.

ADVERSE DRUG REACTIONS

1. Drug Allergy (IgE-Mediated Immediate Hypersensitivity Reactions)

Prick skin testing for most low-molecular-weight drugs is not validated and is interpretable only if the test is positive at a nonirritating concentration. Testing for IgE-mediated allergy to penicillin (PCN) is validated; skin testing with the metabolic determinants of PCN has a high (more than 98%) negative predictive value. Referral of individuals with a listed PCN allergy to an allergist for evaluation is worthwhile because more than 90% have either lost sensitization or do not have a true PCN allergy. Such patients may then safely receive beta-lactam antibiotics, including penicillins and cephalosporins. Allergy testing to non-PCN drugs is more limited; an allergist may provide guidance about whether re-challenging with the drug would be advisable.

Shenoy ES et al. Evaluation and management of penicillin allergy: a review. JAMA. 2019;321:188. [PMID: 30644987]

2. Non-IgE–Mediated Anaphylactic Drug Reactions

Non-IgE–mediated anaphylaxis induced by drugs resembles immediate hypersensitivity reactions but is not mediated by allergen-IgE cross-linking on mast cells or basophils. Mechanisms include direct mast cell activation (eg, opioids, vancomycin [vancomycin flushing syndrome], neuromuscular blocking agents, fluoroquinolones), complement activation–related pseudoallergy (possible mechanism for heparin or liposomal drug infusions [polyethylene glycol)/COVID mRNA vaccines], or IgG-mediated mechanisms. Contrary to IgE-mediated reactions, these reactions can often be prevented by prophylactic medical regimens.

A. Radiocontrast Media Reactions

Reactions to radiocontrast media are not usually IgE antibody–mediated, yet they are clinically similar to anaphylaxis and can be life-threatening. If a patient has had an anaphylactoid reaction to conventional radiocontrast media, the risk for a second reaction upon re-exposure may be as high as 30%. Patients with a history of atopy are at increased risk.

Management includes use of low-osmolality contrast preparations and prophylactic administration of prednisone (50 mg orally every 6 hours beginning 13 hours before the procedure) and diphenhydramine (25–50 mg orally, intramuscularly or intravenously 60 minutes before the procedure). Using lower-osmolality radiocontrast media in combination with the pretreatment regimen decreases the incidence of recurrent reactions to less than 1%.

B. Vancomycin Flushing Syndrome

Vancomycin flushing syndrome causes non-IgE–mediated anaphylaxis comprised of flushing, pruritus, and erythema of the upper body. Initially described as a vancomycin-infusion reaction, it can also occur after intravenous infusion of opioids. The reaction is related to the rate of drug administration resulting in direct activation of mast cells. Management includes administration of an antihistamine such as diphenhydramine, 25–50 mg intravenously or intramuscularly, and re-initiation of the vancomycin infusion at no more than half the former rate. In patients who have previously experienced a vancomycin infusion reaction, premedication with an H_1-antagonist (eg, diphenhydramine) and H_2-antagonist (eg, cimetidine) is recommended 1 hour before the infusion. Although rare, anaphylaxis with vancomycin use can occur. Vancomycin skin testing has not been validated as a diagnostic tool. Induction of tolerance to vancomycin is possible for patients with anaphylaxis without an acceptable alternative antibiotic.

Broyles AD et al. Practical guidance for the evaluation and management of drug hypersensitivity: specific drugs. J Allergy Clin Immunol Pract. 2020;8:S16. [PMID: 33039007]

DELAYED DRUG HYPERSENSITIVITY

Type IV delayed hypersensitivity typically occurs 48–72 hours after contact with the antigen.

1. Drug Exanthems

The clinical manifestation of drug exanthems is vast (see Chapter 6), ranging from common morbilliform rashes to severe cutaneous adverse reactions (SCARs) (eg, Stevens-Johnson syndrome [SJS]/toxic epidermal necrolysis [TEN], drug reaction with eosinophilia and systemic symptoms [DRESS], acute generalized exanthematous pustulosis [AGEP]). Given the broad range of cutaneous findings, the differential diagnosis includes miliaria, lichen planus, folliculitis, pityriasis rosea, tinea corporis, and mycosis fungoides. While many drugs can cause exanthems, there are no commercially available laboratory or other diagnostic tests to reliably confirm these adverse reactions.

Management consists of immediate cessation of suspected medications and monitoring for symptom resolution. Systemic corticosteroids may be indicated for extensive dermatitis or other organ involvement.

Phillips EJ et al. Controversies in drug allergy: testing for delayed reactions. J Allergy Clin Immunol. 2019;143:66. [PMID: 30573342]

2. Severe Cutaneous Adverse Reactions (SCARs)

Potentially life-threatening, systemic drug-induced hypersensitivity reactions most commonly occur with exposure to anticonvulsants and sulfonamides, although other classes of medications (other antimicrobials, antifungals, allopurinol, NSAIDs, and antidepressants) have been implicated. Included in these severe delayed drug hypersensitivity reactions are SJS/TEN, DRESS and AGEP.

Stevens-Johnson Syndrome/Toxic Epidermal Necrolysis (SJS/TEN)

SJS and TEN comprise a spectrum of disease that are differentiated by the severity of disease (see Chapter 6). Drugs and infections are the main etiologies and include anticonvulsants, sulfonamide antibiotics, NSAIDs, and allopurinol, and *Mycoplasma pneumoniae* and herpes simplex virus. Allopurinol hypersensitivity is increased with the HLA-B*58:01 allele, the prevalence of which is highest in Han Chinese, Korean, and Thai persons, as well as in African Americans. Testing for the HLA-B*58:01 allele before starting allopurinol is conditionally recommended for these patients. Universal testing for HLA-B*58:01 is not recommended.

Symptoms start 4–28 days after initiation of an implicated medication or infection and include fever and influenza-like symptoms that precede the onset of cutaneous involvement by a few days. Skin lesions begin as painful round purpuric blisters/bullae with two regions ("atypical target" lesions) on the face and trunk and spread to the extremities. At least 90% of patients have mucosal involvement of the eyes, mouth, or genitalia, or all of the above.

Management involves immediate cessation of the suspected medications and supportive care (eg, fluid replacement, nutrition support and monitoring for infection). Antibiotics for suspected infection are recommended. Adjunctive therapies are controversial (eg, intravenous immunoglobulin [IVIG], corticosteroids), while others (eg, cyclosporine, TNF inhibitors) demonstrate promise.

Drug Reaction with Eosinophilia and Systemic Symptoms (DRESS)/Drug-Induced Hypersensitivity Syndrome (DIHS)

DRESS typically includes eosinophilia, lymphocytosis, and systemic symptoms such as fever and lymph node enlargement, along with rash. Recent classification of DRESS and DIHS indicates that they likely form a continuum of disease with DIHS representing a more severe form of DRESS with HHV-6. A limited number of drugs are implicated in induction of DRESS including anticonvulsants, sulfonamide antibiotics (eg, sulfasalazine), allopurinol, minocycline, dapsone, and vancomycin.

The onset of DRESS typically occurs 2–6 weeks after drug initiation. DRESS often begins with pruritus and fever soon followed by a maculopapular rash with facial and periorbital edema and lymphadenopathy. Rash affects the face, trunk, and upper and lower extremities most commonly although the rash tends to generalize into an exfoliative dermatitis or erythroderma. Mucocutaneous involvement is uncommon. The most common organ damage in DRESS is hepatitis; however; renal, pulmonary, and cardiac involvement may also occur.

Laboratory abnormalities include leukocytosis with eosinophilia (greater than 1.5×10^9/L), atypical lymphocytosis, elevated hepatic transaminases (more than two times above the upper limits of normal) and alkaline phosphatase, and increased serum creatinine, pyuria, and proteinuria (indicative of interstitial nephritis). The most common skin biopsy findings are a dense, perivascular lymphocytic infiltrate in the papillary dermis with eosinophils and dermal edema.

Management consists of discontinuation of causative medications and initiation of systemic corticosteroids. A dose of 1.0–1.5 mg/kg of oral prednisone is recommended as a starting dose, followed by a gradual taper occurring over 3–6 months after laboratory normalization and stabilization. Additional supportive therapies include antipyretics for fever, topical steroids for skin lesions, or fluid and electrolyte replacement in the case of more severe exfoliative dermatitis.

Acute Generalized Exanthematous Pustulosis (AGEP)

AGEP is characterized by hundreds of small, pruritic, sterile pustules on an erythematous base distributed mainly on the trunk and intertriginous areas. The pathogenesis of AGEP results from drug-specific activation of CD4+ and CD8+ T cells that migrate to the dermis and epidermis. At this site in the skin, the CD8+ T cells release cytotoxic perforin/granzyme B as well as engaging Fas on keratinocytes leading to keratinocyte cell death/

apoptosis. Additionally, the production of interferon-γ and granulocyte/macrophage colony stimulating factor increases neutrophil survival allowing for pustule formation.

Onset of AGEP occurs within hours to days following the initiation of the culprit drug. In addition to pustules, mucosal involvement is minimal to none and, if present, is only found in a single site such as the lips or buccal mucosa. Many patients will have fever and neutrophilia (more than 7.5×10^6/mL).

Treatment of AGEP includes cessation of the suspected drug with resolution of symptoms within a few days. The area of skin involved desquamates as the patient recovers from AGEP. While uncommon, mortality occurs in less than 5% of patients. Wet dressings and antiseptic solutions applied while the patient has active pustules is recommended while antibiotics should be used only if there is pustular superinfection. The utility of other treatments such as systemic corticosteroids is unclear.

Zhang J et al. Current perspectives on severe drug eruption. Clin Rev Allergy Immunol. 2021;61:282. [PMID: 34273058]

3. Other Delayed Drug Hypersensitivity Reactions

Aspirin- and NSAID-Exacerbated Respiratory Disease

Aspirin- and NSAID-exacerbated respiratory disease is caused by aberrant arachidonic acid metabolism.

Patients typically have increased airway responsiveness, bronchospasm, rhinorrhea, and nasal congestion. Chronic rhinosinusitis with nasal polyps and asthma is called "Samter's triad." Ocular, cutaneous, and gastric symptoms may also occur. Diagnosis is largely based on history and clinical findings. A positive aspirin challenge can demonstrate NSAID hypersensitivity and may suggest benefit from nasal polypectomy and aspirin desensitization. Long-term aspirin therapy following desensitization has been shown to reduce the need for nasal polypectomy and asthma therapy. Referral to an allergist is appropriate for aspirin desensitization. Treatment may also include montelukast or inhibition of 5-LOX with zileuton.

White AA et al. Aspirin-exacerbated respiratory disease. N Engl J Med. 2018;379:1060. [PMID: 30207919]

PRIMARY IMMUNODEFICIENCY DISORDERS IN ADULTS

Primary immunologic deficiency diseases are estimated to affect 1 in 4000 individuals; most are genetically determined and present in early childhood. Nonetheless, several important immunodeficiency disorders present in adulthood, most notably the antibody deficiency syndromes: selective IgA deficiency, common variable immunodeficiency (CVID), and specific (functional) antibody deficiency (Table 20–14). Antibody deficiency

Table 20–14. Selected primary immunodeficiency syndromes.

Disease	Clinical Presentation	Diagnosis[1]	Treatment
Complement disorders	"Early" complement component (C1–C4) deficiencies: autoimmune diseases "Late" complement component (C5–C8) deficiencies: recurrent meningococcal or gonococcal infections	Screen with CH50 and AH50. Obtain individual serum complement levels if abnormal. **Genetic testing if complement level absent.**	Prompt administration of antibiotics and *Neisseria* vaccination if C5–C8 deficient. Immune suppression if C1–4 deficient to treat organ specific autoimmunity.
Good syndrome	Current or past thymoma, recurrent severe sinopulmonary infections, may also have opportunistic infections.	**Hypogammaglobulinemia (IgG, IgM, IgA), absent B cells on flow cytometry**, may present with pure red cell aplasia or cytopenias. **Chest film consistent with thymoma.**	IgG-RT (subcutaneously or intravenously) 300 mg–500 mg/kg/month
Hereditary angioedema	Unpredictable swelling of face, lips, tongue, hands, feet; no urticaria; GI tract swelling causing severe abdominal pain	**Decreased C1 esterase inhibitor serum level and/or function,** decreased serum C4 level.	Prophylactic treatment: Danazol, tranexamic acid Acute treatment: C1 esterase inhibitor product, kallikrein inhibitor, bradykinin receptor antagonist
Granulocyte disorders	Recurrent invasive skin and soft tissue infections, abscesses requiring incision and drainage Common organisms are *Staphylococcus aureus*, gram-negative bacilli, *Nocardia, Aspergillus*	CBC with differential to evaluate neutrophil count. **Dihydrorhodamine assay confirming defective oxidative burst. Genetic testing confirming diagnosis.**	Antimicrobial prophylaxis; interferon for chronic granulomatous disease

[1]Key diagnostic findings in bold.

predisposes patients to recurrent serious bacterial infections, particularly of the respiratory tract, including refractory chronic rhinosinusitis, bronchitis, pneumonia, and bronchiectasis. Patients are most susceptible to infections with encapsulated bacteria (eg, *Haemophilus influenzae* type b, *Streptococcus pneumoniae, Neisseria meningitides*). However, any part of the innate or adaptive immune system can be defective, which results in infections with different spectra of organisms depending on the severity of the immune defect.

1. Selective IgA Deficiency

Selective IgA deficiency is the most common primary immunodeficiency disorder and is characterized by undetectable serum IgA levels (lower than 7 mg/dL) with normal levels of IgG and IgM (Table 20–14); its prevalence is about 1 in 500 individuals, with a higher prevalence in White persons. Most affected individuals are asymptomatic. A minority of patients have recurrent bacterial infections such as sinusitis, otitis, bronchitis, and GI infections. Selective IgA deficiency can be associated with an increased incidence of atopic and autoimmune disorders, including Graves disease, SLE, juvenile rheumatoid arthritis, type 1 diabetes mellitus, and celiac disease.

Some individuals with undetectable levels of serum IgA may have high titers of anti-IgA IgG or IgE antibodies and are at risk for anaphylactic reactions to IgA following exposure through infusions of plasma (or other blood transfusions). Treatment with commercial immune globulin replacement therapy (IgG-RT) is not indicated for patients with selective IgA deficiency and may result in anaphylaxis in preparations with detectable amounts of IgA in the preparation. Notably, IgG-RT does not treat IgA deficiency since there is little IgA present in IgG-RT products.

When to Refer

- Refer patients with undetectable serum IgA and recurrent sinopulmonary infections, celiac disease, giardiasis, or a family history of immunodeficiency to an immunologist.

2. Common Variable Immunodeficiency (CVID)

ESSENTIALS OF DIAGNOSIS

- Frequent, severe sinopulmonary infections secondary to humoral immune deficiency.
- Two or more low serum immunoglobulin levels (IgG, IgA, IgM) and deficient functional antibody responses to vaccination.
- Secondary causes for hypogammaglobulinemia and recurrent sinopulmonary infections have been ruled out.

General Considerations

CVID is a heterogeneous immunodeficiency disorder clinically characterized by an increased incidence of recurrent severe sinopulmonary infections with hypogammaglobulinemia. Approximately half of CVID patients will also have autoimmune phenomena with or without neoplastic disease. The onset is generally in adolescence or early adulthood, but it can occur at any age, mostly due to delay in diagnosis. Most cases are sporadic; about 10–20% are familial. Thus, routine immunoglobulin screening of family members without severe symptoms is not advised, albeit patients with CVID may have family members with a higher incidence of autoimmune disease or IgA deficiency. Since the genetic defect is not known, patients with CVID and their offspring are not recommended to undergo genetic testing unless advised by an immunologist.

Clinical Findings

A. Symptoms and Signs

Increased susceptibility to serious infections, especially with encapsulated organisms, is the hallmark of the disease. Virtually all patients suffer from recurrent bacterial sinusitis, bronchitis, and otitis, but it is the recurrent pneumonia that sets these individuals apart from patients with severe atopy. Infections may be prolonged or associated with unusual complications such as meningitis, empyema, or sepsis. Bronchiectasis occurs in at least 25% of patients who are not treated with IgG-RT and is a leading cause of morbidity. Recurrent viral infections are not prototypic of the disease, albeit varicella-zoster reactivation, CMV reactivation, and increased symptomatic disease from other herpes viruses and *Candida* can occur in some patients.

GI infections and autoimmunity are commonly associated with CVID. Many patients will develop an inflammatory sprue-like syndrome, with diarrhea, steatorrhea, malabsorption, protein-losing enteropathy, and hepatosplenomegaly. Norovirus and *Giardia* can be problematic, so infectious and inflammatory etiologies should be considered. Paradoxically, there is an increased incidence of autoimmune disease (20%) in these patients, although they often do not display the usual serologic markers as they are hypogammaglobulinemic. Autoimmune cytopenias are most common, but autoimmune endocrinopathies, seronegative rheumatic disease, and the aforementioned GI disorders are also commonly seen. Lymph nodes may be enlarged in CVID patients, yet biopsies show marked reduction in plasma cells. Noncaseating granulomas are frequently found in the spleen, liver, lungs, or skin. There is an increased propensity for the development of B-cell neoplasms (50- to 400-fold increased risk of lymphoma) and gastric carcinomas.

B. Laboratory Findings

The serum IgG level is reduced at least two standard deviations below normal in all patients. Either IgA or IgM is also reduced two standard deviations below normal; it is common that IgA is undetectable. Demonstration of functional or quantitative defects in antibody production is essential and is typically performed by checking antibody response to polysaccharide (Pneumovax-23, *H influenzae* type b) and protein antigens (tetanus, diphtheria). The diagnosis is made in patients who have reduced serum immunoglobulins and poor antibody response to vaccines, after exclusion of secondary causes as highlighted (eg, proteinuria, protein-losing enteropathy, drug effects such as rituximab and other immunosuppressants, antiepileptics, and hematologic malignancies).

The absolute B-cell count in the peripheral blood can be normal. A subset of CVID patients have concomitant T-cell immunodeficiency with increased numbers of activated CD8 cells, splenomegaly, and decreased delayed-type hypersensitivity.

Differential Diagnosis

See secondary causes of hypogammaglobulinemia, below. Secondary causes of recurrent sinopulmonary infections include COPD, current or past prolonged smoking, chronic sinusitis, cystic fibrosis, Kartagener syndrome, and colonization with multi-drug–resistant bacteria.

Treatment

In addition to IgG-RT, patients should be treated aggressively with antibiotics at the first sign of infection. Since antibody deficiency predisposes patients to high-risk pyogenic infections, antibiotic coverage should cover encapsulated bacteria. Infections with other microorganisms can develop including viruses, parasites, and extracellular gram-positive or gram-negative bacteria (such as *S aureus* or *P aeruginosa*). The current standard of care for preventive therapy is treatment with subcutaneous IgG-RT, with a typical monthly dose of 300–600 mg/kg. Subcutaneous injections of IgG offer the convenience of self-administration at home, lower incidence of adverse effects, and can be administered every 1–4 weeks. Adjustment of the dosage or infusion interval is made primarily based on clinical responses in addition to serum IgG levels. Such therapy is essential for decreasing the incidence of potentially life-threatening infections, increasing quality of life, and reducing the progression of lung disease, which can be a severe complication in patients who are not treated with IgG-RT. IgG-RT can be administered intravenously as well, but this is becoming less common due to the improved cost, ease of administration, fewer systemic side effects, and more stable IgG levels achieved with subcutaneous administration.

When to Refer

- Refer patients with low serum immunoglobulins and recurrent serious or unusual infections to a clinical immunologist with expertise in immunodeficiency.
- The presence of bronchiectasis without a known underlying cause such as cystic fibrosis or Kartagener syndrome should raise the suspicion of a primary immunodeficiency and would warrant further evaluation by a clinical immunologist.

3. Specific (Functional) Antibody Deficiency

Specific antibody deficiency is characterized by decreased or absent IgG antibody response to vaccines in the setting of normal or mildly decreased serum immunoglobulin levels. The clinical spectrum can range from mild symptoms that can be managed with antibiotics and vaccination to more rarely, recurrent infections with features very similar to CVID. Since this can be a nuanced diagnosis, recommendations are to refer to a clinical immunologist for diagnosis and treatment recommendations.

4. Immunoglobulin Subclass Deficiency

There are four subclasses of IgG: IgG1, IgG2, IgG3, and IgG4. A low level of at least one IgG subclass has been found incidentally in 2% of the population. Thus, low or absent IgG subclass levels alone are not sufficient for a diagnosis of immunodeficiency, and IgG-RT is not clinically indicated unless other functional impairments in the immune system are identified.

5. Secondary Hypogammaglobulinemia

Secondary causes of hypogammaglobulinemia, rather than from a primary genetic defect, are more likely to occur in the older population due to an increase in comorbid conditions. Some malignancies, immunosuppressants, antipsychotic medications, chronic diarrhea, sepsis, nephrosis, and HIV have known associations with hypogammaglobulinemia. The principle therapy of secondary hypogammaglobulinemia is treatment of the underlying condition or removal of the offending medication. If hypogammaglobulinemia is persistent or severe with recurrent infections, consultation with an allergist immunologist is recommended to determine whether treatment should include IgG-RT, vaccination boosters, and antibiotic prophylaxis.

Bonilla FA et al; Joint Task Force on Practice Parameters, representing the American Academy of Allergy, Asthma & Immunology; the American College of Allergy, Asthma & Immunology; and the Joint Council of Allergy, Asthma & Immunology. Practice parameter for the diagnosis and management of primary immunodeficiency. J Allergy Clin Immunol. 2015;136:1186. [PMID: 26371839]

Cinetto F et al. The broad spectrum of lung diseases in primary antibody deficiencies. Eur Respir Rev. 2018;27:180019. [PMID: 30158276]

Odineal DD et al. The epidemiology and clinical manifestations of autoimmunity in selective IgA deficiency. Clin Rev Allergy Immunol. 2020;58:107. [PMID: 31267472]

Verbsky JW et al. Rituximab and antimetabolite treatment of granulomatous and lymphocytic interstitial lung disease in common variable immunodeficiency. J Allergy Clin Immunol. 2021;147:704. [PMID: 32745555]

Electrolyte & Acid-Base Disorders

Nayan Arora, MD
J. Ashley Jefferson, MD, FRCP

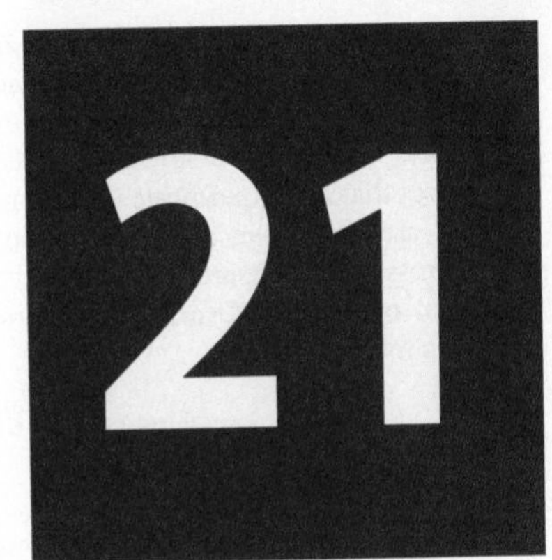

ASSESSMENT OF THE PATIENT

The pathophysiology of all electrolyte disorders is rooted in basic principles of total body water and its distribution across fluid compartments. The optimal evaluation and treatment of fluid and electrolyte disorders requires a careful interpretation of serum and urine chemistries in conjunction with a thorough history and physical examination. While classic teaching has focused on physical examination to determine a patient's volume status, such an approach can be challenging because of limitations in accurate bedside analysis of volume status.

A. Body Water and Fluid Distribution

Total body water depends on the relative proportions of muscle and fat in the body. Total body water is typically estimated as 50% of body weight in women and 60% in men, as women, on average, have a higher proportion of fat to body weight (Table 21–1). Total body water also tends to decrease with age due to declining muscle mass. Approximately two-thirds of total body water is located in the intracellular compartment and one-third is located in the extracellular compartment. The extracellular compartment is further divided into the interstitial fluid volume (15% of body weight) and the plasma fluid volume (5% of body weight).

Changes in total body water content are best evaluated by documenting changes in body weight. Extracellular volume (ECV) may be assessed by physical examination (eg, blood pressure, pulse, jugular venous distention, edema). Quantitative assessments of ECV and intravascular volume may be invasive (ie, central venous pressure or pulmonary wedge pressure) or noninvasive (ie, inferior vena cava diameter and right atrial pressure by echocardiography). Intracellular volume (ICV) is assessed using the serum sodium concentration.

Table 21–1. Total body water (as percentage of body weight) in relation to age and sex.

Age	Male	Female
18–40	60%	50%
41–60	60–50%	50–40%
Over 60	50%	40%

B. Serum Electrolytes

In health, serum electrolytes are maintained within a narrow range by the kidneys (homeostasis). The serum level of an electrolyte may be normal, elevated, or decreased but may not correlate with the total body levels of that electrolyte due to shift of water or electrolytes into and out of cells.

C. Evaluation of Urine

The urine concentration of an electrolyte is helpful to determine whether the kidney is excreting or retaining the electrolyte in response to high or low serum levels. A 24-hour urine collection for daily electrolyte excretion remains the gold standard for assessment of renal electrolyte handling; however, it can be cumbersome, as well as technically challenging in certain patients. A more convenient method to determine renal electrolyte handling is the use of fractional excretion (FE) of an electrolyte X (FE_x) calculated from a spot urine sample and serum sample, using creatinine (Cr):

$$FE_x(\%) = \frac{urine_x \times serum_{Cr}}{serum_x \times urine_{Cr}} \times 100$$

A low fractional excretion indicates renal reabsorption (electrolyte retention), while a high fractional excretion indicates renal wasting (electrolyte excretion). Thus, the fractional excretion helps determine whether the kidney's response is appropriate for a specific electrolyte disorder.

D. Serum Osmolality

Total solute concentration is measured by osmolality in millimoles per kilogram. Osmolarity is measured in millimoles of solute per liter of solution. The terms are often used interchangeably in clinical medicine. Plasma osmolality is the total concentration of all the solutes contained in plasma, both electrolytes and nonelectrolytes, and normally ranges between 285 mmol/L and 295 mmol/L. Differences in osmole concentration across cell membranes lead to movement of water to the region of higher osmolality, stimulation of thirst, and secretion of ADH. Substances that easily permeate cell membranes (eg, urea, ethanol) are ineffective osmoles and do not cause fluid shifts across fluid compartments.

Serum osmolality (Osm) can be estimated using the following formula:

$$\text{Osm} = 2(\text{Na}^+ \text{mEq/L}) + \frac{\text{Glucose mg/dL}}{18} + \frac{\text{BUN mg/dL}}{2.8}$$

(*Note:* dividing urea by 2.8 converts mg/dL to mmol/L; dividing glucose by 18 converts mg/dL to mmol/L)

Sodium is the major extracellular cation; doubling the serum sodium in the formula for estimated osmolality accounts for corresponding anions. A discrepancy between measured and estimated osmolality of greater than 10 mmol/kg suggests an osmolal gap, which is the presence of unmeasured osmoles such as ethanol, methanol, isopropanol, and ethylene glycol (see Table 38–5).

DISORDERS OF SODIUM CONCENTRATION

HYPONATREMIA

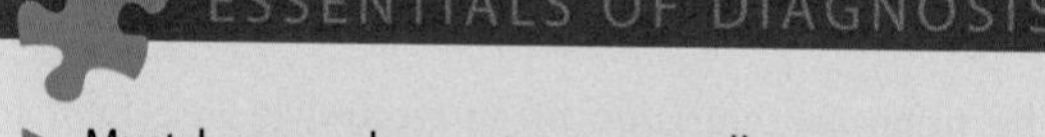

- Must know volume status as well as serum and urine osmolality to determine etiology.
- Hyponatremia usually reflects excess water retention rather than sodium deficiency. The serum sodium concentration is not a measure of total body sodium.
- Hyponatremia in hospitalized patients commonly is caused by administration of hypotonic fluids.

General Considerations

Hyponatremia is defined as a serum sodium concentration less than 135 mEq/L (135 mmol/L) and is the most common electrolyte abnormality encountered in clinical practice. Hyponatremia represents an excess of water relative to sodium in the plasma leading to a reduction in plasma osmolality and subsequent movement of water from the extracellular fluid into the intracellular fluid. Acutely, this movement of water can result in cerebral edema, increasing the risk of seizures and even brain herniation.

Chronic hyponatremia is often asymptomatic or present with mild confusion, nausea, or falls; cerebral adaptation occurs as the brain cells excrete intracellular osmoles to limit cell swelling. In this setting, over-rapid correction of chronic hyponatremia may produce profound neurologic abnormalities (osmotic demyelination syndrome).

A common misconception is that hyponatremia is secondary to a deficiency in total body sodium, when in reality it usually reflects an excess of total body water. The basic pathophysiologic principle is that more water (oral or intravenous) is ingested than the kidney can excrete (commonly due to the action of ADH). A diagnostic algorithm separates the causes of hyponatremia using serum osmolality, urine sodium, and volume status (Figure 21–1).

Etiology

A. Isotonic and Hypertonic Hyponatremia

Hyponatremia is typically associated with hypoosmolality with two exceptions: pseudohyponatremia and hypertonic hyponatremia.

1. Pseudohyponatremia—This represents a rare laboratory artifact in patients with marked hypertriglyceridemia or hypergammaglobulinemia. In these settings, there is an increase in the solid components of plasma, relative to plasma water, resulting in a lower sodium per given volume. This issue has become less prevalent since most laboratories use direct ion selective electrodes without blood dilution. Consult the clinical laboratory if this condition is suspected.

2. Hypertonic hyponatremia—The best clinical examples of this situation are hyperglycemia, and less commonly, mannitol infusion. Both glucose and mannitol are active osmoles, increasing the osmolality of the extracellular fluid, which pulls water from inside cells into the extracellular space. Note, this leads to a reduction in intracellular volume, and cerebral edema is not caused by hyponatremia in this setting; however, cerebral edema may occur in the treatment phase due to over-rapid correction of hyperglycemia and injudicious intravenous fluids. The increased tonicity will also stimulate thirst and vasopressin release, further contributing to water retention. To determine whether the hyponatremia can be entirely attributed to hyperglycemia, a sodium correction factor is often used. Many guidelines recommend using a decrease in the serum sodium concentration of 1.6 mEq/L (1.6 mmol/L) for every 100 mg/dL (5.5 mmol/L) rise in plasma glucose above normal.

B. Hypotonic Hyponatremia

Most cases of hyponatremia are hypotonic, highlighting sodium's role as the predominant extracellular osmole. The presence of hypotonic hyponatremia indicates that water intake exceeds the kidney's excretional capacity. The next step is to classify hypotonic cases as ADH dependent or independent based on the kidney's ability to excrete dilute urine.

1. ADH-independent causes—In rare circumstances, hypotonic hyponatremia can occur when the kidney's ability to excrete free water is intact (urine osmolality less than 100 mOsm/kg).

A. PSYCHOGENIC POLYDIPSIA—This condition develops where excess water intake overwhelms the kidney's capacity to excrete adequate dilute urine. Patients will have

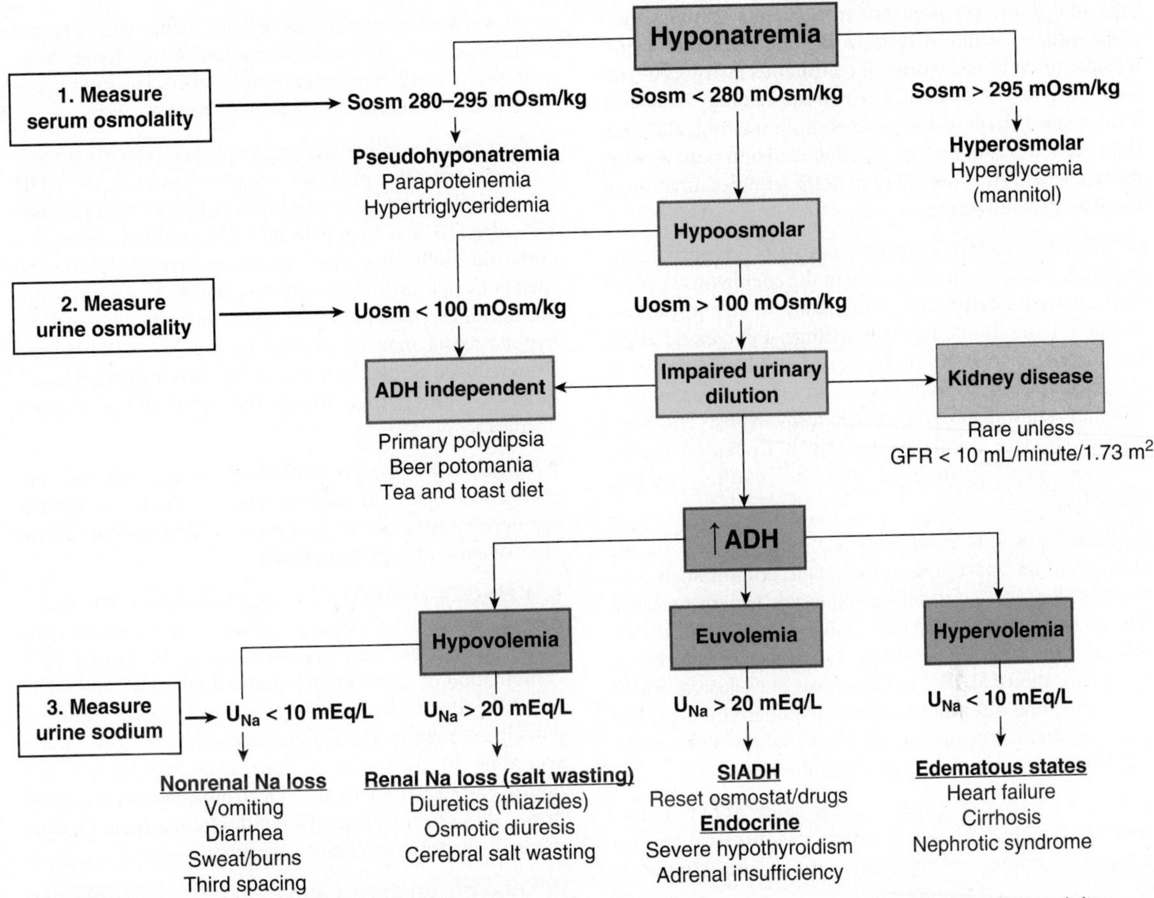

▲ **Figure 21–1.** A diagnostic algorithm for the causes of hyponatremia using serum osmolality, urine osmolality, and urine sodium. SIADH, syndrome of inappropriate antidiuretic hormone.

appropriately suppressed ADH, reflected by a urine osmolality less than 100 mOsm/kg. Polydipsia occurs primarily in patients with psychiatric disorders. Psychiatric medications may also interfere with water excretion or increase thirst through anticholinergic side effects, further increasing water intake.

B. Beer potomania and the "tea and toast" diet—Malnourished patients who consume a low protein diet with large quantities of beer, which is generally very low in sodium (beer potomania), or those who consume a low protein ("tea and toast") diet may have a marked reduction in free water excretion due to insufficient dietary solute intake. The kidney's ability to excrete free water is dependent not only on ADH suppression, but also on solute delivery to the distal tubules. With a typical Western diet generating 1000 mOsm of solute per day, normal kidneys can dilute urine to 50 mOsm/kg, allowing a maximum urine volume of 20 L. By contrast, with a low protein diet generating 200 mOsm per day, urinary output would be limited to a maximum of 4 L per day.

C. Renal impairment—Patients with advanced renal impairment (GFR less than 15 mL/minute/1.73 m^2), whether due to severe CKD or AKI, may be unable to dilute their urine (can often only achieve a minimum urine osmolality of 200–250 mOsm/L even with maximal ADH suppression) and are prone to develop water retention and hyponatremia. This can occur in the setting of normal or high plasma osmolality due to accumulation of urea. This differs from hypertonic hyponatremia because urea is an ineffective osmole and is freely permeable across cell membranes, only minimally pulling water into the plasma space.

2. ADH-dependent causes—The most common cause of hypotonic hyponatremia involves a failure to suppress ADH action. This can either be **appropriate** in the setting of hypovolemia, or a reduced effective arterial volume secondary to cirrhosis or heart failure (hypervolemia), or **inappropriate,** in the absence of hypovolemia or edematous states, which is known as the syndrome of inappropriate ADH secretion (SIADH).

A. Hypovolemic hyponatremia—Hypovolemic hyponatremia occurs with renal or extrarenal volume loss (sodium and water) and subsequent hypotonic fluid replacement (Figure 21–1). The reduced blood pressure results in an increase in ADH secretion by the pituitary, limiting free water excretion. In this setting, the body sacrifices serum osmolality to preserve intravascular volume.

Cerebral salt wasting is a rare subset of hypovolemic hyponatremia that occurs with intracranial disease (eg, infections, cerebrovascular accidents, tumors, and neurosurgery). Clinical features include refractory hypotension, often in the setting of continuous infusion of isotonic or hypertonic saline. The pathophysiology is unclear but has been attributed to renal sodium wasting, although there is uncertainty as to whether cerebral salt wasting represents a distinct entity or SIADH with desalination of the administered saline.

B. Hypervolemic hyponatremia—Hypervolemic hyponatremia commonly occurs in the edematous states of cirrhosis and heart failure, and rarely in nephrotic syndrome (Figure 21–1). In these settings, a decreased effective arterial blood volume (typically low blood pressure) occurs despite an overall increase in extracellular volume (edema) resulting in ADH secretion. In cirrhosis and heart failure, effective circulating volume is decreased due to systemic vasodilation and reduced cardiac output, respectively.

C. SIADH—In this condition, ADH is secreted in the absence of an appropriate physiologic stimuli such as a decreased effective circulating volume or hyperosmolality. The major causes of SIADH (Table 21–2) are disorders affecting the CNS or the lungs (eg, cancer or infections) and medications. SIADH is a diagnosis of exclusion, which involves ruling out other causes of hyponatremia (eg, low effective circulating volume, decreased solute intake, cortisol deficiency, and severe hypothyroidism).

D. Reset osmostat—This is a rare cause of hyponatremia in which patients regulate vasopressin release around a lower, or hypotonic, set point. Diagnosis involves documentation of dilute urine when serum sodium is lowered by administration of free water; however, this is rarely done in clinical practice. The mild hypo-osmolality of pregnancy is a form of reset osmostat.

Table 21–2. Common causes of syndrome of inappropriate ADH secretion.

CNS disorders
Stroke
Hemorrhage
Infection
Trauma
Inflammatory and demyelinating diseases
Pulmonary lesions
Infections (viral, bacterial, fungal)
Malignancies
Many but particularly small cell carcinoma of the lung
Drugs (this is only a partial list as many have been implicated)
Antidepressants: SSRIs, tricyclics, MAO inhibitors
Antineoplastics: cyclophosphamide, ifosfamide, methotrexate
Anticonvulsants: carbamazepine, sodium valproate, lamotrigine
Neuroleptics: haloperidol, fluphenazine, trifluoperazine thioridazine, thiothixene
NSAIDs
Methylenedioxymethamphetamine (MDMA; ecstasy)
Amiodarone
Ciprofloxacin
Opioids
Others
HIV
Pain, postoperative, stress
Hereditary
Idiopathic

E. Adrenal insufficiency and hypothyroidism—Cortisol normally provides negative feedback on ADH release, and therefore cortisol deficiency can lead to uninhibited ADH and hyponatremia. Concomitant mineralocorticoid deficiency may result in hyperkalemia and metabolic acidosis. Hyponatremia due to hypothyroidism has been described in the context of myxedema coma; the hyponatremia may be due to appropriate ADH release from reduced cardiac output and concurrent adrenal insufficiency, rather than from the absence of thyroid hormone.

F. Nausea, pain, and surgery—Nausea and pain are potent stimulators of ADH release. Severe hyponatremia can develop after elective surgery in healthy patients due to excessive use of hypotonic fluids.

G. Exercise-associated hyponatremia—Hyponatremia during or after exercise, especially endurance events such as triathlons and marathons, may be caused by a combination of excessive hypotonic fluid intake and ADH secretion (due to hypovolemia, pain, or nausea). Current guidelines suggest that endurance athletes drink water according to thirst rather than according to specified hourly rates of fluid intake. Electrolyte-containing sport drinks do not protect against hyponatremia since they are markedly hypotonic relative to serum.

H. Thiazide diuretics and other medication—Thiazides may induce hyponatremia, typically in older patients, within a few weeks of initiating therapy, and may be exacerbated by increased thirst and low solute intake. The mechanism appears to be a combination of water intake and a mild diuretic-induced volume contraction leading to ADH secretion. Loop diuretics do not cause hyponatremia as frequently due to impairment of the medullary concentration gradient, limiting the ability of ADH to promote water retention.

NSAIDs increase ADH by inhibiting prostaglandin formation. SSRIs (eg, fluoxetine, paroxetine, and citalopram) can also cause hyponatremia, especially in geriatric patients. Enhanced secretion or action of ADH may result from increased serotonergic tone.

Use of 3,4-methylenedioxymethamphetamine (MDMA, also known as ecstasy) can lead to hyponatremia and severe neurologic symptoms, including seizures, cerebral edema, and brainstem herniation. MDMA and its metabolites increase ADH release from the hypothalamus. Polydipsia may contribute to hyponatremia since MDMA users typically increase fluid intake to prevent hyperthermia.

Clinical Findings

A. Symptoms and Signs

Whether hyponatremia is symptomatic depends on both its severity and acuity. **Acute hyponatremia** (defined as lasting less than 48 hours) can result in marked neurologic symptoms, even with relatively modest hyponatremia, due to acute brain cell swelling and subsequent rise in intracranial pressure. Early symptoms include headache and decrease in attentiveness, which can lead to lethargy, disorientation, and nausea. The most serious symptoms include marked confusion and decreased levels of consciousness, vomiting, seizures, coma, brainstem herniation, and death. **Chronic hyponatremia,** defined as lasting longer than 48 hours, is often diagnosed on routine electrolyte measurements; patients are often asymptomatic as the brain has adapted to the surrounding hypotonicity. Subtle abnormalities, such as mild concentration and cognitive deficits, as well as gait disturbances that can lead to falls, may be present.

Clinical evaluation starts with a history of medications, changes in fluid intake (polydipsia, anorexia, intravenous fluid rates and composition), and fluid output (nausea and vomiting, diarrhea, ostomy output, polyuria, oliguria, insensible losses). The physical examination should attempt to categorize volume status (see Body Water and Fluid Distribution, above). The next determination is why ADH is being released and conditions in which release may be halted abruptly, which can impact the approach to therapy.

B. Laboratory Findings

The initial laboratory assessment should include serum and urine electrolytes and serum and urine osmolality. The severity of hyponatremia can be classified as mild (130–134 mEq/L), moderate (125–129 mEq/L), or severe (less than 125 mEq/L), with complications of untreated hyponatremia and rapid/overcorrection most commonly occurring in patients with severe hyponatremia. In clinical practice ADH levels are not measured; urine osmolality is used as a surrogate for ADH activity. Urine osmolality should be checked not only at the time of diagnosis but may also be useful if checked serially during therapy. Bedside assessment of volume status is often insensitive; therefore, a urine sodium may help differentiate between hypovolemia and euvolemia, particularly in nonedematous patients (Figure 21–1). The etiology of most cases of hyponatremia will be apparent by appropriate interpretation of the above laboratory values, in addition to patient history and assessment of volume status. Additional testing, such as thyroid and adrenal function tests, may be warranted in the appropriate context.

SIADH is a clinical diagnosis characterized by (1) hyponatremia; (2) decreased plasma osmolality (less than 280 mOsm/kg); (3) absence of heart, kidney, or liver disease; (4) normal thyroid and adrenal function (see Chapter 26); and (5) urine sodium usually over 20 mEq/L. Patients with SIADH may have low BUN (less than 10 mg/dL [3.6 mmol/L]) and hypouricemia (less than 4 mg/dL [238 mcmol/L]), which are not only dilutional but result from increased urea and uric acid clearances in response to the volume-expanded state.

Treatment

The initial treatment of hyponatremia is contingent on two primary factors, the acuity of onset and the severity of symptoms. **In patients with documented acute hyponatremia, ie, onset within 48 hours, sodium can be corrected at the rate at which it fell. In general, most cases are chronic and therefore need to be corrected more slowly to minimize risk of osmotic demyelination.**

A. Symptomatic Hyponatremia

If a patient has hyponatremia and severe symptoms (eg, seizures, confusion), regardless of etiology, then emergent treatment with hypertonic saline should commence. A relatively small increase in serum sodium of 4–5 mEq/L is generally sufficient to promptly reverse severe neurologic symptoms and decrease intracranial pressure. This can be accomplished most effectively by using boluses of 100 mL of 3% NaCl over 10 minutes, which can be repeated twice if needed. Each bolus might be predicted to raise the serum sodium by 1–2 mEq/L. In patients with less severe symptoms, an intravenous infusion of 3% NaCl (0.5–2 mL/kg/hour) may be used.

The importance of frequent laboratory monitoring—every 1–2 hours—during treatment of hyponatremia cannot be overemphasized.

B. Chronic Hyponatremia

The cornerstone of therapy in most patients with chronic hyponatremia, regardless of etiology, is restricting fluid intake below the level of urinary output. However, if the urine remains concentrated (greater than 300 mOsm/kg), this therapy alone may be insufficient, and other measures to increase free water excretion should be considered. Loop diuretics (with or without salt tablets) are frequently used since they impair the medullary concentration gradient thereby limiting renal concentration; despite this physiologic principle, this therapy has not been shown to be superior to fluid restriction alone. Other options include vasopressin receptor antagonists (vaptans), and oral urea.

Vaptans impair ADH action by inhibiting the vasopressin type 2 (V_2)-receptors in the collecting duct, thereby inducing a water diuresis. While a logical target for therapy in refractory hyponatremia, these agents have not been shown to improve hard outcomes and are associated with risks of liver toxicity and sodium overcorrection. If these agents are used, they should generally be avoided in patients with cirrhosis, duration should be limited to 30 days, and fluid restriction should concurrently be lifted to reduce the risk of excessive serum sodium correction. An alternative option is the use of oral urea to induce an osmotic diuresis, which enhances free water clearance. The disadvantage of palatability has been addressed by combining urea with sodium bicarbonate, citric acid, and sucrose in commercially available formulations.

Osmotic demyelination and correction rate—Iatrogenic osmotic demyelination syndrome is the result of overly rapid correction of serum sodium in patients with chronic hyponatremia. Previously called central pontine myelinolysis, osmotic demyelination syndrome may also occur outside the brainstem. Demyelination generally occurs 2–6 days after inappropriate sodium correction and presents with profound neurologic deficits that are often irreversible. Risk factors for osmotic demyelination syndrome include the severity of hyponatremia (majority less than 120 mEq/L), alcohol use disorder (alcoholism), liver disease, malnutrition, and concurrent hypokalemia.

The optimal correction rate for hyponatremia is debated, though consensus guidelines suggest a correction not to exceed 8 mEq/L in a 24-hour period. It should be emphasized that this represents a limit and not a goal. In fact, in patients who are deemed at high risk for osmotic demyelination syndrome based on criteria detailed above, a goal of 4–6 mEq/L/day is appropriate. If rapid discontinuation of the effects of vasopressin are anticipated, particularly in patients who are at high risk for osmotic demyelination syndrome, prophylactic use of intravenous desmopressin acetate (DDAVP) to prevent a water diuresis should be considered. In the event of overcorrection, free water, with or without DDAVP, should be infused to lower the serum sodium to an acceptable level.

C. Isotonic and Hypertonic Hyponatremia

Pseudohyponatremia from hypertriglyceridemia or hyperproteinemia requires no therapy except confirmation with the clinical laboratory. Hypertonic hyponatremia from translocational hyponatremia due to hyperglycemia or mannitol can be managed with glucose correction or mannitol discontinuation (if possible).

D. Hypotonic Hyponatremia

In addition to the considerations discussed above, patients with **hypovolemic hyponatremia** require fluid resuscitation. Data from 2018 suggest that balanced crystalloid solutions (lactated Ringer solution) may be a superior choice for resuscitation over normal saline, particularly in ICU patients; however, these results have not been substantiated in more recent trials. The correction of the volume depletion removes the stimulus for ADH and permits renal excretion of a dilute urine. Great care must be taken because the rapid renal excretion of the excess water may correct the serum sodium level too quickly.

When to Refer

- Nephrology consultation should be considered in patients with hyponatremia of uncertain cause or in refractory or complicated cases.
- Aggressive therapies with hypertonic saline, V_2-antagonists, or dialysis mandate specialist consultation.
- Consultation may be necessary with severe liver or heart disease.

When to Admit

Hospital admission is necessary for severe or symptomatic patients or those requiring aggressive therapies (such as hypertonic saline, initiating vaptans) for close monitoring and frequent laboratory testing.

Krisanapan P et al. Efficacy of furosemide, oral sodium chloride, and fluid restriction for treatment of syndrome of inappropriate antidiuresis (SIAD): an open label randomized controlled study (The EFFUSE-FLUID trial). Am J Kidney Dis. 2020;76:203. [PMID: 32199708]

Sterns RH. Treatment of severe hyponatremia. Clin J Am Soc Nephrol. 2018;13:641. [PMID: 29295830]

Zampieri FG et al. Effect of intravenous fluid treatment with a balanced solution vs. 0.9% saline solution on mortality in critically ill patients: the BaSICS randomized clinical trial. JAMA. 2021;326:1. [PMID: 34375394]

HYPERNATREMIA

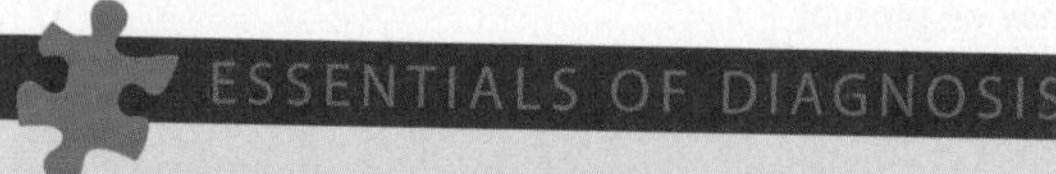

- Increased thirst and water intake are the main defense against hypernatremia.
- Urine osmolality helps differentiate renal from nonrenal water loss.

General Considerations

Hypernatremia is defined as a sodium concentration greater than 145 mEq/L. All patients with hypernatremia have hyperosmolality, unlike hyponatremic patients who can have a low, normal, or high serum osmolality. Hypernatremia develops when there is a relative loss of water that is inadequately compensated for by water ingestion. Rarely, administration of excess sodium in relation to water contributes to hypernatremia. This is most often encountered in critically ill patients when large amounts of hypertonic fluid are administered.

The primary responses to hypernatremia are stimulation of thirst (to increase water intake) and increased secretion of ADH (to minimize water loss in the urine). Cells in the hypothalamus can sense minimal changes in serum osmolarity, triggering the thirst mechanism and subsequent intake of water. It is nearly impossible to develop hypernatremia in the context of an intact thirst mechanism with appropriate access to water.

Clinical Findings

A. Symptoms and Signs

Acute, severe hypernatremia (serum sodium greater than 160 mEq/L) can manifest as lethargy, irritability, and weakness sometimes progressing to hyperthermia, delirium, seizures, and coma. Irreversible neurologic damage may occur if the hypernatremia is left untreated. Because water shifts from the cells to the intravascular space to protect volume status, symptoms may be delayed. Symptoms in older adults may not be specific.

B. Laboratory Findings

The first steps in evaluating patients with hypernatremia are assessing the urine volume, osmolality, and the osmole excretion rate. The latter can be calculated by multiplying the urine osmolality with urine volume. The copeptin test is discussed below.

C. Etiology

The initial step is to determine whether the patient with hypernatremia is oliguric, ie, urine flow less than 0.5 mL/minute, or nonoliguric. Patients who are nonoliguric can be further subdivided by measurement of a urine osmolality.

1. The oliguric patient (urine flow less than 0.5 mL/minute)— This is found in several scenarios.

A. REDUCED WATER INTAKE—Hypernatremia will develop in patients with reduced water intake secondary to the inability to communicate and/or limited access to water.

B. NONRENAL WATER LOSSES—Nonrenal sites of water loss include sweat, GI tract, and the respiratory tract. This is most commonly seen in patients with diarrhea or in febrile patients on a ventilator.

C. SHIFT OF WATER INTO CELLS—Rarely, hypernatremia may manifest from a shift of water into cells due to the intracellular gain of an effective osmole. This may be seen with seizures or rhabdomyolysis.

2. The nonoliguric patient (urine flow greater than 0.5 mL/minute)—

A. URINE OSMOLALITY LESS THAN 250 MOSM/KG—Hypernatremia in the setting of dilute urine is characteristic of diabetes insipidus (DI) or release of a vasopressinase. Central DI results from inadequate ADH release from the pituitary (stroke, tumor, infiltration). In nephrogenic DI, ADH levels are normal or even elevated, but the kidneys are less sensitive to the effects. Common causes include lithium therapy, post-relief of urinary obstruction, chronic interstitial nephritis, hypercalcemia, and hypokalemia. Central and nephrogenic DI can be distinguished by the response to exogenous DDAVP administration while polyuric. An innovative test to assist in the differentiation of patients with hypotonic polyuria is the measurement of **copeptin,** a C-terminal peptide synthesized with vasopressin, which mirrors its concentration over a wide range of plasma osmolalities. Elevated levels of copeptin in the setting of hypernatremia suggest the presence of vasopressin and therefore exclude a diagnosis of central DI. Vasopressin is unstable in isolated plasma, and levels are not helpful.

B. URINE OSMOLALITY GREATER THAN 300 MOSM/KG—Patients with an elevated urine osmolality and a high urine volume have an osmotic diuresis. Both glucose and urea in the urine can promote polyuria associated with an increased free water excretion.

Treatment

Treatment of hypernatremia includes both correcting the cause of the fluid loss, and replacing the water electrolyte deficit.

A. Choice of Fluid for Replacement

In general, the treatment of hypernatremia requires induction of a positive water balance by administration of hypotonic fluids, either intravenously or enterally or a combination of both. Because it can be difficult to correct large water deficits via the GI tract alone, the most common strategy is infusion of 5% dextrose in water (distilled water is contraindicated due to the development of hemolysis). Although there appears to be little risk in the rapid correction of hypernatremia in adults, be cautious when infusing large amount of 5% dextrose in water due to the risk of hyperglycemia and subsequent development of an osmotic diuresis, which can aggravate hypernatremia. In patients who are concurrently volume depleted, priority should be to restore euvolemia using isotonic fluids (eg, 0.9% normal saline), followed by hypotonic fluids to correct any remaining free water deficit. In the rare situation when hypernatremia is due to excess sodium balance (sodium ingestion or intravenous hypertonic saline), diuretics may be administered to enhance sodium excretion.

B. Calculation of Water Deficit

Fluid replacement should include correcting the free water deficit and adding maintenance fluid to replace ongoing and anticipated fluid losses.

1. Acute hypernatremia—This is relatively rare and generally encountered in patients with diabetes insipidus who do not have access to water, or even less commonly, in patients with salt poisoning; rapid restoration of water balance is indicated. Infusion of 0.5% dextrose in water is initiated at a rate of 3–6 mL/kg/hour until the serum sodium is below 145 mEq/L, then the infusion is slowed until the serum sodium normalizes (140 mEq/L). Desmopressin is needed to reduce urine water losses in patients with central diabetes insipidus. Rarely, renal replacement therapy may be needed in patients with acute hypernatremia and severe kidney injury.

2. Chronic hypernatremia—Restoration of water balance with either intravenous 5% dextrose in water or oral rehydration in clinically stable patients with adequate ability to tolerate oral intake should be initiated based on water deficit. The water deficit is the amount of water calculated to restore the sodium concentration to normal (140 mEq/L). Total body water (TBW) (Table 21–1) correlates with muscle mass and therefore decreases with advancing age, cachexia, and dehydration and, on average, is lower in women than in men. Current TBW equals 40–60% current body weight. This equation provides a guide for initial therapy and does not negate the need for repeated measurements to assess response to treatment.

$$\text{Water deficit (L)} = \text{Current TBW} \times \frac{S_{Na} - 140}{140}$$

It should be emphasized that the water deficit represents a static period in time and a critical mistake that is often made when considering the volume of water needed to restore sodium balance is failure to incorporate ongoing water loss via urinary output and insensible losses. Insensible losses can be estimated as 500–1000 mL daily; however, they can vary significantly. The proportion of urine volume that is free water can be estimated by calculating the electrolyte free water (EFW) clearance via the equation below.

$$C_{EFW}\,(L) = \text{Urine volume} \times \left(1 - \frac{U_{Na} + U_K}{S_{Na}}\right)$$

3. Rate of sodium correction—Although it would be appealing to apply similar principles for patients with hyponatremia to patients with hypernatremia, this practice is not supported by the literature. Adverse neurologic symptoms from overly rapid correction of hypernatremia have only been described in children. A slow rate of correction is usually recommended on the basis of osmotic brain adaptation that occurs with chronic hypernatremia and corresponding theoretical risk of cerebral edema if hypernatremia is corrected too quickly. However, a relatively large retrospective study found no evidence of morbidity or mortality with rapid correction of hypernatremia in critically ill patients with admission or hospital-acquired hypernatremia. Despite this, common clinical practice is to limit correction of chronic hypernatremia to below 12 mEq/L in 24 hours given the absence of data to suggest slow correction rates are harmful. However, if this rate is inadvertently exceeded, the serum sodium should not be raised. In patients with acute hypernatremia, the serum sodium should be corrected to normal (ie, 140 mEq/L) within 24 hours.

4. Treatment of the underlying cause—The underlying cause of the hypernatremia should be identified and addressed. For patients who have central DI, vasopressin deficiency should be replaced by administration of DDAVP.

When to Refer

Patients with refractory or unexplained hypernatremia should be referred for nephrology consultation.

When to Admit

- Patients with symptomatic hypernatremia require hospitalization for evaluation and treatment.
- Significant comorbidities or concomitant acute illnesses, especially if contributing to hypernatremia, may necessitate hospitalization.

Chauhan K et al. Rate of correction of hypernatremia and health outcomes in critically ill patients. Clin J Am Soc Nephrol. 2019;14:656. [PMID: 30948456]

Fenske W et al. A copeptin-based approach in the diagnosis of diabetes insipidus. N Engl J Med. 2018;379:428. [PMID: 30067922]

Seay NW et al. Diagnosis and management of disorders of body tonicity-hyponatremia and hypernatremia: Core Curriculum 2020. Am J Kidney Dis. 2020;75:272. [PMID: 31606238]

DISORDERS OF POTASSIUM CONCENTRATION

HYPOKALEMIA

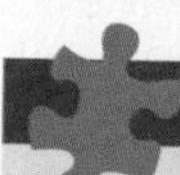

ESSENTIALS OF DIAGNOSIS

- Serum potassium < 3.5 mEq/L (3.5 mmol/L).
- Severe hypokalemia may induce arrhythmias and rhabdomyolysis.
- Assessment of urine potassium excretion (urine potassium to creatinine ratio) can distinguish renal from nonrenal loss of potassium.

General Considerations

Hypokalemia can result from insufficient dietary potassium intake, intracellular shifting of potassium from the extracellular space, or potassium loss (renal or extrarenal) (Table 21–3). A low dietary potassium intake is usually not sufficient as the kidneys can lower urine potassium excretion to very low levels (less than 15 mEq/L).

Table 21–3. Causes of hypokalemia.

Decreased potassium intake
Potassium shift into the cell
Alkalosis
Beta-adrenergic agonists
Insulin release (postprandial, exogenous, insulinoma)
Hypokalemic periodic paralysis
Renal potassium loss with metabolic acidosis
Proximal and distal RTAs
Toluene inhalation (glue sniffing)
Renal potassium loss with metabolic alkalosis
Normal/low blood pressure
Bartter syndrome
Gitelman syndrome
Magnesium deficiency
Vomiting
Loop/thiazide diuretics
High blood pressure
Elevated renin and aldosterone
Malignant hypertension
Renin-producing tumor
Renal artery stenosis
Depressed renin and elevated aldosterone
Adrenal adenoma
Glucocorticoid remediable aldosteronism
Adrenal hyperplasia
Depressed renin and aldosterone
Cushing syndrome
Black licorice
Apparent mineralocorticoid excess
Liddle syndrome
Increased GI losses
Diarrhea
Laxative abuse

RTA, renal tubular acidosis.

Shift of potassium into cells is increased by insulin and beta-adrenergic stimulation. Excess potassium excretion by the kidneys is usually due to increased aldosterone action in the setting of preserved delivery of sodium to the distal nephron. Magnesium is an important regulator of potassium handling and low levels lead to persistent renal excretion of potassium; hypokalemia is often refractory to treatment until the magnesium deficiency is corrected. Loop diuretics (eg, furosemide) cause substantial renal potassium and magnesium losses.

Clinical Findings

A. Symptoms and Signs

Hypokalemia is usually asymptomatic but when severe may lead to muscle weakness and cardiac arrhythmias. Involvement of GI smooth muscle may result in constipation or ileus. Rhabdomyolysis with associated AKI can be seen with serum potassium less than 2.5 mEq/L. Hypokalemia may additionally present as polyuria and polydipsia due to diminished concentrating ability of the kidney (nephrogenic DI) and chronic hypokalemia can lead to kidney disease (tubulointerstitial nephritis).

B. Laboratory Findings

Transient hypokalemia is generally secondary to intracellular shift, while sustained hypokalemia is secondary to potassium wasting or, rarely, inadequate intake. Assessment of renal potassium excretion can help distinguish renal from nonrenal causes of hypokalemia. A 24-hour urine collection is the most accurate method for assessing renal handling of potassium, with a level less than 25 mEq/day compatible with appropriate renal potassium retention, and higher values corresponding to renal potassium wasting. A more immediate assessment can be made by measuring a urine potassium to creatinine ratio (U_K/U_{Cr}) on a spot urine sample (Figure 21–2). In the setting of hypokalemia, a U_K/U_{Cr} ratio less than 13 mEq/g (or 1.5 mEq/mmol) is suggestive of a nonrenal etiology, most commonly GI losses, intracellular potassium shifts, or inadequate dietary intake, whereas higher values imply renal potassium wasting.

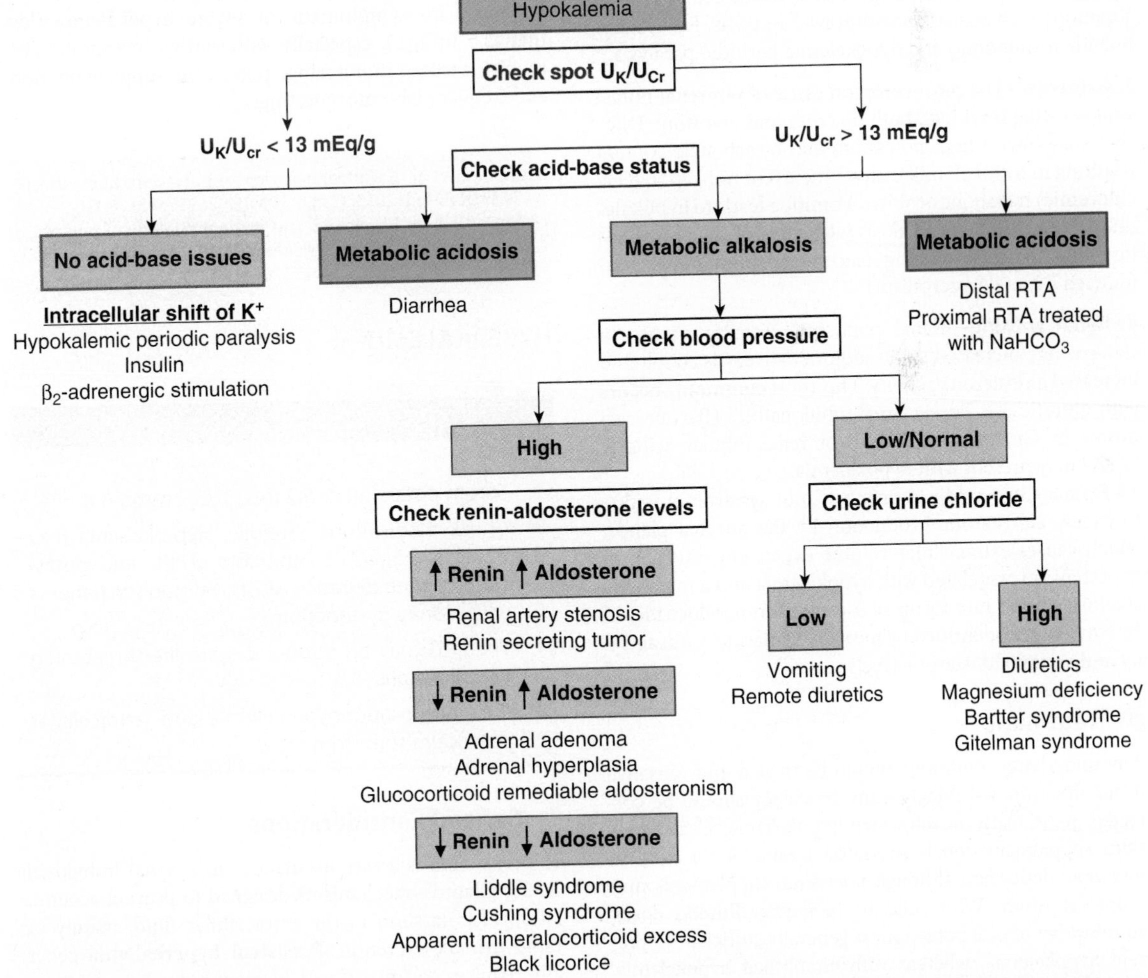

▲ **Figure 21–2.** Differentiating renal from nonrenal causes of hypokalemia using a spot urine potassium and a spot urine creatinine. $NaHCO_3$, sodium bicarbonate; RTA, renal tubular acidosis; U_K/U_{Cr}, urine potassium to creatinine ratio.

C. ECG

Hypokalemia leads to a characteristic progression of ECG changes, initially T wave flattening, subsequently ST depressions and T wave inversions, ultimately leading to U waves as the hypokalemia becomes more severe. There is significant interpatient variability in the degree of hypokalemia and corresponding ECG findings; therefore, typical ECG patterns may not be observed in all patients.

Etiology

1. Inadequate dietary intake—While the kidney can excrete urine that is virtually free of sodium, there continues to be a small amount of potassium excretion even in the setting of diets completely devoid of potassium. With extreme potassium free diets, such as anorexia nervosa and alcohol use disorder, the hypokalemia is worsened by concurrent magnesium depletion.

2. Intracellular shift—The most important determinants of intracellular potassium shifts are postprandial insulin and catecholamine release. These physiologic conditions can be exacerbated by beta-adrenergic–agonist administration, as well as high adrenergic states, which can be seen in situations such as alcohol withdrawal and MIs. Rare causes include insulinomas and hypokalemic periodic paralysis.

3. GI losses—The most common cause of nonrenal potassium wasting is GI loss, both diarrhea and vomiting. Diarrhea may have a high potassium and bicarbonate content resulting in hypokalemia with a concurrent nongap (hyperchloremic) metabolic acidosis. Vomiting leads to hypokalemia with a metabolic alkalosis with most of the potassium loss due to renal wasting (secondary to hypovolemia-induced hyperaldosteronism).

4. Renal wasting—Renal potassium wasting occurs in states where increased distal sodium delivery is coupled to increased aldosterone activity. This most commonly occurs with diuretic use. Rarely, renal tubulopathies (Bartter syndrome or Gitelman syndrome) or renal tubular acidosis (RTA) may present with hypokalemia.

Primary hyperaldosteronism (Conn syndrome) is due to excess aldosterone production by the adrenal glands, which causes extracellular volume expansion resulting in hypertension associated with hypokalemia and a metabolic alkalosis. Other rare forms of increased mineralocorticoid activity may be identified by measuring plasma renin activity and serum aldosterone levels.

Treatment

Any underlying conditions should be treated and causative drugs discontinued. Magnesium deficiency should be corrected, particularly in refractory hypokalemia. Oral potassium supplementation is the safest treatment for mild to moderate deficiency, although potassium supplements may cause GI upset. With mild to moderate diuretic doses, 20 mEq/day of oral potassium is generally sufficient to prevent hypokalemia, whereas with established hypokalemia, 40–100 mEq/day over a period of days to weeks may be needed to treat hypokalemia and fully replete potassium stores.

Intravenous potassium is reserved for severe hypokalemia (less than 3.0 mEq/L) and requires careful monitoring due to the risk of transient hyperkalemia. Potassium chloride may be given through a peripheral intravenous line at rates up to 10–15 mEq/hour diluted in 0.5% or 0.9% normal saline, but higher rates (up to 20 mEq/hour) require central access due to the risk of peripheral vein irritation. In the event of concurrent metabolic acidosis, potassium repletion should take precedence over alkali administration as correction of the acidosis will result in intracellular shift of potassium, further decreasing extracellular potassium concentration. Similarly, potassium should be given in a saline, rather than dextrose, solution since dextrose would stimulate insulin release and, hence, intracellular shift.

When to Refer

Patients with unexplained hypokalemia, refractory or persistent hypokalemia, or suggestive alternative diagnoses (eg, aldosteronism or hypokalemic periodic paralysis) should be referred for nephrology consultation.

When to Admit

Patients with symptomatic or severe hypokalemia (less than 2.5 mEq/L), especially with cardiac manifestations, require cardiac monitoring, potassium supplementation, and frequent laboratory testing.

Gumz ML et al. An integrated view of potassium homeostasis. N Engl J Med. 2015;373:60. [PMID: 26132942]

Palmer BF et al. Physiology and pathophysiology of potassium homeostasis: Core Curriculum 2019. Am J Kidney Dis. 2019;74:682. [PMID: 31227226]

HYPERKALEMIA

ESSENTIALS OF DIAGNOSIS

- Serum potassium > 5.2 mEq/L (5.2 mmol/L).
- Check medications carefully. Hyperkalemia may develop from ACE inhibitors, ARBs, and potassium-sparing diuretics, most commonly in patients with kidney dysfunction.
- The ECG may be normal despite life-threatening hyperkalemia.
- Rule out pseudohyperkalemia and extracellular potassium shift from cells.

General Considerations

Hyperkalemia is a rare occurrence in normal individuals due to adaptive mechanisms designed to prevent accumulation of potassium in the extracellular fluid, mainly via rapid urinary excretion. **Persistent hyperkalemia** generally requires an impairment in renal potassium excretion due to impaired secretion of or hyporesponsiveness to aldosterone, impaired delivery of sodium and water to the

Table 21–4. Causes of hyperkalemia.

Pseudohyperkalemia
Marked thrombocytosis or leukocytosis with release of intracellular K^+
Repeated fist clenching during phlebotomy, tourniquet application, use of small-bore needles during lab draw
Extracellular shift of K^+
Metabolic acidosis
Insulin deficiency
Hyperglycemia
Alpha-adrenergic stimulation
Tissue injury (rhabdomyolysis, hemolysis, tumor lysis)
Hyperkalemic periodic paralysis
Drugs (digoxin overdose, succinylcholine)
Kidney disease, acute and chronic
Renal secretory defects (may or may not have reduced kidney function): interstitial nephritis, SLE, sickle cell disease, amyloidosis, obstructive nephropathy, kidney transplant
Hypoaldosteronism
Addison disease
Type IV renal tubular acidosis
Heparin
Ketoconazole
Drugs that inhibit potassium excretion
Spironolactone, eplerenone, drospirenone, NSAIDs, ACE inhibitors, angiotensin II receptor blockers, triamterene, amiloride, trimethoprim, pentamidine, cyclosporine, tacrolimus
Excessive intake of K^+
Especially in patients with diminished kidney excretion

distal nephron, or kidney disease (acute or chronic) (Table 21–4). **Transient hyperkalemia** suggests shift of potassium from inside cells into the extracellular fluid, which can occur in the context of tissue damage (rhabdomyolysis, tumor lysis, massive hemolysis, and trauma) or metabolic acidosis.

Clinical Findings

A. Symptoms and Signs

The symptoms of hyperkalemia are due to impaired neuromuscular transmission. The most serious manifestations are cardiac conduction abnormalities and neuromuscular manifestations, such as muscle weakness, which may be profound. This generally occurs with potassium concentrations above 7 mEq/L, though it can vary depending on the acuity in development of hyperkalemia. **Hyperkalemic period paralysis** is a rare genetic disorder characterized by episodes of painless muscle weakness precipitated by potassium ingestion, rest after heavy exercise, and cold exposure. Hyperkalemia additionally impairs urinary ammonium excretion and may lead to metabolic acidosis.

B. ECG

ECG is an unreliable method for detecting hyperkalemia; clinical studies show poor correlation between serum potassium and cardiac manifestations. The rapidity in development of hyperkalemia may correlate with the development of ECG changes. Typical sequential changes on the ECG are peaking of the T waves, ST-segment depression, and widening of the PR and QRS intervals. As the QRS continues to widen, sine waves may develop, which are concerning for imminent ventricular fibrillation and ultimately asystole.

Etiology

1. Increased potassium release from cells—

A. Pseudohyperkalemia—This condition arises during specimen collection due to fist clenching, application of tourniquets, or using small bore needles. The presence of hemolysis in the processed sample suggests these etiologies. A more striking example occurs with marked thrombocytosis (greater than 500,000/mcL [500×10^9/L]) or leukocytosis (greater than 100,000/mcL [100×10^9/L]), particularly leukemic cells. Centrifugation or transport via a pneumatic tube system causes significant cell destruction. If this condition is suspected, a noncentrifuged whole blood sample that is walked to the laboratory is required for confirmation.

B. Tissue breakdown—Tissue damage results in release of intracellular potassium to the extracellular space. Common clinical examples include tumor lysis syndrome, crush injuries, and severe hemolysis. Hyperkalemia is more common when concurrent renal impairment is present.

C. Hyperglycemia—Patients with uncontrolled diabetes may have hyperkalemia, even in the setting of a low total body potassium, due to a combination of insulin deficiency and hyperosmolarity from hyperglycemia.

D. Metabolic acidosis—Acidosis results in potassium shifting out of the intracellular fluid due to buffering of hydrogen ions into cells. Serum potassium concentration rises approximately 0.7 mEq/L for every decrease of 0.1 pH unit. This effect is not seen with organic acidosis, such as lactic acidosis or ketoacidosis.

2. Impaired kidney excretion—

A. AKI—A rapid reduction in kidney function leads to poor renal excretion of potassium and does not allow sufficient time for nonrenal adaptive mechanisms to take effect. Hyperkalemia occurs more commonly in oliguric patients.

B. CKD—The ability to maintain normal serum potassium is generally preserved until GFR declines to less than 20–30 mL/minute/1.73 m^2. This is primarily due to adaptive mechanisms, particularly increases in potassium excretion by remaining functioning nephrons and by increased GI tract potassium excretion. Hyperkalemia with more modest decreases in GFR is often due to medications that disrupt the renin-angiotensin-aldosterone system, which are commonly used in these patients.

C. Low effective circulating volume—Volume depletion and the edematous states of cirrhosis and heart failure can cause hyperkalemia due to a decrease in distal delivery of sodium and water, which impairs potassium excretion.

D. Reduced aldosterone action—Mineralocorticoid deficiency from Addison disease may cause hyperkalemia due to a decreased renal excretion of potassium. Mineralocorticoid resistance due to genetic disorders, interstitial kidney disease, or urinary tract obstruction also leads to hyperkalemia.

3. Medications—A number of medications can be implicated in the development of hyperkalemia and a careful review of a patient's medication list is imperative. Common medications include ACE inhibitors, ARBs, and NSAIDs, which reduce aldosterone release. Concomitant use of aldosterone antagonists (spironolactone or eplerenone) or medications that directly block the sodium channels of the principal cells (amiloride, triamterene, or trimethoprim) further increase the risk of hyperkalemia. Beta-blockers can cause mild hyperkalemia by interfering with potassium uptake by cells, a phenomenon more commonly observed with nonselective beta-blockers. Heparin inhibits aldosterone production in the adrenal glands. Calcineurin inhibitors, such as cyclosporine and tacrolimus, can induce hyperkalemia, partly stimulating the sodium chloride co-transporter in the distal nephron impairing distal sodium delivery. These medications should be used cautiously in patients with renal impairment, and laboratory monitoring is indicated within 1–2 weeks of drug initiation or dosage increase.

Treatment

The diagnosis should be confirmed by repeat laboratory testing to rule out spurious hyperkalemia, especially in the absence of medications that cause hyperkalemia or in patients without kidney disease. The initial treatment is determined by the presence of signs and symptoms as well as the severity in plasma potassium elevation. In all patients, exogenous sources of potassium should be eliminated, medications that can impair potassium excretion discontinued, volume depletion corrected, and metabolic acidosis improved.

In emergency situations (cardiac toxicity, muscle weakness, or potassium greater than 6.5 mEq/L), initial therapy should be intravenous calcium gluconate to stabilize the myocardium in order to protect against arrhythmias, followed by therapies to shift potassium into cells. Insulin and beta-agonists shift potassium intracellularly within 10–15 minutes of administration but have a short duration of action (1–2 hours) (Table 21–5). Sodium bicarbonate may help shift potassium into cells in patients with a concurrent metabolic acidosis. Once the patient is stabilized, therapies are focused on potassium excretion.

Potassium excretion may be enhanced with the use of loop diuretics. Patiromer and sodium zirconium cyclosilicate are potassium-binding drugs that may be used to treat chronic hyperkalemia. Studies have demonstrated that these drugs are well tolerated and effective in patients with hyperkalemia who have either CKD or heart failure and take at least one medication that inhibits the renin-angiotensin-aldosterone system. Small studies have suggested utility in acute hyperkalemia as well. If administered for hyperkalemic emergency, sodium zirconium cyclosilicate is preferred due to its more rapid onset of action. Sodium polystyrene (Kayexalate) has been used for decades although its efficacy and safety have been questioned. It may not increase potassium excretion greater than laxatives alone and has been associated with colonic necrosis, both with and without sorbitol coadministration; sodium polystyrene is contraindicated in patients with risk factors for colonic necrosis, such as bowel obstruction, ileus, and postoperative state. Hemodialysis may be necessary to remove potassium in patients with acute or chronic kidney injury, particularly in patients who are oliguric.

When to Refer

- Nephrology consultation should be obtained for patients with hyperkalemia from kidney disease.
- Transplant patients may need adjustment of their immunosuppression regimen by transplant specialists.

When to Admit

Patients with severe hyperkalemia (greater than 6 mEq/L), any degree of hyperkalemia associated with ECG changes, or concomitant illness that may worsen hyperkalemia (eg, tumor lysis, rhabdomyolysis, metabolic acidosis) should be sent to the emergency department for immediate treatment.

Kovesdy CP et al. Potassium homeostasis in health and disease: a scientific workshop cosponsored by the National Kidney Foundation and the American Society of Hypertension. J Am Soc Hypertens. 2017;11:783. [PMID: 29030153]

Peacock FW et al. Emergency potassium normalization treatment including sodium zirconium cyclosilicate: a phase II, randomized, double-blind, placebo-controlled study (ENERGIZE). Acad Emerg Med. 2020;27:475. [PMID: 32149451]

Rafique Z et al. Patiromer for treatment of hyperkalemia in the emergency department: a pilot study. Acad Emerg Med. 2020;27:54. [PMID: 31599043]

DISORDERS OF CALCIUM CONCENTRATION

The normal total plasma (or serum) calcium concentration is 8.5–10.5 mg/dL (2.1–2.6 mmol/L). Ionized calcium (normal: 4.6–5.3 mg/dL [1.16–1.31 mmol/L]) is the physiologically active portion and is necessary for muscle contraction and nerve function. In most situations, measuring total calcium concentration is sufficient since changes mirror that seen in ionized calcium concentration; exceptions include patients with hypoalbuminemia and certain acid-base disorders.

HYPOCALCEMIA

ESSENTIALS OF DIAGNOSIS

- Usually asymptomatic but can cause cramps or tetany if severe.
- Decreased serum parathyroid hormone (PTH), vitamin D, or magnesium levels.
- Despite a low total serum calcium, calcium metabolism is likely normal if ionized calcium level is normal.

Table 21–5. Treatment of hyperkalemia.

Treatment of Hyperkalemia

Emergent/Stabilizing Therapy

Modality	Mechanism of Action	Onset	Duration	Prescription	K^+ Removed From Body
Calcium	Antagonizes cardiac conduction abnormalities	0–5 minutes	1 hour	Intravenous: calcium gluconate 10%, 5–30 mL, or calcium chloride 5%, 5–30 mL	None
Bicarbonate	Distributes K^+ into cells	15–30 minutes	1–2 hours	Intravenous: $NaHCO_3$, 50–100 mEq **Note:** Sodium bicarbonate may not be effective in ESKD patients; dialysis is more expedient and effective. Some patients may not tolerate the additional sodium load of bicarbonate therapy.	None
Insulin	Distributes K^+ into cells	15–60 minutes	4–6 hours	Intravenous: regular insulin, 5–10 units, plus glucose 50%, 25 g	None
Albuterol	Distributes K^+ into cells	15–30 minutes	2–4 hours	Nebulized albuterol, 10–20 mg in 4 mL normal saline, inhaled over 10 minutes **Note:** Much higher doses are necessary for hyperkalemia treatment (10–20 mg) than for airway disease (2.5 mg).	None

Nonemergent/Excretory Therapy

Modality	Mechanism of Action	Onset of Action	Prescription	K^+ Removed From Body
Loop diuretic	Renal K^+ excretion	0.5–2 hours	Intravenous: furosemide, 40–160 mg	Variable
Patiromer	Ca^{2+}-K^+ cation exchange resin	~7 hours	Oral: 4.2–16.8 g once or twice daily	Mean 0.75 mEq/L
Sodium zirconium cyclosilicate	Selective potassium cation trapping agent	1 hour	Oral: 10 g up to three times daily	0.7 mEq/L per 10 g dose
Sodium polystyrene sulfonate (eg, Kayexalate)	Ion-exchange resin binds K^+	1–3 hours	Oral: 15–60 g in 20% sorbitol (60–240 mL) Rectal: 30–60 g in 20% sorbitol **Note:** Resins with sorbitol may cause bowel necrosis and intestinal perforation, especially in patients with abnormal bowel function.	0.5–1 mEq/g resin
Hemodialysis[1]	Extracorporeal K^+ removal	1–8 hours	**Note:** A fast and effective therapy for hyperkalemia, hemodialysis can be delayed by vascular access placement and equipment and/or staff availability. Serum K can be rapidly corrected within minutes, but post-dialysis rebound can occur.	25–50 mEq/hour
Peritoneal dialysis	Peritoneal K^+ removal	1–4 hours	Frequent exchanges	50–70 mEq/24 hours

[1]Can be both acute immediate and urgent treatment of hyperkalemia.
Reproduced with permission from Cogan MG. *Fluid and Electrolytes: Physiology and Pathophysiology*. McGraw-Hill, 1991.

Table 21–6. Causes of hypocalcemia.

Decreased intake or absorption
Malabsorption
Small bowel bypass, short bowel
Vitamin D deficit (decreased absorption, decreased production of 25-hydroxyvitamin D or 1,25-dihydroxyvitamin D)
Increased loss
Alcohol use disorder
CKD
Diuretic therapy
Endocrine disease
Hypoparathyroidism, genetic or acquired (including hypo- and hypermagnesemia)
Post-parathyroidectomy (hungry bone syndrome)
Pseudohypoparathyroidism
Calcitonin secretion with medullary carcinoma of the thyroid
Familial hypocalcemia
Associated diseases
Pancreatitis
Rhabdomyolysis
Septic shock
Physiologic causes
Decreased serum albumin[1]
Decreased end-organ response to vitamin D
Hyperphosphatemia
Aminoglycoside antibiotics, plicamycin, loop diuretics, foscarnet

[1]Ionized calcium concentration is normal.

General Considerations

The most common cause of low total serum calcium is hypoalbuminemia. When serum albumin concentration is lower than 4 g/dL (40 g/L), serum Ca^{2+} concentration is reduced by 0.8–1 mg/dL (0.20–0.25 mmol/L) for every 1 g/dL (10 g/L) of albumin. True hypocalcemia (decreased ionized calcium) implies insufficient action of PTH or active vitamin D. Important causes of hypocalcemia are listed in Table 21–6.

The most common cause of hypocalcemia is advanced CKD, in which decreased production of calcitriol and hyperphosphatemia both play a role (see Chapter 22). Rarely, primary hypoparathyroidism due to mutations of the calcium-sensing receptor inappropriately suppressing PTH release leads to hypocalcemia (see Chapter 26). Magnesium depletion reduces both PTH release and tissue responsiveness to PTH, causing hypocalcemia. Hypocalcemia in pancreatitis is a marker of severe disease. Elderly hospitalized patients with hypocalcemia and hypophosphatemia, with or without an elevated PTH level, are likely vitamin D deficient.

Clinical Findings

A. Symptoms and Signs

The hallmark sign of severe hypocalcemia (ionized calcium below 1 mmol/L) is tetany from increased neuromuscular irritability. Laryngospasm with stridor can obstruct the airway. Convulsions, perioral and peripheral paresthesias, and abdominal pain can develop. Less pronounced symptoms include fatigue, anxiety, and depression. Classic physical findings include Chvostek sign (contraction of the facial muscle in response to tapping the facial nerve) and Trousseau sign (carpal spasm occurring with occlusion of the brachial artery by a blood pressure cuff). QT prolongation predisposes to ventricular arrhythmias, though serious dysrhythmias are rare.

B. Laboratory Findings

Serum calcium concentration is low (less than 8.5 mg/dL [2.1 mmol/L]). In true hypocalcemia, the ionized serum calcium concentration is also low (less than 4.6 mg/dL [1.15 mmol/L]). Serum phosphate is usually elevated in hypoparathyroidism or in advanced CKD, whereas it is suppressed in vitamin D deficiency.

Serum magnesium concentration is commonly low. In respiratory alkalosis, total serum calcium is normal but ionized calcium is low. The ECG shows a prolonged QT interval.

Treatment

A. Severe, Symptomatic Hypocalcemia

In the presence of tetany, arrhythmias, or seizures, intravenous calcium gluconate is indicated. Because of the short duration of action, continuous calcium infusion is usually required. Ten to 15 milligrams of calcium per kilogram body weight, or six to eight 10-mL vials of 10% calcium gluconate (558–744 mg of calcium), are added to 1 L of D_5W and infused over 4–6 hours. By monitoring the serum calcium frequently (every 4–6 hours), the infusion rate is adjusted to maintain the serum calcium at 7–8.5 mg/dL. See Chapter 26 for further discussion of the treatment of hypoparathyroidism.

B. Asymptomatic Hypocalcemia

Oral calcium (1–2 g of elemental calcium) and vitamin D preparations, including active vitamin D sterols, are used. Calcium carbonate is well tolerated and less expensive than many other calcium tablets. A check of urinary calcium excretion is recommended after the initiation of therapy because chronic hypercalciuria (urine calcium excretion greater than 300 mg or 7.5 mmol per day) or urine calcium:creatinine ratio greater than 0.3 may impair kidney function in these patients. The low serum calcium associated with hypoalbuminemia does not require replacement therapy. If serum magnesium is low, therapy must include magnesium replacement, which by itself often corrects hypocalcemia.

When to Refer

Patients with complicated hypocalcemia from hypoparathyroidism, familial hypocalcemia, or CKD require referral to an endocrinologist or nephrologist.

When to Admit

Patients with tetany, arrhythmias, seizures, or other symptoms of hypocalcemia require immediate therapy.

Aberegg SK. Ionized calcium in the ICU: should it be measured and corrected? Chest. 2016;149:846. [PMID: 26836894]

Schafer AL et al. Hypocalcemia: diagnosis and treatment. In: Feingold KR et al, editors. Endotext. 2016. [PMID: 25905251]

HYPERCALCEMIA

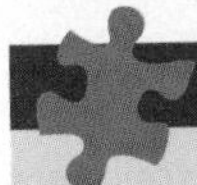

ESSENTIALS OF DIAGNOSIS

- Most common causes: primary hyperparathyroidism and malignancy-associated hypercalcemia.
- Asymptomatic, mild hypercalcemia (> 10.5 mg/dL [2.6 mmol/L]) is usually due to primary hyperparathyroidism.
- Symptomatic, severe hypercalcemia (> 13 mg/dL [3.2 mmol/L]) is usually due to malignancy-associated hypercalcemia.

General Considerations

Important causes of hypercalcemia are listed in Table 21–7. Primary hyperparathyroidism and malignancy account for 90% of cases. Primary hyperparathyroidism is the most common cause of hypercalcemia (usually mild) in ambulatory patients. Hypercalcemia above 14 mg/dL is most often associated with malignancy and is rare with primary hyperparathyroidism. Tumor production of PTH-related proteins (PTHrP) is the most common paraneoplastic endocrine syndrome, accounting for most cases of hypercalcemia in inpatients. The neoplasm is clinically apparent in nearly all cases when the hypercalcemia is detected, and the prognosis is poor. Granulomatous diseases, such as sarcoidosis and tuberculosis, cause hypercalcemia via overproduction of active vitamin D (1,25 dihydroxyvitamin D_3). Patients with mild hypercalcemia and normal to slightly elevated PTH levels should be assessed for familial hypocalciuric hypercalcemia.

Milk-alkali syndrome has had a resurgence due to calcium ingestion for prevention of osteoporosis and treatment of dyspepsia. Heavy calcium carbonate intake causes hypercalcemic AKI, likely from renal afferent vasoconstriction as well as from volume depletion due to its diuretic effect. The decreased GFR impairs bicarbonate excretion, while hypercalcemia stimulates proton secretion and bicarbonate reabsorption. Metabolic alkalosis decreases calcium excretion, maintaining hypercalcemia.

Table 21–7. Causes of hypercalcemia.

Increased intake or absorption
Milk-alkali syndrome
Vitamin D or vitamin A excess
Endocrine disorders
Primary hyperparathyroidism
Secondary or tertiary hyperparathyroidism (usually associated with hypocalcemia)
Acromegaly
Adrenal insufficiency
Pheochromocytoma
Thyrotoxicosis
Neoplastic diseases
Tumors producing PTH-related proteins (ovary, kidney, lung)
Plasma cell myeloma (elaboration of osteoclast-activating factor)
Lymphoma (occasionally from production of calcitriol)
Miscellaneous causes
Thiazide diuretics
Granulomatous diseases (production of calcitriol)
Paget disease of bone
Hypophosphatasia
Immobilization
Familial hypocalciuric hypercalcemia
Complications of kidney transplantation
Lithium intake

PTH, parathyroid hormone.

Clinical Findings

A. Symptoms and Signs

The history and physical examination should focus on the duration of hypercalcemia and evidence for a neoplasm. Hypercalcemia may affect GI, kidney, and neurologic function. Mild hypercalcemia (below 12 mg/dL) is often asymptomatic. Moderate hypercalcemia (12–14 mg/dL) may be tolerated if it is longstanding yet tends to be symptomatic if acute. Severe hypercalcemia (above 14 mg/dL) is frequently symptomatic. Common symptoms include anxiety, lethargy, constipation, anorexia, and cognitive changes, which can progress to lethargy and stupor in severe cases. Pancreatitis from calcium deposition in the pancreatic duct is a rare complication. Polyuria and dehydration may occur from impaired renal concentrating ability. Other symptoms include renal colic and hematuria from nephrolithiasis. Acute hypercalcemia can shorten the QT interval, though clinically relevant arrhythmias are rare.

B. Laboratory Findings

The serum ionized calcium exceeds 1.32 mmol/L (correct for serum albumin if ionized calcium is unavailable [see Hypocalcemia, above]). Check serum PTH to determine if hypercalcemia is PTH-mediated or non-PTH mediated.

PTH should be completely suppressed in the presence of hypercalcemia if kidney function is normal. Therefore, "normal" levels of PTH with hypercalcemia do not rule out hyperparathyroidism. Asymptomatic patients with mild hypercalcemia and PTH in the normal or slightly elevated range should have a 24-hour urine calcium or spot urine calcium to creatinine ratio checked for familial hypocalciuric hypercalcemia. If PTH is appropriately suppressed (typically below 20 pg/mL) PTHrP and vitamin D and its metabolites should be measured. Causes of a suppressed PTH and PTHrP with low or normal 25-OH and 1,25-OH vitamin D_3 levels include plasma cell myeloma, vitamin A intoxication, thyrotoxicosis, and immobilization. Hypocalciuria (below 100 mg/day) occurs in familial hypocalciuric hypercalcemia, thiazide diuretic use, and milk-alkali syndrome. Hypophosphatemia is more common with primary hyperparathyroidism and humoral hypercalcemia of malignancy (elevated PTHrP). In patients with an elevated 1,25-OH vitamin D_3, a chest radiograph may assess for the presence of granulomatous disease.

Treatment

Until the primary cause can be identified and treated, therapy is initiated to promote immediate reduction in serum calcium. Asymptomatic patients with mild hypercalcemia (below 12 mg/dL) do not require immediate therapy; patients should be cautioned to avoid measures that exacerbate hypercalcemia, such as volume depletion and thiazide diuretics. Patient with symptomatic hypercalcemia, a sudden rise in serum calcium above 12 mg/dL and those with severe hypercalcemia (above 14 mg/dL) should receive immediate therapy. Begin treatment with 0.9% normal saline, 200–300 mL/hour, until euvolemia is achieved (lactated Ringer is generally avoided because it contains a small amount of calcium). Loop diuretics to enhance renal calcium excretion should generally be avoided due to possible complications, such as nephrolithiasis. These agents were used more commonly in the era of more aggressive volume administration, ie, beyond that needed to achieve euvolemia, and prior to the wide availability of more effective medications, such as bisphosphonates and calcitonin. Loop diuretics may be carefully used in the context of preventing or managing volume overload, particularly in patients with heart failure or kidney dysfunction.

Calcitonin, 4–8 IU/kg intramuscularly or subcutaneously every 6–12 hours, enhances renal excretion of calcium and decreases bone resorption by interfering with osteoclast activity. Calcitonin efficacy is limited to 48 hours because of tachyphylaxis.

Bisphosphonates are the treatment of choice for hypercalcemia secondary to excessive bone resorption. Denosumab, a monoclonal antibody against RANKL, inhibits osteoclasts, reducing bone resorption and serum calcium levels; this medication is an option when hypercalcemia is refractory to bisphosphonate therapy or when bisphosphonates are contraindicated (ie, severe renal impairment). The calcimimetic agent cinacalcet suppresses PTH secretion and decreases serum calcium concentration; it has been recommended for use in patients with symptomatic or severe primary hyperparathyroidism who are unable to undergo parathyroidectomy and patients with inoperable parathyroid carcinoma. (See Chapters 26 and 39.) Hemodialysis using a low calcium dialysate is an effective therapy for hypercalcemia refractory to the above therapies. Hypercalcemia in granulomatous disease is from overproduction of calcitriol; prednisone inhibits calcitriol synthesis and reduces serum calcium levels within 2–5 days.

Typically, if dialysis patients do not receive proper supplementation of calcium and active vitamin D, hypocalcemia and hyperphosphatemia develop. Conversely, hypercalcemia can develop in severe tertiary hyperparathyroidism with high PTH levels, or from excess vitamin D supplementation. Hypercalcemia in dialysis patients usually occurs when there is hyperphosphatemia; metastatic calcification may occur.

When to Refer

- Patients may require referral to an oncologist or endocrinologist depending on the cause of hypercalcemia.
- Patients with granulomatous diseases (eg, tuberculosis and other chronic infections, granulomatosis with polyangiitis, sarcoidosis) may require assistance from infectious disease specialists, rheumatologists, or pulmonologists.

When to Admit

- Patients with symptomatic or severe hypercalcemia require immediate treatment.
- Unexplained hypercalcemia with associated conditions, such as AKI or suspected malignancy, may require urgent treatment and expedited evaluation.

Carrick AI et al. Rapid fire: hypercalcemia. Emerg Med Clin North Am. 2018;36:549. [PMID: 30037441]

Villalba-Ferrer F et al. Hypercalcemic crisis due to primary hyperparathyroidism resistant to medical treatment. Cir. 2020;88:13. [PMID: 33284269]

Zagzag J et al. Hypercalcemia and cancer: differential diagnosis and treatment. CA Cancer J Clin. 2018;68:377. [PMID: 30240520]

DISORDERS OF PHOSPHORUS CONCENTRATION

Plasma phosphorus is mainly inorganic phosphate and represents a small fraction (less than 0.2%) of total body phosphate. Important determinants of plasma inorganic phosphate are renal excretion, intestinal absorption, and shift between the intracellular and extracellular spaces. The kidney is the most important regulator of the serum phosphate level. PTH decreases reabsorption of phosphate in the proximal tubule while 1,25-dihydroxyvitamin D increases reabsorption. Renal proximal tubular reabsorption of phosphate is decreased by hypertension, corticosteroids, metabolic acidosis, and proximal tubular dysfunction (as in Fanconi syndrome). Fibroblast growth factor 23 (FGF23) is a potent phosphaturic hormone. Intestinal absorption of phosphate is facilitated by active vitamin D. Cellular phosphate uptake is stimulated by various factors and conditions, including alkalemia, insulin, epinephrine, refeeding syndrome, hungry bone syndrome, and accelerated cell proliferation.

Phosphorus metabolism and homeostasis are intimately related to calcium metabolism.

HYPOPHOSPHATEMIA

ESSENTIALS OF DIAGNOSIS

- Severe hypophosphatemia may cause tissue hypoxia and rhabdomyolysis.
- Renal loss of phosphate can be diagnosed by calculating the fractional excretion of phosphate (FE_{PO_4}).
- PTH and FGF23 are the major factors that increase urine phosphate.

General Considerations

The etiology of hypophosphatemia can be categorized as decreased intestinal absorption, increased urinary excretion, or transcellular shift (Table 21–8). Hypophosphatemia may occur in the presence of normal phosphate stores. Serum phosphate levels decrease transiently after food intake, which stimulates endogenous insulin release. In patients with depleted phosphate stores, such as alcoholic or malnourished patients, carbohydrate intake can induce severe hypophosphatemia (refeeding syndrome). Acute respiratory alkalosis can lower serum phosphate concentrations by stimulating glycolysis. Several drugs can impair intestinal absorption of phosphate, particularly calcium-, magnesium-, and aluminum-containing antacids. Elevated PTH causes hypophosphatemia by inhibiting reabsorption in the kidney. Vitamin D deficiency decreases intestinal phosphate and calcium absorption with the resultant hypocalcemia stimulating PTH release, increasing urinary phosphate excretion. Generalized dysfunction in the proximal tubule (Fanconi syndrome) is characterized by hypophosphatemia, metabolic acidosis, glucosuria, and aminoaciduria. Mutations in FGF23 are associated with urinary phosphorous wasting with rickets or osteomalacia.

Table 21–8. Causes of hypophosphatemia.

Decreased intestinal absorption
Starvation
Absorption blocked by oral antacids or phosphate binders
Parenteral alimentation with inadequate phosphate content
Malabsorption syndrome, small bowel bypass
Vitamin D–deficient and vitamin D–resistant osteomalacia
Increased urinary excretion
Hyperparathyroidism (primary or secondary)
Hyperthyroidism
Renal tubular defects with excessive phosphaturia (congenital, Fanconi syndrome induced by monoclonal gammopathy, heavy metal poisoning), alcohol use disorder
Hypokalemic nephropathy
Inadequately controlled diabetes mellitus
Hypophosphatemic rickets
Phosphaturic medications: intravenous iron, acetazolamide, tenofovir
Phosphatonins of oncogenic osteomalacia (eg, FGF23 production)
Transcellular shift of phosphorus
Increased insulin secretion (ie, during refeeding)
Anabolic steroids, estrogen, oral contraceptives, beta-adrenergic agonists, xanthine derivatives
Hungry bone syndrome
Acute respiratory alkalosis
Salicylate poisoning
Other
Electrolyte abnormalities
Hypercalcemia
Hypomagnesemia
Metabolic alkalosis
Abnormal losses followed by inadequate repletion
Diabetes mellitus with acidosis, particularly during aggressive therapy
Recovery from starvation or prolonged catabolic state
Chronic alcohol use disorder, particularly during restoration of nutrition; associated with hypomagnesemia
Recovery from severe burns

FGF23, fibroblast growth factor 23.

Clinical Findings

A. Symptoms and Signs

Phosphorous is a key ingredient component of adenosine triphosphate (ATP), and clinical manifestations are related to ATP deficiency. Symptoms are rare until blood phosphate levels fall below 1.0 mg/dL and are more prominent with acute declines. Symptoms include weakness, paresthesias, and encephalopathy (irritability, confusion, dysarthria, seizures, and coma). Respiratory failure or failure to wean from mechanical ventilation may occur because of diaphragmatic weakness. Decreased myocardial contractility is uncommon but a serious manifestation. Chronic severe depletion may cause anorexia, pain in muscles and bones, and fractures.

B. Laboratory Findings

While the etiology of hypophosphatemia is often revealed from the patient's history and review of medications, urinary phosphate excretion can distinguish between renal and nonrenal causes. Phosphate excretion can be determined by a 24-hour urine collection or by calculation of the $FEPO_4$. The normal renal response to hypophosphatemia is to decrease urinary phosphate excretion to less than 100 mg/day and $FEPO_4$ less than 5%. Renal wasting of phosphate (or increased $FEPO_4$) occurs most commonly with hyperparathyroidism and Fanconi syndrome (Table 21–8). The clinical usefulness of serum FGF23 levels is undetermined except in uncommon diseases.

Other clinical features may be suggestive of hypophosphatemia, such as hemolytic anemia and rhabdomyolysis. Fanconi syndrome may present with any combination of uricosuria, aminoaciduria, normoglycemic glucosuria, normal anion gap metabolic acidosis, and phosphaturia. In chronic hypophosphatemia, radiographs and bone biopsies show changes resembling osteomalacia.

Treatment

Hypophosphatemia can be prevented by including phosphate in repletion and maintenance fluids. Moderate hypophosphatemia (greater than 1 mg/dL) and asymptomatic patients should be treated with oral phosphate, typically 40–80 mmol divided into three or four doses over 24 hours. Patients with severe hypophosphatemia (below 1 mg/dL), symptomatic patients, and those who cannot tolerate oral therapy should be treated with intravenous replacement. Hypocalcemia, hypotension, hyperphosphatemia, and ECG abnormalities can be seen with intravenous therapy, which can be avoided by providing moderate doses. A typical dose is 15 mmol over 2 hours; the rate should be decreased if hypotension occurs and monitoring of plasma phosphate and calcium every 6 hours is necessary. Magnesium deficiency often coexists and should be treated.

Contraindications to phosphate replacement include hypoparathyroidism, advanced CKD, tissue damage and necrosis, and hypercalcemia. When an associated hyperglycemia is treated, phosphate accompanies glucose into cells, and hypophosphatemia may ensue.

When to Refer

- Patients with refractory hypophosphatemia with increased urinary phosphate excretion may require evaluation by an endocrinologist (eg, for hyperparathyroidism and vitamin D disorders) or a nephrologist (eg, for renal tubular defects).
- Patients with decreased GI absorption may require referral to a gastroenterologist.

When to Admit

Patients with severe or refractory hypophosphatemia will require intravenous phosphate.

García Martín A et al. Phosphate disorders and clinical management of hypophosphatemia and hyperphosphatemia. Endocrinol Diabetes Nutr. 2020;67:205. [PMID: 31501071]

HYPERPHOSPHATEMIA

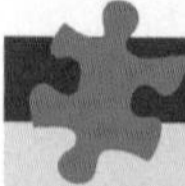

ESSENTIALS OF DIAGNOSIS

- Advanced CKD is the most common cause.
- Hyperphosphatemia in the presence of hypercalcemia imposes a high risk of metastatic calcification.

General Considerations

The two most common etiologies of hyperphosphatemia are decreased kidney clearance from CKD and transcellular shift. Increased dietary intake of phosphates in the setting of advanced CKD can cause hyperphosphatemia. Phosphate-containing laxatives taken as preparation for a GI procedure can cause hyperphosphatemia in patients with impaired kidney function and are less commonly used. Rapid cell breakdown from tumor lysis syndrome, rhabdomyolysis, and massive hemolysis releases intracellular phosphate. Hyperphosphatemia from insulin deficiency can occur in diabetic ketoacidosis (DKA). These patients, however, are typically phosphate depleted and are at risk for developing hypophosphatemia with insulin therapy. Other causes are listed in Table 21–9.

Clinical Findings

A. Symptoms and Signs

Acute hyperphosphatemia is generally asymptomatic, and symptoms are generally associated with concurrent hypocalcemia.

B. Laboratory Findings

In addition to elevated phosphate, blood chemistry abnormalities are those of the underlying disease.

Table 21–9. Causes of hyperphosphatemia.

Massive load of phosphate into the extracellular fluid
Exogenous sources
Hypervitaminosis D
Laxatives or enemas containing phosphate
Intravenous phosphate supplement
Endogenous sources
Rhabdomyolysis (especially if CKD coexists)
Tumor lysis by chemotherapy, particularly lymphoproliferative diseases
Metabolic acidosis (lactic acidosis, ketoacidosis)
Respiratory acidosis (phosphate incorporation into cells is disturbed)
Decreased excretion into urine
CKD
AKI
Hypoparathyroidism
Pseudohypoparathyroidism
Acromegaly
Pseudohyperphosphatemia
Plasma cell myeloma
Hyperbilirubinemia
Hypertriglyceridemia
Hemolysis in vitro

Treatment

Treatment is directed at the underlying cause. Acute hyperphosphatemia with *symptomatic* hypocalcemia and ECG changes (QTc prolongation) can be life-threatening. Intravenous calcium (1–2 g of calcium gluconate over 10–20 minutes) can be given in this situation, though it should be avoided in asymptomatic patients due to the risk of vascular calcification. Hemodialysis may be necessary in patients with impaired kidney function. In chronic hyperphosphatemia, dietary phosphate intake should be decreased and absorption reduced with oral phosphate binders, such as calcium acetate, calcium carbonate, sevelamer, or ferric citrate.

When to Admit

Patients with acute severe hyperphosphatemia require hospitalization for emergent therapy, possibly including dialysis. Concomitant illnesses, such as AKI or cell lysis, may necessitate admission.

Floege J. Phosphate binders in chronic kidney disease: an updated narrative review of recent data. J Nephrol. 2020;33:497. [PMID: 31865608]

Rahmani B et al. Current understanding of tumor lysis syndrome. Hematol Oncol. 2019;37:537. [PMID: 31461568]

DISORDERS OF MAGNESIUM CONCENTRATION

Normal plasma magnesium concentration is 1.7–2.1 mg/dL (0.7–0.85 mmol/L). Similar to calcium, only the ionized form is metabolically active. The primary source of magnesium excretion is via the kidney. Magnesium's physiologic effects on the nervous system resemble those of calcium.

Altered magnesium concentration usually provokes an associated alteration of Ca^{2+}. Both hypomagnesemia and hypermagnesemia can decrease PTH secretion or action. Severe hypermagnesemia (greater than 5 mg/dL [2.1 mmol/L]) suppresses PTH secretion with consequent hypocalcemia; this disorder is typically seen only in patients receiving magnesium therapy for preeclampsia. Severe hypomagnesemia causes PTH resistance in end organs and eventually decreased PTH secretion in severe cases.

HYPOMAGNESEMIA

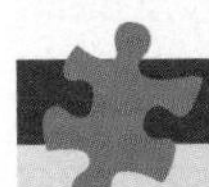

ESSENTIALS OF DIAGNOSIS

- Serum concentration of magnesium may be normal even in the presence of magnesium depletion. Check urinary magnesium excretion if renal magnesium wasting is suspected.
- Causes neurologic symptoms and arrhythmias.
- Associated with hypocalcemia.

General Considerations

Causes of hypomagnesemia are listed in Table 21–10. Hypomagnesemia and hypokalemia share many etiologies, including diarrhea, alcohol use disorder, and diuretic use. Hypomagnesemia causes renal potassium wasting which is refractory to potassium replacement until magnesium is repleted. Hypomagnesemia also suppresses PTH release and causes end-organ resistance to PTH and low 1,25-dihydroxyvitamin D levels. The resultant hypocalcemia is refractory to calcium replacement until the magnesium is normalized. Normomagnesemia does not exclude magnesium depletion because only 1% of total body magnesium is in the extracellular fluid; magnesium repletion should be considered in patients with risk factors for hypomagnesemia and refractory hypokalemia or hypocalcemia. There is an FDA warning about hypomagnesemia for patients taking PPIs. The presumed mechanism is decreased intestinal magnesium absorption, but it is not clear why this complication develops in only a small fraction of patients taking these medications. The potassium binder patiromer can cause hypomagnesemia by binding magnesium in the colon.

Table 21–10. Causes of hypomagnesemia.

Diminished absorption or intake
Malabsorption, chronic diarrhea, laxative abuse
PPIs
Prolonged GI suction
Small bowel bypass
Malnutrition
Alcohol use disorder
Total parenteral alimentation with inadequate Mg^{2+} content
Increased renal loss
Diuretic therapy (loop diuretics, thiazide diuretics)
Hyperaldosteronism, Gitelman syndrome
Hyperparathyroidism, hyperthyroidism
Hypercalcemia
Volume expansion
Tubulointerstitial diseases
Transplant kidney
Drugs (aminoglycoside, cetuximab, cisplatin, amphotericin B, pentamidine)
Others
Diabetes mellitus
Post-parathyroidectomy (hungry bone syndrome)
Respiratory alkalosis
Pregnancy

Clinical Findings

A. Symptoms and Signs

Because hypomagnesemia causes hypokalemia and hypocalcemia, it is difficult to determine whether symptoms are from hypomagnesemia or from potassium and calcium depletion. Marked neuromuscular and CNS hyperirritability may produce tremors, cramps, Trousseau and Chvostek signs, confusion, disorientation, and coma. Weakness is common. Cardiovascular manifestations include hypertension, tachycardia, and ventricular arrhythmias, including torsades de pointes.

B. Laboratory Findings

Urinary excretion of magnesium exceeding 10–30 mg/day or a fractional excretion greater than 3% indicates renal magnesium wasting. Hypocalcemia and hypokalemia are often present. The ECG may show widening of the QRS complex, peaked T waves with ultimate diminution, and a prolonged PR interval. PTH secretion is often suppressed (see Hypocalcemia).

Treatment

Magnesium oxide, 250–500 mg orally once or twice daily, is useful for treating chronic hypomagnesemia. Symptomatic hypomagnesemia requires intravenous magnesium sulfate 1–2 g over 5–60 minutes mixed in either dextrose 5% or 0.9% normal saline. Torsades de pointes in the setting of hypomagnesemia can be treated with 1–2 g of magnesium sulfate in 10 mL of dextrose 5% solution pushed intravenously over 15 minutes. Severe, non–life-threatening deficiency can be treated at a rate to 1–2 g/hour over 3–6 hours. Intravenous magnesium inhibits renal reabsorption and patients will demonstrate increased renal wasting during therapy. Serum levels must be monitored daily and dosage adjusted to keep the concentration from rising above 3 mg/dL (1.23 mmol/L). Tendon reflexes may be checked for hyporeflexia of hypermagnesemia. K^+ and Ca^{2+} replacement may be required, but patients with hypokalemia and hypocalcemia of hypomagnesemia do not recover without magnesium supplementation.

Patients with normal kidney function can excrete excess magnesium; hypermagnesemia should not develop with replacement dosages. In patients with CKD, magnesium replacement should be done cautiously to avoid hypermagnesemia. Reduced doses (50–75% dose reduction) and more frequent monitoring (at least twice daily) are indicated.

Gommers LM et al. Hypomagnesemia in type 2 diabetes: a vicious circle? Diabetes. 2016;65:3. [PMID: 26696633]

HYPERMAGNESEMIA

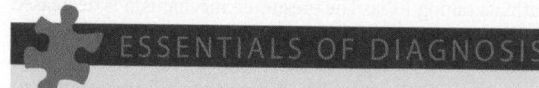

- Often associated with advanced CKD and chronic intake of magnesium-containing drugs.

General Considerations

Hypermagnesemia is almost always the result of advanced CKD and impaired magnesium excretion. Antacids and laxatives are underrecognized sources of magnesium. Pregnant patients may have severe hypermagnesemia from intravenous magnesium for preeclampsia and eclampsia. Magnesium replacement should be done cautiously in patients with CKD; dose reductions up to 75% may be necessary to avoid hypermagnesemia.

Clinical Findings

A. Symptoms and Signs

Muscle weakness, decreased deep tendon reflexes, mental obtundation, and confusion are characteristic manifestations. Weakness, flaccid paralysis, ileus, and hypotension are noted. Serious findings include respiratory muscle paralysis, complete heart block, and cardiac arrest.

B. Laboratory Findings and ECG

Serum Mg^{2+} is elevated. In the common setting of CKD, BUN, creatinine, potassium, phosphate, and uric acid may all be elevated. Serum Ca^{2+} is often low. The ECG may show increased PR interval, broadened QRS complexes, and QT prolongation.

Treatment

Exogenous sources of magnesium should be discontinued. Calcium antagonizes Mg^{2+} and may be given intravenously as calcium chloride, 500 mg or more at a rate of 100 mg (4.1 mmol) per minute. Hemodialysis may be necessary to remove magnesium, particularly with severe kidney disease.

Long-term use of magnesium hydroxide and magnesium sulfate should be avoided in patients with advanced stages of CKD.

Broman M et al. Analysis of hypo- and hypermagnesemia in an intensive care unit cohort. Acta Anaesthesiol Scand. 2018;62:648. [PMID: 29341068]

ACID-BASE DISORDERS

To best evaluate acid-base status, a blood gas and chemistry panel are required. Venous blood pH, typically 0.03–0.04 units lower than arterial blood pH, closely approximates arterial blood pH. An arterial blood gas should be obtained if more accurate assessment of blood pH and Pco_2 is required. Bicarbonate (HCO_3^-) is calculated from the Henderson-Hasselbalch equation below; therefore, the bicarbonate value in the electrolyte panel is typically used.

$$pH = 6.1 + \log \frac{HCO_3^-}{0.03 \times Pco_2}$$

Primary acid-base disorders are secondary to changes in either serum bicarbonate or Pco_2. The first step is to look at the pH of a blood gas (venous or arterial). If changes in pH are secondary to changes in HCO_3^-, a metabolic disorder is present. If changes in pH are secondary to changes in Pco_2, a respiratory disorder is present. If the pH is < 7.40, the primary process is acidosis, either respiratory (Pco_2 greater than 40 mm Hg) or metabolic (HCO_3^- less than 24 mEq/L). If the pH is > 7.40, the primary process is alkalosis, either respiratory (Pco_2 less than 40 mm Hg) or metabolic (HCO_3^- greater than 24 mEq/L). Normally, the kidneys compensate for respiratory acid-base disorders and the lungs compensate for metabolic disorders in order to maintain pH in a narrow physiologic range. For example, with metabolic acidosis (low pH, low HCO_3^-), alveolar ventilation increases (Pco_2 decreases), returning pH close to the normal range. Similarly, with respiratory acidosis (low pH, high Pco_2), the kidneys excrete H^+ (HCO_3^- increase) to return the pH close to normal range. Such compensation can only bring the pH toward normal, though it can never completely correct it. In order to normalize pH, the primary disorder must be corrected.

One respiratory or metabolic disorder with its appropriate compensatory response is a simple acid-base disorder. A mixed acid-base disorder is when multiple simple disorders are present simultaneously. Diagnosing an acid-base disorder requires a systematic approach (see box Step-by-Step Analysis of Acid-Base Status). Once the primary disorder has been identified, the clinician should assess whether the compensatory response is appropriate (Table 21–11). An inadequate or an exaggerated response indicates the presence of another primary acid-base disturbance.

STEP-BY-STEP ANALYSIS OF ACID-BASE STATUS

Step 1: Look at the pH on a blood gas to determine the primary disorder, either acidemia or alkalemia.

Step 2: Look at the serum HCO_3^- value to determine if the primary disorder is metabolic.

Step 3: Calculate the anion gap (see Table 21–12).

Step 4: Calculate the delta gap.

Step 5: Evaluate magnitude of compensation (see Table 21–11).

Step 6: Examine the patient to determine whether the clinical signs are compatible with the acid-base analysis.

Table 21–11. Primary acid-base disorders and expected compensation.

Disorder	Primary Defect	Compensatory Response	Magnitude of Compensation
Respiratory acidosis			
Acute	↑ P_{CO_2}	↑ HCO_3^-	↑ HCO_3^- 1 mEq/L per 10 mm Hg ↑ P_{CO_2}
Chronic	↑ P_{CO_2}	↑ HCO_3^-	↑ HCO_3^- 3.5 mEq/L per 10 mm Hg ↑ P_{CO_2}
Respiratory alkalosis			
Acute	↓ P_{CO_2}	↓ HCO_3^-	↓ HCO_3^- 2 mEq/L per 10 mm Hg ↓ P_{CO_2}
Chronic	↓ P_{CO_2}	↓ HCO_3^-	↓ HCO_3^- 5 mEq/L per 10 mm Hg ↓ P_{CO_2}
Metabolic acidosis	↓ HCO_3^-	↓ P_{CO_2}	↓ P_{CO_2} 1.3 mm Hg per 1 mEq/L ↓ HCO_3^-
Metabolic alkalosis	↑ HCO_3^-	↑ P_{CO_2}	↑ P_{CO_2} 0.7 mm Hg per 1 mEq/L ↑ HCO_3^-

The serum anion gap should subsequently be calculated (see below) for two reasons. First, it helps identify the cause of a metabolic acidosis, and second, to identify the presence of a gap metabolic acidosis, which may be present even without a decreased serum bicarbonate concentration. In patients with metabolic acidoses, clinicians should calculate the **delta gap**, which is the difference between the change in anion gap and the change in bicarbonate, to determine if there is a mixed anion gap or nonanion gap metabolic acidosis. In increased anion gap acidoses, there should be roughly a millimole for millimole decrease in HCO_3^- as the anion gap increases. The corrected serum HCO_3^- should be calculated by adding the change in serum anion gap to the serum HCO_3^-. A value higher or lower than normal (24 mEq/L) indicates the concomitant presence of metabolic alkalosis or normal anion gap metabolic acidosis, respectively.

Seifter JL et al. Disorders of acid-base balance: new perspectives. Kidney Dis (Basel). 2017;2:170. [PMID: 28232934]

METABOLIC ACIDOSIS

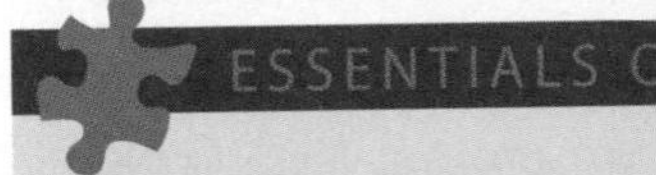

ESSENTIALS OF DIAGNOSIS

- Decreased HCO_3^- with acidemia (low blood pH).
- Classified into increased anion gap acidosis and normal anion gap acidosis.
- Lactic acidosis, ketoacidosis, and toxins produce metabolic acidoses with the largest anion gaps.
- Normal anion gap acidosis is mainly caused by GI HCO_3^- loss or RTA.

General Considerations

The hallmark of metabolic acidosis is low serum bicarbonate concentration from loss of bicarbonate or gain of acid (Table 21–12); the anion gap detects an increase in plasma anions other than from measured bicarbonate and chloride.

Many clinicians use 12 mEq/L as the normal serum anion gap (range 4–12 mEq/L due to differences in analyzer methods).

$$\text{Anion Gap} = Na^+ - (HCO_3^- + Cl^-)$$

If serum potassium is included in the formula, the range for anion gap increase by about 4 mEq/L:

$$\text{Anion gap} = (Na^+ + K^+) - (HCO_3^- + Cl^-)$$

The principle unmeasured anion usually responsible for the anion gap is albumin. The expected anion gap must be adjusted for hypoalbuminemia; the anion gap decreases by approximately 2.5 mEq/L for every 1 g/dL reduction in the serum albumin concentration.

$$\text{Corrected serum anion gap} = (\text{measured serum anion gap}) + (2.5 \times [4.0 - \text{serum albumin}])$$

In metabolic acidosis from a gain of acid, the anion gap will increase because the addition of acid includes the addition of anions. In nongap or hyperchloremic metabolic acidosis, the anion gap is normal because the rise in chloride parallels the fall in bicarbonate.

INCREASED ANION GAP ACIDOSIS

A gap metabolic acidosis is secondary to the addition of acid, either exogenous or endogenous. The major causes are lactic acidosis, ketoacidosis, kidney disease, and ingestions (Table 21–12). A useful mnemonic for the differential diagnosis of increased anion gap metabolic acidosis is GOLDMARK (glycols [ethylene glycol and propylene glycol], oxoproline, L-lactate, D-lactate, methanol, aspirin, renal failure, and ketoacidosis) (Table 21–13).

A. Lactic Acidosis

Lactic acidosis is a common cause of metabolic acidosis, producing an elevated anion gap and decreased serum pH when present without other acid-base disturbances. Lactate is formed from pyruvate in anaerobic glycolysis. Normally, lactate levels remain low (1 mEq/L) because of metabolism of lactate principally by the liver through gluconeogenesis or oxidation via the Krebs cycle. In lactic acidosis, lactate levels are at least 4–5 mEq/L but commonly significantly higher. There are three types of lactic acidosis.

Table 21–12. Anion gap in metabolic acidosis.[1]

Decreased (< 6 mEq/L)
Hypoalbuminemia (decreased unmeasured anion)
Plasma cell dyscrasias
Monoclonal protein (cationic paraprotein accompanied by chloride and bicarbonate)
Bromide intoxication
Increased (> 12 mEq/L)
Metabolic anion
Diabetic ketoacidosis
Alcoholic ketoacidosis
Lactic acidosis
CKD (advanced stages) (PO_4^{3-}, SO_4^{2-})
Starvation ketoacidosis
Drug or chemical anion
Salicylate intoxication
Methanol (formic acid)
Ethylene glycol (oxalic acid)
5-Oxoproline acidosis from acetaminophen toxicity
Normal (4–12 mEq/L)
Loss of HCO_3^-
Diarrhea
Recovery from diabetic ketoacidosis
Pancreatic fluid loss, ileostomy (unadapted)
Carbonic anhydrase inhibitors
Chloride retention
Renal tubular acidosis
Ileal loop bladder
Administration of HCl equivalent or NH_4Cl
Arginine and lysine in parenteral nutrition

[1]Reference ranges for anion gap may vary based on laboratory methods.

Type A (hypoxic) lactic acidosis is most common, resulting from tissue hypoxia, usually from septic, cardiogenic, or hemorrhagic shock; mesenteric ischemia; respiratory failure; and carbon monoxide poisoning. These conditions increase peripheral lactic acid production and decrease hepatic metabolism of lactate as liver perfusion declines.

Type B lactic acidosis is secondary to impaired mitochondrial oxygen utilization and may be due to metabolic causes (eg, diabetes mellitus, liver disease, kidney disease, thiamine deficiency, D-lactic acidosis, leukemia, or lymphoma) or toxins (eg, ethanol, methanol, ethylene glycol, cyanide, isoniazid, or metformin). Propylene glycol can cause lactic acidosis from decreased liver metabolism; it is used as a vehicle for intravenous medications, such as nitroglycerin, etomidate, and diazepam. Parenteral nutrition without thiamine causes severe refractory lactic acidosis from deranged pyruvate metabolism.

D-Lactic acidosis may develop in patients with short bowel syndrome due to carbohydrate malabsorption and subsequent fermentation by colonic bacteria. Metabolic acidosis occurs after meals and is associated with neurologic changes (confusion, slurred speech, and ataxia). A specific D-lactic acid assay is required as the standard lactic acid assay only detects the L-isomer.

B. Ketoacidosis

All forms of ketoacidosis share the physiologic state of insulin deficiency and glucagon excess, which shifts the body's primary fuel source from glucose to fatty acid metabolism. There are three types of ketones: acetone, acetoacetate, and beta-hydroxybutyrate.

Table 21–13. Common causes and therapy for increased anion gap metabolic acidosis.

Cause	Treatment
Lactic acidosis	Therapy aimed at correcting the underlying cause. Treatment of type A requires improving perfusion and matching oxygen consumption with fluids, packed red cells, vasopressors, and inotropes as needed. Treatment of type B generally requires removal of the offending agent or supplementing key cofactors of anaerobic metabolism.
D-Lactic acidosis	Sodium bicarbonate may be administered in the setting of severe acidemia. Specific antimicrobial agents (metronidazole, neomycin) can be utilized in patients with short gut syndrome. A low carbohydrate diet can be effective by decreasing substrate delivery to the distal colon. Fecal transplant has been utilized successfully in patients unresponsive to conventional therapies.
Ketoacidosis Diabetes mellitus Starvation Alcoholic	Therapy involves correction of the state of insulin deficiency and glucagon excess. In diabetic ketoacidosis, this requires administration of exogenous insulin, generally with a continuous infusion. In starvation and alcoholic ketoacidosis, dextrose-containing fluids will stimulate endogenous insulin release. In all groups, correction of volume depletion with isotonic fluids as well as judicious repletion of electrolytes (particularly potassium and phosphorous) are imperative.
Kidney failure	Supplemental alkali therapy (sodium bicarbonate or sodium citrate). Hemodialysis when necessary.
Ingestions	
Ethylene glycol Methanol	See Chapter 38.
Salicylic acid	See Chapter 38.
Pyroglutamic acid (5-Oxoproline)	Therapy is directed at the underlying cause. Generally requires withdrawal of the offending agent (acetaminophen) and sodium bicarbonate therapy for severe acidemia. *N*-Acetylcysteine may be effective in restoring glutathione stores.

1. Diabetic ketoacidosis (DKA)—DKA is characterized by hyperglycemia and metabolic acidosis with an increased anion gap from absolute or relative insulin deficiency:

$$H^+ + B^- + NaHCO_3 \leftrightarrow CO_2 + NaB + H_2O$$

where B^- is beta-hydroxybutyrate or acetoacetate, the ketones responsible for the increased anion gap. DKA may have an additional lactic acidosis from tissue hypoperfusion and increased anaerobic metabolism. The anion gap in DKA is generally large, often more than 20 mEq/L, though it can be variable. The elevated serum glucose leads to a marked osmotic diuresis with sizeable losses of sodium, water, and potassium.

Correction of ketoacidosis can be assessed by measurement of serum beta-hydroxybutyrate, pH, or by normalization of the anion gap. Urine ketones are detected by nitroprusside testing, results of which are rapidly available. However, urinary nitroprusside tests detect both acetoacetate and acetone (albeit to a lesser extent) but do not detect beta-hydroxybutyrate. Direct measurement of serum beta-hydroxybutyrate is preferred and can be used to monitor response to therapy.

2. Fasting ketoacidosis—Hepatic generation of ketones may occur as a normal response to fasting from relative hypoinsulinemia. Mild ketosis often occurs after 12–14 hours of fasting, peaking after 20–30 hours. The level of acidosis is generally small; overt ketoacidosis can occur in patients who consume very low carbohydrate diets.

3. Alcoholic ketoacidosis—Chronically malnourished patients who consume large quantities of alcohol may develop alcoholic ketoacidosis. Alcohol metabolism decreases gluconeogenesis, resulting in hepatic production of beta-hydroxybutyrate and, to a lesser degree, acetoacetate. Mixed acid-base disorders, such as metabolic alkalosis from vomiting, and respiratory alkalosis from alcohol withdrawal, aspiration, or cirrhosis are common.

In both of the above conditions, hypoglycemia, or stimulation of the sympathetic nervous system, suppresses insulin release allowing ketosis to occur. Patients with these disorders are able to sufficiently produce endogenous insulin and therefore do not require exogenous insulin administration. Treatment should commence with glucose administration to stimulate insulin release and suppress ketogenesis. Potassium should be repleted prior to glucose administration as insulin release will cause intracellular potassium shift, risking hypokalemia.

C. Toxins

(See also Chapter 38.) Multiple toxins and drugs increase the anion gap by increasing endogenous acid production. Common examples include methanol (metabolized to formic acid), ethylene glycol (glycolic and oxalic acid), and salicylates (salicylic acid and lactic acid). The latter can cause a mixed disorder of metabolic acidosis with respiratory alkalosis. In toluene poisoning, the metabolite hippurate is rapidly excreted by the kidney and may present as a normal anion gap acidosis. Isopropanol, which is metabolized to acetone, increases the osmolar gap, but not the anion gap. Long-term acetaminophen use, even at therapeutic doses, can result in an elevated anion gap acidosis from accumulation of 5-oxoproline.

D. Uremic Acidosis

As the GFR drops below 15–30 mL/minute/1.73 m^2, the kidneys are increasingly unable to synthesize ammonium (NH_4). The reduced excretion of H^+ (as NH_4Cl) and accumulation of organic anions from decreased excretion (eg, phosphate and sulfate) results in an increased anion gap metabolic acidosis.

NORMAL ANION GAP ACIDOSIS

The two major causes of hyperchloremic metabolic acidosis are HCO_3^- loss from the GI tract or defects in renal acidification (RTA) (Table 21–12 and Table 21–14).

Table 21–14. Hyperchloremic, normal anion gap metabolic acidoses.

			Distal H^+ Secretion			
	Renal Defect	Serum [K^+]	Urine pH	Titratable Acid	Urinary Anion Gap	Treatment
GI HCO_3^- loss	None	↓	< 5.5	↑↑	Negative	Na^+, K^+, and HCO_3^- as required
Renal tubular acidosis						
I. Distal	Distal H^+ secretion	↓	> 5.3	↓	Positive	$NaHCO_3$ (1–3 mEq/kg/day)
II. Proximal	Proximal HCO_3^- reabsorption	↓	Variable	Normal	Positive	$NaHCO_3$ or $KHCO_3$ (10–15 mEq/kg/day), thiazide
IV. Hyporeninemic hypoaldosteronism	Distal Na^+ reabsorption, K^+ secretion, and H^+ secretion	↑	Variable	↓	Positive	Fludrocortisone (0.1–0.5 mg/day), dietary K^+ restriction, furosemide (40–160 mg/day), $NaHCO_3$ (1–3 mEq/kg/day)

Reproduced with permission from Cogan MG. *Fluid and Electrolytes: Physiology and Pathophysiology*. McGraw-Hill, 1991.

The compensatory increase in serum chloride (hyperchloremia) maintains electroneutrality and a normal anion gap. The urinary anion gap can help differentiate between these causes.

A. GI HCO_3^- Loss

The GI tract secretes bicarbonate at multiple sites. The most common cause of a non-anion gap metabolic acidosis from the GI tract is diarrhea (loss of bicarbonate rich stool fluid). An infrequent cause is a ureterosigmoidostomy, where ureters are implanted into the sigmoid colon for urinary diversion. Unlike the bladder, colonic mucosa secretes bicarbonate in exchange for chloride, resulting in metabolic acidosis. More commonly, a neobladder is created using a loop of bowel (generally ileum or colon), which has significantly decreased the incidence of metabolic acidosis, though it can still occur when contact time between urine and mucosa is increased, typically as a result of an anastomotic stricture.

B. Renal Tubular Acidosis

Hyperchloremic acidosis with a normal anion gap and normal (or near normal) GFR, in the absence of diarrhea, defines RTA. The defect is either an inability to excrete H^+ as ammonium (inadequate generation of new HCO_3^-) or inadequate reabsorption of filtered HCO_3^-. Three major types can be differentiated by the clinical setting, urinary pH, urinary anion gap, and serum K^+ level.

1. Distal RTA (type I)—This disorder is characterized by inability to excrete H^+ by the distal nephron. The urine cannot be fully acidified (urine pH > 5.5), despite systemic acidosis. Urinary ammonium excretion is therefore decreased and the urinary anion gap is positive. Voltage dependent distal RTA (dRTA) is due to a defect in sodium reabsorption, which impairs hydrogen secretion by failure to generate a negative lumen potential. This is seen in obstructive uropathy; sickle cell disease; or medications, such as amiloride. This disorder also prevents the excretion of potassium, resulting in hyperkalemia. Classic distal RTA (the most common cause) is secondary to a congenital or acquired decrease in the number of functional H^+ pumps, which reduces H^+ secretion by alpha intercalated cells. This is associated with hypokalemia due to enhanced K^+ excretion from a lack of competition from H^+ in the tubular fluid. This form of dRTA is commonly due to Sjögren syndrome, SLE, plasma cell myeloma, toluene inhalation (glue sniffing), Wilson disease, and lithium. dRTA can also be caused by destruction of tubular integrity (eg, amphotericin B). This type of dRTA is also associated with hypokalemia as destruction of the tubular membrane allows potassium to freely flow down its concentration gradient into the tubular lumen. In all types of dRTA, buffering of acid by release of bicarbonate and calcium from bone results in hypercalciuria, which in addition to low urinary citrate from increased reabsorption, results in the often encountered complication of nephrolithiasis.

2. Proximal RTA (type II)—Proximal RTA is due to a defect in the ability of the proximal tubule to reabsorb filtered HCO_3^-. The maximal rate of bicarbonate reabsorption is set by the tubular maximum (Tm), which is normally 26–28 mEq/L. The hallmark of a proximal RTA (pRTA) is a decrease in the Tm for bicarbonate, typically to 14–20 mEq/L. Therefore, this is a self-limited disease with serum bicarbonate levels predicated on the severity of the proximal defect and the ability of the distal nephron to reabsorb bicarbonate. This essentially creates a new steady state, when the Tm is equivalent to the serum HCO_3^- level, where the urine is acidic (no impairment of distal H^+ secretion) and the urine anion gap is negative (no impairment of ammonium excretion). Bicarbonaturia, and hence an alkaline urine (greater than 5.5), only occurs when the bicarbonate level exceeds the Tm, which has implications in treatment. Fanconi syndrome is pRTA with other proximal reabsorption defects resulting in glucosuria, aminoaciduria, phosphaturia, and uricosuria. The most common cause of pRTA is proximal tubular toxicity from the monoclonal immunoglobulin light chains in plasma cell myeloma. Other causes include heavy metals; Sjögren syndrome; cystinosis; Wilson disease; and various medications, such as acetazolamide, topiramate, tenofovir, and ifosfamide. The increased delivery of HCO_3^- to the distal nephron enhances K^+ secretion, and hypokalemia results when a patient is treated with HCO_3^- without adequate K^+ supplementation. Similar to dRTA, bone loss from persistent acidosis is common. Untreated children can develop rickets, while adult patients can develop osteomalacia. Unlike dRTA, nephrolithiasis is uncommon in pRTA because of the increased citrate in the urine, which increases calcium solubility.

3. Hyporeninemic hypoaldosteronemic RTA (type IV)—Type IV is the most common RTA in clinical practice. This is primarily a disorder of hyperkalemia secondary to a decrease in aldosterone, which inhibits ammonium production. The clinical presentation is a hyperkalemic nongap metabolic acidosis. Common causes include diabetic nephropathy and tubulointerstitial renal diseases. In patients with these disorders, drugs, such as ACE inhibitors, ARBs, spironolactone, and NSAIDs, can worsen the hyperkalemia and acidosis.

C. Other Causes of Nongap Acidosis

A dilutional acidosis may occur when the extracellular volume is rapidly expanded with normal saline since it contains neither bicarbonate nor sodium salts that can be metabolized to bicarbonate. Concerns have been raised regarding potential harm from volume expansion with normal saline. In clinical practice, balanced crystalloid solutions, such as lactated Ringer solution, are more commonly used.

1. Urine anion gap—The normal kidney response to a metabolic acidosis is to increase NH_4Cl excretion to enhance H^+ removal. The daily urinary excretion of NH_4Cl can be increased from 30 mEq at baseline to

200–300 mEq in response to acidosis. Urine ammonium excretion can be estimated using the following urine anion gap equation:

$$\text{Urine anion gap} = U_{Na} + U_K - U_{Cl}$$

The urinary anion gap may help differentiate between GI and renal causes of hyperchloremic acidosis. If the cause is GI HCO_3^- loss (diarrhea), renal acidification remains intact and NH_4Cl excretion increases appropriately (urinary anion gap will be negative). In a distal RTA, ammonium excretion is impaired and the urinary anion gap is positive. In proximal (type II) RTA, the primary problem is impaired HCO_3^- reabsorption, leading to increased HCO_3^- excretion rather than decreased NH_4Cl excretion and the urinary anion gap is often negative until treatment is initiated with exogenous bicarbonate therapy.

2. Urine osmolal gap—When large amounts of other anions (eg, hippurate in toluene poisoning, beta-hydroxybutyrate, acetoacetate) are present in the urine, the urinary anion gap may not be reliable. In this situation, the urine osmolal gap may be a better indicator of NH_4^+ excretion, which can be estimated as 50% of the urinary osmolal gap where urine concentrations and osmolality are in mmol/L. A urine osmolal gap below 150 mOsmol/kg suggests impaired ammonium excretion, whereas a urine osmolal gap above 400 mOsmol/kg suggests an intact renal response to acidosis.

$$\text{Urine osmolal gap} = U_{osm} - 2(U_{Na} + U_K) + U_{urea} + U_{glucose}$$

Clinical Findings

A. Symptoms and Signs

Symptoms of metabolic acidosis are mainly those of the underlying disorder. Compensatory hyperventilation is an important clinical sign and may be misinterpreted as a primary respiratory disorder; Kussmaul breathing (deep, regular, sighing respirations) may be seen with severe metabolic acidosis.

B. Laboratory Findings

Blood pH, serum HCO_3^-, and P_{CO_2} are decreased. Anion gap may be normal (hyperchloremic metabolic acidosis) or increased. Hyperkalemia may be seen.

Treatment

A. Increased Anion Gap Acidosis

Treatment is aimed at the underlying disorder, such as insulin and fluid therapy for diabetes and appropriate volume resuscitation to restore tissue perfusion (see Table 21–13). $NaHCO_3$ therapy is controversial in the treatment of increased anion gap metabolic acidoses and is usually reserved for severe cases (arterial pH < 7.1–7.2). Large amounts of $NaHCO_3$ may have deleterious effects, including hypernatremia, hyperosmolality, volume overload, and worsening of intracellular acidosis.

B. Normal Anion Gap Acidosis

Treatment of RTA is mainly achieved by administration of alkali (bicarbonate or citrate) to correct metabolic abnormalities and prevent nephrocalcinosis and CKD.

Large amounts of oral alkali ($NaHCO_3$ or $KHCO_3$ 10–15 mEq/kg/day) (Table 21–14) may be required to treat proximal RTA because much of the administered alkali is excreted into the urine. This can exacerbate hypokalemia and a mixture of sodium and potassium salts is often required. Treatment of type I distal RTA requires less alkali (1–2 mEq/kg/day) than proximal RTA, and potassium supplementation is typically required.

For type IV RTA, dietary potassium restriction may be necessary and potassium-retaining drugs should be withdrawn. Loop diuretics may be beneficial. Fludrocortisone may be effective in some cases without significant volume expansion. In some cases, oral alkali supplementation (1–2 mEq/kg/day) may be required.

When to Refer

Most clinicians will refer patients with renal tubular acidoses to a nephrologist for evaluation and possible alkali therapy.

When to Admit

Patients will require emergency department evaluation or hospital admission depending on the severity of the acidosis and underlying conditions.

Chávez-Iñiguez JS et al. The Case | Severe hypokalemia and metabolic acidosis. Kidney Int. 2018;93:1255. [PMID: 29680030]

Palmer BF et al. Electrolyte and acid-base disturbances in patients with diabetes mellitus. N Engl J Med. 2015;373:548. [PMID: 26244308]

Palmer BF et al. Salicylate toxicity. N Engl J Med. 2020;382:2544. [PMID: 32579814]

Sharma S et al. Comprehensive clinical approach to renal tubular acidosis. Clin Exp Nephrol. 2015;19:556. [PMID: 25951806]

METABOLIC ALKALOSIS

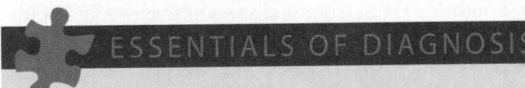

- High HCO_3^- with alkalemia (high pH).
- Evaluate effective circulating volume by physical examination.
- Urinary chloride concentration differentiates saline-responsive alkalosis from saline-unresponsive alkalosis.

General Considerations

Metabolic alkalosis is characterized by high serum HCO_3^- levels. The development of metabolic alkalosis requires its "generation" from loss of acid or gain of alkali, and its

Table 21–15. Metabolic alkalosis.

Chloride-Responsive (U_{Cl} < 20 mEq/L)	Chloride-Unresponsive (U_{Cl} > 20 mEq/L)
Excessive body bicarbonate content	**Excessive body bicarbonate content**
Renal alkalosis	Normotensive
Diuretic therapy (after diuretic effect has ceased)	Bartter syndrome (renal salt wasting and secondary hyperaldosteronism)
Poorly reabsorbable anion therapy: carbenicillin, penicillin, sulfate, phosphate	Severe potassium depletion
Posthypercapnia	Refeeding alkalosis
GI alkalosis	Hypercalcemia and hypoparathyroidism
Loss of HCl from vomiting or nasogastric suction	Hypertensive
Intestinal alkalosis: chloride diarrhea	Endogenous mineralocorticoids
$NaHCO_3$ (baking soda)	Primary aldosteronism
Sodium citrate, lactate, gluconate, acetate	Hyperreninism
Transfusions	Adrenal enzyme (11-beta-hydroxylase and 17-alpha- hydroxylase) deficiency
Antacids	Liddle syndrome
Normal body bicarbonate content	Exogenous alkali
"Contraction alkalosis"	Exogenous mineralocorticoids
	Licorice

Reproduced with permission from Narins RG et al. Diagnostic strategies in disorders of fluid, electrolyte and acid-base homeostasis. *Am J Med*. 1982;72(3):496–520.

"maintenance" from the kidney's inability to excrete excess bicarbonate.

The causes of metabolic alkalosis are classified into two groups based on chloride responsiveness and are generally distinguished using urine chloride values (Table 21–15). The compensatory increase in Pco_2 rarely exceeds 55 mm Hg; higher Pco_2 values imply a superimposed primary respiratory acidosis.

A. Chloride-Responsive Metabolic Alkalosis (U_{Cl}^- less than 20 mEq/L)

Chloride-responsive metabolic alkalosis involves the loss of chloride and extracellular volume. In vomiting and nasogastric suction, loss of acid (HCl) generates the alkalosis and volume contraction from chloride loss maintains the alkalosis. Distally acting diuretics that cause chloride loss, eg, loop and thiazide diuretics, are a common cause of metabolic alkalosis. U_{Cl}^- levels can be unreliable in these settings since these diuretics increase U_{Cl}^-. These disorders cause concurrent hypokalemia, which can exacerbate metabolic alkalosis by stimulating H^+ secretion and ammoniagenesis. In respiratory acidosis, the kidneys compensate by increasing renal HCO_3^- retention, which causes volume expansion and hence NaCl excretion. If the hypercapnia is corrected rapidly, the kidneys will attempt to correct the alkalosis by excreting HCO_3^-; if sufficient Cl^- is unavailable, bicarbonaturia will halt and metabolic alkalosis will persist. This process has been termed **posthypercapneic metabolic alkalosis.**

In alkalosis, bicarbonaturia causes obligatory sodium excretion as the accompanying cation and U_{Na} levels are unreliable markers of extracellular volume.

B. Chloride-Unresponsive Alkalosis (U_{Cl}^- more than 20 mEq/L)

1. Excess mineralocorticoid activity—Mineralocorticoids act directly in the collecting duct to stimulate sodium reabsorption and hydrogen and potassium excretion. The effects on hydrogen excretion are important in the generation of a metabolic alkalosis. Table 21–15 lists important causes of excess mineralocorticoid activity. These disorders are typically associated with hypertension, hypokalemia, metabolic alkalosis, and mild hypernatremia.

2. Bartter and Gitelman syndromes—Metabolic alkalosis, hypokalemia, and normotension are features of both Bartter and Gitelman syndromes.

3. Alkali administration with decreased GFR—The normal kidney has a substantial capacity for bicarbonate excretion; therefore, metabolic alkalosis usually only develops with HCO_3^- intake (eg, intensive antacid therapy) when there is CKD. In milk-alkali syndrome, sustained heavy ingestion of absorbable antacids and milk causes hypercalcemic kidney injury and metabolic alkalosis. Volume contraction from renal hypercalcemic effects exacerbates the alkalosis.

Clinical Findings

A. Symptoms and Signs

There are no characteristic symptoms or signs. However, hypopnea can be present in severe cases. Concomitant hypokalemia may cause weakness and hyporeflexia. An increase in mortality occurs with a pH > 7.48.

B. Laboratory Findings

The arterial blood pH and bicarbonate are elevated. With respiratory compensation, the arterial Pco_2 is increased. Serum potassium and chloride are decreased. The urine Cl^- can differentiate between chloride-responsive (less than 20 mEq/L) and unresponsive (greater than 20 mEq/L) causes.

Treatment

Mild alkalosis is generally well tolerated. Severe or symptomatic alkalosis (pH > 7.60) requires urgent treatment.

A. Chloride-Responsive Metabolic Alkalosis

Therapy for chloride-responsive alkalosis involves volume expansion with chloride salts, generally in the form of intravenous normal saline, until a euvolemic state has been achieved. This reduces proximal tubular bicarbonate reabsorption and increases distal tubular delivery of chloride, where it is exchanged for bicarbonate by the luminal Cl^-/HCO_3^- pendrin. In edematous patients with a contraindication to volume expansion (eg, heart failure), the carbonic anhydrase inhibitor acetazolamide can be given (250–500 mg orally twice daily) to increase renal bicarbonate excretion. Hypokalemia should be corrected by administering oral KCl.

B. Chloride-Unresponsive Metabolic Alkalosis

Therapy for chloride-unresponsive metabolic alkalosis requires therapy targeted to the underlying cause (see Chapter 26).

Emmett M. Metabolic alkalosis: a brief pathophysiologic review. Clin J Am Soc Nephrol. 2020;15:1848. [PMID: 32586924]

RESPIRATORY ACIDOSIS (Hypercapnia)

General Considerations

Respiratory acidosis results from hypoventilation and subsequent hypercapnia. Both pulmonary and extrapulmonary disorders can cause hypoventilation.

Acute respiratory acidosis is associated with only a modest increase in bicarbonate since serum bicarbonate is an ineffective buffer because of impaired elimination of carbon dioxide. After 6–12 hours, the primary increase in Pco_2 evokes a renal compensation to excrete more acid and to generate more HCO_3^-. Complete metabolic compensation by the kidney takes several days. In acute respiratory acidosis, HCO_3^- increases by 1 mEq/L for every 10 mm Hg increase in Pco_2.

Chronic respiratory acidosis is generally seen in patients with underlying lung disease, such as COPD. Renal excretion of acid as NH_4Cl results in a compensatory metabolic alkalosis. In this situation, HCO_3^- increases by 3 mEq/L for every 10 mm Hg increase in Pco_2.

Clinical Findings

A. Symptoms and Signs

With acute onset, somnolence, confusion, mental status changes, asterixis, and myoclonus may develop. Severe hypercapnia increases cerebral blood flow, cerebrospinal fluid pressure, and intracranial pressure; papilledema and seizures may be seen.

B. Laboratory Findings

Arterial pH is low and Pco_2 is increased. Serum HCO_3^- is elevated but does not fully correct the pH. Respiratory etiologies of respiratory acidosis usually have a wide A-a difference; a relatively normal A-a difference in the presence of respiratory acidosis is highly suggestive of global hypoventilation.

Treatment

If opioid overdose is a possible diagnosis or there is no other obvious cause for hypoventilation, the clinician should consider a diagnostic and therapeutic trial of intravenous naloxone (see Chapter 38). Noninvasive or mechanical ventilation may be necessary.

Adrogué HJ et al. Alkali therapy for respiratory acidosis: a medical controversy. Am J Kidney Dis. 2020;75:265. [PMID: 31473018]

RESPIRATORY ALKALOSIS

General Considerations

Respiratory alkalosis is always a disorder of hyperventilation, reducing the Pco_2 and increasing serum pH (Table 21–16). In pregnancy, progesterone stimulates the respiratory center, producing an average Pco_2 of 30 mm Hg

Table 21–16. Causes of respiratory alkalosis.

Hypoxia
Decreased inspired oxygen tension
High altitude
Ventilation/perfusion inequality
Hypotension
Severe anemia
CNS-mediated disorders
Voluntary hyperventilation
Anxiety-hyperventilation syndrome
Neurologic disease
Cerebrovascular accident (infarction, hemorrhage)
Infection
Trauma
Tumor
Pharmacologic and hormonal stimulation
Salicylates
Nicotine
Xanthines
Pregnancy (progesterone)
Liver failure
Gram-negative septicemia
Recovery from metabolic acidosis
Heat exposure
Pulmonary disease
Interstitial lung disease
Pneumonia
PE
Pulmonary edema
Mechanical overventilation

Reproduced with permission from Gennari FJ. Respiratory acidosis and alkalosis. In: Narins RG, ed. *Maxwell and Kleeman's Clinical Disorders of Fluid and Electrolyte Metabolism*, 5th ed. McGraw-Hill, 1994.

Table 21–17. Replacement guidelines for sweat and GI fluid losses.

	Average Electrolyte Composition				Replacement Guidelines per Liter Lost				
	Na^+ (mEq/L)	K^+ (mEq/L)	Cl^- (mEq/L)	HCO_3^- (mEq/L)	0.9% Saline (mL)	0.45% Saline (mL)	D_5W (mL)	KCl (mEq/L)	7.5% $NaHCO_3$ (45 mEq HCO_3^-/amp)
Sweat	30–50	5	30–50			500	500	5	
Gastric secretions	20	10	10			300	700	20	
Pancreatic juice	130	5	35	115		400	600	5	2 amps
Bile	145	5	100	25	600		400	5	0.5 amp
Diarrhea[1]	140	15	110–115	40–45					

[1]In the absence of diarrhea, colonic fluid Na^+ levels are low (40 mEq/L).

and respiratory alkalosis. Salicylates directly stimulate respiration and aspirin toxicity should be suspected when both respiratory alkalosis and an anion gap metabolic acidosis are present, particularly with alkalemia. Symptoms of acute respiratory alkalosis are related to decreased cerebral blood flow induced by the disorder.

Determination of appropriate metabolic compensation may reveal an associated metabolic disorder.

As in respiratory acidosis, the metabolic compensation is greater if the respiratory alkalosis is chronic (see Table 21–11). In acute respiratory alkalosis, HCO_3^- decreases by 2 mEq/L for every 10 mm Hg decrease in PCO_2, whereas in chronic respiratory alkalosis, HCO_3^- decreases by 4 mEq/L for every 10 mm Hg decrease in PCO_2.

Clinical Findings

A. Symptoms and Signs

In acute cases (hyperventilation), there is light-headedness, anxiety, perioral numbness, and paresthesias. Tetany occurs from a low ionized calcium, since severe alkalosis increases calcium binding to albumin.

B. Laboratory Findings

Arterial blood pH is elevated, and PCO_2 is low. Serum bicarbonate is decreased in chronic respiratory alkalosis.

Treatment

Treatment is directed toward the underlying cause. In acute hyperventilation syndrome from anxiety, the traditional treatment of breathing into a paper bag should be discouraged because it does not correct PCO_2 and may decrease PO_2. Reassurance may be sufficient for the anxious patient, but sedation may be necessary if the process persists. Hyperventilation is usually self-limited since muscle weakness caused by the respiratory alkalemia will suppress ventilation. Rapid correction of chronic respiratory alkalosis may result in metabolic acidosis as PCO_2 is increased with a previous compensatory decrease in HCO_3^-. The severity of hypocapnia in critically ill patients has been associated with adverse outcomes.

Scheiner B et al. Acid-base disorders in liver disease. J Hepatol. 2017;67:1062. [PMID: 28684104]

FLUID MANAGEMENT

Daily parenteral maintenance fluids and electrolytes for an average adult of 70 kg would include at least 2 L of water in the form of 0.45% saline with 20 mEq/L of potassium chloride. Patients with hypoglycemia, starvation ketosis, or ketoacidosis being treated with insulin may require 5% dextrose-containing solutions. Guidelines for GI fluid losses are shown in Table 21–17.

Weight loss or gain is the best indication of water balance. Insensible water loss should be considered in febrile patients. Water loss increases by 100–150 mL/day for each degree of body temperature over 37°C.

In patients requiring maintenance and possibly replacement of fluid and electrolytes by parenteral infusion, the total daily ration should be administered continuously over 24 hours to ensure optimal utilization.

If intravenous fluids are the only source of water, electrolytes, and calories for longer than a week, parenteral nutrition containing amino acids, lipids, trace metals, and vitamins may be indicated. (See Chapter 29.)

Balanced crystalloid-like lactated Ringer solution, rather than normal saline, is the resuscitation fluid of choice in most settings (see Chapter 12). Excessive fluid resuscitation and maintenance are complications in hospitalized patients, especially those with critical illness or AKI. These complications have been associated with worsened outcomes, such as prolonged mechanical ventilation, dependence on dialysis, and longer hospitalization with increased mortality.

Moritz ML et al. Maintenance intravenous fluids in acutely ill patients. N Engl J Med. 2015;373:1350. [PMID: 26422725]
Vincent JL. Fluid management in the critically ill. Kidney Int. 2019;96:52. [PMID: 30926137]
Yoo MS et al. Association of positive fluid balance at discharge after sepsis management with 30-day readmission. JAMA Netw Open. 2021;4:e216105. [PMID: 34086036]

Kidney Disease

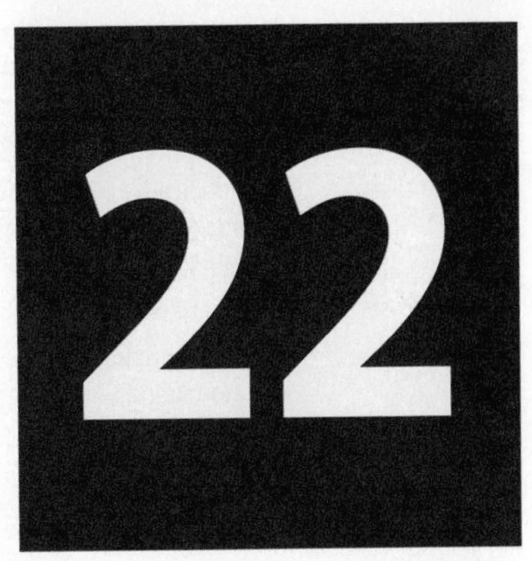

Tonja C. Dirkx, MD
Tyler B. Woodell, MD, MCR

Although some patients with kidney disease experience hypertension, edema, nausea, or hematuria that may lead to its discovery, kidney disease is often discovered incidentally during a routine medical evaluation. The initial approach to kidney disease is to assess the cause and severity of renal abnormalities. In all cases, this evaluation includes (1) estimation of disease duration, (2) careful examination of the urine, and (3) assessment of the GFR. The history and physical examination, though equally important, are variable among renal syndromes—thus, specific symptoms and signs are discussed under each disease entity.

ASSESSMENT OF KIDNEY DISEASE

Kidneys may be damaged by a variety of injuries. Data helpful in the evaluation of kidney disease include estimation of disease duration, eGFR, examination of the urine, and quantification of urinary protein excretion. Additionally, renal imaging (most often ultrasonography) can be helpful. Kidney biopsy may be performed in select cases as noted below, particularly when glomerular disease is suspected.

Disease Duration

Kidney disease can be acute or chronic. AKI is worsening of kidney function over hours to days, resulting in retention of waste products (such as urea nitrogen) and creatinine in the blood. Retention of these substances is called azotemia. CKD is the loss of kidney function over months to years. Differentiating between AKI and CKD is important for diagnosis and treatment, and certain clues may help distinguish the two. For instance, oliguria is only observed in AKI, whereas anemia (from low kidney erythropoietin production) suggests CKD. Additionally, small kidney size on imaging is more consistent with CKD, whereas normal to large kidney size can be seen with both AKI and CKD.

Urinalysis

Examination of the urine can provide important clues when evaluating kidney disease. A urine specimen should be collected midstream or by bladder catheterization and examined within 1 hour after collection to avoid destruction of formed elements. UA includes dipstick examination followed by microscopy if the dipstick has positive findings. The dipstick examination measures urinary pH, specific gravity, protein, hemoglobin, glucose, ketones, bilirubin, nitrites, and leukocyte esterase. Microscopy of centrifuged urinary sediment permits examination of formed elements—crystals, cells, casts, and infectious organisms. A bland (normal) sediment is common, especially in CKD and acute nonparenchymal disorders, such as limited effective blood flow to the kidney or urinary obstruction. Urinary casts form when urine flow is slow, leading to precipitation of Tamm-Horsfall mucoprotein in the renal tubule; if there are many red or white blood cells in the urine, cellular casts may form. The presence of protein on dipstick examination suggests underlying glomerular disease. If the glomerular basement membrane (GBM) is damaged (eg, by inflammation), RBCs may leak into the urinary space and appear dysmorphic. Thus, proteinuria, dysmorphic hematuria, and RBCs casts are highly suggestive of glomerulonephritis. If proteinuria is significant, it is classified as nephrotic-range; significant proteinuria accompanied by lipiduria may indicate nephrotic syndrome. Granular casts (also called "muddy brown casts") and renal tubular epithelial cells alone or in casts are hallmarks of ATN. WBCs (including neutrophils and eosinophils), WBC casts (Table 22–1), and proteinuria of varying degree can be seen with pyelonephritis and interstitial nephritis; pyuria alone can indicate UTI.

A. Proteinuria

Proteinuria is defined as excessive protein excretion in the urine, generally greater than 150 mg/24 hours in adults. Proteinuria more than 1–2 g/day is usually a sign of underlying glomerular kidney disease, whereas proteinuria less than 1 g/day can be due to multiple causes along the nephron segment, as listed below. Proteinuria can be accompanied by other clinical abnormalities—abnormal GFR, abnormal urine sediment, or evidence of systemic illness (eg, fever, rash, vasculitis).

Table 22–1. Significance of specific urinary casts.

Type	Significance
Hyaline casts	Not indicative of kidney disease Concentrated urine, febrile disease, diuretic therapy, after strenuous exercise
Red cell casts	Glomerulonephritis
White cell casts	Indicative of infection or inflammation Pyelonephritis, interstitial nephritis
Renal tubular cell casts	ATN, interstitial nephritis
Granular (muddy brown) casts	Nonspecific; can indicate ATN
Broad waxy casts	Indicative of stasis in enlarged collecting tubules CKD

There are several reasons proteinuria may develop: (1) **Functional proteinuria** is a benign process stemming from stressors such as acute illness, exercise, and "orthostatic proteinuria." The latter condition, generally found in people under 30 years of age, usually causes protein excretion less than 1 g/day. The orthostatic nature of the proteinuria is confirmed by measuring an 8-hour overnight supine urinary protein excretion, which should be less than 50 mg. (2) **Overload proteinuria** occurs when the reabsorptive capacity of tubules is overwhelmed, which can result from excess production of low-molecular-weight plasma proteins (eg, Bence Jones proteins associated with plasma cell myeloma). In the case of plasma cell myeloma, protein electrophoresis from serum or urine will exhibit a discrete, monoclonal protein spike. Other examples of overload proteinuria include myoglobinuria in rhabdomyolysis and hemoglobinuria in hemolysis. (3) **Glomerular proteinuria** results from effacement of epithelial cell foot processes that results in increased glomerular permeability with increased filtration of albumin, as classically occurs in diabetic nephropathy. Protein electrophoresis will exhibit a large albumin spike indicative of increased albumin permeability across the damaged GBM. (4) **Tubular proteinuria** occurs due to faulty reabsorption of normally filtered proteins in the proximal tubule, such as beta-2-microglobulin. Causes may include ATN, toxic injury (lead, aminoglycosides, and certain antiretrovirals), drug-induced interstitial nephritis, and hereditary metabolic disorders (eg, Wilson disease and Fanconi syndrome).

Evaluation of proteinuria by urine dipstick does not actually measure protein, but instead detects the negative electrochemical charge that characterizes albumin. As a result, positively charged Bence Jones proteins are missed with dipstick analysis. Bence Jones proteins can be detected by the addition of sulfosalicylic acid to the urine specimen or, more commonly, directly measuring urine protein.

Because of limitations with dipstick analysis, the recommended approach for quantitative investigation of urine protein excretion requires direct urine protein measurement. This can be measured precisely from a timed urine collection (typically 24 hours) or more simply estimated from a random urine sample. In a random urine sample the ratio of urine protein-to-creatinine concentration ($[U_{protein}]/[U_{creatinine}]$) correlates with a 24-hour urine protein collection (less than 0.2 is normal and corresponds to excretion of less than 200 mg/24 hours). In a 24-hour collection, proteinuria above 150 mg is abnormal and above 3.5 g is classified as nephrotic-range. A kidney biopsy may be indicated to determine the cause of abnormal proteinuria, particularly if accompanied by abnormal GFR or hematuria. The clinical sequelae of proteinuria are discussed in the section on Nephrotic Spectrum Glomerular Diseases.

B. Hematuria

Hematuria (ie, blood in the urine) is considered clinically significant if there are more than three RBCs per high-power field on at least two occasions. It is usually detected incidentally on urine dipstick or following an episode of macroscopic ("gross") hematuria. The diagnosis must be confirmed via microscopic examination, as false-positive dipstick tests can be caused by myoglobin, oxidizing agents, beets and rhubarb, hydrochloric acid, and bacteria. Transient hematuria is common but is less often clinically significant in patients younger than 40 years due to lower risk for malignancy.

Hematuria may be due to renal or extrarenal causes. Extrarenal causes are addressed in Chapter 23. Renal causes account for approximately 10% of cases and are classified as either glomerular or extraglomerular. Glomerular causes include glomerulonephritis (eg, immunoglobulin A [IgA] nephropathy, lupus nephritis), thin basement membrane disease and other hereditary disorders (eg, Alport syndrome). Extraglomerular sources include cysts; calculi; interstitial nephritis; and, most worrisome, genitourinary neoplasms from the kidney, prostate, or bladder (see Chapter 39).

Glomerular Filtration Rate

The GFR provides a useful measure of kidney function at the level of the glomerulus and can either be measured directly using biomarkers (most commonly creatinine) or estimated using validated formulae. The GFR measures the amount of plasma ultrafiltered across the glomerular capillaries per unit time and reflects the kidneys' ability to filter fluids and substances, including medications; it is an important factor when determining drug dosing. Daily GFR in normal individuals is variable, with a range of 150–250 L/24 hours or 100–120 mL/minute/1.73 m^2 of body surface area. Patients with kidney disease can have decreased GFR from any process that causes loss of functioning glomeruli. However, they can also have normal or increased GFR, either from glomerular hyperfiltration or disease at a different segment of the nephron, interstitium, or vascular supply.

GFR can be measured by determining the renal clearance of plasma substances that are not bound to plasma proteins, are freely filterable across the glomerulus, and are neither secreted nor reabsorbed along the renal tubules. The renal clearance of a substance is defined as:

$$C = \frac{U \times \dot{V}}{P}$$

where C is the clearance, U and P are the respective urine and plasma concentrations of the substance, and $\dot{V}$ is volume of urine per unit time (typically mL/minute). In clinical practice, the clearance of endogenous creatinine (termed **creatinine clearance**) is the primary way to measure GFR. The creatinine clearance (C_{cr}) is approximately 100 mL/minute in healthy young women and 120 mL/minute in healthy young men. The creatinine clearance declines by an average of 0.8 mL/minute/year after age 40 years as part of the aging process. Creatinine is a product of muscle metabolism produced at a relatively constant rate and cleared by renal excretion. It is freely filtered by the glomerulus and not reabsorbed by the renal tubules. Creatinine is not a perfect indicator of GFR for the following reasons: (1) a small amount is normally eliminated by tubular secretion, and it progressively increases as GFR declines (thus overestimating GFR); (2) in more advanced kidney disease, gut microorganisms degrade creatinine; (3) dietary meat intake and muscle mass affect plasma creatinine levels; (4) medications such as aspirin, dolutegravir, probenecid, and trimethoprim reduce tubular secretion of creatinine, increasing the plasma creatinine concentration and falsely underestimating GFR; and (5) GFR measurement assumes a stable plasma creatinine concentration over a 24-hour period, so creatinine clearance estimation is inaccurate when values are changing during the development of and recovery from AKI.

One way to measure creatinine clearance is to perform a timed urine collection and determine the plasma creatinine level midway through the collection. An incomplete or prolonged urine collection is a common source of error. The completeness of the collection can be estimated by comparing the amount of creatinine excreted in the collection to that expected over a 24-hour period, which should be constant:

$$U_{cr} \times \dot{V} = 15 - 20 \text{ mg/kg for healthy young women}$$
$$U_{cr} \times \dot{V} = 20 - 25 \text{ mg/kg for healthy young men}$$

Given the tedious nature of timed urine collections for measuring GFR, GFR is more commonly estimated (denoted eGFR) using equations that have been validated using patient characteristics (such as age, sex, and weight) and plasma creatinine levels. The Kidney Disease Improving Global Outcomes workgroup recommends eGFR equations as the primary method for determining GFR. The recommended eGFR equation is the 2021 CKD-Epidemiology (EPI) Collaboration creatinine equation. The Cockcroft-Gault formula is commonly used to determine drug dosing, but it is no longer recommended since it was developed before the standardization of used creatinine assays. The 2021 CKD-EPI equation (and others) can be accessed using several web-based calculators (eg, https://www.kidney.org/professionals/kdoqi/gfr_calculator). **Cystatin C** is another endogenous marker of GFR that is filtered freely at the glomerulus, produced at a relatively constant rate, and less dependent than creatinine on muscle mass. It is reabsorbed and partially metabolized in the renal tubular epithelial cells. Adding the measurement of cystatin C to serum creatinine improves the accuracy of eGFR. A large meta-analysis showed that cystatin C alone or in combination with serum creatinine is a stronger predictor of important clinical events, such as ESKD or death, than serum creatinine alone. However, because cystatin C is not universally available or standardized across assays, it remains a complementary rather than the primary biomarker for estimating GFR.

BUN is another index used in assessing kidney function. It is synthesized mainly in the liver and is the end product of protein catabolism. Urea is freely filtered by the glomerulus, but about 30–70% is reabsorbed in the renal tubules. As such, it underestimates GFR. Renal urea reabsorption increases (in conjunction with increased sodium reabsorption) in hypovolemic patients (who, therefore, have an increased BUN). A normal BUN:creatinine ratio is approximately 10:1, although this varies between individuals. With volume depletion, the ratio can increase to 20:1 or higher. Other causes of increased BUN include increased catabolism (GI bleeding, cell lysis, and corticosteroid usage), increased dietary protein, and decreased renal perfusion prompting increased sodium (and therefore BUN) reabsorption (eg, heart failure, renal artery stenosis) (Table 22–2). Reduced BUN levels are seen in liver disease and in the syndrome of inappropriate ADH (SIADH).

In summary, creatinine and urea clearances overestimate and underestimate GFR, respectively. Because each of these estimates becomes more inaccurate as kidney disease advances, a more accurate measure of GFR as patients approach ESKD is the average of the creatinine and urea clearances.

KIDNEY BIOPSY

Indications for percutaneous needle biopsy include (1) unexplained decline in GFR; (2) unexplained proteinuria or hematuria, or both; (3) previously identified and treated lesions to guide future therapy; (4) systemic diseases associated with kidney dysfunction, such as SLE, anti-GBM disease, and granulomatosis with polyangiitis; and (5) kidney transplant dysfunction, to evaluate for transplant rejection or other abnormalities. Kidney biopsies should only be performed if the results will influence the treatment plan or facilitate discussion about prognosis. Relative contraindications include a solitary or ectopic kidney

Table 22–2. Conditions affecting BUN independently of GFR.

Increased BUN
Reduced effective circulating blood volume (prerenal azotemia)
Catabolic states (GI bleeding, corticosteroid use)
High-protein diets
Tetracycline
Decreased BUN
Liver disease
Malnutrition
Sickle cell anemia
SIADH

SIADH, syndrome of inappropriate ADH.

(exception for transplant allografts), horseshoe kidney, ESKD, congenital anomalies, and multiple cysts. Absolute contraindications include an uncorrected bleeding disorder; severe uncontrolled hypertension; renal infection or neoplasm; hydronephrosis; or uncooperative patients, including those who are unable to lie flat for the procedure.

Percutaneous kidney biopsies are generally safe. The major risk is bleeding, which may occur up to 72 hours post biopsy. More than half of patients will have at least a small hematoma; approximately 1–5% of patients will experience significant bleeding requiring a blood transfusion. Anticoagulation should be held for 5–7 days post biopsy if possible. The risks of nephrectomy and mortality are about 0.06–0.08%. When a percutaneous needle biopsy is technically not feasible and kidney tissue is deemed clinically essential, a closed biopsy via interventional radiologic techniques or open biopsy under general anesthesia can be performed.

Cavanaugh C et al. Urine sediment examination in the diagnosis and management of kidney disease: Core Curriculum 2019. Am J Kidney Dis. 2019;73:258. [PMID: 30249419]

Delgado C et al. A unifying approach for GFR estimation: recommendations of the NKF-ASN Task Force on reassessing the inclusion of race in diagnosing kidney disease. J Am Soc Nephrol. 2021;32:2994. [PMID: 34556489]

Inker LA et al. New creatinine- and cystatin C-based equations to estimate GFR without race. N Engl J Med. 2021;385:1737. [PMID: 34554658]

Inker LA et al. Measurement and estimation of GFR for use in clinical practice: Core Curriculum 2021. Am J Kidney Dis. 2021;78:736. [PMID: 34518032]

ACUTE KIDNEY INJURY

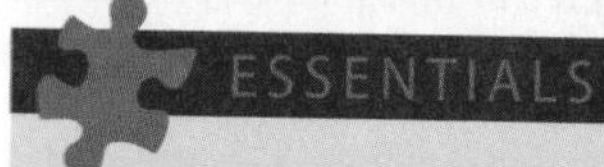

ESSENTIALS OF DIAGNOSIS

- Rapid increase in serum creatinine.
- Oliguria may be present.
- Symptoms and signs depend on cause and severity.

General Considerations

AKI is defined as an absolute increase in serum creatinine by 0.3 mg/dL or more within 48 hours, or a relative increase of 1.5 times baseline or more that is known or presumed to have occurred within 7 days. AKI is characterized as oliguric if urine production is less than roughly 400–500 mL/day. AKI is characterized by an inability to maintain acid-base, fluid, and electrolyte balance, and to excrete nitrogenous wastes. **Stage 1** is a 1.5- to 1.9-fold increase in serum creatinine or a decline in urinary output to less than 0.5 mL/kg/hour over 6–12 hours; **stage 2** is a 2.0- to 2.9-fold increase in serum creatinine or decline in urinary output to less than 0.5 mL/kg/hour over 12 hours or longer; **stage 3** is a 3.0-fold or greater increase in serum creatinine, an increase in serum creatinine to greater than or equal to 4 mg/dL, a decline in urinary output to less than 0.3 mL/kg/hour for 24 hours or longer, anuria for 12 hours or longer, or initiation of kidney replacement therapy. In the absence of functioning kidneys, serum creatinine will typically increase by 1–1.5 mg/dL daily, although with certain conditions such as rhabdomyolysis serum creatinine can increase more rapidly. Using the AKI stage definition above, AKI is estimated to occur in approximately 20% of all hospitalized patients and 65% of patients in the ICU. Observed rates of AKI in the hospital setting are increasing over time.

Clinical Findings

A. Symptoms and Signs

Although most patients will not experience any symptoms or exhibit any signs of AKI, accumulation of waste products can cause nonspecific symptoms and signs collectively termed **uremia**: nausea, vomiting, malaise, and altered sensorium. More commonly, patients experience symptoms and signs of the underlying disease causing their AKI (eg, lupus). Elevated blood pressure can occur, and fluid homeostasis is often impaired. Hypovolemia can cause states of low blood flow to the kidneys, sometimes termed **prerenal azotemia,** whereas hypervolemia can result from intrinsic or postrenal disease. Pericardial effusions can develop with uremia and may result in cardiac tamponade; a pericardial friction rub can be present, signaling pericarditis. With hyperkalemia, ventricular tachycardia and other tachyarrhythmias can occur. The lung examination may reveal rales in the presence of hypervolemia. AKI can cause nonspecific diffuse abdominal pain and ileus. Platelet dysfunction with bleeding and clotting disorders can occur. The neurologic examination sometimes reveals encephalopathic changes with asterixis and confusion; with profound uremia, seizures may ensue.

B. Laboratory Findings

By definition, elevated serum creatinine (and often BUN) levels are present, though these elevations do not distinguish AKI from CKD. Metabolic acidosis (due to decreased clearance of organic and inorganic acids) is often noted. Hyperkalemia can occur from impaired renal potassium excretion or from shifting of potassium from cells into the blood as a result of metabolic acidosis. With hyperkalemia, ECG can reveal peaked T waves, PR prolongation, and QRS widening. A long QT segment can occur with hypocalcemia. Hyperphosphatemia occurs when phosphorus cannot be secreted by damaged tubules. Anemia can occur as a result of decreased erythropoietin production over weeks, and platelet dysfunction is common.

Classification & Etiology

AKI is commonly divided into three anatomic categories: prerenal causes (kidney hypoperfusion), intrinsic kidney disease, and postrenal causes (obstruction to urinary outflow). Identifying the cause is the first step toward treatment (Table 22–3).

Table 22–3. Classification and differential diagnosis of AKI.

	Prerenal Azotemia	Postrenal Azotemia	Intrinsic Renal Disease		
			ATN	Acute Glomerulonephritis	Acute Interstitial Nephritis
Etiology	Poor renal perfusion	Obstruction of the urinary tract	Ischemia, nephrotoxins	Immune complex–mediated, pauci-immune, anti-GBM–related, monoclonal immunoglobulin–mediated, C3 glomerulopathy	Allergic reaction; drug reaction; infection; autoimmune disease
Serum BUN:Cr ratio	> 20:1	> 20:1	< 20:1	> 20:1	< 20:1
U_{Na} (mEq/L)	< 20	Variable	> 20	< 20	Variable
FE_{Na} (%)	< 1	Variable	> 1 (when oliguric)	< 1	Variable
Urine osmolality (mOsm/kg)	> 500	< 400	250–300	Variable	Variable
Urinary sediment	Benign or hyaline casts	Normal or red cells, white cells, or crystals	Granular (muddy brown) casts, renal tubular cell casts	Red cells, dysmorphic red cells, and red cell casts	White cells, white cell casts, with or without eosinophils

BUN:Cr, blood urea nitrogen:creatinine ratio; FE_{Na}, fractional excretion of sodium; GBM, glomerular basement membrane; U_{Na}, urinary concentration of sodium.

A. Prerenal Causes

Prerenal causes are the most common etiology of AKI, accounting for 40–80% of cases. Prerenal azotemia is a physiologic response to renal hypoperfusion. If reversed quickly with restoration of renal blood flow (eg, fluid resuscitation), renal parenchymal damage often does not occur. If hypoperfusion persists, prerenal azotemia can develop into intrinsic kidney injury.

Decreased renal perfusion can occur in several ways, such as a decrease in intravascular volume, a change in vascular resistance, or low cardiac output. Causes of volume depletion include hemorrhage (eg, from trauma), GI losses, excessive diuresis, and extravascular fluid sequestration (eg, pancreatitis, burns, and peritonitis).

Changes in systemic vascular resistance can occur with sepsis, anaphylaxis, anesthesia, and afterload-reducing drugs. Blockade of the renin-angiotensin-aldosterone system, such as with ACE inhibitors, limits efferent renal arteriolar constriction out of proportion to afferent arteriolar constriction and thereby decreases GFR. NSAIDs minimize afferent arteriolar vasodilation by inhibiting prostaglandin-mediated signals. NSAIDs may have deleterious effects on renal perfusion in states of low effective arterial volume (eg, cirrhosis and heart failure) when prostaglandins normally are recruited to increase renal blood flow. Epinephrine, norepinephrine, high-dose dopamine, anesthetic agents, and calcineurin inhibitors also can cause renal vasoconstriction. Renal artery stenosis causes increased resistance and decreased renal perfusion.

Low cardiac output results in a state of low effective renal arterial blood flow. This occurs with heart failure (including cardiogenic shock), PE, and pericardial tamponade. Arrhythmias and valvular disorders can also reduce cardiac output. In the intensive care setting, positive pressure ventilation will decrease venous return and, in effect, cardiac output.

When GFR falls acutely, it is important to determine whether AKI is due to prerenal or intrinsic causes. History, physical examination, and laboratory data may be helpful in distinguishing these causes. In prerenal AKI, the BUN:creatinine ratio often exceeds 20:1 due to increased urea reabsorption by functioning tubules. In oliguric patients, another useful index is the fractional excretion of sodium (FE_{Na}). With decreased GFR, the kidney reabsorbs salt and water avidly if there is no intrinsic tubular dysfunction. Thus, oliguric patients with prerenal AKI should have a low fractional excretion of sodium (less than 1%). Oliguric patients with intrinsic kidney dysfunction typically have a high FE_{Na} (greater than 1–2%), indicating loss of tubular cells' ability to reabsorb sodium. The FE_{Na} is calculated as follows: FE_{Na} = clearance of Na^+/GFR = clearance of Na^+/C_{cr}:

$$FE_{Na} = \frac{Urine_{Na} / Serum_{Na}}{Urine_{cr} / Serum_{cr}} \times 100\%$$

The equation was created and validated to differentiate *oliguric* ATN and prerenal AKI; its utility in nonoliguric patients is limited. Because diuretics act by increasing sodium excretion, a high FE_{Na} within 12–24 hours after diuretic administration cannot be meaningfully interpreted. In contrast, a low FE_{Na} *despite* receiving diuretics offers strong evidence of prerenal states in oliguric patients. Given the limitations of FE_{Na} calculations, urine microscopy is a much more valuable tool for determining cause of AKI. Patients with prerenal azotemia typically have bland urine sediments, though some have hyaline casts. In contrast, patients with ATN often have renal tubular epithelial cells or muddy brown casts.

Treatment of prerenal AKI depends on the underlying cause, but achievement of euvolemia, attention to serum electrolytes, and avoidance of nephrotoxic drugs are benchmarks of therapy. This involves careful assessment of volume status, cardiac function, diet, and drug dosing.

B. Postrenal Causes

Postrenal causes of AKI are the least common, accounting for approximately 5–10% of cases, but are important to detect because of their reversibility. Postrenal AKI occurs when urinary flow from both kidneys, or a single functioning kidney, is obstructed. Obstruction leads to elevated intraluminal pressure and resultant kidney parenchymal damage, with marked effects on renal blood flow and tubular function.

Postrenal AKI can occur from obstruction at the level of the urethra, bladder, ureters, or renal pelvises. In men, benign prostatic hyperplasia is the most common cause. Patients taking anticholinergic drugs are at risk for urinary retention. Obstruction can also be caused by bladder, prostate, and cervical cancers; retroperitoneal fibrosis; and neurogenic bladder (eg, from diabetes mellitus). Less common causes include blood clots, bilateral ureteral stones, urethral stones or strictures, and bilateral papillary necrosis.

Obstruction can be constant or intermittent, and partial or complete. Obstruction may cause anuria but may also cause polyuria in the setting of partial obstruction with resultant tubular dysfunction and inability to reabsorb salt and water. Patients may endorse lower abdominal or back pain, and on examination may have an enlarged prostate, distended bladder, or mass detected.

Laboratory examination may initially reveal high urine osmolality, low urine sodium, high BUN:creatinine ratio, and low FE_{Na} (as tubular function may not be compromised initially). These indices are similar to a prerenal state because extensive intrinsic renal damage has not yet occurred. After several days, however, the urine sodium increases as the kidneys fail and are unable to concentrate urine (isosthenuria). Urine sediment is generally bland, though hematuria may be seen if the obstruction is due to stones, blood clots, or papillary necrosis.

Patients with AKI due to suspected postrenal causes should undergo bladder catheterization and ultrasonography to assess for hydroureter, hydronephrosis, or large bladder volume. After reversal of the underlying process, some patients experience significant increased urinary output (called postobstructive diuresis). In such settings, care should be taken to avoid volume depletion or electrolyte derangements. Prompt treatment of obstruction within days by catheters, stents, or other surgical procedures can result in partial or complete reversal of AKI.

C. Intrinsic Acute Kidney Injury

Intrinsic renal disorders account for up to 50% of all cases of AKI. Intrinsic dysfunction is considered after prerenal and postrenal causes have been excluded. The potential sites of injury are the tubules, interstitium, vasculature, and glomeruli. Intrinsic AKI is discussed in greater detail in the following sections.

▶ When to Refer

- If a patient has signs of AKI that have not reversed over 1–2 weeks, or if the degree of AKI is concerning (eg, doubling of creatinine) and without an immediately reversible cause such as obstruction.
- If a patient has signs of urinary tract obstruction, the patient should be referred to a urologist.

▶ When to Admit

The patient should be admitted if there is sudden loss of kidney function resulting in abnormalities that cannot be handled expeditiously in an outpatient setting (eg, hyperkalemia, volume overload, uremia) or an acute intervention is needed, such as emergent urologic procedures or dialysis.

Kellum JA et al. Acute kidney injury. Nat Rev Dis Primers. 2021;15;7:52. [PMID: 34267223]

Ostermann et al. Recommendations on acute kidney injury biomarkers from the Acute Disease Quality Initiative Consensus Conference: a consensus statement. JAMA Netw Open. 2020;3:e2019209. [PMID: 33021646]

ACUTE TUBULAR NECROSIS

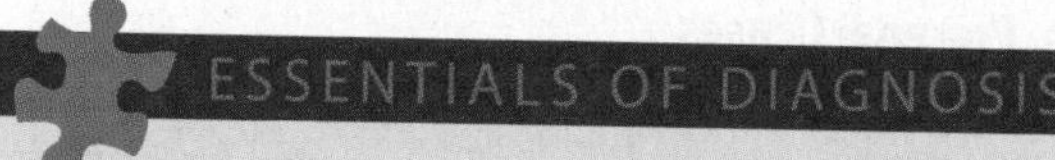

- ▶ AKI.
- ▶ Ischemic or toxic insult, or underlying sepsis.
- ▶ Urine sediment with granular (muddy brown) casts and renal tubular epithelial cells is pathognomonic but not essential.

▶ General Considerations

AKI due to tubular damage is called **acute tubular necrosis (ATN)** and accounts for approximately 85% of intrinsic AKI. The two major causes of ATN are ischemia and nephrotoxin exposure. Ischemic ATN is characterized not only by inadequate GFR but also by renal blood flow that is inadequate to maintain parenchymal cellular perfusion. Renal tubular damage can be caused by low effective arterial blood flow to the kidneys in the setting of prolonged hypotension or hypoxemia, such as volume depletion or shock. Underlying sepsis is an independent risk factor for ATN, even in the absence of hemodynamic compromise. Prolonged renal hypoperfusion can occur with major surgical procedures, and may be exacerbated by vasodilating anesthetic agents.

A. Exogenous Nephrotoxins

Exogenous nephrotoxins more commonly cause ATN than endogenous nephrotoxins.

Aminoglycosides cause ATN in up to 25% of hospitalized patients receiving therapeutic levels of the drugs. Nonoliguric AKI typically occurs after 5–10 days of exposure. Predisposing factors include underlying kidney disease, volume depletion, and advanced age. Monitoring drug levels is important, and troughs are helpful in predicting renal toxicity.

Amphotericin B is typically nephrotoxic after a dose of 2–3 g. This causes a type 1 (distal) renal tubular acidosis with severe vasoconstriction and tubular damage, which can lead to hypokalemia and nephrogenic diabetes insipidus. **Vancomycin**, intravenous **acyclovir**, and **cephalosporins** are also known to cause or be associated with ATN.

Radiographic contrast media may be directly nephrotoxic. Contrast nephropathy is the third leading cause of incident AKI in hospitalized patients and is thought to result from the synergistic combination of direct renal tubular epithelial cell toxicity and renal medullary ischemia. The combination of preexisting diabetes mellitus and CKD is associated with the greatest risk (15–50%) of contrast nephropathy. Other risk factors include advanced age; volume depletion; heart failure; plasma cell myeloma; repeated doses of contrast; and recent exposure to other nephrotoxic agents, including NSAIDs and ACE inhibitors. Lower volumes of contrast with low osmolality are recommended in high-risk patients. Toxicity usually occurs within 24–48 hours after the radiocontrast study. Nonionic contrast media may be less toxic, but this has not been well proven. Prevention of contrast nephropathy is the goal when using these agents. The mainstay of prophylaxis is 1–3 mL/kg or 500–1000 mL of intravenous 0.9% (normal) saline over 6 hours both before and after the contrast administration—cautiously in patients with preexisting cardiac dysfunction; oral intake of fluids is an acceptable alternative for outpatient studies. Isotonic intravenous volume repletion is superior to hypotonic intravenous solutions, and both are superior to oral solutions in small studies. Other nephrotoxic agents should be avoided the day before and after dye administration. Alternative prophylactic strategies involving *N*-acetylcysteine, sodium bicarbonate, mannitol, and furosemide do not show benefit over 0.9% (normal) saline administration. In fact, furosemide may lead to increased rates of kidney dysfunction in this setting.

Calcineurin inhibitor toxicity (from tacrolimus or cyclosporine) is usually dose dependent. It causes distal tubular dysfunction (a type 4 renal tubular acidosis) and severe vasoconstriction. Regular blood level monitoring is important to prevent both acute and chronic nephrotoxicity. Kidney function usually improves after reducing the dose or stopping the drug.

Other exogenous nephrotoxins include antineoplastics, such as cisplatin and organic solvents, and heavy metals such as mercury, cadmium, and arsenic. Herbal medicines are also increasingly recognized as potentially nephrotoxic. Finally, although ACE inhibitors and ARBs have many long-term benefits for patients with CKD, they may cause or contribute to ischemic ATN at times of prolonged hypotension or volume depletion.

B. Endogenous Nephrotoxins

Endogenous nephrotoxins include pigment-containing products (myoglobin and hemoglobin), uric acid, and paraproteins. These products can cause direct tubular toxicity, resulting in ATN. The most common type of pigment nephropathy is rhabdomyolysis, caused by release of myoglobin from muscle. Massive intravascular hemolysis with release of hemoglobin is seen in transfusion reactions and in certain hemolytic anemias. Reversal of the underlying disorder and volume resuscitation are mainstays of treatment.

Hyperuricemia can occur in the setting of rapid cell turnover and lysis. Chemotherapy for germ cell and hematologic malignancies (leukemia and lymphoma) is the primary cause; spontaneous tumor lysis syndrome can also occur, though is less common. ATN results from intratubular precipitation of uric acid crystals; serum uric acid levels often exceed 15–20 mg/dL and urine uric acid levels are typically greater than 600 mg/24 hours. A urine uric acid to urine creatinine ratio greater than 1.0 identifies individuals at risk for ATN. Allopurinol or rasburicase can be used prophylactically, and rasburicase with or without dialysis is often used for treatment in established cases.

Paraproteins seen in plasma cell myeloma can cause direct tubular toxicity and tubular obstruction. Other renal complications from plasma cell myeloma include hypercalcemia and renal tubular dysfunction, including type 2 (proximal) renal tubular acidosis (see Plasma Cell Myeloma below).

Clinical Findings

A. Symptoms and Signs

See Acute Kidney Injury.

B. Laboratory Findings

Hyperkalemia and hyperphosphatemia are commonly present. The BUN:creatinine ratio is usually less than 20:1 because tubular function is not intact, as described in the general section on AKI (Table 22–3). Urinary output can be oliguric or nonoliguric, with oliguria portending a worse prognosis. Urine sodium concentration and FE_{Na} are typically elevated, indicative of tubular dysfunction. Urine microscopy may show evidence of acute tubular damage; the presence of two or more granular casts or renal tubular epithelial cells is strongly predictive of ATN but has a low negative predictive value (see Table 22–1). Although not usually performed in cases of ATN, kidney biopsy is sometimes helpful in cases of diagnostic uncertainty.

Treatment

Treatment of ATN is aimed at hastening recovery and avoiding complications. Preventive measures should be taken to avoid volume overload and hyperkalemia. A prospective randomized controlled trial did not show benefit of loop diuretics on either recovery from AKI or death. Use of diuretics in critically ill patients with AKI should be used only when otherwise clinically indicated (eg, in states of volume overload). Although nonresponsiveness to a trial of high-dose diuretics (called "furosemide stress test") has been shown to predict future need for acute dialysis in this population.

Ultrafiltration is generally reserved for patients with AKI in need of volume removal who are unresponsive to diuretics, with the recognition that this has not been shown to improve survival. A randomized controlled trial did not show benefit on mortality with plasma ultrafiltration compared with intravenous diuretics in patients with decompensated heart failure. Dietary protein restriction of 0.6 g/kg/day curbs the risk of metabolic acidosis. Hypocalcemia and hyperphosphatemia can be treated with dietary modification and phosphate-binding agents taken with meals. Examples include calcium carbonate (500–1500 mg orally), calcium acetate (667 mg orally), sevelamer carbonate (800–1600 mg orally), and lanthanum carbonate (1000 mg orally). Hypocalcemia should not be treated in patients with rhabdomyolysis unless they are symptomatic. Hypermagnesemia can occur because of reduced magnesium excretion by the renal tubules, so magnesium-containing antacids and laxatives should be avoided in these patients. Dosages of all medications must be adjusted for drugs eliminated by the kidney.

Indications for dialysis in AKI from ATN or other intrinsic disorders include life-threatening "AEIOUs" (Acid-base or Electrolyte disturbances [eg, hyperkalemia] refractory to medical management; Intoxications from certain drugs, volume; Overload unresponsive to diuresis; and Uremic complications [eg, encephalopathy, pericarditis, and seizures]). In critically ill patients, less severe but worsening abnormalities may also be indications for dialytic support. Unfortunately, there is no evidence that more intensive or earlier initiation of renal replacement therapy for patients with AKI confers survival benefit.

Course & Prognosis

The clinical course of ATN is often divided into three phases: initial injury, maintenance, and recovery. The maintenance phase is expressed as either oliguric (urinary output less than 500 mL/day) or nonoliguric. Nonoliguric ATN is associated with better outcomes than oliguric ATN; conversion from oliguric to nonoliguric states with the use of diuretics does not alter prognosis. While dopamine has sometimes been used for this purpose, numerous studies have shown that its use in this setting is not beneficial. Average duration of the maintenance phase is 1–3 weeks, but some cases last several months. Cellular repair and removal of tubular debris occur during this period. The recovery phase can be heralded by diuresis, due both to inability of recovering renal tubules to reabsorb salt and water appropriately and to solute-induced diuresis from accumulated BUN. As GFR begins to rise, BUN and serum creatinine fall.

The mortality rate associated with AKI in hospitalized patients is 20–50% and up to 70% in ICU patients requiring dialysis due to additional comorbid illnesses. Increased mortality is associated with advanced age, severe underlying disease, and multisystem organ failure. Leading causes of death are infections, fluid and electrolyte disturbances, and worsening of underlying disease.

When to Refer

- When uncertainty exists as to the cause of or treatment for AKI.
- For fluid, electrolyte, and acid-base abnormalities that are recalcitrant to interventions.
- Nephrology referral improves outcomes in AKI.

When to Admit

A patient with symptoms or signs of AKI that require immediate intervention, such as administration of intravenous fluids or dialytic therapy, or that require a team approach that cannot be coordinated as an outpatient.

Bouchard J et al. Timing of kidney support therapy in acute kidney injury: what are we waiting for? Am J Kidney Dis. 2022;79:417. [PMID: 34461167]

STARRT-AKI Investigators; Canadian Critical Care Trials Group; Australian and New Zealand Intensive Care Society Clinical Trials Group; United Kingdom Critical Care Research Group; Canadian Nephrology Trials Network; Irish Critical Care Trials Group, Bagshaw SM et al. Timing of initiation of renal-replacement therapy in acute kidney injury. N Engl J Med. 2020;383:240. [PMID: 32668114]

RHABDOMYOLYSIS

ESSENTIALS OF DIAGNOSIS

- Associated with crush injuries to muscle, immobility, drug toxicities, and hypothermia.
- Characterized by serum elevations in muscle enzymes, including creatine kinase, and marked electrolyte abnormalities.
- Release of myoglobin leads to direct renal toxicity.

General Considerations

Rhabdomyolysis is a syndrome of acute skeletal muscle necrosis leading to myoglobinuria and markedly elevated creatine kinase levels. ATN is a common complication due to filtration of excess myoglobin, which leads to tubular obstruction from pigmented casts and intrarenal vasoconstriction. Rhabdomyolysis can result from crush injuries, prolonged immobility, seizures, substance abuse (eg, cocaine), and medications (especially statins); concomitant volume depletion in these settings increases risk of rhabdomyolysis. In patients taking statins, the risk of rhabdomyolysis is increased in the presence of kidney or liver disease, diabetes, or hypothyroidism. Concurrent use of statins (except pravastatin or rosuvastatin) and drugs that inhibit cytochrome P450 (including protease inhibitors, erythromycin or clarithromycin, itraconazole, diltiazem, and verapamil) as well as concurrent use of niacin and fibrate-containing therapy also increase the risk.

Clinical Findings

A. Symptoms and Signs

Patients with rhabdomyolysis may have myalgias or weakness or both, though it is not uncommon for them to be asymptomatic. Urine may appear dark.

B. Laboratory Findings

Rhabdomyolysis of clinical importance commonly occurs when serum creatine kinase exceeds 16,000–50,000 IU/L; one study showed that 58% of patients with AKI attributed to rhabdomyolysis had creatine kinase levels greater than 16,000 IU/L, while only 11% of patients without AKI had creatine kinase values greater than 16,000 IU/L. Often, there are elevated serum levels of other skeletal muscle enzymes including AST, ALT, and LD. The acute, significant elevations in muscle enzymes peak quickly and usually resolve within days once the inciting injury has resolved.

The classic laboratory finding in rhabdomyolysis is a urine dipstick test that is positive for "blood" but without RBCs on microscopy; a false-positive result is due to detection of myoglobin rather than hemoglobin. Additionally, clinically meaningful rhabdomyolysis causes injured muscle cells to release intracellular components, leading to electrolyte derangements (including hyperkalemia, hyperphosphatemia, hyperuricemia, and hypocalcemia).

Treatment

The mainstay of treatment is aggressive volume repletion with 0.9% normal saline (ie, more than 4 L/day) and removal of offending medications if thought to have caused the disorder. Adjunctive treatments with mannitol and alkalization of the urine have not been proven to change outcomes in human trials. As patients recover, calcium can translocate from tissues to plasma, so early exogenous calcium administration for hypocalcemia is not recommended unless the patient is symptomatic or the level becomes exceedingly low in an unconscious patient; calcium repletion can cause precipitation of calcium phosphate given the frequently concurrent hyperphosphatemia.

Myopathic complications of statins usually resolve within several weeks of discontinuing the drug.

When to Refer

Clinically meaningful rhabdomyolysis requires immediate attention and inpatient management, so affected patients should not be referred to outpatient nephrology clinics unless to follow-up after a hospital admission.

When to Admit

Patients whose serum creatine kinase levels are greater than 15,000–20,000 IU/L or patients with AKI or electrolyte derangements should be admitted for fluid repletion and serial monitoring of creatine kinase and electrolytes.

Long B et al. An evidence-based narrative review of the emergency department evaluation and management of rhabdomyolysis. Am J Emerg Med. 2019;37:518. [PMID: 30630682]

Safitri N et al. A narrative review of statin-induced rhabdomyolysis: molecular mechanism, risk factors, and management. Drug Healthc Patient Saf. 2021;8;13:211. [PMID: 34795533]

INTERSTITIAL NEPHRITIS

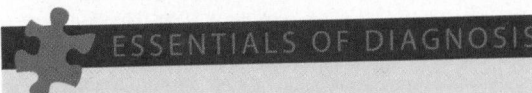

- Fever.
- Transient maculopapular rash.
- Acute or chronic in nature.
- Pyuria, WBC casts, and hematuria.

General Considerations

Acute interstitial nephritis accounts for 10–15% of cases of intrinsic AKI. An interstitial inflammatory response with edema and possible tubular damage is the typical pathologic finding.

Although drugs account for over 70% of cases, acute interstitial nephritis also occurs in infectious diseases, autoimmune disorders, or idiopathically. The most common drugs implicated are penicillins and cephalosporins, immune checkpoint inhibitors, sulfonamides and sulfonamide-containing diuretics, NSAIDs, PPIs, rifampin, and allopurinol. Infectious causes include streptococcal infections, leptospirosis, cytomegalovirus, histoplasmosis, and Rocky Mountain spotted fever. SLE, Sjögren syndrome, sarcoidosis, and cryoglobulinemia can also cause interstitial nephritis, though they are more classically associated with glomerulonephritis.

Clinical Findings

Clinical features may include fever (more than 80% of cases), rash (25–50%), arthralgias, and peripheral blood eosinophilia (80%). The classic triad of fever, rash, and arthralgias is present in only 10–15% of cases. Urine microscopy often reveals white cells (70%), red cells (50%), and white cell casts (15%). Proteinuria is often present, particularly in NSAID-induced interstitial nephritis, but is usually modest (less than 2 g/24 hour). Evaluation for eosinophiluria is not advised as it is neither sensitive nor specific for interstitial nephritis. Although the clinical history and laboratory data often suggest the diagnosis, kidney biopsy is sometimes needed.

Treatment & Prognosis

Acute interstitial nephritis often carries a good prognosis, with recovery occurring over weeks to months. Urgent dialytic therapy may be necessary in up to one-third of patients before resolution, but patients rarely progress to ESKD. Those with prolonged oliguria and advanced age have a worse prognosis. Treatment consists of supportive measures and prompt removal of the inciting agent. If kidney injury persists despite removal of the culprit drug, corticosteroids should be considered, although data to support their use are limited, and their efficacy is diminished if started more than 1–2 weeks after onset of AKI. Short-term, high-dose methylprednisolone (0.25–0.5 g/day intravenously for 1–4 days) or prednisone (60 mg/day orally for

4–6 weeks) followed by a prednisone taper can be used in severe cases of drug-induced interstitial nephritis.

Perazella MA et al. Immune checkpoint inhibitor nephrotoxicity: what do we know and what should we do? Kidney Int. 2020;97:62. [PMID: 31685311]

GLOMERULONEPHRITIS

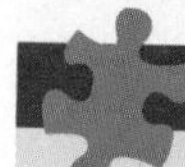

ESSENTIALS OF DIAGNOSIS

- Hematuria, subnephrotic proteinuria.
- Red cell casts pathognomonic but not required for diagnosis.
- Dependent edema and hypertension.
- AKI.

General Considerations

Acute glomerulonephritis is an uncommon cause of AKI, accounting for about 5% of cases. Pathologically, inflammatory glomerular lesions are seen. These include mesangioproliferative, focal and diffuse endocapillary proliferative, and crescentic lesions. The larger the percentage of glomeruli involved and the more severe the lesion, the higher the risk of a poor clinical outcome.

Glomerulonephritides are classified into five pathophysiologic processes, which are characterized by serologic analysis. Markers include anti-GBM antibodies, antineutrophil cytoplasmic antibodies (ANCAs), and other immune markers of disease.

Immune complex glomerulonephritis occurs when autoantibodies develop and combine with antigens to form immune complexes that deposit within glomeruli. There are several distinct immune complex glomerulonephritides, including IgA nephropathy, infection-related glomerulonephritis, lupus nephritis, and cryoglobulinemic glomerulonephritis (often associated with hepatitis C virus [HCV]).

Anti-GBM–associated acute glomerulonephritis is either confined to the kidney or associated with pulmonary hemorrhage. The latter is called "Goodpasture syndrome." Injury is related to autoantibodies against type IV collagen in the GBM.

Pauci-immune acute glomerulonephritis is a form of small-vessel vasculitis associated with ANCAs, causing kidney disease without direct immune complex deposition or antibody binding. Tissue injury is believed to be due to cell-mediated immune processes. An example is granulomatosis with polyangiitis, a systemic necrotizing vasculitis of small arteries and veins associated with intravascular and extravascular granuloma formation. In addition to glomerulonephritis, these patients can have upper airway, pulmonary, and skin manifestations. Cytoplasmic ANCA (c-ANCA) is the common staining pattern. Microscopic polyangiitis is another pauci-immune vasculitis causing glomerulonephritis, and is more commonly associated with perinuclear staining (p-ANCA).

ANCA-associated and anti-GBM–associated acute glomerulonephritides have poor outcomes unless treatment is started early.

Monoclonal immunoglobulin–mediated glomerulonephritis is characterized by the deposition of a monoclonal immunoglobulin in glomeruli, the tubular basement membrane, or both. Immunofluorescent or immunohistochemical staining of kidney biopsies detects monotypic immunoglobulin deposits. Many cases occur in the setting of an identifiable monoclonal gammopathy, but this is not always the case. Serum protein electrophoresis, immunofixation, and free light chain analysis are important diagnostic tests to perform when monoclonal immunoglobulin–mediated glomerulonephritis is suspected or confirmed.

C3 glomerulopathy results from predominant C3 deposition in the glomeruli with or without minimal deposition of immunoglobulins. It is also identified by immunofluorescence or immunohistochemistry. The pathogenesis of C3 glomerulonephropathy stems from abnormalities in regulation of the alternative pathway of complement. Measurement of serum C3 levels may be helpful, but normal levels do not rule out C3 glomerulopathy.

Other vascular causes of glomerulonephritis include hypertensive emergencies and the thrombotic microangiopathies such as hemolytic-uremic syndrome and thrombotic thrombocytopenic purpura (see Chapter 14).

Clinical Findings

A. Symptoms and Signs

Patients with acute glomerulonephritis are often hypertensive and edematous with an abnormal urinary sediment. Patients may experience extrarenal signs that reflect systemic manifestations of their disease (eg, rash in patients with lupus; coughing or sinus congestion in patients with ANCA glomerulonephritis). Macroscopic hematuria is uncommon (in contrast to microscopic hematuria), but may occur in select cases (eg, IgA nephropathy).

B. Laboratory Findings

Serum creatinine can rise over days to months, depending on the rapidity of the underlying process. The BUN:creatinine ratio is not a reliable marker of kidney function and is more reflective of the patient's underlying volume status. Dipstick and microscopic evaluation reveal evidence of hematuria and subnephrotic proteinuria; there may be cellular elements such as dysmorphic red cells, red cell casts, and white cells. Red cell casts are specific for glomerulonephritis, and a detailed search on urine microscopy is warranted.

Serum complement levels (C3, C4) may be low in immune complex glomerulonephritis (except for IgA nephropathy) or C3 glomerulopathy and normal in pauci-immune, anti-GBM–related, and most monoclonal immunoglobulin–mediated glomerulonephritides. Other tests that may be appropriate include ASO titers, anti-GBM antibody levels, ANCAs, antinuclear antibody titers, cryoglobulins, hepatitis serologies, serum protein electrophoresis, immunofixation, serum free light chains, blood cultures, and renal ultrasound. With few exceptions, a kidney biopsy is ultimately necessary to confirm the diagnosis, irrespective of laboratory data.

Treatment

Treatment is tailored to the specific type and severity of glomerulonephritis. It may include high-dose corticosteroids, rituximab, cytotoxic agents (such as cyclophosphamide), antiproliferative agents (eg, mycophenolate), and calcineurin inhibitors (eg, tacrolimus). Plasma exchange can be used in Goodpasture syndrome as a temporizing measure until chemotherapy can take effect. Treatment and prognosis for specific diseases are discussed below.

Geetha D et al. ANCA-associated vasculitis: Core Curriculum 2020. Am J Kidney Dis. 2020;75:124. [PMID: 31358311]

Kant S et al. Advances in understanding of pathogenesis and treatment of immune-mediated kidney disease: a review. Am J Kidney Dis. 2022;79:582. [PMID: 34508831]

Pesce F et al. Glomerulonephritis in AKI: from pathogenesis to therapeutic intervention. Front Med (Lausanne). 2021;7: 582272. [PMID: 33738291]

Prapa P et al. IgA nephropathy: Core Curriculum 2021. Am J Kidney Dis. 2021;78:429. [PMID: 34247883]

COVID-19 & THE KIDNEY

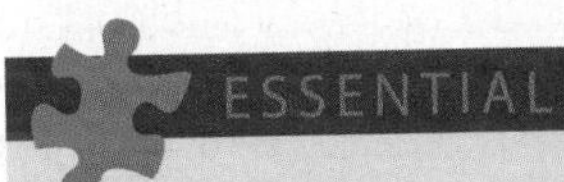

ESSENTIALS OF DIAGNOSIS

- Broad array of clinical presentation and kidney pathology.

Clinical Findings & Treatment

Nearly 30% of patients hospitalized with COVID-19 and 50% of critically ill patients are affected by AKI, which is associated with poorer prognosis. Many causes of AKI are described in patients with COVID-19, but the most common is ATN related to a high inflammatory state (termed "cytokine storm") and to states of prolonged hypotension and volume depletion.

UA may reveal hematuria, reflecting endothelial injury and fibrin thrombi that are commonly observed on biopsy. An emerging entity is COVID-19–associated collapsing glomerulopathy, which is a type of focal segmental glomerulosclerosis that predominantly affects Black patients, due to the increased prevalence of high-risk *APOL1* genetic variants (see section on Nephrotic Spectrum Glomerular Diseases below). Collapsing glomerulopathy presents with nephrotic syndrome. Treatment of COVID-19–related AKI is largely supportive; approximately 20% of patients require kidney replacement therapy. Corticosteroids have been used in COVID-19–associated collapsing glomerulopathy with reported success, but there is a lack of trial data or long-term follow-up to date to confirm efficacy.

Kudose S et al. Longitudinal outcomes of COVID-19-associated collapsing glomerulopathy and other podocytopathies. J Am Soc Nephrol. 2021;32:2958. [PMID: 34670811]

May RM et al. A multi-center retrospective cohort study defines the spectrum of kidney pathology in Coronavirus 2019 Disease (COVID-19). Kidney Int. 2021;100:1303. [PMID: 34352311]

Ng JH et al. Outcomes among patients hospitalized with COVID-19 and acute kidney injury. Am J Kidney Dis. 2021;77:204. [PMID: 32961245]

Ronco C et al. Management of acute kidney injury in patients with COVID-19. Lancet Respir Med. 2020;8:738. [PMID: 32416769]

CARDIORENAL SYNDROME

ESSENTIALS OF DIAGNOSIS

- **Cardiac dysfunction:** acute or chronic heart failure, ischemic injury, or arrhythmias.
- **Kidney disease:** acute or chronic, depending on the type of cardiorenal syndrome.

General Considerations

Cardiorenal syndrome is a pathophysiologic disorder of the heart and kidneys wherein acute or chronic deterioration of one organ results in the acute or chronic deterioration of the other. This syndrome is classified into five types as a matter of convention. Achieving euvolemia is the overarching therapeutic goal regardless of type (see Heart Failure section in Chapter 10).

Type 1 is defined by AKI stemming from acute cardiac disease. Type 2 is CKD due to chronic cardiac disease. Type 3 is acute cardiac disease as a result of AKI. Type 4 is chronic cardiac decompensation from CKD. Type 5 consists of heart and kidney dysfunction due to other acute or chronic systemic disorders (such as sepsis). Although novel agents are being examined, the mainstay of treatment is to address the primary underlying heart or kidney dysfunction. Medical diuresis achieves similar decongestion with lower rates of adverse events compared to extracorporeal therapies (eg, ultrafiltration).

Jentzer JC et al. Contemporary management of severe acute kidney injury and refractory cardiorenal syndrome: JACC council perspectives. J Am Coll Cardiol. 2020;76:1084. [PMID: 32854844]

Ricci Z et al. Cardiorenal syndrome. Crit Care Clin. 2021;37:335. [PMID: 33752859]

CHRONIC KIDNEY DISEASE

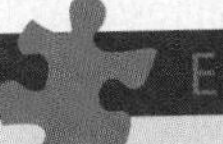

ESSENTIALS OF DIAGNOSIS

- Decline in the GFR over months to years.
- Persistent proteinuria or abnormal renal morphology may be present.
- Hypertension in most cases.
- Bilateral small or echogenic kidneys on ultrasound in advanced disease.
- Symptoms and signs of uremia when nearing end-stage disease.

Table 22–4. Stages of CKD: a clinical action plan.[1,2]

Stage[3]	Description	GFR (mL/minute/1.73 m^2)	Action
1	Kidney damage with normal or ↑↑ GFR	≥ 90	Diagnosis and treatment of underlying etiology if possible. Treatment of comorbid conditions. Estimate progression, work to slow progression. CVD risk reduction.
2	Kidney damage with mildly ↓ GFR	60–89	
3a	Mildly-moderately ↓ GFR	45–59	As above, and evaluating and treating complications.
3b	Moderately-severely ↓ GFR	30–44	
4	Severely ↓ GFR	15–29	Preparation for ESKD.
5	ESKD	< 15 (or dialysis)	Dialysis, transplant, or palliative care.

[1]Based on National Kidney Foundation, KDOQI, and KDIGO Chronic Kidney Disease Guidelines.
[2]CKD is defined as either kidney damage or GFR < 60 mL/minute/1.73 m^2 for 3 or more months. Kidney damage is defined as pathologic abnormalities or markers of damage, including abnormalities in blood or urine tests or imaging studies.
[3]At all stages, persistent albuminuria confers added risk for CKD progression and CVD in the following gradations: < 30 mg/day = lowest added risk, 30–300 mg/day = mildly increased risk, > 300–1000 mg/day = moderately increased risk, > 1000 mg/day = severely increased risk.
Reproduced with permission from Kidney Disease: Improving Global Outcomes (KDIGO) CKD Work Group. KDIGO 2012 Clinical Practice Guideline for the Evaluation and Management of Chronic Kidney Disease. *Kidney Int.* 2013;3(1)(Suppl):1–150.

General Considerations

CKD affects at least 10% of Americans. Many are unaware of the condition because the disease is asymptomatic until it nears end stage. The National Kidney Foundation's staging system helps clinicians formulate practice plans (Table 22–4). Over 70% of cases of late-stage CKD (stage 5 CKD and ESKD) in the United States are due to diabetes mellitus or hypertension/vascular disease. Glomerulonephritis, cystic diseases, chronic tubulointerstitial diseases, and other urologic diseases account for the remainder (Table 22–5). Genetic polymorphisms of the *APOL-1* gene have been shown to be associated with an increased risk of the development of CKD in persons of sub-Saharan African ancestry.

CKD usually leads to a progressive decline in kidney function even if the inciting cause can be identified and treated or removed. Destruction of nephrons leads to compensatory hypertrophy and supranormal GFR of the remaining nephrons in order to maintain overall homeostasis. As a result, the serum creatinine may remain relatively normal even in the face of significant loss of renal mass and is, therefore, an insensitive marker for early renal damage and scarring. In addition, compensatory hyperfiltration leads to overwork injury in the remaining nephrons, which in turn causes progressive glomerular sclerosis and interstitial fibrosis. ARBs, ACE inhibitors, and SGLT2 inhibitors help reduce hyperfiltration injury may slow the progression of proteinuric CKD.

CKD is an independent risk factor for CVD, however proteinuric CKD confers the highest risk. Many patients with stage 3 CKD die of underlying CVD prior to progression to ESKD.

Clinical Findings

A. Symptoms and Signs

Stages 1–4 CKD are asymptomatic. Symptoms develop slowly with the progressive decline in GFR, are

Table 22–5. Causes of CKD.

Glomerular Diseases
Primary glomerular diseases
Focal segmental glomerulosclerosis
Membranoproliferative glomerulonephritis
IgA nephropathy
Membranous nephropathy
Alport syndrome (hereditary nephritis)
Secondary glomerular diseases
Diabetic nephropathy
Renal amyloidosis
Postinfectious glomerulonephritis
HIV-associated nephropathy
Collagen-vascular diseases (eg, SLE)
HCV-associated membranoproliferative glomerulonephritis
Tubulointerstitial Nephritis
Drug hypersensitivity
Heavy metals
Analgesic nephropathy
Reflux/chronic pyelonephritis
Sickle cell nephropathy
Idiopathic
Cystic Diseases
Polycystic kidney disease
Medullary cystic disease
Obstructive Nephropathies
Prostatic disease
Nephrolithiasis
Retroperitoneal fibrosis/tumor
Congenital/reflux
Vascular Diseases
Hypertensive nephrosclerosis
Renal artery stenosis

HCV, hepatitis C virus.

nonspecific, and do not manifest until kidney disease is far advanced (GFR less than 5–10 mL/minute/1.73 m^2). At this point, the accumulation of metabolic waste products, or uremic toxins, results in the **uremic syndrome**. General symptoms of uremia may include fatigue, anorexia, nausea, and a metallic taste in the mouth. Neurologic symptoms such as memory impairment, insomnia, restless legs, and twitching may be due to uremia. Generalized pruritus (without rash) may occur, as may decreased libido and menstrual irregularities. Pericarditis, a rare complication of CKD, may present with pleuritic chest pain. Medications that are cleared by the kidneys will accumulate as kidney function worsens and toxicity may ensue; an important example is insulin and an increasing risk of significant hypoglycemia if doses are not appropriately reduced.

The most common physical finding in CKD is hypertension; this is due in part to impaired sodium excretion. It is often present in early stages of CKD and tends to worsen with CKD progression. In later stages of CKD, sodium retention may lead to clinically apparent volume overload. With a profound decrease in GFR (less than 5–10 mL/minute/1.73 m^2) signs of uremia are seen, including a generally sallow and ill appearance, halitosis (uremic fetor), and encephalopathic signs of decreased mental status, asterixis, myoclonus, and possibly seizures.

Symptoms and signs of uremia warrant immediate hospital admission and nephrology consultation for initiation of dialysis. The uremic syndrome is ameliorated with dialytic therapy.

In any patient with kidney disease, it is important to identify and correct all possibly reversible insults or exacerbating factors (Table 22–6). Urinary obstruction, hypovolemia, hypotension, nephrotoxins (such as NSAIDs, aminoglycosides, or PPIs), severe or emergent hypertension, and heart failure exacerbation should be excluded.

B. Laboratory Findings

CKD is usually defined by an abnormal GFR persisting for at least 3 months. Persistent proteinuria or abnormalities on renal imaging (eg, polycystic kidneys or a single kidney) are also diagnostic of CKD, even when eGFR is normal. Multiple measurements of eGFR over time demonstrate rates of progression. Although rates of progression can be variable (eg, a smooth linear slope, or stair-stepping pattern), any acute decline in eGFR should prompt an evaluation for potentially reversible renal insults. Anemia, hyperphosphatemia, hypocalcemia, hyperkalemia, and metabolic acidosis are common complications of advanced CKD. The urinary sediment may show broad waxy casts as a result of dilated, hypertrophic nephrons. If proteinuria is present, it should be quantified as described above. This can help narrow the differential diagnosis of the etiology of the CKD (Table 22–5); for example, glomerular diseases tend to present with protein excretion of more than 1 g/day. Additionally, higher urinary protein excretion is associated with more rapid progression of CKD and increased risk of cardiovascular mortality.

C. Imaging

The finding of small, echogenic kidneys bilaterally (less than 9–10 cm) by ultrasonography suggests the chronic scarring of advanced CKD. Large kidneys can be seen with adult polycystic kidney disease, diabetic nephropathy, HIV-associated nephropathy, plasma cell myeloma, amyloidosis, and obstructive uropathy.

Inker LA et al. Measurement and estimation of GFR for use in clinical practice: Core Curriculum 2021. Am J Kidney Dis. 2021;78:736. [PMID: 34518032]

Complications

The complications of CKD tend to occur at relatively predictable stages of disease as noted in Figure 22–1.

A. Cardiovascular Complications

Patients with CKD experience greater morbidity and mortality from CVD in comparison to the general population. Roughly 80% of patients with CKD die before reaching ESKD, primarily of CVD. Of those undergoing dialysis, 45% will die of a cardiovascular cause. The mechanisms for enhanced cardiovascular mortality in CKD are complex and include abnormal phosphorus and calcium homeostasis, increased burden of oxidative stress and inflammation, increased vascular reactivity, LVH, and coexistent conditions such as hypertension and diabetes mellitus.

1. Hypertension—Hypertension is the most common complication of CKD; it tends to be progressive and salt-sensitive. Hyperreninemic states and exogenous erythropoietin administration can exacerbate hypertension.

As with other patient populations, control of hypertension should focus on both pharmacologic and nonpharmacologic therapy (eg, diet, exercise, weight loss, treatment of obstructive sleep apnea). CKD results in disturbed sodium homeostasis such that the ability of the kidney to adjust to variations in sodium and water intake becomes limited as GFR declines. A low-salt diet (2 g/day) is often essential to control blood pressure and help avoid overt volume overload. Diuretics are nearly always needed to help control

Table 22–6. Reversible causes of kidney injury.

Reversible Factors	Diagnostic Clues
Obstruction	Post-void residual, bladder catheterization, renal ultrasound
Extracellular fluid volume depletion or significant hypotension relative to baseline	Blood pressure and pulse, including orthostatic pulse
Hypercalcemia	Serum electrolytes, calcium, phosphate
Nephrotoxic agents	Drug history
Severe/urgent hypertension	Blood pressure, chest radiograph
Heart failure exacerbation	Physical examination, chest radiograph

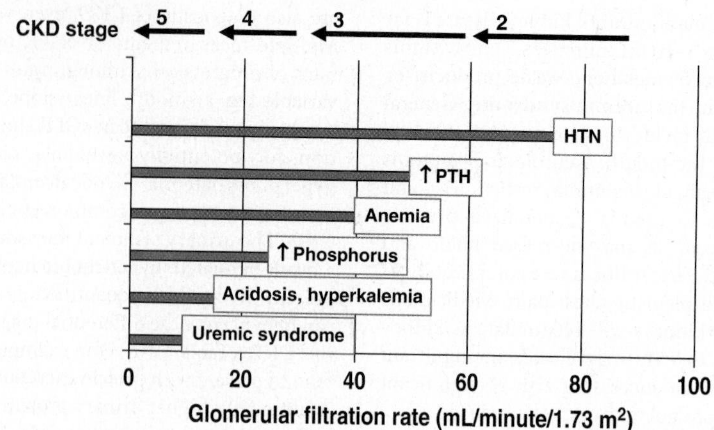

▲ **Figure 22–1.** Complications of CKD by stage and GFR. Complications arising from CKD tend to occur at the stages depicted, although there is considerable variability noted in clinical practice. HTN, hypertension; PTH, parathyroid hormone. (Reproduced with permission from William Bennett, MD.)

hypertension (see Table 11–8). Thiazides work well in earlier CKD, but loop diuretics may be more effective in those with a GFR less than 30 mL/minute/1.73 m^2. Addition of an SGLT2 inhibitor can promote further diuresis and may require down-titration of the baseline diuretic regimen to prevent volume contraction. Likewise decreases in dietary sodium intake may result in hypovolemia and AKI unless diuretic doses are reduced. Initial drug therapy for proteinuric patients should include ACE inhibitors or ARBs (see Table 11–6). For nonproteinuric CKD these drugs have not shown evidence of superiority over other drug classes. When these agents are initiated or their dose increased, serum creatinine and potassium must be checked within 7–14 days. A rise in serum creatinine greater than 30% from baseline mandates drug dose reduction or cessation. Hyperkalemia also may warrant drug cessation, except in patients who can reliably follow a low-potassium diet, adhere to a potassium-binding resin and be monitored closely. An ACE inhibitor and ARB should not be used in combination. CKD is a common cause of refractory hypertension for which agents from multiple classes are often needed. Current guidelines differ with respect to blood pressure goals in CKD; those from the Joint National Commission suggest a goal of less than 140/90 mm Hg, while the American Heart Association and other international bodies suggest less than 130/80 mm Hg. Patients with CKD are at risk for renal hypoperfusion and AKI with overtreatment of hypertension; it is prudent, therefore, to individualize the approach to blood pressure control for each patient.

2. CAD—Patients with CKD are at higher risk for death from CVD than the general population. Traditional modifiable risk factors for CVD, such as hypertension, tobacco use, and hyperlipidemia, should be aggressively treated. Uremic vascular calcification involving disordered phosphorus homeostasis and other mediators may also be a cardiovascular risk factor.

3. Heart failure—CKD complications result in increased cardiac workload due to hypertension, volume overload, and anemia. Patients may also have accelerated rates of atherosclerosis and vascular calcification resulting in vessel stiffness. These factors contribute to LVH and heart failure with preserved EF, which is common in CKD. Over time, heart failure with decreased EF may develop. Diuretic therapy, in addition to fluid and salt restriction, is usually necessary; diuretic dose escalation may be needed as kidney function declines. ACE inhibitors and ARBs can be used for patients with advanced CKD with close monitoring of blood pressure as well as for hyperkalemia and worsening kidney function; mineralocorticoid receptor antagonists may be used with similar precautions, especially when eGFR is less than 30 mL/minute/1.73 m^2. SGLT2 inhibitors improve outcomes for both heart failure and CKD.

4. Atrial fibrillation—Patients with advanced CKD and ESKD suffer increased rates of atrial fibrillation, which approach 20% in patients receiving dialysis. Those with CKD stages 1 to 4 should be treated as the general population, however anticoagulation for prevention of thromboembolic events is challenging due to competing risks of bleeding and clotting as well as a lack of data supporting its routine use. DOACs may be safer and more effective than vitamin K antagonists for thromboembolic prophylaxis for non-valvular atrial fibrillation.

5. Pericarditis—Pericarditis rarely develops in uremic patients; typical findings include pleuritic chest pain and a friction rub. Because cardiac tamponade can occur with uremic pericarditis, hospitalization and initiation of hemodialysis are mandatory.

Fay KS et al. Resistant hypertension in people with CKD: a review. Am J Kidney Dis. 2021;77:110. [PMID: 32712185]

Gómez-Fernández P et al. Oral anticoagulation in chronic kidney disease with atrial fibrillation. Nefrologia (Engl Ed). 2021;41:137. [PMID: 33308848]

Jankowski J et al. Cardiovascular disease in chronic kidney disease: pathophysiologic insights and therapeutic options. Circulation. 2021;143:1157. [PMID: 33720773]

Ott C et al. Diagnosis and treatment of arterial hypertension 2021. Kidney Int. 2022;101:36. [PMID: 34757122]

Packer M et al; EMPEROR-Reduced Trial Investigators. Cardiovascular and renal outcomes with empagliflozin in heart failure. N Engl J Med. 2020;383:1413. [PMID: 32865377]

Tantisattamo E et al. Reconciling systolic blood pressure intervention trial with Eighth Joint National Commission: a nuanced view of optimal hypertension control in the chronic kidney disease population. Curr Opin Nephrol Hypertens. 2022;31:57. [PMID: 34750334]

B. Metabolic Bone Disease

The metabolic bone disease of CKD refers to the complex disturbances of calcium and phosphorus metabolism, parathyroid hormone (PTH), active vitamin D, and fibroblast growth factor-23 (FGF-23) homeostasis (see Chapter 21 and Figure 22–2). A typical pattern seen as early as CKD stage 3 is relative hyperphosphatemia and hypocalcemia, and hypovitaminosis D, resulting in secondary hyperparathyroidism. These abnormalities can contribute to vascular calcification and may be responsible in part for the accelerated CVD and excess mortality seen in the CKD population. Epidemiologic studies show an association between elevated phosphorus levels and increased risk of cardiovascular mortality in early CKD through ESKD. As yet, there are no intervention trials suggesting the best course of treatment in these patients; control of mineral and PTH levels per current guidelines is discussed below.

Bone disease, or renal osteodystrophy, in advanced CKD is common and there are several types of lesions. Renal osteodystrophy can be diagnosed only by bone biopsy, which is rarely done. The most common bone disease, osteitis fibrosa cystica, is a result of secondary hyperparathyroidism and the osteoclast-stimulating effects of PTH. This is a high-turnover disease with bone resorption and subperiosteal lesions; it can result in bone pain and proximal muscle weakness. Adynamic bone disease, or low bone turnover, is becoming more common; it may result iatrogenically from suppression of PTH or via spontaneously low PTH production. Osteomalacia is characterized by lack of bone mineralization. In the past, osteomalacia was associated with aluminum toxicity—either as a result of chronic ingestion of prescribed aluminum-containing phosphorus binders or from high levels of aluminum in impure dialysate water. Currently, osteomalacia is more likely to result from hypovitaminosis D; there is also theoretical risk of osteomalacia associated with use of bisphosphonates in advanced CKD.

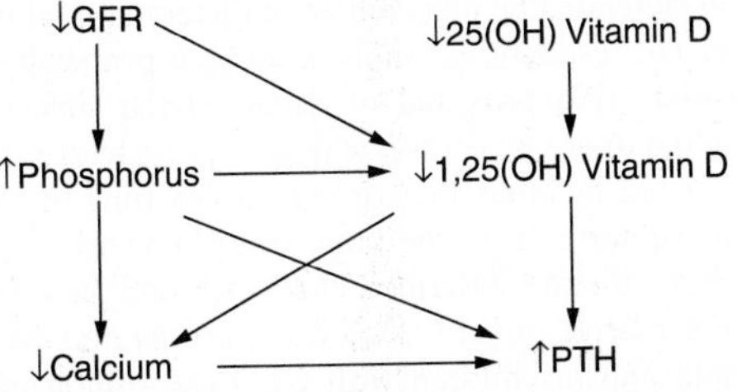

▲ **Figure 22–2.** Mineral abnormalities of CKD. Decline in GFR and loss of renal mass lead directly to increased serum phosphorus and hypovitaminosis D. Both of these abnormalities result in hypocalcemia and hyperparathyroidism. Many CKD patients also have nutritional 25(OH) vitamin D deficiency. PTH, parathyroid hormone.

All of the above entities increase the risk of fractures. Treatment may involve correction of calcium, phosphorus, and 25-OH vitamin D levels toward normal values, and mitigation of hyperparathyroidism. Understanding the interplay between these abnormalities can help target therapy (Figure 22–2). Declining GFR leads to phosphorus retention. This results in hypocalcemia as phosphorus complexes with calcium, deposits in soft tissues, and stimulates PTH. Loss of renal mass and low 25-OH vitamin D levels often seen in CKD patients result in low 1,25(OH) vitamin D production by the kidney. Because 1,25(OH) vitamin D is a suppressor of PTH production, hypovitaminosis D also leads to secondary hyperparathyroidism.

The first step in treatment of metabolic bone disease is control of hyperphosphatemia. This involves dietary phosphorus restriction initially (see section on dietary management), followed by the administration of oral phosphorus binders if targets are not achieved. Oral phosphorus binders block absorption of dietary phosphorus in the gut and are thus given with meals. These should be titrated to maintain a near-normal serum phosphorus level. Calcium-containing binders (calcium carbonate, 650 mg/tablet, or calcium acetate, 667 mg/capsule, used at doses of one to three pills per meal) are relatively inexpensive but may contribute to positive calcium balance and vascular calcification; overt hypercalcemia may also occur. Current guidelines suggest limiting their use in favor of the non–calcium-containing binders sevelamer carbonate (800–3200 mg/meal) and lanthanum carbonate (500–1000 mg/meal). Iron-based phosphorus binders, including ferric citrate and sucroferric oxyhydroxide, may be considered when other binders are not tolerated either due to hypercalcemia or constipation. They should be avoided in patients with iron overload. Aluminum hydroxide is a highly effective phosphorus binder but can cause osteomalacia and neurologic complications when used long-term; it can be used in the acute setting for severe hyperphosphatemia or for short periods (eg, 3 weeks) in CKD patients.

Once serum phosphorus levels are controlled, and 25-OH vitamin D stores are replete(d), active vitamin D (1,25[OH] vitamin D, or calcitriol) or other vitamin D analogs are used to treat secondary hyperparathyroidism in advanced CKD and ESKD. Monitoring for calcitriol-induced hypercalcemia and hyperphosphatemia is important; therapy should be dose-reduced or discontinued if either occur. Typical calcitriol dosing is 0.25 or 0.5 mcg orally daily or every other day. Cinacalcet targets the calcium-sensing receptors of the parathyroid gland and suppresses PTH production. Cinacalcet, 30–90 mg orally once a day, can be used if elevated serum phosphorus or calcium levels prohibit the use of vitamin D analogs; because it can cause serious hypocalcemia, close monitoring is required. Optimal PTH levels in CKD are not known, but because skeletal resistance to PTH develops with uremia, relatively high levels are targeted in advanced CKD to avoid adynamic bone disease. Expert guidelines suggest goal PTH levels near or just above the upper limit of normal for moderate CKD, and twofold to ninefold the upper limit of normal for ESKD.

Evenepoel P et al. European Consensus Statement on the diagnosis and management of osteoporosis in chronic kidney disease stages G4-G5D. Nephrol Dial Transplant. 2021;36:42. [PMID: 33098421]

Scialla JJ et al. State-of-the-art management of hyperphosphatemia in patients with CKD: an NKF-KDOQI controversies perspective. Am J Kidney Dis. 2021;77:132. [PMID: 32771650]

C. Hematologic Complications

1. Anemia—The anemia of CKD is primarily due to decreased erythropoietin production but is often multifactorial. If often becomes clinically significant during stage 3 disease. The approach to a patient with CKD and anemia begins with ensuring that the bone marrow can respond to erythropoietin. Thus, thyroid function tests, serum vitamin B_{12} levels, and iron stores (ferritin and iron saturation) should be checked in the initial evaluation. CKD is also associated with high levels of hepcidin, which blocks GI iron absorption and mobilization of iron from body stores; this results in a functional iron deficiency or "anemia of chronic disease." In CKD, serum ferritin below 100–200 ng/mL or iron saturation less than 20% is suggestive of iron deficiency. Iron stores may be repleted with oral or parenteral iron; iron therapy usually is withheld if the serum ferritin is greater than 500–800 ng/mL, even if the iron saturation is less than 20%. Oral therapy with ferrous sulfate, gluconate, or fumarate, 325 mg once daily, is the initial therapy in pre-ESKD CKD; higher doses will result in increasing hepcidin levels. For those who do not respond due to poor GI absorption or lack of tolerance, intravenous iron (eg, iron sucrose or iron gluconate) may be necessary.

Erythropoiesis-stimulating agents (ESAs, eg, recombinant erythropoietin [epoetin alfa or beta] and darbepoetin) are used to treat the anemia of CKD if other treatable causes are excluded. Initiation of an ESA is usually considered when hemoglobin (Hgb) values are less than 9 g/dL; there is little benefit of ESA at Hgb values above 9 g/dl. Typical ESA starting doses are epoetin alfa 50–100 U/kg once or twice a week; darbepoetin 0.45 mcg/kg every 2–4 weeks; and epoetin beta 60–100 mcg every 2–4 weeks. These agents can be given intravenously (eg, to the hemodialysis patient) or subcutaneously (to both the predialysis or dialysis patient); subcutaneous dosing of epoetin alfa is roughly 30% more effective than intravenous dosing. ESAs should be titrated to an Hgb of 10–11 g/dL for optimal safety; studies show that targeting a higher Hgb increases the risk of stroke and possibly other cardiovascular events. When titrating doses, Hgb levels should rise no more than 1 g/dL every 3–4 weeks. Other concerns regarding ESA use include possible exacerbation of HTN and acceleration of underlying malignancy growth.

2. Coagulopathy—Bleeding diathesis may occur in stage 4–5 CKD due to platelet dysfunction or severe anemia.

Treatment of bleeding diathesis is required only in patients who are symptomatic. Raising the Hgb to 9–10 g/dL can reduce risk of bleeding via improved clot formation. Desmopressin (25 mcg intravenously every 8–12 hours for two doses) is a short-lived but effective treatment for platelet dysfunction and it is often used in preparation for surgery or kidney biopsy; hyponatremia is a potential adverse effect of this treatment. Dialysis improves platelet function in uremic patients.

Babitt JL et al. Controversies in optimal anemia management: conclusions from a Kidney Disease: Improving Global Outcomes (KDIGO) conference. Kidney Int. 2021;99:1280. [PMID: 33839163]

Raichoudhury R et al. Treatment of anemia in difficult-to-manage patients with chronic kidney disease. Kidney Int Suppl (2011). 2021;11:26. [PMID: 33777493]

D. Hyperkalemia

Potassium balance generally remains intact in CKD until stages 4–5. However, hyperkalemia may occur at earlier stages when certain conditions are present, such as type 4 renal tubular acidosis (seen in patients with diabetes mellitus), high potassium diets, or medications that decrease renal potassium secretion (amiloride, triamterene, spironolactone, eplerenone, finerenone, NSAIDs, ACE inhibitors, ARBs) or block cellular potassium uptake (beta-blockers). Other causes include acidemic states and any type of cellular destruction causing release of intracellular contents, such as hemolysis and rhabdomyolysis.

Treatment of acute hyperkalemia is discussed in Chapter 21 (see Table 21–5). Cardiac monitoring is indicated for any ECG changes seen with hyperkalemia or a serum potassium level greater than 6.0–6.5 mEq/L or mmol/L. Chronic hyperkalemia is best treated with dietary potassium restriction (2 g/day) and minimization or elimination of any medications that may impair renal potassium excretion, as noted above. Loop diuretics may be administered for their kaliuretic effect as long as the patient is not volume-depleted, and oral potassium-binding resins may be considered.

Palmer BF et al. Clinical management of hyperkalemia. Mayo Clin Proc. 2021;96:744. [PMID: 33160639]

E. Acid-Base Disorders

Damaged kidneys are unable to excrete the 1 mEq/kg/day of acid generated by metabolism of dietary animal protein intake. The resultant metabolic acidosis is primarily due to decreased GFR; proximal or distal tubular defects may contribute to or worsen the acidosis. Excess hydrogen ions are buffered by bone; the consequent leaching of calcium and phosphorus from the bone contributes to the metabolic bone disease described above. Chronic acidosis can increase muscle protein catabolism, accelerate CKD progression, and in children with CKD can inhibit growth. Reduction of dietary animal protein, increase in fruit and vegetable intake, and the administration of oral sodium bicarbonate (in titrated doses of 0.5–1.0 mEq/kg/day divided twice daily) may bring serum bicarbonate levels toward normal. Citrate salts increase the absorption of dietary aluminum and should be avoided in CKD.

Hultin S et al. Recent evidence on the effect of treatment of metabolic acid on the progression of kidney disease. Curr Opin Nephrol Hypertens. 2021;30:467. [PMID: 34009141]

F. Neurologic Complications

Uremic encephalopathy, resulting from the aggregation of uremic toxins, does not occur until GFR falls below 5–10 mL/minute/1.73 m^2. Symptoms begin with difficulty in concentrating and can progress to lethargy, confusion, seizure, and coma. Physical findings may include altered mental status, weakness, and asterixis. These findings improve with dialysis.

Other neurologic complications of advanced CKD may include peripheral neuropathies (stocking-glove or isolated mononeuropathies), erectile dysfunction, autonomic dysfunction, and restless leg syndrome. These may not improve with dialysis therapy.

G. Endocrine Disorders

Hypothyroidism is common in CKD. Men with advanced CKD may experience decreased libido and erectile dysfunction; women may have menstrual disturbances and anovulatory cycles. During pregnancy, a serum creatinine greater than 1.4 mg/dL is associated with more rapid CKD progression. However, poor outcomes of pregnancy are not increased in women with creatinine less than 1.4 mg/dL and fetal survival is not compromised unless CKD is advance.

Treatment

A. Slowing Progression

Treatment of the underlying cause of CKD is vital. Control of diabetes should be aggressive in early CKD; but in advanced CKD the glycemic targets may need to be relaxed due to increased risk of hypoglycemia. Blood pressure control is vital to slow progression of all forms of CKD. In proteinuric patients, agents that block the renin-angiotensin-aldosterone system are important; mineralocorticoid receptor blockade can also be considered in earlier stages of proteinuric CKD. SGLT2 inhibitor can slow CKD progression; even in those without diabetes, an initial eGFR decline is seen several weeks after initiation and should be followed by stabilization. Management of traditional cardiovascular risk factors is vital. Risks for AKI should be minimized or avoided, including long-term use of NSAIDs and avoidance of PPIs, when possible. Treatment of metabolic acidosis may be helpful.

Chen TK et al. Reducing kidney function decline in patients with CKD: Core Curriculum 2021. Am J Kidney Dis. 2021;77:969. [PMID: 33892998]

Heerspink HJL et al; DAPA-CKD Trial Committees and Investigators. Dapagliflozin in patients with chronic kidney disease. N Engl J Med. 2020;383:1436. [PMID: 32970396]

Kelly JT et al. Lifestyle interventions for preventing and ameliorating CKD in primary and secondary care. Curr Opin Nephrol Hypertens. 2021;30:538. [PMID: 34602599]

B. Dietary Management

Patients with CKD should be evaluated by a renal nutritionist. Patient-specific recommendations should be made concerning protein, salt, water, potassium, and phosphorus intake to help manage CKD progression and complications.

1. Protein restriction—There is increasing interest in plant-based diets for the treatment of CKD. Reduced intake of animal protein to 0.6–0.8 g/kg/day may slow CKD progression. However, significant protein restriction is not advisable in those with cachexia or low serum albumin in the absence of the nephrotic syndrome.

2. Salt and water restriction—In advanced CKD, the kidney is unable to adapt to large changes in sodium intake. Intake of greater than 3–4 g/day can lead to hypertension and hypervolemia, whereas intake of less than 1 g/day can lead to volume depletion and hypotension. A goal of 2 g/day of sodium is reasonable for most patients. Daily fluid restriction to 2 L may be needed if volume overload is present.

3. Potassium restriction—Restriction is needed once the GFR has fallen below 10–20 mL/minute/1.73 m^2, or earlier if the patient is hyperkalemic. Patients should receive detailed lists describing potassium content of foods and should limit their intake to less than 50–60 mEq/day (2 g/day). An aggressive bowel regimen should be instituted for patients with hyperkalemia (more than two bowel movements daily), since a higher percentage of potassium is excreted through the GI tract as GFR declines. Potassium-binding resins may be used (see section on Hyperkalemia).

4. Phosphorus restriction—Guidelines suggest lowering elevated serum phosphorus levels toward normal in all stages of CKD. Dietary phosphate restriction to 800–1000 mg/day is the first step. Processed foods and cola beverages are often preserved with highly bioavailable phosphorus and should be avoided. Foods rich in phosphorus such as eggs, dairy products, nuts, beans, and meat may also need to be limited, although care must be taken to avoid protein malnutrition. When GFR is less than 20–30 mL/minute/1.73 m^2, dietary restriction is rarely sufficient to reach target levels, and phosphorus binders are usually required (see section on Metabolic Bone Disease).

Joshi S et al. Plant-based diets for kidney disease: a guide for clinicians. Am J Kidney Dis. 2021;77:287. [PMID: 33075387]

MacLaughlin HL et al. Nutrition in kidney disease: Core Curriculum 2022. Am J Kidney Dis. 2022;79:437. [PMID: 34862042]

McMahon EJ et al. Altered dietary salt intake for people with chronic kidney disease. Cochrane Database Syst Rev. 2021; 6:CD010070. [PMID: 34164803]

C. Medication Management

Many drugs are excreted by the kidney; dosages should be adjusted for GFR. Decreased renal elimination of insulin in advanced CKD confers risk for hypoglycemia in treated diabetic patients. Doses of oral hypoglycemics and insulin may need reduction. The risk of lactic acidosis with metformin is due to both dose and eGFR; it should be discontinued when eGFR is less than 30 mL/minute/1.73 m^2.

Magnesium-containing medications, such as laxatives or antacids, and phosphorus-containing medicines (eg, cathartics) should be avoided. Active morphine metabolites can accumulate in advanced CKD; this problem is not encountered with other opioid agents. Drugs with potential nephrotoxicity (NSAIDs, intravenous contrast, as well as others noted in the Acute Kidney Injury section) should be avoided. PPIs should be used only when medically necessary.

Vondracek SF et al. Principles of kidney pharmacotherapy for the nephrologist: Core Curriculum 2021. Am J Kidney Dis. 2021;78:442. [PMID: 34275659]

D. Treatment of ESKD

When GFR declines to 5–10 mL/minute/1.73 m^2, renal replacement therapy (hemodialysis, peritoneal dialysis, or kidney transplantation) is required to sustain life. Patient education is important in understanding which mode of therapy is most suitable, as is timely preparation for treatment. Referral to a nephrologist has been shown to improve mortality and should take place in late stage 3 CKD or when the GFR is declining rapidly. Preparation for ESKD treatment requires a team approach with the involvement of dieticians, social workers, primary care clinicians, and nephrologists. For much older patients, or those with multiple debilitating or life-limiting comorbidities, dialysis therapy may not meaningfully prolong life, and the option of palliative care should be discussed with the patient and family. Conversely, for patients who are otherwise relatively healthy, evaluation for possible kidney transplantation should be considered prior to initiation of dialysis.

1. Dialysis—Dialysis initiation should be considered when GFR is near 10 mL/minute/1.73 m^2 and uremic symptoms are present. Other indications for dialysis, which may occur when GFR is 10–15 mL/minute/1.73 m^2, are fluid overload unresponsive to diuresis and refractory hyperkalemia.

A. HEMODIALYSIS—Vascular access for hemodialysis can be accomplished by an arteriovenous fistula (the preferred method) or prosthetic graft; creation of dialysis access should be considered well before dialysis initiation. An indwelling catheter is used when there is no useable vascular access. Because catheters confer a high risk of bloodstream infection, they should be considered a temporary measure. Native fistulas typically last longer than prosthetic grafts but require a longer time after surgical construction for maturation (6–8 weeks for a fistula versus 2 weeks for a graft). Infection, thrombosis, and aneurysm formation are complications seen more often in grafts than fistulas. *Staphylococcus* species are the most common cause of soft tissue infections and bacteremia.

Treatment at a hemodialysis center typically occurs three times a week. Sessions last 3–5 hours, depending on patient size and type of dialysis access. Home hemodialysis is often performed more frequently (3–6 days per week for shorter sessions) and requires a trained helper. Results of trials comparing quotidian modalities (nocturnal and frequent home hemodialysis) to conventional in-center dialysis have not thus far shown significant mortality differences, but there may be improvements in blood pressure control, mineral metabolism, and quality of life.

B. PERITONEAL DIALYSIS—With peritoneal dialysis, the peritoneal membrane is the "dialyzer."

There are different kinds of peritoneal dialysis: continuous ambulatory peritoneal dialysis (CAPD), in which the patient exchanges the dialysate four to six times a day manually; and continuous cyclic peritoneal dialysis (CCPD), which utilizes a cycler machine to automatically perform exchanges at night.

The most common complication of peritoneal dialysis is peritonitis. Peritonitis may present with nausea and vomiting, abdominal pain, diarrhea or constipation, and fever. The normally clear dialysate becomes cloudy; and a diagnostic peritoneal fluid cell count greater than 100 WBC/mcL (0.1×10^9/L) with a differential of greater than 50% polymorphonuclear neutrophils is present. *Staphylococcus aureus* is the most common infecting organism, but streptococci and gram-negative species may also be causative. Empiric intraperitoneal administration of either vancomycin or a first-generation cephalosporin (cefazolin) plus a third-generation cephalosporin (ceftazidime) should be instituted with the first signs of peritonitis and subsequently tailored based on culture results.

2. Kidney transplantation—Many patients with ESKD are otherwise healthy enough to be suitable for transplantation, although standard criteria for recipient selection are lacking between transplant centers. Two-thirds of kidney allografts come from deceased donors, with the remainder from living related or unrelated donors. Over 100,000 patients are on the waiting list for a deceased donor transplant in the United States; the average wait is 3–7 years, depending on geographic location and recipient blood type.

3. Medical management of ESKD—As noted above, some patients are not candidates for kidney transplantation and may not benefit from dialysis. Frail older adults may die soon after dialysis initiation; those who do not may nonetheless rapidly lose functional status in the first year of treatment. The decision to initiate dialysis in patients with limited life expectancy should be weighed against possible deterioration in quality of life. For patients with ESKD who elect not to undergo dialysis or who withdraw from dialysis, progressive uremia with gradual suppression of sensorium results in a painless death within days to months. Involvement of a palliative care team is essential.

Gelfand S et al. Kidney supportive care: core curriculum 2020. Am J Kidney Dis. 2020;75:793. [PMID: 32173108]

Hariharan S et al. Long-term survival after kidney transplantation. N Engl J Med. 2021;385:729. [PMID: 34407344]

Teitelbaum I. Peritoneal dialysis. N Engl J Med. 2021;385:1786. [PMID: 34731538]

Zarantonello D et al. Novel conservative management of chronic kidney disease via dialysis-free interventions. Curr Opin Nephrol Hypertens. 2021;30:97. [PMID: 33186220]

Prognosis in ESKD

Compared with kidney transplant recipients and age-matched controls, mortality is higher for patients undergoing dialysis. There is likely little difference in survival for well-matched peritoneal versus hemodialysis patients.

Patients undergoing dialysis have an average life expectancy of 3–5 years, but survival for as long as 25 years may be achieved depending on comorbidities. Overall 5-year survival is estimated at 40%. Survival rates on dialysis depend on the underlying disease process. Five-year Kaplan-Meier survival rates vary from 37% for patients with diabetes to 54% for patients with glomerulonephritis. The most common cause of death is cardiac disease (more than 50%). Other causes include infection, cerebrovascular disease, and malignancy.

When to Refer

- A patient with stage 3–5 CKD should be referred to a nephrologist for management in conjunction with the primary care provider.
- A patient with other forms of CKD such as those with proteinuria greater than 1 g/day or polycystic kidney disease should be referred to a nephrologist at earlier stages.

When to Admit

- Admission should be considered for decompensation of problems related to CKD, such as worsening of acid-base status, electrolyte abnormalities, and volume overload, that cannot be appropriately treated in the outpatient setting.
- Admission is appropriate when a patient needs to start dialysis and is not stable for its outpatient initiation.

Clark-Cutaia MN et al. Disparities in chronic kidney disease-the state of the evidence. Curr Opin Nephrol Hypertens. 2021;30:208. [PMID: 33464006]

Kalantar-Zadeh K et al. Chronic kidney disease. Lancet. 2021;398:786. [PMID: 34175022]

Shlipak MG et al. The case for early identification and intervention of chronic kidney disease: conclusions from a Kidney Disease: Improving Global Outcomes (KDIGO) controversies conference. Kidney Int. 2021;99:34. [PMID: 33127436]

Thurlow JS et al. Global Epidemiology of end-stage kidney disease and disparities in kidney replacement therapy. Am J Nephrol. 2021;52:98. [PMID: 33752206]

RENAL ARTERY STENOSIS

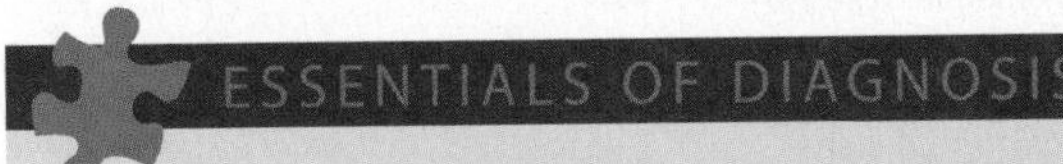

- Produced by atherosclerotic occlusive disease (80–90% of patients) or fibromuscular dysplasia (10–15%).
- Hypertension.
- AKI in patients starting ACE inhibitor therapy if stenosis is bilateral.

General Considerations

Approximately 5% of Americans with hypertension suffer from renal artery stenosis. Atherosclerotic ischemic renal disease accounts for most cases of renal artery stenosis. It typically occurs among persons over 45 years of age with additional risk factors such as CKD, diabetes mellitus, and tobacco use. Fibromuscular dysplasia is a less common cause of renal artery stenosis that most commonly occurs in young women.

Clinical Findings

A. Symptoms and Signs

Patients with atherosclerotic ischemic renal disease may have refractory hypertension, new-onset hypertension (in an older patient), pulmonary edema with poorly controlled blood pressure, and AKI upon starting an ACE inhibitor or ARB. Physical examination may reveal an audible abdominal bruit on the affected side. Unexplained hypertension in a woman younger than 40 years should raise suspicion for fibromuscular dysplasia.

B. Laboratory Findings

BUN and serum creatinine may be elevated if there is significant renal ischemia. Patients with bilateral renal artery stenosis may have hypokalemia, a finding that reflects activation of the renin-angiotensin-aldosterone system in response to reduced blood flow (a "prerenal" state).

C. Imaging

Abdominal ultrasound can reveal either asymmetric kidney size if one renal artery is primarily affected, or small hyperechoic kidneys if both are affected.

Screening with Doppler ultrasonography, CT angiography, or magnetic resonance angiography (MRA) is recommended if a corrective procedure would be performed when a positive test result is found. **Doppler ultrasonography** is highly sensitive and specific (85% and 92%, respectively) and relatively inexpensive but is extremely operator and patient dependent.

CT angiography consists of intravenous contrast injection with digital subtraction arteriography. The sensitivities from various studies range from 77% to 98%, with specificities of 90–94%.

MRA is an excellent but expensive way to screen for renal artery stenosis, particularly in those with atherosclerotic disease. Sensitivity is 77–100% and specificity ranges from 71% to 96%. The imaging agent for MRA (gadolinium) has been associated with nephrogenic systemic fibrosis, which is discussed elsewhere under Nephrogenic Systemic Fibrosis.

Renal angiography is the gold standard for diagnosis, but it is more invasive than the three screening tests discussed above. Thus, it is performed after a positive screening test. Lesions are most commonly found in the proximal third or ostial region of the renal artery. The risk of atheroembolic phenomena after angiography ranges from 5% to 10%. Fibromuscular dysplasia has a characteristic "beads-on-a-string" appearance on angiography.

Treatment

Treatment of atherosclerotic ischemic renal disease is controversial. Options include medical management, angioplasty with or without stenting, and surgical bypass. Two large randomized trials showed that vascular intervention is no better than optimal medical management in patients with renal artery stenosis, except in select circumstances (eg, patients with recurrent episodes of flash pulmonary edema). Angioplasty might reduce the number of antihypertensive medications but does not significantly change the progression of CKD. Stenting produces significantly better results than angioplasty. However, blood pressure and serum creatinine are similar at 6 months with medical management as with either angioplasty or stents.

Treatment of fibromuscular dysplasia with percutaneous transluminal angioplasty is often curative, which is in stark contrast to treatments for atherosclerotic disease.

Fay KS et al. Resistant hypertension in people with CKD: a review. Am J Kidney Dis. 2021;77:110. [PMID: 32712185]

Prince M et al. Renal revascularization in resistant hypertension. Prog Cardiovasc Dis. 2020;63:58. [PMID: 31821813]

Sharma S et al. Renovascular disease and mesenteric vascular disease. Cardiol Clin. 2021;39:527. [PMID: 34686265]

GLOMERULAR DISEASES

The glomerulus is a histologically complex structure consisting of the epithelial cells [podocytes], basement membrane, capillary endothelium, and mesangium. A variety of different insults can occur within these structures causing different patterns of injury. Examples of injuries that can affect any or all of the constituents of the glomerulus are (1) overwork injury, as in CKD; (2) an inflammatory process, such as SLE; (3) a podocyte protein mutation, as in hereditary focal segmental glomerulosclerosis (FSGS); or (4) a deposition disease, as in diabetes or amyloidosis. Different glomerular patterns of injury tend to cause different clinical syndromes or findings, which may help narrow the differential diagnosis; however, when a glomerular disease is suspected, a kidney biopsy may be needed to clarify the etiology.

Classification

Glomerular diseases can be classified in one of two clinical spectra—the nephritic spectrum and the nephrotic spectrum (Figure 22–3). Differentiating between a clinical presentation within the nephritic spectrum versus the nephrotic spectrum is important because it helps narrow the differential diagnosis of the underlying glomerular disease (Tables 22–7 and 22–8).

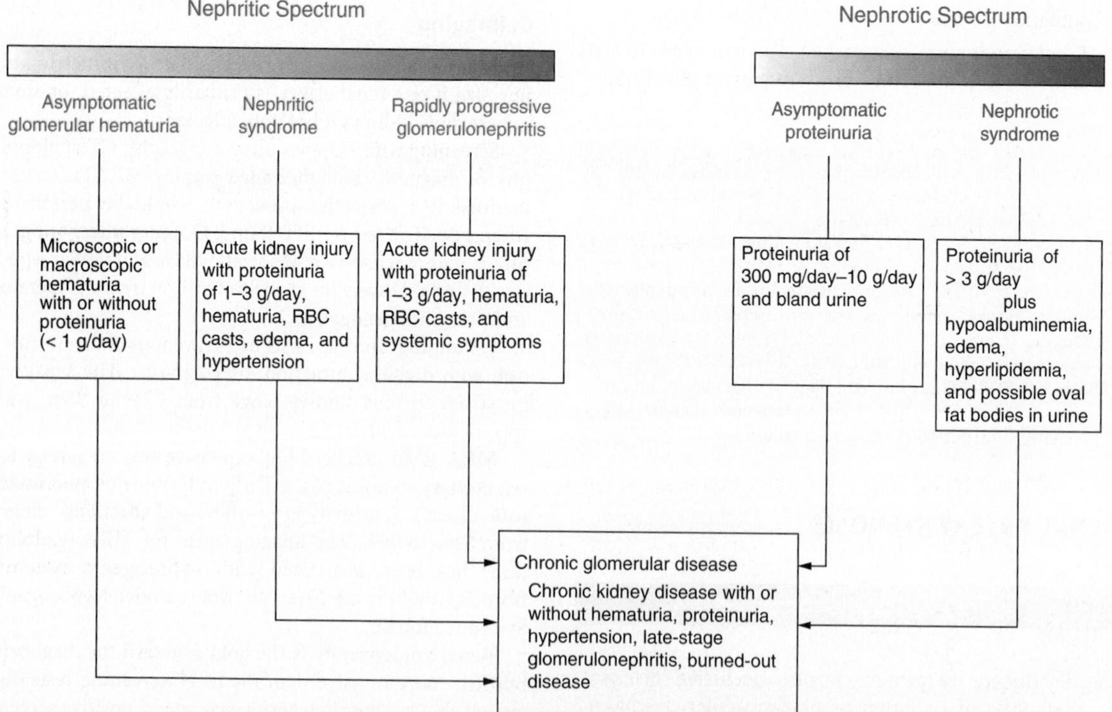

▲ **Figure 22–3.** Glomerular diseases present within one of the clinical spectra shown; the exact presentation is determined by the severity of the underlying disease and the pattern of injury. Nephritic diseases are characterized by the presence of an active urine sediment with glomerular hematuria and often with proteinuria. Nephrotic spectrum diseases are proteinuric with bland urine sediments (no cells or cellular casts). All glomerular diseases may progress to a chronic, scarred state. (Reproduced with permission from Megan Troxell, MD, PhD.)

Table 22–7. Classification and findings in glomerulonephritis: nephritic spectrum presentations.

	Typical Presentation	Association/Notes	Serology
Postinfectious glomerulonephritis	Children: abrupt onset of nephritic syndrome and AKI but can present anywhere in nephritic spectrum	Streptococci, other bacterial infections (eg, staphylococci, endocarditis, shunt infections)	Rising ASO titers, low complement levels
IgA nephropathy (Berger disease) and Henoch-Schönlein purpura, systemic IgA vasculitis	Classically: gross hematuria with respiratory tract infection, but can present anywhere in nephritic spectrum; Henoch-Schönlein purpura with vasculitic rash and GI hemorrhage	Abnormal IgA glycosylation in both primary (familial predisposition) and secondary disease (associated with cirrhosis, HIV, celiac disease) Henoch-Schönlein purpura in children after an inciting infection	No serologic tests helpful; complement levels are normal
Pauci-immune (granulomatosis with polyangiitis, eosinophilic granulomatosis with polyangiitis, polyarteritis, idiopathic crescentic glomerulonephritis)	Classically: crescentic or RPGN, but can present anywhere in nephritic spectrum; may have respiratory tract/sinus symptoms in granulomatosis with polyangiitis	See Figure 22–5	ANCAs: MPO or PR3 titers high; complement levels normal
Anti-GBM glomerulonephritis; Goodpasture syndrome	Classically: crescentic or RPGN, but can present anywhere in nephritic spectrum; pulmonary hemorrhage in Goodpasture syndrome	May develop as a result of respiratory irritant exposure (chemicals or tobacco use)	Anti-GBM antibody titers high; complement levels normal
Cryoglobulin-associated glomerulonephritis	Often acute nephritic syndrome; often with systemic vasculitis including rash and arthritis	Most commonly associated with chronic hepatitis C; may occur with other chronic infections or some connective tissue diseases	Cryoglobulins positive; rheumatoid factor may be elevated; complement levels low
MPGN	Classically: acute nephritic syndrome, but can also have nephrotic syndrome features	Most patients are < 30 years old Immune complex MPGN most common C3 glomerulonephritis	Low complement levels, may have findings of underlying infection or paraproteinemia
Hepatitis C infection	Anywhere in nephritic spectrum	Can cause MPGN pattern of injury or cryoglobulinemic glomerulonephritis; membranous nephropathy pattern of injury uncommon	Low complement levels; positive hepatitis C serology; rheumatoid factor may be elevated
SLE	Anywhere in nephritic spectrum, depending on pattern/severity of injury	Treatment depends on clinical course and International Society of Nephrology and Renal Pathology Society classification on biopsy	High ANA and anti-double-stranded DNA titers; low complement levels

ANA, antinuclear antibodies; ANCAs: antineutrophil cytoplasmic antibodies; ASO, antistreptolysin O; GBM, glomerular basement membrane; MPGN, membranoproliferative glomerulonephritis; MPO, myeloperoxidase; PR3, proteinase 3; RPGN, rapidly progressive glomerulonephritis.

At the "least severe" end of the **nephritic spectrum**, the findings of asymptomatic glomerular hematuria (ie, dysmorphic RBCs with or without some proteinuria [less than 1 g/day]) are characteristic. The mid-portion of the spectrum is the nephritic *syndrome*, which comprises glomerular hematuria, subnephrotic proteinuria (less than 3 g/day), edema, and elevated creatinine. The "most severe" and clinically urgent end of the spectrum are the rapidly progressive glomerulonephritides (RPGNs).

The **nephrotic spectrum** is comprised of diseases that present primarily with proteinuria of at least 0.5–1 g/day and a bland urine sediment (no cells or cellular casts). At the more severe end of the nephrotic spectrum is the nephrotic *syndrome*, consisting of nephrotic-range proteinuria (greater than 3 g/day), hypoalbuminemia, edema, hyperlipidemia, and urinary oval fat bodies.

Glomerular diseases can also be classified according to whether they cause renal abnormalities alone (primary renal disease) or whether the renal abnormalities result from a systemic disease (secondary renal disease).

Further evaluation prior to kidney biopsy may include serologic testing for systemic diseases that can result in glomerular damage (Figure 22–4).

Cavanaugh C et al. Urine sediment examination in the diagnosis and management of kidney disease: Core Curriculum 2019. Am J Kidney Dis. 2019;73:258. [PMID: 30249419]

Table 22–8. Classification and findings in glomerulonephritis: nephrotic spectrum presentations.

Disease	Typical Presentation	Association/Notes
Minimal change disease (nil disease; lipoid nephrosis)	Child with sudden onset of full nephrotic syndrome	Children: associated with allergy or viral infection Adults: associated with Hodgkin disease, NSAIDs
Membranous nephropathy	Anywhere in nephrotic spectrum, but nephrotic syndrome not uncommon; particular predisposition to hypercoagulable state	Primary (idiopathic) may be associated with antibodies to PLA_2R Secondary may be associated with non-Hodgkin lymphoma, carcinoma (GI, renal, bronchogenic, thyroid), gold therapy, penicillamine, SLE, chronic hepatitis B or C infection
Focal and segmental glomerulosclerosis	Anywhere in nephrotic spectrum; children with congenital disease have nephrotic syndrome	Children: congenital disease with podocyte gene mutation, or in spectrum of disease with minimal change disease Adults: associated with heroin abuse, HIV infection, reflux nephropathy, obesity, pamidronate, podocyte protein mutations, *APOL1* mutations
Amyloidosis	Anywhere in nephrotic spectrum	AL: plasma cell dyscrasia with Ig light chain overproduction and deposition; check SPEP/UPEP AA: serum amyloid protein A overproduction and deposition in response to chronic inflammatory disease (rheumatoid arthritis, IBD, chronic infection)
Diabetic nephropathy	High GFR (hyperfiltration) → microalbuminuria → frank proteinuria → decline in GFR	Diabetes diagnosis precedes diagnosis of nephropathy by years
HIV-associated nephropathy	Heavy proteinuria, often nephrotic syndrome, progresses to ESKD relatively quickly	Usually seen in antiviral treatment-naïve patients (rare in antiretroviral therapy era), predilection for those of sub-Saharan African descent (*APOL1* mutations)
Membranoproliferative glomerulonephropathy (MPGN)	Classically presents with acute nephritic syndrome, some may also exhibit nephrotic features	Immune complex MPGN are idiopathic or secondary to infections, paraproteinemia, or systemic autoimmune disease; C3 glomerulopathies are due to alternative complement pathway dysregulation

PLA_2R, phospholipase A_2 receptor; SPEP/UPEP, serum and urine protein electrophoresis.

Kant S et al. Advances in understanding of pathogenesis and treatment of immune-mediated kidney disease: a review. Am J Kidney Dis. 2022;79:582. [PMID: 34508831]

Rovin BH et al. Executive summary of the KDIGO 2021 Guideline for the Management of Glomerular Diseases. Kidney Int. 2021;100:753. [PMID: 34556300]

NEPHRITIC SPECTRUM GLOMERULAR DISEASES

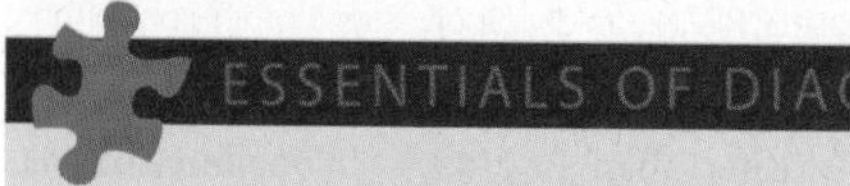

- **Asymptomatic glomerular hematuria**
  - –Hematuria with dysmorphic RBCs
  - –Proteinuria < 1 g/day
- **More severe cases: nephritic syndrome**
  - –Glomerular hematuria (and RBC casts if glomerular bleeding is heavy)
  - –Proteinuria of 1–3 g/day
  - –Hypertension
  - –Edema
  - –Rising creatinine over days to months
- **Most severe cases: rapidly progressive glomerulonephritis**
  - –AKI with rising creatinine over days to months
  - –Glomerular hematuria (and RBC casts)
  - –Proteinuria of 1–3 g/day
  - –Systemic symptoms
  - –Hypertension and edema uncommon

General Considerations

"Glomerulonephritis" is a term given to diseases in the nephritic spectrum and usually signifies an inflammatory process causing renal dysfunction. It may be acute (developing over days to weeks), with or without resolution, or may be chronic and indolent with progressive scarring. As noted above, diseases within the nephritic spectrum may present with glomerular hematuria and proteinuria, with nephritic syndrome, or with RPGN (Figure 22–3).

Clinical Findings

A. Symptoms and Signs

Nephritic syndrome usually leads to an acute decrease in GFR. The resultant sodium retention can lead to

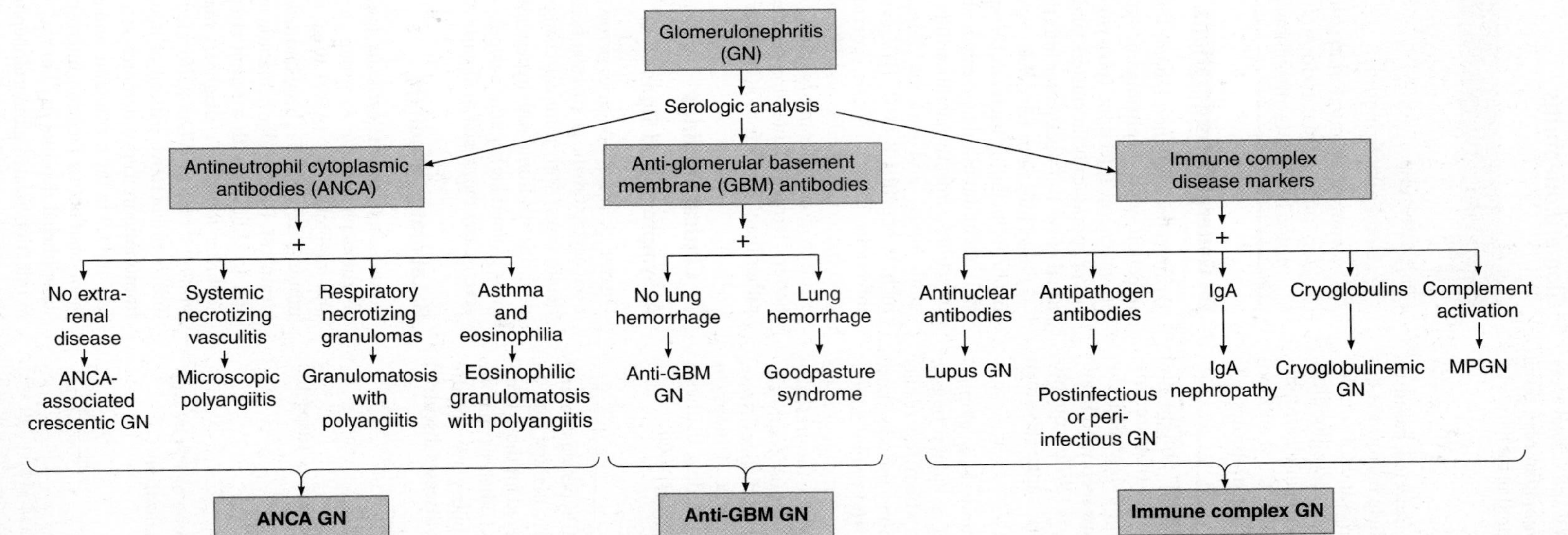

▲ **Figure 22–4. Serologic analysis of patients with glomerulonephritis. MPGN, membranoproliferative glomerulonephritis.** (Reproduced with permission from Greenberg A et al. *Primer on Kidney Diseases*. Academic Press, Elsevier, 1994, and Jennette JC, Falk RJ. Diagnosis and management of glomerulonephritis and vasculitis presenting as acute renal failure. *Med Clin North Am*. 1990;74(4):893–908.)

hypertension and edema, which is first seen in regions of low tissue pressure such as the periorbital and scrotal areas. Heavy bleeding from glomerular inflammation may result in gross hematuria (smoky or cola-colored urine).

B. Laboratory Findings

1. Serologic testing—Serologic tests (selected based on the history and physical examination) help narrow the differential diagnosis. These may include C3 and C4 complement levels, antinuclear antibodies, cryoglobulins, hepatitis serologies, serum and urine protein electrophoreses, serum free light chains, ANCAs, anti-GBM antibodies, and antipathogen antibodies (eg, antistreprolysin O titers) (Figure 22–4).

2. UA—The urine dipstick is positive for protein and blood. Urinary microscopy reveals RBCs that are misshapen or dysmorphic from traversing a damaged glomerular filtration barrier. RBC casts are seen with heavy glomerular bleeding and tubular stasis. When quantified, proteinuria is usually subnephrotic range (less than 3 g/day).

3. Biopsy—Definitive diagnosis of the underlying glomerular disease cannot be made without a kidney biopsy. Candidates for biopsy are patients for whom test results would influence management; exceptions include those with advanced underlying CKD, those who cannot adhere to medical therapy, those for whom immunosuppressive therapy is not appropriate, or those for whom the presentation is "classic" for a particular disease (eg, poststreptococcal glomerulonephritis, childhood minimal change disease, and diabetic nephropathy). The major risk of biopsy is bleeding. Contraindications include a bleeding diathesis, thrombocytopenia, and uncontrolled hypertension.

Treatment

General measures include treatment of hypertension and fluid overload, if present. Antiproteinuric therapy with an ACE inhibitor or ARB should be considered for those without AKI. For those with profound AKI, dialysis may be needed. The inflammatory glomerular injury may require immunosuppressive agents (see specific diseases discussed below).

When to Refer

Any patient in whom a glomerulonephritis is suspected should be referred to a nephrologist.

When to Admit

Any suspicion of acute nephritic syndrome or RPGN warrants consideration of immediate hospitalization.

Lamba P et al. Nephritic syndrome. Prim Care. 2020;47:615. [PMID: 33121632]

Medjeral-Thomas NR et al. Complement and kidney disease, new insights. Curr Opin Nephrol Hypertens. 2021;30:310. [PMID: 33767058]

1. Infection-Related & Postinfectious Glomerulonephritis

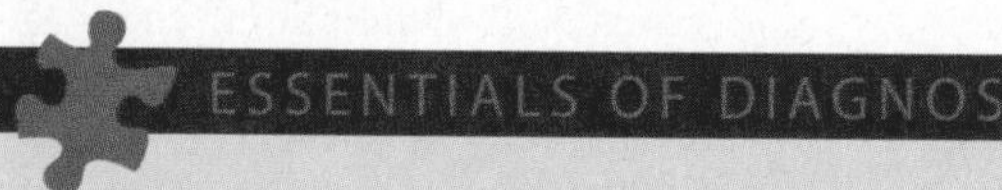

- Proteinuria.
- Glomerular hematuria.
- Symptoms occur during course of some infections (eg, pneumonia, endocarditis) or 1–3 weeks after some infections (often pharyngitis or impetigo).

General Considerations

Postinfectious glomerulonephritis is most often due to infection with nephritogenic group A beta-hemolytic streptococcal infections (pharyngitis or impetigo). It can occur sporadically, in clusters, and during epidemics, with usual onset 1–3 weeks after infection (average 7–10 days).

Other infections have been associated with glomerulonephritis including bacteremia (especially *S aureus*), bacterial pneumonias, deep-seated abscesses, gram-negative infections, infective endocarditis, and shunt infections; viral, fungal, and parasitic causes of glomerulonephritis include hepatitis B or C, HIV, cytomegalovirus infection, infectious mononucleosis, coccidioidomycosis, malaria, mycobacteria, syphilis, and toxoplasmosis. These entities result in glomerular injury during active infection, and are better termed "infection-related glomerulonephritis" rather than "postinfectious glomerulonephritis."

Clinical Findings

A. Symptoms and Signs

Disease presentation varies across the nephritic spectrum from asymptomatic glomerular hematuria (especially in epidemic cases) with minimal change in kidney function, to nephritic syndrome with hypertension, edema, and perhaps gross glomerular hematuria (smoky-colored urine); the most severe cases may result in oliguric AKI requiring dialysis.

B. Laboratory Findings

Serum complement levels are low. In postinfectious glomerulonephritis due to group A streptococcal infection, anti-streptolysin O (ASO) titers can be high unless the immune response has been blunted with previous antibiotic treatment. Glomerular hematuria and proteinuria are present. In children with a recent streptococcal infection and nephritic features, a diagnosis may be made empirically without a biopsy. When performed, kidney biopsy shows a diffuse proliferative pattern of injury on light microscopy. Immunofluorescence demonstrates granular deposition of IgG and C3 in the mesangium and along the capillary basement membrane. Electron microscopy shows large, dense subepithelial deposits or "humps." Kidney biopsy findings in infection-related glomerulonephritis are varied and may show overlap with immune complex membranoproliferative glomerulonephritis or C3 glomerulonephritis.

Treatment

Any active infection should be identified and treated appropriately; otherwise, treatment for postinfectious glomerulonephritis is supportive. Antihypertensives, salt restriction, and diuretics should be used if needed. Corticosteroids have not been shown to improve outcomes. Prognosis depends on the severity of the glomerular injury and age of the patient. Children are more likely to fully recover; adults are more prone to the development of severe disease (RPGN with crescent formation) and CKD.

Rodriguez-Iturbe B. Autoimmunity in acute poststreptococcal GN: a neglected aspect of the disease. J Am Soc Nephrol. 2021;32:534. [PMID: 33531351]

Satoskar AA et al. Epidemiology, pathogenesis, treatment and outcomes of infection-associated glomerulonephritis. Nat Rev Nephrol. 2020;16:32. [PMID: 31399725]

2. IgA Nephropathy

ESSENTIALS OF DIAGNOSIS

- Proteinuria: minimal to nephrotic-range.
- Glomerular hematuria: microscopic is common; macroscopic (gross) after infection.
- Positive IgA staining on kidney biopsy.

General Considerations

IgA nephropathy (Berger disease) results from glomerular mesangial deposition of immune complexes made up of aberrantly glycosylated IgA (a heritable condition) and IgG autoantibodies against these abnormal molecules. IgA nephropathy can be a primary (renal-limited) disease or secondary to hepatic cirrhosis, celiac disease, and infections such as HIV and cytomegalovirus.

IgA nephropathy is the most common primary glomerular disease worldwide, particularly in Asia. It is most often seen in children and young adults, with males affected two to three times more commonly than females.

Clinical Findings

The classic presentation of IgA nephropathy is an episode of gross hematuria associated with a mucosal viral infection, often of the upper respiratory tract. The urine becomes red or smoky-colored 1–2 days after illness onset—in contradistinction to the latent period seen in postinfectious glomerulonephritis. IgA nephropathy can present clinically anywhere along the nephritic spectrum from asymptomatic microscopic hematuria with minimal proteinuria and preserved eGFR to RPGN (Figure 22–3). Rarely, nephrotic syndrome can be present.

There are no serologic tests that aid in this diagnosis; serum complements are normal. The typical pattern of injury seen on kidney biopsy is a focal glomerulonephritis with mesangial proliferation; immunofluorescence demonstrates diffuse mesangial IgA and C3 deposits.

Treatment

The disease course of primary IgA nephropathy varies widely, and the treatment approach is tailored to the risk for progression. Patients with low risk for progression (no hypertension, normal GFR, minimal proteinuria) can be monitored annually. Patients at higher risk (proteinuria greater than 1.0 g/day, decreased GFR, or hypertension or any combination of these three conditions) should be treated with an ACE inhibitor or ARB. Therapy should be titrated to reduce proteinuria to less than 1 g/day and to control blood pressure in the range of 125/75 mm Hg to 130/80 mm Hg. SGLT2-inhibitors may be added to standard care in the well-selected patient. There are conflicting data regarding the efficacy of corticosteroids for reducing proteinuria and slowing progression; however, they may be considered for patients with GFR greater than 30 mL/minute/1.73 m^2 and persistent proteinuria greater than 1 g/day despite maximal ACE inhibitor or ARB. For the rare patient with IgA nephropathy and a rapidly progressive clinical course with crescent formation on biopsy, cyclophosphamide and corticosteroid therapy should be considered (see section on ANCA-associated vasculitis below). Kidney transplantation is an excellent option for patients with ESKD, but recurrent disease has been documented in 30% of patients 5–10 years posttransplant.

Prognosis

Approximately one-third of patients experience spontaneous clinical remission. Progression to ESKD occurs in 20–40% of patients. The most unfavorable prognostic indicator is proteinuria greater than 1 g/day; others include hypertension, reduced eGFR on presentation, and the biopsy findings of tubulointerstitial fibrosis and glomerulosclerosis.

Cambier A et al. New therapeutic perspectives for IgA nephropathy in children. Pediatr Nephrol. 2021;36:497. [PMID: 32040630]

Pattrapornpisut P et al. IgA nephropathy: Core Curriculum 2021. Am J Kidney Dis. 2021;78:429. [PMID: 34247883]

Rovin BH et al. Executive summary of the KDIGO 2021 Guideline for the Management of Glomerular Diseases. Kidney Int. 2021;100:753. [PMID: 34556300]

3. IgA Vasculitis (Henoch-Schönlein Purpura)

IgA vasculitis, or Henoch-Schönlein purpura, is a systemic small-vessel leukocytoclastic vasculitis associated with IgA subclass 1 deposition in vessel walls. It is most common in children and is often associated with an inciting infection or medication exposure. It classically presents with palpable purpura in the lower extremities and buttock area, arthralgias, abdominal symptoms (nausea, colic, and melena), and AKI with nephritic urine sediment. The renal pattern of injury is an IgA nephropathy. Most patients with microscopic hematuria and minimal proteinuria recover fully over several weeks. Progressive CKD and possibly ESKD are more likely to develop in adults and in those with both nephritic and nephrotic syndromes. Although several treatment regimens of various immunosuppressive agents have been clinically tested, none is proven to alter the course of severe nephritis. Rituximab treatment and plasma exchange have been successful for severe disease according to several case reports, but clinical trials are lacking. Rapidly progressive disease with crescent formation on biopsy may be treated as in ANCA-associated vasculitis (see section below). Further details about IgA vasculitis are provided in Chapter 20.

Hastings MC et al. IgA vasculitis with nephritis: update of pathogenesis with clinical implications. Pediatr Nephrol. 2022;37:719. [PMID: 33818625]

Maritati F et al. Adult-onset IgA vasculitis (Henoch-Schönlein): update on therapy. Presse Med. 2020;49:104035. [PMID: 32645417]

4. Pauci-Immune Glomerulonephritis (ANCA-Associated)

Pauci-immune necrotizing glomerulonephritis is caused by the following ANCA-associated vasculitides (AAVs): granulomatosis with polyangiitis, microscopic polyangiitis, and eosinophilic granulomatosis with polyangiitis (formerly Churg-Strauss disease; see Chapter 20). ANCA-associated glomerulonephritis can also present as a kidney-limited disease without systemic vasculitis. The pathogenesis of these entities appears to involve cytokine-primed neutrophils that present the cytoplasmic antigens proteinase 3 or myeloperoxidase on their surfaces. Circulating ANCAs bind to these antigens and activate a neutrophil respiratory burst with consequent vascular damage; primed neutrophils also appear to activate the alternative complement pathway. Immunofluorescence of kidney biopsy specimens demonstrates lack of immunoglobulin or complement deposition, hence the term "pauci-immune." Renal involvement classically presents as an RPGN, but more indolent presentations can be seen. Most cases of AAV are idiopathic, but others may be linked to an infection (including COVID-19), environmental exposure (silica), or to a drug (hydralazine or levamisole).

Clinical Findings

A. Symptoms and Signs

Symptoms of a systemic inflammatory disease, including fever, malaise, and weight loss, may be present, sometimes for months prior to diagnosis. In addition to the glomerular inflammatory signs of hematuria and proteinuria, vasculitic involvement of dermal capillaries and nerve arterioles may result in purpura and mononeuritis multiplex, respectively. Ninety percent of patients with granulomatosis with polyangiitis have upper (especially sinus) or lower respiratory tract symptoms with nodular lesions that can cavitate and bleed. Hemoptysis is a concerning sign for possible alveolar hemorrhage and usually warrants hospitalization and aggressive immunosuppression.

B. Laboratory Findings

Serologically, ANCA subtype analysis is done to determine whether antiproteinase-3 antibodies (PR3-ANCA) or antimyeloperoxidase antibodies (MPO-ANCA) are present. Most patients with granulomatosis with polyangiitis are PR3 positive; the remainder are MPO positive or, more rarely, do not demonstrate circulating ANCA. Microscopic angiitis is generally associated with MPO-ANCA. Renal biopsy demonstrates necrotizing lesions and crescents on light microscopy; immunofluorescence is negative for immune complex deposition.

Treatment

Treatment should be instituted early if aggressive disease is present. Induction therapy of high-dose corticosteroids (methylprednisolone, 1–2 g/day intravenously for 3 days, followed by prednisone, 1 mg/kg orally for 1 month, with a slow taper over the next 6 months) and cytotoxic agents (cyclophosphamide, 0.5–1 g/m^2 intravenously per month or 1.5–2 mg/kg orally for 3–6 months) is followed by long-term azathioprine or mycophenolate mofetil. Rituximab has been shown to be noninferior to cyclophosphamide for induction and is also used in refractory or relapsing cases and as an alternative to azathioprine for maintenance of remission. Plasma exchange is likely helpful in conjunction with induction therapy for cases complicated by pulmonary hemorrhage. In a 2021 randomized controlled trial of patients with AAV who were treated with either cyclophosphamide or rituximab, remission rates were similar (noninferior) with the oral complement inhibitor avacopan compared with oral glucocorticoids.

Prognosis

Without treatment, prognosis is extremely poor. With aggressive treatment, complete remission can be achieved in 75% of patients. Prognosis depends on the extent of renal involvement before treatment is started and may be worse in those with PR3-associated disease. ANCA titers may be monitored to follow treatment efficacy; rising titers may herald relapse.

Geetha D et al. ANCA-associated vasculitis: Core Curriculum 2020. Am J Kidney Dis. 2020;75:124. [PMID: 31358311]

Jayne DRW et al; ADVOCATE Study Group. Avacopan for the treatment of ANCA-associated vasculitis. N Engl J Med. 2021;384:599. [PMID: 33596356]

5. Anti-Glomerular Basement Membrane Glomerulonephritis & Goodpasture Syndrome

Autoantibodies to epitopes of the GBM cause a glomerulonephritis (anti-GBM disease); concomitant immune attack on alveolar basement membranes results in pulmonary hemorrhage as well (Goodpasture syndrome) (Figure 22–4). Anti-GBM–associated glomerulonephritis accounts for 10–20% of patients with acute RPGN. The incidence peaks in the third decade of life during which time males are predominantly affected and lung involvement is more common, and again in the sixth and seventh decades with less gender specificity and pulmonary involvement. Goodpasture syndrome has been associated with pulmonary infection, tobacco use, and exposure to hydrocarbon solvents or alemtuzumab; HLA-DR2 and -B7 antigens may predispose as well.

Clinical Findings

A. Symptoms and Signs

The onset of disease may be preceded by an upper respiratory tract infection; hemoptysis, dyspnea, and possible respiratory failure may ensue. Other findings are consistent with an RPGN, although rare cases may present with much milder forms of the nephritic spectrum of disease (eg, glomerular hematuria and proteinuria with minimal kidney dysfunction).

B. Laboratory Findings

Chest radiographs may demonstrate pulmonary infiltrates if pulmonary hemorrhage is present. Serum complement levels are normal. Circulating anti-GBM antibodies are present in over 90% of patients. A small percentage of patients have elevated ANCA titers; these patients should be treated with plasma exchange as for anti-GBM disease. Kidney biopsy typically shows crescent formation with light microscopy, with linear IgG staining along the GBM with immunofluorescence.

Treatment

Patients with pulmonary hemorrhage and strong clinical suspicion of Goodpasture syndrome should be treated emergently—possibly prior to confirming the diagnosis with serology and kidney biopsy. Treatment is a combination of plasma exchange therapy daily for up to 2 weeks to remove circulating antibodies, and administration of corticosteroids and cyclophosphamide to prevent formation of new antibodies and control the inflammatory response. Rituximab has been used in a small number of patients with refractory disease. Patients with oliguric AKI or who require dialysis upon presentation have a poor prognosis. Anti-GBM antibody titers should decrease as the clinical course improves.

Rovin BH et al. Executive summary of the KDIGO 2021 Guideline for the Management of Glomerular Diseases. Kidney Int. 2021;100:753. [PMID: 34556300]

6. Membranoproliferative Glomerulonephritis & C3 Glomerulopathies

MPGN is a relatively rare pattern of glomerular injury that can present anywhere along the nephritic spectrum from asymptomatic glomerular hematuria to acute nephritic syndrome with bouts of gross hematuria to RPGN; nephrotic syndrome can also be seen. MPGN is classified pathologically and mechanistically into immune complex– and C3-related disease. Etiologies of immune complex–mediated MPGN include chronic infection (most commonly HCV, but also bacterial and parasitic infections), a paraproteinemia, or an underlying autoimmune disease (such as lupus); it can also be idiopathic (especially in children and young adults). In these cases, the pathogenesis is likely a chronic antigenemia leading to classical complement pathway activation with immune complex deposition; however, some cases may result from alternative complement pathway dysregulation. C3 glomerulopathies are caused by several inherited or acquired abnormalities in the alternative complement pathway. Both types result in low circulating C3 complement; C4 is low in immune complex disease. Light microscopy of both types shows varying degrees of mesangial hypercellularity, endocapillary proliferation and capillary wall remodeling resulting in double contours of the GBM ("tram track" appearance). Immunofluorescence and electron microscopy provide distinguishing information. Immune complex–mediated MPGN reveals C3 and IgG or IgM staining (or both) on immunofluorescence; electron microscopy demonstrates mesangial and subepithelial deposits. C3 glomerulonephritis is distinguished by lack of immunoglobulin staining on immunofluorescence, but can appear similar to immune complex disease with respect to light and electron microscopy. An additional but rare type of C3 glomerular injury is "dense deposit disease" based on thick ribbon-like deposits seen on electron microscopy. Together, dense deposit disease and C3 glomerulonephritis are termed "C3 glomerulopathies."

Treatment of immune complex MPGN should be directed at any identifiable underlying cause; idiopathic immune complex disease treatment is controversial and controlled trial data are lacking. For those with mild disease, ACE inhibitors and ARBs should be used. For severe disease, a combination of oral cyclophosphamide or mycophenolate mofetil plus corticosteroids could be considered; rituximab is also sometimes used. Those with RPGN and crescents on biopsy may be treated the same as those with ANCA-associated disease provided secondary causes have been ruled out. Despite therapy, most will progress to ESKD. Treatment for the C3 glomerulopathies is in evolution as novel therapies to target the dysregulated alternative complement cascade are being explored; small, uncontrolled series suggest a possible benefit of eculizumab in some patients; others may respond to mycophenolate mofetil. Less favorable prognostic findings include dense deposit disease, early decline in GFR, hypertension, and persistent nephrotic syndrome. All types of MPGN recur with high frequency after kidney transplantation; however, dense deposit disease recurs more commonly. Plasma exchange, with or without eculizumab, has been used with mixed results to treat posttransplant recurrence of MPGN.

Caravaca-Fontán F et al. Update on C3 glomerulopathy: a complement-mediated disease. Nephron. 2020;144:272. [PMID: 32369815]

Noris M et al. Membranoproliferative glomerulonephritis: no longer the same disease and may need very different treatment. Nephrol Dial Transplant. 2021 Oct 1. [Epub ahead of print] [PMID: 34596686]

7. Cryoglobulin-Associated Glomerulonephritis

Essential (mixed) cryoglobulinemia is a vasculitis caused by cold-precipitable immunoglobulins (cryoglobulins). The most common underlying etiology is HCV infection; in these cases, there is clonal expansion of B lymphocytes, which produce IgM rheumatoid factor. Immune complexes form from rheumatoid factor, HCV antigen, and polyclonal anti-HCV IgG form deposit in vessels and incite inflammation. Other overt or occult infections (eg, viral, bacterial, and fungal) as well as some autoimmune diseases and lymphoproliferative disorders can cause cryoglobulinemic vasculitis.

Patients exhibit purpuric and necrotizing skin lesions in dependent areas, arthralgias, fever, and hepatosplenomegaly. Serum complement levels are low and rheumatoid factor is often elevated. Kidney biopsy may show several different patterns of injury; there may be crescent formation, glomerular capillary thrombi, or MPGN (see above). Treatment consists of aggressively targeting the causative infection. Pulse corticosteroids, plasma exchange, rituximab, and cytotoxic agents have been used when there is little risk of exacerbating the underlying infection or when no infection is present. See also Hepatitis C Virus–Associated Kidney Disease.

Kolopp-Sarda MN et al. Cryoglobulinemic vasculitis: pathophysiological mechanisms and diagnosis. Curr Opin Rheumatol. 2021;33:1. [PMID: 33186245]

8. Hepatitis C Virus–Associated Kidney Disease

Kidney disease can occur in the setting of HCV infection. The three patterns of kidney injury associated with HCV are secondary MPGN (most common), cryoglobulinemic glomerulonephritis, and membranous nephropathy. The clinical presentation driven by the underlying pattern of injury. Many patients have elevated serum transaminases and an elevated rheumatoid factor. Hypocomplementemia is common, with C4 typically more reduced than C3; complement levels and rheumatoid factor tend to be normal if there is a membranous pattern of injury.

Treatment

Viral eradication with direct-acting antiviral agents is the cornerstone of treatment of HCV-associated kidney disease (see Chapter 16). Therapy with rituximab and possibly corticosteroids and plasmapheresis should be initiated in patients with severe vasculitis prior to the initiation of antiviral therapy.

Cohen-Bucay A et al. Progress in hepatitis C virus management in chronic kidney disease. Curr Opin Nephrol Hypertens. 2021;30:493. [PMID: 34054074]
Zignego AL et al. Impact of direct acting antivirals on hepatitis C virus-related cryoglobulinemic syndrome. Minerva Gastroenterol (Torino). 2021;67:218. [PMID: 33793154]

9. Systemic Lupus Erythematosus

Renal involvement occurs in 35–90% of patients who have SLE, with higher estimates encompassing subclinical disease. Rates of lupus nephritis are highest in the non-White population. The pathogenesis may be caused by autoantibodies against nucleosomes; antibody/nucleosome complexes then bind to components of the glomerulus to form immune complex glomerular disease. See Chapter 20 for further discussion of SLE.

The term "lupus nephritis" encompasses many possible patterns of renal injury—most cases present within the nephritic spectrum (class I–IV). Nonglomerular syndromes include tubulointerstitial nephritis and vasculitis. All patients with SLE should have routine urinalyses to monitor for the appearance of hematuria or proteinuria. If urinary abnormalities are detected, kidney biopsy is often performed. The International Society of Nephrology and Renal Pathology Society classification of renal glomerular lesions is class I, minimal mesangial nephritis; class II, mesangial proliferative nephritis; class III, focal (less than 50% of glomeruli affected with capillary involvement) proliferative nephritis; class IV, diffuse (greater than 50% of glomeruli affected with capillary involvement) proliferative nephritis; class V, membranous nephropathy; and class VI, advanced sclerosis without residual disease activity. Classes III and IV, the most severe forms of lupus nephritis, are further classified as active or chronic, and global or segmental, which confers additional prognostic value.

Treatment

Individuals with **class I** and **class II lesions** generally require no treatment; corticosteroids or calcineurin inhibitors should be considered for those with class II lesions with nephrotic-range proteinuria. Transformation of these types to a more active lesion may occur and is usually accompanied by an increase in lupus serologic activity (eg, rising titers of anti–double-stranded DNA antibodies and falling C3 and C4 levels) and increasing proteinuria or falling GFR. Repeat biopsy in such patients is recommended. Hydroxychloroquine should be considered for all patients with lupus nephritis, regardless of histological class.

Patients with extensive **class III lesions** and all **class IV lesions** should receive aggressive immunosuppressive therapy. Poor prognostic indicators include elevated serum creatinine, lower complement levels, male sex, presence of antiphospholipid antibodies, nephrotic-range proteinuria, sub-Saharan African descent (possibly in association with *APOL1* risk alleles), and poor response to therapy. Immunosuppressive therapy for class V lupus nephritis is indicated if superimposed proliferative lesions exist. Class VI lesions should not be treated.

Treatment of class III or IV lupus nephritis consists of induction therapy, followed by maintenance therapy. Induction therapy includes corticosteroids (eg, methylprednisolone 1 g intravenously daily for 3 days followed by prednisone, 1 mg/kg orally daily with subsequent taper over 6–12 months) in combination with either cyclophosphamide or mycophenolate mofetil. Data suggest that Black and Hispanic patients respond more favorably to mycophenolate mofetil than cyclophosphamide; in addition, mycophenolate mofetil has a more favorable side-effect profile than cyclophosphamide and should be favored when preservation of fertility is a consideration. Mycophenolate mofetil induction is typically given at 2–3 g orally daily, then tapered to 1–2 g/day for maintenance. Cyclophosphamide induction regimens vary but usually involve monthly intravenous pulse doses (500–1000 mg/m^2) for 6 months. Induction is followed by daily oral mycophenolate mofetil or azathioprine maintenance therapy; mycophenolate mofetil may be superior to azathioprine maintenance and causes few adverse effects. Add-on therapy with calcineurin inhibitors may also be considered; voclosporin may offer advantages over older calcineurin inhibitors, but its use with cyclophosphamide has not been studied. With standard therapy, remission rates with induction vary from 80% for partial remission to 50–60% for full remission; it may take more than 6 months to see these effects. Relapse is common and rates of disease flare are higher in those who do not experience complete remission; similarly, progression to ESKD is more common in those who relapse more frequently, or in whom no remission has been achieved. The use of add-on B-cell-targeted therapy with rituximab or belimumab for class III, IV, or V disease, or all of the above, may be considered. Pure class V disease is treated with mycophenolate mofetil with or without rituximab.

The levels of various disease activity markers (double-stranded DNA antibodies, serum C3, C4, CH_{50} levels) and the urinary protein levels and sediment activity can be useful in monitoring response to treatment; however, repeat renal biopsy yields more reliable information regarding disease activity and may be used to guide maintenance therapy withdrawal. Patients with SLE who undergo dialysis have a favorable prospect for long-term survival; systemic lupus symptoms may become quiescent with the development of ESKD. Patients with SLE undergoing kidney transplants can have recurrent renal disease, although rates are relatively low.

Furie R et al. Two-year, randomized, controlled trial of belimumab in lupus nephritis. N Engl J Med. 2020;383:1117. [PMID: 32937045]

Gasparotto M et al. Lupus nephritis: clinical presentations and outcomes in the 21st century. Rheumatology. 2020;59:v39. [PMID: 33280015]

Mok CC et al. Long-term outcome of a randomized controlled trial comparing tacrolimus with mycophenolate mofetil as induction therapy for active lupus nephritis. Ann Rheum Dis. 2020;79:1070. [PMID: 32448782]

Parikh SV et al. Update on lupus nephritis: Core Curriculum 2020. Am J Kidney Dis. 2020;76:265. [PMID: 32220510]

Rovin BH et al. Efficacy and safety of voclosporin versus placebo for lupus nephritis (AURORA 1): a double-blind, randomized, multicentre, placebo-controlled, phase 3 trial. Lancet. 2021;397:2070. [PMID: 33971155]

NEPHROTIC SPECTRUM GLOMERULAR DISEASES

ESSENTIALS OF DIAGNOSIS

- Proteinuria with bland urine sediment (few if any cells or cellular casts).
- Nephrotic syndrome (if present) manifestations:
  - –Nephrotic-range proteinuria (urine protein excretion > 3 g per 24 hours).
  - –Hypoalbuminemia (albumin < 3 g/dL).
  - –Peripheral edema.
  - –Hyperlipidemia.
  - –Oval fat bodies may be seen in the urine.

General Considerations

In American adults, the most common cause of nephrotic spectrum glomerular disease is diabetes mellitus. Other causes include minimal change disease, FSGS, membranous nephropathy, and amyloidosis. Clinical presentations along the nephrotic spectrum vary based on etiology, with diabetic nephropathy and secondary FSGS typically on the less severe end (bland UA and proteinuria), and minimal change disease, membranous nephropathy and amyloidosis presenting with the full nephrotic syndrome. Serum creatinine may be abnormal at the time of presentation, depending on the severity and chronicity of the disease.

Clinical Findings

A. Symptoms and Signs

Patients with simple proteinuria do not manifest symptoms of kidney disease. In those with the nephrotic *syndrome*, peripheral edema is present—most likely due both to sodium retention and hypoalbuminemia-induced low plasma oncotic pressure. Edema may develop solely in dependent regions, such as the lower extremities, or it may become generalized and include periorbital edema. Dyspnea due to pulmonary edema, pleural effusions, and diaphragmatic compromise due to ascites can occur.

B. Laboratory Findings

1. UA—Proteinuria occurs as a result of podocytopathy and variable alterations of the GBM. The urine dipstick is a good screening test for albuminuria; if positive, urinary protein excretion should be quantified (see earlier Proteinuria section). A spot urine protein to urine creatinine ratio gives a reasonable approximation of grams of protein excreted per day; a 24-hour urine sample for protein excretion is rarely needed.

Microscopically, the urinary sediment has relatively few cellular elements or casts. However, if marked hyperlipidemia is present, urinary oval fat bodies may be seen. They appear as "grape clusters" under light microscopy and "Maltese crosses" under polarized light.

2. Blood chemistries—The nephrotic syndrome results in hypoalbuminemia (less than 3 g/dL [30 g/L]). Hyperlipidemia occurs in over 50% of patients with early nephrotic syndrome, due to falling oncotic pressure that triggers increased hepatic lipid production and to decreased clearance of very LDLs with resultant hypertriglyceridemia. Hyperlipidemia becomes more frequent and worsens as the severity of the nephrotic syndrome increases. An elevated erythrocyte sedimentation rate may be seen as a result of increased levels of fibrinogen. Heavy urinary excretion of binding proteins may result in deficiencies of vitamin D, zinc, and copper.

Laboratory testing to help elucidate the underlying cause of the glomerular disease includes complement levels, serum and urine protein electrophoresis, serum free light chains, antinuclear antibodies, PLA_2R antibody titers, HbA_{1c}, and serologic testing for hepatitis B and C, HIV, and syphilis.

3. Kidney biopsy—Kidney biopsy is often performed in adults with new-onset idiopathic nephrotic syndrome if a primary renal disease that may require immunosuppressive therapy is suspected. Chronically and significantly decreased GFR indicates irreversible kidney disease mitigating the usefulness of kidney biopsy. In the setting of long-standing diabetes mellitus type 1 or 2, proteinuric renal disease is rarely biopsied unless atypical features (such as significant glomerular hematuria or cellular casts) are also present, or if there is other reason to suspect an additional renal lesion.

Treatment

A. Protein Loss

In those with subnephrotic proteinuria, dietary protein restriction may be helpful in slowing progression of kidney disease (see CKD section).

In both diabetic and nondiabetic patients, anti-proteinuric therapy also slows progression of kidney disease. Useful agents include ACE inhibitors, ARBs, mineralocorticoid receptor antagonists, and SGLT2 inhibitors. They can be used in patients with reduced GFR as long as significant hyperkalemia (potassium greater than 5.2–5.5 mEq/L or mmol/L) does not occur and serum creatinine rises less than 30% after drug initiation or dose titration; patients should be monitored closely to avoid AKI and hyperkalemia. Combination therapy of an ARB and an ACE inhibitor is not recommended. SGLT2 inhibitors should not be used in conjunction with immunosuppression. MRA is not recommended when eGFR is less than 30 mL/minute.

B. Edema

Dietary salt restriction is essential for managing edema; most patients also require diuretic therapy. A combination of loop and thiazide diuretics may be needed for refractory fluid retention. Larger doses often are required because delivery of diuretics to the kidney is reduced with hypoalbuminemia and decreased GFR.

C. Hyperlipidemia

Hypercholesterolemia and hypertriglyceridemia occur as noted above. Dietary modification and exercise should be advocated; however, effective lipid-lowering usually require pharmacologic treatment (see Chapter 28).

D. Hypercoagulable State

Patients with nephrotic syndrome have urinary losses of antithrombin, protein C and protein S, and increased platelet activation. Patients with serum albumin less than 2 g/dL (20 g/L) have considerable risk for thrombophilia and may develop renal vein thrombosis, PE, and other venous thromboemboli; this is likely with membranous nephropathy. Anticoagulation therapy with warfarin is warranted for at least 3–6 months in patients with evidence of thrombosis in any location and may be required indefinitely for renal vein thrombosis, PE, recurrent thromboemboli, or when ongoing nephrotic syndrome poses a risk of thrombosis recurrence.

When to Refer

Any patient with the nephrotic syndrome should be referred immediately to a nephrologist for volume and blood pressure management, assessment for kidney biopsy, and treatment of the underlying disease. Proteinuria of more than 1 g/24 hours without the nephrotic syndrome also merits nephrology referral, though with less urgency.

When to Admit

Patients with edema refractory to outpatient therapy or rapidly worsening kidney function that may require inpatient interventions should be admitted.

Benzing T et al. Insights into glomerular filtration and albuminuria. N Engl J Med. 2021;384:1437. [PMID: 33852781]

Politano SA et al. Nephrotic syndrome. Prim Care. 2020;47:597. [PMID: 33121631]

Xie Y et al. Clinical implications of estimated glomerular filtration rate dip following sodium-glucose cotransporter-2 inhibitor initiation on cardiovascular and kidney outcomes. J Am Heart Assoc. 2021;10:e020237. [PMID: 34013739]

NEPHROTIC SPECTRUM DISEASE IN PRIMARY RENAL DISORDERS

MINIMAL CHANGE DISEASE

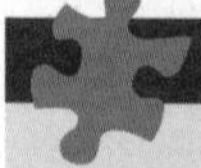

ESSENTIALS OF DIAGNOSIS

- Nephrotic-range proteinuria.
- Kidney biopsy shows no changes on light microscopy.
- Characteristic foot-process effacement on electron microscopy.

General Considerations

Minimal change disease is the most common cause of proteinuric renal disease in children, accounting for about 80% of cases. It often remits upon treatment with a course of corticosteroids. Children with nephrotic syndrome are often treated for minimal change disease empirically without a biopsy diagnosis. Minimal change disease is less common in adults, accounting for 20–25% of cases of primary nephrotic syndrome in those over age 40 years. This entity can be idiopathic but also occurs following viral upper respiratory infections (especially in children), in association with neoplasms such as Hodgkin disease, with drugs (lithium), and with hypersensitivity reactions (especially to NSAIDs and bee stings).

Clinical Findings

A. Symptoms and Signs

Patients present with nephrotic syndrome, which confers susceptibility to infection, tendency toward thromboembolic events, severe hyperlipidemia, and possibly protein malnutrition. Minimal change disease can cause AKI due to renal tubular damage and interstitial edema.

B. Laboratory and Histologic Findings

There is no helpful serologic testing. Biopsy should be considered for children with nephrotic syndrome who exhibit unusual features (such as signs of other systemic illness), or who are steroid-resistant or relapse upon withdrawal of corticosteroid therapy; the latter two conditions may indicate an underlying focal and segmental glomerulosclerosis rather than minimal change disease. When kidney biopsy is performed, glomeruli appear normal on light microscopy and immunofluorescence. On electron microscopy, there is a characteristic effacement of podocyte foot processes. Mesangial cell proliferation may be seen in a subgroup of patients; this finding is associated with more hematuria and hypertension and poor response to standard corticosteroid treatment.

Treatment

Treatment is with prednisone, 60 mg/m^2/day orally; remission in steroid-responsive minimal change disease generally occurs within 4–8 weeks. Adults often require longer courses of therapy than children, requiring up to 16 weeks to achieve a response. Treatment should be continued for several weeks after complete remission of proteinuria, and dosing tapers should be individualized. A significant number of patients relapse and require repeated corticosteroid treatment. Patients with frequent relapses or corticosteroid resistance may require cyclophosphamide, a calcineurin inhibitor (tacrolimus, cyclosporine), or rituximab to induce subsequent remissions. Progression to ESKD is rare. Complications most often arise from prolonged corticosteroid use.

Heybeli C et al. Comparison of treatment options in adults with frequently relapsing or steroid-dependent minimal change disease. Nephrol Dial Transplant. 2021;36:1821. [PMID: 32918483]

FOCAL SEGMENTAL GLOMERULOSCLEROSIS

General Considerations

This relatively common renal pattern of injury results from damage to podocytes; such damage may be a primary/renal-limited disorder or may be secondary to another underlying disease state. Primary causes fall into three categories: (1) heritable abnormalities in any one of several podocyte proteins, or underlying type 4 collagen mutations; (2) polymorphisms in the *APOL1* gene in those of sub-Saharan African ancestry; or (3) increased levels of a circulating permeability factor. Secondary causes include renal overwork injury, obesity, hypertension, chronic urinary reflux, HIV or SARS-CoV-2 infection, or analgesic or bisphosphonate exposure. Genetic testing in primary cases is becoming more common, especially in the pediatric population.

Clinical Findings

In FSGS caused by a primary kidney disease, 80% of children and 50% of adults have overt nephrotic syndrome; however, when it develops due to a secondary cause, nephrotic syndrome is uncommon. Decreased GFR is present in 25–50% of those with FSGS at time of diagnosis.

Diagnosis requires kidney biopsy; there is no helpful serologic test. Light microscopy shows sclerosis of segments of some, but not all, glomeruli. On immunofluorescence, IgM and C3 are seen in the sclerotic lesions, although it is presumed that these immune components are simply trapped in the sclerotic glomeruli and not pathogenetic. As in minimal change disease, electron microscopy shows fusion of epithelial foot processes.

Treatment

Treatment for all forms of FSGS includes diuretics for edema, ACE inhibitors and ARBs to control proteinuria and hypertension, and statins for hyperlipidemia; SGLT2-inhibitors may be considered for those not receiving immunosuppression. Immunosuppression therapy (oral prednisone, 1 mg/kg/day for 4–16 weeks followed by a slow taper) is reserved for nephrotic primary FSGS cases presumed to be due to a circulating permeability factor; in those with steroid-resistance or intolerance, calcineurin inhibitors and mycophenolate mofetil can be considered. Kidney transplantation in this subgroup of FSGS patients is complicated by a relatively high relapse rate and risk of graft loss. Those with *APOL1*-associated and hereditary primary renal disease may not benefit from immunosuppression, although robust clinical trials are lacking. Patients with secondary FSGS do not benefit from immunosuppressive therapy; treatment should be directed at the underlying cause.

DeVriese AS et al. Therapeutic trials in adult FSGS: lessons learned and the road forward. Nat Rev Nephrol. 2021;17:619. [PMID: 34017116]

Friedman DJ et al. APOL1 nephropathy; from genetics to clinical applications. Clin J Am Soc Nephrol. 2021;16:294. [PMID: 32616495]

Hansrivijit P et al. Rituximab for focal segmental glomerulosclerosis and minimal change disease in adults: a systematic review and meta-analysis. BMC Nephrol. 2020;21:134. [PMID: 32293308]

MEMBRANOUS NEPHROPATHY

ESSENTIALS OF DIAGNOSIS

- Varying degrees of proteinuria.
- Most common cause of primary adult nephrotic syndrome.
- Significant risk for hypercoagulable state if nephrotic syndrome present.
- "Spike and dome" pattern on kidney biopsy from subepithelial deposits.
- Secondary causes include hepatitis B virus and carcinomas.

General Considerations

Membranous nephropathy is the most common cause of primary nephrotic syndrome in adults, most often presenting in the fifth and sixth decades. Primary membranous nephropathy is an autoimmune disease with reactivity against several possible podocyte antigens. Secondary disease is associated with infections, (such as hepatitis B and C, endocarditis, and syphilis); underlying carcinomas autoimmune disease (such as SLE, mixed connective tissue disease, and thyroiditis); and certain drugs (such as NSAIDs and captopril). The course of primary disease is highly variable, with spontaneous remission in approximately 30% of patients and progression to ESKD over 3–10 years in 50%. Poorer outcome is associated with concomitant tubulointerstitial fibrosis, male sex, elevated serum creatinine on presentation, hypertension, and proteinuria greater than 10 g/day.

Patients with membranous nephropathy and nephrotic syndrome have a higher risk of hypercoagulable state with thrombosis than nephrosis from other etiologies, including a predisposition to renal vein thrombosis.

Clinical Findings

A. Symptoms and Signs

Patients may be asymptomatic or may have edema or frothy urine. Symptomatic venous thrombosis may be an initial sign. There may be symptoms or signs of an underlying infection or neoplasm (especially lung, stomach, breast, and colon cancers) in secondary membranous nephropathy.

B. Laboratory Findings

Hypoalbuminemia and hyperlipidemia are characteristic laboratory findings in the nephrotic syndrome. Evaluation for secondary causes including serologic testing for SLE, syphilis, and viral hepatitides, and age- and risk-appropriate cancer screening should be performed. Elevated titer of circulating PLA_2R antibodies is generally considered diagnostic for primary membranous nephropathy and may eliminate the need for kidney biopsy. Kidney biopsy findings in membranous nephropathy include increased capillary wall thickness without inflammatory changes or cellular proliferation; when stained with silver methenamine, a "spike and dome" pattern results from projections of excess GBM between the subepithelial immune complex deposits. Immunofluorescence shows IgG and C3 staining along capillary loops. Electron microscopy shows a discontinuous pattern of dense deposits along the subepithelial surface of the basement membrane.

Treatment

Secondary causes must be considered prior to consideration of treatment. Primary disease treatment depends on the risk of renal disease progression. Roughly 30% of patients present with subnephrotic proteinuria (less than 3 g/day) and most have a good prognosis with conservative management, including antiproteinuric therapy with ACE inhibitor or ARB if blood pressure is greater than 125/75 mm Hg. Spontaneous remission may develop even in those with heavy proteinuria (about 30% of cases). Thus, use of immunosuppressive agents should be limited to those at highest risk for progression and with salvageable renal function. Patients with nephrotic syndrome despite 6 months of conservative management and serum creatinine less than 3.0 mg/dL (265 mcmol/L) may elect therapy with rituximab or with corticosteroids and cyclophosphamide for 6 months. Calcineurin inhibitors with or without corticosteroids may be considered as well. Reduction in proteinuria may take up to 6 months, especially with rituximab-based regimens. Patients with primary membranous nephropathy are excellent candidates for transplant.

Alsharhan L et al. Membranous nephropathy: Core Curriculum 2021. Am J Kidney Dis. 2021;77:440. [PMID: 33487481]

Ronco R et al. Membranous nephropathy: current understanding of various causes in light of new target antigens. Curr Opin Nephrol Hypertens. 2021;30:287. [PMID: 33480620]

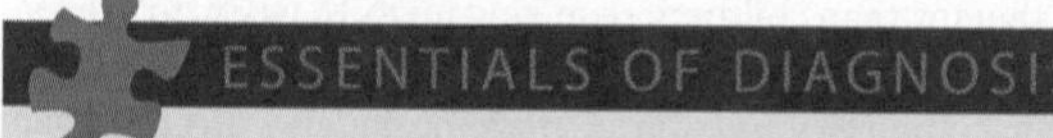

NEPHROTIC SPECTRUM DISEASE FROM SYSTEMIC DISORDERS

DIABETIC NEPHROPATHY

ESSENTIALS OF DIAGNOSIS

- Evidence of diabetes mellitus, typically over 10 years.
- Albuminuria usually precedes decline in GFR.
- Other end-organ damage, such as retinopathy, is common.

General Considerations

Diabetic nephropathy is the most common cause of ESKD in the United States. The incidence is approximately 30% in both type 1 and type 2 diabetes mellitus. ESKD is much more likely to develop in persons with type 1 diabetes mellitus, in part due to fewer comorbidities and deaths before ESKD ensues. With the current epidemic of obesity and type 2 diabetes mellitus, rates of diabetic nephropathy will continue to increase. Those with a family history of kidney disease are at higher risk. Mortality rates are higher for diabetics with kidney disease compared to those without CKD.

Clinical Findings

Diabetic nephropathy develops about 10 years after the onset of diabetes mellitus. It may be present at the time type 2 diabetes mellitus is diagnosed. The first stage of classic diabetic nephropathy is hyperfiltration with an increase in GFR, followed by the development of microalbuminuria (30–300 mg/day). With progression, albuminuria increases to greater than 300 mg/day and can be detected on a urine dipstick as overt proteinuria; the GFR subsequently declines over time. Yearly screening for microalbuminuria is recommended for all diabetic patients to detect disease at its earliest stage; however, diabetic nephropathy can, less commonly present as nonproteinuric CKD.

The most common lesion in diabetic nephropathy is diffuse glomerulosclerosis, but nodular glomerulosclerosis (Kimmelstiel-Wilson nodules) is pathognomonic. The kidneys are usually enlarged. Kidney biopsy is not required in most patients unless atypical findings are present, such as sudden onset of proteinuria, nephritic spectrum features (see above), massive proteinuria (greater than 10 g/day), urinary cellular casts, or rapid decline in GFR.

Patients with diabetes are prone to other renal diseases. These include papillary necrosis, chronic interstitial nephritis, and type 4 (hyporeninemic hypoaldosteronemic) renal tubular acidosis. Patients are more susceptible to AKI from many insults, including intravenous contrast material and concomitant use of an ACE inhibitor or ARB with NSAID.

Treatment

With the onset of microalbuminuria, aggressive treatment is necessary. Strict glycemic control should be emphasized early in diabetic nephropathy, with recognition of risk of hypoglycemia as CKD becomes advanced (see CKD section). Recommended blood pressure goals should be tailored to the individual patient: based on the ACCORD trial, those with microalbuminuria (30–300 mg/day) and preserved GFR and those with significant CVD likely derive little benefit from blood pressure lowering much below 140/90 mm Hg, although the 2017 guidelines from the American Heart Association advocate treatment to 130/80 mm Hg or less. Those with overt proteinuria (especially more than 1 g/day) benefit from a goal of less than 130/80 mm Hg. ACE inhibitors and ARBs in those with microalbuminuria lower the rate of progression to overt proteinuria and slow progression to ESKD by reducing intraglomerular pressure and via antifibrotic effects; these agents are not absolutely indicated in diabetic patients without albuminuria. Diabetic patients, especially with advanced CKD, are at relatively high risk for AKI and hyperkalemia with inhibition of the renin-angiotensin system, so monitoring for hyperkalemia or a decline in GFR more than 30% within ~2 weeks of the initiation or uptitration of this therapy is prudent, with dose reduction or discontinuation of therapy if these complications are encountered. *Combination ARB and ACE inhibitor therapy is not recommended due to lack of efficacy and increased adverse events of hyperkalemia and AKI.* In addition to their cardioprotective effects, the SGLT inhibitors, including canagliflozin, empagliflozin, and dapagliflozin, slow progression of diabetic nephropathy; their use is limited to those with type 2 diabetes mellitus with eGFR greater than 30 mL/minute/1.73 m^2. Use of these agents may require reduction in diuretic dosing in those patients requiring natriuresis, and initial monitoring to ensure that eGFR stabilizes after an initial small/expected decline. Mineralocorticoid receptor antagonism can be considered for blood pressure and proteinuria management in type 2 DM with careful monitoring for hyperkalemia. Treatment of other cardiovascular risk factors and obesity is crucial. Many with diabetes have multiple comorbid conditions; therefore, in patients with ESKD who progress to dialysis, mortality over the first 5 years is high. Patients who are relatively healthy, however, benefit from renal transplantation.

De Boer IH et al. Executive summary of the 2020 KDIGO Diabetes Management in CKD Guideline: evidence-based advances in monitoring and treatment. Kidney Int. 2020; 98:839. [PMID: 32653403]

Hahr AJ et al. Management of diabetes mellitus in patients with CKD: Core Curriculum 2022. Am J Kidney Dis. 2021 Sep 29. [Epub ahead of print] [PMID: 34600745]

Oliva-Damaso N et al. Glomerular diseases in diabetic patients: implications for diagnosis and management. J Clin Med. 2021;10:1855. [PMID: 33923227]

Tuttle KR et al. SLGT2 inhibition for CKD and cardiovascular disease in type 2 diabetes: report of a scientific workshop sponsored by the National Kidney Foundation. Am J Kidney Dis. 2021;77:94. [PMID: 33121838]

HIV-ASSOCIATED NEPHROPATHY

HIV-associated nephropathy usually presents with nephrotic syndrome and declining GFR in patients with active HIV infection. Most who present with HIV-associated nephropathy are of sub-Saharan African descent with *APOL1* risk alleles (see section on Focal Segmental Glomerulosclerosis). HIV-associated nephropathy is usually associated with low CD4 counts and AIDS, but it can also be the initial presentation of HIV disease. Persons living with HIV are at risk for other kidney diseases, such as toxicity from antiretroviral medications (eg, tenofovir disoproxil fumarate), vascular disease, and diabetes, or an immune complex–mediated glomerular disease (HIV-immune complex disease).

Classic HIV-associated nephropathy is characterized by an FSGS pattern of injury with glomerular collapse; severe tubulointerstitial damage may also be present.

HIV-associated nephropathy is less common in the era of HIV screening and more effective antiretroviral therapy. Small, uncontrolled studies have shown that antiretroviral therapy slows progression of disease. ACE inhibitors or ARBs can be used to control blood pressure and proteinuria. Kidney biopsy is necessary for diagnosis and to rule out other causes of kidney dysfunction. Patients who progress to ESKD and are otherwise healthy are good candidates for kidney transplantation.

Hughes C. Renal adverse drug reactions. Curr Opin HIV AIDS. 2021;16:303. [PMID: 34459469]

Naicker S. HIV/AIDS and chronic kidney disease. Clin Nephrol. 2020;93:87. [PMID: 31397267]

RENAL AMYLOIDOSIS

Amyloidosis is a relatively rare cause of nephrotic syndrome. It is caused by tissue deposition of an overproduced and abnormally-folded protein (amyloid). Several different proteins can form amyloid fibrils with renal deposition.

Primary amyloidosis, or AL amyloidosis, is the most common form and is due to a plasma cell dyscrasia causing overproduction and deposition of monoclonal Ig light chains (see Chapter 13). Secondary amyloidosis, or AA amyloidosis, can rarely occur in chronic inflammatory disease such as rheumatoid arthritis, IBD, or chronic infection; in these cases, there is deposition of an acute phase reactant, serum amyloid A protein. Other less common forms of amyloidosis may also be encountered.

Proteinuria, decreased GFR, and nephrotic syndrome are presenting symptoms and signs of renal involvement in amyloidosis; evidence of other organ involvement, such as the heart, is common. Serum and urine protein electrophoresis should be done as screening tests; if a monoclonal spike is found on either, serum free light chains should be quantified and the kappa:lambda ratio assessed. Amyloid-affected kidneys are often larger than 10 cm. Pathologically, glomeruli are filled with amorphous deposits that show green birefringence with Congo red staining.

AL amyloidosis progresses to ESKD in an average of 2–3 years. Five-year overall survival is less than 20%, with worse prognosis in those with advanced cardiac involvement. Standard treatment is a combination of melphalan, corticosteroids, and the proteosome inhibitor bortezomib; addition of daratumumab shows promise. Melphalan and autologous stem cell transplantation are associated with a high (45%) mortality rate but can induce remission in 80% of survivors; however, few patients are eligible for this treatment. In AA amyloidosis, remission can occur if the underlying disease is successfully treated. Renal transplantation is an option.

Hogan JJ et al. Dysproteinemia and the kidney: Core Curriculum 2019. Am J Kidney Dis. 2019;74:822. [PMID: 31331759]

Kastritis E et al; ANDROMEDA Trial Investigators. Daratumumab-based treatment for immunoglobulin light-chain amyloidosis. N Engl J Med. 2021;385:46. [PMID: 34192431]

Law S et al. Advances in diagnosis and treatment of cardiac and renal amyloidosis. Cardiol Clin. 2021;39:389. [PMID: 34247752]

Palladini G et al. Management of AL amyloidosis in 2020. Hematology Am Soc Hematol Educ Program. 2020;2020:363. [PMID: 33275753]

TUBULOINTERSTITIAL DISEASES

Tubulointerstitial disease may be acute or chronic. Acute disease is most commonly associated with medications, infectious agents, and systemic rheumatologic disorders. Interstitial edema, infiltration with polymorphonuclear neutrophils, and accompanying ATN can be seen. (See Acute Kidney Injury, above, and Table 22–9.) Chronic disease is associated with insults from an acute factor or progressive insults without any obvious acute cause. Interstitial fibrosis and tubular atrophy are present, with a mononuclear cell predominance. The chronic disorders are described below.

Table 22–9. Causes of acute tubulointerstitial nephritis (abbreviated list).

Drug Reactions
Antibiotics
Beta-lactam antibiotics: methicillin, penicillin, ampicillin, cephalosporins
Ciprofloxacin
Erythromycin
Sulfonamides (trimethoprim-sulfamethoxazole, loop and thiazide diuretics)
Tetracycline
Vancomycin
Ethambutol
Rifampin
NSAIDs
Diuretics
Thiazides
Furosemide
Other
Allopurinol
Cimetidine
Phenytoin
PPIs
Systemic Infections
Bacteria
Streptococcus
Corynebacterium diphtheriae
Legionella
Viruses
Epstein-Barr
Other
Mycoplasma
Rickettsia rickettsii
Leptospira icterohaemorrhagiae
Toxoplasma
Idiopathic
Tubulointerstitial nephritis-uveitis

CHRONIC TUBULOINTERSTITIAL DISEASES

ESSENTIALS OF DIAGNOSIS

- Kidney size is small and contracted.
- Decreased urinary concentrating ability.
- Hyperchloremic metabolic acidosis.
- Reduced GFR.

General Considerations

The most common cause of *chronic* tubulointerstitial disease is **obstructive uropathy**, which may result from prolonged or recurrent obstruction. The major causes are prostate disease in men; ureteral calculus in a single functioning kidney; bilateral ureteral calculi; carcinoma of the cervix, colon, or bladder; and retroperitoneal tumors or fibrosis.

The second most common cause is nephropathy from **vesicoureteral reflux**. Vesicoureteral reflux is primarily a childhood disorder that occurs when urine passes retrograde from the bladder to the kidneys during voiding, a result of an incompetent vesicoureteral sphincter. Urine can extravasate into the interstitium, triggering an inflammatory response that leads to fibrosis over time. The inflammatory response is due to either bacteria or normal urinary components.

Analgesic nephropathy can occur in patients who ingest large quantities of pain medication. Drugs of concern are paracetamol, aspirin, and other NSAIDs; acetaminophen is a possible but less certain culprit. Phenacetin historically was a common culprit, but is now scarcely available. Ingestion of at least 1 g/day for 3 years of these analgesics is considered necessary for kidney dysfunction to develop, however many patients underestimate their analgesic use. This disorder occurs most frequently in individuals who are using analgesics for chronic headaches, muscular pains, and arthritis; female sex, older age, and malnutrition are risk factors for analgesic nephropathy. Tubulointerstitial inflammation and papillary necrosis are seen on pathologic examination. Papillary tip and inner medullary concentrations of some analgesics are tenfold higher than in the renal cortex. Aspirin and other NSAIDs can cause damage through intermediate metabolites, which can lead to cell necrosis. These drugs also decrease medullary blood flow (via inhibition of prostaglandin synthesis) and decrease glutathione levels, which are necessary for detoxification.

Environmental exposure to **heavy metals**—such as lead, cadmium, mercury, and bismuth—occurs infrequently now in the United States but can cause tubulointerstitial disease. Individuals at risk for lead-induced tubulointerstitial disease are those with occupational exposure (eg, welders who work with lead-based paint) and drinkers of alcohol distilled in automobile radiators ("moonshine" whiskey users). Lead is filtered by the glomerulus and is transported across the proximal convoluted tubule, where it accumulates and causes cell damage. Fibrosed arterioles and cortical scarring also lead to damaged kidneys.

A form of chronic tubulointerstitial disease disproportionately affecting male agricultural workers in Central America is an important cause of ESKD. While the exact pathophysiology is still unknown, the term **Mesoamerican nephropathy** is applied to reflect the geographic region in which this disease occurs. Affected individuals tend to be 30–50 years of age without diabetes, hypertension, or other causes of kidney disease who work under hot conditions, particularly in sugar cane or cotton fields, and are thus susceptible to dehydration.

Clinical Findings

A. General Findings

Polyuria is common because tubular damage leads to nephrogenic diabetes insipidus, possibly from vasopressin insensitivity. Volume depletion can also occur as a result of a salt-wasting defect in some individuals.

Patients can become hyperkalemic both because the GFR is lower and the distal tubules become aldosterone resistant. Renal tubular acidosis is common and develops through three mechanisms: (1) reduced ammoniagenesis in the proximal tubules, (2) inability to reabsorb bicarbonate in the proximal tubules, and (3) inability to secrete protons in the distal tubules, which is needed for urinary acidification. A type 1 or type 4 renal tubular acidosis is more commonly observed in tubulointerstitial disease, except in the case of heavy metal exposure where direct proximal tubular damage leads to a proximal (type 2) renal tubular acidosis. In contrast to acute interstitial nephritis, the UA in chronic tubulointerstitial disease is often nonspecific; a few cells or broad waxy casts may be seen, but UA often is bland. Proteinuria is typically less than 2 g/day, owing to inability of the proximal tubule to reabsorb freely filterable proteins.

B. Specific Findings

1. Obstructive uropathy—In partial obstruction, patients can exhibit polyuria (from tubular damage) or oliguria (due to decreased GFR). Azotemia and hypertension (due to increased renin-angiotensin production) are usually present. Abdominal, rectal, and genitourinary examinations may be helpful in detecting a distended bladder or large prostate. UA is often bland, but may show hematuria, pyuria, or bacteriuria. Abdominal ultrasound may detect mass lesions, hydroureter, and hydronephrosis but may overlook 5% of cases. CT scanning or MRI can be considered if suspicion remains despite a normal ultrasound.

2. Vesicoureteral reflux—Vesicoureteral reflux is typically diagnosed in young children with a history of recurrent UTIs but can also develop after kidney transplantation. Renal ultrasound can show renal scarring and hydronephrosis. Most damage occurs before age 5, and progressive deterioration to ESKD is common.

3. Analgesics—Patients can exhibit hematuria, mild proteinuria, polyuria (from tubular damage), anemia (from GI bleeding or erythropoietin deficiency), and sterile pyuria. Sloughed papillae can be found in the urine when papillary necrosis occurs and can lead to obstruction. Although classically diagnosed by IVP, papillary necrosis is more commonly detected by CT imaging.

4. Heavy metals—Proximal tubular damage from lead exposure can cause decreased secretion of uric acid, resulting in hyperuricemia and saturnine gout. Patients commonly are hypertensive. Diagnosis is established with a calcium disodium edetate (EDTA) chelation test performed on a timed urine collection. Urine excretion of greater than 600 mg of lead following 1 g of EDTA indicates excessive lead exposure. The proximal tubular dysfunction from cadmium can cause hypercalciuria and nephrolithiasis.

5. Mesoamerican nephropathy—In addition to low-grade proteinuria, hyperuricemia and hypokalemia are consistently (but not universally) identified among affected individuals. Although not pathognomonic, areas of glomerular ischemia (despite mild vascular disease) that accompany chronic tubulointerstitial injury on kidney biopsy are highly suggestive of Mesoamerican nephropathy.

6. Balkan nephropathy—Patients commonly develop proteinuria, glycosuria, acidosis, and suffer urinary concentrating defects. Notably, urothelial carcinomas are present in approximately 50% of affected individuals at time of diagnosis.

Treatment

Treatment depends first on identifying the disorder responsible for kidney dysfunction. Interstitial fibrosis on biopsy reflects irreversible damage, the degree of which is directly associated with the likelihood of ESKD progression. Treatment is directed at medical management of risk factors for disease progression, such as hypertension and proteinuria. Tubular dysfunction may require bicarbonate supplementation to treat metabolic acidosis or phosphorus and potassium restriction.

If hydronephrosis is present, the obstruction should be promptly relieved. Prolonged obstruction leads to further tubular damage—particularly in the distal nephron—which may become irreversible. Although surgical correction of reflux may be indicated in select instances, this will unlikely prevent deterioration toward ESKD if fibrosis is extensive.

Patients in whom lead nephropathy is suspected should continue chelation therapy with EDTA if there is minimal evidence of irreversible renal damage, and continued exposure should be avoided.

Treatment of analgesic nephropathy requires cessation of all analgesics. Stabilization of or improvement in kidney function may occur if significant interstitial fibrosis is not present. Ensuring volume repletion during exposure to analgesics may also have some beneficial effects.

Patients with Mesoamerican nephropathy should be counseled to remain adequately hydrated and, if possible, minimize heat exposure. NSAIDs should be avoided due to their hemodynamic effects (reduced renal blood flow and glomerular filtration), which may exacerbate renal injury in states of volume depletion and hot climates.

When to Refer

- Patients with stage 3–5 CKD should be referred to a nephrologist when tubulointerstitial diseases are suspected. Other select cases of stage 1–2 CKD should also be referred, for example if renal tubular acidosis is present.
- Patients with urologic abnormalities should be referred to a urologist.

Murugapoopathy V et al. A primer on congenital anomalies of the kidneys and urinary tracts (CAKUT). Clin J Am Soc Nephrol. 2020;15:723. [PMID: 32188635]

CYSTIC DISEASES OF THE KIDNEY

Renal cysts are epithelium-lined cavities filled with fluid or semisolid material that develop primarily from renal tubular elements. One or more simple cysts are found in 50% of individuals over the age of 50 years. They are rarely symptomatic and have little clinical significance. In contrast, generalized cystic diseases are associated with cysts scattered throughout the cortex and medulla of both kidneys and can progress to ESKD (Table 22–10).

SIMPLE OR SOLITARY CYSTS

Simple cysts account for 65–70% of all renal masses. They are generally found at the outer cortex and contain fluid that is consistent with an ultrafiltrate of plasma. Most are found incidentally on ultrasonographic examination. Simple cysts are typically asymptomatic but can become infected.

Table 22–10. Clinical features of renal cystic disease.

	Simple Renal Cysts	Acquired Renal Cysts	Autosomal Dominant Polycystic Kidney Disease	Medullary Sponge Kidney	Medullary Cystic Kidney
Prevalence	Common	Dialysis patients	1:1000	1:5000	Rare
Inheritance	None	None	Autosomal dominant	None	Autosomal dominant
Age at onset	...	...	20–40 years	40–60 years	Adulthood
Kidney size	Normal	Small	Large	Normal	Small
Cyst location	Cortex and medulla	Cortex and medulla	Cortex and medulla	Collecting ducts	Corticomedullary junction
Hematuria	Occasional	Occasional	Common	Rare	Rare
Hypertension	None	Variable	Common	None	None
Associated complications	None	Adenocarcinoma in cysts	Hepatic cysts, UTIs, renal calculi, cerebral aneurysms	Renal calculi, UTIs	Polyuria, salt-wasting
Kidney failure	Never	Always	Frequently	Never	Always

The major objective with simple cysts is to differentiate them from malignancy, abscess, or polycystic kidney disease. Cystic disease can develop in dialysis patients and has the potential to progress to malignancy. Ultrasound and CT scanning are recommended to evaluate these masses. Simple cysts must display three sonographic features to be considered benign: (1) echo free, (2) sharply demarcated with smooth walls, and (3) an enhanced back wall (indicating good transmission through the cyst). Complex cysts can have thick walls, calcifications, solid components, and mixed echogenicity. On CT scan, simple cysts should have smooth thin walls that are sharply demarcated and should not enhance with contrast media. Renal cell carcinoma will enhance but typically is of lower density than healthy parenchyma. Arteriography can also be used to evaluate a mass preoperatively. Renal cell carcinoma is hypervascular in 80%, hypovascular in 15%, and avascular in 5% of cases.

If a cyst has questionable imaging characteristics or is of uncertain significance, periodic reevaluation is recommended. Urologic consultation and surgical exploration may be considered. Benign cysts do not require any specific follow-up, though changes in clinical presentation should prompt repeat imaging.

Zeng SE et al. Ultrasound, CT, and MR Imaging for evaluation of cystic renal masses. J Ultrasound Med. 2022;41:807. [PMID: 34101225]

AUTOSOMAL DOMINANT POLYCYSTIC KIDNEY DISEASE

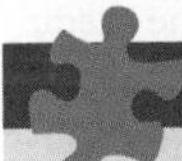

ESSENTIALS OF DIAGNOSIS

- Multiple cysts in both kidneys; number of cysts depends on patient age.
- Combination of hypertension and large palpable kidneys suggestive of disease.
- Autosomal dominant chromosomal abnormalities present in some patients.

General Considerations

Autosomal dominant polycystic kidney disease is the most common monogenic kidney disease, affecting over 12 million individuals worldwide. ESKD develops by age 60 in up to 50% of patients. The disease has variable penetrance but accounts for 5–10% of all ESKD cases globally. At least two genes account for this disorder: *PKD1* on the short arm of chromosome 16 (85–90% of patients) and *PKD2* on chromosome 4 (10–15%). Patients with the *PKD2* mutation have slower progression of disease and longer life expectancy than those with *PKD1*. Other sporadic cases without these mutations are also recognized.

Clinical Findings

Abdominal or flank pain and hematuria (either microscopic or gross) are present in most patients. A history of UTIs and nephrolithiasis is common. A family history of autosomal dominant polycystic kidney disease is present in 75% of cases, and more than 50% of patients have hypertension that may precede clinical manifestations. Patients have large kidneys that may be palpable on abdominal examination. The combination of hypertension and an abdominal mass should raise suspicion for the disease. Forty to 50 percent have concurrent hepatic cysts; pancreatic and splenic cysts may occur. Despite development of CKD, hemoglobin is often normal as a result of cystic erythropoietin production. UA may show hematuria and subnephrotic proteinuria. In patients with an established family history of autosomal dominant polycystic kidney disease, ultrasonography confirms the diagnosis—two or more cysts in patients under age 30 years (sensitivity of 88.5%), two or more cysts in each kidney in patients aged 30–59 years (sensitivity of 100%), and four or more cysts in each kidney in patients aged 60 years or older are diagnostic for autosomal dominant polycystic kidney disease. Importantly, these criteria do *not* apply to individuals without a known family history; patients without a known family history of polycystic kidney disease require additional diagnostic evaluation including CT scanning, which reveals innumerable cysts in cases of polycystic kidney disease (Figure 22–5); the presence of multiple hepatic cysts can aid in establishing the diagnosis. In some cases, genetic testing for *PKD1* and *PKD2* mutations may be required.

Complications & Treatment

A. Pain

Abdominal or flank pain may be caused by infection, cyst rupture or hemorrhage, or nephrolithiasis. Bed rest and analgesics are recommended. Cyst decompression can help with chronic pain.

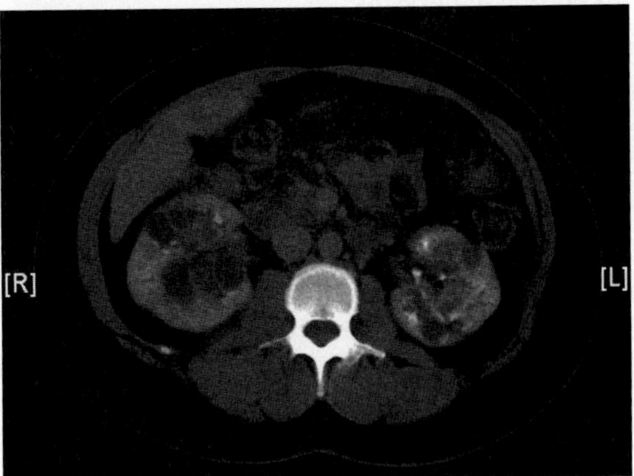

▲ **Figure 22–5.** Polycystic kidney disease. CT scan showing bilateral polycystic kidneys in a 43-year-old woman who presented with newly diagnosed hypertension and microscopic hematuria. (Used, with permission, from Michael Freckleton, MD, in Usatine RP, Smith MA, Mayeaux EJ Jr, Chumley H. *The Color Atlas of Family Medicine*, 2nd ed. McGraw-Hill, 2013.)

B. Hematuria

Gross hematuria is most commonly due to cystic rupture into the renal pelvis, but it can also be caused by a kidney stone or UTI. Hematuria typically resolves within 7 days with bed rest and hydration.

C. Renal Infection

An infected renal cyst should be suspected in patients who have flank pain, fever, and leukocytosis. Importantly, UA may be normal if the cyst does not communicate directly with the urinary tract. CT scans can be helpful because an infected cyst may have increased wall thickness. Bacterial cyst infections are difficult to treat. Antibiotics with cystic penetration are the agents of choice (eg, fluoroquinolones [ciprofloxacin, 500 mg every 12 hours, or levofloxacin, 500 mg once daily if GFR normal], or trimethoprim-sulfamethoxazole double-strength tablet twice daily).

D. Nephrolithiasis

Up to 20% of patients have kidney stones, primarily calcium oxalate. Hydration (2–3 L/day) is recommended in order to prevent precipitation of stones.

E. Hypertension

At time of presentation, 50% of patients have hypertension and most others will develop it during the course of the disease. Cyst-induced ischemia appears to cause activation of the renin-angiotensin system, and cyst decompression can lower blood pressure temporarily. Hypertension should preferentially be treated with ACE inhibitors or ARBs if tolerated. Intensive blood pressure control (goal less than or equal to 110/75 mm Hg) is recommended in adults younger than 50 years of age with eGFR greater than 60 mL/minute/1.73 m^2; for all other affected individuals, goal blood pressure is less than or equal to 130/85 mm Hg.

F. Cerebral Aneurysms

About 10–15% of patients have arterial aneurysms in the circle of Willis. Screening arteriography is not recommended unless the patient has a family history of aneurysms, is employed in a high-risk profession (eg, airline pilot), or is undergoing elective surgery with a high risk of developing moderate to severe perioperative hypertension.

G. Other Complications

Cardiovascular problems include mitral valve prolapse in up to 25% of patients, aortic aneurysms, and aortic valve abnormalities. Colonic diverticula are more common in patients with polycystic kidneys.

Prognosis

Kidney size, reported as total kidney volume, is the best predictor of kidney function decline in patients with autosomal dominant polycystic kidney disease, and can be measured via CT or MRI using the Mayo Classification system (www.mayo.edu/research/documents/pkd-center-adkpkd-classification/doc-20094754). Those at high risk according to this classification system may benefit from treatments that delay cyst growth. Vasopressin receptor antagonists decrease the rate of change in total kidney volume and eGFR decline, and one such medication (tolvaptan) is FDA-approved for the treatment of autosomal dominant polycystic kidney disease. Liberal ingestion of water will have the same physiologic effect on vasopressin, and patients should be encouraged to drink at least 2 L of water daily. Other agents such as octreotide, sirolimus, and tyrosine kinase inhibitors decrease the rate of cyst growth but not the decline in kidney function and are thus not routinely used. Avoidance of caffeine may prevent cyst formation due to effects on G-coupled proteins.

Chebib FT et al. Assessing risk of rapid progression in autosomal dominant polycystic kidney disease and special considerations for disease-modifying therapy. Am J Kidney Dis. 2021;78:282. [PMID: 33705818]

Nobakht N et al. Advances in autosomal dominant polycystic kidney disease: a clinical review. Kidney Med. 2020;2:196. [PMID: 32734239]

MEDULLARY SPONGE KIDNEY

Medullary sponge kidney is a disease involving the distal nephron that affects less than 1% of the general population. Although present at birth, it is not usually diagnosed until the third or fourth decade. It is thought to occur due to disruption of the ureteric bud-metanephric mesenchyme interface, often resulting from autosomal dominant mutations in genes responsible for urogenital development. Kidneys have marked, irregular enlargement of the medullary and papillary collecting ducts. This is associated with diffuse medullary cysts, giving a "Swiss cheese" appearance in these regions.

Clinical Findings

Nephrolithiasis is the most common clinical presentation of medullary sponge kidney, affecting up to 70% of patients. Other presentations may include hematuria (either gross or microscopic) or recurrent UTIs. Common abnormalities include decreased urinary concentrating ability, nephrocalcinosis, and, less commonly, type 1 (distal) renal tubular acidosis. The diagnosis is established clinically through laboratory data and imaging characteristics. CT imaging is the preferred imaging study, which shows cystic dilatation of the distal collecting tubules with a striated appearance, and calcifications in the renal collecting system. Similar findings on ultrasound may also support the diagnosis.

Treatment

Treatment for medullary sponge kidney is supportive and aimed at underlying abnormalities such as nephrolithiasis and acidosis. Adequate fluid intake (2 L/day) helps reduce risk of stone formation. If hypercalciuria is present, thiazide diuretics are recommended because they decrease calcium excretion. Alkali therapy is recommended if renal tubular acidosis is present.

Prognosis

Medullary sponge kidney is generally considered a benign condition unless there are complications from recurrent UTIs, nephrolithiasis, or uncontrolled acidosis.

Pisani I et al. Ultrasound to address medullary sponge kidney: a retrospective study. BMC Nephrol. 2020;21:430. [PMID: 33046028]

MULTISYSTEM DISEASES WITH VARIABLE KIDNEY INVOLVEMENT

PLASMA CELL MYELOMA

Plasma cell myeloma is a malignancy of plasma cells (see Chapter 13) that can cause a variety of kidney disorders. Injury is due to the toxic effects of monoclonal immunoglobulins or light chain components produced by plasma cells. Cast nephropathy (formally called "myeloma kidney") is the most common kidney disease in plasma cell myeloma and occurs when light chains (Bence Jones protein) overwhelm the reabsorptive capacity of the tubules, leading to precipitation in the distal nephron and tubular obstruction. Plasma cell myeloma may also cause Fanconi syndrome, a type 2 (proximal) renal tubular acidosis characterized by hypophosphatemia and inappropriate glycosuria. Proteinuria in cast nephropathy is exclusively tubular; hence, urine dipstick findings are minimal since glomerular proteinuria is not present. Hypercalcemia and hyperuricemia are frequently seen. Another kidney disorder in patients with plasma cell myeloma is glomerular amyloidosis with nephrotic syndrome; in these patients, urine dipstick is positive due to glomerular epithelial cell foot-process effacement and albumin "spilling" into the Bowman capsule; hematuria may or may not be present. Other conditions resulting in kidney disease include plasma cell infiltration of the renal parenchyma and hyperviscosity syndrome compromising renal blood flow. The presence of myeloma-related kidney disease does not itself preclude use of contrast dye for imaging studies; standard precautions for the use of intravenous contrast and gadolinium in patients with reduced GFR apply to patients with myeloma-related kidney disease. Therapy for AKI (see Acute Kidney Injury, above) attributed to plasma cell myeloma includes correction of hypercalcemia; volume repletion; and chemotherapy for the underlying malignancy, typically with bortezomib-based agents. Plasmapheresis and hemodialysis are sometimes considered to reduce the burden of circulating free light chains, but results have been equivocal and their use is controversial.

Bridoux F et al. Management of acute kidney injury in symptomatic multiple myeloma. Kidney Int. 2021;99:570. [PMID: 33440212]

Małyszko J et al. KDIGO Controversies Conference on onco-nephrology: kidney disease in hematological malignancies and the burden of cancer after kidney transplantation. Kidney Int. 2020;98:1407. [PMID: 33276867]

SICKLE CELL DISEASE

Kidney disease associated with sickle cell disease is most commonly due to sickling of RBCs in the renal medulla because of low oxygen tension and hypertonicity. Congestion and stasis lead to hemorrhage, interstitial inflammation, and papillary infarcts with resultant necrosis. Clinically, hematuria is common, and proteinuria can be present as well, portending a poorer prognosis; both sickle cell trait and disease are associated with a faster decline in eGFR compared to those without the trait or disease. Damage to renal capillaries also leads to diminished concentrating ability. Isosthenuria (urine osmolality equal to that of serum) is routine, and patients can easily become dehydrated. Sickle cell glomerulopathy is less common but inexorably progresses to ESKD. Its primary clinical manifestation is proteinuria. Treatment centers on control of sickle cell disease and ensuring adequate fluid intake.

Lemes RPG et al. Sickle cell disease and the kidney: pathophysiology and novel biomarkers. Contrib Nephrol. 2021;199:114. [PMID: 34343995]

Olaniran KO et al. Kidney function decline among black patients with sickle cell trait and sickle cell disease: an observational cohort study. J Am Soc Nephrol. 2020;31:393. [PMID: 31810990]

TUBERCULOSIS

Renal tuberculosis usually results from hematogenous spread and is an underdiagnosed entity. Up to 20% of patients with extrapulmonary tuberculosis have urogenital involvement, of which the kidney is most commonly affected. Its classic manifestation is the presence of microscopic pyuria without bacterial growth on urine culture—or "sterile pyuria." More often, other bacteria are also present, and microscopic hematuria may coexist. Urine cultures were once the gold standard for diagnosis, but the advent of urine nucleic acid testing for tuberculosis has increased sensitivity. Characteristic findings on imaging include papillary necrosis and cavitation of the renal parenchyma. Ureteral strictures or calcifications may also be present. Kidney biopsy is not usually needed to confirm the diagnosis but reveals granulomatous inflammation and tubulointerstitial nephritis. Prompt initiation of antituberculosis treatment is indicated, without which progression to ESKD is common due to chronic inflammation and obstruction.

Kamra E et al. Current updates in diagnosis of male urogenital tuberculosis. Expert Rev Anti Infect Ther. 2021;19:1175. [PMID: 33688791]

Kulchavenya E et al. Challenges in urogenital tuberculosis. World J Urol. 2020;38:89. [PMID: 30997530]

Mantica G et al. Genitourinary tuberculosis: a comprehensive review of a neglected manifestation in low-endemic countries. Antibiotics (Basel). 2021;10:1399. [PMID: 34827337]

GOUT & THE KIDNEY

The kidney is the primary organ for excretion of uric acid. Patients with proximal tubular dysfunction have decreased excretion of uric acid and are more prone to gouty arthritis attacks. Depending on the pH and uric acid concentration, deposition can occur in the tubules, the interstitium, or the urinary tract. The more alkaline pH of the interstitium causes urate salt deposition, whereas the acidic environment of the tubules and urinary tract causes uric acid crystal deposition at high concentrations.

Three disorders can develop: (1) uric acid nephrolithiasis, (2) acute uric acid nephropathy, and (3) chronic urate nephropathy. Kidney disease in uric acid nephrolithiasis stems from obstructive uropathy. Acute uric acid nephropathy presents with direct tubulointerstitial toxicity from uric acid crystals and distal tubule obstruction caused by precipitation of uric acid crystals. Chronic urate nephropathy is caused by deposition of urate crystals in the alkaline medium of the interstitium, which leads to fibrosis and atrophy.

Treatment between gouty attacks involves avoidance of food and drugs causing hyperuricemia (see Chapter 20), adequate fluid intake, and urate-lowering therapy (eg, allopurinol or febuxostat). The three disorders mentioned above are seen in both "overproducers" and "underexcretors" of uric acid. The latter situation may seem counterintuitive; however, these patients have acidic urine, which enables precipitation of relatively insoluble uric acid crystals. For those with uric acid nephrolithiasis, fluid intake should exceed 3 L/day, and use of a urinary alkalinizing agent can be considered. Patients with hyperuricemia but no history of gout or uric acid nephrolithiasis have not been shown to benefit from urate-lowering therapy.

Badve SV et al; CKD-FIX Study Investigators. Effects of allopurinol on the progression of chronic kidney disease. N Engl J Med. 2020;382:2504. [PMID: 32579811]

Dalbeth N et al. Gout. Lancet. 2021;397:1843. [PMID: 33798500]

Goldberg A et al. Mini review: reappraisal of uric acid in chronic kidney disease. Am J Nephrol. 2021;52:837. [PMID: 34673651]

NEPHROGENIC SYSTEMIC FIBROSIS

Nephrogenic systemic fibrosis is a multisystem disorder seen exclusively in patients with advanced CKD (primarily with an eGFR less than 15 mL/minute/1.73 m^2, but rarely 15–29 mL/minute/1.73 m^2), AKI, and after kidney transplantation. Histopathologically, there is an increase in dermal spindle cells positive for CD34 and procollagen I. Collagen bundles with mucin and elastic fibers are also noted.

Nephrogenic systemic fibrosis was first recognized in hemodialysis patients in 1997 and has been strongly linked to use of select contrast agents containing gadolinium. Incidence following exposure to historical ("group I") gadolinium agents is approximately 1–4% in the highest risk (ESKD) population and lower in patients with less severe kidney disease. This incidence has decreased over time due to limiting use of gadolinium in patients with CKD and AKI, and the development of safer gadolinium preparations with different molecular structures that have not been associated with NSF ("group II" agents). There is an FDA warning regarding avoidance of group I gadolinium agents for patients with an eGFR less than 30 mL/minute/1.73 m^2.

Clinical Findings

Nephrogenic systemic fibrosis affects several organ systems, including the skin, muscles, lungs, and cardiovascular system. The most common manifestation is a debilitating fibrosing skin disorder that can range from skin-colored to erythematous papules, which coalesce to brawny patches. The skin can be thick and woody in areas and is painful out of proportion to findings on examination.

Treatment

No treatment has proven definitively effective; a preventive approach of avoiding group I gadolinium exposure in high-risk patients is paramount. Case reports and series describe potential benefit of corticosteroids, photopheresis, plasmapheresis, and sodium thiosulfate, but their true efficacy is unknown. CT is preferred to MRI with gadolinium when similar diagnostic information can be gleaned. If gadolinium absolutely must be used in patients on dialysis, practice guidelines recommend using a group II agent at no more than the standard dose. Hemodialysis immediately after exposure to gadolinium previously was advised but is not considered necessary for group II agents.

Weinreb JC et al. Use of intravenous gadolinium-based contrast media in patients with kidney disease: consensus statements from the American College of Radiology and the National Kidney Foundation. Kidney Med. 2021;3:142. [PMID: 33604544]

Rudnick MR et al. Risks and options with gadolinium-based contrast agents in patients with CKD: a review. Am J Kidney Dis. 2021;77:517. [PMID: 32861792]

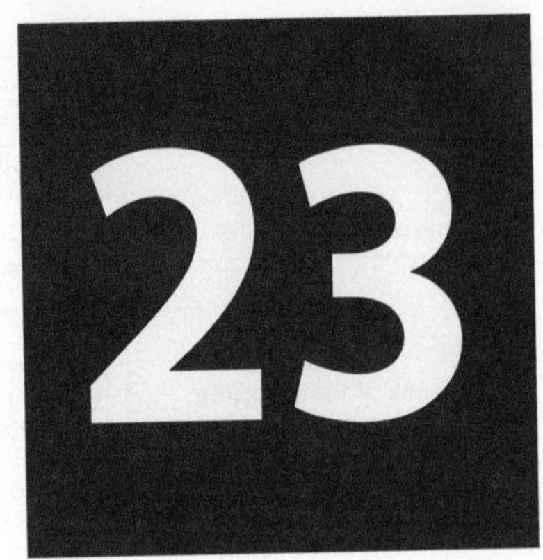

Urologic Disorders

Mathew Sorensen, MD, MS, FACS
Thomas J. Walsh, MD, MS
Brian J. Jordan, MD

HEMATURIA

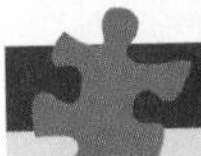

ESSENTIALS OF DIAGNOSIS

- Gross hematuria requires evaluation: the upper urinary tract should be imaged, and the lower tract evaluated by cystoscopy.
- In microscopic hematuria, the workup should be risk stratified.

General Considerations

An **upper tract source** (kidneys and ureters) can be identified in 10% of patients with gross or microscopic hematuria. For upper tract sources, stone disease accounts for 40%, medical kidney disease (medullary sponge kidney, glomerulonephritis, papillary necrosis) for 20%, renal cell carcinoma for 10%, and urothelial cell carcinoma of the ureter or renal pelvis for 5%. Medication ingestion and associated medical problems may provide diagnostic clues. Analgesic use (papillary necrosis), cyclophosphamide (chemical cystitis), antibiotics (interstitial nephritis), diabetes mellitus, sickle cell trait or disease (papillary necrosis), a history of stone disease, or malignancy should all be investigated. The **lower tract source** of gross hematuria (in the absence of infection) is most commonly from bleeding prostatic varices or urothelial carcinoma of the bladder. Microscopic hematuria in men is most commonly from benign prostatic hyperplasia (13%), kidney stones (6%), or urethral stricture (1.4%). The presence of hematuria in patients receiving antiplatelet or anticoagulation therapy cannot be presumed to be due to the medication; a complete evaluation is warranted consisting of upper tract imaging, cystoscopy, and urine cytology **(see Chapter 39 for Bladder Cancer, Cancers of the Ureter & Renal Pelvis, Renal Cell Carcinoma, and Other Primary Tumors of the Kidney)**.

Clinical Findings

A. Symptoms and Signs

If gross hematuria occurs, a description of the timing (initial, terminal, total) may provide a clue to the localization of disease. Associated symptoms (ie, renal colic, irritative voiding symptoms, or constitutional symptoms) should be investigated. The history should be focused on risk factors for urothelial cancer (age, male sex, smoking history, history of gross hematuria, irritative lower urinary tract voiding symptoms, history of cyclophosphamide or ifosfamide chemotherapy, family history of urothelial carcinoma or Lynch syndrome, occupational exposure to benzene chemicals or aromatic amines, history of chronic indwelling foreign body in the urinary tract) and on nonmalignant causes. The physical examination should look for signs of systemic disease (fever, rash, lymphadenopathy, abdominal or pelvic masses) as well as signs of medical kidney disease (hypertension, volume overload). The urologic evaluation may demonstrate an enlarged prostate, flank mass, or urethral disease. The evaluation of patients with hematuria and their risk stratification should not be influenced by whether they are taking any antiplatelet or anticoagulant agents.

B. Laboratory Findings

Initial laboratory investigations include a UA and urine culture. Microhematuria is defined as three or more RBCs per high-power field on a microscopic evaluation of the urine. The degree of microscopic hematuria is important in risk stratification according to the 2020 American Urological Association (AUA) hematuria guidelines (Figure 23–1). A positive dipstick reading for heme merits microscopic examination to confirm or refute the diagnosis of hematuria but is not enough to warrant workup on its own. If UA and culture are suggestive of a UTI, follow-up UA after treatment of the infection is important to ensure resolution of the hematuria. An estimate of kidney function should be obtained since renal insufficiency may influence the methods of further evaluation and management (eg, ability to obtain contrast imaging) of patients with hematuria. Urine cytology and other urinary-based markers are not routinely recommended in the evaluation of asymptomatic microscopic hematuria.

C. Risk Stratification

Following initial evaluation, clinicians should categorize patients with microscopic hematuria as low, intermediate, or high risk for a urothelial malignancy (Figure 23–1).

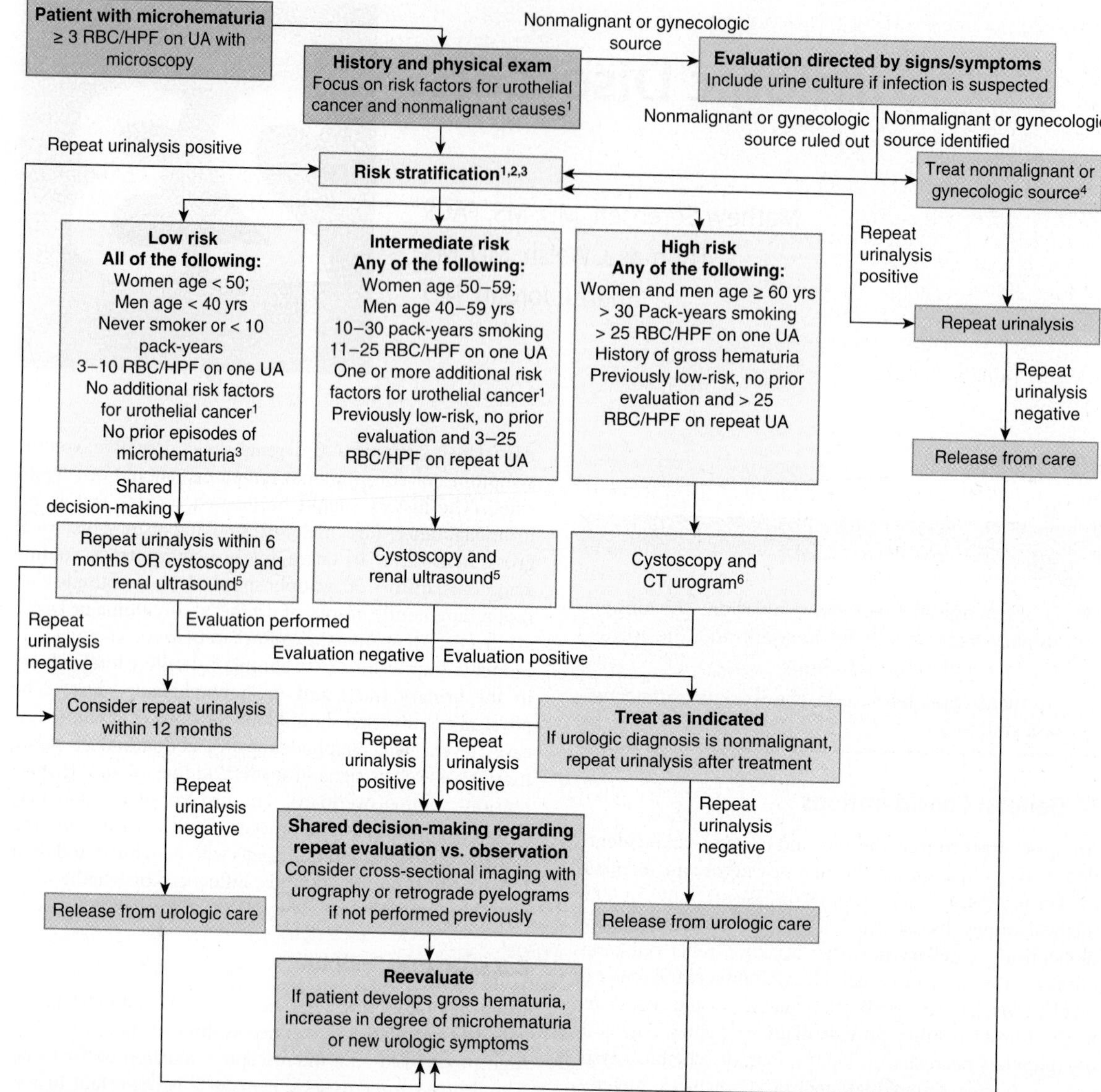

1. Main risk factors for urothelial cancer are those in the AUA risk stratification system (age, male sex, smoking, degree of microhematuria and history of gross hematuria). Additional risk factors for urothelial carcinoma include but are not limited to irritative lower urinary tract voiding symptoms, history of cyclophosphamide or ifosfamide chemotherapy, family history of urothelial carcinoma or Lynch syndrome, occupational exposures to benzene chemicals or aromatic amines, history of chronic indwelling foreign body in the urinary tract.
2. If medical kidney disease is suspected, consider nephrologic evaluation, but pursue concurrent risk-based urological evaluation.
3. Patients may be low-risk at first presentation with microhematuria, but may be considered intermediate- or high-risk if found to have persistent microhematuria.
4. There are nonmalignant and gynecologic sources of hematuria that do not require treatment and/or may confound the diagnosis of microhematuria. Clinicians can consider catheterized urine specimen in women with vaginal atrophy or pelvic organ prolapse. Clinicians must use careful judgment and patient engagement to decide whether to pursue microhematuria evaluation in the setting of chronic conditions that do not require treatment, such as the aforementioned gynecologic conditions, nonobstructing stones or BPH.
5. Clinician may perform cross-sectional imaging with urography or retrograde pyelograms if hematuria persists after negative renal ultrasound.
6. If contraindications to CT urogram, MR urogram or noncontrast imaging plus retrograde pyelograms.

▲ **Figure 23–1. Microscopic hematuria: algorithmic approach to risk stratification of patients as low risk, intermediate risk, and high risk for urothelial malignancy. HPF, high-powered field.** (Reproduced with permission from Barocas DA, Boorjian SA, Alvarez RD, et al. Microhematuria: AUA/SUFU Guideline. J Urol. 2020;204(4):778-786. doi:10.1097/JU.0000000000001297s.)

D. Evaluation

Patients with gross hematuria should have both complete evaluation of the upper tract by a CT-intravenous pyelogram (CT-IVP), or a magnetic resonance urogram (MR-urogram) with and without contrast, and evaluation of the bladder by cystoscopy. No imaging study adequately evaluates the bladder.

Low-risk patients with microscopic hematuria should undertake a shared decision-making approach with their clinician to decide between repeat urinalyses over the next 6 months or proceeding immediately with cystoscopy and renal ultrasound. If microscopic hematuria persists on a repeat UA, then patients who did not initially undergo cystoscopy should be reclassified as intermediate- or high-risk and undergo both upper tract imaging according to their risk group, and lower tract evaluation by cystoscopy.

Intermediate-risk patients should undergo both upper tract imaging with renal ultrasound and lower tract evaluation by cystoscopy.

High-risk patients should undergo upper tract evaluation with CT-IVP (preferred), MR-urogram (if CT-IVP contraindicated), and cystoscopic evaluation of the bladder. If there are contraindications to CT-IVP and MR-urogram, clinicians may perform noncontrast axial imaging along with retrograde pyelography at the time of cystoscopy.

Follow-Up

In patients with negative hematuria evaluations, it is typically recommended that a UA with microscopy be repeated at 6–12 months. Patients with a negative follow-up UA require no further evaluation. If microscopic hematuria persists or recurs on follow-up urinalyses, then providers should engage patients with shared decision-making regarding repeat evaluation. However, patients who develop gross hematuria or increased severity of microscopic hematuria should be referred for repeat upper and lower tract evaluation.

When to Refer

In the absence of a clear benign etiology (such as an infection, menstruation, vigorous exercise, acute stone event, medical renal disease, viral illness, trauma, or recent urologic procedure), hematuria (either gross or microscopic) requires evaluation.

Barocas DA et al. Microhematuria: AUA/SUFU Guideline. J Urol. 2020;204:778. [PMID: 32698717]

Judge C et al. Management of patients with microhematuria. JAMA. 2021;326:563. [PMID: 34374732]

Peterson LM. Hematuria. Prim Care. 2019;46:265. [PMID: 31030828]

Yecies T et al. Evaluation of the risks and benefits of computed tomography urography for assessment of gross hematuria. Urology. 2019;133:40. [PMID: 31255539]

GENITOURINARY TRACT INFECTIONS

UTIs are among the most common entities encountered in medical practice. In acute infections, a single pathogen is usually found, whereas two or more pathogens are often seen in chronic infections. Coliform bacteria are responsible for most non-nosocomial, uncomplicated UTIs, with *Escherichia coli* being the most common. Such infections typically are sensitive to a wide variety of orally administered antibiotics and respond quickly. Nosocomial infections often are due to more resistant pathogens and may require parenteral antibiotics. Renal infections are of particular concern because if they are inadequately treated, loss of kidney function may result. A urine culture is recommended for patients with suspected UTI and ideally should be obtained before the initiation of antibiotic therapy. Previously, a colony count greater than 10^5/mL was considered the criterion for UTI; however, up to 50% of women with symptomatic infections may have lower counts. In addition, the presence of pyuria correlates poorly with the diagnosis of UTI, and thus UA alone is not adequate for diagnosis. With respect to treatment, tissue infections (pyelonephritis, prostatitis) require therapy for 1–2 weeks, while mucosal infections (cystitis) require only 1–3 days of therapy.

1. Acute Cystitis

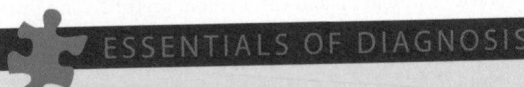

- Irritative voiding symptoms.
- Patient usually afebrile.
- Positive urine culture; blood cultures may also be positive.

General Considerations

Acute cystitis is an infection of the bladder, most commonly due to the coliform bacteria (especially *E coli*) and occasionally gram-positive bacteria (enterococci). The route of infection is typically ascending from the urethra. Viral cystitis due to adenovirus is sometimes seen in children but is rare in immunocompetent adults. Uncomplicated cystitis in men is rare and implies a pathologic process such as infected stones, prostatitis, or chronic urinary retention requiring further investigation.

Clinical Findings

A. Symptoms and Signs

Irritative voiding symptoms (frequency, urgency, dysuria) and suprapubic discomfort are common. Women may experience gross hematuria, and symptoms may often appear following sexual intercourse. Physical examination may elicit suprapubic tenderness, but examination is often unremarkable. Systemic toxicity is absent.

B. Laboratory Findings

UA shows pyuria, bacteriuria, and varying degrees of hematuria. The degree of pyuria and bacteriuria does not necessarily correlate with the severity of symptoms. Urine culture is positive for the offending organism, but colony counts exceeding 10^5/mL are not required for the diagnosis. Patients with asymptomatic bacteriuria or colonization are expected to have positive urine cultures but do not require treatment except in pregnant women. Patients with long-term urinary catheters (indwelling urinary [Foley] or suprapubic catheter) or urostomy urinary diversions are expected to be colonized with bacteria, and thus, UA and urine culture are most helpful in directing therapy rather than determining whether symptomatic infection exists.

C. Imaging

Because uncomplicated cystitis is rare in men, elucidation of the underlying problem with appropriate investigations, such as abdominal ultrasonography, postvoid residual testing, and cystoscopy, is warranted. Follow-up imaging using CT scanning is warranted if pyelonephritis, recurrent infections, or anatomic abnormalities are suspected.

Differential Diagnosis

In women, infectious processes such as vulvovaginitis and pelvic inflammatory disease can usually be distinguished by pelvic examination and UA. In men, urethritis and prostatitis may be distinguished by physical examination (urethral discharge or prostatic tenderness).

Noninfectious causes of cystitis-like symptoms include pelvic irradiation, chemotherapy (cyclophosphamide), bladder carcinoma, interstitial cystitis, voiding dysfunction disorders, bladder irritants, and psychosomatic disorders.

Prevention

The risk of developing a UTI can be reduced by drinking plenty of fluid and completely emptying the bladder frequently. Women in whom UTIs tend to develop after intercourse should be advised to void before, and especially after intercourse, and may benefit from a postcoital single-dose of antibiotic. Postmenopausal women with recurrent UTIs (three or more episodes per year) treated with vaginal estrogen either as a cream or ring have a significant reduction in infections. Daily cranberry tablets may reduce the risk of cystitis, although data are conflicting. Prophylactic antibiotics are generally discouraged. Before institution of antibiotic prophylaxis, a thorough urologic evaluation is warranted to exclude any anatomic abnormality (eg, stones, reflux, fistula). An initial course of 6–12 months of prophylactic antibiotics can be offered, although the benefits of prophylactic antibiotics should be weighed against the risks associated with expected bacterial resistance.

The risk of acquiring a catheter-associated UTI in hospitalized patients can be minimized by using indwelling catheters only when necessary, implementing systems to ensure removal of catheters when no longer needed, using antimicrobial catheters in high-risk patients, using external collection devices (condom catheters) in select men, identifying significant postvoid residuals by ultrasound, maintaining proper insertion techniques, and utilizing alternatives such as intermittent catheterization.

Treatment

Uncomplicated cystitis in women can be treated with short-term antimicrobial therapy, which consists of single-dose therapy or 1–7 days of therapy. Fosfomycin, nitrofurantoin, and trimethoprim-sulfamethoxazole are the medications of choice for uncomplicated cystitis (Table 23–1). The US FDA advises restricting fluoroquinolone use for uncomplicated infections. Local patterns of bacterial resistance should be consulted to identify best treatment options. Some antibiotics may be ineffective because of the emergence of resistant organisms. A review of the literature proposed that acute uncomplicated cystitis in women can be diagnosed without office evaluation or urine culture, and that appropriate first-line therapies include trimethoprim-sulfamethoxazole (160/800 mg twice daily for 3 days), nitrofurantoin (100 mg twice daily for 5–7 days), or fosfomycin trometamol (3 g single dose). In men, uncomplicated UTI is rare; thus, the duration of antibiotic therapy depends on the underlying etiology. Hot sitz baths or urinary analgesics (phenazopyridine, 200 mg orally three times daily) may provide additional symptomatic relief. Postmenopausal women with recurrent cystitis can be treated with vaginal estrogen cream 0.5 g nightly for 2 weeks and then twice weekly thereafter.

Prognosis

Infections typically respond rapidly to therapy, and failure to respond suggests resistance to the selected medication or anatomic abnormalities requiring further investigation.

When to Refer

- Suspicion or radiographic evidence of anatomic abnormality.
- Evidence of urolithiasis.
- Recurrent cystitis due to bacterial persistence.

Babikar A et al. Fosfomycin for treatment of multidrug-resistant pathogens causing urinary tract infection: a real-world perspective and review of the literature. Diagn Microbiol Infect Dis. 2019;95:114856. [PMID: 31307867]

Ferrante KL et al. Vaginal estrogen for the prevention of recurrent urinary tract infection in postmenopausal women: a randomized clinical trial. Female Pelvic Med Reconstr Surg. 2021;27:112. [PMID: 31232721]

Gill CM et al. A review of nonantibiotic agents to prevent urinary tract infections in older women. J Am Med Dir Assoc. 2020;21:46. [PMID: 31227473]

Kim DK et al. Reappraisal of the treatment duration of antibiotic regimens for acute uncomplicated cystitis in adult women: a systematic review and network meta-analysis of 61 randomised clinical trials. Lancet Infect Dis. 2020;20:1080. [PMID: 32446327]

Lee RA et al. Appropriate use of short-course antibiotics in common infections: best practice advice from the American College of Physicians. Ann Intern Med. 2021;174:822. [PMID: 33819054]

Nicolle LE et al. Clinical practice guideline for the management of asymptomatic bacteriuria: 2019 update by the Infectious Diseases Society of America. Clin Infect Dis. 2019;68:1611. [PMID: 31506700]

2. Acute Pyelonephritis

ESSENTIALS OF DIAGNOSIS

- Fever.
- Flank pain.
- Irritative voiding symptoms.
- Positive urine culture.

Table 23–1. Empiric therapy for UTIs.

Diagnosis	Antibiotic	Route	Duration	Cost per Duration Noted[1]
Acute cystitis[a]				
	First-line:			
	Trimethoprim-sulfamethoxazole, 160/800 mg, (one DS tablet) every 12 hours[2]	Oral	3 days	$2.25
	Nitrofurantoin (macrocrystals), 100 mg every 12 hours	Oral	5 days	$27.70
	Fosfomycin, 3 g packet once	Oral	1 day	$72.00
	Second-line:			
	Ciprofloxacin, 250 mg every 12 hours[3]	Oral	3 days	$26.64
	Levofloxacin, 250–500 mg daily[3]	Oral	3 days	$46.80
	Alternative agents:			
	Cephalexin, 500 mg every 6–12 hours	Oral	7 days	$33.88
	Amoxicillin/clavulanate, 500/125 mg every 12 hours	Oral	3 days	$10.16
	Cefpodoxime, 100 mg every 12 hours	Oral	3 days	$40.44
Acute pyelonephritis[a]				
	Hospitalized:			
	Ampicillin, 1 g every 6 hours, plus gentamicin, 1 mg/kg every 8 hours	Intravenous	14 days	$153.11, not including intravenous supplies
	Ceftriaxone, 1 g daily	Intravenous	14 days	$25.62
	Ciprofloxacin, 400 mg every 12 hours[3]	Intravenous	14 days	$77.28
	Non-hospitalized:			
	Initial intravenous dose[4]:			
	Ceftriaxone, 1 g	Intravenous	Once	$1.83
	Ciprofloxacin, 400 mg[3]	Intravenous	Once	$2.76
	Gentamicin, 5 mg/kg	Intravenous	Once	$4.29
	Followed by one of these oral regimens:			
	Ciprofloxacin, 500 mg every 12 hours[3]	Oral	7 days	$4.48
	Levofloxacin, 750 mg daily[3]	Oral	5 days	$123.05
	Trimethoprim-sulfamethoxazole, 160/800 mg (one DS tablet) every 12 hours[2]	Oral	14 days	$10.44
Acute bacterial prostatitis[b]				
	Hospitalized:			
	Ampicillin, 2 g every 6 hours, plus gentamicin, 1.5 mg/kg every 8 hours	Intravenous	Until afebrile	$15.22/day, not including intravenous supplies
	Followed by one of these outpatient oral regimens:			
	Trimethoprim-sulfamethoxazole, 160/800 mg (one DS tablet) every 12 hours[2]	Oral	3 weeks	$15.67/3 weeks
	Ciprofloxacin, 250–500 mg every 12 hours[3]	Oral	3 weeks	$13.44/3 weeks

(continued)

Table 23–1. Empiric therapy for UTIs. (continued)

Diagnosis	Antibiotic	Route	Duration	Cost per Duration Noted[1]
Chronic bacterial prostatitis[b]				
	First-line:			
	Ciprofloxacin, 500 mg every 12 hours[3]	Oral	1–3 months	$19.20/month
	Levofloxacin, 750 mg daily[3]	Oral	28 days	$689.08
	Second-line:			
	Doxycycline, 100 mg twice daily	Oral	4–12 weeks	$74.52/month
	Azithromycin, 500 mg daily	Oral	4–12 weeks	$81.98/month
	Clarithromycin, 500 mg daily	Oral	4–12 weeks	$117.00/month
Acute epididymitis[c]				
Sexually transmitted (under age 35)	Ceftriaxone, 500 mg as single dose, **plus** Doxycycline, 100 mg every 12 hours	Intramuscular Oral	Once 10 days	$1.16/500 mg $24.84 (10 days)
Sexually transmitted in men who practice insertive anal sex	Ceftriaxone, 250 mg as single dose **plus** Levofloxacin, 500 mg daily[3] **or**	Intramuscular Oral	Once 10 days	$0.90/250 mg $156.00 (10 days)
Non–sexually transmitted, usually enteric organisms (over age 35)	Levofloxacin, 500 mg daily[3]	Oral	10 days	$156.00 (10 days)

[1]Average wholesale price (AWP, for AB-rated generic when available) for quantity listed. Source: IBM Micromedex® Red Book (electronic version) IBM Watson Health, Greenwood Village, Colorado, USA. Available at https://www-micromedexsolutions-com.proxy.hsl.ucdenver.edu/ (cited: March 27, 2022). AWP may not accurately represent the actual pharmacy cost because wide contractual variations exist among institutions.
[2]Increasing resistance noted (up to 20%).
[3]FDA advises restricting fluoroquinolone use for some uncomplicated infections, including uncomplicated UTIs, because of mental health side effects including disturbances in attention, disorientation, agitation, nervousness, memory impairment, and delirium; musculoskeletal side effects of risks of tendinitis and tendon rupture; neuromuscular side effects of peripheral neuropathy and worsening of myasthenia gravis; and endocrine side effect of coma from hypoglycemia.
[4]Infectious Diseases Society of America (IDSA) recommends an initial 24-hour intravenous dose of antibiotic when local resistance of the selected oral regimen exceeds 10%. Please refer to local antibiograms.
Sources:
[a]Treatment regimens based upon Gupta K et al. Treatment of acute uncomplicated cystitis and pyelonephritis in women: a 2010 update by the Infectious Diseases Society of America and European Society for Microbiology and Infectious Diseases. Clin Infect Dis. 2011;52:e103; and Lee RA et al; Scientific Medical Policy Committee of the American College of Physicians. Appropriate use of short-course antibiotics in common infections: Best Practice Advice From the American College of Physicians. Ann Intern Med. 2021;174:822.
[b]Treatment regimens based upon Sharp VJ et al. Prostatitis: diagnosis and treatment. Am Fam Physician. 2010;82:397.
[c]Treatment regimens based upon Workowski KA et al; Centers for Disease Control and Prevention. Sexually transmitted diseases treatment guidelines, 2021. MMWR Recomm Rep. 2021;70:1.

General Considerations

Acute pyelonephritis is an infectious inflammatory disease involving the kidney parenchyma and renal pelvis. Gram-negative bacteria are the most common causative agents including *E coli*, *Proteus*, *Klebsiella*, *Enterobacter*, and *Pseudomonas*. Gram-positive bacteria are less commonly seen but include *Enterococcus faecalis* and *Staphylococcus aureus*. The infection usually ascends from the lower urinary tract—with the exception of *S aureus*, which usually is spread by a hematogenous route.

Clinical Findings

A. Symptoms and Signs

Symptoms include fever, flank pain, shaking chills, and irritative voiding symptoms (urgency, frequency, dysuria). Associated nausea and vomiting and diarrhea are common. Signs include fever and tachycardia. Costovertebral angle tenderness is usually pronounced.

B. Laboratory Findings

CBC shows leukocytosis and a left shift. UA shows pyuria, bacteriuria, and varying degrees of hematuria. White cell casts may be seen. Urine culture demonstrates growth of the offending organism, and blood culture may also be positive.

C. Imaging

In complicated pyelonephritis, renal ultrasound may show hydronephrosis from a stone or other source of obstruction. CT scan may demonstrate decreased perfusion of the kidney or focal areas within the kidney and nonspecific perinephric fat stranding.

Differential Diagnosis

The differential diagnosis includes acute cystitis or a lower urinary source. Acute intra-abdominal disease such as appendicitis, cholecystitis, pancreatitis, or diverticulitis must be distinguished from pyelonephritis. A normal UA is usually seen in GI disorders; however, on occasion, inflammation from adjacent bowel (appendicitis or diverticulitis) may result in hematuria or sterile pyuria. Abnormal liver biochemical tests or elevated amylase levels may assist in the differentiation. Lower-lobe pneumonia is distinguishable by the abnormal chest radiograph.

In men, the main differential diagnosis for acute pyelonephritis also includes acute epididymitis and acute prostatitis. Physical examination and the location of the pain should permit this distinction.

Complications

Sepsis with shock can occur with acute pyelonephritis. In diabetic patients, emphysematous pyelonephritis resulting from gas-producing organisms may be life-threatening if not adequately treated. Healthy adults usually recover complete kidney function, yet if coexistent kidney disease is present, scarring or chronic pyelonephritis may result. Inadequate therapy could result in abscess formation.

Treatment

Urine and blood cultures are obtained to identify the causative agent and to determine antimicrobial sensitivity. In the inpatient setting, intravenous ampicillin and an aminoglycoside are initiated prior to obtaining sensitivity results (Table 23–1). In the outpatient setting, empiric therapy may be initiated (Table 23–1). Antibiotics are adjusted according to sensitivities. If local antibiograms demonstrate local resistance rates for the oral regimen exceed 10%, an initial 24-hour intravenous dose of antibiotic is required. Fevers may persist for up to 72 hours even with appropriate antibiotics; failure to respond within 48 hours warrants imaging (CT or ultrasound) to exclude complicating factors that may require intervention (such as a perinephric abscess or an obstructing stone). Catheter drainage may be necessary in the face of urinary retention and nephrostomy drainage if there is ureteral obstruction. In inpatients, intravenous antibiotics are continued for 24 hours after the fever resolves, and oral antibiotics are then given to complete a 14-day course of therapy.

Prognosis

With prompt diagnosis and appropriate treatment, acute pyelonephritis carries a good prognosis. Complicating factors, underlying kidney disease, and increasing patient age may lead to a less favorable outcome.

When to Refer

- Evidence of complicating factors (urolithiasis, obstruction).
- Failure of clinical improvement in 48 hours.

When to Admit

- Severe infections or complicating factors, evidence of sepsis, or need for parenteral antibiotics.
- Need for radiographic imaging or drainage of urinary tract obstruction.

Bader MS et al. Treatment of urinary tract infections in the era of antimicrobial resistance and new antimicrobial agents. Postgrad Med. 2020;132:234. [PMID: 31608743]

Johnson JR et al. Acute pyelonephritis in adults. N Engl J Med. 2018;378:1162. [PMID: 29562155]

Kolman KB. Cystitis and pyelonephritis: diagnosis, treatment and prevention. Prim Care. 2019;46:191. [PMID: 31030820]

Wagenlehner FME et al; EPIC Study Group. Once-daily plazomicin for complicated urinary tract infections. N Engl J Med. 2019;380:729. [PMID: 30786187]

3. Acute Bacterial Prostatitis

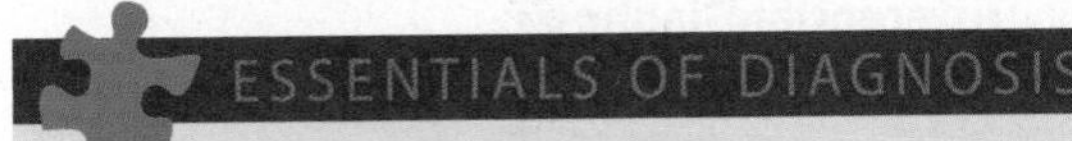

- Fever.
- Irritative voiding symptoms.
- Perineal or suprapubic pain; exquisite tenderness common on rectal examination.
- Positive urine culture.

General Considerations

Acute bacterial prostatitis is usually caused by gram-negative rods, especially *E coli* and *Pseudomonas* species, and less commonly by gram-positive organisms (eg, enterococci). The most likely routes of infection include ascent up the urethra and reflux of infected urine into the prostatic ducts. Lymphatic and hematogenous routes are probably rare.

Clinical Findings

A. Symptoms and Signs

Perineal, sacral, or suprapubic pain, fever, and irritative voiding are common. Varying degrees of obstructive symptoms may occur as the acutely inflamed prostate swells, which may lead to urinary retention. High fevers and a warm and often exquisitely tender prostate are detected on examination. Care should be taken to perform a gentle rectal examination, since vigorous manipulations may result in septicemia. Prostatic massage is contraindicated.

B. Laboratory Findings

CBC shows leukocytosis and a left shift. UA shows pyuria, bacteriuria, and varying degrees of hematuria. Urine or expressed prostatic secretions cultures will demonstrate the offending pathogen (Table 23–2).

Table 23–2. Clinical characteristics of prostatitis and chronic pelvic pain syndrome.

Findings	Acute Bacterial Prostatitis	Chronic Bacterial Prostatitis	Chronic Nonbacterial Prostatitis	Chronic Pelvic Pain Syndrome
Fever	+	–	–	–
UA	+	–	–	–
Expressed prostate secretions	Contraindicated	+ WBC + Culture	+ WBC – Culture	– WBC – Culture
Postprostatic massage urine specimen	Contraindicated	+ Culture	– Culture	– Culture

C. Imaging

Acute prostatitis can progress to prostatic abscess and a pelvic CT or transrectal ultrasound is indicated in patients who do not respond to antibiotics in 24–48 hours.

Differential Diagnosis

Acute pyelonephritis or acute epididymitis should be distinguishable by the location of pain as well as by physical examination. Acute diverticulitis is occasionally confused with acute prostatitis; however, the history and UA should permit clear distinction. Urinary retention from prostatic enlargement is distinguishable by initial or follow-up rectal examination and postvoid residual bladder scan.

Treatment

Hospitalization may be required, and parenteral antibiotics (ampicillin and aminoglycoside) should be initiated until organism sensitivities are available (Table 23–1). After the patient is afebrile for 24–48 hours, oral antibiotics (eg, quinolones if organism is sensitive) are used to complete 4–6 weeks of therapy. If urinary retention develops, an in-and-out catheterization to relieve the initial obstruction or short-term (12 hours) small indwelling urinary catheter is appropriate.

Prognosis

Acute bacterial prostatitis is relatively simple to treat, since bacteria are eradicated with appropriate antibiotic therapy. Progression to chronic bacterial prostatitis is rare.

When to Refer

- Evidence of urinary retention.
- Evidence of chronic prostatitis.

When to Admit

- Signs of sepsis.
- Need for surgical drainage of bladder or prostatic abscess.

Kwan ACF et al. Fosfomycin for bacterial prostatitis: a review. Int J Antimicrob Agents. 2020;56:106106. [PMID: 32721595]

Lupo F et al. Is bacterial prostatitis a urinary tract infection? Nat Rev Urol. 2019;16:203. [PMID: 30700862]

Shakur A et al. Prostatitis: imaging appearances and diagnostic considerations. Clin Radiol. 2021;76:416. [PMID: 33632522]

Xiong S et al. Pharmacological interventions for bacterial prostatitis. Front Pharmacol. 2020;11:504. [PMID: 32425775]

4. Chronic Bacterial Prostatitis

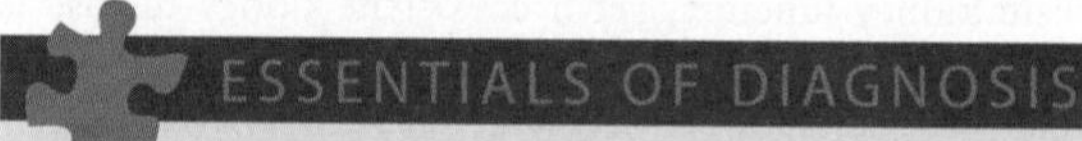

- Irritative voiding symptoms.
- Perineal or suprapubic discomfort, often dull and poorly localized.
- Abnormal expressed prostatic secretions and positive culture.

General Considerations

Although chronic bacterial prostatitis may evolve from acute bacterial prostatitis or recurrent UTI, over half of affected men have no history of acute infection. Gram-negative rods are the most common etiologic agents, but only one gram-positive organism (*Enterococcus*) is associated with chronic infection. Routes of infection are the same as discussed for acute infection.

Clinical Findings

A. Symptoms and Signs

Clinical manifestations are variable. Most patients have varying degrees of irritative voiding symptoms, urethral pain, and obstructive urinary symptoms. Low back and perineal pain are common. Many patients (25–43%) report a history of UTIs. Physical examination is often unremarkable, although the prostate may feel normal, boggy, or indurated. A postvoid residual urine volume should be measured to evaluate for urinary retention.

B. Laboratory Findings

UA is normal unless a secondary cystitis is present. Expressed prostatic secretions or a postprostatic massage voided urine or both demonstrate increased numbers of leukocytes (greater than 5–10 per high-power field) and bacterial growth when cultured (Table 23–2). Culture of the secretions and the postprostatic massage urine specimen is necessary to make the diagnosis. Leukocyte and bacterial counts from expressed prostatic secretions do not correlate with severity of symptoms. If no organisms are identified on culture, then nonbacterial prostatitis, chronic pelvic pain, or interstitial cystitis should be suspected.

C. Imaging

Imaging tests are typically not necessary.

Differential Diagnosis

Chronic urethritis may mimic chronic prostatitis, although cultures of the fractionated urine may localize the source of infection to the initial specimen, which comes from the urethra. Cystitis may be secondary to prostatitis, but urine samples after prostatic massage may localize the infection to the prostate. Other chronic prostatic conditions, such as nonbacterial prostatitis, chronic pelvic pain, or interstitial cystitis, are distinguished from chronic bacterial prostatitis by examination and culture of prostatic secretions and postprostatic massage urine sample. Anal disease may share some of the symptoms of prostatitis, but physical examination should distinguish between the two.

Treatment

As in acute prostatitis, if patients are febrile or systemically ill, they may require admission and initial intravenous therapy with broad-spectrum antibiotics, such as ampicillin plus gentamicin, a third-generation cephalosporin, or a fluoroquinolone (Table 23–1). Therapy would then continue with oral trimethoprim-sulfamethoxazole, fluoroquinolone, or extended-spectrum beta-lactamase antibiotic based on culture and sensitivities of expressed prostatic secretion or postprostatic massage urine. The optimal duration of therapy remains controversial, ranging from 4 to 6 weeks. Symptomatic relief may be provided by anti-inflammatory agents (indomethacin, ibuprofen), hot sitz baths, and alpha-blockers (tamsulosin, alfuzosin, silodosin).

Prognosis

Chronic bacterial prostatitis may be recurrent, can be difficult to cure, and often requires repeated courses of therapeutic antibiotics.

When to Refer

- Persistent symptoms.
- Consideration of enrollment in clinical trials.

Su ZT et al. Management of chronic bacterial prostatitis. Curr Urol Rep. 2020;21:29. [PMID: 32488742]

Zaidi N et al. Management of chronic prostatitis. Curr Urol Rep. 2018;19:88. [PMID: 30167899]

5. Nonbacterial Chronic Prostatitis/Chronic Pelvic Pain Syndrome

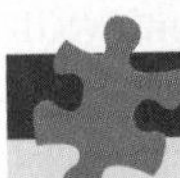

ESSENTIALS OF DIAGNOSIS

- Irritative voiding symptoms.
- Perineal or suprapubic discomfort, similar to that of chronic bacterial prostatitis.
- Presence of WBCs in expressed prostatic secretions but negative culture.

General Considerations

Nonbacterial chronic prostatitis and chronic pelvic pain syndromes are incompletely understood with symptoms due to interrelated cascade of inflammatory, immunologic, endocrine, muscular, neuropathic, and psychologic mechanisms. There are a variety of subtypes based on the most pronounced symptoms. Chronic perineal, suprapubic, or pelvic pain is the most common presenting symptom, although men may report pain in the testes, groin, and low back. Pain during or after ejaculation is one of the most prominent and bothersome symptoms in many patients. Psychosocial factors (depression, anxiety, catastrophizing, poor social support, stress) also likely play an important role in the exacerbation of chronic pelvic pain symptoms. Because the cause of nonbacterial prostatitis remains unknown, the diagnosis is usually one of exclusion, and treatment may require multimodal therapy. Quality of life is greatly decreased for many patients with chronic nonbacterial prostatitis and chronic pelvic pain syndrome.

Clinical Findings

A. Symptoms and Signs

The clinical presentation is identical to that of chronic bacterial prostatitis; however, no history of UTIs is typically present. The National Institutes of Health Chronic Prostatitis Symptom Index (NIH-CPSI) has been validated to quantify symptoms of chronic nonbacterial prostatitis or chronic pelvic pain syndrome.

B. Laboratory Findings

Increased numbers of leukocytes are typically seen in expressed prostatic secretions, but cultures of both expressed prostatic secretions and postprostatic urine specimens are negative.

Differential Diagnosis

The major distinction is from chronic bacterial prostatitis. The absence of positive cultures makes the distinction (Table 23–2). In older men with irritative voiding symptoms and negative cultures, bladder cancer must be excluded. Urinary cytologic examination and cystoscopy are warranted.

Treatment

Multimodal therapy is recommended according to the various modes of patient presentation. Patients with voiding symptoms are treated with alpha-blockers (tamsulosin, alfuzosin, silodosin). Antibiotics are used to treat newly diagnosed, antimicrobial-naive patients. Psychosocial disorders are treated with cognitive behavioral therapy, antidepressants, anxiolytics, and, if necessary, referral to mental health specialists. Neuropathic pain is treated with gabapentinoids, amitriptyline, neuromodulation, acupuncture, and if necessary, referral to a pain management specialist (see Chapter 5). Pelvic floor muscle dysfunction may respond to diazepam, biofeedback, physical therapy (Kegel exercises), pelvic shock wave lithotripsy, and heat therapy. Sexual dysfunction with pain is treated with sexual therapy and phosphodiesterase-5 inhibitors (avanafil, sildenafil, tadalafil, vardenafil). Surgery is not recommended for chronic prostatitis.

Prognosis

Annoying, recurrent symptoms are common, but serious sequelae have not been identified.

Doiron RC et al. Male CP/CPPS: where do we stand? World J Urol. 2019;37:1015. [PMID: 30864007]

Doiron RC et al. Management of chronic prostatitis/chronic pelvic pain syndrome. Can Urol Assoc J. 2018;12:S161. [PMID: 29875042]

Doiron RC et al. The evolving clinical picture of chronic prostatitis/chronic pelvic pain syndrome (CP/CPPS): a look at 1310 patients over 16 years. Can Urol Assoc J. 2018;12:196. [PMID: 29485036]

Franco JVA et al. Non-pharmacological interventions for treating chronic prostatitis/chronic pelvic pain syndrome. Cochrane Database Syst Rev. 2018;1:CD012551. Update in: Cochrane Database Syst Rev 2018;5:CD012551. [PMID: 29372565]

Franco JVA et al. Pharmacological interventions for treating chronic prostatitis/chronic pelvic pain syndrome: a Cochrane systematic review. BJU Int. 2020;125:490. [PMID: 31899937]

Pena VN et al Diagnostic and management strategies for patients with chronic prostatitis and chronic pelvic pain syndrome. Drugs Aging. 2021;38:845. [PMID: 34586623]

6. Acute Epididymitis

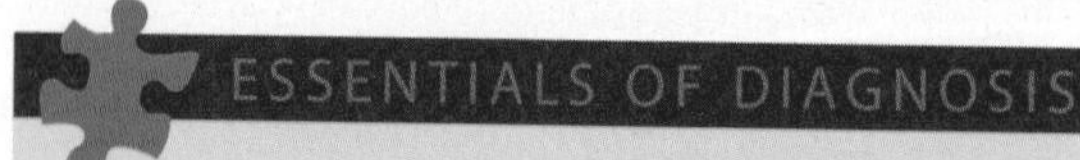

- Fever.
- Irritative voiding symptoms.
- Painful enlargement of epididymis.

General Considerations

Most cases of acute epididymitis are infectious and can be divided into one of two categories that have different age distributions and etiologic agents. **Sexually transmitted forms** typically occur in men under age 35 years, are associated with urethritis, and result from *Chlamydia trachomatis* or *Neisseria gonorrhoeae*. **Men who practice insertive anal intercourse** may have acute epididymitis from sexually transmitted and enteric organisms. **Non–sexually transmitted forms** typically occur in men aged 35 years or older, are associated with UTIs and prostatitis, and are caused by enteric gram-negative rods. The route of infection is probably via the urethra to the ejaculatory duct and then down the vas deferens to the epididymis. Amiodarone has been associated with self-limited epididymitis in a dose-dependent phenomenon.

Clinical Findings

A. Symptoms and Signs

Symptoms may follow chronic dysfunctional voiding, urinary retention, sexual activity, or trauma. Associated symptoms of urethritis (pain at the tip of the penis and urethral discharge) or cystitis (irritative voiding symptoms) may occur. Pain develops in the scrotum and may radiate along the spermatic cord or to the flank. Scrotal swelling and tenderness are usually apparent. Severe cases may develop systemic symptoms such as fever. Early in the course, the epididymis may be distinguishable from the testis; however, later the two may appear as one enlarged, tender mass. A reactive hydrocele may develop. The prostate may be tender on rectal examination.

B. Laboratory Findings

A CBC shows leukocytosis and a left shift. In the sexually transmitted variety, Gram staining of a smear of urethral discharge may be diagnostic of gram-negative intracellular diplococci (*N gonorrhoeae*). White cells without visible organisms on urethral smear signify nongonococcal urethritis, and *C trachomatis* is the most likely responsible pathogen. In the non–sexually transmitted variety, UA shows pyuria, bacteriuria, and varying degrees of hematuria. Urine cultures will demonstrate the offending pathogen.

C. Imaging

Scrotal ultrasound may aid in the diagnosis if examination is difficult because of the presence of a large hydrocele or because questions exist regarding the diagnosis.

Differential Diagnosis

Tumors generally cause painless enlargement of the testis. UA is negative, and examination reveals a normal epididymis. Scrotal ultrasound is helpful to define the pathology. Testicular torsion usually occurs in prepubertal males but is occasionally seen in young adults. Acute onset of symptoms and a negative UA favor testicular torsion or torsion of one of the testicular or epididymal appendages. Prehn sign (elevation of the scrotum improves pain from epididymitis) may be suggestive but is not reliable in its diagnosis. A distal ureteral stone often presents with referred pain into the ipsilateral groin and scrotum, but the scrotum is not tender to palpation and a scrotal ultrasound is normal.

Treatment

Bed rest, ice, and scrotal elevation are important in the acute phase. Treatment is directed toward the identified pathogen (Table 23–1). The sexually transmitted variety in patients under age 35 is treated with a single intramuscular injection of ceftriaxone 250 mg plus 10 days of oral doxycycline 100 mg four times daily; in addition, any sexual partners from the preceding 60 days must be evaluated and treated as indicated. Men who practice insertive anal intercourse receive a single intramuscular injection of ceftriaxone 250 mg and 10 days of an oral fluoroquinolone (ciprofloxacin 500 mg twice daily) to cover sexually transmitted and enteric organisms. Non–sexually transmitted forms are treated for 10 days with a fluoroquinolone, at which time evaluation of the urinary tract is warranted to identify underlying disease. Symptoms and signs of epididymitis that do not subside within 3 days require reevaluation of the diagnosis and therapy.

Prognosis

Prompt treatment usually results in a favorable outcome. If significant scrotal swelling has developed, this may take 4 weeks to resolve. Delayed or inadequate treatment may result in epididymo-orchitis, decreased fertility, or abscess formation.

When to Refer

- Persistent symptoms and infection despite antibiotic therapy.
- Signs of sepsis or abscess formation.

Centers for Disease Control and Prevention (CDC). Sexually Transmitted Infections Treatment Guidelines, 2021: epididymitis. https://www.cdc.gov/std/treatment-guidelines/epididymitis.htm

Louette A et al. Treatment of acute epididymitis: a systematic review and discussion of the implications for treatment based on etiology. Sex Transm Dis. 2018;45:e104. [PMID: 30044339]

INTERSTITIAL CYSTITIS

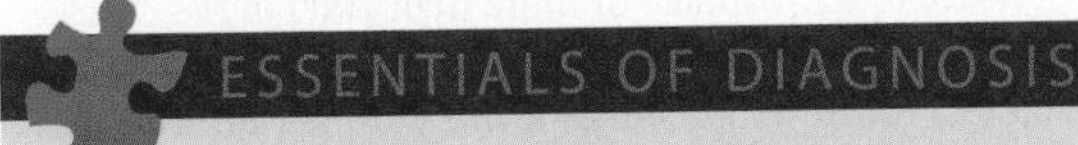

- Pain with bladder filling; urinary urgency and frequency.
- Submucosal petechiae or ulcers on cystoscopic examination.
- Diagnosis of exclusion.

General Considerations

Interstitial cystitis (painful bladder syndrome) is characterized by pain with bladder filling that is relieved by emptying and is often associated with urgency and frequency with a dramatic exaggeration of normal sensations. This is a diagnosis of exclusion, and patients must have a negative urine culture and cytology and no other obvious cause such as radiation cystitis, chemical cystitis (cyclophosphamide), vaginitis, urethral diverticulum, or genital herpes. Up to 40% of patients referred to urologists for interstitial cystitis may actually be found to have a different diagnosis after careful evaluation. What was once considered a bladder disorder is now considered a chronic pain syndrome.

Population-based studies have demonstrated a prevalence of between 18 and 40 per 100,000 people. Both sexes are involved, but most patients are women, with a mean age of 40 years at onset. Patients with interstitial cystitis are more likely to report bladder problems in childhood, especially women. Up to 50% of patients may experience spontaneous remission of symptoms, with a mean duration of 8 months without treatment.

The etiology of interstitial cystitis is unknown, and it is most likely not a single disease but rather several diseases with similar symptoms. Associated diagnoses include severe allergies, irritable bowel syndrome, or IBD. Theories regarding the cause of interstitial cystitis include increased epithelial permeability, neurogenic causes (sensory nervous system abnormalities), and autoimmunity.

Clinical Findings

A. Symptoms and Signs

Pain, pressure, or discomfort with bladder filling that is relieved with urination, and urgency, frequency, and nocturia are the most common symptoms. Patients should be asked about exposure to pelvic radiation or treatment with cyclophosphamide. Examination should exclude genital herpes, vaginitis, or a urethral diverticulum.

B. Laboratory Findings

UA, urine culture, and urinary cytology are obtained to examine for infectious causes and bladder malignancy; in interstitial cystitis, they are all normal. Urodynamic testing can be done to assess bladder sensation and compliance and to exclude detrusor instability.

C. Cystoscopy

Cystoscopy may reveal glomerulations (submucosal hemorrhage) with hydrodistention of the bladder. Total bladder capacity should be determined. Biopsy of any suspicious lesions should be performed to exclude other causes such as carcinoma, eosinophilic cystitis, and tuberculous cystitis. The presence of submucosal mast cells is *not* needed to make the diagnosis of interstitial cystitis.

Differential Diagnosis

Exposures to radiation or cyclophosphamide are discovered by the history. Bacterial cystitis, genital herpes, or vaginitis can be excluded by UA, culture, and physical examination. A urethral diverticulum may be suspected if palpation of the urethra demonstrates an indurated mass that results in the expression of pus from the urethral meatus. Urethral carcinoma presents as a firm mass on palpation.

Treatment

There is no cure for interstitial cystitis, but most patients achieve symptomatic relief from one of several approaches, including hydrodistention, where approximately 20–30% of patients notice symptomatic improvement following this maneuver. Amitriptyline (10–75 mg/day orally) is often used as first-line medical therapy in patients with interstitial cystitis. Both central and peripheral mechanisms may contribute to its activity. Nifedipine (30–60 mg/day orally) and other calcium channel blockers have also demonstrated some activity in patients with interstitial cystitis. Pentosan polysulfate sodium (Elmiron) is an oral synthetic sulfated polysaccharide that helps restore integrity to the epithelium of the bladder in a subset of patients, and it has been evaluated in a placebo-controlled trial. Other options include intravesical instillation of dimethyl sulfoxide and heparin. Intravesical bacillus Calmette-Guérin is not beneficial. Patients with very small bladder capacities (less than 200 mL) are unlikely to respond to medical therapy.

Further treatment modalities include transcutaneous electric nerve stimulation, acupuncture, stress reduction, exercise, biofeedback, massage, and pelvic floor relaxation. Surgical therapy for interstitial cystitis should be considered only as a last resort and may require cystourethrectomy with urinary diversion.

When to Refer

Persistent and bothersome symptoms in the absence of identifiable cause.

Chen PY et al. Comparative safety review of current pharmacological treatments for interstitial cystitis/ bladder pain syndrome. Expert Opin Drug Saf. 2021;20:1049. [PMID: 33944647]

Colemeadow J et al. Clinical management of bladder pain syndrome/interstitial cystitis: a review on current recommendations and emerging treatment options. Res Rep Urol. 2020;12:331. [PMID: 32904438]

Lopez SR et al. Current standard of care in treatment of bladder pain syndrome/interstitial cystitis. Ther Adv Urol. 2021;13:17562872211022478. [PMID: 34178118]

Marcu I et al. Interstitial cystitis/bladder pain syndrome. Semin Reprod Med. 2018;36:123. [PMID: 30566978]

URINARY STONE DISEASE

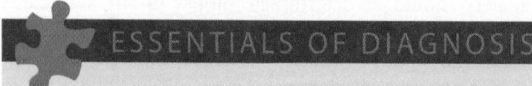

- Severe flank pain.
- Nausea and vomiting.
- Identification on noncontrast CT or ultrasonography.

General Considerations

Urinary stone disease is exceeded in frequency as a urinary tract disorder only by infections and prostatic disease. It is estimated to afflict 240,000–720,000 Americans per year. The prevalence of kidney stones has increased to 8.8%, or 1 in 11 Americans, representing a 70% increase over the last 15 years. While men are more frequently affected by urolithiasis than women, with a ratio of 1.5:1, the prevalence of stones in women is increasing. Initial presentation usually occurs in the third through fifth decades, and more than 50% of patients will have recurrent stones.

Stone formation requires saturated urine that is dependent on solute concentration, ionic strength, pH, and complexation. There are five major types of urinary stones: **calcium oxalate**, **calcium phosphate**, **struvite** (magnesium ammonium phosphate), **uric acid**, and **cystine.** The most common types are those composed of calcium oxalate or phosphate (85%), and for that reason most urinary stones are radiopaque on plain abdominal radiographs. Although pure uric acid stones are radiolucent, uric acid stones may be composed of a combination of uric acid and calcium oxalate and thus may be partially radiopaque. Cystine stones frequently have a smooth-edged ground-glass appearance and are faintly radiolucent, similar to struvite stones.

Geographic factors contribute to the development of stones. High humidity and elevated temperatures appear to be contributing factors, and the incidence of symptomatic ureteral stones is greatest in such areas during hot summer months. Higher incidence of stones has also been associated with sedentary lifestyle, obesity, hypertension, insulin resistance and poor glycemic control, carotid calcification, and CVD.

Many commonly prescribed medications increase the risk of formation of kidney stones, including carbonic anhydrase inhibitors (topiramate, zonisamide, acetazolamide), systemic corticosteroids (prednisone), antiretroviral protease inhibitors (indinavir and others), gout medications (probenecid), diuretics (furosemide, bumetanide, torsemide, triamterene), decongestants (guaifenesin, ephedrine), and laxatives (if abused for weight loss). The risk of stones from calcium supplementation is controversial. Thus, if calcium supplementation is medically necessary, it is recommended that the calcium supplement be taken with meals, and that total calcium intake (diet plus supplementation) not exceed 2000 mg daily. Dietary calcium intake should not be restricted unless excessive (a daily intake of more than 2000 mg).

Inadequate hydration is another very important dietary factor in the development of urinary stones. Efforts should be made to avoid dehydration. Patients who form kidney stones should be encouraged to drink enough fluid to keep their urine clear or light yellow at all times, with a goal of at least 2500 mL of urine produced daily, which typically requires over 3000 mL (85 oz) intake per day. Excess animal protein and salt intake (over 3500 mg daily) as well as restricted dietary calcium intake are other important stone risk factors.

Genetic factors may contribute to urinary stone formation. While approximately 50% of calcium-based stones are thought to have a heritable component, other stone types are better characterized genetically. For example, cystinuria is an autosomal recessive disorder. Homozygous individuals have markedly increased excretion of cystine and frequently have numerous recurrent episodes of urinary stones. Distal renal tubular acidosis may be transmitted as a hereditary trait, and urolithiasis occurs in up to 75% of affected patients.

Clinical Findings

A. Symptoms and Signs

Obstructing urinary stones usually present with acute, unremitting, and severe colic. Pain most often occurs suddenly and may awaken patients from sleep. It is typically localized to the flank and may be associated with nausea and vomiting. In sharp contrast to patients with an acute abdomen, patients with kidney stones are constantly moving, trying to find a comfortable position. The pain may occur episodically and may radiate anteriorly over the abdomen. As the stone progresses down the ureter, the pain may be referred into the ipsilateral groin. As the stone traverses the uretero-vesicular junction, patients may report marked urinary urgency and frequency and in men, pain may radiate to the tip of the penis; this can be confused as a symptom of a UTI. After the stone passes into the bladder, there is immediate relief of symptoms, and then the stone passes harmlessly through the urethra. Stone size does not correlate with the severity of the symptoms but does impact the duration and likelihood of successfully passing it. If the stone fails to pass and obstruction persists, patients may note a deceptive improvement in symptoms. As many as 25% of patients with resolution of pain will have a persistent stone and thus follow-up imaging is recommended in all patients if the stone has not been witnessed to pass.

B. Laboratory Findings

Regardless of symptom severity, UA usually reveals microscopic or gross hematuria (~90%). However, the absence of microhematuria does not exclude urinary stones. A persistent urinary pH < 5.5 may suggest a uric acid stone, while a persistent urinary pH > 7.2 may suggest a struvite (infection-related) or calcium phosphate stone. Caution should be taken in interpreting a single spot urine pH as it fluctuates significantly through the day. Patients with calcium oxalate–based stones typically have a normal urinary pH.

C. Metabolic Evaluation

Stone analysis on recovered stones can facilitate counseling for prevention of recurrence. Patients with uncomplicated first-time stones should undergo dietary counseling as outlined below and can be offered an optional complete metabolic evaluation.

General dietary counseling includes encouraging patients to augment their fluid intake to increase their urine volume (goal urinary output of greater than 2500 mL/day). This typically requires a fluid intake of 3000 mL/day or more. Patients who form kidney stones should reduce their sodium intake (goal less than 3500 mg/day), and reduce their animal protein intake (eggs, fish, chicken, pork, and beef). Detailed medical and dietary history, serum chemistries, and UA should be obtained for all patients with newly diagnosed nephrolithiasis. A serum parathyroid hormone level should be checked when hyperparathyroidism is suspected as the cause of calcium oxalate or calcium phosphate stones, and a serum uric acid should be obtained to exclude severe hyperuricemia, which can lead to uric acid stones as well as crystal deposition in the kidneys or heart. A 24-hour urine collection to determine urinary volume, creatinine, pH, calcium, uric acid, oxalate, phosphate, sodium, and citrate excretion is recommended for interested patients with their first stone, for all patients who have recurrent stones, and for patients at high risk for recurrence. Results are used to personalize medical management to individual patient risk factors.

D. Imaging

Noncontrast CT is the most accurate imaging modality for evaluating flank pain given its superior sensitivity and specificity over other tests; however, ultrasonography (which does not use ionizing radiation) is a safe and effective alternative for initial evaluation of renal colic and one that can be used in the emergency department with good accuracy. If the CT scan is used, it should be obtained in the prone position to help differentiate distal ureterovesicular stones from those that have already passed into the urinary bladder. A "low-dose" imaging protocol should be used when available and repeated CT scans should be minimized due to the substantial cumulative radiation exposure that patients with recurrent stones can face. Stone density can be estimated with Hounsfield units (HU) on CT scans to help determine stone type. All stones, whether radiopaque or radiolucent on plain abdominal radiographs, will be visible on noncontrast CT except the rare calculus caused by the protease inhibitor indinavir. A plain abdominal radiograph (kidney, ureter, and bladder [KUB]) and renal ultrasound examination will diagnose up to 80% of stones. Since more than 60% of patients with acute renal colic will have a stone in the distal 4 cm of the ureter, attention should be directed to that region when examining radiographs and ultrasonographic studies. Pain from a kidney stone is due to the dilatation of the ureter and kidney from the obstruction, and thus small nonobstructing kidney stones are typically not associated with pain.

Medical Treatment & Prevention

To reduce the recurrence rate of urinary stones, dietary modification is important. Metabolic evaluation often identifies a modifiable risk factor that can further reduce stone recurrence rates. If no medical treatment is provided, stones will generally recur in 50% of patients within 5 years. Some stone types (eg, uric acid, cystine) are more prone to rapid recurrence than others. An increased fluid intake to dilute the urine and prevent dehydration is the most important dietary risk factor to reduce stone recurrence and may diminish the risk by 50%. Increasing fluid intake to ensure a voided volume of 2.5 L/day is recommended (normal average voided volume is 1.6 L/day). Urine should be clear or light yellow at each void. Medical therapy should be tailored to the patient's metabolic workup and the activity of their stone disease. Routine follow-up every 6–8 months and annual imaging (preferably with ultrasonography) will help encourage medical compliance, assess for interval stone formation or growth, and permit adjustments in medical therapy based on repeat metabolic studies.

A. General Dietary Recommendations

A 24-hour urinary sodium level of greater than 150 mmol/day indicates excessive sodium intake. **Sodium intake** should not exceed 3500 mg daily. Excessive sodium intake will increase renal sodium and calcium excretion, increase urinary monosodium urates (that can act as a nidus for stone growth), increase the relative saturation of calcium phosphate, and decrease urinary citrate excretion. All of these factors encourage stone growth.

A urinary sulfate level of greater than 20 mEq/day indicates excessive animal protein intake. **Animal protein intake** should be spread out through the day, not all consumed during any individual meal, and is best limited to 1 g/kg/day. An increased protein load during an individual meal can lead to acidic urine and may also increase calcium, oxalate, and uric acid excretion and decrease urinary citrate excretion.

Dietary calcium intake should *not* be restricted in an effort to decrease stone formation because it may paradoxically lead to increased stone formation due to increased oxalate absorption and consequent hyperoxaluria.

B. Calcium Nephrolithiasis

1. Hypercalciuria—Elevated urinary calcium levels (greater than 4 mg/kg/day or greater than 250 mg/day for males and greater than 200 mg/day for females) lead to hypercalciuric calcium nephrolithiasis. Hypercalciuria can be caused by absorptive, resorptive, and renal disorders; however, the categorization system provided below is not routinely used in clinical practice. Thiazide diuretics decrease renal calcium excretion; after primary hyperparathyroidism has been excluded, thiazide diuretics should be offered to patients with high urinary calcium and recurrent calcium stones. Chlorthalidone and indapamide are first-line agents since they can be administered once a day, while hydrochlorothiazide for hypercalciuria should be administered twice a day. Patients should be encouraged to increase their dietary potassium intake by increasing the intake of fruits and vegetables. All patients respond to thiazide diuretics with decreases in urinary calcium unless they have primary hyperparathyroidism or are nonadherent with taking the medication. Clinicians should periodically test patients taking thiazide diuretics for hypokalemia, since they may require potassium supplementation.

Absorptive hypercalciuria is secondary to increased absorption of calcium at the level of the small bowel, predominantly in the jejunum. Absorptive hypercalciuria can be diet-dependent, independent of calcium intake, or due to renal phosphate leak. Oral calcium load testing is no longer performed.

Resorptive hypercalciuria, or primary hyperparathyroidism, is typically due to a parathyroid adenoma. Hypercalcemia, elevated serum parathyroid hormone level, hypophosphatemia, and elevated urinary calcium level are present. Appropriate surgical resection of the parathyroid adenoma is curative in 75% of patients with kidney stones due to primary hyperparathyroidism. Medical management is typically reserved for patients who are not good surgical candidates.

Renal hypercalciuria is the most common form of hypercalciuria and occurs when the renal tubules are unable to efficiently reabsorb filtered calcium. Spilling calcium in the urine may result in secondary hyperparathyroidism with normal serum calcium. A thiazide diuretic is an effective long-term therapy in patients with this disorder because it corrects the urinary calcium losses and is associated with an increase in bone mineral density of approximately 1% per year while receiving therapy.

2. Hyperuricosuria—**Hyperuricosuric calcium nephrolithiasis** is defined by elevated urinary uric acid levels (greater than 800 mg/day for men and greater than 750 mg/day for women). It is usually secondary to dietary purine excess or endogenous uric acid metabolic defects. Excess uric acid in the urine can lead to uric acid stones if the urine pH is low, or to calcium stones at higher urine pH due to formation of a monosodium urate crystal that then calcifies in a process known as heterogenous nucleation. Dietary purine restriction can reduce hyperuricosuria in 85% of cases. Patients with hyperuricosuria, normocalciuria, and recurrent calcium oxalate stones can be successfully treated with allopurinol. However, allopurinol is not first-line treatment of uric acid stones; urinary alkalinization is (see below).

3. Hyperoxaluria—**Hyperoxaluric calcium nephrolithiasis** (greater than 40 mg/day of urinary oxalate) is usually due to either an intestinal malabsorption disorder or a mismatch in dietary calcium and oxalate intake. Patients with a history of chronic diarrhea, IBD, malabsorption, or gastric bypass surgery are at risk for hyperoxaluria. In these disorders, increased intestinal fat or bile (or both) combine with calcium to form a soap-like product. Calcium is therefore unavailable to bind to oxalate, leading to free oxalate absorption. Even a small increase in free oxalate absorption significantly increases risk of stone formation. If the diarrhea or steatorrhea cannot be effectively curtailed, oral calcium should be increased with meals, either by ingesting dairy products or by taking low-dose calcium carbonate supplements (250 mg). When dietary calcium and oxalate intake are consumed concurrently, they are unable to be absorbed systemically since they bind together in the intestinal tract. But if dietary calcium is restricted, or if dietary oxalate is excessive, free oxalate is rapidly absorbed and excreted in the urine, leading to hyperoxaluric calcium nephrolithiasis. Treatment includes adhering to a diet containing moderate calcium intake (1000–1200 mg daily). If dietary calcium increases do not reach 1000 mg daily, low-dose calcium carbonate (250 mg) or calcium citrate (950 mg) can be consumed with meals. Treatment also involves avoiding high-oxalate-containing foods (baked potatoes with skins, sweet potatoes. French fries, okra, cocoa powder, grits, beets, spinach, rhubarb, almonds, cashews, miso soup, and Stevia sweetener). NOTE: High-dose ascorbic acid (greater than 2000 mg/day) will substantially increase urinary oxalate levels.

4. Hypocitraturia—Urinary citrate is the most important inhibitor of stone formation. Urinary citrate binds to calcium in solution, thereby decreasing available calcium for precipitation and subsequent stone formation. Low urine citrate levels (less than 450 mg/day) increase the risk of stones. **Hypocitraturic calcium nephrolithiasis** is usually idiopathic. Urinary citrate excretion is influenced by systemic acid-base balance and serum potassium levels, and thus, hypocitraturia occurs secondary to any metabolic acidemia (chronic diarrhea, distal renal tubular acidosis), or with systemic potassium losses (long-term treatment with thiazide or loop diuretics). Usually, effective treatment in these situations is potassium citrate supplementation: a typical dose is 40–60 mEq total daily intake, divided into two or three daily doses. Alternatively, oral lemonade has been shown to modestly increase urinary citrate, but this must be consumed several times every day since oral citrate is cleared from the urine in 6–8 hours.

C. Uric Acid Calculi

Urinary pH is the most important contributor to uric acid stone formation, and thus first-line efforts to prevent hyperuricosuria should focus on alkalinizing the urine with oral potassium citrate or sodium bicarbonate. Efforts to decrease urinary uric acid (with allopurinol 300 mg/day orally) should be reserved for patients continuing to form stones despite adequate urinary alkalinization. In patients who form pure uric acid stones, urine pH is consistently less than 5.5. Increasing the urinary pH dramatically increases uric acid solubility, leading to prevention of stone formation (with urine pH > 6.0) and even to stone dissolution (with urine pH > 6.5). Nitrazine pH test strips (which turn blue with alkaline urine pH > 6.0) are often useful to some patients in reinforcing adherence to urinary alkalinization efforts. Less common contributors to uric acid stone formation include hyperuricemia, myeloproliferative disorders, chemotherapy for malignancies with rapid cell turnover or cell death, abrupt and dramatic weight loss, and uricosuric medications (probenecid).

D. Struvite Calculi

Struvite stones are composed of magnesium-ammonium-phosphate and are typically visible on plain radiographs. They are most common in women with recurrent UTIs with urease-producing organisms, including *Proteus, Pseudomonas, Providencia*, and, less commonly, *Klebsiella, Staphylococcus*, and *Mycoplasma* (but not *E coli*). Clinically, they rarely present with colic from a ureteral stone. Instead, a struvite stone is discovered as a large staghorn calculus forming a cast of the renal collecting system. Urinary pH is high, routinely above 7.2. Struvite stones are relatively soft and amenable to percutaneous removal. Appropriate perioperative antibiotics are required. They can recur rapidly, and efforts should be taken to remove all of the stone and then to prevent further UTIs.

E. Cystine Calculi

Cystine stones are caused by a genetic metabolic defect resulting in abnormal excretion of cystine. These stones are exceptionally challenging to manage medically. Prevention involves markedly increasing fluid intake during the day and night to achieve a urinary volume of 3–4 L/day, decreasing sodium and dietary cystine intake, and increasing urinary alkalinization (typically with high-dose potassium citrate) with a goal urinary pH > 7.0. Patients whose cystine stones do not respond to these measures may be treated with disulfide inhibitors such as tiopronin (alpha-mercaptoproprionylglycine) or penicillamine. There are no known inhibitors of cystine calculi.

Medical Expulsion & Surgical Treatment

Signs of infection, including associated fever, tachycardia, hypotension, and elevated WBC, may indicate a UTI behind the obstructing stone. Any obstructing stone with associated infection is a **medical emergency** requiring urology consultation and prompt drainage of the kidney with a ureteral stent or a percutaneous nephrostomy tube. Antibiotics alone are inadequate and only used as an adjunct to drainage of the infected urine behind the obstruction.

In the acute setting, forcing intravenous fluids will not push stones down the ureter. Forced diuresis can actually be counterproductive and exacerbate pain; instead, a euvolemic state should be achieved.

A. Ureteral Stones

Ureteral stones are usually discovered at three sites: the ureteropelvic junction, the crossing of the ureter over the iliac artery, or the ureterovesicular junction. Stones smaller than 5–6 mm in diameter on a plain abdominal radiograph usually pass spontaneously. Medical expulsive therapy with alpha-blockers (eg, tamsulosin, 0.4 mg orally once daily) in combination with an anti-inflammatory agent (eg, ibuprofen 600 mg orally three times per day), with or without a short course of a low-dose oral corticosteroid (eg, prednisone 10 mg orally daily for 5–10 days), may increase the rate of spontaneous stone passage and appears to be most effective for distal stones greater than 5 mm. Attempted medical expulsive therapy with effective pain medications and imaging follow-up is appropriate for a few weeks. If the stone fails to pass within 4 weeks, the patient has fever, intolerable pain, or persistent nausea or vomiting, or the patient must return to work or anticipates travel, then surgical intervention is indicated.

Stones in the mid and distal ureter that require surgical removal are best managed with ureteroscopic stone extraction. Ureteroscopic stone extraction involves placement of a small endoscope through the urethra and bladder and into the ureter. Under direct vision, basket extraction or laser fragmentation followed by fragment extraction is performed. A ureteral stent is often placed temporarily to allow drainage of the kidney while the swelling and inflammation from the stone and procedure resolve.

Extracorporeal shock wave lithotripsy (ESWL) can be offered as second-line therapy. ESWL utilizes an external energy source focused on the stone with the aid of fluoroscopy or ultrasonography. ESWL is typically performed under anesthesia or sedation as an outpatient procedure with the goal of stone fragmentation. Most stone fragments then pass uneventfully within 2 weeks. Occasionally after ESWL, stone fragments obstruct the ureter. Conservative management usually results in spontaneous resolution of the obstruction with eventual passage of the stone fragments. Fragments that have not passed within 6 weeks are unlikely to do so without intervention. ESWL is strictly contraindicated in pregnant patients as well as in those with untreated UTI, in those with an uncorrected coagulopathy, or in those who must continue receiving anticoagulant or antiplatelet therapy. A ureteral stent is typically not necessary with ESWL.

Proximal ureteral stones can be treated with ESWL or ureteroscopy. ESWL is less successful with larger stones and those that are very dense. In cases of ESWL failure, ureteroscopic extraction is required.

B. Renal Calculi

Patients with small, asymptomatic, renal calculi, without UTI or obstruction, may not warrant surgical treatment. If surveillance is undertaken, the patient should be monitored with serial abdominal radiographs or renal ultrasonographic examinations every 3–12 months. If the calculi grow or become symptomatic, intervention is indicated. ESWL is most effective for stones less than 1 cm in size in the lower pole of the kidney or less than 2 cm in size elsewhere in the kidney. ESWL is less effective for stones that are very hard (cystine stones, calcium oxalate stones greater than 1000–1200 Hounsfield units on CT scan) and for obese patients (skin-to-stone distance greater than 10–12 cm). Ureteroscopy and laser lithotripsy are effective for multiple stones and larger stones, although very large stones may require multiple treatment sessions. Stones larger than 15–20 mm and staghorn calculi (large-branched stones occupying at least two renal calices) are best treated via percutaneous nephrolithotomy. Percutaneous nephrolithotomy is performed by inserting a needle into the appropriate renal calyx and dilating a tract large enough to allow a nephroscope to pass directly into the kidney. In this fashion, larger and more complex kidney stones can be inspected, fragmented, and removed. In unusual cases, laparoscopic, robotic-assisted, or open stone removal may be considered. Perioperative antibiotic coverage should be given for any stone procedure, ideally based on preoperative urine culture results.

When to Refer

- Evidence of urinary obstruction.
- Urinary stone with associated flank pain.
- Anatomic abnormalities, solitary kidney, or CKD.
- Concomitant pyelonephritis or recurrent UTI.

When to Admit

- Intractable nausea and vomiting or pain.
- Obstructing stone with fever or other signs of infection.

Bishop K et al. Nephrolithiasis. Prim Care. 2020;47:661. [PMID: 33121635]

Corbo J et al. Kidney and ureteral stones. Emerg Med Clin North Am. 2019;37:637. [PMID: 31563199]

Dai JC et al. Innovations in ultrasound technology in the management of kidney stones. Urol Clin North Am. 2019;46:273. [PMID: 30961860]

Li JK et al. Updates in endourological management of urolithiasis. Int J Urol. 2019;26:172. [PMID: 30575154]

Lovegrove CE et al. Natural history of small asymptomatic kidney and residual stones over a long-term follow-up: systematic review over 25 years. BJU Int. 2022;129:442. [PMID: 34157218]

Mayans L. Nephrolithiasis. Prim Care. 2019;46:203. [PMID: 31030821]

Strilchuk L et al. Safety and tolerability of available urate-lowering drugs: a critical review. Expert Opin Drug Saf. 2019;18:261. [PMID: 30915866]

Yuzhakov S et al. 24-hour urine calcium oxalate supersaturation risk correlates with computerized tomography volumetric calcium oxalate stone growth. J Urol. 2021;206:1438. [PMID: 34288713]

MALE SEXUAL DYSFUNCTION & ERECTILE DYSFUNCTION

ESSENTIALS OF DIAGNOSIS

- Erectile dysfunction is a common condition that negatively impacts quality of life when left untreated.
- Most erectile dysfunction is caused by arterial insufficiency, may be an early sign of CVD, and requires evaluation and treatment.
- Peyronie disease is a common, benign fibrotic disorder of the penis that causes pain, penile deformity, and sexual dysfunction.

General Considerations

Male **sexual dysfunction** is manifested in a variety of ways, and patient history is critical to the proper classification and treatment. A **loss of libido** may indicate androgen deficiency or depression. **Erectile dysfunction** is the consistent inability to attain or maintain a sufficiently rigid penile erection for sexual intercourse. More than half of men aged 40–70 years have erectile dysfunction and its incidence increases with age. **Erectile dysfunction** may result from neurological, vascular, hormonal, or psychological causes. Concurrent medical problems may damage one or more of the mechanisms. Normal male erection is a neurovascular event that requires an intact autonomic and somatic nerve supply to the penis, arterial blood flow supplied by the paired cavernosal arteries, and smooth and striated musculature of the corpora cavernosa and pelvic floor. Erection is initiated by nerve impulses in the pelvic plexus leading to an increase in arterial flow, active relaxation of the smooth muscle within the sinusoids of the corpora cavernosa, elevation of hydraulic pressure within the corpora and a subsequent increase in venous outflow resistance. Contraction of the ischiocavernosus muscle causes further rigidity of the penis with intracavernosal pressures exceeding systolic blood pressure. Nitric oxide is the key neurotransmitter that initiates and sustains erections.

The most common cause of erectile dysfunction is a decrease in arterial flow resultant from progressive vascular disease. Endothelial dysfunction results from the decreased bioavailability of nitric oxide with subsequent impairment of arterial vasodilation. In some men, erectile dysfunction may be a manifestation of endothelial dysfunction, which precedes more severe atherosclerotic CVD. Many medications, especially antihypertensive, antidepressant, antipsychotic, and opioid agents, are associated with erectile dysfunction.

Anejaculation is the loss of seminal emission and may result from androgen deficiency, or from sympathetic denervation as a result of spinal cord injury, diabetes mellitus or pelvic or retroperitoneal surgery or radiation. **Retrograde ejaculation** may occur as a result of age-related prostate enlargement or mechanical disruption of the bladder neck due to congenital abnormalities, transurethral prostate surgery, pelvic radiation, sympathetic denervation, or treatment with alpha-blockers. **Premature ejaculation** is the distressing, recurrent ejaculation with minimal stimulation before a person desires. Primary premature ejaculation may be treated with behavioral modification, sexual health counseling, local anesthetic agents, and systemic medications used alone or in combination. Secondary premature ejaculation is due to erectile dysfunction and responds to treatment of the underlying disorder. **Peyronie disease** is a fibrotic disorder of the tunica albuginea of the corpora cavernosa of the penis resulting in varying degrees of penile pain, curvature, or deformity. Peyronie disease affects up to 10% of men and is more common with increased age. Ten percent of men improve spontaneously, 50% will stabilize, and the remainder will progress if left untreated. Penile deformity can impair normal sexual function and impact self-esteem.

Priapism is prolonged penile erection in the absence of sexual stimulation that may result in ischemic injury of the corpora cavernosa from venous congestion, blood coagulation within the cavernous sinuses, and complete cessation of arterial inflow (low flow or "ischemic" priapism). Ischemic priapism is a medical emergency requiring immediate medical or surgical intervention to avoid irreversible penile damage. Ischemic priapism may be caused by RBC dyscrasias, drug use, and treatments for erectile dysfunction, such as phosphodiesterase type 5 inhibitors (listed in the Vasoactive Therapy section below).

Clinical Findings

A. Symptoms and Signs

Erectile dysfunction should be distinguished from problems with penile deformity, libido, orgasm, and ejaculation. The severity, intermittency, and timing of erectile dysfunction should be noted. The history should include inquiries about dyslipidemia, hypertension, depression, neurologic disease, diabetes mellitus, kidney disease, endocrine disorders, and cardiac or peripheral vascular disease. Pelvic trauma, surgery, or irradiation increases a man's likelihood of erectile dysfunction. Histories of prostate cancer treatment or Peyronie disease should be elicited. In the absence of other medical history, the onset of erectile dysfunction may be the first sign of endothelial dysfunction and further cardiovascular risk stratification should be considered. Medication use should be reviewed. Special attention should be given to the use of nitrate-containing medications. Alcohol, tobacco, marijuana, and other recreational drug use are associated with an increased risk of sexual dysfunction. The use of pornography to maintain sexual arousal should be elicited.

During the physical examination, vital signs, body habitus (obesity), and secondary sexual characteristics should be assessed. Basic cardiovascular and neurologic examinations should be performed. The genitalia should be examined, noting the stretched length of the penis, fibrosis of the penile shaft, and any abnormalities in size or consistency of either testicle.

B. Laboratory Findings

Laboratory evaluation should be performed in select cases based on patient history and physical examination findings. Possible testing includes serum lipid profile, glucose, and total testosterone. Patients with an abnormal total testosterone should have measurement of free testosterone and LH to distinguish hypothalamic-pituitary dysfunction from primary testicular failure.

Treatment

Treatment of men suffering from sexual dysfunction should be patient centered and goal oriented. Lifestyle modification and reduction of cardiovascular risk factors are important and should include smoking cessation; reduction of alcohol intake; diet; exercise; and treatment of diabetes, dyslipidemia, and hypertension. Men who have a psychogenic component to their erectile dysfunction or who are experiencing emotional distress will benefit from sexual health therapy or psychological counseling.

A. Hormonal Replacement

In men with hypogonadism who have undergone complete endocrinologic evaluation, restoration of normal testosterone levels may improve sexual function (see Male Hypogonadism in Chapter 26.)

B. Vasoactive Therapy

1. Oral agents—Sildenafil, vardenafil, tadalafil, and avanafil prevent the degradation of cGMP and increase blood flow into the penis. These medications have variable durations of onset, activity, and side effects; each agent should be tried until the one that is most effective with the fewest side effects is identified. Each medication should be initiated at the lowest dose and titrated to achieve the desired effect. These medications are contraindicated in patients taking nitroglycerin or nitrates, since there may be exaggerated cardiac preload reduction causing hypotension and syncope.

The combination of PDE-5 inhibitors and alpha-receptor blockers (prescribed for lower urinary tract symptoms) may cause a larger reduction in systemic blood pressure than when PDE-5 inhibitors are used alone. However, these two classes of medication may be safely used in combination if they are initiated and titrated in a stepwise fashion.

2. Injectable or suppository medications—Injection of prostaglandin E_2 into the corpora cavernosa is an acceptable form of treatment for erectile dysfunction. Injections are performed using a tuberculin-type syringe or a metered-dose injection device. The base and lateral aspect of the penis is used as the injection site to avoid injury to the superficial blood and nerve supply located dorsally. Complications include priapism, penile pain, bruising, fibrosis, and infection. Prostaglandin E_2 (alprostadil urethral) can also be delivered via an intraurethral suppository. Prostaglandin E_2 is often compounded with papaverine, phentolamine, or atropine in order to increase effectiveness. Patients using such compounded agents should be cautioned about the risk of priapism and variability of drug effect due to differences in compounding.

C. Vacuum Erection Device

The vacuum erection device creates negative pressure around the penis, drawing blood into the corpora cavernosa. Once tumescence is achieved, an elastic constriction band is placed around the penile base to prevent loss of erection. Such devices are effective but may cause penile discomfort and numbness leading to a high rate of disuse. Serious complications are rare.

D. Penile Prosthetic Surgery

Penile prostheses are surgically implanted into the paired corpora cavernosa and may be inflatable or semi-rigid (malleable). Inflatable prostheses are self-contained hydraulic devices that result in normal appearance and function. Inflatable prosthetics are used most commonly because they emulate the tumescence and detumescence of the normal erection. This therapy is appropriate for patients who have not achieved a satisfactory response to other therapies.

E. Medical and Surgical Therapy for Peyronie Disease

Injectable collagenase *Clostridium histolyticum* is the only FDA-approved medication for the treatment of Peyronie disease. Collagenase enzymatically digests disordered collagen fibers after injection into the penile plaque. Surgical treatment is an alternative for men with compromised sexual function due to severe curvature, with lesions causing penile instability, or with inadequate results from collagenase. The choice of corrective procedure should be tailored to each patient after a detailed evaluation of disease severity and sexual function.

When to Refer

- Patients with unsatisfactory response to oral medications.
- Patients with Peyronie disease or other penile deformity.
- Patients with a history of pelvic surgery, radiation, or perineal trauma.
- Patients with priapism for emergent intervention to allow restoration of penile perfusion.

Capogrosso P et al. Male sexual dysfunctions in the infertile couple—recommendations from the European Society of Sexual Medicine (ESSM). Sex Med. 2021;9:100377. [PMID: 34090242]

Corona G et al. Erectile dysfunction and cardiovascular risk: a review of current findings. Expert Rev Cardiovasc Ther. 2020;18:155. [PMID: 32192361]

Fernandez-Crespo RE et al. Sexual dysfunction among men who have sex with men: a review article. Curr Urol Rep. 2021;22:9. [PMID: 33420894]

Gabrielson AT et al. Collagenase *Clostridium histolyticum* in the treatment of urologic disease: current and future impact. Sex Med Rev. 2018;6:143. [PMID: 28454897]

MacDonald SM et al. Physiology of erection and pathophysiology of erectile dysfunction. Urol Clin North Am. 2021;48:513. [PMID: 34602172]

Salonia A et al. European Association of Urology Guidelines on Sexual and Reproductive Health—2021 update: male sexual dysfunction. Eur Urol. 2021;80:333. [PMID: 34183196]

Terentes-Printzios D et al. Interactions between erectile dysfunction, cardiovascular disease and cardiovascular drugs. Nat Rev Cardiol. 2021;19:59. [PMID: 34331033]

MALE INFERTILITY

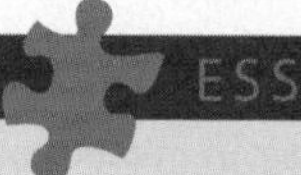

ESSENTIALS OF DIAGNOSIS

- Infertility is common, and male factors are present in 50% of cases.
- Causes include sexual dysfunction, decreased or absent sperm production or function, or obstruction of the male genital tract.
- Abnormal semen quality is a risk factor for infertility and may indicate poor health or increased risk of certain health conditions.

General Considerations

Infertility is disease that results in the failure of a couple to conceive a child after 12 months of sexual intercourse without contraceptive use. It affects 15–20% of US couples and half of cases result from male factors. The evaluation of both partners is critical for optimizing treatment. Following a detailed history and physical examination, a semen analysis should be performed at least twice, on two separate occasions (Figure 23–2). Because spermatogenesis requires approximately 75 days, it is important to review

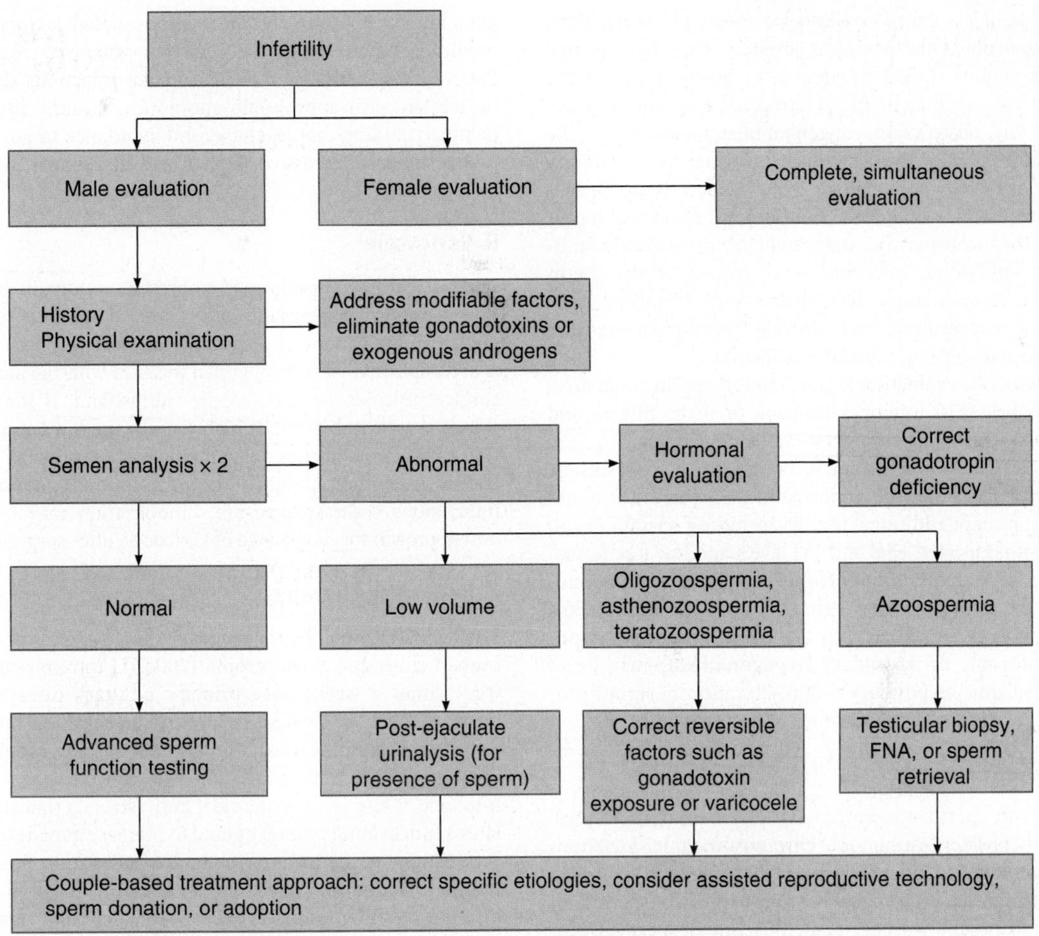

▲ **Figure 23–2.** Couple-based approach to evaluation and treatment of male factor infertility. FNA, fine-needle aspiration.

health events and gonadotoxic exposures from the preceding 3 months. Male infertility is associated with a higher risk of testicular germ cell cancer and with a higher rate of medical comorbidity. These men should be counseled and screened appropriately and taught testicular self-examination.

Clinical Findings

A. Symptoms and Signs

The history should include prior testicular insults (torsion, cryptorchidism, trauma), infections (mumps orchitis, epididymitis, sexually transmitted infections), environmental factors (excessive heat, radiation, chemotherapy, prolonged pesticide exposure), medications (testosterone, finasteride, cimetidine, SSRIs, and spironolactone may affect spermatogenesis; phenytoin may lower FSH; sulfasalazine and nitrofurantoin affect sperm motility; tamsulosin causes retrograde ejaculation), and other drugs (alcohol, tobacco, marijuana). Sexual function, frequency and timing of intercourse, use of lubricants, and each partner's previous fertility are important. Past medical and surgical history should be surveyed for chronic disease, including obesity, cardiovascular, thyroid, or liver disease (decreased spermatogenesis); diabetes mellitus (decreased spermatogenesis, retrograde or anejaculation); or radical pelvic or retroperitoneal surgery (absent seminal emission secondary to sympathetic nerve injury).

Physical examination should assess features of hypogonadism: underdeveloped sexual characteristics, diminished male pattern hair distribution (axillary, body, facial, pubic), body habitus, gynecomastia, and obesity. Testicular size should be noted (normal size approximately 4.5 × 2.5 cm, volume 18 mL). **Varicoceles** are abnormally dilated, refluxing veins of the pampiniform plexus that can be identified in the standing position by gentle palpation of the spermatic cord and, on occasion, may only be appreciated with the Valsalva maneuver. The vasa deferentia and epididymides should be palpated (absence of all or part of one or both of the vasa deferentia may indicate the presence of congenital bilateral or unilateral absence of the vasa deferentia).

B. Laboratory Findings

Semen analysis should be performed after 2–5 days of ejaculatory abstinence. The specimen should be analyzed within 1 hour after collection. Abnormal sperm concentrations are less than 15 million/mL (**oligozoospermia** is the presence of less than 15 million sperm/mL in the ejaculate; **azoospermia** is the complete absence of sperm). Normal semen volume should be equal to or greater than 1.5 mL (lesser volumes may be due to retrograde ejaculation, ejaculatory duct obstruction, congenital bilateral absence of the vasa deferentia, or hypogonadism). Normal sperm motility and morphology demonstrate greater than 39% motile cells and greater than 3% normal morphology. Abnormal motility (asthenozoospermia) may result from varicocele, antisperm antibodies, infection, abnormalities of the sperm flagella, or ejaculatory duct obstruction. Abnormal morphology may result from a varicocele, infection, or exposure to gonadotoxins (eg, tobacco, marijuana).

Endocrine evaluation is warranted if sperm concentration is below 10 million sperm/mL or if the history and physical examination suggest an endocrinologic origin. Initial testing should include serum total and free testosterone and FSH. Specific abnormalities in these hormones should prompt additional testing, including serum LH and prolactin. Elevated FSH and LH levels and low free testosterone levels (**hypergonadotropic** or **primary hypogonadism**) are associated with primary testicular failure. Low FSH and LH associated with low free testosterone (**hypogonadotropic** or **secondary hypogonadism**) may be of hypothalamic or pituitary origin. Elevation of serum prolactin may indicate the presence of prolactinoma.

C. Genetic Testing

Men with sperm concentrations less than 1 million/mL should consider testing for Y chromosome microdeletions and karyotypic abnormalities. Gene deletions from the long arm of the Y chromosome may cause azoospermia or oligozoospermia with age-related decline in spermatogenesis that is transmissible to male offspring. When small (5 mL), firm testes are identified, karyotyping may reveal Klinefelter syndrome. Partial or complete absence of the vasa deferentia should prompt testing for gene pathogenic variants associated with cystic fibrosis.

D. Imaging

Scrotal ultrasound aids in characterizing the testes and may detect a testicular mass or varicocele. Men with low ejaculate volume and no evidence of retrograde ejaculation may undergo transrectal ultrasound to evaluate the prostate and seminal vesicles. MRI of the sella turcica should be performed in men with elevated prolactin or hypogonadotropic hypogonadism to evaluate the anterior pituitary gland. MRI of the pelvis and scrotum should be considered in men for whom the testes cannot be identified in the scrotum by physical examination or ultrasound. Men with unilateral absence of the vas deferens should have abdominal ultrasound or CT to exclude absence of the ipsilateral kidney.

Treatment

A. General Measures

Education about intercourse timing in relation to the woman's ovulatory cycle as well as the avoidance of spermicidal lubricants should be discussed. In cases of gonadotoxic exposure or medication-related factors, the offending agent should be removed whenever feasible. Patients with active genitourinary tract infections should be treated with appropriate antibiotics. Healthy lifestyle habits, including diet, exercise, and avoidance of gonadotoxins (tobacco, excessive alcohol, and marijuana), should be reinforced.

B. Varicocele

Varicocelectomy is performed to prevent retrograde blood flow in abnormal spermatic cord veins and improves semen quality and likelihood of pregnancy. Surgical ligation, which is accomplished via a subinguinal incision with the aid of a surgical microscope and Doppler ultrasound, is the gold standard approach given its high success and low complication rates. Percutaneous venographic embolization of varicoceles is another approach but incurs both radiation and intravenous contrast exposure. Embolization may be the best approach for recurrence of varicocele after surgery.

C. Endocrine Therapy

Hypogonadotropic hypogonadism may be treated with human chorionic gonadotropin (2000 IU intramuscularly three times a week) once primary pituitary disease has been excluded or treated. If sperm concentration fails to rise after 12 months, recombinant FSH therapy should be initiated (150 IU subcutaneously three times a week). Clomiphene citrate is a nonsteroidal anti-estrogen that stimulates a functioning pituitary gland to increase gonadotropin production. Anastrazole inhibits aromatization of testosterone to estradiol, thereby enhancing gonadotropin production. While studied extensively in men, neither clomiphene nor anastrazole are approved by the US FDA for treatment of male infertility. Therefore, men should be counseled appropriately before using either medication.

D. Ejaculatory Dysfunction Therapy

Patients with retrograde ejaculation may benefit from alpha-adrenergic agonists (pseudoephedrine, 60 mg orally three times a day) or imipramine (25 mg orally three times a day). Medical failures may require the collection of postejaculation urine for intrauterine insemination. Anejaculation can be treated with vibratory stimulation or electroejaculation in select cases.

E. Ductal Obstruction

Obstruction of the vas deferens after vasectomy may be treated by microsurgical vasectomy reversal or by surgical sperm retrieval in combination with in vitro fertilization. While somewhat dependent on the duration of vasectomy, overall, microsurgical vasectomy reversal is highly successful in returning sperm to the ejaculate.

F. Assisted Reproductive Techniques

Intrauterine insemination and in vitro fertilization (with or without intracytoplasmic sperm injection) are alternatives for patients in whom other means of treating reduced sperm concentration, motility, or functionality have failed.

Intrauterine insemination should be performed only when adequate numbers of motile sperm are noted in an ejaculate sample. With the use of intracytoplasmic sperm injection, some men with azoospermia may still initiate a pregnancy by surgical retrieval of sperm from the testicle, epididymis, or vas deferens.

When to Refer

- Couples with infertility or who are concerned about their fertility potential.
- Men with known genital insults, genetic diagnoses, or syndromes that preclude natural fertility.
- Reproductive-aged men with newly diagnosed cancer or other disease that may require cytotoxic therapies with interest in fertility preservation.

Agarwal A et al. Male infertility. Lancet. 2021;397:319. [PMID: 33308486]
Farsimadan M et al. Bacterial infection of the male reproductive system causing infertility. J Reprod Immunol. 2020;142:103183. [PMID: 32853846]
Hehemann MC. Evaluation of the impact of marijuana use on semen quality: a prospective analysis. Ther Adv Urol. 2021;13:17562872211032484. [PMID: 34367341]
Minhas S et al. European Association of Urology Guidelines on Male Sexual and Reproductive Health: 2021 update on male infertility. Eur Urol. 2021;80:603. [PMID: 34511305]
Punjani N et al. Technological advancements in male infertility microsurgery. J Clin Med. 2021;10:4259. [PMID: 34575370]
Sharma A et al. Male infertility due to testicular disorders. J Clin Endocrinol Metab. 2021;106:e442. [PMID: 33295608]

BENIGN PROSTATIC HYPERPLASIA

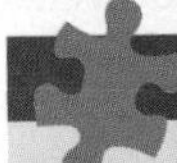

ESSENTIALS OF DIAGNOSIS

- Obstructive or irritative voiding symptoms.
- Enlarged prostate size on rectal examination.
- Absence of UTI, neurologic disorder, stricture disease, prostatic or bladder malignancy.

General Considerations

Benign prostatic hyperplasia (BPH) is the most common benign tumor in men, and its incidence is age related. The prevalence of histologic BPH in autopsy studies rises from approximately 20% in men aged 41–50 years, to 50% in men aged 51–60, and to greater than 90% in men over 80 years of age. Although clinical evidence of disease occurs less commonly, symptoms of prostatic obstruction are also age related. At age 55 years, approximately 25% of men report obstructive voiding symptoms. At age 75 years, 50% of men report a decrease in the force and caliber of the urinary stream.

Risk factors for the development of BPH are poorly understood. Studies have shown that genetic and hereditary factors play a role in some patients. Investigation has also demonstrated insulin resistance and metabolic syndrome as independent risk factors for developing BPH. Other research involving chronic inflammation, growth factor–mediated disease progression, as well as androgen- and estrogen-mediated pathways have shed some insight into the pathophysiology of the disease.

Clinical Findings

A. Symptoms

The symptoms of BPH can are either obstructive or irritative. **Obstructive symptoms** include hesitancy, decreased force and caliber of the stream, sensation of incomplete bladder emptying, double voiding (urinating a second time within 2 hours), straining to urinate, and postvoid dribbling. **Irritative symptoms** include urgency, frequency, and nocturia.

The AUA symptom index (Table 23–3) is an important tool used in the evaluation of patients to establish a baseline and to monitor response to treatment or disease progression over time. Those with significant nocturia should be assessed for 24-hour polyuria or nocturnal polyuria. A simple frequency-volume chart is a useful tool to identify these patients. An estimation of postvoid residual can provide important information on bladder emptying and the need for more urgent intervention.

A detailed history focusing on the urinary tract should be obtained to exclude other possible causes of symptoms such as prostate cancer, UTI, neurogenic bladder, or urethral stricture. A focused medical history may also reveal other comorbidities that can directly affect urinary symptoms such as diabetes mellitus, heart failure, Parkinson disease, and obstructive sleep apnea.

B. Signs

A physical examination, including DRE, and a focused neurologic examination should be performed on all patients. The size and consistency of the prostate should be noted, but prostate size does not correlate well with the severity of symptoms or the degree of obstruction. BPH usually results in a smooth, firm, elastic enlargement of the prostate. Induration, if detected, must alert the clinician to the possibility of cancer, and further evaluation is needed (ie, PSA testing, transrectal ultrasound, and biopsy). Examination of the lower abdomen should be performed to assess for a distended bladder.

C. Laboratory Findings

UA should be performed to exclude infection or hematuria. Clinicians should consider obtaining a serum PSA test, particularly in patients whose life expectancy is longer than 10 years. PSA certainly increases the ability to detect prostate cancer over DRE alone; however, because there is much overlap between levels seen in BPH and prostate cancer, its use remains controversial (see Chapter 39).

D. Imaging

Urologists are advised to consider prostate volume assessment before surgical intervention to determine the

Table 23–3. American Urological Association symptom index for benign prostatic hyperplasia.[1]

Questions to Be Answered	Not at All	Less Than One Time in Five	Less Than Half the Time	About Half the Time	More Than Half the Time	Almost Always
1. Over the past month, how often have you had a sensation of not emptying your bladder completely after you finish urinating?	0	1	2	3	4	5
2. Over the past month, how often have you had to urinate again less than 2 hours after you finished urinating?	0	1	2	3	4	5
3. Over the past month, how often have you found you stopped and started again several times when you urinated?	0	1	2	3	4	5
4. Over the past month, how often have you found it difficult to postpone urination?	0	1	2	3	4	5
5. Over the past month, how often have you had a weak urinary stream?	0	1	2	3	4	5
6. Over the past month, how often have you had to push or strain to begin urination?	0	1	2	3	4	5
7. Over the past month, how many times did you most typically get up to urinate from the time you went to bed at night until the time you got up in the morning?	0	1	2	3	4	5

[1]Sum of seven circled numbers equals the symptom score. Symptom score (severity): 0–7 (mild); 8-19 (moderate); 20–35 (severe). Patients who score 8 points or higher should consult their physician. See text for explanation.

most appropriate approach (eg, TURP versus simple prostatectomy for a very large gland). This assessment can be done with cystoscopy; transrectal or abdominal ultrasound; or cross-sectional imaging of the pelvis, if it is available.

E. Cystoscopy

Cystoscopy is not required to determine the need for treatment but may assist in determining the surgical approach in patients opting for invasive therapy.

F. Additional Tests

Uroflowmetry and postvoid residual should be assessed before surgical treatment of the prostate and can be useful in tracking response to treatments. Cystometrograms and urodynamic profiles should be reserved for patients with unclear etiology of symptoms, suspected neurologic disease, or those who have not responded to prostate surgery.

Differential Diagnosis

A history of prior urethral instrumentation, urethritis, sexually transmitted infections, or trauma should be elucidated to exclude urethral stricture or bladder neck contracture. Hematuria and pain are commonly associated with bladder stones. Carcinoma of the prostate may be detected by abnormalities on DRE or an elevated PSA (see Chapter 39). A UTI can mimic the irritative symptoms of BPH and can be readily identified by UA and culture; however, a UTI can also be a complication of BPH. Carcinoma of the bladder, especially carcinoma in situ, may also present with irritative voiding; however, UA usually shows evidence of hematuria (see Chapter 39). Patients with a neurogenic bladder may also have many of the same symptoms and signs as those with BPH; however, a history of neurologic disease, stroke, diabetes mellitus, or back injury may be obtained, and diminished perineal or lower extremity sensation or alterations in rectal sphincter tone or in the bulbocavernosus reflex might be observed on examination. Simultaneous alterations in bowel function (constipation) might also suggest the possibility of a neurologic disorder.

Treatment

Clinical practice guidelines exist for the evaluation and treatment of patients with BPH. Following evaluation as outlined above, patients may be offered various forms of therapy for BPH. Patients are advised to consult with their primary care clinicians and make an educated decision on the basis of the relative efficacy and side effects of the treatment options (Table 23–4).

Patients with mild symptoms (AUA scores 0–7) and relatively low bother scores may be managed by watchful waiting only. Medical therapy is appropriate for those with significant bother attributed to their symptoms. Surgery should be considered for patients who have moderate to severe symptoms and those whose medical therapy has failed. Failure of medical therapy is defined as a lack of

Table 23–4. Summary of benign prostatic hyperplasia treatment outcomes.[1]

Outcome	Rezūm	TUIP	Open Surgery	TURP	Watchful Waiting	Alpha-Blockers	Finasteride[2]
Chance for improvement[1]	—	78–83%	94–99.8%	75–96%	31–55%	59–86%	54–78%
Degree of symptom improvement (% reduction in symptom score)	47%	73%	79%	85%	Unknown	51%	31%
Morbidity and complications[1]	3.7–16.9%	2.2–33.3%	7–42.7%	5.2–30.7%	1–5%	2.9–43.3%	8.8–13.6%
Death within 30–90 days[1]	0%	0.2–1.5%	1–4.6%	0.5–3.3%	0.8%	0.8%	0.8%
Total incontinence[1]	0%	0.1–1.1%	0.3–0.7%	0.7–1.4%	2%	2%	2%
Need for operative treatment for surgical complications[1]	< 2%	1.3–2.7%	0.6–14.1%	0.7–10.1%	0	0	0
Erectile dysfunction[1]	0%	3.9–24.5%	4.7–39.2%	3.3–34.8%	3%	3%	2.5–5.3%
Retrograde ejaculation	3–6%	6–55%	36–95%	25–99%	0	4–11%	0
Loss of work in days	—	7–21	21–28	7–21	1	3.5	1.5
Hospital stay in days	0%	1–3	5–10	3–5	0	0	0

[1]90% CI.
[2]Most of the data reviewed for finasteride are derived from three trials that have required an enlarged prostate for entry. The chance of improvement in men with symptoms yet minimally enlarged prostates may be much less, as noted from the VA Cooperative Trial.
TUIP, transurethral incision of the prostate; TURP, transurethral resection of the prostate.

efficacy in relief of symptoms, a progression of symptoms despite medical treatment, or the presence of medication side effects or adverse reactions. Surgery may be indicated in patients who experience more serious sequelae of BPH, such as recurrent UTIs, recurrent gross hematuria attributed to the prostate, bladder stones, refractory urinary retention (failing at least one attempt at catheter removal), or obstructive nephropathy; however, medical management should be tried before proceeding to surgery.

A. Watchful Waiting

In the absence of worrisome sequalae from BPH, lower urinary tract symptoms do not necessarily require treatment if they are not significantly bothersome. Quality of life metrics are important considerations and must be balanced with the risks of available treatments. The risk of progression or complications is uncertain since retrospective studies on the natural history of BPH are inherently subject to bias, relating in part to patient selection and to the type and extent of follow-up. However, experts feel that patients with non-bothersome symptoms are unlikely to develop serious health problems due to BPH. Reassurance and observation are appropriate for these patients. In contrast, men with progressive symptoms and large prostates have a higher chance of developing urinary retention or requiring surgical intervention in the future. A large, randomized study compared finasteride with placebo in men with moderate to severely symptomatic disease and enlarged prostates on DRE. Patients in the placebo arm demonstrated a 7% risk of developing urinary retention over 4 years.

B. Medical Therapy

1. Alpha-blockers—Alpha-adrenergic receptors are ubiquitous, but the prostate and bladder neck have high levels of alpha-1a-receptors. Activation of these receptors results in increased prostatic smooth muscle tone, urethral constriction, and impaired urine flow. Blocking these receptors leads to smooth muscle relaxation and reduced resistance at the bladder outlet. Alpha-blockade has been shown to result in both objective and subjective degrees of improvement in the symptoms and signs of BPH in some patients. Alpha-blockers can be classified according to their receptor selectivity (Table 23–5) as well as their half-life.

Several nonselective alpha-blockers previously utilized in the treatment of BPH have fallen out of favor for more selective medications. Terazosin and doxazosin can still be offered but require dose titration and have higher rates of orthostatic hypotension and dizziness; prazosin and phenoxybenzamine are not used in treatment of BPH.

Alpha-1a-receptors are localized to the prostate and bladder neck and are the predominant adrenoreceptor expressed by stromal smooth muscle cells. Selective blockade with tamsulosin, alfuzosin, or silodosin results in fewer systemic side effects than nonselective alpha-blocker

Table 23–5. Alpha-blockade for benign prostatic hyperplasia.

Agent	Action	Oral Dose
Terazosin	Alpha-1-blockade	1–10 mg daily
Doxazosin	Alpha-1-blockade	1–8 mg daily
Tamsulosin	Alpha-1a-blockade	0.4 or 0.8 mg daily
Alfuzosin	Alpha-1a-blockade	10 mg daily
Silodosin	Alpha-1a-blockade	4 or 8 mg daily
Tadalafil	Phosphodiesterase type 5 inhibitor	5 mg daily

therapy, thus obviating the need for dose titration. The typical dose of tamsulosin is 0.4 mg orally daily taken 30 minutes after a meal. Alfuzosin is a long-acting alpha-1a-blocker; its dose is 10 mg orally once daily with food, and it does not require titration. Silodosin is the most selective alpha-blocker to the prostate, with the lowest rate of orthostasis. It can be started at 4 mg or 8 mg orally once daily. Several randomized, double-blind, placebo-controlled trials have been performed comparing terazosin, doxazosin, tamsulosin, and alfuzosin with placebo. All agents have demonstrated safety and efficacy. Floppy iris syndrome, a complication of cataract surgery, can occur in patients taking both nonselective alpha-blockers and alpha-1a-blockers. Retrograde ejaculation is not uncommon with these medications.

2. 5-Alpha-reductase inhibitors—Finasteride and dutasteride block the conversion of testosterone to dihydrotestosterone. These medications impact the epithelial component of the prostate, resulting in reduction in size of the gland and improvement in symptoms. There is a 20–30% reduction in gland size with maximum benefit after 6–12 months of treatment.

Several randomized, double-blind, placebo-controlled trials have been performed comparing finasteride with placebo. Efficacy, safety, and durability are well established. However, symptomatic improvement is seen only in men with enlarged prostates (greater than 40 mL by ultrasonographic examination). Side effects include decreased libido, decrease in volume of ejaculate, and erectile dysfunction. Gynecomastia is also a rare adverse effect. Serum PSA is reduced by approximately 50% in patients receiving finasteride therapy, but the % free PSA is unchanged. Therefore, in order to compare with pre-finasteride PSA levels, the serum PSA of a patient taking finasteride should be doubled.

A report suggests that finasteride therapy may decrease the incidence of urinary retention and the need for operative treatment in men with enlarged prostates and moderate to severe symptoms. The larger the prostate over 40 mL, the greater the relative-risk reduction. However, optimal identification of appropriate patients for prophylactic therapy remains to be determined. Dutasteride is a dual 5-alpha-reductase inhibitor (inhibiting both 5-alpha-reductase types 1 and 2) that appears to be similar to finasteride in its effectiveness; its dose is 0.5 mg orally daily.

Both finasteride and dutasteride have been shown to be effective chemopreventive agents for prostate cancer in large, randomized clinical trials. A 25% risk reduction was observed in men with both low and high risk for prostate cancer. However, despite the strength of the evidence for 5-alpha-reductase inhibitors in reducing the risk of prostate cancer, an FDA advisory committee recommended against labeling these agents for prostate cancer chemoprevention, citing the potential increased risk of high-grade tumors in these studies (1.8% versus 1.0% for finasteride and 1% versus 0.5% for dutasteride), isolated risk reduction in low-grade tumors, and inability to apply the findings to the general population. Moreover, the FDA has included the increased risk of high-grade prostate cancer in the labels of all 5-alpha-reductase inhibitors.

3. Phosphodiesterase-5 inhibitor—Tadalafil is approved by the FDA to treat the symptoms and signs of BPH (Table 23–5); it is also approved to treat urinary symptoms and erectile dysfunction in men. The data from two randomized, double-blind, placebo-controlled trials demonstrated significant improvements in standardized measurements of urinary function between 2 and 4 weeks after initiating treatment at 5 mg once daily, with minimal adverse effects.

4. Combination therapy—The Medical Therapy of Prostatic Symptoms (MTOPS) trial was a large, randomized, placebo-controlled trial comparing finasteride, doxazosin, the combination of the two, and placebo in 3047 men observed for a mean of 4.5 years. Long-term combination therapy with doxazosin and finasteride was safe and reduced the risk of overall clinical progression of BPH significantly more than did treatment with either medication alone. Combination therapy and finasteride alone reduced the long-term risk of acute urinary retention and the need for invasive therapy. Combination therapy had the risks of additional side effects and the cost of two medications. Newer studies have also shown benefit with the combination of alpha-blockers and tadalafil.

C. Transurethral Surgical Therapy

Most cases of BPH requiring surgery can be managed with transurethral or minimally invasive techniques. This remains an area of active research and innovation with several new technologies available. An overview of all the surgical options and decision-making was published by the AUA (Figure 23–3).

1. Transurethral resection of the prostate (TURP)—TURP has long been considered the gold standard treatment for surgical treatment of BPH, and it often requires a 1- to 2-day hospital stay. Most head-to-head surgical studies comparing TURP with minimally invasive therapies show symptom scores and flow rate improvements are superior following TURP compared with any minimally invasive therapy. The risks of TURP include retrograde ejaculation (75%), erectile dysfunction (less than 5%), and urinary incontinence (less than 1%). Potential complications include (1) bleeding; (2) urethral stricture or bladder neck contracture; and (3) perforation of the prostate capsule with extravasation. Transurethral resection syndrome, a hypervolemic, hyponatremic state resulting from absorption of the hypotonic irrigating solution associated with monopolar TURP is very rare with the increased use of bipolar TURPs (using saline irrigation). Clinical manifestations of the syndrome include nausea, vomiting, confusion, hypertension, bradycardia, and visual disturbances.

2. Transurethral incision of the prostate (TUIP)—Men with moderate to severe symptoms and small prostates (less than 30 g) often have posterior commissure hyperplasia or an "elevated bladder neck." These patients will often benefit from incision of the prostate. The procedure is more rapid and less morbid than TURP. Outcomes in well-selected patients are comparable, although a lower rate of retrograde ejaculation has been reported (25%).

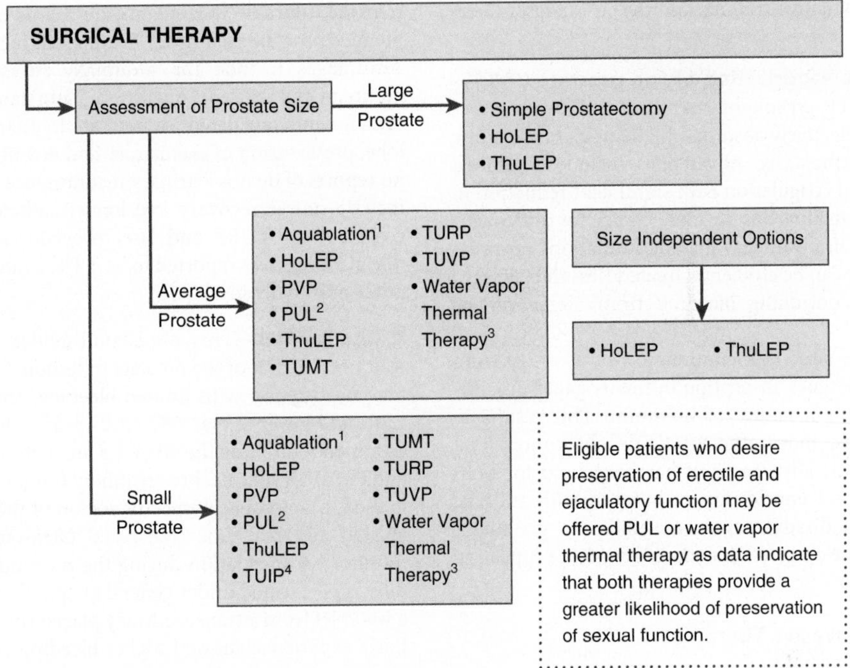

MEDICALLY COMPLICATED PATIENTS

In patients who are at higher risk for bleeding, such as those taking anticoagulation drugs, therapies with a lower need for blood transfusion, such as HoLEP, PVP and ThuLEP, should be considered. For additional information on the use of anticoagulation and antiplatelet therapy in surgical patients, refer to the ICUD/AUA review on Anticoagulation and Antiplatelet Therapy in Urologic Practice.

[1]Eligibility for an aquablation procedure is dependent upon prostate volume > 30/< 80 g.
[2]Eligibility for a PUL procedure is dependent upon absence of obstructing midline prostate tissue and prostate volume < 80 g.
[3]Eligibility for a Water Vapor Thermal Therapy procedure is dependent upon prostate volume < 80 g.
[4]Eligibility for a TUIP procedure is dependent upon prostate volume < 30 g.

▲ **Figure 23–3. Surgical management of lower urinary tract symptoms attributed to benign prostatic hyperplasia. HoLEP, holmium laser enucleation of the prostate; PUL, prostatic urethral lift; PVP, photoselective vaporization of the prostate; ThuLEP, thulium laser enucleation of the prostate; TUIP, transurethral incision of the prostate; TUMT, transurethral microwave therapy; TURP, transurethral resection of the prostate; TUVP, transurethral vaporization of the prostate.** (Reproduced with permission from Foster HE, Dahm P, Kohler TS, et al. Surgical Management of Lower Urinary Tract Symptoms Attributed to Benign Prostatic Hyperplasia: AUA Guideline Amendment 2019. *J Urol.* 2019;202(3):592–598. doi:10.1097/JU.0000000000000319.)

3. Transurethral electrovaporization of the prostate (TUVP)—TUVP is a technical electrosurgical modification of the standard TURP. A variety of energy delivery surfaces including a spherical rolling electrode (rollerball), grooved roller electrode (vaportrode), or hemi-spherical mushroom electrode (button) are used to deliver high current densities resulting in heat vaporization of prostatic tissue. For larger prostates, this procedure usually takes longer than a standard TURP, but it has comparable efficacy with lower transfusion requirements.

4. Laser vaporization of the prostate—Various laser technologies now exist; they vary based on the wavelength and energy produced and the technique of tissue removal. Initial laser technologies relying on tissue coagulation have essentially been abandoned in favor of lasers that result in vaporization of tissue. The laser fiber is placed in direct contact with the prostate tissue, which is then vaporized. An immediate defect is obtained in the prostatic urethra, similar to that seen during TURP. Advantages to such laser therapy include minimal blood loss, rare occurrence of transurethral resection syndrome, ability to treat patients during anticoagulant therapy, and ability to operate on outpatients. Disadvantages are the lack of tissue for pathologic examination, variable effectiveness, more frequent irritative voiding, and the cost of laser fibers and generators.

Photoselective vaporization of the prostate (PVP)— The original KTP greenlight laser used a 532-nm wavelength that is selectively absorbed by hemoglobin, leading to improved hemostasis. Advantages include combined vaporization and coagulation with significant reduction in tissue volume, making this an ideal choice for anticoagulated patients. Disadvantages include limitations on prostate volume that can be efficiently treated (less than 80 mL) and difficulty controlling bleeding from larger venous channels.

The thulium laser is a continuous wave of 2013-nm energy that undergoes absorption in the irrigant but without the intermittent nature of holmium. This results in cleaner incisions, more efficient tissue absorption, and similar hemostatic advantages. It has been used for both resection-type and enucleation techniques with success. Advantages and disadvantages are similar to greenlight PVP, although the cleaner incisions make it more appealing for surgeons.

D. Minimally Invasive Therapies

Treatment for BPH has been an area of active research and innovation with numerous minimally invasive surgical therapies, often able to be delivered in an office setting. Minimally invasive surgical therapies include prostatic urethral lift, water vapor thermal therapy (Rezūm), and Aquablation. Prior attempts at stents were unsuccessful, but a new temporary urethral stent (iTIND) is being investigated. Older techniques such as transurethral microwave therapy (TUMT) or transurethral needle ablation (TUNA) have fallen out of favor due to lower efficacy, durability and high re-treatment rates.

1. Prostatic urethral lift (UroLift)—The UroLift system uses permanent nitinol and stainless-steel implants placed under cystoscopic guidance to retract the lateral lobes of the prostate and mechanically open the prostatic urethra. The procedure is FDA-approved and can be performed under local anesthesia in the clinic. The ideal candidate has primarily lateral lobe hyperplasia and a prostate volume under 80 mL. Short-term data show improved symptoms and voiding flows, preservation of ejaculatory function, and no de novo erectile dysfunction. Re-treatment rates within 5 years have been reported to be as high as 13.6%.

2. Water vapor thermal therapy (Rezūm)—This minimally invasive, FDA-approved technique uses a transurethral device to deliver water vapor into the prostatic tissue. As the steam condenses back into water, it releases large amounts of stored thermal energy leading to tissue necrosis and resorption of tissue over 1–3 months. This procedure is done in the clinic or ambulatory surgery setting with local anesthesia; it requires 3–7 days of catheterization. In contrast to the UroLift procedure, there is a significant reduction in prostate volume over time. Results from a 5-year randomized, controlled trial reported significant objective improvement in lower urinary tract symptoms as early as 2 weeks postprocedure, improvement that remained durable throughout the 5-year period. Recommended prostate volume for Rezūm treatment is 30–80 mL. Advantages include the minimally invasive, outpatient nature of the procedure with no significant bleeding risk even for anticoagulated patients, ability to treat the median lobe, preservation of ejaculatory and erectile function, and no reports of de novo urinary incontinence. Disadvantages include slower recovery and longer catheterization times compared to TURP and laser procedures. Re-treatment rate at 5 years was reported to be 4.4%, a rate far lower than other minimally invasive options.

3. Aquablation—This ultrasound-guided, robot-assisted waterjet ablation of the prostate is designed to relieve prostatic obstruction with limited bleeding, shorter operative time, and lower sexual side-effect profile. It is offered as a treatment option by the AUA for prostates between 30 mL and 80 mL in volume. Pre-treatment transrectal ultrasound is used to map out the specific region of the prostate to be ablated and real-time transrectal ultrasound is used to monitor tissue ablation during the procedure. The procedure is performed under general or spinal anesthesia using a water jet from a transurethrally placed robotic handpiece. Early experience showed higher bleeding and transfusion rates than comparable methods, necessitating the use of electrocautery or traction from a three-way catheter to obtain hemostasis. Short-term data show improvements in urinary flow rate, postvoid residual volume, and quality of life, but long-term data on durability are pending.

4. Prostate artery embolization (PAE)—Initially described in the 1970s to control bleeding, embolization of the prostatic arteries bilaterally has been shown to reduce prostate volume and recent data shows some relief of urinary symptoms. Selective embolization using 100–500 mcm microspheres results in a low risk of non-target ischemia. The available data are limited, and as such, the AUA does not recommend prostatic artery embolization as a standard treatment option, but it can be considered in selected patients, particularly those with larger glands who are not candidates for other available treatments.

E. Enucleation

1. Simple prostatectomy—When the prostate is very large, a simple prostatectomy by an open or robotic enucleation approach may be considered. What size is "too large" depends on the surgeon's experience with TURP. Glands over 100 g are usually considered for enucleation. In addition to size, other relative indications for open prostatectomy include when there is a concomitant bladder diverticulum or stone, and when dorsal lithotomy positioning of the patient is not possible.

Simple prostatectomy can be performed with either a suprapubic or retropubic approach. Simple suprapubic prostatectomy is performed transvesically and is the operation of choice if there is concomitant bladder pathology (eg, bladder stones). These operations can also be performed via robotic-assisted laparoscopic techniques with shorter hospital stays, less blood loss, and decreased need for a suprapubic catheter.

2. Laser enucleation—Holmium or **thulium laser enucleation of the prostate** (**HoLEP** or **ThuLEP**) is a technique of enucleating the adenomatous lobes intact and morcellating the tissue within the bladder. Advantages of HoLEP compared with other methods include ability to treat all prostate sizes, low re-treatment rates, few complications, and shorter duration of catheterization. This technique is an attractive alternative to open simple prostatectomy for very large glands greater than 100 mL) with comparable outcomes. However, due to the steep learning curve for operators, it is not as widely available as other techniques.

When to Refer

- Urinary retention.
- Patient dissatisfaction with medical therapy.
- Need for further evaluation (cystoscopy) or surgical intervention.

Das AK et al. Office-based therapies for benign prostatic hyperplasia: a review and update. Canad J Urol. 2019;26:2. [PMID: 31481142]

Parsons JK et al. Surgical management of lower urinary tract symptoms attributed to benign prostatic hyperplasia: AUA Guideline Amendment 2020. J Urol. 2020;204:799. [PMID: 32698710]

Roehrborn CG et al. Aquablation of the prostate: a review and update. Can J Urol. 2019;26:20. [PMID: 31481145]

Sun F et al. Transurethral procedures in the treatment of benign prostatic hyperplasia: a systematic review and meta-analysis of effectiveness and complications. Medicine (Baltimore). 2018;97:e13360. [PMID: 30572440]

CANCERS OF THE GENITOURINARY TRACT

(See Chapter 39 for Cancers of the Genitourinary Tract: Prostate Cancer, Bladder Cancer, Cancers of the Ureter & Renal Pelvis, Renal Cell Carcinoma, & Testicular Cancers.)

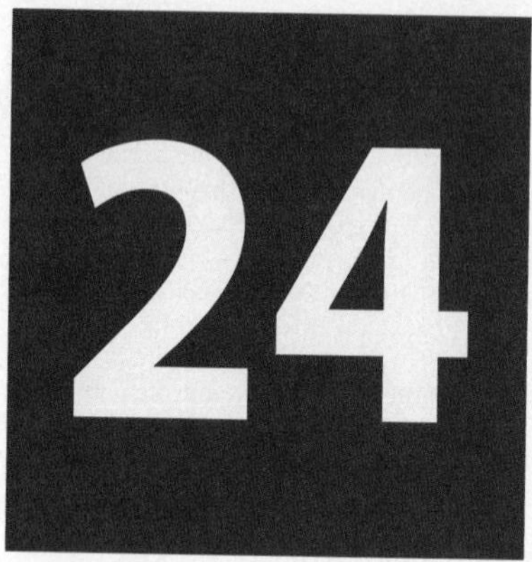

Nervous System Disorders

Vanja C. Douglas, MD
Michael J. Aminoff, MD, DSc, FRCP

HEADACHE

Headache is such a common complaint and can occur for so many different reasons that its proper evaluation may be difficult. New, severe, or acute headaches are more likely than chronic headaches to relate to an intracranial disorder; the approach to such headaches is discussed in Chapter 2. **Chronic headaches** may be primary or secondary to another disorder. Common **primary** headache syndromes include migraine, tension-type headache, and cluster headache. Important **secondary** causes to consider include intracranial lesions, head injury, cervical spondylosis, dental or ocular disease, temporomandibular joint dysfunction, sinusitis, hypertension, depression, and a wide variety of general medical disorders. Although underlying structural lesions are not present in most patients presenting with headache, it is nevertheless important to bear this possibility in mind. About one-third of patients with brain tumors, for example, present with a primary complaint of headache.

1. Migraine

ESSENTIALS OF DIAGNOSIS

- Headache, usually pulsatile, lasting 4–72 hours.
- Pain is typically, but not always, unilateral.
- Nausea, vomiting, photophobia, and phonophobia are common accompaniments.
- Pain is aggravated with routine physical activity.
- An aura of transient neurologic symptoms (commonly visual) may precede head pain.
- Commonly, head pain occurs with no aura.

General Considerations

The pathophysiology of migraine probably relates to neuronal dysfunction in the trigeminal system resulting in release of vasoactive neuropeptides such as calcitonin gene–related peptide leading to neurogenic inflammation, sensitization, and headache. Migraine aura is hypothesized to result from cortical spreading depression, a wave of neuronal and glial depolarization that moves slowly across the cerebral cortex corresponding to the clinical symptoms (ie, occipital cortex and visual aura). Migraine often exhibits a complex, polygenic pattern of inheritance. Sometimes, an autosomal dominant inheritance pattern is apparent, as in **familial hemiplegic migraine,** in which attacks of lateralized weakness represent the aura.

Clinical Findings

Typical migrainous headache is a lateralized throbbing headache that occurs episodically following its onset in adolescence or early adult life. In many cases, the headaches do not conform to this pattern, although their associated features and response to antimigrainous medications nevertheless suggest a similar basis. In this broader sense, migrainous headaches may be lateralized or generalized, may be dull or throbbing, and are sometimes associated with anorexia, nausea, vomiting, photophobia, phonophobia, osmophobia, cognitive impairment, and blurring of vision. They usually build up gradually and last several hours or longer. Focal disturbances of neurologic function (**migraine aura**) may precede or accompany the headaches. Visual disturbances occur commonly and may consist of field defects (**scotoma**); of luminous visual hallucinations such as stars, sparks, unformed light flashes (**photopsia**), geometric patterns, or zigzags of light; or of some combination of field defects and luminous hallucinations (**scintillating scotomas**). Other focal disturbances such as aphasia or numbness, paresthesias, clumsiness, dysarthria, dysequilibrium, or weakness in a circumscribed distribution may also occur.

In rare instances, the neurologic or somatic disturbance accompanying typical migrainous headaches becomes the sole manifestation of an attack ("**migraine aura without headache**"). Very rarely, the patient may be left with a permanent neurologic deficit following a migrainous attack, and migraine with aura is a risk factor for stroke.

Patients often give a family history of migraine. Attacks may be triggered by emotional or physical stress, lack or excess of sleep, missed meals, specific foods (eg, chocolate), alcoholic beverages, bright lights, loud noise, menstruation, or use of oral contraceptives.

An uncommon variant is **migraine with brainstem aura,** in which blindness or visual disturbances throughout both visual fields are accompanied or followed by dysarthria, dysequilibrium, tinnitus, and perioral and distal paresthesias and are sometimes followed by transient loss or impairment of consciousness or by a confusional state. This, in turn, is followed by a throbbing (usually occipital) headache, often with nausea and vomiting.

In **recurrent painful ophthalmoplegic neuropathy** (previously ophthalmoplegic migraine), lateralized pain—often about the eye—is accompanied by nausea, vomiting, and diplopia due to transient external ophthalmoplegia. The ophthalmoplegia is due to third nerve palsy, sometimes with accompanying sixth nerve involvement, and may outlast the orbital pain by several days or even weeks. The ophthalmic division of the fifth nerve has also been affected in some patients. The condition is rare and a diagnosis of exclusion; more common causes of a painful ophthalmoplegia are internal carotid artery aneurysms and diabetes.

Treatment

Management of migraine consists of avoidance of any precipitating factors, together with prophylactic or symptomatic pharmacologic treatment if necessary.

A. Symptomatic Therapy

During acute attacks, rest in a quiet, darkened room may be helpful until symptoms subside. A simple analgesic (eg, aspirin, acetaminophen, ibuprofen, or naproxen) taken immediately often provides relief, but prescription medication is sometimes necessary. *To prevent medication overuse, use of simple analgesics should be limited to 15 days or less per month, and, in general, other medications should be limited to no more than 10 days per month.*

1. Ergotamines—Cafergot, a combination of ergotamine tartrate (1 mg) and caffeine (100 mg), is often particularly helpful; one or two tablets are taken at the onset of headache or warning symptoms, followed by one tablet every 30 minutes, if necessary, up to six tablets per attack and no more than 10 days per month. Cafergot given rectally (one-half to one suppository containing 2 mg of ergotamine) or dihydroergotamine mesylate (0.5–1 mg intravenously or 1–2 mg subcutaneously or intramuscularly) may be useful when vomiting precludes use of oral medications. Ergotamine-containing preparations should be avoided during pregnancy, in patients with CVD or its risk factors, and in patients taking potent CYP 3A4 inhibitors.

2. Serotonin agonists—Triptans are 5-$HT_{1b/1d}$ receptor agonists that inhibit release of vasoactive neuropeptides. Sumatriptan is a rapidly effective agent for aborting attacks when given subcutaneously by an autoinjection device (4–6 mg once subcutaneously, may repeat once after 2 hours if needed; maximum dose 12 mg/24 hours). Nasal and oral preparations are available but may be less effective due to slower absorption. Zolmitriptan is available in oral and nasal formulations. The dose is 5 mg orally or in one nostril once; this may be repeated once after 2 hours. The maximum dose for both formulations is 10 mg/24 hours. Other triptans are available, including rizatriptan (5–10 mg orally at onset, may repeat every 2 hours twice [maximum dose 30 mg/24 hours]); naratriptan (1–2.5 mg orally at onset, may repeat once after 4 hours [maximum dose 5 mg/24 hours]); almotriptan (6.25–12.5 mg orally at onset, may repeat once after 2 hours [maximum dose 25 mg/24 hours]); frovatriptan (2.5 mg orally at onset, may repeat once after 2 hours [maximum dose 7.5 mg/24 hours]); and eletriptan (20–40 mg orally at onset; may repeat once after 2 hours [maximum dose 80 mg/24 hours]). Eletriptan is useful for immediate therapy, and frovatriptan, which has a longer half-life, may be worthwhile for patients with prolonged attacks or attacks provoked by menstrual periods. Patients often experience greater benefit when the triptan is combined with naproxen (500 mg orally).

Triptans may cause nausea and vomiting. They should probably be avoided in women who are pregnant, and in patients with hemiplegic or basilar migraine, a history of stroke or transient ischemic attack, or uncontrolled hypertension. In patients whose hypertension is controlled, triptans are commonly used safely, although caution is advised. *Triptans are contraindicated in patients with coronary or peripheral vascular disease and Prinzmetal angina.*

Lasmiditan (50–200 mg taken once at headache onset; no more than one dose in 24 hours) is a 5-HT_{1F} receptor agonist approved for use in the United States that lacks the vasoconstrictive properties of triptans and can be given safely to patients with cardiovascular risk factors. Dizziness and somnolence are common side effects, and patients should not drive within 8 hours of administration.

3. Calcitonin gene–related peptide antagonists—Rimegepant sulfate (75 mg orally dissolved tablet taken once at headache onset; maximum dose 75 mg/24 hours) and ubrogepant (50 or 100 mg orally at headache onset, may repeat once after 2 hours [maximum dose 200 mg/24 hours]) are both calcitonin gene–related peptide antagonists that achieve pain freedom in 20% and pain relief in 60% of patients within 2 hours. Hypersensitivity reactions may occur immediately or several days after administration with rimegepant.

4. Other agents—Prochlorperazine is effective and may be administered rectally (25 mg suppository), intravenously or intramuscularly (5–10 mg), or orally (5–10 mg). Intravenous metoclopramide (10–20 mg) is also particularly useful in the emergency department setting. Various butalbital-containing combination oral analgesics risk overuse and dependence and should only be used as a last resort. Opioid analgesics should be *avoided* because of high rates of rebound headache and the tendency to develop medication overuse headache.

5. Neuromodulation—Sham-controlled trials show that single-pulse transcranial magnetic stimulation aborts migraine with aura, and noninvasive vagus nerve stimulation, transcutaneous trigeminal nerve stimulation, and remote electrical stimulation applied to the upper arm abort migraine with or without aura. Transcranial magnetic stimulation is contraindicated in patients with epilepsy.

B. Preventive Therapy

Preventive treatment may be necessary if migraine headaches occur *more frequently than two or three times a month* or significant disability is associated with attacks. Avoidance of triggers and maintenance of homeostasis with regular sleep, meals, and hydration should not be neglected; a headache diary may be useful to identify triggers. Some more common agents used for prophylaxis are listed in Table 24–1. The medication chosen first will vary with the individual patient, depending on factors such as comorbid

Table 24–1. Pharmacologic prophylaxis of migraine (listed in alphabetical order within classes).

Medication	Usual Adult Oral Daily Dose	Selected Side Effects and Comments
Antiepileptic[1]		
Topiramate[2]	100 mg (divided twice daily)	Somnolence, nausea, dyspepsia, irritability, dizziness, ataxia, nystagmus, diplopia, glaucoma, renal calculi, weight loss, hypohidrosis, hyperthermia.
Valproic acid[2]	500–1000 mg (divided twice daily)	Nausea, vomiting, diarrhea, drowsiness, alopecia, weight gain, hepatotoxicity, thrombocytopenia, tremor, pancreatitis.
Cardiovascular		
Candesartan[2,3]	8–32 mg once daily	Dizziness, cough, diarrhea, fatigue.
Guanfacine[3]	1 mg once daily	Dry mouth, somnolence, dizziness, constipation, erectile dysfunction.
Propranolol[2,4]	80–240 mg (divided twice to four times daily)	Fatigue, dizziness, hypotension, bradycardia, depression, insomnia, nausea, vomiting, constipation.
Verapamil[3,5]	120–240 mg (divided three times daily)	Headache, hypotension, flushing, edema, constipation. May aggravate atrioventricular nodal heart block and heart failure.
Antidepressant[6]		
Amitriptyline[3,7]	10–150 mg at bedtime	Sedation, dry mouth, constipation, weight gain, blurred vision, edema, hypotension, urinary retention.
Venlafaxine[3]	37.5–150 mg extended-release once daily	Nausea, somnolence, dry mouth, dizziness, diaphoresis, sexual dysfunction, anxiety, weight loss.
Monoclonal antibodies against calcitonin gene–related peptide		
Eptinezumab	100 mg intravenously every 3 months	Hypersensitivity reaction during infusion, nasopharyngitis.
Erenumab	70–140 mg subcutaneously once monthly	Injection site reactions, constipation, muscle cramps, antibody development.
Fremanezumab	225 mg subcutaneously once monthly	Injection site reactions, antibody development.
Galcanezumab	120 mg subcutaneously daily × 2 doses, followed by 120 mg monthly	Injection site reactions, antibody development.
Calcitonin gene–related peptide receptor antagonists		
Atogepant	10–30 mg once daily	Nausea, constipation, fatigue.
Rimegepant	75 mg once every other day	Hypersensitivity, nausea.
Other		
Acupuncture		More rapid pain relief and fewer side effects than pharmacologic treatment.
Botulinum toxin A	Intramuscular injection	Injection site reaction, hypersensitivity, muscle weakness.
Coenzyme Q10	300 mg once daily	
Magnesium citrate	200–300 mg twice daily	Diarrhea, nausea.
Memantine[3]	5 mg once daily to 10 mg twice daily	Somnolence, sedation, nausea.
Riboflavin	400 mg once daily	Yellow-orange discoloration of urine.
Transcutaneous supraorbital neurostimulation	20 minutes daily	Transient paresthesia at site of stimulation.

[1]Gabapentin and possibly other antiepileptics have also been used successfully.
[2]Caution or avoid during pregnancy.
[3]Not FDA-approved for this indication.
[4]Other beta-adrenergic antagonists such as atenolol, metoprolol, nadolol, and timolol are similarly effective.
[5]Other calcium channel antagonists (eg, nimodipine, nicardipine, and diltiazem) may also help.
[6]Depression is commonly comorbid with migraine disorder and may warrant separate treatment.
[7]Other tricyclic antidepressants (eg, nortriptyline and imipramine) may help similarly.

obesity, depression, anxiety, hypertension, and patient preference. Several medications may have to be tried in turn before headaches are brought under control. Once a medication has been found to help, it should be continued for several months. If the patient remains headache-free, the dose may be tapered and the medication eventually withdrawn. Transcutaneous supraorbital neurostimulation reduced the number of migraine days per month in a sham-controlled randomized trial and is approved in the United States. In **chronic migraine** (at least 15 days per month with headaches lasting 4 hours per day or longer), acupuncture is as effective as prophylactic pharmacologic treatment, and botulinum toxin type A reduces headache frequency. Certain neurostimulation techniques look promising as preventive treatment as well as having a role in treatment of acute attacks. These include single-pulse transcranial magnetic stimulation, vagus nerve stimulators, and implantable occipital nerve stimulation, but critical appraisal is necessary.

2. Tension-Type Headache

This is the most common type of primary headache disorder. Patients frequently complain of pericranial tenderness, poor concentration, and other nonspecific symptoms, in addition to headaches that are often vise-like or tight in quality but not pulsatile. Headaches may be exacerbated by emotional stress, fatigue, noise, or glare. The headaches are usually generalized, may be most intense about the neck or back of the head, and are not associated with focal neurologic symptoms. There is diagnostic overlap with migraine.

Abortive therapy with simple analgesics is usually effective. Anti-migraine preparations are not recommended unless the patient has comorbid migraine headaches. Tricyclic antidepressants, such as amitriptyline, are supported for headache prophylaxis by randomized trial evidence and often are tried first. Treatment of comorbid anxiety or depression is important. Behavioral therapies that may be effective include biofeedback and relaxation training.

3. Cluster Headache

Cluster headache affects predominantly middle-aged men. The pathophysiology is unclear but may relate to activation of cells in the ipsilateral hypothalamus, triggering the trigeminal autonomic vascular system. There is often no family history of headache or migraine. Episodes of severe unilateral periorbital pain occur daily for several weeks and are often accompanied by one or more of the following: ipsilateral nasal congestion, rhinorrhea, lacrimation, redness of the eye, and Horner syndrome (ptosis, pupillary meiosis, and facial anhidrosis or hypohidrosis). During attacks, patients are often restless and agitated. Episodes typically occur at night, awaken the patient, and last between 15 minutes and 3 hours. Spontaneous remission then occurs, and the patient remains well for weeks or months before another bout of closely spaced attacks. Bouts may last for 4 to 8 weeks and may occur up to several times per year. During a bout, many patients report alcohol triggers an attack; others report that stress, glare, or ingestion of specific foods occasionally precipitates attacks. In occasional patients, remission does not occur. This variant has been referred to as **chronic cluster headache**. In longstanding cases, Horner syndrome may persist between attacks.

Cluster headache is one of the **trigeminal autonomic cephalgias,** which include hemicrania continua, paroxysmal hemicrania, and short-lasting neuralgiform headache attacks with conjunctival injection and tearing. Similar to cluster headache, the other trigeminal autonomic cephalgias consist of unilateral periorbital pain associated with ipsilateral autonomic symptoms; they are distinguished from cluster headache by different attack duration and frequency and their exquisite responsiveness to indomethacin.

Treatment of an individual attack with oral medications is generally unsatisfactory, but subcutaneous (6 mg) or intranasal (20 mg/spray) sumatriptan or inhalation of 100% oxygen (12–15 L/minute for 15 minutes via a nonrebreather mask) may be effective. Zolmitriptan (5- and 10-mg nasal spray) is also effective. Dihydroergotamine (0.5–1 mg intramuscularly or intravenously) or viscous lidocaine (1 mg of 4–6% solution intranasally) is sometimes effective.

Various prophylactic agents include oral medications such as lithium carbonate (start at 300 mg daily, titrating according to serum levels and treatment response up to a typical total daily dose of 900–1200 mg, divided three or four times), verapamil (start at 240 mg daily, increase by 80 mg every 2 weeks to 960 mg daily, with routine ECG to monitor the PR interval), topiramate (100–400 mg daily), and galcanezumab (300 mg subcutaneously monthly until end of cluster period). As there is often a delay before these medications are effective, transitional therapy is often used. Prednisone (60–100 mg daily for 5 days followed by gradual withdrawal over 7–10 days) is effective in 70–80% of patients, and suboccipital corticosteroid injection about the greater occipital nerve is effective in 75%. Ergotamine tartrate can be given as rectal suppositories (0.5–1 mg at night or twice daily), by mouth (2 mg daily), or by subcutaneous injection (0.25 mg three times daily for 5 days per week). Electrical stimulation of the vagus nerve at headache onset successfully aborts pain in 30–50% of attacks, and twice daily prophylactic stimulation reduces attack number in chronic cluster headache; this treatment is approved in the United States. In Europe, sphenopalatine ganglion stimulation is approved for treatment of cluster headache based on efficacy in one randomized sham-controlled study. Electrical stimulation of the occipital nerve by an implantable device reduces headache frequency in chronic cluster headache, although it does not have regulatory approval.

4. Posttraumatic Headache

A variety of nonspecific symptoms may follow closed head injury, regardless of whether consciousness is lost (see Head Injury). Headache is often a conspicuous feature. It usually appears within a day or so following injury, may worsen over the ensuing weeks, and then gradually subsides. It is usually a constant dull ache, with superimposed throbbing that may be localized, lateralized, or generalized. Headaches are sometimes accompanied by nausea, vomiting, or scintillating scotomas and often respond to simple analgesics; severe headaches may necessitate preventive treatment as outlined for migraine.

5. Primary Cough Headache

Severe head pain may be produced by coughing (and by straining, sneezing, and laughing) but, fortunately, usually lasts for a few minutes or less. Intracranial lesions, usually in the posterior fossa (eg, Arnold-Chiari malformation), are present in about 10% of cases, and brain tumors or other space-occupying lesions may present in this way. Accordingly, *CT scanning or MRI should be undertaken in all patients.*

The disorder is usually self-limited, although it may persist for several years. For unknown reasons, symptoms sometimes clear completely after lumbar puncture. Indomethacin (75–150 mg daily orally) may provide relief. Similar activity-triggered headache syndromes include primary exertional headache and primary headache associated with sexual activity.

6. Headache Due to Giant Cell (Temporal or Cranial) Arteritis

This topic is discussed in Chapter 20.

7. Headache Due to Intracranial Mass Lesion

Intracranial mass lesions of all types may cause headache owing to displacement of vascular structures and other pain-sensitive tissues. While pain and location are nonspecific, headache may be worse upon lying down, awaken the patient at night, or peak in the morning after overnight recumbency. *The key feature prompting brain imaging is a new or worsening headache in middle or later life.* Other features suggesting an intracranial lesion include signs or symptoms of infection or malignancy such as fever, night sweats, and weight loss; immunocompromise; or history of malignancy. Signs of focal or diffuse cerebral dysfunction or of increased intracranial pressure (eg, papilledema) also necessitate investigation.

8. Medication Overuse (Analgesic Rebound) Headache

In many patients with **chronic daily headaches,** medication overuse is responsible. Patients have chronic pain or severe headache unresponsive to medication (typically defined as no effect after having been used regularly for more than 3 months). Ergotamines, triptans, medications containing butalbital, and opioids cause medication overuse headache when taken on more than 10 days per month; acetaminophen, acetylsalicylic acid, and NSAIDs may also be offenders if taken on more than 15 days per month. Whether newer medications such as lasmiditan and the calcitonin gene–related peptide antagonists cause overuse headaches is unknown; nevertheless, their use is also generally restricted to 10 days per month. Dopamine antagonists are unlikely to cause overuse headache, but their use should also be limited to prevent drug-induced parkinsonism or dyskinesia. Early initiation of a migraine preventive therapy permits withdrawal of analgesics and eventual relief of headache.

9. Headache Due to Other Neurologic Causes

Cerebrovascular disease may be associated with headache, but the mechanism is unclear. Headache may occur with internal carotid artery occlusion or carotid dissection and after carotid endarterectomy. Acute severe headache (**"thunderclap"**) accompanies subarachnoid hemorrhage, carotid or vertebral artery dissection, cerebral venous thrombosis, ischemic or hemorrhagic stroke, reversible cerebral vasoconstriction syndrome, hypertensive crisis, posterior reversible leukoencephalopathy syndrome, pituitary apoplexy, spontaneous intracranial hypotension, vasculitis, and meningeal infections; accompanying focal neurologic signs, impairment of consciousness, and signs of meningeal irritation indicate the need for further investigations. Headaches are also a feature of idiopathic intracranial hypertension (pseudotumor cerebri).

Dull or throbbing headache is a frequent sequela of lumbar puncture and may last for several days. It is aggravated by the erect posture and alleviated by recumbency. The mechanism is unclear, but the headache is commonly attributed to leakage of cerebrospinal fluid through the dural puncture site. Its incidence may be reduced if an atraumatic needle (instead of a beveled, cutting needle) is used for the lumbar puncture.

▶ When to Refer

- Thunderclap onset.
- Increasing headache unresponsive to simple measures.
- History of trauma, hypertension, fever, visual changes.
- Presence of neurologic signs or of scalp tenderness.

▶ When to Admit

Suspected subarachnoid hemorrhage or other structural intracranial lesion.

VanderPluym JH et al. Acute treatments for episodic migraine in adults: a systematic review and meta-analysis. JAMA. 2021;325:2357 [PMID: 34128998]

Vukovic-Cvetkovic V et al. Neurostimulation for the treatment of chronic migraine and cluster headache. Acta Neurol Scand. 2019;139:4. [PMID: 30291633]

FACIAL PAIN

1. Trigeminal Neuralgia

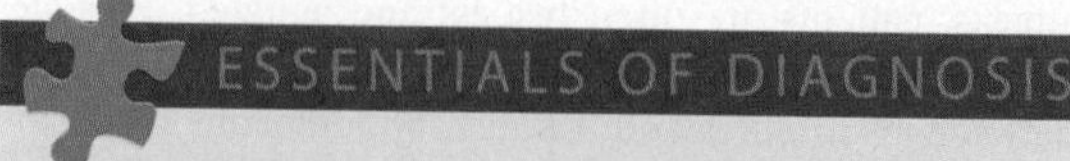

- Brief episodes of stabbing facial pain.
- Pain is in the territory of the second and third division of the trigeminal nerve.
- Pain exacerbated by touch.

General Considerations

Trigeminal neuralgia ("tic douloureux") is most common in middle and later life. It affects women more frequently than men. Pain may be due to an anomalous artery or vein impinging on the trigeminal nerve.

Clinical Findings

Momentary episodes of sudden lancinating facial pain commonly arise near one side of the mouth and shoot toward the ipsilateral ear, eye, or nostril. The pain may be triggered by such factors as touch, movement, drafts, and eating. To lessen the likelihood of triggering further attacks, many patients try to hold the face still while talking. Spontaneous remissions for several months or longer may occur. As the disorder progresses, however, the episodes of pain become more frequent, remissions become shorter and less common, and a dull ache may persist between the episodes of stabbing pain. Symptoms remain confined to the distribution of the trigeminal nerve (usually the second or third division) on one side only.

Differential Diagnosis

The characteristic features of the pain in trigeminal neuralgia usually distinguish it from other causes of facial pain. Neurologic examination shows no abnormality except in a few patients in whom trigeminal neuralgia is symptomatic of some underlying lesion, such as multiple sclerosis or a brainstem neoplasm, in which case the finding will depend on the nature and site of the lesion. Multiple sclerosis must be suspected in a patient younger than 40 years in whom trigeminal neuralgia is the presenting symptom, even if there are no other neurologic signs. Bilateral symptoms should also prompt further investigation. Brain MRI need only be obtained when a secondary cause is suspected; it is usually normal in classic trigeminal neuralgia.

Treatment

The medications most helpful for treatment are oxcarbazepine (although not approved by the FDA for this indication) or carbamazepine, with monitoring by serial blood counts and liver biochemical tests. If these medications are ineffective or cannot be tolerated, phenytoin should be tried. (Doses and side effects of these medications are shown in Table 24–2.) Baclofen (10–20 mg orally three or four times daily), topiramate (50 mg orally twice daily), or lamotrigine (400 mg orally daily) may also be helpful, either alone or in combination with one of these other agents. Gabapentin may also relieve pain, especially in patients who do not respond to conventional medical therapy and those with multiple sclerosis. Depending on response and tolerance, up to 3600 mg daily orally is given in divided doses.

For neuralgia refractory to medical treatment, several surgical treatment options are available that provide initial pain relief in at least 80% of patients. Microvascular surgical decompression with separation of the anomalous vessel (usually not visible on CT scans, MRI, or arteriograms) from the nerve root produces long-term relief of symptoms in roughly 75% of patients. Three less invasive techniques are based on destruction of nociceptive trigeminal nerve fibers, which causes sensory loss in addition to symptom relief in half of patients: (1) radiofrequency rhizotomy produces long-term pain relief in 60% of patients, (2) percutaneous balloon compression of the trigeminal ganglion in 67%, and (3) stereotactic radiosurgery to the trigeminal nerve root in 45%. In older patients with a limited life expectancy, radiofrequency rhizotomy and stereotactic radiosurgery are sometimes preferred because both can be performed without general anesthesia and have few complications. Surgical exploration is inappropriate in patients with trigeminal neuralgia due to multiple sclerosis, but the less invasive techniques are sometimes helpful.

2. Atypical Facial Pain

Facial pain without the typical features of trigeminal neuralgia is generally a constant, often burning pain that may have a restricted distribution at its onset but soon spreads to the rest of the face on the affected side and sometimes involves the other side, the neck, or the back of the head as well. The disorder is especially common in middle-aged women, many of them depressed, but it is not clear whether depression is the cause of or a reaction to the pain. Simple analgesics should be given a trial, as should tricyclic antidepressants, carbamazepine, oxcarbazepine, and phenytoin; the response is often disappointing. Opioid analgesics pose a danger of addiction. Attempts at surgical treatment are not indicated.

3. Glossopharyngeal Neuralgia

Glossopharyngeal neuralgia is an uncommon disorder in which pain similar in quality to that in trigeminal neuralgia occurs in the throat, about the tonsillar fossa, and sometimes deep in the ear and at the back of the tongue. The pain may be precipitated by swallowing, chewing, talking, or yawning and is sometimes accompanied by syncope. In most instances, no underlying structural abnormality is present; multiple sclerosis is sometimes responsible. Oxcarbazepine and carbamazepine are the treatments of choice and should be tried before any surgical procedures are considered. Microvascular decompression is often effective and is generally preferred over destructive surgical procedures such as partial rhizotomy in medically refractory cases.

4. Postherpetic Neuralgia

Postherpetic neuralgia develops in about 15% of patients who have herpes zoster (shingles). This complication seems especially likely to occur in older or immunocompromised persons, when the rash is severe, and when the first division of the trigeminal nerve is affected. It also relates to the duration of the rash before treatment is instituted. A history of shingles and the presence of cutaneous scarring resulting from shingles aid in the diagnosis. Severe pain with shingles correlates with the intensity of postherpetic symptoms.

Acyclovir (800 mg five times daily) or valacyclovir (1000 mg three times daily), when *given within 72 hours* of rash onset, reduces the incidence of postherpetic neuralgia by almost half; systemic corticosteroids do *not* help prevent postherpetic neuralgia (see Chapter 6). Management of the established complication is with simple analgesics. If they fail to help, a trial of a tricyclic antidepressant (eg, amitriptyline or nortriptyline, up to 100–150 mg daily orally) is often effective. Other patients respond to gabapentin (up to 3600 mg daily orally) or pregabalin (up to 600 mg/daily orally). Subcutaneous injection of botulinum toxin A into the affected region produced sustained pain relief in 87% of patients in a small placebo-controlled trial. Topical application of capsaicin cream may be helpful, as may topical lidocaine (5%). The administration of **recombinant zoster vaccine** to patients over the age of 50 years is important in reducing the likelihood of herpes zoster or reducing the severity of postherpetic neuralgia should a reactivation occur.

5. Facial Pain Due to Other Causes

Facial pain may be caused by temporomandibular joint dysfunction in patients with malocclusion, abnormal bite, or faulty dentures. There may be tenderness of the masticatory muscles, and sometimes pain begins at the onset of chewing. This pattern differs from that of jaw (masticatory) claudication, a symptom of giant cell arteritis, in which pain develops progressively with mastication. Treatment of the underlying joint dysfunction relieves symptoms.

A relationship of facial pain to chewing or temperature changes may suggest a dental disturbance. The cause is sometimes not obvious, and diagnosis requires careful dental examination and radiographs. Sinusitis and ear infections causing facial pain are usually recognized by a history of respiratory tract infection, fever, and, in some instances, nasal or aural discharge. There may be localized tenderness. Radiologic evidence of sinus infection or mastoiditis is confirmatory.

Glaucoma is an important ocular cause of facial pain, usually localized to the periorbital region.

On occasion, pain in the jaw may be the principal manifestation of angina pectoris. Precipitation by exertion and radiation to more typical areas suggests a cardiac origin.

When to Refer

- Worsening pain unresponsive to simple measures.
- Continuing pain of uncertain cause.
- For consideration of surgical treatment (trigeminal or glossopharyngeal neuralgia).

Bendtsen L et al. Advances in diagnosis, classification, pathophysiology, and management of trigeminal neuralgia. Lancet Neurol. 2020;19:784. [PMID: 32822636]

EPILEPSY

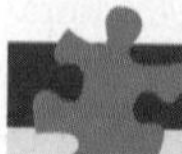

ESSENTIALS OF DIAGNOSIS

- Recurrent unprovoked seizures.
- Characteristic electroencephalographic changes accompany seizures.
- Mental status abnormalities or focal neurologic symptoms may persist for hours postictally.

General Considerations

The term “epilepsy” denotes any disorder characterized by *recurrent unprovoked seizures.* A seizure is a transient disturbance of cerebral function due to an abnormal paroxysmal neuronal discharge in the brain. Epilepsy is relatively common, affecting approximately 0.5% of the population in the United States.

Patients with recurrent seizures provoked by a readily reversible cause, such as withdrawal from alcohol or drugs, hypoglycemia, hyperglycemia, or uremia, are not considered to have epilepsy.

Classification of Epilepsy

According to the International League Against Epilepsy classification system, recurrent seizures should be classified first by seizure type, second by epilepsy type, and third, if possible, by epilepsy syndrome. The etiology of recurrent seizures should be sought at each stage of classification (see Etiology of Epilepsy).

A. Seizure Types

The International League Against Epilepsy distinguishes seizures affecting only part of the brain (focal seizures) from those that are generalized.

1. Focal-onset seizures—The initial clinical and electroencephalographic manifestations of focal (partial) seizures indicate that only a restricted part of one cerebral hemisphere has been activated. The ictal manifestations depend on the area of the brain involved. Focal seizures are classified by motor or nonmotor onset as well as by whether awareness is impaired.

A. MOTOR VERSUS NONMOTOR ONSET—Seizures with motor onset may be **clonic, tonic, atonic, myoclonic,** or **hyperkinetic,** or may manifest as **automatisms** or **epileptic spasms**. The most commonly observed focal motor seizures consist of clonic jerking or automatisms. Nonmotor seizures may be manifested by **sensory symptoms** (eg, paresthesias or tingling, gustatory, olfactory, visual or auditory sensations), **behavior arrest**, **cognitive symptoms** (eg, speech arrest, déjà vu, jamais vu), **emotional symptoms** (eg, fear), or **autonomic symptoms or signs** (eg, abnormal epigastric sensations, sweating, flushing, pupillary dilation). Focal sensory and motor seizures may spread (or “march”) to different parts of the limb or body depending on their cortical representation and were previously called “simple partial” seizures.

B. AWARE VERSUS IMPAIRED AWARENESS—Awareness is defined as knowledge of self and environment and of events occurring during a seizure. Impaired awareness may be preceded, accompanied, or followed by the various motor and nonmotor symptoms mentioned above. Such seizures were previously called “complex partial” seizures.

C. FOCAL TO BILATERAL TONIC-CLONIC—Focal seizures sometimes involve loss of awareness and evolve to bilateral tonic-clonic seizures, in a process previously called “secondary generalization.”

2. Generalized onset seizures—Generalized seizures are thought to originate in or rapidly spread to involve bilateral cortical networks. In some cases, the distinction between focal and generalized onset can only be made by electroencephalogram (EEG). Generalized seizures are classified into those with motor or nonmotor features. Awareness is typically lost with generalized seizures but may be retained partially in the briefest absence attacks and some myoclonic seizures.

A. NONMOTOR (ABSENCE) SEIZURES—These are characterized by impairment of consciousness, sometimes with mild clonic, tonic, myoclonic, or atonic components (ie, reduction or loss of postural tone), autonomic components (eg, enuresis), or accompanying automatisms. Onset and termination of attacks are abrupt. If attacks occur during conversation, the patient may miss a few words or may break off in midsentence for a few seconds. The impairment of external awareness is so brief that the patient is unaware of it. **Absence ("petit mal") seizures** almost always begin in childhood and frequently cease by the age of 20 years or are then replaced by other forms of generalized seizure. Electroencephalographically, such attacks are associated with bursts of bilaterally synchronous and symmetric 3-Hz spike-wave activity. A normal background in the electroencephalogram and normal or above-normal intelligence imply a good prognosis for the ultimate cessation of these seizures. **Atypical absence seizures** may demonstrate more marked changes in tone, or attacks may have a more gradual onset and termination than in typical absence seizures. They commonly occur in patients with multiple seizure types, may be accompanied by developmental delay or mental retardation, and are associated with slower spike-wave discharges than those in typical absence attacks.

B. MOTOR SEIZURES—Types of generalized motor seizures include **tonic-clonic, clonic, tonic, myoclonic, myoclonic-tonic-clonic, myoclonic-atonic, atonic,** and **epileptic spasms.** During tonic-clonic seizures there is sudden loss of consciousness, the patient becomes rigid and falls to the ground, and respiration is arrested. This tonic phase, which usually lasts for under 1 minute, is followed by a clonic phase in which there is jerking of the body musculature that may last for 2 or 3 minutes and is then followed by a stage of flaccid coma. During the seizure, the tongue or lips may be bitten, urinary or fecal incontinence may occur, and the patient may be injured. Immediately after the seizure, the patient may recover consciousness, drift into sleep, have a further convulsion without recovery of consciousness between the attacks **(status epilepticus),** or after recovering consciousness have a further convulsion **(serial seizures).** In other cases, patients may behave in an abnormal fashion in the immediate postictal period, without subsequent awareness or memory of events **(postepileptic automatism)**. Headache, disorientation, confusion, drowsiness, nausea, soreness of the muscles, or some combination of these symptoms commonly occurs postictally. Myoclonic seizures consist of single or multiple myoclonic jerks. Atonic seizures consist of very brief (less than 2 seconds) loss of muscle tone and often result in falls **(epileptic drop attacks)**. **Epileptic spasms** are sudden flexion or extension of truncal muscles; these seizures usually manifest during infancy.

3. Unknown onset seizures—In some circumstances, seizures cannot be classified because of incomplete information or because they do not fit into any category. Generally, with additional information from the history or from video-EEG telemetry, the seizure onset can be correctly classified.

B. Epilepsy Types

The International League Against Epilepsy classifies epilepsy by the seizure type. Thus, epilepsy may be **focal, generalized,** or **combined generalized and focal.** The EEG may be helpful in facilitating classification.

C. Epilepsy Syndromes

Epilepsy syndromes are defined by constellations of seizure types, EEG findings, and imaging features, and often also depend on age at onset and comorbidities. Not every patient with epilepsy can be given a syndromic diagnosis. Several well-known epilepsy syndromes exist but are beyond the scope of this chapter.

Etiology of Epilepsy

In parallel to classifying the seizure type, epilepsy type, and epilepsy syndrome (if applicable), the cause of the patient's seizures should be sought. The International League Against Epilepsy lists six broad etiologic categories; sometimes a patient's seizures have more than one etiology.

A. Structural Etiology

1. Pediatric age groups—Congenital abnormalities and perinatal injuries may result in seizures presenting in infancy or childhood.

2. Mesial temporal sclerosis—Hippocampal sclerosis is a recognized cause of focal and secondarily generalized seizures of uncertain etiology.

3. Trauma—Trauma is an important cause of seizures at any age, but especially in young adults. Posttraumatic epilepsy is more likely to develop if the dura mater was penetrated and generally becomes manifest within 2 years following the injury. Seizures developing in the first week after head injury do not necessarily imply that future attacks will occur. There is *no* evidence that prophylactic anticonvulsant medication treatment reduces the incidence of posttraumatic epilepsy.

4. Tumors and other space-occupying lesions—Neoplasms may lead to seizures at any age, but they are an especially important cause of seizures in middle and later life, when the incidence of neoplastic disease increases. Seizures are commonly the initial symptoms of the tumor and often are focal in character. They are most likely to occur with structural lesions involving the frontal, parietal, or temporal regions. *Tumors must be excluded by imaging studies (MRI preferred over CT) in all patients with onset of* *seizures after 20 years of age, focal seizures or signs, or a progressive seizure disorder.*

5. Vascular diseases—Stroke and other vascular diseases become increasingly frequent causes of seizures with advancing age and are the most common cause of seizures with onset at age 60 years or older.

6. Degenerative disorders—Alzheimer disease and other degenerative disorders are a cause of seizures in later life.

B. Genetic Etiology

This category encompasses a broad range of disorders, for which the age at onset ranges from the neonatal period to adolescence or even later in life. Monogenic disorders tend to exhibit an autosomal dominant pattern of inheritance, and where the mutation is known, the responsible gene often encodes a neuronal ion channel. A genetic etiology may also underpin certain epilepsies with a metabolic or structural basis.

C. Infectious Etiology

Infectious diseases must be considered in all age groups as potentially reversible causes of seizures. Seizures may occur with an acute infective or inflammatory illness, such as bacterial meningitis or herpes encephalitis, or in patients with more longstanding or chronic disorders, such as neurosyphilis or cerebral cysticercosis. In patients with AIDS, seizures may result from CNS toxoplasmosis, cryptococcal meningitis, secondary viral encephalitis, or other infective complications. Seizures are a common sequela of supratentorial brain abscess, developing most frequently in the first year after treatment.

D. Metabolic Etiology

Inborn errors of metabolism and other inherited conditions may cause epilepsy as one of their manifestations (eg, pyridoxine deficiency, mitochondrial disease); these disorders typically present during childhood.

E. Immune Etiology

Autoimmune diseases such as SLE and autoimmune limbic encephalitis may cause epilepsy; often the epilepsy can be cured with immunotherapy and lifelong antiepileptic medication treatment is not necessary.

F. Unknown Etiology

In many cases, the cause of epilepsy cannot be determined.

Clinical Findings

A. Symptoms and Signs

Nonspecific changes such as headache, mood alterations, lethargy, and myoclonic jerking alert some patients to an impending seizure hours before it occurs. These **prodromal symptoms** are distinct from the **aura;** the aura that may precede a generalized seizure by a few seconds or minutes is itself a part of the seizure indicating focal onset from a restricted part of the brain.

In most patients, seizures occur unpredictably at any time and without any relationship to posture or ongoing activities. Occasionally, however, they occur at a particular time (eg, during sleep) or in relation to external precipitants such as lack of sleep, missed meals, emotional stress, menstruation, alcohol ingestion (or alcohol withdrawal), or use of certain recreational drugs. Fever and nonspecific infections may also precipitate seizures in patients with epilepsy. In a few patients, seizures are provoked by specific stimuli such as flashing lights or a flickering television set **(photosensitive epilepsy),** music, or reading.

Clinical examination between seizures shows no abnormality in patients with idiopathic epilepsy, but in the immediate postictal period, extensor plantar responses may be seen. The presence of lateralized or focal signs postictally suggests that seizures may have a focal origin. In patients with symptomatic epilepsy, the findings on examination will reflect the underlying cause.

B. Imaging

MRI is indicated for patients with focal neurologic symptoms or signs, focal seizures, or electroencephalographic findings of a focal disturbance. It should also be performed in patients with clinical evidence of a progressive disorder and in those with new onset of seizures after the age of 20 years because of the possibility of an underlying neoplasm. CT is generally less sensitive than MRI in detecting small structural brain abnormalities but may be used when MRI is contraindicated or unavailable.

C. Laboratory Studies

Initial investigations after a first seizure should include CBC, serum glucose, electrolytes, creatinine, calcium, magnesium, and liver biochemical tests to exclude various causes of provoked seizures and to provide a baseline for subsequent monitoring of long-term effects of treatment. Routine laboratory investigations are *not* usually necessary after recurrent seizures in patients with known epilepsy. A lumbar puncture may be necessary when any sign of infection is present or in the evaluation of new-onset seizures in the acute setting.

D. Electroencephalography

Electroencephalography may support the clinical diagnosis of epilepsy (by demonstrating paroxysmal abnormalities containing spikes or sharp waves), provide a guide to prognosis, and help classify the seizure disorder. Classification of the disorder is important for determining the most appropriate anticonvulsant medication with which to start treatment. For example, absence and focal seizures with impaired awareness may be difficult to distinguish clinically, but the electroencephalographic findings and treatment of choice differ in these two conditions. Finally, by localizing the epileptogenic source, the electroencephalographic findings are important in evaluating candidates for surgical treatment.

Differential Diagnosis

The distinction between the various disorders likely to be confused with generalized seizures is usually based on the history. *The importance of obtaining an eyewitness account of the attacks cannot be overemphasized.*

A. Differential Diagnosis of Focal Seizures

1. TIAs—These are distinguished from seizures by their longer duration, lack of spread, and negative (eg, weakness or numbness) rather than positive (eg, convulsive jerking or paresthesias) symptoms. Level of consciousness, which is unaltered, does not distinguish them.

2. Migraine aura—Migraine aura may produce positive or negative symptoms, tends to spread slowly from one part of the body to another (over minutes rather than seconds), and is usually longer in duration (minutes to hours). It is usually, but not always, followed by a typical migraine headache.

3. Panic attacks—These may be hard to distinguish from focal seizures unless there is evidence of an anxiety disorder between attacks and the attacks have a clear relationship to external circumstances.

4. Rage attacks—These are situational and lead to goal-directed aggressive behavior.

B. Differential Diagnosis of Generalized Seizures

1. Syncope—Syncopal episodes usually occur in relation to postural change, emotional stress, instrumentation, pain, or straining. They are typically preceded by pallor, sweating, nausea, and malaise and lead to loss of consciousness accompanied by flaccidity; recovery occurs rapidly with recumbency, and there is no postictal headache or confusion. In some instances, however, motor accompaniments and urinary incontinence may simulate a seizure.

2. Cardiac disease—Cerebral hypoperfusion due to a disturbance of cardiac rhythm should be suspected in patients with known cardiac or vascular disease or in older patients who present with episodic loss of consciousness. Prodromal symptoms are typically absent. Cardiac rhythm monitoring may be necessary to establish the diagnosis; external event recorders or implantable loop recorders may be valuable if the disturbances of consciousness are rare. A relationship of attacks to physical activity and the finding of a systolic murmur are suggestive of aortic stenosis.

3. Brainstem ischemia—Loss of consciousness is preceded or accompanied by other brainstem signs. Basilar artery migraine and vertebrobasilar vascular disease are discussed elsewhere in this chapter.

4. Psychogenic nonepileptic seizure (PNES)—Simulating an epileptic seizure, a PNES may occur due to a conversion disorder or malingering. Many patients also have epileptic seizures or a family history of epilepsy. A history of childhood physical or sexual abuse is common. Although a PNES tends to occur at times of emotional stress, this may also be the case with epileptic seizures.

Clinically, the attacks superficially resemble tonic-clonic seizures, but there may be obvious preparation before a PNES. Moreover, there is usually no tonic phase; instead, there may be an asynchronous thrashing of the limbs and the attack rarely leads to injury. Eyes are often forcibly closed during PNES, unlike epileptic seizures, in which they are typically open. Consciousness may be normal or "lost," but in the latter context, the occurrence of goal-directed behavior or of shouting, swearing, etc, indicates that it is feigned. Postictally, there are no changes in behavior or neurologic findings.

Often, clinical observation is insufficient to discriminate epileptic from nonepileptic seizures and **video electroencephalographic monitoring** is required. Elevation of serum prolactin level to at least twice the upper limit of normal can be seen between 10 and 20 minutes after a seizure or syncopal event but not after a PNES. However, prolactin measurement has limited clinical utility because levels are normal after an epileptic seizure in roughly half of patients and a baseline prolactin must be drawn 6 hours after the attack.

Treatment

A. General Measures

For patients with epilepsy, medication is prescribed with the goal of preventing further attacks and is usually continued until there have been no seizures for at least 2 years. Patients should be advised to avoid situations that could be dangerous or life-threatening if further seizures should occur. Legislation may require clinicians to report to the state authorities any patients with seizures or other episodic disturbances of consciousness; *driving cessation for 6 months* or as legislated is appropriate following an unprovoked seizure.

1. Choice of medication—Medication selection depends on seizure type (Table 24–2). The dose of the selected anticonvulsant is gradually increased until seizures are controlled or side effects prevent further increases. If seizures continue despite treatment at the maximal tolerated dose, a second medication is added and the dose increased depending on tolerance; the first medication is then gradually withdrawn. In most patients with seizures of a single type, satisfactory control can be achieved with a single anticonvulsant. Treatment with two medications may further reduce seizure frequency or severity but usually only at the cost of greater toxicity. Treatment with more than two medications is almost always unhelpful unless the patient is having seizures of different types. Other factors to consider in selecting an anticonvulsant include likely side effects, teratogenicity, interactions with other medications and oral contraceptives, and route of metabolism.

All antiepileptics are potentially teratogenic, although the teratogenicity of the newer antiseizure medications is less clear. Nevertheless, antiepileptic medication must be given to pregnant women with epilepsy to prevent seizures, which can pose serious risk to the fetus from trauma, hypoxia, or other factors.

2. Monitoring—Individual differences in drug metabolism cause a given dose of a medication to produce different blood concentrations in different patients, and this will affect the therapeutic response. In general, *the dose of an*

Table 24–2. Medication treatment for seizures in adults (in alphabetical order within classes).

Medication	Usual Adult Daily Oral Dose	Minimum No. of Daily Doses	Time to Steady-State Medication Levels	Optimal Medication Level and Laboratory Monitoring[1]	Selected Side Effects and Idiosyncratic Reactions
Generalized or Focal Seizures					
Brivaracetam[2,3]	50–100 mg	2	1–2 days	CBC, liver biochemical tests	Somnolence, fatigue, ataxia, vertigo, psychosis, leukopenia, hypersensitivity (bronchospasm and angioedema).
Cannabidiol[4]	5–20 mg/kg	2	11–13 days	Liver biochemical tests at baseline, 1, 3, and 6 months	Somnolence, fatigue, anorexia, weight loss, anemia, diarrhea, rash, sleep disorder, infections. Elevation in liver enzymes may occur; reduce dose in hepatic impairment.
Carbamazepine[2,3,5,6]	400–1600 mg (immediate- or extended-release)	2	3–4 days	4–8 mcg/mL CBC, liver biochemical tests, BUN/Cr	Nystagmus, dysarthria, diplopia, ataxia, drowsiness, nausea, blood dyscrasias, hepatotoxicity, hyponatremia, Stevens-Johnson syndrome.[7] May exacerbate myoclonic seizures.
Cenobamate[2,3]	200–400 mg	1	14 days	Liver biochemical tests, potassium	Multiorgan hypersensitivity, QT shortening, somnolence, dizziness, cognitive dysfunction, blurred vision.
Clobazam[8]	10–40 mg	2	7–10 days		Lethargy and somnolence, ataxia, insomnia, dysarthria, aggression, constipation, fever, Stevens-Johnson syndrome.
Clorazepate[3]	22.5–90 mg	2	10 days		Sedation, dizziness, confusion, ataxia, depression, dependency/abuse.
Eslicarbazepine[2,3]	400–1200 mg	1	4 days	Serum sodium and chloride; liver biochemical tests	As for carbamazepine.
Ezogabine[3]	300–1200 mg	3	2–3 days	ECG to assess QT interval	Dizziness, somnolence, confusion, vertigo, nausea, ataxia, psychiatric disturbances, prolonged QT interval, retinal abnormalities.[9]
Felbamate[2,3,8,10]	1200–3600 mg	3	4–5 days	CBC and reticulocytes, liver biochemical tests	Anorexia, nausea, vomiting, headache, insomnia, weight loss, dizziness, hepatotoxicity, fatal aplastic anemia. Reserved for refractory epilepsy.
Gabapentin[3]	900–3600 mg	3	1 day		Sedation, fatigue, ataxia, nystagmus, weight loss.
Lacosamide[2,3,5]	100–400 mg	2	3 days	ECG if known cardiac conduction problems or severe cardiac disease	Vertigo, diplopia, nausea, headache, fatigue, ataxia, tremor, anaphylactoid reactions, PR prolongation, cardiac dysrhythmia, suicidality.
Lamotrigine[2,3,5,8]	100–500 mg	2	4–5 days		Sedation, skin rash, visual disturbances, dyspepsia, ataxia.
Levetiracetam[2,3,5,11]	1000–3000 mg	2	2 days		Somnolence, ataxia, headache, behavioral changes.
Oxcarbazepine[2,3]	900–1800 mg	2	2–3 days	Serum sodium	As for carbamazepine.
Perampanel[2,3,5]	4–12 mg	1	3 weeks		Dizziness, somnolence, irritability, weight gain, falls, ataxia, dysarthria, blurred vision.
Phenobarbital[2,3,5,6]	100–200 mg	1	14–21 days	10–40 mcg/mL CBC, liver biochemical tests, BUN/Cr	Drowsiness, nystagmus, ataxia, skin rashes, learning difficulties, hyperactivity.

(*continued*)

Table 24–2. Medication treatment for seizures in adults (in alphabetical order within classes). (continued)

Medication	Usual Adult Daily Oral Dose	Minimum No. of Daily Doses	Time to Steady-State Medication Levels	Optimal Medication Level and Laboratory Monitoring[1]	Selected Side Effects and Idiosyncratic Reactions
Phenytoin[2,3,5,6]	200–400 mg	1	5–10 days	10–20 mcg/mL CBC, liver biochemical tests, folate	Nystagmus, ataxia, dysarthria, sedation, confusion, gingival hyperplasia, hirsutism, megaloblastic anemia, blood dyscrasias, skin rashes, fever, SLE, lymphadenopathy, peripheral neuropathy, dyskinesias. May exacerbate myoclonic seizures.
Pregabalin[3]	150–300 mg	2	2–4 days		Somnolence, dizziness, poor concentration, weight gain, thrombocytopenia, skin rashes, anaphylactoid reactions.
Primidone[2,3,5,6]	750–1500 mg	3	4–7 days	5–12 mcg/mL CBC	Sedation, nystagmus, ataxia, vertigo, nausea, skin rashes, megaloblastic anemia, irritability.
Rufinamide[8]	800–3200 mg	2	2 days		Somnolence, headache, dizziness, suicidality, Stevens-Johnson syndrome, leukopenia, shortened QT interval, nausea, vomiting.
Tiagabine[3]	32–56 mg	2	2 days		Somnolence, anxiety, dizziness, poor concentration, tremor, diarrhea.
Topiramate[2,3,5,6,8]	200–400 mg	2	4 days	Serum bicarbonate, BUN/Cr in older patients	Somnolence, nausea, dyspepsia, irritability, dizziness, ataxia, nystagmus, diplopia, glaucoma, renal calculi, weight loss, hypohidrosis, hyperthermia.
Valproic acid[2,3,12,13]	1500–2000 mg	2–3	2–4 days	50–100 mcg/mL CBC, liver biochemical tests	Nausea, vomiting, diarrhea, drowsiness, alopecia, weight gain, hepatotoxicity, thrombocytopenia, tremor, pancreatitis. Teratogenic; avoid in women of childbearing age.
Vigabatrin[3,14]	3000 mg	2	2 days		Somnolence, anorexia, nausea, vomiting, agitation, hostility, confusion, suicidality, neutropenia, Stevens-Johnson syndrome, permanent visual field loss.[7]
Zonisamide[3]	200–600 mg	1	14 days	BUN/Cr, serum bicarbonate	Somnolence, ataxia, anorexia, nausea, vomiting, rash, confusion, renal calculi. Do not use in patients with sulfonamide allergy.
Absence Seizures					
Clonazepam[8,11,12,15,16]	0.04–0.2 mg/kg	2	7–10 days	20–80 ng/mL CBC, liver biochemical tests	Drowsiness, ataxia, irritability, behavioral changes, exacerbation of tonic-clonic seizures.
Ethosuximide[12]	500–1500 mg	2	5–10 days	40–100 mcg/mL CBC, liver biochemical tests, UA	Nausea, vomiting, anorexia, headache, lethargy, unsteadiness, blood dyscrasias, SLE, urticaria, pruritus.
Valproic acid[2,3,12,13]	1500–2000 mg	2–3	2–4 days	See above	Nausea, vomiting, diarrhea, drowsiness, alopecia, weight gain, hepatotoxicity, thrombocytopenia, tremor, pancreatitis.
Myoclonic Seizures					
Clonazepam[8,11,12,15,16]	0.04–0.2 mg/kg	2	7–10 days	See above	Drowsiness, ataxia, irritability, behavioral changes, exacerbation of tonic-clonic seizures.
Levetiracetam[2,3,5,11]	1000–3000 mg	2	2 days		Somnolence, ataxia, headache, behavioral changes.

(*continued*)

Table 24–2. Medication treatment for seizures in adults (in alphabetical order within classes). (continued)

Medication	Usual Adult Daily Oral Dose	Minimum No. of Daily Doses	Time to Steady-State Medication Levels	Optimal Medication Level and Laboratory Monitoring[1]	Selected Side Effects and Idiosyncratic Reactions
Valproic acid[2,3,12,13]	1500–2000 mg	2–3	2–4 days	See above	Nausea, vomiting, diarrhea, drowsiness, alopecia, weight gain, hepatotoxicity, thrombocytopenia, tremor, pancreatitis.

Cr, creatinine. Note that many factors influence optimal dose of these drugs including age, tolerance, and concomitant medication.
[1]Patients starting treatment with any antiepileptic drug should be monitored for new or worsening depression or suicidal thoughts, especially during the first weeks of therapy. Baseline measurement of creatinine clearance is advisable in renally metabolized drugs.
[2]Approved as monotherapy for focal-onset seizures.
[3]Approved as adjunctive therapy for focal-onset seizures.
[4]Approved for treatment of seizures in Lennox-Gastaut syndrome, Dravet syndrome, and tuberous sclerosis complex.
[5]Approved as adjunctive therapy for primary generalized tonic-clonic seizures.
[6]Approved as initial monotherapy for primary generalized tonic-clonic seizures.
[7]Carriers of the HLA-B*1502 allele are at higher risk for Stevens-Johnson syndrome. Patients of Asian ancestry should be tested for this allele prior to initiation of therapy.
[8]Approved as adjunctive therapy for Lennox-Gastaut syndrome.
[9]Regular ophthalmologic examination is recommended.
[10]Not to be used as a first-line drug; when used, blood counts should be performed regularly (every 2–4 weeks). Should be used only in selected patients because of risk of aplastic anemia and hepatic failure. It is advisable to obtain written informed consent before use.
[11]Approved as adjunctive therapy for myoclonic seizures.
[12]Approved as monotherapy and adjunctive therapy for absence seizures.
[13]Approved as adjunctive therapy for patients with multiple seizure types including absence seizures.
[14]Approved as monotherapy for infantile spasms.
[15]Approved as monotherapy for Lennox-Gastaut syndrome.
[16]Approved as monotherapy for myoclonic seizures.

antiepileptic agent is increased, depending on tolerance, to achieve the desired clinical response regardless of the serum drug level. When a dose is reached that either controls seizures or is the maximum tolerated, then a steady-state trough drug level may be obtained for future reference; rechecking this level may be appropriate during pregnancy, if a breakthrough seizure occurs, a dose change occurs, or another (potentially interacting) medication is added to the regimen. A laboratory's therapeutic range for a medication is only a guide; many patients achieve good seizure control with no adverse effect at serum levels that exceed the stipulated range, and in these cases no dose adjustment is needed. The most common cause of a lower concentration of medication than expected for the prescribed dose is suboptimal patient adherence. Adherence can be improved by limiting to a minimum the number of daily doses. Recurrent seizures or status epilepticus may result if medications are taken erratically, and in some circumstances nonadherent patients may be better off without any medication. All anticonvulsants have side effects, and many require baseline and regular laboratory monitoring (Table 24–2).

3. Discontinuance of medication—Only when adult patients have been seizure-free for 2 years should withdrawal of medication be considered. Unfortunately, there is no way of predicting which patients can be managed successfully without treatment, although seizure recurrence is more likely in (1) patients with a longer duration of epilepsy prior to remission, (2) those with a shorter duration of remission, (3) those who initially did not respond to therapy, (4) those with seizures having focal features or of multiple types, (5) those with onset during adulthood, and (6) those with continuing electroencephalographic abnormalities. Dose reduction should be gradual (over weeks or months), and medications should be withdrawn one at a time. If seizures recur, treatment is reinstituted with the previously effective regimen.

4. Surgical treatment—Patients with seizures refractory to two or more medications may be candidates for operative treatment. Surgical resection is most efficacious when there is a single well-defined seizure focus, particularly in the temporal lobe. Among well-chosen patients, up to 70% remain seizure-free after extended follow-up. Additional surgical techniques for medically refractory epilepsy approved in the United States include laser interstitial thermal therapy, deep brain stimulation, responsive cortical stimulation, and vagus nerve stimulation.

B. Special Circumstances

1. Solitary seizures—In patients who have had only one seizure or a flurry of seizures over a brief period of several hours, investigation as outlined earlier should exclude an underlying cause requiring specific treatment. An electroencephalogram should be obtained, preferably within 24 hours after the seizure. Prophylactic anticonvulsant treatment is generally not required unless further attacks occur or investigations reveal underlying pathology. The risk of seizure recurrence varies in different series between about 30% and 70%, with higher risk of recurrence in patients with structural brain lesions or abnormalities on electroencephalogram. Epilepsy should *not* be diagnosed based on a solitary seizure. If seizures occur in the context of transient, nonrecurrent systemic disorders such as hyponatremia or hypoglycemia, the diagnosis of epilepsy is inaccurate, and long-term prophylactic anticonvulsant treatment is unnecessary.

2. Alcohol withdrawal seizures—The characteristic alcohol withdrawal seizure pattern is one or more generalized tonic-clonic seizures that may occur within 48 hours or so of withdrawal from alcohol after a period of high or prolonged intake. If the seizures have consistently focal features, the possibility of an associated structural abnormality, often traumatic in origin, must be considered. Treatment with anticonvulsants is generally not required for alcohol withdrawal seizures, since they are self-limited. Benzodiazepines are effective and safe for preventing further seizures. Status epilepticus may complicate alcohol withdrawal and is managed along conventional lines. Further attacks will not occur if the patient abstains from alcohol.

3. Tonic-clonic status epilepticus—Poor adherence to the anticonvulsant regimen is the most common cause; however, any disorder that can cause a single seizure may be responsible. The mortality rate may be as high as 20%, and among survivors the incidence of neurologic and cognitive sequelae is high. The prognosis relates to the underlying cause as well as the length of time between onset of status epilepticus and the start of effective treatment.

Status epilepticus is a medical emergency. Initial management includes maintenance of the airway and 50% dextrose (25–50 mL) intravenously in case hypoglycemia is responsible. If seizures continue, an intravenous bolus of lorazepam, 4 mg, is given at a rate of 2 mg/minute and repeated once after 10 minutes if necessary; alternatively, 10 mg of midazolam is given intramuscularly, and again after 10 minutes if necessary. Diazepam can also be given rectally as a gel (0.2 mg/kg). These measures are usually effective in halting seizures for a brief period. Respiratory depression and hypotension may complicate the treatment and are treated as in other circumstances, including intubation and mechanical ventilation and admission to an ICU.

Regardless of the response to lorazepam or midazolam, fosphenytoin or phenytoin should be administered intravenously. Fosphenytoin (18–20 mg phenytoin equivalents [PE]/kg) is rapidly and completely converted to phenytoin following intravenous administration and is preferred because it is less likely to cause reactions at the infusion site, can be given with all common intravenous solutions, and may be administered at a faster rate (150 mg PE/minute). When fosphenytoin is not available, phenytoin (18–20 mg/kg) is given intravenously at a rate of 50 mg/minute. Phenytoin is best injected directly but can also be given in saline; it precipitates, however, if injected into glucose-containing solutions. Because arrhythmias may develop during rapid administration of fosphenytoin or phenytoin, electrocardiographic monitoring is prudent. Hypotension may occur, especially if diazepam has also been given. Alternatively or additionally, intravenous valproate (loading dose 20–40 mg/kg over 15 minutes, maximum dose 3000 mg) or levetiracetam (loading dose 60 mg/kg over 15 minutes, maximum dose 4500 mg) is used for status epilepticus. Although neither is approved by the FDA for this indication, both were equivalent to fosphenytoin in a randomized trial. Due to the teratogenicity of valproate, it should be avoided in women who may be pregnant.

If seizures continue, phenobarbital is then given in a loading dose of 10–20 mg/kg intravenously by slow or intermittent injection (50 mg/minute). Respiratory depression and hypotension are especially common with this therapy.

If these measures fail, general anesthesia with ventilatory assistance may be required; some experts recommend proceeding directly to general anesthesia if convulsions do not cease after the initial 18–20 PE/kg fosphenytoin load. Intravenous midazolam may provide control of refractory status epilepticus; the suggested loading dose is 0.2 mg/kg, followed by 0.05–0.2 mg/kg/hour. Propofol (1–2 mg/kg as an intravenous bolus, followed by infusion at 2–15 mg/kg/hour depending on response) may also be used, as may pentobarbital (5–15 mg/kg intravenously, followed by 0.5–4 mg/kg/hour).

After status epilepticus is controlled, an oral medication program for the long-term management of seizures is started, and investigations into the cause of the disorder are pursued.

4. Nonconvulsive status epilepticus—In some cases, status epilepticus presents not with convulsions, but with a fluctuating abnormal mental status, confusion, impaired responsiveness, and automatism. Electroencephalography establishes the diagnosis. The treatment approach outlined above applies to any type of status epilepticus, although intravenous anesthesia is usually not necessary. The prognosis is a reflection of the underlying cause rather than of continuing seizures.

When to Refer

- Behavioral episodes of uncertain nature.
- Seizures are difficult to control with monotherapy.
- There is a progressive neurologic disorder.

When to Admit

- Status epilepticus.
- Frequent seizures requiring rapid medication titration and electroencephalographic monitoring.
- For inpatient monitoring when PNES is suspected.

Ahmad S et al. Surgical treatments of epilepsy. Semin Neurol. 2020;40:696. [PMID: 33176368]

Marson A et al. The SANAD II study of the effectiveness and cost-effectiveness of levetiracetam, zonisamide, or lamotrigine for newly diagnosed focal epilepsy: an open-label, non-inferiority, multicentre, phase 4, randomized controlled trial. Lancet. 2021;397:1363. [PMID: 33838757]

Marson A et al. The SANAD II study of the effectiveness and cost-effectiveness of valproate versus levetiracetam for newly diagnosed generalized and unclassifiable epilepsy: an open-label, non-inferiority, multicentre, phase 4, randomized controlled trial. Lancet. 2021;397:1375. [PMID: 33838758]

DYSAUTONOMIA

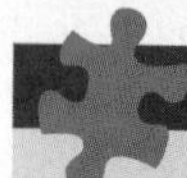

ESSENTIALS OF DIAGNOSIS

- Postural hypotension or abnormal heart rate regulation.
- Abnormalities of sweating, intestinal motility, sexual function, or sphincter control.
- Syncope may occur.
- Symptoms occur in isolation or any combination.

General Considerations

Dysautonomia may occur as a result of pathological processes in the central or peripheral nervous system. It is manifested by a variety of symptoms related to abnormalities of blood pressure regulation, thermoregulatory sweating, GI function, sphincter control, sexual function, respiration, and ocular function. The differential diagnosis depends on the time course of autonomic dysfunction and whether dysautonomia is an isolated symptom or associated with central or peripheral neurologic symptoms and signs.

A. Causes in the Central Nervous System

Disease at certain sites, regardless of its nature, may lead to dysautonomic symptoms. Postural hypotension, which is usually the most troublesome and disabling symptom, may result from spinal cord transection and other myelopathies (eg, due to tumor or syringomyelia) above the T6 level or from brainstem lesions such as syringobulbia and posterior fossa tumors. Sphincter or sexual disturbances may result from cord lesions at any level. Certain primary degenerative disorders are responsible for dysautonomia occurring in isolation (pure autonomic failure) or in association with more widespread abnormalities (multisystem atrophy) that may include parkinsonism, pyramidal symptoms, and cerebellar deficits. Postural hypotension is also a prominent symptom of idiopathic Parkinson disease and dementia with Lewy bodies.

B. Causes in the Peripheral Nervous System

A pure autonomic neuropathy may occur acutely or subacutely after a viral infection or as a paraneoplastic disorder related usually to small cell lung cancer, particularly in association with certain antibodies, such as anti-Hu or those directed at neuronal nicotinic ganglionic acetylcholine receptors. Dysautonomia is often conspicuous in patients with Guillain-Barré syndrome, manifesting with marked hypotension or hypertension or cardiac arrhythmias that may have a fatal outcome. It may also occur with diabetic, uremic, amyloidotic, and various other metabolic or toxic neuropathies; in association with leprosy or Chagas disease; and as a feature of certain hereditary neuropathies with autosomal dominant or recessive inheritance or an X-linked pattern. Autonomic symptoms are prominent in the crises of hepatic porphyria. Small fiber neuropathies may underlie some cases of postural orthostatic tachycardia syndrome (POTS) due to impaired contractility in denervated venules and resulting preload failure (see below). Patients with botulism or the Lambert-Eaton myasthenic syndrome may have constipation, urinary retention, and a sicca syndrome as a result of impaired cholinergic function.

Clinical Findings

A. Symptoms and Signs

Dysautonomic symptoms include syncope, postural hypotension, paroxysmal hypertension, persistent tachycardia without other cause, facial flushing, hypohidrosis or hyperhidrosis, vomiting, constipation, diarrhea, dysphagia, abdominal distention, disturbances of micturition or defecation, erectile dysfunction, apneic episodes, and declining night vision. In syncope, prodromal malaise, nausea, headache, diaphoresis, pallor, visual disturbance, loss of postural tone, and a sense of weakness and impending loss of consciousness are followed by actual loss of consciousness. It is usually accompanied by hypotension and bradycardia and may occur in response to emotional stress, postural hypotension, vigorous exercise in a hot environment, obstructed venous return to the heart, acute pain or its anticipation, fluid loss, and a variety of other circumstances. Although the patient is usually flaccid, some motor activity is not uncommon, and urinary (and rarely fecal) incontinence may also occur, thereby simulating a seizure. Recovery is rapid once the patient becomes recumbent, but headache, nausea, and fatigue commonly persist.

B. Evaluation of the Patient

The extent and severity of autonomic dysfunction should be determined, and the presence of associated neurologic symptoms and signs ascertained. Bedside testing of autonomic function includes examination of pupillary reactivity, examination of the skin for areas of excessive or reduced sweating and of the hands and feet for color or temperature changes, as well as assessment of blood pressure and heart rate in the supine position and 2 minutes after standing. With dysautonomia, *postural hypotension is not accompanied by a compensatory rise in heart rate.* Specialized tests include the cardiovascular response to the Valsalva maneuver and deep respiration, tilt-table testing, the thermoregulatory sweat test, the quantitative sudomotor axon reflex test, and the quantitative direct and indirect axon reflex test. Tests of GI motility and urodynamics may be helpful when symptoms of dysmotility, incontinence, or urinary retention are present.

The neurologic examination should focus on detecting signs of parkinsonism, cerebellar dysfunction, disorders of neuromuscular transmission, and peripheral neuropathy. All patients should be tested for vitamin B_{12} deficiency and diabetes. Patients with acute or subacute isolated dysautonomia should undergo testing for ganglionic acetylcholine receptor, anti-Hu, voltage-gated potassium channel complex, and voltage-gated calcium channel antibodies. For those with evidence of peripheral neuropathy, nerve conduction studies; electromyography; and testing for HIV, amyloidosis, Sjögren syndrome, and Fabry disease are indicated. If there is evidence of central pathology, imaging studies will exclude a treatable structural cause. If the neurologic examination is normal, reversible, non-neurologic causes of symptoms must be considered. Isolated postural hypotension and syncope may relate to a reduced cardiac output, paroxysmal cardiac dysrhythmias, volume depletion, various medications, and endocrine and metabolic disorders such as Addison disease, hypothyroidism or hyperthyroidism, pheochromocytoma, and carcinoid syndrome.

Treatment

The most disabling symptoms are usually postural hypotension and syncope. Abrupt postural change, prolonged recumbency, heavy meals, and other precipitants should be avoided. Medications associated with postural hypotension should be discontinued or reduced in dose. Treatment may include wearing waist-high elastic hosiery, salt supplementation, sleeping in a semierect position (which minimizes the natriuresis and diuresis that occur during recumbency), ingestion of 500 mL water 30 minutes before arising, and fludrocortisone (0.1–0.5 mg orally daily). Vasoconstrictor agents may be helpful and include midodrine (2.5–10 mg orally three times daily), droxidopa (100–600 mg orally three times daily), and ephedrine (15–30 mg orally three times daily). Other agents that have been used occasionally or experimentally are dihydroergotamine, yohimbine, pyridostigmine, atomoxetine, and clonidine; refractory cases may respond to erythropoietin (epoetin alfa) or desmopressin. Patients must be monitored for recumbent hypertension. Postprandial hypotension is helped by caffeine. There is no satisfactory treatment for disturbances of sweating, but an air-conditioned environment is helpful in avoiding extreme swings in body temperature.

When to Refer

- When the diagnosis is uncertain.
- When symptoms persist despite conventional treatment.

Shibao CA et al. Management of orthostatic hypotension, postprandial hypotension, and supine hypertension. Semin Neurol. 2020;40:515. [PMID: 33058087]

POSTURAL ORTHOSTATIC TACHYCARDIA SYNDROME (POTS)

Clinical Findings

In POTS, orthostatic symptoms (tremulousness, lightheadedness, palpitations, visual disturbances, weakness, fatigue, anxiety, hyperventilation, nausea) develop with a significant tachycardia (an increase of 30 beats/minute or more or a heart rate of 120 beats/minute or more) within 10 minutes of standing, in the absence of postural hypotension or an autonomic neuropathy. POTS is more common in women than men and in patients between 20 and 50 years of age. Other medical problems causing a tachycardia must be excluded.

Its pathophysiology is uncertain but may involve cardiac deconditioning; impaired peripheral vasoconstriction due to peripheral sympathetic denervation, leading to venous pooling in the legs on standing and a compensatory tachycardia ("**neuropathic POTS**"); or an exaggerated sympathetic response to standing, with markedly elevated levels of plasma norepinephrine causing the tachycardia ("**hyperadrenergic POTS**"). Other possible mechanisms include hypovolemia, possibly from impaired function of the renin-angiotensin system ("**volume dysregulation POTS**") and excessive mast cell activation leading to inappropriate release of histamine during physical activity. Psychological mechanisms have also been invoked. POTS may be associated with joint hypermobility syndrome and mitral valve prolapse, and it may follow pregnancy, surgery, trauma, chemotherapy, vaccinations, or viral infections.

Treatment

Management may involve volume repletion, a high salt diet and copious fluids, postural and psychophysiologic training, and a graduated exercise program. Medication treatment may include a beta-blocking agent (eg, propranolol 10–40 mg three times daily or metoprolol 12.5–50 mg twice daily), phenobarbital (15 mg in the morning, 60 mg at night), or clonidine (0.2 mg twice daily) for patients with hyperadrenergic POTS; and midodrine, droxidopa, pyridostigmine, or fludrocortisone at the doses described for postural hypotension if a neuropathic basis for symptoms is suspected. The long-term prognosis is unclear but approximately 50% of patients recover within 3 years.

TRANSIENT ISCHEMIC ATTACKS

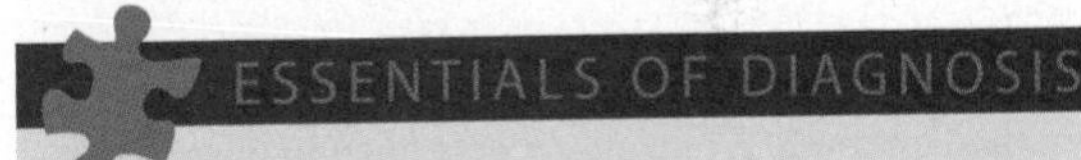

- Focal neurologic deficit of acute onset.
- Clinical deficit resolves completely within 24 hours.
- Risk factors for vascular disease often present.

General Considerations

Transient ischemic attacks (TIAs) are characterized by *focal ischemic cerebral neurologic deficits that last for less than 24 hours* (usually less than 1–2 hours). About 30% of patients with stroke have a history of TIAs and 5–10% of patients with TIAs will have a stroke within 90 days. The natural history of attacks is variable. Some patients will have a major stroke after only a few attacks, whereas others may have frequent attacks for weeks or months without having a stroke. The risk of stroke is high in the first 3 months after an attack, particularly in the first month and especially within the first 48 hours. The stroke risk is greater in patients older than 60 years, in patients with diabetes, or after TIAs that last longer than 10 minutes and with symptoms or signs of weakness, speech impairment, or gait disturbance. In general, carotid ischemic attacks are more liable than vertebrobasilar ischemic attacks to be followed by stroke.

Urgent intervention in TIA patients reduces rates of subsequent stroke, and *the condition should be treated with a similar sense of urgency as unstable angina.*

Etiology

An important cause of transient cerebral ischemia is embolization. In many patients with these attacks, a source is readily apparent in the heart or a major extracranial artery to the head, and emboli sometimes are visible in the retinal arteries. An embolic phenomenon explains why separate attacks may affect different parts of the territory supplied by the same major vessel. Cardiac causes of embolic ischemic attacks include atrial fibrillation, heart failure, infective and nonbacterial thrombotic endocarditis, atrial myxoma, and mural thrombi complicating MI. Atrial septal defects and patent foramen ovale may permit venous thromboemboli to reach the brain (**paradoxical emboli**). An ulcerated plaque on a major artery to the brain may serve as a source of emboli. In the anterior circulation, atherosclerotic changes occur most commonly in the region of the carotid bifurcation extracranially; these changes may cause a bruit. Atherosclerosis also affects the vertebrobasilar system and the major intracranial vessels including the middle and anterior cerebral arteries.

Less common abnormalities of blood vessels that may cause TIAs include fibromuscular dysplasia, which affects particularly the cervical internal carotid artery; atherosclerosis of the aortic arch; inflammatory arterial disorders such as giant cell arteritis, polyarteritis, and granulomatous angiitis; Fabry disease; and meningovascular syphilis. Critical stenosis of a major extracranial or intracranial artery may cause TIA, especially in the setting of hypotension.

Hematologic causes of TIA include polycythemia, sickle cell disease, hyperviscosity syndromes, and the antiphospholipid antibody syndrome. Severe anemia may also lead to transient focal neurologic deficits in patients with preexisting cerebral arterial disease.

The **subclavian steal syndrome** may lead to transient vertebrobasilar ischemia. Symptoms develop when there is localized stenosis or occlusion of one subclavian artery proximal to the source of the vertebral artery, so that blood is "stolen" from the vertebral artery to supply the arm. A bruit in the supraclavicular fossa, unequal radial pulses, and a difference of 20 mm Hg or more between the systolic blood pressures in the arms should suggest the diagnosis in patients with vertebrobasilar TIAs.

Clinical Findings

A. Symptoms and Signs

The symptoms of TIAs vary markedly among patients; however, the symptoms in a given individual tend to be constant in type. Onset is abrupt and without warning, and recovery usually occurs rapidly, often within a few minutes. The specific symptoms depend on the arterial distribution affected, as outlined in the subsequent section on stroke. Of note, TIA *rarely* causes of loss of consciousness or acute confusion but is often erroneously blamed for such symptoms.

B. Imaging

CT or MRI scan is indicated within 24 hours of symptom onset, in part to exclude the possibility of a small cerebral hemorrhage or a cerebral tumor masquerading as a TIA. MRI with diffusion-weighted sequences is particularly sensitive for revealing acute or subacute infarction, which is seen in up to one-third of cases despite resolution of clinical symptoms and indicates a high risk of subsequent stroke. Noninvasive imaging of the cervical vasculature should also be performed; carotid duplex ultrasonography is useful for detecting significant stenosis of the internal carotid artery, and MR or CT angiography permits broader visualization of cervical and intracranial vasculature.

C. Laboratory and Other Studies

Clinical and laboratory evaluation must include assessment for hypertension, heart disease, hematologic disorders, diabetes mellitus, hyperlipidemia, and peripheral vascular disease. It should include CBC, fasting blood glucose and serum cholesterol determinations, and may include serologic tests for syphilis and HIV infection. An ECG should be obtained. Echocardiography with agitated saline contrast is performed if a cardioembolic source is likely, and blood cultures are obtained if endocarditis is suspected. Ambulatory ECG monitoring is indicated to detect paroxysmal atrial fibrillation and, if the cause of the TIA remains elusive, *extended monitoring* may detect paroxysmal atrial fibrillation in up to 20% of patients.

Differential Diagnosis

Focal seizures usually cause abnormal motor or sensory phenomena such as clonic limb movements, paresthesias, or tingling, rather than weakness or loss of feeling. Symptoms generally spread ("march") up the limb and may lead to a generalized tonic-clonic seizure.

Classic migraine is easily recognized by the visual premonitory symptoms, followed by nausea, headache, and photophobia, but less typical cases may be hard to distinguish. Patients with migraine are typically younger, commonly have a history of episodes since adolescence, and report that other family members have a similar disorder.

Focal neurologic deficits may occur during periods of hypoglycemia in diabetic patients receiving insulin or oral hypoglycemic agent therapy.

Treatment

A. Medical Measures

Medical treatment is aimed at preventing further attacks and stroke. Treat diabetes mellitus, hematologic disorders, and hypertension, preferably with an ACE inhibitor or ARB. Among patients with atherosclerosis and LDL greater than 100 mg/dL, atorvastatin 80 mg orally once daily should be started. The LDL should be measured every 3 to 12 months, and ezetimibe (10 mg once orally once daily) added if necessary to lower the LDL to less than 70 mg/dL. In patients with at least two major atherosclerotic cardiovascular events (ischemic stroke, acute coronary syndrome or MI, peripheral arterial disease) or one major such event and multiple risk factors (age over 64 years, cardiac bypass surgery or percutaneous coronary intervention, heterozygous familial hypercholesterolemia, diabetes, hypertension, CKD, or active tobacco smoking), a proprotein convertase subtilisin/kexin type 9 inhibitor (eg, evolocumab or alirocumab) can be added. Cigarette smoking should be stopped, and cardiac sources of embolization should be treated appropriately. Weight reduction and regular physical activity should be encouraged when appropriate. An antiplatelet or anticoagulant should be started as soon as imaging has established the absence of hemorrhage.

1. Hospitalization—Hospitalization should be considered for patients seen within a week of the attack, when they are at increased risk for early recurrence. One commonly used method to assess recurrence risk is the **ABCD² score;** points are assigned for each of the following criteria: age 60 years or older (1 point), blood pressure 140/90 mm Hg or higher (1 point), clinical symptoms of focal weakness (2 points) or speech impairment without weakness (1 point), duration of 60 minutes or longer (2 points) or 10–59 minutes (1 point), or diabetes mellitus (1 point). *An ABCD² score of 4 or more points has been suggested as a threshold for hospital admission.* The **ABCD²I** (with an additional 3 points for any abnormal diffusion-weighted MRI finding or any infarct [new or old] on noncontrast CT) has been proposed as a better predictor of subsequent stroke risk. Admission is also advisable for patients with crescendo attacks, symptomatic carotid stenosis, or a known cardiac source of emboli or hypercoagulable state; such hospitalization facilitates early intervention for any recurrence and rapid institution of secondary prevention measures.

2. Anticoagulation—The chief indication for anticoagulation after TIA is atrial fibrillation. Patients with mechanical heart valves, left atrial or ventricular thrombus, LV assist devices, and the antiphospholipid antibody syndrome should also receive anticoagulation therapy. Treatment is with warfarin (target INR 2.0–3.0); bridging warfarin with heparin is *not* necessary, but some experts advocate treatment with aspirin until the INR becomes therapeutic. For long-term anticoagulation in the setting of atrial fibrillation in patients without moderate to severe mitral stenosis (Chapter 10) or a mechanical heart valve, apixaban (2.5–5 mg orally twice daily), dabigatran (150 mg orally twice daily), edoxaban (60 mg orally daily), and rivaroxaban (20 mg orally daily) are *preferred options over warfarin.* Combination antiplatelet-anticoagulation therapy is only indicated in select patients with mechanical heart valves or those with a separate indication for antiplatelet therapy such as a cardiac stent. In patients with cardiomyopathy and an EF under 35% without atrial fibrillation, warfarin (target INR 2.0–3.0) reduces ischemic stroke risk compared to aspirin but results in a roughly equivalent increase in the risk of major hemorrhage; treatment in this population should therefore be individualized.

3. Antiplatelet therapy—All patients in whom anticoagulation is not indicated should be treated with antiplatelet therapy to reduce the frequency of TIAs and the incidence of stroke. Dual antiplatelet therapy should be initiated within 12 hours after a high-risk TIA (ABCD² score ≥ 4) or minor stroke (defined by a National Institutes of Health Stroke Scale of 3 or less) with an oral loading dose of clopidogrel (300–600 mg) followed by 75 mg/day orally plus aspirin (50–325 mg daily orally) for 21 days, followed by monotherapy with aspirin (81 mg daily orally), aspirin combined with extended-release dipyridamole (200 mg twice daily orally), or clopidogrel (75 mg daily orally). Dual antiplatelet therapy with aspirin and clopidogrel for 90 days after a TIA or stroke due to 70–99% stenosis of an intracranial artery is also recommended. Cilostazol (100 mg twice daily) had similar efficacy as aspirin at long-term stroke prevention in an Asian population with less risk of hemorrhage. Combining clopidogrel with aspirin beyond 90 days increases the risk of hemorrhagic complications and is *not* recommended.

B. Surgical or Endovascular Measures

1. Carotid revascularization—When arteriography reveals a surgically accessible high-grade stenosis (70–99% in luminal diameter) on the side appropriate to carotid ischemic attacks, operative treatment (**carotid endarterectomy**) or **endovascular intervention** reduces the risk of ipsilateral carotid stroke, especially when TIAs are of recent onset (less than 1 month) and when the perioperative morbidity and mortality risk is estimated to be less than 6%. Endovascular therapy carries a slightly higher procedural stroke risk than endarterectomy in patients older than 70 years and is generally reserved for younger patients whose neck anatomy is unfavorable for surgery. Patients with symptomatic carotid stenosis of 50–69% derive moderate benefit from intervention, but surgery is not indicated for mild stenosis (less than 50%).

2. Closure of patent foramen ovale—Carefully selected patients with patent foramen ovale (PFO) and right-to-left shunt benefit from PFO closure and antiplatelet therapy. Patients should be considered for PFO closure if they are between 18 and 60 years old; have had a cryptogenic stroke or TIA; and do not have uncontrolled diabetes, hypertension, or a specific indication for long-term anticoagulation. A cryptogenic stroke does not have an identified mechanism, such as large artery atherosclerosis (greater than or equal to 30–50% stenosis of the intracranial or cervical arteries or a plaque greater than or equal to 4 mm thick in the aortic arch), known cardioembolic source (eg, atrial fibrillation), small vessel arteriolosclerosis (eg, lacunar stroke smaller than 1.5 cm in diameter), hypercoagulable state, or dissection. Patients with moderate to large interatrial shunts or associated atrial septal aneurysms appear to benefit most from PFO closure. See also Chapter 10.

3. Left atrial appendage closure—The left atrial appendage is the source of embolism in most patients with atrial fibrillation. Several randomized trials showed percutaneous left atrial appendage closure was equivalent to anticoagulation in preventing stroke and systemic embolization, and several devices are approved for this indication in the United States and Europe. The procedure should be considered in patients with a contraindication to long-term anticoagulation, although short-term anticoagulation (45 days) followed by dual antiplatelet therapy (4.5 months) and then indefinite aspirin monotherapy is usually necessary after device placement.

When to Refer

All patients should be referred for urgent investigation and treatment to prevent stroke.

When to Admit

If seen within a week of a TIA, patients should be considered for admission when they have an $ABCD^2$ score of 4 points or more, when outpatient evaluation is impractical, or when there are multiple attacks, carotid stenosis of greater than 70%, or other concern for early recurrence or stroke.

Kleindorfer DO et al. 2021 Guideline for the prevention of stroke in patients with stroke and transient ischemic attack. Stroke. 2021;52:e364. [PMID: 34024117]

STROKE

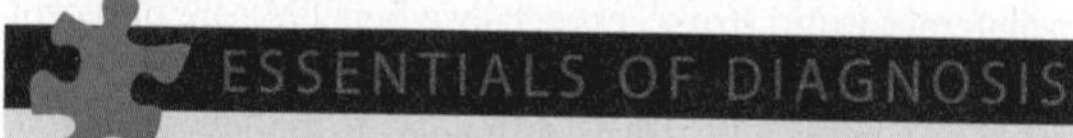

- Sudden onset of neurologic deficit of cerebrovascular origin.
- Patient often has hypertension, diabetes mellitus, tobacco use, atrial fibrillation, or atherosclerosis.
- Distinctive neurologic signs reflect the region of the brain involved.

General Considerations

In the United States, stroke is the fifth leading cause of death and a leading cause of disability. Risk factors for stroke include hypertension, diabetes mellitus, hyperlipidemia, cigarette smoking, cardiac disease, HIV infection, trigeminal herpes zoster, recreational drug abuse, heavy alcohol consumption, and a family history of stroke.

Strokes are subdivided pathologically into **infarcts** and **hemorrhages.** The distinction may be difficult clinically; CT scanning is essential to clarify the pathologic basis (Table 24–3).

1. Lacunar Infarction

Lacunar infarcts are small lesions (usually less than 1.5 cm in diameter) that occur in the distribution of short penetrating arterioles in the basal ganglia, pons, cerebellum, internal capsule, thalamus, and, less commonly, the deep cerebral white matter (Table 24–3). Lacunar infarcts are associated with poorly controlled hypertension or diabetes and have been found in several clinical syndromes, including contralateral pure motor hemiparesis or pure hemisensory deficit, ipsilateral ataxia with hemiparesis, and dysarthria with clumsiness of the hand. The neurologic deficit may progress over 24–36 hours before stabilizing.

Early mortality and risk of stroke recurrence is higher for patients with nonlacunar than lacunar infarcts. The prognosis for recovery from the deficit produced by a lacunar infarct is usually good, with partial or complete resolution occurring over the following 4–6 weeks in many instances. Treatment is as described for TIA and cerebral infarction.

2. Cerebral Infarction

Thrombotic or embolic occlusion of a major vessel leads to cerebral infarction. Causes are identical to the disorders predisposing to TIAs. The resulting deficit depends on the particular vessel involved and the extent of any collateral circulation. Cerebral ischemia leads to release of excitatory and other neuropeptides that may augment calcium flux into neurons, thereby leading to cell death and increasing the neurologic deficit.

Clinical Findings

A. Symptoms and Signs

Onset is usually abrupt, and there may then be very little progression except that due to brain swelling. Clinical evaluation should always include examination of the heart for murmurs and rhythm irregularities. Auscultating over the carotid or subclavian vessels may reveal a bruit but is not sensitive enough to substitute for vascular imaging.

1. Obstruction of carotid circulation—Occlusion of the **anterior cerebral artery** distal to its junction with the anterior communicating artery causes weakness and cortical sensory loss in the contralateral leg and sometimes mild weakness of the arm, especially proximally. There may be a contralateral grasp reflex, paratonic rigidity, abulia (lack of initiative), or frank confusion. Urinary incontinence is not uncommon, particularly if behavioral disturbances are conspicuous. Bilateral anterior cerebral infarction is especially likely to cause marked behavioral changes and memory disturbances. Unilateral anterior cerebral artery occlusion proximal to the junction with the anterior communicating artery is generally well tolerated because of the collateral supply from the other side.

Middle cerebral artery occlusion leads to contralateral hemiplegia, hemisensory loss, and homonymous hemianopia (ie, bilaterally symmetric loss of vision in half of the visual fields), with the eyes deviated to the side of the lesion. If the dominant hemisphere is involved, global aphasia is also present. It may be impossible to distinguish this clinically from occlusion of the internal carotid artery. With occlusion of either of these arteries, there may also be considerable swelling of the hemisphere during the first 72 hours. For example, an infarct involving one cerebral hemisphere may lead to such swelling that the function of the other hemisphere or the rostral brainstem is disturbed and coma results. Occlusions of different branches of the

Table 24–3. Features of the major stroke subtypes.

Stroke Type and Subtype	Clinical Features	Diagnosis	Treatment
Ischemic Stroke			
Lacunar infarct	Small (< 1.5 cm) lesions in the basal ganglia, pons, cerebellum, or internal capsule; less often in deep cerebral white matter; prognosis generally good; clinical features depend on location but may worsen over first 24–36 hours.	MRI with diffusion-weighted sequences usually defines the area of infarction; CT is insensitive acutely but can be used to exclude hemorrhage.	Antiplatelet; control risk factors (hypertension, tobacco use, hypercholesterolemia, and diabetes mellitus).
Carotid circulation obstruction	See text—signs vary depending on occluded vessel.	Noncontrast CT to exclude hemorrhage but findings may be normal during first 6–24 hours of an ischemic stroke; diffusion-weighted MRI is gold standard for identifying acute stroke; electrocardiography, carotid duplex studies, echocardiography, blood glucose, CBC, and tests for hyperlipidemia are indicated; ambulatory ECG monitoring, including extended monitoring in selected instances; CTA, MRA, or conventional angiography in selected cases; tests for hypercoagulable states in selected cases.	0–4.5 hours: intravenous thrombolytics (approved in United States up to 3 hours and in Europe up to 4.5 hours). 0–6 hours: endovascular mechanical embolectomy. 6–24 hours: endovascular mechanical embolectomy in select cases. Secondary prevention: antiplatelet agent is first-line therapy; anticoagulation without heparin bridge for cardioembolic strokes due to atrial fibrillation and other select cases when no contraindications exist; control risk factors as above.
Vertebrobasilar occlusion	See text—signs vary based on location of occluded vessel.	As for carotid circulation obstruction.	As for carotid circulation obstruction.
Hemorrhagic Stroke			
Spontaneous intracerebral hemorrhage	Commonly associated with hypertension; also with bleeding disorders, amyloid angiopathy. Hypertensive hemorrhage is located commonly in the basal ganglia, pons, thalamus, cerebellum, and less commonly the cerebral white matter.	Noncontrast CT is superior to MRI for detecting bleeds of < 48 hours duration; laboratory tests to identify bleeding disorder: angiography may be indicated to exclude aneurysm or AVM in younger patients without hypertension. Do *not* perform lumbar puncture.	Lower systolic blood pressure to 140 mm Hg; cerebellar bleeds or hematomas with gross mass effect may require urgent surgical evacuation. AVM: surgical resection indicated to prevent further bleeding; other modalities to treat nonoperable AVMs available at specialized centers.
Subarachnoid hemorrhage	Present with sudden onset of worst headache of life, may lead rapidly to loss of consciousness; signs of meningeal irritation often present; etiology usually aneurysm or AVM, but 20% have no source identified.	CT to confirm diagnosis but may be normal in rare instances; if CT negative and suspicion high, perform lumbar puncture to look for RBCs or xanthochromia; angiography to determine source of bleed in candidates for treatment.	Lower systolic blood pressure to < 140 mm Hg immediately. Aneurysm: prevent further bleeding by clipping aneurysm or coil embolization; nimodipine helps prevent vasospasm; once aneurysm has been obliterated intravenous fluids and induced hypertension to prevent vasospasm; angioplasty may also reverse symptomatic vasospasm. AVM: as above.

AVMs, arteriovenous malformations; CTA, computed tomography angiography; MRA, magnetic resonance angiography.

middle cerebral artery cause more limited findings. For example, involvement of the superior division in the dominant hemisphere leads to a predominantly expressive (**Broca**) aphasia and to contralateral paralysis and loss of sensations in the arm, the face and, to a lesser extent, the leg. Inferior branch occlusion in the dominant hemisphere produces a receptive (**Wernicke**) aphasia and a homonymous visual field defect. With involvement of the nondominant hemisphere, speech and comprehension are preserved, but there may be a left hemispatial neglect syndrome or constructional and visuospatial deficits.

Occlusion of the **ophthalmic or central retinal artery** leads to sudden painless visual loss with retinal pallor and a macular cherry red spot on fundoscopic examination. Sudden, transient vision loss in one eye (**amaurosis fugax**) is a TIA in this arterial territory.

2. Obstruction of vertebrobasilar circulation—Occlusion of the **posterior cerebral artery** may lead to a thalamic syndrome in which contralateral hemisensory disturbance occurs, followed by the development of spontaneous pain and hyperpathia. There is often a macular-sparing homonymous hemianopia and sometimes a mild, usually temporary, hemiparesis. Involuntary movements may occur if the subthalamic nucleus is involved and alexia if the infarct involves the left occipital lobe and the splenium of the corpus callosum. Occlusion of the main artery beyond the origin of its penetrating branches may lead solely to a macular-sparing hemianopia.

Vertebral artery occlusion below the origin of the anterior spinal and posterior inferior cerebellar arteries may be clinically silent because the circulation is maintained by the other vertebral artery. If the remaining vertebral artery is congenitally small or severely atherosclerotic, however, a deficit similar to that of basilar artery occlusion is seen unless there is good collateral circulation from the anterior circulation through the circle of Willis. An obstruction of the **posterior inferior cerebellar artery** or an obstruction of the **vertebral artery just before it branches** to this vessel leads to the **lateral medullary syndrome,** characterized by vertigo and nystagmus (vestibular nucleus), ipsilateral spinothalamic sensory loss involving the face (trigeminal nucleus and tract), dysphagia (nucleus ambiguus), limb ataxia (inferior cerebellar peduncle), and Horner syndrome (descending sympathetic fibers), combined with contralateral spinothalamic sensory loss involving the limbs.

Occlusion of **both vertebral arteries** or the **basilar artery** leads to coma with pinpoint pupils, flaccid quadriplegia and sensory loss, and variable cranial nerve abnormalities. With partial basilar artery occlusion, there may be diplopia, visual loss, vertigo, dysarthria, ataxia, weakness or sensory disturbances in some or all of the limbs, and discrete cranial nerve palsies. In patients with hemiplegia of pontine origin, the eyes are often deviated to the paralyzed side, whereas in patients with a hemispheric lesion, the eyes commonly deviate from the hemiplegic side. When the small paramedian arteries arising from the basilar artery are occluded, contralateral hemiplegia and sensory deficit occur in association with an ipsilateral cranial nerve palsy at the level of the lesion.

Occlusion of any of the major **cerebellar arteries** produces vertigo, nausea, vomiting, nystagmus, and ipsilateral limb ataxia. Contralateral spinothalamic sensory loss in the limbs may also be present. Deafness due to cochlear infarction may follow occlusion of the anterior inferior cerebellar artery, which may also cause ipsilateral facial spinothalamic sensory loss and weakness. Massive cerebellar infarction may lead to obstructive hydrocephalus, coma, tonsillar herniation, and death.

B. Imaging

A CT scan of the head (without contrast) should be performed immediately, before the administration of aspirin or other antithrombotic agents, to exclude cerebral hemorrhage (Table 24–3). CT is relatively insensitive to acute ischemic stroke within the first 6–12 hours, and subsequent MRI with diffusion-weighted sequences helps define the distribution and extent of infarction as well as exclude tumor or other differential considerations. CT angiography of the head and neck should be performed to identify large vessel occlusions amenable to endovascular therapy in patients presenting within 6 hours of stroke onset and should be considered in those presenting between 6 and 24 hours, together with CT perfusion studies. Regardless of timing of presentation, imaging of the cervical vasculature is indicated as part of a search to identify the source of the stroke. In patients with a PFO and otherwise cryptogenic stroke, the intracranial vasculature must be imaged to rule out large vessel atherosclerosis before PFO closure can be considered.

C. Laboratory and Other Studies

Investigations should include a CBC, blood glucose determination, and fasting lipid panel. Serologic tests for syphilis and HIV infection may be included depending on the circumstances. Screening for antiphospholipid antibodies (lupus anticoagulants, anticardiolipin, and anti-beta$_2$-glycoprotein antibodies); the factor V Leiden mutation; abnormalities of protein C, protein S, or antithrombin; or a prothrombin gene mutation is indicated only if a hypercoagulable disorder is suspected (eg, a young patient without apparent risk factors for stroke) or needs to be ruled out if PFO closure is under consideration. While elevated serum homocysteine is a risk factor for stroke, lowering homocysteine levels with vitamin supplementation has not been shown to decrease stroke risk, and therefore, routinely checking homocysteine is *not* recommended. Electrocardiography or continuous cardiac monitoring for at least 24 hours will help exclude a recent MI or a cardiac arrhythmia that might be a source of embolization. While atrial fibrillation will be discovered in approximately 10% of patients with ischemic stroke during their hospitalization, it is estimated that an arrhythmia will be found in an additional 10% with prolonged ambulatory ECG monitoring after discharge; this testing is indicated in cases where atrial fibrillation is suspected (eg, nonlacunar stroke and left atrial enlargement on echocardiography or lack of intracranial or carotid atherosclerosis) but has not been demonstrated. Echocardiography (with agitated saline contrast) should be performed in cases of nonlacunar stroke to exclude valvular disease, right-to-left shunting, and cardiac thrombus. Blood cultures should be performed if endocarditis is suspected but are not required routinely. Examination of the cerebrospinal fluid is not always necessary but may be helpful if cerebral vasculitis or another inflammatory or infectious cause of stroke is suspected, but it should be delayed until after CT or MRI to exclude any risk for herniation due to mass effect.

Treatment

Management is divided into acute and chronic phases: the first is aimed at minimizing disability and the second at preventing recurrent stroke. A combination of thrombolysis and endovascular therapies is available to patients who present within 24 hours of stroke onset, determined by when the patient was last normal.

Intravenous thrombolytic therapy with recombinant tissue plasminogen activator (rtPA, alteplase; 0.9 mg/kg to a maximum of 90 mg, with 10% given as a bolus over 1 minute and the remainder over 1 hour) improves the chance of recovery without significant disability at 90 days from 26% to 39% if given within 3 hours from stroke onset; it is still effective up to 4.5 hours from stroke onset. Treatment should be initiated as soon as possible; *outcome is directly related to the time from stroke onset to treatment.* Intravenous thrombolysis is approved in Europe for use up to 4.5 hours from stroke onset but only for up to 3 hours in the United States, although off-label use during the 3- to 4.5-hour window is standard. In patients with systolic pressure greater than 185 mm Hg or diastolic pressure greater than 110 mm Hg, the blood pressure should be lowered to less than 185/110 mm Hg with intravenous labetalol or nicardipine to enable rtPA administration. Due to the risk of hemorrhage, rtPA should not be used beyond 4.5 hours, or in other situations where it is medically contraindicated, although some evidence suggests patients with ischemic but not infarcted tissue identified by automated perfusion imaging or MRI may be treated up to 9 hours after onset or upon awakening with stroke symptoms.

Several randomized trials have demonstrated an increased likelihood of achieving functional independence after **endovascular mechanical embolectomy** by stent retrievers as an adjunct to intravenous rtPA. Patients with large vessel occlusion (about 20% of patients with acute ischemic stroke) in whom treatment can be initiated within 6 hours of stroke onset are eligible for embolectomy, as are patients who present between 6 and 24 hours and have a large ischemic penumbra identified by perfusion CT, perfusion MRI, or diffusion-weighted MRI.

Early management of a completed stroke otherwise requires general supportive measures. Management in a **stroke care unit** has been shown to improve outcomes, likely due to early rehabilitation and prevention of medical complications. During the acute stage, there may be marked brain swelling and edema, with symptoms and signs of increasing intracranial pressure, an increasing neurologic deficit, or herniation syndrome. Elevated intracranial pressure is managed by head elevation and osmotic agents such as mannitol. Maintenance of an adequate cerebral perfusion pressure helps prevent further ischemia. Early decompressive hemicraniectomy (within 48 hours of stroke onset) for malignant middle cerebral artery infarctions reduces mortality and improves functional outcome. Attempts to lower the blood pressure of hypertensive patients during the acute phase (ie, within 72 hours) of a stroke should generally be *avoided* unless the purpose is to enable the safe administration of rtPA, as there is loss of cerebral autoregulation, and lowering the blood pressure may further compromise ischemic areas. However, if the systolic pressure exceeds 220 mm Hg, it can be lowered using intravenous labetalol or nicardipine with continuous monitoring to 170–200 mm Hg, and then after 72 hours, it can be reduced further to less than 140/90 mm Hg. Blood pressure augmentation is usually not necessary in patients with relative hypotension but maintenance of hydration with intravenous fluids if necessary is important.

Prophylactic and medical measures are discussed in the section on TIAs and should guide management. Once hemorrhage has been excluded by CT, **aspirin** (325 mg orally daily) is started immediately unless the patient received thrombolysis, in which case aspirin is initiated after a follow-up CT has ruled out thrombolytic-associated hemorrhage at 24 hours. **Dual antiplatelet therapy** should be used for 21 days in patients with minor stroke (National Institutes of Health Stroke Scale of 3 or less). **Anticoagulant** medications are started when indicated, as discussed in the section on TIAs. There is generally *no* advantage in delay, and the common fear of causing hemorrhage into a previously infarcted area is misplaced, since there is a far greater risk of further embolism to the cerebral circulation if treatment is withheld.

Physical therapy has an important role in the management of patients with impaired motor function. Passive movements at an early stage will help prevent contractures. As cooperation increases and some recovery begins, active movements will improve strength and coordination. In all cases, early mobilization and active rehabilitation are important. **Occupational therapy** may improve morale and motor skills, while **speech therapy** may help expressive aphasia or dysarthria. Because of the risk for dysphagia following stroke, access to food and drink is typically restricted until an appropriate swallowing evaluation; the head of the bed should be kept elevated to prevent aspiration. Urinary catheters should *not* be placed and, if placed, removed within 24–48 hours.

Prognosis

The prognosis for survival after cerebral infarction is better than after cerebral or subarachnoid hemorrhage. Patients receiving treatment with rtPA are at least 30% more likely to have minimal or no disability at 3 months than those not treated by this means. Those treated with mechanical embolectomy are also at least 30% more likely to achieve functional independence. Loss of consciousness after a cerebral infarct implies a poorer prognosis than otherwise. The extent of the infarct governs the potential for rehabilitation. Patients who have had a cerebral infarct are at risk for additional strokes and for MIs. The prophylactic measures discussed earlier reduce this risk. Antiplatelet therapy reduces the recurrence rate by 30% among patients with stroke without a cardiac cause who are not candidates for carotid endarterectomy. Nevertheless, the cumulative risk of recurrence of noncardioembolic stroke is still 3–7% annually. Management is focused on palliative care when meaningful recovery from massive strokes is unlikely (see Chapter 5).

When to Refer

All patients should be referred.

When to Admit

All patients should be hospitalized, preferably in a stroke care unit.

Powers WJ et al. Guidelines for the early management of patients with acute ischemic stroke: 2019 update to the 2018 guidelines for the early management of acute ischemic stroke: a guideline for healthcare professionals from the American Heart Association/American Stroke Association. Stroke. 2019;50:e344. [PMID: 31662037]

3. Intracerebral Hemorrhage

Spontaneous, nontraumatic intracerebral hemorrhage in patients with no angiographic evidence of an associated vascular anomaly (eg, aneurysm or angioma) is usually due to hypertension. The pathologic basis for hemorrhage is probably the presence of microaneurysms that develop on perforating vessels in hypertensive patients. Hypertensive intracerebral hemorrhage occurs most frequently in the basal ganglia, pons, thalamus, and cerebellum, and less commonly in the cerebral white matter. Hemorrhage may extend into the ventricular system or subarachnoid space, and signs of meningeal irritation are then found. In older adults, cerebral amyloid angiopathy is another important and frequent cause of hemorrhage, which is usually lobar in distribution, sometimes recurrent, and associated with a better immediate prognosis than hypertensive hemorrhage. Arteriovenous malformations are an important cause of intracerebral hemorrhage in younger patients.

Other causes of nontraumatic intracerebral hemorrhage include hematologic and bleeding disorders (eg, leukemia, thrombocytopenia, hemophilia, or disseminated intravascular coagulation), anticoagulant therapy, liver disease, high alcohol intake, cocaine and methamphetamine abuse, herpes simplex encephalitis, vasculitis, Moyamoya disease, reversible cerebral vasoconstriction syndrome, and primary or secondary brain tumors. There is also an association with advancing age and male sex. Bleeding is primarily into the subarachnoid space when it occurs from an intracranial aneurysm, but it may be partly intraparenchymal as well. Hemorrhage can also occur into arterial and venous cerebral infarcts.

Clinical Findings

A. Symptoms and Signs

With hemorrhage into the cerebral hemisphere, consciousness is initially lost or impaired in about one-half of patients. Vomiting occurs very frequently at the onset of bleeding, and headache is sometimes present. Focal symptoms and signs then develop, depending on the site of the hemorrhage. With hypertensive hemorrhage, there is generally a rapidly evolving neurologic deficit with hemiplegia or hemiparesis. A hemisensory disturbance is also present with more deeply placed lesions. With lesions of the putamen, loss of conjugate lateral gaze may be conspicuous. With thalamic hemorrhage, there may be a loss of upward gaze, downward or skew deviation of the eyes, lateral gaze palsies, and pupillary inequalities.

Cerebellar hemorrhage may present with sudden onset of nausea and vomiting, dysequilibrium, ataxia of gait, limbs, or trunk; headache; and loss of consciousness that may terminate fatally within 48 hours. Pontine hemorrhage causes some combination of lateral conjugate gaze palsies to the side of the lesion; small reactive pupils; contralateral hemiplegia; peripheral facial weakness; and periodic respiration. These signs may be bilateral with larger pontine hemorrhage, and the patient may become locked in, with quadriplegia and preserved consciousness.

B. Imaging

CT scanning (without contrast) is important not only in confirming that hemorrhage has occurred but also in determining the size and site of the hematoma. MRI is equally sensitive when magnetic susceptibility weighted sequences (eg, gradient echo) are used. If the patient's condition permits further intervention, CT angiography, MR angiography, or cerebral angiography may be undertaken to determine whether an aneurysm or arteriovenous malformation is present. In patients under age 55 with lobar hemorrhage and no history of hypertension, a contrast-enhanced MRI may indicate a nonhypertensive cause, such as an underlying neoplasm.

C. Laboratory and Other Studies

A CBC, platelet count, prothrombin and partial thromboplastin times, liver biochemical tests, and kidney function tests may reveal a predisposing cause for the hemorrhage. *Lumbar puncture is contraindicated* because it may precipitate a herniation syndrome in patients with a large hematoma, and CT scanning is superior in detecting intracerebral hemorrhage.

Treatment

Patients should be admitted to an ICU for observation and supportive care. The systolic blood pressure should be lowered to 140 mm Hg with intravenous labetalol or nicardipine, although randomized trials targeting systolic blood pressures of less than 140 mm Hg and less than 180 mm Hg have not shown a difference in outcomes. Thrombocytopenia should be treated with platelet transfusion; the specific threshold for treatment and the goal platelet count after transfusion vary with patient characteristics and provider experience. Coagulopathies should be reversed using fresh frozen plasma, prothrombin complex concentrates, vitamin K, or specific reversal agents (eg, protamine for heparin; idarucizumab for dabigatran; and andexanet alfa or 4-factor prothrombin complex concentrates for apixaban, betrixaban, edoxaban, and rivaroxaban). Hemostatic therapy with recombinant activated factor VII in patients without underlying coagulopathy has not improved survival or functional outcome. Intracranial pressure may require monitoring and osmotic therapy. Ventricular drainage may be required in patients with intraventricular hemorrhage and acute hydrocephalus. Decompression may be helpful when a superficial hematoma in cerebral white matter is exerting a mass effect and causing incipient herniation. In patients with cerebellar hemorrhage who are deteriorating neurologically or who have brainstem compression or hydrocephalus, prompt surgical evacuation of the hematoma is appropriate because spontaneous unpredictable deterioration may otherwise lead to a fatal outcome and because operative treatment may lead to complete resolution of the clinical deficit. The treatment of underlying structural lesions or bleeding disorders depends on their nature. There is no specific treatment for cerebral amyloid angiopathy.

When to Refer

All patients should be referred.

When to Admit

All patients should be hospitalized.

Hostettler IC et al. Intracerebral hemorrhage: an update on diagnosis and treatment. Expert Rev Neurother. 2019;19:679. [PMID: 31188036]

4. Spontaneous Subarachnoid Hemorrhage

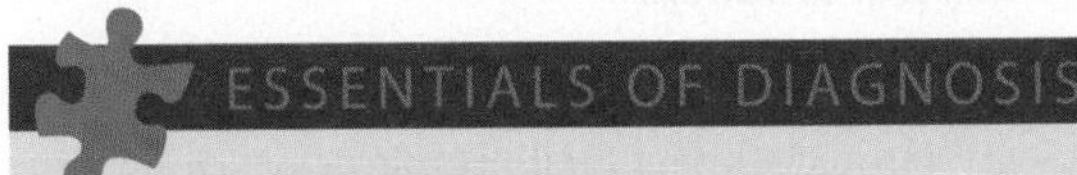

- Sudden ("thunderclap") severe headache.
- Signs of meningeal irritation usually present.
- Obtundation is common.
- Focal deficits frequently absent.

General Considerations

Between 5% and 10% of strokes are due to subarachnoid hemorrhage. **Trauma** is the most common cause of subarachnoid hemorrhage, the prognosis of which depends on the severity of the head injury. Spontaneous (nontraumatic) subarachnoid hemorrhage frequently results from the rupture of an **arterial saccular ("berry") aneurysm** or from an **arteriovenous malformation.**

Clinical Findings

A. Symptoms and Signs

Subarachnoid hemorrhage has a characteristic clinical picture. Its onset is with sudden ("**thunderclap**") headache of a severity never experienced previously by the patient. This may be followed by nausea and vomiting and by a loss or impairment of consciousness that can either be transient or progress inexorably to deepening coma and death. If consciousness is regained, the patient is often confused and irritable and may show other symptoms of an altered mental status. Neurologic examination generally reveals nuchal rigidity and other signs of meningeal irritation, except in deeply comatose patients.

Most aneurysms are asymptomatic until they rupture, but they may cause a focal neurologic deficit by compressing adjacent structures. Occasional patients with aneurysms have headaches, sometimes accompanied by nausea and neck stiffness, a few hours or days before massive subarachnoid hemorrhage occurs. This has been attributed to "warning leaks" of a small amount of blood from the aneurysm.

A higher risk of subarachnoid hemorrhage is associated with older age, female sex, non-White ethnicity, hypertension, tobacco smoking, high alcohol consumption (exceeding 150 g per week), previous symptoms, posterior circulation aneurysms, and larger aneurysms. Focal neurologic signs are usually absent but, when present, may relate either to a focal intracerebral hematoma (from arteriovenous malformations) or to ischemia in the territory of the vessel with a ruptured aneurysm.

B. Imaging

A CT scan (preferably with CT angiography) should be performed immediately to confirm that hemorrhage has occurred and to search for clues regarding its source. It is preferable to use MRI because it is faster and more sensitive in detecting hemorrhage in the first 24 hours. CT findings sometimes are normal in patients with suspected hemorrhage, and the cerebrospinal fluid must then be examined for the presence of blood or xanthochromia before the possibility of subarachnoid hemorrhage is discounted.

Cerebral arteriography is undertaken to determine the source of bleeding. In general, bilateral carotid and vertebral arteriography are necessary because aneurysms are often multiple, while arteriovenous malformations may be supplied from several sources. The procedure allows an interventional radiologist to treat an underlying aneurysm or arteriovenous malformation by various techniques. If arteriograms show no abnormality, the examination should be repeated after 2 weeks because vasospasm or thrombus may have prevented detection of an aneurysm or other vascular anomaly during the initial study. CT or MR angiography may also be revealing but is less sensitive than conventional arteriography.

C. Laboratory and Other Studies

The cerebrospinal fluid demonstrates an elevated RBC count. Subarachnoid hemorrhage can be differentiated from a traumatic lumbar puncture by the lack of clearing of RBCs from the first and fourth tube of cerebrospinal fluid or by the presence of xanthochromia, which occurs due to lysis of RBCs and takes at least 2 hours to develop. The absolute RBC count is also helpful: in the absence of xanthochromia, an RBC count of less than 2000×10^6/L is very unlikely to be due to subarachnoid hemorrhage. Electrocardiographic evidence of arrhythmias or myocardial ischemia has been well described and probably relates to excessive sympathetic activity. Peripheral leukocytosis and transient glycosuria are also common findings.

Treatment

All patients should be hospitalized and seen by a neurologist. The measures outlined below in the section on stupor and coma are applied to comatose patients. Conscious patients are confined to bed, advised against any exertion or straining, treated symptomatically for headache and anxiety, and given laxatives or stool softeners. The systolic blood pressure should be lowered to 140 mm Hg until the aneurysm is treated definitively. Seizure prophylaxis is not necessary unless a convulsion has occurred (see Table 24–2). Patients are generally hospitalized for at least 14 days to monitor, prevent, and treat vasospasm.

The major aim of treatment is to prevent further hemorrhage. The risk of further hemorrhage from a ruptured aneurysm is greatest within a few days of the first hemorrhage; approximately 20% of patients will have further bleeding within 2 weeks and 40% within 6 months. Definitive treatment, ideally within 2 days of the hemorrhage, requires surgical clipping of the aneurysm or endovascular treatment by coil embolization; the latter is sometimes feasible even for inoperable aneurysms and has a lower morbidity than surgery.

Complications

Spontaneous subarachnoid hemorrhage may result in severe complications, so monitoring is necessary, usually in an ICU. Hemiplegia or other focal deficit sometimes may follow aneurysmal bleeding after a delay of 2–14 days due to focal arterial spasm. The etiology of **vasospasm** is uncertain and likely multifactorial, and it sometimes leads to significant cerebral ischemia or infarction and may further aggravate any existing increase in intracranial pressure. Transcranial Doppler ultrasound may be used to screen noninvasively for vasospasm, but conventional arteriography is required to document and treat vasospasm when the clinical suspicion is high. Nimodipine has been shown to reduce the incidence of ischemic deficits from arterial spasm; a dose of 60 mg every 4 hours orally for 21 days is given prophylactically to all patients. After surgical obliteration of all aneurysms, symptomatic vasospasm may also be treated by intravascular volume expansion and induced hypertension; transluminal balloon angioplasty of involved intracranial vessels is also helpful.

Acute hydrocephalus, which sometimes occurs due to cerebrospinal fluid outflow disruption by the subarachnoid blood, should be suspected if the patient deteriorates clinically; a repeat CT scan should be obtained. Acute hydrocephalus frequently causes intracranial hypertension severe enough to require temporary, and less commonly prolonged or permanent, intraventricular cerebrospinal fluid shunting. **Cerebral salt-wasting** is another complication of subarachnoid hemorrhage that may develop abruptly during the first several days of hospitalization. The resulting hyponatremia and cerebral edema may exacerbate intracranial hypertension and may require carefully titrated treatment with oral sodium chloride or intravenous hyperosmotic sodium solution. Daily measurement of the serum sodium level allows for the early detection of this complication. **Hypopituitarism** may occur as a late complication of subarachnoid hemorrhage.

Etminan N et al. Neurovascular disease, diagnosis, and therapy: subarachnoid hemorrhage and cerebral vasospasm. Handb Clin Neurol. 2021;176:135. [PMID: 33272393]

5. Intracranial Aneurysm

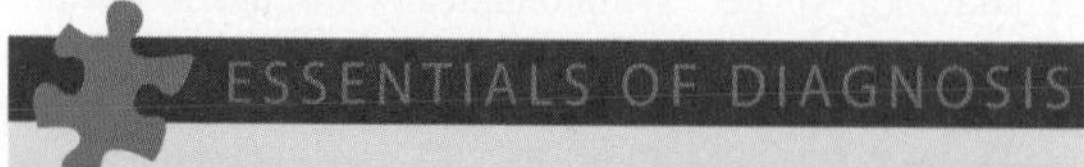

- Subarachnoid hemorrhage or focal deficit.
- Abnormal imaging studies.

General Considerations

Saccular aneurysms (**"berry" aneurysms**) tend to occur at arterial bifurcations, are frequently multiple (20% of cases), and are usually asymptomatic. They are associated with polycystic kidney disease, Moyamoya disease, familial aldosteronism type 1, and coarctation of the aorta. Risk factors for aneurysm formation include cigarette smoking, hypertension, and female sex. Most aneurysms are located on the anterior part of the circle of Willis—particularly on the anterior or posterior communicating arteries, at the bifurcation of the middle cerebral artery, and at the bifurcation of the internal carotid artery. Mycotic aneurysms resulting from septic embolism occur in more distal vessels and often at the cortical surface. The most significant complication of intracranial aneurysms is a subarachnoid hemorrhage, which is discussed in the preceding section.

Clinical Findings

A. Symptoms and Signs

Aneurysms may cause a focal neurologic deficit by compressing adjacent structures. However, most are asymptomatic or produce only nonspecific symptoms until they rupture, at which time subarachnoid hemorrhage results. Its manifestations, complications, and management were outlined in the preceding section.

B. Imaging

Definitive evaluation is by digital subtraction angiography (bilateral carotid and vertebral studies), which generally indicates the size and site of the lesion, sometimes reveals multiple aneurysms, and may show arterial spasm if rupture has occurred. Visualization by CT or MR angiography is not usually adequate if operative treatment is under consideration because lesions may be multiple and small lesions are sometimes missed, but these modalities can be used to screen patients who have two or more first-degree relatives with intracranial aneurysms.

Treatment

The major aim of treatment is to prevent hemorrhage. Management of ruptured aneurysms was described in the section on subarachnoid hemorrhage. Symptomatic but unruptured aneurysms merit prompt treatment, either surgically or by endovascular techniques. The decision to treat or monitor asymptomatic aneurysms discovered incidentally is complicated and depends on aneurysm size, location, risk factors for rupture, and treatment-related morbidity; risk scores to guide decision-making are available.

When to Refer

All patients should be referred.

When to Admit

- All patients with a subarachnoid hemorrhage.
- All patients for detailed imaging.
- All patients undergoing surgical or endovascular treatment.

Hackenberg KAM et al. Neurovascular disease, diagnosis, and therapy: brain aneurysms. Handb Clin Neurol. 2021;176:121. [PMID: 33272392]

6. Arteriovenous Malformations

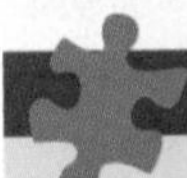

ESSENTIALS OF DIAGNOSIS

- Sudden onset of subarachnoid and intracerebral hemorrhage.
- Distinctive neurologic signs reflect the region of the brain involved.
- Signs of meningeal irritation in patients presenting with subarachnoid hemorrhage.
- Seizures or focal deficits may occur.

General Considerations

Arteriovenous malformations are congenital vascular malformations that result from a localized maldevelopment of part of the primitive vascular plexus and consist of abnormal arteriovenous communications without intervening capillaries. They vary in size, ranging from massive lesions that are fed by multiple vessels and involve a large part of the brain to lesions so small that they are hard to identify at arteriography, surgery, or autopsy. In approximately 10% of cases, there is an associated arterial aneurysm, while 1–2% of patients presenting with aneurysms have associated arteriovenous malformations. Clinical presentation may relate to hemorrhage from the malformation or an associated aneurysm or may relate to cerebral ischemia due to diversion of blood by the anomalous arteriovenous shunt or due to venous stagnation. Regional maldevelopment of the brain, compression or distortion of adjacent cerebral tissue by enlarged anomalous vessels, and progressive gliosis due to mechanical and ischemic factors may also be contributory.

Clinical Findings

Most cerebral arteriovenous malformations are supratentorial, usually lying in the territory of the middle cerebral artery. Up to 70% bleed at some point in their natural history, most commonly before the patient reaches the age of 40 years. Arteriovenous malformations that have bled once are more likely to bleed again, at an approximate rate of 4.5% annually. A higher risk of bleeding is also observed if there is an associated aneurysm, deep venous drainage, or deep brain location; size of the malformation and sex are not associated with risk of hemorrhage.

A. Symptoms and Signs

Initial symptoms consist of hemorrhage in 30–60% of cases, recurrent seizures in 20–40%, headache in 5–25%, and miscellaneous complaints (including focal deficits) in 10–15%. Hemorrhage is commonly intracerebral as well as into the subarachnoid space and is fatal in about 10% of cases. Seizures are more likely with frontal or parietal arteriovenous malformations. Headaches are especially likely when the external carotid arteries are involved in the malformation. These sometimes simulate migraine, but more commonly are nonspecific in character, with nothing about them to suggest an underlying structural lesion. Brainstem and cerebellar arteriovenous malformations may cause obstructive hydrocephalus.

In patients presenting with subarachnoid hemorrhage, examination may reveal an abnormal mental status and signs of meningeal irritation. Additional findings may help localize the lesion and sometimes indicate that intracranial pressure is increased. A cranial bruit always suggests the possibility of a cerebral arteriovenous malformation, but bruits may also be found with aneurysms, meningiomas, acquired arteriovenous fistulas, and arteriovenous malformations involving the scalp, calvarium, or orbit. Bruits are best heard over the ipsilateral eye or mastoid region and are of some help in lateralization but of no help in localization. Absence of a bruit *does not exclude* the possibility of arteriovenous malformation.

B. Imaging

In patients with suspected hemorrhage, CT scanning indicates whether subarachnoid or intracerebral bleeding has recently occurred, helps localize its source, and may reveal the arteriovenous malformation. When intracranial hemorrhage is confirmed but the source of hemorrhage is not evident on the CT scan, arteriography is necessary to exclude aneurysm or arteriovenous malformation. MR and CT angiography are not sensitive enough for this purpose. Even if the findings on CT scan suggest arteriovenous malformation, arteriography is required to establish the nature of the lesion with certainty and to determine its anatomic features so that treatment can be planned. The examination must generally include bilateral opacification of the internal and external carotid arteries and the vertebral arteries.

In patients presenting without hemorrhage, CT scan or MRI usually reveals the underlying abnormality, and MRI frequently also shows evidence of old or recent hemorrhage that may have been asymptomatic. The nature and detailed anatomy of any focal lesion identified by these means are delineated by angiography, especially if operative treatment is under consideration.

Treatment

Surgical treatment to prevent further hemorrhage is justified in patients with arteriovenous malformations that have bled, provided that the lesion is accessible and the patient has a reasonable life expectancy. Surgical treatment is also appropriate if intracranial pressure is increased and to prevent further progression of a focal neurologic deficit. In patients presenting solely with seizures, anticonvulsant treatment is usually sufficient (Table 24–2), and operative treatment is unnecessary unless seizures cannot be controlled medically.

Definitive operative treatment consists of excision of the arteriovenous malformation if it is surgically accessible. Stereotactic radiosurgery is used to treat inoperable cerebral arteriovenous malformations. Arteriovenous malformations that are inoperable because of their location are sometimes treated solely by embolization; although the risk of hemorrhage is not reduced, neurologic deficits may be stabilized or even reversed by this procedure. Embolization is more commonly performed as an adjunct to surgery or radiosurgery; it is also used to treat aneurysms associated with the arteriovenous malformations.

When to Refer

All patients should be referred.

When to Admit

- All patients with a subarachnoid or cerebral hemorrhage.
- All patients for detailed imaging.
- All patients undergoing surgical or endovascular treatment.

Rutledge C et al. Brain arteriovenous malformations. Handb Clin Neurol. 2021;176:171. [PMID: 33272394]

7. Intracranial Venous Thrombosis

Intracranial venous thrombosis may occur in association with intracranial or maxillofacial infections, hypercoagulable states, polycythemia, sickle cell disease, cyanotic congenital heart disease, and in pregnancy or during the puerperium. Genetic factors are also important. Cases of intracranial venous thrombosis with thrombocytopenia and antiplatelet factor 4 antibodies have rarely been observed after administration of SARS-CoV-2 adenoviral vector vaccines. The disorder is characterized by headache, focal or generalized convulsions, drowsiness, confusion, increased intracranial pressure, and focal neurologic deficits—and sometimes by evidence of meningeal irritation. The diagnosis is confirmed by CT or MR venography or angiography.

Treatment includes anticonvulsants if seizures have occurred (Table 24–2) and—if necessary—measures to reduce intracranial pressure. Anticoagulation with dose-adjusted intravenous heparin or weight-adjusted subcutaneous low-molecular-weight heparin, followed by oral warfarin anticoagulation for 6 months reduces morbidity and mortality of venous sinus thrombosis. Dabigatran showed similar efficacy to warfarin in one randomized trial and may be an acceptable alternative. Measurement of antiplatelet factor 4 antibodies and treatment with a non-heparin anticoagulant has been suggested in cases following SARS-CoV-2 vaccination; some experts also recommend intravenous immunoglobulin (1 g/kg daily for 2 days). Concomitant intracranial hemorrhage related to the venous thrombosis does not contraindicate anticoagulant therapy. In cases refractory to anticoagulation, endovascular techniques including catheter-directed thrombolytic therapy (urokinase) and thrombectomy are sometimes helpful but may increase the risk for major hemorrhage.

When to Refer

All patients should be referred.

When to Admit

All patients should be hospitalized.

Ferro JM et al; RE-SPECT CVT Study Group. Safety and efficacy of dabigatran etexilate vs dose-adjusted warfarin in patients with cerebral venous thrombosis: a randomized clinical trial. JAMA Neurol. 2019;76:1457. [PMID: 31479105]
Furie KL et al; American Heart Association/American Stroke Association Stroke Council Leadership. Diagnosis and management of cerebral venous sinus thrombosis with vaccine-induced immune thrombotic thrombocytopenia. Stroke. 2021;52:2478. [PMID: 33914590]

8. Spinal Cord Vascular Diseases

ESSENTIALS OF DIAGNOSIS

- Sudden onset of back or limb pain and neurologic deficit in limbs.
- Motor, sensory, or reflex changes in limbs depending on level of lesion.
- Imaging studies distinguish between infarct and hematoma.

Infarction of the Spinal Cord

Infarction of the spinal cord is rare. It typically occurs in the territory of the anterior spinal artery because this vessel, which supplies the anterior two-thirds of the cord, is itself supplied by only a limited number of feeders. Infarction usually results from interrupted flow in one or more of these feeders, eg, with aortic dissection, aortic aneurysm, aortography, polyarteritis, severe hypotension, or after surgical repair of the thoracic or abdominal aorta. The paired posterior spinal arteries, by contrast, are supplied by numerous arteries at different levels of the cord. Spinal cord hypoperfusion may lead to a central cord syndrome with distal weakness of lower motor neuron type and loss of pain and temperature appreciation, with preserved posterior column function.

Since the anterior spinal artery receives numerous feeders in the cervical region, infarcts almost always occur caudally. Clinical presentation is characterized by acute onset of flaccid, areflexive paraplegia that evolves after a few days or weeks into a spastic paraplegia with extensor plantar responses. There is an accompanying dissociated sensory loss, with impairment of appreciation of pain and temperature but preservation of sensations of vibration and joint position.

The risk of spinal cord infarction in the setting of abdominal aortic surgery and thoracic endovascular repair may be reduced by intraoperative cerebrospinal fluid drainage through a catheter placed in the lumbar subarachnoid space to reduce intraspinal pressure. If signs of infarction are noted after surgery, blood pressure augmentation for 24–48 hours in addition to lumbar drainage has been noted anecdotally to improve outcomes. Treatment is otherwise symptomatic.

Epidural or Subdural Hemorrhage

Epidural or subdural hemorrhage may lead to sudden severe back pain followed by an acute compressive myelopathy necessitating urgent spinal MRI or myelography and surgical evacuation. It may occur in patients with bleeding disorders or those who are taking anticoagulants, sometimes following trauma or lumbar puncture. Epidural hemorrhage may also be related to a vascular malformation or tumor deposit.

Spinal Dural Arteriovenous Fistulae

Spinal dural arteriovenous fistulae are congenital lesions that present with spinal subarachnoid hemorrhage or myeloradiculopathy. Since most of these malformations are located in the thoracolumbar region, they lead to motor and sensory disturbances in the legs and to sphincter disorders. Pain in the legs or back is often severe. Examination reveals an upper, lower, or mixed motor deficit in the legs; sensory deficits are also present and are usually extensive, although occasionally they are confined to a radicular distribution. Cervical spinal dural arteriovenous fistulae lead also to symptoms and signs in the arms. Spinal MRI may not detect the spinal dural arteriovenous fistula, although most cases show either T2 hyperintensity in the cord or perimedullary flow voids. Myelography (performed with the patient prone and supine) may detect serpiginous filling defects due to enlarged vessels. Selective spinal arteriography is required to confirm the diagnosis and plan treatment. Most lesions are extramedullary, are posterior to the cord (lying either intradurally or extradurally), and can be treated easily by ligation of feeding vessels and excision of the fistulous anomaly or by embolization procedures. Delay in treatment may lead to increased and irreversible disability or to death from recurrent subarachnoid hemorrhage.

When to Refer

All patients should be referred.

When to Admit

All patients should be hospitalized.

Goyal A et al. Outcomes following surgical versus endovascular treatment of spinal dural arteriovenous fistula: a systematic review and meta-analysis. J Neurol Neurosurg Psychiatry. 2019;90:1139. [PMID: 31142659]

INTRACRANIAL & SPINAL MASS LESIONS

1. Primary Intracranial Tumors

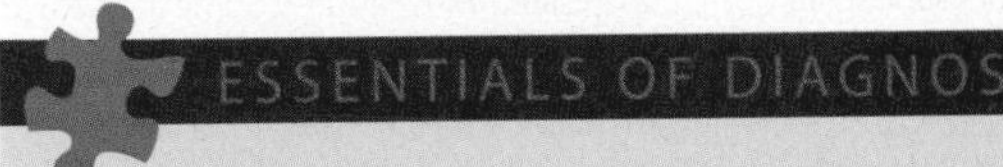

- Generalized or focal disturbance of cerebral function, or both.
- Increased intracranial pressure in some patients.
- Neuroradiologic evidence of space-occupying lesion.

General Considerations

Roughly one-third of all primary intracranial neoplasms (Table 24–4) are meningiomas, one-quarter are gliomas, and the remainder are pituitary adenomas (see Chapter 26), neurofibromas, and other tumors. Certain

Table 24–4. Primary intracranial tumors (listed by major histology grouping and by incidence within each group).

Tumor	Clinical Features	Treatment and Prognosis
Tumors of Meninges		
Meningioma	Originates from the dura mater or arachnoid; compresses rather than invades adjacent neural structures. Increasingly common with advancing age. Tumor size varies greatly. Symptoms vary with tumor site—eg, unilateral proptosis (sphenoidal ridge); anosmia and optic nerve compression (olfactory groove). Tumor is usually benign and readily detected by CT scanning; may lead to calcification and bone erosion visible on plain radiographs of skull.	Treatment is surgical. Tumor may recur if removal is incomplete.
Tumors of Neuroepithelial Origin		
Glioblastoma multiforme	Presents commonly with nonspecific complaints and increased intracranial pressure. As it grows, focal deficits develop. O^6-methylguanine-DNA methyltransferase promoter methylation positivity (seen in 40% of cases) and isocitrate dehydrogenase 1/2 mutations (seen in 10% of cases) carry better prognosis.	Course is rapidly progressive, with poor prognosis (< 20% survival at 2 years). Total surgical removal is usually not possible. Radiation therapy and temozolamide may prolong survival. Tumor treatment fields added to temozolamide after completion of radiation therapy prolong survival.
Astrocytoma	Presentation similar to glioblastoma multiforme but course more protracted, often over several years. Cerebellar astrocytoma may have a more benign course. Isocitrate dehydrogenase 1/2 mutations (seen in most cases) carry better prognosis in grade II and III tumors.	Prognosis is variable. By the time of diagnosis, total excision is usually impossible; tumor may be radiosensitive and temozolamide is also helpful in grade II and III tumors. In cerebellar astrocytoma, total surgical removal is often possible.

(continued)

Table 24–4. Primary intracranial tumors (listed by major histology grouping and by incidence within each group). (continued)

Tumor	Clinical Features	Treatment and Prognosis
Ependymoma	Glioma arising from the ependyma of a ventricle, especially the fourth ventricle; leads to early signs of increased intracranial pressure. Arises also from central canal of cord.	Tumor is best treated surgically if possible. Radiation therapy may be used for residual tumor.
Oligodendroglioma	Slow-growing. Usually arises in cerebral hemisphere in adults. Calcification may be visible on skull radiograph. Co-deletion of 1p/19q and isocitrate dehydrogenase 1/2 mutation required for diagnosis.	Treatment is surgical and usually successful. Radiation and chemotherapy (temozolamide or procarbazine, lomustine, and vincristine) are used in grade II and III tumors.
Brainstem glioma	Presents during childhood with cranial nerve palsies and then with long tract signs in the limbs. Signs of increased intracranial pressure occur late.	Tumor is inoperable; treatment is by irradiation and shunt for increased intracranial pressure.
Neuronal and mixed neuronal-glial tumors	Slow-growing; usually arise in cerebral hemispheres; often associated with seizures. Some are benign (eg, dysembryoblastic neuroepithelial tumors) and some have malignant potential (eg, ganglioglioma).	Resection is not always necessary for benign tumors unless seizures are medically refractory but is indicated for those with malignant potential.
Medulloblastoma	Seen most frequently in children. Generally arises from roof of fourth ventricle and leads to increased intracranial pressure accompanied by brainstem and cerebellar signs. May seed subarachnoid space. Wingless activated tumors carry best prognosis (> 90% 5-year survival).	Treatment consists of surgery combined with radiation therapy and chemotherapy; 5-year survival exceeds 70%. Wingless activated tumors may require less aggressive treatment.
Pineal tumor	Presents with increased intracranial pressure, sometimes associated with impaired upward gaze (Parinaud syndrome) and other deficits indicative of midbrain lesion.	Ventricular decompression by shunting is followed by surgical approach to tumor; irradiation is indicated if tumor is malignant. Prognosis depends on histopathologic findings and extent of tumor.
Tumors of the Sellar Region		
Pituitary adenoma	Functioning adenomas present with symptoms of hormone secretion; nonfunctioning adenomas present with symptoms of local mass effect (eg, bitemporal hemianopsia, hypopituitarism) or are found incidentally.	Prolactin-secreting adenomas are treated with bromocriptine or cabergoline. Others are surgically resected. Pituitary hormone replacement may be required.
Craniopharyngioma	Originates from remnants of Rathke pouch above the sella, depressing the optic chiasm. May present at any age but usually in childhood, with endocrine dysfunction and bitemporal visual field defects.	Treatment is surgical, but total removal may not be possible. Radiation may be used for residual tumor.
Germ cell tumors (germinomas and nongerminomatous germ cell tumors)	Two most common locations are pineal and suprasellar regions. The pineal region presentation is as described in pineal tumors, above. Suprasellar tumors present with hypothalamic and pituitary dysfunction such as diabetes insipidus, delayed or precocious puberty, or growth hormone deficiency.	Germinomas are treated with radiation; prognosis is good for localized tumors. Chemotherapy is added for nongerminomatous germ cell tumors.
Tumors of Cranial and Spinal Nerves		
Acoustic neurinoma (also referred to as acoustic neuroma)	Ipsilateral hearing loss is most common initial symptom. Subsequent symptoms may include tinnitus, headache, vertigo, facial weakness or numbness, and long tract signs. (May be familial and bilateral when related to neurofibromatosis.) Most sensitive screening tests are MRI and brainstem auditory evoked potential.	Treatment is excision by translabyrinthine surgery, craniectomy, or a combined approach. Outcome is usually good.
Lymphomas		
Primary cerebral lymphoma	Associated with AIDS and other immunodeficient states. Presentation may be with focal deficits or with disturbances of cognition and consciousness. May be indistinguishable from cerebral toxoplasmosis.	Treatment is high-dose methotrexate and corticosteroids followed by radiation therapy. Prognosis depends on CD4 count at diagnosis.
Unclassified		
Cerebellar hemangioblastoma	Presents with dysequilibrium, ataxia of trunk or limbs, and signs of increased intracranial pressure. Sometimes familial. May be associated with retinal and spinal vascular lesions, polycythemia, and renal cell carcinoma.	Treatment is surgical. Radiation is used for residual tumor.

tumors, especially neurofibromas, hemangioblastomas, and retinoblastomas, may have a familial basis, and congenital factors bear on the development of craniopharyngiomas. Tumors may occur at any age, but certain gliomas show particular age predilections.

Clinical Findings

A. Symptoms and Signs

Intracranial tumors typically present with headache, seizures, or focal neurologic deficits. New headaches or symptoms of elevated intracranial pressure, such as headaches awaking a patient from sleep or worsening with Valsalva maneuver, cough, or recumbency, are suggestive of brain tumor. Intracranial tumors may also lead to a generalized disturbance of cerebral function with personality changes, intellectual decline, emotional lability, nausea, and malaise.

1. Frontal lobe lesions—Tumors of the frontal lobe often lead to progressive intellectual decline, slowing of mental activity, personality changes, and contralateral grasp reflexes. They may lead to expressive aphasia if the posterior part of the left inferior frontal gyrus is involved. Anosmia may also occur as a consequence of pressure on the olfactory nerve. Precentral lesions may cause focal motor seizures or contralateral pyramidal deficits.

2. Temporal lobe lesions—Tumors of the uncinate region may be manifested by seizures with olfactory or gustatory hallucinations, motor phenomena such as licking or smacking of the lips, and some impairment of external awareness without actual loss of consciousness. Temporal lobe lesions also lead to depersonalization, emotional changes, behavioral disturbances, sensations of déjà vu or jamais vu, micropsia or macropsia (objects appear smaller or larger than they are), visual field defects (crossed upper quadrantanopia), and auditory illusions or hallucinations. Left-sided lesions may lead to dysnomia and receptive aphasia, while right-sided involvement sometimes disturbs the perception of musical notes and melodies.

3. Parietal lobe lesions—Tumors in this location characteristically cause contralateral disturbances of sensation and may cause sensory seizures, sensory loss or inattention, or some combination of these symptoms. The sensory loss is cortical in type and involves postural sensibility and tactile discrimination, so that the appreciation of shape, size, weight, and texture is impaired. Objects placed in the hand may not be recognized (astereognosis). Extensive parietal lobe lesions may produce contralateral hyperpathia and spontaneous pain (thalamic syndrome). Involvement of the optic radiation leads to a contralateral homonymous field defect that sometimes consists solely of lower quadrantanopia. Lesions of the left angular gyrus cause **Gerstmann syndrome** (a combination of alexia, agraphia, acalculia, right-left confusion, and finger agnosia), whereas involvement of the left submarginal gyrus causes ideational apraxia. Anosognosia (the denial, neglect, or rejection of a paralyzed limb) is seen in patients with lesions of the nondominant (right) hemisphere. Constructional apraxia and dressing apraxia may also occur with right-sided lesions.

4. Occipital lobe lesions—Tumors of the occipital lobe characteristically produce contralateral homonymous hemianopia or a partial field defect. With left-sided or bilateral lesions, there may be visual agnosia both for objects and for colors, while irritative lesions on either side can cause unformed visual hallucinations. Bilateral occipital lobe involvement causes cortical blindness in which there is preservation of pupillary responses to light and lack of awareness of the defect by the patient. There may also be loss of color perception, prosopagnosia (inability to identify a familiar face), simultagnosia (inability to integrate and interpret a composite scene as opposed to its individual elements), and Balint syndrome (failure to turn the eyes to a particular point in space, despite preservation of spontaneous and reflex eye movements). The denial of blindness or a field defect constitutes Anton syndrome.

5. Brainstem and cerebellar lesions—Brainstem lesions lead to cranial nerve palsies, ataxia, incoordination, nystagmus, and pyramidal and sensory deficits in the limbs on one or both sides. Intrinsic brainstem tumors, such as gliomas, tend to produce an increase in intracranial pressure only late in their course. Cerebellar tumors produce marked ataxia of the trunk if the vermis cerebelli is involved and ipsilateral appendicular deficits (ataxia, incoordination, and hypotonia of the limbs) if the cerebellar hemispheres are affected.

6. Herniation syndromes—If the pressure is increased in a particular cranial compartment, brain tissue may herniate into a compartment with lower pressure. The most familiar syndrome is herniation of the temporal lobe uncus through the tentorial hiatus, which causes compression of the third cranial nerve, midbrain, and posterior cerebral artery. The earliest sign of this is ipsilateral pupillary dilation, followed by stupor, coma, decerebrate posturing, and respiratory arrest. Another important herniation syndrome consists of displacement of the cerebellar tonsils through the foramen magnum, which causes medullary compression leading to apnea, circulatory collapse, and death.

7. False localizing signs—Tumors may lead to neurologic signs other than by direct compression or infiltration, thereby leading to errors of clinical localization. These false localizing signs include third or sixth nerve palsy and bilateral extensor plantar responses produced by herniation syndromes, and an extensor plantar response occurring ipsilateral to a hemispheric tumor as a result of compression of the opposite cerebral peduncle against the tentorium.

B. Imaging

MRI with gadolinium enhancement is the preferred method to detect the lesion and to define its location, shape, and size; the extent to which normal anatomy is distorted; and the degree of any associated cerebral edema or mass effect. CT scanning with radiocontrast enhancement could be performed; however, it is less helpful than MRI for small lesions or tumors in the posterior fossa. The characteristic appearance of meningiomas on MRI or CT scanning is virtually diagnostic, ie, a lesion in a typical site (parasagittal and sylvian regions, olfactory groove, sphenoidal ridge, tuberculum sellae) that appears as a homogeneous area of increased density in noncontrast scans and enhances uniformly with contrast. Additional MRI sequences that may be helpful in differentiating gliomas from other intracranial pathology include perfusion imaging, magnetic resonance spectroscopy, and diffusion-weighted imaging, although none are specific enough to obviate the need for tissue sampling. Arteriography is largely reserved for presurgical embolization of highly vascular tumors. In patients with normal hormone levels and an intrasellar mass, angiography is sometimes necessary to distinguish with confidence between a pituitary adenoma and an arterial aneurysm.

C. Laboratory and Other Studies

When glial neoplasms are suspected, biopsy is necessary for definitive histologic diagnosis and molecular analysis. The World Health Organization classifies glial tumors by both histology and genetic characteristics. Lumbar puncture is rarely necessary; the findings are seldom diagnostic, and the procedure carries the risk of causing a herniation syndrome. Suspected intracranial germ cell tumors are an exception. If lumbar puncture can be performed safely, cytology and determination of alpha-fetoprotein and beta-human chorionic gonadotropin should be performed in cerebrospinal fluid; tumor markers should be examined in serum as well.

▶ Treatment

Treatment depends on the type and site of the tumor (Table 24–4) and the condition of the patient. Some benign tumors, especially meningiomas discovered incidentally during brain imaging for another purpose, may be monitored with serial annual imaging. For symptomatic tumors, complete surgical removal may be possible if the tumor is extra-axial (eg, meningioma, acoustic neuroma) or is not in a critical or inaccessible region of the brain (eg, cerebellar hemangioblastoma). Surgery also permits the diagnosis to be verified and may be beneficial in reducing intracranial pressure and relieving symptoms even if the neoplasm cannot be completely removed. Clinical deficits are sometimes due in part to obstructive hydrocephalus, in which case simple surgical shunting procedures often produce dramatic benefit. In patients with malignant gliomas, survival correlates to the extent of initial resection.

Radiation therapy increases median survival rates regardless of any preceding surgery, and its combination with chemotherapy provides additional benefit. Indications for irradiation in the treatment of patients with other primary intracranial neoplasms depend on tumor type and accessibility and the feasibility of complete surgical removal. Long-term neurocognitive deficits may complicate radiation therapy. Temozolomide is a commonly used oral and intravenous chemotherapeutic for gliomas. In patients with glioblastoma with methylated methylguanine-DNA methyltransferase (MGMT) promoter, combination therapy with lomustine and temozolomide improved median survival from 31 to 48 months in a randomized controlled trial. The addition of low-intensity, 200 kHz frequency alternating electric fields (tumor treatment fields) delivered extracranially at least 18 hours daily, improves progression-free survival by 2.7 months and median survival by 4.9 months compared to temozolomide alone in glioblastoma. Bevacizumab is approved in the United States but not in Europe for use in recurrent high-grade glioma. Combination therapy with procarbazine, lomustine, and vincristine improves median survival when given with radiation to patients with isocitrate dehydrogenase–mutant astrocytoma and isocitrate dehydrogenase–mutant, p1/19q co-deleted oligodendroglioma.

Corticosteroids help reduce cerebral edema and are usually started before surgery. Herniation is treated with intravenous dexamethasone (10–20 mg as a bolus, followed by 4 mg every 6 hours) and intravenous mannitol (20% solution given in a dose of 1.5 g/kg over about 30 minutes).

Anticonvulsants are also commonly administered in standard doses (see Table 24–2) but are not indicated for prophylaxis in patients who have no history of seizures. For those patients with difficult to treat symptoms or those needing help with advance care planning, specialty palliative care consultation is appropriate (see Chapter 5).

▶ When to Refer

All patients should be referred.

▶ When to Admit

- All patients with increased intracranial pressure.
- All patients requiring biopsy, surgical treatment, or shunting procedures.

Bell EH et al. Comprehensive genomic analysis in NRG oncology/RTOG 9802: a phase III trial of radiation versus radiation plus procarbazine, lomustine (CCNU), and vincristine in high-risk low-grade glioma. J Clin Oncol. 2020;38:3407. [PMID: 32706640]

Herrlinger U et al; Neurooncology Working Group of the German Cancer Society. Lomustine-temozolomide combination therapy versus standard temozolomide therapy in patients with newly diagnosed glioblastoma with methylated MGMT promoter (CeTeG/NOA-09): a randomised, open-label, phase 3 trial. Lancet. 2019;393:678. [PMID: 30782343]

2. Metastatic Intracranial Tumors

A. Cerebral Metastases

Metastatic brain tumors present in the same way as other cerebral neoplasms, ie, with increased intracranial pressure, with focal or diffuse disturbance of cerebral function, or with both of these manifestations. Indeed, in patients with a single cerebral lesion, the metastatic nature of the lesion may become evident only on histopathologic examination. In other patients, there is evidence of widespread metastatic disease, or an isolated cerebral metastasis develops during treatment of the primary neoplasm.

The most common source of intracranial metastasis is carcinoma of the lung; other primary sites are the breast, kidney, skin (melanoma), and GI tract. Most cerebral metastases are located supratentorially. Laboratory and radiologic studies used to evaluate patients with metastases are those described for primary neoplasms. They include MRI and CT scanning performed both with and without contrast. Lumbar puncture is necessary only in patients with suspected carcinomatous meningitis. In patients with verified cerebral metastasis from an unknown primary, investigation is guided by symptoms and signs. In women, mammography is indicated; in men under 50, germ cell origin is sought.

Treatment of brain metastases is rapidly evolving and a multidisciplinary approach between neurosurgery, radiation oncology, oncology, and palliative care is necessary. In patients with only a single, surgically accessible cerebral metastasis who are otherwise well (ie, a high level of functioning and little or no evidence of extracranial disease), it may be possible to remove the lesion and then treat with irradiation; the latter may also be selected as the sole treatment. Systemic immunotherapy may also be an acceptable initial option in select cases. In patients with multiple metastases or widespread systemic disease, stereotactic radiosurgery, whole-brain radiotherapy, or both may help in some instances; systemic chemotherapy or immunotherapy may be options in others, but in many, treatment is palliative only. Memantine (5 mg once daily orally titrated by 5 mg weekly to 10 mg twice daily) reduced cognitive toxicity associated with whole-brain radiotherapy in a randomized trial and is recommended; this effect can be augmented through intensity modulated radiation therapy with hippocampal avoidance.

Brown PD et al. Hippocampal avoidance during whole-brain radiotherapy plus memantine for patients with brain metastases: phase III trial NRG oncology CC001. J Clin Oncol. 2020;38:1019. [PMID: 32058845]

B. Leptomeningeal Metastases (Carcinomatous Meningitis)

The neoplasms metastasizing most commonly to the leptomeninges are carcinoma of the breast and lung, lymphomas, and leukemia (see Chapter 39). Leptomeningeal metastases lead to multifocal neurologic deficits, which may be associated with infiltration of cranial and spinal nerve roots, direct invasion of the brain or spinal cord, obstructive or communicating hydrocephalus, or some combination of these factors.

The diagnosis is confirmed by examination of the cerebrospinal fluid. Findings may include elevated cerebrospinal fluid pressure, pleocytosis, increased protein concentration, and decreased glucose concentration. Cytologic studies may indicate that malignant cells are present; if not, lumbar puncture should be repeated at least twice to obtain further samples for analysis.

CT scans showing contrast enhancement in the basal cisterns or showing hydrocephalus without any evidence of a mass lesion support the diagnosis. Gadolinium-enhanced MRI is more sensitive and frequently shows enhancing foci in the leptomeninges. Myelography may show deposits on multiple nerve roots.

Treatment is by irradiation to symptomatic areas, combined with intrathecal chemotherapy in select patients. The long-term prognosis is poor—only about 10% of patients survive for 1 year—and palliative care is therefore important (see Chapter 5).

3. Intracranial Mass Lesions in Patients with AIDS

Primary cerebral lymphoma is a common complication in patients with AIDS. This leads to disturbances in cognition or consciousness, focal motor or sensory deficits, aphasia, seizures, and cranial neuropathies. Similar clinical disturbances may result from **cerebral toxoplasmosis,** which is also a common complication in patients with AIDS (see Chapters 31 and 35). Neither CT nor MRI findings distinguish these two disorders and serologic tests for toxoplasmosis are unreliable in patients with AIDS. *Toxoplasma gondii* DNA detected by PCR in the spinal fluid is specific but not sensitive for toxoplasmosis, and the finding of Epstein-Barr virus DNA suggests lymphoma but is not specific enough to initiate treatment. Accordingly, for neurologically stable patients, a trial of treatment for toxoplasmosis with pyrimethamine and sulfadiazine is recommended for 3 weeks; the imaging studies are then repeated, and if any lesion has improved, the regimen is continued indefinitely. If any lesion does not improve, cerebral biopsy is necessary (see also Chapter 31). Primary cerebral lymphoma in patients with AIDS is treated with corticosteroids, high-dose methotrexate, and antiretroviral therapy. Rituximab may be used in some patients. Whole-brain irradiation may not be necessary.

Cryptococcal meningitis is a common opportunistic infection in patients with AIDS. Clinically, it may resemble cerebral toxoplasmosis or lymphoma, but cranial CT scans are usually normal (see Chapter 36).

4. Primary & Metastatic Spinal Tumors

Approximately 10% of spinal tumors are intramedullary. Ependymoma is the most common type of intramedullary tumor; the remainder are other types of glioma. Extramedullary tumors may be extradural or intradural in location. Among the primary extramedullary tumors, neurofibromas and meningiomas are relatively common, benign, and may be intradural or extradural. Carcinomatous metastases, lymphomatous or leukemic deposits, and myeloma are usually extradural; in the case of metastases, the prostate, breast, lung, and kidney are common primary sites.

Tumors may lead to spinal cord dysfunction by direct compression, by ischemia secondary to arterial or venous obstruction and, in the case of intramedullary lesions, by invasive infiltration.

Clinical Findings

A. Symptoms and Signs

Symptoms usually develop insidiously. Pain is often conspicuous with extradural lesions; is characteristically aggravated by coughing or straining; may be radicular, localized to the back, or felt diffusely in an extremity; and may be accompanied by motor deficits, paresthesias, or numbness, especially in the legs. Bladder, bowel, and sexual dysfunction may occur. When sphincter disturbances occur, they are usually particularly disabling. Pain, however, often precedes specific neurologic symptoms from epidural metastases.

Examination may reveal localized spinal tenderness. A segmental lower motor neuron deficit or dermatomal sensory changes (or both) are sometimes found at the level of the lesion, while an upper motor neuron deficit and sensory disturbance are found below it.

B. Imaging

MRI with contrast or CT myelography is used to identify and localize the lesion. The combination of known tumor elsewhere in the body, back pain, and either abnormal plain films of the spine or neurologic signs of cord compression is an indication to perform this on an *urgent* basis.

C. Laboratory Findings

The cerebrospinal fluid is often xanthochromic and contains a greatly increased protein concentration with normal cell content and glucose concentration.

Treatment

Intramedullary tumors are treated by decompression and surgical excision (when feasible) and by irradiation. The prognosis depends on the cause and severity of cord compression before it is relieved.

Treatment of epidural spinal metastases consists of surgical decompression, radiation, or both. Dexamethasone is also given in a high dosage (eg, 10–96 mg once intravenously, followed by 4–25 mg four times daily for 3 days orally or intravenously, followed by rapid tapering of the dosage, depending on initial dose and response) to reduce cord swelling and relieve pain. Radiation alone is often all that is required in patients with radiosensitive tumors. Surgical decompression is reserved for patients with tumors that are unresponsive to irradiation or who have previously been irradiated, for those with spinal instability, and for patients in whom there is some uncertainty about the diagnosis. The long-term outlook is poor, but treatment may at least delay the onset of major disability.

Lawton AJ et al. Assessment and management of patients with metastatic spinal cord compression: a multidisciplinary review. J Clin Oncol. 2019;37:61. [PMID: 30395488]

5. Brain Abscess

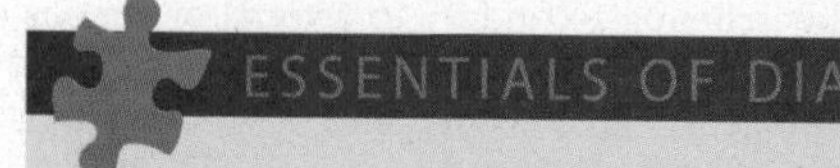

- Signs of expanding intracranial mass.
- Signs of primary infection or congenital heart disease are sometimes present.
- Fever may be absent.

General Considerations

Brain abscess presents as an intracranial space-occupying lesion and arises as a sequela of dental, ear or nose infection, may be a complication of infection elsewhere in the body, or may result from infection introduced intracranially by trauma or surgical procedures. The most common infective organisms are streptococci, staphylococci, and anaerobes; mixed infections also occur.

Clinical Findings

A. Symptoms and Signs

Headache, drowsiness, inattention, confusion, and seizures are early symptoms, followed by signs of increasing intracranial pressure and then a focal neurologic deficit. There may be little or no systemic evidence of infection.

B. Imaging and Other Investigations

A CT scan of the head characteristically shows an area of contrast enhancement surrounding a low-density core. Similar abnormalities may be found in patients with metastatic neoplasms. MRI findings often permit earlier recognition of focal cerebritis or an abscess. Stereotactic needle aspiration may enable a specific etiologic organism to be identified. Examination of the cerebrospinal fluid does not help in diagnosis and may precipitate a herniation syndrome. Peripheral leukocytosis is sometimes present.

Treatment

Treatment consists of intravenous antibiotics combined with surgical drainage (aspiration or excision), if necessary, to reduce the mass effect or sometimes to establish the diagnosis. Abscesses smaller than 2 cm can often be cured medically. Broad-spectrum antibiotics, selected based on risk factors and likely organisms, are used if the infecting organism is unknown (see Chapter 33). An initial empiric multi-antibiotic regimen typically includes ceftriaxone (2 g intravenously every 12 hours), metronidazole (15 mg/kg intravenous loading dose, followed by 7.5 mg/kg intravenously every 6 hours), and vancomycin (1 g intravenously every 12 hours). The regimen is altered once culture and sensitivity data are available. Antimicrobial treatment is usually continued parenterally for 6–8 weeks and is followed by oral treatment for certain infections, such as nocardiosis, actinomycosis, fungal infections, and tuberculosis. The patient should be monitored by serial CT scans or MRI every 2 weeks and at deterioration. Dexamethasone (4–25 mg four times daily intravenously or orally, depending on severity, followed by tapering of dose, depending on response) may reduce any associated edema, but intravenous mannitol is sometimes required.

Bodilsen J. Risk factors for brain abscess: a nationwide, population-based, nested case-control study. Clin Infect Dis. 2020;71:1040. [PMID: 31641757]

NONMETASTATIC NEUROLOGIC COMPLICATIONS OF MALIGNANT DISEASE

A variety of nonmetastatic neurologic complications of malignant disease can be recognized. **Metabolic encephalopathy** due to electrolyte abnormalities, infections, drug overdose, or the failure of some vital organ may be reflected by drowsiness, lethargy, restlessness, insomnia, agitation, confusion, stupor, or coma. The mental changes are usually associated with tremor, asterixis, and multifocal myoclonus. The electroencephalogram is generally diffusely slowed. Laboratory studies are necessary to detect the cause of the encephalopathy, which must then be treated appropriately.

Immune suppression resulting from either the malignant disease or its treatment (eg, by chemotherapy) predisposes patients to brain abscess, progressive multifocal leukoencephalopathy, meningitis, herpes zoster infection, and other opportunistic infectious diseases. Moreover, an overt or occult cerebrospinal fluid fistula, as occurs with some tumors, may also increase the risk of infection. MRI or CT scanning aids in the early recognition of a brain abscess, but metastatic brain tumors may have a similar appearance. Examination of the cerebrospinal fluid is essential in the evaluation of patients with meningitis and encephalitis but is of no help in the diagnosis of brain abscess.

Cerebrovascular disorders that cause neurologic complications in patients with systemic cancer include nonbacterial thrombotic endocarditis, septic embolization, and cerebral infarcts due to malignancy-induced hypercoagulability. Cerebral, subarachnoid, or subdural hemorrhages may occur in patients with myelogenous leukemia and may be found in association with metastatic tumors, especially melanoma. Spinal subdural hemorrhage sometimes occurs after lumbar puncture in patients with marked thrombocytopenia.

Disseminated intravascular coagulation occurs most commonly in patients with acute promyelocytic leukemia or with some adenocarcinomas and is characterized by a fluctuating encephalopathy, often with associated seizures, that frequently progresses to coma or death. There may be few accompanying neurologic signs. **Venous sinus thrombosis,** which usually presents with convulsions and headaches, may also occur in patients with leukemia or lymphoma. Examination commonly reveals papilledema and focal or diffuse neurologic signs. Anticonvulsants, anticoagulants, and medications to lower the intracranial pressure may be of value.

Autoimmune paraneoplastic disorders occur when the immune system reacts against neuronal antigens expressed by tumor cells. The clinical manifestations depend on the autoantibody. Symptoms may precede those due to the neoplasm itself. Several distinct syndromes are common, each associated with specific antibodies and tumors (Table 24–5). Identification of an antibody is not always possible in a suspected autoimmune paraneoplastic condition, and a search for an underlying neoplasm should be undertaken. Treatment of the neoplasm offers the best hope for stabilization or improvement of the neurologic symptoms, which often are not completely reversible. Specific treatment of the antibody-mediated symptoms by intravenous immunoglobulin (IVIG) administration, plasmapheresis, corticosteroids, or other immunosuppressive regimens is frequently attempted despite limited evidence of efficacy. Many of the disorders listed in Table 24–5 can occur either as paraneoplastic phenomena or in isolation; when they occur in the absence of a tumor, the response to immunotherapy is typically more favorable.

Autoimmune disorders may also be triggered as a result of cancer immunotherapy; encephalitis, hypophysitis, meningitis, transverse myelitis, acute and chronic inflammatory demyelinating polyneuropathy, autonomic neuropathy, myasthenia gravis, and myositis have all been described.

Graus F et al. Updated diagnostic criteria for paraneoplastic neurological syndromes. Neurol Neuroimmunol Neuroinflamm. 2021;8:e1014. [PMID: 34006622]

IDIOPATHIC INTRACRANIAL HYPERTENSION (Pseudotumor Cerebri)

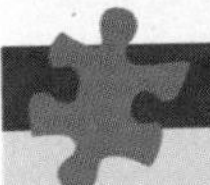

ESSENTIALS OF DIAGNOSIS

- Headache, worse on straining.
- Visual obscurations or diplopia may occur.
- Examination reveals papilledema.
- Abducens palsy is commonly present.

General Considerations

There are many causes of this disorder. Thrombosis of the transverse venous sinus as a complication of otitis media or chronic mastoiditis is one cause, and sagittal sinus thrombosis may lead to a clinically similar picture. Other causes include chronic pulmonary disease, SLE, uremia, endocrine disturbances such as hypoparathyroidism, hypothyroidism, or Addison disease, vitamin A toxicity, and the use of tetracycline or oral contraceptives. Cases have also followed withdrawal of corticosteroids after long-term use. In most instances, however, no specific cause can be found, and the disorder remits spontaneously after several months. This idiopathic variety occurs most commonly among overweight women aged 20–44. In all cases, screening for a space-occupying lesion of the brain is important.

Clinical Findings

A. Symptoms and Signs

Symptoms consist of headache, diplopia, and other visual disturbances due to papilledema and abducens nerve dysfunction. Pulse-synchronous tinnitus may also occur. Examination reveals papilledema and some enlargement of the blind spots, but patients otherwise look well.

B. Imaging

Investigations reveal no evidence of a space-occupying lesion. CT or MRI may show small or normal ventricles, an

Table 24–5. Autoimmune paraneoplastic disorders and their associated antibodies and tumors (listed in alphabetical order).

Syndrome	Clinical Features	Associated Antibodies	Typical Associated Tumors
Anti-NMDA receptor–associated encephalitis	Paranoia, delusions, behavioral disturbance, seizure, orofacial dyskinesias, athetosis, dysautonomia, hypoventilation	NMDA receptor[1]	Ovarian teratoma, lung, breast, ovary, testicle
Autoimmune necrotizing myopathy	Weakness	SRP,[1] HMGCR[1]	Lung, breast, GI, bladder
Autonomic neuropathy	Postural hypotension, gastroparesis	Hu, ganglionic AChR[1]	
Cerebellar degeneration	Ataxia, dysarthria, nystagmus	GAD65,[1] KLHL11, mGluR1,[1] NIF,[1] Ri, Tr, VGCC,[1] Yo	Lung, breast, thymus, ovary, testicle, Hodgkin lymphoma
Dermatomyositis	Weakness, heliotrope skin rash	TIF-1 gamma	Lung, breast, ovary, GI, lymphoma
Lambert-Eaton myasthenic syndrome	Fatiguable weakness, ptosis, diplopia, dry mouth, constipation	VGCC[1]	Lung
Limbic encephalitis/encephalomyelitis	Short-term memory loss, hallucinations, seizures, behavioral disturbance, encephalopathy	AMPA receptor,[1] Caspr2,[1] CV2/CRMP5, DPPX,[1] $GABA_A$ receptor,[1] $GABA_B$ receptor,[1] GAD65,[1] GFAP,[1] Hu, LGI1,[1] Ma2, mGluR5,[1] NIF,[1] thyroglobulin[1]/thyroperoxidase[1]	Lung, breast, thymus, ovary, testicle, Hodgkin lymphoma
Myasthenia gravis	Fatiguable weakness, ptosis, diplopia	AChR,[1] LRP4,[1] MuSK[1]	Thymus
Myelitis	Paraparesis, bowel and bladder dysfunction; sensory level	Amphiphysin,[1] aquaporin 4,[1] CRMP-5, GFAP,[1] Hu, MOG,[1] Yo	Lung, breast, lymphoma, leukemia, thyroid, renal
Opsoclonus/myoclonus	Erratic, conjugate saccadic eye movements and limb myoclonus	Ri	Lung, breast, ovary, testicle, neuroblastoma (children)
Retinopathy	Vision loss	Anti-recoverin, anti-retinal bipolar cell	Small cell lung, melanoma
Sensorimotor neuropathy	Numbness with or without weakness; may be mild and chronic or acute and severe	Hu, MAG	
Sensory neuronopathy	Pain, numbness, sensory ataxia, hearing loss	Hu	Small cell lung
Stiff person syndrome	Co-contraction of antagonist and agonist muscles	Amphiphysin,[1] GAD65,[1] GlyR[1]	Small cell lung, breast, thymus, lymphoma

AChR, acetylcholine receptor; AMPA, alpha-amino-3-hydroxy-5-methylisoxazole-4-propionic acid; Caspr2, contactin associated protein-like 2; CRMP, collapsin response-mediator protein; DPPX, dipeptidyl-peptidase-like protein-6; GABA, gamma-aminobutyric acid; GAD, glutamic acid decarboxylase; GFAP, glial fibrillary acidic protein; GlyR, glycine receptor; HMGCR, 3-hydroxy-3-methylglutaryl-coenzyme A reductase; KLHL11, kelch-like protein 11; LGI1, leucine rich glioma inactivated; LRP4, LDL receptor-related protein 4; mGluR, metabotropic glutamate receptor; MAG, myelin-associated glycoprotein; MOG, myelin oligodendrocyte glycoprotein; MuSK, muscle-specific tyrosine kinase; NIF, neuronal intermediate filament; NMDA, *N*-methyl-D-aspartate; SRP, signal recognition particle; TIF-1, human transcription intermediary factor-1; VGCC, voltage-gated calcium channel.

[1]Can occur in absence of tumor.

empty sella turcica, tortuous optic nerves, distension of the optic nerve sheath, and posterior globe flattening. MR venography is important in screening for thrombosis of the intracranial venous sinuses. In some cases, stenosis of one or more of the venous sinuses will be observed.

C. Laboratory Findings

Lumbar puncture is necessary to confirm the presence of intracranial hypertension, but the cerebrospinal fluid is normal. Laboratory studies help exclude some of the other causes mentioned earlier.

Treatment

Untreated intracranial hypertension sometimes leads to secondary optic atrophy and permanent visual loss. Acetazolamide (250–500 mg orally three times daily, increasing slowly to a maintenance dose of up to 4000 mg daily, divided two to four times daily) reduces formation of cerebrospinal fluid. Like acetazolamide, the antiepileptic medication topiramate (Table 24–2) is a carbonic anhydrase inhibitor and was shown to be similarly effective in an open-label study; topiramate has the added benefit of causing weight loss. Furosemide (20–40 mg daily) may be helpful as adjunct therapy. Corticosteroids (eg, prednisone

60–80 mg daily) are sometimes prescribed, but side effects and the risk of relapse on withdrawal have discouraged their use. Weight loss is important: bariatric surgery led to a decrease in both intracranial pressure and weight at 2 years compared with a community weight management program in a randomized trial and may be considered in patients with a BMI of 35 or greater. Repeated lumbar puncture to lower the intracranial pressure by removal of cerebrospinal fluid is effective as a temporizing measure, but pharmacologic approaches to treatment provide better long-term relief. Treatment is monitored by checking visual acuity and visual fields, funduscopic appearance, and pressure of the cerebrospinal fluid. The disorder may worsen after a period of stability, indicating the need for long-term follow-up.

If medical treatment fails to control the intracranial pressure, surgical placement of a lumboperitoneal or ventriculoperitoneal shunt or optic nerve sheath fenestration should be undertaken to preserve vision. Venous sinus stenting is an increasingly accepted therapeutic option for dural venous sinus stenosis.

In addition to the above measures, any specific cause of intracranial hypertension requires appropriate treatment. Thus, hormone therapy should be initiated if there is an underlying endocrine disturbance. Discontinuing the use of tetracycline, oral contraceptives, or vitamin A will allow for resolution of intracranial hypertension due to these agents. If corticosteroid withdrawal is responsible, the medication should be reintroduced and then tapered more gradually.

When to Refer

All patients should be referred.

When to Admit

All patients with worsening vision requiring surgical treatment should be hospitalized.

Kalyvas A et al. A systematic review of surgical treatments of idiopathic intracranial hypertension (IIH). Neurosurg Rev. 2021;44:773. [PMID: 32335853]

Mollan SP et al. Effectiveness of bariatric surgery vs community weight management intervention for the treatment of idiopathic intracranial hypertension: a randomized controlled trial. JAMA Neurol. 2021;78:678. [PMID: 33900360]

SELECTED NEUROCUTANEOUS DISEASES

Because the nervous system develops from the epithelial layer of the embryo, a number of congenital diseases include both neurologic and cutaneous manifestations. Among these disorders, three are discussed below, and von Hippel-Lindau disease is discussed in Chapter 26.

1. Tuberous Sclerosis

Tuberous sclerosis may occur sporadically or on a familial basis with autosomal dominant inheritance. Neurologic presentation is with seizures and progressive psychomotor delay beginning in early childhood. The cutaneous abnormality adenoma sebaceum becomes manifest usually between 5 and 10 years of age and typically consists of reddened nodules on the face (cheeks, nasolabial folds, sides of the nose, and chin) and sometimes on the forehead and neck. Other typical cutaneous lesions include subungual fibromas, shagreen patches (leathery plaques of subepidermal fibrosis, situated usually on the trunk), and leaf-shaped hypopigmented spots. Associated abnormalities include retinal lesions and tumors, benign rhabdomyomas of the heart, lung cysts, benign tumors in the viscera, and bone cysts.

The disease is slowly progressive and leads to increasing mental deterioration. Anticonvulsants are indicated to control seizures. Everolimus, a mammalian target of rapamycin (mTOR) inhibitor, is approved in the United States and Europe for medically refractory epilepsy and subependymal giant cell astrocytomas due to tuberous sclerosis.

2. Neurofibromatosis

Neurofibromatosis may occur either sporadically or on a familial basis with autosomal dominant inheritance. Two distinct forms are recognized: **Type 1 (Recklinghausen disease)** is characterized by multiple hyperpigmented macules, Lisch nodules, and neurofibromas, and results from mutations in the *NF1* gene on chromosome 17. **Type 2** is characterized by bilateral eighth nerve tumors, often accompanied by other intracranial or intraspinal tumors, and is associated with mutations in the *NF2* (merlin) gene on chromosome 22.

Neurologic presentation is usually with symptoms and signs of tumor. Multiple neurofibromas characteristically are present and may involve spinal or cranial nerves, especially the eighth nerve. Examination of the superficial cutaneous nerves usually reveals palpable mobile nodules. In some cases, there is marked overgrowth of subcutaneous tissues (**plexiform neuromas**), sometimes with an underlying bony abnormality. Associated cutaneous lesions include axillary freckling and patches of cutaneous pigmentation (**café au lait spots**). Malignant degeneration of neurofibromas occasionally occurs and may lead to peripheral sarcomas. Meningiomas, gliomas (especially optic nerve gliomas), bone cysts, pheochromocytomas, scoliosis, and obstructive hydrocephalus may also occur. Selumetinib (25 mg/m^2 orally twice daily), a mitogen-activated protein kinase inhibitor, causes plexiform neurofibromas to shrink by at least 20% in two-thirds of patients and is approved by the FDA for treatment of inoperable plexiform neurofibromas in children 2 years of age and older. Studies in adults are ongoing.

3. Sturge-Weber Syndrome

Sturge-Weber syndrome consists of a congenital, usually unilateral, cutaneous capillary angioma involving the upper face, leptomeningeal angiomatosis, and, in many patients, choroidal angioma. It has no sex predilection and usually occurs sporadically. The cutaneous angioma sometimes has a more extensive distribution over the head and neck and is often quite disfiguring, especially if there is associated overgrowth of connective tissue. Focal or generalized seizures are the usual neurologic presentation and may commence at any age. There may be contralateral homonymous hemianopia, hemiparesis and hemisensory disturbance, ipsilateral glaucoma, and mental subnormality. Skull radiographs taken after the first 2 years of life usually reveal gyriform ("tramline") intracranial calcification, especially in the parieto-occipital region, due to mineral deposition in the cortex beneath the intracranial angioma.

Treatment is aimed at controlling seizures pharmacologically (Table 24–2), but surgical treatment may be necessary. Ophthalmologic advice should be sought concerning the management of choroidal angioma and of increased intraocular pressure.

MOVEMENT DISORDERS

1. Essential (Familial) Tremor

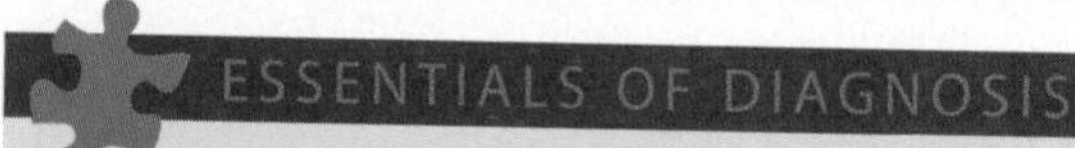

- Postural tremor of hands, head, or voice.
- Family history common.
- May improve temporarily with alcohol.
- No abnormal findings other than tremor.

General Considerations

The cause of essential tremor is uncertain, but it is sometimes inherited in an autosomal dominant manner. Various responsible genes have been identified.

Clinical Findings

Tremor may begin at any age and is enhanced by emotional stress. The tremor usually involves one or both hands, the head, or the hands and head, while the legs tend to be spared. The tremor is *not present at rest* but emerges with action. Examination reveals no other abnormalities. Ingestion of a small quantity of alcohol commonly provides remarkable but short-lived relief by an unknown mechanism.

The tremor typically becomes more conspicuous with time. Occasionally, it interferes with manual skills and leads to impairment of handwriting. Speech may also be affected if the laryngeal muscles are involved.

Treatment

Treatment is often unnecessary. When it is required because of disability, propranolol (60–240 mg daily orally) may be helpful. Long-term therapy is typical; however, intermittent therapy is sometimes useful in patients whose tremor becomes exacerbated in specific predictable situations. Primidone may be helpful when propranolol is ineffective, but patients with essential tremor are often very sensitive to it. Therefore, the starting dose is 50 mg daily orally, and the daily dose is increased by 50 mg every 2 weeks depending on the patient's response; a maintenance dose of 125 mg three times daily orally is commonly effective. Occasional patients do not respond to these measures but are helped by alprazolam (up to 3 mg daily orally in divided doses), topiramate (titrated up to a dose of 400 mg daily orally in divided doses over about 8 weeks), or gabapentin (1800 mg daily orally in divided doses). Botulinum toxin A may reduce tremor, but adverse effects include dose-dependent weakness of the injected muscles.

Disabling tremor unresponsive to medical treatment may be helped by high-frequency thalamic stimulation ("deep brain stimulation") on one or both sides, according to the laterality of symptoms. Focused transcranial ultrasound thalamotomy using MRI guidance is also effective, as is stereotactic radiosurgery for unilateral upper extremity tremor.

When to Refer

- When refractory to first-line treatment with propranolol or primidone.
- When additional neurologic signs are present (ie, parkinsonism).

When to Admit

Patients requiring surgical treatment (deep brain stimulator placement) should be hospitalized.

Ondo WG. Current and emerging treatments of essential tremor. Neurol Clin. 2020;38:309. [PMID: 32279712]

2. Parkinson Disease

ESSENTIALS OF DIAGNOSIS

- Any combination of tremor, rigidity, bradykinesia, and progressive postural instability ("parkinsonism").
- Cognitive impairment is sometimes prominent.

General Considerations

Parkinsonism is a relatively common disorder that occurs in all ethnic groups, with an approximately equal sex distribution. The most common variety, idiopathic Parkinson disease, begins most often between 45 and 65 years of age and is a progressive disease.

Etiology

Parkinsonism may rarely occur on a familial basis, and the parkinsonian phenotype may result from mutations of several different genes. Postencephalitic parkinsonism is becoming increasingly rare. Exposure to certain toxins (eg, manganese dust, carbon disulfide) and severe carbon monoxide poisoning may lead to parkinsonism. Reversible parkinsonism may develop in patients receiving neuroleptic medications (see Chapter 25), reserpine, or metoclopramide. Only rarely is hemiparkinsonism the presenting feature of a progressive space-occupying lesion.

In idiopathic Parkinson disease, dopamine depletion due to degeneration of the dopaminergic nigrostriatal system leads to an imbalance of dopamine and acetylcholine, which are neurotransmitters normally present in the corpus striatum. Treatment of the motor disturbance is directed at redressing this imbalance by blocking the effect of acetylcholine with anticholinergic medications or by the administration of levodopa, the precursor of dopamine. Prior use of ibuprofen is associated with a *decreased* risk of developing Parkinson disease; age, family history, male sex, ongoing herbicide/pesticide exposure, and significant prior head trauma are risk factors.

Clinical Findings

Tremor, rigidity, bradykinesia, and **postural instability** are the cardinal motor features of parkinsonism and may be present in any combination. Nonmotor manifestations include affective disorders (depression, anxiety, and apathy), psychosis, cognitive changes, fatigue, sleep disorders, anosmia, autonomic disturbances, sensory complaints or pain, and seborrheic dermatitis. Dementia or mild cognitive impairment will eventually develop in many patients.

The tremor of about four to six cycles per second is *most conspicuous at rest*, is enhanced by emotional stress, and is often less severe during voluntary activity. Although it may ultimately be present in all limbs, the tremor is commonly confined to one limb or to the limbs on one side for months or years before it becomes more generalized. In some patients, tremor is absent.

Rigidity (an increase in resistance to passive movement) is responsible for the characteristically flexed posture seen in many patients, but the most disabling symptoms of parkinsonism are due to bradykinesia, manifested as a slowness of voluntary movement and a reduction in automatic movements such as swinging of the arms while walking. Curiously, however, effective voluntary activity may briefly be regained during an emergency (eg, the patient is able to leap aside to avoid an oncoming motor vehicle).

Clinical diagnosis of the well-developed syndrome is usually simple. The patient has a relatively immobile face with widened palpebral fissures, infrequent blinking, and a fixity of facial expression. Seborrhea of the scalp and face is common. There is often mild blepharoclonus, and a tremor may be present about the mouth and lips. Repetitive tapping (about twice per second) over the bridge of the nose produces a sustained blink response (**Myerson sign**). Other findings may include saliva drooling from the mouth, perhaps due to impairment of swallowing; soft and poorly modulated voice; a variable rest tremor and rigidity in some or all of the limbs; slowness of voluntary movements; impairment of fine or rapidly alternating movements; and micrographia. There is typically no muscle weakness (provided that sufficient time is allowed for power to be developed) and no alteration in the tendon reflexes or plantar responses. It is difficult for the patient to arise from a sitting position and begin walking. The gait itself is characterized by small shuffling steps and a loss of the normal automatic arm swing; there may be unsteadiness on turning, difficulty in stopping, and a tendency to fall.

Differential Diagnosis

Diagnostic problems may occur in mild cases, especially if tremor is minimal or absent. For example, mild hypokinesia or slight tremor is commonly attributed to old age. Depression, with its associated expressionless face, poorly modulated voice, and reduction in voluntary activity, can be difficult to distinguish from mild parkinsonism, especially since the two disorders may coexist. The family history, the character of the tremor, and lack of other neurologic signs should distinguish essential tremor from parkinsonism. Wilson disease can be distinguished by its early age at onset, the presence of other abnormal movements, Kayser-Fleischer rings, and chronic hepatitis, and by increased concentrations of copper in the tissues. Huntington disease presenting with rigidity and bradykinesia may be mistaken for parkinsonism unless the family history and accompanying dementia are recognized. In multisystem atrophy (previously called the Shy-Drager syndrome), autonomic insufficiency (leading to postural hypotension, anhidrosis, disturbances of sphincter control, erectile dysfunction, etc) may be accompanied by parkinsonism, pyramidal deficits, lower motor neuron signs, or cerebellar dysfunction. In progressive supranuclear palsy, bradykinesia and rigidity are accompanied by a supranuclear disorder of eye movements, pseudobulbar palsy, pseudo-emotional lability (**pseudobulbar affect**), and axial dystonia. Creutzfeldt-Jakob disease may be accompanied by features of parkinsonism, but progression is rapid, dementia is usual, myoclonic jerking is common, ataxia and pyramidal signs may be conspicuous, and the MRI and electroencephalographic findings are usually characteristic. In corticobasal degeneration, asymmetric parkinsonism is accompanied by conspicuous signs of cortical dysfunction (eg, apraxia, sensory inattention, dementia, aphasia). Diffuse Lewy body disease is characterized by prominent visual hallucinations and cognitive impairment that begin before or within 1 year of onset of the motor features of parkinsonism.

Treatment

Treatment is symptomatic. There is great interest in developing disease-modifying therapies, but trials of several putative neuroprotective agents have shown no benefit. Trials of various gene therapies have provided promising results but are not yet complete at the start of 2022.

A. Medical Measures

Medication is not required early in the course of Parkinson disease, but the nature of the disorder and the availability of medical treatment for use when necessary should be discussed with the patient.

1. Amantadine—Patients with mild symptoms but no disability may be helped by amantadine (100 mg orally two to three times daily [immediate release] or once daily [extended release]). This medication improves all of the clinical features of parkinsonism, but its mode of action is unclear. Side effects are uncommon but may include restlessness, confusion, depression, skin rashes, edema, nausea, constipation, anorexia, postural hypotension, and disturbances of cardiac rhythm. It also ameliorates dyskinesias resulting from long-term levodopa therapy.

2. Levodopa—Levodopa, which is converted in the body to dopamine, improves all of the major features of parkinsonism, including bradykinesia, but *does not stop progression* of the disorder. The most common early side effects of levodopa are nausea, vomiting, and hypotension, but cardiac arrhythmias may also occur. Dyskinesias, restlessness, confusion, and other behavioral changes tend to occur somewhat later and become more common with time. **Levodopa-induced dyskinesias** may take any conceivable form, including chorea, athetosis, dystonia, tremor, tics, and myoclonus. An even later complication is the **wearing off effect** or the **on-off phenomenon,** in which abrupt but transient fluctuations in the severity of parkinsonism occur unpredictably but frequently during the day. *The "off" period of marked bradykinesia* has been shown to relate in some instances to falling plasma levels of levodopa. During the *"on" phase,* dyskinesias are often conspicuous but mobility is increased. However, such response fluctuations may relate to advancing disease rather than to levodopa therapy itself.

Carbidopa, which inhibits the enzyme responsible for the breakdown of levodopa to dopamine, does not cross the blood-brain barrier. When levodopa is given in combination with carbidopa, the extracerebral breakdown of levodopa is diminished. This reduces the amount of levodopa required daily for beneficial effects, and it lowers the incidence of nausea, vomiting, hypotension, and cardiac irregularities. Such a combination does not prevent the development of response fluctuations and the incidence of other side effects (dyskinesias or psychiatric complications) may actually be increased.

Sinemet, a commercially available preparation that contains carbidopa and levodopa in a fixed ratio (1:10 or 1:4), is generally used. Treatment is started with a small dose—eg, one tablet of Sinemet 25/100 (containing 25 mg of carbidopa and 100 mg of levodopa) three times daily—and gradually increased depending on the response. Sinemet CR is a controlled-release formulation (containing 25 or 50 mg of carbidopa and 100 or 200 mg of levodopa). It is mainly useful when taken at bedtime to lessen motor disability upon awakening. A formulation of carbidopa/levodopa (Rytary) containing both immediate- and delayed-release beads provides a smoother response in patients with fluctuations. The commercially available combination of levodopa with both carbidopa and entacapone (Stalevo) may also be helpful in this context and is discussed in the following section on COMT inhibitors. Response fluctuations are also reduced by keeping the daily intake of protein at the recommended minimum and taking the main protein meal as the last meal of the day. A continuous infusion of a carbidopa-levodopa enteral suspension through a percutaneous gastrojejunostomy tube by a portable infusion pump reduces "off" time in patients with advanced Parkinson disease. Levodopa can also be taken by inhalation (Inbrija) as a rescue medication for patients developing severe akinesia (off periods). Benefit occurs about 10 minutes after inhalation. Side effects include cough, upper respiratory tract infection, nausea, and discolored sputum.

The dyskinesias and behavioral side effects of levodopa are dose-related, but reduction in dose may eliminate any therapeutic benefit. Levodopa-induced dyskinesias may also respond to amantadine.

Levodopa therapy is contraindicated in patients with psychotic illness or narrow-angle glaucoma. It should not be given to patients taking MAO inhibitors or within 2 weeks of their withdrawal, because hypertensive crises may result. Sudden discontinuation of levodopa can precipitate neuroleptic malignant syndrome and should be avoided.

3. Dopamine agonists—Dopamine agonists, such as pramipexole and ropinirole, act directly on dopamine receptors, and their use in parkinsonism is associated with a lower incidence of the response fluctuations and dyskinesias that occur with long-term levodopa therapy. They are effective in both early and advanced stages of Parkinson disease. They are often given either before the introduction of levodopa or with a low dose of Sinemet 25/100 (carbidopa 25 mg and levodopa 100 mg, one tablet three times daily) when dopaminergic therapy is first introduced; the dose of Sinemet is kept constant, while the dose of the agonist is gradually increased.

Pramipexole is started at a dosage of 0.125 mg three times daily orally, and the dose is built up gradually to between 0.5 and 1.5 mg three times daily. Ropinirole is begun at 0.25 mg three times daily orally and gradually increased; most patients require between 2 and 8 mg three times daily for benefit. Extended-release, once-daily formulations of pramipexole and ropinirole have similar efficacy and tolerability as the immediate release versions. Rotigotine is a dopamine agonist absorbed transdermally from a skin patch; it is started at 2 mg once daily and increased weekly by 2 mg daily until achieving an optimal response, up to a maximum of 8 mg daily. Adverse effects of these various agonists include fatigue, somnolence, nausea, peripheral edema, dyskinesias, confusion, and postural hypotension. Less commonly, an irresistible urge to sleep may occur, sometimes in inappropriate and hazardous circumstances. Impulse control disorders involving gambling, shopping, or sexual activity also occur. Local skin reactions may occur with the rotigotine patch. The **dopamine agonist withdrawal syndrome** develops occasionally in patients in whom a dopamine agonist is tapered. It consists of a combination of distressing physical and psychological symptoms that are refractory to levodopa and other dopaminergic medications and may persist for months or longer. There is no effective treatment. The dopamine agonist should be reintroduced and tapered more gradually if possible.

4. Selective MAO inhibitors—Rasagiline, a selective MAO-B inhibitor, has a clear symptomatic benefit in some patients at a daily oral dose of 1 mg, taken in the morning;

it may also be used for adjunctive therapy in patients with response fluctuations to levodopa. Selegiline (5 mg orally with breakfast and lunch) and safinamide (50 mg orally daily, increased to 100 mg daily after 14 days) are also approved as adjunctive treatments. By inhibiting the metabolic breakdown of dopamine, these medications may improve fluctuations or declining response to levodopa.

Studies have suggested (but failed to show conclusively) that rasagiline may slow the progression of Parkinson disease, and it appears to delay the need for other symptomatic therapies. For these reasons, rasagiline is often started early, particularly for patients who are young or have mild disease.

5. COMT inhibitors—Catecholamine-*O*-methyltransferase (COMT) inhibitors reduce the metabolism of levodopa to 3-*O*-methyldopa and thereby alter the plasma pharmacokinetics of levodopa, leading to more sustained plasma levels and more constant dopaminergic stimulation of the brain. Treatment with entacapone or tolcapone results in reduced response fluctuations, with a greater period of responsiveness to administered levodopa. Tolcapone is given in a dosage of 100 mg or 200 mg three times daily orally, and entacapone is given as 200 mg with each dose of Sinemet. Opicapone, a long-acting, peripherally selective COMT inhibitor, is taken once daily (50 mg) at bedtime at least 1 hour before and after eating. The dose of Sinemet taken concurrently may have to be reduced by up to one-third to avoid side effects. Diarrhea is sometimes troublesome. Because rare cases of fulminant hepatic failure have followed its use, tolcapone should be avoided in patients with preexisting liver disease. Serial liver biochemical tests should be performed at 2-week intervals for the first year and at longer intervals thereafter in patients receiving the medication—as recommended by the manufacturer. Serious hepatotoxicity has not been reported with entacapone or opicapone.

Stalevo is the commercial preparation of levodopa combined with both carbidopa and entacapone. It is best used in patients already stabilized on equivalent doses of carbidopa/levodopa and entacapone. It is priced at or below the price of the individual ingredients (ie, carbidopa/levodopa and entacapone) and has the added convenience of requiring fewer tablets to be taken daily. It is available in three strengths: Stalevo 50 (12.5 mg of carbidopa, 50 mg of levodopa, and 200 mg of entacapone), Stalevo 100 (25 mg of carbidopa, 100 mg of levodopa, and 200 mg of entacapone), and Stalevo 150 (37.5 mg of carbidopa, 150 mg of levodopa, and 200 mg of entacapone).

6. Istradefylline—This adenosine A_{2A} receptor antagonist (20–40 mg orally once daily) is given to patients taking levodopa or a dopamine agonist to reduce off time; total off time is typically reduced by less than 1 hour per day.

7. Anticholinergic medications—Anticholinergics are more helpful in alleviating tremor and rigidity than bradykinesia. Trihexyphenidyl and benztropine are commonly used formulations. Treatment is started with a small dose and gradually increased until benefit occurs or side effects limit further increments. If treatment is ineffective, the medication is gradually withdrawn and another preparation then tried. However, these medications are often poorly tolerated, especially in older adults.

Side effects limit the routine use of these medications, and include dryness of the mouth, nausea, constipation, palpitations, cardiac arrhythmias, urinary retention, confusion, agitation, restlessness, drowsiness, mydriasis, increased intraocular pressure, and defective accommodation. Anticholinergic medications are contraindicated in patients with prostatic hyperplasia, narrow-angle glaucoma, or obstructive GI disease and are often tolerated poorly by older adults. They are best avoided whenever cognitive impairment or a predisposition to delirium exists.

8. Antipsychotics—Confusion and psychotic symptoms may occur as a side effect of dopaminergic therapy or as a part of the underlying illness. Pimavanserin (34 mg once daily), a serotonin(2A) agonist, is approved by the FDA specifically for treating the psychosis of Parkinson disease. This may also respond to the atypical antipsychotic agents clozapine and quetiapine, which have few extrapyramidal side effects and do not block the effects of dopaminergic medication. Clozapine may rarely cause marrow suppression, and weekly blood counts are therefore necessary for patients taking it. The patient is started on 6.25 mg at bedtime and the dosage increased to 25–100 mg/day as needed. In low doses, it may also improve iatrogenic dyskinesias. *Typical antipsychotic agents and the second-generation antipsychotic agents risperidone and olanzapine may cause worsening of motor symptoms and should be avoided.*

B. General Measures

Physical therapy, occupational therapy, and speech therapy helps many patients. Cognitive impairment and psychiatric symptoms may be helped by a cholinesterase inhibitor, such as rivastigmine (3–12 mg orally daily or 4.6 or 9.5 mg/24 hours transdermally daily). Affective disorders, which may be particularly conspicuous during off periods, should be treated by antidepressants or antianxiety agents as necessary. The quality of life can often be improved by the provision of simple aids to daily living, eg, rails or banisters placed strategically about the home, special table cutlery with large handles, nonslip rubber table mats, and devices to amplify the voice.

C. Stimulation and Ablative Treatments

High-frequency stimulation of the subthalamic nuclei or globus pallidus internus may benefit many of the motor features of the disease but does not affect its natural history. Electrical stimulation of the brain has the advantage over ablative thalamotomy and pallidotomy procedures of being reversible and of causing minimal or no damage to the brain, and is therefore the preferred surgical approach to treatment. It is reserved for patients without cognitive impairment or psychiatric disorder who have a good response to levodopa, but in whom dyskinesias or response fluctuations are problematic. It frequently takes 3–6 months after surgery to adjust stimulator programming and to achieve optimal results. Side effects include depression, apathy, impulsivity, executive dysfunction, and decreased verbal fluency in a subset of patients. Focused ultrasound thalamotomy or stereotactic radiosurgery may help patients with medically refractory tremor-predominant parkinsonism who are reluctant to undergo surgery.

When to Refer

All patients should be referred.

When to Admit

Patients requiring surgical treatment should be admitted.

Jankovic J et al. Parkinson's disease: etiopathogenesis and treatment. J Neurol Neurosurg Psychiatry. 2020;91:795. [PMID: 32576618]

Mitchell KT et al. Surgical treatment of Parkinson disease. Neurol Clin. 2020;38:293. [PMID: 32279711]

3. Huntington Disease

ESSENTIALS OF DIAGNOSIS

- Gradual onset and progression of chorea and dementia or behavioral change.
- Family history of the disorder.
- Responsible gene identified on chromosome 4.

General Considerations

Huntington disease is characterized by *chorea and dementia.* It is inherited in an autosomal dominant manner and occurs throughout the world, in all ethnic groups, with a prevalence rate of about 5 per 100,000. There is an expanded and unstable CAG trinucleotide repeat in the huntingtin gene at 4p16.3; longer repeat lengths correspond to an earlier age of onset and faster disease progression.

Clinical Findings

A. Symptoms and Signs

Clinical onset is usually between 30 and 50 years of age. The disease is progressive and usually leads to a fatal outcome within 15–20 years. The initial symptoms may consist of either abnormal movements or intellectual changes, but ultimately both occur. The earliest mental changes are often behavioral, with irritability, moodiness, antisocial behavior, or a psychiatric disturbance, but a more obvious dementia subsequently develops. The dyskinesia may initially be no more than an apparent fidgetiness or restlessness, but eventually choreiform movements and some dystonic posturing occur. A parkinsonian syndrome with progressive rigidity and akinesia (rather than chorea) sometimes occurs in association with dementia, especially in cases with childhood onset. The diagnosis is established with a widely available genetic test, although such testing should be pursued under the guidance of a licensed genetic counselor.

B. Imaging

CT scanning or MRI usually demonstrates cerebral atrophy and atrophy of the caudate nucleus in established cases. PET has shown reduced striatal metabolic rate.

Differential Diagnosis

Chorea developing with no family history of choreoathetosis should not be attributed to Huntington disease, at least not until other causes of chorea have been excluded clinically and by appropriate laboratory studies. Nongenetic causes of chorea include stroke, SLE and antiphospholipid antibody syndrome, paraneoplastic syndromes, infection with HIV, and various medications. In younger patients, self-limiting Sydenham chorea develops after group A streptococcal infections on rare occasions. If a patient presents solely with progressive intellectual failure, it may not be possible to distinguish Huntington disease from other causes of dementia unless there is a characteristic family history or a dyskinesia develops.

Huntington disease–like (HDL) disorders resemble Huntington disease but are caused by other genetic mutations. A clinically similar autosomal dominant disorder **(dentatorubral-pallidoluysian atrophy),** manifested by chorea, dementia, ataxia, and myoclonic epilepsy, is uncommon except in persons of Japanese ancestry. Treatment is as for Huntington disease.

Treatment

There is no cure for Huntington disease; progression cannot be halted; and treatment is purely symptomatic, although studies of antisense oligonucleotides inhibiting production of mutant huntingtin protein are ongoing. The reported biochemical changes suggest a relative underactivity of neurons containing GABA and acetylcholine or a relative overactivity of dopaminergic neurons. Tetrabenazine, an FDA-approved medication that interferes with the vesicular storage of biogenic amines, is widely used to treat the dyskinesia. The starting dose is 12.5 mg twice or three times daily orally, increasing by 12.5 mg every 5 days depending on response and tolerance; the usual maintenance dose is 25 mg three times daily. Side effects include depression, postural hypotension, drowsiness, and parkinsonian features; tetrabenazine should not be given within 14 days of taking MAO inhibitors and is not indicated for the treatment of levodopa-induced dyskinesias. Deutetrabenazine is also FDA-approved for reducing chorea in Huntington disease and may have fewer side effects than tetrabenazine but direct comparisons are lacking. The starting dose is 6 mg once daily orally, increased to 6 mg twice daily after 1 week and by 6-mg increments weekly thereafter, to a maximum of 24 mg twice daily. Treatment with medications blocking dopamine receptors, such as phenothiazines or haloperidol, may control the dyskinesia and any behavioral disturbances. Haloperidol treatment is usually begun with a dose of 1 mg once or twice daily orally, which is then increased every 3 or 4 days depending on the response; alternatively, atypical antipsychotic agents such as quetiapine (increasing from 25 mg daily orally up to 100 mg twice daily orally as tolerated) may be tried.

Amantadine in a dose of 200 mg to 400 mg daily orally is sometimes helpful for chorea. Deep brain stimulation has been used successfully to treat chorea in a small number of patients. Behavioral disturbances may respond to clozapine. Attempts to compensate for the relative GABA deficiency by enhancing central GABA activity or to compensate for the relative cholinergic underactivity by giving choline chloride have not been therapeutically helpful.

Offspring should be offered genetic counseling. Genetic testing permits presymptomatic detection and definitive diagnosis of the disease.

When to Refer

All patients should be referred.

Tabrizi SJ et al; Phase 1–2a IONIS-HTTRx Study Site Teams. Targeting huntingtin expression in patients with Huntington's disease. N Engl J Med. 2019;380:2307. [PMID: 31059641]

4. Idiopathic Torsion Dystonia

ESSENTIALS OF DIAGNOSIS

- Dystonic movements and postures.
- Normal birth and developmental history. No other neurologic signs.
- Investigations (including CT scan or MRI) reveal no cause of dystonia.

General Considerations

Idiopathic torsion dystonia may occur sporadically or on a hereditary basis, with autosomal dominant, autosomal recessive, and X-linked recessive modes of transmission. Symptoms may begin in childhood or later and persist throughout life.

Clinical Findings

The disorder is characterized by the onset of abnormal movements and postures in a patient with a normal birth and developmental history, no relevant past medical illness, and no other neurologic signs. Investigations (including CT scan) reveal no cause for the abnormal movements. Dystonic movements of the head and neck may take the form of torticollis, blepharospasm, facial grimacing, or forced opening or closing of the mouth. The limbs may also adopt abnormal but characteristic postures. The age at onset influences both the clinical findings and the prognosis. With onset in childhood, there is usually a family history of the disorder, symptoms commonly commence in the legs, and progression is likely until there is severe disability from generalized dystonia. In contrast, when onset is later, a positive family history is unlikely, initial symptoms are often in the arms or axial structures, and severe disability does not usually occur, although generalized dystonia may ultimately develop in some patients. If all cases are considered together, about one-third of patients eventually become so severely disabled that they are confined to chair or bed, while another one-third are affected only mildly.

Differential Diagnosis

Perinatal anoxia, birth trauma, and kernicterus are common causes of dystonia, but abnormal movements usually then develop before the age of 5, the early development of the patient is usually abnormal, and a history of seizures is not unusual. Moreover, examination may reveal signs of mental retardation or pyramidal deficit in addition to the movement disorder. Dystonic posturing may also occur in Wilson disease, Huntington disease, or parkinsonism; as a sequela of encephalitis lethargica or previous neuroleptic medication therapy; and in certain other disorders. In these cases, diagnosis is based on the history and accompanying clinical manifestations.

Treatment

Idiopathic torsion dystonia usually responds poorly to medications. A distinct variety of dystonia is remarkably responsive to levodopa; therefore, a levodopa trial is warranted in all patients. Both autosomal dominant and recessive forms have been described. Failing this, diazepam, baclofen, carbamazepine, amantadine, or anticholinergic medication such as trihexyphenidyl or benztropine (in high dosage) is occasionally helpful; if not, a trial of treatment with tetrabenazine, phenothiazines, or haloperidol may be worthwhile. In each case, the dose has to be individualized, depending on response and tolerance. However, the doses of these latter medications that are required for benefit lead usually to mild parkinsonism. Pallidal deep brain stimulation is helpful for disabling generalized dystonia and has a lower morbidity than stereotactic thalamotomy, which is sometimes helpful in patients with predominantly unilateral limb dystonia. Potential adverse events of deep brain stimulation include cerebral infection or hemorrhage, broken leads, affective changes, and dysarthria.

When to Refer

All patients should be referred.

When to Admit

Patients requiring surgical treatment should be admitted.

Rodrigues FB et al. Deep brain stimulation for dystonia. Cochrane Database Syst Rev. 2019;1:CD012405. [PMID: 30629283]

5. Focal Torsion Dystonia

A number of the dystonic manifestations that occur in idiopathic torsion dystonia may also occur as isolated phenomena. They are best regarded as focal dystonias that either occur as formes frustes of idiopathic torsion dystonia in patients with a positive family history or represent a focal manifestation of the adult-onset form of that disorder when there is no family history. Medical treatment is generally unsatisfactory. A trial of the medications used in idiopathic torsion dystonia is worthwhile, however, since a few patients do show some response. In addition, with restricted dystonias such as blepharospasm or torticollis, local injection of botulinum A toxin into the overactive muscles may produce worthwhile benefit for several weeks or months and can be repeated as needed.

Both **blepharospasm** and **oromandibular dystonia** may occur as an isolated focal dystonia. The former is characterized by spontaneous involuntary forced closure of the eyelids for a variable interval. Oromandibular dystonia is manifested by involuntary contraction of the muscles about the mouth causing, for example, involuntary opening or closing of the mouth, roving or protruding tongue movements, and retraction of the platysma. **Cervical dystonia** (spasmodic torticollis), usually with onset between 25 and 50 years of age, is characterized by a tendency for the neck to twist to one side. This initially occurs episodically, but eventually the neck is held to the side. Some patients have a sensory trick ("geste antagoniste") that lessens the dystonic posture, eg, touching the side of the face. Spontaneous resolution may occur in the first year or so. The disorder is otherwise usually lifelong. Local injection of botulinum A toxin provides benefit in most cases. Deep brain stimulation of the globus pallidus interna is an option if medical treatment and botulinum toxin injection are unsuccessful.

Writer's cramp is characterized by dystonic posturing of the hand and forearm when the hand is used for writing and sometimes when it is used for other tasks, eg, playing the piano or using a screwdriver or eating utensils. Medication treatment is usually unrewarding, and patients are often best advised to learn to use the other hand for activities requiring manual dexterity. Injections of botulinum A toxin are helpful in some instances.

Rodrigues FB et al. Botulinum toxin type A therapy for cervical dystonia. Cochrane Database Syst Rev. 2020;11:CD003633. [PMID: 33180963]

6. Myoclonus

Occasional myoclonic jerks may occur in anyone, especially when drifting into sleep. **General or multifocal myoclonus** is common in patients with idiopathic epilepsy and is especially prominent in certain hereditary disorders characterized by seizures and progressive intellectual decline, such as the lipid storage diseases. It is also a feature of subacute sclerosing panencephalitis and Creutzfeldt-Jakob disease. Generalized myoclonic jerking may accompany uremic and other metabolic encephalopathies, result from therapy with levodopa or tricyclic antidepressants, occur in alcohol or drug withdrawal states, or follow anoxic brain damage. It also occurs on a hereditary or sporadic basis as an isolated phenomenon in otherwise healthy subjects.

Segmental myoclonus is a rare manifestation of a focal spinal cord lesion. It may also be the clinical expression of **epilepsia partialis continua**, a disorder in which a repetitive focal epileptic discharge arises in the contralateral sensorimotor cortex, sometimes from an underlying structural lesion. An electroencephalogram is often helpful in clarifying the epileptic nature of the disorder, and CT or MRI scan may reveal the causal lesion.

Myoclonus may respond to certain anticonvulsant medications, especially valproic acid or levetiracetam, or to one of the benzodiazepines, particularly clonazepam (see Table 24–2). It may also respond to piracetam (up to 16.8 g daily; not available in the United States). Myoclonus following anoxic brain damage is often responsive to oxitriptan (5-hydroxytryptophan), the precursor of serotonin, and sometimes to clonazepam. Oxitriptan is given in gradually increasing doses up to 1–1.5 mg daily. In patients with segmental myoclonus, a localized lesion should be searched for and treated appropriately.

7. Wilson Disease

In this metabolic disorder, abnormal movement and posture may occur with or without coexisting signs of liver involvement. Psychiatric and neuropsychological manifestations are common. Wilson disease is discussed in Chapter 16.

8. Drug-Induced Abnormal Movements

Medications may produce a wide variety of abnormal movements, including tremor, parkinsonism, akathisia (ie, motor restlessness), acute dystonia, chorea, myoclonus, and tardive dyskinesias or dystonia. Medication-induced tremor is usually postural with a low amplitude and high frequency, and may occur with beta-2 adrenergic agonists, sympathomimentics, serotonergic agents, glucocorticoids, thyroid hormone, antiseizure medications, antiarrhythmics, antipsychotics, chemotherapeutics, immunosuppressants, hypoglycemic agents, and other medications such as lithium, caffeine, and theophylline.

Drug-induced parkinsonism is usually bilateral at onset, tends to have a lower incidence of tremor, and is poorly responsive to levodopa. It may be caused by antidopaminergic medications (eg, typical and atypical antipsychotics, antiemetics, central monoamine depleting agents), serotonergic agents, calcium channel blockers, and lithium.

Chorea may develop in patients receiving antidopaminergic medications (eg, typical and atypical antipsychotics, antiemetics), levodopa, dopamine agonists, anticholinergic medications, certain antiseizure medications, lithium, amphetamines, or oral contraceptives.

Acute dystonia may be produced by antidopaminergic medications (eg, phenothiazines and their derivatives, butyrephenones, metoclopramide) and dopaminergic medications (eg, levodopa, bromocriptine), serotonergic agents, phenytoin, carbamazepine, and lithium. Dyskinesias related to psychiatric medications are discussed in Chapter 25. With the exception of tardive dyskinesia and dystonia, the movement disorder usually resolves with withdrawal of the offending substance, but parkinsonism may take many months to do so. When severe, acute dystonia and akathisia are treated with intravenous or intramuscular benztropine or diphenhydramine, and drug-induced parkinsonism with oral benztropine.

9. Restless Legs Syndrome

This common disorder, affecting 1–5% of people, may occur as a primary (idiopathic) disorder or in relation to Parkinson disease, pregnancy, iron deficiency anemia, or peripheral neuropathy (especially uremic or diabetic). It may have a hereditary basis, and several genetic loci have been associated with the disorder. Restlessness and curious sensory disturbances lead to an irresistible urge to move the limbs, especially during periods of relaxation; movement of the limbs provides relief. The urge occurs exclusively in the evening and at night or is worse at night than during the day. Most patients also have **periodic limb movements of sleep** and one-third have periodic limb movements during relaxed wakefulness; both consist of brief involuntary flexion at the ankle, knee, and hip. Disturbed nocturnal sleep and excessive daytime somnolence may result. Ferritin levels should always be measured; treatment with oral iron sulfate in patients with ferritin levels less than or equal to 75 mcg/L (13.4 mcmol/L) and transferrin saturation below 45% should be attempted prior to initiation of other pharmacotherapies. In patients who do not respond to or are ineligible for iron therapy, gabapentin enacarbil (300–1200 mg orally each evening), gabapentin (starting with 300 mg orally daily, increasing to approximately 1800 mg daily, depending on response and tolerance), or pregabalin (150–300 mg orally divided twice to three times daily) should be tried next. Therapy with nonergot dopamine agonists, such as pramipexole (0.125–0.5 mg orally once daily), ropinirole (0.25–4 mg orally once daily 2–3 hours before bedtime), or rotigotine (1–3 mg/24 hours transdermal patch once daily) is helpful but may lead to an augmentation of symptoms. Levodopa also is helpful but also leads to augmentation, so its use is generally reserved for those who do not respond to other measures. Extended-release oxycodone-naloxone (2.5–5 mg to 5–10 mg orally twice daily) is useful in patients with severe symptoms or those who are refractory to first-line therapies.

Silber MH et al; Scientific and Medical Advisory Board of the Restless Legs Syndrome Foundation. The management of restless legs syndrome: an updated algorithm. Mayo Clin Proc. 2021;96:1921. [PMID: 34218864]

10. Gilles De La Tourette Syndrome

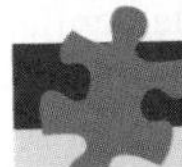

ESSENTIALS OF DIAGNOSIS

- Multiple motor and phonic tics.
- Symptoms begin before age 18 years.
- Tics occur frequently for at least 1 year.
- Tics vary in number, frequency, and nature over time.

Clinical Findings

Simple tics occur transiently in up to 25% of children, remit within weeks to months, and do not require treatment. Tourette syndrome is a more complex disorder. **Motor tics** are the initial manifestation in 80% of cases and most commonly involve the face, whereas in the remaining 20%, the initial symptoms are **phonic tics;** ultimately a combination of different motor and phonic tics develop in all patients. Tics are preceded by an urge that is relieved upon performance of the movement or vocalization; they can be temporarily suppressed but eventually the urge becomes overwhelming. These are noted first in childhood, generally between the ages of 2 and 15. Motor tics occur especially about the face, head, and shoulders (eg, sniffing, blinking, frowning, shoulder shrugging, head thrusting). Phonic tics commonly include grunts, barks, hisses, throat-clearing, and coughs, and sometimes also verbal utterances, including coprolalia (obscene speech). There may also be echolalia (repetition of the speech of others), echopraxia (imitation of others' movements), and palilalia (repetition of words or phrases). Some tics may be self-mutilating in nature, such as nail-biting, hair-pulling, or biting of the lips or tongue. The disorder is chronic, but the course may be punctuated by relapses and remissions. Obsessive-compulsive disorder (OCD) and attention deficit hyperactivity disorder (ADHD) are commonly associated and may be more disabling than the tics themselves. A family history is sometimes obtained.

Examination usually reveals no abnormalities other than the tics. In addition to OCD, psychiatric disturbances may occur because of the associated cosmetic and social embarrassment. The diagnosis of the disorder is often delayed for years, the tics being interpreted as psychiatric illness or some other form of abnormal movement. Patients are thus often subjected to unnecessary treatment before the disorder is recognized. The tic-like character of the abnormal movements and the absence of other neurologic signs should differentiate this disorder from other movement disorders presenting in childhood. Wilson disease, however, can simulate the condition and should be excluded.

Treatment

Treatment is symptomatic and may need to be continued indefinitely. Habit reversal training or other forms of behavioral therapy can be effective alone or in combination with pharmacotherapy. Alpha-adrenergic agonists, such as clonidine (start 0.05 mg orally at bedtime, titrating to 0.3–0.4 mg orally daily, divided three to four times per day) or guanfacine (start 0.5 mg orally at bedtime, titrating to a maximum of 3–4 mg orally daily, divided twice daily), are first-line therapies because of a favorable side-effect profile compared with typical antipsychotics, and are FDA-approved therapies for the disorder. They also have the advantage of improving the symptoms of concomitant ADHD. When a typical antipsychotic is required in cases of severe tics, haloperidol is generally regarded as the medication of choice. It is started in a low dose (0.25 mg daily orally) that is gradually increased (by 0.25 mg every 4 or 5 days) until there is maximum benefit with a minimum of side effects or until side effects limit further increments. A total daily oral dose of between 2 mg and 8 mg is usually optimal, but higher doses are sometimes necessary. Aripiprazole (2.5–20 mg orally daily), fluphenazine (1–15 mg orally daily), pimozide (1–10 mg orally daily), and risperidone (1–6 mg daily orally) are alternatives; haloperidol, aripiprazole, and pimozide are FDA-approved for Tourette syndrome. Typical antipsychotics can cause significant weight gain and carry a risk of tardive dyskinesias and other long-term, potentially irreversible motor side effects. Therefore, many specialists favor the use of tetrabenazine (12.5–25 mg orally three times daily), which is approved for Tourette syndrome in Canada but not the United States. Trials of deutetrabenazine have shown mixed results. Small, randomized trials or observational studies have reported benefit from topiramate, nicotine, tetrahydrocannabinol, baclofen, and clonazepam. Other medications, including valbenazine and ecopipam, are being studied for the treatment of tics.

Injection of botulinum toxin type A at the site of the most distressing tics is sometimes worthwhile and has fewer side effects than systemic antipsychotic therapy. Bilateral high-frequency deep brain stimulation at various sites has been helpful in some, otherwise intractable, cases.

When to Refer

All patients should be referred.

When to Admit

Patients undergoing surgical (deep brain stimulation) treatment should be admitted.

Pringsheim T et al. Practice guideline recommendations summary: treatment of tics in people with Tourette syndrome and chronic tic disorders. Neurology. 2019;92:896. [PMID: 31061208]

DEMENTIA

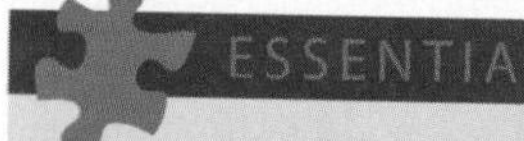

ESSENTIALS OF DIAGNOSIS

- Progressive intellectual decline.
- Not due to delirium or psychiatric disease.
- Age is the main risk factor, followed by family history and vascular disease risk factors.

General Considerations

Dementia is a progressive decline in intellectual function that is severe enough to compromise social or occupational functioning. **Mild cognitive impairment** describes a decline that has *not* resulted in a change in the level of function. Although a few patients identify a precipitating event, most experience an insidious onset and gradual progression of symptoms.

Dementia typically begins after age 60, and the prevalence doubles approximately every 5 years thereafter; in persons aged 85 and older, around half have dementia. The prevalence of Alzheimer dementia is predicted to be 15 million by 2060 in the United States. In most cases, the cause of dementia is acquired, either as a sporadic primary neurodegenerative disease or as the result of another disorder, such as stroke (Table 24–6). Other risk factors for dementia include family history, diabetes mellitus, cigarette smoking, hypertension, obesity, a history of significant head injury, and hearing loss. Vitamin D deficiency and chronic sleep deprivation may also increase the risk of dementia. Dementia is more prevalent among women, but this may be accounted for by their longer life expectancy. Physical activity seems to be protective; education, ongoing intellectual stimulation, and social engagement may also be protective, perhaps by promoting *cognitive reserve,* an improved capacity to compensate for insidious neurodegeneration.

Dementia is distinct from delirium and psychiatric disease. **Delirium** is an acute confusional state that often occurs in response to an identifiable trigger, such as drug or alcohol intoxication or withdrawal (eg, Wernicke encephalopathy, described below), medication side effects (especially medications with anticholinergic properties, antihistamines, benzodiazepines, sleeping aids, opioids, neuroleptics, corticosteroids, and other sedative or psychotropic agents), infection (consider occult UTI or pneumonia in older patients), metabolic disturbance (including an electrolyte abnormality; hypoglycemia or hyperglycemia; or a nutritional, endocrine, renal, or hepatic disorder), sleep deprivation, or other neurologic disease (seizure, including a postictal state, or stroke). Delirium typically involves *fluctuating* levels of arousal, including drowsiness or agitation, and it improves after removal or treatment of the precipitating factor. Patients with dementia are especially susceptible to episodes of delirium, but recognition of dementia is not possible until delirium lifts. For this reason, dementia is typically diagnosed in outpatients who are otherwise medically stable, rather than in acutely ill patients in the hospital.

Psychiatric disease sometimes leads to complaints of impaired cognition (**pseudodementia**). Impaired attention is usually to blame, and in some patients with depression or anxiety, poor focus and concentration may even be a primary complaint. The symptoms should improve with appropriate psychiatric treatment. Mood disorders are commonly seen in patients with neurodegenerative disease and in some cases are an early symptom. There is some evidence that a persistent, untreated mood disorder may predispose to the development of an age-related dementia, and psychiatric symptoms can clearly exacerbate cognitive impairment in patients who already have dementia; therefore, suspicion of dementia should not distract from appropriate screening for and treatment of depression or anxiety.

Clinical Findings

A. Symptoms and Signs

Symptoms and signs of the common causes of dementia are detailed in Table 24–6. Clinicians should be aware that a

Table 24–6. Common causes of age-related dementia (listed by prevalence).

Disorder	Pathology	Clinical Features
Alzheimer disease	Plaques containing beta-amyloid peptide, and neurofibrillary tangles containing tau protein, occur throughout the neocortex.	• Most common age-related neurodegenerative disease; incidence doubles every 5 years after age 60. • Short-term memory impairment is early and prominent in most cases. • Variable deficits of executive function, visuospatial function, and language.
Vascular dementia	Multifocal ischemic change.	• Stepwise or progressive accumulation of cognitive deficits in association with repeated strokes. • Symptoms depend on localization of strokes.
Dementia with Lewy bodies	Histologically indistinguishable from Parkinson disease: alpha-synuclein-containing Lewy bodies occur in the brainstem, midbrain, olfactory bulb, and neocortex. Alzheimer pathology may coexist.	• Cognitive dysfunction, with prominent visuospatial and executive deficits. • Psychiatric disturbance, with anxiety, visual hallucinations, and fluctuating delirium. • Parkinsonian motor deficits with or after other features. • Cholinesterase inhibitors lessen delirium; poor tolerance of neuroleptics and dopaminergics.
Frontotemporal dementia (FTD)	Neuropathology is variable and defined by the protein found in intraneuronal aggregates. Tau protein, TAR DNA-binding protein 43 (TDP-43), or fused-in-sarcoma (FUS) protein account for most cases.	• Peak incidence in the sixth decade; approximately equal to Alzheimer disease as a cause of dementia in patients under 60 years old. • Familial cases result from mutations in genes for tau, progranulin, or others. **Behavioral variant FTD** • Deficits in empathy, social comportment, insight, abstract thought, and executive function. • Behavior is disinhibited, impulsive, and ritualistic, with prominent apathy and increased interest in sex or sweet/fatty foods. • Relative preservation of memory. • Focal right frontal atrophy. • Association with amyotrophic lateral sclerosis. **Semantic variant primary progressive aphasia** • Deficits in word-finding, single-word comprehension, object and category knowledge, and face recognition. • Behaviors may be similar to behavioral variant FTD. • Focal, asymmetric temporal pole atrophy. **Nonfluent/agrammatic variant primary progressive aphasia** • Speech is effortful with dysarthria, phonemic errors, sound distortions, and poor grammar. • Focal extrapyramidal signs and apraxia of the right arm and leg are common; overlaps with corticobasal degeneration. • Focal left frontal atrophy.

patient's insight into a cognitive change may be vague or absent, and *collateral history is essential to a proper evaluation*. As patients age, primary care clinicians should inquire periodically about the presence of any cognitive symptoms.

Symptoms depend on the area of the brain affected. **Short-term memory loss**, involving the repeating of questions or stories and a diminished ability to recall the details of recent conversations or events, frequently results from pathologic changes in the hippocampus. **Word-finding difficulty** often involves difficulty recalling the names of people, places, or objects, with low-frequency words affected first, eventually resulting in speech laden with pronouns and circumlocutions. This problem is thought to arise from pathology at the temporoparietal junction of the left hemisphere. Problems with articulation, fluency, comprehension, or word meaning are anatomically distinct and less common. **Visuospatial dysfunction** may result in poor navigation and getting lost in familiar places, impaired recognition of previously familiar faces and buildings, or trouble discerning an object against a background. The right parietal lobe is one of the brain areas implicated in such symptoms. **Executive dysfunction** may manifest by easy distractibility, impulsivity, mental inflexibility, concrete thought, slowed processing speed, poor planning and organization, or impaired judgment. Localization may vary and could include the frontal lobes or subcortical areas like the basal ganglia or cerebral white matter. **Apathy** or indifference, separate from depression, is common and may have a similar anatomy as executive dysfunction. **Apraxia**, or the loss of learned motor behaviors, may result from dysfunction of the frontal or parietal lobes, especially the left parietal lobe.

The time of symptom onset must be established, but subtle, early symptoms are often apparent only in retrospect. Another event, such as an illness or hospitalization, may lead to new recognition of existing symptoms. Symptoms often accumulate over time, and *the nature of the earliest symptom is most helpful in forming the differential diagnosis.* The history should establish risk factors for dementia, including family history, other chronic illnesses, and vascular disease risk factors. Finally, it is important to document the patient's current capacity to perform **basic and instrumental activities of daily living** (see Chapter 4) and to note the extent of decline from the premorbid level of function. Indeed, *it is this functional assessment that defines the presence and severity of dementia.*

The physical examination is important to identify any occult medical illness. In addition, eye movement abnormalities, parkinsonism, or other motor abnormalities may help identify an underlying neurologic condition. The workup should prioritize the exclusion of conditions that are reversible or require separate therapy. Screening for depression is necessary, along with imaging and laboratory workup, as indicated below.

B. Neuropsychological Assessment

Brief quantification of cognitive impairment is indicated in a patient complaining of cognitive symptoms or if caregivers raise similar concerns. The **Folstein Mini Mental State Exam (MMSE), Montreal Cognitive Assessment (MoCA), Mini-Cog**, and other similar tests are brief, objective, and widely used but have important limitations: they are insensitive to mild cognitive impairment, they may be biased negatively by the presence of language or attention problems, and they do not correlate with functional capacity.

A **neuropsychiatric evaluation** by a trained neuropsychologist or psychometrician may be appropriate. The goal of such testing is to enhance localization by defining the cognitive domains that are impaired as well as to quantify the degree of impairment. There is no standard battery of tests, but a variety of metrics is commonly used to assess the symptom types highlighted above. Assessments are most accurate when a patient is well rested, comfortable, and otherwise medically stable.

C. Imaging

Brain imaging with MRI or CT without contrast is indicated in any patient with a new, progressive cognitive complaint. The goal is to exclude occult cerebrovascular disease, tumor, or other identifiable structural abnormality, rather than to provide positive evidence of a neurodegenerative disease. Global or focal brain atrophy may be worse than expected for age and could suggest a particular neurodegenerative process, but such findings are rarely specific.

PET with fluorodeoxyglucose (FDG) does not confirm or exclude any specific cause of dementia but may be useful as an element of the workup in specific clinical circumstances, such as discriminating between Alzheimer disease and frontotemporal dementia in a patient with some symptoms of each. PET imaging with a radiolabeled ligand for beta-amyloid, one of the pathologic proteins in Alzheimer disease, is highly sensitive to amyloid pathology and may provide positive evidence for Alzheimer disease in a patient with cognitive decline. However, after age 60 or 70, amyloid plaques can accumulate in the absence of cognitive impairment; thus, the specificity of a positive amyloid scan diminishes with age. Single-photon emission CT offers similar information as FDG-PET but is less sensitive. PET imaging with radiolabeled ligands for tau, a pathogenic protein in Alzheimer disease, progressive supranuclear palsy, and some forms of frontotemporal dementia, also may help refine premortem diagnostic accuracy.

D. Laboratory Findings

Serum levels of vitamin B_{12}, free T_4, and TSH should be measured for any patient with cognitive symptoms. A serum rapid plasma reagin (RPR) and testing for HIV should be considered. Other testing should be driven by clinical suspicion, and often includes a CBC, serum electrolytes, glucose, and lipid profile.

Although the presence of one or two ApoE epsilon-4 alleles indicates an increased risk of Alzheimer disease and ApoE genotyping is clinically available, it is of *limited clinical utility.* Finding an ApoE epsilon-4 allele in a young patient with dementia might raise the index of suspicion for Alzheimer disease, but obtaining a genotype in an older patient is unlikely to be helpful, and doing so in an asymptomatic patient as a marker of risk for Alzheimer disease is inappropriate until a preventive therapy becomes available. Spinal fluid protein measurements are also available and may support the diagnosis of Alzheimer disease in the appropriate clinical context; levels of beta-amyloid decrease and tau protein increase in Alzheimer disease, but this testing shares some of the same concerns as amyloid PET imaging.

Differential Diagnosis

In older patients with gradually progressive cognitive symptoms and no other complaint or sign, a neurodegenerative disease is likely (Table 24–6). Decline beginning before age 60, rapid progression, fluctuating course, unintended weight loss, systemic complaints, or other unexplained symptoms or signs raise suspicion for a process other than a neurodegenerative disease. In this case, the differential is broad and includes infection or inflammatory disease (consider a lumbar puncture to screen for cells or antibodies in the spinal fluid), neoplasm or a paraneoplastic condition, endocrine or metabolic disease, drugs or toxins, or other conditions. Normal pressure hydrocephalus is a difficult diagnosis to establish. Symptoms include gait apraxia (sometimes described as a "magnetic" gait, as if the feet are stuck to the floor), urinary incontinence, and dementia. CT scanning or MRI of the brain reveals ventricles that are enlarged in obvious disproportion to sulcal widening and overall brain atrophy.

Treatment

A. Anti-amyloid Therapy

Aducanumab was approved by the FDA despite mixed results in clinical trials, only one of which demonstrated a small reduction in cognitive decline over 1.5 years, and many experts remain skeptical about its utility. Its use is limited to patients with mild cognitive impairment or mild dementia (MMSE 24–30 and clinical dementia rating scale global score of 0.5) and amyloid pathology proven by amyloid PET. Patients and prescribers must adhere to a monitoring regime including frequent brain MRI due to a high risk of complications such as cerebral edema and hemorrhage. Caution should be used in patients with a history of cerebral hemorrhage, evidence of microhemorrhages or superficial siderosis on pretreatment brain MRI, anticoagulant or antiplatelet use other than aspirin, any bleeding disorder, or an ApoE epsilon-4 allele.

B. Nonpharmacologic Approaches

Aerobic exercise (30 minutes several days per week) may reduce the rate of functional decline and decrease the patient's caregiving needs and may reduce the risk of dementia in normal individuals. Maintaining as active a role in the family and community as practically possible is likely to be of benefit, emphasizing activities at which the patient feels confident. Patients with neurodegenerative diseases have a limited capacity to regain lost skills; for instance, memory drills in a patient with Alzheimer disease are more likely to lead to frustration than benefit and studies show that computerized cognitive training does *not* improve cognition or function in patients with dementia. **Vitamin E** (1000 IU twice daily) appears to reduce the rate of functional decline in patients with Alzheimer disease, but does not affect cognition or prevent the development of Alzheimer disease in patients with mild cognitive impairment.

C. Cognitive Symptoms

Cholinesterase inhibitors are first-line therapy for Alzheimer disease and dementia with Lewy bodies (Table 24–6). They provide modest, symptomatic treatment for cognitive dysfunction and may prolong the capacity for independence but do *not* prevent disease progression. Commonly used medications include donepezil (start at 5 mg orally daily for 4 weeks, then increase to 10 mg daily; a 23 mg daily dose is approved for moderate to severe Alzheimer disease, although its modest additional efficacy over the 10 mg dose is overshadowed by an increased risk of side effects); rivastigmine (start at 1.5 mg orally twice daily, then increasing every 2 weeks by 1.5 mg twice daily to a goal of 3–6 mg twice daily; or 4.6, 9.5, or 13.3 mg/24 hours transdermally daily); and galantamine (start at 4 mg orally twice daily, then increasing every 4 weeks by 4 mg twice daily to a goal of 8–12 mg twice daily; a once-daily extended-release formulation is also available). Cholinesterase inhibitors are *not* given for frontotemporal dementia because they may worsen behavioral symptoms. Nausea and diarrhea are common side effects; syncope and cardiac dysrhythmia are uncommon but more serious. An ECG is often obtained before and after starting therapy, particularly in a patient with cardiac disease or a history of syncope.

Memantine (start at 5 mg orally daily, then increase by 5 mg per week up to a target of 10 mg twice daily) is approved for the treatment of moderate to severe Alzheimer disease. In frontotemporal dementia, memantine is ineffective and may worsen cognition. There is some evidence that memantine may improve cognition and behavior among patients with dementia with Lewy bodies.

D. Mood and Behavioral Disturbances

SSRIs are generally safe and well tolerated in older patients with cognitive impairment, and they may be efficacious for the treatment of depression, anxiety, or agitation. Evidence supports the use of citalopram (10–30 mg orally daily) *for agitation;* side effects include QTc prolongation and worsened cognition at the highest dose. Paroxetine should be avoided because it has anticholinergic effects; avoid all tricyclic antidepressants for the same reason. Other antidepressant agents, such as bupropion or venlafaxine, may be tried.

Insomnia is common, and trazodone (25–50 mg orally at bedtime as needed) can be safe and effective. Over-the-counter antihistamine hypnotics must be avoided, along with benzodiazepines, because of their tendency to worsen cognition and precipitate delirium. Other prescription hypnotics such as zolpidem may result in similar adverse reactions.

For agitation, impulsivity, and other behaviors that interfere with safe caregiving, causes of delirium (detailed above) should first be considered. When no reversible trigger is identified, treatment should be approached in a staged manner. Behavioral interventions, such as reorientation and distraction from anxiety-provoking stimuli, are first-line. Ensure that the patient is kept active during the day with both physical exercise and mentally stimulating activities, and that there is adequate sleep at night. Reassess the level of caregiving and consider increasing the time spent directly with an attendant. Next, ensure that appropriate pharmacologic treatment of cognition and mood is optimized. Finally, as a last resort, when other measures prove insufficient and the patient's behaviors raise safety concerns, consider pharmacologic therapy. Citalopram or low doses of an atypical antipsychotic medication such as quetiapine (start 25 mg orally daily as needed, increasing to two to three times daily as needed) can be tried; even though atypical agents cause extrapyramidal side effects less frequently than typical antipsychotics, they should be used with particular caution in a patient at risk for falls, especially if parkinsonian signs are already present. Regularly scheduled dosing of antipsychotics is not recommended, and if implemented should be reassessed on a frequent basis (eg, weekly), with attempts to taper off as tolerated. There is an FDA black box warning against the use of all antipsychotic medications in older patients with dementia because of an *increased risk of death;* the reason for the increased mortality is unclear. The combination of dextromethorphan and quinidine (up to 30/10 mg orally twice daily) has shown promise in early clinical trials.

Special Circumstances

A. Rapidly Progressive Dementia

When dementia develops quickly, with obvious decline over a few weeks to a few months, the syndrome may be classified as a **rapidly progressive dementia.** The differential diagnosis for typical dementias is still relevant, but additional etiologies must be considered, including prion disease; infections; toxins; neoplasms; and autoimmune and inflammatory diseases, including corticosteroid-responsive (Hashimoto) encephalopathy and antibody-mediated paraneoplastic and nonparaneoplastic encephalitis (Table 24–5). Workup should begin with brain MRI with contrast and diffusion-weighted imaging, routine laboratory studies (serum vitamin B_{12}, free T_4, and TSH levels), serum RPR, HIV antibody, Lyme serology, rheumatologic tests (ESR, CRP, and antinuclear antibody), anti-thyroglobulin and anti-thyroperoxidase antibody levels, paraneoplastic and nonparaneoplastic autoimmune antibodies (Table 24–5), and cerebrospinal fluid studies (cell count and differential; protein and glucose levels; protein electrophoresis for oligoclonal bands; IgG index [spinal-fluid-to-serum-gamma-globulin level] ratio; and VDRL). Depending on the clinical context, it may be necessary to exclude Wilson disease (24-hour urine copper level); heavy metal intoxication (urine heavy metal panel); and infectious encephalitis due to atypical bacteria, viruses, fungi, and mycobacteria.

Creutzfeldt-Jakob disease is a relatively common cause of rapidly progressive dementia (see Chapter 32). Family history is important since mutations in *PRNP*, the gene for the prion protein, account for around 15% of cases. Diffusion-weighted MRI is the most helpful diagnostic tool, classically revealing cortical ribboning (a gyral pattern of hyperintensity) as well as restricted diffusion in the caudate and anterior putamen. An electroencephalogram often shows periodic complexes. Real-time quaking induced conversion (RT-QuIC), in which patient cerebrospinal fluid is mixed with recombinant prion protein and aggregation of prion protein is detected, is a sensitive and specific diagnostic test. Reflecting the high rate of neuronal death, cerebrospinal fluid levels of the intraneuronal proteins tau, 14-3-3, and neuron-specific enolase are often elevated, although this finding is neither sensitive nor specific.

B. Driving and Dementia

It is recommended that *any patient with mild dementia or worse should discontinue driving.* Most states have laws regulating driving among cognitively impaired individuals, and many require the clinician to report the patient's diagnosis to the public health department or department of motor vehicles. There is no evidence that driving classes help patients with neurodegenerative diseases.

When to Refer

All patients with new, unexplained cognitive decline should be referred.

When to Admit

Admission to the hospital should only occur when essential in patients with dementia due to increased risk of developing hospital-acquired delirium.

Arvanitakis Z et al. Diagnosis and management of dementia: review. JAMA. 2019;322:1589. [PMID: 31638686]

Law CK et al. Physical exercise attenuates cognitive decline and reduces behavioral problems in people with mild cognitive impairment and dementia: a systematic review. J Physiother. 2020;66:9. [PMID: 31843427]

WERNICKE ENCEPHALOPATHY & KORSAKOFF SYNDROME

Wernicke encephalopathy is characterized by confusion, ataxia, and nystagmus leading to ophthalmoplegia (lateral rectus muscle weakness, conjugate gaze palsies); peripheral neuropathy may also be present. It is *due to thiamine deficiency* and in the United States occurs most commonly in patients with alcohol use disorder. It may also occur in patients with AIDS or hyperemesis gravidarum, and after bariatric surgery. In suspected cases, thiamine (100 mg) is given intravenously immediately and then intramuscularly on a daily basis until a satisfactory diet can be ensured after which the same dose is given orally. Some guidelines recommend initial doses of 200–500 mg intravenously three times daily for the first 5–7 days of treatment. Intravenous glucose given *before* thiamine may precipitate the syndrome or worsen the symptoms. The diagnosis is confirmed by the response in 1 or 2 days to treatment, which must not be delayed while awaiting laboratory confirmation of thiamine deficiency from a blood sample obtained prior to thiamine administration. **Korsakoff syndrome** occurs in more severe cases; it includes anterograde and retrograde amnesia and sometimes confabulation and may not be recognized until after the initial delirium has lifted.

STUPOR & COMA

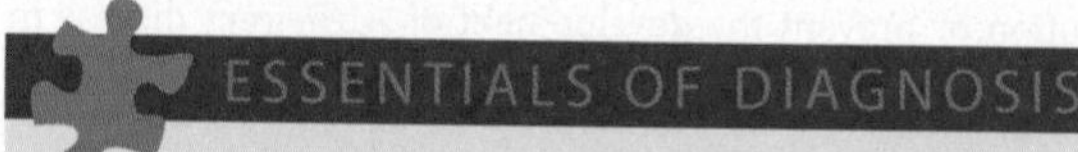

- Level of consciousness is depressed.
- Stuporous patients respond only to repeated vigorous stimuli.
- Comatose patients are unarousable and unresponsive.

General Considerations

The patient who is **stuporous** is unresponsive except when subjected to repeated vigorous stimuli, while the **comatose** patient is unarousable and unable to respond to external events or inner needs, although reflex movements and posturing may be present.

Coma is a major complication of serious CNS disorders. It can result from seizures, hypothermia, metabolic disturbances, meningoencephalitis, or structural lesions causing bilateral cerebral hemispheric dysfunction or a disturbance of the brainstem reticular activating system. A mass lesion involving one cerebral hemisphere may cause coma by compression of the brainstem.

Assessment & Emergency Measures

The diagnostic workup of the comatose patient must proceed concomitantly with management. Supportive therapy for respiration or blood pressure is initiated; in hypothermia, all such patients should be rewarmed before the prognosis is assessed.

The patient can be positioned on one side with the neck partly extended, dentures removed, and secretions cleared by suction; if necessary, the patency of the airways is maintained with an oropharyngeal airway. Blood is drawn for serum glucose, electrolyte, and calcium levels; arterial blood gases; liver biochemical and kidney function tests; and toxicologic studies as indicated. Thiamine (100 mg), followed by dextrose 50% (25 g), and naloxone (0.4–1.2 mg) are given intravenously without delay.

Further details are then obtained from attendants of the patient's medical history, the circumstances surrounding the onset of coma, and the time course of subsequent events. Abrupt onset of coma suggests subarachnoid hemorrhage, brainstem stroke, or intracerebral hemorrhage, whereas a slower onset and progression occur with other structural or mass lesions. Urgent noncontrast CT scanning of the head should be performed to identify intracranial hemorrhage, brain herniation, or other structural lesions that may require immediate neurosurgical intervention, and CT angiogram is important to rule out basilar artery occlusion. A metabolic cause is likely with a preceding intoxicated state or agitated delirium. On examination, attention is paid to the behavioral response to painful stimuli, the pupils and their response to light, the response to touching the cornea with a wisp of sterile gauze, position of the eyes and their movement in response to passive movement of the head and ice-water caloric stimulation, and the respiratory pattern.

A. Response to Painful Stimuli

Purposeful limb withdrawal from painful stimuli implies that sensory pathways from and motor pathways to the stimulated limb are functionally intact. Unilateral absence of responses despite application of stimuli to both sides of the body in turn implies a corticospinal lesion; bilateral absence of responsiveness suggests brainstem involvement, bilateral pyramidal tract lesions, or psychogenic unresponsiveness. Decorticate (flexor) posturing may occur with lesions of the internal capsule and rostral cerebral peduncle and decerebrate (extensor) posturing with dysfunction or destruction of the midbrain and rostral pons. Decerebrate posturing occurs in the arms accompanied by flaccidity or slight flexor responses in the legs in patients with extensive brainstem damage extending down to the pons at the trigeminal level.

B. Ocular Findings

1. Pupils—Hypothalamic disease processes may lead to unilateral Horner syndrome, while bilateral diencephalic involvement or destructive pontine lesions may lead to small but reactive pupils. Ipsilateral pupillary dilation with no direct or consensual response to light occurs with compression of the third cranial nerve, eg, with uncal herniation. The pupils are slightly smaller than normal but responsive to light in many metabolic encephalopathies; however, they may be fixed and dilated following overdosage with atropine or scopolamine, and pinpoint (but responsive) with opioids.

2. Corneal reflex—Touching the cornea with a wisp of sterile gauze or cotton should elicit a blink reflex. The afferent limb of the arc is mediated by the fifth cranial nerve; the efferent limb by the seventh nerve. A unilateral absent corneal reflex implies damage to the ipsilateral pons or a trigeminal deficit. Bilateral loss can be seen with large pontine lesions or in deep pharmacologic coma.

3. Eye movements—Conjugate deviation of the eyes to the side suggests the presence of an ipsilateral hemispheric lesion, a contralateral pontine lesion, or ongoing seizures from the contralateral hemisphere. A mesencephalic lesion leads to downward conjugate deviation. Dysconjugate ocular deviation in coma implies a structural brainstem lesion unless there was preexisting strabismus.

The oculomotor responses to passive head turning and to caloric stimulation relate to each other and provide complementary information. In response to brisk rotation of the head from side to side and to flexion and extension of the head, normally conscious patients with open eyes do not exhibit contraversive conjugate eye deviation (**oculocephalic reflex**) unless there is voluntary visual fixation or bilateral frontal pathology. With cortical depression in lightly comatose patients, a brisk oculocephalic reflex is seen. With brainstem lesions, this oculocephalic reflex becomes impaired or lost, depending on the site of the lesion.

The **oculovestibular reflex** is tested by caloric stimulation using irrigation with ice water. In normal patients, jerk nystagmus is elicited for about 2 or 3 minutes, with the slow component toward the irrigated ear. In unconscious patients with an intact brainstem, the fast component of the nystagmus disappears, so that the eyes tonically deviate toward the irrigated side for 2–3 minutes before returning to their original position. With impairment of brainstem function, the response becomes abnormal and finally disappears. In metabolic coma, oculocephalic and oculovestibular reflex responses are preserved, at least initially.

C. Respiratory Patterns

Diseases causing coma may lead to respiratory abnormalities. **Cheyne-Stokes respiration** (in which episodes of deep breathing alternate with periods of apnea) may occur with bihemispheric or diencephalic disease or in metabolic disorders. **Central neurogenic hyperventilation** occurs with lesions of the brainstem tegmentum; **apneustic breathing** (in which there are prominent end-inspiratory pauses) suggests damage at the pontine level (eg, due to basilar artery occlusion); and **ataxic breathing** (a completely irregular pattern of breathing with deep and shallow breaths occurring randomly) is associated with lesions of the lower pontine tegmentum and medulla.

1. Stupor & Coma Due to Structural Lesions

Supratentorial mass lesions tend to affect brain function in a systematic way. There may initially be signs of hemispheric dysfunction, such as hemiparesis. As coma develops and deepens, cerebral function becomes progressively disturbed, producing a predictable progression of neurologic signs that suggest rostrocaudal deterioration.

Thus, as a supratentorial mass lesion begins to impair the diencephalon, the patient becomes drowsy, then stuporous, and finally comatose. There may be Cheyne-Stokes respiration; small but reactive pupils or an ipsilateral third nerve palsy due to uncal herniation; normal oculocephalic responses with side-to-side head movements but sometimes an impairment of reflex upward gaze with brisk flexion of the head; tonic ipsilateral deviation of the eyes in response to vestibular stimulation with cold water; and initially a positive response to pain but subsequently only decorticate posturing. With further progression, midbrain failure occurs. Motor dysfunction progresses from decorticate to bilateral decerebrate posturing in response to painful stimuli; Cheyne-Stokes respiration is gradually replaced by sustained central hyperventilation; the pupils become middle-sized and fixed; and the oculocephalic and oculovestibular reflex responses become impaired, abnormal, or lost. As the pons and then the medulla fail, the pupils remain unresponsive; oculovestibular responses are unobtainable; respiration is rapid and shallow; and painful stimuli may lead only to flexor responses in the legs. Finally, respiration becomes irregular and stops, the pupils often then dilating widely.

In contrast, a **subtentorial (ie, brainstem) lesion** may lead to an early, sometimes abrupt disturbance of consciousness without any orderly rostrocaudal progression of neurologic signs. Compressive lesions of the brainstem, especially cerebellar hemorrhage, may be clinically indistinguishable from intraparenchymal processes.

2. Stupor & Coma Due to Metabolic Disturbances

Patients with a metabolic cause of coma generally have signs of patchy, diffuse, and symmetric neurologic involvement that cannot be explained by loss of function at any single level or in a sequential manner, although focal or lateralized deficits may occur in hypoglycemia. Pupillary reactivity is usually preserved. Comatose patients with meningitis, encephalitis, or subarachnoid hemorrhage may also exhibit little in the way of focal neurologic signs, however, and clinical evidence of meningeal irritation is sometimes very subtle in comatose patients. Examination of the cerebrospinal fluid in such patients is essential to establish the correct diagnosis, once a CT scan has ruled out a structural lesion posing risk of cerebral herniation.

In patients with coma due to cerebral ischemia and hypoxia, the absence of pupillary light reflexes 24 hours after return of spontaneous circulation indicates that there is little chance of regaining independence; absent corneal reflexes or absent or extensor motor responses at 72 hours also indicate a grim prognosis. Physical findings are less reliable predictors of outcome among those treated with therapeutic hypothermia, although absent corneal or pupillary light reflexes at 72 hours likely indicate a poor prognosis, as do bilaterally absent cortical somatosensory evoked potentials in response to median nerve stimulation after the patient has returned to normothermia.

Treatment of metabolic encephalopathy is of the underlying disturbance and is considered in other chapters. If the cause of the encephalopathy is obscure, all medications except essential ones may have to be withdrawn in case they are responsible for the altered mental status.

3. Brain Death

Brain death occurs when there is complete and irreversible cessation of all brain function; although the organs can be maintained with mechanical ventilation for the purposes of donation, in most countries *the diagnosis of brain death is equivalent to a declaration of death.* To diagnose brain death, the cause of coma must be established, be compatible with a known cause of brain death, and be irreversible. Reversible coma simulating brain death may be seen with hypothermia (temperature lower than 32°C) and overdosage with CNS depressant drugs. These conditions must be excluded by warming the patient and allowing enough time for all sedating medications to be metabolized (ie, at least five half-lives) or by measuring serum levels. Severe blood pressure, electrolyte, acid-base, and endocrine derangements cannot be present.

Finally, a neurologic examination must demonstrate that the patient is comatose (ie, no eye opening and no response to central or peripheral pain); has lost all brainstem reflex responses, including the pupillary, corneal, oculovestibular, oculocephalic, oropharyngeal, and cough reflexes; and has no respiratory drive. The response to pain should be absent or only consist of spinal reflex movements; decerebrate or decorticate posturing is not consistent with brain death. Absence of respiratory drive is demonstrated with an **apnea test** (absence of spontaneous respiratory activity at a PA_{CO_2} of at least 60 mm Hg or after a rise of 20 mm Hg from baseline).

Certain ancillary tests may assist the determination of brain death if the pupillary light reflex cannot be assessed or an apnea test cannot be performed. These include demonstration of an absent cerebral circulation by intravenous radioisotope cerebral angiography or by four-vessel contrast cerebral angiography. If an electroencephalogram, performed according to the recommendations of the American Clinical Neurophysiology Society, is isoelectric, brain death should not be assumed unless brainstem auditory and somatosensory evoked potentials are also performed to assess brainstem function.

4. Persistent Vegetative State

Patients with severe bilateral hemispheric disease may show some improvement from an initially comatose state, so that, after a variable interval, they appear to be awake but lie motionless and without evidence of awareness or higher mental activity. This is called a **"persistent" vegetative state** once it has lasted over 4 weeks and has also been variously referred to as akinetic mutism, apallic state, or coma vigil. Patients in a vegetative state from a medical cause (eg, anoxic brain injury) for more than 3 months and from a traumatic brain injury for more than 12 months are said to be in a **"chronic" vegetative state**, from which a few patients may regain consciousness but remain severely disabled.

5. Minimally Conscious State

In this state, patients exhibit inconsistent evidence of consciousness. There is some degree of functional recovery of behaviors suggesting self- or environmental-awareness, such as basic verbalization or context-appropriate gestures, emotional responses (eg, smiling) to emotional but not neutral stimuli, or purposive responses to environmental stimuli (eg, a finger movement or eye blink apparently to command). Further improvement is manifest by the restoration of communication with the patient. The minimally conscious state may be temporary or permanent. Little information is available about its natural history or long-term outlook, which reflects the underlying cause. The likelihood of useful functional recovery diminishes with time; after 12 months, patients are likely to remain severely disabled and without a reliable means of communication. Prognostication is difficult. Amantadine (100–200 mg orally daily) may hasten recovery when given to patients in a vegetative or minimally conscious state 4–16 weeks after traumatic brain injury.

6. Locked-In Syndrome (De-Efferented State)

Acute destructive lesions (eg, infarction, hemorrhage, demyelination, encephalitis) involving the ventral pons and sparing the tegmentum may lead to a mute, quadriparetic but conscious state in which the patient is capable of blinking and voluntary eye movement in the vertical plane, with preserved pupillary responses to light. Such a patient can mistakenly be regarded as comatose. Clinicians should recognize that "locked-in" individuals are fully aware of their surroundings. The prognosis is usually poor, but recovery has occasionally been reported in some cases, including resumption of independent daily life. A similar condition may occur with severe Guillain-Barré syndrome and has a better prognosis.

Greer DM et al. Determination of brain death/death by neurologic criteria: the world brain death project. JAMA. 2020;324:1078. [PMID: 3276206]

HEAD INJURY

Trauma is the most common cause of death in young people, and head injury accounts for almost half of these trauma-related deaths. Head injury severity ranges from **concussion** to **severe traumatic brain injury (TBI).** Concussion is broadly defined as an alteration in mental status caused by trauma with or without loss of consciousness. The term concussion is often used synonymously with mild TBI. Grades of TBI are traditionally defined by the Glasgow Coma Scale (GCS) measured 30 minutes after injury (Table 24–7).

Head trauma may cause cerebral injury through a variety of mechanisms (Table 24–8). Central to management is determination of which patients need head imaging and observation. Of particular concern is identification of patients with epidural and subdural hematoma, who may present with normal neurologic findings shortly after injury (**lucid interval**) but rapidly deteriorate thereafter, and in whom surgical intervention is life-saving.

Table 24–7. Glasgow Coma Scale.[1]

Points	Eye Opening	Verbal Response	Motor Response
1	None	None	None
2	To pain	Vocal but not verbal	Extension
3	To voice	Verbal but not conversational	Flexion
4	Spontaneous	Conversational but disoriented	Withdraws from pain
5	Spontaneous	Oriented	Localizes pain
6	Spontaneous	Oriented	Obeys commands

[1]GCS score indicating severity of traumatic brain injury: **mild**, 13–15; **moderate**, 9–12; **severe**, ≤ 8.

Reproduced, with permission, from Aminoff MJ et al. *Clinical Neurology*, 9th ed, McGraw-Hill Education, 2015; data from Teasdale G, Jennett B. Assessment of coma and impaired consciousness. A practical scale. *Lancet*. 1974;304:81–84.

▶ Clinical Findings

A. Symptoms and Signs

Common symptoms of concussion that develop acutely include headache, nausea, vomiting, confusion, disorientation, dizziness, and imbalance. A period of amnesia encompassing the traumatic event and a variable period of time leading up to the trauma is typical. Loss of consciousness may occur. Additional symptoms of photophobia, phonophobia, difficulty concentrating, irritability, and sleep and mood disturbances may develop over the following hours to days. Examination is usually normal, although orientation and attention, short-term memory, and reaction time may be impaired. Persistent or progressive decline in the level of consciousness after the initial injury, or focal neurologic findings, suggests the need for urgent imaging and neurosurgical consultation.

Patients should also be examined for signs of scalp lacerations, facial and skull fracture, and neck injury. The clinical signs of basilar skull fracture include bruising about the orbit (**raccoon sign**), blood in the external auditory meatus (**Battle sign**), and leakage of cerebrospinal fluid (which can be identified by its glucose or beta-2-transferrin content) from the ear or nose. Cranial nerve palsies (involving especially the first, second, third, fourth, fifth, seventh, and eighth nerves in any combination) may also occur. The head and neck should be immobilized until imaging can be performed.

B. Imaging and Other Investigations

Recommendations are that head CT be performed in patients with concussion and any of the following: GCS score less than 15, focal neurologic deficit, seizure, coagulopathy, aged 65 or older, skull fracture, persistent headache or vomiting, retrograde amnesia exceeding 30 minutes, intoxication, or soft tissue injury of the head or neck. Otherwise, patients can be sent home as long as a responsible caregiver can check the patient at hourly intervals for the next 24 hours. Patients requiring imaging should be admitted unless the head CT is normal, the GCS score is 15, there have been no seizures, there is no predisposition to bleeding, and they can be monitored by a caregiver at home.

Table 24–8. Acute cerebral sequelae of head injury (listed in alphabetical order).

Sequelae	Clinical Features	Pathology
Acute epidural hemorrhage	Headache, confusion, somnolence, seizures, and focal deficits occur several hours after injury (lucid interval) and lead to coma, respiratory depression, and death unless treated by surgical evacuation.	Tear in meningeal artery, vein, or dural sinus, leading to hematoma visible on CT scan.
Acute subdural hemorrhage	Similar to epidural hemorrhage, but interval before onset of symptoms is longer. Neurosurgical consultation for consideration of evacuation.	Hematoma from tear in veins from cortex to superior sagittal sinus or from cerebral laceration, visible on CT scan.
Cerebral contusion or laceration	Loss of consciousness longer than with concussion. Focal neurologic deficits are often present. May lead to death or severe residual neurologic deficit.	Bruising on side of impact (coup injury) or contralaterally (contrecoup injury). Vasogenic edema, multiple petechial hemorrhages, and mass effect. May have subarachnoid bleeding. Herniation may occur in severe cases. Cerebral laceration specifically involves tearing of the cerebral tissue and pia-arachnoid overlying a contusion.
Cerebral hemorrhage	Generally develops immediately after injury. Clinically resembles hypertensive hemorrhage. Surgery to relieve mass effect is sometimes necessary.	Hematoma, visible on CT scan.
Concussion	A transient, trauma-induced alteration in mental status that may or may not involve loss of consciousness. Symptoms and signs include headache, nausea, disorientation, irritability, amnesia, clumsiness, visual disturbances, and focal neurologic deficit.	Unknown; likely mild diffuse axonal injury and excitotoxic neuronal injury. Cerebral contusion may occur.
Diffuse axonal injury	Persistent loss of consciousness, coma, or persistent vegetative state resulting from severe rotational shearing forces or deceleration.	Imaging may be normal or may show tiny, scattered white matter hemorrhages. Histology reveals torn axons.

Because injury to the spine may have accompanied head trauma, cervical spine radiographs (three views) or CT should always be obtained in comatose patients and in patients with severe neck pain or a deficit possibly related to cord compression.

Treatment

Head injury can often be prevented by helmets, seatbelts, and other protective equipment.

After intracranial bleeding has been excluded clinically or by head CT, treatment of mild TBI is aimed at promoting resolution of postconcussive symptoms and preventing recurrent injury, which increases the risk of chronic neurobehavioral impairment and delays recovery. Rarely, a recurrent concussion while a patient is still symptomatic from a first concussion may lead to fatal cerebral edema (**second impact syndrome**). These observations form the basis of the recommendation that patients at risk for recurrent concussion (eg, athletes) be held out of the risky activity until their concussive symptoms have fully resolved.

In patients hospitalized with moderate or severe TBI, management often requires a multidisciplinary approach due to multiple concomitant injuries. Elevated intracranial pressure can result from diffuse axonal injury or a hematoma requiring surgical evacuation, or from a variety of medical causes. Decompressive craniectomy may reduce otherwise refractory intracranial hypertension but does not improve neurologic outcome. Hypothermia is associated with worsened functional outcomes.

Because bridging veins between the brain and venous sinuses become more vulnerable to shear injury as the brain atrophies, a **subdural hematoma** may develop days or weeks following head injury in older patients or even occur spontaneously. Clinical presentation can be subtle, often with mental changes such as slowness, drowsiness, headache, confusion, or memory disturbance. Focal neurologic deficits such as hemiparesis or hemisensory disturbance are less common. Surgical intervention is indicated if the hematoma is 10 mm or more in thickness or there is a midline shift of 5 mm or more; if there is a decline in GCS score of 2 or more from injury to hospital admission; or if one or both pupils are fixed and dilated.

Scalp lacerations and depressed skull fractures should be treated surgically as appropriate. Simple skull fractures require no specific treatment. If there is any leakage of cerebrospinal fluid, conservative treatment, with elevation of the head, restriction of fluids, and administration of acetazolamide (250 mg orally four times daily), is often helpful; if the leak continues for more than a few days, lumbar subarachnoid drainage may be necessary. Antibiotics are given if infection occurs, based on culture and sensitivity studies; vaccination against pneumococcus is recommended (see Table 30–7). Only very occasional patients require intracranial repair of the dural defect because of persistence of the leak or recurrent meningitis.

Prognosis

Moderate and severe TBI may result in permanent cognitive and motor impairment depending on the severity and location of the initial injury. Initial GCS and head CT findings have prognostic value. Among patients with a GCS score of 8 or less at presentation, mortality approaches 30% and only one-third of survivors regain functional independence. Cognitive impairment tends to affect frontal and temporal lobe function, causing deficits in attention, memory, judgment, and executive function. Behavioral dysregulation, depression, and disinhibition can impair social functioning. Anosmia, presumably due to shearing of fibers from the nasal epithelium, is common.

Epilepsy can develop after TBI, especially with more severe injury. Among patients with severe TBI (typically loss of consciousness for at least 12–24 hours, intracranial hematoma, depressed skull fracture, or cerebral contusion), phenytoin or levetiracetam is typically given for 7 days to reduce the incidence of early posttraumatic seizures; this is done exclusively to minimize acute complications resulting from such seizures and does not prevent the development of posttraumatic epilepsy.

Among patients with mild TBI, symptoms of concussion resolve in most patients by 1 month and in the vast majority by 3 months. Prolonged postconcussive symptoms are uncommon, persisting at 1 year in 10–15% of patients. Risk factors for prolonged postconcussive symptoms include active litigation regarding the injury; repeated concussions; and GCS score of 13 or less at presentation. Headaches often have migrainous features and may respond to tricyclic antidepressants or beta-blockers (see Table 24–1). Opioids should be avoided to minimize the risk of medication overuse headache. Mood symptoms may respond to antidepressants, anxiolytics, and cognitive behavioral therapy.

There appears to be an association between head trauma and the later development of neurodegenerative disease, such as Alzheimer disease, Parkinson disease, or amyotrophic lateral sclerosis (ALS). Normal pressure hydrocephalus may also occur. Repetitive, mild head injury, such as that which occurs in athletes or military personnel, can lead to **chronic traumatic encephalopathy,** a distinct pathologic entity associated with mood and cognitive changes and characterized by the abnormal aggregation of tau or other proteins either focally or globally in the cerebral cortex. Whether chronic traumatic encephalopathy is a static response to recurrent head injury or a progressive neurodegenerative disease is not known, but the severity of neuropathology appears to correlate to lifetime exposure to repetitive head injury.

When to Refer

- Patients with focal neurologic deficits, altered consciousness, or skull fracture.
- Patients with late complications of head injury, eg, posttraumatic seizure disorder or normal pressure hydrocephalus.

When to Admit

- Patients with concussion and GCS score less than 15, predisposition to bleeding, seizure, or no responsible caregiver at home.
- Patients with abnormal head CT.

Mariani M et al. Clinical presentation of chronic traumatic encephalopathy. Semin Neurol. 2020;40:370. [PMID: 32740900]

Misch MR et al. Sports medicine update: concussion. Emerg Med Clin North Am. 2020;38:207. [PMID: 31757251]

MULTIPLE SCLEROSIS

ESSENTIALS OF DIAGNOSIS

- Episodic neurologic symptoms.
- Patient usually < 55 years of age at onset.
- Single pathologic lesion cannot explain clinical findings.
- Multiple foci best visualized by MRI.

General Considerations

This common neurologic disorder, which probably has an autoimmune basis, has its greatest incidence in young adults. Epidemiologic studies indicate that multiple sclerosis is much more common in persons of western European lineage who live in temperate zones. No population with a high risk for multiple sclerosis exists between latitudes 40° N and 40° S. A genetic susceptibility to the disease is present. Pathologically, focal—often perivenular—areas of demyelination with reactive gliosis are found scattered in the white matter of the brain and spinal cord and in the optic nerves. Axonal damage also occurs.

Clinical Findings

A. Symptoms and Signs

The common initial presentation is weakness, numbness, tingling, or unsteadiness in a limb; spastic paraparesis; retrobulbar optic neuritis; diplopia; dysequilibrium; or a sphincter disturbance such as urinary urgency or hesitancy. Symptoms may disappear after a few days or weeks, although examination often reveals a residual deficit.

Several forms of the disease are recognized. In most patients, there is an interval of months or years after the initial episode before new symptoms develop or the original ones recur (**relapsing-remitting disease**). Eventually, however, relapses and usually incomplete remissions lead to increasing disability, with weakness, spasticity, and ataxia of the limbs, impaired vision, and urinary incontinence. The findings on examination at this stage commonly include optic atrophy; nystagmus; dysarthria; and pyramidal, sensory, or cerebellar deficits in some or all of the limbs. In some of these patients, the clinical course changes so that a steady deterioration occurs, unrelated to acute relapses (**secondary progressive disease**). Less commonly, symptoms are steadily progressive from their onset, and disability develops at a relatively early stage (**primary progressive disease**). The diagnosis cannot be made with confidence unless the total clinical picture indicates involvement of *different parts of the CNS at different times.* Fatigue is common in all forms of the disease.

A number of factors (eg, infection) may precipitate or trigger exacerbations. Relapses are reduced in pregnancy but are more likely during the 2 or 3 months following pregnancy, possibly because of the increased demands and stresses that occur in the postpartum period.

B. Imaging

MRI of the brain and cervical cord has a major role in excluding other causes of neurologic dysfunction and in demonstrating the presence of multiple lesions. In T1-weighted images, hypointense "black holes" probably represent areas of permanent axonal damage. Gadolinium-enhanced T1-weighted images may highlight areas of active inflammation with breakdown of the blood-brain barrier, which helps identify newer lesions. T2-weighted images provide information about disease burden or total number of lesions, which typically appear as areas of high signal intensity. CT scans are less helpful than MRI.

In patients with myelopathy alone and no clinical or laboratory evidence of more widespread disease, MRI or myelography is necessary to exclude a congenital or acquired surgically treatable lesion. In patients with mixed pyramidal and cerebellar deficits in the limbs, the foramen magnum region must be visualized to exclude the possibility of Arnold-Chiari malformation, in which parts of the cerebellum and lower brainstem are displaced into the cervical canal.

C. Laboratory and Other Studies

A definitive diagnosis can never be based solely on the laboratory findings. If there is clinical evidence of only a single lesion in the CNS, multiple sclerosis cannot properly be diagnosed unless it can be shown that other regions are affected subclinically. Visual, brainstem auditory, and somatosensory evoked potentials are helpful in this regard, but other disorders may also be characterized by multifocal electrophysiologic abnormalities reflecting disease of central white matter. Certain infections (eg, HIV, Lyme disease, syphilis), connective tissue diseases (eg, SLE, Sjögren syndrome), sarcoidosis, metabolic disorders (eg, vitamin B_{12} deficiency), and lymphoma may therefore require exclusion.

There may be mild lymphocytosis or a slightly increased protein concentration in the cerebrospinal fluid, especially soon after an acute relapse. Elevated IgG in cerebrospinal fluid and discrete bands of IgG (oligoclonal bands) are present in many patients. The presence of such bands is not specific, however, since they have been found in a variety of inflammatory neurologic disorders and occasionally in patients with vascular or neoplastic disorders of the nervous system.

Vitamin D deficiency may be associated with an increased risk of developing multiple sclerosis; randomized trials have *not* shown vitamin D supplementation reduces attack rate or progression in relapsing-remitting disease.

D. Diagnosis

Multiple sclerosis should not be diagnosed unless there is evidence that two or more different regions of the central white matter (*dissemination in space*) have been affected at different times (*dissemination in time*); the most widely used diagnostic algorithm is the 2017 revision to the McDonald criteria. The diagnosis may be made in a patient with two or more typical attacks and objective evidence on clinical examination of two lesions (eg, optic disk atrophy and pyramidal weakness), or objective evidence of one lesion with clear-cut historical evidence the other attack was typical of multiple sclerosis and in a distinct neuroanatomic location, and when no alternative explanation for the patient's presentation has been found. To fulfill the criterion of dissemination in space in a patient with two clinical attacks but objective clinical evidence of only one lesion, MRI should demonstrate at least one lesion in at least two of four typical sites (periventricular, cortical or juxtacortical, infratentorial, or spinal); alternatively, an additional attack localized to a different site suffices. The criterion of dissemination in time in a patient with only one attack can be fulfilled by the simultaneous presence of gadolinium-enhancing and nonenhancing lesions at any time (including at initial examination); the presence of oligoclonal bands unique to the cerebrospinal fluid; a new lesion on follow-up MRI; or a second attack. Lesions in the optic nerve on MRI in patients with optic neuritis cannot be used to fulfill the McDonald criteria for dissemination in space or time. Primary progressive disease requires at least a year of progression, plus two of three of the following: at least one typical brain lesion, at least two spinal lesions, or oligoclonal banding in the cerebrospinal fluid.

In patients with a single clinical event who do not satisfy criteria for multiple sclerosis, a diagnosis of a **clinically isolated syndrome (CIS)** is made. Such patients are at risk for developing multiple sclerosis and are sometimes offered beta-interferon or glatiramer acetate therapy, which may delay progression to clinically definite disease. Follow-up MRI should be considered 6–12 months later to assess for the presence of any new lesion.

Treatment

At least partial recovery from acute exacerbations can reasonably be expected, but further relapses may occur without warning. Some disability is likely to result eventually, but about half of all patients are without significant disability even 10 years after onset of symptoms. Treatments chiefly are aimed at preventing relapses, thereby reducing disability.

Recovery from acute relapses may be hastened by treatment with corticosteroids, but the extent of recovery is unchanged. Intravenous therapy is often given first—typically methylprednisolone 1 g daily for 3 days—followed by oral prednisone at 60–80 mg daily for 1 week with a taper over the ensuing 2–3 weeks, but randomized trials show similar efficacy whether the initial high dose is given orally or intravenously. Long-term treatment with corticosteroids provides no benefit and does not prevent further relapses. Transient exacerbation of symptoms relating to intercurrent infection or heat requires no added treatment.

In patients with relapsing disease, numerous medications have well-established efficacy at *reducing the*

Table 24–9. Treatment of multiple sclerosis (in alphabetical order within categories).[1]

Medication	Dose
Acute Episode, Including Relapse[2]	
Dexamethasone	160 mg orally daily for 3–5 days
Methylprednisolone	1 g intravenously or orally daily for 3–5 days
Plasmapheresis	
Disease-Modifying Therapy (FDA-approved)	
Alemtuzumab (Lemtrada)[3,4]	12 mg intravenously daily for 5 days; 3-day course given 1 year later
Cladribine (Mavenclad)[3,5,6]	1.75 mg/kg orally divided between weeks 1 and 5, repeated once in 1 year
Dimethyl fumarate (Tecfidera)[3,5]	240 mg orally twice daily
Fingolimod (Gilenya)[3,4,5]	0.5 mg orally daily
Glatiramer acetate (Copaxone, Mylan, Glatopa)[5]	20 mg subcutaneously daily or 40 mg subcutaneously three times weekly
Interferon β-1a (Rebif)[5]	44 mcg subcutaneously three times per week
Interferon β-1a (Avonex)[5]	30 mcg intramuscularly once per week
Interferon β-1b (Betaseron, Extavia)[5]	0.25 mg subcutaneously on alternate days
Mitoxantrone[3]	12 mg/m^2 intravenously every 3 months; maximum lifetime dose, 140 mg/m^2
Natalizumab (Tysabri)[3,4]	300 mg intravenously monthly
Ocrelizumab (Ocrevus)[3,4,5,6,7]	300 mg intravenously on day 1 and day 15, followed by 600 mg every 6 months
Ofatumumab (Kesimpta)[3,4,5,6]	20 mg subcutaneously weeks 0, 1, 2, 4, and monthly thereafter
Ozanimod (Zeposia)[3,4,5,6]	0.23 mg orally daily on days 1–4, 0.46 mg daily on days 5–7, and 0.92 mg daily thereafter
Pegylated interferon β-1a (Plegridy)[5]	125 mg subcutaneously once every 2 weeks
Ponesimod (Ponvory)[3,4,5,6]	Titrate from 2 mg orally daily to 5 mg in 1-mg increments every 2 days, then by 1 mg daily to 10 mg by day 12, and then to 20 mg daily on day 15
Siponimod (Mayzent)[3,4,5,6]	0.25 mg orally daily, titrated over 5 or 6 days to 1 or 2 mg orally daily, depending on CYP2C9 genotype
Teriflunomide (Aubagio)[5]	14 mg or 7 mg orally daily

[1]Several of these agents require special monitoring or pretreatment; some should be avoided during pregnancy. Readers should refer to the manufacturer's guidelines.
[2]For corticosteroid-refractory relapses, plasmapheresis may be used.
[3]Relapse prevention for disease activity despite use of first-line treatment.
[4]High disease activity (typically with multiple gadolinium-enhancing lesions on MRI).
[5]Relapse prevention, first-line treatment.
[6]Active secondary progressive disease.
[7]Primary progressive disease.

frequency of attacks (Table 24–9). The initial agent is chosen after considering medication tolerance and risks, patient preference, and disease severity. Glatiramer acetate, an interferon, or dimethyl fumarate is often used initially due to favorable side effect profiles and availability, although the efficacy of early treatment with higher intensity therapy is being explored. In general, the medications most effective in reducing relapses have stronger immunomodulatory effects and more, albeit rare, serious adverse effects. Many of these agents, especially those that deplete or interfere with B-cells, render vaccination ineffective. Prescription of these agents should be managed by a specialist.

Ocrelizumab is the only medication effective in slowing disability progression in primary progressive multiple sclerosis and is approved for this indication by the FDA. For patients with active secondary progressive disease, cladribine, ocrelizumab, ofatumumab, ozanimod, ponesimod, and siponimod can be used. Plasmapheresis is sometimes helpful in patients with severe relapses unresponsive to corticosteroids.

Symptomatic therapy for spasticity, neurogenic bladder, or fatigue may be required. Fatigue is especially common in multiple sclerosis, and modafinil (200 mg orally every morning) is an effective and FDA-approved therapy for this indication. Dalfampridine (an extended-release formulation of 4-aminopyridine administered as 10 mg orally twice daily) is efficacious at improving timed gait in multiple sclerosis. Depression and even suicidality can occur in multiple sclerosis and may worsen with interferon beta-1a therapy; screening and conventional treatment of such symptoms are appropriate.

When to Refer

All patients, but especially those with progressive disease despite standard therapy, should be referred.

When to Admit

- Patients requiring plasma exchange for severe relapses unresponsive to corticosteroids.
- During severe relapses.
- Patients unable to manage at home.

Freedman MS et al. Treatment optimization in multiple sclerosis: Canadian MS working group recommendations. Can J Neurol Sci. 2020;47:437. [PMID: 32654681]

Kappos L et al. Ponesimod compared with teriflunomide in patient with relapsing multiple sclerosis in the active-comparator phase 3 OPTIMUM study. JAMA Neurol. 2021; 78:558. [PMID: 33779698]

NEUROMYELITIS OPTICA

This disorder is characterized by optic neuritis and acute myelitis with MRI changes that extend over at least three segments of the spinal cord. An isolated myelitis or optic neuritis may also occur. Previously known as Devic disease and once regarded as a variant of multiple sclerosis, neuromyelitis optica is associated with a specific antibody marker (NMO-IgG) targeting the water channel aquaporin-4 in 80% of cases, and with antibodies to myelin oligodendrocyte glycoprotein (MOG-IgG) in approximately 33% of NMO-IgG seronegative patients. MRI of the brain typically does not show widespread white matter involvement, but such changes do not exclude the diagnosis. Treatment is by long-term immunosuppression. Three medications are approved by the FDA for treatment of neuromyelitis optica based on placebo-controlled trials demonstrating a reduced annual relapse rate or time to first relapse. Eculizumab is a complement inhibitor, inebilizumab is a humanized anti-CD19 antibody that depletes B-cells, and satralizumab is an interleukin-6 receptor antagonist. Use of eculizumab requires prior immunization against meningococcus. Off-label therapy is with rituximab (two 1-g intravenous infusions spaced by 2 weeks, or four weekly infusions of 375 mg/m^2; re-dosing may occur every 6 months or when CD19/20-positive or CD27-positive lymphocytes become detectable), mycophenolate mofetil (500–1500 mg orally twice daily, titrated until the absolute lymphocyte count falls below 1500/mcL [1.5 × 10^9/L]), or azathioprine (2.5–3 mg/kg orally). Acute relapses are treated with corticosteroids at doses similar to those outlined for multiple sclerosis and with plasma exchange for severe relapses unresponsive to corticosteroids.

Cree BAC et al; N-MOmentum Study Investigators. Inebilizumab for the treatment of neuromyelitis optica spectrum disorder (N-MOmentum): a double-blind, randomized placebo-controlled phase 2/3 trial. Lancet. 2019;394:1352. [PMID: 31495497]

Pittock SJ et al. Eculizumab in aquaporin-4-positive neuromyelitis optica spectrum disorder. N Engl J Med. 2019;381:614. [PMID: 31050279]

VITAMIN E DEFICIENCY

Vitamin E deficiency may produce a disorder somewhat similar to Friedreich ataxia. There is spinocerebellar degeneration involving particularly the posterior columns of the spinal cord and leading to limb ataxia, sensory loss, absent tendon reflexes, slurring of speech, and, in some cases, pigmentary retinal degeneration. The disorder may occur as a consequence of malabsorption or on a hereditary basis (eg, abetalipoproteinemia).

SPASTICITY

The term "spasticity" is commonly used for an upper motor neuron deficit, but it properly refers to a velocity-dependent increase in resistance to passive movement that affects different muscles to a different extent, is not uniform in degree throughout the range of a particular movement, and is commonly associated with other features of pyramidal deficit. It is often a major complication of stroke, cerebral or spinal injury, static perinatal encephalopathy, and multiple sclerosis. Spasticity may be exacerbated by pressure injuries, urinary or other infections, and nociceptive stimuli.

Physical therapy with appropriate stretching programs is important during rehabilitation after the development of an upper motor neuron lesion and in subsequent management of the patient. The aim is to prevent joint and muscle *contractures* and perhaps to modulate spasticity.

Medication management is important also, but treatment may increase functional disability when increased extensor tone is providing additional support for patients with weak legs. Pharmacologic treatment with baclofen (5–10 mg twice daily orally titrated to 80 mg daily), tizanidine (2–8 mg three time daily orally), diazepam (2–10 mg three times daily orally), or dantrolene (25 mg once daily orally, titrated every 3 days as tolerated to a maximum of 100 mg four times daily) is often helpful. Dantrolene is best avoided in patients with poor respiratory function or severe myocardial disease. Cannabinoids are also effective in reducing spasticity, but are associated with side effects, including dizziness, drowsiness, and fatigue. Intramuscular injection of botulinum toxin is used to relax targeted muscles.

In patients with severe spasticity that is unresponsive to other therapies and is associated with marked disability, intrathecal injection of phenol or alcohol may be helpful. Surgical options include implantation of an intrathecal baclofen pump, rhizotomy, or neurectomy. Severe contractures may be treated by surgical tendon release.

MYELOPATHIES IN AIDS

A variety of myelopathies may occur in patients with AIDS. These are discussed in Chapter 31.

MYELOPATHY OF HUMAN T-CELL LEUKEMIA VIRUS INFECTION

Human T-cell leukemia virus (HTLV-1), a human retrovirus, is transmitted by breastfeeding, sexual contact, blood transfusion, and contaminated needles. Most patients are asymptomatic, but after a variable latent period (which may be as long as several years), a myelopathy develops in some instances. The MRI, electrophysiologic, and cerebrospinal fluid findings are similar to those of multiple sclerosis, but HTLV-1 antibodies are present in serum and spinal fluid. There is no specific treatment, but intravenous or oral corticosteroids may help in the initial inflammatory phase of the disease. Prophylactic measures are important. Needles or syringes should not be shared; infected patients should not breastfeed their infants or donate blood, semen, or other tissue. Infected patients should use condoms to prevent sexual transmission.

SUBACUTE COMBINED DEGENERATION OF THE SPINAL CORD

Subacute combined degeneration of the spinal cord is due to **vitamin B_{12} deficiency**, such as occurs in pernicious anemia. It is characterized by myelopathy with spasticity, weakness, proprioceptive loss, and numbness due to degeneration of the corticospinal tracts and posterior columns. Polyneuropathy, mental changes, or optic neuropathy also develop in some patients. Megaloblastic anemia may also occur, but this does *not* parallel the neurologic disorder, and the former may be obscured if folic acid supplements have been taken. Treatment is with vitamin B_{12}. For pernicious anemia, a convenient therapeutic regimen is 1000 mcg cyanocobalamin intramuscularly daily for 1 week, then weekly for 1 month, and then monthly for the remainder of the patient's life. Oral cyanocobalamin replacement is not advised for pernicious anemia when neurologic symptoms are present. A similar syndrome is caused by recreational abuse of inhaled nitrous oxide due to its interference with vitamin B_{12} metabolism. Copper deficiency, caused by malabsorption or excess zinc ingestion, may also be responsible.

SPINAL TRAUMA

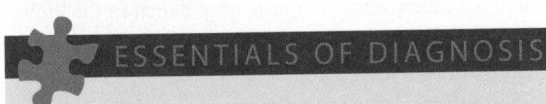

- History of preceding trauma.
- Development of acute neurologic deficit.
- Signs of myelopathy on examination.

General Considerations

While spinal cord damage may result from whiplash injury, severe injury usually relates to fracture-dislocation causing compression or angular deformity of the cord either cervically or in the lower thoracic and upper lumbar regions. Extreme hypotension following injury may also lead to cord infarction.

Clinical Findings

Total cord transection results in immediate flaccid paralysis and loss of sensation below the level of the lesion. Reflex activity is lost for a variable period, and there is urinary and fecal retention. As reflex function returns over the following days and weeks, spastic paraplegia or quadriplegia develops, with hyperreflexia and extensor plantar responses, but a flaccid atrophic (lower motor neuron) paralysis may be found depending on the segments of the cord that are affected. The bladder and bowels also regain some reflex function, permitting urine and feces to be expelled at intervals. As spasticity increases, flexor or extensor spasms (or both) of the legs become troublesome, especially if the patient develops bed sores or a UTI. Paraplegia with the legs in flexion or extension may eventually result.

With lesser degrees of injury, patients may be left with mild limb weakness, distal sensory disturbance, or both. Sphincter function may also be impaired, urinary urgency and urge incontinence being especially common. More particularly, a unilateral cord lesion leads to an ipsilateral motor disturbance with accompanying impairment of proprioception and contralateral loss of pain and temperature appreciation below the lesion (**Brown-Séquard syndrome**). A central cord syndrome may lead to a lower motor neuron deficit at the level of the lesion and loss of pain and temperature appreciation below it, with sparing of posterior column functions. With more extensive involvement, posterior column sensation may also be impaired and pyramidal weakness develops. A radicular deficit may occur at the level of the injury—or, if the cauda equina is involved, there may be evidence of disturbed function in several lumbosacral roots.

Treatment

Treatment of the injury consists of immobilization and—if there is cord compression—early decompressive laminectomy and fusion (within 24 hours). Early treatment with high doses of corticosteroids (eg, methylprednisolone, 30 mg/kg by intravenous bolus, followed by 5.4 mg/kg/hour for 23 hours) may improve neurologic recovery if commenced within 8 hours after injury, although the evidence is limited and some neurosurgical guidelines do not recommend their use. Anatomic realignment of the spinal cord by traction and other orthopedic procedures is important. Subsequent care of the residual neurologic deficit—paraplegia or quadriplegia—requires treatment of spasticity and care of the skin, bladder, and bowels.

When to Refer

All patients with focal neurologic deficits should be referred.

When to Admit

- Patients with neurologic deficits.
- Patients with spinal cord injury, compression, or acute epidural or subdural hematoma.
- Patients with vertebral fracture-dislocation likely to compress the cord.

Ong B et al. Management of the patient with chronic spinal cord injury. Med Clin North Am. 2020;104:263. [PMID: 32035568]

SYRINGOMYELIA

Destruction or degeneration of gray and white matter adjacent to the central canal of the cervical spinal cord leads to cavitation and accumulation of fluid within the spinal cord. The precise pathogenesis is unclear, but many cases are associated with **Arnold-Chiari malformation**, in which there is displacement of the cerebellar tonsils, medulla, and fourth ventricle into the spinal canal, sometimes with accompanying meningomyelocele. In such circumstances, the cord cavity connects with and may merely represent a dilated central canal. In other cases, the cause of cavitation is less clear. There is a characteristic clinical picture, with segmental atrophy, areflexia, and loss of pain and temperature appreciation in a "cape" distribution, owing to the destruction of fibers crossing in front of the central canal in the mid-cervical spinal cord. Thoracic kyphoscoliosis is usually present. With progression, involvement of the long motor and sensory tracts occurs as well, so that a pyramidal and sensory deficit develops in the legs. Upward extension of the cavitation (**syringobulbia**) leads to dysfunction of the lower brainstem and thus to bulbar palsy, nystagmus, and sensory impairment over one or both sides of the face.

Syringomyelia, ie, cord cavitation, may also occur in association with an intramedullary tumor or following severe cord injury, and the cavity then does not communicate with the central canal.

In patients with Arnold-Chiari malformation, CT scans reveal a small posterior fossa and enlargement of the foramen magnum, along with other associated skeletal abnormalities at the base of the skull and upper cervical spine. MRI reveals the syrinx as well as the characteristic findings of the Arnold-Chiari malformation, including the caudal displacement of the fourth ventricle and herniation of the cerebellar tonsils through the foramen magnum. Focal cord enlargement is found at myelography or by MRI in patients with cavitation related to past injury or intramedullary neoplasms.

Treatment of Arnold-Chiari malformation with associated syringomyelia is by suboccipital craniectomy and upper cervical laminectomy, with the aim of decompressing the malformation at the foramen magnum. The cord cavity should be drained and, if necessary, an outlet for the fourth ventricle can be made. In cavitation associated with intramedullary tumor, treatment is surgical, but radiation therapy may be necessary if complete removal is not possible. Posttraumatic syringomyelia is also treated surgically if it leads to increasing neurologic deficits or to intolerable pain.

DEGENERATIVE MOTOR NEURON DISEASES

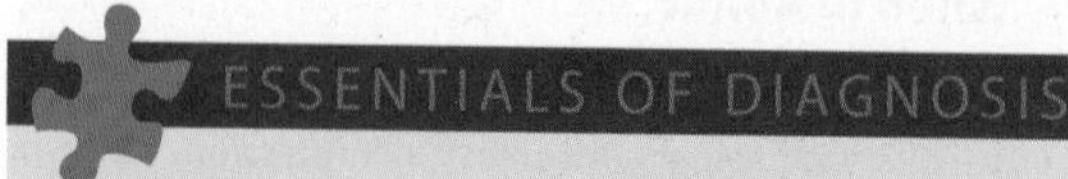

ESSENTIALS OF DIAGNOSIS

- Weakness.
- No sensory loss or sphincter disturbance.
- Progressive course.
- No identifiable underlying cause other than genetic basis in familial cases.

General Considerations

This group of degenerative disorders is characterized clinically by weakness and variable wasting of affected muscles, without accompanying sensory changes.

Motor neuron disease in adults generally commences between 30 and 60 years of age. There is degeneration of the anterior horn cells in the spinal cord, the motor nuclei of the lower cranial nerves, and the corticospinal and corticobulbar pathways. The disorder is usually sporadic, but familial cases may occur and several genetic mutations or loci have been identified. Cigarette smoking may be one risk factor.

Classification

Five varieties have been distinguished on clinical grounds.

A. Progressive Bulbar Palsy

Bulbar involvement predominates owing to disease processes affecting primarily the motor nuclei of the cranial nerves.

B. Pseudobulbar Palsy

Bulbar involvement predominates in this variety also, but it is due to bilateral corticobulbar disease and thus reflects upper motor neuron dysfunction. There may be a "pseudobulbar affect," with uncontrollable episodes of laughing or crying to stimuli that would not normally have elicited such marked reactions.

C. Progressive Spinal Muscular Atrophy

This is characterized primarily by a lower motor neuron deficit in the limbs due to degeneration of the anterior horn cells in the spinal cord.

D. Primary Lateral Sclerosis

There is a purely upper motor neuron deficit in the limbs.

E. Amyotrophic Lateral Sclerosis (ALS)

A mixed upper and lower motor neuron deficit is found in the limbs. This disorder is sometimes associated with cognitive decline (in a pattern consistent with frontotemporal dementia), a pseudobulbar affect, or parkinsonism. Approximately 10% of ALS cases are familial and have been associated with mutations at several different genetic loci, including a hexanucleotide repeat on chromosome 9 that also associates with frontotemporal dementia.

Differential Diagnosis

The spinal muscular atrophies (SMAs) are inherited syndromes caused most often by mutations of the survival motor neuron 1 (*SMN1*) gene on chromosome 5. Different mutations result in more or less severe disruptions of the protein, resulting in an age of onset that ranges from infancy (SMA type I), to early (type II) or late childhood (type III), to adulthood (type IV). X-linked spinal and bulbar muscular atrophy (Kennedy syndrome) is associated with an expanded trinucleotide repeat sequence on the androgen receptor gene and carries a more benign prognosis than other forms of motor neuron disease.

There are reports of juvenile SMA due to hexosaminidase deficiency. Pure motor syndromes resembling motor neuron disease may also occur in association with monoclonal gammopathy or multifocal motor neuropathies with conduction block. A motor neuronopathy may also develop in Hodgkin disease and has a relatively benign prognosis. Infective anterior horn cell diseases (polio virus or West Nile virus infection) can generally be distinguished by the acute onset and monophasic course of the illness, as discussed in Chapter 32. Acute flaccid myelitis following infection with enterovirus may occur, especially in children, without sensory involvement and resembles poliomyelitis. There is no specific treatment.

Clinical Findings

A. Symptoms and Signs

Difficulty in swallowing, chewing, coughing, breathing, and talking (dysarthria) occurs with bulbar involvement. In progressive bulbar palsy, there is drooping of the palate; a depressed gag reflex; pooling of saliva in the pharynx; a weak cough; and a wasted, fasciculating tongue. In pseudobulbar palsy, the tongue is contracted and spastic and cannot be moved rapidly from side to side. Limb involvement is characterized by motor disturbances (weakness, stiffness, wasting, fasciculations) reflecting lower or upper motor neuron dysfunction; there are no objective changes on sensory examination, although there may be vague sensory complaints. The sphincters are generally spared. Cognitive changes or pseudobulbar affect may be present. The disorder is progressive, and ALS is usually fatal within 3–5 years; death usually results from pulmonary infections. Patients with bulbar involvement generally have the poorest prognosis, while patients with primary lateral sclerosis often have a longer survival despite profound quadriparesis and spasticity.

B. Laboratory and Other Studies

Electromyography may show signs of acute and chronic partial denervation with reinnervation. In patients with suspected ALS, the diagnosis should not be made with confidence unless such changes are found in at least three spinal regions (cervical, thoracic, lumbosacral) or two spinal regions and the bulbar musculature. Motor conduction velocity is usually normal but may be slightly reduced, and sensory conduction studies are also normal. Biopsy of a wasted muscle shows the histologic changes of denervation but is not necessary for diagnosis. The serum creatine kinase may be slightly elevated but never reaches the extremely high values seen in some of the muscular dystrophies. The cerebrospinal fluid is normal. To diagnose SMA, molecular genetic testing for pathogenic variants of *SMN1* is available. There are abnormal findings on rectal biopsy and reduced hexosaminidase A in serum and leukocytes in patients with juvenile SMA due to hexosaminidase deficiency.

Treatment

Riluzole, 50 mg orally twice daily, which reduces the presynaptic release of glutamate, increased short-term survival in ALS in randomized trials. Edaravone, a free radical scavenger, slows disease progression in patients with mild disease. It is administered in monthly cycles as a 60 mg intravenous infusion on days 1–14 in the first month and days 1–10 in the subsequent months.

Noninvasive ventilation at least 4 hours per day in patients with a maximal inspiratory pressure less than 60 cm H_2O may prolong survival in ALS. Symptomatic and supportive measures to treat spasticity (discussed earlier), drooling, and dysphagia, prevent contractures, and preserve mobility are important. Drooling is treated with over-the-counter decongestants, anticholinergic medications (such as trihexyphenidyl, amitriptyline, or atropine), botulinum toxin injections into the salivary glands, or use of a portable suction machine. Physical and occupational therapy are helpful throughout the disease course. Combination dextromethorphan/quinidine (20 mg/10 mg, one tablet orally once or twice daily) may relieve symptoms of pseudobulbar affect. A semiliquid diet or gastrostomy tube feeding may be needed if dysphagia is severe; it is advisable to perform the procedure before the forced vital capacity falls below 50% of predicted to minimize the risk of complications. Tracheostomy is sometimes performed if respiratory muscles are severely affected; however, in the terminal stages of these disorders, realistic expectations and advance care planning should be discussed. Information on palliative care is provided in Chapter 5.

Treatment of spinal muscular atrophy takes advantage of the fact that the SMN protein is also encoded by a second gene, *SMN2*, that usually does not translate functional protein due to aberrant splicing. Nusinersen is an antisense oligonucleotide that modulates premessenger RNA splicing of the *SMN2* gene and results in increased production of the full-length protein; it has shown effectiveness in both infants and children with SMA. It is approved for use in all ages and is administered intrathecally (12 mg every 14 days for three doses, then once after a 30-day interval, then once every 4 months). Risdiplam (5 mg orally daily for patients 2 years of age and older weighing more than 20 kg) is a small molecule *SMN2* splicing modifier that also results in production of the full-length protein and is approved for use in infants and adults. Gene therapy with intravenous delivery of an intact *SMN1* gene using a viral vector (onasemnogene abeparvovec) improves ventilator-free survival compared to historical controls and is approved by the FDA for use in children under 2 years of age with biallelic mutations in *SMN1*.

When to Refer

All patients (to exclude other treatable causes of symptoms and signs) should be referred.

When to Admit

Patients may need to be admitted for initiation or titration of noninvasive ventilation, or for periods of increased requirement of noninvasive ventilator support during pulmonary infections.

Baranello G et al; FIREFISH Working Group. Risdiplam in type 1 spinal muscular atrophy. N Engl J Med. 2021;384:915. [PMID: 33626251]

Norris SP et al. Amyotrophic lateral sclerosis: update on clinical management. Curr Opin Neurol. 2020;33:641. [PMID: 32868602]

PERIPHERAL NEUROPATHIES

Peripheral neuropathies can be categorized based on the structure primarily affected. The predominant pathologic feature may be **axonal degeneration (axonal or neuronal neuropathies)** or **paranodal or segmental demyelination.** The distinction may be possible based on neurophysiologic findings. Motor and sensory conduction velocity can be measured in accessible segments of peripheral nerves. In axonal neuropathies, conduction velocity is normal or reduced only mildly and needle electromyography provides evidence of denervation in affected muscles. In demyelinating neuropathies, conduction may be slowed considerably in affected fibers, and in more severe cases, conduction is blocked completely, without accompanying electromyographic signs of denervation.

POLYNEUROPATHIES & MONONEURITIS MULTIPLEX

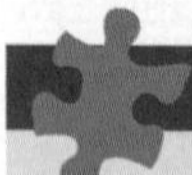

ESSENTIALS OF DIAGNOSIS

- Weakness, sensory disturbances, or both in the extremities.
- Pain is common.
- Depressed or absent tendon reflexes.
- May be family history of neuropathy.
- May be history of systemic illness or toxic exposure.

General Considerations

Diffuse **polyneuropathies** lead to a symmetric sensory, motor, or mixed deficit, often most marked distally. They include the hereditary, metabolic, and toxic disorders; idiopathic inflammatory polyneuropathy (**Guillain-Barré syndrome**); and the peripheral neuropathies that may occur as a nonmetastatic complication of malignant diseases. Involvement of motor fibers leads to flaccid weakness that is most marked distally; dysfunction of sensory fibers causes impaired sensory perception. Tendon reflexes are depressed or absent. Paresthesias, pain, and muscle tenderness may also occur. Multiple mononeuropathies (**mononeuropathy multiplex**) suggest a patchy multifocal disease process such as vasculopathy (eg, diabetes, arteritis), an infiltrative process (eg, leprosy, sarcoidosis), radiation damage, or an immunologic disorder (eg, brachial plexopathy).

Clinical Findings

The cause of polyneuropathy or mononeuritis multiplex is suggested by the history, mode of onset, and predominant clinical manifestations. Laboratory workup includes a CBC, serum protein electrophoresis with reflex to immunofixation or immunotyping, determination of plasma urea and electrolytes, liver biochemical tests, thyroid function tests, vitamin B_{12} level, tests for rheumatoid factor and antinuclear antibody, HBsAg determination, a serologic test for syphilis, fasting blood glucose level and hemoglobin A_{1c}, urinary heavy metal levels, cerebrospinal fluid examination, and chest radiography. These tests should be ordered selectively, as guided by symptoms and signs. Measurement of nerve conduction velocity can confirm the peripheral nerve origin of symptoms and provides a means of following clinical changes, as well as indicate the likely disease process (ie, axonal or demyelinating neuropathy). Cutaneous nerve biopsy may help establish a precise diagnosis (eg, polyarteritis, amyloidosis). In about half of cases, no specific cause can be established; of these, slightly less than half are subsequently found to be familial.

Treatment

Treatment is of the underlying cause, when feasible, and is discussed below under the individual disorders. Physical therapy helps prevent contractures, and splints can maintain a weak extremity in a position of useful function. Anesthetic extremities must be protected from injury. To guard against burns, patients should check the temperature of water and hot surfaces with a portion of skin having normal sensation, measure water temperature with a thermometer, and use cold water for washing or lower the temperature setting of their hot-water heaters. Shoes should be examined frequently during the day for grit or foreign objects in order to prevent pressure lesions.

Patients with polyneuropathies or mononeuritis multiplex are subject to additional nerve injury at pressure points and should therefore avoid such behavior as leaning on elbows or sitting with crossed legs for lengthy periods.

Neuropathic, burning pain may respond to simple analgesics, such as aspirin or NSAIDs, and to gabapentin (300 mg orally three times daily, titrated up to a maximum of 1200 mg orally three times daily as necessary) or pregabalin (50–100 mg orally three times daily). Duloxetine (60 mg orally once or twice daily), venlafaxine (start 37.5 mg orally twice daily, and titrate up to 75 mg orally two to three times daily), or tricyclic antidepressants (eg, amitriptyline 10–150 mg orally at bedtime daily) may be helpful, especially in painful diabetic neuropathy. Medical cannabis may provide some relief, but long-term safety data are lacking. The use of a frame or cradle to reduce contact with bedclothes may be helpful. Many patients experience episodic stabbing pains, which may respond to gabapentin, pregabalin, carbamazepine (start 100 mg orally twice daily, and titrate up to 400 mg orally twice daily), or tricyclic antidepressants. Opioids may be necessary for severe hyperpathia or pain induced by minimal stimuli, but their use generally should be avoided.

Symptoms of autonomic dysfunction are occasionally troublesome. Treatment of postural hypotension is discussed earlier in this chapter. Erectile dysfunction can be treated with phosphodiesterase inhibitors; a flaccid neuropathic bladder may respond to parasympathomimetic medications such as bethanechol chloride, 10–50 mg three or four times daily.

1. Inherited Neuropathies

A. Charcot-Marie-Tooth Disease (HMSN Type I, II)

There are several distinct varieties of Charcot-Marie-Tooth disease, usually with an autosomal dominant mode of inheritance, but occasional cases occur on a sporadic, recessive, or X-linked basis. Clinical presentation may be with foot deformities or gait disturbances in childhood or early adult life. Slow progression leads to the typical features of polyneuropathy, with distal weakness and wasting that begin in the legs, a variable amount of distal sensory loss, and depressed or absent tendon reflexes. Tremor is a conspicuous feature in some instances. **Hereditary motor and sensory neuropathy (HMSN) type I** is characterized by demyelination on electrodiagnostic studies and is usually caused by mutations in the peripheral myelin protein 22 or myelin protein zero gene. In **HMSN type II**, electrodiagnostic studies show axonal loss rather than demyelination; one-third of cases are due to mutations in the gene mitofusin 2.

A similar disorder may occur in patients with progressive distal SMAs, but there is no sensory loss; electrophysiologic investigation reveals that motor conduction velocity is normal or only slightly reduced, and nerve action potentials are normal.

B. Dejerine-Sottas Disease (HMSN Type III)

The disorder may occur on a sporadic, autosomal dominant or, less commonly, autosomal recessive basis. Onset in infancy or childhood leads to a progressive motor and sensory polyneuropathy with weakness, ataxia, sensory loss, and depressed or absent tendon reflexes. The peripheral nerves may be palpably enlarged and are characterized pathologically by segmental demyelination, Schwann cell hyperplasia, and thin myelin sheaths. Electrophysiologically, there is a slowing of conduction, and sensory action potentials may be unrecordable.

C. Friedreich Ataxia

This disorder, the only known **autosomal recessive trinucleotide repeat disease,** is caused most commonly by expansion of a poly-GAA locus in the gene for frataxin on chromosome 9, leading to symptoms in childhood or early adult life. The gait becomes ataxic, the hands become clumsy, and other signs of cerebellar dysfunction develop accompanied by weakness of the legs and extensor plantar responses. Involvement of peripheral sensory fibers leads to sensory disturbances in the limbs and depressed tendon reflexes. There is bilateral pes cavus. Pathologically, there is a marked loss of cells in the posterior root ganglia and degeneration of peripheral sensory fibers. In the CNS, changes are conspicuous in the posterior and lateral columns of the cord. Electrophysiologically, conduction velocity in motor fibers is normal or only mildly reduced, but sensory action potentials are small or absent. Cardiac disease is the most common cause of death.

In the differential diagnosis for Friedreich ataxia are other spinocerebellar ataxias, a growing group of inherited disorders, each involving a different identified gene. These heterogeneous disorders, which frequently (but not exclusively) exhibit an autosomal dominant inheritance pattern and poly-CAG expansion of the affected gene, typically cause cerebellar ataxia and varying combinations of other symptoms (such as peripheral neuropathy, ophthalmoparesis, dysarthria, and pyramidal and extrapyramidal signs).

D. Refsum Disease (HMSN Type IV)

This autosomal recessive disorder is due to a disturbance in phytanic acid metabolism. Pigmentary retinal degeneration is accompanied by progressive sensorimotor polyneuropathy and cerebellar signs. Auditory dysfunction, cardiomyopathy, and cutaneous manifestations may also occur. Motor and sensory conduction velocities are reduced, often markedly, and there may be electromyographic evidence of denervation in affected muscles. Dietary restriction of phytanic acid and its precursors may be helpful therapeutically. Plasmapheresis to reduce stored phytanic acid may help at the initiation of treatment.

E. Porphyria

Peripheral nerve involvement may occur during acute attacks in both **variegate porphyria** and **acute intermittent porphyria.** Motor symptoms usually occur first, and weakness is often most marked proximally and in the upper limbs rather than the lower. Sensory symptoms and signs may be proximal or distal in distribution. Autonomic involvement is sometimes pronounced. The electrophysiologic findings are in keeping with the results of neuropathologic studies suggesting that the neuropathy is axonal in type (see Chapter 40).

F. Familial Amyloid Polyneuropathy

Sensory and autonomic symptoms are especially conspicuous, whereas distal wasting and weakness occur later. The polyneuropathy is axonal and likely results from amyloid deposition within the peripheral nerves due to mutations in the genes encoding transthyretin, apolipoprotein A1, or gelsolin. **Transthyretin amyloidosis** is the most common; is associated with cardiomyopathy, nephropathy, leptomeningeal involvement, and vitreous opacity; and is treatable with liver transplantation, the small interfering ribonucleic acid patisiran (0.3 mg/kg up to 30 mg intravenously once every 3 weeks), or the antisense oligonucleotide inotersen (284 mg subcutaneously weekly). Tafamidis helps transthyretin amyloid cardiomyopathy and may slow the progression of the neuropathy.

2. Neuropathies Associated with Systemic & Metabolic Disorders

A. Diabetes Mellitus

In this disorder, involvement of the peripheral nervous system may lead to symmetric sensory or mixed polyneuropathy, asymmetric motor radiculoneuropathy or plexopathy (diabetic amyotrophy), thoracoabdominal radiculopathy, autonomic neuropathy, or isolated lesions of individual nerves. These may occur singly or in any combination and are discussed in Chapter 27.

B. Uremia

Uremia may lead to a symmetric sensorimotor polyneuropathy that tends to affect the lower limbs more than the upper limbs and is more marked distally than proximally (see Chapter 22). The diagnosis can be confirmed electrophysiologically because motor and sensory conduction velocity is moderately reduced. The neuropathy improves both clinically and electrophysiologically with kidney transplantation and to a lesser extent with chronic dialysis.

C. Alcohol Use Disorder and Nutritional Deficiency

Many patients with alcohol use disorder have an axonal distal sensorimotor polyneuropathy that is frequently accompanied by painful cramps, muscle tenderness, and painful paresthesias and is often more marked in the legs than in the arms. Symptoms of autonomic dysfunction may also be conspicuous. Motor and sensory conduction velocity may be slightly reduced, even in subclinical cases, but gross slowing of conduction is uncommon. Treatment is similar to diabetic polyneuropathy but also includes abstinence from alcohol. A similar distal sensorimotor polyneuropathy is a well-recognized feature of **beriberi** (thiamine deficiency). In vitamin B_{12} deficiency, distal sensory polyneuropathy may develop but is usually overshadowed by CNS manifestations (eg, myelopathy, optic neuropathy, or intellectual changes).

D. Paraproteinemias

A symmetric sensorimotor polyneuropathy that is gradual in onset, progressive in course, and often accompanied by pain and dysesthesias in the limbs may occur in patients (especially men) with **plasma cell myeloma** (formerly multiple myeloma). The neuropathy is of the axonal type in classic lytic myeloma, but segmental demyelination (primary or secondary) and axonal loss may occur in sclerotic myeloma and lead to predominantly motor clinical manifestations. Both demyelinating and axonal neuropathies are also observed in patients with paraproteinemias without myeloma. A small fraction will develop myeloma if serially followed. The demyelinating neuropathy in these patients may be due to the monoclonal proteins reacting to a component of the nerve myelin. The neuropathy of classic plasma cell myeloma is poorly responsive to therapy. The polyneuropathy of **benign monoclonal gammopathy** may respond to immunosuppressant medications and plasmapheresis.

Polyneuropathy may also occur in association with monoclonal gammopathy of unknown significance, macroglobulinemia, and cryoglobulinemia and sometimes responds to plasmapheresis. Many patients with an IgM M-protein will have antibodies to myelin-associated glycoprotein (MAG); these patients may respond to treatment with rituximab. Entrapment neuropathy, such as carpal tunnel syndrome, is more common than polyneuropathy in patients with (nonhereditary) generalized amyloidosis.

3. Neuropathies Associated with Infectious & Inflammatory Diseases

A. Leprosy

Leprosy is an important cause of peripheral neuropathy in certain parts of the world. Sensory disturbances are mainly due to involvement of intracutaneous nerves. In tuberculoid leprosy, they develop at the same time and in the same distribution as the nerve; trunks lying beneath the lesion are also involved. In lepromatous leprosy, there is more extensive sensory loss, and this develops earlier and to a greater extent in the coolest regions of the body, such as the dorsal surfaces of the hands and feet, where the bacilli proliferate most actively. Motor deficits result from involvement of superficial nerves where their temperature is lowest, eg, the ulnar nerve in the region proximal to the olecranon groove, the median nerve as it emerges from beneath the forearm flexor muscle to run toward the carpal tunnel, the peroneal nerve at the head of the fibula, and the posterior tibial nerve in the lower part of the leg; patchy facial muscular weakness may also occur owing to involvement of the superficial branches of the seventh cranial nerve.

Motor disturbances in leprosy are suggestive of multiple mononeuropathy, whereas sensory changes resemble those of distal polyneuropathy. Examination, however, relates the distribution of sensory deficits to the temperature of the tissues; in the legs, for example, sparing frequently occurs between the toes and in the popliteal fossae, where the temperature is higher. Treatment is with antileprotic agents (see Chapter 33).

B. AIDS

A variety of neuropathies occur in patients with HIV (see Chapter 31).

C. Lyme Borreliosis

The neurologic manifestations of Lyme disease include meningitis, meningoencephalitis, polyradiculoneuropathy, mononeuropathy multiplex, and cranial neuropathy. Serologic tests establish the underlying disorder. Lyme disease and its treatment are discussed in depth in Chapter 34.

D. Sarcoidosis

Cranial nerve palsies (especially facial palsy), multiple mononeuropathy and, less commonly, symmetric polyneuropathy may all occur, the latter sometimes preferentially affecting either motor or sensory fibers. Improvement may occur with use of corticosteroids.

E. Polyarteritis

Involvement of the vasa nervorum by the vasculitic process may result in infarction of the nerve. Clinically, one encounters an asymmetric sensorimotor polyneuropathy (mononeuritis multiplex) that pursues a waxing and waning course. Corticosteroids, cyclophosphamide, or rituximab helps, depending on the specific case (Chapter 20).

F. Rheumatoid Arthritis

Compressive or entrapment neuropathies, ischemic neuropathies, mild distal sensory polyneuropathy, and severe progressive sensorimotor polyneuropathy can occur in rheumatoid arthritis (Chapter 20).

4. Neuropathy Associated with Critical Illness

Patients in ICUs with sepsis and multiorgan failure sometimes develop polyneuropathies. This may be manifested initially by unexpected difficulty in weaning patients from a mechanical ventilator and in more advanced cases by wasting and weakness of the extremities and loss of tendon reflexes. Sensory abnormalities are relatively inconspicuous. The neuropathy is axonal in type. Its pathogenesis is obscure, and treatment is supportive. The prognosis is good provided that patients recover from the underlying critical illness. A myopathy may also occur (discussed below).

5. Toxic Neuropathies

Axonal polyneuropathy may follow exposure to industrial agents or pesticides such as acrylamide, organophosphorus compounds, hexacarbon solvents, methyl bromide, and carbon disulfide; metals such as arsenic, thallium, mercury, and lead; and medications such as phenytoin, amiodarone, perhexiline, isoniazid, nitrofurantoin, vincristine, and pyridoxine in high doses. Detailed occupational, environmental, and medical histories and recognition of clusters of cases are important in suggesting the diagnosis. Treatment is by preventing further exposure to the causal agent. Isoniazid neuropathy is prevented by pyridoxine supplementation.

Diphtheritic neuropathy results from a neurotoxin released by the causative organism and is common in many areas. Palatal weakness may develop 2–4 weeks after infection of the throat, and infection of the skin may similarly be followed by focal weakness of neighboring muscles. Disturbances of accommodation may occur about 4–5 weeks after infection and distal sensorimotor demyelinating polyneuropathy after 1–3 months.

6. Neuropathies Associated with Malignant Diseases

A variety of neuropathies have been associated with nonmetastatic complications of malignancy and were discussed earlier.

7. Acute Idiopathic Polyneuropathy (Guillain-Barré Syndrome)

ESSENTIALS OF DIAGNOSIS

- Acute or subacute progressive polyradiculoneuropathy.
- Weakness is more severe than sensory disturbances.
- Acute dysautonomia may be life-threatening.

General Considerations

This acute or subacute polyradiculoneuropathy sometimes follows infective illness, inoculations, or surgical procedures. There is an association with preceding *Campylobacter jejuni* enteritis. The disorder probably has an immunologic basis, but the precise mechanism is unclear.

Clinical Findings

A. Symptoms and Signs

The main complaint is of weakness that varies widely in severity in different patients and often has a proximal emphasis and symmetric distribution. It usually begins in the legs, spreading to a variable extent but frequently involving the arms and often one or both sides of the face. The muscles of respiration or deglutition may also be affected. Sensory symptoms are usually less conspicuous than motor ones, but distal paresthesias and dysesthesias are common, and neuropathic or radicular pain is present in many patients. Autonomic disturbances are also common, may be severe, and are sometimes life-threatening; they include tachycardia, cardiac irregularities, hypotension or hypertension, facial flushing, abnormalities of sweating, pulmonary dysfunction, and impaired sphincter control. The axonal subtypes of the syndrome (**acute motor axonal neuropathy** [AMAN] and **acute motor and sensory axonal neuropathy** [AMSAN]) are caused by antibodies to gangliosides on the axon membrane. The **Miller Fisher syndrome,** another subtype, is characterized by the clinical triad of ophthalmoplegia, ataxia, and areflexia, and is associated with anti-GQ1b antibodies.

B. Laboratory Findings

The cerebrospinal fluid characteristically contains a high protein concentration with a normal cell count, but these changes may take up to 2 weeks to develop; WBC counts greater than 50 cells/mcL (0.05×10^9/L) should prompt consideration of alternative diagnoses. Electrophysiologic studies may reveal marked abnormalities, which do not necessarily parallel the clinical disorder in their temporal course.

Differential Diagnosis

When the diagnosis is made, the history and appropriate laboratory studies should exclude the possibility of porphyric, diphtheritic, or toxic (heavy metal, hexacarbon, organophosphate) neuropathies, and of HIV infection. The temporal course excludes other peripheral neuropathies. Poliomyelitis, botulism, and tick paralysis must also be considered as they cause weakness of acute onset. The presence of pyramidal signs, a markedly asymmetric motor deficit, a sharp sensory level, or early sphincter involvement should suggest a focal cord lesion.

Treatment

Treatment with prednisone is ineffective and may prolong recovery time. Plasmapheresis is of value; it is best performed within the first few days of illness and is particularly useful for clinically severe or rapidly progressive cases or those with ventilatory impairment. IVIG (400 mg/kg/day for 5 days) is equally helpful. Patients should be admitted to ICUs if their forced vital capacity is declining, and intubation is considered if the forced vital capacity reaches 15 mL/kg, the maximum inspiratory pressure reaches −30 mm Hg, or dyspnea becomes evident. Declining oxygen saturation is a late indicator of neuromuscular respiratory failure. Respiratory toilet and chest physical therapy help prevent atelectasis. Marked hypotension may respond to volume replacement or pressor agents. Thromboprophylaxis is important.

Prognosis

Most patients eventually make a good recovery, but this may take many months, and about 20% of patients are left with persisting disability. Approximately 3% of patients with acute idiopathic polyneuropathy have one or more clinically similar relapses, sometimes several years after the initial illness.

When to Refer

All patients should be referred.

When to Admit

All patients should be hospitalized until their condition is stable and there is no respiratory compromise.

Malek E et al. Guillain-Barré syndrome. Semin Neurol. 2019;39:589. [PMID: 31639842]

8. Chronic Inflammatory Polyneuropathy

Chronic inflammatory demyelinating polyneuropathy, an acquired immunologically mediated disorder, is clinically similar to Guillain-Barré syndrome except that it has a relapsing or steadily progressive course over months or years and that autonomic dysfunction is generally less common. It may present as an exclusively motor disorder or with a mixed sensorimotor disturbance. In the relapsing form, partial recovery may occur after some relapses, but in other instances there is no recovery between exacerbations. Although remission may occur spontaneously with time, the disorder frequently follows a progressive downhill course leading to severe functional disability.

Electrodiagnostic studies show marked slowing of motor and sensory conduction, and focal conduction block. Signs of partial denervation may also be present owing to secondary axonal degeneration. Nerve biopsy may show chronic perivascular inflammatory infiltrates in the endoneurium and epineurium, without accompanying evidence of vasculitis. However, a normal nerve biopsy result or the presence of nonspecific abnormalities does not exclude the diagnosis.

Corticosteroids may arrest or reverse the downhill course. Treatment is usually begun with prednisone, 60–80 mg orally daily, continued for 2–3 months or until a definite response has occurred. If no response has occurred despite 3 months of treatment, a higher dose may be tried. In responsive cases, the dose is gradually tapered, but most patients become corticosteroid-dependent, often requiring prednisone, 20 mg daily on alternate days, on a long-term basis. IVIG can be used in place of, or in addition to corticosteroids, and is best used as the initial treatment in pure motor syndromes (2 g/kg over 2–5 days followed by 1 g/kg every 3 weeks); a weekly regimen of 0.2–0.4 g/kg of a 20% subcutaneous immunoglobulin solution is an effective alternative but has not been compared directly to corticosteroids or IVIG. When both IVIG and corticosteroids are ineffective, plasma exchange may be worthwhile. Consistent with the notion that the condition is antibody-mediated, rituximab has shown promise. Immunosuppressant or immunomodulatory medications (such as azathioprine) may be added when the response to other measures is unsatisfactory or to enable maintenance doses of corticosteroids to be lowered. Symptomatic treatment is also important.

Bunschoten C et al. Progress in diagnosis and treatment of chronic inflammatory demyelinating polyneuropathy. Lancet Neurol. 2019;18:784. [PMID: 31076244]

MONONEUROPATHIES

ESSENTIALS OF DIAGNOSIS

- Focal motor or sensory deficit.
- Deficit is in territory of an individual peripheral nerve.

An individual nerve may be injured along its course or may be compressed, angulated, or stretched by neighboring anatomic structures, especially at a point where it passes through a narrow space (**entrapment neuropathy**). The relative contributions of mechanical factors and ischemia to the local damage are not clear. With involvement of a sensory or mixed nerve, pain is commonly felt distal to the lesion. Symptoms never develop with some entrapment neuropathies, resolve rapidly and spontaneously in others, and become progressively more disabling and distressing in yet other cases. The precise neurologic deficit depends on the nerve involved. Percussion of the nerve at the site of the lesion may lead to paresthesias in its distal distribution.

Entrapment neuropathy may be the sole manifestation of subclinical polyneuropathy, and this must be borne in mind and excluded by nerve conduction studies. Such studies are also indispensable for the localization of the focal lesion.

In patients with acute compression neuropathy such as may occur in intoxicated individuals (**Saturday night palsy**), no treatment is necessary. Complete recovery generally occurs, usually within 2 months, presumably because the underlying pathology is demyelination. However, axonal degeneration can occur in severe cases, and recovery then takes longer and may never be complete.

In chronic compressive or entrapment neuropathies, avoidance of aggravating factors and correction of any underlying systemic conditions are important. Local infiltration of the region about the nerve with corticosteroids may be of value; in addition, surgical decompression may help if there is a progressively increasing neurologic deficit or if electrodiagnostic studies show evidence of partial denervation in weak muscles.

Peripheral nerve tumors are uncommon, except in neurofibromatosis type 1, but also give rise to mononeuropathy. This may be distinguishable from entrapment neuropathy only by noting the presence of a mass along the course of the nerve and by demonstrating the precise site of the lesion with appropriate electrophysiologic studies. Treatment of symptomatic lesions is by surgical removal if possible.

1. Carpal Tunnel Syndrome

See Chapter 41.

2. Pronator Teres or Anterior Interosseous Syndrome

The median nerve gives off its motor branch, the anterior interosseous nerve, below the elbow as it descends between the two heads of the pronator teres muscle. A lesion of either nerve may occur in this region, sometimes after trauma or owing to compression from, for example, a fibrous band. With anterior interosseous nerve involvement, there is no sensory loss, and weakness is confined to the pronator quadratus, flexor pollicis longus, and the flexor digitorum profundus to the second and third digits. Weakness is more widespread and sensory changes occur in an appropriate distribution when the median nerve itself is affected. The prognosis is variable. If improvement does not occur spontaneously, decompressive surgery may be helpful.

3. Ulnar Nerve Lesions

Ulnar nerve lesions are likely to occur in the elbow region as the nerve runs behind the medial epicondyle and descends into the cubital tunnel. In the condylar groove, the ulnar nerve is exposed to pressure or trauma. Moreover, any increase in the carrying angle of the elbow, whether congenital, degenerative, or traumatic, may cause excessive stretching of the nerve when the elbow is flexed. Ulnar nerve lesions may also result from thickening or distortion of the anatomic structures forming the cubital tunnel, and the resulting symptoms may also be aggravated by flexion of the elbow, because the tunnel is then narrowed by tightening of its roof or inward bulging of its floor. A severe lesion at either site causes sensory changes in the fifth and medial half of the fourth digits and along the medial border of the hand. There is weakness of the ulnar-innervated muscles in the forearm and hand. With a cubital tunnel lesion, however, there may be relative sparing of the flexor carpi ulnaris muscle. Electrophysiologic evaluation using nerve stimulation techniques allows more precise localization of the lesion.

Initial treatment consists of avoiding pressure on the medial elbow (eg, avoid resting the elbows on arm rests; pad the elbow during sleep) and preventing prolonged elbow flexion, especially at night. Splints are available to keep the elbow from flexing beyond 45 to 90 degrees. If conservative measures are unsuccessful in relieving symptoms and preventing further progression, surgical treatment may be necessary. This consists of nerve transposition if the lesion is in the condylar groove, or a release procedure if it is in the cubital tunnel.

Ulnar nerve lesions may also develop at the wrist or in the palm of the hand, usually owing to repetitive trauma or to compression from ganglia or benign tumors. They can be subdivided depending on their presumed site. Compressive lesions are treated surgically. If repetitive mechanical trauma is responsible, this is avoided by occupational adjustment or job retraining.

4. Radial Nerve Lesions

The radial nerve is particularly liable to compression or injury in the axilla (eg, by crutches or by pressure when the arm hangs over the back of a chair). This leads to weakness or paralysis of all the muscles supplied by the nerve, including the triceps. Sensory changes may also occur but are often surprisingly inconspicuous, being marked only in a small area on the back of the hand between the thumb and index finger. Injuries to the radial nerve in the spiral groove occur characteristically during deep sleep, as in intoxicated individuals, and there is then sparing of the triceps muscle, which is supplied more proximally. The nerve may also be injured at or above the elbow; its purely motor posterior interosseous branch, supplying the extensors of the wrist and fingers, may be involved immediately below the elbow, but then there is sparing of the extensor carpi radialis longus, so that the wrist can still be extended. The superficial radial nerve may be compressed by handcuffs or a tight watch strap.

5. Femoral Neuropathy

The clinical features of femoral nerve palsy consist of weakness and wasting of the quadriceps muscle, with sensory impairment over the anteromedian aspect of the thigh and sometimes also of the leg to the medial malleolus, and a depressed or absent knee jerk. Isolated femoral neuropathy may occur in patients with diabetes or from compression by retroperitoneal neoplasms or hematomas (eg, expanding aortic aneurysm). Femoral neuropathy may also result from pressure from the inguinal ligament when the thighs are markedly flexed and abducted, as in the lithotomy position.

6. Meralgia Paresthetica

The **lateral femoral cutaneous nerve**, a sensory nerve arising from the L2 and L3 roots, may be compressed or stretched in obese or diabetic patients and during pregnancy. The nerve usually runs under the outer portion of the inguinal ligament to reach the thigh, but the ligament sometimes splits to enclose it. Hyperextension of the hip or increased lumbar lordosis—such as occurs during pregnancy—leads to nerve compression by the posterior fascicle of the ligament. However, entrapment of the nerve at any point along its course may cause similar symptoms, and several other anatomic variations predispose the nerve to damage when it is stretched. Pain, paresthesia, or numbness occurs about the outer aspect of the thigh, usually unilaterally, and is sometimes relieved by sitting. The pain stops at the knee, unlike the pain from lower lumbar sciatica that radiates to the foot. Examination shows no abnormalities except in severe cases when cutaneous sensation is impaired in the affected area. Symptoms are usually mild and commonly settle spontaneously. Hydrocortisone injections medial to the anterosuperior iliac spine often relieve symptoms temporarily, while nerve decompression by transposition may provide more lasting relief.

7. Sciatic & Fibular (Common Peroneal) Nerve Palsies

Misplaced deep intramuscular injections are probably still the most common cause of sciatic nerve palsy. Trauma to the buttock, hip, or thigh may also be responsible. The resulting clinical deficit depends on whether the whole nerve has been affected or only certain fibers. In general, the fibular fibers of the sciatic nerve are more susceptible to damage than those destined for the tibial nerve. A sciatic nerve lesion may therefore be difficult to distinguish from fibular neuropathy unless there is electromyographic evidence of involvement of the short head of the biceps femoris muscle. The fibular nerve itself may be compressed or injured in the region of the head and neck of the fibula, eg, by sitting with crossed legs or wearing high boots. There is weakness of dorsiflexion and eversion of the foot, accompanied by numbness or blunted sensation of the anterolateral aspect of the calf and dorsum of the foot.

8. Tarsal Tunnel Syndrome

The tibial nerve, the other branch of the sciatic, supplies several muscles in the lower extremity, gives origin to the sural nerve, and then continues as the posterior tibial nerve to supply the plantar flexors of the foot and toes. It passes through the tarsal tunnel behind and below the medial malleolus, giving off calcaneal branches and the medial and lateral plantar nerves that supply small muscles of the foot and the skin on the plantar aspect of the foot and toes. Compression of the posterior tibial nerve or its branches between the bony floor and ligamentous roof of the tarsal tunnel leads to pain, paresthesias, and numbness over the bottom of the foot, especially at night, with sparing of the heel. Muscle weakness may be hard to recognize clinically. Compressive lesions of the individual plantar nerves may also occur more distally, with clinical features similar to those of the tarsal tunnel syndrome. Treatment is surgical decompression.

When to Refer

- If there is uncertainty about the diagnosis.
- Symptoms or signs are progressing despite treatment.

BELL PALSY

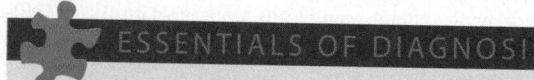

- Sudden onset of lower motor neuron facial palsy.
- Hyperacusis or impaired taste may occur.
- No other neurologic abnormalities.

General Considerations

Bell palsy is an *idiopathic facial paresis of lower motor neuron type* that has been attributed to an inflammatory reaction involving the facial nerve near the stylomastoid foramen or in the bony facial canal. In some instances, this may be due to reactivation of herpes simplex or varicella zoster virus infection in the geniculate ganglion. The disorder is more common in pregnant women and in persons with diabetes mellitus.

Clinical Findings

The facial paresis (Figure 24–1) generally comes on abruptly, but it may worsen over the following day or so. Pain about the ear precedes or accompanies the weakness in many cases but usually lasts for only a few days. The face itself feels stiff and pulled to one side. There may be ipsilateral restriction of eye closure and difficulty with eating and

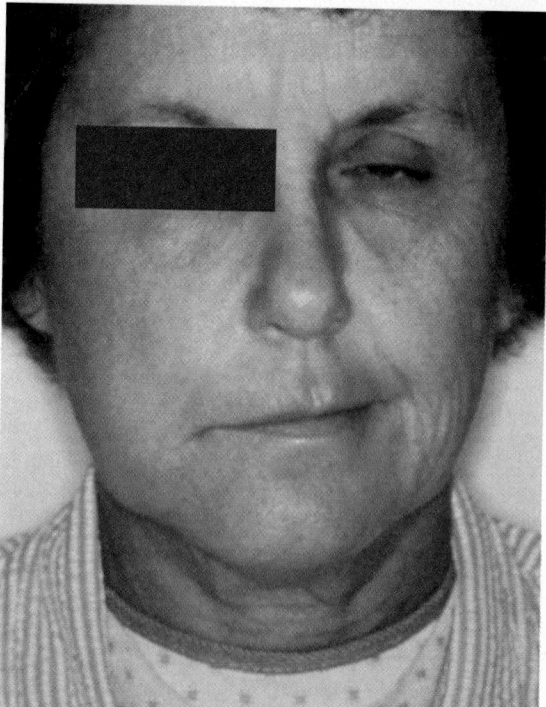

Figure 24–1. Facial palsy caused by an infection with *Borrelia burgdorferi* (Lyme disease). (Public Health Image Library, CDC.)

fine facial movements. A disturbance of taste is common, owing to involvement of chorda tympani fibers, and hyperacusis due to involvement of fibers to the stapedius occurs occasionally. In cases due to herpes zoster infection, vesicles may be observed in the external ear canal.

Differential Diagnosis

Lower motor neuron facial palsy can be differentiated from stroke by clinical examination. A stroke or other central lesion will not cause hyperacusis or disturbance of taste, generally spares the forehead, and is accompanied by other focal deficits. An isolated facial palsy may occur in patients with HIV seropositivity, sarcoidosis, Lyme disease (Figure 24–1; also see Chapter 34), or any process causing an inflammatory reaction in the subarachnoid space, such as meningitis. Whenever facial palsies occur bilaterally, or a facial palsy occurs in conjunction with other neurologic deficits, MRI brain imaging should be undertaken and other investigations considered.

Treatment

Approximately 60% of cases of Bell palsy recover completely without treatment, presumably because the lesion is so mild that it leads merely to conduction block. Treatment with corticosteroids (prednisone 60 mg orally daily for 5 days followed by a 5-day taper, or prednisolone 25 mg orally twice daily for 10 days) increases the chance of a complete recovery at 9–12 months by 12–15%. Treatment with acyclovir or valacyclovir is only indicated when there is evidence of herpetic vesicles in the external ear canal. It is helpful to protect the eye with lubricating drops (or lubricating ointment at night) and a patch if eye closure is not possible. There is no evidence that surgical procedures to decompress the facial nerve are of benefit. Physical therapy may improve facial function.

Gagyor I et al. Antiviral treatment of Bell's palsy (idiopathic facial paralysis). Cochrane Database Syst Rev. 2019;9: CD001869. [PMID: 31486071]

DISCOGENIC NECK PAIN

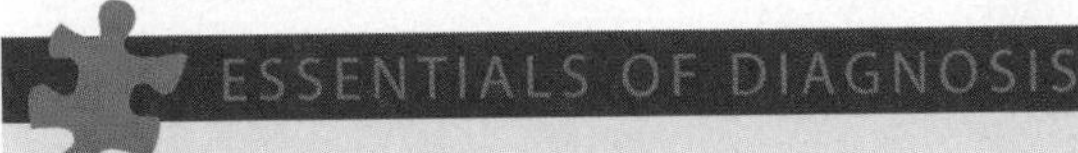

- Neck pain, sometimes radiating to arms.
- Restricted neck movements.
- Motor, sensory, or reflex changes in arms with root involvement.
- Neurologic deficit in legs, gait disorder, or sphincter disturbance with cord involvement.

General Considerations

A variety of congenital abnormalities may involve the cervical spine and lead to neck pain; these include hemivertebrae, fused vertebrae, basilar impression, and instability of the atlantoaxial joint. Traumatic, degenerative, infective, and neoplastic disorders may also lead to pain in the neck. When rheumatoid arthritis involves the spine, it tends to affect especially the cervical region, leading to pain, stiffness, and reduced mobility; displacement of vertebrae or atlantoaxial subluxation may lead to cord compression that can be life-threatening if not treated by fixation. Further details are given in Chapter 41 and discussion here is restricted to disk disease.

1. Acute Cervical Disk Protrusion

Acute cervical disk protrusion leads to pain in the neck and radicular pain in the arm, exacerbated by head movement. With lateral herniation of the disk, motor, sensory, or reflex changes may be found in a radicular (usually C6 or C7) distribution on the affected side (Figure 24–2); with more centrally directed herniations, the spinal cord may also be involved, leading to spastic paraparesis and sensory disturbances in the legs, sometimes accompanied by impaired sphincter function. The diagnosis is confirmed by MRI or CT myelography. In mild cases, the prognosis is good and complete recovery occurs in most patients with conservative therapy. Evidence does not support any specific intervention, and some combination of bed rest, activity restriction, immobilization of the neck in a collar for several weeks, and physical therapy is generally prescribed. If these measures are unsuccessful or the patient has a significant neurologic deficit, surgical removal of the protruding disk may be necessary.

2. Cervical Spondylosis

Cervical spondylosis results from chronic cervical disk degeneration, with herniation of disk material, secondary calcification, and associated osteophytic outgrowths. One or more of the cervical nerve roots may be compressed, stretched, or angulated; and myelopathy may also develop as a result of compression, vascular insufficiency, or recurrent minor trauma to the cord. Patients present with neck pain and restricted head movement, occipital headaches, radicular pain and other sensory disturbances in the arms, weakness of the arms or legs, or some combination of these symptoms. Examination generally reveals that lateral flexion and rotation of the neck are limited. A segmental pattern of weakness or dermatomal sensory loss (or both) may be found unilaterally or bilaterally in the upper limbs, and tendon reflexes mediated by the affected root or roots are depressed. The C5 and C6 nerve roots are most commonly involved, and examination frequently then reveals weakness of muscles supplied by these roots (eg, deltoids, supraspinatus and infraspinatus, biceps, brachioradialis), pain or sensory loss about the shoulder and outer border of the arm and forearm, and depressed biceps and brachioradialis reflexes. Spastic paraparesis may also be present if there is an associated myelopathy, sometimes accompanied by urinary urgency, incontinence, or posterior column or spinothalamic sensory deficits in the legs.

Plain radiographs of the cervical spine show osteophyte formation, narrowing of disk spaces, and encroachment on the intervertebral foramina, but such changes are common

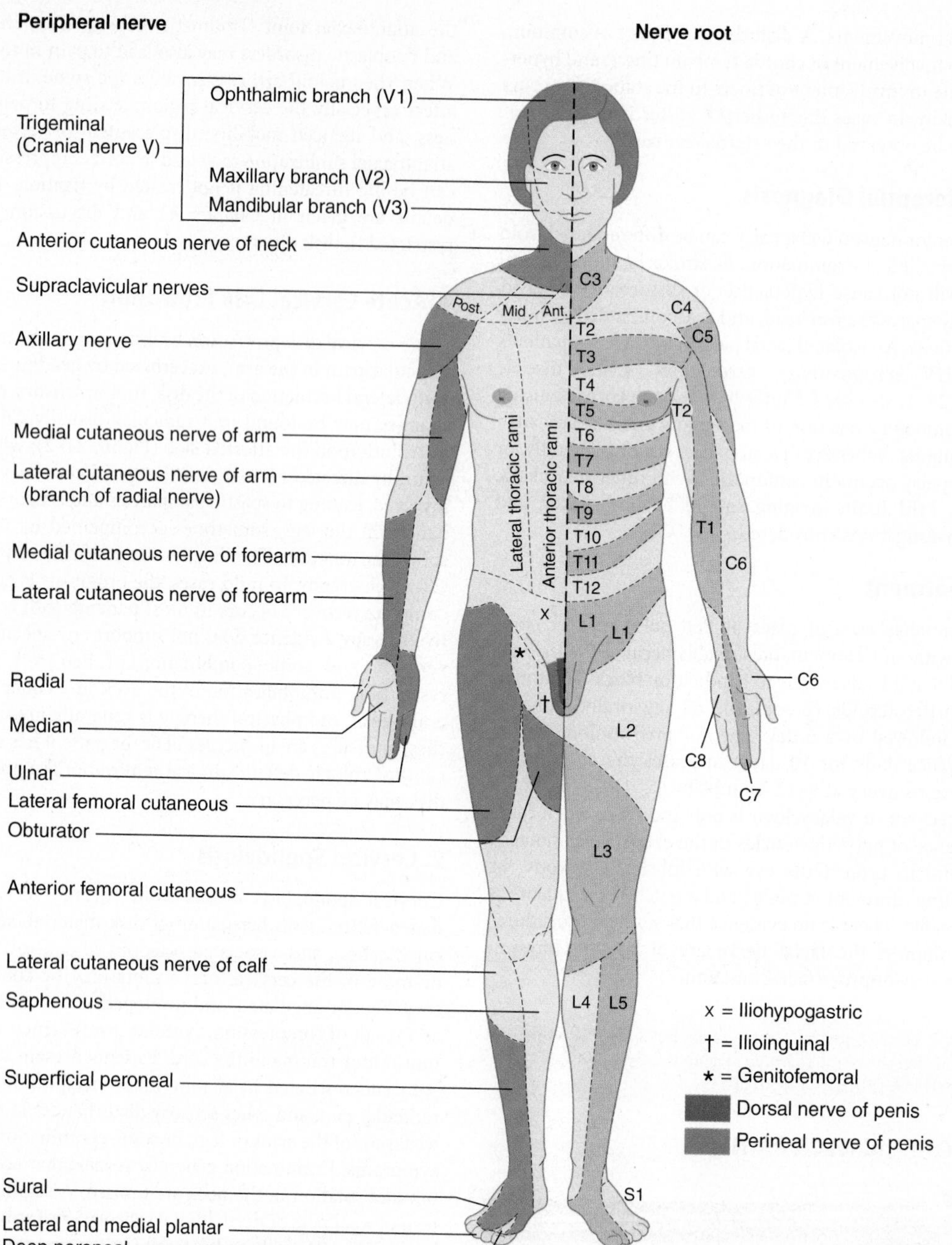

▲ **Figure 24–2.** Cutaneous innervation. The segmental or radicular (root) distribution is shown on the left side of the body and the peripheral nerve distribution on the right side. Segmental maps show differences depending on how they were constructed (single root stimulation or section; local anesthetic injection into single dorsal root ganglia). (Reproduced with permission from Aminoff MJ, Greenberg DA, Simon RP. *Clinical Neurology*, 9th ed. McGraw-Hill Education, 2015.)

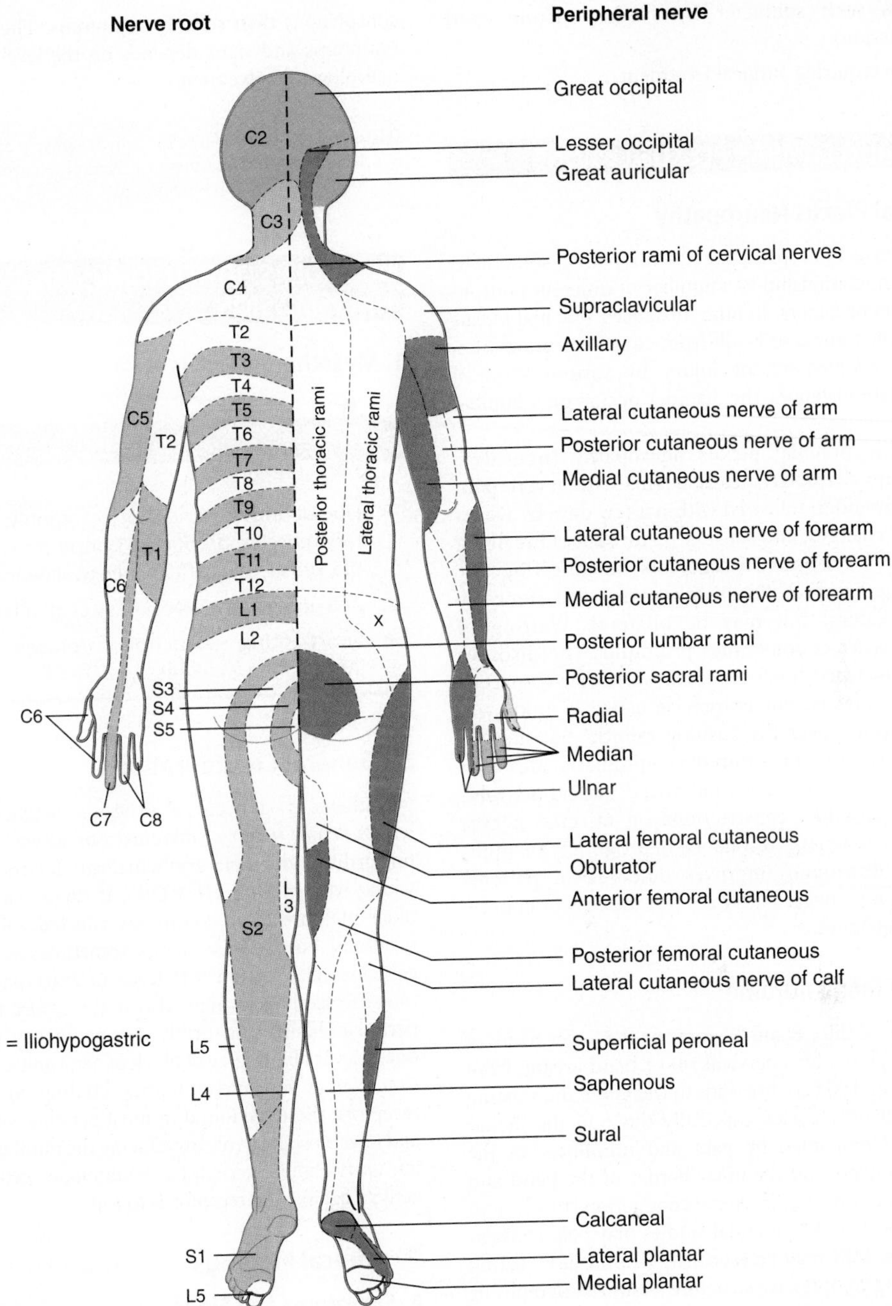

Figure 24–2. (*Continued*)

in middle-aged persons and may be unrelated to the presenting complaint. CT or MRI helps confirm the diagnosis and exclude other structural causes of the myelopathy.

Restriction of neck movements by a cervical collar may relieve pain. Local injection of anesthetics or corticosteroids, for instance by a pain management specialist, may be of benefit. Operative treatment may be necessary to prevent further progression if there is a significant neurologic deficit; if there are bowel or bladder symptoms; or if root pain is severe, persistent, and unresponsive to conservative measures.

When to Refer

- Pain unresponsive to simple measures.
- Patients with neurologic deficits.
- Patients in whom surgical treatment is under consideration.

When to Admit

- Patients with progressive or significant neurologic deficit.

- Patients with sphincter involvement (from cord compression).
- Patients requiring surgical treatment.

BRACHIAL & LUMBAR PLEXUS LESIONS

1. Brachial Plexus Neuropathy

Brachial plexus neuropathy may be idiopathic, sometimes occurring in relationship to a number of different nonspecific illnesses or factors. In other instances, brachial plexus lesions follow trauma or result from congenital anomalies, neoplastic involvement, or injury by various physical agents. In rare instances, the disorder occurs on a familial basis.

Idiopathic brachial plexus neuropathy (**neuralgic amyotrophy**) characteristically begins with severe pain about the shoulder, followed within a few days by weakness, reflex changes, and sensory disturbances involving especially the C5 and C6 segments but affecting any nerve in the brachial plexus. Symptoms and signs are usually unilateral but may be bilateral. Wasting of affected muscles is sometimes profound. The disorder relates to disturbed function of cervical roots or part of the brachial plexus, but its precise cause is unknown. Recovery occurs over the ensuing months but may be incomplete. Treatment is purely symptomatic, although emerging evidence suggests that microsurgical neurolysis of hourglass-like constrictions on affected nerves identified by magnetic resonance neurography or high-resolution ultrasound improves outcome in patients who have not recovered after several months of conservative management.

2. Cervical Rib Syndrome

Compression of the C8 and T1 roots or the lower trunk of the brachial plexus by a cervical rib or band arising from the seventh cervical vertebra leads to weakness and wasting of intrinsic hand muscles, especially those in the thenar eminence, accompanied by pain and numbness in the medial two fingers and the ulnar border of the hand and forearm. Electromyography, nerve conduction studies, and somatosensory evoked potential studies may help confirm the diagnosis. MRI may be especially helpful in revealing the underlying compressive structure. Plain radiographs or CT scanning sometimes shows the cervical rib or a large transverse process of the seventh cervical vertebra, but normal findings do not exclude the possibility of a cervical band. Treatment of the disorder is by surgical excision of the rib or band.

3. Lumbosacral Plexus Lesions

A lumbosacral plexus lesion may develop in association with diseases such as diabetes, cancer, or bleeding disorders or in relation to injury. It occasionally occurs as an isolated phenomenon similar to idiopathic brachial plexopathy (nondiabetic lumbosacral radiculoplexus neuropathy), and pain and weakness then tend to be more conspicuous than sensory symptoms. The distribution of symptoms and signs depends on the level and pattern of neurologic involvement.

Gstoettner C et al. Neuralgic amyotrophy: a paradigm shift in diagnosis and treatment. J Neurol Neurosurg Psychiatry. 2020;91:879. [PMID: 32487526]

DISORDERS OF NEUROMUSCULAR TRANSMISSION

1. Myasthenia Gravis

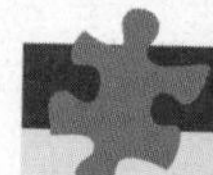

ESSENTIALS OF DIAGNOSIS

- Fluctuating weakness of commonly used voluntary muscles, producing symptoms such as diplopia, ptosis, and difficulty in swallowing.
- Activity increases weakness of affected muscles.
- Short-acting anticholinesterases transiently improve the weakness.

General Considerations

Myasthenia gravis occurs at all ages, *sometimes in association with a thymic tumor or thyrotoxicosis*, as well as in rheumatoid arthritis and lupus erythematosus. It is most common in young women with HLA-DR3; if thymoma is associated, older men are more commonly affected. Onset is usually insidious, but the disorder is sometimes unmasked by a coincidental infection that leads to exacerbation of symptoms. Exacerbations may also occur before the menstrual period and during or shortly after pregnancy. Symptoms are due to a variable degree of block of neuromuscular transmission caused by autoantibodies binding to acetylcholine receptors; these are found in most patients with the disease and have a primary role in reducing the number of functioning acetylcholine receptors. Additionally, cellular immune activity against the receptor is found.

Clinical Findings

A. Symptoms and Signs

Patients present with ptosis, diplopia, difficulty in chewing or swallowing, respiratory difficulties, limb weakness, or some combination of these problems. Weakness may remain localized to a few muscle groups or may become generalized. The external ocular muscles and certain other cranial muscles, including the masticatory, facial, and pharyngeal muscles, are especially likely to be affected, and the respiratory and limb muscles may also be involved. Symptoms often fluctuate in intensity during the day, and this diurnal variation is superimposed on a tendency to longer-term spontaneous relapses and remissions that may last for weeks. Nevertheless, the disorder follows a slowly progressive course and may have a fatal outcome owing to respiratory complications such as aspiration pneumonia.

Clinical examination confirms the weakness and fatigability of affected muscles. In most cases, the extraocular muscles are involved, and this leads to ocular palsies and ptosis, which are commonly asymmetric. Pupillary responses are normal. The bulbar and limb muscles are often weak, but the pattern of involvement is variable. Sustained activity of affected muscles increases the weakness, which improves after a brief rest. Sensation is normal, and there are usually no reflex changes.

Life-threatening exacerbations of myasthenia (so-called **myasthenic crisis**) may lead to respiratory weakness requiring immediate admission to the ICU, where respiratory function can be monitored and ventilator support is readily available.

B. Laboratory and Other Studies

Assay of serum for elevated levels of circulating acetylcholine receptor antibodies is useful because it has a sensitivity of 80–90% for the diagnosis of myasthenia gravis. Certain patients without antibodies to acetylcholine receptors have serum antibodies to muscle-specific tyrosine kinase (MuSK), which should therefore be determined; these patients are more likely to have facial, respiratory, and proximal muscle weakness than those with antibodies to acetylcholine receptors. Other antibodies associated with myasthenia gravis include LDL receptor-related protein 4 (LRP4) and agrin, but tests for these antibodies are not widely commercially available.

Electrophysiologic demonstration of a decrementing muscle response to repetitive 2- or 3-Hz stimulation of motor nerves indicates a disturbance of neuromuscular transmission. Such an abnormality may even be detected in clinically strong muscles with certain provocative procedures. Needle electromyography of affected muscles shows a marked variation in configuration and size of individual motor unit potentials, and single-fiber electromyography reveals an increased jitter, or variability, in the time interval between two muscle fiber action potentials from the same motor unit.

C. Imaging

A CT scan of the chest with and without contrast should be obtained to demonstrate a coexisting thymoma.

Treatment

Anticholinesterase medications provide symptomatic benefit without influencing the course of the disease. Neostigmine, pyridostigmine, or both can be used, the dose being determined on an individual basis. The usual dose of neostigmine is 7.5–30 mg (average, 15 mg) orally taken four times daily; of pyridostigmine, 30–180 mg (average, 60 mg) orally four times daily. Overmedication may temporarily increase weakness. A wide range of medications (eg, aminoglycosides) may exacerbate myasthenia gravis and should be avoided.

Thymectomy should be performed when a thymoma is present. A multicenter randomized trial demonstrated the benefit of thymectomy even in the absence of a radiologically identifiable thymoma, with improved strength, lower immunosuppression requirements, and fewer hospitalizations in the surgically treated group. Thus, *thymectomy should be considered in all patients younger than age 65 unless weakness is restricted to the extraocular muscles.* If the disease is of recent onset and only slowly progressive, operation is sometimes delayed for a year or so, in the hope that spontaneous remission will occur.

Treatment with corticosteroids is indicated for patients who have responded poorly to anticholinesterase medications. Some patients experience transient exacerbation of weakness and even develop respiratory failure within the first 1–2 weeks if corticosteroids are initiated at high doses (eg, prednisone 1 mg/kg/day). Therefore, in stable patients, corticosteroids are introduced gradually in the outpatient setting. Prednisone can be started at 20 mg orally daily and increased by 10 mg increments weekly to a target of 1 mg/kg/day (maximum daily dose 100 mg). For patients hospitalized with severe myasthenia and treated with IVIG or plasmapheresis, the higher dose can be given initially because the more rapid onset of action of the former two therapies mitigates the initial dip in strength due to corticosteroids. Corticosteroids can be prescribed as alternate-day or daily treatment, with alternate-day therapy potentially mitigating side effects. Once the patient has stabilized at the initial high dose, corticosteroids can gradually be tapered to a relatively low maintenance level (eg, 10 mg prednisone orally daily) as improvement occurs; total withdrawal is difficult, however. Treatment with azathioprine may be effective in allowing a lower dose of corticosteroids. The usual dose is 2–3 mg/kg orally daily after a lower initial dose. Other immunosuppressive agents that are used in myasthenia gravis to reduce the corticosteroid dose include mycophenolate mofetil, rituximab, cyclosporine, methotrexate, and tacrolimus. Eculizumab, a complement inhibitor, is approved by the FDA for acetylcholine receptor antibody positive myasthenia in patients who have disease refractory to at least two alternate immunosuppressive therapies. It is administered intravenously (900 mg weekly for four doses, followed by 1200 mg at week 5, and then 1200 mg every 2 weeks). Patients must be vaccinated against meningococcus before receiving eculizumab. A recent trial of efgartigimod, an antibody against the neonatal Fc receptor that inhibits IgG recycling and thus reduces circulating IgG, has shown benefit, and the medication is under review by the FDA as of early 2022.

In patients with major disability, plasmapheresis or IVIG therapy may be beneficial and have similar efficacy. It is also useful for stabilizing patients before thymectomy and for managing acute crisis.

When to Refer

All patients should be referred.

When to Admit

- Patients with acute exacerbation or respiratory involvement.
- Patients requiring plasmapheresis.
- For thymectomy.

Howard Jr JF et al; ADAPT Investigator Study Group. Safety, efficacy, and tolerability of efgartigimod in patient with generalized myasthenia gravis (ADAPT): a multicentre, randomised, placebo-controlled, phase 3 trial. Lancet Neurol. 2021;20:526. [PMID: 34146511]

Muppidi S et al; Regain Study Group. Long-term safety and efficacy of eculizumab in generalized myasthenia gravis. Muscle Nerve. 2019;60:14. [PMID: 30767274]

2. Myasthenic Syndrome (Lambert-Eaton Myasthenic Syndrome)

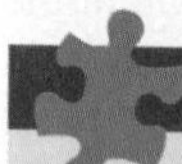

ESSENTIALS OF DIAGNOSIS

- Variable weakness, typically improving with activity.
- Dysautonomic symptoms may also be present.
- A history of malignant disease may be obtained.

Clinical Findings

Myasthenic syndrome *may be associated with small cell carcinoma,* sometimes developing before the tumor is diagnosed, and occasionally occurs with certain autoimmune diseases. There is defective release of acetylcholine in response to a nerve impulse, caused by P/Q-type voltage-gated calcium channel antibodies, and this leads to weakness, especially of the proximal muscles of the limbs. Unlike myasthenia gravis, however, power steadily *increases* with sustained contraction. The diagnosis can be confirmed electrophysiologically, because the muscle response to stimulation of its motor nerve increases remarkably after exercise or if the nerve is stimulated repetitively at high rates (50 Hz), even in muscles that are not clinically weak.

Treatment

Treatment with IVIG, plasmapheresis, and immunosuppressive medication therapy (prednisone and azathioprine) may lead to clinical and electrophysiologic improvement, in addition to therapy aimed at tumor when present. Prednisone is usually initiated in a daily dose of 60–80 mg orally and azathioprine in a daily dose of 2 mg/kg orally. Symptomatic therapy includes the use of potassium channel antagonists; of these, amifampridine is a 3,4-diaminopyridine (15–80 mg/day orally in three divided doses) and is approved in the United States and Europe. Guanidine hydrochloride (25–50 mg/kg/day orally in divided doses) is an alternative and is occasionally helpful in seriously disabled patients, but adverse effects of the medication include marrow suppression. The response to treatment with anticholinesterase medications such as pyridostigmine or neostigmine is usually disappointing.

3. Botulism

The toxin of *Clostridium botulinum* prevents the release of acetylcholine at neuromuscular junctions and autonomic synapses. Botulism occurs most commonly following the ingestion of contaminated home-canned food; outbreaks have also occurred among drug abusers due to wound infection after injection of contaminated heroin. The diagnosis should be suggested by the development of sudden, fluctuating, severe weakness with preserved sensation in a previously healthy person. Symptoms begin within 72 hours following ingestion of the toxin and may progress for several days. Typically, there is diplopia, ptosis, facial weakness, dysphagia, and nasal speech, followed by respiratory difficulty and finally by weakness that appears last in the limbs. Blurring of vision (with unreactive dilated pupils) is characteristic, and there may be dryness of the mouth, constipation (paralytic ileus), and postural hypotension. The tendon reflexes are not affected unless the involved muscles are very weak. If the diagnosis is suspected, the local health authority should be notified and a sample of serum and contaminated food (if available) sent to be assayed for toxin. Support for the diagnosis may be obtained by electrophysiologic studies; with repetitive stimulation of motor nerves at fast rates, the muscle response increases in size progressively.

Patients should be hospitalized in case respiratory assistance becomes necessary. Treatment is with heptavalent antitoxin, in patients without known allergy to horse serum. Potassium channel antagonists may provide symptomatic relief as they do in Lambert-Eaton myasthenic syndrome. Anticholinesterase medications are of no value. Respiratory assistance and other supportive measures should be provided as necessary. Further details are provided in Chapter 33.

4. Disorders Associated with Use of Aminoglycosides

Aminoglycoside antibiotics, eg, gentamicin, may produce a clinical disturbance similar to botulism by preventing the release of acetylcholine from nerve endings, but symptoms subside rapidly as the responsible medication is eliminated from the body. These antibiotics are particularly dangerous in patients with preexisting disturbances of neuromuscular transmission and are therefore best avoided in patients with myasthenia gravis.

MYOPATHIC DISORDERS

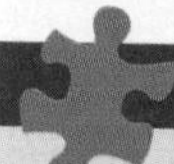

ESSENTIALS OF DIAGNOSIS

- Muscle weakness without sensory loss, often in a characteristic distribution.
- Serum creatine kinase elevated in most cases.
- Age at onset, time course, and inheritance pattern may suggest underlying disorder.

General Considerations

Myopathies can be inherited or acquired. Acquired myopathies often present acutely or subacutely while inherited myopathies are typically insidious in onset. Patients typically complain of *weakness affecting proximal muscles*, such as difficulty climbing stairs, arising from a chair, or reaching overhead, or of head drop. Sensory symptoms are absent. A detailed family history is required.

Examination shows weakness of proximal muscles. In some cases, there is a more specific pattern of weakness (eg, quadriceps and finger flexor weakness in inclusion body myositis). Extraocular muscle involvement is rarely seen, except in certain mitochondrial disorders, oculopharyngeal muscular dystrophy, and hyperthyroidism; when present, it should suggest the possibility of a neuromuscular junction disorder. Reflexes are normal or diminished in proportion to the degree of weakness. Sensation is normal.

Initial testing should include serum creatine kinase determination. Consider testing TSH, cortisol, vitamin D, and calcium. Antibodies specific to certain inflammatory myopathies and connective tissue disease can be checked when these conditions are suspected (see Chapter 20). Electromyography will reveal small motor units and early recruitment; it is helpful in confirming the localization of weakness to the muscle and suggesting a suitable site for biopsy, as does MRI. The electromyographic findings may be normal in corticosteroid and mitochondrial myopathies. Muscle biopsy establishes the diagnosis when inflammatory, mitochondrial, metabolic, or certain inherited myopathies are suspected. In cases where the family history or pattern of weakness suggests a specific genetic disorder, genetic testing can be pursued directly and biopsy may not be needed. Selected common and treatable myopathies are discussed below.

1. Muscular Dystrophies

These inherited myopathic disorders are subdivided by mode of inheritance, age at onset, and clinical features, as shown in Table 24–10. In the **Duchenne type**, pseudohypertrophy of muscles frequently occurs at some stage; intellectual disability is common; and there may be skeletal deformities, muscle contractures, and cardiac involvement.

Table 24–10. Selected muscular dystrophies.[1]

Disorder	Inheritance	Age at Onset (years)	Distribution	Prognosis	Genetic Association
Duchenne type	X-linked recessive	1–5	Pelvic, then shoulder girdle; later, limb and respiratory muscles.	Rapid progression. Death within about 15 years after onset.	Xp21; Dystrophin (loss of functional expression).
Becker	X-linked recessive	5–25	Pelvic, then shoulder girdle.	Slow progression. May have normal life span.	Xp21; Dystrophin (reduced functional expression).
Limb-girdle (Erb)	Autosomal recessive, dominant, or sporadic	10–30	Pelvic or shoulder girdle initially, with later spread to the other.	Variable severity and rate of progression. Possible severe disability in middle life.	Multiple.
Facioscapulohumeral	Autosomal dominant	Any age	Face and shoulder girdle initially; later, pelvic girdle and legs.	Slow progression. Minor disability. Usually normal life span.	4q35.2; Double homeobox protein 4. 18p11.32; Structural maintenance of chromosome's flexible hinge domain-containing protein 1.
Emery-Dreifuss	X-linked recessive or autosomal dominant	5–10	Humeroperoneal or scapuloperoneal.	Variable.	Multiple.
Distal	Autosomal dominant or recessive	40–60	Onset distally in extremities; proximal involvement later.	Slow progression.	Multiple.
Oculopharyngeal	Autosomal dominant	Any age	Ptosis, external ophthalmoplegia, and dysphagia.	Slow progression.	14q11.2–q13; Poly (A)-binding protein-2.
Myotonic dystrophy	Autosomal dominant	Any age (usually 20–40)	Face, neck, distal limbs.	Slow progression.	19q13.32; Myotonin-protein kinase. 3q21.3; Cellular nucleic acid-binding protein.

[1]Not all possible genetic loci are shown.

A genetic defect on the short arm of the X chromosome has been identified in Duchenne dystrophy. The affected gene codes for the protein dystrophin, which is markedly reduced or absent from the muscle of patients with the disease. Dystrophin levels are generally normal in the **Becker** variety, but the protein is qualitatively altered. The diagnosis is usually made with genetic testing; muscle biopsy is needed occasionally. Duchenne muscular dystrophy can be recognized early in pregnancy in about 95% of women by genetic studies; in late pregnancy, DNA probes can be used on fetal tissue obtained for this purpose by amniocentesis. The genes causing some of the other muscular dystrophies are listed in Table 24–10.

Four antisense oligonucleotides are approved by the FDA for treatment of Duchenne muscular dystrophy. Eteplirsen appears to benefit those patients with a dystrophin mutation amenable to exon 51 skipping; golodirsen and viltolarsen benefit those with a mutation amenable to exon 53 skipping; and casimersen benefits those with a mutation amenable to exon 45 skipping. Patients treated with these antisense oligonucleotides had more functional dystrophin on muscle biopsy than controls and a slower rate of disease progression than matched historical controls. Prednisone (0.75 mg/kg orally daily or 10 mg/kg orally given weekly over 2 days) or deflazacort (0.9 mg/kg orally daily) improves muscle strength and function in boys with Duchenne dystrophy, but side effects need to be monitored. Although both corticosteroid preparations cause similar side effects, weight gain at 1 year is less with deflazacort. Prolonged bed rest must be avoided, as inactivity often leads to worsening of the underlying muscle disease. Physical therapy and orthopedic procedures may help counteract deformities or contractures.

2. Myotonic Dystrophy

Myotonic dystrophy, a slowly progressive, dominantly inherited disorder, usually manifests itself in the third or fourth decade but occasionally appears early in childhood. Two types, with a different genetic basis, have been recognized. Myotonia leads to complaints of muscle stiffness and is evidenced by the marked delay that occurs before affected muscles can relax after a contraction. This can often be demonstrated clinically by delayed relaxation of the hand after sustained grip or by percussion of the belly of a muscle. In addition, there is weakness and wasting of the facial, sternocleidomastoid, and distal limb muscles. Associated clinical features include cataracts, frontal baldness, testicular atrophy, diabetes mellitus, cardiac abnormalities, and intellectual changes. Electromyographic sampling of affected muscles reveals myotonic discharges in addition to changes suggestive of myopathy.

It is difficult to determine whether medication therapy for myotonia is safe or effective. When myotonia is disabling, treatment with a sodium channel blocker—such as phenytoin (100 mg orally three times daily), procainamide (0.5–1 g orally four times daily), or mexiletine (150–200 mg orally three times daily)—may be helpful, but the associated side effects, particularly for antiarrhythmic medications, are often limiting. Neither the weakness nor the course of the disorder is influenced by treatment. Cardiac function should be monitored, and pacemaker placement may be considered if there is evidence of heart block.

3. Myotonia Congenita

Myotonia congenita is commonly inherited as a dominant trait. Generalized myotonia without weakness is usually present from birth, but symptoms may not appear until early childhood. Patients complain of muscle stiffness that is enhanced by cold and inactivity and relieved by exercise. Muscle hypertrophy, at times pronounced, is also a feature. A recessive form with later onset is associated with slight weakness and atrophy of distal muscles. Treatment with procainamide, tocainide, mexiletine, or phenytoin may help the myotonia, as in myotonic dystrophy.

4. Mitochondrial Myopathies

The mitochondrial myopathies are a clinically diverse group of disorders that on pathologic examination of skeletal muscle with the modified Gomori stain show characteristic "ragged red fibers" containing accumulations of abnormal mitochondria. Patients may present with progressive external ophthalmoplegia or with limb weakness that is exacerbated or induced by activity. Other patients present with central neurologic dysfunction, eg, myoclonic epilepsy (**myoclonic epilepsy, ragged red fiber syndrome, or MERRF**), or the combination of myopathy, encephalopathy, lactic acidosis, and stroke-like episodes (**MELAS**). Migraine is a common symptom. Systemic features include but are not limited to diabetes mellitus, hearing loss, retinopathy, cardiomyopathy, gastric dysmotility, and short stature. The serum creatine kinase is usually normal. Mitochondrial myopathies result from separate abnormalities of mitochondrial DNA. There are no approved treatments for these disorders, but coenzyme Q10, creatine, and levocarnitine are often prescribed; arginine is also given to patients with MELAS because it reduced frequency and severity of stroke-like episodes in an open-label trial.

5. Acid Maltase Deficiency (Pompe Disease)

This is a glycogen storage disease due to mutations in the gene encoding acid alpha-1,4-glucosidase. Age at presentation ranges from infancy to the late fifties and depends on the degree of residual enzyme activity. The juvenile and adult-onset forms present with slowly progressive proximal weakness that includes respiratory failure. Cardiomyopathy is less common in the adult form. Serum creatine kinase is mildly elevated. Muscle biopsy shows glycogen containing lysosomal vacuoles, but the diagnosis is suggested by detecting reduced acid-1,4-alpha-glucosidase activity on a dried blood spot and then confirmed by genetic testing. Treatment with recombinant alpha-glucosidase (20 mg/kg intravenously every 2 weeks) or avalglucosidase alpha (20–40 mg/kg intravenously every 2 weeks) stabilizes disease progression and results in improvement in respiratory function.

6. Dermatomyositis, Anti-Synthetase Syndromes, Immune-Mediated Necrotizing Myopathies, & Polymyositis

See Chapter 20.

7. Inclusion Body Myositis

This disorder, of unknown cause, begins insidiously, usually after middle age, with progressive proximal weakness of first the lower and then the upper extremities, and affecting facial and pharyngeal muscles. Weakness often begins in the quadriceps femoris in the lower limbs and the forearm flexors in the upper limbs. Distal weakness is usually mild. Serum creatine kinase levels may be normal or increased. The diagnosis is confirmed by muscle biopsy. Anticytosolic 5'-nucleotidase 1A antibodies are detected in one-third of cases and may be associated with a more severe phenotype. Corticosteroid and immunosuppressive therapy is sometimes offered but is usually ineffective, and IVIG therapy is not recommended.

8. Endocrine Myopathies

Myopathy is observed with hypothyroidism, hyperthyroidism, Cushing syndrome and disease, Addison disease, vitamin D deficiency, and both hyperparathyroidism and hypoparathyroidism (the latter mediated by calcium derangements). In hypothyroidism, there may be associated entrapment neuropathies, and examination may show delayed relaxation of tendon reflexes, muscle enlargement, or myoedema. Hyperthyroidism can cause both distal and proximal weakness and rarely a bulbar myopathy. Serum creatine kinase is normal except in hypothyroid myopathy, which can also be painful. Treatment is of the underlying endocrinopathy.

9. Critical Illness Myopathy

Myopathy may occur in association with critical illness, typically in patients who received neuromuscular blocking agents and corticosteroids. It is frequently discovered when patients unexpectedly require prolonged ventilatory support. There can be an associated sensorimotor polyneuropathy. Serum creatine kinase may be elevated initially but has frequently returned to normal or is below normal by the time the condition is suspected. Treatment is supportive.

10. Toxic Myopathies

Myopathy can occur in patients taking aminocaproic acid, amiodarone, chloroquine, colchicine, corticosteroids, cyclosporine, daptomycin, emetine, fibrates, gemcitabine, nucleoside reverse transcriptase inhibitors, or statin medications. Myopathy also occurs with chronic alcohol use disorder, whereas acute reversible muscle necrosis may occur shortly after acute alcohol, cocaine, or methamphetamine intoxication, and with propofol infusion. Inflammatory myopathy may occur in patients taking penicillamine and can be induced by programmed death-1 inhibitors; myotonia may be induced by clofibrate, and preexisting myotonia may be exacerbated or unmasked by depolarizing muscle relaxants (eg, suxamethonium), beta-blockers (eg, propranolol), fenoterol and, possibly, certain diuretics. Valproic acid can precipitate or worsen myopathy in patients with mitochondrial disorders or carnitine palmitoyltransferase II deficiency.

When to Refer

All patients should be referred to establish the diagnosis and underlying cause.

When to Admit

- For respiratory assistance.
- For rhabdomyolysis.

Pasnoor M et al. Approach to muscle and neuromuscular junction disorders. Continuum (Minneap Minn). 2019;25:1536. [PMID: 31794459]

PERIODIC PARALYSIS SYNDROMES

Periodic paralysis may have a familial (dominant inheritance) basis. The syndromes to be described are *channelopathies* that manifest as abnormal, often potassium-sensitive, muscle-membrane excitability and lead clinically to episodes of flaccid weakness or paralysis, sometimes in association with abnormalities of the plasma potassium level. Strength is initially normal between attacks, but progressive myopathic weakness may develop in up to one-third of patients as they age. **Hypokalemic periodic paralysis** is characterized by attacks that tend to occur on awakening, after exercise, or after a heavy meal and may last for several days. Patients should avoid excessive exertion. A low-carbohydrate and low-salt diet may help prevent attacks. An ongoing attack may be aborted by potassium chloride given orally or by intravenous drip, provided the ECG can be monitored and kidney function is satisfactory. In young Asian men, it is commonly associated with hyperthyroidism; treatment of the endocrine disorder prevents recurrences. A nonselective beta-adrenergic blocker may prevent attacks until the endocrine abnormality has been treated. In **hyperkalemic periodic paralysis,** attacks also tend to occur after exercise but usually last for less than 1 hour. They may be terminated by intravenous calcium gluconate (1–2 g) or by intravenous diuretics (furosemide, 20–40 mg), glucose, or glucose and insulin. **Normokalemic periodic paralysis** is similar clinically to the hyperkalemic variety, but the plasma potassium level remains normal during attacks. Several randomized trials support the use of dichlorphenamide (50–100 mg orally twice daily) for prevention of attacks in both hyperkalemic and hypokalemic periodic paralysis; acetazolamide (250–750 mg orally daily) is also effective. Chlorothiazide may also be used to prevent attacks in hyperkalemic periodic paralysis.

When to Refer

All patients should be referred.

Psychiatric Disorders

Kristin S. Raj, MD
Nolan R. Williams, MD
Charles DeBattista, DMH, MD

The fifth edition of the American Psychiatric Association's *Diagnostic and Statistical Manual* (*DSM-5*) is the common language that clinicians use for psychiatric conditions. It utilizes specific criteria with which to objectively assess symptoms for use in clinical diagnosis and communication.

COMMON PSYCHIATRIC DISORDERS

ADJUSTMENT DISORDERS

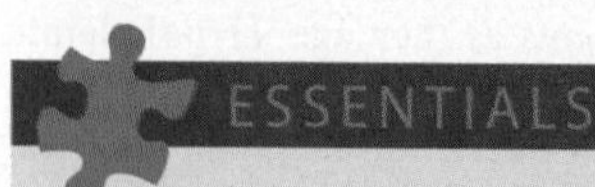

ESSENTIALS OF DIAGNOSIS

- Anxiety or depression in reaction to an identifiable stress, though out of proportion to the severity of the stressor.
- Symptoms are not at the severity of a major depressive episode or with the chronicity of generalized anxiety disorder (GAD).

General Considerations

An individual experiences stress when adaptive capacity is overwhelmed by events. The event may be an insignificant one when objectively considered, and even favorable changes (eg, promotion and transfer) requiring adaptive behavior can produce stress. For everyone, stress is subjectively defined, and the response to stress is a function of each person's personality and physiologic endowment.

Opinion differs about what events are most apt to produce stress reactions. The causes of stress are different at different ages—eg, in young adulthood, the sources of stress are found in the marriage or parent-child relationship, the employment relationship, and the struggle to achieve financial stability; in the middle years, the focus shifts to changing spousal relationships, problems with aging parents, and problems associated with having young adult offspring who themselves are encountering stressful situations; in old age, the principal concerns are apt to be retirement, loss of physical and mental capacity, major personal losses, and thoughts of death.

Clinical Findings

An individual may react to stress by becoming anxious or depressed, by developing a physical symptom, by running away, drinking alcohol, overeating, starting an affair, or in limitless other ways. Common subjective responses are anxiety, sadness, fear, rage, guilt, and shame. Acute and reactivated stress may be manifested by restlessness, irritability, fatigue, increased startle reaction, and a feeling of tension. Inability to concentrate, sleep disturbances (insomnia, bad dreams), and somatic preoccupations sometimes lead to self-medication, most commonly with alcohol or other CNS depressants. Emotional and behavioral distressing symptomatology in response to stress is called **adjustment disorder**, with the major symptom specified (eg, "adjustment disorder with depressed mood, anxiety, mixed depression and anxiety, disturbance of conduct, mixed disturbance of emotions and conduct, or unspecified"). *Even with an identifiable stressor, if the patient meets syndromal criteria for another disorder such as major depression, then the convention would be to diagnose a major depression and not an adjustment disorder with depressed mood.*

Differential Diagnosis

Adjustment disorders are distinguished from anxiety disorders, mood disorders, bereavement, other stress disorders such as PTSD, and personality disorders exacerbated by stress and from somatic disorders with psychic overlay. Unlike many other psychiatric disorders, such as bipolar disorder or schizophrenia, adjustment disorders are *wholly situational* and usually resolve when the stressor resolves or the individual effectively adapts to the situation. Adjustment disorders may have symptoms that overlap with other disorders, such as anxiety symptoms, but they occur in reaction to an identifiable life stressor such as a difficult work situation or romantic breakup. An adjustment disorder that persists and worsens can potentially evolve into another psychiatric disorder such as major depression or GAD. However, that is not the case for most patients.

Patients with adjustment disorders have marked distress after a stressor and significant impairment in social or occupational functioning but not to the degree experienced by patients with a more severe disorder such as major depressive disorder or PTSD. By definition, an adjustment disorder occurs within 3 months of an identifiable stressor.

Treatment

A. Behavioral

Stress reduction techniques include immediate symptom reduction (eg, rebreathing in a bag for hyperventilation) or early recognition and removal from a stress source before full-blown symptoms appear. It is often helpful for the patient to keep a daily log of stress precipitators, responses, and alleviators. Relaxation, mindfulness-based stress reduction, and exercise techniques are also helpful in improving the reaction to stressful events.

B. Social

The stress reactions of life crisis problems are a function of psychosocial upheaval. While it is not easy for the patient to make necessary changes (or they would have been made long ago), it is important for the clinician to establish the framework of the problem, since the patient's denial system may obscure the issues. Clarifying the problem in the patient's psychosocial context allows the patient to begin viewing it within the proper frame and facilitates the difficult decisions the patient eventually must make (eg, change of job).

C. Psychological

Prolonged in-depth psychotherapy is seldom necessary in cases of isolated stress response or adjustment disorder. Supportive psychotherapy (see above) with an emphasis on strengthening of existing coping mechanisms is a helpful approach so that time and the patient's own resiliency can restore the previous level of function. In addition, cognitive behavioral therapy has long been established to treat acute stress and facilitate recovery in patients with an adjustment disorder.

D. Pharmacologic

Judicious use of sedatives (eg, lorazepam, 0.5–1 mg two or three times daily orally) for a limited time and as part of an overall treatment plan can provide relief from acute anxiety symptoms. Problems arise when the situation becomes chronic through inappropriate treatment or when the treatment approach supports the development of chronicity. There are occasions where the short-term use of SSRIs targeting dysphoria and anxiety may be useful.

Prognosis

Return to satisfactory function after a short period is part of the clinical picture of this syndrome. Resolution may be delayed if others' responses to the patient's difficulties are thoughtlessly harmful or if the secondary gains outweigh the advantages of recovery. The longer the symptoms persist, the worse the prognosis. There is also evidence that stress-related disorders are associated with increased risk of autoimmune disease, although this mechanism has yet to be elucidated.

O'Donnell ML et al. Adjustment disorder: current developments and future directions. Int J Environ Res Public Health. 2019;16:2537. [PMID: 31315203]

TRAUMA & STRESSOR-RELATED DISORDERS

ESSENTIALS OF DIAGNOSIS

- Exposure to a traumatic or life-threatening event.
- Flashbacks, intrusive images, and nightmares, often represent reexperiencing the event.
- Avoidance symptoms, including numbing, social withdrawal, and avoidance of stimuli associated with the event.
- Increased vigilance, such as startle reactions and difficulty falling asleep.
- Symptoms impair functioning.

General Considerations

PTSD has been reclassified from an anxiety disorder to a trauma and stressor-related disorder in the *DSM-5*. PTSD is a syndrome characterized by "reexperiencing" a traumatic event (eg, sexual assault, severe burns, military combat) and decreased responsiveness and avoidance of current events associated with the trauma. Studies using cross-sectional surveys have indicated a higher risk for PTSD among frontline workers during the COVID-19 pandemic. The lifetime prevalence of PTSD among adult Americans has been estimated to be 6.8% with a point prevalence of 3.6% and with women having rates twice as high as men. Many individuals with PTSD (20–40%) have experienced other associated problems, including divorce, parenting problems, difficulties with the law, and substance abuse.

Clinical Findings

The key to establishing the diagnosis of PTSD lies in the *history of exposure to a perceived or actual life-threatening event, serious injury, or sexual violence.* This can include serious medical illnesses, and the prevalence of PTSD is higher in people who have experienced serious illnesses such as cancer. The symptoms of PTSD include intrusive thoughts (eg, flashbacks, nightmares), avoidance (eg, withdrawal), negative thoughts and feelings, and increased reactivity. Patients with PTSD can experience physiologic hyperarousal, including startle reactions, illusions, overgeneralized associations, sleep problems, nightmares, dreams about the precipitating event, impulsivity, difficulties in concentration, and hyperalertness. The symptoms may be precipitated or exacerbated by events that are a reminder of the original traumatic event. Symptoms frequently arise after a long latency period (eg, child abuse can result in later-onset PTSD). *DSM-5* includes the requirement that the symptoms persist for at least 1 month. In some individuals, the symptoms fade over months or years, and in others they may persist for a lifetime. Those with comorbid chronic pain tend to have heightened PTSD symptoms compared with those without chronic pain.

Differential Diagnosis

In 75% of cases, PTSD occurs with comorbid depression or panic disorder, and there is considerable overlap in the symptom complexes of all three conditions. Acute stress disorder has many of the same symptoms as PTSD, but symptoms persist for only 3 days to a month after the trauma. The other major comorbidity is alcohol and substance abuse. The **Primary Care-PTSD Screen** (https://www.ptsd.va.gov/professional/assessment/screens/pc-ptsd.asp) and the **PTSD Checklist** (https://www.ptsd.va.gov/professional/assessment/adult-sr/ptsd-checklist.asp#obtain) are two useful screening instruments in primary care clinics or community settings with populations at risk for trauma exposure.

Treatment

A. Psychotherapy

Psychotherapy should be initiated after the diagnosis of PTSD has been established and should be brief (typically 8–12 sessions), once the individual is in a safe environment. Exposure therapy has the strongest evidence in treatment of PTSD among psychotherapies and medications, although those with comorbid depression and refugees may benefit less. Cognitive processing therapy, a form of cognitive behavioral therapy for PTSD, also has strong evidence. In these approaches, the individual confronts the traumatic situation and learns to view and experience it with less hyperarousal over time. Posttraumatic stress syndromes respond to interventions that help patients integrate the event in an adaptive way with some sense of mastery in having survived the trauma. Partner relationship problems are a major area of concern, and it is important to have available a dependable referral source when marriage counseling is indicated.

Treatment of comorbid substance abuse is an essential part of the recovery process for patients with PTSD. In patients with substance use disorders, there are better outcomes when substance abuse treatment is delivered alongside trauma-focused psychotherapy. Support groups and 12-step programs such as Alcoholics Anonymous are often helpful.

Video telepsychiatry for psychotherapy or medication management is widely available. Telepsychiatry allows patients access to resources they may otherwise lack. There is similar efficacy in reduction of PTSD symptoms in women veterans with video teletherapy as with in-person therapy.

B. Pharmacotherapy

SSRIs are helpful in PTSD in ameliorating depression, panic attacks, sleep disruption, and startle responses. Sertraline and paroxetine are approved by the US FDA for this purpose. As SSRIs are the only class of medications approved for the treatment of PTSD they are considered the pharmacotherapy of choice. A 2021 phase 3 randomized placebo-controlled trial reported that MDMA (methylenedioxymethamphetamine, also called ecstasy) significantly enhanced the treatment effects associated with manualized therapy for severe PTSD. Early treatment of anxious arousal with beta-blockers (eg, propranolol, 80–160 mg orally daily) may lessen the peripheral symptoms of anxiety (eg, tremors, palpitations) but has *not* been shown to prevent development of PTSD. Similarly, noradrenergic agents such as clonidine (titrated from 0.1 mg orally at bedtime to 0.2 mg three times a day) have been shown to help with the hyperarousal symptoms of PTSD. The alpha-blocking agent prazosin (2–10 mg orally at bedtime) has mixed evidence for decreasing nightmares and improving quality of sleep in PTSD. Benzodiazepines, such as clonazepam, are generally thought to be *contraindicated* in the treatment of PTSD. The risks of benzodiazepines, including addiction and disinhibition, are thought to outweigh the anxiolytic and sleep benefits in most patients. Trazodone (25–100 mg orally at bedtime) is commonly prescribed as a non–habit forming hypnotic agent. Second-generation antipsychotics have not demonstrated utility in the treatment of PTSD, but agents such as quetiapine 50–300 mg/day may have a limited role in treating agitation and sleep disturbance in PTSD patients.

Prognosis

Approximately half of patients with PTSD experience chronic symptoms. Prognosis is best in those with good premorbid psychiatric functioning. Individuals who experience trauma from a natural disaster (eg, earthquake or hurricane) tend to do better than those who experience a traumatic interpersonal encounter (eg, rape or combat). *The sooner therapy is initiated after the trauma, once a diagnosis of PTSD has been established, the better the prognosis.* However, it is *not* beneficial to begin therapy immediately after a trauma since it does not decrease the rate of progression to PTSD. A study published in 2018 comparing sertraline and prolonged exposure therapy for patients with PTSD demonstrated that patients who received their preferred treatment were more likely to be adherent, respond to treatment, and have lower self-reported PTSD, depression, and anxiety symptoms.

Dutheil F et al. PTSD as the second tsunami of the SARS-Cov-2 pandemic. Psychol Med. 2021;51:1773. [PMID: 32326997]

Guideline Development Panel for the Treatment of PTSD in Adults, American Psychological Association. Summary of the clinical practice guideline for the treatment of posttraumatic stress disorder (PTSD) in adults. Am Psychol. 2019;74:596. [PMID: 31305099]

Johnson SU et al. PTSD symptoms among health workers and public service providers during the COVID-19 outbreak. PLoS One. 2020;15:e0241032. [PMID: 33085716]

Merz J et al. Comparative efficacy and acceptability of pharmacological, psychotherapeutic, and combination treatments in adults with posttraumatic stress disorder: a network meta-analysis. JAMA Psychiatry. 2019;76:904. [PMID: 31188399]

Mitchell JM et al. MDMA-assisted therapy for severe PTSD: a randomized, double-blind, placebo-controlled phase 3 study. Nat Med. 2021;27:1025. [PMID: 33972795]

ANXIETY DISORDERS

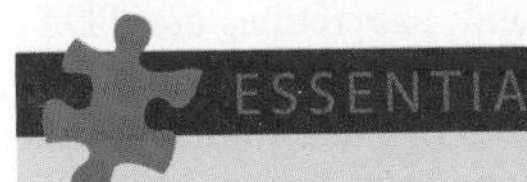

ESSENTIALS OF DIAGNOSIS

- Persistent excessive anxiety or chronic fear and associated behavioral disturbances.
- Somatic symptoms referable to the autonomic nervous system or to a specific organ system (eg, dyspnea, palpitations, paresthesias).
- Not limited to an adjustment disorder.
- Not a result of physical disorders, other psychiatric conditions (eg, schizophrenia), or drug abuse (eg, cocaine).

General Considerations

Stress, fear, and anxiety all tend to be interactive. The principal components of anxiety are **psychological** (tension, fears, difficulty in concentration, apprehension) and **somatic** (tachycardia, hyperventilation, shortness of breath, palpitations, tremor, sweating). Sympathomimetic symptoms of anxiety are both a response to a CNS state and a reinforcement of further anxiety. Anxiety can become *self-generating,* since the symptoms reinforce the reaction, causing it to spiral. Additionally, avoidance of *triggers* of anxiety leads to reinforcement of the anxiety. The person continues to associate the trigger with anxiety and never relearns through experience that the trigger need not always result in fear, or that anxiety will naturally improve with prolonged exposure to an objectively neutral stressor.

Clinical Findings

A. Generalized Anxiety Disorder

Anxiety disorders are the most prevalent psychiatric disorders. About 7% of women and 4% of men will meet criteria for GAD over a lifetime. GAD becomes chronic in many patients and longer than 2 years in over half of patients. Anxiety disorder in older adults is twice as common as dementia and four to six times more common than major depression; it is associated with poorer quality of life and contributes to the onset of disability. The anxiety symptoms of apprehension, worry, irritability, difficulty in concentrating, insomnia, or somatic complaints are present more days than not for at least 6 months. Manifestations can include cardiac (eg, tachycardia, increased blood pressure), GI (eg, increased acidity, nausea, epigastric pain), and neurologic (eg, headache, near-syncope) systems. The focus of the anxiety may be a number of everyday activities.

B. Panic Disorder

Panic attacks are recurrent, unpredictable episodes of intense surges of anxiety accompanied by marked physiologic manifestations. **Agoraphobia**, fear of being in places where escape is difficult, such as open spaces or public places where one cannot easily hide, may be present and may lead the individual to confine his or her life to home. Distressing symptoms and signs such as dyspnea, tachycardia, palpitations, dizziness, paresthesia, choking, smothering feelings, and nausea are associated with feelings of impending doom (alarm response). Although these symptoms may lead to overlap with some of the same bodily complaints found in the somatic symptom disorders, the key to the diagnosis of panic disorder is the psychic pain and suffering the individual expresses. **Panic disorder** is diagnosed when panic attacks are accompanied by a chronic fear of the recurrence of an attack or a maladaptive change in behavior to try to avoid potential triggers of the panic attack. Recurrent **sleep panic attacks** (not nightmares) occur in about 30% of panic disorders. **Anticipatory anxiety** develops in all these patients and further constricts their daily lives. Panic disorder tends to be familial, with onset usually under age 25; it affects 3–5% of the population, and the female-to-male ratio is 2:1. The premenstrual period is one of heightened vulnerability. Patients frequently undergo evaluations for emergent medical conditions (eg, heart attack or hypoglycemia), which are then ruled out before the correct diagnosis is made. GI symptoms (eg, stomach pain, heartburn, diarrhea, constipation, nausea and vomiting) are common, occurring in about one-third of cases. MI, pheochromocytoma, hyperthyroidism, and various recreational drug reactions can mimic panic disorder and should be considered in the differential diagnosis. Patients who have panic disorder can become demoralized, hypochondriacal, agoraphobic, and depressed. These individuals are at increased risk for major depression and suicide. Alcohol abuse (in about 20%) results from self-treatment and is frequently combined with dependence on sedatives. About 25% of panic disorder patients also have obsessive-compulsive disorder (OCD).

C. Phobic Disorders

Simple phobias are fears of a specific object or situation (eg, spiders, height) that are out of proportion to the danger posed, and they tend to be chronic. **Social phobias** are global or specific; in the former, all social situations are poorly tolerated, while the latter group includes **performance anxiety** (eg, fear of public speaking). Agoraphobia is frequently associated with panic attacks, and it often develops in early adult life, making a normal lifestyle difficult. Patients with agoraphobia experience intense fear about common situations, such as being in open spaces (eg, marketplaces), being in enclosed spaces (eg, theaters), standing in line, or being alone outside of their homes.

Treatment

In all cases, underlying medical disorders must be ruled out (eg, cardiovascular, endocrine, respiratory, and neurologic disorders and substance-related syndromes, both intoxication and withdrawal states).

A. Pharmacologic

1. Generalized anxiety disorder—Antidepressants including the SSRIs and SNRIs are first-line treatment and safe and effective in the long-term management of GAD. The antidepressants appear to be as effective as the benzodiazepines without the risks of tolerance or dependence. However, benzodiazepines take effect more quickly if not immediately, which can be beneficial in brief acute management (Table 25–1).

Antidepressants are the first-line medications for sustained treatment of GAD; unlike benzodiazepines, they have the advantage of not causing physiologic dependency problems. *Antidepressants can themselves be anxiogenic when first started*—thus, at the initiation of treatment, patient education and at times concomitant short-term treatment with a benzodiazepine are indicated. SSRIs, such as escitalopram and paroxetine, are FDA-approved. The SNRIs venlafaxine and duloxetine are FDA-approved for the treatment of GAD in usual antidepressant

Table 25–1. Commonly used antianxiety and hypnotic agents (listed in alphabetical order within classes).

Medication	Usual Daily Oral Doses	Usual Daily Maximum Doses	Cost for 30 Days of Treatment Based on Maximum Dosage[1]
Benzodiazepines (used for anxiety)			
Alprazolam (Xanax)[2]	0.5 mg	4 mg	$101.64
Chlordiazepoxide (Librium)[3]	10–20 mg	100 mg	$51.36
Clonazepam (Klonopin)[3]	1–2 mg	10 mg	$152.25
Clorazepate (Tranxene)[3]	15–30 mg	60 mg	$560.40
Diazepam (Valium)[3]	5–15 mg	30 mg	$28.13
Lorazepam (Ativan)[2]	2–4 mg	4 mg	$5.46
Oxazepam (Serax)[2]	10–30 mg	60 mg	$126.00
Benzodiazepines (used for sleep)			
Estazolam (Prosom)[2]	1 mg	2 mg	$29.67
Flurazepam (Dalmane)[3]	15 mg	30 mg	$26.40
Quazepam (Doral)[3]	7.5 mg	15 mg	$779.40
Temazepam (Restoril)[2]	15 mg	30 mg	$26.54
Triazolam (Halcion)[5]	0.125 mg	0.25 mg	$110.00
Miscellaneous (used for anxiety)			
Buspirone (Buspar)[2]	10–30 mg	60 mg	$75.60
Phenobarbital[3]	15–30 mg	90 mg	$22.32
Miscellaneous (used for sleep)			
Eszopiclone (Lunesta)[5]	2–3 mg	3 mg	$350.01
Hydroxyzine (Vistaril)[2]	50 mg	100 mg	$24.53
Lemborexant (Dayvigo)	5 mg	10 mg	$353.10
Ramelteon (Rozerem)	8 mg	8 mg	$365.70
Suvorexant (Belsomra)	5–10 mg	20 mg	$483.90
Zaleplon (Sonata)[6]	5–10 mg	10 mg	$112.37
Zolpidem (Ambien)[5]	5–10 mg	10 mg	$138.60

[1]Average wholesale price (AWP, for AB-rated generic when available) for quantity listed. Source: *IBM Micromedex Red Book (electronic version)*. IBM Watson Health, Greenwood Village, Colorado, USA. Available at: https://www-micromedexsolutions-com.proxy.hsl.ucdenver.edu/ (cited March 27, 2022). AWP may not accurately represent the actual pharmacy cost because wide contractual variations exist among institutions.
[2]Intermediate physical half-life (10–20 hours).
[3]Long physical half-life (> 20 hours).
[4]Intravenously for procedures.
[5]Short physical half-life (1–6 hours).
[6]Short physical half-life (about 1 hour).

doses. Initial daily dosing should start low (37.5–75 mg for venlafaxine and 30 mg for duloxetine) and be titrated upward as needed. Buspirone, sometimes used as an augmenting agent in the treatment of depression and compulsive behaviors, is also effective for generalized anxiety. Buspirone is usually given in a total dose of 30–60 mg/day in divided doses. Higher doses are sometimes associated with side effects of GI symptoms and dizziness. Bupropion may be the most anxiogenic antidepressant and does *not* have evidence in treatment of anxiety disorders. There is a 2- to 4-week delay before antidepressants and buspirone take effect, and *patients require education regarding this lag.* Sleep is sometimes negatively affected. Gabapentin (titrated to doses of 900–1800 mg orally daily, with larger doses at night) and pregabalin appear effective and lack the habit-forming potential of the benzodiazepines. Beta-blockers, such as propranolol, may help reduce peripheral somatic symptoms. Alcohol is the most frequently self-administered drug and should be strongly discouraged.

2. Panic disorder—Antidepressants are the first-line pharmacotherapy for panic disorder. Several SSRIs, including fluoxetine, paroxetine, and sertraline, are approved for the treatment of panic disorder. The SNRI venlafaxine is FDA-approved for treatment of panic disorder. As with GAD, panic disorder is often a chronic condition; the long-term use of benzodiazepines can result in tolerance or even benzodiazepine dependence. While panic disorder often responds to high-potency benzodiazepines such as clonazepam and alprazolam, the best use of these agents is generally early in the course of treatment concurrently with an antidepressant. Once the antidepressant has begun working after 4 or more weeks, the benzodiazepine may be tapered.

Whether the indications for benzodiazepines are anxiety or insomnia, the medications should be used judiciously. The longer-acting benzodiazepines are used for the treatment of alcohol withdrawal and anxiety symptoms; the intermediate medications are useful as sedatives for insomnia (eg, lorazepam), while short-acting agents (eg, midazolam) are used for medical procedures such as endoscopy. In psychiatric disorders, the benzodiazepines are usually given orally; in controlled medical environments (eg, the ICU), where the rapid onset of respiratory depression can be assessed, they often are given intravenously. Because lorazepam does not produce active metabolites and has a half-life of 10–20 hours, it is useful in treating older adult patients or those with liver dysfunction. Ultra–short-acting agents, such as triazolam, have half-lives of 1–3 hours and may lead to rebound withdrawal anxiety. Longer-acting benzodiazepines, such as flurazepam, diazepam, and clonazepam, produce active metabolites, have half-lives of 20–120 hours, and should be avoided in older adults; however, some clinicians prefer clonazepam because of its long half-life and thus ease of dosing to once or twice a day. Medication dosage must be individualized as patients vary widely in their response and effects can be long-lasting. An adequate and scheduled dose early in the course of symptom development will obviate the need for "pill popping," which can contribute to dependency problems.

The side effects of all the benzodiazepine antianxiety agents are patient- and dose-dependent. As the dosage exceeds the levels necessary for sedation, the side effects include disinhibition, ataxia, dysarthria, nystagmus, and delirium. (The patient *should be told not to operate machinery* and drive with caution until he or she is well stabilized without side effects.)

Paradoxical agitation, anxiety, psychosis, confusion, mood lability, and anterograde amnesia have been reported, particularly with the shorter-acting benzodiazepines. These agents produce cumulative clinical effects with repeated dosage (especially if the patient has not had time to metabolize the previous dose), additive effects when given with other classes of sedatives or alcohol, and residual effects after termination of treatment (particularly in the case of medications that undergo slow biotransformation).

Overdosage results in respiratory depression, hypotension, shock syndrome, coma, and death. Flumazenil, a benzodiazepine antagonist, is effective in overdosage. *Overdosage (see Chapter 38) and withdrawal states are medical emergencies.* Serious side effects of chronic excessive dosage are development of tolerance, resulting in increasing dose requirements, and physiologic dependence, resulting in withdrawal symptoms similar in appearance to alcohol and barbiturate withdrawal (withdrawal effects must be distinguished from reemergent anxiety). Abrupt withdrawal of sedative medications may cause serious and even fatal convulsive seizures. Psychosis, delirium, and autonomic dysfunction have also been described. Both duration of action and duration of exposure are major factors related to likelihood of withdrawal.

Common withdrawal symptoms after low to moderate daily use of benzodiazepines are classified as somatic (disturbed sleep, tremor, nausea, muscle aches), psychological (anxiety, poor concentration, irritability, mild depression), or perceptual (poor coordination, mild paranoia, mild confusion). The presentation of symptoms will vary depending on the half-life of the medication. The potential for interactions with benzodiazepines and other medications must be considered.

Antidepressants have been used in conjunction with beta-blockers in resistant cases. Propranolol (40–160 mg/day orally) can mute the peripheral symptoms of anxiety without significantly affecting motor and cognitive performance. They block symptoms mediated by sympathetic stimulation (eg, palpitations, tremulousness) but not nonadrenergic symptoms (eg, diarrhea, muscle tension). Contrary to common belief, *they usually do not cause depression as a side effect* and can be used cautiously in patients with depression.

3. Phobic disorders—Social phobias and agoraphobia may be treated with SSRIs, such as paroxetine, sertraline, and fluvoxamine. In addition, phobic disorders often respond to SNRIs such as venlafaxine. Gabapentin is an alternative to antidepressants in the treatment of social phobia in a dosage of 300–3600 mg/day, depending on response versus sedation. Specific phobias such as performance or test anxiety may respond to moderate doses of beta-blockers, such as propranolol, 20–40 mg 1 hour prior to exposure. Specific phobias tend to respond to behavioral therapies.

B. Behavioral

Behavioral approaches are widely used in various anxiety disorders, often in conjunction with medication. Relaxation techniques can sometimes be helpful in reducing anxiety. Desensitization, by exposing the patient to graded doses of a phobic object or situation, is an effective technique and one that the patient can practice outside the therapy session. Emotive imagery, wherein the patient imagines the anxiety-provoking situation while at the same time learning to relax, helps decrease the anxiety when the patient faces the real-life situation. Physiologic symptoms in panic attacks respond well to relaxation training. *Both GAD and panic disorder appear to respond as well to cognitive behavioral therapy as they do to medications.* Exercise, both aerobic and resistance training, has demonstrated effects in reducing anxiety symptoms across many anxiety disorders as well.

C. Psychological

Cognitive behavioral therapy is the first-line psychotherapy in treatment of anxiety disorders. For anxiety disorders it includes a cognitive component of examining the thoughts associated with the fear and a behavioral technique of exposing the individual to the feared object or situation. The combination of medication and cognitive behavioral therapy is more effective than either alone. **Mindfulness meditation** can also be effective in decreasing symptoms of anxiety. **Group therapy** is the treatment of choice when the anxiety is clearly a function of the patient's difficulties in dealing with social settings. **Acceptance and commitment therapy** have been used with some success in anxiety disorders. It encourages individuals to keep focused on life goals while they "accept" the presence of anxiety in their lives.

D. Social

Peer support groups for panic disorder and agoraphobia have been helpful. Social modification may require measures such as family counseling to aid acceptance of the patient's symptoms and avoid counterproductive behavior in behavioral training. Any help in maintaining the social structure is anxiety-alleviating, and work, school, and social activities should be maintained. School and vocational counseling may be provided by professionals, who often need help from the clinician in defining the patient's limitations.

Prognosis

Anxiety disorders are usually long-standing and may be difficult to treat. All can be relieved to varying degrees with medications and behavioral techniques. The prognosis is better if the commonly observed anxiety-panic-phobia-depression cycle can be broken with a combination of the therapeutic interventions discussed above.

Bandelow B. Current and novel psychopharmacological drugs for anxiety disorders. Adv Exp Med Biol. 2020;1191:347. [PMID: 32002937]

Efron G et al. Remote cognitive behavioral therapy for panic disorder: a meta-analysis. J Anxiety Disord. 2021;79:102385. [PMID: 33774557]

Slee A et al. Pharmacological treatments for generalised anxiety disorder: a systematic review and network meta-analysis. Lancet. 2019;393:768. [PMID: 30712879]

OBSESSIVE-COMPULSIVE DISORDER & RELATED DISORDERS

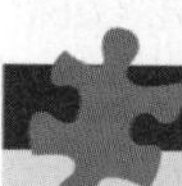

ESSENTIALS OF DIAGNOSIS

- Preoccupations or rituals (repetitive psychologically triggered behaviors) that are distressing to the individual.
- Symptoms are excessive or persistent beyond potentially developmentally normal periods.

General Considerations

OCD is part of a separate category of Obsessive-Compulsive Disorder and Related Disorders in *DSM-5*. In OCD, the irrational idea or impulse repeatedly and unwantedly intrudes into awareness. **Obsessions** (recurring distressing thoughts, such as fears of exposure to germs) and **compulsions** (repetitive actions such as washing one's hands many times or cognitions such as counting rituals) are usually recognized by the individual as unwanted or unwarranted and are resisted, but anxiety often is alleviated only by ritualistic performance of the compulsion or by deliberate contemplation of the intruding idea or emotion. Some patients experience only obsessions, while some experience both obsessions and compulsions. Many patients do not volunteer the symptoms and must be asked about them. There is an overlapping of OCD with some features in other disorders ("**OCD spectrum**"), including tics, trichotillomania (hair pulling), excoriation disorder (skin picking), hoarding, and body dysmorphic disorder. The incidence of OCD in the general population is 2–3% and there is a high comorbidity with major depression: major depression will develop in two-thirds of OCD patients during their lifetime. Male-to-female ratios are similar, with the highest rates occurring in the young, divorced, separated, and unemployed (all high-stress categories). Neurologic abnormalities of fine motor coordination and involuntary movements are common. Under extreme stress, these patients sometimes exhibit paranoid and delusional behaviors, often associated with depression, that can mimic schizophrenia.

Treatment

A. Pharmacologic

OCD responds to serotonergic antidepressants including SSRIs and clomipramine in about 60% of cases and usually requires a longer time to response than depression (up to

12 weeks). Fluoxetine has been widely used but in doses higher than those used in depression (up to 60–80 mg orally daily). The other SSRI medications, such as sertraline, paroxetine, and fluvoxamine, are used with comparable efficacy each with its own side-effect profile. Clomipramine has proved effective in doses equivalent to those used for depression. Plasma levels of clomipramine and its metabolite should be checked 2–3 weeks after a dosing of 50 mg/day has been achieved, with levels kept under 500 ng/mL to avoid toxicity. There is some evidence that antipsychotics, topiramate, memantine, riluzole, *N*-acetylcysteine, lamotrigine, ondansetron, and anti-inflammatory medication (minocycline, celecoxib) may be helpful as adjuncts to the SSRIs in treatment-resistant cases. Preliminary studies have suggested a role for ketamine and esketamine in the treatment of OCD.

B. Behavioral

OCD may respond to a variety of behavioral techniques. One common strategy is **exposure and response prevention.** As in the treatment of simple phobias, exposure and response prevention involves gradually exposing the OCD spectrum patient to situations that the patient fears, such as perceived germs. By gradually exposing patients to increasingly stressful situations and helping them manage their anxiety without performing the unwanted behavior, OCD spectrum patients are often able to develop some mastery over the behaviors.

C. Psychological

In addition to behavioral techniques, OCD may respond to psychological therapies including cognitive behavioral therapy in which the patient learns to identify maladaptive cognitions associated with obsessive thoughts and challenge those cognitions. These cognitions can be identified and gradually replaced with more rational thoughts. **Exposure and response prevention** is a form of cognitive behavioral therapy used in the treatment of OCD. Patients work through a list of their obsessions and compulsions with their therapist by first exposing themselves to the trigger, then working to prevent the habitual thought or compulsion that accompanies it. There is evidence that both cognitive behavioral therapy and exposure and response prevention and medications combined can be more effective than a single intervention alone.

D. Social

OCD can have devastating effects on the ability of a patient to lead a normal life. Educating both the patient and family about the course of illness and treatment options is extremely useful in setting appropriate expectations. Severe OCD is commonly associated with vocational disability, and the clinician may sometimes need to facilitate a leave of absence from work or encourage vocational rehabilitation to get the patient back to work.

E. Procedures

Transcranial magnetic stimulation is an effective FDA-approved therapy for OCD. Psychosurgery has a limited place in selected cases of severe unremitting OCD. Experimental work suggests a role for deep brain stimulation in OCD, and it is FDA-approved on a humanitarian device exemption basis for refractory OCD patients.

▶ Prognosis

OCD is usually a chronic disorder with a waxing and waning course. As many as 40% of patients in whom OCD problems develop in childhood will experience remission as adults. However, it is less common for OCD to remit without treatment when it develops during adulthood.

Beaulieu AM et al. The psychopharmacology algorithm project at the Harvard South Shore Program: an algorithm for adults with obsessive-compulsive disorder. Psychiatry Res. 2019;281:112583. [PMID: 31600606]

Shephard E et al. Toward a neurocircuit-based taxonomy to guide treatment of obsessive-compulsive disorder. Mol Psychiatry. 2021;26:4583. [PMID: 33414496]

Stein DJ et al. Obsessive-compulsive disorder. Nat Rev Dis Primers. 2019;5:52. [PMID: 31371720]

FEEDING & EATING DISORDERS

See Chapter 29.

SOMATIC SYMPTOM DISORDERS (Abnormal Illness Behaviors)

- Prominent physical symptoms may involve one or more organ systems and are associated with distress, impairment, or both.
- Sometimes able to correlate symptom development with psychosocial stresses.
- Combination of biogenetic and developmental patterns.

▶ General Considerations

Any organ system can be affected in somatic symptom disorders. In *DSM-5*, somatic symptom disorders encompass somatic disorders, including conversion disorder, hypochondriasis, somatization disorder, and pain disorder secondary to psychological factors. Vulnerability in one or more organ systems and exposure to family members with somatization problems plays a major role in the development of particular symptoms, and the "functional" versus "organic" dichotomy is a hindrance to good treatment. Clinicians should suspect psychiatric disorders in a number of somatic conditions. For example, 45% of patients describing palpitations had lifetime psychiatric diagnoses including generalized anxiety, depression, panic, and somatic symptom disorders. Similarly, 33–44% of patients who undergo coronary angiography for chest pain but have negative results have been found to have panic disorder.

In any patient presenting with a condition judged to be somatic symptom disorder, depression must be considered in the diagnosis.

Clinical Findings

A. Functional Neurologic Disorder/Conversion Disorder

"Conversion" of psychic conflict into physical neurologic symptoms in parts of the body innervated by the sensorimotor system (eg, paralysis, aphonic) is a disorder that can occur concomitantly with panic disorder or depression. The somatic manifestation that takes the place of anxiety is often paralysis, and in some instances, the dysfunction may have symbolic meaning (eg, arm paralysis in marked anger so the individual cannot use the arm to strike someone). Psychogenic nonepileptic seizures can be difficult to differentiate from intoxication states or panic attacks and can occur in patients who also have epileptic seizures. Lack of postictal confusion, closed eyes during the seizure, ictal crying, and a fluctuating course can suggest nonepileptic seizures; some symptoms such as asynchronous movements or pelvic thrusting can occur in both nonepileptic seizures and frontal lobe seizures (see also Chapter 24). La belle indifférence (an unconcerned affect) is not a significant identifying characteristic, as commonly believed, since individuals even with genuine medical illness may exhibit a high level of denial. It is important to identify physical disorders with unusual presentations (eg, multiple sclerosis, systemic lupus erythematosus).

B. Somatic Symptom Disorder

Somatic symptom disorder is characterized by one or more somatic symptoms that are associated with significant distress or disability. The somatic symptoms are associated with disproportionate and persistent thoughts about the seriousness of the symptoms, a high level of anxiety about health, or excessive time and energy devoted to these symptoms. The patient's focus on somatic symptoms is usually chronic. Panic, anxiety, and depression are often present, and major depression is an important consideration in the differential diagnosis. There is a significant relationship (20%) to a lifetime history of panic-agoraphobia-depression. It usually occurs before age 30 and is 10 times more common in women. Preoccupation with medical and surgical therapy becomes a lifestyle that may exclude other activities. Patients most often first present to primary care physicians and experience reassurance regarding their physical condition as only briefly helpful or dismissive. Patients' complaints of symptoms should always be first carefully medically evaluated.

C. Factitious Disorders

These disorders, in which symptom production is *intentional*, are not somatic symptom conditions in that symptoms are produced consciously, in contrast to the unconscious process of the other somatic symptom disorders. They are characterized by self-induced or described symptoms or false physical and laboratory findings for the purpose of deceiving clinicians or other health care personnel. The deceptions may involve self-mutilation, fever, hemorrhage, hypoglycemia, seizures, and an almost endless variety of manifestations—often presented in an exaggerated and dramatic fashion **(Munchausen syndrome)**. **Factitious disorder imposed on another,** previously termed **Munchausen by proxy**, is diagnosed when someone (often a parent) creates an illness in another person (often a child) for perceived psychological benefit of the first person, such as sympathy or a relationship with clinicians. The duplicity may be either simple or extremely complex and difficult to recognize. The patients are frequently connected in some way with the health professions and there is no apparent external motivation other than achieving the patient role. A poor clinician-patient relationship and "doctor shopping" tend to exacerbate the problem.

Complications

Sedative and analgesic dependency is the most common iatrogenic complication. Patients may pursue medical or surgical treatments that induce iatrogenic problems. Thus, identifying patients with a potential somatic symptom disorder and attempting to limit tests, procedures, and medications that may lead to harm are quite important.

Treatment

A. Medical

Medical support with careful attention to *building a therapeutic clinician-patient relationship is the mainstay of treatment.* It must be accepted that the patient's distress is real. *Every problem not found to have an organic basis is not necessarily a mental disease.* Regular, frequent, short appointments that are not symptom-contingent may be helpful. Medications should *not* be prescribed to replace appointments. One person should be the primary clinician, and consultants should be used mainly for evaluation. An empathic, realistic, optimistic approach must be maintained in the face of the expected ups and downs. Ongoing reevaluation is necessary since somatization can coexist with a concurrent physical illness.

B. Psychological

The primary clinician can use psychological approaches when the patient is ready to make some changes in lifestyle in order to achieve symptomatic relief. This is often best approached with orientation toward pragmatic current changes rather than an exploration of early experiences that the patient frequently fails to relate to current distress. Cognitive behavioral therapy has been shown to be an effective treatment for somatoform disorders by reducing physical symptoms, psychological distress, and disability. Group therapy with other individuals who have similar problems is sometimes of value to improve coping, allow ventilation, and focus on interpersonal adjustment. Hypnosis used early can be helpful in resolving conversion disorders. If the primary clinician has been working with the patient on psychological problems related to the physical illness, the groundwork is often laid for successful psychiatric referral.

For patients who have been identified as having a factitious disorder, early psychiatric consultation is indicated. There are two main treatment strategies for these patients. One consists of a conjoint confrontation of the patient by both the primary clinician and the psychiatrist. The patient's disorder is portrayed as a cry for help, and psychiatric treatment is recommended. The second approach avoids direct confrontation and attempts to provide a face-saving way to relinquish the symptom without overt disclosure of the disorder's origin. Techniques such as biofeedback and self-hypnosis may foster recovery using this strategy.

C. Behavioral

Behavioral therapy is probably best exemplified by **biofeedback** techniques. In biofeedback, the abnormality (eg, increased peristalsis) must be recognized and monitored by the patient and therapist (eg, by an electronic stethoscope to amplify the sounds). This is immediate feedback, and after learning to recognize it, the patient can then learn to identify any change thus produced (eg, a decrease in bowel sounds) and so become a conscious originator of the feedback instead of a passive recipient. Relief of the symptom operantly conditions the patient to utilize the maneuver that relieves symptoms (eg, relaxation causing a decrease in bowel sounds). With emphasis on this type of learning, the patient is able to identify symptoms early and initiate the counter-maneuvers, thus decreasing the symptomatic problem. Migraine and tension headaches have been responsive to biofeedback methods.

Physical-based therapies such as speech/occupational/physical also have strong evidence for improving symptoms in those suffering from functional neurologic disorder.

D. Social

Social endeavors include family, work, and other interpersonal activity. Family members should come for some appointments with the patient so they can learn how best to live with the patient. This is important in treatment of somatic and pain disorders. Peer support groups provide a climate for encouraging the patient to accept and live with the problem. Ongoing communication with the employer may be necessary to encourage long-term continued interest in the employee. Employers can become just as discouraged as clinicians in dealing with employees who have chronic problems.

Prognosis

The prognosis is better if the primary clinician intervenes early before the situation has deteriorated. After the problem has crystallized into chronicity, it is more difficult to effect change.

Gilmour GS et al. Management of functional neurological disorder. J Neurol. 2020;267:2164. [PMID: 32193596]

Liu J et al. The efficacy of cognitive behavioural therapy in somatoform disorders and medically unexplained physical symptoms: a meta-analysis of randomized controlled trials. J Affect Disord. 2019;245:98. [PMID: 30368076]

Scarella TM et al. Illness anxiety disorder: psychopathology, epidemiology, clinical characteristics, and treatment. Psychosom Med. 2019;81:398. [PMID: 30920464]

Toussaint A et al. Detecting DSM-5 somatic symptom disorder: criterion validity of the Patient Health Questionnaire-15 (PHQ-15) and the Somatic Symptom Scale-8 (SSS-8) in combination with the Somatic Symptom Disorder – B Criteria Scale (SSD-12). Psychol Med. 2020;50:324. [PMID: 30729902]

CHRONIC PAIN DISORDERS

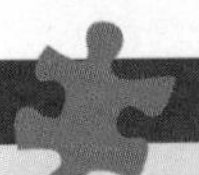

ESSENTIALS OF DIAGNOSIS

- Chronic complaints of pain.
- Symptoms frequently exceed signs.
- Minimal relief with standard treatment.
- History of having seen many clinicians.
- Frequent use of several nonspecific medications.

General Considerations

A problem in the management of pain is the lack of distinction between acute and chronic pain syndromes. Most clinicians are adept at dealing with acute pain problems but face greater challenges in treating a patient with a chronic pain disorder. Patients with chronic pain frequently take many medications, stay in bed a great deal, have seen many clinicians, have lost skills, and experience little joy in work or play. Relationships suffer (including those with clinicians), and life becomes a constant search for relief. The search results in complex clinician-patient relationships that usually include many medication trials, particularly sedatives, with adverse consequences (eg, irritability, depressed mood) related to long-term use. Treatment failures can provoke angry responses and depression from both the patient and the clinician, and the pain syndrome is exacerbated. When frustration becomes too great, a new clinician is found, and the cycle is repeated. The longer the existence of the pain disorder, the more important become the psychological factors of anxiety and depression. As with all other conditions, it is counterproductive to speculate about whether the pain is "real." *It is real to the patient,* and acceptance of the problem must precede a mutual endeavor to alleviate the disturbance.

Clinical Findings

Components of the chronic pain syndrome consist of anatomic changes, chronic anxiety and depression, anger, and changed lifestyle. Usually, the anatomic problem is irreversible, since it has already been subjected to many interventions with increasingly unsatisfactory results. An algorithm for assessing chronic pain and differentiating it from other psychiatric conditions is illustrated in Figure 25–1.

Chronic anxiety and depression produce heightened irritability and overreaction to stimuli. A marked decrease in pain threshold is apparent. This pattern develops into a

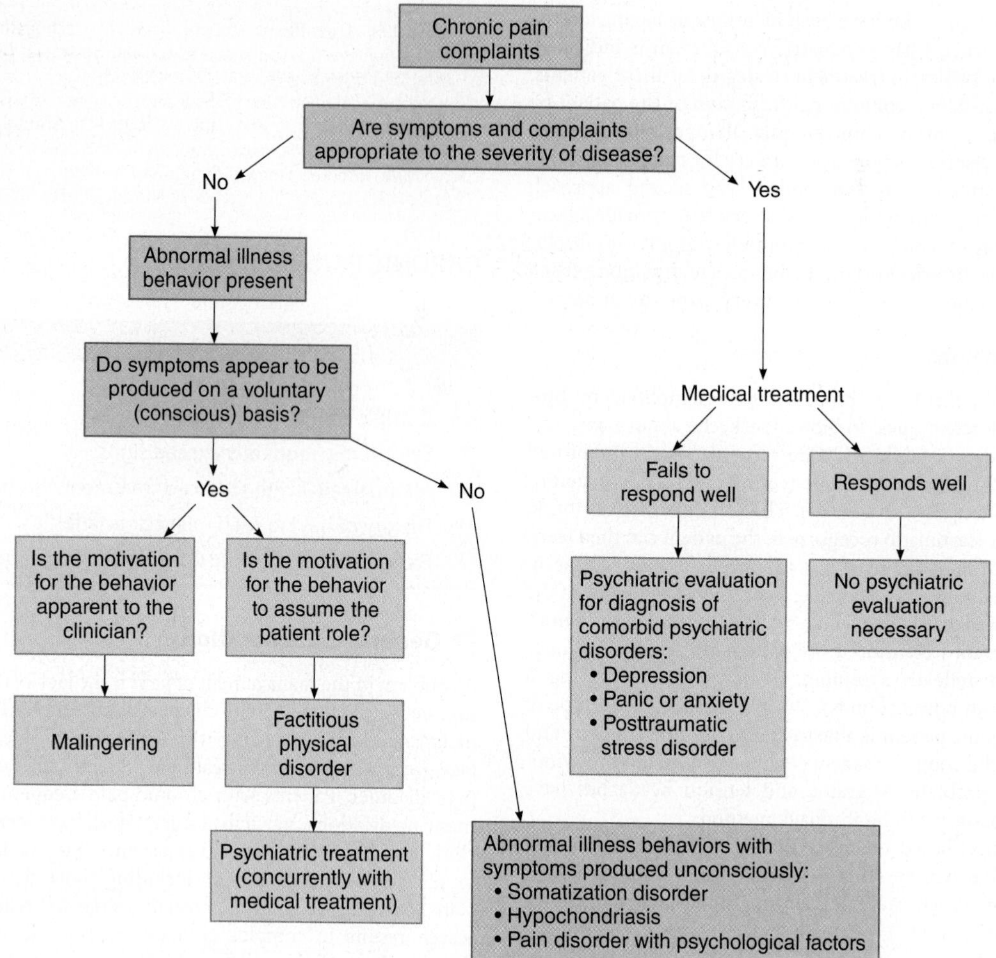

Figure 25–1. Algorithm for assessing psychiatric component of chronic pain. (Reproduced with permission from Eisendrath SJ. Psychiatric aspects of chronic pain. Neurology. 1995;45:S26–S36.)

preoccupation with the body and a constant need for reassurance. Patients may start avoiding usual behaviors when they first develop the pain and chronic avoidance of usual physical functioning can lead to the development of chronic pain. The pressure on the clinician becomes wearing and often leads to covert rejection of the patient, such as not being available or making referrals to other clinicians.

This is perceived by the patient, who then intensifies the effort to find help, and the typical cycle is repeated. Anxiety and depression are seldom discussed, almost as if there is a tacit agreement not to deal with these issues.

Changes in lifestyle involve some of the pain behaviors. These usually take the form of a *family script* in which the patient accepts the role of being sick, and this role then becomes the focus of most family interactions and may become important in maintaining the family, so that neither the patient nor the family wants the patient's role to change. Cultural factors frequently play a role in the behavior of the patient and how the significant people around the patient cope with the problem. Some cultures encourage demonstrative behavior, while others value the stoic role.

Another secondary gain that can maintain the patient in the sick role is financial compensation or other benefits. Frequently, such systems are structured so that they reinforce the maintenance of sickness and discourage any attempts to give up the role. Clinicians unwittingly reinforce this role because of the very nature of the practice of medicine, which is to respond to complaints of illness. Helpful suggestions from the clinician are often met with responses like, "Yes, but…." Medications then become the principal approach, and drug dependency problems may develop.

Treatment

A. Behavioral

The cornerstone of a unified approach to chronic pain syndromes is a **comprehensive behavioral program.** This is necessary to identify and eliminate pain reinforcers, decrease medication use, and use effectively positive reinforcers that shift the focus from the pain. It is critical that the patient be made a partner in the effort to manage and function better in the setting of ongoing pain symptoms.

The clinician must shift from the idea of biomedical cure to ongoing care of the patient. The patient should agree to discuss the pain only with the clinician and not with family members; this tends to stabilize the patient's personal life, since the family is usually tired of the subject. At the beginning of treatment, the patient should be assigned self-help tasks graded up to maximal activity as a means of positive reinforcement. The patient can also be asked to keep a self-rating chart to log accomplishments, so that progress can be measured and remembered. Instruct the patient to record degrees of pain on a self-rating scale in relation to various situations and mental attitudes so that similar circumstances can be avoided or modified.

Avoid positive reinforcers for pain such as marked sympathy and attention to pain. Emphasize a positive response to productive activities, which remove the focus of attention from the pain. Activity is also desensitizing since the patient learns to tolerate increasing activity levels.

Biofeedback techniques (see Somatic Symptom Disorders, above) and hypnosis have been successful in ameliorating some pain syndromes. Hypnosis tends to be most effective in patients with a high level of denial, who are more responsive to suggestion. Hypnosis can be used to lessen anxiety, alter perception of the length of time that pain is experienced, and encourage relaxation. Mindfulness-based stress reduction programs have been useful in helping individuals develop an enhanced capacity to live a higher quality life with persistent pain.

B. Medical

A *single clinician in charge of the comprehensive treatment approach is the highest priority.* Consultations as indicated and technical procedures done by others are appropriate, but the care of the patient should remain in the hands of the primary clinician. Referrals should not be allowed to raise the patient's hopes unrealistically or to become a way for the clinician to reject the case. The attitude of the clinician should be one of honesty, interest, and hopefulness—not for a cure but for control of pain and improved function. If the patient manifests opioid addiction, detoxification may be an early treatment goal.

Medical management of chronic pain is addressed in Chapter 5. *The harms of opioids generally outweigh the benefits in chronic pain management.* A fixed schedule lessens the conditioning effects of these medications. SNRIs (eg, venlafaxine, milnacipran, and duloxetine) and TCAs (eg, nortriptyline) in doses up to those used in depression may be helpful, particularly in neuropathic pain syndromes. Both duloxetine and milnacipran are approved for the treatment of fibromyalgia; duloxetine is also indicated in chronic pain conditions. In general, the SNRIs tend to be safer in overdose than the TCAs; suicidality is often an important consideration in treating patients with chronic pain syndromes. Gabapentin and pregabalin, anticonvulsants with possible applications in the treatment of anxiety disorders, have been shown to be useful in neuropathic pain and fibromyalgia.

In addition to medications, a variety of nonpharmacologic strategies may be offered, including physical therapy and acupuncture.

C. Social

Involvement of family members and other significant persons in the patient's life should be an early priority. The best efforts of both patient and therapists can be unwittingly sabotaged by other persons who may feel that they are "helping" the patient. They frequently tend to reinforce the negative aspects of the chronic pain disorder. The patient becomes more dependent and less active, and the pain syndrome becomes an immutable way of life. The more destructive pain behaviors described by many experts in chronic pain disorders are the results of well-meaning but misguided efforts of family members. Ongoing therapy with the family can be helpful in the early identification and elimination of these behavior patterns.

D. Psychological

Cognitive behavioral therapy, acceptance and commitment therapy, and mindfulness-based therapies have evidence in treatment of chronic pain. Therapy can be used in individual or group settings. A major goal, whether of individual or group therapy, is to gain *patient involvement.* A group can be a powerful instrument for achieving this goal, with the development of group loyalties and cooperation. People will frequently make efforts with group encouragement that they would never make alone. Individual therapy should be directed toward strengthening existing coping mechanisms and improving self-esteem. Teaching patients to challenge expectations induced by chronic pain may lead to improved functioning. As an illustration, many chronic pain patients, making assumptions more derived from acute injuries, *incorrectly believe they will damage themselves by attempting to function.* The rapport between patient and clinician, as in all psychotherapeutic efforts, is a major factor in therapeutic success.

Driscoll MA et al. Psychological interventions for the treatment of chronic pain in adults. Psychol Sci Public Interest. 2021;22:52. [PMID: 34541967]

Williams ACC et al. Psychological therapies for the management of chronic pain (excluding headache) in adults. Cochrane Database Syst Rev. 2020;8:CD007407. [PMID: 32794606]

PSYCHOSEXUAL DISORDERS

The stages of sexual activity include **excitement** (arousal), **orgasm,** and **resolution.** The precipitating excitement or arousal is psychologically determined.

In a well-adjusted person, arousal stimuli lead to vasocongestive and orgasmic responses. These can be considered as separate stages that can produce different syndromes responding to different treatment procedures.

Clinical Findings

There are three major groups of sexual disorders.

A. Paraphilias

In these conditions, the excitement stage of sexual activity is associated with sexual objects or orientations different from those usually associated with adult sexual stimulation. The stimulus may be a woman's shoe, a child, animals, instruments of torture, or incidents of aggression. The pattern of sexual stimulation is usually one that has early psychological roots. When paraphilias are associated with distress, impairment, or risk of harm, they become paraphilic disorders. Some paraphilias or paraphilic disorders include exhibitionism, transvestism, voyeurism, pedophilia, incest, sexual sadism, and sexual masochism.

B. Gender Dysphoria

Gender dysphoria is distress associated with the incongruence between a person's experienced or expressed gender and a person's biological sex. As a disorder, it is defined by significant distress or impairment; those experiencing this incongruence but without the distress would *not* meet criteria for having gender dysphoria. Screening should be done for conditions related to the oppression and stigmatization that transgender people face, including a high risk of suicide.

C. Sexual Dysfunctions

This category includes a large group of vasocongestive and orgasmic disorders. Often, they involve problems of sexual adaptation, education, and technique that are often initially discussed with, diagnosed by, and treated by the primary care provider.

There are two conditions common in men: erectile dysfunction and ejaculation disturbances.

Erectile dysfunction is inability to achieve or maintain an erection firm enough for satisfactory intercourse; patients sometimes use the term incorrectly to mean premature ejaculation. Decreased nocturnal penile tumescence occurs in some depressed patients. Psychological erectile dysfunction is caused by interpersonal or intrapsychic factors (eg, partner disharmony, depression). Organic factors are discussed in Chapter 23.

Ejaculation disturbances include premature ejaculation, inability to ejaculate, and retrograde ejaculation. (Ejaculation is possible in patients with erectile dysfunction.) Ejaculation is usually connected with orgasm, and ejaculatory control is an acquired behavior that is minimal in adolescence and increases with experience. Pathogenic factors are those that interfere with learning control, most frequently sexual ignorance. Intrapsychic factors (anxiety, guilt, depression) and interpersonal maladaptation (partner problems, unresponsiveness of mate, power struggles) are also common. Organic causes include interference with sympathetic nerve distribution (often due to surgery or radiation) and the effects of pharmacologic agents (eg, SSRIs or sympatholytics).

In women, the most common forms of sexual dysfunction are orgasmic disorder and hypoactive sexual desire disorder.

Orgasmic disorder is a complex condition in which there is a general lack of sexual responsiveness. The woman has difficulty in experiencing erotic sensation and does not have the vasocongestive response. Sexual activity varies from active avoidance of sex to an occasional orgasm. **Orgasmic dysfunction**—in which a woman has a vasocongestive response but varying degrees of difficulty in reaching orgasm—is sometimes differentiated from **anorgasmia.** Causes for the dysfunctions include poor sexual techniques, early traumatic sexual experiences, interpersonal disharmony (partner struggles, use of sex as a means of control), and intrapsychic problems (anxiety, fear, guilt). Organic causes include any conditions that might cause pain in intercourse, pelvic pathology, mechanical obstruction, and neurologic deficits.

Hypoactive sexual desire disorder consists of diminished or absent libido in either sex and may be a function of organic or psychological difficulties (eg, anxiety, phobic avoidance). Any chronic illness can reduce desire as can aging. Hormonal disorders, including hypogonadism or use of antiandrogen compounds such as cyproterone acetate, and CKD contribute to deterioration in sexual desire. Alcohol, sedatives, opioids, marijuana, and some medications may affect sexual drive and performance. Menopause may lead to diminution of sexual desire in some women, and testosterone therapy is sometimes warranted as treatment.

Treatment

A. Paraphilias

1. Psychological—Paraphilias, particularly those of a more superficial nature (eg, voyeurism) and those of recent onset, are responsive to psychotherapy in some cases. The prognosis is much better if the motivation comes from the individual rather than the legal system; unfortunately, judicial intervention is frequently the only stimulus to treatment because the condition persists and is reinforced until conflict with the law occurs. Therapies frequently focus on barriers to normal arousal response; the expectation is that the variant behavior will decrease as normal behavior increases.

2. Behavioral—In some cases, paraphilic disorders improve with modeling, role-playing, and conditioning procedures.

3. Social—Although they do not produce a change in sexual arousal patterns or gender role, self-help groups have facilitated adjustment to an often hostile society. Attention to the family is particularly important in helping people in such groups to accept their situation and alleviate their guilt about the role they think they had in creating the problem.

4. Pharmacologic—Medroxyprogesterone acetate, a suppressor of libidinal drive, can be used to mute disruptive sexual behavior in men. Onset of action is usually within 3 weeks, and the effects are generally reversible. Fluoxetine or other SSRIs at depression doses may reduce some of the compulsive sexual behaviors including the paraphilias. A focus of study in the treatment of severe paraphilia has been agonists of luteinizing hormone–releasing hormone (LHRH). Case reports and open label studies suggest that LHRH-agonists may play a role in preventing relapse in some patients with paraphilia.

B. Gender Dysphoria

The Standards of Care for the Health of Transsexual, Transgender, and Gender Nonconforming People is a publication of the World Professional Association for Transgender Health (WPATH), with the goal to provide clinical guidance for health professionals to assist transsexual, transgender, and gender nonconforming people with a path to maximize their health, psychological well-being, and self-fulfillment. The standards of care are based on the best available science and expert professional consensus.

1. Psychological—Individuals with gender dysphoria often find benefit from psychotherapy, providing them with a safe place to explore and understand their thoughts and feelings, and to identify their own specific needs and desires and adjust to a changing life.

2. Social—Peer support groups, parent psychoeducation and support, and community empowerment are important social components of treatment.

3. Medical—Some individuals with gender dysphoria choose to pursue surgery or hormone therapy or both. Medical care can also include gynecologic and urologic care, reproductive options, and voice and communication therapy. Most recommendations prior to surgery include that the individual spends significant time prior living as their desired gender. Rates of suicide fall significantly after surgery but still remain much higher than the general population.

C. Sexual Dysfunction

1. Psychological—The use of psychotherapy by itself is best suited for those cases in which interpersonal difficulties or intrapsychic problems predominate. Anxiety and guilt about parental injunctions against sex may contribute to sexual dysfunction. Even in these cases, however, a combined behavioral-psychological approach usually produces results most quickly. Mindfulness may be beneficial.

2. Behavioral—Syndromes resulting from conditioned responses have been treated by conditioning techniques, with excellent results. Masters and Johnson have used behavioral approaches in all of the sexual dysfunctions, with concomitant supportive psychotherapy and with improvement of the communication patterns of the couple.

3. Social—The proximity of other people (eg, a mother-in-law) in a household is frequently an inhibiting factor in sexual relationships. In such cases, some social engineering may alleviate the problem.

4. Medical—Even if the condition is not reversible, identification of the specific cause helps the patient to accept the condition. Partner disharmony, with its exacerbating effects, may thus be avoided. Of all the sexual dysfunctions, erectile dysfunction is the condition most likely to have an organic basis. Sildenafil, tadalafil, and vardenafil are phosphodiesterase type 5 inhibitors that are effective oral agents for the treatment of penile erectile dysfunction (eg, sildenafil 25–100 mg orally 1 hour prior to intercourse). These agents are effective for SSRI-induced erectile dysfunction in men and in some cases for SSRI-associated sexual dysfunction in women. Use of the medications in conjunction with any nitrates can have significant hypotensive effects leading to death in rare cases. Because of their common effect in delaying ejaculation, the SSRIs have been effective in premature ejaculation.

Flibanserin is a 5-HT_{1A}-agonist/5-HT_2-antagonist that is FDA-approved for the treatment of female hypoactive sexual desire disorder. Women treated with flibanserin have a marginally higher number of sexual events. Patients should be advised that flibanserin interacts with alcohol, causing hypotensive events. Flibanserin is taken 100 mg orally at bedtime to circumvent the side effects of dizziness, sleepiness, and nausea. An intranasal form that may have better bioavailability is being studied.

Bremelanotide is another FDA-approved medication for the treatment of hypoactive sexual desire disorder in premenopausal women; however, the mechanism of action is unclear and subjective improvement is low. Bremelanotide is self-administered by injection to the thigh or abdomen about 45 minutes before anticipated sexual activity. Both flibanserin and bremelanotide have potentially intolerable side effects, and their usage remains low.

Clayton AH et al. Female sexual dysfunction. Med Clin North Am. 2019;103:681. [PMID: 31078200]

Cooper K et al. The phenomenology of gender dysphoria in adults: a systematic review and meta-synthesis. Clin Psychol Rev. 2020;80:101875. [PMID: 32629301]

McMahon CG. Current diagnosis and management of erectile dysfunction. Med J Aust. 2019;210:469. [PMID: 31099420]

Wheeler LJ et al. Female sexual dysfunction: pharmacologic and therapeutic interventions. Obstet Gynecol. 2020;136:174. [PMID: 32541291]

PERSONALITY DISORDERS

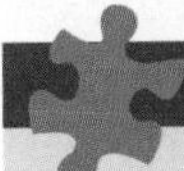

ESSENTIALS OF DIAGNOSIS

- Long history dating back to childhood.
- Recurrent maladaptive behavior.
- Difficulties with interpersonal relationships or society.
- Depression with anxiety when maladaptive behavior fails.

General Considerations

An individual's personality structure, or character, is an integral part of self-image. It reflects genetics, interpersonal influences, and recurring patterns of behavior adopted to cope with the environment. The classification of subtypes of personality disorders depends on the predominant symptoms and their severity. The most severe disorders—those that bring the patient into greatest conflict with society—tend to be antisocial (psychopathic) or borderline.

Classification & Clinical Findings

See Table 25–2.

Table 25–2. Personality disorders: Classification and clinical findings (listed in alphabetical order).

Personality Disorder	Clinical Findings
Antisocial	Selfish, callous, promiscuous, impulsive, unable to learn from experience, often has legal problems.
Avoidant	Fears rejection, hyperreacts to rejection and failure, with poor social endeavors and low self-esteem.
Borderline	Impulsive; has unstable and intense interpersonal relationships; is suffused with anger, fear, and guilt; lacks self-control and self-fulfillment; has identity problems and affective instability; is suicidal (a serious problem—up to 80% of hospitalized borderline patients make an attempt at some time during treatment, and the incidence of completed suicide is as high as 5%); aggressive behavior, feelings of emptiness, and occasional psychotic decompensation.
Dependent	Passive, overaccepting, unable to make decisions, lacks confidence, with poor self-esteem.
Histrionic (hysterical)	Dependent, immature, seductive, egocentric, vain, emotionally labile.
Narcissistic	Exhibitionist, grandiose, preoccupied with power, lacks interest in others, with excessive demands for attention.
Obsessive-compulsive	Perfectionist, egocentric, indecisive, with rigid thought patterns and need for control.
Paranoid	Defensive, oversensitive, secretive, suspicious, hyperalert, with limited emotional response.
Schizoid	Shy, introverted, withdrawn, avoids close relationships.
Schizotypal	Superstitious, socially isolated, suspicious, with limited interpersonal ability, eccentric behaviors, and odd speech.

Differential Diagnosis

Patients with personality disorders tend to experience anxiety and depression when pathologic coping mechanisms fail and may first seek treatment when this occurs. Occasionally, the more severe cases may decompensate into psychosis under stress and mimic other psychotic disorders.

Treatment

A. Social

Social and therapeutic environments such as day hospitals, halfway houses, and self-help communities utilize peer "pressure" to modify the self-destructive behavior. The patient with a personality disorder often has failed to profit from experience, and difficulties with authority can impair the learning experience. The use of peer relationships and the repetition possible in a structured setting of a helpful community enhance the behavioral treatment opportunities and increase learning. When problems are detected early, both the school and the home can serve as foci of intensified social pressure to change the behavior, particularly with the use of behavioral techniques.

B. Behavioral

Dialectical behavioral therapy is a program of individual and group therapy specifically designed for patients with chronic suicidality and borderline personality disorder. It blends mindfulness and a cognitive behavioral model to address self-awareness, interpersonal functioning, affective lability, and reactions to stress.

C. Psychological

Psychological interventions can be conducted in group and individual settings. Group therapy is helpful when specific interpersonal behavior needs to be improved. This mode of treatment also has a place with so-called "acting-out" patients, ie, those who frequently act in an impulsive and inappropriate way. The peer pressure in the group tends to impose restraints on rash behavior. The group also quickly identifies the patient's types of behavior and helps improve the validity of the patient's self-assessment, so that the antecedents of the unacceptable behavior can be effectively handled, thus decreasing its frequency. Individual therapy should initially be supportive, ie, helping the patient to restabilize and mobilize coping mechanisms. If the individual has the ability to observe his or her own behavior, a longer-term and more introspective therapy may be warranted. Psychodynamic psychotherapy can also be an effective treatment, with other specific forms of therapy, including transference-focused psychotherapy, mentalization-based therapy, and schema-focused therapy. The therapist must be able to handle countertransference feelings (which are frequently negative), maintain appropriate boundaries in the relationship, and refrain from premature confrontations and interpretations.

D. Pharmacologic

Hospitalization is indicated in the case of serious suicidal or homicidal danger. In most cases, treatment can be accomplished in the day treatment center or self-help community. Pharmacotherapy can be directed to specific symptom clusters, but there is limited evidence for its efficacy in personality disorders. Antidepressants have improved anxiety, depression, and sensitivity to rejection in some patients with borderline personality disorder. SSRIs also have a role in reducing aggressive behavior in impulsive aggressive patients (eg, fluoxetine 20–60 mg orally daily or sertraline 50–200 mg orally daily). Antipsychotics may be helpful in targeting hostility, agitation, and as adjuncts to antidepressant therapy (eg, olanzapine

[2.5–10 mg/day orally], risperidone [0.5–2 mg/day orally], or haloperidol [0.5–2 mg/day orally, split into two doses]). In some cases, medications are required only for several days and can be discontinued after the patient has regained a previously established level of adjustment; they can also provide ongoing support. Anticonvulsants, including carbamazepine, 400–800 mg orally daily in divided doses, lamotrigine, 50–200 mg/day, and valproate 500–2000 mg/day, have been shown to decrease the severity of behavioral dyscontrol in some personality disorder patients. Patients with a schizotypal personality often improve with antipsychotics, while those with avoidant personality may benefit from strategies that reduce anxiety, including the use of SSRIs and benzodiazepines. **Intermittent explosive disorder** is characterized by episodes of unwarranted anger and sometime violence. Anticonvulsants (such as carbamazepine and phenytoin), fluoxetine, and lithium have been helpful for some patients with intermittent explosive disorder.

Prognosis

Antisocial and borderline categories generally have a guarded prognosis. Those patients with a history of parental abuse and a family history of mood disorder tend to have the most challenging treatments.

Bayes A et al. Differential diagnosis of bipolar II disorder and borderline personality disorder. Curr Psychiatry Rep. 2019;21:125. [PMID: 31749106]

Doering S. Borderline personality disorder in patients with medical illness: a review of assessment, prevalence, and treatment options. Psychosom Med. 2019;81:584. [PMID: 31232916]

SCHIZOPHRENIA SPECTRUM DISORDERS

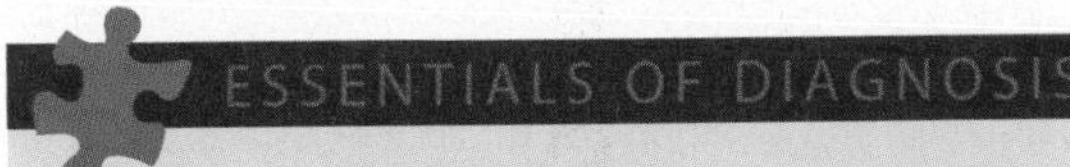

- Social withdrawal, usually slowly progressive, with decrease in emotional expression or motivation or both.
- Deterioration in personal care with disorganized behaviors or decreased reactivity to the environment or both.
- Disorganized thinking, often inferred from speech that switches topics oddly or is incoherent.
- Auditory hallucinations, often of a derogatory nature.
- Delusions, fixed false beliefs despite conflicting evidence, frequently of a persecutory nature.

General Considerations

Schizophrenia is manifested by a massive disruption of thinking, mood, and overall behavior as well as poor filtering of stimuli. The cause of schizophrenia is believed to be multifactorial, with genetic, environmental, and neurotransmitter pathophysiologic components. At present, there is *no laboratory method* for confirming the diagnosis of schizophrenia. There may or may not be a history of a major disruption in the individual's life (failure, loss, physical illness) before gross psychotic deterioration is evident.

Other psychotic disorders on this spectrum are conditions that are similar to schizophrenia in their acute symptoms but have a less pervasive influence over the long term. The patient usually attains higher levels of functioning. The acute psychotic episodes tend to be less disruptive of the person's lifestyle, with a quick return to previous levels of functioning.

Classification

A. Schizophrenia

Schizophrenia is the most common of the psychotic disorders that are characterized by a loss of contact with reality. The term *psychosis* is broad and most often refers to having one or more of the following: paranoia, auditory hallucinations, and delusions. One percent of the population suffers from schizophrenia. Schizophrenia is a chronic disorder that is characterized by increasing social and vocational disability that begins in late adolescence or early adulthood and tends to continue through life. The average age of onset for men is 18 years and for women is 25 years. Symptoms have been classified into positive and negative categories. **Positive symptoms** include hallucinations, delusions, and disorganized speech, which are related to increased dopaminergic (D_2) activity in the mesolimbic region; all patients have at least one or two of these symptoms to meet criteria for diagnosis. There is often a component of paranoia involved. They may also have disorganized behavior. **Negative symptoms** include diminished sociability, restricted affect, and poverty of speech; these symptoms are related to decreased D_2 activity in the mesocortical system. A marked decline in the level of functioning from before the onset of symptoms must last at least 6 months in some form.

B. Delusional Disorder

Delusional disorders are psychoses in which the predominant symptoms are persistent beliefs that are false (delusions) yet remain fixed despite being shown evidence that they are unfounded. Although there is *minimal* impairment of daily functioning and intellectual and occupational activities, social and partner functioning tends to be markedly impacted. Hallucinations are not usually present. The person may have paranoid delusions. Common delusions are of persecution, of one's partner being unfaithful, or of being related to or loved by a well-known person.

C. Schizoaffective Disorder

Schizoaffective disorders are cases that fail to fit comfortably either in the schizophrenia or in the affective categories. These patients usually have affective symptoms (either a major depressive episode, manic episode, or hypomanic episode) that precede or develop concurrently with psychotic manifestations. The psychotic symptoms may linger for some time after resolution of the mood episode but do not remain permanently. Because of this, the long-term prognosis is better than for schizophrenia.

D. Schizophreniform Disorders

Schizophreniform disorders are similar in their symptoms to schizophrenic disorders except that the duration of prodromal, acute, and residual symptoms is longer than 1 month but less than 6 months.

E. Brief Psychotic Disorders

Brief psychotic disorders are defined as psychotic symptoms lasting less than 1 month. They are the result of psychological stress. The shorter duration is significant and correlates with a more acute onset and resolution as well as a much better prognosis.

▶ Clinical Findings

A. Symptoms and Signs

The symptoms and signs of schizophrenia *vary markedly among individuals as well as in the same person at different times.* The patient's appearance may be bizarre, although the usual finding is mildly to moderately unkempt. Motor activity is generally reduced, although extremes ranging from catatonic stupor to frenzied excitement occur. Social behavior is characterized by marked withdrawal coupled with disturbed interpersonal relationships and a reduced ability to experience pleasure. Dependency and a poor self-image are common. Verbal utterances are variable, the language being concrete yet symbolic, with unassociated rambling statements (at times interspersed with mutism) during an acute episode. Neologisms (made-up words or phrases), echolalia (repetition of words spoken by others), and verbigeration (repetition of senseless words or phrases) are occasionally present. Affect is usually flattened, with occasional inappropriateness. *Depression is present in many cases* but may be less apparent during the acute psychotic episode and more obvious during recovery. Depression is sometimes confused with akinetic side effects of antipsychotic medications. It is also related to boredom, which increases symptoms and decreases the response to treatment. Work is generally unavailable and time unfilled, providing opportunities for counterproductive activities such as drug abuse, withdrawal, and increased psychotic symptoms.

Thought content may vary from a paucity of ideas to a rich complex of delusional fantasy with archaic thinking. One frequently notes after a period of conversation that little if any information has been conveyed. Incoming stimuli produce varied responses. In some cases, a simple question may trigger explosive outbursts, whereas at other times there may be no overt response whatsoever (catatonia). When paranoid ideation is present, the patient is often irritable and less cooperative. Delusions (false beliefs) are characteristic of paranoid thinking and usually take the form of a preoccupation with the supposedly threatening behavior exhibited by other individuals. This ideation may cause the patient to adopt active countermeasures such as locking doors and windows, taking up weapons, covering the ceiling with aluminum foil to counteract radar waves, and other unusual efforts. Somatic delusions can revolve around issues of bodily decay or infestation. Perceptual distortions usually include auditory hallucinations—visual hallucinations are more commonly associated with organic mental states—and may include illusions (distortions of reality) such as figures changing in size or lights varying in intensity. Lack of humor, feelings of dread, depersonalization (a feeling of being apart from the self), and fears of annihilation may be present. Any of the above symptoms generate higher anxiety levels, with heightened arousal and occasional panic and suicidal ideation, as the individual fails to cope.

The development of the acute episode in schizophrenia frequently is the end product of a gradual decompensation. Frustration and anxiety appear early, followed by depression and alienation, along with progressive ineffectiveness in day-to-day coping. This often leads to feelings of panic and increasing disorganization, with loss of the ability to test and evaluate the reality of perceptions. The stage of so-called **psychotic resolution** includes delusions, autistic preoccupations, and psychotic insight, with acceptance of the decompensated state. The process can be complicated by using caffeine, alcohol, and other recreational drugs. *Life expectancy of patients with schizophrenia is as much as 20% shorter than that of cohorts in the general population* and is often associated with comorbid conditions such as the metabolic syndrome, which may be induced or exacerbated by the atypical antipsychotic agents.

Polydipsia may produce water intoxication with hyponatremia—characterized by symptoms of confusion, lethargy, psychosis, seizures, and occasionally death—in any psychiatric disorder, but most commonly in schizophrenia.

B. Imaging

A full medical evaluation and CT scan or MRI of the brain should be considered in first episodes of psychosis to rule out organic brain conditions.

Ventricular enlargement and cortical atrophy, as seen on CT scan, have been correlated with chronic course, severe cognitive impairment, and nonresponsiveness to antipsychotic medications. Decreased frontal lobe activity seen on PET scan has been associated with negative symptoms.

▶ Differential Diagnosis

The diagnosis of schizophrenia is best made over time because repeated observations increase the reliability of the diagnosis. When the clinical course has been atypical, the diagnosis of schizophrenia should be reconsidered; cases initially diagnosed as schizophrenia later may be rediagnosed as bipolar disorder, which may respond to mood stabilizers rather than antipsychotics. Some manic episodes can have symptoms that overlap with schizophrenia, including thought disorder, auditory hallucinations, and delusions. However, schizophrenia is less likely to be associated with the decreased need for sleep, increase in goal-directed activity, and overconfidence, all of which are typical symptoms of mania.

Psychotic depressions, brief reactive psychosis, delusional disorder, and any illness with psychotic ideation tend to be confused with schizophrenia, partly because of the incorrect tendency to use the terms interchangeably.

In the early stages of illness, medical disorders such as thyroid dysfunction, adrenal and pituitary disorders, reactions to toxic materials (eg, mercury, PCBs), and other organic mental disorders must be ruled out. Postpartum psychosis is discussed under Mood Disorders. Complex partial seizures, especially when psychosensory phenomena are present, are an important differential consideration. Toxic drug states arising from prescription and over-the-counter medications, street drugs, and herbal products may mimic the psychotic disorders. The chronic use of amphetamines, cocaine, and other stimulants frequently produces a psychosis that is almost identical to the acute paranoid schizophrenic episode. Drug-induced psychoses can have all the positive symptoms of schizophrenia but less commonly the negative symptoms. The presence of formication (sensation of insects crawling on or under the skin) and stereotypy suggests the possibility of stimulant abuse. Phencyclidine, a common street drug, may cause a reaction that is difficult to distinguish from other psychotic disorders. Cerebellar signs, excessive salivation, dilated pupils, and increased deep tendon reflexes should alert the clinician to the possibility of a toxic psychosis. Industrial chemical toxicity (both organic and metallic), degenerative disorders, and metabolic deficiencies must be considered in the differential diagnosis.

Catatonia, a psychomotor disturbance that may involve decreased motor activity, decreased interaction, or excessive and odd motor activity, is frequently assumed to exist solely as a component of schizophrenic disorders. However, it can actually be the end product of a number of illnesses, including a number of organic conditions as well as other psychiatric disorders such as bipolar disorder. Neoplasms, viral and bacterial encephalopathies, CNS hemorrhage, metabolic derangements such as diabetic ketoacidosis, sedative withdrawal, and liver and kidney malfunction have all been implicated. It is particularly important to realize that drug toxicity (eg, overdoses of antipsychotic medications such as fluphenazine or haloperidol) can cause catatonic syndrome, which may be misdiagnosed as a catatonic schizophrenia and inappropriately treated with more antipsychotic medication. Catatonia is also seen in other major psychiatric disorders, including bipolar disorder and major depression.

Treatment

A. Pharmacologic

Antipsychotic medications are the treatment of choice. The relapse rate can be reduced by 50% with proper maintenance antipsychotic therapy. Long-acting, injectable antipsychotics are used in patients who are not adherent to medication recommendations or who do not respond to oral medication, or patients who choose the ease of not taking a daily pill. Side effects are discussed below.

Antipsychotic medications include the **"typical or first-generation"** antipsychotics (haloperidol, chlorpromazine, loxapine, perphenazine, fluphenazine) (dopamine [D_2]-receptor antagonists) and the newer **"atypical or second-generation"** antipsychotics (clozapine, risperidone, olanzapine, quetiapine, aripiprazole, ziprasidone, paliperidone, asenapine, iloperidone, lurasidone, cariprazine, and lumateperone) (Tables 25–3 and 25–4). Generally, increasing milligram potency of the typical antipsychotics is associated with decreasing anticholinergic and adrenergic side effects and increasing extrapyramidal symptoms. There appears to be similar antipsychotic efficacy for first- and second-generation antipsychotics but second-generation antipsychotics may be better tolerated with fewer extrapyramidal side effects, leading to enhanced compliance.

Clozapine, the first "atypical" (novel) antipsychotic medication developed, has dopamine (D_4) receptor–blocking activity as well as central serotonergic, histaminergic, and alpha-blocking activity. It is effective in the treatment of about 30% of psychoses resistant to other antipsychotic medications and may have specific efficacy in decreasing suicidality in patients with schizophrenia. Risperidone is an antipsychotic that blocks some serotonin receptors (5-HT_2) and D_2 receptors. Risperidone causes fewer extrapyramidal side effects than the typical antipsychotics at doses less than 6 mg. It appears to be as effective as haloperidol and possibly as effective as clozapine in treatment-resistant patients without necessitating weekly white cell counts, as required with clozapine therapy. Risperidone-induced hyperprolactinemia, even on low doses, has been reported and more commonly than with other atypical antipsychotics. Risperidone is available in a long-acting injectable preparation.

Olanzapine is a potent blocker of 5-HT_2 and dopamine D_1, D_2, and D_4 receptors. High doses of olanzapine (10–20 mg daily) appear to be more effective than lower doses. The medication is somewhat more effective than haloperidol in the treatment of negative symptoms, such as withdrawal, psychomotor retardation, and poor interpersonal relationships. It is available in an orally disintegrating form for patients who are unable to tolerate standard oral dosing and in an injectable form for the management of acute agitation associated with schizophrenia and bipolar disorder. Olanzapine is available in a long-term injectable preparation, but this formulation tends to be used less commonly than other depot formulations because some patients experience severe sedation and delirium, which occurs in about 0.5–1% of patients.

Quetiapine is an antipsychotic with greater 5-HT_2 relative to D_2 receptor blockade as well as a relatively high affinity for alpha-1 and alpha-2 receptors. It appears to be as efficacious as haloperidol in treating positive and negative symptoms of schizophrenia, with fewer extrapyramidal side effects even at high doses.

Ziprasidone has both anti-dopamine receptor and anti-serotonin receptor effects, with good efficacy for both positive and negative symptoms of schizophrenia. Aripiprazole is a partial agonist at the dopamine D_2 and serotonin 5-HT_1 receptors and an antagonist at 5-HT_2 receptors, and it is effective against positive and negative symptoms of

Table 25–3. Commonly used antipsychotic medications (listed in alphabetical order).

Medication	Usual Daily Oral Dose	Usual Daily Maximum Dose[1]	Cost per Unit	Cost for 30 Days of Treatment Based on Maximum Dosage[2]
Aripiprazole (Abilify)	10–15 mg	30 mg	$0.26/30 mg	$7.92
Asenapine (Saphris)	10–20 mg	20 mg	$2.40/10 mg	$144.00
Cariprazine (Vraylar)	1.5–6 mg	6 mg	$52.48/6 mg	$1574.40
Chlorpromazine (Thorazine; others)	100–400 mg	1 g	$17.86/200 mg	$2679.00
Clozapine (Clozaril)	300–450 mg	900 mg	$1.12/100 mg	$302.40
Fluphenazine (Permitil, Prolixin)[3]	2–10 mg	60 mg	$1.67/10 mg	$300.60
Haloperidol (Haldol)	2–5 mg	60 mg	$2.76/20 mg	$248.40
Iloperidone (Fanapt)	12–24 mg	24 mg	$63.70/12 mg	$3822.00
Loxapine (Loxitane)	20–60 mg	200 mg	$2.57/50 mg	$308.40
Lumateperone (Caplyta)	42 mg	42 mg	$59.27/42 mg	$1778.10
Lurasidone (Latuda)	40–80 mg	80 mg	$56.75/80 mg	$1702.44
Olanzapine (Zyprexa)	5–10 mg	20 mg	$0.95/20 mg	$28.50
Olanzapine/samidorphan (Lybalvi)	5/10 mg	20/10 mg	$55.60/tablet (all strengths)	$1668.00
Paliperidone (Invega)	6–12 mg	12 mg	$13.21/6 mg	$792.60
Perphenazine (Trilafon)[3]	16–32 mg	64 mg	$3.90/16 mg	$468.00
Pimavanserin (Nuplazid)	34 mg	34 mg	$166.92/34 mg	$5007.60
Quetiapine (Seroquel)	200–400 mg	800 mg	$1.68/400 mg	$100.80
Risperidone (Risperdal)[4]	2–6 mg	10 mg	$3.60/2 mg	$540.00
Thiothixene (Navane)[3]	5–10 mg	80 mg	$3.36/10 mg	$806.40
Trifluoperazine (Stelazine)	5–15 mg	60 mg	$2.45/10 mg	$441.00
Ziprasidone (Geodon)	40–160 mg	160 mg	$3.22/80 mg	$193.20

[1]Can be higher in some cases.
[2]Average wholesale price (AWP, for AB-rated generic when available) for quantity listed. Source: *IBM Micromedex Red Book (electronic version)*. IBM Watson Health, Greenwood Village, Colorado, USA. Available at: https://www-micromedexsolutions-com.proxy.hsl.ucdenver.edu/ (cited March 27, 2022). AWP may not accurately represent the actual pharmacy cost because wide contractual variations exist among institutions.
[3]Indicates piperazine structure.
[4]For risperidone, daily doses above 6 mg increase the risk of extrapyramidal syndrome. Risperidone 6 mg is approximately equivalent to haloperidol 20 mg.

schizophrenia. It functions as an antagonist or agonist, depending on the dopaminergic activity at the dopamine receptors, which may decrease side effects. Aripiprazole is available as an acute injectable preparation as well as a long-term injectable preparation that is given once monthly in patients who are unable to adhere to daily oral dosing. Asenapine, approved for the treatment of schizophrenia and bipolar disorder (mixed or manic state), appears to be helpful in treating negative symptoms of schizophrenia. It is available in a transdermal form, which may reduce some side effects associated with the sublingual form. Paliperidone, the active metabolite of risperidone, is available as a capsule and a monthly injection. Lurasidone has been shown to be effective in treating acute decompensation in patients with chronic schizophrenia. Cariprazine is a partial agonist of the D_2 and D_3 receptor and is approved by the FDA for the treatment of schizophrenia and bipolar disorder. Akathisia, weight gain, and insomnia are among the more commonly reported side effects with cariprazine. Because cariprazine is not a potent D_2-antagonist, it is less likely to increase prolactin levels than most antipsychotics. Cariprazine demonstrates greater efficacy in reducing negative symptoms of schizophrenia. Lumateperone, another second-generation antipsychotic, appears to have a favorable metabolic profile and appears to act on glutamate as well as D_2 and 5-HT_2 receptors. Unlike other antipsychotics, it does not require dose titration because the starting dose of 42 mg/day is the therapeutic dose.

Beyond antipsychotics, there is early evidence that cannabidiol (CBD), at a dose of 1000 mg/day, added on to existing antipsychotic treatment, may improve psychotic symptoms in schizophrenia. This agent may represent a new class of treatment for psychotic disorders. The prescription version of CBD was FDA-approved for treatment of rare childhood epilepsy. It is not yet widely used in clinical practice for schizophrenia, perhaps due to cost or off-label usage.

1. Clinical indications—The antipsychotics are used to treat all forms of the schizophrenias as well as drug-induced

Table 25–4. Relative potency and side effects of antipsychotic medications (listed in alphabetical order).

Medication	Chlorpromazine: Drug Potency Ratio	Anticholinergic Effects[1]	Extrapyramidal Effect[1]
Aripiprazole	1:20	1	1
Chlorpromazine	1:1	4	1
Clozapine	1:1	4	—
Fluphenazine	1:50	1	4
Haloperidol	1:50	1	4
Iloperidone	1:25	1	1
Loxapine	1:10	2	3
Lurasidone	1:5	1	2
Olanzapine	1:20	1	1
Perphenazine	1:10	2	3
Quetiapine	1:1	1	1
Risperidone	1:50	1	3
Thiothixene	1:20	1	4
Trifluoperazine	1:20	1	4
Ziprasidone	1:1	1	1

[1]1, weak effect; 4, strong effect.

psychoses, psychotic depression, augmentation of unipolar depression, acute mania, and the prevention of mood cycles in bipolar disorder. They are also effective in Tourette syndrome and behavioral dyscontrol in autistic patients. While frequently used to treat agitation in dementia patients, no antipsychotic has been shown to be reliably effective in this population and may *increase the risk of early mortality in older adult patients with dementia*. The improvement rate for treating positive symptoms with antipsychotics is about 80%. Patients whose behavioral symptoms worsen with use of antipsychotic medications may have an undiagnosed organic condition such as anticholinergic toxicity.

Symptoms that are ameliorated by these medications include hyperactivity, hostility, aggression, delusions, hallucinations, irritability, and poor sleep. Individuals with acute psychosis and good premorbid function respond quite well. The most common cause of failure in the treatment of acute psychosis is inadequate dosage, and the most common cause of relapse is noncompliance.

Although first-generation antipsychotics are efficacious in the treatment of positive symptoms of schizophrenia, such as hallucinations and delusions, second-generation antipsychotics are thought to have efficacy in reducing positive symptoms and some efficacy in treating negative symptoms. Antidepressant medications may be used in conjunction with antipsychotics if significant depression is present. Resistant cases may require concomitant use of lithium, carbamazepine, or valproic acid. The addition of a benzodiazepine medication to the antipsychotic regimen may prove helpful in treating the agitated or catatonic psychotic patient who has not responded to antipsychotics alone—lorazepam, 1–2 mg orally, can produce a rapid resolution of catatonic symptoms and may allow maintenance with a lower antipsychotic dose. Electroconvulsive therapy (ECT) has also been effective in treating catatonia and in treating schizophrenia when used in combination with medications.

2. Dosage forms and patterns—The dosage range is quite broad (Table 25–3). For example, risperidone can be effective for some patients with psychotic features at 0.25–1 mg orally at bedtime, whereas up to 6 mg/day may be used in a young patient with acute schizophrenia. In an acutely distressed, psychotic patient one might use haloperidol, 10 mg intramuscularly, which is absorbed rapidly and achieves an initial tenfold plasma level advantage over equal oral doses. Psychomotor agitation, racing thoughts, and general arousal are quickly reduced. The dose can be repeated every 3–4 hours; when the patient is less symptomatic, oral doses can replace parenteral administration in most cases. In older adults, both atypical (eg, risperidone 0.25–0.5 mg daily or olanzapine 1.25 mg daily) and typical (eg, haloperidol 0.5 mg daily or perphenazine 2 mg daily) antipsychotics often are used effectively for behavioral control but have been linked to premature death in some cases.

After a maintenance dose has been established, most patients can then be maintained on a single daily dose, usually at bedtime. This is appropriate when the sedative effect of the medication is desired for nighttime sleep and undesirable daytime sedative effects can be avoided. For patients who experienced their first psychotic episode, medications should be tapered off after 6 months of stability and then carefully monitored; the rate of relapse is lower for first-episode patients than that of multiple-episode patients.

Psychiatric patients—particularly patients who have paranoia—often neglect to take their medication. In these cases and patients who do not respond to oral medication, long-acting fluphenazine enanthate or decanoate (the latter is slightly longer-lasting and has fewer extrapyramidal side effects) or haloperidol decanoate may be given by deep subcutaneous injection or intramuscularly in the clinician's office with efficacy lasting 7–28 days. The usual dose of the fluphenazine long-acting preparations is 25 mg every 2 weeks, but dosage varies widely from 0.5 mg monthly to 100 mg weekly. Use the smallest effective amount as infrequently as possible.

Intravenous haloperidol, the antipsychotic most commonly used by this route, is often used in critical care units in the management of agitation and delirium. Intravenous haloperidol should be given no faster than 1 mg/minute to reduce cardiovascular side effects, such as torsades de pointes. ECG monitoring should be used whenever haloperidol is being administered intravenously.

Several long-acting formulations of atypical antipsychotic medications also are available, including risperidone (25–50 mg intramuscularly every 2 weeks), paliperidone, aripiprazole, and olanzapine. Concomitant use of a benzodiazepine (eg, lorazepam, 2 mg orally twice daily) may permit reduction of the required dosage of oral or parenteral antipsychotic medication.

Some antipsychotic agents are available for intranasal administration, which may be less traumatic to patients than injectable forms. The intranasal form of loxapine has a more rapid onset of action for the treatment of agitation (about 10 minutes) than either intramuscular or oral antipsychotic agents. However, intranasal loxapine requires the cooperation of the patient and is more expensive than generic antipsychotic injectable preparations.

3. Side effects—For both typical and atypical antipsychotic agents, a range of side effects are reported. The most common anticholinergic side effects include **dry mouth** (which can lead to ingestion of caloric liquids and weight gain or hyponatremia), **blurred near vision, urinary retention** (particularly in older adult men with enlarged prostates), **delayed gastric emptying, esophageal reflux, ileus, delirium,** and precipitation of **acute glaucoma** in patients with narrow anterior chamber angles. Other autonomic effects include **orthostatic hypotension** and **sexual dysfunction**—problems in achieving erection, ejaculation (including retrograde ejaculation), and orgasm in men (approximately 50% of cases) and women (approximately 30%). Delay in achieving orgasm is often a factor in medication noncompliance. **Electrocardiographic changes** occur frequently, but clinically significant arrhythmias are less common. Older adult patients and those with preexisting cardiac disease are at greater risk. The most frequently seen changes include diminution of the T wave amplitude, appearance of prominent U waves, depression of the ST segment, and prolongation of the QT interval (Table 25–5). Ziprasidone can produce QTc prolongation. A pretreatment ECG is indicated for patients at risk for cardiac sequelae (including patients taking other medications that might prolong the QTc interval). In some critical care patients, torsades de pointes has been associated with the use of high-dose intravenous haloperidol (usually greater than 30 mg/24 hours).

Associations have been suggested between the atypical antipsychotics and new-onset **diabetes, hyperlipidemia,** and **weight gain** (Table 25–5). The FDA has noted that the risk of hyperglycemia and new-onset diabetes may *not* be related to weight gain. The risk of diabetes mellitus is increased in patients taking clozapine and olanzapine. Monitoring of weight, fasting blood sugar, and lipids prior to initiation of treatment and at regular intervals thereafter is an important part of medication monitoring. The addition of metformin to olanzapine may improve drug-induced weight gain in patients with drug-naïve, first-episode schizophrenia. **Lactation and menstrual irregularities** are common. Both antipsychotic and antidepressant medications can **inhibit sperm motility. Bone marrow depression** and **cholestatic jaundice** occur rarely; these are hypersensitivity reactions, and they usually appear in the first 2 months of treatment. They subside on discontinuance of the medication. There is cross-sensitivity among all of the phenothiazines, and a medication from a different group should be used when allergic reactions occur.

Clozapine is associated with a 1.6% risk of **agranulocytosis** (higher in persons of Ashkenazi Jewish ancestry);

Table 25–5. Adverse factors associated with atypical antipsychotic medications (listed in alphabetical order).

Medication	Weight Gain	Hyperlipidemia	New-Onset Diabetes Mellitus	QTc Prolongation[1]
Aripiprazole	+/–	–	–	++
Asenapine	+/–	+/–	+/–	+++
Clozapine	+++	+++	+++	+/–
Lurasidone	–	–	–	–
Olanzapine	+++	+++	+++	+/–
Paliperidone	+	+/–	+/–	+++
Quetiapine	++	++	++	+++
Risperidone	++	++	++	+
Ziprasidone	+/–	–	–	+++

[1]QTc prolongation is a side effect of many medications and suggests a possible risk for arrhythmia. Prescriber's Letter 2011;18(12):271207.

hence, monitoring is required with weekly blood counts during the first 6 months of treatment and every other week thereafter. The risk of developing agranulocytosis is approximately 2.5 times higher in patients with a polymorphism for *HLADQB1* gene. Before initiating clozapine, genetic testing may be considered for the *HLADQB1* allele, which increases the risk of developing agranulocytosis 2.5 times higher. Clozapine has been associated with fatal myocarditis and is contraindicated in patients with severe heart disease. In addition, it lowers the seizure threshold and has many side effects, including sedation, severe constipation, hypotension, increased liver biochemical levels, hypersalivation, respiratory arrest, weight gain, and changes in both the ECG and the electroencephalogram. Adynamic ileus is a rare side effect of clozapine that can be fatal; patients should be closely monitored for constipation and treated quickly.

Photosensitivity, retinopathy, and **hyperpigmentation** are associated with use of high dosages of chlorpromazine. Patients on long-term medication should have periodic eye examinations.

The **neuroleptic malignant syndrome (NMS)** is a catatonia-like state manifested by extrapyramidal signs, blood pressure changes, altered consciousness, and hyperpyrexia; it is an uncommon but serious complication of antipsychotic treatment. Muscle rigidity, involuntary movements, confusion, dysarthria, and dysphagia are accompanied by pallor, cardiovascular instability, fever, pulmonary congestion, and diaphoresis and may result in stupor, coma, and death. The cause may be related to a number of factors, including poor antipsychotic medication dosage control, affective illness, decreased serum iron, dehydration, and increased sensitivity of dopamine receptor sites. Lithium in combination with an antipsychotic medication may increase vulnerability, which is already increased in patients with an affective disorder. In most cases, the symptoms develop within the first 2 weeks of antipsychotic drug treatment. The syndrome may occur with small doses of the medications. Intramuscular administration is a risk factor. Elevated creatine kinase and leukocytosis with a shift to the left are present early in about half of cases. Treatment includes controlling fever and providing fluid support. Dopamine agonists such as bromocriptine, 2.5–10 mg orally three times a day, and amantadine, 100–200 mg orally twice a day, have also been useful. Dantrolene, 50 mg intravenously as needed, is used to alleviate rigidity (do not exceed 10 mg/kg/day due to hepatotoxicity risk). There is ongoing controversy about the efficacy of these three agents as well as the use of calcium channel blockers and benzodiazepines. ECT has been used effectively in resistant cases. Clozapine has been used with relative safety and fair success as an antipsychotic medication for patients who have had NMS.

Akathisia is the most common (about 20%) extrapyramidal symptom. It usually occurs early in treatment (but may persist after antipsychotics are discontinued) and is frequently mistaken for anxiety or exacerbation of psychosis. It is characterized by a subjective desire to be in constant motion followed by an inability to sit or stand still and consequent pacing. It may induce suicidality or feelings of fright, rage, terror, or sexual torment. Insomnia is often present. It is crucial to educate patients in advance about these potential side effects so that the patients do not misinterpret them as signs of increased illness. In all cases, reevaluate the dosage requirement or the type of antipsychotic medication. One should inquire also about cigarette smoking, which in women has been associated with an increased incidence of akathisia. Antiparkinsonism medications (such as trihexyphenidyl, 2–5 mg orally three times daily) may be helpful, but first-line treatment often includes a benzodiazepine (such as clonazepam, 0.5–1 mg orally three times daily). In resistant cases, symptoms may be alleviated by propranolol, 30–80 mg/day orally, diazepam, 5 mg orally three times daily, or amantadine, 100 mg orally three times daily.

Acute dystonias usually occur early, although a late (**tardive**) occurrence is reported in patients (mostly men after several years of therapy) who previously had early severe dystonic reactions and a mood disorder. Younger patients are at higher risk for acute dystonias. The most common signs are bizarre muscle spasms of the head, neck, and tongue. Frequently present are torticollis, oculogyric crises, swallowing or chewing difficulties, and masseter spasms. Laryngospasm is particularly dangerous. Back, arm, or leg muscle spasms are occasionally reported. Diphenhydramine, 50 mg intramuscularly, is effective for the acute crisis; one should then give benztropine mesylate, 2 mg orally twice daily, for several weeks, and then discontinue gradually. Few of the extrapyramidal symptoms require long-term use of the antiparkinsonism medications.

Drug-induced parkinsonism is indistinguishable from idiopathic parkinsonism, but it is reversible, occurs later in treatment than the preceding extrapyramidal symptoms, and in some cases appears after antipsychotic withdrawal. The condition includes the typical signs of apathy and reduction of facial and arm movements (akinesia, which can mimic depression), festinating gait, rigidity, loss of postural reflexes, and pill-rolling tremor. Patients with AIDS seem particularly vulnerable to extrapyramidal side effects. High-potency antipsychotics often require antiparkinsonism medications. The antipsychotic dosage should be reduced, and immediate relief can be achieved with antiparkinsonism medications in the same dosages as above. After 4–6 weeks, these antiparkinsonism medications can often be discontinued with no recurrent symptoms. In any of the extrapyramidal symptoms, amantadine, 100–400 mg orally daily, may be used instead of the antiparkinsonism medications. Antipsychotic-induced catatonia is similar to catatonic stupor with rigidity, drooling, urinary incontinence, and cogwheeling. It usually responds slowly to withdrawal of the offending medication and use of antiparkinsonism agents.

Tardive dyskinesia is a syndrome of abnormal involuntary stereotyped movements of the face, mouth, tongue, trunk, and limbs that may occur after months or (usually) years of treatment with antipsychotic agents. The syndrome affects 20–35% of patients who have undergone long-term antipsychotic therapy. Predisposing factors include older age, many years of treatment, cigarette smoking, and diabetes mellitus. There are no clear-cut differences among the antipsychotic medications in the development of tardive dyskinesia. (Although the atypical antipsychotics appear to offer a lower risk of tardive dyskinesia, long-term effects have not been investigated.) However, clozapine is unique in that it has been found to treat antipsychotic-induced tardive dyskinesia. Early manifestations of tardive dyskinesia include fine worm-like movements of the tongue at rest, difficulty in sticking out the tongue, facial tics, increased blink frequency, or jaw movements of recent onset. Later manifestations may include bucco-linguomasticatory movements, lip smacking, chewing motions, mouth opening and closing, disturbed gag reflex, puffing of the cheeks, disrupted speech, respiratory distress, or choreoathetoid movements of the extremities (the last being more prevalent in younger patients). The symptoms do not necessarily worsen and in rare cases may lessen even though antipsychotic medications are continued. The dyskinesias do not occur during sleep and can be voluntarily suppressed for short periods. Stress and movements in other parts of the body will often aggravate the condition.

Early signs of dyskinesia must be differentiated from those reversible signs produced by ill-fitting dentures or nonantipsychotic medications such as levodopa, TCAs, antiparkinsonism agents, anticonvulsants, and antihistamines. Other neurologic conditions such as Huntington chorea can be differentiated by history and examination.

The emphasis should be on prevention of side effects. Use the least amount of antipsychotic medication necessary to improve the psychotic symptoms. Detect early manifestations of dyskinesias. When these occur, gradually discontinue antipsychotic medications, if clinically feasible. Keep the patient off the medications until reemergent psychotic symptoms dictate their resumption, at which point they are restarted in low doses and gradually increased until there is clinical improvement. If antipsychotic medications are restarted, clozapine and olanzapine appear to offer less risk of recurrence. The use of adjunctive agents such as benzodiazepines or lithium may help directly or indirectly by allowing control of psychotic symptoms with a low dosage of antipsychotics. If the dyskinesia syndrome recurs and it is necessary to continue antipsychotic medications to control psychotic symptoms, informed consent should be obtained. Vesicular monoamine transporter 2 (VMAT2) inhibitors, such as valbenazine and deutetetrabenazine, amantadine, vitamin B_6, vitamin E, and propranolol all have had some usefulness in treating the dyskinetic side effects. The VMAT2 inhibitors are considered the treatment of choice for tardive dyskinesia and are the only medications FDA-approved its treatment but are expensive and not covered by many insurance plans.

B. Social

Some individuals with a chronic psychiatric illness may have a history of repeated hospitalizations, a continued low level of functioning, and symptoms that never completely remit. Family rejection and work failure are common. In these cases, board and care homes staffed by personnel experienced in caring for psychiatric patients are most important. There is frequently an inverse relationship between stability of the living situation and the amounts of required antipsychotic medications, since the most salutary environment is one that reduces stimuli. Nonresidential self-help groups such as Recovery, Inc., should be utilized whenever possible. They provide a setting for sharing, learning, and mutual support and are frequently the only social involvement with which this type of patient is comfortable. Vocational rehabilitation and work agencies (eg, Goodwill Industries, Inc.) provide assessment, training, and job opportunities at a level commensurate with the person's clinical condition.

C. Psychological

The need for psychotherapy varies markedly depending on the patient's current status and history. In a person with a single psychotic episode and a previously good level of adjustment, supportive psychotherapy may help the patient reintegrate the experience, gain some insight into antecedent problems, and become a more self-observant individual who can recognize early signs of stress. Research suggests that cognitive behavioral therapy—in conjunction with medication management—has efficacy in the treatment of symptoms of schizophrenia. Cognitive behavioral therapy for psychosis involves helping the individual challenge psychotic thinking and alters response to hallucinations. Similarly, a form of psychotherapy called acceptance and commitment therapy has shown value in helping prevent hospitalizations in schizophrenia. Cognitive remediation therapy is another approach to treatment that may help patients with schizophrenia become better able to focus their disorganized thinking. Family therapy may also help alleviate the patient's stress and to assist relatives in coping with the patient.

D. Behavioral

Hospitalization is sometimes necessary, particularly when the patient's behavior shows gross disorganization. The presence of competent family members or social support lessens the need for hospitalization, and each case should be judged individually. The major considerations are to prevent self-inflicted harm or harm to others and to provide for the patient's basic needs.

Behavioral techniques (see above) are most frequently used in therapeutic settings such as day treatment centers, but they can also be incorporated into family situations or any therapeutic setting. Many behavioral techniques (eg, positive reinforcement—whether it be a word of praise or an approving nod—after some positive behavior) can be a powerful instrument for helping a person learn behaviors that will facilitate social acceptance. Music from portable digital players or smartphones with earphones is one of many ways to divert the patient's attention from auditory hallucinations.

Prognosis

For most patients with any psychosis, the prognosis is good for alleviation of positive symptoms such as hallucinations or delusions treated with medication. Negative symptoms such as diminished affect and sociability are much more difficult to treat but appear mildly responsive to atypical antipsychotics. Cognitive deficits, such as the executive dysfunction that is common to schizophrenia, also do not appear as responsive to antipsychotics as do positive symptoms. Unfortunately, both negative symptoms and cognitive deficits appear to contribute more to long-term disability than do positive symptoms. Unavailability of structured work situations and lack of family therapy or access to other social support are two other reasons why the prognosis is so guarded in such a large percentage of patients.

Artukoglu BB et al. Pharmacologic treatment of tardive dyskinesia: a meta-analysis and systematic review. J Clin Psychiatry. 2020;81:19r12798. [PMID: 32459404]
Correll CU et al. Negative symptoms in schizophrenia: a review and clinical guide for recognition, assessment, and treatment. Neuropsychiatr Dis Treat. 2020;16:519. [PMID: 32110026]
Goff DC et al. Citalopram in first episode schizophrenia: the DECIFER trial. Schizophr Res. 2019;208:331. [PMID: 30709746]
Huhn M et al. Comparative efficacy and tolerability of 32 oral antipsychotics for the acute treatment of adults with multi-episode schizophrenia: a systematic review and network meta-analysis. Lancet. 2019;394:939. [PMID: 31303314]
Keepers GA et al. The American Psychiatric Association practice guideline for the treatment of patients with schizophrenia. Am J Psychiatry. 2020;177:868. [PMID: 32867516]
Tariot PN et al. Trial of pimavanserin in dementia-related psychosis. N Engl J Med. 2021;385:309. [PMID: 34289275]

MOOD DISORDERS (Depression & Mania)

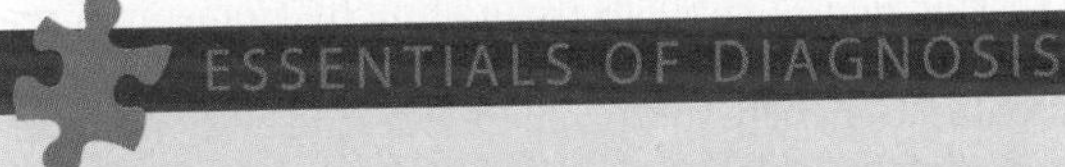

Present in most depressions

- Mood varies from mild sadness to intense despondency and feelings of guilt, worthlessness, and hopelessness.
- Difficulty in thinking, including inability to concentrate, ruminations, and lack of decisiveness.
- Loss of interest, with diminished involvement in work and recreation.
- Somatic complaints such as disrupted, lessened, or excessive sleep; loss of energy; change in appetite; decreased sexual drive.

Present in some severe depressions

- Psychomotor retardation or agitation.
- Delusions of a somatic or persecutory nature.
- Withdrawal from activities.
- Physical symptoms of major severity, eg, anorexia, insomnia, reduced sexual drive, weight loss, and various somatic complaints.
- Suicidal ideation.

Possible symptoms in mania

- Mood ranging from euphoria to irritability.
- Sleep disruption.
- Hyperactivity.
- Racing thoughts.
- Grandiosity or extreme overconfidence.
- Variable psychotic symptoms.

General Considerations

Depression is extremely common, with up to 30% of primary care patients having depressive symptoms. A meta-analysis of studies found a sevenfold increase in depression in communities in Europe and Asia that were heavily impacted by the COVID-19 pandemic. US national surveys show a threefold increase in the prevalence of depressive symptoms, with risk factors including lower income, less than $5000 in savings, and exposure to stressors. Depression may be the final expression of (1) genetic factors (neurotransmitter dysfunction), (2) developmental problems (personality problems, childhood events), or (3) psychosocial stresses (divorce, unemployment). It frequently presents in the form of somatic complaints with negative medical workups. *Although sadness and grief are normal responses to loss, depression is not.*

Mania is often combined with depression and may occur alone, together with depression in a mixed episode, or in cyclic fashion with depression.

Clinical Findings

There are four major types of depression, with similar symptoms in each group.

A. Adjustment Disorder with Depressed Mood

Depressed mood may occur in reaction to some identifiable stressor or adverse life situation, usually loss of a person by death (grief reaction), divorce, etc; financial reversal (crisis); or loss of an established role, such as being needed. Anger is frequently associated with the loss, and this in turn often produces a feeling of guilt. Adjustment disorder by definition occurs within 3 months of the stressor and causes significant impairment in social or occupational functioning. The symptoms range from mild sadness, anxiety, irritability, worry, and lack of concentration, discouragement, and somatic complaints to the more severe symptoms of frank depression. When the full criteria for major depressive disorder are present, that diagnosis should be made and treatment instituted, even when there is a known stressor. One should not neglect treatment for major depression simply because it may appear to be an understandable reaction to a particular stress or difficulty.

B. Depressive Disorders

The subclassifications include major depressive disorder and dysthymia.

1. Major depressive disorder—A major depressive disorder consists of a syndrome of mood, physical and cognitive symptoms that occurs at any time of life. Many consider a physiologic or metabolic aberration to be causative. Complaints vary widely but frequently include a loss of interest and pleasure (**anhedonia**), withdrawal from activities, and feelings of guilt. Also included are inability to concentrate, some cognitive dysfunction, anxiety, chronic fatigue, feelings of worthlessness, somatic complaints (unexplained somatic complaints frequently indicate depression), loss of sexual drive, and thoughts of death. Unemployment has been associated with increase in depression risk. Diurnal variation with improvement as the day progresses is common. Vegetative signs that frequently occur are insomnia, anorexia with weight loss, and constipation. Occasionally, severe agitation and psychotic ideation are present. **Psychotic major depression** occurs up to 14% of all patients with major depression and 25% of patients who are hospitalized with depression. Psychotic symptoms (delusions, paranoia) are more common in depressed persons who are older than 50 years. Paranoid symptoms may range from general suspiciousness to ideas of reference with delusions. The somatic delusions frequently revolve around feelings of impending annihilation or somatic concerns (eg, that the body is rotting away with cancer). Hallucinations are less common than unusual beliefs and tend not to occur independent of delusions.

In addition to psychotic major depression, other subcategories include **major depression with atypical features** that is characterized by hypersomnia, overeating, lethargy, and mood reactivity in which the mood brightens in response to positive events or news. **Melancholic major depression** is characterized by a lack of mood reactivity seen in atypical depression, the presence of a prominent anhedonia, and more severe vegetative symptoms. **Major depression with a seasonal onset (seasonal affective disorder)** is a dysfunction of circadian rhythms that occurs more commonly in the fall and winter months and is believed to be due to decreased exposure to full-spectrum light. Common symptoms include carbohydrate craving, lethargy, hyperphagia, and hypersomnia. **Major depression with peripartum onset** occurs during pregnancy or starts up to 4 weeks after delivery.

Half of depressions associated with the peripartum period start during pregnancy. Most women (up to 80%) experience some mild letdown of mood in the postpartum period. For some of these (10–15%), the symptoms are more severe and similar to those usually seen in serious depression, with an increased emphasis on concerns related to the baby (obsessive thoughts about harming it or inability to care for it). When psychotic symptoms occur, there is frequently associated sleep deprivation, volatility of behavior, and manic-like symptoms. Postpartum psychosis is much less common (less than 2%), often occurs within the first 2 weeks, and requires early and aggressive management. Biologic vulnerability with hormonal changes and psychosocial stressors all play a role. The chances of a second episode are about 25% and may be reduced with prophylactic treatment.

2. Persistent depressive disorder (dysthymia)—Dysthymia is a chronic depressive disturbance. Sadness, loss of interest, and withdrawal from activities over a period of two or more years with a relatively persistent course are necessary for this diagnosis. Generally, the symptoms are milder but longer-lasting than those in a major depressive episode.

3. Premenstrual dysphoric disorder—Depressive symptoms occur during the late luteal phase (last 2 weeks) of the menstrual cycle. (See also Chapter 18.)

C. Bipolar Disorder

Bipolar disorder consists of episodic mood shifts into mania, major depression, hypomania, and mixed mood states. The initial diagnosis of bipolar disorder can be difficult due to its ability to mimic aspects of many other coincident major mental health disorders and a high comorbidity with substance abuse. **Bipolar I** is diagnosed when an individual has manic episodes. For individuals who experience hypomanic episodes without frank mania, the diagnosis is **bipolar II**.

1. Mania—A manic episode is a mood state characterized by elation with hyperactivity, overinvolvement in life activities, increased irritability, flight of ideas, easy distractibility, and little need for sleep. The overenthusiastic quality of the mood and the expansive behavior initially attract others, but the irritability, mood lability with swings into depression, aggressive behavior, and grandiosity usually lead to marked interpersonal difficulties. Activities may occur that are later regretted, eg, excessive spending, resignation from a job, a hasty marriage, sexual acting-out, and exhibitionistic behavior, with alienation of friends and family. Atypical manic episodes can include gross delusions, paranoid ideation of severe proportions, and auditory hallucinations usually related to some grandiose perception. The episodes begin abruptly (sometimes precipitated by life stresses) and may last from several days to months. Generally, the manic episodes are of shorter duration than the depressive episodes. *In almost all cases, the manic episode is part of a broader bipolar disorder.* Patients with four or more discrete episodes of a mood disturbance in 1 year have "**rapid cycling**." Substance abuse, particularly cocaine, can mimic rapid cycling.

2. Cyclothymic disorder—This is a chronic mood disturbance with episodes of subsyndromal depression and hypomania. The symptoms must have at least a 2-year duration and are milder than those that occur in depressive or manic episodes. Occasionally, the symptoms will escalate into a full-blown manic or depressive episode, in which case reclassification as bipolar I or II would be warranted.

D. Mood Disorders Secondary to Illness and Medications

Any illness, severe or mild, can cause significant depression. Conditions such as rheumatoid arthritis, multiple sclerosis, stroke, and chronic heart disease are likely to be associated with depression, as are other chronic illnesses. Depression is common in cancer, as well, with a particularly high degree of comorbidity in pancreatic cancer. Hormonal variations clearly play a role in some depressions. Varying degrees of depression occur at various times in schizophrenic disorders, CNS disease, and organic mental states. Alcohol dependency frequently coexists with serious depression.

Drug-induced depression has occurred with a number of medications. Corticosteroids are commonly associated with mood changes such as depression and hypomania or psychosis. Older antihypertensive medications such as reserpine, methyldopa, guanethidine, and clonidine have been associated with the development of depressive syndromes, as have digitalis, antiparkinsonian medications (eg, levodopa), retinoids, interferon, disulfiram, and anticholinesterase medications. Stimulant use results in a depressive syndrome when the drug is withdrawn. Alcohol, sedatives, and opioids are depressants but, paradoxically, are often used by patients in self-treatment of depression.

Differential Diagnosis

Since depression may be a part of any illness—either reactively or as a secondary symptom—careful attention must be given to personal life adjustment problems and the role of medications. Schizophrenia, partial complex seizures, organic brain syndromes, panic disorders, and anxiety disorders must be differentiated. Thyroid dysfunction and other endocrinopathies should be ruled out. Malignancies are sometimes associated with depressive symptoms and may antecede the diagnosis of tumor. Strokes, particularly dominant hemisphere lesions, can occasionally present with a syndrome that looks like major depression.

Complications

The most important complication is **suicide**, which often includes some elements of aggression. Suicide rates in the general population vary from 9 per 100,000 in Spain to 15 per 100,000 in the United States to 31 per 100,000 in Russia. In individuals hospitalized for depression, the lifetime risk rises to 4–6%. In patients with bipolar I disorder, the risk is higher. Men over the age of 50 are more likely to complete a suicide because of their tendency to use more violent means, particularly guns. On the other hand, women make more attempts but are less likely to complete a suicide. The suicide rate in the younger population, aged 15–35, continues to rise. Patients with cancer, respiratory illnesses, AIDS, and those being maintained on hemodialysis have higher suicide rates. Alcohol use is a significant factor in many suicide attempts.

There are several groups of people who make suicide attempts. One group includes those individuals with acute situational problems. These individuals may be acutely distressed by a recent breakup in a relationship or another type of disappointment or overwhelmed by a stressful situation often with an aspect of public humiliation (eg, victims of cyber-bullying). A suicide attempt in such cases may be an impulsive or aggressive act not associated with significant depression.

Another high-risk group includes individuals with severe depression. Severe depression may be due to conditions such as medical illness (eg, people with AIDS have a suicide rate over 20 times that of the general population) or comorbid psychiatric disorders (eg, panic disorders). Anxiety, panic, and fear are major findings in suicidal behavior. A patient may seem to make a dramatic improvement, but the lifting of depression may be due to the patient's decision to commit suicide. Another high-risk group are individuals with psychotic illness who tend not to verbalize their concerns and are often successful in their suicide attempt, although they make up only a small percentage of the total.

Suicide is 10 times more prevalent in patients with schizophrenia than in the general population, with an increased frequency of jumping from bridges.

The immediate goal of psychiatric evaluation is to assess the current suicidal risk and determine the need for hospitalization versus outpatient management. *A useful question is to ask the person how many hours per day he or she thinks about suicide.* If it is more than 1 hour, the individual is at high risk. Further assessing the risk by inquiring about *intent, plans, means, and suicide-inhibiting factors* (eg, strong ties to children or the church) is essential. Alcohol, hopelessness, delusional thoughts, and complete or nearly complete loss of interest in life or ability to experience pleasure are all positively correlated with suicide attempts. Other risk factors are previous attempts, a family history of suicide, medical or psychiatric illness (eg, anxiety, depression, psychosis), male sex, older age, contemplation of violent methods, a humiliating social stressor, and drug use (including long-term sedative or alcohol use), which contributes to impulsiveness or mood swings. Successful treatment of the patient at risk for suicide cannot be achieved if the patient continues to abuse drugs. An attempt is less likely to be suicidal if small amounts of poison or medication were ingested or scratching of wrists was superficial, if the act was performed near others or with early notification of others, or if the attempt was arranged so that early detection would be anticipated.

The patient's current mood status is best evaluated by direct evaluation of plans and concerns about the future, personal reactions to the attempt, and thoughts about the reactions of others. Measurement of mood is often facilitated by using a standardized instrument such as the **Hamilton** or **Montgomery-Asberg** clinician-administered rating scales or the self-administered **Quick Inventory of Depressive Symptomatology (QIDS-SR 16).** Scales allow for initial assessment as well as ongoing treatment tracking. Suicide risk can be specifically assessed using an instrument such as the **Columbia-Suicide Severity Risk Scale,** https://cssrs.columbia.edu/wp-content/uploads/C-SSRS_Pediatric-SLC_11.14.16.pdf. The patient's immediate resources should also be assessed—people who can be significantly involved (most important), family support, job situation, financial resources, etc.

If hospitalization is not indicated after a suicide attempt, the clinician must formulate and institute a treatment plan or make an adequate referral. (The National Suicide Prevention Lifeline, 1-800-273-8255, may be of assistance.) Medication should be dispensed in small amounts to at-risk patients. Although TCAs and SSRIs are associated with an equal incidence of suicide attempts, the risk of a completed suicide is much higher with TCA overdose. Guns and medications should be removed from the patient's household. Driving should be cautioned against until the patient improves. The problem is often worsened by the long-term complications of the suicide attempt, eg, brain damage due to hypoxia, peripheral neuropathies caused by staying for long periods in one position causing nerve compressions, and medical or surgical problems such as esophageal strictures and tendon dysfunctions.

Treatment of Depression

A. Medical

Milder forms of depression usually do not require medication therapy and can be managed by psychotherapy and the passage of time. In severe cases—particularly when vegetative signs are significant and symptoms have persisted for more than a few weeks—antidepressant medication therapy is often effective. Medication therapy is also suggested by a family history of major depression in first-degree relatives or a past history of prior episodes.

The antidepressant medications may be classified into four groups: (1) the newer antidepressants, including the SSRIs, SNRIs, and bupropion, vilazodone, vortioxetine, and mirtazapine, (2) the TCAs and clinically similar medications, (3) the MAO inhibitors (Table 25–6), and (4) stimulants. ECT and repetitive transcranial magnetic stimulation are procedural treatments for depression. These modalities are described in greater detail below.

Hospitalization is necessary if suicide is a major consideration or if complex treatment modalities are required.

Medication selection is influenced by the history of previous response or lack thereof if that information is available. A positive family history of response to a particular medication may suggest that the patient will respond similarly. If no background information is available, a medication such as sertraline, 25 mg orally daily and increasing gradually up to 200 mg depending on response and side effects, or venlafaxine at 37.5 mg/day and titrated gradually as indicated to a maximum dose of 225 mg/day can be selected and a full trial instituted. During the medication trial, patients should be monitored for worsening mood or suicidal ideation every 1–2 weeks until week 6. The STAR*D trial suggests that if there is no response to the first medication, the best alternatives are to switch to a second agent that may be from the same or different class of antidepressant; if there is partial response to the first agent, another approach is to try augmenting it with a second agent, such as bupropion (150–450 mg/day), lithium (eg, 300–900 mg/day orally), thyroid medication (eg, liothyronine, 25–50 mcg/day orally), or a second-generation antipsychotic (eg, aripiprazole [5–15 mg/day]). The Agency for Health Care Policy and Research has produced clinical practice guidelines that outline one algorithm of treatment decisions (Figure 25–2).

Cognitive issues such as concentration and memory problems are common to depression; the evidence shows that these issues sometimes persist even after depression has remitted, with a higher risk in those individuals who have had more depressive episodes.

Psychotic depression should be treated with a combination of an antipsychotic and an antidepressant such as an SSRI at their usual doses. Mifepristone may have specific and early activity against psychotic depression. ECT is generally regarded as the single most effective treatment for psychotic depression, with remission rates between 60% and 90%.

Major depression with atypical features or seasonal onset can be treated with bupropion or an SSRI with good results. MAO inhibitors appear more effective than TCAs, and an MAO inhibitor may be used if more benign antidepressant strategies prove unsuccessful.

Melancholic depression may respond to ECT, TCAs, and SNRIs, which are preferable to SSRIs. However, SSRIs are often used in the treatment of melancholic depression and are effective in many cases.

Caution: Depressed patients often have suicidal thoughts, and the amount of medication dispensed should be appropriately controlled particularly if prescribing an MAO inhibitor, TCA, and to a lesser extent, venlafaxine. At the same time, *adults with untreated depression are at higher risk for suicide than those who are treated sufficiently to reduce symptoms.* It has been thought that in children and adolescent populations, antidepressants may be associated with some slightly increased risk of suicidality. One meta-analysis indicates that suicidality persists even after symptoms of depression are treated, suggesting other causes such as increased impulsivity among younger patients. After age 25, antidepressants may have neutral or possibly protective effects until age 65 years or older. The older TCAs have a narrow therapeutic index. One advantage of the newer medications is their wider margin of safety. Nonetheless, even with newer agents, because of the possibility of suicidality early in antidepressant treatment, close follow-up is indicated. In all cases of pharmacologic management of depressed states, caution is indicated until the risk of suicide is considered minimal.

1. SSRIs, SNRIs, and atypical antidepressants—SSRIs include fluoxetine, sertraline, paroxetine, fluvoxamine, and citalopram and its enantiomer escitalopram (Table 25–6). The chief advantages of these agents are that they are generally well tolerated, the starting dose is typically a therapeutic dose for most patients, and they have much lower lethality in overdose compared to TCAs or MAO inhibitors. (Notably, citalopram carries a warning regarding QT prolongation in doses above 40 mg, and 20 mg is considered the maximum dose for patients older than 60 years. There is no similar FDA warning for escitalopram.) The SNRIs include venlafaxine, desvenlafaxine, duloxetine, milnacipran, and levomilnacipran. In addition to possessing the strong serotonin reuptake blocking properties of the SSRIs, the SNRIs are also norepinephrine reuptake blockers. The combined serotonergic-noradrenergic properties of these medications may provide benefits in pain conditions such as neuropathy and fibromyalgia as well as conditions such as stress incontinence. The atypical antidepressants are bupropion, nefazodone, trazodone, vilazodone, vortioxetine, and mirtazapine (Table 25–6). All of these antidepressants are effective in the treatment of depression, both typical and atypical. The SSRI medications have been effective in the treatment of panic disorder, bulimia, GAD, OCD, and PTSD.

Most of the medications in this group tend to be activating and are given in the morning so as not to interfere with sleep. Some patients, however, may have sedation, requiring that the medication be given at bedtime. This reaction occurs most commonly with paroxetine, fluvoxamine, and mirtazapine. The SSRIs can be given in

Table 25–6. Commonly used antidepressant medications (listed in alphabetical order within classes).

Medication	Usual Daily Oral Dose (mg)	Usual Daily Maximum Dose (mg)	Sedative Effects[1]	Anticholinergic Effects[1]	Cost per Unit	Cost for 30 Days of Treatment Based on Maximum Dosage[2]
SSRIs						
Citalopram (Celexa)	20	40	< 1	1	$2.33/40 mg	$69.90
Escitalopram (Lexapro)	10	20	< 1	1	$0.62/20 mg	$18.60
Fluoxetine (Prozac, Sarafem)	5–40	80	< 1	< 1	$2.40/20 mg	$288.00
Fluvoxamine (Luvox)	100–300	300	1	< 1	$2.63/100 mg	$236.70
Paroxetine (Paxil)	20–30	50	1	1	$2.64/20 mg	$161.10
Sertraline (Zoloft)	50–150	200	< 1	< 1	$0.55/100 mg	$33.00
SNRIs						
Desvenlafaxine (Pristiq)	50	100	1	< 1	$8.64/100 mg	$259.20
Duloxetine (Cymbalta)	40	60	2	3	$1.72/60 mg	$51.60
Levomilnacipran (Fetzima)	40	120	1	1	$18.19/80 mg	$545.65
Milnacipran (Savella)	100	200	1	1	$8.84/100 mg	$530.56
Venlafaxine XR (Effexor)	150–225	225	1	< 1	$3.82/75 mg	$476.40
Tricyclic and Clinically Similar Compounds						
Amitriptyline (Elavil)	150–250	300	4	4	$2.14/150 mg	$128.40
Amoxapine (Asendin)	150–200	400	2	2	$1.98/100 mg	$237.60
Clomipramine (Anafranil)	100	250	3	3	$1.50/75 mg	$157.80
Desipramine (Norpramin)	100–250	300	1	1	$5.74/100 mg	$516.60
Doxepin (Sinequan)	150–200	300	4	3	$0.65/100 mg	$58.50
Imipramine (Tofranil)	150–200	300	3	3	$1.16/50 mg	$219.60
Maprotiline (Ludiomil)	100–200	300	4	2	$2.34/75 mg	$280.80
Nortriptyline (Aventyl, Pamelor)	100–150	150	2	2	$4.01/75 mg	$240.60
Protriptyline (Vivactil)	15–40	60	1	3	$5.73/10 mg	$1031.40
Trimipramine (Surmontil)	75–200	200	4	4	$16.22/100 mg	$973.20
Monoamine Oxidase Inhibitors						
Phenelzine (Nardil)	45–60	90	...	...	$0.84/15 mg	$151.20
Selegiline transdermal (Emsam)	6 (skin patch)	12	...	...	$76.37/6 mg patch	$2291.04
Tranylcypromine (Parnate)	20–30	50	...	...	$3.60/10 mg	$540.00
Other Compounds						
Bupropion SR (Wellbutrin SR)	300	400[3]	< 1	< 1	$3.38/200 mg	$202.80
Bupropion XL (Wellbutrin XL)	300[4]	450[4]	< 1	< 1	$0.55/300 mg	$32.10
Mirtazapine (Remeron)	15–45	45	4	2	$2.77/30 mg	$84.90
Nefazodone (Serzone)	150–600	600	3	1	$4.98/200 mg	$448.20
Trazodone (Desyrel)	100–300	400	4	< 1	$0.21/100 mg	$25.60
Vilazodone (Viibryd)	10–40	40	1	1	$12.61/40 mg	$378.18
Vortioxetine (Brintellix)	10	20	< 1	< 1	$17.77/20 mg	$532.97

[1]1, weak effect; 4, strong effect.
[2]Average wholesale price (AWP, for AB-rated generic when available) for quantity listed. Source: *IBM Micromedex Red Book (electronic version)*. IBM Watson Health, Greenwood Village, Colorado, USA. Available at: https://www-micromedexsolutions-com.proxy.hsl.ucdenver.edu/ (cited March 27, 2022). AWP may not accurately represent the actual pharmacy cost because wide contractual variations exist among institutions.
[3]200 mg twice daily.
[4]Wellbutrin XL is a once-daily form of bupropion. Bupropion is still available as immediate release, and, if used, no single dose should exceed 150 mg.

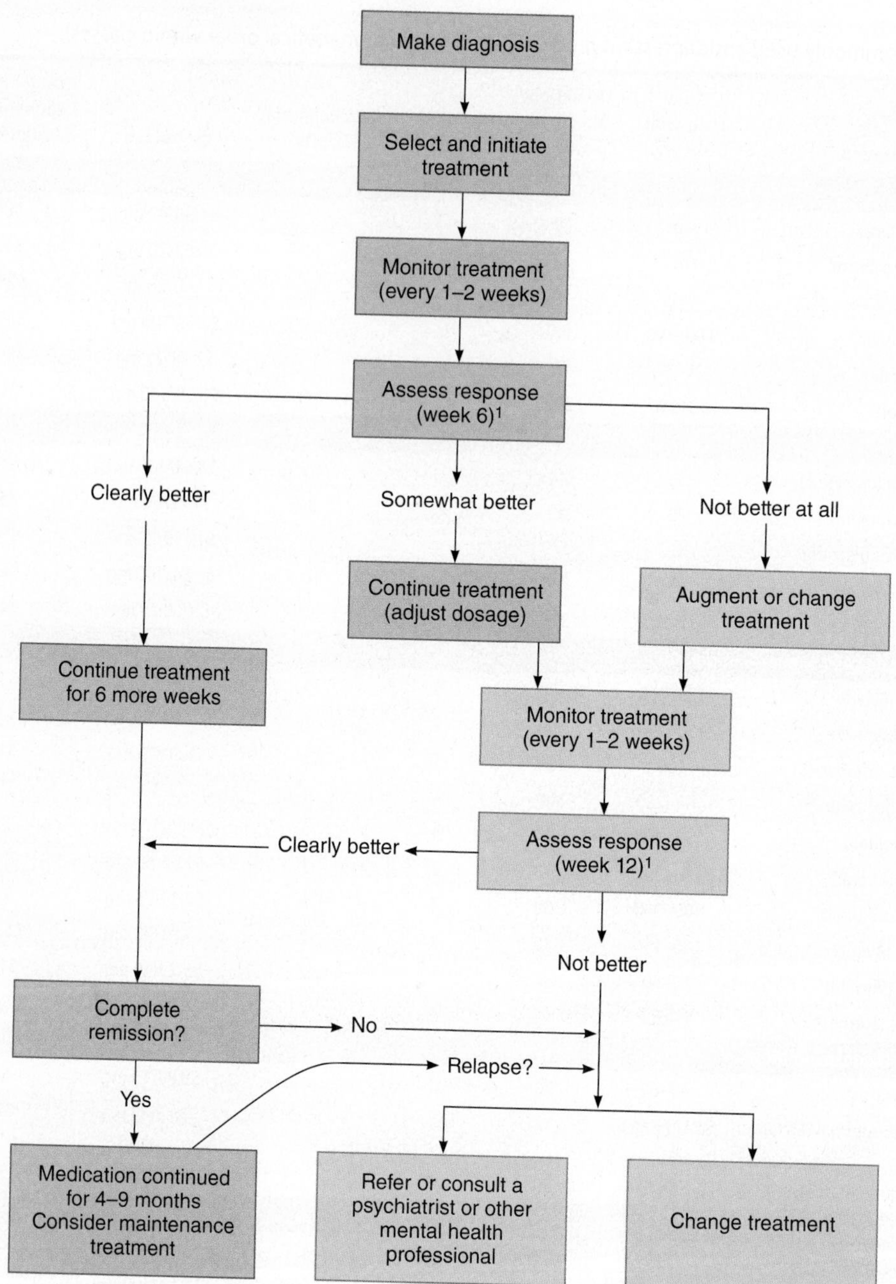

▲ **Figure 25–2.** **Overview of treatment for depression.** (Reproduced from Agency for Health Care Policy and Research: Depression in Primary Care. Vol. 2: Treatment of Major Depression. United States Department of Health and Human Services, 1993.)

once-daily dosage. Nefazodone and trazodone are usually given twice daily. Bupropion and venlafaxine are available in extended-release formulations and can be given once daily. There is usually some delay in response; fluoxetine, for example, requires 2–6 weeks to act in depression, 4–8 weeks to be effective in panic disorder, and 6–12 weeks in treatment of OCD. The starting dose (10 mg) is given for 1 week before increasing to the average daily oral dose of 20 mg for depression, while OCD may require up to 80 mg daily. Some patients, particularly older adults, may tolerate and benefit from as little as 10 mg/day or every other day. The other SSRIs have shorter half-lives and a lesser effect on hepatic enzymes, which reduces their impact on the metabolism of other medications (thus not increasing significantly the serum concentrations of other medications as much as fluoxetine). The shorter half-lives also allow for more rapid clearing if adverse side effects appear. Venlafaxine appears to be more effective with doses greater than 200 mg/day orally, although some individuals respond to doses as low as 75 mg/day.

The side effects common to these medications are headache, nausea, tinnitus, insomnia, and nervousness. Akathisia has been common with the SSRIs; other extrapyramidal symptoms (eg, dystonias) have occurred infrequently but particularly in withdrawal states. Because SSRIs affect platelet serotonin levels, abnormal bleeding can occur. Sertraline and citalopram appear to be the safest agents in this class when used with warfarin. Sexual side effects of erectile dysfunction, retrograde ejaculation, and dysorgasmia are very common with the SSRIs. Oral phosphodiesterase-5 inhibitors (such as sildenafil, 25–50 mg; tadalafil, 5–20 mg; or vardenafil, 10–20 mg taken 1 hour prior to sexual activity) can improve erectile dysfunction in some patients and have been shown to improve other SSRI-induced sexual dysfunction in both men and women. Adjunctive bupropion (75–150 mg orally daily) may also enhance sexual arousal. Cyproheptadine, 4 mg orally prior to sexual activity, may be helpful in countering drug-induced anorgasmia but also is quite sedating and may counter the therapeutic benefits of SSRIs as well. Taking a "drug holiday," ie, skipping a day of medication periodically when sexual activity is anticipated, can also decrease sexual side effects. The SSRIs are strong serotonin uptake blockers and may in high dosage or in combination with MAO inhibitors, including the antiparkinsonian drug selegiline, cause a **"serotonin syndrome."** This syndrome is manifested by rigidity, hyperthermia, autonomic instability, myoclonus, confusion, delirium, and coma. This syndrome can be troublesome in older adults. Research indicates that SSRIs are safer agents to use than TCAs in patients with cardiac disease; the SSRI sertraline is a safe and effective antidepressant treatment in patients with acute MI or unstable angina.

Withdrawal symptoms, including dizziness, paresthesias, dysphoric mood, agitation, and a flu-like state, have been reported for the shorter-acting SSRIs and SNRIs but may occur with other classes including the TCAs and MAO inhibitors. These medications should be discontinued gradually over a period of weeks or months to reduce the risk of withdrawal phenomena.

Most studies show that SSRIs are not associated with birth defects. Paroxetine has some association with a fetal heart defect and should be avoided in favor of other SSRIs during pregnancy. Maternal major mood disorder in pregnancy by itself carries its own risks to the mother and fetus and has been linked to low birth weight and preterm delivery. Postpartum effects of prenatal depression have not been studied. The decision to use SSRIs and other psychotropic agents during pregnancy and postpartum must be a collaborative decision based on a thorough risk-benefit analysis for each individual.

Venlafaxine lacks significant anticholinergic side effects. Nausea, nervousness, and profuse sweating appear to be the major side effects. Venlafaxine appears to have few drug-drug interactions. It does require monitoring of blood pressure because dose-related hypertension may develop in some individuals. Venlafaxine prescribing in the United Kingdom has been restricted to psychiatrists. Desvenlafaxine, a newer form of the medication, is started at its target dose of 50 mg/day orally and does not require upward titration although higher doses have been well studied and some patients benefit from 100 mg/day. Duloxetine may also result in small increases in blood pressure. Common side effects include dry mouth, dizziness, and fatigue. Milnacipran, approved for the treatment of fibromyalgia, and levomilnacipran, approved for the treatment of major depression, carry many of the side effects common to other SNRIs including a mild tachycardia, hypertension, sexual side effects, mydriasis, urinary constriction, and occasional abnormal bleeding. Levomilnacipran is started at 20 mg/day orally then increased to 40 mg/day after 2–3 days. The target dose is 40–120 mg given once daily. Milnacipran is typically started at 12.5 mg/day orally, titrated to 12.5 mg twice daily after 2 days, and then to 25 mg twice daily after 7 days. The target dose is typically 100–200 mg/day given in in two divided doses. While not approved for the treatment of major depression, the evidence suggests that milnacipran, like levomilnacipran, is an effective antidepressant agent.

Nefazodone appears to lack the anticholinergic effects of the TCAs and the agitation sometimes induced by SSRIs. Because nefazodone inhibits the liver's cytochrome P450 3A4 isoenzymes, concurrent use of these medications can lead to serious QT prolongation, ventricular tachycardia, or death. Through the same mechanism of enzyme inhibition, nefazodone can elevate cyclosporine levels sixfold to tenfold. Nefazodone carries an FDA warning given its association with liver failure in rare cases. Pretreatment and ongoing monitoring of liver biochemical enzymes is indicated.

Mirtazapine is thought to enhance central noradrenergic and serotonergic activity with minimal sexual side effects compared with the SSRIs. Its action as a potent antagonist of histaminergic receptors may make it a useful agent for patients with depression and insomnia. It is also an effective antiemetic due to its antagonism of the 5-HT_3 receptor. Its most common adverse side effects include somnolence, increased appetite, weight gain, lipid abnormalities, and dizziness. The labeling for mirtazapine indicated that agranulocytosis was seen in 2 of 2796 patients in premarketing studies. An association of agranulocytosis or a clinically significant neutropenia with the medication appears to be modest. Although it is metabolized by P450 isoenzymes, it is not an inhibitor of this system. It is given in a single oral dose at bedtime starting at 15 mg and titrated up to 45 mg with some evidence that 30 mg may be optimal for most people.

Vortioxetine is an antidepressant that blocks serotonin reuptake, is a partial agonist of the 5-HT_{1A} receptor, and affects a variety of other serotonin receptor sites. The side effects attributed to its serotonergic effects include GI upset and sexual dysfunction. Vortioxetine has demonstrated efficacy in improving some cognitive symptoms of depression and received regulatory approval for this indication in Europe and the United States. Vortioxetine is typically dosed at 10 mg/day orally and may be increased to 20 mg/day.

2. Tricyclic antidepressants (TCAs) and clinically similar medications—TCAs were the mainstay of medication therapy for depression for many years. They have also been effective in panic disorder, pain syndromes, and anxiety states. Specific ones have been studied and found to be effective in OCD (clomipramine), enuresis (imipramine), psychotic depression (amoxapine), and reduction of craving in cocaine withdrawal (desipramine).

TCAs are characterized more by their similarities than by their differences. They tend to affect both serotonin and norepinephrine reuptake; some medications act mainly on the former and others principally on the latter neurotransmitter system. Individuals receiving the same dosages vary markedly in therapeutic drug levels achieved (older adult patients require smaller doses), and determination of plasma drug levels is helpful when clinical response has been disappointing. Nortriptyline is usually effective when plasma levels are between 50 and 150 ng/mL; imipramine at plasma levels of 200–250 ng/mL; and desipramine at plasma levels of 100–250 ng/mL. High blood levels are not more effective than moderate levels and may be counterproductive (eg, delirium, seizures). Patients with GI side effects benefit from plasma level monitoring to assess absorption of the drug. Most TCAs can be given in a single dose at bedtime, starting at low doses (eg, nortriptyline 25 mg orally) and increasing by 25 mg every several days as tolerated until the therapeutic response is achieved (eg, nortriptyline, 100–150 mg) or to maximum dose if necessary (eg, nortriptyline, 150 mg). The most common cause of treatment failure is an inadequate trial. A full trial consists of giving a therapeutic daily dosage for at least 6 weeks. Because of marked anticholinergic and sedating side effects, clomipramine is started at a low dose (25 mg/day orally) and increased slowly in divided doses up to 100 mg/day, held at that level for several days, and then gradually increased as necessary up to 250 mg/day. The TCAs have anticholinergic side effects to varying degrees (amitriptyline 100 mg is equivalent to atropine 5 mg). One must be particularly wary of the effect in older adult men with prostatic hyperplasia. The anticholinergic effects also predispose to other medical problems such as constipation, confusion, heat stroke, or dental problems from xerostomia. Orthostatic hypotension is common, is not dose-dependent, and may not remit with time on medication; this may predispose to falls and hip fractures in older adults.

Cardiac effects of the TCAs are functions of the anticholinergic effect, direct myocardial depression, quinidine-like effect, and interference with adrenergic neurons. These factors may produce altered rate, rhythm, and contractility, particularly in patients with preexisting cardiac disease, such as bundle-branch or bifascicular block. Even relatively small overdoses (eg, 1500 mg of imipramine) have resulted in lethal arrhythmias. Electrocardiographic changes range from benign ST segment and T wave changes and sinus tachycardia to a variety of complex and serious arrhythmias, the latter requiring a change in medication. Because TCAs have class I antiarrhythmic effects, they should be used with caution in patients with ischemic heart disease, arrhythmias, or conduction disturbances. SSRIs or the atypical antidepressants are better initial choices for this population.

TCAs lower the seizure threshold, so this is of particular concern in patients with a propensity for seizures. Loss of libido and erectile, ejaculatory, and orgasmic dysfunction are common and can compromise compliance. Trazodone rarely causes priapism (1 in 9000), but when it occurs, it requires treatment within 12 hours (epinephrine 1:1000 injected into the corpus cavernosum). Delirium, agitation, and mania are infrequent complications of the TCAs but can occur. Sudden discontinuation of some of these medications can produce "cholinergic rebound," manifested by headaches and nausea with abdominal cramps. Overdoses of TCAs are often serious because of the narrow therapeutic index and quinidine-like effects (see Chapter 38).

3. Monoamine oxidase inhibitors—The MAO inhibitors are generally used as third-line medications for depression (after a failure of SSRIs, SNRIs, TCAs, or the atypical antidepressants) because of the dietary and other restrictions required (Table 25–7). They should be considered third-line medications for refractory panic disorder as well as depression; however, this hierarchy has become more flexible since MAO inhibitor skin patches (selegiline) have become available. They deliver the MAO inhibitor to the bloodstream bypassing the GI tract so that dietary restrictions are not necessary in the lowest dosage strength (6 mg/24 hours).

The MAO inhibitors commonly cause symptoms of orthostatic hypotension (which may persist) and sympathomimetic effects of tachycardia, sweating, and tremor. Nausea, insomnia (often associated with intense afternoon drowsiness), and sexual dysfunction are common. Zolpidem 5–10 mg orally at bedtime can ameliorate MAO-induced insomnia. CNS effects include agitation and toxic psychoses. *Dietary limitations* (see Table 25–7) and abstinence from medication products containing phenylpropanolamine, phenylephrine, meperidine, dextromethorphan, and pseudoephedrine are mandatory for MAO-A type inhibitors (those marketed for treatment of depression), since the reduction of available MAO leaves the patient vulnerable to exogenous amines (eg, tyramine in foodstuffs).

4. Other medications and those under investigation—Dextroamphetamine (5–30 mg/day orally) and methylphenidate (10–45 mg/day orally) may be effective for the

Table 25–7. Principal dietary restrictions in MAO inhibitor use.

1. Cheese, except cream cheese and cottage cheese and fresh yogurt
2. Fermented or aged meats such as bologna, salami
3. Broad bean pods such as Chinese bean pods
4. Liver of all types
5. Meat and yeast extracts
6. Red wine, sherry, vermouth, cognac, beer, ale
7. Soy sauce, shrimp paste, sauerkraut

short-term treatment of some depressive symptoms in medically ill and geriatric patients. The stimulants are notable for rapid onset of action (hours) and a paucity of side effects (tachycardia, agitation) in most patients. They are usually given in two divided doses early in the day (eg, 7 am and noon) so as to avoid interfering with sleep. These agents may also be useful as adjunctive agents in refractory depression. Intravenous infusion of the dissociative anesthetic ketamine has been shown to lead to a rapid improvement in depressive symptoms in 50–70% of patients with depression. The effects of a single treatment are short-lived (about 3–7 days). Esketamine nasal spray has been approved by the FDA for the treatment of depression for patients who have been inadequately treated by two other antidepressant medications. However, there are ongoing concerns about long-term use of esketamine or ketamine, including the risk of abuse and longer-term impacts on mood and suicidality. Other NMDA antagonists and opioid system agents continue to be evaluated in the treatment of resistant depression.

Allopregnanolone, a neurosteroid, is an allosteric modulator of GABA-a receptors and is approved for the treatment of postpartum depression. Like ketamine, allopregnanolone is administered intravenously, and the antidepressant effects are rapid. An allopregnanolone infusion is given over 60 hours in a health care facility and was significantly more effective than placebo in treating postpartum depression by the end of the 2.5-day infusion, and benefits were sustained for the 30 days of the study period in three registration trials. The most common side effects of allopregnanolone are headache, dizziness, and somnolence. There is a rare side effect of loss of consciousness that requires the infusion be monitored in a health care facility. There is good reason to believe that GABA-a modulators will be useful in other types of depression, including for addressing anxiety and insomnia in patients with more severe depression. Several orally active GABA-a modulators are in development.

5. Switching and combination therapy— If there has been a partial response, evidence supports medication augmentation. If the therapeutic response has been poor after an adequate trial with the chosen medication, the diagnosis should be reassessed. Assuming that the trial has been adequate and the diagnosis is correct, a trial with a second medication is appropriate. In switching from one group to another, an adequate "washout time" must be allowed. This is critical in certain situations—eg, in switching from an MAO inhibitor to a TCA, allow 2–3 weeks between stopping one medication and starting another; in switching from an SSRI to an MAO inhibitor, allow 4–5 weeks for fluoxetine and at least 2 weeks for other SSRIs. In switching within groups—eg, from one TCA to another (amitriptyline to desipramine, etc)—no washout time is needed, and one can rapidly decrease the dosage of one medication while increasing the other. In clinical practice, adjunctive treatment with lithium, buspirone, or thyroid hormone may be helpful in depression. The adjunctive use of low-dose atypical antipsychotics such as aripiprazole, olanzapine, and quetiapine in the treatment of patients with refractory depression is supported by research. The side effect risk is the same as when treating psychosis. Adding an atypical agent requires monitoring BMI, lipids, and glucose. Combining two antidepressants or adding an antipsychotic to an antidepressant requires caution and is usually reserved for clinicians who feel comfortable managing this or after psychiatric consultation.

6. Maintenance and tapering—When clinical relief of symptoms is obtained, medication is continued for 6–12 months in the same dosage required in the acute stage. Although there is a higher risk of relapse after tapering off medication, there is evidence that cognitive behavioral therapy can prevent symptom relapse and the need for long-term medication. The full dosage should be continued indefinitely when the individual has had three episodes. Major depression generally should be considered a chronic/intermittent disease with most patients having relapses in time and some patients never fully recovering from a depressive episode. If the medication is being tapered, it should be done gradually over several months, monitoring closely for relapse.

7. Drug interactions—There are numerous possible drug interactions that prescribers should consider. Review of potential drug interactions with available online tools or a pharmacist is recommended.

8. Electroconvulsive therapy—ECT is the most effective (about 45–85% remission rate) treatment of severe depression. The mechanism of action is not known, but it is thought to involve major neurotransmitter responses at the cell membrane. In treatment-resistant depression, remission rates from ECT are lower (around 48%). It is particularly effective for the delusions and agitation commonly seen with depression in older adults. It is indicated when medical conditions preclude the use of antidepressants, with nonresponsiveness to these medications, and for extreme suicidality. Comparative controlled studies of ECT in severe depression show that it is more effective than pharmacotherapy. It is also effective in the treatment of mania and catatonia. It has also been shown to be helpful in chronic schizophrenic disorders when clozapine alone is not fully effective.

The most common side effects of ECT are memory disturbance and headache. Memory loss or confusion is usually related to the number and frequency of ECT treatments and proper oxygenation during treatment. Unilateral ECT is associated with less memory loss than bilateral ECT. Both anterograde and retrograde memory loss may occur, but short-term anterograde memory loss is more common. While some memory deficits may persist, memory loss tends to improve in a few weeks after the last ECT treatment.

Increased intracranial pressure is a contraindication. Other problems such as cardiac disorders, aortic aneurysms, bronchopulmonary disease, and venous thrombosis must be evaluated in light of the severity of the medical problem versus the need for ECT. Serious complications arising from ECT occur in less than 1 in 1000 cases. Most of these problems are cardiovascular or respiratory in nature (eg, aspiration of gastric contents, arrhythmias, MI). Poor patient understanding and lack of acceptance of the technique by the public are some of the biggest obstacles to the use of ECT.

9. Phototherapy—Phototherapy is used in major depression with seasonal onset. It consists of indirect eye exposure to a light source of greater than 2500 lux for 2 hours daily or 10,000 lux for 20 minutes daily to increase the photoperiod of the day. Light visors are an adaptation that provides greater mobility and an adjustable light intensity but may not be as effective. The dosage varies, with some patients requiring morning and night exposure. One effect is alteration of biorhythm through melatonin mechanisms.

10. Repetitive transcranial magnetic stimulation—Repetitive transcranial magnetic stimulation (rTMS) is used to treat nonpsychotic treatment-resistant depression and involves the application of electromagnetic pulses to the dorsolateral prefrontal cortex. Its use in depression is approved by the FDA for individuals who have not tolerated or responded to at least one or more standard antidepressant medications. It is usually delivered in a course of 30 sessions over 6 weeks. rTMS neither requires general anesthesia nor is associated with cognitive side effects. Several meta-analyses have demonstrated that in nonpsychotic depression, rTMS is noninferior to ECT. There is a small risk of seizure (1:30,000 in postmarket research), and this is due primarily to operator error. The most common side effects are scalp sensitivity under the coil and transient headache.

11. Other treatments—Vagus nerve stimulation has shown promise in about one-third of extremely refractory cases and is approved by the FDA. Data have demonstrated that the effects plateau around 18 months to 2 years and are durable at 5 years.

B. Psychological

It is often challenging to engage an individual in psychotherapeutic endeavors during the acute stage of a severe depression. While medications may be taking effect, a supportive and behavioral approach to strengthen existing coping mechanisms and appropriate consideration of the patient's continuing need to function at work, to engage in recreational activities, etc, are necessary as the severity of the depression lessens. Therapy during or just after the acute stage may focus on coping techniques, with some practice of alternative choices. Depression-specific psychotherapies help improve self-esteem, increase assertiveness, and lessen dependency. Interpersonal psychotherapy for depression has shown efficacy in the treatment of acute depression, helping patients master interpersonal stresses and develop new coping strategies. Cognitive behavioral therapy for depression addresses patients' patterns of negative thoughts, called cognitive distortions, which lead to feelings of depression and anxiety. Treatment usually includes homework assignments such as keeping a journal of cognitive distortions and of positive responses to them. *The combination of medication therapy plus interpersonal psychotherapy or cognitive behavioral therapy is generally more effective than either modality alone.* It is sometimes helpful to involve the spouse or other significant family members early in treatment. Mindfulness-based cognitive therapy has reduced relapse rates in several randomized controlled trials. In two studies, it was as effective as maintenance medication in preventing relapse. This therapy incorporates meditation and teaches patients to distance themselves from depressive thinking.

C. Social

Flexible use of appropriate social services can be of major importance in the treatment of depression. Since alcohol abuse is often associated with depression, early involvement in alcohol treatment programs such as Alcoholics Anonymous can be important to future success (see Alcohol Use Disorder [Alcoholism]). The structuring of daily activities during severe depression is often quite difficult for the patient, and loneliness is often a major factor. The help of family, employer, or friends is often necessary to mobilize the patient who experiences no joy in daily activities and tends to remain uninvolved and to deteriorate. Insistence on sharing activities will help involve the patient in simple but important daily functions. In some severe cases, the use of day treatment centers or support groups of a specific type (eg, mastectomy groups) is indicated. It is not unusual for a patient to have multiple legal, financial, and vocational problems requiring legal and vocational assistance.

D. Behavioral

When depression is a function of self-defeating coping techniques such as passivity, the role-playing approach can be useful. Behavioral techniques, including desensitization, may be used in problems such as phobias where depression is a by-product. When depression is a regularly used interpersonal style, behavioral counseling to family members or others can help in extinguishing the behavior in the patient. Behavioral activation, a technique of motivating depressed patients to begin engaging in pleasurable activities, has been shown to be a useful depression-specific psychotherapy. Exercise, especially aerobic and supervised by exercise professionals, has evidence in improving depressive symptoms.

Treatment of Bipolar Disorder, Manic & Depressive Episodes

Acute manic or hypomanic symptoms will respond to the mood stabilizers lithium or valproic acid after several days of treatment. Antipsychotics may be used as well for mania. High-potency benzodiazepines (eg, clonazepam) may also be useful adjuncts in managing the agitation and sleep disturbance that are features of manic and hypomanic episodes.

A. Antipsychotics

Acute manic symptoms may be treated initially with a second-generation antipsychotic such as olanzapine (eg, 5–20 mg orally), risperidone (2–3 mg orally), or aripiprazole (15–30 mg) in conjunction with a benzodiazepine if indicated. Alternatively, when behavioral control is immediately necessary, olanzapine in an injectable form (2.5–10 mg intramuscularly) or haloperidol, 5–10 mg orally or intramuscularly repeated as needed until symptoms subside, may be used. The dosage of the antipsychotic may be gradually reduced after lithium or another mood stabilizer is started. Olanzapine, quetiapine, ziprasidone, aripiprazole, and the long-acting injectable risperidone are approved as maintenance treatments for bipolar disorder to prevent subsequent cycles of both mania and depression.

B. Valproic Acid

Valproic acid (divalproex) is a first-line treatment for mania. This issue is particularly important in AIDS or other medically ill patients prone to dehydration or malabsorption with wide swings in serum lithium levels. Valproic acid has also been used effectively in panic disorder and migraine headache. Treatment is often started at a dose of 750 mg/day orally, and dosage is then titrated to achieve therapeutic serum levels. Oral loading in acutely manic bipolar patients in an inpatient setting (initiated at a dosage of 20 mg/kg/day) can safely achieve serum therapeutic levels in 2–3 days. GI symptoms and weight gain are the main side effects. Liver enzyme biochemical tests, CBCs, glucose levels, and weight should be monitored at 2 weeks, 4 weeks, and 3 months initially and annually or more frequently thereafter based on clinical judgment. Significant teratogenic effects are a concern so pregnancy should be ruled out prior to initiation. In utero exposure to valproate has been associated with adversely affecting neural tube development in the fetus and there is an FDA warning to that effect. Thus, alternatives to valproate should be considered in women of childbearing years who might become pregnant.

C. Lithium

Lithium significantly decreases the frequency and severity of both manic and depressive attacks in about 50–70% of patients and is FDA-approved for maintenance and manic episodes.

In addition to its use in bipolar disorder, lithium is sometimes useful in the prophylaxis of recurrent unipolar depressions (perhaps undiagnosed bipolar disorder) and in lowering the risk of suicide. Lithium may ameliorate nonspecific aggressive behaviors and dyscontrol syndromes. Many patients with bipolar disease can be managed long-term with lithium alone, although some will require continued or intermittent use of an antipsychotic or lamotrigine to help prevent depressive episodes. An excellent resource for information is the Lithium Information Center, https://www.uwhealth.org/health/topic/multum/lithium/d00061a1.html.

Before treatment, the clinical workup should include a medical history and physical examination; CBC; T_4, thyroid-stimulating hormone, BUN, serum creatinine, and serum electrolyte determinations; UA; and electrocardiography (in patients over age 45 or with a history of cardiac disease).

1. Dosage—The common starting dosage of lithium carbonate is 300–900 mg daily, with trough blood levels measured after 4–5 days of treatment. A slow-release form or units of different dosage may be used. Lithium citrate is available as a syrup. The dosage is that required to maintain blood levels in the therapeutic range. For acute manic episodes, this ranges from 0.8 mEq/L to 1.2 mEq/L. Although there is controversy about the optimal long-term maintenance dose, many clinicians reduce the acute level to 0.6–1 mEq/L in order to reduce side effects. The dose required to meet this need will vary in different individuals. Augmentation of antidepressants is usually achieved with lower blood levels. Once-a-day dosage is acceptable.

Lithium is readily absorbed, with peak serum levels occurring within 1–3 hours and complete absorption in 8 hours. Half of the total body lithium is excreted in 18–24 hours (95% in the urine). Blood for lithium levels should be drawn 12 hours after the last dose. Serum levels should be measured 4–7 days after initiation of treatment and changes in dose. For maintenance treatment, lithium levels should be monitored initially every 1–2 months but may be measured every 6–12 months in stable, long-term patients. Levels should be monitored more closely when there is any condition that causes volume depletion (eg, diarrhea, dehydration, use of diuretics).

2. Side effects—Early side effects, including mild GI symptoms (take lithium with food and in divided doses), fine tremors (treat with propranolol, 20–60 mg/day orally, only if persistent), slight muscle weakness, and some degree of somnolence, can occur and are usually transient. Moderate polyuria (reduced renal responsiveness to ADH) and polydipsia (associated with increased plasma renin concentration) are often present. Potassium administration can blunt this effect, as may once-daily dosing of lithium. Weight gain (often a result of calories in fluids taken for polydipsia) and leukocytosis not due to infection can occur.

Thyroid side effects include goiter (3%; often euthyroid) and hypothyroidism (10%; concomitant administration of lithium and iodide or lithium and carbamazepine enhances the hypothyroid and goitrogenic effect of either medication). Most clinicians treat lithium-induced hypothyroidism (more common in women) with thyroid hormone while continuing lithium therapy. Changes in the glucose tolerance test toward a diabetes-like curve, nephrogenic diabetes insipidus (usually resolving about 8 weeks after cessation of lithium therapy), nephrotic syndrome, edema, folate deficiency, and pseudotumor cerebri (ophthalmoscopy is indicated if there are complaints of headache or blurred vision) can occur. Thyroid and kidney function should be checked at 4- to 6-month intervals. Hypercalcemia and elevated parathyroid hormone levels occur in some patients. Electrocardiographic abnormalities (principally T wave flattening or inversion) may occur during lithium administration but are not of major clinical significance. Sinoatrial block may occur, particularly in older adults. Lithium alone does not have a significant effect on sexual function, but when combined with benzodiazepines (clonazepam in most symptomatic patients), it causes sexual dysfunction in about 50% of men. Most of these side effects subside when lithium is discontinued; when residual side effects exist, they are usually not serious.

Side effects from long-term lithium therapy include the development of cogwheel rigidity and, occasionally, other extrapyramidal signs. Lithium potentiates the parkinsonian effects of haloperidol. Lithium-induced delirium with therapeutic lithium levels is an infrequent complication usually occurring in older adults and may persist for several days after serum levels have become negligible. Encephalopathy has occurred in patients receiving combined lithium and antipsychotic therapy and in those who have cerebrovascular disease, thus requiring careful evaluation of patients who develop neurotoxic signs at subtoxic blood levels.

Some reports have suggested that the long-term use of lithium may have adverse effects on kidney function (with interstitial fibrosis, tubular atrophy, or nephrogenic diabetes insipidus). Persistent polyuria should require an investigation of the kidney's ability to concentrate urine. A rise in serum creatinine levels is an indication for in-depth evaluation of kidney function and consideration of alternative treatments if the individual can tolerate a change. Incontinence has been reported in women, apparently related to changes in bladder cholinergic-adrenergic balance.

The risk imposed by lithium in pregnancy may be overemphasized. Lithium exposure in early pregnancy minimally increases the frequency of rare congenital anomalies. Mothers who take lithium should use formula to feed their newborn, since concentration in breast milk is one-third to half that in serum.

Frank toxicity usually occurs at blood lithium levels greater than 2 mEq/L. Because sodium and lithium are reabsorbed at the same loci in the proximal renal tubules, any sodium loss (diarrhea, use of diuretics, or excessive perspiration) increases lithium levels. Symptoms and signs include vomiting and diarrhea, the latter exacerbating the problem since more sodium is lost and more lithium is absorbed. Other symptoms and signs, some of which may not be reversible, include tremors, marked muscle weakness, confusion, dysarthria, vertigo, choreoathetosis, ataxia, hyperreflexia, rigidity, lack of coordination, myoclonus, seizures, opisthotonos, and coma. Toxicity is more severe in older adults, who should be maintained on slightly lower serum levels. Lithium overdosage may be accidental or intentional or may occur because of poor monitoring. Significant overdoses of lithium are typically managed with hemodialysis since the medication is excreted completely by the kidneys.

See Chapter 38 for the treatment of patients with massive ingestions of lithium or blood lithium levels greater than 2.5 mEq/L.

3. Drug interactions—Patients receiving lithium should use diuretics with caution and only under close medical supervision. The thiazide diuretics cause increased lithium reabsorption from the proximal renal tubules, resulting in increased serum lithium levels and adjustment of lithium intake must be made to compensate for this. Potential drug interactions of lithium with other medications should be considered; consultation with a pharmacist or online drug interaction tools is recommended.

D. Carbamazepine

Carbamazepine is used in the treatment of bipolar patients who cannot be satisfactorily treated with lithium (nonresponsive, excessive side effects, or rapid cycling). It is often effective at 800–1600 mg/day orally. It has also been used in the treatment of trigeminal neuralgias and alcohol withdrawal as well as in patients with behavioral dyscontrol. It has been used to treat residual symptoms in previous stimulant abusers (eg, PTSD with impulse control problems). Dose-related side effects include sedation and ataxia. Dosages start at 400–600 mg orally daily and are increased slowly to therapeutic levels. Skin rashes and a mild reduction in white count are common. Syndrome of inappropriate antidiuretic hormone secretion occurs rarely. Carbamazepine can be effective in conjunction with lithium, although there have been reports of reversible neurotoxicity with the combination. It also lowers T_4, free T_4, and T_3 levels. Cases of fetal malformation (particularly spina bifida) have been reported along with growth deficiency and developmental delay. Liver biochemical tests and CBCs should be monitored in patients taking carbamazepine. Genetic studies suggest that screening for the HLA-B1502 allele in the Han Chinese population and the HLA-A3101 allele in northern Europeans may help target individuals more susceptible to a serious rash. Oxcarbazepine, a derivative of carbamazepine, does not appear to induce its own metabolism, and is associated with fewer drug interactions, although it may impose a higher risk of hyponatremia. FDA-approved for partial seizures, oxcarbazepine may have efficacy in acute mania. It appears to be a safer alternative to carbamazepine due to its lower risk of hepatotoxicity.

E. Lamotrigine

Lamotrigine is FDA-approved for the maintenance treatment of bipolar disorder. Two double-blind studies support its efficacy in the treatment of acute bipolar depression as adjunctive therapy or as monotherapy, but several other controlled studies failed to demonstrate benefit. Likewise, lamotrigine has *not* proven effective in the management of acute mania. Its metabolism is inhibited by coadministration of valproic acid—doubling its half-life—and accelerated by hepatic enzyme-inducing agents such as carbamazepine. More frequent mild side effects include headache, dizziness, nausea, and diplopia. Rash occurring in 10% of patients may be an indication for immediate cessation of dosing, since lamotrigine has been associated with Stevens-Johnson syndrome (1:1000) and, rarely, toxic epidermal necrolysis. The medication should be stopped for a rash associated with systemic symptoms including fever, lymphadenopathy, and oral mucosa ulcerations, and the patient sent to an emergency department. Any new rash associated with lamotrigine use should be evaluated by a dermatologist. Dosing starts at 25–50 mg/day orally and is titrated upward slowly to decrease the likelihood of rash.

Prognosis

Most depressive episodes are usually time-limited, and the prognosis with treatment is good if a pathologic pattern of adjustment does not intervene. Major affective disorders frequently respond well to a full trial of medication treatment. However, at least 20% of patients will have a more chronic illness lasting two or more years. Many patients do not sustain a complete remission of symptoms and most depressive episodes recur. At least 80% of patients who have a single major depressive episode will have one or more recurrences within 15 years of the index episode. Many patients, therefore, require long-term maintenance therapy with antidepressants.

Mania has a good prognosis with adequate treatment, although patient adherence to treatment is often quite challenging. Few effective medications exist for bipolar depression, which include quetiapine, lurasidone, cariprazine, and the combination of fluoxetine and olanzapine. Many patients with bipolar disorder require treatment with two or more medications such as lithium, antipsychotics, and sleeping agents. Breakthrough manic or depressive episodes are common, even with adherence to maintenance treatments, although maintenance therapy lessens the risk of recurrent episodes.

Breedvelt JJF et al. Continuation of antidepressants vs sequential psychological interventions to prevent relapse in depression. JAMA Psychiatry. 2021;78:868. [PMID: 34009273]

Bueno-Notivol J et al. Prevalence of depression during the COVID-19 outbreak: a meta-analysis of community-based studies. Int J Clin Health Psychol. 2021;21:100196. [PMID: 32904715]

Leader LD et al. Brexanolone for postpartum depression: clinical evidence and practical considerations. Pharmacotherapy. 2019;39:1105. [PMID: 31514247]

ATTENTION-DEFICIT/HYPERACTIVITY DISORDER

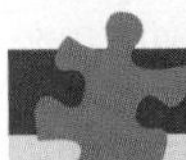

ESSENTIALS OF DIAGNOSIS

- Persistent patterns of inability to sustain attention, excessive motor activity/restlessness/impulsivity, or both.
- Symptoms interfere with daily functioning.
- Symptoms began prior to age 12 and in at least two settings (ie, school/work, home, with friends/family).

Clinical Findings

Attention-deficit/hyperactivity disorder (ADHD) begins in childhood; however symptoms persist into adulthood in two-thirds of patients, with half of those still requiring medication to aid in functioning. The prevalence of ADHD in adults is estimated to be 4–5%. In some patients, ADHD is not diagnosed during childhood because they may not have presented for assessment or were able to compensate for symptoms at the time. The specific presenting symptoms in adulthood tend to be inattention, restlessness, and impulsivity, whereas hyperactivity has often improved. At least five inattention symptoms (such as making careless mistakes, being easily sidetracked, trouble keeping deadlines or with organization, losing belongings, being forgetful in daily chores/tasks) are required to meet criteria for this subtype of ADHD, or five hyperactivity/impulsivity symptoms (such as feeling restless and leaving a seat though expected to remain, feeling "driven by a motor," interrupting others, cannot wait his or her turn) for this subtype. It is often useful to have patients provide questionnaires to other adult observers, including those who knew them during childhood, such as parents. This collateral data can help prevent diagnosing ADHD in someone who is seeking stimulants but without symptomatology as well as aid in making the diagnosis, since evidence shows that many adults who do have ADHD often underreport symptoms.

Treatment

A. Pharmacologic

Stimulants such as methylphenidate and amphetamine are the most effective treatment. These come in short-acting and long-acting formulations. Caution should be used prior to prescribing these mediations to assess for potential substance abuse or diversion as well as for comorbid mood disorders that may not respond well to a stimulant. Atomoxetine, a nonstimulant, is a second-line FDA-approved agent for ADHD. Bupropion also has evidence of efficacy and may be considered in patients in whom a stimulant is contraindicated or in those who also suffer from major depression. Desipramine, a tricyclic antidepressant, can be effective for ADHD and may be considered in patients who have additional needs, such as a concomitant depression or neuropathic pain.

B. Behavioral and Other Treatments

Psychoeducation regarding ADHD should be given to all patients. Many patients are able to implement behavioral changes that either improve their functioning, such as creating calendars and organizational schemes or doing tasks in multiple timed short spurts, or can help them avoid tasks that are challenging for them in favor of complementary tasks they are more suited to (ie, selecting jobs that value more activity rather than sustained focus, or sharing in the chores at home that do not require attention to detail). Cognitive behavioral therapy has some evidence for helping residual symptoms after medication management has been optimized.

Nageye F et al. Beyond stimulants: a systematic review of randomised controlled trials assessing novel compounds for ADHD. Expert Rev Neurother. 2019;19:707. [PMID: 31167583]

AUTISM SPECTRUM DISORDERS

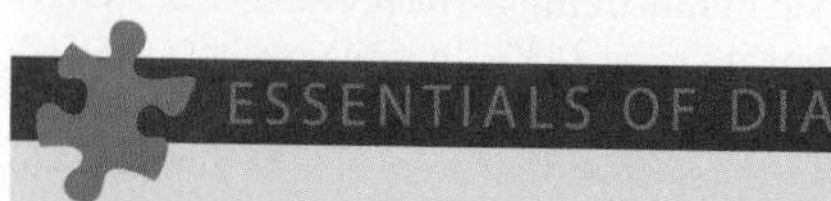

- Persistent issues with social communication and interactions.
- Repetitive behaviors, interests, or activities.
- Symptoms interfere with functioning.
- May or may not have accompanying language or intellectual impairment.

Clinical Findings

Autism spectrum disorder is a neurodevelopmental disorder in which patients suffer from pervasive *difficulties with social communication* and have *repetitive, restricted interests and behaviors*. Autism spectrum disorder affects about 1% of the adult population with an estimated heritability of about 90%. Approximately 20–30% of individuals in whom autism is diagnosed also have a substance use problem as well as a higher risk of ADHD and mood or obsessive-compulsive disorders. The National Institute of Health and Care Excellence (NICE) guidelines recommend that assessment of autism spectrum disorder should be a comprehensive and multidisciplinary approach that includes asking about core autism spectrum disorder difficulties, early development, medical and family history, behavior, education, employment, needs assessment, risks, physical examination with potential laboratory testing, and feedback to the individual.

Treatment

No treatments for the core symptoms of autism spectrum disorder in adults have been validated. Two antipsychotics, risperidone and paliperidone, are approved for treating irritability in patients with autism spectrum disorders. These antipsychotics can help with some of the behavioral symptoms of autism but also carry a risk of metabolic side effects and extrapyramidal symptoms. There is some evidence for therapy, such as applied behavioral analysis, to address social cognitions and behaviors. Use of repetitive transcranial magnetic stimulation and vasopressin for the treatment of autism spectrum disorder are under investigation.

Howes OD et al. Autism spectrum disorder: consensus guidelines on assessment, treatment and research from the British Association for Psychopharmacology. J Psychopharmacol. 2018;32:3. [PMID: 29237331]

SLEEP-WAKE DISORDERS

Sleep consists of two distinct states as shown by electroencephalographic studies: (1) **REM** (rapid eye movement) sleep, also called dream sleep, D state sleep, or paradoxic sleep, and (2) **NREM** (non-REM) sleep, also called S stage sleep, which is divided into stages 1, 2, 3, and 4 and is recognizable by different electroencephalographic patterns. Stages 3 and 4 are "delta" sleep. Dreaming occurs mostly in REM and to a lesser extent in NREM sleep.

Sleep is a cyclic phenomenon, with four or five REM periods during the night accounting for about one-fourth of the total night's sleep (1.5–2 hours). The first REM period occurs about 80–120 minutes after onset of sleep and lasts about 10 minutes. Later REM periods are longer (15–40 minutes) and occur mostly in the last several hours of sleep. Most stage 4 (deepest) sleep occurs in the first several hours.

Age-related changes in normal sleep include an unchanging percentage of REM sleep and a marked decrease in stage 3 and stage 4 sleep, with an increase in wakeful periods during the night. These normal changes, early bedtimes, and daytime naps play a role in the increased complaints of insomnia in older people. Variations in sleep patterns may be due to circumstances (eg, "jet lag") or to idiosyncratic patterns ("night owls") in persons who perhaps because of different "biologic rhythms" habitually go to bed late and sleep late in the morning. Creativity and rapidity of response to unfamiliar situations are impaired by loss of sleep. There are also rare individuals who have chronic difficulty in adapting to a 24-hour sleep-wake cycle (**desynchronization sleep disorder**), which can be resynchronized by altering exposure to light.

The three major sleep disorders are discussed below. Any persistent sleep disorder that is not attributable to another condition should be evaluated by a sleep specialist.

1. Insomnia

Classification & Clinical Findings

Patients may complain of difficulty getting to sleep or staying asleep, intermittent wakefulness during the night, early morning awakening, or combinations of any of these. Transient episodes are usually of little significance. Stress, caffeine, physical discomfort, daytime napping, and early bedtimes are common factors.

Psychiatric disorders are often associated with persistent insomnia. Depression is usually associated with fragmented sleep, decreased total sleep time, earlier onset of REM sleep, a shift of REM activity to the first half of the night, and a loss of slow wave sleep—all of which are nonspecific findings. In manic disorders, a reduced total sleep time and a decreased need for sleep are cardinal features and important early sign of impending mania. In addition to a decreased amount of sleep, manic episodes are characterized by a shortened REM latency and increased REM activity. Sleep-related panic attacks occur in the transition from stage 2 to stage 3 sleep in some patients with a longer REM latency in the sleep pattern preceding the attacks.

Abuse of alcohol may cause or be secondary to the sleep disturbance. There is a tendency to use alcohol as a means of getting to sleep without realizing that it disrupts the normal sleep cycle. Acute alcohol intake produces a decreased sleep latency with reduced REM sleep during the first half of the night. REM sleep is increased in the second half of the night, with an increase in total amount of slow wave sleep (stages 3 and 4). Vivid dreams and frequent awakenings are common. Chronic alcohol abuse increases stage 1 and decreases REM sleep (most medications delay or block REM sleep), with symptoms persisting for many months after the individual has stopped drinking. Acute alcohol or other sedative withdrawal causes delayed onset of sleep and REM rebound with intermittent awakening during the night.

Heavy smoking (more than a pack a day) causes difficulty falling asleep—often independently associated with an increase in coffee drinking. Excess intake of caffeine, cocaine, and other stimulants (eg, over-the-counter cold remedies) near bedtime causes decreased total sleep time—mostly NREM sleep—with some increased sleep latency.

Sedative-hypnotics—specifically, the benzodiazepines, which are the most commonly prescribed medications to promote sleep—tend to increase total sleep time, decrease sleep latency, and decrease nocturnal awakening, with variable effects on NREM sleep. Nonbenzodiazepine hypnotics have similar effects on sleep as do the benzodiazepines, though some evidence shows improved slow wave sleep and less residual next-morning somnolence with nonbenzodiazepines, such as zolpidem. Withdrawal causes just the opposite effects and results in continued use of the medication for the purpose of preventing withdrawal symptoms. Antidepressants decrease REM sleep (with marked rebound on withdrawal in the form of nightmares) and have varying effects on NREM sleep. The effect on REM sleep correlates with reports that REM sleep deprivation produces improvement in some depressions.

Persistent insomnias are also related to a wide variety of medical conditions, particularly delirium, pain, respiratory distress syndromes, uremia, asthma, thyroid disorders, and nocturia due to benign prostatic hyperplasia. Sleep apnea and restless leg movement are described below. Adequate analgesia and proper treatment of medical disorders will reduce symptoms and decrease the need for sedatives.

Treatment

In general, there are two broad classes of treatment for insomnia, and the two may be combined: psychological (cognitive behavioral) and pharmacologic. In situations of acute distress, such as a grief reaction, pharmacologic measures may be most appropriate. *With primary insomnia, however, initial efforts should be psychologically based.* This is true in older adults to avoid the potential adverse reactions of medications. The older population is at risk for complaints of insomnia because sleep becomes lighter and more easily disrupted with aging. Medical disorders that become more common with age may also predispose to insomnia.

A. Psychological

Psychological strategies should include educating the patient regarding good **sleep hygiene:** (1) Go to bed only when sleepy. (2) Use the bed and bedroom only for sleeping and sex. (3) If still awake after 20 minutes, leave the bedroom, pursue a restful activity (such as a bath or meditation), and only return when sleepy. (4) Get up at the same time every morning regardless of the amount of sleep during the night. (5) Discontinue caffeine and nicotine, at least in the evening if not completely. (6) Establish a daily exercise regimen. (7) Avoid alcohol as it may disrupt continuity of sleep. (8) Limit fluids in the evening. (9) Learn and practice relaxation techniques. (10) Establish a bedtime ritual and a routine time for going to sleep. Research suggests that *cognitive behavioral therapy for insomnia is as effective as zolpidem* with benefits sustained 1 year after treatment.

B. Pharmacologic

When the above measures are insufficient, medications may be useful. Lorazepam (0.5 mg orally nightly), temazepam (7.5–15 mg orally nightly), and the nonbenzodiazepine hypnotics zolpidem (5–10 mg orally nightly, with a limit of 5 mg indicated for women) and zaleplon (5–10 mg orally nightly) are often effective for the older population and can be given in larger doses—twice what is prescribed for older patients—in younger patients. Zaleplon is often used to treat insomnia characterized by middle-of-the-night awakening with difficulty falling back to sleep. Eszopiclone (2–3 mg orally) is similar in action to zolpidem and zaleplon and has a longer duration of action. A lower dose of 1 mg is indicated in older adults or those with hepatic impairment. It is important to note that short-acting agents like triazolam or zolpidem may lead to amnestic episodes if used on a daily ongoing basis. Longer-acting agents such as flurazepam (half-life of more than 48 hours) may accumulate in older adults and lead to cognitive slowing, ataxia, falls, and somnolence. In general, it is appropriate to *use medications for short courses of 1–2 weeks.* The medications described above have largely replaced barbiturates as hypnotic agents because of their greater safety in overdose and their lesser hepatic enzyme induction effects. Antihistamines such as diphenhydramine (25 mg orally nightly) or hydroxyzine (25 mg orally nightly) may also be useful for sleep, as they produce no pharmacologic dependency; their anticholinergic effects may, however, produce confusion or urinary symptoms in older adults. Trazodone, an atypical antidepressant, is a non–habit-forming, effective sleep medication in lower than antidepressant doses (25–150 mg orally at bedtime). Priapism is a rare side effect requiring emergent treatment. Doxepin, 3–6 mg per night, is a TCA that is also effective for insomnia. Ramelteon, 8 mg orally at bedtime, is a melatonin receptor agonist that helps with sleep onset and does not appear to have abuse potential. It appears to be safe for ongoing use without the development of tolerance. Melatonin is used in doses of 3–6 mg. While melatonin is effective in reducing sleep latency, it is not usually effective in maintaining sleep. Thus, other strategies or medications are often required for sleep maintenance.

The dual orexin receptor antagonists (DORAs) class of hypnotics are approved to help initiate and maintain sleep. DORAs such as suvorexant and lemborexant may be more effective than other hypnotics for some patients. However, the role of DORAs have not been established relative to other hypnotics and DORAs are more expensive since they are not generically available. DORAs have shown a significant increase in depressive symptoms in a subset of patients, so other hypnotics may be a better choice in depressed patients. The dose of suvorexant is 10–20 mg orally given about 30 minutes before bedtime, while lemborexant is typically given in dosages of 5–10 mg daily.

2. Hypersomnias (Disorders of Excessive Sleepiness)

Classification & Clinical Findings

A. Breathing-Related Sleep Disorders

Obstructive sleep apnea is by far the most common of the breathing-related sleep disorders that include **central sleep apnea** and **sleep-related hypoventilation**. Obstructive sleep apnea hypopnea is characterized by snoring, gasping, or breathing pauses during sleep and five or more apneas or hypopneas per hour or evidence by polysomnography. (See Chapter 9.)

B. Narcolepsy Syndrome

Narcolepsy consists of a tetrad of symptoms: (1) sudden, brief (about 15 minutes) sleep attacks that may occur during any type of activity; (2) cataplexy—sudden loss of muscle tone involving specific small muscle groups or generalized muscle weakness that may cause the person to slump to the floor, unable to move, often associated with emotional reactions and sometimes confused with seizure disorder; (3) sleep paralysis—a generalized flaccidity of muscles with full consciousness in the transition zone between sleep and waking; and (4) hypnagogic hallucinations, visual or auditory, which may precede sleep or occur during the sleep attack. The attacks are characterized by an abrupt transition into REM sleep—a necessary criterion for diagnosis. The disorder begins in early adult life, affects both sexes equally, and usually levels off in severity at about 30 years of age.

REM sleep behavior disorder, characterized by motor dyscontrol and often violent dreams during REM sleep, may be related to narcolepsy.

C. Kleine-Levin Syndrome

This syndrome, which occurs mostly in young men, is characterized by hypersomnic attacks three or four times a year lasting up to 2 days, with hyperphagia, hypersexuality, irritability, and confusion on awakening. It has often been associated with antecedent neurologic insults. It usually remits after age 40.

D. Periodic Limb Movement Disorder

Periodic lower leg movements occur only during sleep with subsequent daytime sleepiness, anxiety, depression, and cognitive impairment. **Restless leg syndrome** includes movements while awake as well.

E. Shift Work Sleep Disorder

Shift work sleep disorder occurs when there is excessive fatigue as a consequence of work occurring during the normal sleep period.

Treatment

Narcolepsy can be managed by daily administration of a stimulant such as dextroamphetamine sulfate, 10 mg orally in the morning, with increased dosage as necessary. Modafinil and its enantiomer armodafinil are schedule IV medications FDA-approved for treating the excessive daytime fatigue of narcolepsy, sleepiness associated with obstructive sleep apnea, as well as for shift work sleep disorder. Usual dosing is 200–400 mg orally each morning for modafinil and 150–250 mg orally in the morning for armodafinil. The exact mechanism of action of modafinil and armodafil is unknown, yet they are thought to be less of an abuse risk than stimulants that are primarily dopaminergic. Common side effects include headache and anxiety; however, modafinil appears to be generally well tolerated. Imipramine, 75–100 mg orally daily, has been effective in treatment of cataplexy but not narcolepsy.

Periodic limb movement disorder and REM sleep behavior disorder can be treated with clonazepam with variable results. There is no treatment for Kleine-Levin syndrome, although lithium can prevent recurrences in some.

Treatment of sleep apnea is discussed in Chapter 9.

3. Parasomnias (Abnormal Behaviors during Sleep)

These disorders (sleep terror, nightmares, sleepwalking, and enuresis) are common in children but less so in adults.

Espie CA et al. Effect of digital cognitive behavioral therapy for insomnia on health, psychological well-being, and sleep-related quality of life: a randomized clinical trial. JAMA Psychiatry. 2019;76:21. [PMID: 30264137]

Krystal AD et al. The assessment and management of insomnia: an update. World Psychiatry. 2019;18:337. [PMID: 31496087]

DISORDERS OF AGGRESSION

Aggression and violence are symptoms rather than diseases and are not necessarily associated with an underlying medical condition. Clinicians are unable to predict dangerous behavior with greater than chance accuracy. Depression, schizophrenia, personality disorders, mania, paranoia, temporal lobe dysfunction, and organic mental states may be associated with acts of aggression. Impulse control disorders are characterized by physical abuse (usually of the aggressor's domestic partner or children), by pathologic intoxication, by impulsive sexual activities, and by reckless driving. Anabolic steroid usage by athletes has been associated with increased tendencies toward violent behavior.

In the United States, a significant proportion of all violent deaths are alcohol related. The ingestion of even small amounts of alcohol can result in pathologic intoxication that resembles an acute organic mental condition. Amphetamines, crack cocaine, and other stimulants are frequently associated with aggressive behavior. Phencyclidine is a drug commonly associated with violent behavior that is occasionally of a bizarre nature, partly due to lowering of the pain threshold. Domestic violence and rape are much more widespread than previously recognized. Awareness of the problem is to some degree due to increasing recognition of the rights of women and the understanding by women that they do not have to accept abuse. Acceptance of this kind of aggressive behavior inevitably leads to more, with the ultimate aggression being murder—20–50% of murders in the United States occur within the family. Police are called more for domestic disputes than all other criminal incidents combined. Children living in such family situations frequently become victims of abuse.

Features of individuals who have been subjected to long-term physical or sexual abuse are as follows: trouble expressing anger, staying angry longer, general passivity in relationships, feeling "marked for life" with an accompanying feeling of deserving to be victimized, lack of trust, and dissociation of affect from experiences. They are prone to express their psychological distress with somatization symptoms, often pain complaints. They may also have symptoms related to posttraumatic stress, as discussed above. The clinician should be suspicious about the origin of any injuries not fully explained, particularly if such incidents recur.

Treatment

A. Psychological

Management of any acutely potentially violent individual includes appropriate psychological maneuvers. Move slowly, talk slowly with clarity and reassurance, and evaluate the situation. Strive to create a setting that is minimally disturbing and eliminate people or things threatening to the violent individual. Do not threaten and do not touch or crowd the person. Allow no weapons in the area (an increasing problem in hospital emergency departments). Proximity to a door is comforting to both the patient and the examiner. Use a negotiator who the violent person can relate to comfortably. Food and drink are helpful in defusing the situation (as are cigarettes for those who smoke). Honesty is important. Make no false promises, bolster the patient's self-esteem, and continue to engage the subject verbally until the situation is under control. This type of individual does better with strong external controls to replace the lack of inner controls over the long term. Close probationary supervision and judicially mandated restrictions can be most helpful. There should be a major effort to help the individual avoid drug use (eg, Alcoholics Anonymous). Victims of abuse are essentially treated as any victim of trauma and, not infrequently, have evidence of PTSD.

B. Pharmacologic

Pharmacologic means are often necessary whether or not psychological approaches have been successful. This is true in the agitated or psychotic patient. The medications of choice in seriously violent or psychotic aggressive states are antipsychotics, given intramuscularly if necessary, every 1–2 hours until symptoms are alleviated. A number of second-generation intramuscular antipsychotics are FDA-approved in the management of acute agitation and include aripiprazole (9.75 mg/1.3 mL), ziprasidone (10 mg/0.5 mL), and olanzapine (10 mg/2 mL). The second-generation antipsychotics appear less likely than first-generation medications like haloperidol (2.5–5 mg) to cause acute extrapyramidal symptoms. However, the second-generation medications appear no more effective than first-generation medications and generally are more expensive. Benzodiazepine sedatives (eg, diazepam, 5 mg orally or intravenously every several hours) can be used for mild to moderate agitation but are sometimes associated with a disinhibition of aggressive impulses similar to alcohol. Chronic aggressive states, particularly in patients with intellectual disabilities and brain damage (rule out causative organic conditions and medications such as anticholinergic medications in amounts sufficient to cause confusion), have been ameliorated with risperidone, 0.5–2 mg/day orally, propranolol, 40–240 mg/day orally, or pindolol, 5 mg twice daily orally (pindolol causes less bradycardia and hypotension than propranolol). Carbamazepine and valproic acid are effective in the treatment of aggression and explosive disorders, particularly when associated with known or suspected brain lesions. Lithium and SSRIs are also effective for some intermittent explosive outbursts. Buspirone (10–45 mg/day orally) is helpful for aggression, particularly in patients with intellectual disabilities.

C. Physical

Physical management is necessary if psychological and pharmacologic means are not sufficient. It requires the active and visible presence of an adequate number of personnel (five or six) to reinforce the idea that the situation is under control despite the patient's lack of inner controls. Such an approach often precludes the need for actual physical restraint. Seclusion rooms and restraints should be used only when necessary (ambulatory restraints are an alternative), and the patient must then be observed at frequent intervals. Narrow corridors, small spaces, and crowded areas exacerbate the potential for violence in an anxious patient.

D. Other Interventions

The treatment of victims (eg, battered women) is challenging and can be complicated by a reluctance to leave the situation. Reasons for staying vary, but common themes include the fear of more violence because of leaving, the hope that the situation may ameliorate (in spite of steady worsening), and the financial aspects of the situation, which are seldom to the woman's advantage. Concerns for the children often finally compel the woman to seek help. An early step is to get the woman into a therapeutic situation that provides the support of others in similar straits. Al-Anon is frequently a valuable asset when alcohol is a factor. The group can support the victim while she gathers strength to consider alternatives without being paralyzed by fear. Many cities offer temporary emergency centers and counseling. Use the available resources, attend to any medical or psychiatric problems, and maintain a compassionate interest. Some states require clinicians to report injuries caused by abuse or suspected abuse to police authorities.

Nash RP et al. Acute pharmacological management of behavioral and emotional dysregulation following a traumatic brain injury: a systematic review of the literature. Psychosomatics. 2019;60:139. [PMID: 30665668]

SUBSTANCE USE DISORDERS

The term "dependency" was previously used to describe a severe form of substance abuse and drug addiction characterized by the triad of: (1) a **psychological dependence or craving** and the behavior involved in procurement of the drug; (2) **physiologic dependence,** with withdrawal symptoms on discontinuance of the drug; and (3) **tolerance,** ie, the need to increase the dose to obtain the desired effects. The terms "dependency" and "abuse" were dropped in *DSM-5* in favor of the single term "substance use disorder," ranging from mild to severe. Many patients could have a severe and life-threatening abuse problem without ever being dependent on a drug. *Substance use disorder is a treatable, chronic medical illness.* Clinicians and health care systems must work against bias toward people with substance use disorder. Medication-assisted treatment is available for a number of substance use disorders and is a key element in their management.

There is accumulating evidence that an impairment syndrome exists in many former (and current) drug users. It is believed that drug use produces damaged neurotransmitter receptor sites and that the consequent imbalance produces symptoms that may mimic other psychiatric illnesses. **"Kindling"**—repeated stimulation of the brain—renders the individual more susceptible to focal brain activity with minimal stimulation. Stimulants and depressants can produce kindling, leading to relatively spontaneous effects no longer dependent on the original stimulus. These effects may be manifested as mood swings, panic, psychosis, and occasionally overt seizure activity. The imbalance also results in frequent job changes, partner problems, and generally erratic behavior. Patients with PTSD frequently have treated themselves with a variety of drugs. Chronic abusers of a wide variety of drugs exhibit cerebral atrophy on CT scans, a finding that may relate to the above symptoms. Early recognition is important, mainly to establish realistic treatment programs that are chiefly symptom-directed.

The clinician faces three problems with substance use disorders: (1) the prescribing of substances such as sedatives, stimulants, or opioids that might produce dependency; (2) the treatment of individuals who have already misused drugs, most commonly alcohol; and (3) the detection of illicit drug use in patients presenting with psychiatric symptoms. The usefulness of **UA for detection of drugs** varies markedly with different drugs and under different circumstances (pharmacokinetics is a major factor) (see also Chapter 5). Water-soluble drugs (eg, alcohol, stimulants, opioids) are eliminated in a day or so. Lipophilic substances (eg, barbiturates, tetrahydrocannabinol) appear in the urine over longer periods of time: several days in most cases, 1–2 months in chronic marijuana users. Sedative drug determinations are quite variable, amount of drug and duration of use being important determinants. False-positives can be a problem related to ingestion of some legitimate medications (eg, phenytoin for barbiturates, phenylpropanolamine for amphetamines, chlorpromazine for opioids) and some foods (eg, poppy seeds for opioids, coca leaf tea for cocaine). Manipulations can alter the legitimacy of the testing. Dilution, either in vivo or in vitro, can be detected by checking urine-specific gravity. Addition of ammonia, vinegar, or salt may invalidate the test, but odor and pH determinations are simple. Hair analysis can determine drug use over longer periods, particularly sequential drug-taking patterns. The sensitivity and reliability of such tests are considered good, and the method may be complementary to UA.

O'Connor EA et al. Screening and behavioral counseling interventions to reduce unhealthy alcohol use in adolescents and adults: updated evidence report and systematic review for the US Preventive Services Task Force. JAMA. 2018;320:1910. [PMID: 30422198]

ALCOHOL USE DISORDER (Alcoholism)

Meshell D. Johnson, MD

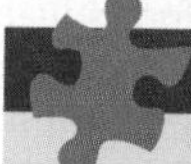

ESSENTIALS OF DIAGNOSIS

- Physiologic dependence as manifested by evidence of withdrawal when intake is interrupted.
- Tolerance to the effects of alcohol.
- Evidence of alcohol-associated illnesses, such as alcoholic liver disease, cerebellar degeneration.
- Continued drinking despite strong medical and social contraindications and life disruptions.
- Impairment in social and occupational functioning.
- Depression.
- Blackouts.

General Considerations

Alcohol use disorder is a syndrome consisting of two phases: **at-risk drinking** and moderate to severe **alcohol misuse.** At-risk drinking is the repetitive use of alcohol, often to alleviate anxiety or solve other emotional problems. A moderate to severe alcohol use disorder is similar to that which occurs following the repeated use of other sedative-hypnotics and is characterized by recurrent use of alcohol despite disruption in social roles (family and work), alcohol-related legal problems, and taking safety risks by oneself and with others. The National Institute on Alcohol Abuse and Alcoholism formally defines at-risk drinking as *more than four drinks per day or 14 drinks per week for men or more than three drinks per day or seven drinks per week for women.* A drink is defined by the CDC as 12 oz of beer, 8 oz of malt liquor, 5 oz of wine, or 1.3 oz or a "shot" of 80-proof distilled spirits or liquor. Individuals with at-risk drinking are at an increased risk for developing or are developing an alcohol use disorder. Alcohol and other drug abuse patients have a much higher prevalence of lifetime psychiatric disorders. While male-to-female ratios in alcoholic treatment agencies remain at 4:1, there is evidence that the rates are converging. Women delay seeking help, and when they do, they tend to seek it in medical or mental health settings. Adoption and twin studies indicate some genetic influence. Ethnic distinctions are important—eg, 40% of Japanese have aldehyde dehydrogenase deficiency and are more susceptible to the effects of alcohol. Depression is often present and should be evaluated carefully. The majority of suicides and intrafamily homicides involve alcohol. Alcohol is a major factor in rapes and other assaults.

There are several screening instruments that may help identify an alcohol use disorder. One of the most useful is the **Alcohol Use Disorder Identification Test (AUDIT)** (see Table 1–7).

Clinical Findings

A. Acute Intoxication

The signs of alcoholic intoxication are the same as those of overdosage with any other CNS depressant: drowsiness, errors of commission, psychomotor dysfunction, disinhibition, dysarthria, ataxia, and nystagmus. For a 70-kg person, an ounce of whiskey, a 4- to 6-oz glass of wine, or a 12-oz bottle of beer (roughly 15, 11, and 13 grams of alcohol, respectively) may raise the level of alcohol in the blood by 25 mg/dL. For a 50-kg person, the blood alcohol level would rise even higher (35 mg/dL) with the same consumption. Blood alcohol levels below 50 mg/dL rarely cause significant motor dysfunction (the legal limit for driving under the influence is commonly 80 mg/dL). Intoxication as manifested by ataxia, dysarthria, and nausea and vomiting indicates a blood level greater than 150 mg/dL, and lethal blood levels range from 350 mg/dL to 900 mg/dL. In severe cases, overdosage is marked by respiratory depression, stupor, seizures, shock syndrome, coma, and death. Serious overdoses are frequently due to a combination of alcohol with other sedatives.

B. Withdrawal

There is a wide spectrum of manifestations of alcohol withdrawal, ranging from anxiety, decreased cognition, and tremulousness, through increasing irritability and hyperreactivity to full-blown delirium tremens (DTs). **Alcohol withdrawal syndrome** can be categorized as mild, moderate, or severe withdrawal, withdrawal seizures, and DTs. Symptoms of mild withdrawal, including tremor, anxiety, tachycardia, nausea, vomiting, and insomnia, begin within 6 hours after the last drink, often before the blood alcohol levels drop to zero, and usually have passed by day two. Severe or major withdrawal occurs 48–96 hours after the last drink and is usually preceded by prolonged heavy alcohol use. Symptoms include disorientation, agitation, diaphoresis, whole body tremor, vomiting, hypertension, and hallucinations (visual > tactile > auditory). Moderate withdrawal symptoms and signs fall between those of minor and major withdrawal. **Withdrawal seizures** can occur as early as 8 hours after the last drink but usually do not manifest more than 48 hours after alcohol cessation. Seizures are more prevalent in persons who have a history of withdrawal syndromes. These seizures are generalized tonic-clonic seizures, are brief in duration, and resolve spontaneously. If withdrawal is untreated, these seizures can recur in about 60% of patients. DTs will develop in approximately half of these patients. If seizures are focal, associated with trauma or fever, or have an onset more than 48 hours after the last drink, another etiology for seizures must be considered. **DT** is the most severe form of alcohol withdrawal. It is an acute organic psychosis that usually manifests 48–72 hours after the last drink but may occur up to 7–10 days later. It is characterized by extreme mental confusion, agitation, tremor, diaphoresis, sensory hyperacuity, visual hallucinations (often of snakes, bugs, etc), and autonomic hyperactivity (tachycardia and hypertension). Complications of DTs include (1) dehydration, (2) electrolyte disturbances (hypokalemia, hypomagnesemia), (3) arrhythmias and seizures, and (4) cardiovascular collapse and death. *The acute withdrawal syndrome is often unexpected,* occurring when the patient has been hospitalized for an unrelated problem, thus presenting as a diagnostic dilemma. Suspect alcohol withdrawal in every unexplained delirium. The mortality rate from DTs, which was upward of 35%, has steadily decreased with early diagnosis and improved treatment.

In addition to the immediate withdrawal symptoms, there is evidence of persistent longer-term ones, including sleep disturbances, anxiety, depression, excitability, fatigue, and emotional volatility. These symptoms may persist for 3–12 months, and in some cases, they become chronic.

C. Alcoholic (Organic) Hallucinosis

This syndrome occurs either during heavy drinking or on withdrawal and is characterized by a paranoid psychosis without the tremulousness, confusion, and clouded sensorium seen in withdrawal syndromes. The patient appears normal except for the auditory hallucinations, which are frequently persecutory and may cause the patient to behave aggressively and in a paranoid fashion.

D. Chronic Alcoholic Brain Syndromes

These encephalopathies are characterized by increasing erratic behavior, memory and recall problems, and emotional instability—the usual signs of organic brain injury due to any cause. Wernicke-Korsakoff syndrome due to thiamine deficiency may develop with a series of episodes. **Wernicke encephalopathy** consists of the triad of confusion, ataxia, and ophthalmoplegia (typically sixth nerve palsy). Early recognition and treatment with thiamine can minimize damage. One of the possible sequelae is **Korsakoff psychosis**, characterized by both anterograde and retrograde amnesia, with confabulation early in the course. Early recognition and treatment with intravenous thiamine and B complex vitamins can minimize damage. Excessive alcohol consumption in men has been associated with faster cognitive decline compared with light to moderate alcohol consumption.

E. Laboratory Findings

Ethanol may contribute to the presence of an otherwise unexplained osmolar gap. There may also be increased serum liver biochemical tests, uric acid, and triglycerides and decreased serum potassium and magnesium. The most definitive biologic marker for chronic alcoholism is carbohydrate deficient transferrin, which can detect heavy use (60 mg/day over 7–10 days) with high specificity. Other useful tests for diagnosing alcohol use disorder are gamma-glutamyl transpeptidase (GGT) measurement (levels greater than 30 units/L are suggestive of heavy drinking) and mean corpuscular volume (MCV) (more than 95 fL in men and more than 100 fL in women). If both are elevated, a serious alcohol problem is likely. Use of other recreational drugs with alcohol skews and negates the significance of these tests.

Differential Diagnosis

The differential diagnosis of alcoholism is essentially between **primary alcohol use disorder** (when no other major psychiatric diagnosis exists) and **secondary alcohol use disorder** (when alcohol is used as self-medication for major underlying psychiatric problems such as schizophrenia or affective disorder). The differentiation is important, since the latter group requires treatment for the specific psychiatric problem. In primary and secondary alcoholism, at-risk drinking can be distinguished from alcohol addiction by taking a careful psychiatric history and evaluating the degree to which recurrent drinking impacts the social role functioning and physical safety of the individual.

The differential diagnosis of alcohol withdrawal includes other sedative withdrawals and other causes of delirium. Acute alcoholic hallucinosis must be differentiated from other acute paranoid states such as amphetamine psychosis or paranoid schizophrenia.

Complications

The medical, economic, and psychosocial problems of alcoholism are staggering. The central and peripheral nervous system complications include chronic brain syndromes, cerebellar degeneration, cardiomyopathy, and peripheral neuropathies. Direct effects on the liver include cirrhosis, esophageal varices, and eventual hepatic failure. Indirect effects include protein abnormalities, coagulation defects, hormone deficiencies, and an increased incidence of liver neoplasms.

Fetal alcohol syndrome includes one or more of the following developmental defects in the offspring of alcoholic women: (1) low birth weight and small size with failure to catch up in size or weight, (2) mental retardation, with an average IQ in the 60s, and (3) a variety of birth defects, with a large percentage of facial and cardiac abnormalities. The risk is appreciably higher with the more alcohol ingested by the mother each day.

Treatment of At-Risk Drinking

A. Psychological

The most important consideration for the clinician is to suspect the problem early and take a nonjudgmental attitude, although this does not mean a passive one. The problem of denial must be faced, preferably with significant family members at the first meeting. This means dealing from the beginning with any enabling behavior of the spouse or other significant people. Enabling behavior allows the patient with an alcohol use disorder to avoid facing the consequences of his or her behavior.

There must be an emphasis on the things that can be done. This approach emphasizes the fact that the clinician cares and strikes a positive and hopeful note early in treatment. Valuable time should not be wasted trying to find out why the patient drinks. The immediate problem to be addressed is how to stop the drinking. Although total abstinence should be the ultimate goal, a **harm reduction model** indicates that gradual progress toward abstinence can be a useful treatment strategy.

Motivational interviewing, a model of counseling that addresses both the patient's ambivalence and motivation for change, may contribute to reduced consumption over time.

B. Social

Encourage the patient to attend **Alcoholics Anonymous** meetings and the spouse to attend **Al-Anon** meetings. Success is usually proportionate to the utilization of Alcoholics Anonymous, religious counseling, and other resources. The patient should be seen frequently for short periods.

Do not underestimate the importance of religion, particularly since the patient with alcohol use disorder is often a dependent person who needs a great deal of support. Early enlistment of the help of a concerned religious adviser can often provide the turning point for a personal conversion to sobriety.

One of the most important considerations is the patient's job—fear of losing a job is one of the most powerful motivations for giving up alcohol. The business community is aware of the problem; about 70% of the Fortune 500 companies offer programs to their employees to help with the problem of alcoholism. Some specific recommendations that can be offered to employers include (1) avoid placement in jobs where the alcoholic patient must be alone, eg, as a traveling buyer or sales executive, (2) use supervision but not surveillance, (3) keep competition with others to a minimum, and (4) avoid positions that require quick decision making on important matters (high-stress situations). In general, commitment to abstinence and avoidance of situations that might be conducive to drinking are most predictive of a good outcome.

C. Medical

Hospitalization is not usually necessary but may be warranted if there are concomitant medical indications. Furthermore, if patients with heavy alcohol use are hospitalized for any other reason, providers must be vigilant for signs and symptoms of alcohol withdrawal.

Because of the many medical complications of alcoholism, a complete physical examination with appropriate laboratory tests is mandatory, with special attention to the liver and nervous system. Use of sedatives as a replacement for alcohol is not desirable.

Disulfiram (250–500 mg/day orally) has been used for many years as an aversive medication to discourage alcohol use. Disulfiram inhibits aldehyde dehydrogenase, causing toxic reactions when alcohol is consumed. The results have generally been of limited effectiveness and depend on the motivation of the individual to be compliant.

Naltrexone, an opiate antagonist, in a dosage of 50 mg orally daily, lowers relapse rates over the 3–6 months after cessation of drinking, apparently by lessening the pleasurable effects of alcohol. One study suggests that naltrexone is most effective when given during periods of drinking in combination with therapy that supports abstinence but accepts the fact that relapses occur. Naltrexone is FDA-approved for maintenance therapy. Studies indicate that it reduces alcohol craving when used as part of a comprehensive treatment program. Acamprosate (333–666 mg orally three times daily) helps reduce craving and maintain abstinence and can be continued even during periods of relapse. Both acamprosate and oral naltrexone have been associated with reduction in return to drinking.

D. Behavioral

Conditioning approaches historically have been used in some settings in the treatment of alcoholism, most commonly as a type of aversion therapy. For example, the patient is given a drink of whiskey and then a shot of apomorphine, and proceeds to vomit. In this way a strong association is built up between the drinking and vomiting. Although this kind of treatment has been successful in some cases, after appropriate informed consent, many people do not sustain the learned aversive response.

Treatment of Hallucinosis & Withdrawal

A. Hallucinosis

Alcoholic hallucinosis, which can occur either during or on cessation of a prolonged drinking period, is not a typical withdrawal syndrome and is handled differently. Since the symptoms are primarily those of a psychosis in the presence of a clear sensorium, they are handled like any other psychosis: hospitalization (when indicated) and adequate amounts of antipsychotic medications. Haloperidol, 5 mg orally twice a day for the first day or so, usually ameliorates symptoms quickly, and the medication can be decreased and discontinued over several days as the patient improves. It then becomes necessary to deal with the chronic alcohol abuse, which has been discussed.

B. Withdrawal

The onset of withdrawal symptoms is usually 6–36 hours, and the peak intensity of symptoms is 48–72 hours after alcohol consumption is stopped. Providing adequate CNS depressants (eg, benzodiazepines) is important to counteract the excitability resulting from sudden cessation of alcohol intake. The choice of a specific sedative is less important than using adequate doses to bring the patient to a level of moderate sedation, and this will vary from person to person.

All patients should be evaluated for their risk of alcohol withdrawal. Mild dependency requires "drying out." For outpatients, in some instances, a short course of tapering long-acting benzodiazepines—eg, diazepam, 20 mg/day orally initially, decreasing by 5 mg daily—may be a useful adjunct. When the history or presentation suggests that patients are actively in withdrawal or at significant risk for withdrawal, they should be hospitalized. Risk factors include a recent drinking history, frequent alcohol consumption, a past history of withdrawal, seizures, hallucinosis, or DTs, a past history of needing medication for detoxification, or a history of benzodiazepine or barbiturate use, abuse, or dependency.

For all hospitalized patients, general management includes ensuring adequate hydration, correction of electrolyte imbalances (particularly magnesium, calcium, and potassium), and administering the vitamins thiamine (100 mg intravenously daily for 3 days then orally daily), folic acid (1 mg orally daily), and a multivitamin orally daily. Thiamine should be given *prior* to any glucose-containing solutions to decrease the risk of precipitating Wernicke encephalopathy or Korsakoff syndrome. Alcohol withdrawal is treated with benzodiazepines. Continual assessment is recommended to determine the severity of withdrawal, and **symptom-driven medication regimens**, which have been shown to prevent undersedation as well as oversedation and to reduce total benzodiazepine usage over fixed-dose schedules, should be used. The severity of withdrawal will determine a patient's level of care. For those at risk for withdrawal and with mild withdrawal symptoms, admission to a medical unit is adequate. For those with moderate withdrawal, a higher acuity hospital environment is recommended. Those with severe withdrawal should be admitted to the ICU.

1. Assessing alcohol withdrawal symptom severity—The **Clinical Institute Withdrawal Assessment for Alcohol, Revised (CIWA-Ar)** is a validated tool that is widely used to determine severity of alcohol withdrawal. This survey assesses symptoms in 10 areas and can be administered relatively quickly (Figure 25–3). One caveat is that the patient must be able to communicate his or her symptoms to the provider. The maximum attainable score is 67. Clinical judgment should be used to determine final dosing of medications to patients who are in alcohol withdrawal because dosing will vary between patients and degrees of withdrawal.

2. Treating alcohol withdrawal symptoms based on CIWA-Ar score—

A. MINIMAL WITHDRAWAL SYMPTOMS (CIWA-AR SCORE LESS THAN 8)—Patients who have a history suggestive of alcohol withdrawal risk with minimal withdrawal symptoms are suitable for withdrawal prophylaxis. The recommended

Patient: ____________ **Date:** ____________ **Time:** ____________ (24 hour clock, midnight = 00:00)

Pulse or heart rate, taken for 1 minute: ____________ **Blood pressure:** ______

NAUSEA AND VOMITING — Ask "Do you feel sick to your stomach? Have you vomited?" Observation.

0 no nausea and no vomiting
1 mild nausea with no vomiting
2
3
4 intermittent nausea with dry heaves
5
6
7 constant nausea, frequent dry heaves and vomiting

TACTILE DISTURBANCES — Ask "Have you any itching, pins and needles sensations, any burning, any numbness, or do you feel bugs crawling on or under your skin?" Observation.

0 none
1 very mild itching, pins and needles, burning, or numbness
2 mild itching, pins and needles, burning, or numbness
3 moderate itching, pins and needles, burning, or numbness
4 moderately severe hallucinations (formications)
5 severe hallucinations
6 extremely severe hallucinations
7 continuous hallucinations

TREMOR — Arms extended and fingers spread apart. Observation.

0 no tremor
1 not visible, but can be felt fingertip to fingertip
2
3
4 moderate, with patient's arms extended
5
6
7 severe, even with arms not extended

AUDITORY DISTURBANCES — Ask "Are you more aware of sounds around you? Are they harsh? Do they frighten you? Are you hearing anything that is disturbing to you? Are you hearing things you know are not there?" Observation.

0 not present
1 very mild harshness or ability to frighten
2 mild harshness or ability to frighten
3 moderate harshness or ability to frighten
4 moderately severe auditory hallucinations
5 severe hallucinations
6 extremely severe hallucinations
7 continuous hallucinations

PAROXYSMAL SWEATS — Observation.

0 no sweat visible
1 barely perceptible sweating, palms moist
2
3
4 beads of sweat obvious on forehead
5
6
7 drenching sweats

VISUAL DISTURBANCES — Ask "Does the light appear to be too bright? Is its color different? Does it hurt your eyes? Are you seeing anything that is disturbing to you? Are you seeing things you know are not there?" Observation.

0 not present
1 very mild photosensitivity
2 mild sensitivity
3 moderate sensitivity
4 moderately severe visual hallucinations
5 severe hallucinations
6 extremely severe hallucinations
7 continuous hallucinations

ANXIETY — Ask "Do you feel nervous?" Observation.

0 no anxiety, at ease
1 mildly anxious
2
3
4 moderately anxious, or guarded, so anxiety is inferred
5
6
7 severely anxious, equivalent…

HEADACHE, FULLNESS IN HEAD — Ask "Does your head feel different? Does it feel like there is a band around your head?" Do not rate for dizziness or lightheadedness. Otherwise, rate severity.

0 not present
1 very mild
2 mild
3 moderate
4 moderately severe
5 severe
6 very severe
7 extremely severe

AGITATION — Observation.

0 normal activity
1 somewhat more than normal activity
2
3
4 moderately fidgety and restless
5
6
7 paces back and forth during most of the interview, or constantly thrashes about

ORIENTATION AND CLOUDING OF SENSORIUM — Ask "What is today's date?… Who am I?" Serial additions: "Please count up by 5's — 0, 5, 10…"

0 oriented and can do serial additions
1 cannot do serial additions or is uncertain about date
2 disoriented for date by no more than 2 calendar days
3 disoriented for date by more than 2 calendar days
4 disoriented for date and place or person

Total **CIWA-Ar** Score ________

Rater's Initials ________

Maximum Possible Score 67

This assessment for monitoring withdrawal symptoms requires approximately 5 minutes to administer. The maximum score is 67 (see instrument). Patients scoring less than 8 (or 10, according to some experts) do not usually need additional medication for withdrawal.

▲ **Figure 25–3.** Alcohol withdrawal assessment. (Reproduced from Sullivan JT et al. Assessment of alcohol withdrawal: The revised clinical institute withdrawal assessment for alcohol scale [CIWA-Ar]. Br J Addict. 1989;84:1353. This scale is not copyrighted and may be used freely.)

benzodiazepine options include chlordiazepoxide or lorazepam orally, tapered over 3 days. The protocol calls for nursing assessment of sedation and withdrawal symptoms (CIWA-Ar) every 6 hours. If prophylactic medication is indicated, a sample tapering regimen may include lorazepam, 1 mg orally every 6 hours for 1 day, then 1 mg orally every 8 hours for 1 day, then 1 mg orally every 12 hours for 1 day, then discontinue; or chlordiazepoxide, 50 mg orally every 6 hours for 1 day, 25 mg orally every 6 hours for 2 days, then discontinue. Avoid chlordiazepoxide in the older patients or in patients with liver disease. Lorazepam is preferred in patients with liver disease. Sedation is assessed 30–60 minutes after each medication dose. The benzodiazepine dose is held for oversedation or if the respiratory rate is less than 10 breaths per minute. For CIWA-Ar score greater than 8, the provider must be notified, because this is suggestive of active withdrawal, and escalation of treatment must occur.

B. Mild withdrawal symptoms (CIWA-Ar score 8–15)—For patients in mild withdrawal, either chlordiazepoxide orally or lorazepam orally or intravenously can be used. Initially, chlordiazepoxide 50 mg orally or lorazepam 1 or 2 mg orally or intravenously is given hourly for 2 hours. Patients must be assessed for level of sedation and withdrawal symptoms (CIWA-Ar) every 4 hours. Dosing is adjusted as necessary to control symptoms without excessive sedation. After the first 2 hours, chlordiazepoxide or lorazepam is given every 4 hours and as needed. Typical dosing may include chlordiazepoxide 25–50 mg orally or lorazepam 0.5–1 mg orally or intravenously every 4 hours as needed. Additional doses of benzodiazepines should be given if the CIWA-Ar score remains between 8 and 15.

C. Moderate withdrawal (CIWA-Ar score 16–20)—For patients in moderate withdrawal, chlordiazepoxide 100 mg orally or lorazepam 3 or 4 mg orally or intravenously is given every hour for the first 2 hours. CIWA-Ar monitoring should occur every 2 hours. Dosing is adjusted to control symptoms without excessive sedation. After initial dosing, continued treatment could include chlordiazepoxide 50 mg orally or lorazepam 1–2 mg orally or intravenously every 2 hours as needed for CIWA-Ar score between 16 and 20, and chlordiazepoxide 25 mg orally or lorazepam 0.5–1 mg orally or intravenously every 2 hours for CIWA-Ar score between 8 and 15. The maximum dose of chlordiazepoxide is 600 mg in 24 hours. Continuous pulse oximetry and cardiac monitoring should be considered. The degree of sedation should be monitored 30–60 minutes after each oral dose of medication and for 15 minutes after each parenteral dose.

D. Severe withdrawal (CIWA-Ar score greater than 20)—Patients with severe withdrawal are at risk for the development of DTs and should be transferred or admitted to the ICU. Intravenous lorazepam can be used to treat severe withdrawal. A potential treatment protocol is to administer lorazepam 1–2 mg intravenously every 15 minutes until the patient is calm and sedated but awake. Initial CIWA-Ar monitoring should occur every 30 minutes. The patient can then receive lorazepam 2 mg orally or intravenously every hour as needed when the CIWA-Ar score is between 16 and 20, and lorazepam 1–2 mg orally or intravenously every hour as needed when the CIWA-Ar score is between 8 and 15. If the patient requires more than 8 mg/hour of lorazepam as an initial dose or continues to demonstrate observable agitation, tremors, tachycardia, or hypertension despite high doses of lorazepam, consider adding dexmedetomidine. Dexmedetomidine, an alpha-2-agonist, produces sedation with minimal effect on respiratory drive. It is not recommended as a sole agent for the treatment of alcohol withdrawal but as adjunctive therapy along with benzodiazepines to decrease the hyperadrenergic output in patients with severe alcohol withdrawal not controlled by benzodiazepines or in patients at risk for respiratory depression from high-dose benzodiazepine administration. The recommended dosing of dexmedetomidine is 0.2–0.7 mcg/kg/hour, with lorazepam 1–2 mg intravenously every 8 hours plus lorazepam 1–2 mg intravenously every hour as needed for agitation. In limited cases of severe withdrawal requiring frequent lorazepam boluses for at least 6 hours, continuous intravenous lorazepam infusion can be considered, but the patient must be monitored extremely carefully for signs of respiratory depression. Continuous pulse oximetry and close observance of the patient's respiratory status are required. Sedation is assessed 15 minutes after each intravenous dose. If withdrawal symptoms are refractory to escalating benzodiazepine usage, despite the addition of dexmedetomidine, escalation to propofol should be considered. Patients receiving large doses of benzodiazepines often require intubation for airway protection, at which time initiation of propofol infusion for sedation, in addition to treatment of refractory alcohol withdrawal, is recommended. Phenobarbital monotherapy for alcohol withdrawal is used at some institutions, but randomized controlled trials comparing the efficacy of phenobarbital over benzodiazepines are needed to inform adoption of new treatment regimens.

In all cases, benzodiazepines should be held if the patient is too sedated or has a respiratory rate less than 10 breaths per minute. Do not bolus lorazepam in doses greater than 4 mg intravenously. Mixing benzodiazepines, eg, chlordiazepoxide orally every 8 hours with lorazepam, is not recommended. Instead, select a single agent and titrate as needed. Once a patient has been stable for 24 hours, the benzodiazepine dose can be reduced by 20% daily until withdrawal is complete.

3. Managing other withdrawal-associated conditions—Meticulous examination for other medical problems is necessary. Alcoholic hypoglycemia can occur with low blood alcohol levels (see Chapter 27). Patients with severe alcohol use disorder commonly have liver disease with associated clotting disorders and are also prone to injury—and the combination all too frequently leads to undiagnosed subdural hematoma.

Phenytoin does *not* appear to be useful in managing alcohol withdrawal seizures per se. Sedating doses of benzodiazepines are effective in treating alcohol withdrawal seizures. Thus, other anticonvulsants are not usually needed unless there is a preexisting seizure disorder.

Chronic brain syndromes secondary to a long history of alcohol intake are not clearly responsive to thiamine and vitamin replenishment. Attention to the social and environmental care of this type of patient is paramount.

4. Initiating psychological and social measures—The psychological and behavioral treatment methods outlined under Treatment of At-Risk Drinking become the primary considerations after successful treatment of alcoholic hallucinosis or withdrawal. Psychological and social measures should be initiated in the hospital prior to discharge. This increases the possibility of continued posthospitalization treatment.

Casper R et al. Which detoxification syndromes are effective for alcohol withdrawal syndrome? J Fam Pract. 2021;70:E16. [PMID: 33760908]

Gupta A et al. Novel targets explored in the treatment of alcohol withdrawal syndrome. CNS Neurol Disord Drug Targets. 2021;20:158. [PMID: 33213357]

Oks M et al. The safety and utility of phenobarbital use for the treatment of severe alcohol withdrawal syndrome in the medical intensive care unit. J Intensive Care Med. 2020;35:844. [PMID: 29925291]

Sullivan SM et al. Comparison of phenobarbital-adjunct versus benzodiazepine-only approach for alcohol withdrawal syndrome in the ED. Am J Emerg Med. 2019;37:1313. [PMID: 30414743]

Wolf C et al. Management of alcohol withdrawal in the emergency department: current perspectives. Open Access Emerg Med. 2020;12:53. [PMID: 32256131]

Yanta J et al. Alcohol withdrawal syndrome: improving outcomes in the emergency department with aggressive management strategies. Emerg Med Pract. 2021;23:1. [PMID: 33729735]

OTHER DRUG & SUBSTANCE USE DISORDERS

A number of recreational drugs and prescription medications may be misused. Treatment for acute intoxication is distinguished from treatment of possible use disorder.

1. Opioids

While the terms "opioids" and "narcotics" both refer to a group of drugs with actions that mimic those of morphine, the term "opioids" is used when discussing medications prescribed in a controlled manner by a clinician and "narcotics" is used to connote illicit drug use. The opioid analgesics can be reversed by the opioid antagonist naloxone.

The clinical symptoms and signs of mild narcotic intoxication include changes in mood, with feelings of euphoria; drowsiness; nausea with occasional emesis; needle tracks; and miosis. The incidence of snorting and inhaling ("smoking") heroin has risen, particularly among cocaine users. Overdosage causes respiratory depression, peripheral vasodilation, pinpoint pupils, pulmonary edema, coma, and death.

Tolerance and withdrawal are major concerns when continued use of opioids occurs, although withdrawal causes only moderate morbidity (similar in severity to a bout of "flu"). Grades of withdrawal are categorized from 0 to 4: **grade 0** includes craving and anxiety; **grade 1,** yawning, lacrimation, rhinorrhea, and perspiration; **grade 2,** previous symptoms plus mydriasis, piloerection, anorexia, tremors, and hot and cold flashes with generalized aching; **grades 3 and 4,** increased intensity of previous symptoms and signs, with increased temperature, blood pressure, pulse, and respiratory rate and depth. In withdrawal from the most severe addiction, vomiting, diarrhea, weight loss, hemoconcentration, and spontaneous ejaculation or orgasm commonly occur.

Treatment for overdosage (or suspected overdosage) is discussed in Chapter 38.

Treatment for withdrawal begins if grade 2 signs develop. If a withdrawal program is necessary, use methadone, 10 mg orally (use parenteral administration if the patient is vomiting), and observe. If signs (piloerection, mydriasis, cardiovascular changes) persist for more than 4–6 hours, give another 10 mg; continue to administer methadone at 4- to 6-hour intervals until signs are not present (rarely greater than 40 mg of methadone in 24 hours). Divide the total amount of medication required over the first 24-hour period by two and give that amount every 12 hours. Each day, reduce the total 24-hour dose by 5–10 mg. Thus, a moderately addicted patient initially requiring 30–40 mg of methadone could be withdrawn over a 4- to 8-day period. Clonidine, 0.1 mg orally several times daily over a 10- to 14-day period, is both an alternative and an adjunct to methadone detoxification; it is not necessary to taper the dose. Clonidine is helpful in alleviating cardiovascular symptoms but does not significantly relieve anxiety, insomnia, or generalized aching. There is a protracted abstinence syndrome of metabolic, respiratory, and blood pressure changes over a period of 3–6 months. Alternative strategies for the treatment of opioid withdrawal have included rapid and ultrarapid detoxification techniques. However, data do not support the use of either method.

Treatment of opioid use disorder is key given evidence of significant morbidity and mortality, including what has been called the "opioid epidemic" in the United States. Opioid use disorder may be treated with medications and psychosocial interventions such as Narcotics Anonymous (NA). Buprenorphine, a partial agonist, is a mainstay of office-based treatment of opiate dependency. Its use requires certified training along with a special license from the Drug Enforcement Agency. Buprenorphine is a mu partial agonist and kappa antagonist. Unlike conventional opioids, buprenorphine may have a role in the treatment of major depression. Recently, a long-acting injectable form demonstrated efficacy.

Methadone maintenance programs are of some value in opioid use disorder. Under carefully controlled supervision, the person with opioid use disorder is maintained on high doses of methadone (40–120 mg daily) that satisfy craving and block the effects of heroin to a great degree.

Opioid antagonists (eg, naltrexone) can also be used successfully for treatment of the patient who has been free of opioids for 7–10 days. Naltrexone blocks the narcotic "high" of heroin when 50 mg is given orally every 24 hours initially for several days and then 100 mg is given every 48–72 hours. A monthly injectable form of naltrexone is available and may enhance compliance. Liver disorders are a major contraindication.

Bohnert ASB et al. Understanding links among opioid use, overdose, and suicide. N Engl J Med. 2019;380:71. [PMID: 30601750]
Haight BR et al; RB-US-13-0001 Study Investigators. Efficacy and safety of a monthly buprenorphine depot injection for opioid use disorder: a multicentre, randomised, double-blind, placebo-controlled, phase 3 trial. Lancet. 2019;393:778. [PMID: 30792007]
Jones CM et al. Naloxone co-prescribing to patients receiving prescription opioids in the Medicare Part D program, United States, 2016–2017. JAMA. 2019;322:462. [PMID: 31386124]
Leshner AI et al. Medication-based treatment to address opioid use disorder. JAMA. 2019;321:2071. [PMID: 31046072]

2. Sedatives (Anxiolytics)

See Anxiety Disorders, this chapter.

3. Psychedelics

Substance use disorder with psychedelics is not common. All of the common psychedelics (LSD, mescaline, psilocybin, dimethyltryptamine, and other derivatives of phenylalanine and tryptophan) can produce similar behavioral and physiologic effects. An initial feeling of tension is followed by emotional release such as crying or laughing (1–2 hours). Later and at higher doses, perceptual distortions occur, with visual illusions and hallucinations, and occasionally there is fear of ego disintegration (2–3 hours). Major changes in time sense and mood lability then occur (3–4 hours). A feeling of detachment and a sense of destiny and control occur (4–6 hours). Of course, reactions vary among individuals, and some of the drugs produce markedly different time frames. Occasionally, the acute episode is terrifying (a "bad trip"), which may include panic, depression, confusion, or psychotic symptoms. Preexisting emotional problems, the attitude of the user, and the setting where the drug is used affect the experience.

Treatment of the acute episode primarily involves protection of the individual from erratic behavior that may lead to injury or death. A structured environment is usually sufficient until the drug is metabolized. In severe cases, antipsychotic medications with minimal side effects (eg, haloperidol, 5 mg intramuscularly) may be given every several hours until the individual has regained control. In cases where "flashbacks" occur (mental imagery from a "bad trip" that is later triggered by mild stimuli such as marijuana, alcohol, or psychic trauma), a short course of an antipsychotic medication—eg, olanzapine, 5–10 mg/day orally, or risperidone, 2 mg/day orally, initially, and up to 20 mg/day and 6 mg/day, respectively—is usually sufficient. Lorazepam or clonazepam, 1–2 mg orally every 2 hours as needed for acute agitation, may be a useful adjunct. An occasional patient may have "flashbacks" for much longer periods and may require small doses of antipsychotic medications over the longer term.

4. Phencyclidine

Phencyclidine (PCP, angel dust, peace pill, hog) is simple to produce and mimics to some degree the traditional psychedelic drugs. PCP is a common deceptive substitute for LSD, tetrahydrocannabinol, and mescaline. It is available in crystals, capsules, and tablets to be inhaled, injected, swallowed, or smoked (it is commonly sprinkled on marijuana).

Treatment for acute intoxication is discussed in Chapter 38.

5. Marijuana

Cannabis sativa, a hemp plant, is the source of marijuana. The drug is usually inhaled by smoking but vaporizing is popular. There is a clinically distinct syndrome associated with "vaping" THC—**vaping-associated lung injury**—that may result in devastating pulmonary effects and a pathologically distinct pathophysiology. Effects occur in 10–20 minutes and last 2–3 hours. "Joints" of good quality contain about 500 mg of marijuana (which contains approximately 5–15 mg of tetrahydrocannabinol with a half-life of 7 days).

With moderate dosage, recreational marijuana (higher in the THC versus CBD component) produces two phases: mild euphoria followed by sleepiness. In the acute state, the user has an altered time perception, less inhibited emotions, psychomotor problems, impaired immediate memory, and conjunctival injection. High doses produce transient psychotomimetic effects. No specific treatment is necessary except in the case of the occasional "bad trip," in which case the person is treated in the same way as for psychedelic usage. Marijuana frequently aggravates existing mental illness and adversely affects motor performance.

Studies of long-term effects have conclusively shown abnormalities in the pulmonary tree. Laryngitis and rhinitis are related to prolonged use, along with chronic obstructive pulmonary disease. Electrocardiographic abnormalities are common, but no chronic cardiac disease has been linked to marijuana use. Long-term usage has resulted in depression of plasma testosterone levels and reduced sperm counts. Abnormal menstruation and failure to ovulate have occurred in some women. Cognitive impairments are common. Health care utilization for a variety of health problems is increased in long-term marijuana smokers. Sudden withdrawal produces insomnia, nausea, myalgia, and irritability. Psychological effects of long-term marijuana usage are still unclear. Urine testing is reliable if samples are carefully collected and tested. Detection periods span 4–6 days in short-term users and 20–50 days in long-term users. At the beginning of 2021, in the United States, marijuana is legal for medical use, recreational use, or both, or decriminalized, in all but six states.

6. Stimulants: Amphetamines & Cocaine

Stimulant misuse is quite common, either alone or in combination with abuse of other drugs. The stimulants include illicit drugs such as methamphetamine ("speed")—one variant is a smokable form called "ice," which gives an intense and long-lasting high—and methylphenidate and dextroamphetamine, which are under prescription control. Moderate usage of any of the stimulants produces hyperactivity, a sense of enhanced physical and mental capacity, and sympathomimetic effects. The clinical picture of acute stimulant intoxication includes sweating, tachycardia, elevated blood pressure, mydriasis, hyperactivity, and an acute brain syndrome with confusion and disorientation. Tolerance develops quickly, and, as the dosage is increased, hypervigilance, paranoid ideation (with delusions of parasitosis), stereotypy, bruxism, tactile hallucinations of insect infestation, and full-blown psychoses occur, often with persecutory ideation and aggressive responses. Stimulant withdrawal is characterized by depression with symptoms of hyperphagia and hypersomnia.

People who have used stimulants chronically (eg, anorexigenics) occasionally become sensitized ("kindling") to future use of stimulants. In these individuals, even small amounts of mild stimulants such as caffeine can cause symptoms of paranoia and auditory hallucinations.

Cocaine is a stimulant. It is a product of the coca plant. The derivatives include seeds, leaves, coca paste, cocaine hydrochloride, and the free base of cocaine. Cocaine hydrochloride is the salt and the most commonly used form. Freebase, a purer (and stronger) derivative called "crack," is prepared by simple extraction from cocaine hydrochloride.

There are various modes of use. Coca leaf chewing involves toasting the leaves and chewing with alkaline material (eg, the ash of other burned leaves) to enhance buccal absorption. One achieves a mild high, with onset in 5–10 minutes and lasting for about an hour. Intranasal use is simply snorting cocaine through a straw. Absorption is slowed somewhat by vasoconstriction (which may eventually cause tissue necrosis and septal perforation); the onset of action is in 2–3 minutes, with a moderate high (euphoria, excitement, increased energy) lasting about 30 minutes. The purity of the cocaine is a major determinant of the high. Intravenous use of cocaine hydrochloride or "freebase" is effective in 30 seconds and produces a short-lasting, intense high of about 15 minutes' duration. The combined use of cocaine and ethanol results in the metabolic production of cocaethylene by the liver. This substance produces more intense and long-lasting cocaine-like effects. Smoking freebase (volatilized cocaine because of the lower boiling point) acts in seconds and results in an intense high lasting several minutes. The intensity of the reaction is related to the marked lipid solubility of the freebase form and produces by far the most severe medical and psychiatric symptoms.

Cardiovascular collapse, arrhythmias, MI, and transient ischemic attacks have been reported. Seizures, strokes, migraine symptoms, hyperthermia, and lung damage may occur, and there are several obstetric complications, including spontaneous abortion, abruptio placentae, teratogenic effects, delayed fetal growth, and prematurity. Cocaine can cause anxiety, mood swings, and delirium, and chronic use can cause the same problems as other stimulants.

Clinicians should be alert to cocaine use in patients presenting with unexplained nasal bleeding or septal perforations, headaches, fatigue, insomnia, anxiety, depression, and chronic hoarseness. Sudden withdrawal of the drug is not life-threatening but usually produces craving, sleep disturbances, hyperphagia, lassitude, and severe depression (sometimes with suicidal ideation) lasting days to weeks.

Treatment for acute intoxication is imprecise and difficult. Since the high is related to blockage of dopamine reuptake, the dopamine agonist bromocriptine, 1.5 mg orally three times a day, alleviates some of the symptoms of craving associated with acute cocaine withdrawal. Treatment of psychosis is the same as that of any psychosis: antipsychotic medications in dosages sufficient to alleviate the symptoms. Any medical symptoms (eg, hyperthermia, seizures, hypertension) are treated specifically. These approaches should be used in conjunction with a structured program for use disorder, most often based on the Alcoholics Anonymous model. Hospitalization may be required if self-harm or violence toward others is a perceived threat (usually indicated by paranoid delusions).

7. Caffeine

Caffeine, along with nicotine and alcohol, is one of the most commonly used drugs worldwide although a caffeine use disorder is not described. Low to moderate doses (30–200 mg/day) tend to improve some aspects of performance (eg, vigilance). The approximate content of caffeine in a (180-mL) cup of beverage is as follows: brewed coffee, 80–140 mg; instant coffee, 60–100 mg; decaffeinated coffee, 1–6 mg; black leaf tea, 30–80 mg; tea bags, 25–75 mg; instant tea, 30–60 mg; cocoa, 10–50 mg; and 12-oz cola drinks, 30–65 mg. A 2-oz chocolate candy bar has about 20 mg. Some herbal teas (eg, "morning thunder") contain caffeine. Caffeine-containing analgesics usually contain approximately 30 mg per unit. Symptoms of caffeinism (usually associated with ingestion of over 500 mg/day) include anxiety, agitation, restlessness, insomnia, a feeling of being "wired," and somatic symptoms referable to the heart and GI tract. It is common for a case of caffeinism to present as an anxiety disorder. It is also common for caffeine and other stimulants to precipitate severe symptoms in compensated schizophrenic and manic-depressive patients. Chronically depressed patients often use caffeine drinks as self-medication. This diagnostic clue may help distinguish some major affective disorders. Discontinuation of caffeine (greater than 250 mg/day) can produce withdrawal symptoms, such as headaches, irritability, lethargy, and occasional nausea.

8. Miscellaneous Drugs & Solvents

The principal over-the-counter drugs of concern are an assortment of antihistaminic agents, frequently in combination with a mild analgesic promoted as cold remedies.

Antihistamines usually produce some CNS depression—thus their use as over-the-counter sedatives. Practically all of the so-called sleep aids are antihistamines. The mixture of antihistamines with alcohol usually exacerbates the CNS effects. Scopolamine and bromides generally have been removed from over-the-counter products.

The abuse of laxatives sometimes can lead to electrolyte disturbances that may contribute to the manifestations of a delirium. The greatest use of laxatives tends to be in older adults and those with eating disorders, both of whom are the most vulnerable to physiologic changes.

Anabolic steroids are abused by people who wish to increase muscle mass for cosmetic reasons or for greater strength. In addition to the medical problems, the practice is sometimes associated with significant mood swings, aggressiveness, and paranoid delusions. Alcohol and stimulant use are higher in these individuals. Withdrawal symptoms of steroid dependency include fatigue, depressed mood, restlessness, and insomnia.

Amyl nitrite is used as an "orgasm expander." The changes in time perception, "rush," and mild euphoria caused by the drug prompted its nonmedical use. Subjective effects last from 5 seconds to 15 minutes. Tolerance develops readily, but there are no known withdrawal symptoms. Abstinence for several days reestablishes the previous level of responsiveness. Long-term effects may include damage to the immune system and respiratory difficulties.

Sniffing of solvents and inhaling of gases (including aerosols) produce a form of inebriation similar to that of the volatile anesthetics. Agents include gasoline, toluene, petroleum ether, lighter fluids, cleaning fluids, paint thinners, and solvents that are present in many household products (eg, nail polish). Typical intoxication states include euphoria, slurred speech, hallucinations, and confusion, and with high doses, acute manifestations are unconsciousness and cardiorespiratory depression or failure; chronic exposure produces a variety of symptoms related to the liver, kidney, bone marrow, or heart. Lead encephalopathy can be associated with sniffing leaded gasoline. In addition, studies of workers chronically exposed to jet fuel showed significant increases in neurasthenic symptoms, including fatigue, anxiety, mood changes, memory difficulties, and somatic complaints. These same problems have been noted in long-term solvent abuse.

The so-called designer drugs are synthetic substitutes for commonly used recreational drugs. Common designer drugs include methyl analogs of fentanyl used as heroin substitutes. MDMA is also a designer drug not only with high abuse potential and purported neurotoxicity but also with therapeutic uses that are being explored. Often not detected by standard toxicology screens, these substances can present a vexing problem for clinicians faced with symptoms from a totally unknown cause.

Volkow ND et al. Prevention and treatment of opioid misuse and addiction: a review. JAMA Psychiatry. 2019;76:208. [PMID: 30516809]

NEUROCOGNITIVE DISORDERS

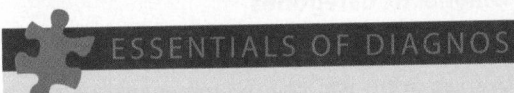

ESSENTIALS OF DIAGNOSIS

- Transient or permanent brain dysfunction with alterations in awareness or attention.
- Cognitive impairment to varying degrees.
- Impaired recall and recent memory, inability to focus attention and problems in perceptual processing, often with psychotic ideation.
- Random psychomotor activity such as stereotypy.
- Emotional disorders frequently present: depression, anxiety, irritability.
- Behavioral disturbances: impulse control, sexual acting-out, attention deficits, aggression, and exhibitionism.

General Considerations

The organic problem may be a primary brain disorder or a secondary manifestation of some general disorder. All of the cognitive disorders show *some degree of impaired thinking* depending on the site of involvement, the rate of onset and progression, and the duration of the underlying brain lesion. Emotional disturbances (eg, depression) are often present as significant comorbidities. The behavioral disturbances tend to be more common with chronicity, more directly related to the underlying personality or CNS vulnerability to drug side effects, and not necessarily correlated with cognitive dysfunction.

The causes of cognitive disorders are listed in Table 25–8.

Clinical Findings

The many manifestations include problems with orientation, short or fluctuating attention span, loss of recent memory and recall, impaired judgment, emotional lability, lack of initiative, impaired impulse control, inability to reason through problems, depression (worse in mild to moderate types), confabulation (not limited to alcohol organic brain syndrome), constriction of intellectual functions, visual and auditory hallucinations, and delusions. Physical findings will vary according to the cause. The electroencephalogram usually shows generalized slowing in delirium.

A. Delirium

Delirium (**acute confusional state**) is a transient global disorder of attention, with clouding of consciousness, usually a result of systemic problems (eg, medications, hypoxemia). See Chapters 4 and 24. Onset is usually rapid. The mental status fluctuates (impairment is usually least in the morning), with varying inability to concentrate, maintain attention, and sustain purposeful behavior. There is a marked deficit of short-term memory and recall. Anxiety and irritability are common. Orientation problems follow the inability to retain information. Perceptual disturbances (often visual hallucinations) and psychomotor restlessness with insomnia are common. "**Sundowning**"—mild to moderate delirium at night—is more common in patients with preexisting dementia and may be precipitated by hospitalization, medications, and sensory deprivation.

B. Dementia

Dementia is characterized by chronicity and deterioration of selective mental functions. See Chapters 4 and 24.

Table 25–8. Etiology of delirium and other cognitive disorders (listed in alphabetical order).

Disorder	Possible Causes
Cardiovascular disorders	MIs, cardiac arrhythmias, cerebrovascular spasms, hypertensive encephalopathy, hemorrhages, embolisms, and occlusions indirectly cause decreased cognitive function.
Collagen-vascular and immunologic disorders	Autoimmune disorders, including SLE, Sjögren syndrome, and AIDS.
Degenerative diseases	Alzheimer disease, Pick disease, multiple sclerosis, parkinsonism, Huntington chorea, normal pressure hydrocephalus.
Endocrine disorders	Thyrotoxicosis, hypothyroidism, adrenocortical dysfunction (including Addison disease and Cushing syndrome), pheochromocytoma, insulinoma, hypoglycemia, hyperparathyroidism, hypoparathyroidism, panhypopituitarism, diabetic ketoacidosis.
Infections	Septicemia; meningitis and encephalitis due to bacterial, viral, fungal, parasitic, or tuberculous organisms or to CNS syphilis; acute and chronic infections due to the entire range of microbiologic pathogens.
Intoxication	Alcohol, sedatives, bromides, analgesics (eg, pentazocine), psychedelic drugs, stimulants, and household solvents.
Long-term effects of alcohol	Wernicke-Korsakoff syndrome.
Medication withdrawal	Withdrawal from alcohol, sedative-hypnotics, corticosteroids.
Medications	Anticholinergic medications, antidepressants, H_2-blocking agents, digoxin, salicylates (long-term use), and a wide variety of other over-the-counter and prescribed medications.
Metabolic disturbances	Fluid and electrolyte disturbances (especially hyponatremia, hypomagnesemia, and hypercalcemia), acid-base disorders, hepatic disease (hepatic encephalopathy), kidney failure, porphyria.
Neoplasms	Primary or metastatic lesions of the CNS, cancer-induced hypercalcemia.
Nutritional deficiencies	Deficiency of vitamin B_1 (beriberi), vitamin B_{12} (pernicious anemia), folic acid, nicotinic acid (pellagra); protein-calorie malnutrition.
Respiratory disorders	Hypoxia, hypercapnia.
Seizure disorders	Ictal, interictal, and postictal dysfunction.
Trauma	Subdural hematoma, subarachnoid hemorrhage, intracerebral bleeding, concussion syndrome.

In all types of dementia, loss of impulse control (sexual and language) is common. **Pseudodementia** is a term previously applied to depressed patients who appear to be demented. These patients are often identifiable by their tendency to complain about memory problems vociferously rather than try to cover them up. They usually say they cannot complete cognitive tasks but with encouragement can often do so. They can be considered to have depression-induced reversible dementia that improves when the depression resolves. In many geriatric patients, however, the depression appears to be an insult that often unmasks a progressive dementia.

C. Amnestic Syndrome

This is a memory disturbance without delirium or dementia. It is usually associated with thiamine deficiency and chronic alcohol use (eg, Korsakoff syndrome). There is an impairment in the ability to learn new information or recall previously learned information.

D. Substance-Induced Hallucinosis

This condition is characterized by persistent or recurrent hallucinations (usually auditory) without the other symptoms usually found in delirium or dementia. Alcohol or hallucinogens are often the cause. There does not have to be any other mental disorder, and there may be complete spontaneous resolution.

Treatment

See Chapters 4 and 24 for detailed discussion.

Atri A. Current and future treatments in Alzheimer's disease. Semin Neurol. 2019;39:227. [PMID: 30925615]

Devlin JW et al. Clinical practice guidelines for the prevention and management of pain, agitation/sedation, delirium, immobility, and sleep disruption in adult patients in the ICU. Crit Care Med. 2018;46:e825. [PMID: 30113379]

PSYCHIATRIC PROBLEMS ASSOCIATED WITH HOSPITALIZATION & ILLNESS

Diagnostic Categories

A. Acute Problems

1. Delirium with psychotic features secondary to the medical or surgical problem, or compounded by effect of treatment.
2. Acute anxiety, often related to ignorance and fear of the immediate problem as well as uncertainty about the future.

3. Anxiety as an intrinsic aspect of the medical problem (eg, hyperthyroidism).
4. Denial of illness, which may present during acute or intermediate phases of illness.

B. Intermediate Problems

1. Depression as a function of the illness or acceptance of the illness, often associated with realistic or fantasied hopelessness about the future.
2. Behavioral problems, often related to denial of illness and, in extreme cases, causing the patient to leave the hospital against medical advice.

C. Recuperative Problems

1. Decreasing cooperation as the patient sees that improvement and compliance are not compelled.
2. Readjustment problems with family, job, and society.

General Considerations

A. Acute Problems

1. "Intensive care unit psychosis"—The ICU environment may contribute to the etiology of delirium. Critical care unit factors include sleep deprivation, increased arousal, mechanical ventilation, and social isolation. Other causes include those common to delirium and require vigorous investigation (see Delirium).

2. Presurgical and postsurgical anxiety states—Anxiety before or after surgery is common and commonly ignored. **Presurgical anxiety** is very common and is principally a fear of death (many surgical patients make out their wills). Patients may be fearful of anesthesia (improved by the preoperative anesthesia interview), the mysterious operating room, and the disease processes that might be uncovered by the surgeon. Such fears frequently cause people to delay examinations that might result in earlier surgery and a greater chance of cure.

The opposite of this is **surgery proneness,** the quest for surgery to escape from overwhelming life stresses. Some polysurgery patients may be classified as having factitious disorders. Dynamic motivations include the need to get medical care as a way of getting dependency needs met, the desire to outwit authority figures, unconscious guilt, or a masochistic need to suffer. Frequent surgery may also be related to a somatic symptom disorder, particularly body dysmorphic disorder (an obsession that a body part is disfigured). More apparent reasons may include an attempt to get relief from pain and a lifestyle that has become almost exclusively medically oriented, with all the risks entailed in such an endeavor.

Postsurgical anxiety states are usually related to pain, procedures, and loss of body image. Acute pain problems are quite different from chronic pain disorders (see Chronic Pain Disorders, this chapter); the former are readily handled with adequate analgesic medication (see Chapter 5). Alterations in body image, as with amputations, ostomies, and mastectomies, often raise concerns about relationships with others.

3. Iatrogenic problems—These usually pertain to medications, complications of diagnostic and treatment procedures, and impersonal and unsympathetic staff behavior. Polypharmacy is often a factor. Patients with unsolved diagnostic problems are at higher risk. They are desirous of relief, and the quest engenders more diagnostic procedures with a higher incidence of complications. The upset patient and family may be very demanding. Excessive demands usually result from anxiety. Such behavior is best handled with calm and measured responses.

B. Intermediate Problems

1. Prolonged hospitalization—Prolonged hospitalization presents unique problems in certain hospital services, eg, burn units or orthopedic services. The acute problems of the severely burned patient are discussed in Chapter 37. The problems often are behavioral difficulties related to length of hospitalization and necessary procedures. For example, in burn units, pain is a major problem in addition to anxiety about procedures. Disputes with staff are common and often concern pain medication or ward privileges. Some patients regress to infantile behavior and dependency. Staff members must agree about their approach to the patient in order to ensure the smooth functioning of the unit.

Denial of illness may present in some patients. Intervention by an authority figure (eg, immediate work supervisor) may help the patient accept treatment and eventually abandon the coping mechanism of denial.

2. Depression—Mood disorders ranging from mild adjustment disorder to major depressive disorder frequently occur during prolonged hospitalizations. A key to the diagnosis of depression in the medical setting is the individual's loss of self-esteem; they often think of themselves as worthless and are guilt ridden. Therapeutic medications (eg, corticosteroids) may be a factor. Depression can contribute to irritability and overt anger. Severe depression can lead to anorexia, which further complicates healing and metabolic balance. It is during this period that the issue of disfigurement arises—relief at survival gives way to concern about future function and appearance.

C. Recuperative Problems

1. Anxiety—Anxiety about return to the posthospital environment can cause regression to a dependent position. Complications increase, and staff forbearance again is tested. Anxiety occurring at this stage usually is handled more easily than previous behavior problems.

2. Posthospital adjustment—Adjustment difficulties after discharge are related to the severity of the deficits and the use of outpatient facilities (eg, physical therapy, rehabilitation programs, psychiatric outpatient treatment). Some patients may experience posttraumatic stress symptoms (eg, from traumatic injuries or even from necessary medical treatments). Lack of appropriate follow-up can contribute to depression in the patient, who may feel that he or she is making poor progress and may have thoughts of "giving up." Reintegration into work, educational, and social endeavors may be slow.

Clinical Findings

The symptoms that occur in these patients are similar to those discussed in previous sections of this chapter, eg, delirium, stress and adjustment disorders, anxiety, and depression. Behavior problems may include lack of cooperation, increased complaints, demands for medication, sexual approaches to nurses, threats to leave the hospital, and actual signing out against medical recommendations. The stress of hospitalization often brings out these more primitive defense mechanisms than the patient displays in daily life.

Complications

Prolongation of hospitalization causes increased expense, deterioration of patient-staff relationships, and increased probabilities of iatrogenic and legal problems. The possibility of increasing posthospital treatment problems is enhanced.

Treatment

A. Medical

The most important consideration by far is to *have one clinician in charge,* a clinician whom the patient trusts and who is able to oversee multiple treatment approaches (see Somatic Symptom Disorders, above). In acute problems, attention must be paid to metabolic imbalance, alcohol withdrawal, and previous drug use—prescribed, recreational, or over-the-counter. Adequate sleep and analgesia are important in enhancing a patient's coping abilities.

Many clinicians are attuned to the early detection of the surgery-prone patient. Plastic and orthopedic surgeons are at particular risk. Appropriate consultations may help detect some problems and mitigate future ones.

Postsurgical anxiety states can be alleviated by personal attention from the surgeon. Anxiety is not so effectively lessened by ancillary medical personnel, whom the patient perceives as lesser authorities, until after the clinician has reassured the patient. "Patient-controlled analgesia" can improve pain control, decrease anxiety, and minimize side effects.

Depression should be recognized early. If moderate to severe, antidepressant medications (see Antidepressant Medications, above) may be prescribed. High levels of anxiety can be lowered with judicious use of anxiolytic agents. Unnecessary medications tend to reinforce the patient's impression that there must be a serious illness or medication would not be required.

B. Psychological

Prepare the patient and family for what is to come. This includes the types of units where the patient will be quartered, the procedures that will be performed, and any disfigurements that will result from surgery. Repetition improves understanding. The nursing staff can be helpful, since patients frequently confide a lack of understanding to a nurse but are reluctant to do so to the physician.

Denial of illness is frequently a block to acceptance of treatment. This too should be handled with family members present (to help the patient face the reality of the situation) in a series of short interviews (for reinforcement). Dependency problems resulting from long hospitalization are best handled by focusing on the changes to come as the patient makes the transition to the outside world. Key figures are teachers, vocational counselors, and physical therapists. Challenges should be realistic and practical and handled in small steps.

Depression is usually related to the loss of familiar hospital supports, and the outpatient therapists and counselors help to lessen the impact of the loss. Some of the impact can be alleviated by anticipating, with the patient and family, the signal features of the common depression to help prevent the patient from assuming a permanent sick role.

Suicide is always a concern when a patient is faced with despair. An honest, compassionate, and supportive approach will help sustain the patient during this trying period.

C. Behavioral

Prior desensitization can significantly allay anxiety about medical procedures. A "dry run" can be done to reinforce the oral description. Cooperation during acute problem periods can be enhanced by the use of appropriate reinforcers such as a favorite nurse or helpful family member. People who are positive reinforcers are even more helpful during the intermediate phases when the patient becomes resistant to the seemingly endless procedures (eg, debridement of burned areas).

Specific situations (eg, psychological dependency on the respirator) can be corrected by weaning with appropriate reinforcers (eg, watching a favorite movie on a media player or laptop when disconnected from the ventilator). Behavioral approaches should be used in a positive and optimistic way for maximal reinforcement.

Relaxation techniques, hypnosis, and attentional distraction can be used to block side effects of a necessary treatment (eg, nausea in cancer chemotherapy).

D. Social

A change in environment requires adaptation. Because of the illness, admission and hospitalization may be more easily handled than discharge. A predischarge evaluation must be made to determine whether the family will be able to cope with the physical or mental changes in the patient. Working with the family while the patient is in the acute stage may presage a successful transition later on.

Development of a new social life can be facilitated by various self-help organizations (eg, the stoma club). Sharing problems with others in similar circumstances eases the return to a social life, which may be quite different from that prior to the illness.

Prognosis

The prognosis is good in all patients who have reversible medical and surgical conditions. It is guarded when there is serious functional loss that impairs vocational, educational, or societal possibilities—especially in the case of progressive and ultimately life-threatening illness.

Cortés-Beringola A et al. Diagnosis, prevention, and management of delirium in the intensive care unit. Am Heart J. 2021;232:164. [PMID: 33253676]

Endocrine Disorders

Paul A. Fitzgerald, MD

DISEASES OF THE HYPOTHALAMUS & PITUITARY GLAND

ANTERIOR HYPOPITUITARISM

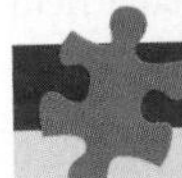

ESSENTIALS OF DIAGNOSIS

- ACTH deficiency: low adrenal secretion of cortisol and epinephrine; normal aldosterone secretion.
- Growth hormone (GH) deficiency: short stature in children; asthenia, obesity, and increased cardiovascular risk in adults.
- Prolactin (PRL) deficiency: postpartum lactation failure.
- TSH deficiency: secondary hypothyroidism.
- LH and FSH deficiency: hypogonadism and infertility in men and women.

General Considerations

The anterior pituitary hormones are GH, PRL, ACTH, TSH, LH, and FSH. The hypothalamus synthesizes hormones that regulate anterior pituitary secretion, including corticotropin-releasing hormone (CRH), growth hormone–releasing hormone, gonadotrophin-releasing hormone (GnRH), thyrotropin-releasing hormone, and somatostatin. The hypothalamus also secretes dopamine that inhibits PRL secretion. These hypothalamic regulatory hormones are transported by a portal venous system down the pituitary stalk to the anterior pituitary. The hypothalamus also synthesizes oxytocin and arginine vasopressin (AVP), also known as ADH. Nerves from the hypothalamus carry oxytocin and AVP to the posterior pituitary, where they are stored and released.

1. Hypopituitarism with mass lesions—

A. Pituitary neuroendocrine tumors—These tumors, also known as pituitary adenomas, can cause anterior hypopituitarism, particularly when they are large macroadenomas (1 cm or larger). Nonfunctioning pituitary neuroendocrine tumors are more likely than functioning pituitary adenomas to grow large enough to cause anterior hypopituitarism; they rarely cause diabetes insipidus.

B. Pituitary metastases—These lesions are usually from breast cancer (45%); about 50% present over 10 years after the primary tumor. Lung cancer accounts for about 21% of pituitary metastases that typically present either before or within 1 year of the primary cancer. Pituitary metastases often present with visual loss or ophthalmoplegia, ACTH deficiency (71%), TSH deficiency (65%), diabetes insipidus (26%), or gonadotropin deficiency (88%).

C. Other mass lesions—These lesions include craniopharyngioma, plasmacytoma, germ cell tumors, glioma, lymphomas, cysts (Rathke cleft, dermoid, epidermoid, arachnoid), meningioma, and hemangiopericytoma.

D. Vascular lesions—These lesions include pituitary tumor apoplexy, cavernous sinus aneurysm, and subarachnoid hemorrhage.

E. Inflammatory/infiltrative lesions—These include granulomatosis with polyangiitis, xanthomatosis, giant cell granuloma, Langerhans cell histiocytosis, sarcoidosis, syphilis, hypophysitis, and tuberculosis. Infectious lesions can be bacterial, fungal, or parasitic. Lymphocytic hypophysitis is an autoimmune disorder that is characterized by infiltration of the infundibulum and pituitary by lymphocytes, macrophages, and plasma cells. Spontaneous lymphocytic hypophysitis is more common in women (71%) and most frequently presents during pregnancy or postpartum. Immune checkpoint inhibitor hypophysitis can be caused by several immunity-enhancing drugs, particularly the anti-CTLA-4 agents ipilimumab and tremelimumab (14%), as well as with the anti-PD-1 agents pembrolizumab and nivolumab (0.5%).

F. Pituitary stalk thickening—This disorder is caused most frequently by lymphocytic hypophysitis, metastases, neurosarcoidosis, or a congenital ectopic posterior pituitary, but the cause is never clinically apparent in many patients. Pituitary stalk damage frequently causes central diabetes insipidus and one or more anterior pituitary hormone deficiencies.

2. Hypopituitarism without mass lesions—

A. CONGENITAL HYPOPITUITARISM—This disorder occurs in syndromes such as septo-optic dysplasia and in patients with various gene mutations that cause a progressive loss of anterior pituitary function in childhood. Prader-Willi syndrome is a genetic disorder where genes on the paternal chromosome 15 are deleted or unexpressed. Kallmann syndrome is caused by various gene mutations that impair the development or migration of GnRH-synthesizing neurons from the olfactory bulb to the hypothalamus. Congenital GH deficiency occurs as an isolated pituitary hormone deficiency in about one-third of cases.

B. ACQUIRED HYPOPITUITARISM—This disorder can result from cranial radiation therapy, pituitary surgery, encephalitis, cerebral malaria, hemochromatosis, autoimmunity, or coronary artery bypass grafting. *Hypopituitarism can occur acutely, usually with severe secondary adrenal insufficiency that may be fatal unless recognized and treated.* Acute hypopituitarism may also be associated with diabetes insipidus.

Bexarotene chemotherapy causes a high rate of pituitary insufficiency with central hypothyroidism. Mitotane therapy for adrenocortical carcinoma causes secondary hypothyroidism in most patients. At least one pituitary hormone deficiency develops in about 25–30% of survivors of moderate to severe **traumatic brain injury** and in about 55% of survivors of **aneurysmal subarachnoid hemorrhage.** Some degree of hypopituitarism, most commonly GH deficiency and hypogonadotropic hypogonadism, occurs in one-third of **ischemic stroke** patients. Other cases of acquired hypopituitarism can be idiopathic or associated with an empty sella on MRI.

Sheehan syndrome refers to hypopituitarism caused by postpartum pituitary necrosis, usually following severe postpartum uterine hemorrhage. It is usually characterized by postpartum amenorrhea and inability to lactate. Hypopituitarism in Sheehan syndrome usually occurs gradually over 10–20 years; the diagnosis is typically delayed an average of 9 years. Manifestations in affected women are typically hyponatremia, hypoglycemia, or anemia. In acute Sheehan syndrome, MRI shows an enlarged pituitary with only a thin rim of enhancement with gadolinium. After 1 year, MRI shows atrophy of the pituitary and a partially empty sella.

C. FUNCTIONAL HYPOPITUITARISM—Functional hypogonadotropic hypogonadism can occur in both women and men secondary to excessive exercise or weight loss. Partial hypogonadotropic hypogonadism commonly develops in men with normal aging, obesity, and serum free testosterone levels that are low or near the lower end of normal reference ranges while serum FSH and LH levels remain normal. Women may develop hypothalamic amenorrhea during periods of severe emotional or physical stress. LH and FSH deficiency with hypogonadotropic hypogonadism occur in serious illness, malnutrition, anorexia nervosa, alcohol use disorder (alcoholism), Cushing syndrome (spontaneous or iatrogenic), and hyperprolactinemia (drug-induced or spontaneous). Partial hypogonadotropic hypogonadism develops in about 63% of long-term opioid (including methadone) users. Opioid use also causes secondary adrenal insufficiency in about 15% of patients but is less likely to cause GH or TSH deficiency. Therapy with GnRH agonists (eg, leuprolide) also causes hypogonadotropic hypogonadism that can persist after therapy is stopped.

Functional GH deficiency can occur with normal aging, malnutrition, and chronic kidney ACTH suppression with functional isolated secondary adrenal insufficiency occurs in patients receiving megesterol acetate, patients on high-dose opioid therapy (15%), and in patients exposed to excess endogenous or exogenous corticosteroids (parenteral, oral, inhaled, or topical). TSH deficiency can be caused by mitotane or bexarotene, resulting in secondary hypothyroidism.

Clinical Findings

When hypopituitarism is caused by a mass lesion or hypophysitis, patients may have headaches or visual field defects. Nonspecific symptoms, such as fatigue, dizziness and hypotension, confusion, cognitive dysfunction, sexual dysfunction, polydipsia, or cold intolerance, can develop. Other symptoms and signs attributable to specific pituitary hormone deficiencies are described below.

A. Symptoms and Signs

1. GH (somatropin) deficiency—Congenital GH deficiency can present in newborns with hypoglycemia, jaundice, and a small penis and later with short stature in childhood.

GH deficiency in adults is often undiagnosed, since maximum height has already been reached and other manifestations are nonspecific. Symptoms vary in severity from mild to severe, resulting in a variable spectrum of nonspecific symptoms that include mild to moderate central obesity, reduced physical and mental energy, impaired concentration and memory, and depression. Patients may also have variably reduced muscle mass, increased LDL cholesterol, and reduced cardiac output with exercise. Chronic GH deficiency leads to osteopenia and an increased risk of fractures. When other more recognizable pituitary hormone deficits are present, there is a high likelihood of concurrent GH deficiency.

2. Gonadotropin deficiency (hypogonadotropic hypogonadism)—In gonadotropin deficiency, insufficiencies of LH and FSH cause hypogonadism and infertility.

Congenital gonadotropin deficiency is characterized by partial or complete lack of pubertal development. The sense of olfaction (smell) is entirely normal in 58% (normosmic isolated hypogonadotropic hypogonadism), or hyposmic or anosmic in 42% (Kallmann syndrome). Patients frequently have abnormal genitalia (25%), kidney anomalies (28%), midline craniofacial defects (50%), neurologic deficits (42%), and musculoskeletal malformations. Some affected women have menarche followed by secondary amenorrhea. Some affected males also have congenital adrenal hypoplasia with X-linked inheritance.

Prader-Willi syndrome presents with cryptorchidism, mental retardation, short stature, hyperflexibility, autonomic dysregulation, cognitive impairment, obesity, hypogonadotropic hypogonadism, or primary hypogonadism.

Acquired gonadotropin deficiency is characterized by the gradual loss of facial, axillary, pubic, and body hair. Men may note diminished libido, erectile dysfunction, muscle atrophy, infertility, and osteopenia. Women have amenorrhea, infertility, and osteoporosis.

3. TSH deficiency—TSH deficiency causes hypothyroidism (see Hypothyroidism, below).

4. ACTH deficiency—Central adrenal insufficiency is caused by ACTH deficiency. There is functional atrophy of the adrenal cortex within 2 weeks of pituitary damage, which results in diminished cortisol. Adrenal mineralocorticoid secretion continues, so manifestations of adrenal insufficiency in hypopituitarism may be less striking than in bilateral adrenal gland destruction (see Primary Adrenal Insufficiency [Addison disease]). Central adrenal insufficiency from pituitary metastases typically presents with nausea, weight loss, and fatigue; these symptoms are often attributed to chemotherapy or to the malignancy itself. Patients with partial ACTH deficiency have some cortisol secretion and may not have symptoms until stressed by illness or surgery.

5. PRL deficiency—This presents in women with failure to lactate in the puerperium.

6. Panhypopituitarism—This condition refers to a deficiency of several or all pituitary hormones. There may be hypogonadotropic hypogonadism (62%), diabetes insipidus (54%), headache (50%), hypothyroidism (48%), ACTH deficiency (47%), GH deficiency (37%), and hyperprolactinemia (36%), which clinicians may mistake for a prolactinoma. Hypopituitarism typically presents in women with amenorrhea.

7. Hypothalamic damage—This can cause obesity and cognitive impairment. Hypopituitarism occurs but usually along with *increased* serum levels of PRL. Local tumor effects can cause headache or optic nerve compression with visual field impairment.

B. Laboratory Findings

Initially, there may be hyponatremia and hypoglycemia, with secondary hypoadrenalism, hypothyroidism, or GH deficiency. Hyponatremia can be caused by hypothyroidism or hypoadrenalism. Patients with lymphocytic hypophysitis frequently have elevated serum antinuclear or anticytoplasmic antibodies. Patients with hypopituitarism without an established etiology should be screened for hemochromatosis with a serum ferritin or iron and transferrin saturation.

Male hypogonadotropic hypogonadism is diagnosed by drawing blood before 10 AM after an overnight fast in men without an acute or subacute illness. Affected men have a low fasting serum total or free serum testosterone with a low or normal serum LH. A serum PRL is also obtained, since hyperprolactinemia of any cause can result in hypogonadism.

Female hypogonadotropic hypogonadism is suspected in nonpregnant women with amenorrhea or oligomenorrhea, who do not have acute illness, hyperthyroidism, or hyperandrogenism. The serum estradiol is low and the serum FSH is low or normal. In nonpregnant women, a serum PRL is obtained, since hyperprolactinemia of any cause can result in hypogonadism. In postmenopausal women, the absence of an elevated serum FSH (in a woman not taking estrogen replacement) indicates gonadotropin deficiency.

Central hypothyroidism is diagnosed with a low serum free thyroxine (FT_4) in the setting of pituitary disease. The serum TSH can be low, normal, or even mildly elevated (oddly). Central hypothyroidism can emerge when patients begin GH replacement, so thyroid levels must be monitored in that setting. Patients undergoing pituitary surgery should be assessed for central hypothyroidism preoperatively and again 6 weeks postoperatively.

Central adrenal insufficiency is diagnosed after withholding corticosteroid replacement for at least 18–24 hours. Blood is drawn at 8–9 AM for baseline plasma ACTH and serum cortisol. A serum cortisol less than 3 mcg/dL (80 nmol/L) usually indicates adrenal insufficiency, whereas an 8–9 AM serum cortisol higher than 15 mcg/dL (400 nmol/L) usually excludes adrenal insufficiency. For 8–9 AM cortisol levels between 3 and 15 mcg/dL, a cosyntropin test is often required. For the cosyntropin test, patients should hold any corticosteroid replacement for at least 18–24 hours. At 8–9 AM, blood is drawn for serum cortisol, ACTH, and dehydroepiandrosterone (DHEA); then cosyntropin (synthetic $ACTH_{1-24}$) 0.25 mg is administered intramuscularly or intravenously. Another serum cortisol is obtained 45 minutes after the cosyntropin injection; a stimulated serum cortisol of less than 20 mcg/dL (550 nmol/L) indicates probable adrenal insufficiency. With gradual pituitary damage and early in the course of ACTH deficiency, patients can have a stimulated serum cortisol of 20 mcg/dL or more (550 nmol/L) but a baseline 8 AM serum cortisol of 5 mcg/dL (138 nmol/L) or less, which is suspicious for adrenal insufficiency. The baseline serum ACTH level is low or normal in secondary hypoadrenalism, distinguishing it from primary adrenal disease. Serum DHEA is a proxy for ACTH; levels are usually low in patients with secondary adrenal deficiency, helping confirm the diagnosis. Hyponatremia may occur, especially when ACTH and TSH deficiencies are both present.

For patients with signs of secondary adrenal insufficiency (hyponatremia, hypotension, pituitary tumor) but borderline cosyntropin test results, treatment can be instituted empirically and the test repeated at a later date.

GH deficiency in adults is difficult to diagnose, since GH secretion is normally pulsatile and serum GH levels are normally undetectable for much of the day. Also, adults (particularly men) physiologically tend to produce less GH when they are over age 50 or have abdominal obesity. Therefore, pathologic GH deficiency is often inferred by symptoms of GH deficiency in the presence of pituitary destruction or other pituitary hormone deficiencies. GH deficiency is present in 96% of patients with three or more other pituitary hormone deficiencies and a low serum IGF-1.

While GH stimulates the production of IGF-1, the serum IGF-1 level is neither a sensitive (about 50%) nor specific test for GH deficiency in adults. Very low serum IGF-1 levels (less than 84 mcg/L) are usually indicative of GH deficiency but also occur in malnutrition, prolonged fasting, oral estrogen, hypothyroidism, uncontrolled diabetes mellitus, and liver failure. A therapeutic trial of GH therapy should be considered for symptomatic patients who have either a serum IGF-1 less than 84 mcg/L or three other pituitary hormone deficiencies.

Provocative GH stimulation testing to help diagnose adult GH deficiency has a sensitivity of only 66%; however, tests are sometimes indicated or required for insurance coverage of GH therapy. In the absence of a serum IGF-1 level less than 84 mcg/L or multiple other pituitary hormone deficiencies, provocative GH-stimulation testing may be indicated for the following patients: (1) young adult patients who have completed GH therapy for childhood GH deficiency and have achieved maximal linear growth; (2) patients who have a hypothalamic or pituitary tumor or who have received surgery or radiation therapy to these areas; and (3) patients who have had prior head trauma, cerebrovascular accident, or encephalitis. When required, such testing usually entails measuring serum GH following provocative stimuli. The single-dose oral macimorelin (Macrilen) GH stimulation test involves the oral administration of macimorelin (a GH secretogogue) to a fasting individual at a dose of 0.5 mg/kg body weight. Blood samples for GH are drawn immediately prior to administration and then at 30, 45, 60, and 90 minutes afterward. A maximum serum GH level below 5.1 ng/mL suggests GH deficiency with 92% sensitivity and 96% specificity. The glucagon stimulation test is a practical alternative to traditional provocative GH stimulation testing to diagnose pathologic GH deficiency or functional GH deficiency due to aging or obesity. It should not be given to patients who are malnourished or who have not eaten for over 48 hours.

C. Imaging

MRI of the hypothalamus and pituitary is indicated when a mass lesion is suspected. MRI can detect lesions of the pituitary, hypothalamus or pituitary stalk, including pituitary adenoma, lymphocytic hypophysitis, neurosarcoidosis, Langerhans cell histiocytosis, craniopharyngioma, germinoma, astrocytoma, and metastatic malignancy. MRI shows pituitary enlargement in 75% of cases of ipilimumab-associated hypophysitis but only 25% of cases of anti-PD-1 agent–induced hypophysitis. MRI is not warranted in cases of functional hypopituitarism associated with severe obesity, drugs, or nutritional disorders.

Differential Diagnosis

The failure to enter puberty may simply reflect a constitutional delay in growth and puberty. Secondary adrenal insufficiency may persist for many months following high-dose corticosteroid therapy and may also be seen with inhaled or topical corticosteroid therapy.

Reversible, second hypothyroidism with suppression of TSH and T_4 can be caused by severe illness, hyperthyroxinemia, and administration of triiodothyronine, mitotane, or bexarotene, resulting in temporary central hypothyroidism. Corticosteroids and megestrol reversibly suppress endogenous ACTH and cortisol secretion.

GH deficiency occurs normally with aging and physiologically with obesity (reversible with sufficient weight loss). Very low serum IGF-1 levels can be seen with prolonged fasting, malnutrition, liver failure, hypothyroidism, and uncontrolled diabetes mellitus.

Complications

During a stressful illness, patients with untreated hypoadrenalism may become febrile and comatose and die of hyponatremia and shock.

Rarely, acute hemorrhage may occur in large pituitary tumors, manifested by rapid loss of vision, headache, and evidence of acute pituitary failure (pituitary apoplexy) requiring emergency decompression of the sella. Among patients with craniopharyngiomas, diabetes insipidus is found in 16% preoperatively and in 60% postoperatively. Hyponatremia often presents abruptly during the first 2 weeks following any pituitary surgery. Conventional radiation therapy for intracranial disorders can result in an increased incidence of small vessel ischemic strokes, second tumors and damaged hypothalamic-pituitary function.

Treatment

A. Corticosteroid Replacement

Long-term therapy is initiated with hydrocortisone 10–25 mg orally in the morning and 5–15 mg in the late afternoon. Other corticosteroids may be used; the dosing and timing must be individually tailored. No mineralocorticoid replacement is required. See Corticosteroid Replacement Therapy-Primary Adrenal Insufficiency (Addison Disease) below.

B. Thyroid Hormone Replacement

Levothyroxine is given to correct hypothyroidism only after the patient is assessed for cortisol deficiency or is already receiving corticosteroids. The typical maintenance dose is about 1.6 mcg/kg body weight, averaging 125 mcg daily with a wide range of 25–300 mcg daily. Because assessment of serum TSH is useless for monitoring patients with hypopituitarism, the optimal replacement dose of levothyroxine is determined clinically by raising or lowering the dose, according to the patient's symptoms and clinical examination. With clinically optimized levothyroxine replacement, serum FT_4 levels are usually in the mid to high-normal range. Some patients do not feel clinically euthyroid until they receive levothyroxine in doses at which the serum FT_4 levels are mildly elevated; however, serum T_3 or FT_3 levels should be in the low-normal range. During pregnancy, clinical status and serum FT_4 or total T_4 levels need to be monitored frequently, since higher doses of levothyroxine are usually required.

C. Gonadotropin Hormone Replacement

Hyperprolactinemia-related hypogonadotropic hypogonadism improves or resolves with treatment. Sex hormone replacement may be required. See Male Hypogonadism and Female Hypogonadism.

Women with panhypopituitarism have profound androgen deficiency caused by the combination of both secondary hypogonadism and adrenal insufficiency. When serum DHEA levels are less than 400 ng/mL, women may also be treated with compounded USP-grade DHEA 50 mg/day orally. DHEA therapy tends to increase pubic and axillary hair and may modestly improve libido, alertness, stamina, and overall psychological well-being.

For men with oligospermia, human chorionic gonadotropin (hCG) (equivalent to LH) may be given at a dosage of 2000–3000 units intramuscularly three times weekly and testosterone replacement discontinued. The dose of hCG is adjusted to normalize serum testosterone levels. After 6–12 months of hCG treatment, if the sperm count remains low, hCG injections are continued along with injections of follitropin beta (synthetic recombinant FSH) or urofollitropins (urine-derived FSH). An alternative for patients with an intact pituitary is the use of leuprolide (GnRH analog) by intermittent subcutaneous infusion. With treatment, testicular volumes increase within 5–12 months, and some spermatogenesis occurs in most cases.

Clomiphene, 25–50 mg/day orally, can sometimes stimulate men's own pituitary gonadotropins (when their pituitary is intact), thereby increasing testosterone and sperm production. For fertility induction in females, ovulation may be induced with clomiphene, 50–100 mg/day orally for 5 days every 2 months. Ovulation induction with FSH and hCG can induce multiple births and should be used only by those experienced with their administration.

D. Human Growth Hormone (hGH) Replacement

Symptomatic adults with GH deficiency may be treated with subcutaneous recombinant human growth hormone (rhGH, somatropin) injections, 0.2 mg/day (0.6 IU/day), administered three times weekly. The dosage of rhGH is increased every 2–4 weeks by increments of 0.1 mg (0.3 IU) until side effects occur or a sufficient salutary response and a normal serum IGF-1 level are achieved. In adults, if the desired effects (eg, improved energy and mentation, reduction in visceral adiposity) are not seen within 3–6 months at maximum tolerated dosage, rhGH therapy is discontinued. Therapy with hGH can bring out central hypothyroidism, so serum FT_4 levels require monitoring when beginning hGH therapy.

RhGH may be safely administered to pregnant women with hypopituitarism at their usual pregestational dose during the first trimester, tapering the dose during the second trimester, and discontinuing rhGH during the third trimester.

Oral estrogen replacement reduces hepatic IGF-1 production. Therefore, prior to commencing rhGH therapy, oral estrogen should be changed to transdermal or transvaginal estradiol.

Treatment of adult GH deficiency usually improves the patient's overall quality of life, with better emotional sense of well-being, increased muscle mass, and decreased visceral fat and waist circumference. Long-term treatment with rhGH does not appear to affect mortality.

Side effects of rhGH therapy may include peripheral edema, hand stiffness, arthralgias and myalgias, paresthesias, carpal tunnel syndrome, tarsal tunnel syndrome, headache, pseudotumor cerebri, gynecomastia, hypertension, and proliferative retinopathy. Treatment with rhGH can also cause sleep apnea, insomnia, dyspnea, sweating, and fatigue. Side effects usually remit promptly after a sufficient reduction in dosage. Replacement therapy with rhGH does not increase the risk of any malignancy or the regrowth of pituitary or brain neoplasms; serum IGF-1 levels should be kept in the normal range.

GH should not be administered during critical illness, since administration of very high doses of rhGH increased mortality in patients receiving intensive care. *There is currently no proven role for GH replacement for the physiologic GH deficiency that is seen with abdominal obesity or normal aging.*

E. Other Treatment

Selective transsphenoidal surgery is usually performed to resect non-prolactinoma pituitary masses and Rathke cleft cysts that cause local symptoms or hypopituitarism. Such surgery reverses hypopituitarism in a minority of cases. Patients with lymphocytic hypophysitis have been treated with corticosteroid therapy and other immunosuppressants without much response and without reversing hypopituitarism.

Prognosis

Functionally, most patients with hypopituitarism do well with hormone replacement. Men with infertility who are treated with hCG/FSH or GnRH are likely to resume spermatogenesis if they have had sexual maturation and have descended testicles with a baseline serum inhibin B level over 60 pg/mL. Women under age 40 years with infertility from hypogonadotropic hypogonadism can usually have successful ovulation induction.

Hypopituitarism resulting from a pituitary tumor may be reversible with dopamine agonists for prolactinomas (see Prolactinoma, below) or with careful selective resection of the tumor. Spontaneous recovery from hypopituitarism associated with pituitary stalk thickening has been reported. Patients can also recover from functional hypopituitarism due to excessive exercise or weight loss if they greatly reduce exercise and gain weight; about half of men regain normal serum testosterone levels. Spontaneous reversal of idiopathic isolated hypogonadotropic hypogonadism occurs in about 10% of patients after several years of hormone replacement therapy (HRT). However, hypopituitarism is usually permanent, and long-term HRT is ordinarily required.

Patients with hypopituitarism have an increased mortality risk, particularly women and those in whom diagnosis was made at a younger age, who have a craniopharyngioma, or who required transcranial surgery or radiation therapy. There is also an increased risk of death from infections with adrenal crisis in patients with untreated secondary insufficiency. Some pituitary tumors are locally invasive. Asymptomatic Rathke cleft cysts may not require surgery but do require endocrine, ophthalmic, and scan surveillance.

de Vries F et al. Opioids and their endocrine effects: a systematic review and meta-analysis. J Clin Endocrinol Metab. 2020;105:1020. [PMID: 31511863]

Dwyer AA et al. Functional hypogonadotropic hypogonadism in men: underlying neuroendocrine mechanisms and natural history. J Clin Endocrinol Metab. 2019;104:3403. [PMID: 31220265]

Lu J et al. Immune checkpoint inhibitor-associated pituitary-adrenal dysfunction. A systematic review and meta-analysis. Cancer Med. 2019;8:7503. [PMID: 31679184]

Melmed S. Pituitary-tumor endocrinopathies. N Engl J Med. 2020;382:937. [PMID: 32130815]

Prete A et al. Hypophysitis. Endotext [Internet]. 2021. [PMID: 30160871]

Prodam F et al. Insights into non-classic and emerging causes of hypopituitarism. Nat Rev Endocrinol. 2021;17:114. [PMID: 33247226]

CENTRAL DIABETES INSIPIDUS

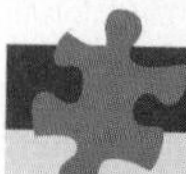

ESSENTIALS OF DIAGNOSIS

- ADH deficiency with polyuria (2–20 L/day) and polydipsia.
- Hypernatremia occurs if fluid intake is inadequate.

General Considerations

Central diabetes insipidus is an uncommon disease caused by a deficiency in vasopressin (ADH) from the posterior pituitary.

Primary central diabetes insipidus (without an identifiable lesion noted on MRI of the pituitary and hypothalamus) accounts for about one-third of all cases of diabetes insipidus. Familial diabetes insipidus occurs as a dominant genetic trait with symptoms developing at about 2 years of age. Central diabetes insipidus may also be idiopathic or due to autoimmunity against hypothalamic AVP-secreting cells. Reversible central diabetes insipidus can occur with administration of ketamine, temozolomide, or the anti-PD-L1 monoclonal antibody avelumab, and in the myelodysplastic preleukemic phase of acute myelogenous leukemia.

Secondary central diabetes insipidus is most commonly due to damage to the hypothalamus or pituitary stalk by tumor, hypophysitis, infarction, hemorrhage, anoxic encephalopathy, or surgical or head trauma. Less commonly, central diabetes insipidus is caused by infection (eg, encephalitis, tuberculosis, syphilis) or granulomas (sarcoidosis or Langerhans cell granulomatosis). Metastases to the pituitary are more likely to cause diabetes insipidus (33%) than are pituitary adenomas (1%).

Clinical Findings

A. Symptoms and Signs

The symptoms of the disease are intense thirst, especially with a craving for ice water, with the volume of ingested fluid varying from 2 L to 20 L daily, and polyuria, with large urine volumes and low urine specific gravity (usually less than 1.006 with ad libitum fluid intake). The urine is otherwise normal. Partial diabetes insipidus presents with less intense symptoms and should be suspected in patients with enuresis. Most patients with diabetes insipidus are able to maintain fluid balance by continuing to ingest large volumes of water. However, in patients without free access to water or with a damaged hypothalamic thirst center and altered thirst sensation, diabetes insipidus may present with hypernatremia and dehydration. Diabetes insipidus is aggravated by administration of high-dose corticosteroids, which increases renal free water clearance.

B. Laboratory Findings

Diagnosis of central diabetes insipidus is a clinical one; there is no single diagnostic laboratory test. Evaluation should include a 24-hour urine collection for volume and creatinine. A urine volume of less than 2 L/24 hours (in the absence of hypernatremia) rules out diabetes insipidus. The patient can be tested during ad libitum fluid intake. A random urine is tested for osmolality. Blood testing includes plasma vasopressin and serum glucose, urea nitrogen, calcium, potassium, sodium, and uric acid.

Plasma AVP levels are usually low (below 1 pg/mL) with both central diabetes insipidus and primary polyuria, whereas plasma AVP levels are normal or elevated (more than 2.5 pg/mL) with nephrogenic diabetes insipidus. Plasma osmolality of 300 mOsm/kg or more implies either central or nephrogenic diabetes insipidus, whereas plasma osmolality of 280 mOsm/kg or less implies primary polydipsia as the diagnosis. Urine osmolality is low (300 mOsm/L or lower) in all three polyuric conditions and is not a helpful test. Hyperuricemia occurs frequently with both central and nephrogenic diabetes insipidus, whereas it is uncommon with primary polydipsia.

A supervised "vasopressin challenge test" may be done: Desmopressin acetate 0.05–0.1 mL (5–10 mcg) intranasally (or 1 mcg subcutaneously or intravenously) is given, with measurement of urine volume for 12 hours before and 12 hours after administration. A serum sodium is obtained at baseline, 12 hours after the desmopressin, and immediately if symptoms of hyponatremia develop. Patients with central diabetes insipidus notice a distinct reduction in thirst and polyuria; serum sodium usually remains normal. The dosage of desmopressin is doubled if the response is marginal. In patients with primary polydipsia, a desmopressin challenge causes no significant reduction in polydipsia. Patients with nephrogenic diabetes insipidus show no response in polydipsia or urine volume.

Another test to distinguish central diabetes insipidus from primary polydipsia involves the carefully supervised hypertonic 3% saline-stimulated measurement of plasma copeptin, the C-terminal fragment of pre-pro-arginine vasopressin. Hypertonic 3% saline is administered intravenously as a 250 mL bolus, followed by a continuous infusion rate of 0.15 mL/kg/minute. Plasma sodium is measured stat every 30 minutes; when the plasma sodium level reaches 150 mmol/L, blood is drawn for plasma copeptin. A level 4.9 pmol/L or less helps confirm the diagnosis of central diabetes insipidus.

C. Imaging

The normal posterior "bright spot" seen on the MRI T1-weighted image is undetectable or small with central diabetes insipidus, whereas it is normal in primary polydipsia and nephrogenic diabetes insipidus. MRI can also detect pathology responsible for central diabetes insipidus. Pituitary MRI must be interpreted cautiously. Normal patients with an "empty sella" frequently lack the posterior pituitary bright spot. Patients with nephrogenic diabetes insipidus may also have an absent or faint pituitary bright spot, due to depletion of AVP in the posterior caused by the high secretion rate of AVP in nephrogenic diabetes insipidus. Also, fat in the marrow of the dorsum sella can be misinterpreted as the posterior pituitary bright spot.

Differential Diagnosis

Central diabetes insipidus must be distinguished from polyuria caused by psychogenic polydipsia, diabetes mellitus, Cushing syndrome, hypercalcemia, hypokalemia, and nocturnal polyuria of Parkinson disease.

Vasopressinase-induced diabetes insipidus may be seen in the last trimester of pregnancy, associated with oligohydramnios, preeclampsia, or liver dysfunction, and in the puerperium. Maternal circulating vasopressin is destroyed by placental vasopressinase; however, synthetic desmopressin is unaffected.

Nephrogenic diabetes insipidus is caused by unresponsiveness of the kidney tubules to the normal secretion of vasopressin. A congenital form is familial and transmitted as an X-linked trait; acquired forms are usually less severe and occur in pyelonephritis, renal amyloidosis, myeloma, potassium depletion, Sjögren syndrome, sickle cell anemia, chronic hypercalcemia, or recovery from ATN. Certain medications (eg, corticosteroids, diuretics, demeclocycline, lithium, foscarnet, or methicillin) may induce nephrogenic diabetes insipidus.

Complications

If water is not readily available, the excessive output of urine will lead to severe dehydration and worsening hypernatremia. Patients with an impaired thirst mechanism are very prone to hypernatremia, as are those with impaired mentation who forget to take their desmopressin. Excessive desmopressin acetate can induce water intoxication and hyponatremia.

Treatment

Mild cases of diabetes insipidus require no treatment other than adequate fluid intake. Reduction of aggravating factors (eg, corticosteroids) will improve polyuria.

Desmopressin acetate is the treatment of choice for central diabetes insipidus and for vasopressinase-induced diabetes insipidus associated with pregnancy or the puerperium. Desmopressin acetate (100 mcg/mL solution) is given intranasally every 12–24 hours as needed for thirst and polyuria. It may be administered via metered-dose nasal inhaler containing 0.1 mL (10 mcg/spray) or via a calibrated rhinal tube. The starting dose is one metered-dose spray or 0.05–0.1 mL every 12–24 hours, and the dose is then individualized according to response. Desmopressin nasal may cause rhinitis or conjunctivitis. If the generic preparation is ineffective, switching to the desmopressin brand may provide relief.

Oral desmopressin is initiated at 0.05 mg twice daily and increased to a maximum of 0.4 mg every 8 hours, if required. Oral desmopressin is particularly useful for patients in whom rhinitis or conjunctivitis develops from the nasal preparation. GI symptoms, asthenia, and mild increases in hepatic enzymes can occur with the oral preparation. Sublingual desmopressin, 60, 120, or 250 mcg, is not available in the United States; hyponatremia has been reported with this formulation.

Desmopressin can be given intravenously, intramuscularly, or subcutaneously in doses of 1–4 mcg every 12–24 hours as needed.

Desmopressin may cause hyponatremia, but this is uncommon if minimum effective doses are used and the patient allows thirst to occur every 1–2 days. Desmopressin can sometimes cause agitation, emotional changes, and depression with an increased risk of suicide. Patients should be monitored by family, friends, and medical staff when desmopressin therapy is started.

Prognosis

Central diabetes insipidus after pituitary surgery or head trauma usually remits after days to weeks but may be permanent if the hypothalamus or upper pituitary stalk is damaged.

Chronic central diabetes insipidus is ordinarily more an inconvenience than a dire medical condition. Hypernatremia can occur, especially when the hypothalamic thirst center is damaged, but diabetes insipidus does not otherwise reduce life expectancy, and the prognosis is that of the underlying disorder. Treatment with desmopressin allows normal sleep and activity.

Christ-Crain M et al. Copeptin in the differential diagnosis of hypotonic polyuria. J Endocrinol Invest. 2020;43:21. [PMID: 31368050]

Devuyst F et al. Central diabetes insipidus and pituitary stalk thickening in adults: distinction of neoplastic from non-neoplastic lesions. Eur J Endocrinol 2020;181:95. [PMID: 32530258]

Gubbi S et al. Diagnostic testing for diabetes insipidus. Endotext [Internet]. 2019. [PMID: 30779536]

Refardt J et al. Diabetes insipidus: an update. Endocrinol Metab Clin North Am. 2020;49:517. [PMID: 32741486]

ACROMEGALY & GIGANTISM

ESSENTIALS OF DIAGNOSIS

- Pituitary neuroendocrine tumor with over secretion of GH.
- **Gigantism:** begins before puberty before closure of epiphyses.
- **Acromegaly:** occurs after puberty with excessive growth of hands, feet, jaw, internal organs.
- Amenorrhea, hypertension, headaches, visual field loss, weakness.
- Soft, doughy, sweaty handshake.
- Elevated serum IGF-1.

General Considerations

GH exerts much of its growth-promoting effects by stimulating the release of IGF-1 from the liver and other tissues.

Acromegaly is a rare condition, with a yearly incidence of about 10 cases per million. It is nearly always caused by a pituitary adenoma. About 70% are macroadenomas (1 cm or larger) when diagnosed. These tumors may be locally invasive, particularly into the cavernous sinus. Less than 1% are malignant. Acromegaly is usually sporadic but may rarely be familial, with less than 3% being due to multiple endocrine neoplasia (MEN) types 1 or 4. Acromegaly may also be seen rarely in McCune-Albright syndrome and Carney complex. Acromegaly is rarely caused by ectopic secretion of growth hormone–releasing hormone or GH secreted by a neuroendocrine tumor or lymphoma.

Clinical Findings

A. Symptoms and Signs

Excessive GH causes tall stature and gigantism if it occurs in youth, before closure of epiphyses. Afterward, acromegaly develops. The manifestations of acromegaly usually present insidiously; median time to diagnosis after symptom onset is 10 years. The hands enlarge and a doughy, moist handshake is characteristic. The fingers widen, causing patients to enlarge their rings. Carpal tunnel syndrome is common. The feet also grow, particularly in shoe width. Facial features coarsen since the bones and sinuses of the skull enlarge; hat size increases. The mandible becomes more prominent, causing prognathism and malocclusion. Tooth spacing widens. Older photographs of the patient can be a useful comparison.

Macroglossia occurs, as does hypertrophy of pharyngeal and laryngeal tissue; this causes a deep, coarse voice and sometimes makes intubation difficult. Snoring and obstructive sleep apnea are common. A goiter may be noted. Hypertension (50%) and cardiomegaly are common. At diagnosis, about 10% of acromegalic patients have a dilated LV and heart failure with reduced EF. Weight gain is typical, particularly of muscle and bone. Insulin resistance is usually present and frequently causes diabetes mellitus (30%). Polyarticular arthralgias and degenerative arthritis are present in about 70% of patients. Overgrowth of vertebral bone can cause spinal stenosis. Colon polyps are found in about 30%, especially in patients with skin papillomas. The skin may also manifest hyperhidrosis, thickening, cystic acne, skin tags, and acanthosis nigricans.

GH-secreting pituitary tumors usually cause some hypogonadism, either by cosecretion of PRL or by direct pressure upon normal pituitary tissue. Decreased libido and erectile dysfunction are common in men and irregular menses or amenorrhea occur in women. Women who become pregnant have an increased risk of gestational diabetes and hypertension. Secondary hypothyroidism sometimes occurs; hypoadrenalism is unusual. Headaches are frequent. Temporal hemianopia may occur as a result of the optic chiasm being impinged by suprasellar extension of the tumor.

B. Laboratory Findings

For screening purposes, a random serum IGF-1 can be obtained. If it is normal for age, acromegaly is ruled out.

For further evaluation, the patient should be fasting for at least 8 hours (except for water), not be acutely ill, and not have exercised on the day of testing. Assay for the following: serum GH, IGF-1 (increased and usually over five times normal in acromegaly), PRL (cosecreted by many GH-secreting tumors), glucose (diabetes mellitus is common in acromegaly), liver enzymes and serum creatinine or urea nitrogen (liver failure or kidney disease can misleadingly elevate GH), serum calcium (to exclude hyperparathyroidism), serum inorganic phosphorus (frequently elevated), serum free T_4, and TSH (secondary hypothyroidism is common in acromegaly; primary hypothyroidism may increase PRL). Acromegaly is excluded if any serum GH is less than 1 mcg/L; however, many normal individuals can have a serum GH above this level. Therefore, the glucose suppression test is usually performed. Glucose syrup (100 g) is administered orally, and serum GH is measured 60 minutes afterward; acromegaly is excluded if the serum GH is suppressed to below 0.4 mcg/L with an ultrasensitive GH assay. The serum IGF-1 and glucose-suppressed GH are usually complementary tests; however, disparities between the two occur in up to 30% of patients.

C. Imaging

MRI shows a pituitary tumor in over 90% of acromegalic patients. MRI is generally superior to CT scanning, especially in the postoperative setting. Radiographs may show an enlarged sella and thickened skull and tufting of the terminal phalanges of the fingers and toes.

Differential Diagnosis

Active acromegaly must be distinguished from familial coarse features, large hands and feet, and isolated prognathism and from inactive ("burned-out") acromegaly in which there has been a spontaneous remission due to infarction of the pituitary adenoma. GH-induced gigantism must be differentiated from familial tall stature and from aromatase deficiency.

Misleadingly high serum GH levels can be caused by exercise or eating just prior to the test; acute illness or agitation; liver failure or kidney disease; malnourishment; diabetes mellitus; or concurrent treatment with oral estrogens, beta-blockers, or clonidine. Acromegaly can be difficult to diagnose during pregnancy, since the placenta produces GH and commercial GH assays may not be able to distinguish between pituitary and placental GH. During normal adolescence, serum IGF-1 is usually elevated and GH may fail to be suppressed.

Complications

Complications include hypopituitarism, hypertension, hyperglycemia, cardiac enlargement, heart failure, and colon polyps. Arthritis of hips, knees, and spine can be troublesome as can carpal tunnel syndrome. Cord compression may occur. Visual field defects may be severe and progressive. Acute loss of vision or cranial nerve palsy may occur if the tumor undergoes spontaneous hemorrhage and necrosis (pituitary apoplexy).

Treatment

A. Pituitary Microsurgery

Transsphenoidal pituitary surgery achieves a remission in about 70% of patients followed over 3 years. With tumors smaller than 2 cm and GH levels below 50 ng/mL, transsphenoidal pituitary surgery is successful in 80% of patients. Extrasellar extension of the pituitary tumor, particularly cavernous sinus invasion, reduces the likelihood of surgical cure. Transsphenoidal surgery is usually well tolerated, but complications occur in about 12% of patients, including infection, cerebrospinal fluid (CSF) leak, and hypopituitarism.

B. Medications

Acromegalic patients with an incomplete biochemical remission after pituitary surgery may benefit from medical therapy with dopamine agonists, somatostatin analogs, tamoxifen, or pegvisomant.

Cabergoline is the oral dopamine agonist of choice. It is most successful for tumors that secrete both PRL and GH but can also be effective for patients with normal serum PRL levels. Cabergoline may be tried as monotherapy for patients with serum IGF-1 levels above normal but less than 2.5 times the upper limit of normal. Cabergoline will shrink one-third of acromegaly-associated pituitary tumors by more than 50%. It appears to be safe during pregnancy. The initial dose is 0.25 mg orally twice weekly, which is gradually increased to a maximum dosage of 1 mg three times weekly (based on serum GH and IGF-1 levels).

Octreotide LAR and **lanreotide** are long-acting somatostatin analogs that are given monthly by subcutaneous injection. They can achieve serum GH levels below 2 ng/mL in 79% of patients and normal serum IGF-1 levels in 53% of patients.

Raloxifene is a selective estrogen receptor modulator (SERM) that may be useful for persistent acromegaly in men and in women who are postmenopausal or who have had breast cancer.

Pegvisomant, a GH receptor antagonist, can be helpful for patients resistant to other treatments, especially when there is associated diabetes mellitus. It blocks hepatic IGF-1 production but does not shrink GH-secreting tumors. Pegvisomant therapy produces symptomatic relief and normalizes serum IGF-1 levels in 63% of patients.

C. Stereotactic Radiosurgery

Acromegalic patients who do not achieve a complete remission with transsphenoidal surgery or medical therapy may be treated with stereotactic radiosurgery: linear accelerator (eg, Cyberknife), gamma knife radiosurgery, and proton beam radiosurgery. Following any pituitary radiation therapy, patients are advised to take lifelong daily low-dose aspirin because of the increased risk of small-vessel stroke. Stereotactic radiosurgery to pituitary tumors causes anterior hypopituitarism in 35–60% of patients within 5 years, so patients must have regular monitoring of their pituitary function.

Prognosis

Acromegaly is usually chronic and progressive unless treated. Spontaneous remissions are rare but have been reported following clinical or subclinical apoplexy (hemorrhage) within the tumor. Patients with acromegaly experience increased mortality from cardiovascular disorders and progressive acromegalic symptoms. Those who are treated and have a random serum GH under 1.0 ng/mL or a glucose-suppressed serum GH under 0.4 ng/mL with normal age-adjusted serum IGF-1 levels have reduced morbidity and mortality.

Postoperatively, normal pituitary function is usually preserved. Soft tissue swelling regresses but bone enlargement is permanent. Hypertension frequently persists despite successful surgery. Adjuvant medical therapy is successful in treating patients who are not cured by pituitary surgery. Gamma knife or cyberknife radiosurgery reduces GH levels an average of 77%, with 20% of patients having a full remission after 12 months. Proton beam radiosurgery produces a remission in about 70% of patients by 2 years and 80% of patients by 5 years. Radiation therapy eventually produces some degree of hypopituitarism in most patients. Patients must receive lifelong follow-up, with regular monitoring of serum GH and IGF-1 levels. Serum GH levels over 5 ng/mL and rising IGF-1 levels usually indicate a recurrent tumor.

Fleseriu M et al. A Pituitary Society update to acromegaly management guidelines. Pituitary. 2021;24:1. [PMID: 33079318]

Giustina A et al. A consensus on the diagnosis and treatment of acromegaly comorbidities: an update. J Clin Endocrinol Metab. 2020;105:dgz096. [PMID: 31606735]

Melmed S et al. A consensus statement on acromegaly therapeutic outcomes. Nat Rev Endocrinol. 2018;14:552. [PMID: 30050156]

Tritos NA et al. All-cause mortality in patients with acromegaly treated with pegvisomant: an ACROSTUDY analysis. Eur J Endocrinol. 2020;182:285. [PMID: 31917681]

HYPERPROLACTINEMIA

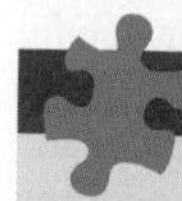

ESSENTIALS OF DIAGNOSIS

- Women: Oligomenorrhea, amenorrhea; galactorrhea; infertility.
- Men: Hypogonadism; decreased libido and erectile dysfunction; infertility.
- Elevated serum PRL.
- CT or MRI may show a pituitary adenoma.

General Considerations

Some causes of hyperprolactinemia are shown in Table 26–1. PRL-secreting pituitary tumors (prolactinomas) are the most common secretory pituitary tumor; they are usually sporadic but may rarely be familial as part of MEN type 1 or 4. Most are microadenomas (smaller than 1 cm), which are more common in women and typically do not grow even with pregnancy or oral contraceptives.

Table 26–1. Causes of hyperprolactinemia.

Physiologic Causes	Pharmacologic Causes	Pathologic Causes
Assay interference Exercise Familial (mutant prolactin receptor) Idiopathic Macroprolactin ("big prolactin") Nipple stimulation Neonatal Pregnancy Sleep (REM phase) Stress (trauma, surgery) Suckling	Amoxapine Amphetamines Anesthetic agents Antipsychotics (conventional and atypical) Androgens Butyrophenones Cimetidine (not famotidine or nizatidine) Cocaine use or withdrawal Domperidone Estrogens Hydroxyzine Licorice (real) Locaserin MAO inhibitors Methyldopa Metoclopramide Opioids Nicotine Phenothiazines Protease inhibitors Progestins Reserpine SSRIs Tricyclic antidepressants Verapamil	Acromegaly Chronic chest wall stimulation (thoracotomy, augmentation or reduction mammoplasty, mastectomy, herpes zoster, chest acupuncture, nipple rings, etc) Hypothalamic or pituitary stalk damage Hypothyroidism Liver disease Multiple sclerosis Optic neuromyelitis Prolactin-secreting tumors Pseudocyesis (false pregnancy) Kidney failure (especially with zinc deficiency) Spinal cord lesions SLE

REM, rapid eye movement.

Aggressive macroprolactinomas (larger than 1 cm) are more common in men and can spread into the cavernous sinuses and suprasellar areas; rarely, they may erode the floor of the sella to invade the paranasal sinuses. Hyperprolactinemia (without a pituitary adenoma) may also be familial.

Clinical Findings

A. Symptoms and Signs

Hyperprolactinemia may cause hypogonadotropic hypogonadism and reduced fertility. Men usually have diminished libido and erectile dysfunction that may not respond to testosterone replacement; gynecomastia sometimes occurs.

About 90% of premenopausal women with prolactinomas experience amenorrhea, oligomenorrhea, or infertility. Estrogen deficiency can cause decreased vaginal lubrication, irritability, anxiety, and depression. Galactorrhea (lactation in the absence of nursing) is common. During pregnancy, clinically significant enlargement of a microprolactinoma (smaller than 10 mm) occurs in less than 3%; clinically significant enlargement of a macroprolactinoma occurs in about 30%.

Pituitary prolactinomas may cosecrete GH and cause acromegaly. Large tumors may cause headaches, visual symptoms, and pituitary insufficiency.

Aside from pituitary tumors, some women secrete an abnormal form of PRL that appears to cause peripartum cardiomyopathy.

B. Laboratory Findings

An elevated serum prolactin level should be verified with a repeat determination, ideally in a different laboratory. Biotin supplements can cause falsely low serum PRL measurements; patients should not take a biotin supplement for at least 8 hours before the blood draw. Evaluate for conditions known to cause hyperprolactinemia, particularly pregnancy (serum hCG), hypothyroidism (serum FT_4 and TSH), kidney disease (BUN and serum creatinine), cirrhosis (liver tests), and hyperparathyroidism (serum calcium). Screen for acromegaly with a random serum IGF-1 level. Men are evaluated for hypogonadism with serum total and free testosterone, LH, and FSH. Women who have amenorrhea are assessed for hypogonadism with serum estradiol, LH, and FSH. Patients with macroprolactinomas or manifestations of possible hypopituitarism should be evaluated for hypopituitarism. Patients with hyperprolactinemia who are relatively asymptomatic and have no apparent cause for hyperprolactinemia should have an assay for macroprolactinemia, which is an increased circulating level of a high molecular weight PRL that is biologically inactive but is detected on assays.

C. Imaging

Patients with hyperprolactinemia not induced by drugs, hypothyroidism, or pregnancy should be examined by pituitary MRI. Small prolactinomas may be demonstrated, but clear differentiation from normal variants is not always possible. In the event that a woman with a macroprolactinoma becomes pregnant and elects not to take dopamine agonists during her pregnancy, MRI is usually not performed since the normal pituitary grows during pregnancy. However, if visual-field defects or other neurologic symptoms develop in a pregnant woman, a limited MRI study should be done, focusing on the pituitary without gadolinium contrast.

Differential Diagnosis

The differential diagnosis for galactorrhea includes the small amount of breast milk that can normally be expressed from the nipple in many parous women. Nipple stimulation from nipple rings, chest surgery, or acupuncture can cause galactorrhea; serum PRL levels may be normal or minimally elevated. Some women can have idiopathic galactorrhea with normal serum PRL levels. Normal breast milk may be various colors besides white. However, bloody galactorrhea requires evaluation for breast cancer.

About 40% of nonfunctional pituitary macroadenomas produce some degree of hyperprolactinemia. These and other lesions and malignancies can be misdiagnosed as prolactinomas. One distinguishing characteristic is that the serum PRL is usually only marginally elevated in the latter tumors, whereas with pituitary macroprolactinomas the serum PRL typically exceeds 100 mcg/L.

Pregnant women have high serum PRL levels, with physiological hyperplastic enlargement of the pituitary on MRI. Increased pituitary size is a normal variant in young women. Primary hypothyroidism can cause hyperprolactinemia and hyperplasia of the pituitary that can be mistaken for a pituitary adenoma. Macroprolactinemia occurs in 3.7% of the general population and accounts for 10–25% of all cases of hyperprolactinemia; pituitary MRI shows a nonpathological abnormality in 22% of such patients.

Treatment

Medications known to increase PRL should be stopped if possible (Table 26–1). Hyperprolactinemia due to hypothyroidism is corrected by levothyroxine.

Women with microprolactinomas who have amenorrhea or who desire contraception may safely take estrogen replacement or oral contraceptives; there is minimal risk of stimulating enlargement of the microadenoma. Patients with infertility and hyperprolactinemia may be treated with a dopamine agonist to improve fertility.

Pituitary macroprolactinomas have a higher risk of progressive growth, particularly during estrogen or testosterone HRT or during pregnancy. Therefore, patients with macroprolactinomas should not be treated with HRT or oral contraceptives unless they are in remission with dopamine agonist medication or surgery.

Pregnant women with macroprolactinomas should continue to receive treatment with dopamine agonists throughout the pregnancy to prevent tumor growth. If dopamine agonists are not used during pregnancy in a woman with a macroprolactinoma, visual field testing is required in each trimester. Measurement of PRL is not useful surveillance for tumor growth due to the fact that PRL increases greatly during normal pregnancy.

A. Dopamine Agonists

Dopamine agonists (cabergoline, bromocriptine, or quinagolide) are the initial treatment of choice for patients with giant prolactinomas and those with hyperprolactinemia desiring restoration of normal sexual function and fertility. Cabergoline is the most effective and usually best-tolerated ergot-derived dopamine agonist. Begin with 0.25 mg orally once weekly for 1 week, then 0.25 mg twice weekly for the next week, then 0.5 mg twice weekly. Further dosage increases may be required monthly, based on serum PRL levels, up to a maximum of 1.5 mg twice weekly. Bromocriptine (1.25–20 mg/day orally) is an alternative. Women who experience nausea with oral preparations may find relief with deep vaginal insertion of cabergoline or bromocriptine tablets; vaginal irritation sometimes occurs. Patients whose tumor is resistant to one dopamine agonist may be switched to another in an effort to induce a remission.

Dopamine agonists are given at bedtime to minimize side effects of fatigue, nausea, dizziness, and orthostatic hypotension, which occur in up to 50% of patients. These symptoms usually improve with dosage reduction and continued use. Dopamine agonists can cause a variety of psychiatric side effects (particularly depression, impulse control disorder, and hypersexuality) that are not dose related and may take weeks to resolve once the drug is discontinued. In doses used for prolactinomas, dopamine agonists have not caused cardiac valvulopathy.

Dopamine agonists do not increase the risk of miscarriage or teratogenicity. Pregnant women with microprolactinomas may safely stop treatment during pregnancy and breastfeeding. However, macroadenomas may enlarge significantly during pregnancy; if therapy is withdrawn, patients must be monitored with serum PRL determinations and computer-assisted visual fields. Women with macroprolactinomas who have responded to dopamine agonists may safely receive oral contraceptives as long as they continue receiving dopamine agonist therapy.

B. Surgical Treatment

Transsphenoidal pituitary surgery may be urgently required for large tumors undergoing apoplexy or those severely compromising visual fields. It is also used electively for patients who do not tolerate or respond to dopamine agonists. Transsphenoidal pituitary surgery is generally well tolerated, with a mortality rate of less than 0.5%. For pituitary microprolactinomas, skilled neurosurgeons are successful in normalizing PRL in 87% of patients and some patients prefer surgery to long-term therapy with dopamine agonists.

Complications, such as CSF leakage, meningitis, stroke, or visual loss, occur in about 3% of cases; sinusitis, nasal septal perforation, or infection complicates about 6.5% of transsphenoidal surgeries. Diabetes insipidus can occur within 2 days postoperatively but is usually mild and self-correcting. Hyponatremia can occur abruptly 4–13 days postoperatively in 21% of patients; symptoms may include nausea, vomiting, headache, malaise, or seizure. It is treated with free water and hypotonic fluid restriction.

C. Stereotactic Radiosurgery

Stereotactic radiosurgery is seldom required for prolactinomas since they usually respond to cabergoline or surgery. It is reserved for patients with macroadenomas that are growing despite treatment with dopamine agonists.

D. Chemotherapy

Some patients with aggressive pituitary macroadenomas or carcinomas are not surgical candidates and do not respond to dopamine agonists or radiation therapy. A small percentage of patients with aggressive tumors respond to the addition of temozolomide or everolimus to cabergoline. Treatment efficacy is determined by PRL measurement and MRI scanning.

Prognosis

Pituitary microprolactinomas are typically indolent, and only 15% grow after diagnosis. However, pituitary macroprolactinomas tend to be more aggressive. Prolactinomas generally respond well to dopamine agonist therapy. Ninety percent of patients with prolactinomas experience a fall in serum PRL to 10% or less of pretreatment levels and 80% achieve a normal serum PRL level. Shrinkage of a pituitary adenoma occurs early, but the maximum effect may take up to 1 year. Nearly half of prolactinomas—even massive tumors—shrink more than 50%. During pregnancy, growth of a pituitary prolactinoma occurs in 3% of women with a microprolactinoma and in 23% of those with a macroprolactinoma. If cabergoline is stopped after 2 years of therapy, hyperprolactinemia recurs in 68% of patients with idiopathic hyperprolactinemia, 79% with microprolactinomas, and 84% with macroprolactinomas.

The 10-year recurrence rate is 13% for pituitary microadenomas after transsphenoidal surgery; pituitary function can be preserved in over 95% of cases. However, the surgical success rate for macroprolactinomas is much lower, and the complication rates are higher.

De Sousa SMC et al. Impulse control disorders in dopamine agonist-treated hyperprolactinemia: prevalence and risk factors. J Clin Endocrinol Metab. 2020;105:dgz076. [PMID: 31580439]

Donoho DA et al. The role of surgery in the management of prolactinomas. Neurosurg Clin N Am. 2019;30:509. [PMID: 31471058]

Glezer A et al. Prolactinomas in pregnancy: considerations before conception and during pregnancy. Pituitary. 2020;23:65. [PMID: 31792668]

Hage C et al. Predictors of the response to dopaminergic therapy in patients with prolactinoma. J Clin Endocrinol Metab. 2020;105:dgaa652. [PMID: 32930718]

Lasolle H et al. Aggressive prolactinomas: how to manage? Pituitary. 2020;23:70. [PMID: 31617128]

NONFUNCTIONING PITUITARY ADENOMAS

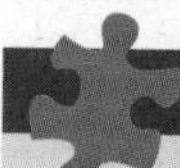

ESSENTIALS OF DIAGNOSIS

- Clinical and biochemical evaluation for pituitary hormone hypersecretion is negative.
- MRI shows a pituitary microadenoma (< 1 cm) or macroadenoma (≥ 1 cm).
- Headache, visual field compromise, and anterior hypopituitarism are common with macroadenomas.
- Elevated serum PRL with macroadenomas may be due to stalk compression.

General Considerations

Nonfunctioning pituitary adenomas are benign neuroendocrine neoplasms that do not produce symptoms from hormone oversecretion. Pituitary nonfunctioning adenomas occur more frequently in men than women and are more common with age. Nonfunctioning pituitary microadenomas (smaller than 1 cm) are common, detected as an incidental finding in 4–37% of brain CT or MR imaging.

Clinical Findings

A. Symptoms and Signs

Nonfunctioning pituitary macroadenomas (1 cm or larger) tend to be more aggressive than functioning pituitary adenomas. Those with nonfunctioning macroadenomas are much more likely to be symptomatic from mass effect with visual field compromise, headache, cranial nerve palsies affecting extraocular muscles, and pituitary apoplexy. Larger macroadenomas frequently cause some hypopituitarism, particularly hypogonadotropic hypogonadism. Nonfunctioning pituitary microadenomas are asymptomatic.

B. Laboratory Findings

1. Pituitary hormone hypersecretion—All patients with a pituitary adenoma require testing for pituitary hormone hypersecretion. Obtain a serum PRL to screen for prolactin hypersecretion; women with hyperprolactinemia are tested for pregnancy with a serum hCG. Testing for Cushing disease or acromegaly should be obtained, if clinically indicated.

2. Anterior hypopituitarism—Men should have following tests: serum free T_4, TSH, morning serum testosterone and free testosterone. Serum LH and FSH should be obtained in men with low serum testosterone, women who are postmenopausal, and younger women with amenorrhea. Serum sodium and glucose should also be obtained in all patients. A serum IGF-1 is drawn to screen for GH deficiency. Younger patients with short stature who have not fused their epiphyses should have a full evaluation for growth hormone deficiency.

3. Pituitary macroadenomas—Patients with a macroadenoma that impinges upon the optic chiasm require formal visual field testing. A cosyntropin stimulation test is performed for patients with hyponatremia or symptoms of possible hypoadrenalism.

C. Imaging

Pituitary dynamic contrast-enhanced MRI (3T) is the imaging modality of choice for the evaluation and follow-up of pituitary adenomas. Nonfunctioning pituitary microadenomas that are smaller than 0.5 cm require no further MRI follow-up. For nonfunctioning pituitary adenomas 0.5 cm or larger, repeat MRI is recommended at 6 months, then yearly for 3 years. If no enlargement is noted, MRI surveillance can then be done less frequently.

Differential Diagnosis

About 29% of pituitary adenomas that are initially diagnosed as incidental turn out to have another etiology; mass lesions that can mimic pituitary adenoma include pituitary craniopharyngiomas, gliomas, meningiomas, skull base osteosarcomas, Rathke cysts, lymphocytic hypophysitis, infection, or metastases. Large normal pituitary glands and physiologic pituitary enlargement during primary hypothyroidism or pregnancy should also be considered; serum prolactin levels are elevated in primary hypothyroidism and pregnancy. Hyperprolactinemia also occurs when there is pituitary stalk compression from pituitary macroadenomas and other mass lesions; with pituitary stalk compression, serum prolactin is typically lower than expected for the size of the pituitary mass.

Treatment

Patients with asymptomatic pituitary nonfunctioning microadenomas ordinarily require no treatment. Surgery is the preferred treatment option for patients whose adenoma is causing mass effect symptoms, premature development of puberty, hormonal deficiencies, or the emergence of symptomatic hormonal hypersecretion. Radiation therapy can be used for select individuals with pituitary macroadenomas.

Prognosis

The prognosis is excellent for patients with nonfunctioning microadenomas smaller than 0.5 cm. Patients with larger nonfunctioning microadenomas also have a very good prognosis but require follow-up. Transsphenoidal surgery is 65% successful in completely resecting pituitary macroadenomas, improves hypopituitarism in 50%, and reverses visual field compromise in 80% of patients. The 6-year postoperative recurrence rate has been reported to be 36% following surgery alone and 13% after surgery plus adjuvant radiation therapy.

Bryl M et al. The quality of life after transnasal microsurgical and endoscopic resection of nonfunctioning pituitary adenoma. Adv Clin Exp Med. 2020;29:921. [PMID: 32745380]

Gerges MM et al. Long-term outcomes after endoscopic endonasal surgery for nonfunctioning pituitary adenomas. J Neurosurg. 2020 Jan 31. [Epub ahead of print] [PMID: 32005016]

Tresoldi AS et al. Clinically nonfunctioning pituitary incidentalomas: characteristics and natural history. Neuroendocrinology. 2020;110:595. [PMID: 31525736]

DISEASES OF THE THYROID GLAND

THYROIDITIS

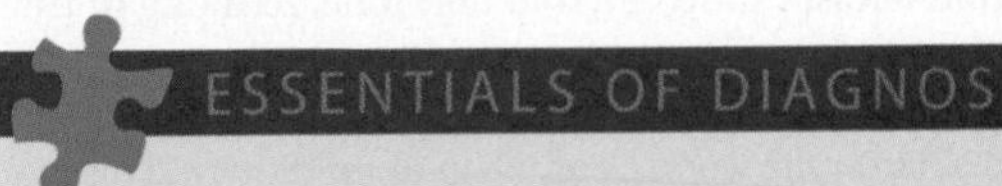

ESSENTIALS OF DIAGNOSIS

Autoimmune thyroiditis

- Chronic lymphocytic (Hashimoto) thyroiditis is the most common thyroiditis and often progresses to hypothyroidism.
- Postpartum thyroiditis and subacute lymphocytic thyroiditis (silent thyroiditis) can cause transient hyperthyroidism due to passive release of stored thyroid hormone.
- Thyroid peroxidase antibodies (TPO Ab) or thyroglobulin antibodies (Tg Ab) are usually high.

Painful subacute thyroiditis (de Quervain thyroiditis)

- Hallmark is tender thyroid gland with painful dysphagia.
- Elevated ESR.
- Viral etiology. Antithyroid antibodies are absent or low, distinguishing it from autoimmune thyroiditis.

Infectious (suppurative) thyroiditis

- Severe, painful thyroid gland.
- Febrile with leukocytosis and elevated ESR.

IgG_4-related thyroiditis (Riedel thyroiditis)

- Most often in middle age or older women.
- Usually part of a systemic fibrosing syndrome.

General Considerations

A. Autoimmune Thyroiditis

Several clinical entities are classified as autoimmune thyroiditis, including chronic lymphocytic thyroiditis, postpartum thyroiditis, and painless (silent) sporadic subacute thyroiditis. Dietary iodine supplementation (especially when excessive) and certain medications can cause autoimmune thyroiditis. The incidence of autoimmune thyroiditis varies by kindred, race, and sex. It is commonly familial. Elevated serum levels of antithyroid antibodies are detectable in the general population in 3% of men and 13% of women. Among United States adults studied, elevated levels of antithyroid antibodies are found in 14.3% of those who self-identify as White, 10.9% as Latinx, and 5.3% as Black. Subclinical thyroiditis is extremely common; autopsy series have found focal thyroiditis in about 40% of women and 20% of men.

1. Chronic lymphocytic thyroiditis—Also known as "Hashimoto thyroiditis," chronic lymphocytic thyroiditis is the most common thyroid disorder in the United States. It is chronic and cell-mediated; T-lymphocyte invasion gives the microscopic appearance of "lymphocytic thyroiditis." Humoral autoimmunity, with detectable serum antithyroid antibodies (TPO Ab or Tg Ab, or both), is present in most but not all affected patients.

2. Postpartum thyroiditis—Postpartum thyroiditis occurs soon after delivery in about 7% of women. The affected thyroid releases stored thyroid hormone, resulting in transient hyperthyroidism (often mild and undiagnosed) followed by hypothyroidism. The thyroid gland is not acutely tender, but some women complain of mild thyroid discomfort. Most women recover normal thyroid function. Women in whom postpartum thyroiditis develops have a 70% chance of recurrence after subsequent pregnancies. It occurs most commonly in women who have high levels of TPO Ab in the first trimester of pregnancy or immediately after delivery. It is also more common in women with preexistent type 1 diabetes mellitus, other autoimmunity, or a family history of autoimmune thyroiditis.

3. Painless (silent) sporadic subacute thyroiditis—This form of autoimmune thyroiditis is similar to postpartum thyroiditis, except that it is not related to pregnancy. Causes include amiodarone and immunotherapy. Hyperthyroidism results from the release of stored thyroid hormone. This accounts for about 1% of cases of thyrotoxicosis and is followed by hypothyroidism that may or may not resolve spontaneously.

4. Other causes—Dietary iodine supplementation (especially when excessive), and certain medications, including tyrosine kinase inhibitors, alemtuzumab, interferon-alpha, interleukin-2, thalidomide, lenalidomide, lithium, amiodarone, and immune checkpoint inhibitors are other causes of autoimmune thyroiditis. Chronic hepatitis C is associated with an increased risk of autoimmune thyroiditis, with 21% of affected patients having antithyroid antibodies and 13% having hypothyroidism.

Autoimmune thyroiditis often progresses to hypothyroidism, which may be linked to thyrotropin receptor–blocking antibodies, detected in 10% of patients with autoimmune thyroiditis. Hypothyroidism is more likely to develop in persons who smoke cigarettes. High serum levels of TPO Ab also predict progression from subclinical to symptomatic hypothyroidism. Although the hypothyroidism is usually permanent, up to 11% of patients experience a remission after several years. Hyperthyroidism can be caused by the destructive release of thyroid hormones (followed by hypothyroidism) or by increased synthesis of thyroid hormones (Graves disease).

Autoimmune thyroiditis is sometimes associated with other endocrine deficiencies as part of autoimmune polyendocrine syndrome type 2 (APS-II). Adults with APS-II are prone to autoimmune thyroiditis, type 1 diabetes mellitus, autoimmune gonadal failure, hypoparathyroidism, and adrenal insufficiency. Thyroiditis is frequently associated with other autoimmune conditions: pernicious anemia, Sjögren syndrome, vitiligo, IBD, celiac disease, and gluten sensitivity.

B. Painful Subacute Thyroiditis

Also called de Quervain thyroiditis, granulomatous thyroiditis, and giant cell thyroiditis, painful subacute thyroiditis is relatively common. Multinucleated giant cells are found on histology in the characteristically tender thyroid gland. Like painless subacute thyroiditis, most affected patients have transient hyperthyroidism, followed by hypothyroidism. Painful subacute thyroiditis is typically associated with viral upper respiratory infection (including COVID-19) and may follow vaccinations, including SARS-CoV-2. Some patients also have antithyroid antibodies. Its incidence peaks in the summer to early autumn. It affects both sexes, but young and middle-aged women are most commonly affected. Subacute thyroiditis can also be a sequelae of a drug-induced hypersensitivity syndrome.

C. Infectious (Suppurative) Thyroiditis

Infectious thyroiditis is rare among immunocompetent patients. It is usually bacterial but mycobacterial, fungal, and parasitic infections can occur, particularly in immunosuppressed individuals.

D. IgG_4-Related Thyroiditis

IgG_4-related thyroiditis, also called Riedel thyroiditis, invasive fibrous thyroiditis, Riedel struma, woody thyroiditis, ligneous thyroiditis, and invasive thyroiditis, is the rarest form of thyroiditis. It is found most frequently in middle-aged or older women and is usually part of a multifocal systemic fibrosis syndrome. It may occur as a thyroid manifestation of IgG_4-related systemic disease.

Clinical Findings

A. Symptoms and Signs

In **autoimmune thyroiditis,** the thyroid gland may be diffusely enlarged, firm, and finely nodular but is frequently not palpable. One thyroid lobe may be asymmetrically enlarged, raising concerns about neoplasm. Although patients may complain of neck tightness, pain and tenderness are not usually present. Other patients have no palpable goiter and no neck symptoms. The thyroid is fibrotic and atrophic in about 10% of cases, particularly in older women.

Symptoms and signs are mostly related to levels of thyroid hormone. Affected patients may have combinations of hyperthyroidism and hypothyroidism. For example, a patient with hypothyroidism might later develop hyperthyroidism that can wax and wane. Depression and chronic fatigue are more common, even after correction of hypothyroidism.

About one-third of patients have mild dry mouth (xerostomia) or dry eyes (keratoconjunctivitis sicca) related to Sjögren syndrome. Associated myasthenia gravis is usually of mild severity, mainly affecting the extraocular muscles and having a relatively low incidence of detectable AChR Ab or thymic disease. Associated celiac disease or gluten intolerance can produce fatigue or depression, sometimes in the absence of GI symptoms.

Postpartum thyroiditis is typically manifested by hyperthyroidism that begins 1–6 months after delivery and persists for only 1–2 months. Then, hypothyroidism tends to develop beginning 4–8 months after delivery.

In painless sporadic thyroiditis, thyrotoxic symptoms are usually mild; a small, nontender goiter may be palpated in about 50% of such patients. The course is similar to postpartum thyroiditis.

Painful subacute thyroiditis presents with an acute, usually painful enlargement of the thyroid gland, often with dysphagia. About 38% of patients have one thyroid lobe involved, while 62% have both lobes involved. Those with bilateral involvement are likely to be more hyperthyroid. The pain may radiate to the ears. Patients usually have a low-grade fever and fatigue. The manifestations may persist for weeks or months and may be associated with malaise. Thyrotoxicosis develops in 50% of affected patients and tends to last for several weeks. Subsequently, hypothyroidism develops that lasts 4–6 months. Normal thyroid function typically returns within 12 months, but persistent hypothyroidism develops in 5% of patients.

Infectious suppurative thyroiditis patients usually are febrile and have severe pain, tenderness, redness, and fluctuation in the region of the thyroid gland. In **IgG4-related thyroiditis,** thyroid enlargement is often asymmetric; the gland is stony hard and adherent to the neck structures, causing signs of compression and invasion, including dysphagia, dyspnea, pain, and hoarseness. Related conditions include retroperitoneal fibrosis, fibrosing mediastinitis, sclerosing cervicitis, subretinal fibrosis, and sclerosing cholangitis.

B. Laboratory Findings

In **autoimmune thyroiditis** (including postpartum thyroiditis), there are usually increased circulating levels of the antithyroid antibodies TPO Ab (90%) or Tg Ab (40%). However, 5% of patients have no detectable antithyroid antibodies. Most patients with thyroiditis caused by immune checkpoint inhibitors have no detectable antithyroid antibodies. Antithyroid antibodies decline during pregnancy and are often undetectable in the third trimester. Once autoimmune thyroiditis has been diagnosed, monitoring of antibody levels is not helpful. If autoimmune thyroiditis leads to inadequate thyroid hormone release, the serum TSH level is elevated and thyroid hormone levels may be normal or decreased (hypothyroidism). Autoimmune thyroiditis may also lead passive release of stored thyroid hormones, resulting in hyperthyroidism increased serum FT_4 levels that are proportionally higher than T_3 levels and suppressed TSH levels. Because T_4 is less active than T_3, the hyperthyroidism seen in autoimmune thyroiditis is usually less severe than with Graves disease.

Patients with autoimmune thyroiditis have a 15% incidence of having serum IgA tissue transglutaminase (tTG) antibody and at least 5% have clinically significant celiac disease.

In **painful subacute thyroiditis,** the ESR is markedly elevated while antithyroid antibody titers are low, distinguishing it from autoimmune thyroiditis. Subacute thyroiditis may result in passive release of stored thyroid hormones, resulting in hyperthyroidism. In **infectious thyroiditis,** both the leukocyte count and ESR are usually elevated.

C. Imaging

Ultrasound typically shows diffuse heterogeneous thyroid density and reduced echogenicity. Ultrasound is useful to distinguish autoimmune thyroiditis from multinodular goiter, thyroid nodules that are suspicious for malignancy, and Graves disease.

Radioiodine (RAI) uptake and scan can help distinguish thyroiditis from Graves disease; painful subacute thyroiditis exhibits a very low RAI uptake. However, RAI uptake may be normal or high with uneven uptake on the scan in chronic autoimmune thyroiditis (euthyroid or hypothyroid); CT or MRI is not useful in diagnosis.

[^{18}F] Fluorodeoxyglucose positron emission tomography (^{18}FDG-PET) scanning frequently shows diffuse thyroid uptake of isotope in cases of thyroiditis. In fact, of ^{18}FDG-PET scans done for any reason, about 3% show such uptake.

D. Fine-Needle Aspiration Cytology

Patients with autoimmune thyroiditis who have a thyroid nodule should have an ultrasound-guided FNA biopsy, since the risk of papillary thyroid cancer is about 8% in such nodules. When infectious (suppurative) thyroiditis is suspected, an FNA biopsy with Gram stain and culture is required. FNA biopsy is usually not required for painful subacute thyroiditis but shows characteristic giant multinucleated cells.

Complications

Autoimmune thyroiditis may lead to hypothyroidism. Hyperthyroidism may develop, either due to the emergence of Graves disease or due to the release of stored thyroid hormone, a condition variably termed "hashitoxicosis" or "painless sporadic thyroiditis." Euthyroid women with high serum TPO Ab may have an increased risk of miscarriage and preterm birth; unfortunately, treatment with levothyroxine fails to improve these risks. Perimenopausal women with high serum levels of TPO Ab have a higher relative risk of depression, independent of ambient thyroid hormone levels.

Subacute and chronic thyroiditis are complicated by the effects of pressure on the neck structures: dyspnea and, in Riedel struma, vocal cord palsy. Papillary thyroid carcinoma or thyroid lymphoma may rarely be associated with chronic thyroiditis and must be considered in the diagnosis of uneven painless enlargements that continue despite treatment; such patients require FNA biopsy. In the suppurative forms of thyroiditis, any complication of infection may occur.

Differential Diagnosis

All types of goiters must be considered in the differential diagnosis of thyroiditis, especially if enlargement is rapid.

Unlike in goiters, in subacute thyroiditis there is very low RAI uptake and the T_4 and T_3 are elevated. Thyroid autoantibody tests have been helpful in the diagnosis of autoimmune thyroiditis, but the tests are not specific (positive in patients with multinodular goiters, malignancy [eg, thyroid carcinoma, lymphoma], and concurrent Graves disease). The subacute and suppurative forms of thyroiditis may resemble any infectious process in or near the neck structures. Chronic thyroiditis may resemble thyroid carcinoma, especially if the enlargement is uneven and if there is pressure on surrounding structures; both disorders may be present in the same gland.

Treatment

A. Hashimoto Autoimmune Thyroiditis

If hypothyroidism is present, levothyroxine should be given in usual replacement doses (0.05–0.2 mg orally daily) (see Hypothyroidism & Myxedema, below). If hyperthyroidism is present, see Hyperthyroidism (Thyrotoxicosis), below.

In patients with a large goiter and normal or elevated serum TSH, an attempt is made to shrink the goiter with levothyroxine in doses sufficient to drive the serum TSH below the reference range while maintaining clinical euthyroidism. Suppressive doses of T_4 tend to shrink the goiter an average of 30% over 6 months. If the goiter does not regress, lower replacement doses of levothyroxine may be given. If the thyroid gland is only minimally enlarged and the patient is euthyroid, regular observation is indicated, since hypothyroidism may develop, often years later.

Dietary supplementation with selenium 200 mcg/day reduces serum levels of TPO Ab. In pregnant women with autoimmune thyroiditis, selenium supplementation at 83 mcg orally daily reduced the usual rebound postpartum increase in antithyroid antibodies without side effects on mother or newborn, but the clinical impact is not known.

B. Painful Subacute Thyroiditis

All treatment is empiric and must be continued for several weeks. Recurrence is common. The drug of choice is aspirin (325–650 mg orally every 4–6 hours, which relieves pain and inflammation) or NSAIDs. For patients with severe pain, prednisone, 20 mg orally daily for about 2 weeks, can be effective. Thyrotoxic symptoms are treated with propranolol, 10–40 mg orally every 6 hours, or propranolol ER, 60–160 mg orally daily. Iodinated contrast agents cause a prompt fall in serum T_3 levels and a dramatic improvement in thyrotoxic symptoms. Ipodate sodium (Bilivist, Oragrafin) or iopanoic acid (Telepaque) is given orally in doses of 500 mg orally daily until serum FT_4 levels return to normal. Transient hypothyroidism is treated with T_4 (0.05–0.1 mg orally daily) if symptomatic.

C. Infectious (Suppurative) Thyroiditis

Treatment is with antibiotics and with surgical drainage when fluctuation is marked. Immunocompromised individuals are particularly at risk. Surgical thyroidectomy may be required.

D. IgG_4-Related Thyroiditis

The treatment of choice is tamoxifen, 20 mg orally twice daily, which must be continued for years. Tamoxifen can induce partial to complete remissions in most patients within 3–6 months. Its mode of action appears to be unrelated to its antiestrogen activity. Short-term corticosteroid treatment may be added for partial alleviation of pain and compression symptoms. Surgical decompression usually fails to permanently alleviate compression symptoms; such surgery is difficult due to dense fibrous adhesions, making surgical complications more likely. Rituximab may be useful for Riedel thyroiditis that is refractory to tamoxifen and corticosteroids.

Prognosis

Patients with Hashimoto autoimmune thyroiditis generally have an excellent prognosis, since the condition either remains stable for years or progresses slowly to hypothyroidism, which is easily treated. Hashimoto autoimmune thyroiditis is occasionally associated with other autoimmune disorders (celiac disease, diabetes mellitus, Addison disease, pernicious anemia, etc). Although 80% of women with postpartum thyroiditis subsequently recover normal thyroid function, permanent hypothyroidism eventually develops in about 50% within 7 years, more commonly in women who are multiparous or who have had a spontaneous abortion. In subacute painful thyroiditis, spontaneous remissions and exacerbations are common; the disease process may smolder for months. Papillary thyroid carcinoma carries a relatively good prognosis when it occurs in patients with autoimmune thyroiditis.

Grani G et al. Contemporary thyroid nodule evaluation and management. J Clin Endocrinol Metab. 2020;105:2869. [PMID: 32491169]

Moleti M et al. Postpartum thyroiditis in women with euthyroid and hypothyroid Hashimoto's thyroiditis antedating pregnancy. J Clin Endocrinol Metab. 2020;105:105. [PMID: 32301483]

Muir CA et al. Thyroid toxicity following immune checkpoint inhibitor treatment in advanced cancer. Thyroid. 2020;30:1458. [PMID: 32264785]

Ralli M et al. Hashimoto's thyroiditis: an update on pathogenic mechanisms, diagnostic protocols, therapeutic strategies, and potential malignant transformation. Autoimmun Rev. 2020;19:102469. [PMID: 32805423]

Zala A et al. Riedel thyroiditis J Clin Endocrinol Metab. 2020;105:dgaa468. [PMID: 32687163]

HYPOTHYROIDISM & MYXEDEMA

ESSENTIALS OF DIAGNOSIS

- Hashimoto autoimmune thyroiditis is the most common cause of hypothyroidism.
- Fatigue, cold intolerance, constipation, weight change, depression, menorrhagia, hoarseness.
- Dry skin, bradycardia, delayed return of deep tendon reflexes.

- FT_4 is usually low.
- TSH elevated in primary hypothyroidism.

General Considerations

Hypothyroidism is common, affecting over 1% of the general population and 5% of individuals over age 60 years. About 85% of affected individuals are women. Thyroid hormone deficiency affects almost all body functions. The degree of severity ranges from mild and unrecognized hypothyroid states to striking myxedema. Maternal hypothyroidism during pregnancy results in offspring with IQ scores that are an average 7 points lower than those of euthyroid mothers. Congenital hypothyroidism occurs in about 1:4000 births; untreated, it causes cretinism with permanent cognitive impairment.

Autoimmune thyroiditis is the most common cause of hypothyroidism. Hypothyroidism also may be due to failure or resection of the thyroid gland itself (primary hypothyroidism) or deficiency of pituitary TSH (secondary hypothyroidism). A hypothyroid phase also occurs in subacute (de Quervain) viral thyroiditis following initial hyperthyroidism.

Goiter (thyroid enlargement) may be present with thyroiditis, iodide deficiency, genetic thyroid enzyme defects, food goitrogens in iodide-deficient areas (eg, turnips, cassavas), or, rarely, peripheral resistance to thyroid hormone or infiltrating diseases (eg, cancer, sarcoidosis). Goitrogenic medications include iodide, propylthiouracil (PTU) or methimazole, sulfonamides, amiodarone, interferon-alpha, interferon-beta, interleukin-2, and lithium. About 50% of patients taking lithium long term have an ultrasound-detectable goiter. Goiter is often absent in patients with autoimmune thyroiditis. Goiter is also usually absent when hypothyroidism is due to destruction of the gland by head-neck or chest-shoulder radiation therapy or ^{131}I therapy. Total thyroidectomy causes hypothyroidism; after hemithyroidectomy, hypothyroidism develops in 22% of patients.

Amiodarone, because of its high iodine content, causes clinically significant hypothyroidism in 15–20% of patients as well as thyrotoxicosis (see Amiodarone-induced thyrotoxicosis, below). Hypothyroidism occurs most often in patients with preexisting autoimmune thyroiditis. The T_4 level is low or low-normal, and the TSH is elevated, usually over 20 mIU/L. Another 17% of patients taking amiodarone are asymptomatic with normal serum T_4 levels despite elevations in serum TSH; they can be closely monitored without levothyroxine therapy. Hypothyroidism may also develop in patients with a high iodine intake from other sources, especially if they have underlying lymphocytic thyroiditis. Some malignancies overexpress thyroid hormone inactivating enzyme (type 3 deiodinase) and cause "consumptive hypothyroidism." This has occurred with large hemangiomas or a heavy tumor burden of colon cancer, basal cell cancer, fibrous tumors, or gastrointestinal stromal tumors (GISTs).

Chemotherapeutic agents that can cause silent thyroiditis include tyrosine kinase inhibitors, denileukin diftitox, alemtuzumab, interferon-alpha, interleukin-2, thalidomide, lenalidomide, and immune checkpoint inhibitors (pembrolizumab, ipilimumab, tremelimumab, and atezolizumab). Thyroiditis usually starts with hyperthyroidism (often unrecognized) and then progresses to hypothyroidism. RAI-based targeted radioisotope therapy can also cause hypothyroidism.

Clinical Findings

A. Symptoms and Signs

1. Common manifestations—Mild hypothyroidism often escapes detection without a screening serum TSH. Patients typically have nonspecific symptoms that include weight gain, fatigue, lethargy, depression, weakness, dyspnea on exertion, arthralgias or myalgias, muscle cramps, menorrhagia, constipation, dry skin, headache, paresthesias, cold intolerance, carpal tunnel syndrome, and Raynaud syndrome. Physical findings can include bradycardia; diastolic hypertension; thin, brittle nails; thinning of hair; peripheral edema; puffy face and eyelids; and skin pallor or yellowing (carotenemia). Delayed relaxation of deep tendon reflexes may be present. Patients often have a goiter that arises due to elevated serum TSH levels or the underlying thyroid pathology.

2. Less common manifestations—Less common symptoms of hypothyroidism include diminished appetite and weight loss, hoarseness, decreased sense of taste and smell, and diminished auditory acuity. Some patients with goiter may complain of dysphagia or neck discomfort. Although most menstruating women have menorrhagia, some women have scant menses or amenorrhea. Physical findings may include loss of eyelash and eyebrow hairs; thickening of the tongue; hard pitting edema; and effusions into the pleural and peritoneal cavities as well as into joints. Galactorrhea may also be present. Cardiac enlargement ("myxedema heart") and pericardial effusions may develop. Psychosis "myxedema madness" can occur from severe hypothyroidism or from toxicity of other drugs whose metabolism is slowed in hypothyroidism. Hypothermia and stupor or "myxedema coma," which is often associated with infection (especially pneumonia), may develop in patients with severe hypothyroidism.

Some hypothyroid patients with autoimmune thyroiditis have symptoms that are not due to hypothyroidism but rather to conditions associated with autoimmune thyroiditis; these include Addison disease, hypoparathyroidism, diabetes mellitus, pernicious anemia, Sjögren syndrome, vitiligo, biliary cirrhosis, gluten sensitivity, and celiac disease.

B. Laboratory Findings

The single best screening test for hypothyroidism is the serum TSH (Table 26–2). In primary hypothyroidism, the serum TSH is increased in a reflex effort to stimulate the failing gland, while the serum FT_4 is low or low-normal. The normal reference range for ultrasensitive TSH levels is generally 0.4–4.0 mIU/L. The normal range of TSH varies with age; for example, the reference range for both children

Table 26–2. Appropriate use of thyroid tests.

	Test	Comment
For screening	Serum TSH	Most sensitive test for primary hypo- and hyperthyroidism
	Free thyroxine (FT_4)	Excellent test
For hypothyroidism	Serum TSH	High in primary and low in secondary hypothyroidism
	Thyroid peroxidase and thyroglobulin antibodies	Elevated in autoimmune (Hashimoto) thyroiditis
For hyperthyroidism	Serum TSH	Suppressed except in TSH-secreting pituitary tumor or pituitary hyperplasia (rare)
	Triiodothyronine (T_3) or free triiodothyronine (FT_3)	Elevated
	^{123}I uptake and scan	Increased uptake; diffuse versus "hot" foci on scan
	Thyroid peroxidase and thyroglobulin antibodies	Elevated in Graves disease
	Thyroid-stimulating immunoglobulin (TSI)	Usually (65%) positive in Graves disease
For thyroid nodules	Fine-needle aspiration (FNA) biopsy	Best diagnostic method for thyroid cancer
	^{123}I uptake and scan	Cancer is usually "cold"; less reliable than FNA biopsy
	^{99m}Tc scan	Vascular versus less vascular
	Ultrasonography	Useful to assist FNA biopsy. Useful in assessing the risk of malignancy (multinodular goiter or pure cysts are less likely to be malignant). Useful to monitor nodules and patients after thyroid surgery for carcinoma.

and elderly patients is higher than the reference range for younger patients.

Other laboratory abnormalities can include hypoglycemia or anemia (with normal or increased mean corpuscular volume). Hyponatremia due to the syndrome of inappropriate ADH secretion (SIADH) or decreased GFR is common. Additional frequent findings include increased serum levels of LDL cholesterol, triglycerides, lipoprotein (a), liver enzymes, creatine kinase, or PRL. In patients with autoimmune thyroiditis, titers of antibodies against thyroperoxidase and thyroglobulin are high; serum antinuclear antibodies may be present but are not usually indicative of lupus.

Subclinical hypothyroidism is defined as the state of having a normal serum FT_4 with a serum TSH that is above the reference range. It occurs most often in persons aged 65 years or older, in whom the prevalence is 13%. Subclinical hypothyroidism is often transient, and serum TSH levels normalize spontaneously in about 60% of cases within 5 years. The likelihood of TSH normalization is higher in patients without antithyroid antibodies and those with a marginally elevated serum TSH. The term "subclinical" is somewhat misleading, since it refers to the serum hormone levels and not the patient's symptoms.

C. Imaging

Radiologic imaging is usually not necessary for patients with hypothyroidism. On CT or MRI, a goiter may be noted in the neck or in the mediastinum (retrosternal goiter). An enlarged thymus is frequently seen in cases of autoimmune thyroiditis. On MRI, the pituitary is often quite enlarged in primary hypothyroidism, due to hyperplasia of TSH-secreting cells.

Differential Diagnosis

The differential diagnosis for subclinical hypothyroidism includes antibody interference with the serum TSH assay, macro-TSH, sleep deprivation, exercise, recovery from nonthyroidal illness, acute psychiatric emergencies, and other conditions and medications that can cause a low serum T_4 or high serum TSH in the absence of hypothyroidism (Table 26–3).

Euthyroid sick syndrome should be considered in patients without known thyroid disease who are found to have a low serum FT_4 with a serum TSH that is not elevated. This syndrome can be seen in patients with severe illness, caloric deprivation, or major surgery. Treatment with levothyroxine is not indicated for patients with euthyroid sick syndrome.

Serum TSH tends to be suppressed in severe nonthyroidal illness, making the diagnosis of concurrent primary hypothyroidism difficult, although the presence of a goiter suggests the diagnosis. The clinician must decide whether such severely ill patients (with a low serum T_4 and low TSH) might have hypothyroidism due to hypopituitarism. Patients without symptoms of prior brain lesion or hypopituitarism are very unlikely to suddenly develop hypopituitarism during an unrelated illness. Patients with diabetes insipidus, hypopituitarism, or other signs of a CNS lesion may be given T_4 empirically.

Patients receiving prolonged dopamine infusions can develop true secondary hypothyroidism caused by dopamine's direct suppression of TSH-secreting cells. Bexarotine and mitotane also cause secondary hypothyroidism in most patients.

Complications

Patients with severe hypothyroidism have an increased susceptibility to bacterial pneumonia. Megacolon has been described in long-standing hypothyroidism. Organic psychoses with paranoid delusions may occur ("myxedema madness"). Rarely, adrenal crisis may be precipitated by thyroid therapy. Rhabdomyolysis may occur and cause kidney dysfunction. Hypothyroidism is a rare cause of

Table 26–3. Factors that may cause aberrations in laboratory tests that may be mistaken for primary hypothyroidism.[1]

Low Serum T_4 or T_3	High Serum TSH

Acute psychiatric illness
Cirrhosis
Familial thyroid-binding globulin deficiency
Laboratory error
Nephrotic syndrome
Severe illness
Drugs
  Androgens
  Antiseizure drugs
    Carbamazepine
    Phenobarbitol
    Phenytoin
  Asparaginase
  Carbamazepine (T_4)
  Chloral hydrate
  Corticosteroids
  Diclofenac (T_3), naproxen (T_3)
  Didanosine
  Fenclofenac
  5-Fluorouracil
  Halofenate
  Imatinib
  Mitotane
  Nicotinic acid
  Oxcarbazepine
  Phenobarbital
  Phenytoin
  Salicylates in large doses (T_3 and T_4)
  Sertraline
  Stavudine
  T_3 therapy (T_4)
	Acute psychiatric illness (transient) (14%)
	Amiodarone
	Anti-mouse antibodies
	Antithyrotropin antibodies
	Anti-TSH receptor antibodies
	Autoimmune disease (assay interference)
	Drugs
	  Amphetamines
	  Atypical antipsychotics
	  Dopamine agonists
	  Heroin
	  Phenothiazines
	Exercise before testing
	Following prolonged primary hypothyroidism
	Heterophile antibodies
	Laboratory error
	Macro-thyrotropin
	Nonadherence to thyroid replacement therapy
	Older adults (especially women)
	Pituitary TSH hypersecretion
	Recovery from acute nonthyroidal illness (transient)
	Strenuous exercise (acute)
	Sleep deprivation (acute)
	TSH resistance

[1]True primary hypothyroidism may coexist.
T_4, levothyroxine; T_3, triiodothyronine.

infertility, which may respond to thyroid replacement. Untreated hypothyroidism during pregnancy often results in miscarriage. Preexistent CAD and heart failure may be exacerbated by levothyroxine therapy.

Myxedema crisis refers to severe, life-threatening manifestations of hypothyroidism. Myxedema crisis particularly affects elderly women and can occur spontaneously in severely hypothyroid patients with prolonged exposure to the cold, with resultant hypothermia. It can also be induced by a stroke, heart failure, infection (particularly pneumonia), or trauma. Metabolism of drugs is slowed in hypothyroidism, and myxedema crisis is often precipitated by the administration of sedatives, antidepressants, hypnotics, anesthetics, or opioids. The drugs further impair cognition and respiratory drive and can precipitate respiratory arrest. Affected patients have impaired cognition, ranging from confusion to somnolence to coma (myxedema coma). Convulsions and abnormal CNS signs may occur. Patients have profound hypothermia, hypoventilation, hyponatremia, hypoglycemia, hypoxemia, hypercapnia, and hypotension. Rhabdomyolysis and AKI may occur. The mortality rate is high.

Treatment

Before beginning therapy with thyroid hormone, the hypothyroid patient requires at least a clinical assessment for adrenal insufficiency and angina. The presence of either condition requires further evaluation and management.

Levothyroxine therapy is given to women attempting pregnancy, young adult patients aged 30 years or younger, patients with serum TSH levels 20 mIU/L or higher, and those with significant symptoms attributable to hypothyroidism. Other patients with subclinical hypothyroidism do not require levothyroxine therapy but must be monitored regularly for the emergence of symptoms.

A. Initial Treatment of Hypothyroidism

Synthetic levothyroxine is the preferred preparation for treating hypothyroidism. Intestinal absorption can vary by up to 15% with different oral levothyroxine preparations, so ideally, the patient should receive a consistent manufacturer's preparation. Lyophilized preparations of levothyroxine are available for reconstitution and intravenous administration, when indicated.

Otherwise healthy young and middle-aged adults with hypothyroidism may be treated initially with levothyroxine in average doses of about 1.6 mcg/kg/day. Lower doses can be used for very mild hypothyroidism, while full doses are given for more symptomatic hypothyroidism. The initial hormonal goal of levothyroxine replacement therapy should be to normalize serum TSH levels. Bedtime levothyroxine administration results in somewhat higher serum T_4 and lower TSH levels than morning administration. Therefore, the administration timing for levothyroxine should be kept constant. After beginning daily administration, significant increases in serum T_4 levels are seen within 1–2 weeks, and near-peak levels are seen within 3–4 weeks.

Pregnant women with overt hypothyroidism or myxedema should be treated immediately with levothyroxine at full replacement doses (see Thyroiditis, Chapter 19).

Patients with stable CAD or those who are over age 60 years are treated with smaller initial doses of levothyroxine, 25–50 mcg orally daily; higher initial doses may be used if such patients are severely hypothyroid. The dose can be increased by 25 mcg every 1–3 weeks until the patient is euthyroid. Ideally, patients with hypothyroidism and unstable CAD or uncontrolled atrial fibrillation should begin levothyroxine replacement following medical or interventional therapy.

Myxedema crisis requires larger initial doses of levothyroxine intravenously, since myxedema itself can interfere with intestinal absorption of oral levothyroxine. Levothyroxine sodium 500 mcg is given intravenously as a loading dose, followed by 50–100 mcg intravenously daily; the lower dose is given to patients with suspected CAD. In patients with severe myxedema crisis, liothyronine (T_3, Triostat) can be given intravenously with a loading bolus of 10–20 mcg, followed by 10 mcg intravenous boluses every 8–12 hours for the first 48 hours. The hypothermic patient is warmed only with blankets since faster warming can precipitate cardiovascular collapse. Hypoglycemic patients are given 5% dextrose intravenously.

Hyponatremia in any hypothyroid patient requires evaluation for adrenal insufficiency. Medications and hypotonic intravenous solutions that can cause or aggravate hyponatremia are discontinued. Patients who are mildly symptomatic with a serum sodium 120–129 mEq/mL are treated with fluid restriction, unless they are dehydrated. Symptomatic patients with a serum sodium 120–129 mEq/mL must be managed as an inpatient and are administered 0.9% NaCl intravenously at 125 mL/hour to correct hypovolemia. Hypothyroid patients with a serum sodium below 120 mEq/mL are treated with boluses of 100 mL of 3% NaCl intravenously with intravenous furosemide 20–40 mg to promote water diuresis; serum sodium levels must be monitored closely and boluses of 3% NaCl can be repeated about every 6 hours until the serum sodium rises to 120 mmol/L or higher. When giving intravenous saline to myxedematous patients, care must be taken to avoid fluid overload.

Patients with hypercapnia require mechanical assistance with ventilation. Opioid medications must be stopped or used in very low doses. Infections must be detected and treated aggressively. Patients in whom concomitant adrenal insufficiency is suspected are treated with hydrocortisone, 100 mg intravenously, followed by 25–50 mg every 6–8 hours.

B. Monitoring and Optimizing Treatment of Hypothyroidism

Regular clinical and laboratory monitoring is critical to determine the optimal levothyroxine dose for each patient. After initiating levothyroxine replacement, serum TSH, FT_4, and FT_3 levels are monitored monthly, and the dose is adjusted with an aim to normalize the serum TSH within 2 months of commencing thyroid replacement therapy. The patient should be prescribed sufficient levothyroxine to restore a clinically euthyroid state; this can usually be attained by maintaining the serum TSH, FT_4, and FT_3 within their reference ranges.

Pregnancy usually increases the levothyroxine dosage requirement; an increase in levothyroxine requirement has been noted as early as the fifth week of pregnancy (see Thyroid Disease, Chapter 19). Postpartum, levothyroxine replacement requirement ordinarily returns to prepregnancy level.

Decreased levothyroxine dose requirements occur in women after delivery, after bilateral oophorectomy or natural menopause, after cessation of oral estrogen replacement, or during therapy with GnRH agonists.

1. Elevated serum TSH level—For most patients, a high serum TSH indicates underreplacement with levothyroxine. However, patient nonadherence to prescribed levothyroxine is surprisingly common; before increasing the levothyroxine dosage, it is important to confirm patient compliance. For patients with CAD or recurrent atrial fibrillation, it may be prudent to administer lower doses of levothyroxine to keep serum TSH in the high-normal or even slightly elevated range.

Levothyroxine should be taken in the morning with water only. Increased levothyroxine dosage requirements (low serum T_4 levels) can occur with drugs that increase the hepatic metabolism of levothyroxine (Table 26–3). Amiodarone can increase or decrease levothyroxine dose requirements. Malabsorption of levothyroxine can be caused by coadministration of binding substances, such as iron (eg, in multivitamins); fiber; raloxifene; sucralfate; aluminum hydroxide antacids; sevelemer; orlistat; bile acid–binding resins (cholestyramine and colesevelam); and calcium, magnesium, milk, coffee, and soy milk, or formula.

Serum TSH may be elevated transiently in acute psychiatric illness, with antipsychotics and phenothiazines, and during recovery from nonthyroidal illness. Autoimmune disease can interfere with the assay and cause false elevations of TSH.

2. Normal serum TSH level—For most patients, the goal of levothyroxine replacement is to maintain the serum TSH in the low normal range (0.4–2.0 mIU/L). However, treated patients with normal serum TSH levels have higher serum LDL cholesterol levels, lower average basal metabolic rate, and lower serum T_3 levels compared to matched euthyroid controls. This appears to explain why some treated patients continue to have subjective symptoms suggestive of mild hypothyroidism, despite normal serum TSH levels. Such patients must be assessed for concurrent conditions, such as an adverse drug reaction, Addison disease, depression, hypogonadism, anemia, celiac disease, or gluten sensitivity. If such conditions are not present or are treated and hypothyroid-type symptoms persist, a serum T_3 or free T_3 level is often helpful. Low serum T_3 levels may reflect inadequate peripheral deiodinase activity to convert inactive T_4 to active T_3. Unless contraindicated by unstable angina, such patients with continued hypothyroid-type symptoms may be carefully administered a slightly higher dose of levothyroxine to suppress the serum TSH while achieving clinical euthyroidism and a serum FT_3 near the low-normal range. For most patients with hypothyroidism, an ideal stable maintenance dose of levothyroxine can usually be found.

Desiccated natural porcine thyroid preparations containing both T_4 and T_3 (eg, Armour Thyroid, Nature-Throid, NP Thyroid) are prescribed by some clinicians. About 65 mg (1 grain) of desiccated thyroid is equivalent to 100 mcg of levothyroxine. Several professional medical societies discourage the use of desiccated thyroid preparations, but some patients prefer them.

3. Low or suppressed serum TSH level—A serum TSH level below the reference range (adults 0.4–4.0 mIU/L) is either "low" (0.1–0.39 mIU/L) or "suppressed" (less than 0.1 mIU/L). Clinically euthyroid patients receiving levothyroxine who have "low" TSH levels do not have increased morbidity. However, a "suppressed" serum TSH often indicates over-replacement with levothyroxine, and such patients may have symptoms of hyperthyroidism with an increased risk for atrial fibrillation, osteoporosis, and clinical hyperthyroidism. A suppressed serum TSH can occur with hypopituitarism, severe nonthyroidal illness, and some medications such as NSAIDs, biotin, opioids, nifedipine, verapamil, and high-dose (short-term) corticosteroids. Aside from the latter circumstances, when the serum TSH is suppressed, the dosage of levothyroxine is reduced. However, some patients feel unmistakably hypothyroid while taking the reduced dose of levothyroxine and have low serum T_3 or free T_3 levels. For such patients, a higher levothyroxine dose may be resumed with close surveillance for atrial fibrillation, osteoporosis, and manifestations of subtle hyperthyroidism.

Prognosis

Patients with mild hypothyroidism caused by autoimmune thyroiditis have a remission rate of 11%. Hypothyroidism caused by interferon-alpha resolves within 17 months of stopping the drug in 50% of patients. With levothyroxine treatment of hypothyroidism, striking transformations take place both in appearance and mental function. Return to a normal state is usually the rule, but relapses will occur if treatment is interrupted. Untreated patients with myxedema crisis have a mortality rate approaching 100%; even with optimal treatment, the mortality rate is 20–50%.

When to Refer

- Difficulty titrating levothyroxine replacement to normal TSH or clinically euthyroid state.
- Any patient with significant CAD needing levothyroxine therapy.

When to Admit

- Suspected myxedema crisis.
- Hypercapnia.

Bridwell RE et al. Decompensated hypothyroidism: a review for the emergency clinician. Am J Emerg Med. 2021;39:207. [PMID: 33039222]

Calissendorff J et al. To treat or not to treat subclinical hypothyroidism, what is the evidence? Medicina (Kaunas). 2020;56:40. [PMID: 31963883]

Ettleson MD et al. Individualized therapy for hypothyroidism: is T4 enough for everyone? J Clin Endocrinol Metab. 2020;105:e3090. [PMID: 32614450]

Li SW et al. Management of overt hypothyroidism during pregnancy. Best Pract Res Clin Endocrinol Metab. 2020;34:101439. [PMID: 32616466]

McDermott MT. Hypothyroidism. Ann Intern Med. 2020;173:ITC1. [PMID: 32628881]

HYPERTHYROIDISM (Thyrotoxicosis)

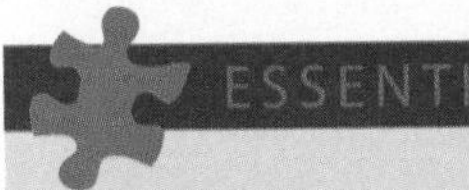

ESSENTIALS OF DIAGNOSIS

- Sweating, weight loss or gain, anxiety, palpitations, loose stools, heat intolerance, menstrual irregularity.
- Tachycardia; warm, moist skin; stare; tremor.
- Graves disease: most common cause of hyperthyroidism; palpable goiter (sometimes with bruit) in most patients; ophthalmopathy also common.
- Amiodarone: most common cause of thyrotoxic crisis ("thyroid storm").
- Suppressed TSH in primary hyperthyroidism; usually increased T_4, FT_4, T_3, FT_3.

General Considerations

The term "thyrotoxicosis" refers to the clinical manifestations associated with elevated serum levels of T_4 or T_3 that are excessive for the individual (hyperthyroidism).

A. Graves Disease

Graves disease (also known as Basedow disease) is the most common cause of thyrotoxicosis. It is an autoimmune disorder, characterized by an increase in synthesis and release of thyroid hormones. Autoantibodies bind to the TSH receptors in the thyroid cell membranes and stimulate the gland to overproduce thyroid hormones. These autoantibodies are known as thyroid-stimulating immunoglobulins (TSI) or thyrotropin receptor antibodies (TRAb). The presence of the latter antibodies distinguishes Graves disease from autoimmune chronic lymphocytic (Hashimoto) thyroiditis since in both conditions serum antithyroid antibodies (TPO Ab or Tg Ab or both) are usually present.

Graves disease is much more common in women than in men (8:1), and its usual onset is between the ages of 20 and 40 years. It may be accompanied by infiltrative ophthalmopathy (Graves exophthalmos) and, less commonly, by infiltrative dermopathy (pretibial myxedema). The thymus gland is typically enlarged and serum antinuclear antibody levels are usually elevated. Many patients with Graves disease have a family history of either Graves disease or Hashimoto autoimmune thyroiditis.

Dietary iodine supplementation can trigger Graves disease. Similarly, patients being treated with potassium iodide or amiodarone (which contains iodine) have an increased risk of developing Graves disease.

Chemotherapy with immune checkpoint inhibitors (ipilimumab, pembrolizumab, tremelimumab, and atezolizumab) and alemtuzumab (for multiple sclerosis) can precipitate Graves disease and cause hyperthyroidism from destructive autoimmune thyroiditis (silent thyroiditis).

Patients with Graves disease have an increased risk of other systemic autoimmune disorders, including Sjögren syndrome, celiac disease, pernicious anemia, Addison disease, alopecia areata, vitiligo, type 1 diabetes mellitus, hypoparathyroidism, myasthenia gravis, and cardiomyopathy.

B. Toxic Multinodular Goiter and Thyroid Nodules

Autonomous hyperfunctioning thyroid nodules that produce hyperthyroidism are known as toxic multinodular goiter (Plummer disease). They are more prevalent among older adults and in iodine-deficient regions. A single hyperfunctioning nodule can also produce hyperthyroidism. Thyroid cancer is found in 5% of patients with toxic multinodular goiter.

C. Autoimmune (Postpartum or Silent) Thyroiditis and Subacute Thyroiditis

These conditions cause thyroid inflammation with release of stored hormone. They all produce a variable triphasic course: variable hyperthyroidism is followed by transient euthyroidism and progression to hypothyroidism (see Thyroiditis, above).

D. Medication-Induced Hyperthyroidism

1. Amiodarone-induced thyrotoxicosis—Amiodarone is 37% iodine by weight and its metabolites have a half-life of about 100 days. In the short term, amiodarone normally increases serum TSH (without hypothyroidism), though usually not over 20 mIU/L. Serum T_4 and FT_4 rise about 40% and may become elevated in clinically euthyroid patients, while serum T_3 levels typically decline. Due to these short-term changes, it is best to not check thyroid function tests during the first 3 months of therapy with amiodarone, unless clinically indicated. After about 3 months, the serum TSH usually normalizes.

Amiodarone-induced thyrotoxicosis is diagnosed when serum TSH levels are suppressed and serum T_3 or FT_3 levels are high or high-normal. Amiodarone-induced thyrotoxicosis is categorized as type 1, type 2, or mixed (27%). Treatment is based on distinguishing type 1 from type 2. Type 1 is caused by the *active* production of excessive thyroid hormone. Type 2 is caused by thyroiditis with the *passive* release of stored thyroid hormone.

In the United States, amiodarone causes thyrotoxicosis in about 3% of patients taking the drug. In Europe and iodine-deficient geographic areas, it induces thyrotoxicosis in about 20%. Thyrotoxicosis can occur at any time during treatment and may develop several months after treatment discontinuation. Amiodarone is the leading cause for thyrotoxic crisis ("thyroid storm"); however, the manifestations can be missed since amiodarone tends to cause bradycardia. Thyroid function tests (TSH, FT_4, T_3) should be checked before starting amiodarone, at 3–6 months, and at least every 6 months thereafter (sooner if clinically indicated).

2. Iodine-induced hyperthyroidism (Basedow disease)—The recommended iodine intake for nonpregnant adults is 150 mcg/day. Higher iodine intake can precipitate hyperthyroidism in patients with nodular goiters, autonomous thyroid nodules, or asymptomatic Graves disease, and less commonly in patients with no detectable underlying thyroid disorder. Common sources of excess iodine include intravenous iodinated radiocontrast dye, certain foods (eg, kelp, nori), topical iodinated antiseptics (eg, povidine iodine), and medications (eg, amiodarone or potassium iodide). Intravenous iodinated radiocontrast dye can rarely induce a painful, destructive subacute thyroiditis, similar to type 2 amiodarone-induced thyrotoxicosis.

3. Tyrosine kinase inhibitors—Silent autoimmune thyroiditis that releases stored thyroid hormone, resulting in hyperthyroidism, develops in about 3% of patients receiving chemotherapy with tyrosine kinase inhibitors (eg, axitinib, sorafenib, sunitinib). While such hyperthyroidism may be subclinical, thyrotoxic crisis has been reported. Hypothyroidism usually follows hyperthyroidism and occurs in 19% of patients taking these drugs.

4. Immune checkpoint inhibitor cancer therapy—Immune checkpoint inhibitor therapy directed against either PD-1/PD-L1 or CTLA-4/B7-1/B7-2 frequently precipitates autoimmune adverse reactions. Thyroid autoimmunity commonly causes thyroiditis, hypothyroidism (primary or secondary), or hyperthyroidism from either passive release of thyroid hormone or active production of thyroid hormone (Graves disease).

E. Pregnancy, hCG-Secreting Trophoblastic Tumors, and Testicular Choriocarcinoma

Human chorionic gonadotropin (hCG) can bind to the thyroid's TSH receptors. Very high levels of serum hCG, particularly during the first 4 months of pregnancy may cause sufficient receptor activation to cause gestational thyrotoxicosis. About 20% of pregnant women have a low serum TSH during pregnancy, but only 1% of such women have clinical hyperthyroidism that requires treatment. Pregnant women are more likely to have hCG-induced thyrotoxicosis if they have high levels of serum asialo-hCG, a subfraction of hCG that has a greater affinity for TSH receptors. Such women are also more likely to suffer from hyperemesis gravidarum. This condition must be distinguished from true Graves disease in pregnancy, which usually predates conception and may be associated with high serum levels of TSI and antithyroid antibodies or with exophthalmos.

F. Rare Causes of Hyperthyroidism

Thyrotoxicosis factitia is due to intentional or accidental ingestion of excessive amounts of exogenous thyroid hormone. Struma ovarii is thyroid tissue contained in about 3% of ovarian dermoid tumors and teratomas. Pituitary TSH hypersecretion by a pituitary thyrotrophe tumor or hyperplasia can rarely cause hyperthyroidism; serum TSH is elevated or inappropriately normal in the presence of true thyrotoxicosis. Metastatic functioning thyroid carcinoma can cause hyperthyroidism in patients with a heavy tumor burden.

High levels of hCG can also cause thyrotoxicosis in some cases of pregnancies with gestational trophoblastic disease (molar pregnancy, choriocarcinoma). Some such pregnancies have produced thyrotoxic crisis. Men have developed hyperthyroidism from high levels of serum hCG secreted by a testicular choriocarcinoma.

▶ Clinical Findings

A. Symptoms and Signs

Thyrotoxicosis can produce nervousness, restlessness, heat intolerance, increased sweating, palpitations, pruritus, fatigue, muscle weakness, muscle cramps, frequent bowel movements, weight change (usually loss), or menstrual irregularities. There may be fine resting finger tremors, moist warm skin, fever, hyperreflexia, fine hair, and onycholysis. Angina or atrial fibrillation may also be present, sometimes in the absence of other thyrotoxic symptoms (apathetic hyperthyroidism). Women with postpartum thyroiditis are often asymptomatic or experience only minor symptoms, such as palpitations, heat intolerance, and irritability. Chronic thyrotoxicosis may cause osteoporosis. Even subclinical hyperthyroidism (suppressed serum

TSH with normal FT_4) may increase the risk of nonvertebral fractures.

Patients with Graves disease usually have a diffusely enlarged thyroid that is frequently asymmetric and often accompanied by a bruit. However, there may be no palpable thyroid enlargement. The thyroid gland in painful subacute thyroiditis is usually moderately enlarged and tender. There is often dysphagia and pain that can radiate to the jaw or ear. With toxic multinodular goiter, there are usually palpable nodules. Patients with silent thyroiditis or postpartum thyroiditis have either no palpable goiter or a small, nontender goiter.

Cardiopulmonary manifestations of thyrotoxicosis commonly include a forceful heartbeat, premature atrial contractions, and sinus tachycardia. Patients often have exertional dyspnea. Atrial fibrillation or atrial tachycardia occurs in about 8% of patients with thyrotoxicosis, more commonly in men, older adults, and those with ischemic or valvular heart disease. The ventricular response from the atrial fibrillation may be difficult to control. Thyrotoxicosis can cause a thyrotoxic cardiomyopathy, and the onset of atrial fibrillation can precipitate heart failure. Echocardiogram reveals pulmonary artery hypertension in about 40% of hyperthyroid patients. Even "subclinical hyperthyroidism" increases the risk for atrial fibrillation and overall mortality. Hemodynamic abnormalities and pulmonary hypertension are reversible with restoration of euthyroidism.

Thyrotoxic crisis or "thyroid storm" is an extreme form of severe thyrotoxicosis and an immediate threat to life. The most common manifestations are cardiac (heart failure, severe sinus tachycardia [60%], ventricular fibrillation [13%], MI, and cardiogenic shock), agitation or delirium (63%), high fever, vomiting, diarrhea, dehydration, and hepatic impairment (52%).

Eye manifestations that occur with hyperthyroidism are discussed in Thyroid Eye Disease, below.

Graves dermopathy (pretibial myxedema) occurs in about 3% of patients with Graves disease. It usually affects the pretibial region but can also affect the dorsal forearms and wrists and dorsum of the feet. It is more common in patients with high levels of serum TSI and severe Graves ophthalmopathy. Glycosaminoglycans accumulation and lymphoid infiltration occur in affected skin, which becomes erythematous with a thickened, rough texture.

Thyroid acropachy is an extreme and unusual manifestation of Graves disease. It presents with digital clubbing, swelling of fingers and toes, and radiographic findings of periostitis involving phalangeal and metacarpal bones. Extremity skin can become very thickened, resembling elephantiasis.

Clinical hyperthyroidism during pregnancy has a prevalence of about 0.2%. It may commence before conception or emerge during pregnancy, particularly the first trimester. Pregnancy can have a beneficial effect on the thyrotoxicosis of Graves disease, with decreasing antibody titers and decreasing serum T_4 levels as the pregnancy advances; about 30% of affected women experience a remission by late in the second trimester. Undiagnosed or undertreated hyperthyroidism carries an increased risk of miscarriage, preeclampsia-eclampsia, preterm delivery, abruptio placenta, maternal heart failure, and thyrotoxic crisis (thyroid storm). Such thyrotoxic crisis can be precipitated by trauma, infection, surgery, or delivery and confers a fetal/maternal mortality rate of about 25%.

Hypokalemic periodic paralysis occurs in about 15% of Asian or American Indian men with thyrotoxicosis and is 30 times more common in men than women. It is marked by sudden symmetric flaccid paralysis, along with hypokalemia and hypophosphatemia, that occurs during hyperthyroidism (often after intravenous dextrose, oral carbohydrates, or vigorous exercise) despite few, if any, of the classic signs of thyrotoxicosis. Attacks last 7–72 hours.

B. Laboratory Findings

Serum FT_4, T_3, FT_3, and T_4, thyroid resin uptake, and FT_4 index are all usually increased. Sometimes the FT_4 level may be normal but with an elevated serum T_3 (T_3 toxicosis). The severity of the elevation of serum FT_4 and FT_3 levels does not always correlate with the severity of thyrotoxic manifestations; patients with thyrotoxic crisis tend to have serum thyroid levels that are not significantly higher than those with less pronounced symptoms. Serum T_4 or T_3 can be elevated in other nonthyroidal conditions (Table 26–4).

Table 26–4. Factors that can cause aberration laboratory tests for hyperthyroidism.

High Serum T_4 or T_3	Low Serum TSH
Laboratory error	Laboratory error
Collection vial contains gel barrier for T_3	African descent (3–4%)
Acute psychiatric problems (30%)	Autonomous thyroid or thyroid nodule
Acute or chronic active hepatitis, primary biliary cirrhosis	Corticosteroids (short-term use)
AIDS (increased TBG)	Drugs
Autoimmunity	Amphetamines
Euthyroid sick	Biotin supplements (certain assays)
Familial thyroid-binding abnormalities	Calcium channel blockers (nifedipine, verapamil)
Familial resistance to thyroid (Refetoff syndrome)	Dopamine
Pregnancy: morning sickness, hyperemesis gravidarum	Dopamine agonists
Drugs	Glucocorticoids
Amiodarone	Metformin
Amphetamines	Somatostatin analogs
Biotin supplements (certain assays)	Thyroid hormone
Clofibrate	Elderly euthyroid
Estrogens (oral)	hCG-secreting trophoblastic tumors
Heparin	Hypopituitarism
Heroin, methadone	Nonthyroidal illness (severe)
Perphenazine	Pregnancy (especially with morning sickness)
Tamoxifen	Suppression after recent therapy for hyperthyroidism
Thyroid hormone therapy (excessive or factitious)	TSH variants not detected by commercial assays

hCG, human chorionic gonadotropin; T_4, levothyroxine; T_3, triiodothyronine; TBG, thyroid-binding globulin.

Serum TSH is suppressed in hyperthyroidism (except in the very rare cases of pituitary inappropriate secretion of thyrotropin). Serum TSH may be misleadingly low in other nonthyroidal conditions (Table 26–4). The term **"subclinical hyperthyroidism"** is used to describe individuals with a low serum TSH but normal serum levels of FT_4 and T_3; in such patients, the overall prevalence of symptomatic hyperthyroidism is 0.7–1.8% in iodine-sufficient patients and 2–15% in patients with iodine deficiency. About two-thirds of patients with subclinical hyperthyroidism have serum TSH levels of 0.1–0.4 mIU/L (mild subclinical hyperthyroidism), while the remainder have serum TSH levels below 0.1 mIU/L (severe subclinical hyperthyroidism).

Hyperthyroidism can cause hypercalcemia, increased liver enzymes, increased alkaline phosphatase, anemia, and neutropenia. Hyperthyroidism also increases urinary magnesium excretion, which can lead to hypomagnesemia, functional hypoparathyroidism with hypocalcemia, and tetany (rarely). Hypokalemia and hypophosphatemia occur in thyrotoxic periodic paralysis.

Problems of diagnosis occur in patients with acute psychiatric disorders; about 30% of these patients have elevated serum T_4 levels without clinical thyrotoxicosis. The TSH is not usually suppressed, distinguishing psychiatric disorder from true hyperthyroidism. T_4 levels return to normal gradually.

In **Graves disease**, serum thyroid-stimulating immunoglobulin (TSI, TSHrAb) is usually detectable (65%). Very high serum TSI levels predispose to Graves ophthalmopathy. TPO Ab or Tg Ab are usually elevated but are nonspecific. Serum antinuclear antibodies are also usually elevated without any evidence of SLE or other rheumatologic disease.

With painful **subacute thyroiditis,** patients often have an increased WBC, ESR, and CRP. About 25% have antithyroid antibodies (usually in low titer) and serum TSI (TSHrAb) levels are normal. Patients with iodine-induced hyperthyroidism have undetectable serum TSI (or TSHrAb), no serum TPO Ab, and an elevated urinary iodine concentration. In thyrotoxicosis factitia, serum thyroglobulin levels are low, distinguishing it from other causes of hyperthyroidism.

With **hyperthyroidism during pregnancy,** women have an elevated serum total T_4 and FT_4 while the TSH is suppressed. An apparent lack of full TSH suppression in hyperthyroidism can be seen due to misidentification of hCG as TSH in certain assays. The serum FT_4 assay is difficult to interpret in pregnancy. Although the serum T_4 is elevated in most pregnant women, values over 20 mcg/dL (257 nmol/L) are encountered only in hyperthyroidism. The T_3 resin uptake, which is low in normal pregnancy because of high thyroxine-binding globulin (TBG) concentration, is normal or high in thyrotoxic persons.

Since high levels of T_4 and FT_4 are normally seen in patients taking **amiodarone,** a suppressed TSH must be present along with a greatly elevated T_4 (greater than 20 mcg/dL [257 nmol/L]) or T_3 (greater than 200 ng/dL [3.1 nmol/L]) in order to diagnose hyperthyroidism. In type 1 amiodarone-induced thyrotoxicosis, the presence of proptosis and serum TSI (TSHrAb) is diagnostic. In type 2 amiodarone-induced thyrotoxicosis, serum levels of interleukin-6 (IL-6) are usually quite elevated.

C. Radioisotope Uptake and Imaging

Note: *All radioisotope testing is contraindicated during pregnancy or breastfeeding.*

Thyroid radioisotope scanning may be performed using either (^{123}I or ^{99m}Tc pertechnetate). Scanning can be helpful in some situations to determine the cause of hyperthyroidism but is unnecessary for diagnosis in patients with obvious Graves disease who have elevated serum TSI or associated Graves ophthalmopathy. A high thyroid RAI uptake is seen in Graves disease and toxic nodular goiter. A low ^{123}I RAI uptake is characteristic of iodine-induced hyperthyroidism and thyroiditis (subacute, silent, or postpartum), distinguishing them from Graves disease.

Patients with Graves disease have increased or normal thyroid uptake of **technetium (Tc-99m) pertechnetate,** whereas those with thyrotoxicosis from thyroiditis (silent, subacute, postpartum) have reduced uptake.

Thyroid ultrasound can be helpful in hyperthyroid patients with palpable thyroid nodules. Thyroid ultrasound shows a variably heterogeneous, hypoechoic gland in thyroiditis. Color flow Doppler sonography is helpful to distinguish type 1 amiodarone-induced thyrotoxicosis (enlarged gland with normal to increased blood flow velocity and vascularity) from type 2 amiodarone-induced thyrotoxicosis (normal gland without increased vascularity).

99mTc-sestamibi scanning usually shows normal or increased uptake with type 1 amiodarone-induced thyrotoxicosis and decreased uptake in type 2.

MRI and CT scanning of the orbits are the imaging methods of choice to visualize Graves ophthalmopathy affecting the extraocular muscles. Imaging is required only in severe or unilateral cases or in euthyroid exophthalmos that must be distinguished from orbital pseudotumor, tumors, and other lesions.

Differential Diagnosis

True thyrotoxicosis must be distinguished from those conditions that elevate serum T_4 and T_3 or suppress serum TSH without affecting clinical status (see Table 26–4). Serum TSH is commonly suppressed in early pregnancy and only about 10% of pregnant women with a low TSH have clinical hyperthyroidism.

States of hypermetabolism without thyrotoxicosis—notably severe anemia, leukemia, polycythemia, cancer, and pheochromocytoma—rarely cause confusion. Acromegaly may also produce tachycardia, sweating, and thyroid enlargement.

The differential diagnosis for thyroid-associated ophthalmopathy includes an orbital tumor (eg, lymphoma) or pseudotumor. Ocular myasthenia gravis is another autoimmune condition that occurs more commonly in Graves disease.

Diabetes mellitus and Addison disease may coexist with thyrotoxicosis and can aggravate the weight loss, fatigue, and muscle weakness seen with hyperthyroidism.

Complications

Hypercalcemia, osteoporosis, and nephrocalcinosis may occur in hyperthyroidism. Decreased libido, erectile dysfunction, diminished sperm motility, and gynecomastia may be noted in men. Other complications include cardiac arrhythmias and heart failure, thyroid crisis, ophthalmopathy, dermopathy, and thyrotoxic hypokalemic periodic paralysis.

Treatment

A. Treatment of Graves Disease

Table 26–5 outlines the treatment options for hyperthyroidism.

1. Propranolol—Propranolol is used for symptomatic relief of tachycardia, tremor, diaphoresis, and anxiety until the hyperthyroidism is resolved. It is the initial treatment of choice for thyrotoxic crisis and effectively treats thyrotoxic hypokalemic periodic paralysis. Treatment usually starts with propranolol ER, which is given every 12 hours for severe hyperthyroidism due to accelerated metabolism of the propranolol; it may be given once daily as hyperthyroidism improves (Table 26–5).

2. Thiourea drugs—Methimazole or PTU is generally used for young adults or patients with mild thyrotoxicosis, small goiters, or fear of isotopes. See Treatment of Hyperthyroidism during Pregnancy-Planning, Pregnancy, and Lactation, below. Elderly patients usually respond particularly well. There is a 50% chance of remission of hyperthyroidism with long-term thiourea therapy. A better likelihood of long-term remission occurs in patients with small goiters, mild hyperthyroidism, those requiring small doses of thiourea, and those with serum TSI (TSHrAb) less than 2 mU/L. Patients whose TPO Ab and Tg Ab remain low after 2 years of therapy have only a 10% rate of relapse. There should be no rush to discontinue thiourea therapy in favor of RAI or surgery, even after years of treatment. Thioureas may be continued long term for patients who are tolerating them well. The exception is women with thyrotoxic Graves disease who are planning pregnancy in the near future; thyroid surgery or RAI should be considered at least 4 months in advance of conception. Thiourea drugs are also useful for preparing nonpregnant hyperthyroid patients for surgery and elderly patients for RAI treatment.

Agranulocytosis (absolute neutrophil count below 500/mcL [0.5×10^9/L]) or pancytopenia may occur abruptly in

Table 26–5. Medications for the treatment of hyperthyroidism.[1]

Medication	Dose and Frequency	Indications
Propranolol ER	Dose: 60–80 mg orally once daily, increasing every 3 days until heart rate < 90 beats per minute. Maximum dose: 320 mg daily	Symptomatic relief of tachycardia, tremor, diaphoresis, anxiety Thyrotoxic crisis Hypokalemic periodic paralysis
Thioureas Methimazole	Initial dose: usually 30–60 mg orally once daily Dose may be divided and given twice daily to avoid GI upset Lower dose of 10–20 mg for very mild symptoms During pregnancy or breastfeeding, dose should not exceed 20 mg daily	Young adults Older adult patients Mild thyrotoxicosis Small goiter Fear of isotopes Precautions during pregnancy[2]
Propylthiouracil (PTU)	Dose: 300–600 mg orally daily in four divided doses During pregnancy or breastfeeding, dose should not exceed 200 mg daily	Precautions during pregnancy[2]
Iodinated contrast agents Iopanoic acid or ipodate sodium	Initial dose: 500 mg orally twice daily for 3 days Maintenance dose: 500 mg once daily	Effective temporary treatment of thyrotoxicosis, especially for patients who are very symptomatic Alternative treatment for patients intolerant of thioureas
Lithium carbonate	Dose: 500–750 mg orally daily in divided doses	Thioureas greatly preferred over lithium Alternative treatment of patients intolerant of thioureas Do not use during pregnancy
Radioactive iodine (RAI, ^{131}I)		Destroys overactive thyroid tissue See text for Precautions Avoid with thyroid eye disease (Graves ophthalmopathy)
Prednisone	Initial dose: 0.5–0.7 mg/kg orally daily After 2 weeks: begin to slowly taper and stop after about 3 months	Type 2 amiodarone-induced thyrotoxicosis

[1]See text for expanded discussion of these agents.
[2]See Treatment of Hyperthyroidism During Pregnancy-Planning, Pregnancy, and Lactation in text.

0.4% of patients taking either methimazole or PTU. All patients receiving thiourea therapy must be informed of the danger of agranulocytosis or pancytopenia and the need to stop the drug and seek medical attention immediately with the onset of any infection or unusual bleeding. Nearly 85% of agranulocytosis cases occur within 90 days of commencing therapy; however, continued long-term vigilance with routine blood tests is required as many cases may be discovered while the patient is asymptomatic. Half of cases are discovered because of fever, pharyngitis, or bleeding. There is a genetic tendency to develop agranulocytosis with thiourea therapy; if a close relative has had this adverse reaction, other therapies should be considered. Agranulocytosis generally remits spontaneously with discontinuation of the thiourea. Recovery has not been improved by filgrastim (granulocyte colony-stimulating factor).

Other common side effects include pruritus, allergic dermatitis, nausea, and dyspepsia. Since the two thiourea drugs are similar, patients who have a major allergic reaction to one should not be given the other.

The patient may become clinically hypothyroid for 2 weeks or more before TSH levels rise. Therefore, the patient's changing thyroid status is best monitored clinically and with serum FT_4 levels. Rapid growth of a goiter usually occurs if prolonged hypothyroidism is allowed to develop; the goiter may sometimes become massive but usually regresses rapidly with reduction or cessation of thiourea therapy or with thyroid hormone replacement.

A. Methimazole—Except during the first trimester of pregnancy, methimazole is generally preferred over PTU since it is more convenient to use and is less likely to cause fulminant hepatic necrosis. Methimazole therapy is also less likely to cause ^{131}I treatment failure. Rare complications peculiar to methimazole include serum sickness, cholestatic jaundice, alopecia, nephrotic syndrome, hypoglycemia, and loss of taste. The dosage is reduced as manifestations of hyperthyroidism resolve and as the FT_4 level falls toward normal. Following ^{131}I therapy, the dose of methimazole is gradually reduced according to frequent thyroid function testing; most patients are able to discontinue methimazole within 1–3 months following RAI therapy.

B. Propylthiouracil—Acute liver failure occurs in about 1 in 1000 patients, making PTU a second-line medication for treating patients with Graves hyperthyroidism. The onset of severe liver toxicity varies from 3 days to 12 months after starting PTU. Therefore, PTU is ordinarily reserved for treating women actively seeking fertility and during the first trimester of pregnancy, when it is preferred over methimazole. See Treatment of Hyperthyroidism During Pregnancy-Planning, Pregnancy, and Lactation, below.

3. Iodinated contrast agents—Iopanoic acid (Telepaque) and ipodate sodium (Bilivist, Oragrafin) are iodinated contrast agents that provide effective temporary treatment for thyrotoxicosis of any cause and are particularly useful for patients who are symptomatically very thyrotoxic. These agents inhibit peripheral 5′-monodeiodination of T_4, thereby blocking its conversion to active T_3. Within 24 hours, serum T_3 levels fall an average of 62%. For patients with **Graves disease,** methimazole is begun first to block iodine organification; the next day, ipodate sodium or iopanoic acid may be added. They offer a therapeutic option for patients with subacute thyroiditis, amiodarone-induced thyrotoxicosis, T_4 overdosage, and for those intolerant to thioureas. Treatment periods of 8 months or more are possible, but efficacy tends to wane with time. In Graves disease, thyroid RAI uptake may be suppressed during treatment but typically returns to pretreatment uptake by 7 days after discontinuation of the drug, allowing ^{131}I treatment.

4. Lithium carbonate—Thioureas are greatly preferred over lithium for the medical treatment of hyperthyroidism in Graves disease. However, lithium may be used effectively in cases of methimazole or PTU-induced hepatic toxicity or leukopenia. Lithium should not be used during pregnancy.

5. Radioactive iodine (RAI, ^{131}I)—^{131}I therapy destroys overactive thyroid tissue (either diffuse or toxic nodular goiter). Adolescent and adult patients who have been treated with ^{131}I in adulthood do not have an increased risk of subsequent thyroid cancer, leukemia, or offspring with congenital abnormalities. Conflicting evidence has shown either no increased risk or a slightly increased risk of subsequent solid tumor malignancies following ^{131}I treatment for hyperthyroidism.

Precautions: Because radiation is harmful to the fetus and children, *RAI should not be given to pregnant or lactating women or to mothers who lack childcare. Women are advised to avoid pregnancy for at least 4 months following ^{131}I therapy. A pregnancy test should be obtained within 48 hours before therapy for any woman with childbearing potential. Men have been found to have abnormal spermatozoa for up to 6 months following ^{131}I therapy and are advised to use contraceptive methods during that time.*

Patients may receive ^{131}I while being symptomatically treated with propranolol ER, which is then reduced in dosage as hyperthyroidism resolves. A higher rate of ^{131}I treatment failure has been reported in patients with Graves disease who have been receiving methimazole or PTU. However, therapy with ^{131}I will usually be effective if the methimazole is discontinued at least 3–4 days before RAI therapy and if the therapeutic dosage of ^{131}I is adjusted (upward) according to RAI uptake on the pretherapy scan. Prior to ^{131}I therapy, patients are instructed against receiving intravenous iodinated contrast and should consume a low-iodine diet.

The presence of Graves ophthalmopathy is a relative contraindication to ^{131}I therapy. Following ^{131}I treatment for hyperthyroidism, Graves ophthalmopathy appears or worsens in 15% of patients (23% in cigarette smokers and 6% in nonsmokers) and improves in none. Among patients receiving prednisone following ^{131}I treatment, preexistent ophthalmopathy worsens in none and improves in 67%. Therefore, patients with Graves ophthalmopathy who are to be treated with ^{131}I should be considered for prophylactic prednisone (20–40 mg orally daily) for 2 months following administration of ^{131}I, particularly in patients who have severe orbital involvement.

Cigarette use increases the risk of having a flare in ophthalmopathy following ^{131}I treatment and also reduces the effectiveness of prednisone treatment. Patients who smoke cigarettes are strongly encouraged to quit prior to ^{131}I treatment. Smokers receiving ^{131}I should be considered for prophylactic prednisone.

FT_4 levels may sometimes drop within 2 months after ^{131}I treatment, but then rise again to thyrotoxic levels, at which time thyroid RAI uptake is low. This phenomenon is caused by a release of stored thyroid hormone from injured thyroid cells and does not indicate a treatment failure. In fact, serum FT_4 then falls abruptly to hypothyroid levels.

There is a high incidence of hypothyroidism in the months to years after ^{131}I, even when low activities are given. Patients with Graves disease treated with ^{131}I also have an increased lifetime risk of developing hyperparathyroidism, particularly when ^{131}I therapy was administered in childhood or adolescence. Lifelong clinical follow-up is mandatory, with measurements of serum TSH, FT_4, and calcium when indicated.

6. Thyroid surgery—Surgery may be indicated for patients with Graves disease who are intolerant to thioureas, women planning pregnancy in the near future, patients who choose not to have RAI therapy, and patients with Graves ophthalmopathy. The surgical procedure of choice is a total resection of one lobe and a subtotal resection of the other lobe, leaving about 4 g of thyroid tissue (Hartley–Dunhill operation).

Patients are ordinarily rendered euthyroid preoperatively with a thiourea drug (Table 26–5). Propranolol ER is given until the heart rate is less than 90 beats per minute and continued until the serum T_3 (or free T_3) is normal preoperatively. The patient should be euthyroid by the time of surgery.

The risks of subtotal or total thyroidectomy includes damage to a recurrent laryngeal nerve, with resultant vocal fold paralysis. Hypoparathyroidism also occurs; serum calcium levels must be checked postoperatively.

B. Treatment of Toxic Solitary Thyroid Nodules

Toxic solitary thyroid nodules are usually benign but may rarely be malignant. If a nonsurgical therapy is elected, the nodule should be evaluated with a fine-needle aspiration (FNA) biopsy. **Medical therapy** for hyperthyroidism caused by a single hyperfunctioning thyroid nodule may be treated symptomatically with propranolol ER and methimazole or PTU, as in Graves disease (Table 26–5). The dose of methimazole should be adjusted to keep the TSH slightly suppressed, so the risk of TSH-stimulated growth of the nodule is reduced. **Surgical treatment** is usually recommended for patients under age 40 years, for healthy older patients with toxic solitary thyroid nodules, and for nodules that are suspicious for malignancy. Patients are made euthyroid with a thiourea preoperatively and given several days of iodine, ipodate sodium, or iopanoic acid before surgery. Postoperative hypothyroidism usually resolves spontaneously, but permanent hypothyroidism occurs in about 14% of patients by 6 years after surgery. **^{131}I therapy** may be offered to patients with a toxic solitary nodule who are over age 40 or in poor health (see **Precautions** for RAI use, above). RAI should not be given to women with Graves disease within 3 months prior to a planned conception. If the patient has been receiving methimazole preparatory to ^{131}I, the TSH should be kept slightly suppressed in order to reduce the uptake of ^{131}I by the normal thyroid. Nevertheless, permanent hypothyroidism occurs in about one-third of patients by 8 years after ^{131}I therapy. The nodule remains palpable in 50% and may grow in 10% of patients after ^{131}I.

C. Treatment of Toxic Nodular Goiter

Medical therapy for patients with toxic nodular goiter consists of propranolol ER (while hyperthyroid) and a thiourea, as in Graves disease (Table 26–5). Thioureas (methimazole or PTU) reverse hyperthyroidism but do not shrink the goiter. There is a 95% recurrence rate if the drug is stopped.

Surgical therapy is the definitive treatment for a large toxic nodular goiter, following therapy with a thiourea to render them euthyroid. Surgery is particularly indicated to relieve pressure symptoms or for cosmetic indications. Patients with toxic nodular goiter are not treated preoperatively with potassium iodide. Total or near-total thyroidectomy is recommended, since surgical pathology reveals unsuspected differentiated thyroid cancer in 18.3% of cases.

^{131}I therapy may be used to treat patients with toxic nodular goiter. See **Precautions** for RAI use, above. Any suspicious nodules should be evaluated beforehand for malignancy with FNA cytology. Patients are rendered euthyroid with methimazole, which is stopped 3–4 days before a repeat ^{131}I therapy.

Meanwhile, the patient follows a low-iodine diet in order to enhance the thyroid gland's uptake of ^{131}I, which may be relatively low in this condition (compared to Graves disease). Relatively high doses of ^{131}I are usually required; hypothyroidism or recurrent thyrotoxicosis typically occurs, so patients must be monitored closely. Peculiarly, in about 5% of patients with diffusely nodular toxic goiter, the administration of ^{131}I therapy may induce Graves disease. Also, Graves ophthalmopathy has occurred rarely following ^{131}I therapy for multinodular goiter.

D. Treatment of Hyperthyroidism from Thyroiditis

Patients with thyroiditis (subacute, postpartum, or silent) are treated with propranolol during the hyperthyroid phase, which usually subsides spontaneously within weeks to months. For symptomatic relief, begin propranolol ER until the heart rate is less than 90 beats per minute (Table 26–5). Ipodate sodium or iopanoic acid, 500 mg orally daily, promptly corrects elevated T_3 levels and is continued for 15–60 days until the serum FT_4 level normalizes. Thioureas are ineffective since thyroid hormone production is actually low in this condition. Patients are monitored carefully for the development of hypothyroidism and treated with levothyroxine as needed.

With subacute thyroiditis, pain can usually be managed with NSAIDs and corticosteroids, but opioid analgesics are sometimes required.

E. Treatment of Hyperthyroidism During Pregnancy-Planning, Pregnancy, and Lactation

Due to the increased risk of congenital anomalies with every thiourea, all women who are planning to become pregnant are encouraged to consider definitive therapy with ^{131}I or surgery well before conception. Both men and women who are planning pregnancy should not have ^{131}I treatment within about 4 months of conception. See **Precautions** for RAI use, above. Dietary iodine must not be restricted for such women to protect the fetus from iodine deficiency.

First-trimester fetal exposure to thioureas (methimazole or PTU) increases the risk of birth defects by about 2%. The fetal anomalies associated with PTU are typically less severe than those associated with methimazole; therefore, PTU is the preferred thiourea for women actively seeking fertility and during the first trimester of pregnancy, despite the very low risk for hepatic necrosis with PTU. Therefore, women should be treated with PTU immediately prepregnancy and through the first trimester; during pregnancy, the dose of PTU is kept below 200 mg daily to avoid goitrous hypothyroidism in the infant. PTU can be switched to methimazole in the second trimester (see Thiourea drugs, above). Thiourea should be given in the smallest dose possible, permitting mild subclinical hyperthyroidism to occur, since it is usually well tolerated. About 30% of women with Graves disease experience a remission by the late second trimester.

Both PTU and methimazole cross the placenta and can induce hypothyroidism, with fetal TSH hypersecretion and goiter. Fetal ultrasound at 20–32 weeks' gestation can visualize any fetal goiter, allowing fetal thyroid dysfunction to be diagnosed and treated. Thyroid hormone administration to the mother does not prevent hypothyroidism in the fetus, since T_4 and T_3 do not freely cross the placenta. Fetal hypothyroidism is rare if the mother's hyperthyroidism is controlled with small daily doses of PTU (50–150 mg/day orally) or methimazole (5–15 mg/day orally). Serum total T_4 levels during pregnancy should be kept at about 1.5× the prepregnancy level. Maternal serum TSI levels over 500% at term predict an increased risk of neonatal Graves disease in the infant.

Subtotal thyroidectomy is indicated for pregnant women with Graves disease or for fertile women of reproductive age who are sexually active and decline contraceptives, under the following circumstances: (1) severe adverse reaction to thioureas; (2) high dosage requirement for thioureas (methimazole greater than or equal to 30 mg/day or PTU greater than or equal to 450 mg/day); or (3) uncontrolled hyperthyroidism due to nonadherence to thiourea therapy. Surgery is best performed during the second trimester.

Both methimazole and PTU are secreted in breast milk but not in amounts that affect the infant's thyroid hormone levels. No adverse reactions to these drugs have been reported in breast-fed infants. See Table 26–5 for recommended doses. It is recommended that the medication be taken just after breastfeeding.

F. Treatment of Amiodarone-Induced Thyrotoxicosis

Patients with either type 1 or type 2 amiodarone-induced thyrotoxicosis require treatment with propranolol ER for symptomatic relief and methimazole (Table 26–5). After two doses of methimazole, iopanoic acid or sodium ipodate may be added to the regimen to further block conversion of T_4 to T_3 until the thyrotoxicosis is resolved. If iopanoic acid or sodium ipodate is not available, the alternative is potassium perchlorate; it is given in doses of less than or equal to 1000 mg daily (in divided doses) for a course not to exceed 30 days to avoid the complication of aplastic anemia. Amiodarone may be withdrawn but this does not have a significant therapeutic impact for several months because of its long half-life. For patients with type 1 amiodarone-induced thyrotoxicosis, therapy with ^{131}I may be successful, but only for those with sufficient RAI uptake. Patients with clear-cut type 2 amiodarone-induced thyrotoxicosis are usually also treated with prednisone for about 2 weeks and then slowly tapered and finally withdrawn after about 3 months. Subtotal thyroidectomy should be considered for patients with amiodarone-induced thyrotoxicosis that is resistant to treatment.

G. Treatment of Complications

1. Thyroid eye disease—See Thyroid Eye Disease (Graves Ophthalmopathy below).

2. Cardiac complications—

A. SINUS TACHYCARDIA—Treatment consists of treating the thyrotoxicosis. A beta-blocker such as propranolol is used in the interim unless there is an associated cardiomyopathy.

B. ATRIAL FIBRILLATION—Hyperthyroidism must be treated immediately. Other drugs, including digoxin, beta-blockers, and anticoagulants, may be required. Electrical cardioversion is unlikely to convert atrial fibrillation to normal sinus rhythm while the patient is thyrotoxic. Spontaneous conversion to normal sinus rhythm occurs in 62% of patients with return of euthyroidism, but that likelihood decreases with age. Following conversion to euthyroidism, there is a 60% chance that atrial fibrillation will recur, despite normal thyroid function tests. Those with persistent atrial fibrillation may have elective cardioversion following anticoagulation 4 months after resolution of hyperthyroidism.

(1) Digoxin—Digoxin is used to slow a rapid ventricular response to thyrotoxic atrial fibrillation; it must be used in larger than normal doses. Digoxin doses are reduced as hyperthyroidism is corrected.

(2) Beta-blockers—Beta-blockers may also reduce the ventricular rate, but they must be used with caution, particularly in patients with heart failure with reduced EF. An initial trial of a short-duration beta-blocker should be considered, such as esmolol intravenously. If a beta-blocker is used, doses of digoxin must be reduced.

(3) Anticoagulants—Dabigatran malabsorption has been reported in thyrotoxicosis-induced diarrhea. The doses of warfarin required in thyrotoxicosis are smaller than normal because of an accelerated plasma clearance of

vitamin K–dependent clotting factors. Higher warfarin doses are usually required as hyperthyroidism subsides.

c. Heart failure—Thyrotoxicosis can cause high-output heart failure due to extreme tachycardia, cardiomyopathy, or both. Aggressive treatment of the hyperthyroidism is required in either case.

Heart failure may also occur as a result of low-output dilated cardiomyopathy. It is uncommon and may be caused by an idiosyncratic severe toxic effect of hyperthyroidism upon certain hearts. Cardiomyopathy may occur at any age and without preexisting cardiac disease. See Chapter 10 for treatment of heart failure and dilated cardiomyopathy. The patient should be rendered euthyroid. However, the heart failure usually persists despite correction of the hyperthyroidism.

d. Apathetic hyperthyroidism—Apathetic hyperthyroidism may present with angina pectoris. Treatment is directed at reversing the hyperthyroidism as well as providing standard antianginal therapy. PCI or coronary artery bypass grafting can often be avoided by prompt diagnosis and treatment.

3. Thyrotoxic crisis or "thyroid storm"—ICU admission is required. A thiourea drug is given (eg, methimazole, 15–25 mg orally every 6 hours, or PTU, 150–250 mg orally every 6 hours). Ipodate sodium (500 mg/day orally) can be helpful if begun 1 hour *after* the first dose of thiourea. Iodide is given 1 hour later as potassium iodide (10 drops three times daily orally). Propranolol is given in a dosage of 0.5–2 mg intravenously every 4 hours or 20–120 mg orally every 6 hours. Hydrocortisone is usually given in doses of 50 mg orally every 6 hours, with rapid dosage reduction as the clinical situation improves. Plasmapheresis has been successfully used in refractory cases to directly remove thyroid hormone. Aspirin is avoided since it displaces T_4 from thyroxine-binding globulin (TBG), raising FT_4 serum levels. For refractory cases, emergency surgical thyroidectomy is an option.

Supportive care is usually required, including vasopressors, mechanical ventilation, dialysis, and extracorporeal membrane oxygenation (ECMO) for cardiogenic shock.

4. Hyperthyroidism from postpartum thyroiditis—Propranolol ER is given during the hyperthyroid phase followed by levothyroxine during the hypothyroidism phase.

5. Graves dermopathy—Treatment involves application of a topical corticosteroid (eg, fluocinolone) with nocturnal plastic occlusive dressings. Compression stockings may improve any associated edema.

6. Thyrotoxic hypokalemic periodic paralysis—Therapy with oral propranolol, 3 mg/kg in divided doses, normalizes the serum potassium and phosphate levels and reverses the paralysis within 2–3 hours. No intravenous potassium or phosphate is usually required. Intravenous dextrose and oral carbohydrate aggravate the condition and are to be avoided. Therapy is continued with propranolol, 60–80 mg orally every 8 hours (or propranolol ER daily at equivalent daily dosage), along with a thiourea drug (eg, methimazole) to treat the hyperthyroidism.

7. Thyroid acropachy—This rare complication of Graves disease is often mild and may not require therapy. More severe cases are treated with systemic immunosuppressant therapy that may include intravenous immune globulin and rituximab.

Prognosis

Mild **Graves disease** may sometimes subside spontaneously. Graves disease that presents in early pregnancy has a 30% chance of spontaneous remission before the third trimester. The ocular, cardiac, and psychological complications can become serious and persistent even after treatment. Permanent hypoparathyroidism and vocal cord palsy are risks of surgical thyroidectomy. Recurrences are common following thiourea therapy but also occur after low-dose ^{131}I therapy or subtotal thyroidectomy. With adequate treatment and long-term follow-up, the results are usually good. However, despite treatment for hyperthyroidism, women experience an increased long-term risk of death from thyroid disease, CVD, stroke, and fracture of the femur. Posttreatment hypothyroidism is common. It may occur within a few months or up to several years after RAI therapy or subtotal thyroidectomy. Patients with thyrotoxic crisis have a high mortality rate despite treatment.

Subclinical hyperthyroidism generally subsides spontaneously. Progression to symptomatic thyrotoxicosis occurs at a rate of 1–2% per year in patients without a goiter and at a rate of 5% per year in patients with a multinodular goiter. Most patients do well without treatment and the serum TSH usually reverts to normal within 2 years. Most such patients do not have accelerated bone loss. However, if a baseline bone density shows significant osteopenia, bone densitometry may be performed periodically. In persons over age 60 years, serum TSH is suppressed (below 0.1 mIU/L) in 3% and mildly low (0.1–0.4 mIU/L) in 9%. The chance of developing atrial fibrillation is 2.8% yearly in elderly patients with a suppressed TSH and 1.1% yearly in those with mildly low TSH. Asymptomatic persons with very low serum TSH are monitored closely but are not treated unless atrial fibrillation or other manifestations of hyperthyroidism develop.

When to Admit

- Thyroid crisis.
- Hyperthyroidism-induced atrial fibrillation with severe tachycardia.
- Thyroidectomy.

Brancatella A et al. Management of thyrotoxicosis induced by PD1 or PD-L1 blockade. J Endocr Soc. 2021;5:bvab093. [PMID: 34337277]

Gronich N et al. Cancer risk after radioactive iodine treatment for hyperthyroidism: a cohort study. Thyroid. 2020;30:243. [PMID: 31880205]

Kahaly GJ. Management of Graves thyroidal and extrathyroidal disease: an update. J Clin Endocrinol Metab. 2020;105:3704. [PMID: 32929476]

McDermott MT. Hyperthyroidism. Ann Intern Med. 2020;172:ITC49 [PMID: 32252086]

Ylli D et al. Evaluation and treatment of amiodarone-induced thyroid disorders. J Clin Endocrinol Metab. 2021;106:226. [PMID: 33159436]

Yu W et al. Side effects of PTU and MMI in the treatment of hyperthyroidism: a systematic review and meta-analysis. Endocr Pract. 2020;26:207. [PMID: 31652102]

THYROID EYE DISEASE

General Considerations

Thyroid eye disease (Graves ophthalmopathy) is a syndrome of clinical and orbital imaging abnormalities caused by deposition of mucopolysaccharides and infiltration with chronic inflammatory cells of the orbital tissues, particularly the extraocular muscles. In patients with Graves disease, 20–40% have clinically apparent eye disease; about 5–10% of patients experience severe exophthalmos. The severity of eye disease is not closely correlated with the severity of thyrotoxicosis; clinical or laboratory evidence of thyroid dysfunction and thyroid antibodies may not be detectable at presentation or even on long-term follow-up, but their absence requires consideration of other disease entities.

Thyroid eye disease has an early inflammatory stage, typically lasting 18–36 months, where there is active lymphocytic infiltration into retrobulbar tissues. The active inflammatory stage then tends to evolve to a chronic, fibrotic, "burned out" stage in which treatment of the exophthalmos is medically resistant to glucocorticoid treatment. Aggravation of thyroid eye disease has occurred after ^{131}I treatment (see Radioactive iodine, above) or during therapy with thiazolidinediones (eg, pioglitazone); the presence of thyroid eye disease is a relative contraindication to ^{131}I treatment. Cigarette smoking increases the severity of thyroid eye disease, and ethanol injection of thyroid nodules have been reported to be followed by severe disease.

Clinical Findings

The primary clinical features of thyroid eye disease of any etiology include upper eyelid retraction, lid lag with downward gaze, and a staring appearance. There can be proptosis, conjunctival chemosis, episcleral inflammation, and weakness of upward gaze. Corneal drying may occur with inadequate lid closure. Eye changes may sometimes be asymmetric or unilateral. Resulting symptoms are cosmetic abnormalities and surface irritation. Patients with severe exophthalmos can experience diplopia from extraocular muscle entrapment and optic nerve compression, causing progressive loss of color vision, visual acuity, and visual fields (inferior especially).

Symptoms of active retrobulbar inflammation include (1) retrobulbar aching, (2) orbital inflammation and edema worse after recumbent sleep, (3) edematous or erythematous eyelids, (4) conjunctival redness or chemosis (edema), (5) recent progression in exophthalmos, (6) recent diplopia or strabismus, and (7) recent loss of visual acuity.

Exophthalmometry should be performed on all patients with Graves disease to document their degree of exophthalmos and detect progression of orbitopathy. The protrusion of the eye beyond the orbital rim is measured with a prism instrument (Hertel exophthalmometer). Maximum normal eye protrusion varies between kindreds and races, being about 24 mm for Black, 20 mm for White, and 18 mm for Asian patients.

The primary imaging features are enlargement of the extraocular muscles, usually affecting both orbits.

Differential Diagnosis

The clinical and imaging abnormalities of thyroid eye disease may be mimicked by congenital proptosis, asymmetry in orbital protrusion, or dural carotid-cavernous sinus fistula. Ocular myasthenia and thyroid eye disease are associated and may coexist, with the presence of ptosis rather than lid retraction being more characteristic of the former.

Treatment

General eye protective measures include wearing glasses to protect the protruding eye and taping the lids shut during sleep if corneal drying is a problem. Methylcellulose drops and gels ("artificial tears") may also help. Patients with mild thyroid eye disease may be treated with selenium 100 mcg orally twice daily, which may slow its progression.

The Mourits clinical activity score helps grade the severity of thyroid eye disease. Therapy in addition to selenium is warranted for active thyroid eye disease with a clinical activity point score greater than or equal to 3.

Therapy with intravenous pulse methylprednisolone, 500 mg weekly for 6 weeks, then 250 mg weekly for 6 weeks, begun promptly for active thyroid eye disease, is superior to oral prednisone. If oral prednisone is used, 40–60 mg daily with dosage reduction over several weeks must be given promptly. Higher initial daily prednisone doses of 80–120 mg are used when there is optic nerve compression.

Corticosteroid-resistant acute thyroid eye disease may be treated with monoclonal antibodies that reduce immune-mediated inflammation. Teprotumumab or tocilizumab is administered intravenously; rituximab may be given by retro-orbital injection.

Progressive active exophthalmos may be treated with retrobulbar radiation therapy over 2 weeks. Prednisone in high doses is given concurrently. Patients who respond well to orbital radiation include those with signs of acute inflammation, recent exophthalmos (less than 6 months), or optic nerve compression. Patients with chronic proptosis and orbital muscle restriction respond less well.

Diplopia should be treated conservatively (eg, with prisms) in the active stages of the disease and only by surgery when the disease has been static for at least 6 months. For severe cases, orbital decompression surgery may save vision, though diplopia often persists postoperatively. Tarsorrhaphy or canthoplasty can frequently help protect the cornea and provide improved appearance.

When to Refer

All patients with thyroid eye disease should be referred to an ophthalmologist, urgently if there is reduced vision.

Douglas RS et al. Teprotumumab for the treatment of active thyroid eye disease. N Engl J Med. 2020;382:341. [PMID: 31971679]

Pouso-Diz JM et al. Thyroid eye disease: current and potential medical management. Int Ophthalmol. 2020;40:1035. [PMID: 31919775]

Taylor PN et al. New insights into the pathogenesis and nonsurgical management of Graves orbitopathy. Nat Rev Endocrinol. 2020;16:104. [PMID: 31889140]

THYROID NODULES & MULTINODULAR GOITER

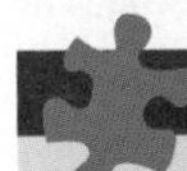

ESSENTIALS OF DIAGNOSIS

- Single or multiple thyroid nodules are commonly palpated by the patient or clinician or discovered incidentally on imaging studies.
- Thyroid function tests recommended.
- FNA cytology for thyroid nodules ≥ 1 cm or for smaller nodules when prior head-neck or chest-shoulder radiation.
- Ultrasound guidance improves FNA diagnosis for palpable and nonpalpable nodules.
- Clinical follow-up required.

General Considerations

Thyroid nodules are extremely common. Palpable nodules occur in 4–7% of all adults. They are much more common in women than men and become more prevalent with age. About 87% of palpable thyroid nodules (1 cm or larger) are benign adenomas, colloid nodules, or cysts, but some are primary thyroid malignancies or (less frequently) metastatic malignancy. On MRI, incidental small thyroid nodules are found in about 50% of adults. Thyroid nodules 1 cm or larger warrant follow-up and further testing for function and malignancy; an occasional smaller nodule requires follow-up if it has high-risk characteristics on ultrasound or if the patient is at high-risk for thyroid cancer due to prior head-neck radiation therapy during childhood.

Most patients with a thyroid nodule are euthyroid, but there is a high incidence of hypo- or hyperthyroidism. Patients with multiple thyroid nodules have the same overall risk of thyroid cancer as patients with solitary nodules. The risk of malignancy is also higher for large solitary nodules and if there is hoarseness or vocal fold paralysis, adherence to the trachea or strap muscles, cervical lymphadenopathy. The presence of autoimmune thyroiditis does not reduce the risk of malignancy; a nodule of 1 cm or larger in a gland with thyroiditis carries an 8% chance of malignancy.

Clinical Findings

Table 26–6 illustrates how to evaluate thyroid nodules based on the index of suspicion for malignancy.

A. Symptoms and Signs

Most small thyroid nodules cause no symptoms. They may sometimes be detected only by having the patient swallow during inspection and palpation of the thyroid.

A thyroid nodule or multinodular goiter can grow to become visible and of concern to the patient. Large nodular goiters can become a cosmetic embarrassment. Nodules can grow large enough to cause discomfort, hoarseness, or dysphagia. Nodules that cause ipsilateral recurrent laryngeal nerve palsy are more likely to be malignant. Retrosternal large multinodular goiters can cause dyspnea due to tracheal compression. Large substernal goiters may cause superior vena cava syndrome, manifested by facial erythema and jugular vein distention that progress to cyanosis and facial edema when both arms are kept raised over the head.

Table 26–6. Clinical evaluation of thyroid nodules.[1]

Clinical Evidence	Low Index of Suspicion	High Index of Suspicion
History	Family history of goiter; residence in area of endemic goiter	Previous therapeutic radiation of head, neck, or chest; hoarseness
Physical characteristics	Older women; soft nodule; multinodular goiter	Young adults, men; solitary, firm nodule; vocal fold paralysis; enlarged lymph nodes; distant metastatic lesions
Serum factors	High titer of thyroid peroxidase antibody; hypothyroidism; hyperthyroidism	Elevated serum calcitonin
Fine-needle aspiration biopsy	Colloid nodule or adenoma	Papillary carcinoma, follicular lesion, medullary or anaplastic carcinoma
Scanning techniques		
Uptake of ^{123}I	Hot nodule	Cold nodule
Ultrasonogram	Cystic lesion	Solid lesion
Radiograph	Shell-like calcification	Punctate calcification
Response to levothyroxine therapy	Regression after 0.05–0.1 mg/day for 6 months or more	Increase in size

[1]Clinically suspicious nodules should be evaluated with fine-needle aspiration biopsy.

Goiters and thyroid nodules may be associated with hypothyroidism (autoimmune thyroiditis, endemic goiter) or hyperthyroidism (Graves disease, toxic nodular goiter, subacute thyroiditis, and thyroid cancer with metastases).

B. Laboratory Findings

A serum TSH and FT_4 determine if the thyroid is hyperfunctioning. Patients with a subnormal serum TSH must have a radionuclide (^{123}I or ^{99m}Tc pertechnetate) thyroid scan to examine whether the nodule is hyperfunctioning; hyperfunctioning nodules are usually, but not always, benign. Serum calcitonin is obtained if a medullary thyroid carcinoma is suspected in a patient with a family history of medullary thyroid carcinoma or MEN types 2 or 3.

C. Imaging

Neck ultrasonography should be performed and is generally preferred over CT and MRI (see Fine-Needle Aspiration of Thyroid Nodules, below). CT scanning is helpful for larger thyroid nodules and multinodular goiter; it can determine the degree of tracheal compression and the degree of extension into the mediastinum. Thyroid nodules that are moderately to markedly hypoechoic are more likely to be malignant than nodules that are mildly hypoechoic. Nodules with heterogenous hypoechogenicity are also more likely to be malignant than nodules that hyperechoic.

RAI (^{123}I or ^{131}I) scans are not helpful for assessing whether a thyroid nodule is benign or malignant. Hyperfunctioning (hot) nodules are ordinarily benign (but may rarely be malignant). RAI uptake and scanning are helpful mainly for assessing the etiology of hyperthyroidism (eg, hyperfunctioning nodule).

D. Incidentally Discovered Thyroid Nodules

Thyroid nodules are frequently discovered as an incidental finding, with an incidence that depends on the imaging modality: ultrasound, 30%; MRI, 50%; CT, 13%; and ^{18}FDG-PET, 2%. When MRI, CT, and ^{18}FDG-PET detect a thyroid nodule, an ultrasound is performed to better determine the nodule's risk for malignancy and the need for FNA cytology, and to establish a baseline for ultrasound follow-up. The malignancy risk is about 13–17% for nodules discovered incidentally on CT, MRI, or ultrasound and 25–50% for nodules discovered incidentally by ^{18}FDG-PET. However, most such malignancies are very low grade. For incidentally discovered thyroid nodules of borderline concern, follow-up thyroid ultrasound in 3–6 months may be helpful; growing lesions should be assessed with FNA cytology or resected.

E. Fine-Needle Aspiration of Thyroid Nodules

FNA is the best method to assess a thyroid nodule for malignancy. FNA can be done while patients continue taking anticoagulants or aspirin. For multinodular goiters, the four largest nodules (1 cm or larger) are usually biopsied to minimize the risk of missing a malignancy.

Thyroid nodules are classified for malignancy risk according to their appearance on ultrasound. High-risk nodules (80% malignancy risk) have microcalcifications, irregular margins, extrathyroidal extension, extrusion of soft tissue into a calcified rim, or are taller than wide; such nodules require FNA if they are 1 cm or larger. Intermediate-risk nodules (15% malignancy risk) are hypoechoic and solid; they also usually require FNA if they are 1 cm or larger. Low-risk nodules (7% malignancy risk) are partially cystic with eccentric solid areas; they require biopsy if they are 1.5 cm or larger. Very low-risk nodules (below 3% malignancy risk) are those that are spongiform or simple cysts; FNA is optional if they are 2 cm or larger. Using ultrasound guidance for FNA biopsy improves the diagnostic accuracy for both palpable and nonpalpable thyroid nodules. FNA cytology is typically reported using The Bethesda System for Reporting Thyroid Cytopathology (TBSRTC), which divides results into six categories:

1. **Nondiagnostic or unsatisfactory:** The malignancy risk is 1–4%. The usual management is a repeat FNA under ultrasound guidance.
2. **Benign:** The malignancy risk is about 2.5%. The usual management is clinical follow-up with palpation or ultrasound at 6- to 18-month intervals.
3. **Atypia of undetermined significance (AUS):** The malignancy risk is about 14%, higher with sonographic features of malignancy. The usual management is clinical correlation and a repeat FNA.
4. **Suspicious for follicular neoplasm (SFN) or follicular neoplasm (FN):** The malignancy risk is about 25%, higher when Hürthle cells are present and in patients over age 50. The usual management is thyroid lobectomy.
5. **Suspicious for malignancy (SFM):** The malignancy risk is about 70%. The usual management is thyroid lobectomy or near-total thyroidectomy.
6. **Malignant:** The malignancy risk is about 99%. The usual management is a near-total thyroidectomy.

Surveillance and Treatment

All thyroid nodules, including those that are benign, need to be monitored by regular periodic palpation and ultrasound every 6 months initially. After several years of stability, yearly examinations are sufficient. Thyroid nodules should be rebiopsied if growth occurs. Excessive iodine intake should be minimized; a toxic multinodular goiter and hyperthyroidism may develop in patients who have had exposure to large amounts of iodine, either orally (eg, amiodarone) or intravenously (eg, radiographic contrast).

Patients with hyperthyroidism caused by thyroid nodules or multinodular goiter may be treated with propranolol, thioureas, surgery, or radioiodine.

A. Levothyroxine Suppression Therapy

Patients with nodules larger than 2 cm and elevated or normal TSH levels may be considered for TSH suppression with levothyroxine (starting doses of 50 mcg orally daily). Levothyroxine suppression therapy is not recommended if the serum TSH is low or for small benign thyroid nodules if the serum TSH level is normal. Levothyroxine suppression therapy is more successful in iodine-deficient areas.

Long-term levothyroxine suppression of TSH tends to keep nodules from enlarging but only 20% shrink more than 50%. Thyroid nodule size increased in 29% of patients treated with levothyroxine versus 56% of patients not receiving levothyroxine. Levothyroxine suppression also reduces the emergence of new nodules: 8% with levothyroxine and 29% without levothyroxine. Levothyroxine suppression therapy is not usually given to patients with ischemic heart disease, since it increases the risk for angina and atrial fibrillation.

Levothyroxine suppression needs to be carefully monitored, since it carries a 17% risk of inducing hyperthyroidism. All patients receiving levothyroxine suppression therapy should have serum TSH levels monitored at least annually, with the levothyroxine dose adjusted to keep the serum TSH mildly suppressed (between 0.1 mIU/L and 0.8 mIU/L).

B. Surgery

Total thyroidectomy is required for thyroid nodules that are malignant on FNA biopsy. More limited thyroid surgery is indicated for benign nodules with indeterminate or suspicious cytologic test results, compression symptoms, discomfort, or cosmetic embarrassment. Surgery may also be used to remove hyperfunctioning "hot" thyroid adenomas or toxic multinodular goiter causing hyperthyroidism.

C. Radiofrequency and Alcohol Ablation

Ultrasound-guided radiofrequency ablation is a therapeutic option for cytology-proven benign thyroid nodules that are 3 cm or larger and predominantly solid. Radiofrequency ablation shrinks such nodules by about 67% after 6 months, improving pressure symptoms and dysphagia in most patients and reducing the size of cosmetically embarrassing thyroid nodules. Side effects include mild neck discomfort, swelling, bruising, and dysphagia that generally resolves within 5 days. Radiofrequency ablation of thyroid nodules close to the vagus nerve may cause temporary vasovagal hypotension. Radiofrequency ablation–induced damage to the recurrent laryngeal nerve can cause hoarseness. Radiofrequency ablation–induced rupture of a thyroid nodule presents as acute neck swelling and pain; most such patients recover spontaneously, but some may require neck aspiration or surgical incision and drainage. Ultrasound-guided alcohol ablation can be useful for predominantly cystic thyroid nodules that are unassociated with Graves disease. However, recurrence is common.

D. Radioiodine (^{131}I) Therapy

^{131}I is a treatment option for hyperthyroid patients with toxic thyroid adenomas, multinodular goiter, or Graves disease. See **Precautions** for RAI use, above. Therapy with ^{131}I shrinks benign nontoxic thyroid nodules by an average of 40% by 1 year and 59% by 2 years after ^{131}I therapy. Nodules that shrink after ^{131}I therapy generally remain palpable and become firmer; they may develop unusual cytologic characteristics on FNA biopsy. ^{131}I therapy may be used to shrink large multinodular goiters but may rarely induce Graves disease. Hypothyroidism may occur years after ^{131}I therapy; it is advisable to assess thyroid function every 3 months for the first year, every 6 months thereafter, and immediately for symptoms of hypo- or hyperthyroidism.

Prognosis

Benign thyroid nodules may involute but usually persist or grow slowly. About 90% of thyroid nodules will increase their volume by 15% or more over 5 years. Growth is more common with multinodular goiter and larger nodules and in men; nodules are less likely to grow when they are solitary or cystic and when patients are over age 60. Cytologically benign nodules that grow are unlikely to be malignant; in one series, only 1 of 78 rebiopsied nodules was found to be malignant. Patients with very small (less than 1 cm), incidentally discovered, nonpalpable thyroid nodules that have a benign ultrasound appearance require no FNA cytology and only yearly palpation and clinical follow-up, whereas such small nodules that have a slightly suspicious ultrasound appearance may require FNA cytology or thyroid ultrasound every 1–2 years.

Le JY et al. Ultrasound malignancy risk stratification of thyroid nodules based on the degree of hypoechogenicity and echotexture. Eur Radiol. 2020;30:1653. [PMID: 31732777]

Maxwell C et al. Clinical diagnostic evaluation of thyroid nodules. Endocrinol Metab Clin North Am. 2019;48:61. [PMID: 30717911]

THYROID CANCER

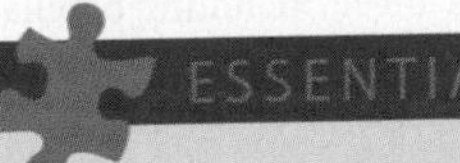

ESSENTIALS OF DIAGNOSIS

- Painless swelling in region of thyroid.
- Thyroid function tests are usually normal.
- Possible history of childhood irradiation to head and neck region.
- Positive thyroid FNA cytology.

General Considerations

The incidence of thyroid cancer in the United States is 53,000/year and increasing annually, probably as a result of the wider use of ultrasound, CT, MRI, and PET that may detect small thyroid malignancies. Thyroid cancer mortality has been stable, accounting for about 2000 deaths in the United States annually. The incidence of differentiated (papillary and follicular) thyroid carcinomas increases with age (Table 26–7) with a 3:1 female:male ratio. In routine autopsy series, thyroid papillary microcarcinoma (10 mm or smaller) is found with the surprising frequency of 11.5%. Most thyroid cancers remain microscopic and indolent. However, larger thyroid cancers (palpable or 1 cm or larger) are more malignant and require treatment.

Pure papillary (and mixed papillary-follicular) carcinoma comprises 80% of all thyroid cancers. It usually presents as a single thyroid nodule but can arise out of a multinodular goiter. Papillary thyroid carcinoma is commonly multifocal, with other foci usually arising de novo

Table 26–7. Some characteristics of thyroid cancer.

	Papillary	Follicular	Medullary	Anaplastic
Incidence	Most common	Common	Uncommon	Uncommon
Average age (years)	42	50	50	57
Females	70%	72%	56%	56%
Invasion				
Juxtanodal	+++++	+	++++++	+++
Blood vessels	+	+++	+++	+++++
Distant sites	+	+++	++	++++
^{123}I uptake	+	++++	0	0
10-year disease-specific survival	97%	92%	78%	7.3%

rather than a result of intraglandular metastases. The tumor involves both lobes in 30% of patients.

Papillary thyroid carcinoma is the least aggressive thyroid malignancy. It tends to grow slowly and often remains confined to the thyroid and regional lymph nodes for years. In about 80% of patients, there are microscopic metastases to cervical lymph nodes. The malignancy may become more aggressive in patients over age 45 years and most particularly in older adults. The cancer may invade the trachea and local muscles and spread to the lungs.

Childhood exposure to head and neck radiation therapy poses a particular threat because of an increased lifetime risk of developing thyroid cancer, including papillary carcinoma. These cancers may emerge 10–40 years after exposure, with a peak occurrence 20–25 years later.

Papillary thyroid carcinoma can occur in familial syndromes as an autosomal dominant trait, caused by loss of various tumor suppressor genes.

Microscopic "micropapillary" carcinoma (1 mm or smaller and invisible on thyroid ultrasound) is a variant of normal, being found in 24% of thyroidectomies performed for benign thyroid disease. The overwhelming majority of these microscopic foci never become clinically significant. The surgical pathology report of such tiny papillary carcinomas does not warrant aggressive measures. All that may be required is yearly follow-up with palpation of the neck and mild TSH suppression by thyroxine.

Follicular thyroid carcinoma and its variants (eg, Hürthle cell carcinoma) account for about 14% of thyroid malignancies; follicular carcinomas are generally more aggressive than papillary carcinomas. Most absorb iodine, making diagnostic scanning and treatment with ^{131}I after total thyroidectomy possible. Poorly differentiated and Hürthle cell (oncocytic) variants are associated with a high risk of metastasis and recurrence and do not take up RAI.

Medullary thyroid carcinoma represents 2–3% of thyroid cancers. They arise from thyroid parafollicular cells that can secrete calcitonin, prostaglandins, serotonin, ACTH, CRH, and other peptides that may cause symptoms and can be used as tumor markers. About one-third are sporadic, one-third are familial, and one-third are associated with MEN type 2A or 2B. Medullary thyroid carcinoma is often caused by an activating mutation of the *ret* protooncogene on chromosome 10. Mutation analysis of the *ret* protooncogene exons 10, 11, 13, 14, and 16 detects most mutations causing MEN 2A and MEN 2B and the mutations causing familial medullary thyroid carcinoma. Discovery of a medullary thyroid carcinoma makes genetic analysis mandatory.

Anaplastic thyroid carcinoma represents about 2% of thyroid cancers. It is the most aggressive thyroid carcinoma and metastasizes early to surrounding nodes and distant sites. It usually presents in an older patient as a rapidly enlarging mass in a multinodular goiter. This tumor does not concentrate iodine, which precludes the therapeutic use of RAI.

Other thyroid malignancies represent about 3% of thyroid cancers. Primary thyroid lymphomas are most commonly diffuse large B-cell lymphomas (50%), mucosa-associated lymphoid tissue lymphoma (23%), or mixed type; other types include follicular, small lymphocytic, and Burkitt lymphoma and Hodgkin disease. Cancers may sometimes metastasize to the thyroid, particularly bronchogenic, breast, renal carcinoma, and melanoma.

Clinical Findings

A. Symptoms and Signs

Thyroid carcinoma usually presents as a palpable, firm, nontender thyroid nodule. Most thyroid carcinomas are asymptomatic, but large thyroid cancers can cause neck discomfort, dysphagia, or hoarseness (due to pressure on the recurrent laryngeal nerve). **Papillary thyroid cancer** presents with palpable lymph node involvement in 10%; it may invade the trachea and local muscles. Occult metastases to the lung occur in 10–15%. **Follicular thyroid carcinoma** commonly metastasizes to neck nodes, bones, and lung, but nearly every organ can be involved.

Medullary thyroid carcinoma typically metastases to local nodes and adjacent muscle and trachea as well as mediastinal lymph nodes. Metastases may appear in the bones, lungs, adrenals, or liver. It frequently causes flushing and diarrhea (30%), which may be the initial clinical features. Cushing syndrome develops in 5% of patients from tumor secretion of ACTH or CRH.

Anaplastic thyroid carcinoma is more apt to be advanced at the time of diagnosis, presenting with signs of pressure or invasion of surrounding tissue, resulting in dysphagia, hoarseness, or recurrent laryngeal nerve palsy or dyspnea due to lung metastases.

B. Laboratory Findings

FNA biopsy is discussed in Thyroid Nodules, above. Thyroid function tests are generally normal unless there is concomitant thyroiditis. However, with a heavy tumor burden, functioning follicular or papillary thyroid carcinomas can sometimes secrete enough thyroid hormone to produce thyrotoxicosis and suppress the serum TSH.

Serum thyroglobulin is high in most metastatic papillary and follicular tumors, making this a useful marker for recurrent or metastatic disease. Caution must be exercised for the following reasons: (1) Circulating Tg Ab can cause erroneous thyroglobulin determinations. However, declining levels of Tg Ab are a good prognostic sign after treatment. (2) Thyroglobulin levels may be misleadingly elevated in thyroiditis, which often coexists with carcinoma. (3) Certain thyroglobulin assays falsely report the continued presence of thyroglobulin after total thyroidectomy and tumor resection, causing undue concern about possible metastases.

Serum calcitonin is usually elevated in medullary thyroid carcinoma, making this a marker for metastatic disease. Serum calcitonin may be elevated in thyroiditis; pregnancy; kidney disease; hypergastrinemia; hypercalcemia; and other malignancies, particularly neuroendocrine tumors (including pheochromocytomas, carcinoid tumors) and carcinomas of the lung, pancreas, breast, and colon. Serum calcitonin and carcinoembryonic antigen (CEA) determinations should be obtained before surgery, then regularly in postoperative follow-up: every 4 months for 5 years, then every 6 months for life. Serum calcitonin levels greater than 250 ng/L (73 pmol/L) or rising levels of calcitonin are the best indication of recurrence or metastatic disease. Serum CEA levels also are elevated with medullary thyroid carcinoma but are not specific for this cancer.

C. Imaging

1. Ultrasound of the neck—Ultrasound of the neck should be performed on all patients with thyroid cancer for the initial diagnosis and for follow-up. Ultrasound is useful in determining the size and location of the malignancy as well as the location of any neck metastases.

2. Radioactive iodine scanning—RAI (^{131}I or ^{123}I) thyroid and whole-body scanning is used after thyroidectomy for differentiated thyroid cancer utilizing the protocol described later. (See Radioactive Iodine (^{131}I) Therapy for Differentiated Thyroid Cancer, below.) Medullary thyroid cancer does not avidly uptake RAI.

3. CT and MRI scanning—CT scanning may demonstrate metastases and is particularly useful for localizing and monitoring lung metastases but is less sensitive than ultrasound for detecting metastases within the neck. Medullary carcinoma in the thyroid, nodes, and liver may calcify, but lung metastases rarely do so. MRI is particularly useful for imaging bone metastases.

4. PET scanning—PET scanning is especially helpful for detecting thyroid cancer metastases that do not have sufficient iodine uptake to be visible on RAI scans. Thyroid cancer metastases may be detected with ^{18}FDG-PET whole-body scanning. The sensitivity of ^{18}FDG-PET scanning for differentiated thyroid cancer is enhanced if the patient is hypothyroid or receiving thyrotropin, which increases the metabolic activity of differentiated thyroid cancer. Patients with medullary thyroid cancer are monitored with MRI and ^{18}FDG PET/CT scanning. ^{68}Ga-DOTATATE-PET imaging is superior for detecting medullary thyroid cancer metastases in certain patients, particularly those with very high serum calcitonin levels (above 500 pg/mL). Although ^{68}Ga-DOTATATE-PET is more specific for neuroendocrine tumors, other malignancies express somatostatin receptors and can have misleading uptake on this scan, including non-Hodgkin lymphoma, meningioma, breast cancer, thyroid adenoma, and papillary thyroid carcinoma.

Differential Diagnosis

Head-neck RAI uptake is seen in normal thyroid, salivary glands, nasal mucosa, thyroglossal duct remnants, and sinusitis.

Negative RAI scans are common in early metastatic differentiated thyroid carcinoma. Negative RAI scans also occur frequently with advanced metastatic thyroid carcinoma, making it difficult to detect and to distinguish from nonthyroidal neoplasms. An elevated serum thyroglobulin in patients with a negative RAI scan should arouse suspicion for metastases that are not avid for RAI. Medullary thyroid carcinoma does not concentrate iodine.

Complications

Hyperthyroidism can develop in patients with a heavy tumor burden. One-third of medullary thyroid carcinomas secrete serotonin and prostaglandins, producing flushing and diarrhea. The management of patients with medullary carcinomas may be complicated by the coexistence of pheochromocytomas or hyperparathyroidism.

Treatment of Differentiated Thyroid Carcinoma

A. Surgical Treatment

Surgical removal is the treatment of choice for thyroid carcinomas. Neck ultrasound is obtained preoperatively, since suspicious cervical lymphadenopathy is detected in about 25%.

For papillary and follicular thyroid carcinoma smaller than 1 cm, surgery involves lobectomy alone in patients under age 45 years who have no history of head and neck irradiation and no evidence of lymph node metastasis on ultrasonography. Other patients should have a total or near total thyroidectomy.

For differentiated papillary and follicular carcinoma larger than 1 cm or with evidence of metastases, a total thyroidectomy is performed with limited removal of cervical lymph nodes. Surgery consists of a thyroid lobectomy for an indeterminate "follicular lesion" that is 4 cm or smaller. For indeterminate follicular lesions larger than 4 cm that are at higher risk for being malignant, a bilateral thyroidectomy is performed as the initial surgery.

The advantage of near-total thyroidectomy for differentiated thyroid carcinoma is that multicentric foci of carcinoma are more apt to be resected. Also, there is less normal thyroid tissue to compete with uptake of residual cancer of ^{131}I administered later for scans or treatment. A central neck lymph node dissection is performed at the time of thyroidectomy for patients with nodal metastases that are clinically evident. A lateral neck dissection is performed for patients with biopsy-proven lateral cervical lymphadenopathy. Levothyroxine, 0.05–0.1 mg orally daily, is begun immediately postoperatively. About 2–4 months after surgery, patients require reevaluation and often ^{131}I therapy.

Following surgical resection, permanent injury to one recurrent laryngeal nerve (rarely both) occurs in 1–7% of patients, temporary laryngeal nerve palsies in 5%, and hypoparathyroidism (usually temorary) in 20%. Thyroidectomy requires at least an overnight hospital admission, since late bleeding, airway problems, and tetany can occur. *Ambulatory thyroidectomy is potentially dangerous and should not be done.* Following surgery, staging (Table 26–8) should be done to help determine prognosis and to plan therapy and follow-up.

In pregnant women with thyroid cancer, surgery is usually delayed until after delivery, except for fast-growing tumors that may be resected after 24 weeks' gestation; there has been no difference in survival or tumor recurrence rates in women who underwent surgery during or after their pregnancy. Differentiated thyroid carcinoma does not behave more aggressively during pregnancy. However, compared to nonpregnant women, there is a higher risk of complications in pregnant women undergoing thyroid surgery.

Table 26–8. Staging and prognosis for patients with papillary thyroid carcinoma using MACIS scoring.

Total Score[1] - Stage	Percentage of Patients with Papillary Thyroid Carcinoma	20-Year Survival
< 6.0 = Stage I	74.2%	96–99%
6.0–6.99 = Stage II	8.5%	68–89%
7.0–7.99 = Stage III	9.2%	55–56%
≥ 8.0 = Stage IV	8.1%	17–24%

[1]Total score = 3.1 (if aged ≤ 39 years) *or* 0.08 × age (if aged ≥ 40 years) + 0.3 × tumor size (cm), + 1 (if incompletely resected), + 1 (if locally invasive), + 3 (if distant metastases).
MACIS, metastases, age, complete resection, invasion, size.

B. Active Surveillance for Papillary Thyroid Microcarcinoma

Most papillary thyroid microcarcinomas that are less than 1 cm are indolent with an excellent prognosis. Conservative management therefore may be warranted for patients who have a limited life expectancy, a high surgical risk, or very low-risk tumors. Surveillance protocol used in some medical centers consists of clinical examination and neck ultrasound every 6 months.

C. Levothyroxine Suppression of TSH

Levothyroxine is prescribed for differentiated thyroid cancer in doses to achieve a target serum TSH: (1) For initial TSH suppression in patients with stage II–IV disease, the target serum TSH is below 0.1 mIU/L while avoiding clinical hyperthyroidism. (2) For initial TSH suppression in patients with stage I disease and for 5–10 years after remission in previously stage II–IV patients, the target TSH is between 0.1 and 0.5 mIU/L. (3) For patients who are free of disease and at low risk for recurrence, the target TSH is 0.5–2 mIU/L.

D. Radioactive Iodine (^{131}I) Therapy for Differentiated Thyroid Cancer

Following thyroidectomy ^{131}I therapy is recommended for two indications: (1) ablation of thyroid remnants in patients at high risk for recurrence and (2) treatment of metastatic thyroid cancer. ^{131}I is usually administered 2–4 months after surgery. However, the indications and optimal activity (dose) for ^{131}I therapy for differentiated thyroid cancer remain controversial, since the prognosis for most patients is overwhelmingly good.

Before receiving ^{131}I therapy, patients should follow a low-iodine diet for at least 2 weeks. Patients must not be given amiodarone or intravenous radiologic contrast dyes containing iodine. Despite restriction of dietary iodine, differentiated thyroid cancer frequently lacks sufficient RAI avidity to allow RAI therapy.

1. RAI thyroid remnant ablation—A low activity[1] of 30 mCi (1.1 GBq) ^{131}I is sometimes given for "remnant ablation" of residual normal thyroid tissue after surgery for differentiated thyroid cancer in patients without known metastases. However, ^{131}I remnant ablation is not required for patients with low-risk stage I papillary thyroid carcinomas or carcinomas that are smaller than 1 cm (whether unifocal or multifocal), except for patients with unfavorable histopathology (tall-cell, columnar cell, insular cell, Hürthle cell, or diffuse sclerosing subtypes).

2. RAI treatment of metastases—Therapy with ^{131}I improves survival and reduces recurrence rates of differentiated thyroid cancer for patients with stage III–IV cancer

[1]The amount of RAI radioactivity given in a procedure is referred to as radioactivity or "activity" and is expressed as Curies (Ci) or Becquerels (Bq), whereas the term "dose" is reserved to describe the amount of radiation absorbed by a given organ or tumor and is expressed as Gray (Gy) or radiation-absorbed dose (RAD).

and those with stage II cancer having gross extrathyroidal extension. RAI therapy is also given to patients with stage II cancer who have distant metastases, a primary tumor larger than 4 cm, or primary tumors 1–4 cm with lymph node metastases or other high-risk features. Brain metastases do not usually respond to ^{131}I and are best resected or treated with gamma knife radiosurgery. About 70% of small lung metastases resolve following ^{131}I therapy; however, larger pulmonary metastases have only a 10% remission rate.

Staging with RAI scanning or ^{18}FDG-PET/CT scanning assists with determining the activity of ^{131}I to be administered. Patients with differentiated thyroid carcinoma who have little or no uptake of RAI into metastases (about 35% of cases) should not be treated with ^{131}I. Patients with asymptomatic, stable, RAI-resistant metastases should receive levothyroxine to suppress serum TSH and should be carefully monitored for tumor progression.

Some patients have elevated serum thyroglobulin levels but a negative whole-body RAI scan and a negative neck ultrasound. In such patients, an ^{18}F-FDG PET/CT scan is obtained. If all scans are negative, the patient has a good prognosis and empiric therapy with ^{131}I is not useful.

3. Recombinant human TSH (rhTSH)-stimulated ^{131}I therapy—Recombinant human thyroid-stimulating hormone (rhTSH, Thyrogen) can be given to increase the sensitivity of serum thyroglobulin for residual cancer and to increase the uptake of ^{131}I into residual thyroid tissue (thyroid remnant "ablation") or cancer.

Thyrogen should not be administered to patients with an intact thyroid gland because it can cause severe thyroid swelling and hyperthyroidism. Hyperthyroidism can also occur in patients with significant metastases or residual normal thyroid. Other side effects include nausea (11%) and headache (7%). Thyrotropin has caused neurologic deterioration in 7% of patients with CNS metastases.

4. Thyroid-withdrawal stimulated ^{131}I therapy—Thyroid withdrawal is sometimes used because of its lower cost than rhTSH, despite the discomforts of becoming hypothyroid. Levothyroxine is withdrawn for 14 days and the patient is allowed to become hypothyroid; high levels of endogenous TSH stimulate the uptake of RAI and production of thyroglobulin by thyroid cancer or residual thyroid. Just prior to ^{131}I therapy, the following blood tests are obtained: serum TSH to confirm it is greater than 30 mU/L, serum hCG in reproductive-age women to screen for pregnancy, and serum thyroglobulin as a tumor marker. Three days after ^{131}I therapy, levothyroxine therapy may be resumed at full replacement dose.

5. Side effects from ^{131}I therapy—National Cancer Institute surveillance data of patients with differentiated thyroid cancer, treated with only surgery, have a 5% increased risk of developing a second non-thyroid malignancy. Patients with thyroid cancer who also receive ^{131}I therapy have a further increased risk of developing a second non-thyroid malignancy (especially leukemia and lymphoma). The risk of second cancers peaks about 5 years following ^{131}I therapy.

^{131}I therapy can cause gastritis, temporary oligospermia, sialadenitis, and xerostomia. Radioiodine therapy can cause neurologic decompensation in patients with thyroid brain metastases; such patients are treated with prednisone 30–40 mg orally daily for several days before and after ^{131}I therapy. Cumulative doses of ^{131}I over 500 mCi (18.5 GBq) can cause infertility, pancytopenia (4%), leukemia (0.3%), and pulmonary fibrosis.

E. Other Therapies for Differentiated Thyroid Cancer

Patients with osteolytic metastases to bone from differentiated thyroid cancer may be treated with one of two anti-bone resorptive drugs: (1) zoledronic acid, 4 mg intravenously; or (2) denosumab, 120 mg subcutaneously. These drugs must be used judiciously; there is an increased risk of atypical femur fractures and osteonecrosis of the jaw with prolonged therapy with either drug.

Patients with aggressive differentiated thyroid cancers may have metastases that are refractory to ^{131}I therapy. Recurrence in the neck may be treated with surgical debulking and external beam radiation therapy. Patients with RAI-refractory differentiated thyroid cancer metastases that are advanced and rapidly progressive may be treated with tyrosine kinase inhibitors.

Treatment of Other Thyroid Malignancies

Medullary thyroid carcinoma is best treated with surgery for the primary tumor and metastases. Patients with a *ret* protooncogene mutation should have a prophylactic total thyroidectomy, ideally by age 6 years (MEN 2A) or at age 6 months (MEN 2B). Medullary thyroid carcinoma does not respond to ^{131}I therapy or chemotherapy. Patients should be monitored closely, with serum calcitonin levels checked about every 3 months. Since medullary thyroid carcinoma can be indolent, patients should be considered for chemotherapy only if they have rapidly progressive metastases, as evidenced by a doubling time of serum calcitonin or CEA doubling time less than 2 years. ^{177}Lu-DOTATATE peptide receptor radionuclide therapy (PRRT, Lutathera) is an option for patients with progressive medullary thyroid carcinoma metastases that are very avid for ^{68}Ga-DOTATATE on diagnostic imaging or demonstrate SSTR2a receptor expression on immunohistochemical staining. Vandetanib and cabozantinib are approved for use against rapidly progressive metastatic medullary thyroid carcinoma; both require close observation to avoid toxicity. Patients with medullary thyroid carcinoma and diabetes should not receive diabetic therapy with glucagon-like peptide-1 (GLP-1) agonists because they may stimulate the growth of medullary thyroid carcinoma.

Anaplastic thyroid carcinoma is treated with local resection and radiation. It does not respond to ^{131}I therapy. Anaplastic thyroid cancers with mTOR mutations may be inhibited by everolimus. In patients with $BRAF^{V600E}$ mutant anaplastic thyroid cancer, combined BRAF and MEK inhibition with dabrafenib and trametinib has induced durable responses.

Thyroid mucosa-associated lymphoid tissue lymphomas have a low risk of recurrence after simple thyroidectomy. Patients with other thyroid lymphomas are best treated with external radiation therapy; chemotherapy is added for extensive lymphoma (Table 39–2).

External beam radiation therapy may be delivered to bone metastases, especially those that are without radioiodine uptake or are RAI-refractory. Local neck radiation therapy may also be given to patients with anaplastic thyroid carcinoma. Brain metastases can be treated with gamma knife radiosurgery.

Follow-Up

Most recurrences of differentiated thyroid carcinoma are within 5–10 years after thyroidectomy. All patients require at least a yearly thyroid ultrasound and serum thyroglobulin level (while taking levothyroxine). Patients at higher risk usually require at least two annual consecutively negative stimulated serum thyroglobulin determinations less than 1 ng/mL and normal RAI scans (if done) and neck ultrasound scans before they are considered to be in remission. The first surveillance occurs with stimulated postoperative serum thyroglobulin, ^{131}I therapy, and post-therapy scanning about 2–4 and 9–12 months after surgery. Serum thyroglobulin and RAI scanning are stimulated by either rhTSH or thyroid hormone withdrawal according to the protocols described above for ^{131}I treatment. Patients need not have repeated ^{131}I therapies if persistent RAI uptake is confined to the thyroid bed, neck ultrasounds appear normal, and stimulated serum thyroglobulin levels remain less than 2 ng/mL. Patients with differentiated thyroid carcinoma must be monitored long term for recurrent or metastatic disease. Further RAI or other scans may be required for patients with more aggressive differentiated thyroid cancer, prior metastases, rising serum thyroglobulin levels, or other evidence of metastases.

1. Levothyroxine suppression for differentiated thyroid cancer—Patients who have had a thyroidectomy for differentiated thyroid cancer must take levothyroxine replacement for life. Serum TSH should be suppressed below 0.1–0.5 mIU/L for low-risk patients with stage I disease, below 0.1 mIU/L for patients with stage II disease, and below 0.05 mIU/L for patients with stage III–IV disease. (See Table 26–8.)

Patients who are considered cured should nevertheless be treated with sufficient levothyroxine to keep the serum TSH less than 2 mIU/L. To achieve suppression of serum TSH, the levothyroxine dose required may be such that serum FT_4 levels may be slightly elevated; in that case, measurement of serum T_3 or free T_3 can be useful to ensure the patient is not frankly hyperthyroid. Thyrotoxicosis can be caused by over-replacement with levothyroxine or by the growth of functioning metastases. Patients receiving levothyroxine suppression therapy should have periodic bone densitometry.

2. Serum thyroglobulin—Thyroglobulin is produced by normal thyroid tissue and by most differentiated thyroid carcinomas. After a total or near-total thyroidectomy and ^{131}I remnant ablation, thyroglobulin becomes a useful marker for residual or metastatic tumor in for patients with differentiated papillary or follicular thyroid cancer, particularly for patients who do not have serum Tg Ab. In patients receiving levothyroxine following thyroidectomy (with TSH suppression), baseline thyroglobulin levels are insensitive for detection of residual or recurrent disease. Therefore, *stimulated* serum thyroglobulin measurements should be used. Following stimulation by either rhTSH or levothyroxine withdrawal, serum thyroglobulin levels 2 ng/mL or higher indicate the need for a repeat neck ultrasound and further scanning with RAI or ^{18}FDG-PET (see ^{131}I Treatment).

3. Neck ultrasound—Neck ultrasound should be used in all patients with thyroid carcinoma at 3 months postoperatively and regularly thereafter. Ultrasound is more sensitive for lymph node metastases than either CT or MRI scanning. Ultrasound-guided FNA biopsy should be performed on suspicious lesions.

4. Radioactive iodine (RAI: ^{131}I or ^{123}I) neck and whole-body scanning—Despite its limitations, RAI scanning has traditionally been used to detect metastatic differentiated thyroid cancer and to determine whether it is amenable to treatment with ^{131}I. RAI scanning is particularly useful for high-risk patients and those with persistent Tg Ab that make serum thyroglobulin determinations unreliable.

Following total or near-total thyroidectomy, about 65% of metastases are detectable by RAI scanning after optimal preparation. The combination of rhTSH-stimulated scanning and thyroglobulin levels detects a thyroid remnant or cancer with a sensitivity of 84%. The presence of Tg Ab renders the serum thyroglobulin determination uninterpretable. It is reasonable to perform a rhTSH-stimulated scan and thyroglobulin level 2–3 months after the initial neck surgery. If the scan is negative and the serum thyroglobulin is less than 2 ng/mL, low-risk patients may not require further scanning but should continue to be monitored with neck ultrasound and serum thyroglobulin levels every 6–12 months. In about 21% of low-risk patients, rhTSH stimulates serum thyroglobulin to above 2 ng/mL; such patients have a 23% risk of local neck metastases and a 13% risk of distant metastases. The rhTSH-stimulated RAI neck and whole-body scan detects only about half of these metastases because they are small or not avid for iodine. For higher-risk patients, the rhTSH-stimulated thyroglobulin and RAI scan may be repeated about 1 year after surgery and then again if warranted.

Some patients have persistent RAI uptake in the neck on diagnostic scanning but have no visible tumor on neck ultrasound; such patients do not require additional RAI therapy, especially if the serum thyroglobulin level is very low.

5. Positron emission tomography scanning—^{18}FDG-PET scanning is particularly useful for detecting differentiated thyroid cancer metastases in patients with a detectable serum thyroglobulin (especially serum thyroglobulin levels greater than 10 ng/mL and rising) who have a normal whole-body RAI scan and an unrevealing neck ultrasound. It is also sensitive for detecting metastases from medullary thyroid carcinoma. ^{18}FDG-PET scanning can be combined with a CT scan; the resultant ^{18}FDG-PET/CT fusion scan is

60% sensitive for detecting metastases that are not visible by other methods. This scan is less sensitive for small brain metastases.

^{68}Ga-DOTATATE-PET scanning is useful for staging patients with medullary thyroid carcinoma. It is also useful to determine whether a patient can be treated with PRRT.

6. Other scanning—Thallium-201 (^{201}Tl) scans may be useful for detecting metastatic differentiated thyroid carcinoma when the ^{131}I scan is normal but serum thyroglobulin is elevated. MRI scanning is particularly useful for imaging metastases in the brain, mediastinum, or bones. CT scanning is useful for imaging and monitoring pulmonary metastases.

Prognosis

1. Papillary thyroid carcinoma—This cancer has an overall mortality rate of 3%. It is best staged using the MACIS (metastasis, age, completeness of resection, invasion, size) scoring system (Table 26–8). ^{18}FDG-PET scanning independently predicts survival. Unlike other forms of cancer, patients with papillary thyroid carcinoma who have palpable lymph node metastases do not have a particularly increased mortality rate; however, their risk of local recurrence is increased. The following characteristics imply a worse prognosis: age over 45 years, male sex, bone or brain metastases, macronodular (greater than 1 cm) pulmonary metastases, and lack of ^{131}I uptake into metastases. The best prognosis has been with the follicular variant of papillary thyroid cancer.

2. Follicular thyroid carcinoma—The mortality rate of follicular thyroid carcinoma is 3.4 times higher than that of papillary carcinoma. Both follicular carcinoma and its more aggressive Hürthle cell variant tend to present at a more advanced stage than papillary carcinoma. Patients with primary tumors larger than 1 cm who undergo limited thyroid surgery (subtotal thyroidectomy or lobectomy) have a 2.2-fold increased mortality over those having total or near-total thyroidectomies. Patients who have not received ^{131}I ablation have mortality rates that are increased twofold by 10 years and threefold by 25 years (over those who have received ablation). The risk of cancer recurrence is twofold higher in men than in women and 1.7-fold higher in multifocal than in unifocal tumors.

Patients with a normal ^{18}FDG-PET scan have a 98% 5-year survival. Five-year survival is 95% with local metastases, 70% with regional (supraclavicular, mediastinal) metastases, and 35% with distant metastases.

3. Medullary thyroid carcinoma—This cancer is more aggressive than differentiated thyroid cancer but is typically indolent. However, medullary thyroid carcinoma with a somatic *RET* codon M918T mutation has a poorer prognosis. The overall 10-year survival rate is 90% when the tumor is confined to the thyroid, 70% for those with metastases to cervical lymph nodes, and 20% for those with distant metastases. When postoperative serum calcitonin levels are above 500 pg/mL (146 pmol/L), distant metastases are likely. Patients with metastatic medullary thyroid carcinoma whose serum calcitonin doubling time is over 2 years also have a relatively good prognosis.

4. Other thyroid carcinomas—**Lymphoma** has a 5-year survival of nearly 100% if localized and 63% if there is extension beyond the thyroid. **Anaplastic thyroid carcinoma** carries a 1-year survival rate of 10% and a 5-year survival rate of 5%.

Grani G et al. Contemporary thyroid nodule evaluation and management. J Clin Endocrinol Metab. 2020;105:2869. [PMID: 32491169]

Grossrubatscher E et al. Advances in the management of medullary thyroid carcinoma: focus on peptide receptor radionuclide therapy. J Clin Med. 2020;9:3507. [PMID: 33138305]

Schlumberger M et al. Current practice in patients with differentiated thyroid cancer. Nat Rev Endocrinol. 2021;17:176. [PMID: 33339988]

Singh Ospina N et al. Thyroid nodules: diagnostic evaluation based on thyroid cancer risk assessment. BMJ. 2020;368:l6670. [PMID: 31911452]

Tiedje V et al. Therapeutic breakthroughs for metastatic thyroid cancer. Nat Rev Endocrinol. 2020;16:77. [PMID: 31819229]

Zhang C et al. Total thyroidectomy versus lobectomy for papillary thyroid cancer: a systematic review and meta-analysis. Medicine (Baltimore). 2020;99:e19073. [PMID: 32028431]

IODINE DEFICIENCY DISORDER & ENDEMIC GOITER

ESSENTIALS OF DIAGNOSIS

- Common in regions with low-iodine diets.
- High rate of congenital hypothyroidism and cretinism.
- Goiters may become multinodular and enlarge.
- Most adults with endemic goiter are euthyroid; however, some are hypo- or hyperthyroid.

General Considerations

Moderate iodine deficiency during gestation and infancy can cause manifestations of hypothyroidism, deafness, and short stature and lower a child's intelligence quotient by 10–15 points. Even mild-to-moderate iodine deficiency appears to impair a child's perceptual reasoning and global cognitive index. Severe iodine deficiency increases the risk of miscarriage and stillbirth. Cretinism occurs in about 0.5% of live births in iodine-deficient areas.

Although iodine deficiency is the most common cause of endemic goiter, there are other natural goitrogens, including certain foods (eg, sorghum, millet, maize, cassava), mineral deficiencies (selenium, iron, zinc), and water pollutants, which can themselves cause goiter or aggravate a goiter proclivity caused by iodine deficiency. In iodine-deficient patients, cigarette smoking can induce goiter growth. Pregnancy aggravates iodine deficiency. Some individuals are particularly susceptible to goiter owing to congenital partial defects in thyroid enzyme activity.

Clinical Findings

A. Symptoms and Signs

Endemic goiters may become multinodular and very large. Growth often occurs during pregnancy, increasing the size of thyroid nodules and causing new nodules; compressive symptoms may occur.

Substernal goiters are usually asymptomatic but can cause tracheal compression, respiratory distress, dysphagia, superior vena cava syndrome, palsies of the phrenic or recurrent laryngeal nerves, or Horner syndrome. The incidence of significant malignancy is less than 1%.

Some patients with endemic goiter may become hypothyroid. Others may become thyrotoxic as the goiter grows and becomes more autonomous, especially if iodine is added to the diet.

B. Laboratory Findings

The serum T_4 and TSH are generally normal. TSH is low in hyperthyroidism if a multinodular goiter has become autonomous and there is sufficient iodine for thyroid hormone synthesis. TSH increases with hypothyroidism. Thyroid RAI uptake is usually elevated, but it may be normal if iodine intake has improved. Serum antithyroid antibodies are usually either undetectable or in low titers. Serum thyroglobulin is often elevated above 13 mcg/L.

Differential Diagnosis

Endemic goiter must be distinguished from other forms of nodular goiter that may coexist in an endemic region.

Prevention

The daily minimum dietary requirement for iodine is 150 mcg daily in nonpregnant adults and 250 mcg daily for pregnant or lactating women. Iodized salt contains iodine at about 20 mg per kg salt. Other sources of iodine include commercial bread, milk, and seafood. Initiating iodine supplementation in an iodine-deficient area greatly reduces the emergence of new goiters but causes an increased frequency of hyperthyroidism during the first year.

Treatment

Most patients with iodine-deficient goiter are euthyroid. Dietary iodine supplementation is recommended to avoid hypothyroidism but has proven ineffective in shrinking such goiters. Thyroidectomy may be required for cosmesis, compressive symptoms, or thyrotoxicosis. There is a high goiter recurrence rate in iodine-deficient geographic areas, so near-total thyroidectomy is preferred when surgery is indicated.

Complications

Dietary iodine supplementation increases the risk of autoimmune thyroid dysfunction, which may cause hypo- or hyperthyroidism. High-dose iodine supplementation may precipitate thyrotoxicosis. Suppression of TSH by administering levothyroxine carries the risk of inducing hyperthyroidism, particularly in patients with autonomous multinodular goiters. Levothyroxine suppression should not be started in patients with a low TSH level. Treating patients with ^{131}I for large multinodular goiter may shrink the gland; however, Graves disease develops in some patients 3–10 months following therapy.

Dineva M et al. Systematic review and meta-analysis of the effects of iodine supplementation on thyroid function and child neurodevelopment in mildly-to-moderately iodine deficient pregnant women. Am J Clin Nutr. 2020;112:389. [PMID: 32320029]

DISEASES OF THE PARATHYROIDS

HYPOPARATHYROIDISM & PSEUDOHYPOPARATHYROIDISM

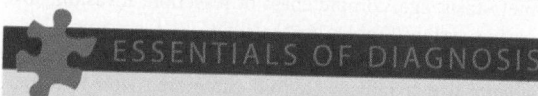

- Tetany, carpopedal spasms, tingling of lips and hands, muscle cramps, irritability.
- Chvostek sign and Trousseau phenomenon.
- Hypocalcemia with low serum PTH; serum phosphate high; alkaline phosphatase normal; urine calcium excretion reduced.
- Serum magnesium may be low.

General Considerations

Acquired hypoparathyroidism is most commonly caused by anterior neck surgery, occurring after total thyroidectomy in about 25% of patients transiently, and in about 4% of patients permanently. The risk of permanent postoperative hypoparathyroidism can be reduced during thyroid surgery by taking parathyroid glands with suspected vascular damage and autotransplanting them into the sternocleidomastoid muscle. Permanent hypoparathyroidism may occur after the resection of multiple parathyroid adenomas.

Transient hypothyroidism may occur after surgical removal of a single parathyroid adenoma for primary hyperparathyroidism due to suppression of the remaining normal parathyroids and accelerated remineralization of the skeleton ("hungry bone syndrome").

All patients undergoing thyroidectomy or parathyroidectomy must be observed closely overnight. Hypocalcemia can be quite severe, particularly in patients with preoperative hyperparathyroid bone disease and vitamin D or magnesium deficiency.

Autoimmune hypoparathyroidism may be isolated or combined with other endocrine deficiencies. Autoimmune polyendocrine syndrome type I (APS-I) is also known as autoimmune polyendocrinopathy-candidiasis-ectodermal dystrophy (APECED). Hypoparathyroidism can also occur in SLE caused by antiparathyroid antibodies.

Parathyroid deficiency may also be the result of damage from heavy metals such as copper (Wilson disease) or iron (hemochromatosis, transfusion hemosiderosis), granulomas, Riedel thyroiditis, tumors, infection, and neck irradiation.

Magnesium deficiency causes functional hypoparathyroidism. Although mild hypomagnesemia stimulates PTH secretion, more profound hypomagnesemia (below 1.2 mg/dL) inhibits PTH secretion. Hypomagnesemia also causes resistance to PTH in bone and renal tubules. Correction of hypomagnesemia results in rapid disappearance of the condition. **Hypermagnesemia** also suppresses PTH secretion due to stimulation of the glands calcium-sensing receptor (CaSR).

Congenital hypoparathyroidism causes hypocalcemia beginning in infancy. However, it may not be diagnosed for many years. Since hypoparathyroidism can be familial, screening is suggested for family members of any patient with idiopathic hypoparathyroidism.

Clinical Findings

A. Symptoms and Signs

Symptoms of hypoparathyroidism depend on the severity of hypocalcemia as well as its rate of development. Patients with acute hypocalcemia after parathyroidectomy may manifest severe symptoms, despite having mildly low or low-normal serum calcium levels. Patients with chronic severe hypocalcemia may have few symptoms. **Neuromuscular irritability** presents with perioral numbness, paresthesias of the feet or hands, myalgias, muscle cramping, generalized muscle spasms with tetany, hyperactive reflexes, and laryngospasm that can cause respiratory stridor. Chvostek sign (facial muscle contraction on tapping the facial nerve in front of the tragus) is present in 70% of patients with hypocalcemia and in about 15% of individuals who are normocalcemic. Trousseau sign (flexion of the wrist and metacarpal-phalangeal joints with adduction of the fingers after application of a sphygmomanometer cuff inflated to over systolic blood pressure for 3 minutes) is present in over 90% of patients with hypocalcemia but in only about 1% of normocalcemic individuals. **Cardiovascular** manifestations of acute hypocalcemia include bradycardia, ventricular arrhythmias, and impaired ventricular EF. **CNS** manifestations include seizures as well as psychiatric changes, irritability, fatigue, and cognitive impairment. **Ophthalmic** manifestations of severe hypocalcemia include papilledema and cataracts. **Renal** manifestations of chronic hypoparathyroidism occur due to hypercalciuria and include nephrolithiasis, nephrocalcinosis, and kidney disease. **Dermatologic** manifestations include dry, rough skin; dry hair; scalp and eyebrow hair loss; and brittle fingernails with transverse grooves. Chronic hypocalcemia with hyperphosphatemia can cause calcifications in soft tissues, such as joints, skin, and arteries.

B. Laboratory Findings

Serum calcium is low, serum phosphate high, urinary calcium low, and alkaline phosphatase normal. Because serum calcium is largely bound to albumin, the serum *ionized* calcium may be determined in patients with hypoalbuminemia. Alternatively, the serum calcium level can be corrected for serum albumin level as follows:

$$\text{"Corrected" serum } Ca^{2+} = \text{Serum } Ca^{2+} \text{ mg/dL} + (0.8 \times [4.0 - \text{Albumin g/dL}])$$

Serum PTH levels are usually low or not elevated in the presence of hypocalcemia. Serum magnesium levels should always be measured.

C. Imaging

CT scanning of the brain may reveal calcifications of the basal ganglia and other areas in over 50% of patients with chronic hypocalcemia. The bones may appear denser than normal and bone mineral density (BMD) is usually increased, particularly in the lumbar spine. Cutaneous calcification may occur.

D. Other Examinations

Slit-lamp examination may show early posterior lenticular cataract formation. The ECG may show heart block, a prolonged QTc interval, and ST-T changes suggestive of an MI.

Complications

Acute tetany with stridor, especially if associated with vocal cord palsy, may lead to respiratory obstruction requiring tracheostomy. Seizures are common in untreated patients. Hypocalcemia can also cause heart failure and dysrhythmias. Ossification of the paravertebral ligaments may occur with nerve root compression; surgical decompression may be required. Overtreatment with vitamin D and calcium may produce nephrocalcinosis and impairment of kidney function. There may be associated autoimmunity causing celiac disease, pernicious anemia, or Addison disease.

Differential Diagnosis

Paresthesias, muscle cramps, or tetany due to respiratory alkalosis, in which the serum calcium is normal, can be confused with hypocalcemia. In fact, hyperventilation tends to accentuate hypocalcemic symptoms.

Hypocalcemia may be caused by certain medications: loop diuretics, plicamycin, phenytoin, foscarnet, denosumab, and bisphosphonates. Hypocalcemia may also be due to malabsorption of calcium, magnesium, or vitamin D. Hypocalcemia may develop in patients with osteoblastic metastatic carcinomas (especially breast, prostate) instead of the expected hypercalcemia. Hypocalcemia with hyperphosphatemia (simulating hypoparathyroidism) is seen in azotemia but may also be caused by large doses of intravenous, oral, or rectal phosphate preparations and by chemotherapy of responsive lymphomas or leukemias.

Hypocalcemia with hypercalciuria may be due to a familial autosomal dominant syndrome involving a mutation in the calcium-sensing receptor; patients have serum PTH levels that are in the normal range, distinguishing it from hypoparathyroidism. Such patients are hypercalciuric; treatment with calcium and vitamin D may cause nephrocalcinosis.

Congenital pseudohypoparathyroidism is a group of disorders characterized by hypocalcemia due to resistance to PTH. Subtypes are caused by different mutations involving the renal PTH receptor, the receptor's G protein, or adenylyl cyclase.

Treatment

A. Prophylaxis Against Severe Postoperative Hypocalcemia

Post-thyroidectomy hypocalcemia can be detected early by closely monitoring serum PTH and calcium. If the serum calcium falls below 8.0 mg/dL (2.0 mmol/L) with a serum PTH below 10–15 pg/mL (1.0–1.5 pmol/L) after thyroid or parathyroid surgery, the patient is at high risk for hypocalcemia and can be prophylactically treated with calcitriol and calcium. An oral prophylactic regimen is calcitriol, 0.25–1 mcg twice daily, and calcium carbonate (with meals), 500–1000 mg twice daily.

B. Emergency Treatment for Acute Hypocalcemia (Hypoparathyroid Tetany)

1. Airway—Be sure an adequate airway is present.

2. Intravenous calcium gluconate—Calcium gluconate, 10–20 mL of 10% solution intravenously, may be given *slowly* until tetany ceases. Ten to 50 mL of 10% calcium gluconate may be added to 1 L of 5% glucose in water or saline and administered by slow intravenous drip. The rate should be adjusted so that the serum calcium is maintained in the range of 8–9 mg/dL (2–2.25 mmol/L).

3. Oral calcium—Oral calcium salts should be given as soon as possible to supply 1–2 g of elemental calcium daily. Liquid calcium carbonate, 500 mg/5 mL, contains 40% calcium and may be especially useful; it should be given with meals.

4. Vitamin D preparations—(Table 26–9) Vitamin D therapy should be started as soon as oral calcium is begun. 1,25-Dihydroxycholecalciferol (calcitriol) has a very rapid onset of action and is not as long-lasting as vitamin D_3 if hypercalcemia occurs. Begin calcitriol at a dose of 0.25 mcg (1000 IU) orally each morning and titrate upward to near normocalcemia. Ultimately, doses of 0.5–4 mcg/day may be required.

5. Magnesium—If hypomagnesemia (serum magnesium less than 1.8 mg/dL or less than 0.8 mmol/L) is present, it must be corrected to treat the resulting hypocalcemia. For critical hypomagnesemia (serum magnesium less than 1.0 mg/dL or less than 0.45 mmol/L), 50% magnesium sulfate solution (5 g/10 mL) is diluted in 250 mL 0.9% saline or 5% dextrose in water and given by an intravenous infusion of 5 g over 3 hours, with further dosing based on serum magnesium levels. Long-term oral magnesium replacement may be given as magnesium oxide 500 mg (60% elemental magnesium) tablets, one to three times daily.

C. Maintenance Treatment of Hypoparathyroidism

Patients with mild hypoparathyroidism may require no therapy but need close monitoring for manifestations of hypocalcemia. Therapy is ordinarily required for symptomatic hypocalcemia or serum calcium below 8.0 mg/dL (2 mmol/L).

Vitamin D, calcium, and magnesium therapy: Patients with hypoparathyroidism have a reduced renal tubular reabsorption of calcium and are thus prone to hypercalciuria and kidney stones if the serum calcium is normalized with calcium and vitamin D therapy. Therefore, the goal is to maintain the serum calcium in a slightly low but asymptomatic range of 8–8.6 mg/dL (2–2.15 mmol/L). It is prudent to monitor urine calcium with "spot" urine determinations and keep the level below 30 mg/dL (7.5 mmol/L), if possible. Hypercalciuria may respond to oral hydrochlorothiazide, 25 mg daily, usually given with a potassium supplement. Serum magnesium should be monitored and kept in the normal range with supplemental magnesium, if required. Serum phosphate should also be monitored and the serum calcium × phosphate product kept below 55 mg^2/dL^2 (4.4 $mmol^2/L^2$).

Calcium supplements can be given in doses of 800–1000 mg orally daily. Calcium carbonate (40% elemental calcium) is best absorbed at the low gastric pH that occurs with meals. Calcium citrate (21% elemental calcium) is absorbed with or without meals and is a better choice for patients taking PPIs or H_2-blockers; it causes less GI

Table 26–9. Vitamin D preparations used in the treatment of hypoparathyroidism.

	Available Preparations	Daily Dose	Duration of Action
Calcitriol (Rocaltrol)	0.25 mcg (1000 IU) and 0.5 mcg (2000 IU) capsules; 1 mcg/mL oral solution; 1 mcg/mL for injection	0.25–3 mcg divided into 2 doses daily	3–5 days
Alfacalcidol	0.25 mcg, 0.5 mcg, and 1 mcg capsules	0.25 mcg with calcitriol, 0.5–3.0 mcg (divided into 2 doses) without calcitriol	3–5 days
Cholecalciferol (vitamin D_3)	400 IU/mL liquid, 1000–50,000 IU capsules (not available commercially in United States; may be compounded)	400–4000 IU with calcitriol, 10,000–100,000 IU without calcitriol	4–8 weeks
Ergocalciferol, ergosterol (vitamin D_2, calciferol)	8000 IU/mL liquid, 50,000 IU capsules	400–4000 IU with calcitriol, 50,000–200,000 IU without calcitriol	1–2 weeks

intolerance than calcium carbonate. Calcium supplements are given orally in divided doses to provide 800–1200 mg elemental calcium daily.

Vitamin D analogs are generally required for patients with chronic hypoparathyroidism (Table 26–9). The dosage of vitamin D preparations required to maintain target serum calcium levels can vary over time. In hypoparathyroidism, there is a deficiency in renal 1-hydroxylation of vitamin D; therefore, vitamin D analogs that are already 1-hydroxylated (activated) (such as calcitriol and alphacalcidol) are usually used. Monitoring serum calcium, serum phosphate, and serum 25-(OH) vitamin D levels is recommended at least every 3–4 months. Vitamin D_3 may be required in doses of 1000–5000 units daily to maintain serum 25-(OH) vitamin D above 30 ng/mL.

For patients with recurrent hypocalcemia despite treatment with active vitamin D analogs, the use of cholecalciferol (vitamin D_3, derived from skin exposed to sunlight or diet supplements) or ergocalciferol (vitamin D_2 derived from plants) is a treatment option (Table 26–9). These vitamin D preparations have a biologic duration of action of 4–6 weeks; if hypercalcemia develops, it may persist for weeks after the preparation is discontinued. Severe hypercalcemia requires treatment with hydration and prednisone. Despite the risk of prolonged hypercalcemia, cholecalciferol and ergocalciferol usually produce more stable serum calcium levels than the shorter-acting preparations.

Recombinant human parathyroid hormone (rhPTH) is identical to native PTH and FDA approved as an adjunct to calcium and vitamin D analogs to control symptomatic hypocalcemia in patients with hypoparathyroidism. It must be given by subcutaneous injection every 1–2 days. Side effects of rhPTH include nausea, vomiting, diarrhea, arthralgias, and paresthesias. Osteosarcoma have occurred in rats receiving very high doses. The expense of rhPTH limits its use.

Transplantation of cryopreserved parathyroid tissue, removed during prior surgery, restores normocalcemia in about 23% of cases.

Hypoparathyroidism in pregnancy presents special challenges. Maternal hypocalcemia can adversely affect the skeletal development of the fetus and cause compensatory hyperparathyroidism in the newborn. Maternal hypercalcemia can suppress fetal parathyroid development, resulting in neonatal hypocalcemia. This requires very close clinical and biochemical monitoring during pregnancy.

Prognosis

Patients with mild hypoparathyroidism generally do well. Periodic serum calcium levels are required, since changes may call for modification of the treatment schedule. Hypercalcemia that develops in patients with seemingly stable, treated hypoparathyroidism may be a presenting sign of Addison disease.

Despite optimal therapy, patients with moderate-to-severe hypoparathyroidism have an overall reduced quality of life. Chronically affected patients frequently develop calcifications in their kidneys and basal ganglia. They have an increased risk of calcium kidney stones and kidney dysfunction as well as seizures, mood and psychiatric disorders, and a reduced overall sense of well-being. Therapy with rhPTH may prevent or improve these manifestations.

Bilezikian JP. Hypoparathyroidism. J Clin Endocrinol Metab. 2020;105:1722. [PMID: 32322899]

Gafni RI et al. Hypoparathyroidism. N Engl J Med. 2019;380:1738. [PMID: 31042826]

HYPERPARATHYROIDISM

ESSENTIALS OF DIAGNOSIS

- Often found incidentally by routine blood testing.
- Renal calculi, polyuria, hypertension, constipation, fatigue, mental changes.
- Bone pain; rarely, cystic lesions and pathologic fractures.
- Elevated serum PTH, serum and urine calcium, and urine phosphate; serum phosphate low to normal; alkaline phosphatase normal to elevated.

General Considerations

Primary hyperparathyroidism is the most common cause of hypercalcemia, with an estimated prevalence of 0.89% of the US population, but it is underdiagnosed and undertreated. It occurs at all ages but most commonly in the seventh decade and in women (74%).

Parathyroid glands vary in number and location, and ectopic parathyroid glands have been found within the thyroid gland, high in the neck or carotid sheath, the retroesophageal space, and the thymus or mediastinum. Hyperparathyroidism is usually caused by a single parathyroid adenoma (80%), and less commonly by hyperplasia or adenomas of two or more parathyroid glands (20%), or carcinoma (less than 1%). When hyperparathyroidism presents before age 30 years, there is a higher incidence of multiglandular disease (36%) and parathyroid carcinoma (5%). The size of the parathyroid adenoma correlates with the serum PTH level.

Hyperparathyroidism is familial in about 5–10% of cases; hyperparathyroidism presenting before age 45 has a higher chance of being familial. Parathyroid hyperplasia commonly arises in MEN types 1, 2 (2A), and 4. (See Table 26–12.)

Hyperparathyroidism results in the excessive excretion of calcium and phosphate by the kidneys. PTH stimulates renal tubular reabsorption of calcium; however, hyperparathyroidism causes hypercalcemia and an increase in calcium in the glomerular filtrate that overwhelms tubular reabsorption capacity, resulting in hypercalciuria. At least 5% of renal calculi are associated with this disease. Diffuse parenchymal calcification (nephrocalcinosis) is seen less commonly.

Parathyroid carcinoma is a rare cause of hyperparathyroidism, accounting for less than 1% of hyperparathyroidism. Local recurrence is the rule if surgical margins are positive. Distant metastases arise most commonly in the lungs but also in bones, liver, brain, and mediastinum. Although parathyroid carcinoma is typically indolent, an increasing tumor burden is associated with critically severe hypercalcemia and death.

Secondary and tertiary hyperparathyroidism usually occurs with CKD, in which hyperphosphatemia and decreased renal production of 1,25-dihydroxycholecalciferol (1,25[OH]$_2$D$_3$) frequently result in a decrease in ionized calcium. The parathyroid glands are stimulated by the hypocalcemia (secondary hyperparathyroidism) and over time may become enlarged and autonomous (tertiary hyperparathyroidism). Renal osteodystrophy is the bone disease of this disorder (see Disorders of Mineral Metabolism, Chapter 22). Secondary hyperparathyroidism also develops in patients with a deficiency in vitamin D. Serum calcium levels are typically in the normal range but may become borderline elevated over time with tertiary hyperparathyroidism.

Clinical Findings

A. Symptoms and Signs

Hypercalcemia is often discovered incidentally by routine chemistry panels. Many patients are asymptomatic or have mild symptoms that may be elicited only upon questioning. Parathyroid adenomas are usually small, located deeply in the neck, and almost never palpable; when a mass is palpated, it usually turns out to be an incidental thyroid nodule.

Symptomatic patients are said to have problems with "bones, stones, abdominal groans, psychic moans, with fatigue overtones."

1. Skeletal manifestations—Low bone density is typically most prominent at the distal one-third of the radius, a site of mostly cortical bone. Lumbar (trabecular) spine bone density is often spared and is higher compared to the distal radius. Hip bones are a mixture of trabecular and cortical bone, and femur bone density tends to be midway between the lumbar spine and distal radius. Postmenopausal women are prone to asymptomatic vertebral fractures, but severe bone demineralization is uncommon in mild hyperparathyroidism. More commonly, patients experience arthralgias and bone pain, particularly involving the legs. Severe chronic hyperparathyroidism can cause **osteitis fibrosa cystica**, which is the replacement of calcified bone matrix with fibrous tissue forming cystic brown tumors of bone that can be palpable in the jaw.

2. Hypercalcemic manifestations—Mild hypercalcemia may be asymptomatic. However, symptom severity is not entirely predicted by the level of serum calcium or PTH; even mild hypercalcemia can cause significant symptoms, particularly depression, constipation, and bone and joint pain. **Neuromuscular** manifestations include paresthesias, muscle cramps and weakness, and diminished deep tendon reflexes. **Neuropsychiatric** manifestations include malaise, headache, fatigue, insomnia, irritability, and depression. Patients may have cognitive impairment that can vary from intellectual weariness to severe disorientation, psychosis, or stupor. **Cardiovascular** manifestations include hypertension, palpitations, prolonged P-R interval, shortened Q-T interval, bradyarrhythmias, heart block, asystole, and sensitivity to digitalis. Overall cardiovascular mortality is increased in patients with chronic moderate to severe hypercalcemia. **Renal** manifestations include polyuria and polydipsia from hypercalcemia-induced nephrogenic diabetes insipidus. Among all patients with newly discovered hyperparathyroidism, calcium-containing renal calculi have occurred or are detectable in about 18%. Patients with asymptomatic hyperparathyroidism have a 5% incidence of asymptomatic calcium nephrolithiasis. **GI** symptoms include anorexia, nausea, heartburn, vomiting, abdominal pain, weight loss, constipation, and obstipation. Pancreatitis occurs in 3%. **Dermatologic** symptoms may include pruritus. Calcium may precipitate in the corneas ("band keratopathy"), in extravascular tissues (calcinosis), and in small arteries, causing small vessel thrombosis and skin necrosis (calciphylaxis).

3. Normocalcemic primary hyperparathyroidism—Patients with normocalcemic primary hyperparathyroidism generally have few symptoms. However, on average, such patients have a slightly more atherogenic lipid panel and higher blood pressures (systolic blood pressure 10 mm Hg higher and diastolic blood pressure 7 mm Hg higher) than controls. Also, affected patients can have very subtle symptoms, such as mild fatigue, that may not be appreciated as abnormal.

4. Hyperparathyroidism during pregnancy—Pregnant women having mild hyperparathyroidism with a serum calcium below 11.0 mg/dL (less than 2.75 mmol/L) generally tolerate pregnancy well with normal outcomes. However, the majority of pregnant women with more severe hypercalcemia experience complications such as nephrolithiasis, hyperemesis, pancreatitis, muscle weakness, and cognitive changes. About 30% of affected women experience preeclampsia and two-thirds of eclamptic women have preterm delivery. Hypercalcemic crisis may occur, especially postpartum. About 80% of fetuses experience complications of maternal hyperparathyroidism, including fetal demise, preterm delivery, and low birth weight. Newborns have hypoparathyroidism that can be permanent.

5. Parathyroid carcinoma—Hyperparathyroidism with a large palpable neck mass, or vocal fold paralysis from recurrent laryngeal nerve palsy, raises concern for parathyroid carcinoma. Some cases present with smaller tumors, less severe hypercalcemia, and benign-appearing histologic features. *FNA biopsy is not recommended because it may seed the biopsy tract with tumor and cytologic distinction between benign and malignant tumors is problematic.* Parathyroid carcinoma is more frequent in patients with hyperparathyroidism–jaw tumor syndrome as well as patients with MEN 1 and MEN 2A. Therefore, patients should have genetic testing.

B. Laboratory Findings

The hallmark of primary hyperparathyroidism is hypercalcemia, with the serum adjusted total calcium greater than

10.5 mg/dL (2.6 mmol/L). The adjusted total calcium = measured serum calcium in mg/dL + [0.8 × (4.0 – patient's serum albumin in g/dL)]. Serum ionized calcium levels are elevated (above 1.36 mmol/L).

To confirm the diagnosis of hyperparathyroidism, assess urinary calcium excretion. In primary hyperparathyroidism, the urine calcium excretion is normal (100–300 mg/day [25–75 mmol/day]) or high. Low urine calcium excretions (below 100 mg/day [25 mmol/day]) in the absence of thiazide diuretics occur in only 4% of cases of primary hyperthyroidism and raise the differential diagnosis of familial hypocalciuric hypercalcemia.

In primary hyperparathyroidism, serum phosphate may be less than 2.5 mg/dL (0.8 mmol/L) due to an excessive loss of phosphate in the urine (25% of cases). A serum calcium:phosphate (Ca/P) ratio above 2.5 (mg/dL) or above 2.17 (mmol/L) helps confirm the diagnosis of primary hyperparathyroidism. The alkaline phosphatase is elevated only if bone disease is present. The plasma chloride and uric acid levels may be elevated. Serum 25-OH vitamin D levels should be measured, since vitamin D deficiency is common in patients with hyperparathyroidism. Serum 25-OH vitamin D levels below 20 mcg/L (50 nmol/L) can aggravate hyperparathyroidism and its bone manifestations.

Elevated serum levels of intact PTH confirm the diagnosis of hyperparathyroidism. Parathyroid carcinoma must always be suspected in patients with a serum calcium of 14.0 mcg/dL (3.5 mmol/L) or more and a serum PTH 5 or more times the upper limit of normal.

Patients with low bone density, normal serum calcium, and an elevated serum PTH must be evaluated for causes of secondary hyperparathyroidism (eg, vitamin D or calcium deficiency, hyperphosphatemia, CKD). In the absence of secondary hyperparathyroidism, patients with an elevated serum PTH but normal serum calcium have **normocalcemic hyperparathyroidism.** Such individuals require monitoring since hypercalcemia develops in about 19% of patients over 3 years of follow-up.

Genetic testing is recommended for patients with documented primary hyperparathyroidism who are younger than age 40, have a family history of hyperparathyroidism, or have multiglandular disease.

C. Imaging

Parathyroid imaging is not necessary for the diagnosis of hyperparathyroidism but is performed for most patients prior to parathyroid surgery.

Ultrasound should scan the neck from the mandible to the superior mediastinum in an effort to locate ectopic parathyroid adenomas. Ultrasound has a sensitivity of 79% for single adenomas but only 35% for multiglandular disease. Ultrasound is useful for the surgeon to localize parathyroid adenomas while also assessing the vocal folds.

Sestamibi scintigraphy with ^{99m}Tc-sestamibi and single-photon emission computed tomography (SPECT) is most useful for localizing parathyroid adenomas. However, false-positive scans are common, caused by thyroid nodules, thyroiditis, or cervical lymphadenopathy. Sestamibi-SPECT imaging improves sensitivity for single parathyroid adenomas. Small benign thyroid nodules are discovered incidentally in nearly 50% of patients with hyperparathyroidism who have imaging with ultrasound or MRI.

^{18}F-flurocholine PET/MRI is a useful scan for patients with primary hyperparathyroidism and negative or discordant localization imaging on neck ultrasound and sestamibi scanning. This scan correctly localizes a parathyroid adenoma in about 75% of cases.

Conventional CT and MRI imaging are not usually required prior to a first neck surgery for hyperparathyroidism. However, a four-dimensional CT (4D-CT) is useful for preoperative imaging when ultrasonography and sestamibi scans are negative. It can also be helpful for patients who have had prior neck surgery and for those with ectopic parathyroid glands. MRI may also be useful for repeat neck operations and when ectopic parathyroid glands are suspected. MRI shows better soft tissue contrast than CT.

Noncontrast CT scanning of the kidneys in patients with hyperparathyroidism can visualize calcium-containing stones. However, for patients with mild and apparently asymptomatic hyperparathyroidism, only about 5% are found to have unsuspected nephrolithiasis.

Bone density measurements by dual energy x-ray absorptiometry (DXA) are helpful in determining the amount of cortical bone loss in patients with hyperparathyroidism. DXA should include three areas: distal radius (cortical), hip (cortical and trabecular), and lumbar vertebrae (trabecular). Vertebral bone density is usually not diminished in hyperparathyroidism.

Complications

Pathologic long bone fractures are a complication of hyperparathyroidism. UTI due to stone and obstruction may lead to kidney disease and uremia. If the serum calcium level rises rapidly, clouding of sensorium, kidney disease, and rapid precipitation of calcium throughout the soft tissues may occur (calciphylaxis). Peptic ulcer and pancreatitis may be intractable before surgery. Insulinomas or gastrinomas may be associated, as well as pituitary tumors (MEN type 1). Pseudogout may complicate hyperparathyroidism both before and after surgical removal of tumors. Hypercalcemia during gestation produces neonatal hypocalcemia.

In tertiary hyperparathyroidism due to CKD, high serum calcium and phosphate levels may cause calciphylaxis; calcification of arteries can result in painful ischemic necrosis of skin and gangrene, cardiac arrhythmias, and respiratory failure.

Differential Diagnosis

Artifactual hypercalcemia is common, so a confirmatory serum calcium level should be drawn after an overnight fast along with a serum protein, albumin, and triglyceride while ensuring that the patient is well-hydrated. Hypercalcemia may be due to high serum protein concentrations; in the presence of very high or low serum albumin concentrations, an adjusted serum calcium or a serum ionized calcium is more dependable than the total serum calcium concentration. Hypercalcemia may also be seen with dehydration.

Hypercalcemia of malignancy occurs most frequently with breast, lung, pancreatic, uterine, and renal cell carcinoma, and paraganglioma. Most of these tumors secrete PTH-related protein (PTHrP) that has structural homologies to PTH and causes bone resorption and hypercalcemia similar to those caused by PTH. Serum PTH levels are low or low-normal while serum PTHrP levels are elevated; phosphate is often low. Other tumors can secrete excessive 1,25 $(OH)_2$ vitamin D_3, particularly lymphoproliferative and ovarian malignancies. Plasma cell myeloma causes hypercalcemia in older individuals. Other hematologic cancers associated with hypercalcemia include monocytic leukemia, T-cell leukemia and lymphoma, and Burkitt lymphoma. The clinical features of malignant hypercalcemia can closely simulate hyperparathyroidism.

Pseudohyperparathyroidism of pregnancy presents with hypercalcemia during pregnancy. It is caused by hypersensitivity of the breasts to PRL. The breasts become abnormally enlarged and secrete excessive amounts of PTHrP that causes hypercalcemia. Treatment with dopamine agonists reverses the hypercalcemia.

Sarcoidosis and other granulomatous disorders, such as tuberculosis, berylliosis, histoplasmosis, coccidioidomycosis, leprosy, and foreign-body granuloma, can cause hypercalcemia. Sarcoid granulomas can secrete PTHrP, but granulomas secrete $1,25(OH)_2D_3$ and serum levels of $1,25(OH)_2D_3$ are usually elevated in the presence of hypercalcemia. However, in hypercalcemia with disseminated coccidiomycosis, serum $1,25(OH)_2D_3$ levels may not be elevated. Serum PTH levels are usually low.

Dietary factors can cause hypercalcemia. Excessive calcium, vitamin D, or vitamin A ingestion can cause hypercalcemia, especially in patients who concurrently take thiazide diuretics, which reduce urinary calcium loss. Hypercalcemia is reversible following withdrawal of calcium and vitamin D supplements. In vitamin D intoxication, hypercalcemia may persist for several weeks. Serum levels of 25-hydroxycholecalciferol ($25[OH]D_3$) are helpful to confirm the diagnosis. A brief course of corticosteroid therapy may be necessary if hypercalcemia is severe. A severely carbohydrate-restricted ketogenic diet can also cause hypercalcemia with a low serum PTH.

Familial hypocalciuric hypercalcemia (FHH) is an uncommon autosomal dominant inherited disorder Reduced function of the CaSR causes the parathyroid glands to falsely "sense" hypocalcemia and inappropriately release excessive amounts of PTH. The renal tubule CaSRs are also affected, causing hypocalciuria.

Adults with hypercalcemia due to FHH are either asymptomatic or have nonspecific complaints such as fatigue, weakness, or cognitive issues. Recurrent pancreatitis can occur.

FHH is characterized by a mildly elevated serum calcium that is usually below 11.0 mg/dL (2.75 mmol/L) and a low urine calcium excretion that is usually less than 50 mg/24 hours (13 mmol/24 hours). FHH is confirmed with genetic testing for *FHH* gene mutations. These patients do not normalize their hypercalcemia after subtotal parathyroid removal and should not be subjected to surgery. Cinacalcet, a calcimimetic, may be helpful.

Prolonged immobilization at bed rest commonly causes hypercalcemia, particularly in adolescents, critically ill patients, and patients with extensive Paget disease of bone. Hypercalcemia develops in about one-third of acutely ill patients being treated in ICUs, particularly patients with AKI. Serum calcium elevations are typically mild but may reach 15 mg/dL (3.75 mmol/L). Serum PTH levels are usually slightly elevated, consistent with mild hyperparathyroidism but may be suppressed or normal.

Rare causes of hypercalcemia include untreated adrenal insufficiency. Modest hypercalcemia is occasionally seen in patients taking thiazide diuretics or lithium; the PTH level may be inappropriately nonsuppressed with hypercalcemia. Hyperthyroidism causes increased turnover of bone and occasional hypercalcemia. Bisphosphonates can increase serum calcium in 20% and serum PTH becomes high in 10%, mimicking hyperparathyroidism. Other causes of hypercalcemia are shown in Table 21–7.

Treatment

A. "Asymptomatic" Primary Hyperparathyroidism

Normocalcemic or mild hyperparathyroidism should be considered "asymptomatic" only after obtaining a detailed patient medical history. Many patients may not recognize subtle manifestations, such as cognitive slowing, having become accustomed to them over years. It is important to assess blood pressure, serum BUN and creatinine, and to determine the presence of nephrolithiasis or nephrocalcinosis by radiography, ultrasonography, or CT of the kidneys. Truly asymptomatic patients may be closely monitored and advised to keep active, avoid immobilization, and drink adequate fluids. For postmenopausal women with hyperparathyroidism, estrogen replacement therapy reduces serum calcium by an average of 0.75 mg/dL (0.19 mmol/L) and slightly improves bone density. For patients with hypercalciuria (more than 400 mg daily) or calcium nephrolithiasis, hydrochlorthiazide may be used in doses of 12.5–25 mg daily to reduce calciuria; however, serum calcium must be monitored carefully. Parathyroidectomy does not improve the bone density of patients with osteoporosis who have normocalcemia or normocalcemic hyperparathyroidism.

Affected patients should avoid large doses of thiazide diuretics, vitamin A, and calcium-containing antacids or supplements. Serum calcium and albumin are checked at least twice yearly, kidney function and urine calcium once yearly, and three-site bone density (lumbar vertebrae, hip, and distal radius) every 2 years. Rising serum calcium should prompt further evaluation and determination of serum PTH levels.

If it is not clear whether a patient with primary hyperparathyroid is symptomatic, it is reasonable to consider a trial of medical therapy with cinacalcet.

B. Medical Measures

1. Fluids—Hypercalcemia is treated with a large fluid intake unless contraindicated. Severe hypercalcemia requires hospitalization and intensive hydration with intravenous saline.

2. CaSR activators—Cinacalcet is a calcimimetic agent that binds to sites of the parathyroid glands' extracellular CaSRs to increase the glands' affinity for extracellular calcium, thereby decreasing PTH secretion. Cinacalcet may be used as the initial therapy for patients with hyperparathyroidism or for failed surgical parathyroidectomy. For primary hyperparathyroidism with mild hypercalcemia, begin cinacalcet (15 mg orally [one-half of a 30-mg tablet]) and monitor the serum calcium weekly; increase the dose every 2 weeks if hypercalcemia persists until the patient becomes normocalcemic, which is successful in about 65% of sporadic cases and 80% of familial cases. Patients with parathyroid carcinoma and severe hypercalcemia are treated with cinacalcet in addition to the bisphosphonate, zoledronic acid. For parathyroid cancer, cinacalcet is administered in doses of 30 mg orally twice daily, increased progressively to 60 mg twice daily, then 90 mg twice daily to a maximum of 90 mg every 6–8 hours. Cinacalcet is usually well tolerated but may cause nausea and vomiting (11%), myalgia, or malaise. Cinacalcet does not usually correct hypercalciuria. Hypocalcemia has occurred, even at 30 mg/day. About 50% of azotemic patients with secondary or tertiary hyperparathyroidism have hypercalcemia that is resistant to vitamin D analogs; begin cinacalcet 30 mg orally daily to a maximum of 250 mg daily, with dosage adjustments to keep the serum PTH in the range of 150–300 pg/mL (15.8–31.6 pmol/L). Etelcalcetide also activates the parathyroid glands' CaSR and reduces hypercalcemia in dialysis patients; it is given intravenously at the end of hemodialysis sessions, thereby avoiding the GI side effects of cinacalcet.

3. Bisphosphonates—Intravenous bisphosphonates are potent inhibitors of bone resorption and can temporarily treat the hypercalcemia of hyperparathyroidism. Pamidronate in doses of 30–90 mg (in 0.9% saline) is administered intravenously over 2–4 hours. Zoledronic acid 5 mg is administered intravenously over 15–20 minutes. These drugs cause a gradual decline in serum calcium over several days that may last for weeks to months. Such intravenous bisphosphonates are used generally for patients with severe hyperparathyroidism in preparation for surgery. Oral bisphosphonates, such as alendronate, are not effective for treating the hypercalcemia or hypercalciuria of hyperparathyroidism. However, oral alendronate has been shown to improve BMD in the trabecular bone of the lumbar spine and hip (not distal radius) and may be used for asymptomatic patients with hyperparathyroidism who have a low BMD. It may also be combined with cinacalcet for the medical treatment of osteoporosis in patients with persistent hyperparathyroidism.

4. Denosumab—For patients with severe hypercalcemia due to parathyroid carcinoma, denosumab 120 mcg subcutaneously monthly may be effective. However, high-dose denosumab increases the risk of jaw osteonecrosis and serious infections.

5. Vitamin D and vitamin D analogs—

a. Primary hyperparathyroidism—For patients with vitamin D deficiency, vitamin D replacement may be beneficial to patients with hyperparathyroidism. Aggravation of hypercalcemia does not ordinarily occur. Serum PTH levels may fall with vitamin D replacement in doses of 800–2000 IU daily or more to achieve serum 25-OH vitamin D levels 30 ng/mL or more (50 nmol/L or more).

b. Secondary and tertiary hyperparathyroidism associated with azotemia—See Disorders of Mineral Metabolism, Kidney Disease.

6. Other measures—Estrogen replacement reduces hypercalcemia slightly in postmenopausal women with hyperparathyroidism. Similarly, oral raloxifene (60 mg/day) may be given to postmenopausal women with hyperparathyroidism; it reduces serum calcium an average of 0.4 mg/dL (0.1 mmol/L), while having an anti-estrogenic effect on breast tissue. Beta-blockers, such as propranolol, may also be useful for preventing the adverse cardiac effects of hypercalcemia. Parathyroid carcinoma metastases may be treated with radiofrequency ablation or arterial embolization.

C. Surgical Parathyroidectomy

Parathyroidectomy is recommended for patients with hyperparathyroidism who are symptomatic or who have nephrolithiasis or parathyroid bone disease. During pregnancy, parathyroidectomy is performed in the second trimester for women who are symptomatic or have a serum calcium above 11 mg/dL (2.75 mmol/L).

Some patients with seemingly asymptomatic hyperparathyroidism may be surgical candidates for other reasons such as (1) serum calcium 1 mg/dL (0.25 mmol/L) above the upper limit of normal, (2) urine calcium excretion greater than 400 mg/day (10 mmol/day), (3) eGFR less than 60 mL/minute/1.73 m^2, (4) nephrolithiasis or nephrocalcinosis, (5) cortical bone density (wrist, hip, or distal radius) indicating osteoporosis (T score below –2.5) or previous fragility bone fracture, (6) relative youth (under age 50 years), (7) difficulty ensuring medical follow-up, or (8) pregnancy.

Surgery for patients with "asymptomatic" hyperparathyroidism may improve cortical BMD and confer modest benefits in social and emotional well-being and overall quality of life in comparison to similar patients being monitored without surgery. Cognitive function may benefit with improvements in nonverbal abstraction and memory.

Preoperative parathyroid imaging has been used in an attempt to allow unilateral minimally invasive neck surgery (see Imaging, above). The reported success rates vary considerably. Even in patients with concordant sestamibi and ultrasound scans, and an intraoperative PTH drop of more than 50%, hyperparathyroidism may persist postoperatively in up to 15% of patients.

Without preoperative localization studies, bilateral neck exploration is usually advisable for the following: (1) patients with a family history of hyperparathyroidism, (2) patients with a personal or family history of MEN, and (3) patients wanting an optimal chance of success with a single surgery. Parathyroid glands are often supernumerary (five or more) or ectopic (eg, intrathyroidal, carotid sheath, mediastinum).

For patients with MEN type 1, the optimal surgical management is subtotal parathyroidectomy. Recurrent hyperparathyroidism develops in 18%, and the rate of postoperative hypoparathyroidism is high. In such cases, a parathyroid gland may be transplanted into a neck muscle, from which it may be easily removed if hyperparathyroidism persists. About 30% of patients with successful parathyroid surgery continue to have an elevated serum PTH postoperatively, despite normal serum calcium levels; this is sometimes due to vitamin D deficiency.

Parathyroid hyperplasia is commonly seen with secondary or tertiary hyperparathyroidism associated with uremia. Cinacalcet is an alternative to surgery. When surgery is performed, a subtotal parathyroidectomy is optimal; three and one-half glands are usually removed, and a metal clip is left to mark the location of residual parathyroid tissue.

Parathyroid carcinoma surgery consists of en bloc resection of the tumor and ipsilateral thyroid lobe with care to avoid rupturing the tumor capsule. If the surgical margins are not clear of tumor, postoperative neck radiation therapy may be given. Local and distant metastases may be debulked or irradiated. Preoperative MRI scanning is required to delineate the tumor. Zoledronic acid or denosumab is given preoperatively. Severe hypercalcemia requires multiple medical measures, including hydration, furosemide, cinacalcet, zoledronic acid, or denosumab. Radiation therapy can be given for localized tumor. Osseous metastases must be distinguished from benign brown tumors caused by hyperparathyroidism; biopsy may be required. Chemotherapy has been ineffective for patients with distant metastases. Immunotherapy with anti-hPTH monoclonal antibodies is a treatment option.

Complications—Serum PTH levels fall below normal in 70% of patients within hours after successful surgery, commonly causing hypocalcemic paresthesias or even tetany. Hypocalcemia tends to occur the evening after surgery or on the next day. Frequent postoperative monitoring of serum calcium (or serum calcium plus albumin) is advisable beginning the evening after surgery. Once hypercalcemia has resolved, liquid or chewable calcium carbonate is given orally to reduce the likelihood of hypocalcemia. Symptomatic hypocalcemia is treated with larger doses of calcium; calcitriol (0.25–1 mcg daily orally) may be added, with the dosage depending on symptom severity. Magnesium salts are sometimes required postoperatively, since adequate magnesium is required for functional recovery of the remaining suppressed parathyroid glands.

In about 12% of patients having successful parathyroid surgery, PTH levels rise above normal (while serum calcium is normal or low) by 1 week postoperatively. This secondary hyperparathyroidism is probably due to "hungry bones" and is treated with calcium and vitamin D preparations. Such therapy is usually needed only for 3–6 months but is required long term by some patients.

Hyperthyroidism commonly occurs immediately following parathyroid surgery. It is caused by release of stored thyroid hormone during surgical manipulation of the thyroid. In symptomatic patients, short-term treatment with propranolol may be required for several days.

Prognosis

Patients with symptomatic hyperparathyroidism usually experience worsening disease (eg, nephrolithiasis) unless they have treatment. Conversely, the majority of completely asymptomatic patients with a serum calcium below 11.0 mg/dL (2.75 mmol/L) remain stable with follow-up. However, worsening hypercalcemia, hypercalciuria, and reductions in cortical BMD develop in about one-third of asymptomatic patients. Therefore, asymptomatic patients must be monitored carefully and treated with oral hydration and mobilization.

Surgical removal of apparently single sporadic parathyroid adenomas is successful in 94%. Patients with MEN 1 undergoing subtotal parathyroidectomy may experience long remissions, but hyperparathyroidism frequently recurs. Despite treatment for hyperparathyroidism, hypertension is usually not reversed and patients remain at increased risk for all-cause mortality, CVD, renal calculi, and kidney dysfunction.

Spontaneous cure due to necrosis of the tumor is exceedingly rare. The bones, in spite of severe cyst formation, deformity, and fracture, will heal if hyperparathyroidism is successfully treated. The presence of pancreatitis increases the mortality rate. Acute pancreatitis usually resolves with correction of hypercalcemia, whereas subacute or chronic pancreatitis tends to persist. Kidney damage may progress even after removal of a parathyroid adenoma.

Parathyroid carcinoma is associated with 5- and 10-year survival rates of 78% and 49%, respectively. A positive surgical margins or metastases predict a very poor 5-year survival. Metastases are relatively radiation-resistant, but additional therapies such as radiofrequency ablation or arterial embolization may be palliative.

When to Refer

Refer to parathyroid surgeon for parathyroidectomy.

When to Admit

Patients with severe hypercalcemia for intravenous hydration.

Carpenter TO et al. Case 32-2021: a 14-year-old girl with swelling of the jaw and hypercalcemia. N Engl J Med. 2021;385:1604. [PMID: 34670047]

Davis C et al. Hyperparathyroidism in pregnancy. BMJ Case Rep. 2020;13:e232653. [PMID: 32066577]

Rodrigo JP et al. Parathyroid cancer: an update. Cancer Treat Rev. 2020;86:102012. [PMID: 32247225]

Zhu CY et al. Diagnosis and management of primary hyperparathyroidism. JAMA. 2020;323:1186. [PMID: 32031566]

METABOLIC BONE DISEASE

BMD is typically expressed in g/cm^2, for which there are different normal ranges for each bone and for each type of DXA-measuring machine. The "Z score" expresses an individual's BMD as the number of standard deviations from age-matched, race-matched, and sex-matched means. The "T score" reports BMD as the number of standard deviations from young sex-matched means. Patients with a low T score are said to have "osteopenia" or "osteoporosis," although osteomalacia is also frequently present. Any BMD classification is somewhat arbitrary and there is no

BMD fracture threshold; instead, fracture risk increases about twofold for each standard deviation drop in BMD. The World Health Organization has established criteria for defining osteopenia and osteoporosis based on the T score: T score greater than or equal to −1.0, normal; T score −1.0 to −2.5, osteopenia ("low bone density"); T score less than −2.5, osteoporosis; T score less than −2.5 with a fracture, severe osteoporosis.

Fracture Risk Assessment Tool (FRAX) helps predict an individual's 10-year risk of hip or other major osteoporotic fracture. FRAX is particularly useful for treatment decisions in patients with osteopenia and takes into consideration age, sex, BMD, and other risk factors. The National Osteoporosis Foundation recommends treatment for individuals with osteopenia (T score between −1.0 and −2.5) who have a computed 10-year hip fracture risk of at least 3% or a 10-year risk of any major fracture of at least 20%. However, the FRAX model has limitations since it only considers femoral neck BMD and not vertebral BMD. Also, FRAX does not consider the dose of exposure to corticosteroids, race, alcohol, smoking, or an individual's proclivity to falls; treatment decisions must always be individualized. FRAX is available at https://www.sheffield.ac.uk/FRAX/tool.aspx/.

Black DM et al. Treatment-related changes in bone mineral density as a surrogate biomarker for fracture risk reduction: meta-regression analyses of individual patient data from multiple randomised controlled trials. Lancet Diabetes Endocrinol. 2020;8:672. [PMID: 32707115]

DeSapri KT et al. To scan or not to scan? DXA in postmenopausal women. Cleve Clin J Med. 2020;87:205. [PMID: 32238375]

OSTEOPENIA

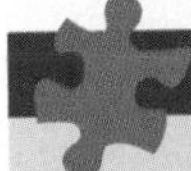

ESSENTIALS OF DIAGNOSIS

- Patients are typically asymptomatic.
- Bone density below that for young normal adults but less severe than osteoporosis.
- Diagnosis is by DXA.
- Fracture risk determined with FRAX tool.

General Considerations

Osteopenia is less severe than osteoporosis, with T scores between −1.0 and −2.4 (see above). There is no absolute fracture threshold for BMD, and most patients with bone fractures are found to have osteopenia rather than osteoporosis. Patients who are identified as osteopenic require an evaluation for causes of osteoporosis or osteomalacia and monitoring for worsening BMD.

Clinical Findings

A. Symptoms and Signs

Patients with osteopenia are typically asymptomatic. However, bone pain can be present, particularly with osteomalacia. Osteopenia predisposes to low-impact and pathological fractures of vertebrae, hips, wrists, metatarsals, and ribs.

B. Laboratory Findings

Patients with moderate to severe osteopenia (T scores between −1.5 and −2.4) require an evaluation for underlying causes of osteoporosis and osteomalacia. Testing should include a serum BUN, creatinine, albumin, calcium, phosphate, alkaline phosphatase, and 25-OH vitamin D; a CBC is also recommended. A serum PTH is obtained if the serum calcium is abnormal.

C. DXA Bone Densitometry and FRAX

Osteopenia is diagnosed by DXA bone densitometry with T scores of −1.0 to −2.4. The frequency of surveillance DXA testing for postmenopausal women and older adult men should be based on the T scores: every 5 years for T scores −1.0 to −1.5, every 3–5 years for T scores −1.5 to −2.0, and every 1–2 years for T scores below −2.0. Patients requiring high-dose long-term prednisone therapy should have DXA surveillance every 1–2 years. FRAX score (see above) should be determined with each DXA BMD determination.

Prevention & Treatment

Patients with osteopenia require adequate vitamin D intake to achieve serum 25-OH vitamin D levels above 30 ng/mL (75 nmol/L). Calcium supplementation is not usually required, except for patients with unusually low dietary calcium intake. Lifestyle modifications may be required, including smoking cessation, alcohol moderation, strength training and weight-bearing exercise. Balance exercises such as tai chi may help prevent falls. Other fall prevention measures include reduction of tranquilizer and alcohol consumption, visual or walking aids when warranted, removal of home tripping hazards, and adequate night lighting.

Pharmacologic therapy is not usually required for patients with osteopenia. However, pharmacologic intervention treatments (see osteoporosis) may be required for patients who require long-term high-dose prednisone, for patients with fragility fractures, and for those whose FRAX score indicates a 10-year risk for fracture above 20% or hip fracture risk above 3%.

OSTEOPOROSIS

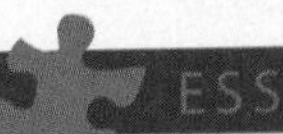

ESSENTIALS OF DIAGNOSIS

- Fracture propensity of spine, hip, pelvis, and wrist.
- Asymptomatic until a fracture has occurred.
- Serum PTH, calcium, phosphorus, and alkaline phosphatase usually normal.
- Serum 25-hydroxyvitamin D levels often low as a comorbid condition.

General Considerations

Osteoporosis is characterized by a loss of bone matrix (osteoid) that reduces bone integrity and bone strength, predisposing to an increased risk of fragility and fracture. In the United States, osteoporosis causes over 1.5 million fractures annually. White women age 50 years and older (who do not receive estrogen replacement) have a 46% risk of sustaining an osteoporotic fracture during the remainder of their lives. Vertebral fractures are the most common fracture; they are usually diagnosed incidentally on radiographs or CT scanning.

Largely due to a reduction in smoking, the age-adjusted risk for hip fracture has declined in the United States in recent years. However, the risk for fragility fractures remains high and varies with ethnicity, sex, and age. The lifetime risk of hip fracture is 12.1% in White women and 4.6% in White men. The risks are lower in Latinx women and men and lower yet in Chinese women and men (with similar gender differences). Black adults also have a lower risk for fracture due to higher BMD and hip morphology that is less fracture-prone. There is much less ethnic variability for vertebral fractures. The prevalence of vertebral fractures in women older than 65 years is 70% for White women, 68% for Japanese women, 55% for Mexican women, and 50% in Black women.

Osteoporosis can be caused by a variety of factors (Table 26–10); the most common include aging, sex hormone deficiency, alcohol use disorder, cigarette smoking, long-term PPI therapy, and high-dose corticosteroid administration. Women who consume cola beverages for a prolonged time are at increased risk for osteoporosis of the hip. Hypogonadal men frequently develop osteoporosis. Anti-androgen therapy for prostate cancer can cause osteoporosis, and such men should be monitored with bone densitometry.

Table 26–10. Causes of osteoporosis.[1]

Aging	**Medications (long-term)**
Alcohol use disorder (alcoholism)	Aromatase inhibitors
Cigarette smoking	Corticosteroids
Cola consumption in women (hip)	GnRH inhibitors
Ethnicity: White	Heparin
Female sex	Pioglitazone
Genetic disorders	PPIs
Aromatase deficiency	SSRIs (older adults)
Collagen disorders	SGLT2 inhibitors
Ehlers-Danlos syndrome	Vitamin A excess, vitamin D excess
Homocystinuria	**Underweight (BMI < 18.5)**
Hypophosphatasia	**Miscellaneous conditions**
Idiopathic juvenile and adult osteoporosis	Anorexia nervosa
Marfan syndrome	Celiac disease
Osteogenesis imperfecta	Copper deficiency
Hormone deficiency	Cystic fibrosis
Estradiol (women)	Diabetes mellitus (uncontrolled)
Testosterone (men)	HIV infection
Hormone excess	Hyponatremia (chronic)
Cushing syndrome	IBD
Hyperparathyroidism	Liver disease (chronic)
Thyrotoxicosis	Mastocytosis (systemic)
Low physical activity and immobilization	Primary biliary cholangitis
Malignancy, especially plasma cell myeloma	Protein-calorie malnutrition
	Rheumatoid arthritis
	Thalassemia major
	Vitamin C deficiency

[1]See Table 26–11 for causes of osteomalacia.

Clinical Findings

A. Symptoms and Signs

Osteoporosis is usually asymptomatic until fractures occur, which may present as backache of varying degrees of severity or as a spontaneous fracture, collapse of a vertebra, or spinal kyphosis. Loss of height is common. Vertebral fractures and hip fractures are associated with increased mortality, pain, reduced independence, and diminished quality of life. Once osteoporosis is identified, a directed history and physical examination must be performed to determine its cause (Table 26–10).

B. Laboratory Findings

DXA bone densitometry is required to diagnose osteoporosis (T score less than –2.5) (see above). **Laboratory testing** is required to screen for secondary causes of osteoporosis or concomitant osteomalacia. For patients with a low bone densitometry, obtain serum determinations for BUN, creatinine, albumin, serum calcium, phosphate, alkaline phosphatase, and 25-hydroxyvitamin D (25HD, 25-hydroxycalciferol). A serum PTH is obtained if the serum calcium is abnormal. A low serum alkaline phosphatase (below 40 units/L in adults) may indicate hypophosphatasia. A CBC is obtained and is usually normal; for patients with anemia, screen for plasma cell myeloma with a serum protein electrophoresis and screen for intestinal malabsorption, where indicated. Serum 25HD levels below 20 ng/mL (50 nmol/L) are considered frank vitamin D deficiency. Lesser degrees of vitamin D insufficiency (serum 25HD levels in the range of 20–30 ng/mL [50–75 nmol/L]) may also slightly increase the risk for hip fracture. Test for thyrotoxicosis, hypogonadism, and celiac disease, if clinically warranted.

Differential Diagnosis

Osteopenia and fractures can be caused by osteomalacia and bone marrow neoplasia such as plasma cell myeloma or metastatic bone disease. Hypophosphatasia also causes diminished bone density. These conditions coexist in many patients and cannot be distinguished with bone densitometry.

Prevention & Treatment

A. Nonpharmacologic Measures

For prevention and treatment of osteoporosis, the diet should be adequate in protein, total calories, calcium, and vitamin D. Pharmacologic corticosteroid (oral, parenteral, or inhaled) should be reduced or discontinued if possible. Cigarette smoking cessation is essential. Excessive alcohol intake must be avoided. Exercise is strongly recommended to increase both bone density and strength, thereby reducing the risk of fractures due to frailty falls. Walking increases the bone density at both the spine and hip. Resistance exercise increases spine density. Other fall prevention measures include adequate home lighting, handrails on stairs, handholds in bathrooms, and physical therapy training in fall prevention and balance exercises. Patients who have weakness or balance problems must use a cane or a walker; rolling walkers should have a brake mechanism. Medications that cause orthostasis, dizziness, or confusion should be avoided.

B. Pharmacologic Measures

Treatment is indicated for most patients with osteoporosis, particularly those who have had recent fragility fractures, women with previous fragility fractures of the hip or vertebra, or a DXA T score between −2.5 and −1.0 with FRAX-determined 10-year hip fracture risk greater than 3% or major osteoporotic fracture risk greater than 20% (see above). Osteoporosis treatment reduces fracture risk but does not improve overall mortality.

1. Vitamin D and calcium—Deficiency of vitamin D or calcium causes osteomalacia, rather than osteoporosis, but they often coexist and cannot be distinguished by DXA bone densitometry; it is crucial to ensure sufficient vitamin D and calcium intake. Recommended daily vitamin D intake of 600–800 IU/day is difficult to achieve by diet (unless high in fish) and sun exposure, particularly during winter months and for patients with intestinal malabsorption or during prolonged hospitalization or nursing home care. Oral vitamin D_3 (cholecalciferol) is given either as a universal supplement of 800–2000 IU/day or in doses titrated to achieve 25-hydroxvitamin D (25-OHD) serum levels greater than or equal to 20 ng/mL (50 nmol/L) for most of the population. However, the 25-OHD serum levels should be maintained at 30 ng/mL (75 nmol/L) or higher for those "at risk": pregnant women, older adults, and those with osteoporosis or fragility fractures. Doses of vitamin D_3 above 4000 IU daily in adults are generally not advised (except in patients with intestinal malabsorption), since GI side effects or hypercalcemia may occur. There are early observational data that imply an increased all-cause mortality at 25-OHD serum levels that are either excessively low or high, so the optimal therapeutic range for 25-OHD serum levels appears to be about 30–50 ng/mL (75–125 nmol/L).

A total elemental calcium intake at least 1000 mg/day is recommended for all adults and 1200 mg/day for postmenopausal women and men older than 70 years. Many individuals do not consume this amount of calcium, but a large prospective study of osteopenic postmenopausal women showed no improvement in BMD with high calcium consumption, and most cohort studies have shown no association between dietary calcium intake and fracture risk. Calcium supplementation (1 g/day or more) has not been shown to reduce the risk of hip or forearm fractures and reduces vertebral fractures by only 14% reduction. Therefore, normal and osteopenic individuals do not require calcium supplementation. Calcium supplements are reserved for patients with intestinal malabsorption or calcium-deficient diets (ie, low intake of dairy products, dark leafy greens, sardines, tofu, or fortified foods). Calcium citrate does not require acid for absorption and is preferred for patients receiving acid blockers. Calcium carbonate should be taken with food to enhance calcium absorption. Calcium supplements are usually taken along with vitamin D_3, and many commercial supplements contain the combination. Although calcium supplements are usually tolerated, some patients experience intestinal bloating and constipation. Taking calcium supplements with meals can reduce the risk of nephrolithiasis.

2. Sex hormones—Sex hormone replacement can prevent osteoporosis in hypogonadal women and men but is not an effective therapy for established osteoporosis. Low-dose transdermal systemic estrogen prevents osteoporosis in women with hypogonadism, including young patients with anorexia nervosa (see Hormone Replacement Therapy). Testosterone replacement or low-dose transdermal estradiol therapy prevents osteoporosis in men with severe testosterone deficiency (see Male Hypogonadism).

3. Bisphosphonates—Bisphosphonate therapy is indicated for patients with osteoporosis in the spine, total hip, or femoral neck or for patients with a pathologic spine fracture or a low-impact hip fracture. Bisphosphonates include intravenous zoledronic acid or pamidronate and oral alendronate, risedronate, or ibandronate. Ibandronate reduces vertebral fracture risk but not nonvertebral fracture risk. Bisphosphonates all work similarly, inhibiting osteoclast-induced bone resorption. They increase bone density significantly and all reduce the incidence of vertebral fractures; all but ibandronate have been demonstrated to also reduce the risk of nonvertebral fractures. Bisphosphonates have also been effective in preventing corticosteroid-induced osteoporosis. To ensure intestinal absorption, oral bisphosphonates must be taken in the morning with at least 8 oz of plain water at least 40 minutes before consumption of anything else. The patient must remain upright after taking bisphosphonates to reduce the risk of esophagitis. No dosage adjustments are required for patients with creatinine clearances above 35 mL/minute. Bisphosphonates are excreted in urine and serum phosphate levels should be monitored in patients with kidney disease; bisphosphonates are relatively contraindicated in patients with CrCl below 35 mL/minute. Bone density falls in 18% of patients during their first year of treatment with bisphosphonates, but 80% of such patients gain bone density with continued bisphosphonate treatment. The half-life of bisphosphonates in bone is about 10 years. Therefore, after 3 years, a DXA bone densitometry may be obtained. If the patient's T score has risen above −2.5 and the patient has a relatively low fracture risk, the patient may have a bisphosphonate "drug holiday" for 3–5 years. However, for patients with continued osteoporosis and a high fracture risk, the bisphosphonate may be continued another 2 years. The usual treatment course with bisphosphonates is 3–5 years due to the increasing risk of atypical femoral fractures after that time.

Alendronate is administered orally once weekly as either a 70-mg standard tablet (Fosamax) or a 70-mg effervescent pH-buffered tablet (Binosto) that is easier to swallow for some patients and may reduce esophageal injury. **Risedronate** (Actonel) may be given once monthly as a 150-mg tablet. Risedronate is favored for women of childbearing age, since it has a shorter half-life and less bone retention than other bisphosphonates. Both medications reduce the risk of vertebral and nonvertebral fractures, but alendronate appears to be superior to risedronate in preventing nonvertebral fractures. **Ibandronate sodium** (Boniva) is taken once monthly in a dose of 150 mg orally. It reduces the risk of vertebral fractures but not nonvertebral fractures; its effectiveness has not been directly compared with other bisphosphonates.

For patients who cannot take oral bisphosphonates, intravenous bisphosphonates are available. They should not be given to patients with a creatinine clearance below 35 mL/minute. **Zoledronic acid** (Reclast) is a third-generation bisphosphonate and a potent osteoclast inhibitor. The dose is 5 mg intravenously over at least 15–30 minutes every 12 months. In a study of postmenopausal women with osteoporosis, once yearly intravenous zoledronic acid reduced the 3-year incidence of hip fractures by 41% (from 2.5% to 1.4%) and clinical vertebral fractures by 77% (from 2.6% to 0.5%). **Pamidronate** (Aredia) is given in doses of 30–60 mg by slow intravenous infusion in normal saline solution every 3–6 months.

SIDE EFFECTS OF BISPHOSPHONATES—**Oral bisphosphonates** can cause nausea, chest pain, and hoarseness. Erosive esophagus can occur, particularly in patients with hiatal hernia and gastroesophageal reflux. Although no increased risk of esophageal cancer has been conclusively demonstrated, the FDA recommends that oral bisphosphonates not be used by patients with Barrett esophagus.

Intravenous bisphosphonate therapy can cause side effects that are collectively known as the acute-phase response. This occurs in 42% of patients after the first infusion of zoledronic acid, usuallywithin the first few days following the infusion; these side effects include fever, chills, or flushing (20%); musculoskeletal pain (20%); nausea, vomiting, or diarrhea (8%); nonspecific symptoms, such as fatigue, dyspnea, edema, headache, or dizziness (22%); and ocular inflammation (0.6%). Symptoms are transient, lasting several days and usually resolving spontaneously. They typically recur with subsequent doses but diminish in intensity with time. Symptoms may be treated with acetaminophen or NSAIDs. Loratadine may reduce musculoskeletal pain. The acute-phase response is usually less severe with intravenous pamidronate than with zoledronic acid; thus, intravenous pamidronate can replace zoledronic acid for subsequent treatments. Patients who experience an especially severe acute-phase response can be given prophylactic corticosteroids and ondansetron prior to subsequent bisphosphonate infusions. Intravenous zoledronic acid has caused seizures that may be idiosyncratic or due to hypocalcemia.

Osteonecrosis of the jaw is a rare complication of bisphosphonate therapy. A painful, necrotic, nonhealing lesion of the mandible or maxilla occurs, particularly after tooth extraction. The risk is increased with older age, in women, and in patients concomitantly receiving chemotherapy or corticosteroid therapy. About 95% of jaw osteonecrosis cases have occurred with intravenous high-dose therapy with zoledronic acid or pamidronate for patients with osteolytic metastases. Only about 5% of cases have occurred in patients receiving oral bisphosphonates or once-yearly bisphosphonate infusions for osteoporosis. The incidence of osteonecrosis is estimated to be about 1:100,000 patients treated for osteoporosis with oral bisphosphonates versus1:100 in patients being treated for cancer with intravenous bisphosphonates. The risk for osteonecrosis of the jaw with dental surgery can be approximated preoperatively with a serum level of C-telopeptide. Bisphosphonates reduce C-telopeptide levels. There appears to be minimal risk of osteonecrosis with serum C-telopeptide levels greater than or equal to 150 pg/mL, moderate risk with levels of 100–149 pg/mL, and higher risk with levels less than 100 pg/mL. Patients receiving bisphosphonates must receive regular dental care and try to avoid dental extraction. If dental surgery is required, bisphosphonate therapy is ordinarily stopped 3 months before the surgery and resumed about 1 month afterward if the bone has healed.

Atypical low-impact "chalkstick" fractures of the femoral shaft are an uncommon complication of bisphosphonate therapy. Asian women, however, experience a relative risk of atypical femur fracture that is 4.8 times higher than White women. In more than 52,000 postmenopausal women taking bisphosphonates for 5 years or longer, a subtrochanteric fracture occurred in 0.22% during the subsequent 2 years; 27% of such fractures were bilateral. About 70% of affected patients had prodromal thigh pain prior to the fracture. The risk for atypical femoral fractures is particularly increased among Asian women, patients taking high-dose corticosteroids, and those receiving bisphosphonate treatment for more than 5 years. Teriparatide (a PTH analog) may be helpful to promote healing of such fractures. Despite this potential complication, the benefits of bisphosphonates outweigh the risks, particularly in non-Asian women. In a large cohort analysis, for every 10,000 women taking bisphosphonates for 3 years, 149 hip fractures were prevented and 2 atypical femur fractures occurred in White women, while 91 hip fractures were prevented and 8 atypical femur fractures occurred in Asian women.

In patients taking bisphosphonates, hypercalcemia is seen in 20% and serum PTH levels increase above normal in 10%, mimicking primary hyperparathyroidism. Hypocalcemia occurs frequently, resulting in secondary hyperparathyroidism; such patients may be treated with oral calcium salt supplements (500–1000 mg/day) and with oral vitamin D_3 (starting at 1000 units/day).

4. Denosumab—Denosumab (Prolia) is a monoclonal antibody that inhibits the proliferation and maturation of preosteoclasts into mature osteoclast bone-resorbing cells. It is indicated for treatment of osteoporosis, major fragility fractures, or osteopenia with a high FRAX score in both men and women. It is also used for patients with high fracture risk who are receiving sex hormone suppression therapy for breast cancer or prostate cancer. Treatment reduces vertebral fractures by 68% and hip fractures by 40%. Denosumab is administered in doses of 60 mg subcutaneously every 6 months. Unlike bisphosphonates, denosumab can be given to patients with severe kidney disease. It has been relatively well tolerated, with an 8% incidence of flu-like symptoms. It can decrease serum calcium and should not be administered to patients with hypocalcemia. Other side effects include hypercholesterolemia, eczema and dermatitis, and pancreatitis. Denosumab may slightly increase the risk of serious infections (particularly ear, nose, throat, and GI), so it is not recommended for patients receiving immunosuppressants or high-dose corticosteroid therapy. *In premenopausal women, denosumab should be used with great caution and with birth control, since denosumab has caused fetal teratogenicity in animal studies.* With prolonged use, denosumab predisposes to atypical femoral fractures and osteonecrosis of the jaw and is additive to bisphosphonates in that regard.

Compared to oral bisphosphonates, denosumab appears to be slightly superior at improving BMD of the spine, total femur, and femoral neck and at reducing fracture risk after 2 years of therapy. Compared to intravenous zoledronic acid, denosumab has been somewhat superior at increasing BMD at the total femur and femoral neck, but the two have similar efficacy at improving spine BMD.

The effects of denosumab on bone wane quickly after 6 months, and patients can experience a dramatic increased risk of multiple vertebral fractures within 1–2 years following discontinuation of denosumab. Therefore, denosumab must be given on-schedule without drug holidays. Denosumab should not be discontinued without substituting another antiresorptive agent (bisphosphonate, estradiol, or selective estrogen receptor modulator [SERM]) or other therapy.

5. PTH and PTHrP analogs—Teriparatide (Forteo) and **abaloparatide** (Tymlos) are analogs of PTH and PTHrP, respectively. They are indicated only for patients with osteoporosis who are at very high fracture risk, particularly those who have sustained severe or multiple vertebral fractures. These analogs are anabolic agents that stimulate the production of new collagenous bone matrix, particularly in vertebral trabecular bone that must be mineralized. Patients receiving teriparatide or abaloparatide must have sufficient intake of vitamin D and calcium. When given in a sequence with an antiresorptive agent, the preferred sequence is to first give a course of PTH/PTHrP analog therapy followed by a bisphosphonate or denosumab.

The teriparatide dose is 20 mg or 40 mg daily, and the abaloparatide dose is 80 mg daily; both are given subcutaneously daily for up to 2 years. These drugs dramatically improve bone density in most bones except the distal radius. They may also be used to promote healing of atypical femoral chalkstick fractures associated with bisphosphonate therapy. The recommended dose should not be exceeded, since both drugs have caused osteosarcoma in rats when administered long-term in very high doses. Due to the potential risk for osteosarcoma, patients are excluded from receiving teriparatide or abaloparatide if they have an increased risk of osteosarcoma due to the following: Paget disease of bone, unexplained elevations in serum alkaline phosphatase, prior radiation therapy to bones, open epiphyses, or a past history of osteosarcoma or chondrosarcoma. Side effects may include injection site reactions, orthostatic hypotension, arthralgia, muscle cramps, depression, or pneumonia. Hypercalcemia can occur and manifest as nausea, constipation, asthenia, or muscle weakness. These drugs are approved for only a 2-year course of treatment.

Teriparatide and abaloparatide should not be used for patients with hypercalcemia. Similarly, they should be used with caution in patients if they are also taking corticosteroids and thiazide diuretics along with oral calcium supplementation because hypercalcemia may develop.

Following a 2-year course of teriparatide or abaloparatide, bisphosphonates should be given to retain the improved bone density. Alternatively, for very severe osteoporosis, these drugs may be administered along with denosumab; combined treatment for 2 years is more effective than any other single therapy, but adverse effects of fatigue, joint pain, and nausea are very common.

6. Selective estrogen receptor modulators (SERMs)— These agents can prevent osteoporosis but are not effective therapy for established osteoporosis. Raloxifene 60 mg/day orally may be taken by postmenopausal women in place of estrogen for prevention of osteoporosis. Bone density increases about 1% over 2 years in postmenopausal women versus 2% increases with estrogen replacement. It reduces the risk of vertebral fractures by about 40% but does not appear to reduce the risk of nonvertebral fractures. Unlike estrogen, raloxifene does not reduce hot flushes; in fact, it often intensifies them. It does not relieve vaginal dryness. Unlike estrogen, however, raloxifene does not cause endometrial hyperplasia, uterine bleeding, or cancer, nor does it cause breast soreness. The risk of breast cancer is reduced 76% in women taking raloxifene for 3 years. Since it is a potential teratogen, it is relatively contraindicated in women capable of pregnancy. Raloxifene increases the risk for thromboembolism and should not be used by women with such a history. Leg cramps can also occur. Tamoxifen is commonly administered to women for up to 5 years after resection of breast cancer that is estrogen receptor–positive. Tamoxifen has opposite effects on bone density in premenopausal versus postmenopausal women. In premenopausal women, tamoxifen causes a *loss* of vertebral bone mineral density of −1.44% yearly, whereas in postmenopausal women, tamoxifen causes an *increase* in vertebral bone mineral density of +1.17% yearly. Bazedoxifene is available as a fixed-dose combination of conjugated estrogens with a SERM (bazedoxifene) (0.45 mg/20 mg [Duavee]). It is FDA approved for the prevention of osteoporosis in postmenopausal women with an intact uterus. However, unlike raloxifene, it has not been shown to reduce the risk of breast cancer. Women taking this combination medication long-term experience an increased risk of thromboembolic events.

7. Calcitonin—Nasal salmon calcitonin is used primarily for its analgesic effect for the pain of acute osteoporotic vertebral compression fractures. It is ineffective for chronic pain. Its analgesic effect may be seen within 2–4 weeks. If it appears to be effective for analgesia, it is continued for up to 3 months. The usual dose is one spray (200 IU) once daily in alternating nostrils. Rhinitis and epistaxis occur commonly; less common reactions include flu-like symptoms, allergy, arthralgias, back pain, headache, and hypocalcemia. An injectable form (100 IU subcutaneously or intramuscularly every 1–2 days) can be used for vertebral fracture pain when the nasal formulation is not tolerated due to local reactions. Because its anti-osteoporosis effect is modest, calcitonin is only used in patients who cannot tolerate other therapies. Calcitonin increases the overall risk of malignancy by about 1.1%, particularly hepatic cancer, and has been withdrawn from the market in Canada and Europe.

8. Romosozumab—Romosozumab (Evenity) is an injectable monoclonal antibody that inhibits sclerostin, increasing new bone formation and decreasing bone resorption. In one large cohort of women with osteoporosis and fragility fractures, romosozumab treatment for 12 months followed by alendronate for 12 months resulted in a 48% lower risk of vertebral fractures and a 38% lower risk of hip fracture compared to women receiving alendronate alone. The dose is 210 mg subcutaneously monthly for up to 12 months. It is reserved for patients with very severe osteoporosis, such as those with multiple vertebral fractures. It should only be given to patients with a low risk of coronary disease or stroke since it may slightly increase the risk of adverse cardiovascular events.

Prognosis

Osteoporosis should ideally be prevented since it can be only partially reversed. Measures noted above are reasonably effective in preventing and treating osteoporosis and reducing fracture risk.

Black DM et al. Atypical femur fracture risk versus fragility fracture prevention with bisphosphonates. N Engl J Med. 2020;383:743. [PMID: 32813950]

Camacho PM et al. American Association of Clinical Endocrinologists/American College of Endocrinology Clinical Practice Guidelines for the diagnosis and treatment of postmenopausal osteoporosis—2020 update. Endocr Pract. 2020;26:1. [PMID: 32427503]

Ensrud KE et al. Anabolic therapy for osteoporosis. JAMA. 2021;326:350. [PMID: 34313699]

Shoback D et al. Pharmacological management of osteoporosis in postmenopausal women: an Endocrine Society guideline update. J Clin Endocrinol Metab. 2020;105:587. [PMID: 32068863]

RICKETS & OSTEOMALACIA

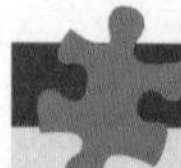

ESSENTIALS OF DIAGNOSIS

- Low bone density from defective mineralization.
- Caused by deficiency in calcium, phosphorus, or low alkaline phosphatase.
- **Rickets:** defective bone mineralization in childhood or adolescence before epiphyseal fusion.
- **Osteomalacia:** defective bone mineralization in adults with fused epiphyses.
- Painful proximal muscle weakness (especially pelvic girdle); bone pain.
- Low serum 25-hydroxy-vitamin D (25-OHD), hypocalcemia, hypocalciuria, hypophosphatemia, secondary hyperparathyroidism.
- Classic radiologic features may be present.

General Considerations

Defective mineralization of the growing skeleton in childhood causes permanent bone deformities (rickets). Defective skeletal mineralization in adults is known as osteomalacia. It is caused by inadequate calcium or phosphate mineralization of bone osteoid.

Etiology

Causes of osteomalacia are listed in Table 26–11.

A. Vitamin D Deficiency

Vitamin D deficiency is the most common cause of osteomalacia; its incidence is increasing throughout the world as a result of diminished exposure to sunlight caused by urbanization with use of automobile and public transportation,

Table 26–11. Causes of osteomalacia.[1]

Vitamin disorders
Insufficient sunlight exposure
Kidney: CKD, nephrotic syndrome, kidney transplantation
Liver disease
Nutritional deficiency of vitamin D
Malabsorption: aging, excess wheat bran, bariatric surgery, pancreatic enzyme deficiency, orlistat
Vitamin D–dependent rickets types I and II
Phenytoin, carbamazepine, valproate, or barbiturate therapy (long-term)
Dietary calcium deficiency
Phosphate deficiency
Adefovir therapy
Fanconi syndrome, renal tubular acidosis, and alcohol use disorder (alcoholism)
Intestinal malabsorption
Nutritional deficiency of phosphorus
Phosphate-binding antacid therapy
Renal loss
Tumoral hypophosphatemic osteomalacia
X-linked hypophosphatemic rickets
Other disorders, including paraproteinemias, glycogen storage diseases, neurofibromatosis, Wilson disease
Inhibitors of mineralization
Aluminum
Bisphosphonates
Disorders of bone matrix
Axial osteomalacia
Hypophosphatasia
Fibrogenesis imperfecta

[1]See Table 26–10 for causes of osteoporosis.

living at high latitudes, winter season, institutionalization, sunscreen use, or very modest dressing. About 36% of adults in the United States are deficient in vitamin D.

Other risk factors for vitamin D deficiency include the following: pregnancy, age over 65 years, obesity, dark skin, malnutrition, and intestinal malabsorption Patients with severe nephrotic syndrome lose large amounts of vitamin D–binding protein in the urine.

Anticonvulsants (eg, phenytoin, carbamazepine, valproate, phenobarbital) inhibit the hepatic production of 25-OHD and sometimes cause osteomalacia. Phenytoin can also directly inhibit bone mineralization.

Vitamin D–dependent rickets type I is caused by a rare autosomal recessive disorder with a defect in the renal enzyme 1-alpha-hydroxylase leading to defective synthesis of $1,25(OH)_2D$.

Vitamin D–dependent rickets type II (hereditary $1,25[OH]_2D$-resistant rickets) is caused by a genetic defect in the $1,25(OH)_2D$ receptor.

B. Calcium Deficiency

The total daily consumption of calcium should be at least 1000 mg daily. Patients who have deficient calcium intake develop rickets (childhood) or osteomalacia (adulthood) despite sufficient vitamin D. A nutritional deficiency of calcium can occur in any severely malnourished patient. Some degree of calcium deficiency is common in older adults, since intestinal calcium absorption declines with age. Ingestion of excessive wheat bran also causes calcium malabsorption.

C. Phosphate Deficiency

Osteomalacia develops in patients with hypophosphatemia due to lack of sufficient phosphate to mineralize bone osteoid. Such patients typically have musculoskeletal pain and muscle weakness and are prone to fractures.

1. Genetic disorders—Fibroblast growth factor-23 (FGF23) is a phosphaturic factor (phosphatonin) that is secreted by bone osteoblasts in response to elevated serum phosphate levels. Various genetic mutations can result in high serum FGF23 levels, causing hypophosphatemia and bone mineral depletion.

2. Tumor-induced osteomalacia—This is a rare paraneoplastic syndrome that can be caused by a variety of mesenchymal tumors (87% benign) secrete FGF23 and cause marked hypophosphatemia and hyperphosphaturia due to renal phosphate wasting. Such tumors are usually phosphaturic mesenchymal tumors (70%); other tumors include hemangiopericytomas, osteosarcomas, and giant cell tumors. Such tumors are often small and difficult to find, frequently lying in the sinuses or extremities.

3. Other causes of hypophosphatemia—Hypophosphatemia can be caused by alcohol use disorder (alcoholism), poor nutrition, and prolonged parenteral nutrition. Tenofovir therapy (tenofovir disoproxil fumarate more so than tenofovir alafamide) can cause renal phosphate wasting and hypophosphatemia. Severe hypophosphatemia can occur with refeeding after starvation. Hypophosphatemia can also be caused by chelation of phosphate in the gut by aluminum hydroxide antacids, calcium acetate (Phos-Lo), or sevelamer hydrochloride (Renagel). Excessive renal phosphate losses are also seen in proximal renal tubular acidosis, Fanconi syndrome, and in some women using oral contraceptives.

D. Aluminum Toxicity

Bone mineralization is inhibited by aluminum. Osteomalacia may occur in patients receiving long-term renal hemodialysis with tap water dialysate or from aluminum-containing antacids used to reduce phosphate levels.

E. Hypophosphatasia

Hypophosphatasia refers to a severe deficiency of bone alkaline phosphatase. It is a rare genetic cause of osteomalacia that is commonly misdiagnosed as osteoporosis.

It can present in adulthood with premature loss of teeth, metatarsal stress fractures, thigh pain due to femoral pseudofractures, or arthritis due to chondrocalcinosis. Bone density is low. Serum alkaline phosphatase is low (below 40 U/L in adults and often less than 20 U/L in severe cases). The differential diagnosis is asymptomatic hypophosphatasia and other causes of low serum alkaline phosphatase, such as early pregnancy, hypothyroidism, myeloma, severe anemia, or vitamin D intoxication.

F. Fibrogenesis Imperfecta Ossium

This rare condition sporadically affects middle-aged patients, who present with progressive bone pain and pathologic fractures. Bones have a dense "fishnet" appearance on radiographs. Serum alkaline phosphatase levels are elevated. Some patients have a monoclonal gammopathy, indicating a possible plasma cell dyscrasia causing an impairment in osteoblast function and collagen disarray.

Clinical Findings

Neonates and young children with hypocalcemia may have spasms and convulsions. Older children and adolescents can have bone pain and muscle weakness and may develop the skeletal deformities of classic rickets, such as delayed longitudinal growth, deformities at epiphyses leading to thickened wrists and ankles, and bowed legs or knock-knees (adolescents). Kyphoscoliosis or lumbar lordosis is common. Thickening at the costochondral joints can cause widening of the chest and deformities known as a "rachitic rosary."

In adults, osteomalacia is initially asymptomatic. Nonspecific complaints include fatigue, reduced endurance and muscle strength, and pain in the bones involving their shoulders ribs, low back, and thighs develop. Pathologic fractures can occur with little or no trauma.

Hypocalcemia causes a reduced quality of life, with fatigue, irritability, depression, anxiety, cognitive impairment, lethargy, and paresthesias in the circumoral area, hands, and feet. More severe manifestations include muscle weakness or cramps, carpopedal spasm, convulsions, tetany, laryngospasm, and stridor. Hypophosphatemia can cause severe major muscle weakness, reduced endurance, dysphagia, diplopia, cardiomyopathy, and respiratory muscle weakness. Patients may also have impaired cognition.

Diagnostic Tests

DXA BMD is used to determine the presence of low bone density that can be due to osteoporosis, osteomalacia, or both. Serum is obtained for calcium, albumin, phosphate, alkaline phosphatase, PTH, and 25-OHD determinations. Vitamin D *deficiency* is defined as a serum 25-OHD less than 20 ng/mL (50 nmol/L). Vitamin D *insufficiency* is defined as a serum 25-OHD between 20 ng/mL and 30 ng/mL (50–75 nmol/L). Patients with severe osteomalacia typically have chronic severe vitamin D deficiency (serum 25-OHD under 12 ng/mL [25 nmol/L]).

$1,25(OH)_2D_3$ may be low even when $25(OH)D_2$ levels are normal. In one series of biopsy-proved osteomalacia, alkaline phosphatase was elevated in 94% of patients; the calcium or phosphorus was low in 47% of patients; $25(OH)D_3$ was low in 29% of patients; and urinary calcium was low in 18% of patients. Pseudofractures were seen in 18% of patients. Radiographs may show diagnostic features. Bone densitometry helps document the degree of osteopenia.

Oral contraceptives can cause renal hypophosphatemia in some women, so a drug holiday from oral contraceptives is warranted. Patients with otherwise unexplained hypophosphatemia should have a measurement of serum or plasma fibroblast growth factor 23 (FGF-23). Patients with high FGF23 levels can have genetic testing for X-linked hypophosphatemic rickets (*PHEX*), autosomal dominant hypophosphatemic rickets (*FGF23*), and autosomal recessive hypophosphatemic rickets (*DMP1*). In hypophosphatemic patients without such mutations, searching for a tumor causing tumor-induced osteomalacia is reasonable, particularly in patients with bone pain or fractures. Such tumors are typically small and may be located anywhere, so they are best localized using a whole-body DOTATATE-PET/CT scan.

Patients with hypophosphatasia have low serum levels of alkaline phosphatase (below 40 units/L in adults and below 20 units/L in severe cases). However, immediately following a fracture, serum alkaline phosphatase rises and may obscure the diagnosis. The diagnosis of hypophosphatasia is further suggested by a 24-hour urine assay for phosphoethanolamine or serum pyridoxal 5-phosphate (B_6) level; these substrates for tissue-nonspecific alkaline phosphatase are always elevated in patients with hypophosphatasia. The diagnosis is confirmed with genetic testing for mutations in the *ALPL* gene.

Differential Diagnosis

Osteomalacia often coexists with osteoporosis. The relative contribution of the two entities to diminished bone density may not be apparent until treatment since a dramatic rise in bone density is often seen with therapy for osteomalacia. Phosphate deficiency must be distinguished from hypophosphatemia seen in hyperparathyroidism.

Prevention & Treatment

Humans naturally receive about 90% of their vitamin D from sunlight. To obtain adequate vitamin D, the face, arms, hands, or back must have sun exposure without sunscreen for 15 minutes at least twice weekly. In sunlight-deprived individuals (eg, veiled women, confined patients, or residents of higher latitudes during winter), vitamin D_3, 1000 IU daily, should be given prophylactically. Patients receiving long-term phenytoin therapy should also receive vitamin D_3 supplementation. The main natural food source of vitamin D is fish, particularly salmon, mackerel, cod liver oil, and sardines or tuna canned in oil. Most commercial cow's milk is fortified with vitamin D at about 400 IU (10 mcg) per quart; however, yogurt and cottage cheese may contain little to no vitamin D_3.

Many vitamin supplements contain plant-derived vitamin D_2, which has variable biologic availability. Therefore, it is prudent to recommend that patients take a dedicated vitamin D_3 supplement from a reliable manufacturer.

Severe vitamin D deficiency can be treated with ergocalciferol (D_2), 50,000 IU orally once weekly for 8 weeks. Some patients require long-term supplementation with D_2 of up to 50,000 IU weekly. The alternative is to treat vitamin D–deficient patients with daily cholecalciferol D_3 at doses of at least 2000 IU daily. High daily doses of vitamin D_3 (10,000 IU/day for adults) are sometimes required for patients with obesity, intestinal malabsorption, or following gastric bypass surgery; rarely, severe malabsorption may require 25,000–100,000 IU daily. Patients with steatorrhea may respond better to oral $25(OH)D_3$ (calcifediol), 50–100 mcg/day. Serum levels of 25-OHD should be monitored, and the dosage of vitamin D adjusted to maintain serum 25-OHD levels above 30 ng/mL. The Endocrine Society recommends a target range of serum 25-OHD of 40–60 ng/mL. Serum 25-OHD levels above this range provide no additional benefit and may actually cause *reduce* bone strength.

The addition of calcium supplements to vitamin D is unnecessary for the prevention of osteomalacia in most otherwise well-nourished patients. Patients with malabsorption or poor nutrition should receive supplementation with calcium citrate (eg, Citracal), 0.4–0.6 g elemental calcium per day, or calcium carbonate (eg, OsCal, Tums), 1–1.5 g elemental calcium per day with meals.

In hypophosphatemic rickets or osteomalacia, nutritional deficiencies are corrected, aluminum-containing antacids are discontinued, and patients with renal tubular acidosis are given bicarbonate therapy.

For patients with tumoral hypophosphatemia, resection of the tumor normalizes serum phosphate levels but about 20% experience recurrence, usually in the same location. With both tumoral and genetic FGF23-related hypophosphatemia, therapy with burosumab improves osteomalacia.

Patients with hypophosphatasia may be treated with asfotase alfa (Strensiq). Teriparatide can improve bone pain and fracture healing. Bisphosphonates are contraindicated.

Burt LA et al. Effect of high-dose vitamin D supplementation on volumetric bone density and bone strength: a randomized clinical trial. JAMA. 2019;322:736. [PMID: 31454046]

PAGET DISEASE OF BONE (Osteitis Deformans)

ESSENTIALS OF DIAGNOSIS

- Often asymptomatic.
- Bone pain may be the first symptom.
- Kyphosis, bowed tibias, large head, deafness, and frequent fractures.
- Serum calcium and phosphate normal; elevated alkaline phosphatase and urinary hydroxyproline.
- Dense, expanded bones on radiographs.

General Considerations

Paget disease of bone is manifested by one or more bony lesions having high bone turnover and disorganized osteoid formation. The involved bone first has increased osteoclast activity, causing lytic lesions that may progress at about 1 cm/year. Increased osteoblastic activity follows, producing a high rate of disorganized bone formation. Involved bones become vascular, weak, and deformed. Eventually, there is a final burned-out phase with markedly reduced bone cell activity and abnormal bones that may be enlarged with skeletal deformity.

The prevalence of Paget disease has declined by about 36% over the past 20 years. It is most common in the United Kingdom and in areas of European migration, and it is rare in Africa, India, Asia, and Scandinavia. In the United States, Paget disease affects about 1% of White persons over age 55 years, with its prevalence increasing with age over 40 years. Most cases are discovered incidentally during radiology imaging or because of incidentally discovered elevations in serum alkaline phosphatase.

Clinical Findings

A. Symptoms and Signs

Paget disease is often mild and asymptomatic. Only 27% of affected individuals are symptomatic at the time of diagnosis. Paget disease involves multiple bones (polyostotic) in 72% and only a single bone (monostotic) in 28%. It occurs most commonly in the pelvis, vertebrae, femur, humerus, and skull. The disease typically involves affected bones simultaneously and tends not to involve additional bones during its course. Pain, often described as aching, deep, and worse at night, is the usual initial symptom. It may occur in the involved bone or in an adjacent joint, which can be involved with degenerative arthritis. Paget disease typically affects long bones proximally and then advances distally, with bone pain at the osteolytic front being aggravated by weight bearing. Joint surfaces (such as the knee) can be involved and cause arthritic pain. The bones can become soft, leading to bowed tibias, kyphosis, and frequent "chalkstick" fractures with slight trauma. If the skull is involved, the patient may report headaches and an increased hat size; half such patients have dilated scalp veins, the "scalp vein sign." Involvement of the petrous temporal bone frequently damages the cochlea, causing hearing loss, tinnitus, or vertigo. Increased vascularity over the involved bones causes increased warmth.

B. Laboratory Findings

Serum alkaline phosphatase is often markedly elevated and its source is bone (rather than liver). About 40% of patients have normal serum alkaline phosphatase levels, particularly those with monostotic involvement. Bone alkaline phosphatase is less useful for following the effectiveness of therapy. Other markers for bone turnover are serum N-terminal propeptide of type 1 collagen (NTx) and serum beta C-terminal propeptide of type 1 collagen (betaCTx). However, such bone turnover markers may overestimate or underestimate the response to treatment. Serum calcium may be elevated, particularly if the patient is at bed rest. A serum 25-OH vitamin D determination should be obtained to screen for vitamin D deficiency, which can also present with an increased serum alkaline phosphatase and bone pain.

C. Imaging

Initial radiographic lesions of Paget disease are typically osteolytic, with focal radiolucencies ("osteoporosis circumscripta") in the skull or advancing flame-shaped lytic lesions in long bones. In vertebrae, the lesions may display a "clover" or "heart" appearance, helping distinguish them from bone metastases. Bone lesions may subsequently become sclerotic and have a mixed lytic and sclerotic appearance. The affected bones eventually become thickened and deformed. Technetium-99m pyrophosphate bone scans are helpful in delineating activity of bone lesions and finding additional lesions in other locations.

Differential Diagnosis

Rare familial types of sclerosing bone dysplasias share phenotypic homologies with Paget disease of bone. The differential diagnosis also includes myelofibrosis, intramedullary osteosclerosis, Erdheim-Chester disease, Langerhans cell histiocytosis, and sickle cell disease.

Paget disease must be differentiated from primary bone lesions (eg, osteogenic sarcoma, plasma cell myeloma, and fibrous dysplasia) and from secondary bone lesions (eg, osteitis fibrosa cystica and metastatic carcinoma to bone). Fibrogenesis imperfecta ossium is a rare symmetric disorder that can mimic the features of Paget disease; serum alkaline phosphatase is likewise elevated. This condition may be associated with paraproteinemias.

Complications

If immobilization occurs, hypercalcemia and renal calculi may develop. With severe polyostotic disease, the increased vascularity may give rise to high-output heart failure. Arthritis frequently develops in joints adjacent to involved bone.

Extensive skull involvement may cause cranial nerve palsies from impingement of the neural foramina.

Skull involvement can also cause a vascular steal syndrome with somnolence or ischemic neurologic events; the optic nerve may be affected, resulting in loss of vision. Jaw involvement can cause the teeth to spread intraorally and become misaligned. Vertebral collapse can cause compression of spinal cord or spinal nerves, resulting in radiculopathy or paralysis. Vertebral involvement can also cause a vascular steal syndrome with paralysis. Surgery for fractured long bones is often complicated by excessive blood loss from these vascular lytic lesions.

Sarcoma or giant cell tumor develops in less than 1% of long-standing lesions. Sarcomatous change is suggested by a marked increase in bone pain, sudden rise in alkaline phosphatase, and appearance of a new lytic lesion.

Treatment

Asymptomatic patients may require only clinical surveillance. However, treatment with bisphosphonates should be considered for asymptomatic patients who have significant involvement of the skull, long bones, or vertebrae. Patients must be monitored carefully before, during, and after treatment with clinical examinations and serial serum alkaline phosphatase determinations.

Zoledronic acid is the treatment of choice. Administered intravenously as a single 5-mg dose, it normalizes the serum alkaline phosphatase in 89% of patients by 6 months and in 98% by 2 years.

Zoledronic acid should be administered prior to total arthroplasty for a Paget-involved joint or before osteotomy for lower extremity bowing in order to reduce the risk of intraoperative hemorrhaging and loosening of the prosthesis postoperatively. For patients with paraplegia due to vertebral involvement, intravenous zoledronic acid should be given while neurosurgical consultation is obtained.

Patients frequently experience a paradoxical increase in pain at sites of disease soon after commencing bisphosphonate therapy; this "first dose effect" usually subsides with further treatment. Following intravenous zoledronic acid, patients frequently experience fever, fatigue, myalgia, bone pain, and ocular problems. Serious side effects are rare but include seizures, uveitis, and acute kidney disease. Asthma may occur in aspirin-sensitive patients. Hypocalcemia is common and may be severe, especially if intravenous bisphosphonates are given along with loop diuretics. Therefore, it is advisable to administer calcium and vitamin D supplements, especially during the first 2 weeks following treatment. Any vitamin D deficiency should be corrected before prescribing a bisphosphonate.

Oral bisphosphonate regimens are inferior to intravenous zoledronic acid for therapy of Paget disease. Patients who cannot tolerate bisphosphonates may be treated with calcitonin.

Prognosis

The prognosis is good, but relapse can occur after an initial successful treatment with bisphosphonate. By 6.5 years after initial therapy, the recurrence rate is 12.5% after treatment with zoledronic acid and 62% after risedronate. Patients must be monitored long term, measuring serum alkaline phosphatase at least yearly. In general, the prognosis is worse the earlier in life the disease starts. Fractures usually heal well. In the severe forms, marked deformity, intractable pain, and high-output heart failure occur if not treated with bisphosphonates. Osteosarcoma that arises at sites of Paget disease results in a 2-year survival of only 25%.

Hsu E. Paget's disease of bone: updates for clinicians. Curr Opin Endocrinol Diabetes Obes. 2019;26:329. [PMID: 31574000]

Ralston SH et al. Diagnosis and management of Paget's disease of bone in adults: a clinical guideline. J Bone Miner Res. 2019; 34:579. [PMID: 30803025]

DISEASES OF THE ADRENAL CORTEX

PRIMARY ADRENAL INSUFFICIENCY (Addison Disease)

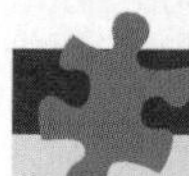

ESSENTIALS OF DIAGNOSIS

- Deficiency of cortisol and mineralocorticoid from destruction of the adrenal cortex.
- Weakness, vomiting, diarrhea; abdominal pain, arthralgias; amenorrhea.
- Increased skin pigmentation, especially of creases, pressure areas, and nipples.
- Hypovolemic hypotension.
- Hyponatremia; hyperkalemia; hypoglycemia; eosinophilia.
- Elevated plasma ACTH level; cosyntropin unable to stimulate serum cortisol to ≥ 20 mcg/dL (550 nmol/L).
- **Acute adrenal crisis:** above manifestations become critical, with fever, shock, confusion, coma, death.

General Considerations

Primary adrenal insufficiency (Addison disease) is caused by dysfunction or absence of the adrenal cortices. Secondary adrenal insufficiency is caused by deficient secretion of ACTH. Addison disease refers to a chronic deficiency of cortisol caused by adrenocortical insufficiency; plasma ACTH and alpha-MSH levels are consequently elevated, causing pigmentation that ranges from none to strikingly dark.

Addison disease is an uncommon disorder. In the United States, the prevalence is about 90–140 cases per million and the annual incidence is about 5–6 cases per million. Patients with destruction of the adrenal cortices or with classic 21-hydroxylase deficiency also have mineralocorticoid deficiency, typically with hyponatremia, volume depletion, and hyperkalemia. In contrast, mineralocorticoid deficiency is not present in patients with familial corticosteroid deficiency, Allgrove syndrome, or secondary adrenal insufficiency.

Acute adrenal (Addisonian) crisis is an emergency caused by insufficient cortisol. Crisis may occur in the course of treatment of chronic adrenal insufficiency, or it may be the presenting manifestation of adrenal insufficiency. Acute adrenal crisis is more commonly seen in primary adrenal insufficiency than in secondary adrenal insufficiency. It is usually precipitated by one of the following: (1) severe stress (eg, infection, trauma, surgery, hyperthyroidism, or prolonged fasting), or minor stress (vaccinations) in patients with latent or treated adrenal insufficiency; (2) hyperthyroidism or prescription of thyroid hormone to patients with untreated adrenal insufficiency; (3) nonadherence to glucocorticoid replacement or sudden withdrawal of adrenocortical hormone in patients with chronic primary or secondary adrenal insufficiency; (4) bilateral adrenalectomy or removal of a functioning adrenal tumor that had suppressed the other adrenal gland; (5) sudden destruction of the pituitary gland (pituitary necrosis) or damage to both adrenals (by trauma, hemorrhage, anticoagulant therapy, thrombosis, infection or, rarely, metastatic carcinoma); or (6) administration of intravenous etomidate (used for rapid anesthesia induction or intubation).

Etiology

Autoimmunity is the most common cause of Addison disease in industrialized countries, accounting for about 90% of spontaneous cases; adrenal function decreases over several years as it progresses to overt adrenal insufficiency. Over half the cases of autoimmune Addison disease occur as part of an autoimmune polyendocrine syndrome (APS-1, APS-2). Addison disease can also occur following treatment for malignancies with PD-1 immune checkpoint inhibitors.

Bilateral adrenal infiltrative diseases cause primary adrenal insufficiency. Causative neoplasms include lymphomas, breast cancer, and lung cancer. Causative infections include tuberculosis, coccidiomycosis, histoplasmosis, cytomegalovirus, cryptococcus, and syphilis.

Infections of the adrenal glands, particularly with cytomegalovirus, are found in nearly half of patients with untreated HIV at autopsy. However, a much lower percentage have clinical Addison disease. The diagnosis of adrenal insufficiency in HIV patients is often problematic. A cortisol resistance syndrome has been described in patients with HIV, and a revision of normal range for the cosyntropin test for these patients has been advocated (normal peak cortisol over 22 mcg/dL). Also, isolated hyperkalemia occurs commonly in HIV patients, particularly during therapy with pentamidine; this is usually due to isolated hypoaldosteronism and responds to mineralocorticoid (fludrocortisone) therapy alone.

Bilateral adrenal hemorrhage may occur with sepsis, heparin-associated thrombocytopenia, anticoagulation, or the antiphospholipid antibody syndrome. It may occur in association with major surgery or trauma, presenting about 1 week later with pain, fever, and shock. It may also occur spontaneously and present with flank pain. Meningococcemia may be associated with purpura and adrenal insufficiency secondary to adrenal infarction (Waterhouse-Friderichsen syndrome).

Adrenoleukodystrophy is an X-linked peroxisomal disorder causing accumulation of very long-chain fatty acids in the adrenal cortex, testes, brain, and spinal cord. Adrenal insufficiency ultimately occurs in 80% of affected patients and accounts for one-third of cases of Addison disease in boys. It presents most commonly in childhood or adolescence but can manifest at any age.

Congenital adrenal insufficiency occurs in several conditions. Familial corticosteroid deficiency is an autosomal recessive disease that is caused by mutations in the adrenal ACTH receptor (melanocortin 2 receptor, MC2R). It is characterized by isolated cortisol deficiency and ACTH resistance and may present with neonatal hypoglycemia, frequent infections, and dark skin pigmentation. Triple A (Allgrove) syndrome is caused by a mutation in the *AAAS* gene that encodes a protein known as ALADIN (***al***achrima, ***a***chalasia, a***d***renal ***i***nsufficiency, ***n***eurologic disorder). Cortisol deficiency usually presents in infancy but may not occur until the third decade of life.

Congenital adrenal hyperplasia is caused by various genetic defects in the enzymes responsible for steroid synthesis. Due to defective cortisol synthesis, patients have variable degrees of adrenal insufficiency and increased levels of ACTH that causes hyperplasia of the adrenal cortex. The most common enzyme defect is *P450c21 (21-hydroxylase deficiency).*

Drugs that cause primary adrenal insufficiency include mitotane, abiraterone acetate, and the tyrosine kinase inhibitors lenvatinib and vandetanib. **Rare causes** of adrenal insufficiency include lymphoma, metastatic carcinoma, scleroderma, amyloidosis, and hemochromatosis.

Clinical Findings

A. Symptoms and Signs

The onset of symptoms can occur suddenly but usually develops gradually over months or years. The diagnosis is often delayed, since many early symptoms are nonspecific. Over 90% of patients complain of fatigue, reduced stamina, weakness, anorexia, and weight loss. Over 80% of affected patients present with symptoms of orthostatic hypotension (aggravated by dehydration caused by nausea or vomiting), lightheadedness with standing, salt craving, and eventually hyperpigmentation of skin and gums. Abdominal pain, nausea, and vomiting eventually develop in most patients; diarrhea can occur, aggravating dehydration and hypotension. Fevers and lymphoid tissue hyperplasia may also occur. Patients often have significant pain: arthralgias, myalgias, chest pain, abdominal pain, back pain, leg pain, or headache. Psychiatric symptoms include anxiety, irritability and depression; by the time of diagnosis, over 40% of patients have been told that their symptoms were psychological. Cerebral edema can cause headache, vomiting, gait disturbance, and intellectual dysfunction that may progress to coma. Hypoglycemia can occur and worsen the patient's weakness and mental functioning. Patients treated long-term for adrenal insufficiency appear to be more prone to pneumonia and GI and UTIs.

Skin hyperpigmentation due to increased pituitary secretion of alpha-MSH varies among affected patients (eg, from none to increased freckling to diffuse darkening that resembles a suntan or a bronze appearance). Sun-exposed areas darken the most, but nonexposed areas darken as well. Hyperpigmentation is often especially prominent over the knuckles, elbows, knees, posterior neck, palmar creases, gingival mucosa, and vermilion border of the lips. Nail beds may develop longitudinal pigmented bands. Nipples and areolas tend to darken. The skin also darkens in pressure areas, such as the belt or brassiere lines and the buttocks. Skin folds and new scars may also become pigmented. Conversely, patches of autoimmune vitiligo can be found in about 10% of patients. Scant axillary and pubic hair typically develops in women.

In pregnancy, undiagnosed adrenal insufficiency is rare, since the condition tends to cause anovulation and reduced fertility.. Undiagnosed adrenal insufficiency can cause intrauterine growth retardation and fetal loss. Pregnant women with undiagnosed adrenal insufficiency can experience shock from adrenal crisis, particularly during the first trimester, concurrent illness, labor, or postpartum.

Patients with preexistent type 1 diabetes experience more frequent hypoglycemia with the onset of adrenal insufficiency, such that their insulin dosage must be reduced.

Acute adrenal crisis is an immediate threat to life. Affected patients have magnified symptoms of chronic adrenal insufficiency and experience an acute deterioration in their health, typically with acute GI symptoms and fever that can mimic an abdominal emergency. Infections (lower respiratory, urinary, or GI) are common triggers for acute adrenal crisis. Patients also frequently experience back pain, arthralgias, and profound fatigue. They may have delirium or coma, sometimes aggravated by hypoglycemia. Adrenal crisis is marked by orthostatic dizziness and hypotension (blood pressure below 100 mm Hg systolic or 20 mm Hg lower than their basline). Reversible cardiomyopathy and heart failure can also occur, causing hypotension that can progress to life-threatening shock that does not respond to intravenous fluids and vasopressors.

B. Laboratory Findings

Typically, there is mild anemia, moderate neutropenia, lymphocytosis, and eosinophilia (total eosinophil count over 300/mcL). Among patients with chronic adrenal insufficiency, the serum sodium is usually low (88%) and the potassium elevated (64%). However, patients with vomiting or diarrhea may not be hyperkalemic. Fasting hypoglycemia is common. Hypercalcemia may be present.

A plasma cortisol less than 3 mcg/dL (83 nmol/L) at 8 AM is diagnostic, especially if accompanied by simultaneous elevation of the plasma ACTH level greater than 200 pg/mL (44 pmol/L). The diagnosis is confirmed by a simplified cosyntropin stimulation test: (1) Synthetic $ACTH_{1-24}$ (cosyntropin), 0.25 mg, is given intramuscularly. (2) Serum cortisol is obtained 45 minutes after cosyntropin is administered. Normally, serum cortisol rises to at least 20 mcg/dL (550 pmol/L), whereas patients with adrenal insufficiency have stimulated serum cortisol levels less than 20 mcg/dL (550 pmol/L). For patients receiving corticosteroid treatment, hydrocortisone must not be given for at least 8 hours before the test. Other corticosteroids (eg, prednisone, dexamethasone) do not interfere with specific assays for cortisol. Cosyntropin is usually well tolerated, but infrequent (less than 5%) side effects have included hypersensitivity reactions with nausea, headache, dizziness, dyspnea, palpitations, flushing, edema, and local injection site reactions.

One or more serum anti-adrenal antibodies are found in about 50% of cases of autoimmune Addison disease. The sensitivity of four serum anti-adrenal antibodies is as follows: cytoplasmic antibodies (26%), 21-hydroxylase antibodies (21%), 17-hydroxylase antibodies (21%), and side-chain cleavage antibodies (16%). Antibodies to thyroid (45%) and other tissues may also be present.

Elevated plasma renin activity (PRA) indicates the presence of depleted intravascular volume and the need for fludrocortisone administration. Serum epinephrine levels are low in untreated patients with adrenal insufficiency.

Salt-wasting congenital adrenal hyperplasia due to 21-hydroxylase deficiency is usually diagnosed at birth. The specific diagnosis requires elevated serum levels of 17-OH progesterone.

Young men with idiopathic Addison disease are screened for X-linked adrenoleukodystrophy by determining plasma very long-chain fatty acid levels; affected patients have high levels.

In acute adrenal crisis, blood, sputum, or urine cultures may be positive if bacterial infection is the precipitating cause.

C. Imaging

When adrenal insufficiency is not clearly autoimmune, a CT scan of the adrenal glands should be obtained. The adrenals are enlarged in about 85% of cases related to metastatic or granulomatous disease. Adrenal calcifications occur in 50% of tuberculous Addison cases but are also seen with hemorrhage, fungal infection, pheochromocytoma, and melanoma. Small, noncalcified adrenals are seen in autoimmune Addison disease.

Differential Diagnosis

Patients with secondary adrenal insufficiency due to ACTH deficiency have normal mineralocorticoid production and do not develop hyperkalemia (see Hypopituitarism). In contrast to Addison disease, patients with secondary adrenal insufficiency have normal to decreased skin pigmentation that has been described as "alabaster skin." Hemochromatosis also causes bronze skin hyperpigmentation, and hemochromatosis may in fact be the cause of Addison disease. Acute adrenal crisis must be distinguished from other causes of shock (eg, septic, hemorrhagic, cardiogenic).

The constitutional symptoms may be mistaken for cancer, anorexia nervosa, or emotional stress. Acute adrenal insufficiency must be distinguished from an acute abdomen in which neutrophilia is the rule, whereas in adrenal insufficiency there is lymphocytosis and eosinophilia.

The neurologic manifestations of Allgrove syndrome and adrenoleukodystrophy (especially in women) may mimic multiple sclerosis. Hyperkalemia can be caused by hyporeninemic hypoaldosteronism from type IV renal tubular acidosis. Hyperkalemia is also seen with rhabdomyolysis, hyperkalemic paralysis, and some drugs (eg, ACE inhibitors, spironolactone, and drospirenone) (see Chapter 21).

Hyponatremia is seen in many other conditions (eg, hypothyroidism, diuretic use, heart failure, cirrhosis, vomiting, diarrhea, severe illness, or major surgery) (see Figure 21–1). Nearly 40% of critically ill patients have low serum cortisol levels due to low serum albumin levels; their total serum cortisol levels may be low but their serum free cortisol levels are normal.

Complications

Any of the complications of the underlying disease (eg, tuberculosis) are more likely to occur in adrenal insufficiency, and intercurrent infections may precipitate an acute adrenal crisis. Associated autoimmune diseases are common (see above).

Treatment

A. General Measures

Patients and family members must be thoroughly educated about adrenal insufficiency. *Patients are advised to wear a medical alert bracelet or medal reading, "Adrenal insufficiency—takes hydrocortisone."* They need to be provided with a dose escalation schedule for increased corticosteroids for illness, accidents, or prior to minor surgical procedures and for increased fludrocortisone for hot weather or prolonged strenuous exercise. Corticosteroids and fludrocortisone must be prescribed in liberal amounts with automatic refills to avoid the patient's running out of medication. It is also advisable to prescribe a routine antiemetic such as ondansetron ODT 8-mg tablets to be taken every 8 hours for nausea. Parenteral hydrocortisone (Solu-Cortef) 100 mg is also prescribed for patient self-injection in the event of vomiting. Patients must receive advance instructions to seek medical attention at an emergency facility immediately in the event of vomiting or severe illness. All infections should be treated immediately and vigorously, with hydrocortisone administered at appropriately increased doses.

B. Specific Therapy

Replacement therapy should include corticosteroids with mineralocorticoids for primary adrenal insufficiency. In mild cases, corticosteroids alone may be adequate.

1. Corticosteroid replacement therapy—Maintenance therapy for most patients with Addison disease is 15–30 mg of hydrocortisone orally daily in two divided doses (10–20 mg in the morning; 5–10 mg in the evening) or three divided doses (eg, 10 mg at 7 AM, 10 mg at 1 PM, and 5 mg at 7 PM). Some patients respond better to prednisone or methylprednisolone in doses of about 3–6 mg daily in divided doses. Adjustments in dosage are made according to the clinical response. The corticosteroid dose should be kept at the lowest level at which the patient feels clinically well.

Patients with partial ACTH deficiency (basal morning serum cortisol above 8 mg/dL [220 mmol/L]) require hydrocortisone replacement in lower doses of about 5 mg orally twice daily or even 10 mg every morning. Some patients feel better with the substitution of prednisone (2–7.5 mg/day orally) or methylprednisolone (2–6 mg/day orally), given in divided doses. Fludrocortisone is not required. Additional corticosteroid must be given during stress, (eg, infection, trauma, or surgical procedures). For mild illness or mild-moderate surgical stress, corticosteroid doses are doubled or tripled. For severe illness, trauma, or major surgical stress, hydrocortisone 100 mg is given intravenously, followed by 200 mg daily, given as either a continuous intravenous infusion or as 50 mg boluses given every 6 hours intravenously or intramuscularly and then reduced to usual doses as the stress subsides.

Plenadren MR (5- or 20-mg modified-release tablets) is a once-daily dual-release oral preparation of hydrocortisone that may be administered in the morning (usual dose range is 20–30 mg daily). Preliminary studies indicate that plenadren may improve quality of life in some patients with adrenal insufficiency. It is not available in the United States but is available in Canada and elsewhere.

Patients must be monitored carefully for clinical signs of over- or under-replacement of corticosteroid replacement therapy. A proper corticosteroid dose usually results in clinical improvement. Fatigue may also be an indication of suboptimal dosing of medication, electrolyte imbalance, or concurrent hypothyroidism or diabetes mellitus. A WBC count with a differential can be useful, since a relative neutrophilia and lymphopenia can indicate corticosteroid over replacement, and vice versa. Serum ACTH levels vary substantially and should not be used to determine dosing.

Caution: Increased corticosteroid dosing is required in circumstances of infection, trauma, surgery, stressful diagnostic procedures, or other forms of stress. For severe stress of major illness, surgery, or delivery, a maximum stress dose of hydrocortisone is given as 50–100 mg intravenously or intramuscularly, followed by 50 mg every 6 hours (continuous intravenous infusion or boluses), then reduced over several days. However, following major trauma, increased doses of replacement hydrocortisone may be required for up to several weeks. Lower doses, oral or parenteral, are used for less severe stress. For immunizations that are given with an adjuvant, such as varicella zoster (Shingrix), there is sufficient local inflammation that increased doses of hydrocortisone are recommended for 5 days following the immunization. The dose is reduced back to normal as the stress subsides. Decreased corticosteroid dosing is required when medications are prescribed that inhibit corticosteroid metabolism by blocking the isoenzyme CYP34A, particularly the antifungals ketoconazole or itraconazole, the antidepressant nefazodone, anti-HIV protease inhibitors, and cobicistat. Rifampin increases hydrocortisone clearance, necessitating increased corticosteroid dosing. During the third trimester of pregnancy, corticosteroid requirements are higher, so usual corticosteroid doses are increased by 50%.

2. Mineralocorticoid replacement therapy—Fludrocortisone acetate has a potent sodium-retaining effect. The dosage is 0.05–0.3 mg orally daily or every other day. In the presence of postural hypotension, hyponatremia, or hyperkalemia, the dosage is increased. Similarly, in patients with fatigue, an elevated PRA indicates the need for a higher replacement dose of fludrocortisone. If edema, hypokalemia, or hypertension ensues, the dose is decreased. During treatment with hydrocortisone with maximum doses appropriate for stress, fludrocortisone replacement is not required. Some patients cannot tolerate fludrocortisone and must substitute NaCl tablets to replace renal sodium loss.

3. DHEA replacement therapy—DHEA is given to some women with adrenal insufficiency. In a double-blind clinical trial, women taking DHEA 50 mg orally each morning experienced an improved sense of well-being, increased muscle mass, and a reversal in bone loss at the femoral neck. Older women who receive DHEA should be monitored for androgenic effects. Because over-the-counter preparations have variable potencies, it is best to have the pharmacy formulate this with pharmaceutical-grade micronized DHEA.

4. Treatment of hyperandrogenism in women with congenital adrenal hyperplasia—See Hirsutism & Virilization.

5. Treatment of acute adrenal crisis—If acute adrenal crisis is suspected but the diagnosis of adrenal insufficiency is not yet established, intravenous access must be established. Blood is drawn for cultures, plasma ACTH, serum cortisol, serum glucose, BUN, creatinine, and electrolyte levels. A UA is obtained to screen for a UTI. Without waiting for the results, treatment is initiated *immediately* with hydrocortisone, 100 mg by intravenous bolus followed by 50 mg intravenously every 6 hours as either intravenous boluses or a continuous intravenous infusion. The hydrocortisone dosage may then be reduced according to the clinical picture and laboratory test results.

Intravenous fluids are administered as either 0.9% normal saline or 0.9% normal saline/5% dextrose solutions. A volume of 2–3 L is given quickly and then the intravenous rate is reduced according to clinical parameters and frequent serum electrolytes and glucose determinations. When intravenous saline is stopped, mineralocorticoid replacement is commenced with fludrocortisone, starting with 0.1 mg orally daily and adjusted according to serum electrolyte determinations.

Since bacterial infection frequently precipitates acute adrenal crisis, broad-spectrum antibiotics should be administered empirically while waiting for the results of initial cultures (Table 30–5). The patient must also be treated for electrolyte abnormalities, hypoglycemia, and dehydration, as indicated.

When the patient can take food by mouth, hydrocortisone is administered orally in doses of 10–20 mg every 6 hours, and the dosage is reduced to maintenance levels as needed. Most patients ultimately require hydrocortisone twice daily (10–20 mg in the morning; 5–10 mg in the evening). Mineralocorticoid replacement is not needed when large amounts of hydrocortisone are given, but as its dose is reduced, it is usually necessary to add fludrocortisone acetate, 0.05–0.2 mg orally daily. Some patients never require fludrocortisone or become edematous at doses of more than 0.05 mg once or twice weekly. Once the crisis has passed, the patient must be evaluated to assess the degree of permanent adrenal insufficiency and to establish the cause, if possible.

Prognosis

The life expectancy of patients with Addison disease is reasonably normal, as long as they are compliant with their medications and knowledgeable about their condition. Adrenal crisis can occur in patients who stop their medication or who experience stress such as infection, trauma, or surgery without appropriately higher doses of corticosteroids. Cushing syndrome can develop, imposing its own risks, in patients who take excessive doses of corticosteroid replacement.

Rapid treatment is usually lifesaving in acute adrenal crisis. However, if adrenal crisis is unrecognized and untreated, shock that is unresponsive to fluid replacement and vasopressors can result in death.

Merke DP et al. Congenital adrenal hyperplasia due to 21-hydroxylase deficiency. N Engl J Med. 2020;383:124861. [PMID: 32966723]

Prete A et al. Prevention of adrenal crisis: cortisol responses to major stress compared to stress dose hydrocortisone delivery. J Clin Endocrinol Metab. 2020;105:2262. [PMID: 32170323]

Rushworth RL et al. Adrenal crisis. N Engl J Med. 2019;381:852. [PMID: 31461595]

Saverino S et al. Autoimmune Addison's disease. Best Pract Res Clin Endocrinol Metab. 2020;34:101379. [PMID: 32063488]

CUSHING SYNDROME (Hypercortisolism)

ESSENTIALS OF DIAGNOSIS

- Central obesity, muscle wasting, hirsutism, purple striae.
- Psychological changes.
- Osteoporosis, hypertension, poor wound healing.
- Hyperglycemia, leukocytosis, lymphocytopenia, hypokalemia.
- Elevated serum cortisol and urinary free cortisol. Lack of normal suppression by dexamethasone.

General Considerations

The term Cushing "syndrome" refers to the manifestations of excessive corticosteroids, commonly due to supraphysiologic doses of corticosteroid drugs and rarely due to spontaneous production of excessive cortisol by the adrenal cortex. Cases of spontaneous Cushing syndrome are rare, with an incidence of 2.6 new cases yearly per million population in the United States.

A. Cushing Disease with Elevated ACTH Levels

About 68% of cases are due to Cushing "disease," caused by a benign ACTH-secreting pituitary adenoma that is typically smaller than 5 mm and usually located in the anterior pituitary (94%); however, about 6% of such adenomas are ectopic in locations such as the cavernous sinus, sphenoid sinus, ethmoid sinus, or posterior pituitary. Cushing disease is at least three times more frequent in women than men.

About 7% of cases are due to nonpituitary ACTH-secreting neuroendocrine neoplasms that produce ectopic ACTH. Ectopic locations include the lungs (55%), pancreas (9%), mediastinum-thymus (8%), adrenal (6%), GI tract (5%), thyroid (4%), and other sites (13%). About 15% of cases are due to ACTH from a source that cannot be initially located.

B. Cushing Disease with Normal or Low ACTH

About 25% of cases are due to excessive *autonomous* secretion of cortisol by the adrenals. Cortisol secretion is independent of ACTH, and plasma ACTH levels are usually low or low-normal. Most such cases are due to a unilateral adrenal tumor. Benign adrenal adenomas are generally small and produce mostly cortisol; adrenocortical carcinomas are usually large when discovered and can produce excessive cortisol as well as androgens but may be nonsecretory. ACTH-independent macronodular adrenal hyperplasia can also produce hypercortisolism due to the adrenal cortex cells' abnormal stimulation by hormones such as catecholamines, arginine vasopressin, serotonin, hCG/LH, or gastric inhibitory polypeptide; in the latter case, hypercortisolism may be intermittent and food-dependent, and plasma ACTH levels may not be completely suppressed. Bilateral primary pigmented adrenal macronodular adrenocortical disease may be an isolated condition or part of the Carney complex, an autosomal dominant condition with additional features consisting of myxomas of the heart and skin with spotty skin pigmentation and facial freckles.

Clinical Findings

A. Symptoms and Signs

The manifestations of Cushing syndrome vary considerably. Early in the course of the disease, patients frequently complain of nonspecific symptoms, such as fatigue or reduced endurance but may have few, if any, of the physical stigmata described below. Most patients eventually develop central obesity with a plethoric "moon face," "buffalo hump," supraclavicular fat pads, protuberant abdomen, and thin extremities. Muscle atrophy causes weakness, with difficulty standing up from a seated position or climbing stairs. Patients may also experience backache, headache, hypertension, osteoporosis, avascular necrosis of bone, acne, superficial skin infections, and oligomenorrhea or amenorrhea in women or erectile dysfunction in men. Patients may have thirst and polyuria (with or without glycosuria), renal calculi, glaucoma, purple striae (especially around the thighs, breasts, and abdomen), and easy bruisability. Unusual bacterial or fungal infections are common. Wound healing is impaired. Mental symptoms may range from diminished ability to concentrate to increased lability of mood to frank psychosis. Patients are susceptible to opportunistic infections. Hyperpigmentation is common with ectopic ACTH-secreting neoplasms that tend to produce very high plasma ACTH levels; hyperpigmentation is uncommon with pituitary Cushing disease.

Adrenal carcinomas usually have gross metastases by the time of diagnosis. Microscopic metastases are not visible by scanning but can be inferred from the presence of detectable cortisol levels following removal of the primary adrenal tumor in patients with a cortisol-secreting carcinoma and Cushing syndrome. The ENSAT staging system is used: stage 1 is a localized tumor 5 cm or smaller; stage 2, a localized tumor larger than 5 cm; stage 3, tumor with local metastases; and stage 4, tumor with distant metastases.

B. Laboratory Findings

Glucose tolerance is impaired as a result of insulin resistance. Polyuria is present as a result of increased free water clearance; diabetes mellitus with glycosuria may worsen it. Patients with Cushing syndrome often have leukocytosis with relative granulocytosis and lymphopenia. Hypokalemia may be present, particularly in cases of ectopic ACTH secretion.

1. Diagnostic tests for hypercortisolism—Testing for hypercortisolism involves determining whether the following characteristics of Cushing syndrome are present: (1) lack of cortisol diurnal variation, (2) reduced suppressibility of cortisol by dexamethasone, (3) increased cortisol production rate, and (4) suppression of plasma ACTH by hypercortisolism from an adrenal nodule. Conflicting results are common.

Late-night (10–11 PM) salivary cortisol determinations are particularly useful, especially for ACTH-dependent hypercortisolism. Normal late-night salivary cortisol levels are less than 150 ng/dL (4.0 nmol/L). Late-night salivary cortisol levels that are consistently greater than 250 ng/dL (7.0 nmol/L) are considered abnormal. The late-night salivary cortisol test has a relatively high sensitivity and specificity for Cushing syndrome.

The **overnight dexamethasone suppression test** is an easy screening test for hypercortisolism and is particularly sensitive for mild ACTH-independent hypercortisolism from an adrenal nodule. Dexamethasone 1 mg is given orally at 11 PM and serum collected for cortisol determination at 8 AM the next morning; a cortisol level less than 1.8 mcg/dL (50 nmol/L) excludes Cushing syndrome with some certainty. However, 8% of established patients with pituitary Cushing disease have dexamethasone-suppressed cortisol levels less than 2 mcg/dL (55 nmol/L). Several antiseizure drugs and rifampin accelerate the metabolism of dexamethasone, causing a lack of cortisol suppression by dexamethasone. Estrogens—during pregnancy or as oral contraceptives or HRT—may also cause lack of dexamethasone suppressibility.

A 24-hour urinary free cortisol and creatinine is usually used to confirm hypercortisolism in patients with a high late-night salivary cortisol or an abnormal dexamethasone suppression test. A high 24-hour urine free cortisol (greater than 50 mcg/day or 140 nmol/day in adults), or free cortisol to creatinine ratio of greater than 95 mcg cortisol/g creatinine, helps confirm hypercortisolism. However, many patients with mild hypercortisolism have a urinary free cortisol that is misleadingly within the reference range. A misleadingly high urine free cortisol excretion occurs with high fluid intake. In pregnancy, urine free cortisol is increased, while 17-hydroxycorticosteroids remain normal and diurnal variability of serum cortisol is normal.

2. Diagnostic tests for the source of hypercortisolism— Once hypercortisolism is confirmed, a plasma ACTH and plasma DHEAS are obtained. A plasma ACTH below 6 pg/mL (1.3 pmol/L), with a low serum DHEAS, indicates a probable adrenal tumor, whereas higher levels are produced by pituitary or ectopic ACTH-secreting tumors. Certain ACTH assays suffer interference and report low-normal plasma ACTH levels in patients with ACTH-independent hypercortisolism. Serum dehydroepiandrosterone sulfate (DHEAS) levels can be used as a proxy for ACTH, since DHEAS secretion is ACTH-dependent; levels below the reference range and particularly below 40 mcg/dL (1.1 mcmol/L) imply ACTH-independent hypercortisolism.

C. Imaging

In ACTH-independent Cushing syndrome, CT of the adrenals usually detects a mass lesion, which is most often an adrenal adenoma. Adrenocortical carcinomas can usually be distinguished from benign adrenal adenomas since they are generally larger (average 11 cm) and many have metastases that are visible on preoperative scans.

In ACTH-dependent Cushing syndrome, MRI of the pituitary gland demonstrates a pituitary lesion in about 50% of cases. When the pituitary MRI is normal or shows a tiny (less than 5 mm) irregularity that may be incidental, selective catheterization of the inferior petrosal sinus veins draining the pituitary is performed. ACTH levels in the inferior petrosal sinus that are more than twice the simultaneous peripheral venous ACTH levels are indicative of pituitary Cushing disease.

When inferior petrosal sinus ACTH concentrations are not above the requisite levels, a search for an ectopic source of ACTH is undertaken. Location of ectopic sources of ACTH begins with CT scanning of the chest and abdomen, with special attention to the lungs (for carcinoid or small cell carcinomas), the thymus, the pancreas, and the adrenals. In patients with ACTH-dependent Cushing syndrome, chest masses should not be assumed to be the source of ACTH, since opportunistic infections are common. It is prudent to biopsy a chest mass to confirm the pathologic diagnosis prior to resection.

For Cushing syndrome due to ectopic ACTH, CT scanning fails to detect the source of ACTH in about 34% of cases. In such cases, the most sensitive (82%) scanning technique is whole-body imaging with ^{68}Ga-somatostatin receptor-PET/CT (^{68}Ga-DOTATOTATE-PET/CT).

Differential Diagnosis

Alcoholic patients can have hypercortisolism and many clinical manifestations of Cushing syndrome. Pregnant women have elevated serum ACTH levels, increased urine free cortisol, and high serum cortisol levels due to high serum levels of cortisol-binding globulin. Critically ill patients frequently have hypercortisolism, usually with suppression of serum ACTH. Depressed patients also have hypercortisolism that can be nearly impossible to distinguish biochemically from Cushing syndrome but without clinical signs of Cushing syndrome. Cushing syndrome can be misdiagnosed as anorexia nervosa (and vice versa) owing to the muscle wasting and extraordinarily high urine free cortisol levels found in anorexia. Patients with severe obesity frequently have an abnormal dexamethasone suppression test, but the urine free cortisol is usually normal, as is diurnal variation of serum cortisol. Patients with familial cortisol resistance have hyperandrogenism, hypertension, and hypercortisolism without actual Cushing syndrome. Excessive ingestion of gamma-hydroxybutyric acid (GHB, sodium oxybate) can also induce ACTH-dependent Cushing syndrome that resolves after the drug is stopped.

Some adolescents develop violaceous striae on the abdomen, back, and breasts; these are known as "striae distensae" and are not indicative of Cushing syndrome. Patients receiving antiretroviral therapy for HIV-1 infection frequently develop partial lipodystrophy with thin extremities and central obesity with a dorsocervical fat pad ("buffalo hump") causing pseudo-Cushing syndrome.

Treatment

Patients must receive treatment for cortisol-dependent comorbidities, including osteoporosis, psychiatric disorders, diabetes mellitus, hypertension, hypokalemia, muscle weakness, and infections. Bone densitometry is recommended for all patients and treatment is commenced for patients with osteoporosis.

A. Surgical Therapy

Pituitary Cushing disease is best treated with transsphenoidal selective resection of the pituitary adenoma, even when the pituitary MRI is normal or inconclusive. With an experienced pituitary neurosurgeon, remission rates range from 80% to 90%. Postoperative hyponatremia occurs frequently; serum sodium should be monitored often for the first 2 weeks postoperatively. The patient should be screened for secondary hypothyroidism with a serum free T_4 within 1–2 weeks after surgery. After successful pituitary surgery, the rest of the pituitary usually returns to normal function; however, the pituitary corticotrophs remain suppressed and require 6–36 months to recover normal function. Therefore, patients receive empiric replacement-dose hydrocortisone postoperatively. Postoperative secondary adrenal insufficiency is a mark of successful pituitary surgery; screening may include a morning serum cortisol 8 hours following the prior evening dose of hydrocortisone. The cosyntropin test becomes abnormal by 2 weeks following successful pituitary surgery. Patients with secondary adrenal insufficiency and their families require patient education about the condition and must continue corticosteroid replacement until a cosyntropin stimulation test is normal. A pituitary MRI is obtained about 3 months postoperatively and repeated as indicated for clinical evidence of recurrent Cushing disease or Nelson syndrome, the progressive enlargement of ACTH-secreting pituitary tumors following bilateral adrenalectomy.

Cushing disease may persist after pituitary surgery, particularly when there has been cavernous sinus involvement. After apparent successful pituitary surgery, Cushing disease recurs in 16% after a mean of 38 months. Patients must have repeated evaluations for recurrent Cushing disease for years postoperatively. For patients with persistent or recurrent Cushing disease, repeat transsphenoidal pituitary surgery may be warranted if the recurrent tumor is visible and deemed resectable. Otherwise, bilateral laparoscopic adrenalectomy is usually the best treatment option, particularly for patients with very severe disease, since it renders an immediate remission in a condition with significant morbidity and mortality. Residual or recurrent ACTH-secreting pituitary tumors may also be treated with stereotactic radiosurgery, which normalizes urine free cortisol in 70% of patients within a mean of 17 months, compared with a 23% remission rate with conventional radiation therapy. Pituitary radiosurgery can also be used to treat Nelson syndrome.

Ectopic ACTH-secreting tumors should be surgically resected. If the tumor cannot be localized or is metastatic, laparoscopic bilateral adrenalectomy is usually recommended. Medical treatment with an oral combination of mitotane (3–5 g/24 hours), ketoconazole (0.4–1.2 g/24 hours), and metyrapone (3–4.5 g/24 hours) often suppresses the hypercortisolism.

B. Medical Therapy

For patients with Cushing syndrome who decline surgery or for whom surgery has been unsuccessful, treatment with osilodrostat orally twice daily can normalize urine free cortisol and improve the manifestations of hypercortisolism. **Osilodrostat** reduces cortisol synthesis by blocking the adrenal enzyme 11B-hydroxylase. Adverse effects include adrenal insufficiency, a prolonged cardiac QT interval, hirusutism, and acne. Mineralocorticoid hypertension can be treated with spironolactone, eplerenone, and dihydropyridine calcium channel blockers. Women with hyperandrogenism may be treated with flutamide. Cabergoline, 0.5–3.5 mg orally twice weekly, reduced hypercortisolemia in 40% of patients with Cushing disease in one small study. Pasireotide, a multireceptor-targeting somatostatin analog, is a treatment option for refractory ACTH-secreting pituitary tumors causing Cushing disease or Nelson syndrome. Ketoconazole inhibits adrenal steroidogenesis and is another treatment option when given in doses of about 200 mg orally every 6 hours; however, it is marginally effective and can cause liver toxicity. Metyrapone can suppress hypercortisolism; required median oral daily doses are 1250–1500 mg/day in divided doses. It may be combined with ketoconazole. Metyrapone also may be used for patients with secretory adrenocortical carcinoma whose hypercortisolism is not fully controlled with mitotane.

Metastatic ACTH-producing tumors that are visible with Octreoscan or ^{68}Ga-DOTATATE-PET imaging have somatostatin receptors. Such tumors may respond to therapy with somatostatin analogs; pasireotide LAR (60 mg intramuscularly every 28 days) or octreotide LAR (30–40 mg intramuscularly every 28 days) slows progression of the malignancy and reduces ACTH secretion in up to half such patients. Potassium-sparing diuretics are often helpful. Radionuclide therapy with several cycles of ^{177}Lu-DOTATATE has produced remissions in some patients.

Patients who are successfully surgically treated for Cushing syndrome typically develop "cortisol withdrawal syndrome," even when given replacement corticosteroids for adrenal insufficiency. Manifestations can include hypotension, nausea, fatigue, arthralgias, myalgias, pruritus, and flaking skin. Increasing the hydrocortisone replacement to 30 mg orally twice daily can improve these symptoms; the dosage is then reduced slowly as tolerated.

Benign adrenal adenomas may be resected laparoscopically if they are smaller than 6 cm; cure is achieved in most patients. However, most patients experience prolonged secondary adrenal insufficiency. Patients with bilateral adrenal macronodular hyperplasia usually require bilateral adrenalectomies and an evaluation for Carney complex that can be confirmed with a genetic evaluation for activating mutations in the gene *PRKAR1A* or genetic changes at chromosome 2p16.

Adrenocortical carcinomas are resected surgically. If the adrenocortical carcinoma was functional, postoperative secondary adrenal insufficiency is a good prognostic sign, with an increased chance that the tumor was completely resected without metastases; however, detectable postoperative cortisol levels predict metastases, even if no metastases are detectable on scans.

Patients with secretory adrenocortical carcinomas are usually treated with mitotane postoperatively, particularly if metastases are visible or cortisol is detectable postoperatively. Patients with nonsecretory metastatic adrenocortical carcinomas have also responded to mitotane. Mitotane is typically given for 2–5 years postoperatively. It is given orally with meals, beginning with 0.5 g twice daily, increasing to 1 g twice daily within 2 weeks, with subsequent increased doses every 2–3 weeks to reach serum levels of 14–20 mcg/mL. Unfortunately, only half the patients are able to reach these levels due to side effects. Mitotane can cause hypogonadism, can suppress TSH and cause hypothyroidism, and can cause primary adrenal insufficiency. Replacement hydrocortisone or prednisone should be started when mitotane doses reach 2 g daily. The replacement dose of oral hydrocortisone starts at 15 mg in the morning and 10 mg in the afternoon but must often be doubled or tripled because mitotane increases cortisol metabolism and cortisol-binding globulin levels; the latter can artifactually raise serum cortisol levels. Combined chemotherapy with etoposide, doxorubicin, cisplatin, and mitotane (EDP-M) appears to be the most effective regimen for recurrent or metastatic adrenocortical carcinoma.

Prognosis

The manifestations of Cushing syndrome regress with time, but patients may have residual cognitive or psychiatric impairment, muscle weakness, osteoporosis, and sequelae from vertebral fractures. Continued impaired quality of life is more common in women compared to men. Younger patients have a better chance for full recovery.

Patients with Cushing syndrome from a benign adrenal adenoma experience a 5-year survival of 95% and a 10-year survival of 90%, following a successful adrenalectomy. Patients with Cushing disease from a pituitary adenoma experience a similar survival if their pituitary surgery is successful, which can be predicted if the postoperative nonsuppressed serum cortisol is less than 2 mcg/dL (55 nmol/L). Following successful treatment, overall mortality remains particularly higher for patients with older age at diagnosis, higher preoperative ACTH concentrations, and longer duration of hypercortisolism. Patients in remission from Cushing disease continue to experience a higher mortality rate than expected, particularly from ischemic heart disease and from cerebral infarction, bacterial infections, and suicide.

Patients who have a complete remission after transsphenoidal surgery have about a 15–20% chance of recurrence over the next 10 years. Recurrence of hypercortisolism may occur as a result of growth of an adrenal remnant stimulated by high levels of ACTH. The prognosis for patients with ectopic ACTH-producing tumors depends on the aggressiveness and stage of the particular tumor. Patients with ACTH of unknown source have a 5-year survival rate of 65% and a 10-year survival rate of 55%.

In patients with adrenocortical carcinoma, 5-year survival rates of treated patients have correlated with the ENSAT stage. For stage 1, the 5-year survival was 81%; for stage 2, 61%; for stage 3, 50%; and for stage 4, 13%.

Complications

Following bilateral adrenalectomy for Cushing disease, a pituitary adenoma may enlarge progressively (Nelson syndrome), causing local destruction (eg, visual field impairment, cranial nerve palsy) and hyperpigmentation. Following successful therapy for Cushing syndrome, secondary adrenal insufficiency occurs and requires long-term corticosteroid replacement. Five years after successful surgery, secondary hypoadrenalism resolves in about 58% of patients with pituitary Cushing disease, 82% of those with ectopic ACTH, and only 38% of those who had an adrenal tumor.

When to Refer

Dexamethasone suppression test is abnormal.

When to Admit

- Transsphenoidal hypophysectomy.
- Adrenalectomy.
- Resection of ectopic ACTH-secreting tumor.

Barbot M et al. Cushing's syndrome: overview of clinical presentation, diagnostic tools and complications. Best Pract Res Clin Endocrinol Metab. 2020;34:101380. [PMID: 32165101]

Fleseriu M et al. Consensus on diagnosis and management of Cushing's disease: a guideline update. Lancet Diabetes Endocrinol. 2021;9:847. [PMID: 34687601]

Galm BP et al. Accuracy of laboratory tests for the diagnosis of Cushing syndrome. J Clin Endocrinol Metab. 2020;105:2081. [PMID: 32133504]

Pivonello R et al. Efficacy and safety of osilodrostat in patients with Cushing's disease (LINC 3): a multicentre phase III study with a double-blind, randomised withdrawal phase. Lancet Diabetes Endocrinol. 2020;8:748. [PMID: 32730798]

Ragnarsson O. Cushing's syndrome: disease monitoring: recurrence, surveillance with biomarkers or imaging studies. Best Pract Res Clin Endocrinol Metab. 2020;34:101382. [PMID: 32139169]

PRIMARY ALDOSTERONISM

ESSENTIALS OF DIAGNOSIS

- Hypertension may be severe or drug-resistant.
- Hypokalemia (in minority of patients) may cause polyuria, polydipsia, muscle weakness.
- Low plasma renin; elevated plasma and urine aldosterone levels.

General Considerations

Primary aldosteronism (hyperaldosteronism) refers to renin-independent, inappropriately high and nonsuppressible aldosterone secretion and is associated with adverse cardiovascular disorders. Although most affected patients have hypertension, some may be normotensive. The prevalence of primary aldosteronism is 5–10% in hypertensive patients and at least 20% in patients with resistant hypertension. Primary aldosteronism should be suspected when the patient has early-onset hypertension or stroke (before age 50 years). Primary aldosteronism and cases of low renin essential hypertension may overlap, making distinguishing between them difficult. Patients of all ages may be affected, but the peak incidence is between 30 years and 60 years. Excessive aldosterone production increases sodium retention; increases renal potassium excretion, which can lead to hypokalemia; and suppresses plasma renin. Cardiovascular events are more prevalent in patients with aldosteronism (35%) than in those with essential hypertension (11%).

Primary aldosteronism is most frequently caused by bilateral adrenal cortical hyperplasia (75%) that is more common in men with a 4:1 ratio, peaking between ages 50 and 60. Primary aldosteronism may be also caused by a unilateral aldosterone-producing adrenal cortical adenoma (Conn syndrome, 25%) that is more common in women with a 2:1 ratio, peaking between ages 30 and 50. It is important to distinguish the two, since a unilateral aldosteronoma (Conn syndrome) may be cured by surgical resection, whereas patients with bilateral adrenal hyperplasia are treated medically.

Clinical Findings

A. Symptoms and Signs

Primary aldosteronism is the most common cause of refractory hypertension in youths and middle-aged adults. Patients have hypertension that is typically moderate but may be severe. Some patients have only diastolic hypertension, without other symptoms and signs. Edema is rarely seen in primary aldosteronism. Hypokalemia can produce muscle weakness, paresthesias with tetany, headache, polyuria, and polydipsia.

B. Laboratory Findings

Plasma potassium should be determined in hypertensive individuals. However, hypokalemia, once thought to be the hallmark of hyperaldosteronism, is present in only 37% of affected patients: 50% of those with an aldosterone-producing adenoma and 17% of those with adrenal hyperplasia. An elevated serum bicarbonate (HCO_3) concentration indicates metabolic alkalosis and is commonly present.

Testing for primary aldosteronism should be considered for all hypertensive patients with any of the following: (1) sustained hypertension above 150/100 mm Hg on 3 different days; (2) hypertension resistant to three conventional antihypertensive drugs, including a diuretic; (3) controlled blood pressure requiring four or more antihypertensive drugs; (4) hypokalemia, particularly when unrelated to diuretics; (5) personal or family history of early-onset hypertension or cerebrovascular accident at age 40 or younger; (6) first-degree relative with primary aldosteronism; (7) presence of an adrenal mass; and (8) low PRA.

For at least 2 weeks prior to testing, patients should have any hypokalemia corrected, consume a diet high in NaCl (more than 6 g/day) and, ideally, withhold certain medications: diuretics, ACE inhibitors and ARBs (stimulate PRA), beta-blockers, clonidine, NSAIDs (suppress PRA), and oral estrogens and contraceptives. Medications that are allowed include extended-release verapamil, hydralazine, terazosin, and doxazosin.

For blood testing, the patient should be out of bed for at least 2 hours and seated for 15–60 minutes before the blood draw, which should preferably be obtained between 8 AM and 10 AM. The blood should be drawn slowly with a syringe and needle (rather than a vacutainer) at least 5 seconds after tourniquet release and without fist clenching. Plasma potassium, rather than the routine serum potassium, should be measured in cases of unexpected hyperkalemia. Plasma potassium levels must be normal since hypokalemia suppresses aldosterone. For practical purposes, the same blood draw can be used for simultaneous assays for plasma potassium, serum aldosterone, and PRA. Patients with primary aldosteronism have a suppressed PRA below or near 1.0 ng/mL/hour. Suppressed PRA with a serum aldosterone concentration greater than 15 ng/dL (420 pmol/L) indicates probable primary hyperaldosteronism. Serum aldosterone (ng/dL) to PRA (ng/mL/hour) ratios less than 24 exclude primary aldosteronism; ratios between 24 and 30 are indeterminate; ratios between 30 and 64 are suspicious; a ratio above 64 helps confirm the diagnosis of primary aldosteronism. To help confirm the diagnosis of aldosteronism, especially for patients with a suppressed PRA but lower serum aldosterone levels, a 24-hour urine is collected in an acidified container for aldosterone, cortisol, and creatinine; urine aldosterone greater than 12 mcg/24 hours (33 nmol/24 hours) confirms primary aldosteronism with 93% specificity.

Genetic testing is recommended for patients with confirmed primary aldosteronism by age 20 years and those with a family history of primary aldosteronism or stroke at young age (under age 40). The testing is for familial corticosteroid-remediable aldosteronism.

C. Imaging

Some patients with undiagnosed primary aldosteronism are incidentally found to have an adrenal nodule (incidentaloma) during abdominal or chest imaging. All patients with biochemically confirmed primary aldosteronism require a thin-section CT scan of the adrenals to screen for a rare adrenal carcinoma. In the absence of a large adrenal carcinoma, adrenal CT scanning cannot reliably distinguish unilateral from bilateral aldosterone excess, having both a sensitivity and specificity of 78% for unilateral aldosteronism. Therefore, the decision to perform a unilateral adrenalectomy should not be based solely on the adrenal CT scan. Adrenal vein sampling is often required.

D. Adrenal Vein Sampling

Bilateral selective adrenal vein sampling is invasive, expensive, and not widely available. Adrenal vein sampling has a sensitivity of 95% and a specificity of 100% but only when performed by an experienced radiologist. This procedure entails a 0.6% risk of major complications.

The procedure (and surgery) may not be required for patients whose blood pressure is well controlled with spironolactone or eplerenone and for those with familial hyperaldosteronism. It is indicated only if surgery is contemplated in order to direct the surgeon to the correct adrenal gland. In such cases, adrenal vein sampling can be useful to identify the adrenal to be removed when there is no visible adrenal adenoma on CT imaging. Adrenal vein sampling can also help avoid mistaken removal of an incidental nonsecreting adrenal adenoma. Adrenal vein sampling is not required in patients who have a classic adrenal adenoma (Conn syndrome), which is characterized by spontaneous hypokalemia and a unilateral adrenal adenoma 10 mm or larger on CT.

Before this procedure, the patient must be properly prepared (see Laboratory Findings). However, patients with a persistently suppressed PRA may continue mineralocorticoid blockade. Lateralization is present when the aldosterone:cortisol ratio from one adrenal vein is at least four times that from the opposite adrenal vein.

Aldosterone hypersecretion that is lateralized to one adrenal usually indicates that adrenal has a unilateral aldosteronoma or hyperplasia, particularly when aldosterone secretion from the contralateral adrenal is suppressed.

Differential Diagnosis

The differential diagnosis of primary aldosteronism includes other causes of hypokalemia in patients with essential hypertension, especially diuretic therapy; chronic depletion of intravascular volume stimulates renin secretion and secondary hyperaldosteronism (see Table 21–3).

Apparent mineralocorticoid excess syndrome may be caused by real (black) licorice (derived from anise) or anise-flavored drinks (sambuca, pastis), which contain glycyrrhizinic acid. Abiraterone, a drug therapy for prostate cancer, causes hypertension and hypokalemia. Similarly, posaconazole, an oral antifungal drug, can cause pseudohyperaldosteronism with hypertension and hypokalemia.

Oral contraceptives may increase aldosterone secretion in some patients. Renal vascular disease can cause severe hypertension with hypokalemia but PRA is high. Excessive adrenal secretion of other corticosteroids (besides aldosterone), certain congenital adrenal enzyme disorders, and primary cortisol resistance may also cause hypertension with hypokalemia. The differential diagnosis also includes Liddle syndrome, an autosomal dominant cause of hypertension and hypokalemia resulting from excessive sodium absorption from the renal tubule; renin and aldosterone levels are low.

Complications

Cardiovascular complications occur more frequently in primary aldosteronism than in idiopathic hypertension. Following unilateral adrenalectomy for Conn syndrome, suppression of the contralateral adrenal may result in temporary postoperative hypoaldosteronism, characterized by hyperkalemia and hypotension.

Treatment

The **unilateral adrenal adenoma** of Conn syndrome is usually treated by laparoscopic adrenalectomy. During pregnancy, such surgery is best performed during the second trimester. Long-term medical therapy is an option for unilateral hyperaldosteronism, if adequate blood pressure control can be maintained.

Bilateral adrenal hyperplasia is best treated with medical therapy. Medical treatment must include a potassium-sparing diuretic, particularly spironolactone, eplerenone, or amiloride. Spironolactone is the most effective drug but also has antiandrogen activity and men frequently experience breast tenderness, gynecomastia, or reduced libido; initial dose is 12.5–25 mg orally once daily and may be titrated to 200 mg daily. Spironolactone might lead to undervirilization of male infants and is contraindicated in pregnancy; reproductive-age women are cautioned to use contraception during therapy. Eplerenone, 25–50 mg orally twice daily, is favored during pregnancy (FDA pregnancy category B) and for men, since it does not have antiandrogen effects. Blood pressure must be monitored daily when beginning these anti-mineralocorticoid medications; significant drops in blood pressure have occurred when these drugs are added to other antihypertensives. Other antihypertensive drugs may be required, particularly amlodipine, and ACE inhibitors or ARBs. Corticosteroid-remediable aldosteronism is very rare, but may respond well to suppression with low-dose corticosteroids.

Prognosis

The hypertension from unilateral adrenal adenoma is reversible in about two-thirds of cases but persists or returns despite surgery in the remainder. The prognosis is much improved by early diagnosis and treatment. Only 2% of aldosterone-secreting adrenal tumors are malignant.

Hundemer GL et al. Management of endocrine disease: the role of surgical adrenalectomy in primary aldosteronism. Eur J Endocrinol. 2020;183:R185. [PMID: 33077688]

Mehdi A et al. Our evolving understanding of primary aldosteronism. Cleve Clin J Med. 2021;188:221. [PMID: 33795246]

Turcu AF et al. Approach to the patient with primary aldosteronism: utility and limitations of adrenal vein sampling. J Clin Endocrinol Metab. 2021;106:1195. [PMID: 33382421]

PHEOCHROMOCYTOMA & PARAGANGLIOMA

ESSENTIALS OF DIAGNOSIS

- "Attacks" of headache, perspiration, palpitations, anxiety. Multisystem crisis.
- Hypertension: sustained but often paroxysmal, especially during surgery or delivery; may be orthostatic.
- Elevated plasma free fractionated metanephrines.

General Considerations

Both pheochromocytomas and non–head-neck paragangliomas are rare tumors. The yearly incidence is about 2–6 cases/million; however, many cases are undiagnosed during life since the prevalence of pheochromocytomas and paragangliomas in autopsy series is 1 in 2000. These tumors may be located in either or both adrenals; anywhere along the sympathetic nervous chain; and sometimes in the mediastinum, heart, or bladder. Pheochromocytomas arise from the adrenal medulla and usually secrete both epinephrine and norepinephrine. Paragangliomas ("extra-adrenal pheochromocytomas") arise from sympathetic paraganglia and frequently metastasize. About 50% of paragangliomas secrete norepinephrine; the rest are nonfunctional or secrete only dopamine, normetanephrine, or chromogranin A (CgA).

These tumors are dangerous and deceptive, causing death in at least one-third of patients prior to diagnosis. They account for less than 0.4% of hypertension cases. The incidence is higher in hypertensive children and patients with moderate to severe hypertension, particularly in the presence of suspicious symptoms of headache, significant palpitations, or diaphoretic episodes. Nearly 50% of cases are discovered incidentally on imaging studies. They account for about 4% of adrenal incidentalomas.

Nonsecretory paragangliomas arise in the head or neck, particularly in the carotid body, jugular-tympanic region, or vagal body; only about 4% secrete catecholamines.

About 40% of patients with pheochromocytomas or paragangliomas harbor a germline mutation in 1 of at least 16 known susceptibility genes that predispose to the tumor, usually in an autosomal dominant manner with incomplete penetrance. Genetic testing is recommended for all patients with these tumors.

von Hippel–Lindau (VHL) disease type 2 is associated with a 30% lifetime incidence of pheochromocytoma that can present as early as age 5 years or later in adulthood. The pheochromocytomas in VHL are less likely to be malignant (3.5%) compared to pheochromocytomas without VHL (about 10%). They are also less likely to metastasize than paragangliomas, where there is a 20–25% risk of metastasis. About 25% of these patients are asymptomatic and normotensive at diagnosis. The condition is also associated with hemangiomas of the retina, cerebellum, brainstem, and spinal cord; hyperparathyroidism; pancreatic cysts; endolymphatic sac tumors; cystadenomas of the adnexa or epididymis; pancreatic neuroendocrine tumors; and renal cysts, adenomas, and carcinomas; inheritance is autosomal dominant.

MEN 2 (MEN 2A) is associated with pheochromocytomas, medullary thyroid carcinoma, hyperparathyroidism, and cutaneous lichen amyloidosis. Pheochromocytomas are often silent in MEN 2; at diagnosis, only about 50% have symptoms and fewer are hypertensive. The lack of symptoms may be due to earlier diagnosis through yearly screening of mutation carriers. **MEN 3 (MEN 2B)** may be familial, but usually arises from a de novo *ret* mutation; MEN 3 is associated with pheochromocytoma (50%), aggressive medullary thyroid carcinoma, mucosal neuromas, and Marfan-like habitus.

von Recklinghausen neurofibromatosis type 1 (NF-1) is associated with an increased risk of pheochromocytomas/paragangliomas as well as cutaneous neurofibromas, optic and brainstem gliomas, astrocytomas, vascular anomalies, hamartomas, malignant nerve sheath tumors, and smooth-bordered café au lait spots.

Clinical Findings

A. Symptoms and Signs

Clinical manifestations of pheochromocytoma and paraganglioma depend on the manner in which the tumor is discovered. Pheochromocytomas may be relatively asymptomatic when they are diagnosed preemptively by screening members of kindreds harboring germline mutations that predispose to these tumors. Similarly, patients with pheochromocytomas discovered incidentally on CT scanning may have few symptoms. However, other pheochromocytomas can be lethal unless they are diagnosed and treated appropriately. Catastrophic hypertensive crisis and fatal cardiac arrhythmias can occur spontaneously or may be triggered by needle biopsy or manipulation of the mass, glucagon injection, vaginal delivery, trauma, anesthesia, or surgery (both unrelated to the tumor or for its removal). Exercise, bending, lifting, or emotional stress can trigger paroxysms. Bladder paragangliomas may present with paroxysms during micturition. Certain drugs can precipitate attacks: decongestants, amphetamines, cocaine, epinephrine, corticosteroids, fluoxetine and other SSRIs, metoclopramide, MAO inhibitors, caffeine, nicotine, and ionic intravenous contrast.

Clinical manifestations of pheochromocytoma typically include hypertension (81%) that may be paroxysmal or sustained, headache (60%), palpitations (60%), or diaphoresis (52%). About 60% of patients have episodic nonspecific "spells." Other symptoms include anxiety (often with a sense of impending doom), weakness/fatigue, dyspnea, nausea/vomiting, tremor, dizziness, chest pain, abdominal pain, paresthesias, or constipation. Vasospasm during an attack can cause Raynaud syndrome, mottled cyanosis, or facial pallor. As the attack subsides, facial flushing and drenching sweats can occur. Epinephrine secretion by an adrenal pheochromocytoma can cause episodic tachyarrhythmias and sometimes orthostatic hypotension or even syncope. Cardiac manifestations include acute coronary syndrome, cardiomyopathy, heart failure, and potentially fatal dysrhythmias. Catecholamine-induced cardiomyopathy can present with shock. Confusion, psychosis, paresthesias, seizures, transient ischemic attacks, or stroke may occur with cerebrovascular vasoconstriction or hemorrhagic stroke. Abdominal pain, nausea, vomiting, and even ischemic bowel can occur. Patients may experience increased appetite, loss of weight, numbness, or fevers. During pregnancy, pheochromocytomas can produce hypertension and proteinuria, mimicking eclampsia; vaginal delivery can produce hypertensive crisis followed by postpartum shock. Painful bony metastases may be a presenting symptom of metastatic pheochromocytoma. A minority of patients are normotensive and asymptomatic, particularly when the tumor is nonsecretory or discovered at an early stage.

Pheochromocytomas can also rarely produce other "ectopic" peptide hormones, resulting in Cushing syndrome (ACTH), Verner-Morrison syndrome (VIP), or hypercalcemia (PTHrP). **Multisystem crisis** can occur, with manifestations of severe hyper- or hypotension, acute respiratory distress syndrome (ARDS), cardiomyopathy with acute heart failure, kidney dysfunction, liver failure, and death. Multisystem crisis can occur spontaneously, or it may be provoked by surgery, vaginal delivery, or treatment of metastatic disease.

B. Laboratory Findings

Pheochromocytomas are rare tumors, but they are deadly; a missed diagnosis can be catastrophic. However, less than 1% of biochemical evaluations in patients with suspicious symptoms lead to a diagnosis of pheochromocytoma. More commonly, testing yields misleading minor elevations in tumor markers, particularly when levels are less than three times the upper limit of normal.

Plasma fractionated free metanephrines is the most sensitive test for secretory pheochromocytomas and paragangliomas. Free metanephrines are lower when the patient is supine than when ambulatory. For practicality, the blood specimen is usually obtained after the patient sits quietly in the laboratory for at least 15 minutes. The test is 97% sensitive for secretory tumors, so normal levels rule out secretory pheochromocytoma and paraganglioma with some certainty. The exceptions are patients who are being monitored because they harbor a germline mutation for familial pheochromocytoma; such patients with a pheochromocytoma are often asymptomatic early on and frequently have normal testing or only mild elevations in plasma metanephrines. However, for other patients with severe hypertension or "spells" caused by a pheochromocytoma, plasma fractionated free metanephrines are ordinarily at least three times the upper limit of normal. Such testing has a false-positive rate of 17%, usually with less dramatic elevations in plasma metanephrines. False-positive test results should be suspected when the ratio of normetanephrine to norepinephrine is less than 0.52 or the ratio of metanephrine to epinephrine is less than 4.2. In such cases, it is best to repeat biochemical testing under optimal conditions, eg, after eliminating potentially recovery from illness, treating sleep apnea, or eliminating potentially interfering drugs. Such drugs (including tricyclic antidepressants, antipsychotics, levodopa, MAO inhibitors, and antidepressants that are norepinephrine reuptake inhibitors) should ideally be discontinued for at least 2 weeks before retesting. Patients may be retested while lying supine in a quiet room for 30–90 minutes before the blood is drawn. Most patients with marginal elevations in plasma fractionated free metanephrines require confirmation with a 24-hour urine for fractionated metanephrines and creatinine.

Urinary fractionated metanephrines and creatinine effectively confirm most pheochromocytomas that were detected by elevated plasma fractionated free metanephrines. A 24-hour urine specimen is obtained, although an overnight or shorter collection may be used; patients with pheochromocytomas generally have more than 2.2 mcg of total metanephrine per milligram of creatinine, and more than 135 mcg total catecholamines per gram creatinine. Urinary assay for total metanephrines is about 97% sensitive for detecting functioning pheochromocytomas.

Plasma fractionated catecholamines may be helpful to confirm whether an adrenal tumor is a secretory pheochromocytoma. The test may also be useful for normotensive patients with a paraganglioma; the tumor may secrete only dopamine, which can be followed as a tumor marker.

Serum CgA is elevated in about 85% of patients with pheochromocytoma or paraganglioma and the levels correlate with tumor size, being higher in patients with metastatic disease. Serum CgA must be assayed in the fasting state, since levels rise after meals. Misleading elevated CgA levels also occur in patients with azotemia or hypergastrinemia, and in those treated with corticosteroids or PPIs. Serum CgA is not specific for pheochromocytoma, so its measurement is not very useful for the initial diagnosis.

Clonidine suppression testing can help distinguish whether elevated plasma free normetanephrine levels are physiologic or indicative of pheochromocytoma. Plasma fractionated free metanephrines are measured before the administration of clonidine (0.3 mg orally) and 3 hours afterward. A fall of plasma normetanephrine into the normal range or a fall of greater than 40% from baseline helps rule out the presence of a tumor.

Hyperglycemia is present in about 35% of patients but is usually mild. Proteinuria is present in about 10–20% of patients. Leukocytosis is common. Erythrocytosis or eosinophilia can occur. The ESR is sometimes elevated. PRA may be increased by catecholamines.

C. Imaging

1. CT and MRI scanning—When an adrenal pheochromocytoma is suspected, a *noncontrast* CT scan of the abdomen is performed, with thin sections through the adrenals. *Glucagon should not be used during scanning, since it can provoke hypertensive crisis in patients with a pheochromocytoma.*

MRI scanning has the advantage of not requiring intravenous contrast dye; its lack of radiation makes it the imaging of choice during pregnancy and for serial imaging. Both CT and MRI scanning have a sensitivity of about 90% for adrenal pheochromocytoma and a sensitivity of 95% for adrenal tumors over 0.5 cm. However, both CT and MRI are less sensitive for detecting recurrent tumors, metastases, and extra-adrenal paragangliomas. If no adrenal tumor is found, the scan is extended to include the entire abdomen, pelvis, and chest.

2. Nuclear imaging—^{68}**Ga-DOTATOC-PET** scanning is the most sensitive scan, detecting about 90% of pheochromocytomas, paragangliomas, and metastases. However, it is not entirely specific for these tumors. PET imaging gives crisper imaging than scintigraphy. Nuclear imaging is usually combined with volumetric imaging (CT or MRI) to determine the precise size and location of tumors.

^{18}**FDG-PET** scanning detects about 54% of metastases but is more sensitive for patients with *SDHB* germline mutations. However, ^{18}FDG-PET scanning is not specific for pheochromocytoma or paraganglioma.

^{123}**I-MIBG** whole-body scintigraphy can lateralize and confirm adrenal pheochromocytomas with a sensitivity of over 90%, but is only about 67% sensitive for extra-adrenal (paraganglioma) tumors and metastases and is also less sensitive for MEN 2– or MEN 3–related pheochromocytomas. ^{123}I-MIBG scintigraphy is also less sensitive for particularly aggressive tumors. Prior to the scan, the patient is given KI to competitively inhibit the uptake of free ^{123}I into the thyroid. Also, drugs that reduce ^{123}I-MIBG uptake should be avoided. Drug interference is suspected in negative ^{123}I-MIBG scans that do not show normal uptake in salivary glands.

Differential Diagnosis

Conditions that mimic pheochromocytoma include thyrotoxicosis, labile essential hypertension, myocarditis, glomerulonephritis or other renal lesions, eclampsia, acute intermittent porphyria, hypogonadal vascular instability (hot flushes), anxiety attacks, cocaine or amphetamine use, and clonidine withdrawal. Patients taking nonselective MAO inhibitor antidepressants can have hypertensive crisis after eating foods that contain tyramine. Patients with erythromelalgia can have hypertensive crises. Renal artery stenosis can cause severe hypertension. Plasma fractionated free metanephrines can be elevated in sleep apnea or with stressful illness. On CT scan, adrenal pheochromocytomas must be distinguished from adrenal adenomas and other masses. ^{123}I-MIBG scintigraphy uptake in the adrenal glands can be physiologic uptake and can sometimes occur in benign adrenal adenomas.

Complications

All the complications of severe hypertension may be encountered. In addition, a catecholamine-induced cardiomyopathy may develop. Severe heart failure and cardiovascular collapse may develop in patients during a paroxysm. Sudden death may occur due to cardiac arrhythmia. ARDS and multisystem crisis can occur acutely and thus the initial manifestation of pheochromocytoma may be hypotension or even shock. Hypertensive crises with sudden blindness or cerebrovascular accidents are not uncommon.

After removal of the tumor, a state of severe hypotension and shock (resistant to epinephrine and norepinephrine) may ensue with precipitation of AKI or MI. Hypotension and shock may occur from spontaneous infarction or hemorrhage of the tumor.

Pheochromocytomas and paragangliomas may metastasize. Cells can also be seeded within the peritoneum, either spontaneously or as a complication during surgical resection. Such seeding of the abdomen can lead to multifocal recurrent intra-abdominal tumors, a condition known as pheochromocytomatosis.

Medical Treatment

Patients must receive adequate treatment for hypertension and tachyarrhythmias prior to surgery for pheochromocytoma/paraganglioma. Patients are advised to measure their blood pressures daily and immediately during paroxysms. Some patients with pheochromocytoma or paraganglioma are not hypertensive and do not require preoperative antihypertensive management. Alpha-blockers or calcium channel blockers can be used, either alone or in combination. Blood pressure should be controlled before cardioselective beta-blockers are added for control of tachyarrhythmias. Normotensive patients with pheochromocytoma or sympathetic paraganglioma do not require preoperative alpha blockade, which increases their requirement for vasopressors and colloid after the tumor resection.

Alpha-blockers are typically administered in preparation for surgery. Phenoxybenzamine is a long-acting nonselective alpha-blocker with a half-life of 24 hours; it is given initially in a dosage of 10 mg orally every 12 hours, increasing gradually by about 10 mg/day about every 3 days until hypertension is controlled. Maintenance doses range from 10 mg/day to 120 mg/day. Doxazosin (half-life 22 hours), a selective alpha-1-blocker, may also be used in doses of 2–32 mg daily. Optimal alpha-blockade is achieved when supine arterial pressure is below 140/90 mm Hg or as low as possible for the patient to have a standing arterial pressure above 80/45 mm Hg.

Calcium channel blockers (nifedipine ER or nicardipine ER) are very effective and are usually added to alpha-blockers but may be used alone. Nifedipine ER is initially given orally at a dose of 30 mg/day, increasing the dose gradually to a maximum of 60 mg twice daily. Calcium channel blockers are superior to phenoxybenzamine for long-term use, since they cause less fatigue, nasal congestion, and orthostatic hypotension. However, they should not be used for patients with severe heart failure. For acute hypertensive crisis (systolic blood pressure higher than 170 mm Hg), a nifedipine 10-mg capsule may be chewed and swallowed. Nifedipine is quite successful for treating acute hypertension in patients with pheochromocytoma/paraganglioma, even at home; it is reasonably safe as long as the blood pressure is carefully monitored.

Beta-blockers (eg, metoprolol XL) are often required after institution of alpha-blockade or calcium channel blockade. *The use of a beta-blocker as initial antihypertensive therapy has resulted in an "unopposed alpha" status that causes paradoxical worsening of hypertension.* Labetalol has combined alpha- and beta-blocking activity and is an effective agent but can cause paradoxical hypertension if used as the initial antihypertensive agent. Labetalol can also interfere with catecholamine determinations in some laboratories and reduces the tumor's uptake of radioisotopes, such that it must be discontinued for at least 4–7 days before ^{123}I-MIBG or ^{18}FDG-PET scanning or therapy with high-dose ^{131}I-MIBG.

Surgical Treatment

Surgical removal of pheochromocytomas or abdominal paragangliomas is the treatment of choice. For surgery, a team approach—endocrinologist, anesthesiologist, and surgeon—is critically important. Laparoscopic surgery is preferred, but large and invasive tumors require open laparotomy. Patients with small familial or bilateral pheochromocytomas may undergo selective resection of the tumors, sparing the adrenal cortex; however, there is a recurrence rate of 10% over 10 years.

Prior to surgery, blood pressure control should be maintained for a minimum of 4–7 days or until optimal cardiac status is established. It may take a week or even months to correct ECG changes in patients with catecholamine myocarditis, and it may be prudent to defer surgery until then in such cases. Patients must be very closely monitored during surgery to promptly detect sudden changes in blood pressure or cardiac arrhythmias.

Autotransfusion of 1–2 units of blood at 12 hours preoperatively plus generous intraoperative volume replacement reduces the risk of postresection hypotension and shock caused by desensitization of the vascular alpha-1-receptors. Shock is treated with intravenous saline or colloid and high doses of intravenous norepinephrine. Intravenous 5% dextrose is infused postoperatively to prevent hypoglycemia.

Pheochromocytoma in Pregnancy

Although rare, pheochromocytoma must always be considered in women with hypertension or tachycardia who are planning pregnancy. Susceptible members of known kindreds with familial pheochromocytoma syndromes should be screened for pheochromocytoma *while planning* pregnancy, even if totally asymptomatic. During pregnancy, women with hypertension, heart failure, or pulmonary edema should be screened for pheochromocytoma. Untreated pheochromocytoma results in mortality rates of 25% for the mother and 50% in the fetus. The diagnosis is typically delayed, since hypertension, tachycardia, abdominal pain, and chest pains are often attributed to preeclampsia and pregnancy itself. A suspicion for pheochromocytoma is confirmed with elevated fasting plasma free fractionated metanephrines drawn at rest. MRI is preferred over ultrasound to detect an adrenal mass. In diagnosed cases, the mother should have genetic testing for germline mutations associated with pheochromocytoma. Affected women with hypertension are treated with phenoxybenzamine, calcium channel blockade (nifedipine or nicardipine), or both. Beta-blockers should be used judiciously, since they can cause intrauterine growth retardation. The optimal time for laparoscopic surgical removal of a pheochromocytoma is during the second trimester and before 24 weeks, gestation. Women with a pheochromocytoma diagnosed after 28 weeks' gestation are best treated medically until they can have an elective cesarean section at 38 weeks' gestation.

Metastatic Pheochromocytoma & Paraganglioma

Surgical histopathology for pheochromocytoma and paraganglioma cannot reliably determine whether a tumor is malignant. Only the presence of metastases defines malignancy, hence the WHO endocrine tumor classification uses the term "metastatic pheochromocytoma" to replace "malignant pheochromocytoma." Therefore, all pheochromocytomas and paragangliomas must be approached as possibly malignant. It is essential to recheck blood pressure and plasma fractionated metanephrine levels about 4–6 weeks postoperatively, at least every 6 months for 5 years, then yearly for life and immediately if hypertension, suspicious symptoms, or metastases become evident.

About 15% of pheochromocytomas and up to 50% of abdominal paragangliomas are eventually found to metastasize. Of patients with metastases, about 35% are detected when the primary tumor is discovered. Other metastases become clinically apparent 5.5 years (range 0.3–53 years) after initial diagnosis. Since some metastases are indolent, it is important to tailor treatment according to the tumor's aggressiveness. Most surgeons resect the main tumor and larger metastases (debulking). Some asymptomatic, indolent metastases may be kept under close surveillance without treatment.

A. Chemotherapy

The most common chemotherapy regimen combines intravenous cyclophosphamide, vincristine, and dacarbazine (Table 39–3). About one-third of patients experience some degree of temporary remission. Another chemotherapy regimen uses temozolomide, which is usually the best-tolerated chemotherapy and is particularly effective for metastatic pheochromocytoma or paraganglioma in patients with *SDHB* germline mutations. Sunitinib, a tyrosine kinase inhibitor, can also produce remissions. Metyrosine reduces catecholamine synthesis but does not slow the growth of metastases.

B. Targeted Radioisotope Therapy

1. ^{131}I-MIBG—About 60% of patients with metastatic pheochromocytoma or paraganglioma have tumors with sufficient uptake of ^{123}I-MIBG on diagnostic scanning to allow for therapy with high-activity ^{131}I-MIBG. Azedra (^{131}Idobenguanine) is FDA-approved for treating patients with metastatic pheochromocytoma or paraganglioma. Medications that reduce MIBG uptake must be avoided, particularly labetalol, phenothiazines, tricyclics, and sympathomimetics.

2. Peptide receptor radionuclide treatment (PRRT)—This therapy uses a radioisotope-tagged somatostatin analog against neuroendocrine tumors that express somatostatin receptors. ^{177}Lu-DOTATATE (Lutathera) is FDA-approved for treating patients with metastatic gastroenteropancreatic neuroendocrine tumors (GEP-NETs); it is being used off-label and on protocol to treat patients with metastatic pheochromocytoma and paraganglioma tumors, 90% of which are avid for PRRT. The objective response rate is 25%, and the short-term disease control rate is 84%.

C. Treatment for Bone Metastases

Patients with significant osteolytic bone metastases may be treated with external beam radiation therapy. Patients with vertebral metastases and spinal cord compression require surgical decompression and kyphoplasty. Intravenous zoledronic acid or subcutaneous denosumab may also be administered to patients with osteolytic bone metastases.

Prognosis

The prognosis is good for patients with pheochromocytomas that are resected before causing cardiovascular damage. Hypertension usually resolves after successful surgery but may persist or return in 25% of patients despite successful surgery. In such cases, biochemical reevaluation is required to detect a possible second or metastatic pheochromocytoma.

The surgical mortality is under 3% with the use of laparoscopic surgical techniques, intraoperative monitoring, and preoperative blood pressure control with alpha-blockers or calcium channel blockers.

Even if no metastases are evident at the time of surgery, lifetime surveillance is indicated for detection of possible later metastases. Patients with metastatic pheochromocytoma or paraganglioma have an extremely variable prognosis. Some metastases are indolent for several decades after the primary tumor diagnosis. Metastases from head-neck paragangliomas are particularly slow-growing. However, some of these tumors are extremely aggressive. Rapid disease progression has been associated with male sex, older age, larger primary tumor size, dopamine hypersecretion, failure to undergo primary tumor resection, very high tumor burden, and metastases that are visible at the time of primary tumor diagnosis.

Granberg D et al. Metastatic pheochromocytomas and abdominal paragangliomas. J Clin Endocrinol Metab. 2021;106:e1937. [PMID: 33462603]
Groeben H et al. International multicentre review of perioperative management and outcome for catecholamine producing tumours. Br J Surg. 2020;107:e170. [PMID: 31903598]
Jasim S et al. Metastatic pheochromocytoma and paraganglioma: management of endocrine manifestations, surgery and ablative procedures, and systemic therapies. Best Pract Res Clin Endocrinol Metab. 2020;34:101354. [PMID: 31685417]
Olson KR et al. Case 9-2021: a 16-year-old boy with headache, abdominal pain, and hypertension. N Engl J Med. 2021;384:1145. [PMID: 33761211]

INCIDENTALLY DISCOVERED ADRENAL MASSES

Adrenal incidentalomas are defined as adrenal nodules that are discovered incidentally on abdominal imaging obtained for other reasons. Their incidence increases with age, being found on 1–7% (average 4%) of all CT or MRI scans. About 75% are nonfunctioning adrenal adenomas; however, 14% secrete increased cortisol or aldosterone, resulting in Cushing syndrome or aldosteronism, respectively, and 7% are pheochromocytomas. Another 4% of incidentalomas represented metastases or adrenal adenocarcinomas. The differential diagnosis for incidentally discovered adrenal masses also includes adrenal infection, hemorrhage, and cysts.

Autonomous cortisol secretion typically results in Cushing syndrome withlow or low-normal plasma ACTH and serum DHEAS. Patients should be further assessed with a 1 mg dexamethasone suppression test (DST). (See Cushing Syndrome for details.) On the DST, an 8 AM serum cortisol greater than or equal to 1.8 mcg/dL (50 nmol/L) indicates either Cushing syndrome or mild autonomous cortisol excess and a level greater than or equal to 3 mcg/dL (83 nmol/L) portends an increased mortality risk, even without clinical manifestations of Cushing syndrome).

Patients with hypertension are screened for primary aldosteronism with a PRA and serum aldosterone (see Primary Aldosteronism).

All patients with an adrenal incidentaloma should be screened for pheochromocytoma with plasma fractionated free metanephrines, except those whose nodules meet all the following criteria: (1) normotensive, (2) nodule density on unenhanced CT density 10 HU or less, (3) size 3 cm diameter or less, and (4) morphology not suspicious. (See Pheochromocytoma.)

Surgical resection is recommended in adrenal incidentalomas larger than 4 cm, unless it is an unmistakably benign myelolipoma, hemorrhage, or adrenal cyst. Smaller adrenal incidentalomas are usually observed after endocrine testing. Suspicion for malignancy in smaller adrenal incidentalomas is increased in patients under age 40 or and lesions that have suspicious features (heterogeneity or irregularity). A *noncontrast* CT should be performed to determine the density of the mass. Over 99% of adrenal pheochromocytomas and adrenocarcinomas have a density of 10 HU or more; patients with adrenal incidentalomas with densities of 10 HU or more that are not resected require both clinical follow-up and CT follow-up in 6–12 months.

Jason DS et al. Evaluation of an adrenal incidentaloma. Surg Clin North Am. 2019;99:721. [PMID: 31255202]
Kebebew E et al. Adrenal incidentaloma. N Engl J Med. 2021;384:1542. [PMID: 33882207]
Kjellbom A et al. Association between mortality and levels of autonomous cortisol secretion by adrenal incidentalomas: a cohort study. Ann Intern Med. 2021;174:1041. [PMID: 34029490]

GASTROENTEROPANCREATIC NEUROENDOCRINE TUMORS (GEP-NETS) & CARCINOID TUMORS

ESSENTIALS OF DIAGNOSIS

- GEP-NETs are neuroendocrine tumors that originate in the GI tract.
- About 60% of GEP-NETs are nonsecretory or secretory without clinical manifestations; they may be detected incidentally or may present with weight loss, abdominal pain, or jaundice.
- Carcinoid tumors arise from the intestines or lung, secrete serotonin, and may metastasize.

General Considerations

GEP-NETs are neuroendocrine tumors (NETs) that arise from the stomach, intestines, or endocrine pancreas.

The reported incidence of GEP-NETs has increased to about 37 per million yearly in the United States due to the incidental detection of small tumors on abdominal scans. About 40% are functional, producing hormones that also serve as tumor markers, important for diagnosis and follow-up. At presentation, 65% of GEP-NETs are unresectable or metastatic. Up to 25% of GEP-NETs are associated with one of four different inherited disorders: MEN 1, VHL, NF-1, and tuberous sclerosis complex. In MEN 1, GEP-NETs are usually gastrinomas, carcinoids, or nonfunctioning tumors and are a common cause of death. In VHL, GEP-NETs are usually benign and multiple.

Insulinomas are the most common functional type of GEP-NET and are usually small, intrapancreatic, and benign (90%). Insulinomas are solitary in 95% of sporadic cases but are multiple in about 90% of cases arising in MEN 1. (See Chapter 27.)

Gastrinomas are often malignant (about 50%) and metastasize to the liver. Gastrinomas are typically found in the duodenum (49%), pancreas (24%), or lymph nodes (11%). Sporadic gastrinoma is rarely suspected at the onset of symptoms; typically, there is a 5-year delay in diagnosis. About 22% of gastrinomas arise in patients with MEN 1, who usually present at a younger age, often with multiple tumors; hyperparathyroidism can occur many years before or after the discovery of a gastrinoma.

Glucagonomas are rare and usually malignant, despite their benign histologic appearance. They usually arise as a large intrapancreatic tumor with 60% having liver metastases apparent by the time of diagnosis. Besides glucagon, they usually secrete additional hormones, including gastrin.

Somatostatinomas are very rare and usually single. They arise in the pancreas (50%) or small intestine. They secrete somatostatin.

VIPomas are quite rare and usually single intrapancreatic tumors with metastases usually evident (80%) at diagnosis. They produce vasoactive intestinal polypeptide (VIP).

Cholecystokinin-producing tumors (CCKomas) are rare tumors of the endocrine pancreas.

Carcinoid tumors can arise from the small bowel (53%, particularly terminal ileum), colon (12%), esophagus through duodenum (6%), or lung (bronchial carcinoid [5%]). About 20% of cases present with metastases without a known primary location. Carcinoids are multiple in about 28% of cases. Although tumors are usually indolent, metastases are common, particularly to liver, lymph nodes, and peritoneum.

Clinical Findings

A. Symptoms and Signs

Nonfunctioning tumors typically present with mass effect and metastases, such as pancreatitis, jaundice, abdominal pain, or weight loss.

Insulinomas secrete insulin and present with the symptoms of fasting hypoglycemia. (See Chapter 27.)

Gastrinomas usually present with peptic ulcer disease—abdominal pain (75%), heartburn (44%), bleeding (25%)—or weight loss (17%) (Zollinger-Ellison syndrome). Endoscopy usually shows hyperplastic gastric rugae (94%).

Glucagonomas usually present with weight loss caused by glucagon-stimulated protein hepatic gluconeogenesis and related protein catabolism. Other common manifestations include diarrhea, nausea, peptic ulcer, hypoaminoacidemia, or necrolytic migratory erythema, known as "glucagonoma syndrome." Diabetes mellitus develops in about 35% of patients. The median survival is 34 months after diagnosis.

Somatostatinomas can present with a classic triad of symptoms: diabetes mellitus due to its inhibition of insulin and glucagon secretion; cholelithiasis due to its inhibition of gallbladder motility; and steatorrhea due to its inhibition of pancreatic exocrine function. Diarrhea, hypochlorhydria, and anemia can also occur.

VIPomas present with profuse ***w****atery* ***d****iarrhea* (unremitting), ***h****ypokalemia*, and ***a****chlorhydria* ("WDHA"), the so-called Verner-Morrison syndrome.

CCKomas may present with liver metastases and symptoms of diarrhea, peptic ulcer disease, and weight loss.

Carcinoid tumors can produce "carcinoid syndrome": episodes of abdominal pain, diarrhea, bronchospasm, and weight loss. Dry skin and flushing typically affect the upper chest, neck, and face and lasts from 30 seconds to 30 minutes, although flushing with bronchial carcinoids can persist for days. Although abdominal pain and diarrhea may occur at the same time as flushing, they usually occur at other times. Flushing can be unprovoked or precipitated by exercise, anesthesia, emotional stimuli, or foods (bananas, tomatoes, cheese, kiwi, eggplant, and alcohol). However, the full-blown carcinoid syndrome occurs with only about 10% of tumors. Other manifestations include carcinoid heart disease caused by endocardial fibrotic plaques. Tumor-induced fibrosis can also occur in the retroperitoneum causing ureteral obstruction or in the penis causing Peyronie disease. Pellagra (glossitis, confusion, dry skin), which results from the conversion of tryptophan (a precursor to niacin) to serotonin by tumor cells, may develop in affected patients with widespread metastases.

Bronchial carcinoids secrete serotonin and can produce carcinoid syndrome even without hepatic metastases. Foregut carcinoids secrete serotonin that is hepatically metabolized and therefore produce carcinoid syndrome only when they have metastasized to the liver. Appendiceal carcinoids are typically discovered incidentally during appendectomy; hemicolectomy is required if the tumor is 2 cm or larger or has unfavorable histopathology. Cecal carcinoids often present with intestinal obstruction or intestinal bleeding. Hindgut carcinoids rarely produce serotonin and do not cause carcinoid syndrome.

Ectopic hormones can be secreted by GEP-NETs. Ectopic ACTH secretion from bronchial carcinoids or pancreatic neuroendocrine tumors (pNETs) can produce Cushing syndrome.

B. Laboratory Findings

About 40% of GEP-NETs are functional, producing hormones that serve as tumor markers, which are important for diagnosis and follow-up. Insulinomas produce insulin, proinsulin and C-peptide. Gastrinomas secrete gastrin. Glucagonomas secrete glucagon and other hormones, including gastrin. For carcinoid tumors, serum serotonin may be elevated along with urinary 5-hydroindoleacetic acid (5-HIAA). Patients with CCKomas may have elevated serum levels of cholecystokinin and CgA.

C. Imaging

Localization of GEP-NETs and their metastases is best done with PET scanning using ^{68}Ga-DOTATATE, a radiolabeled somatostatin analog. For hepatic metastases, MRI is more sensitive than CT.

For insulinomas, preoperative localization studies are less successful and have the following sensitivities: ultrasonography 25%, CT 25%, endoscopic ultrasonography 27%, transhepatic portal vein sampling 40%, and arteriography 45%. Nearly all insulinomas can be successfully located at surgery by the combination of intraoperative palpation (sensitivity 55%) and ultrasound (sensitivity 75%), and ^{68}Ga-DOTATATE-PET (sensitivity 90%). Tumors may be located in the pancreatic head or neck (57%), body (15%), or tail (19%) or in the duodenum (9%). MRI is used to screen members of kindreds with genetic syndromes that predispose them to GEP-NETs.

Treatment

Surgery is the primary initial treatment for most GEP-NETs and is a reasonable option even for patients with stage IV disease. The aggressiveness of the surgery may vary from conservative debulking to radical resection and even liver transplantation. However, incidentally discovered nonfunctioning pNETS that are asymptomatic and smaller than 2 cm are increasingly being monitored without surgery. Another treatment option for pNETs is endoscopic ultrasound-guided radiofrequency ablation (EUS-RFA) that induces thermal necrosis of the tumor.

With gastrinomas, the gastric hyperacidity of Zollinger-Ellison syndrome is treated with a PPI (see Chapter 15).

Tumor visualization on ^{68}Ga-DOTATATE-PET imaging indicates that they may respond to long-acting preparations of somatostatin analogs, including lanreotide (Somatuline Depot) and octreotide (Sandostatin LAR Depot). Subcutaneous injections of octreotide LAR 20–30 mg are required every 4 weeks. Treatment improves symptoms in patients with functioning tumors and also appears to improve progression-free survival in patients with either functioning or nonfunctioning GEP-NETs. Enlarging hepatic metastases may be embolized with ^{90}Y-labeled resin or glass microspheres. For patients with progressive metastatic disease, chemotherapy (eg, everolimus) improves progression-free survival when added to somatostatin analog therapy (Table 39–2). Patients with GEP-NETs that continue to progress may be treated with PRRT, usually with four separate infusions of ^{177}Lu-DOTATE (Lutathera).

Prognosis

The prognosis for patients with GEP-NETs is variable, depending on the tumor grade and stage. Patients with well- or moderately well-differentiated GEP-NETs (Ki-67, a marker for cellular proliferation, less than 20%) have a better survival than those with poorly differentiated tumors. Smaller tumors without detectable metastases have a much lower chance of recurrence after surgery. However, most patients with GEP-NETs are stage IV with hepatic metastases by the time of diagnosis. Nevertheless, low-grade metastases may be indolent or slow-growing and may respond to octreotide or lanreotide. The overall prognosis for patients with GEP-NETs is much better than that for adenocarcinomas that arise from the same organs. The prognosis is worse for patients with serum pancreastatin levels above 500 pmol/L, since it correlates with the amount of hepatic metastases.

The surgical complication rate for GEP-NETs is about 40%, with patients commonly developing fistulas and infections. Extensive pancreatic resection may cause diabetes mellitus. EUS-RFA is effective for most patients with pNETs up to 3 cm, even those with multiple tumors. Patients with insulinomas usually experience correction of hypoglycemia within 1 hour following this procedure. However, the long-term response rate is unknown. For patients with gastrinomas, the 5-, 10-, and 20-year survival rates with MEN 1 are 94%, 75%, and 58%, respectively, while the survival rates for patients with sporadic gastrinomas are 62%, 50%, and 31%, respectively. Decreased overall survival has been noted with the following: higher stage and grade of tumor, male sex, age over 60 years, unmarried status, nonfunctioning tumor, location of tumor in pancreatic head, and lack of surgical treatment.

Bonds M et al. Neuroendocrine tumors of the pancreatobiliary and gastrointestinal tracts. Surg Clin North Am. 2020;100:635. [PMID: 32402306]

MULTIPLE ENDOCRINE NEOPLASIA (MEN)

MEN TYPES 1–4

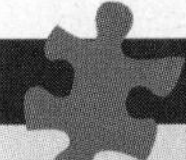

ESSENTIALS OF DIAGNOSIS

- **MEN 1:** tumors of the parathyroid glands, endocrine pancreas and duodenum, anterior pituitary, adrenal, thyroid; carcinoid tumors; lipomas and facial angiofibromas.
- **MEN 2:** medullary thyroid cancer, hyperparathyroidism, pheochromocytoma, Hirschsprung disease.
- **MEN 3:** medullary thyroid cancer, pheochromocytoma, Marfan-like habitus, mucosal neuromas, intestinal ganglioneuroma, delayed puberty.
- **MEN 4:** tumors of the parathyroid glands, anterior pituitary gland, adrenal gland, ovary, testicle, kidney.

Syndromes of MEN are inherited as autosomal dominant traits that cause a predisposition to the development of tumors of two or more different endocrine glands (Table 26–12). MEN syndromes are caused by germline mutations and tumors arising when additional somatic mutations occur in predisposed organs. Patients with MEN should have genetic testing so that their first-degree relatives may then be tested for the specific mutation.

1. MEN 1

Multiple endocrine neoplasia type 1 (MEN 1, Wermer syndrome) is a tumor syndrome with a prevalence of 2–10 per 100,000 persons in the United States. About 90% of affected patients harbor a detectable germline mutation in the *menin* gene.

The presentation of MEN 1 is variable, even in the same kindred. Affected patients are prone to many different tumors, particularly involving the parathyroids, endocrine pancreas and duodenum, and anterior pituitary (Table 26–12). Incidental adrenal nodules are found in about 50% of affected patients but are rarely secretory. The initial biochemical manifestations (usually hypercalcemia) can often be detected as early as age 14–18 years in patients with a MEN 1 gene mutation, although clinical manifestations usually present in the third or fourth decade.

Hyperparathyroidism is the first clinical manifestation of MEN 1 in two-thirds of affected patients, but it may present at any time of life.

GEP-NETs and carcinoids occur in up to 70% of patients with MEN 1. The GEP-NETs may secrete only pancreatic polypeptide or be nonsecretory altogether

Table 26–12. Multiple endocrine neoplasia (MEN) syndromes: incidence of tumor types.

Tumor Type	MEN 1	MEN 2 (MEN 2A)	MEN 3 (MEN 2B)	MEN 4
Parathyroid	95%	20–50%	Rare	Common
Pancreatic	54%			Common
Pituitary	42%			Common
Medullary thyroid carcinoma		> 90%	80%	
Pheochromocytoma	Rare	20–35%	60%	
Mucosal and GI ganglioneuromas		Rare	> 90%	
Subcutaneous lipoma	30%			
Adrenocortical adenoma	30%			Common
Thoracic carcinoid	15%			
Thyroid adenoma	55%			Common
Facial angiofibromas and collagenomas	85%			
Breast cancer	27%			

(20–55%). Gastrinomas occur in about 40% of patients with MEN 1. Concurrent hypercalcemia, due to hyperparathyroidism in MEN 1, stimulates gastrin and worsens gastric acid secretion; control of the hypercalcemia often reduces serum gastrin levels and gastric acid secretion. Carcinoid tumors can arise in the lung or abdomen and can metastasize, especially to the liver.

Insulinomas occur in about 10% of patients with MEN 1. Extrapancreatic neuroendocrine tumors are common in MEN 1; they are frequently malignant and include carcinoid tumors (usually in foregut locations [69%], such as the lung, thymus, duodenum, or stomach).

Pituitary adenomas are the presenting tumor in 29% of patients with MEN 1 and eventually are found in about 42% of patients with MEN 1. About 42% of pituitary adenomas are nonsecretory. Nonsecretory pituitary microadenomas (less than 1 cm and detected on routine MRI screening) are usually indolent; 25% of nonsecretory pituitary adenomas are macroadenomas (1 cm or more) and more aggressive.

Adrenal adenomas or hyperplasia occur in about 40% of patients with MEN 1; 50% are bilateral. They are generally benign and nonfunctional. These adrenal lesions are ACTH-independent.

Thymic neuroendocrine tumors occur in 3.4% of affected patients, with a 10-year survival of 25%. Lung neuroendocrine tumors occur in 13%, with a 10-year survival of 71%.

Benign thyroid adenomas or multinodular goiter occurs in 55% of MEN 1 patients

Nonendocrine tumors occur commonly in MEN 1, particularly small head-neck angiofibromas (85%) and lipomas (30%). Collagenomas are common (70%), presenting as firm dermal nodules. Breast cancer risk is increased over two-fold. Breast cancer tends to present earlier; cancer surveillance is recommended in women beginning by age 40 years, optimally using MRI. Affected patients may also be more prone to meningiomas, breast cancer, colorectal cancers, prostate cancer, and malignant melanomas.

Overall, patients with MEN 1 have an increased mortality rate with a mean life expectancy of only 55 years.

2. MEN 2 (formerly MEN 2A)

Multiple endocrine neoplasia type 2 (MEN 2A, Sipple syndrome) is a rare autosomal-dominant tumor syndrome that arises in patients with a germline gain-of-function *ret* protooncogene mutation. Genetic testing identifies about 95% of affected individuals.

Medullary thyroid carcinoma (greater than 90%); hyperparathyroidism (30%), with hyperplasia or adenomas of multiple parathyroid glands developing in most cases; pheochromocytomas (30%), which are often bilateral and frequently asymptomatic; and Hirschsprung disease may develop. No patients with MEN 2 should receive therapy for diabetes with glucagon-like peptide 1 (GLP 1) agonists that may increase the risk for medullary thyroid carcinoma. Before any surgical procedure, MEN 2 (2A) carriers should be screened for pheochromocytoma (see above) and for medullary thyroid carcinoma.

3. MEN 3 (formerly MEN 2B)

Multiple endocrine neoplasia type 3 (MEN 2B) is a familial, autosomal dominant multiglandular syndrome that is also caused by a germline gain-of-function mutation of the *ret* protooncogene. MEN 3 (2B) is characterized by mucosal neuromas (in more than 90% of cases) with bumpy and enlarged lips and tongue, Marfan-like habitus (75% of cases), and adrenal pheochromocytomas (60%) that are rarely malignant and often bilateral. Patients also have intestinal abnormalities (75%) such as intestinal ganglioneuromas, skeletal abnormalities (87%), and delayed puberty (43%). Medullary thyroid carcinoma (80%) is aggressive and presents early in life.

4. MEN 4

Multiple endocrine neoplasia type 4 (MEN 4) is a rare autosomal-dominant familial tumor syndrome caused by germline mutations in the gene *CDKN1B*. Affected patients are particularly prone to parathyroid adenomas (80%), pituitary adenomas (less aggressive than those seen with MEN 1), pancreatic neuroendocrine tumors, and adrenal tumors. Unlike patients with MEN 1, those with MEN 4 are also prone to renal tumors, testicular cancer, neuroendocrine cervical carcinoma, and primary ovarian failure.

Kiernan CM et al. Surgical management of multiple endocrine neoplasia 1 and multiple endocrine neoplasia 2. Surg Clin North Am. 2019;99:693. [PMID: 31255200]

McDonnell JE et al. Multiple endocrine neoplasia: an update. Intern Med J. 2019;49:954. [PMID: 31387156]

DISEASES OF THE TESTES & MALE BREAST

MALE HYPOGONADISM

ESSENTIALS OF DIAGNOSIS

- Diminished libido and erections.
- Fatigue, depression, reduced exercise endurance.
- Testes small or normal in size.
- Low serum total testosterone or free testosterone.
- Hypogonadotropic hypogonadism: low or normal serum LH and FSH.
- Hypergonadotropic hypogonadism: testicular failure, high serum LH and FSH.

General Considerations

Male hypogonadism is caused by deficient testosterone secretion by the testes. It may be due to (1) insufficient gonadotropin secretion by the pituitary (hypogonadotropic); (2) pathology in the testes (hypergonadotropic); or (3) both (Table 26–13). Partial male hypogonadism may be difficult to distinguish from the physiologic reduction in serum testosterone seen in normal aging, obesity, and illness.

Etiology

A. Hypogonadotropic Hypogonadism (Low Testosterone with Normal or Low LH)

A deficiency in FSH and LH may be isolated or associated with other pituitary hormonal abnormalities. (See Hypopituitarism.) Hypogonadotropic hypogonadism can be primary, defined as failure to enter puberty by age 14, or it can be acquired. Causes of primary hypogonadotropic hypogonadism include hypopituitarism, isolated hypogonadotropic hypogonadism, or simple constitutional delay of growth and puberty. Causes of acquired hypogonadotropic hypogonadism include genetic conditions (eg, Kallmann syndrome or *PROKR2* mutations, X-linked congenital adrenal hypoplasia, 17-ketosteroid reductase deficiency, Prader-Willis syndrome), which account for about 40% of cases of isolated and idiopathic disease with a serum testosterone level less than 150 ng/dL (5.2 nmol/L) (Table 26–13).

Partial male hypogonadotropic hypogonadism is defined as a serum testosterone in the range of 150–300 ng/dL (5.2–10.4 nmol/L). The main causes of acquired partial male hypogonadotropic hypogonadism include obesity, poor health, or normal aging, such that it is termed **age-related hypogonadism**. However, other causes need to be excluded, including pituitary or hypothalamic tumors. Spermatogenesis is usually preserved.

B. Hypergonadotropic Hypogonadism (Testicular Failure with High LH)

A failure of the testicular Leydig cells to secrete adequate testosterone causes a rise in LH and FSH. Acquired conditions that can cause testicular failure are listed in Table 26–13. Male hypergonadotropic hypogonadism can be caused by XY gonadal dysgenesis, partial 17-ketosteroid reductase deficiency and a congenital partial deficiency in the steroidogenic enzyme CYP17 (17-hydroxylase). Abiraterone acetate, a drug for prostate cancer, inhibits CYP17. In men who have had a unilateral orchiectomy for cancer, the remaining testicle frequently fails, even in the absence of radiation or chemotherapy.

Table 26–13. Causes of male hypogonadism.

Hypogonadotropic (Low or Normal LH)	Hypergonadotropic (High LH)
Aging	Aging
Alcohol	Autoimmunity
Chronic illness	Anorchia (bilateral)
Constitutional delay of growth and puberty	Chemotherapy
Cushing syndrome	Idiopathic
Drugs	Klinefelter syndrome
Estrogen	Leprosy
GnRH agonist (leuprolide)	Lymphoma
Ketoconazole	Male climacteric
Marijuana	Myotonic dystrophy
Opioids (oral, injected, or intrathecal)	Noonan syndrome
Prior androgens	Orchiectomy (bilateral or unilateral)
Spironolactone	Orchitis
Genetic conditions[1]	Radiation or radioisotope therapy
Granulomatous diseases	Sertoli cell-only syndrome
Hemochromatosis	Testicular trauma
Hypopituitarism	Tuberculosis
Hypothalamic or pituitary tumors	Uremia
Hypo-, hyperthyroidism	Viral infections (mumps)
Idiopathic	XY gonadal dysgenesis
Kidney disease	
Lymphocytic hypophysitis	
Major medical or surgical illnesses	
Malnourishment	
Obesity (BMI > 30)	

[1]See text for discussion.
GnRH, gonadotropin-releasing hormone.

Klinefelter syndrome (47,XXY and its variants) is the most common chromosomal abnormality among males, with an incidence of about 1:500 (see Chapter 40). Although puberty occurs at the normal time, the degree of virilization is variable. Serum testosterone is usually low and gonadotropins are elevated. Other common findings include tall stature and abnormal body proportions that are unusual for hypogonadal men (eg, height more than 3 cm greater than arm span).

XY gonadal dysgenesis describes several conditions that result in the failure of the testes to develop normally. *SRY* is a gene on the Y chromosome that initiates male sexual development. Mutations in *SRY* result in testicular dysgenesis. Affected individuals lack testosterone, which results in sex reversal: female external genitalia with a blind vaginal pouch, no uterus, and intra-abdominal dysgenetic gonads. Affected individuals appear as normal girls until their lack of pubertal development and amenorrhea leads to the diagnosis. Intra-abdominal rudimentary testes have an increased risk of developing a malignancy and are usually resected.

C. Androgen Insensitivity

Partial resistance to testosterone is a rare condition in which phenotypic males have variable degrees of apparent hypogonadism, hypospadias, cryptorchism, and gynecomastia. Serum testosterone levels are normal.

Clinical Findings

A. Symptoms and Signs

Hypogonadism that is congenital or acquired during childhood presents as delayed puberty. Men with acquired hypogonadism have variable manifestations, known as "testosterone deficiency syndrome." Most men experience decreased libido. Others complain of erectile dysfunction, poor morning erection, or hot sweats. Men often have depression, fatigue, or decreased ability to perform vigorous physical activity. The presenting complaint may also be infertility, gynecomastia, headache, fracture, or other symptoms related to the cause or result of the hypogonadism. The patient's history often gives a clue to the cause (Table 26–13).

Physical signs associated with hypogonadism may include decreased body, axillary, beard, or pubic hair, but only after years of severe hypogonadism. Men with hypogonadism lose muscle mass and gain weight due to an increase in subcutaneous fat. Examination should include measurements of arm span and height. Testicular size should be assessed with an orchidometer (normal volume is about 10–25 mL; normal length is 3–5 cm). Testicular size may decrease but usually remains within the normal range in men with postpubertal hypogonadotropic hypogonadism, but it may be diminished with testicular injury or Klinefelter syndrome. The testes must be palpated for masses and examined for evidence of trauma, infiltrative lesions (eg, lymphoma), or infection (eg, leprosy, tuberculosis).

B. Laboratory Findings

Serum testosterone circulates as 'free' hormone and hormone bound to sex hormone–binding globulin. Serum total and free testosterone levels in men are highest at age 20–30 years. Thereafter, serum testosterone levels decline variably by an average of 1–2% annually; serum free testosterone levels decline even faster since sex hormone–binding globulin increases with age. In evaluating laboratory values for total and free testosterone, it is important to compare with age-adjusted reference ranges.

The evaluation for hypogonadism begins with a morning (before 10 AM) total testosterone and free testosterone measurement. Total testosterone levels are low if they are confirmed to be less than 240 ng/dL (8.3 nmol/L). Serum *free* testosterone below 35 pg/mL (120 pmol/L) is considered low for men ages 18–69 or below 30 pg/mL (100 pg/L) for men ages 70 and over. Normal ranges for serum testosterone have been derived from nonfasting morning blood specimens, which tend to be the highest of the day. A low serum testosterone or free testosterone should be verified with a repeat morning nonfasting assay, along with serum LH and PRL levels.

The main conditions that contribute to a decline in serum testosterone with aging include obesity, illness, and opioids. After age 70, LH levels tend to rise, indicating a contribution of primary gonadal dysfunction with advancing age. Testing for serum free testosterone is especially important for detecting hypogonadism in elderly men, who generally have high levels of sex hormone binding globulin. Serum LH levels are high in patients with hypergonadotropic hypogonadism but low or inappropriately normal in men with hypogonadotropic hypogonadism or normal aging. High serum estradiol levels are seen in men with obesity-related hypogonadotropic hypogonadism.

Testosterone stimulates erythropoiesis in men, causing the normal RBC range to be higher in men than in women; mild anemia is common in men with hypogonadism. For men with long-standing severe male hypogonadism, osteoporosis is common, so a bone densitometry is recommended.

1. Hypogonadotropic hypogonadism—A serum PRL determination is obtained to screen for a pituitary prolactinoma (see Table 26–1). Men with no discernible cause for hypogonadotropic hypogonadism should be screened for hemochromatosis. Adult men with hypogonadotropic hypogonadism should have an MRI of the pituitary/hypothalamus to search for a mass lesion in presence of one or more of the following: (1) severe hypogonadism (total testosterone below 150 ng/mL [5.2 nmol/L]), (2) elevated serum PRL, (3) other pituitary hormone deficiencies, or (4) symptoms of a mass lesion (headaches or visual field deficits).

2. Hypergonadotropic hypogonadism—Men with hypergonadotropic hypogonadism have low serum testosterone levels with a compensatory increase in FSH and LH. Klinefelter syndrome can be confirmed by karyotyping or by measurement of leukocyte XIST. Testicular biopsy is usually reserved for younger patients in whom the reason for primary hypogonadism is unclear.

Treatment

Testosterone replacement is reasonable for boys who have not entered puberty by age 14 years. It is also beneficial for most men with primary testicular failure (hypergonadotropic hypogonadism). Testosterone replacement or gonadal stimulation therapy is also warranted for men with severe hypogonadotropic hypogonadism of any etiology with serum testosterone levels less than 150 ng/mL (5.2 nmol/L). Testosterone therapy should also be considered for men with low or low-normal serum testosterone or free testosterone, along with elevated serum LH levels. For other men without elevated serum LH levels and an average of at least two morning serum total testosterone levels below 275 ng/dL (9.5 nmol/L, "physiologic hypogonadism"), a trial of testosterone therapy may be considered, particularly if they have at least three of the following six symptoms: erectile dysfunction, poor morning erection, low libido, depression, fatigue, and inability to perform vigorous activity. Testosterone replacement should be continued only if patients clearly derive clinical benefit from therapy. Therapy can be adjusted with an aim to improve clinical symptoms while maintaining normal serum levels of testosterone or free testosterone. Men with physiologic low-normal serum testosterone levels above 325 ng/dL (11.3 nmol/L) are unlikely to benefit from testosterone therapy.

Drug interactions can occur. Testosterone should be administered cautiously to men receiving coumadin, since the combination can increase the INR and risk of bleeding. Similarly, testosterone therapy can increase serum levels of cyclosporine, tacrolimus, and tolvaptan. Testosterone can predispose to hypoglycemia in diabetic men receiving insulin or oral hypoglycemic agents, so close monitoring of blood sugars is advisable during initiation of testosterone therapy.

Men with severe osteoporosis may require treatment with bisphosphonates and vitamin D, in addition to testosterone replacement therapy.

A. Therapies for Male Hypogonadism

1. Testosterone topical gels—Topical testosterone is usually applied once daily in the morning after showering. One or two fingers are used to apply the gel evenly to skin, followed by hand washing. Topical testosterone should not be applied to the breast or genitals. The gel should be allowed to air-dry (about 10 minutes) before dressing. Before close contact with people, a shirt must be worn or the areas of application washed with soap and water to prevent transfer of testosterone to them. The patient should avoid swimming, showering, or washing the application area for at least 2 hours following application. Table 26–14 lists topical testosterone formulations and dosages.

The serum testosterone level should be determined about 14 days after starting therapy; if the level remains below normal or the clinical response is inadequate, the daily dose may be increased to 1.5–2 times the initial dose. Serum testosterone levels vary considerably during the day after topical testosterone gel application, such that a single serum testosterone level may not accurately reflect the average serum testosterone for that individual.

2. Transdermal testosterone patches—Testosterone transdermal systems (skin patches) are applied to nongenital skin. Androderm (2 or 4 mg/day) patches may be applied at bedtime in doses of 4–8 mg; they adhere tightly to the skin and may cause skin irritation.

3. Parenteral testosterone—The dose and injection intervals are adjusted according to the patient's clinical response and serum testosterone levels drawn just before the next injection is due. A target serum testosterone level of 500 ng/dL (17.3 nmol/L) is suggested. **Testosterone cypionate** has been in use for decades; it is an intramuscular testosterone formulation that is available in solutions containing

Table 26–14. Topical testosterone formulations and recommended daily doses.

Medication	Available Formulations	Recommended Daily Dose and Suggestion Application Site
Testosterone 1% gel	*Packets:* 12.5 mg/1.25 g, 25 mg/2.5 g, or 50 mg/5 g *Tubes:* 50 mg/5 g	50–100 mg
Testosterone 2% gel	*Pump:* 10 mg/0.5 g actuation	40–70 mg
Androgel 1% gel	*Packets:* 25 mg/2.5 g, 50 mg/5 g *Pump:* 12.5 mg per actuation	50–100 mg Apply to the shoulders
Androgel 1.6% gel	*Pump:* 20.25 mg per actuation	40.5–81 mg
Testim 1% gel	*Tubes:* 50 mg/5 g	50–100 mg Apply to shoulders, upper arms, or abdomen
Fortesta 2% gel	*Pump:* 10 mg per actuation	40–70 mg Apply to shoulders, upper arms, or abdomen
Testogel (not available in the United States)	*Sachet:* 50 mg/5 g	Apply to shoulders, upper arms, or abdomen
Axiron 2% solution	*Pump:* 30 mg per actuation	30–60 mg Apply to each axilla daily
Vogelxo 1% gel	*Packets or tubes:* 50 mg/5 g *Pump:* 12.5 mg/1.25 g per actuation	50–100 mg Apply to the shoulders

200 mg/mL. Its main advantage is low cost. The usual dose is 200 mg every 2 weeks or 300 mg every 3 weeks. It is usually injected into the gluteus medius muscle in the upper lateral buttock, alternating sides. The injection technique must include sterile precautions and draw-back prior to injection to ensure against intravenous injection, which can result in pulmonary oil embolism.

Testosterone pellets (Testopel) are a long-lasting depot testosterone formulation that is available as individual vials containing a single 75-mg implantable pellet in each vial. With sterile technique, the skin of the upper-outer buttock is anesthetized with lidocaine; using a trochar, the pellets are injected subcutaneously in doses of 150–450 mg every 3–6 months as an in-office procedure.

Testosterone undecanoate (Aveed) is a long-lasting depot testosterone formulation that is restricted to qualified health care facilities. It is usually injected into the gluteus medius muscle in the upper lateral buttock, alternating sides. A serum testosterone level is measured before the fourth dose; if the serum testosterone remains low, the dosing interval is shortened to every 10 weeks.

Caution: Testosterone undecanoate injections have caused serious pulmonary oil microembolism reactions that present with cough, dyspnea, tight throat, chest pain, and syncope. Anaphylaxis can also occur. *Patients must be observed in the health care setting for 30 minutes after the injection in order to provide appropriate medical care for the complication.*

4. Buccal testosterone—Testosterone buccal tablets (Striant) are placed between the upper lip and gingivae. One or two 30-mg tablets are thus retained and changed every 12 hours. They should not be chewed or swallowed. It is not available in the United States.

5. Testosterone nasal gel—Intranasal gel testosterone (Natesto) is self-administered by a metered-dose nasal pump: one pump actuation (5.5 mg) into each nostril three times daily. The nasal pump needs to be primed by inverting it and pressing the pump 10 times before it is used the first time. It should not be used concurrently with intranasal sympathomimetic decongestants. Adverse effects include nasopharyngitis, sinusitis, bronchitis, epistaxis, nasal discomfort, and headache.

6. Clomiphene citrate—Men with functional hypogonadotropic hypogonadism usually respond well to clomiphene citrate that is administered orally in doses that are titrated to achieve the desired clinical response with a serum testosterone level of about 500 ng/dL (17.3 nmol/L). Begin with clomiphene 25 mg on alternate days and increased to 50 mg on alternate days if necessary, with a maximum dose of 50 mg daily. Serum testosterone levels usually normalize while spermatogenesis usually improves.

7. Gonadotropins—Patients with hypogonadotropic hypogonadism may require therapy with gonadotropins, particularly to induce fertility. Men may receive hCG 1000 units subcutaneously three times weekly for 6 months; if the semen analysis shows inadequate sperm, FSH 75 units subcutaneously three times weekly is added. Many men prefer long-term therapy with hCG over testosterone therapy, but cost is an issue.

8. Oral testosterone undecanoate—An oral preparation of testosterone undecanoate (Jatenzo) is available in capsules of 158 mg, 198 mg, and 237 mg and should be taken with food. The starting dose is 237 mg twice daily and can be increased to a maximum of 792 mg daily, with adjustments according to clinical response and serum testosterone levels obtained 3–4 hours (peak) after an oral dose. Serum testosterone falls to low levels by 12 hours after an oral dose; dosing every 8 hours may produce more consistent serum testosterone levels. Side effects are those of nonoral testosterone with additional side effect including GI intolerance and an increase in systolic blood pressure (average 4 mm Hg).

9. Weight loss—When hypogonadotropic hypogonadism is due to morbid obesity, significant weight loss will improve serum testosterone levels. The rise in serum testosterone is proportionate to the weight loss.

B. Benefits of Testosterone Replacement Therapy

Testosterone therapy given for the indications listed under Treatment, above, usually benefits men with low serum testosterone and at least three manifestations of hypogonadism. Replacement testosterone therapy can improve overall mood, sense of well-being, sexual desire, and erectile function. It also increases physical vigor and muscle strength. Testosterone replacement improves exercise endurance and stair climbing ability. Long-term testosterone replacement causes significant weight loss and a reduction in waist circumference. After 2 years of testosterone replacement, muscle mass increases about 4.5%, while fat mass decreases by about 9.1%. Appropriate testosterone replacement therapy also appears to improve longevity.

C. Risks of Testosterone Replacement or Stimulation Therapy

Testosterone therapy does not appear to increase the risk of prostate cancer or BPH above that of normal men, provided serum testosterone levels are maintained in the normal reference range. However, testosterone therapy is contraindicated in the presence of active prostate cancer. Hypogonadal men who have had a prostatectomy for low-grade prostate cancer, and who have remained in complete remission for several years, may have testosterone therapy given cautiously while monitoring serum PSA levels.

Erythrocytosis is more common with intramuscular injections of testosterone enanthate than with transcutaneous testosterone. Testosterone replacement has not been considered to significantly increase the risk of thromboembolic events in most hypogonadal men. However, one large medical database study has found a correlation between testosterone therapy and thromboembolic events, particularly in men with a prior history of vascular events and in men being prescribed testosterone without proper documentation of hypogonadism.

Testosterone therapy tends to aggravate sleep apnea in older men, likely through CNS effects. Surveillance for sleep apnea is recommended during testosterone therapy and a formal evaluation is recommended for all high-risk patients with snoring, obesity, partner's report of apneic episodes, nocturnal awakening, unrefreshing sleep with daytime fatigue, or hypertension.

Testosterone therapy frequently increases acne that is usually mild and tolerated; topical antiacne therapy or a reduction in testosterone replacement dosage may be required. Increases in intraocular pressure have occurred during testosterone therapy. During the initiation of testosterone replacement therapy, gynecomastia develops in some men, which usually is mild and tends to resolve spontaneously; switching from testosterone injections to testosterone transdermal gel may help this condition.

D. Risks of Performance-Enhancing Anabolic Steroids

Performance-enhancing agents, particularly androgenic anabolic steroids, are used by up to 2% of young athletes and by 20–65% of power sport athletes. They are often used as part of a "stacking" polypharmacy that may include nandrolone decanoate, dimethandrolone, testosterone propionate, or testosterone enanthate. These androgens are usually illegal, often contaminated by toxic substances (such as arsenic), and can produce toxic hepatitis, dependence, aggression, depression, dyslipidemias, gynecomastia, acne, male pattern baldness, hepatitis, thromboembolism, and cardiomyopathy. Arsenic contamination can cause multiorgan failure and death.

Prognosis of Male Hypogonadism

If hypogonadism is due to a pituitary lesion, the prognosis is that of the primary disease (eg, tumor, necrosis). The prognosis for restoration of virility is good if testosterone is given. In one large study, cardiovascular risk was reduced in hypogonadal men over age 40 who were receiving testosterone replacement therapy to maintain serum testosterone levels within the normal reference range.

Diem SJ et al. Efficacy and safety of testosterone treatment in men: an evidence report for a clinical practice guideline by the American College of Physicians. Ann Intern Med. 2020;172:1184. [PMID: 31905375]

Glintborg D et al. Testosterone replacement therapy of opioid-induced male hypogonadism improved body composition but not pain perception; a double-blind, randomized, and placebo-controlled trial. Eur J Endocrinol. 2020;182:539. [PMID: 32213659]

McGriff SC et al. Optimal endocrine evaluation and treatment of male infertility. Urol Clin North Am. 2020;47:139. [PMID: 32272985]

Salter CA et al. Guideline of guidelines: testosterone therapy for testosterone deficiency. BJU Int. 2019;124:722. [PMID: 31420972]

Walker RF et al. Association of testosterone therapy with risk of venous thromboembolism among men with and without hypogonadism. JAMA Intern Med. 2020;180:190. [PMID: 31710339]

CRYPTORCHISM

Cryptorchidism is found in 1–2% of males after 1 year of age but must be distinguished from retractile testes, which require no treatment. Infertility or subfertility occurs in up to 75% of men with bilateral cryptorchism and in 50% of men with unilateral cryptorchism. Some patients have underlying hypogonadism, including hypogonadotropic hypogonadism.

For a testis that is not palpable, it is important to locate the testis and bring it into the scrotum or prove its absence. About one-third of nonpalpable testes are located within the inguinal canal, one-third are intra-abdominal, and one-third are absent. Ultrasound can detect an inguinal testis. If ultrasound is negative, MRI is performed to locate the testis.

The lifetime risk of testicular neoplasia is 0.002% in healthy males. The risk of malignancy is higher for cryptorchid testes (0.06%) and for intra-abdominal testes (5%). Orchiopexy decreases the risk of neoplasia when performed before 10 years of age. For bilateral undescended testes, boys with early orchiopexy (before age 13 years) appear to have relatively normal fertility, whereas boys with delayed orchiopexy may have reduced fertility. With a unilateral undescended testis, about 50% descend spontaneously and early orchiopexy does not improve fertility, so orchiopexy is usually delayed until after puberty. For intra-abdominal testes, orchiectomy after puberty is usually the best option.

Hildorf S et al. Fertility potential is compromised in 20% to 25% of boys with nonsyndromic cryptorchidism despite orchiopexy within the first year of life. J Urol. 2020;203:832. [PMID: 31642739]

GYNECOMASTIA

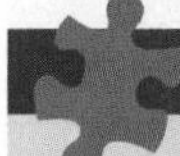

ESSENTIALS OF DIAGNOSIS

- Palpable enlargement of the male breast, often asymmetric or unilateral.
- Glandular gynecomastia: typically tender.
- Fatty gynecomastia: typically nontender.
- Must be distinguished from carcinoma or mastitis.

General Considerations

Gynecomastia is defined as the presence of palpable glandular breast tissue in males. Gynecomastia is a common condition, and its incidence is increasing in all age groups. The causes are multiple and diverse (Table 26–15). Pubertal gynecomastia develops in 60% of boys, more commonly teenagers who are overweight; the swelling usually subsides spontaneously within a year. About 20% of adult gynecomastia is caused by drug therapy. It can develop in HIV-infected men treated with antiretroviral therapy, especially

Table 26–15. Causes of gynecomastia.

Physiologic causes	Anti-androgens
Aging	Antipsychotics (first- and second-generation)
Neonatal period, puberty	Antiretroviral agents
Obesity	Calcium channel blockers (rare)
Endocrine diseases	Chorionic gonadotropin
Androgen insensitivity syndrome	Cimetidine
Aromatase excess syndrome (sporadic or familial)	Clomiphene
Diabetic lymphocytic mastitis	Diazepam
Hyperprolactinemia	Digitalis preparations
Hyper- or hypothyroidism	Dutasteride, finasteride
Klinefelter syndrome	Estrogens (oral or topical)
Male hypogonadism (primary or secondary)	Ethionamide
Partial 17-ketosteroid reductase deficiency	Famotidine (rare)
Systemic diseases	Fenofibrate (rare)
Chronic liver disease	GH
CKD	GnRH analogs
Hansen disease	Hydroxyzine
Neurologic disorders	Isoniazid
Refeeding after starvation	Ketoconazole
Spinal cord injury	Lavender and tea tree oil (topical)
Neoplasms	Marijuana
Adrenal tumors	Methadone
Bronchogenic carcinoma	Methyldopa
Breast carcinoma	Metoclopramide
Ectopic hCG: CNS germinoma, lung, hepatocellular, gastric, renal carcinomas	Metronidazole
Pituitary prolactinoma	Opioids
Testicular hCG-secreting tumors	Phenothiazines
Drugs (partial list)	Progestins
Alcohol	PPIs (uncommon)
Alkylating chemotherapeutic agents	SSRIs
Amiodarone	Soy ingestion
Anabolic steroids	Statins (rare)
Androgens (testosterone)	Spironolactone (common)
	Sunitinib
	Tea tree oil (topical)
	Tricyclics

GH, growth hormone; GnRH, gonadotropin-releasing hormone.

efavirenz or didanosine, and in athletes who abuse androgens and anabolic steroids. Fatty pseudogynecomastia is common among elderly men, particularly when there is associated weight gain. True glandular gynecomastia can be the first sign of a serious disorder in older men (Table 26–15).

Clinical Findings

A. Symptoms and Signs

The male breasts must be palpated to distinguish firm true glandular gynecomastia from softer fatty pseudogynecomastia in which only adipose tissue is felt. The breasts are best examined both seated and supine. Using the thumb and forefinger as pincers, the subareolar tissue is compared to nearby adipose tissue. Fatty tissue is usually diffuse and nontender. True glandular enlargement beneath the areola may be tender. Pubertal gynecomastia is characterized by tender discoid enlargement of breast tissue 2–3 cm in diameter beneath the areola. The following characteristics are worrisome for malignancy: asymmetry; location not immediately below the areola; unusual firmness; or nipple retraction, bleeding, or discharge. The examination must also include an assessment of masculinization, examination of the testes for size and masses, and examination of the penis for hypospadias.

B. Laboratory Findings

In the presence of true glandular gynecomastia, laboratory studies should include liver biochemical tests, serum BUN, and creatinine. Endocrine testing, including serum testosterone, free testosterone, LH, FSH, TSH, and FT_4, is obtained to determine whether primary hypogonadism (low serum testosterone, high LH), secondary hypogonadism (low serum testosterone, low or normal LH), or androgen resistance may be present. High serum testosterone levels plus high LH levels characterize partial androgen insensitivity syndrome. A serum PRL is obtained to screen for hyperprolactinemia and pituitary/hypothalamic lesions. Serum beta-hCG and estradiol levels are obtained to screen for malignancy-associated gynecomastia. Detectable levels of beta-hCG implicate a testicular tumor (germ cell or Sertoli cell) or other malignancy (usually lung or liver). Increased serum estradiol levels may result from testicular tumors, increased beta-hCG, liver disease, obesity, adrenal tumors (rare), true hermaphroditism (rare), or aromatase gene gain-of-function mutations (rare). A karyotype for Klinefelter syndrome is obtained in men with persistent gynecomastia without obvious cause.

C. Imaging and Biopsy

Investigation of unclear cases should include bilateral mammography and a chest CT to search for bronchogenic or metastatic carcinoma. Benign mammographic findings make malignancy very unlikely. Suspicious mammographic findings require ultrasound-guided FNA and cytologic examination to distinguish gynecomastia from benign lesions (pseudogynecomastia, lipoma, posttraumatic hematoma/fat necrosis, epidermal inclusion cyst), lymphoma, and male breast cancer. Male breast cancer and gynecomastia may coexist.

Men with a high serum hCG or estradiol levels should have the test confirmed with repeat testing. Confirmed increased levels warrant a testicular ultrasound. If the testicular ultrasound is normal, high serum estradiol levels may warrant a CT of the adrenal glands; high serum hCG levels may warrant additional CT scanning to detect rare hCG-secreting carcinomas of the lung, mediastinum, liver, stomach, or kidney.

Treatment

Pubertal gynecomastia often resolves spontaneously within 1–2 years. Drug-induced gynecomastia resolves within months in most patients after the offending drug is removed. Patients with painful or persistent gynecomastia may be treated with medical therapy, usually for 9–12 months.

Selective estrogen receptor modulator (SERM) therapy is effective for true glandular gynecomastia. Raloxifene, 60 mg orally daily, may be more effective than tamoxifen.

Aromatase inhibitor (AI) therapy is also reasonably effective; anastrozole, 1 mg orally daily, reduces breast volume significantly over 6 months in adolescents. Serum estradiol levels fall slightly while serum testosterone levels rise. Long-term AI therapy in adolescents is not recommended because of the possibility of inducing osteoporosis and of delaying epiphyseal fusion, which could cause an increase in adult height.

Testosterone therapy for men with hypogonadism may improve or worsen preexistent gynecomastia.

Radiation therapy has been used prophylactically to prevent gynecomastia in men with prostate cancer being treated with antiandrogen therapy.

Surgical correction is reserved for patients with persistent or severe gynecomastia.

Ali SN et al. Which patients with gynaecomastia require more detailed investigation? Clin Endocrinol (Oxf). 2018;88:360. [PMID: 29193251]

HIRSUTISM & VIRILIZATION

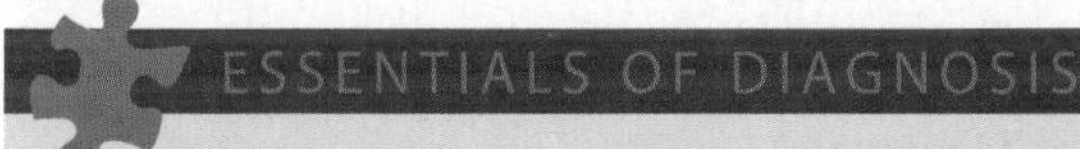

ESSENTIALS OF DIAGNOSIS

- Hirsutism, acne, menstrual disorders.
- Virilization: muscularity, androgenic alopecia, deepening voice, clitoromegaly.
- Rarely, a palpable pelvic tumor.
- Serum DHEAS and androstenedione elevated in adrenal disorders; variable in others.
- Serum testosterone is often elevated.

General Considerations

Hirsutism is defined as cosmetically unacceptable terminal hair growth that appears in women in a male pattern. Significant hirsutism affects about 5–10% of non-Asian women of reproductive age and over 40% of women at some point during their life. The amount of hair growth deemed unacceptable depends on a woman's ethnicity and cultural norms. Virilization is defined as the development of male physical characteristics in women, such as pronounced muscle development, deep voice, male pattern baldness, and more severe hirsutism.

Etiology

Hirsutism may be idiopathic or familial or be caused by the following disorders: polycystic ovary syndrome (PCOS), ovarian hyperthecosis, steroidogenic enzyme defects, neoplastic disorders; or rarely by medications, acromegaly, or ACTH-induced Cushing disease.

A. Idiopathic or Familial

Most women with hirsutism or androgenic alopecia have no detectable hyperandrogenism; hirsutism may be considered normal in the context of their genetic background. Such patients may have elevated serum levels of androstenediol glucuronide, a metabolite of dihydrotestosterone that is produced by skin in cosmetically unacceptable amounts.

B. Polycystic Ovary Syndrome (Hyperthecosis, Stein-Leventhal Syndrome)

PCOS is a common functional disorder of the ovaries of unknown etiology (see Chapter 18). It accounts for at least 50% of all cases of hirsutism associated with elevated serum testosterone levels.

A diagnosis of PCOS must meet three criteria: (1) androgen excess with clinical hyperandrogenism or elevated serum free or total testosterone; (2) ovarian dysfunction with oligoanovulation or polycystic ovary morphology; and (3) absence of other causes of testosterone excess or anovulation such as pregnancy, thyroid dysfunction, 21-hydroxylase deficiency, neoplastic testosterone secretion, Cushing syndrome, or hyperprolactinemia.

Affected women usually have signs of hyperandrogenism, including hirsutism, acne, or male-pattern thinning of scalp hair; this persists after natural menopause. However, women of East Asian ancestry are less likely to exhibit hirsutism. Most women also have elevated serum testosterone or free testosterone levels. About 70% of affected women have polycystic ovaries on pelvic ultrasound and 50% have oligomenorrhea or amenorrhea with anovulation. Of note, about 30% of women with PCOS do *not* have cystic ovaries and 25–30% of normal menstruating women *have* cystic ovaries.

Obesity and high serum insulin levels (due to insulin resistance) contribute to the syndrome in 70% of women. The serum LH:FSH ratio is often greater than 2.0. Both adrenal and ovarian androgen hypersecretion are commonly present.

C. Steroidogenic Enzyme Defects

Congenital adrenal steroidogenic enzyme defects result in reduced cortisol secretion with a compensatory increase in ACTH that causes adrenal hyperplasia. The most common enzyme defect is 21-hydroxylase deficiency, with a prevalence of about 1:18,000.

Partial deficiency in adrenal 21-hydroxylase can present in women as hirsutism. About 2% of patients with adult-onset hirsutism have been found to have a partial defect in adrenal 21-hydroxylase. The phenotypic expression is delayed until adolescence or adulthood.

D. Neoplastic Disorders

Ovarian tumors are uncommon causes of hirsutism (0.8%) and include arrhenoblastomas, Sertoli-Leydig cell tumors, dysgerminomas, and hilar cell tumors. Adrenal carcinoma, a rare cause of Cushing syndrome and hyperandrogenism, can be quite virilizing. Pure androgen-secreting adrenal tumors occur very rarely; about 50% are malignant.

E. Rare Causes of Hirsutism & Virilization

Acromegaly and ACTH-induced Cushing syndrome are rare causes of hirsutism and virilization. Porphyria cutanea tarda can cause periorbital hair growth in addition to dermatitis in sun-exposed areas. Maternal virilization during pregnancy may result from a luteoma of pregnancy, hyperreactio luteinalis, or polycystic ovaries. In postmenopausal women, diffuse stromal Leydig cell hyperplasia is a rare cause of hyperandrogenism. Acquired hypertrichosis lanuginosa, which is diffuse fine lanugo hair growth on the face and body along with stomatologic symptoms, is usually associated with an internal malignancy, especially colorectal cancer, and may regress after tumor removal. Pharmacologic causes include minoxidil, cyclosporine, phenytoin, anabolic steroids, interferon, cetuximab, diazoxide, and certain progestins.

Clinical Findings

A. Symptoms and Signs

Modest androgen excess from any source increases sexual hair (chin, upper lip, abdomen, and chest) and increases sebaceous gland activity, producing acne. Menstrual irregularities, anovulation, and amenorrhea are common. If androgen excess is pronounced, defeminization (decrease in breast size, loss of feminine adipose tissue) and virilization (frontal balding, muscularity, clitoromegaly, and deepening of the voice) occur. Virilization points to the presence of an androgen-producing neoplasm.

Hirsutism is quantitated using the Ferriman-Gallwey score; hirsutism is graded from 0 (none) to 4 (severe) in nine areas of the body (maximum possible score is 36) (https://education.endocrine.org/ferriman-gallwey-hirsutism-system). Scores below 8 are considered mild hirsutism and normal variants. Scores of 8–15 indicate moderate hirsutism. Scores over 15 indicate severe hirsutism. Of note, the normal score is lower in Asian women and higher in Mediterranean women.

A pelvic examination may disclose clitoromegaly or ovarian enlargement that may be cystic or neoplastic. Hypertension may be present in Cushing syndrome, adrenal 11-hydroxylase deficiency, or cortisol resistance syndrome.

B. Laboratory Testing and Imaging

Serum androgen testing is mainly useful to screen for rare occult adrenal or ovarian neoplasms. Testing is warranted for women with moderate to severe hirsutism, mild hirsutism with menstrual disturbances, and women with worsening hirsutism despite therapy.

Serum is assayed for total testosterone and free testosterone. A serum testosterone level greater than 200 ng/dL (6.9 nmol/L) or free testosterone greater than 40 ng/dL (140 pmol/L) indicates the need for a manual pelvic examination and ultrasound. If that is negative, an adrenal CT scan is performed. A serum androstenedione level greater than 1000 ng/dL (34.9 nmol/L) also points to an ovarian or adrenal neoplasm.

Patients with a serum DHEAS greater than 700 mcg/dL (35 nmol/L) have an adrenal source of androgen. This usually is due to adrenal hyperplasia and rarely to adrenal carcinoma. Patients with any clinical signs of Cushing syndrome should receive a screening test (eg, 1-mg overnight dexamethasone suppression test) (see Cushing Syndrome, above).

Screening for nonclassical "late-onset" congenital adrenal hyperplasia (CAH) due to 21-hydroxylase deficiency is warranted for women with (1) high serum testosterone or free testosterone levels and (2) hirsutism with normal serum testosterone levels who are at high risk for CAH due to having a family history of hirsutism or being a member of a high-risk ethnic group (eg, Ashkenazi Jews, Croatians, Iranians, Yupik Inuit). The evaluation requires an early morning blood draw for serum 17-hydroxyprogesterone, ideally during the follicular (early) phase of the menstrual cycle or on a random day for women with irregular menses or amenorrhea. Patients with CAH usually have a baseline 17-hydroxyprogesterone level greater than 300 ng/dL (9.1 nmol/L). Serum levels of FSH and LH are elevated if amenorrhea is due to ovarian failure. An LH:FSH ratio greater than 2.0 is common in patients with PCOS. On abdominal ultrasound, about 25–30% of normal young women have polycystic ovaries, so the appearance of ovarian cysts on ultrasound is not helpful. Pelvic ultrasound or MRI usually detects virilizing tumors of the ovary. However, small virilizing ovarian tumors may not be detectable on imaging studies; selective venous sampling for testosterone may be used for diagnosis in such patients.

Treatment

Any drugs causing hirsutism (see above) should be stopped. Any underlying medical causes of hirsutism (eg, Cushing syndrome, acromegaly) should be treated.

A. Laser and Topical Treatments

Local treatment of facial hirsutism is by shaving or depilatories, waxing, electrolysis, or bleaching. Eflornithine (Vaniqa) 13.9% topical cream retards hair growth when applied twice daily to unwanted facial hair; improvement is noted within 4–8 weeks. Eflornithine may be used during laser therapy for a more dramatic response. However, local skin irritation may occur. Hirsutism returns with discontinuation, unless it is given with laser therapy.

Laser therapy (photoepilation) can be a very effective treatment for facial hirsutism, particularly for women with dark hair and light skin. For women of color, a longer-wavelength laser such as Nd:YAG or diode laser given with skin cooling is used. In such women, laser removal of facial hair significantly improves hirsutism. Repeated laser treatments are usually required. Accidental eye injuries have been reported; eye shields should be used during treatments. Laser therapy is not recommended for Middle Eastern and Mediterranean women with facial hirsutism, since they have a particularly increased risk of paradoxical hypertrichosis with laser therapy.

Topical minoxidil may be used to treat androgenic alopecia and is mildly effective when applied to the scalp twice daily. Only the 2% formulation is FDA-approved for women.

B. Medications

Oral contraceptives are warranted as an initial therapy for women with hirsutism who are not actively pursuing pregnancy. To reduce the risk of DVT, an oral contraceptive is recommended with a low-dose of estradiol (20 mcg) and a progestin having a relatively low risk of venous thrombosis (norethindrone, norgestimate, levonorgestrel). A favored formulation for daily use contains norethindrone 1 mg with ethinyl estradiol 20 mcg. Nevertheless, such oral contraceptives confer over twofold increased risk of DVT. Also, levonorgestrel causes insulin resistance, so its use is problematic in women with polycystic ovary syndrome. Oral contraceptives that contain particularly antiandrogenic progestins such as desogestrel (Azurette, Kariva), drospirenone (Yaz, Gianvi), norgestimate (Ortho Tri-Cyclen Lo), or cyproterone acetate (Diane 35, not available in United States) more effectively reduce hirsutism and acne; however, such antiandrogenic oral contraceptives confer a fourfold risk of DVT, and their use is discouraged in high-risk patients.

Cyproterone acetate is a unique progestin that is used to treat women with hirsutism worldwide, except in the United States, where it is not FDA-approved. Cyproterone acetate blocks androgen receptors as well as 5-alpha-reductase activity while also suppressing testosterone levels. It is typically prescribed as an oral contraceptive in a dose of 2 mg with ethinyl estradiol 35 mcg.

Combined oral contraceptives are relatively contraindicated for women who are predisposed to thromboembolism, such as women who are smokers or who have migraines, women who are over age 39 years or who are obese, those with hypertension or a personal history of thromboembolism. Metabolic syndrome and hypertriglyceridemia are seen, particularly with antiandrogenic progestins.

Spironolactone is effective for reducing hirsutism, acne, and androgenic alopecia in women. It may be taken in doses of 100–200 mg orally daily (taken as a single dose or in two divided doses) on days 5–25 of the menstrual cycle or daily if used concomitantly with an oral contraceptive. Spironolactone is contraindicated in pregnancy, so reproductive-age women must use reliable contraception during this therapy. Hyperkalemia is an uncommon side effect, but serum potassium should be checked 1 month after beginning therapy or after dosage increases. Spironolactone should be avoided or used cautiously in women with kidney disease or who are taking an ACE inhibitor or ARB. Spironolactone should not be given with an oral contraceptive containing drospirenone because the progestin has an anti-mineralocorticoid effect that predisposes to hyperkalemia. Side effects of spironolactone include breast tenderness, menstrual irregularity, headaches, nausea, and fatigue, which may improve with continued treatment or dose reduction; paradoxical scalp hair loss has been reported at higher doses.

Flutamide and **bicalutamide** inhibit testosterone binding to androgen receptors and also suppress serum testosterone. They should only be used as a last resort for women with severe hirsutism/virilization and only with very close monitoring for hepatic toxicity and strict contraceptive precautions due to risks of fetal malformations.

Finasteride inhibits 5-alpha-reductase, the enzyme that converts testosterone to active dihydrotestosterone in the skin. Due to inconsistent reduction in hirsutism and androgenic alopecia and risk ofpseudohermaphroditism in male infants if mistakenly taken during pregnancy, finasteride for hirsutism is strongly discouraged.

Metformin alone is ineffective in improving hirsutism but can enhance the anti-hirsutism effect of spironolactone. Start metformin at a dose of 500 mg/day with breakfast for 1 week, then increased to 500 mg with breakfast and dinner. If this dose is clinically insufficient but tolerated, the dose may be increased to 850–1000 mg twice daily with meals. Although metformin reduces insulin resistance, it does not cause hypoglycemia in nondiabetic patients. **GLP-1 agonist** therapy reduced weight and serum testosterone levels in women with PCOS in one short-term study. However, an effect on hirsutism has not been demonstrated clinically.

Simvastatin can reduce hirsutism in women with PCOS. In one study, simvastatin 20 mg orally daily was given to women receiving an oral contraceptive for PCOS. Besides improving their serum lipid profiles, women receiving simvastatin had greater decreases in hirsutism and serum free testosterone levels than the women receiving an oral contraceptive alone. Atorvastatin also reduced serum testosterone by an average of 25% in women with PCOS.

Glucocorticoid replacement is necessary for women with classical congenital adrenal hyperplasia (21-hydroxylase deficiency) with hirsutism and adrenal insufficiency that requires glucocorticoid and mineralocorticoid replacement. However, women with partial "late-onset" 21-hydroxylase deficiency are not cortisol deficient and do not require glucocorticoid replacement. Glucocorticoids are ineffective in reducing hirsutism in these women. However, replacement doses of glucocorticoids (prednisone, methylprednisolone) may be indicated to normalize menses and for ovulation induction.

GnRH agonist therapy has been successful in treating postmenopausal women with severe ovarian hyperandrogenism when laparoscopic oophorectomy is contraindicated or declined by the patient.

C. Surgery

Androgenizing tumors of the adrenal or ovary are resected laparoscopically. Postmenopausal women with severe hyperandrogenism should undergo laparoscopic bilateral oophorectomy (if CT scan of the adrenals and ovaries is normal), since small hilar cell tumors of the ovary may not be visible on scans. Women with classic salt-wasting congenital adrenal hyperplasia and infertility or treatment-resistant hyperandrogenism may be treated with laparoscopic bilateral adrenalectomy.

Fraison E et al. Metformin versus the combined oral contraceptive pill for hirsutism, acne and menstrual pattern in polycystic ovary syndrome. Cochrane Database Syst Rev. 2020;8:CD005552. [PMID: 32794179]

Martin KA et al. Evaluation and treatment of hirsutism in premenopausal women: an Endocrine Society clinical practice guideline. J Clin Endocrinol Metab. 2018;103:1233. [PMID: 29522147]

AMENORRHEA & MENOPAUSE

PRIMARY AMENORRHEA

Menarche ordinarily occurs between ages 11 and 15 years (average in the United States: 12.7 years) (see also Chapter 18). The failure of any menses to appear is termed "primary amenorrhea," and evaluation is commenced either (1) at age 14 years if neither menarche nor any breast development has occurred or if height is in the lowest 3% for ethnicity, or (2) at age 16 years if menarche has not occurred.

Etiology of Primary Amenorrhea

The etiologies for primary amenorrhea include hypothalamic-pituitary causes, hyperandrogenism, ovarian causes (gonadal dysgenesis, Müllerian dysgenesis), disorders of sexual development (pseudohermaphroditism), uterine causes, and pregnancy.

A. Hypothalamic-Pituitary Causes (With Low or Normal FSH)

The most common cause of primary amenorrhea is a variant of normal known as constitutional delay of growth and puberty, which accounts for about 30% of delayed puberty cases. There is a strong genetic basis for this condition; over 50% of girls with it have a family history of delayed puberty. However, constitutional delay of growth and puberty is a diagnosis of exclusion.

A genetic deficiency of GnRH and gonadotropins may be isolated or associated with other pituitary deficiencies or diminished olfaction (Kallmann syndrome). Hypothalamic lesions, particularly craniopharyngioma, may be present. Pituitary tumors may be nonsecreting or may secrete PRL or GH. Cushing syndrome may be caused by corticosteroid treatment, a cortisol-secreting adrenal tumor, or an ACTH-secreting pituitary tumor. Hypothyroidism can delay adolescence. Head trauma or encephalitis can cause gonadotropin deficiency. Primary amenorrhea may also be caused by severe illness, vigorous exercise (eg, ballet dancing, running), stressful life events, dieting, or anorexia nervosa; however, these conditions should not be assumed to account for amenorrhea without a full endocrinologic evaluation.

B. Uterine Causes (With Normal FSH)

Müllerian agenesis (Mayer-Rokitansky-Küster-Hauser syndrome) results in a missing uterus and variable degrees of upper vaginal hypoplasia. It is the most common cause of permanent primary amenorrhea. Affected women have intact ovaries and undergo an otherwise normal puberty.

An imperforate hymen is occasionally the reason for the absence of visible menses.

C. Ovarian Causes (With High FSH)

Gonadal dysgenesis (Turner syndrome and variants) is a frequent cause of primary amenorrhea. Autoimmune ovarian failure is another cause. Rare deficiencies in certain ovarian steroidogenic enzymes are causes of primary hypogonadism without virilization: 3-beta-hydroxysteroid dehydrogenase deficiency (adrenal insufficiency with low serum 17-hydroxyprogesterone) and P450c17 deficiency (hypertension and hypokalemia with high serum 17-hydroxyprogesterone).

D. Hyperandrogenism (With Low or Normal FSH)

Polycystic ovaries and ovarian tumors can secrete excessive testosterone. Excess testosterone can also be secreted by adrenal tumors or by adrenal hyperplasia caused by steroidogenic enzyme defects such as P450c21 deficiency (salt-wasting) or P450c11 deficiency (hypertension). Androgenic steroid abuse may also cause this syndrome.

E. 46,XY Disorders of Sexual Development (Pseudohermaphroditism)

Complete androgen insensitivity syndrome is caused by homozygous inactivating mutations in the androgen receptor. 46,XY individuals with complete androgen insensitivity syndrome are born with normal external female genitalia, although some may have labial or inguinal swellings due to cryptorchid testes. Affected individuals are phenotypic girls and experience normal breast development at puberty, but fail to develop sexual hair and have primary amenorrhea.

Partial androgen insensitivity syndrome in 46,XY individuals results in variable degrees of ambiguous genitalia.

F. Pregnancy (With High hCG)

Pregnancy may be the cause of primary amenorrhea even when the patient denies having had sexual intercourse.

Clinical Findings

A. Symptoms and Signs

Headaches or visual field abnormalities implicate a hypothalamic or pituitary tumor. Signs of pregnancy may be present. Blood pressure elevation, acne, and hirsutism should be noted. Short stature may be seen with an associated GH or thyroid hormone deficiency. Short stature with manifestations of gonadal dysgenesis indicates Turner syndrome. Olfactory deficits are seen in Kallmann syndrome. Obesity and short stature may be signs of Cushing syndrome. Tall stature may be due to eunuchoidism or acromegaly. Hirsutism or virilization suggests excessive testosterone.

An external pelvic examination plus a rectal examination should be performed to assess hymen patency and the presence of a uterus.

B. Laboratory and Radiologic Findings

The initial endocrine evaluation should include serum FSH, LH, PRL, total and free testosterone, TSH, FT_4, and beta-hCG (pregnancy test). Patients who are virilized or hypertensive require serum electrolyte determinations and further hormonal evaluation (see Hirsutism & Virilization, above). MRI of the hypothalamus and pituitary is used to evaluate teens with primary amenorrhea and low or normal FSH and LH—especially those with high PRL levels. Pelvic duplex/color sonography is very useful. Girls who have a normal uterus and high FSH without the classic features of Turner syndrome may require a karyotype to diagnose X chromosome mosaicism.

Treatment

Treatment of primary amenorrhea is directed at the underlying cause. Girls with permanent hypogonadism are treated with HRT.

Varughese R et al. Fifteen-minute consultation: a structured approach to the child with primary amenorrhea. Arch Dis Child Educ Pract Ed. 2021;106:18. [PMID: 32561551]

SECONDARY AMENORRHEA

General Considerations

Secondary amenorrhea is defined as the absence of menses for 3 consecutive months in women who have passed menarche. Menopause is defined as the terminal episode of naturally occurring menses; it is a retrospective diagnosis, usually made after 12 months of amenorrhea.

Etiology & Clinical Findings

The causes of secondary amenorrhea include pregnancy, hypothalamic-pituitary causes, hyperandrogenism, uterine causes, premature ovarian failure, and menopause.

A. Pregnancy (High hCG)

Pregnancy is the most common cause for secondary amenorrhea in premenopausal women. The differential diagnosis includes rare ectopic secretion of hCG by a choriocarcinoma or bronchogenic carcinoma.

B. Hypothalamic-Pituitary Causes (With Low or Normal FSH)

The hypothalamus must release GnRH in a pulsatile manner for the pituitary to secrete gonadotropins. GnRH pulses occurring more than once per hour favor LH secretion, while less frequent pulses favor FSH secretion. In normal ovulatory cycles, GnRH pulses in the follicular phase are rapid and favor LH synthesis and ovulation; ovarian luteal progesterone is then secreted that slows GnRH pulses, causing FSH secretion during the luteal phase. Most women with hypothalamic amenorrhea have a persistently low frequency of GnRH pulses.

Secondary "hypothalamic" amenorrhea may be caused by stressful life events such as school examinations or leaving home. Such women usually have a history of normal sexual development and irregular menses since menarche. Amenorrhea may also be the result of strict dieting, vigorous exercise, organic illness, or anorexia nervosa. Intrathecal infusion of opioids causes amenorrhea in most women. These conditions should not be assumed to account for amenorrhea without a full physical and endocrinologic evaluation. Young women in whom the results of evaluation and progestin withdrawal test are normal have noncyclic secretion of gonadotropins resulting in anovulation. Such women typically recover spontaneously but should have regular evaluations and a progestin withdrawal test about every 3 months to detect loss of estrogen effect.

PRL elevation may cause amenorrhea. Pituitary tumors or other lesions may cause hypopituitarism. Corticosteroid excess suppresses gonadotropins.

C. Hyperandrogenism (With Low-Normal FSH)

Elevated serum levels of testosterone can cause hirsutism, virilization, and amenorrhea. In PCOS, GnRH pulses are persistently rapid, favoring LH synthesis with excessive androgen secretion; reduced FSH secretion impairs follicular maturation. Progesterone administration can slow the GnRH pulses, thus favoring FSH secretion that induces follicular maturation. Rare causes of secondary amenorrhea include adrenal P450c21 deficiency, ovarian or adrenal malignancies, and Cushing syndrome. Anabolic steroids also cause amenorrhea.

D. Uterine Causes (With Normal FSH)

Infection of the uterus commonly occurs following delivery or dilation and curettage but may occur spontaneously. Endometritis due to tuberculosis or schistosomiasis should be suspected in endemic areas. Endometrial scarring may result, causing amenorrhea (Asherman syndrome). Such women typically continue to have monthly premenstrual symptoms. The vaginal estrogen effect is normal.

E. Menopause (With High FSH)

Early menopause refers to primary ovarian failure that occurs before age 45. It affects approximately 5% of women. About 1% of women experience **premature menopause** that is defined as ovarian failure before age 40; about 30% of such cases are due to autoimmunity against the ovary. X chromosome mosaicism accounts for 8% of cases of premature menopause. Other causes include surgical bilateral oophorectomy, radiation therapy for pelvic malignancy, and chemotherapy. Women who have undergone hysterectomy are prone to premature ovarian failure even though the ovaries were left intact. Myotonic dystrophy, galactosemia, and mumps oophoritis are additional causes. Early or premature menopause is frequently familial. Ovarian failure is usually irreversible. Women with premature menopause, compared to women with normal menopause, have a 50% increased risk of coronary disease, a 23% increased risk of stroke, and a 12% increased overall mortality.

Laboratory findings in premature menopause—An elevated hCG overwhelmingly indicates pregnancy; false-positive testing may occur very rarely with ectopic hCG secretion (eg, choriocarcinoma or bronchogenic carcinoma).

Further laboratory evaluation for women who are not pregnant includes serum PRL, FSH and LH (both elevated in menopause), and TSH. Hyperprolactinemia or hypopituitarism (without obvious cause) should prompt an MRI study of the pituitary region. Routine testing of kidney and liver function (BUN, serum creatinine, bilirubin, alkaline phosphatase, and ALT) is also performed. A serum testosterone level is obtained in hirsute or virilized women.

Treatment

Nonpregnant women without any laboratory abnormality may receive a 10-day course of a progestin (eg, medroxyprogesterone acetate, 10 mg/day); absence of withdrawal menses typically indicates a lack of estrogen or a uterine abnormality. (See Treatment section of Normal Menopause, below.)

NORMAL MENOPAUSE

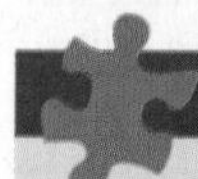

ESSENTIALS OF DIAGNOSIS

- Menopause is a retrospective diagnosis after 12 months of amenorrhea.
- Approximately 80% of women experience hot flushes and night sweats.
- High FSH and low estradiol help confirm the diagnosis.

General Considerations

Normal menopause refers to primary ovarian failure that occurs after age 45. "Climacteric" is defined as the period of natural physiologic decline in ovarian function, generally occurring over about 10 years. By about age 40 years, the remaining ovarian follicles are those that are the least sensitive to gonadotropins. Increasing titers of FSH are required to stimulate estradiol secretion. Estradiol levels may actually rise during early climacteric.

The normal age for menopause in the United States ranges between 48 and 55 years, with an average of about 51.5 years. Serum estradiol levels fall and the remaining estrogen after menopause is estrone, derived mainly from peripheral aromatization of adrenal androstenedione. Such peripheral production of estrone is enhanced by obesity and liver disease. Individual differences in estrone levels partly explain why the symptoms noted above may be minimal in some women but severe in others.

Clinical Findings

A. Symptoms and Signs

1. Cessation of menstruation—Menstrual cycles generally become irregular as menopause approaches. Anovulatory cycles occur more often, with irregular cycle length and occasional menorrhagia. Menstrual flow usually diminishes in amount owing to decreased estrogen secretion, resulting in less abundant endometrial growth. Finally, cycles become longer, with missed periods or episodes of spotting only. When no bleeding has occurred for 1 year, the menopausal transition can be said to have occurred. Any bleeding after 6 months from the cessation of menses warrants investigation by endometrial curettage or aspiration to rule out endometrial cancer.

2. Vasomotor symptoms—Hot flushes (feelings of intense heat over the trunk and face, with flushing of the skin and sweating) occur in over 80% of women as a result of the decrease in ovarian hormones. Hot flushes can begin before the cessation of menses. Menopausal vasomotor symptoms last longer than previously thought, and there are ethnic differences in the duration of symptoms. Vasomotor symptoms last more than 7 years in more than 50% of the women. Hot flushes occur more frequently at night, causing sweating and insomnia that result in fatigue on the following day.

3. Genitourinary syndrome of menopause (GSM)—Decreased estrogen secretion results in less vaginal lubrication and vulvovaginal atrophy with dryness, dyspareunia, burning, and pruritus. Estrogen deficiency also causes urinary frequency, urgency, dysuria, and an increased risk of UTIs. GSM does not improve over time, in contrast to hot flushes. Pelvic examination reveals pale, smooth vaginal mucosa and a small cervix and uterus. The ovaries are not normally palpable after menopause.

4. Other menopausal manifestations—Over 60% of women experience cognitive problems, particularly during the menopausal transition. There is an increased incidence of sleep disturbance and mood changes. Postmenopausal osteoporosis presents later in menopause with fragility fractures of long bones and vertebrae.

B. Laboratory Findings

No laboratory testing is required to diagnose normal menopause when amenorrhea occurs at the expected age. The expected age of menopause correlates with a woman's mother's age at menopause and varies among different kindreds and ethnic groups. An elevated serum FSH with a low or low-normal serum estradiol helps confirm the diagnosis..

Treatment

A. Non-Estrogen Treatments

Women with night sweats should sleep in a cool room and avoid the use of down comforters. Eliminating triggers for hot flushes, such as smoking, alcohol, caffeine, and hot spicy foods, may be helpful. Slow, deep breathing can ameliorate hot flushes. **Aerobic training** for 50 minutes four times weekly reduced all menopausal symptoms except vaginal dryness in a randomized controlled trial. **Clinical hypnosis** reduced hot flushes over 12 weeks in one study. Acupuncture may help alleviate symptoms in some women. Vaginal lubricants can be used daily or 2 hours before intercourse.

For women with severe hot flushes who cannot take estrogen, SSRIs may offer modest relief effective within a week; escitalopram (10–20 mg orally daily) or paroxetine

(7.5 mg orally daily) can reduce hot flushes significantly, but they must not be used by women taking tamoxifen because SSRIs inhibit the conversion of tamoxifen to its active metabolite. Venlafaxine extended release (75 mg orally daily) may also be effective and does not have a drug interaction with tamoxifen. Sexual dysfunction has not been as significant with the latter drugs when used for vasomotor symptoms, compared to their use for depression. Gabapentin is also effective in oral doses titrated up to 200–800 mg every 8 hours. Side effects such as drowsiness, dizziness, and headache, which are most pronounced during the first 2 weeks of therapy, often improve within 4 weeks. An herb, black cohosh, may possibly relieve hot flushes. Tamoxifen and raloxifene offer bone protection but aggravate hot flushes. Women with low serum testosterone levels may experience hypoactive sexual desire disorder that may respond to low-dose testosterone replacement.

B. Estrogen Replacement Therapy—Benefits

Estrogen replacement therapy (ERT) improves overall survival for women who begin ERT before age 60 or within 10 years of menopause. In the California Teachers Study, ERT in such women was associated with a dramatic 46% reduction in all-cause mortality, particularly CVD. Also, a 20-year study of 8801 women living in a retirement community found that ERT was associated with improved survival. Age-adjusted mortality rates were 56.4 (per 1000 person-years) among nonusers and 50.4 among women who had used estrogen for 15 years or longer. The reduction in CVD among younger postmenopausal women taking ERT may be explained by the reduction in serum levels of atherogenic lipoprotein(a) with ERT, with or without a progestin. Improvement in serum HDL cholesterol is greatest with unopposed estrogen but is also seen with the addition of a progestin. The survival advantage diminishes with age; no reduction in mortality was noted in the group of women aged 85–94 years. Nevertheless, other benefits can be reasons to continue ERT beyond the first 10 years of menopause.

Other benefits of even low-dose ERT include the improvement in hot flushes and the prevention of postmenopausal osteoporosis and a 33% reduction in hip fractures. The WHI study found that women who received ERT experienced six fewer fractures/year per 10,000 women compared with placebo. ERT improves vaginal moisture and enhances libido is in some women. ERT may also improve sleep disturbances and mild cognitive dysfunction, which are common menopausal symptoms. Unopposed estrogen improves perimenopause-related depression, but the addition of a progestin may negate this effect. Estrogen replacement may also help the joint pains, generalized body pain, and reduced physical function experienced by some women at the time of menopause. ERT also increases facial skin moisture and thickness and reduces seborrhea but does not prevent skin wrinkling.

Low-dose estrogen alone appears to have a negligible effect on breast cancer risk, with studies variably finding a decreased risk (Women's Health Initiative, WHI) or an increased risk of breast cancer (California Teachers Study). However, combined daily estrogen and progestin increases the long-term risk for breast cancer. Transdermal estradiol replacement does not increase the risk of thromboembolic disease or stroke, whereas oral estrogens increase such risk.

In light of these considerations, estrogen replacement is most commonly prescribed for women who are younger than age 60 years and within the first 5–10 years of menopause, when symptoms are worst and the benefits are greatest. Transdermal estrogen is favored over oral therapy to reduce the risk of thromboembolism. In women with an intact uterus, estrogen replacement without a progestin risks endometrial hypertrophy and dysfunctional uterine bleeding. The addition of a progestin, however, increases the risk of breast cancer. Therefore, only the smallest effective dose of estrogen should be used to avoid the need for progestins or use them in lower doses or intermittently. Also, progestin may be delivered directly to the uterus with progesterone-eluting intrauterine devices. The prescription of estrogen replacement to women up to 65 years of age is generally accepted. The American College of Obstetricians and Gynecologists and the North American Menopause Society have recommended that the decision to continue estrogen replacement past aged 65 should include an assessment of risks and benefits, particularly including relief from hot flushes, prevention of osteoporosis, and improved sense of well-being.

C. Estrogen Replacement Therapy—Risks

Oral ERT increases the risk of arterial and venous thrombotic events in a dose-dependent manner, although the absolute risk is small. The WHI study found that women who received long-term conventional oral combined HRT had an increased risk of DVT (3.5 per 1000 person-years) compared with women receiving placebo (1.7 per 1000 person-years). Oral estrogen also increases the risk of ischemic stroke by about 30%. Oral estrogen causes a particularly increased risk for thromboembolic disease among older women and those with increased stroke proclivity (current smokers and those with hypertension, atrial fibrillation, prior thromboembolic event). Long-term use of oral conjugated estrogens in women over age 65 has been associated with poorer cognitive performance, perhaps due to small strokes. Transdermal or vaginal estrogen administration avoids this risk. Urinary stress incontinence appears to be increased by conventional-dose oral estrogen replacement, whereas topical vaginal estrogen may have a beneficial effect. Estrogen replacement may cause mastalgia that typically responds to dose reduction. Estrogen replacement also appears to increase the risk of seizures in women with epilepsy. ERT can stimulate the growth of untreated large pituitary prolactinomas. Oral estrogens and SERMs also increase the risk of GERD. Oral ERT can increase the size of hepatic hemangiomas, but significant enlargement is uncommon. Conventional doses of ERT carry higher risks than lower doses. The risks for ERT also depend on whether estrogen is administered alone (unopposed ERT) or with a progestin (combined ERT).

1. Risks of ERT without progestin (unopposed ERT)—The California Teachers Study reported an *increased breast* *cancer risk* among such women while the WHI study reported that postmenopausal women taking unopposed estrogen had a *reduced breast cancer risk.* Women taking lower-dose unopposed estrogen therapy are expected to have a lower long-term risk of breast cancer compared to women taking high-dose estrogens.

Conventional-dose unopposed conjugated estrogen replacement (0.625–1.25 mg daily) increases the risk of endometrial hyperplasia and dysfunctional uterine bleeding, which often prompts patients to stop the estrogen. However, lower-dose unopposed estrogen confers a much lower risk of dysfunctional uterine bleeding. Recurrent dysfunctional bleeding necessitates a pelvic examination and possibly an endometrial biopsy. There has been considerable concern that unopposed estrogen replacement might increase the risk for endometrial carcinoma. However, a Cochrane Database Review found no increased risk of endometrial carcinoma in a review of 30 randomized controlled trials. Therefore, lower-dose unopposed estrogen replacement does not appear to confer any significant increased risk for endometrial cancer.

The risk of stroke among women taking a conventional dose of unopposed estrogen is increased; the risk is about 44 strokes per 10,000 person-years versus about 32 per 10,000 person-years in women taking placebo. However, transdermal or transvaginal ERT does not appear to increase the risk of stroke.

Oral estrogens can cause hypertriglyceridemia, particularly in women with preexistent hyperlipidemia, rarely resulting in pancreatitis. Postmenopausal estrogen therapy also slightly increases the risk of gallstones and cholecystitis. These side effects may be reduced or avoided by using transdermal or vaginal estrogen replacement.

2. Risks of ERT with a progestin (combined ERT)—Long-term conventional-dose oral combined HRT increases breast density and the risk for abnormal mammograms (9.4% versus 5.4% for placebo). There is also a higher risk of breast cancer (8 cases per 10,000 women/year versus 6.5 cases per 10,000 women/year for placebo). The implicated progestins have been medroxyprogesterone acetate and norethisterone, so prescribing has shifted to bio-identical progesterone. The increased risk of breast cancer is highest shortly after menopause (about 2 cases per 1000 women annually). This increased risk for breast cancer appears to mostly affect relatively thin women with a BMI less than 24.4. The Iowa Women's Health Study reported an increase in breast cancer with HRT only in women consuming more than 1 oz of alcohol weekly. No accelerated risk of breast cancer has been seen in users of HRT who have benign breast disease or a family history of breast cancer. Women in whom new-onset breast tenderness develops with combined HRT have an increased risk of breast cancer, compared with women without breast tenderness. Women receiving combined HRT experience no increased overall mortality and no increased overall or specific cancer mortality.

The Women's Health Initiative Mental Study (WHIMS) followed the effect of combined conventional-dose oral HRT on cognitive function in women 65–79 years old. HRT did not protect these older women from cognitive decline. In fact, they experienced an increased risk for severe dementia at a rate of 23 more cases/year for every 10,000 women over age 65 years. It is unknown whether this finding applies to younger postmenopausal women.

In the WHI study, women receiving conventional-dose combined oral HRT experienced an increased risk of stroke (31 strokes per 10,000 women/year versus 26 strokes per 10,000 women/year for placebo). Stroke risk was also increased by hypertension, diabetes, and smoking.

Women taking combined oral estrogen–progestin replacement do not experience an increased risk of ovarian cancer. They do experience a slightly increased risk of developing asthma.

Progestins may cause moodiness, particularly in women with a history of premenstrual dysphoric disorder. Cycled progestins may trigger migraines in certain women. Many other adverse reactions have been reported, including breast tenderness, alopecia, and fluid retention. Contraindications to the use of progestins include thromboembolic disorders, liver disease, breast cancer, and pregnancy.

D. Hormone Replacement Therapy Agents

Hormone replacement needs to be individualized. Ideally, in women with an intact uterus, very low-dose transdermal estradiol may be used alone or with intermittent progestin or a progesterone-eluting intrauterine device to reduce the risk of endometrial hyperplasia, while avoiding the need for daily oral progestin. Vaginal estrogen can be added if low-dose systemic estradiol replacement is insufficient to relieve symptoms of vulvovaginal atrophy. Women who have had a hysterectomy may receive transdermal estrogen at whatever is the lowest dose that adequately relieves symptoms. However, some women cannot find sufficient relief with transdermal estradiol and must use an oral preparation.

1. Transdermal estradiol—Estradiol can be delivered systemically with different systems of skin patches, mists, or gels. Transdermal estradiol works for most women, but some women have poor transdermal absorption. If a woman has a skin reaction to an estradiol patch, then a gel or mist may be tried at different doses until the ideal formulation is found.

A. Estradiol patches mixed with adhesive—These systems tend to cause minimal skin irritation. Generic estradiol transdermal is available as a patch that is replaced biweekly (0.025, 0.0375, 0.05, 0.075, or 0.1 mg/day) or weekly (0.025, 0.0375, 0.05, 0.06, 0.075, or 0.1 mg/day). Brand products include: Vivelle-Dot (0.025 mg/day) or Minivivelle (0.0375, 0.05, 0.075, or 0.1 mg/day) or Alora (0.025, 0.05, 0.075, or 0.1 mg/day), replaced twice weekly; Climara (0.025, 0.0375, 0.05, 0.06, 0.075, or 0.1 mg/day), replaced weekly; and Menostar (0.014 mg/day), replaced weekly. This type of estradiol skin patch can be cut in half and applied to the skin without proportionately greater loss of potency. Minivivelle patches are the smallest.

B. Estradiol mists, gels, and lotion—Evamist is a topical mist dispenser that dispenses 1.53 mg estradiol/spray;

1–3 sprays are applied to the inner forearm daily; a single daily spray may provide sufficiently low-dose estradiol to possibly obviate the need for daily progestin in women with an intact uterus. EstroGel 0.06% in a metered-dose pump dispenses 0.75 mg estradiol per actuation (dose: half to 2 actuations/day). Elestrin 0.06% in a metered-dose pump dispenses 0.52 mg estradiol per activation (dose: half to 2 actuations/day). These gels are applied daily to one arm from the wrist to the shoulder after bathing. Divigel 0.1% gel (0.25, 0.5, 0.75 1 g/packet) is applied to the upper-inner thigh or inner arm daily. Estrasorb 2.5% is available in 1.74-g pouches (4.35 mg estradiol); 1–2 pouches of lotion are applied to the thigh/calf daily. To avoid spreading topical estradiol to others, the hands should be washed and precautions taken to avoid prolonged skin contact with children. Application of sunscreen prior to estradiol gel has been reported to *increase* the transdermal absorption of estradiol.

C. Estradiol patches with progestin mixed with adhesive—These preparations mix estradiol with either norethindrone acetate or levonorgestrel. Combipatch (0.05 mg E with 0.14 mg norethindrone acetate daily or 0.05 mg E with 0.25 mg norethindrone acetate daily) is replaced twice weekly. Climara Pro (0.045 mg E with 0.015 mg levonorgestrel daily) is replaced once weekly. The addition of a progestin reduces the risk of endometrial hyperplasia, but breakthrough bleeding occurs commonly. The combined patch increases the risk of breast cancer. Scalp hair loss, acne, weight gain, skin reactions, and poor skin adherence have been reported with these patches.

2. Oral estrogen—

A. Oral estrogen-only preparations—These preparations include conjugated equine estrogens that are available as Premarin (0.3, 0.45, 0.625, 0.9, and 1.25 mg), conjugated plant-derived estrogens (eg, Menest, 0.3, 0.625, and 2.5 mg), and conjugated synthetic estrogens (Cenestin: 0.3, 0.45, 0.625, 0.9, and 1.25 mg; and Enjuvia: 0.3, 0.45, 0.625, 0.9, and 1.25 mg). Other preparations include estradiol (0.5, 1, and 2 mg) and estropipate (0.75, 1.5, and 3 mg).

B. Oral estrogen plus progestin preparations—Conjugated equine estrogens with medroxyprogesterone acetate are available as Prempro (0.3/1.5, 0.45/1.5, 0.625/2.5, and 0.625 mg/5 mg); conjugated equine estrogens for 14 days cycled with conjugated equine estrogens plus medroxyprogesterone acetate for 14 days are available as Premphase (0.625/0, then 0.625 mg/5 mg); estradiol with norethindrone acetate (0.5/0.1 and 1 mg/0.5 mg); ethinyl estradiol with norethindrone acetate is available as Femhrt (2.5/0.5 and 5 mcg/1 mg) and Jinteli (5 mcg/1 mg); estradiol with drospirenone is available as Angeliq (0.5/0.25, and 1.0 mg/0.5 mg); estradiol with norgestimate is available as Prefest (estradiol 1 mg/day for 3 days, alternating with 1 mg estradiol/0.09 mg norgestimate daily for 3 days); estradiol with progesterone is available as Bijuva (1 mg/100 mg) capsules. Oral contraceptives can also be used for combined HRT.

3. Vaginal estrogen—Vaginal estrogen is intended to deliver estrogen directly to local tissues and is moderately effective in reducing symptoms of urogenital atrophy, while minimizing systemic estrogen exposure. Some estrogen is absorbed systemically and can relieve menopausal symptoms. Vaginal estrogen can be used without a break at low doses or in women who have had a hysterectomy. To reduce the risk of endometrial proliferation and dysfunctional bleeding, manufacturers recommend that these preparations be used for only 3–6 months and for only 3 out of every 4 weeks in women with an intact uterus, since vaginal estrogen can cause endometrial proliferation. However, most clinicians use them for longer periods and without cycling. Vaginal estrogen can be administered in three different ways: creams, tablets, and rings.

A. Estrogen vaginal creams—These creams are administered intravaginally with a measured-dose applicator daily for 2 weeks for atrophic vaginitis, then administered one to three times weekly. *Conjugated equine estrogens* are available as Premarin Vaginal (0.625 mg/g cream), dosed as 0.25–2 g cream administered vaginally one to three times weekly. *Estradiol* is available as Estrace Vaginal (0.1 mg/g cream), 1 g cream administered vaginally one to two times weekly.

B. Estradiol vaginal tablets and softgel inserts—*Vagifem and Yuvafem* (generic equivalent) are available as 10 mcg tablets. *Imvexxy* is a softgel vaginal insert (4 mcg or 10 mcg estradiol in a coconut oil base). Either preparation can be administered intravaginally daily for 2 weeks for atrophic vaginitis, then twice weekly. Prasterone (Intrarosa) is available as a 6.5 mg vaginal insert that is used daily. Vaginal preparations are usually inserted at bedtime.

C. Estradiol vaginal rings—These rings are inserted manually into the upper third of the vagina, worn continuously, and replaced every 3 months. Only a small amount of the released estradiol enters the systemic circulation. Vaginal rings do not usually interfere with sexual intercourse. If a ring is removed or descends into the introitus, it may be washed in warm water and reinserted. Estring (2 mg estradiol/ring) releases 17-beta-estradiol 7.5 mcg/day with only 8% entering the systemic circulation, resulting in mean serum estradiol concentrations of only about 10 pg/mL; it is most effective for local vaginal symptoms. Femring releases estradiol acetate that is quickly hydrolyzed to estradiol and is available in two strengths: 12.4 mg/ring releases estradiol acetate 0.05 mg/day or 24.8 mg/ring releases estradiol acetate 0.1 mg/day, resulting in mean serum estradiol concentrations of about 40 pg/mL and 80 pg/mL, respectively; it is effective for both systemic and local vaginal symptoms. Both rings are replaced every 90 days. For women with postmenopausal urinary urgency and frequency, even the low-dose Estring can successfully reduce urinary symptoms and vaginal dryness.

D. Estradiol with progestin vaginal rings—Nuva Ring releases a mixture of ethinyl estradiol 0.015 mg/day and etonogestrel 0.12 mg/day. It is a contraceptive vaginal ring that is placed in the vagina on or before day 5 of the menstrual cycle, left for 3 weeks, removed for 1 week, and then replaced.

4. Estradiol injections—Parenteral estradiol should be used only for particularly severe menopausal symptoms when other measures have failed or are contraindicated. Estradiol cypionate (Depo-Estradiol 5 mg/mL) may be administered intramuscularly in doses of 1–5 mg every 3–4 weeks. Estradiol valerate (20 or 40 mg/mL) may be administered intramuscularly in doses of 10–20 mg every 4 weeks. Women with an intact uterus should receive progestin for the last 10 days of each cycle.

5. Oral progestins—For a woman with an intact uterus, long-term conventional-dose unopposed systemic estrogen therapy can cause endometrial hyperplasia, which typically results in dysfunctional uterine bleeding and might rarely lead to endometrial cancer. Progestin therapy transforms proliferative into secretory endometrium, causing a possible menses when given intermittently or no bleeding when given continuously.

The type of progestin preparation, its dosage, and the timing of administration may be tailored to the given situation. Progestins may be given daily, monthly, or at longer intervals. When given episodically, progestins are usually administered for 7- to 14-day periods. Bedtime administration may improve sleep. Some women find that progestins produce adverse effects, such as irritability, nausea, fatigue, or headache; long-term progestins given with estrogen replacement increase the risk for breast cancer.

Oral progestins are available in different formulations: Micronized progesterone (100 mg and 200 mg/capsule) may carry a reduced risk of breast cancer, vascular thromboembolism, and reduced adverse effects on mood and lipid levels compared to other progestins, according to observational studies. Other progestins include medroxyprogesterone (2.5, 5.0, and 10 mg/tablet), norethindrone acetate (5 mg/tablet), and norethindrone (0.35 mg/tablet). Topical progesterone (20–50 mg/day) may reduce hot flushes in women who are intolerant to oral HRT. It may be applied to the upper arms, thighs, or inner wrists daily. It may be compounded as micronized progesterone 250 mg/mL in a transdermal gel. Its effects upon the breast and endometrium are unknown. Progesterone is also available as vaginal gels (eg, Prochieve, 4% = 45 mg/applicatorful, and 8% = 90 mg/applicatorful) that are typically given for secondary amenorrhea and administered vaginally every other day for six doses.

6. Vaginal progesterone—Vaginal progesterone minimizes dysfunctional uterine bleeding while reducing systemic progesterone exposure. Crinone and Prochieve contain 4% and 8% gel with 45 mg and 90 mg per applicatorful, respectively. Endometrin comes as a 100 mg vaginal insert. Administered twice weekly with daily estrogen, most women experience no endometrial hypertrophy or dysfunctional uterine bleeding.

7. Progestin-releasing intrauterine devices—Intrauterine devices that release progestins can be useful for women receiving ERT, since they can reduce the incidence of dysfunctional uterine bleeding and endometrial carcinoma without exposing women to the significant risks of systemic progestins. The Mirena intrauterine device releases levonorgestrel and is inserted into the uterus by a clinician within 7 days of the onset of menses. It is equally effective at reducing endometrial hyperplasia as cycled medroxyprogesterone acetate and is associated with less hirsutism. It remains effective for up to 5 years. Parous women are generally better able to tolerate the Mirena intrauterine device than nulliparous women.

8. Selective estrogen receptor modulators—SERMs (eg, raloxifene, ospemifene, tamoxifen) are an alternative to estrogen replacement for hypogonadal women at risk for osteoporosis who prefer not to take estrogens because of their contraindications (eg, breast or uterine cancer) or side effects (see Osteoporosis, above). Raloxifene (Evista) does not reduce hot flushes, vaginal dryness, skin wrinkling, or breast atrophy; it does not improve cognition. However, in doses of 60 mg/day orally, it inhibits bone loss without stimulating effects upon the breasts. In fact, it reduces the risk of invasive breast cancer by about 50%. Raloxifene does not stimulate the endometrium and actually reduces the risk of endometrial carcinoma, so concomitant progesterone therapy is not required. Raloxifene slightly increases the risk of venous thromboembolism (though less so than tamoxifen), so it should not be used by women at prolonged bed rest or otherwise prone to thrombosis. Ospemifene (Osphena) is a SERM that has unique estrogen-like effects on the vaginal epithelium and is indicated for the treatment of postmenopausal dyspareunia when other therapies are ineffective. Given orally in doses of 60 mg/day, it commonly aggravates hot flushes but has an estrogenic effect upon bone and slows bone loss in menopause. It does not usually cause endometrial hypertrophy. Ospemifene has unknown long-term effects upon the breast.

9. Androgen replacement therapy in women—In premenopausal women, serum testosterone levels decline with age. Between 25 and 45 years of age, women's testosterone levels fall 50%. After natural menopause, the ovaries remain a significant source for testosterone and serum testosterone levels do not fall abruptly. In contrast, very low serum testosterone levels are found in women after bilateral oophorectomy, autoimmune ovarian failure, or adrenalectomy, and in hypopituitarism. Testosterone deficiency contributes to hot flushes, loss of sexual hair, muscle atrophy, osteoporosis, and diminished libido, also known as hypoactive sexual desire disorder (see Chapter 25). Selected women may be treated with low-dose testosterone that result in physiologic premenopausal serum testosterone levels. In women with hypoactive sexual desire disorder, low-dose testosterone therapy improves libido, sexual responsiveness, and orgasmic function. Methyltestosterone can be compounded into capsules and taken orally in doses of 1.25–2.5 mg daily. Testosterone can also be compounded as a cream containing 1 mg/mL, with 1 mL applied to the abdomen daily. Methyltestosterone also is available combined with esterified estrogens: 1.25 mg methyltestosterone/0.626 mg esterified estrogens or 2.5 mg methyltestosterone/1.25 mg esterified estrogens. The latter formulations are convenient but carry the same disadvantages as oral estrogen—particularly an increased risk of thromboembolism.

Side effects of low-dose testosterone therapy are usually minimal but may include erythrocytosis, emotional changes, hirsutism, acne, an adverse effect on lipids, and potentiation of warfarin anticoagulation therapy. Low-dose testosterone therapy tends to reduce both triglyceride and HDL cholesterol levels. Hepatocellular neoplasms and peliosis hepatis, rare complications of oral androgens at higher doses, have not been reported with oral methyltestosterone doses of 2.5 mg or less daily.

Vaginal androgen is an option for postmenopausal women who are experiencing vaginal dryness and reduced sexual satisfaction. It is also an option for women who cannot use systemic or vaginal estrogen due to breast cancer. Testosterone cream 150–300 mcg (formulated) is administered vaginally daily for 2 weeks and then three times weekly. It improves sexual satisfaction while reducing vaginal dryness and dyspareunia without increasing systemic estrogen or testosterone levels. Prasterone 0.5% vaginal (Intrarosa), a formulation of DHEA, is available as a 6.5 mg tablet that is inserted vaginally nightly at bedtime. It is indicated for relief of moderate to severe dyspareunia of menopause. However, it is contraindicated in women with breast cancer.

Caution: *Androgens should not be given to women with liver disease or during pregnancy or breastfeeding.* Testosterone replacement therapy for women should be used judiciously, since long-term prospective clinical trials are lacking. An analysis of the Nurses' Health Study found that women who had been taking conjugated equine estrogens plus methyltestosterone experienced an increased risk of breast cancer, so breast cancer screening is recommended.

E. Surgical Menopause

The abrupt hormonal decrease resulting from bilateral oophorectomy generally results in severe vasomotor symptoms and rapid onset of dyspareunia and osteoporosis unless treated. If not contraindicated, estrogen replacement is generally started immediately after surgery. Either transdermal estradiol or an oral estrogen may be used. (See above.) No progestin is required in women who have had a hysterectomy.

Anagostis P et al. Menopause symptom management in women with dyslipidemias: an EMAS clinical guide. Maturitas. 2020;135:82. [PMID: 32209279]

Chlebowski RT et al. Association of menopausal hormone therapy with breast cancer incidence and mortality during long-term follow-up of the Women's Health Initiative randomized controlled clinical trials. JAMA. 2020;324:369. [PMID: 32721007]

Davis SR et al. Global consensus position statement on the use of testosterone therapy for women. J Clin Endocrinol Metab. 2019;104:4660. [PMID: 31498871]

Greendale GA et al. The menopause transition and cognition. JAMA. 2020;325:149. [PMID: 32163094]

Kingsberg SA et al. Clinical effects of early or surgical menopause. Obstet Gynecol. 2020;135:853. [PMID: 32168205]

Pinkerton JV. Hormone therapy for postmenopausal women. N Engl J Med. 2020;382:446. [PMID: 31995690]

TURNER SYNDROME (Gonadal Dysgenesis)

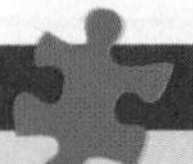

ESSENTIALS OF DIAGNOSIS

- Short stature with normal GH levels.
- Primary amenorrhea or early ovarian failure.
- Epicanthal folds, webbed neck, short fourth metacarpals.
- Renal and cardiovascular anomalies.

Turner syndrome comprises a group of X chromosome disorders that are associated with spontaneous abortion, primary hypogonadism, short stature, and other phenotypic anomalies (Table 26–16). It affects 1–2% of fetuses, of which about 97% abort, accounting for about 10% of all spontaneous abortions. Nevertheless, it affects about 1 in every 2500 live female births. Patients with the classic syndrome (about 50% of cases) lack one of the two X chromosomes (45,XO karyotype). About 12% of patients harbor mosaicism for Y chromosome sequences. Other patients with Turner syndrome have X chromosome abnormalities, such as ring X or Xq (X/abnormal X) or X chromosome deletions affecting all or some somatic cells (mosaicism, XX/XO).

1. Classic Turner Syndrome (45,XO Gonadal Dysgenesis)

Clinical Findings

A. Symptoms and Signs

Features of Turner syndrome are variable and may be subtle in girls with mosaicism. Turner syndrome may be diagnosed in infant girls at birth, since they tend to be small and may exhibit severe lymphedema. Evaluation for childhood short stature often leads to the diagnosis. Girls and women with Turner syndrome have an increased risk of aortic coarctation and bicuspid aortic valves; these cardiac abnormalities are more common in patients with a webbed neck. Typical manifestations in adulthood include short stature, hypogonadism, webbed neck, high-arched palate, wide-spaced nipples, hypertension, and kidney abnormalities (Table 26–16). Emotional disorders are common. Affected women are also more prone to autoimmune disease, particularly thyroiditis, IBD, and celiac disease.

Hypogonadism presents as "delayed adolescence" (primary amenorrhea, 80%) or early ovarian failure (20%); girls with 45,XO Turner (blood karyotyping) who enter puberty are typically found to have mosaicism if other tissues are karyotyped.

B. Laboratory Findings

Hypogonadism is confirmed in girls who have high serum levels of FSH and LH. A blood karyotype showing 45,XO (or X chromosome abnormalities or mosaicism) establishes the diagnosis. GH and IGF-1 levels are normal.

Table 26–16. Manifestations of Turner syndrome.

Affected Systems	Symptom, Sign, or Condition
Head and neck features	High-arched palate (35%) Low posterior hairline (40%) Micrognathia (60%) Pterygium colli (webbed neck 40%)
Eye abnormalities	Cataracts, corneal opacities Epicanthal folds (20%) Strabismus (15%) Ptosis (10%)
Ear abnormalities	Conductive hearing loss (30%) and recurrent otitis media (60%) Low-set and posteriorly rotated ears
Cardiovascular anomalies	Aortic dilation or aneurysm (25% with bicuspid aortic valve) Bicuspid aortic valve (30%) with aortic stenosis or regurgitation Coarctation (14%) and cystic medial necrosis of aorta Hypertension (50%, idiopathic or due to coarctation or kidney disease) Partial anomalous pulmonary venous return (18%)
GI disorders	Achlorhydria Celiac disease (8%) Colon carcinoma Hepatic transaminases, elevated (65%) IBD (3%) Telangiectasias with bleeding
Kidney abnormalities (60%)	Horseshoe kidney (10%), duplication or abnormal positioning of renal pelvis or ureters (15%)
Gonadal abnormalities	Gonadal dysgenesis (primary amenorrhea 80%) or early ovarian failure (20%)
Skeletal and extremity abnormalities	Short stature (98%) Broad (shield) chest (30%) with wide-spaced hypoplastic nipples Cubitus valgus of arms (50%) and knock knees (35%) Lymphedema of hands and feet (30%) Madelung wrist deformity (5%) Osteopenia (65%) Scoliosis (10%) Short fourth metacarpals (40%)
CNS disorders	Emotional immaturity (40%) Learning disabilities and ADHD (40%) Sensorineural hearing loss
Skin and nail disorders	Hyperconvex nails Keloid formation Pigmented nevi
Associated conditions	Autoimmune (Hashimoto) thyroiditis (37%) Diabetes mellitus (10%) or glucose intolerance (35%) Dyslipidemia Hyperuricemia Neuroblastoma (1%) Obesity Rheumatoid arthritis

ADHD, attention-deficit/hyperactivity disorder.

C. Imaging

A transthoracic ultrasound and MRI scan of the chest and abdomen should be done in all patients with Turner syndrome to determine whether cardiac, aortic, and renal abnormalities are present.

▶ Treatment

For short stature, GH therapy should be started early, ideally by age 4–6 and before age 12 years. GH is given subcutaneously in doses of 50 mcg/kg/day or 4.5 IU/m^2/day; the GH dose is titrated to keep the serum IGF-I levels within 3 SD above the mean for age. Rarely, GH treatment causes pseudotumor cerebri. The oral androgen oxandrolone (0.03–0.05 mg/kg/day) is added after age 10 for girls whose growth is inadequate with GH therapy alone. After age 12 years, estrogen therapy is begun with low doses of transdermal estradiol, with a gradual increase in dose over 2–3 years. Progesterone is added after 2 years of estrogen therapy or if menstrual bleeding occurs.

Complications & Surveillance

Women with Turner syndrome have a reduced life expectancy due in part to their increased risk of diabetes mellitus (types 1 and 2), hypertension, dyslipidemia, and osteoporosis. Annual surveillance should include a blood pressure determination and laboratory evaluations that include a serum TSH, liver enzymes, BUN, creatinine, and fasting serum lipids and glucose. Celiac disease screening (serum TTG IgA Ab) is warranted every 2–5 years for school-age girls and then whenever indicated clinically. Audiology exams are recommended every 1–5 years. Bone mineral densitometries should be measured periodically for women over age 18 years.

Bicuspid aortic valves are common and are associated with an increased risk of infective endocarditis, aortic valvular stenosis or regurgitation, and ascending aortic root dilation and dissection. The risk of aortic dissection is increased more than 100-fold in women with Turner syndrome, particularly those with pronounced neck webbing and shield chest. Patients with aortic root enlargement are usually treated with beta-blockade and serial imaging.

Partial anomalous pulmonary vein connections can lead to left-to-right shunting of blood. Adults with Turner syndrome also have a high incidence of ECG abnormalities, such as long QT syndrome.

Patients with the classic 45,XO karyotype have a high risk of renal structural abnormalities, whereas those with 46,X/abnormal X are more prone to malformations of the urinary collecting system.

2. Turner Syndrome Variants

A. 46,X (Abnormal X) Karyotype

Patients with small distal short arm deletions of the X chromosome (Xp-) that include the *SHOX* gene often have short stature and skeletal abnormalities but have a low risk of ovarian failure. Patients with deletions of the long arm of the X chromosome (distal to Xq24) often have amenorrhea without short stature or other features of Turner syndrome. Abnormalities or deletions of other genes located on both the long and short arms of the X chromosome can produce gonadal dysgenesis with few other somatic features.

B. 45,XO/46,XX and 45,XO/46,XY Mosaicism

45,XO/46,XX mosaicism results in a modified form of Turner syndrome. Such girls tend to be taller and may have more gonadal function and fewer other manifestations of Turner syndrome.

45,XO/46,XY mosaicism can produce some manifestations of Turner syndrome. Patients may have ambiguous genitalia or male infertility with an otherwise normal phenotype. Germ cell tumors, such as gonadoblastomas and seminomas, develop in about 10% of patients with 45,XO/46,XY mosaicism; most such tumors are benign.

Kruszka P et al. Turner syndrome in diverse populations. Am J Med Genet A. 2020;182:303. [PMID: 31854143]

CLINICAL USE OF CORTICOSTEROIDS

Prolonged treatment with high-dose corticosteroids causes toxic effects that can be life threatening. Besides oral and parenteral administration, transdermal and inhaled corticosteroids have some systemic absorption and can cause similar adverse effects. Patients should be thoroughly informed of the major possible side effects of treatment: insomnia, cognitive and personality changes, weight gain with central obesity, skin thinning and bruising, striae, muscle weakness, polyuria, renal calculi, diabetes mellitus, glaucoma, cataracts, sex hormone suppression, candidiasis, and opportunistic infections (Table 26–17). Prolonged high-dose corticosteroids also increase the risk of hypertension, dyslipidemia, MI, stroke, atrial fibrillation or flutter, and heart failure. Gastric ulceration is more common with high-dose corticosteroids, particularly when patients take NSAIDs concurrently. High-dose inhaled corticosteroids predispose to oral thrush and pulmonary nontuberculous mycobacterial infection. To reduce risks, the dosage and duration of corticosteroid administration must be minimized. Immediately following inhaled corticosteroids, proper mouth-washing and gargling can reduce systemic absorption.

Prolonged oral, inhaled, intravenous, or high-dose topical corticosteroid therapy commonly suppresses pituitary ACTH secretion, causing secondary adrenal insufficiency. Adrenal crisis occurs in 5–10% of such patients yearly with an estimated 6% associated mortality.

Most corticosteroids (dexamethasone, prednisone, hydrocortisone, deflazacort, budesonide) are metabolized by the enzyme CYP34A. When drugs that inhibit CYP34A are administered along with even modest doses of corticosteroids (oral, inhaled, intravenous), the blood levels of the corticosteroids rise and can cause iatrogenic Cushing syndrome and secondary adrenal insufficiency. Medications that strongly inhibit CYP34A include itraconazole, ketoconazole, nefazodone, protease inhibitors and cobicistat.

In pregnancy, corticosteroids taken by the mother are transmitted across the placenta to the fetus, causing adverse effects on fetal growth and development as well as childhood cognition and behavior. Therefore, women who are to receive high-dose corticosteroids should be screened for pregnancy and counseled to use contraception.

Osteoporotic fractures (especially vertebral) ultimately occur in about 40% of patients receiving long-term corticosteroid therapy. Osteoporotic fractures can occur even in patients receiving long-term corticosteroid therapy at relatively low doses (eg, 5–7.5 mg prednisone daily). The risk of vertebral fractures increases 14-fold and the risk of hip fractures increases 3-fold. Patients at increased risk for corticosteroid osteoporotic fractures include those who are over age 60 or who have a low BMI, pretreatment osteoporosis, a family history of osteoporosis, or concurrent disease that limits mobility. Avascular necrosis of bone (especially hips) develops in about 15% of patients who receive corticosteroids at high doses (eg, prednisone 15 mg daily or more) for more than 1 month with cumulative prednisone doses of 10 g or more.

Table 26–17. Management of patients receiving systemic corticosteroids.

Recommendations for prescribing
- Do not administer systemic corticosteroids unless absolutely indicated or more conservative measures have failed.
- Keep dosage and duration of administration to the minimum required for adequate treatment.

Monitoring recommendations
- Screen for tuberculosis with a purified protein derivative (PPD) test or interferon gamma release assay before commencing long-term corticosteroid therapy.
- Screen for pregnancy in reproductive age women; recommend contraceptive measures.
- Screen for diabetes mellitus before treatment and then every 3–4 months.
- Screen for hypertension before treatment and every 3–4 months.
- Screen for glaucoma and cataracts before treatment, 3 months after treatment inception, and then at least yearly.
- Monitor plasma potassium for hypokalemia and treat as indicated.
- Obtain bone densitometry before treatment and then periodically. Treat osteoporosis.
- Weigh daily. Use dietary measures to avoid obesity and optimize nutrition.
- Measure height frequently and obtain bone densitometry by DXA every 1–2 years to document the degree of axial spine demineralization and compression.
- Watch for fungal or yeast infections of skin, nails, mouth, vagina, and rectum, and treat appropriately.
- With dosage reduction, watch for signs of adrenal insufficiency or corticosteroid withdrawal syndrome.

Patient information
- Prepare the patient and family for possible adverse effects on mood, memory, and cognitive function.
- Teach the patient about the symptoms of hyperglycemia.
- Inform the patient about other possible side effects, particularly weight gain, osteoporosis, and aseptic necrosis of bone.
- Counsel to avoid smoking and excessive ethanol consumption.

Prophylactic measures
- Institute a vigorous physical exercise and isometric regimen tailored to each patient's abilities or disabilities.
- Administer calcium (1 g elemental calcium) and vitamin D_3, 400–800 units orally daily.
  –Check spot morning urine for calcium; alter dosage to keep urine calcium concentration < 30 mg/dL (< 7.5 mmol/L).
  –If the patient is receiving thiazide diuretics, check for hypercalcemia, and administer only 500 mg elemental calcium daily.
- If the patient has preexistent osteoporosis or has been receiving corticosteroids for ≥ 3 months, consider prophylaxis:
  –Bisphosphonate such as alendronate (70 mg every week orally), zoledronic acid (5 mg every year intravenously) for up to 3–5 years; Or
  –Teriparatide, 20 mcg subcutaneously daily for up to 2 years
- Avoid prolonged bed rest that will accelerate muscle weakness and bone mineral loss. Ambulate early after fractures.
- Avoid elective surgery, if possible. Vitamin A in a daily dose of 20,000 units orally for 1 week may improve wound healing, but it is not prescribed in pregnancy.
- Fall prevention strategies: walking assistance (cane, walker, wheelchair, handrails) when required due to weakness or balance problems; avoid activities that could cause falls or other trauma.
- For ulcer prophylaxis, if administering corticosteroids with NSAIDs, prescribe a PPI (not required for corticosteroids alone). Avoid large doses of antacids containing aluminum hydroxide (many popular brands) because aluminum hydroxide binds phosphate and may cause a hypophosphatemic osteomalacia that can compound corticosteroid osteoporosis.
- Treat hypogonadism.
- Treat infections aggressively. Consider unusual pathogens.
- Treat edema as indicated.

Bisphosphonates (eg, alendronate) prevent the development of osteoporosis among patients receiving prolonged courses of corticosteroids (Table 26–17). For patients who are unable to tolerate oral bisphosphonates (due to esophagitis, hiatal hernia, or gastritis), parenteral bisphosphonates can be used. Denosumab inhibits bone resorption but may increase the risk of infection compared to bisphosphonates; therefore, the use of denosumab is not recommended for patients receiving high-dose corticosteroid therapy who are already at an increased risk for infection.

The PTH/PTHrP analogs teriparatide and abaloparatide are anabolic agents that are also effective against corticosteroid-induced osteoporosis. They can be given for a 2-year course and increase bone density more effectively than bisphosphonates. For patients who are currently receiving corticosteroid therapy, however, these analogs increase the risk of hypercalcemia and must be used with great caution; they are most useful for patients with osteoporosis who have stopped high-dose corticosteroid therapy. Following a 2-year course of therapy with these analogs, bone loss and fractures occur quickly after discontinuation, so such therapy is usually followed by bisphosphonate therapy in patients with a history of fracture or osteoporosis by bone densitometry. (See Osteoporosis.) It is wise to follow an organized treatment plan such as the one outlined in Table 26–17.

Buttgereit F. Views on glucocorticoid therapy in rheumatology: the age of convergence. Nat Rev Rheumatol. 2020;16:239. [PMID: 32076129]

Chotiyarnwong P et al. Pathogenesis of glucocorticoid-induced osteoporosis and options for treatment. Nat Rev Endocrinol. 2020;16:437. [PMID: 32286516]

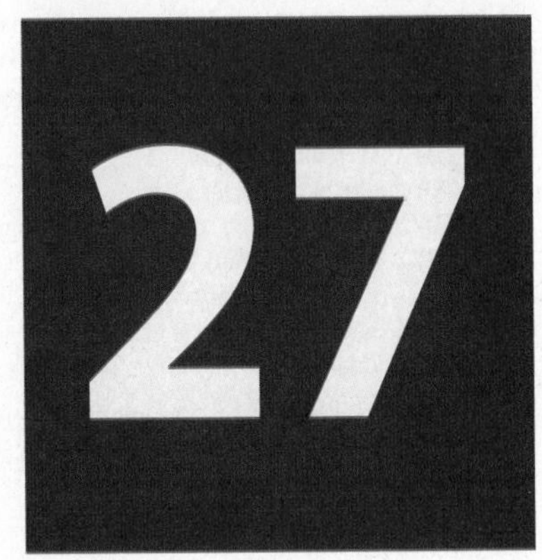

Diabetes Mellitus & Hypoglycemia

Umesh Masharani, MB, BS, MRCP (UK)

DIABETES MELLITUS

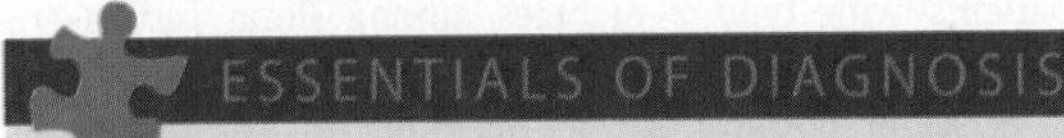

ESSENTIALS OF DIAGNOSIS

Type 1 diabetes

- Polyuria, polydipsia, and weight loss with random plasma glucose of ≥ 200 mg/dL (11.1 mmol/L).
- Plasma glucose of ≥ 126 mg/dL (7.0 mmol/L) after an overnight fast, documented on more than one occasion.
- Ketonemia, ketonuria, or both.
- Islet autoantibodies are frequently present.

Type 2 diabetes

- Many patients are over 40 years of age and have obesity.
- Polyuria and polydipsia. Ketonuria and weight loss are uncommon at time of diagnosis. Candidal vaginitis may be an initial manifestation.
- Plasma glucose of ≥ 126 mg/dL after an overnight fast on more than one occasion. Two hours after 75 g oral glucose, diagnostic values are ≥ 200 mg/dL (11.1 mmol).
- HbA_{1c} ≥ 6.5%.
- Hypertension, dyslipidemia, and atherosclerosis are often associated.

Epidemiologic Considerations

An estimated 34.2 million people (10.5%) in the United States have diabetes mellitus, of whom approximately 5–10% have type 1 diabetes and most of the rest have type 2 diabetes. A third group designated as "other specific types" by the American Diabetes Association (ADA) (Table 27–1) number in the thousands.

Classification & Pathogenesis

A. Type 1 Diabetes Mellitus

This form of diabetes is due to autoimmune destruction of pancreatic islet B cell. The rate of pancreatic B cell destruction is variable, being rapid in some individuals and slow in others. It occurs at any age but most commonly arises in children and young adults with a peak incidence at age 10–14 years. Type 1 diabetes is usually associated with ketosis in its untreated state. Exogenous insulin is therefore required to reverse the catabolic state, prevent ketosis, reduce the hyperglucagonemia, and reduce blood glucose.

Family members of diabetic probands are at increased lifetime risk for developing type 1 diabetes mellitus. A child whose mother has type 1 diabetes has a 3% risk of developing the disease and a 6% risk if the child's father has it. The risk in siblings is related to the number of HLA haplotypes that the sibling shares with the diabetic proband. If one haplotype is shared, the risk is 6% and if two haplotypes are shared, the risk increases to 12–25%. The highest risk is for monozygotic twins, where the concordance rate is 25–50%.

Some patients with a milder expression of type 1 diabetes mellitus initially retain enough B cell function to avoid ketosis, but as their B cell mass diminishes later in life, dependence on insulin therapy develops. Islet cell antibody surveys among northern Europeans indicate that up to 15% of patients with "type 2" diabetes may have this mild form of type 1 diabetes (**latent autoimmune diabetes of adulthood; LADA**). Evidence for environmental factors playing a role in the development of type 1 diabetes include the observation that the disease is more common in Scandinavian countries and becomes progressively less frequent in countries nearer to the equator. Also, the risk for type 1 diabetes increases when individuals who normally have a low risk emigrate to the Northern Hemisphere. For example, Pakistani children born and raised in Bradford, England, have a higher risk for developing type 1 diabetes compared with children who lived in Pakistan all their lives.

Table 27–1. Other specific types of diabetes mellitus.

Genetic defects of pancreatic B cell function
MODY 1 (HNF-4alpha); rare
MODY 2 (glucokinase); less rare
MODY 3 (HNF-1alpha); accounts for two-thirds of all MODY
MODY 4 (PDX1); very rare
MODY 5 (HNF-1beta); very rare
MODY 6 (neuroD1); very rare
Mitochondrial DNA
Wolfram syndrome
Genetic defects in insulin action
Type A insulin resistance
Leprechaunism
Rabson-Mendenhall syndrome
Lipoatrophic diabetes
Diseases of the exocrine pancreas
Endocrinopathies
Drug- or chemical-induced diabetes
Other genetic syndromes (Down, Klinefelter, Turner, others) sometimes associated with diabetes

HNF, hepatic nuclear factor; MODY, maturity-onset diabetes of the young; PDX1, pancreatic duodenal homeobox 1.

Which environmental factor is responsible for the increased risk is not known. Breastfeeding in the first 6 months of life appears to be protective. There is accumulating evidence that improvements in public health and reduced infections (especially parasitic) lead to immune system dysregulation and development of autoimmune disorders such as asthma and type 1 diabetes.

Check point inhibitor immunotherapies, such as nivolumab, pembrolizumab, and ipilimumab, can precipitate autoimmune disorders, including type 1 diabetes. The onset of diabetes can be rapid and the patients frequently have diabetic ketoacidosis at presentation. Autoantibodies against islet antigens are only present in about 50% of patients. Patients receiving these drugs should be carefully monitored for the development of diabetes.

Approximately 5% of subjects have no evidence of pancreatic B cell autoimmunity to explain their insulinopenia and ketoacidosis. This subgroup has been classified as "idiopathic type 1 diabetes" and designated as "type 1B." Although only a minority of patients with type 1 diabetes fall into this group, most of these individuals are of Asian or African origin. About 4% of the West Africans with ketosis-prone diabetes are homozygous for a mutation in *PAX-4 (Arg133Trp)*—a transcription factor that is essential for the development of pancreatic islets.

B. Type 2 Diabetes Mellitus

Type 2 diabetes is due to non-immune causes of pancreatic B cell loss with variable degree of tissue insensitivity to insulin, that is, insulin resistance. The residual beta cell function is sufficient to prevent ketoacidosis but is inadequate to prevent the hyperglycemia. This form of diabetes used to occur predominantly in adults, but it is now more frequently encountered in children and adolescents.

Genetic and environmental factors combine to cause both the beta cell loss and the insulin resistance. Most epidemiologic data indicate strong genetic influences, since in monozygotic twins over 40 years of age, concordance develops in over 70% of cases within a year whenever type 2 diabetes develops in one twin. Genome studies have identified 143 risk variants and putative regulator mechanisms for type 2 diabetes. A significant number of the identified loci appear to code for proteins that have a role in beta cell function or development. One of the genetic loci with the largest risk effect is *TCF7L2*. This gene codes for a transcription factor involved in the WNT signaling pathway that is required for normal pancreatic development.

Obesity is the most important environmental factor causing insulin resistance. The degree and prevalence of obesity vary among different racial groups with type 2 diabetes. While obesity is apparent in no more than 30% of Chinese and Japanese patients with type 2 diabetes, it is found in 60–70% of North Americans, Europeans, or Africans with type 2 diabetes and approaches 100% of patients with type 2 diabetes among Pima Indians or Pacific Islanders from Nauru or Samoa.

Visceral obesity, due to accumulation of fat in the omental and mesenteric regions, correlates with insulin resistance; subcutaneous abdominal fat seems to have less of an association with insulin insensitivity. "Metabolic obesity" is a term used to describe increased visceral fat in patients with type 2 diabetes without overt obesity. Exercise may affect the deposition of visceral fat as suggested by CT scans of Japanese wrestlers, whose extreme obesity is predominantly subcutaneous. Their daily vigorous exercise program prevents accumulation of visceral fat, and they have normal serum lipids and euglycemia despite daily intakes of 5000–7000 kcal and development of massive subcutaneous obesity.

C. Other Specific Types of Diabetes Mellitus

1. Maturity-onset diabetes of the young (MODY)—This subgroup of monogenic disorders is characterized by non-insulin requiring diabetes with autosomal dominant inheritance and an age at onset of 25 years or younger. Patients do not have obesity and their hyperglycemia is due to impaired glucose-induced secretion of insulin. Six types of MODY have been described (Table 27–1). Except for MODY 2, in which a glucokinase gene is defective, all other types involve mutations of a nuclear transcription factor that regulates islet gene expression. Patients younger than 30 years with endogenous insulin production (urinary C-peptide/creatinine ratio of 0.2 nmol/mmol or higher) and negative autoantibodies are candidates for genetic screening for MODY. The enzyme glucokinase is a rate-limiting step in glycolysis and determines the rate of adenosine triphosphate (ATP) production from glucose and the insulin secretory response in the beta cell. MODY 2, due to glucokinase mutations, is usually quite mild, associated with only slight fasting hyperglycemia and few if any microvascular diabetic complications. MODY 3, due to mutations in hepatic nuclear factor 1 alpha, is the most common form, accounting for two-thirds of all MODY cases. Initially, patients with MODY 3 are responsive to sulfonylurea therapy but the clinical course is of progressive beta cell failure and eventual need for insulin therapy. Mutations in both alleles of glucokinase present with more severe neonatal diabetes. Mutation in one allele of the pancreatic duodenal homeobox 1 (PDX1) causes diabetes usually at a later age (~ 35 years) than other forms of MODY; mutations in both alleles of PDX1 cause pancreatic agenesis.

2. Diabetes mellitus associated with a mutation of mitochondrial DNA— Diabetes due to mutations of mitochondrial DNA occurs in less than 2% of patients with diabetes. The most common cause is the A3243G mutation in the gene coding for the tRNA (Leu, UUR). Diabetes usually develops in these patients in their late 30s, and characteristically, they also have hearing loss (maternally inherited diabetes and deafness [MIDD]).

3. Wolfram syndrome—Wolfram syndrome is an autosomal recessive neurodegenerative disorder first evident in childhood. It consists of diabetes insipidus, diabetes mellitus, optic atrophy, and deafness, hence the acronym DIDMOAD. It is due to mutations in a gene named *WFS1*, which encodes a 100.3 KDa transmembrane protein localized in the endoplasmic reticulum. Cranial diabetes insipidus and sensorineural deafness develop during the second decade in 60–75% of patients. Ureterohydronephrosis, neurogenic bladder, cerebellar ataxia, peripheral neuropathy, and psychiatric illness develop later in many patients.

4. Autosomal recessive syndromes—Homozygous mutations in a number of pancreatic transcription factors, *NEUROG3, PTF1A, RFX6*, and *GLI-similar 3 (GLIS3)*, cause neonatal or childhood diabetes. Homozygous *PTF1A* mutations result in absent pancreas and cerebellar atrophy; *NEUROG3* mutations cause severe malabsorption and diabetes before puberty. Homozygous mutations in *RFX6* cause the Mitchell-Riley syndrome characterized by absence of all islet cell types apart from pancreatic polypeptide cells, hypoplasia of the pancreas and gallbladder, and intestinal atresia. *GLIS3* gene plays a role in transcription of insulin gene, and homozygous mutations cause neonatal diabetes and congenital hypothyroidism. The gene *EIF2AK3* encodes PKR-like ER kinase (PERK), which controls one of the pathways of the unfolded protein response. Absence of PERK leads to inadequate response to ER stress and accelerated beta cell apoptosis. Patients with mutation in this gene have neonatal diabetes, epiphyseal dysplasia, developmental delay, and liver and kidney dysfunction (Wolcott-Rallison syndrome).

5. Diabetes mellitus secondary to other causes—Endocrine tumors secreting growth hormone, glucocorticoids, catecholamines, glucagon, or somatostatin can cause glucose intolerance (Table 27–2). In the first four of these situations, peripheral responsiveness to insulin is impaired. With excess of glucocorticoids, catecholamines, or glucagon, increased hepatic output of glucose is a contributory factor; in the case of catecholamines, decreased insulin release is an additional factor in producing carbohydrate intolerance, and with somatostatin, inhibition of insulin secretion is the major factor. Diabetes mainly occurs in individuals with underlying defects in insulin secretion, and hyperglycemia typically resolves when the hormone excess is resolved.

Table 27–2. Secondary causes of hyperglycemia.

Hyperglycemia due to tissue insensitivity to insulin
Medications (corticosteroids, sympathomimetic drugs, niacin, alpelisib, sirolimus)
Hormonal tumors (acromegaly, Cushing syndrome, glucagonoma, pheochromocytoma)
Liver disease (cirrhosis, hemochromatosis)
Muscle disorders (myotonic dystrophy)
Adipose tissue disorders (lipodystrophy, truncal obesity)
Hyperglycemia due to reduced insulin secretion
Medications (thiazide diuretics, phenytoin, pentamidine, calcineurin inhibitors, atypical antipsychotics)
Hormonal tumors (somatostatinoma, pheochromocytoma)
Pancreatic disorders (pancreatitis, hemosiderosis, hemochromatosis)

High-titer anti-insulin receptor antibodies that inhibit insulin binding cause a clinical syndrome characterized by severe insulin resistance, glucose intolerance or diabetes mellitus, and acanthosis nigricans. These patients usually have other autoimmune disorders.

Many drugs are associated with carbohydrate intolerance or frank diabetes (Table 27–2). The drugs act by decreasing insulin secretion or by increasing insulin resistance or both. Cyclosporine and tacrolimus impair insulin secretion; sirolimus principally increases insulin resistance. These agents contribute to the development of new-onset diabetes after transplantation. Corticosteroids increase insulin resistance but may also have an effect on beta cell function; in a case control study and a large population cohort study, oral corticosteroids doubled the risk for development of diabetes. Thiazide diuretics and beta-blockers modestly increase the risk for diabetes. Treating the hypokalemia due to thiazides may reverse the hyperglycemia. Atypical antipsychotics, particularly olanzapine and clozapine, are associated with increased risk of glucose intolerance. These drugs cause weight gain and insulin resistance but may also impair beta cell function; an increase in rates of diabetic ketoacidosis (DKA) has been reported. Alpelisib is a phosphatidylinositol-3-kinase (PI3K) inhibitor used in combination with fulvestrant for hormone receptor–positive, HER2-negative, *PIK3CA*-mutated breast cancer. PI3K is a component of the insulin signaling pathway, and hyperglycemia is a common side effect of alpelisib treatment.

Chronic pancreatitis or subtotal pancreatectomy reduces the number of functioning B cells and can result in a metabolic derangement similar to that of genetic type 1 diabetes except that a concomitant reduction in pancreatic A cells may reduce glucagon secretion so that relatively lower doses of insulin replacement are needed.

Metabolic Syndrome (Insulin Resistance Syndrome)

The term metabolic syndrome has been advocated to identify individuals who were at higher risk for development of diabetes and CVD. Criteria included waist circumference, glucose levels, blood pressure, triglycerides, and HDL cholesterol. There is, however, no unifying pathophysiologic basis for the syndrome, and in 2010, a WHO expert committee reported that the syndrome lacked utility as a diagnostic or management tool. They observed that there was only modest association between metabolic syndrome and CVD, and the definition was outperformed by traditional cardiovascular risk prediction algorithms such as the Framingham risk score. Similarly, fasting glucose conveys a greater risk of incident diabetes than the metabolic syndrome. There is also no evidence that hyperinsulinemia and insulin resistance play a direct role in these metabolic abnormalities.

Clinical Trials About Optimum Diabetic Glucose Control

Findings of the Diabetes Control and Complications Trial in type 1 diabetes and of the United Kingdom Prospective Diabetes Study in type 2 diabetes have confirmed the beneficial effects of improved glycemic control in both type 1 and type 2 diabetes.

A. Type 1 Diabetes

The Diabetes Control and Complications Trial (DCCT), a long-term therapeutic study involving 1441 patients with type 1 diabetes mellitus, reported that "near" normalization of blood glucose resulted in a delay in the onset and a major slowing of the progression of established microvascular and neuropathic complications of diabetes.

In half of the patients, a mean HbA_{1c} of 7.2% (normal: less than 6%) and a mean blood glucose of 155 mg/dL (8.6 mmol/L) were achieved using intensive therapy, while in the conventionally treated group, HbA_{1c} averaged 8.9% with an average blood glucose of 225 mg/dL (12.5 mmol/L). Over the study period, which averaged 7 years, there was an approximately 60% reduction in risk between the two groups in regard to diabetic retinopathy, nephropathy, and neuropathy. The intensively treated group also had a nonsignificant reduction in the risk of macrovascular disease of 41% (95% CI, –10% to 68%). Intensively treated patients had a threefold greater risk of serious hypoglycemia as well as a greater tendency toward weight gain. However, there were no deaths definitely attributable to hypoglycemia in any persons in the DCCT study, and no evidence of posthypoglycemic cognitive damage was detected.

The general consensus of the ADA is that intensive insulin therapy associated with comprehensive self-management training should be standard therapy in patients with type 1 diabetes mellitus after the age of puberty. Exceptions include those with advanced chronic kidney disease and older adults since the detrimental risks of hypoglycemia outweigh the benefits of tight glycemic control in these groups.

B. Type 2 Diabetes

The United Kingdom Prospective Diabetes Study (UKPDS), a multicenter study, was designed to establish whether the risk of macrovascular or microvascular complications could be reduced by intensive blood glucose control with oral hypoglycemic agents or insulin and whether any particular therapy was more beneficial than the other for patients with type 2 diabetes.

Intensive treatment with either sulfonylureas, metformin, combinations of those two, or insulin achieved mean HbA_{1c} levels of 7%. This level of glycemic control decreased the risk of microvascular complications (retinopathy and nephropathy) in comparison with conventional therapy (mostly diet alone), which achieved mean levels of HbA_{1c} of 7.9%. Weight gain occurred in intensively treated patients except when metformin was used as monotherapy. No adverse cardiovascular outcomes were noted regardless of the therapeutic agent. In the subgroup of patients who were overweight or had obesity, metformin therapy was more beneficial than diet alone in reducing the number of patients who suffered MIs and strokes. Hypoglycemic reactions occurred in the intensive treatment groups, but only one death from hypoglycemia was documented during 27,000 patient-years of intensive therapy.

Tight control of blood pressure (median value 144/82 mm Hg vs 154/87 mm Hg) substantially reduced the risk of microvascular disease and stroke but not MI. In fact, reducing blood pressure by this amount had substantially greater impact on microvascular outcomes than that achieved by lowering HbA_{1c} from 7.9% to 7%. An epidemiologic analysis of the UKPDS data showed that every 10 mm Hg decrease in mean systolic blood pressure was associated with 11% reduction in risk for MI. More than half of the patients needed two or more medications for adequate therapy of their hypertension, and there was no demonstrable advantage of ACE inhibitor therapy over therapy with beta-blockers with regard to diabetes end points. Use of a calcium channel blocker added to both treatment groups appeared to be safe over the long term in this population with diabetes despite some controversy in the literature about its safety in patients with diabetes.

Findings from the UKPDS support that glycemic control to levels of HbA_{1c} to 7% show benefit in reducing total diabetes end points, including a 25% reduction in microvascular disease as compared with HbA_{1c} levels of 7.9%. This reassures those who have questioned whether the value of intensive therapy, so convincingly shown by the DCCT in type 1 diabetes, can safely be extrapolated to older patients with type 2 diabetes. It also argues against the concept of a "threshold" of glycemic control since in this group there was a benefit from this modest reduction of HbA_{1c} below 7.9% whereas in the DCCT a threshold was suggested in that further benefit was less apparent at HbA_{1c} levels below 8%.

Probably the most striking implication of the UKPDS is the benefit of intensive control of blood pressure to patients with hypertension and type 2 diabetes. There was no demonstrable advantage of ACE inhibitor therapy on outcome despite several short-term reports in smaller populations, which have implied that these drugs have special efficacy in reducing glomerular pressure beyond their general antihypertensive effects. Moreover, slow-release nifedipine showed no evidence of cardiac toxicity in this study despite some previous reports claiming that calcium channel blockers may be hazardous in patients with diabetes. The greater benefit in diabetes end points from antihypertensive than from antihyperglycemic treatments may be that the difference between the mean blood pressures achieved (144/82 mm Hg versus 154/87 mm Hg) is therapeutically more influential than the slight difference in HbA_{1c} (7% versus 7.9%). Greater hyperglycemia in the control group would most likely have rectified this discrepancy in outcomes.

Diabetes Prevention Trials

A. Prevention of Type 1 Diabetes

At the time of diagnosis of type 1 diabetes, there remains significant B cell pancreatic function. This explains why soon after diagnosis, the diabetes goes into partial clinical remission and little or no insulin is required ("honeymoon"). The clinical remission is short-lived, however, and eventually patients lose all B cell function and have more labile glucose control. Studies have been performed to prolong this partial clinical remission using immunomodulatory agents. The CD3 complex is the major signal-transducing element of the T cell receptor, and the anti-CD3 antibodies are believed to modulate the autoimmune response by selectively inhibiting the pathogenic T cells or by inducing regulatory T cells. Clinical trials of humanized monoclonal antibodies against CD3, hOKT-3gamma (Ala-Ala) (teplizumab), and ChAglyCD3 (otelixizumab) delayed but did not completely arrest the decline in insulin production in patients with newly diagnosed type 1 diabetes. A similar clinical trial using teplizumab was undertaken in relatives (who did not have diabetes) of patients with type 1 diabetes who had two or more diabetes-related antibodies and glucose intolerance. In the 5 years after randomization, 43% of the patients receiving teplizumab and 72% of the placebo group developed diabetes.

B. Prevention of Type 2 Diabetes

The Diabetes Prevention Program studied whether treatment with either diet and exercise or metformin could prevent the onset of type 2 diabetes in overweight men and women aged 25–85 years who had impaired glucose tolerance. Intervention with a low-fat diet and 150 minutes of moderate exercise (equivalent to a brisk walk) per week reduced the risk of progression to type 2 diabetes by 71%. Participants who took metformin 850 mg twice daily reduced their risk of developing type 2 diabetes by 31%, but this intervention was relatively ineffective in those who had a lesser degree of obesity or were in the older age group. Eighty-eight percent of the persons in the Diabetes Prevention Program elected to continue follow-up in the Diabetes Prevention Program Outcome Study. At 15 years of follow-up, the cumulative incidence of diabetes was 55% in the lifestyle group and 62% in the control group.

Clinical Findings

A. Symptoms and Signs

1. Type 1 diabetes—A characteristic symptom complex of hyperosmolality and hyperketonemia from the accumulation of circulating glucose and fatty acids typically occurs in patients with type 1 diabetes. When absolute insulin deficiency is of acute onset, there is abrupt increase in urination, thirst, blurred vision, weight loss, paresthesias, and altered level of consciousness. Ketoacidosis exacerbates the dehydration and hyperosmolality by producing anorexia and nausea and vomiting, interfering with oral fluid replacement.

a. Increased urination and thirst—These symptoms are consequences of osmotic diuresis secondary to sustained hyperglycemia. The diuresis results in a loss of glucose as well as free water and electrolytes in the urine.

b. Blurred vision—As the lenses are exposed to hyperosmolar fluids, blurred vision often develops.

c. Weight loss—Despite normal or increased appetite, weight loss is a common feature of type 1 when it develops subacutely. The weight loss is initially due to depletion of water, glycogen, and triglycerides; thereafter, reduced muscle mass occurs as amino acids are diverted to form glucose and ketone bodies. Loss of subcutaneous fat and muscle wasting are features of more slowly developing insulin deficiency. Lowered plasma volume produces symptoms of postural hypotension, which is a serious prognostic sign. Total body potassium loss and the general catabolism of muscle protein contribute to the weakness.

d. Paresthesias—Paresthesias may be present at the time of diagnosis, particularly when the onset is subacute. They reflect a temporary dysfunction of peripheral sensory nerves, which clears as insulin replacement restores glycemic levels closer to normal, suggesting neurotoxicity from sustained hyperglycemia.

e. Level of consciousness—The patient's level of consciousness can vary depending on the degree of hyperosmolality. When insulin deficiency develops relatively slowly and sufficient water intake is maintained, patients remain relatively alert and physical findings may be minimal. When vomiting occurs in response to worsening ketoacidosis, dehydration progresses and compensatory mechanisms become inadequate to keep serum osmolality below 320–330 mOsm/L. Stupor or even coma may occur when the serum osmolality exceeds 320–330 mOsm/L. The fruity breath odor of acetone further suggests the diagnosis of DKA.

2. Type 2 diabetes—While increased urination and thirst may be presenting symptoms in some patients with type 2 diabetes, many other patients have an insidious onset of hyperglycemia and are asymptomatic initially. This is particularly true in patients with obesity, whose diabetes may be detected only after glycosuria or hyperglycemia is noted during routine laboratory studies. Occasionally, when the disease has been occult for some time, patients may have evidence of neuropathic or cardiovascular complications at the time of presentation. Hyperglycemic hyperosmolar coma can also be present when the serum osmolality exceeds 320–330 mOsm/L; in these cases, patients are profoundly dehydrated, hypotensive, lethargic, or comatose but without the Kussmaul respirations of ketoacidosis.

A. Skin manifestations—Chronic skin infections are common. Generalized pruritus and symptoms of vaginitis are frequently the initial complaints of women. Diabetes should be suspected in women with chronic candidal vulvovaginitis. Balanoposthitis (inflammation of the foreskin and glans in uncircumcised males) may occur.

Other skin findings include acanthosis nigricans. which is associated with significant insulin resistance. The skin in the axilla, groin, and back of neck is hyperpigmented and hyperkeratotic (Figure 27–1). Eruptive xanthomas on the flexor surface of the limbs and on the buttocks and lipemia retinalis due to hyperchylomicronemia can occur in patients with uncontrolled type 2 diabetes who also have a familial form of hypertriglyceridemia.

B. Body habitus—Patients who are overweight or have obesity frequently have type 2 diabetes. Even those who do not have significant obesity often have characteristic localization of fat deposits on the upper segment of the body (particularly the abdomen, chest, neck, and face) and relatively less fat on the appendages, which may be quite muscular. This centripetal fat distribution is characterized by a high waist circumference; a waist circumference larger than 40 inches (102 cm) in men and 35 inches (88 cm) in women is associated with an increased risk of diabetes. Mild hypertension is often present in patients with diabetes and obesity.

C. Obstetrical complications—Type 2 diabetes should be considered in women who have delivered babies larger than 9 lb (4.1 kg) or have had polyhydramnios, preeclampsia, or unexplained fetal losses.

B. Laboratory Findings

1. Urine glucose—A convenient method to detect glucosuria is the paper strip impregnated with glucose oxidase and a chromogen system (Clinistix, Diastix), which is sensitive to as little as 100 mg/dL (5.5 mmol) glucose in urine. A normal renal threshold for glucose as well as reliable bladder emptying are essential for interpretation.

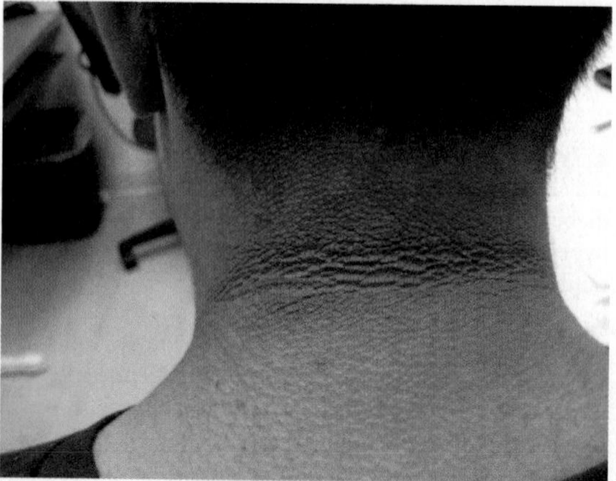

▲ **Figure 27–1.** Acanthosis nigricans of the nape of the neck, with typical dark and velvety appearance. (Used, with permission, from Umesh Masharani, MB, BS, MRCP [UK].)

Nondiabetic glycosuria (renal glycosuria) is a benign asymptomatic condition wherein glucose appears in the urine despite a normal amount of glucose in the blood, either basally or during a glucose tolerance test. Its cause may vary from mutations in the *SGLT2* gene coding for sodium-glucose transporter 2 (familial renal glycosuria) to one associated with dysfunction of the proximal renal tubule (Fanconi syndrome, CKD), or it may merely be a consequence of the increased load of glucose presented to the tubules by the elevated GFR during pregnancy. As many as 50% of pregnant women normally have demonstrable sugar in the urine, especially during the third and fourth months. This sugar is practically always glucose except during the late weeks of pregnancy, when lactose may be present.

2. Urine and blood ketones—Qualitative detection of ketone bodies can be accomplished by nitroprusside tests (Acetest or Ketostix). Although these tests do not detect beta-hydroxybutyric acid, which lacks a ketone group, the semiquantitative estimation of ketonuria thus obtained is nonetheless usually adequate for clinical purposes. Many laboratories measure beta-hydroxybutyric acid, and there are meters available (Precision Xtra; Nova Max Plus) for patient use that measures beta-hydroxybutyric acid levels in capillary glucose samples. Beta-hydroxybutyrate levels greater than 0.6 mmol/L require evaluation. Patients with levels greater than 3.0 mmol/L, equivalent to very large urinary ketones, require hospitalization.

3. Plasma or serum glucose—The glucose concentration is 10–15% higher in plasma or serum than in whole blood because structural components of blood cells are absent. A plasma glucose level of 126 mg/dL (7 mmol/L) or higher on more than one occasion after at least 8 hours of fasting is diagnostic of diabetes mellitus (Table 27–3). Fasting plasma glucose levels of 100–125 mg/dL (5.6–6.9 mmol/L) are associated with increased risk of diabetes (impaired fasting glucose tolerance).

4. Oral glucose tolerance test—If the fasting plasma glucose level is less than 126 mg/dL (7 mmol/L) when diabetes is nonetheless suspected, then a standardized oral glucose tolerance test may be done (Table 27–3). In order to optimize insulin secretion and effectiveness, especially when patients have been on a low-carbohydrate diet, a minimum of 150–200 g of carbohydrate per day should be included in the diet for 3 days preceding the test. The patient should eat nothing after midnight prior to the test day. On the morning of the test, patients are then given 75 g of glucose in 300 mL of water. The glucose load is consumed within 5 minutes. The test is performed in the morning because of diurnal variation in oral glucose tolerance; patients should not smoke or be active during the test.

Blood samples for plasma glucose are obtained at 0 and 120 minutes after ingestion of glucose. Table 27–3 provides diagnostic criteria for diabetes mellitus based on the oral glucose tolerance test. A fasting value of 126 mg/dL (7 mmol/L) or higher or a 2-hour value of greater than 200 mg/dL (11.1 mmol/L) is diagnostic of diabetes mellitus. Patients with a 2-hour value of 140–199 mg/dL (7.8–11.1 mmol/L) have impaired glucose tolerance.

Table 27–3. Criteria for the diagnosis of diabetes.

	Normal Glucose Tolerance[1]	Impaired Glucose Tolerance[1]	Diabetes Mellitus[2]
Fasting plasma glucose mg/dL (mmol/L)	< 100 (5.6)	100–125 (5.6–6.9)	≥ 126 (7.0)
Plasma glucose mg/dL (mmol/L) 2 hours after glucose load	< 140 (7.8)	≥ 140–199 (7.8–11.0)	≥ 200 (11.1)
HbA_{1c} (%)	< 5.7	5.7–6.4	≥ 6.5

[1]See text for the oral glucose tolerance test protocol.
[2]A fasting plasma glucose ≥ 126 mg/dL (7.0 mmol) is diagnostic of diabetes if confirmed by *repeat testing*. A fasting plasma glucose ≥ 126 mg/dL (7.0 mmol) and HbA_{1c} ≥ 6.5% on the *same sample* is also diagnostic of diabetes.

False-positive results may occur in patients who are malnourished, bedridden, or afflicted with an infection or severe emotional stress.

5. Glycated hemoglobin (hemoglobin A_1) measurements—Hemoglobin becomes glycated by ketoamine reactions between glucose and other sugars and the free amino groups on the alpha and beta chains. Only glycation of the N-terminal valine of the beta chain imparts sufficient negative charge to the hemoglobin molecule to allow separation by charge dependent techniques. These charge-separated hemoglobins are collectively referred to as hemoglobin A_1 (HbA_1). The major form of HbA_1 is hemoglobin A_{1c} (HbA_{1c}) where glucose is the carbohydrate. HbA_{1c} comprises 4–6% of total hemoglobin A. Since HbA_{1c} circulates within RBCs whose life span lasts up to 120 days, it generally reflects the state of glycemia over the preceding 8–12 weeks, thereby providing an improved method of assessing diabetic control. The HbA_{1c} value, however, is weighted to more recent glucose levels (previous month) and this explains why significant changes in HbA_{1c} are observed with short-term (1 month) changes in mean plasma glucose levels. Measurements should be made in patients with either type of diabetes mellitus at 3- to 4-month intervals. In patients monitoring their own blood glucose levels, HbA_{1c} values provide a valuable check on the accuracy of monitoring. In patients who do not monitor their own blood glucose levels, HbA_{1c} values are essential for adjusting therapy. The A_{1c} Derived Average Glucose Study reported that the relationship between average glucose in the previous 3 months and HbA_{1c} was (28.7 × HbA_{1c}) – 46.7. There is, however, substantial individual variability; for HbA_{1c} values between 6.9% and 7.1%, the glucose levels range from 125 mg/dL to 205 mg/dL (6.9–11.4 mmol/L; 95% CIs). For HbA_{1c} of 6%, the mean glucose levels range from 100 mg/dL to 152 mg/dL (5.5–8.5 mmol/L); and for 8% they range from 147 mg/dL to 217 mg/dL (8.1–12.1 mmol/L). For this reason, caution should be exercised in estimating average glucose levels from measured HbA_{1c}.

The accuracy of HbA_{1c} values can be affected by hemoglobin variants or traits. In patients with high levels of hemoglobin F, immunoassays give falsely low values of HbA_{1c}. The National Glycohemoglobin Standardization Program website (www.ngsp.org) has information on the impact of frequently encountered hemoglobin variants and traits on the results obtained with the commonly used HbA_{1c} assays.

Any condition that shortens erythrocyte survival or decreases mean erythrocyte age (eg, recovery from acute blood loss, hemolytic anemia) will falsely lower HbA_{1c}, irrespective of the assay method used because of the extended time that it takes circulating hemoglobin to be glycosylated. Intravenous iron and erythropoietin therapy for treatment of anemia in CKD also falsely lower HbA_{1c} levels. Alternative methods such as fructosamine (see below) should be considered for these patients. Vitamins C and E are reported to falsely lower test results possibly by inhibiting glycation of hemoglobin. Conditions that increase erythrocyte survival such as splenectomy for hereditary spherocytosis will falsely raise HbA_{1c} levels. Iron deficiency anemia is also associated with higher HbA_{1c} levels.

HbA_{1c} is endorsed by the ADA as a diagnostic test for type 1 and type 2 diabetes (Table 27–3). A cutoff value of 6.5% (48 mmol/mol) was chosen because the risk for retinopathy increases substantially above this value. *The advantages of using the HbA_{1c} to diagnose diabetes is that there is no need to fast;* it has lower intraindividual variability than the fasting glucose test and the oral glucose tolerance test; and it provides an estimate of glucose control for the preceding 2–3 months. People with HbA_{1c} levels of 5.7–6.4% (39–46 mmol/mol) should be considered at high risk for developing diabetes (prediabetes). This test is not appropriate to use in populations with high prevalence of hemoglobinopathies or in conditions with increased red cell turnover.

6. Serum fructosamine—Serum fructosamine is formed by nonenzymatic glycosylation of serum proteins (predominantly albumin). Since serum albumin has a much shorter half-life than hemoglobin, serum fructosamine generally reflects the state of glycemic control for only the preceding 1–2 weeks. Reductions in serum albumin (eg, nephrotic state, protein-losing enteropathy, or hepatic disease) will lower the serum fructosamine value. When abnormal hemoglobins or hemolytic states affect the interpretation of glycohemoglobin or when a narrower time frame is required, such as for ascertaining glycemic control at the time of conception in a woman with diabetes who has recently become pregnant, serum fructosamine assays offer some advantage. Normal values vary in relation to the serum albumin concentration and are 200–285 mcmol/L when the serum albumin level is 5 g/dL. HbA_{1c} values and serum fructosamine are highly correlated. Serum fructosamine levels of 300, 367, and 430 mcmol/L approximate to HbA_{1c} values of 7%, 8%, and 9%, respectively. Substantial individual variability exists, though, when estimating the likely HbA_{1c} value from the fructosamine measurement.

7. Glycated albumin—This is the specific measurement of glycosylated form of albumin. It has the same advantages and disadvantages as serum fructosamine measurements.

8. Self-monitoring of blood glucose—Capillary blood glucose measurements performed by patients themselves, as outpatients, are extremely useful. A large number of blood glucose meters are available. All are accurate, but they vary with regard to speed, convenience, size of blood samples required, reporting capability, and cost. Popular models include those manufactured by LifeScan (One Touch), Bayer Corporation (Contour), Roche Diagnostics (Accu-Chek), and Abbott Laboratories (Precision, FreeStyle). These blood glucose meters are relatively inexpensive, ranging from \$20 to \$80 each. Test strips remain a major expense, costing about \$0.25 to \$1.50 apiece. The meters also come with a lancet device and disposable 26- to 33-gauge lancets. Another meter uses a test cartridge to automatize the blood sampling and glucose measurement (Pogo automatic meter, Intuity Medical); the patient simply places a finger on the testing platform and presses a button to get a glucose reading. Most meters can store from 100 to 1000 glucose values in their memories and have capabilities to download the values into a computer or smartphone. Educating the patient in correct sampling and measuring procedures will help ensure the accuracy of data obtained by home glucose monitoring.

The clinician should be aware of the limitations of the self-monitoring glucose systems. The strips have limited lifespans and improper storage (high temperature; open vial) can affect their function. Patients should also be advised not to use expired strips. Increases or decreases in hematocrit can decrease or increase the measured glucose values. Meters and the test strips are calibrated over the glucose concentrations ranging from 60 mg/dL (3.3 mmol/L) to 160 mg/dL (8.9 mmol/L) and the accuracy is not as good for higher and lower glucose levels. When the glucose is less than 60 mg/dL (3.3 mmol/L), the difference between the meter and the laboratory value may be as much as 20%. Glucose oxidase–based amperometric systems underestimate glucose levels in the presence of high oxygen tension. This may be important in the critically ill who are receiving supplemental oxygen; under these circumstances, a glucose dehydrogenase–based system may be preferable. Glucose-dehydrogenase pyrroloquinoline quinone (GDH-PQQ) systems may report falsely high glucose levels in patients who are receiving parenteral products containing nonglucose sugars such as maltose, galactose, or xylose or their metabolites. Some meters are approved for measuring glucose in blood samples obtained at alternative sites such as the forearm and thigh. There is, however, a 5- to 20-minute lag in the glucose response on the arm with respect to the glucose response on the finger. Forearm blood glucose measurements could therefore result in a delay in detection of rapidly developing hypoglycemia. Impaired circulation to the fingers (for example, in patients with Raynaud disease) will artificially lower fingerstick glucose measurements (pseudohypoglycemia).

9. Continuous glucose monitoring systems—Continuous glucose monitoring systems measure glucose concentrations in the interstitial fluid. These systems, manufactured by Medtronic MiniMed, DexCom systems, and Abbott Diagnostics, involve the patient inserting a subcutaneous sensor (rather like a small wire) that measures glucose concentrations continuously in the interstitial fluid for 7–14 days. The DexCom and MiniMed systems transmit glucose data wirelessly to smartphones or to the screens of insulin pumps. Directional arrows indicate rate and direction of change of glucose levels, and alerts can be set for dangerously low or high glucose values. The wearer also gains insight into how particular foods and activities affect their glucose level. The FreeStyle Libre (Abbott Diagnostics) sensor system requires the patient to hold a reading device or a smartphone close to the sensor patch for about a second to see the real-time glucose value. The MiniMed system requires calibration with periodic fingerstick glucose levels, which is not necessary for the Dexcom and Freestyle Libre systems. The factory calibrated systems use a calibration function that automatically corrects for sensor drift over the subsequent 10–14 days; it is inadvisable to reset the sensor and attempt to use it for longer than the recommended time frame. A 6-month randomized controlled study of patients with type 1 diabetes showed that adults (25 years and older) using these continuous glucose monitoring systems had improved glycemic control without an increase in the incidence of hypoglycemia. A randomized controlled study of continuous glucose monitoring during pregnancy showed improved glycemic control in the third trimester, lower (more normal) birth weight, and reduced risk of macrosomia. Summaries of the continuous glucose monitoring data collected over 2–12 weeks can be very helpful. The percentage of "time in range" (glucose levels 70–180 mg/day [3.9–10 mmol/L]), glucose levels that are low or high, and their variability can be assessed. There is a strong correlation between glucose levels that are 70% "time in range" and an HbA_{1c} of approximately 7%. All patients with type 1 diabetes and patients with type 2 diabetes who are on agents that can cause hypoglycemia should be encouraged to use these systems.

10. Lipoprotein abnormalities in diabetes—Circulating lipoproteins are just as dependent on insulin as is the plasma glucose. In type 1 diabetes, moderately deficient control of hyperglycemia is associated with only a slight elevation of LDL cholesterol and serum triglycerides and little if any change in HDL cholesterol. Once the hyperglycemia is corrected, lipoprotein levels are generally normal. However, in patients with type 2 diabetes, a distinct "diabetic dyslipidemia" is characteristic of the insulin resistance syndrome. Its features are a high serum triglyceride level (300–400 mg/dL [3.4–4.5 mmol/L]), a low HDL cholesterol (less than 30 mg/dL [0.8 mmol/L]), and a qualitative change in LDL particles, producing a smaller dense particle whose membrane carries supranormal amounts of free cholesterol. These smaller dense LDL particles are more susceptible to oxidation, which renders them more atherogenic. Measures designed to correct the obesity and hyperglycemia, such as exercise, diet, and hypoglycemic therapy, are the treatment of choice for diabetic dyslipidemia, and in occasional patients in whom normal weight was achieved, all features of the lipoprotein abnormalities cleared. Since primary disorders of lipid metabolism may coexist with diabetes, persistence of lipid abnormalities after restoration of normal weight and blood glucose should prompt a diagnostic workup and possible pharmacotherapy of the lipid disorder. Chapter 28 discusses these matters in detail.

American Diabetes Association. *Standards of Medical Care in Diabetes—2022*. Diabetes Care. https://diabetesjournals.org/care/issue/45/Supplement_1

Treatment

A. Diet

A well-balanced, nutritious diet remains a fundamental element of therapy. There is no specific recommendation on the percentage of calories that should come from carbohydrate, protein, and fat. The macronutrient proportions should be individualized based on the patient's eating patterns, preferences, and metabolic goals. In general, most patients with diabetes consume about 45% of their total daily calories in the form of carbohydrates, 25–35% in the form of fat, and 10–35% in the form of protein. In patients with type 2 diabetes, limiting the carbohydrate intake and substituting some of the calories with monounsaturated fats, such as olive oil, rapeseed (canola) oil, or the oils in nuts and avocados, can lower triglycerides and increase HDL cholesterol. A Mediterranean-style eating pattern (a diet supplemented with walnuts, almonds, hazelnuts, and olive oil) has been shown to improve glycemic control and lower combined endpoints for cardiovascular events and stroke. In those patients with obesity and type 2 diabetes, weight reduction by caloric restriction is an important goal of the diet (see Chapter 29). Patients with type 1 diabetes or type 2 diabetes who take insulin should be taught "carbohydrate counting," so they can administer their insulin bolus for each meal based on its carbohydrate content.

The current recommendations for saturated fats and dietary cholesterol intake for people with diabetes are the same as for the general population. Saturated fats should be limited to less than 10% of daily calories and dietary cholesterol intake should be less than 300 mg/day. For those patients with kidney disease, dietary protein should be maintained at the recommended daily allowance of 0.8 g/kg/day. Exchange lists for meal planning can be obtained from the American Diabetes Association and its affiliate associations or from the American Dietetic Association (http://www.eatright.org), 216 W. Jackson Blvd., Chicago, IL 60606 (312-899-0040).

1. Dietary fiber—Plant components such as cellulose, gum, and pectin are indigestible by humans and are termed dietary "fiber." Insoluble fibers such as cellulose or hemicellulose, as found in bran, tend to increase intestinal transit and may have beneficial effects on colonic function. In contrast, soluble fibers such as gums and pectins, as found in beans, oatmeal, or apple skin, tend to retard nutrient absorption rates so that glucose absorption is slower and hyperglycemia may be slightly diminished. Although its recommendations do not include insoluble fiber supplements such as added bran, the ADA recommends food such as oatmeal, cereals, and beans with relatively high soluble fiber content as staple components of the diet . High soluble fiber content in the diet may also have a favorable effect on blood cholesterol levels.

2. Glycemic index—The glycemic index of a carbohydrate containing food is determined by comparing the glucose excursions after consuming 50 g of test food with glucose excursions after consuming 50 g of reference food (white bread):

$$\text{Glycemic index} = \frac{\text{Blood glucose area under the curve (3h) for test food}}{\text{Blood glucose area under the curve (3h) for reference food}} \times 100$$

Eating low glycemic index foods results in lower glucose levels after meals. Low glycemic index foods have values of 55 or less and include many fruits, vegetables, grainy breads, pasta, and legumes. High glycemic index foods have values of 70 or greater and include baked potato, white bread, and white rice. Glycemic index is lowered by the presence of fats and protein when food is consumed in a mixed meal. Even though it may not be possible to accurately predict the glycemic index of a particular food in the context of a meal, it is reasonable to choose foods with low glycemic index.

3. Artificial and other sweeteners—Saccharin (Sweet N Low), sucralose (Splenda), acesulfame potassium (Sweet One), and rebiana (Truvia) are "artificial" sweeteners that can be used in cooking and baking. Aspartame (NutraSweet) lacks heat stability, so it cannot be used in cooking. None of these sweeteners raise blood glucose levels.

Fructose represents a "natural" sugar substance that is a highly effective sweetener, induces only slight increases in plasma glucose levels, and does not require insulin for its metabolism. However, because of potential adverse effects of large amounts of fructose on raising serum cholesterol, triglycerides, and LDL cholesterol, it does not have any advantage as a sweetening agent in the diabetic diet. This does not preclude, however, ingestion of fructose-containing fruits and vegetables or fructose-sweetened foods in moderation.

Sugar alcohols, also known as polyols or polyalcohol, are commonly used as sweeteners and bulking agents. They occur naturally in a variety of fruits and vegetables but are also commercially made from sucrose, glucose, and starch. Examples are sorbitol, xylitol, mannitol, lactitol, isomalt, maltitol, and hydrogenated starch hydrolysates. They are not as easily absorbed as sugar, so they do not raise blood glucose levels as much. Therefore, sugar alcohols are often used in food products that are labeled as "sugar free," such as chewing gum, lozenges, hard candy, and sugar-free ice cream. However, if consumed in large quantities, they will raise blood glucose and can cause bloating and diarrhea.

B. Medications for Treating Hyperglycemia

The medications for treating type 2 diabetes are listed in Table 27–4.

1. Medications that primarily stimulate insulin secretion by binding to the sulfonylurea receptor on the beta cell—

A. SULFONYLUREAS—The primary mechanism of action of the sulfonylureas is to stimulate insulin release from pancreatic B cells and is used in patients with type 2 diabetes.

Table 27–4. Medications for treatment of type 2 diabetes mellitus (oral doses unless otherwise noted).

Drug	Tablet Size	Daily Dose	Duration of Action
Sulfonylureas			
Acetohexamide (Dymelor) (not available in United States)	250 and 500 mg	0.25–1.5 g as single dose or in two divided doses	8–24 hours
Chlorpropamide (Diabinese)	100 and 250 mg	0.1–0.5 g as single dose	24–72 hours
Gliclazide (not available in United States)	80 mg	40–80 mg as single dose; 160–320 mg as divided dose	12 hours
Glimepiride (Amaryl)	1, 2, and 4 mg	*Usual dose:* 1–4 mg once daily *Maximal dose:* 8 mg once daily	Up to 24 hours
Glipizide			
(Glucotrol)	5 and 10 mg	*Usual dose:* 2.5–10 mg twice daily 30 minutes before meals *Maximal dose:* 20 mg twice daily	6–12 hours
(Glucotrol XL)	2.5, 5, and 10 mg	*Usual dose:* 2.5–10 mg once daily *Maximal dose:* 20 mg once daily	Up to 24 hours
Glyburide			
(Dia Beta, Micronase)	1.25, 2.5, and 5 mg	1.25–20 mg as single dose or in two divided doses	Up to 24 hours
(Glynase)	1.5, 3, and 6 mg	1.5–12 mg as single dose or in two divided doses	Up to 24 hours
Tolazamide (Tolinase)	100, 250, and 500 mg	0.1–1 g as single dose or in two divided doses	Up to 24 hours
Tolbutamide (Orinase)	250 and 500 mg	0.5–2 g in two or three divided doses	6–10 hours
Meglitinide Analogs			
Mitiglinide (available in Japan)	5 and 10 mg	5 or 10 mg three times daily before meals	2 hours
Repaglinide (Prandin)	0.5, 1, and 2 mg	*Usual dose:* 0.5 to 4 mg three times daily 15 minutes before meals *Maximal dose:* 16 mg daily	3 hours
D-Phenylalanine Derivative			
Nateglinide (Starlix)	60 and 120 mg	60 or 120 mg three times daily before meals	4 hours
Biguanides			
Metformin (Glucophage)	500, 850, and 1000 mg	500–850 mg with meals two or three times daily; 850–1000 mg with breakfast and dinner	4 hours
Metformin, extended release (Glucophage XR)[1]	500, 750, and 1000 mg	500–2000 mg once daily	Up to 24 hours
Thiazolidinediones			
Pioglitazone (Actos)	15, 30, and 45 mg	15–45 mg daily	Up to 24 hours
Rosiglitazone (Avandia)	2, 4, and 8 mg	4–8 mg daily (can be divided)	Up to 24 hours
Alpha-Glucosidase Inhibitors			
Acarbose (Precose)	25, 50, and 100 mg	25–100 mg three times daily just before meals	4 hours
Miglitol (Glyset)	25, 50, and 100 mg	25–100 mg three times daily just before meals	4 hours
Voglibose (not available in United States)	0.2 and 0.3 mg	0.2–0.3 mg three times daily just before meals	4 hours
GLP-1 Receptor Agonists			
Dulaglutide (Trulicity)	0.75-, 1.5-mg single-dose pen or prefilled syringe	*Usual dose:* 0.75 mg subcutaneously once weekly *Maximal dose:* 1.5 mg subcutaneously once weekly	1 week
Exenatide (Byetta)	1.2 mL and 2.4 mL prefilled pens delivering 5 mcg and 10 mcg doses	5 mcg subcutaneously twice daily within 1 hour of breakfast and dinner. Increase to 10 mcg subcutaneously twice daily after about a month. **AVOID** if eGFR < 30 mL/minute/1.73 m^2	6 hours

(*continued*)

Table 27–4. Medications for treatment of type 2 diabetes mellitus (oral doses unless otherwise noted). (continued)

Drug	Tablet Size	Daily Dose	Duration of Action
Exenatide, long-acting release (Byetta LAR, Bydureon)	2 mg (powder)	Suspend in provided diluent and inject subcutaneously.	1 week
Liraglutide (Victoza)	Prefilled, multi-dose pens delivering 0.6 mg, 1.2 mg, or 1.8 mg	*Initial dose:* 0.6 mg subcutaneously once daily. Increase to 1.2 mg after a week if no adverse reactions. *Maximal dose:* 1.8 mg subcutaneously once daily	24 hours
Lixisenatide (Adlyxin, Lyxumia)	3-mL prefilled pens delivering 10 or 20 mcg	*Initial dose:* 10 mcg daily. Increase to 20 mcg daily after 2 weeks.	24 hours
Semaglutide (Ozempic, Rybelsus)	Prefilled pens delivering 0.25 mg, 0.5 mg, or 1 mg 1-, 3-, 7-, and 14-mg tablets	*Initial dose:* 0.25 mg weekly for 1 month and increase to 0.5 mg weekly if no adverse reactions. *Maximal dose:* 1 mg weekly *Initial dose:* 3 mg for 1 month and then increase to 7 mg. Take fasting daily with water and wait 30 minutes to eat. *Maximal dose:* 14 mg	1 week Daily
DPP-4 Inhibitors			
Alogliptin (Nesina)	6.25, 12.5, and 25 mg	25 mg once daily if eGFR ≥ 60 mL/minute/1.73 m^2; 12.5 mg daily if eGFR 30–59 mL/minute/1.73 m^2; 6.25 mg daily if eGFR < 30 mL/minute/1.73 m^2	24 hours
Linagliptin (Tradjenta)	5 mg	5 mg daily	24 hours
Saxagliptin (Onglyza)	2.5 and 5 mg	2.5 mg or 5 mg once daily if eGFR > 50 mL/minute/1.73 m^2. 2.5 mg daily if eGFR ≤ 50 mL/minute/1.73 m^2 or if also taking drugs that are strong CYP3A4/5 inhibitors such as ketoconazole	24 hours
Sitagliptin (Januvia)	25, 50, and 100 mg	100 mg once daily if eGFR > 50 mL/minute/1.73 m^2; 50 mg once daily if eGFR 30–50 mL/minute/1.73 m^2; 25 mg once daily if eGFR < 30 mL/minute/1.73 m^2	24 hours
Vildagliptin (Galvus) (not available in United States)	50 mg	50 mg once or twice daily. **AVOID** if eGFR ≤ 60 mL/minute/1.73 m^2 or AST/ALT three times upper limit of normal	24 hours
SGLT2 Inhibitors			
Canagliflozin (Invokana)	100 and 300 mg	*Usual dose:* 100 mg daily. 300 mg can be used if normal eGFR, resulting in lowering the HbA_{1c} an additional ~ 0.1–0.25%. **AVOID** if eGFR < 45 mL/minute/1.73 m^2	24 hours
Dapagliflozin (Farxiga)	5 and 10 mg	10 mg daily	24 hours
Empagliflozin (Jardiance)	10 and 25 mg	*Usual dose:* 10 mg daily *Maximal dose:* 25 mg	24 hours
Ertugliflozin (Steglatro)	5 and 15 mg	*Usual dose:* 5 mg daily *Maximal dose:* 15 mg	24 hours
Other			
Pramlintide (Symlin)	5-mL vial containing 0.6 mg/mL; also available as prefilled pens. Symlin pen 60 or Symlin pen 120	For insulin-treated type 2 patients, start at 60-mcg dose subcutaneously three times daily (10 units on U100 insulin syringe). Increase to 120 mcg three times daily (20 units on U100 insulin syringe) if no nausea for 3–7 days. Give immediately before meal. For type 1 patients, start at 15 mcg three times daily (2.5 units on U100 insulin syringe) and increase by increments of 15 mcg to a maximum of 60 mcg three times daily, as tolerated. To avoid hypoglycemia, lower insulin dose by 50% on initiation of therapy.	2 hours

They are metabolized by the liver, and apart from acetohexamide, whose metabolite is more active than the parent compound, the metabolites of all the other sulfonylureas are weakly active or inactive. The metabolites are excreted by the kidney and, in the case of the second-generation sulfonylureas, partly excreted in the bile.

Hypoglycemia is a common adverse reaction with the sulfonylureas. Weight gain is also common, especially in the first year of use. The mechanisms of the weight gain include improved glucose control and increased food intake in response to hypoglycemia. Idiosyncratic reactions are rare, with skin rashes or hematologic toxicity (leukopenia, thrombocytopenia) occurring in less than 0.1% of users.

(1) First-generation oral sulfonylureas (tolbutamide, tolazamide, acetohexamide, chlorpropamide)—Tolbutamide is probably best administered in divided doses (eg, 500 mg before each meal and at bedtime); however, some patients require only one or two tablets daily with a maximum dose of 3000 mg/day.

Because of its short duration of action (about 6–10 hours, which is independent of kidney function), tolbutamide is relatively safe to use in kidney disease. Prolonged hypoglycemia has been reported rarely with tolbutamide, mostly in patients receiving antibacterial sulfonamides (sulfisoxazole), or the oral azole antifungal medications to treat candidiasis.

Tolazamide, acetohexamide, and chlorpropamide are rarely used. Chlorpropamide has a prolonged biologic effect, and severe hypoglycemia can occur especially in older adults as their renal clearance declines with aging. Its other side effects include alcohol-induced flushing and hyponatremia due to increased vasopressin secretion and action.

(2) Second-generation sulfonylureas (glyburide, glipizide, gliclazide, glimepiride)—Glyburide, glipizide, gliclazide, and glimepiride are 100–200 times more potent than tolbutamide. These medications should be used with caution in patients with CVD or in older patients, in whom prolonged hypoglycemia would be especially dangerous.

The usual starting dose of **glyburide** is 2.5 mg/day, and the average maintenance dose is 5–10 mg/day given as a single morning dose; maintenance doses higher than 20 mg/day are not recommended. Glyburide is metabolized in the liver and the metabolic products have hypoglycemic activity. This probably explains why assays specific for the unmetabolized compound suggest a plasma half-life of only 1–2 hours, yet the biologic effects of glyburide are clearly persistent 24 hours after a single morning dose in patients with diabetes.

Glyburide can cause prolonged hypoglycemia and should not be used in older patients or in patients with liver failure or CKD. Flushing has rarely been reported after ethanol ingestion.

The recommended starting dose of glipizide is 5 mg/day, with up to 15 mg/day given as a single daily dose before breakfast. When higher daily doses are required, they should be divided and given before meals. The maximum recommended dose is 40 mg/day, although doses above 10–15 mg probably provide little additional benefit. For maximum effect in reducing postprandial hyperglycemia, glipizide should be ingested 30 minutes before meals, since rapid absorption is delayed when the medication is taken with food.

At least 90% of glipizide is metabolized in the liver to inactive products, and 10% is excreted unchanged in the urine. Glipizide therapy should therefore not be used in patients with liver failure. Because of its lower potency and shorter duration of action, it is preferable to glyburide in elderly patients and for those patients with kidney disease. Glucotrol-XL provides extended release of glipizide during transit through the GI tract with greater effectiveness in lowering prebreakfast hyperglycemia than the shorter-duration immediate-release standard glipizide tablets. However, this formulation appears to have sacrificed its lower propensity for severe hypoglycemia compared with longer-acting glyburide without showing any demonstrable therapeutic advantages over glyburide.

Gliclazide (not available in the United States) is another intermediate duration sulfonylurea with a duration of action of about 12 hours. The recommended starting dose is 40–80 mg/day with a maximum dose of 320 mg. Doses of 160 mg and above are given as divided doses before breakfast and dinner. The medication is metabolized by the liver; the metabolites and conjugates have no hypoglycemic effect. An extended-release preparation is available.

Glimepiride has a long duration of effect with a half-life of 5 hours allowing once or twice daily dosing. Glimepiride achieves blood glucose lowering with the lowest dose of any sulfonylurea compound. A single daily dose of 1 mg/day has been shown to be effective, and the maximal recommended dose is 8 mg. It is completely metabolized by the liver to relatively inactive metabolic products.

B. Meglitinide analogs—Repaglinide is structurally similar to glyburide but lacks the sulfonic acid-urea moiety. It acts by binding to the sulfonylurea receptor and closing the adenosine triphosphate (ATP)-sensitive potassium channel. It is rapidly absorbed from the intestine and then undergoes complete metabolism in the liver to inactive biliary products, giving it a plasma half-life of less than 1 hour. The medication therefore causes a brief but rapid pulse of insulin. The starting dose is 0.5 mg three times a day 15 minutes before each meal. The dose can be titrated to a maximum daily dose of 16 mg. Like the sulfonylureas, repaglinide can be used in combination with metformin. Hypoglycemia is the main side effect. Like the sulfonylureas, repaglinide causes weight gain. Metabolism is by cytochrome P450 3A4 isoenzyme, and other medications that induce or inhibit this isoenzyme may increase or inhibit (respectively) the metabolism of repaglinide. The medication may be useful in patients with kidney impairment or in older adults.

Mitiglinide is a benzylsuccinic acid derivative that binds to the sulfonylurea receptor and is similar to repaglinide in its clinical effects. It is approved for use in Japan.

C. D-phenylalanine derivative—Nateglinide stimulates insulin secretion by binding to the sulfonylurea receptor and closing the ATP-sensitive potassium channel. It is rapidly absorbed from the intestine, reaching peak plasma levels within 1 hour. It is metabolized in the liver and has a plasma half-life of about 1.5 hours. Like repaglinide, it causes a brief rapid pulse of insulin, and when given before a meal it reduces the postprandial rise in blood glucose. For most patients, the recommended starting and maintenance dose is 120 mg three times a day before meals. Use 60 mg in patients who have mild elevations in HbA_{1c}. Like the other insulin secretagogues, its main side effects are hypoglycemia and weight gain.

2. Medications that primarily lower glucose levels by their actions on the liver, muscle, and adipose tissue—

A. Metformin—Metformin is the first-line therapy for patients with type 2 diabetes. It can be used alone or in conjunction with other oral agents or insulin in the treatment of patients with type 2 diabetes. It is ineffective in patients with type 1 diabetes.

Metformin's therapeutic effects primarily derive from reducing hepatic gluconeogenesis. Metformin has a half-life of 1.5–3 hours and is not bound to plasma proteins or metabolized, being excreted unchanged by the kidneys.

Metformin use should be reassessed when the serum creatinine exceeds 130 mcmol/L (1.5 mg/dL) or the eGFR falls below 45 mL/minute/1.73 m^2. The medication should be stopped if the serum creatinine exceeds 150 mcmol/L (1.7 mg/dL) or the eGFR is below 30 mL/minute/1.73 m^2. Patients with liver failure or persons with excessive alcohol intake should not receive this medication because of the risk of lactic acidosis.

The maximum dosage of metformin is 2550 mg, although little benefit is seen above a total dose of 2000 mg. It is important to begin with a low dose and increase the dosage very gradually in divided doses—taken with meals—to reduce minor GI upsets (anorexia, nausea, vomiting, abdominal discomfort, diarrhea), which occur in up to 20% of patients. A common schedule would be one 500-mg tablet three times a day with meals or one 850- or 1000-mg tablet twice daily at breakfast and dinner. Up to 2000 mg of the extended-release preparation can be given once a day. Lower doses should be used in patients with eGFRs between 30 and 45 mL/minute/1.73 m^2 and in the older adults who are at higher risk for AKI from reduced renal functional reserve.

The GI side effects are dose-related, tend to occur at onset of therapy, and often are transient. However, in 3–5% of patients, therapy may have to be discontinued because of persistent diarrheal discomfort. Patients switching from immediate-release metformin to comparable dose of extended-release metformin may experience fewer GI side effects.

Hypoglycemia does not occur with therapeutic doses of metformin, which permits its description as a "euglycemic" or "antihyperglycemic" medication rather than an oral hypoglycemic agent. Dermatologic or hematologic toxicity is rare. Metformin interferes with the calcium dependent absorption of vitamin B_{12}-intrinsic complex in the terminal ileum; vitamin B_{12} deficiency can occur after many years of metformin use. *Periodic screening with vitamin B_{12} levels should be considered*, especially in patients with peripheral neuropathy (which may be erroneously attributed to diabetic neuropathy) or if a macrocytic anemia develops. Increased intake of dietary calcium may prevent the metformin-induced B_{12} malaborption.

Lactic acidosis has been reported as a side effect but is uncommon with metformin in contrast to phenformin. Almost all reported cases have involved persons with associated risk factors that should have contraindicated its use (kidney, liver, or cardiorespiratory insufficiency and alcoholism). AKI can occur rarely in patients taking metformin who receive radiocontrast agents. Metformin therapy should therefore be temporarily halted on the day of radiocontrast administration and restarted a day or two later after confirmation that kidney function has not deteriorated.

B. Thiazolidinediones—Two medications of this class, rosiglitazone and pioglitazone, are available for clinical use. These medications sensitize peripheral tissues to insulin. They bind the nuclear receptor peroxisome proliferator-activated receptor gamma (PPAR-gamma) and affect the expression of a number of genes. Like the biguanides, this class of medications does not cause hypoglycemia.

Both rosiglitazone and pioglitazone are effective as monotherapy and in combination with sulfonylureas or metformin or insulin, lowering HbA_{1c} by 1–2%. When used in combination with insulin, they can result in a 30–50% reduction in insulin dosage, and some patients can come off insulin completely. The oral dosage of rosiglitazone is 4–8 mg daily and of pioglitazone, 15–45 mg daily; the medications do not have to be taken with food. Rosiglitazone is primarily metabolized by the CYP 2C8 isoenzyme and pioglitazone is metabolized by CYP 2C8 and CYP 3A4.

The combination of a thiazolidinedione and metformin has the advantage of not causing hypoglycemia. Patients inadequately managed on sulfonylureas can do well on a combination of sulfonylurea and rosiglitazone or pioglitazone.

These medications have some additional effects apart from glucose lowering. Rosiglitazone therapy is associated with increases in total cholesterol, LDL cholesterol (15%), and HDL cholesterol (10%). There is a reduction in free fatty acids of about 8–15%. The changes in triglycerides are generally not different from placebo. Pioglitazone in clinical trials lowered triglycerides (9%) and increased HDL cholesterol (15%) but did not cause a consistent change in total cholesterol and LDL cholesterol levels. A prospective randomized comparison of the metabolic effects of pioglitazone and rosiglitazone showed similar effects on HbA_{1c} and weight gain. Small prospective studies have demonstrated that treatment with these medications leads to improvements in the biochemical and histologic features of nonalcoholic fatty liver disease. The thiazolidinediones also may limit vascular smooth muscle proliferation after injury, and there are reports that pioglitazone can reduce neointimal proliferation after coronary stent placement. In one double-blind, placebo-controlled study, rosiglitazone was shown to be associated with a decrease in the ratio of urinary albumin to creatinine excretion.

Safety concerns and some troublesome side effects limit the use of this class of medication.

Edema occurs in about 3–4% of patients receiving monotherapy with rosiglitazone or pioglitazone. The edema occurs more frequently (10–15%) in patients receiving concomitant insulin therapy and may result in heart failure. The medications are contraindicated in individuals with diabetes and New York Heart Association class III and IV cardiac status. Thiazolidinediones have also been reported as being associated with new-onset or worsening macular edema. Apparently, this is a rare side effect, and most of these patients also had peripheral edema. The macular edema resolved or improved once the medication was discontinued.

Troglitazone, the first medication in this class, was withdrawn from clinical use because of medication-associated fatal liver failure. Although rosiglitazone and pioglitazone have not been reported to cause liver injury, the FDA recommends that they should not be used in patients with clinical evidence of active liver disease or pretreatment elevation of the ALT level that is 2.5 times greater than the upper limit of normal. Liver biochemical tests should be performed on all patients prior to initiation of treatment and periodically thereafter.

An increase in fracture risk in women (but not men) has been reported with both rosiglitazone and pioglitazone. The fracture risk is in the range of 1.9 per 100 patient-years with the thiazolidinedione as opposed to 1.1 per 100 patient-years on comparison treatment. In at least one study of rosiglitazone, the fracture risk was increased in premenopausal as well as postmenopausal women.

Other side effects include anemia, which occurs in 4% of patients treated with these medications; it may be due to a dilutional effect of increased plasma volume rather than a reduction in red cell mass. Weight gain occurs, especially when the medication is combined with a sulfonylurea or insulin. Some of the weight gain is fluid retention, but there is also an increase in total fat mass. Clinical studies have reported conflicting results regarding an association of bladder cancer with pioglitazone use. A 10-year observational cohort study of patients taking pioglitazone failed to find an association with bladder cancer. A large multipopulation pooled analysis (1.01 million persons over 5.9 million person-years) also failed to find an association between cumulative exposure of pioglitazone or rosiglitazone and incidence of bladder cancer. Another population-based study, however, generating 689,616 person-years of follow-up did find that pioglitazone but not rosiglitazone was associated with an increased risk of bladder cancer.

3. Medications that affect absorption of glucose—Alpha-glucosidase inhibitors competitively inhibit the alpha-glucosidase enzymes in the gut that digest dietary starch and sucrose. Two of these medications—acarbose and miglitol—are available for clinical use in the United States. Voglibose, another alpha-glucosidase inhibitor, is available in Japan, Korea, and India. Acarbose and miglitol are potent inhibitors of glucoamylase, alpha-amylase, and sucrase but have less effect on isomaltase and hardly any on trehalase and lactase.

A. Acarbose—The recommended starting dose of acarbose is 50 mg orally twice daily, gradually increasing to 100 mg three times daily. For maximal benefit on postprandial hyperglycemia, acarbose should be given with the first mouthful of food ingested. In patients with diabetes, acorbose reduces postprandial hyperglycemia by 30–50%, and its overall effect is to lower the HbA_{1c} by 0.5–1%.

The principal adverse effect, seen in 20–30% of patients, is flatulence. In 3% of cases, troublesome diarrhea occurs. This GI discomfort tends to discourage excessive carbohydrate consumption and promotes improved compliance of patients with type 2 diabetes with their diet prescriptions. When acarbose is given alone, there is no risk of hypoglycemia. However, if combined with insulin or sulfonylureas, it might increase the risk of hypoglycemia from these agents. A slight rise in hepatic aminotransferases has been noted in clinical trials with acarbose (5% vs 2% in placebo controls, and particularly with doses greater than 300 mg/day). The levels generally return to normal on stopping the medication.

B. Miglitol—Miglitol is similar to acarbose in terms of its clinical effects. It is indicated for use in diet- or sulfonylurea-treated patients with type 2 diabetes. Therapy is initiated at the lowest effective dosage of 25 mg orally three times a day. The usual maintenance dose is 50 mg three times a day, although some patients may benefit from increasing the dose to 100 mg three times a day. GI side effects occur as with acarbose. The medication is not metabolized and is excreted unchanged by the kidney. Miglitol should not be used in ESKD, when its clearance would be impaired.

4. Incretins—Oral glucose provokes a threefold to fourfold higher insulin response than an equivalent dose of glucose given intravenously. This is because the oral glucose causes a release of gut hormones, principally glucagon-like peptide 1 (GLP-1) and glucose-dependent insulinotropic polypeptide (GIP1), that amplify the glucose-induced insulin release. This "incretin effect" of GLP-1 secretion (but not GIP1 secretion) is reduced in patients with type 2 diabetes; when GLP-1 is infused in patients with type 2 diabetes, it stimulates insulin secretion and lowers glucose levels. GLP-1, unlike the sulfonylureas, has only a modest insulin stimulatory effect at normoglycemic concentrations. This means that GLP-1 has a lower risk for hypoglycemia than the sulfonylureas.

In addition to its insulin stimulatory effect, GLP-1 has a number of other pancreatic and extrapancreatic effects. It suppresses glucagon secretion and so may ameliorate the hyperglucagonemia that is present in people with diabetes and improve postprandial hyperglycemia. GLP-1 acts on the stomach, delaying gastric emptying; the importance of this effect on glucose lowering is illustrated by the observation that antagonizing the deceleration of gastric emptying markedly reduces the glucose lowering effect of GLP-1. GLP-1 receptors are present in the CNS and may play a role in the anorectic effect of the drugs. Patients with type 2 diabetes undergoing GLP-1 infusion are less hungry; it is unclear whether this is mainly due to a deceleration of gastric emptying or whether there is a CNS effect as well.

A. GLP-1 receptor agonists—GLP-1's half-life is only 1–2 minutes. It is rapidly proteolyzed by dipeptidyl peptidase 4 (DPP-4) and by other enzymes, such as endopeptidase 24.11, and is also cleared quickly by the kidney. The native peptide, therefore, cannot be used therapeutically. Five GLP-1 receptor agonists with longer half-lives, exenatide, liraglutide, dulaglutide, lixisenatide, and semaglutide, are available for clinical use. Tirzepatide, a dual GLP-1 and GIP receptor agonist, has been reported in a large clinical trial of patients with type 2 diabetes to reduce weight and improve glucose control.

Exenatide (Exendin 4) is a GLP-1 receptor agonist isolated from the saliva of the Gila monster (a venomous lizard) that is more resistant to DPP-4 action and cleared by the kidney. Its half-life is 2.4 hours, and its glucose lowering effect is about 6 hours. Exenatide is dispensed as two fixed-dose pens (5 mcg and 10 mcg). It is injected 60 minutes before breakfast and before dinner. Patients with type 2 diabetes should be prescribed the 5 mcg pen for the first month and, if tolerated, the dose can then be increased to 10 mcg twice a day. The medication is not recommended in patients with eGFR less than 30 mL/minute/1.73 m^2. In clinical trials, adding exenatide therapy to patients with type 2 diabetes already taking metformin or a sulfonylurea, or both, further lowered the HbA_{1c} value by 0.4% to 0.6% over a 30-week period. These patients also experienced a weight loss of 3–6 pounds. Exenatide LAR is a once-weekly preparation that is dispensed as a powder (2 mg). It is suspended in the provided diluent just prior to injection. In comparative clinical trials, the long-acting drug lowers the HbA_{1c} level a little more than the twice daily drug. Low-titer antibodies against exenatide develop in over one-third (38%) of patients, but the clinical effects are not attenuated. High-titer antibodies develop in a subset of patients (~6%), and in about half of these cases, an attenuation of glycemic response has been seen.

Liraglutide is a soluble fatty acid acylated GLP-1 analog. The half-life is approximately 12 hours, allowing the medication to be injected once a day. The dosing is initiated at 0.6 mg daily, increased after 1 week to 1.2 mg daily. Some patients may benefit from increasing the dose to 1.8 mg. In clinical trials lasting 26 and 52 weeks, adding liraglutide to the therapeutic regimen (metformin, sulfonylurea, thiazolidinedione) of patients with type 2 diabetes further lowered the HbA_{1c} value. Depending on the dose and design of the study, the HbA_{1c} decline was in the range of 0.6% to 1.5%. The patients had sustained weight loss of 1–6 pounds. Liraglutide at a dose of 3 mg daily has been approved for weight loss.

In a postmarketing multinational study of 9340 patients with type 2 diabetes with known CVD, the addition of liraglutide was associated with a lower primary composite outcome of death from cardiovascular causes, nonfatal MI, or nonfatal stroke (hazard ratio 0.87, $P = 0.01$). Patients taking liraglutide had lower HbA_{1c} levels, weight loss of 2.3 kg, lower systolic blood pressure, and fewer episodes of severe hypoglycemia.

Dulaglutide consists of two GLP-1 analog molecules covalently linked to an Fc fragment of human IgG_4. The GLP-1 molecule has amino acid substitutions that resist DPP-4 action. The half-life of dulaglutide is about 5 days. The usual dose is 0.75 mg weekly by subcutaneous injection. The maximum recommended dose is 1.5 mg weekly. Dulaglutide monotherapy and combination therapy lowers HbA_{1c} by about 0.7% to 1.6%. Weight loss ranged from 2 pounds to 7 pounds.

Lixisenatide is a synthetic analog of exendin 4 (deletion of a proline and addition of 6 lysines to the C-terminal region) with a half-life of 3 hours. It is dispensed as two fixed-dose pens (10 mcg and 20 mcg). The 10-mcg dose is injected once daily before breakfast for the first 2 weeks, and if tolerated, the dose is then increased to 20 mcg daily. Its clinical effect is about the same as exenatide with HbA_{1c} lowering in the 0.4–0.6% range. Weight loss ranges from 2 pounds to 6 pounds. Antibodies to lixisenatide occur frequently (70%) and ~2.4% with the highest antibody titers have attenuated glycemic response.

Semaglutide is a synthetic analog of GLP-1 with a drug half-life of about 1 week. It has an alpha-aminoisobutyric acid substitution at position 8 that makes the molecule resistant to DPP4 action and a C-18 fatty di-acid chain attached to lysine at position 26 that binds to albumin, which accounts for the drug's long half-life. Semaglutide is dispensed either subcutaneously or orally. There are two pens for subcutaneous injection: one pen delivers a 0.25-mg or 0.5-mg dose and the other pen delivers a 1-mg dose. The recommended dosing is 0.25 mg weekly for 4 weeks and if tolerated the dose is then increased to 0.5 mg per week. The 1-mg per week dose can provide additional glucose lowering effect. Semaglutide monotherapy and combination therapy lowers HbA_{1c} from 1.5% to 1.8%.

Oral semaglutide is co-formulated with sodium N-[8 (2-hydroxylbenzoyl) amino] caprylate, which results in a complex that is more lipophilic and resistant to proteolysis The patient must take oral semaglutide fasting with a glass of water and then wait half an hour before eating, drinking, or taking other medicines. The recommended starting dose is 3 mg daily for the first month, with the dose increased to 7–14 mg daily as tolerated and as needed for glucose control.

Side effects—The most frequent adverse reactions of the GLP-1 receptor agonists are nausea (11–40%), vomiting (4–13%), and diarrhea (9–17%). The reactions are more frequent at the higher doses. In clinical trials about 1–5% of participants withdrew from the studies because of the GI symptoms.

The GLP-1 receptor agonists have been associated with increased risk of pancreatitis. The pancreatitis was severe (hemorrhagic or necrotizing) in 6 instances, and 2 of these patients died. In the liraglutide and dulaglutide clinical trials, there were 13 and 5 cases of pancreatitis in the drug-treated groups versus 1 and 1 case in the comparator groups, respectively. This translates to about 1.4–2.2 vs 0.6–0.9 cases of pancreatitis per 1000 patient-years. *Patients taking GLP-1 receptor agonists should be advised to seek immediate medical care if they experience unexplained persistent severe abdominal pain.*

There have been rare reports of AKI in patients taking exenatide. Some of these patients had preexisting kidney disease, and others had one or more risk factors for kidney disease. A number of the patients reported nausea, vomiting, and diarrhea, and it is possible that these side effects caused volume depletion and contributed to the development of the kidney injury. Liraglutide, semaglutide, and dulaglutide are metabolized by proteolysis and are preferred choices in patients with kidney failure.

GLP-1 receptor agonists stimulate C-cell neoplasia and cause medullary thyroid carcinoma in rats. Human C-cells express very few GLP-1 receptors, and the relevance to human therapy is unclear. The medications, however, should not be used in patients with personal or family history of medullary thyroid carcinoma or multiple endocrine neoplasia (MEN) syndrome type 2.

B. DPP-4 INHIBITORS—An alternate approach to the use of GLP-1 receptor agonists is to inhibit the enzyme DPP-4 and prolong the action of endogenously released GLP-1 and GIP. Four oral DPP-4 inhibitors, sitagliptin, saxagliptin, linagliptin, and alogliptin, are available in the United States for the treatment of type 2 diabetes. An additional DPP-4 inhibitor, vildagliptin, is available in Europe. Other DPP-4 inhibitors—gemigliptin, anagliptin, teneligliptin, trelagliptin, omarigliptin, evogliptin, and gosogliptin—have been approved outside the United States and European Union (Korea, India, Thailand, Japan, Russia, and several South American countries).

Sitagliptin, when used alone or in combination with other diabetes medications, lowers HbA_{1c} by approximately 0.5%. The usual dose is 100 mg once daily, but the dose is reduced to 50 mg daily if the calculated creatinine clearance is 30–50 mL/minute and to 25 mg for clearances less than 30 mL/minute. **Saxagliptin**, when added to the therapeutic regimen (metformin, sulfonylurea, thiazolidinedione) of patients with type 2 diabetes, further lowered the HbA_{1c} value by about 0.7–0.9%. The dose is 2.5 mg or 5 mg orally once a day. The 2.5-mg dose should be used in patients with eGFR less than 50 mL/minute/1.73 m^2.

Alogliptin lowers HbA_{1c} by about 0.5–0.6% when added to metformin, sulfonylurea, or pioglitazone. The usual dose is 25 mg orally daily. The 12.5-mg dose is used in patients with eGFR of 30–60 mL/minute/1.73 m^2; and 6.25 mg for clearance less than 30 mL/minute/1.73 m^2. **Linagliptin** lowers HbA_{1c} by about 0.4–0.6% when added to metformin, sulfonylurea, or pioglitazone. The dose is 5 mg orally daily, and since, it is primarily excreted unmetabolized via the bile, no dose adjustment is needed in patients with kidney disease. **Vildagliptin** lowers HbA_{1c} by about 0.5–1% when added to the therapeutic regimen of patients with type 2 diabetes. The dose is 50 mg once or twice daily.

Side effects—The main adverse effect of DPP-4 inhibitors appears to be a predisposition to nasopharyngitis or upper respiratory tract infection. Hypersensitivity reactions, including anaphylaxis, angioedema, and exfoliative skin conditions (such as Stevens-Johnson syndrome), have been reported. There have also been reports of pancreatitis, but the frequency of the event is unclear. Cases of liver failure have been reported with the use of alogliptin, but it is uncertain if alogliptin was the cause. The medication, however, should be discontinued in the event of liver failure. Rare cases of hepatic dysfunction, including hepatitis, have been reported with the use of vildagliptin; and liver biochemical testing is recommended quarterly during the first year of use and periodically thereafter. Saxagliptin may increase the risk of heart failure. In a post-marketing study of 16,492 patients with type 2 diabetes, heart failure occurred in 3.5% in the saxagliptin group and 2.8% in the placebo group (hazard ratio 1.27). Patients with the highest risk of heart failure were those who had a history of heart failure or had elevated levels of N-terminal of the prohormone BNP (NT-pBNP) or had kidney impairment. In a large post-marketing study, alogliptin, like saxagliptin, was associated with a slightly increased rate of heart failure. The FDA has issued a warning that the DPP-4 inhibitors can occasionally cause joint pains that resolve after stopping the drug.

5. Sodium-glucose co-transporter 2 inhibitors—Glucose is freely filtered by the kidney glomeruli and is reabsorbed in the proximal tubules by the action of sodium-glucose co-transporters (SGLT). Sodium-glucose co-transporter 2 (SGLT2) accounts for about 90% of glucose reabsorption and its inhibition causes glycosuria in people with diabetes, lowering plasma glucose levels. The oral SGLT2 inhibitors canagliflozin, dapagliflozin, empagliflozin, and ertugliflozin are approved for clinical use in the United States. Sotagliflozn is a combined SGLT2 and SGLT1 inhibitor that is available in Europe for use in persons with type 1 diabetes. These agents reduce the threshold for glycosuria from a plasma glucose threshold of about a 180 mg/dL to about 40 mg/dL; and lower HbA_{1c} by 0.5–1% when used alone or in combination with other oral agents or insulin. The efficacy is higher at higher HbA_{1c} levels when more glucose is excreted as a result of SGLT2 inhibition. The loss of calories results in modest weight loss of 2–5 kg.

Canagliflozin is dosed at 100 mg daily but up to 300 mg daily can be used in patients with normal kidney function. The dose of **dapagliflozin** is 10 mg daily but 5 mg daily is the recommended initial dose in patients with hepatic failure. The usual dosage of **empagliflozin** is 10 mg daily but a higher dose of 25 mg daily can be used. The recommended starting dose of **ertugliflozin** is 5 mg, but the dose can be increased to 15 mg daily if additional glucose lowering is needed.

Empagliflozin was evaluated in a multinational study of 7020 patients with type 2 diabetes with known CVD; the addition of empagliflozin was associated with a lower primary composite outcome of death from cardiovascular causes, nonfatal MI, or nonfatal stroke (hazard ratio 0.86, $P = 0.04$). The mechanisms regarding the benefit remain unclear. Weight loss, lower blood pressure, and diuresis may have played a role since there were fewer deaths from heart failure in the treated group whereas the rates of MI were unaltered. A similar multinational study was performed with the addition of canagliflozin. This was a study of 10,142 patients with type 2 diabetes with known or at increased risk for CVD. The canagliflozin treated group had a lower primary composite outcome of death from cardiovascular causes, nonfatal MI, or nonfatal stroke (hazard ratio 0.86, $P = 0.02$). In a 2019 heart failure study of 4744 patients with NYHA class II, III, or IV heart failure and EF of less 40%, dapagliflozin reduced the cumulative incidence of worsening heart failure or cardiovascular death (hazard ratio 0.74, $P < 0.001$). Forty-two percent of the patients had diabetes; the findings in patients with and without diabetes were the same. Both empagliflozin and canagliflozin show benefit in terms of progression of albuminuria and kidney injury, possibly by lowering glomerular hyperfiltration. In a 2019 multinational study of 4401 patients with type 2 diabetes and albuminuric CKD (eGFR 30–89 mL/minute/1.73 m^2 with albumin [mg] to creatinine [g] ratio > 300 to 5000) and taking an ACE inhibitor or angiotensin receptor blocker, canagliflozin reduced the risk of ESKD, the doubling of serum creatinine, and of renal death. In a 2020 multinational study of 4304 patients with CKD, dapagliflozin reduced the risk of ESKD or death from renal and cardiovascular causes. A third of the patients in the study did not have diabetes and had benefit.

Side effects—As might be expected, the efficacy of the SGLT2 inhibitors is reduced in CKD. They can also increase creatinine and decrease eGFR, especially in patients with kidney impairment. Their use is generally not recommended in patients with eGFR less than 45 mL/minute/1.73 m^2 and are contraindicated in patients with eGFR less than 30 mL/minute/1.73 m^2. The study of dapagliflozin in CKD, however, noted that the drug is safe and beneficial in patients with eGFR as low as 25 mL/minute/1.73 m^2. The main side effects are increased incidence of genital mycotic infections and UTIs affecting ~8–9% of patients. Cases of necrotizing fasciitis of the perineum (Fournier gangrene) have been reported. There have also been reports of cases of pyelonephritis and septicemia requiring hospitalization. The glycosuria can cause intravascular volume contraction and hypotension.

One multinational study with canagliflozin showed an increased risk of amputations, especially of the toes (hazard ratio 1.97). This finding has not been observed in other studies of this drug or with other SGLT2 inhibitors.

Canagliflozin causes a decrease in bone mineral density at the lumbar spine and the hip. In a pooled analysis of eight clinical trials (mean duration 68 weeks), a 30% increase in fractures was observed in patients taking canagliflozin. All SGLT2 inhibitors cause a modest increase in LDL cholesterol levels (3–8%).

Cases of DKA have been reported with off-label use of SGLT2 inhibitors in patients with type 1 diabetes. Type 1 patients are taught to give less insulin if their glucose levels are not elevated. SGLT2 inhibitors lower glucose levels by changing the renal threshold and not by insulin action. Type 1 patients taking an SGLT2 inhibitor, because the glucose levels are not elevated, may either withhold or reduce their insulin doses to such a degree as to induce ketoacidosis. *SGLT2 inhibitors should not be used in patients with type 1 diabetes and in those patients labeled as having type 2 diabetes but who are very insulin deficient and ketosis-prone.*

6. Others—Pramlintide is a synthetic analog of islet amyloid polypeptide (IAPP or amylin). When given subcutaneously, it delays gastric emptying, suppresses glucagon secretion, and decreases appetite. It is approved for use both in type 1 diabetes and in insulin-treated type 2 diabetes. In 6-month clinical studies with type 1 and insulin-treated type 2 patients, those taking the medication had an approximately 0.4% reduction in HbA_{1c} and about 1.7 kg weight loss compared with placebo. The HbA_{1c} reduction was sustained for 2 years but some of the weight was regained. The medication is given by injection immediately before the meal. Hypoglycemia can occur, and it is recommended that the short-acting or premixed insulin doses be reduced by 50% when the medication is started. Since the medication slows gastric emptying, recovery from hypoglycemia can be a problem because of delay in absorption of fast-acting carbohydrates. Nausea is the other main side effect, affecting 30–50% of persons, but tends to improve with time. In patients with type 1 diabetes, the initial dose of pramlintide is 15 mcg before each meal and titrated up by 15-mcg increments to a maintenance dose of 30 mcg or 60 mcg before each meal. In patients with type 2 diabetes, the starting dose is 60 mcg premeals increased to 120 mcg in 3 to 7 days if no significant nausea occurs.

Bromocriptine, a dopamine 2 receptor agonist, has been shown to modestly lower HbA_{1c} by 0.1–0.5% when compared to baseline and 0.4–0.5% compared to placebo. Common side effects are nausea, vomiting, dizziness, and headache.

Colesevelam, the bile acid sequestrant, when added to metformin or sulfonylurea or insulin, lowered HbA_{1c} 0.3–0.4% when compared to baseline and 0.5–0.6% compared to placebo. HbA_{1c} lowering, however, was not observed in a single monotherapy clinical trial comparing colesevelam to placebo. Colesevelam use is associated with ~20% increase in triglyceride levels. Other adverse effects include constipation and dyspepsia.

With their modest glucose lowering and significant side effects, using bromocriptine or colesevelam to treat diabetes is not recommended.

7. Medication combinations—Several medication combinations are available in different dose sizes, including glyburide and metformin (Glucovance); glipizide and metformin (Metaglip); repaglinide and metformin (PrandiMet); rosiglitazone and metformin (Avandamet); pioglitazone and metformin (ACTOplusMet); rosiglitazone and glimepiride (Avandaryl); pioglitazone and glimepiride (Duetact); sitagliptin and metformin (Janumet); saxagliptin and metformin XR (Kombiglyze XR); linagliptin and metformin (Jentadueto); alogliptin and metformin (Kazano); alogliptin and pioglitazone (Oseni); dapagliflozin and metformin (Xigduo); canagliflozin and metformin (Invokamet); empagliflozin and metformin (Synjardy); empagliflozin and linagliptin (Glyxambi); empagliflozin, linagliptin, and metformin (Trijardy); ertugliflozin and metformin (Segluormet); ertugliflozin and sitagliptin (Steglujan); insulin degludec and liraglutide (Xultophy); and insulin glargine and lixisenatide (Soliqua). These medication combinations, however, limit the clinician's ability to optimally adjust dosage of the individual medications and for that reason are not recommended.

C. Insulin

Insulin is indicated for patients with type 1 diabetes as well as for patients with type 2 diabetes with insulinopenia whose hyperglycemia does not respond to diet therapy

Table 27–5. Summary of bioavailability characteristics of the insulins.

Insulin Preparations[1]	Onset of Action	Peak Action	Effective Duration
Insulins lispro, aspart,[2,3] glulisine	5–15 minutes	1–1.5 hours	3–4 hours
Human regular	30–60 minutes	2 hours	6–8 hours
Human NPH	2–4 hours	6–7 hours	10–20 hours
Insulin glargine	0.5–1 hour	Flat	~24 hours
Insulin detemir	0.5–1 hour	Flat	17 hours
Insulin degludec	0.5–1.5 hours	Flat	More than 42 hours
Technosphere inhaled insulin	5–15 minutes	1 hour	3 hours

[1]Insulin administered subcutaneously unless otherwise noted.
[2]Insulin aspart formulated with niacinamide (FiAsp) has an ~10-minute faster onset of action.
[3]Insulin lispro formulated with treprostinil and citrate (Lyumjev, lispro-aabc) has an 11-minute faster onset of action.

either alone or combined with other hypoglycemic medications.

1. Characteristics of available insulin preparations— Human insulin is dispensed as either regular (R) or NPH (N) formulations. Six analogs of human insulin—three rapidly acting (insulin lispro, insulin aspart, insulin glulisine) and three long-acting (insulin glargine, insulin detemir, and insulin degludec)—are available for clinical use. Insulin preparations differ with respect to the time of onset and duration of their biologic action (Table 27–5). All currently available insulins contain less than 10 ppm of proinsulin and are labeled as "purified." These purified insulins preserve their potency, so that refrigeration is recommended but not crucial. During travel, reserve supplies of insulin can be readily transported for weeks without losing potency if protected from extremes of heat or cold. All the insulins in the United States are available in a concentration of 100 U/mL (U100) and dispensed in 10-mL vials or 0.3-mL cartridges or prefilled disposable pens.

2. Insulin preparations— See Table 27–6. The rapidly acting insulin analogs and the long-acting insulins are designed for subcutaneous administration, while regular insulin and insulin aspart can also be given intravenously.

A. Short-acting insulin preparations—

(1) Regular insulin—Regular insulin is a short-acting soluble crystalline zinc insulin whose effect appears within 30 minutes after subcutaneous injection and lasts 5–7 hours when usual quantities are administered. Intravenous infusions of regular insulin are particularly useful in the treatment of DKA and during the perioperative management of patients with diabetes who require insulin. For markedly insulin-resistant persons who would otherwise require large volumes of insulin solution, a U500 preparation of human regular insulin is available both in a vial form and a disposable pen. A U500 insulin syringe should be used if the vial form is dispensed. U500 regular insulin is much more expensive than the U100 concentration and is rarely needed.

(2) Rapidly acting insulin analogs—Insulin lispro (Humalog, Admelog) is an insulin analog where the proline at position B28 is reversed with the lysine at B29. Insulin aspart (Novolog) is a single substitution of proline by aspartic acid at position B28. In insulin glulisine (Apidra) the asparagine at position B3 is replaced by lysine and the lysine in position B29 by glutamic acid. These three analogs have less of a tendency to form hexamers, in contrast to human insulin. When injected subcutaneously, the analogs quickly dissociate into monomers and are absorbed very rapidly, reaching peak serum values in as soon as 1 hour—in contrast to regular human insulin, whose hexamers require considerably more time to dissociate and

Table 27–6. Insulin preparations available in the United States.[1]

Rapidly acting human insulin analogs
- Insulin lispro (Humalog, Lyumjev, Lilly; Admelog, Sanofi)
- Insulin aspart (Novolog, FiAsp, Novo Nordisk)
- Insulin glulisine (Apidra, Sanofi Aventis)

Short-acting regular insulin
- Regular insulin (Lilly, Novo Nordisk)
- Technosphere inhaled regular insulin (Afrezza)

Intermediate-acting insulins
- NPH insulin (Lilly, Novo Nordisk)

Premixed insulins
- 70% NPH/30% regular (70/30 insulin—Lilly, Novo Nordisk)
- 75% NPL/25% insulin lispro (Humalog Mix 75/25—Lilly)
- 50% NPL/50% insulin lispro (Humalog Mix 50/50—Lilly)
- 70% insulin aspart protamine/30% insulin aspart (Novolog Mix 70/30—Novo Nordisk)
- 70% insulin degludec/30 insulin aspart (Ryzodeg, Novo Nordisk)

Long-acting human insulin analogs
- Insulin glargine (Lantus [U100], Toujeo [U300], Sanofi Aventis; Basaglar [U100], Lilly)
- Insulin detemir (Levemir, Novo Nordisk)
- Insulin degludec (Tresiba, Novo Nordisk)

[1]All insulins available in the United States are recombinant human or human insulin analog origin. All the above insulins are dispensed at U100 concentration. There is an additional U500 preparation of regular insulin; U300 preparation of insulin glargine; U200 preparation of insulin lispro; and U200 preparation of insulin degludec. NPH, neutral protamine Hagedorn.

become absorbed. The amino acid changes in these analogs do not interfere with their binding to the insulin receptor, with the circulating half-life, or with their immunogenicity, which are all identical with that of human regular insulin. An insulin aspart formulation (FiAsp) that contains niacinamide (vitamin B_3) has a more rapid initial absorption and its onset of action is about 10 minutes faster than the standard insulin aspart formulation. Because of this more rapid onset of action, the 1-hour (but not 2-hour) postprandial glucose excursions are lower compared to the standard formulation. Similarly, an insulin lispro formulation (Lyumjev) containing trepostinil to induce local vasodilation and citrate to increase vascular permeability has 11 minutes faster onset of action and lower 1- and 2-hour postprandial glucose excursions compared to the standard insulin lispro formulation.

Clinical trials have demonstrated that the optimal times of preprandial subcutaneous injection of comparable doses of the rapidly acting insulin analogs and of regular human insulin are 20 minutes and 60 minutes, respectively, before the meal. The quicker onset of action with the rapidly acting insulin analogs allows the patient to inject insulin 15–20 minutes before eating rather than wait for 60 minutes as needed for regular insulin. Another desirable feature of rapidly acting insulin analogs is that their duration of action remains at about 4 hours for most commonly used dosages. This contrasts with regular insulin, whose duration of action is significantly prolonged when larger doses are used.

The rapidly acting analogs are commonly used in pumps. In a double-blind crossover study comparing insulin lispro with regular insulin in insulin pumps, persons using insulin lispro had lower HbA_{1c} values and improved postprandial glucose control with the same frequency of hypoglycemia. In the event of pump failure, however, users of the rapidly acting insulin analogs will have more rapid onset of hyperglycemia and ketosis.

While insulin aspart has been approved for intravenous use (eg, in hyperglycemic emergencies), there is no advantage in using insulin aspart over regular insulin by this route. A U200 concentration of insulin lispro is available in a disposable prefilled pen. The only advantage of the U200 over the U100 insulin lispro preparation is that it delivers the same dose in half the volume.

B. Long-Acting Insulin Preparations—

(1) NPH (neutral protamine Hagedorn or isophane) insulin—NPH is an intermediate-acting insulin whose onset of action is delayed to 2–4 hours, and its peak response is generally reached in about 6–7 hours. The onset of action is delayed by combining 2 parts soluble crystalline zinc insulin with 1 part protamine zinc insulin. This produces equivalent amounts of insulin and protamine, so that neither is present in an uncomplexed form ("isophane"). Because its duration of action is often less than 24 hours (with a range of 10–20 hours), most patients require at least two injections daily to maintain a sustained insulin effect. Occasional vials of NPH insulin have tended to show unusual clumping of their contents or "frosting" of the container, with considerable loss of bioactivity. This instability is rare and occurs less frequently if NPH human insulin is refrigerated when not in use and if bottles are discarded after 1 month of use.

(2) Insulin glargine—In this insulin, the asparagine at position 21 of the insulin A chain is replaced by glycine and two arginines are added to the carboxyl terminal of the B chain. The arginines raise the isoelectric point of the molecule closer to neutral, making it more soluble in an acidic environment. In contrast, human insulin has an isoelectric point of pH 5.4. Insulin glargine is a clear insulin, which, when injected into the neutral pH environment of the subcutaneous tissue, forms microprecipitates that slowly release the insulin into the circulation. This insulin lasts for about 24 hours without any pronounced peaks and is given once a day to provide basal coverage. This insulin cannot be mixed with the other human insulins because of its acidic pH. When this insulin was given as a single injection at bedtime to type 1 patients in clinical trials, fasting hyperglycemia was better controlled with less nocturnal hypoglycemia when compared to NPH insulin.

A more concentrated form of insulin glargine (U300) is available as an insulin pen. In clinical trials in type 1 patients, U300 use did not result in better control or reduce the rates of hypoglycemia. Although limited clinical data suggest that insulin glargine is safe in pregnancy, it is not approved for this use.

(3) Insulin detemir—In this insulin analog, the threonine at position B30 has been removed and a 14-C fatty acid chain (tetradecanoic acid) is attached to the lysine at position 29 by acylation. Its prolonged action is due to dihexamerization and binding of hexamers and dimers to albumin at the injection site as well as binding of the monomer via its fatty acid side chain to albumin in the circulation. The affinity of insulin detemir is fourfold to fivefold lower than that of human soluble insulin and therefore the U100 formulation of insulin detemir has an insulin concentration of 2400 nmol/mL compared with 600 nmol/mL for NPH. The duration of action for insulin detemir is about 17 hours at therapeutically relevant doses. It is recommended that the insulin be injected once or twice a day to achieve a stable basal coverage. It has been approved for use during pregnancy.

(4) Insulin degludec—In this insulin analog, the threonine at position B30 has been removed, and the lysine at position B29 is conjugated to hexdecanoic acid via a gamma-L-glutamyl spacer. In the vial, in the presence of phenol and zinc, the insulin is in the form of dihexamers but when injected subcutaneously, it self associates into large multihexameric chains consisting of thousands of dihexamers. The chains slowly dissolves in the subcutaneous tissue and insulin monomers are steadily released into the systemic circulation. The half-life of insulin degludec is 25 hours. Its onset of action is in 30–90 minutes and its duration of action is more than 42 hours. It is recommended that the insulin be injected once or twice a day to achieve a stable basal coverage. Insulin degludec is available in two concentrations, U100 and U200, and dispensed in prefilled disposable pens.

(5) Insulin icodec—This is an insulin analog that is suitable for once weekly injection and is in phase 3 clinical trials.

c. Mixed insulin preparations—Patients with type 2 diabetes can sometimes achieve reasonable glucose control with just prebreakfast and predinner injections of mixtures of short acting and NPH insulins. The regular insulin or rapidly acting insulin analog is withdrawn first, then the NPH insulin and then injected immediately. Stable premixed insulins (70% NPH and 30% regular) are available as a convenience to patients who have difficulty mixing insulin because of visual problems or impairment of manual dexterity (Table 27–6). Premixed preparations of insulin lispro and NPH insulins are unstable; stability is achieved by replacing the NPH insulin with NPL (neutral protamine lispro). This insulin has the same duration of action as NPH insulin. Premixed combinations of NPL and insulin lispro (75% NPL/25% insulin lispro mixture [Humalog Mix 75/25] and 50% NPL/50% insulin lispro mixture [Humalog Mix 50/50]) are available for clinical use. Similarly, a 70% insulin aspart protamine/30% insulin aspart (NovoLog Mix 70/30) is available. The main advantages of these mixtures are that they can be given within 15 minutes of starting a meal and they are superior in controlling the postprandial glucose rise after a carbohydrate-rich meal. These benefits have not translated into improvements in HbA_{1c} levels when compared with the usual 70% NPH/30% regular mixture. The longer-acting insulin analogs, insulin glargine and insulin detemir, cannot be mixed with either regular insulin or the rapidly acting insulin analogs. Insulin degludec, however, can be mixed and is available as 70% insulin degludec/30% insulin aspart and is injected once or twice a day.

3. Methods of insulin administration—

a. Insulin syringes and needles—Plastic disposable syringes are available in 1-mL, 0.5-mL, and 0.3-mL sizes. Three lengths of needles are available: 6 mm, 8 mm, and 12.7 mm. Long needles are preferable in patients with obesity to reduce variability of insulin absorption. The needles are of 28, 30, and 31 gauges. The 31-gauge needles are almost painless. "Disposable" syringes may be reused until blunting of the needle occurs (usually after three to five injections). Sterility adequate to avoid infection with reuse appears to be maintained by recapping syringes between uses. Cleansing the needle with alcohol may not be desirable since it can dissolve the silicone coating and can increase the pain of skin puncturing.

b. Sites of injection—Any part of the body covered by loose skin can be used, such as the abdomen, thighs, upper arms, flanks, and upper buttocks. Preparation with alcohol is not required prior to injection as long as the skin is clean. Rotation of sites is recommended to avoid delayed absorption when fibrosis or lipohypertrophy occurs from repeated use of a single site. Regular insulin is absorbed more rapidly when injected in the deltoid or abdomen compared to thighs and buttocks. Exercise can increase absorption when the injection site is adjacent to the exercise muscle. For most patients, the abdomen is the recommend region for injection because it provides adequate area in which to rotate sites. The effect of anatomic regions appears to be much less pronounced with the analog insulins.

c. Insulin pen injector devices—Insulin pens (Novo Nordisk, and Owen Mumford) eliminate the need for carrying insulin vials and syringes. Smart pens (Companion Medical) that are linked to cell phones can be used to remind the user to take their insulin before meals, calculate doses, and keep track of timing of the doses. Cartridges of insulin lispro and insulin aspart are available for the reusable pens. Disposable prefilled pens are also available for regular insulin (U100 and U500), insulin lispro, insulin aspart, insulin glulisine, insulin detemir, insulin glargine, insulin degludec, NPH, 70% NPH/30% regular, 75% NPL/25% insulin lispro, 50% NPL/50% insulin lispro, 70% insulin aspart protamine/30% insulin aspart, and 70% insulin degludec/30% insulin aspart. Pen needles are available in 29, 31, and 32 gauges and 4-, 5-, 6-, 8-, and 12.7-mm lengths (Novofine; BD).

d. Insulin pumps—In the United States, Medtronic MiniMed, Insulet, and Tandem make battery operated continuous subcutaneous insulin infusion (CSII) pumps. SOOIL makes a pump that is available in Europe and Asia. These pumps are small (about the size of a pager) and easy to program. They offer many features, including the ability to set a number of different basal rates throughout the 24 hours and to adjust the time over which bolus doses are given. They also are able to detect pressure build-up if the catheter is kinked. The catheter connecting the insulin reservoir to the subcutaneous cannula can be disconnected, allowing the patient to remove the pump temporarily (eg, for bathing). Ominpod (Insulet Corporation) is an insulin infusion system in which the insulin reservoir and infusion set are integrated into one unit (pod), so there is no catheter (electronic patch pump). The pod, placed on the skin, delivers subcutaneous basal and bolus insulin based on wirelessly transmitted instructions from a personal digital assistant. The great advantage of continuous subcutaneous insulin infusion (CSII) is that it allows for establishment of a basal profile tailored to the patient allowing for better overnight and between meals glucose control. The ability to adjust the basal insulin infusion makes it easier for the patient to manage glycemic excursions that occur with exercise. The pumps have software that can assist the patient to calculate boluses based on glucose reading and carbohydrates to be consumed. They keep track of the time elapsed since the last insulin bolus; the patient is reminded of this when he or she attempts to give additional correction bolus before the effect of the previous bolus has worn off ("insulin on board" feature). This feature reduces the risk of overcorrecting and subsequent hypoglycemia.

CSII therapy is appropriate for patients with type 1 diabetes who are motivated, mechanically inclined, educated about diabetes (diet, insulin action, treatment of hypoglycemia and hyperglycemia), and willing to monitor their blood glucose four to six times a day. Known complications of CSII include ketoacidosis, which can occur when insulin delivery is interrupted, and skin infections. Another disadvantage is its cost and the time needed of the clinician and staff to initiate therapy. Almost all patients use rapid-acting insulin analogs in their pumps.

V-go (Valeritas) is a mechanical patch pump designed specifically for people with type 2 diabetes who use a basal/bolus insulin regimen. The device is preset to deliver one of three fixed and flat basal rates (20, 30, or 40 units) for 24 hours (at which point it must be replaced) and there is a button that delivers two units per press to help cover meals.

E. Closed loop systems—Control algorithms have been devised to use glucose data from the continuous glucose monitoring systems to automatically deliver insulin by continuous subcutaneous insulin infusion pump. These closed loop systems (artificial pancreas) have been shown in clinical studies to improve nighttime glucose control, modestly lower HbA_{1c} levels, and reduce the risk of nocturnal hypoglycemia. The MiniMed 770 G and the Tandem Control-IQ, are approved for clinical use in the United States. CamAPS FX is available in the United Kingdom and in Europe. The MiniMed 770 G closed loop system uses glucose data from a sensor to automatically adjust basal insulin doses every 5 minutes, targeting a sensor glucose level of 120 mg/dL (6.7 mmol/L). Insulin delivery is suspended when the sensor glucose level falls below or is predicted to fall below target level. The glucose target can be adjusted up to 150 mg/dL (8.3 mmol/L) for physical activity. The Tandem Control-IQ targets a sensor glucose level of 112.5 mg/dL (6.25 mmol/L). The CamAPS FX has a default target of 104 mg/dL (5.8 mmol/L) but can be customized to targets between 79–198 mg/dL (4.4 to 11 mmol/L). This system also adapts to prandial and diurnal patterns. The patient is still responsible for bolusing insulin for meals and snacks. There are also Do-It-Yourself closed loop systems using free open-source software. One such system, called the "Loop," uses the Dexcom G6 sensor, the iPhone, and the Omnipod insulin pump. The "Loop" controller is downloaded on to the iPhone, and it uses the Dexcom G6 sensor glucose measurements (also on the iPhone) to automatically adjust basal insulin delivery on the Omnipod pump. Many patients with type 1 diabetes use these Do-It-Yourself systems, but they are not approved for use by the FDA. Successful use of these systems requires proficiency at using both the insulin pump and continuous glucose monitor. The systems are expensive; the insulin pump, which needs to be replaced every 4 years, costs about $6000 and the pump supplies are $1500 per year. The continuous glucose monitoring system costs approximately $4000 per year.

F. Inhaled insulin—Technosphere insulin (Afrezza) is a dry-powder formulation of recombinant human regular insulin that can be inhaled. It consists of 2- to 2.5-mcm crystals of the excipient fumaryl diketopiperazine that provide a large surface area for adsorption of proteins like insulin. The technosphere insulin is rapidly absorbed with peak insulin levels reached in 12–15 minutes and declining to baseline in 3 hours; the median time to maximum effect with inhaled insulin is approximately 1 hour and declines to baseline by about 3 hours. In contrast, the median time to maximum effect with subcutaneous insulin lispro is about 2 hours and declines to baseline by 4 hours. In clinical trials, technosphere insulin combined with basal insulin was as effective in glucose lowering as rapid-acting insulin analogs combined with basal insulin. It is formulated as a single-use, color-coded cartridge delivering 4, 8, or 12 units immediately before the meal. The manufacturer provides a dose conversion table; patients injecting up to 4 units of rapid-acting insulin analog should use the 4-unit cartridge. Those injecting 5 to 8 units should use the 8-unit cartridge. If the dose is 9–12 units of rapid-acting insulin premeal then one 4-unit cartridge and one 8-unit cartridge or one 12-unit cartridge should be used. The inhaler is about the size of a referee's whistle.

The most common adverse reaction of the inhaled insulin is a cough, affecting about 27% of patients. A small decrease in pulmonary function (forced expiratory volume in 1 second [FEV_1]) is seen in the first 3 months of use, which persists over 2 years of follow-up. Inhaled insulin is contraindicated in patients who smoke cigarettes and in those with chronic lung disease, such as asthma and COPD. Spirometry should be performed to identify potential lung disease prior to initiating therapy. During clinical trials, there were two cases of lung cancer in patients who were taking inhaled insulin and none in the comparator-treated patients. All the patients in whom lung cancer developed had a history of prior cigarette smoking. Cases of lung cancer were also reported in cigarette smokers using a previously available inhaled insulin preparation (Exubera). The incidence rate in the Exubera-treated group was 0.13 per 1000 patient-years, whereas it was 0.03 per 1000 patient-years in the comparator-treated group.

D. Transplantation

1. Pancreas transplantation—All patients with ESKD and type 1 diabetes who are candidates for a kidney transplant should be considered potential candidates for a pancreas transplant. Eligibility criteria include age younger than 55 and minimal cardiovascular risk. Contraindications include noncorrectable CAD, extensive peripheral vascular disease, and significant obesity (weight greater than 100 kg). The pancreas transplant may occur at the same time as kidney transplant or after kidney transplant. Patients undergoing simultaneous pancreas and kidney transplantation have an 83% chance of pancreatic graft survival at 1 year and 69% at 5 years. Solitary pancreatic transplantation in the absence of a need for kidney transplantation is considered only in those rare patients who do not respond to all other insulin therapeutic approaches and who have frequent severe hypoglycemia, or who have life-threatening complications related to their lack of metabolic control. Solitary pancreas transplant graft survival is 78% at 1 year and 54% at 5 years.

2. Islet transplantation—Total pancreatectomy is curative for severe pain syndrome associated with chronic pancreatitis. The pancreatectomy, however, results in surgical diabetes. Harvesting islets from the removed pancreas and autotransplanting them into the liver (via portal vein) can prevent the development of diabetes or result in "mild" diabetes (partial islet function) that is easier to manage. Since the islets are autologous, no immunosuppression is required. The number of islets transplanted is the main predictor of insulin independence.

People with type 1 diabetes can become insulin independent after receiving islets isolated from a donor pancreas (alloislet transplant). The islets are infused into the portal vein using a percutaneous transhepatic approach, and they lodge in the liver releasing insulin in response to physiologic stimuli. Long-term immunosuppression is necessary to prevent allograft rejection and to suppress the autoimmune process that led to the disease in the first place. Insulin independence for more than 5 years has been demonstrated in patients who got anti-CD3 antibody or anti-thymocyte globulin induction immunosuppression and calcineurin inhibitors, mTor inhibitors, and mycophenolate mofetil as maintenance immunosuppression. One major limitation is the need for more than one islet infusion to achieve insulin independence because of significant loss of islets during isolation and the period prior to engraftment. Stem cell–derived beta cells or islets may solve the problem of islet availability.

Boughton CK et al. New closed-loop insulin systems. Diabetologia. 2021;64:1007. [PMID: 33550442]
Kristensen SL et al. Cardiovascular, mortality, and kidney outcomes with GLP-1 receptor agonists in patients with type 2 diabetes: a systematic review and meta-analysis of cardiovascular outcome trials. Lancet Diabetes Endocrinol. 2019;7:776. [PMID: 31422062]
McGuire DK et al. Association of SGLT2 inhibitors with cardiovascular and kidney outcomes in patients with type 2 diabetes: a meta-analysis. JAMA Cardiol. 2021;6:148. [PMID: 33031522]

Steps in the Management of Diabetes

A. Distinguishing the Types of Diabetes

An attempt should be made to characterize the diabetes as type 1 or type 2 or other specific types such as MODY, based on the clinical features present and on whether or not ketonuria accompanies the glycosuria. Features that suggest end-organ insulin insensitivity to insulin, such as visceral obesity, acanthosis nigricans, or both, must be identified. The family history should document the incidence of diabetes in other members of the family and also the age at onset, association with obesity, the need for insulin, and whether there were complications. Measurement of GAD65, IAA, ICA 512, and zinc transporter 8 antibodies can help distinguish between type 1 and type 2 diabetes (Table 27–7). Many patients with newly diagnosed type 1 diabetes still have significant endogenous insulin production, and C-peptide levels do not reliably distinguish between type 1 and type 2 diabetes.

Table 27–7. Diagnostic sensitivity and specificity of autoimmune markers in patients with newly diagnosed type 1 diabetes mellitus.

	Sensitivity	Specificity
Islet cell antibodies (ICA)	44–100%	96%
Glutamic acid decarboxylase (GAD65)	70–90%	99%
Insulin (IAA)	40–70%	99%
Tyrosine phosphatase (IA-2, ICA 512)	50–70%	99%
Zinc transporter 8 (ZnT8)	50–70%	99%

B. Patient Education (Self-Management Training)

Since diabetes is a lifelong disorder, education of the patient and the family is probably the most important obligation of the clinician who provides care. The best persons to manage a disease that is affected so markedly by daily fluctuations in environmental stress, exercise, diet, and infections are the patients themselves and their families. The "teaching curriculum" should include explanations by the clinician or nurse of the nature of diabetes and its potential acute and chronic hazards and how they can be recognized early and prevented or treated. Self-monitoring of blood glucose should be emphasized, especially in patients with diabetes who require insulin, and instructions must be given on proper testing and recording of data.

Patients taking insulin should have an understanding of the actions of basal and bolus insulins. They should be taught to determine whether the basal dose is appropriate and how to adjust the rapidly acting insulin dose for the carbohydrate content of a meal. Patients and their families and friends should be taught to recognize signs and symptoms of hypoglycemia and how to treat low glucose reactions. Strenuous exercise can precipitate hypoglycemia, and patients must therefore be taught to reduce their insulin dosage in anticipation of strenuous activity or to take supplemental carbohydrate. Injection of insulin into a site farthest away from the muscles most involved in the exercise may help ameliorate exercise-induced hypoglycemia, since insulin injected in the proximity of exercising muscle may be more rapidly mobilized. Exercise training also increases the effectiveness of insulin, and insulin doses should be adjusted accordingly. Infections can cause insulin resistance, and patients should be instructed on how to manage the hyperglycemia with supplemental rapidly acting insulin.

Advice on personal hygiene, including detailed instructions on foot and dental care, should be provided. All infections (especially pyogenic ones) provoke the release of high levels of insulin antagonists, such as catecholamines or glucagon, and thus bring about a marked increase in insulin requirements. Patients who are taking oral agents may decompensate and temporarily require insulin. Patients should be told about community agencies, such as Diabetes Association chapters, that can serve as a continuing source of instruction.

Finally, vigorous efforts should be made to persuade patients with newly diagnosed diabetes who smoke to give up the habit, since large vessel peripheral vascular disease and debilitating retinopathy are less common in nonsmoking patients with diabetes.

C. Medications

Treatment must be individualized on the basis of the type of diabetes and specific needs of each patient. However, certain general principles of management can be outlined for hyperglycemic states of different types.

1. Type 1 diabetes—A combination of rapidly acting insulin analogs and long-acting insulin analogs allows for more physiologic insulin replacement. Table 27–8 illustrates a regimen with a rapidly acting insulin analog and long-acting basal insulin that might be appropriate for a 70-kg person with type 1 diabetes eating meals providing standard carbohydrate intake and moderate to low fat content.

Insulin glargine or insulin degludec is usually given once in the evening to provide 24-hour coverage. There are occasional patients in whom insulin glargine does not last for 24 hours, and in such cases, it needs to be given twice a day. Insulin detemir usually has to be given twice a day to get adequate 24-hour basal coverage. Alternatively, small doses of NPH (~3–4 units) can be given with each meal to provide daytime basal coverage with a larger dose at night.

CSII by portable battery-operated "open loop" devices allow the setting of different basal rates throughout the 24 hours and permit bolus dose adjustments by as little as 0.05-unit increments. The 24-hour basal dosage is usually based on age and body weight. An adolescent might need as much as 0.4 unit/kg/day; a young adult (less than 25 years), 0.35 unit per/kg/day; and an older adult, 0.25 unit/kg/day. For example, a 70-kg, 30-year-old person may require a basal rate of 0.7 unit per hour throughout the 24 hours with the exception of 3 AM to 8 AM, when 0.8 unit per hour might be appropriate (given the "**dawn phenomenon**"—reduced tissue sensitivity to insulin between 5 AM and 8 AM). The meal bolus varies based on the time of day and the person's age. Adolescents and young adults usually require 1 unit for about 10 g of carbohydrate. Older adults usually require about 1 unit for 15 g of carbohydrate. The correction factor—how much insulin is needed to lower glucose levels by 50 mg/dL—can be calculated from the insulin-to-carbohydrate ratios. For example, if 1 unit is required for 15 g of carbohydrate, then 1 unit will lower glucose levels by 50 mg/dL. If 1.5 units of insulin are required for 15 g of carbohydrate (that is, 1 unit for 10 g carbohydrate), then 1.5 units of insulin will lower glucose levels by 50 mg/dL (that is, 1 unit will lower glucose level by 33 mg/dL). For a 70-kg, 30-year-old person, bolus ratios of 1 unit for 12–15 g of carbohydrate plus 1 unit for 50 mg/dL of blood glucose over a target value of 120 mg/dL would be reasonable starting point. Further adjustments to basal and bolus dosages would depend on the results of blood glucose monitoring. One of the more difficult therapeutic problems in managing patients with type 1 diabetes is determining the proper adjustment of insulin dose when the prebreakfast blood glucose level is high. Occasionally, the prebreakfast hyperglycemia is due to the **Somogyi effect**, in which nocturnal hypoglycemia leads to a surge of counterregulatory hormones to produce high blood glucose levels by 7 AM. However, a more common cause for prebreakfast hyperglycemia is the waning of circulating insulin levels by the morning.

Table 27–8. Examples of intensive insulin regimens using rapidly acting insulin analogs (insulin lispro, aspart, or glulisine) and long-acting insulin analogs (insulin detemir, or insulin glargine or degludec) in a 70-kg man with type 1 diabetes.[1–3]

	Pre-breakfast	Pre-lunch	Pre-dinner	At Bedtime
Rapidly acting insulin analog	5 units	4 units	6 units	
Insulin detemir[3]	6–7 units			8–9 units
OR				
Rapidly acting insulin analog	5 units	4 units	6 units	—
Insulin glargine or degludec[3]		—		15–16 units

[1]Assumes that patient is consuming approximately 75 g carbohydrate at breakfast, 60 g at lunch, and 90 g at dinner.
[2]The dose of rapidly acting insulin can be raised by 1 or 2 units if extra carbohydrate (15–30 g) is ingested or if premeal blood glucose is > 170 mg/dL (9.4 mmol/L).
[3]Insulin glargine or insulin detemir must be given as a separate injection.

The diagnosis of the cause of prebreakfast hyperglycemia can be facilitated by self-monitoring of blood glucose at 3 AM in addition to the usual bedtime and 7 AM measurements or by analyzing data from the continuous glucose monitor. This is required for only a few nights, and when a particular pattern emerges from monitoring blood glucose levels overnight, appropriate therapeutic measures can be taken. The Somogyi effect can be treated by lowering the basal insulin dose at bedtime or by eating a snack at bedtime. When a waning insulin level is the cause, then either increasing the evening basal insulin dose or shifting it from dinnertime to bedtime (or both) can be effective.

The currently available closed loop systems enable patients to achieve close to normal glucose levels in the morning with a low risk of nocturnal hypoglycemia and improve overall glucose control. All patients with type 1 diabetes who have good self-management skills should be using these systems.

2. Type 2 diabetes—Therapeutic recommendations are based on the relative contributions of beta cell insufficiency and insulin insensitivity in individual patients. The possibility that the individual patient has a specific etiologic cause for their diabetes should always be considered, especially when the patient does not have a family history of type 2 diabetes or does not have any evidence of central obesity or insulin resistance. Such patients should be evaluated for other types of diabetes such as LADA or MODY (Table 27–1). Patients with LADA should be prescribed insulin when the disease is diagnosed and treated like patients with type 1 diabetes. Importantly, many patients with type 2 diabetes mellitus have a progressive loss of beta cell function and will require additional therapeutic interventions with time.

A. WEIGHT REDUCTION—One of the primary modes of therapy in patients with obesity and type 2 diabetes is weight reduction. Normalization of glycemia can be achieved by weight loss and improvement in tissue sensitivity to insulin. A combination of caloric restriction, increased exercise, and behavior modification is required if a weight reduction program is to be successful. Understanding the risks associated with the diagnosis of diabetes may motivate the patient to lose weight.

For selected patients, medical or surgical options for weight loss should be considered. The GLP-1 receptor agonists can be prescribed at doses approved for weight loss (liraglutide 3 mg daily or semaglutide 2.4 mg weekly). Other medical options include orlistat, phentermine/topiramate, and naltrexone/extended-release bupropion (see Chapter 29).

Bariatric surgery (Roux-en-Y, gastric banding, gastric sleeve, biliopancreatic diversion/duodenal switch) typically results in substantial weight loss and improvement in glucose levels. A meta-analysis examining the impact of bariatric surgery on patients with diabetes and BMI of 40 kg/m^2 or greater noted that 82% of patients had resolution of clinical and laboratory manifestations of diabetes in the first 2 years after surgery and 62% remained free of diabetes more than 2 years after surgery. The improvement was most marked in the procedure that caused the greatest weight loss (biliopancreatic diversion/duodenal switch). There was, however, a high attrition of patients available for follow-up, and there was little information about different ethnic types. Weight regain does occur after bariatric surgery, and it can be expected that 20–25% of the lost weight will be regained over 10 years. The impact of this weight gain on diabetes recurrence depends principally on the degree of beta cell dysfunction.

Patients with type 2 diabetes without obesity frequently have increased visceral adiposity—the so-called metabolic obesity in people with normal body weight. There is less emphasis on weight loss, but exercise remains an important aspect of treatment.

B. Glucose-lowering agents—Figure 27–2 outlines the treatment approach based on a consensus algorithm by the American Diabetes Association and the European Association for the Study of Diabetes. The current recommendation is to start metformin therapy at diagnosis and not wait to see whether the patient can achieve target glycemic control with weight management and exercise. See discussion of the individual medications, above.

When diabetes is not well controlled with initial therapy (usually metformin), then a second agent should be added. Presence of cardiovascular or kidney disease, or both, will determine the choice of the second agent. Liraglutide, semaglutide, empagliflozin, canagliflozin, and dapagliflozin have improved cardiovascular outcomes. The SGLT2 inhibitors are especially beneficial in patients with heart failure or diabetic nephropathy, or both. The need for weight loss should lead to the use of GLP-1 receptor agonists in patients with obesity and with or without CAD. SGLT2 inhibitors also promote modest weight loss and should be prescribed in the patient with heart failure or diabetic nephropathy. Sulfonylureas have been available for many years and their use in combination with metformin is well established. They do, however, have the propensity of causing hypoglycemia and weight gain. In patients who experience hyperglycemia after a carbohydrate-rich meal (such as dinner), a short-acting secretagogue (repaglinide or nateglinide) before meals may suffice to get the glucose

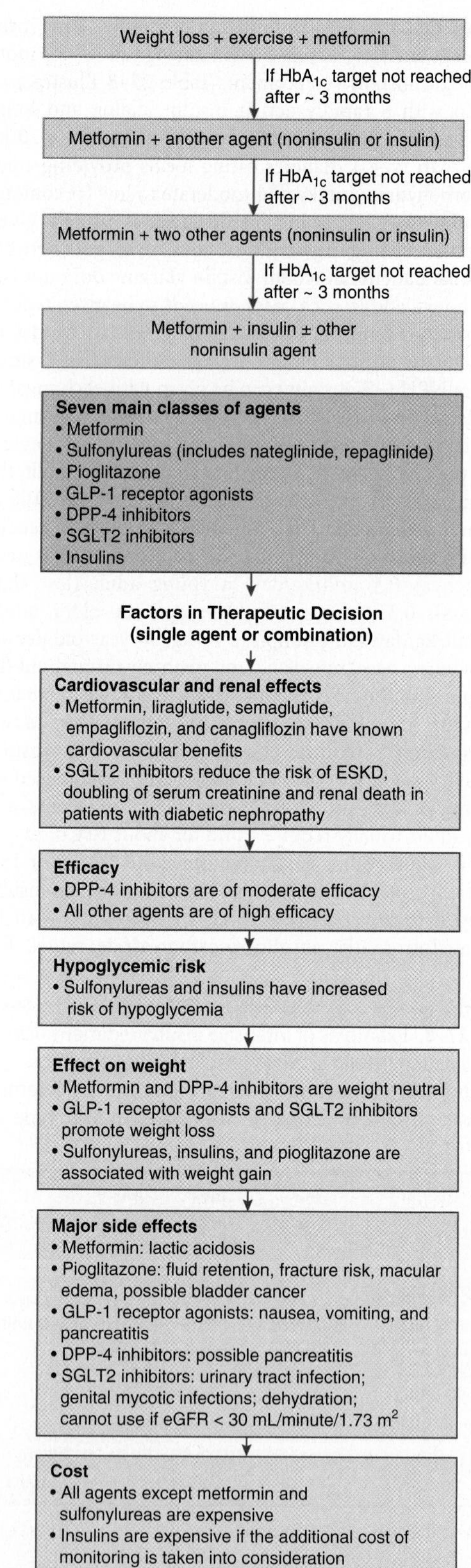

▲ **Figure 27–2.** Algorithm for the treatment of type 2 diabetes based on the 2018 recommendations of the consensus panel of the American Diabetes Association/European Association for the Study of Diabetes.

levels into the target range. Patients with severe insulin resistance may be candidates for pioglitazone. Pioglitazone may also reduce the risk for recurrent stroke in patients who have a history of stroke or transient ischemic attack. If two agents are inadequate, then a third agent is added. The combination of metformin, a GLP-1 receptor agonist, and an SGLT2 inhibitor should be considered in patients with obesity, heart disease, and kidney disease, although data regarding efficacy of such combined therapy are limited.

When the combination of oral agents (and injectable GLP-1 receptor agonists) fails to achieve euglycemia in patients with type 2 diabetes, then insulin treatment should be instituted. Various insulin regimens may be effective. One proposed regimen is to continue the oral agents (and injectable GLP-1 receptor agonists) and then simply add a bedtime dose of NPH or long-acting insulin analog (insulin glargine, detemir, or degludec) to reduce excessive nocturnal hepatic glucose output and improve fasting glucose levels. If the patient does not achieve target glucose levels during the day, then daytime insulin treatment can be initiated. A convenient insulin regimen under these circumstances is a split dose of 70/30 NPH/regular mixture (or Humalog Mix 75/25 or NovoLogMix 70/30) before breakfast and before dinner. If this regimen fails to achieve satisfactory glycemic goals or is associated with unacceptable frequency of hypoglycemic episodes, then a more intensive regimen of multiple insulin injections can be instituted as in patients with type 1 diabetes. Metformin principally reduces hepatic glucose output, and it is reasonable to continue with this medication when insulin therapy is instituted. Pioglitazone, which improves peripheral insulin sensitivity, can be used together with insulin but this combination is associated with more weight gain and peripheral edema. Sulfonylureas, GLP-1 receptor agonists, DPP-4 inhibitors, and SGLT2 inhibitors also have been shown to be of continued benefit and may be continued. Weight-reducing interventions should continue even after initiation of insulin therapy and may allow for simplification of the therapeutic regimen in the future.

D. Acceptable Levels of Glycemic Control

A reasonable aim of therapy is to approach normal glycemic excursions without provoking severe or frequent hypoglycemia. Table 27–9 summarizes blood glucose and HbA_{1c} goals for different patient groups. *The UKPDS study demonstrated that blood pressure control was as significant or more significant than glycemic control in patients with type 2 diabetes regarding the prevention of microvascular as well as macrovascular complications.*

E. Complications of Insulin Therapy

1. Hypoglycemia—Hypoglycemic reactions are the most common complications that occur in patients with diabetes who are treated with insulin. The signs and symptoms of hypoglycemia may be divided into those resulting from stimulation of the autonomic nervous system and those from neuroglycopenia (insufficient glucose for normal CNS function). When the blood glucose falls to around 54 mg/dL (3 mmol/L), the patient starts to experience both sympathetic (tachycardia, palpitations, sweating, tremulousness) and parasympathetic (nausea, hunger) nervous system symptoms. If these autonomic symptoms are ignored and the glucose levels fall further (to around 50 mg/dL [2.8 mmol/L]), then neuroglycopenic symptoms appear, including irritability, confusion, blurred vision, tiredness, headache, and difficulty speaking. A further decline in glucose can lead to loss of consciousness or even a seizure.

2. Hypoglycemic unawareness—With repeated episodes of hypoglycemia, there is adaptation, and autonomic

Table 27–9. Glycemic targets for different groups of adults with diabetes.

	Blood Glucose mg/dL (mmol/L) Targets	HbA_{1C} % (mmol/mol) Targets
Nonpregnant healthy adults	Premeal glucose 90–130 (5–7.2) 1-hour peak < 180 (10) 2-hour peak < 150 (8.3)	< 7 (53). Aim for < 6.5 (48) if it can be achieved without significant hypoglycemia or polypharmacy
Pregnant women	Premeal glucose ≤ 95 (5.3) 1-hour peak ≤ 140 (7.8) 2-hour peak ≤ 120 (6.7)	6–6.5 (42–48). Aim for < 6 (42) if possible without significant hypoglycemia
Older adults		
Healthy	Premeal 90–130 (5–7.2) Bedtime 90–150 (5–8.3)	< 7.5 (58)
Frail with limited life expectancy	Premeal 100–180 (5.6–10) Bedtime 110–200 (6.1–11.1)	< 8.5 (69)
Patients with history of severe hypoglycemia	Premeal 90–150 (5–8.3) Bedtime 100–180 (5.6–10)	< 8 (64)
Hospitalized patients	140–180 (7.8–10)	—
Patients with CKD	Glycemic targets in CKD are the same as those without CKD. HbA_{1c} and fructosamine values may not be accurate in ESKD, and greater reliance should be placed on the home glucose measurements	

symptoms do not occur until the blood glucose levels are much lower and so the first symptoms are often due to neuroglycopenia. This condition is referred to as "hypoglycemic unawareness." It has been shown that hypoglycemic unawareness can be reversed by keeping glucose levels high for a period of several weeks.

Except for sweating, most of the sympathetic symptoms of hypoglycemia are blunted in patients receiving beta-blocking agents. Though not absolutely contraindicated, these medications must be used with caution in patients with diabetes who require insulin, and beta-1-selective blocking agents are preferred.

Hypoglycemia can occur in a patient taking sulfonylureas, repaglinide, and nateglinide, particularly if the patient is elderly, has kidney or liver disease, or is taking certain other medications that alter metabolism of the sulfonylureas (eg, sulfonamides or warfarin). It occurs more frequently with the use of long-acting sulfonylureas than with shorter-acting agents. Otherwise, hypoglycemia in insulin-treated patients occurs as a consequence of three factors: behavioral issues, impaired counterregulatory systems, and complications of diabetes.

Behavioral issues include injecting too much insulin for the amount of carbohydrates ingested. Drinking alcohol in excess, especially on an empty stomach, can also cause hypoglycemia. In patients with type 1 diabetes, hypoglycemia can occur during or even several hours after exercise, and so glucose levels need to be monitored and food and insulin adjusted. Some patients do not like their glucose levels to be high, and they treat every high glucose level aggressively. These individuals who "stack" their insulin—that is, give another dose of insulin before the first injection has had its full action—can develop hypoglycemia.

Counterregulatory issues resulting in hypoglycemia include impaired glucagon response, sympatho-adrenal responses, and cortisol deficiency. Patients with diabetes of greater than 5 years in duration lose their glucagon response to hypoglycemia. As a result, they are at a significant disadvantage in protecting themselves against falling glucose levels. Once the glucagon response is lost, their sympatho-adrenal responses take on added importance. Unfortunately, aging, autonomic neuropathy, or hypoglycemic unawareness due to repeated low glucose levels further blunts the sympatho-adrenal responses. Occasionally, Addison disease develops in persons with type 1 diabetes mellitus; when this happens, insulin requirements fall significantly, and unless insulin dose is reduced, recurrent hypoglycemia will develop.

Complications of diabetes that increase the risk for hypoglycemia include autonomic neuropathy, gastroparesis, and ESKD. The sympathetic nervous system is an important system alerting the individual that the glucose level is falling by causing symptoms of tachycardia, palpitations, sweating, and tremulousness. Failure of the sympatho-adrenal responses increases the risk of hypoglycemia. In addition, in patients with gastroparesis, if insulin is given before a meal, the peak of insulin action may occur before the food is absorbed causing the glucose levels to fall. Finally, in ESKD, hypoglycemia can occur presumably because of decreased insulin clearance as well as loss of renal contribution to gluconeogenesis in the postabsorptive state.

To prevent and treat insulin-induced hypoglycemia, a patient with diabetes should carry glucose tablets or juice at all times. For most episodes, ingestion of 15 grams of carbohydrate is sufficient to reverse the hypoglycemia. The patient should be instructed to check the blood glucose in 15 minutes and treat again if the glucose level is still low. *A parenteral (1 mg) or nasal inhalation (3 mg) glucagon emergency kit should be provided to every patient with diabetes who is receiving insulin therapy.* Family or friends should be instructed how to inject it subcutaneously or intramuscularly into the buttock, arm, or thigh or administer a nasal dose in the event that the patient is unconscious or refuses food. The medication can occasionally cause vomiting, and the unconscious patient should be turned on his or her side to protect the airway. Glucagon mobilizes glycogen from the liver, raising the blood glucose by about 36 mg/dL (2 mmol/L) in about 15 minutes. After the patient recovers consciousness, additional oral carbohydrate should be given. *People with diabetes receiving hypoglycemic medication therapy should also wear an identification MedicAlert bracelet or necklace or carry a card in his or her wallet (1-800-ID-ALERT, www.medicalert.org).*

Medical personnel treating severe hypoglycemia can give 50 mL of 50% glucose solution by rapid intravenous infusion. If intravenous access is not available, 1 mg of glucagon can be injected intramuscularly or 3 mg given by nasal spray.

3. Immunopathology of insulin therapy—At least five molecular classes of insulin antibodies are produced during the course of insulin therapy in diabetes, including IgA, IgD, IgE, IgG, and IgM. With the switch to human and purified pork insulin, the various immunopathologic syndromes such as insulin allergy, immune insulin resistance, and lipoatrophy have become quite rare since the titers and avidity of these induced antibodies are generally quite low.

A. Insulin allergy—Insulin allergy, or immediate-type hypersensitivity, is a rare condition in which local or systemic urticaria is due to histamine release from tissue mast cells sensitized by adherence of anti-insulin IgE antibodies. In severe cases, anaphylaxis results. When only human insulin has been used from the onset of insulin therapy, insulin allergy is exceedingly rare. Antihistamines, corticosteroids, and even desensitization may be required, especially for systemic hypersensitivity.

B. Immune insulin resistance—A low titer of circulating IgG anti-insulin antibodies that neutralize the action of insulin to a small extent develops in most insulin-treated patients. With the old animal insulins, a high titer of circulating antibodies sometimes developed, resulting in extremely high insulin requirements—often more than 200 units daily. This is now rarely seen with the switch to human or highly purified pork insulins and has not been reported with the analogs.

C. Lipodystrophy—Atrophy of subcutaneous fatty tissue leading to disfiguring excavations and depressed areas may rarely occur at the site of injection. This complication results from an immune reaction, and it has become rarer with the development of human and highly purified insulin preparations. Lipohypertrophy, on the other hand, is a consequence of the pharmacologic effects of insulin being deposited in the same location repeatedly. It can occur with purified insulins as well. Rotation of injection sites will prevent lipohypertrophy.

Rodriguez-Gutierrez R et al. Benefits and harms of intensive glycemic control in patients with type 2 diabetes. BMJ. 2019;367:l5887. [PMID: 31690574]

Chronic Complications of Diabetes

Late clinical manifestations of diabetes mellitus include a number of pathologic changes that involve small and large blood vessels, cranial and peripheral nerves, the skin, and the lens of the eye. These lesions lead to hypertension, ESKD, blindness, autonomic and peripheral neuropathy, amputations of the lower extremities, MI, and cerebrovascular accidents. These late manifestations correlate with the duration of the diabetic state subsequent to the onset of puberty. In type 1 diabetes, ESKD develops in up to 40% of patients, compared with less than 20% of patients with type 2 diabetes. Proliferative retinopathy ultimately develops in both types of diabetes but has a slightly higher prevalence in type 1 patients (25% after 15 years' duration). In patients with type 1 diabetes, complications from ESKD are a major cause of death, whereas patients with type 2 diabetes are more likely to have macrovascular diseases leading to MI and stroke as the main causes of death. Cigarette use adds significantly to the risk of both microvascular and macrovascular complications in diabetes.

A. Ocular Complications

1. Diabetic cataracts—Premature cataracts occur in patients with diabetes and seem to correlate with both the duration of diabetes and the severity of chronic hyperglycemia. Nonenzymatic glycosylation of lens protein is twice as high in patients with diabetes as in age-matched persons without diabetes and may contribute to the premature occurrence of cataracts.

2. Diabetic retinopathy—The two main categories of diabetic retinopathy, nonproliferative and proliferative, are discussed in Chapter 7.

3. Glaucoma—Glaucoma occurs in approximately 6% of persons with diabetes. It is responsive to the usual therapy for open-angle disease. Neovascularization of the iris in patients with diabetes can predispose to closed-angle glaucoma, but this is relatively uncommon except after cataract extraction, when growth of new vessels has been known to progress rapidly, involving the angle of the iris and obstructing outflow.

B. Diabetic Nephropathy

Diabetic nephropathy is initially manifested by albuminuria; subsequently, as kidney function declines, urea and creatinine accumulate in the blood (see Chapter 22). An albumin-creatinine ratio in an early morning spot urine collected upon awakening is the preferred method to assess albumin excretion. In the early morning spot urine, a ratio of albumin (mcg/L) to creatinine (mg/L) of less than 30 mcg/mg creatinine is normal, and a ratio of 30–300 mcg/mg creatinine suggests abnormal microalbuminuria. At least two early morning spot urine collections over a 3- to 6-month period should be abnormal before a diagnosis of microalbuminuria is justified. Short-term hyperglycemia, exercise, UTIs, heart failure, and acute febrile illness can cause transient albuminuria and so testing for microalbuminuria should be postponed until resolution of these problems.

Subsequent ESKD can be predicted by persistent urinary albumin excretion rates exceeding 30 mcg/mg creatinine. Glycemic control as well as a protein diet of ~0.8 g/kg/day may reduce both the hyperfiltration and the elevated microalbuminuria in patients in the early stages of diabetes and those with incipient diabetic nephropathy. Antihypertensive therapy also decreases microalbuminuria. Evidence from some studies supports a specific role for ACE inhibitors in reducing intraglomerular pressure in addition to their lowering of systemic hypertension. An ACE inhibitor (captopril, 50 mg twice daily) in normotensive patients with diabetes impedes progression to proteinuria and prevents the increase in albumin excretion rate. SGLT2 therapy should be instituted in patients with type 2 diabetes who have progression of kidney disease despite taking optimal antihypertensive therapy, which includes an ACE inhibitor or angiotensin receptor blocker.

C. Diabetic Neuropathy

Diabetic neuropathies are the most common complications of diabetes, affecting up to 50% of older patients with type 2 diabetes.

1. Peripheral neuropathy—

A. DISTAL SYMMETRIC POLYNEUROPATHY—This is the most common form of diabetic peripheral neuropathy where loss of function appears in a stocking-glove pattern and is due to an axonal neuropathic process. Longer nerves are especially vulnerable, hence the impact on the foot. Both motor and sensory nerve conduction is delayed in the peripheral nerves, and ankle jerks may be absent.

Sensory involvement usually occurs first and is generally bilateral, symmetric, and associated with dulled perception of vibration, pain, and temperature. The pain can range from mild discomfort to severe incapacitating symptoms. The sensory deficit may eventually be of sufficient degree to prevent patients from feeling pain. Patients who have a sensory neuropathy should therefore be examined with a 5.07 Semmes-Weinstein filament and those who cannot feel the filament must be considered at risk for unperceived neuropathic injury.

The denervation of the small muscles of the foot can result in clawing of the toes and displacement of the submetatarsal fat pads anteriorly. These changes, together with the joint and connective tissue changes, alter the biomechanics of the foot and increase plantar pressures. This combination of decreased pain threshold, abnormally high foot pressures, and repetitive stress (such as from walking) can lead to calluses and ulcerations in the high-pressure

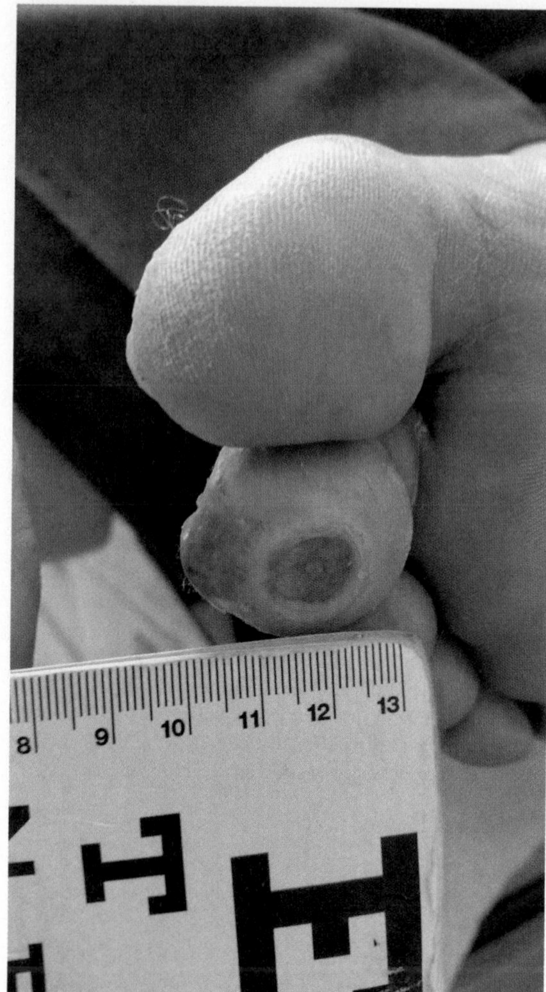

▲ **Figure 27–3.** Neuropathic foot ulcer in a patient with diabetes.

areas such as over the metatarsal heads (Figure 27–3). Peripheral neuropathy, autonomic neuropathy, and trauma also predisposes to the development of **Charcot arthropathy.** An acute case of Charcot foot arthropathy presents with pain and swelling, and if left untreated, leads to a "rocker bottom" deformity and ulceration. The early radiologic changes show joint subluxation and periarticular fractures. As the process progresses, there is frank osteoclastic destruction leading to deranged and unstable joints particularly in the midfoot. Not surprisingly, the key issue for the healing of neuropathic ulcers in a foot with good vascular supply is mechanical unloading. In addition, any infection should be treated with debridement and appropriate antibiotics; healing duration of 8–10 weeks is typical. Occasionally, when healing appears refractory, platelet-derived growth factor (becaplermin [Regranex]) should be considered for local application. Once ulcers are healed, therapeutic footwear is key to preventing recurrences. Custom molded shoes are reserved for patients with significant foot deformities. Other patients with neuropathy may require accommodative insoles that distribute the load over as wide an area as possible. Patients with foot deformities and loss of their protective threshold should get regular care from a podiatrist. Patients should be educated on appropriate footwear and those with loss of their protective threshold should be instructed to inspect their feet daily for reddened areas, blisters, abrasions, or lacerations.

In some patients, hypersensitivity to light touch and occasionally severe "burning" pain, particularly at night, can become physically and emotionally disabling. Nortriptyline or desipramine in doses of 25–150 mg/day orally may provide dramatic relief for pain from diabetic neuropathy, often within 48–72 hours. Patients often attribute the benefit to having a full night's sleep. Mild to moderate morning drowsiness is a side effect that generally improves with time or can be lessened by giving the medication several hours before bedtime. This medication should not be continued if improvement has not occurred after 5 days of therapy. Amitriptyline, 25–75 mg orally at bedtime, can also be used but has more anticholinergic effects. Tricyclic antidepressants, in combination with fluphenazine (3 mg daily in three divided doses) have been shown in two studies to be efficacious in painful neuropathy, with benefits unrelated to relief of depression. Gabapentin (900–1800 mg orally daily in three divided doses) has also been shown to be effective in the treatment of painful neuropathy and should be tried if the tricyclic medications prove ineffective. Pregabalin, a congener of gabapentin, has been shown in an 8-week study to be more effective than placebo in treating painful diabetic peripheral neuropathy. However, this medication was not compared with an active control. Also, because of its abuse potential, it is categorized as a schedule V controlled substance. Duloxetine (60–120 mg), a serotonin and norepinephrine reuptake inhibitor, is approved for the treatment of painful diabetic neuropathy. Capsaicin, a topical irritant, is effective in reducing local nerve pain; it is dispensed as a cream (Zostrix 0.025%, Zostrix-HP 0.075%) to be rubbed into the skin over the painful region two to four times daily. Gloves should be used for application since hand contamination could result in discomfort if the cream comes in contact with eyes or sensitive areas such as the genitalia. Application of a 5% lidocaine patch over an area of maximal pain has been reported to be of benefit. It is approved for treatment of postherpetic neuralgia.

Diabetic neuropathic cachexia is a syndrome characterized by a symmetric peripheral neuropathy, profound weight loss (up to 60% of total body weight), and painful dysesthesias affecting the proximal lower limbs, the hands, or the lower trunk. Treatment is usually with insulin and analgesics. The prognosis is generally good, and patients typically recover their baseline weight with resolution of the painful sensory symptoms within 1 year.

B. Isolated peripheral neuropathy—Involvement of the distribution of only one nerve ("mononeuropathy") or of several nerves ("mononeuropathy multiplex") is characterized by sudden onset with subsequent recovery of all or most of the function. This neuropathology has been attributed to vascular ischemia or traumatic damage. Cranial and femoral nerves are commonly involved, and motor abnormalities predominate. The patient with cranial nerve involvement usually has diplopia and single third, fourth, or sixth nerve weakness on examination but the pupil is spared. A full recovery of function occurs in 6–12 weeks. Diabetic amyotrophy presents with onset of severe pain in the front of the thigh. Within a few days or weeks of the onset of pain, weakness and wasting of the quadriceps develops. As the weakness appears, the pain tends to improve. Management includes analgesia and improved diabetes control. The symptoms improve over 6–18 months.

2. Autonomic neuropathy—Neuropathy of the autonomic system occurs principally in patients with diabetes of long duration. It affects many diverse visceral functions including blood pressure and pulse, GI activity, bladder function, and erectile dysfunction. Treatment is directed specifically at each abnormality. Insulin neuritis or treatment-induced neuropathy of diabetes occurs occasionally in patients with poor glucose control and whose glucose levels improve rapidly in days or a few weeks. Symptoms include severe sensory neuropathic pains and sometimes autonomic functions. These symptoms improve over a few months.

A. GI SYSTEM—Involvement of the GI system may be manifested by nausea, vomiting, postprandial fullness, reflux or dysphagia, constipation or diarrhea (or both), and fecal incontinence. Gastroparesis should be considered in patients with type 1 diabetes in whom unexpected fluctuations and variability in their blood glucose levels develops after meals. Metoclopramide has been of some help in treating diabetic gastroparesis. It is given in a dose of 10 mg orally three or four times a day, 30 minutes before meals and at bedtime. Drowsiness, restlessness, fatigue, and lassitude are common adverse effects. Tardive dyskinesia and extrapyramidal effects can occur, especially when used for longer than 3 months, and the FDA has cautioned against the long-term use of metoclopramide.

Erythromycin appears to bind to motilin receptors in the stomach and has been found to improve gastric emptying over the short term in doses of 250 mg three times daily, but its effectiveness seems to diminish over time. In selected patients, injections of botulinum toxin into the pylorus can reduce pylorus sphincter resistance and enhance gastric emptying. Gastric electrical stimulation has been reported to improve symptoms and quality of life indices in patients with gastroparesis refractory to pharmacologic therapy.

Diarrhea associated with autonomic neuropathy has occasionally responded to broad-spectrum antibiotic therapy (such as rifaximin, metronidazole, amoxicillin/clavulanate, ciprofloxacin, or doxycycline), although it often undergoes spontaneous remission. Refractory diabetic diarrhea is often associated with impaired sphincter control and fecal incontinence. Therapy with loperamide, 4–8 mg daily, or diphenoxylate with atropine, two tablets up to four times a day, may provide relief. In more severe cases, tincture of paregoric or codeine (60-mg tablets) may be required to reduce the frequency of diarrhea and improve the consistency of the stools. Clonidine has been reported to lessen diabetic diarrhea; however, its usefulness is limited by its tendency to lower blood pressure in these patients who already have autonomic neuropathy, resulting in orthostatic hypotension. Constipation usually responds to stimulant laxatives such as senna.

B. GENITOURINARY SYSTEM—Incomplete emptying of the bladder can sometimes occur. Bethanechol in doses of 10–50 mg orally three times a day has occasionally improved emptying of the atonic urinary bladder. Catheter decompression of the distended bladder has been reported to improve its function, and considerable benefit has been reported after surgical severing of the internal vesicle sphincter.

Erectile dysfunction can result from neurologic, psychological, or vascular causes, or a combination of these causes. The phosphodiesterase type 5 (PDE5) inhibitors sildenafil (Viagra), vardenafil (Levitra), and tadalafil (Cialis) have been shown in placebo-controlled clinical trials to improve erections in response to sexual stimulation. The recommended dose of sildenafil for most patients is one 50-mg tablet taken approximately 1 hour before sexual activity. The peak effect is at 1.5–2 hours, with some effect persisting for 4 hours. Patients with diabetes mellitus using sildenafil reported 50–60% improvement in erectile function. The maximum recommended dose is 100 mg. The recommended dose of both vardenafil and tadalafil is 10 mg. The doses may be increased to 20 mg or decreased to 5 mg based on efficacy and side effects. Tadalafil has been shown to improve erectile function for up to 36 hours after dosing. Low doses are available for daily use. In clinical trials, only a few adverse effects have been reported—transient mild headache, flushing, dyspepsia, and some altered color vision. Priapism can occur with these medications, and patients should be advised to seek immediate medical attention if an erection persists for longer than 4 hours. The PDE5 inhibitors potentiate the hypotensive effects of nitrates and their use is contraindicated in patients who are concurrently using organic nitrates in any form. *Caution is advised for men who have suffered a heart attack, stroke, or life-threatening arrhythmia within the previous 6 months; men who have resting hypotension or hypertension; and men who have a history of heart failure or have unstable angina.* Rarely, a decrease in vision or permanent visual loss has been reported after PDE5 inhibitor use.

Intracorporeal injection of vasoactive medications causes penile engorgement and erection. Medications most commonly used include papaverine alone, papaverine with phentolamine, and alprostadil (prostaglandin E_1). Alprostadil injections are relatively painless, but careful instruction is essential to prevent local trauma, priapism, and fibrosis. Intraurethral pellets of alprostadil avoid the problem of injection of the medication.

External vacuum therapy (Erec-Aid System) is a nonsurgical treatment consisting of a suction chamber operated by a hand pump that creates a vacuum around the penis. This draws blood into the penis to produce an erection that is maintained by a specially designed tension ring inserted around the base of the penis and which can be kept in place for up to 20–30 minutes. While this method is generally effective, its cumbersome nature limits its appeal.

Surgical implants of penile prostheses remain an option for those patients in whom the nonsurgical approaches are ineffective.

c. **Orthostatic hypotension**—Use of Jobst fitted stockings, tilting the head of the bed, and arising slowly from the supine position can be helpful in treating symptoms of orthostatic hypotension. When such measures are inadequate, treatment with fludrocortisone 0.1–0.2 mg orally daily can be considered. This medication, however, can result in supine hypertension and hypokalemia. The alpha-agonist midodrine (10 mg orally three times a day) can also be used.

D. Cardiovascular Complications

1. Heart disease—Microangiopathy occurs in the heart of patients with diabetes and may explain the etiology of congestive cardiomyopathies in those who do not have demonstrable CAD. More commonly, however, heart disease in patients with diabetes is due to coronary atherosclerosis. MI is three to five times more common in patients with diabetes and is the leading cause of death in patients with type 2 diabetes. CVD risk is increased in patients with type 1 diabetes as well, although the absolute risk is lower than in patients with type 2 diabetes. Premenopausal women who normally have lower rates of CAD lose this protection once diabetes develops. The increased risk in patients with type 2 diabetes reflects the combination of hyperglycemia, hyperlipidemia, abnormalities of platelet adhesiveness, coagulation factors, hypertension, oxidative stress, and inflammation. Large intervention studies of risk factor reduction in diabetes are lacking, but it is reasonable to assume that reducing these risk factors would have a beneficial effect. Lowering LDL cholesterol reduces first events in patients without known coronary disease and secondary events in patients with known coronary disease. These intervention studies included some patients with diabetes, and the benefits of LDL cholesterol lowering was apparent in this group. The National Cholesterol Education Program clinical practice guidelines have designated diabetes as a coronary risk equivalent and have recommended that patients with diabetes should have an LDL cholesterol goal of less than 100 mg/dL (2.6 mmol/L). Lowering LDL cholesterol to 70 mg/dL (1.8 mmol/L) may have additional benefit and is a reasonable target for most patients with type 2 diabetes who have multiple risk factors for CVD.

Aspirin at a dose of 81–325 mg daily is effective in reducing cardiovascular morbidity and mortality in patients who have a history of MI or stroke (secondary prevention). For primary prevention, a 2018 randomized study of 15,480 persons with diabetes but no evident CVD observed that 100 mg of aspirin reduced the first vascular event of MI, stroke or transient ischemic attack or death from vascular event (excluding intracranial hemorrhage) (rate ratio 0.88; 95% CI 0.79 to 0.97). There were, however, more major bleeding events, especially GI, in the aspirin group (rate ratio 1.29; 95% CI 1.09 to 1.52). Thus, for primary prevention, the use of aspirin should only be considered for patients with diabetes who have high cardiovascular risk and low bleeding risk and generally not for adults older than 70 years. Based on the Early Treatment Diabetic Retinopathy Study (ETDRS), there does not appear to be a contraindication to aspirin use to achieve cardiovascular benefit in patients with diabetes who have proliferative retinopathy. Aspirin also does not seem to affect the severity of vitreous/preretinal hemorrhages or their resolution.

2. Hypertension—The ADA recommends lowering systolic blood pressure to less than 140 mm Hg and diastolic pressure to less than 90 mm Hg in patients with diabetes. The systolic target of 130 mm Hg or less and diastolic target of 80 mm Hg or less are recommended for the younger patient if they can be achieved without undue treatment burden. The Systolic Blood Pressure Intervention Trial (SPRINT) reported that treating to a systolic blood pressure of less than 120 mm Hg reduced cardiovascular events by 25% and death from cardiovascular causes by 43% during 3.26 years of follow-up. People with diabetes, however, were excluded from this study, and it is unclear if the results are applicable to this population. Patients with type 2 diabetes who already have CVD or microalbuminuria should be considered for treatment with an ACE inhibitor. More clinical studies are needed to address the question of whether patients with type 2 diabetes who do not have CVD or microalbuminuria would specifically benefit from ACE inhibitor treatment.

3. Peripheral vascular disease—Atherosclerosis is markedly accelerated in the larger arteries. It is often diffuse, with localized enhancement in certain areas of turbulent blood flow, such as at the bifurcation of the aorta or other large vessels. Clinical manifestations of peripheral vascular disease include ischemia of the lower extremities, erectile dysfunction, and intestinal angina.

The incidence of **gangrene of the feet** in patients with diabetes is 30 times that in age-matched controls. The factors responsible for its development, in addition to peripheral vascular disease, are small vessel disease, peripheral neuropathy with loss of both pain sensation and neurogenic inflammatory responses, and secondary infection. In two-thirds of patients with ischemic gangrene, pedal pulses are not palpable. In the remaining one-third who have palpable pulses, reduced blood flow through these vessels can be demonstrated by plethysmographic or Doppler ultrasound examination. Prevention of foot injury is imperative. Agents that reduce peripheral blood flow such as tobacco should be avoided. Control of other risk factors such as hypertension is essential. Beta-blockers are relatively contraindicated because of presumed negative peripheral hemodynamic consequences but data that support this are lacking. Cholesterol-lowering agents are useful as adjunctive therapy when early ischemic signs are detected and when dyslipidemia is present. Patients should be advised to seek immediate medical care if a diabetic foot ulcer develops. Improvement in peripheral blood flow with endarterectomy and bypass operations is possible in certain patients.

E. Skin and Mucous Membrane Complications

Chronic pyogenic infections of the skin may occur, especially in patients with poorly controlled diabetes. Candidal infection can produce erythema and edema of intertriginous areas below the breasts, in the axillas, and between the fingers. It causes vulvovaginitis in women with chronically uncontrolled diabetes who have persistent glucosuria and is a frequent cause of pruritus. While antifungal creams containing miconazole or clotrimazole offer immediate relief of vulvovaginitis, recurrence is frequent unless glucosuria is reduced.

In some patients with type 2 diabetes, poor glycemic control can cause severe hypertriglycemia, which can present as eruptive cutaneous xanthomas and pancreatitis. The skin lesions appear as yellow morbilliform eruptions 2–5 mm in diameter with erythematous areolae. They occur on extensor surfaces (elbows, knees, buttocks) and disappear after triglyceride levels are reduced.

Necrobiosis lipoidica diabeticorum is usually located over the anterior surfaces of the legs or the dorsal surfaces of the ankles. They are oval or irregularly shaped plaques with demarcated borders and a glistening yellow surface and occur in women two to four times more frequently than in men. Pathologically, the lesions show degeneration of collagen, granulomatous inflammation of subcutaneous tissues and blood vessels, capillary basement membrane thickening and obliteration of vessel lumina. The condition is associated with type 1 diabetes, although it can occur in patients with type 2 diabetes, and also in patients without diabetes. First-line therapy includes topical and subcutaneous corticosteroids. Improving glycemic control may help the condition.

"Shin spots" (diabetic dermopathy) are not uncommon in adults with diabetes. They are brownish, rounded, painless atrophic lesions of the skin in the pretibial area.

F. Bone and Joint Complications

Long-standing diabetes can cause progressive stiffness of the hand secondary to contracture and tightening of skin over the joints (diabetic cheiroarthropathy), frozen shoulder (adhesive capsulitis), carpal tunnel syndrome, and Dupuytren contractures. These complications are believed to be due to glycosylation of collagen and perhaps other proteins in connective tissue. There may also be an inflammatory component.

Data on bone mineral density and fracture risk in people with diabetes are contradictory. Patients with type 2 diabetes do appear to be at increased risk for nonvertebral fractures. Women with type 1 diabetes have an increased risk of fracture when compared with women without diabetes. Other factors, such as duration of diabetes, and diabetes complications, such as neuropathy and kidney disease, likely affect both the bone mineral density and fracture risk.

Diffuse idiopathic skeletal hyperostosis (DISH) is characterized by ossification of the anterior longitudinal ligaments of the spine and various extraspinal ligaments. It causes stiffness and decreased range of spinal motion. The peripheral joints most commonly affected are the metacarpophalangeal joints, elbows, and shoulders. Diabetes, obesity, hypertension, and dyslipidemia are risk factors for this condition.

Hyperuricemia and acute and tophaceous gout are more common in type 2 diabetes.

Bursitis, particularly of the shoulders and hips, occurs more frequently than expected in patients with diabetes.

ASCEND Study Collaborative Group et al. Effects of aspirin for primary prevention in persons with diabetes mellitus. N Engl J Med. 2018;379:1529. [PMID: 30146931]

Grennan D. Diabetic foot ulcers. JAMA. 2019;321:114. [PMID: 30620372]

Hinchliffe RJ et al; International Working Group on the Diabetic Foot (IWGDF). Guidelines on diagnosis, prognosis, and management of peripheral artery disease in patients with foot ulcers and diabetes (IWGDF 2019 update). Diabetes Metab Res Rev. 2020;36:e3276. [PMID: 31958217]

Selvarajah D et al. Diabetic peripheral neuropathy: advances in diagnosis and strategies for screening and early intervention. Lancet Diabetes Endocrinol. 2019;7:938. [PMID: 31624024]

Shen JI et al. Evidence for and against ACC/AHA 2017 guideline for target systolic blood pressure of < 130 mm Hg in persons with type 2 diabetes. Curr Cardiol Rep. 2019;21:149. [PMID: 31760494]

Special Situations

A. Diabetes Management in the Hospital

Hospitalized patients are generally not eating as usual and they are often fasting for procedures, which makes it challenging to use outpatient oral or insulin regimens. There may be an increase in the adverse reactions of diabetes medicines (eg, thiazolidinediones can cause fluid retention and worsen heart failure); metformin should not be used in patients with significant chronic kidney or liver disease or those getting contrast for radiographic studies; and SGLT2 inhibitors may be associated with increased risk of diabetic ketoacidosis. The data on the use of continuous glucose monitors, insulin pumps, and hybrid closed loop systems in hospitalized patients are insufficient. Whether patients stay on these systems in the hospital will depend on their severity of illness and access to specialist care. In general, decisions regarding insulin dosing should be made based on capillary blood glucose measurements and not on the data from continuous glucose monitors. Patients should be transitioned to a conventional basal bolus subcutaneous insulin regimen if they are unable to manage their pump and/or continuous glucose monitor because of their illness or if they refuse to follow the institutional guidelines on using the pump or continuous monitor (eg, giving themselves insulin boluses and not informing the clinical staff). The systems have to be removed if the patient is getting an MRI.

On the **general medical and surgical inpatient services**, most patients are treated with subcutaneous insulin regimens. Limited cross-sectional and prospective studies suggest that the best glucose control is achieved on a combination of basal and bolus regimen with 50% of daily insulin needs provided by intermediate- or long-acting insulins. Standardized order sets can reduce errors, and they often include algorithms for recognition and treatment of hypoglycemia (see http://ucsfinpatientdiabetes.pbworks.com for examples). Oral medicines, especially metformin and sulfonylureas, can be resumed as the patient is being prepared for hospital discharge.

In the **ICUs**, glucose levels are controlled most frequently using insulin infusions (http://ucsfinpatientdiabetes.pbworks.com). Patients receiving total parenteral nutrition can have insulin added to the bag. Standard total parenteral nutrition contains 25% dextrose so an infusion rate of 50 mL/hour delivers 12.5 g of dextrose per hour.

Based on the evidence available, ICU patients with diabetes and new-onset hyperglycemia with blood glucose levels above 180 mg/dL (10 mmol/L) should be treated with insulin, aiming for target glucose levels between 140 mg/dL (7.8 mmol/L) and 180 mg/dL (10 mmol/L). In the ICU setting, aiming for blood glucose levels close to 100 mg/dL (5.6 mmol/L) is not beneficial and may even be harmful. When patients leave the ICU, target glucose values between 100 mg/dL (5.6 mmol/L) and 180 mg/dL (10 mmol/L) may be appropriate, although this view is based on clinical observations rather than conclusive evidence.

Preoperative and perioperative diabetic management strategies are discussed in Chapter 3.

The morbidity and mortality in hospitalized patients with diabetes are twice those of patients without diabetes. Those with new-onset hyperglycemia (ie, those without a preadmission diagnosis of diabetes) have even higher mortality—almost eightfold that of patients without diabetes in one study. These observations have led to the question of whether tight glycemic control in the hospital improves outcomes.

B. Diabetes in Pregnancy

See Chapter 19.

DIABETIC COMA

Coma may be due to causes not directly related to diabetes. Diabetic coma requires differentiation (Table 27–10): (1) Hypoglycemic coma from excessive insulin or oral hypoglycemic agents. (2) Hyperglycemic coma with either severe insulin deficiency (DKA) or mild to moderate insulin deficiency (hyperglycemic hyperosmolar state). (3) Lactic acidosis, particularly when patients with diabetes have severe infections or cardiovascular collapse.

DIABETIC KETOACIDOSIS

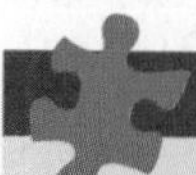

ESSENTIALS OF DIAGNOSIS

- Hyperglycemia > than 250 mg/dL (13.9 mmol/L).
- Metabolic acidosis with blood pH < 7.3; serum bicarbonate < 15 mEq/L.
- Serum positive for ketones.

General Considerations

Diabetic ketoacidosis (DKA) is a disorder primarily of type 1 diabetes but can occur in patients with type 2 diabetes who have severe illness, such as sepsis or trauma. DKA may be the initial manifestation of type 1 diabetes or may result from increased insulin requirements in patients with type 1 diabetes during the course of infection, trauma, MI, or surgery. It is a life-threatening medical emergency. The National Data Group reports an annual incidence of five to eight episodes of DKA per 1000 persons with diabetes. DKA is one of the more common serious complications of insulin pump therapy, occurring in approximately 1 per 80 patient-months of treatment. Many patients who monitor capillary blood glucose regularly ignore urine ketone measurements, which signals the possibility of insulin leakage or pump failure before serious illness develops. Poor compliance, either for psychological reasons or because of inadequate education, is the most common cause of recurrent DKA.

Table 27–10. Laboratory diagnosis of diabetic coma.

	Urine Glucose	Urine Ketones	Plasma Glucose	Serum Bicarbonate	Serum Ketones
Related to Diabetes					
Hypoglycemia	0[1]	0 or +	Low	Normal	0
Diabetic ketoacidosis	++++	++++	High	Low	++++
Hyperglycemic hyperosmolar state coma	++++	0 or +	High	Normal or slightly low	0
Lactic acidosis	0 or +	0 or +	Normal or low or high	Low	0 or +
Unrelated to Diabetes					
Alcohol or other toxic drugs	0 or +	0 or +	May be low	Normal or low[2]	0 or +
Cerebrovascular accident or head trauma	+ or 0	0	Often high	Normal	0
Uremia	0 or +	0	High or normal	Low	0 or +

[1]Leftover urine in bladder might still contain glucose from earlier hyperglycemia.
[2]Alcohol can elevate plasma lactate as well as keto acids to reduce pH.

Clinical Findings

A. Symptoms and Signs

The appearance of DKA is usually preceded by a day or more of polyuria and polydipsia associated with marked fatigue, nausea, and vomiting.

If untreated, mental stupor ensues that can progress to coma. Drowsiness is fairly common, but frank coma only occurs in about 10% of patients. On physical examination, evidence of dehydration in a stuporous patient with rapid deep breathing and a "fruity" breath odor of acetone strongly suggests the diagnosis. Hypotension with tachycardia indicates profound fluid and electrolyte depletion, and mild hypothermia is usually present. Abdominal pain and even tenderness may be present in the absence of abdominal disease. Conversely, cholecystitis or pancreatitis may occur with minimal symptoms and signs.

B. Laboratory Findings

Typically, the patient with moderately severe DKA has a plasma glucose of 350–900 mg/dL (19.4–50 mmol/L), serum ketones at a dilution of 1:8 or greater or beta-hydroxybutyrate more than 4 nmol/L, hyperkalemia (serum potassium level of 5–8 mEq/L), mild hyponatremia (serum sodium of approximately 130 mEq/L), hyperphosphatemia (serum phosphate level of 6–7 mg/dL [1.9–2.3 mmol/L]), and elevated BUN and serum creatinine levels (Table 27–10). Acidosis may be severe (pH ranging from 6.9 to 7.2 and serum bicarbonate ranging from 5 mEq/L to 15 mEq/L); PCO_2 is low (15–20 mm Hg) related to compensatory hyperventilation. Fluid depletion is marked, typically about 100 mL/kg. Lactate levels are usually elevated and higher than 2 mmol/L in more than 50 % of the patients. The hyperlactatemia is not due to hypoxia or sepsis and reflects metabolic fuel use in the insulin deficient state. Higher glucose levels and lower pH levels are associated with higher lactate levels. In euglycemic ketoacidosis, the patient can have severe acidosis and fluid depletion but the plasma glucose levels are only modestly elevated, usually less than 250 mg/day (13.9 mmol/L). This condition is seen in patients in whom DKA develops while receiving treatment with SGLT2 inhibitors. Ketoacidosis with lower glucose levels also occurs in pregnancy and may reflect the expanded plasma volume and the increased GFR.

The difference between venous and arterial pH is 0.02 to 0.15 pH units and venous and arterial bicarbonate is 1.88 mEq/L. These small differences will not affect the diagnosis or the management of DKA, and there is no need to collect arterial blood for measuring the acid-base status.

The hyperkalemia occurs despite total body potassium depletion because of the shift of potassium from the intracellular to extracellular spaces that occurs in systemic acidosis. The average total body potassium deficit resulting from osmotic diuresis, acidosis, and GI losses is about 3–5 mEq/kg. Similarly, despite the elevated serum phosphate, total body phosphate is generally depleted. Serum sodium is generally reduced due to loss of sodium ions (7–10 mEq/kg) by polyuria and vomiting and because severe hyperglycemia shifts intracellular water into the interstitial compartment. For every 100 mg/dL of plasma glucose, serum sodium decreases by 1.6 mEq/L (5.56 mmol/L). The decrease in serum sodium may be greater when patients have more severe hyperglycemia (greater than 400 mg/dL, 22.2 mmol/L) and a correction factor of 2.4 mEq/L may be used. Hypertriglyceridemia should be considered if the corrected sodium is very low. Serum osmolality can be directly measured by standard tests of freezing point depression or can be estimated by calculating the molarity of sodium, chloride, and glucose in the serum. A convenient method of estimating effective serum osmolality is as follows (normal values are 280–300 mOsm/kg):

$$\text{mOsm/kg} = 2\,[\text{measured Na}^+] + \frac{\text{Glucose (mg/dL)}}{18}$$

These calculated estimates are usually 10–20 mOsm/kg lower than values measured by standard cryoscopic techniques. CNS depression or coma occurs when the effective serum osmolality exceeds 320–330 mOsm/L. Coma in a patient with diabetes with a lower osmolality should prompt a search for the cause of coma other than hyperosmolality (see Table 27–10 and Chapter 24).

Ketoacidemia represents the effect of insulin lack at multiple enzyme loci. Insulin lack associated with elevated levels of growth hormone, catecholamines, and glucagon contributes to increases in lipolysis from adipose tissue and in hepatic ketogenesis. In addition, reduced ketolysis by insulin-deficient peripheral tissues contributes to the ketoacidemia. The only true "keto" acid present in diabetic ketoacidosis is acetoacetic acid which, along with its by-product acetone, is measured by nitroprusside reagents (Acetest and Ketostix). The sensitivity for acetone, however, is poor, requiring over 10 mmol/L, which is seldom reached in the plasma of ketoacidotic patients—although this detectable concentration is readily achieved in urine. Thus, in the plasma of ketotic patients, only acetoacetate is measured by these reagents. The more prevalent beta-hydroxybutyric acid has no ketone group and is therefore not detected by conventional nitroprusside tests. This takes on special importance in the presence of circulatory collapse during DKA, wherein an increase in lactic acid can shift the redox state to increase beta-hydroxybutyric acid at the expense of the readily detectable acetoacetic acid. Bedside diagnostic reagents are then unreliable, suggesting no ketonemia in cases where beta-hydroxybutyric acid is a major factor in producing the acidosis. Combined glucose and ketone meters (Precision Xtra, Nova Max Plus) that measure blood beta-hydroxybutyrate concentration on capillary blood are available. Many clinical laboratories also offer direct blood beta-hydroxybutyrate measurement.

Nonspecific elevations of serum amylase and lipase occur in about 16–25% of cases of DKA, and an imaging study may be necessary if the diagnosis of acute pancreatitis is being seriously considered. Leukocytosis as high as 25,000/mcL (25×10^9/L) with a left shift may occur with or without associated infection. The presence of an elevated or even a normal temperature can suggest the presence of an infection since patients with DKA are generally hypothermic if uninfected.

Treatment

Patients with **mild DKA** are alert and have pH levels between 7.25 and 7.30 and beta-hydroxybutyrate levels of 3–4 mmol/L; those with **moderate ketoacidosis** are either alert or a little drowsy and have pH levels between 7.0 and 7.24 and beta-hydroxybutyrate levels of 4–8 mmol/L; and those with **severe ketoacidosis** are stuporose and have a pH < 7.0 and beta-hydroxybutyrate levels of greater than 8 mmol/L. Patients with mild ketoacidosis can be treated in the emergency department, but those with moderate or severe ketoacidosis require admission to the ICU or step-down unit. Therapeutic goals are to restore plasma volume and tissue perfusion, reduce blood glucose and osmolality toward normal, correct acidosis, replenish electrolyte losses, and identify and treat precipitating factors. Gastric intubation is recommended in the comatose patient to prevent vomiting and aspiration that may occur as a result of gastric atony, a common complication of DKA. An indwelling urinary catheter may also be necessary. In patients with preexisting heart or kidney failure or those in severe cardiovascular collapse, a central venous pressure catheter should be inserted to evaluate the degree of hypovolemia and to monitor subsequent fluid administration.

A comprehensive flow sheet that includes vital signs, serial laboratory data, and therapeutic interventions (eg, fluids, insulin) should be meticulously maintained by the clinician responsible for the patient's care. Plasma glucose should be recorded hourly and electrolytes and pH at least every 2–3 hours during the initial treatment period. Bedside glucose meters should be used to titrate the insulin therapy. The patient should not receive sedatives or opioids in order to avoid masking signs and symptoms of impeding cerebral edema (see Complications & Prognosis, below).

A. Fluid Replacement

In most patients, the fluid deficit is 4–5 L. Initially, 0.9% saline solution is the solution of choice to help re-expand the contracted vascular volume and should be started in the emergency department as soon as the diagnosis is established. The saline should be infused rapidly to provide 1 L/hour over the first 1–2 hours. After the first 2 L of fluid have been given, the intravenous infusion should be at the rate of 300–400 mL/hour. Use 0.9% ("normal") saline unless the serum sodium is greater than 150 mEq/L, when 0.45% ("half normal") saline solution should be used. The volume status should be carefully monitored clinically. Failure to give enough volume replacement (at least 3–4 L in 8 hours) to restore normal perfusion is one of the most serious therapeutic shortcomings adversely influencing satisfactory recovery. Excessive fluid replacement (more than 5 L in 8 hours) may contribute to acute respiratory distress syndrome or cerebral edema. When blood glucose falls to approximately 250 mg/dL (13.9 mmol/L), the fluids should be changed to a 5% glucose-containing solution to maintain serum glucose in the range of 250–300 mg/dL (13.9–16.7 mmol/L). This will prevent the development of hypoglycemia and will also reduce the likelihood of cerebral edema, which could result from too rapid decline of blood glucose.

B. Insulin Replacement

Immediately after initiation of fluid replacement, regular insulin can be given intravenously in a loading dose of 0.1 unit/kg as a bolus to prime the tissue insulin receptors. Following the initial bolus, intravenous doses of insulin as low as 0.1 unit/kg/hour are continuously infused or given hourly as an intramuscular injection; this is sufficient to replace the insulin deficit in most patients. A prospective randomized study showed that a bolus dose is not required if patients are given hourly insulin infusion at 0.14 unit/kg. Replacement of insulin deficiency helps correct the acidosis by reducing the flux of fatty acids to the liver, reducing ketone production by the liver, and also improving removal of ketones from the blood. Insulin treatment reduces the hyperosmolality by reducing the hyperglycemia. It accomplishes this by increasing removal of glucose through peripheral utilization as well as by decreasing production of glucose by the liver. This latter effect is accomplished by direct inhibition of gluconeogenesis and glycogenolysis as well as by lowered amino acid flux from muscle to liver and reduced hyperglucagonemia.

The insulin infusion should be "piggy-backed" into the fluid line so the rate of fluid replacement can be changed without altering the insulin delivery rate. If the plasma glucose level fails to fall at least 10% in the first hour, a repeat loading dose (0.1 or 0.14 unit/kg) is recommended. Rarely, a patient with immune insulin resistance is encountered, and this requires doubling the insulin dose every 2–4 hours if hyperglycemia does not improve after the first two doses of insulin. The insulin dose should be adjusted to lower the glucose concentration by about 50–70 mg/dL/hour (2.8–3.9 mmol/L). If clinical circumstances prevent use of an insulin infusion, then the insulin can be given intramuscularly. An initial 0.15 unit/kg of regular insulin is given intravenously, and at the same time, the same size dose is given intramuscularly. Subsequently, regular insulin is given intramuscularly hourly at a dose of 0.1 unit/kg until the blood glucose falls to around 250 mg/dL, when the insulin can be given subcutaneously. Patients who normally take insulin glargine or insulin detemir can be given their usual maintenance doses during the initial treatment of their DKA. The continuation of their subcutaneous basal insulins means that lower doses of intravenous insulin will be needed, and there will be a smoother transition from intravenous insulin infusion to the subcutaneous regimen.

C. Potassium

Total body potassium loss from polyuria and vomiting may be as high as 200 mEq. However, because of shifts of potassium from cells into the extracellular space as a consequence of acidosis, serum potassium is usually normal to slightly elevated prior to institution of treatment. As the acidosis is corrected, potassium flows back into the cells, and hypokalemia can develop if potassium replacement is not instituted. If the patient is not uremic and has an adequate urinary output, potassium chloride in doses of 10–30 mEq/hour should be infused during the second and third hours after beginning therapy as soon as the acidosis starts to resolve. Replacement should be started sooner if the initial serum potassium is inappropriately normal or low and should be delayed if serum potassium fails to respond to initial therapy and remains above 5 mEq/L, as in cases of CKD. Occasionally, a patient may present with a serum potassium level less than 3.5 mEq/L, in which case insulin therapy should be delayed until the potassium level is corrected to greater than 3.5 mEq/L. An ECG can help monitor the patient's potassium status: High peaked T waves are a sign of hyperkalemia, and flattened T waves with U waves are a sign of hypokalemia. Foods high in potassium content should be prescribed when the patient has recovered sufficiently to take food orally. Tomato juice has 14 mEq of potassium per 240 mL, and a medium-sized banana provides about 10 mEq.

D. Sodium Bicarbonate

The use of sodium bicarbonate in the management of DKA has been questioned since clinical benefit was not demonstrated in one prospective randomized trial and because of the following potentially harmful consequences: (1) development of hypokalemia from rapid shift of potassium into cells if the acidosis is overcorrected; (2) tissue anoxia from reduced dissociation of oxygen from hemoglobin when acidosis is rapidly reversed (leftward shift of the oxygen dissociation curve); and (3) cerebral acidosis resulting from lowering of cerebrospinal fluid pH. It must be emphasized, however, that these considerations are less important when very severe acidosis exists. Therefore, it is recommended that bicarbonate be administered in DKA if the arterial blood pH is 7.0 or less, with careful monitoring to prevent overcorrection. One or two ampules of sodium bicarbonate (one ampule contains 44 mEq/50 mL) should be added to 1 L of 0.45% saline with 20 mEq KCl or to 400 mL of sterile water with 20 mEq KCl and infused over 1 to 2 hours. (**Note:** Addition of sodium bicarbonate to 0.9% saline would produce a markedly hypertonic solution that could aggravate the hyperosmolar state already present.) It can be repeated until the arterial pH reaches 7.1, but *it should not be given if the pH is 7.1 or greater* since additional bicarbonate would increase the risk of rebound metabolic alkalosis as ketones are metabolized. Alkalosis shifts potassium from serum into cells, which could precipitate a fatal cardiac arrhythmia.

E. Phosphate

Phosphate replacement is seldom required in treating DKA. However, if severe hypophosphatemia of less than 1 mg/dL (0.32 mmol/L) develops during insulin therapy, a small amount of phosphate can be replaced per hour as the potassium salt. Three randomized studies, though, in which phosphate was replaced in patients with DKA did not show any apparent clinical benefit from phosphate administration. Moreover, attempts to use potassium phosphate as the sole means of replacing potassium have led to a number of reported cases of severe hypocalcemia with tetany. To minimize the risk of inducing tetany from too-rapid replacement of phosphate, the average deficit of 40–50 mmol of phosphate should be replaced intravenously at a rate *no greater than 3–4 mmol/hour* in a 60- to 70-kg person. A stock solution (Abbott) provides a mixture of 1.12 g KH_2PO_4 and 1.18 g K_2HPO_4 in a 5-mL single-dose vial (this equals 22 mmol of potassium and 15 mmol of phosphate). One-half of this vial (2.5 mL) should be added to 1 L of either 0.45% saline or 5% dextrose in water. Two liters of this solution, infused at a rate of 400 mL/hour, will correct the phosphate deficit at the optimal rate of 3 mmol/hour while providing 4.4 mEq of potassium per hour. (Additional potassium should be administered as potassium chloride to provide a total of 10–30 mEq of potassium per hour, as noted above.) If the serum phosphate remains below 2.5 mg/dL (0.8 mmol/L) after this infusion, a repeat 5-hour infusion can be given.

F. Hyperchloremic Acidosis During Therapy

Because of the considerable loss of keto acids in the urine during the initial phase of therapy, substrate for subsequent regeneration of bicarbonate is lost and correction of the total bicarbonate deficit is hampered. A portion of the bicarbonate deficit is replaced with chloride ions infused in large amounts as saline to correct the dehydration. In most patients, as the ketoacidosis clears during insulin replacement, a hyperchloremic, low-bicarbonate pattern emerges with a normal anion gap. This is a relatively benign condition that reverses itself over the subsequent 12–24 hours once intravenous saline is no longer being administered. Using a balanced electrolyte solution with a pH of 7.4 and 98 mEq/L chloride such as Plasma-lyte instead of normal saline (pH ~5.5; chloride 154 mEq/L) has been reported to prevent the hyperchloremic acidosis.

G. Treatment of Associated Infection

Antibiotics are prescribed as indicated (Table 30–5). Cholecystitis and pyelonephritis may be particularly severe in these patients.

H. Transition to Subcutaneous Insulin Regimen

Once the DKA is controlled and the patient is awake and able to eat, subcutaneous insulin therapy can be initiated. The patient with type 1 diabetes may have persistent significant tissue insulin resistance and may require a total daily insulin dose of approximately 0.6 unit/kg. The amount of insulin required in the previous 8 hours can also be helpful in estimating the initial insulin doses. Half the total daily dose can be given as a long-acting basal insulin and the other half as short-acting insulin premeals. The patient should receive subcutaneous basal insulin and rapid-acting insulin analog with the first meal and the insulin infusion discontinued an hour later. The overlap of the subcutaneous insulin action and insulin infusion is necessary to prevent relapse of the DKA. In patients with preexisting diabetes, giving their basal insulin by subcutaneous injection at initiation of treatment simplifies the transition from intravenous to subcutaneous regimen. The increased insulin resistance is only present for a few days, and it is important to reduce both the basal and bolus insulins to avoid hypoglycemia. A patient with new-onset type 1 diabetes usually still has significant beta cell function and may not need any basal insulin and only very low doses of rapid-acting insulin before meals after recovery from the ketoacidosis. Patients with type 2 diabetes and DKA due to severe illness may initially require insulin therapy but can often transition back to oral agents during outpatient follow-up.

Complications & Prognosis

Low-dose insulin infusion and fluid and electrolyte replacement combined with careful monitoring of patients' clinical and laboratory responses to therapy have dramatically reduced the mortality rates of DKA to less than 5% in individuals under 40 years of age. However, this complication remains a significant risk in the aged who have mortality rates greater than 20% and in patients in profound coma in whom treatment has been delayed. Acute MI and infarction of the bowel following prolonged hypotension worsen the outlook. A serious prognostic sign is ESKD, and prior kidney dysfunction worsens the prognosis considerably because the kidney plays a key role in compensating for massive pH and electrolyte abnormalities. Symptomatic cerebral edema occurs primarily in the pediatric population. Risk factors for its development include severe baseline acidosis, rapid correction of hyperglycemia, and excess volume administration in the first 4 hours. Onset of headache or deterioration in mental status during treatment should lead to consideration of this complication. Intravenous mannitol at a dosage of 1–2 g/kg given over 15 minutes is the mainstay of treatment. Excess crystalloid infusion can precipitate pulmonary edema. Acute respiratory distress syndrome is a rare complication of treatment of DKA.

After recovery and stabilization, patients should be instructed on how to recognize the early symptoms and signs of ketoacidosis. Urine ketones or capillary blood beta-hydroxybutyrate should be measured in patients with signs of infection or in insulin pump-treated patients when capillary blood glucose remains unexpectedly and persistently high. When heavy ketonuria and glycosuria persist on several successive examinations, supplemental rapid-acting insulin should be administered and liquid foods such as lightly salted tomato juice and broth should be ingested to replenish fluids and electrolytes. The patient should be instructed to contact the clinician if ketonuria persists, and especially if there is vomiting and inability to keep down fluids. Recurrent episodes of severe ketoacidosis often indicate poor compliance with the insulin regimen, and these patients will require intensive counseling.

Fayfman M et al. Management of hyperglycemic crises: diabetic ketoacidosis and hyperglycemic hyperosmolar state. Med Clin North Am. 2017;101:587. [PMID: 28372715]

Islam T et al. Guidelines and controversies in the management of diabetic ketoacidosis—a mini-review. World J Diabetes. 2018;9:226. [PMID: 30588284]

Karslioglu French E et al. Diabetic ketoacidosis and hyperosmolar hyperglycemic syndrome: review of acute decompensated diabetes in adult patients. BMJ. 2019;365:l114. [PMID: 31142480]

Modi A et al. Euglycemic diabetic letoacidosis: a review. Curr Diabetes Rev. 2017;13:315. [PMID: 27097605]

HYPERGLYCEMIC HYPEROSMOLAR STATE

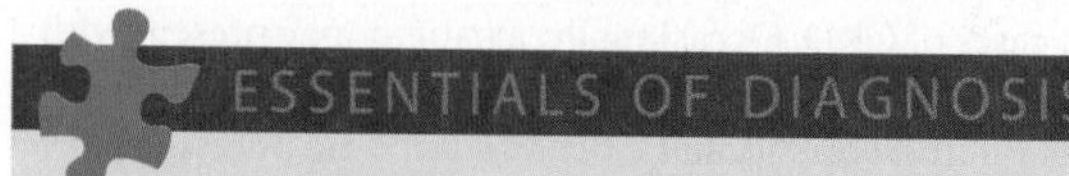

- Hyperglycemia > 600 mg/dL (33.3 mmol/L).
- Serum osmolality > 310 mOsm/kg.
- No acidosis; blood pH > 7.3.
- Serum bicarbonate > 15 mEq/L.
- Normal anion gap (< 14 mEq/L).

General Considerations

This second most common form of hyperglycemic coma is characterized by severe hyperglycemia in the absence of significant ketosis, with hyperosmolality and dehydration. It occurs in patients with mild or occult diabetes, and most patients are typically middle-aged to elderly. Accurate figures are not available as to its true incidence, but from data on hospital discharges it is rarer than DKA even in older age groups. Underlying CKD or heart failure is common, and the presence of either worsens the prognosis. A precipitating event such as infection, MI, stroke, or recent operation is often present. Certain medications such as phenytoin, diazoxide, corticosteroids, and diuretics have been implicated in its pathogenesis, as have procedures associated with glucose loading such as peritoneal dialysis.

Pathogenesis

A partial or relative insulin deficiency may initiate the syndrome by reducing glucose utilization of muscle, fat, and liver while inducing hyperglucagonemia and increasing hepatic glucose output. With massive glycosuria, obligatory water loss ensues. If a patient is unable to maintain adequate fluid intake because of an associated acute or chronic illness or has suffered excessive fluid loss, marked dehydration results. As the plasma volume contracts, kidney function becomes impaired, limiting the urinary glucose losses and exacerbating the hyperglycemia. Severe hyperosmolality develops that causes mental confusion and finally coma. It is not clear why ketosis is virtually absent under these conditions of insulin insufficiency, although reduced levels of growth hormone may be a factor, along with portal vein insulin concentrations sufficient to restrain ketogenesis.

Clinical Findings

A. Symptoms and Signs

Onset may be insidious over a period of days or weeks, with weakness, polyuria, and polydipsia. The lack of features of DKA (eg, vomiting, rapid deep breathing, acetone odor) may retard recognition of the syndrome and delay therapy until dehydration becomes more profound than in ketoacidosis. Reduced intake of fluid is not an uncommon historical feature, due to either inappropriate lack of thirst, nausea, or inaccessibility of fluids to elderly, bedridden patients. A history of ingestion of large quantities of glucose-containing fluids, such as soft drinks or orange juice, can occasionally be obtained. Lethargy and confusion develop as serum osmolality exceeds 310 mOsm/kg, and convulsions and coma can occur if osmolality exceeds 320–330 mOsm/kg. Physical examination confirms the presence of profound dehydration in a lethargic or comatose patient without Kussmaul respirations.

B. Laboratory Findings

Severe hyperglycemia is present, with blood glucose values ranging from 800 mg/dL to 2400 mg/dL (44.4 mmol/L to 133.2 mmol/L) (Table 27–10). In mild cases, where dehydration is less severe, dilutional hyponatremia as well as urinary sodium losses may reduce serum sodium to 120–125 mEq/L, which protects to some extent against extreme hyperosmolality. However, as dehydration progresses, serum sodium can exceed 140 mEq/L, producing serum osmolality readings of 330–440 mOsm/kg. Ketosis and acidosis are usually absent or mild. Prerenal azotemia is the rule, with serum urea nitrogen elevations over 100 mg/dL (35.7 mmol/L) being typical.

Treatment

A. Fluid Replacement

Fluid replacement is of paramount importance in treating the nonketotic hyperglycemic state. Fluid deficit may be as much as 6–10 L.

If hypovolemia is present as evidenced by hypotension and oliguria, fluid therapy should be initiated with 0.9% saline. In all other cases, 0.45% saline appears to be preferable as the initial replacement solution because the body fluids of these patients are markedly hyperosmolar. As much as 4–6 L of fluid may be required in the first 8–10 hours. Careful monitoring of the patient is required for proper sodium and water replacement. An important end point of fluid therapy is to restore urinary output to 50 mL/hour or more. Once blood glucose reaches 250 mg/dL (13.9 mmol/L), fluid replacement should include 5% dextrose in either water, 0.45% saline solution, or 0.9% saline solution. The rate of dextrose infusion should be adjusted to maintain glycemic levels of 250–300 mg/dL (13.9–16.7 mmol/L) in order to reduce the risk of cerebral edema.

B. Insulin

Less insulin may be required to reduce the hyperglycemia in nonketotic patients as compared to those with diabetic ketoacidotic coma. In fact, fluid replacement alone can reduce hyperglycemia considerably by correcting the hypovolemia, which then increases both glomerular filtration and renal excretion of glucose. Insulin treatment should therefore be delayed unless the patient has significant ketonemia (beta-hydroxybutyrate more than 1 mmol/L). Start the insulin infusion rate at 0.05 unit/kg/hour (bolus is not needed) and titrate to lower blood glucose levels by 50–70 mg/dL per hour (2.8–3.9 mmol/L/hour). Once the patient has stabilized and the blood glucose falls to around 250 mg/dL (13.9 mmol/L), insulin can be given subcutaneously.

C. Potassium

With the absence of acidosis, there may be no initial hyperkalemia unless associated ESKD is present. This results in less severe total potassium depletion than in DKA, and less potassium replacement is therefore needed. However, because initial serum potassium is usually not elevated and because it declines rapidly as a result of insulin's effect on driving potassium intracellularly, it is recommended that potassium replacement be initiated earlier than in ketotic patients, assuming that no CKD or oliguria is present. Potassium chloride (10 mEq/L) can be added to the initial bottle of fluids administered if the patient's serum potassium is not elevated.

D. Phosphate

If severe hypophosphatemia (serum phosphate less than 1 mg/dL [0.32 mmol/L]) develops during insulin therapy, phosphate replacement can be given as described for ketoacidotic patients (at 3 mmol/hour).

Complications & Prognosis

The severe dehydration and low output state may predispose the patient to complications such as MI, stroke, PE, mesenteric vein thrombosis, and disseminated intravascular coagulation. Fluid replacement remains the primary approach to the prevention of these complications. Low-dose heparin prophylaxis is reasonable but benefits of routine anticoagulation remain doubtful. Rhabdomyolysis is a recognized complication and should be looked for and treated.

The overall mortality rate of hyperglycemic hyperosmolar state coma is more than ten times that of DKA, chiefly because of its higher incidence in older patients, who may have compromised cardiovascular systems or associated major illnesses and whose dehydration is often excessive because of delays in recognition and treatment. (When patients are matched for age, the prognoses of these two hyperglycemic emergencies are reasonably comparable.) When prompt therapy is instituted, the mortality rate can be reduced from nearly 50% to that related to the severity of coexistent disorders.

After the patient is stabilized, the appropriate form of long-term management of the diabetes must be determined. Insulin treatment should be continued for a few weeks but patients usually recover sufficient endogenous insulin secretion to make a trial of diet or diet plus oral agents worthwhile. When the episode occurs in a patient who has known diabetes, then education of the patient and caregivers should be instituted. They should be taught how to recognize situations (nausea and vomiting, infection) that predispose to recurrence of the hyperglycemic, hyperosmolar state, as well as detailed information on how to prevent the escalating dehydration that culminates in hyperosmolar coma (small sips of sugar-free liquids, increase in usual hypoglycemic therapy, or early contact with the clinician).

Fayfman M et al. Management of hyperglycemic crises: diabetic ketoacidosis and hyperglycemic hyperosmolar state. Med Clin North Am. 2017;101:587. [PMID: 28372715]

Scott AR; Joint British Diabetes Societies (JBDS) for Inpatient Care; JBDS hyperosmolar hyperglycaemic guidelines group. Management of hyperosmolar hyperglycaemic state in adults with diabetes. Diabet Med. 2015;32:714. [PMID: 25980647]

LACTIC ACIDOSIS

ESSENTIALS OF DIAGNOSIS

- Severe metabolic acidosis with compensatory hyperventilation.
- Blood pH < 7.30.
- Serum bicarbonate < 15 mEq/L.
- Anion gap > 15 mEq/L.
- Absent serum ketones.
- Serum lactate > 5 mmol/L.

General Considerations

Lactic acidosis is characterized by accumulation of excess lactic acid in the blood. Normally, the principal sources of this acid are the erythrocytes (which lack enzymes for aerobic oxidation), skeletal muscle, skin, and brain. Conversion of lactic acid to glucose and its oxidation principally by the liver but also by the kidneys represent the chief pathways for its removal. Hyperlactatemia and acidosis occur when lactate production exceeds lactate consumption. Causes include tissue hypoxia, disorders that increase epinephrine levels (severe asthma with excess beta-adrenergic agonist use, cardiogenic or hemorrhagic shock, pheochromocytoma), and drugs that impair oxidative phosphorylation (antiretroviral agents and propofol). Most cases of metformin-associated lactic acidosis occur in patients in whom there were contraindications to the use of metformin, in particular kidney failure. Metformin levels are usually greater than 5 mcg/L when metformin is implicated as the cause of lactic acidosis. Other causes of lactic acidosis include several inborn errors of metabolism and the MELAS syndrome (mitochondrial encephalopathy, lactic acidosis, and stroke-like episodes). D-Lactic acidosis can occur in patients with short bowel syndrome when unabsorbed carbohydrates are presented as substrate for fermentation by colonic bacteria.

Clinical Findings

A. Symptoms and Signs

The main clinical feature of lactic acidosis is marked hyperventilation. When lactic acidosis is secondary to tissue hypoxia or vascular collapse, the clinical presentation is variable, being that of the prevailing catastrophic illness. However, in the idiopathic, or spontaneous, variety, the onset is rapid (usually over a few hours), blood pressure is normal, peripheral circulation is good, and there is no cyanosis.

B. Laboratory Findings

Plasma bicarbonate and blood pH are quite low, indicating the presence of severe metabolic acidosis. Ketones are usually absent from plasma and urine or at least not prominent. The first clue may be a high anion gap (serum sodium minus the sum of chloride and bicarbonate anions [in mEq/L] should be no greater than 15). A higher value indicates the existence of an abnormal compartment of anions. If this cannot be clinically explained by an excess of keto acids (diabetes), inorganic acids (uremia), or anions from medication overdosage (salicylates, methyl alcohol, ethylene glycol), then lactic acidosis is probably the correct diagnosis. (See also Chapter 21.) In the absence of azotemia, hyperphosphatemia may be a clue to the presence of lactic acidosis for reasons that are not clear. The diagnosis is confirmed by a plasma lactic acid concentration of 5 mmol/L or higher (values as high as 30 mmol/L have been reported). Normal plasma values average 1 mmol/L, with a normal lactate/pyruvate ratio of 10:1. This ratio is greatly exceeded in lactic acidosis.[1]

Treatment

Aggressive treatment of the precipitating cause of lactic acidosis is the main component of therapy, such as ensuring adequate oxygenation and vascular perfusion of tissues. Empiric antibiotic coverage for sepsis should be given after culture samples are obtained in any patient in whom the cause of the lactic acidosis is not apparent (Table 30–5).

Alkalinization with intravenous sodium bicarbonate to keep the pH above 7.2 has been recommended by some in the emergency treatment of lactic acidosis; as much as 2000 mEq in 24 hours has been used. However, there is no evidence that the mortality rate is favorably affected by administering bicarbonate, and its use remains controversial. Hemodialysis may be useful in cases where large sodium loads are poorly tolerated and in cases associated with metformin toxicity.

Prognosis

The mortality rate of spontaneous lactic acidosis is high. The prognosis in most cases is that of the primary disorder that produced the lactic acidosis.

DeFronzo R et al. Metformin-associated lactic acidosis: current perspectives on causes and risk. Metabolism. 2016;65:20. [PMID: 26773926]

[1]In collecting samples, it is essential to rapidly chill and separate the blood in order to remove red cells, whose continued glycolysis at room temperature is a common source of error in reports of high plasma lactate. Frozen plasma remains stable for subsequent assay.

THE HYPOGLYCEMIC STATES

Spontaneous hypoglycemia in adults is of two principal types: fasting and postprandial. Symptoms begin at plasma glucose levels in the range of 60 mg/dL (3.3 mmol/L) and impairment of brain function at approximately 50 mg/dL (2.8 mmol/L). Fasting hypoglycemia is often subacute or chronic and usually presents with neuroglycopenia as its principal manifestation; postprandial hypoglycemia is relatively acute and is often heralded by symptoms of neurogenic autonomic discharge (sweating, palpitations, anxiety, tremulousness).

Differential Diagnosis (Table 27–11)

Fasting hypoglycemia may occur in certain endocrine disorders, such as hypopituitarism, Addison disease, or myxedema; in disorders related to liver malfunction, such as acute alcoholism or liver failure; and in instances of ESKD, particularly in patients requiring dialysis. These conditions are usually obvious, with hypoglycemia being only a secondary feature. When fasting hypoglycemia is a primary manifestation developing in adults without apparent endocrine disorders or inborn metabolic diseases from childhood, the principal diagnostic possibilities include (1) hyperinsulinism, due to either pancreatic B cell tumors or iatrogenic or surreptitious administration of insulin or sulfonylurea; and (2) hypoglycemia due to extrapancreatic tumors.

Postprandial (reactive) hypoglycemia may occur after GI surgery and is particularly associated with the dumping syndrome after gastrectomy and Roux-en-Y gastric bypass surgery. Occult diabetes very occasionally presents with postprandial hypoglycemia.

Alcohol-related hypoglycemia is due to hepatic glycogen depletion combined with alcohol-mediated inhibition of gluconeogenesis. It is most common in malnourished individuals with excessive alcohol intake but can occur in anyone who is unable to ingest food after an acute alcoholic episode followed by gastritis and vomiting.

Immunopathologic hypoglycemia is an extremely rare condition in which anti-insulin antibodies or antibodies to insulin receptors develop spontaneously.

Table 27–11. Common causes of hypoglycemia in adults.[1]

Fasting hypoglycemia
Pancreatic B cell tumor
Surreptitious administration of insulin or sulfonylureas
Extrapancreatic tumors
Postprandial hypoglycemia
Gastric surgery
Occult diabetes mellitus
Alcohol-related hypoglycemia
Immunopathologic hypoglycemia
Idiopathic anti-insulin antibodies (which release their bound insulin)
Antibodies to insulin receptors (which act as agonists)
Drug-induced hypoglycemia

[1]In the absence of clinically obvious endocrine, kidney, or liver disorders and exclusive of diabetes mellitus treated with hypoglycemic agents.

HYPOGLYCEMIA DUE TO PANCREATIC B CELL TUMORS

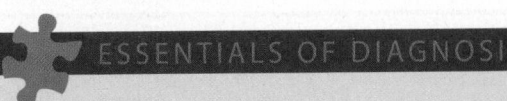

- Hypoglycemic symptoms—often neuroglycopenic (confusion, blurred vision, anxiety, convulsions).
- Immediate recovery upon administration of glucose.
- Blood glucose 40–50 mg/dL (2.2–2.8 mmol/L) with a serum insulin level of ≥ 6 microunits/mL.

General Considerations

Fasting hypoglycemia in an otherwise healthy, well-nourished adult is rare and is most commonly due to an adenoma of the islets of Langerhans. Ninety percent of such tumors are single and benign, but multiple adenomas can occur as well as malignant tumors with functional metastases. Adenomas may be familial, and multiple adenomas have been found in conjunction with tumors of the parathyroids and pituitary (MEN type 1 [MEN 1]). Over 99% of insulinomas are located within the pancreas and less than 1% in ectopic pancreatic tissue.

Clinical Findings

A. Symptoms and Signs

The most important prerequisite to diagnosing an insulinoma is simply to consider it, particularly in relatively healthy-appearing persons who have fasting hypoglycemia associated with some degree of CNS dysfunction such as confusion or abnormal behavior. A delay in diagnosis can result in unnecessary treatment for epilepsy or psychiatric disorders and may cause irreversible brain damage. In long-standing cases, obesity can result as a consequence of overeating to relieve symptoms.

The so-called Whipple triad is characteristic of hypoglycemia regardless of the cause. It consists of (1) a history of hypoglycemic symptoms, (2) an associated low plasma glucose level (40–50 mg/dL), and (3) relief of symptoms upon ingesting fast-acting carbohydrates in approximately 15 minutes. The hypoglycemic symptoms in insulinoma often develop in the early morning or after missing a meal. Occasionally, they occur after exercise.

Patients typically complain of neuroglycopenic symptoms such as blurred vision or diplopia, headache, feelings of detachment, slurred speech, and weakness. Personality and mental changes vary from anxiety to psychotic behavior, and neurologic deterioration can result in convulsions or coma. Hypoglycemic unawareness is very common and adrenergic symptoms of palpitations and sweating may be blunted. With the ready availability of home blood glucose–monitoring systems, patients sometimes present with documented fingerstick blood glucose levels in the 40s and 50s at time of symptoms. Access to sulfonylureas or insulin

Table 27–12. Diagnostic criteria for insulinoma after a 72-hour fast.

Laboratory Test	Result
Plasma glucose	< 45 mg/dL (2.5 mmol/L)
Plasma insulin (RIA)	≥ 6 microunits/mL (36 pmol/L)
Plasma insulin (ICMA)	≥ 3 microunits/mL (18 pmol/L)
Plasma C-peptide	≥ 200 pmol/L (0.2 nmol/L, 0.6 ng/mL)
Plasma proinsulin	≥ 5 pmol/L
Beta-hydroxybutyrate	≤ 2.7 mmol/L
Sulfonylurea screen (including repaglinide and nateglinide)	Negative

ICMA, immunochemiluminometric assays; RIA, radioimmunoassay.

should be explored—does a family member have diabetes, or does the patient or family member work in the medical field? Medication-dispensing errors should be excluded—has the patient's prescription medication changed in shape or color? Patients with insulinoma or factitious hypoglycemia usually have a normal physical examination.

B. Laboratory Findings

B cell adenomas do not reduce secretion of insulin in the presence of hypoglycemia, and the critical diagnostic test is to demonstrate inappropriately elevated serum insulin, proinsulin, and C-peptide levels, at a time when plasma glucose level is below 45 mg/dL or when the patient has neuroglycopenic symptoms.

The diagnostic criteria for insulinoma after a 72-hour fast are listed in Table 27–12. Other causes of hyperinsulinemic hypoglycemia include factitious administration of insulin or sulfonylureas. Factitious use of insulin will result in suppression of endogenous insulin secretion and low C-peptide levels. In patients who have injected insulin, the insulin/C-peptide ratio (pmol/L) will be greater than 1. An elevated circulating proinsulin level in the presence of fasting hypoglycemia is characteristic of most B cell adenomas and does not occur in factitious hyperinsulinism. Thus, C-peptide levels (by immunochemiluminometric assays [ICMA]) of greater than 200 pmol/L and proinsulin levels (by radioimmunoassay [RIA]) of greater than 5 pmol/L are characteristic of insulinomas. In patients with insulinoma, plasma beta-hydroxybutyrate levels are suppressed to 2.7 mmol/L or less. No single hormone measurement (insulin, proinsulin, C-peptide) is 100% sensitive and specific for the diagnosis of insulinoma, and insulinoma cases have been reported with insulin levels below 3 microunits/mL (ICMA assay) or proinsulin level below 5 pmol/L. These hormonal assays are also not standardized, and there can be significant variation in the test results. Therefore, the diagnosis should be based on multiple biochemical parameters.

In patients with epigastric distress, a history of renal calculi, or menstrual or erectile dysfunction, a serum calcium, gastrin, or prolactin level may be useful in screening for MEN 1 associated with insulinoma.

C. Diagnostic Tests

If the history is consistent with episodic spontaneous hypoglycemia, patients should be given a home blood glucose monitor and advised to monitor blood glucose levels at the time of symptoms and before consumption of carbohydrates, if this can be done safely. Patients with insulinomas frequently report fingerstick blood glucose levels between 40 mg/dL (2.2 mmol/L) and 50 mg/dL (2.8 mmol/L) at the time of symptoms. The diagnosis, however, cannot be made based on a fingerstick blood glucose. It is necessary to have a low laboratory glucose concomitantly with elevated plasma insulin, proinsulin, and C-peptide levels and a negative sulfonylurea screen. When patients give a history of symptoms after only a short period of food withdrawal or with exercise, then an outpatient assessment can be attempted. The patient should be brought by a family member to the office after an overnight fast and observed in the office. Activity such as walking should be encouraged and fingerstick blood glucose measured repeatedly during observation. If symptoms occur or fingerstick blood glucose is below 50 mg/dL (2.8 mmol/L), then samples for plasma glucose, insulin, C-peptide, proinsulin, sulfonylurea screen, serum ketones, and antibodies to insulin should be sent. If outpatient observation does not result in symptoms or hypoglycemia and if the clinical suspicion remains high, then the patient should undergo an inpatient supervised 72-hour fast. A suggested protocol for the supervised fast is shown in Table 27–13.

Table 27–13. Suggested hospital protocol for supervised fast in diagnosis of insulinoma.

(1) Place intravenous cannula and obtain baseline plasma glucose, insulin, proinsulin, beta-hydroxybutyrate, and C-peptide measurements at onset of fast.
(2) Permit only calorie-free and caffeine-free fluids and encourage supervised activity (such as walking).
(3) Obtain fingerstick glucose measurements every 4 hours until values < 60 mg/dL are obtained. Then increase the frequency of fingersticks to 1–2 hours, and when capillary glucose value is < 45 mg/dL send a venous blood sample to the laboratory for plasma glucose.[1] Check frequently for manifestations of neuroglycopenia.
(4) At 48 hours into the fast, send a venous blood sample for plasma glucose, insulin, proinsulin, C-peptide, beta-hydroxybutyrate, and sulfonylurea measurement.
(5) If symptoms of hypoglycemia occur **or** if a laboratory value of serum glucose is < 45 mg/dL, **or** if 72 hours have elapsed, conclude the fast with a final blood sample for plasma glucose,[1] insulin, proinsulin, C-peptide, beta-hydroxybutyrate, and sulfonylurea measurements. Then give oral fast-acting carbohydrate followed by a meal. If the patient is confused or unable to take oral agents, administer 50 mL of 50% dextrose intravenously over 3–5 minutes. Do not conclude a fast based simply on a capillary blood glucose measurement—wait for the laboratory glucose value—unless the patient is very symptomatic and it would be dangerous to wait.

[1]Glucose sample should be collected in sodium fluoride containing tube on ice to prevent glycolysis and the plasma separated immediately upon receipt at the laboratory. Arrange for the laboratory to run the glucose samples "stat."

In 30% of patients with insulinoma, the blood glucose levels often drop below 45 mg/dL (2.5 mmol/L) after an overnight fast, but some patients require up to 72 hours to develop symptomatic hypoglycemia. However, the term "72-hour fast" is actually a misnomer in most cases since the fast should be immediately terminated as soon as symptoms appear and laboratory confirmation of hypoglycemia is available. In normal male subjects, the blood glucose does not fall below 55–60 mg/dL (3.1–3.3 mmol/L) during a 3-day fast. In contrast, in normal premenopausal women, the plasma glucose can reach values as low as 35 mg/dL (1.9 mmol/L). In these cases, however, the women are not symptomatic, presumably owing to the development of sufficient ketonemia to supply energy needs to the brain. Insulinoma patients, on the other hand, become symptomatic when plasma glucose drops to subnormal levels, since inappropriate insulin secretion restricts ketone formation. Moreover, the demonstration of a nonsuppressed insulin level of 3 microunits/mL or more using an ICMA assay (greater than 6 microunits/mL using an RIA assay) in the presence of hypoglycemia suggests the diagnosis of insulinoma. If hypoglycemia does not develop in a male patient after fasting for up to 72 hours—and particularly when this prolonged fast is terminated with a period of moderate exercise—insulinoma must be considered an unlikely diagnosis.

An oral glucose tolerance test is of no value in the diagnosis of insulin-secreting tumors. HbA_{1c} levels may be low but there is considerable overlap with normal patients and no particular value is diagnostic.

D. Preoperative Localization of B Cell Tumors

After the diagnosis of insulinoma has been unequivocally made by clinical and laboratory findings, studies to localize the tumor should be initiated. Most tumors are in the pancreas, and ectopic cases are rare.

Because of the small size of these tumors (averaging 1.5 cm in diameter in one large series), imaging studies do not necessarily identify all of them. A pancreatic dual phase helical CT scan with thin section can identify 82–94% of the lesions. MRI scans with gadolinium can be helpful in detecting a tumor in 85% of cases. One case report suggests that diffusion-weighted MRI can be useful for detecting and localizing small insulinomas, especially for those with no hypervascular pattern. PET/CT scans using gallium-labeled somatostatin analogs such as DOTA-1-NaI3-octreotide (DOTA-NOC), which have a higher affinity for somatostatin receptor subtypes 2, 3, and 5, have been reported to be useful in localizing the tumors. Insulinomas express GLP-1 receptors, and radiolabeled GLP-1 receptor agonists such as Lys(40)(Ahx-hydrazinonicotinamide [HYNIC]-[(99m)Tc)NH(2)]-exendin-4 for SPECT/CT have also been reported to visualize the tumors. If the imaging study is normal, then an endoscopic ultrasound should be performed. In experienced hands, about 80–90% of tumors can be detected with this procedure. Fine-needle aspiration of the identified lesion can be attempted to confirm the presence of a neuroendocrine tumor. If the tumor is not identified or the imaging result is equivocal, then the patient should undergo selective calcium-stimulated angiography, which has been reported to localize the tumor to a particular region of the pancreas approximately 90% of the time. In this test, angiography is combined with injections of calcium gluconate into the gastroduodenal, splenic, and superior mesenteric arteries, and insulin levels are measured in the hepatic vein effluent. The procedure is performed after an overnight fast. Calcium stimulates insulin release from insulinomas but not normal islets, and so a step-up from baseline in insulin levels (twofold or greater) regionalizes the source of the hyperinsulinism to the head of the pancreas for the gastroduodenal artery, the uncinate process for the superior mesenteric artery, and the body and tail of the pancreas for the splenic artery calcium infusions. These studies combined with careful intraoperative ultrasonography and palpation by a surgeon experienced in insulinoma surgery identifies up to 98% of tumors.

Treatment

The treatment of choice for insulin-secreting tumors is surgical resection. While waiting for surgery, patients should be given oral diazoxide. Divided doses of 300–400 mg/day usually suffice, although an occasional patient may require up to 800 mg/day. Side effects include edema due to sodium retention, gastric irritation, and mild hirsutism. Hydrochlorothiazide, 25–50 mg daily, can be used to counteract the sodium retention and edema as well potentiate diazoxide's hyperglycemic effect.

In patients with a single benign pancreatic B cell adenoma, 90–95% have a successful cure at the first surgical attempt when intraoperative ultrasound is used by a skilled surgeon. Diazoxide should be administered on the day of the surgery because it reduces the risk of hypoglycemia during surgery. Typically, it does not mask the glycemic rise indicative of surgical cure. Blood glucose should be monitored throughout surgery, and 5% or 10% dextrose infusion should be used to maintain euglycemia. In cases where the diagnosis has been established but no adenoma is located after careful palpation and use of intraoperative ultrasound, it is no longer advisable to blindly resect the body and tail of the pancreas, since a nonpalpable tumor missed by ultrasound is most likely embedded within the fleshy head of the pancreas that is left behind with subtotal resections. Most surgeons prefer to close the incision and schedule a selective arterial calcium stimulation with hepatic venous sampling to locate the tumor site prior to a repeat operation. Laparoscopy using ultrasound and enucleation has been successful with a single tumor of the body or tail of the pancreas, but open surgery remains necessary for tumors in the head of the pancreas.

In patients with inoperable functioning islet cell carcinoma with and without hepatic metastasis and in approximately 5–10% of MEN 1 cases when subtotal removal of the pancreas has failed to produce cure, the treatment approach is the same as for other types of pancreatic neuroendocrine tumors (pNETs). Diazoxide is the treatment of choice in preventing hypoglycemia. Frequent carbohydrate feedings (every 2–3 hours) can also be helpful, although weight gain can become a problem. Somatostatin analogs, octreotide or lanreotide, should be considered if diazoxide is ineffective or if there is tumor progression. Surgery or embolization (bland, chemo- and radio-) or thermal ablation (radiofrequency, microwave, and cryoablation) can be used to reduce tumor burden and also provide symptomatic relief. Chemotherapy regimens that can be considered include combination of streptozocin, 5-fluorouracil, and doxorubicin; capecitabine and oxaliplatin; and capecitabine and temozolomide (see Table 39–3). Targeted therapies against multiple steps in the PI3K/AKT/mTor pathway have been shown to be helpful. Everolimus, an inhibitor of mTor, is approved for treatment of advanced pNETs. Sunitinib has been shown to slow growth of pNETs. Treatment with radioisotopes (indium-111, yttrium-90, or lutetium-177) linked to a somatostatin analog has been reported to show benefit in a proportion of patients.

NONISLET CELL TUMOR HYPOGLYCEMIA

These rare causes of hypoglycemia include mesenchymal tumors such as retroperitoneal sarcomas, hepatocellular carcinomas, adrenocortical carcinomas, and miscellaneous epithelial-type tumors. The tumors are frequently large and readily palpated or visualized on CT scans or MRI.

In many cases the hypoglycemia is due to the expression and release of an incompletely processed insulin-like growth factor 2 (IGF-2) by the tumor.

The diagnosis is supported by laboratory documentation of serum insulin levels below 5 microunit/mL with plasma glucose levels of 45 mg/dL (2.5 mmol/L) or lower. Values for growth hormone and IGF-1 are also decreased. Levels of IGF-2 may be increased but often are "normal" in quantity, despite the presence of the immature, higher-molecular-weight form of IGF-2, which can be detected only by special laboratory techniques.

Not all the patients with nonislet cell tumor hypoglycemia have elevated pro-IGF-2. Ectopic insulin production has been described in bronchial carcinoma, ovarian carcinoma, and small cell carcinoma of the cervix. Hypoglycemia due to IgF-1 released from a metastatic large cell carcinoma of the lung has also been reported. GLP-1–secreting tumors (ovarian and pNETs) can also cause hypoglycemia by stimulating insulin release from normal pancreatic islets.

The prognosis for these tumors is generally poor, and surgical removal should be attempted when feasible. Dietary management of the hypoglycemia is the mainstay of medical treatment, since diazoxide is usually ineffective.

POSTPRANDIAL HYPOGLYCEMIA

1. Hypoglycemia Following Gastric Surgery

Hypoglycemia sometimes develops in patients who have undergone gastric surgery (eg, gastrectomy, vagotomy, pyloroplasty, gastrojejunostomy, Nissan fundoplication, Billroth II procedure, and Roux-en-Y), especially when they consume foods containing high levels of readily absorbable carbohydrates. This late dumping syndrome occurs about 1–3 hours after a meal and is a result of rapid delivery of high concentration of carbohydrates in the proximal small bowel and rapid absorption of glucose. The hyperinsulinemic response to the high carbohydrate load causes hypoglycemia. Excessive release of GI hormones such as GLP-1 likely play a role in the hyperinsulinemic response. The symptoms include lightheadedness, sweating, confusion and even loss of consciousness after eating a high carbohydrate meal. To document hypoglycemia, the patient should consume a meal that leads to symptoms during everyday life. An oral glucose tolerance test is not recommended because many normal persons have false-positive test results. There have been case reports of insulinoma in patients with hypoglycemia following Roux-en-Y surgery. It is unclear how often this occurs. A careful history may identify patients who have a history of hypoglycemia with exercise or missed meals, and these individuals may require a formal 72-hour fast to rule out an insulinoma.

Treatment for secondary dumping includes dietary modification, but this may be difficult to sustain. Patients can try more frequent meals with smaller portions of less rapidly digested carbohydrates. Alpha-glucosidase therapy may be a useful adjunct to a low carbohydrate diet. Octreotide 50 mcg administered subcutaneously two or three times a day 30 minutes prior to each meal has been reported to improve symptoms due to late dumping syndrome. Treatment with exendin 9-39, a GLP-1 receptor agonist, may prevent post gastric bypass hypoglycemia. SGLT2 inhibitors may ameliorate the postprandial glucose rise, the subsequent insulin response, and hypoglycemia. There is a report of a patient with Roux-en-Y surgery who had complete resolution of both hyperglycemia and hypoglycemia when she was given canagliflozin. Various surgical procedures to delay gastric emptying have been reported to improve symptoms but long-term efficacy studies are lacking.

2. Functional Alimentary Hypoglycemia

Patients have symptoms suggestive of increased sympathetic activity, including anxiety, weakness, tremor, sweating or palpitations after meals. Physical examination and laboratory tests are normal. It is not recommended that patients with symptoms suggestive of increased sympathetic activity undergo either a prolonged oral glucose tolerance test or a mixed meal test. Instead, the patients should be given home blood glucose monitors (with memories) and instructed to monitor fingerstick glucose levels at the time of symptoms. Only patients who have symptoms when their fingerstick blood glucose is low (less than 50 mg/dL) and who have resolution of symptoms when the glucose is raised by eating rapidly released carbohydrate need additional evaluation. Patients who do not have evidence for low glucose levels at time of symptoms are generally reassured by their findings. Counseling and support should be the mainstays in therapy, with dietary manipulation only an adjunct.

3. Occult Diabetes

This condition is characterized by a delay in early insulin release from pancreatic B cells, resulting in initial exaggeration of hyperglycemia during a glucose tolerance test. In response to this hyperglycemia, an exaggerated insulin release produces a late hypoglycemia 4–5 hours after ingestion of glucose. These patients frequently have obesity and a family history of diabetes mellitus.

Patients with this type of postprandial hypoglycemia often respond to reduced intake of refined sugars with multiple, spaced, small feedings high in dietary fiber. In patients with obesity, treatment is directed at weight reduction to achieve ideal weight. These patients should be considered to have prediabetes or early diabetes (type 1 or 2) and advised to have periodic medical evaluations.

4. Autoimmune Hypoglycemia

Patients with autoimmune hypoglycemia have early postprandial hyperglycemia followed by hypoglycemia 3–4 hours later. The hypoglycemia is attributed to a dissociation of insulin-antibody immune complexes, releasing free insulin.

The disorder is associated with methimazole treatment for Graves disease, although it can also occur in patients treated with various other sulfhydryl-containing medications (captopril, penicillamine) as well as other drugs such as hydralazine, isoniazid, and procainamide. In addition, it has been reported in patients with autoimmune disorders such as rheumatoid arthritis, SLE, and polymyositis as well as in plasma cell myeloma and other plasma cell dyscrasias where paraproteins or antibodies cross-react with insulin. There is also an association with the HLA class II alleles (DRB1*0406, DQA1*0301, and DQB1*0302). These alleles are 10 to 20 times more common in Japanese and Korean populations, which explains why the disorder has been reported mostly in Japanese patients.

High titers of insulin autoantibodies, usually IgG class, can be detected. Insulin, proinsulin, and C-peptide levels may be elevated, but the results may be erroneous because of the interference of the insulin antibodies with the immunoassays for these peptides.

In most cases, the hypoglycemia is transient and usually resolves spontaneously within 3–6 months of diagnosis, particularly when the offending medications are stopped. The most consistent therapeutic benefit in management of this syndrome has been achieved by dietary treatment with small, frequent low-carbohydrate meals. Prednisone (30–60 mg orally daily) has been used to lower the titer of insulin antibodies.

FACTITIOUS HYPOGLYCEMIA

Factitious hypoglycemia may be difficult to document. A suspicion of self-induced hypoglycemia is supported when the patient is associated with the health professions or has access to diabetic medications taken by a member of the family who has diabetes. The triad of hypoglycemia, high immunoreactive insulin, and suppressed plasma C-peptide immunoreactivity is pathognomonic of exogenous insulin administration. Insulin and C-peptide are secreted in a 1:1 molar ratio. A large fraction of the endogenous insulin is cleared by the liver, whereas C-peptide, which is cleared by the kidney, has a lower metabolic clearance rate. For this reason, the molar ratio of insulin and C-peptide in a hypoglycemic patient should be less than 1.0 in cases of insulinoma and is greater than 1.0 in cases of exogenous insulin administration (see Hypoglycemia Due to Pancreatic B Cell Tumors, above). When sulfonylureas, repaglinide, and nateglinide are suspected as a cause of factitious hypoglycemia, a plasma level of these medications to detect their presence may be required to distinguish laboratory findings from those of insulinoma.

HYPOGLYCEMIA DUE TO INSULIN RECEPTOR ANTIBODIES

Hypoglycemia due to insulin receptor autoantibodies is an extremely rare syndrome; most cases have occurred in women often with a history of autoimmune disease. Almost all of these patients have also had episodes of insulin-resistant diabetes and acanthosis nigricans. Their hypoglycemia may be either fasting or postprandial and is often severe and is attributed to an agonistic action of the antibody on the insulin receptor. Balance between the antagonistic and agonistic effects of the antibodies determines whether insulin-resistant diabetes or hypoglycemia occurs. Hypoglycemia was found to respond to corticosteroid therapy but not to plasmapheresis or immunosuppression.

MEDICATION- & ETHANOL-INDUCED HYPOGLYCEMIA

A number of medications apart from diabetic medications can occasionally cause hypoglycemia. Common offenders include the fluoroquinolones such as gatifloxacin and levofloxacin, pentamidine, quinine, ACE inhibitors, salicylates and beta-adrenergic blocking agents. The fluoroquinolones, particularly gatifloxacin, have been associated with both hypoglycemia and hyperglycemia. It is thought that the drug acts on the ATP sensitive potassium channels in the beta cell. Hypoglycemia is an early event, and hyperglycemia occurs several days into therapy. Intravenous pentamidine is cytotoxic to beta cells and causes acute hyperinsulinemia and hypoglycemia followed by insulinopenia and hyperglycemia. Fasting patients taking noncardioselective beta-blockers can have an exaggerated hypoglycemic response to starvation. The beta-blockade inhibits fatty acids and gluconeogenesis substrate release and reduces plasma glucagon response. Therapy with ACE inhibitors increases the risk of hypoglycemia in patients who are taking insulin or sulfonylureas presumably because these drugs increase sensitivity to circulating insulin by increasing blood flow to the muscle. Some opioids cause hypoglycemia. Tramadol use has been associated with increased risk of hospitalization for hypoglycemia. Methadone overdose has also been reported to cause hypoglycemia and a rapid dose escalation of methadone in cancer patients can lower glucose levels.

Ethanol-associated hypoglycemia may be due to hepatic alcohol dehydrogenase activity depleting NAD. The resultant change in the redox state—increase in NADH to NAD^+ ratio—causes a partial block at several points in the gluconeogenic pathway. With prolonged starvation, glycogen reserves become depleted within 18–24 hours and hepatic glucose output becomes totally dependent on gluconeogenesis. Under these circumstances, a blood concentration of ethanol as low as 45 mg/dL (9.8 mmol/L) can induce profound hypoglycemia by blocking gluconeogenesis. Neuroglycopenia in a patient whose breath smells of alcohol may be mistaken for alcoholic stupor. Prevention consists of adequate food intake during ethanol ingestion. Therapy consists of glucose administration to replenish glycogen stores until gluconeogenesis resumes.

When sugar-containing soft drinks are used as mixers to dilute alcohol in beverages (gin and tonic, rum and cola), there seems to be a greater insulin release than when the soft drink alone is ingested and a tendency for more of a late hypoglycemic overswing to occur 3–4 hours later. Prevention would consist of avoiding sugar mixers while ingesting alcohol and ensuring supplementary food intake to provide sustained absorption.

Lipid Disorders

Michael J. Blaha, MD, MPH

The "Lipid Hypothesis" of CVD—stating that cholesterol is causal in the development of atherosclerotic CVD (ASCVD) and that lowering cholesterol is associated with lower cardiovascular event rates—is widely accepted throughout the medical community. For patients with known CVD (secondary prevention), studies have shown that cholesterol lowering leads to a consistent reduction in total mortality and in recurrent cardiovascular events in men and women; other studies have documented lowered mortality and events in middle-aged and older patients. Among patients without CVD (primary prevention), the data are generally consistent, with rates of cardiovascular events, heart disease mortality, and all-cause mortality differing among studies. Treatment guidelines have been designed to assist clinicians in selecting patients for cholesterol-lowering therapy based predominantly on their overall risk of developing CVD as well as their baseline cholesterol levels.

There are several genetic disorders that provide insight into the pathogenesis of lipid-related diseases. **Familial hypercholesterolemia,** rare in the homozygous state (about one per million), causes markedly high LDL levels and early CVD. The most common genetic defects involve absent or defective LDL receptors, resulting in unregulated LDL metabolism, genetic pathogenic variants of apolipoprotein B, or gain of function in proprotein convertase subtilisin/kexin type 9 (PCSK9), a protein that regulates breakdown of LDL receptors. Patients with two abnormal genes (homozygotes) have extremely high levels—up to eight times normal—and present with atherosclerotic disease in childhood. Patients with two abnormal genes (homozygotes) may require liver transplantation or plasmapheresis to correct their severe lipid abnormalities; early treatment with statins appears to confer lifetime benefits in such patients. Those with one defective gene (heterozygotes) have LDL concentrations up to two or three times normal; persons with this condition may develop CVD in their 30s or 40s.

Another rare condition is caused by an abnormality of lipoprotein lipase, the enzyme that enables peripheral tissues to take up triglyceride from chylomicrons and very-low-density lipoprotein (VLDL) particles. Patients with this condition, one cause of **familial chylomicronemia syndrome,** have marked hypertriglyceridemia with recurrent pancreatitis and hepatosplenomegaly in childhood.

Numerous other genetic abnormalities of lipid metabolism are named for the abnormality noted when serum is electrophoresed (eg, dysbetalipoproteinemia, characterized by elevated levels of remnant lipoproteins) or from polygenic combinations of lipid abnormalities in families (eg, familial combined hyperlipidemia).

When to Refer

- Known genetic lipid disorders.
- Striking family history of hyperlipidemia or premature atherosclerosis.
- Extremely high serum LDL cholesterol, triglycerides, and/or lipoprotein(a), as well as extremely low serum HDL cholesterol.

Chyzhyk V et al. Familial chylomicronemia syndrome: a rare but devastating autosomal recessive disorder characterized by refractory hypertriglyceridemia and recurrent pancreatitis. Trends Cardiovasc Med. 2020;30:80. [PMID: 31003756]

Hegele RA et al. Rare dyslipidaemias, from phenotype to genotype to management: a European Atherosclerosis Society task force consensus statement. Lancet Diabetes Endocrinol. 2020;8:50. [PMID: 31582260]

Khera AV et al. What is familial hypercholesterolemia, and why does it matter? Circulation. 2020;141:1760. [PMID: 32479201]

Mortensen MB et al. Elevated LDL cholesterol and increased risk of myocardial infarction and atherosclerotic cardiovascular disease in individuals aged 70-100 years: a contemporary primary prevention cohort. Lancet. 2020;396:1644. [PMID: 33186534]

Sniderman AD et al. Apolipoprotein B particles and cardiovascular disease: a narrative review. JAMA Cardiol. 2019;4:1287. [PMID: 31642874]

LIPID FRACTIONS & THE RISK OF CORONARY HEART DISEASE

In serum, cholesterol is carried primarily on three different lipoproteins—the VLDL, LDL, and HDL molecules. Total cholesterol equals the sum of these three components:

$$\text{Total cholesterol} = \text{HDL cholesterol} + \text{VLDL cholesterol} + \text{LDL cholesterol}$$

Using these assumptions, the Friedewald equation states that LDL cholesterol can be estimated as:

$$\text{LDL cholesterol} = \text{Total cholesterol (mg/dL)} - \text{HDL cholesterol (mg/dL)} - \frac{\text{Triglycerides (mg/dL)}}{5}$$

When using SI units, the formula becomes

$$\text{LDL cholesterol} = \text{Total cholesterol (mmol/L)} - \text{HDL cholesterol (mmol/L)} - \frac{\text{Triglycerides (mmol/L)}}{2.2}$$

Modern research has questioned several of the assumptions underlying the Friedewald equation, particularly the assumption that VLDL is always best estimated as triglycerides/5, which is inaccurate when triglycerides are above 150 mg/dL and when LDL cholesterol is less than 70 mg/dL. Therefore, many commercial laboratories have switched to the Martin-Hopkins equation, which uses a flexible factor for deriving VLDL from triglycerides (as opposed to always using 5). The Martin-Hopkins equation reduces the systematic underestimation of LDL cholesterol when triglycerides are greater than 150 mg/dL and LDL is less than 70 mg/dL and is more accurate in estimating LDL from nonfasting blood specimens.

Non-HDL cholesterol is increasingly recognized as an important measure of the total quantity of apolipoprotein B–containing atherogenic lipid particles. Non-HDL cholesterol is calculated as: total cholesterol – HDL cholesterol. Advantages of calculating non-HDL cholesterol are that it is directly measured, requires no additional cost, is less sensitive to fasting status, and is a better predictor of cardiovascular risk compared to LDL cholesterol.

Lipoprotein(a), a subfraction of LDL that is largely genetically determined, has also been recognized as a causal factor in atherosclerosis. One-time measurement of lipoprotein(a) in patients with a strong family history, with manifestations of early ASCVD, or with familial hypercholesterolemia is useful. The National Lipid Association also recommends cascade screening in family members of those with severe hypercholesterolemia, including elevated lipoprotein(a). Values greater than 50 mg/dL or greater than 100 nmol/L are considered elevated. The 2019 European Society of Cardiology/European Atherosclerosis Society (ESC/EAS) guidelines recommend one-time lipoprotein(a) measurement for all adults to identify those with very high values (greater than 180 mg/dL or greater than 430 nmol/L). Novel antisense oligonucleotide therapies associated with nearly 80% reduction in lipoprotein(a) are being tested in phase 3 cardiovascular outcomes trials of patients with prior MI and high lipoprotein(a). Lipoprotein(a) is increasingly measured and used as a risk-enhancing factor favoring early and more aggressive statin treatment.

It is difficult to assign a "normal" range for serum lipids. This is because our cholesterol values are vastly higher than our evolutionary ancestors (whose LDL cholesterol may have been 30–50 mg/dL) and because mean values vary across the world. Mean LDL cholesterol levels are currently declining in the United States, including in youths. There is no evidence available that adult cholesterol levels can be "too low"; that is, there is no evidence that very low LDL cholesterol is linked with any side effects (eg, cognitive dysfunction).

Reyes-Soffer G et al. Lipoprotein(a): a genetically determined, causal, and prevalent risk factor for atherosclerotic cardiovascular disease: a Scientific Statement from the American Heart Association. Arterioscler Thromb Vasc Biol. 2022;42:e48. [PMID: 34647487]

Sampson M et al. A new equation for calculation of low-density lipoprotein cholesterol in patients with normolipidemia and/or hypertriglyceridemia. JAMA Cardiol. 2020;5:540. [PMID: 32101259]

Sathiyakumar V et al. Fasting versus nonfasting and low-density lipoprotein cholesterol accuracy. Circulation. 2018;137:10. [PMID: 29038168]

Wilson DP et al. Use of lipoprotein(a) in clinical practice: a biomarker whose time has come. A scientific statement from the National Lipid Association. J Clin Lipidol. 2019;13:374. [PMID: 31147269]

THERAPEUTIC EFFECTS OF LOWERING CHOLESTEROL

Reducing cholesterol levels in healthy middle-aged men without CHD (in **primary prevention studies**) reduces risk in direct proportion to the reduction in LDL cholesterol. Treated adults have clinically important reductions in the rates of MIs, new cases of angina, need for coronary artery bypass or other revascularization procedures, peripheral artery disease, and stroke. The West of Scotland Study showed a 31% decrease in MIs in middle-aged men treated with pravastatin compared with placebo. The Air Force/Texas Coronary Atherosclerosis Prevention Study (AFCAPS/TexCAPS) study showed similar results with lovastatin. As with any primary prevention interventions, large numbers of healthy patients need to be treated to prevent a single event. The numbers of patients needed to treat (NNT) to prevent one nonfatal MI or one CAD death in these two studies were 46 and 50, respectively. The Anglo-Scandinavian Cardiac Outcomes Trial (ASCOT) study of atorvastatin in persons with hypertension and other risk factors but without CHD demonstrated a 36% reduction in CHD events. The Justification for the Use of Statins in Prevention: An Intervention Trial Evaluating Rosuvastatin (JUPITER) study showed a 44% reduction in a combined end point of MI, stroke, revascularization, hospitalization for unstable angina, or death from cardiovascular causes in both men and women. The NNT for 1 year to prevent one event was 169. The Heart Outcomes Prevention Evaluation (HOPE-3) trial of rosuvastatin showed a 24% reduction in cardiovascular events. The NNT over 5.6 years was 91.

Primary prevention studies have found a less consistent effect on total mortality. The West of Scotland Study found a 20% decrease in total mortality. The AFCAPS/TexCAPS study with lovastatin showed no difference in total mortality. The Antihypertensive and Lipid-Lowering Treatment to Prevent Heart Attack Trial (ALLHAT-LLT) also showed no reduction either in all-cause mortality or in

CHD events when pravastatin was compared with usual care. Persons treated with atorvastatin in the ASCOT study had a 13% reduction in mortality, but the result was not statistically significant. The JUPITER trial demonstrated a statistically significant 20% reduction in death from any cause. The NNT for 1 year was 400. The HOPE-3 trial showed a 7% reduction in all-cause mortality, but the result was not statistically significant.

In **secondary prevention studies** among patients with established CVD, the mortality benefits of cholesterol lowering are clearer. Major trials with statins have shown significant reductions in cardiovascular events, cardiovascular deaths, and all-cause mortality in men and women with CAD. The NNT to prevent a nonfatal MI or a CAD death in these studies was between 12 and 34. Aggressive cholesterol lowering with these agents causes regression of atherosclerotic plaques in some patients, reduces the progression of atherosclerosis in saphenous vein grafts, and can slow or reverse carotid artery atherosclerosis. Results with other classes of medications, particularly those with little effect on LDL or the LDL receptor, have been less consistent. The benefits and adverse effects of cholesterol lowering may be specific to each type or mechanism of drug; the clinician cannot assume that the effects of new drugs with novel mechanisms of action will generalize to other classes of medication.

The disparities in absolute event lowering between primary and secondary prevention studies highlight a critical aspect of clinical cholesterol lowering. The net benefits from cholesterol lowering depend on the underlying risk of ASCVD as well as the competing risks of other diseases. In middle-aged patients with atherosclerosis and high cholesterol, morbidity and mortality rates are high, and measures that reduce cholesterol-related risk are more likely to provide a robust net benefit to the patient. In older patients with little atherosclerosis and lower cholesterol levels, there may be no meaningful net benefit to cholesterol lowering.

Arnett DK et al. 2019 ACC/AHA guideline on the primary prevention of cardiovascular disease: executive summary: a report of the American College of Cardiology/American Heart Association Task Force on Clinical Practice Guidelines. J Am Coll Cardiol. 2019;74:1376. [PMID: 30894319]

Grundy SM et al. 2018 AHA/ACC/AACVPR/AAPA/ABC/ACPM/ADA/AGS/APhA/ASPC/NLA/PCNA guideline on the management of blood cholesterol: executive summary. Circulation. 2019;139:e1046. [PMID: 30565953]

Michos ED et al. Lipid management for the prevention of atherosclerotic cardiovascular disease. N Engl J Med. 2019;381:1557. [PMID: 31618541]

Ray KK et al. Pharmacological lipid-modification therapies for prevention of ischaemic heart disease: current and future options. Lancet. 2019;394:697. [PMID: 31448741]

SECONDARY CONDITIONS THAT AFFECT LIPID METABOLISM

Several factors, including drugs, can influence serum lipids. These are important for two reasons: abnormal lipid levels (or changes in lipid levels) may be the presenting sign of some of these conditions, and correction of the underlying condition may obviate the need to treat an

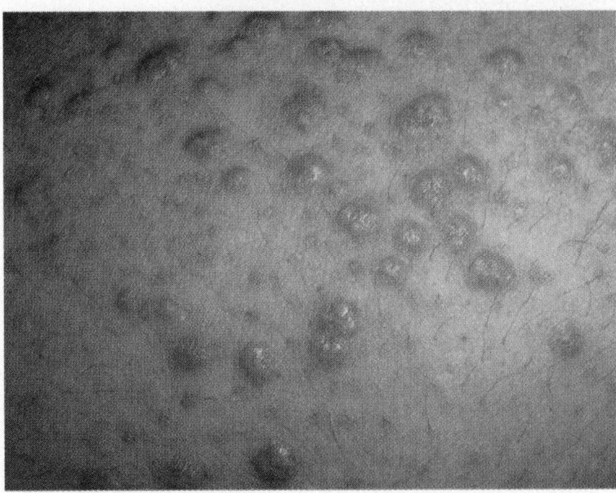

▲ **Figure 28–1. Eruptive xanthomas on the arm of a man with untreated hyperlipidemia and diabetes mellitus.** (Reproduced with permission from Richard P. Usatine, MD, in Usatine RP, Smith MA, Mayeaux EJ Jr, Chumley H. *The Color Atlas of Family Medicine*, 2nd ed. McGraw-Hill, 2013.)

apparent lipid disorder. Thyroid disease, particularly hypothyroidism, is associated with a high LDL. Poorly controlled diabetes mellitus and alcohol use, in particular, are commonly associated with high triglyceride levels that decline with improvements in glycemic control or reduction in alcohol use, respectively. Thus, secondary causes of high blood lipids should be considered in each patient with a lipid disorder before lipid-lowering therapy is started. In most instances, special testing is not needed: a history and physical examination are sufficient.

CLINICAL PRESENTATIONS

Most patients with high cholesterol levels have no specific symptoms or signs. The vast majority of patients with lipid abnormalities are detected by the laboratory, either as part of the workup of a patient with CVD or as part of a preventive screening strategy. Extremely high levels of chylomicrons or VLDL particles (triglyceride level above 1000 mg/dL or 10 mmol/L) result in the formation of **eruptive xanthomas** (Figure 28–1) (red-yellow papules, especially on the buttocks). High LDL concentrations result in **tendinous xanthomas** on certain tendons (Achilles, patella, back of the hand). Such xanthomas usually indicate one of the underlying genetic hyperlipidemias. **Lipemia retinalis** (cream-colored blood vessels in the fundus) is seen with extremely high triglyceride levels (above 2000 mg/dL or 20 mmol/L).

SCREENING & TREATMENT OF HIGH BLOOD CHOLESTEROL

While screening of all children for cholesterol disorders remains controversial, all adults should have their lipids checked before middle age. Patients with documented atherosclerosis and diabetes mellitus deserve the most scrutiny of their lipids since these patients are at the highest risk for suffering additional manifestations in the near term and thus have the most to gain from lipid lowering.

Additional risk reduction measures for atherosclerosis are discussed in Chapter 10; lipid lowering should be just one aspect of a program to reduce the progression and effects of atherosclerosis.

The best screening and treatment strategy for adults who do not have ASCVD is less clear. Several algorithms have been developed to guide the clinician in treatment decisions, but management decisions must always be individualized based on the patient's risk to maximize net benefit.

The 2018 American Heart Association/American College of Cardiology (AHA/ACC)/Multi-society guidelines recommend screening of all adults aged 20 years or older for high blood cholesterol. The 2016 USPSTF guidelines recommend beginning at age 20 years only if there are other cardiovascular risk factors such as tobacco use, diabetes, hypertension, obesity, or a family history of premature CVD. For men without other risk factors, screening is recommended beginning at age 35 years. For women and for men aged 20 to 35 without increased risk, the USPSTF makes no recommendation for or against routine screening for lipid disorders. Although there is no established interval for screening, screening can be repeated every 5 years for those with average or low risk and more often for those whose levels are close to therapeutic thresholds.

Individuals without CVD should have their 10-year risk of CVD calculated, with lifetime risk also considered. Although those with LDL cholesterol greater than 190 mg/dL (4.91 mmol/L) are recommended for treatment independent of their 10-year risk of CVD, all other patients are recommended for treatment based on their overall cardiovascular risk. While other calculators (such as SCORE2 or QRISK) may be more appropriate for other parts of the world, the best method for estimating 10-year risk in the United States is the Pooled Cohort Equations. First introduced in the 2013 ACC/AHA guidelines, the Pooled Cohort Equations include separate equations for White and Black patients and estimate the 10-year risk of heart attack, stroke, and cardiovascular death. This represents an improvement over the older Framingham 10-year calculator, which includes CHD but not stroke risk. The ACC/AHA risk estimator can be found at https://www.cvriskcalculator.com/, and mobile apps are available for download. While it has been shown to overestimate risk in some modern populations, including those of at least moderate socioeconomic status, the ACC/AHA risk estimator remains an excellent starting point for a risk discussion. Recalibrated versions of the calculator are available for countries across the world. The LIFE-CVD model is the best for illustrating lifetime risk and benefit of therapy (https://www.u-prevent.com/calculators/lifeCvd).

Shared decision-making is a central part of cholesterol management in primary prevention. Therefore, the 2018 AHA/ACC/Multi-society guidelines and the 2019 ACC/AHA primary prevention guidelines identify a set of "**risk-enhancing factors**" that might influence a clinician and patient to favor cholesterol-lowering treatment. Table 28–1 lists these risk-enhancing factors that may be considered, particularly for patients at borderline to intermediate risk (5–20% 10-year cardiovascular risk).

Table 28–1. Risk-enhancing factors that help identify patients who may benefit most from lipid-lowering therapy: 2018 AHA/ACC/Multi-society guidelines.

Family history of premature disease (males, age < 55 years; females, age < 65 years)
Primary hypercholesterolemia (LDL cholesterol, 160–189 mg/dL [4.1–4.8 mmol/L]; non–HDL cholesterol, 190–219 mg/dL [4.9–5.6 mmol/L])
Metabolic syndrome
CKD (not ESKD)
Chronic inflammatory conditions, such as psoriasis, rheumatoid arthritis, or HIV/AIDS
History of preeclampsia or of premature menopause before age 40 years
High-risk race/ethnicities (eg, South Asian ancestry)
Persistently high triglycerides ≥ 175 mg/dL
Elevated high-sensitivity CRP (≥ 2.0 mg/L)
Elevated lipoprotein(a) (≥ 50 mg/dL or ≥ 125 nmol/L)
Elevated apolipoprotein B (≥ 130 mg/dL)
Ankle brachial index < 0.9

AHA/ACC, American Heart Association/American College of Cardiology.

Importantly, the 2018 AHA/ACC/Multi-society guidelines, the 2019 ACC/AHA primary prevention guidelines, and the 2020 Endocrine Society guidelines also identify the **coronary artery calcium score** as the single best test for additional risk stratification. The coronary calcium score is a simple noncontrast cardiac-gated CT scan that takes about 10–15 minutes to do, is associated with approximately 1 mSv of radiation, and costs between $50 and $300, although some centers have begun offering the test for free. As opposed to the risk-enhancing factors, which may incline a clinician and patient toward treatment, the coronary artery calcium score may also help identify patients who are unlikely to benefit from cholesterol-lowering therapy. For example, when the coronary artery calcium score is zero in the absence of smoking or diabetes, the patient is low risk and less likely to receive net benefit from therapy; instead, the coronary artery calcium score can be repeated in approximately 3 years for higher-risk patients and 7 years for lower-risk patients. In 2021, the National Lipid Association published a comprehensive clinical practice statement on coronary artery calcium testing. The USPSTF does not endorse calcium scoring as a broad screening test; rather it says the test should be reserved for situations in which additional data will inform shared decision-making and potentially change a therapeutic decision.

Statins are nearly always the first-line therapy. Treatment decisions are based on the presence of clinical CVD or diabetes, LDL cholesterol greater than 190 mg/dL (4.91 mmol/L), patient age, and the estimated 10-year risk of developing CVD. The 2018 AHA/ACC/Multi-society guidelines define four groups of patients who benefit from statin medications: (1) individuals with clinical ASCVD; (2) individuals with primary elevation of LDL cholesterol greater than 190 mg/dL (4.91 mmol/L); (3) individuals aged 40–75 with diabetes and LDL greater than or equal to 70 mg/dL (1.81 mmol/L); and (4) individuals aged 40–75 without clinical ASCVD or diabetes, with LDL 70–189 mg/dL

(1.81–4.91 mmol/L), and estimated 10-year CVD risk of 7.5% or higher.

Ezetimibe and PCSK9 inhibitors have the strongest recommendations as second-line therapy for patients with (1) CVD whose LDL on statin therapy remains above the 70 mg/dL treatment threshold or (2) possible familial hypercholesterolemia with baseline LDL greater than 190 mg/dL (4.91 mmol/L) whose LDL remains above the 100 mg/dL treatment threshold. In high-risk patients, ezetimibe therapy is favored in part due to reduced cost, while in very high-risk patients, PCSK9 inhibitor therapy should be considered.

Screening & Treatment in Older Patients

Meta-analysis of evidence relating cholesterol to CVD in older adults suggests that cholesterol is a somewhat weaker risk factor for CVD for persons over age 75 years. The 2018 AHA/ACC/Multi-society guidelines suggest continuing statin treatment in patients over age 75 who have CVD. The guidelines, however, suggest selectively treating patients over the age of 75 who do not have evidence of CVD. Individual patient decisions to discontinue statin therapy should be based on overall functional status and life expectancy, comorbidities, and patient preference and should be made in context with overall therapeutic goals and end-of-life decisions.

Arnett DK et al. 2019 ACC/AHA guideline on the primary prevention of cardiovascular disease: executive summary: a report of the American College of Cardiology/American Heart Association Task Force on Clinical Practice Guidelines. J Am Coll Cardiol. 2019;74:1376. [PMID: 30894319]

Grundy SM et al. 2018 AHA/ACC/AACVPR/AAPA/ABC/ACPM/ADA/AGS/APhA/ASPC/NLA/PCNA guideline on the management of blood cholesterol: executive summary. Circulation. 2019;139:e1046. [PMID: 30565953]

Jaspers NEM et al. Prediction of individualized lifetime benefit from cholesterol lowering, blood pressure lowering, antithrombotic therapy, and smoking cessation in apparently healthy people. Eur Heart J. 2020;41:1190. [PMID: 31102402]

Mach F et al. 2019 ESC/EAS Guidelines for the management of dyslipidaemias: lipid modification to reduce cardiovascular risk. Eur Heart J. 2020;41:111. [PMID: 31504418]

Orringer CE, Blaha MJ et al. The National Lipid Association scientific statement on coronary artery calcium scoring to guide preventive strategies for ASCVD risk reduction. J Clin Lipidol. 2021;15:33. [PMID: 33419719]

Pallazola VA et al. A clinician's guide to healthy eating for cardiovascular disease prevention. Mayo Clin Proc Innov Qual Outcomes. 2019;3:251. [PMID: 31485563]

Wilkins JT et al. Novel lipid-lowering therapies to reduce cardiovascular risk. JAMA. 2021;326:266. Erratum in: JAMA. 2021;326:1637. [PMID: 34283191]

TREATMENT OF HIGH LDL CHOLESTEROL

Reduction of LDL cholesterol with statins is just one part of a program to reduce the risk of CVD. Other measures—including diet, exercise, smoking cessation, hypertension control, weight loss, diabetes control, and antithrombotic therapy—are also of central importance. For example, exercise (and weight loss) may reduce the LDL cholesterol and increase the HDL.

The use of medications to raise the HDL cholesterol has not been demonstrated to provide additional benefit. For example, cholesteryl ester transfer protein inhibitors are a class of medicines being investigated to raise HDL levels; however, agents in this class have not been shown to be effective in so doing. The addition of niacin to statins has also been carefully studied in the AIM-HIGH study and the HPS2-THRIVE study in patients at high risk for CVD and shown not to produce any further benefit (ie, to decrease parameters of cardiovascular risk).

Pappa E et al. Cardioprotective properties of HDL: structural and functional considerations. Curr Med Chem. 2020;27:2964. [PMID: 30714519]

Preiss D et al. Lipid-modifying agents, from statins to PCSK9 inhibitors: JACC focus seminar. J Am Coll Cardiol. 2020;75:1945. [PMID: 32327106]

Diet Therapy

Studies of nonhospitalized adults have reported only modest cholesterol-lowering benefits of individual dietary therapies, typically in the range of a 5–10% decrease in LDL cholesterol, and even less over the long term. The effect of diet therapies, however, may be additive; some patients will have striking reductions in LDL cholesterol—up to a 25–30% decrease—whereas others will have clinically important increases. Thus, the results of diet therapy should be assessed about 4 weeks after initiation.

Several nutritional approaches to diet therapy are available. Most Americans eat over 35% of calories as fat, of which 15% is saturated fat. A traditional cholesterol-lowering diet recommends reducing total fat to 25–30% and saturated fat to less than 7% of calories, with complete elimination of trans fats. These diets replace fat, particularly saturated fat, with carbohydrate. Other diet plans, including the Dean Ornish Diet and most vegetarian diets, restrict fat even further. Low-fat, high-carbohydrate diets may, however, result in insulin resistance, elevated triglycerides, and reductions in HDL cholesterol.

An alternative strategy is the Mediterranean diet, which maintains total fat at approximately 35–40% of total calories but replaces saturated fat with monounsaturated fat such as that found in canola oil and in olives, peanuts, avocados, and their oils. This diet is equally effective at lowering LDL cholesterol and is less likely to lead to reductions in HDL cholesterol. Several studies have suggested that this diet may also be associated with reductions in endothelial dysfunction, insulin resistance, and markers of vascular inflammation and may result in better resolution of the metabolic syndrome than traditional cholesterol-lowering diets. A clinical trial demonstrated reduced cardiovascular events in persons on a Mediterranean diet supplemented with additional nuts or extra-virgin olive oil compared to persons on a less intensive standard Mediterranean diet.

Other dietary changes may also result in beneficial changes in blood lipids. Soluble fiber, such as that found in oat bran or psyllium, may reduce LDL cholesterol by 5–10%. Plant stanols and sterols can reduce LDL cholesterol by 10%. Intake of garlic, soy protein, vitamin C, and pecans may also yield modest reductions of LDL cholesterol. Because oxidation of LDL cholesterol is a potential initiating event in atherogenesis, diets rich in antioxidants, found primarily in fruits and vegetables, may be helpful (see Chapter 29). Studies have suggested that when all of these elements are combined into a single dietary prescription, the impact of diet on LDL cholesterol may approach that of statin medications, lowering LDL cholesterol by close to 30%.

Arnett DK et al. 2019 ACC/AHA guideline on the primary prevention of cardiovascular disease: executive summary: a report of the American College of Cardiology/American Heart Association Task Force on Clinical Practice Guidelines. J Am Coll Cardiol. 2019;74:1376. [PMID: 30894319]

Grundy SM et al. 2018 AHA/ACC/AACVPR/AAPA/ABC/ACPM/ADA/AGS/APhA/ASPC/NLA/PCNA guideline on the management of blood cholesterol: executive summary. Circulation. 2019;139:e1046. [PMID: 30565953]

Lichtenstein AH et al. 2021 Dietary guidance to improve cardiovascular health: a scientific statement from the American Heart Association. Circulation. 2021;144:e472. [PMID: 34724806]

Vadiveloo M et al. Rapid diet assessment screening tools for cardiovascular disease risk reduction across healthcare settings: a scientific statement from the American Heart Association. Circ Cardiovasc Qual Outcomes. 2020;13:e000094. [PMID: 32762254]

Table 28–2. Indications for high-intensity and moderate-intensity statins: recommendations of the 2018 AHA/ACC/Multi-society guidelines.

Indications	Treatment Recommendation
Presence of clinical ASCVD	High-intensity statin **or** moderate-intensity statin if over age 75 years
Primary elevation of LDL cholesterol ≥ 190 mg/dL (4.91 mmol/L)	High-intensity statin
Age 40–75 years[1] Presence of diabetes LDL ≥ 70 mg/dL (1.81 mmol/L)	Moderate-intensity statin **or** high-intensity statin if 10-year CVD risk ≥ 7.5% or other risk-enhancing criteria[1]
Age 40–75 years No clinical ASCVD or diabetes LDL 70–189 mg/dL (1.81–4.91 mmol/L) Estimated 10-year CVD risk ≥ 7.5% or coronary artery calcium score ≥ 100 or ≥ 75th percentile	Treat with moderate- to high-intensity statin

[1]Diabetes duration > 10 years, microalbuminuria, CKD, and ankle brachial index < 0.9 favor aggressive treatment even for patients aged 20–39 years.

AHA/ACC, American Heart Association/American College of Cardiology; ASCVD, atherosclerotic CVD.

Pharmacologic Therapy

There are eight classes of medications currently available for consideration in patients who require drug treatment of an elevated cholesterol (statins, ezetimibe, PCSK9 inhibitors, omega-3 fatty acids, bempedoic acid, bile-acid–binding resins, fibrates, and niacin). As discussed above, statins are the cornerstone of nearly all medical regimens, and current guidelines define four groups of patients who benefit from statin medications (adults with diabetes mellitus, those with existing ASCVD, LDL cholesterol greater than 190 mg/dL, or 10-year risk of ASCVD greater than 7.5%). For LDL cholesterol, the evidence is strongest for ezetimibe and PCSK9 inhibitors; for triglycerides, the evidence is strongest for adding prescription-grade omega-3 fatty acid preparations. There is less evidence for cholesterol absorption inhibitors, fibrates, and niacin. Bempedoic acid, an inhibitor of adenosine triphosphate citrate lyase (ACL)—the enzyme two steps upstream from HMG-CoA reductase, the target of statins—was approved by the FDA in 2020 and represents an additional option for further LDL lowering.

A. Statins (Hydroxymethylglutaryl-Coenzyme A [HMG-CoA] Reductase Inhibitors)

The statins (HMG-CoA reductase inhibitors) work by inhibiting the rate-limiting enzyme in the formation of cholesterol. Cholesterol synthesis in the liver is reduced, with a compensatory increase in hepatic LDL receptors (so that the liver can take more of the cholesterol that it needs from the blood) and a reduction in the circulating LDL cholesterol level by 50% or more at the highest doses. There are also modest increases in HDL levels, substantial decreases in triglyceride levels, and marked reductions in high-sensitivity CRP levels.

The 2018 AHA/ACC/Multi-society guidelines divide statins into two categories: "high-intensity" and "moderate-intensity" statins (Table 28–2). High-intensity statins lower LDL cholesterol by approximately 50%. Examples include high-dose atorvastatin 40–80 mg/day and rosuvastatin 20–40 mg/day (Table 28–3). Moderate-intensity statins lower LDL cholesterol by approximately 30–50%. Examples include pitavastatin 2–4 mg/day, simvastatin 20–40 mg/day, and pravastatin 40–80 mg/day, as well as low-dose atorvastatin 10–20 mg/day and rosuvastatin 5–10 mg/day. All statins are given once daily in the morning or evening.

Statin-associated muscle aches, with normal serum creatine kinase levels, occur in up to 10% of patients, and often such patients can tolerate the statin upon rechallenge. The SAMSON trial demonstrated the importance of the nocebo effect with perceived statin intolerance (reported side effects being due to patient expectations); in this trial, 90% of the symptoms associated with statin rechallenge were also noted with placebo. The Statin-Associated Muscle Symptom Clinical Index (SAMS-CI) is a useful tool to help differentiate statin-related symptoms from symptoms unrelated to statins. More serious, but very uncommon, muscle disease includes myositis and rhabdomyolysis, with moderate and marked elevations of serum creatine kinase

Table 28–3. Effects of selected lipid-modifying drugs (listed alphabetically).

Drug	Lipid-Modifying Effects			Regimens	Cost for 30 Days of Treatment (for Suggested Dose)[1]
	LDL	HDL	Triglyceride		
Alirocumab (Praluent)[2]	−45 to −60%	±	±	*Initial:* 75 mg once subcutaneously every 2 weeks *Maximum:* 150 mg once subcutaneously every 2 weeks	$556.20 (75 mg subcutaneously every 2 weeks)
Atorvastatin (Lipitor)	−25 to −40%	+5 to 10%	↓↓	*Initial:* 10 mg orally once *Maximum:* 80 mg orally once	$8.49 (20 mg orally once)
Bempedoic acid (Nexletol)	−17 to −20%	−6%	±	*Initial:* 180 mg orally once *Maximum:* 180 mg orally once	$461.32
Cholestyramine (Questran, others)	−15 to −25%	+5%	±	*Initial:* 4 g orally twice a day *Maximum:* 24 g orally divided	$56.23 (8 g orally divided)
Colesevelam (WelChol)	−10 to −20%	+10%	±	*Initial:* 625 mg, 6–7 tablets orally once *Maximum:* 625 mg, 6–7 tablets orally once	$673.82 (6 tablets orally once)
Colestipol (Colestid)	−15 to −60%	+5%	±	*Initial:* 5 g orally twice a day *Maximum:* 30 g orally divided	$300.00 (10 g orally divided)
Evinacumab (Evkeeza)[3]	−47%	−52%	↓↓	*Initial:* 15 mg/kg intravenously every 4 weeks *Maximum:* 15 mg/kg intravenously every 4 weeks	$46,000.00/1200 mg vial
Evolocumab (Repatha)[2]	−50 to −60%	±	±	*Initial:* 140 mg subcutaneously once every 2 weeks *Maximum:* 420 mg subcutaneously once monthly	$605.60 (140 mg subcutaneously every 2 weeks)
Ezetimibe (Zetia)	−15 to −20%	+5%	±	*Initial:* 10 mg orally once *Maximum:* 10 mg orally once	$250.91 (10 mg orally once)
Fenofibrate (Tricor, others)	−10 to −15%	+15 to 25%	↓↓	*Initial:* 48 mg orally once *Maximum:* 145 mg orally once	$37.20 (145 mg orally once)
Fenofibric acid (Trilipix)	−10 to −15%	+15 to 25%	↓↓	*Initial:* 45 mg orally once *Maximum:* 135 mg orally once	$160.05 (135 mg orally once)
Fluvastatin (Lescol)	−20 to −30%	+5 to 10%	↓	*Initial:* 20 mg orally once *Maximum:* 40 mg orally once	$149.89 (20 mg orally once)
Gemfibrozil (Lopid, others)	−10 to −15%	+15 to 20%	↓↓	*Initial:* 600 mg orally once *Maximum:* 1200 mg orally divided	$24.73 (600 mg orally twice a day)
Inclisiran (Leqvio)[2]	−50 to −52%	+5% to 6%	↓	*Initial:* 284 mg subcutaneously at baseline and 3 months *Maintenance:* 284 mg subcutaneously every 6 months	$650.00 (284 mg every 6 months)
Lomitapide (Juxtapid)[3,4]	−40 to −50%	−7%	↓↓	*Initial:* 5 mg orally once *Maximum:* 60 mg orally once	$57,476.62 (any dose)
Lovastatin (Mevacor, others)	−25 to −40%	+5 to 10%	↓	*Initial:* 10 mg orally once *Maximum:* 80 mg orally divided	$71.16 (20 mg orally once)
Niacin (OTC, Niaspan)[2]	−15 to −25%	+25 to 35%	↓↓	*Initial:* 100 mg orally once *Maximum:* 3–4.5 g orally divided	$10.80 (1.5 g orally twice a day, OTC) $449.40 (2 g Niaspan)
Omega-3 fatty acid ethyl esters (Lovaza)			↓↓	*Initial:* 4 g orally once *Maximum:* 4 g orally once	$248.40 (4 g orally daily)
Omega-3 fatty acid icosapent ethyl (Vascepa)			↓↓	*Initial:* 2 g orally twice *Maximum:* 2 g orally twice	$425.26 (2 g orally twice day)

(*continued*)

Table 28–3. Effects of selected lipid-modifying drugs (listed alphabetically). (continued)

Drug	Lipid-Modifying Effects			Regimens	Cost for 30 Days of Treatment (for Suggested Dose)[1]
	LDL	HDL	Triglyceride		
Pitavastatin (Livalo, Zypitamag)	−30 to −40%	+10 to 25%	↓↓	*Initial:* 2 mg orally once *Maximum:* 4 mg orally once	$384.00 (2 mg orally once)
Pravastatin (Pravachol)	−25 to −40%	+5 to 10%	↓	*Initial:* 20 mg orally once *Maximum:* 80 mg orally once	$74.85 (20 mg orally once)
Rosuvastatin (Crestor)	−40 to −50%	+10 to 15%	↓↓	*Initial:* 10 mg orally once *Maximum:* 40 mg orally once	$43.20 (20 mg orally once)
Simvastatin (Zocor, others)	−25 to −40%	+5 to 10%	↓↓	*Initial:* 5 mg orally once *Maximum:* 80 mg orally once	$4.67 (10 mg orally once)

[1]Average wholesale price (AWP, for AB-rated generic when available) for quantity listed. Source: *IBM Micromedex Red Book (electronic version).* IBM Watson Health, Greenwood Village, Colorado, USA. Available at: https://www-micromedexsolutions-com.proxy.hsl.ucdenver.edu/(cited: March 28, 2022). AWP may not accurately represent the actual pharmacy cost because wide contractual variations exist among institutions.
[2]Also associated with reduction in lipoprotein(a).
[3]Restricted to patients with homozygous familial hypercholesterolemia.
[4]FDA Black Box warning regarding hepatotoxicity. Can only be prescribed in the context of a Food and Drug Administration Risk Evaluation and Mitigation Strategies plan.
± variable, if any; others, indicates availability of less expensive generic preparations; OTC, over the counter.

levels, respectively. Such muscle disease occurs more often when the statin is taken with niacin or a fibrate, as well as with erythromycin, antifungal medications, nefazodone, or cyclosporine. Simvastatin at the highest approved dose (80 mg) is associated with an elevated risk of muscle injury or myopathy; this dose should be used only in patients who have been taking simvastatin at a lower dose for longer than 1 year without muscle toxicity. Liver disease, with elevations of serum transaminases, is another uncommon side effect of statin therapy and is again more common in patients who are also taking fibrates or niacin. Manufacturers of statins recommend monitoring liver enzymes before initiating therapy and as clinically indicated thereafter; current guidelines do not recommend routine monitoring. Finally, statin therapy is associated with a 10% increase in risk of developing diabetes mellitus in at-risk individuals (eg, those with the metabolic syndrome).

B. Ezetimibe

Ezetimibe inhibits the intestinal absorption of dietary and biliary cholesterol across the intestinal wall by inhibiting a cholesterol transporter. The dose of ezetimibe is 10 mg/day orally. Ezetimibe reduces LDL cholesterol between 15% and 20% when used as monotherapy, reduces high-sensitivity CRP, and can further reduce LDL in patients taking statins in whom the therapeutic goal has not been reached. While beneficial effects of ezetimibe monotherapy on cardiovascular outcomes are available from only a large open-label trial, the double-blind IMPROVE-IT trial showed that adding ezetimibe to a statin resulted in a small incremental 5–10% relative risk reduction in detrimental cardiovascular outcomes. At the end of 7 years of study, patients taking ezetimibe-simvastatin had a 2% absolute reduction in cardiovascular events compared to patients taking simvastatin alone. Current guidelines recommend adding ezetimibe therapy to maximally tolerated statin therapy in patients at high risk for CVD whose LDL cholesterol remains above the treatment threshold of 70 mg/dL.

C. Proprotein Convertase Subtilisin/Kexin Type 9 (PCSK9) Inhibitors

As of 2021, available PCSK9 inhibitors are fully human monoclonal antibodies that inhibit PCSK9-mediated LDL-receptor degradation and lower LDL cholesterol levels by 50–60% and lipoprotein(a) by up to 20–30%. Two agents, alirocumab and evolocumab, are FDA-approved for use in patients with familial hypercholesterolemia or in patients with CVD already on maximal doses of agents in other classes but who require further lowering of LDL cholesterol. These medications are injected subcutaneously every 2–4 weeks. No significant increase in adverse events has been observed compared to placebo. The FOURIER (Further Cardiovascular Outcomes Research with PCSK9 Inhibition in Subjects with Elevated Risk) trial compared evolocumab with placebo in 27,564 patients with established atherosclerotic disease already taking statin therapy; participants were monitored for a median of 2.2 years. LDL cholesterol was reduced by 59%. Patients receiving the evolocumab plus statin had a 15% reduction in the primary composite endpoint of cardiovascular death, MI, stroke, hospital admission for unstable angina, or coronary revascularization and a 20% reduction in the secondary outcome of cardiovascular death, MI, or stroke. The ODYSSEY-OUTCOMES study randomized 18,924 patients with recent acute coronary syndrome to alirocumab or placebo, demonstrating a 15% reduction in the primary composite cardiovascular endpoint and a 15%

reduction in all-cause mortality in secondary statistical testing after median 2.8-year follow-up.

However, despite these encouraging results from multiple clinical trials, their very high cost meant that initial cost-effectiveness models found that these PCSK9 inhibitors were not cost-effective. After marked price reductions in 2018 and 2019, PCSK9 inhibitors moved closer to being cost-effective; however, most guidelines indicate that their relatively high cost must still remain part of any consideration regarding their use. Current guidelines recommend addition of PCSK9 inhibitors to statins at maximally tolerated doses in patients at very high risk for CVD when on-treatment LDL cholesterol remains above 70 mg/dL (or above 100 mg/dL in patients with familial hypercholesterolemia). Patients considered to be at very high-risk for CVD include those with recent acute coronary syndrome within 12 months; multiple prior MIs or strokes; significant unrevascularized CAD; and polyvascular disease (CAD plus cerebrovascular or peripheral vascular disease).

At the end of 2021, the FDA approved the novel PCSK9 inhibitor inclisiran, which uses silencing RNA technology to reduce liver production of PCSK9 protein by approximately 80%. Inclisiran had already been approved for use in Europe and England. After an initial subcutaneous dose and another one at 3 months, inclisiran can be administered subcutaneously every 6 months (two doses annually). This regimen produces sustained LDL cholesterol reductions of approximately 51%. Twice-yearly dosing is novel for lipid-lowering therapy; inclisiran enables new delivery strategies, including in-clinic administration. The results of the large cardiovascular outcomes trial testing inclisiran, called ORION-4, will be available in 2023 or 2024. Results of earlier trials (ORION-10, -11, and -12) of treatment of heterozygous familial hypercholesterolemia and of elevated LDL cholesterol. were published in 2020 (see references below).

D. Omega-3 Fatty Acid Preparations

Omega-3 fatty acids are essential fatty acids that must be consumed in the diet and are a prominent feature of Mediterranean-style diets. In pharmacologic doses, omega-3 fatty acid preparations can lower triglycerides by up to 30%, with modest reductions in apolipoprotein-B–containing lipoproteins and high-sensitivity CRP. Pharmacologic therapy should be differentiated from dietary omega-3 fatty acid supplements. The former is an FDA-approved product usually given at a much higher dose; dietary supplements are variable, the supporting evidence is much weaker, and they are not currently regulated.

There is modest evidence from meta-analyses that omega-3 fatty acid supplementation reduces MIs, although with no reduction in total or cardiovascular mortality. Omega-3 ethyl esters have not been associated with cardiovascular event reduction when added to statin therapy.

In contrast, icosapent ethyl, which is a highly purified eicosapentaenoic acid (EPA) only preparation, was shown to reduce cardiovascular deaths, nonfatal MIs, nonfatal strokes, coronary revascularizations, and unstable angina by 25% in statin-treated patients with triglycerides greater than 135 mg/dL in the 8179 person REDUCE-IT randomized clinical trial compared to a mineral oil placebo. The mechanism of action of icosapent ethyl is not yet clear but likely involves multiple mechanisms beyond lipid lowering, including antiplatelet activity, anti-inflammatory activity, and arrhythmia prevention. In 2019, the FDA approved icosapent ethyl for the broad indication of CVD event–lowering in patients with triglycerides over 150 mg/dL and either established CVD or diabetes mellitus plus two or more additional risk factors for CVD. However, there remains controversy about the efficacy of omega-3 therapies, since the 2020 STRENGTH trial showed no CVD benefit of omega-3 carboxylic acids; it remains unclear if this result was due to a different omega-3 fatty acid preparation, to a much smaller benefit of omega-3 fatty acids preparations than originally demonstrated, or to chance.

E. Bempedoic Acid

Like statins, bempedoic acid targets cholesterol synthesis in the liver, ultimately resulting in upregulation of expression of the LDL receptor. Bempedoic acid is a small-molecule inhibitor of ACL, an enzyme that is upstream of the mechanism of statins (inhibition of HMG-CoA reductase). Bempedoic acid lowers LDL approximately 17–20% on top of the lowering produced by moderate- to high-intensity statins. Bempedoic acid is also marketed in combination with ezetimibe; this combination provides approximately 38% LDL reduction on top of background lipid-lowering therapy. Treatment with bempedoic acid may mildly decrease both high-sensitivity CRP (hsCRP) and risk of diabetes mellitus. Patients treated with bempedoic acid should be monitored for hyperuricemia and potential onset or worsening of gout. Bempedoic acid also appears to modestly increase the risk of tendon rupture. Bempedoic acid should not be used with more than 20 mg of simvastatin daily or 40 mg of pravastatin daily.

F. Bile Acid–Binding Resins

The bile acid–binding resins include cholestyramine, colesevelam, and colestipol. In the pre-statin era, treatment with these agents reduced the incidence of coronary events in middle-aged men by about 20%, with no significant effect on total mortality. The resins work by binding bile acids in the intestine. The resultant reduction in the enterohepatic circulation causes the liver to increase its production of bile acids, using hepatic cholesterol. Thus, hepatic LDL-receptor activity increases, with a decline in plasma LDL levels. The triglyceride level tends to increase in some patients treated with bile acid–binding resins; these resins should be used with caution in patients with elevated triglycerides and not at all in patients who have triglyceride levels above 500 mg/dL. The clinician can anticipate a reduction of 15–25% in the LDL cholesterol level, with insignificant effects on the HDL level. Resins are the only lipid-modifying medication considered safe in pregnancy.

These agents may interfere with the absorption of fat-soluble vitamins (thereby complicating the management of patients receiving warfarin) and may bind other drugs in the intestine. They often cause GI symptoms, such as constipation and gas.

G. Fibric Acid Derivatives

The fibrates are peroxisome proliferative-activated receptor-alpha (PPAR-alpha) agonists that result in significant reductions of plasma triglycerides and increases in HDL cholesterol. They reduce LDL levels by about 10–15% (although the result is variable) and triglyceride levels by about 40% and raise HDL levels by about 15–20%. The fibric acid derivatives or fibrates approved for use in the United States are gemfibrozil and fenofibrate. Ciprofibrate and bezafibrate are also available for use internationally.

Gemfibrozil monotherapy reduced CHD rates in hypercholesterolemic middle-aged men free of coronary disease in the Helsinki Heart Study. The effect was observed only among those who also had lower HDL cholesterol levels and high triglyceride levels. In a Veterans Affairs study, gemfibrozil monotherapy was also shown to reduce cardiovascular events in men with existing CHD whose primary lipid abnormality was a low HDL cholesterol.

However, fibrates have not been shown to reduce cardiovascular events in all statin-treated patients with CVD or diabetes. For example, in the ACCORD study, addition of fenofibrate to statin in patients with diabetes and mild triglyceride elevations resulted in no benefit.

The usual dose of gemfibrozil is 600 mg once or twice a day. Side effects include cholelithiasis, hepatitis, and myositis. The incidence of the latter two conditions may be higher among patients also taking other lipid-lowering agents. Fenofibrate, 48–145 mg daily, has slightly fewer side effects than gemfibrozil.

H. Niacin (Nicotinic Acid)

Niacin reduces the production of VLDL particles, with secondary reduction in LDL and increases in HDL cholesterol levels. The average effect of full-dose niacin therapy is a 15–25% reduction in LDL cholesterol and a 25–35% increase in HDL cholesterol.

There is very little evidence to support the use of niacin in the modern era. In two large pivotal clinical trials, AIM-HIGH and HPS2-THRIVE, extended-release niacin did not reduce cardiovascular events when added to statin therapy in high-risk patients. Therefore, niacin should be rarely used.

Treatment Algorithms

For patients who require a lipid-modifying medication, an HMG-CoA reductase inhibitor (statin) is recommended. In patients with CVD, this should be at its maximally tolerated dose.

Combination therapy is indicated for (1) patients with familial hypercholesterolemia with on-treatment LDL cholesterol that is above 100 mg/dL; (2) patients with advanced subclinical atherosclerosis (coronary artery calcium scores greater than 300 or even greater than 1000) or existing CVD with on-treatment LDL cholesterol that remains above 70 mg/dL; and (3) many high-risk patients with triglycerides greater than 150 mg/dL or non-HDL cholesterol greater than 100 mg/dL.

Patients with heterozygous familial hypercholesterolemia or premature CVD may need two or more medications to get below the treatment threshold, while those without CVD (primary prevention) less commonly need multiple medications. The 2018 AHA/ACC/Multi-society guidelines recommend addition of ezetimibe in high-risk patients, while reserving PCSK9 inhibitor therapy for very high-risk patients or those taking maximally tolerated statin therapy and ezetimibe with LDL cholesterol still not below 70 mg/dL (Figure 28–2). Notably, the 2019 ESC guidelines have endorsed an LDL cholesterol treatment goal of less than 55 mg/dL in very high-risk patients, which uniquely include patients with at least two 50% coronary artery stenoses identified by coronary CT angiography, or in the carotid arteries on ultrasound. These guidelines further endorse an LDL goal of less than 40 mg/dL in the highest-risk patients with multiple recent CVD events. Other guidelines, including the American Diabetes Association and the National Lipid Association, have endorsed the use of icosapent ethyl in high-risk patients with CVD or diabetes and on-treatment triglycerides greater than 150 mg/dL.

Patients with homozygous familial hypercholesterolemia may need plasmapheresis and/or special lipid-lowering therapies uniquely approved for this population (Table 28–3).

Di Minno A et al. Efficacy and safety of bempedoic acid in patients with hypercholesterolemia: systematic review and meta-analysis of randomized controlled trials. J Am Heart Assoc. 2020;9:e016262. [PMID: 32689862]

Grundy SM et al. 2018 AHA/ACC/AACVPR/AAPA/ABC/ACPM/ADA/AGS/APhA/ASPC/NLA/PCNA guideline on the management of blood cholesterol: executive summary. Circulation. 2019;139:e1046. [PMID: 30565953]

Mach F et al. 2019 ESC/EAS Guidelines for the management of dyslipidaemias: lipid modification to reduce cardiovascular risk. Eur Heart J. 2020;41:111. [PMID: 31504418]

Nicholls SJ et al. Effect of high-dose omega-3 fatty acids vs corn oil on major adverse cardiovascular events in patients at high cardiovascular risk: the STRENGTH randomized clinical trial. JAMA. 2020;324:2268. [PMID: 33190147]

Nurmohamed NS et al. New and emerging therapies for reduction of LDL-cholesterol and apolipoprotein B: JACC Focus Seminar 1/4. J Am Coll Cardiol. 2021;77:1564. [PMID: 33766264]

Raal FJ et al; ORION-9 Investigators. Inclisiran for the treatment of heterozygous familial hypercholesterolemia. N Engl J Med. 2020;382:1520. [PMID: 32197277]

Ray KK et al; ORION-10 and ORION-11 Investigators. Two phase 3 trials of inclisiran in patients with elevated LDL cholesterol. N Engl J Med. 2020;382:1507. [PMID: 32187462]

Wood FA et al. N-of-1 trial of a statin, placebo, or no treatment to assess side effects. N Engl J Med. 2020;383:2182. [PMID: 33196154]

HIGH BLOOD TRIGLYCERIDES

Patients with very high levels of serum triglycerides (greater than 1000 mg/dL) are at risk for pancreatitis. The pathophysiology is not certain since pancreatitis never

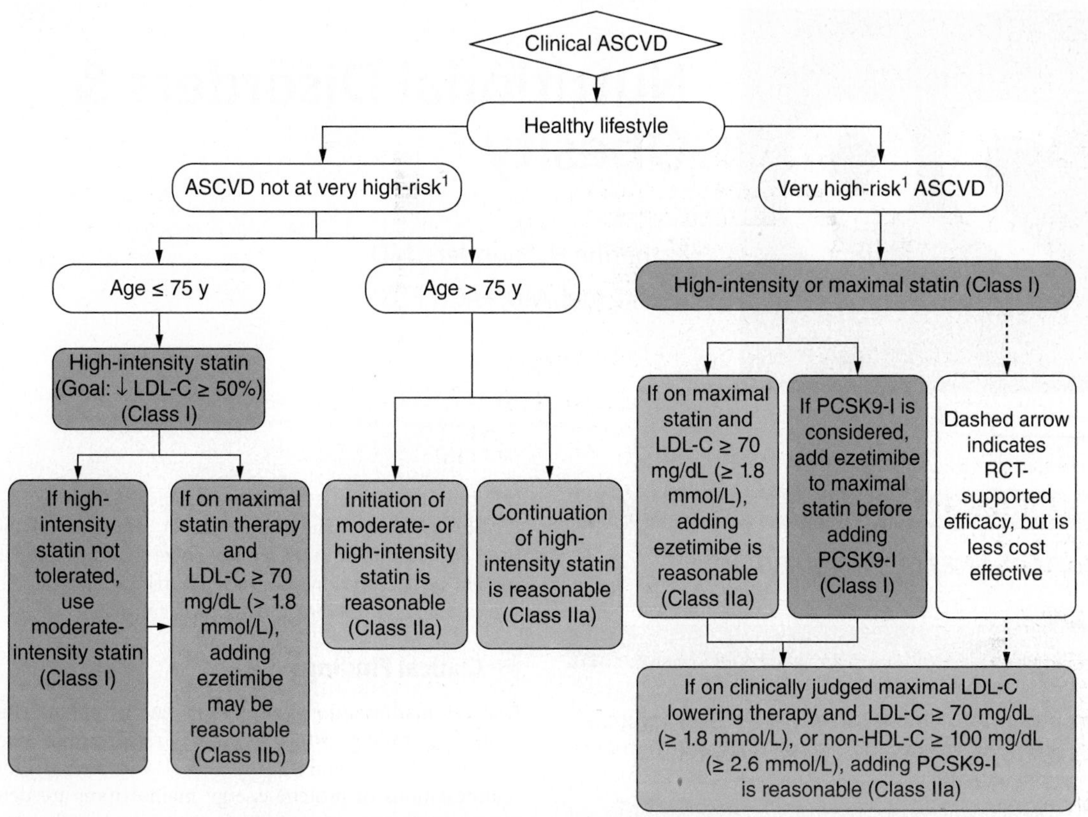

[1]Very high-risk groups include patients with recent acute coronary syndrome within 12 months; multiple prior MIs or strokes; significant unrevascularized CAD; and polyvascular disease (coronary + cerebrovascular or peripheral vascular)
(Class I = Strong recommendation [benefit >>> risk]; Class IIa = Moderately strong recommendation [benefit >> risk]; Class IIb = Weak recommendation [benefit > risk])
HDL-C, high-density lipoprotein cholesterol; LDL-C, low-density lipoprotein cholesterol; PCSK9-I, proprotein convertase subtilisin/kexin type 9 inhibitor; RCT, randomized controlled trial.

▲ **Figure 28–2.** Clinical treatment algorithm for patients with atherosclerotic CVD. (Reprinted with permission Circulation. 2019;139:e1082–e1143. ©2018 American Heart Association, Inc.)

develops in some patients with very high triglyceride levels. Most patients with congenital abnormalities in triglyceride metabolism present in childhood; hypertriglyceridemia-induced pancreatitis first presenting in adults is more commonly due to an acquired problem in lipid metabolism.

Although there are no clear triglyceride levels that predict pancreatitis, most clinicians treat fasting levels above 500 mg/dL (5 mmol/L). The risk of pancreatitis may be more related to the triglyceride level following consumption of a fatty meal. Because postprandial increases in triglyceride are inevitable if fat-containing foods are eaten, fasting triglyceride levels in persons prone to pancreatitis should be kept well below that level.

The primary therapy for high triglyceride levels is dietary, avoiding alcohol, simple sugars, refined starches, and saturated and trans fatty acids, and restricting total calories. Control of secondary causes of high triglyceride levels may also be helpful. In patients with fasting triglycerides greater than or equal to 500 mg/dL (5 mmol/L) despite adequate dietary compliance—and certainly in those with a previous episode of pancreatitis—therapy with a triglyceride-lowering drug (eg, statins, omega-3 preparations, or fibric acid derivatives) is indicated. Combinations of these medications may also be used.

Drug treatment for patients with triglycerides greater than 150 mg/dL (1.5 mmol/L) is reserved for those with established CVD with well-controlled LDL cholesterol on maximally tolerated therapy with statins or other agents. Data are strongest for icosapent ethyl.

Orringer CE et al. National Lipid Association Scientific Statement on the use of icosapent ethyl in statin-treated patients with elevated triglycerides and high or very-high ASCVD risk. J Clin Lipidol. 2019;13:860. [PMID: 31787586]

Packard CJ et al. Causes and consequences of hypertriglyceridemia. Front Endocrinol (Lausanne). 2020;11:252. [PMID: 32477261]

Simha V. Management of hypertriglyceridemia. BMJ. 2020;371:m3109. [PMID: 33046451]

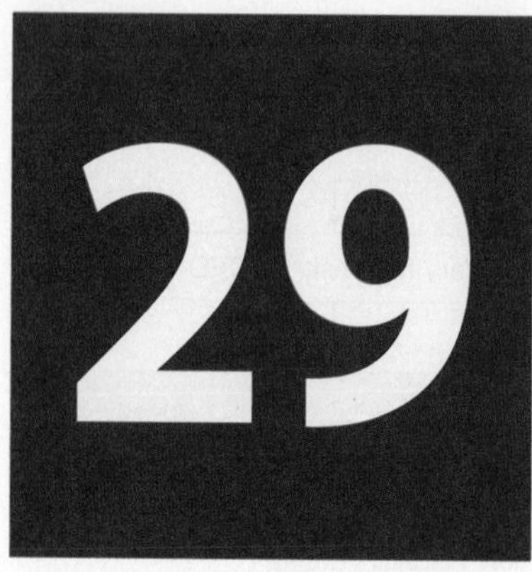

Nutritional Disorders & Obesity

Katherine H. Saunders, MD
Leon I. Igel, MD, FACP, FTOS

NUTRITIONAL DISORDERS

PROTEIN–ENERGY MALNUTRITION

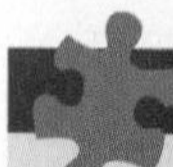

ESSENTIALS OF DIAGNOSIS

- Inadequate intake of energy and/or protein, increased nutrient losses, or increased nutrient requirements.
- **Kwashiorkor:** caused by protein deficiency
- **Marasmus:** caused by combined protein and energy deficiency.
- Protein–calorie malnutrition may be mild, moderate, or severe.
- Protein loss correlates with weight loss.
- 35–40% total body weight loss can be fatal.

General Considerations

Protein–energy malnutrition occurs as a result of a relative or absolute deficiency of energy and protein. It may be primary, due to inadequate food intake; secondary, as a result of other illness and associated inflammation; or a combination of both. For many developing nations, primary protein–energy malnutrition remains a significant health problem. There are two distinct syndromes: **kwashiorkor**, which is caused by a deficiency of protein in the presence of adequate energy, and **marasmus**, which is caused by combined protein and energy deficiency.

In industrialized societies, malnutrition is more often a sequela of other diseases/illnesses, than to pure starvation. Although there is no universally accepted definition of malnutrition, there are a number of internationally recognized malnutrition assessment tools that have been developed in an effort to standardize malnutrition identification and promote nutrition interventions. Examples include the Subjective Global Assessment (SGA), the American Society for Parenteral and Enteral Nutrition (ASPEN) and Academy of Nutrition and Dietetics (AND) Criteria, and the European Society for Parenteral and Enteral Nutrition (ESPEN) Criteria. The ASPEN/AND criteria are widely used and unique in that they recognize the role of inflammation in the development of malnutrition and therefore propose an etiology-based diagnostic approach.

Clinical Findings

Clinical manifestations of protein–energy malnutrition range from mild growth restriction in children and weight loss in adults to several distinct clinical syndromes. Clinical manifestations of protein–energy malnutrition are determined by the patient's nutritional status prior to illness, the disease process itself, associated treatments, and the severity of the malnutrition.

Performing a nutrition-focused physical assessment is essential to determine clinical manifestations of protein–energy malnutrition. Wasting begins with weight loss and can be seen in adipose tissue, muscle mass, or both. Cachexia is defined as loss of lean body mass only, irrespective of adipose tissues changes, and is associated with inflammation and protein catabolism. Muscle mass depletion is seen in the temples, clavicles, shoulders, scapula, hands, thigh, and calf. Subcutaneous body fat loss may be evident in the orbital area, triceps, and rib cage. Dependent edema, ascites, or anasarca may develop and can be assessed on a physical exam. Laboratory studies may be unremarkable—serum albumin, for example, tends to be normal in patients with malnutrition related to social, behavioral, or environmental etiologies; however, levels decline in the presence of inflammation and tend to be low in patients who have malnutrition related to acute and chronic diseases. Overall albumin is not considered a good marker of malnutrition and should not be used as part of diagnosis. Similarly, laboratory assessment of micronutrient deficiencies may not be reliable.

Treatment

The treatment of protein–energy malnutrition should be a slow process and requires great care, especially in more chronic and severe cases. In early treatment, the focus should be on prevention of refeeding syndrome, which is defined as a range of electrolyte alterations occurring as a result of the provision of calories (glucose) after a period of decreased or absent caloric intake. Patients who are refed too quickly are at risk for developing heart failure due to fluid and electrolyte shifts.

Initial efforts should be directed at correcting fluid and electrolyte abnormalities, particularly phosphorus, potassium, and magnesium. The second phase of treatment is directed at cautiously repleting calories, protein, and micronutrients. Although patients can receive adequate amounts of protein, this may be difficult to achieve with the conservative initiation and advancement of total calories. Depending on the severity of malnutrition, patients may benefit from as little as 5–20 kcal/kg/day for the first few days with advancement of calories as tolerated over the next 7 days. Once out of the initial refeeding window, most patients should receive at least 30–35 kcal/kg/day and 1.5 g protein/kg/day, although some may require significantly more depending on their BMI and severity of malnutrition. All patients should receive additional thiamine 100 mg daily for at least 5–7 days.

Refeeding edema is benign but must be differentiated from heart failure. Changes in renal sodium reabsorption and poor skin and blood vessel integrity may result in dependent edema. Treatment includes elevation of the edematous area and sodium restriction, if appropriate. Diuretics should not be used.

Nutrition screening is essential for identifying patients who are malnourished or at risk for becoming malnourished. These patients require a formal nutrition assessment with targeted interventions and close monitoring throughout a hospital stay.

Ponzo V et al. The refeeding syndrome: a neglected but potentially serious condition for inpatients. A narrative review. Intern Emerg Med. 2021;16:49. [PMID: 33074463]

Reber E et al. Nutritional risk screening and assessment. J Clin Med. 2019;8:E1065. [PMID: 31330781]

OBESITY

ESSENTIALS OF DIAGNOSIS

- Disorder of energy homeostasis; BMI ≥ 30.
- Central obesity (abdomen and flank) is a greater health risk than excess weight in the lower body (buttocks and thighs).
- Associated comorbid conditions include type 2 diabetes mellitus, hypertension, hyperlipidemia, heart disease, stroke, and obstructive sleep apnea.

Definition & Measurement

Obesity is a multifactorial, chronic disease characterized by an accumulation of visceral and subcutaneous fat, which promotes adipocyte dysfunction. Obesity predisposes to a wide variety of comorbid conditions. **BMI** typically correlates with excess adipose tissue but does not reflect body composition. It is calculated by dividing body weight in kilograms by height in meters squared (kg/m^2). The National Institutes of Health defines a normal BMI as 18.5–24.9. Overweight is defined as BMI 25–29.9. Class I obesity is 30–34.9, class II is 35–39.9, and class III is 40 and above. Central obesity (excess adipose tissue around the waist and flank) is a greater health risk than lower body obesity (adipose tissue in the thighs and buttocks). Patients with obesity and increased abdominal circumference (greater than 102 cm or 40 inches in men and 88 cm or 35 inches in women) or high waist–hip ratios (greater than 1.0 in men and 0.85 in women) have a greater risk of weight-related comorbid conditions and early death than patients with the same BMI and lower ratios. Visceral fat within the abdominal cavity is more hazardous to health than subcutaneous fat around the abdomen. Over 40% of Americans have obesity.

Health Consequences of Obesity

Obesity is associated with significant increases in both morbidity and mortality, and many disorders occur with greater frequency in patients with obesity. Obesity-related comorbidities include many leading causes of preventable death such as heart disease, stroke, type 2 diabetes, and many cancers. Over 200 health conditions ranging from hypertension and CAD to thromboembolic and skin disorders are more prevalent in patients with obesity. Patients with higher BMI have increased surgical and obstetric risks and higher rates of major depression and binge-eating disorder. Most patients with excess weight have experienced weight bias.

Etiology

Both genetic and environmental factors contribute to the development of obesity. Twin studies demonstrate that genetics account for 40–90% of variation in BMI, although only a small percentage is due to single gene mutations. Most obesity develops from interactions of multiple genes, environmental factors, and behavior. The rapid increase in obesity in the last several decades points to major roles for environmental and behavioral factors.

Medical Evaluation of the Patient with Obesity

Medical history should determine the age at onset of weight gain, recent weight changes, family history of obesity, occupational history, eating and exercise behavior, previous weight loss experience, and psychosocial factors, including assessment for mood and eating disorders.

Physical examination should assess BMI, degree and distribution of body fat, and overall nutritional status. Signs of secondary causes of obesity should be pursued; however, less than 1% of patients have an identifiable cause. Cushing syndrome is an example that can be diagnosed by physical examination and laboratory testing in patients with unexplained weight gain (see Chapter 26). All patients should be screened for weight-related comorbid conditions, including obstructive sleep apnea. Blood pressure, waist circumference, fasting glucose, comprehensive metabolic profile, lipid panel, and hemoglobin A_{1c} should be measured as well as other laboratory tests as clinically indicated.

Treatment

Weight loss of 5–10% body weight is sufficient in many patients with obesity to achieve clinically relevant improvements in many risk factors, and the risk reduction appears to be "dose-related." Magnitude of weight loss at 1 year is strongly associated with improvements in many parameters including blood sugar, blood pressure, triglycerides, and HDL cholesterol.

Successful treatment of obesity requires a multidisciplinary approach to counteract the body's resistance to weight loss. Diet, physical activity, and behavioral modifications are the cornerstone of weight management. Many **dietary strategies** can be effective for weight loss. Recommendations should be tailored to a patient's preferences as dietary adherence is associated with greater weight loss. Dietary instructions should emphasize intake of predominantly "unprocessed" foods, with special attention to limiting foods that provide large amounts of calories without other nutrients, such as ultra-processed foods, sugary drinks, fast food, junk food, and sweets. A Mediterranean diet can be a good option for patients at high cardiovascular risk, since it has been shown to reduce the incidence of major cardiovascular events. A low-glycemic-index diet can curb hunger and decrease cravings by reducing blood sugar fluctuations. Meal replacement diets can also facilitate weight loss. Registered dietitians can provide dietary education and customize diet plans.

Long-term changes in eating behavior are required to maintain weight loss and **behavior modification** strategies support weight loss maintenance. It is important to emphasize meal planning and self-monitoring, including weighing at regular intervals. Some patients maintain a food log to track caloric intake. Self-monitoring aids in behavioral change and provides the practitioner with additional data to guide recommendations. Patients can learn to recognize "eating cues" (eg, emotional, situational) and how to avoid or control them. Weight maintenance can be more challenging than initial weight loss, so it is important to continue self-monitoring and regular follow-up to ensure adherence to a treatment plan.

Physical activity offers several advantages for patients trying to achieve and maintain weight loss. Aerobic exercise increases daily energy expenditure and partially prevents the decrease in basal energy expenditure (BEE) resulting from weight loss. It is useful for long-term weight maintenance and helps preserve lean body mass. The combination of exercise and diet results in greater weight loss than diet or exercise alone. Higher intensity exercise is associated with more weight loss. Up to 1 hour of moderate exercise per day is associated with long-term weight maintenance in individuals who have successfully lost weight.

The American College of Sports Medicine recommends 150 minutes of moderate-intensity aerobic physical activity (such as tennis or brisk walking) per week, 75 minutes of vigorous-intensity aerobic exercise (such as jogging or swimming laps) per week, or an equivalent combination of moderate- and vigorous-intensity aerobic activity. Exercise should be spread throughout the week. Resistance training is also recommended at least twice per week. Exercise physiologists and physical therapists can provide additional support for patients.

Medications can have unpredictable and variable effects on patients' weight, so it is important to review patients' medication regimens and balance their benefits against the probability of weight gain. Multiple medications are associated with weight gain, including corticosteroids, contraceptives (and other hormonal agents), and certain antidiabetic, antihypertensive, antidepressant, antipsychotic, antiepileptic, and antihistamine agents. Table 29–1 provides an overview of weight-gaining medications as well as potential alternatives. When possible, clinicians should prescribe weight-neutral– or weight-loss–promoting medications. If there are no alternatives, weight gain can be prevented or lessened by selecting the lowest clinically effective dose for the shortest duration.

Weight loss achieved by lifestyle modification alone is often limited and difficult to maintain. Reduced calorie intake and increased energy expenditure are counteracted by adaptive physiologic responses. Appetite increases and resting metabolic rate (RMR) decreases disproportionately to what would be expected based on changes in body composition. As a result, patients may require antiobesity medications, bariatric surgery, devices, or endoscopic bariatric therapies to achieve and maintain significant weight loss.

Antiobesity medications (Table 29–2) can be considered in patients with a BMI 30 or higher or a BMI 27 or higher with weight-related comorbidities. Some agents affect mechanisms regulating appetite through serotonergic, dopaminergic, or noradrenergic pathways. Medications approved for weight management should be viewed as additions to diet and exercise for patients who have been unsuccessful with lifestyle changes alone. The six most widely prescribed antiobesity medications approved by the FDA are phentermine, orlistat, phentermine/topiramate extended-release (ER), naltrexone sustained-release (SR)/bupropion SR, liraglutide 3.0 mg, and semaglutide 2.4 mg. Table 29–2 provides an overview of these medications. In addition to producing weight loss, each medication improves biomarkers including blood sugar, blood pressure, and lipids. Three of the agents approved since 2012 have stopping rules, which provide weight loss thresholds after 12–16 weeks of treatment under which medication discontinuation is suggested.

Phentermine is the most commonly prescribed adrenergic agonist and antiobesity medication in the United States. In a 28-week controlled trial, participants taking phentermine 15 mg daily lost an average of 6.0 kg compared with 1.5 kg among those assigned to placebo. The maximum recommended dosage of phentermine is 37.5 mg daily, but the dosage should be individualized to the lowest effective dose.

Orlistat works in the GI tract to inhibit intestinal lipase, thus reducing dietary fat absorption. It may thereby cause steatorrhea, fecal urgency, abdominal discomfort, and reduced absorption of fat-soluble vitamins. Orlistat is

Table 29–1. Medications and their effects on weight.

Drug Class	Result: Weight Gain	Result: Weight Neutral (or Minor Weight Gain)	Result: Weight Loss
Antidiabetics	Insulin Meglitinides Sulfonylureas Thiazolidinediones	Alpha-glucosidase inhibitors Bromocriptine Colesevelam DPP-4 inhibitors	GLP-1 agonists Metformin Pramlintide SGLT2 inhibitors
Antihypertensives	Alpha-adrenergic blockers Beta-adrenergic blockers (atenolol, metoprolol, nadolol, propranolol)	ACE inhibitors ARBs Beta-adrenergic blockers (carvedilol, nebivolol) Calcium channel blockers Thiazides	
Antidepressants	Lithium MAO inhibitors Mirtazapine SNRIs (duloxetine, venlafaxine) SSRIs (citalopram, paroxetine) Tricyclic antidepressants (amitriptyline, desipramine, doxepin, imipramine, nortriptyline)	SSRIs (fluoxetine, sertraline)	Bupropion
Antipsychotics	Clozapine Haloperidol Olanzapine Quetiapine Risperidone	Lurasidone Ziprasidone	
Antiepileptics	Carbamazepine Gabapentin Pregabalin Valproic acid	Lamotrigine Levetiracetam Phenytoin	Topiramate Zonisamide
Contraceptives	Medroxyprogesterone acetate	Barrier methods IUDs Surgical sterilization	
Antihistamines	First-generation antihistamines	Second- and third-generation antihistamines	
Steroids	Glucocorticoids	Inhaled steroids Topical steroids	

DPP-4, dipeptidyl peptidase-4; GLP-1, glucagon-like peptide-1; IUD, intrauterine device; SGLT2, sodium-glucose co-transporter 2.
Reproduced with permission from Igel LI et.al. Practical use of pharmacotherapy for obesity. Gastroenterology. 2017;152(7):1765–1779.

associated with a 9.6% weight loss after 1 year compared with 5.6% with placebo. The recommended dose is 120 mg (Xenical, prescription-strength) or 60 mg (Alli, over-the-counter) three times per day with each main meal containing fat.

The combination of **phentermine** and **topiramate ER** (3.75 mg/23 mg orally daily for 14 days, then 7.5 mg/46 mg orally daily, to a maximum dosage of 15 mg/92 mg orally daily) targets two different weight-regulation mechanisms simultaneously. In a 56-week clinical trial, participants taking 15/92 mg lost significantly more weight (9.8%) than those assigned to 7.5/46 mg (7.8%) or placebo (1.2%). There is a potential increased risk of orofacial clefts in infants exposed to topiramate during the first trimester of pregnancy.

The combination of **naltrexone SR** and **bupropion SR** (8 mg/90 mg, increasing from 1 tablet orally daily by 1 additional daily tablet each week to a maximum of 2 tablets twice daily) reduces both appetite and food cravings by targeting two areas of the brain: the arcuate nucleus of the hypothalamus and the mesolimbic dopamine reward circuit. Naltrexone 32 mg/bupropion 360 mg is associated with a 6.1% reduction in body weight compared to 1.3% with placebo after 56 weeks. As with all antidepressants, bupropion carries a black box warning related to a potential increase in suicidality among patients under age 24 years during the early phase of treatment.

Liraglutide 3.0 mg and **semaglutide 2.4 mg** are two glucagon-like peptide-1 (GLP-1) receptor agonists approved by the FDA for the treatment of obesity. Liraglutide was initially FDA-approved in 2010 for the treatment of type 2 diabetes at doses up to 1.8 mg subcutaneously daily and in 2017 for cardiovascular risk reduction in patients with type 2 diabetes and established CVD. Liraglutide 3.0 mg was approved by the FDA for weight loss in 2014. It is initiated at a dose of 0.6 mg subcutaneously daily and increased by 0.6 mg each week to a maximum of 3.0 mg subcutaneously daily. Liraglutide 3.0 mg is

Table 29–2. Medications tested in clinical trials for treatment of obesity.

Medication	Mechanism, Dosage, and Available Formulations	Trial and Duration	Trial Arms	Weight Loss (%)	Most Common Adverse Events	Good Candidates	Poor Candidates
Phentermine (Adipex,[1] Lomaira[2]) Schedule IV controlled substance NOTE: approved for short-term use (up to 3 months)	Adrenergic agonist 8–37.5 mg daily (8 mg dose can be prescribed up to three times daily) Capsule, tablet	Aronne LJ et al[3] 28 weeks	15 mg daily 7.5 mg daily Placebo (topiramate extended-release and phentermine/topiramate extended-release arms excluded)	6.06* 5.45* 1.71	Dry mouth, insomnia, dizziness, irritability	Younger patients who need assistance with appetite suppression	Patients with uncontrolled hypertension, active or unstable coronary disease, hyperthyroidism, glaucoma, anxiety, insomnia, or general sensitivity to stimulants Patients with a history of drug abuse or recent MAO inhibitor use Patients who are pregnant
Orlistat (Alli,[4] Xenical[5])	Lipase inhibitor 60–120 mg three times daily with meals Capsule	XENDOS[6] 208 weeks	120 mg three times daily Placebo	9.6 (week 52)* 5.25 (week 208)* 5.61 (week 52) 2.71 (week 208)	Fecal urgency, oily stool, flatus with discharge, fecal incontinence	Patients with hypercholesterolemia and/or constipation who can limit their intake of dietary fat	Patients with malabsorption syndromes or other GI conditions that predispose to GI upset/diarrhea Patients who cannot modify the fat content of their diets Patients who are pregnant
Phentermine/Topiramate Extended-release (Qsymia)[7] Schedule IV controlled substance	Adrenergic agonist/neurostabilizer 3.75/23–15/92 mg daily (dose titration) Capsule	EQUIP[8] 56 weeks CONQUER[9] 56 weeks SEQUEL[10] 108 weeks (52-week extension of CONQUER trial)	15/92 mg daily 3.75/23 mg daily Placebo 15/92 mg daily 7.5/46 mg daily Placebo 15/92 mg daily 7.5/46 mg daily Placebo	10.9* 5.1* 1.6 9.8* 7.8* 1.2 (weeks 0–56) 10.5* 9.3* 1.8 (weeks 0–108)	Paresthesias, dizziness, dysgeusia, insomnia, constipation, dry mouth	Younger patients who need assistance with appetite suppression	Patients with uncontrolled hypertension, active or unstable coronary disease, hyperthyroidism, glaucoma, anxiety, insomnia, or general sensitivity to stimulants Patients with a history of drug abuse or recent MAO inhibitor use Patients with a history of nephrolithiasis Patients who are pregnant or trying to conceive

Naltrexone/Bupropion sustained-release (Contrave)[11]	Opioid receptor antagonist/dopamine and norepinephrine reuptake inhibitor 8/90 mg daily to 16/180 mg twice daily Tablet	COR-I[12] 56 weeks	16/180 mg twice daily 8/180 mg twice daily Placebo	6.1* 5.0* 1.3	Nausea, vomiting, constipation, headache, dizziness, insomnia, dry mouth	Patients who describe cravings for food and/or addictive behaviors related to food; patients who are trying to quit smoking, reduce alcohol intake, and/or who have concomitant depression	Patients with uncontrolled hypertension, uncontrolled pain, recent MAO inhibitor use, history of seizures, or any condition that predisposes to seizure, such as anorexia/bulimia nervosa, abrupt discontinuation of alcohol, benzodiazepines, barbiturates, or antiepileptic drugs Patients who are pregnant
		COR-II[13] 56 weeks	16/180 mg twice daily Placebo	6.4* 1.2			
		COR-BMOD[14] 56 weeks	16/180 mg twice daily Placebo	9.3* 5.1			
		COR-DIABETES[15] 56 weeks	16/180 mg twice daily Placebo	5.0* 1.8			
Liraglutide 3.0 mg (Saxenda)[16]	GLP-1 receptor agonist 0.6–3.0 mg daily Prefilled pen for subcutaneous injection	SCALE Obesity and Prediabetes[17] 56 weeks	3.0 mg daily Placebo	8.0* 2.6	Nausea, vomiting, diarrhea, constipation, dyspepsia, abdominal pain	Patients who report inadequate meal satiety, and/or have type 2 diabetes, prediabetes, or impaired glucose tolerance Patients requiring use of concomitant psychiatric medications	Patients with a history of pancreatitis, personal/family history of MTC or MEN2 Patients with an aversion to needles Patients who are pregnant
		SCALE Diabetes[18] 56 weeks	3.0 mg daily	6*			
		SCALE Maintenance[19] 56 weeks (after initial ≥ 5% weight loss with low-calorie diet)	1.8 mg daily Placebo 3.0 mg daily Placebo	4.7* 2.0 6.2* 0.2			
Semaglutide 2.4 mg (Wegovy)	GLP-1 receptor agonist 0.25–2.4 mg weekly Prefilled pen for subcutaneous injection	STEP 1[20] 68 weeks STEP 2[21] 68 weeks STEP 3[22] 68 weeks STEP 4[23] 68 weeks (after 20-week run in with semaglutide titrated to 2.4 mg weekly)	Placebo 2.4 mg weekly Placebo 1.0 mg weekly 2.4 mg weekly Placebo 2.4 mg weekly Placebo 2.4 mg weekly	2.4 14.9* 3.4 7.0* 9.4* 5.7 16.0* +6.9 (weight gain after discontinuation of semaglutide) 7.9* (additional weight loss beyond 20 weeks)	Nausea, vomiting, diarrhea, constipation, dyspepsia, abdominal pain	Patients who report inadequate meal satiety, and/or have type 2 diabetes, prediabetes, or impaired glucose tolerance Patients requiring use of concomitant psychiatric medications	Patients with a history of pancreatitis, personal/family history of MTC or MEN2 Patients with an aversion to needles Patients who are pregnant

(*continued*)

Table 29–2. Medications tested in clinical trials for treatment of obesity. (continued)

*$P < 0.001$ versus placebo.

[1]Adipex [package insert]. Tulsa, OK: Physicians Total Care, Inc; 2012.

[2]Lomaira [package insert]. Newtown, PA: KVK-TECH, INC; 2016.

[3]Aronne LJ et al. Evaluation of phentermine and topiramate versus phentermine/topiramate extended-release in obese adults. Obesity (Silver Spring). 2013;21:2163.

[4]Alli [package insert]. Moon Township, PA: GlaxoSmithKline Consumer Healthcare, LP; 2015.

[5]Xenical [package insert]. South San Francisco, CA: Genentech USA, Inc; 2015.

[6]Torgerson JS et al. XENical in the prevention of diabetes in obese subjects (XENDOS) study: a randomized study of orlistat as an adjunct to lifestyle changes for the prevention of type 2 diabetes in obese patients. Diabetes Care. 2004;27:155.

[7]Qsymia [package insert]. Mountain View, CA: VIVUS, Inc; 2012.

[8]Allison DB et al. Controlled-release phentermine/topiramate in severely obese adults: a randomized controlled trial (EQUIP). Obesity (Silver Spring). 2012;20:330.

[9]Gadde KM et al. Effects of low-dose, controlled-release, phentermine plus topiramate combination on weight and associated comorbidities in overweight and obese adults (CONQUER): a randomised, placebo-controlled, phase 3 trial. Lancet. 2011;377:1341.

[10]Garvey WT et al. Two-year sustained weight loss and metabolic benefits with controlled-release phentermine/topiramate in obese and overweight adults (SEQUEL): a randomized, placebo-controlled, phase 3 extension study. Am J Clin Nutr. 2012;95:297.

[11]Contrave [package insert]. Deerfield, IL: Takeda Pharmaceuticals America, Inc; 2014.

[12]Greenway FL et al. Effect of naltrexone plus bupropion on weight loss in overweight and obese adults (COR-I): a multicentre, randomised, double-blind, placebo-controlled, phase 3 trial. Lancet. 2010;376:595.

[13]Apovian CM et al. A randomized, phase 3 trial of naltrexone SR/bupropion SR on weight and obesity-related risk factors (COR-II). Obesity (Silver Spring). 2013;21:935.

[14]Wadden TA et al. Weight loss with naltrexone SR/bupropion SR combination therapy as an adjunct to behavior modification: the COR-BMOD trial. Obesity (Silver Spring). 2011;19:110.

[15]Hollander P et al. Effects of naltrexone sustained-release/bupropion sustained-release combination therapy on body weight and glycemic parameters in overweight and obese patients with type 2 diabetes. Diabetes Care. 2013;36:4022.

[16]Saxenda [package insert]. Plainsboro, NJ: Novo Nordisk; 2014.

[17]Pi-Sunyer X et al. A randomized, controlled trial of 3.0 mg of liraglutide in weight management. N Engl J Med. 2015;373:11.

[18]Davies MJ et al. Efficacy of liraglutide for weight loss among patients with type 2 diabetes: the SCALE Diabetes randomized clinical trial. JAMA. 2015;314:687.

[19]Wadden TA et al. Weight maintenance and additional weight loss with liraglutide after low-calorie-diet induced weight loss: the SCALE Maintenance randomized study. Int J Obes (Lond). 2013;37:1443.

GLP-1, glucagon-like peptide-1; MEN2, multiple endocrine neoplasia syndrome type 2; MTC, medullary thyroid carcinoma.

Reproduced with permission from Saunders KH et.al, Obesity pharmacotherapy. Med Clin North Am. 2018;102(1):135–148.

[20]Wilding JPH et al. Once-weekly semaglutide in adults with overweight or obesity. N Engl J Med. 2021;384:989.

[21]Davies M et al. STEP 2 Study Group. Semaglutide 2.4 mg once a week in adults with overweight or obesity, and type 2 diabetes (STEP 2): a randomised, double-blind, double-dummy, placebo-controlled, phase 3 trial. Lancet. 2021;397(10278):971.

[22]Wadden TA et al.; STEP 3 Investigators. Effect of subcutaneous semaglutide vs placebo as an adjunct to intensive behavioral therapy on body weight in adults with overweight or obesity: The STEP 3 randomized clinical trial. JAMA. 2021;325:1403.

[23]Rubino Det al. Supplement to: Effect of continued weekly subcutaneous semaglutide vs placebo on weight loss maintenance in adults with overweight or obesity: The STEP 4 randomized clinical trial. JAMA. 2021;325:1414.

associated with 8.0% weight loss compared to 2.6% with placebo after 56 weeks.

Semaglutide 1.0 mg was initially FDA-approved for the treatment of type 2 diabetes in 2017 and in 2020 for cardiovascular risk reduction in patients with type 2 diabetes and known heart disease. In 2021, **semaglutide 2.4 mg** was FDA-approved for the treatment of obesity. It is initiated at a dose of 0.25 mg subcutaneously weekly and titrated to a maximum dose of 2.4 mg weekly. In a 68-week clinical trial, semaglutide 2.4 mg was associated with 14.9% weight loss compared to 2.4% weight loss with placebo. There is a boxed warning that both liraglutide and semaglutide may cause thyroid C-cell tumors (including medullary thyroid carcinoma) in rodents. There is no evidence of GLP-1 receptor agonists causing C-cell tumors in humans.

Bariatric surgery is the most effective treatment for obesity. It is associated with significant and sustained weight loss, reduced obesity-related comorbidities, and improved quality of life. Bariatric surgery is associated with lower incidence of cardiovascular events, decreased number of cardiovascular deaths, and reduced overall mortality compared to usual care. The two most common bariatric procedures in the United States are the sleeve gastrectomy and the Roux-en-Y gastric bypass. The laparoscopic adjustable gastric band and other bariatric surgical procedures are performed less frequently. Bariatric surgery can be considered in patients with a BMI 40 or higher or with a BMI 35 or higher with one or more obesity-related complications who are motivated but failed to achieve sufficient weight loss following lifestyle modification, with or without pharmacotherapy. Long-term medical follow-up, lifestyle changes, and adherence to a vitamin regimen are crucial to the success of bariatric surgery. Some patients have difficulty maintaining weight loss and regain some portion of the lost weight. Despite the known benefits of bariatric surgery, less than 1% of eligible patients undergo a weight-loss surgery. This is likely due to limited patient knowledge of the health benefits of surgery, limited provider comfort in recommending surgery, and inadequate insurance coverage.

Sleeve gastrectomy involves removing approximately 70% of the stomach body and antrum along the greater curvature. The fundus of the stomach, which secretes ghrelin, a hormone that stimulates appetite, also is removed. Sleeve gastrectomy is associated with approximately 25% total body weight loss after 1 year. Because this procedure is mainly restrictive (versus the Roux-en-Y gastric bypass, which is also malabsorptive), there is a lower risk of nutritional deficiencies. In general, sleeve gastrectomy is associated with fewer complications than the Roux-en-Y gastric bypass. Early adverse events include bleeding, leakage along the staple line, stenosis, and vomiting. Late complications include gastroesophageal reflux, nutritional deficiencies, and stomach expansion, leading to decreased restriction. Unlike Roux-en-Y gastric bypass, sleeve gastrectomy is not reversible.

The **Roux-en-Y gastric bypass** involves a staple partition across the proximal stomach with attachment of a small proximal stomach to a jejunal limb, thus bypassing the remainder of the stomach, duodenum, and the proximal jejunum. Roux-en-Y gastric bypass is associated with approximately 30% total body weight loss at 1 year and greater improvements in comorbid disease markers compared to the sleeve gastrectomy. Roux-en-Y gastric bypass is associated with a lower rate of gastroesophageal reflux than sleeve gastrectomy and can even alleviate gastroesophageal reflux in patients who have it. It is often recommended over sleeve gastrectomy for patients with type 2 diabetes because it leads to greater long-term remission. Early adverse events associated with Roux-en-Y gastric bypass include obstruction, stricture, leak, and failure of the staple partition of the upper stomach. Late adverse events include nutritional deficiencies (eg, vitamins B_1, B_{12}, D, and iron) and anastomosis ulceration. Dumping syndrome can develop at any time. Roux-en-Y gastric bypass is technically a reversible procedure; however, it is generally only reversed in extreme circumstances.

The **laparoscopic adjustable gastric band** is an inflatable device that is placed around the fundus of the stomach to create a small pouch. This procedure is associated with 15–20% total body weight loss at 1 year. Laparoscopic adjustable gastric band is reversible and less invasive than the other two procedures, but it is associated with more complications and less weight loss than sleeve gastrectomy and Roux-en-Y gastric bypass. As a result, the band only accounts for 1% of bariatric procedures performed in the United States, and many bands are ultimately removed due to complications.

Patients who cannot achieve clinically meaningful weight loss with antiobesity medications and who do not undergo bariatric surgery fall into a "treatment gap." Several **devices and endoscopic procedures** are available that are reversible, minimally invasive, and potentially more effective than antiobesity medications. In addition, they may be less expensive and safer than bariatric surgery for poor surgical candidates. The five FDA-approved devices include two intragastric balloons (Orbera and Obalon), the AspireAssist aspiration device, superabsorbent hydrogel capsules (Plenity), and the TransPyloric Shuttle device. The endoscopic sleeve gastroplasty is a newer option that has gained popularity. It uses an endoscopic suturing device to reduce the cavity of the stomach, mimicking the surgical sleeve gastrectomy without the need for surgical resection.

When to Refer

- Patients with a BMI greater than or equal to 30 or a BMI greater than or equal to 27 with weight-related comorbidities may be referred to an obesity medicine specialist.
- Patients with a BMI greater than or equal to 40 (or greater than or equal to 35 with obesity-related morbidities) who have not achieved sufficient weight loss to address health goals following behavioral treatment, with or without pharmacotherapy, may be referred to a bariatric surgeon.

Arterburn DE et al. Benefits and risks of bariatric surgery in adults: a review. JAMA. 2020;324:879. [PMID: 32870301]
Bray GA et al. Evidence-based weight loss interventions: individualized treatment options to maximize patient outcomes. Diabetes Obes Metab. 2021;23(Suppl 1):50. [PMID: 32969147]
Carlsson LMS et al. Life expectancy after bariatric surgery in the Swedish Obese Subjects study. N Engl J Med. 2020;383:1535. [PMID: 33053284]
Doumouras AG et al. Association between bariatric surgery and all-cause mortality: a population-based matched cohort study in a universal health care system. Ann Intern Med. 2020;173:694. [PMID: 32805135]
Grönroos S et al. Effect of laparoscopic sleeve gastrectomy vs Roux-en-Y gastric bypass on weight loss and quality of life at 7 years in patients with morbid obesity: the SLEEVEPASS randomized clinical trial. JAMA Surg. 2021;156:137. [PMID: 33295955]
Tchang BG, Saunders KH, Igel LI. Best practices in the management of overweight and obesity. Med Clin North Am. 2021;105:149. [PMID: 33246516]

EATING DISORDERS

ANOREXIA NERVOSA

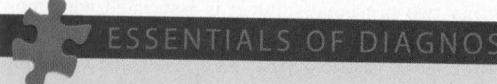

- Restriction of calorie intake leading to underweight BMI (BMI < 18.5).
- Intense fear of gaining weight or behavior that prevents weight gain.
- Distorted perception of body image, with undue influence of weight on self-worth.
- Denial of the medical seriousness of underweight status.

General Considerations

Anorexia nervosa is characterized by underweight BMI, intense fear of gaining weight, and distorted perception of body image. Anorexia nervosa typically begins in the years between adolescence and young adulthood. Ninety percent of patients are female, most of middle and upper socioeconomic status.

The prevalence of anorexia nervosa is greater than previously suggested since prior diagnostic criteria were more restrictive and individuals with anorexia often conceal their illness. Many adolescents have mild versions of the disorder without severe weight loss. The American Psychiatric Association's *Diagnostic and Statistical Manual of Mental Disorders*, fifth edition (*DSM-5*) classifies the severity of anorexia according to BMI: mild, BMI 17–18.49; moderate, BMI 16–16.99; severe, BMI 15–15.99; extreme, BMI less than 15.

There are two subtypes of anorexia nervosa: binge-eating/purging type and restricting type. The binge-eating/purging subtype is characterized by recurrent episodes of binge-eating or purging (ie, self-induced vomiting and/or abuse of diuretics, laxatives, enemas, cathartics). The restricting subtype is characterized by dieting, fasting, or excessive exercising without associated binge-eating or purging.

The cause of anorexia nervosa is not known. Although multiple endocrinologic abnormalities exist in patients with anorexia nervosa, most authorities believe they are secondary to malnutrition and not the primary disorder. Most experts favor a primary psychiatric origin, but no hypothesis explains all cases. The patient characteristically comes from a family whose members are highly goal-oriented. Patients are often perfectionistic in behavior and exhibit obsessional personality characteristics. Obsessional preoccupation with food is also common.

Clinical Findings

A. Symptoms and Signs

Patients with anorexia nervosa may exhibit severe emaciation and frequently complain of cold intolerance or constipation. Bradycardia, hypotension, and hypothermia may be present in severe cases. Examination demonstrates loss of body fat, dry and scaly skin, and increased lanugo body hair. Parotid enlargement and edema may also occur. In females of reproductive age, cessation of menstruation is common.

B. Laboratory Findings

Laboratory findings are variable but may include anemia, leukopenia, electrolyte abnormalities, and elevations of BUN and serum creatinine. Serum cholesterol levels are often increased. Endocrine abnormalities include depressed levels of LH and FSH and impaired response of LH to gonadotropin-releasing hormone.

Diagnosis & Differential Diagnosis

The diagnosis is based on weight loss to a BMI less than 18.5, distorted body image, and fear of weight gain or of loss of control over food intake. Other medical or psychiatric illnesses that can account for anorexia and weight loss must be excluded.

Behavioral features required for the diagnosis include intense fear of gaining weight, disturbance of body image, and refusal to exceed a minimal normal weight.

The differential diagnosis includes bulimia nervosa, binge-eating disorder, endocrine and metabolic disorders (eg, panhypopituitarism, Addison disease, hyperthyroidism, and diabetes mellitus), GI disorders (eg, Crohn disease and gluten enteropathy), chronic infections (eg, tuberculosis), cancers (eg, lymphoma), and rare CNS disorders (eg, hypothalamic tumor).

Treatment

The goal of treatment is restoration of normal body weight and improvement in psychological comorbidities. Hospitalization may be necessary. Treatment programs conducted by experienced teams successfully restore normal weight in approximately two-thirds of cases. The remainder continue to experience difficulties with underweight, eating behaviors, and associated psychiatric conditions. Two to 6% of patients die of the complications of the disorder or commit suicide.

Various treatment methods have been used without clear evidence of superiority of one over another. Supportive care by clinicians and family is the most important feature of any therapy. Cognitive-behavioral therapy, intensive psychotherapy, and family therapy may be tried. A variety of medications including tricyclic antidepressants, SSRIs, and lithium carbonate are effective in some cases; however, clinical trial results have been disappointing. Patients with severe malnutrition must be hemodynamically stabilized and may require enteral or parenteral feeding. Forced feedings should be reserved for life-threatening situations, since the goal of treatment is to reestablish normal eating behavior.

When to Refer

- Adolescents and young adults with otherwise unexplained profound weight loss should be evaluated by a psychiatrist or eating disorders specialist.
- All patients with diagnosed anorexia nervosa should be co-managed with a psychiatrist or eating disorders specialist.

When to Admit

- Signs of hypovolemia, major electrolyte disorders, and severe protein–energy malnutrition.
- Failure to improve with outpatient management.

Jansingh A et al. Developments in the psychological treatment of anorexia nervosa and their implications for daily practice. Curr Opin Psychiatry. 2020;33:534. [PMID: 32796187]

Muratore AF et al. Current therapeutic approaches to anorexia nervosa: state of the art. Clin Ther. 2021;43:85. [PMID: 33293054]

Voderholzer U et al. Medical management of eating disorders: an update. Curr Opin Psychiatry. 2020;33:542. [PMID: 32925184]

BULIMIA NERVOSA

ESSENTIALS OF DIAGNOSIS

- Uncontrolled episodes of binge-eating at least once weekly for 3 months.
- Recurrent inappropriate compensatory behavior to prevent weight gain such as self-induced vomiting, laxatives, diuretics, fasting, or excessive exercise.
- Excessive concern with body weight and body shape, with undue influence of weight on self-worth.

General Considerations

Bulimia nervosa is the episodic uncontrolled ingestion of large quantities of food followed by recurrent inappropriate compensatory behavior to prevent weight gain, such as self-induced vomiting, diuretic or cathartic use, strict dieting, or vigorous exercise.

Like anorexia nervosa, bulimia nervosa is predominantly a disorder of young, White, middle- and upper-class women. It is more difficult to detect than anorexia, and some studies have estimated that the prevalence may be as high as 19% in college-aged women.

Clinical Findings

Patients with bulimia nervosa typically consume large quantities of easily ingested high-calorie foods, usually in secrecy. Some patients may have several such episodes per day over multiple days; others report regular and persistent patterns of binge-eating. Binging is usually followed by vomiting, cathartics, or diuretics and accompanied by feelings of guilt or depression. Periods of binging may be followed by intervals of self-imposed starvation. Body weight may fluctuate but generally remains within 20% of normal BMI.

Family and psychological conditions are generally similar to those of patients with anorexia nervosa. Patients with bulimia, however, have a higher incidence of obesity, greater use of cathartics and diuretics, and more impulsive or antisocial behavior. Menstruation is typically preserved.

Medical complications are numerous. Gastric dilatation and pancreatitis have been reported after binges. Vomiting can result in poor dentition, pharyngitis, esophagitis, aspiration, and electrolyte abnormalities. Cathartic and diuretic abuse can also cause electrolyte abnormalities or dehydration. Constipation is common.

Treatment

Treatment of bulimia nervosa requires supportive care and psychotherapy. Individual, group, family, and behavioral therapy have all been utilized. Antidepressant medications may be helpful. The best results have been with fluoxetine and other SSRIs. Although death from bulimia is rare, the long-term psychiatric prognosis in severe bulimia is worse than that in anorexia nervosa.

When to Refer

All patients with diagnosed bulimia should be co-managed with a psychiatrist or eating disorders specialist.

Hagan KE et al State of the art: the therapeutic approaches to bulimia nervosa. Clin Ther. 2021;43:40. [PMID: 33358256]

Himmerich H et al. Pharmacological treatment of eating disorders, comorbid mental health problems, malnutrition and physical health consequences. Pharmacol Ther. 2021;217:107667. [PMID: 32858054]

Nitsch A et al. Medical complications of bulimia nervosa. Cleve Clin J Med. 2021;88:333. [PMID: 34078617]

Treasure J et al. Eating disorders. Lancet. 2020;395:899. [PMID: 32171414]

DISORDERS OF VITAMIN METABOLISM

THIAMINE (B_1) DEFICIENCY

Most thiamine deficiency in the United States is due to alcohol use disorder, with poor dietary intake of thiamine and impaired thiamine absorption, metabolism, and storage.

It is also associated with malabsorption (eg, following bariatric surgery), dialysis, and other causes of chronic protein–calorie undernutrition. Thiamine depletion can be precipitated when patients with low thiamine are given a large carbohydrate load, such as an intravenous dextrose infusion.

Clinical Findings

Early manifestations of thiamine deficiency include anorexia, muscle cramps, paresthesia, and irritability. Advanced deficiency primarily affects the cardiovascular system ("wet beriberi") or the nervous system ("dry beriberi"). Wet beriberi occurs in thiamine deficiency accompanied by severe physical exertion and high carbohydrate intake. Dry beriberi occurs in thiamine deficiency accompanied by inactivity and low-calorie intake.

Wet beriberi is characterized by marked peripheral vasodilation resulting in high-output heart failure with dyspnea, tachycardia, cardiomegaly, pulmonary edema, and peripheral edema with warm extremities mimicking cellulitis.

Dry beriberi involves both the peripheral and the CNS. Peripheral nerve involvement is typically a symmetric motor and sensory neuropathy with pain, paresthesia, and loss of reflexes. Legs are affected more than arms. CNS involvement results in Wernicke-Korsakoff syndrome. Wernicke encephalopathy consists of nystagmus progressing to ophthalmoplegia, truncal ataxia, and confusion. Korsakoff syndrome includes amnesia, confabulation, and impaired learning.

Diagnosis

In most instances, the clinical response to empiric thiamine therapy is used to support a diagnosis of thiamine deficiency. The most commonly used biochemical tests measure thiamine concentration directly, while other assays measure erythrocyte transketolase activity and urinary thiamine excretion. Normal thiamine values typically range from 70 nmol/L to 180 nmol/L.

Treatment

Thiamine deficiency is treated with large parenteral doses of thiamine. Fifty to 100 mg/day is initially administered intravenously, followed by daily oral doses of 5–10 mg/day. All patients should simultaneously receive therapeutic doses of other water-soluble vitamins. Treatment results in complete resolution in one-fourth of patients immediately and another one-fourth over days, but half have only partial or no benefit.

When to Refer

Patients with signs of dry beriberi or Wernicke-Korsakoff syndrome should be referred to a neurologist. Patients with signs of wet beriberi should be referred to a cardiologist.

THIAMINE TOXICITY

There is no known toxicity of thiamine.

Smith TJ et al. Thiamine deficiency disorders: a clinical perspective. Ann N Y Acad Sci. 2021;1498:9. [PMID: 33305487]

RIBOFLAVIN (B_2) DEFICIENCY

Clinical Findings

Riboflavin deficiency usually occurs in combination with other vitamin deficiencies. Dietary inadequacy, interactions with medications, alcohol use disorder, and other causes of protein–calorie undernutrition are the most common causes.

Manifestations of riboflavin deficiency include cheilosis, angular stomatitis, glossitis, seborrheic dermatitis, weakness, corneal vascularization, and anemia.

Diagnosis

Riboflavin deficiency can be confirmed by measuring the riboflavin-dependent enzyme erythrocyte glutathione reductase. Urinary riboflavin excretion and serum levels of plasma and red cell flavins can also be measured.

Treatment

When suspected, riboflavin deficiency is usually treated empirically with foods such as meat, fish, and dairy products or with oral preparations of the vitamin. Administration of 5–15 mg/day until clinical findings resolve is usually adequate. Riboflavin can also be given parenterally.

RIBOFLAVIN TOXICITY

There is no known toxicity of riboflavin.

NIACIN DEFICIENCY

"Niacin" is a generic term for nicotinic acid and other derivatives with similar nutritional activity. Unlike most other vitamins, niacin can be synthesized from the amino acid tryptophan. Niacin is an essential component of the coenzymes nicotinamide adenine dinucleotide (NAD) and nicotinamide adenine dinucleotide phosphate (NADP), which are involved in many oxidation-reduction reactions. The major food sources of niacin are proteins containing tryptophan and numerous cereals, vegetables, and dairy products.

Historically, niacin deficiency occurred when corn, which is relatively deficient in both tryptophan and niacin, was the major source of calories. Niacin deficiency is more commonly due to alcohol use disorder and nutrient–drug interactions. Niacin deficiency can also occur in inborn errors of metabolism. Niacin in the form of nicotinic acid is used therapeutically for the treatment of hypercholesterolemia and hypertriglyceridemia. Niacinamide (the form of niacin generally used to treat niacin deficiency) does not exhibit the lipid-lowering effects of nicotinic acid.

Clinical Findings

As with other B vitamins, early manifestations of niacin deficiency are nonspecific—anorexia, weakness, irritability, mouth soreness, glossitis, stomatitis, and weight loss.

More advanced deficiency results in the classic triad of pellagra: dermatitis, diarrhea, and dementia. The dermatitis is symmetric, involving sun-exposed areas. Skin lesions are dark, dry, and scaly. The dementia begins with insomnia, irritability, and apathy and progresses to confusion, memory loss, hallucinations, and psychosis. The diarrhea can be severe and may result in malabsorption due to atrophy of the intestinal villi. Advanced pellagra can result in death.

Diagnosis

In early deficiency, diagnosis requires a high index of suspicion. Low levels may be found in patients with generalized undernutrition. In advanced cases, the diagnosis of pellagra can be made clinically. Niacin can be measured in serum or plasma.

Treatment

Niacin deficiency can be effectively treated with oral niacin, usually given as nicotinamide (10–150 mg/day).

NIACIN TOXICITY

At the high doses of niacin used to treat hyperlipidemia, side effects are common. These include cutaneous flushing (partially prevented by pretreatment with aspirin, 81–325 mg/day, and use of ER nicotinic acid preparations) and gastric irritation. Elevation of liver enzymes, hyperglycemia, and gout are less common side effects.

Handelsman Y et al. Consensus statement by the American Association of Clinical Endocrinologists and American College of Endocrinology on the management of dyslipidemia and prevention of cardiovascular disease algorithm—2020 executive summary. Endocr Pract. 2020;26:1196. [PMID: 33471721]

Simha V. Management of hypertriglyceridemia. BMJ. 2020; 371:m3109. [PMID: 33046451]

VITAMIN B_6 DEFICIENCY

Vitamin B_6 deficiency most commonly occurs as a result of alcohol use disorder or interactions with medications, especially isoniazid, and oral contraceptives. A number of inborn errors of metabolism and other pyridoxine-responsive syndromes, particularly pyridoxine-responsive anemia, are not clearly due to vitamin deficiency but commonly respond to high doses of the vitamin. Patients with common variable immunodeficiency may have concomitant vitamin B_6 deficiency.

Clinical Findings

Vitamin B_6 deficiency results in clinical symptoms similar to those of other B vitamin deficiencies, including mouth soreness, glossitis, cheilosis, weakness, and irritability. Severe deficiency can result in peripheral neuropathy, anemia, and seizures.

Diagnosis

The diagnosis of vitamin B_6 deficiency can be confirmed by measurement of pyridoxal phosphate in blood.

Treatment

Vitamin B_6 deficiency can be treated effectively with vitamin B_6 supplements (10–20 mg/day orally). Some patients taking medications that interfere with pyridoxine metabolism (such as isoniazid) may need doses as high as 50–100 mg/day orally to prevent vitamin B_6 deficiency. This is true for patients who are more likely to have diets marginally adequate in vitamin B_6, such as older patients and patients with alcohol use disorder. Inborn errors of metabolism and pyridoxine-responsive syndromes often require doses up to 600 mg/day orally.

VITAMIN B_6 TOXICITY

A sensory neuropathy, at times irreversible, can occur in patients receiving large doses of vitamin B_6 (200–2000 mg/day).

VITAMIN B_{12} & FOLATE

Vitamin B_{12} (cobalamin) and folate are reviewed in Chapter 13.

VITAMIN C (Ascorbic Acid) DEFICIENCY

Most cases of vitamin C deficiency in the United States are due to dietary inadequacy in older patients and patients with alcohol use disorder. Patients with chronic illnesses such as cancer and CKD and individuals who smoke cigarettes are also at risk.

Clinical Findings

Early manifestations of vitamin C deficiency are nonspecific and include malaise and weakness. In more advanced stages, the typical features of scurvy develop. Manifestations include perifollicular hemorrhages, perifollicular hyperkeratotic papules, petechiae, purpura, splinter hemorrhages, bleeding gums, hemarthroses, and subperiosteal hemorrhages. Anemia is common, and wound healing is impaired. The late stages of scurvy are characterized by edema, oliguria, neuropathy, intracerebral hemorrhage, and death.

Diagnosis

The diagnosis of advanced scurvy can be made clinically based on skin lesions in the proper clinical setting. Atraumatic hemarthrosis is also highly suggestive. The diagnosis can be confirmed with decreased plasma ascorbic acid levels, typically below 0.2 mg/dL.

Treatment

Adult scurvy can be treated with ascorbic acid 300–1000 mg/day orally. Improvement generally occurs within days.

VITAMIN C TOXICITY

Very large doses of vitamin C can cause gastric irritation, flatulence, or diarrhea. Oxalate kidney stones are of theoretical concern because ascorbic acid is metabolized to oxalate, but stone formation has not been frequently reported. Vitamin C can also confound common diagnostic tests by causing false-negative results for some fecal occult blood tests and both false-negative and false-positive results for urine glucose.

VITAMIN A DEFICIENCY

Clinical Findings

Vitamin A deficiency is one of the most common vitamin deficiency syndromes, particularly in developing countries. In certain regions, it is the most common cause of blindness. In the United States, it is usually due to fat malabsorption syndromes or mineral oil laxative abuse and occurs most commonly in older adults and patients with malabsorptive conditions.

Night blindness is the earliest symptom. Dryness of the conjunctiva (xerosis) and the development of small white patches on the conjunctiva (Bitot spots) are early signs. Ulceration and necrosis of the cornea (keratomalacia), perforation, endophthalmitis, and blindness are late manifestations. Xerosis and hyperkeratinization of the skin and loss of taste may also occur.

Diagnosis

Abnormalities of dark adaptation are strongly suggestive of vitamin A deficiency. Serum levels below the normal range of 30–65 mg/dL are commonly seen in advanced deficiency.

Treatment

Night blindness, poor wound healing, and other signs of deficiency can be effectively treated with vitamin A 30,000 IU orally daily for 1 week.

VITAMIN A TOXICITY

Excess intake of beta-carotene (hypercarotenosis) results in staining of the skin a yellow-orange color but is otherwise benign. Skin changes are most marked on the palms and soles, while scleras remain white, clearly distinguishing hypercarotenosis from jaundice.

Excessive vitamin A (hypervitaminosis A), on the other hand, can be quite toxic. Chronic toxicity usually occurs after ingestion of daily doses of over 50,000 IU/day for more than 3 months. Early manifestations include dry, scaly skin, hair loss, mouth sores, painful hyperostosis, anorexia, and vomiting. More serious findings include hypercalcemia; increased intracranial pressure with papilledema, headaches, and decreased cognition; and hepatomegaly, which can progress to cirrhosis. Acute toxicity can result from ingestion of excessive doses of vitamin A via medications or supplements. Manifestations include nausea, vomiting, abdominal pain, headache, papilledema, and lethargy.

The diagnosis can be confirmed by elevations of serum vitamin A levels. The only treatment is withdrawal of vitamin A from the diet. Most symptoms and signs improve rapidly.

Carazo A et al. Vitamin A update: forms, sources, kinetics, detection, function, deficiency, therapeutic use and toxicity. Nutrients. 2021;13:1703. [PMID: 34069881]

VITAMIN D

Vitamin D is reviewed in Chapter 26.

VITAMIN E DEFICIENCY

Clinical Findings

Clinical deficiency of vitamin E is most commonly due to severe malabsorption or abetalipoproteinemia in adults and chronic cholestatic liver disease, biliary atresia, or cystic fibrosis in children. Manifestations of deficiency include areflexia, disturbances of gait, decreased vibration and proprioception, and ophthalmoplegia.

Diagnosis

Plasma vitamin E levels can be measured; normal levels are 0.5–0.7 mg/dL or higher. Since vitamin E is normally transported in lipoproteins, the serum level should be interpreted in relation to circulating lipid levels.

Treatment

The optimal therapeutic dose of vitamin E has not been defined. Large doses, often administered parenterally, can be used to improve the neurologic complications seen in abetalipoproteinemia and cholestatic liver disease. Vitamin E supplementation may also provide benefit in patients with nonalcoholic fatty liver disease.

VITAMIN E TOXICITY

Clinical trials have suggested an increase in all-cause mortality with high dose (greater than 400 IU/day) vitamin E supplements. Large doses of vitamin E can also increase the vitamin K requirement and result in bleeding in patients taking oral anticoagulants.

Sherf-Dagan S et al. Vitamin E status among bariatric surgery patients: a systematic review. Surg Obes Relat Dis. 2021;17:816. [PMID: 33323330]

VITAMIN K

Vitamin K is reviewed in Chapter 14.

DIET THERAPY

Specific therapeutic diets can complement the medical management of most common illnesses. Dietary modifications can be difficult to sustain, and patients may benefit from the support of a registered dietitian or other provider who can offer guidance. Eliciting a food recall is a helpful strategy to provide insight into a patient's dietary preferences and restrictions and provides information about nutrient content in the current diet. Ongoing food tracking can improve dietary adherence and there are many online programs and applications that facilitate this activity.

Therapeutic diets can be divided into three groups: (1) diets that alter food consistency, (2) diets that restrict or modify dietary components, and (3) diets that supplement dietary components.

DIETS THAT ALTER CONSISTENCY

Clear Liquid Diet

This diet provides adequate water, 500–1000 kcal as simple sugar, and some electrolytes. It is fiber-free and requires minimal digestion or intestinal motility.

A clear liquid diet is useful for patients with resolving postoperative ileus, acute gastroenteritis, partial intestinal obstruction, and in preparation for diagnostic GI procedures. It is commonly used as the first diet for patients who have been taking nothing by mouth for a long period. Because of the low calorie and minimal protein content of the clear liquid diet, it is used only for short durations.

Full Liquid Diet

The full liquid diet provides adequate water and can be designed to provide sufficient calories and protein. Vitamins and minerals—especially folic acid, iron, and vitamin B_6—may be inadequate and should be provided in the form of supplements. Dairy products, protein shakes, and soups are used to supplement clear liquids. Commercial oral supplements can also be incorporated into the diet or used alone.

This diet is low in residue and can be used in patients with difficulty chewing or swallowing, with partial obstructions, or in preparation for certain diagnostic procedures. Full liquid diets are commonly used following clear liquid diets in patients who have been taking nothing by mouth for a long period.

Soft Diets

Soft diets are designed for patients unable to chew or swallow hard food. Easily masticated foods are used, and most raw fruits and vegetables, coarse breads, and cereals are eliminated. Soft diets are commonly used to assist in progression from full liquid diets to regular diets in postoperative patients, patients who are too weak or those whose dentition is too poor for a regular diet, head and neck surgical patients, and patients with esophageal strictures. The soft diet can be designed to meet all nutritional requirements.

DIETS THAT RESTRICT NUTRIENTS

Diets can be designed to restrict (or eliminate) virtually any nutrient or food component. The most commonly used restricted diets are those that limit sodium, fat, carbohydrate, and protein. Other restrictive diets include gluten restriction in gluten enteropathy, potassium and phosphate reduction in CKD, and elimination of certain allergens for food allergies.

Sodium-Restricted Diets

Low-sodium diets can be useful in the management of hypertension and in conditions in which sodium retention and edema are prominent features, particularly heart failure, chronic liver disease, and CKD. Sodium restriction may be beneficial with or without diuretic therapy. When used in conjunction with diuretics, sodium restriction may allow lower dosages of diuretic medications and may prevent side effects. For example, sodium restriction decreases diuretic-related potassium losses by reducing distal tubule sodium delivery.

Typical American diets contain 4–6 g (175–260 mEq) of sodium per day. A no-added-salt diet contains approximately 3 g (132 mEq) of sodium per day. Further restriction can be achieved with diets of 2 or 1 g of sodium per day. Diets with more severe restriction are difficult to adhere to and are rarely used. National Academies of Sciences, Engineering, and Medicine guidelines recommend 2.3 g of sodium per day (approximately 1 teaspoon of salt).

Dietary sodium includes sodium naturally occurring in foods, sodium added during food processing, and sodium added during cooking and at the table. Approximately 80% of dietary intake in American diets is from processed and pre-prepared foods. Diets designed for 2.3 g of sodium per day require elimination of most processed foods, added salt, and foods with high sodium content. Many patients with mild hypertension will achieve significant reductions in blood pressure (approximately 5 mm Hg diastolic) with this degree of sodium restriction.

Diets allowing 1 g of sodium require further restriction of commonly consumed foods. Special "low-sodium" products are available to facilitate such diets. These diets are difficult for most people to follow and are generally reserved for hospitalized patients, most commonly those with heart failure, CKD, or severe liver disease and ascites.

Fat-Restricted Diets & Low–Saturated Fat Diets

Traditional fat-restricted diets are useful in the treatment of fat malabsorption syndromes. Such diets will improve the symptoms of diarrhea with steatorrhea independent of the primary physiologic abnormality by limiting the quantity of fatty acids that reach the colon. The degree of fat restriction necessary to control symptoms must be individualized. Patients with severe malabsorption can be limited to 40–60 g of fat per day. Diets containing 60–80 g of fat per day can be designed for patients with less severe abnormalities.

Fat-restricted diets that specifically restrict saturated fats are the mainstay of dietary treatment of hyperlipidemia with elevated LDL cholesterol (see Chapter 28). Similar diets are often recommended for the prevention of CAD (see Chapter 10). The large Women's Health Initiative Dietary Modification Trial, however, did not show significant benefit of a low-fat diet on weight control or prevention of CVD or cancer. In contrast, a study of Mediterranean diets, supplemented by nuts or extra-virgin olive oil, demonstrated a reduction in cardiovascular events. Plant-based diets, defined by low frequency of animal food consumption, have been increasingly recommended for their health benefits. Numerous studies have found diets enriched with high-quality plant foods, such as whole grains, fruits, vegetables, and nuts, to be associated with lower risk of cardiovascular end points.

The aim of low-fat diets is to restrict total fat to less than 30% of calories and saturated fat to 7% of calories. More extreme restriction offers little further advantage in modification of serum lipids. Low-fat diets can be augmented with the addition of plant stanols and sterols and with soluble dietary fiber to further reduce serum lipids.

Carbohydrate-Restricted Diets

Low-carbohydrate diets restrict carbohydrate intake to at most 50–100 g/day. Consumption of foods that contain higher protein and fat with lower carbohydrate content has been shown to promote satiety. Carbohydrate-restricted diets, including low-glycemic-index diets (see Chapter 27), can be helpful for patients with type 2 diabetes and other forms of insulin resistance to reduce both blood sugar and weight. Several studies investigating the efficacy of low-fat versus low-carbohydrate diets for weight loss show no clear benefit of one versus the other.

Protein-Restricted Diets

Protein-restricted diets are most commonly used in patients with hepatic encephalopathy due to chronic liver disease and in patients with advanced CKD in order to slow the progression of early disease and to decrease symptoms of uremia in more severe disease.

Protein restriction is intended to limit the production of nitrogenous waste products. Energy intake must be adequate to facilitate the efficient use of dietary protein. A sufficient quantity of proteins (at least 0.6 g/kg/day in most patients) must be provided to meet minimal requirements. Patients with encephalopathy who do not respond to this degree of restriction are unlikely to respond to more severe restriction.

DIETS THAT SUPPLEMENT NUTRIENTS

High-Fiber Diets

Dietary fiber is a diverse group of plant constituents that is resistant to digestion by the human digestive tract. Guidelines suggest that adult men should eat 30–38 g of fiber per day and adult women 21–25 g/day. Typical US diets, however, contain about half of that amount. Epidemiologic evidence suggests that populations consuming greater quantities of fiber have a lower incidence of certain GI disorders, including diverticulitis and, in some studies, colon cancer as well as a lower risk of CVD. A meta-analysis of 22 studies suggested that each 7 g of dietary fiber was associated with a 9% decrease in first cardiovascular event.

Diets high in dietary fiber (21–38 g/day) are commonly used in the management of a variety of GI disorders such as irritable bowel syndrome and recurrent diverticulitis. Diets high in fiber, particularly soluble fiber, may also be useful to reduce blood sugar in patients with diabetes and to reduce cholesterol levels in patients with hypercholesterolemia. Good sources of soluble fiber are oats, nuts, seeds, legumes, and most fruits. Foods with insoluble fiber include whole wheat, brown rice, other whole grains, and most vegetables. For some patients, the addition of psyllium or methylcellulose may be a useful adjunct to increase dietary fiber.

High-Potassium Diets

Potassium-supplemented diets are used most commonly to compensate for potassium losses caused by diuretics. Although potassium losses can be partially prevented by using lower doses of diuretics, concurrent sodium restriction, and potassium-sparing diuretics, some patients require additional potassium to prevent hypokalemia. High-potassium diets may also have a direct antihypertensive effect. Typical American diets contain about 3 g (80 mEq) of potassium per day. High-potassium diets commonly contain 4.5–7 g (120–180 mEq) of potassium per day.

Most fruits, vegetables, and their juices contain high concentrations of potassium. Supplemental potassium can also be provided with potassium-containing salt substitutes or as potassium chloride in solution, capsules, or effervescent tablets.

High-Calcium Diets

Adequate intake of dietary calcium has been recommended for the prevention of postmenopausal osteoporosis, the prevention and treatment of hypertension, and the prevention of colon cancer. The Women's Health Initiative, however, suggested that calcium and vitamin D supplementation did not prevent fractures or colon cancer. Observational studies have also suggested that calcium supplements, especially when taken without vitamin D, may be associated with an increased risk of CHD. The recommended dietary allowance for the total calcium intake (from food and supplements) in adults ranges from 1000 mg/day to 1200 mg/day. Average American daily intakes are approximately 700 mg/day.

Dairy products are the primary dietary sources of calcium in the United States. An 8-ounce glass of milk, for example, contains approximately 300 mg of calcium. Patients with lactose intolerance who cannot tolerate liquid dairy products may be able to drink lactose-free milk, take supplemental lactase enzyme supplements, or tolerate nonliquid products such as yogurt and aged cheeses. Leafy green vegetables also contain high concentrations of calcium.

Chawla S et al. The effect of low-fat and low-carbohydrate diets on weight loss and lipid levels: a systematic review and meta-analysis. Nutrients. 2020;12:3774. [PMID: 33317019]

Papadaki A et al. The effect of the Mediterranean diet on metabolic health: a systematic review and meta-analysis of controlled trials in adults. Nutrients. 2020;12:3342. [PMID: 33143083]

Zhubi-Bakija F et al. The impact of type of dietary protein, animal versus vegetable, in modifying cardiometabolic risk factors: a position paper from the International Lipid Expert Panel (ILEP). Clin Nutr. 2021;40:255. [PMID: 32620446]

NUTRITIONAL SUPPORT

Jonathan A. Waitman, MD
Sarah Adler Fink, RD, CDN, CNSC

Nutritional support is the provision of nutrients to patients who cannot meet their nutritional requirements by intake of standard diets alone. Nutrients may be delivered enterally via oral nutrition supplements and feeding tubes, or parenterally using lines or catheters inserted directly into veins. Nutritional support techniques permit adequate nutrition delivery; however, their use should be considered only when likely to improve a patient's outcomes.

INDICATIONS FOR NUTRITIONAL SUPPORT

Nutritional support is indicated in patients who are malnourished or at risk of malnourishment. Common indications for enteral nutrition include dysphagia, mechanical ventilation preventing oral nutrition intake, the need to feed the gut distal to an obstruction or high-output fistula, and hypermetabolic disease states, such as burns and trauma. Parenteral nutrition is required when enteral nutrition is contraindicated, or when the GI tract has diminished function due to underlying conditions, including small bowel obstructions, paralytic ileus, short bowel syndrome, and fistulae. In most other conditions, it has been difficult to prove the efficacy of nutritional support over treatment without such support.

The ASPEN has published recommendations for the rational use of nutritional support. These emphasize the need to individualize the decision to begin nutritional support, weighing the risks, benefits, and costs. The guidelines also highlight the need to perform comprehensive nutrition assessments to identify patients who may benefit from aggressive nutrition interventions.

Nutritional Support Methods

Selection of the most appropriate nutritional support method involves consideration of GI function, the anticipated duration of nutritional support, and the ability of each method to meet the patient's nutritional requirements. The method chosen should meet the patient's nutritional needs with the lowest risk and cost. For most patients, enteral feeding is safer and less expensive and offers significant physiologic advantages. An algorithm for selection of the most appropriate nutritional support method is presented in Figure 29–1.

Prior to initiating specialized enteral nutritional support, efforts should be made to supplement food intake. Attention to patient food preferences, liberalizing diet orders, timing of meals in relation to diagnostic procedures and required medications, and the use of foods brought to the hospital by family and friends can often increase oral intake. Patients unable to eat enough at regular mealtimes to meet nutritional requirements can be given **oral supplements** as snacks or to replace low-calorie beverages. Oral supplements with different nutritional compositions are available to meet the specific needs of various clinical conditions. Formulations vary in fiber and lactose content, caloric density, protein level, and electrolyte concentrations.

Patients with functioning GI tracts who are unable to take adequate oral nutrition or safely swallow are appropriate for enteral nutritional support (tube feeding). Short-term enteral access devices can be placed into the nose or mouth and terminate in the stomach or small bowel. Examples are orogastric, nasogastric, nasoduodenal, and nasojejunal tubes. Bedside placement of short-term enteral access devices is typically successful; however, it may be difficult to achieve post-pyloric placement. Some patients will require fluoroscopic or endoscopic guidance to insert the feeding tube distal to the gastric pylorus. Correct feeding tube placement should always be confirmed radiographically prior to initiation of feeding. Long-term enteral access devices are placed directly into the stomach or small bowel, called tube enterostomies. Percutaneous gastrostomies, jejunostomies, and gastrojejunostomies can be placed by an endoscopist, interventional radiologist, or surgeon.

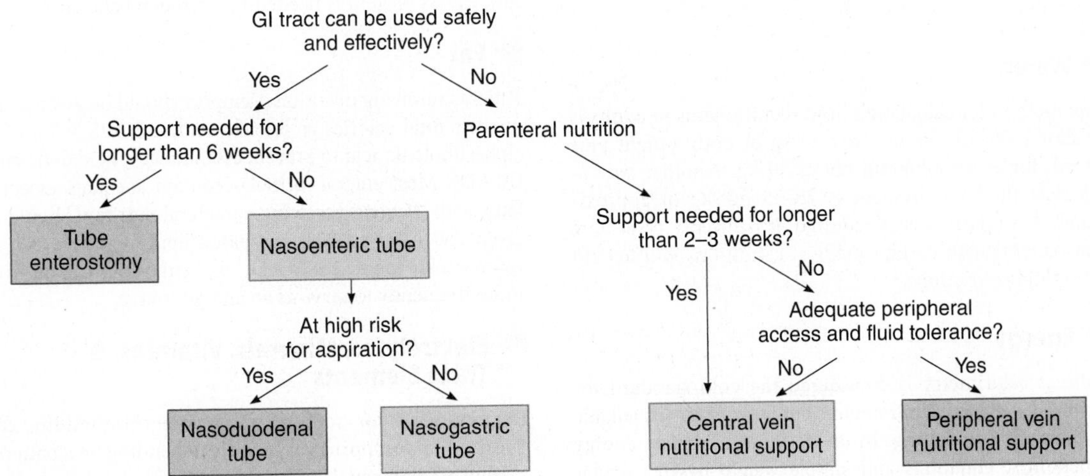

Figure 29–1. Nutritional support method decision tree.

When selecting the appropriate enteral access device, one should consider the anticipated duration of use and the patient anatomy, aspiration risk, and quality of life. Patients who are at increased risk of aspiration may benefit from small bowel feeding; however, this may not prevent aspiration, particularly if the pylorus is patulous. Patients fed via the stomach can receive bolus, intermittent or cycled, or continuous tube feeding. Patients fed via the small bowel require pump-assisted continuous or cycled tube feeding; bolus feeds are prohibited.

Patients who require nutritional support but whose GI tracts are impaired are candidates for **parenteral nutritional support**. The preferred site of parenteral nutrition delivery is via a central vein (most commonly the subclavian vein), but peripheral vein administration may be appropriate in some patients.

Central vein nutritional support is reserved for patients who are malnourished and require nutritional support for greater than 7 days. It is delivered via intravenous catheters placed percutaneously using aseptic technique. Proper placement in the superior vena cava is documented radiographically before the solution is infused. Catheters must be carefully maintained by experienced nursing personnel to prevent infection and other catheter-related complications.

Peripheral vein nutritional support is most commonly used in patients who are not malnourished and will require short-term parenteral nutritional support. Peripheral vein nutritional support is administered via standard intravenous lines. Serious adverse events are infrequent, but there is a high incidence of phlebitis, infiltration of intravenous lines, and volume overload.

NUTRITIONAL REQUIREMENTS

Prior to initiation of nutritional support, the patient's estimated nutritional requirements should be determined. In most situations, solutions of equal nutrient value can be designed for delivery via enteral and parenteral routes, but differences in absorption should be considered. A complete nutritional support solution must contain water, carbohydrates, amino acids, fat, electrolytes, vitamins, and minerals.

Water

One method for calculating fluid requirements in adults is to allot 1500 mL for the first 20 kg of body weight plus 20 mL for every kilogram above 20 kg. Another way to calculate fluid requirement is 25–35 mL/kg or approximately 1 mL/kcal energy required. It is important to note that patients with certain medical conditions will benefit from fluid restrictions.

Energy

Indirect calorimetry is considered the gold standard for estimating energy requirements, but it may not be available in every clinical setting. In its absence, predictive energy expenditure equations and simple weight-based calculations can be utilized.

The most widely used and validated predictive energy expenditure equations for healthy individuals include the Harris-Benedict Equation and Mifflin-St. Jeor Equation, which calculate RMR with the addition of stress and/or activity factors. The Penn State Equation is the recommended predictive equation for critically ill patients due to its superior accuracy. This formula calculates RMR combined with dynamic physiological variables such as maximum temperature in a 24-hour period and minute ventilation. Different versions of the equation exist for patients above 60 years in age or with BMI greater than 30. Actual body weight should be used for all predictive equations.

Energy requirements can also be estimated by multiplying actual body weight in kilograms by 25–35 kcal/kg/day. This method is simple and easy to use, but validation studies have shown an accuracy rate of less than 50%.

The above methods provide imprecise estimates of actual energy expenditure, especially for markedly underweight, overweight, and critically ill patients who are ideal candidates for indirect calorimetry. Studies using indirect calorimetry have demonstrated that as many as 30–40% of patients will have measured expenditures 10% above or below estimated values.

In standard diets and balanced nutritional support solutions, carbohydrates provide the greatest amount of energy compared to the other macronutrients; however, protein and fat are required in optimal amounts to provide the body energy and assist with other functions.

Protein

Protein and energy requirements are closely related. If adequate calories are provided, stable and non-stressed patients should receive 0.8–1.2 g/kg/day of protein. Patients under moderate to severe stress require at least 1.5 g/kg/day, although patients with trauma and burns may need closer to 2.5 g/kg/day. Actual weight should be used for normal and underweight patients while adjusted body weight is used for patients with obesity.

Patients who are receiving protein without adequate calories will catabolize protein for energy rather than utilizing it for protein synthesis. Thus, when energy intake is low, excess protein is needed for nitrogen balance.

Fat

Patients receiving nutritional support should be given 2–4% of their total calories as linoleic acid and 0.25–0.5% of as alpha-linolenic acid to prevent essential fatty acid deficiency (EFAD). Most enteral formulas contain adequate essential fatty acids. Patients receiving parenteral nutrition should be given 250 mL of a 20% soy-based lipid emulsion at least twice weekly to prevent EFAD. Lipid emulsions can be given more frequently to serve as an energy source.

Electrolytes, Minerals, Vitamins, & Trace Elements

Requirements for sodium, potassium, magnesium, calcium, and phosphorus vary widely depending on a patient's cardiovascular, renal, endocrine, and GI status as well as measurements of serum concentration.

Patients receiving enteral nutritional support should receive adequate vitamins and minerals according to recommended daily allowances. Most enteral formulations provide sufficient vitamins, minerals, electrolytes, and trace elements as long as adequate volumes are administered. Certain formulas, like those intended for patients with renal disease, have a lower electrolyte profile.

Patients receiving parenteral nutritional support typically require 1–2 mEq/kg/day of sodium and potassium; 10–15 mEq/day of calcium; 8–20 mEq/day of magnesium; and 20–40 mmol/day of phosphorus.

Parenteral formulations also contain the trace elements zinc, copper, manganese, selenium, and chromium. Patients with diarrhea may require additional zinc supplementation to replace fecal losses. Copper and manganese may be excluded from a parenteral formulation in patients with liver disease due to impaired excretion and risk for toxicity. It is important to note that trace element products do not contain iron, so patients on long-term parenteral nutrition may require additional iron supplementation.

Vitamins are provided daily in the parenteral nutrition solution. Injectable multivitamin products for use in adults contain vitamins A, D, E, K, B_1, B_2, B_6, B_{12}, niacinamide, dexpanthenol, biotin, folic acid, and ascorbic acid.

ENTERAL NUTRITIONAL SUPPORT SOLUTIONS

Patients who require enteral nutritional support in an acute care setting receive commercially prepared enteral formulas (Table 29–3). Most enteral formulations have been designed to provide adequate proportions of water, energy, protein, and micronutrients. Some formulas contain less free water for patients who require fluid restrictions. Modular products are also available to provide specific macronutrients (eg, protein, carbohydrate, and fat) to supplement commercially available formulas for patients with unique nutrition requirements.

Enteral formulas can generally be classified as standard (polymeric), peptide-based (elemental or semi-elemental) or disease-specific. The classification is generally based on the overall composition of the formula and its contained macronutrients. Most enteral formulas are lactose-free.

Standard polymeric formulas are generally isotonic, have moderate amounts of intact macronutrients and may contain fiber. Normal digestive and absorptive capacity are needed for the use of polymeric formulas. Isotonic formulas contain 1 kcal/mL, whereas concentrated formulas contain 1.2–2 kcal/mL. Standard polymeric formulas are well tolerated in most patients.

Semi-elemental and elemental formulas are designed for patients with impaired GI function who have demonstrated malabsorption and maldigestion with standard polymeric formulas. Elemental formulas contain free amino acids, whereas semi-elemental formulas contain partially hydrolyzed oligopeptides. Elemental formulas contain minimal amounts of fat, typically in the form of medium chain triglycerides, which can increase the risk of EFAD when used long term in patients. Elemental formulas are hypertonic and can result in severe diarrhea.

Table 29–3. Enteral formulations.

Standard products
Blenderized commercially prepared (eg, Compleat Regular, Compleat Modified[1], Liquid Hope, Real Food Blends, Kate Farms)
Intact protein, lactose-free, low-residue:
1 kcal/mL (eg, Isosource 1.0, Osmolite 1.0, Nutren 1.0[1])
1.5 kcal/mL (eg, Isosource 1.5, Osmolite 1.5, Nutren 1.5)
2 kcal/mL (eg, TwoCal HN, Nutren 2.0, Resource 2.0)
Intact protein, lactose-free, high-residue:
1 kcal/mL (eg, Jevity,[1] Nutren with fiber,[1] Fibersource HN)
"Disease-specific" products
Advanced CKD: with adjusted protein content, fluid concentration and electrolytes (eg, Nepro, Nepro with Carb Steady, Suplena with Carb Steady, Novosource Renal, Renalcal)
Type 2 diabetes: with lower carbohydrate content (eg, Glucerna 1.0, 1.2, or 1.5, Nutren Glytrol, Diabetisource AC)
Malabsorption: with partially or fully hydrolyzed nutrients (eg, Peptamen, Peptamen 1.5, Peptamen AF, Peptamen with Prebio, Peptamen Intense VHP, Tolerex, Vital 1.0 and 1.5, Vital AF 1.2, Vital High Protein, Vivonex T.E.N., Vivonex RTF, Vivonex Plus)
Respiratory failure: with > 50% calories from fat (eg, Pulmocare, Nutren Pulmonary, Oxepa)
Hepatic encephalopathy: with high amounts of branched-chain amino acids (eg, Nutri-Hep)
Wound healing: with high protein content (eg, Promote, Replete, Perative)
Modular products
Protein (eg, ProMod, ProStat Sugar Free, Beneprotein, Unjury)
Carbohydrate (eg, Polycose, SolCarb)
Fat (eg, MCT Oil, Microlipid)

[1]Isotonic.

Disease-specific enteral formulas have been designed for patients with diabetes, kidney disease, hepatic encephalopathy, and respiratory failure. However, they have not been shown to be superior to standard polymeric formulas for most patients.

When initiating enteral nutrition, a continuous pump-infusion is generally preferred. In critically ill patients, enteral nutrition is commonly started at 10–40 mL/hour and advanced to goal rate by 10–20 mL/hour every 8–12 hours. Stable non-critically ill patients can tolerate enteral nutrition at goal rate; however, this is not appropriate in patients at risk for refeeding syndrome who benefit from more conservative initiation and advancement. In patients with long-term enteral access devices, transitioning to bolus feeds or cycled/nocturnal feeds can improve quality of life.

COMPLICATIONS OF ENTERAL NUTRITIONAL SUPPORT

Enteral nutrition is the preferred feeding method in patients with functional GI tracts, however complications occur in 10–15%. Minor mechanical complications are common and include tube occlusion and dislodgment. Common GI complications include diarrhea, nausea, vomiting, and constipation. GI bleeding from feeding tube placement may occur but is less common. Diarrhea is the most common complication. Diarrhea may be caused by the formula itself (ie, intolerance to a hyperosmotic load or to a specific component in the formula), medications, infections, or related to a primary disease of the intestine. All possibilities should be considered before attributing diarrhea to the enteral nutrition.

One of the most serious complications of enteral nutritional support is the risk of aspiration. Aspiration is best prevented by identifying patients who are at risk and utilizing protocols to reduce risk that include elevating the head of bed to 30 degrees, checking gastric residual volumes every 4 hours, utilizing promotility agents, and placing post-pyloric feeding tubes, as appropriate.

Metabolic complications during enteral nutritional support are less likely to be caused by the enteral nutrition itself and more likely related to underlying conditions that predispose patients to metabolic alterations. The most common complications include refeeding syndrome, electrolyte derangements, hyperglycemia, and dehydration.

Berger MM. Nutrition and micronutrient therapy in critical illness should be individualized. JPEN J Parenter Enteral Nutr. 2020;44:1380. [PMID: 32829498]

PARENTERAL NUTRITIONAL SUPPORT SOLUTIONS

The parenteral nutrition formulation is a complex solution containing up to 40 different nutrients. The basic parenteral solution is composed of dextrose, amino acids, lipids, electrolytes, minerals, trace elements, vitamins, and water. Medications can also be added. Most commercial solutions contain the monohydrate form of dextrose that provides 3.4 kcal/g. Crystalline amino acids are used in parenteral nutrition formulations to provide protein and provide 4 kcal/g when oxidized. Lipid emulsions are available in 20% and 30% concentrations, which provide 2 kcal/mL and 3 kcal/mL respectively. The 30% concentration is approved only for compounding within a 3-in-1 admixture.

Parenteral nutrition administered via a central vein allows for administration of hyperosmolar solution (more than 1800 mOsm/L) and adequate nutrition delivery. The dextrose, amino acids, and electrolytes contribute to the osmotic load and can be given in higher concentrations as compared to peripheral parenteral nutrition. Lipid emulsions are isotonic and can be given via a central or peripheral vein.

Solutions with lower osmolarities (less than 900 mOsm/L) must be administrated via peripheral veins. Solutions for peripheral infusion usually contain 5–10% dextrose and 3% amino acids. These lower osmolarity solutions result in a high incidence of thrombophlebitis and line infiltration. These solutions may provide adequate protein for some patients, but inadequate total energy from dextrose, depending on volume limitations. Additional energy can be provided with lipid emulsions since these solutions are isotonic and well tolerated by peripheral veins.

Lipid emulsions can prevent EFAD and provide energy to patients on parenteral nutrition. There are four lipid emulsion products available for use in the United States. Two formulations are composed of long-chain triglycerides, derived from either 100% soybean oil, or 50% safflower oil and 50% soybean oil. The third formulation, Smoflipid, was created due to concerns about the high content of proinflammatory omega-6 polyunsaturated fatty acids in traditional lipid emulsions. Smoflipid is composed of 30% soybean oil, 30% medium-chain triglycerides, 25% olive oil, and 15% fish oil. The fourth emulsion, Clinolipid, is composed of 80% olive oil and 20% soybean oil. For all lipid emulsions, providers should follow manufacturer dosing recommendations to prevent complications associated with excessive fat administration or EFAD.

Parenteral nutrition solutions should be initiated at half of the estimated energy requirement, or approximately 100–150 g dextrose for the first 24 hours; they are increased daily as tolerated to prevent hyperglycemia and electrolyte abnormalities in patients at risk for refeeding syndrome. Amino acids and lipid emulsions can be started at target goals.

Alsharif DJ et al. Effect of supplemental parenteral nutrition versus enteral nutrition alone on clinical outcomes in critically ill adult patients: a systematic review and meta-analysis of randomized controlled trials. Nutrients. 2020;12:2968. [PMID: 32998412]

COMPLICATIONS OF PARENTERAL NUTRITIONAL SUPPORT

Parenteral nutrition is considered a high-risk nutrition therapy, which can result in mechanical, infectious, and metabolic complications, for which patients require close monitoring for prevention, detection, and treatment.

Catheter-related complications can occur during insertion or while the catheter is in place. Pneumothorax, arterial laceration, air emboli, and brachial plexus injury can occur during catheter placement. Radiographic imaging must be performed to confirm proper placement of central venous access prior to initiating parenteral nutrition. Additional catheter-related complications include thrombotic occlusions and non-thrombotic occlusions caused by drug-nutrient interactions, precipitates, and residue.

Catheter-related bloodstream infections are the most serious of all complications. Patients with indwelling central vein catheters in whom fever develops without an apparent source should have their lines removed or changed immediately, at which time the catheter tip should be cultured, and empiric antibiotics initiated. Quantitative tip cultures and blood cultures narrow antibiotic therapy. Catheter-related sepsis occurs in 2–3% of patients even if optimal efforts are made to prevent infection. "Central line bundles" are evidence-based practices designed to reduce the incidence of central line–associated infections.

Metabolic complications of central vein nutritional support include hyperglycemia, hypoglycemia, EFAD, hypertriglyceridemia, fluid and electrolyte abnormalities, hepatobiliary disorders, and metabolic bone disease. A skilled nutritional support clinician is needed to safely prescribe, monitor, and address potential parenteral nutrition–associated complications. Examples of metabolic complications and suggested solutions are outlined in Table 29–4.

Kaegi-Braun N et al. Evaluation of nutritional support and in-hospital mortality in patients with malnutrition. JAMA Netw Open. 2021;4:e2033433. [PMID: 33471118]

Table 29–4. Metabolic complications of parenteral nutritional support.

Complication	Common Causes	Possible Solutions
Hyperglycemia	Too rapid infusion of dextrose, "stress," corticosteroids	Decrease glucose infusion; insulin; replacement of dextrose with fat
Hyperosmolar nonketotic dehydration	Severe, undetected hyperglycemia	Insulin, hydration, potassium
Hyperchloremic metabolic acidosis	High chloride administration	Decrease chloride
Azotemia	Excessive protein administration	Decrease amino acid concentration
Hypophosphatemia, hypokalemia, hypomagnesemia	Extracellular to intracellular shifting with refeeding	Increase solution concentration and provide repletion outside of parenteral nutrition bag; do not advance dextrose further
Liver enzyme abnormalities	Lipid trapping in hepatocytes, fatty liver	Decrease dextrose and lipid to a more balanced solution, cycle parenteral nutrition
Acalculous cholecystitis	Biliary stasis	Encourage oral diet or tube feeding as able
Zinc deficiency	Diarrhea, small bowel fistulas	Increase concentration
Copper deficiency	Biliary fistulas	Increase concentration

Santacruz E et al. Infectious complications in home parenteral nutrition: a long-term study with peripherally inserted central catheters, tunneled catheters, and ports. Nutrition. 2019;58:89. [PMID: 30391696]

PATIENT MONITORING DURING NUTRITIONAL SUPPORT

Every patient receiving enteral or parenteral nutritional support should be monitored closely. Formal nutritional support teams composed of a physician, a nurse, a dietitian, and a pharmacist have been shown to decrease the rate of complications.

Patients should be monitored both for the adequacy of treatment and to prevent complications or detect them early when they occur. Because estimates of nutritional requirements are imprecise, frequent reassessment is necessary. Daily intakes should be recorded and compared with estimated requirements. Body weight, hydration status, and overall clinical status should be followed. Patients who do not appear to be responding as anticipated should have an indirect calorimetry study performed if possible and be evaluated for nitrogen balance by means of the following equation:

$$\text{Nitrogen balance} = \frac{\text{24-hour protein intake (g)}}{6.25} - \left(\text{24-hour urinary nitrogen (g)} + 4\right)$$

Patients who are receiving calorie prescriptions comparable to the results of the indirect calorimetry study and who have positive nitrogen balances can be continued on their current regimens, whereas patients not meeting their energy targets or who have negative nitrogen balances should receive moderate increases in calorie and protein, and then be reassessed. Monitoring for metabolic complications includes daily measurements of basic metabolic panels, magnesium, and phosphorus levels. Once the patient is stabilized on the goal nutritional support regimen, laboratory values can be checked 1–2 times per week. Patients on parenteral nutrition should receive weekly liver function tests and triglyceride levels. Vitamins and trace elements should be obtained every 3–6 months in patients receiving long-term nutritional support.

Hellerman Itzhaki M et al. Advances in medical nutrition therapy: parenteral nutrition. Nutrients. 2020;12:717. [PMID: 32182654]

Lambell KJ et al. Nutrition therapy in critical illness: a review of the literature for clinicians. Crit Care. 2020;24:35. [PMID: 32019607]

30 Common Problems in Infectious Diseases & Antimicrobial Therapy

Monica Fung, MD, MPH
Peter V. Chin-Hong, MD
B. Joseph Guglielmo, PharmD
Katherine Gruenberg, PharmD

COMMON PROBLEMS IN INFECTIOUS DISEASES

FEVER OF UNKNOWN ORIGIN (FUO)

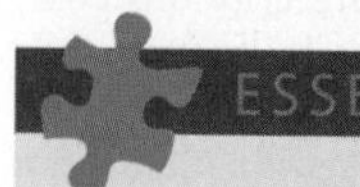

ESSENTIALS OF DIAGNOSIS

- Illness of at least 3 weeks in duration.
- Fever > 38.3°C on several occasions.
- Diagnosis has not been made after three outpatient visits or 3 days of hospitalization.

General Considerations

The intervals specified in the criteria for the diagnosis of FUO are arbitrary ones intended to exclude patients with protracted but self-limited illnesses and to allow time for the usual radiographic, serologic, and cultural studies to be performed. The criteria for FUO are met when a diagnosis has not been made after three outpatient visits or 7 days of hospitalization.

Added categories of FUO include complications of current health care scenarios: (1) **Hospital-associated FUO** refers to the hospitalized patient with fever of 38.3°C or higher on several occasions, due to a process not present or incubating at the time of admission, in whom initial cultures are negative and the diagnosis remains unknown after 1 week of investigation (see Health Care–Associated Infections below); (2) **Neutropenic FUO** includes patients with fever of 38.3°C or higher on several occasions with less than 500 neutrophils per microliter in whom initial cultures are negative and the diagnosis remains uncertain after 3 days (see Chapter 2 and Infections in the Immunocompromised Patient, below); (3) **HIV-associated FUO** pertains to HIV patients with HIV and fever of 38.3°C or higher who have been febrile for 4 weeks or more as an outpatient or 3 days as an inpatient, in whom the diagnosis remains uncertain after 3 days of investigation with at least 2 days for cultures to incubate (see Chapter 31). Although not usually considered separately, **FUO in solid organ transplant recipients** and **FUO in the returning traveler** are common scenarios, each with a unique differential diagnosis, and are also discussed in this chapter.

For a general discussion of fever, see the section on fever and hyperthermia in Chapter 2.

A. Common Causes

Most cases represent unusual manifestations of common diseases and not rare or exotic diseases—eg, tuberculosis, endocarditis, gallbladder disease, and HIV (primary infection or opportunistic infection) are more common causes of FUO than Whipple disease or familial Mediterranean fever.

B. Age of Patient

In adults, infections (25–40% of cases) and cancer (25–40% of cases) account for the majority of FUOs. In children, infections are the most common cause of FUO (30–50% of cases) and cancer a rare cause (5–10% of cases). Autoimmune disorders occur with equal frequency in adults and children (10–20% of cases), but the diseases differ. Juvenile rheumatoid arthritis is particularly common in children, whereas SLE, granulomatosis with polyangiitis, and polyarteritis nodosa are more common in adults. Still disease, giant cell arteritis, and polymyalgia rheumatica occur exclusively in adults. In adults over 65 years of age, multisystem immune-mediated diseases such as temporal arteritis, polymyalgia rheumatica, sarcoidosis, rheumatoid arthritis, and granulomatosis with polyangiitis account for 25–30% of all FUOs.

C. Duration of Fever

The cause of FUO changes dramatically in patients who have been febrile for 6 months or longer. Infection, cancer, and autoimmune disorders combined account for only 20% of FUOs in these patients. Instead, other entities such as granulomatous diseases (granulomatous hepatitis, Crohn disease, ulcerative colitis) and factitious fever become important causes. One-fourth of patients who say they have been febrile for 6 months or longer actually have no true fever or underlying disease. Instead, the usual normal circadian variation in temperature (temperature

0.5–1°C higher in the afternoon than in the morning) is interpreted as abnormal. Patients with **episodic** or **recurrent fever** (ie, those who meet the criteria for FUO but have fever-free periods of 2 weeks or longer) are similar to those with **prolonged fever**. Infection, malignancy, and autoimmune disorders account for only 20–25% of such fevers, whereas various miscellaneous diseases (Crohn disease, familial Mediterranean fever, allergic alveolitis) account for another 25%. *Approximately 50% of cases remain undiagnosed but have a benign course with eventual resolution of symptoms.*

D. Immunologic Status

In the neutropenic patient, fungal infections and occult bacterial infections are important causes of FUO. In the patient taking immunosuppressive medications (particularly organ transplant patients), cytomegalovirus (CMV) infections are a frequent cause of fever, as are fungal infections, nocardiosis, *Pneumocystis jirovecii* pneumonia, and mycobacterial infections.

E. Classification of Causes of FUO

Most patients with FUO will fit into one of five categories.

1. Infection—Both systemic and localized infections can cause FUO. Tuberculosis and endocarditis are the most common systemic infections associated with FUO, but mycoses, viral diseases (particularly infection with Epstein-Barr virus and CMV), toxoplasmosis, brucellosis, Q fever, cat-scratch disease, salmonellosis, malaria, and many other less common infections have been implicated. Primary infection with HIV or opportunistic infections associated with AIDS—particularly mycobacterial infections—can also present as FUO. The most common form of localized infection causing FUO is an occult abscess. Liver, spleen, kidney, brain, and bone abscesses may be difficult to detect. A collection of pus may form in the peritoneal cavity or in the subdiaphragmatic, subhepatic, paracolic, or other areas. Cholangitis, osteomyelitis, UTI, dental abscess, or paranasal sinusitis may cause prolonged fever.

2. Neoplasms—Many cancers can present as FUO. The most common are lymphoma (both Hodgkin and non-Hodgkin) and leukemia. Posttransplant lymphoproliferative disorders may also present with fever. Other diseases of lymph nodes, such as angioimmunoblastic lymphoma and Castleman disease, can also cause FUO. Primary and metastatic tumors of the liver are frequently associated with fever, as are renal cell carcinomas. Atrial myxoma is an often forgotten neoplasm that can result in fever. Chronic lymphocytic leukemia and multiple myeloma are rarely associated with fever, and the presence of fever in patients with these diseases should prompt a search for infection.

3. Autoimmune disorders—Still disease, SLE, cryoglobulinemia, and polyarteritis nodosa are the most common causes of autoimmune-associated FUO. Giant cell arteritis and polymyalgia rheumatica are seen almost exclusively in patients over 50 years of age and are nearly always associated with an elevated ESR (greater than 40 mm/hour).

4. Miscellaneous causes—Many other conditions have been associated with FUO but less commonly than the foregoing types of illness. Examples include thyroiditis, sarcoidosis, Whipple disease, familial Mediterranean fever, recurrent pulmonary emboli, alcoholic hepatitis, drug fever, and factitious fever.

5. Undiagnosed FUO—Despite extensive evaluation, the diagnosis remains elusive in 15% or more of patients. Of these patients, the fever abates spontaneously in about 75% with no diagnosis; in the remainder, more classic manifestations of the underlying disease appear over time.

Clinical Findings

Because the evaluation of a patient with FUO is costly and time-consuming, it is imperative to first document the presence of fever. This is done by observing the patient while the temperature is being taken to ascertain that fever is not factitious (self-induced). Associated findings that accompany fever include tachycardia, chills, and piloerection. A thorough history—including family, occupational, social (sexual practices, use of injection drugs), dietary (unpasteurized products, raw meat), exposures (animals, chemicals), and travel—may give clues to the diagnosis. Repeated physical examination may reveal subtle, evanescent clinical findings essential to diagnosis.

A. Laboratory Tests

In addition to routine laboratory studies, blood cultures should always be obtained, preferably when the patient has not taken antibiotics for several days, and should be held by the laboratory for 2 weeks to detect slow-growing organisms. Cultures on special media are requested if *Legionella*, *Bartonella*, or nutritionally deficient streptococci are possible pathogens. "Screening tests" with immunologic or microbiologic serologies ("febrile agglutinins") are of low yield and should *not* be done. If the history or physical examination suggests a specific diagnosis, specific serologic tests with an associated fourfold rise or fall in titer may be useful. Because infection is the most common cause of FUO, other body fluids are usually cultured, ie, urine, sputum, stool, cerebrospinal fluid, and morning gastric aspirates (if one suspects tuberculosis). Direct examination of blood smears may establish a diagnosis of malaria or relapsing fever (*Borrelia*).

B. Imaging

All patients with FUO should have a chest radiograph. Studies such as sinus CT, upper GI series with small bowel follow-through, barium enema, proctosigmoidoscopy, and evaluation of gallbladder function are reserved for patients who have symptoms, signs, or a history that suggest disease in these body regions. CT scan of the abdomen and pelvis is also frequently performed and is particularly useful for looking at the liver, spleen, and retroperitoneum. When the CT scan is abnormal, the findings often lead to a specific diagnosis. A normal CT scan is not quite as useful; more invasive procedures such as biopsy or exploratory laparotomy may be needed. The role of MRI in the investigation of FUO has not been evaluated. In general, however, MRI is better than CT for detecting lesions of the nervous system and is useful in diagnosing various vasculitides. Ultrasound is sensitive for detecting lesions of the kidney, pancreas, and biliary tree. Echocardiography should be used if one is considering endocarditis or atrial myxoma. Transesophageal echocardiography is more sensitive than surface echocardiography for detecting valvular lesions, but even a negative transesophageal study does not exclude endocarditis (10% false-negative rate). The usefulness of radionuclide studies in diagnosing FUO is variable. Some experts use PET if CT scans (chest and abdominal) are nondiagnostic early in the investigation of FUO. However, more studies are needed before this practice can be more fully integrated into clinical practice. In general, radionuclide scans are plagued by high rates of false-positive and false-negative results that are not useful when used as screening tests and, if done at all, are limited to those patients whose history or examination suggests local inflammation or infection.

C. Biopsy

Invasive procedures are often required for diagnosis. Any abnormal finding should be aggressively evaluated: Headache calls for lumbar puncture to rule out meningitis; skin rash should be biopsied for cutaneous manifestations of collagen vascular disease or infection; and enlarged lymph nodes should be aspirated or biopsied for neoplasm and sent for culture. Bone marrow aspiration with biopsy is a relatively low-yield procedure (15–25%; except in patients with HIV, in whom mycobacterial infection is a common cause of FUO), but the risk is low and the procedure should be done if other less invasive tests have not yielded a diagnosis, particularly in persons with hematologic abnormalities. Liver biopsy will yield a specific diagnosis in 10–15% of patients with FUO and should be considered in any patient with abnormal liver tests even if the liver is normal in size. CT scanning and MRI have decreased the need for exploratory laparotomy; however, surgical visualization and biopsies should be considered when there is continued deterioration or lack of diagnosis.

▶ Treatment

Although an empiric course of antimicrobials is sometimes considered for FUO, it is *rarely* helpful and may impact infectious diseases diagnoses (eg, by reducing the sensitivity of blood cultures).

▶ When to Refer

- Any patient with FUO and progressive weight loss and other constitutional signs.
- Any immunocompromised patient (eg, transplant recipients and patients with HIV).
- Infectious diseases specialists may also be able to coordinate and interpret specialized testing (eg, Q fever serologies) with outside agencies, such as the US CDC.

▶ When to Admit

- Any patient who is rapidly declining with weight loss where hospital admission may expedite workup.
- If FUO is present in immunocompromised patients, such as those who are neutropenic from recent chemotherapy or those who have undergone transplantation (particularly in the previous 6 months).

David A et al. Fever of unknown origin in adults. Am Fam Physician. 2022;105:137. [PMID: 35166499]
Haidar G et al. Fever of unknown origin. N Engl J Med. 2022;386:463. [PMID: 35108471]
Wright WF et al. Fever of unknown origin (FUO)—a call for new research standards and updated clinical management. Am J Med. 2022;135:173. [PMID: 34437835]
Yenilmez E et al. Fever of unknown origin (FUO) on a land on cross-roads between Asia and Europa: a multicentre study from Turkey. Int J Clin Pract. 2021;75:e14138. [PMID: 33683769]

INFECTIONS IN THE IMMUNOCOMPROMISED PATIENT

ESSENTIALS OF DIAGNOSIS

- Fever and other symptoms may be blunted because of immunosuppression.
- A contaminating organism in an immunocompetent individual may be a pathogen in an immunocompromised one.
- The interval since transplantation and the degree of immunosuppression can narrow the differential diagnosis.
- Empiric broad-spectrum antibiotics may be appropriate in high-risk patients whether or not symptoms are localized.

▶ General Considerations

Immunocompromised patients have defects in their natural defense mechanisms resulting in an increased risk for infection. In addition, infection is often severe, rapidly progressive, and life threatening. Organisms that are not usually problematic in the immunocompetent person may be important pathogens in the compromised patient (eg, *Staphylococcus epidermidis, Corynebacterium jeikeium, Propionibacterium acnes, Bacillus* species). Therefore, culture results must be interpreted with caution, and isolates should not be disregarded as solely contaminants. Although the type of immunodeficiency is associated with specific infectious disease syndromes, *nearly any pathogen can cause infection in any immunosuppressed patient at any time.* Thus, a systematic evaluation is required to identify a specific organism.

A. Impaired Humoral Immunity

Defects in humoral immunity are often congenital, although hypogammaglobulinemia can occur in multiple myeloma, chronic lymphocytic leukemia, small lymphocyte lymphoma, and in patients who have undergone splenectomy. Patients with ineffective humoral immunity lack opsonizing antibodies and are at particular risk for infection with **encapsulated organisms**, such as *Haemophilus influenzae, Neisseria meningitides*, and *Streptococcus pneumoniae*. Although rituximab is normally thought of as being linked to impaired cellular immunity, it has been associated with the development of *Pneumocystis jirovecii* infection and progressive multifocal leukoencephalopathy (PML) as well as with hepatitis B reactivation.

B. Granulocytopenia (Neutropenia)

Granulocytopenia is common following hematopoietic stem cell transplantation and among patients with solid tumors—as a result of myelosuppressive chemotherapy—and in acute leukemias. *The risk of infection begins to increase when the absolute granulocyte count falls below 1000/mcL, with a dramatic increase in frequency and severity when the granulocyte count falls below 100/mcL.* The infection risk is also increased with a rapid rate of decline of neutrophils and with a prolonged period of neutropenia. The granulocytopenic patient is particularly susceptible to infections with gram-negative enteric organisms, *Pseudomonas*, gram-positive cocci (particularly *Staphylococcus aureus* and viridans streptococci), *Candida, Aspergillus*, and other fungi that have recently emerged as pathogens such as *Scedosporium, Fusarium*, and the mucormycoses.

C. Impaired Cellular Immunity

Patients with cellular immune deficiency encompass a large and heterogeneous group, including patients with HIV infection (see Chapter 31); patients with lymphoreticular malignancies, such as Hodgkin disease; and patients receiving immunosuppressive medications, such as corticosteroids, cyclosporine, tacrolimus, and other cytotoxic medications. This latter group—those who are immunosuppressed as a result of medications—includes patients who have undergone solid organ transplantation, many patients receiving therapy for solid tumors, and patients receiving prolonged high-dose corticosteroid treatment (eg, for asthma, temporal arteritis, SLE). Patients taking tumor necrosis factor (TNF) inhibitors, such as etanercept and infliximab, are also included in this category. Patients with cellular immune dysfunction are susceptible to infections by a large number of organisms, particularly ones that replicate intracellularly. Examples include bacteria, such as *Listeria, Legionella, Salmonella*, and *Mycobacterium;* viruses, such as herpes simplex, varicella, and CMV; fungi, such as *Cryptococcus, Coccidioides, Histoplasma*, and *Pneumocystis;* and protozoa, such as *Toxoplasma*.

D. Hematopoietic Cell Transplant Recipients

The length of time it takes for complications to occur in hematopoietic cell transplant recipients can be helpful in determining the etiologic agent. In the **early (preengraftment) posttransplant period (days 1–21)**, patients will become severely neutropenic for 7–21 days. Patients are at risk for gram-positive (particularly catheter-related) and gram-negative bacterial infections, as well as herpes simplex virus, respiratory syncytial virus, and fungal infections. In contrast to solid organ transplant recipients, the source of fever is unknown in 60–70% of hematopoietic cell transplant patients. **Between 3 weeks and 3 months posttransplant**, infections with CMV, adenovirus, *Aspergillus*, and *Candida* are most common. *P jirovecii* pneumonia is possible, particularly in patients who receive additional immunosuppression for treatment of graft-versus-host disease. Patients continue to be at risk for infectious complications **beyond 3 months following transplantation**, particularly those who have received allogeneic transplantation and those who are taking immunosuppressive therapy for chronic graft-versus-host disease. Varicella-zoster is common, and *Aspergillus* and CMV infections are increasingly seen in this period as well.

E. Solid Organ Transplant Recipients

The length of time it takes for infection to occur following solid organ transplantation can also be helpful in determining the infectious origin. **Immediate postoperative infections** often involve the transplanted organ. Following lung transplantation, pneumonia and mediastinitis are particularly common; following liver transplantation, intra-abdominal abscess, cholangitis, and peritonitis may be seen; after kidney transplantation, UTIs, perinephric abscesses, and infected lymphoceles can occur.

Most infections that occur in the **first 2–4 weeks posttransplant** are related to the operative procedure and to hospitalization itself (wound infection, intravenous catheter infection, UTI from an indwelling urinary catheter) or are related to the transplanted organ. In rare instances, donor-derived infections (eg, West Nile virus, tuberculosis) may present during this time period. Compensated organ transplants obtained abroad through "medical tourism" can introduce additional risk of infections, which vary by country and by transplant setting. Infections that occur **between the first and sixth months** are often related to immunosuppression. During this period, reactivation of viruses, such as herpes simplex, varicella-zoster, and CMV is quite common. Opportunistic infections with fungi (eg, *Candida, Aspergillus, Cryptococcus, Pneumocystis*), *Listeria monocytogenes, Nocardia*, and *Toxoplasma* are also common. **After 6 months**, if immunosuppression has been reduced to maintenance levels, infections that would be expected in any population occur. Patients with poorly functioning allografts receiving long-term immunosuppression therapy continue to be at risk for opportunistic infections.

F. Tumor Necrosis Factor Inhibitor Recipients

Patients taking TNF inhibitors (infliximab, etanercept, adalimumab, certolizumab pegol, golimumab) have specific defects that increase risk of bacterial, mycobacterial (particularly tuberculosis), viral (HBV reactivation and HCV progression), and fungal infections (*Pneumocystis*, molds, and endemic mycoses). Infection risk may be highest shortly after therapy is initiated (within the first 3 months) and with a higher dose of medications.

G. Recipients of Other Biologics

In addition to TNF inhibitors, other biologics target a variety of immunologic pathways that are involved in immunologic mediated disease and in cancer replication. Disruption of these pathways include, but are not limited to impact on B cells, T cells, complement, and leukocytes. *This may result in not only serious infections, but the development of autoimmune disease and malignancies as well.* Some medications have been observed to have specific associations with opportunistic infections (eg, natalizumab and PML, or eculizumab and meningococcal disease). Other biologics such as chimeric antigen receptor T (CAR-T) cells may have unintended infectious risks that are currently unknown, or may have adverse effects that mimic infection (eg, cytokine release syndrome). Checkpoint inhibitors (eg, anti-PD-1 and CTLA antibodies) used for the treatment of advanced malignancies also may have effects that mimic infection via immune enhancement. Prolonged immunosuppression used to treat immune-associated adverse events in CAR-T and checkpoint inhibitor therapy (eg, TNF inhibitors and corticosteroids) can then result in opportunistic and other infections. As more biologics are developed and used, clinicians must remain vigilant for the possibility of serious infectious disease risk.

H. Other Immunocompromised States

A large group of patients who are not specifically immunodeficient are at increased risk for infection due to debilitating injury (eg, burns or severe trauma), invasive procedures (eg, chronic central intravenous catheters, indwelling urinary catheters, dialysis catheters), CNS dysfunction (which predisposes patients to aspiration pneumonia and pressure injuries), obstructing lesions (eg, pneumonia due to an obstructed bronchus, pyelonephritis due to nephrolithiasis, cholangitis secondary to cholelithiasis), and use of broad-spectrum antibiotics. Patients with diabetes mellitus have alterations in cellular immunity, resulting in mucormycosis, emphysematous pyelonephritis, and foot infections.

Clinical Findings

A. Laboratory Findings

Routine evaluation includes CBC with differential, chest radiograph, and blood cultures; urine and respiratory cultures should be obtained if indicated clinically or radiographically. Any focal complaints (localized pain, headache, rash) should prompt imaging and cultures appropriate to the site.

Patients who remain febrile without an obvious source should be evaluated for viral infection (serum CMV antigen test or PCR), abscesses (which usually occur near previous operative sites), candidiasis involving the liver or spleen, or aspergillosis. Serologic evaluation may be helpful if toxoplasmosis or an endemic fungal infection (coccidioidomycosis, histoplasmosis) is a possible cause. Antigen-based assays may be useful for the diagnosis of aspergillosis (detected by galactomannan level in serum or bronchoalveolar lavage fluid), or other invasive fungal disease, including *Pneumocystis* infection (serum [1→3]-beta-D-glucan level).

B. Special Diagnostic Procedures

Special diagnostic procedures should also be considered. The cause of pulmonary infiltrates can be easily determined with simple techniques in some situations—eg, induced sputum yields a diagnosis of *Pneumocystis* pneumonia in 50–80% of patients with AIDS with this infection. In other situations, more invasive procedures may be required (bronchoalveolar lavage, transbronchial biopsy, open lung biopsy). Skin, liver, or bone marrow biopsy may be helpful in establishing a diagnosis. Next-generation DNA-sequencing analysis (eg, of plasma, bronchoalveolar lavage, cerebrospinal fluid) is an increasingly used and validated option for diagnosis of infectious diseases in immunocompromised persons.

Differential Diagnosis

Transplant rejection, organ ischemia and necrosis, thrombophlebitis, and lymphoma (posttransplant lymphoproliferative disease) may all present as fever and must be considered in the differential diagnosis.

Prevention

While prophylactic antimicrobial medications are used commonly, the optimal medications or dosage regimens are debated. *Hand washing is the simplest and most effective means of decreasing hospital-associated infections*, especially in the compromised patient. Invasive devices such as central and peripheral lines and indwelling urinary catheters are potential sources of infection. Some centers use laminar airflow isolation or high-efficiency particulate air (HEPA) filtering in hematopoietic cell transplant patients. Rates of infection and episodes of febrile neutropenia, but not mortality, are decreased if colony-stimulating factors are used (typically in situations where the risk of febrile neutropenia is 20% or higher) during chemotherapy or during stem-cell transplantation.

A. *Pneumocystis* & Herpes Simplex Infections

Trimethoprim-sulfamethoxazole (TMP-SMZ), one double-strength tablet orally three times a week, one double-strength tablet twice daily on weekends, or one single-strength tablet daily, can prevent *Pneumocystis* infections. In patients allergic to TMP-SMZ, dapsone, 50 mg orally daily or 100 mg three times weekly, is recommended. Glucose-6-phosphate dehydrogenase (G6PD) levels should be assessed before dapsone is instituted. Acyclovir prevents herpes simplex infections in bone marrow and solid organ transplant recipients and is given to seropositive patients who are not receiving ganciclovir or valganciclovir for CMV prophylaxis. The usual dose is 200 mg orally three times daily for 4 weeks (hematopoietic cell transplants) to 12 weeks (solid organ transplants).

B. CMV

The two approaches to CMV prevention are **universal prophylaxis** or **preemptive therapy.** Among solid organ transplant recipients (liver, kidney, heart, lung), the strategy chosen depends on the serologic status of the donor and recipient and the organ transplanted, which determines the level of immunosuppression sought after transplant. The greatest risk of developing CMV disease is in seronegative recipients who receive organs from seropositive donors. These high-risk patients usually receive prophylaxis with oral valganciclovir for 3–6 months, potentially longer in lung transplant recipients. Other solid organ transplant recipients (seropositive recipients) are at lower risk for developing CMV disease but still usually receive either prophylaxis with oral valganciclovir for 3 months or preemptive management in which they are monitored for the presence of CMV by PCR. If CMV is detected, then therapy is instituted with treatment-dose oral valganciclovir for a minimum of 2–3 weeks. The lowest-risk group for the development of CMV disease is in seronegative patients who receive organs from seronegative donors. Typically, no CMV prophylaxis is used in this group. Ganciclovir and valganciclovir also prevent herpes virus reactivation. Because immunosuppression is increased during periods of rejection, patients treated for rejection either receive CMV prophylaxis or are monitored preemptively during rejection therapy.

Recipients of hematopoietic cell transplants are more severely immunosuppressed than recipients of solid organ transplants, are at greater risk for developing serious CMV infection (usually CMV reactivation), and thus usually receive more aggressive prophylaxis. Like in solid organ transplant recipients, all high-risk patients (seropositive patients who receive allogeneic transplants) may receive oral valganciclovir or letermovir to day 100. Because valganciclovir is associated with significant bone marrow toxicity, letermovir is being used increasingly. Because of the possibility of bone marrow toxicity and the expense, many clinicians traditionally preferred the preemptive approach over the universal prophylaxis approach for recipients of hematopoietic stem cell transplants. However, while this preemptive approach is effective, it does miss a small number of patients in whom CMV disease would have been prevented had prophylaxis been used. Other preventive strategies include use of CMV-negative or leukocyte-depleted blood products for CMV-seronegative recipients.

C. Other Organisms

Routine decontamination of the GI tract to prevent bacteremia in the neutropenic patient is *not* recommended. The use of prophylactic antibiotics in the afebrile, asymptomatic neutropenic patient is debated, although many centers have adopted this strategy. Rates of bacteremia are decreased, but overall mortality is not affected and emergence of resistant organisms takes place. Use of intravenous immunoglobulin is reserved for the small number of patients with severe hypogammaglobulinemia following hematopoietic stem cell transplantation and should not be routinely administered to all transplant patients.

Prophylaxis with antifungal agents to prevent invasive mold (primarily *Aspergillus*) and yeast (primarily *Candida*) infections is routinely used, but the optimal agent, dose, and duration are also debated. Lipid-based preparations of amphotericin B as well as systemic fluconazole, voriconazole, or posaconazole are all prophylactic options in the neutropenic patient. Voriconazole and posaconazole are superior to amphotericin for documented *Aspergillus* infections, and posaconazole prophylaxis (compared with fluconazole) results in fewer cases of invasive aspergillosis among allogeneic stem cell transplant recipients with graft-versus-host disease; thus, one approach to prophylaxis is to use oral fluconazole (400 mg/day) for patients at low risk for developing fungal infections (autologous stem cell transplants) and oral voriconazole (200 mg twice daily) or oral posaconazole (200 mg suspension three times daily or 300 mg [three 100-mg tablets] sustained-release tablets once daily) for those at high risk (allogeneic transplants, graft-versus-host disease) at least until engraftment (usually 30 days). In solid organ transplant recipients, the risk of invasive fungal infection varies considerably (1–2% in liver, pancreas, and kidney transplants and 6–8% in heart and lung transplants). Whether universal prophylaxis or observation with preemptive therapy is the best approach has not been determined. Although fluconazole is effective in preventing yeast infections, emergence of fluconazole-resistant *Candida* and molds (*Fusarium, Aspergillus, Mucor*) has raised concerns about its routine use as a prophylactic agent in the general solid organ transplant population. However, liver transplant recipients with additional risk factors, such as having undergone a choledochojejunostomy, having had a high transfusion requirement, or having developed kidney disease, may benefit from abbreviated postoperative *Candida* prophylaxis.

Given the high risk of reactivation of tuberculosis in patients taking TNF inhibitors, *all patients should be screened for latent tuberculosis infection (LTBI)* with a tuberculin skin test or an interferon-gamma release assay prior to the start of therapy. If LTBI is diagnosed, treatment with the TNF inhibitors should be delayed until treatment for LTBI is completed. There is also a marked risk of reactivation of hepatitis B and hepatitis C in patients taking TNF inhibitors; patients should also be screened for these viruses when TNF inhibitor treatment is being considered. Providers should also ensure that patients' vaccinations are up-to-date before starting TNF inhibitors therapy.

Treatment

A. General Measures

Because infections in the immunocompromised patient can be rapidly progressive and life-threatening, diagnostic procedures must be performed promptly, and empiric therapy is usually instituted.

While reduction or discontinuation of immunosuppressive medication may jeopardize the viability of the transplanted organ, this measure may be necessary if the infection is life-threatening. Hematopoietic growth factors (granulocyte and granulocyte-macrophage colony-stimulating factors) stimulate proliferation of bone marrow stem cells, resulting in an increase in peripheral leukocytes. These agents shorten the period of neutropenia and have been associated with reduction in infection.

B. Specific Measures

Antimicrobial medication therapy ultimately should be tailored to culture results. While combinations of antimicrobials are used with the intent of providing synergy or preventing resistance, the primary reason for empiric combination therapy is broad-spectrum coverage of all likely pathogens.

Empiric therapy is often instituted at the earliest sign of infection in the immunosuppressed patient because prompt therapy favorably affects outcome, particularly in febrile neutropenia. The antibiotic or combination of antibiotics used depends on the degree of immune compromise and the site of infection. For example, in the febrile neutropenic patient, an **algorithmic approach** to therapy is often used. Febrile neutropenic patients should be empirically treated with broad-spectrum agents active against selected gram-positive bacteria, *Pseudomonas aeruginosa*, and other aerobic gram-negative bacilli (such as cefepime 2 g every 8 hours intravenously). The addition of vancomycin, 10–15 mg/kg/dose intravenously every 12 hours, should be considered in those patients with suspected infection due to methicillin-resistant *S aureus* (MRSA), *S epidermidis*, enterococcus, and resistant viridans streptococci. Continued neutropenic fever necessitates broadening of antibacterial coverage from cefepime to agents such as imipenem 500 mg every 6 hours or meropenem 1 g every 8 hours intravenously with or without tobramycin 5–7 mg/kg intravenously every 24 hours, along with an additional gram-negative agent (ciprofloxacin or tobramycin) if patient is critically ill or unstable. Antifungal agents (such as voriconazole, 200 mg intravenously or orally every 12 hours, or caspofungin, 50 mg daily intravenously) should be added if fevers continue after 5–7 days of broad-spectrum antibacterial therapy. While the traditional approach was to continue antibiotics until resolution of neutropenia, *current evidence supports earlier discontinuation of antibiotics in the neutropenic patient who becomes afebrile for 72 hours if no signs or symptoms of infection persist.*

Patients with fever and low-risk neutropenia (neutropenia expected to persist for less than 10 days, no comorbid complications requiring hospitalization, and cancer adequately treated) can be treated with oral antibiotic regimens, such as ciprofloxacin, 750 mg every 12 hours, plus amoxicillin-clavulanic acid, 500 mg every 8 hours. Antibiotics are usually continued as long as the patient is neutropenic even if a source is not identified. In the organ transplant patient with interstitial infiltrates, the main concern is infection with *Pneumocystis* or *Legionella* species, so that empiric treatment with a macrolide or fluoroquinolone (*Legionella*) and TMP-SMZ, 15 mg/kg/day orally or intravenously (*Pneumocystis*), would be reasonable in those patients not receiving TMP-SMZ prophylaxis. If the patient does not respond to empiric treatment, a decision must be made to add more antimicrobial agents or perform invasive procedures to make a specific diagnosis. By making a definite diagnosis, therapy can be specific, thereby reducing selection pressure for resistance and superinfection.

When to Refer

- Any immunocompromised patient with an opportunistic infection.
- Patients with potential drug toxicities and drug interactions related to antimicrobials where alternative agents are sought.
- Patients with latent tuberculosis, HBV, and HCV infection in whom therapy with TNF inhibitors is planned.

When to Admit

Immunocompromised patients who are febrile, or those without fevers in whom an infection is suspected, particularly in the following groups: solid-organ or hematopoietic stem cell transplant recipient (particularly in the first 6 months), neutropenic patients, patients receiving TNF inhibitors, and transplant recipients who have had recent rejection episodes (including graft-versus-host disease).

Alghamdi W et al. Hepatitis C positive organ transplantation to negative recipients at a multiorgan Canadian transplant centre: ready for prime time. BMC Gastroenterol. 2022;22:34. [PMID: 35078405]

Baden LR et al. NCCN Clinical Practice Guidelines in Oncology: Prevention and treatment of cancer-related infections, version 1.2021. https://www.nccn.org/guidelines/guidelines-detail?category=3&id=1457

Casto AM et al. Diagnosis of infectious diseases in immunocompromised hosts using metagenomic next generation sequencing-based diagnostics. Blood Rev. 2022;53:100906. [PMID: 34802773]

Chiu Y-M et al. Infection risk in patients undergoing treatment for inflammatory arthritis: non-biologics versus biologics. Expert Rev Clin Immunol. 2020;16:207. [PMID: 31852268]

Duan H et al. The diagnostic value of metagenomic next-generation sequencing in infectious diseases. BMC Infect Dis. 2021;21:6. [PMID: 33435894]

Donnelly JP et al. Revision and update of the consensus definitions of invasive fungal disease from the European Organization for Research and Treatment of Cancer and the Mycoses Study Group Education and Research Consortium. Clin Infect Dis. 2020;71:1367. [PMID: 31802125]

Durand CM et al. Four-week direct-acting antiviral prophylaxis for kidney transplantation from hepatitis C-viremic donors to hepatitis C-negative recipients: an open-label nonrandomized study. Ann Intern Med. 2021;174:137. [PMID: 32894697]

Haidar G et al. Cytomegalovirus infection in solid organ and hematopoietic cell transplantation: state of the evidence. J Infect Dis. 2020;221(Suppl 1):S23. [PMID: 32134486]

Kahn JA. The use of organs from hepatitis C virus-viremic donors into uninfected recipients. Curr Opin Organ Transplant. 2020;25:620. [PMID: 33105203]

Limaye AP et al. Progress and challenges in the prevention, diagnosis, and management of cytomegalovirus infection in transplantation. Clin Microbiol Rev. 2020;34:e00043. [PMID: 33115722]

HEALTH CARE–ASSOCIATED INFECTIONS

ESSENTIALS OF DIAGNOSIS

- Acquired during the course of receiving health care treatment for other conditions.
- Most cases are preventable.
- Hospital-associated infections are defined as not being present or incubating at the time of hospital admission and developing ≥ 48 hours after admission.
- Hand washing is the most effective prevention and should be done routinely even when gloves are worn.

General Considerations

Worldwide, approximately 10% of patients acquire a health care–associated infection, resulting in prolongation of the hospital stay, increase in cost of care, and significant morbidity and mortality. The most common infections are UTIs, usually associated with indwelling urinary catheters or urologic procedures; bloodstream infections, most commonly from indwelling catheters but also from secondary sites, such as surgical wounds, abscesses, pneumonia, the genitourinary tract, and the GI tract; pneumonia in intubated patients or those with altered levels of consciousness; surgical wound infections; MRSA infections; and *Clostridioides difficile* infection. There has been hospital-associated transmission of SARS-CoV-2.

Some general principles are helpful in preventing, diagnosing, and treating health care–associated infections:

1. Many infections are a direct result of the use of *invasive devices* for monitoring or therapy, such as intravenous catheters, indwelling urinary catheters, shunts, surgical drains, catheters placed by interventional radiology for drainage, nasogastric tubes, and orotracheal or nasotracheal tubes for ventilatory support. *Early removal of such devices reduces the possibility of infection.*
2. Patients in whom health care–associated infections develop are often critically ill, have been hospitalized for extended periods, and have received several courses of broad-spectrum antibiotic therapy. As a result, health care–associated infections are often due to *multidrug resistant pathogens* and differ from those encountered in community-acquired infections. For example, *S aureus* and *S epidermidis* (a frequent cause of prosthetic device infection) are often resistant to methicillin and most cephalosporins (ceftaroline is the only active cephalosporin against MRSA) and require vancomycin for therapy; *Enterococcus faecium* resistant to ampicillin and vancomycin; gram-negative infections caused by *Pseudomonas, Citrobacter, Enterobacter, Acinetobacter, Stenotrophomonas*, extended-spectrum beta-lactamases (ESBL)–producing *E coli*, *Klebsiella*, and carbapenem-resistant Enterobacteriaceae (CRE) may be resistant to most antibacterials. When choosing antibiotics to treat the seriously ill patient with a health care–associated infection, antimicrobial history and the "local ecology" must be considered. In the most seriously ill patients, broad-spectrum coverage with vancomycin and a carbapenem with or without an aminoglycoside is recommended. Once a pathogen is isolated and susceptibilities are known, the most narrow-spectrum, least toxic, most cost-effective regimen should be used.

Widespread use of antimicrobial medications contributes to the selection of drug-resistant organisms; thus, *every effort should be made to limit the spectrum of coverage and unnecessary duration*. All too often, unreliable or uninterpretable specimens are obtained for culture that result in unnecessary use of antibiotics. The best example of this principle is the diagnosis of line-related or bloodstream infection in the febrile patient. To avoid unnecessary use of antibiotics, thoughtful consideration of culture results is mandatory. A positive wound culture without signs of inflammation or infection, a positive sputum culture without pulmonary infiltrates on chest radiograph, or a positive urine culture in a catheterized patient without symptoms or signs of pyelonephritis are all likely to represent *colonization*, not infection.

Clinical Findings

A. Symptoms and Signs

Catheter-associated infections have a variable presentation, depending on the type of catheter used (peripheral or central venous catheters, nontunneled or tunneled). Local signs of infection may be present at the insertion site, with pain, erythema, and purulence. Fever is often absent in uncomplicated infections and, if present, may indicate more disseminated disease such as bacteremia, cellulitis and septic thrombophlebitis. Often signs of infection at the insertion site are absent.

1. Fever in an ICU patient—Fever complicates up to 70% of patients in ICUs, and the etiology of the fever may be infectious or noninfectious. Common infectious causes include catheter-associated infections, hospital-acquired and ventilator-associated pneumonia (see Chapter 9), surgical site infections, UTIs, and sepsis. Clinically relevant sinusitis is relatively uncommon in the patient in the ICU.

An important noninfectious cause is thromboembolic disease. Fever in conjunction with refractory hypotension and shock may suggest sepsis; however, adrenal insufficiency, thyroid storm, and transfusion reaction may have a similar clinical presentation. Drug fever is difficult to diagnose and is usually a diagnosis of exclusion unless there are other signs of hypersensitivity, such as a typical maculopapular rash (most common with beta-lactams).

2. Fever in the postoperative patient—Postoperative fever is very common and noninfectious fever resolves spontaneously. Timing of the onset of the fever in relation to the surgical procedure may be of diagnostic benefit.

A. IMMEDIATE FEVER (IN THE FIRST FEW HOURS AFTER SURGERY)—Immediate fever can be due to medications that were given perioperatively, to surgical trauma, or to infections that were present before surgery. Necrotizing fasciitis due to group A streptococci or mixed organisms may present in this period. **Malignant hyperthermia** is rare and presents 30 minutes to several hours following inhalational anesthesia and is characterized by extreme hyperthermia, muscle rigidity, rhabdomyolysis, electrolyte abnormalities, and hypotension. Aggressive cooling and dantrolene are the mainstays of therapy. Aspiration of acidic gastric contents during surgery can result in a chemical pneumonitis (**Mendelson syndrome**) that develops rapidly, is transient, and does not require antibiotics. Fever due to surgical trauma usually resolves in 2–3 days; however, it may be longer in more complicated operative cases and in patients with head trauma.

B. ACUTE FEVER (WITHIN 1 WEEK OF SURGERY)—Acute fever is usually due to common causes of hospital-associated infections, such as ventilator-associated pneumonia (including aspiration pneumonia in patients with decreased gag reflex) and line infections. Noninfectious causes include alcohol withdrawal, gout, PE, and pancreatitis. Atelectasis following surgery is commonly invoked as a cause of postoperative fever but *there is no good evidence to support a causal association between the presence or degree of atelectasis and fever.*

c. Subacute fever (at least 1 week after surgery)—Surgical site infections commonly present at least 1 week after surgery. The type of surgery that was performed predicts specific infectious etiologies. Patients undergoing cardiothoracic surgery may be at higher risk for pneumonia and deep and superficial sternal wound infections. Meningitis without typical signs of meningismus may complicate neurosurgical procedures. Postoperative deep abdominal abscesses may require drainage.

B. Laboratory Findings

Blood cultures are universally recommended, and chest radiographs are frequently obtained. A properly prepared sputum Gram stain and semi-quantitative sputum cultures may be useful in selected patients where there is a high pretest probability of pneumonia but multiple exclusion criteria probably limit generalizability in most patients, such as immunocompromised patients and those with drug resistance. Other diagnostic strategies will be dictated by the clinical context (eg, transesophageal echocardiogram in a patient with *S aureus* bacteremia).

Any fever in a patient with a central venous catheter should prompt the collection of blood. The best method to evaluate bacteremia is to gather *at least two peripherally obtained blood cultures.* Blood cultures from unidentified sites, a single blood culture from any site, or a blood culture through an existing line will often be positive for coagulase-positive staphylococci, particularly *S epidermidis*, often resulting in the inappropriate use of vancomycin. *Unless two separate venipuncture cultures are obtained—not through catheters—interpretation of results is impossible*, and unnecessary therapy often results. Each "pseudobacteremia" increases bacterial resistance pressure, laboratory costs, antibiotic use, and length of stay. Microbiologic evaluation of the removed catheter can sometimes be helpful, but only in addition to (not instead of) blood cultures drawn from peripheral sites. The **differential time to positivity** measures the difference in time that cultures simultaneously drawn through a catheter and a peripheral site become positive. A positive test (at least 120 minutes' difference in time) supports a catheter-related bloodstream infection, while a negative test suggests catheters may be retained.

Complications

Complications such as septic thrombophlebitis, endocarditis, or metastatic foci of infection (particularly with *S aureus*) may be suspected in patients with persistent bacteremia and fever despite removal of the infected catheter. Additional studies such as venous Doppler studies, transesophageal echocardiogram, and chest radiographs may be indicated, and 4–6 weeks of antibiotics may be needed. In the case of septic thrombophlebitis, anticoagulation with heparin is also recommended if there are no contraindications.

Differential Diagnosis

Although most fevers are due to infections, about 25% of patients will have fever of noninfectious origin, including drug fever, nonspecific postoperative fevers (tissue damage or necrosis), hematoma, pancreatitis, PE, MI, and ischemic bowel disease.

Prevention

The concept of **universal precautions** emphasizes that all patients are treated as though they have a potential bloodborne transmissible disease, and thus all body secretions are handled with care to prevent spread of disease. Body substance isolation requires use of gloves whenever a health care worker anticipates contact with blood or other body secretions. *Even though gloves are worn, health care workers should routinely wash their hands, since it is the easiest and most effective means of preventing hospital-associated infections.* Application of a rapid drying, alcohol-based antiseptic is simple, takes less time than traditional hand washing with soap and water, is more effective at reducing hand colonization, and promotes compliance with hand decontamination. For prevention of transmission of *C difficile* infection, hand washing is *more* effective than alcohol-based antiseptics. Consequently, even after removing gloves, providers should always wash hands in cases of proven or suspected *C difficile* infection.

Peripheral intravenous lines should be replaced no more frequently than every 3–4 days. Some clinicians replace only when clinically indicated or if the line was put in emergently. Arterial lines and lines in the central venous circulation (including those placed peripherally) can be left in place indefinitely and are changed or removed when they are clinically suspected of being infected, when they are nonfunctional, or when they are no longer needed. Using sterile barrier precautions (including cap, mask, gown, gloves, and drape) is recommended while inserting central venous catheters. Antibiotic-impregnated (minocycline plus rifampin or chlorhexidine plus silver sulfadiazine) venous catheters reduce line infections. Silver alloy–impregnated indwelling urinary catheters reduce the incidence of catheter-associated bacteriuria, but not consistently catheter-associated UTIs. Best practices to prevent ventilator-associated pneumonia include avoiding intubation if possible, minimizing and daily interruption of sedation, pooling/draining of subglottic secretions above the tube cuff, and elevating the head of the bed. Silver-coated endotracheal tubes may reduce the incidence of ventilator-associated pneumonia but has limited impact on hospital stay duration or mortality, so they are not generally recommended. Catheter-related UTIs and intravenous catheter-associated infections are not Medicare-reimbursable conditions in the United States. Preoperative skin preparation with chlorhexidine and alcohol (versus povidone-iodine) reduces the incidence of infection following surgery. Another strategy that can prevent surgical-site infections is the identification and treatment of *S aureus* nasal carriers with 2% mupirocin nasal ointment and chlorhexidine soap. Daily bathing of ICU patients with chlorhexidine-impregnated washcloths versus soap and water results in lower incidence of health care–associated infections and colonization. Selective decontamination of the digestive tract with nonabsorbable or parenteral antibiotics, or both, may prevent hospital-acquired pneumonia and decrease mortality but is in limited use because of the concern of the development of antibiotic resistance. **Prevention bundles** (implementing more than one intervention concomitantly) are commonly used as a practical strategy to enhance care.

Attentive nursing care (positioning to prevent pressure injuries, wound care, elevating the head during tube feedings to prevent aspiration) is critical in preventing hospital-associated infections. In addition, monitoring of high-risk areas by hospital epidemiologists is critical in the prevention of infection. Some guidelines advocate rapid screening (active surveillance cultures) for MRSA on admission to acute care facilities among certain subpopulations of patients (eg, those recently hospitalized, admission to the ICU, patients undergoing hemodialysis). However, outside the setting of an MRSA outbreak, it is not clear whether this strategy decreases the incidence of hospital-associated MRSA infections.

Vaccines, including hepatitis A, hepatitis B, and the varicella, pneumococcal, influenza, and SARS-CoV-2 vaccinations, are important adjuncts. (See section below titled Immunization Against Infectious Diseases.)

Treatment

A. Fever in an ICU Patient

Unless the patient has a central neurologic injury with elevated intracranial pressure or has a temperature higher than 41°C, there is less physiologic need to maintain euthermia. Empiric broad-spectrum antibiotics (see Table 30–5) are recommended for neutropenic and other immunocompromised patients and in patients who are clinically unstable.

B. Catheter-Associated Infections

Factors that inform treatment decisions include the type of catheter, the causative pathogen, the availability of alternate catheter access sites, the need for ongoing intravascular access, and the severity of disease.

In general, catheters should be removed if there is purulence at the exit site; if the organism is *S aureus*, gram-negative rods, or *Candida* species; if there is persistent bacteremia (more than 48 hours while receiving antibiotics); or if complications, such as septic thrombophlebitis, endocarditis, or other metastatic disease, exist. Central venous catheters may be exchanged over a guidewire provided there is no erythema or purulence at the exit site and the patient does not appear to be septic. Methicillin-resistant, coagulase-negative staphylococci are the most common pathogens; thus, empiric therapy with vancomycin, 15 mg/kg/dose intravenously twice daily, should be given assuming normal kidney function. Empiric gram-negative coverage should be used in patients who are immunocompromised or who are critically ill (see Table 30–5).

Antibiotic treatment duration depends on the pathogen and the extent of disease. For uncomplicated bacteremia, 5–7 days of therapy is usually sufficient for coagulase-negative staphylococci, even if the original catheter is retained. Fourteen days of therapy are generally recommended for uncomplicated bacteremia caused by gram-negative rods, *Candida* species, and *S aureus*. **Antibiotic lock therapy** involves the instillation of supratherapeutic concentrations of antibiotics with heparin in the lumen of catheters. The purpose is to achieve adequate concentrations of antibiotics to kill microbes in the biofilm. Antibiotic lock therapy can be used for catheter-related bloodstream infections caused by both gram-positive and gram-negative bacterial pathogens and when the catheter is being retained in a salvage situation.

When to Refer

- Any patient with multidrug-resistant infection.
- Any patient with fungemia, *S aureus* bacteremia, or persistent bacteremia of any organism.
- Patients whose catheters cannot be removed.
- Patients with multisite infections.
- Patients with impaired or fluctuating kidney function for assistance with dosing of antimicrobials.
- Patients with refractory or recurrent *C difficile* infection.

Bassetti M et al. Post-operative abdominal infections: epidemiology, operational definitions, and outcomes. Intensive Care Med. 2020;46:163. [PMID: 31701205]

File TM Jr et al. The role of antibiotic stewardship and telemedicine in the management of multidrug-resistant infections. Infect Dis Clin North Am. 2020;34:903. [PMID: 33131574]

Johnson S et al. Clinical practice guideline by the Infectious Diseases Society of America (IDSA) and Society for Healthcare Epidemiology of America (SHEA): 2021 focused update guidelines on management of *Clostridioides difficile* infection in adults. Clin Infect Dis. 2021;73:e1029. [PMID: 34164674]

Kelly CR et al. ACG clinical guidelines: prevention, diagnosis, and treatment of *Clostridioides difficile* Infections. Am J Gastroenterol. 2021;116:1124. [PMID: 34003176]

Khanna S. Advances in *Clostridioides difficile* therapeutics. Expert Rev Anti Infect Ther. 2021;19:1067. [PMID: 33427531]

Lai CC et al. Increased antimicrobial resistance during the COVID-19 pandemic. Int J Antimicrob Agents. 2021;57:106324. [PMID: 33746045]

Mancuso G. Bacterial antibiotic resistance: the most critical pathogens. Pathogens. 2021;10:1310. [PMID: 34684258]

Slimings C et al. Antibiotics and healthcare facility-associated *Clostridioides difficile* infection: systematic review and meta-analysis 2020 update. J Antimicrob Chemother. 2021;76:1676. [PMID: 33787887]

Stewart S et al. Epidemiology of healthcare-associated infection reported from a hospital-wide incidence study: considerations for infection prevention and control planning. J Hosp Infect. 2021;114:10. [PMID: 34301392]

INFECTIONS OF THE CENTRAL NERVOUS SYSTEM

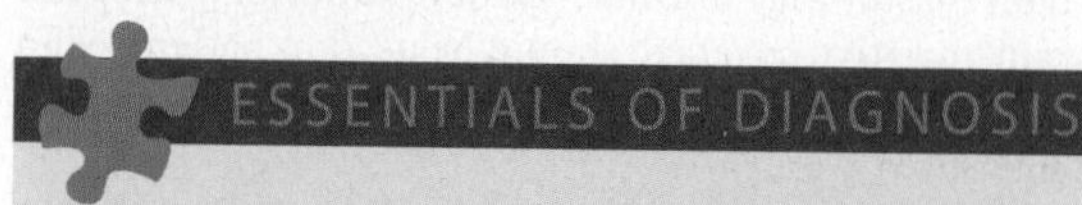

- CNS infection is a medical emergency.
- Symptoms and signs common to all CNS infections include headache, fever, sensorial disturbances, neck and back stiffness, positive Kernig and Brudzinski signs, and cerebrospinal fluid abnormalities.

General Considerations

Infections of the CNS can be caused by almost any infectious agent, including bacteria, mycobacteria, fungi, spirochetes, protozoa, helminths, and viruses.

Etiologic Classification

CNS infections can be divided into several categories that usually can be readily distinguished from each other by cerebrospinal fluid examination as the first step toward etiologic diagnosis (Table 30–1).

A. Purulent Meningitis

Patients with bacterial meningitis usually seek medical attention within hours or 1–2 days after onset of symptoms. The organisms responsible depend primarily on the age of the patient as summarized in Table 30–2. The diagnosis is usually based on the Gram-stained smear (positive in 60–90%) or culture (positive in over 90%) of the cerebrospinal fluid.

B. Chronic Meningitis

The presentation of chronic meningitis is less acute than purulent meningitis. Patients with chronic meningitis usually have a history of symptoms lasting weeks to months. The most common pathogens are *Mycobacterium tuberculosis*, atypical mycobacteria, fungi (*Cryptococcus, Coccidioides, Histoplasma*), and spirochetes (*Treponema pallidum* and *Borrelia burgdorferi*). The diagnosis is made by culture or in some cases by serologic tests (cryptococcosis, coccidioidomycosis, syphilis, Lyme disease).

C. Aseptic Meningitis

Aseptic meningitis—a much more benign and self-limited syndrome than purulent meningitis—is caused principally by viruses, especially herpes simplex virus and the enterovirus group (including coxsackieviruses and echoviruses). Infectious mononucleosis may be accompanied by aseptic meningitis. Leptospiral infection is also usually placed in the aseptic group because of the lymphocytic cellular response and its relatively benign course. This type of meningitis also occurs during secondary syphilis and disseminated Lyme disease. Prior to the routine administration of measles-mumps-rubella (MMR) vaccines, mumps was the most common cause of viral meningitis. Drug-induced aseptic meningitis has been reported with NSAIDs, sulfonamides, and certain monoclonal antibodies.

D. Encephalitis

Encephalitis (due to herpesviruses, arboviruses, rabies virus, flaviviruses [West Nile encephalitis, Japanese encephalitis], and many others) produces disturbances of the sensorium, seizures, and many other manifestations. Patients are more ill than those with aseptic meningitis. Cerebrospinal fluid may be entirely normal or may show

Table 30–1. Typical cerebrospinal fluid findings in various CNS diseases (listed in alphabetical order after Normal).

Diagnosis	Cells/mcL	Glucose (mg/dL)	Protein (mg/dL)	Opening Pressure
Normal	0–5 lymphocytes	45–85[1]	15–45	70–180 mm H_2O
Aseptic meningitis, viral meningitis, or meningoencephalitis[2]	25–2000 (0.025–2.0 × 10^9/L), mostly lymphocytes[3]	Normal or low	High (> 50)	Slightly elevated
Granulomatous meningitis (mycobacterial, fungal)[3]	100–1000 (0.1–1.0 × 10^9/L), mostly lymphocytes[3]	Low (< 45)	High (> 50)	Moderately elevated
"Neighborhood reaction"[4]	Variably increased	Normal	Normal or high	Variable
Purulent meningitis (bacterial)[5] community-acquired	200–20,000 (0.2–20 × 10^9/L) polymorphonuclear neutrophils	Low (< 45)	High (> 50)	Markedly elevated
Spirochetal meningitis	100–1000 (0.1–1.0 × 10^9/L), mostly lymphocytes[3]	Normal	High (> 50)	Normal to slightly elevated

[1]Cerebrospinal fluid glucose must be considered in relation to blood glucose level. Normally, cerebrospinal fluid glucose is 20–30 mg/dL lower than blood glucose, or 50–70% of the normal value of blood glucose.
[2]Viral isolation from cerebrospinal fluid early; antibody titer rise in paired specimens of serum; PCR for herpesvirus.
[3]Polymorphonuclear neutrophils may predominate early.
[4]May occur in mastoiditis, brain abscess, epidural abscess, sinusitis, septic thrombus, brain tumor. Cerebrospinal fluid culture results usually negative.
[5]Organisms in smear or culture of cerebrospinal fluid; counterimmunoelectrophoresis or latex agglutination may be diagnostic.

Table 30–2. Initial antimicrobial therapy for purulent meningitis of unknown cause.

Population	Usual Microorganisms	Standard Therapy
18–50 years	*Streptococcus pneumoniae, Neisseria meningitidis*	Vancomycin[1] **plus** ceftriaxone[2]
Over 50 years	*S pneumoniae, N meningitidis, Listeria monocytogenes*, gram-negative bacilli, group B streptococcus	Vancomycin[1] **plus** ampicillin,[3] **plus** ceftriaxone[2]
Impaired cellular immunity	*L monocytogenes*, gram-negative bacilli, *S pneumoniae*	Vancomycin[1] **plus** ampicillin,[3] **plus** cefepime[4]
Postsurgical or posttraumatic	*Staphylococcus aureus, S pneumoniae*, aerobic gram-negative bacilli, coagulase-negative staphylococci,[5] diphtheroids (eg, *Propionibacterium acnes*)[5] (uncommon)	Vancomycin[1] **plus** cefepime[4]

[1]Given to cover highly penicillin- or cephalosporin-resistant pneumococci. The dose of vancomycin is 15–20 mg/kg/dose intravenously every 8–12 hours. Doses should be adjusted to achieve a target area under the curve (AUC) between 400 and 600 mg*hour/L for confirmed methicillin-resistant *Staphylococcus aureus* (MRSA). Vancomycin should be stopped if the causative organism is susceptible to ceftriaxone.
[2]Ceftriaxone can often be used safely in most patients with a history of low risk (eg, not IgE-mediated) penicillin allergy. Aztreonam can be considered for empiric coverage of gram-negative bacilli in patients with type 1 IgE-mediated penicillin and cephalosporin allergy. The usual dose of ceftriaxone is 2 g intravenously every 12 hours. If the organism is susceptible, penicillin 4 million units intravenously every 4 hours is given.
[3]In severely ill patients, ampicillin is used when *L monocytogenes* infection is a consideration. For confirmed infection due to *L monocytogenes*, gentamicin is sometimes added to ampicillin. (For patients with type 1 IgE-mediated penicillin allergy, trimethoprim-sulfamethoxazole [TMP-SMZ] in a dosage of 15–20 mg/kg/day of TMP in three or four divided doses can be considered.) The dose of ampicillin is 2 g intravenously every 4 hours with normal kidney function.
[4]Cefepime is given in a dose of 2 g intravenously every 8 hours.
[5]Primarily associated with presence of hardware.

some lymphocytes and, in some instances (eg, herpes simplex), red cells as well. Influenza has been associated with encephalitis, but the relationship is not clear. An autoimmune form of encephalitis associated with *N*-methyl-D-aspartate receptor antibodies should be suspected in younger patients with encephalitis and associated seizures, movement disorders, and psychosis.

E. Partially Treated Bacterial Meningitis

Previous effective antibiotic therapy given for 12–24 hours will decrease the rate of positive cerebrospinal fluid Gram stain results by 20% and culture by 30–40% but will have little effect on cell count, protein, or glucose. Occasionally, previous antibiotic therapy will change a predominantly polymorphonuclear response to a lymphocytic pleocytosis, and some of the cerebrospinal fluid findings may be similar to those seen in aseptic meningitis.

F. Neighborhood Reaction

As noted in Table 30–1, this term denotes a purulent infectious process in close proximity to the CNS that spills some of the products of the inflammatory process—WBCs or protein—into the cerebrospinal fluid. Such an infection might be a brain abscess, osteomyelitis of the vertebrae, epidural abscess, subdural empyema, or bacterial sinusitis or mastoiditis.

G. Noninfectious Meningeal Irritation

Carcinomatous meningitis, sarcoidosis, SLE, chemical meningitis, and certain medications—NSAIDs, OKT3, TMP-SMZ, and others—can also produce symptoms and signs of meningeal irritation with associated cerebrospinal fluid pleocytosis, increased protein, and low or normal glucose. Meningismus with normal cerebrospinal fluid findings occurs in the presence of other infections such as pneumonia and shigellosis.

H. Brain Abscess

Brain abscess presents as a space-occupying lesion; symptoms may include vomiting, fever, change of mental status, or focal neurologic manifestations. When brain abscess is suspected, a CT scan should be performed. If positive, lumbar puncture should *not* be performed since results rarely provide clinically useful information and herniation can occur. The bacteriology of brain abscess is usually polymicrobial and includes *S aureus*, gram-negative bacilli, streptococci, and mouth anaerobes (including anaerobic streptococci and *Prevotella* species).

I. Health Care–Associated Meningitis

This infection may arise as a result of invasive neurosurgical procedures (eg, craniotomy, internal or external ventricular catheters, external lumbar catheters), complicated head trauma, or hospital-acquired bloodstream infections. Outbreaks have been associated with contaminated epidural or paraspinal corticosteroid injections. In general, the microbiology is distinct from community-acquired meningitis, with gram-negative organisms (eg, *Pseudomonas*), *S aureus*, and coagulase-negative staphylococci and, in the outbreaks associated with contaminated corticosteroids, mold and fungi (*Exserohilum rostratum* and *Aspergillus fumigatus*) playing a larger role.

Clinical Findings

A. Symptoms and Signs

The classic triad of fever, stiff neck, and altered mental status has a low sensitivity (44%) for bacterial meningitis.

However, nearly all patients with bacterial meningitis have at least two of the following symptoms—fever, headache, stiff neck, or altered mental status.

B. Laboratory Tests

Evaluation of a patient with suspected meningitis includes a blood count, blood culture, lumbar puncture followed by careful study and culture of the cerebrospinal fluid, and a chest film. The fluid must be examined for cell count, glucose, and protein, and a smear stained for bacteria (and acid-fast organisms when appropriate) and cultured for pyogenic organisms and for mycobacteria and fungi when indicated. Latex agglutination tests can detect antigens of encapsulated organisms (*S pneumoniae, H influenzae, N meningitidis*, and *Cryptococcus neoformans*) but are rarely used except for detection of *Cryptococcus* or in partially treated patients. PCR testing of cerebrospinal fluid has been used to detect bacteria (*S pneumoniae, H influenzae, N meningitidis, M tuberculosis, B burgdorferi*, and *Tropheryma whipplei*) and viruses (herpes simplex, varicella-zoster, CMV, Epstein-Barr virus, and enteroviruses) in patients with meningitis. The greatest experience is with PCR for herpes simplex, varicella-zoster, and JC virus. These tests are very sensitive (greater than 95%) and specific. In addition to its use in meningitis, molecular methods such as PCR and next-generation sequencing are being used increasingly for the diagnosis of encephalitis, transverse myelitis, and brain abscess. In general, molecular diagnostic tests may provide a more sensitive and rapid alternative to traditional culture and serology methods. However, it is difficult to ascertain the true sensitivity of many molecular tests for CNS infections given the absence of a gold standard. In some cases, tests to detect several organisms may not be any more sensitive than culture (or serology), but the *real value is the rapidity* with which results are available, ie, hours compared with days or weeks.

C. Lumbar Puncture and Imaging

Since performing a lumbar puncture in the presence of a space-occupying lesion (brain abscess, subdural hematoma, subdural empyema, necrotic temporal lobe from herpes encephalitis) may result in brainstem herniation, *a CT scan is performed prior to lumbar puncture if a space-occupying lesion is suspected on the basis of papilledema, seizures, or focal neurologic findings.* Other indications for CT scan are an immunocompromised patient or moderately to severely impaired level of consciousness. If delays are encountered in obtaining a CT scan and bacterial meningitis is suspected, blood cultures should be drawn and antibiotics and corticosteroids administered even before cerebrospinal fluid is obtained for culture to avoid delay in treatment (Table 30–1). *Antibiotics given within 4 hours before obtaining cerebrospinal fluid probably do not affect culture results.* MRI with contrast of the epidural injection site and surrounding areas is recommended (sometimes repeatedly) for those with symptoms following a possibly contaminated corticosteroid injection to exclude epidural abscess, phlegmon, vertebral osteomyelitis, discitis, or arachnoiditis.

Treatment

Although it is difficult to prove with existing clinical data that early antibiotic therapy improves outcome in bacterial meningitis, prompt therapy is still recommended. In purulent meningitis, the identity of the causative microorganism may remain unknown or doubtful for a few days and initial antibiotic treatment as set forth in Table 30–2 should be directed against the microorganisms most common for each age group.

The duration of therapy for bacterial meningitis varies depending on the etiologic agent: *H influenzae*, 7 days; *N meningitidis*, 3–7 days; *S pneumoniae*, 10–14 days; *L monocytogenes*, 14–21 days; and gram-negative bacilli, 21 days.

For adults with pneumococcal meningitis, dexamethasone 10 mg administered intravenously 15–20 minutes before or simultaneously with the first dose of antibiotics and continued every 6 hours for 4 days decreases morbidity and mortality. Patients most likely to benefit from corticosteroids are those infected with gram-positive organisms (*S pneumoniae* or *S suis*), and those who are HIV negative. It is unknown whether patients with meningitis due to *N meningitidis* and other bacterial pathogens benefit from the use of adjunctive corticosteroids. Increased intracranial pressure due to brain edema often requires therapeutic attention. Hyperventilation, mannitol (25–50 g intravenously as a bolus), and even drainage of cerebrospinal fluid by repeated lumbar punctures or by placement of intraventricular catheters have been used to control cerebral edema and increased intracranial pressure. Dexamethasone (4 mg intravenously every 4–6 hours) may also decrease cerebral edema.

Therapy of brain abscess consists of drainage (excision or aspiration) in addition to 3–4 weeks of systemic antibiotics directed against isolated organisms. An empiric regimen often includes metronidazole, 500 mg intravenously or orally every 8 hours, plus ceftriaxone, 2 g intravenously every 12 hours (CNS dosing), with or without vancomycin, 10–15 mg/kg/dose intravenously every 12 hours. Vancomycin trough serum levels should be greater than 15 mcg/mL in such patients; however, achievement of an area under the curve/minimal inhibitory concentration (AUC/MIC) ratio of 400–600 is a better predictor of outcome and should be used in confirmed MRSA abscesses. In cases where abscesses are smaller than 2 cm, where there are multiple abscesses that cannot be drained, or if an abscess is located in an area where significant neurologic sequelae would result from drainage, antibiotics for 6–8 weeks can be used without drainage.

In addition to antibiotics, in cases of health care–associated meningitis associated with an external intraventricular catheter, the probability of cure is increased if the catheter is removed. In infections associated with internal ventricular catheters, removal of the internal components and insertion of an external drain is recommended. After collecting cerebrospinal fluid, epidural aspirate, or other specimens for culture, routine empiric treatment for other pathogens (as above) is recommended until the specific cause of the patient's CNS or parameningeal infection has been identified. In addition, early consultation with a neurosurgeon is recommended for those found to have an epidural abscess, phlegmon, vertebral osteomyelitis, discitis, or arachnoiditis to discuss possible surgical management (eg, debridement).

Therapy of other types of meningitis is discussed elsewhere in this book (fungal meningitis, Chapter 36; syphilis and Lyme borreliosis, Chapter 34; tuberculous meningitis, Chapter 33; herpes encephalitis, Chapter 32).

When to Refer

- Patients with acute meningitis, particularly if culture negative or atypical (eg, fungi, syphilis, Lyme disease, *M tuberculosis*), or if hospital acquired, associated with an intraventricular catheter, or if the patient is immunosuppressed.
- Patients with chronic meningitis.
- All patients with brain abscesses and encephalitis.
- Patients with suspected hospital-acquired meningitis (eg, in patients who have undergone recent neurosurgery or epidural or paraspinal corticosteroid injection).
- Patients with recurrent meningitis.

When to Admit

- Patients with suspected acute meningitis, encephalitis, and brain or paraspinous abscess should be admitted for urgent evaluation and treatment.
- There is less urgency to admit patients with chronic meningitis; these patients may be admitted to expedite diagnostic procedures and coordinate care, particularly if no diagnosis has been made in the outpatient setting.

Bystritsky RJ et al. Infectious meningitis and encephalitis. Neurol Clin. 2022;40:77. [PMID: 34798976]

Hasbun R. Healthcare-associated ventriculitis: current and emerging diagnostic and treatment strategies. Expert Rev Anti Infect Ther. 2021;19:993. [PMID: 33334204]

Hurt WJ et al. Combination therapy for HIV-associated cryptococcal meningitis—a success story. J Fungi (Basel). 2021;7:1098. [PMID: 34947080]

Richie MB. Autoimmune meningitis and encephalitis. Neurol Clin. 2022;40:93. [PMID: 34798977]

ANIMAL & HUMAN BITE WOUNDS

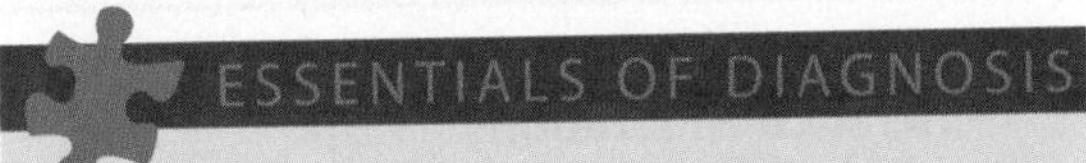

ESSENTIALS OF DIAGNOSIS

- Cat and human bites have higher rates of infection than dog bites.
- Hand bites are particularly concerning for the possibility of closed-space infection.
- Antibiotic prophylaxis indicated for noninfected bites of the hand and hospitalization required for infected hand bites.
- All infected wounds need to be cultured to direct therapy.

General Considerations

About 1000 dog bite injuries require emergency department attention each day in the United States, most often in urban areas. Dog bites occur most commonly in the summer months. Biting animals are usually known by their victims, and most biting incidents are provoked (ie, bites occur while playing with the animal or after surprising the animal while eating or waking it abruptly from sleep). Failure to elicit a history of provocation is important, because *an unprovoked attack raises the possibility of rabies.* Human bites are usually inflicted by children while playing or fighting; in adults, bites are associated with alcohol use and closed-fist injuries that occur during fights.

The animal inflicting the bite, the location of the bite, and the type of injury inflicted are all important determinants of whether they become infected. Cat bites are more likely to become infected than human bites—between 30% and 50% of all cat bites become infected. Infections following human bites are variable. Bites inflicted by children rarely become infected because they are superficial, and bites by adults become infected in 15–30% of cases, with a particularly high rate of infection in closed-fist injuries. Dog bites, for unclear reasons, become infected only 5% of the time. Bites of the head, face, and neck are less likely to become infected than bites on the extremities. "Through and through" bites (eg, involving the mucosa and the skin) have an infection rate similar to closed-fist injuries. Puncture wounds become infected more frequently than lacerations, probably because the latter are easier to irrigate and debride.

The bacteriology of bite infections is polymicrobial. Following dog and cat bites, over 50% of infections are caused by aerobes and anaerobes and 36% are due to aerobes alone. Pure anaerobic infections are rare. *Pasteurella* species are the single most common isolate (75% of infections caused by cat bites and 50% of infections caused by dog bites). Other common aerobic isolates include streptococci, staphylococci, *Moraxella*, and *Neisseria;* the most common anaerobes are *Fusobacterium*, *Bacteroides*, *Porphyromonas*, and *Prevotella*. The median number of isolates following human bites is four (three aerobes and one anaerobe). Like dog and cat bites, infections caused by most human bites are a mixture of aerobes and anaerobes (54%) or are due to aerobes alone (44%). Streptococci and *S aureus* are the most common aerobes. *Eikenella corrodens* (found in up to 30% of patients), *Prevotella*, and *Fusobacterium* are the most common anaerobes. Although the organisms noted are the most common, innumerable others have been isolated—including *Capnocytophaga* (dog and cat), *Pseudomonas*, and *Haemophilus*—emphasizing the point that *all infected bites should be cultured* to define the microbiology.

HIV can be transmitted from bites (either from biting or receiving a bite from a patient with HIV) but has rarely been reported.

Treatment

A. Local Care

Vigorous cleansing and irrigation of the wound as well as debridement of necrotic material are the most important factors in decreasing the incidence of infections. Radiographs should be obtained to look for fractures and the presence of foreign bodies. Careful examination to assess the extent of the injury (tendon laceration, joint space penetration) is critical to appropriate care.

B. Suturing

If wounds require closure for cosmetic or mechanical reasons, suturing can be done. However, *one should never suture an infected wound*, and wounds of the hand should generally not be sutured since a closed-space infection of the hand can result in loss of function.

C. Prophylactic Antibiotics

Prophylaxis is indicated in high-risk bites and in high-risk patients. **Cat bites in any location and hand bites by any animal, including humans, should receive prophylaxis.** Individuals with certain comorbidities (diabetes, liver disease) are at increased risk for severe complications and should receive prophylaxis even for low-risk bites, as should patients without functional spleens who are at increased risk for overwhelming sepsis (primarily with *Capnocytophaga* species). Amoxicillin-clavulanate (Augmentin) 500 mg orally three times daily for 5–7 days is the regimen of choice. For patients with serious allergy to penicillin, a combination of clindamycin 300 mg orally three times daily together with one of the following is recommended for 5–7 days: doxycycline 100 mg orally twice daily, or double-strength TMP-SMZ orally twice daily, or a fluoroquinolone (ciprofloxacin 500 mg orally twice daily or levofloxacin 500–750 mg orally once daily). Moxifloxacin, a fluoroquinolone with good aerobic and anaerobic activity, may be suitable as monotherapy at 400 mg orally once daily for 5–7 days. Agents such as dicloxacillin, cephalexin, macrolides, and clindamycin should not be used alone because they lack activity against *Pasteurella* species. TMP-SMZ has poor activity against anaerobes and should only be used in combination with clindamycin.

Because the risk of HIV transmission is so low following a bite, routine postexposure prophylaxis is *not* recommended. Each case should be evaluated individually and consideration for prophylaxis should be given to those who present within 72 hours of the incident, the source is known to be HIV infected, and the exposure is high risk.

D. Antibiotics for Documented Infection

For wounds that are infected, antibiotics are clearly indicated. How they are given (orally or intravenously) and the need for hospitalization are individualized clinical decisions. The most commonly encountered pathogens require treatment with ampicillin-sulbactam (Unasyn), 1.5–3.0 g intravenously every 6–8 hours; or amoxicillin-clavulanate (Augmentin), 500 mg orally three times daily; or ertapenem, 1 g intravenously daily. For the patient with severe penicillin allergy, a combination of clindamycin, 600–900 mg intravenously every 8 hours, plus a fluoroquinolone (ciprofloxacin, 400 mg intravenously every 12 hours; levofloxacin, 500–750 mg intravenously once daily) is indicated. Duration of therapy is usually 2–3 weeks unless complications such as septic arthritis or osteomyelitis are present; if these complications are present, therapy should be extended to 4 and 6 weeks, respectively.

E. Tetanus and Rabies

All patients must be evaluated for the need for tetanus (see Chapter 33) and rabies (see Chapter 32) prophylaxis.

When to Refer

- If septic arthritis or osteomyelitis is suspected.
- For exposure to bites by dogs, cats, reptiles, amphibians, and rodents.
- When rabies is a possibility.

When to Admit

- Patients with infected hand bites.
- Deep bites, particularly if over joints.

Desai AN. Dog bites. JAMA. 2020;323:2535. [PMID: 32573671]

Greene SE et al. Infectious complications of bite injuries. Infect Dis Clin North Am. 2021;35:219. [PMID: 33494873]

Haskell MG et al. Animal-encounter fatalities, United States, 1999–2016: cause of death and misreporting. Public Health Rep. 2020;135:831. [PMID: 32933400]

Kheiran A et al. Cat bite: an injury not to underestimate. J Plast Surg Hand Surg. 2019;53:341. [PMID: 31287352]

SEXUALLY TRANSMITTED DISEASES

ESSENTIALS OF DIAGNOSIS

- All sexually transmitted diseases (STDs) have subclinical or latent periods, and patients may be asymptomatic.
- Simultaneous infection with several organisms is common.
- All patients who seek STD testing should be screened for syphilis and HIV.
- Partner notification and treatment are important to prevent further transmission and reinfection of the index case.

General Considerations

The most common STDs are gonorrhea,* syphilis,* HPV-associated condyloma acuminatum, chlamydial genital infections,* herpesvirus genital infections, trichomonas

*Reportable to public health authorities.

vaginitis, chancroid,* granuloma inguinale, scabies, louse infestation, and bacterial vaginosis (among women who have sex with women). However, shigellosis*; hepatitis A, B, and C*; amebiasis; giardiasis*; cryptosporidiosis*; salmonellosis*; and campylobacteriosis may also be transmitted by sexual (oral-anal) contact, especially in men who have sex with men. Ebola virus and Zika virus have both been associated with sexual transmission. Both homosexual and heterosexual contact are risk factors for the transmission of HIV (see Chapter 31). All STDs have *subclinical* or *latent phases* that play an important role in long-term persistence of the infection or in its transmission from infected (but largely asymptomatic) persons to other contacts. *Simultaneous infection by several different agents is common.*

Infections typically present in one of several ways, each of which has a defined differential diagnosis, which should prompt appropriate diagnostic tests.

A. Genital Ulcers

Common etiologies include herpes simplex virus, primary syphilis, and chancroid. Other possibilities include lymphogranuloma venereum (see Chapter 33), granuloma inguinale caused by *Klebsiella granulomatis* (see Chapter 33), as well as lesions caused by infection with Epstein-Barr virus and HIV. Noninfectious causes are Behçet disease (see Chapter 20), neoplasm, trauma, drugs, and irritants.

B. Urethritis With or Without Urethral Discharge

The most common infections causing urethral discharge are *Neisseria gonorrhoeae* and *Chlamydia trachomatis*. *N gonorrhoeae* and *C trachomatis* are also frequent causes of prostatitis among sexually active men. Other sexually transmitted infections that can cause urethritis include *Mycoplasma genitalium* and, less commonly, *Ureaplasma urealyticum* and *Trichomonas vaginalis*. Noninfectious causes of urethritis include reactive arthritis with associated urethritis.

C. Vaginal Discharge

Common causes of vaginitis are bacterial vaginosis (caused by overgrowth of anaerobes such as *Gardnerella vaginalis*), candidiasis, and *T vaginalis* (see Chapter 18). Less common infectious causes of vaginitis include HPV-associated condylomata acuminata and group A streptococcus. Noninfectious causes are physiologic changes related to the menstrual cycle, irritants, and lichen planus. Even though *N gonorrhoeae* and *C trachomatis* are frequent causes of cervicitis, they *rarely* produce vaginal discharge.

▶ Screening & Prevention

All persons who seek STD testing should undergo routine screening for HIV infection, using rapid HIV testing (if patients may not follow up for results obtained by standard methods) or nucleic acid amplification followed by confirmatory serology (if primary HIV infection may be a possibility) as indicated. Most algorithms now start with an antigen/antibody combination HIV-1/2 immunoassay with a confirmatory HIV-1/HIV-2 antibody differentiation immunoassay. Patients in whom certain STDs have been diagnosed and treated (chlamydia or gonorrhea, and trichomonas in women) are at a high risk for reinfection and should be encouraged to be rescreened for STDs at 3 months following the initial STD diagnosis.

Asymptomatic patients often request STD screening at the time of initiating a new sexual relationship. Routine HIV testing and hepatitis B serology testing should be offered to all such patients. In sexually active women who have not been recently screened, cervical Papanicolaou testing and nucleic acid amplification testing of a urine specimen for gonorrhea and chlamydia are recommended. Among men who have sex with men, additional screening is recommended for syphilis; hepatitis A; urethral, pharyngeal, and rectal gonorrhea; as well as urethral and rectal chlamydia. Nucleic acid amplification testing is recommended for gonorrhea or chlamydia. There are no recommendations to screen heterosexual men for urethral chlamydia, but this could be considered in STD clinics, adolescent clinics, or correctional facilities. The periodicity of screening thereafter depends on sexual risk, but most screening should be offered at least annually to sexually active adults (particularly to those 25 years old and under). Clinicians should also evaluate transgender men and women for STD screening, based on current anatomy and behaviors practiced. If not immune, *hepatitis B vaccination is recommended for all sexually active adults*, and hepatitis A vaccination in men who have sex with men. Persons between the ages of 9 and 26 should be routinely offered vaccination against HPV (9-valent).

The risk of developing an STD following a sexual assault is difficult to accurately ascertain given high rates of baseline infections and poor follow-up. Victims of assault have a high baseline rate of infection (*N gonorrhoeae*, 6%; *C trachomatis*, 10%; *T vaginalis*, 15%; and bacterial vaginosis, 34%), and the risk of acquiring infection as a result of the assault is significant but is often lower than the preexisting rate (*N gonorrhoeae*, 6–12%; *C trachomatis*, 4–17%; *T vaginalis*, 12%; syphilis, 0.5–3%; and bacterial vaginosis, 19%). Victims should be evaluated within 24 hours after the assault, and nucleic acid amplification tests for *N gonorrhoeae* and *C trachomatis* should be performed. Vaginal secretions are obtained for *Trichomonas* wet mount and culture, or point-of-care testing. If a discharge is present, if there is itching, or if secretions are malodorous, a wet mount should be examined for *Candida* and bacterial vaginosis. In addition, a blood sample should be obtained for immediate serologic testing for syphilis, hepatitis B, and HIV. Follow-up examination for STDs should be repeated within 1–2 weeks, since concentrations of infecting organisms may not have been sufficient to produce a positive test at the time of initial examination. If prophylactic treatment was given (may include postexposure hepatitis B vaccination without hepatitis B immune globulin; treatment for chlamydial, gonorrheal, or trichomonal infection; and emergency contraception), tests should be repeated only if the victim has symptoms. If prophylaxis was not administered, the individual should be seen in 1 week so that any positive tests can be treated. Follow-up serologic testing for syphilis and HIV infection should be performed in 6, 12, and 24 weeks if the initial tests are negative. The usefulness of presumptive therapy is controversial, with some feeling that all patients should receive it and others that it should be limited to those in whom follow-up cannot be ensured or to patients who request it.

Although seroconversion to HIV has been reported following sexual assault when this was the only known risk, this risk is believed to be low. The likelihood of HIV transmission from vaginal or anal receptive intercourse when the source is known to be HIV positive is 1 per 1000 and 5 per 1000, respectively. Although prophylactic antiretroviral therapy has not been studied in this setting, the Department of Health and Human Services recommends the prompt institution of *postexposure prophylaxis with antiretroviral therapy* if the person seeks care within 72 hours of the assault, the source is known to be HIV positive, and the exposure presents a substantial risk of transmission.

In addition to screening asymptomatic patients with STDs, other strategies for preventing further transmission include evaluating sex partners and administering preexposure vaccination of preventable STDs to individuals at risk; other strategies include the consistent use of male and female condoms and **male circumcision**. Adult male circumcision has been shown to decrease the transmission of HIV by 50%, and of herpes simplex virus and HPV by 30% in heterosexual couples in sub-Saharan Africa. For each patient, there are one or more sexual contacts who require diagnosis and treatment. Prompt treatment of contacts by giving antibiotics to the index case to distribute to all sexual contacts (**patient-delivered therapy**) is an important strategy for preventing further transmission and to prevent reinfection of the index case.

Note that vaginal spermicides and condoms containing nonoxynol-9 provide *no* additional protection against STDs. Early initiation of antiretroviral therapy in HIV-infected individuals can prevent HIV acquisition in an uninfected sex partner. Also, preexposure prophylaxis with a once-daily pill containing emtricitabine plus tenofovir disoproxil fumarate (TDF) has been shown to be effective in preventing HIV infection among high-risk men who have sex with men, heterosexual women and men, transgender women, and persons who inject drugs.

When to Refer

- Patients with a new diagnosis of HIV.
- Patients with persistent, refractory, or recurrent STDs, particularly when drug resistance is suspected.

Ambrosioni J et al. Primary HIV-1 infection in users of pre-exposure prophylaxis. Lancet HIV. 2021;8:e166. [PMID: 33316212]

Centers for Disease Control and Prevention (CDC). *Sexually Transmitted Disease Surveillance 2019*. Atlanta: US Department of Health and Human Services; 2021. https://www.cdc.gov/std/statistics/2019/default.htm

Dombrowski JC et al. Doxycycline versus azithromycin for the treatment of rectal chlamydia in men who have sex with men: a randomized controlled trial. Clin Infect Dis. 2021;35:824. [PMID: 33606009]

Inciarte A et al; Sexual Assault Victims Study Group. Postexposure prophylaxis for HIV infection in sexual assault victims. HIV Med. 2020;21:43. [PMID: 31603619]

Michienzi SM et al. Evidence regarding rapid initiation of antiretroviral therapy in patients living with HIV. Curr Infect Dis Rep. 2021;23:7. [PMID: 33824625]

St Cyr S et al. Update to CDC's treatment guidelines for gonococcal infection, 2020. MMWR Morb Mortal Wkly Rep. 2020;69:1911. [PMID: 33332296]

Tuddenham S et al. Diagnosis and treatment of sexually transmitted infections: a review. JAMA. 2022;327:161. [PMID: 35015033]

US Preventive Services Task Force; Krist AH et al. Behavioral counseling interventions to prevent sexually transmitted infections: US Preventive Services Task Force recommendation statement. JAMA. 2020;324:674. [PMID: 32809008]

Workowski KA et al. Sexually transmitted infections treatment guidelines, 2021. MMWR Recomm Rep. 2021;70:1. [PMID: 34292926]

INFECTIONS IN PERSONS WHO INJECT DRUGS

ESSENTIALS OF DIAGNOSIS

- Common infections that occur with greater frequency in persons who inject drugs include:
  - Skin infections, aspiration pneumonia, tuberculosis.
  - Hepatitis A, B, C, D; STDs; HIV/AIDS.
  - Pulmonary septic emboli, infective endocarditis.
  - Osteomyelitis and septic arthritis.

General Considerations

There is a high incidence of infection among persons with opioid use disorder, particularly among people who inject drugs. Increased risk of infection is likely associated with poor hygiene and colonization with potentially pathogenic organisms, contamination of drugs and equipment, increased sexual risk behaviors, and impaired immune defenses. The use of parenterally administered recreational drugs has increased enormously in recent years, fueled in part by an epidemic of prescription opioid misuse and abuse. More than 2 million persons in North America are estimated to have used injection drugs in the past year.

Skin infections are associated with poor hygiene and use of nonsterile technique when injecting drugs. *S aureus* (including community-acquired methicillin-resistant strains) and oral flora (streptococci, *Eikenella, Fusobacterium, Peptostreptococcus*) are the most common organisms, with enteric gram-negatives generally more likely seen in those who inject into the groin. Cellulitis and subcutaneous abscesses occur most commonly, particularly in association with subcutaneous ("skin-popping") or intramuscular injections and the use of cocaine and heroin mixtures (probably due to ischemia). Myositis, clostridial myonecrosis, and necrotizing fasciitis occur infrequently but are life-threatening. Wound botulism in association with black tar heroin occurs sporadically but often in clusters.

Aspiration pneumonia and its complications (lung abscess, empyema, brain abscess) result from altered consciousness associated with drug use. Mixed aerobic and anaerobic mouth flora are usually involved.

Tuberculosis also occurs in persons who use drugs, and infection with HIV has fostered the spread of tuberculosis in this population. Morbidity and mortality rates are increased in individuals with HIV and tuberculosis. Classic radiographic findings are often absent; tuberculosis is suspected in any patient with infiltrates who does not respond to antibiotics.

Hepatitis is very common among persons who inject drugs and is transmissible both by the parenteral (hepatitis B, C, and D) and by the fecal-oral route (hepatitis A). Multiple episodes of hepatitis with different agents can occur. Hepatitis C has also been associated with non-injection heroin use as well as intranasal use of other drugs, likely secondary to blood on shared straws.

Pulmonary septic emboli may originate from venous thrombi or right-sided endocarditis.

STDs are not directly related to drug use, but the practice of exchanging sex for drugs has resulted in an increased frequency of STDs. Syphilis, gonorrhea, and chancroid are the most common.

HIV/AIDS has a high incidence among persons who inject drugs and their sexual contacts and among the offspring of infected women (see Chapter 31).

Infective endocarditis in persons who inject drugs is most commonly caused by *S aureus*, *Candida* (usually *C albicans* or *C parapsilosis*), *Enterococcus faecalis*, other streptococci, and gram-negative bacteria (especially *Pseudomonas* and *Serratia marcescens*). See Chapter 33.

Other vascular infections include septic thrombophlebitis and mycotic aneurysms. Mycotic aneurysms resulting from direct trauma to a vessel with secondary infection most commonly occur in femoral arteries and less commonly in arteries of the neck. Aneurysms resulting from hematogenous spread of organisms frequently involve intracerebral vessels and thus are seen in association with endocarditis.

Osteomyelitis and **septic arthritis** involving vertebral bodies, sternoclavicular joints, the pubic symphysis, the sacroiliac joints, and other sites usually results from hematogenous distribution of injected organisms or septic venous thrombi. Pain and fever precede radiographic changes, sometimes by several weeks. While *S aureus*—often methicillin-resistant—is most common, *Serratia, Pseudomonas, Candida* (often not *C albicans*), and other pathogens rarely encountered in spontaneous bone or joint disease are found in persons who inject drugs.

Treatment

A common and difficult clinical problem is management of a person known to inject drugs who presents with fever. In general, after obtaining appropriate cultures (blood, urine, and sputum if the chest radiograph is abnormal), empiric therapy is begun. If the chest radiograph is suggestive of a community-acquired pneumonia (consolidation), therapy for outpatient pneumonia is begun with ceftriaxone, 1 g intravenously every 24 hours, plus either azithromycin (500 mg orally or intravenously every 24 hours) or doxycycline (100 mg orally or intravenously twice daily). If the chest radiograph is suggestive of septic emboli (nodular infiltrates), therapy for presumed endocarditis is initiated, usually with vancomycin 15 mg/kg/dose every 12 hours intravenously (due to the high prevalence of MRSA and the possibility of enterococcus). If the chest radiograph is normal and no focal site of infection can be found, endocarditis is presumed. While awaiting the results of blood cultures, empiric treatment with vancomycin is started. If blood cultures are positive for organisms that frequently cause endocarditis in drug users (see above), endocarditis is presumed to be present and treated accordingly. In the instance of confirmed methicillin-susceptible *S aureus* infection, vancomycin should be discontinued and treatment initiated with cefazolin or an antistaphylococcal penicillin. If blood cultures are positive for an organism that is an unusual cause of endocarditis, evaluation for an occult source of infection should go forward. In this setting, a transesophageal echocardiogram may be quite helpful since it is 90% sensitive in detecting vegetations and a negative study is strong evidence against endocarditis. If blood cultures are negative and the patient responds to antibiotics, therapy should be continued for 7–14 days (oral therapy can be given once an initial response has occurred). In every patient, careful examination for an occult source of infection (eg, genitourinary, dental, sinus, gallbladder) should be done. Clinicians also can have a significant role to play in integrating treatment of opioid use disorder when patients present with infectious disease complications. This includes screening for opioid use disorder, undergoing specific training for and prescribing opioid use disorder medications, treatment of withdrawal symptoms, and linkage to community-based treatment after hospital discharge.

When to Refer

- Any patient with suspected or proven infective endocarditis.
- Patients with persistent bacteremia.

When to Admit

- Persons who inject drugs with fever.
- Patients with abscesses or progressive skin and soft tissue infection that require debridement.

Appa A et al. Comparative 1-year outcomes of invasive *Staphylococcus aureus* infections among persons with and without drug use: an observational cohort study. Clin Infect Dis. 2022;74:263. [PMID: 33904900]

Dhanani M et al. Antibiotic therapy completion for injection drug use-associated infective endocarditis at a center with routine addiction medicine consultation: a retrospective cohort study. BMC Infect Dis. 2022;22:128. [PMID: 35123439]

Marks LR et al. Infectious complications of injection drug use. Med Clin North Am. 2022;106:187. [PMID: 34823730]

Pericàs JM et al. Prospective cohort study of infective endocarditis in people who inject drugs. J Am Coll Cardiol. 2021;77:544. [PMID: 33538252]

Weimer MB et al. The need for multidisciplinary hospital teams for injection drug use-related infective endocarditis. J Addict Med. 2021 Sep 10. [Epub ahead of print] [PMID: 34510088]

ACUTE INFECTIOUS DIARRHEA

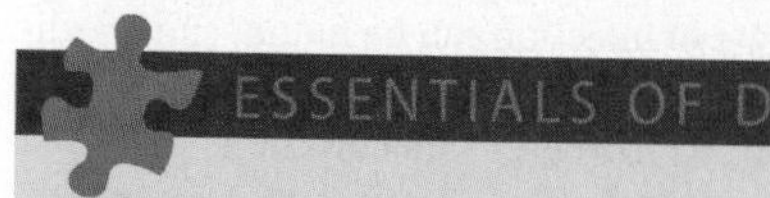

ESSENTIALS OF DIAGNOSIS

- Acute diarrhea: lasts < 2 weeks.
- Chronic diarrhea: lasts > 2 weeks.
- Mild diarrhea: ≤ 3 stools per day.
- Moderate diarrhea: ≥ 4 stools per day with local symptoms (abdominal cramps, nausea, tenesmus).
- Severe diarrhea: ≥ 4 stools per day with systemic symptoms (fever, chills, dehydration).

General Considerations

Acute diarrhea can be caused by a number of different factors, including emotional stress, food intolerance, inorganic agents (eg, sodium nitrite), organic substances (eg, mushrooms, shellfish), medications, and infectious agents (including viruses, bacteria, and protozoa) (Table 30–3). From a diagnostic and therapeutic standpoint, it is helpful to classify infectious diarrhea into syndromes that produce inflammatory or bloody diarrhea and those that are noninflammatory, nonbloody, or watery. In general, the term "**inflammatory diarrhea**" suggests colonic involvement by invasive bacteria or parasites or by toxin production. Patients complain of frequent bloody, small-volume stools, often associated with fever, abdominal cramps, tenesmus, and fecal urgency. Common causes of this syndrome include *Shigella, Salmonella, Campylobacter, Yersinia*, invasive strains of *Escherichia coli*, and other Shiga-toxin–producing strains of *E coli* (STEC), *Entamoeba histolytica*, and *C difficile*. Tests for fecal leukocytes or the neutrophil marker lactoferrin are frequently positive, and definitive etiologic diagnosis requires stool culture. **Noninflammatory diarrhea** is generally milder and is caused by viruses or toxins that affect the small intestine and interfere with salt and water balance, resulting in large-volume watery diarrhea, often with nausea, vomiting, and cramps. Common causes of this syndrome include viruses (eg, rotavirus, norovirus, astrovirus, enteric adenoviruses), vibriones (*Vibrio cholerae, Vibrio parahaemolyticus*), enterotoxin-producing *E coli, Giardia lamblia*, cryptosporidia, and agents that can cause food-borne gastroenteritis. In developed countries, viruses (particularly norovirus) are an important cause of hospitalizations due to acute gastroenteritis among adults.

The term **food poisoning** denotes diseases caused by toxins present in consumed foods. When the incubation period is short (1–6 hours after consumption), the *toxin is usually preformed*. Vomiting is usually a major complaint, and fever is usually absent. Examples include intoxication from *S aureus* or *Bacillus cereus*, and toxin can be detected in the food. When the incubation period is longer—between 8 hours and 16 hours—the organism is present in the food and *produces toxin after being ingested*. Vomiting is less prominent, abdominal cramping is frequent, and fever is often absent. The best example of this disease is that due to *Clostridium perfringens*. Toxin can be detected in food or stool specimens.

The inflammatory and noninflammatory diarrheas discussed above can also be transmitted by food and water and usually have incubation periods between 12 and 72 hours. *Cyclospora*, cryptosporidia, and *Isospora* are protozoans capable of causing disease in both immunocompetent and immunocompromised patients. Characteristics of disease include profuse watery diarrhea that is prolonged but usually self-limited (1–2 weeks) in the immunocompetent patient but can be chronic in the compromised host. Epidemiologic features may be helpful in determining etiology. Recent hospitalization or antibiotic use suggests *C difficile;* recent foreign travel suggests *Salmonella, Shigella, Campylobacter, E coli*, or *V cholerae;* undercooked hamburger suggests STEC; outbreak in long-term care facility, school, or cruise ship suggests norovirus (including newly identified strains, eg, GII.4 Sydney); and fried rice consumption is associated with *B cereus* toxin. Prominent features of some of these causes of diarrhea are listed in Table 30–3.

Treatment

A. General Measures

In general, *most cases of acute gastroenteritis are self-limited and do not require therapy other than supportive measures.* Treatment usually consists of replacement of fluids and electrolytes and, very rarely, management of hypovolemic shock and respiratory compromise. In mild diarrhea, increasing ingestion of juices and clear soups is adequate. In more severe cases of dehydration (postural lightheadedness, decreased urination), oral glucose-based rehydration solutions can be used (Ceralyte, Pedialyte).

B. Specific Measures

In immunocompetent adults, empiric antimicrobial therapy for bloody diarrhea while waiting for results is recommended only with the following circumstances: (1) documented fever, abdominal pain, bloody diarrhea, and bacillary dysentery (frequent scant bloody stools, fever, abdominal cramps, tenesmus) presumptively due to *Shigella*; and (2) returning travelers with a temperature of at least 38.5°C or signs of sepsis.

Either a fluoroquinolone or azithromycin should be used as empiric antimicrobial therapy for bloody diarrhea. Empiric antibacterial treatment should be considered in immunocompromised people with severe illness and bloody diarrhea. Loperamide may be given to immunocompetent adults with acute watery diarrhea but should be avoided with *Shigella* infection or in suspected or proven toxic megacolon. Therapeutic recommendations for specific agents can be found elsewhere in this book.

Table 30–3. Acute bacterial diarrheas and "food poisoning" (listed in alphabetical order).

Organism	Incubation Period	Vomiting	Diarrhea	Fever	Associated Foods	Diagnosis	Clinical Features and Treatment
Bacillus cereus (diarrheal toxin)	10–16 hours	±	+++	–	Toxin in meats, stews, and gravy.	Clinical. Food and stool can be tested for toxin.	Abdominal cramps, watery diarrhea, and nausea lasting 24–48 hours. Supportive care.
Bacillus cereus (preformed toxin)	1–8 hours	+++	±	–	Reheated fried rice causes vomiting or diarrhea.	Clinical. Food and stool can be tested for toxin.	Acute onset, severe nausea and vomiting lasting 24 hours. Supportive care.
Campylobacter jejuni	2–5 days	±	+++	+	Raw or undercooked poultry, unpasteurized milk, water.	Stool culture on special medium.	Fever, diarrhea that can be bloody, cramps. Usually self-limited in 2–10 days. Treat with azithromycin. Fluoroquinolones can be used if susceptibility is confirmed. May be associated with Guillain-Barré syndrome.
Clostridium botulinum	12–72 hours	±	–	–	Clostridia grow in anaerobic acidic environment, eg, canned foods, fermented fish, foods held warm for extended periods.	Stool, serum, and food can be tested for toxin. Stool and food can be cultured.	Diplopia, dysphagia, dysphonia, respiratory embarrassment. Treatment requires clear airway, ventilation, and intravenous polyvalent antitoxin (see text). Symptoms can last for days to months.
Clostridioides difficile	Usually occurs after 7–10 days of antibiotics. Can occur after a single dose or several weeks after completion of antibiotics.	–	+++	++	Associated with antibacterial drugs; clindamycin and beta-lactams most commonly implicated. Fluoroquinolones associated with hypervirulent strains.	Stool tested for toxin.	Abrupt onset of diarrhea that may be bloody; fever. Vancomycin 125 mg orally four times per day or fidaxomicin 200 mg twice daily for 10 days.
Clostridium perfringens	8–16 hours	±	+++	–	Clostridia grow in rewarmed meat and poultry dishes and produce an enterotoxin.	Stools can be tested for enterotoxin or cultured.	Abrupt onset of profuse diarrhea, abdominal cramps, nausea; vomiting occasionally. Recovery usual without treatment in 24–48 hours. Supportive care; antibiotics not needed.
Enterohemorrhagic *Escherichia coli*, including STEC	1–8 days	+	+++	–	Undercooked beef, especially hamburger; unpasteurized milk and juice; raw fruits and vegetables.	STEC can be cultured on special medium. Other toxins can be detected in stool.	Usually abrupt onset of diarrhea, often bloody; abdominal pain. In adults, it is usually self-limited to 5–10 days. In children, it is associated with HUS. Antibiotic therapy may increase risk of HUS. Plasma exchange may help patients with STEC-associated HUS.
Enterotoxigenic *E coli*	1–3 days	±	+++	±	Water, food contaminated with feces.	Stool culture. Special tests required to identify toxin-producing strains.	Watery diarrhea and abdominal cramps, usually lasting 3–7 days. In travelers, fluoroquinolones shorten disease.

(*continued*)

Table 30–3. Acute bacterial diarrheas and "food poisoning" (listed in alphabetical order). (continued)

Organism	Incubation Period	Vomiting	Diarrhea	Fever	Associated Foods	Diagnosis	Clinical Features and Treatment
Noroviruses and other caliciviruses	12–48 hours	++	+++	+	Shellfish and fecally contaminated foods touched by infected food handlers.	Clinical diagnosis with negative stool cultures. PCR available on stool.	Nausea, vomiting (more common in children), diarrhea (more common in adults), fever, myalgias, abdominal cramps. Lasts 12–60 hours. Supportive care.
Rotavirus	1–3 days	++	+++	+	Fecally contaminated foods touched by infected food handlers.	Immunoassay on stool.	Acute onset, vomiting, watery diarrhea that lasts 4–8 days. Supportive care.
Salmonella species	1–3 days	–	++	+	Eggs, poultry, unpasteurized milk, cheese, juices, raw fruits and vegetables.	Routine stool culture.	Gradual or abrupt onset of diarrhea and low-grade fever. No antimicrobials unless high risk (see text) or systemic dissemination is suspected. If susceptibility is confirmed, treatment with ceftriaxone, ciprofloxacin, TMP-SMZ, or amoxicillin is recommended. Prolonged carriage can occur.
Shigella species (mild cases)	24–48 hours	±	+	+	Food or water contaminated with human feces. Person to person spread.	Routine stool culture.	Abrupt onset of diarrhea, often with blood and pus in stools, cramps, tenesmus, and lethargy. Stool cultures are positive. Azithromycin, ciprofloxacin, and ceftriaxone are drugs of choice. Avoid fluoroquinolones if the ciprofloxacin MIC is 0.12 mcg/mL or greater even if the laboratory report identifies the isolate as susceptible. Do not give opioids. Often mild and self-limited.
Staphylococcus (preformed toxin)	1–8 hours	+++	±	±	Staphylococci grow in meats, dairy, and bakery products and produce enterotoxin.	Clinical. Food and stool can be tested for toxin.	Abrupt onset, intense nausea and vomiting for up to 24 hours, recovery in 24–48 hours. Supportive care.
Vibrio cholerae	24–72 hours	+	+++	–	Contaminated water, fish, shellfish, street vendor food.	Stool culture on special medium.	Abrupt onset of liquid diarrhea in endemic area. Needs prompt intravenous or oral replacement of fluids and electrolytes. Doxycycline is drug of choice if antibiotics are indicated. Ciprofloxacin, azithromycin, or ceftriaxone are alternatives.
Vibrio parahaemolyticus	2–48 hours	+	+	±	Undercooked or raw seafood.	Stool culture on special medium.	Abrupt onset of watery diarrhea, abdominal cramps, nausea and vomiting. Recovery is usually complete in 2–5 days.
Yersinia enterocolitica	24–48 hours	±	+	+	Undercooked pork, contaminated water, unpasteurized milk, tofu.	Stool culture on special medium.	Severe abdominal pain (appendicitis-like symptoms), diarrhea, fever. Polyarthritis, erythema nodosum in children. If severe, give TMP-SMZ. Alternatives are cefotaxime and ciprofloxacin. Without treatment, self-limited in 1–3 weeks.

HUS, hemolytic-uremic syndrome; MIC, minimum inhibitory concentration; STEC, Shiga-toxin–producing *E coli* strains; TMP-SMZ, trimethoprim-sulfamethoxazole.

Fleckenstein JM et al. Acute bacterial gastroenteritis. Gastroenterol Clin North Am. 2021;50:283. [PMID: 34024442]
Lucero Y et al. Norovirus: facts and reflections from past, present, and future. Viruses. 2021;13:2399. [PMID: 34960668]
Mattison CP et al. Non-norovirus viral gastroenteritis outbreaks reported to the National Outbreak Reporting System, USA, 2009–2018. Emerg Infect Dis. 2021;27:560. [PMID: 33496216]
Meier JL. Viral acute gastroenteritis in special populations. Gastroenterol Clin North Am. 2021;50:305. [PMID: 34024443]

INFECTIOUS DISEASES IN THE RETURNING TRAVELER

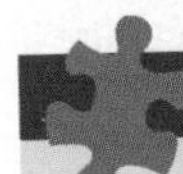

ESSENTIALS OF DIAGNOSIS

- Most infections are common and self-limited.
- Identify patients with transmissible diseases that require isolation.
- The incubation period may be helpful in diagnosis.
  - Less than 3 weeks following exposure may suggest dengue, leptospirosis, and yellow fever.
  - More than 3 weeks suggests typhoid fever, malaria, and tuberculosis.

General Considerations

The differential diagnosis of fever in the returning traveler is broad, ranging from self-limited viral infections to life-threatening illness. The evaluation is best done by identifying whether a particular syndrome is present, then refining the differential diagnosis based on an exposure history. The travel history should include directed questions regarding geography (rural versus urban, specific country and region visited), time of year, animal or arthropod contact, unprotected sexual intercourse, ingestion of untreated water or raw foods, historical or pretravel immunizations, and adherence to malaria prophylaxis.

Etiologies

The most common infectious causes of fever—excluding simple causes such as upper respiratory infections, bacterial pneumonia and UTIs—in returning travelers are malaria (see Chapter 35), diarrhea (see next section), and dengue (see Chapter 32). Others include mononucleosis (associated with Epstein-Barr virus or cytomegalovirus), respiratory infections, including seasonal influenza, influenza A/H1N1 "swine" influenza, and influenza A/H5N1 or A/H7N9 "avian" influenza (see Chapter 32); leptospirosis (see Chapter 34); typhoid fever (see Chapter 33); and rickettsial infections (see Chapter 32). In recent years, coronaviruses have emerged as particularly significant regional and global outbreaks of various sizes (SARS-CoV, MERS-CoV, and the massive global pandemic from SARS-CoV-2). Foreign travel is increasingly recognized as a risk factor for colonization and disease with resistant pathogens, such as ESBL-producing gram-negative organisms. Systemic febrile illnesses without a diagnosis also occur commonly, particularly in travelers returning from sub-Saharan Africa or Southeast Asia.

A. Fever and Rash

Potential etiologies include dengue, Ebola, Chikungunya, and Zika viruses, viral hemorrhagic fever, leptospirosis, meningococcemia, yellow fever, typhus, *Salmonella typhi*, and acute HIV infection.

B. Pulmonary Infiltrates

Tuberculosis, ascaris, *Paragonimus*, and *Strongyloides* can all cause pulmonary infiltrates.

C. Meningoencephalitis

Etiologies include *N meningitidis*, leptospirosis, arboviruses, rabies, and (cerebral) malaria.

D. Jaundice

Consider hepatitis A, yellow fever, hemorrhagic fever, leptospirosis, and malaria.

E. Fever Without Localizing Symptoms or Signs

Malaria, typhoid fever, acute HIV infection, rickettsial illness, visceral leishmaniasis, trypanosomiasis, and dengue are possible etiologies.

F. Traveler's Diarrhea

See next section.

Clinical Findings

Fever and rash in the returning traveler should prompt blood cultures and serologic tests based on the exposure history. The workup of a pulmonary infiltrate should include the placement of a PPD or use of an interferon-gamma release assay, examination of sputum for acid-fast bacilli and possibly for ova and parasites. Patients with evidence of meningoencephalitis should receive lumbar puncture, blood cultures, thick/thin smears of peripheral blood, history-guided serologies, and a nape biopsy (if rabies is suspected). Jaundice in a returning traveler should be evaluated for hemolysis (for malaria), and the following tests should be performed: liver biochemical tests, thick/thin smears of peripheral blood, and directed serologic testing. The workup of traveler's diarrhea is presented in the following section. Finally, patients with fever but no localizing signs or symptoms should have blood cultures performed. Routine laboratory studies usually include CBC with differential, electrolytes, liver biochemical tests, UA, and blood cultures. Thick and thin peripheral blood smears should be done (and repeated in 12–24 hours if clinical suspicion remains high) for malaria if there has been travel to endemic areas. Other studies are directed by the results of history, physical examination, and initial laboratory tests. They may include stool for ova and parasites, chest radiograph, HIV test, and specific serologies (eg, dengue, leptospirosis, rickettsial disease, schistosomiasis, *Strongyloides*). Bone marrow biopsy to diagnose typhoid fever could be helpful in the appropriate patient. Increasingly, next-generation sequencing of plasma or body fluids such as cerebrospinal fluid is used as an adjunctive modality for diagnosis when traditional methods have not yielded a diagnosis.

When to Refer

Travelers with fever, particularly if immunocompromised.

When to Admit

Any evidence of hemorrhage, respiratory distress, hemodynamic instability, and neurologic deficits.

Buss I et al. Aetiology of fever in returning travellers and migrants: a systematic review and meta-analysis. J Travel Med. 2020;27:taaa207. [PMID: 33146395]
Camprubí-Ferrer D et al. Causes of fever in returning travelers: a European multicenter prospective cohort study. J Travel Med. 2022;29:taac002 [PMID: 35040473]
Masuet-Aumatell C et al. Typhoid fever infection—antibiotic resistance and vaccination strategies: a narrative review. Travel Med Infect Dis. 2021;40:101946. [PMID: 33301931]

TRAVELER'S DIARRHEA

ESSENTIALS OF DIAGNOSIS

- Usually a benign, self-limited disease occurring about 1 week into travel.
- Prophylaxis *not* recommended unless there is a comorbid disease (inflammatory bowel syndrome, HIV, immunosuppressive medication).
- Single-dose therapy of a fluoroquinolone usually effective if significant symptoms develop.

General Considerations

Whenever a person travels from one country to another—particularly if the change involves a marked difference in climate, social conditions, or sanitation standards and facilities—diarrhea may develop within 2–10 days. Bacteria cause 80% of cases of traveler's diarrhea, with enterotoxigenic *E coli*, *Shigella* species, and *Campylobacter jejuni* being the most common pathogens. Less common are *Aeromonas*, *Salmonella*, noncholera vibriones, *E histolytica*, and *G lamblia*. Contributory causes include unusual food and drink, change in living habits, occasional viral infections (adenoviruses or rotaviruses), and change in bowel flora. Chronic watery diarrhea may be due to amebiasis or giardiasis or, rarely, tropical sprue.

Clinical Findings

A. Symptoms and Signs

There may be up to ten or even more loose stools per day, often accompanied by abdominal cramps and nausea, occasionally by vomiting, and rarely by fever. The stools are usually watery and not associated with fever when caused by enterotoxigenic *E coli*. With invasive bacterial pathogens (*Shigella, Campylobacter, Salmonella*), stools can be bloody and fever may be present. The illness usually subsides spontaneously within 1–5 days, although 10% remain symptomatic for 1 week or longer, and symptoms persist for longer than 1 month in 2%. Traveler's diarrhea is also a significant risk factor for developing irritable bowel syndrome.

B. Laboratory Findings

In patients with fever and bloody diarrhea, stool culture is indicated, but in most cases, cultures are reserved for those who do not respond to antibiotics.

Prevention

A. General Measures

Avoidance of fresh foods and water sources that are likely to be contaminated is recommended for travelers to developing countries, where infectious diarrheal illnesses are endemic.

B. Specific Measures

Because not all travelers will have diarrhea and because most episodes are brief and self-limited, the recommended approach is to *provide the traveler with a supply of antimicrobials.* Prophylaxis is recommended for those with significant underlying disease (IBD, AIDS, diabetes mellitus, heart disease in older adults, conditions requiring immunosuppressive medications) and for those whose full activity status during the trip is so essential that even short periods of diarrhea would be unacceptable.

Prophylaxis is started upon entry into the destination country and is continued for 1 or 2 days after leaving. For stays of more than 3 weeks, prophylaxis is not recommended because of the cost and increased toxicity. For prophylaxis, several oral antimicrobial once-daily regimens are effective, such as ciprofloxacin, 500 mg, or rifaximin, 200 mg. Bismuth subsalicylate is effective but turns the tongue and the stools black and can interfere with doxycycline absorption, which may be needed for malaria prophylaxis; it is rarely used.

Treatment

For most individuals, the affliction is short-lived, and symptomatic therapy with loperamide is all that is required, provided the patient is not systemically ill (fever 39°C or higher) and does not have dysentery (bloody stools), in which case antimotility agents should be avoided. Packages of oral rehydration salts to treat dehydration are available over the counter in the United States (Infalyte, Pedialyte, others) and in many foreign countries.

When treatment is necessary, in areas where toxin-producing bacteria are the major cause of diarrhea (Latin America and Africa), loperamide (4 mg oral loading dose, then 2 mg after each loose stool to a maximum of 16 mg/day) with a single oral dose of ciprofloxacin (750 mg), levofloxacin (500 mg), or ofloxacin (200 mg) cures most cases of traveler's diarrhea. If diarrhea is associated with bloody stools or persists despite a single dose of a fluoroquinolone, 1000 mg of azithromycin should be taken. In pregnant women and in areas where invasive bacteria more commonly cause diarrhea (Indian subcontinent, Asia, especially Thailand where fluoroquinolone-resistant *Campylobacter* is prevalent), azithromycin is the medication of choice. Rifaximin, a nonabsorbable agent, is also approved for therapy of traveler's diarrhea at a dose of 200 mg orally three times per day or 400 mg twice a day for 3 days. Because luminal concentrations are high, but tissue levels are insufficient, it should not be used in situations where there is a high likelihood of invasive disease (eg, fever, systemic toxicity, or bloody stools).

When to Refer

- Cases refractory to treatment.
- Persistent infection.
- Immunocompromised patient.

When to Admit

Patients who are severely dehydrated or hemodynamically unstable should be admitted to the hospital.

Gefen-Halevi S et al. Persistent abdominal symptoms in returning travelers: clinical and molecular findings. J Travel Med. 2022 Feb 3. [Epub ahead of print] [PMID: 35134178]

Sridhar S et al. Antimicrobial-resistant bacteria in international travelers. Curr Opin Infect Dis. 2021;34:423. [PMID: 34267046]

ANTIMICROBIAL THERAPY

SELECTED PRINCIPLES OF ANTIMICROBIAL THERAPY

Specific steps (outlined below) are required when considering antibiotic therapy for patients. Medications within classes, medications of first choice, and alternative medications are presented in Table 30–4.

A. Etiologic Diagnosis

Based on the organ system involved, the organism causing infection can often be predicted. See Tables 30–5 and 30–6.

B. "Best Guess"

Select an empiric regimen that is likely to be effective against the suspected pathogens.

Table 30–4. Medication of choice for suspected or documented microbial pathogens (listed in alphabetical order, within classes).

Suspected or Proved Etiologic Agent	Medication(s) of First Choice	Alternative Medication(s)
Gram-Negative Cocci		
Moraxella catarrhalis	Cefuroxime, amoxicillin-clavulanic acid	Ceftriaxone, cefuroxime axetil, a fluoroquinolone,[1] a macrolide,[2] a tetracycline,[3] TMP-SMZ[4]
Neisseria gonorrhoeae (gonococcus)	Ceftriaxone + azithromycin or doxycycline	Cefixime + azithromycin or doxycycline[5]
Neisseria meningitidis (meningococcus)	Penicillin[6]	Ceftriaxone, ampicillin
Gram-Positive Cocci		
Enterococcus faecalis	Ampicillin ± gentamicin[7] Ampicillin ± ceftriaxone	Vancomycin ± gentamicin
Enterococcus faecium	Vancomycin ± gentamicin[7]	Linezolid,[8] quinupristin-dalfopristin,[8] daptomycin,[8] tigecycline,[8] tedizolid,[8] oritavancin[8]
Staphylococcus, methicillin-susceptible	Cefazolin or Penicillinase-resistant penicillin[10]	Vancomycin, a cephalosporin,[9] clindamycin, amoxicillin-clavulanic acid, ampicillin-sulbactam
Staphylococcus, methicillin-resistant	Vancomycin	TMP-SMZ,[4] doxycycline, minocycline, linezolid,[8] tedizolid,[8] daptomycin,[8] televancin,[8] dalbavancin,[8] oritavancin,[8] ceftaroline, delafloxacin
Streptococcus, hemolytic, groups A, B, C, G	Penicillin[6]	Macrolide,[2] a cephalosporin,[9] vancomycin, clindamycin
Streptococcus pneumoniae[11] (pneumococcus)	Penicillin[6]	A cephalosporin,[9] vancomycin, clindamycin, a tetracycline,[3] respiratory fluoroquinolones[1]
Viridans streptococci	Penicillin[6]	Cephalosporin,[9] vancomycin

(*continued*)

Table 30–4. Medication of choice for suspected or documented microbial pathogens (listed in alphabetical order, within classes). (continued)

Suspected or Proved Etiologic Agent	Medication(s) of First Choice	Alternative Medication(s)
Gram-Negative Rods		
Acinetobacter	Imipenem, meropenem	Tigecycline, minocycline, doxycycline, aminoglycosides,[12] colistin, cefiderocol
Bacteroides, GI strains	Metronidazole	Ampicillin-sulbactam, piperacillin-tazobactam, ertapenem
Brucella	Doxycycline + rifampin[3]	TMP-SMZ[4] ± gentamicin; ciprofloxacin + rifampin
Burkholderia mallei (glanders)	Streptomycin + tetracycline[3]	Chloramphenicol + streptomycin
Burkholderia pseudomallei (melioidosis)	Ceftazidime	Tetracycline,[3] TMP-SMZ,[4] amoxicillin-clavulanic acid, imipenem or meropenem
Campylobacter jejuni	Azithromycin	A fluoroquinolone[1]
Enterobacter	Ertapenem, imipenem, meropenem, cefepime	Aminoglycoside, a fluoroquinolone,[1] TMP-SMZ[4]
Escherichia coli (uncomplicated outpatient urinary infection)	Nitrofurantoin, fosfomycin	Fluoroquinolones,[1] TMP-SMZ,[4] oral cephalosporin
Escherichia coli (sepsis)[13]	Cefotaxime, ceftriaxone	Ertapenem,[13] imipenem[13] or meropenem,[13] aminoglycosides,[12] aztreonam, ticarcillin-clavulanate, piperacillin-tazobactam, ceftazidime-avibactam,[13,15] ceftolozane-tazobactam,[13,14] meropenem/vaborbactam,[15] imipenem/cilastatin-relebactam[13,14,15]
Haemophilus (respiratory infections, otitis)	Ampicillin-clavulanate	Doxycycline, azithromycin, ceftriaxone, cefuroxime, cefuroxime axetil, TMP-SMZ[4]
Haemophilus (serious infection)	Ceftriaxone	Aztreonam
Helicobacter pylori	PPI, clarithromycin, amoxicillin, and metronidazole	PPI, clarithromycin, and amoxicillin **or** metronidazole
Klebsiella[13]	Ceftriaxone	TMP-SMZ,[4] aminoglycoside,[12] ertapenem,[13] imipenem[13] or meropenem,[13] a fluoroquinolone,[1] aztreonam, ticarcillin-clavulanate, piperacillin-tazobactam, ceftazidime-avibactam,[13] ceftolozane-tazobactam,[13,14] meropenem/vaborbactam,[15] imipenem/cilastatin-relebactam[13,14,15]
Legionella species (pneumonia)	Azithromycin, or fluoroquinolones[1] ± rifampin	Doxycycline ± rifampin
Prevotella, oropharyngeal strains	Clindamycin	Metronidazole
Proteus mirabilis	Ampicillin	TMP-SMZ,[4] a fluoroquinolone,[1] a cephalosporin[9]
Proteus vulgaris and other species (*Morganella, Providencia*)	Ceftriaxone	Ertapenem, imipenem or meropenem, TMP-SMZ,[4] a fluoroquinolone[1]
Pseudomonas aeruginosa	Piperacillin-tazobactam or ceftazidime or cefepime, or imipenem or meropenem or doripenem or aztreonam (any one of the previous agents) ± aminoglycoside[12]	Ciprofloxacin (or levofloxacin) ± piperacillin-tazobactam; ciprofloxacin (or levofloxacin) ± ceftazidime; ciprofloxacin (or levofloxacin) ± cefepime; ceftazidime-avibactam[13]; ceftolozane-tazobactam,[13] cefiderocol, imipenem/cilastatin-relebactam, meropenem/vaborbactam
Salmonella (bacteremia)	Ceftriaxone	A fluoroquinolone[1]
Serratia	Carbapenem	TMP-SMZ,[4] a fluoroquinolone,[1] ceftriaxone
Shigella	Azithromycin, ciprofloxacin, or ceftriaxone	TMP-SMZ[4]
Vibrio (cholera, sepsis)	A tetracycline[3]	TMP-SMZ,[4] a fluoroquinolone[1]
Yersinia pestis (plague)	Streptomycin ± a tetracycline[3]	Chloramphenicol, TMP-SMZ[5]
Gram-Positive Rods		
Actinomyces	Penicillin[6]	Tetracycline,[3] clindamycin
Bacillus (including anthrax)	Penicillin[6]	A macrolide,[2] a fluoroquinolone[1]
Clostridium (eg, gas gangrene, tetanus)	Penicillin[6]	Metronidazole, clindamycin, imipenem, or meropenem
Corynebacterium diphtheria	Macrolide[2]	Penicillin[6]
Corynebacterium jeikeium	Vancomycin	Linezolid
Listeria	Ampicillin ± aminoglycoside[12]	TMP-SMZ[4]

(*continued*)

Table 30–4. Medication of choice for suspected or documented microbial pathogens (listed in alphabetical order, within classes). (continued)

Suspected or Proved Etiologic Agent	Medication(s) of First Choice	Alternative Medication(s)
Acid-Fast Rods		
Mycobacterium avium complex	Clarithromycin or azithromycin + ethambutol, ± rifabutin	Amikacin, ciprofloxacin
Mycobacterium fortuitum-chelonei	Cefoxitin + clarithromycin	Amikacin, rifampin, sulfonamide, doxycycline, linezolid
Mycobacterium kansasii	INH + rifampin ± ethambutol	Clarithromycin, azithromycin, ethionamide, cycloserine
Mycobacterium leprae	Dapsone + rifampin ± clofazimine	Minocycline, ofloxacin, clarithromycin
Mycobacterium tuberculosis[16]	Isoniazid (INH) + rifampin + pyrazinamide ± ethambutol	Other antituberculous drugs (see Tables 9–14 and 9–15)
Nocardia	TMP-SMZ[4]	Minocycline, imipenem or meropenem, linezolid
Spirochetes		
Borrelia burgdorferi (Lyme disease)	Doxycycline, amoxicillin, cefuroxime axetil	Ceftriaxone, penicillin, azithromycin
Borrelia recurrentis (relapsing fever)	Doxycycline[3]	Penicillin[6]
Leptospira	Penicillin[6]	Doxycycline,[3] ceftriaxone
Treponema pallidum (syphilis)	Penicillin[6]	Doxycycline, ceftriaxone
Treponema pertenue (yaws)	Penicillin[6]	Doxycycline
Mycoplasmas	**Azithromycin or doxycycline**	**A fluoroquinolone[1]**
Chlamydiae		
C pneumoniae	Doxycycline[3]	Azithromycin, a fluoroquinolone[1,17]
C psittaci	Doxycycline	Chloramphenicol
C trachomatis (urethritis or pelvic inflammatory disease)	Doxycycline or azithromycin	Levofloxacin, ofloxacin
Rickettsiae	**Doxycycline[3]**	**Chloramphenicol, a fluoroquinolone[1]**

[1]Fluoroquinolones include ciprofloxacin, levofloxacin, moxifloxacin, and others. Gemifloxacin, levofloxacin, and moxifloxacin, the so-called respiratory fluoroquinolones, demonstrate the most reliable activity against penicillin-resistant *S pneumoniae* and other respiratory infection pathogens. Delafloxacin is predictably active against methicillin-resistant *S aureus* (MRSA).
[2]Azithromycin is the preferred macrolide due to increased safety profile and minimal drug interaction potential.
[3]All tetracyclines have similar activity against most microorganisms. Minocycline (the most active tetracycline) and doxycycline are more active than tetracycline against *S aureus*.
[4]TMP-SMZ is a mixture of 1 part trimethoprim and 5 parts sulfamethoxazole.
[5]Test of cure required if ceftriaxone not used.
[6]Penicillin G is preferred for parenteral injection; penicillin V for oral administration.
[7]Addition of gentamicin indicated only for severe enterococcal infections (eg, endocarditis, meningitis).
[8]Linezolid, tedizolid, daptomycin, televancin, dalbavancin, and oritavancin should be reserved for the treatment of vancomycin-resistant isolates or in patients intolerant of vancomycin.
[9]Most intravenous cephalosporins (with the exception of ceftazidime) are active against streptococci and methicillin-susceptible staphylococci.
[10]Parenteral nafcillin or oxacillin; oral dicloxacillin, cloxacillin, or oxacillin.
[11]Infections caused by isolates with intermediate resistance may respond to high dose penicillin or ceftriaxone or the respiratory fluoroquinolones (gemifloxacin, levofloxacin, and moxifloxacin). Infections caused by highly penicillin-resistant isolates should be treated with vancomycin. Penicillin-resistant pneumococci are often resistant to macrolides, tetracyclines, and TMP-SMZ.
[12]Aminoglycosides—gentamicin, tobramycin, amikacin, netilmicin, plazomicin—should be chosen on the basis of local patterns of susceptibility.
[13]Extended beta-lactamase–producing (ESBL) isolates should be treated with a carbapenem. If a carbapenem cannot be used, ceftazidime-avibactam or possibly ceftolozane-tazobactam can be considered.
[14]Ceftolozane-tazobactam, cefiderocol, imipenem/cilastatin-relebactam and occasionally ceftazidime-avibactam may be active against multidrug-resistant *P aeruginosa*.
[15]Consider in cases of infection due to carbapenemase-producing *Enterobacteriaceae*.
[16]Resistance is common and susceptibility testing must be performed.
[17]Ciprofloxacin has inferior antichlamydial activity compared with levofloxacin or ofloxacin.
±, alone or combined with.

Table 30–5. Examples of initial antimicrobial therapy for acutely ill, hospitalized adults pending identification of causative organism (listed in alphabetical order).

Suspected Clinical Diagnosis	Likely Etiologic Diagnosis	Medication of Choice
Brain abscess	Mixed anaerobes, pneumococci, streptococci	Ceftriaxone, 2 g intravenously every 12 hours **plus** metronidazole, 500 mg orally/intravenous every 8 hours, **plus** vancomycin, 15–20 mg/kg intravenously every 8–12 hours[1]
Endocarditis, acute (including injection drug user)	*Staphylococcus aureus*, *Enterococcus faecalis*, viridans streptococci	Vancomycin, 15–20 mg/kg/dose intravenously every 8-12 hours[1]
Fever in neutropenic patient receiving cancer chemotherapy	*S aureus*, *Pseudomonas*, *Klebsiella*, *Escherichia coli*	Cefepime, 2 g intravenously every 8 hours. If concerned for MRSA infection, add vancomycin 15–20 mg/kg intravenously every 8–12 hours[1]
Intra-abdominal sepsis (eg, postoperative, peritonitis, cholecystitis)	Gram-negative bacteria, *Bacteroides*, anaerobic bacteria, enterococcus	Piperacillin-tazobactam, 4.5 g intravenously every 6–8 hours, **or** ertapenem, 1 g every 24 hours
Meningitis, bacterial, age > 50 years, community-acquired	Pneumococcus, meningococcus, *Listeria monocytogenes*,[2] gram-negative bacilli, group B streptococcus	Ampicillin, 2 g intravenously every 4 hours, **plus** ceftriaxone, 2 g intravenously every 12 hours, **plus** vancomycin, 15–20 mg/kg intravenously every 8–12 hours[1]
Meningitis, bacterial, community-acquired	*Streptococcus pneumoniae* (pneumococcus),[3] *Neisseria meningitidis* (meningococcus)	Ceftriaxone, 2 g intravenously every 12 hours,[3] **plus** vancomycin, 15–20 mg/kg intravenously every 8–12 hours[1]
Meningitis, postoperative (or posttraumatic)	*S aureus*, gram-negative bacilli, coagulase-negative staphylococci, diphtheroids (eg, *Propionibacterium acnes*) (uncommon) pneumococcus (in posttraumatic)	Vancomycin, 15–20 mg/kg intravenously every 8–12 hours[1], **plus** cefepime, 2 g intravenously every 8 hours
Osteomyelitis	*S aureus*, secondarily gram-negative aerobes	Vancomycin 15–20 mg/kg intravenously every 8–12 hours,[1] **plus** ceftriaxone 2 g intravenously every 24 hours
Pneumonia, acute, community-acquired, non-ICU hospital admission	Pneumococci, *Mycoplasma pneumoniae*, *Legionella*, *Chlamyodophila pneumoniae*	Ceftriaxone, 1 g intravenously every 24 hours or ampicillin-sulbactam 1.5–3 g intravenously every 6 hours) **plus** azithromycin, 500 mg intravenously every 24 hours; **or** a respiratory fluoroquinolone[4] alone
Pneumonia, postoperative or nosocomial	*S aureus*, mixed anaerobes, gram-negative bacilli	Cefepime, 2 g intravenously every 8 hours; **or** ceftazidime, 2 g intravenously every 8 hours; **or** piperacillin-tazobactam, 4.5 g intravenously every 6–8 hours; **or** imipenem, 500 mg intravenously every 6 hours; **or** meropenem, 1 g intravenously every 8 hours **plus** tobramycin, 5–7 mg/kg intravenously every 24 hours; **or** ciprofloxacin, 400 mg intravenously every 8 hours; **or** levofloxacin, 750 mg intravenously every 24 hours **plus** vancomycin, 15–20 mg/kg/dose intravenously every 8–12 hours[1]
Pyelonephritis with flank pain and fever (recurrent UTI)	*E coli*, *Klebsiella*, *Enterobacter*, *Pseudomonas*	Ceftriaxone, 1 g intravenously every 24 hours; **or** if culture results confirm susceptibility, ciprofloxacin, 400 mg intravenously every 12 hours (500 mg orally); **or** levofloxacin, 500 mg once daily (intravenously/orally)
Septic arthritis	*S aureus*, *N gonorrhoeae*	Ceftriaxone, 1–2 g intravenously every 24 hours
Septic thrombophlebitis (eg, intravenous tubing, intravenous shunts)	*S aureus*, gram-negative aerobic bacteria	Vancomycin, 15 mg/kg/dose intravenously every 12 hours[1], **plus** ceftriaxone, 1 g intravenously every 24 hours

[1]Vancomycin serum levels should be monitored. Select drug interval based on estimated kidney function and dose rounded to nearest 250 mg.
[2]TMP-SMZ can be used to treat *Listeria monocytogenes* in patients allergic to penicillin in a dosage of 15–20 mg/kg/day of TMP in three or four divided doses.
[3]Including penicillin-resistant isolates.
[4]Levofloxacin 750 mg/day, moxifloxacin 400 mg/day.

Table 30–6. Examples of empiric choices of antimicrobials for adult outpatient infections (listed in alphabetical order, except for syphils).

Suspected Clinical Diagnosis	Likely Etiologic Agents	Medications of Choice	Alternative Medications
Acute sinusitis	*Streptococcus pneumoniae, Haemophilus influenzae, Moraxella catarrhalis*	Amoxicillin-clavulanate,[1] 875 mg orally twice daily for 5–7 days	For patients allergic to penicillin, doxycycline, 100 mg twice daily for 5–7 days
Aspiration pneumonia	Mixed oropharyngeal flora, including anaerobes	Clindamycin, 300 mg orally four times daily for 5–7 days	Amoxicillin 500 mg orally three times daily for 5–7 days
Cystitis (uncomplicated)	*Escherichia coli, Staphylococcus saprophyticus, Klebsiella pneumoniae, Proteus* species, other gram-negative rods or enterococci	Nitrofurantoin monohydrate macrocrystals 100 mg twice daily for 5–7 days (unless pregnant); fosfomycin 3 g orally as a single dose	Cephalexin, 500 mg orally four times daily for 7 days, for uncomplicated cystitis. Due to increasing bacterial resistance, TMP-SMZ and fluoroquinolones are **not** recommended as first-line therapy for empiric treatment
Erysipelas, impetigo, nonpurulent cellulitis, ascending lymphangitis	Group A streptococcus	Penicillin V, 250–500 mg orally four times daily for 5–7 days	Cephalexin, 500 mg orally four times daily for 5–7 days
Furuncle with surrounding cellulitis	*Staphylococcus aureus*	Dicloxacillin, 500 mg orally four times daily for 5–7 days for MSSA. For CA-MRSA: TMP-SMZ[2] one to two double-strength tablet twice daily for 5–7 days; **or** clindamycin 300 mg orally three to four times daily for 5–7 days	Cephalexin, 500 mg orally four times daily for 5–7 days for MSSA. For CA-MRSA, doxycycline, 100 mg orally twice daily, is a reasonable alternative
Gastroenteritis	*Salmonella, Shigella, Campylobacter, Entamoeba histolytica*	See footnote 3	
Otitis media	*S pneumoniae, H influenzae, M catarrhalis*	Amoxicillin, 500 mg–1 g orally three times daily for 7–10 days	Amoxicillin-clavulanate,[1] 875 mg orally twice daily; **or** cefuroxime, 500 mg orally twice daily; **or** cefpodoxime, 200–400 mg daily; **or** doxycycline, 100 mg twice daily
Pelvic inflammatory disease	*Neisseria gonorrhoeae, Chlamydia trachomatis*, anaerobes, gram-negative rods	Ceftriaxone 500 mg intramuscularly once plus doxycycline 100 mg orally twice daily for 14 days **plus** metronidazole 500 mg orally twice daily for 14 days; **or** cefoxitin 2 g intramuscularly once **plus** probenecid 1 g orally once, **plus** doxycycline 100 mg orally twice daily for 14 days **plus** metronidazole 500 mg orally twice daily for 14 days	—
Pharyngitis	Group A streptococcus	Penicillin V, 500 mg orally four times daily, **or** amoxicillin, 500 mg–1 g orally three times daily for 10 days	For patients with history of mild penicillin allergy, cephalexin, 500 mg orally four times daily for 10 days; for patients with IgE-mediated reaction, clindamycin, 300 mg orally four times daily for 10 days; **or** azithromycin, 500 mg on day 1 and 250 mg on days 2–5
Pneumonia	*S pneumoniae, Mycoplasma pneumoniae, Legionella pneumophila, Chlamydophila pneumoniae*	Amoxicillin, 1 g three times daily **or** Doxycycline, 100 mg orally twice daily	For patients at high risk for infection due to resistant pneumococci: amoxicillin-clavulanate **or** cefpodoxime **or** cefuroxime + macrolide or doxycycline **or** a respiratory fluoroquinolone[4]

(*continued*)

Table 30–6. Examples of empiric choices of antimicrobials for adult outpatient infections (listed in alphabetical order, except for syphils). (continued)

Suspected Clinical Diagnosis	Likely Etiologic Agents	Medications of Choice	Alternative Medications
Pyelonephritis	*E coli, K pneumoniae, Proteus* species, *S saprophyticus*	Fluoroquinolones[5] for 7 days if prevalence of resistance among uropathogens is < 10%	TMP-SMZ,[2] one to two double-strength tablets twice daily for 7–14 days for susceptible pathogens. Oral beta-lactams are less effective than fluoroquinolones or TMP-SMZ
Urethritis, epididymitis	*N gonorrhoeae, C trachomatis*	Ceftriaxone, 500 mg intramuscularly once for *N gonorrhoeae*; doxycycline, 100 mg orally twice daily for 7 days, for *C trachomatis*	Gentamicin 240 mg intramuscularly once **or** cefixime 800 mg orally once for *N gonorrhoeae*[6] Alternatives for *C trachomatis* include azithromycin 1 g orally once **or** levofloxacin 500 mg orally once daily for 7 days
Syphilis			
Early syphilis (primary, secondary, or latent of < 1 year's duration)	*Treponema pallidum*	Benzathine penicillin G, 2.4 million units intramuscularly once	Doxycycline, 100 mg orally twice daily for 2 weeks. Ceftriaxone, 1 g intravenously or intramuscularly once daily for 10 days
Latent syphilis of > 1 year's duration or cardiovascular syphilis	*T pallidum*	Benzathine penicillin G, 2.4 million units intramuscularly once a week for 3 weeks (total: 7.2 million units)	Doxycycline, 100 mg orally twice daily for 4 weeks
Neurosyphilis	*T pallidum*	Aqueous penicillin G, 18–24 million units/day intravenously for 10–14 days	—

[1]Amoxicillin-clavulante is available as a combination of amoxicillin, 250 mg, 500 mg, or 875 mg, plus 125 mg of clavulanic acid. Augmentin XR is a combination of amoxicillin 1 g and clavulanic acid 62.5 mg.
[2]TMP-SMZ is a fixed combination of 1 part trimethoprim and 5 parts sulfamethoxazole. Single-strength tablets: 80 mg TMP, 400 mg SMZ; double-strength tablets: 160 mg TMP, 800 mg SMZ.
[3]The diagnosis should be confirmed by culture before therapy. *Salmonella* gastroenteritis generally does not require therapy. For susceptible *Shigella* isolates, give ciprofloxacin, 500 mg orally twice daily for 5 days. For *Campylobacter* infection, give azithromycin, 1 g orally for one dose, or ciprofloxacin, 500 mg orally twice daily for 5 days. For *E histolytica* infection, give metronidazole, 750 mg orally three times daily for 5–10 days, followed by an intraluminally active drug such as paromomycin 10 mg/kg orally three times daily for 7 days.
[4]Fluoroquinolones with activity against *S pneumoniae*, including penicillin-resistant isolates, include levofloxacin (500–750 mg orally once daily), moxifloxacin (400 mg orally once daily), or gemifloxacin (320 mg orally once daily). Use fluoroquinolones as medication of choice if recent non-fluoroquinolone antibiotic use within 3 months.
[5]Fluoroquinolones and dosages include ciprofloxacin, 500 mg orally twice daily; ofloxacin, 400 mg orally twice daily; and levofloxacin, 500 mg orally daily.
[6]Test of cure recommended if ceftriaxone is not used.
CA-MRSA, community-acquired methicillin-resistant *Staphylococcus aureus*; MRSA, methicillin-resistant *S aureus*; MSSA, methicillin-susceptible *S aureus*; TMP-SMZ, trimethoprim-sulfamethoxazole.

C. Laboratory Control

Specimens for laboratory examination should be obtained before institution of therapy to determine susceptibility.

D. Clinical Response

Based on clinical response and other data, the laboratory reports are evaluated and then the desirability of changing the regimen is considered. If the specimen was obtained from a normally sterile site (eg, blood, cerebrospinal fluid, pleural fluid, joint fluid), the recovery of a microorganism in significant amounts is meaningful even if the organism recovered is different from the clinically suspected agent, and this may force a change in treatment. Isolation of unexpected microorganisms from the respiratory tract, GI tract, or surface lesions (sites that have a complex flora) may represent colonization or contamination, and cultures must be critically evaluated before medications are abandoned that were judiciously selected on a "best guess" basis.

E. Drug Susceptibility Tests

Some microorganisms are predictably inhibited by certain medications; if such organisms are isolated, they need not be tested for drug susceptibility. For example, all group A hemolytic streptococci are inhibited by penicillin. Other organisms (eg, enteric gram-negative rods) are variably susceptible and generally require susceptibility testing whenever they are isolated. Organisms that once had predictable susceptibility patterns are now associated with resistance and require testing. Examples include the pneumococci, which may be resistant to multiple medications (including penicillin, macrolides, and tetracyclines); the enterococci, which may be resistant to penicillin, aminoglycosides, and vancomycin; and ESBL producing–*E coli* resistant to third-generation cephalosporins, aminoglycosides, and fluoroquinolones.

When culture and susceptibility results have been finalized, clinicians must use the most narrow-spectrum agent and the shortest duration possible to decrease the selection pressure for antibacterial resistance.

Antimicrobial drug susceptibility tests may be performed on solid media as disk diffusion tests, in broth, in tubes, in wells of microdilution plates, or as E-tests (strips with increasing concentration of antibiotic). The latter three methods yield results expressed as MIC. In most infections, the MIC is the appropriate in vitro test to guide selection of an antibacterial agent. When there appear to be marked discrepancies between susceptibility testing and clinical response, the following possibilities must be considered:

1. Selection of an inappropriate medication, medication dosage, or route of administration.
2. Failure to drain a collection of pus or to remove a foreign body.
3. Failure of a poorly diffusing drug to reach the site of infection (eg, CNS) or to reach intracellular phagocytosed bacteria.
4. Superinfection in the course of prolonged chemotherapy.
5. Emergence of drug resistance in the original pathogen or superinfection with a new more resistant organism.
6. Participation of two or more microorganisms in the infectious process, of which only one was originally detected and used for medication selection.
7. Inadequate host defenses, including immunodeficiencies and diabetes mellitus.
8. Noninfectious causes, including drug fever, malignancy, and autoimmune disease.

F. Promptness of Response

Response depends on a number of factors, including the patient (immunocompromised patients respond slower than immunocompetent patients), the site of infection (deep-seated infections such as osteomyelitis and endocarditis respond more slowly than superficial infections such as cystitis or cellulitis), the pathogen (virulent organisms such as *S aureus* respond more slowly than viridans streptococci; mycobacterial and fungal infections respond slower than bacterial infections), and the duration of illness (in general, the longer the symptoms are present, the longer it takes to respond). Thus, depending on the clinical situation, persistent fever and leukocytosis several days after initiation of therapy may not indicate improper choice of antibiotics but may be due to the natural history of the disease being treated. In most infections, either a bacteriostatic or a bactericidal agent can be used. In some infections (eg, infective endocarditis and meningitis), a bactericidal agent should be used. When potentially toxic medications (eg, aminoglycosides, flucytosine) are used, serum levels of the medication are measured to minimize toxicity and ensure appropriate dosage. In patients with altered renal or hepatic clearance of medications, the dosage or frequency of administration must be adjusted; it is best to measure levels in older adults, in morbidly obese patients, or in those with altered kidney function when possible and adjust therapy accordingly.

G. Duration of Antimicrobial Therapy

Generally, effective antimicrobial treatment results in reversal of the clinical and laboratory parameters of active infection and marked clinical improvement. However, varying periods of treatment may be required for cure. Key factors include (1) the type of infecting organism (bacterial infections generally can be cured more rapidly than fungal or mycobacterial ones), (2) the location of the process (eg, endocarditis and osteomyelitis require prolonged therapy), and (3) the immunocompetence of the patient.

H. Adverse Reactions and Toxicity

These include hypersensitivity reactions, direct toxicity, superinfection by drug-resistant microorganisms, and drug interactions. If the infection is life-threatening and treatment cannot be stopped, the reactions are managed symptomatically or another medication is chosen that does not cross-react with the offending one (Table 30–4). If the infection is less serious, it may be possible to stop all antimicrobials and monitor the patient closely.

I. Route of Administration

Intravenous therapy is preferred for acutely ill patients with serious infections (eg, endocarditis, meningitis, sepsis, severe pneumonia) when dependable levels of antibiotics are required for successful therapy. Certain medications (eg, doxycycline, fluconazole, voriconazole, rifampin, metronidazole, TMP-SMZ, and fluoroquinolones) are so well absorbed that they generally can be administered orally in seriously ill—but not hemodynamically unstable—patients.

Food does not significantly influence the bioavailability of most oral antimicrobial agents. However, the tetracyclines (particularly tetracycline) and the quinolones chelate multivalent cations resulting in decreased oral bioavailability. Posaconazole suspension should always be administered with food.

A major complication of intravenous antibiotic therapy is infection due to the manipulation of the intravenous catheter. Peripheral catheters are changed every 48–72 hours to decrease the likelihood of catheter-associated infection, and antimicrobial-coated central venous catheters (minocycline and rifampin, chlorhexidine and sulfadiazine) have been associated with a decreased incidence of these infections. Most of these infections present with local signs of infection (erythema, tenderness) at the insertion site. In a patient with fever who is receiving intravenous therapy, the catheter must always be considered a potential source.

Small-gauge (20–23F) peripherally inserted silicone or polyurethane catheters (Per Q Cath, A-Cath, Ven-A-Cath, and others) are associated with a low infection rate and can be maintained for 3–6 months without replacement. Such catheters are ideal for long-term outpatient antibiotic therapy.

J. Cost of Antibiotics

The cost of these agents can be substantial. In addition to acquisition costs and monitoring costs (drug levels, liver biochemical tests, electrolytes, etc), the cost of treating adverse reactions, the cost of treatment failure and superinfection, and the costs associated with drug administration must be considered.

K. Antimicrobial Stewardship

Antimicrobial stewardship is a critically important tool intended to optimize clinical outcomes while minimizing unintended consequences of antimicrobial use. These consequences include drug toxicity, superinfection, emergence of bacterial resistance, and impact upon the human microbiome. **The Infectious Diseases Society of America recommends establishment of an antimicrobial stewardship team at all acute care facilities.** The core members of a stewardship team should include an infectious diseases physician and a clinical pharmacist with infectious diseases training. If possible, the addition of a clinical microbiologist, an information system specialist, an infection control professional, and a hospital epidemiologist would be preferable. Key strategies for a stewardship team, as well as the individual prescriber, should include questions associated with the "Four Moments of Antibiotic Decision Making": (1) Does this patient have an infection that requires antibiotics? (2) Have the appropriate cultures been ordered before starting antibiotics? (3) After a few days of empiric antibiotics have passed, can antibiotics be stopped? Can therapy be narrowed? Can therapy be switched from intravenous to oral? (4) What duration of antibiotic therapy is necessary for this patient's diagnosis? Stewardship interventions centered upon one or more of the above questions have been demonstrated to decrease the risk of *C difficile* and *Candida* superinfection as well as attenuate the negative impact of antibiotics on the human microbiome.

Kadri SS et al. U.S. efforts to curb antibiotic resistance—are we saving lives? N Engl J Med. 2020;383:806. [PMID: 32846058]

Kelly CR et al. ACG clinical guidelines: prevention, diagnosis, and treatment of *Clostridioides difficile* infections. Am J Gastroenterol. 2021;116:1124. [PMID: 34003176]

Tamma PD et al. Rethinking how antibiotics are prescribed: incorporating the 4 moments of antibiotic decision making into clinical practice. JAMA. 2019;321:139. [PMID: 30589917]

HYPERSENSITIVITY

Penicillin Allergy

All penicillins are cross-sensitizing and cross-reacting. Skin tests using penicilloyl-polylysine and undegraded penicillin can identify most individuals with IgE-mediated reactions (eg, hives, bronchospasm). In those patients with positive reaction to skin tests, the incidence of subsequent immediate severe reactions associated with penicillin administration is high. A history of a penicillin reaction in the past is often *not* reliable. Only a small proportion (less than 5%) of patients with a stated history of penicillin allergy experience an adverse reaction when challenged with the medication. The decision to administer penicillin or related medications (other beta-lactams) to patients with an allergic history depends on the severity of the reported reaction, the severity of the infection being treated, and the availability of alternative medications. For patients with a history of severe reaction (anaphylaxis), alternative medications should be used. In the rare situations when there is a strong indication for using penicillin (eg, syphilis in pregnancy) in allergic patients, desensitization can be performed. If the reaction is mild (nonurticarial rash), the patient may be rechallenged with penicillin or may be given another beta-lactam antibiotic.

Allergic reactions include anaphylaxis, serum sickness (urticaria, fever, joint swelling, angioedema 7–12 days after exposure), skin rashes, fever, interstitial nephritis, eosinophilia, hemolytic anemia, other hematologic disturbances, and vasculitis. The incidence of hypersensitivity to penicillin is estimated to be 1–5% among adults in the United States. Life-threatening anaphylactic reactions are very rare (0.05%). Ampicillin produces maculopapular skin rashes more frequently than other penicillins, but many ampicillin (and other beta-lactam) rashes are not allergic in origin. The nonallergic ampicillin rash usually occurs after 3–4 days of therapy, is maculopapular, is more common in patients with coexisting viral illness (especially Epstein-Barr infection), and resolves with continued therapy. The maculopapular rash may or may not reappear with rechallenge. Beta-lactams can induce nephritis with primary tubular lesions associated with anti-basement membrane antibodies.

If the intradermal test described below is negative, desensitization is not necessary, and a full dose of the penicillin may be given. If the test is positive, alternative medications should be strongly considered. If that is not feasible, desensitization is necessary.

Patients with a history of allergy to penicillin are also at an increased risk for having a reaction to cephalosporins or carbapenems. A common approach to these patients is to assess the severity of the reaction. If an IgE-mediated reaction to penicillin can be excluded by history, a cephalosporin can be administered. When the history justifies concern about an immediate-type reaction, penicillin skin testing should be performed. If the test is negative, the cephalosporin or carbapenem can be given. If the test is positive, there is a 5–10% chance of cross-reactivity with cephalosporins, and the decision whether to use cephalosporins depends on the availability of alternative agents and the severity of the infection. While carbapenems were considered highly cross-reactive with penicillins, the cross-reactivity appears to be minimal (1%).

Caruso C et al. Beta-lactam allergy and cross-reactivity: a clinician's guide to selecting an alternative antibiotic. J Asthma Allergy. 2021;14:31. [PMID: 33500632]

Collins CD et al. Impact of an antibiotic side-chain-based cross-reactivity chart combined with enhanced allergy assessment processes for surgical prophylaxis antimicrobials in patients with beta-lactam allergies. Clin Infect Dis. 2021;72:1404. [PMID: 32155264]

Leone M et al. Beta-lactam allergy labeling in intensive care units: an observational, retrospective study. Medicine (Baltimore). 2021;100:e26494. [PMID: 34232182]

IMMUNIZATION AGAINST INFECTIOUS DISEASES

RECOMMENDED IMMUNIZATION FOR ADULTS

Immunization is one of the most important tools (along with sanitation) used to prevent morbidity and mortality from infectious diseases. In general, the administration of most vaccinations induces a durable antibody response (**active immunity**). In contrast, **passive immunization** occurs when preformed antibodies are given (eg, immune globulin from pooled serum), resulting in temporary protection, which is a less durable response. The two variants of active immunization are **live attenuated vaccines** (which are believed to result in an immunologic response more like natural infection) and **inactivated or killed vaccines.**

The schedule of vaccinations varies based on the risk of the disease being prevented by vaccination, whether a vaccine has been given previously, the immune status of the patient (probability of responding to vaccine) and safety of the vaccine (live versus killed product, as well as implications for the fetus in pregnant women). Recommendations for healthy adults as well as special populations based on medical conditions are summarized in Table 30–7, which can be accessed online at https://www.cdc.gov/vaccines/schedules. Recommendations for SARS-CoV-2 vaccinations and boosters are being updated regularly.

1. Healthy Adults

Vaccination recommendations are made by the Advisory Committee on Immunization Practices (ACIP) of the US CDC (Table 30–7). Characteristics of selected COVID-19 vaccines can be found online and in Chapter 32.

2. Pregnant Women

Given the uncertainty of risks to the fetus, vaccination during pregnancy is *generally avoided* with the following exceptions: tetanus (transfer of maternal antibodies across the placenta is important to prevent neonatal tetanus), diphtheria, and influenza. Live vaccines are avoided during pregnancy.

Influenza can be a serious infection if acquired in pregnancy, and *all pregnant women should be offered influenza (inactivated) vaccination.* The live attenuated (intranasal) influenza vaccine is *not* recommended during pregnancy.

3. Adults with HIV

Patients with HIV have impaired cellular and B-cell responses. Inactivated or killed vaccinations can generally be given without any consequence, but the recipient may not be able to mount an adequate antibody response. Live or attenuated vaccines are generally avoided with some exceptions (ie, in patients with $CD4^+$ T lymphocytes greater than 200 cells/mcL [0.2×10^9/L]). Guidelines for vaccinating patients with HIV have been issued jointly by the CDC, the US National Institutes of Health, and the HIV Medical Association of the Infectious Diseases Society of America. Timing of vaccination is important to optimize response. If possible, vaccination should be given early in the course of HIV disease or following immune reconstitution.

4. Hematopoietic Cell Transplant Recipients

Hematopoietic cell transplant (HCT) recipients have varying rates of immune reconstitution following transplantation, depending on (1) the type of chemotherapy or radiotherapy used pretransplant (in autologous HCT), (2) the preparative regimen used for the transplant, (3) whether graft-versus-host disease is present, and (4) the type of immunosuppression used posttransplantation (in allogeneic HCT). Vaccines may not work immediately in the posttransplant period. B cells may take 3–12 months to return to normal posttransplant, and naïve T cells that can respond to new antigens appear only 6–12 months posttransplant. B cells of posttransplant patients treated with rituximab may take up to 6 months to fully recover after the last dose of the medication. Vaccines are therefore administered 6–12 months following transplantation with a minimum of 1 month between doses to maximize the probability of response.

5. Solid Organ Transplant Recipients

Solid organ transplant recipients demonstrate a broad spectrum of immunosuppression, depending on the reason for and type of organ transplantation and the nature of the immunosuppression (including T-cell-depleting agents during treatment of organ rejection). These factors affect the propensity for infection posttransplantation and the ability to develop antibody responses to vaccination. In many cases, the time between placing a patient on a transplant list and undergoing the transplantation takes months or years. Providers should take this opportunity to ensure that indicated *vaccines are given during this pretransplant period to optimize antibody responses.* If this is not possible, most experts give vaccines 3–6 months following transplantation. Live vaccines are contraindicated in the posttransplant period.

RECOMMENDED IMMUNIZATIONS FOR TRAVELERS

Individuals traveling to other countries frequently require immunizations in addition to those routinely recommended and may benefit from chemoprophylaxis against various diseases. Vaccinations against yellow fever and

Table 30–7. Recommended adult immunization schedule—United States, 2022.

Vaccine	19–26 years	27–49 years	50–64 years	≥65 years
Influenza inactivated (IIV4) or **Influenza recombinant** (RIV4)	1 dose annually			
or				
Influenza live, attenuated (LAIV4)	1 dose annually			
Tetanus, diphtheria, pertussis (Tdap or Td)	1 dose Tdap each pregnancy; 1 dose Td/Tdap for wound management (see notes) 1 dose Tdap, then Td or Tdap booster every 10 years			
Measles, mumps, rubella (MMR)	1 or 2 doses depending on indication (if born in 1957 or later)			
Varicella (VAR)	2 doses (if born in 1980 or later)		2 doses	
Zoster recombinant (RZV)	2 doses for immunocompromising conditions (see notes)		2 doses	
Human papillomavirus (HPV)	2 or 3 doses depending on age at initial vaccination or condition	27 through 45 years		
Pneumococcal (PCV15, PCV20, PPSV23)	1 dose PCV15 followed by PPSV23 OR 1 dose PCV20 (see notes)			1 dose PCV15 followed by PPSV23 OR 1 dose PCV20
Hepatitis A (HepA)	2 or 3 doses depending on vaccine			
Hepatitis B (HepB)	2, 3, or 4 doses depending on vaccine or condition			
Meningococcal A, C, W, Y (MenACWY)	1 or 2 doses depending on indication, see notes for booster recommendations			
Meningococcal B (MenB)	2 or 3 doses depending on vaccine and indication, see notes for booster recommendations 19 through 23 years			
***Haemophilus influenzae* type b** (Hib)	1 or 3 doses depending on indication			

Legend:
- Recommended vaccination for adults who meet age requirement, lack documentation of vaccination, or lack evidence of past infection
- Recommended vaccination for adults with an additional risk factor or another indication
- Recommended vaccination based on shared clinical decision-making
- No recommendation/Not applicable

Vaccine	Pregnancy	Immuno-compromised (excluding HIV infection)	HIV infection CD4 percentage and count		Asplenia, complement deficiencies	End-stage renal disease, or on hemodialysis	Heart or lung disease; alcoholism[1]	Chronic liver disease	Diabetes	Health care personnel[2]	Men who have sex with men
			<15% or <200 mm³	≥15% and ≥200 mm³							
IIV4 or RIV4	1 dose annually										
or LAIV4	Contraindicated					Precaution				or 1 dose annually	
Tdap or Td	1 dose Tdap each pregnancy	1 dose Tdap, then Td or Tdap booster every 10 years									
MMR	Contraindicated*	Contraindicated		1 or 2 doses depending on indication							
VAR	Contraindicated*	Contraindicated			2 doses						
RZV		2 doses at age ≥19 years			2 doses at age ≥50 years						
HPV	Not Recommended*	3 doses through age 26 years			2 or 3 doses through age 26 years depending on age at initial vaccination or condition						
Pneumococcal (PCV15, PCV20, PPSV23)		1 dose PCV15 followed by PPSV23 OR 1 dose PCV20 (see notes)									
HepA	2 or 3 doses depending on vaccine										
HepB	3 doses (see notes)	2, 3, or 4 doses depending on vaccine or condition									
MenACWY	1 or 2 doses depending on indication, see notes for booster recommendations										
MenB	Precaution	2 or 3 doses depending on vaccine and indication, see notes for booster recommendations									
Hib		3 doses HSCT[3] recipients only			1 dose						

Recommended vaccination for adults who meet age requirement, lack documentation of vaccination, or lack evidence of past infection

Recommended vaccination for adults with an additional risk factor or another indication

Recommended vaccination based on shared clinical decision-making

Precaution—vaccination might be indicated if benefit of protection outweighs risk of adverse reaction

Contraindicated or not recommended—vaccine should not be administered.

*Vaccinate after pregnancy.

No recommendation/ Not applicable

(continued)

Table 30–7. Recommended adult immunization schedule—United States, 2022. (continued)

NOTES

For vaccine recommendations for persons 18 years of age or younger, see the Recommended Child/Adolescent Immunization Schedule.

Additional Information

COVID-19 Vaccination

Advisory Committee on Immunization Practices (ACIP) recommends use of COVID-19 vaccines for everyone ages 5 and older. COVID-19 vaccine and other vaccines may be administered on the same day.

***Haemophilus influenzae* type b vaccination**

Special situations

- Anatomical or functional asplenia (including sickle cell disease): 1 dose if previously did not receive Hib; if elective splenectomy, 1 dose, preferably at least 14 days before splenectomy
- Hematopoietic stem cell transplant (HSCT): 3-dose series 4 weeks apart starting 6–12 months after successful transplant, regardless of Hib vaccination history

Hepatitis A vaccination

Routine vaccination

- Not at risk but want protection from hepatitis A (identification of risk factor not required): 2-dose series HepA (Havrix 6–12 months apart or Vaqta 6–18 months apart [minimum interval: 6 months]) or 3-dose series HepA-HepB (Twinrix at 0, 1, 6 months [minimum intervals: dose 1 to dose 2: 4 weeks / dose 2 to dose 3: 5 months])

Special situations

- At risk for hepatitis A virus infection: 2-dose series HepA or 3-dose series HepA-HepB as above
- Chronic liver disease (eg, persons with hepatitis B, hepatitis C, cirrhosis, fatty liver disease, alcoholic liver disease, autoimmune hepatitis, ALT or AST level greater than twice the upper limit of normal)
- HIV infection
- Men who have sex with men
- Injection or noninjection drug use
- Persons experiencing homelessness
- Work with hepatitis A virus in research laboratory or with nonhuman primates with hepatitis A virus infection
- Travel in countries with high or intermediate endemic hepatitis A (HepA-HepB [Twinrix] may be administered on an accelerated schedule of 3 doses at 0, 7, and 21–30 days, followed by a booster dose at 12 months)
- Close, personal contact with international adoptee (eg, household or regular babysitting) in first 60 days after arrival from country with high or intermediate endemic hepatitis A (administer dose 1 as soon as adoption is planned, at least 2 weeks before adoptee's arrival)
- Pregnancy if at risk for infection or severe outcome from infection during pregnancy
- Settings for exposure, including health care settings targeting services to injection or noninjection drug users or group homes and nonresidential day care facilities for developmentally disabled persons (individual risk factor screening not required)

Hepatitis B vaccination

Routine vaccination

- Not at risk but want protection from hepatitis B (identification of risk factor not required): 2- or 3-dose series (2-dose series Heplisav-B at least 4 weeks apart [2-dose series HepB only applies when 2 doses of Heplisav-B are used at least 4 weeks apart] or 3-dose series Engerix-B or Recombivax HB at 0, 1, 6 months [minimum intervals: dose 1 to dose 2: 4 weeks / dose 2 to dose 3: 8 weeks / dose 1 to dose 3: 16 weeks]) or 3-dose series HepA-HepB (Twinrix at 0, 1, 6 months [minimum intervals: dose 1 to dose 2: 4 weeks / dose 2 to dose 3: 5 months])

Special situations

- At risk for hepatitis B virus infection: 2-dose (Heplisav-B) or 3-dose (Engerix-B, Recombivax HB) series or 3-dose series HepA-HepB (Twinrix) as above
- Chronic liver disease (eg, persons with hepatitis C, cirrhosis, fatty liver disease, alcoholic liver disease, autoimmune hepatitis, ALT or AST level greater than twice upper limit of normal)
- HIV infection
- Sexual exposure risk (eg, sex partners of hepatitis B surface antigen [HBsAg]-positive persons; sexually active persons not in mutually monogamous relationships; persons seeking evaluation or treatment for a sexually transmitted infection; men who have sex with men)
- Current or recent injection drug use
- Percutaneous or mucosal risk for exposure to blood (eg, household contacts of HBsAg-positive persons; residents and staff of facilities for developmentally disabled persons; health care and public safety personnel with reasonably anticipated risk for exposure to blood or blood-contaminated body fluids; hemodialysis, peritoneal dialysis, home dialysis, and predialysis patients; persons with diabetes mellitus age younger than 60 years, shared clinical decision-making for persons age 60 years or older)

- Incarcerated persons
- Travel in countries with high or intermediate endemic hepatitis B
- Pregnancy if at risk for infection or severe outcome from infection during pregnancy (Heplisav-B not currently recommended due to lack of safety data in pregnant women)

HPV vaccination

Routine vaccination

- HPV vaccination recommended for all persons through age 26 years: 2- or 3-dose series depending on age at initial vaccination or condition:
- Age 15 years or older at initial vaccination: 3-dose series at 0, 1–2 months, 6 months (minimum intervals: dose 1 to dose 2: 4 weeks / dose 2 to dose 3: 12 weeks / dose 1 to dose 3: 5 months; repeat dose if administered too soon)
- Age 9–14 years at initial vaccination and received 1 dose or 2 doses less than 5 months apart: 1 additional dose
- Age 9–14 years at initial vaccination and received 2 doses at least 5 months apart: HPV vaccination series complete, no additional dose needed
- Interrupted schedules: If vaccination schedule is interrupted, the series does not need to be restarted
- No additional dose recommended after completing series with recommended dosing intervals using any HPV vaccine

Shared clinical decision-making

- Some adults age 27–45 years: Based on shared clinical decision-making, 2- or 3-dose series as above

Special situations

- Age ranges recommended above for routine and catch-up vaccination or shared clinical decision-making also apply in special situations
- Immunocompromising conditions, including HIV infection: 3-dose series as above, regardless of age at initial vaccination
- Pregnancy: HPV vaccination not recommended until after pregnancy; no intervention needed if vaccinated while pregnant; pregnancy testing not needed before vaccination

Influenza vaccination

Routine vaccination

- Persons age 6 months or older: 1 dose any influenza vaccine appropriate for age and health status annually
- For additional guidance, see www.cdc.gov/flu/professionals/index.htm

Special situations

- Egg allergy, hives only: 1 dose any influenza vaccine appropriate for age and health status annually
- Egg allergy–any symptom other than hives (eg, angioedema, respiratory distress): 1 dose any influenza vaccine appropriate for age and health status annually. If using an influenza vaccine other than RIV4 or ccIIV4, administer in medical setting under supervision of health care provider who can recognize and manage severe allergic reactions.
- Severe allergic reactions to any vaccine can occur even in the absence of a history of previous allergic reaction. Therefore, all vaccine providers should be familiar with the office emergency plan and certified in CPR.
- A previous severe allergic reaction to any influenza vaccine is a contraindication to future receipt of the vaccine.
- LAIV4 should not be used in persons with the following conditions or situations:
- History of severe allergic reaction to any vaccine component (excluding egg) or to a previous dose of any influenza vaccine
- Immunocompromised due to any cause (including medications and HIV infection)
- Anatomic or functional asplenia
- Close contacts or caregivers of severely immunosuppressed persons who require a protected environment
- Pregnancy
- Cranial CSF/oropharyngeal communications
- Cochlear implant
- Received influenza antiviral medications oseltamivir or zanamivir within the previous 48 hours, peramivir within the previous 5 days, or baloxavir within the previous 17 days
- Adults 50 years or older
- History of Guillain-Barré syndrome within 6 weeks after previous dose of influenza vaccine: Generally, should not be vaccinated unless vaccination benefits outweigh risks for those at higher risk for severe complications from influenza

(continued)

Table 30–7. Recommended adult immunization schedule—United States, 2022. (continued)

Measles, mumps, and rubella vaccination
Routine vaccination
- No evidence of immunity to measles, mumps, or rubella: 1 dose
- Evidence of immunity: Born before 1957 (health care personnel, see below), documentation of receipt of MMR vaccine, laboratory evidence of immunity or disease (diagnosis of disease without laboratory confirmation is not evidence of immunity)

Special situations
- Pregnancy with no evidence of immunity to rubella: MMR contraindicated during pregnancy; after pregnancy (before discharge from health care facility), 1 dose
- Nonpregnant women of childbearing age with no evidence of immunity to rubella: 1 dose
- HIV infection with CD4 count ≥ 200 cells/mL for at least 6 months and no evidence of immunity to measles, mumps, or rubella: 2-dose series at least 4 weeks apart; MMR contraindicated for HIV infection with CD4 count < 200 cells/mL
- Severe immunocompromising conditions: MMR contraindicated
- Students in postsecondary educational institutions, international travelers, and household or close, personal contacts of immunocompromised persons with no evidence of immunity to measles, mumps, or rubella: 2-dose series at least 4 weeks apart if previously did not receive any doses of MMR or 1 dose if previously received 1 dose MMR
- Health care personnel:
- Born in 1957 or later with no evidence of immunity to measles, mumps, or rubella: 2-dose series at least 4 weeks apart for measles or mumps or at least 1 dose for rubella
- Born before 1957 with no evidence of immunity to measles, mumps, or rubella: Consider 2-dose series at least 4 weeks apart for measles or mumps or 1 dose for rubella

Meningococcal vaccination
Special situations for MenACWY
- Anatomical or functional asplenia (including sickle cell disease), HIV infection, persistent complement component deficiency, complement inhibitor (eg, eculizumab, ravulizumab) use: 2-dose series MenACWY-D (Menactra, Menveo or MenQuadfi) at least 8 weeks apart and revaccinate every 5 years if risk remains
- Travel in countries with hyperendemic or epidemic meningococcal disease, microbiologists routinely exposed to *Neisseria meningitidis*: 1 dose MenACWY (Menactra, Menveo or MenQuadfi) and revaccinate every 5 years if risk remains
- First-year college students who live in residential housing (if not previously vaccinated at age 16 years or older) and military recruits: 1 dose MenACWY (Menactra, Menveo or MenQuadfi)
- For MenACWY booster dose recommendations for groups listed under "Special situations" and in an outbreak setting (eg, in community or organizational settings and among men who have sex with men) and additional meningococcal vaccination information, see www.cdc.gov/mmwr/volumes/69/rr/rr6909a1.htm

Shared clinical decision-making for MenB
- Adolescents and young adults age 16–23 years (age 16–18 years preferred) not at increased risk for meningococcal disease: Based on shared clinical decision-making, 2-dose series MenB-4C (Bexsero) at least 1 month apart or 2-dose series MenB-FHbp (Trumenba) at 0, 6 months (if dose 2 was administered less than 6 months after dose 1, administer dose 3 at least 4 months after dose 2); MenB-4C and MenB-FHbp are not interchangeable (use same product for all doses in series)

Special situations for MenB
- Anatomical or functional asplenia (including sickle cell disease), persistent complement component deficiency, complement inhibitor (eg, eculizumab, ravulizumab) use, microbiologists routinely exposed to *Neisseria meningitidis*: 2-dose primary series MenB-4C (Bexsero) at least one month apart or
- MenB-4C (Bexsero) at least 1 month apart or 3-dose primary series MenB-FHbp (Trumenba) at 0, 1–2, 6 months (if dose 2 was administered at least 6 months after dose 1, dose 3 not needed); MenB-4C and MenB-FHbp are not interchangeable (use same product for all doses in series); 1 dose MenB booster 1 year after primary series and revaccinate every 2–3 years if risk remains
- Pregnancy: Delay MenB until after pregnancy unless at increased risk and vaccination benefits outweigh potential risks
- For MenB booster dose recommendations for groups listed under "Special situations" and in an outbreak setting (eg, in community or organizational settings and among men who have sex with men) and additional meningococcal vaccination information, see www.cdc.gov/mmwr/volumes/69/rr/rr6909a1.htm

Pneumococcal vaccination
Routine vaccination
- Age 65 years or older who have not previously received a pneumococcal conjugate vaccine or whose previous vaccination history is unknown:
  -1 dose PCV15 or 1 dose PCV20
  -If PCV15 is used, this should be followed by a dose of PPSV23 given at least 1 year after the PCV15 dose
  -A minimum interval of 8 weeks between PCV15 and PPSV23 can be considered for adults with an immunocompromising condition,* cochlear implant, or cerebrospinal fluid leak to minimize the risk of invasive pneumococcal disease caused by serotypes unique to PPSV23 in these vulnerable groups.
- For guidance for patients who have already received a previous dose of PCV13 and/or PPSV23, see www.cdc.gov/mmwr/volumes/71/wr/mm7104a1.htm.

Special situations

- Age 19–64 years with certain underlying medical conditions or other risk factors** who have not previously received a pneumococcal conjugate vaccine or whose previous vaccination history is unknown:
  - -1 dose PCV15 or 1 dose PCV20
  - -If PCV15 is used, this should be followed by a dose of PPSV23 given at least 1 year after the PCV15 dose
  - -A minimum interval of 8 weeks between PCV15 and PPSV23 can be considered for adults with an immunocompromising condition,* cochlear implant, or cerebrospinal fluid leak to minimize the risk of invasive pneumococcal disease caused by serotypes unique to PPSV23 in these vulnerable groups.
- For guidance for patients who have already received a previous dose of PCV13 and/or PPSV23, see www.cdc.gov/mmwr/volumes/71/wr/mm7104a1.htm.

*Note: Immunocompromising conditions include CKD, nephrotic syndrome, immunodeficiency, iatrogenic immunosuppression, generalized malignancy, HIV, Hodgkin disease, leukemia, lymphoma, plasma cell myeloma, solid organ transplants, congenital or acquired asplenia, sickle cell disease, or other hemoglobinopathies.

**Note: Underlying medical conditions or other risk factors include alcohol use disorder, chronic heart/liver/lung disease, CKD, cigarette smoking, cochlear implant, congenital or acquired asplenia, cerebrospinal fluid leak, diabetes mellitus, generalized malignancy, HIV, Hodgkin disease, immunodeficiency, iatrogenic immunosuppression, leukemia, lymphoma, plasma cell myeloma, nephrotic syndrome, solid organ transplants, or sickle cell disease, or other hemoglobinopathies.

Tetanus, diphtheria, and pertussis vaccination

Routine vaccination

- Previously did not receive Tdap at or after age 11 years: 1 dose Tdap, then Td or Tdap every 10 years

Special situations

- Previously did not receive primary vaccination series for tetanus, diphtheria, or pertussis: At least 1 dose Tdap followed by 1 dose Td or Tdap at least 4 weeks after Tdap and another dose Td or Tdap 6–12 months after last Td or Tdap (Tdap can be substituted for any Td dose, but preferred as first dose), Td or Tdap every 10 years thereafter
- Pregnancy: 1 dose Tdap during each pregnancy, preferably in early part of gestational weeks 27–36
- Wound management: Persons with 3 or more doses of tetanus-toxoid-containing vaccine: For clean and minor wounds, administer Tdap or Td if more than 10 years since last dose of tetanus-toxoid-containing vaccine; for all other wounds, administer Tdap or Td if more than 5 years since last dose of tetanus-toxoid-containing vaccine. Tdap is preferred for persons who have not previously received Tdap or whose Tdap history is unknown. If a tetanus-toxoid-containing vaccine is indicated for a pregnant woman, use Tdap. For detailed information, see www.cdc.gov/mmwr/volumes/69/wr/mm6903a5.htm

Varicella vaccination

Routine vaccination

- No evidence of immunity to varicella: 2-dose series 4–8 weeks apart if previously did not receive varicella-containing vaccine (VAR or MMRV [measles-mumps-rubella-varicella vaccine] for children); if previously received 1 dose varicella-containing vaccine, 1 dose at least 4 weeks after first dose
- Evidence of immunity: U.S.-born before 1980 (except for pregnant women and health care personnel [see below]), documentation of 2 doses varicella-containing vaccine at least 4 weeks apart, diagnosis or verification of history of varicella or herpes zoster by a health care provider, laboratory evidence of immunity or disease

Special situations

- Pregnancy with no evidence of immunity to varicella: VAR contraindicated during pregnancy; after pregnancy (before discharge from health care facility), 1 dose if previously received 1 dose varicella-containing vaccine or dose 1 of 2-dose series (dose 2: 4–8 weeks later) if previously did not receive any varicella-containing vaccine, regardless of whether U.S.-born before 1980
- Health care personnel with no evidence of immunity to varicella: 1 dose if previously received 1 dose varicella-containing vaccine; 2-dose series 4–8 weeks apart if previously did not receive any varicella-containing vaccine, regardless of whether U.S.-born before 1980
- HIV infection with CD4 count ≥200 cells/mm^3 with no evidence of immunity: Vaccination may be considered (2 doses 3 months apart); VAR contraindicated for HIV infection with CD4 count <200 cells/mm^3
- Severe immunocompromising conditions: VAR contraindicated

Zoster vaccination

Routine vaccination

- Age 50 years or older: 2-dose series RZV (Shingrix) 2–6 months apart (minimum interval: 4 weeks; repeat dose if administered too soon), regardless of previous herpes zoster or history of zoster vaccine live (ZVL, Zostavax) vaccination (administer RZV at least 2 months after ZVL)

Special situations

- Pregnancy: Consider delaying RZV until after pregnancy if RZV is otherwise indicated.
- Severe immunocompromising conditions (including HIV infection with CD4 count <200 cells/mm^3): Recommended use of RZV under review

Table 30–8. Adverse effects and contraindications to commonly used vaccines in adults (listed in alphabetical order).

Vaccine	Adverse Effects	Contraindications[1]
Haemophilus influenzae type b (Hib)	Minimal Consist mainly of pain at the injection site	Any severe allergic reaction (eg, anaphylaxis) after a previous dose or to a vaccine component.
Hepatitis A	Minimal Consist mainly of pain at the injection site	Any severe allergic reaction (eg, anaphylaxis) after a previous dose or to a vaccine component.
Hepatitis B	Minimal Consist mainly of pain at the injection site	Any severe allergic reaction (eg, anaphylaxis) after a previous dose or to a vaccine component.
HPV	Minimal Consist mainly of mild to moderate localized pain, erythema, swelling Systemic reactions, mainly fever, seen in 4% of recipients	Any severe allergic reaction (eg, anaphylaxis) after a previous dose or to a vaccine component.
Influenza (intramuscular inactivated and intranasal live attenuated vaccines)	**Intramuscular, inactivated vaccine:** Local reactions (erythema and tenderness) at the site of injection are common, but fevers, chills, and malaise (which last in any case only 2–3 days) are rare. **Either inactivated or live attenuated vaccine:** A potential association between Guillain-Barré syndrome (3000–6000 cases per year in the United States, usually following respiratory infections) and vaccination with intramuscular, inactivated influenza vaccine has been reported (possibly, 1–2 persons per million persons vaccinated), but this rate is lower than the risk of the syndrome developing after influenza itself (given that approximately 750 persons per million adults are hospitalized annually with influenza, and many more cases remain as outpatients). Influenza vaccination may be associated with multiple false-positive serologic tests to HIV, HTLV-1, and hepatitis C, but it is self-limited, lasting 2–5 months.	Contraindication to both inactivated and live attenuated vaccine: History of Guillain-Barré syndrome, especially within 6 weeks of receiving a previous influenza vaccine. Any severe allergic reaction (eg, anaphylaxis) after a previous dose or to a vaccine component, including egg protein.[2] Intranasal, live attenuated vaccine (FluMist) should not be used in: • People 50 years of age and over • Immunosuppressed individuals and those on immunosuppressive therapy • Household members of immunosuppressed individuals • Health care workers, or others with close contact with immunosuppressed persons • Presence of reactive airway disease (eg, asthma) or chronic underlying metabolic (eg, kidney), pulmonary, or heart diseases (use intramuscular inactivated vaccine) • Pregnancy[3] It is recommended that salicylates should be avoided for 6 weeks following vaccination (to prevent Reye syndrome).
Measles, mumps, and rubella (MMR)[4]	Fever will develop in about 5–15% of unimmunized individuals, and a mild rash will develop in about 5% 5–12 days after vaccination. Fever and rash are self-limited, lasting only 2–3 days. Local swelling and induration are particularly common in individuals previously vaccinated with inactivated vaccine.	Pregnancy[5] Known severe immunodeficiency (eg, from hematologic and solid cancers, receipt of chemotherapy, congenital immunodeficiency, long-term immunosuppressive therapy [eg, > 2 weeks of prednisone 20 mg daily or higher]), other disease- or therapy-related immune suppression, or patients with HIV infection who are severely immunocompromised. May be used in asymptomatic individuals with HIV whose CD4 count is > 200/mcL (0.2×10^9/L). Severe allergic reaction (eg, anaphylaxis) to a previous dose or to a vaccine component (eg, neomycin or to related agents such as streptomycin).

Meningococcal, oligosaccharide conjugate; (MCV4 or MenACWY [Menactra, Menveo]; meningococcal polysaccharide conjugate MPSV4 [Menomune]); meningococcal group B, recombinant (MenB [Bexsero, Trumenba])	Minor reactions (fever, redness, swelling, erythema, pain) occur slightly more commonly with MCV4. Major reactions are rare. A potential association between Guillain-Barré syndrome (3000–6000 cases per year in the United States, usually following respiratory infections) and vaccination with MCV4 has been reported, but current recommendations favor continued use of MCV4, since the benefits of preventing the serious consequences of meningococcal infection outweigh the theoretical risk of Guillain-Barré syndrome.	Any severe allergic reaction (eg, anaphylaxis) to a previous dose or to a vaccine component (eg, persons with history of adverse reaction to diphtheria toxoid should not receive meningococcal oligosaccharide conjugate and polysaccharide conjugate vaccines since the protein conjugate used in them is diphtheria toxoid).
Pneumococcal conjugate (PCV13 [Prevnar]); pneumococcal polysaccharide (PPSV23) [Pneumovax])	Mild local reactions (erythema and tenderness) occur in up to 50% of recipients, but systemic reactions are uncommon. Similarly, revaccination at least 5 years after initial vaccination is associated with mild self-limited local but not systemic reactions.	Any severe allergic reaction (eg, anaphylaxis) after a previous dose or to a vaccine component (eg, for PCV13 to any vaccine containing diphtheria toxoid).
Tetanus, diphtheria, and pertussis (DTP, Tdap); tetanus, diphtheria (Td)	Minimal Consist mainly of pain at the injection site	Any severe allergic reaction (eg, anaphylaxis) after a previous dose or to a vaccine component. For pertussis-containing vaccines: any history of unexplained encephalopathy (eg, coma, decreased level of consciousness, or prolonged seizures) within 7 days of administration of a previous dose of Tdap or diphtheria and tetanus toxoids and pertussis (DTP) or diphtheria and tetanus toxoids and acellular pertussis (Tdap) vaccine.
Varicella	Can occur as late as 4–6 weeks after vaccination. Tenderness and erythema at the injection site are seen in 25%, fever in 10–15%, and a localized maculopapular or vesicular rash in 5%; a diffuse rash, usually with five or fewer vesicular lesions, develops in a smaller percentage. Spread of virus from vaccinees to susceptible individuals is possible, but the risk of such transmission even to immunocompromised patients is small, and disease, when it develops, is mild and treatable with acyclovir.	Known severe immunodeficiency (eg, from hematologic and solid cancers, receipt of chemotherapy, congenital immunodeficiency, long-term immunosuppressive therapy [eg, > 2 weeks of prednisone 20 mg daily or higher; other immunosuppressive medications], other disease- or therapy-related immune suppression, or patients with HIV infection who are severely immunocompromised). Pregnancy. Severe allergic reaction (eg, anaphylaxis) after a previous dose or to a vaccine component (eg, neomycin). For theoretical reasons, it is recommended that salicylates should be avoided for 6 weeks following vaccination (to prevent potential for Reye syndrome).
Zoster	Mild and limited to local reactions Although it is theoretically possible to transmit the virus to susceptible contacts, no such cases have been reported.	Known severe immunodeficiency (eg, from hematologic and solid cancers, receipt of chemotherapy, congenital immunodeficiency, long-term immunosuppressive therapy [eg, > 2 weeks of prednisone 20 mg daily or higher; other immunosuppressive medications], other disease- or therapy-related immune suppression, or patients with HIV infection who are severely immunocompromised. May be used in asymptomatic individuals with HIV whose CD4 count is > 200/mcL [0.2×10^9/L]). Pregnancy. Any severe allergic reaction (eg, anaphylaxis) after a previous dose or to a vaccine component (eg, gelatin or neomycin).

[1]Adapted from Centers for Disease Control and Prevention. Contraindications and precautions to commonly used vaccines in adults. General recommendations on immunization: recommendations of the Advisory Committee on Immunization Practices. https://www.cdc.gov/vaccines/hcp/acip-recs/general-recs/contraindications.html, accessed March 12, 2021; and from Hamborsky J et al (editors). Appendix A. Epidemiology and prevention of vaccine preventable diseases. 13th edition. Washington, DC, Public Health Foundation, 2015. Available at www.cdc.gov/vaccines/pubs/pinkbook/index.html.

[2]The vaccine has typically been prepared using embryonated chicken eggs. However, a new vaccine using mammalian cell culture is now FDA approved.

[3]The inactivated influenza vaccine can be given during any trimester.

[4]MMR vaccine can be safely given to patients with a history of egg allergy even when severe.

[5]Although vaccination of pregnant women is *not* recommended, with the currently available RA27/3 vaccine strain, the congenital rubella syndrome does not occur in the offspring of those inadvertently vaccinated during pregnancy or within 3 months before conception.

meningococcus are the only ones required by certain countries. These and other travel-specific vaccines are listed at http://wwwnc.cdc.gov/travel/destinations/list.

Various vaccines can be given simultaneously at different sites. Some, such as cholera, plague, and typhoid vaccine, cause significant discomfort and are best given at different times. In general, live attenuated vaccines (measles, mumps, rubella, yellow fever, and oral typhoid vaccine) should not be given to immunosuppressed individuals or household members of immunosuppressed people or to pregnant women. Immunoglobulin should not be given for 3 months before or at least 2 weeks after live virus vaccines, because it may attenuate the antibody response.

Chemoprophylaxis of malaria is discussed in Chapter 35.

VACCINE SAFETY

Most vaccines are safe to administer. In general, it is recommended that the use of live vaccines be avoided in immunocompromised patients, including pregnant women. Vaccines are generally not contraindicated in the following situations: mild, acute illness with low-grade fevers (less than 40.5°C); concurrent antibiotic therapy; soreness or redness at the site; and family history of adverse reactions to vaccinations. Absolute contraindications to vaccines are rare (Table 30–8).

Centers for Disease Control and Prevention (CDC). Adult immunization schedules—United States, 2022. https://www.cdc.gov/vaccines/schedules/hcp/imz/adult.html

Centers for Disease Control and Prevention (CDC). CDC Yellow Book 2020. Health information for international travel. https://wwwnc.cdc.gov/travel/page/yellowbook-home-2020

Centers for Disease Control and Prevention (CDC). Vaccine safety. https://www.cdc.gov/vaccinesafety/index.html

Danziger-Isakov L et al. Vaccination of solid organ transplant candidates and recipients: guidelines from the American society of transplantation infectious diseases community of practice. Clin Transplant. 2019;33:e13563. [PMID: 31002409]

Freedman MS et al. Advisory Committee on Immunization Practices recommended immunization schedule for adults aged 19 years or older—United States, 2021. MMWR Morb Mortal Wkly Rep. 2021;70:193. [PMID: 33571173]

Grohskopf LA et al. Prevention and control of seasonal influenza with vaccines: recommendations of the Advisory Committee on Immunization Practices—United States, 2020-21 influenza season. MMWR Recomm Rep. 2020;69:1. [PMID: 32820746]

Kobayashi M et al. Use of 15-valent pneumococcal conjugate vaccine and 20-valent pneumococcal conjugate vaccine among U.S. adults: updated recommendations of the Advisory Committee on Immunization Practices—United States, 2022. MMWR Morb Mortal Wkly Rep. 2022;71:109. [PMID: 35085226]

Leibovici Weissman Y et al. Clinical efficacy and safety of high dose trivalent influenza vaccine in adults and immunosuppressed populations—a systematic review and meta-analysis. J Infect. 2021;83:444. [PMID: 34425161]

HIV Infection & AIDS

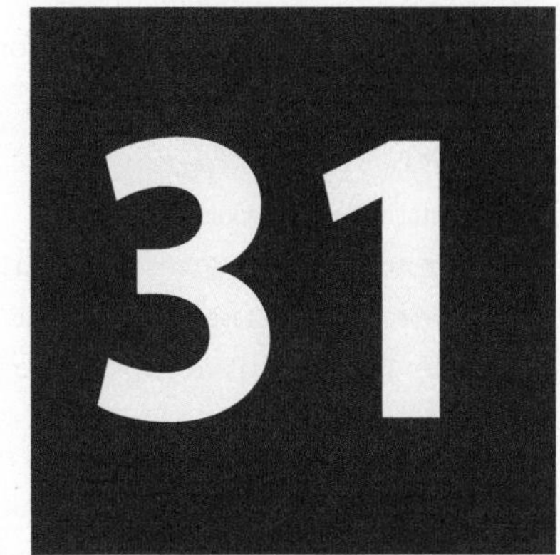

Monica Gandhi, MD
Matthew A. Spinelli, MD, MAS
Mitchell H. Katz, MD

ESSENTIALS OF DIAGNOSIS

- Modes of transmission: sexual contact with an infected person, parenteral exposure to infected blood (needle sharing, very rarely with transfusion), perinatal exposure.
- Prominent systemic complaints: sweats, diarrhea, weight loss, and wasting.
- Opportunistic infections due to diminished cellular immunity—often life-threatening.
- Aggressive cancers, particularly non-Hodgkin lymphoma.
- Neurologic manifestations, including dementia, aseptic meningitis, and neuropathy.

General Considerations

The CDC AIDS case definition (Table 31–1) includes opportunistic infections and malignancies that rarely occur in the absence of severe immunodeficiency (eg, *Pneumocystis* pneumonia, CNS lymphoma, cytomegalovirus retinitis). It also classifies persons as having AIDS if they have a positive HIV antibody test and certain infections and malignancies that can occur in immunocompetent hosts but that are more common among persons living with HIV infection (eg, pulmonary tuberculosis, invasive cervical cancer). Several nonspecific conditions, including dementia and wasting (documented weight loss)—in the presence of a positive HIV test—are also classified as AIDS. The definition includes criteria for both definitive and presumptive diagnoses of certain infections and malignancies. Finally, persons with a positive HIV test whose CD4 lymphocyte count drops below 200 cells/mcL or a CD4 lymphocyte percentage below 14% are considered to have AIDS.

Inclusion of persons with low CD4 counts as AIDS cases reflects the recognition that *immunodeficiency is the defining characteristic of AIDS*. The choice of a cutoff point at 200 cells/mcL is supported by several cohort studies showing that AIDS will develop within 3 years in over 80% of persons with counts below this level in the absence of effective antiretroviral therapy (ART). Fortunately, the prognosis of persons living with HIV/AIDS has dramatically improved due to the development of effective ART. One consequence is that fewer persons living with HIV ever develop an infection or malignancy or have a low enough CD4 count to classify them as having AIDS, which means that the CDC definition has become a less useful measure of the impact of HIV/AIDS in the United States. Conversely, persons in whom AIDS had been diagnosed based on a serious opportunistic infection, malignancy, or immunodeficiency may now be markedly healthier, with high CD4 counts, due to the use of ART. Therefore, the Social Security Administration, as well as most social service agencies, now focus on functional assessment for determining eligibility for benefits rather than the simple presence or absence of an AIDS-defining illness.

Epidemiology

The modes of transmission of HIV are similar to those of hepatitis B, in particular with respect to sexual, parenteral, and vertical transmission. Although certain sexual practices (eg, receptive anal intercourse) confer higher risk than other sexual practices (eg, insertive vaginal intercourse), it is difficult to quantify per-contact risks. The reason is that studies of sexual transmission of HIV show that most people at risk for HIV infection engage in a variety of sexual practices or have sex with multiple persons, or both, only some of whom may actually be living with HIV. Thus, it is difficult to determine which practice with which person actually resulted in HIV transmission.

Nonetheless, the best available estimates indicate that the risk of HIV transmission with receptive anal intercourse is 138 per 10,000 exposures, with insertive anal intercourse being 11 per 10,000 exposures. Receptive vaginal intercourse results in HIV transmission in 8 per 10,000 exposures, with insertive vaginal intercourse being 4 per 10,000 exposures, and a much lower risk with insertive or receptive oral intercourse.

A number of *cofactors* are known to increase the risk of HIV transmission during a given encounter, including the presence of ulcerative or inflammatory sexually

Table 31–1. CDC AIDS case definition for surveillance of adults and adolescents.

Definitive AIDS Diagnoses (with or without laboratory evidence of HIV infection)
1. Candidiasis of the esophagus, trachea, bronchi, or lungs.
2. Cryptococcosis, extrapulmonary.
3. Cryptosporidiosis with diarrhea persisting > 1 month.
4. Cytomegalovirus disease of an organ other than liver, spleen, or lymph nodes.
5. Herpes simplex virus infection causing a mucocutaneous ulcer that persists > 1 month; or bronchitis, pneumonitis, or esophagitis of any duration.
6. Kaposi sarcoma in a patient < 60 years of age.
7. Lymphoma of the brain (primary) in a patient < 60 years of age.
8. *Mycobacterium avium* complex or *Mycobacterium kansasii* disease, disseminated (at a site other than or in addition to lungs, skin, or cervical or hilar lymph nodes).
9. *Pneumocystis jirovecii* pneumonia.
10. Progressive multifocal leukoencephalopathy.
11. Toxoplasmosis of the brain.
Definitive AIDS Diagnoses (with laboratory evidence of HIV infection)
1. Coccidioidomycosis, disseminated (at a site other than or in addition to lungs or cervical or hilar lymph nodes).
2. HIV encephalopathy.
3. Histoplasmosis, disseminated (at a site other than or in addition to lungs or cervical or hilar lymph nodes).
4. Isosporiasis with diarrhea persisting > 1 month.
5. Kaposi sarcoma at any age.
6. Lymphoma of the brain (primary) at any age.
7. Other non-Hodgkin lymphoma of B cell or unknown immunologic phenotype.
8. Any mycobacterial disease caused by mycobacteria other than *Mycobacterium tuberculosis*, disseminated (at a site other than or in addition to lungs, skin, or cervical or hilar lymph nodes).
9. Disease caused by extrapulmonary *M tuberculosis*.
10. Salmonella (nontyphoid) septicemia, recurrent.
11. HIV wasting syndrome.
12. CD4 lymphocyte count < 200 cells/mcL or a CD4 lymphocyte percentage < 14%.
13. Pulmonary tuberculosis.
14. Recurrent pneumonia.
15. Invasive cervical cancer.
Presumptive AIDS Diagnoses (with laboratory evidence of HIV infection)
1. Candidiasis of esophagus: (a) recent onset of retrosternal pain on swallowing; and (b) oral candidiasis.
2. Cytomegalovirus retinitis. A characteristic appearance on serial ophthalmoscopic examinations.
3. Mycobacteriosis. Specimen from stool or normally sterile body fluids or tissue from a site other than lungs, skin, or cervical or hilar lymph nodes, showing acid-fast bacilli of a species not identified by culture.
4. Kaposi sarcoma. Erythematous or violaceous plaque-like lesion on skin or mucous membrane.
5. *Pneumocystis jirovecii* pneumonia: (a) a history of dyspnea on exertion or nonproductive cough of recent onset (within the past 3 months); and (b) chest film evidence of diffuse bilateral interstitial infiltrates or gallium scan evidence of diffuse bilateral pulmonary disease; and (c) arterial blood gas analysis showing an arterial oxygen partial pressure < 70 mm Hg or a low respiratory diffusing capacity < 80% of predicted values or an increase in the alveolar-arterial oxygen tension gradient; and (d) no evidence of a bacterial pneumonia.
6. Toxoplasmosis of the brain: (a) recent onset of a focal neurologic abnormality consistent with intracranial disease or a reduced level of consciousness; and (b) brain imaging evidence of a lesion having a mass effect or the radiographic appearance of which is enhanced by injection of contrast medium; and (c) serum antibody to toxoplasmosis or successful response to therapy for toxoplasmosis.
7. Recurrent pneumonia: (a) more than one episode in a 1-year period; and (b) acute pneumonia (new symptoms, signs, or radiologic evidence not present earlier) diagnosed on clinical or radiologic grounds by the patient's clinician.
8. Pulmonary tuberculosis: (a) apical or miliary infiltrates and (b) radiographic and clinical response to antituberculous therapy.

transmitted diseases, trauma, menses, and the absence of male circumcision.

The risk of acquiring HIV infection from a needlestick with blood infected with HIV is estimated at 1 in 300. Factors known to increase the risk of transmission include depth of penetration, hollow bore needles, visible blood on the needle, and advanced stage of disease in the source. The risk of HIV transmission from a mucosal splash with infected blood is unknown but is assumed to be significantly lower.

The risk of acquiring HIV infection from injection drug use with sharing of needles from a person living with HIV is estimated at 63 per 10,000 exposures. Use of clean needles markedly decreases the chance of HIV transmission but does not eliminate it if other drug paraphernalia are shared (eg, cookers).

When blood transfusion from a donor with HIV occurs, the risk of transmission is 93%. Fortunately, since 1985, blood donor screening for HIV has been universally practiced in the United States. Also, persons who have recently engaged in behaviors that might result in HIV acquisition (eg, sex with a person at risk for HIV, injection drug use) are not allowed to donate. This essentially eliminates donations from persons who have acquired HIV but have not yet developed antibodies (ie, persons in the "window" period). HIV antigen and viral load testing have been added to the screening of blood to further lower the chance of HIV transmission. With these precautions, the chance of HIV transmission with receipt of blood transfusion in the United States is about 1:2,000,000.

Between 13% and 40% of children born to a mother living with HIV contract HIV infection when the mother has not received treatment or when the child has not received perinatal HIV prophylaxis. The risk is higher with vaginal than with cesarean delivery; higher among mothers with high viral loads; and higher among those who breastfeed their children. The combination of prenatal HIV testing and counseling, ART for mothers living with HIV during pregnancy and for the infant immediately after birth, scheduled cesarean delivery if the mother has a viral load that is unknown or greater than 1000 copies/mL at delivery, and avoidance of breastfeeding has reduced the rate of perinatal transmission of HIV to less than 1% in the United States and Europe (https://clinicalinfo.hiv.gov/en/guidelines/perinatal/introduction).

HIV has not been shown to be transmitted by respiratory droplet spread, by vectors such as mosquitoes, or by casual nonsexual contact. Saliva, sweat, stool, and tears are *not* considered infectious fluids.

More than 1.3 million adults and adolescents in the United States are estimated to be living with HIV, 14% of whom are undiagnosed. Young people (aged 13–24 years) are the most likely to not know they are infected. In 2019, there were 34,800 newly diagnosed HIV infections in the United States; 82% male sex at birth (28,400) and 18% female sex at birth (6400). Men who have sex with men accounted for 66% of the new diagnoses (23,199). Black and Latinx people accounted for 41% and 29% of new infections, respectively. Heterosexual contacts accounted for 23% (8004) of new HIV diagnoses, and injection drug users (including men who have sex with men and use injection drugs) accounted for 11% (3900) of new HIV diagnoses. Among persons living with HIV in the United States, the prevalence of infection in non-White people is *staggeringly higher* compared with White people. The rate of infection per 100,000 people was 42 for Black people, 21 for people of multiple races, 22 for Latinx people, and 6 for White people.

In general, the progression of HIV-related illness is similar in men and women, although women generally have lower viral loads then men early in infection. There are other important differences. Women are at risk for gynecologic complications of HIV, including recurrent candidal vaginitis, pelvic inflammatory disease, and cervical dysplasia and carcinoma. Violence directed against women, pregnancy, and frequent occurrence of drug use and poverty all complicate the treatment of women living with HIV.

Worldwide there are an estimated 37.7 million persons living with HIV, with heterosexual spread being the most common mode of transmission for men and women. The reason for the greater risk for transmission with heterosexual intercourse in Africa and Asia than in the United States may relate to cofactors such as general health status, the presence of genital ulcers, relative lack of male circumcision, the number of sexual partners, and different HIV serotypes. It was estimated that in 2019, 66% of Americans living with HIV received some HIV care and 57% were virally suppressed. Worldwide, 67% of individuals living with HIV are on ART and 59% are virally suppressed.

Centers for Disease Control and Prevention. HIV Surveillance Report, 2019; vol.32. http://www.cdc.gov/hiv/library/reports/hiv-surveillance.html. Published May 2021.

US Department of Health and Human Services. HIV Basics. https://www.hiv.gov/hiv-basics

World Health Organization. Number of people (all ages) living with HIV: estimates by WHO region. Updated 2020. https://apps.who.int/gho/data/node.main.620?lang=en

Pathophysiology

Clinically, the syndromes caused by HIV infection are usually explicable by one of three known mechanisms: immunodeficiency, autoimmunity, and allergic and hypersensitivity reactions.

A. Immunodeficiency

Immunodeficiency is a direct result of the effects of HIV upon immune cells as well as the indirect impact of a generalized state of inflammation and immune activation due to chronic viral infection. A spectrum of infections and neoplasms is seen, as in other congenital or acquired immunodeficiency states. Two remarkable features of HIV immunodeficiency are the low incidence of certain infections such as listeriosis and aspergillosis and the frequent occurrence of certain neoplasms such as lymphoma or Kaposi sarcoma. This latter complication has been seen primarily in men who have sex with men or in bisexual men, and its incidence steadily declined through the first

15 years of the epidemic. A herpesvirus (HHV-8) is the cause of Kaposi sarcoma.

B. Autoimmunity and Allergic & Hypersensitivity Reactions

Autoimmunity can occur as a result of disordered cellular immune function or B lymphocyte dysfunction. Examples of both lymphocytic infiltration of organs (eg, lymphocytic interstitial pneumonitis) and autoantibody production (eg, immunologic thrombocytopenia) occur. These phenomena may be the only clinically apparent disease or may coexist with obvious immunodeficiency. Moreover, people living with HIV appear to have higher rates of allergic reactions to unknown allergens as seen with eosinophilic pustular folliculitis ("itchy red bump syndrome") as well as increased rates of hypersensitivity reactions to medications (for example, the fever and sunburn-like rash seen with trimethoprim-sulfamethoxazole reactions).

▶ Clinical Findings

The complications of HIV-related infections and neoplasms *affect virtually every organ*. The general approach to the people living with HIV with symptoms is to evaluate the organ systems involved, aiming to diagnose treatable conditions rapidly. As shown in Figure 31–1, the CD4 lymphocyte count level enables the clinician to focus on the diagnoses most likely to be seen at each stage of immunodeficiency. Certain infections may occur at any CD4 count, while others rarely occur unless the CD4 lymphocyte count has dropped below a certain level. For example, a patient with a CD4 count of 600 cells/mcL, cough, and fever may have a bacterial pneumonia but would be very unlikely to have *Pneumocystis jirovecii* pneumonia.

A. Symptoms and Signs

Many individuals living with HIV infection remain asymptomatic for years even without ART, with a mean time of approximately 10 years between infection and development of AIDS. When symptoms occur, they may be remarkably protean and nonspecific. Since virtually all the findings may be seen with other diseases, a combination of complaints is more suggestive of HIV infection than any one symptom.

Physical examination may be entirely normal. Abnormal findings range from completely nonspecific to highly specific for HIV infection. Some opportunistic infections specific for HIV infection include oral hairy leukoplakia of the tongue, disseminated Kaposi sarcoma, and cutaneous bacillary angiomatosis. Generalized lymphadenopathy, which is nonspecific, is common early in infection.

The specific presentations and management of the various complications of HIV infection are discussed under the Complications section below.

Dillon SM et al. Gut innate immunity and HIV pathogenesis. Curr HIV/AIDS Rep. 2021;18:128. [PMID: 33687703]

Sonti S et al. HIV-1 persistence in the CNS: mechanisms of latency, pathogenesis and an update on eradication strategies. Virus Res. 2021;303:198523. [PMID: 34314771]

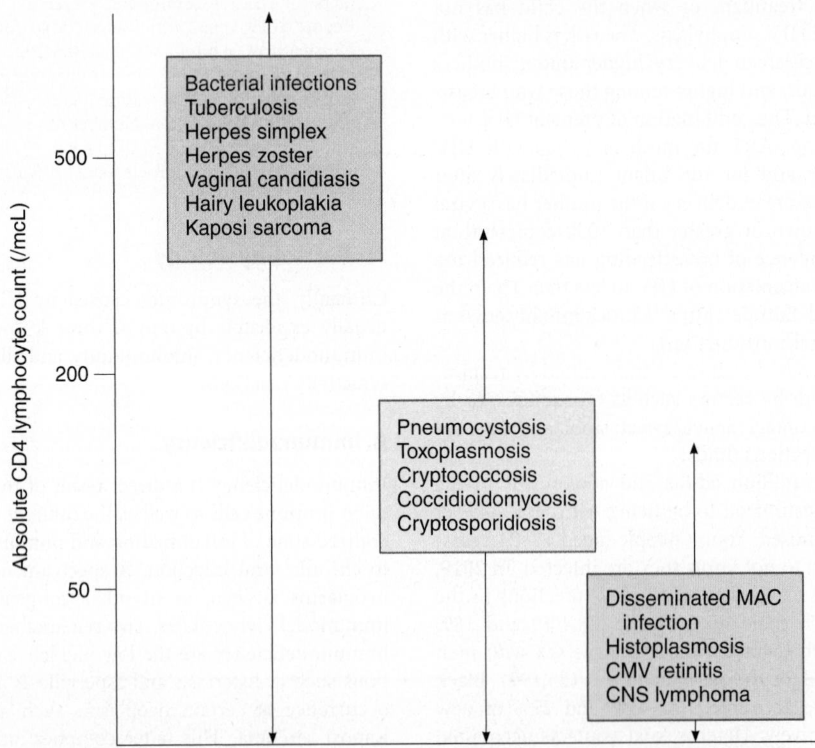

▲ **Figure 31–1.** Relationship of CD4 count to development of opportunistic infections. MAC, *Mycobacterium avium* complex; CMV, cytomegalovirus.

B. Laboratory Findings

Specific tests for HIV include antibody, antigen, and viral load detection (Table 31–2). Initial testing for HIV should be done using a **fourth-generation HIV antigen/antibody immunoassay**. It detects HIV-1 and HIV-2 antibodies and HIV-1 p24 antigen. Reactive specimens are then tested with an **HIV-1/HIV-2 differentiation immunoassay** to confirm infection and to distinguish HIV-1 from HIV-2. For patients who are reactive on both tests, the sensitivity and specificity for chronic HIV approach 100%. Patients who have a reactive HIV antigen/antibody immunoassay but a negative HIV-1/HIV-2 differentiation immunoassay should have a **HIV-1 viral load test (nucleic acid test)**; those with positive viral loads despite a negative differentiation assay are likely having acute HIV infection. Persons who are reactive on the initial test and then negative on the confirmatory test and have nondetectable viral loads are presumed to have a false-positive test, which may occur with recent influenza vaccination, autoantibodies (eg, with collagen vascular or autoimmune diseases), or alloantibodies from pregnancy. With fourth-generation tests, antibodies will be detectable in 99% of persons within 6 weeks after infection, with the median time to detection of about 2 weeks.

Rapid HIV antibody tests of blood or oral fluid provide results within 10–20 minutes and can be performed in clinician offices, including by personnel without laboratory training and without a Clinical Laboratory Improvement Amendment (CLIA)–approved laboratory. Persons who test positive on a rapid test require confirmation with a standard testing as above. Rapid testing is particularly helpful in settings where a result is needed immediately (eg, a woman in labor who has not recently been tested for HIV; with use of intramuscular cabotegravir or HIV prevention) or when the patient is unlikely to return for a result. Rapid HIV home tests that allow the testers to learn their status privately by simply swabbing along their gum lines are also available (www.oraquick.com).

Nonspecific laboratory findings with HIV infection may include anemia, leukopenia (particularly lymphopenia), and thrombocytopenia in any combination, elevation of the ESR, polyclonal hypergammaglobulinemia, and hypocholesterolemia. Cutaneous anergy is common with immunosuppression.

The absolute **CD4 lymphocyte count** is the most widely used marker to provide prognostic information and to guide therapy decisions (Table 31–2). As counts decrease, the risk of serious opportunistic infection over the subsequent 3–5 years increases. There are many limitations to using the CD4 count, including diurnal variation, depression with intercurrent illness or vaccination for another pathogen, and intra-laboratory and interlaboratory variability. Therefore, *the trend is more important than a single determination* and the CD4 percentage can circumvent some of the limitations of a single absolute CD4 count. The frequency of performance of counts depends on the patient's health status and whether or not they are receiving ART. All patients regardless of CD4 count should be offered ART and the CD4 count monitored regularly until virologic suppression achieved; regular CD4 monitoring after the achievement of a CD4 count greater than 350 cells/mm^3 and virologic suppression is not necessary. Initiation of *Pneumocystis jirovecii* prophylactic therapy is recommended when the CD4 count drops below 200 cells/mcL, with prophylaxis of *Toxoplasma gondii* recommended in those who are IgG-positive for the pathogen with CD4

Table 31–2. Commonly ordered tests for HIV infection.

Test	Significance
HIV-1/2 antigen/antibody immunoassay	Detects antibodies for HIV-1 and HIV-2 along with HIV-1 p24 antigen. Positive specimens require testing with HIV-1/HIV-2 antibody differentiation assay.
HIV-1/HIV-2 antibody differentiation immunoassay	Serves as confirmatory test and differentiates HIV-1 and HIV-2. Tests that are reactive on HIV-1/2 antigen/antibody immunoassay but negative on this confirmatory test should have a HIV-1 viral load test. Sensitivity and specificity of combination of reactive antigen/antibody immunoassay and positive differentiation assay approach 100% for chronic infection.
HIV rapid antibody test	Screening test for HIV. Produces results in 10–20 minutes. Can be performed by personnel with limited training. Sensitivity and specificity for chronic infection are > 99%. Positive results must be confirmed with standard HIV testing using the HIV-1/2 antigen/antibody immunoassay and the HIV-1/HIV-2 antibody differentiation assay.
HIV-1 viral load tests	This nucleic acid test measures the amount of actively replicating HIV virus. Patients who have a negative result on the HIV-1/2 antigen/antibody immunoassay or the HIV-1/HIV-2 antibody differentiation assay, or both, but have a positive HIV viral load are likely experiencing acute HIV infection; however, caution is warranted when the test result shows low-level viremia (ie, < 1000 copies/mL) as this may represent a false-positive result. Besides its use in diagnosing acute HIV infection, HIV viral load is the most accurate indicator of viral activity and response to treatment.
Absolute CD4 lymphocyte count	Best test for determining stage of HIV infection. Risk of progression to an AIDS opportunistic infection or malignancy is high with CD4 count is < 200 cells/mcL in the absence of treatment.
CD4 lymphocyte percentage	Percentage may be more reliable than the CD4 count. Risk of progression to an AIDS opportunistic infection or malignancy is high with percentage < 14% in the absence of treatment.

count less than 100 cells/mcL. Initiation of *Mycobacterium avium* prophylaxis is now only recommended in the rare cases of individuals with CD4 counts less than 50 cells/mcL who do not initiate ART (eg, due to patient refusal). The percentage of CD4 lymphocytes can be a more reliable indicator of prognosis than the absolute counts (with a percentage less than 14% roughly predictive of a CD4 count less than 200 cells/mm^3), particularly in the setting of acute illness. While the CD4 count measures immune dysfunction, it does not provide a measure of how actively HIV is replicating in the body. HIV viral load tests assess the level of viral replication and provide useful prognostic information that is independent of the information provided by CD4 counts. **The goal of ART is virologic suppression below or at the limits of detection of the assay.**

Differential Diagnosis

HIV infection may mimic a variety of other medical illnesses. Specific differential diagnosis depends on the mode of presentation. In patients presenting with constitutional symptoms such as weight loss and fevers, differential considerations include cancer, chronic infections such as tuberculosis and endocarditis, and endocrinologic diseases such as hyperthyroidism. When pulmonary processes dominate the presentation, acute and chronic lung infections must be considered as well as other causes of diffuse interstitial pulmonary infiltrates, including SARS-CoV-2 infection (COVID-19). When neurologic disease is the mode of presentation, conditions that cause mental status changes or neuropathy—eg, alcohol use disorder (alcoholism), liver disease, kidney dysfunction, thyroid disease, and vitamin deficiency—should be considered. If a patient presents with headache and a cerebrospinal fluid (CSF) pleocytosis, other causes of chronic meningitis enter the differential. When diarrhea is a prominent complaint, infectious enterocolitis, antibiotic-associated colitis, IBD, and malabsorptive syndromes must be considered.

Complications

A. Systemic Complaints

Fever, night sweats, and weight loss are common symptoms in people living with HIV and may occur without a complicating opportunistic infection. Patients with persistent fever and no localizing symptoms should nonetheless be carefully examined and evaluated with a chest radiograph (*Pneumocystis* pneumonia can present with subtle respiratory symptoms), bacterial blood cultures if the fever is greater than 38.0°C, serum cryptococcal antigen, and mycobacterial cultures of the blood. Abdominal CT scans can be considered to evaluate occult intrabdominal infections or cancers. If these studies are normal, patients should be observed closely. Antipyretics are useful to prevent dehydration.

Centers for Disease Control and Prevention. 2018 quick reference guide: recommended laboratory HIV testing algorithm for serum or plasma specimens. https://stacks.cdc.gov/view/cdc/50872

Erlandson KM et al. HIV and aging: reconsidering the approach to management of comorbidities. Infect Dis Clin North Am. 2019;33:769. [PMID: 31395144]

Pahwa S et al. NIH Workshop on HIV-associated comorbidities, coinfections, and complications: summary and recommendation for future research. J Acquir Immune Defic Syndr. 2021;86:11. [PMID: 33306561]

1. Weight changes—Weight loss is a particularly distressing complication of long-standing HIV infection. Patients typically have *disproportionate loss of muscle mass*, with maintenance or less substantial loss of fat stores. The mechanism of HIV-related weight loss is not completely understood but appears to be multifactorial, with some of the older thymidine analog medications implicated. In the setting of the newer medications, weight gain has been seen with ART, with the mechanisms and interactions currently being examined.

A. PRESENTATION—Patients with AIDS frequently suffer from anorexia, nausea, and vomiting, all of which contribute to weight loss by decreasing caloric intake. In some cases, these symptoms are secondary to a specific infection, such as viral hepatitis. In other cases, however, evaluation of the symptoms yields no specific pathogen, and it is assumed to be due to a primary effect of HIV. Malabsorption also plays a role in decreased caloric intake. Patients may suffer diarrhea from infections with bacterial, viral, or parasitic agents.

Exacerbating the decrease in caloric intake, many patients with AIDS have an increased metabolic rate. This increased rate has been shown to exist even among asymptomatic people living with HIV, but it accelerates with disease progression and secondary infection. Patients with AIDS with secondary infections also have decreased protein synthesis, which makes maintaining muscle mass difficult.

B. MANAGEMENT—Several strategies have been developed to slow AIDS wasting. In the long term, nothing is as effective as ART, since it treats the underlying HIV infection. In the short term, effective fever control decreases the metabolic rate and may slow the pace of weight loss, as does treating any underlying opportunistic infection. Food supplementation with high-calorie drinks and appetite stimulants may enable patients with low appetite to maintain their intake.

Two pharmacologic approaches for increasing appetite and weight gain are the progestational agent megestrol acetate liquid suspension (400–800 mg orally daily in divided doses) and the antiemetic agent dronabinol (2.5–5 mg orally three times a day), but *neither of these agents increases lean body mass.* Side effects from megestrol acetate are rare, but thromboembolic phenomena, edema, nausea, vomiting, and rash have been reported. In 3–10% of patients using dronabinol, euphoria, dizziness, paranoia, and somnolence and even nausea and vomiting have been reported. Dronabinol contains only one of the active ingredients in marijuana, and many patients report better relief of nausea and improvement of appetite with **medical cannabis** (THC is thought to be more effective than CBD;

administered via smoking, vaporization, essential oils, or cooked in food). In the United States, 36 states and the District of Columbia have legalized medical marijuana, and 18 states have legalized recreational (nonmedical) use. However, the use and sale of marijuana are still illegal under federal law.

Saeteaw M et al. Efficacy and safety of pharmacological cachexia interventions: systematic review and network meta-analysis. BMJ Support Palliat Care. 2021;11:75. [PMID: 33246937]

2. Nausea—Nausea leading to weight loss is sometimes due to esophageal candidiasis. Patients with oral candidiasis and nausea should be empirically treated with an oral antifungal agent. Patients with weight loss due to nausea of unclear origin may benefit from use of antiemetics or promotility agents prior to meals (prochlorperazine, 10 mg three times daily; metoclopramide, 10 mg three times daily; or ondansetron, 8 mg three times daily). Dronabinol (5 mg three times daily) or medical cannabis can also be used to treat nausea. Depression and adrenal insufficiency are two potentially treatable causes of weight loss.

Unal E et al. Cannabinoids: a guide for use in the world of gastrointestinal disease. J Clin Gastroenterol. 2020;54:769. [PMID: 31789770]

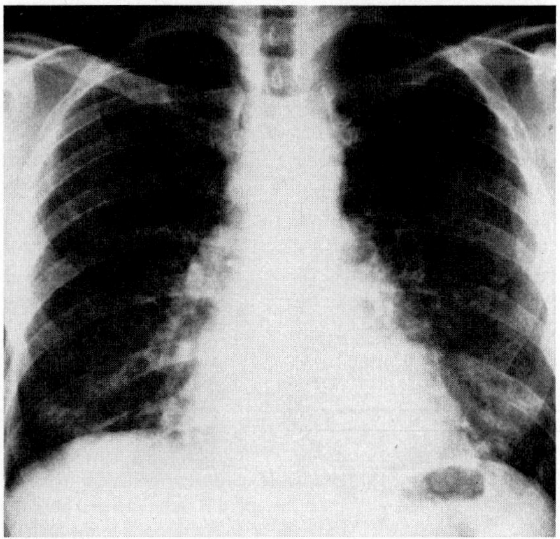

▲ **Figure 31–2.** ***Pneumocystis* pneumonia** in a Haitian woman suspected of having underlying HIV/AIDS. Typical chest radiograph showing bilateral diffuse interstitial infiltrates extending out from the hilar areas. (Reproduced, with permission, from Grippi MA, Elias JA, Fishman JA et al (editors). *Fishman's Pulmonary Diseases and Disorders*, 5th ed. McGraw-Hill, 2015.)

B. Pulmonary Disease

1. *Pneumocystis* pneumonia—(See also Chapter 36.) *P jirovecii* pneumonia is the most common opportunistic infection associated with AIDS. *Pneumocystis* pneumonia may be difficult to diagnose because the symptoms—fever, cough, and shortness of breath—are nonspecific. Furthermore, the severity of symptoms ranges from fever and no respiratory symptoms through mild cough or dyspnea to frank respiratory distress.

Hypoxemia may be severe, with a Po_2 less than 60 mm Hg. The cornerstone of diagnosis is the chest radiograph or CT scan (Figure 31–2). Diffuse or perihilar infiltrates are most characteristic, but only two-thirds of patients with *Pneumocystis* pneumonia have this finding. Normal chest radiographs are seen in 5–10% of patients with *Pneumocystis* pneumonia, although sensitivity may be increased with CT scanning, while the remainder have diffuse ground glass opacities. Severe cases can lead to pneumothoraces. Large pleural effusions are uncommon with *Pneumocystis* pneumonia; their presence suggests bacterial pneumonia, other infections such as tuberculosis, or pleural Kaposi sarcoma.

Definitive diagnosis can be obtained in 50–80% of cases by Wright-Giemsa stain or direct fluorescence antibody (DFA) test of induced sputum. Sputum induction is performed by having patients inhale an aerosolized solution of 3% saline produced by an ultrasonic nebulizer. Patients should not eat for at least 8 hours and should not use toothpaste or mouthwash prior to the procedure since they can interfere with test interpretation. The next step for patients with negative sputum examinations in whom *Pneumocystis* pneumonia is still suspected should be bronchoalveolar lavage. This technique establishes the diagnosis in over 95% of cases.

In patients with symptoms suggestive of *Pneumocystis* pneumonia but with negative or atypical chest radiographs and negative sputum examinations, other diagnostic tests may provide additional information in deciding whether to proceed to bronchoalveolar lavage. Elevation of serum LD occurs in 95% of cases of *Pneumocystis* pneumonia, but the specificity of this finding is at best 75%. A normal serum beta-glucan test makes *Pneumocystis* pneumonia unlikely, although a variety of factors can cause a false-positive serum beta-glucan test. Either a normal diffusing capacity of carbon monoxide (DL_{CO}) or a high-resolution CT scan of the chest that demonstrates no interstitial lung disease makes the diagnosis of *Pneumocystis* pneumonia very unlikely. In addition, a CD4 count greater than 250 cells/mcL within 2 months prior to evaluation of respiratory symptoms makes a diagnosis of *Pneumocystis* pneumonia unlikely; only 1–5% of cases occur above this CD4 count level (see Figure 31–1). This is true even if the patient previously had a CD4 count lower than 200 cells/mcL but has had an increase with ART. Pneumothoraces can be seen in people living with HIV with a history of *Pneumocystis* pneumonia.

Trimethoprim-sulfamethoxazole is the preferred treatment of *Pneumocystis* pneumonia (Table 31–3). In addition to specific anti-*Pneumocystis* treatment, corticosteroid therapy has been shown to improve the course of patients with moderate to severe *P jirovecii* pneumonia (Pao_2 less than 70 mm Hg on room air or alveolar-arterial O_2 gradient greater or equal to 35 mm Hg) when administered within 72 hours of the start of anti-*Pneumocystis* treatment. Steroids should be started as early as possible after

Table 31–3. Treatment of AIDS-related opportunistic infections and malignancies[1] (listed in alphabetical order).

Infection or Malignancy	Treatment	Complications[2]
Cryptococcal meningitis	Preferred regimen: Induction: Liposomal amphotericin B, 3–4 mg/kg/day intravenously, with flucytosine, 25 mg/kg/dose orally four times daily for minimum of 2 weeks (adjust flucytosine dose for kidney function), then fluconazole, 400 mg orally daily for a minimum of 8 weeks (consolidation), then 200 mg orally daily to complete a minimum of 1 year of therapy (maintenance)	Liposomal amphotericin: fever, chills, hypokalemia, kidney disease Flucytosine: bone marrow suppression, kidney disease, hepatitis Fluconazole: hepatitis
	Induction: Amphotericin B, 0.7–1.0 mg/kg/day intravenously, with flucytosine, 25 mg/kg/dose orally four times daily for a minimum of 2 weeks (adjust flucytosine dose for kidney function), then fluconazole, 400 mg orally daily for a minimum of 8 weeks (consolidation), then 200 mg orally daily to complete a minimum of 1 year of therapy (maintenance)	Amphotericin: fever, chills, hypokalemia, kidney disease Flucytosine: bone marrow suppression, kidney disease, hepatitis Fluconazole: hepatitis
	Fluconazole, used alone, is inferior to amphotericin B as induction therapy; it is recommended only for patients who cannot tolerate or do not respond to the preferred regimen above. If used for primary induction therapy, give fluconazole, 1200 mg orally daily, with flucytosine, 25 mg/kg/dose orally four times daily for a minimum of 2 weeks (adjust flucytosine dose for kidney function), then 400 mg orally daily for a minimum of 8 weeks (consolidation), then 200 mg orally daily to complete a minimum of 1 year of therapy.	Hepatitis
Cytomegalovirus retinitis (immediate sight-threatening)	Preferred regimen: First-line therapy is oral valganciclovir, 900 mg orally twice a day with food for 21 days followed by 900 mg daily (maintenance). For sight-threatening infections involving the macula or optic nerve, add intravitreal ganciclovir (2 mg/injection) or foscarnet (2.4 mg/injection) for 1–4 doses/day for 7–10 days	For valganciclovir: neutropenia, anemia, thrombocytopenia (avoid in patients with hemoglobin < 8 g/dL, neutrophil count below 500 cells/mcL [0.5×10^9/L] or platelet count below 25,000/mcL [25×10^9/L]). Potentially embryotoxic.
	Ganciclovir, 10 mg/kg/day intravenously in two divided doses for 14–21 days, followed by 5 mg/kg daily (maintenance)	Neutropenia, anemia, thrombocytopenia Adjust ganciclovir dose for kidney function. Potentially embryotoxic.
	Foscarnet, 90 mg/kg intravenously every 12 hours for 14 days, followed by 90–120 mg/kg once daily	Nausea, hypokalemia, hypocalcemia, hyperphosphatemia, azotemia Adjust foscarnet dose for kidney function.
	Cidofovir, 5 mg/kg/week intravenously for 2 weeks, then 5 mg/kg every other week with probenecid, 2 g orally 3 hours before dose, 1 g orally 2 hours after dose, and 1 g orally 8 hours after dose	Nephrotoxicity (to reduce likelihood, pre- and post-saline hydration, along with probenecid), ocular hypotony, anterior uveitis, neutropenia Avoid in patients with sulfa allergy because of cross hypersensitivity with probenecid
Esophageal candidiasis or recurrent vaginal candidiasis	Fluconazole, 100–200 mg orally daily for 14–21 days for esophageal disease and > 7 days for recurrent vaginal disease	Hepatitis, development of azole resistance. Fluconazole should *not* be given to women who are or may be pregnant because of risk of spontaneous abortion.
Herpes simplex infection	Acyclovir, 400 mg orally three times daily for 5–10 days; or acyclovir, 5 mg/kg intravenously every 8 hours for severe cases	Resistant herpes simplex with long-term therapy
	Valacyclovir, 1 g orally twice daily for 5–10 days	Nausea
	Famciclovir, 500 mg orally twice daily for 5–10 days	Nausea
	Foscarnet, 40 mg/kg intravenously every 8 hours, for acyclovir-resistant cases	Nausea, hypokalemia, hypocalcemia, hyperphosphatemia, azotemia Adjust foscarnet dose for kidney function
Herpes zoster	Preferred regimen: Valacyclovir, 1000 mg orally three times daily for 7–10 days	Nausea
	Preferred regimen: Famciclovir, 500 mg orally three times daily for 7–10 days	Nausea
	Acyclovir, 800 mg orally five times daily for 7–10 days. Intravenous therapy at 10 mg/kg every 8 hours for extensive cutaneous or visceral disease until clinical improvement, then switch to oral therapy to complete a 10- to 14-day course. For ocular involvement, consult an ophthalmologist immediately.	Nausea

(*continued*)

Table 31–3. Treatment of AIDS-related opportunistic infections and malignancies[1] (listed in alphabetical order). (continued)

Infection or Malignancy	Treatment	Complications[2]
Kaposi sarcoma		
Mild to moderate	Initiation or optimization of antiretroviral treatment	Side effects of antiretroviral treatment
Advanced disease	Chemotherapy (eg, doxorubicin or daunorubicin)	Bone marrow suppression, cardiac toxicity
	Pomalidomide, 5 mg/day orally on days 1–21 of every 28-day cycle; alternative to chemotherapy	Fatigue, asthenia, dyspnea, anemia, neutropenia; contraindicated in pregnancy
Mycobacterium avium complex infection	Clarithromycin, 500 mg orally twice daily, or azithromycin, 600 mg once daily with ethambutol, 15 mg/kg/day orally (maximum, 1 g). May also add:	Clarithromycin: hepatitis, nausea, diarrhea Ethambutol: hepatitis, optic neuritis
	Rifabutin, 300 mg orally daily	Rash, hepatitis, uveitis
Non-Hodgkin lymphoma	Combination chemotherapy (eg, R-CHOP and G-CSF). CNS disease: Radiation treatment with dexamethasone for edema	Nausea, vomiting, anemia, neutropenia, thrombocytopenia, cardiac toxicity (with doxorubicin)
Pneumocystis jirovecii infection[3]	Preferred regimen: Trimethoprim-sulfamethoxazole, 15 mg/kg/day (based on trimethoprim component) intravenously or one double-strength tablet orally three times a day for 21 days. Add prednisone when $Pao_2 < 70$ mm Hg on room air or alveolar-arterial O_2 gradient > 35 mm Hg: 40 mg orally twice a day on days 1–5, 40 mg orally daily on days 6–10, 20 mg orally daily on days 11–21	Nausea, neutropenia, anemia, hepatitis, rash, Stevens-Johnson syndrome
	Pentamidine, 3–4 mg/kg/day intravenously for 21 days plus prednisone when indicated as above	Hypotension, hypoglycemia, anemia, neutropenia, pancreatitis, hepatitis
	Primaquine, 30 mg/day orally, and clindamycin, 600 mg every 8 hours orally, for 21 days plus prednisone when indicated as above	Primaquine: hemolytic anemia in G6PD-deficient patients,[3] methemoglobinemia, neutropenia, colitis Clindamycin: rash, nausea, abdominal pain, colitis
	Not recommended for severe disease: Trimethoprim, 15 mg/kg/day orally in three divided doses, with dapsone, 100 mg/day orally, for 21 days,[3] plus prednisone when indicated as above	Nausea, rash, hemolytic anemia in G6PD[3]-deficient patients; methemoglobinemia (weekly levels should be < 10% of total hemoglobin)
	Not recommended for severe disease: Atovaquone, 750 mg orally twice daily with food for 21 days, plus prednisone when indicated as above	Rash, elevated aminotransferases, anemia, neutropenia
Toxoplasmosis	Preferred regimen: Pyrimethamine, 200 mg orally as loading dose, followed by 50 mg daily (weight ≤ 60 kg) or 75 mg daily (weight > 60 kg), combined with sulfadiazine, 1000 mg orally four times daily (weight ≤ 60 kg) or 1500 mg orally four times daily (weight > 60 kg), and leucovorin, 10–25 mg orally daily, for at least 6 weeks. Longer courses are necessary for extensive disease or incomplete clinical or radiographic resolution. Maintenance therapy with pyrimethamine, 25–50 mg orally, plus sulfadiazine, 2000–4000 mg in two to four divided doses, plus leucovorin, 10–25 mg orally daily. Long-term treatment should be maintained until immune reconstitution with antiretroviral treatment occurs.	Pyrimethamine: leukopenia, anorexia, vomiting Sulfadiazine: nausea, vomiting, Stevens-Johnson syndrome
	For patients who are intolerant of sulfa who cannot be desensitized: Substitute clindamycin, 600 mg intravenously or orally every 6 hours, for the sulfadiazine in the above regimen	Clindamycin: rash, nausea, abdominal pain, colitis
	If pyrimethamine not available: Trimethoprim-sulfamethoxazole, 10 mg/kg/day (based on trimethoprim component)	Nausea, neutropenia, anemia, hepatitis, rash, Stevens-Johnson syndrome

[1]Recommendations drawn from Centers for Disease Control and Prevention. Guidelines for the prevention and treatment of opportunistic infections in HIV-infected adults and adolescents. February 11, 2020. Downloaded from https://aidsinfo.nih.gov/guidelines on February 14, 2020.
[2]List of complications is not exhaustive.
[3]Prior to use of primaquine or dapsone, check glucose-6-phosphate dehydrogenase (G6PD) level in Black patients and those of Mediterranean origin.
G-CSF, granulocyte colony-stimulating factor (filgrastim); R-CHOP, rituximab, cyclophosphamide, doxorubicin, vincristine, prednisolone.

initiation of treatment, using prednisone 40 mg orally twice daily for days 1–5, 40 mg daily for days 6–10, and 20 mg daily for days 11–21 (for patients who cannot take oral medication, intravenous methylprednisolone can be substituted at 75% of the oral dose). The mechanism of action is presumed to be a decrease in alveolar inflammation.

Fishman JA. *Pneumocystis jirovecii*. Semin Respir Crit Care Med. 2020;41:141. [PMID: 32000290]

Shibata S et al. Pneumocystis pneumonia in HIV-1-infected patients. Respir Investig. 2019;57:213. [PMID: 30824356]

Tasaka S. Recent advances in the diagnosis and management of *Pneumocystis* pneumonia. Tuberc Respir Dis (Seoul). 2020;83: 132. [PMID: 32185915]

US Department of Health and Human Services. Guidelines for the prevention and treatment of opportunistic infections in adults and adolescents with HIV. 2020. https://clinicalinfo.hiv.gov/en/guidelines/adult-and-adolescent-opportunistic-infection/whats-new-guidelines

2. Other infectious pulmonary diseases—Other infectious causes of pulmonary disease in patients with AIDS include bacterial, mycobacterial, and viral etiologies.

A. BACTERIAL—*Community-acquired pneumonia is the most common cause of pulmonary disease in people living with HIV*. The incidence of pneumococcal pneumonia with septicemia and *Haemophilus influenzae* pneumonia is higher among people living with HIV. *Pseudomonas aeruginosa* is an important respiratory pathogen in advanced disease and, more rarely, pneumonia from *Rhodococcus equi* infection can occur sometimes along with concomitant brain abscesses. Since B-cell dysfunction is more common early on in HIV infection, recurrent bacterial infections can be one clue of a new diagnosis.

B. MYCOBACTERIAL—The incidence of infection with *Mycobacterium tuberculosis* has markedly increased in metropolitan areas because of HIV infection as well as homelessness. Tuberculosis occurs in an estimated 4% of persons in the United States who have AIDS. Patients with active tuberculosis and CD4 counts above 350 cells/mcL are likely to present with upper lobe and hilar infiltrates and paratracheal adenopathy, findings similar to persons without HIV (Figure 31–3). With advanced immunodeficiency, lower lobe, middle lobe, interstitial, and miliary infiltrates are more common, along with mediastinal adenopathy and extrapulmonary involvement. Although a purified protein derivative (PPD) test or an **interferon-gamma release assay (IGRA,** including the QuantiFERON and T-SPOT tests) should be performed on all people living with HIV in whom a diagnosis of tuberculosis is being considered, the lower the CD4 cell count, the greater the likelihood of falsely negative PPD or IGRA test results or of indeterminate IGRA test results.

In cases of active tuberculosis, treatment of people living with HIV is similar to that of people without HIV. However, *rifampin should not be given to patients receiving a boosted protease inhibitor (PI) regimen*. In these cases, rifabutin may be substituted, but it may require dosing modifications depending on the antiretroviral regimen. Tenofovir alafenamide should not be used with a rifampin and should be substituted for tenofovir disoproxil

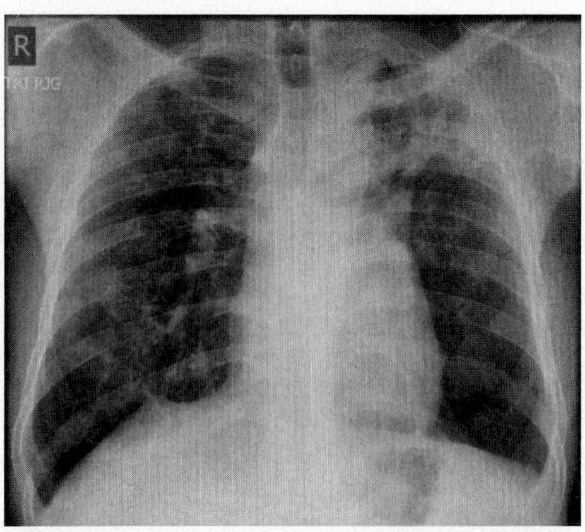

▲ **Figure 31–3.** A 36-year-old man with **pulmonary tuberculosis.** There is an opacification of a portion of the left upper lung in association with a cavity, findings consistent with pulmonary tuberculosis. Also, there is an infiltrate in the right lung. The extent of his disease raises the specter that he has underlying HIV/AIDS. (Reproduced with permission from Richard P. Usatine, MD, in Usatine RP, Smith MA, Mayeaux EJ Jr, Chumley H. *The Color Atlas of Family Medicine*, 3rd ed. McGraw-Hill, 2019)

fumarate. Dolutegravir may be given with rifampin but should be dose adjusted to twice daily. Multidrug-resistant tuberculosis has been a major problem in several metropolitan areas of the developed world, and reports from South Africa of "extremely resistant" tuberculosis in patients with AIDS are a growing global concern. Noncompliance with prescribed antituberculous medications is a major risk factor. Several of the reported outbreaks appear to implicate nosocomial spread. *The emergence of medication resistance makes it essential that antibiotic sensitivities be performed on all positive cultures*. Medication therapy should be individualized. Patients with multidrug-resistant *M tuberculosis* infection should receive at least three medications to which their organism is sensitive.

Atypical mycobacteria can cause pulmonary disease in patients with AIDS with or without preexisting lung disease and responds variably to treatment. Distinguishing between *M tuberculosis* and atypical mycobacteria requires culture of sputum specimens. DNA probes allow for presumptive identification usually within days of a positive culture. While awaiting definitive diagnosis, clinicians should err on the side of treating patients as if they have *M tuberculosis* infection unless the risk of atypical mycobacteria is very high (eg, a person without risk for tuberculosis exposure with a CD4 count under 50 cells/mcL—see Figure 31–1). Clinicians may wait for definitive diagnosis if the person is smear-negative for acid-fast bacilli, clinically stable, and not living in a communal setting.

Blanc FX et al; STATIS ANRS 12290 Trial Team. Systematic or test-guided treatment for tuberculosis in HIV-infected adults. N Engl J Med. 2020;382:2397. [PMID: 32558469]

Kerkhoff AD et al. Virtual CROI 2020: tuberculosis and coinfections in HIV infection. Top Antivir Med. 2020;28:455. [PMID: 32886465]

Lapinel NC et al. Prevalence of non-tuberculous mycobacteria in HIV-infected patients admitted to hospital with pneumonia. Int J Tuberc Lung Dis. 2019;23:491. [PMID: 31064629]

Western Cape Department of Health in collaboration with the National Institute for Communicable Diseases, South Africa. Risk factors for Coronavirus Disease 2019 (COVID-19) death in a population cohort study from the Western Cape Province, South Africa. Clin Infect Dis. 2021;73:e2005. [PMID: 32860699]

c. Viral (SARS-CoV-2 and other)—COVID-19, the illness caused by SARS-CoV-2, causes a very wide spectrum of illness, ranging from no symptoms to a mild upper respiratory tract illness with fever and cough, to a clinical triad of fever, cough, and dyspnea, to pneumonia, to acute respiratory distress syndrome (ARDS), and even to fulminant multisystem organ failure and death. Chest radiographs and CT scans may be normal early in the disease course, then may show nonspecific diffuse ground glass opacities, multilobar infiltrates, and consolidations, some progressing to full-blown ARDS (see Chapter 32).

People living with HIV have a greater propensity for severe COVID-19 disease, in part related to higher rates of medical comorbidities (eg, CVD, lung disease, long-term smoking), although low CD4 counts and virologic nonsuppression also portend higher risk. People living with HIV should be considered a priority group for preventive strategies, including boosting the initial vaccination series, and early treatment approaches such as with monoclonal antibodies or antivirals.

Persons living with HIV should not alter their ART regimens or add medications for the purpose of possibly preventing or treating SARS-CoV-2 infection. During COVID-19 surges, persons living with HIV may need additional assistance with food, housing, transportation, and childcare.

For persons living with HIV in self-isolation or quarantine due to SARS-CoV-2 exposure, clinicians should devise a plan to evaluate patients if they develop COVID-19–related persistent fever, cough, or dyspnea, including possible transfer to a health care facility for care. When a person living with HIV is hospitalized for presumed COVID-19, ART should be continued.

Isolation of cytomegalovirus (CMV) from bronchoalveolar lavage fluid occurs commonly in patients with AIDS but does not establish a definitive diagnosis. Diagnosis of CMV pneumonia requires biopsy; response to treatment is poor. Histoplasmosis, coccidioidomycosis, and cryptococcal disease as well as more common respiratory viral infections should also be considered in the differential diagnosis of unexplained pulmonary infiltrates.

Centers for Disease Control and Prevention. What to know about HIV and COVID-19. Updated 2021 Feb 1. https://www.cdc.gov/coronavirus/2019-ncov/need-extra-precautions/hiv.html

Tesoriero JM et al. COVID-19 outcomes among persons living with or without diagnosed HIV infection in New York State. JAMA Netw Open. 2021;4:e2037069. [PMID: 33533933]

US Department of Health and Human Services. Interim guidance for COVID-19 and persons with HIV. https://clinicalinfo.hiv.gov/en/guidelines/covid-19-and-persons-hiv-interim-guidance/interim-guidance-covid-19-and-persons-hiv. Updated 2021 Feb 26.

3. Noninfectious pulmonary diseases—

a. Presentation—Noninfectious causes of lung disease include Kaposi sarcoma, non-Hodgkin lymphoma, interstitial pneumonitis, primary effusion lymphoma, and increasingly, in the current ART era, lung cancer. Some of these cancers (eg, lymphoma, Kaposi sarcoma) have an underlying viral etiology. In patients with known Kaposi sarcoma, pulmonary involvement complicates the course in approximately one-third of cases. However, pulmonary involvement is rarely the presenting manifestation of Kaposi sarcoma. Non-Hodgkin lymphoma may involve the lung as the sole site of disease, but more commonly involves other organs as well, especially the brain, liver, and GI tract. Both of these processes may show nodular or diffuse parenchymal involvement, pleural effusions, and mediastinal adenopathy on chest radiographs.

Nonspecific interstitial pneumonitis may mimic *Pneumocystis* pneumonia. Lymphocytic interstitial pneumonitis seen in lung biopsies has a variable clinical course. Typically, these patients present with several months of mild cough and dyspnea; chest radiographs show interstitial infiltrates. Many patients with this entity undergo transbronchial biopsies in an attempt to diagnose *Pneumocystis* pneumonia. Instead, the tissue shows interstitial inflammation ranging from an intense lymphocytic infiltration (consistent with lymphoid interstitial pneumonitis) to a mild mononuclear inflammation.

b. Management—Corticosteroids may be helpful in some cases refractory to ART.

Marcus JL et al. Comparison of overall and comorbidity-free life expectancy between insured adults with and without HIV infection, 2000-2016. JAMA Netw Open. 2020;3:e207954. [PMID: 32539152]

4. Sinusitis—Chronic sinusitis can be a frustrating problem for people living with HIV. Symptoms include sinus congestion and discharge, headache, and fever. Some patients may have radiographic evidence of sinus disease on sinus CT scan in the absence of significant symptoms.

C. Central Nervous System Disease

CNS disease in people living with HIV can be divided into intracerebral space-occupying lesions, encephalopathy, meningitis, and spinal cord processes. Many of these complications have declined markedly in prevalence in the era of effective ART. Cognitive declines, however, may be more common in persons with HIV, especially as they age (older than 50 years), even those who are taking fully suppressive ART.

Stephens RJ et al. Central nervous system infections in the immunocompromised adult presenting to the emergency department. Emerg Med Clin North Am. 2021;39:101. [PMID: 33218652]

1. Toxoplasmosis—Toxoplasmosis used to be one of the most common CNS space-occupying lesion in people living with HIV. Headache, focal neurologic deficits, seizures, or altered mental status may be presenting symptoms. The diagnosis is usually made presumptively based on the characteristic appearance of cerebral imaging studies in an individual known to be seropositive for *Toxoplasma*. Typically, toxoplasmosis appears as multiple contrast-enhancing lesions on CT scan. Lesions tend to be peripheral, with a predilection for the basal ganglia.

Single lesions are atypical of toxoplasmosis. When a single lesion has been detected by CT scanning, MRI scanning may reveal multiple lesions because of its greater sensitivity. If a patient has a single lesion on MRI and is neurologically stable, clinicians may pursue a 2-week empiric trial of toxoplasmosis therapy. A repeat scan should be performed at 2 weeks. If the lesion has not diminished in size, biopsy of the lesion should be performed. A positive *Toxoplasma* serologic test does *not* confirm the diagnosis because many people living with HIV have detectable titers without having active disease. Conversely, less than 3% of patients with toxoplasmosis have negative titers. Therefore, negative *Toxoplasma* titers in a patient with HIV infection and a space-occupying lesion should be a cause for aggressively pursuing an alternative diagnosis. The preferred treatment of toxoplasmosis is with pyrimethamine and sulfadiazine (Table 31–3). If pyrimethamine is not available, patients can be treated with oral trimethoprim-sulfamethoxazole.

Vidal JE. HIV-related cerebral toxoplasmosis revisited: current concepts and controversies of an old disease. J Int Assoc Provid AIDS Care. 2019;18:2325958219867315. [PMID: 31429353]

2. CNS lymphoma—Primary non-Hodgkin lymphoma is the second most common CNS space-occupying lesion in people living with HIV. Symptoms are similar to those with toxoplasmosis. While imaging techniques cannot distinguish these two diseases with certainty, lymphoma more often is solitary. Other less common lesions should be suspected if there is preceding bacteremia, positive tuberculin test, fungemia, or injection drug use. These include bacterial abscesses, cryptococcomas, tuberculomas, and *Nocardia* lesions.

Stereotactic brain biopsy should be strongly considered if lesions are solitary or do not respond to toxoplasmosis treatment, especially if they are easily accessible. Diagnosis of lymphoma is important because many patients benefit from treatment (radiation therapy). A positive PCR assay of CSF for Epstein-Barr virus (EBV) DNA is consistent with a diagnosis of lymphoma; recent data show that PCR for EBV DNA in CSF was 100% sensitive and 98.5% specific for AIDS-associated primary CNS lymphoma, making it useful as a diagnostic tumor marker.

Cinque P et al. Epstein-Barr virus DNA in cerebrospinal fluid from patients with AIDS-related primary lymphoma of the central nervous system. Lancet. 1993;342:398. [PMID: 8101902]

Kimani SM et al. Epidemiology of haematological malignancies in people living with HIV. Lancet HIV. 2020;7:e641. [PMID: 32791045]

3. HIV-associated dementia and neurocognitive disorders—Patients with HIV-associated dementia typically have difficulty with cognitive tasks (eg, memory, attention), exhibit diminished motor function, and have emotional or behavioral problems. Patients may first notice a deterioration in their handwriting. The manifestations of dementia may wax and wane, with persons exhibiting periods of lucidity and confusion over the course of a day. The diagnosis of HIV-associated dementia is one of exclusion based on a brain imaging study and on spinal fluid analysis that excludes other pathogens. Neuropsychiatric testing is helpful in distinguishing patients with dementia from those with depression. Many patients improve with effective ART. However, slowly progressive neurocognitive deficits may still develop in patients taking ART as they age.

Metabolic abnormalities may also cause changes in mental status: hypoglycemia, hyponatremia, hypoxia, and drug overdose are important considerations in this population. Other less common infectious causes of encephalopathy include progressive multifocal leukoencephalopathy (discussed below), CMV, syphilis, and herpes simplex encephalitis.

Avedissian SN et al. Pharmacologic approaches to HIV-associated neurocognitive disorders. Curr Opin Pharmacol. 2020;54:102. [PMID: 33049585]

Rosca EC et al. Montreal Cognitive Assessment (MoCA) for HIV-associated neurocognitive disorders. Neuropsychol Rev. 2019;29:313. [PMID: 31440882]

4. Cryptococcal meningitis—Cryptococcal meningitis typically presents with fever and headache. Less than 20% of patients have meningismus. Diagnosis is based on a positive latex agglutination test of serum that detects cryptococcal antigen (or "CrAg") or positive culture of spinal fluid for *Cryptococcus*. Seventy to 90% of patients with cryptococcal meningitis have a positive serum CrAg. Thus, a negative serum CrAg test makes a diagnosis of cryptococcal meningitis unlikely and can be useful in the initial evaluation of a patient with headache, fever, and normal mental status. Treatment has three phases: induction, consolidation, and maintenance. Induction treatment is given for a minimum of 2 weeks plus evidence of clinical improvement and a negative CSF culture on repeat lumbar puncture. The preferred induction treatment is liposomal amphotericin with flucytosine (Table 31–3), followed by an oral fluconazole treatment, and then secondary prophylaxis. Prophylaxis can be stopped if the patient is asymptomatic, has a CD4 cell count of greater than 100/mcL for at least 3 months, and has suppressed viral load on effective ART.

Boyer-Chammard T et al. Recent advances in managing HIV-associated cryptococcal meningitis. F1000Res. 2019;8:743. [PMID: 31275560]

Lawrence DS. Emerging concepts in HIV-associated cryptococcal meningitis. Curr Opin Infect Dis. 2019;32:16. [PMID: 30507673]
Skipper C et al. Diagnosis and management of central nervous system cryptococcal infections in HIV-infected adults. J Fungi (Basel). 2019;5:E65. [PMID: 31330959]

5. Meningococcal meningitis—People living with HIV infection are at increased risk for meningococcal disease. Treatment is the same as in people without infection. Therefore, the Advisory Committee on Immunization Practices recommends the meningococcal conjugate vaccine (serogroups A, C, W, and Y) for all persons aged 2 months or older with HIV infection.

6. HIV meningitis and HIV myelopathy—HIV meningitis, characterized by lymphocytic pleocytosis of the spinal fluid with negative culture, is common early in HIV infection. Spinal cord function may also be impaired in individuals with HIV infection. HIV myelopathy presents with leg weakness and incontinence. Spastic paraparesis and sensory ataxia are seen on neurologic examination. Myelopathy is usually a late manifestation of HIV disease, and most patients will have concomitant HIV encephalopathy. Pathologic evaluation of the spinal cord reveals vacuolation of white matter. Because HIV myelopathy is a diagnosis of exclusion, symptoms suggestive of myelopathy should be evaluated by lumbar puncture to rule out CMV polyradiculopathy (described below) and an MRI or CT scan to exclude epidural lymphoma.

Leffert J et al. HIV-vacuolar myelopathy: an unusual early presentation in HIV. Int J STD AIDS. 2021;32:205. [PMID: 33323068]

7. Progressive multifocal leukoencephalopathy (PML)—PML is a viral infection (with the JC polyomavirus) of the white matter of the brain seen in patients with very advanced HIV infection. It typically results in focal neurologic deficits such as aphasia, hemiparesis, and cortical blindness. Imaging studies are strongly suggestive of the diagnosis if they show non-enhancing white matter lesions without mass effect; the diagnosis is verified by JC virus positivity via PCR in the CSF. Patients can stabilize or improve after the institution of effective ART. In the setting of wide-scale ART and because PML occurs at very low CD4 counts, the prevalence of this condition is now rare.

Abrão CO et al. AIDS-related progressive multifocal leukoencephalopathy. Rev Soc Bras Med Trop. 2020;54:e02522020. [PMID: 33338109]
Cortese I et al. Progressive multifocal leukoencephalopathy and the spectrum of JC virus-related disease. Nat Rev Neurol. 2021;17:37. [PMID: 33219338]

D. Peripheral Nervous System

A. PRESENTATION—Peripheral nervous system syndromes include inflammatory polyneuropathies, sensory neuropathies, and mononeuropathies.

An **inflammatory demyelinating polyneuropathy** similar to Guillain-Barré syndrome can occur in people living with HIV, usually prior to frank immunodeficiency. The syndrome in many cases improves with plasmapheresis, supporting an autoimmune basis of the disease. CMV can cause an ascending polyradiculopathy characterized by lower extremity weakness and a neutrophilic pleocytosis on spinal fluid analysis with a negative bacterial culture. Transverse myelitis can be seen with herpes zoster or CMV.

Peripheral neuropathy is common among people living with HIV. Patients typically complain of numbness, tingling, and pain in the lower extremities. Symptoms are disproportionate to findings on gross sensory and motor evaluation. Beyond HIV infection itself, the most common cause is prior ART with a thymidine analog, such as stavudine or didanosine (although both are very rarely used now). Unfortunately, medication-induced neuropathy was not always reversed when the offending agent was discontinued. Patients with advanced disease may also develop peripheral neuropathy even if they have never taken ART. Evaluation should rule out other causes of sensory neuropathy such as alcohol use disorder, thyroid disease, diabetes, vitamin B_{12} deficiency, and syphilis.

B. MANAGEMENT—Treatment of peripheral neuropathy is aimed at symptomatic relief. Patients should be initially treated with gabapentin (start at 300 mg at bedtime and increase to 300–900 mg orally three times a day) or other co-analgesics for neuropathic pain (see Chapter 5). Opioid analgesics should be avoided because the condition tends to be chronic and patients are likely to become dependent on these agents without significant improvement in their functional status.

Julian T et al. Human immunodeficiency virus-related peripheral neuropathy: a systematic review and meta-analysis. Eur J Neurol. 2021;28:1420. [PMID: 33226721]

E. Rheumatologic and Bone Manifestations

Arthritis, involving single or multiple joints, with or without effusion, has been commonly noted in people living with HIV. Involvement of large joints is most common. Although the cause of HIV-related arthritis is unknown, most patients will respond to NSAIDs. Patients with a sizable effusion, especially if the joint is warm or erythematous, should have the joint aspirated, followed by culture of the fluid to rule out suppurative arthritis as well as fungal and mycobacterial disease.

Several **rheumatologic syndromes**, including reactive arthritis, psoriatic arthritis, sicca syndrome, and SLE, have been reported in people living with HIV (see Chapter 20). However, it is unclear if the prevalence is greater than in the general population. Cases of avascular necrosis of the femoral heads have been reported sporadically, generally in the setting of advanced disease with long-standing infection and in patients receiving long-term ART. The etiology is not clear but is probably multifactorial in nature.

Osteoporosis and **osteopenia** appear to be more common in people living with HIV with chronic infection and perhaps associated with long-term use of ART. Vitamin D deficiency appears to be quite common among people living with HIV and monitoring vitamin D levels and instituting replacement therapy for detected deficiency are recommended. Bone mineral density scans for postmenopausal women with HIV and men over the age of 50 years are also recommended.

Thomsen MT et al. Prevalence of and risk factors for low bone mineral density assessed by quantitative computed tomography in people living with HIV and uninfected controls. J Acquir Immune Defic Syndr. 2020;83:165. [PMID: 31929404]

Vega LE et al. Human immunodeficiency virus infection (HIV)-associated rheumatic manifestations in the pre- and post-HAART eras. Clin Rheumatol. 2020;39:2515. [PMID: 32297034]

F. Myopathy

Myopathies are infrequent in the era of effective ART but can be related to either HIV infection or ART, particularly with use of the older agent zidovudine (azidothymidine [AZT]). Proximal muscle weakness is typical, and patients may have varying degrees of muscle tenderness. Given its long-term toxicities, zidovudine is no longer recommended when alternative treatments are available. Integrase strand transferase inhibitors rarely have been associated with myopathy.

G. Retinitis

In people living with HIV, complaints of visual changes must be evaluated immediately by an ophthalmologist familiar with the manifestations of HIV disease. **CMV retinitis,** characterized by perivascular hemorrhages and white fluffy exudates, is the most common retinal infection in patients with AIDS, usually with CD4 counts greater than 50 cells/mm^3, and can be rapidly progressive (Figure 31–4). In contrast, cotton wool spots, which are also common in people living with HIV, are benign, remit spontaneously, and appear as small indistinct white spots without exudation or hemorrhage. Other rare retinal processes include other herpesvirus infections or toxoplasmosis. Choice of treatment for CMV retinitis (Table 31–3) depends on severity and location of lesions, and the patient's overall condition and circumstances.

Ballard B et al. CMV retinitis. EyeWiki. 2020 Oct 22. https://eyewiki.org/CMV_Retinitis#General_treatment

Heiden D et al. Active cytomegalovirus retinitis after the start of antiretroviral therapy. Br J Ophthalmol. 2019;103:157. [PMID: 30196272]

Tang Y et al. Clinical features of cytomegalovirus retinitis in HIV infected patients. Front Cell Infect Microbiol. 2020;10:136. [PMID: 32318357]

Wons J et al. HIV-induced retinitis. Ocul Immunol Inflamm. 2020;28:1259. [PMID: 32966142]

H. Oral Lesions

A. Presentation—**Oral candidiasis** can be bothersome to patients, many of whom report an unpleasant taste or mouth dryness. The two most common forms of oral candidiasis seen are pseudomembranous (removable white plaques) and erythematous (red friable plaques). **Angular cheilitis**—fissures at the sides of the mouth—is usually due to *Candida* as well

Hairy leukoplakia is caused by the Epstein-Barr virus. The lesion is not usually troubling to patients and sometimes regresses spontaneously. Hairy leukoplakia is commonly seen as a white lesion on the lateral aspect of the tongue. It may be flat or slightly raised, is usually corrugated, and has vertical parallel lines with fine or thick ("hairy") projections (see Figure 8–6). Unlike oral candidiasis, this lesion cannot be scraped off, a distinguishing feature in the physical examination.

The presence of oral candidiasis or hairy leukoplakia is significant for several reasons. First, these lesions are highly suggestive of HIV infection in patients who have no other obvious cause of immunodeficiency. Second, several studies have indicated that patients with candidiasis have a high rate of progression to AIDS even with statistical adjustment for CD4 count.

Gingival disease is common in people living with HIV and is thought to be due to an overgrowth of microorganisms. **Aphthous ulcers** are painful and may interfere with eating.

Other lesions seen in the mouths of people living with HIV include **Kaposi sarcoma** (usually on the hard palate) and **warts**.

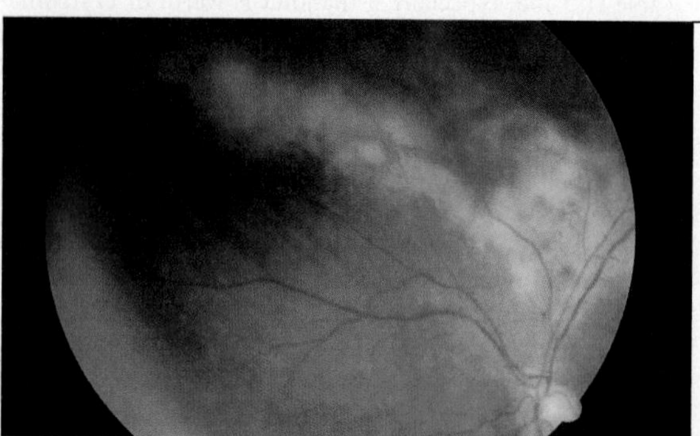

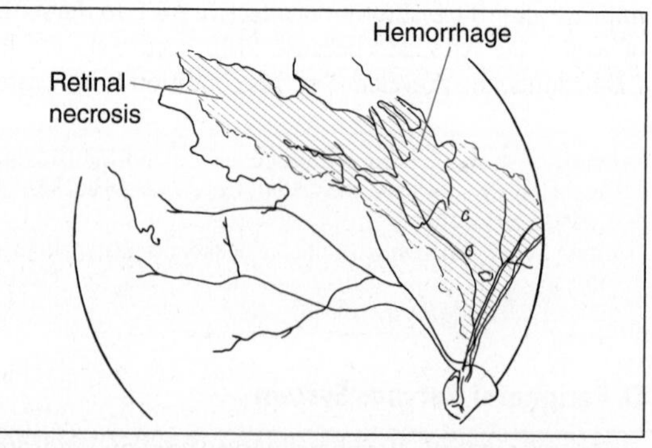

▲ **Figure 31–4. CMV retinitis.** **Retina has classic "pizza pie" or "cheese and ketchup" appearance, with hemorrhages and dirty white, granular appearing retinal necrosis adjacent to major vessels (see diagrammatic map).** (Diagram reproduced with permission from Knoop KJ, Stack LB, Storrow AB, Thurman RJ. *The Atlas of Emergency Medicine*, 5th ed. McGraw Hill, 2021.)

b. Management—Treatment of oral candidiasis is with topical agents such as clotrimazole 10-mg troches (one troche four or five times a day). Patients with candidiasis who do not respond to topical antifungals can be treated with fluconazole (50–100 mg orally once a day for 3–7 days). Angular cheilitis can be treated topically with ketoconazole cream (2%) twice a day.

Gingival disease usually responds to professional dental cleaning and chlorhexidine rinses. A particularly aggressive gingivitis or periodontitis will develop in some people living with HIV; these patients should be given antibiotics that cover anaerobic oral flora (eg, metronidazole, 250 mg four times a day for 4 or 5 days) and referred to oral surgeons with experience with these entities.

Aphthous ulcers can be treated with fluocinonide (0.05% ointment mixed 1:1 with plain Orabase and applied six times a day to the ulcer). For lesions that are difficult to reach, patients should use dexamethasone swishes (0.5 mg in 5 mL elixir three times a day). The pain of the ulcers can be relieved with use of an anesthetic spray (10% lidocaine).

Indrastiti RK et al. Oral manifestations of HIV: can they be an indicator of disease severity? (A systematic review). Oral Dis. 2020;26:133. [PMID: 32862546]

Tappuni AR. The global changing pattern of the oral manifestations of HIV. Oral Dis. 2020;26:22. [PMID: 32862536]

I. Gastrointestinal Manifestations

1. Candidal and other esophagitis—(See also Chapter 15.) **Esophageal candidiasis** is a common AIDS complication. In a patient with characteristic symptoms, empiric antifungal treatment is begun with fluconazole (100–200 mg orally daily for 14–21 days). Improvement in symptoms should be apparent within 1–2 days of antifungal treatment. If there is no improvement, fungal culture to exclude fluconazole resistance, and further evaluation to identify other causes of esophagitis (herpes simplex, CMV) is recommended.

Hoversten P et al. Risk factors, endoscopic features, and clinical outcomes of cytomegalovirus esophagitis based on a 10-year analysis at a single center. Clin Gastroenterol Hepatol. 2020;18:736. [PMID: 31077832]

Mohamed AA et al. Diagnosis and treatment of esophageal candidiasis: current updates. Can J Gastroenterol Hepatol. 2019;2019:3585136. [PMID: 31772927]

2. Hepatic disease—

a. Presentation—Autopsy studies have demonstrated that the liver is a frequent site of infections and neoplasms in people living with HIV. However, many of these infections are not clinically symptomatic. Mild elevations of alkaline phosphatase and aminotransferases are often noted on routine chemistry panels. **Mycobacterial disease, CMV, hepatitis B virus, hepatitis C virus,** and **lymphoma** cause liver disease and can present with varying degrees of nausea, vomiting, right upper quadrant abdominal pain, and jaundice. Sulfonamides, imidazole medications, antituberculous medications, pentamidine, clarithromycin, and didanosine have also been associated with hepatitis. *The thymidine analog medications in the nucleoside reverse transcriptase inhibitor (NRTI) class can cause lactic acidosis and hepatic steatosis, which can be fatal.* However, these medications, especially didanosine and stavudine, are rarely used in ART regimens any longer. Finally, people living with HIV with chronic hepatitis may have more rapid progression of liver disease because of the concomitant immunodeficiency or hepatotoxicity of ART. Percutaneous liver biopsy may be helpful in diagnosing liver disease, but some common causes of liver disease (eg, *M avium* complex, lymphoma) can be determined by less invasive measures (eg, blood culture, biopsy of a more accessible site).

b. Management—With patients living longer as a result of advances in ART, advanced liver disease and hepatic failure due to chronic active hepatitis B or hepatitis C, or both, are increasing causes of morbidity and mortality. People living with HIV who also have **hepatitis B** infection should be treated with antiretroviral regimens that include medications with activity against both viruses (tenofovir disoproxil fumarate [TDF] or tenofovir alafenamide [TAF], lamivudine, or emtricitabine). It is important to be extremely cautious about discontinuing these medications in coinfected patients as sudden discontinuation could lead to a fatal flare of hepatitis B infection. **Nonalcoholic fatty liver disease** is a growing concern among people living with HIV, particularly given concerns for weight gain and insulin resistance with integrase inhibitors. Treatment involves lifestyle modification, avoidance of alcohol, and optimization of diabetes control. If nonalcoholic steatohepatitis (NASH) with fibrosis is identified on biopsy, vitamin E therapy can be considered.

Hepatitis C is more virulent in persons living with HIV and should be treated using the new HCV direct-acting antivirals (see Table 16–6). Prior to treatment, the patient's HCV viral load and HCV genotype should be determined. Depending on the genotype and the proposed treatment regimen, HCV resistance testing is recommended. For example, HCV resistance testing is recommended for patients with genotype 1a (the most common hepatitis C genotype in the United States) who are being considered for treatment with elbasvir/grazoprevir because substitutions in certain amino acid positions confer resistance. Because the appropriate treatment regimen depends on genotype, resistance profile, whether the patient is treatment-naïve, as well as whether the patient has cirrhosis (and, if so, whether it is compensated or decompensated), clinicians should check the guidelines of the American Association for the Study of Liver Disease (ASLD)/Infectious Diseases Society of America (IDSA) (https://www.hcvguidelines.org/) to see the recommended regimens (see also Tables 16–6 and 16–7). Costs of the different regimens vary by purchaser, and many clinicians choose the least expensive of the recommended regimens.

Although the recommended regimens are the same for people living with HIV, potential drug interactions with ART may complicate treatment. Clinicians should check the guidelines of the AASLD/IDSA and US Department of Health and Human Services or the guidelines of the University of Liverpool to determine interactions between proposed hepatitis C regimen and HIV regimen.

Liver transplants have been performed successfully in people living with HIV. This strategy is most likely to be successful in persons who have CD4 counts greater than 100 cells/mcL and nondetectable viral loads.

Lake JE et al. Expert panel review on nonalcoholic fatty liver disease in persons with human immunodeficiency virus. Clin Gastroenterol Hepatol. 2022;20:256. [PMID: 33069882]
Patel SV et al. Real-world efficacy of direct acting antiviral therapies in patients with HIV/HCV. PLoS One. 2020;15:e0228847. [PMID: 32053682]
University of Liverpool. HEP drug interactions. https://www.hep-druginteractions.org

3. Biliary disease—Cholecystitis presents with manifestations similar to those seen in immunocompetent hosts but is more likely to be acalculous. **Sclerosing cholangitis** and **papillary stenosis** have also been reported in people living with HIV. Typically, the syndrome presents with severe nausea, vomiting, and right upper quadrant pain. Liver enzymes generally show alkaline phosphatase elevations disproportionate to elevation of the aminotransferases. Although dilated ducts can be seen on ultrasound, the diagnosis is made by endoscopic retrograde cholangiopancreatography, which reveals intraluminal irregularities of the proximal intrahepatic ducts with "pruning" of the terminal ductal branches. Stenosis of the distal common bile duct at the papilla is commonly seen. CMV, *Cryptosporidium*, and microsporidia are thought to play inciting roles in this syndrome, but these conditions are rarely seen unless the patient is suffering with very advanced HIV-related immunodeficiency.

Velásquez JN et al. Multimethodological approach to gastrointestinal microsporidiosis in HIV-infected patients. Acta Parasitol. 2019;64:658. [PMID: 31286356]

4. Enterocolitis—

A. PRESENTATION—**Enterocolitis** is a common problem in people living with HIV. Organisms known to cause enterocolitis include bacteria (*Campylobacter*, *Salmonella*, *Shigella*), viruses (CMV, adenovirus, SARS-CoV-2), and protozoans (*Cryptosporidium*, *Entamoeba histolytica*, *Giardia*, *Isospora*, microsporidia). HIV itself may cause enterocolitis. Several of the organisms causing enterocolitis in people living with HIV also cause diarrhea in immunocompetent persons. However, people living with HIV tend to have more severe and more chronic symptoms, including high fevers and severe abdominal pain that can mimic acute abdominal catastrophes. Bacteremia and concomitant biliary involvement are also more common with enterocolitis in people living with HIV. Relapses of enterocolitis following adequate therapy have been reported with both *Salmonella* and *Shigella* infections.

Because of the wide range of agents known to cause enterocolitis, a stool culture and multiple stool examinations for ova and parasites (including modified acid-fast staining for *Cryptosporidium*) should be performed. Those patients who have *Cryptosporidium* in one stool with improvement in symptoms in less than 1 month should not be considered to have AIDS, as *Cryptosporidium* is a cause of self-limited diarrhea in HIV-negative persons. More commonly, people living with HIV with *Cryptosporidium* infection have persistent enterocolitis with profuse watery diarrhea.

B. MANAGEMENT—To date, no consistently effective treatments have been developed for *Cryptosporidium* infection except to improve immune function through the use of effective ART. The diarrhea can be treated symptomatically with diphenoxylate with atropine (one or two tablets orally three or four times a day). Those who do not respond may be given paregoric with bismuth (5–10 mL orally three or four times a day). Octreotide in escalating doses (starting at 0.05 mg subcutaneously every 8 hours for 48 hours) has been found to ameliorate symptoms in approximately 40% of patients with cryptosporidia, although the benefit is often short-lived. Paromomycin has been shown to have benefit in small randomized clinical trials. However, only nitazoxanide (500–1000 mg twice daily) is FDA-approved for treatment of cryptosporidiosis in children and adults as an effective anti-parasitic treatment. Finally, durable remission almost always requires immune reconstitution with ART.

Patients with a negative stool examination and persistent symptoms should be evaluated with colonoscopy and biopsy. Patients whose symptoms last longer than 1 month with no identified cause of diarrhea are considered to have a presumptive diagnosis of HIV enteropathy. Patients may respond to institution of effective ART or octreotide. Upper endoscopy with small bowel biopsy is not recommended as a routine part of the evaluation.

Sparks BS et al. Treatment of *Cryptosporidium*: what we know, gaps, and the way forward. Curr Trop Med Rep. 2015;2:181. [PMID: 26568906]

5. Other disorders—Two other important GI abnormalities in people with advanced AIDS are **gastropathy** and **malabsorption**. It has been documented that some people living with HIV do not produce normal levels of stomach acid and therefore are unable to absorb medications that require an acid medium. This decreased acid production may explain, in part, the susceptibility of people living with HIV to *Campylobacter*, *Salmonella*, and *Shigella*, all of which are sensitive to acid concentration. There is no evidence that *Helicobacter pylori* is more common in people living with HIV.

A malabsorption syndrome occurs commonly in patients with AIDS. It can be due to infection of the small bowel with *M avium* complex, *Cryptosporidium*, or microsporidia.

J. Endocrinologic Manifestations

Hypogonadism is probably the most common endocrinologic abnormality in men living with HIV. The adrenal gland is also a commonly afflicted endocrine gland in patients with AIDS. Abnormalities demonstrated on autopsy include infection (especially with CMV and *M avium* complex), infiltration with Kaposi sarcoma, and injury from hemorrhage and presumed autoimmunity. The prevalence of clinically significant adrenal insufficiency is low. Patients with suggestive symptoms should undergo a cosyntropin stimulation test.

Although frank deficiency of cortisol is rare, an isolated defect in mineralocorticoid metabolism may lead to salt-wasting and hyperkalemia. Such patients should be treated with fludrocortisone (0.1–0.2 mg orally daily).

Patients with AIDS appear to have abnormalities of thyroid function tests different from those of patients with other chronic diseases. Patients with AIDS have been shown to have high levels of triiodothyronine (T_3), thyroxine (T_4), and thyroid-binding globulin and low levels of reverse triiodothyronine (rT_3). The causes and clinical significance of these abnormalities are unknown.

Maffezzoni F et al. Hypogonadism and bone health in men with HIV. Lancet HIV. 2020;7:e782. [PMID: 33128905]
Pezzaioli LC et al. The importance of SHBG and calculated free testosterone for the diagnosis of symptomatic hypogonadism in HIV-infected men: a single-centre real-life experience. Infection. 2021;49:295. [PMID: 33289905]
Santi D et al. The prevalence of hypogonadism and the effectiveness of androgen administration on body composition in HIV-infected men: a meta-analysis. Cells. 2021;10:2067. [PMID: 34440836]

K. Skin Manifestations

The skin manifestations that commonly develop in people living with HIV can be grouped into viral, bacterial, fungal, neoplastic, and nonspecific dermatitides.

Coates SJ et al. What's new in HIV dermatology? F1000Res. 2019;8:980. [PMID: 31297183]

1. Viral dermatitides—

A. Herpes simplex infections—These infections (Figure 31–5) occur more frequently, tend to be more severe, and are more likely to disseminate in patients with AIDS than in immunocompetent persons. Because of the risk of progressive local disease, *all herpes simplex attacks should be treated* for 5–10 days with acyclovir (400 mg orally three times a day), famciclovir (500 mg orally twice daily), or valacyclovir (500 mg orally twice daily) (Table 31–3). To avoid the complications of attacks, many clinicians recommend suppressive therapy for people living with HIV with a history of recurrent herpes. Options for suppressive therapy include acyclovir (400 mg orally twice daily), famciclovir (250 mg orally twice daily), and valacyclovir (500 mg orally daily). Long-term suppressive herpes prophylaxis with acyclovir does not reduce HIV transmission between heterosexual men and women from developing countries.

James C et al. Herpes simplex virus: global infection prevalence and incidence estimates, 2016. Bull World Health Organ. 20201;98:315. [PMID: 32514197]

B. Herpes zoster—This is a common manifestation of HIV infection. Patients with herpes zoster infections should be treated for 7–10 days with famciclovir (500 mg orally three times a day) or valacyclovir (500 mg three times a day). Acyclovir can also be used, but it requires very frequent dosing (800 mg orally four or five times per day for 7 days). Vesicular lesions should be cultured if there is any question about their origin, since herpes simplex responds to much lower doses of acyclovir. Disseminated zoster and cases with ocular involvement should be treated with intravenous (10 mg/kg every 8 hours for 7–10 days) rather than oral acyclovir. *The recombinant zoster vaccine (Shingrix, two doses administered 2–6 months apart) should be given to people living with HIV*. Because it is not a live virus like the previous zoster vaccine (Zostavax), it is not contraindicated in patients with immune deficiency but, based on other vaccines, people living with HIV are likely to develop more robust immune response to the vaccine when their CD4 count is greater than 200/mcL.

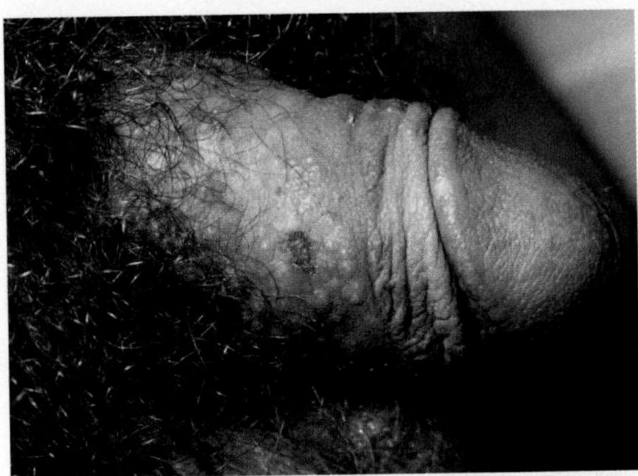

▲ Figure 31–5. Herpes simplex viral skin infection, frequently found in men living with HIV. Shown are grouped vesicles typical of herpes simplex on the penis, with both intact vesicles of initial eruption and visible crusts of resolving lesions. (Reproduced, with permission, from Eric Kraus, MD, in: Usatine RP, Smith MA, Mayeaux EJ Jr, Chumley H. *The Color Atlas and Synopsis of Family Medicine*, 3rd ed. McGraw-Hill, 2019.)

Harbecke R et al. Herpes zoster vaccines. J Infect Dis. 2021; 224:S429. [PMID: 34590136]

C. Molluscum contagiosum—This infection is caused by a pox virus and is seen in people living with HIV, as in other immunocompromised patients. The characteristic umbilicated fleshy papular lesions have a propensity for spreading widely over the patient's face and neck (Figure 31–6) and should be treated with topical liquid nitrogen.

Murphy M et al. Non-HPV perianal and anorectal sexually transmitted viral infections. Clin Colon Rectal Surg. 2019; 32:340. [PMID: 31507343]

2. Bacterial dermatitides—

A. Staphylococcal infection—*Staphylococcus* is the most common bacterial cause of skin disease in

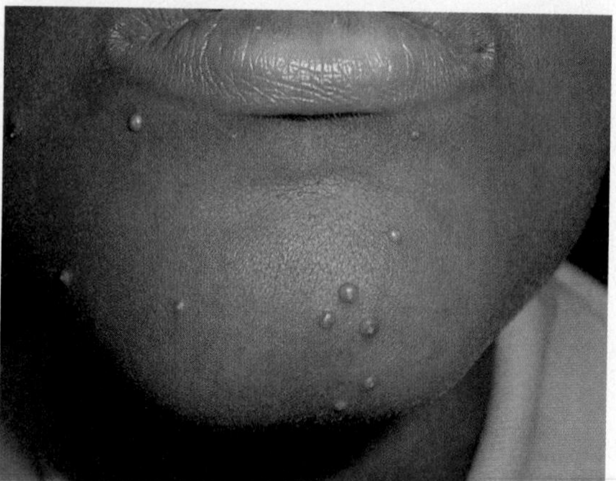

▲ **Figure 31–6. Molluscum contagiosum.** Extensive molluscum contagiosum lesions on the face of a young woman, suggestive she may have HIV. (Reproduced with permission from Richard P. Usatine, MD, in Usatine RP, Smith MA, Mayeaux EJ Jr, Chumley H. *The Color Atlas of Family Medicine*, 3rd ed. McGraw-Hill, 2019.)

people living with HIV; it usually presents as **folliculitis, superficial abscesses (furuncles),** or **bullous impetigo.** These lesions should be treated aggressively since sepsis can occur. Folliculitis is initially treated with topical clindamycin or mupirocin, and patients may benefit from regular washing with an antibacterial soap such as chlorhexidine. Intranasal mupirocin and cleaning intact skin with chlorhexidine soap, has been used successfully for staphylococcal decolonization in other settings. In people living with HIV with recurrent staphylococcal infections, weekly intranasal mupirocin should be considered in addition to topical care and systemic antibiotics. Abscesses often require incision and drainage. Patients may need antistaphylococcal antibiotics as well. Due to high frequency of methicillin-resistant *Staphylococcus aureus* (MRSA) skin infections in people living with HIV, *coverage of MRSA in empiric regimens is necessary*. Recommendations for empiric treatment are either (1) trimethoprim-sulfamethoxazole (one double-strength tablet orally twice daily); (2) doxycycline (100 mg orally twice daily); or (3) linezolid (600 mg orally twice daily) with close follow-up.

Hatlen TJ et al. Staphylococcal skin and soft tissue infections. Infect Dis Clin North Am. 2021;35:81. [PMID: 33303329]

Sabbagh P et al. The global and regional prevalence, burden, and risk factors for methicillin-resistant *Staphylococcus aureus* colonization in HIV-infected people: a systematic review and meta-analysis. Am J Infect Control. 2019;47:323. [PMID: 30170767]

B. Bacillary angiomatosis—It is caused by two closely related organisms: *Bartonella henselae* and *Bartonella quintana*. The epidemiology of these infections suggests zoonotic transmission from fleas of infected domestic cats (*henslae*) or contact with human body louse feces (*quintana*). The most common manifestation is raised, reddish, highly vascular skin lesions that can mimic lesions of Kaposi sarcoma. Fever is a common manifestation of this infection; involvement of bone, lymph nodes, liver (peliosis hepatis) and endocarditis have also been reported. The infection is treated with doxycycline, 100 mg orally twice daily and rifampin, 300 mg orally twice daily for a prolonged period depending on the seriousness of the infection. Patients who are seriously ill with visceral involvement or endocarditis may require at least 6 months of therapy.

Ding F et al. Clinical and echocardiographic characteristics of Bartonella infective endocarditis: an 8-year single-centre experience in the United States. Heart Lung Circ. 2022;31:350. [PMID: 34456130]

3. Fungal rashes—

A. Rashes due to dermatophytes and Candida—Most fungal rashes afflicting patients with AIDS are due to dermatophytes and *Candida*. While particularly common in the inguinal region, they may occur anywhere on the body. Fungal rashes generally respond well to topical clotrimazole (1% cream twice a day) or ketoconazole (2% cream twice a day).

B. Seborrheic dermatitis—This is more common in people living with HIV. Scrapings of seborrhea have revealed *Malassezia furfur (Pityrosporum ovale)*, implying that the seborrhea is caused by this fungus. A consistent finding is that seborrhea responds well to topical clotrimazole (1% cream) as well as hydrocortisone (1% cream).

Moreno-Coutiño G et al. Isolation of *Malassezia* spp. in HIV-positive patients with and without seborrheic dermatitis. An Bras Dermatol. 2019;94:527. [PMID: 31777352]

Wikramanayake TC et al. Seborrheic dermatitis—looking beyond *Malassezia*. Exp Dermatol. 2019;28:991. [PMID: 31310695]

4. Neoplastic dermatitides—See Chapter 6 and the Kaposi sarcoma section below.

5. Nonspecific dermatitides—

A. Xerosis—This condition presents in people living with HIV with severe pruritus. The patient may have no rash, or nonspecific excoriations from scratching. Treatment is with emollients (eg, absorption base cream) and antipruritic lotions (eg, camphor 9.5% and menthol 0.5%).

B. Psoriasis—Psoriasis can be very severe in people living with HIV. Phototherapy, topical retinoids, and etretinate (0.25–9.75 mg/kg/day orally in divided doses) may be used for recalcitrant cases in consultation with a dermatologist.

L. HIV-Related Malignancies

Four cancers are currently included in the CDC classification of AIDS: Kaposi sarcoma, non-Hodgkin lymphoma, primary lymphoma of the brain, and invasive cervical carcinoma. Epidemiologic studies have shown that between 1973 and 1987, among single men in San Francisco, the risk of Kaposi sarcoma increased more than 5000-fold and the risk of non-Hodgkin lymphoma more than 10-fold. The increase in incidence of malignancies is probably a function of impaired cell-mediated immunity. In the current treatment era, cancers not classified as AIDS-related, such as lung cancer, are being increasingly diagnosed in aging people living with HIV despite optimal ART. *Cohort studies suggest that adults living with HIV are at increased risk for a variety of cancers compared with age-matched adults who do not have HIV.* Mortality secondary to malignancies represents an increasing cause of death in people with HIV.

Chiao EY et al. The effect of non-AIDS-defining cancers on people living with HIV. Lancet Oncol. 2021;22:e240. [PMID: 34087151]

Pumpalova YS et al. The impact of HIV on non-AIDS defining gastrointestinal malignancies: a review. Semin Oncol. 2021;48:226. [PMID: 34593219]

Vangipuram R et al. AIDS-associated malignancies. Cancer Treat Res. 2019;177:1. [PMID: 30523619]

1. Kaposi sarcoma—

A. PRESENTATION—Lesions may appear anywhere; careful examination of the eyelids, conjunctiva, pinnae, palate, and toe webs is mandatory to locate potentially occult lesions. In light-skinned individuals, Kaposi lesions usually appear as purplish, nonblanching lesions that can be papular or nodular. In dark-skinned individuals, the lesions may appear browner. In the mouth, lesions are most often palatal papules, though exophytic lesions of the tongue and gingivae may also be seen. Kaposi lesions may be confused with other vascular lesions such as angiomas and pyogenic granulomas. Pulmonary Kaposi sarcoma can present with chronic cough, hemoptysis, or both and is associated with peribronchovascular nodules on CT scan. It can be diagnosed via bronchoscopy following visualization of the typical lesions. Kaposi sarcoma lesions can occur shortly after initiating ART, especially in patients starting ART who have advanced immunodeficiency. In this situation, Kaposi sarcoma is likely to be an immune reconstitution reaction (see Inflammatory Reactions, below). Kaposi sarcoma can also cause visceral disease (eg, GI, pulmonary).

B. MANAGEMENT—Patients with mild to moderate forms of Kaposi sarcoma do not require specific treatment as the lesions usually resolve with effective ART. However, it should be noted that the lesions may flare when ART is first initiated—probably as a result of an immune reconstitution process. Advanced disease is treated with combination chemotherapy (Table 31–3).

Alves CGB et al. Clinical and laboratory profile of people living with HIV/AIDS with oral Kaposi sarcoma. AIDS Res Hum Retroviruses. 2021;37:870. [PMID: 34538064]

Gouveia-Moraes F et al. Conjunctival Kaposi's sarcoma. N Engl J Med. 2021;385:e36. [PMID: 34525288]

Ngalamika O et al. Antiretroviral therapy for HIV-associated cutaneous Kaposi's sarcoma: clinical, HIV-related, and sociodemographic predictors of outcome. AIDS Res Hum Retroviruses. 2021;37:368. [PMID: 33386064]

2. Non-Hodgkin lymphoma—

A. PRESENTATION—Non-Hodgkin lymphomas in HIV-infected persons tends to be very aggressive. These malignancies are usually of B-cell origin and characterized as diffuse large-cell tumors. Over 70% of the malignancies are extranodal.

B. MANAGEMENT—The prognosis of patients with systemic non-Hodgkin lymphoma depends primarily on the degree of immunodeficiency at the time of diagnosis. Patients with high CD4 counts do markedly better than those diagnosed with lower CD4 counts. Patients with primary CNS lymphoma typically are treated with high-dose methotrexate-based chemotherapy with or without rituximab in concert with a hematologist or oncologist.

Kimani SM et al. Epidemiology of haematological malignancies in people living with HIV. Lancet HIV. 2020;7:e641. [PMID: 32791045]

Lurain K et al. Treatment of HIV-associated primary CNS lymphoma with antiretroviral therapy, rituximab, and high-dose methotrexate. Blood. 2020;136:2229. [PMID: 32609814]

3. Hodgkin disease—Although Hodgkin disease is not included as part of the CDC definition of AIDS, studies have found that HIV infection is associated with a fivefold increase in the incidence of Hodgkin disease. HIV-infected persons with Hodgkin disease are more likely to have mixed cellularity and lymphocyte depletion subtypes of Hodgkin disease and to seek medical attention at an advanced stage of disease.

Perricone AJ et al. Cytodiagnostic sensitivity of fine needle aspiration biopsy for Hodgkin's lymphoma is decreased in patients with human immunodeficiency virus infection. Acta Cytol. 2019;63:352. [PMID: 31234174]

Re A et al. HIV and lymphoma: from epidemiology to clinical management. Mediterr J Hematol Infect Dis. 2019;11:e2019004. [PMID: 30671210]

4. Anal dysplasia and squamous cell carcinoma—These lesions have been strongly correlated with previous infection by HPV and noted in both men and women living with HIV. Although many of the men who have sex with men who are living with HIV report a history of anal warts or have visible warts, a significant percentage have silent papillomavirus infection. Cytologic (using Papanicolaou smears) and papillomavirus DNA studies can easily be performed on specimens obtained by anal swab. Because of the risk of progression from dysplasia to cancer in immunocompromised patients, **regular anal cytologic examinations in people with HIV should be performed**. An anal Papanicolaou smear is performed by rotating a moistened Dacron swab about 2 cm into the anal canal. The swab is immediately inserted into a cytology bottle. In the large ANCHOR study presented at the 2022 Conference on Retroviruses and Opportunistic Infections (CROI), which involved nearly 4500 individuals with anal high-grade squamous intraepithelial lesions (HGSIL), nine patients who were assigned to aggressive therapy (mostly office-based electrocautery) developed anal cancer compared with 21 of those in an active monitoring group, representing a 57% decrease in relative risk over the median 25.8-month follow-up period. This pivotal study will change care toward more aggressive screening for HGSIL and treatment to prevent progression to anal cancer.

HPV also appears to play a causative role in **cervical dysplasia** and **carcinoma** in women living with HIV (discussed below).

Cimic A et al. Importance of anal cytology and screening for anal dysplasia in individuals living with HIV with an emphasis on women. Cancer Cytopathol. 2019;127:407. [PMID: 31145557]

Goddard SL et al; Study for the Prevention of Anal Cancer (SPANC) Research Team. Prevalence and association of perianal and intra-anal warts with composite high-grade squamous intraepithelial lesions among gay and bisexual men: baseline data from the Study of the Prevention of Anal Cancer. AIDS Patient Care STDS. 2020;34:436. [PMID: 32955927]

Palefsky J et al. Treatment of anal high-grade squamous intraepithelial lesions to prevent anal cancer. CROI 2022 (special session)

Power Foley M et al. Management of anal intraepithelial neoplasia and anal squamous cell carcinoma at a tertiary referral centre with a dedicated infectious diseases unit: an 18-year review. Int J Colorectal Dis. 2020;35:1855. [PMID: 32500433]

M. Gynecologic Manifestations

Vaginal candidiasis, cervical dysplasia and neoplasia, and pelvic inflammatory disease are more common in women living with HIV than in women without HIV. These manifestations also tend to be more severe when they occur in association with HIV infection. Therefore, women living with HIV need frequent gynecologic care. **Vaginal candidiasis** may be treated with topical agents or a single dose of oral fluconazole (150 mg) (see Chapter 36). Recurrent vaginal candidiasis should be treated with fluconazole (100–200 mg) for at least 7 days. However, fluconazole increases the risk of spontaneous abortion and should not be given to women who are or may be pregnant.

The incidence of **cervical dysplasia** in women living with HIV is 40%. Because of this finding, *recommended screening for women living with HIV is more extensive than for women without HIV* (see Chapter 18). For women younger than age 30 years, a Papanicolaou smear should be performed within a year of the onset of sexual activity, but no later than age 21 years. If normal, Papanicolaou smears should be performed yearly. After three negative examinations, screening should be done every 3 years. HPV DNA testing of the cervical specimen is not recommended for women younger than age 30 years.

For women aged 30 years or older, screening should continue beyond age 65 years (unlike the general population). There are two accepted screening protocols: cytology alone and cytology with HPV DNA co-testing. A Papanicolaou smear is done when HIV is diagnosed and every 12 months thereafter, and after three negative smears, ongoing screening can be performed every 3 years. Alternatively, a Papanicolaou smear with co-testing for HPV DNA can be performed when HIV is diagnosed or starting when patients are 30 years old. If Papanicolaou smear is normal and HPV test is negative, then the next screening can be in 3 years.

The management of abnormal Papanicolaou tests and positive HPV tests is the same in infected women as in uninfected women. Treatment should follow the consensus guidelines in the references below.

While **pelvic inflammatory disease** appears to be more common in women living with HIV, the bacteriology of this condition appears to be the same as among women without HIV. Women living with HIV who have pelvic inflammatory disease should be treated with the same regimens as women without HIV (see Chapter 18).

Castle PE et al. Cervical cancer prevention and control in women living with human immunodeficiency virus. CA Cancer J Clin. 2021;71:505. [PMID: 34499351]

Strickler HD et al. Primary HPV and molecular cervical cancer screening in US women living with HIV. Clin Infect Dis. 2021;72:1529. [PMID: 32881999]

N. Coronary Artery Disease

People living with HIV are at higher risk for CAD than age- and sex-matched controls. Part of this increase in CAD may be due to changes in lipids caused by antiretroviral agents (see below), including several of the PIs and tenofovir alafenamide. Some data suggest abacavir may be associated with MI, possibly related to increased platelet aggregation, although this has not been found in all studies. Some of the risk appears to be due to HIV infection, independent of its therapy. It is important that clinicians pay close attention to this issue because MIs tend to present at a younger age in individuals with HIV than in individuals without HIV. People living with HIV with symptoms of CAD such as chest pain or dyspnea should be rapidly evaluated. Clinicians should aggressively treat conditions that result in increased risk of heart disease, especially smoking, hypertension, hyperlipidemia, obesity, diabetes mellitus, and sedentary lifestyle.

Hsue PY et al. HIV infection and coronary heart disease: mechanisms and management. Nat Rev Cardiol. 2019;16:745. [PMID: 31182833]

Patel AA et al. Coronary artery disease in patients with HIV infection: an update. Am J Cardiovasc Drugs. 2021;21:411. [PMID: 33184766]

O. Inflammatory Reactions (Immune Reconstitution Inflammatory Syndromes)

With initiation of ART, some patients experience inflammatory reactions that appear to be associated with immune reconstitution as indicated by a rapid increase in CD4 count. These inflammatory reactions may present with generalized signs of fevers, sweats, and malaise with or without more localized manifestations that usually represent unusual presentations of opportunistic infections. For example, vitreitis has developed in patients with CMV retinitis after they have been treated with ART.

M avium can present as focal even suppurative lymphadenitis or granulomatous masses in patients receiving ART. Tuberculosis may paradoxically worsen with new or evolving pulmonary infiltrates and lymphadenopathy.

PML and cryptococcal meningitis may also behave atypically. Clinicians should be alert to these syndromes, which are most often seen in patients who have initiated ART in the setting of advanced disease and who show rapid increases in CD4 counts with treatment. The diagnosis of **immune reconstitution inflammatory syndrome (IRIS)** is one of exclusion and can be made only after recurrence or new opportunistic infection has been ruled out as the cause of the clinical deterioration. Management of IRIS is conservative and supportive with use of corticosteroids only for severe reactions. Most authorities recommend that ART be continued unless the IRIS reaction is life-threatening.

Sereti I. Immune reconstruction inflammatory syndrome in HIV infection: beyond what meets the eye. Top Antivir Med. 2020;27:106. [PMID: 32224502]

Sereti I et al. Prospective international study of incidence and predictors of immune reconstitution inflammatory syndrome and death in people living with human immunodeficiency virus and severe lymphopenia. Clin Infect Dis. 2020;71:652. [PMID: 31504347]

Prevention

A. Primary Prevention

Until a safe and effective HIV vaccine is available, prevention of HIV infection will depend on HIV testing and counseling, including precautions regarding sexual practices and injection drug use, initiation of ART as a prevention tool for transmission to others, preexposure and postexposure use of antiretrovirals, perinatal management including antiretroviral treatment of the mother, screening of blood products, and infection control practices in the health care setting.

1. HIV testing and counseling—Primary care clinicians should routinely obtain a sexual history and provide risk factor assessment of their patients. Because approximately 13% of people living with HIV in the United States do *not* know they have infection, **the USPSTF recommends that clinicians screen for HIV infection in adolescents and adults ages 15 to 65 years at least once in a lifetime**. Younger adolescents and older adults who are at increased risk should also be screened, with repeat screening as often as indicated for anyone at ongoing risk. Clinicians should review the risk factors for HIV infection with the patient and discuss HIV prevention strategies and safer needle use as well as the meaning of a positive test. Although the CDC recommends "opt-out" testing in medical settings, some states require specific written consent. For persons whose test results are positive, it is critically important that they be connected to medical care. *Most public health guidelines and HIV specialists advocate for initiating care and treatment the same day that someone tests positive, including patients in safety-net settings* (see C. Antiviral Treatment, below). Referrals for partner-notification services, social services, mental health services, and HIV prevention services should also be provided.

For patients whose test results are negative, clinicians should review HIV prevention strategies, needle use practices, or both. Pre-exposure prophylaxis and postexposure prophylaxis are highly effective HIV prevention strategies and are reviewed below. To prevent sexual transmission of HIV, only **latex or polyurethane condoms** should be used, along with a water-soluble lubricant. Although nonoxynol-9, a spermicide, kills HIV, it is *contraindicated* because in some patients it may cause genital ulcers that could facilitate HIV transmission. Patients should be counseled that condoms are not 100% effective. They should be made familiar with the use of condoms, including, specifically, the advice that condoms must be used every time, that space should be left at the tip of the condom as a receptacle for semen, that intercourse with a condom should not be attempted if the penis is only partially erect, that men should hold on to the base of the condom when withdrawing the penis to prevent slippage, and that condoms should not be reused. Women as well as men having sex with men should understand how to use condoms to be sure that their partners are using them correctly. Several randomized trials in Africa demonstrated that **male circumcision** significantly reduced HIV incidence in men and, eventually, in female partners. This has led to circumcision roll-out programs across the African continent.

Persons using injection drugs should be cautioned not to share **needles or other drug paraphernalia**. When sterile needles are not available, bleach does appear to inactivate HIV and can be used to clean needles. Pre-exposure prophylaxis is an effective prevention option if clean needles are not readily available (see below).

Beksinska M et al. Male and female condoms: their key role in pregnancy and STI/HIV prevention. Best Pract Res Clin Obstet Gynaecol. 2020;66:55. [PMID: 32007451]

Coffey S… Gandhi M. RAPID antiretroviral therapy: high virologic suppression rates with immediate antiretroviral therapy initiation in a vulnerable urban clinic population. AIDS. 2019;33:825. Erratum in: AIDS. 2019;33:2113. [PMID: 30882490]

2. ART for decreasing transmission of HIV to others (treatment as prevention)—Besides preventing progression of HIV disease, effective ART decreases the risk of HIV transmission between sexual partners. Among serodiscordant couples (men who have sex with men or heterosexual), stably suppressing HIV with ART completely eliminated the risk of HIV transmission to the uninfected partner in three large cohort studies. Although HIV-negative persons in stable long-term partnerships with persons living with HIV represent only one group of at-risk persons, increasing the use of ART among the population of people living with HIV appears to decrease community-wide transmission of HIV. *Despite major improvements in effectiveness and tolerability of ART, only about 60% of people living with HIV in the United States are virally suppressed.* Persons in whom the HIV virus remains consistently suppressed (less than 200 copies/mL) do not transmit HIV *sexually*. The efficacy of treatment as prevention for transmission via injection drug use is less clear; people living with HIV or at risk of HIV should be encouraged to avoid sharing injection equipment to prevent forward transmission.

Cobb DA et al. Long-acting approaches for delivery of antiretroviral drugs for prevention and treatment of HIV: a review of recent research. Expert Opin Drug Deliv. 2020;17:1227. [PMID: 32552187]

Cohen MS et al. Prevention of HIV transmission and the HPTN 052 Study. Annu Rev Med. 2020;71:347. [PMID: 31652410]

Saag MS et al. Antiretroviral drugs for treatment and prevention of HIV infection in adults: 2020 recommendations of the International Antiviral Society—USA Panel. JAMA. 2020;324:1651. [PMID: 33052386]

3. Preexposure ART prophylaxis—Several large randomized double-blind placebo-controlled trials demonstrated that administering tenofovir disoproxil fumarate/emtricitabine (TDF/FTC) can reduce the risk of sexual transmission of HIV among uninfected individuals at high risk for infection; one study was of HIV-negative men and transgender women who have sex with men, and two studies were conducted in heterosexual couples. Preexposure tenofovir has also been shown to reduce HIV infection among injection drug users from Thailand. In addition, real-world studies and demonstration projects of men who have sex with men and cisgender women, where adherence with emtricitabine/TDF has been adequate (high efficacy with an average of at least four doses/week), have found **preexposure prophylaxis (PrEP)** to be highly effective in preventing HIV infection. Subsequent trials and open-label studies have also shown high efficacy with the use of event-based dosing (two tablets 2 to 24 hours prior to sex, and then one tablet 24 hours later, and a final tablet 24 hours after that) for TDF/FTC among men who have sex with men. And, finally, tenofovir alafenamide TAF/FTC was also shown to be noninferior to TDF/FTC among men who have sex with men and transgender women so is approved for non-vaginal sex. TAF/FTC is associated with lower bone and renal toxicity than TDF/FTC but increased weight gain and dyslipidemia. Emtricitabine/TAF has not been studied among cisgender women or with the use of event-based PrEP dosing (ie, 2-1-1 dosing). Cabotegravir, a long-acting medication for PrEP, was approved by the FDA in 2022 for use as PrEP as an injectable medication, every 8 weeks. This medication has been shown to be superior to oral TDF/FTC in preventing HIV infection among men who have sex with men, transgender women who have sex with men, and cisgender women in sub-Saharan Africa.

CDC guidelines recommend offering PrEP to persons at "substantial risk" for HIV. Risk for HIV is a combination of the likelihood of having a partner who is living with HIV and the likelihood that the behavior (eg, type of intercourse, shared needles) puts them at risk of HIV transmission. Men who have sex with men, and transgender women are the groups with the highest HIV seroprevalence in the United States, and they are likely to have partners who may be living with HIV or of unknown HIV status. Those who have receptive anal intercourse have the highest risk of HIV because the behavior is more efficient at transmitting HIV than other sexual practices. People who use drugs are also at high risk for HIV infection if they do not consistently use clean needles or if they trade drugs for sex. It can be hardest to assess the risk of heterosexual people who are not at risk from drug use because it requires assessing the likelihood that their partners have HIV risks. However, it is important to assess risk as accurately as possible among cisgender women in order to offer PrEP when indicated. Factors known to increase the risk of HIV transmission and therefore make PrEP a good choice for particular groups of patients are shown in Table 31–4.

Finally, for PrEP to be effective, patients need to have adequate adherence, particularly around the time of exposure. Following results of the 2-1-1 event-based dosing protocol showing high efficacy among men who have sex with men, taking a double dose on the first day 2–24 hours prior to sex is recommended to shorten the time to maximum protection. This approach has not been studied among transgender women, heterosexuals, and people who inject drugs. Based on pharmacology modelling, it takes at least 7–10 days for PrEP to reach maximum efficacy for receptive vaginal sex. Men who have sex with men and transgender women study participants who took at least four daily doses in a week were protected as well as those who took the drug every day, indicating that occasional missed doses do not render the treatment ineffective. PrEP demonstration projects conducted in cisgender women show similar findings. For patients preparing to stop PrEP, dosing should be continued for at least 2 days beyond the last exposure for men who have sex with men based on the 2-1-1 protocol. It is not clear how long other groups should continue PrEP following the last exposure, with some clinicians recommending 28 days based on postexposure prophylaxis studies.

Recommendations on initial and follow-up assessments are shown in Table 31–4. TDF/FTC is contraindicated for persons with kidney disease (creatinine clearance less than 60 mL/minute) because of the small risk of kidney toxicity with TDF. Decreases in bone mineral density have been documented in persons taking TDF/FTC for PrEP at 24 weeks; whether this decrease will have clinical significance is unknown, and declines appear to reverse after stopping PrEP. For men who have sex with men and have creatinine clearance less than 60 mL/minute but greater than 30 mL/minute, or osteoporosis/osteopenia (or at risk for these conditions), clinicians may opt to use TAF/FTC.

High rates of sexually transmitted infections (STIs) have also been seen in persons taking PrEP, indicating the importance of regular follow-up in patients using PrEP. Regular asymptomatic STI screening and subsequent treatment among PrEP users (including rectal and pharyngeal testing for people exposed at those sites) can make substantial impact on the worsening non-HIV STI epidemic. Some patients are reluctant to use insurance to cover the cost of the medication for fear of revealing that they are at risk for HIV; without insurance, the cost is high. Programs are available from the medication manufacturer to cover the cost of treatment for low-income uninsured persons and to cover insurance copays for insured patients. Increasing availability of generic emtricitabine/TDF is expected to further decrease costs. Finally, latex or polyurethane condoms will prevent other STIs and pregnancy.

Table 31–4. Recommendations for preexposure prophylaxis (PrEP) of HIV infection.

Patients for whom PrEP should definitely be considered as a good option for HIV prevention
Sexually active men who have sex with men, male-to-female transgender persons, and heterosexuals and bisexual women who are likely to have partners with HIV risks
Injection drug users
Factors that increase the likelihood that PrEP is a good option
Patient has receptive anal intercourse
Patient has a partner with a known HIV infection without durable virologic suppression, or a partner of unknown HIV status
Patient has a history of STDs
Patient has a high number of sex partners
Patient is a commercial sex worker
Patient with inconsistent or no condom use
Patient who has been incarcerated or who has partners that have been incarcerated
Patient is from or whose partners are from an area where HIV incidence is high
Patient who is sharing needles or related paraphernalia ("works")
Initial assessment before prescribing PrEP
HIV antibody test to confirm HIV-negative
Symptom review to exclude primary HIV infection (eg, no history of acute illness with fever and rash in prior month)
STD tests: syphilis; gonorrhea (at risk site-specific); and chlamydia (at risk site-specific)
Serum creatinine and eGFR[1]
Confirm immunity to HBV or vaccinate if nonimmune[2]
Pregnancy test
Discuss that PrEP does not protect against other STDs and may have side effects
Counsel patients that they can use latex or polyurethane condoms to prevent STDs and clean needles to prevent bacterial infections and hepatitis C, in addition to PrEP
Assess illicit substance use and offer treatment, if needed
Discuss importance of adherence to daily medication or 2-1-1 PrEP around the time of exposures
PrEP prescription
Emtricitabine/TDF (Truvada) 1 tablet orally daily, 90-day prescription supply recommended. (Double dose is recommended on day 1 for men who have sex with men but would shorten the time to therapeutic drug levels in any patient)
Emtricitabine/TAF (Descovy) 1 tablet orally daily, 90-day prescription supply recommended (men who have sex with men and transgender women only)
Follow-up assessment
HIV test every 3 months
Serum creatinine every 6–12 months
Pregnancy test every 3 months
STD tests: syphilis, gonorrhea (at risk site-specific); and chlamydia (at risk site-specific)
Assess and support medication adherence
Reinforce benefits of using latex or polyurethane condoms and clean needles with PrEP
Assess substance use and offer treatment, if needed

[1]Emtricitabine/TDF is contraindicated if creatinine clearance < 60 mL/minute.

[2]Persons with HBV infection may experience HBV reactivation and liver damage if emtricitabine/TDF is stopped.

HBV, hepatitis B virus; STD, sexually transmitted disease; TDF, tenofovir disoproxil fumarate.

PrEP checklists for providers and patients are available at https://www.cdc.gov/hiv/risk/prep/index.html (Last reviewed August 6, 2021).

Chou R et al. Pre-exposure prophylaxis for the prevention of HIV infection: evidence report and systematic review for the U.S. Preventive Services Task Force. JAMA. 2019;321:2214. [PMID: 31184746]

Hillis A et al. Pre-exposure prophylaxis (PrEP) for HIV prevention among men who have sex with men (MSM): a scoping review on PrEP service delivery and programming. AIDS Behav. 2020;24:3056. [PMID: 32274670]

Joseph Davey DL; PrEP in Pregnancy Working Group. Emerging evidence from a systematic review of safety of pre-exposure prophylaxis for pregnant and postpartum women: where are we now and where are we heading? J Int AIDS Soc. 2020;23:e25426. [PMID: 31912985]

Vanhamel J et al. The current landscape of pre-exposure prophylaxis service delivery models for HIV prevention: a scoping review. BMC Health Serv Res. 2020;20:704. [PMID: 32736626]

4. Postexposure prophylaxis for sexual and drug use exposures to HIV—The goal of **postexposure prophylaxis** is to reduce or prevent local viral replication prior to dissemination such that the infection can be aborted. Although there is no prior clinical trial showing that administration of antiretroviral medications following a sexual or parenteral drug use exposure reduces the likelihood of infection, there is suggestive data from animal models, perinatal experience, and a case-control study of health care workers who experienced a needle stick.

Treatment of persons who have been exposed to HIV should be *within 72 hours*, but sooner is better. All exposed persons should first receive HIV testing to exclude the possibility that they already have infection. If rapid tests are not available, treatment should begin pending the results of a standard HIV test.

The choice of antiretroviral agents and the duration of treatment are the same as those for exposures that occur through the occupational route; the preferred regimen is tenofovir 300 mg with emtricitabine 200 mg daily with dolutegravir 50 mg once daily or raltegravir 400 mg twice a day. In contrast to those with occupational exposures, some individuals may present very late after exposure. Because the likelihood of success declines with length of time from HIV exposure, treatment is *not* recommended after more than 72 hours after exposure. In addition, because the psychosocial issues involved with postexposure prophylaxis for sexual and drug use exposures are complex, it should be offered with prevention counseling. Counseling should focus on how to prevent future exposures. Individuals with ongoing risk for HIV infection should be considered candidates for PrEP, sometimes called PEP-to-PrEP. Clinicians needing more information on postexposure prophylaxis for occupational or nonoccupational exposures should contact the National Clinicians' Post-Exposure Prophylaxis Hotline (1-888-448-4911; http://nccc.ucsf.edu/clinician-consultation/pep-post-exposure-prophylaxis/).

Atim M et al; Dean Street Collaborative Group. Post-exposure prophylaxis in the era of pre-exposure prophylaxis. HIV Med. 2020;21:668. [PMID: 32902098]

Centers for Disease Control and Prevention. HIV, HIV Basics, Prevention, PEP (Post-Exposure Prophylaxis). 2020 Oct 21. https://www.cdc.gov/hiv/basics/pep.html

DeHaan E. Post-exposure prophylaxis (PEP) to prevent HIV infection [Internet]. Baltimore (MD): Johns Hopkins University; 2020. [PMID: 33026756]
Heendeniya A et al. Antiretroviral medications for the prevention of HIV infection: a clinical approach to preexposure prophylaxis, postexposure prophylaxis, and treatment as prevention. Infect Dis Clin North Am. 2019;33:629. [PMID: 31239092]
O'Connell KA et al. HIV post-exposure prophylaxis in the emergency department: an updated assessment and opportunities for HIV prevention identified. Am J Emerg Med. 2020: S0735-6757(20)30888-3 [PMID: 33069548]

5. Prevention of perinatal transmission of HIV—Prevention of perinatal transmission of HIV begins by offering HIV counseling and testing to all women who are pregnant or considering pregnancy. Women living with HIV who are pregnant should start ART with at least three medications as quickly as possible. The recommended regimens include a dual-NRTI combination and either dolutegravir or ritonavir-boosted darunavir. Cesarean delivery should be planned if HIV viral load is greater than 1000 copies/mL or unknown near the time of delivery and one or more antiretroviral medications administered to the newborn for 6 weeks to reduce the risk of perinatal acquisition. In places with full access to infant formula, breastfeeding is usually discouraged.

Dettinger JC et al. Perinatal outcomes following maternal preexposure prophylaxis (PrEP) use during pregnancy: results from a large PrEP implementation program in Kenya. J Int AIDS Soc. 2019;22:e25378. [PMID: 31498563]
Joseph Davey DL et al; PrEP in Pregnancy Working Group. Emerging evidence from a systematic review of safety of preexposure prophylaxis for pregnant and postpartum women: where are we now and where are we heading? J Int AIDS Soc. 2020;23:e25426. [PMID: 31912985]

6. Prevention of HIV transmission in health care settings—In health care settings, **universal body fluid precautions** should be used, including use of gloves when handling body fluids and the addition of gown, mask, and goggles for procedures that may result in splash or droplet spread, and use of specially designed needles with sheath devices to decrease the risk of needle sticks.

Epidemiologic studies show that needle sticks occur commonly among health care professionals, especially among surgeons performing invasive procedures, inexperienced hospital house staff, and medical students. Efforts to reduce needle sticks should focus on avoiding recapping needles and use of safety needles whenever doing invasive procedures under controlled circumstances. The risk of HIV transmission from a needle stick with blood from a patient with HIV infection is approximately 1:300, although determinants of risk include deep punctures, large inoculum, and source patients with high viral loads. The risk from mucous membrane contact and contact to non-intact skin is 1:1000 or less.

Health care professionals who sustain needle sticks should be counseled and offered **HIV testing** as soon as possible. HIV testing is done to establish a negative baseline in case there is a subsequent conversion. Follow-up testing is usually performed at 6 weeks and 3 months. With the patient's permission, their blood can be tested for HIV, with postexposure prophylaxis and further follow-up discontinued for the healthcare worker if the source patient tests negative.

A case-control study by the CDC indicates that administration of zidovudine following a needle stick decreases the rate of HIV seroconversion by 79%. Therefore, *clinicians should be offered ART as soon as possible after exposure and continued for 4 weeks.* Modern antiretrovirals have not been studied, but the efficacy is expected to be higher with more potent and better-tolerated integrase inhibitor-based three-drug regimens. The preferred regimen is TDF 300 mg with emtricitabine 200 mg (Truvada) daily with dolutegravir 50 mg once daily or raltegravir 400 mg twice a day. Clinicians who have exposures to persons who are likely to have antiretroviral medication resistance (eg, persons receiving therapy who have detectable viral loads) should have their therapy individualized, using at least two medications to which the source is unlikely to be resistant.

Centers for Disease Control and Prevention. Human Immunodeficiency Virus (HIV) and Occupational Exposure. September 5, 2019. https://www.cdc.gov/hiv/workplace/healthcareworkers.html

7. Prevention of transmission of HIV through blood or blood products—Current efforts in the United States to screen blood and blood products have lowered the risk of HIV transmission with transfusion of a unit of blood to 1:2,000,000. Use of blood and blood products should be judicious and only when clinically indicated.

8. HIV vaccine—Primate model data have suggested that development of a protective vaccine may be possible, but clinical trials in humans have been disappointing. Only one vaccine trial has shown any degree of efficacy. In this randomized, double-blind, placebo-controlled trial, a recombinant canarypox vector vaccine plus two booster injections of a recombinant gp120 vaccine reduced the risk of HIV among a primarily heterosexual population in Thailand, but efficacy was too low (31%) for widespread use. A mosaic HIV vaccine resulted in a strong immune response among adult humans and protection against infection with an HIV-like virus in rhesus monkeys. Unfortunately, initial results from a phase 2b trial (Imbokodo Study) did not show efficacy, and it was discontinued, although a phase 3 study (Mosaico) using a different formulation is ongoing in Latin America, North America, and Europe. Finally, the first human trial of an mRNA vaccine against HIV/AIDS launched in 2022. Prior vaccine candidates for HIV have not managed to elicit broadly neutralizing antibodies and T cells against the virus, but preliminary work with the mRNA vaccine developed for HIV shows the development of both. Moreover, preliminary evidence in a small group of macaques shows good effectiveness in preventing simian HIV with the adapted mRNA HIV vaccine.

Pitisuttithum P et al. Prophylactic HIV vaccine: vaccine regimens in clinical trials and potential challenges. Expert Rev Vaccines. 2020;19:133. [PMID: 31951766]

Zhang P et al. A multiclade env–gag VLP mRNA vaccine elicits tier-2 HIV-1-neutralizing antibodies and reduces the risk of heterologous SHIV infection in macaques. Nat Med. 2021;27:2234. [PMID: 34887575]

B. Secondary Prevention

In the era prior to the development of effective ART, cohort studies of individuals with documented dates of seroconversion demonstrate that AIDS developed within 10 years in approximately 50% of untreated seropositive persons. With currently available treatment, progression of disease has been markedly decreased. In addition to ART, prophylactic regimens can prevent opportunistic infections and improve survival. Prophylaxis and early intervention prevent several infectious diseases, including tuberculosis and syphilis, which are transmissible to others. Recommendations for screening tests, vaccinations, and prophylaxis are listed in Table 31–5.

1. Tuberculosis—Because of the increased occurrence of tuberculosis among people living with HIV, all such individuals should undergo an intradermal PPD test or an IGRA blood test at baseline and yearly thereafter if they remain at risk of exposure (eg, incarcerated, living in congregate settings). Those with a positive PPD (defined for people living with HIV as greater than 5 mm of induration) or a positive IGRA assay (results that are reported as positive and not negative or indeterminate) should be clinically evaluated for active tuberculosis, including by a chest radiograph. Patients with an infiltrate in any location, especially if accompanied by mediastinal adenopathy, should have sputum sent for acid-fast staining. Patients with active tuberculosis should be treated as outlined in Chapter 9 (see Tables 9–14 and 9–15). Patients with a positive PPD or IGRA assay, and a normal chest radiograph or negative sputum evaluation for active tuberculosis are classified as having latent tuberculosis infection. Patients with latent tuberculosis infection who have not been previously treated for (active or latent) tuberculosis should receive once-weekly isoniazid (900 mg orally weekly for patients greater

Table 31–5. Health care maintenance and monitoring of people living with HIV.

For all individuals living with HIV:

- CD4 counts every 3–6 months (can decrease to every 12 months if viral load suppressed on ART for 2 years and CD4 count > 300 cells/mcL, optional if consistently above 500 cells/mcL)
- Viral load tests every 3–6 months and 2–4 weeks following a change in therapy
- Genotypic resistance testing at baseline and if viral load not fully suppressed and patient taking ART
- CBC, chemistry profile, transaminases and total bilirubin, at baseline and every 3–6 months
- UA at baseline and annually during ART (every 6 months if ART regimen includes TDF)
- Glucose or hemoglobin A_{1c} at baseline and annually during ART
- Lipid panel at baseline, 4–8 weeks after starting or changing an ART regimen that affects lipids, and annually for everyone over 40 years of age
- PPD or IGRA at baseline and annually if at high risk for exposure to persons with active TB
- Latent TB infection treatment for those with positive PPD or IGRA, normal chest radiograph, and no history of treatment for active or latent TB
- RPR or VDRL at entry and periodically based on sexual activity
- Toxoplasma IgG serology at baseline
- Hepatitis serologies: hepatitis A antibody, hepatitis B surface antigen, hepatitis B surface antibody, hepatitis B core antibody, hepatitis C antibody
- Pneumococcal vaccine
- Meningococcal vaccine
- Herpes zoster vaccine[1]
- Inactivated influenza vaccine annually in season
- Hepatitis A vaccine for those without immunity to hepatitis A
- Hepatitis B vaccine for those who are hepatitis B surface antigen and antibody negative. (Use 40 mcg formulation at 0, 1, and 6 months; repeat if no immunity 1 month after three-vaccine series.)
- Combined tetanus, diphtheria, pertussis vaccine
- COVID-19 vaccination
- HPV vaccine for women aged 26 years or younger living with HIV
- *Haemophilus influenzae* type b vaccination
- Bone mineral density monitoring for postmenopausal women and men aged 50 years or older
- Papanicolaou smears annually; if three smears are negative, can switch to longer intervals (see Complications, Section M. Gynecologic Manifestations)
- Consider anal swabs for cytologic evaluation

For individuals living with HIV with CD4 < 200 cells/mcL:

- *Pneumocystis jirovecii* prophylaxis (see Treatment, Section A. Prophylaxis for Complications of HIV Infection and Table 31–6)

For individuals living with HIV with CD4 < 100 cells/mcL and Toxoplasma IgG-positive:

- Ensure current prophylaxis covers toxoplasma, and if not, add toxoplasma prophylaxis (see Treatment, Section A. Prophylaxis for Complications of HIV Infection and Table 31–6)

[1]Consider in patients age > 50 years with history of varicella immunity and T cells > 200 cells/mcL.

ART, antiretroviral therapy; CMV, cytomegalovirus; IgG, immunoglobulin G; IGRA, interferon-gamma release assay; INH, isoniazid; PPD, purified protein derivative; RPR, rapid plasma reagin; TB, tuberculosis; TDF, tenofovir disoproxil fumarate; VDRL, Venereal Disease Research Laboratories.

than 50 kg) and rifapentine (900 mg orally weekly for patients greater than 50 kg) for 12 weeks. Other preferred regimens are rifampin daily (10 mg/kg; maximum and usual adult dose is 600 mg orally daily) for 4 months, although all people living with HIV should be evaluated for drug interactions, including with ART and 3 months of once daily rifampin and isoniazid once daily (300 mg orally daily). The World Health Organization also recommends 1 month of daily isoniazid and daily rifapentine (300 mg daily for a weight of less than 35 kg, 450 mg daily for a weight of 35 to 45 kg, and 600 mg for a weight of more than 45 kg) as a short-course regimen. An alternative, less preferred regimen given low completion rates, is 9 months of daily isoniazid. In patients with advanced immunodeficiency, both the PPD and IGRA assay are more likely to be falsely negative or (for IGRA assay) indeterminant. Therefore, it may be worth obtaining a chest radiograph, tuberculosis sputum evaluation, or both in people at high risk of tuberculosis, and retesting patients with initially low CD4 counts once they have received ART and have immune reconstitution (CD4 count greater than or equal to 200 cells/mcL).

Khan PY et al. Transmission of drug-resistant tuberculosis in HIV-endemic settings. Lancet Infect Dis. 2019;19:e77. [PMID: 30554996]

Peters JS et al. Advances in the understanding of *Mycobacterium tuberculosis* transmission in HIV-endemic settings. Lancet Infect Dis. 2019;19:e65. [PMID: 30554995]

2. Syphilis—Because of the increased number of cases of syphilis among men who have sex with men, including those living with HIV, all such men should be screened for syphilis by a syphilis enzyme immunoassay, rapid plasma reagin (RPR) or Venereal Disease Research Laboratories (VDRL) test every 3–6 months. Increases of syphilis cases among people living with HIV are of particular concern because these individuals are at increased risk for reactivation of syphilis and progression to tertiary syphilis despite standard treatment. People living with HIV may lose fluorescent treponemal antibody absorption (FTA-ABS) reactivity after treatment for syphilis, particularly if they have low CD4 counts. Thus, *in this population, a nonreactive treponemal test does not rule out a past history of syphilis.* People living with HIV should be evaluated carefully for otic, ophthalmic, or any other neurologic symptoms after a diagnosis of syphilis, with lumbar puncture pursued if there are neurologic symptoms, assuming empiric treatment is not pursued due to the presence of unexplained ophthalmic or otic symptoms. CSF cell count and CSF-VDRL should be examined in these cases. Those without neurologic symptoms or a normal CSF evaluation are treated as having early latent syphilis (prior syphilis evaluation within 1 year or symptoms of early syphilis) with one dose of benzathine penicillin G, 2.4 million units intramuscularly. Those with unknown or greater than 1 year since a prior syphilis evaluation are treated as late latent syphilis (benzathine penicillin G, 2.4 million units intramuscularly weekly for 3 weeks). Those with a pleocytosis or a positive CSF-VDRL test are treated as having neurosyphilis (aqueous penicillin G, 2–4 million units intravenously every 4 hours for 10–14 days). Given higher rates of clinical failure, people living with HIV should be evaluated for treatment response, with non-response defined as lack of four-fold decrease in titers in 1 year after early latent syphilis treatment or 2 years after late latent syphilis treatment. These individuals should be evaluated for neurosyphilis, particularly if there is no clinical evidence of reinfection. For a more detailed discussion of this topic, see Chapter 34.

Ren M et al. Deciphering the serological response to syphilis treatment in men living with HIV. AIDS. 2020;34:2089. [PMID: 32773482]

3. Immunizations—Patients living with HIV should receive immunizations as outlined in Table 31–5. Patients without evidence of hepatitis B surface antigen or surface antibody should receive hepatitis B vaccination, using the 40-mcg formulation (the higher dose is to increase the chance of developing protective immunity) or using the new two-dose CpG-adjuvanted hepatitis B vaccine (Heplisav-B). Although the CpG-adjuvanted vaccine was not specifically studied among people living with HIV, it has demonstrated greater immune responses in other populations, with a clinical trial among immunocompromised patients ongoing. If the patient does not have immunity 1 month after series completion, then the series should be repeated. People living with HIV should also receive the standard inactivated vaccines such as tetanus, diphtheria, and pertussis boosters that would be given to uninfected persons. **Most live vaccines, such as yellow fever vaccine, should be avoided in people with CD4+ T-cell counts less than 200 cells/mcL.** Measles vaccination, while a live virus vaccine, appears relatively safe when administered to patients with HIV and should be given if the patient has never had measles or been adequately vaccinated. The new recombinant adjuvanted herpes zoster vaccine (Shingrix), two doses 2–6 months apart, is recommended for people living with HIV with CD4 counts greater than 200 cells/mcL. However, it is not known if it is efficacious in preventing herpes zoster in this population. COVID-19 vaccinations in the United States are safe for people living with HIV, although efficacy data are limited.

Garrido HMG et al. Immunogenicity of pneumococcal vaccination in HIV infected individuals: a systematic review and meta-analysis. EClinicalMedicine. 2020;29: 100576. [PMID: 33294820]

Lee JH et al. Systematic review and meta-analysis of immune response of double dose of hepatitis B vaccination in HIV-infected patients. Vaccine. 2020;38:3995. [PMID: 32334887]

4. Other measures—Sexually transmitted infection screening should continue as there are high rates of syphilis, gonorrhea, and chlamydia infection among people living with HIV. Substance abuse treatment should be recommended for persons with substance use disorders, as this can improve adherence and treatment engagement. They should be warned to avoid consuming raw meat, eggs, or shellfish to avoid infections with *Toxoplasma,*

Table 31–6. *Pneumocystis jirovecii* prophylaxis, in order of preference.

Medication	Dose	Side Effects	Limitations
Trimethoprim-sulfamethoxazole	One double-strength tablet three times a week to one tablet daily	Rash, neutropenia, hepatitis, Stevens-Johnson syndrome	Hypersensitivity reaction is common but, if mild, it may be possible to treat through.
Dapsone	50–100 mg orally daily or 100 mg two or three times per week	Anemia, nausea, methemoglobinemia, hemolytic anemia	Less effective than above. Glucose-6-phosphate dehydrogenase (G6PD) level should be checked prior to therapy. Check methemoglobin level after 1 month of treatment.
Atovaquone	1500 mg orally daily with a meal	Rash, diarrhea, nausea	Less effective than suspension trimethoprim-sulfamethoxazole; equal efficacy to dapsone, but more expensive.
Aerosolized pentamidine	300 mg monthly	Bronchospasm (pretreat with bronchodilators); rare reports of pancreatitis	Apical *P jirovecii* pneumonia, extrapulmonary *P jirovecii* infections, pneumothorax.

Campylobacter, and *Salmonella*. Those with CD4+ counts less than 200 cells/mcL should wash their hands thoroughly after cleaning cat litter or should forgo this household chore to avoid possible exposure to toxoplasmosis. To reduce the likelihood of infection with *Bartonella* species, patients should avoid activities that might result in cat scratches or bites.

Because of the emotional impact of HIV infection and subsequent illness, many patients will benefit from supportive counseling.

Treatment

Treatment for HIV infection can be broadly divided into the following categories: (1) prophylaxis for opportunistic infections, malignancies, and other complications of HIV infection; (2) treatment of opportunistic infections, malignancies, and other complications of HIV infection; and (3) treatment of the HIV infection itself with ART.

A. Prophylaxis for Complications of HIV Infection

In general, decisions about prophylaxis of opportunistic infections are based on the CD4 count, recent HIV viral load, and a history of having had the infection in the past. In the era prior to ART, patients who started taking prophylactic regimens were maintained on them indefinitely. However, studies have shown that *in patients with robust improvements in immune function—as measured by increases in CD4 counts above the levels that are used to initiate treatment—prophylactic regimens can safely be discontinued.*

Because individuals living with advanced HIV infection are susceptible to a number of opportunistic pathogens, the use of agents with activity against more than one pathogen is preferable.

1. Prophylaxis against *Pneumocystis* pneumonia— Patients with CD4 counts below 200 cells/mcL, a CD4 lymphocyte percentage below 14%, or oral candidiasis should be offered primary prophylaxis for *Pneumocystis* pneumonia. Patients with a history of *Pneumocystis* pneumonia should receive secondary prophylaxis until their viral load is undetectable and they have maintained a CD4 count of 200 cells/mcL or more while receiving ART for longer than 3 months. Regimens for *Pneumocystis* prophylaxis are given in Table 31–6.

2. Prophylaxis against *M avium* complex infection— Prophylaxis against *M avium* complex is no longer recommended in most individuals who are initiating ART, including in those with CD4+ counts less than 50 cells/mcL. The incidence of *M avium* complex infection is very low among those on ART. In rare cases where individuals delay ART (eg, due to patient refusal) whose CD4 counts fall to below 50 cells/mcL, prophylaxis against *M avium* complex infection should be offered. Clarithromycin (500 mg orally twice daily) and azithromycin (1200 mg orally weekly) are the recommended regimens. The azithromycin regimen is generally preferred based on high compliance and low cost. Prophylaxis against *M avium* complex infection may be discontinued in patients who initiate ART.

3. Prophylaxis against toxoplasmosis—Toxoplasmosis prophylaxis is desirable in patients with a positive IgG toxoplasma serology and CD4 counts below 100 cells/mcL. Trimethoprim-sulfamethoxazole (one double-strength tablet daily) offers good protection against toxoplasmosis, as does a combination of pyrimethamine, 25 mg orally once a week, plus dapsone, 50 mg orally daily, plus leucovorin, 25 mg orally once a week. A glucose-6-phosphate dehydrogenase (G6PD) level should be checked prior to dapsone therapy, and a methemoglobin level should be checked at 1 month. Prophylaxis can be discontinued when the CD4 cells have increased to greater than 200 cells/mcL for more than 3 months.

B. Treatment of Complications of HIV Infection

Treatment of common AIDS-related complications is detailed above and in Table 31–3. In the era prior to the use of ART, patients required lifelong treatment for many infections, including CMV retinitis, toxoplasmosis, and cryptococcal meningitis. However, *among patients who have a good response to ART, maintenance therapy for some opportunistic infections can be terminated.* For example, in consultation with an ophthalmologist, maintenance treatment for CMV infection can be discontinued when persons receiving ART have had a sustained increase in CD4 count to greater than 100 cells/mcL for at least 3–6 months. Similar results have been observed in patients with *M avium* complex bacteremia, who have completed a year or more of therapy for *M avium* complex and have an increase in their CD4 count to 100 cells/mcL for greater than 6 months while receiving ART. Cessation of secondary prophylaxis for *Pneumocystis* pneumonia is described above.

Treating patients with repeated episodes of the same opportunistic infection can pose difficult therapeutic challenges. For example, patients with second or third episodes of *Pneumocystis* pneumonia may have developed allergic reactions to standard treatments with a prior episode. Fortunately, there are several alternatives available for the treatment of *Pneumocystis* infection. Trimethoprim with dapsone and primaquine with clindamycin are two combinations that often are tolerated in patients with a prior allergic reaction to trimethoprim-sulfamethoxazole and intravenous pentamidine.

Adjunctive treatments—Epoetin alfa (erythropoietin) is approved for use in people living with HIV with anemia, including those with anemia secondary to zidovudine use. As zidovudine is rarely used now, especially at high doses, the use of epoetin alfa has also decreased. An erythropoietin level less than 500 mU/mL should be demonstrated before starting therapy. The starting dose of epoetin alfa is 8000 units subcutaneously three times a week. Hypertension is the most common side effect.

Human G-CSF (filgrastim) and granulocyte-macrophage colony-stimulating factor (GM-CSF [sargramostim]) have been shown to increase the neutrophil counts of people living with HIV. Because of the high cost of this therapy, the dosage should be closely monitored and minimized, aiming for a neutrophil count of 1000/mcL (1.0×10^9/L). When the medication is used for indications other than cytotoxic chemotherapy, one or two doses at 5 mcg/kg per week subcutaneously are usually sufficient.

C. Antiretroviral Therapy

The availability of agents that in combination suppress HIV replication (Table 31–7) has had a profound impact on the natural history of HIV infection. Indeed, *with the advent of effective ART, the life expectancy of people living with HIV approaches that of people without infection when treatment is initiated early in the course of the disease and maintained.*

The recognition that HIV damages the immune system from the beginning of infection, even when the damage is not easily measured by conventional tests, combined with the greater potency, the improved side-effect profile, and the decreased pill burden of modern HIV regimens, have led to the recommendation to **start treatment as soon as possible for all people living with HIV, including patients having acute HIV infection, regardless of CD4 count.** The START trial demonstrated that immediate treatment is associated with a greater than 50% reduction in risk for serious illness or death, compared to delaying treatment until the CD4 count falls below 350 cells/mcL. The TEMPRANO trial showed that individuals immediately initiating ART versus delaying treatment for CD4 count to fall below 500 cells/mcL had lower rates of severe illness.

Rapid initiation programs have been created, where treatment can be started on the same day that patients test positive for HIV, so patients can start receiving treatment promptly and avoid being lost to follow-up. The clinician should provide sufficient resources to help patients cope with these major events in a short time, receive sufficient insurance and benefits coverage, and connect to other social services resources (ie, food assistance, housing, etc). If treatment is started before the results of resistance testing are available, a nonnucleoside reverse transcriptase inhibitor (NNRTI) should not be used given the possibility of transmitted drug resistance. Recommended regimens for initiating treatment before resistance testing results are available include (1) dolutegravir plus TAF/emtricitabine or TDF/emtricitabine (or lamivudine), (2) bictegravir/TAF/emtricitabine, or (3) boosted darunavir plus TAF/emtricitabine or TDF/emtricitabine (or lamivudine). Also, patients requiring abacavir as part of their regimen should not start treatment prior to the results of HLA-B*5701 allele testing or hepatitis B testing.

Once a decision to initiate therapy has been made, several important principles should guide therapy. *The primary goal of therapy should be complete suppression of viral replication as measured by the serum viral load.* Partially suppressive combinations should be avoided. Similarly, if toxicity develops, it is preferable to change the offending medication given availability of multiple effective and well-tolerated medications.

Although the HIV treatment protocol has traditionally included three medications from at least two different classes, *several two-drug regimens using medications from at least two different classes have been shown to be effective.* A combination of dolutegravir plus lamivudine (Table 31–8) has been shown to be noninferior to dolutegravir plus TDF and emtricitabine as initial therapy in patients with HIV viral load of less than 500,000 copies/mL. A second exception is the coformulation of dolutegravir and rilpivirine (Table 31–8); this combination is FDA approved as an alternative treatment for patients who have been successfully virally suppressed for at least 6 months, have no history of treatment failure, and are not resistant to either of the two component agents. A third approved two-drug regimen is cabotegravir with rilpivirine as an intramuscular injection given every 4 or 8 weeks.

The presence of an acute opportunistic infection in most cases does not preclude the initiation of ART. Randomized trials compared early initiation of ART (within 2 weeks of starting treatment for an opportunistic infection or tuberculosis) with ART that was deferred until after treatment of the opportunistic infection was completed (6 weeks after its start); results demonstrated that early initiation reduced death or AIDS progression by 50%. The reduced progression rates were related to more rapid improvements in CD4 counts in patients with

Table 31–7. Antiretroviral therapy agents by class (in alphabetical order within classes).

Medication	Dose	Common Side Effects	Special Monitoring[1]	Cost[2]	Cost/Month
Nucleoside Reverse Transcriptase Inhibitors (NRTIs)					
Abacavir (Ziagen)	600 mg orally once daily	Rash, fever—if occur, rechallenge may be fatal	No special monitoring	$9.64/300 mg	$578.56
Emtricitabine (Emtriva)	200 mg orally once daily	Skin discoloration palms/soles (mild)	No special monitoring	$19.31/200 mg	$579.38
Lamivudine (Epivir)	150 mg orally twice daily or 300 mg daily	Rash, peripheral neuropathy	No special monitoring	$7.15/150 mg	$429.10
Zidovudine (AZT) (Retrovir)	600 mg orally daily in two divided doses	Anemia, neutropenia, nausea, malaise, headache, insomnia, myopathy	CBC with differential 4–8 weeks after starting AZT	$0.90/300 mg	$54.00
Nucleotide Reverse Transcriptase Inhibitors (NRTIs)					
Tenofovir alafenamide (TAF)/emtricitabine (Descovy)	25 mg of TAF with 200 mg of emtricitabine once daily	Weight gain; dyslipidemia; lower but still present risk of nephrotoxicity and bone resorption	Creatinine at baseline, at 2–8 weeks, then every 3–6 months; UA and urine glucose and protein at baseline and repeated as clinically indicated; HBsAg, liver enzymes at baseline, at 2–8 weeks, then every 3–6 months, continue for months after discontinuation; consider bone densitometry	$81.55/tablet	$2446.60
Tenofovir (TDF) (Viread)	300 mg orally once daily	Kidney dysfunction, bone resorption, GI distress	Creatinine at baseline, at 2–8 weeks, then every 3–6 months; UA and urine glucose and protein at baseline and repeated as clinically indicated; consider bone densitometry	$5.57/300 mg	$167.18
Nonnucleoside Reverse Transcriptase Inhibitors (NNRTIs)					
Doravirine (Pifeltro)	100 mg daily	Headache, fatigue, abdominal pain	No special monitoring	$63.89/100 mg	$1916.64
Efavirenz (Sustiva)	600 mg orally daily	Neurologic disturbances, rash, hepatitis	No special monitoring	$35.77/600 mg	$1073.18
Etravirine (Intelence)	200 mg orally twice daily	Rash, peripheral neuropathy	No special monitoring	$13.41/100 mg	$1609.11
Nevirapine (Viramune)	200 mg orally daily for 2 weeks, then 200 mg orally twice daily	Rash	No special monitoring	$10.80/200 mg	$648.00
Rilpivirine (Edurant)	25 mg daily	Depression, rash	No special monitoring	$51.44/25 mg	$1543.10

(*continued*)

Table 31–7. Antiretroviral therapy agents by class (in alphabetical order within classes). (continued)

Medication	Dose	Common Side Effects	Special Monitoring[1]	Cost[2]	Cost/Month
Protease Inhibitors (PIs)					
Atazanavir (Reyataz)	400 mg orally once daily or 300 mg atazanavir with 100 mg ritonavir daily	Hyperbilirubinemia	Bilirubin level every 3–4 months	$25.05/200 mg or $50.09/300 mg	$1502.76 (plus cost of ritonavir) $1502.76 (plus cost of ritonavir)
Atazanavir/cobicistat (Evotaz)	300 mg of atazanavir with 150 mg of cobicistat orally once daily	Hyperbilirubinemia	Bilirubin level every 3–4 months	$64.22/tablet	$1926.56
Darunavir/cobicistat (Prezcobix)	800 mg of darunavir and 150 mg of cobicistat orally once daily	Rash	No special monitoring	$89.09/tablet	$2672.56
Darunavir/ritonavir (Prezista/Norvir)	**PI-experienced patients:** 600 mg of darunavir and 100 mg of ritonavir orally twice daily **For PI-naïve patients:** 800 mg of darunavir and 100 mg of ritonavir orally daily	Rash	No special monitoring	$38.97/600 mg (darunavir) $77.94/800 mg (darunavir)	$2338.22 (plus cost of ritonavir) $2338.22 (plus cost of ritonavir)
Lopinavir/ritonavir (Kaletra)	400 mg/100 mg orally twice daily	Diarrhea	No special monitoring	$9.22/200 mg (Kaletra)	$1105.95
Ritonavir (Norvir)	600 mg orally twice daily or in lower doses (eg, 100 mg orally once or twice daily) for boosting other PIs	GI distress, peripheral paresthesias	No special monitoring	$9.26/100 mg	$3333.60 ($277.80–555.60 in lower doses)
Entry Inhibitors					
Enfuvirtide (Fuzeon)	90 mg subcutaneously twice daily	Injection site pain and allergic reaction	No special monitoring	$71.71/90 mg	$4302.67
Integrase Inhibitors					
Bictegravir	50 mg orally daily. No longer marketed as a single agent; used in antiretroviral combination (Table 31–8)	Diarrhea, nausea, headache	No special monitoring	No longer marketed as a single agent	No longer marketed as a single agent
Dolutegravir (Tivicay)	Treatment-naïve or integrase-naïve patients: 50 mg daily When administered with efavirenz, fosamprenavir/ritonavir, tipranavir/ritonavir, or rifampin: 50 mg twice daily When administered to integrase-experienced patients with suspected integrase resistance: 50 mg twice daily	Hypersensitivity, insomnia, fatigue, headache, rash	No special monitoring	$80.45/50 mg	$2413.66/50 mg daily or $4827.32/50 mg twice daily
Elvitegravir	No longer marketed as a single agent; used in antiretroviral combinations (Table 31–8)	Diarrhea, headache	No special monitoring	No longer marketed as a single agent	No longer marketed as a single agent

(*continued*)

Table 31–7. Antiretroviral therapy agents by class (in alphabetical order within classes). (continued)

Medication	Dose	Common Side Effects	Special Monitoring[1]	Cost[2]	Cost/Month
Raltegravir (Isentress)	400 mg orally twice daily	Diarrhea, nausea, headache	No special monitoring	$36.43/400 mg	$2185.92
Cabotegravir	Oral regimen of 30 mg daily with rilpivirine 25 mg daily for 1 month; then intramuscular loading dose of 600 mg with rilpivirine 900 mg intramuscularly in separate buttock injections; followed by monthly intramuscular injections of 400 mg with 600 mg rilpivirine thereafter	Injection site reactions with intramuscular dose	No special monitoring		Monthly maintenance regimen $4440.00
Entry and Fusion Inhibitors					
Enfuvirtide (Fuzeon)	90 mg subcutaneously twice daily	Injection site pain and allergic reaction	No special monitoring	$71.71/90 mg	$4302.67
Maraviroc (Selzentry)	150 mg orally twice daily or 300 mg orally twice daily	Cough, fever, rash	No special monitoring	$32.66 (for either dose)	$1959.70 (for either dose)
Ibalizumab (Trogarzo)	Loading dose of 2000 mg intravenously over 30 minutes; maintenance dose of 800 mg intravenously every 2 weeks thereafter	Diarrhea, dizziness, nausea, rash, elevated creatinine, lymphopenia	Monthly CBC, creatinine, bilirubin, glucose, lipase	$3211.20/400 mg	$12,844.80
Attachment Inhibitor					
Fostemsavir	600 mg orally twice a day	Nausea	No special monitoring	$160.56/600 mg	$9633.49

[1]Standard monitoring is CBC and differential, basic chemistries, serum aminotransferases, and total bilirubin every 3–6 months, UA at baseline and annually during antiretroviral treatment, fasting glucose or hemoglobin A_{1c} at baseline and annually during antiretroviral treatment, and fasting lipid profile at baseline, 4–8 weeks after starting an antiretroviral treatment regimen that affects lipids, and annually for everyone over 40 years of age.
[2]Average wholesale price (AWP, for AB-rated generic when available) for quantity listed. Source: IBM Micromedex Red Book (electronic version). IBM Watson Health, Greenwood Village, Colorado, USA. Available at: https://www-micromedexsolutions-com.proxy.hsl.ucdenver.edu/ (cited March 29, 2022). AWP may not accurately represent the actual pharmacy cost because wide contractual variations exist among institutions.

advanced immunodeficiency. Furthermore, IRIS and other adverse events were no more frequent in the early ART arm.

Several randomized studies have also demonstrated improved clinical outcomes in HIV/tuberculosis coinfected patients who initiate ART early in the setting of active treatment for tuberculosis and whose CD4 counts are less than 50 cells/mcL. The exception to early ART in the setting of active infections may be in patients with a CNS-associated infection, such as cryptococcal or tuberculosis meningitis. Several studies from low-income countries have shown high mortality rates with early ART initiation in this setting.

An initial antiretroviral regimen should be chosen to minimize side effects. For hospitalized patients, initiating treatment in patients with opportunistic infections requires close coordination between inpatient and outpatient clinicians to ensure that treatment is continued once patients are discharged.

D. Choosing an Antiretroviral Treatment Regimen

HIV antiretroviral medications can be grouped into six major categories: nucleoside and nucleotide reverse transcriptase inhibitors (NRTIs); nonnucleoside reverse transcriptase inhibitors (NNRTIs); PI; integrase inhibitors; entry and fusion inhibitors; and attachment inhibitors.

1. Nucleoside and nucleotide reverse transcriptase inhibitors (NRTI)—There are currently six NRTI agents available (counting TDF and TAF as separate agents) for use. The choice of which agent to use depends primarily on the patient's prior treatment experience, results of resistance testing, medication side effects, other underlying conditions, and convenience of formulation. However, most clinicians use fixed-dose combinations (see Table 31–8) of including either emtricitabine/TDF, emtricitabine/TAF, or abacavir/lamivudine (ABC/lamivudine), all of which can be given once a day. Abacavir should be

Table 31–8. Fixed-dose antiretroviral combinations (alphabetical order by brand name).

Name	Components	Dosing and Special Considerations	Cost per Month
Atripla	TDF 300 mg Emtricitabine 200 mg Efavirenz 600 mg	One pill daily constitutes a complete ART regimen.	$302.40
Biktarvy	Emtricitabine 200 mg TAF 25 mg Bictegravir 50 mg	One pill daily constitutes a complete ART regimen. One of the recommended initial treatment regimens.	$4300.56
Complera	TDF 300 mg Emtricitabine 200 mg Rilpivirine 25 mg	One pill daily constitutes a complete ART regimen. Only for patients with HIV viral load < 100,000/mL.	$3913.84
Delstrigo	TDF 300 mg Lamivudine 300 mg Doravirine 100 mg	One pill daily constitutes a complete ART regimen.	$2917.08
Descovy	TAF 25 mg Emtricitabine 200 mg	One pill daily along with an NNRTI, PI, integrase inhibitor, or maraviroc (entry inhibitor). The difference between Descovy and Truvada is that Descovy has a different form of tenofovir (TAF) that appears to have less effect on kidney function and bone mineral density than the form of tenofovir (TDF) in Truvada. Descovy is approved for use as a single agent for PrEP in men (not studied in women).	$2446.60
Dovato	Dolutegravir 50 mg Lamivudine 300 mg	One pill daily constitutes a complete ART regimen in adults with no prior antiviral treatment and no known substitutions associated with resistance to either component.	$3182.63
Epzicom	Abacavir 600 mg Lamivudine 300 mg	One pill daily along with an NNRTI, PI, integrase inhibitor, or maraviroc (entry inhibitor).	$1550.05
Genvoya	TAF 10 mg Emtricitabine 200 mg Elvitegravir 150 mg Cobicistat 150 mg	One pill daily constitutes a complete ART regimen. Although it contains four medications, one component (cobicistat) is a medication booster only. The only difference between Stribild and Genvoya is that Genvoya has a different form of tenofovir (TAF) that appears to be safer than tenofovir TDF with less effect on kidney function and bone mineral density.	$4300.56
Juluca	Dolutegravir 50 mg Rilpivirine 25 mg	One pill daily with a meal for patients who have been virologically suppressed (viral load < 50 copies/mL) on a stable ART regimen for ≥ 6 months and no history of treatment failure or resistance to dolutegravir or rilpivirine.	$3755.30
Odefsey	TAF 25 mg Emtricitabine 200 mg Rilpivirine 25 mg	One pill daily constitutes a complete ART regimen. Only for patients with no history of HIV viral load ≥ 100,000 copies/mL. Or for replacement of stable antiretroviral regimen in patients fully suppressed for > 6 months, with no history of treatment failure, and with no known resistance to components of the drug combination.	$3913.84
Stribild	TDF 300 mg Emtricitabine 200 mg Elvitegravir 150 mg Cobicistat 150 mg	One pill daily constitutes a complete ART regimen. Although it contains four medications, one component (cobicistat) is a medication booster only.	$4511.29
Symtuza	TAF 10 mg Emtricitabine 200 mg Darunavir 800 mg Cobicistat 150 mg	One pill daily constitutes a complete ART regimen. Although it contains four medications, one component (cobicistat) is a medication booster only. One of the recommended initial treatment regimens.	$5150.92
Triumeq	Abacavir 600 mg Lamivudine 300 mg Dolutegravir 50 mg	One pill constitutes a complete ART regimen. One of the recommended initial treatment regimens.	$4006.87
Trizivir	Abacavir 300 mg Lamivudine 150 mg Zidovudine 300 mg	One tablet twice daily with an NNRTI, PI, integrase inhibitor, or maraviroc (entry inhibitor). Although it contains three medications it *does not* constitute a complete ART regimen.	$1931.64
Truvada	TDF 300 mg Emtricitabine 200 mg	One pill daily with an NNRTI, PI, integrase inhibitor, or maraviroc (entry inhibitor). TDF is the most commonly used NRTI backbone. Truvada is approved for use as a single agent for PrEP.	$70.07

ART, antiretroviral therapy; NNRTI, non-nucleoside reverse transcriptase inhibitor (eg, delavirdine, efavirenz, etravirine, nevirapine, rilpivirine); NRTI, nucleoside/nucleotide reverse transcriptase inhibitor (eg, abacavir, didanosine, emtricitabine, lamivudine, stavudine, tenofovir, zidovudine); PI, protease inhibitor; PrEP, preexposure prophylaxis; TAF, tenofovir alafenamide; TDF, tenofovir disoproxil fumarate.
Average wholesale price (AWP, for AB-rated generic when available) for quantity listed. Source: Source: IBM Micromedex Red Book (electronic version). IBM Watson Health, Greenwood Village, Colorado, USA. Available at: https://www-micromedexsolutions-com.proxy.hsl.ucdenver.edu/ (cited March 29, 2022). AWP may not accurately represent the actual pharmacy cost because wide contractual variations exist among institutions.

given only to HLA-B*5701-negative persons. In patients with viral loads greater than 100,000 copies/mL, ABC/lamivudine was less effective than emtricitabine/TDF when combined with efavirenz or ritonavir-boosted atazanavir. However, ABC/lamivudine appears to be equally efficacious as emtricitabine/TDF in patients with viral loads greater than 100,000 copies/mL when combined with dolutegravir or raltegravir. In some studies, abacavir increased risks of MI, and therefore should be avoided in patients at high risk for CVD. Zidovudine/lamivudine (AZT/lamivudine) is rarely used and usually reserved for second- or third-line regimens because of toxicity and dosing schedule. Of the available agents, zidovudine is the most likely to cause anemia or neutropenia. As of 2020, stavudine and didanosine are no longer available due to increased toxicity. Emtricitabine, TDF, TAF, and lamivudine have activity against hepatitis B. TDF, TAF, emtricitabine, abacavir, and lamivudine can be administered once daily. Information specific to each medication is given below and in Table 31–7.

A. Zidovudine—Zidovudine was the first approved antiviral medication for HIV infection. It is administered at a dose of 300 mg orally twice daily. A combination of zidovudine 300 mg and lamivudine 150 mg (Combivir) is available. Approximately 40% of patients experience subjective side effects that usually remit within 6 weeks. The common dose-limiting side effects are anemia and neutropenia, which require ongoing laboratory monitoring. Long-term use has been associated with lipoatrophy.

B. Lamivudine—Lamivudine is a safe and well-tolerated agent. The dosage is 150 mg orally twice daily or 300 mg orally once a day. The dose should be reduced in patients with CKD, although toxicity is not anticipated. There are no significant side effects with lamivudine; it has activity against hepatitis B, though HBV resistance to it is an increasing problem, and it is always given with tenofovir in the setting of HIV/hepatitis B coinfection.

C. Emtricitabine—Emtricitabine is dosed at 200 mg orally once daily. Emtricitabine also has activity against hepatitis B. Its dosage should be reduced in patients with CKD.

D. Abacavir—Abacavir is dosed at 600 mg once daily. Prior to initiation of abacavir, patients should undergo testing for HLA typing. Those with the B*5701 allele should not be treated with abacavir because the likelihood of a hypersensitivity reaction developing is high; the reaction is characterized by a flu-like syndrome with rash and fever that worsens with successive doses. Unfortunately, the absence of this allele does not guarantee that the patient will avoid the hypersensitivity reaction. Individuals in whom the hypersensitivity reaction develops should *not* be rechallenged with this agent because subsequent hypersensitivity reactions can be fatal. Abacavir, specifically recent use, has also been associated with an increased risk of MI in some cohort studies, generally in patients who have underlying risks for CVD. Abacavir is usually prescribed as a fixed-dose combination pill with lamivudine for use as a once-daily pill (Epzicom; Table 31–8).

E. Tenofovir—Tenofovir is the only licensed nucleotide analog. It comes in two forms: TDF and tenofovir alafenamide (TAF). TDF is available for use both in the form of a single pill at an oral dose of 300 mg once daily and as an oral fixed-dose combination pill with emtricitabine 200 mg (Truvada; Table 31–8) once daily. Several other single-tablet once-a-day complete regimens include TDF (Atripla, Complera, Stribild) (Table 31–8). Tenofovir is active against hepatitis B, including isolates that have resistance to lamivudine. TDF is associated with a clinically modest loss of kidney function, a small increased risk of AKI, and increased rate of bone resorption. In patients taking boosted therapy (eg, therapy including cobicistat or ritonavir), TAF appears to cause fewer problems with kidney dysfunction and bone loss and is the preferred choice.

TAF attains higher levels in cells with a much lower plasma level. For this reason, it appears to cause less harm to kidneys and less bone resorption. TAF should not be used with rifamycins. TDF appears to be associated with lower lipid levels, and TAF seems to be associated with greater weight gain when combined with integrase inhibitors.

If tenofovir (both TDF and TAF) cannot be avoided in patients with creatinine clearance below 60 mL/minute, their kidney function should be monitored very closely. TAF is preferred in individuals with creatinine clearances between 30–60 mL/minute. It is recommended that the serum creatinine be checked at baseline, at 2–8 weeks, and then every 3–6 months and that a UA and urine glucose and protein be checked at baseline and monitored periodically as clinically indicated.

2. Nonnucleoside reverse transcriptase inhibitors—
NNRTIs inhibit reverse transcriptase at a site different from that of the nucleoside and nucleotide agents described above. The major advantage of NNRTIs is that four of them (efavirenz, rilpivirine, doravirine, and nevirapine) have potencies comparable to that of PIs (next section), at least for patients with viral loads under 100,000 copies/mL—with lower pill burden and fewer side effects. However, they have lower barrier to resistance when compared to PIs and integrase inhibitors. Unlike PIs, they do *not* cause lipodystrophy; patients with cholesterol and triglyceride elevations who are switched from a PI to an NNRTI may have improvement in their lipids. The resistance patterns of NNRTIs are distinct from those of the PIs. Because these agents may cause alterations in the clearance of PIs, dose modifications may be necessary when these two classes of medications are administered concomitantly. There is a high degree of cross-resistance among the "first-generation" NNRTIs, such that resistance to one medication in this class uniformly predicts resistance to other medications. However, the "second-generation" NNRTIs etravirine, rilpivirine, and doravirine can have consistent antiviral activity in patients with prior exposure and resistance to nevirapine or efavirenz, although genotypic analysis is needed first in these contexts. In particular, the *K103N* mutation does not have an impact on etravirine, doravirine, or rilpivirine. There is no therapeutic reason for using more than one NNRTI at the same time. Delavirdine is no longer available in the United States.

A. Efavirenz—Efavirenz can be given once daily in a single dose (600 mg orally) and is available in a once-daily fixed-dose combination with TDF and emtricitabine in a single pill (Atripla; Table 31–8). The major side effects are rash and psychiatric/neurologic complaints, with patients reporting symptoms ranging from lack of concentration and strange dreams to delusions and mania. These side effects tend to wane over time, usually within a month or so; however, there are some patients who cannot tolerate these effects, especially if they persist longer than a month. Participant level data from four randomized trials of efavirenz regimens versus non-efavirenz containing regimens found increased suicidality (hazard ratio of 2.6) among those taking efavirenz. As a result of these neuropsychiatric side effects, efavirenz is no longer a preferred regimen. Administration of efavirenz with food, especially fatty food, may increase its serum levels and consequent neurotoxicity. Therefore, it should be taken on an empty stomach; taking before bedtime may also reduce patients' experience of neuropsychiatric symptoms.

B. Doravirine—Dosed at 100 mg orally daily, this drug can be taken with or without food. Two 48-week phase 3 studies showed that, in previously untreated individuals, doravirine, when used with two NRTIs resulted in similar levels of viral suppression as efavirenz plus two NRTIs or darunavir/ritonavir plus two NRTIs. It is also available as a single-pill combination with TDF and lamivudine (Delstrigo; Table 31–8). It is well tolerated. In cases of virologic failure, NNRTI cross-resistance may develop.

C. Rilpivirine—This medication, dosed at 25 mg once daily, is equal in efficacy to efavirenz in patients with HIV viral loads below 100,000 copies/mL. Rilpivirine should not be used in patients with baseline viral loads of 100,000 copies/mL or greater or those with CD4 counts below 200 cells/mcL because of greater risk of viral failure. As is true of efavirenz, rilpivirine is available in a once-daily fixed-dose combination with TDF and emtricitabine (Complera; Table 31–8) and with TAF and emtricitabine (Odefsey; Table 31–8) to be taken with a meal. It is also available in a two-drug regimen with dolutegravir (Juluca; Table 31–8). PPIs should not be given with rilpivirine. Rilpivirine has fewer neurologic side effects than efavirenz. The FDA has approved a long-acting formulation of rilpivirine for monthly intramuscular injections to be given with the integrase inhibitor cabotegravir (see below).

D. Nevirapine—The dose of nevirapine is 400 mg orally daily (extended release), but it is initiated at a dose of 200 mg once a day to decrease the incidence of rash, which is as high as 40% when full doses are begun immediately. If rash develops while the patient is taking 200 mg daily, liver enzymes should be checked and the dose should not be increased until the rash resolves. Patients with mild rash and no evidence of hepatotoxicity can continue to be treated with nevirapine. Nevirapine should not be used in treatment-naïve women with CD4 counts greater than 250 cells/mcL or in males with CD4 counts greater than 400 cells/mcL because they have greater risk of hepatotoxicity. In general, because of the risk of fatal hepatotoxicity, *nevirapine should be used only when there is not a better alternative.*

E. Etravirine—Etravirine is an NNRTI approved for the treatment of patients with prior NNRTI intolerance or resistance. Etravirine has been shown to be effective in treatment-experienced patients even when some degree of NNRTI resistance is present, making it a true "second-generation" medication in this class. Etravirine dosage is one 200 mg tablet twice daily or 400 mg once daily. The most common side effects are nausea and rash; rarely, the rash can be severe (toxic epidermal necrolysis). Patients with signs of severe rash or hypersensitivity reactions should immediately discontinue the medication. Prior rash due to treatment with one of the other NNRTIs does not make rash more likely with etravirine. Etravirine should not be taken by people with severe liver disease or administered with tipranavir/ritonavir, fosamprenavir/ritonavir, atazanavir/ritonavir, full-dose ritonavir, or PIs without low-dose ritonavir.

3. Protease inhibitors—Four PIs—ritonavir, lopinavir (in combination with ritonavir), atazanavir, and darunavir—are still available (with others used rarely). PIs are potent suppressors of HIV replication and are administered as part of a combination regimen.

All of the PIs—to differing degrees—are metabolized by the cytochrome P450 system, and each can inhibit and induce various P450 isoenzymes. Therefore, medication interactions are common and difficult to predict. Clinicians should consult the product inserts before prescribing PIs with other medications. Medications that are known to induce the P450 system, such as rifampin, should be avoided.

The fact that the PIs are dependent on metabolism through the cytochrome P450 system has led to the use of ritonavir to *boost* the medication levels of other PIs, allowing use of lower doses and simpler dosing schedules of these PIs. A second boosting agent, cobicistat, is coformulated with the PI atazanavir (Evotaz) and darunavir (Prescobix). Similar to ritonavir, cobicistat also inhibits liver enzymes that metabolize other HIV medications.

When choosing which PI to use, prior patient experience, resistance patterns, side effects, and ease of administration are the major considerations. Unfortunately, all PIs, with the exception of unboosted atazanavir have been linked to a constellation of metabolic abnormalities, including elevated cholesterol levels, elevated triglyceride levels, insulin resistance, diabetes mellitus, and changes in body fat composition (eg, abdominal obesity). The lipid abnormalities and body habitus changes are referred to as **lipodystrophy.** Although lipodystrophy is commonly associated with PIs, it has been seen also in people living with HIV who have never been treated with these agents. In particular, the lipoatrophy effects seen in patients receiving ART appears to be more related to the nucleoside toxicity and in particular to the thymidine analogs (ie, zidovudine).

Of the different manifestations of lipodystrophy, the dyslipidemias that occur are of particular concern because of the likelihood that increased levels of cholesterol and triglycerides will result in increased prevalence of heart disease. All patients taking PIs should have fasting serum cholesterol, LDL cholesterol, and triglyceride levels assessed. Clinicians should assess for CHD (see Chapter 28) and consider initiating dietary changes or medication therapy (or both). PIs inhibit statin metabolism. Lovastatin and simvastatin should be avoided. In general, the least interaction is with pravastatin (20 mg daily orally). Atorvastatin (10 mg daily orally) or rosuvastatin (5 mg/day orally initially; maximum 10 mg/day) may also be used cautiously. Patients with persistently elevated fasting serum triglyceride levels of 500 mg/dL or more who do not respond to dietary intervention should be treated with one of the statin medications, followed by gemfibrozil (600 mg twice daily prior to the morning and evening meals). PIs are associated with abnormalities in cardiac conduction, especially prolongation of the PR interval.

A. **Ritonavir**—Use of this potent PI at full dose (600 mg orally twice daily) has been limited by its inhibition of the cytochrome P450 pathway causing a large number of drug-drug interactions and by its frequent side effects of fatigue, nausea, and paresthesias. However, it is widely used in lower dose (eg, 100 mg daily to 100 mg twice daily) as a booster of other PIs.

B. **Lopinavir/r**—Lopinavir/r is lopinavir (200 mg) coformulated with a low dose of ritonavir (50 mg) to maximize the bioavailability of lopinavir. The usual dose is lopinavir 400 mg with ritonavir 100 mg (two tablets) orally twice daily with food. When given along with efavirenz or nevirapine, a higher dose (600 mg/150 mg—three tablets) is usually prescribed. The most common side effect is diarrhea, and lipid abnormalities are frequent. Because of these side effects, lopinavir/r has fallen off the list of medications recommended as part of first-line treatment regimens.

C. **Atazanavir**—Atazanavir is available alone and coformulated with cobicistat (Evotaz). Atazanavir can be dosed as 400 mg (two 200-mg capsules) daily with food or it can be dosed as 300 mg in combination with 100 mg of ritonavir once daily with food. When coformulated with cobicistat, it is dosed at 300-mg atazanavir and 150-mg cobicistat. The most common side effect is mild hyperbilirubinemia that resolves with discontinuation of the medication. Nephrolithiasis and cholelithiasis have also been reported with this PI. Both tenofovir and efavirenz lower the serum concentration of atazanavir. Therefore, when either of these two medications is used with atazanavir, it should be boosted by administering ritonavir or given coformulated with cobicistat. PPIs are contraindicated in patients taking atazanavir because atazanavir requires an acidic pH to remain in solution.

D. **Darunavir**—Darunavir has impressive antiviral activity in the setting of significant PI resistance and in treatment-naïve patients. It is formulated by itself and coformulated with cobicistat (Prezcobix). When formulated without cobicistat it requires boosting with ritonavir. For initial treatment of HIV or for treatment-experienced patients without darunavir-related resistance mutations, daily dosing is 800 mg of darunavir with 100 mg of ritonavir or with 150 mg of cobicistat. Darunavir 800 mg is also available in a coformulated tablet with emtricitabine, TAF, and cobicistat (Symtuza, Table 31–8). For patients with PI resistance (with mutations known to impact darunavir), darunavir should be dosed at 600 mg orally twice daily, with ritonavir, 100 mg orally twice daily. Darunavir has a safety profile similar to other PIs, such as ritonavir-boosted lopinavir, but is generally better tolerated. Like tipranavir, darunavir is a sulfa-containing medication, and its use should be closely monitored in patients with sulfa allergy.

4. Integrase inhibitors—Integrase inhibitors slow HIV replication by blocking the HIV integrase enzyme needed for the virus to multiply. They are now the *preferred regimens for initiating therapy* because of the combination of efficacy, ease of administration, and low incidence of side effects. Five integrase inhibitors are currently available: raltegravir; elvitegravir; dolutegravir; bictegravir; and cabotegravir, which is given via injections along with injections of rilpivirine every 4 or 8 weeks. Clinical trials of available integrase inhibitors reveal a consistent pattern of more rapid decline in viral load compared with more standard PI/r or NNRTI-based regimens. Integrase inhibitors are effective (when combined with other active medications) in the treatment of people living with HIV with documented resistance to each of the three main classes of antiretroviral medications (nucleoside analogs, PIs, NNRTIs). Avoid administering oral integrase inhibitors with antacids or other medications with divalent cations (Ca^{2+}, Mg^{2+}, Al^{2+}, Fe^{2+}) because chelation of the integrase inhibitor by the cation reduces absorption. When these medications must be taken with integrase inhibitors, they should either be taken together with food or the integrase inhibitor taken 2 hours before divalent cations.

A. **Raltegravir**—The dose of raltegravir is 400 mg orally twice daily or 1200 mg orally once daily (two pills of 600 mg). It has been found to be superior to efavirenz and ritonavir-boosted darunavir and ritonavir-boosted atazanavir. Common side effects are diarrhea, nausea, and headache, but overall, it is well tolerated and has the additional advantage over PI-based regimens and efavirenz-based regimens in that it appears to have little impact on lipid profiles or glucose metabolism. Given the higher barrier to resistance with good tolerability of once-daily dosing, second-generation integrase inhibitors (dolutegravir, bictegravir), raltegravir is now rarely used.

B. **Elvitegravir**—Elvitegravir is not manufactured as a single agent. It can be prescribed in a once-a-day combination pill (Stribild) that contains 125 mg of elvitegravir and 150 mg of cobicistat, a boosting agent, along with standard doses of TDF and emtricitabine (Table 31–8). Stribild has been shown to be noninferior to two preferred first-line regimens: Atripla and boosted atazanavir with emtricitabine/TDF. The main side effect of Stribild is an increase in serum creatinine levels that has been shown to be related to the cobicistat inhibition of tubular secretion of creatinine by the kidney and is thought to be nonpathologic and reversible. However, because of this effect, Stribild is recommended in patients with estimated creatinine clearance greater than 70 mL/minute. A UA should be done at baseline and at initial follow-up to look for proteinuria and glycosuria, which are signs of tubulopathy. Diarrhea and rash may also occur, although overall the medication is well tolerated. Elvitegravir is also coformulated with emtricitabine and TAF along with cobicistat boosting in a single once-a-day pill (Genvoya, Table 31–8). Given the higher barrier to resistance and decreased drug interactions of second-generation integrase inhibitors (dolutegravir, bictegravir), elvitegravir is now rarely used.

c. Dolutegravir—Dolutegravir shows excellent potency and tolerability and is dosed once a day in most circumstances. It has been shown to be superior to efavirenz and darunavir. Unlike elvitegravir, dolutegravir does not require a boosting agent and has fewer drug-drug interactions. Similar to cobicistat, it inhibits tubular secretion of creatinine by the kidney, resulting in small increases in serum creatinine levels. The standard dosage used in treatment-naïve, integrase-naïve patients is 50 mg/day. It is available combined with abacavir and lamivudine in a single once a day tablet (Triumeq, Table 31–8). In patients receiving efavirenz, tipranavir/ritonavir, or rifampin, the dose should be increased to 50 mg twice daily. It should also be dosed at 50 mg twice daily in integrase-experienced patients in whom dolutegravir resistance is documented or suspected. Indeed, when combined with other active medications, it has been shown to provide some activity in patients with integrase resistance who have not responded to prior raltegravir- or elvitegravir-containing regimens. Dolutegravir has demonstrated impressive results in clinical trials of treatment-naïve patients, in terms of effectiveness, tolerability, and high barrier to resistance, when compared with NNRTI, boosted PI, and raltegravir-containing regimens. Dolutegravir is coformulated in combination with rilpivirine (Juluca, Table 31–8) for use as a once-a-day (to be taken with a meal) treatment for patients who are virologically suppressed (viral load less than 50 copies/mL) on a stable regimen for at least 6 months, with no history of treatment failures or resistance to either of the two agents.

d. Bictegravir—Bictegravir is dosed once daily, does not require boosting, and has a high barrier to resistance. It is dosed at 50 mg daily. It has been shown to be noninferior to dolutegravir. It is not available as a single agent but is marketed as a fixed-dose combination of bictegravir with emtricitabine and TAF (Biktarvy, Table 31–8).

e. Cabotegravir—Cabotegravir is an integrase inhibitor that has been approved for use in the United States, Canada, and in the European Union. Cabotegravir comes in two forms: an oral tablet and an injectable formulation. In both forms, it is intended to be given with rilpivirine. The oral form is meant only for the first month of therapy to ensure that the patient is able to tolerate the medication before injecting it in its long-acting formulation. Oral dosing is 30 mg daily of cabotegravir with 25 mg daily of rilpivirine. However, given few adverse events with injectable cabotegravir and rilpivirine (outside of injection reactions), the oral lead-in is optional. When given intramuscularly in combination with rilpivirine, the cabotegravir and rilpivirine are given as separate injections at the same time, one in each buttock. The first intramuscular loading doses are cabotegravir 600 mg and rilpivirine 900 mg. Thereafter, monthly intramuscular dosing is 400 mg of cabotegravir and 600 mg of rilpivirine. The advantage of this combination is that it is complete therapy for patients in whom the viral load is stable and suppressed (less than 50 copies) on their current regimen, which is then stopped in favor of cabotegravir/rilpivirine. Additionally, the combination of cabotegravir 600 mg and rilpivirine 900 mg given every 8 weeks via injection has been approved. The most common side effect is injection site reactions.

5. Entry and fusion inhibitors—

a. Enfuvirtide—Enfuvirtide (Fuzeon) is known as a fusion inhibitor; it blocks the entry of HIV into cells by blocking the fusion of the HIV envelope to the cell membrane. The addition of enfuvirtide to an optimized antiretroviral regimen improved CD4 counts and lowered viral loads in heavily pretreated patients with multidrug-resistant HIV. Unfortunately, resistance to enfuvirtide develops rapidly in patients receiving a nonsuppressive treatment regimen. The dose is 90 mg by subcutaneous injection twice daily; unfortunately, painful injection site reactions develop in most patients, which makes long-term use problematic.

b. Maraviroc—Maraviroc is a CCR5 co-receptor antagonist. Medications in this class prevent the virus from entering uninfected cells by blocking the CCR5 co-receptor. Before starting therapy, a viral tropism assay should be performed because this class of entry inhibitors is only active against "CCR5-tropic virus." This form of the HIV-1 virus tends to predominate early in infection, while so-called dual/mixed tropic virus (which utilizes either R5 or CXCR4 co-receptors) emerges later as infection progresses. Approximately 50–60% of previously treated people living with HIV have circulating CCR5-tropic HIV. The medication has been shown to be effective in people living with HIV who have CCR5-tropic virus and ongoing viral replication despite being heavily treated. The dose of maraviroc is 150–300 mg orally twice daily, based on the other medications the patient is taking at the time—in combination with a ritonavir-boosted PI, 150 mg daily of maraviroc has been used successfully. Common side effects are cough, fever, rash, musculoskeletal problems, abdominal pain, and dizziness; however, maraviroc is generally well tolerated with limited impact on serum lipids.

c. Ibalizumab—A newer treatment for HIV, ibalizumab is a monoclonal antibody that blocks the entry of HIV into the CD4 cell by blocking the CD4 receptor. Given as an intravenous infusion therapy along with other oral HIV medications, it is used as rescue therapy for patients with multidrug-resistant HIV that is not controlled by other treatments. It is given every 2 weeks. Common side effects include diarrhea, dizziness, nausea, rash, elevations in creatinine, and lymphopenia.

6. Attachment inhibitor—

Fostemavir—The active metabolite of fostemavir, temsavir, binds to the viral envelope glycoprotein 120, near to the CD4 binding site, such that the virus does not attach to the

CD4 cells and cannot enter them. With its unique mechanism, it has no cross-resistance with other antiretrovirals. Unlike maraviroc, it is effective regardless of HIV-1 tropism. It is FDA approved for use in heavily treatment-experienced adults with multidrug-resistant HIV-1 infection who are not responding to their current regimen. The dosage of fostemavir is 600 mg orally twice daily, along with an optimized regimen of other antiretroviral medications. It should not be used in conjunction with drugs that are strong P450 (CYP)3A inducers, such as rifampin, phenytoin, and St John's wort.

7. Constructing an initial regimen—Guidelines for starting ART are shown in Table 31–9. The regimens with the strongest evidence all contain integrase inhibitors. This reflects their high efficacy, high barrier to resistance, tolerability, low pill burden, and safety profile. The two

Table 31–9. Recommended and alternative initial antiretroviral therapy regimens (alphabetical order).

Regimen	Advantages	Disadvantages
Recommended Initial Regimens		
Bictegravir + TAF + emtricitabine (Biktarvy)	Single pill once-a-day regimen Low risk of resistance Noninferior to dolutegravir	Less experience than with dolutegravir
Dolutegravir (50 mg daily)[1] + Either: emtricitabine/TDF or emtricitabine/TAF or lamivudine/TDF or lamivudine/TAF	Has activity in some patients with integrase resistance Once-a-day regimen Dolutegravir plus either abacavir/lamivudine or emtricitabine/TDF is superior to darunavir/ritonavir plus either of the NRTI backbones	Dolutegravir has an increased risk of infant neural tube defects and therefore its use in women of reproductive age should be carefully considered and undertaken only with "double" contraceptive measures and written informed consent. No single tablet available When used in patients with integrase resistance or combined with certain other medications, requires twice-a-day dosing
Dolutegravir + abacavir + lamivudine (Triumeq)	Single pill once-a-day regimen Low risk of resistance Superior to Atripla Dolutegravir plus either abacavir/lamivudine or emtricitabine/TDF is superior to darunavir/ritonavir plus either of the NRTI backbones	Dolutegravir has an increased risk of infant neural tube defects, and therefore, its use in premenopausal women should be carefully considered and undertaken only with "double" contraceptive measures and written informed consent. Abacavir should be used only in HLA-B*5701-negative persons Should not be used in patients with hepatitis B coinfection When used in patients with integrase resistance or combined with certain other medications, requires twice-a-day dosing Fixed-dose combination should not be used in patients with creatinine clearance < 50 mL/minute
Dolutegravir + lamivudine (Dovato)	Only recommended initial two-drug regimen Single pill once-a-day regimen	Not for use in patients with HIV RNA > 500,000 copies/mL, or patients initiating therapy during an opportunistic infection, or patients with hepatitis B coinfection, or patients in whom antiretroviral therapy is being started prior to results of HIV genotypic resistance testing or hepatitis B testing. Dolutegravir has an increased risk of infant neural tube defects, and therefore, its use in women of reproductive age should be carefully considered and undertaken only with "double" contraceptive measures and written informed consent.
Other Integrase Inhibitor Regimens		
Raltegravir (400 mg twice daily or 1200 mg once daily) + Either: emtricitabine/TDF or emtricitabine/TAF or lamivudine/TDF or lamivudine/TAF	Fewest drug interactions of integrase inhibitors	Lower barrier to resistance than bictegravir and dolutegravir Requires twice-a-day dosing or taking two pills once a day No single tablet available

(continued)

Table 31–9. Recommended and alternative initial antiretroviral therapy regimens (alphabetical order). (continued)

Regimen	Advantages	Disadvantages
Alternative Initial Regimens That Are Non–Integrase Inhibitor-Based		
Darunavir (800 mg daily) with cobicistat + Either: emtricitabine/TDF or emtricitabine/TAF or lamivudine/TDF or lamivudine/TAF (boosted PI regimen)	Single tablet once-a-day regimen (with emtricitabine and TAF, Symtuza)	Cobicistat boosting causes similar drug-drug interactions as ritonavir; increases in serum creatinine (nonpathologic)
Darunavir (800 mg daily) with ritonavir (100 mg daily) boosting + Either: emtricitabine/TDF or emtricitabine/TAF or lamivudine/TDF or lamivudine/TAF (boosted PI regimen)	Potent boosted PI Can be given once daily Limited risk of resistance with poor adherence	Not available as a single tablet May cause rash in patients with sulfa allergy Ritonavir boosting required Has metabolic side effects
Doravirine with Either: emtricitabine/TDF or emtricitabine/TAF or lamivudine/TDF or lamivudine/TAF	Avoids the use of both integrase inhibitors and PIs Available as a single pill with lamivudine and TDF (Delstrigo) Does inhibit or induce the cytochrome P450 3A4 enzyme	In cases of viral virologic failure, NNRTI cross-resistance may develop.
Rilpivirine/emtricitabine/TDF (Complera) or with emtricitabine/TAF (Odefsey) Non-integrase, non-PI regimens	Single tablet once-a-day regimens Noninferior to Atripla in patients with baseline viral load < 100,000/mcL Limited metabolic side effects	Requires taking with a meal Cannot be used with PPIs Use only in patients with viral loads < 100,000 copies/mL and CD4 counts > 200 cells/mcL Do not use in patients with viral loads > 100,000 copies/mL or CD4 counts < 200 cells/mcL

[1]Usual medication doses are supplied when not part of a fixed-dose preparation.
NNRTI, non-nucleoside reverse transcriptase inhibitor (eg, delavirdine, efavirenz, etravirine, nevirapine, rilpivirine); NRTI, nucleoside/nucleotide reverse transcriptase inhibitor (eg, abacavir, didanosine, emtricitabine, lamivudine, stavudine, tenofovir, zidovudine); PI, protease inhibitor; TAF, tenofovir alafenamide; TDF, tenofovir disoproxil fumarate.

best-tolerated, high barrier to resistance integrase inhibitors are bictegravir and dolutegravir and so they form the backbone of the recommended regimens. Integrase inhibitors are typically given with a backbone of two NRTIs (although see discussion of two-drug therapy below). With respect to nucleoside and nucleotide reverse transcriptase inhibitors (NRTIs), the most commonly used combination is TDF or TAF with emtricitabine or lamivudine. From an efficacy standpoint, there is no difference between TDF or TAF; for patients on a boosted regimen (ie, one including cobicistat or ritonavir), those with renal dysfunction or osteoporosis or osteopenia (or risk for these conditions) should receive TAF. However, TAF is associated with increased weight gain and dyslipidemia, so TDF may be considered in individuals with obesity or dyslipidemia. Also, choosing between TDF and TAF may depend on convenience: which one is coformulated with other desired partner drugs. Emtricitabine and lamivudine are essentially the same from the point of view of efficacy and side effects. The next most commonly used two-drug NRTI backbone is abacavir and lamivudine (coformulated as part of epizcom or with dolutegravir in triumeq). Given the need to perform B*5701 allele and hepatitis B testing, abacavir-containing regimens are not appropriate for rapid ART initiation.

The only two-drug regimen approved for initial ART is dolutegravir plus lamivudine, which is available as a single

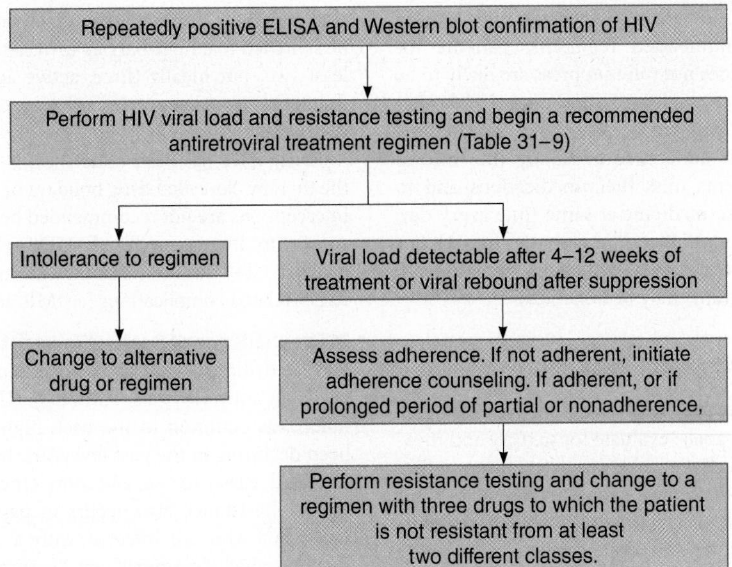
Repeatedly positive ELISA and Western blot confirmation of HIV
Perform HIV viral load and resistance testing and begin a recommended antiretroviral treatment regimen (Table 31–9)
Intolerance to regimen
Viral load detectable after 4–12 weeks of treatment or viral rebound after suppression
Change to alternative drug or regimen
Assess adherence. If not adherent, initiate adherence counseling. If adherent, or if prolonged period of partial or nonadherence,
Perform resistance testing and change to a regimen with three drugs to which the patient is not resistant from at least two different classes.

▲ **Figure 31–7.** Approach to monitoring initial and subsequent antiretroviral therapy.

pill for once-a-day treatment (Dovato, Table 31–8). (All other recommended first-line initial regimens contain three medications, sometimes with a fourth agent as a booster.) This two-drug regimen is not recommended for patients with high HIV viral load (greater than 500,000 copies/mL), or for patients with HBV coinfection (because of development of resistance by the hepatitis B virus to lamivudine when used as monotherapy with possibility of severe flares of hepatitis), or for patients for whom the results from HIV resistance or HBV testing are not yet available. There is also concern about its use in patients with CD4 cell counts less than 200/mL. Dolutegravir/rilpivirine (Juluca) and injectable cabotegravir/rilpivirine (Cabenuva) are only approved in the setting of prior virologic suppression without prior treatment failure or drug resistance.

Studies have shown dolutegravir/abacavir/lamivudine to be superior to efavirenz/TDF/emtricitabine and have shown dolutegravir to be superior to ritonavir-boosted darunavir (both combined with either abacavir/lamivudine or TDF/emtricitabine). A network meta-analysis adjusting for NRTI backbone found that dolutegravir had superior efficacy in suppressing viral load compared with regimens containing ritonavir-boosted atazanavir, ritonavir-boosted darunavir, efavirenz, or ritonavir-boosted lopinavir. Discontinuation due to adverse events was also statistically lower with the dolutegravir regimens.

The medication combinations incorporating the integrase inhibitor raltegravir have done well in comparative studies. Among treatment-naïve patients, raltegravir in combination with TDF/emtricitabine is as effective as efavirenz/TDF/emtricitabine for daily treatment and has fewer side effects. In a 5-year follow-up to the double-blind trial, the raltegravir arm outperformed the efavirenz combination regimen largely due to better long-term tolerability. Furthermore, the CD4 response appeared better in patients treated with the raltegravir combination.

Some studies have shown a potential very small increase in neural tube defects in the offspring of women taking dolutegravir at conception in settings where routine folate supplementation does not occur. As any possible teratogenicity of dolutegravir is thought to represent an integrase class-effect, the risk of neural tube defects has been shown to be smaller than initially documented, and health outcomes are superior with integrase inhibitors compared with alternatives, dolutegravir is still recommended as part of the first-line regimen in women of reproductive age. Elvitegravir/cobicistat and other drugs boosted with cobicistat should not be used during pregnancy and there are limited data on the safety of bictegravir in pregnancy.

The emergence of generic antiretroviral medications is also likely to affect prescribing choices when equally effective regimens are available at different costs. There are generic versions available for abacavir, atazanavir, efavirenz, lamivudine, and TDF. But how this will affect the costs patients pay can be very difficult to determine because of complicated copay rules.

For patients who cannot take an integrase inhibitor, alternative regimens are recommended (Table 31–9).

Resistance testing should be performed prior to starting ART. Of people with newly diagnosed infections in some urban areas of the United States, 8–10% have transmitted drug resistance (most commonly to NNRTIs followed by NRTIs).

The most important determinant of treatment efficacy is adherence to the regimen. Therefore, it is vitally important that the regimen chosen be one to which the patient can easily adhere (Figure 31–7). In general, patients are more compliant if their medication regimens (Table 31–9) offer complete therapy in one pill that needs to be taken only once a day, do not require special timing with regard to meals, can be taken at the same time as other medications, do not require refrigeration or special preparation, and do not have bothersome side effects. Given the high level of effectiveness of recommended regimens, patients for whom the viral load does not fully suppress are likely to be encountering adherence challenges. Pharmacists and other specially trained clinicians can be very effective in helping patients improve their adherence by taking the time to understand why patients miss their medications and to problem solve (eg, take medicine at same time every day, keep a supply in the car or at work in case they forget). For certain populations (eg, unstably housed individuals), specially tailored programs may be beneficial.

E. Monitoring Antiretroviral Treatment

1. Goals of monitoring ART—Monitoring of ART (Figure 31–7) has two goals: evaluate for *toxicity* and measure *efficacy* using objective markers to determine whether to maintain or change regimens. Laboratory evaluation for toxicity depends on the specific medications in the combination but generally should be done approximately every 3–6 months once a patient is on a stable regimen. Patients who are intolerant of their initial regimen should be changed to one of the other initial recommended or alternative regimens in Table 31–9. The second aspect of monitoring is to measure HIV viral load, the objective marker of efficacy. The HIV viral load should be repeated 2–4 weeks after the initiation or change of antiretroviral regimen and every 3–6 months thereafter in clinically stable patients. With integrase regimens, a two-log10 reduction is expected within 2 weeks of starting therapy, and approximately 80% of patients will have undetectable HIV viral load at 1 month. All patients should have undetectable viral loads by 3 months; if not, the usual problem is nonadherence (see below). CD4+ counts are most useful in determining the immunologic response to ART, although the response can vary significantly, and determining whether opportunistic infection prophylaxis can be discontinued. CD4+ counts should be monitored approximately every 3–6 months in individuals newly initiating ART. For those who have consistently suppressed HIV viral loads over the first 1–2 years of therapy with a CD4+ count greater than 300 cells/mcL, monitoring can occur yearly, and is optional in those with CD4+ counts greater than 500 cells/mcL.

2. The challenge of medication adherence—In a patient who is adherent to an integrase inhibitor regimen, viral load should drop by 100-fold within 2 weeks. For patients in whom viral loads do not decrease adequately, or who have viral rebound after suppression, the major question facing the clinician is whether the patient is nonadherent or has resistance to the regimen, or both. Patients who are having trouble adhering to their treatment should receive adherence counseling. In patients who are adherent or who have missed enough doses to make resistance possible, resistance testing should be performed. Based on the results of resistance testing, if there is no treatment-emergent resistance, and the patient is tolerating the regimen well, the patient should continue the regimen with assessment of potential barriers to adherence (ie, mental health, substance use, medication coverage, or housing challenges). If resistance has emerged, the patient should be switched to a high-barrier-to-resistance regimen with at least two, but ideally three, active agents (ie, three-drug dolutegravir, bictegravir, or boosted darunavir-based regimen).

Once ART has been initiated, it is not advisable to stop the therapy. So-called drug holidays or structured treatment interruptions are not recommended because they have been shown to increase risk of AIDS-related complications, increase CD4 declines, and increase morbidity from non–AIDS-related complications (eg, MIs and liver failure).

3. The challenge of medication resistance—Resistance to HIV-1 medication has been documented for all currently available antiretrovirals. Although HIV medication resistance was common in the past, high-level resistance has been declining in the past few years, likely related to better tolerated, easier to use, and more efficacious antiretroviral agents. Resistance also occurs in patients who are ART-naïve but who are infected with a medication-resistant strain—called **"primary" or "transmitted" medication resistance.** Cohort studies of ART-naïve patients entering care in North America and Western Europe show that roughly 8–10% of people with a recent infection have a medication-resistant strain of HIV-1.

In addition to being part of a standard baseline evaluation, resistance testing is recommended for patients who are receiving ART and have suboptimal viral suppression (typically a viral load greater than 500 copies/mL is needed for resistance testing be performed). *Both genotypic and phenotypic resistance tests are commercially available, and in randomized controlled studies, their use has been shown to result in improved short-term virologic outcomes compared to making treatment choices without resistance testing.* Furthermore, multiple retrospective studies have conclusively demonstrated that resistance tests provide prognostic information about virologic response to newly initiated therapy that cannot be gleaned from standard clinical information (ie, treatment history, examination, CD4 count, and viral load tests).

Because of the complexity of resistance tests, many clinicians require expert interpretation of results. In the case of genotypic assays, results may show that the mutations that are selected for during ART are medication-specific or contribute to broad cross-resistance to multiple medications within a therapeutic class. An example of a medication-specific mutation for the reverse transcriptase inhibitors would be the *M184V* mutation that is selected for by lamivudine or emtricitabine therapy—this mutation causes resistance only to those two medications. Conversely, the thymidine analog mutations ("TAMs") of *M41L, D67N, K70R, L210W, T215Y/F,* and *T219Q/K/E* are selected for by either prior zidovudine or stavudine therapy, but cause resistance to all the medications in the class and often extend to the nucleotide inhibitor tenofovir when three or more of these TAMs are present. The combination of *M184V* and *K65R* is important to know as it causes resistance to all NRTIs except zidovudine and would typically necessitate change to an NRTI-sparing regimen. The most common mutations associated with medication resistance and cross-resistance patterns for NRTIs, NNRTIs, PIs, and integrase inhibitors can be found at https://hivdb.stanford.edu (see specific references below). Phenotypic resistance testing can provide complementary data and is usually provided with an interpretation about susceptibility to the virus. Proviral DNA testing is increasingly used in individuals with suppressed HIV viral loads but concerns that prior resistance may exist impacting a preferred alternate regimen, although proviral DNA resistance testing and historical standard genotypic testing are sometimes not concordant, complicating their interpretation.

Furthermore, both methods of resistance testing are limited by the fact that they may measure resistance in only some of the viral strains present in an individual. Resistance results may also be misleading if a patient is not taking antiretroviral medications at the time of testing because the dominant virus is likely the wild-type, even if there are resistant viruses in the body that can become dominant with the selective pressure of antivirals. Thus, resistance results do not replace a careful history of what medications a patient has taken in the past and for how long. Also, the results of resistance testing should be viewed cumulatively—ie, if resistance is reported to an agent on one test, it should be presumed to be present thereafter even if subsequent tests do not give the same result.

Stanford University HIV Drug Resistance Database Home Page (https://hivdb.stanford.edu/) provides Genotypic Resistance Interpretation Algorithm, HIVdb Program, version 9.0, February 22, 2021 (https://hivdb.stanford.edu/hivdb/by-mutations/); Genotype-Phenotype Correlations (https://hivdb.stanford.edu/pages/genotype-phenotype.html); Genotype-Treatment Correlations (https://hivdb.stanford.edu/pages/genotype-rx.html); Genotype-Clinical Outcome Correlations (https://hivdb.stanford.edu/pages/genotype-clinical.html)

F. Constructing Antiretroviral Treatment Regimens for Patients with Resistance

In designing second-line regimens for patients with resistance to initial therapy, *the goal is to identify three medications from at least two different classes to which the virus is not resistant*. Even without resistance testing, certain forms of cross-resistance between medications within a class can be assumed. For example, the resistance patterns of raltegravir and elvitegravir are overlapping, and patients with treatment-emergent resistance to these regimens potentially harboring resistance to second-generation integrase inhibitors such as bictegravir and dolutegravir. Fostemsavir, an attachment inhibitor, and ibalizumab, a monoclonal antibody, are specifically FDA-approved for heavily treated adults with multidrug-resistant HIV who are not responding to their existing regimen. They are used in combination with other antiretroviral drugs.

In constructing regimens, toxicities should be nonoverlapping and agents that are either virologically antagonistic or incompatible in terms of drug-drug interactions should be avoided. For example, dolutegravir and etravirine should not be coadministered without inclusion of a ritonavir-boosted PI, as etravirine will reduce the plasma concentrations of dolutegravir. The combination of TDF and boosted PIs should ideally be avoided given the potential for increased tenofovir toxicity with this regimen. Coformulated TAF and boosted PI regimens (ie, emtricitabine/TAF/darunavir or Symtuza) are preferred in this setting given these are the only formulations where a lower dose of TAF is available (10 mg versus typical 25 mg dose). Lamivudine and emtricitabine are essentially the same medication and so are not used together.

Given the availability of new class medications and new generation medications, *a combination of ART can successfully treat virtually all patients*—no matter how much resistance is present.

Course & Prognosis

With improvements in therapy, patients who are adherent with treatment should have near normal life spans. A population-based study conducted in Denmark found that people aged 25 years living with HIV without hepatitis C had a life expectancy similar to that of a 25-year-old without HIV. Unfortunately, not all people living with HIV have access to treatment. *Studies consistently show less access to treatment for Black people living with HIV and those experiencing homelessness or who inject drugs.* For patients whose disease progresses even though they are receiving appropriate treatment, palliative care must be provided (see Chapter 5), with attention to pain control, spiritual needs, and family (biologic and chosen) dynamics.

When to Refer

- People living with HIV in whom viral loads cannot be fully suppressed on one of the initial recommended regimens should be treated in consultation with a specialist.
- Specialty consultation is particularly important for those patients with detectable viral loads on ART; those intolerant of standard medications; those in need of systemic chemotherapy; and those with complicated opportunistic infections, particularly when invasive procedures or experimental therapies are needed.

When to Admit

Admit patients with opportunistic infections who are acutely ill (eg, who are febrile, who have had rapid change of mental status, or who are in respiratory distress) or who require intravenous medications.

Cahn P et al; GEMINI Study Team. Dolutegravir plus lamivudine versus dolutegravir plus tenofovir disoproxil fumarate and emtricitabine in antiretroviral-naive adults with HIV-1 infection (GEMINI-1 and GEMINI-2): week 48 results from two multicentre, double-blind, randomised, non-inferiority, phase 3 trials. Lancet. 2019;393:143. [PMID: 30420123]

Kozal M et al. Fostemsavir in adults with multidrug-resistant HIV-1 infection. N Engl J Med. 2020;382:1232. [PMID: 32212519]

Panel on Opportunistic Infections in Adults and Adolescents with HIV. Guidelines for the prevention and treatment of opportunistic infections in adults and adolescents with HIV: recommendations from the Centers for Disease Control and Prevention, the National Institutes of Health, and the HIV Medicine Association of the Infectious Diseases Society of America. https://clinicalinfo.hiv.gov/sites/default/files/guidelines/documents/Adult_OI.pdf. Updated 2020 May 26.

Saag MS et al. Antiretroviral drugs for treatment and prevention of HIV infection in adults: 2020 recommendations of the International Antiviral Society-USA Panel. JAMA. 2020;324:1651. [PMID: 33052386]

Swindells S et al. Long-acting cabotegravir and rilpivirine for maintenance of HIV-1 suppression. N Engl J Med. 2020;382:1112. [PMID: 32130809]

Panel on Opportunistic Infections in Adults and Adolescents with HIV. Guidelines for the prevention and treatment of opportunistic infections in adults and adolescents with HIV: recommendations from the Centers for Disease Control and Prevention, the National Institutes of Health, and the HIV Medicine Association of the Infectious Diseases Society of America. https://clinicalinfo.hiv.gov/sites/default/files/guidelines/documents/Adult_OI.pdf. Updated 2020 May 26.

Viral & Rickettsial Infections

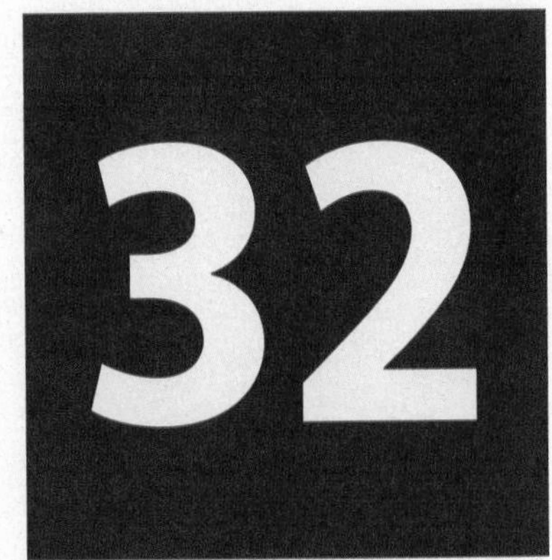

Christine Akamine, MD
Eva Clark, MD, PhD
Wayne X. Shandera, MD

VIRAL DISEASES

HUMAN HERPESVIRUSES

1. Herpesviruses 1 & 2

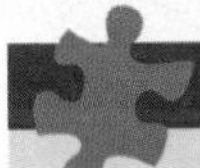

ESSENTIALS OF DIAGNOSIS

- Spectrum of illness: stomatitis, urogenital lesions, Bell palsy, encephalitis.
- Variable intervals between exposure and clinical disease since herpes simplex virus (HSV) causes both primary (often subclinical) and reactivation disease.

General Considerations

HSV-1 and HSV-2 affect primarily the oral and genital areas, respectively. Asymptomatic shedding of either virus is common, but it is more common with HSV-2 and from genital areas, with most infected individuals shedding virus at least once a month, which may be responsible for transmission. Individuals with asymptomatic HSV-2–infection shed the virus less often than those with symptomatic infection. Clinical disease typically indicates reactivation. Total and subclinical shedding of HSV-2 virus decrease after the first year of initial infection, although viral shedding continues for years thereafter.

Although HSV-2 is the most common cause of genital ulcers in the developed world, epidemiologic studies show that HSV-1 is a more common cause of both genital and oral lesions than HSV-2 in young women in the United States. Most persons with HSV-2 infection in the United States are unaware that they are infected.

HSV-2 seropositivity is associated with higher risk of HIV acquisition (it is threefold higher among persons who are HSV-2 seropositive than among those who are HSV-2 seronegative), and HSV-2 reactivates more often in advanced HIV infection. HIV replication is increased by interaction with HSV proteins. Suppression of HSV-2 decreases HIV plasma levels and genital tract shedding of HIV, which can contribute to a reduction in the sexual transmission of HIV.

Clinical Findings

A. Symptoms and Signs

1. Mucocutaneous disease—See Chapter 6 for HSV-1 mucocutaneous disease (**"herpes labialis"** or **"gingivostomatitis"**). Digital lesions (whitlows) (Figure 32–1) are an occupational hazard in medicine and dentistry. Contact sports (eg, wrestling) are associated with outbreaks of skin infections (**"herpes gladiatorum"**).

Vesicles form moist, painful ulcers after several days and epithelialize over 1–2 weeks if untreated. Primary infection is usually more severe than recurrences but may be asymptomatic. Recurrences often involve fewer lesions, tend to be labial, heal faster, and are triggered by stress, fever, infection, sunlight, chemotherapy (eg, fludarabine, azathioprine), among other undetermined factors.

HSV-2 lesions largely involve the genital tract. The virus typically remains latent in the presacral ganglia and shedding of HSV-2 can occur for years after acquisition (see Chapter 6). Occasionally, lesions arise in the perianal region or on the buttocks and upper thighs. Dysuria, cervicitis, and urinary retention may occur in women. Urethritis may occur in men. Proctitis and extensive, ulcerating, weeping sacral lesions may be presenting symptoms in people living with HIV infection with low CD4 counts. Large ulcerations and atypical lesions suggest drug-resistant isolates.

2. Ocular disease—HSV can cause uveitis, keratitis, blepharitis, and keratoconjunctivitis (see Chapter 7). Lesions limited to the epithelium usually heal without affecting vision, whereas stromal involvement can cause uveitis, scarring, and eventually blindness. HSV is the second most common infectious cause of acute retinal necrosis, after varicella-zoster virus (VZV).

3. Neonatal and congenital infection—Rarely, either HSV-1 or HSV-2 can infect the fetus and induce congenital malformations (organomegaly, bleeding, and CNS abnormalities). Neonatal transmission during delivery, however, is more common than intrauterine infection. The global

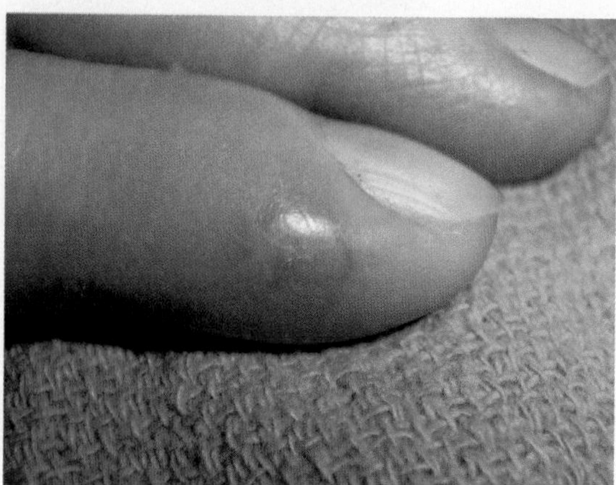

▲ **Figure 32–1.** Herpetic whitlow. (Reproduced with permission from Richard P. Usatine, MD, in Usatine RP, Smith MA, Mayeaux EJ Jr, Chumley H. *The Color Atlas of Family Medicine*, 2nd ed. McGraw-Hill, 2013.)

rate of neonatal herpes is estimated to be about 10 cases per 100,000 live births. Maternal infection during the third trimester is associated with the highest risk of neonatal transmission, but about 70% of these infections are asymptomatic or unrecognized. Invasive fetal monitoring and vacuum or forceps delivery increase the risk of herpesvirus transmission.

4. CNS disease—Traditionally, herpes simplex encephalitis is associated with HSV-1 infection and aseptic meningitis with HSV-2 infection. Both viruses, however, can cause encephalitis. Encephalitis presents with nonspecific symptoms: a flu-like prodrome, followed by headache, fever, behavioral and speech disturbances, and focal or generalized seizures. The temporal lobe is often involved. Untreated disease and presentation with coma carry a high mortality. Ischemic stroke, although infrequent, can complicate the course of HSV meningitis or encephalitis, or can happen in isolation due to HSV-induced cerebral vasculitis. Many survivors suffer neurologic sequelae, which are observed more frequently among patients with HSV-1 infection. Both HSV-1 and HSV-2 can cause mild, nonspecific neurologic symptoms and are also associated with benign recurrent lymphocytic (Mollaret) meningitis. Hyponatremia is a predictive marker for encephalitis before lumbar puncture data are available.

5. Disseminated infection—Disseminated HSV infection occurs in the setting of immunosuppression, either primary or iatrogenic, or rarely with pregnancy. In disseminated disease, skin lesions are not always present. Disseminated skin lesions are a particular complication in patients with atopic eczema (**eczema herpeticum**) and burns. Pneumonia can occur regardless of immune status.

6. Bell palsy—HSV-1 is a cause of Bell palsy (facial nerve paralysis) (see also Chapter 24).

7. Esophagitis and proctitis—HSV-1 can cause esophagitis in immunocompromised patients, particularly those with AIDS. The lesions are smaller and deeper than those observed in patients with cytomegalovirus (CMV) esophagitis or with other herpesviruses known to cause esophagitis in immunocompromised persons. Rarely HSV esophagitis is accompanied by significant upper GI hemorrhage. Proctitis occurs mainly in men who have sex with men.

8. Erythema multiforme—HSVs are a leading cause of erythema multiforme minor ("**herpes-associated erythema multiforme**") and of the more severe condition Stevens-Johnson syndrome/toxic epidermal necrolysis (see also Chapter 6).

9. Other—HSV infection causes approximately 1% of cases of acute liver failure, particularly in pregnant women and immunosuppressed patients. The mortality of such rare fulminant hepatitis is nearly 75%. An HSV lower respiratory tract infection of unknown clinical significance is common in mechanically ventilated patients. Evidence suggests that this finding is usually an indicator rather than the cause of a poor clinical condition. HSV-1 pneumonia is associated with high morbidity in patients with solid tumors. HSV-1 is reported to be a cause of perinephric abscess, febrile neutropenia, chronic urticaria, and esophagitis and enteritis in SLE. HSV is also associated with *Helicobacter pylori*–negative upper GI tract ulcers.

B. Laboratory Findings

1. Mucocutaneous disease—See Chapter 6.

2. Ocular disease—Herpes keratitis is diagnosed by branching (dendritic) ulcers that stain with fluorescein. The extent of epithelial injury in herpes keratitis correlates well with PCR positivity. Uveitis from HSV is often diagnosed clinically, although PCR assays (including a new multiplex assay that includes VZV) on anterior chamber aspirated material may assist in making the diagnosis.

3. Encephalitis and recurrent meningitis—Cerebrospinal fluid (CSF) pleocytosis is common, with a similar increase in the number of red cells, although CSF findings may be atypical in immunosuppressed patients. HSV real-time PCR of the CSF is a rapid, sensitive, and specific tool for early diagnosis and can be included in a multiple rapid array panel. Viral detection by this method can be used if the clinical picture is consistent, especially if initial studies are negative. Antibodies to HSV in CSF can confirm the diagnosis but appear late in disease. Viral culture shows a sensitivity of only 10%. MRI scanning is often a useful adjunct showing increased signal in the temporal and frontal lobes (thalamic signal changes are associated with worse functional outcome). Temporal lobe seizure foci may be shown on electroencephalograms (EEGs).

4. Esophagitis, proctitis, and other GI disease—Esophagitis is diagnosed by endoscopic biopsy with real-time PCR and cultures. Proctitis may be diagnosed by rectal swab for PCR, culture, or both. Complicated cases may require biopsy. Concomitant hepatitis and colitis have been reported with herpes simplex. In pregnancy, HSV hepatitis is infrequently (18% in one series) associated with a rash and carries a mortality up to 39%.

5. Pneumonia—Pneumonia is diagnosed by clinical, pathologic, and radiographic findings. The CT findings include diffuse or multifocal areas of ground-glass attenuation or consolidative changes or both and are best confirmed by using high-resolution CT techniques.

Treatment & Prophylaxis

Medications that inhibit replication of HSV-1 and HSV-2 include acyclovir and related compounds, foscarnet, cidofovir, and trifluridine and vidarabine (both for keratitis) (Table 32–1). Agents under study include helicase-primase inhibitors (IM-250) with promising preliminary data as of early 2022. Brincidofovir, a lipid conjugate of cidofovir, shows in vitro activity against HSV/VZV and is effective in preliminary studies in hematopoietic cell transplant recipients as HSV/VZV prophylaxis.

A. Mucocutaneous Disease

See Chapter 6.

B. Keratitis and Uveitis

For the treatment of acute epithelial keratitis, oral antiviral agents such as valacyclovir or famciclovir are first-line therapies (see Chapter 7). The usage of topical corticosteroids may exacerbate the infection, although systemic corticosteroids may help with selected cases of stromal infection. Long-term treatment (more than 1 year) with acyclovir at a dosage of 800 mg/day orally decreases recurrence rates of keratitis, conjunctivitis, or blepharitis due to HSV.

Uveitis is best managed with oral systemic (not topical) acyclovir, although HSV resistance among people living with HIV infection is reported because of the diversity of the HSV species often present.

C. Neonatal Disease

Counseling (but not serologic screening) should be offered to pregnant mothers. The use of maternal antenatal suppressive therapy with acyclovir (typically, 400 mg orally three times daily) beginning at 36 weeks' gestation decreases the presence of detectable HSV, the rates of recurrence at delivery, and the need for cesarean delivery. Cesarean delivery is recommended for pregnant women with active genital lesions or typical prodromal symptoms.

D. Encephalitis and Meningitis

Because of the need for rapid treatment to decrease mortality and neurologic sequelae, intravenous acyclovir (10 mg/kg every 8 hours for 10 days or more, adjusting for kidney disease) should be started in those patients with suspected HSV encephalitis, *stopping only if another diagnosis is established*. If the PCR of CSF is negative but clinical suspicion remains high, treatment should be continued for 10 days because the false-negative rate for PCR can be as high as 25% (especially in children) and acyclovir is relatively nontoxic. Acyclovir resistance in a case of herpes simplex encephalitis is reported. Herpes simplex viral load does not appear to correlate with outcome of meningitis, and it is not recommended to follow viral load over time.

Long-term neurologic sequelae of HSV encephalitis are common, and late pediatric relapse is recognized. Aseptic meningitis may also require a course of intravenous acyclovir or valacyclovir. Long-term oral prophylaxis with valacyclovir, however, does not appear to prevent recurrences of aseptic meningitis with HSV-2.

E. Disseminated Disease

Disseminated disease responds best to parenteral acyclovir when treatment is initiated early.

F. Bell Palsy

Prednisolone, 25 mg orally twice daily for 10 days started within 72 hours of onset, significantly increases the rate of recovery. Data on antiherpes agents are equivocal, and therefore, HSV assays are *not* routinely recommended; according to one study, valacyclovir (but not acyclovir), 1 g orally daily for 5 days, plus corticosteroid therapy may be beneficial if started within 7 days of symptom onset. In patients with severe or complete facial paralysis, such antiviral therapy is often administered but without proof of efficacy.

G. Esophagitis and Proctitis

Patients with esophagitis should receive either intravenous acyclovir (5–10 mg/kg every 8 hours) or oral acyclovir (400 mg five times daily) through resolution of symptoms, typically 3–5 days; however, longer treatment may be necessary for immunosuppressed patients. Maintenance therapy for AIDS patients is also with acyclovir (400 mg orally three to five times daily). Proctitis is treated with similar dosages and usually responds within 5 days, although in patients living with HIV, higher doses (up to 5 g/day) intravenously in five or six divided doses may be needed for severe lesions.

H. Erythema Multiforme

Suppressive therapy with oral acyclovir (400 mg twice a day for 6 months) decreases the recurrence rate of HSV-associated erythema multiforme. Valacyclovir (500 mg orally twice a day) may be effective in cases unresponsive to acyclovir.

Prevention

Besides antiviral suppressive therapy (see Erythema multiforme, above and in Chapter 6), prevention also requires counseling and the use of condom barrier precautions during sexual activity. Disclosure to sexual partners of HSV-seropositive status is associated with about a 50% reduction in HSV-2 acquisition. Male circumcision is associated with a lower incidence of acquiring HSV-2 infection.

Preventing spread to hospital staff and other patients from cases with mucocutaneous, disseminated, or genital disease requires isolation and usage of hand washing and gloving–gowning precautions. Staff with active lesions (eg, whitlows) should not have contact with patients. No herpes

Table 32–1. Agents for viral infections (listed in alphabetical order).[1]

Drug	Dosing[2]	Spectrum	Toxicities
Acyclovir	**HSV and VZV infections:** 400 mg orally three times daily or 200 mg orally five times daily; 30 mg/kg/day or 10 mg/kg every 8 hours intravenously for 7 days **Acute herpes encephalitis:** 10 mg/kg intravenously every 8 hours for 14–21 days	HSV, VZV	Neurotoxic reactions, reversible kidney dysfunction, local reactions
Baloxavir	40 mg dose if patient is 40 to < 80 kg 80 mg if patient is ≥ 80 kg Only use for patients 12 years or older	Influenza A and B strains	Diarrhea and bronchitis
Cidofovir	5 mg/kg intravenously weekly for 2 weeks, then every other week	CMV	Neutropenia, kidney disease, ocular hypotonia
Famciclovir	**Acute VZV:** 500 mg orally three times daily for 7 days **Genital or cutaneous HSV-1/HSV-2:** 250 mg three times daily for 7–10 days; 125 mg twice daily for 5 days for recurrences (500 mg twice daily for 7 days if HIV-positive)	HSV, VZV	Early angioedema; later rarely, GI symptoms, headaches, rashes
Foscarnet	**Induction:** 90 mg/kg intravenously (90- to 120-minute infusion) every 12 hours or 60 mg/kg intravenously (minimum 1-hour infusion) every 8 hours over 2–3 weeks depending on clinical response **Maintenance:** 90–120 mg/kg intravenously (2-hour infusion) once daily	HSV resistant to acyclovir, CMV, VZV, HIV-1	Nephrotoxicity, genital ulcerations, calcium disturbances
Ganciclovir	**Induction:** 5 mg/kg intravenously every 12 hours for 14–21 days **Maintenance:** 6 mg/kg/day intravenously for 5 days each week	CMV	Neutropenia, thrombocytopenia, CNS side effects
Idoxuridine	Topical, 0.1% every 1–2 hours for 3–5 days (not available in the United States)	HSV keratitis	Local reactions
Interferon alfa-2b	**HBV infection:** 10 million IU subcutaneously three times weekly or 5 million U daily[1] **Condylomata:** 1 million IU intralesionally in up to five warts three times weekly for 3 weeks	HBV, HCV, HPV	Influenza-like syndrome, myelosuppression, neurotoxicity
Interferon alfa-n3	**Refractory or recurring external condylomata acuminata:** 0.05 mL (250,000 IU) per wart intralesionally twice weekly for up to 8 weeks; 0.5 mL (2.5 million IU) is the maximum dose per treatment session	HPV, HCV	Local reactions Influenza-like syndrome, myelosuppression, neurotoxicity
Oseltamivir	75 mg orally twice daily for 5 days	Influenza A and B	Dose needs to be adjusted for kidney dysfunction
Palivizumab	15 mg/kg intramuscularly every month in RSV season	RSV	Upper respiratory infection symptoms
Penciclovir	Topical 1% cream every 2 hours for 4 days	HSV	Local reactions
Peramivir	Intravenous, 600-mg single dose	Uncomplicated influenza A	Nausea, vomiting, diarrhea, neutropenia
Remdesivir	Intravenous, 200 mg first day followed by 100 mg/day for 4 days for non-ICU patients, 9 more days for ICU patients	COVID-19	Transaminitis, fatigue, headaches, nausea
Ribavirin	**RSV infection:** one vial (6 g) dissolved and delivered through a Small Particle Aerosol Generator (SPAG-2) over a continuous 12- to 18-hour period daily for 5 consecutive days	RSV, severe influenza A or B, Lassa fever	Wheezing, hemolytic anemia
Trifluridine	Topical, 1% drops every 2 hours to 9 drops/day	HSV keratitis	Local reactions
Valacyclovir	**Acute VZV:** 1 g orally three times daily for 7 days **Primary genital HSV-1/HSV-2:** 1 g twice daily for 10 days **Recurrent genital HSV-1/HSV-2:** 500 mg twice daily for 3 days **Suppressive therapy:** 1 g daily; 500 mg if fewer than 9 recurrences/year (Dose depends on immune status and number of recurrences.)	VZV, HSV	Thrombotic thrombocytopenic purpura or hemolytic-uremic syndrome in AIDS
Valganciclovir	900 mg orally twice daily for 3 weeks; 900 mg daily as maintenance	CMV	See ganciclovir
Zanamivir	5 mg inhalations twice daily for 5 days	Uncomplicated influenza A and B	Bronchospasm in patients with asthma

Sources: Data from Drugs.com and Lexicomp Online.

[1]Agents used exclusively in the management of HIV infection and AIDS are found in Chapter 31. Agents used in the management of HBV and HCV infections are found in Chapter 16.

[2]Dosing varies considerably by indication and may require adjustment based on patient's clinical state and type of viral infection. Consultation with a pharmacist is recommended.

CMV, cytomegalovirus; CSF, cerebrospinal fluid; HBV, hepatitis B virus; HCV, hepatitis C virus; HSV, herpes simplex virus; RSV, respiratory syncytial virus; VZV, varicella-zoster virus.

vaccine is publicly available, although several vaccine candidates have undergone early clinical trials. An mRNA vaccine against HSV-2 that expresses HSV-2 glycoproteins C, D, and E in lipid nanoparticles has completed phase 1 trials as of early 2022.

Cruz AT et al. Predictors of invasive herpes simplex virus infection in young infants. Pediatrics. 2021;148:e2021050052. [PMID: 34446535]
Cully M. Antiviral therapy targets latent HSV infections. Nat Rev Drug Discov. 2021;20:586. [PMID: 34175893]
Pittet LF et al. Postnatal exposure to herpes simplex virus: to treat or not to treat? Pediatr Infect Dis J. 2021;40:S16. [PMID: 32773663]
Sarton B et al. Assessment of magnetic resonance imaging changes and functional outcomes among adults with severe herpes simplex encephalitis. JAMA Netw Open. 2021;4:e2114328. [PMID: 34313743]

2. Varicella (Chickenpox) & Herpes Zoster (Shingles)

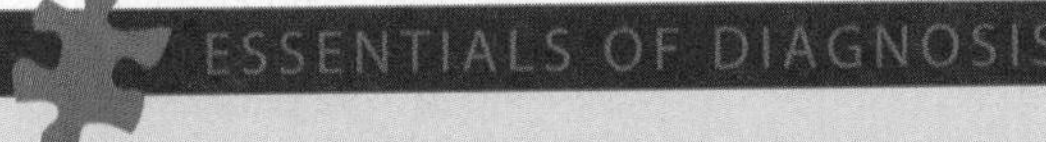

ESSENTIALS OF DIAGNOSIS

- **Varicella rash:** pruritic, centrifugal, papular changing to vesicular ("dew drops on a rose petal"), pustular, and finally crusting.
- **Zoster rash:** tingling, pain, eruption of vesicles in a dermatomal distribution, evolving to pustules and then crusting.

General Considerations

Disease manifestations of VZV, or human herpesvirus (HHV)-3, include chickenpox (varicella) and shingles (herpes zoster). Chickenpox generally presents during childhood; has an incubation period of 10–20 days (average 2 weeks); and is highly contagious, spreading by inhalation of infective droplets or contact with lesions.

The incidence and severity of herpes zoster ("**shingles**"), which *affects up to 30% of persons during their lifetime*, increases with age due to an age-related decline in immunity against VZV. More than half of all patients in whom herpes zoster develops are older than 60 years, and the incidence of herpes zoster reaches 10 cases per 1000 patient-years by age 80 (by which time 50% are infected with VZV). The annual incidence in the United States of 1 million cases is increasing as the population ages. Populations at increased risk for varicella-zoster–related diseases include immunosuppressed persons and persons receiving biologic agents.

Clinical Findings

A. Varicella

1. Symptoms and signs—Fever and malaise are mild in children and more marked in adults. The pruritic rash begins prominently on the face, scalp, and trunk, and later involves the extremities (Table 32–2). Maculopapules change within a few hours to vesicles that become pustular and eventually form crusts (Figures 32–2 and 32–3). New lesions may erupt for 1–5 days, so that different stages of

Table 32–2. Diagnostic features of some acute exanthems (listed in alphabetical order).

Disease	Prodromal Signs and Symptoms	Nature of Eruption	Other Diagnostic Features	Laboratory Tests
Atypical measles	Same as measles.	Maculopapular centripetal rash, becoming confluent.	History of measles vaccination.	Measles antibodies present in past, with titer rise during illness.
Chikungunya fever	2–4 (sometimes 1–12) days, fever, headaches, abdominal complaints, myalgias, arthralgias.	Maculopapular, centrally distributed, pruritus, can be bullous with sloughing in children, occasional facial edema and petechiae.	History of mosquito bites, epidemiologic factors.	ELISA-based IgM or IgG (fourfold increase in titers); PCR and cultures are infrequently available.
Eczema herpeticum	None.	Vesiculopustular lesions in area of eczema.		HSV isolated in cell culture. Multinucleated giant cells in smear of lesion.
Ehrlichiosis	Headache, malaise.	Rash in one-third, similar to Rocky Mountain spotted fever.	Pancytopenia, elevated liver biochemical tests.	PCR, immunofluorescent antibody.
Enterovirus infections	1–2 days of fever, malaise.	Maculopapular rash resembling rubella, rarely papulovesicular or petechial.	Aseptic meningitis.	Virus isolation from stool or CSF; complement fixation titer rise.

(*continued*)

Table 32–2. Diagnostic features of some acute exanthems (listed in alphabetical order). (continued)

Disease	Prodromal Signs and Symptoms	Nature of Eruption	Other Diagnostic Features	Laboratory Tests
Erythema infectiosum (erythroparvovirus)	None. Usually in epidemics.	Red, flushed cheeks; circumoral pallor; maculopapules on extremities.	"Slapped face" appearance.	WBC count normal.
Exanthema subitum (HHV-6, 7; roseola)	3–4 days of high fever.	As fever falls, pink maculopapules appear on chest and trunk; fade in 1–3 days.		WBC count low.
Infectious mononucleosis (EBV)	Fever, adenopathy, sore throat.	Maculopapular rash resembling rubella, rarely papulovesicular.	Splenomegaly, tonsillar exudate.	Atypical lymphocytes in blood smears; heterophile agglutination (Monospot test).
Kawasaki disease	Fever, adenopathy, conjunctivitis.	Cracked lips, strawberry tongue, maculopapular polymorphous rash, peeling skin on fingers and toes.	Edema of extremities. Angiitis of coronary arteries.	Thrombocytosis, electrocardiographic changes.
Measles (rubeola)	3–4 days of fever, coryza, conjunctivitis, and cough.	Maculopapular, brick red; begins on head and neck; spreads downward and outward, in 5–7 days rash brownish, desquamating. See Atypical measles, above.	Koplik spots on buccal mucosa.	WBC count low. Virus isolation in cell culture. Antibody tests by hemagglutination inhibition or neutralization.
Meningococcemia	Hours of fever, vomiting.	Maculopapules, petechiae, purpura.	Meningeal signs, toxicity, shock.	Cultures of blood, CSF. WBC count high.
Rocky Mountain spotted fever	3–4 days of fever, vomiting.	Maculopapules, petechiae, initial distribution centripetal (extremities to trunk, including palms).	History of tick bite.	Indirect fluorescent antibody; complement fixation.
Rubella	Little or no prodrome.	Maculopapular, pink; begins on head and neck, spreads downward, fades in 3 days. No desquamation.	Lymphadenopathy, postauricular or occipital.	WBC count normal or low. Serologic tests for immunity and definitive diagnosis (hemagglutination inhibition).
Scarlet fever	One-half to 2 days of malaise, sore throat, fever, vomiting.	Generalized, punctate, red; prominent on neck, in axillae, groin, skin folds; circumoral pallor; fine desquamation involves hands and feet.	Strawberry tongue, exudative tonsillitis.	Group A beta-hemolytic streptococci in cultures from throat; antistreptolysin O titer rise.
Smallpox	Fever, malaise, prostration.	Maculopapules to vesicles to pustules to scars (lesions develop at the same pace).	Centrifugal rash; fulminant sepsis in small percentage of patients, GI and skin hemorrhages.	Contact CDC[1] for suspicious rash; EM and gel diffusion assays.
Typhus	3–4 days of fever, chills, severe headaches.	Maculopapules, petechiae, initial distribution centrifugal (trunk to extremities).	Endemic area, lice.	Complement fixation.
Varicella (chickenpox)	0–1 day of fever, anorexia, headache.	Rapid evolution of macules to papules, vesicles, crusts; all stages simultaneously present; lesions superficial, distribution centripetal.	Lesions on scalp and mucous membranes.	Specialized complement fixation and virus neutralization in cell culture. Fluorescent antibody test of smear of lesions.

[1]https://www.cdc.gov/smallpox/index.html

CSF, cerebrospinal fluid; EBV, Epstein-Barr virus; EM, electron microscopy; HHV, human herpesvirus; HSV, herpes simplex virus; Ig, immunoglobulin.

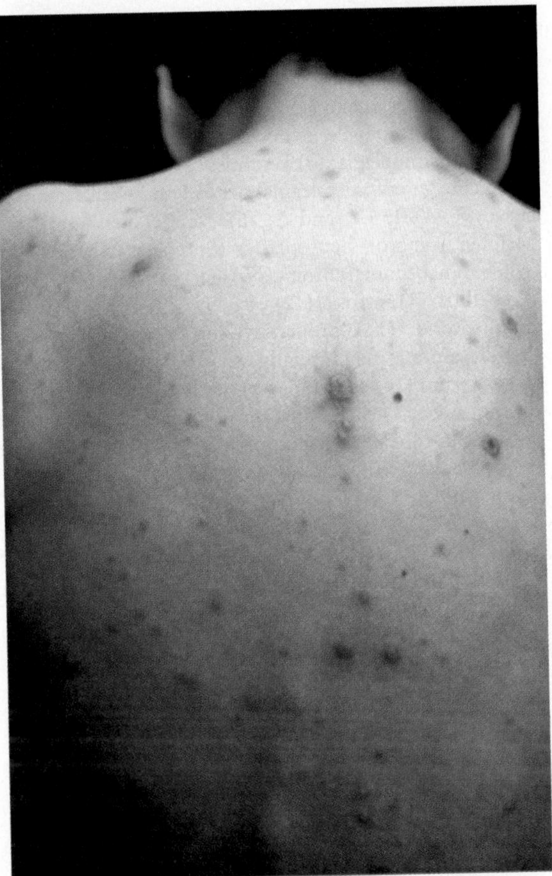

▲ **Figure 32–2.** Primary varicella (chickenpox) skin lesions. (Public Health Image Library, CDC.)

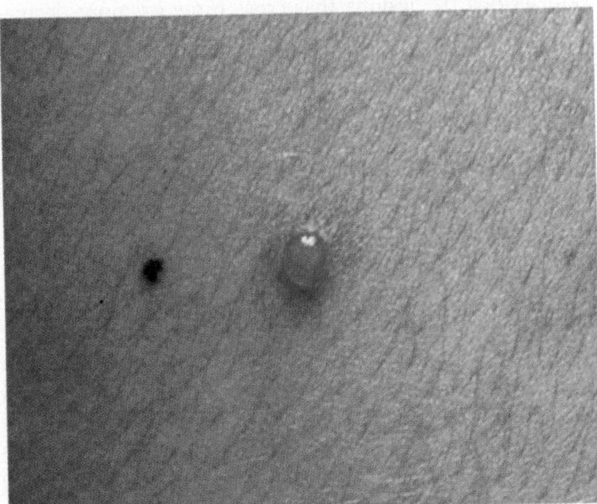

▲ **Figure 32–3.** Chickenpox (varicella) with classic "dew drop on rose petal" appearance. (Reproduced with permission from Richard P. Usatine, MD, in Usatine RP, Smith MA, Mayeaux EJ Jr, Chumley H. *The Color Atlas of Family Medicine*, 2nd ed. McGraw-Hill, 2013.)

the eruption are usually present simultaneously. The crusts slough in 7–14 days. The vesicles and pustules are superficial and elliptical, with slightly serrated borders. Pitted scars are frequent. Although the disease is often mild, complications (such as secondary bacterial infection, pneumonitis, and encephalitis) occur in about 1% of cases and often lead to hospitalization.

Varicella is more severe in older patients and immunocompromised persons. In the latter, atypical presentations, including widespread dissemination in the absence of skin lesions, are often described. After the primary infection, the virus remains dormant in cranial nerve sensory ganglia and spinal dorsal root ganglia. *Latent VZV will reactivate as herpes zoster in about 30% of persons.* The risk of Guillain-Barré syndrome is somewhat higher for at least 2 months after an acute herpes zoster attack.

2. Laboratory findings—Diagnosis is usually made clinically, with confirmation by direct immunofluorescent antibody staining or PCR of scrapings from lesions, both of which are more sensitive than culture. Multinucleated giant cells are usually apparent on a Tzanck smear of material from the vesicle base. Leukopenia and subclinical transaminase elevation are often present, and thrombocytopenia occasionally occurs. Although elevation of varicella IgM is occasionally used to diagnose a primary VZV infection, the assay has poor performance and is generally not recommended. The exception is that varicella antibody tested in the CSF is useful for identifying CNS involvement if VZV vasculopathy is suspected but CSF VZV DNA PCR is negative. A varicella skin test and interferon-gamma enzyme-linked immunospot (ELISPOT) can screen for VZV susceptibility.

B. Herpes Zoster

Herpes zoster ("shingles") usually occurs among adults, but cases are reported among infants and children. Shingles incidence rises markedly with age because of immunosenescence and loss of specific immunity to VZV, with rates of 8 to 12 per 1000 person-years in individuals older than 80 years. Skin lesions typically develop into clusters of vesicles over 3–5 days and can be painful or pruritic. Superficial sensory symptoms such as pain are often severe and commonly *precede* the appearance of rash by several days. Lesions follow a dermatomal distribution, with thoracic and lumbar roots being the most common. In most cases, a single unilateral dermatome is involved, but occasionally, neighboring and distant areas are involved. If lesions cover three or more dermatomes, disease is considered to be disseminated. Lesions eventually dry and crust over; in untreated immunocompetent individuals they take 2–4 weeks to heal and can leave hyperpigmented macular scars. Lesions on the tip of the nose, inner corner of the eye, and root and side of the nose **(Hutchinson sign)** indicate involvement of the trigeminal nerve **(herpes zoster ophthalmicus).** Facial palsy and lesions of the external ear with or without tympanic membrane involvement, vertigo and tinnitus, or deafness signify geniculate ganglion involvement **(Ramsay Hunt syndrome** or **herpes zoster oticus).** Shingles is a particularly common and serious complication among immunosuppressed patients.

Complications

A. Varicella

Secondary bacterial skin superinfections, particularly with group A *Streptococcus* and *Staphylococcus aureus*, are the most common complications. Cellulitis, erysipelas, and scarlet fever are described. Bullous impetigo and necrotizing fasciitis are less often seen. Other associations with varicella include epiglottitis, necrotizing pneumonia, osteomyelitis, septic arthritis, epidural abscess, meningitis, endocarditis, pancreatitis, giant cell arteritis, IBD, and purpura fulminans. Toxic shock syndrome can also develop.

Interstitial VZV pneumonia is more common in adults (especially cigarette smokers, people living with HIV, and pregnant women) and may result in acute respiratory distress syndrome (ARDS). After healing, numerous densely calcified lesions are seen throughout the lung fields on chest radiographs.

Historically, neurologic complications developed in about 1 in 2000 children. Cerebellar ataxia occurs at a frequency of 1:4000 in the young. A limited course and complete recovery are the rule. Encephalitis is similarly infrequent, occurs mostly in adults, and is characterized by delirium, seizures, and focal neurologic signs. The rates for both mortality and long-term neurologic sequelae are about 10%. Ischemic strokes in the wake of acute VZV infection present at a mean of 4 months after rashes and may be due to an associated vasculitis. Multifocal encephalitis (described without a rash in solid organ transplant recipients), ventriculitis, myeloradiculitis, arterial aneurysm formation, Ramsay Hunt syndrome, an optic neuritis (with zoster ophthalmicus), and arteritis are also described in immunosuppressed individuals, especially those living with HIV. When seizures develop in immunosuppressed patients, especially those taking corticosteroids, disseminated zoster should be considered.

Clinical hepatitis is uncommon and mostly presents in the immunosuppressed patient but can be fulminant and fatal. **Reye syndrome** (fatty liver with encephalopathy) also complicates varicella (and other viral infections, especially influenza B virus), usually in childhood, and is associated with aspirin therapy (see Influenza, below).

When contracted during the first or second trimesters of pregnancy, varicella carries a miniscule risk of congenital malformations, including cicatricial lesions of an extremity, growth retardation, microphthalmia, cataracts, chorioretinitis, deafness, and cerebrocortical atrophy. If varicella develops around the time of delivery, the newborn is at risk for disseminated disease. VZV is a greater risk to the pregnant mother.

B. Herpes Zoster

Postherpetic neuralgia occurs in 10–13% of patients who have herpes zoster and are older than 60 years. The pain can be prolonged and debilitating. Risk factors for postherpetic neuralgia include advanced age, female sex, the presence of a prodrome, and severity of rash or pain but not family history.

Other complications include the following: (1) bacterial skin superinfections; (2) herpes zoster ophthalmicus, which occurs with involvement of the trigeminal nerve, is a *sight-threatening complication* (especially when it involves the iris), and is a marker for vasculopathic stroke over the ensuing year (Hutchinson sign is a marker of ocular involvement in people living with HIV); (3) rarely, unilateral ophthalmoplegia; (4) keratitis; (5) involvement of the geniculate ganglion of cranial nerve VII as well as cranial nerves V, VIII, IX, and X; (6) aseptic meningitis; (7) peripheral motor neuropathy; (8) transverse myelitis, which can become chronic; (9) encephalitis; (10) acute cerebellitis; (11) stroke; (12) vasculopathy; (13) acute retinal necrosis; (14) progressive outer retinal necrosis (largely among people living with HIV); (15) temporal arteritis; and (16) sacral meningoradiculitis (Elsberg syndrome). Visceral dissemination in immunocompromised patients is rare and fatal over half the time. VZV is a major cause of Bell palsy in patients who are HSV seronegative.

Diagnosis of neurologic complications requires the detection of VZV DNA in CSF or the detection of VZV DNA in tissue. **Zoster sine herpete** (pain without rash) can also be associated with most of the above complications. A molecular assays can help distinguish HSV from VZV for patients with keratitis.

Varicella-zoster increases maternal but not fetal morbidity, and pregnant women should be advised to avoid exposure to VZV.

Treatment

A. General Measures

In general, patients with varicella should be isolated until primary lesions have crusted. The skin is kept clean. Pruritus can be relieved with antihistamines, calamine lotion, and colloidal oatmeal baths. Fever can be treated with acetaminophen (*not* aspirin). Fingernails can be closely cropped to avoid skin excoriation and infection. Hospitalized individuals with open, disseminated herpes zoster skin lesions (ie, lesions that cross three or more dermatomes) should be placed on both contact and airborne isolation until lesions crust over.

B. Antiviral Therapy

1. Varicella—Uncomplicated disease in otherwise healthy children and adolescents does not require antiviral therapy. Acyclovir, 20 mg/kg (up to 800 mg per dose) orally four times daily for 5–7 days, should be given within the first 24 hours after the onset of varicella rash and should be considered for patients older than 12 years, secondary household contacts (disease tends to be more severe in secondary cases), patients with chronic cutaneous and cardiopulmonary diseases, and children receiving long-term therapy with salicylates (to decrease the risk of Reye syndrome). *Acyclovir hastens defervescence and healing of lesions but does not impact complication rates.* Famciclovir is not approved for anyone under 18 years of age. Valacyclovir can be given between ages 2 and 18 at a dose of 20 mg/kg (max 1 g) three times daily for 5 days. NSAID use in children with varicella infection appears to be associated with an increase in bacterial infections.

In immunocompromised patients, in pregnant women during the third trimester, and in patients with extracutaneous disease (encephalitis, pneumonitis), antiviral therapy with high-dose acyclovir (30 mg/kg/day in three divided doses intravenously for at least 7 days, 10 days for encephalitis) should be started once the diagnosis is suspected. The oral alternative is 800 mg four times daily for 5–10 days, based on disease state treated. Corticosteroids may be useful in the presence of pneumonia. Prolonged prophylactic acyclovir is important to prevent VZV reactivation in profoundly immunosuppressed patients. Adjuvant treatment with VSV-specific immunoglobulins for patients with pneumonia is advocated by some experts.

2. Herpes zoster—For uncomplicated herpes zoster, valacyclovir or famciclovir is preferable to acyclovir due to dosing convenience and higher drug levels in the body (Table 32–1). *Therapy should start within the first 72 hours of the onset of the lesions* and be continued for 7 days or until the lesions crust over. *Antiviral therapy reduces the duration of herpetic lesions and associated episodes of acute pain but does not decrease the risk of postherpetic neuralgia.* Corticosteroids (a tapering course starting at 60 mg/day, for 2–3 weeks) are safe in immunocompetent patients and may be useful in the acute management of disease to hasten the resolution of acute lesions. Corticosteroids do *not* prevent the development of postherpetic neuralgia.

Intravenous acyclovir is used for extradermatomal complications of zoster. Adjunctive therapy may be considered in retinal disease (eg, vitreal foscarnet infections) and acute herpes zoster (eg, sorivudine, a topical antiviral). In cases of prolonged or repeated acyclovir use, immunosuppressed patients may require a switch to intravenous foscarnet due to the development of acyclovir-resistant VZV infections. VZV associated with the Ramsay Hunt syndrome is more resistant to antiviral therapy.

C. Treatment of Postherpetic Neuralgia

Once established, postherpetic neuralgia is difficult to treat, and less than half of patients achieve adequate pain relief. This condition may respond to neuropathic pain agents such as gabapentin or lidocaine patches. Tricyclic antidepressants and capsaicin cream are also widely used and effective; use of opioids in managing neuropathic pain is controversial and based on limited evidence, and their long-term use should be avoided. The epidural injection of corticosteroids and local anesthetics appears to modestly reduce herpetic pain at 1 month but, as with oral corticosteroids, is not effective for prevention of long-term postherpetic neuralgia. Transcutaneous electrical nerve stimulation or pulsed radiofrequency is reportedly successful. Gabapentin appears to show efficacy as a preventive medication in reducing the risk of postherpetic neuralgia in patients with diabetes and neuropathy.

Prognosis

The total duration of varicella from onset of symptoms to disappearance of crusts rarely exceeds 2 weeks. Fatalities are rare except in immunosuppressed patients.

Herpes zoster resolves in 2–6 weeks. Antibodies persist longer and at higher levels than with primary varicella. Eye involvement with herpes zoster necessitates periodic future examinations.

Prevention

Health care workers should be screened for varicella and vaccinated if seronegative. Patients with active varicella or herpes zoster are promptly separated from seronegative patients. For patients with varicella, airborne and contact isolation is recommended, whereas for those with zoster, contact precautions are sufficient. For immunosuppressed patients with zoster, precautions should be the same as if the patient had varicella. Exposed serosusceptible patients should be placed in isolation and exposed serosusceptible employees should stay away from work for 8–21 days after exposure. Health care workers with zoster should receive antiviral agents during the first 72 hours of disease and withdraw from work until lesions are crusted. The need for postexposure prophylaxis should be assessed.

A. Varicella

1. Vaccination—Universal childhood vaccination against varicella is effective. The varicella vaccine is *live and attenuated*, safe, and over 98.1% effective when given after 13 months of age. A single antigen live attenuated vaccine (VARIVAX, VARILRIX) or a quadrivalent measles, mumps, rubella, and varicella (MMRV) vaccine (ProQuad) is available (the combination is immunogenic). The first dose of the single antigen vaccine should be administered at 12–18 months of age and the second at 4–6 years. Alternatively, the MMRV vaccine can be given as a first dose at 12–15 months of age and the second dose before elementary school entry. *Aspirin should be avoided for at least 6 weeks after vaccination because of the risk of Reye syndrome.* The single antigen vaccine is safe and well tolerated, but the quadrivalent MMRV vaccine is associated with a small risk of febrile seizures 5–12 days after vaccination among infants aged 12–23 months. Because of this risk, the CDC recommends using separate varicella and measles, mumps, and rubella (MMR) vaccines for the first dose in children younger than 48 months old. Rashes, when secondary to the varicella vaccine, appear 15–42 days after vaccination. Rare cases of keratitis are associated with zoster and varicella vaccines.

For serosusceptible individuals older than 13 years, two doses of varicella vaccine (single antigen) administered 4–8 weeks apart are recommended. For those who received a single dose in the past, a *catch-up second dose* is advised, especially in the epidemic setting (where it is effective when it can be given during the first 5 days postexposure). Household contacts of immunocompromised patients should adhere to these recommendations. Susceptible pregnant women (who should not be vaccinated with live varicella or zoster vaccines during pregnancy) need to receive the first dose of single antigen vaccine before discharge after delivery and the second dose 4–8 weeks later. The Advisory Committee on Immunization Practices (ACIP) recommends administration of the single-agent varicella vaccine as two doses 3 months apart to children living with HIV aged 12 months or older with CD4 cell percentage greater than 15% and adolescents and adults with CD4 cell counts 200/mcL or higher.

The vaccine may also be given to patients with impaired humoral immunity, to patients receiving corticosteroids, to pediatric oncology patients receiving chemotherapy, and to patients with juvenile rheumatoid arthritis who receive methotrexate. Patients receiving high doses of corticosteroids for over 2 weeks may be vaccinated a month after discontinuation of the therapy. Patients with leukemia, lymphoma, or other malignancies whose disease is in remission and who have not undergone chemotherapy for at least 3 months may be vaccinated. Kidney and liver transplant patients should be vaccinated if they are susceptible to varicella.

The incidence of varicella in the United States is significantly reduced with the varicella vaccine. Although uncommon, the varicella vaccine, like any of the live varicella-zoster vaccines, has the potential to reactivate and cause clinical disease. It is thought that vaccination against varicella provides *less* protection against future zoster than does natural varicella infection. The incidence of varicella-associated group A streptococcal infection and varicella neurologic complications are both diminished with the advent of varicella vaccination.

The FDA no longer maintains a registry for exposed pregnant women because of the low rate of such incidents and the general safety of varicella vaccines. Incidents can be reported to Merck (877-888-4231) or through the Vaccine Adverse Events Registry System Vaccine (https://vaers.hhs.gov/index).

2. Postexposure—Postexposure vaccination is recommended for unvaccinated persons without other evidence of immunity. **Varicella-zoster immune globulin** available in the United States only as VariZIG should be considered for susceptible exposed patients (for up to 10 days after exposure but as soon as feasible) who should not receive the vaccine, including immunosuppressed patients, neonates from mothers with varicella around the time of delivery, exposed premature infants born from serosusceptible mothers at greater than 28 weeks' gestation, and neonates born at less than 28 weeks' gestation regardless of maternal serostatus. Varicella and zoster vaccines are not recommended for pregnant women.

No controlled studies have evaluated the use of acyclovir in this setting. VariZIG is given by intramuscular injection in a dosage of 125 IU/10 kg, to a maximum of 625 IU with a weight-based (2-kg cutoff) minimum dose of 62.5 or 125 IU), with a repeat identical dose in 3 weeks if a high-risk patient remains exposed. VariZIG has no place in therapy of established disease; however, it reduces severity of varicella in high-risk children or adults (ie, those with impaired immunity and infants exposed peripartum) if given within 4 days of exposure. Varicella vaccination should be delayed at least 5 months after VariZIG administration. If VariZIG is not available, standard pooled intravenous immunoglobulin (IVIG) (400 mg/kg given in one dose) can be given. Acyclovir (40–80 mg/kg) for 5 days or the varicella vaccine (if not contraindicated) can also be given as postexposure prophylaxis within 3 days of exposure. Either of these options offers an efficacy of 70–85% compared with 90% efficacy for VariZIG.

Further information may be obtained by calling the CDC's Immunization Information Hotline (1-800-232-4636).

B. Herpes Zoster

Shingrix, HZ/su (GlaxoSmithKline Biologics), an adjuvanted recombinant subunit vaccine, is approved by the FDA for VZV, and is recommended for individuals 50 years of age and older. *Shingrix is preferred over the older live attenuated VZV vaccine* (ZOSTAVAX, see below). Shingrix is particularly effective in reducing the incidence of herpes zoster infection and postherpetic neuralgia in adults 70 years of age and older; immunosenescence to the vaccine does not appear to occur in older patients; in fact, strong, persistent immune responses are seen more than 7 years after initial vaccination. It can also be used in immunosuppressed patients. Two doses of the vaccine given 2 months apart had 97% efficacy in preventing herpes zoster. Shingrix also is safe in people living with HIV and with immune restoration (typically CD4 cell counts above 50/mcL), recipients of autologous stem cell transplants, and adults with autoimmune disease taking immunosuppressive therapy.

The older live attenuated VZV vaccine, ZOSTAVAX (19,400 plaque forming units [pfu] of Oka/Merck strain) contains at least 14 times the concentration of varicella virus found in VARIVAX. ZOSTAVAX has been recommended for persons 60 years and older because it reduces the incidence of herpes zoster by 33–55% in the first 3 years after vaccination and reduces the incidence of postherpetic neuralgia by 55–67%. The efficacy of ZOSTAVAX wanes over time, from 69% in the first year after vaccination to 45% by the third year. ZOSTAVAX is safe but only moderately immunogenic among people living with HIV and with a CD4 cell count of at least 200/mcL. Decreased efficacy occurs in patients older than 70, and this vaccine should not be given to immunosuppressed persons. Nonetheless, hematologic oncology patients taking anti-CD20 monoclonal antibodies may be successfully vaccinated with ZOSTAVAX. An increased risk of herpes zoster during a 6-week interval following vaccination is reported among patients taking immunosuppressant medications. This vaccine provides protection for about 3 years.

Even if the person has had a prior episode of herpes zoster, either of the two zoster vaccines has efficacy and can be administered. No specific recommendations exist regarding how long to wait between a zoster outbreak and administering the vaccine; the CDC recommends waiting at least until the outbreak has resolved. Concurrent administration of the adjuvanted recombinant subunit vaccine or the live attenuated VZV vaccine with pneumococcal vaccine is safe. This policy is based on CDC analysis of data, although some experts including original statements of the manufacturer of ZOSTAVAX (Merck & Co.) contend that the two vaccines should be separated by 4 weeks. If a varicella vaccine is mistakenly administered to an adult instead of the adjuvanted recombinant subunit vaccine or the live attenuated zoster vaccine, the dose should be considered invalid, and the patient should be administered a dose of zoster vaccine at the same visit. The zoster vaccine cannot be used in children in place of varicella vaccine; if the vaccine is accidentally given to a child, the event should be reported to the CDC.

Boutry C et al. The adjuvanted recombinant zoster vaccine confers long-term protection against herpes zoster: interim results of an extension study of the pivotal phase iii clinical trials (ZOE-50 and ZOE-70). Clin Infect Dis. 2022;74:1459. [PMID: 34283213]

Cohen E. Herpes zoster and postherpetic neuralgia. Clin Infect Dis. 2021;73:e3218. [PMID: 32829389]

Ghanavatian S et al. Premedication with gabapentin significantly reduces the risk of postherpetic neuralgia in patients with neuropathy. Mayo Clin Proc. 2019;94:484. [PMID: 30718068]

Tseng HF et al. The epidemiology of herpes zoster in immunocompetent, unvaccinated adults ≥50 years old: incidence, complications, hospitalization, mortality, and recurrence. J Infect Dis. 2020;222:798. [PMID: 31830250]

Wu CY et al. Efficacy of pulsed radiofrequency in herpetic neuralgia: a meta-analysis of randomized controlled trials. Clin J Pain. 2020;36:887. [PMID: 32701526]

3. Epstein-Barr Virus & Infectious Mononucleosis

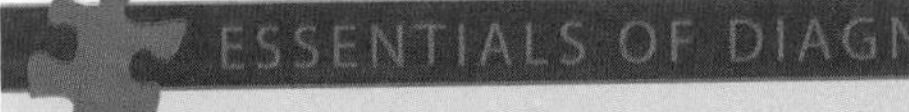

- Malaise, fever, and (exudative) sore throat.
- Palatal petechiae, lymphadenopathy, splenomegaly; occasionally, a maculopapular rash.
- Positive heterophile agglutination test (Monospot).
- Atypical large lymphocytes in blood smear; lymphocytosis.
- Complications: hepatitis, myocarditis, neuropathy, encephalitis, airway obstruction from adenitis, hemolytic anemia, thrombocytopenia.

General Considerations

Epstein-Barr virus (EBV, or human herpes virus-4 [HHV-4]) is one of the most ubiquitous human viruses, infecting more than 95% of the adult population worldwide and persisting for the lifetime of the host. **Infectious mononucleosis** is a common manifestation of EBV and may occur at any age. In the United States the incidence of EBV infection is declining, although prevalence of EBV remains high for those aged 12–19 years. In the developing world, infectious mononucleosis occurs at younger ages and tends to be less symptomatic. Rare cases in older adults occur usually without the full symptomatology. EBV is largely transmitted by saliva but can also be recovered from genital secretions. Saliva may remain infectious during convalescence, for 6 months or longer after symptom onset. The incubation period lasts several weeks (30–50 days). Patients with immunodeficiency disorders are at risk for the full spectrum of EBV-associated disorders.

Clinical Findings

A. Symptoms and Signs

Fever, exudative sore throat, fatigue, malaise, anorexia, and myalgia typically occur in the early phase of the illness. Physical findings include lymphadenopathy (discrete, nonsuppurative, slightly painful, especially along the posterior cervical chain), transient upper lid edema (**Hoagland sign**), and splenomegaly (in up to 50% of patients and sometimes massive). A maculopapular or occasionally petechial rash occurs in less than 15% of patients unless ampicillin is given. Conjunctival hemorrhage, exudative pharyngitis, uvular edema, tonsillitis, or gingivitis may occur and soft palatal petechiae may be noted.

Other manifestations include hepatitis, interstitial pneumonitis (sometimes with pleural involvement), cholestasis, gastritis, kidney disease (mostly interstitial nephritis), epiglottitis, and nervous system involvement in 1–5% (mononeuropathies and occasionally aseptic meningitis, encephalitis, cerebellitis, peripheral and optic neuritis, transverse myelitis, or Guillain-Barré syndrome). Vaginal ulcers are rare but may be present. Airway obstruction from lymph node enlargement can occur. Complications of acute disease are more common among older adults.

B. Laboratory Findings

An initial phase of granulocytopenia is followed within 1 week by lymphocytic leukocytosis (greater than 50% of all leukocytes) with atypical lymphocytes (larger than normal mature lymphocytes, staining more darkly, and showing vacuolated, foamy cytoplasm and dark nuclear chromatin) comprising more than 10% of the leukocyte count. Hemolytic anemia, with antibodies, occurs occasionally as does thrombocytopenia (at times marked and life-threatening).

Diagnosis is made based on characteristic manifestations and serologic evidence of infection (the **heterophile sheep cell agglutination [HA] antibody tests** or the correlated **mononucleosis spot test [Monospot]**). These tests usually become positive within 4 weeks after onset of illness and are specific but often not sensitive in early illness. Heterophile antibodies may be absent in young children and in as many as 20% of adults. During acute illness, immunoglobulin M (IgM) antibody to EB virus capsid antigen (VCA) rises and falls, and immunoglobulin G (IgG) antibody to VCA rises and persists for life. Antibodies (IgG) to EBV nuclear antigen (EBNA) appear after 4 weeks of onset and also persist. Absence of IgG and IgM VCA or the presence of IgG EBNA should make one reconsider the diagnosis of acute EBV infection.

Differential Diagnosis

CMV infection, toxoplasmosis, acute HIV infection, secondary syphilis, HHV-6 infection, rubella, and drug hypersensitivity reactions may be indistinguishable from infectious mononucleosis due to EBV, but exudative pharyngitis is usually absent and the heterophile antibody tests are negative. With acute HIV infection, rash and mucocutaneous ulceration are common but atypical lymphocytosis is much less common. Heterophile-negative infectious mononucleosis with nonsignificant lymphocytosis (especially if rash or mucocutaneous ulcers are present) should prompt investigation for acute HIV infection. CMV, toxoplasmosis, and, on occasion, EBV can cause heterophile-negative infectious mononucleosis with atypical lymphocytosis. *Mycoplasma* infection may also present as pharyngitis, though lower respiratory symptoms usually predominate. A hypersensitivity syndrome induced by carbamazepine or phenytoin may mimic infectious mononucleosis.

The differential diagnosis of acute exudative pharyngitis includes gonococcal and streptococcal infections, and infections with adenovirus and herpes simplex. Head and neck soft tissue infections (pharyngeal and tonsillar abscesses) may occasionally be mistaken as the lymphadenopathy of mononucleosis.

Complications

Secondary bacterial pharyngitis can occur and is often streptococcal. Splenic rupture (0.5–1%) is a rare but dramatic complication, and a history of preceding trauma can be elicited in 50% of the cases. Acalculous cholecystitis, fulminant hepatitis with massive necrosis, pericarditis, and myocarditis are also infrequent complications of acute EBV infection. Rarely, severe chronic EBV-associated disorder causes chronic fatigue, fevers, multiorgan failure, chronic pneumonia, and lymphoproliferative diseases.

Treatment

A. General Measures

Over 95% of patients with acute EBV-associated infectious mononucleosis recover without specific antiviral therapy. Treatment is symptomatic with NSAIDs or acetaminophen and warm saline throat irrigations or gargles three or four times daily. Acyclovir decreases viral shedding but shows no clinical benefit. Corticosteroid therapy, although widespread, is *not* recommended in uncomplicated cases; its use is reserved for impending airway obstruction from enlarged lymph nodes, hemolytic anemia, and severe thrombocytopenia. The value of corticosteroid therapy in impending splenic rupture, pericarditis, myocarditis, and nervous system involvement is less well established. If a throat culture grows beta-hemolytic streptococci, a 10-day course of penicillin or azithromycin is indicated. Ampicillin and amoxicillin are avoided because of the frequent association with rash (90%), although one study indicates that the incidence of drug hypersensitivity is much lower than previously reported.

B. Treatment of Complications

Hepatitis, myocarditis, and encephalitis are treated symptomatically. Rupture of the spleen requires splenectomy and is most often caused by deep palpation of the spleen or vigorous activity. *Patients should avoid contact or collision sports for at least 4 weeks to decrease the risk of splenic rupture (even if splenomegaly is not detected by physical examination, which can be insensitive).*

Prognosis & Prevention

In uncomplicated cases, fever disappears in 10 days and lymphadenopathy and splenomegaly in 4 weeks. The debility sometimes lingers for 2–3 months.

Death is uncommon and is usually due to splenic rupture, hypersplenic phenomena (severe hemolytic anemia, thrombocytopenic purpura), or encephalitis.

4. Other EBV-Associated Conditions

EBV is associated with certain malignancies, including several types of lymphomas. EBV viral antigens are found in more than 90% of patients with endemic (African) Burkitt lymphoma and nasopharyngeal carcinoma. Risk factors for Burkitt lymphoma include a history of malaria (which may decrease resistance to EBV infection), while risk factors for nasopharyngeal carcinoma include long-term heavy cigarette smoking and seropositive EBV serologies (VCA and deoxyribonuclease [Dnase]). VCA-IgA in peripheral blood is a sensitive and specific predictor for nasopharyngeal carcinoma in an endemic area. Among Hodgkin lymphoma patients, EBV seropositivity is common when the disease is found in the developing world or is associated with HIV infection, when pathologic specimens show mixed cellularity, and when patients are younger than 10 years or older than 45 years at onset of the lymphoma. EBV-seropositive patients have a worse prognosis for early stages of Hodgkin lymphoma.

Age is a major determinant of the type of tumor associated with EBV. T- and NK-cell lymphomas caused by chronic active EBV infections are more frequent in childhood, while peripheral T-cell lymphomas and diffuse large B-cell lymphomas are more common in older patients due to waning immunity. EBV is also associated with leiomyomas in children with AIDS and with nasal T-cell lymphomas.

PCR for EBV DNA is useful in the evaluation of malignancies associated with EBV. For instance, detection of EBV DNA in CSF shows a sensitivity of 90% and specificity of nearly 100% for the diagnosis of primary CNS lymphoma in patients with AIDS.

Many therapies, including traditional chemotherapies as well as immunotherapies, have been trialed or are under study for EBV-associated lymphomas, though none yet have been clearly successful.

Both primary disseminated and reactivated EBV infections are a concern in individuals with compromised cellular immunity, including those post-organ transplantation. Chronic EBV infection is associated with aberrant cellular immunity (a low frequency of EBV-specific $CD8^+$ T cells), an X-linked lymphoproliferative syndrome (Duncan disease), lymphomatoid granulomatosis, and a fatal T-cell lymphoproliferative disorder in children. Posttransplant EBV infection/reactivation and sequelae are particularly concerning, including **posttransplant lymphoproliferative disorders (PTLD)** in patients who are donor organ EBV-positive and recipient negative. The main risk factor for both early PTLD (less than 1-year posttransplantation) and late PTLD (more than 1 year after transplantation) remains controversial. PTLD is associated with EBV particularly in children. EBV serostatus, however, is *not* associated with overall survival among patients with PTLD. CD30 and EBV viral load monitoring are prognostic markers for EBV-associated PTLD in high-risk patients. The role of antiviral prophylaxis for preventing PTLD remains unclear. The 2019 guidelines by the American Society of Transplantation Infectious Disease Community of Practice emphasize the importance of reduction of iatrogenic immunosuppression for PTLD but also note that rituximab and cytotoxic chemotherapy are useful for EBV-positive, CD20-positive lymphoproliferative states.

When to Admit

Presence of severe complications of EBV disease including the following:

- Acute meningitis, encephalitis, or Guillain-Barré syndrome.
- Severe thrombocytopenia; significant hemolysis.
- Potential splenic rupture.
- Airway obstruction from severe adenitis.
- Pericarditis.
- Abdominal findings mimicking an acute abdomen.

Kerr JR. Epstein-Barr virus (EBV) reactivation and therapeutic inhibitors. J Clin Pathol. 2019;72:651. [PMID: 31315893]

Stocker N et al. Pre-emptive rituximab treatment for Epstein-Barr virus reactivation after allogeneic hematopoietic stem cell transplantation is a worthwhile strategy in high-risk recipients: a comparative study for immune recovery and clinical outcomes. Bone Marrow Transplant. 2020;55:586. [PMID: 31562397]

Yoon SE et al. A phase II study of ibrutinib in combination with rituximab-cyclophosphamide-doxorubicin hydrochloride-vincristine sulfate-prednisone therapy in Epstein-Barr virus-positive, diffuse large B cell lymphoma (54179060LYM2003: IVORY study): results of the final analysis. Ann Hematol. 2020;99:1283. [PMID: 32333154]

5. Cytomegalovirus Disease

ESSENTIALS OF DIAGNOSIS

- Mononucleosis-like syndrome.
- Frequent pathogen seen in populations with compromised cellular immunity, such as transplant populations.
- Diverse clinical syndromes in HIV (retinitis, esophagitis, pneumonia, encephalitis).
- Most important infectious cause of congenital abnormalities.

General Considerations

Most CMV infections are asymptomatic. After primary infection, the virus remains latent in most body cells. Seroprevalence in adults of high-income countries is about 60–80% but is higher in low- and middle-income countries. The virus can be isolated from a variety of tissues under nonpathogenic conditions. Transmission occurs through sexual contact, breastfeeding, blood products, or transplantation; it may also occur person to person (eg, day care centers) or be congenital. Serious disease occurs primarily in immunocompromised persons, including those post-organ transplant, with AIDS, and with IBD.

Three recognizable clinical syndromes exist: (1) perinatal disease and CMV inclusion disease, (2) diseases in immunocompetent persons, and (3) diseases in immunocompromised persons. *Congenital CMV infection is the most common congenital infection in high-income countries* (about 0.6% of live births, with higher rates in underdeveloped areas and among lower socioeconomic groups). Transmission is much higher from mothers with primary disease than those with reactivation (40% versus 0.2–1.8%). About 10% of infected newborns will be symptomatic with CMV inclusion disease.

In immunocompetent persons, acute CMV infection is the most common cause of the mononucleosis-like syndrome with negative heterophile antibodies. In critically ill immunocompetent adults, CMV reactivation is associated with prolonged hospitalization and death.

CMV is usually disseminated in persons with compromised cellular immunity, leading to a number of different clinical manifestations, described below. Solid organ and bone marrow transplant patients are at highest risk for disease from CMV reactivation for a year after allograft transplantation (but especially during the first 100 days posttransplantation) and in particular when graft-versus-host disease is present or when the donor is CMV-seropositive and the recipient is seronegative. Depending on the serostatus of the donor and recipient, disease may present as primary infection or reactivation. The risk of CMV disease is proportionate to the degree of immunosuppression and manifestations may differ by the cause. CMV may contribute to transplanted organ dysfunction, which often mimics organ rejection.

Clinical Findings

A. Symptoms and Signs

1. Perinatal disease and CMV inclusion disease—CMV inclusion disease in infected newborns is characterized by hepatitis, thrombocytopenia, microcephaly, periventricular CNS calcifications, mental retardation, and motor disability. Hearing loss develops in more than 50% of infants who are symptomatic at birth, making CMV a leading cause of pediatric hearing loss. Most infected neonates are asymptomatic, but neurologic deficits may ensue later in life, including hearing loss in 15% and cognitive impairment in 10–20%. Perinatal infection acquired through breastfeeding or blood products typically has a benign clinical course.

2. Disease in immunocompetent persons—Acute CMV infection is characterized by fever, malaise, myalgias, arthralgias, and splenomegaly. Unlike in EBV mononucleosis, exudative pharyngitis or cervical lymphadenopathies are uncommon, but cutaneous rashes (including the typical maculopapular rash after exposure to ampicillin) are common. The mean duration of symptoms is 7–8 weeks. Complications include mucosal GI damage, encephalitis, severe hepatitis, thrombocytopenia (on occasion, refractory), the Guillain-Barré syndrome, pericarditis, and myocarditis. The risk of Guillain-Barré syndrome developing after primary CMV infection is estimated to be 0.6–2.2 cases per 1000 primary infection, similar to that seen with *Campylobacter jejuni* infection. A mononucleosis-like syndrome due to CMV can also occur post splenectomy, often years later and associated with a protracted fever, marked lymphocytosis, and impaired anti-CMV IgM response.

3. Disease in immunocompromised persons—Distinguishing between CMV *infection* (with evidence of CMV replication) and CMV *disease* (evidence for systemic symptoms or organ invasion by pathologic diagnosis) is important. In addition to people living with HIV, those who have undergone transplantation (solid organ or hematopoietic stem cell) show a wide spectrum of disease including ocular, GI (eg, colitis, esophagitis, and acute cholecystitis), kidney, and CNS disease, as outlined above. CMV viremia, assessed with "viral loads," serves as an important predictor of disease presence.

A. CMV RETINITIS—A funduscopic examination reveals neovascular, proliferative lesions ("pizza-pie" retinopathy). Immune restoration with ART is associated with CMV vitritis and cystoid macular edema.

B. GI AND HEPATOBILIARY CMV—Esophagitis presents with odynophagia. Gastritis can occasionally cause bleeding, and small bowel disease may mimic IBD or may present as ulceration or perforation. Colonic CMV disease causes diarrhea, hematochezia, abdominal pain, fever, and weight loss and may mimic IBD. CMV hepatitis commonly complicates liver transplantation and appears to be increased in those with hepatitis B or hepatitis C viral infection.

C. RESPIRATORY CMV—CMV pneumonitis is characterized by cough, dyspnea, and relatively little sputum production. Concomitant infection with *Pneumocystis jirovecii* occurs among patients regardless of HIV status.

D. NEUROLOGIC CMV—Neurologic syndromes associated with CMV include polyradiculopathy, transverse myelitis, ventriculoencephalitis (suspected with ependymitis), and focal encephalitis. These manifestations are more prominent in patients with advanced AIDS in whom the encephalitis has a subacute onset.

B. Laboratory Findings

1. Mothers and newborns—Pregnant women should be tested for CMV viremia every 3 months if found to be seropositive during the first trimester. Congenital CMV disease is confirmed by presence of the virus in amniotic fluid or an IgM assay from fetal blood. Amniocentesis is less reliable before 21 weeks' gestation (due to inadequate fetal urinary development and release into the amniotic fluid), but amniocentesis is attendant with greater risk when performed after 21 weeks' gestation. PCR assays of dried blood samples from newborns, micro-ELISA, shell-vial culture, or culture of urine, saliva, or blood specimens obtained during the first 3 weeks of life are used to diagnose congenital CMV infection.

2. Immunocompetent persons—The acute mononucleosis-like syndrome is characterized by initial leukopenia; within 1 week, it is followed by absolute lymphocytosis with atypical lymphocytes. Abnormal liver biochemical tests are common in the first 2 weeks of the disease (often 2 weeks after the fever). Detection of CMV DNA, specific IgM, or a fourfold increase of specific IgG levels supports the diagnosis of acute infection.

3. Immunocompromised persons—CMV retinitis is diagnosed on the basis of the characteristic ophthalmoscopic findings. In people living with HIV, negative CMV serologies lower the possibility of the diagnosis but do *not* eliminate it. Cultures alone are of little use in diagnosing AIDS-related CMV infections since viral shedding of CMV is common. Detection of CMV by quantitative DNA PCR of the CSF should be used to diagnose CNS infection since cultures are not specific for disease.

Detection of CMV by quantitative DNA PCR is also used in posttransplant patients to guide both treatment and prevention and should be interpreted in the context of clinical and pathologic findings. CMV DNA levels are internationally standardized and have replaced conventional CMV antigenemia tests in many settings. The PCR is sensitive in predicting clinical disease. Serial PCR should be performed and compared using the same specimen type (ie, whole blood or plasma). To assist in the diagnosis of CMV pneumonia, bronchoalveolar lavage fluid can be tested to quantify CMV DNA levels with a viral load assay. Rapid shell-vial cultures detect early CMV antigens with fluorescent antibodies in 24–48 hours. Shell-vial cultures are more useful on bronchoalveolar lavage fluid than in routine blood monitoring. CMV colitis can occur in the absence of a detectable viremia. The CMV-specific ELISPOT assay is used in some centers to evaluate risk of CMV infection, control of CMV infection, or both in stem cell transplant recipients.

C. Imaging

The chest radiographic findings of CMV pneumonitis are consistent with interstitial pneumonia.

D. Biopsy

Tissue confirmation is especially useful in diagnosing CMV pneumonitis and CMV GI disease; the diagnosis of colonic CMV disease is made by mucosal biopsy showing characteristic CMV histopathologic findings of intranuclear ("owl's eye") and intracytoplasmic inclusions. In situations where histopathologic or immunohistochemical findings are not seen but CMV colitis is suspected, CMV DNA PCR can be used to identify additional cases.

Treatment & Prognosis

In immunocompetent persons, CMV infection is usually self-limited, and no specific antiviral therapy is needed. In contrast, in immunocompromised persons, treatment of CMV disease is necessary. All types of CMV disease in immunocompromised patients (particularly those with AIDS or after solid organ transplant) typically are treated initially with intravenous ganciclovir (recommended dose is 5 mg/kg every 12 hours, although this needs to be adjusted for kidney function) until two CMV PCRs 1 week apart are negative (usually 14–21 days). Oral valganciclovir (900 mg every 12 hours), which also needs to be adjusted for kidney function, is an acceptable alternative in patients with non–life-threatening disease.

Pneumonia due to CMV in hematopoietic stem cell transplant recipients is treated even more aggressively, with 5 mg/kg of ganciclovir intravenously every 12 hours for 21 days followed by 5 mg/kg daily for 3–4 weeks plus CMV immunoglobulin (500 mg/kg) or CMV immunoglobulin (150 mg/kg) twice per week for 2 weeks and then once weekly for an additional 4 weeks.

CMV infections in immunosuppressed patients require a reduction of immunosuppression when possible (especially for muromonab, azathioprine, or mycophenolate mofetil; data are less consistent for alemtuzumab used for graft-versus-host disease and not consistently associated with a risk of CMV disease). Secondary prophylaxis (ie, continuation of CMV therapy after initial treatment) is typically maintained until immune restoration (with two CD4 cell counts greater than 100/mcL present for at least 6 months in the setting of HIV infection). Prolonged prophylaxis may be necessary in other immunosuppressed patients, such as those receiving tumor necrosis factor (TNF) inhibitors.

Foscarnet and cidofovir are reserved for treatment of resistant infections. Filociclovir (also known as cyclopropavir or MBX-400) is a methylenecyclopropane nucleoside analog that completed phase 1 clinical trials for the treatment of CMV-related disease in transplant patients but has not been advanced further, as of early 2022. Other agents that may be useful in resistant CMV infections include CMV immunoglobulin, maribavir, leflunomide, sirolimus-based therapy, artesunate, and adoptive immunotherapy. Rare cases of post–hematopoietic stem cell transplant CMV meningoencephalitis have been treated successfully using adoptive T cells against CMV.

Treatment of CMV retinitis is discussed in Chapter 7.

Prevention

Two live vaccines (based on the fibroblast-adapted AD169 and Towne CMV strains, respectively) were shown to be safe and well tolerated in clinical trials. However, the Towne vaccine was not effective in preventing primary infection or viral reactivation in kidney transplant patients or in seronegative women. A vaccine candidate based on a replication-defective AD169 virus (named V160) has been shown to be safe and immunogenic in seronegative adults; phase 3 trials are underway.

A major source of CMV for pregnant women is their own young children, particularly those in childcare. These women can decrease their risk of contracting primary CMV just before pregnancy or during pregnancy by practicing hand hygiene after changing diapers and after contact with respiratory secretions; avoiding kissing young children on the face; and avoiding sharing utensils, food, and cleansing objects that have been in contact with children's secretions. CMV serologic tests are being evaluated to diagnose primary maternal CMV infection and are under review for use as a screening tool during the first trimester of pregnancy. Early antiviral therapy with valaciclovir is under study to prevent vertical transmission of CMV.

ART is effective in preventing CMV infections in people living with HIV. Primary prevention is best accomplished by good hand hygiene and use of barrier methods during sexual contacts with persons who are members of high-prevalence groups (ie, men who have sex with men, injection drug users, and those who have exposure to children in childcare settings).

The use of *leukocyte-depleted blood products* effectively reduces the incidence of CMV disease in patients who have undergone transplantation. Prophylactic and preemptive strategies (eg, antiviral agents only when antigen detection or PCR assays show evidence of active CMV replication) appear equally effective in preventing invasive disease and mortality after hematopoietic stem cell transplant. The appropriate management of transplant patients is based on the serostatus of the donor and the recipient. All effective anti-CMV therapies can serve as prophylactic agents for CMV-seropositive transplants or for CMV-seronegative recipients of CMV-positive organ transplants. Starting CMV prophylaxis 7–14 days after transplant may help reduce late-onset CMV end-organ disease. The typical dose for valganciclovir prophylaxis is 450 mg orally twice daily, although a prospective trial in kidney transplant recipients indicated that prophylaxis with low-dose valganciclovir (450 mg/day, three times a week for 6 months) seemed to be effective. Acyclovir may also be used. Letermovir is useful in prophylaxis against CMV infections in adult allogenic hematopoietic stem cell transplant recipients. It is given as 480 mg orally daily with dose adjustments for cyclosporine administration and for advanced kidney dysfunction (less than a creatinine clearance of 10 mL/minute). Major side effects reported to date include cough, diarrhea, headache, nausea, stomach pain, weakness, and vomiting. Recommended duration of CMV prophylaxis in posttransplant patients and in other immunocompromised patients varies by the type of transplant.

CMV immune globulin may also be useful in reducing the incidence of bronchiolitis obliterans in the bone marrow transplant population and is used in some centers as part of the prophylaxis in kidney, liver, and lung transplantation patients. CMV immune globulin as prophylaxis is not recommended in hematopoietic stem cell transplant recipients.

When to Refer

- People with AIDS with retinitis, esophagitis, colitis, hepatobiliary disease, or encephalitis.
- Organ and hematopoietic stem cell transplants with suspected reactivation CMV.

When to Admit

- Escalating CMV viral load at the onset of illness.
- Risk of colonic perforation.
- Evaluation of unexplained, advancing encephalopathy.
- Initiation of treatment with intravenous anti-CMV agents.

Chemaly AF et al. Cytomegalovirus (CMV) cell-mediated immunity and CMV infection after allogeneic hematopoietic cell transplantation: The REACT Study. Clin Infect Dis. 2020;71:2365. [PMID: 32076709]

Hussein ITM et al. The discovery and development of filociclovir for the prevention and treatment of human cytomegalovirus-related disease. Antiviral Res. 2020;176:104710. [PMID: 31940473]

Seo E et al. Immunologic monitoring of cytomegalovirus (CMV) enzyme-linked immune absorbent spot (ELISPOT) for controlling clinically significant CMV infection in pediatric allogeneic hematopoietic stem cell transplant recipients. PloS One. 2021;16:e0246191. [PMID: 33544726]

Shahar-Nissan K et al. Valaciclovir to prevent vertical transmission of cytomegalovirus after maternal primary infection during pregnancy: a randomised, double-blind, placebo-controlled trial. Lancet. 2020;396:779. [PMID: 32919517]

US Department of Health and Human Services (HHS). AIDSinfo. Guidelines for the prevention and treatment of opportunistic infections in adults and adolescents with HIV. Cytomegalovirus. 2019 Jun 26:K1–15. https://aidsinfo.nih.gov/contentfiles/lvguidelines/adult_oi.pdf

6. Human Herpesviruses 6, 7, & 8

HHV-6 is a B-cell lymphotropic virus that is the principal cause of **exanthema subitum** (roseola infantum, sixth disease). Primary HHV-6 infection occurs most commonly in children under 2 years of age and is a major cause of infantile febrile seizures (21% in one recent series). HHV-6 is also associated with encephalitis (symptoms may include insomnia, seizures, and hallucinations), autoimmune (Hashimoto) thyroiditis, myocarditis, and acute liver failure. Primary infection in immunocompetent adults is not common but can produce a mononucleosis-like illness. The lymphadenitis may be confused with lymphoma. Pathologically, HHV-6 is associated with mesial temporal sclerosis, which may lead to mesial temporal lobe epilepsy, and HHV-6 is associated with epilepsy syndromes. Reactivation of HHV-6 in immunocompetent adults is rare and can present as encephalitis. Imaging studies in HHV-6 encephalitis typically show lesions in the hippocampus, amygdala, and limbic structures.

Infection during pregnancy and congenital transmission is recognized. Most cases of reactivation occur in immunocompromised persons. Reactivation is associated with graft rejection, graft-versus-host disease, and bone marrow suppression in transplant patients and with encephalitis and pneumonitis in AIDS patients. In recipients of hematopoietic stem cell transplants, HHV-6 may cause fever. It is also associated with an HHV-6–induced encephalitis (diagnosed with multiplex PCR assays) that is correlated strongly with umbilical cord hematopoietic cell transplants (although HHV-6 is not associated with survival in such patients and surveillance for the virus may not be needed).

HHV-6 is on occasion also associated with drug-induced hypersensitivity syndromes. HHV-6 may cause fulminant hepatic failure and acute decompensation of chronic liver disease in children. Purpura fulminans and corneal inflammation are reported. Two variants (A and B) of HHV-6 have been identified. HHV-6B is the predominant strain found in both normal and immunocompromised persons. Ganciclovir, cidofovir, and foscarnet (but not acyclovir) appear to be clinically active against HHV-6. Adoptively transferred virus-specific T-cell therapy is also being developed for treatment of HHV-6 and other viral infections in hematopoietic stem cell transplant recipients.

HHV-7 is a T-cell lymphotropic virus that is associated with roseola seizures and, rarely, encephalitis, even in immunocompetent adults. Pregnant women are often infected. Infection with HHV-7 is synergistic with CMV in kidney transplant recipients.

HHV-8 (see also Chapter 31) is associated with a spectrum of related syndromes including Kaposi sarcoma, primary effusion lymphoma, multicentric Castleman disease (MCD), HHV-8+ diffuse large cell lymphoma (DLBCL), germinotropic lymphoproliferative disorder (GLPD), and Kaposi sarcoma inflammatory cytokine syndrome (KICS). HHV-8 infection is endemic in Africa; transmission seems to be primarily horizontal in childhood from intrafamilial contacts and continues through adulthood possibly by nonsexual routes.

Ceasarman E et al. KSHV/HHV8-mediated hematologic diseases. Blood. 2021;139:1013. [PMID: 34479367]

Cosme I et al. Human herpes virus 6 detection in children with suspected central nervous system infection. Pediatr Infect Dis J. 2020;39:e469. [PMID: 32925539]

MAJOR VACCINE-PREVENTABLE VIRAL INFECTIONS

1. Measles

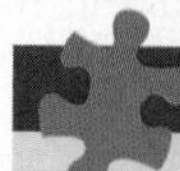

ESSENTIALS OF DIAGNOSIS

- Onset of prodrome 7–18 days after exposure in an unvaccinated patient.
- Prodrome: fever, coryza, cough, conjunctivitis, malaise, irritability, photophobia, Koplik spots.
- Rash: brick red, maculopapular; appears 3–4 days after onset of prodrome; begins on the face and proceeds "downward and outward," affecting the palms and soles last.
- Leukopenia.

General Considerations

Measles is a reportable acute systemic paramyxoviral infection transmitted by direct contact with infectious droplets or by airborne spread. It is highly contagious with communicability greatest during the pre-eruptive and catarrhal stages but continues 4 days after the appearance of rash. Measles elimination is defined as the absence of endemic measles virus transmission in an area for 12 months or longer. Measles remains a major cause of mortality with more than 140,000 estimated deaths globally in 2018, mostly in children younger than 5 years old.

In 2020, there was more than an 80% decrease in reported measles cases. This is likely due to the deterioration of existing surveillance, testing, and reporting of measles. The World Health Organization (WHO) previously considered measles eradicated in most countries worldwide, including the Americas. Many countries, however, are reporting ongoing measles outbreaks, including the Democratic Republic of the Congo, Nigeria, Pakistan, Somalia, Afghanistan, Burkina Faso, Côte d'Ivoire, Ethiopia, Niger, and India. During 2019, measles outbreaks occurred in countries with high vaccination coverage, including the United States, Israel, Thailand, Tunisia, New Zealand, and many European countries and the Pacific Islands. For 2020, the WHO European Region reported a total of 12,205 measles cases; this is compared to 104,554 cases and 42 deaths in 2019.

Most measles cases in the United States are due to either travel to endemic areas or exposure to individuals who have not been vaccinated against measles. *Intentional undervaccination continues to undermine measles elimination programs, and many measles vaccination campaigns have been halted by COVID-19.* Over 22 million infants did not receive their first dose of the measles vaccine in 2020, the largest deficit in two decades, which increases the likelihood of major outbreaks.

Clinical Findings

A. Symptoms and Signs

The incubation period for measles is 10–14 days. The illness starts with a prodromal phase manifested by high-grade fever (often as high as 40–40.6°C), malaise, coryza (nasal obstruction, sneezing, and sore throat resembling upper respiratory infections), persistent cough, and conjunctivitis (redness, swelling, photophobia, and discharge). These symptoms intensify over 2–4 days before onset of the rash and peak on the first day of the rash. The fever persists through the early rash (about 5–7 days) (Table 32–2).

The characteristic measles rash appears on the face and behind the ears. Initial lesions are pinhead-sized papules that coalesce to form a brick red, irregular, blotchy maculopapular rash. The rash spreads to the trunk and extremities, including the palms and soles. It lasts for 3–7 days and fades in the same manner it appeared. Other findings include pharyngeal erythema, tonsillar exudate, moderate generalized lymphadenopathy, and, at times, splenomegaly.

Koplik spots (small, irregular, and red with whitish center on the mucous membranes) are pathognomonic of measles (Figure 32–4). They appear about 2 days before the rash and last 1–4 days as tiny "table salt crystals" on the palatal or buccal mucosa opposite the molars.

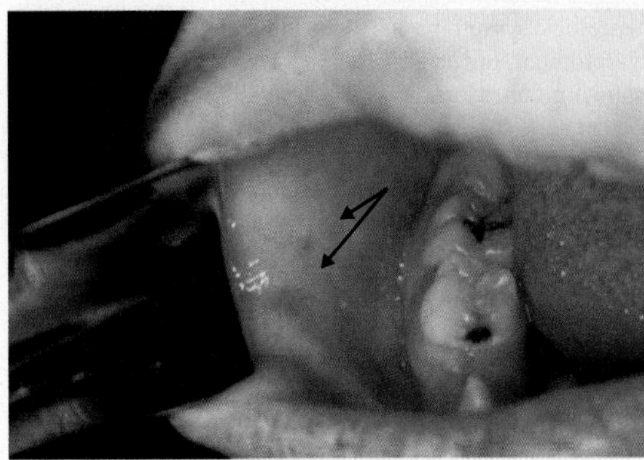

Figure 32–4. Very small, bright red spots on the buccal mucosa indicative of Koplik spots. (Public Health Image Library, CDC.)

B. Laboratory Findings

Leukopenia is usually present unless secondary bacterial complications exist. A lymphocyte count under 2000/mcL (2.0×10^9/L) is a poor prognostic sign. Thrombocytopenia is common. Proteinuria is often observed.

Detection of IgM measles antibodies with ELISA or a fourfold rise in serum hemagglutination inhibition antibody supports the diagnosis. IgM assays can be falsely negative the first few days of infection and falsely positive in the presence of rheumatoid factor or with acute rubella, erythrovirus (formerly parvovirus B19), or HHV-6 infection.

Measles virus is technically difficult to culture. Real-time reverse transcriptase–PCR (RT-PCR), available from the CDC and some public health laboratories, can help establish a diagnosis promptly.

Differential Diagnosis

Measles is usually diagnosed clinically but may be mistaken for Kawasaki disease and other exanthematous infections (Table 32–2). Frequent difficulty in establishing a diagnosis suggests that measles may be more prevalent than is recognized.

Complications

A. Respiratory Tract Disease

Early in the course of the disease, bronchopneumonia or bronchiolitis due to the measles virus may occur in up to 5% of patients and result in serious respiratory difficulties. Bronchiectasis may occur in up to a quarter of unvaccinated children. The incidence of severe respiratory disease may be increased among immunocompromised children and pregnant women.

B. Central Nervous System

Postinfectious encephalomyelitis occurs in 0.05–0.1% of cases, with higher rates occurring in adolescents. It is an acute demyelinating disease that usually starts 3–7 days after the rash. Seizures, coma, and other neurologic symptoms and signs may develop. Treatment is symptomatic and supportive. Virus isolation from the CNS is uncommon. Mortality is 10–20%, and morbidity includes 33% of survivors left with neurologic deficits.

Measles inclusion body encephalitis is another form of neurologic complication that results in neurologic deterioration and death within months of the acute illness among patients with impaired cellular immunity. Treatment is supportive, including stopping immunosuppressants when feasible. Interferon and ribavirin are variably successful.

Subacute sclerosing panencephalitis is a very rare, fatal CNS complication that occurs 5–15 years after infection. It is characterized by progressive deterioration of motor and cognitive function leading to death. It is more common in boys of rural backgrounds who are infected with measles before 2 years of age.

C. Other Complications

Immediately following measles, secondary bacterial infection, particularly otitis media (the most common complication), cervical adenitis, and pneumonia, occurs in about 15% of patients. Keratoconjunctivitis is a serious complication that caused blindness before the widespread use of measles vaccine and vitamin A supplementation. Diarrhea and protein-losing enteropathy (prodromal rectal Koplik spots may occur) are significant complications among malnourished children, although the mortality associated with diarrhea is primarily 1 week prior to and 4 weeks after the measles rash, with no longer-term mortality shown with measles-associated diarrhea. Some data implicate the measles virus in the pathogenesis of rheumatoid arthritis.

Treatment

Treatment is symptomatic, including antipyretics and fluids as needed. *Vitamin A supplementation for children reduces pediatric morbidity and measles-associated mortality.* Data are less substantial for adult supplementation, although many advocate megadose vitamin A given to the mother at the time of delivery in order to boost infant levels of the vitamin.

Measles virus is susceptible to ribavirin and other antivirals in vitro. Ribavirin is used in selected severe cases of pneumonitis, but insufficient data prevent recommending antiviral use. Zinc has a role in the maintenance of normal immune functions, but routine zinc supplementation to children with measles is *not* recommended, again for lack of data.

Prognosis

It is estimated that 23.2 million deaths were prevented between 2000 and 2018 by use of measles vaccination. In the United States, the case fatality rate is around 2 per 1000 reported cases, with deaths principally due to respiratory and neurologic complications. Deaths in the developing world are mainly related to acute diarrhea and protein-losing enteropathy. Pregnant women with measles may be at increased risk for death. Historically famines are particularly associated with high measles mortality.

Prevention

The measles vaccine is a *live* vaccine that is available worldwide as part of the trivalent MMR vaccine or the quadrivalent MMRV vaccine. Because measles is highly contagious, the vaccine coverage rates must exceed 95% to prevent outbreaks. Illness confers permanent immunity. One vaccine dose is about 93% effective. Two doses of vaccine are estimated to be 97% protective. In the United States, based on the National Immunization Survey, 91.6% of children received one or more doses of MMR in 2017–2018 by 24 months of age and more than 90% of adolescents aged 13–17 years received two or more doses of MMR in 2020. These data suggest considerable geographic disparity. Clustering of unvaccinated individuals increases the likelihood of an outbreak.

At 6 months of age, more than 99% of infants of vaccinated women and 95% of infants of naturally immune women lose maternal antibodies. The susceptibility to measles is 2.4-fold higher if the vaccine is given prior to 15 months (with impact of waning maternal antibody levels). In the United States, children receive their first vaccine dose of MMR vaccine at 12–15 months of age (https://www.cdc.gov/vaccines/schedules/hcp/imz/child-adolescent.html). The second dose is given at age 4–6 years, prior to school entry.

Older children, teens, and adults without evidence of immunity should receive two MMR doses separated by 28 days. For individuals born before 1957, herd immunity is assumed. Persons at high risk for measles exposure (teachers, health care workers, post–high school students, travelers to developing countries) should also receive two vaccination doses at least 28 days apart. Immigrants and refugees should be screened and vaccinated if necessary. The MMRV vaccines may be used in place of the traditional MMR vaccine.

MMR and MMRV vaccine should *not* be administered to pregnant women, patients with anaphylactic reactions to neomycin, and patients with known primary or acquired immunodeficiency. Asymptomatic patients living with HIV infection with CD4 cell counts higher than 200/mcL should receive the MMR vaccine but not the MMRV vaccine.

Repeated studies fail to show an association between vaccination and autism. MMR vaccine can cause fever and transient rash. Severe allergic reactions are rare. Quadrivalent MMRV vaccine is associated with an increased risk of febrile seizures that appears to be age-related; the risk is highest when MMRV is given to infants between 12 and 23 months of age. Postimmunization seizures appear in whole genome studies to be associated with an interferon receptor and a measles receptor. Immune thrombocytopenia is a documented side effect. Rare cases of postimmunization encephalitis are reported.

In case of an outbreak, when susceptible individuals are exposed to measles, MMR vaccine can prevent disease if given within 3 days of exposure. Immunoglobulin should be administered within 6 days of exposure in any high-risk person exposed to measles, followed by active immunization 3 months later. All infants less than 1 year of age should receive intramuscular immunoglobulin (0.5 mL/kg, maximum dose 15 mL). For infants between 6 months and 12 months of age, MMR vaccination with repeat at 15 months can be given in place of intramuscular immunoglobulin. Pregnant women and severely immunocompromised persons who are exposed to active measles cases should receive IVIG (400 mg/kg).

Patients with measles should be isolated for 4 days after the onset of rash. In the hospital setting, patients with measles should be placed under airborne precautions.

When to Refer

- Any suspect cases should be reported to public health authorities.
- HIV infection.
- Pregnancy.

When to Admit

- Meningitis, encephalitis, or myelitis.
- Severe pneumonia.
- Diarrhea that significantly compromises fluid or electrolyte status.

Di Pietrantonj C et al. Vaccines for measles, mumps, rubella, and varicella in children. Cochrane Database Syst Rev. 2020;4:CD004407. [PMID: 32309885]

Hill HA. Vaccination coverage by age 24 months among children born in 2017 and 2018 — National Immunization Survey-Child, United States, 2018–2020. MMWR Morb Mortal Wkly Rep. 2021;70. [PMID: 31622284]

Rana MS, Alam MM, Ikram A, et al. Emergence of measles during the COVID-19 pandemic threatens Pakistan's children and the wider region. Nat Med. 2021;27:1127. [PMID: 34183836]

Walker TY et al. National, regional, state, and selected local area vaccination coverage among adolescents aged 13–17 years—United States, 2018. MMWR Morb Mortal Wkly Rep. 2019; 68:718. [PMID: 31437143]

2. Mumps

ESSENTIALS OF DIAGNOSIS

- Exposure 12–25 days before onset.
- Painful, swollen salivary glands, usually parotid.
- Frequent involvement of testes, pancreas, and meninges in unvaccinated individuals.
- Mumps can occur in appropriately vaccinated persons in highly vaccinated communities.

General Considerations

Mumps is a paramyxoviral disease spread by respiratory droplets. Children are most commonly affected; however, in outbreaks, infection can affect patients in their second or third decades of life. Mumps can spread rapidly in congregate settings, such as colleges and schools. The incubation period is 12–25 days (average, 16–18 days). The mumps virus spreads through direct contact with respiratory secretions or saliva or infected surfaces. Transmission can also be airborne or via droplets. Up to one-third of affected individuals have subclinical infection, which is still transmissible. Since the MMR vaccine was introduced in 1989, the mumps case rate has decreased by more than 99%, with only a few hundred cases reported most years.

Unfortunately, the mumps case rate started to increase in late 2015. From January 2016 to June 2017, 9200 cases were reported, including a large outbreak of close to 3000 cases in one Arkansas community. In 2019, 3474 mumps cases were reported. In 2020 the number of cases decreased, and data reported to the CDC showed 616 cases of mumps. It is thought that COVID-19 measures, including masking and social distancing, are the likely reason for this decrease. A combination of factors contributes to outbreaks, including efficacy of vaccines; waning individual immunity; and crowded conditions, which promote transmission.

Clinical Findings

A. Symptoms and Signs

Mumps is more serious in adults than in children and appears to occur more commonly in male children, adolescents, and adults. *Parotid tenderness* and *overlying facial edema* (Figure 32–5) are the most common physical findings and typically develop within 48 hours of the prodromal symptoms. Usually, one parotid gland enlarges before the other, but unilateral parotitis occurs in 25% of patients. The parotid duct (orifice of Stensen) may be red and swollen. Trismus may result from parotitis. The parotid glands return to normal within 1 week. Involvement of other salivary glands (submaxillary and sublingual) occurs in 10% of

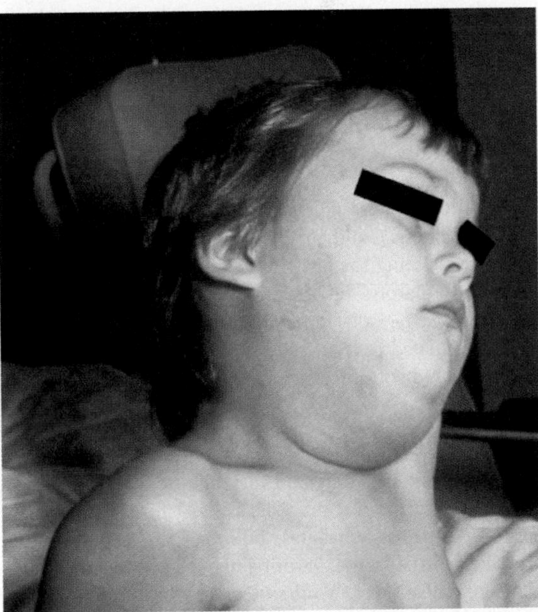

Figure 32–5. Mumps. (Public Health Image Library, CDC.)

cases. Fever and malaise are variable but often minimal in young children. The entire course of mumps rarely exceeds 2 weeks.

The testes are the most common extra salivary disease site in adults. High fever, testicular swelling, and tenderness (unilateral in 75% of cases) denote *orchitis*, which usually develops 7–10 days after the onset of parotitis. In the mumps outbreaks that occurred between 2006 and 2010 in the United States, complications from mumps were rare; 3.3–10% of adolescent and men developed orchitis (which occurred less frequently in persons who have received two doses of vaccine). Lower abdominal pain and ovarian enlargement suggest oophoritis, which is usually unilateral and occurs in less than 1% of postpubertal women.

Other rare complications, occurring in less than 1% of cases, are meningitis, encephalitis, Guillain-Barré syndrome, hearing loss, priapism or testicular infarction from orchitis, pancreatitis, thyroiditis, keratitis, neuritis, hepatitis, myocarditis, thrombocytopenia, migratory arthralgias, and nephritis. No mumps-related deaths have occurred in the United States in recent outbreaks. A rare cause of mumps is iodine exposure in medical procedures ("iodide mumps").

B. Laboratory Findings

Mild leukopenia with relative lymphocytosis may be present. Elevated serum amylase usually reflects salivary gland involvement rather than pancreatitis. Mild kidney injury is found in up to 60% of patients.

The characteristic clinical picture usually suffices for diagnosis. An elevated serum IgM is considered diagnostic. Repeat testing 2–3 weeks after the onset of symptoms is recommended if the first assay is negative because the rise in IgM may be delayed, especially in vaccinated persons. A fourfold rise in complement-fixing antibodies to mumps virus in paired serum IgG also confirms infection. Anti-mumps IgM and IgG in the CSF can confirm the diagnosis of mumps-associated meningitis. Nucleic acid amplification techniques, such as RT-PCR, are more sensitive than viral cultures and are available from some commercial laboratories, selected state laboratories, and the CDC. Diagnostic yield is highest if collected during the first 3 days of illness. Confirmatory diagnosis of mumps is also made by isolating the virus preferably from a swab of the duct of the parotid or other affected salivary gland. The virus can also be isolated from CSF early in aseptic meningitis. Vaccinated persons may shed virus for shorter periods compared with those who are unvaccinated.

Differential Diagnosis

Swelling of the parotid gland may be due to calculi in the parotid ducts, tumors, or cysts. Other causes include sarcoidosis, cirrhosis, diabetes, bulimia, pilocarpine usage, and Sjögren syndrome. Parotitis may be produced by pyogenic organisms (eg, *S aureus*, gram-negative organisms [particularly in debilitated individuals with poor oral intake]), drug reaction (phenothiazines, propylthiouracil), and other viruses (HIV, influenza A, parainfluenza, EBV infection, coxsackieviruses, adenoviruses, HHV-6). Swelling of the parotid gland must be differentiated from inflammation of the lymph nodes located more posteriorly and inferiorly than the parotid gland.

Treatment

Treatment is symptomatic. Topical compresses may relieve parotid discomfort. Some clinicians advocate IVIG for complicated disease (eg, thrombocytopenia), although its definitive role is unproven. No specific treatment exists for orchitis.

Prevention

Vaccination is the most effective way to prevent mumps.

The vaccination schedule, indications, and contraindications are described in the measles section. The mumps vaccine component of the MMR is less effective than the measles and rubella components. One dose is 78% (range: 49–92%) protective. Two doses of the vaccine are 88% (range: 66–95%) effective. Rare reported complications of mumps vaccination include immune thrombocytopenic purpura and aseptic meningitis.

A study evaluating the effect of a third dose of MMR vaccine after a mumps outbreak showed that the attack rate was significantly lower among students who received a third dose compared with two doses, especially if the second dose was given more than 13 years prior to the outbreak. The CDC recommends a third dose of vaccine in case of an outbreak.

Suspected cases should be isolated. For outbreak control, the most important step is to vaccinate all susceptible individuals. The MMR vaccine is *not* effective in preventing the disease in unvaccinated patients who already have been exposed to the virus. In the health care setting, the following steps should be taken: implement droplet and standard precautions, isolate patients until swelling subsides (about 9 days from onset), and provide vaccination to health care workers with no evidence of immunity.

When to Refer

Any suspect cases should be reported to public health authorities.

When to Admit

- Trismus; meningitis; encephalitis; myocarditis; pancreatitis.
- Severe testicular pain; priapism.
- Severe thrombocytopenia.

Deal A et al; European Society of Clinical Microbiology and Infectious Diseases Study Group for Infections in Travellers and Migrants (ESGITM). Migration and outbreaks of vaccine-preventable disease in Europe: a systematic review. Lancet Infect Dis. 2021;21:e387. [PMID: 34626552]

Kaaijk P et al. A third dose of measles-mumps-rubella vaccine to improve immunity against mumps in young adults. J Infect Dis. 2020;221:902. [PMID: 31112277]

3. Rubella

ESSENTIALS OF DIAGNOSIS

- Exposure 14–21 days before onset.
- No prodrome in children, mild prodrome in adults; mild symptoms (fever, malaise, coryza) coincide with, or precede by up to 5 days, the eruption of rash.
- Posterior cervical and postauricular lymphadenopathy 5–10 days before rash.
- Fine maculopapular rash of 3 days' duration; face to trunk to extremities.
- Leukopenia, thrombocytopenia.

General Considerations

Rubella is a systemic disease caused by a togavirus transmitted by inhalation of infective droplets. It is moderately communicable. Infection usually confers permanent immunity. The incubation period is 14–21 days. The disease is transmissible from 1 week before the rash appears until 15 days afterward.

The last cases of endemic rubella and **congenital rubella syndrome** were reported in 2009 from the Americas region. Each year in the United States, fewer than 10 cases of rubella are reported, all of which are due to the arrival of infected persons from other countries. In 2015, the WHO declared that the Americas were the first region to be free of rubella and congenital rubella syndrome. Some European countries face a challenge with lower immunization coverage among refugees and migrants. Worldwide, cases are decreasing due to widespread implementation of rubella-containing vaccines; as of January 2020, the vaccine was added to the national vaccine schedule in 173 of 195 (89%) countries, though it is important to note that extensive variation in the rate of national coverage exists. On the other hand, the number of cases of congenital rubella syndrome remains high, particularly in Africa and Southeast Asia. The increase in congenital rubella syndrome may be secondary to an increase in surveillance and reporting of congenital rubella cases. The WHO set a goal to eliminate rubella in at least five of the six regions (all but the Western Pacific region, which includes China) by 2020, although progress has been hampered by lack of resources.

Clinical Findings

A. Postnatal Rubella

Rubella is a common childhood disease; most cases are asymptomatic. The clinical picture of rubella is difficult to distinguish from other viral illnesses, such as infectious mononucleosis, measles, echovirus infections, and coxsackievirus infections. Fever and malaise, usually mild, accompanied by tender suboccipital adenitis, may precede the eruption by 1 week. Early posterior cervical and postauricular lymphadenopathy is common. A fine, pink maculopapular rash appears and fades from the face, trunk, and extremities in rapid progression (2–3 days), usually lasting 1 day in each area (Table 32–2).

B. Congenital Rubella

The principal importance of rubella lies in its devastating effects on the fetus in utero causing fetal death, preterm delivery, and teratogenic effects. The severity of symptoms is directly related to the gestational age; fetal infection during the first trimester leads to congenital rubella in at least 80% of fetuses; however, an infection during the fourth month can lead to 10% risk of a single congenital defect. In the second trimester of pregnancy, deafness is the primary complication.

C. Laboratory Findings

When rubella is suspected, the diagnosis requires serologic confirmation. Diagnosis of acute rubella infection is based on elevated IgM antibody, fourfold or greater rise in IgG antibody titers, or isolation of the virus. Serosensitivity to rubella is thought to change with subsequent pregnancies, although data from Hong Kong (lower immunity) and the United Kingdom (higher immunity) differed in their findings.

IgM is detectable in 50% of persons on day 1 of the rash but in most on day 5 after rash onset. Antibody testing can be performed on sera or saliva. An isolated IgM-positive test does not necessarily imply acute infection. IgM antibodies can persist after an infection or could be false-positive due to cross-reactivity with other antigens such as EBV, CMV, erythrovirus, and rheumatoid factor. This distinction is very important to make when infection is suspected in pregnancy. High-avidity anti-rubella IgG assays can distinguish between recent and remote infection. Low-avidity IgG is observed in acute rubella infections and lasts up to 3 months postinfection. After 3 months, low-avidity antibodies are replaced by high-avidity antibodies indicating remote infection.

The CDC can test for virus by RT-PCR from throat swabs, oral fluids, or nasopharyngeal secretions. The timing of sample collection is important and is best if collected within the first 3 days of an acute illness and within 3 months in case of congenital rubella syndrome. After 3 months of age, up to 50% of infants with congenital rubella syndrome will not shed the virus.

Complications

Complications of rubella are rare aside from the congenital rubella syndrome. Polyarticular arthritis and arthralgia occur more commonly in adult women; involve the fingers, wrists, and knees; and usually subside within 7 days but may persist for weeks. Hemorrhagic manifestations due to thrombocytopenia and vascular damage occur more commonly in children, unlike other complications. Hepatitis has been reported. Encephalitis, another rare complication, occurs more commonly in adults and has a high mortality rate.

Treatment

Rubella infection, including complications, is treated symptomatically.

Prevention

Patients with rubella should be isolated for 7 days after rash onset.

In the United States, monovalent rubella vaccine is not produced. *Live attenuated* rubella virus vaccine is included in the MMR or MMRV vaccine. It is recommended that the first dose be given between 12 months and 15 months. The second dose is given between age 4 and 6 years, prior to school entry. More details on scheduling, side effects, and contraindications are explained in the measles section. It is important that girls are immune to rubella prior to menarche. In the United States, about 80% of 20-year-old women are immune to rubella.

Rubella vaccine is safe and highly efficacious; a single dose of MMR vaccine is about 97% effective at preventing rubella.

The immune status of pregnant women should be evaluated because antibody titers fall in about 10% of vaccinated individuals within 12 years of vaccination. While no evidence exists for adverse outcomes with MMR immunization of pregnant women, it is still recommended that women avoid pregnancy for at least 4 weeks after vaccination. Opportunities should be made available to vaccinate all women of childbearing age.

The administration of live vaccines to immunocompromised patients is controversial. In patients receiving immunosuppressive therapy as well as in patients who have undergone solid organ or bone marrow transplantation, seroconversion is higher to rubella compared with measles, mumps, and varicella. In addition, response to live attenuated vaccines may be lessened due to presence of antibodies from IVIG or other blood products.

Safety is another concern when administering live attenuated vaccines to immunocompromised patients. Because MMR vaccine is contraindicated in solid organ transplant recipients, current evidence recommends that seronegative patients receive one or two doses of the MMR vaccine at least 4 weeks prior to solid organ transplantation. Patients who have undergone bone marrow transplant lose antigen-specific antibodies and should be revaccinated regardless of their vaccination history. The revised guidelines recommend MMR and varicella vaccines be given to seronegative patients without graft-versus-host disease 2 years after hematopoietic stem cell transplantation.

Prognosis

Rubella typically is a mild illness and rarely lasts more than 3–4 days. Congenital rubella has a high fetal mortality rate, and the associated congenital defects are largely permanent.

When to Refer

- Pregnancy.
- Meningitis/encephalitis.
- Significant vaccination reactions.
- Any suspect cases should be reported to public health authorities.

O'Connor P. Progress toward rubella elimination—World Health Organization European Region, 2005–2019. MMWR Morb Mortal Wkly Rep. 2021;70. [PMID: 34111057]

Patel MK, Antoni S, Danovaro-Holliday MC, et al. The epidemiology of rubella, 2007–18: an ecological analysis of surveillance data. Lancet Glob Health. 2020;8:e1399. [PMID: 33069300]

Plotkin SA. Rubella eradication: not yet accomplished, but entirely feasible. J Infect Dis. 2021;224:S360. [PMID: 34590132]

4. Poliomyelitis

ESSENTIALS OF DIAGNOSIS

- Incubation period 7–14 days after exposure.
- Headache, stiff neck, fever, vomiting, sore throat.
- Lower motor neuron lesion (flaccid myelitis) with decreased deep tendon reflexes and muscle wasting; sensation intact.

General Considerations

Poliomyelitis virus, an enterovirus, is highly contagious through fecal-oral route, especially during the first week of infection. Three wild poliovirus serotypes exist; however, only wild poliovirus type 1 has remained endemic since 2012. Pakistan and Afghanistan currently are the only countries with endemic wild type poliovirus transmission. Unfortunately, there has been a concerning uptick in the numbers of both wild and vaccine-derived polio cases. In 2020, 56 cases of wild poliovirus type 1 were reported from Afghanistan and 84 cases from Pakistan. As of November 10, 2021, there has only been one reported case of wild poliovirus type 1 in Afghanistan and one case in Pakistan. In 2020, 101 cases of vaccine-derived polio were reported, derived mostly from type 2 attenuated live oral poliovirus vaccine (OPV). As of May 5, 2021, 75 cases of vaccine-derived polio were reported in 2021.

Cases of acute flaccid myelitis (formerly acute flaccid paralysis) resembling polio but not due to poliomyelitis virus are being reported (see Acute Flaccid Myelitis, below).

Clinical Findings

A. Symptoms and Signs

At least 95% of infections are asymptomatic. Patients who become symptomatic can present with abortive poliomyelitis, nonparalytic poliomyelitis, or paralytic poliomyelitis. Post-poliomyelitis syndrome is the constellation of symptoms that affect polio survivors and is not infectious.

1. Abortive poliomyelitis—Nonspecific symptoms of this minor illness include fever, headache, vomiting, diarrhea, constipation, and sore throat lasting 2–3 days.

2. Nonparalytic poliomyelitis—In addition to the above symptoms, signs of meningeal irritation and muscle spasm occur in the absence of frank paralysis.

3. Paralytic poliomyelitis—Characterized as a flaccid asymmetric paralysis affecting mostly the proximal muscles of the lower extremities; the febrile period is present over 2–3 days. Sensory loss is very rare. Paralytic poliomyelitis is divided into two forms, which may coexist: (1) **spinal poliomyelitis** involving the muscles innervated by the spinal nerves, and (2) **bulbar poliomyelitis** involving the muscles supplied by the cranial nerves (especially nerves IX and X) and of the respiratory and vasomotor centers. The most life-threatening aspect of bulbar poliomyelitis is respiratory paralysis. The incidence of paralytic poliomyelitis is higher when infections are acquired later in life.

4. Post-poliomyelitis syndrome—The syndrome presents with signs of chronic and new denervation. The most frequent symptoms are progressive muscle limb paresis with muscle atrophy, with fasciculations and fibrillation during rest activity. The restless leg syndrome is also reported.

B. Laboratory Findings

The virus may be recovered from throat washings (early) and stools (early and late), and PCR of washings, stool, or CSF can also facilitate diagnosis. CSF findings include the following: (1) normal or slightly increased pressure and protein, (2) glucose is not decreased, and (3) WBC count usually less than 500/mcL (0.5×10^9/L) and are principally lymphocytes after the first 24 hours. CSF findings are normal in 5% of patients. Neutralizing and complement-fixing antibodies appear during the first or second week of illness. Serologic testing cannot distinguish between wild type and vaccine-related virus infections.

Differential Diagnosis

Acute inflammatory polyneuritis (Guillain-Barré syndrome), Japanese encephalitis virus infection, West Nile virus infection, and tick paralysis may resemble poliomyelitis. In Guillain-Barré syndrome (see Chapter 24), the weakness is more symmetric and ascending in most cases, but the Miller Fisher variant of Guillain-Barré is similar to bulbar poliomyelitis. Paresthesia is uncommon in poliomyelitis but common in Guillain-Barré syndrome. The CSF usually has high protein content but normal cell count in Guillain-Barré syndrome. While no evidence of poliomyelitis infection exists in acute flaccid myelitis that resembles polio, enteroviruses are isolated in some cases of acute flaccid myelitis.

Treatment

In the acute phase of paralytic poliomyelitis, patients should be hospitalized. In cases of respiratory weakness or paralysis, intensive care is needed. Intensive physiotherapy may help recover some motor function with paralysis. Attention to psychological disorders in longstanding disease is also important.

Immunodeficient individuals have prolonged excretion of poliovirus leading to virus circulation and threatening the polio eradication efforts.

Immune modulators, such as prednisone, interferon, and IVIG, do *not* show any clear benefit in the treatment of post-poliomyelitis syndrome.

Prognosis

The death-to-case ratio for paralytic polio ranges between 2% and 30%, depending on age. Bulbar poliomyelitis carries a mortality rate of up to 75%.

Prevention

Given the epidemiologic distribution of poliomyelitis and the continued concern about vaccine-associated disease with the trivalent live OPV, the inactive (Salk) parenteral vaccine (IPV) is currently used in the United States for all four recommended doses (at ages 2 months, 4 months, 6–18 months, and at 4–6 years). Inactivated vaccine is also routinely used elsewhere in the developed world where one dose is often administered, although immunogenicity is improved with additional doses.

Because most of circulating vaccine-derived poliovirus and vaccine-associated poliomyelitis are live OPV type 2, the WHO replaced worldwide the trivalent live OPV (containing types 1, 2, and 3) with the bivalent live OPV (type 1 and 3) in 2016. *The goal is to replace all live OPV with inactive parenteral vaccination to eliminate poliovirus circulation.* The advantages of oral vaccination are the ease of administration, low cost, effective local GI and circulating immunity, and herd immunity. Monovalent OPV type 2 (mOPV2) as well as the trivalent OPV are used for control in countries with vaccine-derived type 2 outbreaks. A novel oral polio vaccine type 2 (nOPV2) has been developed in response to the ongoing circulating vaccine-derived type 2 poliovirus outbreaks and has been shown to be safe and immunogenic in previously immunized adults. Studies so far have shown that nOPV2 is more genetically stable than the mOPV2 and therefore less prone to reverting to neurovirulence. The nOPV2 was recommended for initial use under the WHO's Emergency Use Listing Procedure in November 2020.

Routine immunization of adults in the United States is *no longer recommended* because of the low incidence of the disease. Vaccination should be considered for adults not vaccinated within the prior decade who are exposed to poliomyelitis or who plan to travel to endemic areas and adults engaged in high-risk activities (eg, laboratory workers handling stools).

When to Refer

Any suspicious cases should be referred to public health authorities.

Bigouette JP. Progress toward polio eradication—Worldwide, January 2019–June 2021. MMWR Morb Mortal Wkly Rep. 2021;70. [PMID: 34437527]

Coster ID et al. Safety and immunogenicity of two novel type 2 oral poliovirus vaccine candidates compared with a monovalent type 2 oral poliovirus vaccine in healthy adults: two clinical trials. Lancet. 2021;397:39. [PMID: 33308429]

5. Acute Flaccid Myelitis

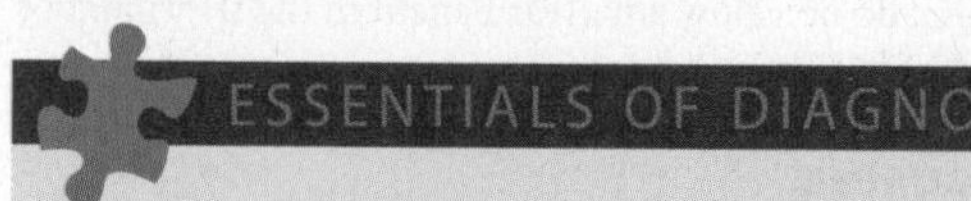

- Viral illness precedes neurologic signs.
- Flaccid paralysis usually affects upper limbs or all four limbs.
- Enterovirus is commonly isolated; poliomyelitis must be ruled out.

General Considerations

Before widespread polio vaccination in the 1950s, polio was the most common cause of acute flaccid myelitis (also known as acute flaccid paralysis). More recently, nonpolio enteroviruses are most often the cause of acute flaccid myelitis. This disease has been reported throughout Africa (20 countries), the Eastern Mediterranean region (5 countries), intermittently in Europe (Germany and France), and the United States (50 states and the District of Colombia). The CDC began surveillance for acute flaccid myelitis in 2014. Since then, there have been three outbreaks in the United States. The largest to date occurred in 2018, with 238 confirmed cases; most had a preceding viral illness in the month before presentation of neurologic signs. The neurologic signs most commonly involved the upper limbs or all four limbs. The most commonly associated viruses were enterovirus A71 and enterovirus D68. In all instances, poliomyelitis was ruled out but an exact cause for the acute flaccid myelitis was not always determined.

Clinical Findings

Acute flaccid myelitis is usually a childhood disease; the average age of presentation is 5 years. Cases usually present in late summer or early fall. The three clinical stages of acute flaccid myelitis are prodromal illness, acute neurologic injury, and convalescence.

A. Symptoms and Signs

The prodrome typically consists of fever, upper respiratory symptoms, and GI symptoms. One to four weeks later, neurologic symptoms begin and usually manifest as flaccid limb weakness with decreased reflexes. Fever may recur, and the patient experiences myalgia and flaccid weakness in one or more limbs. Upper extremities are affected more often than lower extremities. Once new neurologic symptoms have subsided, the convalescent phase can last for months to years. During this time, patients may experience residual muscle weakness and atrophy.

B. Laboratory Findings

Cerebrospinal fluid analysis shows pleocytosis (WBC count greater than 5/mcL [0.005×10^9/L]) often paired with elevated protein level (and a normal glucose concentration).

All individuals with suspected acute flaccid myelitis should be tested for enteroviruses (including D68 and A71) and rhinovirus from relevant anatomic sites. Testing for arboviruses, adenovirus, and herpesviruses should also be considered. All suspected cases should be reported to the state health department, the CDC, or both.

C. Imaging

MRIs of the brain and spinal cord should be accompanied by lumbar puncture. MRI typically shows disease of the central gray matter within the spinal cord in the location of the anterior horn cells.

Treatment

No specific treatment exists for acute flaccid myelitis. Management consists of supportive care. Many adjunctive therapies have been used, including IVIG, high-dose corticosteroids, and plasmapheresis, but none have shown efficacy. Neurologists specializing in the management of acute flaccid myelitis can be contacted through the AFM Physician Consult and Support Portal at https://bit.ly/2Y2U3VR.

Long-term therapy during the convalescent phase should include physical therapy and any other necessary forms of physical rehabilitation.

Prevention

An effective enterovirus-A71 vaccine has been developed for children and is in phase 3 trials.

Guan X et al. Effectiveness and safety of an inactivated enterovirus 71 vaccine in children aged 6–71 months in a phase IV study. Clin Infect Dis. 2020;71:2421. [PMID: 31734699]

Murphy OC et al. Acute flaccid myelitis: cause, diagnosis, and management. Lancet Lond Engl. 2021; 397:334. [PMID: 33357469]

OTHER NEUROTROPIC VIRUSES

1. Rabies

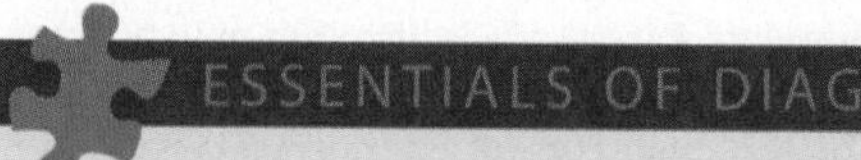

- History of animal bite.
- Paresthesias, hydrophobia, rage alternating with calm.
- Convulsions, paralysis, thick tenacious saliva.

General Considerations

Rabies is a viral (rhabdovirus) encephalitis transmitted by infected saliva that enters the body by an animal bite or an open wound. Worldwide, over 17 million cases of animal bites are reported every year, and it is estimated that about 59,000 deaths annually are attributable to rabies. Rabies is endemic in over 150 countries; it is estimated that over 40% of the world's population lives in areas without rabies surveillance. Most cases of rabies occur in rural areas of Africa and Asia. India has the highest incidence, accounting for 36% of global deaths (http://www.who.int/rabies/epidemiology/en/). In developing countries, more than 90% of human cases and 99% of human deaths from rabies are secondary to bites from infected dogs. Rabies among travelers to rabies-endemic areas is usually associated with animal injuries (including dogs in North Africa and India, cats in the Middle East, and nonhuman primates in sub-Saharan Africa and Asia), with most travel-associated cases occurring within 10 days of arrival. Rabies-free areas include much of Western Europe, Australia, New Zealand, Japan, and the state of Hawaii in the United States. A map outlining these areas is available with Wikimedia Commons (https://commons.wikimedia.org/wiki/File:Rabies_Free_Countries_and_Territories.svg).

In the United States, domestically acquired rabies cases are rare (approximately 92% of cases are associated with wildlife) but probably underreported. Reports largely from the East Coast show an increase in rabies among cats, with about 1% of tested cats showing rabies seropositivity. The annual caseload in the United States is 1–3 cases (https://www.cdc.gov/rabies/location/usa/surveillance/human_rabies.html). Between 1960 and 2018, a total of 125 human rabies cases were reported in the United States. These included 36 cases (28%) with a history of dog bites during international travel. The remaining 89 cases (72%) were acquired in the United States, most often by bats.

Surveillance for animal rabies in 2018 showed 4951 animal and three human cases occurring in 49 states and Puerto Rico. *Wild animals accounted for 92.7% of cases, and among wild animals, bats were the most common animal (33%).* Wildlife reservoirs, with each species having its own rabies variant(s), follow a unique geographic distribution in the United States: raccoons on the East Coast; skunks in the Midwest, Southwest, and California; and foxes in the Southwest and in Alaska. However, some areas have all three wildlife reservoirs (eg, the hill country of Texas) https://www.cdc.gov/rabies/location/usa/surveillance/wild_animals.html.

Raccoons, bats, and skunks accounted for 86.6% of the rabid animals found in the United States in 2018; other rabid animals include foxes, cats, cattle, and dogs. Rodents and lagomorphs (eg, rabbits) are unlikely to spread rabies because they cannot survive the disease long enough to transmit it (woodchucks and groundhogs are exceptions). Wildlife epizootics present a constant public health threat in addition to the danger of reintroducing rabies to domestic animals. Vaccination is the key to controlling rabies in small animals and preventing rabies transmission to human beings.

The virus enters the salivary glands of dogs 5–7 days before their death from rabies, thus limiting their period of infectivity. Less common routes of transmission include contamination of mucous membranes with saliva or brain tissue, aerosol transmission, and corneal transplantation. Recognized mutations in rabies virus proteins can subvert the host immune system. Transmission through solid organ and vascular segment transplantation from donors with unrecognized infection is also reported. A number of transplantation-associated cases are reported, including two clusters in the United States. Postexposure prophylaxis can be administered in these patients and may prevent development of disease.

The incubation period may range from 10 days to many years but is usually 3–7 weeks depending in part on the distance of the wound from the CNS. The virus travels via the nerves to the brain, multiplies there, and then migrates along the efferent nerves to the salivary glands. Rabies virus infection forms cytoplasmic inclusion bodies similar to Negri bodies. These Negri bodies are thought to be the sites of viral transcription and replication.

Clinical Findings

A. Symptoms and Signs

While patients usually report an animal bite, bat bites may not be recognized. The prodromal syndrome consists of pain at the site of the bite in association with fever, malaise, headache, nausea, and vomiting. The skin is sensitive to changes of temperature, especially air currents (aerophobia). Percussion myoedema (a mounding of muscles after a light pressure stimulus) can be present and persist throughout the disease. Abnormal sexual behavior is also a recognized presenting symptom of rabies; such behavior includes priapism and frequent ejaculation in men and hypersexuality in women.

The CNS stage begins about 10 days after the prodrome and may be either encephalitic ("furious") or paralytic ("dumb"). The **encephalitic form** (about 80% of the cases) produces the classic rabies manifestations of delirium alternating with periods of calm, extremely painful laryngeal spasms on attempting drinking (hydrophobia), autonomic stimulation (hypersalivation), and seizures. In the less common **paralytic form**, an acute ascending paralysis resembling Guillain-Barré syndrome predominates with relative sparing of higher cortical functions initially. Both forms progress relentlessly to coma, autonomic nervous system dysfunction, and death.

B. Laboratory Findings

Biting animals that appear well should be quarantined and observed for 10 days. Sick or dead animals should be tested for rabies. A wild animal, if captured, should be sacrificed and the head shipped on ice to the nearest laboratory qualified to examine the brain for evidence of rabies virus. *When the animal cannot be examined, raccoons, skunks, bats, and foxes should be presumed to be rabid.*

Direct fluorescent antibody testing of skin biopsy material from the posterior neck of the potentially infected animal (where hair follicles are highly innervated) has a sensitivity of 60–80%.

Quantitative RT-PCR, nucleic acid sequence-based amplification, direct rapid immunohistochemical test, and viral isolation from the patient's CSF or saliva are advocated as definitive diagnostic assays. Antibodies can be detected in the serum and the CSF. Pathologic specimens often demonstrate round or oval eosinophilic inclusion bodies (Negri bodies) in the cytoplasm of neuronal cells, but the finding is neither sensitive nor specific. MRI signs are diffuse and nonspecific.

Treatment & Prognosis

Management requires intensive care with attention to the airway, maintenance of oxygenation, and control of seizures. Universal precautions are essential. Corticosteroids are of no use. Survival is rare, and data are insufficient to provide estimate of success.

If postexposure prophylaxis (discussed below) is given expediently, before clinical signs develop, it is nearly 100% successful in prevention of disease. Once the symptoms have appeared, death almost inevitably occurs after 7 days, usually from respiratory failure. Most deaths occur in persons with unrecognized disease who do not seek medical care or in individuals who do not receive postexposure prophylaxis. The very rare cases in which patients recover without intensive care are referred to as "abortive rabies."

Prevention

Immunization of household dogs and cats and active immunization of persons with significant animal exposure (eg, veterinarians) are important. The most important decisions, however, concern animal bites. Animals that are frequent sources of infection to travelers are dogs, cats, and nonhuman primates.

In the developing world, education, surveillance, and animal (particularly dog) vaccination programs (at recurrent intervals) are preferred over mass destruction of dogs, which is followed typically by invasion of susceptible feral animals into urban areas. In some Western European countries, campaigns of oral vaccination of wild animals led to the elimination of rabies in wildlife.

A. Local Treatment of Animal Bites and Scratches

Thorough cleansing, debridement, and repeated flushing of wounds with soap and water are important. Rabies immune globulin (RIG) or antiserum should be given as stated below. Wounds caused by animal bites should not be sutured.

B. Postexposure Immunization

The decision to treat should be based on the circumstances of the bite, including the extent and location of the wound, the biting animal, the history of prior vaccination, and the local epidemiology of rabies. *Any contact or suspect contact with a bat, skunk, or raccoon is usually deemed a sufficient indication to warrant prophylaxis.* Consultation with state and local health departments is recommended. Postexposure treatment including both immune globulin and vaccination should be administered as promptly as possible when indicated.

For patients who had not received rabies vaccination prior to possible exposure, the optimal form of **passive immunization** is human RIG (HRIG), 20 IU/kg, administered once, although recent data from Côte d'Ivoire questions its utility. As much as possible of the full dose should be infiltrated around the wound, with any remaining injected intramuscularly at a site distant from the wound. Finger spaces can be safely injected without development of a compartment syndrome. If HRIG is not available and appropriate tests for horse serum sensitivity are done, equine rabies antiserum (40 IU/kg) can be used.

Two vaccines containing inactivated rabies viruses are licensed for **active immunization** and available for use in humans in the United States: a human diploid cell vaccine (Immovax) and a purified chick embryo cell vaccine (RabAvert). Several postexposure prophylaxis strategies are recommended. The most commonly used one is the "abbreviated Essen" strategy, where either of the current vaccines is given as four intramuscular injections of 1 mL in the deltoid or, in small children, into the anterolateral thigh muscles on days 0, 3, 7, and 14 after exposure (the fifth dose at 28 days after exposure is no longer recommended except among immunosuppressed patients). The vaccine should not be given in the gluteal area due to suboptimal response. An alternative intramuscular vaccination strategy that takes only 1 week, with injections on days 0, 3, and 7 after exposure with a Vero cell vaccine (Verorab), was reportedly successful in achieving adequate neutralizing titers at days 14 and 28 in a study from Thailand; this vaccine is not currently available in the United States. Several new rabies vaccines are undergoing phase 1 clinical trials, including replication-defective chimpanzee adenovirus vaccines (ChAd155-RG and ChAdOx2 RabG) and a mRNA vaccine (CreVac CV7202).

An alternative to RIG, a monoclonal antibody cocktail referred to as SYN023 and developed by a Taiwanese company with Chinese and American support, is being studied as a promising effective agent, although it reduces RIG efficacy if given simultaneously.

The WHO supports an intradermal vaccination strategy using Verorab and the inactivated rabies virus vaccine Rabipur (an alternative formulation of the purified chick embryo cell) (0.1 mL per intradermal injection) for regions of the world where vaccine is in short supply; either vaccine can be given at two sites on days 0, 3, 7, and 28. A review from 2019 confirms the suitability of Verrab for rabies prophylaxis.

Rabies vaccines and HRIG should never be given in the same syringe or at the same site. Allergic reactions to the vaccine are rare and include a report of sudden unilateral sensorineural hearing loss and immune thrombocytopenic purpura, although local reactions (pruritus, erythema, tenderness) occur in about 25% and mild systemic reactions (headaches, myalgias, nausea) in about 20% of recipients. Rare cases of postimmunization encephalitis have been reported. Intradermal vaccines appear to be better tolerated than intramuscular vaccines, especially among young children (while titers achieved with intramuscular vaccinations are higher, the titers achieved with intradermal vaccination are deemed sufficient for protection against clinical rabies). The vaccines are commercially available or can be obtained through health departments. Adverse reactions to HRIG seem to be more frequent in women and rare in young children.

In patients with history of past vaccination, the need for HRIG is eliminated (HRIG is in short supply worldwide), but postexposure vaccination is still required. The vaccine should be given 1 mL in the deltoid twice (on days 0 and 3). Neither the passive nor the active form of postexposure prophylaxis is associated with fetal abnormalities and thus pregnancy is not considered a contraindication to vaccination. Peripartum rabies transmission occurs but is rare. Neonates may also receive both forms of postexposure prophylaxis at birth.

The WHO has a program to eliminate dog-transmitted human rabies by 2030.

C. Preexposure Immunization

Preexposure prophylaxis with three injections of human diploid cell (Immovax) vaccine intramuscularly (1 mL on days 0, 7, and 21 or 28) is recommended for persons at high risk for exposure: veterinarians (who should have rabies antibody titers checked every 2 years and be boosted with 1 mL intramuscularly); animal handlers; laboratory workers; Peace Corps workers; and travelers with stays over 1 month to remote areas in endemic countries in Africa, Asia, and Latin America. An intradermal route is also available (0.1 mL on days 0, 7, and 21 over the deltoid) but not in the United States. Intradermal administration of a double dose of 0.1 mL on days 0 and 7 is safe and as effective as the three-dose schedule. Immunosuppressive illnesses and agents including corticosteroids as well as antimalarials—in particular chloroquine—may diminish the antibody response. Children have been successfully coimmunized against influenza (with a quadrivalent vaccine) at either the 7- or 28-day rabies immunization. A single-dose regimen for preexposure prophylaxis with supplemental topical imiquimod is being studied in Belgium and shows promising results

A single-dose booster at 10 years after initial immunization increases the level of antibody titers. Unfortunately, data from travel services indicate that only a small proportion of travelers with anticipated lengthy stays in rabies-impacted areas receive the vaccine as recommended.

When to Refer

Suspicion of rabies requires contact with public health personnel to initiate appropriate passive and active prophylaxis and observation of suspect cases. A set of guidelines to determine need for treatment based on type of exposure is available at the WHO website: https://www.who.int/news-room/fact-sheets/detail/rabies.

When to Admit

- Respiratory, neuromuscular, or CNS dysfunction consistent with rabies.
- Patients with suspect rabies require initiation of therapy until the disease is ruled out in suspect animals, and this requires coordination of care based on likelihood of patient compliance, availability of inpatient and outpatient facilities, and response of local public health teams.

Chao TY et al. In vivo efficacy of SYN023, an anti-rabies monoclonal antibody cocktail, in post-exposure prophylaxis animal models. Trop Med Infect Dis. 2020;5:31. [PMID: 32098049]

Moulenat T et al. Purified Vero cell rabies vaccine (PVRV, Verorab®): a systematic review of intradermal use between 1985 and 2019. Trop Med Infect Dis. 2020;5:40. [PMID: 32156005]

Pieracci EG et al. Vital Signs: trends in human rabies deaths and exposures—United States, 1938–2018. MMWR Morb Mortal Wkly Rep. 2019;68:524. [PMID: 31194721]

Soentjens P et al. Preexposure intradermal rabies vaccination: a noninferiority trial in healthy adults on shortening the vaccination schedule from 28 to 7 Days. Clin Infect Dis. 2019;68:607. [PMID: 29939243]

2. Arbovirus Encephalitides

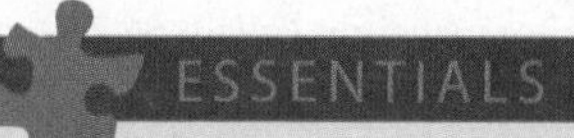

ESSENTIALS OF DIAGNOSIS

- Acute febrile illness; rash may be present; stiff neck progressing to stupor, coma, and convulsions.
- Upper motor neuron lesion signs: exaggerated deep tendon reflexes, absent superficial reflexes, and spastic paralysis.
- CSF opening pressure and protein are often increased with lymphocytic pleocytosis.

General Considerations

The arboviruses are arthropod-borne viral pathogens carried by mosquitoes or ticks that produce clinical manifestations in humans. The **mosquito-borne pathogens** include togaviruses (most of which are of the genus *Alphavirus,* including Western, Eastern, Venezuelan equine encephalitis, chikungunya, and Mayaro virus), flaviviruses (West Nile, St. Louis encephalitis [whose epidemiology shows a westward migration in the United States], Japanese encephalitis, Murray Valley encephalitis, dengue, Zika, yellow fever, and Rocio viruses), and orthobunyaviruses (the California serogroup viruses, including the Jamestown Canyon [seen largely in northeastern states], La Crosse [seen in the upper Midwest and mid-Atlantic primarily], and Keystone viruses). The **tick-borne** causes of encephalitis include the flaviviruses Powassan virus (North American Northeast and Great Lakes) and tick-borne encephalitis virus (Europe and Asia), as well as the Colorado tick fever reovirus. Only those viruses causing primarily encephalitis in the United States are discussed here. The most commonly encountered arboviruses from 2019 in the United States are West Nile virus (971 cases, 83% of arboviral disease), the La Crosse virus (556 cases, 5%), Jamestown Canyon virus (45 cases, 4%), Powassan virus (43 cases, 4%), and Eastern equine encephalitis, 38 cases, 3%). Rarer causes of domestic arboviruses were St. Louis encephalitis virus (17 cases, 1%) and four ungrouped California encephalitis cases. Of these cases, 802 (68%) were considered neuroinvasive. A cluster of four cases of Eastern equine encephalitis occurred in Eastern Connecticut in 2019.

West Nile virus is the leading cause of domestically acquired arboviral disease in the United States. West Nile virus disease is a nationally notifiable condition. Among the 971 cases reported in 2019, based on preliminary data from the CDC from 43 states and the District of Columbia, 633 (65%) were classified as neuroinvasive disease. The states reporting the most cases of neuroinvasive disease are in the west and southwest and include California (147 cases), Arizona (132 cases), Colorado (52 cases), Nevada (34 cases), and New Mexico (30 cases). Asymptomatic seroconversion is the norm and is not reported.

Outbreaks with West Nile infection tend to occur between mid-July and early September. Climatic factors, including elevated mean temperatures and rainfall, correlate with increased West Nile infection. West Nile virus circulates between mosquitoes (mainly *Culex* species) and birds. In case of West Nile virus outbreak, infected birds develop high level viremia that leads to substantial avian mortality and a high incidence of mosquito infection. Infected mosquitoes bite and infect people and other mammals. However, humans and other mammals are "dead end" hosts since they do not transmit the virus on to other biting mosquitoes; only dengue and Venezuelan equine encephalitis viruses produce viremias high enough to allow continued transmission to other mosquitoes and ticks between humans and vectors. Human-to-human transmission is usually related to blood transfusion and organ transplantation. Since 2003, all blood donations in the United States are screened with nucleic acid amplification assays for West Nile virus. Eastern equine encephalitis is now also shown to be transmitted by organ transplantation. The Powassan encephalitis virus has been transmitted via renal transplantation.

Clinical Findings

A. Symptoms and Signs

West Nile virus infection has an incubation period of 2–14 days. The infection is symptomatic in about 20% of the cases and less than 1% progress to neuroinvasive disease, including meningitis, encephalitis, and flaccid paralysis. The case fatality rate is 3–15% in symptomatic patients.

Symptoms include acute febrile illness, and a nonpruritic maculopapular rash is variably present. Meningitis is indistinguishable from other viral meningitis. West Nile virus encephalitis presents with fever and altered mental status. Other signs include tremors, seizures, cranial nerve palsies, Bell palsy, and other pathologic reflexes. Acute flaccid (poliomyelitis-like) paralysis, which is asymmetric and can involve facial and respiratory muscles, is a well-known complication and is less commonly seen with other arboviruses infection. West Nile virus can also present as Guillain-Barré syndrome with radiculopathy. The disease manifestations associated with West Nile virus infection are strongly age-dependent: the acute febrile syndrome and mild neurologic symptoms are more common in the young, aseptic meningitis and poliomyelitis-like syndromes are seen in middle-aged persons, and frank encephalopathy is seen more often in older adults. All forms of disease tend to be severe in immunocompromised persons in whom neuroinvasive manifestations and associated high mortality are more apt to develop. Other risk factors for development of neuroinvasive disease and increased mortality include Black race, diabetes, CKD, and hepatitis C virus infection.

Host genetic variation in the interferon response pathway is associated with both risk for symptomatic West Nile virus infection and increased likelihood of West Nile virus disease progression. Quasispecies intrahost variation is also documented for Eastern equine encephalitis.

B. Laboratory Findings

The peripheral WBC count is typically normal. Usually, a CSF lymphocytic pleocytosis is present, and polymorphonuclear cells predominate early. The diagnosis of arboviral encephalitides depends on serologic tests. For West Nile virus, an IgM capture ELISA in serum or CSF is almost always positive by the time the disease is clinically evident, and the presence of IgM in CSF indicates neuroinvasive disease. Documentation of a fourfold increase in acute/convalescent IgG titers is confirmatory for all arboviruses. Antibodies to arboviruses persist for life, and the presence of IgG in the absence of a rising titer of IgM may indicate past exposure rather than acute infection. Serologic tests are available commercially and through local and state health departments. Cross-reactivity exists among the different flaviviruses, so a plaque reduction assay may be needed to definitively distinguish between West Nile fever, St. Louis encephalitis, and others. PCR assays (available through state laboratories and the CDC) can be used to detect viral RNA in serum, CSF, or tissue early after illness onset and may be particularly useful in immunocompromised patients with abnormal antibody responses. Blood products are best screened using nucleic acid assays. MRI of the brain may reveal leptomeningeal, basal ganglia, thalamic, or periventricular enhancement.

Differential Diagnosis

Mild forms of encephalitis must be differentiated from aseptic meningitis, lymphocytic choriomeningitis, and nonparalytic poliomyelitis. A concurrent outbreak of West Nile and St. Louis encephalitis in 2015 in Maricopa County, Arizona, showed that distinguishing the two clinically may be difficult.

Severe forms of arbovirus encephalitides are to be differentiated from other causes of viral encephalitis (HSV, mumps virus, poliovirus or other enteroviruses, HIV), encephalitis accompanying exanthematous diseases of childhood (measles, varicella, infectious mononucleosis, rubella), encephalitis following vaccination or infection (a demyelinating type seen after rabies, measles, pertussis vaccination), toxic encephalitis (from drugs, poisons, or bacterial toxins such as *Shigella dysenteriae* type 1), Reye syndrome, and severe forms of stroke, brain tumors, brain abscess, autoimmune processes such as lupus cerebritis, and intoxications. In the California Encephalitis Project, anti-*N*-methyl-D-aspartate receptor (anti-NMDAR) encephalitis is a more common cause of encephalitis than viral diseases, especially in the young, with 65% of cases of encephalitis due to anti-NMDAR occurring among patients 18 or younger.

Complications

Bronchial pneumonia, urinary retention and infection, prolonged weakness, and pressure injuries may occur. Retinopathy occurs in 24% of patients with a history of West Nile virus infection and is associated with increased risk in those with encephalitis. Individuals with chronic symptoms after West Nile virus infection may show persistent kidney infection for up to 6 years with West Nile virus RNA present in urine; kidney infection may lead to progressive renal pathology.

Treatment

Although specific antiviral therapy is not available for most causative entities, vigorous supportive measures can be helpful. Some studies suggest improved outcomes with the use of IVIG enriched with West Nile virus antibody; however, a randomized, controlled trial of IVIG did *not* show a benefit.

Prognosis

Although most infections are mild or asymptomatic, the prognosis is always guarded, especially at the extremes of age. Most fatalities occur with neuroinvasive disease. The majority of patients with non-neuroinvasive West Nile virus disease or West Nile virus meningitis recover completely, but a syndrome of fatigue, malaise, and weakness can linger for weeks or months. Patients who recover from West Nile virus encephalitis or poliomyelitis often have residual neurologic deficits. The recovery of persons with severe neurologic compromise may take 6 months or longer. The sequelae of West Nile virus infection include a poliomyelitis-like syndrome, cognitive complaints, movement disorders, epilepsy, and depression; and they may become apparent late in the course of what appears to be a successful recovery.

Another entity (nonprimary infection), characterized by elevated serum IgG, absent serum IgM, and occasional detection of West Nile virus RNA in blood or CSF, is associated with underlying psychiatric disorders, hospitalization during times not associated with peak West Nile transmission, fever, and increased in-hospital mortality.

The long-term prognosis is generally better for Western equine than for Eastern equine or St. Louis encephalitis.

Prevention

Mosquito avoidance (repellents, protective clothing, and insecticide spraying) is effective prevention. Laboratory precautions are indicated for handling all these pathogens. No human vaccine is currently available for the arboviruses prevalent in North America. A chimeric live attenuated West Nile virus vaccine is tested in phase 2 clinical trials and is shown to be safe and immunogenic in healthy adults. No licensed treatment protects against the other arboviral encephalitis.

McDonald E et al. West Nile virus and other domestic nationally notifiable arboviral diseases—United States, 2018. MMWR Morb Mortal Wkly Rep. 2019;68:673. [PMID: 31393865]

Stromberg ZR et al. Vaccine advances against Venezuelan, eastern, and western equine encephalitis viruses. Vaccines (Basel). 2020;8:273. [PMID: 32503232]

Vahey GM et al. West Nile virus and other domestic nationally notifiable arboviral diseases—United States, 2019. MMWR Morb Mortal Wkly Rep 2021;70:1069. [PMID: 34383731]

3. Japanese Encephalitis

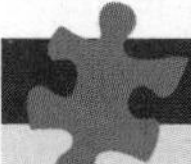

ESSENTIALS OF DIAGNOSIS

- Most important vaccine-preventable cause of encephalitis in the Asia-Pacific region.
- The virus is transmitted by mosquitoes, especially *Culex* species.
- Wide symptom spectrum; most infections asymptomatic.

General Considerations

The Japanese encephalitis virus is a flavivirus akin to those causing West Nile infection and St. Louis encephalitis. It is the most common cause of encephalitis in East Asia with over 68,000 estimated annual cases and up to 20,400 annual deaths. It is geographically confined to East Asia and the Western Pacific. Most cases occur in the summer and late fall, although in tropical and subtropical areas transmission occurs throughout the year. Major outbreaks every 2–15 years often correlate with patterns of agricultural development. The virus is transmitted by mosquitoes, especially *Culex* species. Areas with high endemicity tend to be warm-temperate, semitropical or tropical areas with high annual rainfalls. Wading birds (such as herons) and pigs more commonly sustain the infection as reservoirs in nature, since the viremia in humans is transient and not usually high enough to sustain transmission. In endemic countries, Japanese encephalitis is primarily a disease of children. Travelers to major urban areas for less than 1 month are at minimal risk for Japanese encephalitis. Transmission by blood transfusion is documented.

Clinical Findings

A. Symptoms and Signs

The median incubation period is 5–15 days. Most persons asymptomatically seroconvert. The 1% of patients in whom disease develops report sudden-onset headaches, nausea, and vomiting, followed by mental status changes, parkinsonian movement disorders, and in a smaller percentage, seizures, typically in children.

Japanese encephalitis most closely resembles St. Louis encephalitis and West Nile encephalitis, although epidemiologic data readily distinguish these infections in most instances. The clinical course is less severe in patients with a history of dengue virus infection.

B. Laboratory Findings and Diagnosis

The disease should be suspected in persons with symptoms of CNS infection who recently visited or who reside in an endemic area.

Common laboratory abnormalities include leukocytosis, mild anemia, and hyponatremia. CSF typically has a mild to moderate pleocytosis with a lymphocytic predominance, slightly elevated protein, and normal glucose.

Diagnosis is confirmed by finding anti-Japanese encephalitis virus IgM in CSF or serum using ELISA. Definitive diagnosis requires fourfold increase in virus-specific IgG confirmed by plaque reduction neutralization assay. Because of low levels of viremia in humans, RT-PCR is not recommended. A point-of-care simple diagnostic assay is needed.

In severe disease, brain imaging reveals thalamic lesions, with the hippocampus, midbrain, basal ganglia, and cerebral cortex affected to varying degrees.

Complications

A variety of cognitive, neurologic, and psychiatric complications, including memory impairment and intellectual impairment in adults and children, are recognized to occur in as many as 30–50% of survivors and to persist at least 1–2 years after the acute infection. Opsoclonus myoclonus syndrome is rarely reported. The mortality is as high as 20–30%.

Severe complications appear to be associated with upregulation of certain inflammasome genes.

Treatment

Treatment is supportive, including antipyretics, analgesics, bed rest, and fluids. Corticosteroids may result in clinical improvement of opsoclonus myoclonus syndrome.

Prevention

Using mosquito repellents; wearing long sleeves, long pants, and socks; and using air-conditioned facilities and bed nets are essential means of protection.

In the United States, formalin inactivated Vero cell culture-derived Japanese encephalitis vaccine (IXIARO) is licensed for the prevention of Japanese encephalitis in non-pregnant persons 2 months of age or older. Travelers who plan to spend more than 1 month in endemic areas should receive the vaccine. Vaccine should also be considered for travelers who plan to spend less than 1 month in endemic areas but who are at increased risk for Japanese encephalitis (based on season, location, activities). Primary vaccination requires two doses administered 28 days apart, to be completed more than 1 week before travel. For adults, a booster dose is recommended in case of potential reexposure or of continued risk for infection if the primary series of the vaccine was administered over a 1 year before.

At least eight effective types of vaccine against Japanese encephalitis are available worldwide, including live attenuated and inactivated vaccines. The benefits of a third dose of the vaccine are established among Korean children. The risk of serious reactions, including potential encephalitis with live vaccines, is low and decreases with age. Rare reported neurologic reactions are not definitively associated with vaccination. The CV (ChimeriVax-JE, marketed as IMOJEV) vaccine from India is shown in Taiwan to be particularly safe. No studies exist detailing the safety of IXIARO in pregnant women. Therefore, administration of this vaccine to pregnant women should be deferred, unless the risk of infection outweighs the risk of vaccine complications.

Bharucha T et al. A need to raise the bar—a systematic review of temporal trends in diagnostics for Japanese encephalitis virus infection, and perspectives for future research. Int J Infect Dis. 2020;95:444. [PMID: 32205287]

Hills SL et al. Japanese encephalitis vaccine: recommendations of the Advisory Committee on Immunization Practices. MMWR Recomm Rep. 2019;68:1. [PMID: 31518342]

Kwak BO et al. Immunogenicity and safety of the third booster dose of the inactivated Japanese encephalitis vaccine in Korean children: a prospective multicenter study. Vaccine. 2021;39:1929. [PMID: 33712352]

World Health Organization. Japanese encephalitis: fact sheet. May 2019. https://www.who.int/news-room/fact-sheets/detail/japanese-encephalitis

4. Tick-Borne Encephalitis

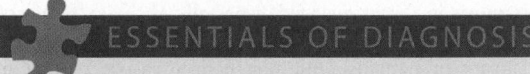

- Flaviviral encephalitis found in Eastern, Central, and occasionally Northern Europe and Asia.
- Transmitted via ticks or ingestion of unpasteurized milk.
- Long-term neurologic sequelae in 2–25% of cases.
- Therapy is largely supportive.
- Prevention: avoid tick exposure, pasteurize milk, and vaccinate.

General Considerations

Tick-borne encephalitis (TBE) is a flaviviral infection caused by TBE virus with three subtypes: **European**, **Siberian**, and **Far Eastern.** The principal reservoirs and vectors for TBE virus are ticks with small rodents as the amplifying host; humans are an accidental host. The vectors for most cases are *Ixodes ricinus* (European subtype) and *Ixodes persulcatus* (Siberian and Far Eastern subtype) but *Dermatocenter reticularis* is also a vector. Infection results from tick bites during outdoor activities in forested areas (it is known to predominate in a "beech climate"), predominantly in the late spring through fall. Ingestion of unpasteurized milk from viremic livestock (goats, sheep, and cattle) is also a recognized mode of transmission. Transmission by transplantation of solid organs is reported leading to fatal outcomes. TBE is endemic in certain parts of Europe (where its prevalence has been expanding in recent years), Asia (principally China but a few cases from Japan as well), and where a variety of subtypes extend beyond the original three (Western, Siberian, and Far Eastern). The WHO reports 10,000–12,000 cases per year, a number considered a gross underestimate, with the actual number of reported cases annually fluctuating significantly depending on surveillance, human activities, socioeconomic factors, ecology, and climate. The incubation period is 7–14 days for tick-borne exposures but only 3–4 days for milk ingestion.

Powassan virus is the only North American member of the tick-borne encephalitides. Its vector is several *Ixodes* species ticks. Most cases occur in older men (median age, 62; all deaths have occurred in persons over age 50), primarily from Northeast and North Central states (especially Minnesota, New York, and Wisconsin). It is also reported from Canada and Russia. Most reported cases are neuroinvasive with presentations including acute encephalitis and aseptic meningitis. The incubation period can range from 1 to 5 weeks, although pinpointing the date of actual exposure is often difficult.

Alkhurma hemorrhagic fever is also caused by a flavivirus first uncovered in Jeddah, Saudi Arabia, in 1995 and is reemerging in the Middle East with occurrences in tourists to Egypt, Djibouti, and possibly India. Its extent of geographic distribution is currently unknown.

Clinical Findings

A. Symptoms and Signs

Most cases are subclinical, and many resemble an influenza-like syndrome with 2–10 days of fever (usually with malaise, headache, and myalgias). In some cases, the disease is biphasic where the initial flu-like period is followed by a 1- to 21-day symptom-free interval followed by a second phase with fevers and neurologic symptoms (cases from Asia appear not to show this biphasic pattern). The neurologic manifestations range from febrile headache to aseptic meningitis and encephalitis with or without myelitis (preferentially of the cervical anterior horn) and spinal paralysis (usually flaccid). A myeloradiculitic form can also develop but is less common. Peripheral facial palsies, sometimes bilateral, tend to occur infrequently late in the course of infection, usually after encephalitis and generally are associated with a favorable outcome within 30–90 days. The main sequela of disease is paresis. Other causes of long-term morbidity include protracted cognitive dysfunction and persistent spinal nerve paralysis.

The **post-encephalitic syndrome** is characterized by headache, difficulties concentrating, balance disorders, dysphasia, hearing defects, and chronic fatigue. A progressive motor neuron disease and partial continuous epilepsy are complications. Longstanding psychiatric complications are reported and include attention deficits, slowness of thought and learning impairment, depression, lability, and mutism.

Mortality in TBE is usually a consequence of brain edema or bulbar involvement.

B. Laboratory Findings and Diagnosis

Leukopenia alternating with leukocytosis can be seen. Abnormal CSF findings include an inconsistent pleocytosis that may persist for up to 4 months. Hyponatremia is more commonly seen than with other viral encephalitides. Neuroimaging might show hyperintense lesions in the thalamus, brainstem, and basal ganglia, and cerebral atrophy.

When neurologic symptoms develop, the TBE virus is typically no longer detectable in blood and CSF samples. Virus detection by RT-PCR in ticks from TBE patients, if available, can help with the diagnosis. TBE virus IgM and IgG are detected by ELISA when neurologic symptoms occur.

Cross-reactivity with other flaviviruses or a vaccinated state may require confirmation by detection of TBE virus–specific antibodies by plaque reduction neutralization tests.

Differential Diagnosis

The differential diagnosis includes other causes of aseptic meningitis, such as enteroviral infections; poliomyelitis (no longer reported from Eastern Europe); herpes simplex encephalitis; and a variety of tick-borne pathogens, including tularemia, the rickettsial diseases, babesiosis, Lyme disease, and other flaviviral infections. Coinfections are documented with *Anaplasma, Babesia,* and *Borrelia* infections.

Treatment

No specific antiviral treatment is available, and therapy is largely supportive. Recombinant antibody therapy is under development.

Prognosis

The three subtypes of TBE have different prognoses. The European subtype is usually milder with up to 2% mortality and 30% neuroinvasive disease. The Siberian subtype is associated with 3% mortality and chronic, progressive disease. The Far Eastern subtype is usually more severe with up to 40% mortality and higher likelihood of neurologic involvement. All three subtypes are more severe among older adults compared with children. Coinfection with *Borrelia burgdorferi* (the agent of Lyme disease; transmitted by the same tick vector) may result in more severe disease.

Prevention

Four inactivated TBE virus vaccines for adults and children are licensed: three in Europe and one in China. TicoVac (known as FSME-Immun in Europe) was approved for use in the United States in 2021. The vaccine is safe and effective and should provide cross-protection against all three TBE virus subtypes. The initial vaccination schedule requires two to three doses given over 6 or more months with boosters every 1–5 years (10 years in Switzerland and Finland), with the interval dependent on the vaccine and national guidelines. Breakthrough TBE in vaccinated individuals is reported, especially among recipients who are over 50 years of age and among persons who are immunosuppressed, such as those receiving anti-TNF therapy or methotrexate, indicating the need for a modified immunization strategy in such patients. Data support adding an extra booster vaccine dose for individuals aged 50 years and older. Neuritis and neuropathies of peripheral nerves (plexus neuropathy—paresis of lower limb muscles, polyradiculopathy) are recognized complications of TBE vaccination. The vaccine is indicated for those residing and traveling to endemic areas (and the disease is now extending to higher altitudes with climate change).

The low popular support for the vaccine in endemic countries is responsible for limited abilities to control the disease. Other prevention recommendations include avoidance of tick exposure and pasteurization of cow and goat milk.

Hansson KE et al. Tick-borne encephalitis (TBE) vaccine failures: a ten-year retrospective study supporting the rationale for adding an extra priming dose in individuals at age 50 years. Clin Infect Dis. 2020;70:245. [PMID: 30843030]

Kunze U et al. Report of the 21st Annual Meeting of the International Scientific Working Group on Tick-Borne Encephalitis (ISW-TBE): TBE – record year 2018. Ticks Tick Borne Dis. 2020;11:101287. [PMID: 31522919]

Ličková M et al. Dermacentor reticulatus is a vector of tick-borne encephalitis virus. Ticks Tick Borne Dis. 2020;11: 101414. [PMID: 32173297]

5. Lymphocytic Choriomeningitis

ESSENTIALS OF DIAGNOSIS

- "Influenza-like" prodrome of fever, chills, and cough, followed by a meningeal phase.
- Aseptic meningitis: stiff neck, headache, vomiting, lethargy.
- CSF: slight increase of protein, lymphocytic pleocytosis (500–3000/mcL [0.5–3.0 × 10^9/L]).
- Complement-fixing antibodies within 2 weeks.

General Considerations

The lymphocytic choriomeningitis virus is an arenavirus (related to the pathogen causing Lassa fever, discussed below) that primarily infects the CNS. Its main reservoir is the house mouse (*Mus musculus*), and the prevalence of LCM correlates with the expansion of rodents. Other rodents (such as rats, guinea pigs, porcupines, and even pet hamsters), monkeys, shrews, dogs, and swine are also potential reservoirs. The infected animal sheds lymphocytic choriomeningitis virus in nasal secretions, urine, and feces; transmission to humans probably occurs through aerosolized particles and mucosal exposure, percutaneous inoculation, direct contact, or animal bites.

The disease in humans is underdiagnosed and occurs most often in autumn. The lymphocytic choriomeningitis virus is typically not spread person to person, although vertical transmission is reported, and it is considered to be an underrecognized teratogen. Rare cases related to solid organ transplantation and autopsies of infected individuals are also reported. All reported cases were donor-derived. Outbreaks are uncommon, and usually occur in laboratory settings among those workers with significant rodent exposure.

The ubiquitous nature of its reservoir and the large distribution of the reported cases (reports from Croatia, Czechia, Gabon, and Iraq add to the list of endemic countries), suggest a widespread geographic risk of lymphocytic choriomeningitis virus infection. Serologic surveys in the United States show significant variability in prior infection, from less than 1% in New York to 3–5% in southern and eastern United States.

Clinical Findings

A. Symptoms and Signs

The incubation period is 8–13 days to the appearance of systemic manifestations and 15–21 days to the appearance of meningeal symptoms. Symptoms are biphasic, with a prodromal illness characterized by fever, chills, headache, myalgia, cough, and vomiting, occasionally with lymphadenopathy and maculopapular rash. After 3–5 days, the fever subsides only to return after 2–4 days along with the meningeal phase, characterized by headache, nausea and vomiting, lethargy, and variably present meningeal signs. Arthralgias can develop late in the course. Transverse myelitis, deafness, Guillain-Barré syndrome, and transient and permanent hydrocephalus are reported. Lymphocytic choriomeningitis virus is a well-known, albeit underrecognized, cause of congenital infection frequently complicated with obstructive hydrocephalus, intracerebral calcifications, and chorioretinitis. In fetuses and newborns with ventriculomegaly or other abnormal neuroimaging findings, screening for congenital lymphocytic choriomeningitis may be considered; mothers are asymptomatic half the time. In over one-third of cases, rodent exposure is reported retrospectively. Occasionally, a syndrome resembling the viral hemorrhagic fevers is described in transplant recipients of infected organs and in patients with lymphoma.

B. Laboratory Findings

Leukocytosis or leukopenia and thrombocytopenia may be initially present. During the meningeal phase, CSF analysis frequently shows lymphocytic pleocytosis (total count is often 500–3000/mcL [0.5–3.0 × 10^9/L]) with a slight increase in protein, while a low to normal glucose is seen in at least 25%. The virus may be recovered from the blood and CSF by mouse inoculation. Complement-fixing antibodies appear during or after the second week. Detection of specific IgM by ELISA is widely used. Detection of lymphocytic choriomeningitis virus by PCR is available in research settings.

Differential Diagnosis

The influenza-like prodrome and latent period may distinguish this from other aseptic meningitides, and bacterial and granulomatous meningitis. A history of exposure to mice or other potential vectors is an important diagnostic clue.

Treatment

Treatment is supportive. In several survivors of transplant-associated outbreaks, ribavirin (which is effective against other arenaviruses) has been used successfully along with decreasing immunosuppression.

Prognosis

Complications and fatalities are rare in the general population. The illness usually lasts 1–2 weeks, though convalescence may be prolonged. Congenital infection is more severe with about 30% mortality rate among infected infants, and more than 90% of survivors suffering long-term neurologic abnormalities. Lymphocytic choriomeningitis in solid organ transplant recipients is associated with a poor prognosis; the mortality rate may exceed 80%.

Prevention

Pregnant women should be advised of the dangers to their unborn children inherent in exposure to rodents. Infection risk can be reduced by limiting contact with pet rodents and rodent trappings.

Fornůsková A et al. New perspective on the geographic distribution and evolution of lymphocytic choriomeningitis virus, Central Europe. Emerg Infect Dis. 2021;27:2638. [PMID: 34545789]

Vilibic-Cavlek T et al. Lymphocytic choriomeningitis—emerging trends of a neglected virus: a narrative review. Trop Med. Infect Dis 2021;6:88. [PMID: 34070581]

6. Prion Diseases

ESSENTIALS OF DIAGNOSIS

- Rare in humans.
- Cognitive decline.
- Myoclonic fasciculations, ataxia, visual disturbances, pyramidal and extrapyramidal symptoms.
- Variant form presents in younger persons with prominent psychiatric or sensory symptoms.
- Specific EEG patterns.

General Considerations

The **transmissible spongiform encephalopathies** are a group of fatal neurodegenerative diseases affecting humans and animals. They are caused by proteinaceous infectious particles or **prions.** These agents show slow replicative capacity and long latent intervals in the host. They induce the conformational change ("misfolding") of a normal brain protein (prion protein; PrP[C]) into an abnormal isoform (PrP[Sc]) that accumulates and causes neuronal vacuolation (spongiosis), reactive proliferation of astrocytes and microglia, and, in some cases, the deposition of beta-amyloid oligomeric plaques.

Prion disease can be hereditary, sporadic, or transmissible in humans. **Hereditary** disorders are caused by germ line mutations in the PrP[C] gene causing familial Creutzfeldt-Jakob disease (fCJD), Gerstmann-Sträussler-Scheinker syndrome, and fatal familial insomnia. Another uncommon hereditary disorder is PrP systemic amyloidosis.

Sporadic Creutzfeldt-Jakob disease (sCJD) is the most common of the human prion diseases, accounting for approximately 85% of cases; it has no known cause. Transmissible prion disease is described only for kuru and Creutzfeldt-Jakob disease in its **iatrogenic (iCJD)** and **variant (vCJD)** form. Iatrogenic transmission of CJD is associated with prion contaminated human corneas, dura mater grafts, pituitary-derived growth hormone, gonadotropins, stereotactic electroencephalography, electrodes, and neurosurgical instruments. A subset of cases with a history of neurosurgical intervention shows hyperintense thalamic lesions but no periodic sharp wave complexes on EEG (which may be a presymptomatic sign for most cases of sCJD). Abnormal prion proteins have been detected in the nasal mucosa and urine of patients with Creutzfeldt-Jakob disease, raising health concerns about possibility of transmission.

Kuru, once prevalent in central New Guinea, is now rare, a decline in prevalence that started after the abandonment of cannibalism in the late 1950s (a protective allele of the PrP gene is now identified at codon 127).

More than 200 cases of vCJD (**bovine spongiform encephalopathy** [BSE] or "mad cow disease") were reported in the United Kingdom since the first documented cases there in the mid-1990s. It is far less common in North America, with only four cases reported in the United States (the last one in 2015) and two deaths in Canada from definite or probable vCJD. Of the US-reported cases, none are confirmed to have acquired the disease locally (two of them acquired the infection in the United Kingdom, one in Saudi Arabia, one possibly in a Middle Eastern or Eastern European country). The overall annual incidence of prion disease worldwide is approximately 1–2 persons per million. This disease is characterized by its bovine-to-human transmission through ingestion of meat from cattle infected with BSE. BSE does not spread from animal to animal, and milk and its derived products are not considered infectious. Reports of secondary transmission of vCJD due to blood transfusions from asymptomatic donors are reported in the United Kingdom.

A **chronic wasting disease** also due to a transmissible spongiform encephalopathic agent is increasing; occurs among deer, elk, and moose; and is reported from 26 states including most of Wyoming and parts of Colorado but present in the East and South as well. Although no cases of transmission to humans are documented, transmission in the laboratory to squirrel monkeys has occurred, and the CDC recommends refraining from killing bizarrely acting animals, not handling or eating roadkill, and wearing gloves when dressing wild game. Testing for the virus in game animals may be useful, but its efficacy is not established.

Clinical Findings

A. Symptoms and Signs

Both sCJD and fCJD usually present in the sixth or seventh decade of life, whereas the iCJD form tends to occur in a much younger population. Clinical features of these three forms of disease usually involve mental deterioration (dementia, behavioral changes, loss of cortical function) that is progressive over several months, as well as myoclonus and extrapyramidal (hypokinesia) and cerebellar manifestations (ataxia, dysarthria). Finally, coma ensues, usually associated with an akinetic state and less commonly decerebrate/decorticate posturing. Like iCJD, vCJD usually affects younger patients (averaging ~28 years), but the duration of disease is longer (about 1 year). The degree of organ involvement is often extensive, and the clinical symptoms are unique, mainly characterized by prominent psychiatric and sensory symptoms.

B. Laboratory Findings

CJD should be diagnosed in the proper clinical scenario, in the absence of alternative diagnoses after routine investigations. Abnormalities in CSF are subtle and rarely helpful. The detection of 14-3-3 protein in the CSF is helpful for the diagnosis of sCJD but not in vCJD and fCJD. Its sensitivity and specificity are widely variable among different studies and may be increased with use of tau protein assays. CSF detection of total PrP can differentiate CJD from atypical Alzheimer disease with 82% sensitivity and 91% specificity.

A blood-based assay and PCR in CSF may help with the diagnosis of vCJD with high specificity but 71% sensitivity. The assay as well as 14-3-3 protein assay and a "quaking induced conversion" assay are all available through the National Prion Disease Surveillance Center at Case Western University in Cleveland. Other referral laboratories with variable availability of assays include state health departments, academic centers, and the National Prion Clinics in the United Kingdom. It is also recognized that the presence of a variant with low titers ("very low peripheral prion colonization") in peripheral tissue, including frequently biopsied tonsillar tissue, may be responsible for the underrecognition of vCJD. A skin biopsy using a prion "real-time quaking induced conversion" (RT-QuIC) is under study and may be emerging as the most sensitive diagnostic tool for sCJD, showing 89% sensitivity and 100% specificity.

Probable diagnosis requires the presence of rapidly progressive dementia plus two of four clinical features (myoclonus, visual or cerebellar signs, pyramidal/extrapyramidal signs, and akinetic mutism) as well as a positive laboratory assay (typical EEG, positive 14-3-3 CSF assay with duration under 2 years) and MRI high signal in the caudate or putamen on diffusion-weighted imaging, or both, or fluid-attenuated inversion recovery (FLAIR) imaging. In sCJD, the EEG typically shows a pattern of paroxysms with high voltages and slow waves, while the MRI is characteristic for bilateral areas of increased signal intensity, predominantly in the caudate and putamen. MRI findings of cortical and subcortical atrophy occur in both fast and slow progressors. An MRI can improve early diagnosis of sCJD because clinical findings are often missed. When an experienced neuroradiologist or a prion disease expert reviews the MRI, diagnostic sensitivity of MRI for sCJD increases to 91%.

Differential Diagnosis

Autoimmune encephalitis can have a similar clinical picture. The presence of high-titer autoantibodies (eg, to the NMDA receptor) in the CSF is consistent with autoimmune encephalitis. A presentation suggesting cerebrovascular accident can also be seen with sCJD, complicating the diagnostic profile.

Treatment & Prevention

CJD does not have a specific treatment. Once symptoms appear, the infection invariably leads to death. Flupirtine (an analgesic medication) is sometimes useful in slowing the associated cognitive decline but does not affect survival. Quinacrine (mepacrine) was not shown to improve survival for people with sCJD. Antibodies against PrP are also proposed as a therapeutic strategy. Studies are in progress to identify epitopes for vaccine development, but no promising candidates exist to date.

Iatrogenic CJD can be prevented by limiting patient exposure to potentially infectious sources as mentioned above. Prevention of vCJD relies on monitoring livestock for possible infection. The American Red Cross does not accept blood donations from persons with a family history of CJD or with a history of dural grafts or pituitary-derived growth hormone injections.

An international referral and database for CJD is available at http://www.cjdsurveillance.com.

Flones I et al. Mitochondrial respiratory chain deficiency correlates with the severity of neuropathology in sporadic Creutzfeldt-Jakob disease. Acta Neuropathol Commun. 2020; 8:50. [PMID: 32299489]

Mammana A et al. Detection of prions in skin punch biopsies of Creutzfeldt–Jakob disease patients. Ann Clin Transl Neurol. 2020;7:559. [PMID: 32141717]

Younes K et al. Selective vulnerability to atrophy in sporadic Creutzfeldt-Jakob disease. Ann Clin Transl Neurol. 2021; 8:1183. [PMID: 33949799]

7. Progressive Multifocal Leukoencephalopathy (PML)

PML is a rare demyelinating CNS disorder caused by the reactivation of two polyoma viruses, the **JC virus** (John Cunningham virus or JCV) and, less commonly, the **BK virus** (associated with nephropathy). The JC virus usually causes its primary infection during childhood with about 80% of adults typically being seropositive. The virus remains latent in the kidneys, lymphoid tissues, epithelial cells, peripheral blood leukocytes, bone marrow, and possibly brain until *reactivation* occurs and symptoms become evident. This reactivation is usually seen in adults with impaired cell-mediated immunity, especially AIDS patients (5–10% of whom develop PML and who comprise 46% of cases in a German series), as well as those with idiopathic CD4 lymphopenia syndrome. It is also reported among those with lymphoproliferative and myeloproliferative disorders; in those with granulomatous, inflammatory, and rheumatic diseases (SLE and rheumatoid arthritis in particular); in those who have undergone solid and hematopoietic cell transplantation; and occasionally in those who have other medical states, including cirrhosis and kidney disease. Diagnostic criteria that use clinical, imaging, pathologic, and virologic manifestations of JCV are available from the American Academy of Neurology.

Medication-associated PML is described with the use of natalizumab, rituximab, infliximab, alemtuzumab, azathioprine with corticosteroids, cyclophosphamide, and mycophenolate mofetil. Natalizumab, a monoclonal antibody used in the treatment of multiple sclerosis, is associated with the risk of PML developing in 4 per 1000 treated patients, with the rate increasing with duration of therapy. The risk of clinical PML appears to increase up to 36 months of therapy and levels off thereafter. The mean interval between use of the medication to the diagnosis of PML is 5.5 months. JCV is detected in the CSF of up to one-half of all patients treated with natalizumab. An immune reconstitution inflammatory state (IRIS) may follow cessation of natalizumab or other monoclonal antibody therapy, although the JCV presence and the residual neurologic deficits may not clear for years after therapy is stopped. The risk of developing PML associated with rituximab is at least 1 in 25,000 exposed patients with cases reported in various autoimmune conditions treated with rituximab (SLE, rheumatoid arthritis, multiple sclerosis). Although the exact relationship between latent JCV and frank PML remains unclear, higher JC viral loads are detected among patients who are immunosuppressed and among those who have HIV infection with lower CD4 cell counts.

Clinical Findings

A. Symptoms and Signs

JCV causes lytic infection of oligodendrocytes in the white matter and symptoms presenting subacutely reflect the diverse areas of CNS involvement. Symptoms include altered mental status, aphasia, ataxia, hemiparesis or hemiplegia, and visual field disturbances. Seizures occur in about 18% and status epilepticus is seen with a particular PnP variant (E200K). Involvement of cranial nerves and the cervical spine is rare.

B. Laboratory Findings

Quantitative PCR for JCV in CSF is used for diagnosis in patients with compatible clinical and radiologic findings. Persistent JC viremia and increasing urinary JCV DNA may be predictive of PML. An anti-JCV IgG was higher 6 months before diagnosis but was not predictive of PML in a cohort of people living with HIV infection. Serum neurofilament levels are increased natalizumab-treated patients with multiple sclerosis who develop PML compared with those who do not and may provide prognostic utility (specificity 67% specificity 80%).

C. Imaging

MRI of the brain shows multifocal areas of white matter demyelination without mass effect or, usually, contrast enhancement. These findings may not be distinguishable from IRIS. Increased uptake of methionine with concomitant decreased uptake of fluorodeoxyglucose in PET may be helpful for diagnosis. In people living with HIV, a syndrome of cerebellar degeneration is described. Case reports attest to the variability of MRI findings and should not be relied upon solely for diagnosis.

Treatment & Prevention

Limiting the immunosuppressed state without inducing an IRIS represents the mainstay of therapy for HIV-associated PML. Treatment of HIV with ART reduces the incidence of PML, improves the clinical symptoms, reverses some of the radiographic abnormalities, and improves the 1-year mortality rate, regardless of baseline CD4 cell count. Immune recovery can induce worsening of the clinical picture in a small number of cases. Immune reconstitution syndromes do not alter mortality but are associated with a form of PML called **non-determined leukoencephalopathy** associated with a chemokine polymorphism. Significant neurologic sequelae to PML infections are the rule and deficits may persist for years. The 24-month mortality in a German series from 2020 was 44%.

Decreasing immunosuppression in patients without HIV but with PML (eg, patients with multiple sclerosis or those who have undergone transplant) is also important. Cidofovir may be beneficial in non–HIV-related cases, while corticosteroids may be useful with immune reconstitution. Because the JCV infects cells through serotonin receptors, some clinicians recommend the use of risperidone and mirtazapine. Anecdotal reports show that premature stopping of natalizumab in multiple sclerosis may itself lead to IRIS states and that the combination of teriflunomide with interferon may hold PML symptoms in abeyance while allowing for control of underlying multiple sclerosis. Plasma exchange, which theoretically reduces the plasma level of agents associated with PML, may be useful in natalizumab-associated PML but is associated with a high risk of IRIS. In patients post-kidney transplantation, a preinduction regimen with IVIG and rituximab and transplantation with lymphocyte-depleted cells appears to reduce the risk of PML. Titers of JC antibody are not shown to significantly increase prior to clinical onset of PML in patients who have undergone solid organ transplantation.

More recently, programmed cell death protein (PD-1) inhibitor therapy (also known as "immune checkpoint inhibitor") is being evaluated for use in PML. The PD-1 inhibitor pembrolizumab reduced JC viral load and increases CD4+ and CD8+ activity against the virus in a preliminary set of eight patients with PML with different predisposing conditions. In addition, allogeneic BK virus-specific T cells are useful in lowering JC viral load.

Beck ES et al. Checkpoint inhibitors for the treatment of JC virus-related progressive multifocal leukoencephalopathy. Curr Opin Virol. 2020;40:19. [PMID: 32279025]

Fissolo N et al. Serum neurofilament levels and PML risk in patients with multiple sclerosis treated with natalizumab. Neurol Neuroimmunol Neuroinflamm. 2021;8:e1003. [PMID: 33903203]

Graf LM et al. Clinical presentation and disease course of 37 consecutive cases of progressive multifocal leukoencephalopathy (PML) at a German tertiary-care hospital: a retrospective observational study. Front Neurol. 2020;12:632535. [PMID: 33613439]

8. Human T-Cell Lymphotropic Virus (HTLV)

HTLV-1 and -2 are retroviruses that infect CD4 and CD8 T cells, respectively, where they persist as a lifelong latent infection. HTLV-1 currently infects approximately 20 million individuals worldwide. It is endemic to many regions in the world including southern Japan, the Caribbean, much of sub-Saharan Africa, South America, Eastern Europe, and Oceania. The Caribbean basin and southwestern Japan show the highest prevalence of infection (4–37%). Conversely, HTLV-2 is mainly found in native populations of South (1–58%), Central (8–10%), and North America (2–13%) as well as African pygmy tribes. In some areas of Africa (eg, Malawi), HTLV-2 seroprevalence is higher than HTLV-1 seroprevalence.

In the United States, studies done in blood donors show a seroprevalence of HTLV-1 of 0.005% and HTLV-2 of 0.014%, a decline since the early 1990s. The virus is transmitted horizontally (sex), vertically (intrauterine, peripartum, and prolonged breastfeeding), and parenterally (injection drug use and blood transfusion). Hence, a higher prevalence is seen among injection drug users. Coinfection with HIV-1 occurs (in less than 5% in a series from Spain) but is often underrecognized. Transmission via organ transplant has been reported. Disease may flare when biologic agents are used for rheumatoid conditions. HTLV-1 infection is associated with **HTLV-1 adult T-cell lymphoma/leukemia** (ATL) and **HTLV-1–associated myelopathy/tropical spastic paraparesis (HAM/TSP).** In contrast, HTLV-2 is significantly less pathogenic, with few reported cases of HAM/TSP as well as other neurologic manifestations. The causative association of HTLV-1 with ATL, attributed to the virally encoded oncoprotein *tax*, is well established.

Clinical Findings

A. Symptoms and Signs

The lifetime risk of developing ATL among HTLV-1 seropositive persons is estimated to be 3% in women and 7% in men, with an incubation period of at least 15 years. The mean age at diagnosis of ATL is 40–50 years in Central and South America and 60 years in Japan.

ATL clinical syndromes may be classified as chronic, acute (leukemic), smoldering, or lymphomatous. A primary cutaneous tumor is also described (with appearance ranging from papular lesions to exfoliative erythroderma) and shows a worse prognosis compared with the smoldering type. Clinical features of ATL include diffuse lymphadenopathy, maculopapular skin lesions that may evolve into erythroderma, periodontitis, a bronchoalveolar disorder, organomegaly, lytic bone lesions, and hypercalcemia. Opportunistic infections, such as *P jirovecii* pneumonia and cryptococcal meningitis, are common.

HAM/TSP, associated with both HTLV-1 and HTLV-2, develops in 0.3–4% of seropositive individuals and is more common in women and in older individuals. A chronic inflammation of the CNS and spinal cord leads to intense and progressive motor weakness and symmetric spastic paraparesis, bilateral facial palsies, cognitive impairment, falls, nociceptive low back pain, and paraplegia with hyperreflexia. Bladder and sexual disorders (eg, dyspareunia, erectile dysfunction), sensory disturbances, and constipation are also common. Both viruses can also induce motor abnormalities, such as leg weakness, impaired tandem walk, and vibration sense, without overt HTLV-associated myelopathy.

Studies from Brazil show that a subset of chronically inflamed patients with HTLV-1 infections may be asymptomatic and are recognized as having an "intermediate syndrome" that may progress to full blown myelopathy.

HTLV-1 seropositivity is associated with an increased risk of tuberculosis, *Strongyloides stercoralis* hyperinfection, crusted scabies, and infective dermatitis. Inflammatory states associated with HTLV-1 infection include arthropathy, recurrent facial palsies, polymyositis, uveitis, and sicca, but inconsistently Sjögren syndrome, vasculitis, cryoglobulinemia, infiltrative pneumonitis, and ichthyosis. Bronchioloalveolar carcinoma is increased in frequency in the presence of HTLV-1.

HTLV-2 appears to cause a myelopathy that is milder and slower to progress than HAM. All-cause and cancer mortality are higher among HTLV-2 seropositive patients.

HTLV-1/HIV coinfection is associated both with higher CD4 cell counts and a higher risk of HAM.

B. Laboratory Findings

The peripheral smear can show atypical lymphoid cells with basophilic cytoplasm and convoluted nuclei (flower cells). The diagnostic standard is evidence of clonal integration of the proviral DNA genome into tumor cell. The identification of HTLV-1 antibodies supports the diagnosis. Serum neopterin levels may indicate disease activity. An HTLV-1 provirus load in peripheral blood mononuclear cells and CSF cells and an HTLV-1 mRNA load are proposed as markers of HAM risk and progression. HTLV positivity is associated with erythrocytosis, lymphocytosis (HTLV-2), and thrombocytosis (HTLV-1).

Treatment, Prevention, & Prognosis

No vaccine or antiviral therapy currently exists for the prevention and treatment of HTLV infections.

Management of ATL consists mainly of chemotherapy (such as CHOP and EPOCH regimens), followed by allogeneic stem cell transplantation. Immunotherapies are increasingly used, including monoclonal antibodies (eg, the anti-CCR4 inhibitor mogamulizumab, anti-CD25 agents), spleen tyrosine kinase and Janus kinase (JAK) inhibitors (eg, cerdulatinib and ruxolitinib), and PD-1/immune checkpoint inhibitors (eg, nivolumab).

A chemotherapy regimen in Japan using eight different agents shows a higher response rate than traditional biweekly CHOP (40% versus 25%). A clinical trial is underway evaluating lenalidomide plus EPOCH (NCT04301076). Combination therapy with interferon-alpha is used with success. Prophylaxis against infections is needed in ATL because patients show a profound immunodeficiency. Patients who are coinfected with HIV-1 and HTLV reportedly do respond to ART.

HAM is treated with a variety of immune-modulating agents (including corticosteroids) without consistent results. Modalities of therapy, none of which are uniformly accepted as a mainstay, include combination therapy with the antiretroviral raltegravir alone or in combination with zidovudine; interferon-alpha; and a combination of prednisolone, pegylated interferon, and sodium valproate; pentoxifylline, cyclosporine, and the retinoid tamibarotene. Small, uncontrolled studies suggest plasmapheresis results in improvement in gait and sensory disturbance among some patients and improvement in muscle pain with pulsed methylprednisolone. Mogamulizumab has shown mixed results against T-cell lymphoma. A clinical trial evaluating tamibarotene (AM80H, also known as retinobenzoic acid) has been initiated in Japan without any results to date.

Screening of the blood supply for HTLV-1 is required in the United States. HTLV-1 and HTLV-2 have significant serologic cross-reactivity, but PCR can distinguish the two. Improved assays to screen organ donors for HTLV-1 and -2 infections are needed, although such screening is not currently required. Antenatal screening and avoiding breastfeeding (where the virus can be transmitted) are also important preventive measures.

Champs APS. Cognitive impairment in HTLV-1-associated myelopathy, proviral load and inflammatory markers. Int J Infect Dis. 2019;84:121. [PMID: 31085316]

Hirons A et al. Human T-cell lymphotropic virus type-1: a lifelong persistent infection, yet never truly silent. Lancet Infect Dis. 2021;21:e2. [PMID: 32986997]

Kannagi M et al. Impact of host immunity on HTLV-1 pathogenesis: potential of Tax-targeted immunotherapy against ATL. Retrovirology. 2019;16:23. [PMID: 31438973]

Keikha M et al. Molecular targeting of PD-1 signaling pathway as a novel therapeutic approach in HTLV-1 infection. Microb Pathog. 2020;144:104198. [PMID: 32283259]

Marino-Merlo F et al. Antiretroviral therapy in HTLV-1 infection: an updated overview. Pathogens. 2020;9:342. [PMID: 32369988]

VIRAL HEMORRHAGIC FEVERS

1. Ebola Viral Disease (EVD)

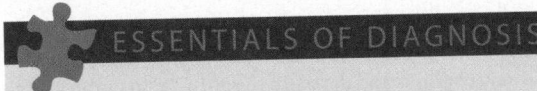

- Early-stage EVD: a nonspecific febrile illness.
- Later stage EVD: severe GI symptoms, then neurologic symptoms and hypovolemic shock.
- Hemorrhagic manifestations are late-stage manifestations.
- Uveitis is prominent.
- Travel and contact history from an Ebola-affected country raise suspicion.
- Virus is detected via RT-PCR.

General Considerations

Genus *Ebolavirus* is a single-stranded RNA virus in the Filoviridae family. Four different species of *Ebolavirus* have been identified to cause human disease. Fruit bats are possible reservoirs for *Ebolavirus*. Zoonotic transmission to humans occurs via contact with the reservoir or an infected primate. *Ebolavirus can continue to be transmitted among humans who have direct contact with infected body fluids.* To acquire EVD, the virus must enter the body via mucous membranes, nonintact skin, sexual intercourse, breastfeeding, or needlesticks. Traditional burial practices in some African communities (which entail considerable contact with the corpse) and unprotected direct care of persons with EVD are associated with highest transmission risk. *Ebolavirus* has been detected in semen up to 9 months after recovery from infection.

EVD has a 2–21-day incubation period. Prior to manifestation of symptoms, *Ebolavirus* is not transmissible. Even at symptom onset, the risk of transmission is low but increases over time.

The first Ebola outbreak occurred in 1976 as a simultaneous epidemic in the Democratic Republic of Congo and South Sudan. Subsequent outbreaks were confined to the Democratic Republic of Congo, Uganda, and Sudan until March 2014 when the first Ebola case in West Africa was identified in Guinea. *Zaire ebolavirus* was the associated species. This Ebola outbreak grew to be larger than all prior Ebola outbreaks combined. The number of EVD cases spread rapidly; there were at least 10 affected countries, especially Guinea, Liberia, and Sierra Leone. Many cases and deaths in these countries occurred among health care workers. In the United States, 11 persons were treated for Ebola; most were health care workers who were evacuated to the United States, and four cases were diagnosed in the United States. In total, approximately 30 distinct outbreaks of Ebola have occurred since 1976, mostly in Africa. The estimated case fatality rate is 60%.

Clinical Findings

A. Symptoms and Signs

At symptom onset, early-stage EVD most typically presents as a nonspecific febrile illness. Along with fever, patients tend to experience headache, weakness, dizziness, malaise, fatigue, myalgia, and arthralgia. After 3–5 days, patients with later stage EVD may develop abdominal pain, severe nausea, vomiting, and diarrhea accompanying the febrile illness. This stage of the illness may continue for a week, during which time neurologic symptoms gain prominence. Encephalitis is commonly observed and manifested as confusion, slowed cognition, agitation, and occasional seizures. Hypovolemic shock develops in most patients, but hemorrhagic manifestations (GI bleeding, diffuse mucosal bleeding, conjunctival bleeding) develop in only 1–5% of patients. Respiratory symptoms are not typical for EVD, although interstitial pneumonia and respiratory failure are reported.

B. Laboratory Findings

During the first few days of symptoms, diagnosis may be made via several modalities, including antigen-capture ELISA, IgM ELISA, RT-PCR, or virus isolation. Blood samples obtained within the first 3 days of illness and tested by a molecular method should be repeated if results are negative and clinical symptoms and signs persist. RNA levels peak a median of 7 days after illness onset. Later in the disease course or after recovery, IgM and IgG serologic tests may be sent. After about 10 days, IgM antibodies begin to develop, and, after approximately 2 weeks, an IgG antibody response develops. Postmortem diagnosis may be made by using immunohistochemistry, RT-PCR, or virus isolation. The WHO recommends automated or semi-automated nucleic acid tests (NATs) of EDTA-anticoagulated whole blood from symptomatic patients for routine diagnostic management, and rapid antigen detection tests in areas where NATs are not available. Oral fluid can be used for diagnostics when blood collection is not possible. **Importantly, patient samples are extreme biohazard risks and should be handled accordingly using appropriate personal protective equipment.**

Given that filoviruses infect dendritic cells and then hepatocytes and renal cortical cells, laboratory findings typically include a low platelet count (and a thrombotic thrombocytopenic purpura syndrome has been postulated with the probable cause multifactorial), leukopenia, and transaminitis (AST greater than ALT). As nonspecific symptoms progress to a severe systemic inflammatory response, coagulopathy with evidence of platelet dysfunction and disseminated intravascular coagulopathy (DIC) often develops. Whether DIC is a common cause of bleeding has not yet been firmly established because clinical measurements of fibrinogen, prothrombin time, fibrin-split products, and platelets are not routinely taken in the communities where most outbreaks have occurred. Additional observed laboratory abnormalities include hypoalbuminemia, electrolytes imbalance, and increased serum creatinine level. Elevated BUN, AST, and creatinine upon presentation are associated with higher mortality.

Differential Diagnosis

The differential diagnosis varies with the stage of illness. Early-stage EVD is commonly mistaken for malaria, typhoid, and other viral illnesses. As GI symptoms develop, health providers should also consider viral hepatitis, toxins, leptospirosis, and rickettsial diseases. In later stage EVD, bacterial, viral, and parasitic illnesses, including cholera and, in children, rotavirus infection can present with severe gastroenteritis and shock. Encephalitis must be differentiated from the confusion associated with uremia. Hemorrhagic manifestations raise suspicion for EVD but could be due to leukemia, thrombotic thrombocytopenic purpura, hemolytic-uremic syndrome, or DIC. Travel and contact history are crucial when considering the differential diagnosis in areas where Ebola is not endemic.

Complications

Hypovolemic shock and multiorgan failure are the most common complications of EVD. Hemorrhage can occur in late stages. Rhabdomyolysis is reported frequently and may explain many of the associated laboratory abnormalities. Coinfections with malaria or bacteria (or both) are important considerations and can occur before presentation and during treatment of EVD. The virus is known to persist in immunologically privileged sites, such as the CNS, eye, and testes; however, viral relapse is uncommon. Post-EVD musculoskeletal pain, headache, auditory symptoms including hearing loss, and ocular symptoms (uveitis being the most common ocular finding) may develop. EVD survivors exhibit high rates of neuropsychological long-term sequelae including depression, anxiety, insomnia, and PTSD.

Treatment

Treatment is primarily supportive. Several studies have shown that *intravenous fluids* can reduce the mortality rates to less than 50%. Despite the wide availability of oral rehydration salts, mortality is high, ranging from 25% to 90%. In these studies, the amount of intravenous fluid replacement was relatively less than what would be used in countries with more developed health systems. Among patients treated in the United States or Europe, almost all received intravenous fluids, electrolyte supplementation, and empiric antibiotic therapy. Invasive or noninvasive mechanical ventilation and continuous renal replacement therapy are necessary in many cases. This increased level of intervention likely contributed to the decreased mortality (19%) among these patients. The use of individual air-conditioned biosecure cubicles is preferred to the burdensome protective equipment used during the 2014 West African outbreaks and allows for more time spent with patients.

While administration of convalescent plasma does not result in improved survival, several monoclonal antibodies do. Two monoclonal antibody cocktails (Inmazeb [previously known as REGTN-EB3] and Ebanga) were approved for the treatment of infection with the *Zaire ebolavirus* species in adults and children by the United States in 2020.

Aside from supportive treatment and experimental therapeutics, patients typically receive empiric antimalarial agents in endemic areas and broad-spectrum antibiotics.

Prognosis

Children under 5 years of age and adults older than 40 have a high risk of death from EVD. Pregnancy is a risk factor for severe illness and death. In the 2014–2016 outbreak, the average maternal mortality was 86%. Immunosuppressed patients had shorter incubation time, rapid progression of disease, and poor outcomes. A higher baseline viral load was a strong predictor of mortality. In general, poor overall medical care confers a poor prognosis. Among survivors, protective antibodies persist for at least 10 years.

Prevention

Risk reduction should focus on preventing wildlife to human transmission and reducing human-to-human transmission by surveillance, early detection and isolation of cases, contact tracing, containment measures (disinfection, hygiene, and sanitation), strict droplet and contact precautions in health care setting, and reduction of sexual transmission in Ebola survivors. The WHO recommends that *men avoid sexual activity or use barrier protection* during intercourse for 12 months from onset of symptoms or until their semen tests negative twice for Ebola virus.

The recombinant vesicular stomatitis virus (rVSV)-based vaccine expressing Z ebolavirus (ZEBOV) glycoprotein (rVSV-ZEBOV, marketed as Ervebo by Merck) is the only Ebola vaccine candidate that has demonstrated clinical effectiveness. It is effective in disease prevention as soon as 10 days from vaccine administration and seems to generate a long-lived immune response. Side effects, such as fever, myalgia, chills, fatigue, headaches, and oligoarthritis, develop in most people who received the vaccine. rVSV-ZEBOV was approved by the European Medicines Agency (EMA) on November 11, 2019, and by the US FDA on December 19, 2019. A second vaccine, an adenovirus/vaccinia virus vector vaccine (marketed as Zabdeno-and-Mvabea), was approved by the EMA in 2020. It is actually a two-dose series of two different vaccines, Ad26.ZEBOV (replication-incompetent recombinant adenovirus 26 expressing the ZEBOV [Mayinga strain] glycoprotein) and MVA-BN-Filo (a nonreplicating modified vaccinia Ankara-Bavarian Nordic virus vector expressing the glycoproteins of Zaire and Sudan ebolaviruses, Marburg virus, and the nucleoprotein of Tai Forest virus), given about 8 weeks apart. This vaccine is not considered appropriate for use in situations where immediate protection is needed, such as during an outbreak. Thus, in an outbreak setting, rVSV-ZEBOV is preferred.

Risk stratification may be useful in deciding when and to whom to administer antiviral postexposure prophylaxis. A high-risk exposure is defined as penetrating sharps injury from used device or through contaminated gloves or clothing, direct contact with an infected patient (alive or deceased) or their bodily fluids with broken skin or mucous membranes such as eyes, nose, or mouth. The rVSV-ZEBOV vaccine was used in the setting of postexposure prophylaxis among health care workers and found to be effective, but the evidence is limited to case series. The vaccine-mediated immunity requires an average of 10 days to develop and might not be fast enough in certain cases to prevent infection.

The use of antiviral agents in postexposure prophylaxis is another alternative that, to date, also shows no clear survival benefit.

When to Admit

Persons living in or returning from a country with high rates of Ebola transmission should be monitored for 21 days and admitted to a health care facility when symptoms meeting the WHO case definition of a suspected EVD case develop, in accordance with the screening protocol designated by the respective country's governmental health decision-making body.

Bond NG et al. Post-Ebola syndrome presents with multiple overlapping symptom clusters: evidence from an ongoing cohort study in Eastern Sierra Leone. Clin Infect Dis. 2021;73:1046. [PMID: 33822010]

Choi MJ et al. Use of Ebola vaccine: Recommendations of the Advisory Committee on Immunization Practices, United States, 2020. MMWR Recomm Rep. 2021;70:1. [PMID: 33417593]

Kawuki J et al. Impact of recurrent outbreaks of Ebola virus disease in Africa: a meta-analysis of case fatality rates. Public Health. 2021;195:89. [PMID: 34077889]

2. Other Hemorrhagic Fevers

This diverse group of illnesses results from infection with one of several single-stranded RNA viruses (members of the families Arenaviridae, Bunyaviridae, Filoviridae, Flaviviridae, and Nairoviridae). Flaviviruses, such as the pathogens causing dengue and yellow fever, and Filoviridae, causing EVD, are discussed in separate sections.

Lassa fever is a rodent-associated disease caused by an Old World *arenavirus*. Rodents shed the virus in urine and droppings and transmit the virus to humans either by direct contact with these materials, ingestion, or inhalation of aerosolized particles. Lassa fever is mostly endemic in West Africa, where 100,000 to 300,000 cases and 5000 deaths are seen annually. Case fatality rates in hospitalized patients in West Africa are up to 50%. Other arenaviruses include the Junin virus (cause of Argentine hemorrhagic fever), the Machupo virus (cause of Bolivian hemorrhagic fever), the Chaparé virus (cause of Chaparé hemorrhagic fever, which also occurs in Bolivia), the Guanarito mammarenavirus (GTOV; cause of Venezuelan hemorrhagic fever), the Brazilian mammarenavirus (cause of Brazilian hemorrhagic fever), and the Lujo virus.

The **bunyavirus hemorrhagic fevers** include hantaviruses (discussed separately), Crimean-Congo hemorrhagic fever, Rift Valley fever, and several newly emerging viruses such as the one that causes severe fever with thrombocytopenia syndrome.

Crimean-Congo hemorrhagic fever (CCHF) is a disease transmitted from ticks and livestock. Human-to-human transmission can occur in the community or hospital setting by contact with infected body secretions. The geographic distribution is widespread with cases reported from Africa, Asia, the Middle East, Eastern Europe, particularly the East Mediterranean region.

Rift Valley fever is transmitted from livestock animals, infected mosquitoes, and flies. No human-to-human transmission is reported. Risk factors for acquiring Rift Valley fever include working with abortive animal tissue; slaughtering, skinning, or sheltering animals; and drinking unpasteurized milk. Rift Valley fever causes outbreaks in Africa and, more recently, the Arabian Peninsula.

A new bunyavirus was identified in 2009 in central and northeastern China and was named for its symptoms:

severe fever with thrombocytopenia syndrome (SFTS) virus. SFTS is transmitted by tick bite (Ixodidae family, including the tick *Haemaphysalis longicornis,* which is found in Asia as well as among animals [rarely humans] in the eastern United States). It may also be transmitted between humans through direct contact with infected blood or secretions. Another virus (**Heartland virus**), identified in the United States, is similar to the SFTS virus. Transmission occurs via the Lone Star tick (*Amblyomma americanum*). The virus appears to be amplified in deer and raccoons. In the United States, most cases are reported from the Midwest and southern states. More recently a novel *Orthonairovirus*, named **Songling virus** (SGLV), was identified in northeastern China. SGLV causes a febrile illness often associated with headache and is likely transmitted by ticks.

Clinical Findings

A. Symptoms and Signs

The incubation period varies between species, ranging from 2 to 21 days. The clinical symptoms in the early phase of a viral hemorrhagic fever are indistinguishable from other viral illnesses. Due to lack of specific symptoms on presentation, viral hemorrhagic fevers are an important cause to consider in fever of unknown origin in children in endemic areas. The late phase is more specific and is characterized by organ failure, altered mental status, and hemorrhage. Exanthems and mucosal lesions can occur.

In advanced stages, significant edema, pleural effusion, and fewer hemorrhagic manifestations compared with EVD can develop in patients with Lassa fever and Lujo virus infection. Hearing loss in various degrees is the most common complication of Lassa fever infection. Mortality in pregnant patients during the third trimester and fetal mortality are very high.

CCHF has more prominent hemorrhagic manifestations. Patients have red eyes, flushed face, red throat, and petechiae that progress to severe uncontrollable bleeding. Severe headaches are common in CCHF and correlate with the severity of vascular damage, vasodilatation, and cytokine release.

Rift Valley fever disease can present with three distinct syndromes: (1) ocular disease; retinitis is the most common complication and permanent vision loss develops in 1–10% of patients; (2) meningoencephalitis occurs in less than 1% of cases; these patients have headache, coma, or seizures 1–4 weeks after initial symptoms and a low mortality but a high morbidity with neurologic deficits that can be severe; and (3) hemorrhagic fever; patients present 2–4 days after illness and show evidence of severe liver impairment and later hemorrhages; the hemorrhagic state occurs in less than 1% of patients, but the case fatality ratio of such patients reaches about 50%.

B. Laboratory Findings

Laboratory features usually include thrombocytopenia, leukopenia (although with Lassa fever leukocytosis is noted), anemia, elevated liver biochemical tests, and abnormalities consistent with DIC.

Special care should be taken for handling clinical specimens of suspected cases. Laboratory personnel should be warned about the diagnostic suspicion, and, in the United States, the CDC should be contacted for guidance. The diagnosis may be made by antigen detection (by ELISA), culture of the virus (the "gold standard" for Lassa virus diagnosis), PCR, or demonstration of a fourfold rise in antibody titer. CCHF is best diagnosed with an IgM serology, although IgG ELISA or immunofluorescence and quantitative RT-PCR are nearly as effective. Isolation of the viruses in culture requires a biosafety level 4 laboratory. Serologic assays are attendant with early false-negative and late false-positive assays.

Differential Diagnosis

The differential diagnosis for hemorrhagic fever includes meningococcemia or other septicemias, rickettsial infection, dengue, typhoid fever, and malaria. SFTS differential diagnosis includes anaplasmosis, hemorrhagic fever with renal syndrome, or leptospirosis. The likelihood of acquiring hemorrhagic fevers among travelers is low.

Treatment & Prevention

Patients should be placed in private rooms with standard contact and droplet precautions. Barrier precautions to prevent contamination of skin or mucous membranes should also be adopted by health care providers. Airborne precautions should be considered in patients with significant pulmonary involvement or undergoing procedures that stimulate cough.

Supportive care is the mainstay of therapy. No antiviral medication is approved for use against Lassa virus, but ribavirin may be effective in vitro and in vivo. Early diagnosis and management can reduce mortality.

Convalescent plasma is routinely used to treat patients with Argentine hemorrhagic fever.

Postexposure prophylaxis with ribavirin in the management CCHF appears to be effective; however, little data exist to support its efficacy for Lassa fever and other arenaviruses. The antitrypanosomal agent suramin may be effective against the Rift Valley fever virus. Sorafenib, a tyrosine kinase inhibitor approved for treatment of renal cell and hepatocellular carcinoma, has antiviral activity against Rift Valley fever virus. A combination of monoclonal antibodies that cross-react with the glycoproteins of Lassa virus has been tested in macaques with promising results.

An inactivated vaccine is available for Rift Valley fever but is not licensed and is not commercially available. No vaccines are approved for other viruses causing viral hemorrhagic fever. Several vaccines have been developed for Lassa virus but only two have entered clinical trials. A one-dose vaccine for Lassa virus that consists of a measles vector simultaneously expressing LASV glycoprotein and nucleoprotein was successfully tested in monkeys and has completed a phase 1 clinical trial involving 60 human participants. A second vaccine (rVSVΔG-LASV-GPC) started phase 1 clinical trials in 2021.

The main method of preventing Rift Valley fever is vaccination of susceptible livestock before outbreaks occur.

Several vaccines have been developed for Rift Valley fever control in livestock, but only one, the Smithburn vaccine (a live attenuated virus), is produced commercially and used in East Africa. An inactivated vaccine has been developed for humans but is neither licensed nor commercially available.

When to Admit

- Persons with symptoms of any hemorrhagic fever and who have been in possible endemic area should be isolated for diagnosis and symptomatic treatment.
- Isolation is particularly important because diseases due to some of these agents, such as Lassa virus, are highly transmissible to health care workers.

Mateo M et al. Vaccines inducing immunity to Lassa virus glycoprotein and nucleoprotein protect macaques after a single shot. Sci Transl Med. 2019;11:eaaw3163. [PMID: 31578242]

Tucker CJ et al. Reanalysis of the 2000 Rift Valley fever outbreak in Southwestern Arabia. PLoS One. 2020;15:e0233279. [PMID: 33315866]

3. Dengue

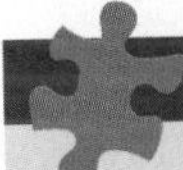

ESSENTIALS OF DIAGNOSIS

- Incubation period 7–10 days.
- Sudden onset of high fever, chills, severe myalgias and arthralgias, headache, and retroorbital pain.
- Severe dengue is defined by the presence of plasma leakage, hemorrhage, or organ involvement.
- Signs of hemorrhage such as ecchymoses, GI bleeding, and epistaxis appear later in the disease.

General Considerations

Dengue virus belongs to the genus *Flavivirus* and has four distinct serotypes that can cause infection. Infection with one serotype does not confer immunity to the other serotypes. Dengue is transmitted primarily from human to human by the bite of the *Aedes* mosquito. Health care–associated transmission (needlestick or mucocutaneous exposure) and vertical transmission occur rarely. Transmission via bone marrow and solid organ transplant is also known to occur. The WHO reports that dengue is currently endemic in 128 countries, mostly in tropical and subtropical regions with more than 3 billion persons at risk for infection. An estimated 100–400 million cases of dengue fever occur annually. Case numbers have increased over the last two decades; this surge of cases is associated with climatic factors, travel, and urbanization. Thus, along with malaria, *dengue is one of the two most common vector-borne diseases of humans*. Dengue is also the *second overall cause of a febrile illness (after malaria and excluding common upper respiratory viral infections) in travelers returning from developing countries.*

Most dengue cases occur in Asia (about 70% of cases) and Latin America. As of September 30, 2021, 1,182,721 cases are reported. Most are from Brazil (813,881), Vietnam (48,256), Peru (35,699), Philippines (32,555), and Réunion (29,618). Bangladesh, Yemen, and Colombia also report several thousands of cases in 2021.

Dengue has been a nationally notifiable condition in the United States since 2010. Even though dengue is endemic in Northern Mexico and the *Aedes* mosquito is common in the southern states, outbreaks are uncommon in the continental United States. Most cases occur in travelers, immigrants, or inhabitants of US territories that are endemic to the dengue virus. Puerto Rico experiences periodic large outbreaks, as did Hawaii in 2015 and 2016. As of September 1, 2021, 32 dengue cases were reported in the United States and 367 in US territories (primarily Puerto Rico).

The incubation period is usually 7–10 days. When the virus is introduced into susceptible populations, usually by viremic travelers from endemic countries, epidemic attack rates range from 50% to 70%.

Clinical Findings

A. Symptoms and Signs

A history of travel to a dengue-endemic area within 14 days of symptom onset is helpful in establishing a diagnosis. Most infected patients are asymptomatic. Only 20% develop symptoms ranging from mild disease (**dengue fever**) to severe hemorrhagic fever to fatal shock (**dengue shock syndrome**). In 1997 the WHO classified symptomatic dengue into dengue fever, dengue hemorrhagic fever, and dengue shock syndrome. The 2009 WHO classification of dengue is the following: dengue without warning signs; dengue with warning signs; and severe dengue. This classification was criticized for lacking clarity and mixing distinct disease phenotypes within each category and was not adopted by all countries.

After the incubation period, the febrile phase begins abruptly with nonspecific symptoms, high fever, chills, facial flushing, malaise, retroorbital eye pain, generalized body pain, and arthralgia. Some patients might have maculopapular rash, sore throat, and conjunctival injection. Not all patients have all symptoms or fever. Mild hemorrhagic manifestations can be seen. Most of the patients will recover, and fever is usually cleared by day 8.

A subset of patients, especially those with suboptimally controlled type 2 diabetes, may progress to severe dengue, which is defined by the presence of plasma leakage, hemorrhage, or organ involvement. Hematocrit increase may be the earliest sign and an indicator of the severity of plasma leakage. Pleural effusion and ascites can develop and may be detected by lateral decubitus chest radiograph or ultrasound before clinical detection. Increasing liver size, persistent vomiting, and severe abdominal pain are indications of plasma leakage. Signs of hemorrhage such as ecchymoses, GI bleeding, and epistaxis appear. Severe organ involvement may develop, such as hepatitis, encephalitis, and myocarditis.

Shock develops in patients when a critical volume of plasma is lost through leakage. Decrease in the level of consciousness, hypothermia, hypoperfusion resulting in metabolic acidosis, progressive organ impairment, and DIC leading to severe hemorrhage should raise concern for shock. AKI in dengue largely occurs with shock syndrome and shows a high mortality.

B. Laboratory Findings

Leukopenia is characteristic, and elevated transaminases are found frequently in dengue fever. Thrombocytopenia, fibrinolysis, and hemoconcentration occur more often in the hemorrhagic form of the disease. In other forms of disease, especially in children, anemia is more common. The ESR is normal in most cases.

The nonspecific nature of the illness mandates laboratory verification for diagnosis, usually with IgM and IgG ELISAs after the febrile phase. Virus is recovered from the blood by PCR or detection of the specific viral protein NS1 by ELISA during the first few days of infection. Immunohistochemistry for antigen detection in tissue samples and dried blood spots can also be used. Thrombocytopenia and blood vessel fragility in remote settings can be assessed with a tourniquet test. General evaluation recommendations include testing for infecting serotype and monitoring platelet count and serum albumin, AST, and ALT during the febrile phase of illness to monitor for development of severe disease.

Differential Diagnosis

Distinguishing between dengue and other causes of febrile illness in endemic areas is difficult. Fevers due to dengue are more often associated with neutropenia and thrombocytopenia and with myalgias, arthralgias/arthritis, and lethargy among adults. Chikungunya is more apt to develop a chronic arthritis. The arboviral encephalitides require additional epidemiologic information and serologic data to make the diagnosis. Influenza and malaria are easily confused early in disease, although the rhinitis and malaise should help distinguish influenza, and the cyclicity of fevers and presence of splenomegaly should suggest malaria.

Complications

Usual complications include pneumonia, bone marrow failure, hepatitis, iritis, retinal hemorrhages and maculopathy, orchitis, and oophoritis. Neurologic complications (such as encephalitis, Guillain-Barré syndrome, phrenic neuropathy, subdural hematoma, cerebral vasculitis, and transverse myelitis) are less common. Acute disseminated encephalomyelitis has been linked with infection and the live dengue vaccine. Bacterial superinfection can occur. Oral complications include acute gingivitis, palatal bleeding, tongue plaques, xerostomia, and rarely osteonecrosis of the jaw.

Maternal infection poses a risk of hemorrhage in both the mother and the infant if infection occurs near term. Severe dengue is a risk factor for obstetric complications, cesarean delivery, fetal distress, and maternal morbidity.

Treatment

No specific therapeutic options are available for the clinical management of dengue besides supportive care. Treatment entails the appropriate use of volume replacement, blood products, and vasopressors. Acetaminophen is recommended for analgesic and antipyretic treatment. NSAID usage should be minimized and preferably avoided to decrease the risk of gastritis and bleeding, particularly in patients with a predilection for hemorrhage or with abnormalities in platelets, liver function, or clotting factors.

Platelet counts do not usefully predict clinically significant bleeding. Platelet transfusions may be considered for severe thrombocytopenia (less than 10,000/mcL [10.0×10^9/L]) or for patients who are bleeding. However, benefit in the absence of bleeding may not be observed, and harm may be caused by delay in count recovery. Monitoring vital signs and blood volume may help in anticipating the complications of dengue hemorrhagic fever or shock syndrome.

Repurposed medications, such as chloroquine, statins, and balapiravir, have not shown clear therapeutic benefit. Research is focusing on monoclonal antibodies as a therapeutic option as well as medications, including peptide agents that target structural and nonstructural proteins of dengue virus essential to its replication.

Prognosis

Although fatalities occur with severe disease, the estimated mortality (2.5% of severe cases) appears to be diminishing, likely due to improved recognition of the disease and wider availability of supportive treatment. Causes of death include hemorrhagic fever (seen with recurrent disease) and occasionally fulminant hepatitis. Thrombocytopenia and acute hepatitis are predictors of severe dengue and higher mortality. AKI in dengue shock syndrome portends poor prognosis. In general, the more severe forms of disease (hemorrhagic fever and shock) occur more often in Asia than in the Americas. Comorbidities of CVD, diabetes, stroke, pulmonary disease, kidney disease, and older age are associated with more severe dengue.

Prevention

Preventive measures should be encouraged, such as control of mosquitoes by screening and insect repellents including long-lasting insecticides, particularly during early morning and late afternoon exposures. Screening blood transfusions for dengue is important, especially in endemic areas.

Dengvaxia (CYD-TDV), a recombinant, live, attenuated, tetravalent dengue vaccine, is FDA-approved for children 9–16 years old with previous history of dengue infection and who live in endemic areas. It was first licensed in 2015 and is approved in more than 20 countries. Dengvaxia trials reported overall 56% efficacy; however, efficacy was lower in younger age groups, seronegative individuals at the time of vaccination, and those infected with dengue serotype 2. The vaccine is given as a 0-, 6-, and 12-month series, although a two-dose schedule is likely efficacious. Serious side effects were no more common than in placebo recipients. Vaccination is indicated for those between ages 9 and 45 years. However, Dengvaxia carries an increased risk of severe dengue in those who experience their first natural dengue infection after vaccination (those who were seronegative at the time of vaccination). Thus, the WHO recommends limiting the vaccine to those who have had at least one dengue infection prior to vaccination and, for countries considering using Dengvaxia as part of their dengue control program, recommends prevaccination screening using dengue serology. Pregnant women and immunosuppressed persons should *not* be vaccinated. Another tetravalent dengue vaccine, a two-dose TAK-003, is currently in phase 3 clinical trials and has shown promising results (73.3% efficacy; NCT02747927).

Since 2011, researchers have been injecting a bacterium that blocks mosquitoes' ability to transmit dengue (*Wolbachia pipientis*) into the eggs of *Aedes aegypti* mosquitoes. In a recent randomized controlled trial in Indonesia, *A aegypti* infected with *W pipientis* were introduced into several geographic clusters; the incidence of symptomatic dengue and number of dengue hospitalizations were reduced in these geographic clusters compared with control clusters.

Coronel-Martínez DL et al. Immunogenicity and safety of simplified vaccination schedules for the CYD-TDV dengue vaccine in healthy individuals aged 9-50 years (CYD65): a randomised, controlled, phase 2, non-inferiority study. Lancet Infect Dis. 2021;21:517. [PMID: 33212067]

Sangkaew S et al. Risk predictors of progression to severe disease during the febrile phase of dengue: a systematic review and meta-analysis. Lancet Infect Dis. 2021;21:1014. [PMID: 33640077]

Utarini A et al. Efficacy of Wolbachia-infected mosquito deployments for the control of dengue. N Engl J Med. 2021;384:2177. [PMID: 34107180]

4. Hantaviruses

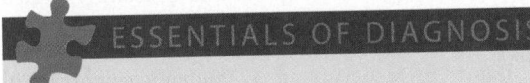

- Transmitted by rodents and cause two clinical syndromes.
- **Hemorrhagic fever with renal syndrome (HFRS):** mild to severe illness.
- **Hantavirus pulmonary syndrome (HPS):** 40% mortality rate.

General Considerations

Hantaviruses are enveloped RNA bunyaviruses naturally hosted in rodents, moles, and shrews. Globally, hantaviruses infect more than 200,000 people annually, and their collective mortality rate is about 35–40%. Hantavirus infection in humans can cause several disease syndromes. HFRS is primarily caused by Dobrava-Belgrade virus, Puumala virus, Seoul virus, and Hantaan virus in Asia and Europe. These viruses are called Old World hantaviruses. *Nephropathia epidemica* is a milder form of HFRS. Puumala virus is the most prevalent pathogen and is present throughout Europe. The HPS, also known as hantavirus cardiopulmonary syndrome, is caused mainly by Sin Nombre virus and Andes virus, the New World Hantaviruses in Americas. While they share many clinical features, a specific strain is not associated with a specific syndrome and overlap is seen between the syndromes. The primary reservoirs include the field mouse for Hantaan virus HFRS, the bank vole for Puumala virus, and the deer mouse for SNV-HPS.

Aerosols of virus-contaminated rodent urine and feces are thought to be the main vehicle for transmission to humans. Person-to-person transmission is observed only with the Andes virus. *Occupation is the main risk factor for transmission of all hantaviruses*: animal trappers, forestry workers, laboratory personnel, farmers, and military personnel are at highest risk. Climate change appears to be impacting the incidence of hantavirus infection mainly through effects on reservoir ecology.

Clinical Findings

A. Symptoms and Signs

Vascular leakage is the hallmark of the disease for both syndromes, with kidneys being the main target with variants associated with HFRS and the lungs with variants associated with HPS.

1. HFRS—HFRS manifests as mild, moderate, or severe illness depending on the causative strain. A 2- to 3-week incubation period is followed by a protracted clinical course, typically consisting of five distinct phases: febrile period, hypotension, oliguria, diuresis, and convalescence phase. Various degrees of kidney involvement are usually seen. Puumala virus infection is often referred to as nephropathia epidemica. Thromboembolic phenomena are also recognized complications. A secondary hemophagocytic lymphohistiocytosis can be seen with HFRS. Pulmonary edema is not typically seen but when present usually occurs in the final stages of disease (oliguric and diuretic phase). Encephalitis and pituitary involvement are rare findings with hantavirus infection, although a few cases are reported with Puumala virus infection. Patients may have persistent hematuria, proteinuria, or hypertension up to 35 months after infection. Smoking appears to exacerbate the viremia with the Puumala virus infection, and bradycardia can also be prominent.

2. HPS—The clinical course of HPS is divided into a febrile prodrome, a cardiopulmonary stage, oliguric and diuretic phase, followed by convalescence. A 14- to 17-day incubation period is followed by a prodromal phase, typically lasting 3–6 days, that is associated with myalgia; malaise; abdominal pain along with nausea, vomiting, and diarrhea; headache; chills; and fever of abrupt onset. An ensuing cardiopulmonary phase is characterized by the acute onset of pulmonary edema. In this stage, cough is generally present, abdominal pain and symptoms as above may dominate the clinical presentation, and in severe cases, significant myocardial depression occurs. AKI and myositis may occur. Sequelae include neuropsychological impairments in some HPS survivors.

B. Laboratory Findings

Laboratory features include hemoconcentration and elevation in LD, serum lactate, and hepatocellular enzymes. Early thrombocytopenia and leukocytosis (as high as 90,000 cells/mcL [90.0 × 10^9/L] in HPS) are seen in both HFRS and HPS. In HPS, immunoblasts (activated lymphocytes with plasmacytoid features) can be seen in blood, lungs, kidneys, bone marrow, liver, and spleen.

An indirect fluorescent assay and enzyme immunoassay are available for detection of specific IgM or low-avidity IgG virus-specific antibodies. A quantitative RT-PCR is available; however, the viremia of human hantavirus infections is short-term, and therefore, viral RNA cannot be readily detected in the blood or urine of patients unless for the more readily detected early viremia of the Andes variant.

A plaque reduction neutralization test remains a gold standard serologic assay and distinguishes between the different hantavirus species, although cross-reaction between Old and New World viruses exists. This test needs to be performed in a laboratory with appropriate biosafety (level 3).

▶ Differential Diagnosis

The differential diagnosis of the acute febrile syndrome seen with HFRS or early HPS includes scrub typhus, leptospirosis, and dengue. HPS requires differentiation from other respiratory infections caused by such pathogens as SARS-CoV-2, *Legionella, Chlamydia*, and *Mycoplasma*. Coxsackievirus infection should also be considered in the differential diagnosis.

▶ Treatment

Treatment is mainly supportive. Cardiorespiratory support with vasopressors is frequently needed; extracorporeal membrane oxygenation may be required in severe cases of HPS. Intravenous ribavirin is used in HFRS (Hantaan virus) with some success in decreasing the severity of the kidney injury. Its effectiveness in HPS, however, is not established.

▶ Prevention

Because infection is thought to occur by inhalation of rodent waste, prevention is aimed at eradication of rodents in houses and avoidance of exposure to rodent excreta, including forest service facilities. Climatic changes often require particular attention to rodent populations in parks. Inactivated vaccines are used in several Asian countries where patients are at risk for. Vaccines under investigation include a Hantaan/Puumala virus DNA vaccine (delivered via a TriGrid device).

▶ Prognosis

The outcome is highly variable depending on severity of disease. HPS is a more severe disease than HFRS, with a mortality rate of about 40%. In Sin Nombre virus infections, the persistence of elevated IgG titers correlates with a favorable outcome.

Dheerasekara K et al. Hantavirus infection—treatment and prevention. Curr Treat Options Infect Dis. 2020;29:1. [PMID: 33144850]

Munir N et al. Hantavirus diseases pathophysiology, their diagnostic strategies and therapeutic approaches: a review. Clin Exp Pharmacol Physiol. 2020 Sep 7. [Epub ahead of print] [PMID: 32894790]

Song JY et al. Immunogenicity and safety of a modified three-dose priming and booster schedule for the Hantaan virus vaccine (Hantavax): a multi-center phase III clinical trial in healthy adults. Vaccine. 2020;38:8016. [PMID: 33131933]

5. Yellow Fever

ESSENTIALS OF DIAGNOSIS

- Endemic area exposure: tropical and subtropical South America and Africa.
- Sudden onset of severe headache, aching in legs, and tachycardia.
- Brief (1 day) remission, followed by bradycardia, hypotension, jaundice, hemorrhagic tendency.
- Albuminuria, leukopenia, bilirubinemia.

▶ General Considerations

Yellow fever is a zoonotic flavivirus infection transmitted by *Aedes* mosquito bites. The three types of transmission cycles include sylvatic (or jungle; humans working or traveling in the forest are bitten by infected mosquitoes), intermediate (most common type of outbreak in Africa; mosquitoes infect both monkeys and people leading to outbreaks in separate villages), and urban (seen in large epidemics; infected mosquitoes transmit the virus from person to person). Elevated temperatures and increased rainfall are major determinants of transmission.

Yellow fever occurs in 47 endemic countries in Africa and in Central and South America. Around 90% of cases reported every year occur in sub-Saharan Africa. Adults and children are equally susceptible, though attack rates are highest among adult men because of their work habits. Modeling data from Africa in 2013 estimates the annual case load is 84,000 to 170,000 annual cases with 29,000 to 60,000 deaths. The number of people susceptible to infection with yellow fever virus worldwide is estimated to be between 394 million and 473 million.

The last decade has seen a resurgence of yellow fever, likely due to suboptimal vaccination coverage along with waning population-level immunity.

▶ Clinical Findings

A. Symptoms and Signs

Most persons have no illness or only mild illness. The incubation period is 3–6 days in persons in whom symptoms develop.

1. Mild form—Symptoms are malaise, headache, fever, retroorbital pain, nausea, vomiting, and photophobia. Relative bradycardia (a lower than expected heart rate for the degree of body temperature elevation), conjunctival injection, and facial flushing may be present.

2. Severe form—Severe illness develops in about 15%. Initial symptoms are similar to the mild form, but brief fever remission lasting hours to a few days is followed by a "period of intoxication" manifested by fever and relative bradycardia, hypotension, jaundice, hemorrhage (GI, nasal, oral), and delirium that may progress to coma.

B. Laboratory Findings

Leukopenia, elevated liver enzymes, and bilirubin can occur. Proteinuria is present and usually disappears completely with recovery. Bleeding dyscrasias with elevated prothrombin and partial thromboplastin times, decreased platelet count, and presence of fibrin-split products can also occur.

In the early stages of the disease (up to 10 days), diagnosis is confirmed if yellow fever virus RNA is detected by RT-PCR in blood from a person with no history of recent yellow fever vaccination. PCR determinants can distinguish between wild type virus and vaccine-associated strains.

In later stages, serologic diagnosis can be made by using ELISA to measure IgM 3 days after the onset of symptoms; however, yellow fever vaccine and other flaviviruses, including dengue, West Nile, and Zika viruses, may give a false-positive ELISA test result. Thus, the presence of yellow fever virus–specific IgM antibody and negative ELISA panel for other relevant flaviviruses confirm the diagnosis. If ELISA is positive for other flaviviruses, the more specific plaque reduction neutralization assay should be done in reference laboratories, which measures the titer of the neutralizing antibodies in the serum toward the infecting virus.

Differential Diagnosis

It may be difficult to distinguish yellow fever from other viral hepatitides, malaria, leptospirosis, louse-borne relapsing fever, dengue, and other hemorrhagic fevers on clinical evidence alone. *Albuminuria* is a constant feature in yellow fever patients, and its presence helps differentiate yellow fever from other viral hepatitides. Serologic confirmation is often needed.

Treatment

No specific antiviral therapy is available. Treatment is directed toward symptomatic relief and management of complications. A randomized clinical trial of sofosbuvir for treatment of yellow fever is underway in Brazil.

Prognosis

The mortality rate of the severe form is 20–50%, with death occurring most commonly between the sixth and the tenth days. Convalescence is prolonged, including 1–2 weeks of asthenia. Infection confers lifelong immunity to those who recover.

Prevention

Four live attenuated yellow fever virus vaccines (all derived from the 17D strain) are prequalified by the WHO. All are given as a single dose (10-year booster doses are recommended for some groups) and are safe and effective. A single dose of vaccine in the past was considered to provide lifelong immunity. While the 10-year booster dose is no longer recommended for most people, persistent seropositivity at 8 years post vaccination is only 85% (and below 60% in children vaccinated at 9–12 months of age). Thus, at-risk groups with waning immunity and high probability of exposure may consider receiving a second dose of vaccine after 10 years (these groups are listed at https://www.cdc.gov/yellowfever/healthcareproviders/vaccine-info.html).

Yellow fever vaccine is recommended for persons aged over 9 months who are traveling to or living in areas at risk for yellow fever virus transmission. This vaccine should never be given to children under 6 months old due to their higher risk of developing encephalitis related to the vaccine. *The WHO recommends that all endemic countries should include yellow fever vaccine in their national immunization programs and provides a list of countries that require yellow fever vaccination for entry.*

The vaccine is contraindicated in persons with severe egg allergies or who are severely immunocompromised, including patients with primary immunodeficiencies, HIV infection with CD4+ cell count below 200/mcL, thymus disorder with abnormal immune function, malignant neoplasms, transplantation, or immunosuppressive and immunomodulatory therapies. The vaccine should not be given to breastfeeding women or patients over 60 years of age because this age group is at higher risk for viscerotropic and neurologic disease. It should be administered at least 24 hours apart from the measles vaccine. Pregnant women should receive the vaccine only if they cannot defer travel to endemic areas (Chapter 30). Clinicians should be aware of rare but frequently fatal vaccine-induced reactions, including anaphylaxis, yellow fever vaccine–associated viscerotropic disease, and yellow fever vaccine–associated neurologic disease.

A 2017 initiative, the Eliminate Yellow Fever Epidemics (EYE) program, is composed of more than 50 organizations and designed to increase surveillance and control in 40 countries of Africa and the Americas in an attempt to reach a billion at-risk individuals with seroprotection by 2026.

The best personal protective measures are to avoid mosquito bites. If not in an endemic area, the patient should be isolated from mosquitoes to prevent transmission, since blood in the acute phase is potentially infectious.

Juan-Giner A et al. Immunogenicity and safety of fractional doses of yellow fever vaccines: a randomized double-blind, non-inferiority trial. Lancet. 2021;397:119. [PMID: 33422245]

Waters TW et al. Updated yellow fever entry requirements and recommendations from WHO as of August 2020. J Travel Med. 2020;27(7):taaa152. [PMID: 32889538]

OTHER SYSTEMIC VIRAL DISEASES

1. Zika Virus

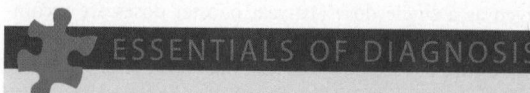

- Most infected persons asymptomatically seroconvert.
- Clinical symptoms are akin to those of chikungunya virus infection but with less arthritis.
- Complications include microcephaly and ocular abnormalities in infants born to mothers infected during pregnancy, as well as Guillain-Barré.
- No effective antiviral or vaccine is available.

General Considerations

Zika virus is a flavivirus, akin to the viruses that cause dengue fever, Japanese encephalitis, and West Nile infection.

The virus was noted in Africa and Asia during the 1950s–1980s, but first spread beyond those two continents during 2007 when an outbreak occurred in Yap State, Federated States of Micronesia. A large outbreak occurred in French Polynesia in 2013. The virus then spread to the Western hemisphere and was first noted in northeastern Brazil in 2015, and 239,742 cases were subsequently reported between 2015 and 2018. Zika virus spread rapidly throughout the Americas, including the United States and worldwide (http://www.who.int/csr/disease/zika/en/). Despite distinct lineages, Zika virus exists as only one serotype.

Aedes species mosquitoes, particularly *Aedes aegypti*, are primarily responsible for transmission of Zika virus. The biodistribution of the species largely determines the area of prevalence for Zika virus. *Aedes* species mosquitoes are found primarily in the southeastern United States, but one species *Aedes albopictus* may be seen as far north as Pennsylvania and New Jersey. Rarely, a few other mosquito species including *Anopheles* and *Culex* may be competent for the Zika virus. Sexual transmission is reported from men and women to partners via vaginal, anal, or oral sex. Vertical transmission from pregnant woman to fetus is prominent. Transmission via platelet transfusion is also reported.

Since the onset of the first reported cases in the United States in 2015, most cases occur in US territories (largely Puerto Rico). The territorial cases are largely locally acquired and the US state cases are largely travel-acquired. The number of annual cases is diminishing markedly in the United States with a peak in 2016 of 4897 travel-associated cases and 224 locally acquired cases (Florida, 218; Texas, 6). The CDC case count for the year 2021, as of November 2, 2021, includes one case (a returning traveler) in the United States and 25 (all locally acquired cases) in the US territories.

Clinical Findings

A. Symptoms and Signs

The incubation period is 3–14 days. The majority (50–80%) of Zika virus infections are asymptomatic. Symptoms include acute-onset fever, maculopapular rash that is usually pruritic, nonpurulent conjunctivitis, and arthralgias, the latter mimicking the symptoms of the chikungunya virus. Rash may outlast the fever but is not always present. Symptoms last up to 7 days. Most infections are asymptomatic. Viral infections most often confused with Zika include dengue and chikungunya virus infections.

B. Laboratory Findings and Diagnostic Studies

Diagnosis is made by detecting viral RNA (nucleic acid testing) in patients presenting with onset of symptoms less than 7 days. Nucleic acid testing can be performed within 14 days of illness onset. Persons being tested 14 days or more after symptom onset should be tested using IgM serology. The Trioplex RT-PCR assay, which detects Zika virus, chikungunya virus, and dengue virus RNA, and the Zika MAC-ELISA, which detects Zika virus IgM antibodies (usually present up to 12 weeks after illness onset), are available. Matched serum and urine specimens should be tested simultaneously. Although not routinely recommended, RT-PCR can be performed on amniotic fluid, CSF, and placental tissue. A positive RT-PCR test definitively makes the diagnosis of Zika virus infection and does not require additional confirmatory testing. A negative test does not exclude the presence of the virus in other tissues and does not rule out infection. Persons with negative NATs and symptoms of Zika infection should undergo further testing for Zika virus IgM antibody and other arboviral infections. Serologic testing for Zika virus should only be conducted by laboratories with experience in performing flavivirus serology.

Recommended serologic assays include enzyme immunoassays and immunofluorescence assays (which detect IgM antibodies using viral lysate, cell culture supernatant, or recombinant proteins) as well as neutralization assays (such as plaque reduction neutralization tests). The Zika MAC-ELISA can be performed on serum or CSF. Anti-Zika IgM antibodies are observed in CSF of children with congenital infection. Neutralizing antibodies can cross-react with dengue and other flaviviruses, so samples testing positive should be sent to public health laboratories for confirmation.

In the United States, testing for asymptomatic pregnant women is not currently recommended by the CDC even after travel to an area with Zika activity. The WHO, however, still recommends testing via IgM antibody for asymptomatic pregnant women who could have had contact with vector-borne or sexually transmitted Zika virus. In areas with active Zika transmission, asymptomatic pregnant women should be tested for IgM antibody as part of routine obstetric care. Persistent Zika virus RNA in serum has been reported in pregnancy. Pregnant women with confirmed or suspected Zika virus infection may be monitored by serial ultrasounds at 3- to 4-week intervals, assessing fetal anatomy and growth. With a declining prevalence of Zika virus infection, positive antibody tests run the risk of more likely being false-positives and thus the need for the outlined assessments exists.

Complications

Two neurologic complications are of particular concern: (1) **congenital microcephaly,** often associated with brain calcifications and other abnormalities, first noted during the outbreak in Brazil; and (2) **Guillain-Barré syndrome,** first noted during the outbreak in French Polynesia. The incidence of Guillain-Barré syndrome is estimated at 2–3 cases per 10,000 Zika virus infections. In addition to microcephaly, Zika causes a spectrum of birth defects of the CNS that collectively are termed **"congenital Zika syndrome."** These include fetal brain disruption sequence, subcortical calcifications, pyramidal and extrapyramidal signs, ocular lesions of chorioretinal atrophy, focal pigmented mottling of the retina, and congenital contractures. Newborns of women infected with Zika virus during pregnancy have a 5–14% risk of congenital Zika syndrome and a 4–6% risk of Zika virus–associated microcephaly. Spontaneous abortions and rare deaths related to Zika virus infection are reported.

As with Ebola virus, the Zika virus can persist in semen for months; in the male reproductive tract the prostate gland and the testes are the presumed reservoirs. Persistence of the virus in the female reproductive tract is possible.

Treatment

No antivirals are approved for treatment of Zika virus; thus, management should focus on supportive care. Aspirin and NSAIDs are avoided during illness caused by the flavivirus dengue because of its propensity to cause hemorrhage. Zika virus infections, however, do not appear to be associated with major hemorrhagic complications.

Prevention

The most effective means is environmental control of mosquitoes and removal of areas where water is stagnant or builds up. Such measures include screens on houses; removal of old tires and debris from endemic areas of infection; and movement toward better living conditions, including air conditioning in impoverished areas. Because of the association between microcephaly and Zika virus infection during pregnancy, *pregnant women are advised to avoid travel to areas where Zika virus is circulating* (http://www.who.int/csr/disease/zika/information-for-travelers/en/). Guidelines for testing of pregnant women potentially exposed are available through the CDC. Infected individuals should refrain from blood donations for several months.

No approved vaccine against Zika virus exists; however, several inactivated vaccine candidates have shown the ability to induce neutralizing antibodies based in phase 1 trials. A phase 2 multicenter randomized trial evaluating Zika virus wild type DNA vaccine is currently undergoing data analysis. Vaccine candidate evaluation has been hampered by the declining incidence of Zika virus.

Giron S et al. Vector-borne transmission of Zika virus in Europe, southern France, August 2019. Eurosurveillance. 2019;24:1900655. [PMID: 31718742]

Kovacs A. Zika, the newest TORCH infectious disease in the Americas. Clin Infect Dis. 2020;70:2673. [PMID: 31346608]

Sánchez-Montalvá A et al. Persistence of Zika virus in body fluids—final report. N Engl J Med. 2019;380:198. [PMID: 30628425]

2. Chikungunya Fever

Chikungunya ("that which bends up" in the Bantu language Kimakonde) fever is an alphavirus infection transmitted to humans by *A aegypti* and *A albopictus* and is considered a classic "arthritogenic" virus. The virus originated with two strains, one in West Africa and the other in East/Central/Southern Africa. The first documented clinical cases in India were derivative of the E/C/S African strains with later reports of outbreaks in Kenya in 2004. Subsequently, there were reports from areas that adjoin the Indian Ocean, Southeast Asia and its neighboring islands (2005–2007), South India (2005), and the island of La Réunion (2005–2006), with further spread including autochthonous cases in Italy and France (2007). In 2013, the first autochthonous case of chikungunya reported in the western hemisphere occurred on Saint Martin in the Caribbean, with isolates derivative of the East/Central/South Africa strains. Despite these differences, only one serotype exists.

For 2021, the CDC reported 17 travel-associated US cases. Chikungunya virus prevalence is ubiquitous in endemic countries in Africa, the Americas, Asia, and Europe.

Among naïve populations, attack rates are often as high as 50%. On Saint Martin, 39% of infections were asymptomatic. Vertical transmission is documented if the mother is viremic during parturition, and transmission does not appear to occur throughout pregnancy as it does with Zika virus. Infectious virus was isolated from saliva, although transmission from oral secretions is not observed among humans. Endemicity of *A aegypti* in the Americas and the introduction of *A albopictus* into Europe and the New World raise concern for further extension of the epidemic. Case reports show that chikungunya virus may coinfect patients with yellow fever virus, plasmodia, Zika virus, and dengue virus.

Clinical Findings

A. Symptoms and Signs

After an incubation period of 1–12 days (estimated median 3), several symptoms begin abruptly, including fever; headache; intestinal complaints, including diarrhea, vomiting, or abdominal pain; myalgias; and arthralgias/arthritis affecting small, large, and axial joints. The simultaneous involvement of more than 10 joints and the presence of tenosynovitis (especially in the wrist) are characteristic. The *stooped posture* of patients gives the disease its name. Joint symptoms persist for 4 months in 33% and linger for years in about 10%. A centrally distributed pigmented or pruritic maculopapular rash is reported in 10–40% of patients; it can be bullous with sloughing in children. Mucosal disease occurs in about 15%. Facial edema and localized petechiae are reported. Neurologic complications, including encephalitis, myelopathy, peripheral neuropathy, Guillain-Barré syndrome, myeloneuropathy, and myopathy, are usually found in persons younger than 5 years or older than 49 years. Encephalitis occurred in 8.6 per 100,000 persons infected in La Réunion during 2005–2006 with 17% mortality and increased risk of encephalitis among those older than 65 years. Hemorrhagic fever–like presentations are unusual. Coinfection with other respiratory viruses and with dengue is common. Some of the neuropathology may be immune-mediated, and these cases are usually in those over age 20 and associated with longer latencies and better outcomes. Death is rare and usually related to underlying comorbidities. The differential diagnosis includes other tropical febrile diseases, such as malaria, leishmaniasis, or dengue.

B. Laboratory Findings

Diagnosis is made epidemiologically and clinically. Mild leukopenia occurs as does thrombocytopenia, which is seldom severe. Elevated inflammatory markers do not correlate well with the severity of arthritis. Radiographs of affected joints are normal during the acute phase. Bone lesions are visible in some patients with chronic symptoms.

Serologic confirmation requires elevated IgM titers or fourfold increase in convalescent IgG levels using an ELISA. RT-PCR and ELISA are commercially available; no ELISA kit is FDA-cleared. Culture techniques (viral isolation in insect or mammalian cell lines or by inoculation of mosquitoes or mice) require BSL 3 (biosafety level 3) containment. Directions on submitting specimens for testing may be obtained from the CDC Arboviral Diseases Branch, 970-221-6400. Suspected cases in the United States should be promptly reported to public health authorities.

Complications & Prognosis

Common complications of chikungunya fever are long-term weakness, asthenia, myalgia, arthralgia, and arthritis, noted to be present in 25–66.5% of cases at 1 year. Risk factors for long-term arthralgias include the existence of such symptoms at 4 months after onset of disease and age over 35 years. Persons with preexisting arthritis are also at increased risk for prolonged symptoms after chikungunya infection with polyarthralgias occasionally lasting for years. Nasal skin necrosis is rarely reported. The Guillain-Barré syndrome is also reported. Comorbid conditions, including hypertension, diabetes, and cardiac diseases, may contribute to severe outcomes; although in some series, patients with significant neurologic complications do not show comorbidities. Severe outcomes and higher mortality are reported among more recent Brazilian cases.

Treatment & Prevention

Treatment is supportive with NSAIDs and corticosteroids. Chloroquine and methotrexate may be useful for managing refractory arthritis. Chronic disease may require disease modifying antirheumatic medications, such as the reports from La Réunion where methotrexate was associated with a positive response. No licensed vaccine exists, although at least 18 vaccines are in trials including inactivated and live attenuated vaccines. A measles-vectored chikungunya virus vaccine (MV-CHIK) demonstrated good immunogenicity and was shown to be safe and effective in a phase 2 clinical trial. Prevention relies on avoidance of mosquito vectors. Transplantation of tissue from immigrants or from travelers to known endemic areas should be discouraged. Prophylaxis with specific chikungunya immunoglobulins may be useful for immunosuppressed persons.

Stegmann-Planchard S et al. Chikungunya, a risk factor for Guillain-Barré syndrome. Clin Infect Dis. 2020;70:1233. [PMID: 31290540]

3. Colorado Tick Fever

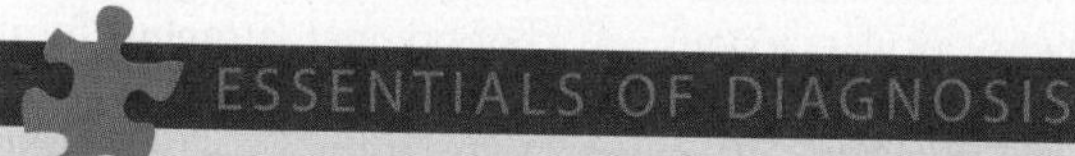

- Onset 1–19 days (average, 4 days) following tick bite.
- Fever, chills, myalgia, headache, prostration.
- Leukopenia, thrombocytopenia.
- Second attack of fever after remission lasting 2–3 days.

General Considerations

Colorado tick fever is a reportable biphasic, febrile illness caused by a reovirus infection transmitted by *Dermacentor andersoni* tick bite. About five cases occur annually, largely among men over age 40. The disease is limited to the western United States and Canada and is most prevalent during the tick season (March to November), typically at 4,000–10,000 feet above sea level in grassy areas. Most cases (90%) report a discrete history of tick bite or exposure. The virus infects the marrow erythrocyte precursors. Blood transfusions can be a vehicle of transmission.

Clinical Findings

A. Symptoms and Signs

The incubation period is 3–6 days, rarely as long as 19 days. The onset is usually abrupt with a high fever. Severe myalgia, headache, photophobia, anorexia, nausea and vomiting, and generalized weakness are prominent. Physical findings are limited to an occasional faint rash. The acute symptoms resolve within a week. Remission is followed in 50% of cases by recurrent fever and a full recrudescence lasting 2–4 days.

The differential diagnosis includes influenza, Rocky Mountain spotted fever, numerous other viral infections, and, in the right setting, relapsing fevers.

B. Laboratory Findings

Leukopenia with a shift to the left and atypical lymphocytes occurs, reaching a nadir 5–6 days after the onset of illness. Thrombocytopenia may occur. An RT-PCR assay may be used to detect early viremia. Detection of IgM by capture ELISA or plaque reduction neutralization is possible after 2 weeks from symptom onset and is the most frequently used diagnostic tool.

Complications

Aseptic meningitis (particularly in children), encephalitis, and hemorrhagic fever occur rarely. Malaise may last weeks to months. Fatalities are very uncommon. Rarely, spontaneous abortion or multiple congenital anomalies may complicate Colorado tick fever infection acquired during pregnancy.

Treatment

No specific treatment is available. Ribavirin has shown efficacy in an animal model. Antipyretics are used, although salicylates should be avoided due to potential bleeding with the thrombocytopenia seen in patients with Colorado tick fever.

Prognosis

The disease is usually self-limited and benign.

Prevention

Tick avoidance is the best prevention. The tick season is primarily from March to November, and the ticks mostly live at high altitudes (over 7000 feet) in sagebrush.

McDonald E et al. Notes from the field: investigation of Colorado tick fever virus disease cases—Oregon, 2018. MMWR Morb Mortal Wkly Rep. 2019;68:289. [PMID: 30921304]

Rodino KG et al. Tick-borne diseases in the United States. Clin Chem. 2020;66:537. [PMID: 32232463]

COMMON VIRAL RESPIRATORY INFECTIONS

1. Severe Acute Respiratory Syndrome—Coronavirus 2019 (SARS-CoV-2)

The COVID-19 pandemic has been both devastating and fast-changing. Several authoritative websites provide current statistics about the impact of the pandemic and current guidelines, including https://www.cdc.gov/coronavirus/2019-ncov/index.html and https://coronavirus.jhu.edu.

ESSENTIALS OF DIAGNOSIS

- Asymptomatic in approximately 85% of adults and most children.
- When symptomatic, adults often have upper respiratory tract illness with fever, cough, upper tract symptoms being more prominent with the omicron variant.
- Advanced pulmonary complications (pneumonia, ARDS) occur with fulminant disease.
- Mortality of 1–21% (varied by geographic area and strain).
- High predilection for older adults, the immunocompromised, those with chronic diseases, those living in crowded conditions.

General Considerations

Coronaviruses are a large family of viruses commonly found in humans as well as many other species of animals, including bats, camels, cattle, cats, white-tailed deer (among whom deer-to-deer transmission is documented), and hamsters. There are four genera of coronaviruses, of which only the alphacoronaviruses (coronavirus NL63 and 229E) and the betacoronaviruses affect humans.

A. Clinical Epidemiology

Data collected from all US states with the observational cohort study *All of Us* show that in early 2020, in five states, cases were serologically identified before official reports of cases and as early as January 7th and 8th in Illinois and Massachusetts, respectively. COVID-19 was declared a pandemic by the WHO on March 11, 2020.

As of March 18, 2022, global cases surpassed 467 million, including more than 6 million deaths from 220 countries and territories. SARS-CoV-2 has surpassed *Mycobacterium tuberculosis* as the global leading single infectious agent cause of death. The 10 countries with the highest number of cases as of March 17, 2022, are the United States, India, Brazil, France, the United Kingdom, Germany, Russia, Turkey, Italy, and Spain. The United States alone reports over 79 million cases and 970,000 deaths. Data on morbidity and mortality rates may be inaccurate since case counts may be grossly underestimated due to high rates of home testing.

Significant increases in deaths attributable to diabetes and heart disease are recorded since the start of the pandemic. Accordingly, the CDC has identified "hotspot counties" where social vulnerability to COVID-19 is greater. Such counties show a higher proportion of racial and ethnic minorities, a greater density of housing units as well as more crowded housing (persons/room). *These data imply that the actual number of deaths caused by COVID-19 may be up to 50% higher than reported.*

B. Transmission

R_0 is the basic reproductive number signifying the number of contacts infected by one infectious individual. Calculations of R_0 for SARS-CoV-2 have varied but the true R_0 likely lies somewhere between 2 and 3. While the case fatality rate was far higher with the 2003 SARS-CoV-1 and with the Middle East respiratory syndrome (MERS) virus, the rate of person-to-person spread and the number of infected cases are much higher with SARS-CoV-2 than with either the SARS or MERS viruses. The reported rates of SARS-CoV-2 transmission are 5% for close contacts and 10–40% for household contacts.

Presymptomatic spread accounts for many cases, and the viral load for SARS-CoV-2 is highest the day before symptoms develop. A CDC telephone survey of infected individuals showed that only 46% reported contact with a known case, and among the known contacts, the most common were family members (46%) or work colleagues (34%).

The incubation period for SARS-CoV-2 ranges from 2 to 24 days with an average of about 5 days. The principal mode of transmission is respiratory droplets, which can be propelled 6 feet or more by sneezing or coughing (and have been documented to be propelled as far as 27 feet). The CDC recommends that airborne precautions be used in health care settings principally for health care providers performing respiratory procedures (such as collecting induced sputum or intubating the patient).

C. Risk Factors

Data from the United States emphasize that the rate of infection is highest among young and middle-aged adults, with nearly 25% of confirmed cases occurring in persons aged 20–29 years, and about 20% of cases in those aged 50–64 years. Data from the southern United States show increases in incidence among persons aged 20–39 precedes the increases among those over age 60 by 4–15 days. *COVID-19 mortality rates are distinctly higher over the age of 50 and in those with medical comorbidities, particularly obesity and diabetes.* Symptomatic disease appears to develop in men more often than in women. Populations at particular risk for infection include health care personnel, people with immunosuppression, pregnant women, and those with genetic susceptibility.

D. Public Health Concerns

Population-level and individual public health precautions remain important in communities where the SARS-CoV-2 continues to circulate or where most community members are unvaccinated or both. Public health strategies vary across the world to minimize the impacts of COVID-19, including recommendations or mandates for social distancing, contact tracing, community activities, travel restrictions, and vaccines. Other factors affecting strategies include the response to multiple conditions, including the prevalence of COVID-19 in a particular communities; the rate and degree of vaccination; the availability of health care resources; and COVID-19 treatments.

E. SARS-CoV-2 Variants

In the spectrum of existing RNA viruses, SARS-CoV-2 mutates relatively infrequently. Nonetheless, several SARS-CoV-2 genetic variants have been identified to date and are categorized as Variants of Concern, Variants of Interest, and Variants under Monitoring.

Clinical Findings

A. Symptoms and Signs

Most individuals with infection are asymptomatic, although the ratio of asymptomatic to symptomatic infection remains unclear and changes as more individuals are tested. Adults can manifest a wide range of symptoms from mild to severe illness that typically begin 2–14 days after exposure to SARS-CoV-2. Symptomatic patients may have cough, fever, chills/rigors, or myalgias. The presence of dyspnea is variable but is common in severe infection. No single symptom should be used as a discriminant for disease. Less frequent symptoms include rhinitis, pharyngitis, abdominal symptoms, such as nausea and diarrhea, headaches, anosmia and cacosmia, and ageusia and cacogeusia. It appears that 15–20% of adults with SARS-CoV-2 infection require hospitalization and 3–5% require critical care.

B. Laboratory Findings

Hematologic findings include neutrophilia, absolute lymphopenia, and an increased neutrophil to lymphocyte ratio. As disease advances, blood chemistry findings often include elevated liver biochemical tests and total bilirubin. Serum markers of systemic inflammation are increased in most patients with severe COVID-19, including LD, ferritin, CRP, procalcitonin, and interleukin 6 (IL-6). A coagulopathy often is seen in severe COVID-19, which is identified by elevated von Willebrand factor (VWF) antigen, elevated D-dimer, and fibrin/fibrinogen degradation products; the prothrombin time, partial thromboplastin time, and platelet counts are usually unaffected initially (see Chapter 14). The entity, referred to as **COVID-19–associated coagulopathy (CAC),** has laboratory findings that differ from traditional DIC. In CAC, fibrinogen levels are higher and platelets levels are more often normal than with DIC. Mortality among hospitalized patients with SARS-CoV-2 correlates with levels of VWF antigen as well as levels of soluble thrombomodulin, suggesting that an endotheliopathy occurs in critically ill patients. Coagulation factor V is increased in COVID-19, and this is a known suppressor of T-cell proliferation and associated with lymphopenia in COVID-19 patients.

C. Diagnostic Studies

The three basic diagnostic studies are PCR molecular tests (most sensitive and specific), rapid antigen detection (cheap and fast but not as sensitive), and antibody testing (useful for confirmation of exposure but with current assays not always able to distinguish vaccination from infection).

Diagnosis of SARS-CoV-2 infection is typically most firmly established using nucleic acid testing.

1. Molecular tests—In general, the reverse transcriptase–PCR (RT-PCR) assays are the standard for diagnosis, and assays based on nucleic acid amplification technology (NAAT), rapid antigen assays, and laminar flow procedures are less sensitive.

2. Antibody tests—A variety of laboratories are producing antibody assays to determine immunity and facilitate decision-making in return-to-work policies.

3. Clinical diagnosis—An unstandardized combination of clinical findings in conjunction with NATs are used to make the formal diagnosis of COVID-19, recognizing that the wide spectrum of clinical findings and the false reassurance of assays are not fully sensitive or specific.

D. Imaging

Early in the disease course, neither chest radiographs nor chest CT scans provide diagnostic utility, since both may be normal, and the nonspecific findings overlap with many respiratory viral infections. Later in the disease course, nonspecific diffuse ground-glass opacities or multilobular infiltrates (which often progress to consolidation), or both, become more common. Chest ultrasonography, MRI, and PET/CT findings tend to confirm the CT findings of an evolving organizing pneumonia. Serial imaging may be useful in identifying the progression of COVID-19–associated pulmonary aspergillosis (discussed below).

Differential Diagnosis

The key element in the differential diagnosis is seasonal influenza infection, which can usually be ruled out by a nasal swab. Concomitant infection with influenza or other respiratory pathogens is possible. Prominent musculoskeletal manifestations, sinusitis, and a sudden onset favor influenza infection, while a more insidious presentation with cough, weakness, malaise, and a gradual worsening of pulmonary symptoms favor SARS-CoV-2 infection.

Complications

Most patients recover without sequelae.

A clinical risk score calculator to predict critical illness in hospitalized patients with COVID-19 called COVID-GRAM has been validated (https://www.mdcalc.com/covid-gram-critical-illness-risk-score); predictors of clinical deterioration include presence of chest film abnormalities, older age, positive cancer history, increased number of comorbidities, presence of certain signs and symptoms (hemoptysis, dyspnea, and decreased consciousness), and presence of certain laboratory abnormalities (increased neutrophil to lymphocyte ratio, increased LD, and increased direct bilirubin). A British predictive scale suggests that eight variables be used at the time of hospitalization to assess the likelihood of death: age, sex, number of comorbidities, respiratory rate, peripheral oxygen saturation, Glasgow coma scale, serum urea level, and CRP. A standardized Quick COVID-19 Severity Index using respiratory rate, pulse oximetry, and oxygen flow rate is available at https://www.mdcalc.com/quick-covid-19-severity-index-qcsi.

1. SARS-CoV-2–related immune activation—A key component distinguishing mild and severe COVID-19 illness is the presence of early bystander CD8 T cells and strong plasmablast responses among patients with mild disease. Those with more severe disease show pronounced systemic inflammation at early presentation, often called a "cytokine storm" in the later phase of illness. (This term is criticized by some experts because cytokine levels in COVID-19 are lower than those in patients with ARDS and lower than those in patients with bacterial sepsis.) Persistent immune activation in predisposed patients can lead to uncontrolled amplification of cytokine production (including IL-6), leading to multiorgan failure and death. The period approximately 17–23 days after infection is identified as a critical point when a unique inflammatory response occurs in critically ill patients whose outcomes are fatal. Inflammatory immunologic abnormalities can persist for 60 or more days.

2. Pulmonary complications—The most common system involved with complications of severe COVID-19 is pulmonary. Some patients progress to ARDS akin to the coronavirus infections that cause SARS and MERS. In a large Veterans Affairs database, the risk for such progression was 19-fold greater among COVID-19 patients than among influenza patients. **COVID-19–related ARDS** is so commonly recognized that it is referred to as "CARDS." CARDS care requires the involvement of intensivists who can provide guidelines for respiratory support, including appropriate oxygen flow and ventilator parameters, prone positioning (which is also useful for nonventilated pulmonary patients), and hydration status. One of the most significant features of poor prognosis in CARDS is the development of pulmonary fibrosis. The presence of a capillary leak syndrome with associated alveolar edema was evaluated in the Netherlands with the tyrosine kinase inhibitor imatinib. This study suggested a preliminary benefit regarding survival and duration of ventilation, although statistical analysis was not fully confirmed and the agent needs further study. A myopathic process involving the diaphragm is also reported among patients with severe pulmonary complications.

The spectrum of pulmonary pathology shows that the most common findings on postmortem examinations are diffuse alveolar congestion, hyaline membrane formation, pneumocyte hyperplasia and necrosis, platelet-fibrin thrombi, interstitial edema, and squamous metaplasia with atypia. Pathologic findings are seen in other organs as well at autopsy.

The use of noninvasive ventilation versus extracorporeal membrane oxygenation (ECMO) is based on severity of disease and likelihood of progressive ARDS. The use of pulmonary consultants is essential, and the data showing various outcomes by use of respiratory modality are complicated by patient selection and the confounding variables determining outcome.

3. Coagulation complications—Many extrapulmonary complications are reported and most of these are likely related to SARS-CoV-2–induced inflammatory reactions. **COVID-19–related coagulopathy** is associated with a particular predisposition to pulmonary emboli and to thrombosis of vessels used for continuous renal replacement therapy and, less often, to thrombosis of extracorporeal membrane oxygenation–associated vessels. The reported incidence of DVT among ICU patients with COVID-19 infection is 6.3% and the incidence of a major bleed is 2.8%. Male sex and high D-dimer levels on day 1 are associated with greater likelihood of thrombotic complications. The presence of antiphospholipid antibodies in over half of patients hospitalized with COVID-19 suggests that autoantibodies may promote coagulation. A component of cell membranes, phosphatidylserine, is thought to have a significant role in the induction of thromboinflammation. Such inflammatory cell remnants are referred to as neutrophil extracellular traps, and preliminary studies suggest that dipyridamole may show both immunomodulatory and antiviral properties and stimulate type I interferon responses. The benefits and risks of anticoagulants in patients hospitalized with COVID-19 are being actively studied and current management recommendations are available at https://www.covid19treatmentguidelines.nih.gov/antithrombotic-therapy/.

In general, outpatients with COVID-19 should not receive anticoagulant or antiplatelet therapy for prevention of venous or arterial thrombosis unless other strong indications are present. Hospitalized patients should be given standard antithrombotic therapy; recommendations differ among specialist societies, with current recommendations advising heparin for moderate but not severe illness. The complexity of vaccine-induced thrombosis and thrombocytopenia management is discussed below. Antiplatelet treatments alone are not recommended.

4. Cardiac complications—Cardiac involvement is unique among coronaviruses pathogenic for humans, with only rare cases of cardiac complications with MERS or SARS and none with human cold viruses. In a multicenter US cohort study, MIs occurred in 14% of patients; survival was infrequent (2.9%) in those with infarction who were older than 80 years. A fulminant myocarditis occurs in about 15% of ICU patients, which can be further complicated by heart failure, cardiac arrhythmias, acute coronary syndrome, stress cardiomyopathy, cardiac aneurysms, vasculitis, and sudden death. Increased plasma ACE-2 concentration is associated with an increased risk of major cardiovascular events.

5. Renal complications—AKI occurs in approximately 12% of patients hospitalized with COVID-19. Of these, more than 20% require renal replacement therapy, which portends mortality (89–100%). Additionally, a collapsing glomerulopathy has been associated with COVID-19, called "**COVID-19–associated nephropathy**" or COVAN, which specifically affects individuals with polymorphisms in the apolipoprotein L1 (*APOL1*) gene. In France, patients with kidney failure caused by SLE show a particularly high rate of complications and mortality (25% versus 15% in patients with SLE versus other COVID-19 renal conditions).

6. GI complications—A particularly strong association exists between acute pancreatitis and SARS-CoV-2 infection. In a prospective international multicenter study based at Newcastle upon Tyne, patients with acute pancreatitis and coexisting SARS-CoV-2 infection are at increased risk for severe pancreatitis, ICU admission, local complications, organ failure, prolonged hospital stay, and higher 30-day mortality.

7. Neurologic complications—Commonly reported neurologic complications are headaches; seizures; strokes; and more often, a loss of taste and smell (ageusia and anosmia). The loss of smell in the absence of significant rhinorrhea or nasal congestion suggests a neurotropism by this coronavirus. SARS-CoV-2–related meningitis as well as other neurologic complications including impairment of consciousness to a comatose state, Guillain-Barré syndrome, and acute hemorrhagic necrotizing encephalopathy are reported. The presence of such neurologic manifestations is associated with higher in-hospital mortality.

While the presence of ACE receptors in brain tissue supports direct CNS involvement, actual isolation of the virus from the CNS is not consistent, and the CNS damage may occur via indirect mechanisms. The NIH has established a databank/biobank to document and track neurologic involvement in COVID-19 infection (the NeuroCOVID Project).

8. Psychiatric complications—Acute psychiatric diagnoses occurring at increased frequency include anxiety, depression, substance use disorder, and PTSD. The CDC currently reports that either anxiety or depression have increased in prevalence from 36.4% to 41.5% with highest rates among adults 18–29 and those with less than high school education. A global review from Australia confirms the high prevalence of anxiety and depression and estimates that in 2020 the number of disability-adjusted life-years lost was 44.5 million for anxiety and 49.4 million for major depression. In an Icelandic study, depression and insomnia were the most prevalent psychiatric symptoms, with anxiety more common among those who were bedridden.

Psychoses otherwise do not appear at increased rates, although eventual development of psychosis among people with no prior or family history is reported among some patients after COVID-19. Suicidal behavior appears to occur in about 6% of patients, and this rate is the same among health care professionals. Data from Australia suggest that the suicide rate is not impacted by COVID-19. Neurologists and psychiatrists express concern that long-term sequelae, including encephalopathy, psychoses, and movement disorders, may follow the pandemic (as they did after the influenza pandemic of 1918). Opioid use disorders are increasing because of the outbreak and are attendant with a decrease in outpatient visits for management and a possible decrease in access to naloxone.

9. Dermatologic complications—Skin manifestations are diverse and on occasion the presenting sign. Approximately 5–20% of patients with COVID-19 are found to have dermatologic symptoms. One review of patients with COVID-19 identified acral lesions as the most common rash type, followed by erythematous maculopapular rashes, vesicular rashes, urticarial rashes, and many others. Such skin manifestations typically last no longer than 2 weeks, although rarely COVID-19–related rashes are reported to last 2–4 weeks.

10. Infectious complications—One systematic review found that approximately 8% of patients hospitalized with COVID-19 have bacterial coinfection or secondary infection.

The higher complication rates among patients who have COVID-19 compared with patients who have influenza include risks for pneumonia, ventilator dependence, pneumothorax, acute myocarditis, stroke, cardiogenic shock, sepsis, and pressure injuries but not for acute MIs, unstable angina, or heart failure.

A unique form of pulmonary aspergillosis, referred to as **COVID-19–associated pulmonary aspergillosis (CAPA)**, increases the morbidity and mortality of patients infected with SARS-CoV-2. Due to the difficulty distinguishing airway colonization from CAPA, debate about many features of this entity remains. CAPA usually responds to voriconazole or isavuconazonium, although in some azole-resistant cases, amphotericin is needed. Diagnosis is facilitated by galactomannan assays when available. In a multinational observational cohort study, 15% of patients hospitalized in an ICU with COVID-19 became infected with *Aspergillus*. However, pathologists in a Canadian study report the incidence of CAPA or an associated invasive mold disease (about 2%) among autopsies of patients with COVID-19 as far lower than anticipated. Clinicians in Arkansas and India have reported an increased incidence of mucormycosis in patients with COVID-19.

11. Endocrine complications—A host of endocrine abnormalities are reported including diabetic ketoacidosis, subacute thyroiditis with clinical thyrotoxicosis, and new-onset Graves disease, or Hashimoto autoimmune thyroiditis. In addition, malnutrition occurs in up to 45% of patients with COVID-19 and significant deficits in a variety of quality of life and functional capacity measures are reported 6 months after infection.

12. Multisystem inflammatory syndrome (MIS)—Inflammatory complications weeks after mild or asymptomatic SARS-CoV-2 infection in adults are increasingly recognized; this syndrome is called **MIS-A.**

13. Postoperative complications—Patients with COVID-19 are at high risk for postoperative complications. In an international cohort study assessing postsurgical outcomes, postoperative severe acute respiratory problems occurred in 71.5% and the 30-day postoperative mortality was 23.8%.

14. Other complications and "long COVID"—Acute musculoskeletal pain is reported in nearly 20%. Hepatic and biliary injury, often acute, and DIC in advanced cases are reported from China. Conjunctivitis is reported from China in about one-third of cases.

The diversity of physical and mental health problems among COVID-19 patients supports the need for tailored rehabilitation services. The long-term sequelae of COVID-19 are being described; a diversity of syndromes appears to characterize these long-term sequelae and are in the process of further definition. A compilation of nine studies of **post-acute COVID-19 syndrome** from the United States, Europe, and China shows a male preponderance (52–67%) and an age range skewed toward upper middle age (mean, 45–63, median 56–71, not all studies giving both values). The most common symptoms were fatigue (32%), smell or taste disorder (22%), dyspnea (16%), headache (12%), memory impairment (11%), hair loss (10%), and sleep disorder (10%). Among patients who tested positive for SARS-CoV-2, female sex (aOR = 1.7) and overweight/obesity (aOR = 1.7) predicted persistent symptoms. Many refer to such complications as **"long COVID"** (also referred to as **PASC** or **post-acute sequelae after SARS-CoV-2**) and attest to a relapsing and remitting nature to the entity as well as a multisystem nature with pulmonary, dermatologic, GI, and neurologic symptoms all variably involved. The prevalence of certain symptoms, in particular, dyspnea, anxiety, and depression (which correlates with limited assets) and, in women, fatigue and muscle weakness, increased. Among students, COVID-19 infection is associated with food insecurity. Rehabilitation programs are essential in the management of long COVID but less than 1% of patients report such usage. Current vaccines are reported to reduce the incidence of long COVID by about half.

The COVID-19 pandemic has resulted in consequential delays in preventive screenings (eg, mammograms), emergency care, and elective surgery. When elective surgery is performed, it should be delayed to about 7 weeks after acute COVID-19 infection since the mortality rate declines from 9.1% in the first 2 weeks following infection to 2% after 7 weeks have passed following acute infection.

The serious psychological sequelae of potentially dying alone, of restricted or impaired access to family or friends (especially in nursing homes), and limited funeral services are all relevant issues with which society is grappling. These important aspects require creativity to find tolerable, safe, and sustainable solutions.

Treatment

Most infections are mild and require no treatment or only supportive therapy. Because of the biphasic nature of advanced cases, the early course should be managed with antiviral agents, and the later inflammatory phase should be managed with anti-inflammatory agents. For the treatment of COVID-19, many medications from various pharmacologic classes are being evaluated in clinical trials and include RNA polymerase inhibitors, corticosteroids, IL-6 receptor inhibitors, JAK inhibitors, interferon therapies, convalescent plasma, monoclonal antibodies, and viral protease inhibitors. As of April 2022, the medications that are the most promising, at least for severe disease, are remdesivir, dexamethasone, tocilizumab, and baricitinib. The WHO (https://www.who.int/publications/i/item/WHO-2019-nCoV-clinical-2021-2), the NIH (https://www.covid19treatmentguidelines.nih.gov/whats-new/), and the Infectious Diseases Society of America (IDSA) (https://www.idsociety.org/practice-guideline/covid-19-guideline-treatment-and-management/) provide current guidance for the management of COVID-19 patients including during screening, outpatient management, and inpatient care.

Prevention

A. Personal and Public Health Measures

In the setting of significant community SARS-CoV-2 transmission, the recommended precautions to prevent SARS-CoV-2 infection include frequent handwashing with soap and water for at least 20 seconds, avoiding touching the face, wearing a cloth face covering in public (and, for health care personnel, wearing an impermeable mask [eg, N95 mask] and face shield if exposure to patients with cough or respiratory secretions, or both, is anticipated), practicing social distancing of at least 6 feet when in public, and isolating cases (in particular, removing infected patients from long-term care facilities, such as nursing homes, and transportation structures, such as cruise ships). Using eye protection (including wearing eyeglasses daily) provides protection from SARS-CoV-2 as well.

For social activities among vaccinated individuals, an easing of masking precautions can be recommended. Masking is still needed for medical and some educational settings and may be recommended for transportation settings.

B. Vaccines

As of March 18, 2022, 35 vaccines have received at least preliminary regulatory authorization and begun to be distributed in one or more countries (https://covid19.trackvaccines.org/vaccines/approved/). Ten are approved for use by the WHO: Moderna, Pfizer, Janssen, Oxford/AstraZeneca, Covishield, Sinopharm, Sinovac, Bharat Biotech, Novavax, and Covovax.

1. Vaccine distribution in the United States—Distribution of the Pfizer and Moderna vaccines began in the United States in December 2020 after these two vaccines received FDA Emergency Use Authorization (EUA). Subsequently the Janssen vaccine also received FDA EUA. The Pfizer vaccine (now marketed as Comirnaty) attained full FDA approval (for people aged 16 and older) on August 23, 2021; additionally, the Pfizer vaccine has EUA for children aged 5–17 years (given as two doses, 10 mcg, 0.2 mL each, 3 weeks apart). The vaccine is safe and associated with no serious adverse effects reported to date. The Janssen vaccine is also available in the United States.

Those with prior infection should still undergo vaccination since immune responses to mild or moderate infections are not always durable (although those with prior infection mount a stronger response to vaccination).

Both the Pfizer and Moderna vaccines require two doses spaced 3–4 weeks apart, and it is recommended that they are followed by a "booster" dose at 5 months. CDC guidelines recommend those with moderate to severe immune deficiency should receive an additional (third) dose 28 days after completing the usual two mRNA vaccine series (prior to any booster vaccines given at 6 months following the initial vaccination series, see below). In contrast, the Janssen vaccine only requires one dose followed by a booster dose at 2 months.

2. Vaccine storage—Notably, one concern for both the Pfizer and Moderna mRNA vaccines is the need for a cold chain; the Pfizer vaccine requires storage at –70°C and the Moderna vaccine can be stored at 2°C to 8°C for up to 30 days after thawing from frozen (between –25°C and –15°C). The available adenovirus-vectored vaccines generally have more flexible storage conditions.

3. Vaccine-associated reactions and complications—Commonly reported side effects post-mRNA vaccine administration include nausea, low-grade fevers, injection site soreness (shown for the Moderna vaccine to be a local delayed hypersensitivity reaction and not a contraindication for further vaccination), headaches (4.5%, both vaccines), and fatigue (as high as 9.7% with the Moderna vaccine, 3.8% with the Pfizer vaccine). Local injection site reactions, fatigue, headache, fever, and muscle pains also are common for the adenovirus-vectored vaccines AstraZeneca and Johnson & Johnson vaccines. Concomitant administration of anti-inflammatory agents, such as paracetamol or ibuprofen, is *not* recommended because antibody responses may be blunted. A promising anti-inflammatory agent in trials is CD24Fc.

The Vaccine Safety Datalink is used to document complications of currently used vaccines. Myocarditis, a rare complication of the mRNA vaccines, has been studied in healthy members of the American military (23 cases among 2.8 million doses). Surveillance data show that myocarditis/pericarditis occurs disproportionately in young adults aged 12–39 years at an excess rate of 6.3 per million doses during the week following vaccination. Rates are slightly higher after the second dose and for younger adolescents. CDC rates are 1 in 12,361 for adolescents 12–15 years old (1 in 144,439 for female teens) and for Israeli adolescents (after the Pfizer BioNTech vaccine) of this age cohort 1 in 16,129.

CDC data show that non–COVID-19 associated death rates among vaccinated people show lower mortality than the rates among unvaccinated people, with appropriate cofactor adjustments (sex, age, race, ethnicity, location), thus confirming the safety profile of COVID-19 vaccines.

A British study outlines a distinct set of patients who are at highest risk for COVID-19 vaccine-related deaths. Among 81 possible vaccine-related deaths (of almost 7 million vaccinated persons), patients with the following conditions or factors had a twofold or greater risk of death: Down syndrome (12.7-fold increase), kidney transplants, sickle cell anemia, nursing home residency, chemotherapy, HIV/AIDS infection, cirrhosis, neurologic conditions, recent solid organ or bone marrow transplantation, dementia, and Parkinson disease.

4. Vaccination rates—As of February 11, 2022, at least 75% (251 million people) of the United States population have received one dose, and 64% (213 million people) are considered fully vaccinated. Considerable regional variation exists, with the highest full vaccination rates in New England and the lowest in the South.

Globally, countries with more people vaccinated than the United States are China, India, and the composite nations of the European Union, although over 70 jurisdictions globally have higher vaccination *rates* than the United States (66%, with corresponding reported estimates for China of 80%; the European Union, 69%; and India, 53%). In the United States, highest rates remain in New England and Hawaii and lowest in the South and Upper Midwest. Rural areas in the United States show considerably lower primary vaccinated rates (58.5% versus 75.4% for urban areas).

5. "Real-world" vaccine efficacy and duration of protective immunity—The CDC reports excellent effectiveness with COVID-19 vaccines, that hospitalization among veterans who received mRNA vaccines was reduced 80% in those over age 60, and that in a nine-state study of all three vaccines used in the United States, at a time of delta variant predominance, the rates of infections were reduced 5-fold and rates of hospitalization and death over 10-fold.

Duration of protection post-SARS-CoV-2 vaccination appears to last for at least 6 months post vaccination. Studies of the Moderna vaccine indicate that vaccine-induced neutralizing antibody activity and CD4 T-cell memory remain high at 6 months post vaccination. Protective immunity generated by the Pfizer vaccine show immunologic maturity and stem cell memory at 6 months, although a recent Israeli study indicated that 6 months after receipt of the second dose of the Pfizer vaccine, humoral responses were significantly decreased among men, those aged 65 years of age or older, and immunosuppressed people. The AstraZeneca vaccine induces high antibodies and good cellular responses at 3 months after a single dose and antibody persistence up to 320 days.

Data are evolving for protection after the third dose, which is better than after the second. The CDC reported that with an mRNA vaccine during the omicron-predominant period, vaccine efficacy against emergency department or urgent care visits was 87–91% during the 2 months after a third dose but decreased to 66–78% by 4 months. Immunity from natural infection reportedly exists for at least 1 year.

Patients with intellectual disabilities should also be prioritized for vaccination in that they show higher than average rates of disease and worse outcomes when infected.

6. Breakthrough SARS-CoV-2 infections post vaccination—While SARS-CoV-2 infection can occur after vaccination, most cases are not severe. Breakthrough cases are often caused by SARS-CoV-2 variants.

The odds of confirmed COVID-19 infection in the CDC's nine-state study are 5.49-fold higher among unvaccinated persons with previous SARS-CoV-2 infection than among vaccinated persons with no such previous infection. Hence, *all eligible persons should be vaccinated, including those previously infected.*

In addition to having a less severe illness course, infected vaccinated persons seem to have a faster decrease in SARS-CoV-2 viral loads after infection compared with unvaccinated persons, indicating that they are able to clear the virus faster.

Since several variants are more transmissible, public implementation of vaccination programs is even more important. Continued surveillance and genomic sequencing are essential to continue to provide comprehensive vaccine coverage and to assess the potential need for booster doses in the future. Programs that provide vaccines to the developing world are one of the most effective way of containing the emergence of more transmissible or pathogenic variants (and the WHO recommends that surplus doses preferentially be given to vaccine deprived areas).

7. Booster vaccine doses—Studies from Israel and Qatar confirm the presence of significant waning immunity 5–6 months after the second dose of the Pfizer vaccine, especially in association with the emergence of the delta variant. Third-dose booster doses of the mRNA vaccines (Pfizer and Moderna) have been commercially available in the United States since September 20, 2021 (the FDA authorized a 5- [Pfizer] or 6- [Moderna] month booster dose of the Pfizer and Moderna vaccines and a 2-month booster dose of the Janssen vaccine, for any adult who has completed primary vaccination). Boosters are given at full dose for the Pfizer vaccine and half dose for the Moderna vaccine.

8. Vaccination of immunocompromised people (third dose and booster dose)—Patients taking certain medications (eg, B-cell depleting therapies such as rituximab and high-dose corticosteroids that deplete antibody levels more than JAK inhibitors, antimetabolites, or TNF inhibitors) or with certain malignancies and immunosuppressive states (especially B-cell disorders) and even autoimmune states may not have a measurable antibody response postvaccination and should be considered as equivalent to being unvaccinated. Despite a failure of humoral response with three doses of SARS-CoV-2 vaccines in such patients (studied in rheumatoid arthritis patients), a third dose is still thought to boost the cellular immune responses. A third dose and a booster dose are recommended by the CDC.

It is important that family and contacts of immunocompromised people be vaccinated. Those with impending iatrogenic immunocompromise should receive SARS-CoV-2 vaccination before receiving immunosuppressive therapy if possible.

9. Vaccination in pregnant and lactating women—Vaccine registry data indicate that mRNA vaccines are safe in pregnant women (including assessment in an Israeli cohort of over 10,000 vaccinated women), thus pregnant women and those planning pregnancy should be targeted for vaccination with the mRNA vaccines. Among vaccinated women, SARS-CoV-2 vaccine antibodies appear in breastmilk by 2 weeks after vaccination and persist for 7 weeks (but vaccine-associated mRNA does not), thus lactating women and their breastfeeding children likely benefit from vaccination.

10. Vaccination, herd immunity, and vaccine hesitancy—To achieve effective herd immunity in a population, vaccination uptake must be relatively high (the threshold for herd immunity is directly related to the virus's transmissibility; eg, with an R_0 of 2.5, herd immunity can be achieved at a 60% threshold, whereas with an R_0 of 6, the threshold for herd immunity increases 84%). Studies on attitudes toward SARS-CoV-2 vaccine acceptance by the general population, however, indicated that a significant portion of the adult population would not accept a SARS-CoV-2 vaccine (including more than 25% of French adults, nearly 15% of Australian adults, and more than 20% of US adults), and this has indeed been the case in the United States as vaccines have become available. *Vaccine hesitancy* research in late 2020 by the CDC showed that highest nonintent to receive vaccines exists among younger adults; women;

non-Hispanic Black adults; adults in nonmetropolitan areas; and adults who are less educated, have lower income, and do not have health insurance. Measures advocated to increase vaccine acceptance by the public include making the vaccine free and accessible, establishing conditions dependent on vaccination (school entry, employment maintenance, flight requirements as has been done by Qantas), announcing public endorsement by trusted leaders, encouraging public documentation of vaccination (stickers), and facilitating access with early sign-up periods.

C. Immunity to SARS-CoV-2

Promising data have been released about naturally acquired immunity to SARS-CoV-2, indicating that robust T- and B-cell immunity develops even after asymptomatic or mild SARS-CoV-2 infection.

The Ethical Issues of Care

Health care workers in their special relationship to society often find themselves in a bind when confronted with the high rate of illness among medical staff and the real risks of employment on the front line. Health care workers show a higher-than-expected rate of mental health conditions, especially anxiety, depression, PTSD, and suicidal ideation, in particular when they are unable to take time off or work 41 hours or more per week. Students enter the health care profession recognizing these risks and such risks are especially great for certain frontline workers. The opting-out of frontline care is a consideration when age or concomitant diseases such as diabetes place providers at particular risk for infection, and in these cases, their ethical obligations can be considered supererogatory (moral but not required). The provision by hospitals of safe working environment and adequate protective gear is an important major corollary obligation.

When to Refer

Even asymptomatic patients and those with atypical manifestations may be shedding and transmitting the virus. Patients in whom the disease is suspected should be tested appropriately and quarantined or triaged based on the severity of their symptoms.

Clinics and hospitals with the resources to screen or test outpatients for SARS-CoV-2 should set up a testing area that is isolated from other patient care areas (and outside or in an "open air" environment if possible). These facilities should also designate separate care areas for patients in whom SARS-CoV-2 infection is confirmed or suspected and provide the necessary personal protective equipment for staff who could potentially be exposed to patients infected with SARS-CoV-2.

When to Admit

Respiratory complications require admission. Progression to respiratory failure and ARDS can be rapid, and any patient in a high-risk category for complications should be admitted for observation and placed under intensive care based on respiratory parameters.

Adhikari EH et al. COVID-19 vaccination in pregnant and lactating women. JAMA. 2021;325:1039. [PMID: 33555297]

Al-Samkari H et al. Thrombosis, bleeding, and the observational effect of early therapeutic anticoagulation on survival in critically ill patients with COVID-19. Ann Intern Med. 2021;174:622. [PMID: 33493012]

Andrasfay T et al. Reductions in 2020 US life expectancy due to COVID-19 and the disproportionate impact on the Black and Latino populations. Proc Natl Acad Sci U S A. 2021;118:e2014746118. [PMID: 33446511]

Beigel JH et al. Remdesivir for the treatment of Covid-19 – final report. N Engl J Med. 2020;383:1813. [PMID: 32445440]

Belay ED et al. Multisystem inflammatory syndrome in adults after SARS-CoV-2 infection and COVID-19 vaccination. Clin Infect Dis. 2021 Nov 28. [Epub ahead of print] [PMID: 34849680]

Bryant-Genevier J et al. Symptoms of depression, anxiety, post-traumatic stress disorder, and suicidal ideation among state, tribal, local, and territorial public health workers during the COVID-19 pandemic – United States, March-April 2021. MMWR Morb Mortal Wkly Rep. 2021;70:1680. [PMID: 34855723]

Cohen MS. Monoclonal antibodies to disrupt progression of early COVID-19 infection. N Engl J Med. 2021;384:289. [PMID: 33471984]

Crook H et al. Long COVID – mechanisms, risk factors, and management. BMJ. 2021;374;n1648. [PMID: 34312178]

Holmes EC et al. The origins of SARS-CoV-2: a critical review. Cell. 2021;184:4848.[PMID: 34480864]

Huang L et al. 1-year outcomes in hospital survivors with COVID-19; a longitudinal cohort study. Lancet. 2021;398:747. [PMID: 34454673]

Loembé MM et al. COVID-10 vaccine access in Africa: global distribution, vaccine platforms, and challenges ahead. Immunity. 2021;54:1353. [PMID: 34260880]

Sidebottom DB et al. Safety and efficacy of antivirals against SARS-CoV-2. BMJ. 2021;375:n2611. [PMID: 34711614]

Woolf SH et al. COVID-19 as the leading cause of death in the United States. JAMA. 2021;325:123. [PMID: 33331845]

2. Respiratory Syncytial Virus (RSV) & Other Paramyxoviruses

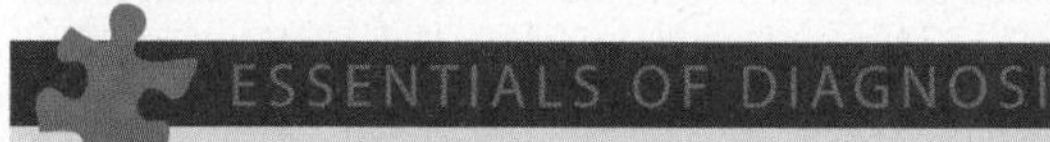

- RSV is a major cause of morbidity and mortality at the extremes of age (< 5 years and > 65 years).
- Treatment is largely supportive.
- No active vaccination for RSV is currently available.

General Considerations

RSV is a paramyxovirus that causes annual outbreaks during the wintertime with usual onset of pulmonary symptoms between mid-October and early January in the continental United States. Outside the United States, RSV usually peaks during wet months in areas with high annual precipitation and during cooler months in hot and dry areas. Infections occur earlier in urban areas.

There are two major subtypes of RSV: A and B; the A subtype may be associated with severe disease. RSV is a frequent cause of hospitalization in US children, with annual hospitalization rates of 6 per 1000 children younger than 5 years. RSV is the most common cause of bronchiolitis and pneumonia in children younger than 1 year in the United States. Prematurity and bronchopulmonary dysplasia are major risk factors for severe disease. Early RSV bronchiolitis in children, along with a family history of asthma, are associated with persistence of airway reactivity later in life.

RSV also causes upper and lower respiratory tract infection in adults, with the virus entering through contact with mucous membranes. RSV occurs with increasing severity in those with comorbid conditions, older adults (accounting for a rate of 4 per 1000 hospitalizations and 14,000 deaths annually), persons with severe combined immunodeficiency, and patients after lung or bone marrow transplantation (because CD8 T cells are not available for viral clearance). An interleukin-1 receptor polymorphism is associated with more severe bronchiolitis. Recurrences occur throughout life. The average incubation period is 5 days. Up to 10% of disease classified as invasive pneumococcal disease is thought to be RSV or influenza.

In immunocompromised patients, such as bone marrow transplant recipients, serious pneumonia can occur, and outbreaks with a high mortality rate (over 70%) are reported.

Other paramyxoviruses important in human disease include human metapneumovirus, parainfluenza virus, and Nipah virus.

Human metapneumovirus is a ubiquitous seasonal virus circulating during late winter to early spring. It is divided into subgroups A and B. Metapneumovirus accounted for 7.3% of childhood (younger than 16 years old) pneumonia in a Norwegian series of 3650 patients in which RSV accounted for 28.7%. Clinical presentations range from mild upper respiratory tract infections to severe lower respiratory tract infections (eg, bronchiolitis, croup, and pneumonia). Lower respiratory tract (sometimes severe) infections are observed among immunocompromised and older adults, especially residents of nursing homes. In lung transplant recipients, human metapneumovirus is a common cause of respiratory illness and may increase the risk of acute and chronic graft rejection. Ribavirin appears to be well tolerated in lung transplant recipients with metapneumovirus infection. The control of RSV infection in modeling studies reduces the incidence of human metapneumovirus infection.

Human parainfluenza viruses (HPIVs) are commonly seen in children and are the most common cause of laryngotracheitis (croup). Four different serotypes are described, and they differ in their clinical presentations as well as epidemiology. HPIV-1 and HPIV-2 are responsible for croup. HPIV-3 is associated with bronchiolitis and pneumonia. HPIV-4 is a less frequently reported pathogen. Reinfections are common throughout life. HPIVs can also cause severe disease in older individuals, immunocompromised persons, and patients with chronic illnesses.

Nipah virus is a highly virulent paramyxovirus first described in 1999. Cases are concentrated mainly in Southeast Asia (Malaysia, Singapore, Bangladesh, and India). Fruit bats are identified as the natural host of the virus. An outbreak of 14 cases, 8 fatal, occurred in Bangladesh associated with drinking date palm sap between 2010 and 2014. Direct pig-human, cow-human, human-human, and nosocomial transmission are reported. Nipah virus causes acute encephalitis with a high fatality rate (67–92%), although respiratory symptoms are also described. Cranial nerve palsies, encephalopathy, and dystonia are among neurologic sequelae (15–32%) seen in infected individuals. Relapses occurring weeks and months after initial infection are described (3.4–7.5%).

Clinical Findings

A. Symptoms and Signs

In RSV bronchiolitis, proliferation and necrosis of bronchiolar epithelium develop, producing obstruction from sloughed epithelium and increased mucus secretion. Signs of infection include low-grade fever, tachypnea, and wheezes. Apnea is a common presenting symptom. Hyperinflated lungs, decreased gas exchange, and increased work of breathing are present. Pulmonary hemorrhage is reported. *In children, RSV is globally a common cause of acute lower respiratory infection and acute and recurrent otitis media.*

B. Laboratory Findings

A rapid diagnosis of RSV infection is made by viral antigen identification of nasal washings using an ELISA or immunofluorescent assay; molecular rapid tests are also used. Multiplex assays in conjunction with other respiratory viruses, most commonly influenza and SARS-CoV-2, are available commercially. RSV viral load assay values at day 3 of infection may correlate with requirement of intensive care and respiratory failure in children.

Human metapneumovirus is best diagnosed by PCR. Tests for rapid detection of viral antigens with immunofluorescence, ELISA, and PCR techniques are widely available for detection of HPIV. Culture may also be used. ELISA (serum and CSF) and PCR (urine and respiratory secretions but not blood) are both used for Nipah virus infection diagnosis.

Treatment & Prevention

Treatment of RSV consists of supportive care, including hydration, humidification of inspired air, antibiotic therapy (to reduce other respiratory morbidity) if concomitant bacterial pneumonia is suspected, and ventilatory support as needed. Neither bronchodilating agents nor corticosteroids show efficacy in bronchiolitis although individual patients with significant bronchospasm or history of asthma may respond to them.

The use of aerosolized ribavirin or RSV-enriched IVIG, or both, can be considered in high-risk patients, such as those with a history of bone marrow transplantation, and appears to lessen mortality.

Several additional agents are under study for treatment of RSV. They include small-molecule RSV fusion inhibitors that bind to the surface F protein (such as JNJ-53718678, presatovir, ziresovir, and sisunatovir). Compounds targeting viral replication also have been under study, including lumicitabine (although its development has been stopped), AZ-27, PC786, JNJ-64417184, and EDP-938.

The prophylactic monoclonal antibody palivizumab, while recommended for and effective in high-risk infants (premature infants less than 32 weeks' gestation as well as infants 32- to 25-weeks' gestation with additional risk factors such as congenital heart and lung diseases and Down syndrome), is not of proven efficacy among adults with RSV. The monoclonal antibody nirsevimab is also effective in preventing RSV-associated lower respiratory tract infections in premature infants.

No RSV vaccine is currently commercially available; however, three vaccine candidates are in phase 3 clinical trials, including two protein subunit vaccines (one by GSK and one by Pfizer) and a recombinant vector vaccine by Janssen (https://www.path.org/resources/rsv-vaccine-and-mab-snapshot/).

Prevention in hospitals entails rapid diagnosis, hand washing contact isolation, and perhaps passive immunization. (Passive immunization is costly but is associated with improved antiviral titers in hematologic stem cell transplant recipients.) The use of conjugated pneumococcal vaccination appears to decrease the incidence of concomitant pneumonia associated with viral infections in children in some countries. Viral shedding averages 11 days and correlates inversely with age and directly with severity of infection.

Therapeutic modalities for human metapneumovirus and parainfluenza virus infections under investigation include intravenous ribavirin administration.

Cunningham S et al. Nebulised ALX-0171 for respiratory syncytial virus lower respiratory tract infection in hospitalised children: a double-blind, randomised, placebo-controlled, phase 2b trial. Lancet Respir Med. 2021;9:21. [PMID: 33002427]

Elawar F et al. Pharmacological targets and emerging treatments for respiratory syncytial virus bronchiolitis. Pharmacol Ther. 2021;220:107712. [PMID: 33121940]

Griffin MP et al; Nirsevimab Study Group. Single-dose nirsevimab for prevention of RSV in preterm infants. N Engl J Med. 2020;383:415. [PMID: 32726528]

Madhi SA et al. Respiratory syncytial virus vaccination during pregnancy and effects in infants. N Engl J Med. 2020;383:426. [PMID: 32726529]

3. Seasonal Influenza

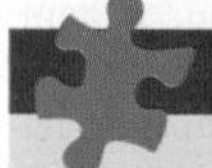

ESSENTIALS OF DIAGNOSIS

- Cases usually in epidemic pattern.
- Onset with fever, chills, malaise, cough, coryza, and myalgias.
- Aching, fever, and prostration out of proportion to catarrhal symptoms.
- Leukopenia.

General Considerations

Influenza (an orthomyxovirus) is a highly contagious disease transmitted by the respiratory route in humans. Transmission occurs primarily by *droplet nuclei* rather than fomites or direct contact. Three types of influenza viruses infect humans. While type A can infect a variety of mammals (humans, swine, horses, etc) and birds, types B and C almost exclusively infect humans. Type A viruses are further divided into subtypes based on the hemagglutinin (H) and the neuraminidase (N) expressed on their surface. Eighteen subtypes of hemagglutinin and 11 subtypes of neuraminidase are identified.

Annual epidemics usually appear in the fall or winter in temperate climates. Up to 5 million cases of severe influenza are estimated by the WHO to occur annually, with up to 0.5 million annual deaths. Influenza epidemics affect 10–20% of the global population on average each year and are typically the result of minor antigenic variations of the virus, or **antigenic drift**, which occur often in influenza A virus. On the other hand, pandemics—associated with higher mortality—appear at longer and varying intervals (decades) as a consequence of major genetic reassortment of the virus (**antigenic shift**) or adaptation of an avian or swine virus to humans (as with the pandemic H1N1 virus of 1918) (https://www.who.int/influenza/surveillance_monitoring/updates/latest_update_GIP_surveillance/en/).

The highly pathogenic avian influenza subtypes are discussed in the next section. The novel swine-origin influenza A (pandemic H1N1) virus emerged in Mexico in 2009 and quickly spread throughout North America and the world causing a pandemic. This virus originated from triple-reassortment of North American swine, human, and avian virus lineages and Eurasian swine virus lineages and replaced the previous H1N1 seasonal virus.

Clinical Findings

A. Symptoms and Signs

Type A and B seasonal influenza viruses produce clinically indistinguishable infections, whereas type C usually causes mild illness. The incubation period is 1–4 days. In unvaccinated persons, uncomplicated influenza often begins abruptly. Symptoms range widely from nearly asymptomatic to a constellation of systemic symptoms (including fever, chills, headache, malaise, and myalgias) and respiratory symptoms (including rhinorrhea, congestion, pharyngitis, hoarseness, nonproductive cough, and substernal soreness). GI symptoms and signs may occur, particularly among young children with influenza B virus infections. Fever lasts 1–7 days (usually 3–5). Older patients especially may present with lassitude and confusion, often without fever or respiratory symptoms. Signs include mild pharyngeal injection, flushed face, and conjunctival redness. Moderate enlargement of the cervical lymph nodes and tracheal tenderness may be observed. The presence of fever (higher than 38.2°C) and cough during influenza season is highly predictive of influenza infection in those older than 4 years.

B. Laboratory Findings

Rapid influenza diagnostic tests for detection of influenza antigens from nasal or throat swabs are widely available, highly specific, and produce fast results but have low sensitivity leading to high false-negative results. Because of this, *the CDC recommends empirically treating patients in whom influenza is suspected.* Testing is not necessary unless the patient is ill enough to require admission to the hospital. Not all commercial rapid influenza diagnostic tests can differentiate between influenza A and influenza B, and none of the available rapid influenza diagnostic tests can provide information on influenza A subtypes. Newer digital immunoassays and rapid nucleic acid amplification tests are more sensitive than traditional rapid influenza diagnostic tests; however, the sensitivity of newer PCR techniques is compromised early in the season during low prevalence periods. A nasopharyngeal swab, nasal aspirate, combined nasopharyngeal swab with oropharyngeal swab, or material from a bronchoalveolar lavage can be tested for any influenza strain. When influenza pneumonia is suspected, lower respiratory tract specimens should be collected and tested for influenza viruses by RT-PCR or the above assays.

Differential Diagnosis

The differential diagnoses for influenza-like infections include a variety of viral respiratory infections (SARS-CoV-2, parainfluenza, RSV, atypical dengue, adenovirus, enterovirus, coronavirus) or other viral infections (flavivirus, CMV, EBV, acute HIV infection), as well as bacterial infections such as mycobacterial infection (atypical pneumonia), pertussis, and Legionnaire disease. Epidemiologic factors can suggest Legionnaire (older adult smokers). Chronicity of cough may suggest adenovirus, mycobacterial, or pertussis infection. Leukocytosis and lymphadenopathy are more often seen with CMV and EBV. Distinguishing influenza from dengue requires attention to rhinitis (influenza) and thrombocytopenia (dengue).

Complications

Hospitalization or ICU admission for influenza is often a consequence of diffuse viral pneumonitis with severe hypoxemia and sometimes shock. Patients with asthma, residents of nursing homes and long-term care facilities, adults aged 65 years or older, persons who have morbid obesity, and persons with underlying medical conditions (pulmonary, renal, cardiovascular, hepatic, hematologic, neurologic, and neurodevelopmental conditions; and immune-deficient conditions, such as HIV, diabetes, and cirrhosis) are at high risk for complications. Infection during pregnancy increases the risk for hospitalization and may be associated with severe illness, sepsis, pneumothorax and respiratory failure, spontaneous abortion, preterm labor, and fetal distress.

Influenza causes necrosis of the respiratory epithelium, increased adherence of bacteria to infected cells, and ciliary dysfunction, which predispose to secondary bacterial infections. Pneumococcal pneumonia is the most common secondary infection, and staphylococcal pneumonia is the most serious. *Haemophilus* spp infections also occur. Other frequent complications are acute sinusitis, otitis media, and purulent bronchitis.

CVDs are a complication of influenza infection, in particular among older adults, and influenza is postulated to be a significant trigger for MI, cerebrovascular disease, and sudden death. Several studies suggest that influenza vaccination has protective effect against major adverse cardiovascular events. Neurologic complications, including seizures and encephalopathy, may occur. Encephalopathic complications of influenza are uncommon.

Reye syndrome is a rare and severe complication of influenza (usually B type) and other viral diseases (especially varicella), particularly in young children. It consists of rapidly progressive hepatic failure and encephalopathy, and the mortality rate is 30%. The pathogenesis is unknown, but the syndrome is associated with aspirin use in the management of viral infections.

Treatment

Treatment is supportive. Antiviral therapy should be considered for all persons with acute illness, in particular those at high risk for developing complications who have a suggestive clinical presentation or with laboratory-confirmed influenza. Clinical trials show a reduction in the duration of symptoms, hospital admissions, as well as secondary complications, such as otitis, sinusitis, or pneumonia, but not mortality when using these agents. Maximum benefit is expected with the earliest initiation of therapy. Although the benefit of antiviral therapy after 48 hours of illness is reduced, it should be initiated if the patient is hospitalized or critically ill. Benefit has been noted up to 4–5 days into illness.

The antiviral treatment of choice should be based on the susceptibility of the circulating virus. Since high levels of resistance to the adamantanes (amantadine and rimantadine) persist among seasonal H1N1 and H3N2 influenza A viruses and these agents are not effective against influenza B viruses, amantadine and rimantadine are not recommended for treatment.

Three neuraminidase inhibitors are FDA-approved for treatment of influenza A and B: oral oseltamivir, inhaled zanamivir, and intravenous peramivir. The CDC recommends treatment with **oral oseltamivir** (75 mg twice daily for 5 days) as the medication of choice for patients of any age, pregnant women, and patients who are hospitalized or have complicated infection. Absorption of oral oseltamivir is considered reliable, except in patients with impaired gastric motility or GI bleeding.

Inhaled zanamivir (10 mg, two inhalations twice daily for 5 days) is indicated for uncomplicated acute influenza in patients 7 years and older, is relatively contraindicated among persons with asthma because of the risk of bronchospasm and is not formulated for use in mechanically ventilated patients. Inhaled zanamivir lacks efficacy in pneumonia, probably due to poor bioavailability in the peripheral lungs.

Intravenous peramivir (600 mg in single dose) is used for outpatient treatment of uncomplicated infection in patients 18 years and older. It is also recommended if concern exists about inadequate oral absorption of oseltamivir. The efficacy of peramivir in patients with severe illness and in patients with influenza B is not well established. Some studies demonstrated that repeated doses for up to 5 days of intravenous peramivir are safe, effective, and shorten the duration of influenza illness.

Resistance to neuraminidase inhibitors (oseltamivir, zanamivir, and peramivir) can occur during or after prolonged use in immunocompromised patients, particularly in persons who have undergone hematopoietic stem cell transplant. Intravenous **zanamivir** is an investigational drug that could be requested for clinical use if concern exists for an oseltamivir-resistant influenza strain. **Laninamivir** is a long-acting inhaled neuraminidase inhibitor used for the treatment of seasonal influenza, including infection caused by oseltamivir-resistant virus. It is licensed in Japan and South Korea but not in the United States.

Baloxavir (a selective inhibitor of influenza cap-dependent endonuclease that is given as a single oral dose) is FDA-approved for treatment of uncomplicated influenza A and B infections and postexposure prophylaxis. It is given as 40 mg or 80 mg orally as a single dose depending on weight (the higher dose for persons 80 kg or more) and should be given within the first 48 hours of infection. Its side effects include diarrhea, headache, and bronchitis. Baloxavir's unique mechanism of action may be beneficial as part of multidrug therapy for resistant or severe disease, however, these are areas of ongoing study. For complicated disease, especially in immunosuppressed patients, the combination of oseltamivir, amantadine, and ribavirin appears to produce faster viral clearance but no definite clinical improvement.

The first class of organosilanes have potent antiviral activity against influenza A viruses that are resistant to amantadine and oseltamivir. **Dapivirine**, an FDA-approved HIV nonnucleoside reverse transcriptase inhibitor, has broad-spectrum antiviral against multiple strains of influenza A and B viruses. Iminosugars are also under study. Updated advice is available at http://www.cdc.gov/flu/index.htm.

Prognosis

The duration of the uncomplicated illness is 1–7 days, and the prognosis is excellent in healthy adults and children. Hospitalization typically occurs in those with underlying medical disease, at the extremes of age, and in pregnant women. *Most fatalities are due to bacterial pneumonia, although exacerbations of other disease processes, in particular cardiac diseases, occur.* Pneumonia resulting from influenza has a high mortality rate among pregnant women and persons with a history of rheumatic heart disease. Mortality among adults hospitalized with influenza ranges from 4% to 8%, although higher mortality (greater than 10–15%) may be seen during pandemics and among immunocompromised individuals. At least 64% of pneumonia and influenza deaths occurred among older persons in the United States, who comprised only 15% of the population.

If the fever recurs or persists for more than 4 days with productive cough and white cell count over 10,000/mcL (10.0×10^9/L), secondary bacterial infection should be suspected.

Prevention

Annual administration of influenza vaccine is the most effective measure for preventing influenza and its complications. Seasonal influenza vaccines can reduce influenza hospitalizations by an estimated 61%. Vaccination of health care workers is associated with decreased mortality among hospitalized patients and those in long-term care facilities. Vaccination prevents influenza illness among pregnant women and their infants during the first months of life.

The ACIP and the American College of Obstetricians and Gynecologists' Committee recommend annual influenza vaccination for all persons over 6 months of age with no contraindications. Vaccination is emphasized for high-risk groups and their contacts and caregivers.

Several Cochrane database analyses have examined the efficacy of the influenza vaccines in select populations. The studied groups include patients with COPD (a documented reduction in exacerbations with inactivated vaccine), older adults (where vaccination shows some efficacy), adults with cancer (weak evidence, some lower mortality and influenza-related outcomes), healthy adults (established efficacy with inactivated vaccine, but only modest effects in pregnant women and newborns), and healthy children (where both live and inactivated vaccines lower the rate of influenza infections).

Other reviews establish the efficacy and safety of influenza vaccination in patients with rheumatoid arthritis, asthma, or myasthenia gravis, and older nursing home patients. Patients with obesity have an impaired response to the influenza vaccine.

Multiple influenza vaccine products are licensed in the United States and available from different manufacturers (see Table 30–8). These include inactivated influenza vaccines (standard- or high-dose, trivalent [IIV3] or quadrivalent [IIV4], adjuvanted or unadjuvanted), recombinant vaccines (trivalent [RIV3] or quadrivalent [RIV4]), and live attenuated influenza vaccine (LAIV4). All trivalent vaccines contain antigens from one strain each of influenza A (H1N1), influenza A (H3N2), and influenza B. Quadrivalent vaccines include an additional influenza B strain. The CDC does not endorse one influenza vaccine product over another, although each influenza vaccine product has different age indications and contraindications. The CDC publishes its annual influenza recommendations in the late summer (www.cdc.gov/mmwr).

LAIV4 (which was not recommended by the CDC during the 2016–2017 and 2017–2018 seasons in the Northern Hemisphere due to concerns about its effectiveness against influenza viruses in prior years) is considered an acceptable option for groups in whom it is indicated.

Adults over the age of 18 years, including pregnant women, can receive any influenza vaccine, with few exceptions. Patients 65 years or older should receive a high-dose trivalent inactivated influenza vaccine containing four times more hemagglutinin than standard dose (Fluzone High Dose), or Fluad, a trivalent inactivated influenza vaccine that contains an adjuvant (MF59), which enhances the immune response to the vaccine. Adults older than 65 years can use any IIV or RIV intramuscular vaccine; in a large, randomized trial, high-dose IIV3 showed superior efficacy over standard-dose IIV3 and may provide better protection. Some data suggest intradermal vaccination is more effective than intramuscular vaccination in older adults.

Based on limited evidence to date, the COVID-19 vaccines can be safely *coadministered* with the inactivated seasonal influenza vaccines with an acceptable reactogenicity profile and without evidence of immunointerference.

For patients with cancer, chemotherapeutic regimens containing rituximab show persistent perturbations of B-cell and Ig synthesis, and these modifications decrease humoral responses to the influenza vaccine. Adjuvanted vaccine is efficacious but has resulted in brief disease exacerbation in persons with psoriatic arthritis taking TNF-alpha inhibitors.

Vaccination is contraindicated for persons with a history of severe allergic reaction to an influenza vaccine. Precautions should be taken if patients report a history of Guillain-Barré syndrome 6 weeks following an influenza vaccine and if patients have a moderate to severe acute illness with or without fever until clinical improvement. Persons with a history of egg allergy with hives only may receive any recommended influenza vaccine. Those with more severe allergic reactions to eggs may receive any recommended vaccine under close observation in a health care facility under the supervision of a provider with experience treating severe allergic reactions. Only the recombinant vaccine and the US cell culture-based inactivated (Flucelvax Quadrivalent, ccIIV4) vaccine are egg-free. Additional vaccine information can be found at http://www.cdc.gov/flu/professionals/vaccination/index.htm.

When antiviral chemoprophylaxis is used, it prevents 70–90% of influenza infections. *Chemoprophylaxis is not routinely recommended and is not recommended prior to exposure to prevent development of resistance.* Chemoprophylaxis may be considered for persons at increased risk for complications from infection who are exposed to an infected patient within 2 weeks of vaccination, for persons unlikely to respond to vaccination because of immunosuppression after exposure to an infected person, for persons for whom vaccination is contraindicated and who are at high risk for complications after exposure to an infected person, and for prevention of infection in residents of institutions during an outbreak. Alternatively, a person can be monitored closely, and antiviral therapy initiated at the first onset of symptoms after exposure. Initiation of chemoprophylaxis is not recommended more than 48 hours after exposure. Patients taking chemoprophylaxis should seek urgent medical care if an influenza-like illness develops.

Chemoprophylaxis against influenza A and B is accomplished with daily administration of the neuraminidase inhibitors oseltamivir (75 mg/day, oral) or zanamivir (10 mg/day, inhaled) to continue through 7 days after last known exposure. For outbreak control in long-term care facilities and hospitals, a minimum of 2 weeks is recommended, including in vaccinated persons if the seasonal vaccine is not well matched to the circulating strain, to continue until 1 week after identification of the last known case. Zanamivir should not be given as chemoprophylaxis to asthmatic persons, nursing home residents, or children younger than 5 years.

Breakthrough infections with influenza occur with neuraminidase inhibitors (in a study with zanamivir) and with vaccination. The efficacy of chemoprophylaxis is proven for individuals and households but not community settings.

Hand hygiene and surgical facemasks appear to prevent household transmission of influenza virus isolates when implemented within 36 hours of recognition of symptoms in an index patient. Such nonpharmaceutical interventions assist in mitigating the spread of pandemic and interpandemic influenza to unvaccinated persons. In one study, patients with seasonal H1N1 influenza infection were infectious from 1 day before to about 7 days following illness onset. Children and immunosuppressed persons exhibit prolonged viral shedding and may be infectious longer. Winter school breaks during periods of high influenza transmission appear to decrease rates of visits to primary care practitioners for influenza illness among children and adults.

Any hospital patient in whom the infection is suspected should be isolated in an individual room with standard and droplet precautions. CDC guidelines recommend the equivalent of N95 masks for aerosol-generating procedures (eg, bronchoscopy, elective intubation, suctioning, administering nebulized medications). For such procedures, an airborne infection isolation room can be used, with air exhausted directly outside or recirculated after filtration by a high efficiency particulate air (HEPA) filter. Strict adherence to hand hygiene with soap and water or an alcohol-based hand sanitizer and immediate removal of gloves and other equipment after contact with respiratory secretions is essential. Precautions should be maintained until 7 days from symptom onset or until 24 hours after symptom resolution, whichever is longer. Postexposure prophylaxis or close monitoring and early treatment should be considered for close contacts of patients who are at high risk for complications of influenza and may be considered for health care personnel, public health workers, or first responders who experienced a recognized, unprotected close contact exposure to a person with influenza virus infection during that person's infectious period.

A regimen of dose-sparing vaccination (to 3.5 mcg) is advocated by some providers to address the extreme shortage of influenza vaccine, particularly in low- and middle-income countries. Dose-sparing vaccination provides adequate vaccination against all components except H3N2.

When to Admit

- Limited availability of supporting services.
- Pneumonia or decreased oxygen saturation.
- Changes in mental status.
- Consider with pregnancy.

Centers for Disease Control and Prevention (CDC). FluView: a weekly U.S. influenza surveillance report. https://www.cdc.gov/flu/weekly

Coadministration of seasonal inactivated influenza and COVID-19 vaccines. Accessed November 18, 2021. https://www.who.int/publications-detail-redirect/WHO-2019-nCoV-vaccines-SAGE_recommendation-coadministration-influenza-vaccines

Cochrane Library. Influenza: evidence from Cochrane Reviews. https://www.cochranelibrary.com/collections/doi/10.1002/14651858.SC000006/full

Cohen C et al. Vaccinating mothers to protect their babies against influenza. J Infect Dis. 2020;221:5. [PMID: 31671176]

Grohskopf LA et al. Prevention and control of seasonal influenza with vaccines: recommendations of the Advisory Committee on Immunization Practices—United States, 2020-21 influenza season. MMWR Recomm Rep. 2020;69:1. [PMID: 32820746]

Ikematsu H et al. Baloxavir marboxil for prophylaxis against influenza in household contacts. N Engl J Med. 2020;383:309. [PMID: 32640124]

4. Avian Influenza

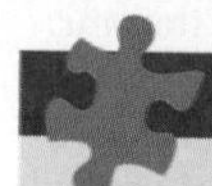

ESSENTIALS OF DIAGNOSIS

- Most human cases occur after exposure to infected poultry.
- Clinically indistinguishable from seasonal influenza.
- Epidemiologic factors assist in diagnosis.
- Rapid antigen assays confirm diagnosis but do not distinguish avian from seasonal influenza.

General Considerations

Zoonotic influenza viruses are distinct from human seasonal influenza viruses and do not easily transmit between humans. In addition, a number of viral genetic changes are required for adaptation to humans. For avian influenza viruses, birds are the natural hosts. Around the world and in North America, avian influenza A outbreaks occur in poultry from time to time (including a 2016 outbreak in Dubois County, Indiana, with avian but no human cases), and the virus has become endemic in poultry in some countries, mostly in Southeast Asia and Egypt. Occasionally, avian influenza viruses may infect humans or other mammals, including domestic cats and dogs. Illness in humans ranges from mild disease to rapid progressive severe disease and death depending on the subtype.

The primary risk factor for human infection is direct or indirect exposure to infected live or dead poultry or contaminated environments, such as live bird markets. Slaughtering and handling carcasses of infected poultry are also risk factors.

The emergence of H5, H7, and H9 avian influenza virus subtypes in humans raises concern that the virus may undergo genetic reassortment or mutations in some of the genes and develop greater human-to-human transmissibility with the potential to produce a global pandemic. All fatal avian influenza virus infections acquire their internal gene segments from H9N2 viruses, the most widespread avian influenza subtype.

Human infections with H5N1 viruses have been reported to WHO from 16 countries, the first report in the Americas was in Canada in 2014, and approximately 60% of the cases have died. Infection with H7N9 avian influenza virus was first reported in China in 2013. Since then, many cases have been reported around the world with an average case fatality rate of 40%. Infections with other H7 avian influenza viruses (H7N2, H7N3, and H7N7) have occurred sporadically around the world. Rare human cases of influenza H9N2 are also reported.

Clinical Findings

A. Symptoms and Signs

Distinguishing avian influenza from regular influenza is difficult. History of exposure to dead or ill birds or live poultry markets in the prior 10 days, recent travel to Southeast Asia or Egypt, or contact with known cases should be investigated. Patients infected by H5N1 or H7N9 avian influenza A viruses have an aggressive clinical course. The symptoms and signs include fever followed by lower respiratory symptoms (cough, dyspnea). Upper respiratory tract symptoms are less common. GI symptoms are reported more frequently in H5N1 infections. Conjunctivitis is reported in influenza H7 infections. Other systems can also be involved leading to neurologic manifestations (encephalopathy, seizure) and liver impairment. Prolonged febrile states and generalized malaise are common. Respiratory failure, multiorgan dysfunction, and septic shock are the usual cause of death. Bacterial superinfections are reported.

For human infections with H7N7 and N9B2 avian influenza virus infections, most cases have been mild with a few cases hospitalized and very few reports of deaths resulting from infection.

B. Laboratory Findings

Commercial rapid antigen tests are not optimally sensitive or specific for detection of H5N1 influenza and should *not* be the definitive test for influenza. More sensitive RT-PCR assays are available through many hospitals and state health departments. Diagnostic yield can be improved by early collection of samples, preferably within 7 days of illness onset. Throat swabs or lower respiratory specimens (such as tracheal aspirate or bronchoalveolar lavage fluid) may provide higher yield of detection than nasal swabs. When highly pathogenic strains, such as H5N1 influenza virus infections, are suspected, extreme care in the handling of these samples must be observed during preliminary testing. Positive samples must then be forwarded to the appropriate public health authorities for further investigation (eg, culture) in laboratories with the adequate level of biosafety (level 3).

Treatment

Persons with severe illness and confirmed and probable cases with mild disease should receive treatment as soon as possible. The first-line recommendation is to use the neuraminidase inhibitor oseltamivir, 75 mg orally twice daily for 5 days administered within 48 hours from onset of illness. Longer courses of therapy (eg, 10 days) should be considered in hospitalized patients with severe illness and persistent viral shedding. Data are lacking for use of inhaled zanamivir or peramivir for severe avian influenza. Overall oseltamivir, by modeling, is associated with a 49%

reduction in mortality from H5N1 avian influenza virus infections. As with seasonal influenza, enteric oseltamivir is well absorbed in critically ill persons without gastric stasis, known malabsorption, or GI bleeding. Daily intravenous peramivir (600 mg, reduced to 200 mg for kidney dysfunction) for a minimum of 5 days and a maximum of 10 or more days (depending on severity of illness) or zanamivir (10 mg inhaled daily for 10 days) may be considered in such patients. Combination therapy with amantadine or rimantadine (in countries where H5N1 influenza virus A strains are likely to be susceptible to adamantanes) may be considered in patients with pneumonia or progressive disease. Resistance of avian H5N1 influenza strains to amantadine and rimantadine is present in most geographic areas. Resistance to neuraminidase inhibitors (oseltamivir, zanamivir, and peramivir) can occur in patients with H5NA and H7N9 avian infection. Successful treatment with administration of convalescent plasma is reported.

Prevention

The most effective method of prevention is *avoidance of exposure*. Persons who work with poultry should practice good hand hygiene and use appropriate personal protective equipment. These workers should also be vaccinated against seasonal influenza since this can reduce the likelihood of coinfection with avian and seasonal influenza. Persons should avoid visiting live poultry markets and should avoid contact with ill birds. No risk exists for acquiring avian influenza through the consumption of well-cooked poultry products. The US government bans the importation of poultry from infected areas. Culling of animals has been effective in ending outbreaks of highly pathogenic avian influenza but is difficult with H7-infected poultry because most are asymptomatic. Policies regarding closure of live poultry markets during avian epidemics are controversial.

Persons with exposure should monitor themselves for 10 days after the last known exposure and should seek prompt medical attention if new fever or respiratory symptoms develop. Postexposure prophylaxis is not recommended in persons working with noninfected birds or who used appropriate personal protective equipment while working with infected birds. For persons with exposure to infected persons, postexposure prophylaxis is recommended for household and family members and may be considered for health care personnel with close unprotected contact. Postexposure prophylaxis regimens include 75 mg of oseltamivir orally or 10 mg inhaled zanamivir twice daily for 5 or 10 days from the last known exposure, depending on the length of the exposure. Careful surveillance for human cases and prudent stockpiling of medications with establishment of an infrastructure for dissemination are essential modalities of control. Nonpharmacologic means of control include masks, social distancing, quarantine, travel limitations, and infrastructure development, particularly for emergency departments.

Vaccines do not provide cross-protection against strains of the H5, H7, and H9 influenza viruses. The US government has prepandemic stockpiles of adjuvanted H5N1 vaccines and H7N9 vaccines that are not available to the public. The highly diverse genetic nature and the rapid evolution of the avian influenza viruses have resulted in the emergence of viruses that are not covered by stockpiled vaccines. The US FDA approved an adjuvanted influenza A (H5N1) monovalent vaccine (Audenz) in January 2020. It is approved for persons 6 months of age and older. An adjuvanted recombinant hemagglutinin H7 vaccine against avian influenza A subtype H7N9 has been shown to be safe and immunogenic in healthy adults.

Because the potential for pandemic influenza for many of the new reassortment viruses is not fully known, continued surveillance is essential, and stockpiling of vaccines, adjuvant, and medications (oseltamivir and zanamivir) is warranted at the public health level.

5. Severe Acute Respiratory Syndrome (SARS-CoV-1)

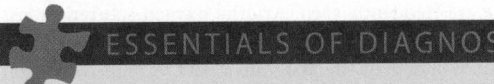

- Mild, moderate, or severe respiratory illness.
- Travel to endemic area within 10 days before symptom onset, including mainland China, Hong Kong, Singapore, Taiwan, Vietnam, and Toronto.
- Persistent fever; dry cough, dyspnea in most.
- Diagnosis confirmed by antibody testing or isolation of virus.
- No specific treatment; mortality as high as 14% in clinically diagnosed cases.

General Considerations

SARS-CoV-1 (previously referred to as "SARS") is a respiratory syndrome caused by a coronavirus, transmitted through direct or indirect contact of mucous membranes with infectious respiratory droplets. The virus is shed in stools, but the role of fecal-oral transmission is unknown. The natural reservoir appears to be the horseshoe bat (which eats and drops fruits ingested by civets, the earlier presumed reservoir and a likely amplifying host), which can carry a variety of different coronavirus strains.

The earliest cases were traced to a health care worker in Guangdong Province in China in late 2002, with rapid spread thereafter throughout Asia and Canada, considered a consequence of spread through travel. The last cases were reported in 2004. The 2003 outbreak involved 8098 probable cases from 29 countries, with 774 fatalities. Nine additional cases associated with a research laboratory were reported in China in 2004 with no further cases reported since then. A 29-base pair deletion evolved during the course of human-to-human transmission, and it is thought to be responsible in part for the abeyance of the outbreak.

Clinical Findings

A. Symptoms and Signs

SARS-CoV-1 is an atypical pneumonia that affects persons in all age groups. Severity ranges from asymptomatic disease to severe respiratory illness. Many subclinical cases probably go undiagnosed. Seasonality, as with influenza, is not established. The incubation period is 2–7 days, and it can be spread to contacts of affected patients for 10 days. The mean time from onset of clinical symptoms to hospital admission is 3–5 days. In all clinical cases, persistent fever is present; chills or rigors (or both), cough, shortness of breath, rales, and rhonchi are the rule. Headache, myalgias, and sore throat are common with watery diarrhea occurring in a subset of patients. Older adult patients may report malaise and delirium, without the typical febrile response.

B. Laboratory Findings and Imaging

Leukopenia (particularly lymphopenia) and low-grade DIC are common. Modest elevations of ALT and creatine kinase are frequently seen. Arterial oxygen saturation less than 95% with associated nonspecific pulmonary infiltrates is evident in 80% of affected individuals. A high-resolution CT scan is abnormal in 67% of patients with initially normal chest radiographs.

Serologic tests, including enzyme immunoassays and fluorescent antibody assays, are available through public health departments at the state level, although seroconversion may not occur until 3 weeks after the onset of symptoms. The detection rates for the virus using conventional RT-PCR are generally low during the first week of illness. Urine, nasopharyngeal aspirate, and stool specimens are positive in 42%, 68%, and 97%, respectively, on day 14 of illness. Viral isolation is technically laborious and time-consuming.

Complications

ARDS, with extensive bilateral consolidation, occurs in about 16% of patients, and about 20–30% of patients require intubation and mechanical ventilation.

Treatment

Severe cases require intensive supportive management. Different agents including, lopinavir/ritonavir, ribavirin, interferon, IVIG, and systemic corticosteroids were used during the 2003 epidemic, but the treatment efficacy of these agents remains inconclusive. In vitro studies with ribavirin show no activity against the virus, and a retrospective analysis of the epidemic in Toronto suggests worse outcomes in patients who received the medication. A 2017 study of alisporivir, a nonimmunosuppressive cyclosporine A analog, alone and in combination with ribavirin, initially showed efficacy in vitro but then did not improve outcomes in a mouse model. A meta-analysis studying the use of Chinese herbs failed to show any efficacy in treating SARS-CoV-1. Many promising treatments for SARS-CoV-1 (such as monoclonal antibodies, convalescent sera of convalescent patients, and antivirals) were put on hold when naturally acquired SARS-CoV-1 cases dwindled. However, many of these treatments are now being re-tested and repurposed for treatment of SARS-CoV-2 infection (see SARS-CoV-2/COVID-19 for additional details).

Prognosis

The overall mortality rate of identified cases is about 14%. Poor prognostic factors include advanced age (mortality rate greater than 50% in those over 65 years of age compared with less than 1% for those under 2 years of age), chronic hepatitis B infection treated with lamivudine, high initial or high peak LD concentration, high neutrophil count on presentation, diabetes mellitus, acute kidney disease, and low counts of CD4 and CD8 on presentation.

Prevention

Health care workers engaged in procedures that involve contact with respiratory droplets are at risk. Isolation of high-risk patients is essential, and simple hygienic measures may help reduce transmission.

Control measures include quarantining in the home for high-risk exposed persons. The tourist industry, in particular hotels with attention to hygiene and quarantine, were significant places for control measure in the past outbreak.

Facemasks are useful for preventing hospital-acquired infection. Continual reporting of suspected cases is crucial, as is awareness of restrictions on international travel. The most cautious modalities include monitoring for 10 days after the last potential exposure and confinement of recovering patients for a similar interval.

Two vaccine candidates are in early stages of development. One is the 218-amino acid residue receptor-binding domain of SARS, expressed in yeast, and it is called RBD219-N1. The other is a single-plasmid DNA vaccine encoding the spike (S) glycoprotein of SARS; it has been shown to be safe in a phase 1 clinical trial.

Sabarimurugan S et al. Comprehensive review on the prevailing COVID-19 therapeutics and the potential of repurposing SARS-CoV-1 candidate drugs to target SARS-CoV-2 as a fast-track treatment and prevention option. Ann Transl Med. 2020;8:1247. [PMID: 33178779]

6. Middle East Respiratory Syndrome–Coronavirus (MERS-CoV)

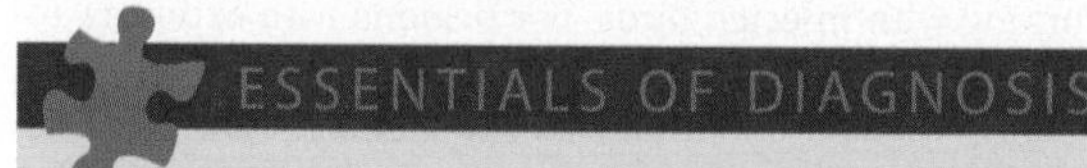

- Mild, moderate, or severe respiratory illness.
- Travel to endemic area, including Saudi Arabia, United Arab Emirates, Qatar, and Jordan, within 14 days before symptom onset.
- Contact with camels reported in many cases.
- Fever, cough, and dyspnea.
- CDC can assist with RT-PCR.
- Supportive treatment; mortality 36–45%.

General Considerations

MERS is a syndrome associated with a coronavirus similar to the cause of SARS. Patients with MERS have had a history of residence or travel in the Middle East, in particular Saudi Arabia, or contact with such patients. The virus is transmitted between humans through direct or indirect contact of mucous membranes with infectious respiratory droplets. The virus is shed in stool, but the role of fecal-oral transmission is unknown. The earliest cases were identified in 2012 in the Kingdom of Saudi Arabia, and 75% of all cases have occurred there. Additional cases have occurred throughout the Middle East, Africa, and Europe, with a reported death rate of 36% (http://www.who.int/emergencies/mers-cov/en/). Only two cases have ever been identified in the United States; both were reported in 2014 in health care providers who lived and worked in Saudi Arabia. As of August 2021, 2578 cases of MERS had been reported to the WHO, including 888 deaths (case fatality rate of 34.4%); most were reported from Saudi Arabia.

So-called super-spreaders are often responsible for propagating the pathogen in the early stages of an outbreak. It is also recognized more often that asymptomatic cases are frequent, especially among children, and they may contribute to disease transmission. Person-to-person transmission can occur within families; hospital-associated cases comprise 10–25% of reported infections. The median incubation period is 5 days (range, 2–14) with the mean age of 50 (range 9 months to 99 years) and 65% occurring among men. Over 90% of patients have an underlying medical condition, including diabetes mellitus (68%), hypertension (34%), or chronic heart or kidney disease. Those with diabetes, kidney disease, chronic lung disease, or other immunocompromising conditions likely are at highest risk for severe disease.

Camels (especially female camels) appear to be the principal reservoir, and several studies show that contact with dromedary herds of camels is greater among cases than controls. Raw camel milk is considered a potential source. Persons who work with camels are more likely to have antibody evidence of past infection.

Clinical Findings

A. Symptoms and Signs

MERS is an acute respiratory syndrome, with the most common symptoms being fever (98%), cough (83%), and dyspnea (72%). Chills and rigors are common (87%). GI symptoms may occur, with diarrhea being most common (26%), followed by nausea and abdominal pain, and may precede respiratory symptoms. Mild and asymptomatic cases are reported.

B. Laboratory Findings and Imaging

Hematologic findings in the largest series to date include thrombocytopenia (36%), lymphopenia (34%), and lymphocytosis (11%). Moderate elevations in LD (49%), AST (15%), and ALT (11%) are recognized. Chest radiograph abnormalities are nearly universal and include increased bronchovascular markings, patchy infiltrates or consolidations, interstitial changes, opacities (reticular and nodular) and pleural effusions, and total lung opacification. Ground-glass opacities and consolidation are most commonly seen. The findings mimic those of many other causes of pneumonia.

Serum serologies and RT-PCR are available through CDC (https://www.cdc.gov/coronavirus/mers/lab/index.html). Highest viral loads are found in lower respiratory tract specimens, including bronchoalveolar lavage fluid, sputum, and tracheal aspirates. These samples are preferred for diagnosis. The CDC recommends sending lower respiratory tract specimens, nasopharyngeal and oropharyngeal swabs, and serum for testing. In confirmed cases, serial sample collection (perhaps every 2–4 days) from multiple sites is recommended to increase understanding of virus shedding kinetics. In cases in which symptom onset occurred more than 14 days prior and symptoms are ongoing, serum should be sent to the CDC for serologic testing and the above specimens should be sent for RT-PCR.

C. Case Definition

A patient with severe illness shows the following characteristics: fever (38°C, 100.4°F or higher) and pneumonia or ARDS (based on clinical or radiologic evidence); and either history of travel in or near the Arabian Peninsula within 14 days before symptom onset; or close contact with a symptomatic traveler in whom fever and acute respiratory illness (not necessarily pneumonia) developed within 14 days after traveling in or near the Arabian Peninsula (above); or is a member of a cluster of patients with severe acute respiratory illness (eg, fever and pneumonia requiring hospitalization) of unknown etiology in which MERS-CoV is being evaluated, in consultation with state and local health departments.

In milder illness, patients have fever and symptoms of respiratory illness (not necessarily pneumonia; eg, cough, shortness of breath) and history of having close contact with a confirmed MERS case as well as a history of being in a health care facility (as a patient, worker, or visitor) within 14 days of symptom onset in a country or territory within the Arabian Peninsula in which recent health care–associated cases of MERS have been identified.

Of note, fever may not be present in certain patients, including the very young, older adults, immunosuppressed individuals, or those taking certain medications.

Complications

Respiratory failure is such a common complication that in a series from Saudi Arabia, 89% of patients required intensive care and mechanical ventilation. Patients with MERS-CoV appear to advance faster to respiratory failure than do those with SARS.

Treatment

Respiratory support is essential. No vaccine or known antiviral therapy exists to combat MERS. Therapies are adapted from SARS treatments, which include interferons, ribavirin, lopinavir-ritonavir, or mycophenolate mofetil. The use of macrolides is not associated with a reduction in mortality. A small retrospective study found improved survival at 14 days with ribavirin and interferon-alpha but not at 28 days.

Prognosis

The overall mortality rate of identified cases is about 36%. Factors associated with mortality include the use of corticosteroids and also the use of continuous renal replacement therapy. A set of radiographic criteria (diffuse involvement, fibrosing sequela) are associated with a worse prognosis and the need for intubation. Advanced age is associated with a poor prognosis. Functional outcomes of survivors are similar to those of other non-MERS severe acute respiratory virus illnesses.

Prevention

Isolation and quarantine of cases is authorized by CDC. Strict infection control measures are essential as well as care and management of household contacts and hospital workers engaged in the care of patients. Travelers to Saudi Arabia (including the many pilgrims to the holy sites) should practice frequent hand washing and avoid contact with those who have respiratory symptoms. Evaluation of patients with suspect symptoms within 14 days of return from Saudi Arabia is essential. Because health care workers engaged in procedures that involve contact with respiratory droplets are at risk, isolation of high-risk patients is essential, as are simple hygienic measures. Limiting the number of hospital contacts and visits is important. Control measures, including quarantining in the home for high-risk exposed persons and the use of facemasks for preventing hospital-acquired infections, are important. Assisting public health authorities with case reporting and surveillance is essential. Postexposure prophylaxis with ribavirin and lopinavir/ritonavir for health care workers is associated with a 40% decrease in the risk of acquiring infection.

Camel workers including slaughterhouse and market workers, veterinarians, and racing personnel should wear facial protection and protective clothing and practice good personal hygiene, including frequent hand washing after touching animals and receive education about the syndrome. Family members of such personnel should not be exposed to work paraphernalia including clothing and shoes and workers should shower at the site of employment rather than the home. Avoidance of direct contact with camels (who may be asymptomatic but who can transmit the virus though nasal or ocular discharge, milk, urine, and feces) is important. Infected camels should be segregated from other livestock and kept off the market, including their meat products, and buried or destroyed.

Arabi YM et al; Saudi Critical Care Trials Group. Macrolides in critically ill patients with Middle East respiratory syndrome. Int J Infect Dis. 2019;81:184. [PMID: 30690213]

Momattin H et al. A systematic review of therapeutic agents for the treatment of the Middle East respiratory syndrome coronavirus (MERS-CoV). Travel Med Infect Dis. 2019;30:9. [PMID: 31252170]

Park SY et al. Post-exposure prophylaxis for Middle East respiratory syndrome in healthcare workers. J Hosp Infect. 2019; 101:42. [PMID: 30240813]

ADENOVIRUS INFECTIONS

General Considerations

At least 88 serotypes of adenovirus are currently described, and these are members of seven species classified A–G with species A-D showing most pathogenic types. About half of these subgroups produce a variety of clinical syndromes. Adenoviruses show a worldwide distribution and occur throughout the year. These infections are usually self-limited or clinically inapparent and occur most commonly among infants, young children, and military recruits and appear to be responsible for about 2–7% of childhood viral respiratory infections and 5–11% of viral pneumonia and bronchiolitis. These infections cause particular morbidity and mortality in immunocompromised persons, such as people living with HIV infection and COPD, as well as in patients who have undergone solid organ and hematopoietic stem cell transplantation or cardiac surgery or in those who have received cancer chemotherapy. A few cases of donor-transmitted adenoviral infection have been reported in past years.

Adenoviruses, although a common cause of human disease, also receive particular recognition through their *role as vectors in gene therapy and vaccine development.*

Clinical Findings

A. Symptoms and Signs

The incubation period is 4–9 days. Clinical syndromes of adenovirus infection, often overlapping, include the following. The common cold (see Chapter 8) is characterized by rhinitis, pharyngitis, and mild malaise without fever. Conjunctivitis is often present. Nonstreptococcal exudative pharyngitis is characterized by fever lasting 2–12 days and accompanied by malaise and myalgia. Lower respiratory tract infection may occur, including bronchiolitis, suggested by cough and rales, or pneumonia. Species B and C, and types 1, 2, 3, 4, 7, 55, and 66 commonly cause acute respiratory disease and atypical pneumonia; coinfections or serial infections are documented to occur. Infections are especially severe in Native American children. Adenovirus B14 is a cause of severe and sometimes fatal pneumonia in those with chronic lung disease but is also seen in healthy young adults and military recruit outbreaks. Viral or bacterial coinfections occur with adenovirus in 15–20% of cases. Pharyngoconjunctival fever is manifested by fever and malaise, conjunctivitis (often unilateral), mild pharyngitis, and cervical adenitis. Epidemic keratoconjunctivitis (transmissible person-to-person, most often species C, types 8, 19, and 37) occurs in adults and is manifested by bilateral conjunctival redness, pain, tearing, and an enlarged preauricular lymph node (multiple types may be involved in a single outbreak). Keratitis may lead to subepithelial opacities (especially with the above types).

Sexually transmitted genitourinary ulcers and urethritis may be caused by species C and D, types 2, 8, and 37. Adenoviruses also cause acute gastroenteritis (types 40 and 41), mesenteric adenitis, acute appendicitis, rhabdomyolysis, and intussusception. Rarely, they are associated with encephalitis, meningitis, cerebellitis, ARDS, acute flaccid myelitis, and pericarditis. Adenovirus is commonly identified in endomyocardial tissue of patients with myocarditis and dilated cardiomyopathy. Risk factors associated with severity of infection include youth, chronic underlying infections, recent transplantation, and serotypes 5 or 21.

Hepatitis (C5 adenovirus), pneumonia, and hemorrhagic cystitis (species B, types 11 and 34) tend to develop in infected liver, lung, or kidney transplant recipients, respectively. Disease states that may develop in hematopoietic stem cell transplant patients include hepatitis, pneumonia, diarrhea, hemorrhagic cystitis, tubulointerstitial nephritis, colitis, and encephalitis.

B. Laboratory Findings and Imaging

Antigen detection assays including direct fluorescence assay or enzyme immunoassay are rapid and show sensitivity of 40–60% compared with viral culture (considered the standard). Samples with negative rapid assays require PCR assays or viral cultures for diagnosis. Quantitative real-time rapid-cycle PCR is useful in distinguishing disease from colonization, especially in hematopoietic stem cell transplant patients. Multiplex nucleic acid amplification assays can test for multiple respiratory viruses simultaneously with increased sensitivity. Adenovirus differs from other viral and bacterial respiratory infections seen on chest CT imaging, appearing as a multifocal consolidation or ground-glass opacity without airway inflammatory findings.

Treatment & Prognosis

Treatment is symptomatic. Ribavirin or cidofovir is used in immunocompromised individuals with occasional success, although cidofovir is attendant with significant renal toxicity. Brincidofovir, the lipid-conjugated prodrug of cidofovir, has better oral bioavailability, is better tolerated, and achieves higher intracellular concentrations of active drug than cidofovir but currently is only available through compassionate use policies since its primary indicated use remains for Ebola virus infections. IVIG is used in immunocompromised patients and can be used in combination with other therapies, but data are still limited. Reduced immunosuppression is often required. Typing of isolates is useful epidemiologically and in distinguishing transmission from endogenous reactivation. Topical steroids or tacrolimus may be used to treat adenoviral keratoconjunctivitis. The commercially available synthetic corticosteroid mifepristone shows some in vitro activity against adenoviruses. Complications of adenovirus pneumonia in children include bronchiolitis obliterans. Deaths are reported on occasion.

The control of epidemic adenoviral conjunctivitis is often difficult and requires meticulous attention to hand hygiene, use of disposable gloves, sterilization of equipment (isopropyl alcohol is insufficient, recommendations of manufacturers are preferred), cohorting of cases, and furloughing of employees. Treatment with a combination of povidone-iodine 1.0% eyedrops and dexamethasone 0.1% eyedrops four times a day can reduce symptoms and expedite recovery. Prolonged shedding of adenovirus type 55 is reported.

Vaccines are not available for general use. Use of live oral vaccines containing attenuated type 4 and type 7 was reinstated in military personnel in 2013 and has been associated with significant decrease in adenoviral disease.

Fu Y et al. Human adenovirus type 7 infection causes a more severe disease than type 3. BMC Infect Dis. 2019;19:36. [PMID: 30626350]

Saha B et al. Recent advances in novel antiviral therapies against human adenovirus. Microorganisms. 2020;8:1284. [PMID: 32842697]

OTHER EXANTHEMATOUS VIRAL INFECTIONS

1. *Erythroparvovirus* Infections

Primate erythroparvovirus 1, more commonly known as **parvovirus B19,** infects human erythroid precursor cells. It is quite widespread (by age 15 years about 50% of children have detectable IgG), and its transmission occurs through respiratory secretions and saliva, through the placenta (vertical transmission with 30–50% of pregnant women nonimmune), and through administration of blood products. The incubation period is 4–14 days. Chronic forms of the infection can occur. Bocavirus, another erythroparvovirus, is a cause of winter acute respiratory disease in children and adults.

Clinical Findings

A. Symptoms and Signs

Parvovirus B19 causes several syndromes and manifests differently in various populations.

1. Children—In children, an exanthematous illness (“**fifth disease**,” **erythema infectiosum**) is characterized by a fiery red “slapped cheek” appearance, circumoral pallor, and a subsequent lacy, maculopapular, evanescent rash on the trunk and limbs. Eosinophilic cellulitis (Well syndrome) is also reported with parvovirus B19, as are microvesicular eruptions and atypical rashes. Parvovirus B19 infection is also one of the most common causes of myocarditis in childhood.

2. Immunocompromised patients—A transient aplastic crisis and pure RBC aplasia may occur, although symptoms and signs may be less classic among the immunocompromised populations. Bone marrow aspirates reveal absence of mature erythroid precursors and characteristic giant pronormoblasts. The parvovirus B19 gene is detected in 16–19% of patients with acute leukemia and chronic myeloid leukemia. Patients undergoing chronic dialysis also show a high prevalence of parvovirus infection.

3. Adults—A limited nonerosive symmetric polyarthritis that mimics lupus erythematosus and rheumatoid arthritis, which may in some cases be a type II mixed cryoglobulinemia, can develop in middle-aged persons (especially women). Rashes, especially facial, are less common in adults.

Chloroquine and its derivatives exacerbate parvovirus B19–associated anemia and are linked with significantly lower hematocrit in hospital admissions in malaria endemic areas. Rare reported presentations include myocarditis with infarction, constrictive pericarditis, chronic dilated cardiomyopathy, uveitis, encephalitis (from India), autoimmune (Hashimoto) thyroiditis, hepatitis and liver failure, pneumonitis, neutropenia, thrombocytopenia, a lupus-like syndrome, glomerulonephritis, CNS vasculitis, papular-purpuric "gloves and socks" syndrome, complications of drug hypersensitivity, and a chronic fatigue syndrome. A subclinical infection is documented among patients with sickle cell disease. Other CNS manifestations of parvovirus B19 include encephalitis, meningitis, stroke (usually in sickle cell anemia patients with aplastic crises), and peripheral neuropathy (brachial plexitis and carpal tunnel syndrome) with occasional chronic residua.

The symptoms of parvovirus B19 infection can mimic those of autoimmune states such as lupus, systemic sclerosis, antiphospholipid syndrome, or vasculitis. In children it may mimic influenza-like illnesses. A more specific entity named relapsing symmetric seronegative synovitis with edema was reported in two cases to be associated serologically with parvovirus B19 infection.

In pregnancy, premature labor, hydrops fetalis, fetal anemia, and fetal loss are reported sequelae. Pregnant women with a recent exposure or with suggestive symptoms should be tested for the disease and carefully monitored if results are positive.

A serosurvey from France suggests parvovirus B19 infection may occur more commonly in patients with schizophrenia.

Metagenomics studies suggest that parvoviruses are associated with some cases of tubulointerstitial fibrosis.

B. Laboratory Findings

The diagnosis is clinical (Table 32–2) but may be confirmed by either an elevated titer of IgM anti-parvovirus B19 antibodies in serum or with PCR in serum or bone marrow. By the time common presenting symptoms manifest, in particular a rash or polyarthropathy in an immunocompetent patient, the viremia may have cleared but IgM antibodies are likely present. In immunocompromised patients, RT-PCR is the optimal test. Autoimmune antibodies (antiphospholipid and antineutrophil cytoplasmic antibodies) can be present and are thought to be a consequence of molecular mimicry. False-positive serologies also occur in the presence of recent IVIG and anti–B-cell therapy. Also, remnant parvovirus B19, from tissue and serum, is thought to explain some false-positive findings. Assays on marrow tissue are indicated only if a marrow is deemed necessary for other hematologic reasons.

▶ Treatment

Treatment in healthy persons is symptomatic (NSAIDs are used to treat arthralgias, and transfusions are used to treat transient aplastic crises). In immunosuppressed patients including those with HIV, IVIG is very effective in the short-term reduction of anemia. Relapses tend to occur about 4 months after administration of IVIG. Administration of IVIG does not reduce encephalitic complications. Intrauterine blood transfusion can be considered in severe fetal anemia, although such transfusions have been linked to impaired neurologic development.

▶ Prevention & Prognosis

Several nosocomial outbreaks are documented. In these cases, standard containment guidelines, including hand washing after patient exposure and avoiding contact with pregnant women, are paramount. Among infected, pregnant women, the presence of hydrops is associated with a poor prognosis. Serologic data show that day care attendants are at higher risk for infection and need practice hygienic principles in particular.

Because transfusion-transmitted parvovirus is very rare, blood banks do *not* routinely screen for parvovirus in the United States or abroad. Most infected donor patients have concomitant antibodies, most recipients have had prior parvovirus infection, and the levels of viremia are considered too low in infected patients to transmit the virus. Transfusion specialists recommend DNA screening of vulnerable patients after transfusion.

The prognosis is generally excellent in immunocompetent individuals. In immunosuppressed patients, persistent anemia may require prolonged transfusion dependence. Remission of parvovirus B19 infection in AIDS patients may occur with ART, though the immune reconstitution inflammatory syndrome is also reported.

Telbivudine, a thymidine analog used in hepatitis B virus infection, appears to show some in vitro activity, in particular with myocarditis, suggesting a potential future commercial role for this compound in parvovirus B19 infections.

Alves ADR et al. High prevalence of parvovirus B19 infection in patients with chronic kidney disease under hemodialysis: a multicenter study. Int J Infect Dis. 2020;100:350. [PMID: 32927082]

Romero Starke K et al. Are daycare workers at a higher risk of parvovirus B19 infection? A systematic review and meta-Analysis. Int J Environ Res Public Health. 2019;16:E1392. [PMID: 30999694]

Sim JY et al. Human parvovirus B19 infection in patients with or without underlying diseases. J Microbiol Immunol Infect. 2019;52:534. [PMID: 31257106]

2. Poxvirus Infections

Among the poxviruses causing disease in humans, the following are the most clinically important: variola/vaccinia, molluscum contagiosum, orf and paravaccinia, and monkeypox.

1. Variola/vaccinia—Smallpox (caused by the variola virus) was a highly contagious disease associated with high mortality and disabling sequelae. Its manifestations include severe headache, acute onset of fever, prostration, and a rash characterized by uniform progression from macules to papules to firm, deep-seated vesicles or pustules. The synchronous progression in smallpox readily differentiates lesions from those of varicella.

Complications of smallpox include bacterial superinfections (cellulitis and pneumonia), encephalitis, and keratitis with corneal ulcerations (risk factor for blindness). Effective vaccination led to its global elimination by 1979 and routine vaccination stopped in 1985. Recommendations to destroy remaining samples of this virus have not been acted upon thus far, and significant concern exists for potential misuse of these repositories in military or terrorist activities.

Smallpox should be considered, in concordance with the CDC Smallpox Response Plan (https://www.cdc.gov/smallpox/bioterrorism-response-planning/community/index.html), in any patient with fever and a characteristic rash for which other etiologies—such as herpes infections (eczema herpeticum may be differentiated from suspect smallpox by appropriate serologic stains and clinical appearance), erythema multiforme, drug reactions, or other infections—are unlikely. Patients with suspected infection should be placed in airborne and contact isolation and the official agency contacted (CDC Poxvirus and Rabies Branch help desk may be reached at 404-639-4129 and the Director's Emergency Operation Center at 770-488-7100).

A needlestick injury case of vaccinia virus infection reported in 2019 from California was treated with the p37 inhibitor tecovirimat and vaccinia immune globulin intravenous (VIGIV) and resolution of a necrotic finger lesion was prolonged (94 days).

Guidelines regarding smallpox vaccination are available at https://www.cdc.gov/smallpox/vaccine-basics/index.html.

2. Molluscum contagiosum—Molluscum contagiosum is caused by a molluscipox virus that may be transmitted sexually or by other close contact. The disease is manifested by pearly, raised, umbilicated skin nodules sparing the palms and soles. Keratoconjunctivitis can occur. Most ocular lesions are typical umbilicated dome-shaped lesions, but a variety of atypical ocular lesions are reported often in immunocompetent patients, more often in women and young adults (mean age 19 years). Rare anal and scalp lesions are reported.

There may be an association with atopic dermatitis or eczema. Molluscum contagiosum is also reported as a complication of therapy with dupilumab for atopic dermatitis. Marked and persistent lesions in patients with AIDS respond readily to combination ART. Treatment options include destructive therapies (curettage, cryotherapy, cantharidin given at least twice and 2–3 weeks apart, 10–15% hydrogen peroxide, 10% potassium hydroxide, and keratolytics [ingenol mebutate and SB206/berdazimer sodium gel are under study], among others), immunomodulators (imiquimod, cimetidine, tuberculin-purified protein derivatives [PPDs], and *Candida* antigen), and antiviral agents (topical cidofovir is effective anecdotally in refractory cases; brincidofovir is approved for the treatment of Ebola but is still off-label for molluscum contagiosum, where it shows some efficacy). No treatment is uniformly effective although cantharidin is better in one study than vehicle alone and imiquimod in another (and considered by some dermatologists the treatment of choice). Multiple courses of therapy are often needed. One meta-analysis recommends natural resolution of lesions if normal immunity can be restored.

3. Orf and paravaccinia—Orf (contagious pustular dermatitis, or ecthyma contagiosa) and paravaccinia (milker's nodules) are occupational diseases acquired by contact with sheep/goats and cattle, respectively. Household meat processing and animal slaughter have been implicated as risk factors. A new poxvirus akin to parapoxviruses was reported in 2015 in two patients from rural Tennessee and Missouri (the latter had also traveled to Tanzania). Orf is a common infection in sheep, goats, and deer. Thus, it is found worldwide, and farmers, veterinarians, and hunters are considered high-risk populations. It progresses through six clinically distinct dermatologic stages and lesions usually heal in 3–6 weeks without scarring. The use of nonporous gloves for persons handling animals is recommended, especially if the persons are immunosuppressed. Molecular tests are used to confirm clinical diagnosis. Although Orf has no specific treatment, it anecdotally responds to imiquimod. A live vaccine is available for animals, and the orfvirus, which has immunomodulatory properties, is increasingly used as a vector and as an oncolytic agent in human vaccine trials.

4. Monkeypox—First identified in 1970, monkeypox is enzootic in the rain forests of equatorial Africa and presents in humans as a syndrome similar to smallpox. The incubation period is about 13 days (range, 6–28 in one Central African Republic outbreak) and limited person-to-person spread occurs. Cultural tribal factors in the Congo are associated with selective risk for acquiring infection. Mortality rates vary from 3% to 11% depending on the immune status of the patient. Secondary attack rates appear to be about 10%. Since 2017, confirmed cases of monkeypox have occurred in Cameroon, Central African Republic, Côte d'Ivoiure, Democratic Republic of the Congo, Republic of the Congo, Gabon, Liberia, Nigeria (where cases occurred after a 40-year hiatus), Sierra Leone, and South Sudan. Risk factors identified from the Democratic Republic of Congo include being bitten by rodents, working as a hunter, and being male over 18 years of age. Travel by Nigerians to Israel, Singapore, and the UK was the source of cases in these areas in 2018–2019. The giant pouched rat is a particular reservoir for disease in Central Africa, although the full spectrum of reservoirs remains unknown.

Confusion with smallpox and varicella occurs; however, both lymphadenopathy (seen in up to 90% of unvaccinated persons) and a febrile prodrome are prominent features in monkeypox infection. The monkeypox rash is distinguished by its deep-seated and well-circumscribed nature, lesions at the same stage of development (unlike varicella but like smallpox), and its centrifugal progression (including palms and soles). Suspected cases should be placed on standard, contact, and droplet precautions; local and state public health officials and the CDC should be notified for assistance with confirmation of the diagnosis (by electron microscopy, viral culture, ELISA, PCR, and a GeneXpert assay referred to as MPX/OPX [monkeypox/orthopox]). No standard or optimized guidelines for the clinical management of monkeypox exist. Cidofovir is effective in vitro against monkeypox, and its less toxic prodrug brincidofovir may be useful as well. Vaccinia immune globulin can be used in selected cases.

Other general precautions that should be taken are avoidance of contact with rodents from endemic areas (whose illness is manifested by alopecia, rash, and ocular or nasal discharge), appropriate care and isolation of humans exposed to such animals within the prior 3 weeks, and veterinary examination and investigation of suspect animals through health departments. Vaccinia immunization (MVA-BN) is effective against monkeypox and is recommended for those aged 18 years or older involved in the investigation of the outbreak and for health care workers caring for those infected with monkeypox if no contraindication exists (outlined above). Postexposure vaccination is also advised for documented contacts of infected persons or animals. US federal agencies prohibit the importation of African rodents.

5. Novel orthopoxviruses—Two cases of a novel orthopoxvirus were identified in the country of Georgia in 2013. Another novel orthopoxvirus was identified in a patient who had undergone kidney transplantation in North America in 2015. The seroprevalence to orthopoxviruses is high in veterinary workers and those with cat exposures.

Centers for Disease Control and Prevention (CDC). Updated interim CDC guidance for use of smallpox vaccine, cidofovir, and vaccinia immune globulin (VIG) for prevention and treatment in the setting of an outbreak of monkeypox infections. http://www.cdc.gov/ncidod/monkeypox/treatmentguidelines.htm

Eichenfield LF et al. Safety and efficacy of VP-102, a proprietary, drug-device combination product containing cantharidin, 0.7% (w/v), in children and adults with molluscum contagiosum: two phase 3 randomized clinical trials. JAMA Dermatol. 2020;156:1315. [PMID: 32965495]

Meyer H et al. Smallpox in the post-eradication era. Viruses. 2020;12:138. [PMID: 31991671]

Overton E et al. MVA-BN as monkeypox vaccine for healthy and immunocompromised. Int J Infect Dis 2020;101:464.

Simpson K et al. Human monkeypox—After 40 years, an unintended consequence of smallpox eradication. Vaccine. 2020; 38:5077. [PMID: 32417140]

Wang R et al. Orf virus: a promising new therapeutic agent. Rev Med Virol. 2019;29:e2013. [PMID: 30370570]

VIRUSES & GASTROENTERITIS

Viruses are responsible for at least 30–40% of cases of infectious diarrhea in the United States. These agents include rotaviruses; caliciviruses, including noroviruses such as Norwalk virus; astroviruses; enteric adenoviruses; and, less often, toroviruses, coronaviruses, picornaviruses (including the Aichi virus), and pestiviruses. Rotaviruses and noroviruses are responsible for most nonbacterial cases of gastroenteritis.

Rotaviruses are reoviruses associated with significant morbidity and mortality. Each year, over 200,000 children die of rotavirus infection worldwide. Children aged 6 months to 2 years are the most affected, although adults are affected occasionally as well. By age 5, virtually every child has been infected with this pathogen. The diverse set of rotaviruses (classified by glycoproteins and protease-sensitive proteins [G-type and P-type antigens], which segregate independently) results in a constellation of serotypes, although only five of these cause over 90% of disease. Rotavirus infections follow an endemic pattern, especially in the tropics and low-income countries, but they peak during the winter in temperate regions. The virus is transmitted by fecal-oral route and can be shed in feces for up to 3 weeks in severe infections. In outbreak settings (eg, day care centers), the virus is ubiquitously found in the environment, and secondary attack rates are between 16% and 30% (including household contacts). Nosocomial outbreaks are reported.

The disease is usually mild and self-limiting. A 2- to 3-day prodrome of fever and vomiting is followed by nonbloody diarrhea (up to 10–20 bowel movements per day) lasting for 1–4 days. It is thought that systemic disease occurs rarely, and unusual reported presentations include cerebellitis and pancreatitis. Patients with gastroenteritis are not routinely tested for rotavirus because the results do not alter treatment. Oral and intravenous rehydration solutions are the primary treatment options.

Vaccines have been highly successful in reducing the global burden of rotavirus. Four oral, live, attenuated rotavirus vaccines—Rotarix (derived from a single common strain of human rotavirus), RotaTeq (a reassorted bovine-human rotavirus), Rotavac (naturally occurring bovine-human reassortant neonatal G9P, also called 116E), and RotaSiil (bovine-human reassortant with human G1, G2, G3 and G4 bovine UK G6P[5] backbone)—are available internationally and WHO prequalified. All four vaccines are considered highly effective in preventing severe GI disease. In the United States, two rotavirus vaccines have been approved since 2006: RotaTeq (given at 2, 4, and 6 months of age) and a live, oral attenuated monovalent human rotavirus vaccine (HRV, Rotarix or RV1; given at 2 and 4 months of age). One advantage of these vaccines is the evidence of *heterotypic immunity* (prevention against rotavirus strains not included in the vaccine). Accordingly, some data suggest that rotavirus vaccination confers herd immunity to children under 1 year of age.

Vaccine coverage is inadequate in the United States for rotavirus (75.3% in the 2017 National Immunization Study). National immunization programs of over 80 countries include rotavirus vaccine, and the different rotavirus vaccines are available commercially in 100 countries.

With the control of rotavirus, **noroviruses**, such as Norwalk virus (one of a variety of small round viruses divided into six genogroups [three causing disease in man] and at least 25 genotypes), are now *the major cause of diarrhea globally*. Noroviruses are a leading cause of foodborne disease in the United States (with food handlers largely responsible and associated foods most often leafy vegetables, fruits, nuts, and mollusks) and are significantly associated with military deployment as well as travel-associated and nosocomial infections.

Norovirus gastroenteritis is responsible for nearly 700 million infections globally annually and up to 20% of all diarrhea in both children and adults, with an estimated 900 deaths annually in the United States (primarily among older adults) and 200,000 deaths globally. The efficacy of the rotavirus vaccination has increased the percentage of gastroenteritis caused by norovirus. The noroviruses appear to evolve by antigenic drift (similar to influenza). While 90% of young adults show serologic evidence of past infection, no long-lasting protective immunity develops, and reinfections are common.

Outbreak environments include long-term care facilities (nursing homes in particular), restaurants, hospitals, schools, day care centers, vacation destinations (including cruise ships), and military bases. Persons at particular risk are younger individuals, older adults, those who are institutionalized, and those who are immunosuppressed. Although transmission is usually fecal-oral, airborne, person to person, and water-borne transmission are also documented. A short incubation period (24–48 hours), a short symptomatic illness (12–60 hours, but up to 5 days in hospital-associated cases), a high frequency (greater than 50%) of vomiting, and absence of bacterial pathogens in stool samples are highly predictive of norovirus gastroenteritis.

RT-PCR of stool samples is used for diagnostic and epidemiologic purposes. Several licensed multiple pathogen platform assays are available, but they are expensive and interpretation of the cause of illness in a given patient may be difficult. Treatment options are similar to rotavirus (see above) and rely mostly on oral and intravenous rehydration. Deaths are rare in the developed world, and the more common associated diseases are aspiration pneumonia, septicemia, and necrotizing enterocolitis.

Outbreak control for both rotavirus and norovirus infections include strict adherence to general hygienic measures. Despite the promise of alcohol-based sanitizers for the control of pathogen transmission, *such cleansers may be relatively ineffective against the noroviruses compared with antibacterial soap and water*, reinforcing the need for new hygienic agents against this prevalent group of viruses. Cohorting of sick patients, contact precautions for symptomatic hospitalized patients, and proper decontamination procedures are crucial. Symptomatic staff should be excluded from work until symptom resolution (or 48–72 hours after this for norovirus disease).

Burnett E et al. Real-world effectiveness of rotavirus vaccines, 2006–19: a literature review and meta-analysis. Lancet Glob Health. 2020;8:e1195. [PMID: 32827481]

Netzler NE et al. Norovirus antivirals: where are we now? Med Res Rev. 2019;39:860. [PMID: 30584800]

ENTEROVIRUSES THAT PRODUCE SEVERAL SYNDROMES

The most famous enterovirus, the poliomyelitis virus, is discussed above under Major Vaccine-Preventable Viral Infections. Other clinically relevant enteroviral infections are discussed in this section.

1. Coxsackievirus Infections

Coxsackievirus infections cause several clinical syndromes. As with other enteroviruses, infections are most common during the summer. Two groups, A and B, are defined either serologically or by mouse bioassay. More than 50 serotypes are identified.

▶ Clinical Findings

A. Symptoms and Signs

The clinical syndromes associated with coxsackievirus infection are summer grippe; herpangina; epidemic pleurodynia; aseptic meningitis and other neurologic syndromes; acute nonspecific pericarditis; myocarditis; hand, foot, and mouth disease; epidemic conjunctivitis; and other syndromes.

1. Summer grippe (A and B)—A febrile illness, principally of children, summer grippe usually lasts 1–4 days. Minor upper respiratory tract infection symptoms are often present.

2. Herpangina (A2–6, 10; B3)—There is sudden onset of fever, which may be as high as 40.6°C, sometimes with febrile convulsions. Other symptoms are headache, myalgia, and vomiting. The sore throat is characterized early by petechiae or papules on the soft palate that ulcerate in about 3 days and then heal. Treatment is symptomatic.

3. Epidemic pleurodynia (Bornholm disease) (B1–5)—Pleuritic pain is prominent. Tenderness, hyperesthesia, and muscle swelling are present over the area of diaphragmatic attachment. Other findings include headache, sore throat, malaise, nausea, and fever. Orchitis and aseptic meningitis occur in less than 10% of patients. Most patients are ill for 4–6 days.

4. Aseptic meningitis (A and B) and other neurologic syndromes—Fever, headache, nausea, vomiting, stiff neck, drowsiness, and CSF lymphocytosis without chemical abnormalities may occur, and pediatric clusters of group B (especially B5) meningitis are reported. Focal encephalitis and transverse myelitis are reported with coxsackievirus group A and acute flaccid myelitis with group B in India. Disseminated encephalitis occurs after group B infection, and acute flaccid myelitis is reported with both coxsackievirus groups A and B.

5. Acute nonspecific pericarditis (B types)—Sudden onset of anterior chest pain, often worse with inspiration and in the supine position, is typical. Fever, myalgia, headache, and pericardial friction rub appear early and are often transient. Evidence for pericardial effusion on imaging studies is often present, and the occasional patient has a paradoxical pulse. Electrocardiographic evidence of pericarditis is often present. Relapses may occur.

6. Myocarditis (B1–5)—Heart failure in the neonatal period secondary to in utero myocarditis and over 20% of adult cases of myocarditis and dilated cardiomyopathy are associated with group B (especially B3) infections.

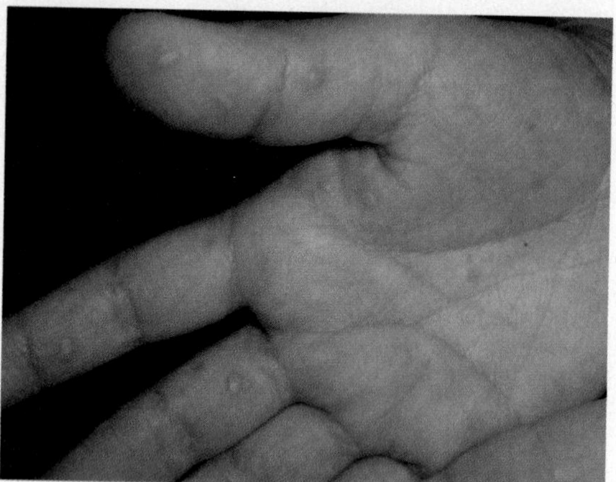

▲ **Figure 32–6.** Rash of hand, foot, and mouth disease. Typical flat, gray, oval vesicular lesions on the ventral hand and fingers. (Reproduced with permission from Richard P. Usatine, MD, in Usatine RP, Smith MA, Mayeaux EJ Jr, Chumley H. *The Color Atlas and Synopsis of Family Medicine*, 3rd ed. McGraw-Hill, 2019.)

7. Hand, foot, and mouth disease (A5, 6, 10, 12, and 16, B5)—This disease can be epidemic. It is characterized by stomatitis, a vesicular rash on hands and feet (Figure 32–6), nail dystrophies, and onychomadesis (nail shedding), with some cases showing higher fevers, long duration, and more severe skin manifestations. Enteroviruses 71 and 33 are also causative agents, the former of usually more severe disease. A16 disease is usually mild. A6 may be atypical but is usually self-limited. Rare fatalities are reported among surveillance programs in China where recombinant patterns between coxsackieviruses and echoviruses are reported.

8. Epidemic conjunctivitis—As with enterovirus 70, the A24 variant of coxsackievirus is associated with acute epidemic hemorrhagic conjunctivitis in tropical areas with outbreaks reported in southern China, Pakistan, southern Sudan, the Comoros, Uganda, Cuba, and Thailand. It is also reported as a cause of corneal endothelitis after cataract surgery.

9. Other syndromes associated with coxsackievirus infections—These include rhabdomyolysis, fulminant neonatal hepatitis (occurs rarely), pancreatitis with concomitant hepatitis and myocarditis (A4), glomerulopathy (group B infections), onychomadesis (B1), neonatal hemophagocytic lymphohistiocytosis (B1), types 1 and 2 diabetes mellitus (mainly group B infections), and thyroid disease (group B4), although definitive causality is not established. A pathogenic role in primary Sjögren syndrome and acute MI has also been proposed for group B coxsackievirus infections. A report of confirmed infective endocarditis due to coxsackievirus B2 in a patient with a prosthetic cardiac patch used in repair of a child with complete atrial ventricular septic defect suggests that viral etiologies of culture-negative infective endocarditis should be considered even in cases of cardiac surgery.

B. Laboratory Findings

Routine laboratory studies show no characteristic abnormalities. Neutralizing antibodies appear during convalescence. The virus may be isolated from throat washings or stools inoculated into suckling mice. Viral culture is expensive, labor intensive, and requires several days for results. A PCR test for enterovirus RNA is available and, although it cannot identify the serotype, may be useful, particularly in cases of meningitis.

▶ Treatment & Prognosis

Treatment is symptomatic. Except for meningitis, myocarditis, pericarditis, diabetes, and rare illnesses such as pancreatitis or poliomyelitis-like states, the most common syndromes caused by coxsackieviruses are benign and self-limited. Two controlled trials showed a potential clinical benefit with pleconaril for patients with enteroviral meningitis although the compassionate use of this medication has stopped (clinicians can contact Schering Plough for updates). Anecdotal reports describe success with IVIG in severe disease. Vaccines against the most common etiologic agents in a given country have been developed, but simultaneous circulation of more than one virus makes coxsackievirus vaccines based on a single agent relatively ineffective.

2. Echovirus Infections

Echoviruses are enteroviruses that produce several clinical syndromes, particularly in children. Infection is most common during summer. Among reported specimens, death ensues in about 3%. Adolescents and men younger than 20 years are more commonly infected than other persons.

Over 30 serotypes of echoviruses are recognized and the most common serotypes for disease are A types 6, 9, 11, 19, 29, 30, and 33 as well as C99. Most can cause aseptic meningitis, which may be associated with a rubelliform rash. Transmission is primarily fecal-oral. Hand washing is an effective control measure in outbreaks of aseptic meningitis. Outbreaks related to fecal contamination of water sources, including drinking water and swimming and bathing pools, were reported previously.

Besides meningitis, other conditions associated with echoviruses range from common respiratory diseases and epidemic diarrhea to myocarditis, a hemorrhagic obstetric syndrome, keratoconjunctivitis, severe hepatitis with coagulopathy, leukocytoclastic vasculitis, encephalitis with sepsis, interstitial pneumonitis, pleurodynia, hemophagocytic syndromes (in children with cancer), sudden deafness, encephalitis, acute flaccid myelitis (a leading cause in India), optic neuritis, uveitis, and septic shock. Echoviruses and enteroviruses are also a common cause of nonspecific exanthems.

As with other enterovirus infections, diagnosis is best established by correlation of clinical, epidemiologic, and laboratory evidence. Cytopathic effects are produced in tissue culture after recovery of virus from throat washings, blood, or CSF. An enterovirus PCR of the CSF can assist in the diagnosis and is associated with a shorter duration of hospitalization in febrile neonates. Fourfold or greater rises in antibody titer signify systemic infection.

Treatment is usually symptomatic, and the prognosis is excellent, although mild paralysis after CNS infection is reported. In vitro data suggest some role for amantadine or ribavirin, but clinical studies supporting these findings are not available.

From a public health standpoint, clustered illnesses, such as among travelers swimming in sewage-infested seawater, suggest point-source exposure. Prevention of fecal-oral contamination and maintenance of pool hygiene through chlorination and pH control are important public health control measures.

Zhang J et al. Identification of a new recombinant strain of echovirus 33 from children with hand, foot, and mouth disease complicated by meningitis in Yunnan, China. Virol J. 2019;16:63. [PMID: 31068194]

3. Enteroviruses 68, 70, 71, & Related Agents

Enteroviruses are nonenveloped, single-stranded viruses in the *Picornaviridae* family. They are divided into 12 species (A to L; human enteroviruses include species A to D). Several distinct clinical syndromes are described in association with enteroviruses.

Enterovirus D68 (EV-D68) is a unique enterovirus that shares epidemiologic characteristics with human rhinovirus and is typically associated with respiratory illness. Several clusters are reported from the Netherlands, Japan, the Philippines, and Thailand. An outbreak throughout the United States was reported during 2014–2015. The outbreak was also associated with cases of acute flaccid myelitis but not definitively linked thus far. The virus is implicated also in aseptic meningitis and encephalitis. After removing public health restrictions targeting SARS-CoV-2 in 2021, an increase in EV-D68 cases was reported, including 139 cases in eight European countries between July and October 2021.

Enterovirus 70 (EV-A70), a ubiquitous virus and responsible for abrupt bilateral eye discharge and subconjunctival hemorrhage with occasional systemic symptoms, is most commonly associated with acute hemorrhagic conjunctivitis.

Enterovirus 71 (EV-A71) almost always occurs in the Asia-Pacific region (but with reports from the United States since the 1980s) and is associated with (1) hand, foot, and mouth disease, which can be severe or even fatal; (2) herpangina; (3) a form of epidemic encephalitis associated on occasion with pulmonary edema; and (4) acute flaccid myelitis mimicking poliomyelitis (see separate section on acute flaccid myelitis).

Human enteroviruses are neurotropic. They may have a role in amyotrophic lateral sclerosis. EV-D68 has been reported in a case of fatal meningitis/encephalitis. A number of nonpolio type C enteroviruses are associated with polio-like syndromes, and surveillance for these is most active in China. Enterovirus infection of the pancreas can trigger cell-mediated autoimmune destruction of beta cells resulting in diabetes. Enterovirus myocarditis can be a serious infection in neonates, complicated by cardiac dysfunction and arrhythmias. An association with hemophagocytosis is also reported.

Mortality is especially high in EV-A71–associated brainstem encephalitis, which is often complicated by pulmonary edema, particularly when it occurs in children younger than 5 years. A complication is autonomic nervous system dysregulation, which may precede the pulmonary edema. Because of lower herd immunity, hand, foot, and mouth disease tends to infect children under age 5 in nonendemic areas. Clinical and epidemiologic findings aided by isolation of the suspect agent from conjunctival scraping for EV-A70; vesicle swabs, body secretions, or CSF for EV-A71; and respiratory secretions for D68 facilitate diagnosis of these enteroviral entities. Enzyme immunoassays and complement fixation tests show good specificity but poor sensitivity (less than 80%). RT-PCR may increase the detection rate in enterovirus infections and is useful in the analysis of CSF samples among patients with meningitis and of blood samples among infants with a sepsis-like illness.

Treatment of these entities remains largely symptomatic. A study in China showed that recombinant human interferon-alpha1b in EV-A71–associated hand, foot, and mouth disease was associated with decreased fever duration, healing time of typical skin or oral mucosal lesions, and EV-A71 viral load. Clinicians report anecdotal success in managing myocarditis with immunoglobulins.

The major complication associated with EV-A70 is the rare development of an acute neurologic illness with motor paralysis akin to poliomyelitis. Treatment of acute flaccid myelitis related to EV-A71 with IVIG does not appear to improve neurologic outcomes. Attention-deficit with hyperactivity occurs in about 20% with confirmed infection.

EV-D68 requires supportive care with particular attention to respiratory support. The CDC's National Enterovirus Surveillance System should receive reports of disease at https://www.cdc.gov/surveillance/ness/ness-sites.html.

Household contacts, especially children under 6 months of age, are at particular risk for EV-A71 acquisition. A commercial disinfectant, Virkon S at 1–2% application, appears to reduce infectivity of fomites. A stage-based supportive treatment for EV-A71 infections, recognizing the potential for late-onset CNS disease and cardiopulmonary failure is important. No EV-A71 vaccine is commercially available in the United States, although vaccines produced in China appear to be successful against EV-A71–associated hand, foot, and mouth disease and herpangina. Decreases in antibody titers suggest booster doses of these vaccines may be needed.

Enterovirus 72 (EV-A72) is another term for hepatitis A virus (see Chapter 16). **Enterovirus EV-A104** is related to rhinoviruses and associated with respiratory illness in reports from Italy and Switzerland.

Hu YL et al. Current status of enterovirus D68 worldwide and in Taiwan. Pediatr Neonatol. 2020;61:9. [PMID: 31706947]

Bodilsen J et al. Enterovirus meningitis in adults: a prospective nationwide population-based cohort study. Neurology. 2021;97:e454. [PMID: 34088872]

4. Human Parechovirus Infection

Human parechovirus is classified among 19 genotypes among a distinct genus of picornaviruses and causes a wide variety of disease in humans, especially in infants. The pathogen mainly affects small children during the summer and early fall, although disease can also occur in older adults. Cases are reported worldwide. Virus type A3 is the most commonly reported isolate in the United States. In a recent Chinese study of children with acute gastroenteritis, 12% tested positive for parechovirus A and the most common genotype was A1b. Clinical presentation is mainly driven by GI and respiratory illness, although otitis, neonatal sepsis, fever without a detectable source, gastroenteritis, flaccid paralysis, myalgias (which may be epidemic), diffuse maculopapular and palmar-plantar rashes, aseptic meningitis, intracranial hemorrhage, seizures, pericarditis, and an acute disseminated encephalitis are described in the literature.

Type A6 typically affects individuals older than 20 years while type A3 is responsible for meningitis/encephalitis, neonatal sepsis (13% of late-onset neonatal sepsis [between 4 and 120 days of life] in one series was due to parechovirus) and was reported in association with necrotizing enterocolitis and hepatitis. It is the most common cause of neonatal meningitis and is the picornavirus most often found in CSF samples of CNS-related infections in very young children. The encephalitis can be severe, and the Guillain-Barré syndrome is also reported with parechovirus type A6. CSF parameters include a normal count in over 90% and an abnormal protein in less than 50%. CNS infection may be seen with virus type A4 as well. Respiratory and GI illnesses are seen with types A4–A6, A10, A13, and A15.

Treatment is largely supportive and rapid identification of the viral antigen by PCR in stools, respiratory samples, and CSF may decrease use of unnecessary antibiotics and shorten hospital stay, although current PCR assays are not always sufficiently sensitive to exclude parechoviruses. Intravenous immunoglobulin was anecdotally successful in one case of parechovirus dilated cardiomyopathy and maternal antibodies to parechovirus type 3 are protective. Reported complications of neonatal cerebral infections include learning disabilities, epilepsy, and cerebral palsy. Because intrafamilial transmission is well documented, diagnosis may help isolate the affected children. Also, diagnosis may prevent the excessive use of antibiotics.

Kabuga AI et al. Human parechovirus are emerging pathogens with broad spectrum of clinical syndromes in adults. J Med Virol. 2020 Aug 6. [Epub ahead of print] [PMID: 32761910]

RICKETTSIAL DISEASES

TYPHUS GROUP

1. Epidemic (Louse-Borne) Typhus

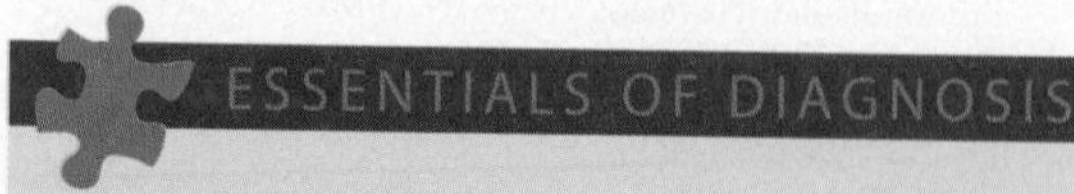

- Prodrome of headache, then chills and fever.
- Severe, intractable headaches, prostration, persistent high fever.
- Macular rash appearing on days 4–7 on the trunk and in the axillae, spreading to the rest of the body but sparing the face, palms, and soles.
- Diagnosis confirmed by complement fixation, microagglutination, or immunofluorescence.

General Considerations

Epidemic louse-borne typhus is caused by *Rickettsia prowazekii*, an obligate parasite of the body louse *Pediculus humanus* (other lice were thought not to contribute although a 2018 report from Turkey suggests *P humanus capitus* may transmit *R prowazekii*) (Table 32–3). Transmission is favored by crowded, unsanitary living conditions, famine, war, or any circumstances that predispose to heavy infestation with lice. After biting a person infected with *R prowazekii*, the louse becomes infected by the organism, which persists in the louse gut and is excreted in its feces. When the same louse bites an uninfected individual, the feces enter the bloodstream when the person scratches the itching wound. Dry, infectious louse feces may also enter via the respiratory tract. Cases can be acquired by travel to pockets of infection (eg, central and northeastern Africa, Central and South America). Outbreaks have been reported from Peru, Burundi, Ethiopia, Turkey, and Russia and are associated with migration of peoples as well as with refugee camps where crowding and poor hygiene may occur. Because of aerosol transmissibility, *R prowazekii* is considered a possible bioterrorism agent. In the United States, cases occur among the homeless, refugees, and the unhygienic, most often in the winter.

R prowazekii can survive in lymphoid and adipose (in endothelial reservoirs) tissues after primary infection, and years later, produce recrudescence of disease (**Brill-Zinsser disease**) without exposure to infected lice. This phenomenon can serve as a point-source for future outbreaks.

An extrahuman reservoir of *R prowazekii* in the United States is flying squirrels, *Glaucomys volans*. Transmission to humans can occur through their ectoparasites, known as sylvatic typhus, usually causing atypical mild disease. Foci of sylvatic typhus are found in the eastern United States and are reported to occur in Brazil, Ethiopia, and Mexico.

Clinical Findings

A. Symptoms and Signs

Prodromal malaise, cough, headache, backache, arthralgia, myalgia, and chest pain begin after an incubation period of 10–14 days, followed by an abrupt onset of chills, high fever, and prostration, with flu-like symptoms progressing to delirium and stupor. The headache is severe, and the fever is prolonged (Table 32–2).

Other findings consist of conjunctivitis, mild vitritis, retinal lesions, optic neuritis, and hearing loss from neuropathy of the eighth cranial nerve, abdominal pain, and often splenomegaly. Flushed faces and macular rash (that may become confluent) appear; the rash appears first in the axillae and then over the trunk, spreading to the

Table 32–3. Rickettsial diseases (listed in alphabetical order, within groups).

Disease	Rickettsial Pathogen	Geographic Areas of Prevalence	Insect Vector	Mammalian Reservoir	Travel Association
Typhus Group					
Endemic (murine) typhus	*Rickettsia typhi*	Worldwide; small foci (United States: southeastern Gulf Coast)	Flea	Rodents, opossums	Often
Epidemic (louse-borne) typhus	*Rickettsia prowazekii*	South America, Northeastern and Central Africa	Louse	Humans, flying squirrels	Rare
Scrub Typhus Group					
Scrub typhus	*Orientia tsutsugamushi*	Southeast Asia, Japan, Australia, Western Siberia	Mite[1]	Rodents	Often
Spotted Fever Group					
African tick bite fever	*Rickettsia africae*	Rural sub-Saharan Africa, Eastern Caribbean	Tick[1]	Cattle	Often
California flea rickettsiosis	*Rickettsia felis*	Worldwide	Flea	Cats, opossums	
Lymphangitis-associated rickettsiosis	*R sibirica mongolitimonae*	Europe, Africa, Mongolia	Tick[1]	Unknown	Unknown
Mediterranean spotted fever, Boutonneuse fever, Kenya tick typhus, South African tick fever, Indian tick typhus	*Rickettsia conorii*	Africa, India, Mediterranean regions	Tick[1]	Rodents, dogs	Often
Queensland tick typhus	*Rickettsia australis*	Eastern Australia	Tick[1]	Rodents, marsupials	Rare
Rocky Mountain spotted fever, Brazilian spotted fever	*Rickettsia rickettsii*	Western Hemisphere; United States (especially mid-Atlantic coast region) Southeastern Brazil	Tick[1]	Rodents, dogs, porcupines, capybaras for Brazilian spotted fever	Rare
Siberian Asian tick typhus	*Rickettsia sibirica*	Siberia, Mongolia	Tick[1]	Rodents	Rare
Tick-borne lymphadenopathy/ *Dermacentor*-borne necrosis erythema lymphadenopathy/scalp eschar neck lymphadenopathy	*R slovaca, R raoultii, Candidatus R rioja*	Europe	Tick	Unknown	Occasional
Transitional Group					
Rickettsialpox	*Rickettsia akari*	United States, Korea, former USSR	Mite[1]	Mice	Occasional
Ehrlichiosis/Anaplasmosis					
Human granulocytic anaplasmosis	*Anaplasma phagocytophilum, Ehrlichia ewingii, Ehrlichia muris eauclairensis*[2] *Neorickettsia sennetsu*[2]	Northeastern United States and upper Midwest (*E muris eauclairensis*) Southeast Asia (*N sennetsu*)	Tick[1]	Rodents, deer, sheep	Occasional
Human monocytic ehrlichiosis	*Ehrlichia chaffeensis, Ehrlichia canis*	Southeastern United States	Tick[1]	Dogs	Occasional
Q fever	*Coxiella burnetii*	Worldwide	None[3]	Cattle, sheep, goats	Occasional

[1]Also serve as arthropod reservoirs by maintaining rickettsiae through transovarian transmission.
[2]Limited data available on exact cell involved in pathogenesis.
[3]Human infection results from inhalation of dust.

extremities on the fifth or sixth day of illness but sparing the palms of hands and soles of feet. In severely ill patients, the rash becomes hemorrhagic, and hypotension becomes marked. Pneumonia, thromboses, vasculitis with major vessel obstruction and gangrene, circulatory collapse, myocarditis, uremia, and seizure may occur. Improvement begins 13–16 days after onset with a rapid drop of fever and typically a spontaneous recovery.

B. Laboratory Findings

The WBC count is variable. Thrombocytopenia, elevated liver enzymes, proteinuria, and hematuria commonly occur. Serum obtained 5–12 days after onset of symptoms usually shows specific antibodies for *R prowazekii* antigens as demonstrated by complement fixation, microagglutination, or immunofluorescence. In primary rickettsial infection, early antibodies are IgM; in recrudescence (Brill-Zinsser disease), early antibodies are predominantly IgG. A PCR test exists, but its availability is limited.

C. Imaging

Radiographs of the chest may show patchy consolidation.

Differential Diagnosis

The prodromal symptoms and the early febrile stage lack enough specificity to permit diagnosis in nonepidemic situations. The rash is sufficiently distinctive for diagnosis, but it may be absent in up to 50% of cases or may be difficult to observe in dark-skinned persons. A variety of other acute febrile diseases should be considered, including typhoid fever, meningococcemia, and measles.

Treatment

Treatment consists of doxycycline 100 mg orally twice daily for 7–10 days or for at least 3 days after the fever subsides. A single dose of 200 mg of doxycycline may be effective; however, some patients may relapse. Chloramphenicol is considered less effective than doxycycline, but it is still the drug of choice in pregnancy.

Prognosis

The prognosis depends greatly on the patient's age and immune status. The mortality rate is 10% in the second and third decades but in the past, it reached 60% in the sixth decade. Brill-Zinsser disease is rarely fatal.

Prevention

Prevention consists of louse control with insecticides, particularly by applying chemicals to clothing or treating it with heat, and frequent bathing.

A deloused and bathed typhus patient is not infectious. The disease is not transmitted from person to person. Patients are infectious from the lice during the febrile period and perhaps 2–3 days after the fever returns to normal.

No vaccine is available for the prevention of *R prowazekii* infection.

Centers for Disease Control and Prevention (CDC). Typhus fevers. https://www.cdc.gov/typhus/healthcare-providers/index.html

2. Endemic (Murine) Typhus

Rickettsia typhi, a ubiquitous pathogen recognized on all continents, is transmitted from rat to rat through the rat flea (Table 32–3). Serosurveys of animals show high prevalence of antibodies to *R typhi* in opossums, followed by dogs and cats. Humans usually acquire the infection in an urban or suburban setting when bitten by an infected flea. Rare human cases in the developed world occur in travelers, usually to Southeast Asia, Africa, or the Mediterranean area, although other pockets of infection are also known to occur in the Andes and the Yucatán. It is increasingly recognized, including in the United States along the Gulf Coast. Sun exposure appears to correlate with increased risk of exposure.

In the United States, the related *Rickettsia felis* cases (a spotted fever rickettsia, discussed below) are mainly reported from Texas and Southern California.

Clinical Findings

A. Symptoms and Signs

The presentation is nonspecific, including fever, headache, myalgia, and chills. Relative bradycardia is reported. Maculopapular rash occurs in around 50% of cases; it is concentrated on the trunk, mostly sparing the palms and soles, and fades rapidly. Rare presentations include pain or painful genital (Lipschutz) ulcers. Untreated infections last an average of 12–15 days.

Even if untreated, endemic typhus is usually self-limited, and the prognosis is excellent. One systematic review including 239 untreated patients from 12 studies reported an overall mortality of 0.4%. The illness may be associated with maternal death, miscarriage, preterm birth, and low birth weight if acquired early during pregnancy.

B. Laboratory Findings

Serologic confirmation may be necessary for differentiation, with complement-fixing or immunofluorescent antibodies detectable within 15 days after onset, with specific *R typhi* antigens. A fourfold rise in serum antibody titers between the acute and the convalescent phase is diagnostic although cut-off values for diagnosis are not standardized. It is important to note that *R typhi* antigens frequently cross-react with those of *R prowazekii*. The PCR can distinguish between these two infections depending on the sample type, the timing of sample collection, bacterial load, and severity of disease. During the first week of illness, PCR is the most sensitive test if samples are taken before doxycycline administration.

Differential Diagnosis

The most common entity in the differential diagnosis is Rocky Mountain spotted fever, usually occurring after rural exposure and with a different rash (centripetal versus centrifugal for epidemic or endemic typhus). Coinfection with *Bartonella henelsae* is reported in 3.8% of a Greek population of all ages. The disease has been confused with COVID and interestingly is, like COVID, associated with a multisystem inflammatory syndrome. Murine typhus also occurs in pregnancy, is often associated with transaminitis, and has usually a favorable prognosis.

Complications

The most common complication is pulmonary, in the form of pneumonia, followed by pleural effusion and respiratory failure. Other complications include neurologic (peripheral facial paralysis, meningitis, ataxia, and seizures), AKI (and a focal segmental glomerulosclerpsis), fulminant myocarditis, and multiorgan failure. Rare complications include ocular findings, DIC, and hemophagocytosis lymphocytosis syndrome. Anemia, thrombocytopenia, leukopenia, hyponatremia, and elevated levels of liver enzymes commonly occur.

Treatment

Doxycycline 100 mg orally twice daily for 3 days (or until the patient is afebrile for 48 hours) is the medication of choice, except during pregnancy. Ciprofloxacin (500–750 mg orally twice a day) and ampicillin (500 mg orally three times a day) are reportedly successful in pregnant women. Azithromycin is frequently used but is likely inferior to doxycycline and is not associated with improved fetal outcomes.

Prevention

Preventive measures are directed at control of rats and ectoparasites (rat fleas) with insecticides, rat poisons, and rat-proofing of buildings.

Prognosis

Endemic typhus is usually a self-limited disease. A large case series from Texas reported a fatality rate of 0.4%.

Dean A et al. Murine typhus in 5 children hospitalized for multisystem inflammatory syndrome in children. Hosp Pediatr. 2021;11:e61. [PMID: 33431429]

Doppler JF et al. A systematic review of the untreated mortality of murine typhus. PLoS Negl Trop Dis. 2020;14:e0008641. [PMID: 32925913]

3. Scrub Typhus (Tsutsugamushi Fever)

ESSENTIALS OF DIAGNOSIS

- Exposure to mites in endemic South and East Asia, the western Pacific (including Korea), and Australia.
- Black eschar at site of the bite, with regional and generalized lymphadenopathy.
- High fever, relative bradycardia, headache, myalgia, and a short-lived macular rash.
- Frequent pneumonitis, encephalitis, and myocarditis.

General Considerations

Scrub typhus is caused by *Orientia tsutsugamushi*, which is a parasite of rodents and is transmitted by larval trombiculid mites (chiggers). Multiple strains exist and are associated with geographic areas. The disease is endemic in Korea; China; Taiwan; Japan; Pakistan; India (where it is reported to be the leading cause of acute febrile illness in central India); Thailand (where scrub typhus is also the leading cause of acute undifferentiated fever); Malaysia; Vietnam; Laos; and Queensland, Australia (Table 32–3), which form an area known as the "tsutsugamushi triangle." Scrub typhus is a cause of acute febrile illness in India and China and is a recognized cause of fever of unknown origin. Cases are also reported in the Middle East, Kenya, and South America. Transmission is often more common at higher altitudes. The mites live on vegetation (grass and brush) but complete their maturation cycle by biting humans who encounter infested vegetation. Risk factors in China include female sex, age between 60 and 69 years, and farming. Therefore, the disease is more common in rural areas, but urban cases have also been described. Vertical transmission occurs, and blood transfusions may transmit the pathogen as well. Rare occupational transmission via inhalation is documented among laboratory workers. Cases among travelers to endemic areas are increasingly recognized.

Clinical Findings

A. Symptoms and Signs

After a 1- to 3-week incubation period, malaise, chills, severe headache, and backache develop. At the site of the bite, a papule evolves into a flat black eschar (the groin and the abdomen being the most common sites followed by the chest and axilla), which is a helpful finding for diagnosis but was only described in 19% of patients in a South Korean series of scrub typhus. The regional lymph nodes are commonly enlarged and tender, and sometimes a more generalized adenopathy occurs. Fever rises gradually during the first week of infection, and the rash is usually macular and primarily on the trunk area. The rash can be fleeting or more severe, peaking at 8 days but lasting up to 21 days after onset of infection. Relative bradycardia, defined as an increase in heart rate of fewer than 10 beats/minute for a 1°C increase in temperature, frequently accompanies scrub typhus infection. The occurrence of relative bradycardia has no effect on clinical outcome. GI symptoms, including nausea, vomiting, and diarrhea, occur in nearly two-thirds of patients and correspond to the presence of superficial mucosal hemorrhage, multiple erosions, or ulcers in the GI tract. AKI and other renal abnormalities are frequently present.

Severe complications, such as pneumonitis, myocarditis, encephalitis or aseptic meningitis, peritonitis, granulomatous hepatitis, hemophagocytic syndrome, immune thrombocytopenia, DIC, cerebrovascular hemorrhage or infarction, cranial nerve palsies, parkinsonian symptoms, an opsoclonus myoclonus syndrome, ataxia, seizures, cerebral venous thrombosis, and cerebellitis. Henoch-Schönlein purpura is a reported complication. ARDS, or hemophagocytosis, may develop during the second or third week. An attack confers prolonged immunity against homologous strains and transient immunity against heterologous strains. Heterologous strains produce mild disease if infection occurs within a year after the first episode.

B. Laboratory Findings

Thrombocytopenia and elevation of liver enzymes, bilirubin, and creatinine are common. Indirect immunofluorescent assay and indirect immunoperoxidase assays are the gold standard for scrub typhus diagnosis. These tests are expensive and have limited availability. An ELISA detecting *Orientia*-specific antibodies in serum is available. PCR (from the eschar or blood) is the most sensitive diagnostic test but remains positive even after initiation of treatment. Culture of the organism from blood obtained in the first few days of illness is another diagnostic modality but requires a specialized BSL 3 laboratory. It is suggested to combine IgM detection by ELISA and conventional PCR to improve the diagnosis of scrub typhus. A new 47-kD antigen appears to have improved diagnostic utility. Future next-generation sequencing may, when available and less expensive, revolutionize diagnosis.

Differential Diagnosis

Leptospirosis, typhoid, dengue, malaria, Q fever, hemorrhagic fevers, tuberculous meningitis, and other rickettsial infections should be considered. The headache may mimic trigeminal neuralgia. Scrub typhus is a recognized cause of obscure tropical fevers, especially in children. The presence of an eschar, lymphocytosis, and elevated CRP may help distinguish scrub typhus from dengue. Coinfection with malaria may exist, although studies are complicated by the variety and reliability of diagnostic tests and the differential public health reporting of the two diseases.

Treatment & Prognosis

Without treatment, fever subsides spontaneously after 2 weeks, but the mortality rate may be 10–30%. The treatment of choice is doxycycline (100 mg orally twice daily) or minocycline (100 mg intravenously twice daily). Patients should be treated for at least 3 days after their fever subsides. Shorter duration of therapy is associated with relapse. A randomized controlled trial comparing doxycycline with rifampin showed that 600 mg of rifampin daily for 5 days is noninferior to 200 mg of daily doxycycline therapy for 5 days. Alternative therapy for pregnant women and patients with doxycycline allergy include chloramphenicol, although chloramphenicol- and tetracycline-resistant strains have been reported from Southeast Asia. Azithromycin is shown to be as effective as doxycycline with fewer side effects, but it is more expensive. Azithromycin may not prevent poor fetal outcomes in infected pregnant women.

Poor prognostic factors include hypotension requiring vasopressors, ICU care, age over 60 years, absence of an eschar (making the diagnosis difficult), pregnancy, and laboratory findings such as leukocytosis or hypoalbuminemia. Most patients recover without neurologic sequelae.

Severe infections correlate with intermediate and high early IgG levels and higher levels of proteases, referred to as granzymes. Pulmonary disease outcome correlates with rapidity of fever clearance and the presence of anemia, facial puffiness, and maculopapular rash.

Prevention

Mite control with repeated application of long-acting miticides and, less so, rodent control can make endemic areas safe. Insect repellents on clothing and skin as well as protective clothing are effective preventive measures. Although chemoprophylaxis with doxycycline has been used, the CDC does not recommend prophylaxis with antibiotics for asymptomatic travelers. No effective vaccines are available.

Kim W et al. Identification of a novel antigen for serological diagnosis of scrub typhus. Am J Trop Med Hyg. 2021;105:1356 [PMID: 34544047]

Pathak S et al. Clinical profile, complications and outcome of scrub typhus in children: a hospital based observational study in central Nepal. PLoS One. 2019;14:e0220905. [PMID: 31408484]

Rajan SJ et al. Scrub typhus in pregnancy: maternal and fetal outcomes. Obstet Med. 2016;9:164. [PMID: 27829876]

Richards AL et al. Scrub typhus: historic perspective and current status of the worldwide presence of Orientia species. Trop Med Infect Dis. 2020;5:49. [PMID: 32244598]

Wangrangsimakul T et al. Scrub typhus and the misconception of doxycycline resistance. Clin Infect Dis. 2020;70:2444. [PMID: 31570937]

SPOTTED FEVERS

1. Rocky Mountain Spotted Fever

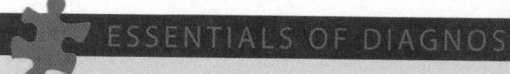

- Exposure to tick bite in an endemic area.
- Influenza-like prodrome followed by fever, severe headache, and myalgias; occasionally, delirium and coma.
- Red macular rash appears between days 2 and 6 of fever, first on the wrists and ankles and then spreading centrally; it may become petechial.
- Mortality over 70% in untreated patients.
- Serial serologic examinations by indirect fluorescent antibody confirm the diagnosis retrospectively.

General Considerations

Rocky Mountain spotted fever (RMSF) is caused by *R rickettsii* and is endemic in parts of the Americas (Table 32–3). In the United States, the numbers of RMSF cases have increased over the last two decades, peaking in 2017 at 6248. Despite its name, most cases of RMSF occur outside the Rocky Mountain area. More than half of US cases are from five states: North Carolina, Tennessee, Oklahoma, Missouri, and Arkansas. Human cases reemerged in northern Mexico in 2008 after decades of quiescence (since the 1940s) and since 2004 have resurged in Panama. As of 2019, 4290 cases were found in the Mexicali area.

R rickettsii is transmitted to humans by the bite of ticks. Several hours of contact between the tick and the human host are required for transmission. Ticks that can transmit the infection include the Rocky Mountain wood tick, *Dermacentor andersoni*, in the western United States, and the American dog tick, *D variabilis*, in the eastern United States. Other hard-bodied ticks transmit the organism in the southern United States and in Central and South America and are responsible for transmitting it among rodents, dogs, porcupines, and other animals. The brown dog tick, *Rhipicephalus sanguineus*, is a vector in eastern Arizona and responsible for many Native American cases. Epidemic RMSF, as described in Arizona and Mexico, is associated with massive local infestations of the brown dog tick in domestic dogs, which may explain why the incidence of RMSF in the three most highly affected communities in an Arizona epidemic from 2003 to 2012 was 150 times the US national average. Needlestick transmission to a nurse is reported from Brazil.

Twenty-five genotypes of *R rickettsii* exist within four different groups, and potential genomic-clinical correlations are underway. Several other rickettsial species cause mild, nonlethal infections in the United States, including *R parkeri*, *R phillipi*, and *R massiliae*. These are discussed in the "tick typhus" section.

A **Brazilian spotted fever** with higher mortality than RMSF is thought to be due to a virulent strain of *R rickettsii*. A host of spotted fever species have been identified from human patients over the last 20 years throughout the world including species from China (*Rickettsia* sp. XY99), Slovakia (*R slovaca*), Morocco (*R aeschlimannii*), Sicily (*R massiiliae*), China, and Egypt (*R sibirica monolitimonae*). Capybaras are a highly mobile vector for the Brazilian disease.

Clinical Findings

A. Symptoms and Signs

RMSF can cause severe multiorgan dysfunction and fatality rates of up to 73% if left untreated, making it *the most serious rickettsial disease*. Two to 14 days (mean, 7 days) after the bite of an infectious tick, symptoms begin with the abrupt onset of high fever, chills, headache, nausea and vomiting, myalgias, restlessness, insomnia, and irritability. The characteristic rash (faint macules that progress to maculopapules and then petechiae) appears between days 2 and 6 of fever. It initially involves the wrists and ankles, spreading *centrally* to the arms, legs, and trunk over the next 2–3 days. Involvement of the palms and soles is characteristic. Eschars are not usually seen and are more suggestive of rickettsial fevers. Facial flushing, conjunctival injection, and hard palate lesions (Figure 32–7) may occur. In about 10% of cases, however, no rash or only a minimal

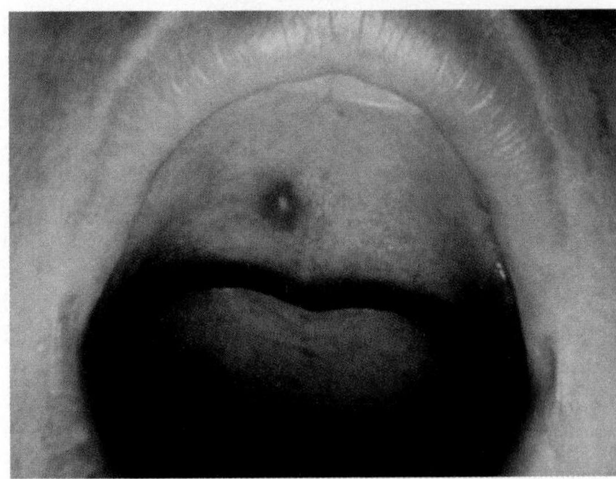

Figure 32–7. Hard palate lesion caused by Rocky Mountain spotted fever. (Public Health Image Library, CDC.)

rash is seen. Cough and pneumonitis may develop, and delirium, lethargy, seizures, stupor, and coma may also appear in more severe cases. Splenomegaly, hepatomegaly, jaundice, myocarditis (which may mimic an acute coronary syndrome), adrenal hemorrhage, polyarticular arthritis, or uremia is occasionally present. ARDS and necrotizing vasculitis, when present, are of greatest concern.

In Sonora, Mexico, during 2015–2016, spontaneous abortions were reported in three of four pregnant women with RMSF.

B. Laboratory Findings

Thrombocytopenia, hyponatremia, elevated aminotransferases, and hyperbilirubinemia are common. CSF may show hypoglycorrhachia and mild pleocytosis. DIC is observed in severe cases. Diagnosis during the acute phase of the illness can be made by immunohistologic or PCR demonstration of *R rickettsii* in skin biopsy specimens (or cutaneous swabs of skin lesions). Performing such studies as soon as skin lesions become apparent and before antibiotics commence maximizes sensitivity.

Serologic studies confirm the diagnosis, but most patients do not mount an antibody response until the second week of illness. The indirect fluorescent antibody IgG test is most commonly used.

Diagnosis is most commonly made serologically and 99% of cases are diagnosed with probable disease. It is important that paired sera (acute and convalescent) be used when possible to establish an acute infection.

Differential Diagnosis

The diagnosis is challenging because early symptoms resemble those of many other infections. The classic triad of fever, rash, and tick bite is rarely recognized, with up to 40% of patients not recalling a tick bite. Moreover, the rash may be confused with that of measles, typhoid, and ehrlichiosis, or—most importantly—meningococcemia. Blood cultures and examination of CSF establish the latter. Coinfections may mask the diagnosis. Some spotted fever rickettsioses may also mimic RMSF but will not be detected by routine serologic testing for RMSF.

Treatment & Prognosis

Treatment with doxycycline (100 mg orally twice daily for 5–7 days or for at least 3 days after the fever subsides) is recommended in all ages and in pregnant women. Although data suggest that doxycycline is *unlikely* to be a teratogen, pregnant women should be counseled regarding potential risks. Chloramphenicol (50–100 mg/kg/day in four divided doses, orally or intravenously for 4–10 days) is the only alternative medication to treat RMSF; however, patients who are treated with chloramphenicol may be at higher risk for death than people treated with a tetracycline. Note that oral formulations of chloramphenicol are not available in the United States and that use of chloramphenicol potentially has adverse risks such as aplastic anemia. Patients usually defervesce within 48–72 hours, and therapy should be continued for at least 3 days after defervescence occurs.

The reported mortality rate for treated patients in the United States is about 3–5%. In the Mexicali outbreak over the last decade, the mortality rate was nearly 18%. The following features are associated with increased mortality: (1) infection in older adults or Native Americans; (2) the presence of atypical clinical features (absence of headache, no history of tick attachment, GI symptoms) and underlying chronic diseases; and (3) a delay in initiation of appropriate antibiotic therapy. The usual cause of death is pneumonitis with respiratory or cardiac failure. A fulminant form of RMSF can be seen in patients with glucose-6-phosphate dehydrogenase deficiency.

Complications include seizures, encephalopathy and encephalitis, peripheral neuropathy, paraparesis, bowel and bladder incontinence, cerebellar and vestibular dysfunction, hearing loss, and motor deficits; these sequelae are reported to last for years after the initial infection. The presence of a “starry sky” pattern signifying multifocal punctate diffuse restricting lesions on T2 MRI imaging should prompt treatment.

Prevention

Protective clothing, tick-repellent chemicals, and the removal of ticks at frequent intervals are helpful measures. The effectiveness of aggressive campaigns to decrease ticks in the community is under investigation in communities with high RMSF attack rates. Prophylactic therapy after a tick bite is not recommended.

Binder AM et al. Diagnostic methods used to classify confirmed and probable cases of spotted fever rickettisoses—United States, 2010–2015. MMWR Morb Mortal Wkly Rep. 2019;68:243. [PMID: 30870409]

Bradshaw MJ et al. Meningoencephalitis due to spotted fever rickettsioses, including Rocky Mountain spotted fever. Clin Infect Dis. 2020;71:188. [PMID: 31412360]

2. Tick Typhus (Rickettsial Fever)

The term “tick typhus” denotes a variety of spotted rickettsial fevers, often named by their geographic location (eg, Mediterranean spotted fever, Queensland tick typhus, Oriental spotted fever, African tick bite fever, Siberian tick typhus, North Asian tick typhus) or by morphology (eg, boutonneuse fever). More than 30 species of spotted fever group rickettsioses are found worldwide (mostly in Europe and Asia), 21 of which are pathogenic in humans (including *R rickettsii*, described above). These illnesses are caused by various rickettsial organisms (eg, *R africae, R australis, R conorii, R japonica, R massiliae, R parkeri, R sibirica*, and *R 364D*) and are transmitted by various tick species. Dogs and wild animals, usually rodents and even reptiles, may serve as reservoirs for rickettsial fevers. Travel is a risk factor for disease, particularly among older adult ecotourists.

Tick-borne rickettsioses are the main source of rickettsial infections in Europe and cause a syndrome similar to that seen in Mediterranean spotted fever. Physicians from Algeria and India report endemic tick typhus, suggesting a pandemicity of tick-borne rickettsioses. Newer recognized species include *R helvetica, R monacensis, R massiliae*, and *R aeschlimannii*. Another described syndrome is tick-borne lymphadenopathy/*Dermacentor*-borne-necrosis-erythema-lymphadenopathy/scalp eschar neck lymphadenopathy associated with *R slovaca, R candidatus, R rioja*, and *R raoultii* and characterized by tick bite, eschar on the scalp, and cervical lymphadenopathy. In an Israeli series of 42 *R conorii* infections, a history of tick bite was rare (5%), eschars were infrequent (12%), and leukocytosis was more common than leukopenia.

The pathogens usually produce an eschar or black spot (tâche noire) at the site of the tick bite that may be useful in diagnosis, though spotless boutonneuse fever occurs. Symptoms include fever, headache, myalgias, and rash. Painful lymphadenopathy or lymphangitis may also occur. Rarely, papulovesicular lesions may resemble rickettsialpox. Endothelial injury produces perivascular edema and dermal necrosis. Regional adenopathy, disseminated lesions, kidney disease splenic rupture, and hepatitis including focal hepatic necrosis are reported. Multifocal retinitis is a reported complication. Neurologic manifestations, including encephalitis, internuclear ophthalmoplegia, vertebral arteritis with associated glossopharyngeal associated dysphagia, coronary involvement, purpura fulminans, and the hemophagocytic syndrome are rare.

The diagnosis is clinical, with serologic or PCR (culture can be used but is less sensitive than either) of the buffy coat of blood, or an eschar if one is available, used for confirmation. Treatment should be started upon clinical suspicion since delayed therapy is the usual cause of increased morbidity. Oral treatment with doxycycline (100 mg twice daily) or chloramphenicol (50–75 mg/kg/day in four divided doses) for 7–10 days is indicated. Caution is advised with the use of ciprofloxacin because it is associated with a poor outcome and increases the severity of disease in Mediterranean spotted fever. Primary care practitioners in endemic areas often include macrolides in the management of acute febrile illnesses to cover for these rickettsial fevers. The combination of azithromycin and rifampin is effective and safe in pregnancy. Prevention entails protective clothing, repellents, and inspection for and removal of ticks. Severe cases may require ICU care for multiorgan failure, respiratory failure in particular; fatalities are reported more often than with scrub typhus. Defervescence (over 48 hours) is reported with severe cases.

Formerly classified as an endemic or murine typhus, the cat-flea typhus, caused by *R felis* is more properly classified as a spotted fever. The causative agent has been linked to the cat flea and opossum exposure. While the diseases appear to be ubiquitous, most cases in the United States (southern Texas, California, and possibly Hawaii) occur in the spring and summer. Treatment is the same as for other rickettsial fevers.

Cases of non-rickettsiae–associated spotted fever tend to have a better prognosis than those due to *R rickettsiae* infection. Treatment for non-rickettsiae–associated spotted fever as well as *R rickettsiae* infection is with a tetracycline, typically doxycycline. Laboratory evidence suggests that these organisms may be less responsive to macrolides.

Bagshaw R et al. The characteristics and clinical course of patients with scrub typhus and Queensland tick typhus infection requiring intensive care unit admission: a 23-year case series from Queensland, tropical Australia. Am J Trop Med Hyg. 2020;103:2472. [PMID: 32959771]

Cohen R et al. Spotted fever group rickettsioses in Israel, 2010–2019. Emerg Infect Dis. 2021;27:2117. [PMID: 34286684]

3. Rickettsialpox

Rickettsialpox is an acute, self-limiting, febrile illness caused by *Rickettsia akari*, a parasite of mice, transmitted by the mite *Liponyssoides sanguineus* (Table 32–3). Rickettsialpox is in the spotted fever group of rickettsia. *R akari* infections are reported globally. Seroprevalence studies among injection drug users in Baltimore show seropositivity as high as 16%. In New York, its association with poverty is very strong. The illness has also been found in farming communities. Crowded conditions and mouse-infested housing allow transmission of the pathogen to humans. The *classic triad of fever, rash, and eschar is found in 99% of cases*. The primary lesion is a painless red papule that appears at variable times but on the average a week after a mite bite. The lesion often vesiculates and forms a black eschar. Lesions of African tick bite fever caused by *R africae* may resemble those of rickettsialpox.

The onset of symptoms—chills, fever, headache, photophobia, and disseminated aches and pains—is sudden. The fever may be followed by a widespread papular eruption 2–4 days later, with an average of 30–40 lesions that spare the palms and soles. The interval from vesiculation to crust formation is about 10 days. Early lesions may resemble those of chickenpox (typically vesicular versus papulovesicular in rickettsialpox). Pathologic findings include dermal edema, subepidermal vesicles, and the essence appears to be lymphocytic and granulocytic vasculitis.

Transient leukopenia and thrombocytopenia and acute hepatitis can occur. A fourfold rise in serum antibody titers to rickettsial antigen, detected by complement fixation or indirect fluorescent assays, is diagnostic and available through the CDC. Conjugated anti-rickettsial globulin can identify antigen in punch biopsies of skin lesions. PCR detection of rickettsial DNA in fresh tissue also appears of value. *R akari* can also be isolated from eschar biopsy specimens. A 44-kD protein is being characterized and appears to specify rickettsialpox.

Treatment consists of oral doxycycline (200 mg loading dose followed by 100 mg twice daily) for 2–5 days or until defervescence. The disease is usually mild and self-limited without treatment, but occasionally, severe symptoms may require hospitalization. Control requires the elimination of mice from human habitations and insecticide applications.

Csicsay F et al. Proteomic analysis of Rickettsia akari proposes a 44-kD-OMP as a potential biomarker for rickettsialpox diagnosis. BMC Microbiol. 2020;20:200. [PMID: 32640994]

Vyas NS et al. Investigating the histopathological findings and immunolocalization of rickettsialpox infection in skin biopsies: a case series and review of the literature. J Cutan Pathol. 2020;47:451. [PMID: 31955452]

OTHER RICKETTSIAL & RICKETTSIAL-LIKE DISEASES

1. Ehrlichiosis & Anaplasmosis

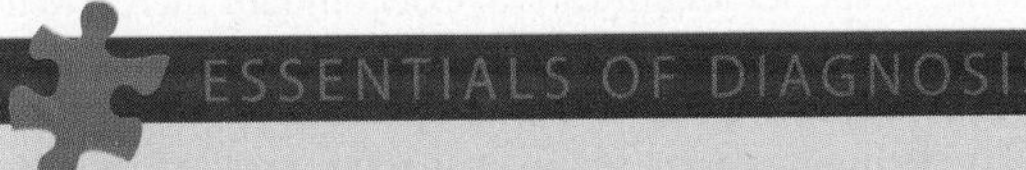

- Infection of monocyte or granulocyte by tick-borne gram-negative bacteria.
- Nine-day incubation period; clinical disease ranges from asymptomatic to life-threatening.
- Malaise, nausea, fever, and headaches.
- US cases of ehrlichiosis typically occur in men aged 60–69 years; US cases of anaplasmosis typically occur in men aged over 40 years; both occur in the summer, with different geographic areas of prevalence.
- Excellent response to therapy with tetracyclines.

General Considerations

Human ehrlichiosis and anaplasmosis are endemic in the United States.

Ehrlichia chaffeensis (Table 32–3), the most common *Ehrlichia* species infecting humans, is seen primarily in the south-central United States (especially Arkansas, Missouri, and Oklahoma) but also reported from Mexico City. *Ehrlichia ewingii* causes human granulocytic ehrlichiosis similar to anaplasmosis and constitutes almost 10% of ehrlichiosis cases; most cases in the United States are reported from the Midwest and Southeast. Human granulocytic anaplasmosis is caused by *Anaplasma phagocytophilum;* most cases in the United States are reported from New England, New York, Minnesota, and Wisconsin. Increasingly, anaplasmosis is being reported from Asia,

South Korea, Mongolia, China (where a new species is identified, *Anaplasma capra*), and Northern Europe.

In North America, the major tick-borne rickettsial disease vectors for these pathogens are (1) the Lone Star tick (*Amblyomma americanus*), which is the vector for *E chaffeensis* and *E ewingii*; (2) the black-legged tick (*Ixodes scapularis*), which is a vector for *B burgdorferi* (Lyme disease), *Babesia microti* (babesiosis), and *A phagocytophilum* (anaplasmosis), and a possible vector for *Ehrlichia muris eauclairensis*; and (3) the western black-legged tick (*Ixodes pacificus*), which is a vector for *A phagocytophilum* along the Pacific coast of the United States. Vectors for European and Asian cases are *Ixodes* species such as *I ricinus* and *I persulcatus*. The principal reservoirs for human monocytic ehrlichiosis and human granulocytic anaplasmosis are the white tail deer and the white-footed mouse, respectively. Other mammals are implicated as well. Transfusion-transmitted anaplasmosis has been reported.

CDC reports indicate that the incidences of human monocytic ehrlichiosis, granulocytic ehrlichiosis and, in particular, anaplasmosis are increasing (the latter in particular in New York and New England); cases are reportable to local and state health departments. Because more than one agent may coexist in the same area, cases of human ehrlichiosis and anaplasmosis may be reported as "human ehrlichiosis/anaplasmosis undetermined" in the absence of species identification. Concomitant increases in tick populations may be responsible for the surge.

The case fatality rate is 1% with *E chaffeensis* infections and 0.3% among cases of human anaplasmosis. Most cases of *E ewingii* infection have occurred among immunocompetent patients. No deaths have been reported from either *E ewingii* or *E muris eauclairensis*.

Clinical Findings

A. Symptoms and Signs

Clinical disease of human monocytic ehrlichiosis ranges from mild to life-threatening. Typically, after a 1- to 2-week incubation period and a prodrome consisting of malaise, rigors, and nausea, high fever and headache develop. A pleomorphic rash may occur. Presentation in immunosuppressed patients (including transplant patients) and older patients tends to be more severe. Rare serious sequelae include acute respiratory failure and ARDS; neurologic complications, the most common being meningoencephalitis and aseptic meningitis; acute kidney disease (which may mimic thrombotic thrombocytopenic purpura); hemophagocytic syndrome; and multiorgan failure.

The clinical manifestations of human granulocytic ehrlichiosis and anaplasmosis are similar to those seen with human monocytic ehrlichiosis. Asymptomatic infection is recognized. Rash, however, is infrequent. If a rash is present, coinfection with other tick-borne diseases or an alternative diagnosis should be suspected. Persistent fever and malaise are reported to occur for 2 or more years. Reported complications of anaplasmosis include hyponatremia, leukopenia, thrombocytopenia, and an acute cerebral infarction.

Coinfection with anaplasmosis and Lyme disease or babesiosis may occur, but the clinical manifestations (including fever and cytopenias) are more severe with anaplasmosis than with Lyme disease. A spirochete, *Borrelia miyamotoi*, may mimic anaplasmosis in its clinical manifestations.

B. Laboratory Findings

Diagnosis can be made by the history of tick exposure followed by a characteristic clinical presentation. Leukopenia, absolute lymphopenia, thrombocytopenia, and transaminitis occur often. Thrombocytopenia occurs more often than leukopenia in human granulocytic ehrlichiosis. Hyponatremia from volume depletion is reported. Examination of peripheral blood with Giemsa stain may reveal characteristic intraleukocytic vacuoles (morulae) in up to 20% of patients. An indirect fluorescent antibody assay is available through the CDC and requires acute and convalescent sera. A PCR assay can be helpful for making the diagnosis early in the disease course. PCR assay is most sensitive in the first week of illness and can be used as a confirmatory test.

Treatment & Prevention

Treatment for human ehrlichiosis and anaplasmosis is with doxycycline, 100 mg twice daily (orally or intravenously) for 10–14 days or until 3 days of defervescence. Rifampin is an alternative in pregnant women. Treatment should not be withheld while awaiting confirmatory serology when suspicion is high. Lack of clinical improvement and defervescence 48 hours after doxycycline initiation suggests an alternate diagnosis. Some patients may continue to have headache, weakness, and malaise for weeks despite adequate treatment. Tick control is the essence of prevention.

Centers for Disease Control and Prevention (CDC). Ehrlichiosis: epidemiology and statistics. https://www.cdc.gov/ehrlichiosis/stats/index.html

Centers for Disease Control and Prevention (CDC). Anaplasmosis: epidemiology and statistics. https://www.cdc.gov/anaplasmosis/stats/index.html

Russell A et al. Epidemiology and spatial emergence of anaplasmosis, New York, USA, 2010-2018. Emerg Infect Dis. 2021;27:2154. [PMID: 34287128]

2. Q Fever (*Coxiella burnetii* Infection)

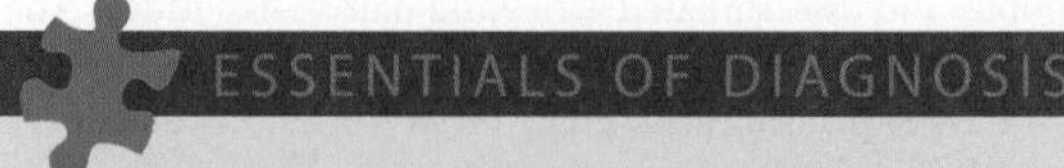

- Exposure to sheep, goats, cattle, or their products; some infections are laboratory acquired.
- Acute or chronic febrile illness: headache, cough, prostration, and abdominal pain.
- Pneumonitis, hepatitis, or encephalopathy; less often, endocarditis, vascular infections, or chronic fatigue syndrome.
- A common cause of culture-negative endocarditis.

General Considerations

Q fever, a reportable and significantly underestimated disease in the United States, is caused by the gram-negative intracellular coccobacillus *C burnetii*. *Coxiella* infections occur globally, mostly in cattle, sheep, and goats, in which they cause mild or subclinical disease (Table 32–3). In these animals, reactivation of the infection occurs during pregnancy and causes abortions or low birth weight offspring. *Coxiella* is resistant to heat and drying and remains infective in the environment for months.

Human infection occurs via inhalation of aerosolized bacteria (in dust or droplets) from feces, urine, milk, or products of conception of infected animals. Ingestion and skin penetration are other recognized routes of transmission. A 2017 outbreak in Spain had an attack rate of 25% (16/64). Animal handlers, slaughterhouse workers, veterinarians, laboratory workers, and other workers exposed to animal products are at risk due to their occupations. In the United States, over 60% of cases do not report an exposure to potentially infectious animals, but cases are more than twice as likely as non-cases to report drinking raw milk.

Human-to-human transmission does *not* seem to occur, but maternal-fetal infection can occur and infection after liver transplant is reported. Rare tick-borne transmission is suspected, but ticks may be important in ruminant transmission. In Europe, 4.8% of ticks carry *C burnetii*.

Clinical Findings

A. Symptoms and Signs

Asymptomatic infection is common. For the remaining cases, a febrile illness develops after an incubation period of 2–3 weeks, usually accompanied by headache, relative bradycardia, prostration, and muscle pains. The clinical course may be acute, chronic (duration 6 months or longer), or relapsing. Pneumonia and granulomatous hepatitis are the predominant manifestations in the acute form (and these may vary in incidence geographically), whereas other less common manifestations include skin rashes (maculopapular or purpuric), fever of unknown origin, myocarditis, pericarditis, aortic aneurysms, aseptic meningitis, encephalitis, orchitis, iliopsoas abscess, spondylodiscitis, tenosynovitis, granulomatous osteomyelitis (more often seen in children), and regional (mediastinal) or diffuse lymphadenopathies.

It has been recommended that the term "*chronic Q fever*" be abandoned to avoid confusion and be replaced with "*persistent localized infections*." The most common presentation in patients with persistent localized infections is culture-negative endocarditis. Risk factors for endocarditis are the immunocompromised state, presence of preexisting valvular conditions, male sex, and age above 40 years. Valvular prosthesis (mechanical or bioprosthesis) represents the most important risk factor. In series of post-cardiac surgery patients with culture-negative endocarditis, Q fever is the most common cause (about 40% of cases). In a Dutch series of 107 patients with Q fever endocarditis risk factors and positive serologies, follow-up at a median of 64 months after initial screening showed that 4.7% went on to develop a persistent localized infection (one person despite an intermediate negative serology), while 23.4% became seronegative, and most (72%) showed a pattern of resolved infection.

The clinical manifestations of endocarditis are nonspecific with fever, night sweats, and weight loss. Rarely, urticaria, edema, erythema nodosum, and arthralgias are reported. Sudden cardiac insufficiency, stroke, or other embolic and mycotic aneurysms can also develop. Vascular infections, particularly of the aorta (causing mycotic aneurysms) and of graft prostheses, are the second most common presentation and are associated with a high mortality (25%). A post–Q fever chronic fatigue syndrome (1 year after acute infection with chronic symptoms) is controversial and of unknown pathophysiology. Cognitive behavioral therapy is effective in reducing fatigue severity in patients with Q fever fatigue syndrome; long-term treatment with doxycycline has not been shown to be effective.

New infection or reactivation of Q fever can occur in pregnant women and is associated with spontaneous abortions, intrauterine growth retardation, intrauterine fetal death, and premature delivery. *C burnetii* infection during the first trimester can cause oligohydramnios.

B. Laboratory Findings

Laboratory examination during the acute phase may show elevated liver biochemical tests and occasional leukocytosis. Patients with acute Q fever usually produce antibodies to *C burnetii* phase II antigen (phase II antigens are formed in vitro from deleted avirulent mutants and are empirically more commonly seen in acute disease, whereas phase I antigens, seen in nature and laboratory infections, are found in the IgG form in chronic disease). A fourfold rise between acute and convalescent sera by indirect immunofluorescence is diagnostic of the infection. Real-time PCR for *C burnetii* DNA is helpful only in early diagnosis of Q fever. *C burnetii* DNA becomes undetectable in serum as serologic responses develop. The positive predictive value of antibodies to phase II antigens in acute disease is at most 65%, and considerable intertest variability exists with phase 2 antigens. Diagnostic tests combining PCR with ELISA (Immuno-PCR) improve the sensitivity and specificity during the first 2 weeks after the onset of symptoms.

While persistent infection can be diagnosed based on serologic tests done at 3- and 6-month intervals (with an IgG titer against phase I antigen of 1:800 or greater), the sensitivity of such serologies is often low, and the diagnosis of Q fever is often made clinically. An automated epifluorescence assay has greater than 95% sensitivity for the detection of phase I antigens in persistent infection. The presence of elevated levels of anticardiolipin antibodies have a high positive predictive value for acute endocarditis.

Diagnosis of Q fever endocarditis is often made at the time of valve replacement with PCR of tissue samples. *C burnetii* may also be isolated from affected valves using the shell-vial technique.

C. Imaging

Radiographs of the chest can show patchy pulmonary infiltrates. *All patients with acute Q fever should be screened for underlying valvular disease with echocardiography.* Initial imaging and follow-up with serial 18-FDG PET/CT scan may be helpful in identifying chronic infection and monitoring treatment response.

Differential Diagnosis

Viral, *Mycoplasma*, and bacterial pneumonias; viral hepatitis; brucellosis; Legionnaire disease; murine or scrub typhus; Kawasaki disease; tuberculosis; psittacosis; and other animal-borne diseases can have similar clinical presentations to Q fever. Q fever should be considered in cases of unexplained fevers with negative blood cultures in association with embolic or cardiac disease. Cases of Q fever can mimic autoimmune disease. Coinfection with typhus and leptospirosis is reported.

Treatment & Prognosis

Doxycycline is the most effective medication against *C burnetii*; doxycycline resistance is rare. Isolates remain susceptible to levofloxacin, moxifloxacin, and to a lesser extent ciprofloxacin. No resistance to sulfamethoxazole-trimethoprim is reported to date.

For acute infection, treatment with doxycycline (100 mg orally twice daily) for 14 days or at least 3 full days after defervescence is recommended. Even in untreated patients, the mortality rate is usually low, except when endocarditis develops.

No consensus guidelines exist for the treatment of persistent *C burnetii* infections. Most experts recommend a combination oral therapy with doxycycline (100 mg twice a day) plus hydroxychloroquine for approximately 18 months for native valve endocarditis and 24 months for prosthetic valve endocarditis. The use of alternative combination regimens with a quinolone or rifampin shows some efficacy.

Serologic responses can be monitored during and after completion of therapy and treatment can be extended in the absence of favorable serologic response. The general variability of serologic data, however, limits their usefulness and providers usually rely on clinical criteria. Patients should be monitored for an extended period of time, generally at least several years per expert opinion, due to risk of relapse.

For patients with endocarditis, clinical cure is possible without valve replacement. Heart valve replacement is *not* associated with better survival, except in the group of patients with a valvular prosthesis. Given the difficulty in treating endocarditis, transthoracic echocardiography is recommended to screen for predisposing valvulopathy in all patients with acute Q fever, and the same therapy for 1 year should be offered in the presence of valvulopathy. In addition, patients undergoing routine valve surgery in endemic countries should be evaluated via Q fever serology and treated if positive.

All infected pregnant women should be given long-term trimethoprim-sulfamethoxazole (320/1600 mg orally for the duration of pregnancy, but not beyond 32 weeks' gestation) to prevent the obstetric complications.

In retrospective studies, an increased risk of diffuse B-cell lymphoma and follicular lymphoma was found in patients with Q fever compared with the general population. Patients with persistent focalized infections were at higher risk for lymphadenitis and progression to lymphoma.

Prevention

Prevention is based on detection of the infection in livestock, with reduction of contact with infected and parturient animals or contaminated dust; special care when working with animal tissues; and effective pasteurization of milk. A whole-cell Q fever vaccine is available in Australia for persons with high-risk exposures (where the overall seroprevalence of antibodies to *Coxiella* is only 19%). Clinicians have reported vaccine failure more than 15 days after vaccination.

The organism is highly transmissible to laboratory workers and culture techniques require a biosafety level 3 setting. *C burnetii* is a category B bioterrorism agent. In the setting of a bioterrorist attack, postexposure prophylaxis with doxycycline 100 mg orally twice a day for 5–7 days should be administered within 8–12 days of exposure. Pregnant women may take trimethoprim-sulfamethoxazole as an alternative.

Buijs SB et al. Long-term serological follow-up after primary Coxiella burnetii infection in patients with vascular risk factors for chronic Q fever. Eur J Clin Microbiol Infect Dis. 2021;40:1569. [PMID: 33566203]

Centers for Disease Control and Prevention (CDC). National Notifiable Diseases Surveillance System (NNDSS): Q Fever (*Coxiella burnetii*) 2009 Case Definition https://wwwn.cdc.gov/nndss/conditions/q-fever/case-definition/2009/

KAWASAKI DISEASE

ESSENTIALS OF DIAGNOSIS

- Fever, conjunctivitis, oral mucosal changes, rash, cervical lymphadenopathy, peripheral extremity changes.
- Elevated ESR and CRP levels.
- Risk for coronary arteritis and aneurysms.

General Considerations

Kawasaki disease is a worldwide multisystem disease. It is also known as the "**mucocutaneous lymph node syndrome**." It occurs mainly in children between the ages of 3 months and 5 years but can occur occasionally in adults as well. Kawasaki disease occurs most often in persons of Asian or native Pacific Islander descent. Its incidence in Japan is twice that of the United States, and it occurs among siblings at twice the incidence of cases and at higher rates among parents of cases. These findings plus the known seasonality (higher incidence in winter and early spring) and occasional epidemic pattern of cases point to the inadequate current understanding of the etiology of this disease.

Kawasaki disease is an acute, self-limiting, mucocutaneous vasculitis characterized by the infiltration of vessel walls with mononuclear cells and later by IgA secreting plasma cells that can result in the destruction of the tunica media and aneurysm formation. The cause remains unknown. Epidemiologic studies show an increased risk with advanced maternal age, mother of foreign birth, maternal group B *Streptococcus* colonization, and early infancy hospitalization for a bacterial illness. Genetic factors are considered to play an important role in the pathogenesis of the disease. Ongoing analyses identify many gene polymorphisms, which significantly correlate with Kawasaki disease susceptibility (at least 23 to disease, and 10 to the presence of coronary aneurysms).

The Kawasaki-like disease, called **multisystem inflammatory syndrome in children (MIS-C)**, is described in the section above on SARS-CoV-2.

Clinical Findings

A. Symptoms and Signs

A clinical diagnosis of classic or "**complete**" **Kawasaki disease** requires the presence of at least 5 days of fever, usually high-grade (over 39°C to 40°C) and four of the following five criteria: (1) bilateral nonexudative conjunctivitis (begins shortly after the onset of fever), (2) oral changes of erythema and cracking of lips, strawberry tongue, and erythema of oral and pharyngeal mucosa (ulcers and pharyngeal exudates are not consistent with Kawasaki disease), (3) peripheral extremity changes (erythema and edema of the hands and feet in the acute phase, or periungual desquamation, or both, within 2 to 3 weeks after the onset of fever), (4) polymorphous rash, and (5) cervical lymphadenopathy (larger than 1.5 cm, usually unilateral; least common of the clinical features). The revised case definition allows the diagnosis on day 4 in the presence of more than four principal clinical criteria, particularly when redness and swelling of the hands and feet are present.

A diagnosis of atypical or "**incomplete**" **Kawasaki disease** can be made in patients with unexplained fever and fewer than four principal criteria if accompanied by compatible laboratory tests or findings of aneurysms detected by echocardiography or angiography.

A wide spectrum of rare diagnostic and recognized presentations includes an erythema multiforme rash, onychomycosis, cervical lymphadenopathy, febrile seizures, cheilitis, torticollis, facial nerve palsy, Beau lines of the nails, inflammation at the site of BCG vaccination, and UTI.

B. Laboratory Findings

Laboratory findings in the acute phase of Kawasaki disease typically include leukocytosis with neutrophilic predominance, anemia, and an elevated ESR and CRP. High platelet counts are characteristic but occur in the second week. N-terminal moiety of BNP (NT-proBNP), likely indicative of myocardial involvement, may be elevated in some patients with Kawasaki disease.

The laboratory components of the CDC's case definition of MIS-C are positivity for current or recent SARS-CoV-2 infection by RT-PCR, serology, or antigen test (or known COVID-19 exposure within the 4 weeks prior to the onset of symptoms) in conjunction with evidence of inflammation (including one or more of the following: elevated CRP, ESR, fibrinogen, procalcitonin, D-dimer, ferritin, lactic acid dehydrogenase, interleukin-6 [IL-6], or neutrophils; or reduced lymphocytes or albumin).

Major complications include arteritis and aneurysms of the coronary vessels. The arteritis begins 6–8 days after the onset of disease, occurs in about 25% of untreated patients, and occasionally causes MI. Coronary complications are more common among patients older than 6 years or younger than 1 year of age; males; and those unresponsive to IVIG, who received a smaller dose of IVIG, or did not receive treatment within 10 days of symptom onset. According to the 2017 American Heart Association definitions of coronary artery aneurysm, such aneurysms developed in 6.4% of patients with Kawasaki disease despite treatment with IVIG and aspirin. While myocarditis can be found in all patients with Kawasaki disease on histologic specimens and is prominent during the acute stage, only a small percentage of patients are clinically symptomatic.

Cardiac complications include left ventricular dysfunction, which usually normalizes promptly with IVIG therapy, and mitral regurgitation, which occurs early and does not appear to persist. Noninvasive diagnosis of coronary complications can be made with CT coronary angiography (the most sensitive test), magnetic resonance angiography, or transthoracic echocardiography (advocated for early screening). Kawasaki shock syndrome is a complication, with an estimated incidence of 7%, possibly caused by decrease in peripheral vascular resistance, myocarditis with or without myocardial ischemia, and capillary leakage.

The multisystemic findings of Kawasaki disease show it to be a systemic disease that affects medium-sized arteries of multiple organs, causing elevations in serum transaminases, interstitial pneumonitis, abdominal pain, vomiting, diarrhea, gallbladder hydrops, pancreatitis, lymphadenopathy, hypoalbuminemia, arrhythmias, aseptic meningitis, acute encephalopathy with biphasic seizures and late reduced diffusion, retinal and choroidal detachment, pulmonary complications (effusions, empyema, pneumothorax), and pyuria. CSF pleocytosis with a mononuclear cell predominance, normal glucose levels, and protein levels is seen in one-third of children who undergo lumbar puncture.

Other diseases with similar presentation that should be considered include measles in unimmunized children as well as other viral infections, such as SARS-CoV-2, adenovirus, scarlet fever, hemophagocytic lymphohistiocytosis syndrome, and toxic shock syndrome; rickettsial infections; or leptospirosis and drug hypersensitivity reactions.

Treatment & Prevention

All patients meeting the diagnostic criteria for Kawasaki disease (complete and incomplete), including patients with recurrent Kawasaki disease, should be treated as soon as the diagnosis is suspected to reduce inflammation and arterial damage.

A single dose of IVIG should be given in the first 10 days of the illness. Patients in whom the diagnosis was made later than the tenth day may still benefit from IVIG treatment if they have elevated inflammatory markers (ESR or CRP), with persistent fever or have coronary artery aneurysms. When IVIG treatment is not given, coronary artery aneurysms occur in 20% of children. Even when treated with IVIG within the first 10 days of illness, coronary artery aneurysms still develop in 5% of patients.

Rare cases of aseptic meningitis are reported with IVIG. Coombs-positive hemolytic anemia, especially in individuals with AB blood type and anaphylactic reactions to immunoglobulins with selective IgA deficiency are other complications associated with IVIG administration.

Although aspirin does not lower the frequency of development of coronary abnormalities, it has important anti-inflammatory activity and antiplatelet activity. Concomitant aspirin with IVIG should be started at 80–100 mg/kg/day orally (divided into four doses and not exceeding 4 g/day) until the patient is afebrile for 48 hours and then reduced to 3–5 mg/kg/day until markers of acute inflammation normalize. A 2019 meta-analysis indicates that low-dose aspirin (3–5 mg/kg/day) may be as effective as the use of high-dose aspirin (30 mg/kg/day or more) for the initial treatment of Kawasaki disease. Since ibuprofen antagonizes the irreversible platelet inhibition induced by aspirin, it should be avoided when aspirin is given.

The use of corticosteroids for children with Kawasaki disease is controversial. According to the 2017 published guidelines by the American Heart Association, single-dose pulse methylprednisolone should not be used routinely for patients with Kawasaki disease. A course of corticosteroid therapy with tapering over 2–3 weeks could be considered in addition to IVIG and aspirin for patients at high-risk for not responding to IVIG.

Resistant Kawasaki disease, defined as having recrudescent or persistent fever at least 36 hours after the end of the first IVIG infusion when no other source of fever is found, develops in about 10–20% of patients. The Egami score is a predictor used in Japan to help determine who will respond to IVIG, although the scoring system has been shown to have lower utility in US cases. The presence of coronary artery abnormalities on the initial echocardiogram and their presence before day 5 of fever predict nonresponse to IVIG in one Israeli study.

Options for refractory cases include a second dose of IVIG (the full validity of which needs further study), high-dose pulse corticosteroids over 3 days with or without a subsequent oral taper course, longer oral tapering course of corticosteroids over 2–3 weeks together with IVIG and aspirin, TNF-alpha blockers such as infliximab, the anti-inflammatory interleukin-1 receptor antagonist anakinra, low-dose methotrexate, and cyclosporine. Immunomodulatory monoclonal antibody therapy and cytotoxic agents or (rarely) plasma exchange should be considered only in highly refractory cases in which other therapy has failed.

The most common serious complication in the acute phase is thrombotic occlusion of a coronary artery aneurysm leading to MI or sudden death. An echocardiogram is recommended within 1–2 weeks and 4–6 weeks after treatment for uncomplicated patients. More frequent imaging is recommended for patients with significant and evolving coronary artery abnormalities. Coronary artery aneurysms with smaller diameter, especially smaller than 6 mm, tend to regress earlier, typically within 6 months of infection.

Anticoagulation with warfarin or low-molecular-weight heparin is indicated, along with aspirin, in patients with rapidly expanding coronary artery aneurysms. Aspirin, a second antiplatelet agent, and anticoagulation with warfarin, low-molecular-weight heparin, or DOACs (which need further study in this population) may be considered for patients with large or giant aneurysms (at least 8 mm) (which correlate with delay in diagnosis) and a recent history of coronary artery thrombosis. Platelets from patients with Kawasaki disease treated with antiplatelet agents do show decreased platelet aggregation function. Systemic arterial aneurysms are also recognized and always occur concomitantly with coronary aneurysms, and large systemic aneurysms show a high rate of regression.

If MI occurs, therapy with thrombolytics, percutaneous coronary intervention, coronary artery bypass grafts, and even cardiac transplantation should be considered. Manifestations of coronary artery aneurysms can occur as late as in the third or fourth decade of life with a study showing a prevalence of 5% coronary sequelae from Kawasaki disease among young adults evaluated with angiography. Calcified coronary aneurysms on CT scans are less likely to regress.

Prognosis

The reported recurrence rate is 3% in one study from Japan. The highest risk of recurrence occurs in the first 2 years after the first episode. The mortality peaks between 15 and 45 days after the onset of fever, at the time of coronary artery vasculitis, thrombocytosis, and a hypercoagulable state.

Over the long-term, the risk for clinical cardiac events in patients with no coronary artery abnormalities is similar to the general population. For patients in whom coronary artery abnormalities developed, the risk for cardiac complications, such as thrombosis, stenosis, MI, and death, ranges between 1% and 48%. Follow-up is especially needed among the subset of patients with neutropenia who have been treated with IVIG. The administration of IVIG is shown to improve left ventricular function. The American Heart Association recommends risk stratification based on the assessment of coronary luminal dimensions by echocardiogram, under cardiologic supervision. The frequency of clinical follow-up, diagnostic testing, reproductive counseling, indications for medical therapy (beta-blockers, statins), and thromboprophylaxis (aspirin and anticoagulation) depends on the individual's risk assessment.

When to Refer

All cases of Kawasaki disease merit referral to specialists.

Centers for Disease Control and Prevention. Multisystem inflammatory syndrome in children. https://www.cdc.gov/coronavirus/2019-ncov/hcp/pediatric-hcp.html#anchor_1589580133375

Rowley AH. Multisystem inflammatory syndrome in children and Kawasaki disease: two different illnesses with overlapping clinical features. J Pediatr. 2020;224:129. [PMID: 32585239]

Schroeder AR et al. COVID-19 and Kawasaki disease: finding the signal in the noise. Hosp Pediatr. 2020;10:e1. [PMID: 32404331]

Selamet Tierney ES et al; International Kawasaki Disease Registry. Variation in pharmacologic management of patients with Kawasaki disease with coronary artery aneurysms. J Pediatr. 2021;240:164. [PMID: 34474088]

Bacterial & Chlamydial Infections

Bryn A. Boslett, MD
Rachel Bystritsky, MD

INFECTIONS CAUSED BY GRAM-POSITIVE BACTERIA

STREPTOCOCCAL INFECTIONS

Group A beta-hemolytic streptococci *(Streptococcus pyogenes)* are the most common bacterial cause of pharyngitis.

1. Pharyngitis & Tonsillitis (see Chapter 8)

2. Acute Rheumatic Fever & Scarlet Fever

General Considerations

Group A streptococci producing erythrogenic toxin may cause scarlet fever in susceptible persons. Acute rheumatic fever may follow recurrent episodes of pharyngitis beginning 1–4 weeks after the onset of symptoms. Effectively controlling rheumatic fever depends on identification and treatment of primary streptococcal infection and secondary prevention of recurrences.

Glomerulonephritis is another rare complication, following a single infection with a nephritogenic strain of streptococcus group A (eg, types 4, 12, 2, 49, and 60), more commonly on the skin than in the throat, and begins 1–3 weeks after the onset of the infection.

Clinical Findings

S pyogenes (group A *Streptococcus* [GAS]) pharyngitis is usually a self-limited condition, lasting 3–5 days.

1. Scarlet fever—Scarlet fever may appear one or two days after the onset of GAS pharyngitis. The rash of scarlet fever (also called scarletina) is diffusely erythematous and resembles a sunburn, and superimposed fine red papules give the skin a sandpaper consistency; it is most intense in the groin and axillas. It blanches on pressure, may become petechial, and fades in 2–5 days, leaving a fine desquamation. The face is flushed, with circumoral pallor, and the tongue is coated with enlarged red papillae (strawberry tongue). The diagnosis is clinical in the setting of streptococcal pharyngitis.

2. Rheumatic fever—The diagnosis of acute rheumatic fever relies on a constellation of signs, symptoms, and laboratory findings, known as the Jones criteria: major criteria include presence of pancarditis, polyarthritis, subcutaneous nodules, erythema marginatum, chorea, and minor criteria include presence of heart block, arthralgia, elevated ESR or CRP, fever, leukocytosis, or history of prior rheumatic fever. At least two major Jones criteria or one major and two minor criteria plus evidence of recent GAS infection by either bacterial culture data, rapid strep testing, or elevated anti-strep antibody titers are required to establish a diagnosis. These complications are more common in children.

Treatment

Antimicrobial therapy of pharyngitis may reduce the risk of complications (see Chapter 8). There is no additional treatment of scarlet fever or acute rheumatic fever beyond that of the underlying streptococcal pharyngitis.

Prevention of Recurrent Rheumatic Fever

Patients who have had rheumatic fever should be treated with a continuous course of antimicrobial prophylaxis for at least 5 years. Effective regimens are erythromycin, 250 mg orally twice daily, or penicillin G, 500 mg orally daily.

Sable C et al. Update on prevention and management of rheumatic heart disease. Pediatr Clin North Am. 2020;67:843. [PMID: 32888685]

van Driel ML et al. Different antibiotic treatments for group A streptococcal pharyngitis. Cochrane Database Syst Rev. 2021;3:CD004406. [PMID: 33728634]

3. Streptococcal Skin Infections

Group A beta-hemolytic streptococci are not normal skin flora. Streptococcal skin infections result from colonization of normal skin by contact with other infected individuals or by preceding streptococcal respiratory infection.

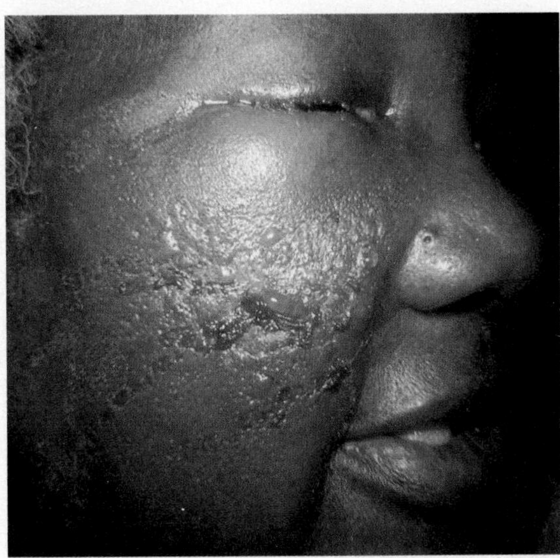

▲ **Figure 33–1.** Erysipelas of the face with edema, bright red erythema, and serosanguineous discharge from the severely swollen cheek. (Public Health Image Library, CDC.)

Clinical Findings

A. Symptoms and Signs

Erysipelas is a painful superficial cellulitis that is well demarcated from the surrounding normal skin and frequently involves the face (Figure 33–1). It affects skin with impaired lymphatic drainage, such as edematous lower extremities or wounds.

Impetigo is a focal, vesicular, pustular lesion with a thick, amber-colored crust with a "stuck-on" appearance (see Chapter 6).

B. Laboratory Findings

Cultures obtained from a wound or pustule are likely to grow group A streptococci. Blood cultures are occasionally positive.

Treatment

Although penicillin is the treatment of choice for streptococcal infections, it may be difficult to differentiate staphylococcal infections from streptococcal infections. In practice, initial therapy for patients with risk factors for *Staphylococcus aureus* (eg, injection drug use, diabetes mellitus, wound infection) should cover this organism. Parenteral therapy with either intravenous nafcillin or cefazolin (which can also be given intramuscularly) is a reasonable choice. In the patient at risk for methicillin-resistant *S aureus* infection or with a serious penicillin allergy (ie, anaphylaxis), intravenous vancomycin or daptomycin should be used (Table 33–1).

Patients who do not require parenteral therapy and in whom *S aureus* infection is less likely may be treated with amoxicillin, 500 mg three times daily or 875 mg twice daily for 7–10 days. A first-generation oral cephalosporin, eg, cephalexin, or clindamycin is an alternative to amoxicillin

Table 33–1. Treatment of common skin and soft tissue infections (SSTIs).

SSTI Type	Common Pathogens	Treatment
Purulent (abscess, furuncle, carbuncle, cellulitis with purulence)	*Staphylococcus aureus*	Incision and drainage is the primary treatment Consider the addition of antibiotics in select situations[1] **Oral antibiotic regimens[2]** Dicloxacillin 500 mg four times daily *or* cephalexin 500 mg four times daily Clindamycin 300 four times daily or 450 mg three times daily *or* trimethoprim-sulfamethoxazole one double-strength tablet twice daily *or* doxycycline (or minocycline) 100 mg twice daily **Intravenous antibiotic regimens[2]** Nafcillin 1–2 g four to six times daily *or* cefazolin 1 g three times daily Vancomycin 1 g twice daily *or* daptomycin 4 mg/kg once daily
Nonpurulent (cellulitis, erysipelas)	Beta-hemolytic streptococci (*S aureus* less likely)	**Oral antibiotic regimens[2]** Amoxicillin 500 mg three times daily or 875 mg twice daily Cephalexin 500 mg four times daily *or* clindamycin 300 mg four times daily[2] **Intravenous antibiotic regimens[2]** Nafcillin 1–2 g four to six times daily *or* cefazolin 1 g three times daily Vancomycin 1 g twice daily *or* daptomycin 4 mg/kg once daily

[1]Antibiotic therapy should be given in addition to incision and drainage for purulent SSTIs if the patient has any of the following: severe or extensive disease, symptoms and signs of systemic illness, purulent cellulitis/wound infection, comorbidities and extremes of age, abscess in area difficult to drain or on face/hand, associated septic phlebitis, or lack of response to incision and drainage alone. Antibiotic doses may vary based on weight and kidney function. Dosages listed assume normal renal and hepatic function, as well as average weight. Reevaluate dosing with renal/hepatic impairment.

[2]Other drugs that are FDA-approved for treating SSTIs include linezolid 600 mg intravenously or orally twice daily for 10–14 days; daptomycin 4 mg/kg intravenously once daily for 7–14 days; tedizolid 200 mg orally once daily for 6 days; tigecycline 100 mg intravenously once followed by 50 mg intravenously twice a day for 5–14 days; ceftaroline 600 mg twice a day for 7–14 days; dalbavancin 1500 mg as a single intravenous dose; oritavancin 1200 mg as a single intravenous dose; telavancin 10 mg/kg intravenously once daily for 7–14 days; and delafloxacin 450 mg orally or 300 intravenously twice daily for 5–14 days.

(Table 33–1). In patients with recurrent cellulitis of the leg, maintenance therapy (for at least 1 year) with penicillin, 250 mg orally twice daily, may reduce relapses.

Rrapi R et al. Cellulitis: a review of pathogenesis, diagnosis, and management. Med Clin North Am. 2021;105:723. [PMID: 34059247]

Stevens DL et al. Practice guidelines for the diagnosis and management of skin and soft tissue infections: 2014 update by the Infectious Diseases Society of America. Clin Infect Dis. 2014;59:147. [PMID: 24947530]

4. Necrotizing Fasciitis

Necrotizing fasciitis is a rapidly spreading infection involving the fascia of deep muscle often involving an extremity, head and neck, perianal, or genital area ("Fournier gangrene"). Some patients have a preceding skin or blunt trauma injury. Patients who are immunosuppressed, have diabetes, are at extremes of age (older adults or neonates), or are affected by liver disease are generally more susceptible.

Distinguishing necrotizing fasciitis from necrotizing myositis may be difficult as skeletal muscle and fascia are involved in both syndromes. Necrotizing fasciitis is most often monomicrobial; the usual causative agent is *S pyogenes* (group A beta-hemolytic streptococci), but it can also be caused by other streptococcal species, and occasionally by *S aureus*. Infections can be polymicrobial (mixed aerobic and anaerobic bacteria). A history of exposure to brackish water or marine life should raise suspicion for *Vibrio vulnificans* or *Aeromonas* species. Patients with burn injuries are susceptible to *Pseudomonas* species. Necrotizing myositis is often caused by *Clostridia* species (clostridial myonecrosis or "gas gangrene"). See Clostridial Diseases, below.

Clinical Findings

A. Symptoms and Signs

The clinical findings at presentation may be those of severe cellulitis, but the presence of systemic toxicity and severe pain, which may be followed by anesthesia of the involved area due to destruction of nerves as infection advances through the fascial planes, is a clue to the diagnosis. Infection can progress rapidly, and pain often subsides as nerves are destroyed. Multiorgan failure is common as infection progresses.

B. Laboratory Findings

Nonspecific serum markers include elevated WBC, ESR, and CRP. Elevated creatine kinase may indicate muscle involvement. Blood cultures and wound cultures should be obtained, as well as tissue cultures from surgical specimens. Histologic specimens may demonstrate extensive tissue destruction, thrombosis of blood vessels, and bacteria spreading along fascial planes.

C. Imaging

CT or MRI of the affected area may show gas in tissues or fascial plane infection. Imaging may also appear normal, so rely on clinical suspicion and surgical evaluation.

Treatment

Surgical exploration is mandatory when the diagnosis is suspected. Early and extensive debridement is essential for survival. Surgical evaluation should not be delayed while awaiting imaging or other diagnostic tests, especially in the setting of rapid progression of clinical manifestations.

Broad-spectrum antibiotic therapy should be initiated whenever the diagnosis is suspected and should cover aerobic and anaerobic organisms. Initial therapy for patients with normal kidney function typically consists of intravenous therapy with a carbapenem (meropenem 2 g every 8 hours or imipenem 1 g every 6 hours) or piperacillin-tazobactam 4.5 g every 6 hours plus an agent with activity against methicillin-resistant *S aureus* (vancomycin, linezolid, or daptomycin) plus clindamycin for its antitoxin and other effects against toxin-producing strains of streptococci and staphylococci. Patients with exposure histories that suggest less common etiologies should have therapy targeted to those organisms. Antibiotic therapy should then be tailored to culture results. Antibiotic therapy should be continued until all infected tissue has been removed and the patient has stabilized; the final duration depends on individual patient factors.

In addition to surgical and antibiotic therapy, the use of intravenous immunoglobulin for streptococcal necrotizing soft tissue infections has been shown to reduce mortality. The dose is 1 g/kg on day 1, followed by 0.5 g/kg on days 2 and 3.

Eckmann C et al. Current management of necrotizing soft-tissue infections. Curr Opin Infect Dis. 2021;34:89. [PMID: 33278180]

5. Other Group A Streptococcal Infections

Arthritis, pneumonia, empyema, endocarditis, and necrotizing fasciitis are relatively uncommon infections that may be caused by group A streptococci. Toxic shock–like syndrome also occurs.

Arthritis generally occurs in association with cellulitis. In addition to intravenous therapy with penicillin G, 2 million units every 4 hours (or cefazolin or vancomycin), frequent percutaneous needle aspiration should be performed to remove joint effusions. Open surgical drainage may be necessary in many cases. Treatment duration is not well studied but is generally 2–4 weeks, with final duration dependent upon clinical improvement and normalization of inflammatory markers (ESR, CRP).

Pneumonia and **empyema** often are characterized by extensive tissue destruction and an aggressive, rapidly progressive clinical course associated with significant morbidity and mortality. High-dose penicillin (4 million units of penicillin G intravenously every 4 hours) and chest tube drainage are indicated for treatment of empyema. Vancomycin is an acceptable substitute in penicillin-allergic patients. Duration of therapy is guided by clinical improvement, with a minimum of 5 days for pneumonia. Adequate drainage is key for the management of empyema and serial imaging is usually necessary to assess for resolution.

Group A streptococci can cause **endocarditis** in rare instances. Endocarditis should be treated with 4 million units of penicillin G intravenously every 4 hours for 4–6 weeks. Vancomycin, 1 g intravenously every 12 hours, is recommended for persons allergic to penicillin.

Any streptococcal infection—and necrotizing fasciitis in particular—can be associated with **streptococcal toxic shock syndrome**, typified by invasion of skin or soft tissues, acute respiratory distress syndrome, and kidney failure. Young persons, older adults, and those with underlying medical conditions are at high risk for invasive disease. Bacteremia occurs in most cases. Skin rash and desquamation may not be present. Mortality rates can be up to 80%. A beta-lactam, such as penicillin, 4 million units intravenously every 4 hours, remains the drug of choice for treatment of serious streptococcal infections, but clindamycin, which is a potent inhibitor of toxin production, should also be administered at a dose of 900 mg every 8 hours intravenously for invasive disease, especially in the presence of shock. Intravenous immune globulin can be considered for streptococcal toxic shock syndrome for possible therapeutic benefit from specific antibody to streptococcal exotoxins in immune globulin preparations. Many dosing regimens have been used, including 0.5 g/kg once daily for 5–6 days or a single dose of 2 g/kg with a repeat dose at 48 hours if the patient remains unstable.

Baddour LM et al. Infective endocarditis in adults: diagnosis, antimicrobial therapy, and management of complications: a scientific statement for healthcare professionals from the American Heart Association. Circulation. 2015;132:1435. [PMID: 26373316]

6. Non–Group A Streptococcal Infections

Non–group A hemolytic streptococci (eg, groups B, C, and G) produce a spectrum of disease similar to that of group A streptococci. The treatment of infections caused by these strains is similar to group A streptococci.

Group B streptococci are an important cause of sepsis, bacteremia, and meningitis in the neonate. Antepartum screening to identify carriers and peripartum antimicrobial prophylaxis are recommended in pregnancy. This organism, part of the normal vaginal flora, may cause septic abortion, endometritis, or peripartum infections and, less commonly, cellulitis, bacteremia, and endocarditis in adults. Treatment of infections caused by group B streptococci is with either penicillin or vancomycin in doses recommended for treatment of group A streptococci skin and soft tissue infections (Table 33–1). Because of in vitro synergism, some experts recommend the addition of low-dose gentamicin, 1 mg/kg every 8 hours, for any serious group B *Streptococcus* infection.

Viridans streptococci, which are nonhemolytic or alpha-hemolytic (ie, producing a green zone of hemolysis on blood agar), are part of the normal oral flora. Although these strains may produce focal pyogenic infection, they are most notable as the leading cause of native valve endocarditis.

Group D streptococci include *Streptococcus gallolyticus* (formerly known as *S bovis*) and the enterococci. *S gallolyticus* is a cause of endocarditis in association with bowel neoplasia or cirrhosis and is treated like viridans streptococci.

ENTEROCOCCAL INFECTIONS

Two species, *Enterococcus faecalis* and *Enterococcus faecium*, are responsible for most human enterococcal infections. Enterococci cause wound infections, UTIs, bacteremia, and endocarditis. Infections caused by penicillin-susceptible strains should be treated with ampicillin 2 g every 4 hours or penicillin 3–4 million units every 4 hours; if the patient is penicillin-allergic, vancomycin 15 mg/kg every 12 hours intravenously can be given. If the patient has endocarditis or meningitis, gentamicin 1 mg/kg every 8 hours intravenously should be added to the regimen for a duration of 2–3 weeks in order to achieve bactericidal activity. In cases of endocarditis, ceftriaxone 2 g every 12 hours may be given instead of gentamicin in combination with the ampicillin, for a duration of 6 weeks.

Resistance to vancomycin, penicillin, and gentamicin is common among enterococcal isolates, especially *E faecium;* it is essential to determine antimicrobial susceptibility of isolates. Infection control measures that may be indicated to limit their spread include isolation, barrier precautions, and avoidance of overuse of vancomycin and gentamicin. Consultation with an infectious disease specialist is strongly advised when treating infections caused by resistant strains of enterococci. Quinupristin/dalfopristin and linezolid are approved by the FDA for treatment of infections caused by vancomycin-resistant strains of enterococci. Daptomycin, tigecycline, tedizolid, and oritavancin are not specifically approved for the treatment for vancomycin-resistant strains of enterococci, although they are frequently active in vitro.

Quinupristin/dalfopristin is not active against strains of *E faecalis* and should be used only for infections caused by *E faecium*. The dose is 7.5 mg/kg intravenously every 8–12 hours. Phlebitis and irritation at the infusion site (often requiring a central line) and an arthralgia-myalgia syndrome are relatively common side effects. Linezolid is active against both *E faecalis* and *E faecium*. The dose is 600 mg twice daily, and both intravenous and oral preparations are available. Its two principal side effects are thrombocytopenia and bone marrow suppression; however, peripheral neuropathy, optic neuritis, and lactic acidosis have been observed with prolonged use (typically greater than 6 weeks) due to mitochondrial toxicity. Emergence of resistance has occurred during therapy with both quinupristin/dalfopristin and linezolid.

Rosselli Del Turco E et al. How do I manage a patient with enterococcal bacteraemia? Clin Microbiol Infect. 2021;27:364. [PMID: 33152537]

PNEUMOCOCCAL INFECTIONS

1. Pneumococcal Pneumonia

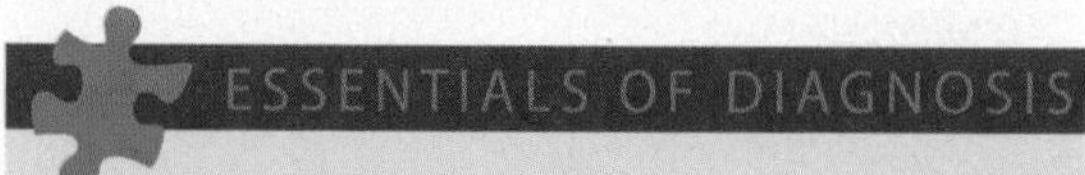

ESSENTIALS OF DIAGNOSIS

- Productive cough, fever, rigors, dyspnea, early pleuritic chest pain.
- Consolidating lobar pneumonia on chest radiograph.
- Gram-positive diplococci on Gram stain of sputum.

General Considerations

Pneumococcus is the most common cause of community-acquired pyogenic bacterial pneumonia. Alcohol use disorder, asthma, HIV infection, sickle cell disease, splenectomy, and hematologic disorders are predisposing factors. Mortality rates remain high in cases of advanced age, multilobar disease, hypoxemia, extrapulmonary complications, and bacteremia.

Clinical Findings

A. Symptoms and Signs

Presenting symptoms and signs include high fever, productive cough, occasional hemoptysis, and pleuritic chest pain. Rigors may occur initially but are uncommon later in the course. Bronchial breath sounds are an early sign.

B. Laboratory Findings

There is often leukocytosis, or occasionally leukopenia, but neither finding should be used to make a decision about hospital admission (see When to Admit, below).

Diagnosis requires isolation of the organism in culture, although the Gram stain of sputum can be suggestive. Sputum and blood cultures, positive in 60% and 25% of cases of pneumococcal pneumonia, respectively, should be obtained prior to initiation of antimicrobial therapy in patients who are admitted to the hospital. A good-quality sputum sample (less than 10 epithelial cells and greater than 25 polymorphonuclear leukocytes per high-power field) shows gram-positive diplococci in 80–90% of cases. A rapid urinary antigen test for *Streptococcus pneumoniae*, with sensitivity of 70–80% and specificity greater than 95%, can assist with early diagnosis. The use of procalcitonin to guide therapy is discussed below.

C. Imaging

Pneumococcal pneumonia classically is a lobar pneumonia with radiographic findings of consolidation and occasionally effusion. Differentiating it from other pneumonias is not possible radiographically or clinically because of significant overlap in presentations.

Complications

Parapneumonic (sympathetic) effusion is common and may cause recurrence or persistence of fever. These sterile fluid accumulations need no specific therapy. Empyema occurs in 5% or less of cases and is differentiated from sympathetic effusion clinically and by the presence of organisms on Gram-stained fluid or positive pleural fluid cultures.

Pneumococcal pericarditis is a rare complication that can cause tamponade. Pneumococcal arthritis also is uncommon. Pneumococcal endocarditis usually involves the aortic valve and often occurs in association with meningitis and pneumonia (sometimes referred to as Austrian or Osler triad). Early heart failure and multiple embolic events are typical.

Treatment

A. Specific Measures

Initial antimicrobial therapy for pneumonia is empiric (see Table 9–9) pending isolation and identification of the causative agent. Once *S pneumoniae* is identified as the infecting pathogen, any of several antimicrobial agents may be used depending on the clinical setting, community patterns of penicillin resistance, and susceptibility of the particular isolate.

1. Outpatient therapy—Uncomplicated pneumococcal pneumonia (ie, arterial Po_2 greater than 60 mm Hg, no coexisting medical problems, and single-lobe disease without signs of extrapulmonary infection) caused by penicillin-susceptible strains of pneumococcus may be treated on an outpatient basis with amoxicillin, 750 mg orally twice daily for 7–10 days. Cephalosporins including cefpodoxime, 200 mg orally twice daily, and cefdinir, 300 mg twice daily, may also be used. For penicillin-allergic patients, alternatives are azithromycin, one 500-mg dose orally on the first day and 250 mg for the next 4 days; clarithromycin, 500 mg orally twice daily for 7 days; doxycycline, 100 mg orally twice daily for 7 days; levofloxacin, 750 mg orally for 5–7 days; or moxifloxacin, 400 mg orally for 7–14 days. Patients should be monitored for clinical response (eg, less cough, defervescence within 2–3 days) because pneumococci have become increasingly resistant to penicillin and the second-line agents.

Outpatients with high-risk comorbid conditions (such as pulmonary disease, diabetes, cardiac disease, or alcohol use disorder) may benefit from broader combination therapy (eg, amoxicillin/clavulanate or cephalosporin *plus* doxycycline or a macrolide), unless a fluoroquinolone (eg, levofloxacin or moxifloxacin) is chosen for monotherapy.

2. Inpatient therapy—Parenteral therapy is generally recommended for the hospitalized patient at least until there has been clinical improvement. Ceftriaxone, 1–2 g intravenously every 24 hours, is effective for strains that are penicillin-susceptible (ie, strains for which the minimum inhibitory concentration [MIC] of penicillin is 2 mcg/mL or less for non-CNS specimens). For serious penicillin allergy or infection caused by a highly penicillin-resistant strain, vancomycin, 1 g intravenously every 12 hours, is effective. Additionally, azithromycin (500 mg orally on the first day and 250 mg for the next 4 days) or doxycycline (100 mg orally twice daily) is typically added for coverage of atypical organisms. Alternatively, a respiratory fluoroquinolone (eg, levofloxacin, 750 mg) can be used. The total duration of therapy is not well defined but 5–7 days is appropriate for patients who have an uncomplicated infection and demonstrate a good clinical response. Corticosteroid use remains controversial in community-acquired pneumonia and should not be administered routinely.

Procalcitonin is a peptide released by human cells in response to exposure to bacterial toxins and is measurable in the serum. In trials, antibiotics have been safely held or withdrawn when the procalcitonin level was normal or decreasing by a substantial amount. Antibiotic consumption is significantly reduced in patients presenting with acute respiratory infections and sepsis when guided by procalcitonin levels; procalcitonin can be used effectively in these settings only when used as a point of care test.

B. Treatment of Complications

Pleural effusions developing after initiation of antimicrobial therapy usually are sterile, and thoracentesis need not be performed if the patient is otherwise improving. Thoracentesis is indicated for an effusion present prior to initiation of therapy and in the patient who has not responded to antibiotics after 3–4 days. Chest tube drainage may be required if pneumococci are identified by culture or Gram stain, especially if aspiration of the fluid is difficult.

Echocardiography should be done if pericardial effusion is suspected. Patients with pericardial effusion who are responding to antibiotic therapy and have no signs of tamponade may be monitored and treated with indomethacin, 50 mg orally three times daily, for pain. In patients with increasing effusion, unsatisfactory clinical response, or evidence of tamponade, pericardiocentesis will determine whether the pericardial space is infected. Infected fluid must be drained either percutaneously (by tube placement or needle aspiration), by placement of a pericardial window, or by pericardiectomy. Pericardiectomy eventually may be required to prevent or treat constrictive pericarditis.

Endocarditis should be treated for 4 weeks with 3–4 million units of penicillin G every 4 hours intravenously; ceftriaxone, 2 g once daily intravenously; or vancomycin, 15 mg/kg every 12 hours intravenously. Mild heart failure due to valvular regurgitation may respond to medical therapy, but moderate to severe heart failure is an indication for prosthetic valve implantation, as are systemic emboli or large friable vegetations as determined by echocardiography.

C. Penicillin-Resistant Pneumococci

Resistance breakpoints for parenterally administered penicillin (1–2 million units every 6 hours) and high-dose oral amoxicillin (2 g twice daily) are as follows: susceptible, penicillin MIC of 2 mcg/mL or less; intermediate, MIC of 4 mcg/mL; resistant, MIC of 8 mcg/mL or more. Note, however, that these breakpoints do not apply to orally administered penicillin, which are the same as for use of penicillin in treatment of meningitis. In cases of pneumococcal pneumonia where the isolate has a penicillin MIC greater than 2 mcg/mL, cephalosporin cross-resistance is common, and a non–beta-lactam antimicrobial, such as vancomycin, 1 g intravenously every 12 hours, or a fluoroquinolone with enhanced gram-positive activity (eg, levofloxacin, 750 mg intravenously or orally once daily, or moxifloxacin, 400 mg intravenously or orally once daily), is recommended. Penicillin-resistant strains of pneumococci may be resistant to macrolides, trimethoprim-sulfamethoxazole, and chloramphenicol, and susceptibility must be documented prior to their use. All blood and cerebrospinal fluid isolates should still be tested for resistance to penicillin.

Prevention

See Chapter 30 for discussion of pneumococcal vaccines. All patients should have screening for smoking cessation.

When to Refer

- Extensive disease.
- Seriously ill patient with pneumonia, particularly in the setting of comorbid conditions (eg, liver disease).
- Progression of pneumonia or failure to improve on antibiotics.
- All patients with suspected pneumococcal endocarditis or meningitis need infectious disease specialist consultation.

When to Admit

- Failure of outpatient pneumonia therapy, including inability to maintain oral intake and medications.
- All patients with pneumococcal pneumonia that is multilobar or is associated with significant hypoxemia.
- Exacerbations of underlying disease (eg, heart failure) by pneumonia that would benefit from hospitalization.
- Risk scores for illness severity using PSI (Pneumonia Severity Index) (https://www.thecalculator.co/health/Pneumonia-Severity-Index-(PSI)-Calculator-977.html) and CURB-65 (Confusion, Urea, Respiratory rate, Blood Pressure, Age ≥ 65 years) (https://www.mdcalc.com/curb-65-score-pneumonia-severity) can aid in the decision about whether to admit a patient.
- All patients in whom pneumococcal endocarditis or meningitis is suspected or documented should be admitted for observation and empiric therapy.

Suaya JA et al. Identification of *Streptococcus pneumoniae* in hospital-acquired pneumonia in adults. J Hosp Infect. 2021;108:146. [PMID: 33176175]

Wunderink RG et al. Advances in the causes and management of community acquired pneumonia in adults. BMJ. 2017;358:j2471. [PMID: 28694251]

2. Pneumococcal Meningitis

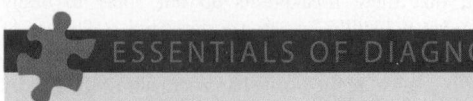

- Fever, headache, altered mental status.
- Meningismus.
- Gram-positive diplococci on Gram stain of cerebrospinal fluid.

General Considerations

S pneumoniae is the most common cause of bacterial meningitis in adults. Head trauma with cerebrospinal fluid leaks, sinusitis, and pneumonia may precede it.

Clinical Findings

A. Symptoms and Signs

The onset is rapid, with fever, headache, meningismus, and altered mentation. Pneumonia may be present. Compared with meningitis caused by the meningococcus, pneumococcal meningitis lacks a rash. Obtundation, focal neurologic deficits, and cranial nerve palsies are more prominent features and may lead to long-term sequelae.

B. Laboratory Findings

The cerebrospinal fluid has WBC count typically greater than 1000/mcL (1.0×10^9/L), over 60% of which are polymorphonuclear leukocytes; the glucose concentration is less than 40 mg/dL (2.22 mmol/L), or less than 50% of the simultaneous serum concentration; and the protein usually exceeds 150 mg/dL (1500 mg/L). Not all cases of meningitis will have these typical findings, and alterations in cerebrospinal fluid analysis may be surprisingly minimal, overlapping with those of aseptic meningitis.

Gram stain of cerebrospinal fluid shows gram-positive cocci in 80–90% of cases, and in untreated cases, blood or cerebrospinal fluid cultures are almost always positive. Urine antigen tests may be positive but are not sufficiently sensitive to exclude the diagnosis.

Treatment

Antibiotics should be given as soon as the diagnosis is suspected. If lumbar puncture must be delayed (eg, while awaiting results of an imaging study to exclude a mass lesion), the patient should be treated empirically with intravenous ceftriaxone, 2 g, plus vancomycin, 15 mg/kg, plus dexamethasone, 0.15 mg/kg administered concomitantly after blood cultures (positive in 50% of cases) have been obtained. Once susceptibility to penicillin has been confirmed, penicillin, 24 million units intravenously daily in six divided doses, or ceftriaxone, 2 g every 12 hours intravenously, is continued for 10–14 days in documented cases.

The best therapy for penicillin-resistant strains is not known. Penicillin-resistant strains (MIC greater than 0.06 mcg/mL) are often cross-resistant to the third-generation cephalosporins as well as other antibiotics. Susceptibility testing is essential for proper management of this infection. If the MIC of ceftriaxone or cefotaxime is 0.5 mcg/mL or less, single-drug therapy with either of these cephalosporins is likely to be effective; when the MIC is 1 mcg/mL or more, treatment with a combination of ceftriaxone, 2 g intravenously every 12 hours, plus vancomycin, 30 mg/kg/day intravenously in two or three divided doses, is recommended. If a patient with a penicillin-resistant organism is slow to respond clinically, repeat lumbar puncture may be indicated to assess bacteriologic response.

Dexamethasone administered with antibiotic to adults has been associated with a 60% reduction in mortality and a 50% reduction in unfavorable outcomes. It is recommended that dexamethasone be given immediately prior to or concomitantly with the first dose of appropriate antibiotic and continued in those with pneumococcal disease every 6 hours thereafter for a total of 4 days. The effect of dexamethasone on outcome of meningitis caused by penicillin-resistant organisms is not known.

Mora Carpio AL et al. Pneumococcal bacteremia and meningitis. N Engl J Med. 2018;379:2063. [PMID: 30462944]

Tansarli GS et al. Diagnostic test accuracy of the BioFire® FilmArray® meningitis/encephalitis panel: a systematic review and meta-analysis. Clin Microbiol Infect. 2020;26:281. [PMID: 31760115]

STAPHYLOCOCCUS AUREUS INFECTIONS

1. Skin & Soft Tissue Infections

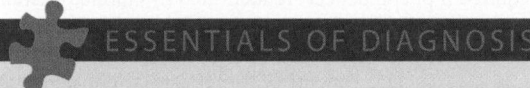

- Localized erythema with induration and purulent drainage.
- Abscess formation.
- Folliculitis commonly observed.
- Gram stain of pus shows gram-positive cocci in clusters; cultures usually positive.

General Considerations

About one-quarter of people are asymptomatic nasal carriers of *S aureus*, which is spread by direct contact. Carriage often precedes infection, which occurs as a consequence of disruption of the cutaneous barrier or impairment of host defenses. *S aureus* tends to cause more purulent skin infections than streptococci; abscess formation is common. The prevalence of methicillin-resistant strains in many communities is high and should influence antibiotic choices when antimicrobial therapy is needed.

Clinical Findings

A. Symptoms and Signs

S aureus skin infections may begin around one or more hair follicles, causing folliculitis; may become localized to form boils (or furuncles); or may spread to adjacent skin

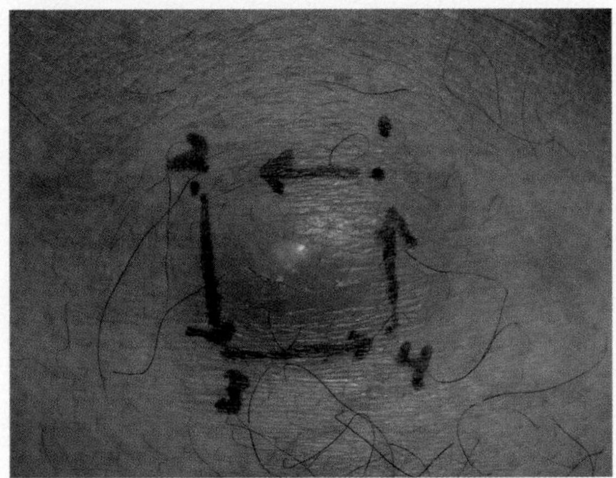

▲ **Figure 33–2.** Methicillin-resistant *Staphylococcus aureus* (MRSA) abscess on the back of the neck. (Reproduced with permission from Richard P. Usatine, MD, in Usatine RP, Smith MA, Mayeaux EJ Jr, Chumley HS. *The Color Atlas and Synopsis of Family Medicine*, 3rd ed. McGraw-Hill, 2019.)

and deeper subcutaneous tissue (ie, a carbuncle). Deep abscesses involving muscle or fascia may occur, often in association with a deep wound or other inoculation or injection (Figure 33–2). Necrotizing fasciitis, a rare form of *S aureus* skin and soft tissues infection, has been reported with community strains of methicillin-resistant *S aureus*.

B. Laboratory Findings

Cultures of the wound or abscess material will almost always yield the organism. In patients with systemic signs of infection, blood cultures should be obtained because of potential bacteremia, endocarditis, osteomyelitis, or metastatic seeding of other sites. Patients who are bacteremic should have blood cultures repeated every 24–28 hours during therapy to exclude persistent bacteremia, an indicator of severe or complicated infection.

▶ Treatment

Proper drainage of abscess fluid or other focal infections is the mainstay of therapy. Incision and drainage alone is highly effective for the treatment of most uncomplicated cutaneous abscesses. A small benefit can be obtained from the addition of antimicrobials following incision and drainage (Table 33–1). In areas where methicillin resistance among community *S aureus* isolates is high, recommended oral antimicrobial agents include clindamycin, trimethoprim-sulfamethoxazole, doxycycline, or minocycline. When the risk of methicillin resistance is low or methicillin susceptibility has been confirmed by testing of the isolate, consider dicloxacillin or cephalexin. Treatment for 5–7 days is sufficient in most cases.

For complicated infections with extensive cutaneous or deep tissue involvement or fever, initial parenteral therapy is often indicated. When methicillin resistance rates are high (above 10%), empiric therapy with vancomycin is a drug of choice. For infections caused by methicillin-susceptible isolates, cefazolin intravenously or intramuscularly or a penicillinase-resistant penicillin such as nafcillin or oxacillin in a dosage of 1.5 g every 6 hours intravenously is preferred. Total duration of therapy for soft tissue infections depends on clinical response and effectiveness of drainage/debridement. Courses of 7 days with early transition to oral therapy are effective in many cases.

Linezolid is FDA-approved for treatment of skin and skin-structure infections as well as hospital-acquired pneumonia caused by methicillin-resistant strains of *S aureus*; it is clinically as effective as vancomycin for these indications. Its considerable cost makes it an unattractive choice for most routine outpatient infections, and its safety in treatment courses lasting longer than 2–3 weeks is not well characterized. Other drugs that are FDA-approved for treating skin and soft tissue infections are listed in Table 33–1. Telavancin is approved for the treatment of hospital-acquired *S aureus* pneumonia but has been associated with nephrotoxicity.

Lin HS et al. Interventions for bacterial folliculitis and boils (furuncles and carbuncles). Cochrane Database Syst Rev. 2021;2:CD013099. [PMID: 33634465]

2. Osteomyelitis

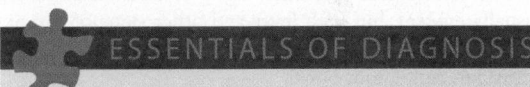

- ▶ Fever associated with pain and tenderness of involved bone.
- ▶ Microbiologic diagnosis often made from blood cultures.
- ▶ Elevated ESR and CRP.
- ▶ Radiographs early in the course are typically negative.

▶ General Considerations

S aureus causes approximately 60% of all cases of osteomyelitis. Osteomyelitis may be caused by (1) hematogenous spread, (2) extension from a contiguous focus of infection or open wound (eg, Open fracture or as a result of surgery), and (3) skin breakdown in the setting of vascular insufficiency. Long bones and vertebrae are the usual sites. Epidural abscess is a common complication of vertebral osteomyelitis and should be suspected if fever and severe back or neck pain are accompanied by radicular pain or symptoms or signs indicative of spinal cord compression (eg, incontinence, extremity weakness, pathologic extremity reflexes).

▶ Clinical Findings

A. Symptoms and Signs

1. Hematogenous osteomyelitis—Osteomyelitis resulting from bacteremia is a disease associated with sickle cell disease, injection drug use, diabetes mellitus, or older adults. Patients with this form of osteomyelitis often present with sudden onset of high fever, chills, and pain and tenderness of the involved bone. The site of osteomyelitis and the causative organism depend on the host. Osteomyelitis in injection drug users develops most commonly in the spine. Although in this setting *S aureus* is most common, gram-negative infections, especially *P aeruginosa* and *Serratia* species, are also frequent pathogens. Among patients with hemoglobinopathies such as sickle cell anemia, osteomyelitis is caused most often by salmonellae; *S aureus* is the second most common cause. Rapid progression to epidural abscess causing fever, pain, and sensory and motor loss is not uncommon. In older patients with hematogenous osteomyelitis, the most common sites are the thoracic and lumbar vertebral bodies. Risk factors for these patients include diabetes, intravenous catheters, and indwelling urinary catheters. These patients often have more subtle presentations, with low-grade fever and gradually increasing bone pain.

2. Osteomyelitis from a contiguous focus of infection— Prosthetic joint replacement or other orthopedic surgery, neurosurgery, and trauma most frequently cause soft tissue infections that can spread to bone. *S aureus* and *Staphylococcus epidermidis* are the most common organisms. Polymicrobial infections, rare in hematogenously spread osteomyelitis, are more common in osteomyelitis due to contiguous spread. Localized signs of inflammation are usually evident, but high fever and other signs of toxicity are usually absent. Septic arthritis and cellulitis can also spread to contiguous bone.

3. Osteomyelitis associated with vascular insufficiency— Patients with diabetes mellitus and vascular insufficiency are susceptible to developing a very challenging form of osteomyelitis. The foot and ankle are commonly affected sites, as well as the hip and sacrum due to pressure injury (formerly called pressure ulcer). Infection originates from an ulcer or other break in the skin that is usually still present but may appear disarmingly unimpressive. Polymicrobial infections are common due to contiguous spread, often involving aerobic gram-negative bacilli and anaerobes. Occasionally, *S aureus* may be found as a single pathogen. Bone pain is often absent or muted by the associated neuropathy. Fever is also commonly absent. Two of the best bedside clues to the presence of osteomyelitis are the ability to easily advance a sterile probe to bone through a skin ulcer and an ulcer area larger than 2 cm^2.

B. Laboratory Findings

The diagnosis is made by isolation of *S aureus* (or another organism) from the blood, bone, or a contiguous focus of a patient with symptoms and signs of focal bone infection. Blood culture will be positive in approximately 60% of untreated cases. The ESR and serum CRP are almost always elevated and can be useful parameters to follow during the course of therapy. Bone biopsy and culture are indicated if blood cultures are sterile. Cultures from overlying ulcers, wounds, or fistulas are unreliable as they will contain skin flora.

C. Imaging

Plain bone films early in the course of infection are often normal but will become abnormal in most cases even with effective therapy. Spinal infection (unlike malignancy) traverses the disk space to involve the contiguous vertebral body. CT is more sensitive than plain bone radiographs and helps localize associated abscesses. Bone scan and gallium scan, each with a sensitivity of approximately 95% and a specificity of 60–70%, are useful in identifying or confirming the site of bone infection. MRI is slightly less sensitive than bone scan but has a specificity of 90%. It is indicated when epidural abscess is suspected in association with vertebral osteomyelitis. ^{18}F-FDG-PET/CT may be useful in the diagnosis of vertebral osteomyelitis as well as the detection of other metastatic sites of infection.

Treatment

Identification of the causative organism and determination of antibiotic susceptibility determines therapy; consultation with an infectious disease specialist is recommended.

Prolonged therapy (4–6 weeks or longer) is recommended for staphylococcal osteomyelitis. Traditionally, intravenous therapy has been preferred, particularly during the acute phase of the infection for patients with systemic toxicity. Intravenous therapy with cefazolin, 2 g every 8 hours, or alternatively, nafcillin or oxacillin, 9–12 g/day in six divided doses, are the drugs of choice for infection with methicillin-sensitive isolates. Patients with infections due to methicillin-resistant strains of *S aureus* or who have severe penicillin allergies should be treated with vancomycin, 30 mg/kg/day intravenously divided in two or three doses. Doses should be adjusted to achieve a vancomycin trough level of 15–20 mcg/mL. Studies have also demonstrated noninferiority of oral regimens following 2 weeks of intravenous therapy. In patients with *S aureus* isolates susceptible to oral agents, combination oral therapy has been shown to be effective if given for 4–6 weeks following 2 weeks of induction therapy with an intravenous agent as above. Levofloxacin, 750 mg orally daily, or ciprofloxacin, 750 mg orally twice daily, in combination with rifampin, 300 mg twice daily, is an oral regimen with the most data supporting efficacy. Trimethoprim-sulfamethoxazole, doxycycline, or clindamycin may be an option for oral therapy.

Surgical treatment is often indicated under the following circumstances: (1) staphylococcal osteomyelitis with associated epidural abscess and spinal cord compression (urgent neurosurgical decompression may be required), (2) other abscesses (psoas, paraspinal), (3) extensive disease, or (4) recurrent or persistent infection despite standard medical therapy. Follow-up imaging may not be needed in patients who demonstrate improvement in symptoms and normalization of inflammatory markers.

Berbari EF et al. 2015 Infectious Diseases Society of America (IDSA) clinical practice guidelines for the diagnosis and treatment of native vertebral osteomyelitis in adults. Clin Infect Dis. 2015;61:e26. [PMID: 26229122]

Li HK et al; OVIVA Trial Collaborators. Oral versus intravenous antibiotics for bone and joint infection. N Engl J Med. 2019;380:425. [PMID: 30699315]

Urish KL et al. Staphylococcus aureus osteomyelitis: bone, bugs, and surgery. Infect Immun. 2020;88:e00932. [PMID: 32094258]

3. Staphylococcal Bacteremia

S aureus readily invades the bloodstream and infects sites distant from the primary site of infection. Whenever *S aureus* is recovered from blood cultures, the possibility of endocarditis, osteomyelitis, or other metastatic deep infection must be considered. Bacteremia that persists for more than 48–96 hours after initiation of therapy is strongly predictive of worse outcome and complicated infection. Given the relatively high risk of infective endocarditis in patients with *S aureus* bacteremia, transesophageal echocardiography is recommended for most patients as a sensitive and cost-effective method for excluding underlying endocarditis. However, transthoracic echocardiography may be sufficient in select patients considered to be at low risk for endocarditis, namely those who meet all the following criteria: (1) no permanent intracardiac device, (2) sterile follow-up blood cultures within 4 days after the initial set, (3) no hemodialysis dependence, (4) nosocomial acquisition of *S aureus* bacteremia, and (5) no clinical signs of infective endocarditis or secondary foci of infection.

Empiric therapy of staphylococcal bacteremia should be with vancomycin, 15–20 mg/kg/dose intravenously every 8–12 hours, or daptomycin, 6 mg/kg/day intravenously, until results of susceptibility tests are known. If the *S aureus* isolate is methicillin-susceptible, treatment should be narrowed to cefazolin, 2 g every 8 hours, or nafcillin or oxacillin, 2 g intravenously every 4 hours. Cefazolin is as effective as nafcillin or oxacillin and has been associated with fewer adverse events during treatment. In patients with methicillin-resistant *S aureus*, treatment should be with vancomycin, 15–20 mg/kg/dose intravenously every 8–12 hours; maintaining a vancomycin trough concentration of 15–20 mcg/mL may improve outcomes and is recommended. Daptomycin 6 mg/kg/day is also an FDA-approved option as long as the patient does not require treatment for concomitant *S aureus* pneumonia. The addition of rifamycins to standard antimicrobial therapy has not been shown to be beneficial in the absence of indwelling prosthetic material and is associated with more adverse events. Duration of therapy for *S aureus* bacteremia is 4–6 weeks of antibiotic therapy but a subset of patients with uncomplicated infection may be able to be treated for 14 days. A patient with uncomplicated bacteremia must meet all the following criteria: (1) infective endocarditis has been excluded, (2) no implanted prostheses are present, (3) follow-up blood cultures drawn 2–4 days after the initial set are sterile, (4) the patient defervesces within 72 hours of initiation of effective antibiotic therapy, and (5) no evidence of metastatic infection is present on examination. When present at the time of diagnosis, central venous catheters should be removed. Vancomycin treatment failures are relatively common, particularly for complicated bacteremia and among infections involving foreign bodies. Improved outcomes have been demonstrated when consultation with an infectious disease specialist is obtained and should be considered in all cases of *S aureus* bacteremia.

Tong SYC et al. Effect of vancomycin or daptomycin with vs without an antistaphylococcal β-lactam on mortality, bacteremia, relapse, or treatment failure in patients with MRSA bacteremia: a randomized clinical trial. JAMA. 2020;323:527. [PMID: 32044943]

4. Toxic Shock Syndrome

S aureus produces toxins that cause three important entities: "scalded skin syndrome" in children, toxic shock syndrome in adults, and enterotoxin food poisoning. Toxic shock syndrome is characterized by abrupt onset of high fever, vomiting, and watery diarrhea. Sore throat, myalgias, and headache are common. Hypotension with kidney and heart failure is associated with a poor outcome. A diffuse macular erythematous rash and nonpurulent conjunctivitis are common, and desquamation, especially of palms and soles, is typical during recovery (Figure 33–3). Fatality rates may be as high as 15%. Although originally associated with tampon use, any focus (eg, nasopharynx, bone, vagina, rectum, abscess, or wound) harboring a toxin-producing *S aureus* strain can cause toxic shock syndrome. Classically, blood cultures are negative because symptoms are due to the effects of the toxin and not systemic infection. Other entities associated with toxic shock include invasive group A streptococcal infection and certain *Clostridium* species (*C perfringens, C sordellii).*

Important aspects of treatment include rapid rehydration, targeted antimicrobials (antistaphylococcal therapy when *S aureus* is implicated) (Table 33–1), management of kidney or heart failure, and addressing sources of toxin, eg, removal of tampon or drainage of abscess. Intravenous clindamycin, 900 mg every 8 hours, is often added to inhibit toxin production. Intravenous immune globulin may be considered, although there are limited data compared with *Streptococcus* toxic shock syndrome (see above).

5. Infections Caused by Coagulase-Negative Staphylococci

Coagulase-negative staphylococci are an important cause of infections of intravascular and prosthetic devices and of wound infection following cardiothoracic surgery.

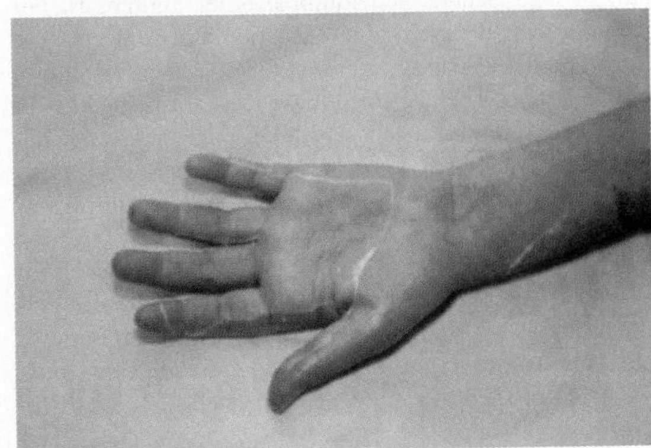

▲ **Figure 33–3.** Marked desquamation due to toxic shock syndrome, which develops late in the disease. (Public Health Image Library, CDC.)

These organisms infrequently cause infections such as osteomyelitis and endocarditis in the absence of a prosthesis. Most human infections are caused by *Staphylococcus epidermidis, S haemolyticus, S hominis, S warnerii, S saprophyticus, S saccharolyticus*, and *S cohnii*. These common hospital-acquired pathogens are less virulent than *S aureus*, and infections caused by them tend to be more indolent.

Because coagulase-negative staphylococci are normal inhabitants of human skin, it is difficult to distinguish infection from contamination, the latter perhaps accounting for three-fourths of blood culture isolates. Infection is more likely if the patient has a foreign body (eg, sternal wires, prosthetic joint, prosthetic cardiac valve, pacemaker, intracranial pressure monitor, cerebrospinal fluid shunt, peritoneal dialysis catheter) or an intravascular device in place. Purulent or serosanguineous drainage, erythema, pain, or tenderness at the site of the foreign body or device suggests infection. Joint instability and pain are signs of prosthetic joint infection. Fever, a new murmur, instability of the prosthesis, and signs of systemic embolization are evidence of prosthetic valve endocarditis.

Infection is also more likely if the same strain is consistently isolated from two or more blood cultures (particularly if samples were obtained at different times) and from the foreign body site. Contamination is more likely when a single blood culture is positive or if more than one strain is isolated from blood cultures. The antimicrobial susceptibility pattern and speciation are used to determine whether one or more strains have been isolated.

Whenever possible, the intravascular device or foreign body suspected of being infected should be removed. However, removal and replacement of some devices (eg, prosthetic joint, prosthetic valve, cerebrospinal fluid shunt) can be a difficult or risky procedure, and it may sometimes be preferable to treat with antibiotics alone, knowing that the probability of cure is reduced and that surgical management may eventually be necessary.

Coagulase-negative staphylococci are commonly resistant to beta-lactams and multiple other antibiotics. For patients with normal kidney function, vancomycin, 1 g intravenously every 12 hours, is the treatment of choice until susceptibility to penicillinase-resistant penicillins or other agents has been confirmed. Duration of therapy has not been established for relatively uncomplicated infections, such as those from intravenous devices, which may be eliminated by simply removing the device. Infection involving bone or a prosthetic valve should be treated for 6 weeks. A combination regimen of vancomycin plus rifampin, 300 mg orally twice daily, plus gentamicin, 1 mg/kg intravenously every 8 hours, is recommended for treatment of prosthetic valve endocarditis caused by methicillin-resistant strains.

Becker K et al. Emergence of coagulase-negative staphylococci. Expert Rev Anti Infect Ther. 2020;18:349. [PMID: 32056452]

CLOSTRIDIAL DISEASES

1. Clostridial Myonecrosis (Gas Gangrene)

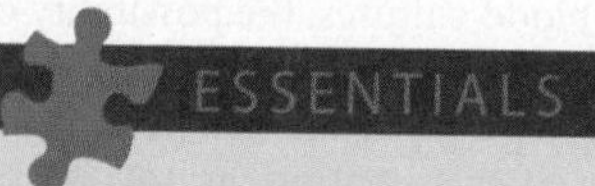

ESSENTIALS OF DIAGNOSIS

- Sudden onset of pain and edema in and around a contaminated wound.
- Prostration and systemic toxicity.
- Brown to blood-tinged watery exudate, with skin discoloration of surrounding area.
- Gas in the tissue by palpation or radiograph.
- Gram-positive rods in culture or smear of exudate.

General Considerations

Gas gangrene or clostridial myonecrosis is a life-threatening muscle infection produced by any one of several clostridia (*Clostridium perfringens, C ramosum, C bifermentans, C histolyticum, C novyi*, etc). Trauma and injection drug use are common predisposing conditions. Toxins produced in devitalized tissues under anaerobic conditions result in shock, hemolysis, and myonecrosis.

Clinical Findings

A. Symptoms and Signs

The onset is usually sudden, with rapidly increasing pain in the affected area, hypotension, and tachycardia. Fever is present but is not proportionate to the severity of the infection. In the last stages of the disease, severe prostration, stupor, delirium, and coma occur.

The wound becomes swollen, and the surrounding skin is pale. There is a foul-smelling brown, blood-tinged serous discharge. As the disease advances, the surrounding tissue changes from pale to dusky and finally becomes deeply discolored, with coalescent, red, fluid-filled vesicles. Gas may be palpable in the tissues.

B. Laboratory Findings

Gas gangrene is a clinical diagnosis, and empiric therapy is indicated if the diagnosis is suspected. Radiographic studies may show gas within the soft tissues, but this finding is not sensitive or specific. The smear shows absence of neutrophils and the presence of gram-positive rods. Anaerobic culture confirms the diagnosis.

Differential Diagnosis

Other bacteria can produce gas in infected tissue, eg, enteric gram-negative organisms, or anaerobes.

Treatment

Adequate surgical debridement and exposure of infected areas are essential, with radical surgical excision often necessary. Penicillin, 2 million units every 3 hours intravenously, is an effective adjunct. Clindamycin may decrease the production of bacterial toxin, and some experts recommend the addition of clindamycin, 600–900 mg every 8 hours intravenously, to penicillin. Hyperbaric oxygen therapy has been used empirically but must be used in conjunction with administration of an appropriate antibiotic and surgical debridement.

Peetermans M et al. Necrotizing skin and soft-tissue infections in the intensive care unit. Clin Microbiol Infect. 2020;26:8. [PMID: 31284035]

Stevens DL et al. Practice guidelines for the diagnosis and management of skin and soft tissue infections: 2014 update by the Infectious Diseases Society of America. Clin Infect Dis. 2014;59:147. [PMID: 24947530]

Yang Z et al. Interventions for treating gas gangrene. Cochrane Database Syst Rev. 2015;12:CD010577. [PMID: 26631369]

2. Tetanus

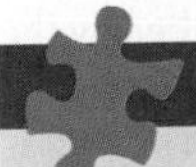

ESSENTIALS OF DIAGNOSIS

- History of wound and possible contamination.
- Jaw muscle stiffness ("lock jaw"), then spasms (trismus).
- Neck stiffness, dysphagia, irritability, hyperreflexia.
- Finally, painful convulsions precipitated by minimal stimuli.

General Considerations

Tetanus is caused by the neurotoxin tetanospasmin, elaborated by *C tetani*. Spores of this organism are ubiquitous in soil and may germinate when introduced into a wound. Tetanospasmin interferes with neurotransmission at spinal synapses of inhibitory neurons. As a result, minor stimuli result in uncontrolled spasms, and reflexes are exaggerated. The incubation period is 5 days to 15 weeks, with the average being 8–12 days.

Most cases occur in unvaccinated individuals. Persons at risk are older adults, migrant workers, newborns, and injection drug users. While puncture wounds are prone to causing tetanus, any wound, including bites or decubiti, may become infected by *C tetani*.

Clinical Findings

A. Symptoms and Signs

The first symptom may be pain and tingling at the site of inoculation, followed by spasticity of the muscles nearby. Stiffness of the jaw, neck stiffness, dysphagia, and irritability are other early signs. Hyperreflexia develops later, with spasms of the jaw muscles (trismus) or facial muscles and rigidity and spasm of the muscles of the abdomen, neck, and back. Painful tonic convulsions precipitated by minor stimuli are common. Spasms of the glottis and respiratory muscles may cause acute asphyxia. The patient is awake and alert throughout the illness. The sensory examination is normal. The temperature is normal or only slightly elevated.

B. Laboratory Findings

The diagnosis of tetanus is made clinically.

Differential Diagnosis

Tetanus must be differentiated from various acute CNS infections such as meningitis. Trismus may occasionally develop with the use of phenothiazines. Strychnine poisoning should also be considered.

Complications

Airway obstruction is common. Urinary retention and constipation may result from spasm of the sphincters. Respiratory arrest and cardiac failure are late events.

Prevention

Active immunization prevents tetanus (see Table 30–7). For primary immunization of adults, Td (tetanus and diphtheria toxoids vaccine) is administered as two doses 4–6 weeks apart, with a third dose 6–12 months later. For one of the three doses, Tdap (tetanus toxoid, reduced-dose diphtheria toxoid, acellular pertussis vaccine) should be substituted for Td. Booster Td doses are given every 10 years or at the time of major injury if it occurs more than 5 years after a dose; a single dose of Tdap is preferred to Td for wound management if the patient has not been previously vaccinated with Tdap. Women should receive Tdap with each pregnancy, preferably between 27 and 36 weeks, with immunization at 27–30 weeks associated with the highest antibody concentrations.

Passive immunization with tetanus immune globulin, 250 units intramuscularly, should be used in nonimmunized individuals and those whose immunization status is uncertain whenever a wound is contaminated or likely to have devitalized tissue. Active immunization with tetanus toxoid vaccine is started concurrently. Table 33–2 provides a guide to prophylactic management.

Treatment

A. Specific Measures

Human tetanus immune globulin, 500 units, should be administered intramuscularly within the first 24 hours of presentation. Whether intrathecal administration has any additional benefit is controversial. An unblinded, randomized trial comparing intramuscular tetanus immune globulin to intramuscular plus intrathecal tetanus immune globulin found clinical benefit in the intrathecal group. However, the exact immune globulin preparation was not specified and the total dose was 4000 units. Tetanus does not produce natural immunity, and a full course of immunization with tetanus toxoid should be administered once the patient has recovered.

B. General Measures

Debridement of wounds should be undertaken if implicated as the source. Metronidazole, 7.5 mg/kg

Table 33–2. Guide to tetanus prophylaxis in wound management.

History of Absorbed Tetanus Toxoid	Clean, Minor Wounds		All Other Wounds[1]	
	Tdap or Td[2]	TIG[3]	Tdap or Td[2]	TIG[3]
Unknown or < 3 doses	Yes	No	Yes	Yes
3 or more doses	No[4]	No	No[5]	No

[1]Examples include wounds contaminated with dirt, feces, soil, or saliva; puncture wounds; avulsions; and wounds from missiles, crushing, burns, and frostbite.
[2]Td indicates tetanus toxoid and diphtheria toxoid vaccine, adult form. Tdap indicates tetanus toxoid, reduced diphtheria toxoid, and acellular pertussis vaccine, which may be substituted as a single dose for Td. Unvaccinated individuals should receive a complete series of three doses, one of which is Tdap.
[3]Human tetanus immune globulin, 250 units intramuscularly.
[4]Yes if more than 10 years have elapsed since last dose.
[5]Yes if more than 5 years have elapsed since last dose. (More frequent boosters are not needed and can enhance side effects.) Tdap has been safely administered within 2 years of Td vaccination, although local reactions to the vaccine may be increased.

administered intravenously or orally every 6 hours (maximum 4 g daily), is preferred and should be administered to all patients. Penicillin, 20 million units intravenously daily in divided doses, is an alternative. Minimal stimuli can provoke spasms, so the patient should be placed at bed rest and monitored under the quietest conditions possible. Sedation, paralysis with curare-like agents, and mechanical ventilation are often necessary. Enteral nutritional support should be given early.

▶ Prognosis

High mortality rates are associated with a short incubation period, early onset of convulsions, and delay in treatment. Contaminated lesions about the head and face are more dangerous than wounds elsewhere.

Pfausler B et al. Toxin-associated infectious diseases: tetanus, botulism and diphtheria. Curr Opin Neurol. 2021;34:432. [PMID: 33840775]

3. Botulism

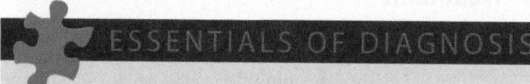

- Recent ingestion of home-canned or smoked foods; recovery of toxin in serum or food.
- Injection drug use.
- Diplopia, dry mouth, dysphagia, dysphonia; muscle weakness leading to respiratory paralysis; normal sensory examination.
- Pupils are fixed and dilated in most cases.

▶ General Considerations

Botulism is a paralytic disease caused by botulinum toxin, which is produced by *Clostridium botulinum*, a ubiquitous, strictly anaerobic, spore-forming bacillus found in soil. Four toxin types—A, B, E, and F—cause human disease. Botulinum toxin is extremely potent and is classified by the CDC as a high-priority agent because of its potential for use as an agent of bioterrorism. Naturally occurring botulism exists in three forms: food-borne botulism, infant botulism, or wound botulism. Food-borne botulism is caused by ingestion of preformed toxin present in canned, smoked, or vacuum-packed foods such as home-canned vegetables, smoked meats, and vacuum-packed fish. Commercial foods have been associated with outbreaks of botulism. Infant botulism (associated with ingestion of honey) and wound botulism (often occurs in association with injection drug use) result from organisms present in the gut or wound that secrete toxin.

▶ Clinical Findings

A. Symptoms and Signs

Twelve to 36 hours after ingestion of the toxin, visual disturbances appear, particularly diplopia and loss of accommodation. Ptosis, cranial nerve palsies with impairment of extraocular muscles, and fixed dilated pupils are characteristic signs. The sensory examination is normal. Other symptoms are dry mouth, dysphagia, and dysphonia. Nausea and vomiting may be present, particularly with type E toxin. The sensorium remains clear and the temperature normal. Paralysis progressing to respiratory failure and death may occur unless mechanical assistance is provided.

B. Laboratory Findings

Toxin in foods and patients' serum can be demonstrated by mouse inoculation and identified with specific antiserum.

▶ Differential Diagnosis

Because the clinical presentation of botulism is so distinctive and the differential diagnosis limited, botulism once considered is not easily confused with other diseases. Cranial nerve involvement may be seen with vertebrobasilar insufficiency, the C. Miller Fisher variant of Guillain-Barré syndrome, myasthenia gravis, or any basilar meningitis (infectious or carcinomatous).

Treatment

If botulism is suspected, the clinician should contact state health authorities or the CDC for advice and help with procurement of equine serum heptavalent botulism antitoxin and for assistance in obtaining assays for toxin in serum, stool, or food. Skin testing is recommended to exclude hypersensitivity to the antitoxin preparation. Antitoxin should be administered as early as possible, ideally within 24 hours of the onset of symptoms, to arrest progression of disease; its administration should not be delayed for laboratory confirmation of the diagnosis. Respiratory failure is managed with intubation and mechanical ventilation. Parenteral fluids or alimentation should be given while swallowing difficulty persists. The removal of unabsorbed toxin from the gut may be attempted. Remnants of suspected foods should be assayed for toxin. Persons who might have eaten the suspected food must be located and observed.

Pfausler B et al. Toxin-associated infectious diseases: tetanus, botulism and diphtheria. Curr Opin Neurol. 2021;34:432. [PMID: 33840775]

LISTERIOSIS

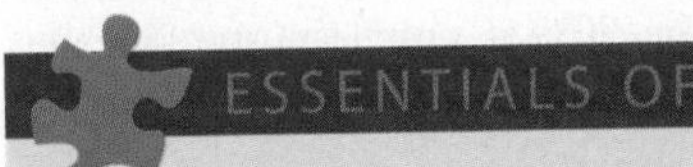

ESSENTIALS OF DIAGNOSIS

- Ingestion of contaminated food product.
- Fever in a pregnant woman in her third trimester.
- Altered mental status and fever in an older or immunocompromised patient.
- Blood and cerebrospinal fluid cultures confirm the diagnosis.

General Considerations

Listeria monocytogenes is a facultative, motile, gram-positive rod. Most cases of infection caused by *L monocytogenes* are sporadic, but outbreaks have been traced to eating contaminated food, including unpasteurized dairy products, hot dogs, delicatessen meats, cantaloupes, and ricotta cheese. Outbreaks have been associated with significant morbidity and mortality in infected persons.

Clinical Findings

Five types of infection are recognized:

1. **Infection during pregnancy**, usually in the last trimester, is a mild febrile illness without an apparent primary focus and may resolve without specific therapy. However, approximately one in five pregnancies complicated by listeriosis result in spontaneous abortion or stillbirth and surviving infants are at risk for clinical neonatal listeriosis.
2. **Granulomatosis infantisepticum** is a neonatal infection acquired in utero, characterized by disseminated abscesses, granulomas, and a high mortality rate.
3. **Bacteremia** with or without sepsis syndrome is an infection of neonates or immunocompromised adults. Presentation is a febrile illness without a recognized source.
4. **Meningitis** caused by *L monocytogenes* affects infants under 2 months of age as well as older adults, ranking third after pneumococcus and meningococcus as common causes of bacterial meningitis. Cerebrospinal fluid shows a *neutrophilic* pleocytosis. Adults with meningitis are often immunocompromised, and cases have been associated with HIV infection and therapy with tumor necrosis factor (TNF) inhibitors such as infliximab.
5. **Focal infections**, including adenitis, brain abscess, endocarditis, osteomyelitis, and arthritis, occur rarely.

Prevention

At-risk patients (eg, pregnant women) should avoid unpasteurized milk products. Smoked seafoods, cold cuts, hot dogs, and meat spreads also carry risk. Thoroughly cook animal source food and wash raw vegetables.

Treatment

Ampicillin, 8–12 g/day intravenously in four to six divided doses (the higher dose for meningitis), is the treatment of choice. Gentamicin, 5 mg/kg/day intravenously once or in divided doses, is synergistic with ampicillin against *Listeria* in vitro and in animal models, and the use of combination therapy may be considered during the first few days of treatment to enhance eradication of organisms. In patients with penicillin allergies, trimethoprim-sulfamethoxazole has excellent intracellular and cerebrospinal fluid penetration and is an appropriate alternative. The dose is 10–20 mg/kg/day intravenously of the trimethoprim component. Mortality and morbidity rates still are high. Therapy should be administered for at least 2–3 weeks. Longer durations—between 3 and 6 weeks—have been recommended for treatment of meningitis, especially in immunocompromised persons.

Lepe JA. Current aspects of listeriosis. Med Clin (Barc). 2020;154:453. [PMID: 32147188]

INFECTIVE ENDOCARDITIS

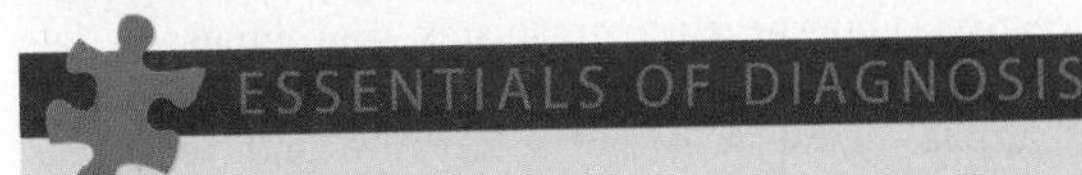

ESSENTIALS OF DIAGNOSIS

- Fever.
- Preexisting organic heart lesion.
- Positive blood cultures.
- Evidence of vegetation on echocardiography.
- Evidence of systemic emboli.

General Considerations

Endocarditis is a bacterial or fungal infection of the valvular or endocardial surface of the heart. The clinical presentation depends on the infecting organism and the valve or valves that are infected. More virulent organisms—*S aureus* in particular—tend to produce a more rapidly progressive and destructive infection. Endocarditis caused by more virulent organisms often presents as an acute febrile illness and is complicated by early embolization, acute valvular regurgitation, and myocardial abscess formation. Viridans strains of streptococci, enterococci, other bacteria, yeasts, and fungi tend to cause a more subacute picture.

Predisposing valvular abnormalities include a variety of congenital disorders such as ventricular septal defect, tetralogy of Fallot, coarctation of the aorta, or patent ductus arteriosus, and rheumatic involvement of any valve, bicuspid aortic valves, calcific or sclerotic aortic valves, hypertrophic subaortic stenosis, mitral valve prolapse. Rheumatic disease is no longer the major predisposing factor in developed countries. Regurgitation lesions are more susceptible than stenotic ones.

The initiating event in native valve endocarditis is colonization of the valve by bacteria or yeast that gain access to the bloodstream. Transient bacteremia is common during dental, upper respiratory, urologic, and lower GI diagnostic and surgical procedures. It is less common during upper GI and gynecologic procedures. Intravascular devices are also a portal of access of microorganisms into the bloodstream. A large proportion of cases of *S aureus* endocarditis are attributable to health care–associated bacteremia.

Native valve endocarditis is usually caused by *S aureus*, viridans streptococci, enterococci, or HACEK organisms (an acronym for *Haemophilus aphrophilus* [now *Aggregatibacter aphrophilus*], *Actinobacillus actinomycetemcomitans* [now *Aggregatibacter actinomycetemcomitans*], *Cardiobacterium hominis, Eikenella corrodens*, and *Kingella* species). *S aureus,* and no longer streptococcal species, is now the leading cause of native valve endocarditis. Gram-negative organisms and fungi account for a small percentage.

In injection drug users, *S aureus* accounts for over 60% of all endocarditis cases and for 80–90% of cases in which the tricuspid valve is infected. Enterococci and streptococci comprise most of the balance in about equal proportions. Other causative organisms are gram-negative aerobic bacilli, fungi, and unusual organisms.

The microbiology of **prosthetic valve endocarditis** is distinctive. Early infections (ie, those occurring within 2 months after valve implantation) are commonly caused by staphylococci—both coagulase-positive and coagulase-negative—gram-negative organisms, and fungi. In late prosthetic valve endocarditis, streptococci are commonly identified, although coagulase-negative and coagulase-positive staphylococci still cause many cases.

Clinical Findings

A. Symptoms and Signs

Virtually all patients have fever at some point in the illness, although it may be very low grade (less than 38°C) in older individuals and in patients with heart failure or kidney failure. Rarely, there may be no fever at all.

The duration of illness typically is a few days to a few weeks. Nonspecific symptoms are common. The initial symptoms and signs of endocarditis may be caused by direct arterial, valvular, or cardiac damage. Although a changing regurgitant murmur is significant diagnostically, it is the exception rather than the rule. Symptoms also may occur as a result of embolization, metastatic infection or immunologically mediated phenomena. These include cough; dyspnea; arthralgias or arthritis; diarrhea; and abdominal, back, or flank pain.

The characteristic peripheral lesions—petechiae (on the palate or conjunctiva or beneath the fingernails), subungual ("splinter") hemorrhages (Figure 33–4), Osler nodes (painful, violaceous raised lesions of the fingers, toes, or feet), Janeway lesions (painless erythematous lesions of the palms or soles), and Roth spots (exudative lesions in the retina)—occur in about 25% of patients. Strokes and major systemic embolic events are present in about 25% of patients and tend to occur before or within the first week of antimicrobial therapy. Hematuria and proteinuria may result from emboli or immunologically mediated glomerulonephritis.

B. Imaging

Chest radiograph may show evidence for the underlying cardiac abnormality and, in right-sided endocarditis, pulmonary infiltrates. The ECG is nondiagnostic, but new

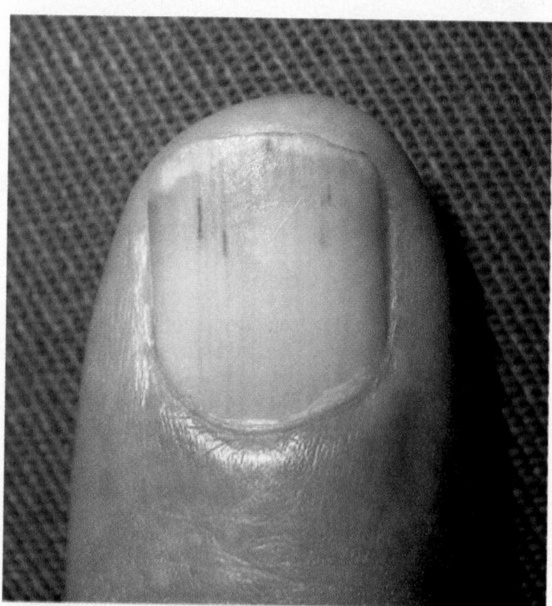

▲ **Figure 33–4.** Splinter hemorrhages appearing as red lineal streaks under the nail plate and within the nail bed, in endocarditis, psoriasis, and trauma. (Reproduced with permission from Richard P. Usatine, MD, in Usatine RP, Smith MA, Mayeaux EJ Jr, Chumley H, Tysinger J. *The Color Atlas of Family Medicine*. McGraw-Hill, 2009.)

conduction abnormalities suggest myocardial abscess formation. Echocardiography is useful in identifying vegetations and other characteristic features suspicious for endocarditis and may provide adjunctive information about the specific valve or valves that are infected. The sensitivity of transthoracic echocardiography is between 55% and 65%; it cannot reliably rule out endocarditis but may confirm a clinical suspicion. Transesophageal echocardiography is 90% sensitive in detecting vegetations and is useful for identifying valve ring abscesses as well as prosthetic valve endocarditis.

C. Diagnostic Studies

1. Blood cultures—Three sets of blood cultures are recommended before starting antibiotics to maximize microbiologic diagnosis; adequate volume is important. Each culture bottle should be filled with 10 mL of blood since half of adults have less than 1 colony forming unit of bacteria per mL blood. The yield of bacteria may be up to 5% higher for every additional milliliter collected. Optimal yield is with two or three sets of cultures from different sites. There is no difference in yield if blood is collected simultaneously or several hours apart.

Approximately 5% of cases will be culture-negative, usually attributable to administration of antimicrobials prior to cultures. If antimicrobial therapy has been administered prior to obtaining cultures and the patient is clinically stable, it is reasonable to withhold antimicrobial therapy for 2–3 days so that appropriate cultures can be obtained. Culture-negative endocarditis may also be due to organisms that require special media for growth (eg, *Legionella, Bartonella, Abiotrophia* species, formerly referred to as nutritionally deficient streptococci), organisms that do not grow on artificial media (*Tropheryma whipplei*, or pathogens of Q fever or psittacosis), or those that may require prolonged incubation (eg, *Brucella*, anaerobes, HACEK organisms). *Bartonella quintana* is an important cause of culture-negative endocarditis.

2. Modified Duke criteria—The Modified Duke criteria are useful for the diagnosis of endocarditis. **Major criteria** include (1) two positive blood cultures for a microorganism that typically causes infective endocarditis or persistent bacteremia, or a single positive blood culture for *Coxiella burnetii* or IgG antibody titer greater than or equal to 1:800; and (2) evidence of endocardial involvement documented by echocardiography showing definite vegetation, myocardial abscess, new partial dehiscence of a prosthetic valve, or new valvular regurgitation (increase or change in murmur is not sufficient). **Minor criteria** include the presence of a predisposing condition; fever of 38°C or higher; vascular phenomena, such as cutaneous hemorrhages, aneurysm, systemic emboli, or pulmonary infarction; immunologic phenomena, such as glomerulonephritis, Osler nodes, Roth spots, or rheumatoid factor; and positive blood cultures not meeting the major criteria or serologic evidence of an active infection. A definite diagnosis can be made with 80% accuracy if two major criteria, one major criterion and three minor criteria, or five minor criteria are fulfilled. A possible diagnosis of endocarditis is made if one major and one minor criterion or three minor criteria are met. If fewer criteria are found, or a sound alternative explanation for illness is identified, or the patient's febrile illness has resolved within 4 days, endocarditis is unlikely.

Complications

The course of infective endocarditis is determined by the degree of damage to the heart, by the site of infection (right-sided versus left-sided, aortic versus mitral valve), by the presence of metastatic foci of infection, by the occurrence of embolization, and by immunologically mediated processes. Destruction of infected heart valves is especially common and precipitous with *S aureus* but can occur with any organism and can progress even after bacteriologic cure. The infection can also extend into the myocardium, resulting in abscesses leading to conduction disturbances, and involving the wall of the aorta, creating sinus of Valsalva aneurysms.

Peripheral embolization to the brain and myocardium may result in infarctions. Embolization to the spleen and kidneys is also common. Peripheral emboli may initiate metastatic infections or may become established in vessel walls, leading to mycotic aneurysms. Right-sided endocarditis (usually the tricuspid valve) causes septic pulmonary emboli, occasionally with infarction and lung abscesses.

Prevention

The American Heart Association recommends antibiotic prophylaxis for infective endocarditis in a relatively small group of patients with predisposing congenital or valvular anomalies (Table 33–3) undergoing select dental procedures, operations involving the respiratory tract, or operations of infected skin, skin structure, or musculoskeletal tissue (Table 33–4). Current antimicrobial recommendations are given in Table 33–5.

Treatment

Empiric regimens for endocarditis while culture results are pending should include agents active against staphylococci, streptococci, and enterococci. Vancomycin 1 g every 12 hours intravenously plus ceftriaxone 2 g every 24 hours provides appropriate coverage pending definitive diagnosis; consultation with an infectious disease expert is strongly recommended when initiating treatment. Intravenous therapy has been the mainstay of treatment for infective endocarditis. Some data, however, support the use of oral antibiotic therapy following 2 weeks of intravenous antibiotic regimens for certain organisms.

A. Viridans Streptococci

For penicillin-susceptible viridans streptococcal endocarditis (ie, MIC 0.1 mcg/mL or less), penicillin G, 18 million units intravenously either continuously or in four to six equally divided doses, or ceftriaxone, 2 g intravenously once daily for 4 weeks, is recommended. The duration of therapy can be shortened to 2 weeks if gentamicin, 3 mg/kg intravenously every 24 hours, is used with penicillin or ceftriaxone. The 2-week regimen is reasonable and can be

Table 33–3. Cardiac conditions with high risk of adverse outcomes from endocarditis for which prophylaxis with dental procedures is recommended.[1,2]

Prosthetic cardiac valve
Previous infective endocarditis
Congenital heart disease (CHD)[3]
Unrepaired cyanotic CHD, including palliative shunts and conduits
Completely repaired congenital heart defect with prosthetic material or device, whether placed by surgery or by catheter intervention, during the first 6 months after the procedure[4]
Repaired CHD with residual defects at the site or adjacent to the site of a prosthetic patch or prosthetic device
Cardiac transplantation recipients in whom cardiac valvulopathy develops

[1]Reprinted with permission Circulation. 2007;116:1736–1754 ©2007 American Heart Association, Inc.
[2]See Table 33–5 for prophylactic regimens.
[3]Except for the conditions listed above, antibiotic prophylaxis is not recommended for other forms of CHD.
[4]Prophylaxis is recommended because endothelialization of prosthetic material occurs within 6 months after procedure.

Table 33–4. Recommendations for administration of bacterial endocarditis prophylaxis for patients according to type of procedure.[1]

Prophylaxis Recommended	Prophylaxis Not Recommended
Dental procedures All dental procedures that involve manipulation of gingival tissue or the periapical region of the teeth or perforation of the oral mucosa, including routine cleaning **Respiratory tract procedures** Only respiratory tract procedures that involve incision of the respiratory mucosa **Procedures on infected skin, skin structure, or musculoskeletal tissue**	**Dental procedures** Routine anesthetic injections through noninfected tissue, taking dental radiographs, placement of removable prosthodontic or orthodontic appliances, adjustment of orthodontic appliances, placement of orthodontic brackets, shedding of deciduous teeth, and bleeding from trauma to the lips or oral mucosa **GI tract procedures** **Genitourinary tract procedures**

[1]Reprinted with permission Circulation.2007;116:1736-1754 ©2007 American Heart Association, Inc.

considered in patients with uncomplicated endocarditis, rapid response to therapy, and no underlying kidney disease. For the patient unable to tolerate penicillin or ceftriaxone, vancomycin, 15 mg/kg intravenously every 12 hours for 4 weeks, is given with a desired trough level of 10–15 mcg/mL. Prosthetic valve endocarditis is treated with a 6-week course of penicillin or ceftriaxone and the clinician can consider adding 2 weeks of gentamicin at the start of therapy.

Viridans streptococci relatively resistant to penicillin (ie, MIC greater than 0.12 mcg/mL but less than or equal to 0.5 mcg/mL) should be treated for 4 weeks. Penicillin G,

Table 33–5. American Heart Association recommendations for endocarditis prophylaxis for dental procedures for patients with cardiac conditions.[1–3]

Oral	Amoxicillin	2 g 1 hour before procedure
Penicillin allergy	Clindamycin	600 mg 1 hour before procedure
	or	
	Cephalexin	2 g 1 hour before procedure (contraindicated if there is history of a beta-lactam immediate hypersensitivity reaction)
	or	
	Azithromycin or clarithromycin	500 mg 1 hour before procedure
Parenteral	Ampicillin	2 g intramuscularly or intravenously 30 minutes before procedure
Penicillin allergy	Clindamycin	600 mg intravenously 1 hour before procedure
	or	
	Cefazolin	1 g intramuscularly or intravenously 30 minutes before procedure (contraindicated if there is history of a beta-lactam immediate hypersensitivity reaction)

[1]Data from the American Heart Association. Circulation. 2007;116:1736.
[2]For patients undergoing respiratory tract procedures involving incision of respiratory tract mucosa to treat an established infection or a procedure on infected skin, skin structure, or musculoskeletal tissue known or suspected to be caused by *S aureus*, the regimen should contain an antistaphylococcal penicillin (eg, nafcillin 2 g intravenously 30 minutes prior to procedure) or cephalosporin (eg, cephalexin or cefazolin, dosed as per above). Vancomycin can be used to treat patients unable to tolerate a beta-lactam or if the infection is known or suspected to be caused by a methicillin-resistant strain of *S aureus*.
[3]See Table 33–3 for list of cardiac conditions.

24 million units intravenously either continuously or in four to six equally divided doses, is combined with gentamicin, 3 mg/kg intravenously every 24 hours for the first 2 weeks. Ceftriaxone may be a reasonable alternative treatment option for isolates that are susceptible to ceftriaxone. In the patient with IgE-mediated allergy to penicillin, vancomycin alone, 15 mg/kg intravenously every 12 hours for 4 weeks, should be administered. Prosthetic valve endocarditis is treated with a 6-week course of penicillin or ceftriaxone plus gentamicin as above.

Endocarditis caused by viridans streptococci with an MIC greater than 0.5 mcg/mL or by *Abiotrophia* species should be treated the same as enterococcal endocarditis.

B. Other Streptococci

Endocarditis caused by *S pneumoniae*, group A streptococci (*S pyogenes*), or groups B, C, and G streptococci is unusual. *S pneumoniae* sensitive to penicillin (MIC less than 0.1 mcg/mL) can be treated with penicillin, 18 million units intravenously either continuously or in four to six equally divided doses, or cefazolin, 6 g intravenously either continuously or in three equally divided doses, or ceftriaxone, 2 g daily intravenously for 4 weeks. High-dose penicillin (24 million units) or a third-generation cephalosporin may be required for the treatment of endocarditis (without meningitis) caused by strains resistant to penicillin (MIC greater than 0.1 mcg/mL). The addition of vancomycin and rifampin to ceftriaxone may be considered in patients with *S pneumoniae* strains with cefotaxime MIC greater than 2 mcg/mL. Group A streptococcal infection can be treated with penicillin or ceftriaxone for 4–6 weeks. Groups B, C, and G streptococci tend to be more resistant to penicillin than group A streptococci, and some experts have recommended adding gentamicin, 3 mg/kg intravenously every 24 hours, to penicillin for the first 2 weeks of a 4- to 6-week course. Endocarditis caused by *S gallolyticus (bovis)* is associated with liver disease, especially cirrhosis, and GI abnormalities, especially colon cancer. Colonoscopy should be performed to exclude the latter.

C. Group D Streptococci (Enterococci)

For enterococcal endocarditis, penicillin or ampicillin alone is inadequate. One recommended regimen is ampicillin, 2 g intravenously every 4 hours, or penicillin G, 18–30 million units intravenously continuously or in six equally divided doses plus gentamicin, 1 mg/kg intravenously every 8 hours. The second recommended regimen is ampicillin (2 g intravenously every 4 hours) plus ceftriaxone 2 g intravenously every 12 hours. The recommended duration of therapy is 4–6 weeks (the longer duration for patients with symptoms for more than 3 months, relapse, or prosthetic valve endocarditis). The combination of ampicillin plus ceftriaxone is recommended for patients with creatinine clearance less than 50 mL/minute or whose enterococcal isolates are resistant to gentamicin. In patients who cannot tolerate penicillin and ampicillin or who have enterococcal isolate resistant to these agents, vancomycin plus gentamicin can be used.

Endocarditis caused by strains resistant to penicillin and vancomycin are difficult to treat and should always be managed with an infectious disease specialist.

D. Staphylococci

For methicillin-susceptible *S aureus* isolates, nafcillin or oxacillin, 12 g intravenously daily given continuously or in four to six divided doses, or cefazolin, 6 g intravenously daily given continuously or in three divided doses for 6 weeks, is the preferred therapy. In cases of brain abscess resulting from methicillin-susceptible *S aureus* endocarditis, nafcillin should be used instead of cefazolin. For patients with history of immediate type hypersensitivity to beta-lactams, a desensitization protocol should be undertaken. For patients with a history of non-anaphylactoid reactions to penicillins, cefazolin should be used. Patients who are infected with methicillin-resistant *S aureus* or who are unable to tolerate beta-lactam therapy should receive vancomycin, 30 mg/kg/day intravenously divided in two or three doses, to achieve a goal trough level of 15–20 mcg/kg, or daptomycin intravenously at greater than or equal to 8 mg/kg/day. Aminoglycoside combination regimens are not recommended. The effect of rifampin with antistaphylococcal drugs is variable, and its routine use is not recommended.

Because coagulase-negative staphylococci—a common cause of prosthetic valve endocarditis—are routinely resistant to methicillin, beta-lactam antibiotics should not be used unless the isolate is demonstrated to be susceptible. A combination of vancomycin, 30 mg/kg/day intravenously divided in two or three doses for 6 weeks; rifampin, 300 mg every 8 hours for 6 weeks; and gentamicin, 3 mg/kg intravenously every 8 hours for the first 2 weeks, is recommended for prosthetic valve infection. If the organism is sensitive to methicillin, either nafcillin or oxacillin or cefazolin can be used in combination with rifampin and gentamicin. Combination therapy with nafcillin or oxacillin (vancomycin or daptomycin for methicillin-resistant strains), rifampin, and gentamicin is also recommended for treatment of *S aureus* prosthetic valve infection.

E. HACEK Organisms

HACEK organisms are slow-growing, fastidious gram-negative coccobacilli or bacilli (*H aphrophilus* [now *A aphrophilus*], *A actinomycetemcomitans, C hominis, E corrodens*, and *Kingella* species) that are normal oral flora and cause less than 5% of all cases of endocarditis. They may produce beta-lactamase, and thus the treatment of choice is ceftriaxone (or another third-generation cephalosporin), 2 g intravenously once daily for 4 weeks. Prosthetic valve endocarditis should be treated for 6 weeks. In the penicillin-allergic patient, experience is limited, but fluoroquinolones have in vitro activity and should be considered.

F. Culture-Negative Endocarditis

Failure to culture microorganisms from patients with suspected infective endocarditis may be due to infection from organisms not recovered in routine microbiology testing or previous administration of antimicrobial agents before blood cultures were obtained. These cases must be managed with the assistance of an infectious disease specialist. Pathogens that are not able to be cultured by commonly used techniques include *Bartonella* species, *Chlamydia* species, *Brucella* species, and *Tropheryma whipplei*. Serologic testing should be performed in patients who have epidemiologic risk factors for these infections. Treatment should be directed at likely pathogens while awaiting serologic results; treatment of patients given prior antimicrobials before cultures were obtained must also consider likely pathogens.

G. Role of Surgery

While many cases can be successfully treated medically, operative management is frequently required. Acute heart failure unresponsive to medical therapy is an indication for valve replacement even if active infection is present. Infections unresponsive to appropriate antimicrobial therapy after 7–10 days (ie, persistent fevers, positive blood cultures despite therapy) are more likely to be eradicated if the valve is replaced. Surgery is nearly always required for cure of fungal endocarditis and is more often necessary with highly resistant bacteria. It is also indicated when the infection involves the sinus of Valsalva or produces septal abscesses. Recurrent infection with the same organism prompts an operative approach, especially with infected prosthetic valves. Continuing embolization presents a difficult problem when the infection is otherwise responding; surgery may be the proper approach. Particularly challenging is a large and fragile vegetation demonstrated by echocardiography in the absence of embolization. Most clinicians favor an operative approach with vegetectomy and valve repair if the patient is a good candidate. Operation without delay may be considered in patients with endocarditis and an embolic stroke who have an indication for surgery. If not urgent or if intracranial hemorrhage is present, a delay of at least 4 weeks should be considered. Embolization after bacteriologic cure does not necessarily imply recurrence of endocarditis.

H. Role of Anticoagulation

Anticoagulation is contraindicated in native valve endocarditis because of an increased risk of intracerebral hemorrhage from mycotic aneurysms or embolic phenomena. The role of anticoagulant therapy during prosthetic valve endocarditis is more controversial. Reversal of anticoagulation may result in thrombosis of the mechanical prosthesis, particularly in the mitral position. Conversely, anticoagulation during active prosthetic valve endocarditis caused by *S aureus* has been associated with fatal intracerebral hemorrhage. One approach is to discontinue anticoagulation during the septic phase of *S aureus* prosthetic valve endocarditis. In patients with *S aureus* prosthetic valve endocarditis complicated by a CNS embolic event, anticoagulation should be discontinued for the first 2 weeks of therapy. Indications for anticoagulation following prosthetic valve implantation for endocarditis are the same as for patients with prosthetic valves without endocarditis (eg, nonporcine mechanical valves and valves in the mitral position).

▶ Response to Therapy

If infection is caused by viridans streptococci, enterococci, or coagulase-negative staphylococci, defervescence occurs in 3–4 days on average; with *S aureus* or *Pseudomonas aeruginosa*, fever may persist for longer. Blood cultures should be obtained every 1–2 days to document sterilization. Other causes of persistent fever are myocardial or metastatic abscess, sterile embolization, superimposed hospital-acquired infection, and drug reaction. Most relapses occur within 1–2 months after completion of therapy. Obtaining one or two blood cultures during this period is prudent.

▶ When to Refer

- Consider consulting an infectious diseases specialist in all cases of suspected infective endocarditis.
- Consult a cardiac surgeon as discussed in the Role of Surgery section above to prevent further embolic disease, heart failure, and other complications, including death.

▶ When to Admit

Patients with infective endocarditis should be hospitalized for expedited evaluation and treatment.

Baddour LM et al. Infective endocarditis in adults: diagnosis, antimicrobial therapy, and management of complications: a scientific statement for healthcare professionals from the American Heart Association. Circulation. 2015;132:1435. [PMID: 26373316]

Goff DA et al. Review of guidelines for dental antibiotic prophylaxis for prevention of endocarditis and prosthetic joint infections and need for dental stewardship. Clin Infect Dis. 2020;71:455. [PMID: 31728507]

Iversen K et al. Partial oral versus intravenous antibiotic treatment of endocarditis. N Engl J Med. 2019;380:415. [PMID: 30152252]

Spellberg B et al. Evaluation of a Paradigm shift from intravenous antibiotics to oral step-down therapy for the treatment of infective endocarditis: a narrative review. JAMA Intern Med. 2020;180:769. [PMID: 32227127]

INFECTIONS CAUSED BY GRAM-NEGATIVE BACTERIA

BORDETELLA PERTUSSIS INFECTION (Whooping Cough)

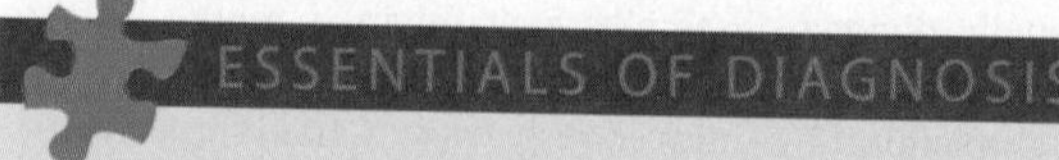

- ▶ Predominantly in infants under age 2 years; adolescents and adults are reservoirs of infection.
- ▶ Two-week prodromal catarrhal stage of malaise, cough, coryza, and anorexia.
- ▶ Paroxysmal cough ending in a high-pitched inspiratory "whoop."
- ▶ Absolute lymphocytosis, often striking; culture confirms diagnosis.

General Considerations

Pertussis is an acute infection of the respiratory tract caused by *B pertussis* that is transmitted by respiratory droplets. The incubation period is 7–17 days. Half of all cases occur before age 2 years. Neither immunization nor disease confers lasting immunity to pertussis. Consequently, adults are an important reservoir of the disease.

Clinical Findings

The symptoms of classic pertussis last about 6 weeks and are divided into three consecutive stages. The catarrhal stage is characterized by its insidious onset, with lacrimation, sneezing, and coryza, anorexia and malaise, and a hacking night cough that becomes diurnal. The paroxysmal stage is characterized by bursts of rapid, consecutive coughs followed by a deep, high-pitched inspiration (whoop). The convalescent stage begins 4 weeks after onset of the illness with a decrease in the frequency and severity of paroxysms of cough. The diagnosis often is not considered in adults, who may not have a typical presentation. Cough persisting more than 2 weeks is suggestive. Infection may also be asymptomatic.

The WBC count is usually 15,000–20,000/mcL (15–20 × 10^9/L) (rarely, as high as 50,000/mcL [50 × 10^9/L] or more), 60–80% of which are lymphocytes. The diagnosis is established by isolating the organism from a nasopharyngeal culture on special medium (eg, Bordet-Gengou agar). PCR assays for *B pertussis* may be available in some clinical or health department laboratories.

Prevention

Acellular pertussis vaccine is recommended for all infants, combined with diphtheria and tetanus toxoids (DtaP). Infants and susceptible adults with significant exposure should receive prophylaxis with an oral macrolide. In recognition of their importance as a reservoir of disease, vaccination of adolescents and adults against pertussis is recommended (see Table 30–7 and www.cdc.gov/vaccines/schedules). Adolescents aged 11–18 years (preferably between 11 and 12 years of age) who have completed the DTP or DtaP vaccination series should receive a single dose of either Tdap product instead of Td (tetanus and diphtheria toxoids vaccine) for booster immunization against tetanus, diphtheria, and pertussis. Tdap, which immunizes against the same bacteria as DtaP, is a booster immunization; Tdap contains the same amount of tetanus toxoid (T) as DtaP but reduced diphtheria toxoid and acellular pertussis (hence the lower case -dap). Adults of all ages (including those older than age 64 years) should receive a single dose of Tdap. In addition, pregnant women should receive a dose of Tdap during each pregnancy regardless of prior vaccination history, ideally between 27 and 36 weeks of gestation, to maximize the antibody response of the woman and the passive antibody transfer to the infant. For any woman who was not previously vaccinated with Tdap and for whom the vaccine was not given during her pregnancy, Tdap should be administered immediately postpartum. The CDC has eliminated the recommendation that a 2-year period window is needed between receiving the Td and Tdap vaccines based on data showing that there is not an increased risk of adverse events.

Treatment

Antibiotic treatment should be initiated in all suspected cases. Treatment options include erythromycin, 500 mg four times a day orally for 7 days; azithromycin, 500 mg orally on day 1 and 250 mg for 4 more days; or clarithromycin, 500 mg orally twice daily for 7 days. Trimethoprim-sulfamethoxazole, 160–800 mg orally twice a day for 7 days, also is effective. Treatment shortens the duration of carriage and may diminish the severity of coughing paroxysms. These same regimens are indicated for prophylaxis of contacts to an active case of pertussis who are exposed within 3 weeks of the onset of cough in the index case.

Craig R et al. Asymptomatic infection and transmission of pertussis in households: a systematic review. Clin Infect Dis. 2020;70:152. [PMID: 31257450]

Wilkinson K et al. Pertussis vaccine effectiveness and duration of protection—a systematic review and meta-analysis. Vaccine. 2021;39:3120. [PMID: 33934917]

OTHER *BORDETELLA* INFECTIONS

Bordetella bronchiseptica is a pleomorphic gram-negative coccobacillus causing kennel cough in dogs. On occasion it causes upper and lower respiratory infection in humans, principally in patients with HIV infection. Infection has been associated with contact with dogs and cats, suggesting animal-to-human transmission. Treatment of *B bronchiseptica* infection is guided by results of in vitro susceptibility tests.

MENINGOCOCCAL MENINGITIS

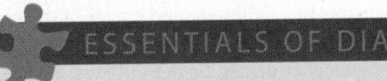

- Fever, headache, vomiting, delirium, convulsions.
- Petechial rash on skin and mucous membranes.
- Neck and back stiffness and positive Kernig and Brudzinski signs are characteristic.
- Purulent spinal fluid with gram-negative intracellular and extracellular diplococci.
- Culture of cerebrospinal fluid, blood, or petechial aspiration confirms the diagnosis.

General Considerations

Meningococcal meningitis is caused by *Neisseria meningitidis* of groups A, B, C, Y, and W-135, among others. Meningitis due to serogroup A is uncommon in the United States. Serogroup B generally causes sporadic cases. Serogroup C meningococcus is the most common cause of epidemic disease in the United States. Up to 40% of persons are nasopharyngeal carriers of meningococci, but disease develops in relatively few of these persons. Infection is transmitted by droplets. The clinical illness may take the form of meningococcemia (a fulminant form of septicemia without meningitis), meningococcemia with meningitis, or meningitis. Recurrent meningococcemia with fever, rash, and arthritis is seen rarely in patients with certain terminal complement deficiencies. Asplenic patients are also at risk.

Clinical Findings

A. Symptoms and Signs

High fever, chills, nausea, vomiting, and headache as well as back, abdominal, and extremity pains are typical. Rapidly developing confusion, delirium, seizures, and coma occur in some. On examination, nuchal and back rigidity are typical. Positive Kernig and Brudzinski signs (Kernig sign is pain in the hamstrings upon extension of the knee with the hip at 90-degree flexion; Brudzinski sign is flexion of the knee in response to flexion of the neck) are specific but not sensitive findings. A petechial rash appearing all over the body, including on mucous membranes, on the lower extremities, and at pressure points, is found in most cases. Petechiae may vary in size from pinpoint lesions to large ecchymoses or even skin gangrene that may later slough.

B. Laboratory Findings

Lumbar puncture typically reveals a cloudy or purulent cerebrospinal fluid, with elevated pressure, increased protein, and decreased glucose content. The fluid usually contains a cell count greater than 1000/mcL (1.0×10^9/L) with polymorphonuclear cells predominating and containing gram-negative intracellular diplococci. The organism is usually demonstrated by smear and culture of the cerebrospinal fluid, oropharynx, blood, or aspirated petechiae. The absence of organisms in a Gram-stained smear of the cerebrospinal fluid sediment does not rule out the diagnosis. The capsular polysaccharide can be demonstrated in cerebrospinal fluid or urine by latex agglutination; this is useful in partially treated patients, although sensitivity is 60–80%.

Disseminated intravascular coagulation is an important complication of meningococcal infection and is typically present in toxic patients with ecchymotic skin lesions.

Differential Diagnosis

Meningococcal meningitis must be differentiated from other meningitides. In small infants and in older adults, fever or stiff neck is often missing, and altered mental status may dominate the picture.

Rickettsial, echovirus, and, rarely, other bacterial infections (eg, staphylococcal infections, scarlet fever) also cause petechial rash.

Prevention

Five meningococcal vaccines are available. There are three vaccines with coverage against meningococcal serogroups A, C, Y, and W-135 and two with coverage against meningococcal serogroup B. The three vaccines effective for meningococcal serogroups A, C, Y, and W-135 are the meningococcal polysaccharide vaccine (MPSV4), indicated for vaccination of persons over age 55; and two conjugate vaccines (MCV4 and MenACWY-CRM), indicated for persons aged 2–55 years. The two vaccines against meningococcal serogroup B are MenB-FHbp and MenB-4C; they are approved for persons aged 10–25 years and are not interchangeable.

The Advisory Committee on Immunization Practices recommends immunization with a dose of MCV4 for preadolescents aged 11–12 with a booster at age 16 (see www.cdc.gov/vaccines/schedules/hcp/child-adolescent.html). For ease of program implementation, persons aged 21 years or younger should have documentation of receipt of a dose of MCV4 not more than 5 years before enrollment to college. If the primary dose was administered before the sixteenth birthday, a booster dose should be administered before enrollment. Vaccine is also recommended as a two-dose primary series administered 2 months apart for persons aged 2 through 54 years with persistent complement deficiency, persons with functional or anatomic asplenia, and for adolescents with HIV infection. All other persons at increased risk for meningococcal disease (eg, military recruits, microbiologists routinely exposed to isolates of *N meningitidis*, or travelers to an epidemic or highly endemic country) should receive a single dose. One of the meningococcal serogroup B vaccines may be administered to persons 10 years of age or older who are at increased risk for meningococcal disease. These persons include those with persistent complement deficiencies; persons with anatomic or functional asplenia; microbiologists; and persons identified to be at increased risk because of a serogroup B meningococcal disease outbreak. Vaccination of persons aged 16–23 years may provide short-term protection against most strains of serogroup B meningococcal disease.

Eliminating nasopharyngeal carriage of meningococci is an effective prevention strategy in closed populations and to prevent secondary cases in household or otherwise close contacts. Rifampin, 600 mg orally twice a day for 2 days, ciprofloxacin, 500 mg orally once, or one intramuscular 250-mg dose of ceftriaxone is effective. Cases of fluoroquinolone-resistant meningococcal infections have been identified in the United States. However, ciprofloxacin remains a recommended empiric agent for eradication of nasopharyngeal carriage. School and work contacts ordinarily need not be treated. Hospital contacts receive therapy only if intense exposure has occurred (eg, mouth-to-mouth resuscitation). Accidentally discovered carriers without known close contact with meningococcal disease do not require prophylactic antimicrobials.

Treatment

Blood cultures must be obtained and intravenous antimicrobial therapy started immediately. This may be done prior to lumbar puncture in patients in whom the diagnosis is not straightforward and for those in whom MR or CT imaging is indicated to exclude mass lesions. Aqueous penicillin G is the antibiotic of choice (24 mU/24 hours intravenously in divided doses every 4 hours). The prevalence of strains of *N meningitidis* with intermediate resistance to penicillin in vitro (MICs 0.1–1 mcg/mL) is increasing, particularly in Europe. Penicillin-intermediate strains thus far remain fully susceptible to ceftriaxone and other third-generation cephalosporins used to treat meningitis, and these should be effective alternatives to penicillin. In penicillin-allergic patients or those in whom *Haemophilus influenzae* or gram-negative meningitis is a consideration, ceftriaxone, 2 g intravenously every 12 hours, should be used. Treatment should be continued in full doses by the intravenous route until the patient is afebrile for 5 days. Shorter courses—as few as 4 days if ceftriaxone is used—are also effective.

When to Admit

All patients with suspected meningococcal infection should be admitted for evaluation and empiric intravenous antibiotic therapy.

Linder KA et al. JAMA patient page. Meningococcal meningitis. JAMA. 2019;321:1014. [PMID: 30860561]

McMillan M et al. Effectiveness of meningococcal vaccines at reducing invasive meningococcal disease and pharyngeal *Neisseria meningitidis* carriage: a systematic review and meta-analysis. Clin Infect Dis. 2021;73:e609. [PMID: 33212510]

INFECTIONS CAUSED BY *HAEMOPHILUS* SPECIES

H influenzae and other *Haemophilus* species may cause sinusitis, otitis, bronchitis, epiglottitis, pneumonia, cellulitis, arthritis, meningitis, and endocarditis. Nontypeable strains are responsible for most disease in adults. Alcohol use disorder, smoking, chronic lung disease, advanced age, and HIV infection are risk factors. *Haemophilus* species colonize the upper respiratory tract in patients with COPD and frequently cause purulent bronchitis.

Beta-lactamase–producing strains are less common in adults than in children. For adults with sinusitis, otitis, or respiratory tract infection, oral amoxicillin, 750 mg twice daily for 10–14 days, is adequate. For beta-lactamase–producing strains, use of the oral fixed-drug combination of amoxicillin, 875 mg, with clavulanate, 125 mg, is indicated. For the penicillin-allergic patient, oral cefuroxime axetil, 250 mg twice daily; or a fluoroquinolone (ciprofloxacin, 500 mg orally twice daily; levofloxacin, 500–750 mg orally once daily; or moxifloxacin, 400 mg orally once daily) for 7 days is effective. Azithromycin, 500 mg orally once followed by 250 mg daily for 4 days, is preferred over clarithromycin when a macrolide is the preferred agent. Trimethoprim-sulfamethoxazole (160/800 mg orally twice daily) can be considered, but resistance rates have been reported to be up to 25%.

In the more seriously ill patient (eg, the toxic patient with multilobar pneumonia), ceftriaxone, 1 g/day intravenously, is recommended pending determination of whether the infecting strain produces beta-lactamase. A fluoroquinolone (see above for dosages) can be used for the penicillin-allergic patients for a 10- to 14-day course of therapy.

Epiglottitis is characterized by an abrupt onset of high fever, drooling, and inability to handle secretions. An important clue to the diagnosis is complaint of a severe sore throat despite an unimpressive examination of the pharynx. Stridor and respiratory distress result from laryngeal obstruction. The diagnosis is best made by direct visualization of the cherry-red, swollen epiglottis at laryngoscopy. Because laryngoscopy may provoke laryngospasm and obstruction, especially in children, it should be performed in an intensive care unit or similar setting, and only at a time when intubation can be performed promptly. Ceftriaxone, 1 g intravenously every 24 hours for 7–10 days, is the drug of choice. Trimethoprim-sulfamethoxazole or a fluoroquinolone (see above for dosage) may be used in the patient with serious penicillin allergy.

Meningitis, rare in adults, is a consideration in the patient who has meningitis associated with sinusitis or otitis. Initial therapy for suspected *H influenzae* meningitis should be with ceftriaxone, 4 g/day in two divided doses, until the strain is proved not to produce beta-lactamase. Meningitis is treated for at least 7 days. Dexamethasone, 0.15 mg/kg intravenously every 6 hours, may reduce the incidence of long-term sequelae, principally hearing loss.

Sriram KB et al. Nontypeable *Haemophilus influenzae* and chronic obstructive pulmonary disease: a review for clinicians. Crit Rev Microbiol. 2018;44:125. [PMID: 28539074]

INFECTIONS CAUSED BY *MORAXELLA CATARRHALIS*

M catarrhalis is a gram-negative aerobic coccus morphologically and biochemically similar to *Neisseria*. It causes sinusitis, bronchitis, and pneumonia. Bacteremia and meningitis have also been reported in immunocompromised patients. The organism frequently colonizes the respiratory tract, making differentiation of colonization from infection difficult. If *M catarrhalis* is the predominant isolate, therapy is directed against it. *M catarrhalis* typically produces beta-lactamase and therefore is usually resistant to ampicillin and amoxicillin. It is susceptible to amoxicillin-clavulanate, ampicillin-sulbactam, trimethoprim-sulfamethoxazole, ciprofloxacin, and second- and third-generation cephalosporins.

LEGIONNAIRES DISEASE

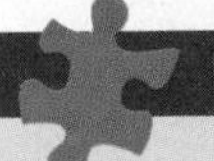

ESSENTIALS OF DIAGNOSIS

- Patients are often immunocompromised, smoke cigarettes, or have chronic lung disease.
- Scant sputum production, pleuritic chest pain, toxic appearance.
- Chest radiograph: focal patchy infiltrates or consolidation.
- Gram stain of sputum: polymorphonuclear leukocytes and no organisms.

General Considerations

Legionella infection ranks among the three or four most common causes of community-acquired pneumonia and is considered whenever the etiology of a pneumonia is in question. Legionnaires disease is more common in persons who smoke cigarettes and in those with chronic lung disease or who are immunocompromised. Outbreaks have been associated with contaminated water sources, such as showerheads and faucets in patient rooms and air conditioning cooling towers.

Clinical Findings

A. Symptoms and Signs

Legionnaires disease is one of the atypical pneumonias, so called because a Gram-stained smear of sputum does not show organisms. However, many features of Legionnaires disease are more like typical pneumonia, with high fevers, toxic appearance, pleurisy, and grossly purulent sputum. Nausea, vomiting, and diarrhea may be prominent. There may be relative bradycardia. Classically, this pneumonia is caused by *Legionella pneumophila*, though other species can cause identical disease.

B. Laboratory Findings

There may be hyponatremia, hypophosphatemia, elevated liver enzymes, and elevated creatine kinase. Culture of *Legionella* species has an 80–90% sensitivity. Testing sputum samples using polymerase chain reaction is as a highly sensitive method for diagnosing *Legionella*. Dieterle silver staining of tissue, pleural fluid, or other infected material is also a reliable method for detecting *Legionella* species. Direct fluorescent antibody stains and serologic testing such as urinary antigen are less sensitive because these will detect only *L pneumophila* serotype 1.

Treatment

Azithromycin (500 mg orally once daily), clarithromycin (500 mg orally twice daily), or a fluoroquinolone (eg, levofloxacin, 750 mg orally once daily), and not erythromycin, are the drugs of choice for treatment of legionellosis. Duration of therapy is 10–14 days, although a 21-day course of therapy is recommended for immunocompromised patients.

Herwaldt LA et al. Legionella: a reemerging pathogen. Curr Opin Infect Dis. 2018;31:325. [PMID: 29794542]

GRAM-NEGATIVE BACTEREMIA & SEPSIS

Gram-negative bacteremia can originate in a number of sites, the most common being the genitourinary system, hepatobiliary tract, GI tract, and lungs. Less common sources include intravenous lines, infusion fluids, surgical wounds, drains, and pressure injuries.

Patients with potentially fatal underlying conditions in the short term such as neutropenia or immunosuppression have a mortality rate of 40–60%; those with serious underlying diseases likely to be fatal in 5 years, such as solid tumors, cirrhosis, and aplastic anemia, die in 15–20% of cases; and individuals with no underlying diseases have a mortality rate of 5% or less.

Clinical Findings

A. Symptoms and Signs

Most patients have fevers and chills, often with abrupt onset. However, 15% of patients are hypothermic (temperature 36.4°C or less) at presentation, and 5% never develop a temperature above 37.5°C. Hyperventilation with respiratory alkalosis and changes in mental status are important early manifestations. Hypotension and shock, which occur in 20–50% of patients, are unfavorable prognostic signs.

B. Laboratory Findings

Neutropenia or neutrophilia, often with increased numbers of immature forms of polymorphonuclear leukocytes, is the most common laboratory abnormality in septic patients. Thrombocytopenia occurs in 50% of patients, laboratory evidence of coagulation abnormalities in 10%, and overt disseminated intravascular coagulation in 2–3%. Both clinical manifestations and the laboratory abnormalities are nonspecific and insensitive, which accounts for the relatively low rate of blood culture positivity (approximately 20–40%). Two sets of blood cultures from separate sites should be obtained starting antimicrobial therapy. The false-negative rate for a single culture of 5–10 mL of blood is 30%. This may be reduced to 5–10% (albeit with a slight false-positive rate due to isolation of contaminants) if a single volume of 30 mL is inoculated into several blood culture bottles. When a patient with presumed septic shock, negative blood cultures, and inadequate explanation for the clinical course responds to antimicrobial agents, therapy should be continued for 10–14 days.

Treatment

Several factors are important in the management of sepsis.

A. Removal of Predisposing Factors

This usually means decreasing or stopping immunosuppressive medications and, in certain circumstances, giving granulocyte colony-stimulating factor (filgrastim; G-CSF) to the neutropenic patient.

B. Identifying the Source of Bacteremia

By simply finding the source of bacteremia and removing it (central venous catheter) or draining it (abscess), a fatal disease becomes easily treatable.

C. Supportive Measures

The use of fluids, vasopressors, and corticosteroids in septic shock is discussed in Chapter 14. Management of disseminated intravascular coagulation is discussed in Chapter 13.

D. Antibiotics

Antibiotics should be given as soon as the diagnosis is suspected, since delays in therapy have been associated with increased mortality rates, particularly once hypotension develops. In general, bactericidal antibiotics should be used and given intravenously to ensure therapeutic serum levels. Penetration of antibiotics into the site of primary infection is critical for successful therapy—ie, if the infection originates in the CNS, antibiotics that penetrate the blood-brain barrier should be used—eg, third- or fourth-generation cephalosporin—but not first-generation cephalosporins or aminoglycosides, which penetrate poorly. Sepsis caused by gram-positive organisms cannot be differentiated on clinical grounds from that due to gram-negative bacteria. Therefore, initial therapy should include antibiotics active against both types of organisms. Administering a beta-lactam prior to vancomycin as the first dose of antibiotic has been shown to improve survival in patients with bloodstream infections.

The number of antibiotics necessary remains controversial and depends on the cause. Table 30–4 provides a guide for empiric therapy. Although a combination of antibiotics is often recommended for "synergism," combination therapy has not been shown to be superior to a single-drug regimen with any of several broad-spectrum antibiotics (eg, a third-generation cephalosporin, piperacillin-tazobactam, carbapenem). If multiple drugs are used initially, the regimen should be modified and coverage narrowed based on the results of culture and sensitivity testing. Rapid molecular diagnostic testing on positive blood cultures can decrease time to species identification and detection of resistance mechanisms.

Goal-directed therapy (see Chapter 12) for gram-negative bacteremia may be treated with as few as 7 days of antibiotic therapy.

Aillet C et al. Bacteraemia in emergency departments: effective antibiotic reassessment is associated with a better outcome. Eur J Clin Microbiol Infect Dis. 2018;37:325. [PMID: 29164361]

Rhodes A et al. Surviving Sepsis Campaign: international guidelines for management of sepsis and septic shock: 2016. Intensive Care Med. 2017;43:304. [PMID: 28101605]

Yahav D et al; Bacteremia Duration Study Group. Seven versus 14 days of antibiotic therapy for uncomplicated gram-negative bacteremia: a noninferiority randomized controlled trial. Clin Infect Dis. 2019;69:1091. [PMID: 30535100]

SALMONELLOSIS

Salmonellosis includes infection by any of approximately 2000 serotypes of salmonellae. Human infections are caused almost exclusively by *S enterica* subsp *enterica*, of which three serotypes—*typhi*, *typhimurium*, and *enteriditis*—are predominantly isolated. Three clinical patterns of infection are recognized: (1) enteric fever, for example, typhoid fever, due to serotype *typhi*; (2) acute enterocolitis, caused by serotype *typhimurium*, among others; and (3) the "septicemic" type, characterized by bacteremia and focal lesions. All types are transmitted by ingestion of the organism, usually from tainted food or drink.

1. Enteric Fever (Typhoid Fever)

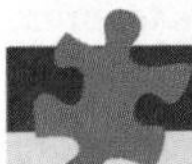

ESSENTIALS OF DIAGNOSIS

- Gradual onset of headache, vomiting, abdominal pain.
- Rose spots, relative bradycardia, splenomegaly, and abdominal distention and tenderness.
- Slow (stepladder) rise of fever to maximum and then slow return to normal.
- Leukopenia; blood, stool, and urine cultures positive for *Salmonella*.

General Considerations

Enteric fever is a clinical syndrome characterized by GI symptoms as well as constitutional symptoms such as fever, malaise, and headache. It may have a long incubation period (6–30 days), and the GI symptoms may resolve but then recur. Progressive infection often evolves with delirium. Enteric fever is caused by typhoidal strains of *Salmonella, S typhi* (typhoid fever) and to a lesser extent S *paratyphi* (subtypes A, B and C). Infection begins when organisms breach the mucosal epithelium of the intestines. Having crossed the epithelial barrier, organisms invade and replicate in macrophages in Peyer patches, mesenteric lymph nodes, and the spleen. Serotypes other than *typhi* usually do not cause invasive disease, presumably because they lack the necessary human-specific virulence factors. Bacteremia occurs, and the infection then localizes principally in the lymphoid tissue of the small intestine. Peyer patches become inflamed and may ulcerate, with involvement greatest during the third week of disease. The organism may disseminate to the lungs, gallbladder, kidneys, or CNS.

Clinical Findings

A. Symptoms and Signs

During the prodromal stage, there is increasing malaise, headache, cough, and sore throat, often with abdominal pain and constipation, while the fever ascends in a stepwise fashion. After about 7–10 days, it reaches a plateau and the patient is much more ill. There may be marked constipation, especially early, or "pea soup" diarrhea; marked abdominal distention occurs as well. If there are no complications, the patient's condition will gradually improve over 7–10 days. However, relapse may occur for up to 2 weeks after defervescence.

During the early prodrome, physical findings are few. Later, splenomegaly, abdominal distention and tenderness, relative bradycardia, and occasionally meningismus appear. The rash (rose spots) commonly appears during the second week of disease. The individual spot, found principally on the trunk, is a pink papule 2–3 mm in diameter that fades on pressure. It disappears in 3–4 days.

B. Laboratory Findings

Unlike with other causes of gram-negative bacteremia, most patients with enteric fever do not have leukocytosis and leukopenia can be observed. Transaminitis is common. Typhoid fever is best diagnosed by blood culture, which is positive in the first week of illness in 80% of patients who have not taken antimicrobials. The rate of positivity declines thereafter, but one-fourth or more of patients still have positive blood cultures in the third week. Cultures of bone marrow occasionally are positive when blood cultures are not. Stool cultures are often negative by the time systemic symptoms develop.

Differential Diagnosis

Enteric fever must be distinguished from other GI illnesses and from other infections that have few localizing findings. Examples include tuberculosis, infective endocarditis, brucellosis, lymphoma, and Q fever. Often there is a history of recent travel to endemic areas; consider viral hepatitis, malaria, or amebiasis.

Complications

Complications occur in about 30% of untreated cases and account for 75% of deaths. Intestinal hemorrhage, manifested by a sudden drop in temperature and signs of shock followed by dark or fresh blood in the stool, or intestinal perforation, accompanied by abdominal pain and tenderness, is most likely to occur during the third week. Appearance of leukocytosis and tachycardia should suggest these complications. Urinary retention, pneumonia, thrombophlebitis, myocarditis, neurologic complications, cholecystitis, nephritis, osteomyelitis, and meningitis are less often observed.

Prevention

Immunization is not always effective but should be considered for household contacts of a typhoid carrier, for travelers to endemic areas, and during epidemic outbreaks. A multiple-dose oral vaccine and a single-dose parenteral vaccine are available. Their efficacies are similar, but oral vaccine causes fewer side effects. Boosters, when indicated, should be given every 5 years and 2 years for oral and parenteral preparations, respectively.

Adequate waste disposal and protection of food and water supplies from contamination are important public health measures to prevent salmonellosis. Carriers cannot work as food handlers.

Treatment

A. Specific Measures

Because of high antimicrobial resistance, fluoroquinolones—such as ciprofloxacin 750 mg orally twice daily or levofloxacin 500 mg orally once daily, 5–7 days for uncomplicated enteric fever and 10–14 days for severe infection—are the agents of choice for treatment of *Salmonella* infections. Ceftriaxone, 2 g intravenously for 7 days, is also effective. Although resistance to fluoroquinolones or cephalosporins occurs uncommonly, the prevalence is increasing, and extensively drug-resistant *S typhi* has emerged in South Asia in recent years. When an infection is caused by a multidrug-resistant strain, select an antibiotic to which the isolate is susceptible in vitro. There is global resistance to ampicillin, chloramphenicol, and trimethoprim-sulfamethoxazole.

B. Treatment of Carriers

Ciprofloxacin, 750 mg orally twice a day for 4 weeks, has proved to be highly effective in eradicating the carrier state. When the isolate is susceptible, treatment of carriage with ampicillin, trimethoprim-sulfamethoxazole, or chloramphenicol may be successful. *Salmonella* may sequester in the gallbladder; cholecystectomy may be required if prolonged antimicrobial therapy fails.

Prognosis

The mortality rate of typhoid fever is about 2% in treated cases. Older or debilitated persons are likely to do worse. With complications, the prognosis is poor. Relapses occur in up to 15% of cases. A residual carrier state frequently persists despite therapy.

Marchello CS et al. A systematic review on antimicrobial resistance among *Salmonella* Typhi worldwide. Am J Trop Med Hyg. 2020;103:2518. [PMID: 32996447]
Wain J et al. Typhoid fever. Lancet. 2015;385:1136. [PMID: 25458731]

2. *Salmonella* Gastroenteritis

By far the most common form of salmonellosis is acute enterocolitis, which is typically caused by non-typhoidal *Salmonella*. The incubation period is 8–48 hours after ingestion of contaminated food or liquid.

Symptoms and signs consist of fever (often with chills), nausea and vomiting, cramping abdominal pain, and diarrhea, which may be grossly bloody, lasting 3–5 days. Differentiation must be made from viral gastroenteritis, food poisoning, shigellosis, amebic dysentery, and acute ulcerative colitis. The diagnosis is made by culturing the organism from the stool. The disease is usually self-limited, but bacteremia with localization in joints or bones may occur, especially in patients with sickle cell disease.

In most cases, treatment of uncomplicated enterocolitis is symptomatic only as most illnesses are self-limited and antimicrobial treatment may prolong bacterial shedding. However, patients who are malnourished or severely ill, patients with sickle cell disease, and patients who are immunocompromised (including those with HIV infection) should be treated with ciprofloxacin, 500 mg orally twice a day; ceftriaxone, 1 g intravenously once daily; trimethoprim-sulfamethoxazole, 160 mg/80 mg orally twice a day; or azithromycin, 500 mg orally once daily for 7–14 days (14 days for immunocompromised patients).

Shane AL et al. 2017 Infectious Diseases Society of America clinical practice guidelines for the diagnosis and management of infectious diarrhea. Clin Infect Dis. 2017;65:1963. [PMID: 29194529]

3. *Salmonella* Bacteremia

Salmonella infection may be manifested by prolonged or recurrent fevers accompanied by bacteremia and local infection in bone, joints, pleura, pericardium, lungs, or other sites. Mycotic aortic aneurysms may also occur. This complication of bacteremia tends to occur in immunocompromised persons, including persons with HIV infection, or in older adults with preexisting aneurysms or atherosclerotic plaques. Serotypes other than typhi usually are isolated. Treatment requires systemic antimicrobial therapy (duration depends on the site of infection) plus drainage of any abscesses. In patients with HIV infection, relapse is common, and lifelong suppressive therapy may be needed. Ciprofloxacin, 750 mg orally twice a day, is effective both for therapy of acute infection and for suppression of recurrence. Incidence of infections caused by drug-resistant strains may be on the rise.

Crump JA et al. Epidemiology, clinical presentation, laboratory diagnosis, antimicrobial resistance, and antimicrobial management of invasive *Salmonella* infections. Clin Microbiol Rev. 2015;28:901. [PMID: 26180063]

SHIGELLOSIS

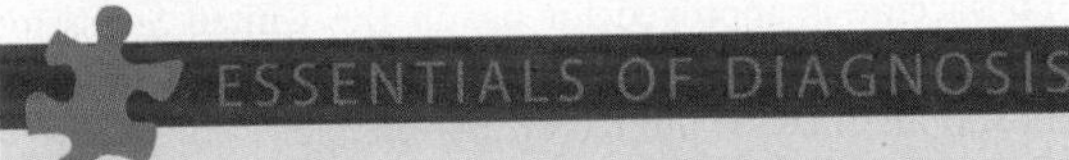

- Diarrhea, often with blood and mucus.
- Crampy abdominal pain and systemic toxicity.
- Leukocytes in stool; positive stool culture.

General Considerations

Shigella dysentery is a common disease, often self-limited and mild but occasionally serious. *S sonnei* is the leading cause in the United States, followed by *S flexneri*. *S dysenteriae* causes the most serious form of the illness. Shigellae are invasive organisms. The infective dose is low at 10^2–10^3 organisms. Shigellosis is highly transmissible via the fecal route including ingestion of contaminated food and water and oral anal sexual contact. There has been a rise in strains resistant to multiple antibiotics.

Clinical Findings

A. Symptoms and Signs

The illness usually starts abruptly, with diarrhea, lower abdominal cramps, and tenesmus. The diarrheal stool often is mixed with blood and mucus. Systemic symptoms are fever, chills, anorexia and malaise, and headache. The abdomen is tender. Sigmoidoscopic examination reveals an inflamed, engorged mucosa with punctate and sometimes large areas of ulceration.

B. Laboratory Findings

The stool shows many leukocytes and red cells. Stool culture is positive for *Shigella* in most cases, but blood cultures grow the organism in less than 5% of cases.

Differential Diagnosis

Bacillary dysentery must be distinguished from *Salmonella* enterocolitis and from disease due to enterotoxigenic *Escherichia coli*, *Campylobacter*, and *Yersinia enterocolitica*. Amebic dysentery may be similar clinically and is diagnosed by finding amoebas in the fresh stool specimen. Ulcerative colitis is another cause of bloody diarrhea.

Complications

Temporary disaccharidase deficiency may follow the diarrhea. Reactive arthritis is an uncommon complication, usually occurring in HLA-B27 individuals infected by *Shigella*. Hemolytic-uremic syndrome occurs rarely.

Treatment

Treatment of dehydration and hypotension is lifesaving in severe cases. Recommended empiric antimicrobial therapy is either a fluoroquinolone (ciprofloxacin, 750 mg orally twice daily for 7–10 days, or levofloxacin, 500 mg orally once daily for 3 days) or ceftriaxone, 1 g intravenously once daily for 5 days. If the isolate is susceptible, trimethoprim-sulfamethoxazole, 160/80 mg orally twice daily for 5 days, or azithromycin, 500 mg orally once daily for 3 days, is also effective. High rates of resistance to amoxicillin make it a less effective treatment option.

Shane AL et al. 2017 Infectious Diseases Society of America clinical practice guidelines for the diagnosis and management of infectious diarrhea. Clin Infect Dis. 2017;65:1963. [PMID: 29194529]

GASTROENTERITIS CAUSED BY *ESCHERICHIA COLI*

E coli causes gastroenteritis by a variety of mechanisms. Enterotoxigenic *E coli* (ETEC) elaborates either a heat-stable or heat-labile toxin that mediates the disease. ETEC is an important cause of traveler's diarrhea (see Chapter 30, Traveler's Diarrhea). Enteroinvasive *E coli* (EIEC) differs from other *E coli* bowel pathogens in that these strains invade cells, causing bloody diarrhea and dysentery similar to infection with *Shigella* species. EIEC is uncommon in the United States. Neither ETEC nor EIEC strains are routinely isolated and identified from stool cultures because there is no selective medium but can be detected on stool-based multiplex-PCR. Antimicrobial therapy, such as ciprofloxacin 500 mg orally twice daily, shortens the clinical course, but the disease is self-limited.

Shiga-toxin–producing *E coli* (STEC) infection can result in asymptomatic carrier stage, nonbloody diarrhea, hemorrhagic colitis, hemolytic-uremic syndrome, or thrombotic thrombocytopenic purpura. Although *E coli* O157:H7 is responsible for most cases of STEC infection in the United States, other STEC strains that cause severe disease (such as *E coli* O104:H4) have been reported in Europe. *E coli* O157:H7 has caused several outbreaks of diarrhea and hemolytic-uremic syndrome related to consumption of undercooked hamburger, raw flour, unpasteurized apple juice, and spinach, while *E coli* O145 was linked to the consumption of contaminated lettuce. Older individuals and young children are most affected, with hemolytic-uremic syndrome being more common in the latter group. STEC identification can be difficult. The CDC recommends that all stools submitted for routine testing from patients with acute community-acquired diarrhea be simultaneously cultured for *E coli* O157:H7 and tested for Shiga toxins to detect non-O157 STEC, such as *E coli* O145. Antimicrobial therapy does not alter the course of the disease and may increase the risk of hemolytic-uremic syndrome. Treatment is primarily supportive. Hemolytic-uremic syndrome or thrombotic thrombocytopenic purpura occurring in association with a diarrheal illness suggests the diagnosis and should prompt evaluation for STEC. Confirmed infections should be reported to public health officials.

Tack D et al. Preliminary incidence and trends of infections with pathogens transmitted commonly through food—Foodborne Diseases Active Surveillance Network, 10 U.S. Sites, 2016–2019. MMWR Morb Mortal Wkly Rep. 2020;69:508. [PMID: 3235295]

CHOLERA

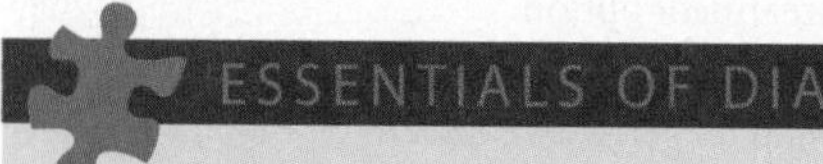

- History of travel in endemic area or contact with infected person.
- Voluminous diarrhea (up to 15 L/day).
- Characteristic "rice water stool."
- Rapid development of marked dehydration.
- Positive stool cultures.

General Considerations

Cholera is an acute diarrheal illness caused by certain serotypes of *Vibrio cholerae*. The disease is toxin-mediated, and fever is unusual. The toxin activates adenylyl cyclase in intestinal epithelial cells of the small intestines, producing hypersecretion of water and chloride ion and a massive diarrhea of up to 15 L/day. Death results from profound hypovolemia. Cholera occurs in epidemics under conditions of crowding, war, and famine (eg, in refugee camps) and where sanitation is inadequate. Infection is acquired by ingestion of contaminated food or water.

Clinical Findings

Cholera is characterized by a sudden onset of severe, frequent watery diarrhea (up to 1 L/hour). The liquid stool is gray; turbid; and without fecal odor, blood, or pus ("rice water stool"). Dehydration and hypotension develop rapidly. Stool cultures are positive, and agglutination of vibrios with specific sera can be demonstrated. Rapid antigen and PCR-based testing is also available.

Treatment

Treatment is primarily by replacement of fluids. In mild or moderate illness, oral rehydration usually is adequate. A simple oral replacement fluid can be made from 1/2 teaspoon of table salt and 6 level teaspoons of sugar added to 1 L of water. Intravenous fluids are indicated for persons with signs of severe hypovolemia and those who cannot take adequate fluids orally. Lactated Ringer infusion is satisfactory.

Antimicrobial therapy will shorten the course of illness and is indicated for severely ill patients. Antimicrobials active against *V cholerae* include tetracycline, ampicillin, trimethoprim-sulfamethoxazole, fluoroquinolones, and azithromycin. Multidrug-resistant strains exist, so susceptibility testing, if available, is advisable. A single 1 g oral dose of azithromycin is effective for severe cholera caused by strains with reduced susceptibility to fluoroquinolones, but resistance is emerging to this drug as well.

Prevention

Oral cholera vaccines are available that confer short-lived, limited protection and may be required for entry into or reentry after travel to some countries. One live attenuated oral vaccine is approved for use in the United States for persons traveling to areas of active cholera transmission, but supplies may be limited or unavailable.

Vaccination programs are expensive and not effective in managing outbreaks of cholera. When outbreaks occur, efforts should be directed toward establishing clean water and food sources and proper waste disposal.

Clemens JD et al. Cholera. Lancet. 2017;390:1539. [PMID: 28302312]

Wong KK et al. Recommendations of the Advisory Committee on Immunization Practices for use of cholera vaccine. MMWR Morb Mortal Wkly Rep. 2017;66:482. [PMID: 28493859]

INFECTIONS CAUSED BY OTHER *VIBRIO* SPECIES

Vibrios other than *V cholerae* that cause human disease are *Vibrio parahaemolyticus*, *V vulnificus*, and *V alginolyticus*. All are halophilic marine organisms. Infection is acquired by exposure to organisms in contaminated, undercooked, or raw crustaceans or shellfish and warm (greater than 20°C [82.4°F]) ocean waters and estuaries. Infections are more common during the summer months from regions along the Atlantic coast and the Gulf of Mexico in the United States and from tropical waters around the world. Oysters are implicated in up to 90% of food-related cases. *V parahaemolyticus* causes an acute watery diarrhea with crampy abdominal pain and fever, typically occurring within 24 hours after ingestion of contaminated shellfish. The disease is self-limited, and antimicrobial therapy is usually not necessary. Patients with chronic liver disease and those who are immunocompromised should be cautioned to avoid eating raw oysters. *V parahaemolyticus* may also cause cellulitis and sepsis, though these findings are more characteristic of *V vulnificus* infection.

V vulnificus and *V alginolyticus*—neither of which is associated with diarrheal illness—are important causes of cellulitis, wound infections, and primary bacteremia following exposure to sea water or ingestion of contaminated shellfish. Cellulitis with or without sepsis may be accompanied by bulla formation and necrosis with extensive soft tissue destruction, at times requiring debridement and amputation. The infection can be rapidly progressive and is particularly severe in immunocompromised individuals—especially those with cirrhosis—with death rates as high as 50%.

Doxycycline 100 mg orally twice daily plus ceftriaxone 2 g intravenously daily for 7–10 days is the drug of choice for treatment of suspected or documented primary bacteremia or cellulitis caused by *Vibrio* species. *V vulnificus* is susceptible in vitro to penicillin, ampicillin, cephalosporins, chloramphenicol, aminoglycosides, and fluoroquinolones, and these agents may also be effective. *V parahaemolyticus* and *V alginolyticus* produce beta-lactamase and therefore are resistant to penicillin and ampicillin, but susceptibilities otherwise are similar to those listed for *V vulnificus*.

Baker-Austin C et al. *Vibrio vulnificus*: new insights into a deadly opportunistic pathogen. Environ Microbiol. 2018;20:423. [PMID: 29027375]

INFECTIONS CAUSED BY *CAMPYLOBACTER* SPECIES

Campylobacter organisms are microaerophilic, motile, gram-negative rods. Two species infect humans: *Campylobacter jejuni*, an important cause of diarrheal disease, and *C fetus* subsp *fetus*, which typically causes systemic infection and less frequently gastroenteritis. Dairy cattle and poultry are an important reservoir for campylobacters. Outbreaks of enteritis have been associated with consumption of raw milk. *Campylobacter* gastroenteritis is associated with fever, abdominal pain, and diarrhea characterized by loose, watery, or bloody stools. The differential diagnosis includes shigellosis, *Salmonella* gastroenteritis, and enteritis caused by *Y enterocolitica* or invasive *E coli*. The disease is self-limited, but its duration can be shortened with antimicrobial therapy. Either azithromycin, 1 g orally as a single dose, or ciprofloxacin, 500 mg orally twice daily for 3 days, is effective therapy. However, *C jejuni* isolates may be resistant to fluoroquinolone, particularly in Southeast Asia, and susceptibility testing should be confirmed.

C fetus causes systemic infections that can be fatal, including primary bacteremia, endocarditis, meningitis, and focal abscesses. It infrequently causes gastroenteritis. Patients infected with *C fetus* are often older, debilitated, or immunocompromised. Closely related species, collectively termed "*campylobacter*-like organisms," cause bacteremia in persons with HIV infection. Systemic infections respond to therapy with gentamicin, carbapenems, ceftriaxone, or ciprofloxacin. Ceftriaxone, meropenem, or chloramphenicol should be used to treat infections of the CNS because of their ability to penetrate the blood-brain barrier.

Heimesaat MM et al. Human Campylobacteriosis—a serious infectious threat in a one health perspective. Curr Top Microbiol Immunol. 2021;431:1. [PMID: 33620646]

Shane AL et al. 2017 Infectious Diseases Society of America clinical practice guidelines for the diagnosis and management of infectious diarrhea. Clin Infect Dis. 2017;65:1963. [PMID: 29194529]

TULAREMIA

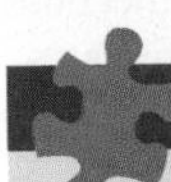

ESSENTIALS OF DIAGNOSIS

- History of contact with rabbits, other rodents, and biting ticks in summer in endemic area.
- Fever, headache, nausea, and prostration.
- Papule progressing to ulcer at site of inoculation.
- Enlarged regional lymph nodes.
- Positive serologic tests or culture of ulcer, lymph node aspirate, or blood.

General Considerations

Tularemia is a zoonotic infection of wild rodents and rabbits caused by *Francisella tularensis*. Humans usually acquire the infection by contact with animal tissues (eg, trapping muskrats, skinning rabbits) or from a tick or insect bite. Hamsters and prairie dogs also may carry the organism. An outbreak of pneumonic tularemia in 2000 on Martha's Vineyard in Massachusetts was linked to lawn-mowing and brush-cutting as risk factors for infection, underscoring the potential for aerosol transmission of the organism. *F tularensis* has been classified as a high-priority agent for potential bioterrorism use because of its virulence and relative ease of dissemination. Infection in humans often produces a local lesion and widespread organ involvement but may be entirely asymptomatic. The incubation period is typically 3–5 days.

Clinical Findings

A. Symptoms and Signs

Fever, headache, and nausea begin suddenly, and a local lesion—a papule at the site of inoculation—develops and soon ulcerates. Regional lymph nodes may become enlarged and tender and may suppurate. The local lesion may be on the skin of an extremity or in the eye. Pneumonia may develop from hematogenous spread of the organism or may be primary after inhalation of infected aerosols. Following ingestion of infected meat or water, an enteric form may be manifested by GI symptoms, stupor, and delirium. In any type of involvement, the spleen may be enlarged and tender and there may be nonspecific rashes, myalgias, and prostration.

B. Laboratory Findings

Culturing the organism from blood or infected tissue requires special media. For this reason and because cultures of *F tularensis* may be hazardous to laboratory personnel, the diagnosis is usually made serologically. A positive agglutination test (greater than 1:80) develops in the second week after infection and may persist for several years.

Differential Diagnosis

Tularemia must be differentiated from rickettsial and meningococcal infections, cat-scratch disease, infectious mononucleosis, and various bacterial and fungal diseases.

Complications

Hematogenous spread may produce meningitis, perisplenitis, pericarditis, pneumonia, and osteomyelitis.

Treatment

Streptomycin is the drug of choice; the recommended dose is 7.5 mg/kg intramuscularly every 12 hours for 7–14 days. Gentamicin, which has good in vitro activity against *F tularensis*, is generally less toxic than streptomycin but some case series report lower treatment success rates. Doxycycline (200 mg/day orally) is also effective but has a higher relapse rate and should only be used for the less seriously ill. A variety of other agents (eg, fluoroquinolones) are active in vitro, but their clinical effectiveness is not well established.

Maurin M et al. Tularaemia: clinical aspects in Europe. Lancet Infect Dis. 2016;16:113. [PMID: 26738841]

PLAGUE

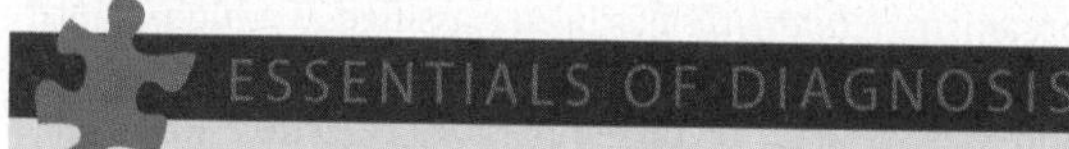

- History of exposure to rodents in endemic area.
- Sudden onset of high fever, muscular pains, and prostration.
- Axillary, cervical, or inguinal lymphadenitis (bubo).
- Pustule or ulcer at inoculation site.
- Pneumonia or meningitis is often fatal.
- Positive smear and culture from bubo and positive blood culture.

General Considerations

Plague is a zoonotic infection carried by wild rodents and caused by *Yersinia pestis*, a small bipolar-staining gram-negative rod. It is endemic in California, Arizona, Nevada, and New Mexico. Worldwide, Madagascar accounts for three-quarters of the global burden. It is transmitted among rodents and to humans by the bites of fleas or from contact with infected animals. Following a fleabite, the organisms spread through the lymphatics to the lymph nodes, which become greatly enlarged (buboes). They may then reach the bloodstream to involve all organs. When pneumonia or meningitis develops, the outcome is often fatal. The patient with pneumonia can transmit the infection to other individuals by droplets. The incubation period is 2–10 days. Because of its extreme virulence, its potential for dissemination and person-to-person transmission, and efforts to develop the organism as an agent of biowarfare, plague bacillus is considered a high-priority agent for bioterrorism.

Clinical Findings

A. Symptoms and Signs

The onset is sudden, with high fever, malaise, tachycardia, intense headache, delirium, and severe myalgias. The patient appears profoundly ill. If pneumonia develops, tachypnea, productive cough, blood-tinged sputum, and cyanosis also occur. There may be signs of meningitis. A pustule or ulcer at the site of inoculation may be observed. Axillary, inguinal, or cervical lymph nodes become enlarged and tender and may suppurate and drain. With hematogenous spread, the patient may rapidly become toxic and comatose, with purpuric spots (black plague) appearing on the skin.

Primary pneumonic plague is a fulminant pneumonitis with bloody, frothy sputum and sepsis. It is usually fatal unless treatment is started within a few hours after onset.

B. Laboratory Findings

The plague bacillus may be found in smears from aspirates of buboes examined with Gram stain. Cultures from bubo aspirate or pus and blood are positive but may grow slowly. In convalescing patients, an antibody titer rise may be demonstrated by agglutination tests.

Differential Diagnosis

The lymphadenitis of plague is most commonly mistaken for the lymphadenitis accompanying staphylococcal or streptococcal infections of an extremity, sexually transmitted diseases such as lymphogranuloma venereum or syphilis, and tularemia. The systemic manifestations resemble those of enteric or rickettsial fevers, malaria, or influenza. The pneumonia resembles other bacterial pneumonias, and the meningitis is similar to those caused by other bacteria.

Prevention

Avoiding exposure to rodents and fleas in endemic areas is the best prevention strategy. Drug prophylaxis may provide temporary protection for persons exposed to the risk of plague infection, particularly by the respiratory route. Doxycycline, 100 mg orally twice daily for 7 days, is effective. No vaccine is available.

Treatment

Therapy should be started immediately once plague is suspected. Either streptomycin (the agent with which there is greatest experience), 1 g every 12 hours intravenously, or gentamicin, 5 mg/kg every 24 hours, is effective.

Alternatively, doxycycline, 100 mg orally twice daily or intravenously every 12 hours, or a fluoroquinolone (ciprofloxacin, levofloxacin or moxifloxacin) may be used. The duration of therapy is 10 days. Patients with plague pneumonia are placed in strict respiratory isolation, and prophylactic therapy is given to any person who came in contact with the patient.

Godfred-Cato S et al. Treatment of human plague: a systematic review of published aggregate data on antimicrobial efficacy, 1939-2019. Clin Infect Dis. 2020;70:S11. [PMID: 32435800]

GONOCOCCAL INFECTIONS

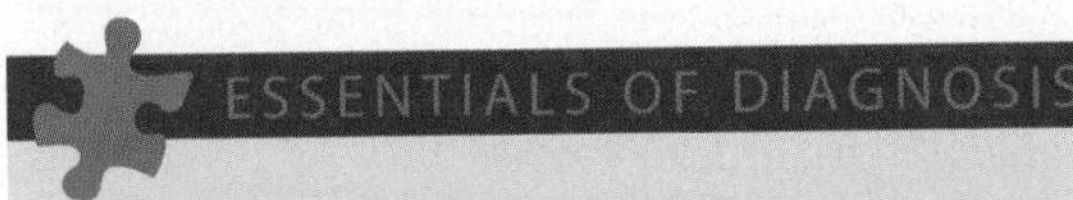

- Purulent, profuse urethral discharge with dysuria, especially in men; yields positive smear.
- **Men:** urethritis, epididymitis, prostatitis, proctitis, pharyngitis.
- **Women:** cervicitis with purulent discharge, or asymptomatic, yielding positive culture; vaginitis, salpingitis, proctitis also occur.
- **Disseminated disease:** fever, rash, tenosynovitis, and arthritis.
- The preferred method of diagnosis is testing with nucleic acid amplification.

General Considerations

Gonorrhea is caused by *Neisseria gonorrhoeae*, a gram-negative diplococcus typically found inside polymorphonuclear cells. It is transmitted during sexual activity and has its greatest incidence in the 15- to 29-year-old age group. The incubation period is usually 2–8 days.

Clinical Findings

A. Urethritis and Cervicitis

1. Men—Initial symptoms seen in men include burning on urination and a serous or milky discharge. One to 3 days later, the urethral pain is more pronounced, and the discharge becomes yellow, creamy, and profuse, sometimes blood-tinged. The disorder may regress and become chronic or progress to involve the prostate, epididymis, and periurethral glands with painful inflammation. Chronic infection leads to prostatitis and urethral strictures. Rectal infection is common in men who have sex with men. Other sites of primary infection (eg, the pharynx) must always be considered. Asymptomatic infection is common and occurs in both sexes.

2. Women—Gonococcal infection in women often presents with dysuria, urinary frequency, and urgency, with a purulent urethral discharge. Vaginitis and cervicitis with inflammation of Bartholin glands are common. Infection may be asymptomatic, with only slightly increased vaginal discharge and moderate cervicitis on examination. Infection may remain as a chronic cervicitis—an important reservoir of gonococci. It can progress to involve the uterus and tubes with acute and chronic salpingitis, with scarring of tubes and sterility. In pelvic inflammatory disease, anaerobes and chlamydia often accompany gonococci. Rectal infection may result from spread of the organism from the genital tract or from anal coitus.

Nucleic acid amplification tests are the preferred method for diagnosing gonorrhea at all sites given their excellent sensitivity and specificity. In women with suspected cervical infection, endocervical or vaginal swabs (clinician- or self-collected) as well as first catch am urine specimen (later specimens have 10% reduced sensitivity) are options. In men with urethral infection, first catch am urine is recommended. Nucleic acid amplification tests are also recommended by the CDC for oropharyngeal and rectal site swab testing. Urine testing does not detect oropharyngeal and rectal gonorrhea unless there is concurrent genital infection. Gram stain of urethral or rectal discharge in men, especially during the first week after onset, shows gram-negative diplococci in polymorphonuclear leukocytes. Gram stain is less often positive in women. Cultures should still be obtained when evaluating a treatment failure to assess for antimicrobial resistance.

B. Disseminated Disease

Systemic complications follow the dissemination of gonococci from the primary site via the bloodstream. Two distinct clinical syndromes—either purulent arthritis or the triad of rash, tenosynovitis, and arthralgias—are commonly observed in patients with disseminated gonococcal infection, although overlap can be seen. The skin lesions can range from maculopapular to pustular or hemorrhagic, which tend to be few in number and peripherally located. The tenosynovitis is often found in the hands and wrists and feet and ankles. These unique findings can help distinguish among other infectious syndromes. The arthritis can occur in one or more joints and may be migratory. Gonococci are isolated by culture from less than half of patients with gonococcal arthritis. Nucleic acid amplification can be performed on synovial fluid, if available, and may be more sensitive for the diagnosis. Rarely, gonococcal endocarditis or meningitis develops.

C. Conjunctivitis

The most common form of eye involvement is direct inoculation of gonococci into the conjunctival sac. In adults, this occurs by autoinoculation of a person with genital infection. The purulent conjunctivitis may rapidly progress to panophthalmitis and loss of the eye unless treated promptly.

Differential Diagnosis

Gonococcal urethritis or cervicitis must be differentiated from nongonococcal urethritis; cervicitis or vaginitis due to *Chlamydia trachomatis*, *Gardnerella vaginalis*, *Trichomonas*, *Candida*, and other pathogens associated with sexually transmitted diseases; and pelvic inflammatory disease, arthritis, proctitis, and skin lesions. Often, several such pathogens coexist in a patient. Reactive arthritis (urethritis, conjunctivitis, arthritis) may mimic gonorrhea or coexist with it.

Prevention

Prevention is based on education and mechanical or chemical prophylaxis. The condom, if properly used, can reduce the risk of infection. Partner notification and referral of contacts for treatment has been the standard method used to control sexually transmitted diseases. Early treatment of contacts can halt the development of symptoms as well. Expedited treatment of sex partners by patient-delivered partner therapy is more effective than partner notification in reducing persistence and recurrence rates of gonorrhea and chlamydia.

Treatment

Therapy typically is administered before antimicrobial susceptibilities are known. The choice of which regimen to use should be based on the national prevalence of antibiotic-resistant organisms. Nationwide, there are strains of gonococci that are resistant to penicillin, tetracycline, or ciprofloxacin. Consequently, these drugs are not considered first-line therapy. Resistance to azithromycin and to ceftriaxone has been reported. All sexual partners should be treated and tested for HIV infection and syphilis, as should the patient.

A. Uncomplicated Gonorrhea

Due to increasing resistance of *N gonorrhoeae* to cephalosporins, the CDC recommends a high dose of intramuscular ceftriaxone when chlamydial infection has been excluded. For uncomplicated gonococcal infections of the cervix, urethra, rectum, and pharynx, the recommended treatment is ceftriaxone (500 mg intramuscularly for patients who weigh less than 105 kg and 1 g intramuscularly for patients who weigh 150 kg or more). Cefixime, 800 mg orally as a single dose, should be used when an oral cephalosporin is the only option. When chlamydial infection has not been excluded, co-treatment of chlamydia with doxycycline 100 mg twice daily for 7 days is recommended. Fluoroquinolones are not recommended for treatment due to high rates of microbial resistance. A single dose of spectinomycin, 1 g intramuscularly, may be used for the penicillin-allergic patient but is not available in the United States.

B. Treatment of Other Infections

Disseminated gonococcal infection (including arthritis and arthritis-dermatitis syndromes) should be treated with ceftriaxone (1 g intravenously daily) until 48 hours after improvement begins, at which time therapy may be switched to an oral agent (eg, cefixime 400 mg orally daily), if susceptibility is confirmed, to complete at least 1 week of antimicrobial therapy. Endocarditis should be treated with ceftriaxone (2 g every 24 hours intravenously) for at least 4 weeks.

Pelvic inflammatory disease requires cefoxitin (2 g intravenously every 6 hours) or cefotetan (2 g intravenously every 12 hours) plus doxycycline (100 mg every 12 hours). Clindamycin (900 mg intravenously every 8 hours) plus gentamicin (administered intravenously as a 2-mg/kg loading dose followed by 1.5 mg/kg every 8 hours) is also effective. Ceftriaxone (500 mg intramuscularly as a single dose) or cefoxitin (2 g intramuscularly) plus probenecid (1 g orally as a single dose) plus doxycycline (100 mg twice a day for 14 days), with metronidazole (500 mg twice daily for 14 days), is an effective outpatient regimen.

De Ambrogi M. International forum on gonococcal infections and resistance. Lancet Infect Dis. 2017;17:1127. [PMID: 29115267]

St Cyr S et al. Update to CDC's treatment guidelines for gonococcal infection, 2020. MMWR Morb Mortal Wkly Rep. 2020;69:1911. [PMID: 33332296]

CHANCROID

Chancroid is a sexually transmitted disease caused by the short gram-negative bacillus *Haemophilus ducreyi*. The incubation period is 3–5 days. At the site of inoculation, a vesicopustule develops that breaks down to form a painful, soft ulcer with a necrotic base, surrounding erythema, and undermined edges. There may be multiple lesions due to autoinoculation. The adenitis is usually unilateral and consists of tender, matted nodes of moderate size with overlying erythema. These may become fluctuant and rupture spontaneously. With lymph node involvement, fever, chills, and malaise may develop. Balanitis and phimosis are frequent complications in men. Women may have no external signs of infection. The diagnosis is established by culturing a swab of the lesion onto a special medium.

Chancroid must be differentiated from other genital ulcers. The chancre of syphilis is clean and painless, with a hard base. Mixed sexually transmitted disease is very common (including syphilis, herpes simplex, and HIV infection), as is infection of the ulcer with fusiforms, spirochetes, and other organisms.

A single dose of either azithromycin, 1 g orally, or ceftriaxone, 250 mg intramuscularly, is effective treatment. Effective multiple-dose regimens are erythromycin, 500 mg orally four times a day for 7 days, or ciprofloxacin, 500 mg orally twice a day for 3 days.

Roett MA. Genital ulcers: differential diagnosis and management. Am Fam Physician. 2020;101:355. [PMID: 32163252]

Romero L et al. Macrolides for treatment of *Haemophilus ducreyi* infection in sexually active adults. Cochrane Database Syst Rev. 2017;12:CD012492. [PMID: 29226307]

GRANULOMA INGUINALE

Granuloma inguinale is a chronic, relapsing granulomatous anogenital infection due to *Klebsiella granulomatis* (previously known as *Calymmatobacterium granulomatis*). The pathognomonic cell, found in tissue scrapings or secretions, is large (25–90 mcm), and contains intracytoplasmic cysts filled with bodies (Donovan bodies) that stain deeply with Wright stain.

The incubation period is 8 days to 12 weeks. The onset is insidious. The lesions occur on the skin or mucous membranes of the genitalia or perineal area. They are relatively painless infiltrated nodules that soon slough. A shallow, sharply demarcated ulcer forms, with a beefy-red friable base of granulation tissue. The lesion spreads by contiguity. The advancing border has a characteristic rolled edge of granulation tissue. Large ulcerations may advance onto the lower abdomen and thighs. Scar formation and healing occur along one border while the opposite border advances.

Superinfection with spirochete-fusiform organisms is common. The ulcer then becomes purulent, painful, foul-smelling, and extremely difficult to treat.

Several therapies are available. Because of the indolent nature of the disease, duration of therapy is relatively long. The following recommended regimens should be given for 3 weeks or until all lesions have healed: azithromycin, 1 g orally once weekly (preferred); doxycycline, 100 mg orally twice daily; or azithromycin, 1 g orally once weekly; or ciprofloxacin, 750 mg orally twice daily; trimethoprim-sulfamethoxazole, 1 double-strength tablet orally twice a day; or erythromycin, 500 mg orally four times a day.

O'Farrell N et al. 2016 European guideline on donovanosis. Int J STD AIDS. 2016;27:605. [PMID: 26882914]

BARTONELLA SPECIES

Bartonella species are responsible for a wide variety of clinical syndromes. **Bacillary angiomatosis**, an important manifestation of bartonellosis, is discussed in Chapter 31. A variety of atypical infections, including retinitis, encephalitis, osteomyelitis, and persistent bacteremia and endocarditis (especially consider in culture-negative endocarditis), have been described.

Trench fever is a self-limited, louse-borne relapsing febrile disease caused by *B quintana*. The disease has occurred epidemically in louse-infested troops and civilians during wars and endemically in residents of scattered geographic areas (eg, Central America). An urban equivalent of trench fever has been described among persons who are homeless. Humans acquire infection when infected lice feces enter sites of skin breakdown. Onset of symptoms is abrupt and fever lasts 3–5 days, with relapses, although isolated febrile episodes and prolonged fevers can also occur. The patient complains of weakness and severe pain behind the eyes and typically in the back and legs. Lymphadenopathy, splenomegaly, and a transient maculopapular rash may appear. Subclinical infection is frequent, and a carrier state is recognized. The differential diagnosis includes other febrile, self-limited states such as dengue, leptospirosis, malaria, relapsing fever, and typhus. Optimal therapy is uncertain.

Cat-scratch disease is an acute infection of children and young adults caused by *Bartonella henselae*. It is transmitted from cats to humans as the result of a scratch or bite. Within a few days, a papule or ulcer will develop at the inoculation site in one-third of patients. One to 3 weeks later, fever, headache, and malaise occur. Regional lymph nodes become enlarged, often tender, and may suppurate. Lymphadenopathy from cat scratches resembles that due to neoplasm, tuberculosis, lymphogranuloma venereum, and bacterial lymphadenitis. The diagnosis is usually made clinically. Special cultures for bartonellae, serology, or excisional biopsy, though rarely necessary, confirm the diagnosis. The biopsy reveals necrotizing lymphadenitis and is itself not specific for cat-scratch disease. Cat-scratch disease is usually self-limited, requiring no specific therapy. Encephalitis occurs rarely.

Disseminated forms of the disease—bacillary angiomatosis, peliosis hepatis, and retinitis—occur most commonly in immunocompromised patients such as persons with late stages of HIV or solid organ transplant recipients. The lesions are vasculoproliferative and histopathologically distinct from those of cat-scratch disease. Unexplained fever in patients with late stages of HIV infection is not uncommonly due to bartonellosis. *B quintana*, the agent of trench fever, can also cause bacillary angiomatosis and persistent bacteremia or endocarditis (which will be "culture-negative" unless specifically sought), the latter two entities being associated with homelessness. Due to the fastidious nature of the organism and its special growth requirements, serologic testing (eg, demonstration of a high antibody titer in an indirect immunofluorescence assay) or nucleic acid amplification tests are often required to establish a diagnosis.

The disseminated forms of the disease (bacillary angiomatosis, peliosis hepatis, and retinitis) require a prolonged course of antibiotic therapy often in combination with a second agent. Bacteremia and endocarditis can be effectively treated with doxycycline (200 mg orally or intravenously in two divided doses per day) plus 2 weeks of either gentamicin (3 mg/kg/day intravenously) or rifampin (600 mg/day orally in two divided doses) followed by doxycycline monotherapy for a total duration of at least 3 months unless valve surgery has been performed, in which case treatment can be shortened to 6 weeks after valve surgery. Relapse may occur.

Okaro U et al. *Bartonella* species, an emerging cause of blood-culture-negative endocarditis. Clin Microbiol Rev. 2017;30:709. [PMID: 28490579]

ANAEROBIC INFECTIONS

Anaerobic infections tend to be polymicrobial and abscesses are common. Pus and infected tissue often are malodorous. Septic thrombophlebitis and metastatic infection are frequent and may require incision and drainage. Diminished blood supply that favors proliferation of anaerobes because of reduced tissue oxygenation may interfere with the delivery of antimicrobials to the site of anaerobic infection. Cultures, unless carefully collected under anaerobic conditions, may yield negative results.

Important types of infections that are most commonly caused by anaerobic organisms are listed below. Treatment of all these infections consists of surgical exploration and judicious excision in conjunction with administration of antimicrobial drugs.

1. Head & Neck Infections

Prevotella melaninogenica (formerly *Bacteroides melaninogenicus*) and anaerobic spirochetes are commonly involved in periodontal infections. These organisms, fusobacteria, and peptostreptococci may cause chronic sinusitis, peritonsillar abscess, chronic otitis media, and mastoiditis. *F necrophorum* has been recognized as a common cause of pharyngitis in adolescents and young adults. *F necrophorum* infection has been associated with septic internal jugular thrombophlebitis (Lemierre syndrome) and causes septic pulmonary embolization. Hygiene, drainage, and surgical debridement are as important in treatment as antimicrobials. Penicillin alone is inadequate treatment for infections from oral anaerobic organisms because of penicillin resistance, usually due to beta-lactamase production. Therefore, ampicillin/sulbactam 1.5–3 g intravenously every 6 hours (if parenteral therapy is required), or amoxicillin/clavulanic acid 875 mg/125 mg orally twice daily, or clindamycin can be used (600 mg intravenously every 8 hours or 300 mg orally every 6 hours). Antimicrobial treatment is continued for a few days after symptoms and signs of infection have resolved. Indolent, established infections (eg, mastoiditis or osteomyelitis) may require prolonged courses of therapy, eg, 4–6 weeks or longer.

2. Chest Infections

Usually in the setting of poor oral hygiene and periodontal disease, aspiration of saliva (which contains 10^8 anaerobic organisms per milliliter in addition to aerobes) may lead to necrotizing pneumonia, lung abscess, and empyema. Polymicrobial infection is the rule, and anaerobes—particularly *P melaninogenica*, fusobacteria, and peptostreptococci—are common etiologic agents. Most pulmonary infections respond to antimicrobial therapy alone. Percutaneous chest tube or surgical drainage is indicated for empyema.

Clindamycin, 600 mg intravenously once, followed by 300 mg orally every 6–8 hours, or ampicillin/sulbactam, 3 g intravenously every 6 hours, followed by amoxicillin/clavulanic acid, 875 mg/125 mg orally twice daily, are preferred regimens. Metronidazole does not cover facultative streptococci, which often are present, and if used, a second agent that is active against streptococci, such as ceftriaxone 1 g intravenously or intramuscularly daily, should be added. Moxifloxacin, 400 mg orally or intravenously once daily, may be used. Because these infections respond slowly, a prolonged course of therapy (eg, 4–6 weeks) is generally recommended.

3. Central Nervous System

Anaerobes are a common cause of brain abscess, subdural empyema, or septic CNS thrombophlebitis. The organisms reach the CNS by direct extension from sinusitis, otitis, or mastoiditis or by hematogenous spread from chronic lung infections. Antimicrobial therapy—eg, ceftriaxone, 2 g intravenously every 12 hours, plus metronidazole, 500 mg intravenously every 8 hours—is an important adjunct to surgical drainage. Duration of therapy is 6–8 weeks but should be based on follow-up imaging. Some small multiple brain abscesses can be treated with antibiotics alone without surgical drainage.

4. Intra-Abdominal Infections

In the colon there are up to 10^{11} anaerobes per gram of content—predominantly *B fragilis*, clostridia, and peptostreptococci. These organisms play a central role in most intra-abdominal abscesses following trauma to the colon, as well as diverticulitis, appendicitis, perirectal abscess, hepatic abscess, and cholecystitis, often in association with aerobic coliform bacteria. The bacteriology includes anaerobes as well as enteric gram-negative rods and on occasion enterococci. Therapy should be directed both against anaerobes and gram-negative aerobes. Agents that are active against *B fragilis* include metronidazole, chloramphenicol, moxifloxacin, tigecycline, ertapenem, imipenem, meropenem, ampicillin-sulbactam, ticarcillin-clavulanic acid, and piperacillin-tazobactam. Resistance to cefoxitin, cefotetan, and clindamycin is increasingly encountered. Most third-generation cephalosporins have poor efficacy.

Table 33–6 summarizes the antibiotic regimens for management of moderate to moderately severe infections (eg, patient hemodynamically stable, good surgical drainage possible or established, low APACHE score, no multiple organ failure) and severe infections (eg, major peritoneal soilage, large or multiple abscesses, patient hemodynamically unstable), particularly if drug-resistant organisms are suspected. An effective oral regimen for patients able to take it is presented also.

Table 33–6. Treatment of anaerobic intra-abdominal infections.

Community-onset

Oral therapy

Moxifloxacin 400 mg every 24 hours

Ciprofloxacin 750 mg twice a day or levofloxacin 750 mg once a day **plus** metronidazole 500 mg every 8 hours

Intravenous therapy

Moderate to moderately severe infections:

Ertapenem 1 g intravenously every 24 hours

or

Ceftriaxone 1 g intravenously every 24 hours plus metronidazole intravenously or orally, 500 mg every 8 hours. If penicillin-allergic, can replace ceftriaxone with ciprofloxacin 400 mg intravenously (or 500 mg orally) every 12 hours

Severe infections:

Imipenem 0.5 g intravenously every 6–8 hours or meropenem 1 g every 8 hours or doripenem 0.5 g every 8 hours or piperacillin/tazobactam 3.75 g every 6 hours

Health care–associated

Intravenous therapy

Imipenem 0.5 g intravenously every 6–8 hours or meropenem 1 g every 8 hours or doripenem 0.5 g every 8 hours or piperacillin/tazobactam 4.5 g every 6 hours

or

Ceftazidime or cefepime 2 g intravenously every 8 hours **plus** metronidazole 500 mg intravenously or orally every 8 hours

5. Female Genital Tract & Pelvic Infections

The normal flora of the vagina and cervix includes several species of bacteroides, peptostreptococci, group B streptococci, lactobacilli, coliform bacteria, and, occasionally, spirochetes and clostridia. These organisms commonly cause genital tract infections and may disseminate from there.

While salpingitis is often caused by gonococci and chlamydiae, tubo-ovarian and pelvic abscesses are associated with anaerobes in most cases. Postpartum infections may be caused by aerobic streptococci or staphylococci, but anaerobes are often found, and the worst cases of postpartum or postabortion sepsis are associated with clostridia and bacteroides. These have a high mortality rate, and treatment requires both antimicrobials directed against anaerobes and coliforms (similar to treatment of anaerobic community-onset intra-abdominal infections, Table 33–6) and abscess drainage or early hysterectomy.

6. Bacteremia & Endocarditis

Anaerobic bacteremia usually originates from the GI tract, the oropharynx, pressure injuries, or the female genital tract. Endocarditis due to anaerobic and microaerophilic streptococci and bacteroides originates from the same sites. Most cases of anaerobic or microaerophilic streptococcal endocarditis can be effectively treated with 12–20 million units of penicillin G intravenously daily for 4–6 weeks, but optimal therapy of other types of anaerobic bacterial endocarditis must rely on laboratory guidance. Propionibacteria, clostridia, and bacteroides occasionally cause endocarditis.

7. Skin & Soft Tissue Infections

Anaerobic infections of the skin and soft tissue usually follow trauma, ischemia, or surgery and are most common in areas that are contaminated by oral or fecal flora. These infections also occur in injection drug users and persons sustaining animal bites. There may be progressive tissue necrosis (Figure 33–5) and a putrid odor.

Several terms, such as bacterial synergistic gangrene, synergistic necrotizing cellulitis, necrotizing fasciitis (see above), and non-clostridial crepitant cellulitis, are used to classify these infections. Although there are some differences in microbiology among them, differentiation on clinical grounds alone is difficult. All are mixed infections caused by aerobic and anaerobic organisms and require aggressive surgical debridement of necrotic tissue for cure.

Broad-spectrum antibiotics active against both anaerobes and gram-positive and gram-negative aerobes (eg, intravenous vancomycin plus piperacillin-tazobactam 4.5 g intravenously every 8 hours) should be instituted empirically and modified by culture results. They are given for about a week after progressive tissue destruction has been controlled and the margins of the wound remain free of inflammation.

de Prost N et al. Therapeutic targets in necrotizing soft tissue infections. Intensive Care Med. 2017;43:1717. [PMID: 28474117]

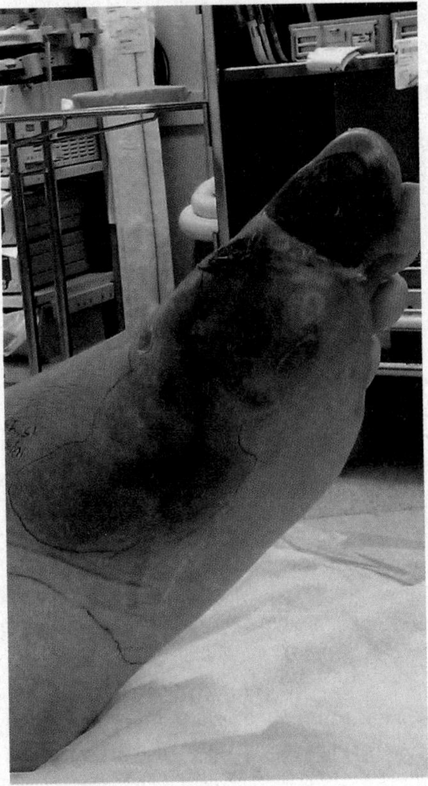

▲ **Figure 33–5.** Left foot gangrene, with plantar extension. (Used, with permission, from Dean SM, Satiani B, Abraham WT. *Color Atlas and Synopsis of Vascular Diseases*. McGraw-Hill, 2014.)

ACTINOMYCOSIS

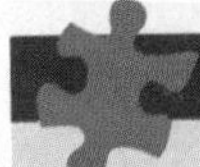

ESSENTIALS OF DIAGNOSIS

- Recent dental infection, abdominal trauma, or intrauterine contraception device placement.
- Chronic pneumonia or indolent cervicofacial or intra-abdominal abscess.
- Sinus tract formation.

General Considerations

Actinomyces israelii and other species of *Actinomyces* occur in the normal flora of the mouth and tonsillar crypts. When introduced into traumatized tissue and associated with other anaerobic bacteria, these actinomycetes become pathogens.

The most common site of infection is the cervicofacial area (about 60% of cases). Infection typically follows extraction of a tooth or other trauma. Lesions may develop in the GI tract or lungs following ingestion or aspiration of the organism from its endogenous source in the mouth. Interestingly, *T whipplei*, the causative agent of Whipple disease, is an actinomycete and therefore is related to the species that cause actinomycosis.

Clinical Findings

A. Symptoms and Signs

1. Cervicofacial actinomycosis—Cervicofacial actinomycosis develops slowly. The area becomes markedly indurated, and the overlying skin becomes reddish or cyanotic. Abscesses eventually draining to the surface persist for long periods. "Sulfur granules"—masses of filamentous organisms—may be found in the pus. There is usually little pain unless there is secondary infection. Trismus indicates that the muscles of mastication are involved. Radiographs may reveal bony involvement. Cervicofacial or thoracic disease may occasionally involve the CNS, most commonly brain abscess or meningitis.

2. Thoracic actinomycosis—Thoracic involvement begins with fever, cough, and sputum production with night sweats and weight loss. Pleuritic pain may be present. Multiple sinuses may extend through the chest wall, to the heart, or into the abdominal cavity. Ribs may be involved. Radiography shows areas of consolidation and in many cases pleural effusion.

3. Abdominal actinomycosis—Abdominal actinomycosis usually causes pain in the ileocecal region, spiking fever and chills, vomiting, and weight loss; it may be confused with Crohn disease. Irregular abdominal masses may be palpated. Pelvic inflammatory disease caused by actinomycetes has been associated with prolonged use of an intrauterine contraceptive device. Sinuses draining to the exterior may develop. CT scanning reveals an inflammatory mass extended to involve bone.

B. Laboratory Findings

The anaerobic, gram-positive organism may be demonstrated as a granule or as scattered branching gram-positive filaments in the pus. Anaerobic culture is necessary to distinguish actinomycetes from *Nocardia* species because specific therapy differs for the two infections. Histopathology examination of affected tissue and bone is useful in identifying organisms that are fastidious and slow to culture.

Treatment

Penicillin G is the drug of choice. Ten to 20 million units are given intravenously for 4–6 weeks, followed by oral penicillin V, 500 mg four times daily. Alternatives include ampicillin, 12 g/day intravenously for 4–6 weeks, followed by oral amoxicillin, 500 mg three times daily, or doxycycline, 100 mg twice daily intravenously or orally. Response to therapy is slow. Therapy should be continued for weeks to months after clinical manifestations have disappeared to ensure cure. Surgical procedures such as drainage and resection may be beneficial. With penicillin and surgery, the prognosis is good. The difficulties of diagnosis, however, may permit extensive destruction of tissue before the diagnosis is identified and therapy is started.

Xu Y et al. Disseminated actinomycosis. N Engl J Med. 2018;379:1071. [PMID: 30207906]

NOCARDIOSIS

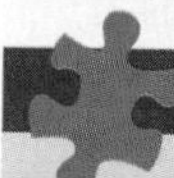

ESSENTIALS OF DIAGNOSIS

- Indolent pneumonia with dissemination to CNS, skin, and bone or primary cutaneous disease.
- Suspect in setting of chronic lung disease or immunocompromised person.

General Considerations

Nocardia species are aerobic filamentous soil bacteria that can cause pulmonary and systemic nocardiosis. Common *Nocardia* species include members of the *Nocardia asteroides* complex and *Nocardia brasiliensis*. Bronchopulmonary abnormalities (eg, bronchiectasis) predispose to colonization, but infection is unusual unless the patient is also receiving systemic corticosteroids or is otherwise immunosuppressed.

Clinical Findings

Pulmonary involvement usually begins with malaise, loss of weight, fever, and night sweats. Cough and production of purulent sputum are the chief complaints. Pulmonary infiltrates may penetrate to the exterior through the chest wall, invading the ribs.

Dissemination involves any organ. Brain abscesses and subcutaneous nodules are most frequent. Cutaneous lesions may mimic actinomycosis. Radiography may show infiltrates accompanied by pleural effusion. Even in the absence of clinical symptoms and signs of CNS infection, clinicians should consider brain imaging in patients with nocardiosis to rule out an occult abscess.

Nocardia species are usually found as delicate, branching, gram-positive filaments. They may be weakly acid-fast, occasionally causing diagnostic confusion with tuberculosis. Identification is made by culture.

Treatment

For isolated primary cutaneous infections, therapy is initiated with trimethoprim-sulfamethoxazole orally or intravenously (5–10 mg/kg/day based on trimethoprim). Surgical procedures such as drainage and resection may be needed as adjunctive therapy for isolated cutaneous disease. A higher dose of 15 mg/kg/day (based on trimethoprim) should be used for disseminated or pulmonary infections. Resistance to trimethoprim-sulfamethoxazole has increased and initiating treatment with two drugs while awaiting antibiotic susceptibilities in cases of disseminated or severe localized disease should be considered. Brain abscesses or pneumonia should be initially treated with combination therapy. Alternative agents or drugs that can be given in combination with trimethoprim-sulfamethoxazole include imipenem, 500 mg intravenously every 6 hours; amikacin, 7.5 mg/kg intravenously every 12 hours; or minocycline, 100–200 mg orally or intravenously twice daily. Consultation with an infectious disease expert is encouraged.

Response may be slow; therapy should be continued for at least 6 months. The prognosis in systemic nocardiosis is poor when diagnosis and therapy are delayed.

Margalit I et al. How do I manage nocardiosis? Clin Microbiol Infect. 2021;27:550. [PMID: 33418019]

INFECTIONS CAUSED BY MYCOBACTERIA

NONTUBERCULOUS MYCOBACTERIAL DISEASES

About 10% of mycobacterial infections are caused by nontuberculous mycobacteria. Nontuberculous mycobacterial infections are among the most common opportunistic infections in advanced HIV disease. These organisms have distinctive laboratory characteristics, occur ubiquitously in the environment, are not communicable from person to person, and are often resistant to standard antituberculous drugs.

1. Pulmonary Infections

Mycobacterium avium complex (MAC) causes a chronic, slowly progressive pulmonary infection resembling tuberculosis in immunocompetent patients who typically have underlying pulmonary disease. Susceptibility testing for macrolide-resistance should be performed on clinical isolates. Pulmonary disease is often classified as nodular, bronchiectatic, or fibrocavitary. Treatment of pulmonary MAC requires a three-drug regimen: clarithromycin (500–1000 mg orally daily) or azithromycin (500 mg orally daily) plus either rifampin (600 mg orally daily) or rifabutin (300 mg orally daily) plus ethambutol (15 mg/kg orally daily). Therapy is continued for at least 12 months after sterilization of cultures.

M kansasii can produce clinical disease resembling tuberculosis, but the illness progresses more slowly. Most such infections occur in patients with preexisting lung disease, though 40% of patients have no known pulmonary disease. Microbiologically, *M kansasii* is similar to *M tuberculosis* and is sensitive to the same drugs except pyrazinamide, to which it is resistant. Therapy with isoniazid, ethambutol, and rifampin for 2 years (or 1 year after sputum conversion) has been successful.

Less common causes of pulmonary disease include *M xenopi, M szulgai, and M malmoense.* These organisms have variable sensitivities, and treatment is based on results of sensitivity tests. The rapidly growing mycobacteria, *M abscessus, M chelonae*, and *M fortuitum*, also can cause pneumonia in the occasional patient.

Nasiri MJ et al. Antibiotic therapy success rate in pulmonary *Mycobacterium avium* complex: a systematic review and meta-analysis. Expert Rev Anti Infect Ther. 2020;18:263. [PMID: 31986933]

2. Lymphadenitis

Most cases of lymphadenitis (scrofula) in adults are caused by *M tuberculosis* and can be a manifestation of disseminated disease. In children, the majority of cases are due to nontuberculous mycobacterial species. Infection with nontuberculous mycobacteria can be successfully treated by surgical excision without antituberculous therapy.

3. Skin & Soft Tissue Infections

Skin and soft tissue infections such as abscesses, septic arthritis, and osteomyelitis can result from direct inoculation or hematogenous dissemination or may occur as a complication of surgery.

M abscessus, M chelonae, and *M fortuitum* are frequent causes of these types of infections. Most cases occur in the extremities and initially present as nodules. Ulceration with abscess formation often follows. The organisms are resistant to the usual antituberculosis drugs and may have susceptibility to clarithromycin, azithromycin, doxycycline, amikacin, cefoxitin, sulfonamides, imipenem, and ciprofloxacin. Given the multidrug-resistance of these organisms, obtaining antibiotic susceptibility testing is recommended. Therapy often includes surgical debridement along with at least two active antibiotics. Antibiotic therapy is usually continued for 3 months, although this must be determined based on clinical response.

M marinum infection ("swimming pool granuloma") presents as a nodular skin lesion following exposure to nonchlorinated water. Therapy is with clarithromycin, doxycycline, minocycline, or trimethoprim-sulfamethoxazole.

M ulcerans infection (Buruli ulcer) is seen mainly in Africa and Australia and produces a large ulcerative lesion. Therapy consists of surgical excision and skin grafting.

4. Disseminated *Mycobacterium avium* Infection

MAC causes disseminated disease in immunocompromised patients, most commonly in patients in the late stages of HIV infection, when the CD4 cell count is less than 50/mcL (see Pulmonary Disease caused by Nontuberculous Mycobacteria, Chapter 9, for a discussion of the infection in immunocompetent persons). Persistent fever and weight loss are the most common symptoms. The organism can usually be cultured from multiple sites, including blood, liver, lymph node, or bone marrow. Blood culture is the preferred means of establishing the diagnosis and has a sensitivity of 98%.

Agents with proved activity against MAC are rifabutin, azithromycin, clarithromycin, and ethambutol. A combination of two or more active agents should be used to prevent rapid emergence of secondary resistance. Clarithromycin, 500 mg orally twice daily, plus ethambutol, 15 mg/kg/day orally as a single dose, with or without rifabutin, 300 mg/day orally, is the treatment of choice. Azithromycin, 500 mg orally once daily, may be used instead of clarithromycin. Insufficient data are available to permit specific recommendations about second-line regimens for patients who cannot tolerate macrolides or those with macrolide-resistant organisms. MAC therapy may be discontinued in patients who have been treated with 12 months of therapy for disseminated MAC, who have no evidence of active disease, and whose CD4 counts exceed 100/mcL (0.1×10^9/L) for 6 months while receiving antiretroviral therapy.

Antimicrobial prophylaxis of MAC prevents disseminated disease and prolongs survival. It is the standard of care to offer it to all patients with HIV infection and CD4 counts of 50/mcL (0.05×10^9/L) or less. In contrast to active infection, single-drug oral regimens of clarithromycin, 500 mg twice daily, azithromycin, 1200 mg once weekly, or rifabutin, 300 mg once daily, are appropriate. Clarithromycin or azithromycin is more effective and better tolerated than rifabutin, and therefore preferred. Primary prophylaxis for MAC infection can be stopped in patients who have responded to antiretroviral combination therapy with elevation of CD4 counts of greater than 100/mcL (0.1×10^9/L) for 3 months.

Panel on Guidelines for the Prevention and Treatment of Opportunistic Infections in Adults and Adolescents with HIV. Guidelines for the Prevention and Treatment of Opportunistic Infections in HIV-infected Adults and Adolescents: Recommendations from the Centers for Disease Control and Prevention, the National Institutes of Health, and the HIV Medicine Association of the Infectious Diseases Society of America. Available at https://clinicalinfo.hiv.gov/en/guidelines/adult-and-adolescent-opportunistic-infection

MYCOBACTERIUM TUBERCULOSIS INFECTIONS

Tuberculosis is discussed in Chapter 9. Further information and expert consultation can be obtained from the Curry International Tuberculosis Center at the website www.currytbcenter.ucsf.edu or by telephone, 510-238-5100.

TUBERCULOUS MENINGITIS

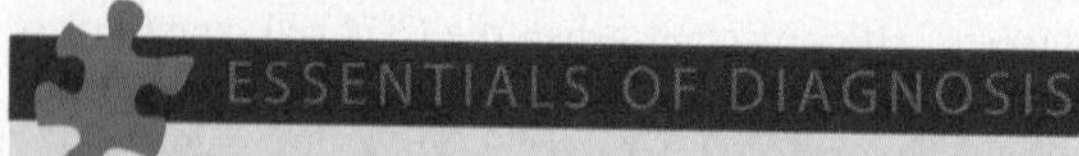

- Gradual onset of listlessness and anorexia.
- Headache, vomiting, and seizures common.
- Cranial nerve abnormalities typical.
- Tuberculosis focus may be evident elsewhere.
- Cerebrospinal fluid shows several hundred lymphocytes, low glucose, and high protein.

General Considerations

Tuberculous meningitis is caused by rupture of a meningeal tuberculoma resulting from earlier hematogenous seeding of tubercle bacilli from a pulmonary focus, or it may be a consequence of miliary spread.

Clinical Findings

A. Symptoms and Signs

The onset is usually gradual, with listlessness, irritability, anorexia, and fever, followed by headache, vomiting, convulsions, and coma. In older patients, headache and behavioral changes are prominent early symptoms. Nuchal rigidity and cranial nerve palsies occur as the meningitis progresses. Evidence of active tuberculosis elsewhere or a history of prior tuberculosis is present in up to 75% of patients.

B. Laboratory Findings

The spinal fluid is frequently yellowish, with increased pressure, cell count 100–500/mcL (0.1–0.5 × 10^9/L) (predominantly lymphocytes, though neutrophils may be present early during infection), increased protein, and decreased glucose. Acid-fast stains of cerebrospinal fluid are often negative, and cultures also may be negative in 15–25% of cases. Nucleic acid amplification tests are valuable tools that allow for rapid diagnosis although sensitivity is only 68–80%. Chest radiographs often reveal abnormalities compatible with tuberculosis but may be normal. The tuberculin skin testing and interferon-gamma release assays do not distinguish between active and latent tuberculosis and are frequently negative in the presence of CNS infection.

Differential Diagnosis

Tuberculous meningitis may be confused with any other type of meningitis, but the gradual onset, the predominantly lymphocytic pleocytosis of the spinal fluid, and evidence of tuberculosis elsewhere often point to the diagnosis. Fungal and other granulomatous meningitides, syphilis, and carcinomatous meningitis are in the differential diagnosis.

Complications

Complications of tuberculous meningitis include seizures, cranial nerve palsies, stroke, and obstructive hydrocephalus with impaired cognitive function. These result from inflammatory exudate primarily of the basilar meninges and arteries.

Treatment

Presumptive diagnosis followed by early, empiric antituberculous therapy is essential for survival and to minimize sequelae. Even if cultures are not positive, a full course of therapy is warranted if the clinical setting is suggestive of tuberculous meningitis.

Regimens that are effective for pulmonary tuberculosis are effective also for tuberculous meningitis (see Table 9–15). Rifampin, isoniazid, and pyrazinamide all penetrate well into cerebrospinal fluid. The penetration of ethambutol is more variable, but therapeutic concentrations can be achieved, and the drug has been successfully used for meningitis. Aminoglycosides penetrate less well. Regimens that do not include both isoniazid and rifampin may be effective but are less reliable and generally must be given for longer periods.

Many authorities recommend the addition of corticosteroids as adjunctive therapy. Dexamethasone, 0.15 mg/kg intravenously or orally four times daily for 1–2 weeks, then discontinued in a tapering regimen over 4 weeks, may be used.

Heemskerk AD et al. Intensified antituberculosis therapy in adults with tuberculous meningitis. N Engl J Med. 2016;374:124. [PMID: 26760084]

Khonga M et al. Xpert MTB/RIF Ultra: a gamechanger for tuberculous meningitis? Lancet Infect Dis. 2018;18:6. [PMID: 28919337]

Prasad K et al. Corticosteroids for managing tuberculous meningitis. Cochrane Database Syst Rev. 2016;4:CD002244. [PMID: 27121755]

INFECTIONS CAUSED BY CHLAMYDIAE

CHLAMYDIA TRACHOMATIS INFECTIONS

1. Lymphogranuloma Venereum

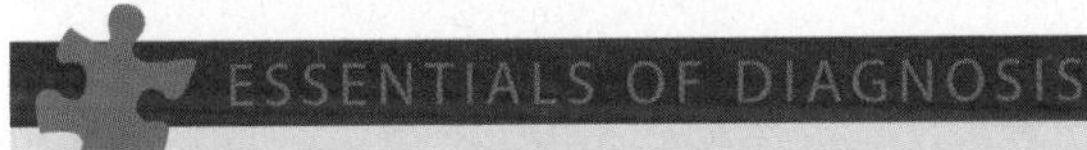

- Evanescent primary genital lesion.
- Inguinal buboes with suppuration and draining sinuses.
- Proctitis and rectal stricture in women or in men who have sex with men.
- Positive complement fixation test.

General Considerations

Lymphogranuloma venereum (LGV) is an acute and chronic sexually transmitted disease caused by *C trachomatis* types L1–L3. The disease is acquired during intercourse or through contact with contaminated exudate from active lesions. The incubation period is 5–21 days. After the genital lesion disappears, the infection spreads to the lymph nodes of the genital and rectal areas. Inapparent infections and latent disease are not uncommon.

Clinical Findings

A. Symptoms and Signs

In men, the initial vesicular or ulcerative lesion (on the external genitalia) is evanescent and often goes unnoticed. Inguinal buboes appear 1–4 weeks after exposure, are often bilateral, and have a tendency to fuse, soften, and break down to form multiple draining sinuses, with extensive scarring. **In women,** the genital lymph drainage is to the perirectal glands. Early anorectal manifestations are proctitis with tenesmus and bloody purulent discharge; late manifestations are chronic cicatrizing inflammation of the rectal and perirectal tissue. These changes lead to obstipation and rectal stricture and, occasionally, rectovaginal and perianal fistulas. They are also seen with anal coitus.

B. Laboratory Findings

The complement fixation antibody testing may be positive (titers greater than 1:64), but cross-reaction with other chlamydiae occurs. Although a positive reaction may reflect remote infection, high titers usually indicate active disease. Nucleic acid detection tests are sensitive but cannot differentiate LGV from non-LGV strains.

Differential Diagnosis

The early lesion of LGV must be differentiated from the lesions of syphilis, genital herpes, and chancroid; lymph node involvement must be distinguished from that due to tularemia, tuberculosis, plague, neoplasm, or pyogenic infection; and rectal stricture must be distinguished from that due to neoplasm and ulcerative colitis.

Treatment

If diagnostic testing for LGV is not available, patients with a clinical presentation suggestive of LGV should be treated empirically. The antibiotic of choice is doxycycline (contraindicated in pregnancy), 100 mg orally twice daily for 21 days. Erythromycin, 500 mg orally four times a day for 21 days, is also effective. Azithromycin, 1 g orally once weekly for 3 weeks, may also be effective.

De Vries HJC et al. 2019 European guideline on the management of lymphogranuloma venereum. J Eur Acad Dermatol Venereol. 2019;33:1821. [PMID: 31243838]

Workowski KA et al; Centers for Disease Control and Prevention (CDC). Sexually transmitted infections treatment guidelines, 2021. MMWR Recomm Rep. 2021;70:1. [PMID: 34292926]

2. Chlamydial Urethritis & Cervicitis

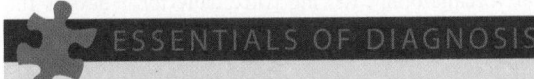

- *C trachomatis*: common cause of urethritis, cervicitis, and postgonococcal urethritis.
- Diagnosis made by nucleic acid amplification of urine or swab specimen.

General Considerations

C trachomatis immunotypes D–K are isolated in about 50% of cases of nongonococcal urethritis and cervicitis. In other cases, *Ureaplasma urealyticum* or *Mycoplasma genitalium* can be grown as a possible etiologic agent. *C trachomatis* is an important cause of postgonococcal urethritis. Coinfection with gonococci and chlamydiae is common, and postgonococcal (ie, chlamydial) urethritis may persist after successful treatment of the gonococcal component.

Occasionally, epididymitis, prostatitis, or proctitis is caused by chlamydial infection. Chlamydiae are a leading cause of infertility in females in the United States.

Clinical Findings

A. Symptoms and Signs

The urethral or cervical discharge due to *C trachomatis* tends to be less painful, less purulent, and watery compared with gonococcal infection. Women infected with chlamydiae may be asymptomatic or may have symptoms and signs of cervicitis, salpingitis, or pelvic inflammatory disease. Long-term sequelae may include ectopic pregnancy and infertility.

B. Laboratory Findings

A patient with clinical signs and symptoms of urethritis or cervicitis is assumed to have chlamydial infection until proven otherwise. The diagnosis should be confirmed, whenever possible, by the FDA-approved, highly sensitive nucleic acid amplification tests for use with urine or vaginal swabs. A negative urine nucleic acid amplification test for chlamydia reliably excludes the diagnosis of chlamydial urethritis or cervicitis and therapy need not be administered. Urine testing does not exclude infection at other sites, such as rectal or pharyngeal disease.

C. Screening

Active screening for chlamydial infection is recommended in certain settings: pregnant women; all sexually active women 25 years of age and under; older women with risk factors for sexually transmitted diseases; and men with risk factors for sexually transmitted diseases, such as men with HIV infection or men who have sex with men.

Treatment

Doxycycline orally 100 mg twice daily for 7 days is the preferred regimen but is contraindicated in pregnancy. A single oral 1-g dose of azithromycin (alternative regimen, preferred in pregnancy), or 500 mg of levofloxacin once daily for 7 days. Presumptively administered therapy still may be indicated for some patients, such as for an individual with gonococcal infection in whom no chlamydial testing was performed or a test other than a nucleic acid amplification test was used to exclude the diagnosis, or an individual for whom a test result is pending but is considered unlikely to follow up, and for sexual contacts of documented cases. As for all patients in whom sexually transmitted diseases are diagnosed, studies for HIV and syphilis should also be performed.

Wiesenfeld HC. Screening for *Chlamydia trachomatis* infections in women. N Engl J Med. 2017;376:765. [PMID: 28225683]
Workowski KA et al; Centers for Disease Control and Prevention (CDC). Sexually transmitted infections treatment guidelines, 2021. MMWR Recomm Rep. 2021;70:1. [PMID: 34292926]

CHLAMYDOPHILA PSITTACI & PSITTACOSIS (Ornithosis)

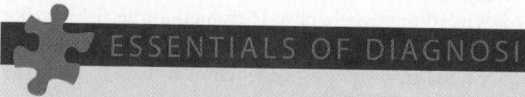

- Fever, chills, and cough; headache common.
- Atypical pneumonia with slightly delayed appearance of signs of pneumonitis.
- Contact with infected bird (psittacine, pigeons, many others) 7–15 days previously.
- Isolation of chlamydiae or rising titer of complement-fixing antibodies.

General Considerations

Psittacosis is acquired from contact with birds (parrots, parakeets, pigeons, chickens, ducks, and many others), which may or may not be ill. The history may be difficult to obtain if the patient acquired infection from an illegally imported bird.

Clinical Findings

The onset is usually rapid, with fever, chills, myalgia, dry cough, and headache. Signs include temperature-pulse dissociation, dullness to percussion, and rales. Pulmonary findings may be absent early. Dyspnea and cyanosis may occur later. Endocarditis, which is culture-negative, may occur. The radiographic findings in typical psittacosis are those of atypical pneumonia, which tends to be interstitial and diffuse in appearance, though consolidation can occur. Psittacosis is indistinguishable from other bacterial or viral pneumonias by radiography.

The organism is rarely isolated from cultures. The diagnosis is usually made serologically; antibodies appear during the second week and can be demonstrated by complement fixation or immunofluorescence. Antibody response may be suppressed by early chemotherapy.

Differential Diagnosis

The illness is indistinguishable from viral, mycoplasmal, or other atypical pneumonias except for the history of contact with birds. Psittacosis is in the differential diagnosis of culture-negative endocarditis.

Treatment

Treatment is with doxycycline 100 mg orally twice daily for 10–21 days. Erythromycin, 500 mg orally every 6 hours, or azithromycin, 500 mg orally on day 1, and then 250 mg once daily for 4 days, may be effective as well.

Hogerwerf L et al. *Chlamydia psittaci* (psittacosis) as a cause of community-acquired pneumonia: a systematic review and meta-analysis. Epidemiol Infect. 2017;145:3096. [PMID: 28946931]

CHLAMYDOPHILA PNEUMONIAE INFECTION

C pneumoniae causes pneumonia and bronchitis. The clinical presentation of pneumonia is that of an atypical pneumonia. The organism accounts for approximately 10% of community-acquired pneumonias, ranking second to *mycoplasma* as an agent of atypical pneumonia.

Like *C psittaci*, strains of *C pneumoniae* are resistant to sulfonamides. Azithromycin, 500 mg orally on day 1 and 250 mg for 4 more days, or doxycycline, 100 mg orally two times a day for 10 days, appears to be effective therapy. Fluoroquinolones, such as levofloxacin (500 mg orally once daily for 7–14 days) or moxifloxacin (400 mg orally once daily for 7–14 days), are active in vitro against *C pneumoniae* and probably are effective. It is unclear whether empiric coverage for atypical pathogens in hospitalized patients with community-acquired pneumonia provides a survival benefit or improves clinical outcome.

Fujita J et al. Where is *Chlamydophila pneumoniae* pneumonia? Respir Investig. 2020;58:336. [PMID: 32703757]

34 Spirochetal Infections

Susan S. Philip, MD, MPH

SYPHILIS

NATURAL HISTORY & PRINCIPLES OF DIAGNOSIS & TREATMENT

Syphilis is a complex infectious disease caused by *Treponema pallidum*, a spirochete capable of infecting almost any organ or tissue in the body and causing protean clinical manifestations (Table 34–1). Transmission occurs most frequently during sexual contact (including oral sex) or via the placenta from mother to fetus (congenital syphilis). The risk of acquiring syphilis after unprotected sex with an individual with infectious syphilis is approximately 30–50%. Rarely, it can also be transmitted through nonsexual contact or blood transfusion. The natural history of acquired syphilis is generally divided into two major stages: early (infectious) syphilis and late syphilis.

Early infectious syphilis includes primary lesions (chancre and regional lymphadenopathy) appearing during primary syphilis, secondary lesions (commonly involving skin and mucous membranes, occasionally bone, CNS, or liver) appearing during secondary syphilis (when dissemination of *T pallidum* produces systemic signs), relapsing lesions during early latency, and congenital lesions. The hallmark of these lesions is an abundance of spirochetes; tissue reaction is usually minimal.

Late (tertiary) syphilis consists of so-called benign (gummatous) lesions involving skin, bones, and viscera; CVD (principally aortitis); and a variety of CNS and ocular syndromes. These forms of syphilis are not contagious. The lesions contain few demonstrable spirochetes, but tissue reactivity (vasculitis, necrosis) is severe and suggestive of hypersensitivity phenomena. Between these stages are symptom-free latent phases. In early latent syphilis, which is defined as the symptom-free interval lasting up to 1 year after initial infection, infectious lesions can recur.

Public health efforts to control syphilis focus on the diagnosis and treatment of early (infectious) cases and their sexual partners.

Nearly half of all cases of syphilis in the United States occur in men who have sex with men. Globally, the World Health Organization (WHO) estimates 5.6 million total incident syphilis infections occur annually, with a prevalence of 1% among pregnant women attending antenatal clinics. Preventing congenital syphilis is a major public health goal for the CDC and WHO.

COURSE & PROGNOSIS

The lesions associated with primary and secondary syphilis are self-limiting, even without treatment, and resolve with few or no residua. Ocular and otologic syphilis have been associated with permanent vision and hearing loss. Tertiary and congenital syphilis may be highly destructive and permanently disabling and may lead to death. While infection is rarely eradicated completely in the absence of treatment, most infections likely remain latent without sequelae, and only a small number of latent infections progress to further disease.

CLINICAL STAGES OF SYPHILIS

1. Primary Syphilis

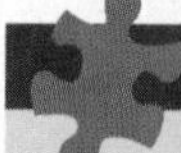

ESSENTIALS OF DIAGNOSIS

- Painless ulcer on genitalia, perianal area, rectum, pharynx, tongue, lip, or elsewhere.
- Fluid expressed from ulcer contains *T pallidum* by immunofluorescence or darkfield microscopy.
- Nontender enlargement of regional lymph nodes.
- Serologic nontreponemal and treponemal tests may be positive.

Clinical Findings

A. Symptoms and Signs

The typical lesion is the chancre at the site or sites of inoculation, most frequently located on the penis (Figure 34–1), labia, cervix, or anorectal region. Anorectal lesions are especially common among men who have sex with men. Chancres also occur occasionally in the oropharynx (lip, tongue, or tonsil) and rarely on the breast or finger

Table 34–1. Stages of syphilis and common clinical manifestations.

Primary syphilis
Chancre: painless ulcer with clean base and firm indurated borders
Regional lymphadenopathy
Secondary syphilis
Skin and mucous membranes
Rash: diffuse (may include palms and soles), macular, papular, pustular, and combinations
Condylomata lata
Mucous patches: painless, silvery ulcerations of mucous membrane with surrounding erythema
Generalized lymphadenopathy
Constitutional symptoms
Fever, usually low-grade
Malaise, anorexia
Arthralgias and myalgias
CNS
Asymptomatic
Symptomatic
Meningitis
Cranial neuropathies (II–VIII)
Other
Ocular: iritis, iridocyclitis
Renal: glomerulonephritis, nephrotic syndrome
Hepatitis
Musculoskeletal: arthritis, periostitis
Tertiary syphilis
Late benign (gummatous): granulomatous lesion usually involving skin, mucous membranes, and bones but any organ can be involved
Cardiovascular
Aortic regurgitation
Coronary ostial stenosis
Aortic aneurysm
Neurosyphilis
Asymptomatic
Meningovascular
Tabes dorsalis
General paresis

Note: CNS involvement may occur at any stage.

or elsewhere. An initial small erosion appears 10–90 days (average, 3–4 weeks) after inoculation then rapidly develops into a painless superficial ulcer with a clean base and firm, indurated margins. This is associated with enlargement of regional lymph nodes, which are rubbery, discrete, and nontender. Healing of the chancre occurs without treatment, but a scar may form, especially with secondary bacterial infection. Multiple chancres may be present, particularly in patients with HIV infection. Although the "classic" ulcer of syphilis has been described as nontender, nonpurulent, and indurated, only 31% of patients have this triad.

B. Laboratory Findings

1. Microscopic examination—In early syphilis, darkfield microscopic examination by a skilled observer of fresh exudate from moist lesions or material aspirated from

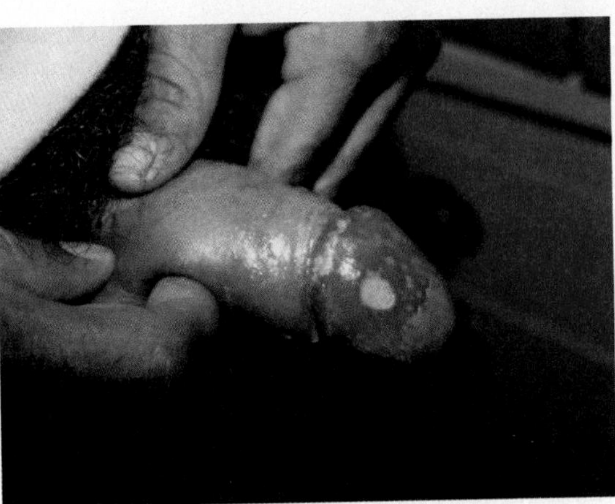

▲ **Figure 34–1. Primary syphilis with a large chancre on the glans of the penis. The multiple small surrounding ulcers are part of the syphilis and not a second disease.** (Reproduced with permission from Richard P. Usatine, MD, in Usatine RP, Smith MA, Mayeaux EJ Jr, Chumley H. *The Color Atlas of Family Medicine*, 2nd ed. McGraw-Hill, 2013.)

regional lymph nodes is up to 90% sensitive for diagnosis but is usually only available in select clinics that specialize in sexually transmitted infections.

An immunofluorescent staining technique for demonstrating *T pallidum* in dried smears of fluid taken from early syphilitic lesions is performed in only a few laboratories.

T pallidum PCR tests are available in selected research, referral, and public health laboratories and have the highest yield in primary and secondary lesions. Organisms can also be detected in blood, especially in congenital and secondary syphilis cases.

2. Serologic tests for syphilis—(Table 34–2.) Serologic tests (the mainstay of syphilis diagnosis) fall into two general categories: (1) Nontreponemal tests detect antibodies

Table 34–2. Percentage of patients with positive serologic tests for syphilis.[1]

Test	Stage		
	Primary	Secondary	Tertiary
VDRL or RPR	75–85%	99–100%	40–95%
FTA-ABS, TPPA, or MHA-TP	69–100%	100%	94–98%
MHA-TP	46–89%	90–100%	NA
EIA or CIA	54–100%	100%	NA

[1]Based on untreated cases.

CIA, chemiluminescence assay; EIA, enzyme immunoassay; FTA-ABS, fluorescent treponemal antibody absorption assay; MHA-TP, microhemagglutination assay for *T pallidum*; RPR, rapid plasma reagin test; TPPA, *T pallidum* particle agglutination; VDRL, Venereal Disease Research Laboratory test.

to lipoidal antigens present in the host after modification by *T pallidum*; and (2) Treponemal tests use live or killed *T pallidum* as antigen to detect antibodies specific for pathogenic treponemes.

A. Nontreponemal antibody tests—The most commonly used nontreponemal antibody tests are the Venereal Disease Research Laboratory (VDRL) and rapid plasma reagin (RPR) tests. A different enzyme immunoassay (EIA)–based screening algorithm is discussed below.

Nontreponemal tests generally become positive 4–6 weeks after infection or 1–3 weeks after the appearance of a primary lesion; they are almost invariably positive in the secondary stage. These tests are nonspecific and may be positive in patients with non–sexually transmitted treponematoses. More important, false-positive serologic reactions are frequently encountered in a wide variety of conditions, including autoimmune diseases, infectious mononucleosis, malaria, febrile diseases, leprosy, injection drug use, infective endocarditis, advanced age, hepatitis C viral infection, and pregnancy. False-positive nontreponemal tests are usually of low titer and transient and may be distinguished from true-positive results by correlating with clinical findings and performing a treponemal-specific antibody test. False-negative results can be seen when very high antibody titers are present (**the prozone phenomenon**). If syphilis is strongly suspected and the nontreponemal test is negative, the laboratory should be instructed to dilute the specimen to detect a positive reaction.

Nontreponemal antibody titers are used to monitor the response to therapy and should decline over time. The rate of decline depends on various factors. In general, persons with repeat infections, higher initial titers, more advanced stages of disease, or HIV infection at the time of treatment have a slower seroconversion rate and are more likely to remain serofast (ie, titers decline but do not become nonreactive). The RPR and VDRL tests are equally reliable, but RPR titers tend to be higher than VDRL titers. Thus, when these tests are used to follow disease activity, the same testing method should be used and preferably performed at the same laboratory.

B. Treponemal antibody tests—These tests measure antibodies capable of reacting with *T pallidum* antigens. The *T pallidum* particle agglutination (TPPA) test and the fluorescent treponemal antibody absorption test (FTA-ABS) are two of the most commonly used treponemal tests. Other treponemal tests include the EIA and chemiluminescence assay (CIA).

In the traditional screening algorithm, the treponemal tests are used to confirm a positive nontreponemal test. Because of their sensitivity, particularly in the late stages of the disease, treponemal tests are also of value when there is clinical evidence of syphilis, but the nontreponemal serologic test for syphilis is negative. Treponemal tests are reactive in many patients with primary syphilis and in almost all patients with secondary syphilis (Table 34–2). Although a reactive treponemal-specific serologic test remains reactive throughout a patient's life in most cases, it may (like nontreponemal antibody tests) revert to negative with adequate therapy. Final decisions about the significance of the results of serologic tests for syphilis must be based on a total clinical appraisal and may require expert consultation.

C. Enzyme immunoassay (EIA)- or chemiluminescence immunoassay (CIA)-based screening algorithms—Newer screening algorithms reverse the traditional test order and begin with an automated treponemal antibody test (eg, EIA or CIA) and then follow-up with a nontreponemal test (RPR or VDRL) if the treponemal test is positive. This algorithm is faster and decreases labor costs to laboratories when compared with traditional screening. The EIAs have sensitivities of 95–100% and specificities of 99–100%.

The reverse algorithms can cause challenges in clinical management. A positive treponemal test with a negative RPR or VDRL may represent prior treated syphilis, untreated latent syphilis, or a false-positive treponemal test. Such results should be evaluated with a second, different treponemal test as a "tie-breaker." Both traditional and reverse algorithms are recognized by the CDC and several international organizations including the International Union Against Sexually Transmitted Infections.

D. Rapid treponemal tests—Both a treponemal and a dual HIV/treponemal rapid point of care test are approved for use in the United States. Other tests are available internationally and are commonly used in limited-resource settings. Sensitivity range is 62–100% and specificity is 83–95%.

3. PCR—In the United States, there are no commercially available, FDA-approved *T pallidum* PCR test kits. However, kits are available as a laboratory-developed test in selected research, referral, and public health laboratories and have the highest yield in primary and secondary lesions. There are no standards for these tests, but PCR has many advantages as a tool for direct detection, including high sensitivity and ability to use a wide range of clinical specimen types, including cerebrospinal fluid. PCR testing of blood has low sensitivity and is not recommended.

4. Cerebrospinal fluid examination (CSF)—See Neurosyphilis section.

Differential Diagnosis

The syphilitic chancre may be confused with genital herpes, chancroid (usually painful and uncommon in the United States), lymphogranuloma venereum, or neoplasm. Simultaneous evaluation for herpes simplex virus types 1 and 2 using PCR or culture should also be done in these cases.

Prevention & Screening

Avoidance of sexual contact is the only completely reliable method of prevention but is an impractical public health measure. Latex or polyurethane condoms are effective only if all infectious lesions are covered. Men who have sex with men should be screened every 6–12 months, and as often as every 3 months in high-risk individuals (those who have multiple encounters with anonymous partners or who have sex in conjunction with the use of drugs). Every pregnant woman should be screened at the first prenatal visit and, in some states with increasing congenital syphilis rates, again in the third trimester. A third screening at delivery is recommended if there are risk indicators, including poverty, sex work, illicit drug use, history of other sexually transmitted diseases, and residence in a community with high syphilis morbidity. Patients treated for other sexually transmitted diseases should also be tested for syphilis, and persons who have known or suspected sexual contact with patients who have syphilis should be evaluated and presumptively treated to abort development of infectious syphilis (see Treating Syphilis Contacts below).

Treatment

A. Antibiotic Therapy

Penicillin remains the preferred treatment for syphilis, since there have been no documented cases of penicillin-resistant *T pallidum* (Table 34–3). In pregnant women, penicillin is the only option that reliably treats the fetus.

The most commonly used alternatives to penicillin for nonpregnant patients include doxycycline and ceftriaxone (although optimum dose and duration for ceftriaxone are not well defined). Azithromycin has been shown to be effective in some parts of the world but should be used with caution; it should not be used at all in men who have sex with men due to demonstrated resistance. All patients treated with a non-penicillin regimen must have close clinical and serologic follow-up.

B. Managing Jarisch–Herxheimer Reaction

The Jarisch–Herxheimer reaction, manifested by fever and aggravation of the existing clinical picture in the hours following treatment, is a cytokine-mediated immunologic reaction to endotoxins released from the killed bacteria. It is most common in early syphilis, particularly secondary syphilis, where it can occur in 66% of cases.

The reaction may be blunted by simultaneous administration of antipyretics, although no proven method of prevention exists. In cases with increased risk of morbidity due to the Jarisch–Herxheimer reaction (including CNS or cardiac involvement and pregnancy), consultation with an infectious disease expert is recommended. Patients should be reminded that the reaction does not signify an allergy to penicillin.

C. Local Measures (Mucocutaneous Lesions)

Local treatment is usually not necessary. No local antiseptics or topical antibiotics should be applied to a lesion until specimens for microscopy have been obtained.

Table 34–3. Recommended treatment for syphilis.[1]

Stage of Syphilis	Treatment	Alternative[2]	Comment
Early			
Primary, secondary, or early latent	Benzathine penicillin G 2.4 million units intramuscularly once	Doxycycline 100 mg orally twice daily for 14 days or Tetracycline 500 mg orally four times daily for 14 days or Ceftriaxone 1 g intramuscularly or intravenously daily for 10 days[3]	HIV testing is recommended at diagnosis or treatment
Late			
Late latent or uncertain duration	Benzathine penicillin G 2.4 million units intramuscularly weekly for 3 weeks	Doxycycline 100 mg orally twice daily for 28 days or Tetracycline 500 mg orally four times daily for 28 days	No routine CSF evaluation needed unless neurologic, otologic, or ocular changes An HIV test should be obtained
Tertiary without neurosyphilis	Benzathine penicillin G 2.4 million units intramuscularly weekly for 3 weeks	Consult with an infectious disease specialist	CSF evaluation and an HIV test are recommended in all patients
Neurosyphilis	Aqueous penicillin G 18–24 million units intravenously daily, given every 3–4 hours or as continuous infusion for 10–14 days	Procaine penicillin, 2.4 million units intramuscularly daily with probenecid 500 mg orally four times daily for 10–14 days or Ceftriaxone 2 g intramuscularly or intravenously daily for 10–14 days	Follow treatment with benzathine penicillin G 2.4 million units intramuscularly weekly for up to 3 weeks Obtain an HIV test

[1]Penicillin is the only documented effective treatment in pregnancy; pregnant patients with true allergy should be desensitized and treated with penicillin according to stage of disease as above.
[2]Patients treated with alternative therapies require close clinical and serologic monitoring.
[3]Fewer data for ceftriaxone treatment; optimal dose or duration not known.
CSF, cerebrospinal fluid.

D. Public Health Measures

Counsel patients with infectious syphilis to abstain from sexual activity for 7–10 days after treatment. All cases of syphilis must be reported to the appropriate local public health agency to identify and treat sexual contacts. In addition, all patients with syphilis who are not known to be infected with HIV should have an HIV test at the time of diagnosis. Those with a negative HIV test should be offered HIV preexposure prophylaxis (HIV PrEP) because syphilis is associated with an increased risk of future HIV acquisition.

E. Treating Syphilis Contacts

Patients who have been sexually exposed to infectious syphilis within the preceding 3 months may be infected but seronegative and, thus, should be treated for early syphilis even if serologic tests are negative. Persons exposed more than 3 months previously should be treated based on serologic results; however, if the patient is unreliable for follow-up, empiric therapy is indicated. Contacts of the persons with syphilis should be evaluated for HIV PrEP.

Follow-Up Care

Because treatment failures and reinfection may occur, patients treated for syphilis should be monitored clinically and serologically with nontreponemal titers every 3–6 months. In primary and secondary syphilis, titers are expected to decrease fourfold by 12 months; however, titers from up to 20% of patients may fail to decrease. Optimal management of these patients is unclear, but at a minimum, close clinical and serologic follow-up is indicated. In patients not infected with HIV, an HIV test should be repeated; a thorough neurologic history and examination should be performed and lumbar puncture considered since unrecognized neurosyphilis can be a cause of treatment failure. If symptoms or signs persist or recur after initial therapy or there is a fourfold or greater increase in nontreponemal titers, the patient has reinfection (more likely) or the therapy failed (if a non-penicillin regimen was used). In those individuals, an HIV test should be performed, a lumbar puncture done (unless reinfection is a certainty), and re-treatment given as indicated above.

2. Secondary Syphilis

ESSENTIALS OF DIAGNOSIS

- Generalized maculopapular rash; condylomata lata in moist skin areas.
- Mucous membrane lesions.
- Generalized nontender lymphadenopathy.
- Fever may be present.
- Meningitis, hepatitis, osteitis, arthritis, iritis.
- Many treponemes in moist lesions by immunofluorescence or darkfield microscopy.
- Positive serologic tests for syphilis.

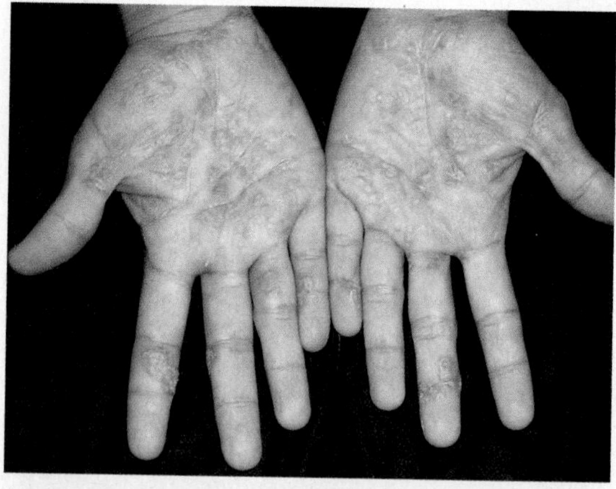

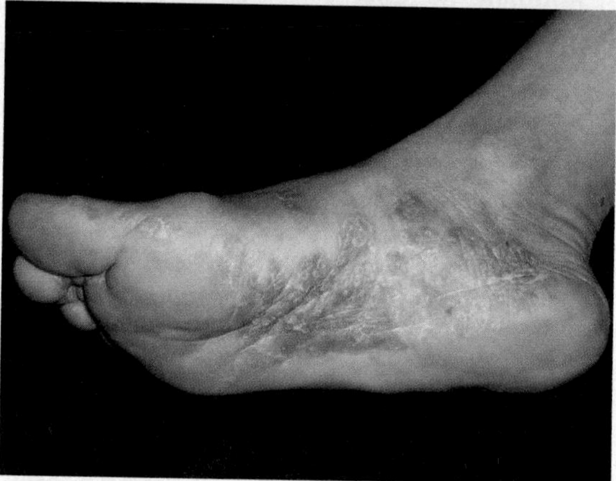

Figure 34–2. Papular squamous eruption of the hands and feet of a woman with secondary syphilis. (Reproduced with permission from Richard P. Usatine, MD, in Usatine RP, Smith MA, Mayeaux EJ Jr, Chumley H. *The Color Atlas of Family Medicine*, 2nd ed. McGraw-Hill, 2013.)

Clinical Findings

The secondary stage of syphilis usually appears a few weeks (or up to 6 months) after development of the chancre, when dissemination of *T pallidum* produces systemic signs (fever, lymphadenopathy) or infectious lesions at sites distant from the site of inoculation. The most common manifestations are skin and mucosal lesions. The skin lesions are nonpruritic, macular, papular, pustular, or follicular (or combinations of any of these types, but generally *not* vesicular) and generalized; involvement of the palms and soles (Figure 34–2) occurs in 80% of cases. Annular lesions simulating ringworm may be observed. Transillumination may help identify faint rashes, or rashes in persons with darker skin color. Mucous membrane lesions may include mucous patches (Figure 34–3), which can be found on the lips, mouth, throat, genitalia, and anus. Specific lesions—condylomata lata (Figure 34–4)—are fused, weeping papules on the moist skin areas and mucous membranes and are sometimes mistaken for genital warts. Unlike the dry rashes, the mucous membrane lesions are highly infectious.

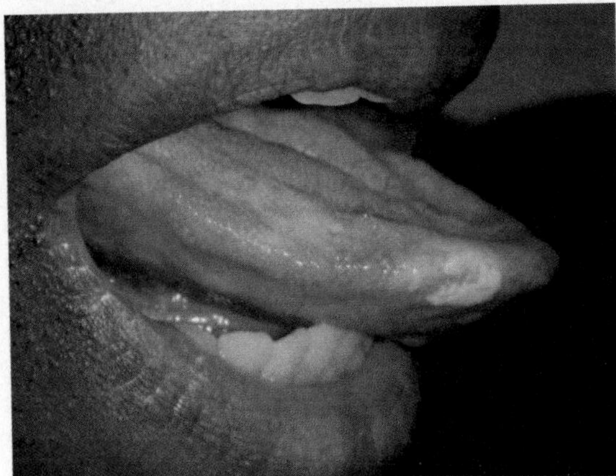

▲ **Figure 34–3.** Secondary syphilis mucous patch of the tongue. (Used with permission from Kenneth Katz, MD, MSc, MSCE.)

Meningeal (aseptic meningitis or acute basilar meningitis), hepatic, renal, bone, and joint invasion may occur, with resulting cranial nerve palsies, jaundice, nephrotic syndrome, and periostitis. Alopecia (moth-eaten appearance) and uveitis may also occur.

The serologic tests for syphilis are positive in almost all cases (see Primary Syphilis and Table 34–2). The moist cutaneous and mucous membrane lesions often show *T pallidum* on darkfield microscopic examination. A transient CSF lymphocytic pleocytosis (cell count usually less than 50–100/mcL [0.05–0.1 × 10^9/L]) is seen in 40% of patients with secondary syphilis. There may be evidence of hepatitis or nephritis (immune complex type) as circulating immune complexes are deposited in blood vessel walls.

Skin lesions may be confused with the infectious exanthems, pityriasis rosea, and drug eruptions. Visceral lesions may suggest nephritis or hepatitis due to other causes.

Treatment

Treatment is as for primary syphilis unless CNS or ocular disease or neurologic signs or symptoms are present, in which case a lumbar puncture should be performed. If examination of the fluid is positive (see Spinal fluid examination for Neurosyphilis, below), treatment for neurosyphilis should be given (Table 34–3). See Primary Syphilis for follow-up care and treatment of contacts.

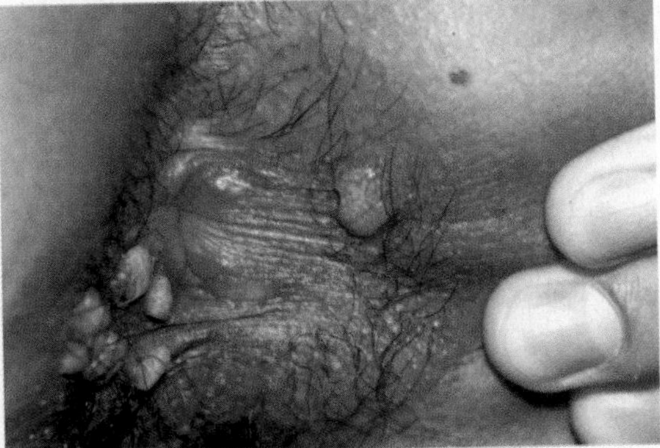

▲ **Figure 34–4.** Secondary syphilis perianal condylomata lata. (Used with permission from Joseph Engelman, MD; San Francisco City Clinic.)

3. Latent Syphilis

ESSENTIALS OF DIAGNOSIS

- **Early latent syphilis:** infection < 1 year.
- **Late latent syphilis:** infection > 1 year.
- No physical signs.
- History of syphilis with inadequate treatment.
- Positive serologic tests for syphilis.

General Considerations

Latent syphilis is the clinically quiescent phase in the absence of primary or secondary lesions; the diagnosis is made by positive serologic tests. **Early latent syphilis** is defined as the first year after primary infection and may relapse to secondary syphilis if undiagnosed or inadequately treated. Relapse is almost always accompanied by a rising titer in quantitative serologic tests; indeed, a rising titer may be the first or only evidence of relapse. About 90% of relapses occur during the first year after infection.

Early latent infection can be diagnosed if there was documented seroconversion or a fourfold increase in nontreponemal titers in the past 12 months; the patient can recall symptoms of primary or secondary syphilis; or the patient had a sex partner with documented primary, secondary, or early latent syphilis.

After the first year of latent syphilis, the patient is said to be in the **late latent stage** and noninfectious to sex partners. Transplacental transmission to a fetus, however, is possible in any phase. A diagnosis of late latent syphilis is justified only when the history and physical examination show no evidence of tertiary disease or neurosyphilis. The latent stage may last from months to a lifetime.

Treatment

Treatment of early latent syphilis and follow-up are the same as for primary syphilis unless CNS disease is present (Table 34–3). Treatment of late latent syphilis is also shown in Table 34–3. The treatment of this stage of the disease is intended to prevent late sequelae. If there is evidence of CNS involvement, a lumbar puncture should be performed and, if positive, the patient should receive treatment for neurosyphilis (see Spinal fluid examination for Neurosyphilis, below). Titers may not decline as rapidly following treatment compared to early syphilis. Nontreponemal serologic tests should be repeated at 6, 12, and 24 months. If titers increase fourfold or if initially high titers (1:32 or higher) fail to decrease fourfold by 12–24 months or if symptoms or signs consistent with syphilis develop, an HIV test should be repeated in patients not known to have an HIV infection, lumbar puncture should be performed, and re-treatment given according to the stage of the disease.

4. Tertiary (Late) Syphilis

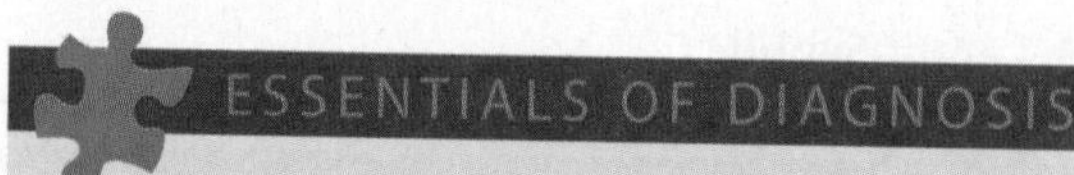

- Infiltrative tumors of skin, bones, liver (gummas).
- Aortitis, aortic aneurysms, aortic regurgitation.
- CNS disorders: meningovascular and degenerative changes, paresthesias, shooting pains, abnormal reflexes, dementia, or psychosis.

General Considerations

This stage may occur at any time after secondary syphilis, even after years of latency, and is rarely seen in developed countries in the modern antibiotic era. Late lesions are thought to represent an immunologic reaction to the organism and are usually divided into two types: (1) a localized hyperproliferative gummatous reaction with a relatively rapid onset and generally prompt response to therapy and (2) diffuse inflammation of a more insidious onset that characteristically involves the CNS and large arteries, may not improve despite treatment, and is often fatal if untreated. Gummas may involve any area or organ of the body but most often affect the skin or long bones. CVD is usually manifested by aortic aneurysm, aortic regurgitation, or aortitis. Various forms of diffuse or localized CNS involvement may occur.

Late syphilis must be differentiated from neoplasms of the skin, liver, lung, stomach, or brain; other forms of meningitis; and primary neurologic lesions.

Although almost any tissue and organ may be involved in late syphilis, the following are the most common types of involvement: skin, mucous membranes, skeletal system, eyes, respiratory system, GI system, cardiovascular system, and nervous system.

Clinical Findings

A. Symptoms and Signs

1. Skin—Cutaneous lesions of late syphilis are of two varieties: (1) multiple nodular lesions that eventually ulcerate (lues maligna) or resolve by forming atrophic, pigmented scars; and (2) solitary gummas that start as painless subcutaneous nodules, then enlarge, attach to the overlying skin, and eventually ulcerate.

2. Mucous membranes—Late lesions of the mucous membranes are nodular gummas or leukoplakia, highly destructive to the involved tissue.

3. Skeletal system—Bone lesions are destructive, causing periostitis, osteitis, and arthritis with little or no associated redness or swelling but often marked myalgia and myositis of the neighboring muscles.

4. Eyes—Late ocular lesions are gummatous iritis, chorioretinitis, optic atrophy, and cranial nerve palsies, in addition to the lesions of CNS syphilis.

5. Respiratory system—Respiratory involvement is caused by gummatous infiltrates into the larynx, trachea, and pulmonary parenchyma, producing discrete pulmonary densities. There may be hoarseness, respiratory distress, and wheezing secondary to the gummatous lesion itself or to subsequent stenosis occurring with healing.

6. GI system—Gummas involving the liver may be benign but can cause cirrhosis. Gastric involvement can consist of diffuse infiltration into the stomach wall or focal lesions that endoscopically and microscopically can be confused with lymphoma or carcinoma. Epigastric pain, early satiety, regurgitation, belching, and weight loss are common symptoms.

7. Cardiovascular system—Cardiovascular lesions (10–15% of tertiary syphilitic lesions) are often progressive, disabling, and life-threatening. CNS lesions are often present concomitantly. Involvement usually starts as an arteritis in the supracardiac portion of the aorta and progresses to one or more of the following: (1) narrowing of the coronary ostia, with resulting decreased coronary circulation, angina, and acute MI; (2) scarring of the aortic valves, producing aortic regurgitation, and eventually heart failure; and (3) weakness of the wall of the aorta, with saccular aneurysm formation (Figure 34–5) and associated pressure symptoms of dysphagia, hoarseness, brassy cough, back pain (vertebral erosion), and occasionally rupture of the aneurysm. Recurrent respiratory infections are common as a result of pressure on the trachea and bronchi.

8. Nervous system (neurosyphilis)—See next section.

Treatment

Treatment of tertiary syphilis (excluding neurosyphilis) is the same as late latent syphilis (Table 34–3); symptoms may not resolve after treatment. Positive serologic tests do not usually become negative.

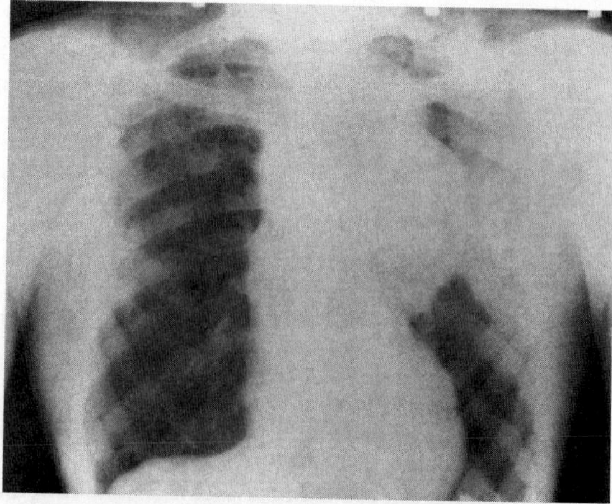

▲ **Figure 34–5.** Ascending saccular aneurysm of the thoracic aorta in tertiary syphilis. (Public Health Image Library, CDC.)

The pretreatment clinical and laboratory evaluation should include neurologic, ocular, cardiovascular, psychiatric, and CSF examinations. In the presence of definite CSF or neurologic abnormalities, treat for neurosyphilis.

5. Neurosyphilis

ESSENTIALS OF DIAGNOSIS

- Can occur at any stage of disease.
- Consider both clinical presentation and laboratory data.
- Perform neurologic examination in all patients; consider CSF evaluation for atypical symptoms or lack of decrease in nontreponemal serology titers.

General Considerations

Neurosyphilis can occur at any stage of disease and can be a progressive, disabling, and life-threatening complication. Asymptomatic CSF abnormalities and meningovascular syphilis occur earlier (months to years after infection, sometimes coexisting with primary and secondary syphilis) than tabes dorsalis and general paresis (2–50 years after infection).

Clinical Findings

A. Classification

1. Asymptomatic neuroinvasion—This form has been reported in up to 40% of patients with early syphilis and is characterized by spinal fluid abnormalities (positive spinal fluid serology, lymphocytic pleocytosis, occasionally increased protein) without symptoms or signs of neurologic involvement. There are no clear data to support that these asymptomatic CSF abnormalities have clinical significance.

2. Meningovascular syphilis—This form is characterized by meningeal involvement or changes in the vascular structures of the brain (or both), producing symptoms of acute or chronic meningitis (headache, irritability); cranial nerve palsies (basilar meningitis); unequal reflexes; irregular pupils with poor light and accommodation reflexes; and when large vessels are involved, cerebrovascular accidents. The CSF shows lymphocytic pleocytosis (cell count of 100–1000/mcL [$0.1–1.0 \times 10^9$/L]) and elevated protein and may have a positive serologic test (CSF VDRL) for syphilis. The symptoms of acute meningitis are rare in late syphilis.

3. Tabes dorsalis—This is a chronic progressive degeneration of the parenchyma of the posterior columns of the spinal cord and of the posterior sensory ganglia and nerve roots. The symptoms and signs are impairment of proprioception and vibration sense, Argyll Robertson pupils (which react poorly to light but accommodate for near focus), and muscular hypotonia and hyporeflexia. Impaired proprioception results in a wide-based gait and inability to walk in the dark. Paresthesias, analgesia, or sharp recurrent pains in the muscles of the leg ("shooting" or "lightning" pains) may occur. Joint damage may occur because of lack of sensory innervation (Charcot joint). The CSF may have a normal or increased lymphocytic cell count, elevated protein, and variable results of serologic tests.

4. General paresis—This is generalized involvement of the cerebral cortex with insidious onset of symptoms. There is usually a decrease in concentrating power, memory loss, dysarthria, tremor of the fingers and lips, irritability, and mild headaches. Most striking is the change of personality; the patient may become slovenly, irresponsible, confused, and psychotic. The CSF findings resemble those of tabes dorsalis. Combinations of the various forms of neurosyphilis (especially tabes and paresis) are not uncommon.

B. Laboratory Findings

See Serologic Tests for Syphilis, above; these tests should also be performed in cases of suspected neurosyphilis.

1. Indications for a lumbar puncture—In early syphilis (primary and secondary syphilis and early latent syphilis), invasion of the CNS by *T pallidum* with CSF abnormalities occurs commonly, but clinical neurosyphilis rarely develops in patients who have received standard therapy. Thus, unless clinical symptoms or signs of neurosyphilis or ocular involvement (uveitis, neuroretinitis, optic neuritis, iritis) are present, a lumbar puncture is not routinely recommended. CSF evaluation is recommended, however, if neurologic or ophthalmologic symptoms or signs are present, if there is evidence of treatment failure (see earlier discussion), or if there is evidence of active tertiary syphilis (eg, aortitis, iritis, optic atrophy, the presence of a gumma).

2. Spinal fluid examination—CSF findings in neurosyphilis are variable. In "classic" cases, there is an elevation of total protein above 46 mg/dL, lymphocytic pleocytosis with a cell count of 5–100/mcL ($0.005–0.1 \times 10^9$/L), and a positive CSF nontreponemal test. VDRL is more sensitive and preferred over RPR. The serum nontreponemal titers will be reactive in most cases. Because the CSF VDRL may be negative in 30–70% of cases of neurosyphilis, *a negative test does not exclude neurosyphilis*, while a positive test confirms the diagnosis. The CSF FTA-ABS is sometimes used; it is a highly sensitive test but lacks specificity, and a high serum titer of FTA-ABS may result in a positive CSF titer in the absence of neurosyphilis.

Treatment

Neurosyphilis is treated with high doses of aqueous penicillin to achieve better penetration and higher drug levels in the CSF than is possible with benzathine penicillin G (Table 34–3). There are limited data for using ceftriaxone to treat neurosyphilis as well, but because other regimens have not been adequately studied, patients with a history of an IgE-mediated reaction to penicillin may require skin testing for allergy to penicillin and, if positive, should be desensitized. Because the 10- to 14-day treatment course for neurosyphilis is less than the 21 days recommended for treatment of late syphilis, CDC guidelines state that clinicians may consider giving an additional 2.4 million units of benzathine penicillin G intramuscularly once weekly for 1–3 weeks at the conclusion of the intravenous treatment.

All patients treated for neurosyphilis should have nontreponemal serologic tests done every 3–6 months. CDC guidelines recommend spinal fluid examinations at 6-month intervals until the CSF cell count is normal; however, there are data to suggest that normalization of serum titers is an acceptable surrogate for CSF response. If the serum nontreponemal titers do not normalize, consider repeating the CSF analysis; expert consultation may be helpful in this scenario. A second course of penicillin therapy may be given if the CSF cell count has not decreased at 6 months or is not normal at 2 years.

6. Syphilis in Patients with HIV Infection

Syphilis is common among individuals with HIV infection. Some data suggest that syphilis coinfection is associated with an increase in HIV viral load and a decrease in CD4 count that normalizes with therapy; other studies have not found an association with HIV disease progression. For optimal patient care as well as prevention of transmission to partners, guidelines for the primary care of patients with HIV infection recommend at least annual syphilis screening.

Interpretation of serologic tests should be the same for persons with or without HIV infection. If the diagnosis of syphilis is suggested on clinical grounds but nontreponemal antibody tests are negative, consider the prozone effect caused by very high titers (see Nontreponemal Antibody Tests, above), or try direct examination of primary or secondary lesions for spirochetes.

Patients with HIV infection and with primary and secondary syphilis should have careful clinical and serologic follow-up at 3-month intervals. The use of antiretroviral therapy has been associated with reduced serologic failure rates after syphilis treatment.

The diagnosis of neurosyphilis in patients with HIV infection is complicated by the fact that mild CSF abnormalities may be found in HIV infection alone. Evaluate patients for visual and hearing changes, since ocular and auditory syphilis may not result in CSF abnormalities. Like in patients without HIV infection, routine lumbar puncture is not recommended in asymptomatic patients; it should be reserved for cases in which neurologic symptoms or signs are present or there is concern for treatment failure. Following treatment, CSF WBC counts should normalize within 12 months regardless of HIV status, while the CSF VDRL may take longer. As discussed above, the same criteria for failure apply to patients with and without HIV infection, and re-treatment regimens are the same.

For all stages and sites of syphilitic infection, treatment does not differ by HIV infection status.

7. Syphilis in Pregnancy

All pregnant women should have a nontreponemal serologic test for syphilis at the time of the first prenatal visit (see Chapter 19). In women who may be at increased risk for syphilis or for populations in which there is a high prevalence of syphilis, additional nontreponemal tests should be performed during the third trimester at 28 weeks and again at delivery. The serologic status of all women who have delivered should be known before discharge from the hospital. Seropositive women should be considered infected and should be treated unless prior treatment with fall in antibody titer is medically documented.

The only recommended treatment for syphilis in pregnancy is penicillin in dosage schedules appropriate for the stage of disease (Table 34–3). Penicillin prevents congenital syphilis in 90% of cases, even when treatment is given late in pregnancy. Women with a history of penicillin allergy should be skin tested and desensitized if necessary. *Tetracycline and doxycycline are contraindicated in pregnancy.*

The infant should be evaluated immediately at birth, and, depending on the likelihood of infection, monitored for clinical and serologic manifestations in the first year of life.

Prevention of Syphilis

A randomized controlled trial of doxycycline postexposure prophylaxis for sexually transmitted infection prevention among men who have sex with men enrolled in a larger HIV PrEP study in France resulted in a 73% reduction in syphilis and 70% reduction in chlamydia. This strategy is not yet recommended, and further trials are underway.

When to Refer

- Consultation with the local public health department may help obtain all prior positive syphilis serologic results and may be helpful in complicated or atypical cases.
- Early (infectious) syphilis cases may be contacted for partner notification and treatment by local public health authorities.

When to Admit

- Pregnant women with syphilis and true penicillin allergy should be admitted for desensitization and treatment.
- Women in late pregnancy treated for early syphilis should have close outpatient monitoring or be admitted because the Jarisch–Herxheimer reaction can induce premature labor.
- Patients with neurosyphilis usually require admission for treatment with aqueous penicillin.

Ghanem KG et al. The modern epidemic of syphilis. N Engl J Med. 2020;382:845. [PMID: 32101666]

Ropper AH. Neurosyphilis. N Engl J Med. 2019;381:1358. [PMID: 31577877]

Workowski KA et al; Centers for Disease Control and Prevention (CDC). Sexually transmitted infections treatment guidelines, 2021. MMWR Recomm Rep. 2021;70:1. [PMID: 34292926]

NON–SEXUALLY TRANSMITTED TREPONEMATOSES

A variety of treponemal diseases other than syphilis occur endemically in many tropical areas of the world. They are distinguished from disease caused by *T pallidum* by their nonsexual transmission via direct skin contact, their relatively high incidence in certain geographic areas and among children, and their tendency to produce less severe visceral manifestations. As in syphilis, skin, soft tissue, and bone lesions may develop, organisms can be demonstrated in infectious lesions with darkfield microscopy or immunofluorescence but cannot be cultured in artificial media; the serologic tests for syphilis are positive; molecular methods such as PCR and genome sequencing are available, but not widely used in endemic areas; the diseases have primary, secondary, and sometimes tertiary stages. Treatment with 2.4 million units of benzathine penicillin G intramuscularly is generally curative in any stage of the non–sexually transmitted treponematoses. In cases of penicillin hypersensitivity, tetracycline, 500 mg orally four times a day for 10–14 days, is usually the recommended alternative. In randomized controlled trials, oral azithromycin (30 mg/kg once) was noninferior to benzathine penicillin G for the treatment of yaws in children.

YAWS

Yaws, the most prevalent of the endemic treponematoses, is largely limited to tropical regions and is caused by *T pallidum* subspecies *pertenue.* It is characterized by granulomatous lesions of the skin, mucous membranes, and bone and is rarely fatal, though if untreated it may lead to chronic disability and disfigurement. Yaws is acquired by direct nonsexual contact, usually in childhood, although it may occur at any age. The "mother yaw," a painless papule that later ulcerates, appears 3–4 weeks after exposure, usually with associated regional lymphadenopathy. Six to 12 weeks later, secondary raised papillomas and papules that weep highly infectious material appear and last for several months or years. Painful ulcerated lesions on the soles are called "crab yaws" because of the resulting gait. Late gummatous lesions may occur, with associated tissue destruction involving large areas of skin and subcutaneous tissues. The late effects of yaws, with bone change, shortening of digits, and contractions, may be confused with similar changes occurring in leprosy. CNS, cardiac, or other visceral involvement is rare. The WHO has set a goal of eliminating yaws using mass treatment with azithromycin in endemic regions.

Frimpong M et al. Multiplex recombinase polymerase amplification assay for simultaneous detection of *Treponema pallidum and Haemophilus ducreyi* in yaws-like lesions. Trop Med Infect Dis. 2020;5:157. [PMID: 33036234]

John LN et al. Trial of three rounds of mass azithromycin administration for yaws eradication. N Engl J Med. 2022;386:47. [PMID: 34986286]

SELECTED SPIROCHETAL DISEASES

RELAPSING FEVER

The infectious organisms in relapsing fever are spirochetes of the genus *Borrelia.* The infection has two forms: tick-borne and louse-borne. The main reservoir for **tick-borne** relapsing fever is rodents, which serve as the source of infection for ticks. Tick-borne relapsing fever may be transmitted transovarially from one generation of ticks to the next. Humans can be infected by tick bites or by rubbing crushed tick tissues or feces into the bite wound. Tick-borne relapsing fever is endemic but is not transmitted from person to person. In the United States, infected ticks are found throughout the western states, but clinical cases are uncommon in humans.

The **louse-borne** form is primarily seen in the developing world, and humans are the only reservoir. Large epidemics may occur in louse-infested populations, and transmission is favored by crowding, malnutrition, and cold climate.

Clinical Findings

A. Symptoms and Signs

There is an abrupt onset of fever, chills, tachycardia, nausea and vomiting, arthralgia, and severe headache. Hepatomegaly and splenomegaly may develop, as well as various types of rashes (macular, papular, petechial) that usually occur at the end of a febrile episode. Delirium occurs with high fever, and there may be various neurologic and psychological abnormalities. The attack terminates, usually abruptly, after 3–10 days. After an interval of 1–2 weeks, relapse occurs, but often it is somewhat milder. Three to ten relapses may occur before recovery in tick-borne disease, whereas louse-borne disease is associated with only one or two relapses.

B. Laboratory Findings

During episodes of fever, large spirochetes are seen in thick and thin blood smears stained with Wright or Giemsa stain. The organisms can be cultured in special media but rapidly lose pathogenicity. The spirochetes can multiply in injected rats or mice and can be seen in their blood.

A variety of anti-*Borrelia* antibodies develop during the illness; sometimes the Weil–Felix test for rickettsioses and nontreponemal serologic tests for syphilis may be falsely positive. Infection can cause false-positive indirect fluorescent antibody and Western blot tests for *Borrelia burgdorferi,* causing some cases to be misdiagnosed as Lyme disease. PCR assays can be performed on blood, CSF, and tissue but are not always available in endemic regions. CSF abnormalities occur in patients with meningeal involvement. Mild anemia and thrombocytopenia are common, but the WBC count tends to be normal.

Differential Diagnosis

The manifestations of relapsing fever may be confused with malaria, leptospirosis, meningococcemia, yellow fever, typhus, or rat-bite fever.

Prevention

Prevention of tick bites (as described for rickettsial diseases) and delousing procedures applicable to large groups can prevent illness. There are no vaccines for relapsing fever.

Postexposure prophylaxis with doxycycline 200 mg orally on day 1 and 100 mg daily for 4 days has been shown to prevent relapsing fever following tick bites in highly endemic areas.

Treatment

In **tick-borne disease**, treatment begins with penicillin G, 3 million units intravenously every 4 hours, or ceftriaxone, 1 g intravenously daily; with clinical improvement, a 10-day course can be completed with 0.5 g of tetracycline or erythromycin given orally four times daily. If CNS invasion is suspected, intravenous penicillin G or ceftriaxone should be continued for 10–14 days. Jarisch–Herxheimer reactions occur commonly following treatment and may be life-threatening, so patients should be closely monitored (see Syphilis, above). All pregnant women with tick-borne disease should be treated for 14 days, ideally with intravenous penicillin or ceftriaxone. For **louse-borne relapsing fevers**, a single dose of tetracycline or erythromycin, 0.5 g orally, or a single dose of procaine penicillin G, 600,000–800,000 units intramuscularly (adults), probably constitutes adequate treatment; however, some experts advocate for longer courses of treatment to prevent persistent infection.

Prognosis

The overall mortality rate is usually about 5%. Fatalities are most common in older, debilitated, or very young patients. With treatment, the initial attack is shortened and relapses are largely prevented.

Talagrand-Reboul E. Relapsing fevers: neglected tick-borne diseases. Front Cell Infect Microbiol. 2018;8:98. [PMID: 29670860]

Warrell DA. Louse-borne relapsing fever (*Borrelia recurrentis* infection). Epidemiol Infect. 2019;147:e106. [PMID: 30869050]

RAT-BITE FEVER

Rat-bite fever is an uncommon acute infectious disease caused by the treponeme *Spirillum minus* (Asia) or the bacteria *Streptobacillus notomytis* (Asia) *or Streptobacillus moniliformis* (North America). It is transmitted to humans from rat bites and from ingesting rat feces. Inhabitants of rat-infested dwellings, owners of pet rats, and laboratory workers are at greatest risk.

Clinical Findings

A. Symptoms and Signs

In *Spirillum* infections, the original rat bite, unless secondarily infected, heals promptly, but one to several weeks later, the site becomes swollen, indurated, and painful. It assumes a dusky purplish hue and may ulcerate. Regional lymphangitis and lymphadenitis, fever, chills, malaise, myalgia, arthralgia, and headache are present. Splenomegaly may occur. A sparse, dusky-red maculopapular rash appears on the trunk and extremities in many cases, and there may be frank arthritis.

After a few days, both the local and systemic symptoms subside, only to reappear several days later. This relapsing pattern of fever for 3–4 days alternating with afebrile periods lasting 3–9 days may persist for weeks. The other features, however, usually recur only during the first few relapses.

S moniliformis infections have similar clinical features as *Spirillum* infections but have a shorter incubation period of up to 7 days and a diffuse rash. Endocarditis, meningitis, and sepsis are rare complications.

B. Laboratory Findings

Leukocytosis is often present, and the nontreponemal test for syphilis is often falsely positive. *S minus* may be identified in darkfield examination of the ulcer exudate or aspirated lymph node material. It has not been cultured in artificial media.

Differential Diagnosis

Rat-bite fever must be distinguished from the rat-bite–induced lymphadenitis and rash of streptobacillary fever. Clinically, the severe arthritis and myalgias seen in streptobacillary disease are rarely seen in disease caused by *S minus*. Reliable differentiation requires an increasing titer of agglutinins against *S moniliformis* or isolation of the causative organism. Other diseases in the differential include tularemia, rickettsial disease, *Pasteurella multocida* infections, and relapsing fever.

Treatment

In acute illness, intravenous penicillin, 1–2 million units every 4–6 hours, is given initially; ceftriaxone 1 g intravenously daily is another option. Once improvement has occurred, therapy may be switched to oral penicillin V 500 mg four times daily, or amoxicillin 500 mg three times daily, to complete 10–14 days of therapy. For the penicillin-allergic patient, tetracycline 500 mg orally four times daily or doxycycline 100 mg twice a day can be used.

Prognosis

The reported mortality rate of about 10% should be markedly reduced by prompt diagnosis and antimicrobial treatment.

Kämmerer T et al. Rat bite fever, a diagnostic challenge: case report and review of 29 cases. J Dtsch Dermatol Ges. 2021;19:1283. [PMID: 34323361]

LEPTOSPIROSIS

ESSENTIALS OF DIAGNOSIS

- Clinical illness can vary from asymptomatic to fatal liver and kidney failure.
- **Anicteric leptospirosis:** more common and milder form of the disease.
- **Icteric leptospirosis (Weil syndrome):** impaired kidney and liver function, abnormal mental status, hemorrhagic pneumonia; 5–40% mortality rate.

General Considerations

Leptospirosis is an acute and sometimes severe treponemal infection that is caused by several species within the genus *Leptospira*. The disease is distributed worldwide, and it is among the most common zoonotic infections. The leptospires enter through minor skin lesions and probably via the conjunctiva. Cases have occurred in international travelers after swimming or rafting in contaminated water, and occupational cases occur among sewer workers, rice planters, abattoir workers, and farmers. Sporadic urban cases have been seen in homeless persons exposed to rat urine.

Clinical Findings

A. Symptoms and Signs

Anicteric leptospirosis, the more common and milder form of the disease, is often biphasic. After an incubation period of 2–20 days, the initial or "septicemic" phase begins with abrupt fever to 39–40°C, chills, abdominal pain, severe headache, and myalgias, especially of the calf muscles. There may be marked conjunctival suffusion. Leptospires can be isolated from blood, CSF, and tissues. Following a 1- to 3-day period of improvement in symptoms and absence of fever, the second or "immune" phase begins; however, in severe disease the phases may appear indistinct. Leptospires are absent from blood and CSF but are still present in the kidney, and specific antibodies appear. A recurrence of symptoms is seen as in the first phase of disease with the onset of meningitis. Uveitis, rash, nausea, vomiting, diarrhea, and adenopathy may occur. A rare but severe manifestation is hemorrhagic pneumonia. The illness is usually self-limited, lasting 4–30 days, and complete recovery is the rule.

Icteric leptospirosis (Weil syndrome) is the more severe form of the disease, characterized by impaired kidney and liver function, abnormal mental status, hemorrhagic pneumonia, hypotension, and a 5–40% mortality rate. Symptoms and signs often are continuous and not biphasic.

Leptospirosis with jaundice must be distinguished from hepatitis, yellow fever, rickettsial disease, and relapsing fever.

B. Laboratory Findings

The leukocyte count may be normal or as high as 50,000/mcL (50×10^9/L), with neutrophils predominating. The urine may contain bile, protein, casts, and red cells. Oliguria is common, and in severe cases uremia may occur. Elevated bilirubin and aminotransferases are seen in 75%, and elevated creatinine (greater than 1.5 mg/dL) (132.6 mcmol/L) is seen in 50% of cases. Serum creatine kinase is usually elevated in persons with leptospirosis and normal in persons with hepatitis. In cases with meningeal involvement, organisms may be found in the CSF during the first 10 days of illness. Early in the disease, the organism may be identified by darkfield examination of the patient's blood (a test requiring expertise since false-positives are frequent in inexperienced hands) or by culture. Cultures take 1–6 weeks to become positive but may remain negative if antibiotics were started before culture was obtained. The organism may also be grown from the urine from the tenth day to the sixth week. Diagnosis is usually made by serologic tests, including the microscopic agglutination test and ELISA. PCR molecular diagnostics appear to be sensitive, specific, positive early in disease, and able to detect leptospiral DNA in blood, urine, CSF, and aqueous humor.

Complications

Myocarditis, aseptic meningitis, AKI, and pulmonary infiltrates with hemorrhage are not common but are the usual causes of death. Iridocyclitis may occur.

Prevention

The mainstay of prevention is avoidance of potentially contaminated food and water.

Prophylaxis with doxycycline (200 mg orally once a week) may be useful if a person is at high risk due to being in an area or season (eg, monsoon flooding) when exposure would be more likely. Human vaccine is used in some limited settings but is not widely available.

Treatment

Many cases are self-limited without specific treatment. Many antibiotics, including penicillin, ceftriaxone, and tetracyclines, show antileptospiral activity; meta-analysis has not demonstrated a clear survival benefit for any antibiotic. Doxycycline (100 mg every 12 hours orally or intravenously), penicillin (eg, 1.5 million units every 6 hours intravenously), and ceftriaxone (1 g daily intravenously) are used in severe leptospirosis. Jarisch–Herxheimer reactions may occur (see Syphilis, above). Although therapy for mild disease is controversial, most clinicians treat with doxycycline, 100 mg orally twice daily for 7 days, or amoxicillin, 50 mg/kg, divided into three doses daily.

Prognosis

Without jaundice, the disease is almost never fatal. With jaundice, the mortality rate is 5% for those under age 30 years and 40% for those over age 60 years.

When to Admit

Patients with jaundice or other evidence of severe disease should be admitted for close monitoring and may require admission to an ICU.

Karpagam KB et al. Leptospirosis: a neglected tropical zoonotic infection of public health importance-an updated review. Eur J Clin Microbiol Infect Dis. 2020;39:835. [PMID: 31898795]

LYME DISEASE (Lyme Borreliosis)

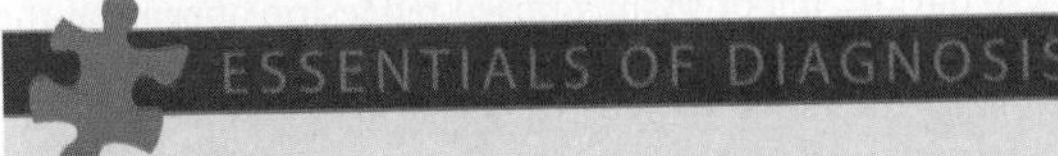

- Erythema migrans: a flat or slightly raised red lesion that expands with central clearing.
- Headache or stiff neck.
- Arthralgias, arthritis, and myalgias; arthritis is often chronic and recurrent.

General Considerations

This illness, named after the town of Old Lyme, Connecticut, is the most common tick-borne disease in the United States and Europe and is caused by genospecies of the spirochete *B burgdorferi*. Most US cases are reported from the mid-Atlantic, northeastern, and north central regions of the country. The true incidence of Lyme disease is not known for several reasons: (1) serologic tests are not standardized (see below); (2) clinical manifestations are nonspecific; and (3) even with reliable testing, serology is insensitive in early disease.

The tick vector of Lyme disease varies geographically and is *Ixodes scapularis* in the northeastern, north central, and mid-Atlantic regions of the United States; *Ixodes pacificus* on the West Coast; *Ixodes ricinus* in Europe; and *Ixodes persulcatus* in Asia. The disease also occurs in Australia. Mice and deer make up the major animal reservoir of *B burgdorferi*, but other rodents and birds may also be infected. Domestic animals such as dogs, cattle, and horses can also develop clinical illness, usually manifested as arthritis.

Under experimental conditions, ticks must feed for 24–36 hours or longer to transmit infections. Most cases are reported in the spring and summer months. In addition, the percentage of ticks infected varies on a regional, and local basis. These are important epidemiologic features in assessing the likelihood that tick exposure will result in disease. Eliciting a history of brushing a tick off the skin (ie, the tick was not feeding) or removing a tick on the same day as exposure (ie, the tick did not feed long enough) decreases the likelihood that infection will develop.

Because the *Ixodes* tick is so small, the bite is usually painless and goes unnoticed. After feeding, the tick drops off in 2–4 days. If a tick is found, it should be removed immediately. The best way to accomplish this is to use fine-tipped tweezers to pull firmly and repeatedly on the tick's mouth part—not the tick's body—until the tick releases its hold. Saving the tick in a bottle of alcohol for future identification may be useful, especially if symptoms develop.

Clinical Findings

The three stages of Lyme disease are classified based on early or late manifestations of the disease and whether it is localized or disseminated.

A. Symptoms and Signs

1. Stage 1, early localized infection—Stage 1 infection is characterized by erythema migrans (see Figure 6–18). About 1 week after the tick bite (range, 3–30 days; median 7–10 days), a flat or slightly raised red lesion appears at the site, which is commonly seen in areas of tight clothing such as the groin, thigh, or axilla. This lesion expands over several days. Although originally described as a lesion that progresses with central clearing ("bulls-eye" lesion), often there is a more homogeneous appearance or even central intensification. About 10–20% of patients either do not have typical skin lesions or the lesions go unnoticed. Most patients with erythema migrans will have a concomitant viral-like illness (the "summer flu") characterized by myalgias, arthralgias, headache, and fatigue. Fever may or may not be present. Even without treatment, the symptoms and signs of erythema migrans resolve in 3–4 weeks. Although the classic lesion of erythema migrans is not difficult to recognize, atypical forms can occur that may lead to misdiagnosis. Southern tick–associated rash illness (STARI) has a similar appearance, but it occurs in geographically distinct areas of the United States.

Completely asymptomatic disease, without erythema migrans or flu-like symptoms, can occur but is very uncommon in the United States.

2. Stage 2, early disseminated infection—Up to 50–60% of patients with erythema migrans are bacteremic and within days to weeks of the original infection, secondary skin lesions develop in about 50% of patients. These lesions are similar in appearance to the primary lesion but are usually smaller. Malaise, fatigue, fever, headache (sometimes severe), neck pain, and generalized achiness are common with the skin lesions. Most symptoms are transient. After hematogenous spread, some patients experience cardiac (4–10% of patients) or neurologic (10–15% of patients) manifestations, including myopericarditis, with atrial or ventricular arrhythmias and heart block. Neurologic manifestations include both the central and peripheral nervous systems. The most common CNS manifestation is aseptic meningitis with mild headache and neck stiffness. The most common peripheral manifestation is a cranial nerve VII neuropathy, ie, facial palsy (usually unilateral but can be bilateral, see Figure 24–1). A sensory or motor radiculopathy and mononeuritis multiplex occur less frequently. Conjunctivitis, keratitis, and, rarely, panophthalmitis can also occur. Rarely, a cutaneous hypopigmented skin lesion called a borrelial lymphocytoma develops.

3. Stage 3, late persistent infection—Stage 3 infection occurs months to years after the initial infection and again primarily manifests itself as musculoskeletal, neurologic, and skin disease. In early reports, musculoskeletal complaints developed in up to 60% of patients, but with early recognition and treatment of disease, this has decreased to less than 10%. The classic manifestation of late disease is a monoarticular or oligoarticular arthritis most commonly affecting the knee or other large weight bearing joints. While these joints may be quite swollen, these patients generally report less pain compared to patients with bacterial septic arthritis. Even if untreated, the arthritis is self-limited, resolving in a few weeks to months. Multiple recurrences are common but are usually less severe than the original disease. Joint fluid reflects an inflammatory arthritis with a mean WBC count of 25,000/mcL (25×10^9/L) with a predominance of neutrophils. Chronic arthritis can develop in about 10% of patients; this pathogenesis may be an immunologic phenomenon rather than persistence of infection.

Rarely, the nervous system (both central and peripheral) can be involved in late Lyme disease. In the United States, a subacute encephalopathy, characterized by memory loss, mood changes, and sleep disturbance, is seen. In Europe, a more severe encephalomyelitis caused by *B garinii* is seen and presents with cognitive dysfunction, spastic paraparesis, ataxia, and bladder dysfunction. Peripheral nervous system involvement includes intermittent paresthesias, often in a stocking glove distribution, or radicular pain.

The cutaneous manifestation of late infection, which can occur up to 10 years after infection, is acrodermatitis chronicum atrophicans. It has been described mainly in Europe after infection with *B afzelii*. There is usually bluish-red discoloration of a distal extremity with associated swelling. These lesions become atrophic and sclerotic with time and eventually resemble localized scleroderma. Cases of diffuse fasciitis with eosinophilia, an entity that resembles scleroderma, have been rarely associated with infection with *B burgdorferi*.

B. Laboratory Findings

The diagnosis of Lyme disease is based on both clinical manifestations and laboratory findings. **The US Surveillance Case Definition specifies a person with exposure to a potential tick habitat (within the 30 days just prior to developing erythema migrans) with (1) erythema migrans diagnosed by a clinician or (2) at least one late manifestation of the disease and (3) laboratory confirmation as fulfilling the criteria for Lyme disease.**

Nonspecific laboratory abnormalities can occur, particularly in early disease. The most common are an elevated ESR of more than 20 mm/hour seen in 50% of cases, and mildly abnormal liver biochemical tests are present in 30%. The abnormal liver biochemical tests are transient and return to normal within a few weeks of treatment. A mild anemia, leukocytosis (11,000–18,000/mcL [$11–18 \times 10^9$/L]), and microscopic hematuria have been reported in 10% or less of patients.

Laboratory confirmation requires serologic tests to detect specific antibodies to *B burgdorferi* in serum, preferably by ELISA and not by indirect immunofluorescence assay (IFA), which is less sensitive and specific and can cause misdiagnosis. A two-test approach is recommended for the diagnosis of active Lyme disease, with all specimens positive or equivocal by ELISA then confirmed with a Western immunoblot assay that can detect both IgM and IgG antibodies or with a different ELISA. A positive immunoblot requires that antibodies are detected against two (for IgM) or five (for IgG) specific protein antigens from *B burgdorferi*.

If a patient with suspected early Lyme disease has negative serologic studies, acute and convalescent titers should be obtained since up to 50% of patients with early disease can be antibody negative in the first several weeks of illness. A fourfold rise in antibody titer would be diagnostic of recent infection. False-negative serologic reactions occur early in illness, and antibiotic therapy early in disease can abort subsequent seroconversion.

The diagnosis of late nervous system Lyme disease is often difficult since clinical manifestations, such as subtle memory impairment, may be difficult to document. Patients with late disease and peripheral neuropathy almost always have positive serum antibody tests, usually have abnormal electrophysiology tests, and may have abnormal nerve biopsies showing perivascular collections of lymphocytes; however, the CSF is usually normal and does not demonstrate local antibody production.

Caution should be exercised in interpreting serologic tests because they are not subject to national standards, and inter-laboratory variation is a major problem. In addition, some laboratories perform tests that are entirely unreliable and should never be used to support the diagnosis of Lyme disease (eg, the Lyme urinary antigen test, immunofluorescent staining for cell wall–deficient forms of *B burgdorferi*, lymphocyte transformation tests, or PCR on inappropriate specimens such as blood or urine). Finally, testing is often done in patients with nonspecific symptoms such as headache, arthralgia, myalgia, fatigue, and palpitations. For these reasons, the CDC and Infectious Diseases Society of America have established guidelines for laboratory evaluation of patients with suspected Lyme disease:

1. The diagnosis of early Lyme disease is clinical (ie, exposure in an endemic area, with clinician-documented erythema migrans) and does *not* require laboratory confirmation. (Tests are often negative at this stage.) If lesions are atypical, serology performed on acute and convalescent sera (collected 14–21 days later) can help confirm the diagnosis.
2. Late disease requires objective evidence of clinical manifestations (recurrent brief attacks of monoarticular or oligoarticular arthritis of the large joints; lymphocytic meningitis, cranial neuritis [facial palsy], peripheral neuropathy or, rarely, encephalomyelitis—but *not* headache, fatigue, paresthesias, or stiff neck alone; atrioventricular conduction defects with or without myocarditis) and laboratory evidence of disease (two-stage testing with ELISA or IFA followed by Western blot or a second ELISA, as described above).
3. Patients with nonspecific symptoms without objective signs of Lyme disease should *not* have serologic testing done. It is in this setting that false-positive tests occur more commonly than true-positive tests.
4. When assessing for CNS Lyme disease in an appropriate clinical syndrome, serum antibody testing is recommended over CSF serology or PCR.
5. While serology is recommended to diagnose Lyme arthritis, PCR can be done on synovial fluid or tissue if needed to confirm the diagnosis and guide treatment.

Erythema migrans is a clinical diagnosis; cultures and PCR of the lesions for *B burgdorferi* are not recommended.

Complications

B burgdorferi infection in pregnant women has *not* been associated with congenital syndromes, unlike other spirochetal illnesses such as syphilis.

Some patients and advocacy groups have claimed either a post–Lyme disease syndrome (in the presence of positive laboratory tests and after appropriate treatment) or "chronic Lyme disease" in which tests may all be negative. Both entities include nonspecific symptoms such as fatigue, myalgias, and cognitive difficulties (see Prognosis below). Expert groups agree that there are no data to support that ongoing infection is the cause of either syndrome.

Prevention

There is no human vaccine available. Simple preventive measures such as avoiding tick-infested areas, covering exposed skin with long-sleeved shirts, tucking long trousers into socks, wearing light-colored clothing, using repellents, and inspecting for ticks after exposure will greatly reduce the number of tick bites.

Prophylactic antibiotic treatment following tick bites is recommended in certain high-risk situations if all of the following criteria are met: (1) a tick identified as an adult or nymphal *I scapularis* has been attached for at least 36 hours; (2) prophylaxis can be started within 72 hours of the time the tick was removed; (3) more than 20% of ticks in the area are known to be infected with *B burgdorferi*; and (4) there is no contraindication to the use of doxycycline (not pregnant, age greater than 8 years, not allergic). The medication of choice for prophylaxis is a single 200-mg dose of doxycycline. If doxycycline is contraindicated, no prophylaxis should be given since short-course prophylactic therapy with other agents has not been studied. The patient should be closely monitored for early disease, and if early disease does develop, appropriate therapy is very effective in preventing long-term sequelae. Individuals who have removed ticks (including those who have had prophylaxis) should be monitored carefully for 30 days for possible coinfections.

Coinfections

Lyme disease, babesiosis (see Chapter 35), and human granulocytic anaplasmosis (see Chapter 32) are endemic in similar areas of the country and are transmitted by the same tick, *I scapularis*. Coinfection with two or all three of these organisms can occur, causing a clinical picture that is not "classic" for any of these diseases. The presence of erythema migrans is highly suggestive of Lyme disease, whereas flu-like symptoms without rash are more suggestive of babesiosis or anaplasmosis. *Coinfection should be considered and excluded in patients who have persistent high fevers 48 hours after starting appropriate therapy for Lyme disease; in patients with persistent symptoms despite resolution of rash; and in those with anemia, leukopenia, or thrombocytopenia.*

Treatment

Recommendations for therapy are outlined in Table 34–4. For erythema migrans, antibiotic therapy shortens the duration of rash and prevents late sequelae. Doxycycline is most commonly used and has the advantage of being active against anaplasmosis, a common coinfection. It has proven effective in shorter courses of 10 days compared to other regimens. Amoxicillin is also effective and is recommended for pregnant or lactating women and for those who cannot tolerate doxycycline.

Isolated facial palsy (without meningitis or peripheral neuropathy) can be treated with doxycycline, amoxicillin, or cefuroxime axetil for 2–3 weeks. Therapy does not affect the rate of resolution of the cranial neuropathy, but it does prevent development of late disease manifestations.

Some clinicians perform lumbar puncture on all patients with facial palsy and others only if there are symptoms or signs of meningitis. If meningitis is present, either parenteral therapy with ceftriaxone, cefotaxime, or penicillin G or oral doxycycline is recommended. The best initial agent will depend on the clinical scenario; patients who initially receive parenteral therapy can be switched to oral therapy to complete 14–21 total days of treatment. Patients with parenchymal brain or spinal cord disease should be treated with intravenous antibiotics.

Atrioventricular block or myopericarditis (or both) can be treated with either oral or parenteral agents for 2–3 weeks. Hospitalization and observation are indicated for symptomatic patients, those with second- or third-degree block, and those with first-degree block with a PR interval of 300 milliseconds or more. Once stabilized, hospitalized patients can be transitioned to one of the oral regimens to complete therapy.

Therapy of arthritis is difficult because some patients do not respond to any therapy, and those who do respond may do so slowly. Oral agents (doxycycline, amoxicillin, or cefuroxime axetil) are as effective as intravenous regimens (ceftriaxone, cefotaxime, or penicillin). A reasonable approach to the patient with Lyme arthritis is to start with oral therapy for 28 days. If there is partial resolution, re-treat with an additional 28 days of the same oral regimen. However, if there has been no response or worsening with initial oral therapy, switch to intravenous ceftriaxone for 14–28 days. If arthritis persists after re-treatment, symptomatic therapy with NSAIDs is recommended. For severe refractory pain, synovectomy may be required.

Acrodermatitis chronicum atrophicans can be treated with oral doxycycline, amoxicillin, or cefuroxime for 21–28 days.

Based on limited data, therapy of Lyme disease in pregnancy should be the same as therapy in other patients, with the exception that doxycycline should not be used.

Clinicians may encounter patients with nonspecific symptoms (such as fatigue and myalgias) and positive serologic tests for Lyme disease who request therapy for their illness. When treating these patients, clinicians must remember (1) that nonspecific symptoms alone are not diagnostic; (2) that serologic tests are fraught with difficulty (as noted above), and in areas where disease prevalence is low, false-positive serologic tests are much more common than true-positive tests; and (3) that parenteral therapy with ceftriaxone for 2–4 weeks is costly and can cause significant adverse effects, including cholelithiasis and *Clostridioides difficile* colitis. Parenteral therapy should be reserved for those most likely to benefit, ie, those with characteristic cutaneous, neurologic, cardiac, or rheumatic manifestations of Lyme disease.

Prognosis

Most patients respond to appropriate therapy with prompt resolution of symptoms within 4 weeks. True treatment failures are thus uncommon, and in most cases, re-treatment or prolonged treatment of Lyme disease is instituted because of misdiagnosis or misinterpretation of serologic results (both IgG and IgM antibodies can persist for prolonged periods despite adequate therapy) rather than inadequate therapy or response. Prolonged courses of antibiotic therapy for nonspecific symptoms that persist after completion of appropriate assessment (and treatment, if necessary) for Lyme disease are not recommended.

Table 34–4. Treatment of Lyme disease.

Manifestations	Medication and Dosage
Tick bite	No treatment in most circumstances (see text); observe
Erythema migrans	Doxycycline, 100 mg orally twice daily for 10 days, or amoxicillin, 500 mg orally three times daily for 14 days, or cefuroxime axetil, 500 mg orally twice daily for 14 days An alternative is azithromycin, 500 mg orally daily for 7 days
Neurologic disease	
Facial palsy (without meningitis)	Doxycycline, 100 mg orally twice daily, or amoxicillin, 500 mg orally three times daily, or cefuroxime axetil, 500 mg orally twice daily for 14–21 days
Other acute neurologic disease (not parenchymal disease of brain or spinal cord)	Ceftriaxone, 2 g intravenously once daily, or penicillin G, 18–24 million units daily intravenously in six divided doses, or cefotaxime, 2 g intravenously every 8 hours—all for 14–21 days or Doxycycline, 100 mg orally twice daily for 14–21 days
Parenchymal brain or spinal cord disease	Ceftriaxone, 2 g intravenously once daily, or penicillin G, 18–24 million units daily intravenously in six divided doses, or cefotaxime, 2 g intravenously every 8 hours—all for 14–28 days
Cardiac disease	
Atrioventricular block and myopericarditis[1]	
Outpatient	Doxycycline, 100 mg orally twice daily for 14–21 days, or amoxicillin, 500 mg orally three times daily for 14–21 days, or cefuroxime axetil, 500 mg orally twice daily for 14–21 days
Inpatient	Ceftriaxone, 2 g intravenously once daily; patients can be switched to an oral agent (doxycycline is first-line therapy) to complete 14–21 days of total antibiotic treatment if clinically improving
Arthritis	Doxycycline, 100 mg orally twice daily for 28 days, or amoxicillin, 500 mg orally three times daily for 28 days, or cefuroxime axetil, 500 mg orally twice daily for 28 days (see text). An oral agent is preferred as initial treatment and can be repeated if needed. If no response to initial treatment, ceftriaxone, 2 g intravenously once daily, can be given for 14–21 days
Acrodermatitis chronicum atrophicans	Doxycycline, amoxicillin, or cefuroxime axetil as above for 21–28 days
"Chronic Lyme disease" or "post–Lyme disease syndrome"	Symptomatic therapy; prolonged antibiotics are *not* recommended

[1]Symptomatic patients, those with second- or third-degree block, and those with first-degree block with a PR interval ≥ 300 milliseconds should be hospitalized for observation.

The long-term outcome of adult patients with Lyme disease is generally favorable, but some patients have chronic complaints. Joint pain, memory impairment, and poor functional status because of pain are common subjective complaints, but physical examination and neurocognitive testing fail to document the presence of these symptoms as objective sequelae.

Immunity is not complete after Lyme disease. Reinfection, although uncommon, is predominantly seen in patients successfully treated for early disease (erythema migrans) in whom antibody titers do not develop. Clinical manifestations and serologic response are similar to an initial infection.

When to Refer

Consultation with an infectious diseases specialist with experience in diagnosing and treating Lyme disease can be helpful in atypical or prolonged cases.

When to Admit

Admission for parenteral antibiotics is indicated for any patient with symptomatic CNS or cardiac disease as well as those with second- or third-degree atrioventricular block, or first-degree block with a PR interval of 300 milliseconds or more.

Cardenas-de la Garza JA et al. Clinical spectrum of Lyme disease. Eur J Clin Microbiol Infect Dis. 2019;38:201. [PMID: 30456435]

Lantos PM et al. Clinical Practice Guidelines by the Infectious Diseases Society of America (IDSA), American Academy of Neurology (AAN), and American College of Rheumatology (ACR): 2020 guidelines for the prevention, diagnosis and treatment of Lyme disease. Clin Infect Dis. 2021;72:e1. [PMID: 33417672]

Protozoal & Helminthic Infections

Philip J. Rosenthal, MD

PROTOZOAL INFECTIONS

AFRICAN TRYPANOSOMIASIS (Sleeping Sickness)

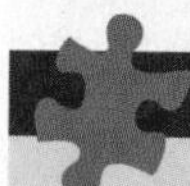

ESSENTIALS OF DIAGNOSIS

- Exposure to tsetse flies; chancre at bite site uncommon.
- **Hemolymphatic disease:** Irregular fever, headache, joint pain, rash, edema, lymphadenopathy.
- **Meningoencephalitic disease:** Somnolence, severe headache, progressing to coma.
- Trypanosomes in blood or lymph node aspirates; positive serologic tests.
- Trypanosomes and increased white cells and protein in cerebrospinal fluid (CSF).

General Considerations

African trypanosomiasis is caused by the hemoflagellates *Trypanosoma brucei rhodesiense* and *Trypanosoma brucei gambiense*. The organisms are transmitted by bites of tsetse flies (genus *Glossina*), which inhabit shaded areas along streams and rivers. Trypanosomes ingested in a blood meal develop over 18–35 days in the fly; when the fly feeds again on a mammalian host, the infective stage is injected. Human disease occurs in rural areas of sub-Saharan Africa from south of the Sahara to about 30 degrees south latitude. *T b gambiense* causes West African trypanosomiasis and is transmitted in the moist sub-Saharan savannas and forests of west and central Africa. *T b rhodesiense* causes East African trypanosomiasis and is transmitted in the savannas of east and southeast Africa.

T b rhodesiense infection is primarily a zoonosis of game animals and cattle; humans are infected sporadically. Humans are the principal mammalian host for *T b gambiense*, but domestic animals can be infected. The number of reported cases has decreased greatly since the 1990s, although cases are reported from over 20 countries. Total incidence has been estimated at less than 5000 cases per year, mostly due to *T b gambiense*, with the largest number in the Democratic Republic of the Congo. Infections are rare among travelers, including visitors to game parks.

Clinical Findings

A. Symptoms and Signs

1. West African trypanosomiasis—Chancres at the site of the bite are uncommon. After an asymptomatic period that may last for months, hemolymphatic disease presents with fever, headache, myalgias, arthralgias, weight loss, and lymphadenopathy, with discrete, nontender, rubbery nodes, referred to as Winterbottom sign when in a posterior cervical distribution. Other common signs are mild splenomegaly, transient edema, and a pruritic erythematous rash. Febrile episodes may be broken by afebrile periods of up to several weeks. The hemolymphatic stage progresses over months to meningoencephalitic disease, with somnolence, irritability, personality changes, severe headache, and parkinsonian symptoms progressing to coma and death.

2. East African trypanosomiasis—Chancres at the bite site are more commonly recognized with *T b rhodesiense* infection, with a painful lesion of 3–10 cm and regional lymphadenopathy that appears about 48 hours after the tsetse fly bite and lasts 2–4 weeks. East African disease follows a much more acute course, with the onset of symptoms usually within a few days of the insect bite. The hemolymphatic stage includes intermittent fever and rash, but lymphadenopathy is less common than with West African disease. Myocarditis can cause tachycardia and death due to arrhythmias or heart failure. If untreated, East African trypanosomiasis progresses over weeks to months to meningoencephalitic disease, somnolence, coma, and death.

B. Laboratory Findings

Diagnosis can be difficult, and definitive diagnosis requires identification of trypanosomes. Microscopic examination of fluid expressed from a chancre or lymph node may show motile trypanosomes or, in fixed specimens, parasites stained with Giemsa. During the hemolymphatic stage, detection of parasites in Giemsa-stained blood smears is common in East African disease but difficult in West African disease. Serial specimens should be examined, since parasitemias vary greatly over time. Meningoencephalitic disease is defined by the World Health Organization (WHO) as CSF showing at least five mononuclear cells per microliter, elevated protein, or presence of trypanosomes. Concentration techniques can aid identification of parasites in blood or CSF. Serologic tests are also available. The card agglutination test for trypanosomes (CATT) has excellent sensitivity and specificity for West African disease and can be performed in the field, but the diagnosis should be confirmed by identification of the parasites. Field-applicable immunochromatographic lateral flow rapid diagnostic tests that cost less than CATT and are simpler to perform are available; combining tests improves sensitivity and specificity. Molecular diagnostic tests, including PCR and field-friendly loop-mediated isothermal amplification (LAMP), are available but are not yet standardized or routinely available.

Treatment

Detection of trypanosomes is a prerequisite for treatment of African trypanosomiasis because of the significant toxicity of available therapies. Treatment recommendations depend on the type of trypanosomiasis (Table 35–1), which is determined by geography, and stage of disease. Fexinidazole is recommended by the WHO as first-line therapy and is FDA-approved for treatment of early and advanced (CNS) West African disease. Eflornithine, suramin, and melarsoprol are available in the United States from the CDC Drug Service (www.cdc.gov/laboratory/drugservice).

A. West African Trypanosomiasis

Fexinidazole is effective and safe when administered orally over 10 days. It is recommended for persons 6 years of age and older, with body weight at least 20 kg, and a CSF leukocyte count below 100/mcL (0.1×10^9/L). Evaluation of the CSF can be avoided if there is no suspicion of severe CNS disease. Fexinidazole greatly simplifies therapy compared with parenteral regimens, but relapse and death after treatment may be more common than after treatment with eflornithine plus nifurtimox. Side effects from fexinidazole include headache, nausea, vomiting, insomnia, anxiety, weakness, tremor, and decreased appetite. For advanced CNS disease (CNS leukocytes more than 100/mcL [0.1×10^9/L]), a combination of intravenous eflornithine (400 mg/kg/day in two doses for 7 days) and oral nifurtimox (15 mg/kg/day in three doses for 10 days) is recommended. Eflornithine, although less toxic than older trypanocidal drugs, can cause GI symptoms, bone marrow suppression, seizures, and alopecia. Alternative therapies include pentamidine and suramin for early disease and melarsoprol for CNS disease, all with serious toxicity concerns.

Table 35–1. Treatment of African trypanosomiasis.

Disease	Stage	Treatment: First Line	Treatment: Alternative
West African	Early	Fexinidazole	Pentamidine Suramin Eflornithine
	CNS involvement	Fexinidazole (< 100 leukocytes/mcL [0.1×10^9/L] in CNS) Eflornithine + nifurtimox	Melarsoprol
East African	Early	Suramin	Pentamidine
	CNS involvement	Melarsoprol	

B. East African Trypanosomiasis

Early disease is treated with suramin; dosing regimens vary (eg, 100–200 mg test dose, then 20 mg/kg [maximum 1 g] intravenously on days 1, 3, 7, 14, and 21 or weekly for five doses). Suramin toxicities include vomiting and, rarely, seizures and shock during infusions as well as subsequent fever, rash, headache, neuropathy, and kidney and bone marrow dysfunction.

Suramin does not enter the CNS, so East African trypanosomiasis involving the CNS is treated with melarsoprol (three series of 3.6 mg/kg/day intravenously for 3 days, with 7-day breaks between the series or a 10-day intravenous course with 0.6 mg/kg on day 1, 1.2 mg/kg on day 2, and 1.8 mg/kg on days 3–10). Immediate side effects of melarsoprol include fever and GI symptoms. The most important side effect is a reactive encephalopathy that can progress to seizures, coma, and death. To help avoid this side effect, corticosteroids are coadministered (dexamethasone 1 mg/kg/day intravenously for 2–3 days or oral prednisolone 1 mg/kg/day for 5 days, and then 0.5 mg/kg/day until treatment completion). Increasing resistance to melarsoprol is a serious concern.

Prevention & Control

Individual prevention in endemic areas should include neutral-colored clothes (eg, long sleeve shirts and pants), insect repellents, and mosquito nets. Control programs focusing on vector elimination and treatment of infected persons and animals have shown good success in many areas but suffer from limited resources.

Büscher P et al. Human African trypanosomiasis. Lancet. 2017;390:2397. [PMID: 28673422]

Hidalgo J et al. Efficacy and toxicity of fexinidazole and nifurtimox plus eflornithine in the treatment of African trypanosomiasis: a systematic review. Cureus. 2021;13:e16881. [PMID: 34513456]

Lutje V et al. Chemotherapy for second-stage human African trypanosomiasis: drugs in use. Cochrane Database Syst Rev. 2021;12:CD015374. [PMID: 34882307]

Mesu VKBK et al. Oral fexinidazole for late-stage African Trypanosoma brucei gambiense trypanosomiasis: a pivotal multicentre, randomised, non-inferiority trial. Lancet. 2018;391:144. [PMID: 29113731]

AMERICAN TRYPANOSOMIASIS (Chagas Disease)

ESSENTIALS OF DIAGNOSIS

Acute stage

- Inflammatory lesion at inoculation site.
- Fever.
- Hepatosplenomegaly; lymphadenopathy.
- Myocarditis.
- Parasites in blood are diagnostic.

Chronic stage

- Heart failure, cardiac arrhythmias.
- Thromboembolism.
- Megaesophagus; megacolon.
- Serologic tests are usually diagnostic.

General Considerations

Chagas disease is caused by *Trypanosoma cruzi*, a protozoan parasite found only in the Americas; it infects wild animals and, to a lesser extent, humans from southern South America to the southern United States. An estimated 6–7 million people are infected, mostly in rural areas, with the highest national prevalence in Bolivia, Argentina, Paraguay, Ecuador, El Salvador, and Guatemala. Control efforts in endemic countries have decreased disease incidence to about 30,000 new infections and 12,000 deaths per year. The disease is often acquired in childhood. In many countries in South America, Chagas disease is the most important cause of heart disease. The vector is endemic in the southern United States where some animals are infected, and a few instances of local transmission have been reported.

T cruzi is transmitted by reduviid (triatomine) bugs infected by ingesting blood from animals or humans who have circulating trypanosomes. Multiplication occurs in the digestive tract of the bug and infective forms are eliminated in feces. Infection in humans occurs when the parasite penetrates the skin through the bite wound, mucous membranes, or the conjunctiva. Transmission can also occur by blood transfusion, organ or bone marrow transplantation, congenital transfer, or ingestion of food contaminated with vector feces. From the bloodstream, *T cruzi* invades many cell types but has a predilection for myocardium, smooth muscle, and CNS glial cells. Multiplication causes cellular destruction, inflammation, and fibrosis, with progressive disease over decades.

Clinical Findings

A. Symptoms and Signs

As many as 70% of infected persons remain asymptomatic. The **acute stage** is seen principally in children and lasts 1–2 months. The earliest findings are at the site of inoculation either in the eye—Romaña sign (unilateral edema, conjunctivitis, and lymphadenopathy)—or in the skin—a chagoma (swelling with local lymphadenopathy). Subsequent findings include fever, malaise, headache, mild hepatosplenomegaly, and generalized lymphadenopathy. Acute myocarditis and meningoencephalitis are rare but can be fatal.

An asymptomatic **latent period** (indeterminate phase) may last for life, but symptomatic disease develops in 10–30% of individuals with infection, commonly many years after infection.

Chronic Chagas disease generally manifests as abnormalities in cardiac and smooth muscle. Cardiac disease includes arrhythmias, heart failure, and embolic disease. Smooth muscle abnormalities lead to megaesophagus and megacolon, with dysphagia, regurgitation, aspiration, constipation, and abdominal pain. These findings can be complicated by superinfections. In immunosuppressed persons, including people living with AIDS and transplant recipients, latent Chagas disease may reactivate; findings have included brain abscesses and meningoencephalitis.

B. Diagnostic Testing

The diagnosis is made by detecting parasites in persons with suggestive findings who have resided in an endemic area. With acute infection, evaluation of fresh blood or buffy coats may show motile trypanosomes, and fixed preparations may show Giemsa-stained parasites. Concentration methods increase diagnostic yields. Trypanosomes may be identified in lymph nodes, bone marrow, or pericardial or spinal fluid. Molecular tests are highly sensitive and can be used to detect parasites in organ transplant recipients or after accidental exposure. When initial tests are unrevealing, xenodiagnosis using laboratory vectors, laboratory culture, or animal inoculation may provide a diagnosis, but these methods are expensive and slow.

Chronic Chagas disease is usually diagnosed serologically. Many serologic assays, including rapid diagnostic tests, are available, but sensitivity and specificity are not ideal; confirmatory assays are advised after an initial positive test, as is standard for blood bank testing in South America. The diagnosis of chronic disease with PCR remains suboptimal.

Treatment

Treatment is inadequate because the two drugs used, benznidazole and nifurtimox, often cause severe side effects, must be used for long periods, and are ineffective against chronic infection. In acute and congenital infections, the drugs can reduce the duration and severity of infection, and apparent cure is achieved in about 70–90% of patients. During the chronic phase of infection, although parasitemia may disappear in up to 70% of patients, treatment does not clearly alter the progression of the disease. In a 2015 trial for Chagas cardiomyopathy, benznidazole significantly reduced parasite detection but not progression of cardiac disease. Nevertheless, there is general consensus that treatment should be considered in all *T cruzi*–infected persons regardless of clinical status or time since infection. In particular, treatment is recommended for acute, congenital, and reactivated infections and for children and young adults with chronic disease. Both drugs are FDA-approved for the treatment of Chagas disease: benznidazole in children 2–12 years old and nifurtimox in children under 18 years of age and weighing at least 2.5 kg.

Benznidazole is generally preferred due to better efficacy and safety profiles. The dose is 5 mg/kg/day orally in two divided doses for 60 days; shorter (2–4 week) regimens offer good efficacy. Its side effects include granulocytopenia, rash, and peripheral neuropathy. The dose of nifurtimox is 8–10 mg/kg orally in four divided doses after meals for 90–120 days. Side effects include GI (anorexia, vomiting) and neurologic (headaches, ataxia, insomnia, seizures) symptoms, which appear to be reversible and to lessen with dosage reduction. For both drugs, some recommendations suggest higher dosing for acute infections. Patients with chronic Chagas disease may also benefit from antiarrhythmic therapy, standard therapy for heart failure, and conservative and surgical management of megaesophagus and megacolon.

▶ Prevention & Control

In South America, a major eradication program based on improved housing, use of residual pyrethroid insecticides and pyrethroid-impregnated bed curtains, and screening of blood donors has achieved striking reductions in new infections. In endemic areas and ideally in donors from endemic areas, blood should not be used for transfusion unless at least two serologic tests are negative.

Bern C et al. Chagas disease in the United States: a public health approach. Clin Microbiol Rev. 2019;33:e00023. [PMID: 31776135]

Pérez-Molina JA et al. Chagas disease. Lancet. 2018;391:82. [PMID: 28673423]

Torrico F et al. New regimens of benznidazole monotherapy and in combination with fosravuconazole for treatment of Chagas disease (BENDITA): a phase 2, double-blind, randomised trial. Lancet Infect Dis. 2021;21:1129. [PMID: 33836161]

LEISHMANIASIS

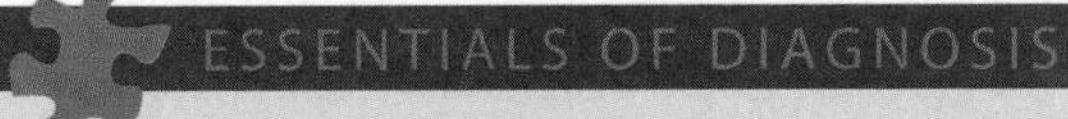

ESSENTIALS OF DIAGNOSIS

- Sand fly bite in an endemic area.
- **Visceral leishmaniasis:** irregular fever, progressive hepatosplenomegaly, pancytopenia, wasting.
- **Cutaneous leishmaniasis:** chronic, painless, moist ulcers or dry nodules.
- **Mucocutaneous leishmaniasis:** destructive nasopharyngeal lesions.
- Amastigotes in macrophages in aspirates, touch preparations, or biopsies.
- Positive culture, serologic tests, PCR, or skin test.

▶ General Considerations

Leishmaniasis is a zoonosis transmitted by bites of sand flies of the genus *Lutzomyia* in the Americas and *Phlebotomus* elsewhere. When sand flies feed on an infected host, the parasitized cells are ingested with the blood meal. Leishmaniasis is caused by about 20 species of *Leishmania;* taxonomy is complex. Clinical syndromes are generally dictated by the infecting species, but some species can cause more than one syndrome.

The estimated annual incidence of disease has been decreasing, with estimates of 600,000 to 1 million annual cases of cutaneous disease and 50,000–90,000 cases of visceral disease. Progress against visceral disease has been greatest on the Indian subcontinent.

Visceral leishmaniasis (kala azar) is caused mainly by *Leishmania donovani* in the Indian subcontinent and East Africa; *Leishmania infantum* in the Mediterranean, Middle East, China, parts of Asia, and Horn of Africa; and *Leishmania chagasi* in South and Central America. Other species may occasionally cause visceral disease. Over 90% of cases occur in seven countries: Brazil, Ethiopia, India, Kenya, Somalia, South Sudan, and Sudan. In each locale, the disease has particular clinical and epidemiologic features. The incubation period is usually 4–6 months (range: 10 days to 24 months). Without treatment, the fatality rate reaches 90%. Early diagnosis and treatment reduce mortality to 2–5%.

About 90% of cases of **cutaneous leishmaniasis occur** in Afghanistan, Pakistan, Syria, Saudi Arabia, Algeria, Iran, Brazil, and Peru. Old World cutaneous leishmaniasis is caused mainly by *Leishmania tropica, Leishmania major,* and *Leishmania aethiopica* in the Mediterranean, Middle East, Africa, Central Asia, and Indian subcontinent. New World cutaneous leishmaniasis is caused by *Leishmania mexicana, Leishmania amazonensis,* and the species listed below for mucocutaneous disease in Central and South America. Mucocutaneous leishmaniasis (espundia) occurs in lowland forest areas of the Americas and is caused by *Leishmania braziliensis, Leishmania panamensis,* and *Leishmania peruviana.*

▶ Clinical Findings

A. Symptoms and Signs

1. Visceral leishmaniasis (kala azar)—Most infections are subclinical, but a small number progress to full-blown disease. A local nonulcerating nodule at the site of the sand fly bite may precede systemic manifestations but usually is inapparent. The onset of illness may be acute, within 2 weeks of infection, or insidious. Symptoms and signs include fever, chills, sweats, weakness, anorexia, weight loss, cough, and diarrhea. The spleen progressively becomes greatly enlarged, firm, and nontender. The liver is somewhat enlarged, and generalized lymphadenopathy may occur. Hyperpigmentation of skin can be seen, leading to the name kala azar ("black fever"). Other signs include skin lesions, petechiae, gingival bleeding, jaundice, edema, and ascites. As the disease progresses, severe wasting and malnutrition are seen; death eventually occurs, often due to secondary infections, within months to a few years. Post-kala azar dermal leishmaniasis may appear after apparent cure in the Indian subcontinent and Sudan. It may simulate leprosy, with hypopigmented macules or nodules developing on preexisting lesions. Viscerotropic leishmaniasis has been reported in small numbers of American military personnel in the Middle East, with mild systemic febrile illnesses after *L tropica* infections.

2. Old World and New World cutaneous leishmaniasis— Cutaneous swellings appears 1 week to several months after sand fly bites and can be single or multiple. Characteristics of lesions and courses of disease vary depending on the leishmanial species and host immune response. Lesions begin as small papules and develop into nonulcerated dry plaques or large encrusted ulcers with well-demarcated raised and indurated margins (Figure 35–1). Satellite lesions may be present. The lesions are painless unless secondarily infected. Local lymph nodes may be enlarged. Systemic symptoms are uncommon, but fever, constitutional symptoms, and regional lymphadenopathy may be seen. For most species, healing occurs spontaneously in months to a few years, but scarring is common.

Leishmaniasis recidivans is a relapsing form of *L tropica* infection associated with hypersensitivity, in which the primary lesion heals centrally, but spreads laterally, with extensive scarring. Diffuse cutaneous leishmaniasis involves spread from a primary lesion, with local dissemination of nodules and a protracted course. Disseminated cutaneous leishmaniasis involves multiple nodular or ulcerated lesions, often with mucosal involvement.

3. Mucocutaneous leishmaniasis (espundia)—In Latin America, mucosal lesions develop in a small percentage of persons infected with *L braziliensis* and some other species, usually months to years after resolution of a cutaneous lesion. Nasal congestion is followed by ulceration of the nasal mucosa and septum, progressing to involvement of the mouth, lips, palate, pharynx, and larynx. Extensive destruction can occur, and secondary bacterial infection is common.

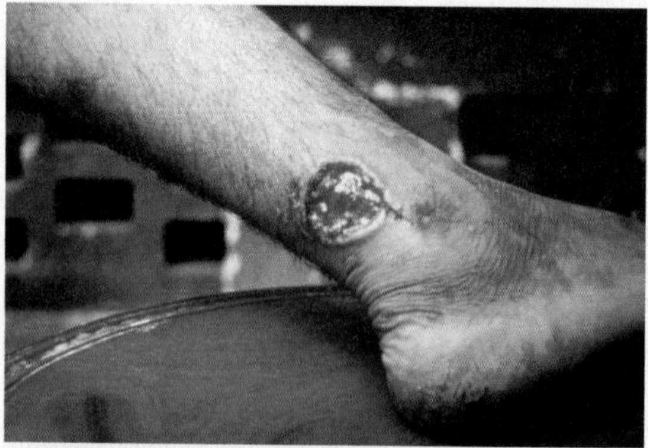

▲ Figure 35–1. Skin ulcer due to cutaneous leishmaniasis. Note the classic morphologic characteristics of this wound with its erythematous, nodular interior, surrounded by a raised border. (From Dr. Mae Melvin, Public Health Image Library, CDC.)

4. Infections in patients with AIDS—Leishmaniasis is an opportunistic infection in persons with AIDS. Visceral leishmaniasis can present late in the course of HIV infection, with fever, hepatosplenomegaly, and pancytopenia. The GI tract, respiratory tract, and skin may also be involved.

B. Laboratory Findings

Identifying amastigotes within macrophages in tissue samples provides a definitive diagnosis. In **visceral leishmaniasis**, fine-needle aspiration of the spleen for culture and tissue evaluation is generally safe and yields a diagnosis in over 95% of cases. Bone marrow aspiration is less sensitive but safer and diagnostic in most cases, and Giemsa-stained buffy coat of peripheral blood may occasionally show organisms. Cultures with media available from the CDC will grow promastigotes within a few days to weeks. Molecular assays can also be diagnostic. Serologic tests may facilitate diagnosis, but none are sufficiently sensitive or specific to be used alone. Numerous antibody-based rapid diagnostic tests are available; these have shown good specificity but limitations in sensitivity outside of India. Antigen-based rapid diagnostic tests may offer improved sensitivity. For **cutaneous lesions**, biopsies should be taken from the raised border of a skin lesion, with samples for histopathology, touch preparation, and culture. The histopathology shows inflammation with mononuclear cells. Macrophages filled with amastigotes may be present, especially early in infection. An intradermal leishmanin (Montenegro) skin test is positive in most individuals with cutaneous disease but negative in those with progressive visceral or diffuse cutaneous disease; this test is not approved in the United States. In **mucocutaneous leishmaniasis**, diagnosis is established by detecting amastigotes in scrapings, biopsy preparations, or aspirated tissue fluid, but organisms may be rare. Cultures from these samples may grow organisms. Serologic studies are often negative, but the leishmanin skin test is usually positive.

▶ Treatment

A. Visceral Leishmaniasis

The treatment of choice for visceral leishmaniasis on the Indian subcontinent is liposomal amphotericin B (approved by the FDA), which is generally effective and well tolerated but expensive. Standard dosing is 3 mg/kg/day intravenously on days 1–5, 14, and 21. Simpler regimens that have shown good efficacy in India include four doses of 5 mg/kg over 4–10 days and a single dose of 15 mg/kg, but efficacies of shorter regimens have been lower outside India. A single infusion of an amphotericin B lipid emulsion, which is more affordable than liposomal preparations, showed excellent efficacy, albeit lower than that of the liposomal formulation. Conventional amphotericin B deoxycholate, which is much less expensive, is also highly effective but with more toxicity. It is administered as a slow intravenous infusion of 1 mg/kg/day for 15–20 days or 0.5–1 mg/kg every second day for up to 8 weeks. Infusion-related side effects with conventional or liposomal amphotericin B include GI symptoms, fever, chills, dyspnea, hypotension, and hepatic and renal toxicity.

Pentavalent antimonials remain the most commonly used drugs to treat leishmaniasis in most areas. Response rates are good outside India, but in India, resistance is a major problem. Two preparations are available, sodium stibogluconate in many other areas and meglumine antimonate in Latin America and francophone countries; the compounds appear to have comparable activities. Sodium stibogluconate is no longer available in the United States. Standard dosing for either antimonial is 20 mg/kg once daily intravenously (preferred) or intramuscularly for 20 days for cutaneous leishmaniasis and 28 days for visceral or mucocutaneous disease. Toxicity increases over time, with development of GI symptoms, fever, headache, myalgias, arthralgias, pancreatitis, and rash. Intramuscular injections can cause sterile abscesses. Monitoring should include serial ECGs, and changes are indications for discontinuation to avoid progression to serious arrhythmias.

The efficacy of amphotericin B is lower in East Africa than in Asia, and the standard treatment is a combination of sodium stibogluconate (20 mg/kg/day intravenously) plus paromomycin (15 mg/kg/day intramuscularly) for 17 days, with demonstrated excellent efficacy; liposomal amphotericin B may be considered in older adults or pregnant women due to toxicity concerns.

Miltefosine is the first oral drug for the treatment of leishmaniasis, and it is registered in India for this indication. It initially demonstrated excellent results in India, but efficacy is decreasing due to drug resistance. It can be administered at a daily oral dose of 2.5 mg/kg in two divided doses for 28 days. A 14-day course plus a single dose of liposomal amphotericin B showed excellent efficacy. A 28-day course of miltefosine (2.5 mg/kg/day) is also effective for the treatment of New World cutaneous leishmaniasis. Vomiting, diarrhea, and elevations in transaminases and kidney function studies are common, but generally short-lived, side effects.

The aminoglycoside paromomycin (11 mg/kg/day intramuscularly for 21 days) was shown to be similarly efficacious to amphotericin B for the treatment of visceral disease in India, where it is approved for this indication. It is much less expensive than liposomal amphotericin B or miltefosine. The drug is well tolerated; side effects include ototoxicity and reversible elevations in liver enzymes.

Combination therapy—The use of drug combinations to improve treatment efficacy, shorten treatment courses, and reduce the selection of resistant parasites has been actively studied. In India, compared with a standard 30-day (treatment on alternate days) course of amphotericin, noninferior efficacy and decreased adverse events were seen with a single dose of liposomal amphotericin plus a 7-day course of miltefosine, a single dose of liposomal amphotericin plus a 10-day course of paromomycin, or a 10-day course of miltefosine plus paromomycin. A combination of sodium stibogluconate and paromomycin is the standard treatment in East Africa.

B. Cutaneous Leishmaniasis

In the Old World, cutaneous leishmaniasis is generally self-healing over some months and does not metastasize to the mucosa, so it may be justified to withhold treatment in regions without mucocutaneous disease if lesions are small and cosmetically unimportant. Lesions on the face or hands are generally treated. New World leishmaniasis has a greater risk of progression to mucocutaneous disease, so treatment is more often warranted, but choice of therapy is complex. Standard therapy is with pentavalent antimonials for 20 days, as described above. Other treatments include those discussed above for visceral disease, azole antifungals, and allopurinol. Alternative therapies increasingly used are miltefosine, which benefits from oral dosing and relatively little toxicity, and amphotericin B, which is widely available. In studies in South America, a 28-day course of miltefosine was superior to a 20-day course of meglumine antimoniate, and oral fluconazole also showed good efficacy. Topical therapy has included intralesional antimony, intralesional pentamidine, paromomycin ointment, cryotherapy, local heat, and surgical removal. Diffuse cutaneous leishmaniasis and related chronic skin processes generally respond poorly to therapy.

C. Mucocutaneous Leishmaniasis

Cutaneous infections from regions where parasites include those that cause mucocutaneous disease (eg, *L braziliensis* in parts of Latin America) should all be treated to help prevent disease progression. Treatment of mucocutaneous disease with antimonials is disappointing, with responses in only about 60% in Brazil. Other therapies listed above for visceral leishmaniasis may also be used, although they have not been well studied for this indication.

Prevention & Control

Personal protection measures for avoidance of sand fly bites include use of insect repellants, fine-mesh insect netting, long sleeves and pants, and avoidance of warm shaded areas where flies are common. Disease control measures include destruction of animal reservoir hosts, mass treatment of humans in disease-prevalent areas, residual insecticide spraying in dwellings, limiting contact with dogs and other domesticated animals, and use of permethrin-impregnated collars for dogs.

Burza S et al. Leishmaniasis. Lancet. 2018;392:951. [PMID: 30126638]

Gedda MR et al. Post kala-azar dermal leishmaniasis: a threat to elimination program. PLoS Negl Trop Dis. 2020;14:e0008221. [PMID: 32614818]

Goswami RP et al. Combination therapy against Indian visceral leishmaniasis with liposomal amphotericin B (Fungisome") and short-course miltefosine in comparison to miltefosine monotherapy. Am J Trop Med Hyg. 2020;103:308. [PMID: 32394874]

Machado PRL et al. A double-blind, randomized trial to evaluate miltefosine and topical granulocyte macrophage colony-stimulating factor in the treatment of cutaneous leishmaniasis caused by *Leishmania braziliensis* in Brazil. Clin Infect Dis. 2021;73:e2465. [PMID: 32894278]

Mann S et al. A review of leishmaniasis: current knowledge and future directions. Curr Trop Med Rep. 2021;8:121. [PMID: 33747716]

MALARIA

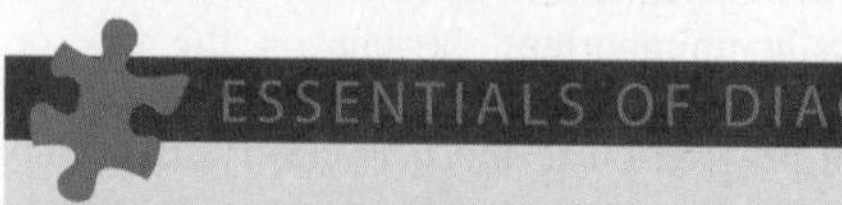

- Exposure to anopheline mosquitoes in a malaria-endemic area.
- Intermittent attacks of chills, fever, and sweating.
- Headache, myalgia, vomiting, splenomegaly; anemia, thrombocytopenia.
- Intraerythrocytic parasites identified in thick or thin blood smears or positive rapid diagnostic tests.
- **Falciparum malaria complications:** cerebral malaria, severe anemia, hypotension, pulmonary edema, AKI, hypoglycemia, acidosis, and hemolysis.

General Considerations

Malaria is the most important parasitic disease of humans, causing hundreds of millions of illnesses and hundreds of thousands of deaths each year. The disease is endemic in most of the tropics, including much of South and Central America, Africa, the Middle East, the Indian subcontinent, Southeast Asia, and Oceania. Transmission, morbidity, and mortality are greatest in Africa, where most deaths from malaria are in young children. Malaria is also common in travelers from nonendemic areas to the tropics. Although the disease remains a major problem, impressive advances have been made in many regions. However, after marked gains, progress appears to have stalled, particularly in Africa, where about 95% of cases occur. The WHO estimated that 241 million cases of malaria occurred in 85 endemic countries in 2020. The WHO changed its methods of estimation of malaria deaths, leading to an increase of past estimates; there were 627,000 estimated deaths in 2020, an increase of 69,000 from 2019, with 47,000 of these excess deaths attributed to service disruptions from the COVID-19 pandemic.

Four species of the genus *Plasmodium* classically cause human malaria. *Plasmodium falciparum* is responsible for nearly all severe disease, since it uniquely infects erythrocytes of all ages and mediates the sequestration of infected erythrocytes in small blood vessels, thereby evading clearance by the spleen. *P falciparum* is endemic in most malarious areas and is by far the predominant species in Africa. *Plasmodium vivax* is about as common as *P falciparum* outside of Africa. *P vivax* uncommonly causes severe disease, although this outcome may be more common than previously appreciated. *Plasmodium ovale* and *Plasmodium malariae* are much less common causes of disease, and generally do not cause severe illness. *Plasmodium knowlesi*, a parasite of macaque monkeys, causes illnesses in humans, including some severe disease, in Southeast Asia.

Malaria is transmitted by the bite of infected female anopheline mosquitoes. During feeding, mosquitoes inject sporozoites, which circulate to the liver, and rapidly infect hepatocytes, causing asymptomatic liver infection. Merozoites are subsequently released from the liver, and they rapidly infect erythrocytes to begin the asexual erythrocytic stage of infection that is responsible for human disease. Multiple rounds of erythrocytic development, with production of merozoites that invade additional erythrocytes, lead to large numbers of circulating parasites and clinical illness. Some erythrocytic parasites also develop into sexual gametocytes, which are infectious to mosquitoes, allowing completion of the life cycle and infection of others.

Malaria may uncommonly be transmitted from mother to infant (congenital malaria), by blood transfusion, and in nonendemic areas by mosquitoes infected after biting infected immigrants or travelers. In *P vivax* and *P ovale*, parasites also form dormant liver hypnozoites, which are not killed by most drugs, allowing subsequent relapses of illness after initial elimination of erythrocytic infections. For all plasmodial species, parasites may recrudesce following initial clinical improvement after suboptimal therapy.

In highly endemic regions, where people are infected repeatedly, antimalarial immunity prevents severe disease in most older children and adults. However, young children, who are relatively nonimmune, are at high risk for severe disease from *P falciparum* infection, and this population is responsible for most deaths from malaria. Pregnant women are also at increased risk for severe falciparum malaria. In areas with lower endemicity, individuals of all ages commonly present with uncomplicated or severe malaria. Travelers, who are generally nonimmune, are at high risk for severe disease from falciparum malaria at any age.

Clinical Findings

A. Symptoms and Signs

An acute attack of malaria typically begins with a prodrome of headache and fatigue, followed by fever. A classic malarial paroxysm includes chills, high fever, and then sweats. Patients may appear to be remarkably well between febrile episodes. Fevers are usually irregular, especially early in the illness, but without therapy may become regular, with 48-hour (*P vivax* and *P ovale*) or 72-hour (*P malariae*) cycles, especially with non-falciparum disease. Headache, malaise, myalgias, arthralgias, cough, chest pain, abdominal pain, anorexia, nausea, vomiting, and diarrhea are common. Seizures may represent simple febrile convulsions or evidence of severe neurologic disease. Physical findings may be absent or include signs of anemia, jaundice, splenomegaly, and mild hepatomegaly. Rash and lymphadenopathy are not typical in malaria, and thus suggestive of another cause of fever.

In the developed world, it is imperative that all persons with suggestive symptoms, in particular fever, who have traveled in an endemic area be evaluated for malaria. The risk for falciparum malaria is greatest within 2 months of return from travel; other species may cause disease many months—and occasionally more than a year—after return from an endemic area.

Severe malaria is principally a result of *P falciparum* infection. It is characterized by signs of severe illness, organ dysfunction, or a high parasite load (peripheral parasitemia greater than 5% or greater than 200,000 parasites/mcL). Severe falciparum malaria can include dysfunction of any organ system, including neurologic abnormalities progressing to alterations in consciousness, repeated seizures, and coma (cerebral malaria); severe anemia; hypotension and shock; noncardiogenic pulmonary edema and acute respiratory distress syndrome; AKI due to ATN or, less commonly, severe hemolysis; hypoglycemia; acidosis; hemolysis with jaundice; hepatic dysfunction; retinal hemorrhages and other fundoscopic abnormalities; bleeding abnormalities, including disseminated intravascular coagulation; and secondary bacterial infections, including pneumonia and *Salmonella* bacteremia. In the developing world, severe malaria and deaths from the disease are mostly in young children, in particular from cerebral malaria and severe anemia. Cerebral malaria is a consequence of a single severe infection while severe anemia follows multiple malarial infections, intestinal helminths, and nutritional deficiencies. In a large trial of African children, acidosis, impaired consciousness, convulsions, renal impairment, and underlying chronic illness were associated with poor outcome.

Uncommon disorders resulting from immunologic responses to chronic infection are massive splenomegaly and, with *P malariae* infection, immune complex glomerulopathy with nephrotic syndrome. People living with HIV are at increased risk for malaria and for severe disease, in particular with advanced immunodeficiency.

B. Laboratory Findings

Giemsa-stained blood smears remain the mainstay of diagnosis. Thick smears provide efficient evaluation of large volumes of blood, but thin smears are simpler for inexperienced personnel and better for discrimination of parasite species (Figure 35–2). Single smears are usually positive in infected individuals, although parasitemias may be very low in nonimmune individuals. If illness is suspected, repeating smears at 8- to 24-hour intervals is appropriate. The severity of malaria correlates only loosely with the quantity of infecting parasites, but high parasitemias (especially greater than 10–20% of erythrocytes infected or greater than 200,000–500,000 parasites/mcL) or the presence of malarial pigment (a breakdown product of hemoglobin) in more than 5% of neutrophils is associated with a particularly poor prognosis.

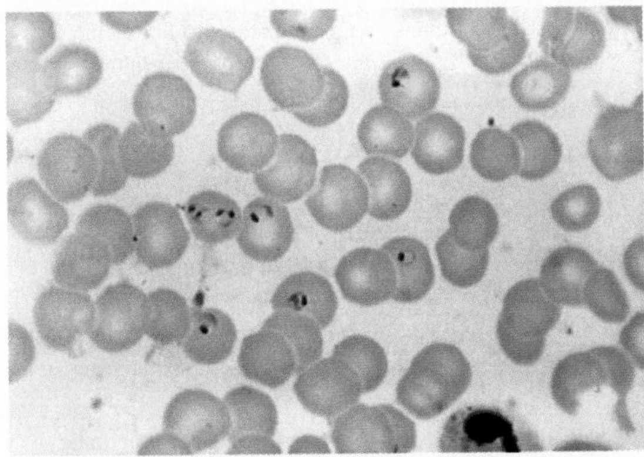

▲ **Figure 35–2.** Thin film Giemsa-stained micrograph with *Plasmodium falciparum* ring forms. (From Steven Glenn, Laboratory & Consultation Division, Public Health Image Library, CDC.)

A second means of diagnosis is rapid diagnostic tests to identify circulating plasmodial antigens. These tests offer sensitivity and specificity near that of high-quality blood smear analysis and are simpler to perform. However, *P falciparum* lacking the most common rapid diagnostic test antigen, histidine-rich protein 2 (HRP2), has been identified in some areas (especially parts of South America and the Horn of Africa), so HRP2-based tests may miss some cases of falciparum malaria.

Serologic tests indicate history of disease but are not useful for diagnosis of acute infection. PCR and related molecular tests (eg, LAMP) are highly sensitive but not available for routine diagnosis. In immune populations, highly sensitive molecular tests, such as PCR, have limited value because subclinical infections, which are not routinely treated, are common.

Other diagnostic findings with uncomplicated malaria include thrombocytopenia, anemia, leukocytosis or leukopenia, liver function abnormalities, and hepatosplenomegaly. Severe malaria can present with the laboratory abnormalities expected for the advanced organ dysfunction discussed above.

▶ Treatment

Malaria is the most common cause of fever in much of the tropics and in travelers seeking medical attention after return from endemic areas. Fevers are often treated presumptively in endemic areas, but treatment should follow definitive diagnosis, especially in nonimmune individuals. Symptomatic malaria is caused only by the erythrocytic stage of infection. Available antimalarial drugs (Table 35–2) act against this stage, except for primaquine and tafenoquine, which act principally against hepatic parasites.

A. Non-Falciparum Malaria

The first-line drug for non-falciparum malaria from most areas remains chloroquine. Due to increasing resistance of *P vivax*, alternative therapies are recommended when resistance is suspected, particularly for infections acquired in Indonesia, Oceania, and South America. These infections can be treated with artemisinin-based combination therapies (ACTs) or other first-line regimens for *P falciparum* infections as discussed below. For *P vivax* or *P ovale*, eradication of erythrocytic parasites with chloroquine should be accompanied by treatment with primaquine or tafenoquine (after evaluating for glucose-6-phosphate dehydrogenase [G6PD] deficiency; see below) to eradicate dormant liver stages (hypnozoites), which may lead to relapses with recurrent erythrocytic infection and malaria symptoms after weeks to months if left untreated. *P malariae* infections need only be treated with chloroquine.

Table 35–2. Major antimalarial drugs.

Drug	Class	Use
Chloroquine	4-Aminoquinoline	Treatment and chemoprophylaxis of infection with sensitive parasites
Amodiaquine	4-Aminoquinoline	Treatment of *Plasmodium falciparum*, optimally in fixed combination with artesunate
Piperaquine	4-Aminoquinoline	Treatment of *P falciparum* in fixed combination with dihydroartemisinin
Quinine	Quinoline methanol	Oral and intravenous[1] (for severe infections) treatment of *P falciparum*
Quinidine	Quinoline methanol	Intravenous therapy of severe infections with *P falciparum*
Mefloquine	Quinoline methanol	Chemoprophylaxis and treatment of infections with *P falciparum*
Primaquine, tafenoquine	8-Aminoquinoline	Radical cure and terminal prophylaxis of infections with *Plasmodium vivax* and *Plasmodium ovale*; alternative for malaria chemoprophylaxis
Sulfadoxine-pyrimethamine (Fansidar)	Folate antagonist combination	Treatment of *P falciparum*, optimally in combination with artesunate; intermittent preventive therapy
Atovaquone-proguanil (Malarone)	Quinone-folate antagonist combination	Treatment and chemoprophylaxis of *P falciparum* infection
Doxycycline	Tetracycline	Treatment (with quinine) of infections with *P falciparum*; chemoprophylaxis
Lumefantrine	Amyl alcohol	Treatment of *P falciparum* malaria in fixed combination with artemether (Coartem)
Pyronaridine	Benzonaphthyridine	Treatment of *P falciparum* malaria in fixed combination artesunate
Artemisinins (artesunate, artemether, dihydroartemisinin)	Sesquiterpene lactone endoperoxides	Treatment of *P falciparum* in oral combination regimens for uncomplicated disease and parenterally for severe malaria

[1]Not available in the United States.
Reproduced with permission from Katzung BG. *Basic & Clinical Pharmacology*. 14th edition. McGraw-Hill, 2018.

B. Uncomplicated Falciparum Malaria

P falciparum is resistant to chloroquine and sulfadoxine-pyrimethamine in most areas, and falciparum malaria should not be treated with these older drugs. ACTs, all including a short-acting artemisinin and longer-acting partner drug, are first-line therapies in nearly all endemic countries. The WHO recommends six ACTs to treat falciparum malaria (Table 35–3). In developed countries, malaria is an uncommon but potentially life-threatening infection of travelers and immigrants. Nonimmune individuals with falciparum malaria should generally be admitted to the hospital due to risks of rapid progression of disease. Several options are available for the treatment of uncomplicated falciparum malaria in the United States (Table 35–4).

C. Severe Malaria

Severe malaria is a medical emergency. Parenteral treatment is indicated for severe malaria, as defined above, and with inability to take oral drugs. With appropriate prompt therapy and supportive care, rapid recoveries may be seen even in very ill individuals.

Intravenous artesunate is FDA-approved and the standard of care for severe malaria. It has demonstrated superior efficacy and better tolerability than quinine. Artesunate is administered intravenously in four doses of 2.4 mg/kg

Table 35–3. WHO recommendations for the treatment of uncomplicated falciparum malaria.

Regimen	Notes
Artemether-lumefantrine (Coartem, Riamet)	Coformulated, first-line therapy in many countries. Approved in the United States.
Artesunate-amodiaquine (ASAQ)	Coformulated, first-line therapy in multiple African countries.
Artesunate-mefloquine	First-line therapy in parts of Southeast Asia and South America but efficacy decreasing in parts of Thailand.
Artesunate-pyronaridine	Coformulated. Most recently approved regimen; used in some Southeast Asian countries.
Artesunate-sulfadoxine-pyrimethamine	First-line in some countries, but efficacy lower than other regimens in most areas.
Dihydroartemisinin-piperaquine	Coformulated. First-line in some countries, but efficacy decreasing in parts of Southeast Asia.

Data from World Health Organization: Guidelines for the Treatment of Malaria. World Health Organization. Geneva 2015.

Table 35–4. Treatment of malaria.

Clinical Setting	Drug Therapy[1]	Alternative Drugs
Chloroquine-sensitive *Plasmodium falciparum* and *Plasmodium malariae* infections	Chloroquine phosphate, 1 g at 0 hours, then 500 mg at 6, 24, and 48 hours or Chloroquine phosphate, 1 g at 0 hours and 24 hours, then 0.5 g at 48 hours	
Plasmodium vivax and *Plasmodium ovale* infections	Chloroquine (as above), then (if G6PD normal) primaquine, 30-mg base daily for 14 days or tafenoquine 300 mg once	For infections from Indonesia, Papua New Guinea, and other areas with suspected resistance: therapies listed for uncomplicated chloroquine-resistant *P falciparum* plus primaquine
Uncomplicated infections with chloroquine-resistant *P falciparum*	Coartem (artemether 20 mg, lumefantrine 120 mg), four tablets twice daily for 3 days or Malarone, four tablets (total of 1 g of atovaquone, 400 mg of proguanil) daily for 3 days or Quinine sulfate, 650 mg three times daily for 3–7 days Plus one of the following (when quinine given for < 7 days) Doxycycline, 100 mg twice daily for 7 days or Clindamycin, 600 mg twice daily for 7 days	Mefloquine, 15 mg/kg once or 750 mg, then 500 mg in 6–8 hours or Dihydroartemisinin-piperaquine[2] (dihydroartemisinin 40 mg, piperaquine 320 mg), 4 tablets daily for 3 days or ASAQ[2] (artesunate 100 mg, amodiaquine 270 mg), two tablets daily for 3 days
Severe or complicated infections with *P falciparum*	Artesunate 2.4 mg/kg intravenously every 12 hours for 1 day, then daily[3]	Quinidine gluconate,[4,5] 10 mg/kg intravenously over 1–2 hours, then 0.02 mg/kg intravenously/minute or Quinidine gluconate,[4,5] 15 mg/kg intravenously over 4 hours, then 7.5 mg/kg intravenously over 4 hours every 8 hours or Quinine dihydrochloride,[2,4,5] 20 mg/kg intravenously over 4 hours, then 10 mg/kg intravenously every 8 hours or Artemether,[2,3] 3.2 mg/kg intramuscularly, then 1.6 mg/kg/day intramuscularly

[1]All dosages are oral and refer to salts unless otherwise indicated. See text for additional information on all agents, including toxicities and cautions. See CDC guidelines (phone: 877-FYI-TRIP; http://www.cdc.gov/malaria/) for additional information and pediatric dosing.
[2]Not available in the United States.
[3]With all parenteral regimens, change to an oral regimen as soon as the patient can tolerate it.
[4]Cardiac monitoring should be in place during intravenous administration of quinidine or quinine.
[5]Avoid loading doses in persons who have received quinine, quinidine, or mefloquine in the prior 24 hours.
G6PD, glucose-6-phosphate dehydrogenase.

over 3 days every 12 hours on day 1, and then daily. If artesunate cannot be obtained promptly, severe malaria should be treated with intravenous quinine (available in most countries but not the United States), intravenous quinidine (no longer available in the United States), or an oral agent until intravenous artesunate is available. In endemic regions, if parenteral therapy is not available, intrarectal administration of artemether or artesunate is also effective. Patients receiving intravenous quinine or quinidine should receive continuous cardiac monitoring; if QTc prolongation exceeds 25% of baseline, the infusion rate should be reduced. Blood glucose should be monitored every 4–6 hours, and 5–10% dextrose may be coadministered to decrease the likelihood of hypoglycemia.

Appropriate care of severe malaria includes maintenance of fluids and electrolytes; respiratory and hemodynamic support; and consideration of blood transfusions, anticonvulsants, antibiotics for bacterial infections, and hemofiltration or hemodialysis. Exchange transfusion is sometimes used for those with high parasitemia (greater than 5–10%), but beneficial effects have not clearly been demonstrated.

D. Antimalarial Drugs

1. Chloroquine—Chloroquine remains the drug of choice for the treatment of sensitive *P falciparum* and other species of malaria parasites (Table 35–4). Chloroquine is active against erythrocytic parasites of all human malaria species. It does not eradicate hepatic stages. Chloroquine-resistant *P falciparum* is widespread in nearly all areas of the world with falciparum malaria, with the exceptions of Central

America west of the Panama Canal and Hispaniola. Chloroquine-resistant *P vivax* has been reported from a number of areas, most notably Southeast Asia and Oceania.

Chloroquine is the drug of choice for the treatment of non-falciparum and sensitive falciparum malaria. It rapidly terminates fever (in 24–48 hours) and clears parasitemia (in 48–72 hours) caused by sensitive parasites. Chloroquine is also the preferred chemoprophylactic agent in malarious regions without resistant falciparum malaria.

Chloroquine is usually well tolerated, even with prolonged use. Pruritus is common, primarily in Africans. Nausea, vomiting, abdominal pain, headache, anorexia, malaise, blurring of vision, and urticaria are uncommon. Dosing after meals may reduce some side effects.

2. Amodiaquine, piperaquine, and pyronaridine—Amodiaquine is a 4-aminoquinoline that is closely related to chloroquine. Amodiaquine has been widely used to treat malaria because of its low cost, limited toxicity, and, in some areas, effectiveness against chloroquine-resistant strains of *P falciparum*. Use of amodiaquine decreased after recognition of rare but serious side effects, notably agranulocytosis, aplastic anemia, and hepatotoxicity. However, serious side effects are rare with short-term use, and artesunate-amodiaquine is one of the standard ACTs recommended to treat falciparum malaria (Table 35–3). Chemoprophylaxis with amodiaquine should be avoided because of increased toxicity with long-term use.

Piperaquine is another 4-aminoquinoline that has been coformulated with dihydroartemisinin in an ACT. Piperaquine is well tolerated, and in combination with dihydroartemisinin offers a highly efficacious therapy for falciparum and vivax malaria. Due to the long half-life of piperaquine (~3 weeks), dihydroartemisinin-piperaquine offers the longest period of posttreatment prophylaxis of available ACTs. However, resistance to piperaquine, with consequent treatment failures of dihydroartemisinin-piperaquine has emerged in Southeast Asia.

Pyronaridine is a benzonaphthyridine active against many drug-resistant strains of *P falciparum*. The combination of artesunate plus pyronaridine has shown excellent efficacy against falciparum and vivax malaria and has been well tolerated, although elevated transaminases can be seen.

3. Mefloquine—Mefloquine is effective against many chloroquine-resistant strains of *P falciparum* and against other malarial species. Although toxicity is a concern, mefloquine is also a recommended chemoprophylactic drug. Resistance to mefloquine has been reported sporadically from many areas, but it appears to be uncommon except in regions of Southeast Asia with high rates of multidrug resistance (especially border areas of Thailand).

For treatment of uncomplicated malaria, mefloquine can be administered as a single dose or in two doses over 1 day. It is used in combination with artesunate for falciparum malaria, although resistance limits efficacy in Southeast Asia. It should be taken with meals and swallowed with a large amount of water. Mefloquine is recommended by the CDC for chemoprophylaxis in all malarious areas except those with no chloroquine resistance (where chloroquine is preferred) and some rural areas of Southeast Asia with a high prevalence of mefloquine resistance.

Side effects with weekly dosing of mefloquine for chemoprophylaxis include nausea, vomiting, dizziness, sleep and behavioral disturbances, epigastric pain, diarrhea, abdominal pain, headache, rash and, uncommonly, seizures and psychosis. There is an FDA black box warning about neuropsychiatric toxicity, possibly including rare, irreversible effects. Mefloquine should be avoided in persons with histories of psychiatric disease or seizures.

Side effects are more common (up to 50% of treatments) with the higher dosages of mefloquine required for treatment. These effects may be lessened by splitting administration into two doses separated by 6–8 hours. Serious neuropsychiatric toxicities (depression, confusion, acute psychosis, or seizures) have been reported in less than 1 in 1000 treatments, but some authorities believe that these are more common. Mefloquine can also alter cardiac conduction, and so it should not be coadministered with quinine. Mefloquine is generally considered safe in young children and pregnant women.

4. Quinine and quinidine—Quinine dihydrochloride and quinidine gluconate are effective therapies for falciparum malaria, especially severe disease, although toxicity concerns complicate therapy (Table 35–4). Quinine acts rapidly against all human malaria parasites. Quinidine, the dextrorotatory stereoisomer of quinine, is at least as effective in the treatment of severe falciparum malaria but is no longer available in the United States.

Resistance of *P falciparum* to quinine is common in some areas of Southeast Asia, where the drug may fail if used alone to treat falciparum malaria. However, quinine still provides at least a partial therapeutic effect in most patients.

Quinine and quinidine are effective treatments for severe falciparum malaria, although intravenous artesunate is the standard of care. The drugs can be administered in divided doses or by continuous intravenous infusion; treatment should begin with a loading dose to rapidly achieve effective plasma concentrations and include cardiac monitoring. Therapy should be changed to an oral agent as soon as the patient has improved and can tolerate oral medications.

In areas without newer combination regimens, oral quinine sulfate is an alternative first-line therapy for uncomplicated falciparum malaria, although poor tolerance may limit compliance. Quinine is commonly used with a second drug (most often doxycycline) to shorten the duration of use (to 3 days) and limit toxicity. Therapeutic dosages of quinine and quinidine commonly cause tinnitus, headache, nausea, dizziness, flushing, and visual disturbances. Hematologic abnormalities include hemolysis (especially with G6PD deficiency), leukopenia, agranulocytosis, and thrombocytopenia. Therapeutic doses may cause hypoglycemia through stimulation of insulin release; this is a particular problem in severe infections and in pregnant patients, who have increased sensitivity to insulin. Overly rapid infusions can cause severe hypotension. ECG abnormalities (QT prolongation) are common, but dangerous arrhythmias are uncommon when the drugs are administered appropriately. Quinine should not be given concurrently with mefloquine and should be used with caution in a patient who has previously received mefloquine.

5. Primaquine and tafenoquine—Primaquine phosphate, a synthetic 8-aminoquinoline, is the drug of choice for the eradication of dormant liver forms of *P vivax* and *P ovale* (Table 35–4). Primaquine is active against hepatic stages of all human malaria parasites. This action is optimal soon after therapy with chloroquine or other agents. Primaquine also acts against erythrocytic stage parasites, although this activity is too weak for the treatment of active disease, and against gametocytes. The addition of a single low dose of primaquine in conjunction with an ACT in G6PD-normal patients with falciparum malaria is a strategy to lower transmission to mosquitoes.

For *P vivax* and *P ovale* infections, chloroquine or other drugs are used to eradicate erythrocytic forms, and if the G6PD level is normal, a 14-day course of primaquine (52.6 mg primaquine phosphate [30 mg base] daily) is initiated to eradicate liver hypnozoites and prevent a subsequent relapse. Some strains of *P vivax*, particularly in New Guinea and Southeast Asia, are relatively resistant to primaquine, and the drug may fail to eradicate liver forms.

Standard chemoprophylaxis does not prevent a relapse of *P vivax* or *P ovale* infections, since liver hypnozoites are not eradicated by chloroquine or other standard treatments. To diminish the likelihood of relapse, some authorities advocate the use of a treatment course of primaquine after the completion of travel to an endemic area. Primaquine can also be used for chemoprophylaxis to prevent *P falciparum* and *P vivax* infection in persons with normal levels of G6PD.

Primaquine in recommended doses is generally well tolerated. It infrequently causes nausea, epigastric pain, abdominal cramps, and headache, especially when taken on an empty stomach. Rare side effects include leukopenia, agranulocytosis, leukocytosis, and cardiac arrhythmias. Standard doses of primaquine may cause hemolysis or methemoglobinemia (manifested by cyanosis), especially in persons with G6PD deficiency or other hereditary metabolic defects. Patients should be tested for G6PD deficiency before primaquine is prescribed. Primaquine should be discontinued if there is evidence of hemolysis or anemia and should be avoided in pregnancy.

Tafenoquine, an 8-aminoquinoline, has a much longer half-life than primaquine. These two medications share the risk of hemolysis with G6PD deficiency and probably other toxicities; tafenoquine should not be used during pregnancy or in those with G6PD deficiency. Tafenoquine is FDA-approved for patients at least 16 years of age for two indications, but with different formulations, marketed by different companies. To eliminate hepatic stages of *P vivax*, a single dose (Krintafel, two 150-mg tablets once daily) is taken with food soon after initiation of primary therapy (with chloroquine or other agents). For malaria chemoprophylaxis, the drug (Arakoda, two 100-mg tablets) is taken once daily for 3 days and then weekly until 1 week after the last exposure.

6. Inhibitors of folate synthesis—Inhibitors of two parasite enzymes involved in folate metabolism, dihydrofolate reductase (DHFR) and dihydropteroate synthase (DHPS), are used, generally in combination regimens, for the treatment and prevention of malaria, although the drugs are rather slow acting and limited by resistance.

Fansidar is a fixed combination of sulfadoxine (500 mg) and pyrimethamine (25 mg). It is not advised for chemoprophylaxis due to rare serious side effects with long-term dosing. For treatment, advantages of sulfadoxine-pyrimethamine include ease of administration (a single oral dose) and low cost. However, resistance is a major problem.

Sulfadoxine-pyrimethamine plus artesunate has shown efficacy for malaria treatment in some areas, in particular India, but is best replaced by more effective ACTs. Sulfadoxine-pyrimethamine is recommended by the WHO for monthly preventive therapy in pregnant women in areas of high endemicity, although its efficacy is limited by resistance. Amodiaquine plus sulfadoxine-pyrimethamine is recommended monthly during the rainy season (known as seasonal malaria chemoprevention [SMC]) for chemoprevention in regions of West Africa with seasonal malaria transmission and limited drug resistance.

7. Artemisinins—Artemisinin (qinghaosu) is a sesquiterpene lactone endoperoxide. The analogs artesunate, artemether, and dihydroartemisinin increase solubility and improve antimalarial efficacy. The WHO encourages availability of oral artemisinins only in coformulated combination regimens.

Artemisinins act very rapidly against all erythrocytic-stage human malaria parasites. Of concern, delayed clearance of parasites and clinical failures have been seen after treatment with artemisinins or ACTs in parts of Southeast Asia, heralding the emergence of artemisinin resistance in this region. Artemisinin resistance is mediated by any of a series of mutations in the *P falciparum* kelch (K13) gene; of great concern, these same mutations and evidence for delayed clearance after treatment with artemisinins were reported in East Africa in 2021.

Artemisinins play a vital role in the treatment of malaria, including multidrug-resistant *P falciparum* malaria. Due to their short plasma half-lives, recrudescence rates are unacceptably high after short-course therapy, leading to approved use only as *initial* therapy for severe malaria and in ACTs for uncomplicated malaria. The ACTs that are most advocated in Africa are artemether plus lumefantrine (Coartem) and artesunate plus amodiaquine (ASAQ), each available as a coformulated product. Artesunate plus mefloquine is not as well tolerated and is used mostly outside of Africa; its efficacy has declined in parts of Southeast Asia. Dihydroartemisinin-piperaquine has shown excellent efficacy and is the first-line regimen in some countries in Southeast Asia, but efficacy has declined in Cambodia due to decreased activity of both components of the regimen. The newest approved ACT, artesunate-pyronaridine, has demonstrated excellent efficacy.

In studies of severe malaria, intravenous artesunate was superior to intravenous quinine in terms of efficacy and tolerability. Thus, the standard of care for severe malaria is intravenous artesunate, although parenteral quinine and quinidine remain acceptable alternatives. Artesunate and artemether have also been effective in the treatment of severe malaria when administered rectally, offering a valuable treatment modality when parenteral therapy is not available.

Artemisinins are very well tolerated. The most commonly reported side effects have been nausea, vomiting, and diarrhea, which may often be due to acute malaria, rather than drug toxicity. Neutropenia, anemia, hemolysis, and elevated levels of liver enzymes have been noted rarely. Hemolysis may occur weeks after therapy with intravenous artesunate. Artemisinins are teratogenic in animals, but with good safety seen in humans, and the importance of effectively treating malaria during pregnancy, the WHO recommends ACTs to treat uncomplicated malaria and intravenous artesunate to treat complicated malaria during all trimesters of pregnancy.

8. Atovaquone plus proguanil (Malarone)—Atovaquone, a hydroxynaphthoquinone, is not effective when used alone, due to rapid development of drug resistance. However, Malarone, a fixed combination of atovaquone (250 mg) and the antifolate proguanil (100 mg), is highly effective for both the treatment and chemoprophylaxis of falciparum malaria, and it is approved for both indications in the United States (Table 35–4). It also appears to be active against other species of malaria parasites. Unlike most other antimalarials, Malarone provides activity against both erythrocytic and hepatic stage parasites.

For treatment, Malarone is given at an adult dose of four tablets daily for 3 days (Table 35–5). For chemoprophylaxis, Malarone must be taken daily. It has an advantage over mefloquine and doxycycline in requiring shorter durations of treatment before and after the period at risk for malaria transmission, due to activity against liver-stage parasites. It should be taken with food.

Malarone is generally well tolerated. Side effects include abdominal pain, nausea, vomiting, diarrhea, headache, and rash, and these are more common with the higher dose required for treatment. Reversible elevations in liver enzymes have been reported. The safety of atovaquone in pregnancy is unknown.

9. Antibiotics—A number of antibacterials in addition to the folate antagonists and sulfonamides are slow-acting antimalarials. None of the antibiotics should be used as single agents for the treatment of malaria due to their slow rate of action.

Doxycycline is commonly used in the treatment of falciparum malaria in conjunction with quinidine or quinine, allowing a shorter and better-tolerated course of those drugs (Table 35–4). Doxycycline is also a standard chemoprophylactic drug. Doxycycline side effects include GI symptoms, candidal vaginitis, and photosensitivity. The drug should be taken while upright with a large amount of water to avoid esophageal irritation. Clindamycin can be used in conjunction with quinine or quinidine in those for whom doxycycline is not recommended, such as children and pregnant women (Table 35–4). The most common toxicities with clindamycin are GI.

10. Lumefantrine—Lumefantrine, an aryl alcohol related to halofantrine, is available only as a fixed-dose combination with artemether (Coartem or Riamet). Oral absorption is

Table 35–5. Drugs for the prevention of malaria in travelers.[1]

Drug	Use[2]	Adult Dosage (all oral)[3]
Chloroquine	Areas without resistant *Plasmodium falciparum*	500 mg weekly
Malarone	Areas with multidrug-resistant *P falciparum*	1 tablet (250-mg atovaquone/100-mg proguanil) daily
Mefloquine	Areas with chloroquine-resistant *P falciparum*	250 mg weekly
Doxycycline	Areas with multidrug-resistant *P falciparum*	100 mg daily
Primaquine[4]	Terminal prophylaxis of *Plasmodium vivax* and *Plasmodium ovale* infections; alternative for *P falciparum* prophylaxis	30-mg base daily: for terminal prophylaxis take for 14 days after travel; for chemoprevention begin 1–2 days before travel, take during travel and for 7 days after travel
Tafenoquine[4]	Alternative for *P falciparum* prophylaxis	200 mg once daily for 3 days and then weekly until 1 week after last exposure

[1]Recommendations may change, as resistance to all available drugs is increasing. See text for additional information on toxicities and cautions. For additional details and pediatric dosing, see CDC guidelines (phone: 800-CDC-INFO; http://wwwnc.cdc.gov/travel/). Travelers to remote areas should consider carrying effective therapy (see text) for use if a febrile illness develops, and they cannot reach medical attention quickly.

[2]Areas without known chloroquine-resistant *P falciparum* are Central America west of the Panama Canal, Haiti, Dominican Republic, Egypt, and most malarious countries of the Middle East. Malarone or mefloquine is currently recommended for other malarious areas except for border areas of Thailand, where doxycycline is recommended.

[3]For drugs other than primaquine, begin 1–2 weeks before departure (except 2 days before for doxycycline and Malarone) and continue for 4 weeks after leaving the endemic area (except 1 week for Malarone). All dosages refer to salts unless otherwise indicated.

[4]Screen for glucose-6-phosphate dehydrogenase deficiency before using primaquine.

Reproduced with permission from Katzung BG. *Basic & Clinical Pharmacology*, 14th edition. McGraw-Hill, 2018.

highly variable and improved when the drug is taken with food. Use of Coartem with a fatty meal is recommended. Coartem is highly effective for the treatment of falciparum malaria, but it requires twice-daily dosing. Despite this limitation, due to its reliable efficacy against falciparum malaria, Coartem is the first-line therapy for malaria in many malarious countries and is the most widely used antimalarial in the world. Coartem is well tolerated; side effects include headache, dizziness, loss of appetite, GI symptoms, and palpitations.

Prevention

Malaria is transmitted by night-biting anopheline mosquitoes. Bed nets, in particular nets treated with permethrin insecticides, are heavily promoted as inexpensive means of antimalarial protection, but effectiveness varies in part due to widespread insecticide resistance. Indoor spraying of insecticides is generally highly effective in Africa but limited by resource constraints.

Extensive efforts are underway to develop malaria vaccines. The RTS,S vaccine, which is based on a sporozoite antigen, has been widely studied; multiple trials showed about 25–50% protection against malaria in children in the year after immunization, but lower levels of protection in very young children, in areas of highest malaria exposure, and over longer periods of time. The RTS,S vaccine, although endorsed by the WHO in 2021 for broad use in children, will probably not be widely available for several years. Seasonal malaria immunization, using the RTS,S vaccine in conjunction with SMC during the high transmission season, has shown good preventive efficacy. The R21 vaccine, with the same antigen as RTS,S but a different adjuvant, showed improved (approximately 75%) protection. Other approaches under study include vaccines containing erythrocytic, liver-stage, and sexual-stage antigens, and use of radiation-attenuated or molecularly attenuated sporozoites.

When travelers from nonendemic to endemic countries are counseled on the prevention of malaria, it is imperative to emphasize measures to prevent mosquito bites (insect repellents, insecticides, and bed nets), since parasites are increasingly resistant to multiple drugs and no chemoprophylactic regimen is fully protective. Chemoprophylaxis is recommended for all travelers from nonendemic regions to endemic areas, although risks vary greatly for different locations, and some tropical areas entail no risk; specific recommendations for travel to different locales are available from the CDC (www.cdc.gov). Recommendations from the CDC include the use of chloroquine for chemoprophylaxis in the few areas with only chloroquine-sensitive malaria parasites (principally the Caribbean and Central America west of the Panama Canal), and Malarone, mefloquine, or doxycycline for other areas (Table 35–5). Primaquine and tafenoquine are also effective but not used as often. In some circumstances, it may be appropriate for travelers to not use chemoprophylaxis but to carry supplies of drugs (ACTs or Malarone) with them in case a febrile illness develops and medical attention is unavailable. Most authorities do not recommend routine terminal prophylaxis with primaquine to eradicate dormant hepatic stages of *P vivax* and *P ovale* after travel, but this may be appropriate for travelers with major exposure to these parasites.

Regular chemoprophylaxis is not a standard management practice in developing world populations due to the expense and potential toxicities of long-term therapy. However, intermittent preventive therapy, whereby at-risk populations receive antimalarial therapy at set intervals, may decrease the incidence of malaria while allowing antimalarial immunity to develop. During pregnancy, intermittent preventive therapy with sulfadoxine-pyrimethamine, provided monthly during the second and third trimesters, has improved pregnancy outcomes. With increasing resistance, the preventive efficacy of sulfadoxine-pyrimethamine is likely falling, and the long-acting ACT dihydroartemisinin-piperaquine is a promising replacement. In areas with seasonal malaria transmission and limited drug resistance, principally the Sahel subregion of West Africa, SMC (monthly amodiaquine plus sulfadoxine-pyrimethamine during the transmission season) is widely practiced.

Prognosis

When treated appropriately, uncomplicated malaria generally responds well, with resolution of fevers within 1–2 days and a mortality of about 0.1%. Severe malaria can commonly progress to death, but many children respond well to therapy. In the developed world, mortality from malaria is mostly in adults, and often follows extended illnesses and secondary complications long after eradication of the malarial infection. Pregnant women are at particular risk during their first pregnancy. Malaria in pregnancy also increases the likelihood of poor pregnancy outcomes, with increased prematurity, low birth weight, and mortality.

When to Refer

Referral to an expert on infectious diseases or travel medicine is important with all cases of malaria in the United States, and in particular for falciparum malaria; referral should not delay initial diagnosis and therapy, since delays in therapy can lead to severe illness or death.

When to Admit

- Admission for non-falciparum malaria is warranted only if specific problems that require hospital management are present.
- Patients with falciparum malaria are generally admitted because the disease can progress rapidly to severe illness; exceptions may be made with individuals who are from malaria-endemic areas, and thus expected to have a degree of immunity, who are without evidence of severe disease, and who are judged able to return promptly for medical attention if their disease progresses.

Ashley EA et al. Malaria. Lancet. 2018;391:1608. [PMID: 29631781]

Balikagala B et al. Evidence of artemisinin-resistant malaria in Africa. N Engl J Med. 2021;385:1163. [PMID: 34551228]

Chandramohan D. Seasonal malaria vaccination with or without seasonal malaria chemoprevention. N Engl J Med. 2021;385:1005 [PMID: 34432975]

Conrad MD, Rosenthal PJ. Antimalarial drug resistance in Africa: the calm before the storm? Lancet Infect Dis. 2019;19:e338. [PMID: 31375467]

Datoo MS et al. Efficacy of a low-dose candidate malaria vaccine, R21 in adjuvant Matrix-M, with seasonal administration to children in Burkina Faso: a randomised controlled trial. Lancet. 2021;397:1809. [PMID: 33964223]

Haston JC et al. Guidance for using tafenoquine for prevention and antirelapse therapy for malaria—United States, 2019. MMWR Morb Mortal Wkly Rep. 2019;68:1062. [PMID: 31751320]

Uwimana A et al. Association of *Plasmodium falciparum kelch13* R561H genotypes with delayed parasite clearance in Rwanda: an open-label, single-arm, multicentre, therapeutic efficacy study. Lancet Infect Dis. 2021;21:1120. [PMID: 33864801]

World Health Organization. *World Malaria Report 2021*. Geneva, Switzerland: WHO, 2020. https://www.who.int/teams/global-malaria-programme/reports/world-malaria-report-2021

BABESIOSIS

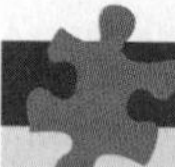

ESSENTIALS OF DIAGNOSIS

- History of tick bite or exposure to ticks.
- Fever, flu-like symptoms, anemia.
- Intraerythrocytic parasites on Giemsa-stained blood smears.
- Positive serologic tests.

General Considerations

Babesiosis is an uncommon intraerythrocytic infection caused mainly by two *Babesia* species and transmitted by *Ixodes* ticks. In the United States, hundreds of cases of babesiosis have been reported, and infection is caused by *Babesia microti,* which also infects wild mammals. Most babesiosis in the United States occurs in the coastal northeast, with some cases also in the upper Midwest, following the geographic range of the vector *Ixodes scapularis*, and Lyme disease and anaplasmosis, which are spread by the same vector. The incidence of the disease appears to be increasing in some areas. Babesiosis is caused by *Babesia divergens* in Europe and by *Babesia venatorum* in China. Babesiosis due to *Babesia duncani* and other Babesia-like organisms have been reported uncommonly from the western United States. Babesiosis can also be transmitted by blood transfusion, but blood supplies are not screened. A survey of a large set of blood samples from endemic regions of the United States identified approximately 0.4% as potentially infectious for *B microti*.

Clinical Findings

A. Symptoms and Signs

Serosurveys suggest that asymptomatic infections are common in endemic areas. With *B microti* infections, symptoms appear one to several weeks after a tick bite; parasitemia is evident after 2–4 weeks. Patients usually do not recall the tick bite. The typical flu-like illness develops gradually and is characterized by fever, malaise, fatigue, headache, anorexia, and myalgia. Other findings may include nausea, vomiting, abdominal pain, arthralgia, sore throat, depression, emotional lability, anemia, thrombocytopenia, elevated transaminases, and splenomegaly. Parasitemia may continue for months to years, with or without symptoms, and the disease is usually self-limited. Severe complications are most likely to occur in older persons or in those who have had splenectomy. Serious complications include respiratory failure, hemolytic anemia, disseminated intravascular coagulation, heart failure, and AKI. In a study of hospitalized patients, the mortality rate was 6.5%. Most recognized *B divergens* infections in Europe have been in patients who have had splenectomy. These infections progress rapidly with high fever, severe hemolytic anemia, jaundice, hemoglobinuria, and AKI, with death rates over 40%.

B. Laboratory Findings

Identification of the intraerythrocytic parasite on Giemsa-stained blood smears establishes the diagnosis. These can be confused with malaria parasites, but the morphology is distinctive. Repeated smears are often necessary because well under 1% of erythrocytes may be infected, especially early in infection, although parasitemias can exceed 10%. Diagnosis can also be made by PCR, which is more sensitive than blood smear. An indirect immunofluorescent antibody test for *B microti* is available from the CDC; antibody is detectable within 2–4 weeks after the onset of symptoms and persists for months, and a fourfold increase in antibody titer between acute and convalescent sera confirms acute infection.

Treatment

Most patients have a mild illness and recover without therapy. Standard therapy for mild to moderate disease is a 7-day course of atovaquone (750 mg orally every 12 hours) plus azithromycin (600 mg orally once daily), which is equally effective and better tolerated than the alternative regimen, a 7-day course of quinine (650 mg orally three times daily) plus clindamycin (600 mg orally three times daily). However, there is more experience using quinine plus clindamycin, and this regimen is recommended by some experts for severe disease. Exchange transfusion has been used successfully in severely ill asplenic patients and those with parasitemia greater than 10%.

Krause PJ. Human babesiosis. Int J Parasitol. 2019;49:165. [PMID: 30690090]

Madison-Antenucci S et al. Emerging tick-borne diseases. Clin Microbiol Rev. 2020;33:e00083–18. [PMID: 31896541]

Renard I et al. Treatment of human babesiosis: then and now. Pathogens. 2021;10:1120. [PMID: 34578153]

TOXOPLASMOSIS

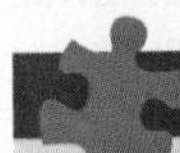

ESSENTIALS OF DIAGNOSIS

- Infection confirmed by isolation of *Toxoplasma gondii* or identification of tachyzoites in tissue or body fluids.

Primary infection

- Fever, malaise, headache, sore throat.
- Lymphadenopathy.
- Positive IgG and IgM serologic tests.

Congenital infection

- After acute infection of seronegative mothers, CNS abnormalities and retinochoroiditis seen in offspring.

Infection in immunocompromised persons

- Reactivation leads to encephalitis, retinochoroiditis, pneumonitis, myocarditis.
- Positive IgG but negative IgM serologic tests.

General Considerations

T gondii, an obligate intracellular protozoan, is found worldwide in humans and in many species of mammals and birds. The definitive hosts are cats. Humans are infected after ingestion of cysts in raw or undercooked meat, ingestion of oocysts in food or water contaminated by cats, transplacental transmission of trophozoites or, rarely, direct inoculation of trophozoites via blood transfusion or organ transplantation. *Toxoplasma* seroprevalence varies widely. It has decreased in the United States to less than 20%, but it is much higher in other countries in both the developed and developing worlds, where it may exceed 80%. In the United States, *T gondii* is estimated to infect 1.1 million persons each year, with resultant chorioretinitis developing in 21,000 and vision loss in 4800.

Clinical Findings

A. Symptoms and Signs

The clinical manifestations of toxoplasmosis may be grouped into four syndromes.

1. Primary infection in the immunocompetent person— After ingestion, *T gondii* infection progresses from the GI tract to lymphatics, and then dissemination. Most acute infections are asymptomatic. About 10–20% are symptomatic after an incubation period of 1–2 weeks. Acute infections in immunocompetent persons typically present as mild, febrile illnesses that resemble infectious mononucleosis. Nontender cervical or diffuse lymphadenopathy may persist for weeks to months. Systemic findings may include fever, malaise, headache, sore throat, rash, myalgias, hepatosplenomegaly, and atypical lymphocytosis. Rare severe manifestations are pneumonitis, meningoencephalitis, hepatitis, myocarditis, polymyositis, and retinochoroiditis. Symptoms may fluctuate; most patients recover spontaneously within a few months.

2. Congenital infection—Congenital transmission occurs as a result of infection, which may be symptomatic or asymptomatic, in a nonimmune woman during pregnancy. Fetal infection follows maternal infection in 30–50% of cases, but this risk varies by trimester: 10–25% during the first, 30–50% during the second, and 60% or higher during the third trimester. In the United States, an estimated 400 to 4000 congenital infections occur yearly. While the risk of fetal infection increases, the risk of severe fetal disease decreases over the course of pregnancy. Early fetal infections commonly lead to spontaneous abortion, stillbirths, or severe neonatal disease, including neurologic manifestations. Retinochoroiditis and other sight-threatening eye lesions may develop. Infections later in pregnancy less commonly lead to major fetal problems. Most infants appear normal at birth, but they may have subtle abnormalities and progress to symptoms and signs of congenital toxoplasmosis later in life.

3. Retinochoroiditis—The most common late presentation of congenital toxoplasmosis is retinochoroiditis, which presents weeks to years after congenital infection, commonly in teenagers or young adults. Retinochoroiditis is also seen in persons who acquire infection early in life, and these patients more often present with unilateral disease. Uveitis is also seen. Disease presents with pain, photophobia, and visual changes, usually without systemic symptoms. Signs and symptoms eventually improve, but visual defects may persist. Rarely, progression may result in glaucoma and blindness.

4. Disease in the immunocompromised person—Reactivated toxoplasmosis occurs in patients with AIDS, cancer, or those given immunosuppressive drugs. In advanced AIDS, the most common manifestation is encephalitis, with multiple necrotizing brain lesions. The encephalitis usually presents subacutely, with fever, headache, altered mental status, focal neurologic findings, and other evidence of brain lesions. Less common manifestations of toxoplasmosis in AIDS are chorioretinitis and pneumonitis. Chorioretinitis presents with ocular pain and alterations in vision. Pneumonitis presents with fever, cough, and dyspnea. Toxoplasmosis can develop in recipients of solid organ or bone marrow transplants due to reactivation or, more rarely, transmission of infection. Reactivation also can occur in those with hematologic malignancies or treated with immunosuppressive drugs. With primary or reactivated disease in those with immunodeficiency due to malignancy or immunosuppressive drugs, toxoplasmosis is similar to that in individuals with AIDS, but pneumonitis and myocarditis are more common.

B. Diagnostic Testing

1. Identification of parasites—Organisms can be seen in tissue or body fluids, although they may be difficult to identify; special staining techniques can facilitate identification. The demonstration of tachyzoites indicates acute infection; cysts may represent either acute or chronic infection. With lymphadenopathy due to toxoplasmosis, examination of lymph nodes usually does not show organisms. Parasite identification can also be made by inoculation of tissue culture or mice. PCR can be used for sensitive identification of organisms in amniotic fluid, blood, CSF, aqueous humor, and bronchoalveolar lavage fluid.

2. Serologic diagnosis—Multiple serologic methods are used, including the Sabin-Feldman dye test, ELISA, indirect fluorescent antibody test, and agglutination tests. IgG antibodies are seen within 1–2 weeks of infection and usually persist for life. IgM antibodies peak earlier than IgG and decline more rapidly, although they may persist for years. In immunocompromised individuals in whom reactivation is suspected, a positive IgG assay indicates distant infection, and thus the potential for reactivated disease; a negative IgG argues strongly against reactivation toxoplasmosis. With reactivation in immunocompromised persons, IgM tests are generally negative.

3. During pregnancy and in newborns—Conversion from a negative to positive serologic test or rising titers are suggestive of acute infection, but tests are not routinely performed during pregnancy. When pregnant women are screened, negative IgG and IgM assays exclude active infection, but indicate the risk of infection during the pregnancy. Positive IgG with negative IgM is highly suggestive of chronic infection, with no risk of congenital disease unless the mother is severely immunocompromised. A positive IgM test is concerning for new infection because of the risk of congenital disease. Confirmatory testing should be performed before consideration of treatment or possible termination of pregnancy due to the limitations of available tests. Tests of the avidity of anti-IgG antibodies can be helpful, but a battery of tests is needed for confirmation of acute infection during pregnancy. When acute infection during pregnancy is suspected, PCR of amniotic fluid offers a sensitive assessment for congenital disease. In newborns, positive IgM or IgA antibody tests are indicative of congenital infection, although the diagnosis is not ruled out by a negative test. Positive IgG assays may represent transfer of maternal antibodies without infection of the infant, but persistence of positive IgG beyond 12 months of age is diagnostic of congenital infection. PCR of blood, CSF, or urine can also be helpful for early diagnosis of congenital disease.

4. In immunocompetent individuals—Individuals with a suggestive clinical syndrome should be tested for IgG and IgM antibodies. Seroconversion, a 16-fold rise in antibody titer, or an IgM titer greater than 1:64 is suggestive of acute infection, although false-positive results may occur. Acute infection can also be diagnosed by detection of tachyzoites in tissue, culture of organisms, or PCR of blood or body fluids. Histologic evaluation of lymph nodes can show characteristic morphology, with or without organisms.

5. In immunodeficient individuals—A presentation consistent with toxoplasmic encephalitis warrants imaging of the brain. CT and MRI scans typically show multiple ring-enhancing cerebral lesions, most commonly involving the corticomedullary junction and basal ganglia. MRI is the more sensitive imaging modality. In patients living with AIDS with a positive IgG serologic test and no recent antitoxoplasma or antiviral therapy, the predictive value of a typical imaging study is about 80%. The other common diagnosis in this setting is CNS lymphoma, which more typically causes a single brain lesion. The differential diagnosis also includes tuberculoma, bacterial brain abscess, fungal abscess, and carcinoma. Diagnosis of CNS toxoplasmosis is most typically made after a therapeutic trial, with clinical and radiologic improvement expected within 2–3 weeks. Definitive diagnosis requires brain biopsy and search for organisms and typical histology. In retinochoroiditis, funduscopic examination shows vitreous inflammatory reaction, white retinal lesions, and pigmented scars. Diagnosis of other clinical entities in immunocompromised individuals is generally based on histology.

Treatment

A. Approach to Treatment

Therapy is generally not necessary in immunocompetent persons, since primary illness is self-limited. However, for severe, persistent, or visceral disease, treatment for 2–4 weeks may be considered. Treatment is appropriate for primary infection during pregnancy because the risk of fetal transmission or the severity of congenital disease may be reduced. For retinochoroiditis, most episodes are self-limited, and opinions vary on indications for treatment. Treatment is often advocated for episodes with decreases in visual acuity, multiple or large lesions, macular lesions, significant inflammation, or persistence for over a month. Immunocompromised patients with active infection must be treated. For those with transient immunodeficiency, therapy can be continued for 4–6 weeks after cessation of symptoms. For those with persistent immunodeficiency, such as patients living with AIDS, full therapy for 4–6 weeks is followed by maintenance therapy with lower doses of drugs. Immunodeficient patients who are asymptomatic but have a positive IgG serologic test should receive long-term chemoprophylaxis.

B. Medications

Drugs for toxoplasmosis are active only against tachyzoites, so they do not eradicate infection. Standard therapy is the combination of pyrimethamine (200-mg loading dose, then 50–75 mg [1 mg/kg] orally once daily) plus sulfadiazine (1–1.5 g orally four times daily), with folinic acid (10–20 mg orally once daily) to prevent bone marrow suppression. Patients should be screened for a history of sulfonamide sensitivity (skin rashes, GI symptoms, hepatotoxicity). To prevent sulfonamide crystal-induced nephrotoxicity, good urinary output should be maintained. Pyrimethamine side effects include headache and GI symptoms. Even with folinic acid therapy, bone marrow suppression may occur; platelet and WBC counts should be monitored at least weekly. A first-line alternative is clindamycin (600 mg orally four times daily) replacing sulfadiazine as the standard therapy regimen. Another alternative is TMP-SMZ. Pyrimethamine is not used during the first trimester of pregnancy due to its teratogenicity. Standard therapy for acute toxoplasmosis during pregnancy is spiramycin (1 g orally three times daily until delivery) to decrease the risk of fetal infection; it reduces the frequency of transmission to the fetus by about 60%. Spiramycin does not cross the placenta, so when fetal infection is documented or for acute infections late in pregnancy (which commonly lead to fetal transmission), treatment with combination regimens as described above is indicated.

Prevention

Prevention of primary infection centers on avoidance of undercooked meat or contact with material contaminated by cat feces, particularly for seronegative pregnant women and immunocompromised persons. Irradiation, cooking to 66°C, or freezing to –20°C kills tissue cysts. Thorough cleaning of hands and surfaces is needed after contact with raw meat or areas contaminated by cats. Oocysts passed in cat feces can remain infective for a year or more, but fresh oocysts are not infective for 48 hours. For best protection, litter boxes should be changed daily and soaked in boiling water for 5 minutes, gloves should be worn when gardening, fruits and vegetables should be thoroughly washed, and ingestion of dried meat should be avoided.

Universal screening of pregnant women for *T gondii* antibodies is conducted in some countries but not the United States. Pregnant women should ideally have their serum examined for IgG and IgM antibody, and those with negative titers should adhere to the prevention measures described above. Seronegative women who continue to have environmental exposure should undergo repeat serologic screening several times during pregnancy.

For immunocompromised individuals, chemoprophylaxis to prevent primary or reactivated infection is warranted. For hematopoietic cell transplant recipients and patients living with advanced AIDS, chemoprophylaxis with TMP-SMZ (one double-strength tablet daily or two tablets three times weekly), used for protection against *Pneumocystis*, is effective against *T gondii*. Alternatives are pyrimethamine plus either sulfadoxine or dapsone (various regimens). In patients living with AIDS, chemoprophylaxis can be discontinued if antiretroviral therapy leads to immune reconstitution.

Elsheikha HM et al. Epidemiology, pathophysiology, diagnosis, and management of cerebral toxoplasmosis. Clin Microbiol Rev. 2020;34:e00115. [PMID: 33239310]

AMEBIASIS

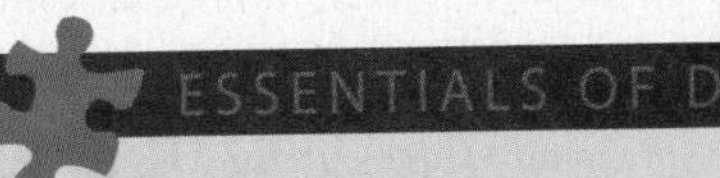

- Organisms or antigen present in stools or abscess aspirate.
- Positive serologic tests with colitis or hepatic abscess, but these may represent prior infections.
- Mild to moderate colitis with recurrent diarrhea.
- Severe colitis: bloody diarrhea, fever, and abdominal pain, with potential progression to hemorrhage or perforation.
- Hepatic abscess: fever, hepatomegaly, and abdominal pain.

General Considerations

The *Entamoeba* complex contains three morphologically identical species: *Entamoeba dispar* and *Entamoeba moshkovskii*, which are avirulent, and *Entamoeba histolytica*, which may be an avirulent intestinal commensal or lead to serious disease. Disease follows penetration of the intestinal wall, resulting in diarrhea, and with severe involvement, dysentery or extraintestinal disease, most commonly liver abscess.

E histolytica infections are present worldwide but are most prevalent in subtropical and tropical areas under conditions of crowding, poor sanitation, and poor nutrition. Of the estimated 500 million persons worldwide infected with *Entamoeba*, most are infected with *E dispar* and an estimated 10% with *E histolytica*. The prevalence of *E moshkovskii* is unknown. Mortality from invasive *E histolytica* infections is estimated at 100,000 per year.

Humans are the only established *E histolytica* host. Transmission occurs through ingestion of cysts from fecally contaminated food or water, facilitated by person-to-person spread, flies and other arthropods as mechanical vectors, and use of human excrement as fertilizer. Urban outbreaks have occurred because of common-source water contamination.

Clinical Findings

A. Symptoms and Signs

1. Intestinal amebiasis—In most infected persons, the organism lives as a commensal, and the carrier is without symptoms. With symptomatic disease, diarrhea may begin within a week of infection, although an incubation period of 2–4 weeks is more common, with gradual onset of abdominal pain and diarrhea. Fever is uncommon. Periods of remission and recurrence may last days, weeks, or longer. Abdominal examination may show distention, tenderness, hyperperistalsis, and hepatomegaly. Microscopic hematochezia is common. More severe presentations include colitis and dysentery, with worse diarrhea

(10–20 stools per day) and bloody stools. With dysentery, physical findings include high fevers, prostration, vomiting, abdominal pain and tenderness, hepatic enlargement, and hypotension. Severe presentations are more common in young children, pregnant women, those who are malnourished, and those receiving corticosteroids. Thus, in endemic regions, corticosteroids should not be started for presumed IBD without first ruling out amebiasis. Fulminant amebic colitis can progress to necrotizing colitis, intestinal perforation, mucosal sloughing, and severe hemorrhage, with mortality rates over 40%. More long-term complications of intestinal amebiasis include chronic diarrhea with weight loss, which may last for months to years; bowel ulcerations; and amebic appendicitis. Localized granulomatous lesions (amebomas) can present after either dysentery or chronic intestinal infection. Clinical findings include pain, obstructive symptoms, and hemorrhage and may suggest intestinal carcinoma.

2. Extraintestinal amebiasis—The most common extraintestinal manifestation is amebic liver abscess. This can occur with colitis, but more frequently presents without history of prior intestinal symptoms. Patients present with the acute or gradual onset of abdominal pain, fever, an enlarged and tender liver, anorexia, and weight loss. Diarrhea is present in a small number of patients. Physical examination may show intercostal tenderness. Abscesses are most commonly single and in the right lobe of the liver, and they are much more common in men. Without prompt treatment, amebic abscesses may rupture into the pleural, peritoneal, or pericardial space, which is often fatal. Amebic infections may rarely occur throughout the body, including the lungs, brain, and genitourinary system.

B. Laboratory Findings

Laboratory studies with intestinal amebiasis show leukocytosis and hematochezia, with fecal leukocytes not present in all cases. With extraintestinal amebiasis, leukocytosis and elevated liver function studies are seen.

C. Diagnostic Testing

Diagnosis is typically made by finding *E histolytica* or its antigen or by serologic tests. However, each method has limitations. Molecular diagnosis is possible from multipathogen panels, which are sensitive and specific but expensive.

1. Intestinal amebiasis—Diagnosis is most commonly made by identifying organisms in the stool. *E histolytica* and *E dispar* cannot be distinguished, but the identification of amebic trophozoites or cysts in a symptomatic patient is highly suggestive of amebiasis. Stool evaluation for organisms is not highly sensitive (~30–50% for amebic colitis), and at least three stool specimens should be evaluated after concentration and staining. Multiple serologic assays are available; these tests are sensitive, although sensitivity is lower (~70% in colitis) early in illness, and they cannot distinguish recent and old disease, as they remain positive for years after infection. Commercially available stool antigen tests (TechLab II, CELISA, QUIK CHEK) can distinguish *E histolytica* from nonpathogenic species and offer improved sensitivity (greater than 90% for colitis). The QUIK CHEK assay is FDA-approved, offers rapid point-of-care diagnosis, and is available in a combined assay for amebiasis, giardiasis, and cryptosporidiosis. Highly sensitive molecular tests are not used routinely but available in some high resource settings within commercial panels for identifying gut pathogens. Colonoscopy of uncleansed bowel typically shows no specific findings in mild intestinal disease; in severe disease, ulcers may be found with intact intervening friable mucosa, resembling IBD. Examination of fresh ulcer exudate for motile trophozoites and for *E histolytica* antigen may yield a diagnosis.

2. Hepatic abscess—Serologic tests for anti-amebic antibodies are almost always positive, except very early in the infection. Thus, a negative test in a suspicious case should be repeated in about a week. The TechLab II antigen test can be used to test serum with good sensitivity if used before the initiation of therapy. Examination of stools for organisms or antigen is frequently negative; the antigen test is positive in ~40% of cases. As imaging studies cannot distinguish amebic and pyogenic abscesses, when a diagnosis is not available from serologic studies, percutaneous aspiration may be indicated, ideally with an image-guided needle. Aspiration typically yields brown or yellow fluid. Detection of organisms in the aspirate is uncommon, but detection of *E histolytica* antigen is very sensitive and diagnostic. The key risk of aspiration is peritoneal spillage leading to peritonitis from amoebas or other (pyogenic or echinococcal) organisms.

D. Imaging

Liver abscesses can be identified by ultrasonography, CT, or MRI, typically with round or oval low-density nonhomogeneous lesions, with abrupt transition from normal liver to the lesion, and hypoechoic centers. Abscesses are most commonly single, but more than one may be present. The right lobe is usually involved.

Treatment

Treatment of amebiasis generally entails the use of metronidazole or tinidazole to eradicate tissue trophozoites and a luminal amebicide to eradicate intestinal cysts (Table 35–6). Asymptomatic infection with *E dispar* does not require therapy. This organism cannot be differentiated morphologically from *E histolytica*, but with negative serology *E dispar* colonization is likely, and treatment is not indicated. Intestinal colonization with *E histolytica* is treated with a luminal agent. Effective luminal agents are diloxanide furoate (500 mg orally three times daily with meals for 10 days), iodoquinol (diiodohydroxyquin; 650 mg orally three times daily for 21 days), and paromomycin (30-mg/kg base orally, maximum 3 g, in three divided doses after meals daily for 7 days). Side effects associated with luminal agents are flatulence with diloxanide furoate, mild diarrhea with iodoquinol, and GI symptoms with paromomycin. Relative contraindications are thyroid disease for iodoquinol and kidney disease for iodoquinol or paromomycin.

Treatment of intestinal amebiasis requires tinidazole (2 g orally once daily for 3–5 days) or metronidazole (750 mg orally three times daily for 10 days) plus a luminal agent (Table 35–6). Tinidazole offers simpler dosing, a more rapid clinical response, and fewer side effects than metronidazole. Side effects from either agent include transient nausea, vomiting, epigastric discomfort, headache, or a metallic taste. A disulfiram-like reaction may occur if alcohol is co-ingested. Metronidazole and tinidazole should be avoided in pregnant or nursing mothers, if possible. Fluid and electrolyte replacement is also important for patients with significant diarrhea. Surgical management of acute complications of intestinal amebiasis is best avoided whenever possible. Successful therapy of severe amebic colitis may be followed by postdysenteric colitis, with continued diarrhea without persistent infection; this syndrome generally resolves in weeks to months.

Amebic liver abscess is also treated with metronidazole or tinidazole plus a luminal agent (even if intestinal infection is not documented; Table 35–6). Metronidazole can be used intravenously when necessary. With failure of initial response to metronidazole or tinidazole, chloroquine, emetine, or dehydroemetine may be added. Needle aspiration may be helpful for large abscesses (over 5–10 cm), in particular if the diagnosis remains uncertain, if there is an initial lack of response, or if a patient is very ill, suggesting imminent abscess rupture. With successful therapy, abscesses disappear slowly (over months).

Prevention & Control

Prevention requires safe water supplies; sanitary disposal of human feces; adequate cooking of food; protection of food from fly contamination; hand washing; and, in endemic areas, avoidance of fruits and vegetables that cannot be cooked or peeled. Water supplies can be boiled, treated with iodine (0.5-mL tincture of iodine per liter for 20 minutes; cysts are resistant to standard concentrations of chlorine), or filtered.

Gupta S at al. Amebiasis and amebic liver abscess in children. Pediatr Clin North Am. 2022;69:79. [PMID: 34794678]

Shirley DT et al. A review of the global burden, new diagnostics, and current therapeutics for amebiasis. Open Forum Infect Dis. 2018;5:ofy161. [PMID: 30046644]

Table 35–6. Treatment of amebiasis.[1]

Clinical Setting	Drugs of Choice and Adult Dosage	Alternative Drugs and Adult Dosage
Asymptomatic intestinal infection	**Luminal agent:** Diloxanide furoate,[2] 500 mg orally three times daily for 10 days or Iodoquinol, 650 mg orally three times daily for 21 days or Paromomycin, 10 mg/kg orally three times daily for 7 days	
Mild to moderate intestinal infection	Metronidazole, 750 mg orally three times daily (or 500 mg intravenously every 6 hours) for 10 days or Tinidazole, 2 g orally daily for 3 days **plus** Luminal agent (see above)	Luminal agent (see above) plus either Tetracycline, 250 mg orally three times daily for 10 days or Erythromycin, 500 mg orally four times daily for 10 days
Severe intestinal infection	Metronidazole, 750 mg orally three times daily (or 500 mg intravenously every 6 hours) for 10 days or Tinidazole, 2 g orally daily for 5 days **plus** Luminal agent (see above)	Luminal agent (see above) plus either Tetracycline, 250 mg orally three times daily for 10 days or Dehydroemetine[2] or emetine,[2] 1 mg/kg subcutaneously or intramuscularly for 3–5 days
Hepatic abscess, ameboma, and other extraintestinal disease	Metronidazole, 750 mg orally three times daily (or 500 mg intravenously every 6 hours) for 10 days or Tinidazole, 2 g orally daily for 5 days **plus** Luminal agent (see above)	Dehydroemetine[2] or emetine,[2] 1 mg/kg subcutaneously or intramuscularly for 8–10 days, followed by (liver abscess only) chloroquine, 500 mg orally twice daily for 2 days, then 500 mg daily for 21 days **plus** Luminal agent (see above)

[1]See text for additional details and cautions.
[2]Not available in the United States.

COCCIDIOSIS (Cryptosporidiosis, Isosporiasis, Cyclosporiasis, Sarcocystosis) & MICROSPORIDIOSIS

ESSENTIALS OF DIAGNOSIS

- Acute diarrhea, especially in children in developing countries.
- Outbreaks of diarrhea secondary to contaminated water or food.
- Prolonged diarrhea in immunocompromised persons.
- Diagnosis mostly by identifying organisms in specially stained stool specimens.

General Considerations

The causes of coccidiosis are *Cryptosporidium* species (*C parvum, C hominis,* and others); *Cystoisospora* (formerly *Isospora*) *belli; Cyclospora cayetanensis;* and *Sarcocystis* species. Microsporidiosis is caused by at least 14 species, most commonly *Enterocytozoon bieneusi* and *Encephalitozoon intestinalis.* These infections occur worldwide, particularly in the tropics and in regions where hygiene is poor. They are causes of endemic childhood gastroenteritis (particularly in malnourished children in developing countries); institutional and community outbreaks of diarrhea; traveler's diarrhea; and acute and chronic diarrhea in immunosuppressed patients, in particular those with AIDS. They are all notable for the potential to cause prolonged diarrhea, often lasting for a number of weeks. Clustering occurs in households, day care centers, and among sexual partners.

The infectious agents are oocysts (coccidiosis) or spores (microsporidiosis) transmitted from person to person or by contaminated drinking or swimming water or food. Ingested oocysts release sporozoites that invade and multiply in enterocytes, primarily in the small bowel. Coccidian oocysts and microsporidian cysts can remain viable in the environment for years.

Cryptosporidiosis is a zoonosis *(C parvum* principally infects cattle), but most human infections are acquired from humans, in particular with *C hominus.* Cryptosporidia are highly infectious and readily transmitted in day care settings and households. They have caused large community outbreaks due to contaminated water supplies (causing about 400,000 illnesses in Milwaukee in 1993 and about 2780 illnesses in Oregon in 2013) and are the leading cause of recreational water–associated outbreaks of gastroenteritis. In the developing world, cryptosporidiosis is a leading cause of childhood diarrhea. In a study of causes of moderate-to-severe diarrhea in Asia and Africa, *Cryptosporidium* was the second most commonly identified pathogen in children under 2 years of age.

C belli and *C cayetanensis* appear to infect only humans. *C cayetanensis* has caused a number of food-borne outbreaks in the United States in recent years, most commonly associated with imported fresh produce. *Sarcocystis* infects many species; humans are intermediate hosts (infected by ingestion of fecal sporocysts) for some species but definitive hosts for *Sarcocystis bovihominis* and *Sarcocystis suihominis* (infected by ingestion of tissue cysts in undercooked beef and pork, respectively).

Clinical Findings

A. Symptoms and Signs

1. Coccidiosis—

A. CRYPTOSPORIDIOSIS—The incubation period appears to be approximately 14 days. In developing countries, disease is primarily in children under 5 years of age, causing 5–10% of childhood diarrhea. Presenting symptoms include acute watery diarrhea, abdominal pain, and cramps, with rapid resolution in most patients; however, symptoms quite commonly persist for 2 weeks or more. In developed countries, most patients are adults. Diarrhea in immunocompetent individuals typically lasts 5–10 days; it is usually watery, with accompanying abdominal pain and cramps, nausea, vomiting, and fever. Relapses may follow initial resolution of symptoms. Mild illness and asymptomatic infection are also common.

Cryptosporidiosis is a well-characterized cause of diarrhea in those with AIDS. It was common before the advent of highly active antiretroviral therapy, particularly with advanced immunosuppression. Clinical manifestations are variable, but patients commonly have chronic diarrhea with frequent foul-smelling stools, malabsorption, and weight loss. Severe, life-threatening watery diarrhea may be seen. Cryptosporidiosis also causes extraintestinal disease with AIDS, including pulmonary infiltrates with dyspnea and biliary tract infection with sclerosing cholangitis and AIDS cholangiopathy.

B. ISOSPORIASIS—The incubation period for *C belli* is about 1 week. In immunocompetent persons, it usually causes a self-limited watery diarrhea lasting 2–3 weeks, with abdominal cramps, anorexia, malaise, and weight loss. Fever is unusual. Chronic symptoms may persist for months. In immunocompromised patients, isosporiasis more commonly causes severe and chronic diarrhea, with complications including marked dehydration, malnutrition, and hemorrhagic colitis. Extraintestinal disease has been reported rarely.

C. CYCLOSPORIASIS—*C cayetanensis* oocysts must undergo a period of sporulation of 7 days or more after shedding before they become infectious. Therefore, person-to-person spread is unlikely, and spread has typically been due to contaminated food (especially fresh produce) and water. The incubation period is 1–11 days. Infections can be asymptomatic. Cyclosporiasis causes an illness similar to that described for the other pathogens included in this section, with watery diarrhea, abdominal cramps, nausea, fatigue, and anorexia. Fever is seen in 25% of cases. Symptoms typically continue for 2 weeks or longer and may persist for months without therapy. Relapses of diarrhea are common. Diarrhea may be preceded by a flu-like prodrome and followed by persistent fatigue. In immunocompromised patients, cyclosporiasis is typically more severe and prolonged, with chronic fulminant watery diarrhea and weight loss.

D. SARCOCYSTOSIS—*Sarcocystis* infection is common in some developing countries but is usually asymptomatic. Infection appears to most commonly follow the ingestion of undercooked beef or pork, leading to the development of cysts in muscle, with myalgias, fever, bronchospasm, pruritic rash, lymphadenopathy, and subcutaneous nodules. Ingestion of fecal sporocysts may lead to GI symptoms.

2. Microsporidiosis—Microsporidia are obligate intracellular protozoans that cause a wide spectrum of diseases. Many infections are of zoonotic origin, but human-to-human transmission has been documented. Infection is mainly by ingestion of spores, but also by direct inoculation of the eyes. In immunocompetent hosts, microsporidian infections most commonly present as self-limited diarrhea. Ocular infections have also been described. Disease from microsporidia is seen mainly in immunocompromised persons, particularly those with AIDS. Infections in people living with AIDS are most commonly with *E bieneusi* and *E intestinalis*. They cause chronic diarrhea, with anorexia, bloating, weight loss, and wasting, especially in those with advanced immunodeficiency. Fever is usually not seen. Other illnesses in immunocompromised persons associated with microsporidians (including the genera *Enterocytozoon, Encephalitozoon, Brachiola, Vittaforma, Pleistophora, Trachipleistophora*, and *Microsporidium*) include biliary tract disease (AIDS cholangiopathy), genitourinary infection with cystitis, kidney disease, hepatitis, peritonitis, myositis, respiratory infections including sinusitis, CNS infections including granulomatous encephalitis, and disseminated infections. Ocular infections with *Encephalitozoon* species cause conjunctivitis and keratitis, presenting as redness, photophobia, and loss of visual acuity.

B. Laboratory Findings

1. Coccidiosis—

A. CRYPTOSPORIDIOSIS—Typically, stool is without blood or leukocytes. Diagnosis is traditionally made by detecting the organism in stool using a modified acid-fast stain; this technique is relatively insensitive, and multiple specimens should be evaluated before ruling out the diagnosis. Of note, routine evaluation for ova and parasites typically does not include a modified acid-fast stain, so this must be specifically requested in many laboratories. Various antigen detection methods, including immunofluorescence microscopy, ELISA, and immunochromatography, offer improved sensitivity and specificity, both over 90% with available assays, and these methods may be considered the optimal means of diagnosis. Molecular diagnostic panels that recognize *Cryptosporidium* and other enteropathogens in stool are available but expensive.

B. ISOSPORIASIS—Diagnosis of isosporiasis is by examination of stool wet mounts or after modified acid-fast staining, in which the organism is clearly distinguishable from other parasites. Other stains also show the organism. Shedding of oocysts may be intermittent, so the sensitivity of stool evaluation is not high, and multiple samples should be examined. The organism may also be identified in duodenal aspirates or small bowel biopsies.

C. CYCLOSPORIASIS—Diagnosis is made by examination of stool wet mounts or after modified acid-fast staining. Multiple specimens may need to be examined to make a diagnosis; concentration of specimens improves sensitivity. The organism can also be identified in small bowel aspirates or biopsy specimens. Molecular assays with high sensitivity and specificity, including multi-pathogen panels, are available.

D. SARCOCYSTOSIS—Eosinophilia and elevated creatine kinase may be seen. Diagnosis is by identification of the acid-fast organisms in stool or by identification of trophozoites or bradyzoites in tissue biopsies.

2. Microsporidiosis—Diagnosis can be made by identification of organisms in specially stained stool, fluid, or tissue specimens, for example with Weber chromotrope-based stain. Electron microscopy is helpful for confirmation of the diagnosis and speciation. PCR and culture techniques are available but not used routinely.

Treatment

Most acute infections with these pathogens in immunocompetent persons are self-limited and do not require treatment. Supportive treatment for severe or chronic diarrhea includes fluid and electrolyte replacement and, in some cases, parenteral nutrition.

1. Coccidiosis—

A. CRYPTOSPORIDIOSIS—Treatment of cryptosporidiosis is challenging. No agent is clearly effective. Modest benefits have been seen in some (but not other) studies, generally in immunocompetent hosts, with nitazoxanide, which is FDA-approved for this indication (500 mg–1 g orally twice daily for 3 days in immunocompetent patients and 2–8 weeks in patients living with advanced AIDS), and paromomycin, a nonabsorbed aminoglycoside (25–35 mg/kg orally for 14 days has been used). Other agents that have been used with mixed success in the treatment of cryptosporidiosis in patients living with AIDS include azithromycin, spiramycin, bovine hyperimmune colostrum, and octreotide. Reversing immunodeficiency with effective antiretroviral therapy is of greatest importance.

B. ISOSPORIASIS—Isosporiasis is effectively treated in immunocompetent and immunosuppressed persons with TMP-SMZ (160 mg/800 mg orally two to four times daily for 10 days, with the higher dosage for patients living with AIDS). An alternative therapy is pyrimethamine (75 mg orally in four divided doses) with folinic acid (10–25 mg/day orally). Maintenance therapy with low-dose TMP-SMZ (160 mg/800 mg daily or three times per week) or Fansidar (1 tablet weekly) prevents relapse in those with persistent immunosuppression.

C. CYCLOSPORIASIS—Cyclosporiasis is also treated with TMP-SMZ (dosing as for isosporiasis). With AIDS, long-term maintenance therapy (160 mg/800 mg three times weekly) helps prevent relapse. For patients intolerant of TMP-SMZ, ciprofloxacin (500 mg orally twice daily for 7 days) showed efficacy, albeit with less ability to clear the organism than TMP-SMZ.

D. Sarcocystosis—For sarcocystosis, no specific treatment is established, but patients may respond to therapy with albendazole or TMP-SMZ.

2. Microsporidiosis—Treatment of microsporidiosis is complex. Infections with most species, including those causing GI and other manifestations, should be treated with albendazole (400 mg orally twice daily for 2–4 weeks), which has activity against a number of species, but relatively poor efficacy (about 50%) against *E bieneusi*, the most common microsporidial cause of diarrhea in patients living with AIDS. Fumagillin, which is used to treat honeybees and fish with microsporidian infections, has shown benefit in clinical trials at a dose of 20 mg three times per day for 14 days; treatment was accompanied by reversible thrombocytopenia. As with cryptosporidiosis, the best means of controlling microsporidiosis in patients living with AIDS is to restore immune function with effective antiretroviral therapy. Ocular microsporidiosis can be treated with topical fumagillin solution (3 mg/mL); this probably should be given with concurrent systemic therapy with albendazole. Adjunctive management may include topical corticosteroids to decrease inflammation and keratoplasty.

Prevention

Water purification is important for control of these infections. Chlorine disinfection is not effective against cryptosporidial oocysts, so other purification measures are needed. Immunocompromised patients should boil or filter drinking water and should consider avoidance of lakes and swimming pools. Routine precautions (hand washing, gloves, disinfection) should prevent institutional patient-to-patient spread. Optimal means of preventing microsporidial infections are not well understood, but water purification and body substance precautions for immunocompromised and hospitalized individuals are likely effective.

Diptyanusa A et al. Treatment of human intestinal cryptosporidiosis: a review of published clinical trials. Int J Parasitol Drugs Drug Resist. 2021;17:128. [PMID: 34562754]

Mathison BA et al. Cyclosporiasis—updates on clinical presentation, pathology, clinical diagnosis, and treatment. Microorganisms. 2021;9:1863. [PMID: 34576758]

Rosenthal BM. Zoonotic sarcocystis. Res Vet Sci. 2021;136:151. [PMID: 33626441]

GIARDIASIS

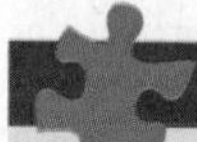

ESSENTIALS OF DIAGNOSIS

- Acute diarrhea may be profuse and watery.
- Chronic diarrhea with greasy, malodorous stools.
- Abdominal cramps, distention, flatulence.
- Cysts or trophozoites in stools.

General Considerations

Giardiasis is a protozoal infection of the upper small intestine caused by the flagellate *Giardia lamblia* (also called *Giardia intestinalis* and *Giardia duodenalis*). The parasite occurs worldwide, most abundantly in areas with poor sanitation. In developing countries, young children are very commonly infected. In the United States and Europe, the infection is the most common intestinal protozoal pathogen; the US estimate is 100,000 to 2.5 million new infections leading to 5000 hospital admissions yearly. Groups at special risk include travelers to *Giardia*-endemic areas, those who swallow contaminated water during recreation or wilderness travel, men who have sex with men, and persons with impaired immunity. Outbreaks are common in households, children's day care centers, and residential facilities, and may occur as a result of contamination of water supplies.

The organism occurs in feces as a flagellated trophozoite and as a cyst. Only the cyst form is infectious by the oral route; trophozoites are destroyed by gastric acidity. Humans are a reservoir for the pathogen; dogs, cats, beavers, and other mammals have been implicated but not confirmed as reservoirs. Under suitable moist, cool conditions, cysts can survive in the environment for weeks to months. Cysts are transmitted as a result of fecal contamination of water or food, by person-to-person contact, or by anal-oral sexual contact. The infectious dose is low, requiring as few as 10 cysts. After the cysts are ingested, trophozoites emerge in the duodenum and jejunum. Epithelial damage and mucosal invasion are uncommon. Hypogammaglobulinemia, low secretory IgA levels in the gut, achlorhydria, and malnutrition favor the development of infection.

Clinical Findings

A. Symptoms and Signs

It is estimated that about 50% of infected persons have no discernable infection, about 10% become asymptomatic cyst passers, and 25–50% develop an acute diarrheal syndrome. Acute diarrhea may clear spontaneously but is commonly followed by chronic diarrhea. The incubation period is usually 1–3 weeks but may be longer. The illness may begin gradually or suddenly. The acute phase may last days or weeks and is usually self-limited. The initial illness may include profuse watery diarrhea, and hospitalization may be required due to dehydration, particularly in young children. Typical symptoms of chronic disease are abdominal cramps, bloating, flatulence, nausea, malaise, and anorexia. Fever and vomiting are uncommon. Diarrhea is usually not severe in the chronic stage of infection; stools are greasy or frothy and foul smelling, without blood, pus, or mucus. The diarrhea may be daily or recurrent; intervening periods may include constipation. Symptoms can persist for weeks to months. Weight loss is frequent.

Chronic disease can include malabsorption, including fat and protein-losing enteropathy and vitamin deficiencies.

B. Laboratory Findings

Most patients seek medical attention after having been ill for over a week, commonly with weight loss of 5 kg or more. Stool is generally without blood or leukocytes. Diagnosis is traditionally made by the identification of trophozoites or cysts in stool. A wet mount of liquid stool may identify motile trophozoites. Stained fixed specimens may show cysts or trophozoites. Cysts may not be detected in the stool at the onset of the illness. Cyst excretion may be prolonged after the self-limited acute phase of infection. Sensitivity of stool analysis is not ideal, estimated at 50–80% for a single specimen and over 90% for three specimens. Sampling of duodenal contents with a string test or biopsy is no longer generally recommended, but biopsies may be helpful in very ill or immunocompromised patients. When giardiasis is suspected, stool antigen assays are simpler and cheaper than repeated stool examinations, but these tests will not identify other stool pathogens. Multiple tests, which identify antigens of trophozoites or cysts in stool, are available. They are generally quite sensitive (85–98%) and specific (90–100%). Molecular diagnostic panels that recognize *Giardia* and other enteropathogens in stool are available but expensive.

Treatment

The treatments of choice for giardiasis are tinidazole (2 g orally once) or metronidazole (250 mg orally three times daily for 5–7 days). The drugs are not universally effective; cure rates for single courses are typically about 80–95%. Toxicities are as described for treatment of amebiasis, but the lower dosages used for giardiasis limit side effects. Albendazole (400 mg orally once daily for 5 days) and nitazoxanide (500 mg orally twice daily for 3 days) both appear to have similar efficacy and fewer side effects compared with metronidazole, although data are limited, and a 2016 meta-analysis suggested superiority in efficacy of tinidazole over albendazole. Nitazoxanide is generally well tolerated but may cause mild GI side effects. Other drugs with activity against *Giardia* include furazolidone (100 mg orally four times a day for 7 days), which is about as effective as the other named drugs but causes GI side effects, and paromomycin (500 mg orally three times a day for 7 days), which appears to have somewhat lower efficacy but, unlike metronidazole, tinidazole, and furazolidone, is safe in pregnancy. Symptomatic giardiasis should always be treated. Treatment of asymptomatic patients should be considered, since they can transmit the infection. With a suggestive presentation but negative diagnostic studies, an empiric course of treatment may be appropriate. Household or day care contacts with an index case should be tested and treated if infected.

Prevention

Community chlorination (0.4 mg/L) of water is relatively ineffective for inactivating cysts, so filtration is required. For wilderness or international travelers, bringing water to a boil for 1 minute or filtration with a pore size less than 1 mcm are adequate. In day care centers, appropriate disposal of diapers and frequent hand washing are essential.

Loderstädt U et al. Antimicrobial resistance of the enteric protozoon *Giardia duodenalis*—a narrative review. Eur J Microbiol Immunol (Bp). 2021;11:29. [PMID: 34237023]

Mmbaga BT et al. *Cryptosporidium* and *Giardia* infections in children: a review. Pediatr Clin North Am. 2017;64:837. [PMID: 28734513]

TRICHOMONIASIS

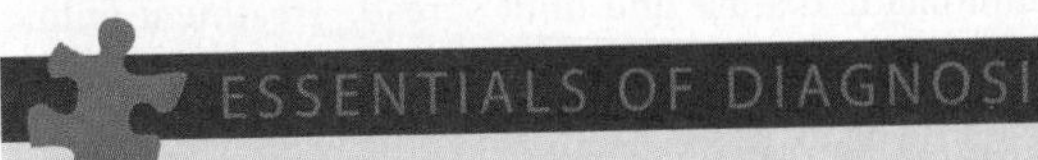

- **Women:** copious vaginal discharge.
- **Men:** nongonococcal urethritis.
- Motile trichomonads on wet mounts.

General Considerations

Trichomoniasis is caused by the protozoan *Trichomonas vaginalis* and is among the most common sexually transmitted diseases, causing vaginitis in women and nongonococcal urethritis in men. It can also occasionally be acquired by other means, since it can survive in moist environments for several hours.

Clinical Findings

A. Symptoms and Signs

T vaginalis is often harbored asymptomatically. For women with symptomatic disease, after an incubation period of 5 days to 4 weeks, a vaginal discharge develops, often with vulvovaginal discomfort, pruritus, dysuria, dyspareunia, or abdominal pain. Examination shows a copious discharge, which is usually not foul smelling but is often frothy and yellow or green in color. Inflammation of the vaginal walls and cervix with punctate hemorrhages are common. Most men infected with *T vaginalis* are asymptomatic, but it can be isolated from about 10% of men with nongonococcal urethritis. In men with trichomonal urethritis, the urethral discharge is generally scantier than with other causes of urethritis.

B. Diagnostic Testing

Diagnosis is traditionally made by identifying the organism in vaginal or urethral secretions. Examination of wet mounts will show motile organisms. Tests for bacterial vaginosis (pH > 4.5, fishy odor after addition of potassium hydroxide) are often positive with trichomoniasis. Newer point-of-care antigen detection and nucleic acid probe hybridization tests and nucleic acid amplification assays offer improved sensitivity compared with wet mount microscopy and excellent specificity.

Treatment

The treatment of choice is tinidazole or metronidazole, each as a 2 g single oral dose. Tinidazole may be better tolerated and active against some resistant parasites. Toxicities of these drugs are discussed in the section on amebiasis. If the large single dose cannot be tolerated, an alternative metronidazole dosage is 500 mg orally twice daily for 1 week. A meta-analysis suggested that a 7-day course of metronidazole (500 mg twice daily) is more effective than a single dose; this regimen is recommended for women living with HIV and may become standard for other groups. All persons with infection should be treated, even if asymptomatic, to prevent subsequent symptomatic disease and limit spread. Treatment failure suggests reinfection, but metronidazole-resistant organisms have been reported. These may be treated with tinidazole, longer courses of metronidazole, intravaginal paromomycin, or other experimental therapies (see Chapter 18).

Van Gerwen OT et al. Recent advances in the epidemiology, diagnosis, and management of *Trichomonas vaginalis* infection. F1000Res. 2019;8:1666. [PMID: 31583080]

HELMINTHIC INFECTIONS

TREMATODE (FLUKE) INFECTIONS

SCHISTOSOMIASIS (Bilharziasis)

ESSENTIALS OF DIAGNOSIS

- History of freshwater exposure in an endemic area.
- **Acute schistosomiasis:** fever, headache, myalgias, cough, urticaria, diarrhea, and eosinophilia.
- **Intestinal schistosomiasis:** abdominal pain, diarrhea, and hepatomegaly, progressing to anorexia, weight loss, and features of portal hypertension.
- **Urinary schistosomiasis:** hematuria and dysuria, progressing to hydronephrosis and urinary infections.
- **Diagnosis:** characteristic eggs in feces or urine; biopsy of rectal or bladder mucosa; positive serology.

General Considerations

Schistosomiasis, which affects more than 200 million persons worldwide, leads to severe consequences in 20 million persons and about 100,000 deaths annually (although estimates vary widely). The disease is caused by six species of trematode blood flukes. Five species cause intestinal schistosomiasis, with infection of mesenteric venules: *Schistosoma mansoni*, which is present in Africa, the Arabian Peninsula, South America, and the Caribbean; *Schistosoma japonicum*, which is endemic in China and Southeast Asia; *Schistosoma mekongi*, which is endemic near the Mekong River in Southeast Asia; and *Schistosoma intercalatum* and *Schistosoma guineensis*, which occur in parts of Africa. *Schistosoma haematobium* causes urinary schistosomiasis, with infection of venules of the urinary tract, and is endemic in Africa and the Middle East. Transmission of schistosomiasis is focal, with greatest prevalence in poor rural areas. Control efforts have diminished transmission significantly in many areas, but high-level transmission remains common in sub-Saharan Africa and some other areas. Prevalence of infection and illness typically peaks at about 15–20 years of age.

Humans are infected with schistosomes after contact with freshwater containing cercariae released by infected snails. Infection is initiated by penetration of skin or mucous membranes. After penetration, schistosomulae migrate to the portal circulation, where they rapidly mature. After about 6 weeks, adult worms mate and migrate to terminal mesenteric or bladder venules, where females deposit their eggs. Some eggs reach the lumen of the bowel or bladder and are passed with feces or urine, while others are retained in the bowel or bladder wall or transported in the circulation to other tissues, in particular the liver. Disease in endemic areas is primarily due to a host response to eggs, with granuloma formation and inflammation, eventually leading to fibrosis. Chronic infection can result in scarring of mesenteric or vesicular blood vessels, leading to portal hypertension and alterations in the urinary tract. In previously uninfected individuals, such as travelers with freshwater contact in endemic regions, acute schistosomiasis may occur, with a febrile illness 2–8 weeks after infection.

Clinical Findings

A. Symptoms and Signs

1. Cercarial dermatitis—Following cercarial penetration, localized erythema develops in some individuals, which can progress to a localized pruritic maculopapular rash that persists for some days. Dermatitis can be caused by human schistosomes and, in nontropical areas, by bird schistosomes that cannot complete their life cycle in humans (swimmer's itch).

2. Acute schistosomiasis (Katayama syndrome)—A febrile illness may develop 2–8 weeks after exposure in persons without prior infection, most commonly after heavy infection with *S mansoni* or *S japonicum*. Presenting symptoms and signs include acute onset of fever; headache; myalgias; cough; malaise; urticaria; diarrhea, which may be bloody; hepatosplenomegaly; lymphadenopathy; and pulmonary infiltrates. Localized lesions may occasionally cause severe manifestations, including CNS abnormalities and death. Acute schistosomiasis usually resolves in 2–8 weeks.

3. Chronic schistosomiasis—Many infected persons have light infections and are asymptomatic, but an estimated 50–60% have symptoms and 5–10% have advanced organ damage. Asymptomatic infected children may suffer from anemia and growth retardation. Symptomatic patients with intestinal schistosomiasis typically experience abdominal pain, fatigue, diarrhea, and hepatomegaly. Over years, anorexia, weight loss, weakness, colonic polyps, and features of portal hypertension develop. Late manifestations include hematemesis from esophageal varices, hepatic failure, and pulmonary hypertension. Urinary schistosomiasis may present within months of infection with hematuria and dysuria, most commonly in children and young adults. Fibrotic changes in the urinary tract can lead to hydroureter, hydronephrosis, bacterial urinary infections and, ultimately, kidney disease or bladder cancer.

B. Laboratory Findings

Microscopic examination of stool or urine for eggs, evaluation of tissue, or serologic tests establish the diagnosis. Characteristic eggs can be identified on smears of stool or urine. The most widely used stool test is the Kato-Katz technique. Quantitative tests that yield more than 400 eggs per gram of feces or 10 mL of urine are indicative of heavy infections with increased risk of complications. Diagnosis can also be made by biopsy of the rectum, colon, liver, or bladder. Serologic tests include an ELISA available from the CDC that is 99% specific for all species but cannot distinguish acute and past infection. Sensitivity of the test is 99% for *S mansoni*, 95% for *S haematobium*, but less than 50% for *S japonicum*. Serology is of limited use in endemic settings but can be helpful in travelers from nonendemic regions. The most widely used point-of-care assays target circulating anodic and cathodic antigens to detect circulating schistosome antigens in serum and urine. Antigen tests have better sensitivity than stool smears, especially for *S mansoni*; sensitivity is lower for *S haematobium*. Molecular tests for schistosomiasis have been developed but are not routinely used for diagnosis. In acute schistosomiasis, leukocytosis and marked eosinophilia may occur; serologic tests may become positive before eggs are seen in stool or urine. After therapy, eggs may be shed in stool or urine for months, and so the identification of eggs in fluids or tissue cannot distinguish past or active disease. With a diagnosis of schistosomiasis, evaluation for the extent of disease is warranted, including liver function studies and imaging of the liver with intestinal disease and ultrasound or other imaging studies of the urinary system in urinary disease.

▶ Treatment

Treatment is indicated for all schistosome infections. In areas where recurrent infection is common, treatment is valuable in reducing worm burdens and limiting clinical complications. The drug of choice for schistosomiasis is praziquantel. The drug is administered for 1 day at an oral dose of 40 mg/kg (in one or two doses) for *S mansoni*, *S haematobium*, *S intercalatum*, and *S guineensis* infections and a dose of 60 mg/kg (in two or three doses) for *S japonicum* and *S mekongi*. Cure rates are generally greater than 80% after a single treatment, and those not cured have marked reduction in the intensity of infection. Praziquantel is active against invading cercariae but not developing schistosomulae. Therefore, the drug may not prevent illness when given after exposure and, for recent infections, a repeat course after a few weeks may be appropriate. Praziquantel may be used during pregnancy. Resistance to praziquantel has been reported. Toxicities include abdominal pain, diarrhea, urticaria, headache, nausea, vomiting, and fever, and may be due both to direct effects of the drug and responses to dying worms. Alternative therapies are oxamniquine for *S mansoni* infection and metrifonate for *S haemotobium* infection. Both drugs have limited availability (they are not available in the United States), and resistance may be a problem. No second-line drug is available for *S japonicum* infections. The antimalarial drug artemether has activity against schistosomulae and adult worms and may be effective in chemoprophylaxis; however, it is expensive, and long-term use in malarious areas might select for resistant malaria parasites. With severe disease, use of corticosteroids in conjunction with praziquantel may decrease complications. Treatment should be followed by repeat examinations for eggs about every 3 months for 1 year after therapy, with re-treatment if eggs are seen.

▶ Prevention

Travelers to endemic areas should avoid freshwater exposure. Vigorous toweling after exposure may limit cercarial penetration. Chemoprophylaxis with artemether has shown efficacy but is not standard practice. Community control of schistosomiasis includes improved sanitation and water supplies, elimination of snail habitats, and intermittent treatment to limit worm burdens.

Aula OP et al. Schistosomiasis with a focus on Africa. Trop Med Infect Dis. 2021;6:109. [PMID: 34206495]

Nelwan ML. Schistosomiasis: life cycle, diagnosis, and control. Curr Ther Res Clin Exp. 2019;91:5. [PMID: 31372189]

LIVER & LUNG FLUKES

FASCIOLIASIS

Infection by *Fasciola hepatica*, the sheep liver fluke, results from ingestion of encysted metacercariae on watercress or other aquatic vegetables. Infection is prevalent in sheep-raising areas in many countries, especially parts of South America, the Middle East, and southern Europe, and it has increasingly been recognized in travelers to these areas. Fasciola gigantica has a more restricted distribution in Asia and Africa and causes similar findings. Eggs are passed from host feces into freshwater, leading to infection of snails, and then deposition of metacercariae on vegetation. In humans, metacercariae excyst, penetrate the peritoneum, migrate through the liver, and mature in the bile ducts, where they cause local necrosis and abscess formation.

Two clinical syndromes are seen, related to acute migration of worms and chronic infection of the biliary tract. Symptoms related to migration of larvae present 6–12 weeks after ingestion. Typical findings are abdominal pain, fever, malaise, weight loss, urticaria, eosinophilia, and leukocytosis. Tender hepatomegaly and elevated liver biochemical tests may be seen. Rarely, migration to other organs may lead to localized disease. The symptoms of worm migration subside after 2–4 months, followed by asymptomatic infection by adult worms or intermittent symptoms of biliary obstruction, with biliary colic and, at times, findings of cholangitis. Early diagnosis is difficult, as eggs are not found in the feces during the acute migratory phase of infection. Clinical suspicion should be based on clinical findings and marked eosinophilia in at risk individuals. CT and other imaging studies show hypodense migratory lesions of the liver. Definitive diagnosis is made by the identification of characteristic eggs in stool. Repeated examinations may be necessary. In chronic infection, imaging studies show masses obstructing the extrahepatic biliary tract. Serologic assays have sensitivity and specificity greater than 90% but cannot distinguish between past and current infection. Antigen tests with excellent sensitivity and specificity are available in veterinary medicine and show promise for humans.

Fascioliasis is unusual among fluke infections such that it does not respond well to treatment with praziquantel. The treatment of choice is triclabendazole, which is available through the CDC under an investigational protocol. Standard dosing of 10 mg/kg orally in a single dose or two doses over 12 hours achieves a cure rate of about 80%, but repeat dosing is indicated if abnormal radiologic findings or eosinophilia do not resolve. Of concern, resistance to triclabendazole has been widely reported in animal infections. The second-line drug for fascioliasis is bithionol (30–50 mg/kg/day orally in three divided doses on alternate days for 10–15 days); this drug is not available in the United States. Treatment with either drug can be accompanied by abdominal pain and other GI symptoms. Other potential therapies are emetine and dehydroemetine, both widely used in the past but quite toxic, and nitazoxanide. Prevention of fascioliasis involves avoidance of ingestion of raw aquatic plants.

CLONORCHIASIS & OPISTHORCHIASIS

Infection by *Clonorchis sinensis*, the Chinese liver fluke, is endemic in areas of Japan, Korea, China, Taiwan, Southeast Asia, and the far eastern part of Russia. An estimated 15 million people are infected (13 million in China); in some communities, prevalence can reach 80%. Opisthorchiasis is principally caused by *Opisthorchis felineus* (regions of the former Soviet Union) or *Opisthorchis viverrini* (Thailand, Laos, Vietnam). Clonorchiasis and opisthorchiasis are clinically indistinguishable. Parasite eggs are shed into water in human or animal feces, where they infect snails, which release cercariae, which infect fish. Human infection follows ingestion of raw, undercooked, or pickled freshwater fish containing metacercariae. These parasites excyst in the duodenum and ascend into the biliary tract, where they mature and remain for many years, shedding eggs in the bile.

Most patients harbor few parasites and are asymptomatic. An acute illness can occur 2–3 weeks after initial infection, with fever, malaise, abdominal pain, anorexia, tender hepatomegaly, urticaria, and eosinophilia. The acute syndrome is difficult to diagnose, since ova may not appear in the feces until 3–4 weeks after onset of symptoms. In chronic heavy infections, findings include abdominal pain, anorexia, weight loss, and tender hepatomegaly. More serious findings can include recurrent bacterial cholangitis and sepsis, cholecystitis, liver abscess, and pancreatitis. An increased risk of cholangiocarcinoma has been documented.

Early diagnosis is presumptive, based on clinical findings and epidemiology. Subsequent diagnosis is made by finding characteristic eggs in stool or duodenal or biliary contents. The stool Kato-Katz test is widely used; performing repeated tests improves sensitivity. Imaging studies show characteristic biliary tract dilatations with filling defects due to flukes. Serologic assays for clonorchiasis with excellent sensitivity are available but cannot distinguish between past and current infection. Molecular tests have been developed but are not widely used.

The drug of choice is praziquantel, 25 mg/kg orally three times daily for 2 days, which provides cure rates over 90% and egg reduction rates of nearly 100%. One day of treatment may be sufficient. Re-treatment may be required, especially in some areas with known decreased praziquantel efficacy. The second-line drug is albendazole (400 mg orally twice daily for 7 days), which appears to be somewhat less effective. Tribendimidine, which is approved in China, has shown efficacy for clonorchiasis similar to that of praziquantel.

PARAGONIMIASIS

Eight species of *Paragonimus* lung flukes cause human disease. The most important is *Paragonimus westermani*. *Paragonimus* species are endemic in East Asia, Oceania, West Africa, and South America, where millions of persons are infected; rare infections caused by *Paragonimus kellicotti* have occurred in North America. Eggs are released into freshwater, where parasites infect snails, and then cercariae infect crabs and crayfish. Human infection follows consumption of raw, undercooked, or pickled freshwater shellfish. Metacercariae then excyst, penetrate the peritoneum, and pass into the lungs, where they mature into adult worms over about 2 months.

Most persons have moderate worm burdens and are asymptomatic. In symptomatic cases, abdominal pain and diarrhea develop 2 days to 2 weeks after infection, followed by fever, cough, chest pain, urticaria, and eosinophilia. Acute symptoms may last for several weeks. Chronic infection can cause cough productive of brown sputum, hemoptysis, dyspnea, and chest pain, with progression to chronic bronchitis, bronchiectasis, bronchopneumonia, lung abscess, and pleural disease. Ectopic infections can cause disease in other organs, most commonly the CNS, where disease can present with seizures, headaches, and focal neurologic findings due to parasite meningitis and to intracerebral lesions.

The diagnosis of paragonimiasis is made by identifying characteristic eggs in sputum or stool or identifying worms in biopsied tissue. Multiple examinations and concentration techniques may be needed. Serologic tests may be helpful; an ELISA available from the CDC has sensitivity and specificity more than 95%. Chest radiographs may show varied abnormalities of the lungs or pleura, including infiltrates, nodules, cavities, and fibrosis, and the findings can be confused with those of tuberculosis. With CNS disease, skull radiographs can show clusters of calcified cysts, and CT or MRI can show clusters of ring-enhancing lesions.

Treatment is with praziquantel (25 mg/kg orally three times daily for 2 days), which provides efficacy of at least 90%. Alternative therapies are bithionol and triclabendazole. As with cysticercosis, for cerebral paragonimiasis, praziquantel should generally be used with corticosteroids. Chronic infection may lead to permanent lung dysfunction and pleural disease requiring drainage procedures.

CESTODE INFECTIONS

NONINVASIVE CESTODE INFECTIONS

The four major tapeworms that cause noninvasive infections in humans are the beef tapeworm *Taenia saginata*, the pork tapeworm *Taenia solium*, the fish tapeworm *Diphyllobothrium latum*, each of which can reach many meters in length, and the dwarf tapeworm *Hymenolepis nana*. *Taenia* and *Hymenolepis* species are broadly distributed, especially in the tropics; *D latum* is most prevalent in temperate regions. Other tapeworms that can cause noninvasive human disease include the rodent tapeworm *Hymenolepis diminuta*, the dog tapeworm *Dipylidium caninum*, and other *Taenia* and *Diphyllobothrium* species. Invasive tapeworm infections, including *T solium* (when infective eggs, rather than cysticerci are ingested) and *Echinococcus* species, will be discussed separately.

1. Beef Tapeworm

Infection is most common in cattle breeding areas. Humans are the definitive host. Gravid segments of *T saginata* are passed in human feces to soil, where they are ingested by grazing animals, especially cattle. The eggs then hatch to release embryos that encyst in muscle as cysticerci. Humans are infected by eating raw or undercooked infected beef. Most individuals infected with *T saginata* are asymptomatic, but abdominal pain and other GI symptoms may be present. Eosinophilia is common. The most common presenting finding is the passage of proglottids in the stool.

2. Pork Tapeworm

T solium is transmitted to pigs that ingest human feces. Humans can be either the definitive host (after consuming undercooked pork, leading to tapeworm infection) or the intermediate host (after consuming food contaminated with human feces containing *T solium* eggs, leading to cysticercosis, which is discussed under Invasive Cestode Infections). As with the beef tapeworm, infection with *T solium* adult worms is generally asymptomatic, but GI symptoms may occur. Infection is generally recognized after passage of proglottids. Autoinfection with eggs can progress to cysticercosis.

3. Fish Tapeworm

Infection with *D latum* follows ingestion of undercooked freshwater fish, most commonly in temperate regions. Eggs from human feces are taken up by crustaceans, these are eaten by fish, which are then infectious to humans. Infection with multiple worms over many years can occur. Infections are most commonly asymptomatic, but nonspecific GI symptoms, including diarrhea, may occur. Diagnosis usually follows passage of proglottids. Prolonged heavy infection can lead to megaloblastic anemia and neuropathy from vitamin B_{12} deficiency, which is due to infection-induced dissociation of the vitamin from intrinsic factor and to utilization of the vitamin by worms.

4. Dwarf Tapeworm

H nana is the only tapeworm that can be transmitted between humans. Infections are common in warm areas, especially with poor hygiene and institutionalized populations. Infection follows ingestion of food contaminated with human feces. Eggs hatch in the intestines, where oncospheres penetrate the mucosa, encyst as cysticercoid larvae, and then rupture after about 4 days to release adult worms. Autoinfection can lead to amplification of infection. Infection with *H nana*, the related rodent tapeworm *H diminuta*, or the dog tapeworm *D caninum* can also follow accidental ingestion of infected insects. *H nana* are dwarf in size relative to other tapeworms but can reach 5 cm in length. Heavy infection is common, especially in children, and can be accompanied by abdominal discomfort, anorexia, and diarrhea.

Laboratory Findings

Diagnosis is usually made based on the identification of characteristic eggs or proglottids in stool. Egg release may be irregular, so examination of multiple specimens or concentration techniques may be needed.

Treatment

The treatment of choice for noninvasive tapeworm infections is praziquantel. A single dose of praziquantel (5–10 mg/kg orally) is highly effective, except for *H nana*, for which the dosage is 25 mg/kg. Treatment of *H nana* is more difficult, as the drug is not effective against maturing cysts. Therefore, a repeat treatment after 1 week and screening after therapy to document cure are appropriate with heavy infections. Therapy can be accompanied by headache, malaise, dizziness, abdominal pain, and nausea.

The alternative therapy for these infections is niclosamide. A single dose of niclosamide (2 g chewed) is effective against *D latum*, *Taenia*, and *D caninum* infections. For *H nana*, therapy is continued daily for 1 week. Niclosamide may cause nausea, malaise, and abdominal pain.

Craig P et al. Intestinal cestodes. Curr Opin Infect Dis. 2007;20:524. [PMID: 17762788]
Panti-May JA et al. Worldwide overview of human infections with *Hymenolepis diminuta*. Parasitol Res. 2020;119:1997. [PMID: 32211990]

INVASIVE CESTODE INFECTIONS

1. Cysticercosis

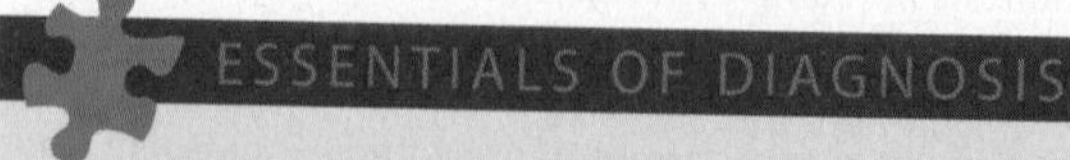

- Exposure to *T solium* through fecal contamination of food.
- Focal CNS lesions; seizures, headache.
- Brain imaging shows cysts; positive serologic tests.

General Considerations

Cysticercosis is due to tissue infection with cysts of *T solium* that develop after humans ingest food contaminated with eggs from human feces, thus acting as an intermediate host for the parasite. Prevalence is high where the parasite is endemic, in particular Mexico, Central and South America, the Philippines, and Southeast Asia. An estimated 20 million persons are infected with cysticerci yearly, leading to about 400,000 persons with neurologic symptoms and 50,000 deaths. Antibody prevalence rates up to 10% are recognized in some endemic areas, and the infection is one of the most important causes of seizures in the developing world and in immigrants to the United States from endemic countries. In Latin America, it is estimated that 0.5–1.5 million people are affected by epilepsy secondary to cysticercosis.

Clinical Findings

A. Symptoms and Signs

Neurocysticercosis can cause intracerebral, subarachnoid, and spinal cord lesions and intraventricular cysts. Single or multiple lesions may be present. Lesions may persist for years before symptoms develop, generally due to local inflammation or ventricular obstruction. Presenting symptoms include seizures, focal neurologic deficits, altered cognition, and psychiatric disease. Symptoms develop more quickly with intraventricular cysts, with findings of hydrocephalus and meningeal irritation, including severe headache, vomiting, papilledema, and visual loss. A particularly aggressive form of the disease, racemose cysticercosis, involves proliferation of cysts at the base of the brain, leading to alterations of consciousness and death. Spinal cord lesions can present with progressive focal findings.

Cysticercosis of other organ systems is usually clinically benign. Involvement of muscles can uncommonly cause discomfort and is identified by radiographs of muscle showing multiple calcified lesions. Subcutaneous involvement presents with multiple painless palpable skin lesions. Involvement of the eyes can present with ptosis due to extraocular muscle involvement or intraocular abnormalities.

B. Laboratory Findings and Imaging

Diagnosis generally requires consideration of both laboratory and imaging findings. The updated Del Brutto diagnostic criteria, which include laboratory and imaging findings, have demonstrated good sensitivity and specificity.

CSF examination may show lymphocytic or eosinophilic pleocytosis, decreased glucose, and elevated protein. Serology plays an important role in diagnosis; both antibody and antigen detection assays are available. ELISAs and related immunoblot assays have excellent sensitivity and specificity, but sensitivity is lower with only single or calcified lesions.

With neuroimaging by CT or MRI, multiple parenchymal cysts are most typically seen. Parenchymal calcification is also common. Performing both CT and MRI is ideal because CT is better for identification of calcification and MRI for smaller and ventricular lesions. Typical findings can be highly suggestive of the diagnosis.

Treatment

The medical management of neurocysticercosis has been controversial because the benefits of cyst clearance must be weighed against potential harm of an inflammatory response to dying worms. Antihelminthic therapy hastens radiologic improvement in parenchymal cysticercosis, but some randomized trials have shown that corticosteroids alone are as effective as specific therapy plus corticosteroids for controlling seizures. Overall, most authorities recommend treatment of active lesions, in particular lesions with a high likelihood of progression, such as intraventricular cysts. At the other end of the spectrum, inactive calcified lesions probably do not benefit from therapy. In addition, cysticidal therapy should be avoided if there is a high risk of hydrocephalus, as with subarachnoid involvement. When treatment is deemed appropriate, standard therapy consists of albendazole (10–15 mg/kg/day orally for 8 days) or praziquantel (50 mg/kg/day orally for 15–30 days). Albendazole is probably preferred, since it has shown better efficacy in some comparisons and since corticosteroids appear to lower circulating praziquantel levels but increase albendazole levels. Increasing the dosage of albendazole to 30 mg/kg/day orally may improve outcomes. Combining albendazole plus praziquantel improved outcomes compared with albendazole alone in patients with multiple viable intraparenchymal cysts. Corticosteroids are usually administered concurrently, but dosing is not standardized. Patients should be observed for evidence of localized inflammatory responses. Anticonvulsant therapy should be provided if needed, and shunting performed if required for elevated intracranial pressure. Surgical removal of cysts may be helpful for some difficult cases of neurocysticercosis and for symptomatic non-neurologic disease.

Del Brutto OH. Twenty-five years of evolution of standard diagnostic criteria for neurocysticercosis. How have they impacted diagnosis and patient outcomes? Expert Rev Neurother. 2020;20:147. [PMID: 31855080]

Garcia HH et al. *Taenia solium* cysticercosis and its impact in neurological disease. Clin Microbiol Rev. 2020;33:e00085–19. [PMID: 32461308]

White AC et al. Diagnosis and treatment of neurocysticercosis: 2017 Clinical Practice Guidelines by the Infectious Diseases Society of America (IDSA) and the American Society of Tropical Medicine and Hygiene (ASTMH). Am J Trop Med Hyg. 2018;98:945. [PMID: 29644966]

World Health Organization. *WHO Guidelines on Management of Taenia Solium neurocysticercosis*. Geneva, Switzerland: WHO, 2021. https://apps.who.int/iris/handle/10665/344802

2. Echinococcosis

ESSENTIALS OF DIAGNOSIS

- History of exposure to dogs or wild canines in an endemic area.
- Large cystic lesions, most commonly of the liver or lung.
- Positive serologic tests.

General Considerations

Echinococcosis occurs when humans are intermediate hosts for canine tapeworms. Infection is acquired by ingesting food contaminated with canine feces containing parasite eggs. The principal species that infect humans are *Echinococcus granulosus*, which causes cystic hydatid disease, and *Echinococcus multilocularis*, which causes alveolar hydatid disease. *E granulosus* is transmitted by domestic dogs in areas with livestock (sheep, goats, camels, and horses) as intermediate hosts, including Africa, the Middle East, southern Europe, South America, Central Asia, Australia, New Zealand, and the southwestern United States. *E multilocularis*, which much less commonly causes human disease, is transmitted by wild canines and is endemic in northern forest areas of the Northern Hemisphere, including central Europe, Siberia, northern Japan, northwestern Canada, and western Alaska. An increase in the fox population in Europe has been associated with an increase in human cases. The disease range has also extended southward in Central Asia and China. Other species that cause limited disease in humans are endemic in South America and China.

After humans ingest parasite eggs, the eggs hatch in the intestines to form oncospheres, which penetrate the mucosa, enter the circulation, and encyst in specific organs as hydatid cysts. *E granulosus* forms cysts most commonly in the liver (65%) and lungs (25%), but the cysts may develop in any organ, including the brain, bones, skeletal muscles, kidneys, and spleen. Cysts are most commonly single. The cysts can persist and slowly grow for many years.

Clinical Findings

A. Symptoms and Signs

Infections are commonly asymptomatic and may be noted incidentally on imaging studies or present with symptoms caused by an enlarging or superinfected mass. Findings may include abdominal or chest pain, biliary obstruction, cholangitis, portal hypertension, cirrhosis, bronchial obstruction leading to segmental lung collapse, and abscesses. Cyst leakage or rupture may be accompanied by a severe allergic reaction, including fever and hypotension. Seeding of cysts after rupture may extend the infection to new areas.

E multilocularis generally causes a more aggressive disease than *E granulosus*, with initial infection of the liver, but then local and distant spread commonly suggesting a malignancy. Symptoms based on the areas of involvement gradually worsen over years, with the development of obstructive findings in the liver and elsewhere.

B. Laboratory Findings

Serologic tests, including ELISA and immunoblot, offer sensitivity and specificity over 80% for *E granulosus* liver infections, but lower sensitivity for involvement of other organs. Serology is somewhat more reliable for *E multilocularis* infections. Serologic tests may also distinguish the two major echinococcal infections.

C. Imaging

Diagnosis is usually based on imaging studies, including ultrasonography, CT, and MRI. In *E granulosus* infection, a large cyst containing multiple daughter cysts that fill the cyst interior is highly suggestive of the diagnosis. In *E multilocularis* infection, imaging shows an irregular mass, often with areas of calcification.

Treatment

The treatment of cystic hydatid disease is with albendazole, often with cautious surgical resection of cysts. When used alone, as in cases where surgery is not possible, albendazole (10–15 mg/kg/day orally) has demonstrated efficacy, with courses of 3 months or longer duration; alternating cycles of treatment and rest may be needed. Mebendazole (40–50 mg/kg/day orally) is an alternative drug, and praziquantel may also be effective. In some cases, medical therapy is begun, with surgery performed if disease persists after some months of therapy. Another approach, in particular with inoperable cysts, is percutaneous puncture, aspiration, injection, and re-aspiration (PAIR). In this approach (which should not be used if cysts communicate with the biliary tract), patients receive antihelminthic therapy, and the cyst is partially aspirated. After diagnostic confirmation by examination for parasite protoscolices, a scolicidal agent (95% ethanol, hypertonic saline, or 0.5% cetrimide) is injected, and the cyst is re-aspirated after about 15 minutes. PAIR includes a small risk of anaphylaxis, which has been reported in about 2% of procedures, but death due to anaphylaxis has been rare. Treatment of alveolar cyst disease is challenging, generally relying on wide surgical resection of lesions. Therapy with albendazole before or during surgery may be beneficial and may also provide improvement or even cure in inoperable cases.

Kikuchi T et al. Human proliferative sparganosis update. Parasitol Int. 2020;75:102036. [PMID: 31841658]

Wen H et al. Echinococcosis: advances in the 21st century. Clin Microbiol Rev. 2019;32:e00075–18. [PMID: 30760475]

INTESTINAL NEMATODE (Roundworm) INFECTIONS

ASCARIASIS

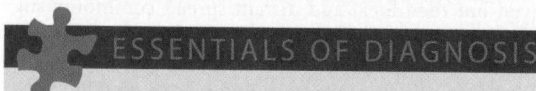

- Transient cough, urticaria, pulmonary infiltrates, eosinophilia.
- Nonspecific abdominal symptoms.
- Eggs in stool; adult worms occasionally passed.

General Considerations

Ascaris lumbricoides is the most common of the intestinal helminths, causing about 800 million infections, 12 million acute cases, and 10,000 or more deaths annually. Prevalence is high wherever there is poor hygiene and sanitation or where human feces are used as fertilizer. Heavy infections are most common in children.

Infection follows ingestion of eggs in contaminated food. Larvae hatch in the small intestine, penetrate into the bloodstream, migrate to the lungs, and then travel via airways back to the GI tract, where they develop to adult worms, which can be up to 40 cm in length, and live for 1–2 years.

Clinical Findings

Most persons with *Ascaris* infection are asymptomatic. In a small proportion of patients, symptoms develop during migration of worms through the lungs, with fever, nonproductive cough, chest pain, dyspnea, and eosinophilia, occasionally with eosinophilic pneumonia. Rarely, larvae lodge ectopically in the brain, kidney, eye, spinal cord, and other sites and may cause local symptoms.

Light intestinal infections usually produce no symptoms. With heavy infection, abdominal discomfort may be seen. Adult worms may also migrate and be coughed up, be vomited, or may emerge through the nose or anus. They may also migrate into the common bile duct, pancreatic duct, appendix, and other sites, which may lead to cholangitis, cholecystitis, pyogenic liver abscess, pancreatitis, obstructive jaundice, or appendicitis. With very heavy infestations, masses of worms may cause intestinal obstruction, volvulus, intussusception, or death. Although severe manifestations of infection are uncommon, the very high prevalence of ascariasis leads to large numbers of individuals, especially children, with important sequelae. Moderate to high worm loads in children are also associated with nutritional abnormalities due to decreased appetite and food intake, and also decreased absorption of nutrients.

The diagnosis of ascariasis is made after adult worms emerge from the mouth, nose, or anus, or by identifying characteristic eggs in the feces, usually with the Kato-Katz technique. Imaging studies demonstrate worms, with filling defects in contrast studies and at times evidence of intestinal or biliary obstruction. Eosinophilia is marked during worm migration but may be absent during intestinal infection.

Treatment

All infections should ideally be treated. Treatments of choice are albendazole (single 400-mg oral dose), mebendazole (single 500-mg oral dose or 100 mg twice daily for 3 days), or pyrantel pamoate (single 11-mg/kg oral dose, maximum 1 g). These drugs are all well tolerated but may cause mild GI toxicity. They are considered safe for children above 1 year of age and in pregnant women, although use in the first trimester is best avoided. An alternative is ivermectin (single 200 mcg/kg oral dose). In endemic areas, reinfection after treatment is common. Intestinal obstruction usually responds to conservative management and antihelminthic therapy. Surgery may be required for appendicitis and other GI complications.

TRICHURIASIS

Trichuris trichiura, the whipworm, infects about 500 million persons throughout the world, particularly in humid tropical and subtropical environments. Infection is heaviest and most frequent in children. Infections are acquired by ingestion of eggs. The larvae hatch in the small intestine and mature in the large bowel to adult worms of about 4 cm in length. The worms do not migrate through tissues.

Most persons with infection are asymptomatic. Heavy infections may be accompanied by abdominal cramps, tenesmus, diarrhea, distention, nausea, and vomiting. The *Trichuris* dysentery syndrome may develop, particularly in malnourished young children, with findings resembling IBD including bloody diarrhea and rectal prolapse.

Trichuriasis is diagnosed by identification of characteristic eggs and sometimes adult worms in stools. Eosinophilia is common. Treatment is typically with albendazole (400 mg/day orally) or mebendazole (200 mg/day orally), for 1–3 days for light infections or 3–7 days for heavy infections, but cure rates are lower than for ascariasis or hookworm infection. An alternative is ivermectin (200 mcg/kg orally once daily for 3 days). Oxantel pamoate (one dose of 15–30 mg/kg) has shown good efficacy in clearing infections; randomized trials showed albendazole plus oxantel pamoate (31% cure; 96% egg reduction) to be superior to mebendazole, and albendazole plus oxantel pamoate (69% cure; 99% egg reduction) and albendazole plus ivermectin (28% cure; 95% egg reduction) to be superior to albendazole plus mebendazole. Oxantel pamoate has low efficacy against *Ascaris* and hookworm infection.

HOOKWORM DISEASE

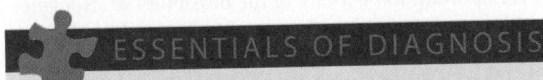

ESSENTIALS OF DIAGNOSIS

- Transient pruritic skin rash and lung symptoms.
- Anorexia, diarrhea, abdominal discomfort.
- Iron deficiency anemia.
- Characteristic eggs and occult blood in the stool.

General Considerations

Infection with the hookworms *Ancylostoma duodenale* and *Necator americanus* is very common, especially in most tropical and subtropical regions. Both worms are broadly distributed. Prevalence is estimated at about 500 million, causing approximately 65,000 deaths each year. The eggs hatch when deposited on warm moist soil, releasing larvae that remain infective for up to one week. With contact, the larvae penetrate skin and migrate in the bloodstream to the pulmonary capillaries. In the lungs, the larvae penetrate into alveoli and then are carried by ciliary action upward to the bronchi, trachea, and mouth. After being swallowed, they reach and attach to the mucosa of the upper small bowel, where they mature to adult worms. *Ancylostoma* infection can also be acquired by ingestion of the larvae in food or water. Hookworms attach to the intestinal mucosa and suck blood. Blood loss is proportionate to the worm burden.

Clinical Findings

A. Symptoms and Signs

Most persons with infection are asymptomatic. A pruritic maculopapular rash (ground itch) may occur at the site of larval penetration, usually in previously sensitized persons. Pulmonary symptoms may be seen during larval migration through the lungs, with dry cough, wheezing, and low-grade fever, but these symptoms are less common than with ascariasis. About 1 month after infection, as maturing worms attach to the small intestinal mucosa, GI symptoms may develop, with epigastric pain, anorexia, and diarrhea, especially in previously unexposed individuals. Persons chronically infected with large worm burdens may have abdominal pain, anorexia, diarrhea, and findings of marked iron deficiency anemia and protein malnutrition. Anemia can lead to pallor, weakness, dyspnea, and heart failure, and protein loss can lead to hypoalbuminemia, edema, and ascites. These findings may be accompanied by impairment in growth and cognitive development in children. Infection with the dog hookworm *Ancylostoma caninum* can uncommonly lead to abdominal pain, diarrhea, and eosinophilia, with intestinal ulcerations and regional lymphadenitis.

B. Laboratory Findings

Diagnosis is based on the demonstration of characteristic eggs in feces; concentration techniques are usually not needed. Microcytic anemia, occult blood in the stool, and hypoalbuminemia are common. Eosinophilia is common, especially during worm migration.

Treatment

Treatment is with albendazole (single 400-mg oral dose) or mebendazole (100 mg orally twice daily for 3 days). Occasional side effects are diarrhea and abdominal pain. Pyrantel pamoate and levamisole are also effective. Anemia should be managed with iron replacement and, for severe symptomatic anemia, blood transfusion. Mass treatment of children with single doses of albendazole or mebendazole at regular intervals limits worm burdens and the extent of disease and is advocated by WHO.

STRONGYLOIDIASIS

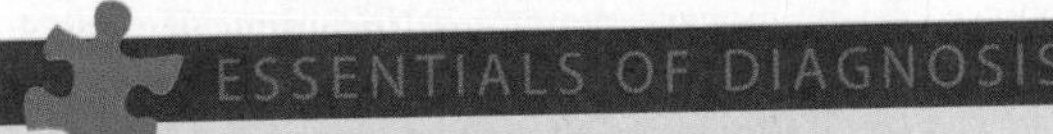

ESSENTIALS OF DIAGNOSIS

- Transient pruritic skin rash and lung symptoms.
- Anorexia, diarrhea, abdominal discomfort.
- Larvae detected in stool.
- Hyperinfection in the immunocompromised; larvae detected in sputum or other fluids.
- Eosinophilia.

General Considerations

Strongyloidiasis is caused by infection with *Strongyloides stercoralis*. Although much less prevalent than ascariasis, trichuriasis, or hookworm infections, strongyloidiasis is nonetheless a significant problem, infecting tens of millions of individuals in tropical and subtropical regions. Infection is also endemic in some temperate regions of North America, Europe, Japan, and Australia. Of particular importance is the predilection of the parasite to cause severe infections in immunocompromised individuals due to its ability to replicate in humans. A related parasite, *Strongyloides fuelleborni*, infects humans in parts of Africa and New Guinea.

Among nematodes, *S stercoralis* is uniquely capable of maintaining its full life cycle both within the human host and in soil. Infection occurs when filariform larvae in soil penetrate the skin, enter the bloodstream, and are carried to the lungs, where they escape from capillaries into alveoli, ascend the bronchial tree, and are then swallowed and carried to the duodenum and upper jejunum, where maturation to the adult stage takes place. Females live embedded in the mucosa for up to 5 years, releasing eggs that hatch in the intestines as free rhabditiform larvae that pass to the ground via the feces. In moist soil, these larvae metamorphose into infective filariform larvae. Autoinfection can occur in humans, when some rhabditiform larvae develop into filariform larvae that penetrate the intestinal mucosa or perianal skin, and enter the circulation. The most dangerous manifestation of *S stercoralis* infection is the **hyperinfection syndrome**, with dissemination of large numbers of filariform larvae to the lungs and other tissues in immunocompromised individuals. Mortality with this syndrome approaches 100% without treatment and has been about 25% with treatment. The hyperinfection syndrome is seen in patients receiving corticosteroids and other immunosuppressive medications; patients with hematologic malignancies, malnutrition, or alcohol use disorder; or persons living with AIDS. The risk seems greatest for those receiving corticosteroids.

Clinical Findings

A. Symptoms and Signs

As with other intestinal nematodes, most infected persons are asymptomatic. An acute syndrome can be seen at the time of infection, with a pruritic, erythematous, maculopapular rash, usually of the feet. These symptoms may be followed by pulmonary symptoms (including dry cough, dyspnea, and wheezing) and eosinophilia after several days, followed by GI symptoms after some weeks, as with hookworm infections. Chronic infection may be accompanied by epigastric pain, nausea, diarrhea, and anemia. Maculopapular or urticarial rashes of the buttocks, perineum, and thighs, due to migrating larvae, may be seen. Large worm burdens can lead to malabsorption or intestinal obstruction. Eosinophilia is common but may fluctuate.

With hyperinfection large numbers of larvae can migrate to many tissues, including the lungs, CNS, kidneys, and liver. GI symptoms can include abdominal pain, nausea, vomiting, diarrhea, and more severe findings related to intestinal obstruction, perforation, or hemorrhage. Bacterial sepsis, probably secondary to intestinal ulcerations, is a common presenting finding. Pulmonary findings include pneumonitis, cough, hemoptysis, and respiratory failure. Sputum may contain adult worms, larvae, and eggs. CNS disease includes meningitis and brain abscesses; the CSF may contain larvae. Various presentations can progress to shock and death.

B. Laboratory Findings

The diagnosis of strongyloidiasis can be difficult, as eggs are seldom found in feces. Diagnosis is usually based on the identification of rhabditiform larvae in the stool or duodenal contents. These larvae must be distinguished from hookworm larvae, which may hatch after stool collection. Repeated examinations of stool or examination of duodenal fluid may be required for diagnosis because the sensitivity of individual tests is only about 30%. Hyperinfection is diagnosed by the identification of large numbers of larvae in stool, sputum, or other body fluids. An ELISA from the CDC offers about 90% sensitivity and specificity, but cross-reactions with other helminths may occur. PCR and related molecular diagnostic methods have improved and are useful diagnostic tests. Eosinophilia and mild anemia are common, but eosinophilia may be absent with hyperinfection. Hyperinfection may include extensive pulmonary infiltrates, hypoproteinemia, and abnormal liver function studies.

C. Screening

It is important to be aware of the possibility of strongyloidiasis in persons with even a distant history of residence in an endemic area, since the infection can be latent for decades. Screening of at-risk individuals for infection is appropriate before institution of immunosuppressive therapy. Screening can consist of serologic tests, with stool examinations in those with positive serologic tests, but consideration of presumptive treatment even if the stool evaluations are negative.

Treatment

Full eradication of *S stercoralis* is more important than with other intestinal helminths due to the ability of the parasite to replicate in humans. The treatment of choice for routine infection is ivermectin (200 mcg/kg orally daily for 1–2 days). Less effective alternatives are albendazole (400 mg orally twice daily for 3 days) and thiabendazole (25 mg/kg orally twice daily for 3 days). For hyperinfection, ivermectin should be administered daily until the clinical syndrome has resolved and larvae have not been identified for at least 2 weeks. Follow-up examinations for larvae in stool or sputum are necessary, with repeat dosing if the infection persists. With continued immunosuppression, eradication may be difficult, and regular repeated therapy (eg, monthly ivermectin) may be required.

ENTEROBIASIS

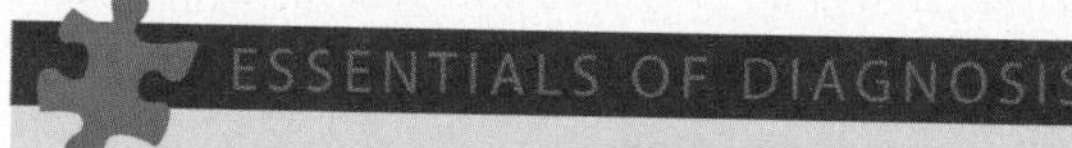

- Nocturnal perianal pruritus.
- Identification of eggs or adult worms on perianal skin or in stool.

General Considerations

Enterobius vermicularis, the pinworm, is a common cause of intestinal infections worldwide, with maximal prevalence in school-aged children. Enterobiasis is transmitted person-to-person via ingestion of eggs after contact with the hands or perianal region of an infected individual, food or fomites that have been contaminated by an infected individual, or infected bedding or clothing. Autoinfection also occurs. Eggs hatch in the duodenum and larvae migrate to the cecum. Females mature in about a month and remain viable for about another month. During this time, they migrate through the anus to deposit large numbers of eggs on the perianal skin. Due to the relatively short life span of these helminths, continuous reinfection, as in institutional settings, is required for long-standing infection.

Clinical Findings

A. Symptoms and Signs

Most individuals with pinworm infection are asymptomatic. The most common symptom is perianal pruritus, particularly at night, due to the presence of the female worms or deposited eggs. Insomnia, restlessness, and enuresis are common in children. Perianal scratching may result in excoriation and impetigo. Many mild GI symptoms have also been attributed to enterobiasis, but associations are not proven. Serious sequelae are uncommon. Rarely, worm migration results in inflammation or granulomatous reactions of the GI or genitourinary tracts. Colonic ulceration and eosinophilic colitis have been reported.

B. Laboratory Findings

Pinworm eggs are usually not found in stool. Diagnosis is made by finding adult worms or eggs on the perianal skin. A common test is to apply clear cellophane tape to the perianal skin, ideally in the early morning, followed by microscopic examination for eggs. The sensitivity of the tape test is reported to be about 50% for a single test and 90% for three tests. Nocturnal examination of the perianal area or gross examination of stools may reveal adult worms, which are about 1 cm in length. Eosinophilia is rare.

Treatment

Treatment is with single oral doses of albendazole (400 mg), mebendazole (100 mg), or pyrantel pamoate (11 mg/kg, to a maximum of 1 g). The dose is repeated in 2 weeks due to frequent reinfection. Other family members with infection should be treated concurrently, and treatment of all close contacts may be appropriate when rates of reinfection are high in family, school, or institutional settings. Standard hand washing and hygiene practices are helpful in limiting spread. Perianal scratching should be discouraged. Washing of clothes and bedding should kill pinworm eggs.

Jourdan PM et al. Soil-transmitted helminth infections. Lancet. 2018;391:252. [PMID: 28882382]

Khurana S et al. diagnostic techniques for soil-transmitted helminths—recent advances. Res Rep Trop Med. 2021;12:181. [PMID: 34377048]

Krolewiecki A et al. Strongyloidiasis: a neglected tropical disease. Infect Dis Clin North Am. 2019;33:135. [PMID: 30712758]

Veesenmeyer AF. Important nematodes in children. Pediatr Clin North Am. 2022;69:129. [PMID: 34794670]

INVASIVE NEMATODE (Roundworm) INFECTIONS

ANGIOSTRONGYLIASIS

Nematodes of rats of the genus *Angiostrongylus* cause two distinct syndromes in humans. *Angiostrongylus cantonensis*, the rat lungworm, causes eosinophilic meningoencephalitis, primarily in Southeast Asia and some Pacific islands, but with multiple recent reports also from the Americas, Hawaii (82 reported cases in 2007–17), and Australia. In one study, *A cantonensis* was responsible for 67% of evaluable cases of eosinophilic meningitis in Vietnam. *Angiostrongylus costaricensis* causes GI inflammation. In both diseases, human infection follows ingestion of larvae within slugs or snails (also crabs, prawns, or centipedes for *A cantonensis*) or on material, such as salads, contaminated by these organisms. Since the parasites are not in their natural hosts, they cannot complete their life cycles, but they can cause disease after migrating to the brain or GI tract. *A cantonensis* can also migrate from the brain to the pulmonary arteries.

Clinical Findings

A. *A cantonensis* Infection

The disease is caused primarily by worm larvae migrating through the CNS and an inflammatory response to dying worms. After an incubation period of 1 day to 2 weeks, presenting symptoms and signs include headache, stiff neck, nausea, vomiting, cranial nerve abnormalities, and paresthesias. Most cases resolve spontaneously after 2–8 weeks, but serious sequelae and death have been reported. The diagnosis is strongly suggested by the finding of eosinophilic CSF pleocytosis (over 10% eosinophils) in a patient with a history of travel to an endemic area. Peripheral eosinophilia may not be present. The diagnosis can be confirmed with PCR, but this may be negative early in disease.

B. *A costaricensis* Infection

Parasites penetrate ileocecal vasculature and develop into adults, which lay eggs, but do not complete their life cycle. Disease is due to an inflammatory response to dying worms in the intestinal tract, with an eosinophilic granulomatous response, at times including vasculitis and ischemic necrosis. Common findings are abdominal pain, vomiting, and fever. Pain is most commonly localized to the right lower quadrant, and a mass may be appreciated, all mimicking appendicitis. Symptoms may recur over months. Uncommon findings are intestinal perforation or obstruction, or disease due to migration of worms to other sites. Many cases are managed surgically, usually for suspected appendicitis. Biopsy of inflamed intestinal tissue may show worms localized to mesenteric arteries and eosinophilic granulomas.

Treatment

Antihelminthic therapy may be harmful for *A cantonensis* infection, since responses to dying worms may worsen with therapy. Some experts, however, recommend prompt therapy for any suspected infection, even for a known accidental snail or slug ingestion in an endemic area, as therapy is likely most beneficial early in the course of disease. Albendazole is probably the best choice, and therapy should be prompt (within 3 weeks of exposure). Corticosteroids are probably appropriate if antihelminthics are provided. Ocular infection is treated surgically. It is not known if antihelminthic therapy is helpful for *A costaricensis* infection.

Ansdell V et al. Guidelines for the diagnosis and treatment of neuroangiostrongyliasis: updated recommendations. Parasitology. 2021;148:227. [PMID: 32729438]

Jarvi S et al. *Angiostrongylus cantonensis* and neuroangiostrongyliasis (rat lungworm disease): 2020. Parasitology. 2021;148:129. [PMID: 33315004]

CUTANEOUS LARVA MIGRANS (Creeping Eruption)

Cutaneous larva migrans is caused principally by larvae of the dog and cat hookworms, *Ancylostoma braziliense* and *A caninum*. Other animal hookworms, gnathostomiasis, and strongyloidiasis may also cause this syndrome. Infections are common in warm areas, including the southeastern United States. They are most common in children. The disease is caused by the migration of worms through skin; the nonhuman parasites cannot complete their life cycles, so only cause cutaneous disease.

Clinical Findings

Intensely pruritic erythematous papules develop, usually on the feet or hands, followed within a few days by serpiginous tracks marking the course of the parasite, which may travel several millimeters per day (Figure 35–3). Several tracks may be present. The process may continue for weeks, with lesions becoming vesiculated, encrusted, or secondarily infected. Systemic symptoms and eosinophilia are uncommon.

The diagnosis is based on the characteristic appearance of the lesions. Biopsy is usually not indicated.

Treatment

Without treatment, the larvae eventually die and are absorbed. Mild cases do not require treatment. Thiabendazole (10% aqueous suspension) can be applied topically three times daily for 5 or more days. Systemic therapy with albendazole (400 mg orally once or twice daily for 3–5 days) or ivermectin (200 mcg/kg orally single dose) is highly effective.

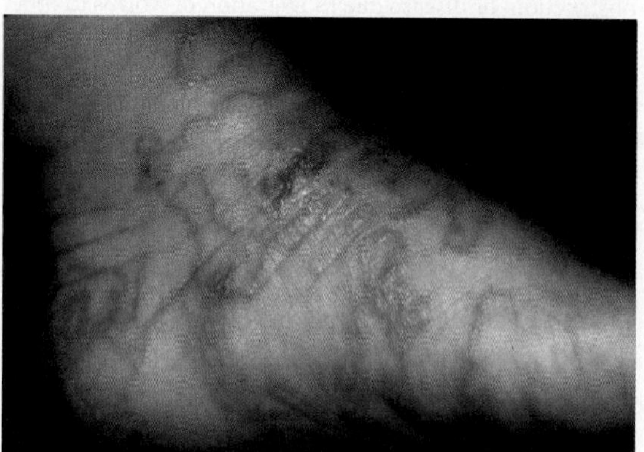

▲ **Figure 35–3.** Cutaneous larva migrans on the foot. (Reproduced with permission from Richard P. Usatine, MD, in Usatine RP, Smith MA, Mayeaux EJ Jr, Chumley H. *The Color Atlas of Family Medicine*, 2nd ed. McGraw-Hill, 2013.)

Kincaid L et al. Management of imported cutaneous larva migrans: a case series and mini-review. Travel Med Infect Dis. 2015;13:382. [PMID: 26243366]

FILARIASIS

LYMPHATIC FILARIASIS

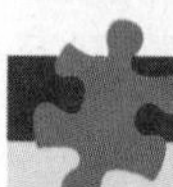

ESSENTIALS OF DIAGNOSIS

- Episodic attacks of lymphangitis, lymphadenitis, and fever.
- Chronic progressive swelling of extremities and genitals; hydrocele; chyluria; lymphedema.
- Microfilariae in blood, chyluria, or hydrocele fluid; positive serologic tests.

General Considerations

Lymphatic filariasis is caused by three filarial nematodes: *Wuchereria bancrofti*, *Brugia malayi*, and *Brugia timori*, and is among the most important parasitic diseases of man. Approximately 120 million people are infected with these organisms in tropical and subtropical countries, about a third of these suffer clinical consequences of the infections, and many are seriously disfigured. *W bancrofti* causes about 90% of episodes of lymphatic filariasis. It is transmitted by *Culex*, *Aedes*, and *Anopheles* mosquitoes and is widely distributed in the tropics and subtropics, including sub-Saharan Africa, Southeast Asia, the western Pacific, India, South America, and the Caribbean. *B malayi* is transmitted by *Mansonia* and *Anopheles* mosquitoes and is endemic in parts of China, India, Southeast Asia, and the Pacific. *B timori* is found only in islands of southeastern Indonesia. *Mansonella* are filarial worms transmitted by midges and other insects in Africa and South America.

Humans are infected by the bites of infected mosquitoes. Larvae then move to the lymphatics and lymph nodes, where they mature over months to thread-like adult worms, and then can persist for many years. The adult worms produce large numbers of microfilariae, which are released into the circulation, and infective to mosquitoes, particularly at night (except for the South Pacific, where microfilaremia peaks during daylight hours).

Clinical Findings

A. Symptoms and Signs

Many infections remain asymptomatic despite circulating microfilariae. Clinical consequences of filarial infection are principally due to inflammatory responses to developing,

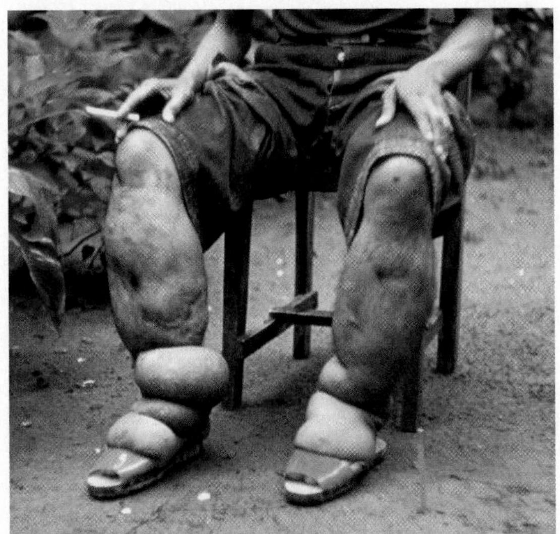

▲ **Figure 35–4.** Elephantiasis of legs due to filariasis. (Public Health Image Library, CDC.)

mature, and dying worms. The initial manifestation of infection is often acute lymphangitis, with fever, painful lymph nodes, edema, and inflammation spreading peripherally from involved lymph nodes (in contrast to bacterial lymphangitis, which spreads centrally). Lymphangitis and lymphadenitis of the upper and lower extremities are common (Figure 35–4); genital involvement, including epididymitis and orchitis, with scrotal pain and tenderness, occurs principally only with *W bancrofti* infection. Acute attacks of lymphangitis last for a few days to a week and may recur a few times per year. Filarial fevers may also occur without lymphatic inflammation.

The most common chronic manifestation of lymphatic filariasis is swelling of the extremities or genitals due to chronic lymphatic inflammation and obstruction. Extremities become increasingly swollen, with a progression over time, including pitting or nonpitting edema or sclerotic changes of the skin that are referred to as elephantiasis. Genital involvement, particularly with *W bancrofti*, occurs more commonly in men, progressing from painful epididymitis to hydroceles that are usually painless but can become very large, with inguinal lymphadenopathy, thickening of the spermatic cord, scrotal lymphedema, thickening and fissuring of the scrotal skin, and occasionally chyluria. Lymphedema of the female genitalia and breasts may also occur.

Tropical pulmonary eosinophilia is a distinct syndrome principally affecting young adult males with either *W bancrofti* or *B malayi* infection, but typically without microfilaremia. This syndrome is characterized by asthma-like symptoms, with cough, wheezing, dyspnea, and low-grade fevers, usually at night. Without treatment, tropical pulmonary eosinophilia can progress to interstitial fibrosis and chronic restrictive lung disease. *Mansonella* can inhabit serous cavities, the retroperitoneum, the eye, or the skin, and cause abnormalities related to inflammation at these sites.

B. Laboratory Findings

The diagnosis of lymphatic filariasis is strongly suggested by characteristic findings of lymphangitis or lymphatic obstruction in persons with risk factors for the disease. The diagnosis is confirmed by finding microfilariae, usually in blood, but microfilariae may be absent, especially early in the disease progression (first 2–3 years) or with chronic obstructive disease. To increase yields, blood samples are obtained at about midnight in most areas, but during daylight hours in the South Pacific. Smears are evaluated by wet mount to identify motile parasites and by Giemsa staining; these examinations can be delayed until the following morning, with storage of samples at room temperature. Of note, the periodicity of microfilaremia is variable, and daytime samples may yield positive results. Microfilariae may also be identified in hydrocele fluid or chylous urine. Eosinophilia is usually absent, except during acute inflammatory syndromes. Serologic tests may be helpful but cannot distinguish past and active infections. Rapid antigen tests with sensitivity and specificity over 90% are available for detection of *W bancrofti*. These can be considered the diagnostic tests of choice and are used to guide control programs. However, cross-reactivity with *Loa* infections has been described. Due to potential severe toxicity, caution is appropriate before treatment with ivermectin for positive *W bancrofti* antigen tests in areas also endemic for *L loa* infection. Multiple molecular tests, including field-friendly LAMP assays, have been developed. Adult worms may also be found in lymph node biopsy specimens (although biopsy is not usually clinically indicated) or by ultrasound of a scrotal hydrocele or lymphedematous breast. When microfilaremia is lacking, especially if sophisticated techniques are not available, diagnoses may need to be made on clinical grounds.

▶ Treatment & Control

A. Drug Treatment

Diethylcarbamazine is the drug of choice, but it cannot cure infections due to its limited action against adult worms. Asymptomatic infection and acute lymphangitis are treated with this drug (2 mg/kg orally three times daily) for 10–14 days, leading to a marked decrease in microfilaremia. Therapy may be accompanied by allergic symptoms, including fever, headache, malaise, hypotension, and bronchospasm, probably due to release of antigens from dying worms. For this reason, treatment courses may begin with a lower dosage, with escalation over the first 4 days of treatment. Single annual doses of diethylcarbamazine (6 mg/kg orally), alone or with ivermectin (400 mcg/kg orally) or albendazole (400 mg orally) may be as effective as longer courses of diethylcarbamazine. Combination therapy with a single dose of each of the three drugs (ivermectin, diethylcarbamazine, and albendazole [IDA]) cleared parasites in more than 95% of persons for 3 years and offered superior clearance compared with two drugs; triple-drug therapy was as safe and well tolerated. When onchocerciasis or loiasis is suspected, it may be appropriate to withhold diethylcarbamazine to avoid severe reactions to dying microfilariae; rather, ivermectin plus albendazole may be given, although these drugs are less active than diethylcarbamazine against adult worms. Appropriate management of advanced obstructive disease is uncertain. Drainage of hydroceles provides symptomatic relief, although they will recur. Therapy with diethylcarbamazine cannot reverse chronic lymphatic changes but is typically provided to lower worm burdens. An interesting approach under study is to treat with doxycycline (100–200 mg/day orally for 4–6 weeks), which kills obligate intracellular *Wolbachia* bacteria, leading to death of adult filarial worms. Doxycycline was also effective at controlling *Mansonella perstans* infection, which does not respond well to standard antifilarial drugs. Secondary bacterial infections must be treated. Surgical correction may be helpful in some cases.

B. Disease Control

Avoidance of mosquitoes is a key measure; preventive measures include the use of screens, bed nets (ideally treated with insecticide), and insect repellents. Community-based treatment with single annual doses of effective drugs offers a highly effective means of control. Combination IDA therapy offers improved efficacy and may become the standard of care for the prevention of lymphatic filariasis.

Dubray CL et al. Safety and efficacy of co-administered diethylcarbamazine, albendazole and ivermectin during mass drug administration for lymphatic filariasis in Haiti: results from a two-armed, open-label, cluster-randomized, community study. PLoS Negl Trop Dis. 2020;14:e0008298. [PMID: 32511226]

King CL et al. A trial of a triple-drug treatment for lymphatic filariasis. N Engl J Med. 2018;379:1801. [PMID: 30403937]

Weil GJ et al. The safety of double- and triple-drug community mass drug administration for lymphatic filariasis: a multicenter, open-label, cluster-randomized study. PLoS Med. 2019;16:e1002839. [PMID: 31233507]

ONCHOCERCIASIS

- Conjunctivitis progressing to blindness.
- Severe pruritus; skin excoriations, thickening, and depigmentation; and subcutaneous nodules.
- Microfilariae in skin snips and on slit-lamp examination; adult worms in subcutaneous nodules.

General Considerations

Onchocerciasis, or river blindness, is caused by *Onchocerca volvulus*. An estimated 37 million persons are infected, of whom 3–4 million have skin disease, 500,000 have severe visual impairment, and 300,000 are blinded. Over 99% of infections are in sub-Saharan Africa, especially the West African savanna, with about half of cases in Nigeria and Congo. In some hyperendemic African villages, close to 100% of individuals are infected, and 10% or more of the population is blind. The disease is also prevalent in the southwestern Arabian Peninsula and Latin America, including southern Mexico, Guatemala, Venezuela, Colombia, Ecuador, and northwestern Brazil. Onchocerciasis is transmitted by simulium flies (blackflies). These insects breed in fast-flowing streams and bite during the day.

After the bite of an infected blackfly, larvae are deposited in the skin, where adults develop over 6–12 months. Adult worms live in subcutaneous connective tissue or muscle nodules for a decade or more. Microfilariae are released from the nodules and migrate through subcutaneous and ocular tissues. Disease is due to responses to worms and to intracellular *Wolbachia* bacteria.

Clinical Findings

A. Symptoms and Signs

After an incubation period of up to 1–3 years, the disease typically produces an erythematous, papular, pruritic rash, which may progress to chronic skin thickening and depigmentation. Itching may be severe and unresponsive to medications, such that more disability-adjusted life-years are lost to onchocercal skin problems than to blindness. Numerous firm, nontender, movable subcutaneous nodules of about 0.5–3 cm, which contain adult worms, may be present. Due to differences in vector habits, these nodules are more commonly on the lower body in Africa but on the head and upper body in Latin America. Inguinal and femoral lymphadenopathy is common, at times resulting in a "hanging groin," with lymph nodes hanging within a sling of atrophic skin. Patients may also have systemic symptoms, with weight loss and musculoskeletal pain.

The most serious manifestations of onchocerciasis involve the eyes. Microfilariae migrating through the eyes elicit host responses that lead to pathology. Findings include punctate keratitis and corneal opacities, progressing to sclerosing keratitis and blindness. Iridocyclitis, glaucoma, choroiditis, and optic atrophy may also lead to vision loss. The likelihood of blindness after infection varies greatly based on geography, with the risk greatest in savanna regions of West Africa.

B. Diagnostic Testing

The diagnosis is made by identifying microfilariae in skin snips, by visualizing microfilariae in the cornea or anterior chamber by slit-lamp examination, by identification of adult worms in a biopsy or aspirate of a nodule or, uncommonly, by identification of microfilariae in urine. Skin snips from the iliac crest (Africa) or scapula (Americas) are allowed to stand in saline for 2–4 hours or longer, and then examined microscopically for microfilariae. Deep punch biopsies are not needed, and if suspicion persists after a skin snip is negative, the procedure should be repeated. Ultrasound may identify characteristic findings suggestive of adult worms in skin nodules. When the diagnosis remains difficult, the Mazzotti test can be used; exacerbation of skin rash and pruritus after a topical or 50-mg oral dose of diethylcarbamazine is highly suggestive of the diagnosis, but this test can elicit severe skin and eye reactions in heavily infected individuals. Eosinophilia is a common but inconsistent finding. Antigen and antibody detection tests are under study.

Treatment & Control

The treatment of choice is ivermectin, which kills microfilariae, but not adult worms, so disease control requires repeat administrations. Treatment is with a single oral dose of 150 mcg/mL, but schedules for re-treatment have not been standardized. One regimen is to treat every 3 months for 1 year, followed by treatment every 6–12 months for the suspected life span of adult worms (about 15 years). Treatment results in marked reduction in numbers of microfilariae in the skin and eyes, although its impact on the progression of visual loss remains uncertain. Toxicities of ivermectin are generally mild; fever, pruritus, urticaria, myalgias, edema, hypotension, and tender lymphadenopathy may be seen, presumably due to reactions to dying worms. Ivermectin should be used with caution in patients also at risk for loiasis, since it can elicit severe reactions including encephalopathy. Moxidectin, which is used for many veterinary parasitic infections, is FDA-approved for the treatment of onchocerciasis. Moxidectin is well tolerated and superior to ivermectin in suppressing skin microfilariae and offers another agent for treatment and control. As with other filarial infections, doxycycline acts against *O volvulus* by killing intracellular *Wolbachia* bacteria. A course of 100 mg/day for 4–6 weeks kills the bacteria and prevents parasite embryogenesis for at least 18 months. Doxycycline shows promise as a first-line agent to treat onchocerciasis because of its improved activity against adult worms compared with other agents and limited toxicity due to the slow action of the drug.

Protection against onchocerciasis includes avoidance of biting flies. Major efforts are underway to control insect vectors in Africa. In addition, mass distribution of ivermectin for intermittent administration at the community level is ongoing, and the prevalence of severe skin and eye disease is decreasing.

Opoku NO et al. Single dose moxidectin versus ivermectin for *Onchocerca volvulus* infection in Ghana, Liberia, and the Democratic Republic of the Congo: a randomised, controlled, double-blind phase 3 trial. Lancet. 2018;392:1207. [PMID: 29361335]

Mycotic Infections

Stacey R. Rose, MD, FACP, FIDSA
Richard J. Hamill, MD

CANDIDIASIS

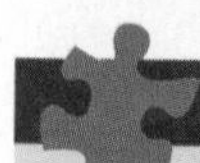

ESSENTIALS OF DIAGNOSIS

- Common normal flora but opportunistic pathogen.
- Typically, mucosal disease, particularly vaginitis and oral thrush/esophagitis.
- Persistent, unexplained oral or vaginal candidiasis: check for HIV or diabetes mellitus.
- (1,3)-Beta-D-glucan results may be positive in candidemia even when blood cultures are negative.

General Considerations

Candida albicans can be cultured from the mouth, vagina, and feces of most people. Cellular immunodeficiency predisposes to mucocutaneous disease. When no other underlying cause is found, persistent oral or vaginal candidiasis should raise suspicion for HIV infection or diabetes. Risk factors for invasive candidiasis include prolonged neutropenia, abdominal surgery, broad-spectrum antibiotic therapy, corticosteroids, kidney disease, and the presence of intravascular catheters. Although *C albicans* remains the most common cause of both mucocutaneous and systemic candidiasis, non-*albicans* strains are of considerable importance in certain contexts and may impact therapy owing to antifungal resistance.

Clinical Findings

A. Mucosal Candidiasis

Vulvovaginal candidiasis occurs in an estimated 75% of women during their lifetime. Risk factors include pregnancy, uncontrolled diabetes mellitus, broad-spectrum antimicrobial treatment, corticosteroid use, and HIV infection. Symptoms include acute vulvar pruritus, burning vaginal discharge, and dyspareunia.

Esophageal candidiasis may present clinically with symptoms of substernal odynophagia, gastroesophageal reflux, or nausea without substernal pain. Oral candidiasis, though often associated, is not invariably present. Diagnosis is best confirmed by endoscopy with biopsy and culture.

B. Candidal Funguria

Most cases of candidal funguria are asymptomatic and represent specimen contamination or bladder colonization (and do not warrant antifungal therapy). However, symptoms and signs of true *Candida* UTIs are indistinguishable from bacterial UTIs and can include urgency, hesitancy, fever, chills, or flank pain.

C. Invasive Candidiasis

Invasive candidiasis can be (1) candidemia (bloodstream infection) without deep-seated infection; (2) candidemia with deep-seated infection (typically eyes, kidney, or abdomen); and (3) deep-seated candidiasis in the absence of bloodstream infection (ie, hepatosplenic candidiasis). Varying ratios of these clinical entities depends on the predominating risk factors for affected patients (ie, neutropenia, indwelling vascular catheters, postsurgical).

The clinical presentation of candidemia varies from minimal fever to septic shock that can resemble a severe bacterial infection. The diagnosis of invasive *Candida* infection is challenging since *Candida* species are often isolated from mucosal sites in the absence of invasive disease while blood cultures are positive only 50% of the time in invasive infection. Consecutively positive (1,3)-beta-D-glucan results may be used to guide empiric therapy in high-risk patients even in the absence of positive blood cultures.

Hepatosplenic candidiasis can occur following prolonged neutropenia in patients with underlying hematologic cancers, but this entity is less common in the era of widespread antifungal prophylaxis. Typically, fever and variable abdominal pain present weeks after chemotherapy when neutrophil counts have recovered. Blood cultures are generally negative, though hepatosplenic abscesses may be seen on abdominal imaging.

D. Candidal Endocarditis

Candidal endocarditis is a rare infection affecting patients with prosthetic heart valves or prolonged candidemia, such as with indwelling catheters. The diagnosis is established definitively by culturing *Candida* from vegetations at the time of valve replacement.

Treatment

A. Mucosal Candidiasis

Vulvovaginal candidiasis can be treated with topical or oral azoles. A single 150-mg oral dose of fluconazole is equivalent to topical treatments with better patient acceptance. Topical azole preparations include clotrimazole, 100-mg vaginal tablet for 7 days, or miconazole, 200-mg vaginal suppository for 3 days. Disease recurrence is common but can be decreased with weekly oral fluconazole therapy (150 mg weekly). Vulvovaginal candidiasis caused by non-*albicans* strains (eg, *Candida glabrata*) may require alternative therapies (such as intravaginal boric acid) in the setting of azole resistance. Oral ibrexafungerp, a highly bioavailable glucan synthase inhibitor, may be used to treat vulvovaginal candidiasis from any disease-causing *Candida* strains, including azole-resistant pathogens.

Treatment of **esophageal candidiasis** depends on the severity of disease. If patients can swallow and take adequate amounts of fluid orally, fluconazole, 200–400 mg orally daily for 14–21 days, is recommended. Patients who are unable to tolerate oral therapy should receive intravenous fluconazole, 400 mg daily, or an echinocandin. Options for patients with fluconazole-refractory disease include oral itraconazole solution, 200 mg daily; oral or intravenous voriconazole, 200 mg twice daily; or an intravenous echinocandin (caspofungin, 70 mg loading dose, then 50 mg/day; anidulafungin, 200 mg/day; or intravenous micafungin, 150 mg/day). Posaconazole tablets, 300 mg/day, may also be considered for fluconazole-refractory disease. Relapse is common with all agents in persons living with HIV without adequate immune reconstitution.

B. Candidal Funguria

Candidal funguria frequently resolves with discontinuance of antibiotics or removal of bladder catheters. Clinical benefit from treatment of asymptomatic candiduria has not been demonstrated, but persistent funguria should raise the suspicion of invasive infection. When symptomatic funguria persists, oral fluconazole, 200 mg/day for 7–14 days, can be used.

C. Invasive Candidiasis

The 2016 Infectious Diseases Society of America guidelines for management of candidemia recommend an intravenous echinocandin as first-line therapy (ie, caspofungin [70 mg once, then 50 mg daily], micafungin [100 mg daily], or anidulafungin [200 mg once, then 100 mg daily]). Intravenous or oral fluconazole (800 mg once, then 400 mg daily) is an acceptable alternative for less critically ill patients without recent azole exposure.

Therapy for candidemia should be continued for 2 weeks after the last positive blood culture and resolution of symptoms and signs of infection. A dilated fundoscopic examination is recommended for patients with candidemia to exclude endophthalmitis and repeat blood cultures should be drawn to demonstrate organism clearance. Susceptibility testing is recommended on all bloodstream *Candida* isolates; once patients have become clinically stable, parenteral therapy can be discontinued and treatment can be completed with oral fluconazole, 400 mg daily for susceptible isolates. Removal or exchange of intravascular catheters is recommended for patients with candidemia in whom the catheter is the suspected source of infection.

Non-*albicans* species of *Candida* often have resistance patterns that are different from *C albicans*. An echinocandin is recommended for treatment of *C glabrata* infection with transition to oral fluconazole or voriconazole reserved for patients whose isolates are susceptible to these agents. For isolates with resistance to azoles and echinocandins, lipid formulation amphotericin B (3–5 mg/kg intravenously daily) may be used. *C krusei* is generally fluconazole-resistant and should be treated with an alternative agent, such as an echinocandin or voriconazole. Health care–associated infections due to multidrug-resistant *Candida auris* may be treated with echinocandins plus environmental source control.

D. Candidal Endocarditis

Best results are achieved with a combination of medical and surgical therapy (valve replacement). Lipid formulation amphotericin B (3–5 mg/kg/day) or high-dose echinocandin (caspofungin 150 mg/day, micafungin 150 mg/day, or anidulafungin 200 mg/day) is recommended as initial therapy. Step-down or long-term suppressive therapy for nonsurgical candidates may be done with fluconazole at 6–12 mg/kg/day for susceptible organisms.

E. Prevention of Invasive Candidiasis

In high-risk patients undergoing induction chemotherapy, hematopoietic stem cell transplantation, liver, small bowel, and pancreas transplantation, prophylaxis with antifungal agents has been shown to prevent invasive fungal infections, although the effect on mortality and the preferred agent(s) remain debated. Although critically ill patients are at higher risk for invasive candidiasis, antifungal prophylaxis has not shown clear clinical benefit.

Al-Dorzi HM et al. Invasive candidiasis in critically ill patients: a prospective cohort study in two tertiary care centers. J Intensive Care Med. 2020;35:542. [PMID: 29628014]

Aslam S et al. Candida infections in solid organ transplantation: guidelines from the American Society of Transplantation Infectious Diseases Community of Practice. Clin Transplant. 2019;33:e13623. [PMID: 31155770]

Gold JAW et al. Treatment practices for adults with candidemia at 9 active surveillance sites—United States, 2017-2018. Clin Infect Dis. 2021;73:1609. [PMID: 34079987]

Pappas PG et al. Clinical practice guideline for the management of candidiasis: 2016 update by the Infectious Diseases Society of America. Clin Infect Dis. 2016;62:e1. [PMID: 26679628]

HISTOPLASMOSIS

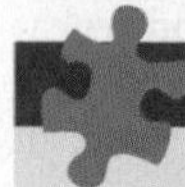

ESSENTIALS OF DIAGNOSIS

- Exposure to bird and bat droppings; common along river valleys (especially the Ohio River and the Mississippi River valleys).
- Most patients asymptomatic; respiratory illness most frequent clinical problem.
- Disseminated disease common in AIDS or other immunosuppressed states; poor prognosis.
- Blood and bone marrow cultures and urine polysaccharide antigen are useful in diagnosis of disseminated disease.

General Considerations

Histoplasmosis is caused by *Histoplasma capsulatum*, a fungus that has been isolated from soil contaminated with bird or bat droppings in endemic areas (central and eastern United States, eastern Canada, Mexico, Central America, South America, Africa, and Southeast Asia). Infection presumably takes place by inhalation of conidia. These convert into small budding cells that are engulfed by phagocytes in the lungs. The organism proliferates and undergoes lymphohematogenous spread to other organs.

Clinical Findings

A. Symptoms and Signs

Most cases of histoplasmosis are asymptomatic or mild and thus go unrecognized. Past infection is recognized by pulmonary and splenic calcification noted on incidental radiographs. Symptomatic infection may present with mild influenza-like illness, often lasting 1–4 days. Moderately severe infections are frequently diagnosed as atypical pneumonia. These patients have fever, cough, and mild central chest pain lasting 5–15 days.

Clinically evident infections occur in several forms: (1) **Acute pulmonary histoplasmosis** frequently occurs in epidemics, often when soil containing infected bird or bat droppings is disturbed. Clinical manifestations can vary from a mild influenza-like illness to severe pneumonia. The illness may last from 1 week to 6 months but is almost never fatal. (2) **Progressive disseminated histoplasmosis** most frequently occurs in patients with underlying HIV infection (with CD4 cell counts usually less than 100 cells/mcL) or other conditions of impaired cellular immunity. Disseminated histoplasmosis has also been reported in patients from endemic areas taking tumor necrosis factor (TNF)-alpha inhibitors. It is characterized by fever and multiple organ system involvement. Chest radiographs may show a miliary pattern. Presentation may be fulminant, simulating septic shock, with death ensuing rapidly unless treatment is provided. Symptoms usually consist of fever, dyspnea, cough, loss of weight, and prostration. Ulcers of the mucous membranes of the oropharynx may be present. The liver and spleen are nearly always enlarged, and all the organs of the body are involved, particularly the adrenal glands; *this results in adrenal insufficiency in about 50% of patients.* GI involvement may mimic IBD. CNS invasion occurs in 5–10% of individuals with disseminated disease. (3) **Chronic pulmonary histoplasmosis** is usually seen in older patients who have underlying chronic lung disease. Chest radiographs show various lesions including complex apical cavities, infiltrates, and nodules. (4) **Complications of pulmonary histoplasmosis** include granulomatous mediastinitis characterized by persistently enlarged mediastinal lymph nodes and fibrosing mediastinitis in which an excessive fibrotic response to *Histoplasma* infection results in compromise of pulmonary vascular structures.

B. Laboratory Findings

Most patients with chronic pulmonary disease show anemia of chronic disease. Bone marrow involvement with pancytopenia may be prominent in disseminated forms. Marked LD and ferritin elevations are also common, as are mild elevations of serum AST.

With pulmonary involvement, sputum culture is rarely positive except in chronic disease; antigen testing of bronchoalveolar lavage fluid may be helpful in acute disease. The combination of urine and serum polysaccharide antigen assays has an 83% sensitivity for the diagnosis of acute pulmonary histoplasmosis.

Blood cultures using lysis centrifugation methods or bone marrow cultures from immunocompromised patients with acute disseminated disease are positive more than 80% of the time but may take several weeks for growth. The urine antigen assay has a sensitivity of greater than 90% for disseminated disease in immunocompromised patients and a declining titer can be used to follow response to therapy. Both cerebrospinal fluid (CSF) antigen and antibody testing should be performed in patients suspected of having meningitis.

Treatment

For progressive localized disease and for mild to moderately severe nonmeningeal disseminated disease in immunocompetent or immunocompromised patients, itraconazole, 200–400 mg/day orally divided into two doses, is the treatment of choice with an overall response rate of approximately 80% (Table 36–1). The oral solution is better absorbed than the capsule formulation, which requires gastric acid for absorption. Therapeutic drug monitoring of itraconazole levels should be performed to assess adequacy of drug absorption. Duration of therapy ranges from weeks to several months depending on the severity of illness. Intravenous liposomal amphotericin B, 3 mg/kg/day, is used in patients with more severe disseminated disease and meningitis. Patients with AIDS-related histoplasmosis require lifelong suppressive therapy with itraconazole, 200 mg/day orally, although secondary prophylaxis may be discontinued if immune reconstitution occurs in response to antiretroviral therapy. Criteria for discontinuing secondary prophylaxis include 1 year of successful antifungal therapy along with a CD4 cell count of greater than 150 cells/mcL and 6 months or more of antiretroviral treatment (ART). There is no clear evidence that antifungal agents are of benefit for patients with fibrosing mediastinitis, although oral itraconazole is often used. Rituximab, in conjunction with corticosteroids, may contribute to slowing progression of the fibrosing process and provide some clinical benefit. Reported outcomes in patients with fibrosing mediastinitis treated with either surgical procedures or nonsurgical intravascular interventions appear to be relatively good in the short term.

Araúz AB et al. Histoplasmosis. Infect Dis Clin North Am. 2021;35:471. [PMID: 34016287]

COCCIDIOIDOMYCOSIS

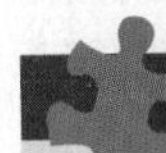

ESSENTIALS OF DIAGNOSIS

- Acute infection: influenza-like illness, fever, backache, headache, fatigue, and cough; erythema nodosum is common.
- Dissemination may result in meningitis, bony lesions, or skin and soft tissue abscesses; common opportunistic infection in AIDS.
- Chest radiograph findings vary from pneumonitis to cavitation.
- Serologic tests useful; large spherules containing endospores demonstrable in sputum or tissues.

General Considerations

Coccidioidomycosis should be considered in the diagnosis of any obscure illness in a patient who has lived in or visited an endemic area. Infection results from the inhalation of arthroconidia of *Coccidioides immitis* or *C posadasii*; both organisms are molds that grow in soil in certain arid regions of the southwestern United States, in Mexico, and in Central and South America. Less than 1% of immunocompetent persons show dissemination, but among these patients, the mortality rate is high.

In patients with AIDS who reside in endemic areas, coccidioidomycosis is a common opportunistic infection. In these patients, disease manifestations range from focal pulmonary infiltrates to widespread miliary disease with multiple organ involvement and meningitis; severity is inversely related to the extent of control of the HIV infection.

Clinical Findings

A. Symptoms and Signs

Symptoms of **primary coccidioidomycosis** occur in about 40% of infections. Symptom onset (after an incubation period of 10–30 days) is usually that of a respiratory tract illness with fever and occasionally chills. Coccidioidomycosis is a common, frequently unrecognized, etiology of community-acquired pneumonia in endemic areas.

Erythema nodosum may appear 2–20 days after onset of symptoms. Persistent pulmonary lesions, varying from cavities and abscesses to parenchymal nodular densities or bronchiectasis, occur in about 5% of diagnosed cases.

Disseminated disease occurs in about 0.1% of White and 1% of non-White patients. Patients who are Filipino or Black are especially susceptible, as are pregnant women of all races. Any organ may be involved. Pulmonary findings usually become more pronounced, with mediastinal lymph node enlargement, cough, and increased sputum production. Lung abscesses may rupture into the pleural space, producing an empyema. Complicated skin and bone infections may develop. Fungemia may occur and is characterized clinically by a diffuse miliary pattern on chest radiograph and by early death. The course may be particularly rapid in immunosuppressed patients. Clinicians caring for immunosuppressed patients in endemic areas need to consider that patients may have latent infection.

Meningitis occurs in 30–50% of cases of dissemination and may result in chronic basilar meningitis. Subcutaneous abscesses and verrucous skin lesions are especially common in fulminating cases. Patients with AIDS with disseminated disease have a higher incidence of miliary infiltrates, lymphadenopathy, and meningitis, but skin lesions are uncommon.

B. Laboratory Findings

In **primary coccidioidomycosis**, there may be moderate leukocytosis and eosinophilia. Serologic testing is useful for both diagnosis and prognosis. The immunodiffusion tube precipitin test and ELISA detect IgM antibodies and are both useful for diagnosis early in the disease process. A persistently rising IgG complement fixation titer (1:16 or more) is suggestive of disseminated disease; immunodiffusion complement fixation titers can be used to assess the adequacy of therapy. Serum complement fixation titers may be low when there is meningitis but no other disseminated disease. In patients with HIV-related coccidioidomycosis, the false-negative rate may reach 30%. Blood cultures are rarely positive.

Patients in whom coccidioidomycosis is diagnosed should undergo evaluation for meningeal involvement when CNS symptoms or neurologic signs are present. Spinal fluid findings include increased cell count with lymphocytosis and reduced glucose. Spinal fluid culture is positive in approximately 30% of meningitis cases. Demonstrable complement-fixing antibodies in spinal fluid are diagnostic of coccidioidal meningitis. These are found in over 90% of cases; *Coccidioides* antigen or (1,3)-beta-D-glucan testing may augment (not replace) CSF antibody testing.

C. Imaging

Radiographic findings vary, but patchy, nodular, and lobar upper lobe pulmonary infiltrates are most common. Hilar lymphadenopathy may be visible and is seen in localized disease; mediastinal lymphadenopathy suggests dissemination. There may be pleural effusions and lytic lesions in bone with accompanying complicated soft tissue collections.

Treatment

General symptomatic therapy should be provided as needed for disease limited to the chest with no evidence of progression. Itraconazole (400 mg orally daily divided into two doses) or fluconazole (200–400 mg or higher orally once or twice daily) should be given for disease in the chest, bones, and soft tissues; however, therapy must be continued for 6 months or longer after the disease is inactive to prevent relapse (Table 36–1). Response to therapy should be monitored by following the clinical response and progressive decrease in serum complement fixation titers.

For progressive pulmonary or extrapulmonary disease, liposomal amphotericin B intravenously should be given, although oral azoles may be used for mild cases. Duration of therapy is determined by a declining complement fixation titer and a favorable clinical response. For meningitis, treatment usually is with high-dose oral fluconazole (400–1200 mg/day), although lumbar or cisternal intrathecal administration of amphotericin B daily in increasing doses up to 1–1.5 mg/day is used initially by some experienced clinicians or in cases refractory to fluconazole. Systemic therapy with liposomal amphotericin B, 3–5 mg/kg/day intravenously, is usually given concurrently with intrathecal therapy, but is not sufficient alone for the treatment of meningeal disease. Once the patient is clinically stable, oral therapy with an azole, usually with fluconazole (400 mg daily) and given lifelong, is the recommended alternative to intrathecal amphotericin B therapy.

Surgical drainage is necessary for management of soft tissue abscesses, necrotic bone, and complicated pulmonary disease (eg, rupture of coccidioidal cavity).

Prognosis

The prognosis for patients with limited disease is good. Serial complement fixation titers should be performed after therapy for coccidioidomycosis; rising titers warrant reinstitution of therapy because relapse is likely. Late CNS complications of adequately treated meningitis include cerebral vasculitis with stroke and hydrocephalus that may require shunting. There may be a benefit from short-term systemic corticosteroids following cerebrovascular events associated with coccidioidal meningitis. Disseminated and meningeal forms still have mortality rates exceeding 50% in the absence of therapy.

Bays DJ et al. Coccidioidomycosis. Infect Dis Clin North Am. 2021;35:453. [PMID: 34016286]

PNEUMOCYSTOSIS (*Pneumocystis Jirovecii* Pneumonia)

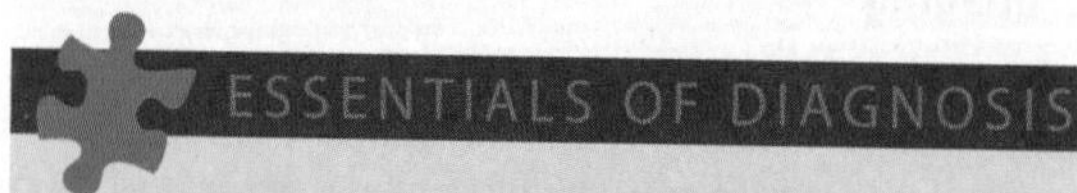

- Fever, dyspnea, dry cough, hypoxia with exertion; often only slight lung physical findings.
- Chest radiograph: diffuse interstitial disease or normal.
- Detection of *P jirovecii* in sputum, bronchoalveolar lavage fluid, or lung tissue; PCR of bronchoalveolar lavage; (1,3)-beta-D-glucan in blood.

General Considerations

Pneumocystis jirovecii, the *Pneumocystis* species that affects humans, is found worldwide.

Overt infection is characterized by a subacute interstitial pneumonia that occurs among older children and adults with abnormal or altered cellular immunity, either due to an underlying condition (eg, AIDS, cancer, malnutrition, hematopoietic stem cell or solid organ transplantation, autoimmune disease) or treatment with immunosuppressive medications (eg, corticosteroids or cytotoxic agents).

Pneumocystis pneumonia occurs in up to 80% of patients with AIDS not receiving prophylaxis and is a major cause of morbidity and mortality. Its incidence increases in direct proportion to the fall in CD4 cells, with most cases occurring at CD4 cell counts less than 200/mcL. In patients without AIDS receiving immunosuppressive therapy, symptoms frequently begin after corticosteroids have been tapered or discontinued.

Clinical Findings

A. Symptoms and Signs

Findings are usually limited to the pulmonary parenchyma. Onset may be subacute, characterized by dyspnea on exertion and nonproductive cough. Pulmonary physical findings may be slight and disproportionate to the degree of illness and radiologic findings; some patients have bibasilar crackles. Without treatment, the course is usually one of rapid deterioration and death. Patients may present with spontaneous pneumothorax, usually in patients with previous episodes or those receiving aerosolized pentamidine prophylaxis. Patients with AIDS will typically have other evidence of HIV-associated disease, including fever, fatigue, and weight loss, for weeks or months preceding the respiratory illness.

B. Laboratory Findings

Arterial blood gas determinations usually show hypoxemia with hypocapnia but may be normal; however, rapid desaturation occurs if patients exercise before samples are drawn. Serum (1,3)-beta-D-glucan levels have reasonable sensitivity but lack specificity as elevated levels occur in other fungal infections. The organism cannot be cultured, and definitive diagnosis depends on morphologic demonstration of the organisms in respiratory specimens using specific stains, such as immunofluorescence. PCR of bronchoalveolar lavage is overly sensitive in that the test can be positive in colonized, uninfected persons; quantitative values may help with identifying infected patients, although precise cutoffs have not been established. A negative PCR from bronchoalveolar lavage rules out disease. Open lung biopsy and needle lung biopsy are infrequently required but may aid in diagnosing a granulomatous form of *Pneumocystis* pneumonia.

C. Imaging

Chest radiographs most often show diffuse "interstitial" infiltration, which may be heterogeneous, miliary, or

Table 36–1. Agents for systemic mycoses.*

Drug	Dosing	Renal Clearance?	CSF Penetration?	Toxicities	Spectrum of Activity
Polyenes					
Amphotericin B	0.3–1.5 mg/kg/day intravenously	No	Poor	Rigors, fever, azotemia, hypokalemia, hypomagnesemia, renal tubular acidosis, anemia	All major pathogens except *Scedosporium*
Amphotericin B lipid complex	5 mg/kg/day intravenously	No	Poor	Fever, rigors, nausea, hypotension, anemia, azotemia, tachypnea	Same as amphotericin B, above
Amphotericin B, liposomal	3–6 mg/kg/day intravenously	No	Poor	Fever, rigors, nausea, hypotension, azotemia, anemia, tachypnea, chest tightness	Same as amphotericin B, above Preferred agent for CNS
Azoles					
Fluconazole	Systemic infection: 400–2000 mg/day intravenously or orally Mucosal infection: 100–200 mg/day orally	Yes	Yes	Nausea, rash, xerosis, alopecia, headache, hepatic enzyme elevations	Mucosal candidiasis (including urinary tract), cryptococcosis, histoplasmosis, coccidioidomycosis
Isavuconazole	200 mg orally or intravenously every 8 hours for six doses (48 hours) as loading dose, followed by 200 mg/day orally or intravenously	No	Low in CSF, high in brain	Nausea, diarrhea, upper abdominal pain, dizziness	Broad range of activity including invasive aspergillosis and mucormycosis (limited data for *Mucorales*)
Itraconazole	Oral solution and capsule formulations available, both dosed at 200 mg three times daily for 3 days, then 200 mg once or twice daily[1]	No	Variable	Nausea, hypokalemia, edema, hypertension, peripheral neuropathy, exacerbation of heart failure	Histoplasmosis, coccidioidomycosis, blastomycosis, paracoccidioidomycosis, mucosal candidiasis (except urinary), sporotrichosis, aspergillosis, chromomycosis
SUBA-itraconazole	130 mg by mouth once daily (two 65-mg capsules)	No	Variable	Nausea, hypokalemia, edema, hypertension, peripheral neuropathy, exacerbation of heart failure	FDA-approved for treatment of histoplasmosis, blastomycosis, aspergillosis
Ketoconazole	200–800 mg/day orally in one or two doses with food or acidic beverage	No	Poor	Anorexia, nausea, suppression of testosterone and cortisol, rash, headache, hepatic enzyme elevations, hepatic failure	Nonmeningeal histoplasmosis and coccidioidomycosis, blastomycosis, paracoccidioidomycosis, mucosal candidiasis (except urinary)
Posaconazole	Delayed-release tablet formulation preferred over oral solution due to more predictable absorption For delayed-release tablet or intravenous formulation: 300 mg twice daily for two doses (1 day) as loading dose followed by 300 mg daily	No	Yes	Nausea, vomiting, abdominal pain, diarrhea, and headache; pseudohyperaldosteronism	Broad range of activity including the *Mucorales*

(*continued*)

Table 36–1. Agents for systemic mycoses.* (continued)

Drug	Dosing	Renal Clearance?	CSF Penetration?	Toxicities	Spectrum of Activity
Azoles (cont.)					
Voriconazole[2]	Systemic infection: 6 mg/kg intravenously every 12 hours for 24 hours loading dose, followed by 4 mg/kg intravenously every 12 hours or 200–300 mg orally every 12 hours Mucosal infection: 200–300 mg orally every 12 hours (no loading dose required)	Yes	Yes	Transient visual disturbances, rash, photosensitivity, fluoride excess with periostitis, peripheral neuropathy, squamous cell skin cancers, hepatic enzyme elevations[1]	All major pathogens except the *Mucorales* and sporotrichosis
Echinocandins					
Anidulafungin	200-mg intravenous loading dose, followed by 100 mg/day intravenously	< 1%	Poor	Diarrhea, hepatic enzyme elevations, histamine-mediated reactions	Mucosal and invasive candidiasis
Caspofungin acetate	70-mg intravenous loading dose, followed by 50 mg/day intravenously	< 50%[3]	Poor	Transient neutropenia; hepatic enzyme elevations when used with cyclosporine	Aspergillosis, mucosal and invasive candidiasis, empiric antifungal therapy in febrile neutropenia
Micafungin sodium	100 mg/day intravenously	No	Poor	Rash, rigors, headache, phlebitis	Mucosal and invasive candidiasis, prophylaxis in hematopoietic stem cell transplantation
Antimetabolite					
Flucytosine (5-FC)	100–150 mg/kg/day orally in four divided doses	Yes	Yes	Leukopenia,[4] rash, diarrhea, hepatitis, nausea, vomiting	Cryptococcosis,[5] candidiasis,[5] chromomycosis
Allylamine					
Terbinafine	250 mg once daily orally	Yes	Poor	Nausea, abdominal pain, taste disturbance, rash, diarrhea, and hepatic enzyme elevations	Dermatophytes, sporotrichosis, chromomycosis, eumycetoma
Triterpenoid (inhibits glucan synthase)					
Ibrexafungerp	300 mg orally every 12 hours for two doses (600 mg total) Dose reduction if concomitant use with CYP3A inhibitors	No	Unknown	Diarrhea, nausea, abdominal pain, dizziness, vomiting; may cause fetal harm (not for use in pregnancy)	Vaginal candidiasis (including azole-resistant strains)

**General information provided, but specific dosing may vary by indication and other patient characteristics; an infectious diseases specialist should be consulted for complex cases.*

[1]Oral solution preferred due to less variable absorption; capsule should be taken with food and acidic beverages to enhance absorption. For severe infections, blood levels should be measured to ensure adequate exposure.

[2]Some authorities advocate therapeutic drug monitoring in patients who are not responding to therapy. Administration with drugs that are metabolized by the cytochrome P450 system is contraindicated or requires careful monitoring of liver function. Intravenous formulation is contraindicated for patients with CrCl < 50 mL/minute because of accumulation of cyclodextrin.

[3]No dosage adjustment required for CKD; dosage adjustment necessary with moderate to severe hepatic dysfunction.

[4]Use should be monitored with blood levels to prevent this or the dose adjusted according to creatinine clearance.

[5]In combination with amphotericin B.

CSF, cerebrospinal fluid.

patchy early in infection. There may also be diffuse or focal consolidation, cystic changes, nodules, or cavitation within nodules. About 5–10% of patients with *Pneumocystis* pneumonia have normal chest films. High-resolution chest CT scans may be quite suggestive of *P jirovecii* pneumonia, helping distinguish it from other causes of pneumonia.

Treatment

It is appropriate to start empiric therapy for *P jirovecii* pneumonia if the disease is suspected clinically; however, in both patients with or without AIDS with mild to moderately severe disease, continued treatment should be based on a proven diagnosis because of clinical overlap with other infections, the toxicity of therapy, and the possible coexistence of other infectious organisms. Initial antimicrobial therapy (typically with TMP-SMX) should be continued for at least 5–10 days before considering changing agents, as fever, tachypnea, and pulmonary infiltrates persist for 4–6 days after starting treatment. Some patients have a transient worsening of their disease during the first 3–5 days, which may be related to an inflammatory response to dead or dying organisms. Early addition of corticosteroids may attenuate this response and improve clinical outcomes (see below).

A. Trimethoprim-Sulfamethoxazole

There are strong data indicating that TMP-SMZ is the optimal first-line therapy for *Pneumocystis* pneumonia. The dosage of TMP-SMZ is 15–20 mg/kg/day (based on trimethoprim component) given orally or intravenously daily in three or four divided doses for 14–21 days. Patients with AIDS have a high frequency of hypersensitivity reactions (approaching 50%), which may include fever, rashes (sometimes severe), malaise, neutropenia, hepatitis, nephritis, thrombocytopenia, hyperkalemia, and hyperbilirubinemia.

B. Primaquine/Clindamycin

Primaquine, 15–30 mg orally daily, plus clindamycin, 600 mg three times orally daily, is the best second-line therapy with superior results when compared with pentamidine. Primaquine may cause hemolytic anemia in patients with glucose-6-phosphate dehydrogenase (G6PD) deficiency.

C. Pentamidine Isethionate

The use of pentamidine has decreased as alternative agents have been studied. This medication is administered intravenously (preferred) or intramuscularly as a single dose of 3–4 mg (salt)/kg/day for 14–21 days. Pentamidine causes side effects in nearly 50% of patients. Hypoglycemia, hyperglycemia, hyponatremia, and nephrotoxicity with azotemia may occur. Inadvertent rapid intravenous infusion may cause precipitous hypotension.

D. Atovaquone

Atovaquone may be used for patients with mild to moderate disease who cannot tolerate TMP-SMZ or other alternative agents, but failure is reported in 15–30% of cases. Mild side effects are common, but no serious reactions have been reported. The dosage is 750 mg orally (taken with a fatty meal) two times daily for 14–21 days.

E. Other Medications

Trimethoprim, 15 mg/kg/day in three divided doses daily, plus dapsone, 100 mg/day, is an alternative oral regimen for mild to moderate disease or for continuation of therapy after intravenous therapy is no longer needed.

F. Prednisone

Based on studies done in patients with AIDS, prednisone is given for moderate to severe pneumonia (when PaO_2 on admission is less than 70 mm Hg or oxygen saturation is less than 90%) in conjunction with antimicrobials. The addition of corticosteroids in such patients is associated with significant reduction in morbidity and mortality; administration of adjunctive corticosteroids within 72 hours is preferred. The dosage of prednisone is 40 mg twice daily orally for 5 days, then 40 mg daily for 5 days, and then 20 mg daily until therapy is completed (total course, 21 days). Observational studies suggest that adjunctive corticosteroids are associated with reduced mortality in patients without AIDS with *Pneumocystis* pneumonia and severe hypoxia (PaO_2 60 mm Hg or less).

Prevention

Primary prophylaxis for *Pneumocystis* pneumonia in patients with HIV should be given to persons with CD4 counts less than 200 cells/mcL, a CD4 percentage below 14%, or weight loss or oral candidiasis. Primary prophylaxis is also beneficial in patients with hematologic malignancy and transplant recipients, and in patients receiving high-dose corticosteroid therapy, although precise recommendations for *Pneumocystis* prophylaxis in these settings have not been established. Persons living with HIV who have a history of *Pneumocystis* pneumonia should receive secondary prophylaxis until they have had a durable virologic response to antiretroviral therapy or maintained a CD4 count of greater than 200 cells/mcL for at least 3–6 months, or both.

Prognosis

In the absence of early and adequate treatment, the fatality rate for *Pneumocystis* pneumonia in immunodeficient persons is nearly 100%. Early treatment reduces the mortality rate to ~10–20% in patients with AIDS. The mortality rate in other immunodeficient patients is still 30–50%, probably because of delays in diagnosis. In immunodeficient patients who do not receive prophylaxis, recurrences are common (30% in AIDS).

Ding L et al. Adjunctive corticosteroids may be associated with better outcome for non-HIV *Pneumocystis* pneumonia with respiratory failure: a systemic review and meta-analysis of observational studies. Ann Intensive Care. 2020;10:34. [PMID: 32198645]

Li R et al. Efficacy and safety of trimethoprim-sulfamethoxazole for the prevention of pneumocystis pneumonia in human immunodeficiency virus-negative immunodeficient patients: a systematic review and meta-analysis. PLoS One. 2021;16:e0248524. [PMID: 33765022]

Panel on Guidelines for the Prevention and Treatment of Opportunistic Infections in Adults and Adolescents with HIV. Guidelines for the Prevention and Treatment of Opportunistic Infections in HIV-infected Adults and Adolescents: Recommendations from the Centers for Disease Control and Prevention, the National Institutes of Health, and the HIV Medicine Association of the Infectious Diseases Society of America. https://clinicalinfo.hiv.gov/sites/default/files/guidelines/documents/Adult_OI.pdf "Pneumocystis Pneumonia" reviewed 2021 Oct.

CRYPTOCOCCOSIS

ESSENTIALS OF DIAGNOSIS

- Most common cause of fungal meningitis.
- Predisposing factors: chemotherapy for hematologic malignancies, Hodgkin lymphoma, corticosteroids, structural lung diseases, transplant recipients, TNF-alpha inhibitors, and AIDS.
- Headache, abnormal mental status; meningismus seen occasionally, although rarely in patients with AIDS.
- Demonstration of capsular polysaccharide antigen or positive culture in CSF is diagnostic.

General Considerations

Cryptococcosis is mainly caused by *Cryptococcus neoformans*, an encapsulated budding yeast that has been found worldwide in soil and on dried pigeon dung. *Cryptococcus gattii* is a closely related species that also causes disease in humans, although *C gattii* may affect more ostensibly immunocompetent persons. It is a major cause of cryptococcosis in the Pacific northwestern region of the United States and may result in more severe disease than *C neoformans*.

Infections are acquired by inhalation. In the lung, the infection may remain localized, heal, or disseminate. Clinically apparent cryptococcal pneumonia rarely develops in immunocompetent persons. Progressive lung disease and dissemination most often occur in the setting of cellular immunodeficiency, including hematologic malignancies under treatment, Hodgkin lymphoma, long-term corticosteroid therapy, solid organ transplant, TNF-alpha inhibitor therapy, or uncontrolled HIV infection.

Clinical Findings

A. Symptoms and Signs

Pulmonary disease ranges from simple nodules to widespread infiltrates leading to respiratory failure. Disseminated disease may involve any organ, but CNS disease predominates. Headache is usually the first symptom of meningitis. Confusion and other mental status changes as well as cranial nerve abnormalities, nausea, and vomiting may be seen as the disease progresses. Nuchal rigidity and meningeal signs occur about 50% of the time but are uncommon in patients with AIDS. Communicating hydrocephalus may complicate the course. *C gattii* infection frequently presents with respiratory symptoms along with neurologic signs caused by space-occupying lesions in the CNS. Primary *C neoformans* infection of the skin may mimic bacterial cellulitis, especially in persons receiving immunosuppressive therapy such as corticosteroids. The immune reconstitution inflammatory syndrome (IRIS), which is paradoxical clinical worsening associated with improved immunologic status, can occur in patients with HIV and transplant recipients with cryptococcosis, as well as patients without AIDS being treated for *C gattii* infection.

B. Laboratory Findings

Respiratory tract disease is diagnosed by culture of respiratory secretions or pleural fluid. For suspected meningeal disease, lumbar puncture is the preferred diagnostic procedure. Spinal fluid findings include increased opening pressure, variable pleocytosis, increased protein, and decreased glucose, although as many as 50% of patients with AIDS have no pleocytosis. Gram stain of the CSF usually reveals budding, encapsulated fungi. In patients with AIDS, the serum cryptococcal antigen is a sensitive screening test for meningitis, being positive in over 95% of cases. Cryptococcal capsular antigen in CSF and culture together establish the diagnosis over 90% of the time. Antigen testing by lateral flow assay has improved sensitivity and specificity over the conventional latex agglutination test and can provide more rapid diagnostic results. MRI is more sensitive than CT in finding CNS abnormalities, such as cryptococcomas.

Treatment

Because of decreased efficacy, initial therapy with an azole alone is not recommended for treatment of acute cryptococcal meningitis. Liposomal amphotericin B, 3–4 mg/kg/day intravenously for 14 days, is the preferred agent for **induction therapy**, followed by an additional 8 weeks of fluconazole, 400 mg/day orally for **consolidation** (Table 36–1). This regimen achieves clinical responses and CSF sterilization in over 70% of patients. The addition of flucytosine has been associated with improved survival, but toxicity is common. Flucytosine is administered orally at a dose of 100 mg/kg/day divided into four equal doses and given every 6 hours. Hematologic parameters should be closely monitored during flucytosine therapy, and it is important to adjust the dose for any decreases in kidney function. Fluconazole (800–1200 mg orally daily) may be given with amphotericin B when flucytosine is not available or patients cannot tolerate it. Frequent, repeated lumbar punctures or ventricular shunting should be performed to relieve high CSF pressures or if hydrocephalus is a complication. *Failure to adequately relieve raised intracranial pressure is a major cause of morbidity and mortality.* Corticosteroids should not be used. The end points for amphotericin B therapy and for switching to **maintenance** with oral fluconazole are a favorable clinical response (decrease in temperature; improvement in headache, nausea, vomiting, and Mini-Mental State Examination scores), improvement in CSF biochemical parameters and, most importantly, conversion of CSF culture to negative.

A similar approach is reasonable for patients with cryptococcal meningitis in the absence of AIDS, although the mortality rate is higher. Therapy is generally continued until CSF cultures become negative. **Maintenance** antifungal therapy is important after treatment of an acute episode in AIDS-related cases, since otherwise the rate of relapse is greater than 50%. Fluconazole, 200 mg/day orally, is the maintenance therapy of choice, decreasing the relapse rate approximately tenfold compared with placebo and threefold compared with weekly amphotericin B in patients whose CSF has been sterilized by the induction therapy. After successful therapy of cryptococcal meningitis, it is possible to discontinue secondary prophylaxis with fluconazole in individuals with AIDS who have had a satisfactory response to antiretroviral therapy (eg, CD4 cell count greater than 100–200 cells/mcL for at least 6 months). Published guidelines suggest that 6–12 months of fluconazole can be used as maintenance therapy in patients without AIDS following successful treatment of the acute illness.

Prognosis

Factors that indicate a poor prognosis include the activity of the predisposing conditions, older age, organ failure, lack of spinal fluid pleocytosis, high initial antigen titer in either serum or CSF, decreased mental status, increased intracranial pressure, and the presence of disease outside the nervous system.

Gushiken AC et al. Cryptococcosis. Infect Dis Clin North Am. 2021;35:493. [PMID: 34016288]

Panel on Guidelines for the Prevention and Treatment of Opportunistic Infections in Adults and Adolescents with HIV. Guidelines for the Prevention and Treatment of Opportunistic Infections in HIV-infected Adults and Adolescents: Recommendations from the Centers for Disease Control and Prevention, the National Institutes of Health, and the HIV Medicine Association of the Infectious Diseases Society of America. https://clinicalinfo.hiv.gov/sites/default/files/guidelines/documents/Adult_OI.pdf "Cryptococcosis" updated 2021 Jul.

ASPERGILLOSIS

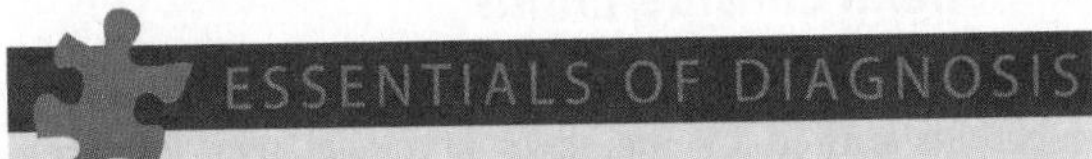

- Most common cause of non-candidal invasive fungal infection in transplant recipients and in patients with hematologic malignancies.
- Risk factors for invasive disease: leukemia, hematopoietic stem cell or solid organ transplantation, corticosteroid use, advanced AIDS, and COVID-19 coinfection.
- Pulmonary, sinus, and CNS are most common disease sites.
- Detection of galactomannan in serum or other body fluids is useful for early diagnosis in at-risk patients.

General Considerations

Aspergillus fumigatus is the usual cause of aspergillosis, though many species of *Aspergillus* may cause a wide spectrum of disease. The lungs, sinuses, and brain are the organs most often involved. Clinical illness results either from an aberrant immunologic response or tissue invasion.

Clinical Findings

A. Symptoms and Signs

1. Allergic forms of aspergillosis—Allergic bronchopulmonary aspergillosis (ABPA) occurs in patients with preexisting asthma or cystic fibrosis. Patients develop worsening bronchospasm and fleeting pulmonary infiltrates. Allergic *Aspergillus* sinusitis produces a chronic sinus inflammation characterized by eosinophilic mucus and noninvasive hyphal elements.

2. Chronic aspergillosis—Chronic pulmonary aspergillosis usually occurs when there is preexisting lung damage without significant immunocompromise. Disease manifestations range from aspergillomas that develop in a lung cavity to chronic fibrosing pulmonary aspergillosis in which most of the lung tissue is replaced with fibrosis. Long-standing (longer than 3 months) pulmonary and systemic symptoms such as cough, shortness of breath, weight loss, and malaise are common.

3. Invasive aspergillosis—Invasive aspergillosis most commonly occurs in profoundly immunodeficient patients, such as those who have undergone hematopoietic stem cell transplantation or have prolonged, severe neutropenia, but it can occur among critically ill immunocompetent patients as well. Tracheobronchitis and pulmonary aspergillosis have also been observed in association with severe COVID-19 infection. Pulmonary disease is most common, with patchy infiltration leading to a severe necrotizing pneumonia. Invasive sinus disease also occurs. At any time, there may be hematogenous dissemination to the CNS, skin, and other organs. Early diagnosis and reversal of any correctable immunosuppression are essential.

B. Laboratory Findings

In ABPA, there is eosinophilia with high levels of IgE and IgG *Aspergillus* precipitins in the blood.

For invasive aspergillosis, definitive diagnosis requires demonstration of *Aspergillus* in tissue or culture from a sterile site; however, given the morbidity of the disease and the low yield of culture, clinicians must maintain a high index of suspicion and use a combination of host, radiologic, and mycologic criteria to yield a probable diagnosis of invasive aspergillosis in at-risk patients. Indirect diagnostic assays include detection of galactomannan in bronchoalveolar lavage fluid or serum or serum assays for (1,3)-beta-D-glucan (though the latter is not specific for *Aspergillus*). To improve the reliability of galactomannan testing, multiple determinations should be done, though sensitivity is decreased in patients receiving anti-mold prophylaxis (ie, voriconazole or posaconazole). Galactomannan levels and Aspergillus DNA PCR can be tested in serum or in bronchoalveolar lavage fluid, which may be more sensitive than serum. Higher galactomannan levels are correlated with increased mortality, and failure of galactomannan levels to fall in response to therapy portends a worse outcome. Isolation of *Aspergillus* from pulmonary secretions does not necessarily imply invasive disease, although its positive predictive value increases with more advanced immunosuppression. Clinical suspicion for invasive aspergillosis should prompt CT scanning of the chest, which may aid in early detection and help direct additional diagnostic procedures. Common radiologic findings include nodules; wedge-shaped infarcts; or a characteristic "halo sign," a zone of diminution of ground glass around a consolidation.

Prevention

The high mortality rate and difficulty in diagnosis of invasive aspergillosis often lead clinicians to institute prophylactic therapy for patients with profound immunosuppression. The best-studied agents include posaconazole (300 mg orally daily) and voriconazole (200 mg orally twice daily). Widespread use of broad-spectrum azoles raises concern for development of breakthrough invasive disease by highly resistant fungi.

Treatment

1. Allergic forms of aspergillosis—Itraconazole is the best-studied agent for the treatment of allergic *Aspergillus* sinusitis with topical corticosteroids being the cornerstone of therapy for ongoing care. For acute exacerbations of ABPA, oral prednisone is begun at a dose of 0.5 mg/kg/day and then tapered slowly over several months. Itraconazole at a dose of 200 mg orally daily for 16 weeks appears to improve pulmonary function and decrease corticosteroid requirements in these patients; voriconazole is an alternative agent.

2. Chronic aspergillosis—The most effective therapy for symptomatic aspergilloma is surgical resection. Other forms of chronic aspergillosis are generally treated with at least 4–6 months of oral azole therapy (itraconazole 200 mg twice daily, voriconazole 200 mg twice daily, or posaconazole 300 mg daily).

3. Invasive aspergillosis—The 2016 Infectious Diseases Society of America guidelines consider voriconazole (6 mg/kg intravenously twice on day 1 and then 4 mg/kg every 12 hours thereafter) as optimal therapy for invasive aspergillosis. However, the 2017 European Society for Clinical Microbiology and Infectious Diseases, the European Confederation of Medical Mycology, and the European Respiratory Society (ESCMID-ECMM-ERS) joint clinical guidelines indicate either isavuconazole (200 mg intravenously every 8 hours for six doses, then 200 mg daily) or voriconazole as first-line therapy. Other alternatives include a lipid formulation amphotericin B (3–5 mg/kg/day), caspofungin (70 mg intravenously on day 1, then 50 mg/day thereafter), micafungin (100–150 mg intravenously daily), and posaconazole oral tablets (300 mg twice daily on day 1, then 300 mg daily thereafter).

Treatment duration may vary depending on the clinical response but 6–12 weeks is generally recommended. Antifungal susceptibility testing of *Aspergillus* isolates is recommended in patients who are unresponsive to therapy or with clinical suspicion for azole resistance. Therapeutic drug monitoring should be considered for both voriconazole and posaconazole given variations in metabolism and absorption.

Surgical debridement is generally done for sinusitis, and can be useful for focal pulmonary lesions, especially for treatment of life-threatening hemoptysis and infections recalcitrant to medical therapy. The mortality rate of pulmonary or disseminated disease in the immunocompromised patient remains high, particularly in patients with refractory neutropenia.

Thompson GR 3rd et al. *Aspergillus* infections. N Engl J Med. 2021;385:1496. [PMID: 34644473]

Ullmann AJ et al. Diagnosis and management of *Aspergillus* diseases: executive summary of the 2017 ESCMID-ECMM-ERS guideline. Clin Microbiol Infect. 2018;24:e1. [PMID: 29544767]

MUCORMYCOSIS

ESSENTIALS OF DIAGNOSIS

- Most common cause of non-*Aspergillus* invasive mold infection.
- Risk factors: uncontrolled diabetes, hematologic malignancy, hematopoietic stem cell or solid organ transplantation, direct inoculation of wounds (trauma, burns), and COVID-19.
- Pulmonary, rhino-orbital-cerebral, and skin are most common disease sites.
- Rapidly fatal without multidisciplinary interventions.

General Considerations

The term "mucormycosis" is applied to opportunistic infections caused by members of the genera *Rhizopus, Mucor, Lichtheimia* (formerly *Absidia*), *Saksenaea, Apophysomyces*, and *Cunninghamella*. Predisposing conditions include hematologic malignancy; hematopoietic or solid organ transplantation; diabetes; iron overload; or treatment with desferoxamine, corticosteroids, or cytotoxic drugs. COVID-19 has been associated with increased rates of mucormycosis, particularly rhino-orbital-cerebral disease. Immunocompetent patients may develop infection due to direct inoculation of wounds such as due to trauma or burns.

Clinical Findings

Invasive disease of the sinuses, orbits, and the lungs may occur. Diabetes is associated with rhino-orbital-cerebral disease, while hematologic malignancy predisposes to pulmonary infection. Necrosis is common due to hyphal tissue invasion that may manifest as ulceration of the palate or hemoptysis. Widely disseminated disease can occur. Biopsy of involved tissue remains the cornerstone of diagnosis; the organisms appear in tissue as broad, branching nonseptate hyphae. Molecular identification (eg, PCR) from tissue or blood may aid in the diagnosis; cultures are frequently negative. A reverse "halo sign" (focal area of ground-glass diminution surrounded by a ring of consolidation) may be seen on chest CT.

Treatment

Optimal therapy of mucormycosis involves reversal of predisposing conditions (if possible), surgical debridement, and prompt antifungal therapy. A prolonged course of intravenous liposomal amphotericin B (5–10 mg/kg with higher doses given for CNS disease) should be started early. Oral posaconazole (300 mg/day) or isavuconazole (200 mg every 8 hours for 1–2 days, then 200 mg daily thereafter) can be used for less severe disease, as step-down therapy after disease stabilization, or as salvage therapy due to poor response to or tolerance of amphotericin. Combination therapy with amphotericin and posaconazole or isavuconazole is not proven but is commonly used because of the poor response to monotherapy. Control of diabetes and other underlying conditions, along with extensive repeated surgical removal of necrotic, nonperfused tissue, is essential. Even when these measures are introduced in a timely fashion, the prognosis remains guarded.

Brunet K et al. Mucormycosis treatment: recommendations, latest advances, and perspectives. J Mycol Med. 2020;30:101007. [PMID: 32718789]

Cornely OA et al. Global guideline for the diagnosis and management of mucormycosis: an initiative of the European Confederation of Medical Mycology in cooperation with the Mycoses Study Group Education and Research Consortium. Lancet Infect Dis. 2019;19:e405. [PMID: 31699664]

Skiada A et al. Epidemiology and diagnosis of mucormycosis: an update. J Fungi (Basel). 2020;6:265. [PMID: 33147877]

BLASTOMYCOSIS

Blastomycosis occurs most often in men infected during occupational or recreational activities outdoors and in a geographically limited area of the south, central, and midwestern United States and Canada. Disease usually occurs in immunocompetent individuals.

Pulmonary infection is most common and may be asymptomatic. With dissemination, lesions most frequently occur in the skin, bones, and urogenital system.

Cough, moderate fever, dyspnea, and chest pain are common. These may resolve or progress, with purulent sputum production, pleurisy, fever, chills, loss of weight, and prostration. Radiologic studies, either chest radiographs or CT scans, usually reveal lobar consolidation or masses.

Raised, verrucous cutaneous lesions are commonly present in disseminated blastomycosis. Bones—often the ribs and vertebrae—are frequently involved. Epididymitis, prostatitis, and other involvement of the male urogenital system may occur. Although they do not appear to be at greater risk for acquisition of disease, infection in people with HIV may progress rapidly, with dissemination common.

Laboratory findings usually include leukocytosis and anemia. The organism is found in clinical specimens, such as expectorated sputum or tissue biopsies, as a 5–20 mcm thick-walled cell with a single broad-based bud. It grows readily on culture. A urinary antigen test is available, but it has considerable cross reactivity with other dimorphic fungi; it may be useful in monitoring disease resolution or progression. A serum enzyme immunoassay based on the surface protein BAD-1 has much better sensitivity and specificity than the urinary antigen test. The quantitative antigen enzyme immunoassay may be helpful in the diagnosis of CNS disease.

Itraconazole, 200–400 mg/day orally for at least 6–12 months, is the therapy of choice for nonmeningeal disease, with a response rate of over 80% (Table 36–1). Liposomal amphotericin B, 3–5 mg/kg/day intravenously, should be given initially for severe disease, treatment failures, or CNS involvement.

Clinical follow-up for relapse should be made regularly for several years so that therapy may be resumed, or another drug instituted.

Mazi PB et al. Blastomycosis. Infect Dis Clin North Am. 2021;35:515. [PMID: 34016289]

SPOROTRICHOSIS

Sporotrichosis is a chronic fungal infection caused by organisms of the *Sporothrix schenckii* complex. It is worldwide in distribution; most patients have had contact with soil, sphagnum moss, or decaying wood. Infection takes place when the organism is inoculated into the skin—usually on the hand, arm, or foot, especially during gardening, or puncture from a rose thorn.

The most common form of sporotrichosis begins with a hard, nontender subcutaneous nodule. This later becomes adherent to the overlying skin and ulcerates. Within a few days to weeks, lymphocutaneous spread along the lymphatics draining this area occurs, which may result in ulceration. Cavitary pulmonary disease occurs in individuals with underlying chronic lung disease.

Disseminated sporotrichosis is rare in immunocompetent persons but may present with widespread cutaneous, lung, bone, joint, and CNS involvement in immunocompromised patients, especially those with cellular immunodeficiencies, including AIDS and alcohol abuse.

Cultures are needed to establish diagnosis. The usefulness of serologic tests is limited, but may be helpful in diagnosing disseminated disease, especially meningitis.

Itraconazole, 200–400 mg orally daily for several months, is the treatment of choice for localized disease and some milder cases of disseminated disease (Table 36–1). Terbinafine, 500 mg orally twice daily, also has good efficacy in lymphocutaneous disease. Amphotericin B intravenously, 0.7–1.0 mg/kg/day, or a lipid amphotericin B preparation, 3–5 mg/kg/day, is used for severe systemic infection. Surgery may be indicated for complicated pulmonary cavitary disease, and joint involvement may require arthrodesis.

The prognosis is good for lymphocutaneous sporotrichosis; pulmonary, joint, and disseminated disease respond less favorably.

Orofino-Costa R et al. Sporotrichosis: an update on epidemiology, etiopathogenesis, laboratory and clinical therapeutics. An Bras Dermatol. 2017;92:606. [PMID: 29166494]

MYCETOMA (Eumycetoma & Actinomycetoma)

Mycetoma is a chronic local, slowly progressive destructive infection that usually involves the foot; it begins in subcutaneous tissues, frequently after implantation of vegetative material into tissues during occupational activities. The infection then spreads to contiguous structures with sinus tracts and extruding grains. Eumycetoma (also known as maduromycosis) is the term used to describe mycetoma caused by true fungi. The disease begins as a papule, nodule, or abscess that over months to years progresses slowly to form multiple abscesses and sinus tracts ramifying deep into the tissue. Secondary bacterial infection may result in large open ulcers. Radiographs may show destructive changes in the underlying bone. Causative species can often be suggested by the color of the characteristic grains and hyphal size within the infected tissues, but definitive diagnosis requires culture.

The prognosis for eumycetoma is poor, though surgical debridement along with prolonged oral itraconazole therapy, 200 mg twice daily, or combination therapy including itraconazole and terbinafine, may result in a response rate of 70% (Table 36–1). The various etiologic agents may respond differently to antifungal agents, so culture results are invaluable. Amputation is necessary in far advanced cases.

Agarwal P et al. Clinical features of mycetoma and the appropriate treatment options. Res Rep Trop Med. 2021;12:173. [PMID: 34267575]

OTHER OPPORTUNISTIC MOLD INFECTIONS

Fungi previously considered to be harmless colonizers, including *Pseudallescheria boydii (Scedosporium apiospermum), Scedosporium prolificans, Fusarium, Paecilomyces, Trichoderma longibrachiatium*, and *Trichosporon*, are now significant pathogens in immunocompromised patients. Opportunistic infections with these agents are seen in patients being treated for hematologic malignancies, in hematopoietic stem cell or organ transplant recipients, and in those receiving broad-spectrum antifungal prophylaxis. Infection may be localized in the skin, lungs, or sinuses, or widespread disease may appear with lesions in multiple organs. Fusariosis should be suspected in severely immunosuppressed persons in whom multiple, painful skin lesions develop; blood cultures are often positive. Sinus infection may cause bony erosion. Infection in subcutaneous tissues following traumatic inoculation may develop as a well-circumscribed cyst or as an ulcer.

Nonpigmented septate hyphae are seen in tissue and are indistinguishable from those of *Aspergillus* when infections are due to *S apiospermum* or species of *Fusarium, Paecilomyces, Penicillium*, or other hyaline molds. The differentiation of *S apiospermum* and *Aspergillus* is particularly important, since the former is uniformly resistant to amphotericin B but may be sensitive to azole antifungals (eg, voriconazole). Treatment of fusariosis may include amphotericin, voriconazole, or combination therapy; there are limited data on the use of isavuconazole or posaconazole for this disease. In addition to antifungal therapy, reversal of underlying immunosuppression is an essential component of treatment for these invasive mold infections.

Infection by melanin-pigmented dematiaceous or "black" molds is designated as phaeohyphomycosis. These black molds (eg, *Exophiala, Bipolaris, Cladophialophora, Curvularia, Alternaria*) are common in the environment, especially on decaying vegetation. In tissues of patients with phaeohyphomycosis, the mold is seen as black or faintly brown hyphae, yeast cells, or both. Culture on appropriate medium is needed to identify the agent. Histologic demonstration of these organisms provides definitive evidence of invasive infection; positive cultures must be interpreted cautiously and not assumed to be contaminants in immunocompromised hosts.

Arcobello JT et al. Phaeohyphomycosis. Semin Respir Crit Care Med. 2020;41:131. [PMID: 32000289]

HOUSEHOLD MOLDS

ESSENTIALS OF DIAGNOSIS

- Molds are very common indoors where moisture exists in enclosed spaces.
- Most common indoor molds are *Cladosporium, Penicillium, Aspergillus*, and *Alternaria*.
- People most at risk for health problems include those with allergies, asthma, and underlying immunocompromising conditions.

Molds are commonly present in homes, particularly in the presence of moisture, and patients will commonly seek assessment for whether their illness is due to molds. Well-established health problems due to molds can be considered in three categories: (1) There is the potential for allergy to environmental mold species, which can manifest in the typical manner with allergic symptoms such as rhinitis and eye irritation. Furthermore, in predisposed individuals, exposure to certain molds can trigger asthma or asthmatic attacks. These types of manifestations are reversible with appropriate therapies. More chronic allergic effects can be seen with disorders such as ABPA (see Allergic Forms of Aspergillosis); (2) Susceptible individuals can develop hypersensitivity reactions upon exposure to mold antigens; these include occupational disorders (eg, farmer's lung and pigeon breeder's disease) as well as hypersensitivity pneumonitis in response to a large antigenic exposure. Affected patients have fever, lymph node swelling, and pulmonary infiltrates. These disease manifestations are transient and improve with removal of the offending antigen; (3) Invasive mold disease (see Invasive Aspergillosis).

At the present time, there are no data to support that mold exposure can induce immune dysfunction. Similarly, the concept of toxic-mold syndrome or cognitive impairment due to inhalation of mycotoxins has not been validated despite scrutiny by expert panels. The presence of mold in the household is typically easily discernable with visual inspection or detection by odor; if present, predisposing conditions should be corrected by individuals experienced in mold remediation.

Several laboratories offer testing for the evaluation of patients who suspect they have a mold-induced disorder, such as testing homes for mold spores, measuring urinary "mycotoxins," and performing serum IgG assays to molds. However, these tests should not be obtained as most are not validated and do not provide meaningful results upon which to make therapeutic decisions.

Borchers AT et al. Mold and human health: a reality check. Clin Rev Allergy Immunol. 2017;52:305. [PMID: 28299723]

Chang C et al. The myth of mycotoxins and mold injury. Clin Rev Allergy Immunol. 2019;57:449. [PMID: 31608429]

Disorders Related to Environmental Emergencies

Jacqueline A. Nemer, MD, FACEP
Marianne A. Juarez, MD

COLD & HEAT

The human body maintains a steady temperature through the balance of internal heat production and environmental heat loss. Heat exchange between the body and environment occurs via four common processes: radiation, evaporation, conduction, and convection. In extreme temperatures, the body's thermoregulation may fail, resulting in the core body temperature moving toward the temperature of the external environment. Cold and heat exposure may cause a wide spectrum of conditions ranging in severity from mild, to potentially life-threatening, to death. Many of these conditions are preventable with appropriate education and planning.

The likelihood and severity of extreme temperature-related conditions depend on physiologic and environmental factors. Physiologic risk factors include extremes of age; cognitive impairment; poor physical conditioning, sedentary lifestyle, or immobility; poor acclimatization; concurrent injury; prior temperature-related injury; and numerous underlying medical conditions, especially those affecting cognition and thermoregulation. Pharmacologic risk factors include medications, holistic or alternative treatments, illicit drugs, tobacco, and alcohol. Medications impacting sweating and the CNS, or affecting cutaneous blood flow, such as peripheral vasoconstrictors or vasodilators, are more likely to worsen temperature-related conditions. Environmental risk factors include changing weather conditions, inadequate clothing or housing (homelessness, or housing with inadequate temperature control), and occupational or recreational exposure.

DISORDERS DUE TO HEAT

ESSENTIALS OF DIAGNOSIS

- Spectrum of preventable heat-related illnesses: heat cramps, heat exhaustion, heat syncope, and heat stroke.
- **Heat stroke:** hyperthermia with cerebral dysfunction in a patient with heat exposure.
- **Best outcome:** early recognition, initiation of rapid cooling, and avoidance of shivering during cooling; delays in cooling result in higher morbidity and mortality in heat stroke patients.
- **Best choice of cooling method:** whichever can be instituted the fastest with the least compromise to the patient.

General Considerations

Heat-related illnesses are among the most commonly seen environmental emergencies presenting to emergency departments. The amount of heat retained in the body is determined by internal metabolic function and environmental conditions, including temperature and humidity. Hyperthermia results from the body's inability to maintain normal internal temperature through heat loss, from either compromised heat dissipation mechanisms or abnormally high heat production. Increased metabolic rate is the most important factor in elevation of body temperature. Heat loss occurs primarily through sweating and peripheral vasodilation. The direct transfer of heat from the skin to the surrounding air, by convection or conduction, occurs with diminishing efficiency as ambient temperature rises, especially above 37.2°C (the point at which heat transfer reverses direction). At normal temperatures, evaporation accounts for approximately 20% of the body's heat loss, but at high temperatures it becomes the primary mechanism for dissipation of heat. This mechanism diminishes as humidity rises.

Heat stress can be caused by a combination of environmental and metabolic heat. Climate change may significantly contribute to the risk of heat-related conditions.

There is a spectrum of preventable heat stress conditions, ranging from mild forms, such as heat cramps, to severe forms, such as heat stroke. Risk factors include longer duration of exertion, hot environment, insufficient acclimatization, and dehydration. Additional risk factors include skin disorders or other medical conditions that inhibit sweat production or evaporation, obesity, prolonged seizures, hypotension, reduced cutaneous blood flow, reduced cardiac output, the use of drugs that increase metabolism or muscle activity or impair sweating, and withdrawal syndromes. Illicit drugs can cause increased muscle activity and thus generate increased body heat.

Classic (nonexertional) heat-related illness may occur in any individual in a hot, relaxing environment with increased severity in individuals with the risk factors mentioned above, despite minimal physical activity.

Heat cramps are exercise-associated painful involuntary muscle contractions during or immediately after exercise. They result from dilutional hyponatremia as sweat losses are replaced with water alone. **Heat exhaustion** is characterized by dehydration, sodium depletion, or isotonic fluid loss with accompanying cardiovascular changes. It results from prolonged strenuous activity in a hot environment without adequate water or salt intake.

Heat syncope is defined as a transient loss of consciousness with spontaneous return to normal mentation. It results from volume depletion and cutaneous vasodilation with subsequent systemic and cerebral hypotension. Exercise-associated postural hypotension is usually the cause of heat syncope and may occur during or immediately following exercise. **Heat stroke** is a severe form of heat-related illness resulting in cerebral dysfunction with core body temperature over 40°C. It may present in one of two forms: classic and exertional. **Classic (nonexertional) heat stroke** occurs in patients with impaired thermoregulatory mechanisms or in extreme environmental conditions. **Exertional heat stroke** occurs in healthy persons undergoing strenuous exertion in a hot or humid environment. Persons at greatest risk are those who are at the extremes of age, chronically debilitated, or taking medications that interfere with heat-dissipating mechanisms.

Clinical Findings

When diagnosing and treating heat-related illnesses, it is necessary to use an internal (rectal, Foley, or esophageal) thermometer since the skin temperature may not accurately reflect core body temperature. **Heat cramps** are painful skeletal muscle contractions and severe muscle spasms with onset during or shortly after exercise. Examination findings typically include stable vital signs; normal or slightly increased core body temperature; moist and cool skin; and tender, hard, lumpy, painful muscles that may be twitching. The diagnosis is made clinically.

Heat exhaustion is diagnosed based on symptoms and clinical findings of a core body temperature slightly elevated but less than 40°C, tachycardia, and moist skin. Symptoms are similar to those of heat cramps and heat syncope. Additional symptoms include nausea, vomiting, malaise, myalgias, hyperventilation, thirst, and weakness. CNS symptoms include headache, dizziness, fatigue, anxiety, paresthesias, impaired judgment, and occasionally psychosis. Heat exhaustion may progress to heat stroke if sweating ceases and mental status declines.

Heat syncope generally occurs in the setting of prolonged vigorous physical activity or prolonged standing in a hot humid environment followed by sudden collapse. Physical examination may reveal cool and moist skin, a weak pulse, and low systolic blood pressure.

Heat stroke is a life-threatening emergency. The hallmark of heat stroke is cerebral dysfunction when the core body temperature is over 40°C. Presenting symptoms include all findings seen in heat exhaustion with additional neurologic symptoms such as dizziness, weakness, emotional lability, confusion, delirium, blurred vision, convulsions, collapse, and unconsciousness. Physical examination findings may be variable and therefore unreliable. Exertional heat stroke may present with sudden collapse and loss of consciousness followed by irrational behavior. Sweating may not be present. Clinicians must be vigilant in monitoring for kidney injury, liver failure, metabolic derangements, respiratory compromise, coagulopathy, and ischemia since initial laboratory findings may be nonspecific.

Treatment

A. Heat Cramps

Move the patient to a shaded, cool environment and provide oral isotonic or hypertonic rehydration solution to replace both electrolytes and water. *Oral salt tablets are not recommended.* Advise the patient to rest for at least 2 days with continued dietary supplementation before returning to work or resuming strenuous activity in the heat.

B. Heat Exhaustion

Move the patient to a shaded, cool environment, provide adequate fluid and electrolyte replacement, and initiate active cooling measures if necessary. Physiologic saline or isotonic glucose solution may be administered intravenously when oral administration is not appropriate. At least 48 hours of rest and rehydration are recommended.

C. Heat Syncope

Treatment is essentially the same as for heat exhaustion: rest and recumbency in a shaded, cool place, and fluid and electrolyte replacement by mouth, or intravenously if necessary.

D. Heat Stroke

Initially, the patient's ABCs (airway, breathing, circulation) must be addressed and stabilized, then treatment is aimed at rapidly reducing the core body temperature within 1 hour while supporting circulation and perfusion. Patients should be placed on pulse oximetry and cardiac monitors while continuing to measure core body temperature and fluid intake and output. The patient should be observed for complications such as hypovolemic or cardiogenic shock, metabolic abnormalities, cardiac arrhythmias, coagulopathy, acute respiratory distress syndrome (ARDS), hypoglycemia, rhabdomyolysis, seizures, organ dysfunction, infection, and severe edema that can progress to a compartment syndrome. Circulatory failure in heat-related illness is mostly due to shock from relative or absolute hypovolemia. Oral or intravenous fluid administration must be provided to ensure adequate urinary output. Clinicians must also assess for and treat concurrent conditions such as infection, trauma, and drug effects.

Choice of cooling method depends on which can be instituted the fastest with the least compromise to the overall care of the patient. Evaporative cooling is preferred for nonexertional heat stroke and conductive-based cooling for exertional heat stroke. **Evaporative cooling** is a noninvasive, effective, quick, and easy way to reduce temperature. This is accomplished by placing the undressed patient in lateral recumbent position or supported in a hands-and-knees position to expose maximum skin surface to the air while the entire undressed body is sprayed with lukewarm water (20°C) and cooled by large fans circulating room air. Addition of inhaled cool air or oxygen may aid in cooling but must not be used alone. **Conductive-based cooling** involves cool fluid infusion, gastric or bladder lavage, ice packs, and immersion into ice water or cool water. Ice water or cold water immersion is the preferred method of cooling for exertional heat stroke in the field when available. Ice packs are most effective when covering the whole body, as opposed to the traditional method of placing them in the axilla and groin only. Intravascular heat exchange catheter systems as well as hemodialysis using cold dialysate (30–35°C) have also been successful in reducing core body temperature.

Shivering must be avoided because it inhibits the effectiveness of cooling by increasing internal heat production. Medications can be used to suppress shivering including magnesium, quick-acting opioid analgesics, benzodiazepines, and quick-acting anesthetic agents. Skin massage is recommended to prevent cutaneous vasoconstriction. *Antipyretics (aspirin, acetaminophen) have no effect on environmentally induced hyperthermia and are contraindicated.* Treatment must be continued until the core body temperature drops to 39°C.

Prevention

Education is necessary to improve prevention and early recognition of heat-related disorders. Individuals may take steps to reduce personal risk factors and to gradually acclimatize to hot environments. For prevention of occupational heat-related illness, a comprehensive preventive program should assess personal risk factors, estimated wet-bulb globe temperature, workload, acclimatization status, and early symptom recognition.

Coaches, athletic trainers, athletes, and parents of young athletes must be educated about heat-related illness, specifically about prevention, risks, symptoms and signs, and treatment. Medical evaluation and monitoring should be used to identify at-risk individuals and weather conditions that increase the risk of heat-related disorders.

Those who are physically active in a hot environment must increase fluid consumption before, during, and after physical activities. Fluid consumption should include balanced electrolyte fluids and water. Water consumption alone may lead to electrolyte imbalance, particularly hyponatremia. *It is not recommended to have salt tablets available for use because of the risk of hypertonic hypernatremia.* Close monitoring of fluid and electrolyte intake and early intervention are recommended in situations necessitating exertion or activity in hot environments.

Prognosis

Mortality is high from heat stroke, most frequently secondary to multiorgan dysfunction. The patient is also at risk for rhabdomyolysis, ARDS, and inflammation even after core temperature has normalized. Following heat stroke, immediate re-exposure to ambient heat must be avoided.

When to Refer

Potential consultants include a surgeon for suspicion of compartment syndrome, nephrologist for kidney injury, and transplant surgeon for fulminant liver failure.

When to Admit

All patients with suspected heat stroke must be admitted to a hospital with intensive care capability for close monitoring.

Epstein Y et al. Heatstroke. N Engl J Med. 2019;380:2449. [PMID: 31216400]

Gauer R et al. Heat-related illnesses. Am Fam Physician. 2019;99:482. [PMID: 30990296]

King MA et al. Influence of prior illness on exertional heat stroke presentation and outcome. PLoS One. 2019;14:e0221329. [PMID: 31430332]

Lipman GS et al. Wilderness Medical Society practice guidelines for the prevention and treatment of heat illness: 2019 update. Wilderness Environ Med. 2019;30:S33. [PMID: 31221601]

ACCIDENTAL SYSTEMIC HYPOTHERMIA

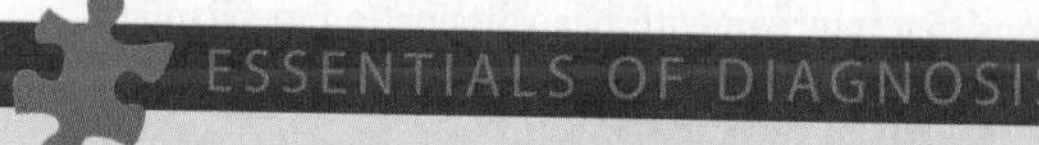

- Systemic hypothermia is a core body temperature < 35°C.
- Accurate core body temperature measurement must be obtained using a low-reading core temperature probe that measures as low as 25°C.
- Core body temperature must be > 32°C before terminating resuscitation efforts.
- Extracorporeal membrane oxygenation (ECMO) or cardiopulmonary bypass may be considered in hypothermic patients with hemodynamic instability or cardiac arrest.

General Considerations

Systemic hypothermia is defined as core body temperature below 35°C. This may be primary, from exposure to prolonged ambient, extremely low temperature, or secondary, due to thermoregulatory dysfunction. Both may be present at the same time.

Hypothermia must be considered in any patient with prolonged exposure to an ambient cold environment, especially in patients with prior cold weather injury as well as the risk factors listed in the Cold & Heat section.

In prolonged or repetitive cold exposure, hypothermia ensues if the body's thermoregulatory responses become impaired.

Clinical Findings

Symptoms and signs of hypothermia are typically nonspecific and markedly variable based on the patient's underlying health and circumstances of cold exposure. All patients must be evaluated for associated conditions including hypoglycemia, trauma, infection, overdose, and peripheral cold injury. Laboratory studies must assess acid-base status; electrolytes, particularly potassium and glucose; kidney, liver, and pancreas function; coagulation; and rhabdomyolysis. Inaccurate laboratory values will occur if the blood sample is warmed to 37°C for testing.

Accurate core body temperature measurements must be obtained using a core temperature probe that measures as low as 25°C. **Stage I hypothermia** is seen when the core body temperature is between 32°C and 35°C and is defined by shivering and possibly poor judgment or coordination but with hemodynamic stability and a normal level of consciousness. **Stage II hypothermia** correlates with core body temperature 28–32°C. Shivering stops; bradycardia, dilated pupils, slowed reflexes, cold diuresis, and confusion and lethargy ensue. The ECG may reveal a J wave or Osborn wave (positive deflection in the terminal portion of the QRS complex, most notable in leads II, V_5, and V_6) (Figure 37–1). When the core body temperature is below 28°C, the likelihood of hemodynamic instability and cardiac arrest increases dramatically. **Stage III hypothermia** (core body temperature 24–28°C) is characterized by loss of consciousness but present vital signs. **Stage IV hypothermia** (core body temperature less than 24°C) is the loss of vital signs. Coma, loss of reflexes, asystole, or ventricular fibrillation may falsely lead the clinician to assume the patient is dead despite reversible hypothermia.

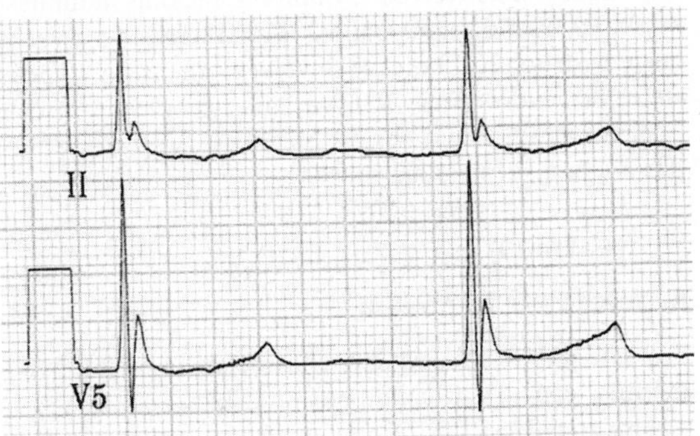

Figure 37–1. ECG shows leads II and V_5 in a patient whose body temperature is 24°C. Note the bradycardia and Osborn waves. These findings become more prominent as the body temperature lowers and gradually resolve with rewarming. Osborn waves have an extra positive deflection in the terminal portion of the QRS complex and are best seen in the inferior and lateral precordial leads (most notably in leads II, V_5, and V_6).

Treatment

Rewarming is the initial, imperative treatment for all hypothermic patients. Resuscitation begins with rapid assessment and support of airway, breathing, and circulation, simultaneously with the initiation of rewarming, and prevention of further heat loss. All cold, wet clothing must be removed and replaced with warm, dry clothing and blankets.

Mild or stage I hypothermia can be treated with **passive external rewarming** (eg, removing and replacing wet clothes with dry ones) or by active external rewarming. In contrast to those with more severe hypothermia, it is safe and recommended for the uninjured patient with mild hypothermia to become physically active to generate heat. **Active external rewarming** is noninvasive, highly effective, and safe for mild hypothermia. It involves applying external heat to the patient's skin. Examples include warm bedding, heated blankets, heat packs, and immersion into a 40°C bath. Warm bath immersion limits the ability to monitor the patient or treat other coexisting conditions. Patients with mild hypothermia and previous good health usually respond well to passive and active external warming.

Stage II and III hypothermia are treated as above with the addition of more aggressive rewarming strategies. This requires close monitoring of vital signs and cardiac rhythm during rewarming. Warm intravenous fluids (38–42°C) are considered minimally invasive and effective.

As hypothermia becomes more severe, there are increased complications of both hypothermia itself and of rewarming. Complications of rewarming occur as colder peripheral blood returns to central circulation. This may result in core temperature afterdrop, rewarming lactic acidosis from shunting lactate into the circulation, rewarming shock from peripheral vasodilation, and hypovolemia, ventricular fibrillation, and other cardiac arrhythmias. Afterdrop can be lessened by active external rewarming of the trunk but not the extremities and by avoiding any muscle movement by the patient. Extreme caution must be taken when handling the hypothermic patient to avoid triggering potentially fatal arrhythmias in a phenomenon known as rescue collapse.

Patients with hemodynamic instability or cardiac arrest should be transferred to a facility with ECMO or cardiopulmonary bypass capability.

Early recognition and advanced management guidelines are needed for patients with stage IV hypothermia. *For hypothermic patients in cardiac arrest, high-quality CPR must be initiated and continued until the patient's core body temperature is at least 32°C.* Below 30°C, arrhythmias and asystole may be refractory to drug therapy until the patient has been rewarmed; therefore, treatment should focus on excellent CPR technique in conjunction with aggressive rewarming of the patient. Epinephrine or vasopressin may be given in cardiac arrest of the severely hypothermic patient. The International Commission for Mountain Emergency Medicine recommends extracorporeal life support as the treatment of choice for patients at high risk for hypothermic cardiac arrest. Extracorporeal life support has been shown to substantially improve survival of patients with unstable circulation or cardiac arrest.

Hypothermic patients with return of spontaneous circulation are at high risk of subsequent multiorgan system failure.

When to Admit

Hypothermia patients must undergo close monitoring for potential complications. This is typically done during an inpatient admission or prolonged emergency department observation.

Dow J et al. Wilderness Medical Society clinical practice guidelines for the out-of-hospital evaluation and treatment of accidental hypothermia: 2019 update. Wilderness Environ Med. 2019;30:S47. [PMID: 31740369]

Pasquier M et al. An evaluation of the Swiss staging model for hypothermia using hospital cases and case reports from the literature. Scand J Trauma Resusc Emerg Med. 2019;27:60. [PMID: 31171019]

HYPOTHERMIA OF THE EXTREMITIES

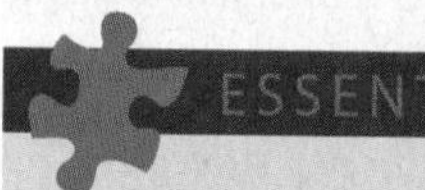

ESSENTIALS OF DIAGNOSIS

- *"Keep warm, keep dry, and keep moving"* to prevent cold-induced injury.
- Rewarming of the extremity suffering cold-induced injury must be performed as soon as possible once there is no risk of refreezing; exercise, rubbing, or massage must be avoided during rewarming.

Clinical Findings

Cold exposure of the extremities produces immediate localized and then generalized vasoconstriction, which may result in a wide range of injuries. Tissue damage occurs because of ischemia and intravascular thromboses, endothelial damage, or actual freezing. Freezing (frostbite) may occur when skin temperatures drop or in the presence of wind, water, immobility, malnutrition, or vascular disease.

For all forms of cold-induced injury to an extremity, caution must be taken to avoid rubbing or massaging the injured area and to avoid applying moisture, ice, or heat. The cold-injured extremity must be protected from trauma, secondary infection, and further cold exposure.

Prevention

"Keep warm, keep dry, and keep moving." For optimal prevention of frostbite, individuals must wear warm, dry clothing. Arms, legs, fingers, and toes must be exercised to maintain circulation. Wet clothing, socks, and shoes must be replaced with dry ones. Risk factors include underlying diseases or medications that decrease tissue perfusion and prolonged cold environmental exposure. Caution must be taken to avoid cramped positions; wet or constrictive clothing; prolonged dependency of the feet; use of tobacco, alcohol, and sedative medications; and exposure to wet, muddy ground and windy conditions.

FROSTNIP & CHILBLAIN (Erythema Pernio)

Frostnip is a superficial nonfreezing injury causing local paresthesias of the involved area that completely resolves with passive external rewarming.

Chilblains, or **erythema pernio,** are inflammatory skin changes caused by exposure to cold without actual freezing of the tissues. These skin lesions may be red or purple papular lesions, which are painful or pruritic, with burning or paresthesias. They may be associated with edema or blistering and aggravated by warmth. With continued exposure, ulcerative or hemorrhagic lesions may appear and progress to scarring, fibrosis, and atrophy. Treatment consists of elevating and passively externally rewarming the affected part.

IMMERSION FOOT OR TRENCH FOOT

Immersion foot (or hand) is caused by prolonged immersion in cold water or mud, usually below 10°C. **Prehyperemic stage** is marked by early symptoms of cold and anesthesia of the affected area. **Hyperemic stage** follows with a hot sensation, intense burning, and shooting pains. **Posthyperemic stage** occurs with ongoing cold exposure; the affected part becomes pale or cyanotic with diminished pulsations due to vasospasm. This may result in blistering, swelling, redness, ecchymoses, hemorrhage, necrosis, peripheral nerve injury, or gangrene.

Treatment consists of air drying and gradual rewarming by exposure to air at room temperature. Affected parts are elevated to aid in removal of edema fluid. Pressure sites are protected with cushions. Bed rest is required until all ulcers have healed.

FROSTBITE

Frostbite is injury from tissue freezing and formation of ice crystals in the tissue. Most tissue destruction follows reperfusion of the frozen tissues resulting in further tissue damage. In mild cases, only the skin and subcutaneous tissues are involved. Symptoms include numbness, prickling, itching, and pallor. With increasing severity, deeper structures become involved; the skin appears white or yellow, loses elasticity, and becomes immobile. Edema, hemorrhagic blisters, necrosis, gangrene, paresthesias, and stiffness may occur.

Treatment

A. Immediate Treatment

Evaluate and treat the patient for associated systemic hypothermia, concurrent conditions, and injury. Early use of systemic analgesics is recommended for nonfrozen injuries. Hydrate the patient to avoid hypovolemia and to improve perfusion.

1. Rewarming—Rapid rewarming at temperatures slightly above normal body temperature may significantly decrease tissue necrosis and reverse the tissue crystallization. **If there is any possibility of refreezing, the frostbitten part must not be thawed.** Ideally, the frozen extremity must not be used, but if required for evacuation, the affected frozen extremity must be padded and splinted to avoid additional injury. Rewarming is best accomplished by warm bath immersion. The frozen extremity is immersed in a moving water bath heated to 37–39°C for approximately 30 minutes until the area becomes soft and pliable to the touch. Water in this temperature range feels warm but not hot to the normal hand or wrist. If warm water is not available, then passive thawing in a warm environment must be allowed. Dry heat is not recommended because it is more difficult to regulate and increases the likelihood of accidental burns. Thawing may cause tenderness and burning pain. Once the frozen part has thawed and returned to normal temperature, discontinue external heat. **In the early stage, rewarming by exercise, rubbing, or friction is contraindicated.** The patient must be kept on bed rest with the affected parts elevated and uncovered at room temperature. Avoid application of casts, occlusive dressings, or bandages. Blisters must be left intact unless signs of infection supervene.

2. Anti-infective measures and wound care—Frostbite increases susceptibility to tetanus and infection. Tetanus prophylaxis status must be verified and updated as needed. Infection risk may be reduced by aseptic wound care. Topical aloe vera cream or gel should be applied to the thawed tissue before application of dressings. Nonadherent sterile gauze and fluffy dressing must be loosely applied to wounds and cushions used for all areas of pressure. Antibiotics should not be administered empirically.

B. Medical and Surgical Treatment Options

Telemedicine may be used so that specialists can provide advice on early field treatment of cold-injured patients in remote areas, thereby improving outcomes. Nonsteroidal anti-inflammatory drugs should be administered (in the absence of contraindications) until frostbite wounds are healed or surgical management occurs. Clinicians must watch for evidence of compartment syndrome and need for fasciotomy. Eschar formation without evidence of infection may be conservatively treated. The underlying skin may heal spontaneously with the eschar acting as a biologic dressing. Rates of amputation have been reduced with intravenous infusions of synthetic prostaglandins and tissue plasminogen activators, and with intra-arterial administration of a thrombolytic within 24 hours of exposure. The rate of tissue salvage decreases with every hour of delay from rewarming to thrombolytic therapy.

C. Follow-Up Care

Patient education must include ongoing care of the cold injury and prevention of future hypothermia and cold injury. Gentle, progressive physical therapy to promote circulation should be instituted as tolerated.

Prognosis

Recovery from frostbite depends on the underlying comorbidities, the extent of initial tissue damage, the rewarming reperfusion injury, and the late sequelae. The involved extremity may be at increased susceptibility for discomfort and injury upon re-exposure to cold. Neuropathic sequelae include pain, numbness, tingling, hyperhidrosis, and cold sensitivity of the extremities. Nerve conduction abnormalities may persist for many years after a cold injury.

When to Admit

- Management of tissue damage, comorbidities, associated injuries.
- Need for hospital-based interventions.
- Psychosocial factors that could compromise patient safety or recovery.

Drinane J et al. Thrombolytic salvage of threatened frostbitten extremities and digits: a systematic review. J Burn Care Res. 2019;40:541. [PMID: 31188429]

Lacey AM et al. An institutional protocol for the treatment of severe frostbite injury—a 6-year retrospective analysis. J Burn Care Res. 2021;42:817. [PMID: 33484248]

McIntosh SE et al. Wilderness Medical Society practice guidelines for the prevention and treatment of frostbite: 2019 update. Wilderness Environ Med. 2019;30:S19. [PMID: 31326282]

Shenaq DS et al. Urban frostbite: strategies for limb salvage. J Burn Care Res. 2019;40:613. [PMID: 30990527]

DROWNING

ESSENTIALS OF DIAGNOSIS

- The first requirement of rescue is immediate rescue breathing and CPR.
- Clinical manifestations include hypoxemia, pulmonary edema, and hypoventilation.
- Patients must be assessed for hypothermia, hypoglycemia, alcohol intake, concurrent injuries, and medical conditions.

General Considerations

Drowning, as defined by the World Health Organization, is any "process resulting in primary respiratory impairment from submersion in a liquid medium." Drowning may result in asphyxiation (from fluid aspiration or laryngospasm), hypoxemia, hypothermia, and acidemia. Outcomes from drowning range from life without morbidity to death. Morbidity may be immediate or delayed. A patient may be deceptively asymptomatic during the initial recovery period only to deteriorate or die from acute respiratory failure within the following 12–24 hours. Disseminated intravascular coagulation may also lead to bleeding after asphyxiation from drowning.

Drowning is a leading cause of death in children worldwide and is highly preventable in all ages with implementation of educational and safety measures. Clinicians must provide patient education and guidance about drowning prevention.

Clinical Findings

A. Symptoms and Signs

The patient's appearance may vary from asymptomatic to marked distress with abnormal vital signs. Symptoms and signs include respiratory difficulty, chest pain, dysrhythmia, hypotension, cyanosis, and hypothermia (from cold water or prolonged submersion). A pink froth from the mouth and nose indicates pulmonary edema. The patient may experience headache, neurologic deficits, and altered level of consciousness.

B. Laboratory Findings

Metabolic acidosis is common and arterial blood gas results may be helpful in determining the degree of injury since initial clinical findings may appear benign. Pao_2 is usually decreased; $Paco_2$ may be increased or decreased; pH is decreased. Bedside blood glucose must be checked rapidly. Other testing is based on clinical scenario.

Prevention

Education and prevention are critical given the high burden of disease from drowning.

Preventive measures must be taken to reduce morbidity and mortality from drowning. Conditions that increase risk of submersion injury include the use of alcohol, psychotropics, and other drugs, inadequate water safety skills, poor physical health, hyperventilation, sudden acute illness, acute trauma, decompression sickness, dangerous water conditions, and environmental hazards (eg, lack of fencing around pools).

Treatment

A. First Aid

1. The first requirement of rescue is immediate basic life support treatment and CPR. At the scene, immediate airway management and measures to combat hypoxemia are critical to improve outcome.
2. Patient must be assessed for hypothermia, hypoglycemia, concurrent medical conditions, and associated trauma.
3. Rescuer must not attempt to drain water from the person's lungs.
4. Resuscitation and basic life support efforts must be continued until core body temperature reaches 32°C.

B. Subsequent Management

1. Ensure optimal ventilation and oxygenation—The onset of hypoxemia exists even in the alert, conscious patient who appears to be breathing normally. Supplemental oxygen should be administered immediately at the highest available concentration to maintain oxygen saturation at 90% or higher.

Serial physical examinations and chest radiographs must be performed to detect possible pneumonitis, atelectasis, and pulmonary edema. Bronchodilators may be used to treat wheezing. Nasogastric suctioning may be necessary to decompress the stomach.

2. Cardiovascular support—Intravascular volume status must be monitored and supported by vascular fluid replacement, vasopressors, or diuretics as needed.

3. Correction of blood pH and electrolyte abnormalities—Metabolic acidosis is present in most persons who drown but typically corrects through adequate ventilation and oxygenation. Glycemic control improves outcome.

4. Cerebral and spinal cord injury—CNS damage may progress despite apparently adequate treatment of hypoxia and shock.

5. Hypothermia—Core body temperature must be measured and managed as appropriate (see Accidental Systemic Hypothermia, above).

Course & Prognosis

Favorable prognosis is related to a duration of submersion less than 5 minutes, with worsening outcomes correlating with increased submersion times. Respiratory damage is often severe in the minutes to hours following a drowning. With appropriate respiratory supportive treatment, patients may improve rapidly over the first few days following the drowning. Long-term complications of drowning may include neurologic impairment, seizure disorder, and pulmonary or cardiac damage. Prognosis is directly correlated with the patient's age, submersion time, rapidity of prehospital resuscitation and subsequent transport to a medical facility, clinical status at time of arrival to hospital, Glasgow Coma Scale score, pupillary reactivity, and overall health assessment (APACHE II score).

When to Admit

Most patients with significant drowning or concurrent medical or traumatic conditions require inpatient monitoring following the event. This includes continuous monitoring of cardiorespiratory, neurologic, renal, and metabolic function. Pulmonary edema may not appear for 24 hours.

Meddings DR et al. Drowning prevention: turning the tide on a leading killer. Lancet Public Health. 2021;6:e692. [PMID: 34310906]

Reynolds JC et al. Long-term survival after drowning-related cardiac arrest. J Emerg Med. 2019;57:129. [PMID: 31262547]

Schmidt AC et al. Wilderness Medical Society clinical practice guidelines for the treatment and prevention of drowning: 2019 update. Wilderness Environ Med. 2019;30:S70. [PMID: 31668915]

THERMAL BURNS

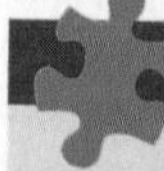

ESSENTIALS OF DIAGNOSIS

- Estimates of the burn location, size, and depth greatly determine the treatment plan.
- The first 48 hours of burn care offer the greatest impact on morbidity and mortality of a burn patient.

Worldwide, burns are a common cause of injury and potential morbidity and mortality. Burn prognosis is affected by the type of environment where the burn occurred. Low-resource settings (wilderness or low-income areas) are associated with delays in and suboptimal access to standard burn treatments.

The first 48 hours after thermal burn injury offer the greatest opportunity to impact the survival of the patient. Early surgical intervention, wound care, enteral feeding, glucose control and metabolic management, infection control, and prevention of hypothermia and compartment syndrome have contributed to significantly lower mortality rates and shorter hospitalizations. Research utilizing several different well-established burn severity scores has shown the importance of patient comorbidities to the prognosis of patients with severe burn injuries.

General Considerations

A. Classification

Burns are classified by extent, depth, patient age, and associated illness or injury. Accurate estimation of burn size and depth is necessary to quantify the parameters of resuscitation.

1. Extent—In adults, the "rule of nines" (Figure 37–2) is useful for rapidly assessing the extent of a burn. It is important to view the entire patient to make an accurate assessment of skin findings on initial and subsequent examinations. One rule of thumb is that the palm of an open hand in adult patients constitutes 1% of total body surface area (TBSA). TBSA is calculated for partial- and full-thickness burns.

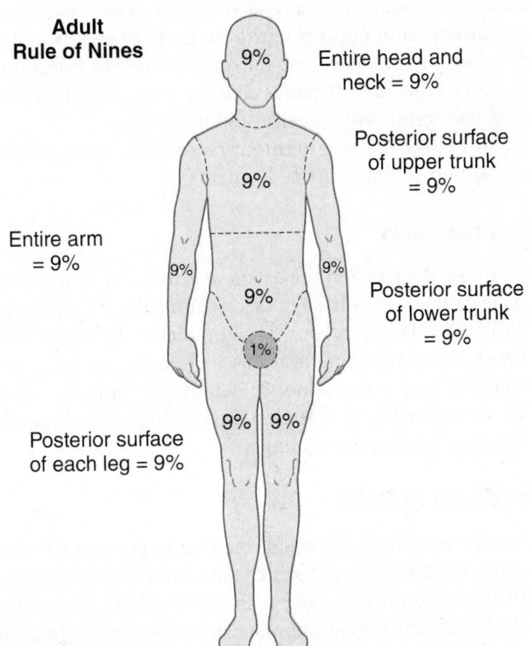

▲ **Figure 37–2.** Estimation of body surface area in burns.

2. Depth—Judgment of depth of injury is difficult. **Superficial burns** may appear red or gray but will demonstrate excellent capillary refill and are not blistered initially. If the wound is blistered and appears pink and wet, this represents a **superficial partial-thickness burn**. **Deep partial-thickness burns** appear white and wet, and bleed if poked; cutaneous sensation is maintained. **Full-thickness burns** result in a loss of adnexal structures and may appear white-yellow or may have a black charred appearance. This stiff, dry skin does not bleed when poked and cutaneous sensation is lost.

Deep partial-thickness and full-thickness burns are treated in a similar fashion. Both require early debridement and grafting to heal appropriately, without which the skin becomes thin and scarred.

B. Survival After Burn Injury

Transfer to a burn unit is determined by large burn size, circumferential burn, or burn involving a joint or high-risk body part, and by comorbidities. Mortality rates have been significantly reduced due to treatment advances including improvements in wound care, treatment of infection, early burn excision, skin substitute usage, and early nutritional support.

C. Associated Injuries or Illnesses

Smoke inhalation, associated trauma, and electrical injuries are commonly associated with burns. Severe burns from any source may result in similar complications (eg, infections, respiratory compromise, multiorgan dysfunction, venous thromboembolism, and GI complications).

D. Systemic Reactions to Burn Injury

Burns greater than approximately 20% of TBSA may lead to systemic metabolic derangements requiring intensive support. The inflammatory cascade can result in shock and coagulopathy.

Treatment

A. Initial Resuscitation

1. Primary survey—Burn patients require a full trauma assessment, starting with "ABCDE" (airway, breathing, circulation, disability, exposure).

A. AIRWAY CONTROL—Serial assessments of airway and breathing are necessary because airway compromise and ARDS may develop, particularly in those with inhalation injury.

B. VASCULAR ACCESS—Vascular access must be obtained on all burn patients.

C. FLUID RESUSCITATION—Patients with burns greater than 15% of TBSA require intravascular fluid administration of large volumes of crystalloid. The most widely recognized guideline for fluid resuscitation is the **Parkland formula** (https://www.mdcalc.com/parkland-formula-burns) in which the fluid requirement in the first 24 hours is estimated as 4 mL/kg × body weight per percentage of body surface area burned. Half the calculated fluid is given in the first 8-hour period from the time of injury, not the time of arrival to medical care. The remaining fluid is delivered over the next 16 hours. An extremely large volume of fluid may be required. Crystalloid solutions alone may be insufficient to restore cardiac preload during the period of burn shock. Conversely, clinicians must watch for clinical signs of volume overload as it may lead to pulmonary complications or to a compartment syndrome from edema. Electrical burns and inhalation injury may increase the fluid requirement.

B. Management

1. Pain control—Pain control is critical in burn injury patients. Treatment is with (oral or intravenous) NSAIDs and opioids (see Chapter 5).

2. Chemoprophylaxis—

A. TETANUS IMMUNIZATION—Verify and update tetanus prophylaxis status in all burn patients. (See Chapter 33.)

B. ANTIBIOTICS—All nonsuperficial wounds need to be covered with topical antibiotics. Prophylaxis with systemic antibiotics is not indicated.

3. Surgical management—

A. ESCHAROTOMY—As tissue swelling occurs, ischemia may develop under any constricting eschar of an extremity, neck, or chest, or in circumferential full-thickness burns of the trunk. Escharotomy incisions can be limb- and life-saving.

B. FASCIOTOMY—Fasciotomy is indicated for any compartment syndrome. Clinicians must frequently monitor patients for development of early signs of a compartment syndrome, particularly in those with circumferential burns.

C. DEBRIDEMENT, DRESSINGS, AND TOPICAL AND SYSTEMIC ANTIBIOTIC THERAPY—Minor burn wounds must be debrided to determine the depth of the burn and then thoroughly cleansed. Thereafter, daily wound care must consist of debridement as needed, topical antibiotics, and wound dressings. Patient compliance and adequate pain control is essential for successful outpatient treatment. The wound must be reevaluated by the treating clinician within 24–72 hours to evaluate for signs of infection.

The goal of burn wound management is to protect the wound from desiccation and avoid further injury or infection. Regular and thorough cleansing of burned areas is of critical importance. Topical antibiotics may be applied after wound cleansing. Silver sulfadiazine is no longer recommended.

It is imperative to closely monitor for and treat systemic infection, since this remains a leading cause of morbidity among patients with major burn injuries. Health care–associated infections are increasingly common.

D. WOUND MANAGEMENT—The goal of therapy after fluid resuscitation is rapid and stable closure of the wound. Wounds that do not heal spontaneously in 7–10 days (eg, deep partial-thickness or full-thickness burns) are best treated by a specialist through excision and autograft to avoid development of granulation and infection. The quality of the skin in regenerated deep partial-thickness burns is marginal because of the very thin dermis that emerges.

Cultured allogeneic keratinocyte grafts can provide rapid early coverage for superficial burn injuries. Skin substitution with cultured grafts may be life-saving for severe burns. Although the replaced dermis has nearly normal histologic dermal elements, there are no adnexal structures present, and very few, if any, elastic fibers.

E. ABDOMINAL COMPARTMENT SYNDROME—Abdominal compartment syndrome is a potentially lethal condition that may develop in severely burned patients, with mortality rates of approximately 60% despite surgical intervention. Diagnosis is confirmed by bladder pressures greater than 30 mm Hg in at-risk patients. Surgical abdominal decompression may improve ventilation and oxygen delivery but may not impact survival.

C. Patient Support

Burn patients require extensive supportive care, both physiologically and psychologically. It is important to maintain normal core body temperature and avoid hypothermia, by maintaining environmental temperature at or above 30°C, in patients with burns over more than 20% of TBSA. Burn patients are at risk for many complications such as respiratory injury, ARDS or respiratory failure unresponsive to maximal ventilatory support, sepsis, multiorgan failure, and venous thromboembolism.

Burn patients have increased metabolic and energy needs for wound healing and require careful assessment and provision of optimal nutrition. Early aggressive nutrition (by parenteral or enteral routes) reduces infections, recovery time, noninfectious complications, length of hospital stay, long-term sequelae, and mortality.

Prevention of long-term scars remains a formidable problem in seriously burned patients.

Prognosis

Prognosis depends on the extent and location of the burn tissue damage, associated injuries, comorbidities, and complications. Hyperglycemia is a predictor of worse outcomes. Common complications include sepsis; gangrene requiring limb amputation; or neurologic, cardiac, cognitive, or psychiatric dysfunction. Psychiatric support may be necessary following burn injury.

When to Refer

Transfer to a burn unit is indicated for large burn size (for partial-thickness burns greater than 10% of TBSA or for full-thickness burns greater than 5% of TBSA), circumferential burn, inhalation injury, or burn involving a joint or high-risk body part (face, hands, feet, genitalia), and for patients with comorbidities.

When to Admit

- All severe burn patients require extensive supportive care, both physiologically and psychologically.
- Significant burns (based on location and extent).
- Patients with significant comorbidities and suboptimal home situations.
- Burn center consultation can advise which patients require transfer and which can be managed via telemedicine/telephone consultation.
- Monitoring includes vital signs, wound care, and observation for potential complications of electrolyte abnormalities, AKI, hepatic failure, cardiopulmonary compromise, hyperglycemia, and infection.

Chao KY et al. Respiratory management in smoke inhalation injury. J Burn Care Res. 2019;40:507. [PMID: 30893426]
Smith RR et al. Analysis of factors impacting length of stay in thermal and inhalation injury. Burns. 2019;45:1593. [PMID: 31130323]
Yeung C et al. Identifying risk factors that increase analgesic requirements at discharge among patients with burn injuries. J Burn Care Res. 2021 Sep 15. [Epub ahead of print] [PMID: 34525191]

ELECTRICAL INJURY

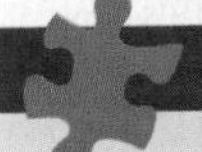

ESSENTIALS OF DIAGNOSIS

- Resuscitation must be initiated at once since clinical findings suggesting death are unreliable.
- Extent of damage from electrical injury is determined by the type, amount, duration, and pathway of electrical current.
- Skin findings may be misleading and are not indicative of the depth of tissue injury.

General Considerations

Electricity-induced injuries are common and yet most are preventable. These injuries occur by exposure to electrical current of low voltage, high voltage, or lightning. Electrical current type is either alternating current or direct current and is measured in volts (V). Electricity causes acute injury by direct tissue damage, muscle tetany, direct thermal injury and coagulation necrosis, and associated trauma.

Alternating current is an electric current that periodically reverses direction in a sine wave pattern and may cause muscle tetany, which prolongs the duration and amount of current exposure. Alternating current can be low voltage or high voltage. Most households and businesses use electric power in the form of alternating current at **low voltages** (less than 1000 V). Low voltage electrical injuries can range from minor to significant damage and death. **High voltage** (greater than 1000 V) alternating current electrical injuries are often related to occupational exposure and associated with deep tissue damage and higher morbidity and mortality. **Direct current** is unidirectional electrical flow (eg, lightning, batteries, and automotive electrical systems). It is more likely to cause a single intense muscle contraction and asystole. **Lightning** differs from other high-voltage electrical shock because lightning delivers a direct current of millions of volts in a fraction of a second.

The extent of damage from electrical injury is determined by the current type, amount (voltage), duration of exposure, pathway of current, tissue resistance, moisture, associated trauma, and comorbidities. Current is the most important determinant of tissue damage and causes direct thermal injury. Tissue resistance varies throughout the body with nerve cells being the most vulnerable and bone the most resistant to electrical current.

Clinical Findings

Electrical burns are of three distinct types: flash (arcing) burns, flame (clothing) burns, and the direct heating effect of tissues by the electrical current.

Skin damage does not correlate with the degree of injury; very minor skin damage may be present with massive internal injuries. Symptoms and signs may range from very subtle to death. The presence of entrance and exit burns signifies an increased risk of deep tissue damage. Current passing through skeletal muscle can cause muscle necrosis and contractions severe enough to result in bone fracture. If the current passes through the heart or brainstem, death may be immediate due to ventricular fibrillation, asystole, or apnea.

Resuscitation must be initiated on all persons who have had an electrical injury since clinical findings of death are deceptive and unreliable.

Complications

Complications may include cardiac or respiratory arrest; dysrhythmias; neurologic dysfunction (eg, autonomic dysfunction [resulting in pupils that are fixed, dilated, or asymmetric]; altered mental status; seizures); paralysis; headache; neuropathy; vascular injury from thrombosis and capillary damage; tissue edema and necrosis; compartment syndrome; associated traumatic injuries (eg, ruptured ear drums, fractures from falls or muscle contractions); pneumothorax; rhabdomyolysis; AKI; hypovolemia from third spacing; infections (with special risk of clostridial infections causing gas gangrene and tetanus); ocular complications (ie, acute or delayed cataract formation); sepsis; gangrene requiring limb amputation; and cognitive or psychiatric dysfunction. Psychiatric support may be necessary following electrical injury.

Treatment

A. Emergency Measures

The patient must be assessed and treated for trauma. The patient must be safely separated from the electrical current prior to initiation of treatments. Resuscitation must be initiated at once since clinical findings suggesting death are unreliable.

B. Hospital Measures

The initial assessment involves airway, breathing, and circulation followed by a full trauma protocol. Fluid resuscitation is important to maintain adequate urinary output (0.5 mL/kg/hour if no myoglobinuria is present; 1.0 mL/kg/hour if myoglobinuria is present). Initial evaluation includes ECG and cardiac monitoring, CBC, electrolytes, kidney function tests, liver chemistries, creatine phosphokinase or urine myoglobin, UA, and cardiac enzymes. ECG does not show typical patterns of ischemia since the electrical damage is epicardial. Patients must be evaluated for hidden trauma, dehydration, hypertension, acid-base disturbances, and neurological as well as psychological damage.

Electrical burn wounds are devastating with wide-ranging and significant complications. Superficial skin may appear deceivingly benign. There must be a high suspicion for extensive deep tissue necrosis which leads to profound tissue swelling, and a high risk of a compartment syndrome.

Pain management is important before, during, and after initial treatment and subsequent rehabilitation.

Prognosis

Prognosis depends on the degree and location of electrical injury, initial tissue damage, associated injuries, comorbidities, and complications.

When to Refer

- Specialists may need to perform fasciotomy for compartment syndrome, debridement of devitalized tissue, or microvascular reconstruction.
- An ophthalmologist should evaluate for possible ocular complications; an otologist should evaluate for tympanic membrane rupture or hearing loss.
- A psychiatrist should assess any psychological impact.

When to Admit

Indications for hospitalization include high-voltage exposure; abnormal cardiac rhythm or ECG changes; large burn size; neurologic, pulmonary, or cardiac symptoms; suspicion of significant deep tissue or organ damage; transthoracic current pathway; history of cardiac disease or other significant comorbidities or injuries; and need for surgery.

Ahmed J et al. Patient outcomes after electrical injury—a retrospective study. Scand J Trauma Resusc Emerg Med. 2021;29:114. [PMID: 34362435]

Delphine D et al. Use of troponin assay after electrical injuries: a 15-year multicentre retrospective cohort in emergency departments. Scand J Trauma Resusc Emerg Med. 2021;29141. [PMID: 34565432]

Stockly OR et al. The impact of electrical injuries on long-term outcomes: a Burn Model System National Database study. Burns. 2020;46:352. [PMID: 31420267]

RADIATION EXPOSURE

ESSENTIALS OF DIAGNOSIS

- Damage from radiation is determined by the radiation type, quantity, and duration, and the patient's bodily location, underlying condition, and accumulated exposures.
- Clinicians and patients must be educated regarding the risks of medical diagnostic radiation weighed against the benefits of the medical imaging needed.

General Considerations

Radiation exposure may occur from environmental, occupational, medical care, accidental, or intentional causes. The extent of damage from radiation exposure depends on the type, quantity, and duration of radiation exposure; the organs exposed; and the patient's age, comorbidities, and accumulated radiation exposures.

Radiation occurs from both nonionizing and ionizing radiation sources. **Nonionizing radiation** is low energy, resulting in injuries related to local thermal damage. **Ionizing radiation** is high energy, causing bodily damage in several ways. Exposure may be external, internal, or both. Radiation exposure triggers multiple metabolic changes resulting in tissue-specific damage.

The International Commission on Radiological Protection (ICRP) website provides the most up-to-date recommendations for protection against ionizing radiation (http://www.icrp.org/index.asp). The World Health Organization (WHO) publishes guidelines on radiation emergencies (https://www.who.int/health-topics/radiation-emergencies#tab=tab_1). These guidelines include recommended interventions during the early, intermediate, and late emergency phases and the management of their psychosocial impact.

Clinical Findings

Radiation exposure results in acute and delayed effects. It is important to obtain the event history, the amount of radiation exposure, and the possibility of coexisting injuries or conditions. Acute effects involve damage of the body's rapidly dividing cells (eg, the mucosa, skin, and bone marrow). Acute findings include mucositis, nausea, vomiting, GI edema and ulcers, skin burns, and bone marrow suppression over hours to days after exposure. Delayed effects include malignancy, reproduction abnormalities, and liver, kidney, CNS, and immune system dysfunction.

Acute radiation syndrome is due to an exposure to high doses of ionizing radiation over a brief time course. The symptom onset is within hours to days depending on the dose. Symptoms include anorexia, nausea, vomiting, weakness, exhaustion, dehydration, lassitude, prostration, anemia, and infection; these symptoms may occur singly or in combination. The CDC offers information regarding acute radiation syndrome (https://www.cdc.gov/nceh/radiation/emergencies/arsphysicianfactsheet.htm).

Treatment for acute radiation exposure includes close monitoring of the GI, cutaneous, hematologic, cardiopulmonary, and cerebrovascular systems from initial exposure and over time.

▶ Therapeutic Radiation Exposure

Radiation therapy has been a successful component in the treatment of many malignancies. Unfortunately, these radiation-treated cancer survivors have a higher risk of a second malignancy; obesity; pulmonary, cardiac, and thyroid dysfunction, as well as an increased overall risk of chronic health conditions and mortality.

▶ Medical Imaging Radiation Exposure

Medical imaging with ionizing radiation exposure has dramatically increased over the past few decades. With the rising use of medical imaging, there is international focus on improving the safety by standardization and regulation of radiation dosing in medical diagnostics and education for clinician and the public.

The American College of Radiology (ACR) provides "ACR Appropriateness Criteria," which are evidence-based guidelines created by expert panels to serve as a reference for best practices for imaging decisions by health care providers (https://www.acr.org/Clinical-Resources/ACR-Appropriateness-Criteria). Clinicians and patients must carefully weigh the risks and benefits of radiation exposure when deciding on an imaging test.

▶ Occupational & Environmental Radiation Exposure

Useful resources for professionals include the CDC "Radiation Emergencies" website (https://www.cdc.gov/nceh/radiation/emergencies/index.htm) and the National Nuclear Security Administration's Radiation Emergency Assistance Center, which provides 24-hour access to expert consultation services (telephone: 1-865-576-1005 or website: https://orise.orau.gov/reacts/).

▶ Treatment

Treatment is focused on decontamination, on management of coexisting conditions or injuries, and on supportive care. Specific supportive treatments are determined by the dose, route, and effects of exposure and associated conditions present.

▶ Prognosis

Prognosis is determined by the radiation dose, duration, and frequency as well as by the underlying condition of the patient. Death following acute radiation exposure is usually due to hematopoietic failure, GI mucosal damage, CNS damage, widespread vascular injury, or secondary infection.

Carcinogenesis is related to the radiation type, total dose, duration, and accumulated exposure, and to the susceptibility of the patient. Radiation-related cancer risks persist throughout the exposed person's life span.

With the increased use of ionizing radiation for medical diagnostics and treatments, there is an iatrogenic increase in radiation-induced cancer risks. There are age-related sensitivities to radiation; pregnant women and younger persons are more susceptible to carcinogenesis.

▶ When to Admit

Most patients with significant ionizing radiation exposure require admission for close monitoring and supportive treatment.

Berrington de Gonzalez A et al. Epidemiological studies of CT scans and cancer risk: the state of the science. Br J Radiol. 2021;94:20210471. [PMID: 34545766]

Jain S. Radiation in medical practice & health effects of radiation: rationale, risks, and rewards. J Family Med Prim Care. 2021;10:1520. [PMID: 34123885]

Khodamoradi E et al. Targets for protection and mitigation of radiation injury. Cell Mol Life Sci. 2020;77:3129. [PMID: 32072238]

ENVIRONMENTAL DISORDERS RELATED TO ALTITUDE

DYSBARISM & DECOMPRESSION SICKNESS

ESSENTIALS OF DIAGNOSIS

- Early recognition of symptoms temporally related to recent altitude or pressure changes. Prompt treatment of decompression illness is extremely important for optimal outcome.
- Patients must also be assessed for hypothermia, hypoglycemia, concurrent injuries, and medical conditions.
- Consultation with diving medicine or hyperbaric oxygen specialist is indicated.

▶ General Considerations

Dysbarism and decompression illness result from altitude changes and effects of environmental pressure on the gases in the body. These are most likely to occur when scuba diving is followed closely by rapid ascent, or when the scuba diver is not adherent to the conservative dive guidelines for dive duration, course, depth, and surface times.

As a diver descends, the gases in the body compress and dissolve throughout areas of the body that are both compressible (lungs, GI tract) and noncompressible (sinuses, joints). As the diver descends further, there is increased pressure on the body's gases and increasing amounts dissolve into the bloodstream and tissues. During the subsequent ascent, these dissolved gases expand within the body, which can cause dysbarism and decompression illness.

Dysbarism results from barotrauma when gas compression or expansion occurs in parts of the body that are noncompressible or have limited compliance. Pulmonary overinflation syndrome is one of the most serious and potentially fatal results of barotrauma. This syndrome is due to an inappropriately rapid ascent causing alveoli rupture and air bubble extravasation into the vital organs or the cerebral circulation.

Decompression illness occurs when the pressure change is too rapid from higher pressure to lower pressure. The result is that gas bubbles form and cause damage on their location (eg, coronary, pulmonary, spinal, or cerebral blood vessels, joints, soft tissues). Decompression illness symptoms depend on the size, number, and location of released gas bubbles. Risk of decompression illness in scuba diving depends on multiple factors: the dive details (depth, duration, number of dives, interval surface time between dives, and water conditions). Patient factors include age, weight, overall health, physical condition, physical exertion, the rate of ascent, and the length of time between the low altitude (scuba dive) and high altitude (ground ascent or air travel). Predisposing factors include obesity, injury, hypoxia, lung, or cardiac disease, right to left cardiac shunt, dehydration, alcohol and medication effects, and panic attacks. Decompression illness may also occur in those who take hot showers after cold dives.

Preventive measures include pre-dive medical screening and dive planning; diver education; strict adherence to dive course, timing, and depths; and a slow and controlled ascent with proper control of buoyancy. Conservative recommendation is to avoid high altitudes (ground ascent or air travel) for at least 24 hours after surfacing from the dive, especially following multiple dives.

Clinical Findings

There is a range of clinical manifestations depending on the location of the gas bubble formation or the compressibility of gases in the body. Symptom onset may be immediate or within minutes or hours up to 48 hours later. Decompression illness symptoms are wide-ranging: pain in the joints; skin pruritus or burning; cardiac; neurologic (symptoms may or may not follow typical neuroanatomic distribution patterns); respiratory compromise; pain in ears or sinuses, or both; and coma and death.

Decompression illness involving the brain and spinal cord may occur by different mechanisms due to air bubbles causing arterial occlusion, venous obstruction, or in situ toxicity.

The clinician must assess for associated conditions of hypothermia, hypoglycemia, hypovolemia, aspiration, near-drowning, trauma, envenomation, or concurrent medical conditions.

Treatment

Early recognition and prompt treatment are extremely important. Decompression illness must be considered if symptoms are temporally related to recent diving or rapid changes in altitude or pressure within the past 48 hours. Continuous administration of 100% oxygen is indicated and beneficial for all patients. Hyperbaric oxygen treatment is commonly recommended for decompression illness symptoms. Immediate consultation with a diving medicine or hyperbaric oxygen specialist is indicated even if mild decompression illness symptoms resolve. NSAIDs, acetaminophen, or aspirin may be given for pain control if there are no contraindications. Opioids must be used very cautiously since these may obscure the response to recompression.

When to Admit

Rapid transportation to a hyperbaric treatment facility for recompression is imperative since this is the recommended treatment by specialists. The Divers Alert Network is an excellent worldwide resource for emergency advice 24 hours daily for the management of diving-related conditions (https://dan.org/).

Garcia-Bustos V et al. Ten-year Spanish cohort of diving-related injuries in a non-hyperbaric tertiary hospital on the Spanish Mediterranean coast. Undersea Hyperb Med. 2021;48:382. [PMID: 34847301]

Mitchell SJ. DCS or DCI? The difference and why it matters. Diving Hyperb Med. 2019;49:152. [PMID: 31523788]

Scarpa A et al. Inner ear disorders in scuba divers: a review. J Int Adv Otol. 2021;17:260. [PMID: 34100753]

HIGH-ALTITUDE ILLNESS

ESSENTIALS OF DIAGNOSIS

- The severity of the high-altitude illness is affected by the rate and height of ascent and the individual's susceptibility.
- Prompt recognition and medical treatment of early findings of high-altitude illness may prevent progression.
- Clinicians must assess other conditions that may coexist or mimic symptoms of high-altitude illness.
- Immediate descent is the definitive treatment for high-altitude cerebral edema and high-altitude pulmonary edema.

General Considerations

As altitude increases, there is a decrease in both barometric pressure and oxygen partial pressure resulting in hypobaric hypoxia. High-altitude illnesses are due to hypobaric hypoxia at high altitudes (usually greater than 2000 meters or 6562 feet). High-altitude illness includes a spectrum of disorders categorized by end-organ effects (mostly cerebral and pulmonary) and exposure duration (acute and long-term). Acute high-altitude illnesses are **acute hypoxia, acute mountain sickness (AMS), high-altitude cerebral edema (HACE),** and **high-altitude pulmonary edema (HAPE).**

Acclimatization occurs as a physiologic response to the increasing altitude and increasing hypobaric hypoxia. High-altitude illness results when the hypoxic stress is greater than the individual's ability to acclimatize. Risk factors for high-altitude illness include increased physical activity with insufficient acclimatization, inadequate education and preparation, individual susceptibility, and previous high-altitude illness. The key determinants of high-altitude illness risk and severity include both individual susceptibility factors and altitudinal factors, such as rate and height of ascent and total change in altitude over time.

Individual susceptibility factors include underlying conditions such as cardiac and pulmonary disease, patent foramen ovale, blood disorders, pregnancy, neurologic conditions, smoking, recent surgery, diabetes mellitus, and many other chronic medical conditions. Those with symptomatic neurologic, cardiac, or pulmonary disease must avoid high altitudes.

Patient assessment for high-altitude illness must also include evaluation for other conditions, which may coexist or may present in a similar manner.

1. High-Altitude–Associated Neurologic Conditions: AMS & HACE

There is a spectrum of neurologic conditions caused by high altitude, ranging from **AMS** to the more serious form, **HACE.**

AMS includes symptoms such as headache (most severe and persistent symptom), lassitude, drowsiness, dizziness, chilliness, nausea and vomiting, and difficulty sleeping. Later symptoms include irritability, difficulty concentrating, anorexia, insomnia, and increased headaches.

HACE includes the severe symptoms of AMS and results from cerebral vasogenic edema and cerebral cellular hypoxia. It usually occurs at elevations above 2500 meters (8202 feet) but may occur at lower elevations. Hallmarks are altered mental status, ataxia, severe lassitude, and encephalopathy. Examination findings may include confusion, ataxia, urinary retention or incontinence, focal neurologic deficits, papilledema, and seizures. Symptoms may progress to obtundation, coma, and death.

▶ Treatment

Definitive treatment is immediate descent of at least 610 meters (2001 feet), and descent must continue until symptoms improve. Descent is essential if the symptoms are persistent, severe, or worsening, or if HACE or HAPE is present. If immediate descent is not possible, portable hyperbaric chambers can provide symptomatic relief, but this must not delay descent.

Initial treatment involves oxygen administration to keep the pulse oximetry S_pO_2 to greater than 90%.

Acetazolamide is an effective medication for both prophylaxis and treatment of mild symptoms of AMS.

Dexamethasone is given for moderate to severe AMS. Dexamethasone is the primary treatment for HACE. Acetazolamide can be added as an adjunct in severe HACE cases. In most individuals, symptoms clear within 24–48 hours. HACE treatment must continue until 24 hours after resolution of symptoms or until descent is completed. Dexamethasone should not be given for longer than 7 days.

It is imperative that the clinician also assess for other conditions that may mimic or coexist with AMS and HACE.

If HAPE symptoms and signs are present along with HACE, nifedipine or a selective phosphodiesterase inhibitor may be added for pulmonary vasodilation. The clinician must be cautious when using combinations of vasodilators.

2. Acute HAPE

HAPE is the leading cause of death from high-altitude illness. The hallmark is markedly elevated pulmonary artery pressure followed by pulmonary edema. Early symptoms may appear within 6–36 hours after arrival at a high-altitude area. These include incessant dry cough, shortness of breath disproportionate to exertion, headache, decreased exercise performance, fatigue, dyspnea at rest, and chest tightness. Recognition of the early symptoms may enable the patient to descend before incapacitating pulmonary edema develops. Strenuous exertion must be avoided. As pulmonary edema worsens, wheezing, orthopnea, and hemoptysis may develop.

Physical findings may include tachycardia, mild fever, tachypnea, cyanosis, prolonged respiration, rales, wheezing, and rhonchi. The clinician must assess for other potential medical conditions because the clinical picture may resemble other entities. Diagnosis is usually clinical; ancillary tests are nonspecific or unavailable on site. Prompt recognition of and medical attention to early symptoms of HAPE may prevent progression.

▶ Treatment

Immediate descent (at least 610 meters [2000 feet]) is essential, although this may not be immediately possible and may not alone improve symptoms.

The patient must be placed at rest, reclined with head elevated. Supplemental oxygen must be administered to maintain pulse oximetry readings of S_pO_2 greater than 90%. Recompression in a portable hyperbaric bag will temporarily reduce symptoms if rapid or immediate descent is not possible but must not delay descent.

Nifedipine can be used as an adjunct if the other therapies (descent, oxygen, or portable hyperbaric chambers) are not available or successful. Selective phosphodiesterase inhibitors may be used for HAPE prevention and may also provide effective symptom relief as an alternative or if nifedipine is not available. Administering nifedipine plus a phosphodiesterase inhibitor as pulmonary vasodilators is not recommended. Treatment for ARDS (see Chapter 9) is required for some patients. If neurologic symptoms are present concurrently with HAPE and do not resolve with improved oxygenation, dexamethasone may be added according to HACE treatment guidelines.

There is an international effort to advance the understanding of HAPE through the research and database registry (https://www.altitude.org).

Prevention of High-Altitude Disorders

Pre-trip preventive measures include participant education, medical preparticipation evaluation, pre-trip planning, optimal physical conditioning before travel, and adequate rest and sleep the day before travel and during the trip. Preventive efforts during ascent include reduced food intake, avoidance of alcohol and tobacco, and limiting any unnecessary physical activity during travel.

Gradual ascent is the most effective way to allow acclimatization. Low-risk ascension rate is 2 or more days to arrive at 2500–3000 meters. The altitude reached during waking hours is not as important as the altitude at which the hiker sleeps.

Drug prophylaxis may be prescribed for AMS and HACE if no contraindications exist. Prophylactic low-dose acetazolamide has been shown to reduce the incidence and severity of AMS and HACE when started 3 days prior to ascent and continued for 48–72 hours at high altitude. Dexamethasone is an alternative prophylactic medication for AMS and HACE.

Individuals with a past history of HAPE should use drug prophylaxis to reduce the risk of recurrence. Nifedipine started the day before ascent and continued through the fourth day at target elevation, or through the seventh day if the ascent rate was faster, is recommended. Salmeterol can be added beginning 24 hours prior to ascent. Salmeterol is used as an adjunct to nifedipine but not as monotherapy.

Phosphodiesterase inhibitors may be beneficial in the treatment of HAPE based on their physiologic effects of decreased pulmonary arterial pressures and pulmonary vasodilation.

When to Admit

- All patients with HACE or HAPE must be hospitalized for further observation.
- Hospitalization must also be considered for any patient who remains symptomatic after treatment and descent.
- Pulmonary symptoms and hypoxia may be worsened by complications such as PE, secondary respiratory infection, bronchospasm, mucous plugging, or acute coronary syndrome.

Luks AM et al. Wilderness Medical Society practice guidelines for the prevention and treatment of acute altitude illness: 2019 update. Wilderness Environ Med. 2019;30:S3. [PMID: 31248818]

Shlim DR. The use of acetazolamide for the prevention of high-altitude illness. J Travel Med. 2020;27:taz106. [PMID: 31897486]

Shroff NA et al. High-altitude illness: updates in prevention, identification, and treatment. Emerg Med Pract. 2021;23:1. [PMID: 34402609]

SAFETY OF AIR TRAVEL & SELECTION OF PATIENTS FOR AIR TRAVEL

The medical safety of air travel depends on the nature and severity of the traveler's preflight condition and factors such as travel duration and frequency of travel, use and frequency of in-flight exercise, cabin altitude pressure, availability of medical supplies, infectious diseases of other travelers, and the presence of health care professionals on board. Air travel passengers are susceptible to a wide range of flight-related problems: pulmonary, venous thromboembolism (VTE), infections, cardiac, GI, ocular, immunologic, syncope, neuropsychiatric, metabolic, trauma, and illicit substance-related conditions. Air travel risks are higher for those air travelers with preexisting medical conditions.

Hypobaric hypoxia is the underlying etiology of most serious medical emergencies in-flight due to cabin altitude. Despite commercial aircraft pressurization requirements, there is significant hypoxemia, dyspnea, gas expansion, and stress in travelers, particularly in those with underlying pulmonary disease.

Any form of prolonged travel involving immobilization is associated with increased risk of VTE. VTE risk is more relevant for those passengers with additional VTE risk factors. Risks for VTE in long-distance travelers include the following: (1) travel involving immobilization for 4 or more hours, (2) hypercoagulable disorders, and (3) acquired risks. Prevention measures may include wearing graduated compression stockings; frequent exercise and position changes during travel; and the use of thromboprophylaxis, such as low-molecular-weight heparin or DOACs (see Chapter 14).

Air travel is not advised for anyone who is "incapacitated" or has any "unstable conditions." The Air Transport Association of America defines an **incapacitated passenger** as "one who is suffering from a physical or mental disability and who, because of such disability or the effect of the flight on the disability, is incapable of self-care; would endanger the health or safety of such person or other passengers or airline employees; or would cause discomfort or annoyance of other passengers." **Unstable conditions** include any condition requiring active treatment immediately. Public Health Travel Restrictions have shown efficacy in preventing commercial air or international travel of persons with certain communicable diseases that pose a public health threat.

Pregnancy

Pregnant travelers have unique travel-related and location-specific risks. A clinician's authorization is required if travel is essential during the ninth month of pregnancy or earlier in a complicated or high-risk pregnancy.

Long travel increases risk of VTE for the pregnant traveler. Pregnant travelers are at higher risk from infection transmission and air travel radiation exposure.

Prevention

Air travel complications may be reduced by the following preventive measures: passenger prescreening, passenger education, and in-flight positioning and activity. Prescreening evaluation is recommended for all high-risk patients including preexisting requirement for oxygen, underlying restrictive or obstructive lung disease, comorbidities worsened by hypoxemia (eg, pulmonary hypertension or underlying cardiac, cerebrovascular, or respiratory disease), previous respiratory distress during air travel, recent pneumothorax, and recent (within 6 weeks) acute respiratory illness. Patients at risk for hypoxia must be assessed prior to air travel to determine if there is a need for supplemental in-flight oxygen.

Air travel education must include risk reduction measures for VTE, infectious diseases, and exacerbations of underlying medical conditions. Patients and clinicians can check the WHO website for the most updated information on travel health risks and infectious diseases (https://www.who.int/travel-advice). Air travel has been associated with an increased risk of transmission of infectious diseases.

All long-distance travelers can reduce VTE risk by avoiding constrictive clothing, staying well-hydrated, changing position frequently, avoiding cramped position, avoiding leg crossing, engaging in frequent (at least every hour) in-flight leg stretching exercises, and walking for 5 minutes every hour. Clinicians must assess those with high risk of VTE prior to air travel to determine whether anticoagulation is indicated (see Table 14–14).

Bellinghausen AL et al. How I do it: assessing patients for air travel. Chest. 2020;S0012-3692:35141. [PMID: 33212136]

Clarke MJ et al. Compression stockings for preventing deep vein thrombosis in airline passengers. Cochrane Database Syst Rev. 2021;4:CD004002. [PMID: 33878207]

Tuite AR et al. Global trends in air travel: implications for connectivity and resilience to infectious disease threats. J Travel Med. 2020;27:taaa070. [PMID: 32374834]

Poisoning

Craig Smollin, MD

INITIAL EVALUATION: POISONING OR OVERDOSE

Patients with drug overdoses or poisoning may initially have no symptoms or they may have varying degrees of overt intoxication. The asymptomatic patient may have been exposed to or may have ingested a lethal dose, but not yet exhibit any manifestations of toxicity. It is important to (1) quickly assess the potential danger, (2) consider gut and skin decontamination to prevent absorption, (3) treat complications if they occur, and (4) observe the asymptomatic patient for an appropriate interval.

Assess the Danger

If the drug or poison is known, its danger can be assessed by consulting a text or computerized information resource or by calling a regional poison control center. (In the United States, dialing 1-800-222-1222 will direct the call to the regional poison control center.) Assessment will usually take into account the dose ingested; the time since ingestion; the presence of any symptoms or clinical signs; preexisting cardiac, respiratory, kidney, or liver disease; and, occasionally, specific serum drug or toxin levels. Be aware that the history given by the patient or family may be incomplete or unreliable.

IMMEDIATE 24-HOUR TOXICOLOGY CONSULTATION

Call your regional poison control center
U.S. toll-free **1-800-222-1222**

Observe the Patient

Asymptomatic or mildly symptomatic patients should be observed for at least 4–6 hours. Longer observation is indicated if the ingested substance is a sustained-release preparation or is known to slow GI motility (eg, opioids, anticholinergics, aspirin) or may cause a delayed onset of symptoms (eg, acetaminophen, colchicine, hepatotoxic mushrooms). After that time, the patient may be discharged if no symptoms have developed. Before discharge, psychiatric evaluation should be performed to *assess suicide risk.* Intentional ingestions in adolescents should raise the possibility of unwanted pregnancy or sexual abuse.

THE SYMPTOMATIC PATIENT

In symptomatic patients, treatment of life-threatening complications takes precedence over in-depth diagnostic evaluation. Patients with mild symptoms may deteriorate rapidly, which is why *all potentially significant exposures should be observed in an acute care facility.* The following complications may occur, depending on the type of poisoning.

COMA

Assessment & Complications

Coma is commonly associated with ingestion of large doses of antihistamines (eg, diphenhydramine), benzodiazepines and other sedative-hypnotic drugs, ethanol, opioids, antipsychotic drugs, or antidepressants. The most common cause of death in comatose patients is respiratory failure, which may occur abruptly. Pulmonary aspiration of gastric contents may also occur, especially in patients who are deeply obtunded or convulsing. Hypoxia and hypoventilation may cause or aggravate hypotension, arrhythmias, and seizures. Thus, *protection of the airway and assisted ventilation are the most important treatment measures for any poisoned patient.*

Treatment

A. Emergency Management

The initial emergency management of coma can be remembered by the mnemonic *ABCD*, for Airway, Breathing, Circulation, and Drugs (dextrose, thiamine, and naloxone or flumazenil), respectively.

1. Airway—Establish a patent airway by positioning, suction, or insertion of an artificial nasal or oropharyngeal airway. If the patient is deeply comatose or if airway reflexes are depressed, perform endotracheal intubation. These airway interventions may not be necessary if the patient is intoxicated by an opioid or a benzodiazepine and responds to intravenous naloxone or flumazenil.

2. Breathing—Clinically assess the quality and depth of respiration and provide assistance, if necessary, with a bag-valve-mask device or mechanical ventilator. Administer supplemental oxygen, if needed. The arterial or venous blood CO_2 tension, or noninvasive end-tidal CO_2 monitoring, is useful in determining the adequacy of ventilation. The arterial blood Po_2 determination may reveal hypoxemia, which may be caused by respiratory depression, bronchospasm, pulmonary aspiration, or noncardiogenic pulmonary edema. Pulse oximetry provides an assessment of oxygenation but is unreliable in patients with methemoglobinemia or carbon monoxide poisoning, unless a pulse oximetry device capable of detecting these forms of hemoglobin is used.

3. Circulation—Measure the pulse and blood pressure and estimate tissue perfusion (eg, by measurement of urinary output, skin signs, arterial blood pH). Place the patient on continuous ECG monitoring. Insert an intravenous line, and draw blood for glucose, electrolytes, serum creatinine and liver tests, and possible quantitative toxicologic testing.

4. Drugs—

A. DEXTROSE AND THIAMINE—Unless promptly treated, severe hypoglycemia can cause irreversible brain damage. Therefore, in all obtunded, comatose, or convulsing patients, give 50% dextrose, 50–100 mL by intravenous bolus, unless a rapid point-of-care blood glucose test rules out hypoglycemia. In patients with alcohol use disorder or malnourishment who may have marginal thiamine stores, give thiamine 100 mg intramuscularly or in the intravenous fluids.

B. OPIOID ANTAGONISTS—Naloxone, 0.4–2 mg intravenously or 2–4 mg by intranasal spray, may reverse opioid-induced respiratory depression and coma. It is *often given empirically* to any comatose patient with depressed respirations. If opioid overdose is strongly suspected, give additional doses of naloxone (up to 5–10 mg may be required to reverse the effects of potent opioids). **Note:** Naloxone has a shorter duration of action (2–3 hours) than most common opioids; *repeated doses* may be required, and continuous observation for at least 3–4 hours after the last dose is mandatory.

C. FLUMAZENIL—Flumazenil, 0.2–0.5 mg intravenously, repeated as needed up to a maximum of 3 mg, may reverse benzodiazepine-induced coma. **Caution:** *In most circumstances, use of flumazenil is not advised as the potential risks outweigh its benefits.* Flumazenil should *not* be given if the patient has coingested a potential convulsant drug, is a user of high-dose benzodiazepines, or has a seizure disorder because its use in these circumstances may precipitate seizures. **Note:** Flumazenil has a short duration of effect (2–3 hours), and recurrent sedation requiring additional doses may occur.

HYPOTHERMIA

Assessment & Complications

Hypothermia commonly accompanies coma due to opioids, ethanol, hypoglycemic agents, phenothiazines, barbiturates, benzodiazepines, and other sedative-hypnotics and CNS depressants. Hypothermic patients may have a barely perceptible pulse and blood pressure. Hypothermia may cause or aggravate hypotension, which will not reverse until the temperature is normalized.

Treatment

Treatment of hypothermia is discussed in Chapter 37. Gradual rewarming is preferred unless the patient is in cardiac arrest.

HYPOTENSION

Assessment & Complications

Hypotension may be due to poisoning by many different drugs, including antihypertensives, beta-blockers, calcium channel blockers, disulfiram (ethanol interaction), iron, trazodone, quetiapine, and other antipsychotic agents and antidepressants. Poisons causing hypotension include cyanide, carbon monoxide, hydrogen sulfide, aluminum or zinc phosphide, arsenic, and certain mushrooms.

Hypotension in the poisoned or drug-overdosed patient may be caused by venous or arteriolar vasodilation, hypovolemia, depressed cardiac contractility, or a combination of these effects.

Treatment

Most hypotensive poisoned patients respond to empiric treatment with repeated 200 mL intravenous boluses of 0.9% saline or other isotonic crystalloid up to a total of 1–2 L; much larger amounts may be needed if the patient is profoundly volume-depleted (eg, as with massive diarrhea due to *Amanita phalloides* mushroom poisoning). Monitoring the central venous pressure can help determine whether further fluid therapy is needed. Consider bedside cardiac ultrasound or pulmonary artery catheterization (or both) to assess central venous pressure. If fluid therapy is not successful after adequate volume replacement, give dopamine or norepinephrine by intravenous infusion.

Hypotension caused by certain toxins may respond to specific treatment. For hypotension caused by overdoses of tricyclic antidepressants or other sodium channel blockers, administer sodium bicarbonate, 50–100 mEq by intravenous bolus injection. Norepinephrine 4–8 mcg/minute by intravenous infusion is more effective than dopamine in some patients with overdoses of tricyclic antidepressants or of drugs with predominantly vasodilating effects. For beta-blocker overdose, glucagon (5–10 mg intravenously) may be of value. For calcium channel blocker overdose, administer calcium chloride, 1–2 g intravenously (repeated doses may be necessary; doses of 5–10 g and more have been given in some cases). High-dose insulin (0.5–1 U/kg/hour intravenously) euglycemic therapy may also be used (see the sections Beta-Adrenergic Blockers and Calcium Channel Blockers, below). Intralipid 20% lipid emulsion has been reported to improve hemodynamics in some cases of intoxication by highly lipid-soluble drugs such as bupivacaine, bupropion, clomipramine, and verapamil. Intravenous methylene blue and extracorporeal membrane oxygenation (ECMO) have been employed in a few refractory cases; ECMO may offer temporary hemodynamic stabilization while the offending drug is eliminated.

Mycyk MB. Extracorporeal membrane oxygenation shows promise for treatment of poisoning some of the time: the challenge to do better by aiming higher. Crit Care Med. 2020;48:1235. [PMID: 32697497]

Nafea OE et al. Comparative effectiveness of methylene blue versus intravenous lipid emulsion in a rodent model of amlodipine toxicity. Clin Toxicol (Phila). 2019;57:784. [PMID: 30729824]

Weiner L et al. Clinical utility of venoarterial-extracorporeal membrane oxygenation (VA-ECMO) in patients with drug-induced cardiogenic shock: a retrospective study of the Extracorporeal Life Support Organizations' ECMO case registry. Clin Toxicol (Phila). 2020;58:705. [PMID: 31617764]

HYPERTENSION

Assessment & Complications

Hypertension may be due to poisoning with amphetamines and synthetic stimulants, anticholinergics, cocaine, performance-enhancing products (eg, containing caffeine, phenylephrine, ephedrine, or yohimbine), MAO inhibitors, and other drugs.

Severe hypertension (eg, diastolic blood pressure greater than 105–110 mm Hg in a person who does not have chronic hypertension) can result in acute intracranial hemorrhage, MI, or aortic dissection.

Treatment

Treat hypertension if the patient is symptomatic or if the diastolic pressure is higher than 105–110 mm Hg—especially if there is no prior history of hypertension.

Hypertensive patients who are agitated or anxious may benefit from a sedative (such as lorazepam, 2–3 mg intravenously) or an antipsychotic drug (eg, haloperidol or olanzapine). For persistent hypertension, administer phentolamine, 2–5 mg intravenously, or nitroprusside sodium, 0.25–8 mcg/kg/minute intravenously. If excessive tachycardia is present, *add* esmolol, 25–100 mcg/kg/minute intravenously, or labetalol, 0.2–0.3 mg/kg intravenously. **Caution:** *Do not give beta-blockers alone, since doing so may paradoxically worsen hypertension in some cases as a result of unopposed alpha-adrenergic stimulation.*

ARRHYTHMIAS

Assessment & Complications

Arrhythmias may occur with a variety of drugs or toxins (Table 38–1). They may also occur as a result of hypoxia, metabolic acidosis, or electrolyte imbalance (eg, hyperkalemia, hypokalemia, hypomagnesemia, or hypocalcemia), or following exposure to chlorinated solvents or chloral hydrate overdose. Atypical ventricular tachycardia (torsades de pointes) is often associated with drugs that prolong the QT interval.

Treatment

Hypoxia or electrolyte imbalance should be sought and treated. If ventricular arrhythmias persist, administer lidocaine or amiodarone at usual antiarrhythmic doses.

Table 38–1. Common toxins or drugs causing arrhythmias (listed in alphabetical order by arrhythmia).[1]

Arrhythmia	Common Causes
Atrioventricular block	Beta-blockers, calcium channel blockers, class Ia antiarrhythmics (including quinidine), carbamazepine, clonidine, digitalis glycosides, lithium
QT interval prolongation and torsades de pointes	Arsenic, class Ia and class III antiarrhythmics, citalopram, droperidol, lithium, methadone, pentamidine, sertraline, sotalol, and many other drugs[2]
Sinus bradycardia	Beta-blockers, calcium channel blockers, clonidine, digitalis glycosides, organophosphates
Sinus tachycardia	Beta-agonists (eg, albuterol), amphetamines, anticholinergics, antihistamines, caffeine, cocaine, pseudoephedrine, tricyclic and other antidepressants
Ventricular premature beats and ventricular tachycardia	Amphetamines, cocaine, ephedrine, caffeine, chlorinated or fluorinated hydrocarbons, digoxin, aconite (found in some Chinese herbal preparations), fluoride, theophylline. QT prolongation can lead to atypical ventricular tachycardia (torsades de pointes)
Wide QRS complex	Class Ia and class Ic antiarrhythmics, phenothiazines (eg, thioridazine), potassium (hyperkalemia), propranolol, tricyclic antidepressants, bupropion, lamotrigine, diphenhydramine (severe overdose)

[1]Arrhythmias may also occur as a result of hypoxia, metabolic acidosis, or electrolyte imbalance (eg, hyperkalemia or hypokalemia, hypocalcemia, hypomagnesemia).
[2]https://crediblemeds.org/

Note: Wide QRS complex tachycardia in the setting of tricyclic antidepressant overdose (or diphenhydramine or class Ia antiarrhythmic drugs) should be treated with sodium bicarbonate, 50–100 mEq intravenously by bolus infusion. **Caution:** *In such cases, avoid class Ia antiarrhythmic agents (eg, procainamide, disopyramide) and amiodarone, which may aggravate arrhythmias caused by tricyclic antidepressants.* Torsades de pointes associated with prolonged QT interval may respond to intravenous magnesium (2 g intravenously over 2 minutes) or overdrive pacing. Treat digitalis-induced arrhythmias with digoxin-specific antibodies.

For tachyarrhythmias induced by chlorinated solvents, chloral hydrate, Freons, or sympathomimetic agents, use propranolol or esmolol (see doses in the Hypertension section, above).

Shakeer SK et al. Chloral hydrate overdose survived after cardiac arrest with excellent response to intravenous β-blocker. Oman Med J. 2019;34:244. [PMID: 31110633]

SEIZURES

Assessment & Complications

Seizures may be caused by many poisons and drugs, including amphetamines, antidepressants (especially tricyclic antidepressants, bupropion, and venlafaxine), antihistamines (especially diphenhydramine), antipsychotics, camphor, synthetic cannabinoids and cathinones, cocaine, isoniazid (INH), chlorinated insecticides, piperazines, tramadol, and theophylline. The onset of seizures may be delayed for up to 18–24 hours after extended-released bupropion overdose.

Seizures may also be caused by hypoxia, hypoglycemia, hypocalcemia, hyponatremia, withdrawal from alcohol or sedative-hypnotics, head trauma, CNS infection, or idiopathic epilepsy.

Prolonged or repeated seizures may lead to hypoxia, metabolic acidosis, hyperthermia, and rhabdomyolysis.

Treatment

Administer lorazepam, 2–3 mg, or diazepam, 5–10 mg, intravenously, or—if intravenous access is not immediately available—midazolam, 5–10 mg intramuscularly. If convulsions continue, administer phenobarbital, 15–20 mg/kg slowly intravenously over no less than 30 minutes. (For drug-induced seizures, phenobarbital is preferred over phenytoin or levetiracetam.) Propofol infusion has also been reported effective for some resistant drug-induced seizures.

Seizures due to a few drugs and toxins may require antidotes or other specific therapies (as listed in Table 38–2).

Table 38–2. Seizures related to toxins or drugs requiring special consideration (listed in alphabetical order by toxin or drug).[1]

Toxin or Drug	Comments
Isoniazid	Administer pyridoxine.
Lithium	May indicate need for hemodialysis.
Methylenedioxymethamphetamine (MDMA; "Ecstasy")	Seizures may also be due to hyponatremia or hyperthermia.
Organophosphates	Administer pralidoxime (2-PAM) and atropine in addition to usual anticonvulsants.
Strychnine	"Seizures" are actually spinally mediated muscle spasms and usually require neuromuscular paralysis and mechanical ventilation.
Theophylline	Seizures indicate need for hemodialysis.
Tricyclic antidepressants	Hyperthermia and cardiotoxicity are common complications of repeated seizures; paralyze early with neuromuscular blockers to reduce muscular hyperactivity.

[1]See text for dosages.

Phillips HN et al. Toxin-induced seizures. Neurol Clin. 2020;38:867. [PMID: 33040866]

Skolnik A et al. The crashing toxicology patient. Emerg Med Clin North Am. 2020;38:841. [PMID: 32981621]

HYPERTHERMIA

Assessment & Complications

Hyperthermia may be associated with poisoning by amphetamines and other synthetic stimulants (cathinones, piperazines), atropine and other anticholinergic drugs, cocaine, salicylates, strychnine, 2,4-dinitrophenol, tricyclic antidepressants, and various other medications. Overdoses of serotonin reuptake inhibitors (eg, fluoxetine, paroxetine, sertraline) or their use in a patient taking an MAO inhibitor may cause agitation, hyperactivity, myoclonus, and hyperthermia (**"serotonin syndrome"**). Antipsychotic agents can cause rigidity and hyperthermia (neuroleptic malignant syndrome). (See Chapter 25.) Malignant hyperthermia is a rare disorder associated with general anesthetic agents.

Hyperthermia is a rapidly life-threatening complication. Severe hyperthermia (temperature higher than 40–41°C) can rapidly cause brain damage and multiorgan failure, including rhabdomyolysis, AKI, and coagulopathy (see Chapter 37).

Treatment

Treat hyperthermia aggressively by removing the patient's clothing, spraying the skin with tepid water, and high-volume fanning. Alternatively, the patient can be placed in an ice water bath (not simply applying ice to selected surfaces). If external cooling is not rapidly effective, as shown by a normal rectal temperature within 30–40 minutes, or if there is significant muscle rigidity or hyperactivity, induce neuromuscular paralysis with a nondepolarizing neuromuscular blocker (eg, rocuronium, vecuronium). Once paralyzed, the patient must be intubated and mechanically ventilated and sedated. While the patient is paralyzed, the absence of visible muscular convulsive movements may give the false impression that brain seizure activity has ceased; bedside electroencephalography may be useful in recognizing continued nonconvulsive seizures.

Dantrolene (2–5 mg/kg intravenously) may be effective for hyperthermia associated with muscle rigidity that does not respond to neuromuscular blockade (ie, malignant hyperthermia). Bromocriptine, 2.5–7.5 mg orally daily, has been recommended for neuroleptic malignant syndrome. Cyproheptadine, 4 mg orally every hour for three or four doses, or chlorpromazine, 25 mg intravenously or 50 mg intramuscularly, has been used to treat serotonin syndrome.

Caroff SN et al. Drug-induced hyperthermic syndromes in psychiatry. Clin Psychopharmacol Neurosci. 2021;19:1. [PMID: 33508784]

Griffiths A et al. 2,4-Dinitrophenol overdose—everything old is new again. J Forensic Leg Med. 2021;79:102148. [PMID: 33706128]

Kuhlwilm L et al. The neuroleptic malignant syndrome—a systematic case series analysis focusing on therapy regimes and outcome. Acta Psychiatr Scand. 2020;142:233. [PMID: 32659853]

Talton CW. Serotonin syndrome/serotonin toxicity. Fed Pract. 2020;37:452. [PMID: 33132683]

ANTIDOTES & OTHER TREATMENT

ANTIDOTES

Give an antidote (if available) when there is reasonable certainty of a specific diagnosis (Table 38–3). Be aware that some antidotes themselves may have serious side effects. The indications and dosages for specific antidotes are discussed in the respective sections for specific toxins.

Hon KL et al. Antidotes for childhood toxidromes. Drugs Context. 2021;10:2020-11-4. [PMID: 34122588]

DECONTAMINATION OF THE SKIN

Corrosive agents rapidly injure the skin and eyes and must be removed immediately. In addition, many toxins are readily absorbed through the skin, and systemic absorption can be prevented only by rapid action.

Table 38–3. Some toxic agents for which there are specific antidotes (listed in alphabetical order).[1]

Toxic Agent	Specific Antidote
Acetaminophen	*N*-acetylcysteine
Anticholinergics (eg, atropine)	Physostigmine
Anticholinesterases (eg, organophosphate pesticides)	Atropine and pralidoxime (2-PAM)
Benzodiazepines	Flumazenil (rarely used)[2]
Carbon monoxide	Oxygen (hyperbaric oxygen of uncertain benefit)
Cyanide	Sodium nitrite, sodium thiosulfate; hydroxocobalamin
Digitalis glycosides	Digoxin-specific Fab antibodies
Heavy metals (eg, lead, mercury, iron) and arsenic	Specific chelating agents
Isoniazid	Pyridoxine (vitamin B_6)
Methanol, ethylene glycol	Ethanol (ethyl alcohol) or fomepizole (4-methylpyrazole)
Opioids	Naloxone, nalmefene
Snake venom	Specific antivenin
Sulfonylurea oral hypoglycemic drugs	Glucose, octreotide

[1]See text for indications and dosages.
[2]May induce seizures in patients with preexisting seizure disorder, benzodiazepine addiction, or concomitant tricyclic antidepressant or other convulsant overdose. If seizures occur, diazepam and other benzodiazepine anticonvulsants will not be effective. As with naloxone, the duration of action of flumazenil is short (2–3 hours) and resedation may occur, requiring repeated doses.

Wash the affected areas with copious quantities of lukewarm water or saline, taking care to limit exposure to health care providers. Wash carefully behind the ears, under the nails, and in skin folds. For oily substances (eg, pesticides), wash the skin at least twice with plain soap and shampoo the hair. Specific decontaminating solutions or solvents (eg, alcohol) are rarely indicated and in some cases may paradoxically *enhance* absorption. For exposure to chemical warfare poisons such as nerve agents or vesicants, some authorities recommend use of a dilute hypochlorite solution (household bleach diluted 1:10 with water), but not in the eyes.

DECONTAMINATION OF THE EYES

Act quickly to prevent serious damage. Flush the eyes with copious amounts of saline or water. (If available, instill local anesthetic drops in the eye before beginning irrigation.) Remove contact lenses if present. Lift the tarsal conjunctiva to look for undissolved particles and to facilitate irrigation. Continue irrigation for 15 minutes or until each eye has been irrigated with at least 1 L of solution. If the toxin is an acid or a base, check the pH of the tears after irrigation, and continue irrigation until the pH is between 7 and 7.4. An amphoteric decontamination solution (Diphoterine, Prevor) is used in some countries for treatment of alkali injuries to the eye.

After irrigation is complete, perform a careful examination of the eye, using fluorescein and a slit lamp or Wood lamp to identify areas of corneal injury. Patients with serious conjunctival or corneal injury should be immediately referred to an ophthalmologist.

GASTROINTESTINAL DECONTAMINATION

Removal of ingested poisons by induced emesis or gastric lavage was a routine part of emergency treatment for decades. However, *prospective randomized studies have failed to demonstrate improved clinical outcome after gastric emptying.* For small or moderate ingestions of most substances, toxicologists often recommend oral **activated charcoal** alone without prior gastric emptying; in some cases, when the interval after ingestion has been more than 1–2 hours and the ingestion is non–life-threatening, even charcoal is withheld (eg, if the estimated benefit is outweighed by the potential risk of pulmonary aspiration of charcoal). Exceptions are large ingestions of anticholinergic compounds and salicylates, which often delay gastric emptying, and ingestion of sustained-release or enteric-coated tablets, which may remain intact for several hours. In these cases, delayed gut decontamination may be indicated.

Gastric emptying is not generally used for ingestion of corrosive agents or petroleum distillates, because further esophageal injury or pulmonary aspiration may result. However, in certain cases, removal of the toxin may be more important than concern over possible complications. Consult a medical toxicologist or regional poison control center (1-800-222-1222) for advice.

A. Activated Charcoal

Activated charcoal effectively adsorbs almost all drugs and poisons. Poorly adsorbed substances include iron, lithium, potassium, sodium, mineral acids, and alcohols.

1. Indications—Activated charcoal can be used for prompt adsorption of drugs or toxins in the stomach and intestine. However, evidence of benefit in clinical studies is lacking. Administration of charcoal, especially if mixed with sorbitol, can provoke vomiting, which could lead to pulmonary aspiration in an obtunded patient.

2. Contraindications—Activated charcoal should *not* be used for comatose or convulsing patients unless it can be given by gastric tube and the airway is first protected by a cuffed endotracheal tube. It is also contraindicated for patients with ileus or intestinal obstruction or those who have ingested corrosives for whom endoscopy is planned.

3. Technique—Administer activated charcoal, 60–100 g orally or via gastric tube, mixed in aqueous slurry. Repeated doses may be given to ensure GI adsorption or to enhance elimination of some drugs.

B. Whole Bowel Irrigation

Whole bowel irrigation uses large volumes of a balanced polyethylene glycol-electrolyte solution to mechanically cleanse the entire intestinal tract. Because of the composition of the irrigating solution, there is no significant gain or loss of systemic fluids or electrolytes.

1. Indications—Whole bowel irrigation is particularly effective for massive iron ingestion in which intact tablets are visible on abdominal radiographs. It has also been used for ingestions of lithium, sustained-release and enteric-coated tablets, and swallowed drug-filled packets.

2. Contraindications—Do not use in patients with suspected intestinal obstruction. Use with caution in patients who are obtunded or have depressed airway protective reflexes.

3. Technique—Administer a balanced polyethylene glycol-electrolyte solution (CoLyte, GoLYTELY) into the stomach via gastric tube at a rate of 1–2 L/hour until the rectal effluent is clear. This may take several hours. It is most effective when patients are able to sit on a commode to pass the intestinal contents.

C. Increased Drug Removal

1. Urinary manipulation—Forced diuresis is hazardous; the risk of complications (fluid overload, electrolyte imbalance) usually outweighs its benefits. Some drugs (eg, salicylates, phenobarbital) are more rapidly excreted with an alkaline urine. To alkalinize the urine, add 100 mEq (two ampules) of sodium bicarbonate to 1 L of 5% dextrose in 0.225% saline (¼ normal saline), and infuse this solution intravenously at a rate of about 150–200 mL/hour. Acidification (sometimes promoted for amphetamines, phencyclidine) is *not* very effective and should not be used.

2. Hemodialysis—The indications for dialysis are as follows: (1) known or suspected potentially lethal amounts of a dialyzable drug (Table 38–4); (2) poisoning with deep coma, apnea, severe hypotension, fluid and electrolyte or acid-base disturbance, or extreme body temperature changes that cannot be corrected by conventional measures; or (3) poisoning in patients with severe kidney, cardiac, pulmonary, or hepatic disease who will not be able to eliminate toxin by the usual mechanisms.

Table 38–4. Recommended use of hemodialysis in selected poisonings (listed in alphabetical order).[1]

Poison	Common Indications[1]
Carbamazepine	Seizures, severe cardiotoxicity; serum level > 60 mg/L
Ethylene glycol	Acidosis, serum level > 50 mg/dL
Lithium	Severe symptoms; level > 4–5 mEq/L, especially if kidney impairment Note: dialysis of uncertain value; consult with medical toxicologist
Methanol	Acidosis, serum level > 50 mg/dL
Phenobarbital	Intractable hypotension, acidosis despite maximal supportive care
Salicylate	Severe acidosis, CNS symptoms, serum level > 100 mg/dL (acute overdose) or > 60 mg/dL (chronic intoxication)
Theophylline	Seizures, severe cardiotoxicity, serum level > 100 mg/L (acute overdose) or > 60 mg/L (chronic intoxication)
Valproic acid	Serum level > 900–1000 mg/L or deep coma, severe acidosis

[1]See text for further discussion of indications.

Continuous renal replacement therapy (including continuous venovenous hemodiafiltration and similar techniques) may be of benefit for elimination of some poisons and has the advantage of gradual removal of the toxin and correction of any accompanying acidosis. Its use has been reported in the management of a variety of poisonings, including lithium intoxication. The Extracorporeal Treatments in Poisoning (EXTRIP) workgroup publishes valuable summary recommendations for several important dialyzable toxins (see https://www.extrip-workgroup.org/recommendations)

3. Repeat-dose charcoal—Repeated doses of activated charcoal, 20–30 g orally or via gastric tube every 3–4 hours, may hasten elimination of some drugs (eg, phenytoin, carbamazepine, dapsone) by absorbing drugs excreted into the gut lumen ("gut dialysis"). However, clinical studies have failed to prove better outcome using repeat-dose charcoal. Sorbitol or other cathartics should *not* be used with each dose, or else the resulting large stool volumes may lead to dehydration or hypernatremia.

Campion GH et al. Extracorporeal treatments in poisonings from four non-traditionally dialysed toxins (acetaminophen, digoxin, opioids and tricyclic antidepressants): a combined single-centre and national study. Basic Clin Pharmacol Toxicol. 2019;124:341. [PMID: 30248244]

Harbord N. Common toxidromes and the role of extracorporeal detoxification. Adv Chronic Kidney Dis. 2020;27:11. [PMID: 32146996]

Zellner T et al. The use of activated charcoal to treat intoxications. Dtsch Arztebl Int. 2019;116:311. [PMID: 31219028]

DIAGNOSIS OF POISONING

The identity of the ingested substance or substances is usually known, but occasionally a comatose patient is found with an unlabeled container or the patient is unable or unwilling to give a coherent history. By performing a directed physical examination and ordering common clinical laboratory tests, the clinician can often make a tentative diagnosis that may allow empiric interventions or may suggest specific toxicologic tests.

Physical Examination

Important diagnostic variables in the physical examination include blood pressure, pulse rate, temperature, pupil size, sweating, muscle tone, level of consciousness, and the presence or absence of peristaltic activity. Poisonings may present with one or more of the following common syndromes.

A. Sympathomimetic Syndrome

The blood pressure and pulse rate are elevated, though with severe hypertension reflex bradycardia may occur. The temperature is often elevated, pupils are dilated, and the skin is sweaty, though mucous membranes are dry. Patients are usually agitated, anxious, or frankly psychotic.

Examples: Amphetamines, cocaine, ephedrine, pseudoephedrine, synthetic cathinones, and cannabinoids.

B. Sympatholytic Syndrome

The blood pressure and pulse rate are decreased, and body temperature is low. The pupils are small or even pinpoint. Patients are usually obtunded or comatose.

Examples: Barbiturates, benzodiazepines and other sedative-hypnotics, gamma-hydroxybutyrate (GHB), clonidine and related antihypertensives, ethanol, opioids.

C. Cholinergic Syndrome

Stimulation of muscarinic receptors causes bradycardia, miosis (constricted pupils), sweating, and hyperperistalsis as well as bronchorrhea, wheezing, excessive salivation, and urinary incontinence. Nicotinic receptor stimulation may produce initial hypertension and tachycardia as well as fasciculations and muscle weakness. Patients are usually agitated and anxious.

Examples: Carbamates, nicotine, organophosphates (including nerve agents), physostigmine.

D. Anticholinergic Syndrome

Tachycardia with mild hypertension is common, and the body temperature is often elevated. Pupils are widely dilated. The skin is flushed, hot, and dry. Peristalsis is decreased, and urinary retention is common. Patients may have myoclonic jerking or choreoathetoid movements. Agitated delirium is frequently seen, and severe hyperthermia may occur.

Examples: Atropine, scopolamine, other naturally occurring and pharmaceutical anticholinergics, antihistamines, tricyclic antidepressants.

Table 38–5. Use of the osmol gap in toxicology.

The osmol gap (Delta osm) is determined by subtracting the calculated serum osmolality from the measured serum osmolality.
$$\text{Calculated osmolality (osm)} = 2[\text{Na}^+ (\text{mEq/L})] + \frac{\text{Glucose (mg/dL)}}{18} + \frac{\text{BUN (mg/dL)}}{2.8}$$
Delta osm = Measured osmolality – Calculated osmolality = 0 ± 10
Serum osmolality may be increased by contributions of exogenous substances such as alcohols and other low-molecular-weight substances. Since these substances are not included in the calculated osmolality, there will be a gap proportionate to their serum concentration. Contact a medical toxicologist or poison control center for assistance in calculating and interpreting the osmol gap.

Reproduced with permission from Stone CK, Humphries RL (editors): *Current Emergency Diagnosis & Treatment*, 5th ed. McGraw-Hill, 2004.

Laboratory Tests

The following clinical laboratory tests are recommended for screening of the overdosed patient: measured serum osmolality and calculated osmol gap (if toxic alcohol ingestion is in the differential diagnosis), electrolytes and anion gap, glucose, creatinine, BUN, creatine kinase (CK), UA (eg, oxalate crystals with ethylene glycol poisoning, myoglobinuria with rhabdomyolysis), and ECG. Quantitative serum acetaminophen and ethanol levels should be determined in all patients with drug overdoses as well as a serum or urine pregnancy test when appropriate.

A. Osmol Gap

The osmol gap (Table 38–5) is increased in the presence of large quantities of low-molecular-weight substances, most commonly ethanol. Other common poisons associated with increased osmol gap are acetone, ethylene glycol, isopropyl alcohol, methanol, and propylene glycol. **Note:** Severe alcoholic ketoacidosis and diabetic ketoacidosis can also cause an elevated osmol gap resulting from the production of ketones and other low-molecular-weight substances.

B. Anion Gap

Metabolic acidosis associated with an elevated anion gap is usually due to an accumulation of lactic acid or other acids (see Chapter 21). Common causes of elevated anion gap in poisoning include carbon monoxide, cyanide, ethylene glycol, propylene glycol, medicinal iron, INH, methanol, metformin, ibuprofen, and salicylates. Massive acetaminophen overdose can cause early-onset anion gap metabolic acidosis.

The osmol gap should also be checked; combined elevated anion and osmol gaps suggests poisoning by methanol or ethylene glycol, though this may also occur in patients with diabetic ketoacidosis and alcoholic ketoacidosis.

Table 38–6. Specific quantitative levels and potential therapeutic interventions (listed in alphabetical order by drug or toxin).[1]

Drug or Toxin	Treatment
Acetaminophen	Specific antidote (*N*-acetylcysteine) based on serum level
Carbon monoxide	High carboxyhemoglobin level indicates need for 100% oxygen, consideration of hyperbaric oxygen
Carbamazepine	High level may indicate need for hemodialysis
Digoxin	On basis of serum digoxin level and severity of clinical presentation, treatment with Fab antibody fragments (eg, DigiFab) may be indicated
Ethanol	Low serum level may suggest nonalcoholic cause of coma (eg, trauma, other drugs, other alcohols); serum ethanol may also be useful in monitoring ethanol therapy for methanol or ethylene glycol poisoning
Iron	Level may indicate need for chelation with deferoxamine
Lithium	Serum levels can guide decision to institute hemodialysis
Methanol, ethylene glycol	Acidosis, high levels indicate need for hemodialysis, therapy with ethanol or fomepizole
Methemoglobin	Methemoglobinemia can be treated with methylene blue intravenously
Salicylates	High level may indicate need for hemodialysis, alkaline diuresis
Theophylline	Immediate hemodialysis or hemoperfusion may be indicated based on serum level
Valproic acid	Elevated levels may indicate need to consider hemodialysis or L-carnitine therapy, or both

[1]Some drugs or toxins may have profound and irreversible toxicity unless rapid and specific management is provided outside of routine supportive care. For these agents, laboratory testing may provide the serum level or other evidence required for administering a specific antidote or arranging for hemodialysis.

C. Toxicology Laboratory Testing

A comprehensive toxicology screen is of little value in the initial care of the poisoned patient because results usually do not return in time to influence clinical management. Specific quantitative levels of certain drugs may be extremely helpful (Table 38–6), however, especially if specific antidotes or interventions (eg, dialysis) would be indicated based on the results.

Many hospitals can perform a quick but limited urine screen for "drugs of abuse" (typically these screens include only opiates, amphetamines, and cocaine, and some add benzodiazepines, barbiturates, methadone, oxycodone, phencyclidine, and tetrahydrocannabinol [marijuana]). There are *numerous false-positive and false-negative results.* For example, synthetic opioids, such as fentanyl, oxycodone, and methadone, are often not detected by routine opiate immunoassays.

Abdominal Imaging

A plain film (or CT scan) of the abdomen may reveal radiopaque iron tablets, drug-filled condoms, or other toxic material. Studies suggest that few tablets are predictably visible (eg, ferrous sulfate, sodium chloride, calcium carbonate, and potassium chloride). Thus, the radiograph is useful only if abnormal.

When to Refer

Consultation with a regional poison control center (1-800-222-1222) or a medical toxicologist is recommended when the diagnosis is uncertain; there are questions about what laboratory tests to order; when dialysis is being considered to remove the drug or poison; or when advice is needed regarding the indications, dose, and side effects of antidotes.

When to Admit

- The patient has symptoms and signs of intoxication that are not expected to clear within a 6- to 8-hour observation period.
- Delayed absorption of the drug might be predicted to cause a later onset of serious symptoms (eg, after ingestion of a sustained-release product).
- Continued administration of an antidote is required (eg, *N*-acetylcysteine for acetaminophen overdose).
- Psychiatric or social services evaluation is needed for suicide attempt or suspected drug abuse.

Nelson LS, Hoffman RS (editors). *Goldfrank's Toxicologic Emergencies*, 11th ed. McGraw-Hill, 2019.

Olson KR, Smollin C (editors). *Poisoning & Drug Overdose*, 8th ed. McGraw-Hill, 2022.

SELECTED POISONINGS

ACETAMINOPHEN

Acetaminophen (paracetamol in the United Kingdom, Europe) is a common analgesic found in many nonprescription and prescription products. After absorption, it is metabolized mainly by glucuronidation and sulfation, with a small fraction metabolized via the P450 mixed-function oxidase system (2E1) to a highly toxic reactive intermediate. This toxic intermediate is normally detoxified by cellular glutathione. With acute acetaminophen overdose (greater than 150–200 mg/kg, or 8–10 g in an average adult), hepatocellular glutathione is depleted and the reactive intermediate attacks other cell proteins, causing necrosis. Patients with enhanced P450 2E1 activity, such as patients who have alcohol use disorder and patients taking

INH, are at increased risk for developing hepatotoxicity. Hepatic toxicity may also occur after overuse of acetaminophen—eg, as a result of taking two or three acetaminophen-containing products concurrently or exceeding the recommended maximum dose of 4 g/day *for several days*. The amount of acetaminophen in US oral prescription combination products (eg, hydrocodone/acetaminophen) is limited by the FDA to no more than 325 mg per tablet.

Clinical Findings

Shortly after ingestion, patients may have nausea or vomiting, but there are usually no other signs of toxicity until 24–48 hours after ingestion, when hepatic aminotransferase levels begin to increase. With severe poisoning, fulminant hepatic necrosis may occur, resulting in jaundice, hepatic encephalopathy, AKI, and death. Rarely, massive ingestion (eg, serum levels greater than 500–1000 mg/L [33–66 mmol/L]) can cause early onset of acute coma, seizures, hypotension, and metabolic acidosis unrelated to hepatic injury.

The diagnosis after acute overdose is based on measurement of the serum acetaminophen level. Plot the serum level versus the time since ingestion on the **acetaminophen nomogram** shown in Figure 38–1. Ingestion of sustained-release products or coingestion of an anticholinergic agent, salicylate, or opioid drug may cause delayed elevation of serum levels, which can make it difficult to interpret the nomogram. In addition, the nomogram cannot be used after chronic or staggered overdose.

Treatment

A. Emergency and Supportive Measures

Administer activated charcoal if it can be given within 1–2 hours of the ingestion. Although charcoal may interfere with absorption of the oral preparation of the antidote acetylcysteine, this is not considered clinically significant.

B. Specific Treatment

If the serum or plasma acetaminophen level falls above the line on the nomogram (Figure 38–1), treatment with *N*-acetylcysteine is indicated; it can be given orally or intravenously. Oral treatment begins with a loading dose of *N*-acetylcysteine, 140 mg/kg, followed by 70 mg/kg every 4 hours. Dilute the solution to about 5% with water, juice, or soda. If vomiting interferes with oral *N*-acetylcysteine administration, consider giving the antidote intravenously. The conventional oral *N*-acetylcysteine protocol in the United States calls for 72 hours of treatment. However, other regimens have demonstrated equivalent success with 20–48 hours of treatment.

The FDA-approved 21-hour intravenous regimen of acetylcysteine (Acetadote) calls for a loading dose of 150 mg/kg given intravenously over 60 minutes, followed by a 4-hour infusion of 50 mg/kg, and a 16-hour infusion of 100 mg/kg. Very large ingestions of acetaminophen (reported ingestions of more than 30 g or if the measured serum acetaminophen level is greater than twice the nomogram line) may require higher dose of *N*-acetylcysteine, and providers should contact a regional poison control center or medical toxicologist for assistance.

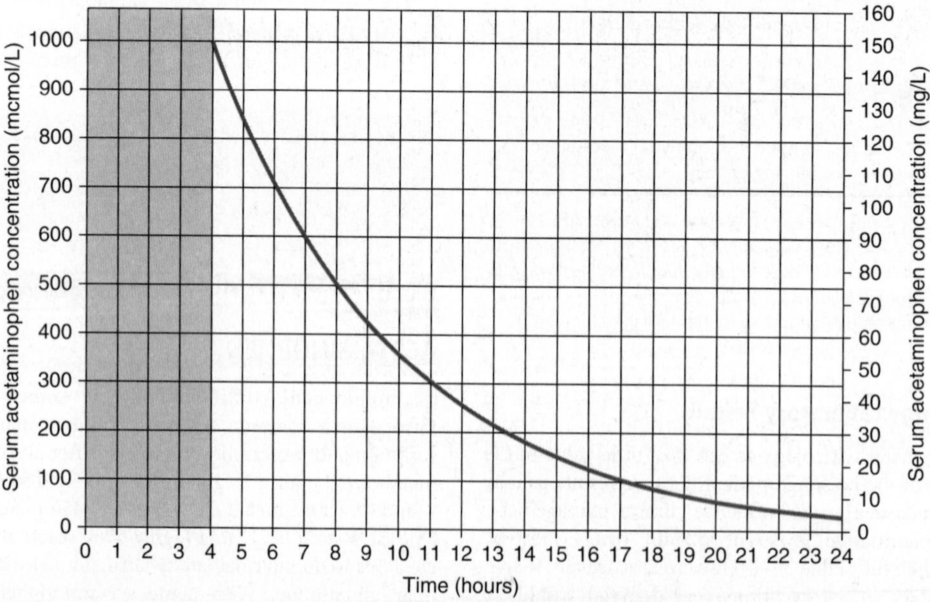

Figure 38–1. Nomogram for prediction of acetaminophen hepatotoxicity following acute overdosage. Patients with serum levels above the line after acute overdose should receive antidotal treatment. (Reproduced with permission from Daly FF, Fountain JS, Murray L, Graudins A, Buckley NA; Panel of Australian and New Zealand clinical toxicologists. Guidelines for the management of paracetamol poisoning in Australia and New Zealand—explanation and elaboration. A consensus statement from clinical toxicologists consulting to the Australasian poisons information centres. Med J Aust. 2008;188(5):296–301.)

Novel simplified intravenous regimens are under investigation and may replace the traditional three-bag dosing described above.

Treatment with *N*-acetylcysteine is most effective if it is started within 8–10 hours after ingestion. Fomepizole, a cytochrome 2E1 inhibitor, has been proposed as an adjunctive therapy, but is not routinely used. Hemodialysis is rarely indicated but might be needed in some patients with massive overdose.

Burnham K et al. A review of alternative intravenous acetylcysteine regimens for acetaminophen overdose. Expert Rev Clin Pharmacol. 2021;14:1267. [PMID: 34187297]
Chiew AL et al. Acetaminophen poisoning. Crit Care Clin. 2021;37:543. [PMID: 34053705]
Chiew AL et al. Updated guidelines for the management of paracetamol poisoning in Australia and New Zealand. Med J Aust. 2020;212:175. [PMID: 31786822]
Hendrickson RG. What is the most appropriate dose of N-acetylcysteine after massive acetaminophen overdose? Clin Toxicol (Phila). 2019;57:686. [PMID: 30777470]
Pourbagher-Shahri AM et al. Use of fomepizole (4-methylpyrazole) for acetaminophen poisoning: a scoping review. Toxicol Lett. 2022;355:47. [PMID: 34785186]

ACIDS, CORROSIVE

The strong mineral acids exert primarily a local corrosive effect on the skin and mucous membranes. Symptoms include severe pain in the throat and upper GI tract; bloody vomitus; difficulty in swallowing, breathing, and speaking; discoloration and destruction of skin and mucous membranes in and around the mouth; and shock. Severe systemic metabolic acidosis may occur both as a result of cellular injury and from systemic absorption of the acid.

Severe deep destructive tissue damage may occur after exposure to hydrofluoric acid because of the penetrating and highly toxic fluoride ion. Systemic hypocalcemia and hyperkalemia may also occur after fluoride absorption, even following skin exposure.

Inhalation of volatile acids, fumes, or gases such as chlorine, fluorine, bromine, or iodine causes severe irritation of the throat and larynx and may cause upper airway obstruction and noncardiogenic pulmonary edema.

▶ Treatment

A. Ingestion

Dilute immediately by giving a glass (4–8 oz) of water to drink. Do *not* give bicarbonate or other neutralizing agents, and do *not* induce vomiting. Some experts recommend immediate cautious placement of a small flexible gastric tube and removal of stomach contents followed by lavage, particularly if the corrosive is a liquid or has important systemic toxicity.

In symptomatic patients, perform flexible endoscopic esophagoscopy to determine the presence and extent of injury. CT scan or plain radiographs of the chest and abdomen may also reveal the extent of injury. Perforation, peritonitis, and major bleeding are indications for surgery. The use of corticosteroids to prevent stricture formation is controversial but may be indicated in select patient populations.

B. Skin Contact

Flood with water for 15 minutes. Use no chemical antidotes; the heat of the reaction may cause additional injury.

For hydrofluoric acid burns, apply 2.5% calcium gluconate gel (prepared by adding 3.5 g calcium gluconate to 5 oz of water-soluble surgical lubricant, eg, K-Y Jelly); then arrange immediate consultation with a plastic surgeon or other specialist. Binding of the fluoride ion may be achieved by injecting 0.5 mL of 5% calcium gluconate per square centimeter under the burned area. (**Caution:** *Do not use calcium chloride.*) Use of a Bier-block technique or intra-arterial infusion of calcium is sometimes required for extensive burns or those involving the nail bed; consult with a hand surgeon or poison control center (1-800-222-1222).

C. Eye Contact

Anesthetize the conjunctiva and corneal surfaces with topical local anesthetic drops (eg, proparacaine). Flood with water for 15 minutes, holding the eyelids open. Check pH with pH 6.0–8.0 test paper, and repeat irrigation, using 0.9% saline, until pH is near 7.0. Check for corneal damage with fluorescein and slit-lamp examination; consult an ophthalmologist about further treatment.

D. Inhalation

Remove from further exposure to fumes or gas. Check skin and clothing. Observe for and treat chemical pneumonitis or pulmonary edema.

Hoffman RS et al. Ingestion of caustic substances. N Engl J Med. 2020;382:1739. [PMID: 32348645]
Hoffman S et al. Dermal hydrofluoric acid toxicity case review: looks can be deceiving. J Emerg Nurs. 2021;47:28. [PMID: 33183770]

ALKALIES

The strong alkalies are common ingredients of some household cleaning compounds and may be suspected by their "soapy" texture. Those with alkalinity above pH 12.0 are particularly corrosive. Disk (or "button") batteries are also a source. Alkalies cause liquefactive necrosis, which is deeply penetrating. Symptoms include burning pain in the upper GI tract, nausea, vomiting, and difficulty in swallowing and breathing. Examination reveals destruction and edema of the affected skin and mucous membranes and bloody vomitus and stools. Radiographs may reveal evidence of perforation or the presence of radiopaque disk batteries in the esophagus or lower GI tract.

▶ Treatment

A. Ingestion

Dilute immediately with a glass of water. Do *not* induce emesis. Some gastroenterologists recommend immediate cautious placement of a small flexible gastric tube and removal of stomach contents followed by gastric lavage after ingestion of liquid caustic substances, to remove residual material. However, others argue that passage of a gastric tube is contraindicated due to the risk of perforation or re-exposure of the esophagus to the corrosive material from vomiting around the tube.

Prompt endoscopy is recommended in symptomatic patients to evaluate the extent of damage; CT scanning may also aid in assessment. If a radiograph reveals ingested disk batteries lodged in the esophagus, immediate endoscopic removal is mandatory.

The use of corticosteroids to prevent stricture formation is controversial but may be indicated in select patient populations.

B. Skin Contact

Wash with running water until the skin no longer feels soapy. Relieve pain and treat shock.

C. Eye Contact

Anesthetize the conjunctival and corneal surfaces with topical anesthetic (eg, proparacaine). Irrigate with water or saline continuously for 20–30 minutes, holding the lids open. Amphoteric solutions may be more effective than water or saline and some are available in Europe (Diphoterine, Prevor). Check pH with pH test paper and repeat irrigation for additional 30-minute periods until the pH is near 7.0. Check for corneal damage with fluorescein and slit-lamp examination; consult an ophthalmologist for further treatment.

Bizrah M et al. An update on chemical eye burns. Eye (Lond). 2019;33:1362. [PMID: 31086244]

AMPHETAMINES & COCAINE

Amphetamines and cocaine are widely used for their euphorigenic and stimulant properties. Both drugs may be smoked, snorted, ingested, or injected. Amphetamines and cocaine produce CNS stimulation and a generalized increase in central and peripheral sympathetic activity. The toxic dose of each drug is highly variable and depends on the route of administration and individual tolerance. The onset of effects is most rapid after intravenous injection or smoking. Amphetamine derivatives and related drugs include methamphetamine ("crystal meth," "crank"), MDMA ("ecstasy"), ephedrine ("herbal ecstasy"), and methcathinone ("cat" or "khat"). Methcathinone derivatives and related synthetic chemicals such as methylenedioxypyrovalerone (MDPV) have become popular drugs of abuse and are often sold as purported "bath salts." Amphetamine-like reactions have also been reported after use of synthetic cannabinoids (eg, "Spice" and "K2"). Nonprescription medications and nutritional supplements may contain stimulant or sympathomimetic drugs such as ephedrine, yohimbine, or caffeine (see also Theophylline & Caffeine section). *Increasingly, amphetamines and cocaine may be adulterated with fentanyl or fentanyl analogs* resulting in unexpected coma, respiratory depression, and death (see also opioids section).

▶ Clinical Findings

Presenting symptoms may include anxiety, tremulousness, tachycardia, hypertension, diaphoresis, dilated pupils, agitation, muscular hyperactivity, and psychosis. Muscle hyperactivity may lead to metabolic acidosis and rhabdomyolysis. In severe intoxication, seizures and hyperthermia may occur. Sustained or severe hypertension may result in intracranial hemorrhage, aortic dissection, or MI; chronic use may cause cardiomyopathy. Ischemic colitis has been reported. Hyponatremia has been reported after MDMA use; the mechanism is not known but may involve excessive water intake, syndrome of inappropriate ADH (SIADH), or both.

The diagnosis is supported by finding amphetamines or the cocaine metabolite benzoylecgonine in the urine. Note that many drugs can give false-positive results on the immunoassay for amphetamines, and most synthetic stimulants do not react with the immunoassay, giving false-negative results.

▶ Treatment

A. Emergency and Supportive Measures

Maintain a patent airway and assist ventilation, if necessary. Treat seizures as described at the beginning of this chapter. Rapidly lower the body temperature in patients who are hyperthermic (temperature higher than 39–40°C). Give intravenous fluids to prevent myoglobinuric kidney injury in patients who have rhabdomyolysis.

B. Specific Treatment

Treat agitation, psychosis, or seizures with a benzodiazepine such as diazepam, 5–10 mg, or lorazepam, 2–3 mg intravenously. Add phenobarbital 15 mg/kg intravenously for persistent seizures. Treat hypertension with a vasodilator drug such as phentolamine (1–5 mg intravenously) or nitroprusside, or a combined alpha- and beta-adrenergic blocker such as labetalol (10–20 mg intravenously). Do *not* administer a pure beta-blocker such as propranolol alone, as this may result in paradoxical worsening of the hypertension as a result of unopposed alpha-adrenergic effects.

Treat tachycardia or tachyarrhythmias with a short-acting beta-blocker such as esmolol (25–100 mcg/kg/minute by intravenous infusion). Treat hyperthermia as described above. Treat hyponatremia as outlined in Chapter 21.

Ciccarone D et al. Understanding stimulant use and use disorders in a new era. Med Clin North Am. 2022;106:81. [PMID: 34823736]

Latif A et al. Is methamphetamine-linked cardiomyopathy an emerging epidemic for new generation? Curr Probl Cardiol. 2021;12:101042. [PMID: 34780869]

Luethi D et al. Designer drugs: mechanism of action and adverse effects. Arch Toxicol. 2020;94:1085. [PMID: 32249347]

Park JN et al. Fentanyl and fentanyl analogs in the illicit stimulant supply: results from U.S. drug seizure data, 2011-2016. Drug Alcohol Depend. 2021;218:108416. [PMID: 33278761]

Stockings E et al. Mortality among people with regular or problematic use of amphetamines: a systematic review and meta-analysis. Addiction. 2019;114:1738. [PMID: 31180607]

ANTICOAGULANTS

Warfarin and related compounds (including ingredients of many commercial rodenticides, the so-called **superwarfarins** such as brodifacoum, difenacoum, and related compounds) inhibit the normal clotting system by blocking hepatic synthesis of vitamin K–dependent clotting factors. After ingestion of "superwarfarins," inhibition of clotting factor synthesis may persist for several weeks or even months after a single dose. DOACs include the direct thrombin inhibitor dabigatran and the factor Xa inhibitors apixaban, edoxaban, and rivaroxaban. Some of these, especially dabigatran, are largely eliminated by the kidney and may accumulate in patients with kidney dysfunction.

Excessive anticoagulation may cause hemoptysis, gross hematuria, bloody stools, hemorrhages into organs, widespread bruising, and bleeding into joint spaces.

Treatment

A. Emergency and Supportive Measures

Discontinue the drug at the first sign of gross bleeding and determine the prothrombin time (INR). The prothrombin time is increased within 12–24 hours (peak 36–48 hours) after overdose of warfarin or "superwarfarins." **Note:** DOACs (dabigatran, apixaban, edoxaban, and rivaroxaban) do *not* predictably alter routine coagulation studies (prothrombin time, partial thromboplastin time, and INR), and these tests are of limited use. Specialized coagulation studies including the hemaclot and ecarin clotting assay and the anti-factor Xa activity may be helpful but are not widely available.

If the patient has ingested an acute overdose, administer activated charcoal.

B. Specific Treatment

1. Warfarin—*In cases of warfarin and "superwarfarin" overdose, do not treat prophylactically with vitamin K*—wait for evidence of anticoagulation (elevated prothrombin time). See Table 14–21 for the management of INR above therapeutic range. Doses of vitamin K as high as 200 mg/day have been required after ingestion of "superwarfarins." Give fresh-frozen plasma, prothrombin complex concentrate, or activated factor VII as needed to rapidly correct the coagulation factor deficit if there is serious bleeding. If the patient is chronically anticoagulated and has strong medical indications for being maintained in that status (eg, prosthetic heart valve), give much smaller doses of vitamin K (1 mg orally) and fresh-frozen plasma (or both) to titrate to the desired prothrombin time. If the patient has ingested brodifacoum or a related superwarfarin, prolonged observation (over weeks) and repeated administration of large doses of vitamin K may be required.

2. DOACs—Vitamin K does not reverse the anticoagulant effects of the DOACs. **Idarucizumab** has been approved by the FDA for reversal of the thrombin inhibitor dabigatran; **andexanet** is approved for reversal of the factor Xa inhibitors apixaban, edoxaban, and rivaroxaban. If specific reversal agents are unavailable, evidence supports the use of prothrombin complex concentrates or activated prothrombin complex concentrates for reversal of factor Xa inhibitors.

Cuker A et al. Reversal of direct oral anticoagulants: guidance from the Anticoagulation Forum. Am J Hematol. 2019;94:697. [PMID: 30916798]

Dobesh PP et al. Antidotes for reversal of direct oral anticoagulants. Pharmacol Ther. 2019;204:107405. [PMID: 31521696]

Gunasekaran K et al. A review of the incidence diagnosis and treatment of spontaneous hemorrhage in patients treated with direct oral anticoagulants. J Clin Med. 2020;9:2984. [PMID: 32942757]

Korobey MJ et al. Efficacy of 4-factor prothrombin complex concentrates in factor Xa inhibitor-associated intracranial bleeding. Neurocrit Care. 2021;34:112. [PMID: 32430804]

Liss DB et al. Antithrombotic and antiplatelet drug toxicity. Crit Care Clin. 2021;37:591. [PMID: 34053708]

ANTICONVULSANTS

Anticonvulsants (carbamazepine, phenytoin, valproic acid, and many newer agents) are widely used in the management of seizure disorders and some are also used for treatment of mood disorders or pain.

Phenytoin can be given orally or intravenously. Rapid intravenous injection of phenytoin can cause acute myocardial depression and cardiac arrest owing to the solvent propylene glycol (fosphenytoin does not contain this diluent). Chronic phenytoin intoxication can occur following only slightly increased doses because of zero-order kinetics and a small toxic-therapeutic window. Phenytoin intoxication can also occur following acute intentional or accidental overdose. The overdose syndrome is usually mild even with high serum levels. The most common manifestations are ataxia, nystagmus, and drowsiness. Choreoathetoid movements have been described.

Carbamazepine intoxication causes drowsiness, stupor and, with high levels, atrioventricular block, coma, and seizures. Dilated pupils and tachycardia are common. Toxicity may be seen with serum levels over 20 mg/L (85 mcmol/L), although severe poisoning is usually associated with concentrations greater than 30–40 mg/L (127–169 mcmol/L). Because of erratic and slow absorption, intoxication may progress over several hours to days.

Valproic acid intoxication produces a unique syndrome consisting of hypernatremia (from the sodium component of the salt), metabolic acidosis, hypocalcemia, elevated serum ammonia, and mild liver aminotransferase elevation. Hypoglycemia may occur as a result of hepatic metabolic dysfunction. Coma with small pupils may be seen and can mimic opioid poisoning. Encephalopathy and cerebral edema can occur.

Gabapentin, levetiracetam, lacosamide, vigabatrin, and zonisamide generally cause somnolence, confusion, and dizziness; there is one case report of hypotension and bradycardia after a large overdose of levetiracetam. Felbamate can cause crystalluria and kidney injury after overdose and may cause idiosyncratic aplastic anemia with therapeutic use. Lamotrigine, topiramate, and tiagabine have been reported to cause seizures after overdose; lamotrigine has sodium channel–blocking properties and may cause QRS prolongation and heart block.

Treatment

A. Emergency and Supportive Measures

For recent ingestions, give activated charcoal orally or by gastric tube. For large ingestions of carbamazepine or valproic acid—especially of sustained-release formulations—consider whole bowel irrigation.

B. Specific Treatment

There are no specific antidotes. Carnitine may be useful in patients with valproic acid–induced hyperammonemia. Consider hemodialysis for massive intoxication with valproic acid or carbamazepine (eg, carbamazepine levels greater than 60 mg/L [254 mcmol/L] or valproic acid levels greater than 800 mg/L [5544 mcmol/L]).

Murty S. Antiepileptic overdose. Indian J Crit Care Med. 2019;23(Suppl 4):S290. [PMID: 32021007]

Pagali S et al. Managing valproic acid toxicity-related hyperammonaemia: an unpredicted course. BMJ Case Rep. 2021;14:e241547. [PMID: 33875509]

Wood KE et al. Correlation of elevated lamotrigine and levetiracetam serum/plasma levels with toxicity: a long-term retrospective review at an academic medical center. Toxicol Rep. 2021;8:1592. [PMID: 34522622]

ANTIPSYCHOTIC DRUGS

Drugs in this group include "conventional" antipsychotics (eg, chlorpromazine, haloperidol, droperidol) and newer "atypical" antipsychotics (eg, risperidone, olanzapine, ziprasidone, quetiapine, aripiprazole). While conventional drugs act mainly on CNS dopamine receptors, atypical drugs also interact with serotonin receptors.

Therapeutic doses of conventional phenothiazines (particularly chlorpromazine) induce drowsiness and mild orthostatic hypotension in as many as 50% of patients. Larger doses can cause obtundation, miosis, severe hypotension, tachycardia, convulsions, and coma. Abnormal cardiac conduction may occur, resulting in prolongation of QRS or QT intervals (or both) and ventricular arrhythmias. Among the atypical agents, quetiapine is more likely to cause coma and hypotension. Hypotension is probably related to blockade of peripheral alpha-adrenergic receptors, causing vasodilatation.

With therapeutic or toxic doses, an acute extrapyramidal dystonic reaction may develop in some patients, with spasmodic contractions of the face and neck muscles, extensor rigidity of the back muscles, carpopedal spasm, and motor restlessness. This reaction is more common with haloperidol and other butyrophenones and less common with newer atypical antipsychotics. Severe rigidity accompanied by hyperthermia and metabolic acidosis ("**neuroleptic malignant syndrome**") may occasionally occur and is life-threatening (see Chapter 25). Atypical antipsychotics have also been associated with weight gain and diabetes mellitus, including diabetic ketoacidosis.

Treatment

A. Emergency and Supportive Measures

Administer activated charcoal for large or recent ingestions. For severe hypotension, treatment with intravenous fluids and vasopressor agents may be necessary. Treat hyperthermia as outlined. Maintain ECG monitoring.

B. Specific Treatment

Hypotension often responds to intravenous saline boluses; cardiac arrhythmias associated with widened QRS intervals on the ECG may respond to intravenous sodium bicarbonate as is given for tricyclic antidepressant overdoses. Prolongation of the QT interval and torsades de pointes are usually treated with intravenous magnesium or overdrive pacing.

For extrapyramidal signs, give diphenhydramine, 0.5–1 mg/kg intravenously, or benztropine mesylate, 0.01–0.02 mg/kg intramuscularly. Treatment with oral doses of these agents should be continued for 24–48 hours.

Bromocriptine (2.5–7.5 mg orally daily) may be effective for mild or moderate neuroleptic malignant syndrome. Dantrolene (2–5 mg/kg intravenously) has also been used for muscle rigidity but is not a true antidote. For severe hyperthermia, rapid neuromuscular paralysis is preferred.

Campleman SL et al; Toxicology Investigators' Consortium (ToxIC). Drug-specific risk of severe QT prolongation following acute drug overdose. Clin Toxicol (Phila). 2020;58:1326. [PMID: 32252558]

Peridy E et al. Quetiapine poisoning and factors influencing severity. J Clin Psychopharmacol. 2019;39:312. [PMID: 31205192]

ARSENIC

Arsenic is found in some pesticides and industrial chemicals and is used as a chemotherapeutic agent. Chronic arsenic poisoning has been associated with contaminated aquifers used for drinking water. Symptoms of acute poisoning usually appear within 1 hour after ingestion but may be delayed as long as 12 hours. They include abdominal pain, vomiting, watery diarrhea, and skeletal muscle cramps. Profound dehydration and shock may occur. In chronic poisoning, symptoms can be vague but often include pancytopenia, painful peripheral sensory neuropathy, and skin changes including melanosis, keratosis, and desquamating rash. Cancers of the lung, bladder, and skin have been reported. Urinary arsenic levels may be falsely elevated after certain meals (eg, seafood) that contain large quantities of a nontoxic form of organic arsenic.

Treatment

A. Emergency Measures

After recent ingestion (within 1–2 hours), perform gastric lavage. Activated charcoal is of uncertain benefit because it binds arsenic poorly. Administer intravenous fluids to replace losses due to vomiting and diarrhea.

B. Antidote

For patients with severe acute intoxication, administer a chelating agent. The preferred drug is 2,3-dimercaptopropanesulfonic acid (DMPS, Unithiol) (3–5 mg/kg intravenously every 4 hours); although there is no FDA-approved commercial formulation of DMPS in the United States, it can be obtained from some compounding pharmacies. An alternative parenteral chelator is dimercaprol (British anti-Lewisite, BAL), which comes as a 10% solution in peanut oil and is given as 3–5 mg/kg intramuscularly every 4–6 hours for 2 days. The side effects include nausea, vomiting, headache, and hypertension. When GI symptoms allow, switch to the oral chelator succimer (dimercaptosuccinic acid, DMSA), 10 mg/kg every 8 hours, for 1 week. Consult a medical toxicologist or regional poison control center (1-800-222-1222) for advice regarding chelation.

Bjørklund G et al. Arsenic intoxication: general aspects and chelating agents. Arch Toxicol. 2020;94:1879. [PMID: 32388818]

Rahaman MS et al. Environmental arsenic exposure and its contribution to human diseases, toxicity mechanism and management. Environ Pollut. 2021;289:117940. [PMID: 34426183]

ATROPINE & ANTICHOLINERGICS

Atropine, scopolamine, belladonna, *Datura stramonium, Hyoscyamus niger*, some mushrooms, tricyclic antidepressants, and antihistamines are antimuscarinic agents with variable CNS effects. Symptoms of toxicity include dryness of the mouth, thirst, difficulty in swallowing, and blurring of vision. Physical signs include dilated pupils, flushed skin, tachycardia, fever, delirium, myoclonus, and ileus. Antidepressants and antihistamines may also induce convulsions.

Antihistamines are commonly available with or without prescription. Diphenhydramine commonly causes delirium, tachycardia, and seizures. Massive diphenhydramine overdose may mimic tricyclic antidepressant cardiotoxic poisoning.

▶ Treatment

A. Emergency and Supportive Measures

Administer activated charcoal. External cooling and sedation, or neuromuscular paralysis in rare cases, are indicated to control high temperatures.

B. Specific Treatment

For severe anticholinergic syndrome (eg, agitated delirium), give physostigmine salicylate, 0.5–1 mg slowly intravenously over 5 minutes, with ECG monitoring; repeat as needed to a total dose of no more than 2 mg. **Caution:** Bradyarrhythmias and convulsions are a hazard with physostigmine administration, and the drug should be avoided in patients with evidence of cardiotoxic effects (eg, QRS interval prolongation) from tricyclic antidepressants or other sodium channel blockers.

Arens AM et al. Adverse effects of physostigmine. J Med Toxicol. 2019;15:184. [PMID: 30747326]

Jayawickreme KP et al. Unknowing ingestion of *Brugmansia suaveolens* leaves presenting with signs of anticholinergic toxicity: a case report. J Med Case Rep. 2019;13:322. [PMID: 31665073]

Saadi R et al. Physostigmine for antimuscarinic toxicity. J Emerg Nurs. 2020;46:126. [PMID: 31918808]

BETA-ADRENERGIC BLOCKERS

There are a wide variety of beta-adrenergic blocking drugs, with varying pharmacologic and pharmacokinetic properties (see Table 11–9). The most toxic beta-blocker is propranolol, which not only blocks beta-1- and beta-2-adrenoceptors but also has direct membrane-depressant and CNS effects.

▶ Clinical Findings

The most common findings with mild or moderate intoxication are hypotension and bradycardia. Cardiac depression from more severe poisoning is often unresponsive to conventional therapy with beta-adrenergic stimulants such as dopamine and norepinephrine. In addition, with propranolol and other lipid-soluble drugs, seizures and coma may occur. Propranolol, oxprenolol, acebutolol, and alprenolol also have membrane-depressant effects and can cause conduction disturbance (wide QRS interval) similar to tricyclic antidepressant overdose.

The diagnosis is based on typical clinical findings. Routine toxicology screening does not usually include beta-blockers.

▶ Treatment

A. Emergency and Supportive Measures

Attempts to treat bradycardia or heart block with atropine (0.5–2 mg intravenously), isoproterenol (2–20 mcg/minute by intravenous infusion, titrated to the desired heart rate), or an external transcutaneous cardiac pacemaker are often ineffective, and specific antidotal treatment may be necessary.

For drugs ingested within an hour of presentation (or longer after ingestion of an extended-release formulation), administer activated charcoal.

B. Specific Treatment

For persistent bradycardia and hypotension, give glucagon, 5–10 mg intravenously, followed by an infusion of 1–5 mg/hour. Glucagon is an inotropic agent that acts at a different receptor site and is therefore not affected by beta-blockade. High-dose insulin (0.5–1 U/kg/hour intravenously) along with glucose supplementation has also been used to reverse severe cardiotoxicity. Membrane-depressant effects (wide QRS interval) may respond to boluses of sodium bicarbonate (50–100 mEq intravenously) as for tricyclic antidepressant poisoning. Vasopressors (norepinephrine and epinephrine) improve hemodynamics and likely survival in case series and animal studies. Intravenous lipid emulsion

(Intralipid 20%, 1.5 mL/kg) has been used successfully in severe propranolol overdose. ECMO should be considered for refractory shock.

Rotella JA et al. Treatment for beta-blocker poisoning: a systematic review. Clin Toxicol (Phila). 2020;58:943. [PMID: 32310006]
St-Onge M. Cardiovascular drug toxicity. Crit Care Clin. 2021;37:563. [PMID: 34053706]

CALCIUM CHANNEL BLOCKERS

In therapeutic doses, nifedipine, nicardipine, amlodipine, felodipine, isradipine, nisoldipine, and nimodipine act mainly on blood vessels, while verapamil and diltiazem act mainly on cardiac contractility and conduction. However, these selective effects can be lost after acute overdose. Patients may present with bradycardia, atrioventricular (AV) nodal block, hypotension, or a combination of these effects. Hyperglycemia is common due to blockade of insulin release. With severe poisoning, cardiac arrest may occur.

Treatment

A. Emergency and Supportive Measures

For ingested drugs, administer activated charcoal. In addition, whole bowel irrigation should be initiated as soon as possible if the patient has ingested a sustained-release product.

B. Specific Treatment

Treat symptomatic bradycardia with atropine (0.5–2 mg intravenously), isoproterenol (2–20 mcg/minute by intravenous infusion), or a transcutaneous cardiac pacemaker. For hypotension, give calcium chloride 10%, 10 mL, or calcium gluconate 10%, 20 mL. Repeat the dose every 3–5 minutes. The optimum (or maximum) dose has not been established, but many toxicologists recommend raising the ionized serum calcium level to as much as twice the normal level. Calcium is most useful in reversing negative inotropic effects and is less effective for AV nodal blockade and bradycardia. High doses of insulin (0.5–1 U/kg intravenous bolus followed by 0.5–1 U/kg/hour infusion) along with sufficient dextrose to maintain euglycemia have been reported to be beneficial, but there are no controlled studies. Vasopressors (norepinephrine and epinephrine) should also be used for refractory hypotension and shock. Infusion of Intralipid 20% lipid emulsion has been reported to improve hemodynamics in animal models and case reports of calcium channel blocker poisoning. Methylene blue (1–2 mg/kg) was reported to reverse refractory shock due to profound vasodilation in a patient with amlodipine poisoning. ECMO has been recommended for refractory shock.

Pellegrini JR et al. "Feeling the blues": a case of calcium channel blocker overdose managed with methylene blue. Cureus. 2021;13(10):e19114. [PMID: 34868762]
Ramanathan K et al. Extracorporeal therapy for amlodipine poisoning. J Artif Organs. 2020;23:183. [PMID: 31552515]
St-Onge M. Cardiovascular drug toxicity. Crit Care Clin. 2021;37:563. [PMID: 34053706]

CARBON MONOXIDE

Carbon monoxide is a colorless, odorless gas produced by the combustion of carbon-containing materials. Poisoning may occur as a result of suicidal or accidental exposure to automobile exhaust, smoke inhalation in a fire, or accidental exposure to an improperly vented gas heater, generator, or other appliance. Carbon monoxide can be generated during degradation of some anesthetic gases by carbon dioxide adsorbents. Carbon monoxide avidly binds to hemoglobin, with an affinity approximately 250 times that of oxygen. This results in reduced oxygen-carrying capacity and altered delivery of oxygen to cells (see also Smoke Inhalation in Chapter 9).

Clinical Findings

At low carbon monoxide levels (carboxyhemoglobin saturation 10–20%), patients may have headache, dizziness, abdominal pain, and nausea. With higher levels, confusion, dyspnea, and syncope may occur. Hypotension, coma, and seizures are common with levels greater than 50–60%. Survivors of acute severe poisoning may develop permanent obvious or subtle neurologic and neuropsychiatric deficits. The fetus and newborn may be more susceptible because of high carbon monoxide affinity for fetal hemoglobin.

Carbon monoxide poisoning should be suspected in any person with severe headache or acutely altered mental status, especially during cold weather, when improperly vented heating systems may have been used. Diagnosis depends on specific measurement of the arterial or venous carboxyhemoglobin saturation, although the level may have declined if high-flow oxygen therapy has already been administered, and levels do not always correlate with clinical symptoms. Routine arterial blood gas testing and pulse oximetry are *not* useful because they give falsely normal Pao_2 and oxyhemoglobin saturation determinations, respectively. (A specialized pulse oximetry device, the Masimo pulse CO-oximeter, is capable of distinguishing oxyhemoglobin from carboxyhemoglobin.)

Treatment

A. Emergency and Supportive Measures

Maintain a patent airway and assist ventilation, if necessary. Remove the patient from exposure. Treat patients with coma, hypotension, or seizures as described at the beginning of this chapter.

B. Specific Treatment

The half-life of the carboxyhemoglobin (CoHb) complex is about 4–5 hours in room air but is reduced dramatically by high concentrations of oxygen. Administer 100% oxygen by tight-fitting high-flow reservoir face mask or endotracheal tube. **Hyperbaric oxygen (HBO)** can provide 100% oxygen under higher than atmospheric pressures, further shortening the half-life; it may also reduce the incidence of subtle neuropsychiatric sequelae. Randomized controlled studies disagree about the benefit of HBO, but commonly recommended indications for HBO in patients with carbon monoxide poisoning include a history of loss of consciousness, CoHb greater than 25%, metabolic acidosis, age over 50 years, and cerebellar findings on neurologic examination.

Casillas S et al. Effectiveness of hyperbaric oxygenation versus normobaric oxygenation therapy in carbon monoxide poisoning: a systematic review. Cureus. 2019;11:e5916. [PMID: 31788375]

Chenoweth JA et al. Carbon monoxide poisoning. Crit Care Clin. 2021;37:657. [PMID: 34053712]

CHEMICAL WARFARE: NERVE AGENTS

Nerve agents used in chemical warfare work by cholinesterase inhibition and are most commonly organophosphorus compounds. Agents such as tabun (GA), sarin (GB), soman (GD), VX, and a group of compounds known as novichoks are similar to insecticides such as malathion but are vastly more potent. They may be inhaled or absorbed through the skin. Systemic effects due to unopposed action of acetylcholine include miosis, salivation, abdominal cramps, diarrhea, and muscle paralysis producing respiratory arrest. Inhalation also produces severe bronchoconstriction and copious nasal and tracheobronchial secretions.

Treatment

A. Emergency and Supportive Measures

Perform thorough decontamination of exposed areas with repeated soap and shampoo washing. Personnel caring for such patients must wear protective clothing and gloves, since cutaneous absorption may occur through normal skin.

B. Specific Treatment

Give atropine in an initial dose of 2 mg intravenously and repeat as needed to reverse signs of acetylcholine excess. (Some patients have required several hundred milligrams.) Treat also with the cholinesterase-reactivating agent pralidoxime, 1–2 g intravenously initially followed by an infusion at a rate of 200–400 mg/hour.

Abbes M et al. Ricin poisoning: a review on contamination source, diagnosis, treatment, prevention and reporting of ricin poisoning. Toxicon. 2021;195:86. [PMID: 33711365]

Agency for Toxic Substances and Disease Registry. Toxic Substances Portal. 2021 Feb 9. https://www.atsdr.cdc.gov/

Grela P et al. How ricin damages the ribosome. Toxins (Basel). 2019;11:241. [PMID: 31035546]

Hulse EJ et al. Organophosphorus nerve agent poisoning: managing the poisoned patient. Br J Anaesth. 2019;123:457. [PMID: 31248646]

Richardson JR et al. Neurotoxicity of pesticides. Acta Neuropathol. 2019;138:343. [PMID: 31197504]

Timperley CM et al. Advice on assistance and protection from the Scientific Advisory Board of the Organisation for the Prohibition of Chemical Weapons: Part 2. On preventing and treating health effects from acute, prolonged, and repeated nerve agent exposure, and the identification of medical countermeasures able to reduce or eliminate the longer-term health effects of nerve agents. Toxicology. 2019;413:13. [PMID: 30500381]

US Department of Labor. Occupational Safety and Health Administration. Safety and Health Guides/Nerve Agents Guide. https://www.osha.gov/SLTC/emergencypreparedness/guides/nerve.html

CLONIDINE & OTHER SYMPATHOLYTIC ANTIHYPERTENSIVES

Overdose with these agents (clonidine, guanabenz, guanfacine, methyldopa) causes bradycardia, hypotension, miosis, respiratory depression, and coma. (Transient hypertension occasionally occurs after acute overdose, a result of peripheral alpha-adrenergic effects in high doses.) Symptoms usually resolve in less than 24 hours, and deaths are rare. Similar symptoms may occur after ingestion of topical nasal decongestants chemically similar to clonidine (oxymetazoline, tetrahydrozoline, naphazoline). Brimonidine and apraclonidine are used as ophthalmic preparations for glaucoma. Tizanidine is a centrally acting muscle relaxant structurally related to clonidine; it produces similar toxicity in overdose.

Treatment

A. Emergency and Supportive Measures

Give activated charcoal. Maintain the airway and support respiration if necessary. Symptomatic treatment is usually sufficient even in massive overdose. Maintain blood pressure with intravenous fluids. Dopamine can also be used. Atropine is usually effective for bradycardia.

B. Specific Treatment

Naloxone is reported to reverse signs and symptoms of clonidine overdose in anecdotal cases and retrospective studies.

Toce MS et al. Clinical effects of pediatric clonidine exposure: a retrospective cohort study at a single tertiary care center. J Emerg Med. 2021;60:58. [PMID: 33036823]

COCAINE

See Amphetamines & Cocaine.

CYANIDE

Cyanide is a highly toxic chemical used widely in research and commercial laboratories and many industries. Its gaseous form, hydrogen cyanide, is an important component of smoke in fires. Cyanide-generating glycosides are also found in the pits of apricots and other related plants. Cyanide is generated by the breakdown of nitroprusside, and poisoning can result from rapid high-dose infusions. Cyanide is also formed by metabolism of acetonitrile, a solvent found in some over-the-counter fingernail glue removers. Cyanide is rapidly absorbed by inhalation, skin absorption, or ingestion. It disrupts cellular function by inhibiting cytochrome oxidase and preventing cellular oxygen utilization.

Clinical Findings

The onset of toxicity is nearly instantaneous after inhalation of hydrogen cyanide gas but may be delayed for minutes to hours after ingestion of cyanide salts or cyanogenic plants or chemicals. Effects include headache, dizziness, nausea, abdominal pain, and anxiety, followed by confusion, syncope, shock, seizures, coma, and death. The odor of "bitter almonds" may be detected on the patient's breath or in vomitus, though this is not a reliable finding. The venous oxygen saturation may be elevated (greater than 90%) in severe poisonings because tissues have failed to take up arterial oxygen.

Treatment

A. Emergency and Supportive Measures

Remove the patient from exposure, taking care to avoid exposure to rescuers. For suspected cyanide poisoning due to nitroprusside infusion, stop or slow the rate of infusion. (Metabolic acidosis and other signs of cyanide poisoning usually clear rapidly.)

For cyanide ingestion, administer activated charcoal. Although charcoal has a low affinity for cyanide, the usual doses of 60–100 g are adequate to bind typically ingested lethal doses (100–200 mg).

B. Specific Treatment

In the United States, there are two available cyanide antidote regimens. The preferred regimen is hydroxocobalamin (Cyanokit, EMD Pharmaceuticals) which directly binds and detoxifies free cyanide. The adult dose is 5 g intravenously (the pediatric dose is 70 mg/kg). **Note:** Hydroxocobalamin causes red discoloration of skin and body fluids that may last several days and can interfere with some laboratory tests.

Poisoning can also be treated with the older cyanide antidote package (Nithiodote), which contains sodium nitrite (to induce methemoglobinemia, which binds free cyanide) and sodium thiosulfate (to promote conversion of cyanide to the less toxic thiocyanate). Administer 3% sodium nitrite solution, 10 mL intravenously, followed by 25% sodium thiosulfate solution, 50 mL intravenously (12.5 g). **Caution:** *Nitrites may induce hypotension and dangerous levels of methemoglobin.*

Hendry-Hofer TB et al. A review on ingested cyanide: risks, clinical presentation, diagnostics, and treatment challenges. J Med Toxicol. 2019;15:128. [PMID: 30539383]

Henretig FM et al. Hazardous chemical emergencies and poisonings. N Engl J Med. 2019;380:1638. [PMID: 31018070]

DIETARY SUPPLEMENTS & HERBAL PRODUCTS

Unlike prescription and over-the-counter pharmaceuticals, dietary supplements do not require FDA approval and do not undergo the same premarketing evaluation of safety and efficacy as drugs, and purveyors may or may not adhere to good manufacturing practices and quality control standards. Supplements may cause illness as a result of intrinsic toxicity, misidentification or mislabeling, drug-herb reactions, or intentional adulteration with pharmaceuticals. If you suspect a dietary supplement or herbal product may be the cause of an otherwise unexplained illness, contact the FDA (1-888-463-6332) or the regional poison control center (1-800-222-1222), or consult the following online database: https://www.fda.gov/food/dietary-supplements.

Table 38–7 lists selected examples of clinical toxicity from some of these products.

Table 38–7. Examples of potential toxicity associated with some dietary supplements and herbal medicines (listed in alphabetical order).

Product	Common Use	Possible Toxicity
Azarcon (Greta)	Mexican folk remedy for abdominal pain, colic	Contains lead
Comfrey	Gastric upset, diarrhea	Contains pyrrolizidine alkaloids, can cause hepatic veno-occlusive disease
Creatine	Athletic performance enhancement	Nausea, diarrhea, abdominal cramps; elevated serum creatinine
Ginkgo	Memory improvement, tinnitus	Antiplatelet effects, hemorrhage; abdominal pain, diarrhea
Ginseng	Immune system; stress	Decreased glucose; increased cortisol
Guarana	Athletic performance enhancement, appetite suppression	Contains caffeine: can cause tremor, tachycardia, vomiting
Kava	Anxiety, insomnia	Drowsiness, hepatitis, skin rash
Ma huang	Stimulant; athletic performance enhancement	Contains ephedrine: anxiety, insomnia, hypertension, tachycardia, seizures
Spirulina	Body building	Niacin-like flushing reaction
Yohimbine	Sexual enhancement	Hallucinations, hypertension, tachycardia
Zinc	Cold/flu symptoms	Nausea, oral irritation, anosmia

Reproduced with permission from Haller C. Herbal and Alternative Products. In: Olson KR (ed.) *Poisoning & Drug Overdose*, 7th edition. McGraw Hill, 2018.

Charen E et al. Toxicity of herbs, vitamins and supplements. Adv Chronic Kidney Dis. 2020;27:67. [PMID: 32147004]

Lim DY et al. Collective exposure to lead from an approved natural product-derived drug in Korea. Ann Occup Environ Med. 2019;31:e20. [PMID: 31620297]

Woo SM et al. Herbal and dietary supplement induced liver injury: highlights from the recent literature. World J Hepatol. 2021;13:1019. [PMID: 34630872]

DIGITALIS & OTHER CARDIAC GLYCOSIDES

Cardiac glycosides paralyze the Na^+-K^+-ATPase pump and have potent vagotonic effects. Intracellular effects include enhancement of calcium-dependent contractility and shortening of the action potential duration. A number of plants (eg, oleander, foxglove, lily-of-the-valley) contain cardiac glycosides. Bufotenin, a cardiotoxic steroid found in certain toad secretions and used as an herbal medicine and a purported aphrodisiac, has pharmacologic properties similar to cardiac glycosides.

Clinical Findings

Intoxication may result from acute single exposure or chronic accidental overmedication, especially in patients with kidney dysfunction taking digoxin. After acute overdosage, nausea and vomiting, bradycardia, hyperkalemia, and AV block frequently occur. Patients in whom toxicity develops gradually during long-term therapy may be hypokalemic and hypomagnesemic owing to concurrent diuretic treatment and more commonly present with ventricular arrhythmias (eg, ectopy, bidirectional ventricular tachycardia, or ventricular fibrillation). Digoxin levels may be only slightly elevated in patients with intoxication from cardiac glycosides other than digoxin because of limited cross-reactivity of immunologic tests.

Treatment

A. Emergency and Supportive Measures

After acute ingestion, administer activated charcoal. Monitor potassium levels and cardiac rhythm closely. Treat bradycardia initially with atropine (0.5–2 mg intravenously) or a transcutaneous external cardiac pacemaker.

B. Specific Treatment

For patients with significant intoxication, administer digoxin-specific antibodies (digoxin immune Fab [ovine]; DigiFab). Estimation of the dose is based on the body burden of digoxin calculated from the ingested dose or the steady-state serum digoxin concentration, as described below. More effective binding of digoxin may be achieved if the dose is given partly as a bolus and the remainder as an infusion over a few hours.

1. From the ingested dose—Number of vials = approximately 1.5–2 × ingested dose (mg).

2. From the serum concentration—Number of vials = serum digoxin (ng/mL) × body weight (kg) × 10^{-2}. **Note:** This is based on the equilibrium digoxin level; after acute overdose, serum levels may be falsely high for several hours before tissue distribution is complete, and overestimation of the DigiFab dose is likely.

3. Empiric dosing—Empiric titration of DigiFab may be used if the patient's condition is relatively stable and an underlying condition (eg, atrial fibrillation) favors retaining a residual level of digitalis activity. Start with one or two vials and reassess the patient's clinical condition after 20–30 minutes. For cardiac glycosides other than digoxin or digitoxin, there is no formula for estimation of vials needed and treatment is entirely based on response to empiric dosing.

Note: After administration of digoxin-specific Fab antibody fragments, serum digoxin levels may be falsely elevated depending on the assay technique.

Chan BS et al. Clinical experience with titrating doses of digoxin antibodies in acute digoxin poisoning. (ATOM-6). Clin Toxicol (Phila). 2022;60:433. [PMID: 34424803]

ETHANOL, BENZODIAZEPINES, & OTHER SEDATIVE-HYPNOTIC AGENTS

The group of agents known as sedative-hypnotic drugs includes a variety of products used for the treatment of anxiety, depression, insomnia, and epilepsy. Besides common benzodiazepines, such as lorazepam, alprazolam, clonazepam, diazepam, oxazepam, chlordiazepoxide, and triazolam, this group includes the newer benzodiazepine-like hypnotics zolpidem, zopiclone, and zaleplon, the muscle relaxants baclofen and carisoprodol, and barbiturates such as phenobarbital. Phenibut, a $GABA_B$ agonist, has gained popularity in recent years, and is associated with CNS depression and a withdrawal syndrome. Ethanol and other selected agents are also popular recreational drugs. All of these drugs depress the CNS reticular activating system, cerebral cortex, and cerebellum.

Clinical Findings

Mild intoxication produces euphoria, slurred speech, and ataxia. Ethanol intoxication may produce hypoglycemia, even at relatively low concentrations, in children and in fasting adults. With more severe intoxication, stupor, coma, and respiratory arrest may occur. Carisoprodol (Soma) commonly causes muscle jerking or myoclonus. *Death or serious morbidity is usually the result of pulmonary aspiration of gastric contents.* Bradycardia, hypotension, and hypothermia are common. Patients with massive intoxication may appear to be dead, with no reflex responses and even absent electroencephalographic activity. Diagnosis and assessment of severity of intoxication are usually based on clinical findings. Ethanol serum levels over 300 mg/dL (0.3 g/dL; 65 mmol/L) can produce coma in infrequent drinkers, while regular drinkers may remain awake at much higher levels.

Treatment

A. Emergency and Supportive Measures

Administer activated charcoal if the patient has ingested a massive dose and the airway is protected. Repeat-dose charcoal may enhance elimination of phenobarbital, but it has not been proved to improve clinical outcome. Hemodialysis may be necessary for patients with severe phenobarbital intoxication.

B. Specific Treatment

Flumazenil is a benzodiazepine receptor-specific antagonist; it has no effect on ethanol, barbiturates, or other sedative-hypnotic agents. If used, flumazenil is given slowly intravenously, 0.2 mg over 30–60 seconds, and repeated in 0.2–0.5 mg increments as needed up to a total dose of 3–5 mg. **Caution:** *Flumazenil should rarely be used because it may induce seizures in patients with preexisting seizure disorder, benzodiazepine tolerance, or concomitant tricyclic antidepressant or other convulsant overdose.* If seizures occur, diazepam and other benzodiazepine anticonvulsants may not be effective. As with naloxone, the duration of action of flumazenil is short (2–3 hours) and resedation may occur, requiring repeated doses.

Doyno CR et al. Sedative-hypnotic agents that impact gamma-aminobutyric acid receptors: focus on flunitrazepam, gamma-hydroxybutyric acid, phenibut, and selank. J Clin Pharmacol. 2021;61(Suppl 2):S114. [PMID: 34396551]
Krause M et al. Toxin-induced coma and central nervous system depression. Neurol Clin. 2020;38:825. [PMID: 33040863]
Peng L et al. Benzodiazepines and related sedatives. Med Clin North Am. 2022;106:113. [PMID: 34823725]

GAMMA-HYDROXYBUTYRATE (GHB)

GHB is a popular recreational drug. It originated as a short-acting general anesthetic and is occasionally used in the treatment of narcolepsy. It gained popularity among bodybuilders for its alleged growth hormone stimulation and found its way into social settings, where it is consumed as a liquid. It has been used to facilitate sexual assault (**"date-rape" drug**). Symptoms after ingestion include drowsiness and lethargy followed by coma with respiratory depression. Muscle twitching and seizures are sometimes observed. Recovery is usually rapid, with patients awakening within a few hours. Other related chemicals with similar effects include butanediol and gamma-butyrolactone (GBL). A prolonged withdrawal syndrome has been described in some heavy users.

▶ Treatment

Monitor the airway and assist breathing if needed. There is no specific treatment. Most patients recover rapidly with supportive care. GHB withdrawal syndrome may require very large doses of benzodiazepines; baclofen has also been used.

Busardò FP et al. Interpreting γ-hydroxybutyrate concentrations for clinical and forensic purposes. Clin Toxicol (Phila). 2019;57:149. [PMID: 30307336]
Marinelli E et al. Gamma-hydroxybutyrate abuse: pharmacology and poisoning and withdrawal management. Arh Hig Rada Toksikol. 2020;71:19. [PMID: 32597141]

HYPOGLYCEMIC DRUGS

Medications used for diabetes mellitus include insulin, sulfonylureas and other insulin secretagogues, alpha-glucosidase inhibitors (acarbose, miglitol), biguanides (metformin), thiazolidinediones (pioglitazone, rosiglitazone), sodium glucose transporter (SGLT2) inhibitors, and peptide analogs (pramlintide, exenatide) or enhancers (sitagliptin) (see Chapter 27). Of these, insulin and the insulin secretagogues are the most likely to cause hypoglycemia. Metformin can cause lactic acidosis, especially in patients with impaired kidney function or after intentional drug overdose. Euglycemic diabetic ketoacidosis has been reported with SGLT2 use. Table 27–4 lists the duration of hypoglycemic effect of oral hypoglycemic agents and Table 27–5 the extent and duration of various types of insulins.

▶ Clinical Findings

Hypoglycemia may occur quickly after injection of short-acting insulins or may be delayed and prolonged, especially if a large amount has been injected into a single area, creating a "depot" effect. Hypoglycemia after sulfonylurea ingestion is usually apparent within a few hours but may be delayed several hours, especially if food or glucose-containing fluids have been given.

▶ Treatment

Give sugar and carbohydrate-containing food or liquids by mouth, or intravenous dextrose if the patient is unable to swallow safely. For severe hypoglycemia, start with D50W, 50 mL intravenously (25 g dextrose); repeat, if needed. Follow up with dextrose-containing intravenous fluids (D5W or D10W) to maintain a blood glucose greater than 70–80 mg/dL.

For hypoglycemia caused by sulfonylureas and related insulin secretagogues, consider use of octreotide, a synthetic somatostatin analog that blocks pancreatic insulin release. A dose of 50–100 mcg octreotide subcutaneously every 6–12 hours can reduce the need for exogenous dextrose and prevent rebound hypoglycemia from excessive dextrose dosing.

Admit all patients with symptomatic hypoglycemia after sulfonylurea overdose. Observe asymptomatic overdose patients for at least 12 hours.

Consider hemodialysis for patients with metformin overdose accompanied by severe lactic acidosis (lactate greater than 20 mmol/L or pH < 7.0).

Baumgartner K et al. Toxicology of medications for diabetes mellitus. Crit Care Clin. 2021;37:577. [PMID: 34053707]
Razavi-Nematollahi L et al. Adverse effects of glycemia-lowering medications in type 2 diabetes. Curr Diab Rep. 2019;19:132. [PMID: 31748838]

ISONIAZID

Isoniazid (INH) is an antibiotic used mainly in the treatment and prevention of tuberculosis. It may cause hepatitis with long-term use, especially in patients with alcohol use disorder and older adults. It produces acute toxic effects by competing with pyridoxal 5-phosphate, resulting in lowered brain gamma-aminobutyric acid (GABA) levels. Acute ingestion of as little as 1.5–2 g of INH can cause toxicity, and severe poisoning is likely to occur after ingestion of more than 80–100 mg/kg.

Clinical Findings

Confusion, slurred speech, and seizures may occur abruptly after acute overdose. Severe lactic acidosis—out of proportion to the severity of seizures—is probably due to inhibited metabolism of lactate. Peripheral neuropathy and acute hepatitis may occur with long-term use.

Diagnosis is based on a history of ingestion and the presence of severe acidosis associated with seizures. INH is not usually included in routine toxicologic screening, and serum levels are not readily available.

Treatment

A. Emergency and Supportive Measures

Seizures may require higher than usual doses of benzodiazepines (eg, lorazepam, 3–5 mg intravenously) or administration of pyridoxine as an antidote.

Administer activated charcoal after large recent ingestion, but with caution because of the risk of abrupt onset of seizures.

B. Specific Treatment

Pyridoxine (vitamin B_6) is a specific antagonist of the acute toxic effects of INH and is usually successful in controlling convulsions that do not respond to benzodiazepines. Give 5 g intravenously over 1–2 minutes or, if the amount ingested is known, give a gram-for-gram equivalent amount of pyridoxine. Patients taking INH are usually given 25–50 mg of pyridoxine orally daily to help prevent neuropathy.

Navalkele B et al. Seizures in an immunocompetent adult from treatment of latent tuberculosis infection: is isoniazid to blame? Open Forum Infect Dis. 2020;7:ofaa144. [PMID: 32462048]

LEAD

Lead is used in a variety of industrial and commercial products, such as firearms ammunition, storage batteries, solders, paints, pottery, plumbing, and gasoline and is found in some traditional Hispanic and Ayurvedic ethnic medicines. *Lead toxicity usually results from chronic repeated exposure and is rare after a single ingestion.* Lead produces a variety of adverse effects on cellular function and primarily affects the nervous system, GI tract, and hematopoietic system.

Clinical Findings

Lead poisoning often goes undiagnosed initially because presenting symptoms and signs are nonspecific and exposure is not suspected. Common symptoms include colicky abdominal pain, constipation, headache, and irritability. Severe poisoning may cause coma and convulsions. Chronic intoxication can cause learning disorders (in children) and motor neuropathy (eg, wrist drop). Lead-containing bullet fragments in or near joint spaces can result in chronic lead toxicity.

Diagnosis is based on measurement of the blood lead level. Whole blood lead levels above 3.5 mcg/dL warrant public health investigation. Levels between 1 and 25 mcg/dL have been associated with subclinical impaired neurobehavioral development in children. Levels of 25–60 mcg/dL may be associated with headache, irritability, subclinical neuropathy, slowed reaction time and other neuropsychiatric effects. Levels of 60–80 mcg/dL are associated with moderate toxicity, and levels greater than 80–100 mcg/dL are often associated with severe poisoning. Other laboratory findings of lead poisoning include microcytic anemia with basophilic stippling and elevated free erythrocyte protoporphyrin.

Treatment

A. Emergency and Supportive Measures

The most critical intervention in the treatment of lead poisoning is identification of and removal from the source of exposure. For patients with encephalopathy, maintain a patent airway and treat coma and convulsions as described at the beginning of this chapter.

For recent acute ingestion, if a large lead-containing object (eg, fishing weight) is still visible in the stomach on abdominal radiograph, whole bowel irrigation, endoscopy, or even surgical removal may be necessary to prevent subacute lead poisoning. (The acidic gastric contents may corrode the metal surface, enhancing lead absorption. Once the object passes into the small intestine, the risk of toxicity declines.)

The US Occupational Safety and Health Administration establishes workplace standards for lead exposure. Contact the regional office for more information. Several states mandate reporting of cases of confirmed lead poisoning.

B. Specific Treatment

The indications for chelation depend on the blood lead level and the patient's clinical state. A medical toxicologist or regional poison control center (1-800-222-1222) should be consulted for advice about selection and use of these antidotes.

1. Severe toxicity—Patients with severe intoxication (encephalopathy or levels greater than 70–100 mcg/dL) should receive edetate calcium disodium (ethylenediaminetetraacetic acid, EDTA), 1500 mg/m^2/kg/day (approximately 50 mg/kg/day) in four to six divided doses or as a continuous intravenous infusion. Some clinicians also add dimercaprol (BAL), 4–5 mg/kg intramuscularly every 4 hours for 5 days, for patients with encephalopathy.

2. Less severe toxicity—Patients with less severe symptoms and asymptomatic patients with blood lead levels between 55 and 69 mcg/dL may be treated with edetate calcium disodium alone in dosages as above. An oral chelator, succimer (DMSA), is available for use in patients with mild to moderate intoxication. The usual dose is 10 mg/kg orally every 8 hours for 5 days, then every 12 hours for 2 weeks.

Centers for Disease Control and Prevention (CDC). Summary of Recommendations for follow-up and case management of children based on initial screening capillary and confirmed venous blood lead levels. Page reviewed 2021. https://www.cdc.gov/nceh/lead/advisory/acclpp/actions-blls.htm

Naranjo VI et al. Lead toxicity in children: an unremitting public health problem. Pediatr Neurol. 2020;113:51. [PMID: 33011642]

Raut TP et al. Acute lead encephalopathy secondary to Ayurvedic medication use: two cases with review of literature. Neurol India. 2021;69:1417. [PMID: 34747829]

LITHIUM

Lithium is widely used for the treatment of bipolar depression and other psychiatric disorders. The only normal route of lithium elimination is via the kidney, so patients with acute or chronic kidney disorders are at risk for accumulation of lithium resulting in gradual onset (chronic) toxicity. Intoxication resulting from chronic accidental overmedication or kidney impairment is more common and usually more severe than that seen after acute oral overdose.

Clinical Findings

Mild to moderate toxicity causes lethargy, confusion, tremor, ataxia, and slurred speech. This may progress to myoclonic jerking, delirium, coma, and convulsions. Recovery may be slow and incomplete following severe intoxication. Laboratory studies in patients with chronic intoxication often reveal an elevated serum creatinine and an elevated BUN/creatinine ratio due to underlying volume contraction. The white blood cell count is often elevated. ECG findings include T-wave flattening or inversion, and sometimes bradycardia or sinus node arrest. Nephrogenic diabetes insipidus can occur with overdose or with therapeutic doses. Dysfunction of the thyroid and parathyroid glands has also been described as a result of prolonged lithium exposure.

Lithium levels may be difficult to interpret. Lithium has a narrow therapeutic window, and chronic intoxication can be seen with levels only slightly above the therapeutic range (0.8–1.2 mEq/L). In contrast, patients with acute ingestion may have transiently high levels (up to 10 mEq/L reported) without any symptoms before the lithium fully distributes into tissues. **Note:** Falsely high lithium levels (as high as 6–8 mEq/L) can be measured if a green-top blood specimen tube (containing lithium heparin) is used for blood collection.

Treatment

After acute oral overdose, consider gastric lavage or whole bowel irrigation to prevent systemic absorption (**Note:** lithium is *not* adsorbed by activated charcoal). In all patients, evaluate kidney function and volume status, and give intravenous saline-containing fluids as needed. Monitor serum lithium levels and seek assistance with their interpretation and the need for dialysis from a medical toxicologist or regional poison control center (1-800-222-1222). Consider hemodialysis if the patient is markedly symptomatic or if the serum lithium level exceeds 4–5 mEq/L, especially if kidney function is impaired. Continuous renal replacement therapy may be an effective alternative to hemodialysis.

Hlaing PM et al. Neurotoxicity in chronic lithium poisoning. Intern Med J. 2020;50:427. [PMID: 31211493]

King JD et al. Extracorporeal removal of poisons and toxins. Clin J Am Soc Nephrol. 2019;14:1408. [PMID: 31439539]

LSD & OTHER HALLUCINOGENS

A variety of substances—ranging from naturally occurring plants and mushrooms to synthetic substances such as phencyclidine (PCP), toluene and other solvents, dextromethorphan, and lysergic acid diethylamide (LSD)—are used for their hallucinogenic properties. The mechanism of toxicity and the clinical effects vary for each substance.

Many hallucinogenic plants and mushrooms produce anticholinergic delirium, characterized by flushed skin, dry mucous membranes, dilated pupils, tachycardia, and urinary retention. Other plants and mushrooms may contain hallucinogenic indoles such as mescaline and LSD, which typically cause marked visual hallucinations and perceptual distortion, widely dilated pupils, and mild tachycardia. PCP, a dissociative anesthetic agent similar to ketamine, can produce fluctuating delirium and coma, often associated with vertical and horizontal nystagmus. Toluene and other hydrocarbon solvents (eg, butane, trichloroethylene, "chemo," etc.) cause euphoria and delirium and may sensitize the myocardium to the effects of catecholamines, leading to fatal dysrhythmias. Other drugs used for their psychostimulant effects include synthetic cannabinoid receptor agonists, *Salvia divinorum*, synthetic tryptamines, and phenylethylamines, and mephedrone and related cathinone derivatives. See https://www.erowid.org/psychoactives/psychoactives.shtml for descriptions of various hallucinogenic substances.

Treatment

A. Emergency and Supportive Measures

Maintain a patent airway and assist respirations if necessary. Treat coma, hyperthermia, hypertension, and seizures as outlined at the beginning of this chapter. For recent large ingestions, consider giving activated charcoal orally or by gastric tube.

B. Specific Treatment

Patients with anticholinergic delirium may benefit from a dose of physostigmine, 0.5–1 mg intravenously, not to exceed 1 mg/minute. Dysphoria, agitation, and psychosis associated with LSD or mescaline intoxication may respond to benzodiazepines (eg, lorazepam, 1–2 mg orally or intravenously) or haloperidol (2–5 mg intramuscularly or intravenously) or another antipsychotic drug (eg, olanzapine or ziprasidone). Monitor patients who have sniffed solvents for cardiac dysrhythmias (most commonly premature ventricular contractions, ventricular tachycardia, ventricular fibrillation); treatment with beta-blockers such as propranolol (1–5 mg intravenously) or esmolol (250–500 mcg/kg intravenously, then 50 mcg/kg/minute by infusion) may be more effective than lidocaine or amiodarone.

Levine M et al. New designer drugs. Emerg Med Clin North Am. 2021;39:677. [PMID: 34215409]

Tamama K et al. Newly emerging drugs of abuse. Handb Exp Pharmacol. 2020;258:463. [PMID: 31595417]

MARIJUANA & SYNTHETIC CANNABINOIDS

Marijuana refers to the crushed dried leaves and flowers of the Cannabis plant. These dried leaves and flowers contain the psychoactive cannabinoid delta-9-tetrahydrocannabinal (THC), which binds to endogenous cannabinoid receptors. Marijuana is usually smoked in cigarettes or pipes but may also be vaporized or added to a variety of foods, beverages, and candies. Resin from the plant may be dried and pressed into blocks called hashish, and solvents may be used to extract THC into highly concentrated oils (butane hash oil). THC has been used medically as an appetite stimulant, as an antiemetic, and in the treatment of a variety of medical conditions. It has now been legalized for both medical and recreational use in an increasing number of US states (https://disa.com/map-of-marijuana-legality-by-state). Toxicity is dose dependent but varies significantly by individual, prior experience, and degree of tolerance. Synthetic cannabinoids ("Spice," "K2," "Black Mamba") are laboratory designed analogs of THC. They have become increasingly popular and are associated with a variety of adverse side effects, including seizures, kidney dysfunction, and serious neuropsychiatric symptoms. Cannabidiol (CBD) is a constituent of Cannabis that does not produce THC-like intoxication. CBD extracts are available over the counter and via the internet for a variety of proposed effects (anti-inflammatory, antioxidant, anxiolysis) and by prescription for some pediatric seizure disorders. Overdoses are typically not dangerous.

▶ Clinical Findings

Onset of symptoms after smoking is usually rapid (minutes) with a duration of effect of approximately 2 hours. Symptoms may be delayed after ingestion and can result in prolonged intoxication (up to 8 hours). Mild intoxication may result in euphoria, palpitations, heightened sensory awareness, altered time perception, and sedation. More severe intoxication may result in anxiety, visual hallucinations, and acute paranoid psychosis. Physical findings include tachycardia, orthostatic hypotension, conjunctival injection, incoordination, slurred speech, and ataxia. Long-term heavy marijuana use is associated with recurrent nausea, abdominal pain, and vomiting, termed the **cannabinoid hyperemesis syndrome.** Children may inadvertently be exposed to marijuana through the consumption of THC-containing candies or other foods. Children may experience more severe symptoms including stupor, coma, and seizures. **E-cigarette or vaping-associated acute lung injury** is a syndrome of diffuse lung injury associated with vaping THC adulterated with vitamin E acetate.

▶ Treatment

A. Emergency and Supportive Measures

Treat anxiety and paranoia with simple reassurance and placement into a calming environment. Benzodiazepines such as lorazepam or diazepam may be used for more severe behavioral and psychomotor symptoms. Hypotension and sinus tachycardia should be treated with intravenous fluids.

B. Specific Treatment

There is no specific antidote available. Consider activated charcoal early after ingestion of large quantities. Topical capsaicin and haloperidol have been used with variable success for the treatment of acute vomiting in patients with cannabinoid hyperemesis syndrome.

Aldy K et al. E-cigarette or vaping product use-associated lung injury (EVALI) features and recognition in the emergency department. J Am Coll Emerg Physicians Open. 2020;1:1090. [PMID: 33145562]

Alves VL et al. The synthetic cannabinoids phenomenon: from structure to toxicological properties. A review. Crit Rev Toxicol. 2020;50:359. [PMID: 32530350]

Kaslow JA et al. E-cigarette and vaping product use-associated lung injury in the pediatric population: a critical review of the current literature. Pediatr Pulmonol. 2021;56:1857. [PMID: 33821574]

Wong K et al. Acute cannabis toxicity. Pediatr Emerg Care. 2019;35:799. [PMID: 31688799]

MERCURY

Mercury poisoning may occur by ingestion of inorganic mercuric salts, organic mercury compounds, or inhalation of metallic mercury vapor. Ingestion of the mercuric salts causes a burning sensation in the throat, discoloration and edema of oral mucous membranes, abdominal pain, vomiting, bloody diarrhea, and shock. Direct nephrotoxicity causes AKI. Inhalation of high concentrations of metallic mercury vapor may cause acute fulminant chemical pneumonia. Chronic mercury poisoning causes weakness, ataxia, intention tremors, irritability, and depression. Exposure to alkyl (organic) mercury derivatives from highly contaminated fish or fungicides used on seeds has caused ataxia, tremors, convulsions, and catastrophic birth defects. Nearly all fish have some traces of mercury contamination; the US Environmental Protection Agency advises consumers to avoid swordfish, shark, king mackerel, and tilefish because they contain higher levels. Fish and shellfish that are generally low in mercury content include shrimp, canned light tuna (not albacore "white" tuna), salmon, pollock, and catfish. Dental fillings composed of mercury amalgam pose a small risk of chronic mercury poisoning and their removal is rarely justified.

Some imported skin lightening creams contain toxic quantities of mercury.

Treatment

A. Acute Poisoning

There is no effective specific treatment for mercury vapor pneumonitis. Remove ingested mercuric salts by lavage and administer activated charcoal. For acute ingestion of mercuric salts, give dimercaprol (BAL) at once, as for arsenic poisoning. Unless the patient has severe gastroenteritis, consider succimer (DMSA), 10 mg/kg orally every 8 hours for 5 days and then every 12 hours for 2 weeks. Unithiol (DMPS) is a chelator that can be given orally or parenterally but is not commonly available in the United States; it can be obtained from some compounding pharmacies. Maintain urinary output. Treat oliguria and anuria if they occur.

B. Chronic Poisoning

Remove from exposure. Neurologic toxicity is not considered reversible with chelation, although some authors recommend a trial of succimer or unithiol (contact a regional poison center or medical toxicologist for advice).

Mudan A...Smollin CG et al. Notes from the field: methylmercury toxicity from a skin lightening cream obtained from Mexico—California 2019. MMWR Morb Mortal Wkly Rep. 2019;68:1166. [PMID: 31856147]

METHANOL & ETHYLENE GLYCOL

Methanol (wood alcohol) is commonly found in a variety of products, including solvents, duplicating fluids, record cleaning solutions, and paint removers. It is sometimes ingested intentionally by patients with alcohol use disorder as a substitute for ethanol and may also be found as a contaminant in bootleg whiskey. Ethylene glycol is the major constituent in most antifreeze compounds. The toxicity of both agents is caused by metabolism to highly toxic organic acids—methanol to formic acid; ethylene glycol to glycolic and oxalic acids. Diethylene glycol is a nephrotoxic solvent that has been improperly substituted for glycerin in various liquid medications (cough syrup, teething medicine, acetaminophen), causing numerous deaths in Haiti, Panama, and Nigeria.

Clinical Findings

Shortly after ingestion of methanol or ethylene glycol, patients usually appear "drunk." The serum osmolality (measured by freezing point depression) is usually increased, but acidosis is often absent early. After several hours, metabolism to toxic organic acids leads to a severe anion gap metabolic acidosis, tachypnea, confusion, convulsions, and coma. Methanol intoxication frequently causes visual disturbances, while ethylene glycol often produces oxalate crystalluria and AKI. **Note:** Point-of-care analytical devices commonly used in the emergency department may falsely measure glycolic acid (a toxic metabolite of ethylene glycol) as lactic acid.

Treatment

A. Emergency and Supportive Measures

For patients presenting within 30–60 minutes after ingestion, empty the stomach by aspiration through a nasogastric tube. Charcoal is not very effective but should be administered if other poisons or drugs have also been ingested.

B. Specific Treatment

Patients with significant toxicity (manifested by severe metabolic acidosis, altered mental status, markedly elevated osmol gap, or evidence of end-organ toxicity) should undergo hemodialysis as soon as possible to remove the parent compound and the toxic metabolites. Treatment with folic acid, thiamine, and pyridoxine may enhance the breakdown of toxic metabolites.

Ethanol blocks metabolism of the parent compounds by competing for the enzyme alcohol dehydrogenase. Fomepizole (4-methylpyrazole; Antizol) blocks alcohol dehydrogenase and is much easier to use than ethanol. If started before onset of acidosis, fomepizole may be used as the sole treatment for ethylene glycol ingestion in some cases. A regional poison control center (1-800-222-1222) should be contacted for indications and dosing.

Gallagher N et al. The diagnosis and management of toxic alcohol poisoning in the emergency department: a review article. Adv J Emerg Med. 2019;3:e28. [PMID: 31410405]
Kraut JA et al. Toxic alcohols. N Engl J Med. 2018;378:270. [PMID: 29342392]
Pohanka M. Antidotes against methanol poisoning: a review. Mini Rev Med Chem. 2019;19:1126. [PMID: 30864518]

METHEMOGLOBINEMIA-INDUCING AGENTS

A large number of chemical agents are capable of oxidizing ferrous hemoglobin to its ferric state (methemoglobin), a form that cannot carry oxygen. Drugs and chemicals known to cause methemoglobinemia include benzocaine (a local anesthetic found in some topical anesthetic sprays and a variety of nonprescription products), aniline, propanil (an herbicide), nitrites, nitrogen oxide gases, nitrobenzene, dapsone, phenazopyridine (Pyridium), and many others. Dapsone has a long elimination half-life and may produce prolonged or recurrent methemoglobinemia. Amyl nitrite and isobutyl nitrite ("poppers") are inhaled as sexual stimulants but can result in methemoglobinemia.

Clinical Findings

Methemoglobinemia reduces oxygen-carrying capacity and may cause dizziness, nausea, headache, dyspnea, confusion, seizures, and coma. The severity of symptoms depends on the percentage of hemoglobin oxidized to methemoglobin; severe poisoning is usually present when methemoglobin fractions are greater than 40–50%. Even at low levels (15–20%), patients appear cyanotic because of the "chocolate brown" color of methemoglobin, but they have normal Po_2 results on arterial blood gas determinations. *Conventional pulse oximetry gives inaccurate oxygen saturation measurements*; the reading is often between 85% and 90%. Severe metabolic acidosis may be present. Hemolysis may occur, especially in patients susceptible to oxidant stress (ie, those with glucose-6-phosphate dehydrogenase deficiency).

Treatment

A. Emergency and Supportive Measures

Administer high-flow oxygen. If the causative agent was recently ingested, administer activated charcoal. Repeat-dose activated charcoal may enhance dapsone elimination.

B. Specific Treatment

Methylene blue enhances the conversion of methemoglobin to hemoglobin by increasing the activity of the enzyme methemoglobin reductase. For symptomatic patients, administer 1–2 mg/kg (0.1–0.2 mL/kg of 1% solution) intravenously. The dose may be repeated once in 15–20 minutes if necessary. Patients with hereditary methemoglobin reductase deficiency or glucose-6-phosphate dehydrogenase deficiency may not respond to methylene blue treatment. In severe cases where methylene blue is not available or is not effective, exchange blood transfusion may be necessary.

Cefalu JN et al. Methemoglobinemia in the operating room and intensive care unit: early recognition, pathophysiology, and management. Adv Ther. 2020;37:1714. [PMID: 32193811]

Hickey TBM et al. Fatal methemoglobinemia: a case series highlighting a new trend in intentional sodium nitrite or sodium nitrate ingestion as a method of suicide. Forensic Sci Int. 2021;326:110907. [PMID: 34298207]

MUSHROOMS

There are thousands of mushroom species that cause a variety of toxic effects. The most dangerous species of mushrooms are *Amanita phalloides* and related species, which contain potent cytotoxins (amatoxins). Ingestion of even a portion of one amatoxin-containing mushroom may be sufficient to cause death.

The characteristic pathologic finding in fatalities from amatoxin-containing mushroom poisoning is acute massive necrosis of the liver.

Clinical Findings

Amatoxin-containing mushrooms typically cause a delayed onset (8–12 hours after ingestion) of severe abdominal cramps, vomiting, and profuse diarrhea, followed in 1–2 days by AKI, hepatic necrosis, and hepatic encephalopathy. Cooking the mushrooms does *not* prevent poisoning.

Monomethylhydrazine poisoning (*Gyromitra* and *Helvella* species) is more common following ingestion of uncooked mushrooms, as the toxin is water-soluble. Vomiting, diarrhea, hepatic necrosis, convulsions, coma, and hemolysis may occur after a latent period of 8–12 hours.

Treatment

A. Emergency Measures

After the onset of symptoms, efforts to remove the toxic agent are probably useless, especially in cases of amatoxin or gyromitrin poisoning, where there is usually a delay of 8–12 hours or more before symptoms occur and patients seek medical attention. However, activated charcoal is recommended for any recent ingestion of an unidentified or potentially toxic mushroom. Administer intravenous fluids liberally to replace massive losses from vomiting and diarrhea; monitor central venous pressure, urinary output, and kidney function tests to help guide volume replacement.

B. Specific Treatment

A variety of purported antidotes (eg, thioctic acid, penicillin, corticosteroids) have been suggested for amatoxin-type mushroom poisoning, but controlled studies are lacking and experimental data in animals are equivocal. Aggressive fluid replacement for diarrhea and intensive supportive care for hepatic failure are the mainstays of treatment. Silymarin (silibinin), a derivative of milk thistle, is commonly used in Europe, but is commercially available in the United States only as an oral nutritional supplement. The European intravenous product (Legalon-SIL) can be obtained in the United States under an emergency IND provided by the FDA. Contact the regional poison control center (1-800-222-1222) for more information. *N*-acetylcysteine has also been used and may provide some benefit. Liver transplant may be the only hope for survival in gravely ill patients—contact a liver transplant center early.

Liu J et al. N-acetylcysteine as a treatment for amatoxin poisoning: a systematic review. Clin Toxicol (Phila). 2020;58:1015. [PMID: 32609548]

White J et al. Mushroom poisoning: a proposed new clinical classification. Toxicon. 2019;157:53. [PMID: 30439442]

Zuker-Herman R et al. Intravenous rifampicin use in the management of amanita phalloides toxicity. Clin Toxicol (Phila). 2021;59:843. [PMID: 33605821]

OPIATES & OPIOIDS

Prescription and illicit opiates and opioids (eg, morphine, heroin, codeine, oxycodone, fentanyl, hydromorphone) are popular drugs of misuse and abuse and the cause of frequent hospitalizations for overdose. These drugs have widely varying potencies and durations of action; for example, *some of the illicit fentanyl derivatives are up to 2000 times more potent than morphine.* Poisonings and fatalities have been reported due to the illicit use of fentanyl and the presence of fentanyl and its derivatives in counterfeit medications. Overdose deaths involving synthetic opioids have accelerated during the COVID-19 pandemic and are a significant public health concern. All of these agents decrease CNS activity and sympathetic outflow by acting on opiate receptors in the brain. Tramadol is an analgesic that is unrelated chemically to the opioids but acts on opioid receptors. Buprenorphine is a partial agonist-antagonist opioid used for the outpatient treatment of both chronic pain and opioid addiction (see Table 5–7). Kratom (*Mitragyna speciosa*) is an herbal supplement with agonist activity at mu opioid receptors. While it has been marketed as a "safe" and natural treatment for patients with opioid use disorder, overdose is associated with both agitation and drowsiness and in severe cases seizures, hallucinations, and respiratory depression.

Clinical Findings

Mild intoxication is characterized by euphoria, drowsiness, and constricted pupils. More severe intoxication may cause hypotension, bradycardia, hypothermia, coma, and respiratory arrest. Pulmonary edema may occur. Death is usually due to apnea or pulmonary aspiration of gastric contents. Methadone may cause QT interval prolongation and torsades de pointes. While the duration of effect for heroin is usually 3–5 hours, methadone intoxication may last for 48–72 hours or longer. Tramadol, dextromethorphan, and meperidine also occasionally cause seizures. With meperidine, the metabolite normeperidine is probably the cause of seizures and is most likely to accumulate with repeated dosing in patients with CKD. Wound botulism has been associated with skin-popping, especially involving "black tar" heroin. Buprenorphine added to an opioid regimen may precipitate acute withdrawal symptoms. Many opioids, including fentanyl, tramadol, oxycodone, and methadone, are not detected on routine urine toxicology "opiate" screening.

Treatment

A. Emergency and Supportive Measures

Protect the airway and assist ventilation. Administer activated charcoal for recent large ingestions.

B. Specific Treatment

Naloxone is a specific opioid antagonist that can rapidly reverse signs of narcotic intoxication. Although it is structurally related to the opioids, it has no agonist effects of its own. If no intravenous access is available, administer naloxone 4 mg intranasally, otherwise administer 0.2–2 mg intravenously and repeat as needed to awaken the patient and maintain airway protective reflexes and spontaneous breathing. Large doses (up to 10 mg) may be required for patients intoxicated by some opioids (eg, codeine, fentanyl derivatives). **Caution:** *The duration of effect of naloxone is only about 2–3 hours; repeated doses may be necessary for patients intoxicated by long-acting drugs such as methadone. Continuous observation for at least 3 hours after the last naloxone dose is mandatory.* The immediate post-overdose period is an important opportunity to discuss harm reduction measures (take-home naloxone, fentanyl testing strips, safe injection practices) and to consider initiation of medications for opioid use disorder (buprenorphine).

Bauman MH et al. U-47700 and its analogs: non-fentanyl synthetic opioids impacting the recreational drug market. Brain Sci. 2020;10:895. [PMID: 33238449]

Lavonas EJ et al. Impact of the opioid epidemic. Crit Care Clin. 2020;36:753. [PMID: 32892827]

Niles JK et al. Notes from the field: testing for nonprescribed fentanyl and percentage of positive test results among patients with opioid use disorder—United States, 2019–2020. MMWR Morb Mortal Wkly Rep 2021;70:1649. [PMID: 34818316]

Peterkin A et al. Current best practices for acute and chronic management of patients with opioid use disorder. Med Clin North Am. 2022;106:61. [PMID: 34823735]

PESTICIDES: CHOLINESTERASE INHIBITORS

Organophosphorus and carbamate insecticides (organophosphates: parathion, malathion, etc; carbamates: carbaryl, aldicarb, etc) are widely used in commercial agriculture and home gardening and have largely replaced older, more environmentally persistent organochlorine compounds such as DDT and chlordane. The organophosphates and carbamates—also called anticholinesterases because they inhibit the enzyme acetylcholinesterase—cause an increase in acetylcholine activity at nicotinic and muscarinic receptors and in the peripheral and CNS. There are a variety of chemical agents in this group, with widely varying potencies. Most of them are poorly water-soluble, are often formulated with an aromatic hydrocarbon solvent such as xylene and are well absorbed through intact skin. Most chemical warfare "nerve agents" (such as GA [tabun], GB [sarin], GD [soman], and VX) are organophosphates.

Clinical Findings

Inhibition of cholinesterase results in abdominal cramps, diarrhea, vomiting, excessive salivation, sweating, lacrimation, miosis, wheezing and bronchorrhea, seizures, and skeletal muscle weakness. Initial tachycardia is usually followed by bradycardia. Profound skeletal muscle weakness, aggravated by excessive bronchial secretions and wheezing, may result in respiratory arrest and death. Symptoms and signs of poisoning may persist or recur over several days, especially with highly lipid-soluble agents such as fenthion or dimethoate.

The diagnosis should be suspected in patients who present with miosis, sweating, and diarrhea. Serum and RBC cholinesterase activity is usually depressed at least 50% below baseline in those patients who have severe intoxication.

Treatment

A. Emergency and Supportive Measures

If the agent was recently ingested, consider gut decontamination by aspiration of the liquid using a nasogastric tube followed by administration of activated charcoal. If the agent is on the person's skin or hair, wash repeatedly with soap or shampoo and water. Providers should take care to avoid skin exposure by wearing gloves and waterproof aprons. Dilute hypochlorite solution (eg, household bleach diluted 1:10) is reported to help break down organophosphate pesticides and nerve agents on equipment or clothing.

B. Specific Treatment

Atropine reverses excessive muscarinic stimulation and is effective for treatment of salivation, bronchial hypersecretion, wheezing, abdominal cramping, and sweating. However, it does not interact with nicotinic receptors at autonomic ganglia and at the neuromuscular junction and has no direct effect on muscle weakness. Administer 2 mg intravenously, and if there is no response after 5 minutes, give repeated boluses in rapidly escalating doses (eg, doubling the dose each time) as needed to dry bronchial secretions and decrease wheezing; as much as several hundred milligrams of atropine have been given to treat severe poisoning.

Pralidoxime (2-PAM, Protopam) is a more specific antidote that reverses organophosphate binding to the cholinesterase enzyme; therefore, it should be effective at the neuromuscular junction as well as other nicotinic and muscarinic sites. It is most likely to be clinically effective if started very soon after poisoning, to prevent permanent binding of the organophosphate to cholinesterase. However, clinical studies have yielded conflicting results regarding the effectiveness of pralidoxime in reducing mortality. Administer 1–2 g intravenously as a loading dose and begin a continuous infusion (200–500 mg/hour, titrated to clinical response). Continue to give pralidoxime as long as there is any evidence of acetylcholine excess. Pralidoxime is of questionable benefit for carbamate poisoning because carbamates have only a transitory effect on the cholinesterase enzyme. Other, unproven therapies for organophosphate poisoning include magnesium, sodium bicarbonate, clonidine, and extracorporeal removal.

Aman S et al. Management of organophosphorus poisoning: standard treatment and beyond. Crit Care Clin. 2021;37:673. [PMID: 34053713]

Hulse EJ et al. Organophosphorus nerve agent poisoning: managing the poisoned patient. Br J Anaesth. 2019;123:457. [PMID: 31248646]

Kharel H et al. The efficacy of pralidoxime in the treatment of organophosphate poisoning in humans: a systematic review and meta-analysis of randomized controlled trials. Cureus. 2020;12:e7174. [PMID: 32257715]

PETROLEUM DISTILLATES & SOLVENTS

Petroleum distillate toxicity may occur from inhalation of the vapor or as a result of pulmonary aspiration of the liquid during or after ingestion. Acute manifestations of aspiration pneumonitis are vomiting, coughing, and bronchopneumonia. Some hydrocarbons—ie, those with aromatic or halogenated subunits—can also cause severe systemic poisoning after oral ingestion. Hydrocarbons can also cause systemic intoxication by inhalation. Vertigo, muscular incoordination, irregular pulse, myoclonus, and seizures occur with serious poisoning and may be due to hypoxemia or the systemic effects of the agents. Chlorinated and fluorinated hydrocarbons (trichloroethylene, Freons, etc) and many other hydrocarbons can cause ventricular arrhythmias due to increased sensitivity of the myocardium to the effects of endogenous catecholamines.

Treatment

Remove the patient to fresh air. For simple aliphatic hydrocarbon ingestion, gastric emptying and activated charcoal are not recommended, but these procedures may be indicated if the preparation contains toxic solutes (eg, an insecticide) or is an aromatic or halogenated product. Observe the patient for 6–8 hours for signs of aspiration pneumonitis (cough, localized crackles or rhonchi, tachypnea, and infiltrates on chest radiograph). Corticosteroids are not recommended. If fever occurs, give a specific antibiotic only after identification of bacterial pathogens by laboratory studies. Because of the risk of arrhythmias, use bronchodilators with caution in patients with chlorinated or fluorinated solvent intoxication. If tachyarrhythmias occur, use esmolol intravenously 25–100 mcg/kg/minute.

Forrester MB. Computer and electronic duster spray inhalation (huffing) injuries managed at emergency departments. Am J Drug Alcohol Abuse. 2020;46:180. [PMID: 31449429]

Jolly G et al. Cardiac involvement in hydrocarbon inhalant toxicity—role of cardiac magnetic resonance imaging: a case report. World J Cardiol. 2021;13:593. [PMID: 34754404]

SALICYLATES

Salicylates (aspirin, methyl salicylate, bismuth subsalicylate, etc) are found in a variety of over-the-counter and prescription medications. Salicylates uncouple cellular oxidative phosphorylation, resulting in anaerobic metabolism and excessive production of lactic acid and heat, and they also interfere with several Krebs cycle enzymes. A *single ingestion* of more than 200 mg/kg of salicylate is likely to produce significant acute intoxication. Poisoning may also occur as a result of *chronic excessive dosing* over several days. Although the half-life of salicylate is 2–3 hours after small doses, it may increase to 20 hours or more in patients with intoxication.

Clinical Findings

Acute ingestion often causes nausea and vomiting, occasionally with gastritis. Moderate intoxication is characterized by hyperpnea (deep and rapid breathing), tachycardia, tinnitus, and elevated anion gap metabolic acidosis. (A normal anion gap sometimes occurs due to salicylate interference with the chemistry analyzer, falsely raising the measured chloride.) Serious intoxication may result in agitation, confusion, coma, seizures, cardiovascular collapse, pulmonary edema, hyperthermia, and death. The prothrombin time is often elevated owing to salicylate-induced hypoprothrombinemia. CNS intracellular glucose depletion can occur despite normal measured serum glucose levels.

Diagnosis of salicylate poisoning is suspected in any patient with metabolic acidosis and is confirmed by measuring the serum salicylate level. Patients with levels greater than 100 mg/dL (1000 mg/L or 7.2 mcmol/L) after an acute overdose are more likely to have severe poisoning. On the other hand, patients with subacute or chronic intoxication may suffer severe symptoms with levels of only 60–70 mg/dL

(4.3–5 mcmol/L). The arterial blood gas typically reveals a respiratory alkalosis with an underlying metabolic acidosis.

Treatment

A. Emergency and Supportive Measures

Administer activated charcoal orally. Gastric lavage followed by administration of extra doses of activated charcoal may be needed in patients who ingest more than 10 g of aspirin. The desired ratio of charcoal to aspirin is about 10:1 by weight; while this cannot always be given as a single dose, it may be administered over the first 24 hours in divided doses every 2–4 hours along with whole bowel irrigation. Give glucose-containing fluids to reduce the risk of cerebral hypoglycemia. Treat metabolic acidosis with intravenous sodium bicarbonate. This is critical because acidosis (especially acidemia, pH < 7.40) promotes greater entry of salicylate into cells, worsening toxicity. **Warning:** *Sudden and severe deterioration can occur after rapid sequence intubation and controlled ventilation if the pH is allowed to fall due to hypercarbia during the apneic period.*

B. Specific Treatment

Alkalinization of the urine enhances renal salicylate excretion by trapping the salicylate anion in the urine. Add 100 mEq (two ampules) of sodium bicarbonate to 1 L of 5% dextrose in 0.2% saline and infuse this solution intravenously at a rate of about 150–200 mL/hour. Unless the patient is oliguric or hyperkalemic, add 20–30 mEq of potassium chloride to each liter of intravenous fluid. Patients who are volume-depleted often fail to produce an alkaline urine (paradoxical aciduria) unless potassium is given.

Hemodialysis may be lifesaving and is indicated for patients with severe metabolic acidosis, markedly altered mental status, or significantly elevated salicylate levels (eg, greater than 100 mg/dL [1000 mg/L or 7.2 mcmol/L] after acute overdose or greater than 60 mg/dL [600 mg/L or 4.3 mcmol/L] with subacute or chronic intoxication).

Bowers D et al. Managing acute salicylate toxicity in the emergency department. Adv Emerg Nurs J. 2019;41:76. [PMID: 30702537]

Palmer BF et al. Salicylate toxicity. N Engl J Med. 2020;382:2544. [PMID: 32579814]

Wiederkehr MR et. Pseudohyperchloremia and negative anion gap—think salicylate! Am J Med. 2021;134:1170. [PMID: 33864761]

SEAFOOD POISONINGS

A variety of intoxications may occur after eating certain types of fish or other seafood. These include scombroid, ciguatera, paralytic shellfish, and puffer fish poisoning. The mechanisms of toxicity and clinical presentations are described in Table 38–8. In most cases, the seafood has a normal appearance and taste (scombroid may have a peppery taste).

Treatment

A. Emergency and Supportive Measures

Caution: *Abrupt respiratory arrest may occur in patients with acute paralytic shellfish and puffer fish poisoning.* Observe patients for at least 4–6 hours. Replace fluid and electrolyte losses from gastroenteritis with intravenous saline or other crystalloid solution.

Table 38–8. Common seafood poisonings (listed in alphabetical order).

Type of Poisoning	Mechanism	Clinical Presentation
Ciguatera	Reef fish ingest toxic dinoflagellates, whose toxins accumulate in fish meat. Commonly implicated fish in the United States are barracuda, jack, snapper, and grouper.	1–6 hours after ingestion, persons develop abdominal pain, vomiting, and diarrhea accompanied by a variety of neurologic symptoms, including paresthesias, reversal of hot and cold sensation, vertigo, headache, and intense itching. Autonomic disturbances, including hypotension and bradycardia, may occur.
Paralytic shellfish poisoning	Dinoflagellates produce saxitoxin, which is concentrated by filter-feeding mussels and clams. Saxitoxin blocks sodium conductance and neuronal transmission in skeletal muscles.	Onset is usually within 30–60 minutes. Initial symptoms include perioral and intraoral paresthesias. Other symptoms include nausea and vomiting, headache, dizziness, dysphagia, dysarthria, ataxia, and rapidly progressive muscle weakness that may result in respiratory arrest.
Puffer fish poisoning	Tetrodotoxin is concentrated in liver, gonads, intestine, and skin. Toxic effects are similar to those of saxitoxin. Tetrodotoxin is also found in some North American newts and Central American frogs.	Onset is usually within 30–40 minutes but may be as short as 10 minutes. Initial perioral paresthesias are followed by headache, diaphoresis, nausea, vomiting, ataxia, and rapidly progressive muscle weakness that may result in respiratory arrest.
Scombroid	Improper preservation of large fish results in bacterial degradation of histidine to histamine. Commonly implicated fish include tuna, mahimahi, bonita, mackerel, and kingfish.	Allergic-like (anaphylactoid) symptoms are due to histamine, usually begin within 15–90 minutes, and include skin flushing, itching, urticaria, angioedema, bronchospasm, and hypotension as well as abdominal pain, vomiting, and diarrhea.

For recent ingestions, it may be possible to adsorb residual toxin in the gut with activated charcoal, 50–60 g orally.

B. Specific Treatment

There is no specific antidote for paralytic shellfish or puffer fish poisoning.

1. Ciguatera—There are anecdotal reports of successful treatment of acute neurologic symptoms with mannitol, 1 g/kg intravenously, but this approach is not widely accepted. Gabapentin 400 mg, three times daily, may also relieve neuropathic symptoms.

2. Scombroid—Antihistamines such as diphenhydramine, 25–50 mg intravenously, and the H_2-blocker cimetidine, 300 mg intravenously, are usually effective.

Chinain M et al. Ciguatera poisoning in French Polynesia: insights into the novel trends of an ancient disease. New Microbes New Infect. 2019;31:100565. [PMID: 31312457]

Warrell DA. Venomous bites, stings, and poisoning: an update. Infect Dis Clin North Am. 2019;33:17. [PMID: 30712761]

SNAKE BITES

The venom of poisonous snakes and lizards may be predominantly **neurotoxic** (coral snake) or predominantly **cytolytic** (rattlesnakes, other pit vipers). Neurotoxins cause respiratory paralysis; cytolytic venoms cause tissue destruction by digestion and hemorrhage due to hemolysis and destruction of the endothelial lining of the blood vessels. The manifestations of rattlesnake envenomation are mostly local pain, redness, swelling, and extravasation of blood. Perioral tingling, metallic taste, nausea and vomiting, hypotension, and coagulopathy may also occur. Thrombocytopenia can persist for several days after a rattlesnake bite. Neurotoxic envenomation may cause ptosis, dysphagia, diplopia, and respiratory arrest.

▶ Treatment

A. Emergency Measures

Immobilize the patient and the bitten part in a neutral position. Avoid manipulation of the bitten area. Transport the patient to a medical facility for definitive treatment. Do *not* give alcoholic beverages or stimulants; do *not* apply ice; do *not* apply a tourniquet. The potential trauma to underlying tissues resulting from incision and suction is not justified in view of the small amount of venom that can be recovered.

B. Specific Antidote and General Measures

1. Pit viper (eg, rattlesnake) envenomation—There are two commercially available antivenins for rattlesnake envenomation (CroFab and Anavip). Depending on the severity of symptoms CroFab is administered in increments of 4–6 vials by slow intravenous drip in 250–500 mL saline. For more serious envenomation with marked local effects and systemic toxicity (eg, hypotension, coagulopathy), higher doses and additional vials may be required. The dosing of Anavip is 10 vials by slow intravenous infusion over 60 minutes initially followed by additional 10-vial increments as needed for more serious envenomations or for progression of symptoms. Monitor vital signs and the blood coagulation profile. Type and cross-match blood. The adequacy of venom neutralization is indicated by improvement in symptoms and signs, and the rate that swelling slows. Prophylactic antibiotics are not indicated after a rattlesnake bite.

2. Elapid (coral snake) envenomation—Give 1–2 vials of specific antivenom as soon as possible. **Note:** Pfizer/Wyeth no longer makes coral snake antivenom in the United States and remaining supplies are dwindling. To locate antisera for this or exotic snakes, call a regional poison control center (1-800-222-1222).

Greene S et al. How should native crotalid envenomation be managed in the emergency department? J Emerg Med. 2021;61:41. [PMID: 33622584]

Greene SC et al. Epidemiology of fatal snakebites in the United States 1989-2018. Am J Emerg Med. 2021;45:309. [PMID: 33046301]

Mascarenas D et al. Comparison of $F(ab')_2$ and Fab antivenoms in rattlesnake envenomation: first year's post-marketing experience with $F(ab')_2$ in New Mexico. Toxicon. 2020;186:42. [PMID: 32763251]

Warrell DA. Venomous bites, stings, and poisoning: an update. Infect Dis Clin North Am. 2019;33:17. [PMID: 30712761]

SPIDER BITES & SCORPION STINGS

Envenomation from most species of spiders in the United States causes only local pain, redness, and swelling. The more venomous black widow spiders (*Latrodectus mactans*) cause generalized muscular pains, muscle spasms, and rigidity. The brown recluse spider (*Loxosceles reclusa*) causes progressive local necrosis as well as hemolytic reactions (rare).

Stings by most scorpions in the United States cause only local pain. Stings by the more toxic *Centruroides* species (found in the southwestern United States) may cause muscle cramps, twitching and jerking, and occasionally hypertension, convulsions, and pulmonary edema. Stings by scorpions from other parts of the world are not discussed here.

▶ Treatment

A. Black Widow Spider Bites

Pain may be relieved with parenteral opioids or muscle relaxants (eg, methocarbamol, 15 mg/kg). Calcium gluconate 10%, 0.1–0.2 mL/kg intravenously, may transiently relieve muscle rigidity, although its effectiveness is unproven. *Latrodectus* antivenom is possibly more effective, but because of concerns about acute hypersensitivity reactions (horse serum–derived), it is often reserved for very young persons, older adults, or those who do not respond promptly to the above measures. Horse serum sensitivity testing is required. (Instruction and testing materials are included in the antivenin kit.)

B. Brown Recluse Spider Bites

Because bites occasionally progress to extensive local necrosis, some authorities recommend early excision of the bite site, whereas others use oral corticosteroids. Anecdotal reports have claimed success with dapsone and colchicine. All of these treatments remain unproven.

C. Scorpion Stings

No specific treatment other than analgesics is required for envenomations by most scorpions found in the United States. An FDA-approved specific antivenom is available for *Centruroides* stings.

Klotz SA et al. Scorpion stings and antivenom use in Arizona. Am J Med. 2021;134:1034. [PMID: 33631163]

Lopes PH et al. Clinical aspects, diagnosis and management of *Loxosceles* spider envenomation: literature and case review. Arch Toxicol. 2020;94:1461. [PMID: 32232511]

Trave I et al. Cutaneous Loxoscelism. JAMA Dermatol. 2020;156:203. [PMID: 31721992]

Warrell DA. Venomous bites, stings, and poisoning: an update. Infect Dis Clin North Am. 2019;33:17. [PMID: 30712761]

THEOPHYLLINE & CAFFEINE

Methylxanthines, including theophylline and caffeine, are nonselective adenosine receptor antagonists. In overdose, toxicity results from the release of endogenous catecholamines with beta-1- and beta-2-adrenergic stimulation. Theophylline may cause intoxication after an acute single overdose, or intoxication may occur as a result of chronic accidental repeated overmedication or reduced elimination resulting from hepatic dysfunction or interacting drug (eg, cimetidine, erythromycin). The usual serum half-life of theophylline is 4–6 hours, but this may increase to more than 20 hours after overdose. Caffeine in energy drinks or herbal or dietary supplement products can produce similar toxicity.

Clinical Findings

Mild intoxication causes nausea, vomiting, tachycardia, and tremulousness. Severe intoxication is characterized by ventricular and supraventricular tachyarrhythmias, hypotension, and seizures. Status epilepticus is common and often intractable to the usual anticonvulsants. After acute overdose (but not chronic intoxication), hypokalemia, hyperglycemia, and metabolic acidosis are common. Seizures and other manifestations of toxicity may be delayed for several hours after acute ingestion, especially if a sustained-release preparation such as Theo-Dur was taken.

Diagnosis is based on measurement of the serum theophylline concentration. Seizures and hypotension are likely to develop in acute overdose patients with serum levels greater than 100 mg/L (555 mcmol/L). Serious toxicity may develop at lower levels (ie, 40–60 mg/L [222–333 mcmol/L]) in patients with chronic intoxication. Serum caffeine levels are not routinely available in clinical practice, but in a study of 51 fatal cases the median level was 180 mg/L (range 33–567 mg/L).

Treatment

A. Emergency and Supportive Measures

After acute ingestion, administer activated charcoal. Repeated doses of activated charcoal may enhance theophylline and caffeine elimination by "gut dialysis." Addition of whole bowel irrigation should be considered for large ingestions involving sustained-release preparations.

Hemodialysis is effective in removing theophylline and is indicated for patients with status epilepticus or markedly elevated serum theophylline levels (eg, greater than 100 mg/L [555 mcmol/L] after acute overdose or greater than 60 mg/L [333 mcmol/L] with chronic intoxication). It has also been used in caffeine overdose. Extracorporeal membrane oxygenation (ECMO) has been used successfully in hemodynamic collapse after caffeine overdose.

B. Specific Treatment

Treat seizures with benzodiazepines (lorazepam, 2–3 mg intravenously, or diazepam, 5–10 mg intravenously) or phenobarbital (10–15 mg/kg intravenously). Phenytoin is not effective. Hypotension and tachycardia—which are mediated through excessive beta-adrenergic stimulation—may respond to beta-blocker therapy even in low doses. Administer esmolol, 25–50 mcg/kg/minute by intravenous infusion, or propranolol, 0.5–1 mg intravenously.

Carreon CC et al. How to recognize caffeine overdose. Nursing. 2019;49:52. [PMID: 30893206]

Kohl BA et al. Acute intentional caffeine overdose treated preemptively with hemodialysis. Am J Emerg Med. 2020;38:692. [PMID: 31785982]

Ou HC et al. A successful experience using labetalol and hemodialysis to treat near-fatal caffeine poisoning: a case report with toxicodynamics. Am J Emerg Med. 2022;55:224.e1. [PMID: 34922795]

Yasuda S et al. Caffeine poisoning successfully treated by venoarterial extracorporeal membrane oxygenation and emergency hemodialysis. Acute Med Surg. 2021;8:e627. [PMID: 33532077]

TRICYCLIC & OTHER ANTIDEPRESSANTS

Tricyclic and related cyclic antidepressants are among the most dangerous drugs involved in suicidal overdose. These drugs have anticholinergic and cardiac depressant properties ("quinidine-like" sodium channel blockade). Tricyclic antidepressants produce more marked membrane-depressant cardiotoxic effects than the phenothiazines.

Newer-generation antidepressants such as trazodone, fluoxetine, citalopram, paroxetine, sertraline, bupropion, venlafaxine, and fluvoxamine are not chemically related to the tricyclic antidepressant agents and, with the exception of bupropion, do not generally produce quinidine-like cardiotoxic effects. However, they may cause seizures in overdoses and serotonin syndrome.

Clinical Findings

Signs of severe intoxication may occur abruptly and without warning within 30–60 minutes after acute tricyclic

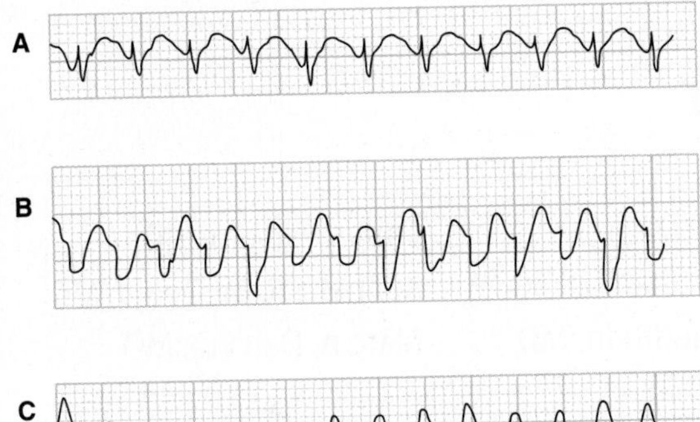

▲ **Figure 38–2.** Cardiac arrhythmias resulting from tricyclic antidepressant overdose. **A:** Delayed intraventricular conduction results in prolonged QRS interval (0.18 seconds). **B** and **C:** Supraventricular tachycardia with progressive widening of QRS complexes mimics ventricular tachycardia. (Reproduced with permission from Benowitz NL, Goldschlager N. Cardiac disturbances in the toxicologic patient. In: Haddad LM, Winchester JF [editors], *Clinical Management of Poisoning and Drug Overdose*, 3rd edition. Saunders/Elsevier, 1998.)

overdose. Anticholinergic effects include dilated pupils, tachycardia, dry mouth, flushed skin, muscle twitching, and decreased peristalsis. Quinidine-like cardiotoxic effects include QRS interval widening (greater than 0.12 seconds; Figure 38–2), ventricular arrhythmias, AV block, and hypotension. Rightward-axis deviation of the terminal 40 milliseconds of the QRS has also been described. Prolongation of the QT interval and torsades de pointes have been reported with several of the newer antidepressants. Seizures and coma are common with severe intoxication. Life-threatening hyperthermia may result from status epilepticus and anticholinergic-induced impairment of sweating. Among newer agents, bupropion and venlafaxine have been associated with a greater risk of seizures.

The diagnosis should be suspected in any overdose patient with anticholinergic side effects, especially if there is widening of the QRS interval or seizures. For intoxication by most tricyclic antidepressants, the QRS interval correlates with the severity of intoxication more reliably than the serum drug level.

Serotonin syndrome should be suspected if agitation, delirium, diaphoresis, tremor, hyperreflexia, clonus (spontaneous, inducible, or ocular), and fever develop in a patient taking serotonin reuptake inhibitors.

Treatment

A. Emergency and Supportive Measures

Observe patients for at least 6 hours and admit all patients with evidence of anticholinergic effects (eg, delirium, dilated pupils, tachycardia) or signs of cardiotoxicity.

Administer activated charcoal and consider gastric lavage after recent large ingestions. All of these drugs have large volumes of distribution and are not effectively removed by hemodialysis procedures.

B. Specific Treatment

Cardiotoxic sodium channel–depressant effects of tricyclic antidepressants may respond to boluses of sodium bicarbonate (50–100 mEq intravenously). Sodium bicarbonate provides a large sodium load that alleviates depression of the sodium-dependent channel. Reversal of acidosis may also have beneficial effects at this site. Maintain the pH between 7.45 and 7.50. Alkalinization does not promote excretion of tricyclic antidepressants. Prolongation of the QT interval or torsades de pointes is usually treated with intravenous magnesium or overdrive pacing. Severe cardiotoxicity in patients with overdoses of lipid-soluble drugs (eg, amitriptyline, bupropion) has reportedly responded to intravenous lipid emulsion (Intralipid), 1.5 mL/kg repeated one or two times if needed. Plasma exchange using albumin and ECMO have been reported to be successful in several cases.

Mild serotonin syndrome may be treated with benzodiazepines and withdrawal of the antidepressant. Moderate cases may respond to cyproheptadine (4 mg orally or via gastric tube hourly for three or four doses) or chlorpromazine (25 mg intravenously). Severe hyperthermia should be treated with neuromuscular paralysis and endotracheal intubation in addition to external cooling measures.

Butt K et al. A peculiar wide complex tachycardia. Circulation. 2019;139:1454. [PMID: 30856002]

Elsamadisi P et al. Delayed cardiotoxicity from a massive nortriptyline overdose requiring prolonged treatment. J Pharm Pract. 2020;33:543. [PMID: 30983469]

Cancer

Sunny Wang, MD
Tiffany O. Dea, PharmD, BCOP
Lawrence S. Friedman, MD
Carling Ursem, MD
Kenneth R. McQuaid, MD
Marc A. Dall'Era, MD

INTRODUCTION TO CANCER

Sunny Wang, MD
Tiffany O. Dea, PharmD, BCOP

Etiology

Cancer is the second most common cause of death in the United States. In 2021, an estimated 1,898,160 cases of cancer were diagnosed, and 608,570 persons died of cancer. Table 39–1 lists the 10 leading cancer types in men and women by site. However, death rates from cancers are declining. Compared with the 1991 overall cancer death rate of 215 per 100,000 population, the 2018 rate of 149 per 100,000 represents a 31% reduction in the overall cancer death rate. Importantly, death rates have declined in all four of the most common cancer types (prostate, breast, lung, and colorectum). Reductions in cancer mortality reflect successful implementation of a broad strategy of prevention, detection, and treatment. Due to these improvements, the number of cancer survivors is increasing. In 2019, an estimated 16.9 million people were alive in whom cancer had been previously diagnosed; that number is projected to grow to 18.9 million in 2024.

Modifiable Risk Factors

Tobacco use is the most common preventable cause of cancer death; at least 30% of all cancer deaths in the United States are directly linked to tobacco use. In 2014, an estimated 167,133 cancer deaths in the United States could be directly attributed to tobacco. Clear evidence links tobacco use to at least 15 cancers. The most dramatic link is with lung cancer; 81% of lung cancer deaths are attributable to smoking.

The prevalence of smoking for US adults based on the 2019 National Health Interview Survey is 14% for adults aged 18 years or older, which is a remarkable reduction from the 1955 peak of 57% for men and the 1965 peak of 34% for women. Cigarettes are the most common form of tobacco used in the United States, though the use of non-cigarette forms of tobacco and of electronic cigarettes is increasing. Electronic cigarette aerosol can contain harmful substances, including nicotine, heavy metals, volatile organic compounds, and carcinogenic substances. The use of flavoring compounds increases the attractiveness of these devices to youth raising the concern that these devices will encourage youth to transition to cigarettes. The percent of US high school students who use e-cigarettes was approximately 1.5% in 2011 and has increased to 21% in 2018.

Tobacco cessation directed toward the individual should start with clinician counseling. Simple, concise advice from a clinician can yield cessation rates of 10–20%. Additive strategies include more intensive counseling; nicotine replacement therapy with patches, gum, lozenges, or inhalers; and prescription medication with bupropion or varenicline (see Chapter 1).

For those Americans who do not use tobacco, the most modifiable cancer risk factors are nutrition and physical activity. Prudent recommendations to reduce cancer risk are to (1) avoid tobacco; (2) be physically active; (3) maintain a healthy weight; (4) consume a diet rich in fruits, vegetables, and whole grains; (5) lower consumption of saturated and trans dietary fats; (6) limit alcohol use; and (7) avoid excess sun exposure.

Another modifiable cancer risk factor is radiation from radiographic studies. A 2009 study reported that the use of CT in diagnostic algorithms exposes individuals to significant radiation doses that may increase their lifetime risk of cancer. Both standardization of CT radiation doses and limiting testing have been important steps in minimizing this risk.

American Cancer Society. Cancer Facts & Figures 2022. https://www.cancer.org/research/cancer-facts-statistics/all-cancer-facts-figures/cancer-facts-figures-2022.html

Centers for Disease Control and Prevention (CDC). Smoking & Tobacco Use: About Electronic Cigarettes (E-Cigarettes). https://www.cdc.gov/tobacco/basic_information/e-cigarettes/about-e-cigarettes.html

Office of Disease Prevention and Health Promotion. Healthy People 2030. Tobacco use objectives: reduce current tobacco use in adults TU01. https://health.gov/healthypeople/objectives-and-data/browse-objectives/tobacco-use/reduce-current-tobacco-use-adults-tu-01

Table 39–1. Estimated 10 most common cancer cases in the United States in men and women (all races).

Rank	Men: Total Cases [N] = 970,250 (100 percent)	Women: Total Cases [N] = 927,910 (100 percent)
1	Prostate 248,530 (26)	Breast 281,550 (30)
2	Lung and bronchus 119,100 (12)	Lung and bronchus 116,660 (13)
3	Colon and rectum 79,520 (8)	Colon and rectum 69,980 (8)
4	Urinary bladder 64,280 (7)	Uterine corpus 66,570 (7)
5	Melanoma 62,260 (6)	Melanoma 43,850 (5)
6	Kidney and renal pelvis 48,780 (5)	Non-Hodgkin lymphoma 35,930 (4)
7	Non-Hodgkin lymphoma 45,630 (5)	Thyroid 32,130 (3)
8	Oral cavity and pharynx 38,800 (4)	Pancreas 28,480 (3)
9	Leukemia 35,530 (4)	Kidney and renal pelvis 27,300 (3)
10	Pancreas 31,950 (3)	Leukemia 25,560 (3)

Data from the American Cancer Society, 2021.

Klein WMP et al. Alcohol and cancer risk: clinical and research implications. JAMA. 2020;323:23. [PMID: 31834355]

Siegel RL et al. Cancer statistics, 2022. CA Cancer J Clin. 2022;72:7. [PMID: 35020204]

Staging

The Tumor, Node, Metastasis (TNM) system is the commonly used classification to stage cancer. Staging is important not only because it correlates with the patient's long-term survival but also because it is used to determine which patients should receive adjuvant or neoadjuvant therapy.

Certain characteristics of cancers, not reflected in the TNM stage, may be used to indicate prognosis and guide treatment. Pathologic features seen on routine histologic examination for some cancers are very important; examples include the Gleason score for prostate cancer, HPV status of oropharyngeal cancer, and grade of sarcomas. Cancer specimens should also be sent for molecular diagnostic testing and programmed death-ligand 1 (PD-L1) expression testing when appropriate.

Liao X et al. The 8th Edition American Joint Committee on Cancer Staging for Hepato-pancreato-biliary Cancer: a review and update. Arch Pathol Lab Med. 2021;145:543. [PMID: 32223559]

Treatment

See Primary Cancer Treatment section below. Table 39–2 outlines treatment choices by cancer type for those responsive to systemic agents, and Table 39–3 provides a listing of common chemotherapeutic agents.

Table 39–2. Treatment choices for cancers responsive to systemic agents.

Diagnosis	Initial Treatment
Acute lymphoblastic leukemia (ALL)	**Induction combination chemotherapy (Philadelphia chromosome–positive):** Cyclophosphamide, vincristine, doxorubicin/daunorubicin, dexamethasone (hyper-CVAD) alternating with cytarabine, methotrexate; add imatinib or dasatinib or nilotinib **Induction combination chemotherapy (Philadelphia chromosome–negative):** Daunorubicin, vincristine, prednisone, pegaspargase, cyclophosphamide; or hyper-CVAD alternating with methotrexate and cytarabine
Acute myeloid leukemia (AML)	**Induction combination chemotherapy:** Cytarabine with daunorubicin or idarubicin, with gemtuzumab ozogamicin (CD33-positive), or with midostaurin (*FLT3*-mutated), or with fludarabine **Alternative chemotherapy for ≥ 60 years old:** Azacitidine, decitabine, or low-dose cytarabine with or without venetoclax; or Liposomal encapsulation of cytarabine and daunorubicin (therapy-related or myelodysplasia-related changes) Ivosidenib (*IDH1* mutation); or Enasidenib (*IDH2* mutation)
Chronic myeloid leukemia (CML)	Nilotinib or dasatinib or imatinib or bosutinib
Chronic lymphocytic leukemia (CLL)	Venetoclax with obinutuzumab, or acalabrutinib with or without obinutuzumab, or ibrutinib
Hodgkin lymphoma	**Combination chemotherapy:** Doxorubicin, bleomycin, vinblastine, dacarbazine (ABVD), or Bleomycin, etoposide, doxorubicin, cyclophosphamide, vincristine, procarbazine, prednisone (BEACOPP)
Non-Hodgkin lymphoma (intermediate and high grade)	**Combination chemotherapy:** Cyclophosphamide, doxorubicin, vincristine, prednisone, rituximab[1] (CHOP-R), or Etoposide, prednisone, vincristine, cyclophosphamide, doxorubicin, rituximab[1] (dose-adjusted R-EPOCH) (for double-/triple-hit)

(continued)

Table 39–2. Treatment choices for cancers responsive to systemic agents. (continued)

Diagnosis	Initial Treatment
Non-Hodgkin lymphoma (low grade)	**Combination chemotherapy:** Bendamustine plus obinutuzumab or rituximab[1], or Cyclophosphamide, vincristine, doxorubicin, prednisone, rituximab[1] (CHOP-R), or Cyclophosphamide, vincristine, prednisone, rituximab[1] (CVP-R), or Lenalidomide, rituximab[1]
Plasma cell myeloma	**Combination chemotherapy (transplant candidates):** Bortezomib, dexamethasone, lenalidomide Followed by autologous or mini-allogeneic stem cell transplantation **Combination chemotherapy (non-transplant candidates):** Bortezomib, lenalidomide, dexamethasone, or Daratumumab, lenalidomide, dexamethasone
Waldenström macroglobulinemia	**Plasmapheresis alone or followed by combination chemotherapy:** Ibrutinib with or without rituximab[1] Bortezomib, dexamethasone, rituximab[1], or Cyclophosphamide, dexamethasone, rituximab[1], or Bendamustine, rituximab[1], or Zanubrutinib
Non–small cell lung cancer	**Combination therapy:** Cisplatin, etoposide, or Paclitaxel, carboplatin, or Cisplatin, gemcitabine or docetaxel (squamous histology), or Cisplatin, pemetrexed (nonsquamous histology), or Carboplatin, albumin-bound paclitaxel, or Dabrafenib/trametinib (*BRAF* V600E mutation), or Carboplatin or cisplatin/pemetrexed/pembrolizumab (nonsquamous); carboplatin/paclitaxel or albumin-bound paclitaxel/pembrolizumab (squamous) Nivolumab/ipilimumab **Single-agent therapy:** Erlotinib, gefitinib, osimertinib, afatinib, or dacomitinib (*EGFR* mutation positive) Crizotinib, alectinib, ceritinib, lorlatinib, or brigatinib (*ALK* mutation positive) Ceritinib, crizotinib, or entrectinib (*ROS1* rearrangement) Larotrectinib or entrectinib (*NTRK* gene fusion positive) Capmatinib or tepotinib (*MET exon 14* skipping mutation) Selpercatinib or pralsetinib (*RET* rearrangement positive) Pembrolizumab, or atezolizumab, or cemiplimab-rwlc (PD-L1 ≥ 50%)
Small cell lung cancer	**Combination therapy:** Cisplatin, etoposide (limited stage) with radiation, or Cisplatin or carboplatin, etoposide, atezolizumab or durvalumab (extensive stage)
Mesothelioma	**Combination therapy:** Cisplatin or carboplatin/pemetrexed with or without bevacizumab, or Nivolumab/ipilimumab
Head and neck cancer	Cisplatin with radiation therapy, or Carboplatin with 5-fluorouracil with radiation therapy, or Docetaxel, cisplatin, 5-fluorouracil, or Pembrolizumab (PD-L1 ≥ 1%), or Pembrolizumab/cisplatin or carboplatin/5-fluorouracil
Esophageal and esophagogastric junction cancer	**Combination therapy:** Cisplatin, 5-fluorouracil or capecitabine, or Paclitaxel, carboplatin, or Oxaliplatin, 5-fluorouracil or capecitabine, or 5-Fluorouracil, leucovorin, oxaliplatin, docetaxel (FLOT) Add trastuzumab for *HER2*-overexpressing metastatic adenocarcinoma
Uterine cancer	**Hormone therapy:** Progestins, tamoxifen, aromatase inhibitors, or fulvestrant **Combination chemotherapy:** Carboplatin, paclitaxel Carboplatin, paclitaxel, trastuzumab (*HER2* positive)
Ovarian cancer	**Combination chemotherapy:** Paclitaxel, carboplatin, with or without bevacizumab, or 5-Fluorouracil/leucovorin or capecitabine, oxaliplatin

(*continued*)

Table 39–2. Treatment choices for cancers responsive to systemic agents. (continued)

Diagnosis	Initial Treatment
Cervical cancer	**With radiation:** Cisplatin or carboplatin **Combination chemotherapy:** Cisplatin or carboplatin, paclitaxel, with or without bevacizumab, add pembrolizumab for PD-L1 positive tumors
Breast cancer	**Adjuvant hormone therapy:** *Premenopausal:* Tamoxifen *Postmenopausal:* Aromatase inhibitors (anastrozole, letrozole, exemestane) **Adjuvant chemotherapy (*HER2* negative):** Doxorubicin, cyclophosphamide, followed by paclitaxel, or Docetaxel, cyclophosphamide, or Olaparib if germline *BRCA 1/2* mutations, or High-risk triple-negative—preoperative pembrolizumab/carboplatin/paclitaxel, followed by pembrolizumab/cyclophosphamide/doxorubicin or epirubicin, followed by adjuvant pembrolizumab **Adjuvant chemotherapy (*HER2* positive):** Docetaxel, carboplatin, trastuzumab with or without pertuzumab, or Paclitaxel, trastuzumab
Testicular cancer	**Combination chemotherapy:** Cisplatin, etoposide (EP), or Bleomycin, etoposide, cisplatin (BEP), or Etoposide, mesna, ifosfamide, cisplatin (VIP)
Kidney (renal cell) cancer	**Clear cell histology:** Axitinib or lenvatinib plus pembrolizumab, or ipilimumab plus nivolumab, or cabozantinib with or without nivolumab **Non–clear cell histology:** Cabozantinib or sunitinib
Bladder cancer	**Combination chemotherapy:** Gemcitabine, cisplatin, or Methotrexate, vinblastine, doxorubicin, cisplatin (MVAC), or Atezolizumab, or pembrolizumab, or gemcitabine plus carboplatin (cisplatin-ineligible)
Prostate cancer	**Hormone therapy:** LH-releasing agonist (leuprolide, goserelin, triptorelin, histrelin) or degarelix with or without an antiandrogen (flutamide, bicalutamide, nilutamide, enzalutamide, apalutamide) or abiraterone **Chemotherapy:** Docetaxel
Thyroid cancer	**Single-agent therapy:** Radioiodine (^{131}I) or lenvatinib, vandetanib (medullary thyroid cancer) or cabozantinib (medullary thyroid cancer)
Stomach (gastric) cancer	**Combination chemotherapy:** 5-Fluorouracil, leucovorin, oxaliplatin, docetaxel (FLOT) (perioperative) 5-Fluorouracil or capecitabine with oxaliplatin or cisplatin Add trastuzumab for *HER2*-overexpressing adenocarcinomas
Pancreatic cancer	**Combination chemotherapy:** Gemcitabine, nab-paclitaxel, or 5-Fluorouracil, leucovorin, irinotecan, oxaliplatin (FOLFIRINOX), or Gemcitabine, capecitabine, or Gemcitabine, cisplatin (for *BRCA1/2* or *PALB2* mutation) **Single-agent chemotherapy:** Gemcitabine
Colon cancer	**Combination chemotherapy:** 5-Fluorouracil, leucovorin, oxaliplatin (FOLFOX) with or without bevacizumab, or Capecitabine, oxaliplatin (CAPEOX) with or without bevacizumab, or 5-Fluorouracil, leucovorin, irinotecan (FOLFIRI) with or without bevacizumab 5-Fluorouracil, leucovorin, oxaliplatin, irinotecan (FOLFOXIRI) with or without bevacizumab Cetuximab or panitumumab added to FOLFOX or FOLFIRI for *KRAS/NRAS/BRAF* wild-type and left-sided tumors Capecitabine or 5-fluorouracil/leucovorin with or without bevacizumab **Single-agent therapy:** Pembrolizumab (deficient mismatch repair [dMMR]/high-level microsatellite instability [MSI-H])
Rectal cancer	5-Fluorouracil or capecitabine or FOLFOX or CAPEOX
Anal cancer	Mitomycin with 5-fluorouracil or capecitabine with radiation Carboplatin, paclitaxel with or without radiation therapy
Carcinoid	Octreotide LAR or lanreotide or everolimus or lutetium Lu 177-dotatate

(*continued*)

Table 39–2. Treatment choices for cancers responsive to systemic agents. (continued)

Diagnosis	Initial Treatment
Soft tissue sarcomas	**Combination chemotherapy:** Doxorubicin, dacarbazine (AD), or Doxorubicin, ifosfamide, mesna (AIM), or Ifosfamide, epirubicin, mesna **Single-agent therapy:** Imatinib or sunitinib or regorafenib (GI stromal tumors) Doxorubicin or epirubicin or liposomal doxorubicin
Melanoma	Pembrolizumab or nivolumab or nivolumab/ipilimumab (non-*BRAF* mutation) Dabrafenib/trametinib or vemurafenib/cobimetinib or encorafenib/binimetinib (*BRAF* mutation)
Hepatocellular cancer	Atezolizumab with bevacizumab

[1]In patients with past hepatitis B virus (HBV) infection, rituximab should be used with anti-HBV agent (eg, entecavir) prophylaxis since HBV reactivation, fulminant hepatitis, and, rarely, death can occur otherwise.

Table 39–3. Common cancer therapeutic agents.

Chemotherapeutic Agent	Usual Adult Dosage	Adverse Effects
Alkylating Agents—Nitrogen Mustards		
Bendamustine (Treanda)	100–120 mg/m^2 intravenously every 3–4 weeks	Acute: hypersensitivity, nausea, vomiting Delayed: myelosuppression, rash, pyrexia, fatigue
Cyclophosphamide (Cytoxan)	500–1000 mg/m^2 intravenously every 3 weeks; 100 mg/m^2/day orally for 14 days every 4 weeks; various doses	Acute: nausea and vomiting Delayed: myelosuppression, alopecia, hemorrhagic cystitis, cardiotoxicity (high dose)
Ifosfamide (Ifex)	1200 mg/m^2 intravenously daily for 5 days every 3 weeks; various doses	Acute: nausea and vomiting Delayed: alopecia, myelosuppression, hemorrhagic cystitis, neurotoxicity
Alkylating Agents—Platinum Analogs		
Carboplatin (Paraplatin)	AUC–based dosing use Calvert equation [Dose (mg) = AUC × (GFR + 25)] AUC = 2–7 mg/mL/minute every 2–4 weeks	Acute: nausea and vomiting Delayed: myelosuppression, electrolyte disturbances, peripheral neuropathy, nephrotoxicity, hypersensitivity
Cisplatin (Platinol)	50–100 mg/m^2 intravenously every 3–4 weeks; 20 mg/m^2/day intravenously for 5 days every 3 weeks; various doses	Acute: nausea and vomiting Delayed: nephrotoxicity, ototoxicity, neurotoxicity, myelosuppression, electrolyte disturbances
Oxaliplatin (Eloxatin)	85–130 mg/m^2 intravenously every 2–3 weeks	Acute: peripheral neuropathy exacerbated by cold, nausea, vomiting, diarrhea Delayed: myelosuppression, elevated transaminases
Alkylating Agents—Triazenes		
Temozolomide (Temodar)	75 mg/m^2 orally daily during radiation for 42 days; 150–200 mg/m^2 orally for 5 days every 4 weeks	Acute: nausea, vomiting, constipation Delayed: myelosuppression, fatigue
Antimetabolites—Folate Antagonists		
Methotrexate (MTX; Trexall)	**Intrathecal:** 12 mg **High dose:** 1000–12,000 mg/m^2 intravenously every 2–3 weeks	Acute: nausea, vomiting, mucositis Delayed: myelosuppression, nephrotoxicity, hepatotoxicity, neurotoxicity, photosensitivity, pulmonary toxicity
Pemetrexed (Alimta)	500 mg/m^2 intravenously every 3 weeks	Acute: nausea, vomiting, diarrhea, rash Delayed: myelosuppression, fatigue, mucositis
Antimetabolites—Purine Analogs		
Fludarabine (Fludara)	25 mg/m^2 intravenously for 5 days every 4 weeks	Acute: fever, nausea, vomiting Delayed: asthenia, myelosuppression, immunosuppression, neurotoxicity, anorexia

(continued)

Table 39–3. Common cancer therapeutic agents. (continued)

Chemotherapeutic Agent	Usual Adult Dosage	Adverse Effects
Antimetabolites—Pyrimidine Analogs		
Azacitidine (Vidaza)	75–100 mg/m² subcutaneously or intravenously for 7 days every 4 weeks	Acute: injection site reaction (subcutaneously), nausea, diarrhea, fever Delayed: myelosuppression, dyspnea, arthralgia
Capecitabine (Xeloda)	1000–1250 mg/m² orally twice a day for 14 days every 3 weeks	Acute: nausea, vomiting, diarrhea Delayed: hand-foot syndrome, mucositis, hyperbilirubinemia, myelosuppression
Cytarabine (Ara-C, Cytosar U)	**Standard dose:** 100 mg/m²/day intravenously via continuous infusion for 7 days **High dose:** 1000–3000 mg/m² intravenously every 12 hours for 2–6 days	Acute: nausea, vomiting, rash, flu-like syndrome Delayed: myelosuppression High-dose: neurotoxicity, ocular toxicities
Decitabine (Dacogen)	15 mg/m² intravenously every 8 hours for 3 days every 8 weeks; 20 mg/m² intravenously daily for 5 days	Acute: nausea, vomiting, hyperglycemia Delayed: myelosuppression, fever, fatigue, cough
Fluorouracil (Adrucil)	400 mg/m² intravenous bolus followed by 2400 mg/m² intravenously over 46 hours every 2 weeks; 1000 mg/m² intravenously via continuous infusion for 4–5 days every 3–4 weeks; various doses	Acute: nausea, vomiting, diarrhea Delayed: myelosuppression, hand-foot syndrome, mucositis, photosensitivity, cardiotoxicity (rare)
Gemcitabine (Gemzar)	1000–1250 mg/m² intravenously on days 1 and 8 every 3 weeks or days 1, 8, 15 every 4 weeks	Acute: nausea, vomiting, rash, flu-like symptoms, fever, diarrhea Delayed: myelosuppression, edema, elevated transaminases
Antimicrotubules—Vinca Alkaloids		
Vincristine (Oncovin)	0.5–1.4 mg/m² intravenously every 3 weeks; various doses; maximum single dose usually limited to 2 mg	Acute: constipation, nausea Delayed: peripheral neuropathy, alopecia
Antimicrotubules—Taxanes		
Docetaxel (Taxotere)	60–100 mg/m² intravenously every 3 weeks	Acute: nausea, vomiting, diarrhea, hypersensitivity, rash Delayed: myelosuppression, asthenia, peripheral neuropathy, alopecia, edema, mucositis
Paclitaxel (Taxol)	135–175 mg/m² intravenously every 3 weeks; 50–80 mg/m² intravenously weekly; various doses	Acute: diarrhea, nausea, vomiting, hypersensitivity Delayed: myelosuppression, peripheral neuropathy, alopecia, mucositis, arthralgia
Paclitaxel protein-bound (Abraxane)	100–125 mg/m² on days 1, 8, 15 every 3–4 weeks; 260 mg/m² intravenously every 3 weeks	Acute: nausea, vomiting, diarrhea Delayed: myelosuppression, peripheral neuropathy, alopecia, asthenia
Enzyme Inhibitors—Anthracyclines		
Daunorubicin (Cerubidine)	30–60 mg/m² intravenously for 3 days	Acute: nausea, vomiting, diarrhea, red/orange discoloration of urine, infusion-related reactions (liposomal products) Delayed: myelosuppression, mucositis, alopecia, hand-foot syndrome (liposomal doxorubicin), cardiotoxicity (dose related)
Doxorubicin (Adriamycin)	45–75 mg/m² intravenously every 3 weeks; various doses	
Idarubicin (Idamycin)	10–12 mg/m² intravenously for 3 days	
Liposomal doxorubicin (Doxil, Lipodox)	20–50 mg/m² intravenously every 3–4 weeks	
Enzyme Inhibitors—Topoisomerase Inhibitors		
Etoposide (Vepesid)	50–100 mg/m² intravenously for 3–5 days every 3 weeks	Acute: nausea, vomiting, diarrhea, hypersensitivity, fever, hypotension Delayed: myelosuppression, alopecia, fatigue
Irinotecan (Camptosar)	180 mg/m² intravenously every other week; various doses	Acute: diarrhea, cholinergic syndrome, nausea, vomiting Delayed: myelosuppression, alopecia, asthenia

(continued)

Table 39–3. Common cancer therapeutic agents. (continued)

Chemotherapeutic Agent	Usual Adult Dosage	Adverse Effects
Targeted Therapy—Monoclonal Antibodies		
Atezolizumab (Tecentriq)	1200 mg intravenously every 3 weeks	Acute: infusion-related reaction Delayed: immune-mediated reactions, fatigue, decreased appetite
Bevacizumab (Avastin)	5–15 mg/kg intravenously every 2–3 weeks	Acute: infusion-related reaction Delayed: hypertension, proteinuria, wound healing complications, GI perforation, hemorrhage
Cetuximab (Erbitux)	Loading dose 400 mg/m^2 intravenously, maintenance dose 250 mg/m^2 intravenously weekly	Acute: infusion-related reaction, nausea, diarrhea Delayed: acneiform skin rash, hypomagnesemia, asthenia, paronychial inflammation, dyspnea
Daratumumab (Darzalex)	16 mg/kg intravenously weekly for weeks 1–8, every 2 weeks for weeks 9–24, and every 4 weeks from week 25 until disease progression	Acute: infusion-related reaction, nausea Delayed: myelosuppression, fatigue, upper respiratory tract infection
Ipilimumab (Yervoy)	1–10 mg/kg intravenously every 3 weeks for a total of four doses	Acute: infusion-related reaction Delayed: immune-related reactions, fatigue
Nivolumab (Opdivo)	240 mg intravenously every 2 weeks or 480 mg every 4 weeks	Acute: vomiting Delayed: fatigue, musculoskeletal pain, rash, pruritus, cough, elevated transaminases
Obinutuzumab (Gazyva)	Cycle 1: 100 mg intravenously on day 1, 900 mg on day 2, 1000 mg on days 8 and 15 of a 28-day cycle; cycles 2–6: 1000 mg intravenously on day 1	Acute: infusion-related reaction, TLS Delayed: myelosuppression, pyrexia, cough, musculoskeletal disorder, potential hepatitis B reactivation
Panitumumab (Vectibix)	6 mg/kg intravenously every 2 weeks	Acute: infusion-related reaction, nausea Delayed: acneiform skin rash, hypomagnesemia, asthenia, paronychia, fatigue, dyspnea
Pembrolizumab (Keytruda)	200 mg intravenously every 3 weeks or 400 mg every 6 weeks	Acute: infusion-related reaction, nausea Delayed: immune-mediated reactions, fatigue, cough
Pertuzumab (Perjeta)	840 mg intravenously once followed by 420 mg intravenously every 3 weeks	Acute: infusion-related reaction, diarrhea, nausea Delayed: fatigue, alopecia, neutropenia, rash, peripheral neuropathy, cardiomyopathy
Rituximab (Rituxan)	375 mg/m^2 intravenously weekly for 4 weeks, or every 3–4 weeks	Acute: infusion-related reaction, TLS Delayed: lymphopenia, asthenia, rash, potential hepatitis B reactivation
Trastuzumab (Herceptin)	Initial dose 4 mg/kg intravenously, then 2 mg/kg intravenously weekly; or initial dose 8 mg/kg, then 6 mg/kg, intravenously every 3 weeks	Acute: headache, nausea, diarrhea, infusion-related reaction Delayed: myelosuppression, pyrexia, cardiomyopathy, pulmonary toxicity (rare)
Targeted Therapy—Kinase Inhibitors		
Acalabrutinib	100 mg orally twice daily	Acute: diarrhea Delayed: myelosuppression, upper respiratory infection, musculoskeletal pain
Alectinib (Alecensa)	600 mg orally twice daily with food	Acute: none Delayed: myelosuppression, fatigue, edema, myalgia, dyspnea, elevated transaminases
Axitinib (Inlyta)	5–10 mg orally twice daily	Acute: diarrhea, nausea, vomiting Delayed: hypertension, fatigue, dysphonia, hand-foot syndrome, elevated transaminases
Bosutinib (Bosulif)	500–600 mg orally once daily with food	Acute: diarrhea, nausea, vomiting Delayed: myelosuppression, rash, abdominal pain, hepatotoxicity, fluid retention

(*continued*)

Table 39–3. Common cancer therapeutic agents. (continued)

Chemotherapeutic Agent	Usual Adult Dosage	Adverse Effects
Targeted Therapy—Kinase Inhibitors (cont.)		
Cobimetinib (Cotellic)	60 mg orally once daily on days 1–21 of a 28-day cycle	Acute: diarrhea, photosensitivity reaction, nausea, vomiting Delayed: myelosuppression, hepatotoxicity, rash, cardiomyopathy (with vemurafenib)
Dabrafenib (Tafinlar)	150 mg orally twice daily without food	Acute: headache Delayed: hyperkeratosis, fever, hand-foot syndrome, hyperglycemia, hypophosphatemia
Dasatinib (Sprycel)	100–180 mg orally once daily	Acute: diarrhea, nausea, vomiting Delayed: myelosuppression, fluid retention, fatigue, dyspnea, musculoskeletal pain, rash
Erlotinib (Tarceva)	100 or 150 mg orally once daily without food	Acute: diarrhea, nausea, vomiting Delayed: acneiform skin rash, fatigue, anorexia, dyspnea
Gefitinib (Iressa)	250 mg orally once daily	Acute: diarrhea Delayed: acneiform skin rash
Ibrutinib (Imbruvica)	420 or 560 mg orally once daily	Acute: diarrhea, nausea Delayed: myelosuppression, fatigue, edema, rash, elevated serum creatinine, hemorrhage
Imatinib (Gleevec)	100–800 mg orally once daily with food	Acute: nausea, vomiting, diarrhea Delayed: edema, muscle cramps, rash, myelosuppression, hepatotoxicity
Lenvatinib (Lenvima)	24 mg orally once daily	Acute: hypertension, nausea, vomiting, diarrhea Delayed: fatigue, arthralgia/myalgia, stomatitis, hand-foot syndrome
Nilotinib (Tasigna)	300 or 400 mg orally twice daily without food	Acute: nausea, vomiting, diarrhea Delayed: rash, fatigue, myelosuppression, prolonged QT interval (rare)
Osimertinib (Tagrisso)	80 mg orally once daily	Acute: diarrhea Delayed: myelosuppression, rash, dry skin, nail toxicity, cardiomyopathy (rare), prolonged QT interval (rare)
Pazopanib (Votrient)	800 mg orally once daily without food	Acute: diarrhea, nausea, vomiting Delayed: hypertension, hair color changes, hepatotoxicity, hemorrhage
Regorafenib (Stivarga)	160 mg orally once daily with food (low-fat breakfast)	Acute: diarrhea Delayed: asthenia, hand-foot syndrome, anorexia, hypertension, mucositis, myelosuppression, hepatotoxicity
Sunitinib (Sutent)	50 mg orally once daily for 4 weeks followed by 2 weeks rest; 37.5 mg orally daily	Acute: diarrhea and nausea Delayed: hypertension, hand-foot syndrome, rash, yellow discoloration of skin, fatigue, hypothyroidism, mucositis, LV dysfunction, bleeding, hepatotoxicity
Trametinib (Mekinist)	2 mg orally once daily without food	Acute: rash, diarrhea Delayed: elevated transaminases, lymphedema, cardiomyopathy
Vemurafenib (Zelboraf)	960 mg orally twice daily	Acute: nausea, hypersensitivity (rare) Delayed: photosensitivity, rash, arthralgia, alopecia, fatigue, prolonged QT interval, cutaneous squamous cell carcinoma
Miscellaneous Agents		
Abiraterone (Zytiga)	1000 mg orally once daily	Acute: diarrhea, edema Delayed: adrenal insufficiency, hepatotoxicity, joint pain, hypokalemia
Bortezomib (Velcade)	1.3 mg/m^2 intravenous bolus or subcutaneously on days 1, 4, 8, 11 followed by a 10-day rest, or weekly for 4 weeks followed by 13-day rest	Acute: nausea, vomiting, diarrhea Delayed: peripheral neuropathy, fatigue, myelosuppression

(*continued*)

Table 39–3. Common cancer therapeutic agents. (continued)

Chemotherapeutic Agent	Usual Adult Dosage	Adverse Effects
Miscellaneous Agents (cont.)		
Lenalidomide (Revlimid)	5–25 mg orally once daily on days 1–21 of 28-day cycle; or continuously	Acute: diarrhea, rash Delayed: myelosuppression, fatigue, venous thromboembolism, potential for birth defects
Mitomycin (Mutamycin)	10–20 mg/m^2 intravenously every 4–8 weeks; 20–40 mg intravesically	Acute: cystitis (intravesically), nausea, vomiting Delayed: myelosuppression, mucositis, anorexia
Venetoclax (Venclexta)	20 mg orally daily during week 1; 50 mg daily during week 2; 100 mg daily during week 3; 200 mg daily during week 4; then 400 mg orally daily thereafter	Acute: diarrhea, nausea, vomiting, TLS Delayed: myelosuppression, upper respiratory infections, fatigue
Antiandrogens		
Apalutamide (Erleada)	240 mg orally once daily	Acute: fatigue, diarrhea Delayed: arthralgia, hot flashes, falls, peripheral edema, seizure (rare)
Bicalutamide (Casodex)	50 mg orally once daily	Acute: none Delayed: hot flashes, back pain, asthenia
Enzalutamide (Xtandi)	160 mg orally once daily	Acute: asthenia, diarrhea Delayed: hot flashes, arthralgia, peripheral edema, seizure (rare)
Selective Estrogen Receptor Modulators		
Tamoxifen (Nolvadex)	20–40 mg orally once daily	Acute: none Delayed: hot flashes, vaginal discharge, menstrual irregularities, arthralgia
Aromatase Inhibitors		
Anastrozole (Arimidex)	1 mg orally once daily	Acute: nausea Delayed: hot flashes, peripheral edema, asthenia, hypercholesterolemia, arthralgia/myalgia, osteoporosis
Exemestane (Aromasin)	25 mg orally once daily	
Letrozole (Femara)	2.5 mg orally once daily	
Pure Estrogen Receptor Antagonist		
Fulvestrant (Faslodex)	500 mg intramuscularly on days 1, 15, 29, then monthly	Acute: injection site reaction, nausea Delayed: hot flashes, bone pain, elevated transaminases
LHRH Analogs		
Goserelin acetate (Zoladex)	3.6 mg subcutaneously every month; 10.8 mg subcutaneously every 3 months	Acute: injection site discomfort Delayed: hot flashes, tumor flare, edema, decreased libido, erectile dysfunction, osteoporosis
Leuprolide (Lupron)	7.5 mg intramuscularly or subcutaneously every month; 22.5 mg intramuscularly or subcutaneously every 3 months; 30 mg intramuscularly or subcutaneously every 4 months; 45 mg intramuscularly or subcutaneously every 6 months	
Triptorelin pamoate (Trelstar)	3.75 mg intramuscularly every 4 weeks; 11.25 mg intramuscularly every 12 weeks; 22.5 mg intramuscularly every 24 weeks	
LHRH Antagonist		
Degarelix (Firmagon)	240 mg subcutaneously once, then 80 mg subcutaneously every 28 days	Acute: injection site reaction Delayed: hot flashes, weight gain, elevated transaminases, QT prolongation

AUC, area under the curve; AV, atrioventricular; CPK, creatine phosphokinase; LHRH, LH-releasing hormone; MCV, mean corpuscular volume; TLS, tumor lysis syndrome.

TYPES OF CANCER

LUNG CANCER

Sunny Wang, MD

BRONCHOGENIC CARCINOMA

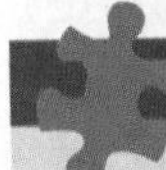

ESSENTIALS OF DIAGNOSIS

- New cough or change in chronic cough.
- Dyspnea, hemoptysis, anorexia, weight loss.
- Enlarging lung nodule or mass; persistent opacity, atelectasis, or pleural effusion on chest radiograph or CT scan.
- Cytologic or histologic findings of lung cancer in sputum, pleural fluid, or biopsy specimen.

General Considerations

Lung cancer is the leading cause of cancer deaths in both men and women. The American Cancer Society (ACS) estimates 235,760 new diagnoses and 131,880 deaths from lung cancer in the United States in 2021, accounting for approximately 12% of new cancer diagnoses and 22% of all cancer deaths. More Americans die of lung cancer than of colorectal, breast, and prostate cancers combined.

Cigarette smoking causes 85–90% of cases of lung cancer. The causal connection between cigarettes and lung cancer is established not only epidemiologically but also through identification of carcinogens in tobacco smoke and analysis of the effect of these carcinogens on specific oncogenes expressed in lung cancer.

Other environmental risk factors for the development of lung cancer include exposure to environmental tobacco smoke, radon, asbestos, diesel exhaust, ionizing radiation, metals (arsenic, chromium, nickel, iron oxide), and industrial carcinogens. A familial predisposition to lung cancer is recognized. Certain diseases are associated with an increased risk of lung cancer, including pulmonary fibrosis, COPD, and sarcoidosis.

The median age at diagnosis of lung cancer in the United States is 71 years; it is unusual under the age of 40 years. The combined relative 5-year survival rate for all stages of lung cancer is 21%.

There are five main histologic categories of bronchogenic carcinoma. **Squamous cell carcinomas** (23% of cases, based on US SEER data 2013–2017) arise from the bronchial epithelium and often present as intraluminal masses. They are usually centrally located and can present with hemoptysis. **Adenocarcinomas** (50% of cases) arise from mucous glands or from any epithelial cell within or distal to the terminal bronchioles. They usually present as peripheral nodules or masses. **Adenocarcinomas in situ** (formerly **bronchioloalveolar cell carcinomas**) spread along preexisting alveolar structures (lepidic growth) without evidence of invasion. **Large cell carcinomas** (1.3% of cases) are a heterogeneous group of undifferentiated cancers that share large cells and do not fit into other categories. Large cell carcinomas are typically aggressive and have rapid doubling times. They present as central or peripheral masses. Cancers that are not better differentiated on pathologic review other than non–small cell carcinomas (NSCLC) or carcinomas not otherwise specified make up about 13% of cases. **Small cell carcinomas** (13% of cases) are tumors of bronchial origin that typically begin centrally, infiltrating submucosally to cause narrowing of the bronchus without a discrete luminal mass. They are aggressive cancers that often involve regional or distant metastasis on presentation.

For purposes of staging and treatment, bronchogenic carcinomas are divided into small cell lung cancer (SCLC) and the other four types, labeled NSCLC. This practical classification reflects different natural histories and treatments. SCLC is prone to early hematogenous spread and has a more aggressive course with a median survival (untreated) of 6–18 weeks.

Clinical Findings

Lung cancer is symptomatic at diagnosis in a majority of patients. The clinical presentation depends on the type and location of the primary tumor, the extent of local spread, and the presence of distant metastases and any paraneoplastic syndromes.

A. Symptoms and Signs

Anorexia, weight loss, or asthenia occurs in 55–90% of patients presenting with a new diagnosis of lung cancer. Up to 60% of patients have a new cough or a change in a chronic cough; 6–31% have hemoptysis; and 25–40% complain of pain, either nonspecific chest pain or pain from bony metastases to the vertebrae, ribs, or pelvis. Local spread may cause endobronchial obstruction with atelectasis and postobstructive pneumonia, pleural effusion (12–33%), change in voice (compromise of the recurrent laryngeal nerve), superior vena cava syndrome (obstruction of the superior vena cava with supraclavicular venous engorgement), and Horner syndrome (ipsilateral ptosis, miosis, and anhidrosis from involvement of the inferior cervical ganglion and the paravertebral sympathetic chain). Distant metastases to the liver are associated with asthenia and weight loss. Brain metastases (10% in NSCLC, more common in adenocarcinoma, and 20–30% in SCLC) may present with headache, nausea, vomiting, seizures, dizziness, or altered mental status.

Paraneoplastic syndromes are patterns of organ dysfunction related to immune-mediated or secretory effects of neoplasms. These syndromes occur in 10–20% of patients with lung cancer. They may precede, accompany, or follow the diagnosis of lung cancer. In patients with small cell carcinoma, the syndrome of inappropriate ADH (SIADH) can develop in 10–15%; in those with squamous cell carcinoma, hypercalcemia can develop in 10%. Digital clubbing is seen in up to 20% of patients at diagnosis (see Figure 6–42). Other common paraneoplastic syndromes include increased ACTH production, anemia, hypercoagulability, peripheral neuropathy, and the Lambert-Eaton myasthenic syndrome. Their recognition is important because treatment of the primary tumor may improve or resolve symptoms even when the cancer is not curable.

B. Laboratory Findings

The diagnosis of lung cancer rests on examination of a tissue or cytology specimen. **Sputum cytology** is highly specific but insensitive; the yield is highest when there are lesions in the central airways. While the diagnostic yield of **CT-guided biopsy** of peripheral nodules approaches 80–90%, the rates of pneumothorax are significant (15–30%), especially in those with emphysema. **Thoracentesis** (sensitivity 50–65%) can be used to establish a diagnosis of lung cancer in patients with malignant pleural effusions. Fine-needle aspiration (FNA) of palpable supraclavicular or cervical lymph nodes is frequently diagnostic.

Fiberoptic bronchoscopy allows visualization of the major airways, cytology brushing of visible lesions or lavage of lung segments with cytologic evaluation of specimens, direct biopsy of endobronchial abnormalities, blind transbronchial biopsy of the pulmonary parenchyma or peripheral nodules, and FNA biopsy of mediastinal lymph nodes. Electromagnetic navigational bronchoscopy allows bronchoscopic approaches to small peripheral nodules. Mediastinoscopy, video-assisted thoracoscopic surgery (VATS), and thoracotomy may be necessary in cases where less invasive techniques fail to yield a diagnosis.

C. Imaging

Nearly all patients with lung cancer have abnormal findings on chest radiography or CT scan (Figure 39–1). These findings are rarely specific for a particular diagnosis. Interpretation of characteristic findings in isolated nodules is described in Chapter 9.

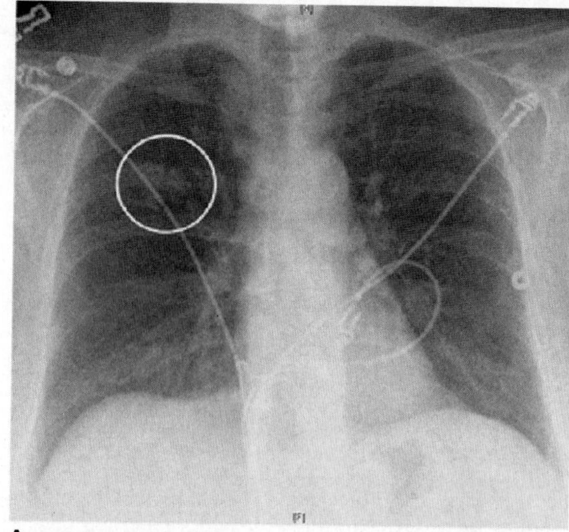

A

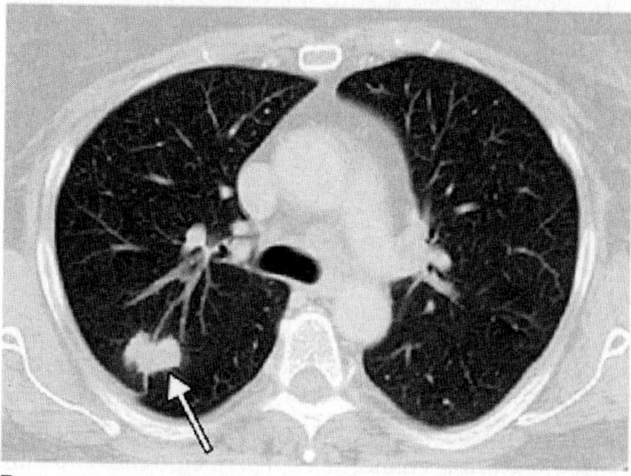

B

▲ **Figure 39–1.** Squamous cell carcinoma of the right lung on chest radiograph **(A)** and CT scan **(B).** (Reproduced, with permission, from Elsayes KM, Oldham SA. *Introduction to Diagnostic Radiology.* McGraw-Hill, 2014.)

D. Special Examinations

1. Staging—Accurate staging is crucial (1) to provide the clinician with information to guide treatment, (2) to provide the patient with accurate information regarding prognosis, and (3) to standardize entry criteria for clinical trials to allow interpretation of results.

Staging of **NSCLC** uses two integrated systems and is continuously updated with the eighth edition of the **American Joint Committee on Cancer (AJCC)/Union for International Cancer Control (UICC)** stage classification for lung cancer in effect since January 2018. The **AJCC TNM international staging system** attempts a physical description of the neoplasm: T describes the size and location of the primary tumor; N describes the presence and location of nodal metastases; and M refers to the presence or absence of distant metastases. These TNM stages are grouped into summary stages I–IV, and these are used to guide therapy. Many patients with stage I and stage II disease are cured through surgery. Patients with stage IIIB and stage IV disease do not benefit from surgery (Table 39–4). Patients with stage IIIA disease have locally invasive disease that may benefit from surgery in selected cases as part of multimodality therapy.

SCLC is traditionally divided into two categories: **limited disease** (30% of cases), when the tumor is limited to the unilateral hemithorax (including contralateral mediastinal nodes); or **extensive disease** (70% of cases), when the tumor extends beyond the hemithorax (including pleural effusion). It is also recommended to stage SCLC according to the TNM staging system.

For both SCLC and NSCLC, a complete examination is essential to exclude obvious metastatic disease to lymph nodes, skin, and bone. A detailed history is essential because the patient's performance status is a powerful predictor of disease course. All patients should have

Table 39–4. Five-year survival rates for non–small cell lung cancer, based on Tumor, Node, Metastasis (TNM) staging.

Stage	TNM Subset	5-Year Survival Rate for Clinical TNM	5-Year Survival Rate for Pathologic TNM
0	Carcinoma in situ		
1A1	T1aN0M0	92%	90%
1A2	T1bN0M0	83%	85%
IA3	T1cN0M0	77%	80%
IB	T2aN0M0	68%	73%
IIA	T2bN0M0	60%	65%
IIB	T1/T2, N1M0 T3N0M0	53%	56%
IIIA	T1/T2, N2M0 T3N1M0 T4, N0/N1, M0	36%	41%
IIIB	T1/T2, N3M0 T3/T4, N2M0	26%	24%
IIIC	T3/T4, N3M0	13%	12%
IVA	Any T, Any N, M1a/M1b	10%	—
IVB	Any T, Any N, M1c	0%	—

Reproduced with permission from Detterbeck FC et al. The Eighth Edition Lung Cancer Stage Classification. Chest. 2017;151(1):193–203 and data from Goldstraw P et al. The IASLC Lung Cancer Staging Project: proposals for revision of the TNM stage groupings in the forthcoming (eighth) edition of the TNM classification for lung cancer. J Thorac Oncol. 2015;11:39.

measurement of a CBC, serum electrolytes, calcium, creatinine, liver biochemical tests, LD, and albumin.

NSCLC patients being considered for surgery require meticulous evaluation to identify those with resectable disease. CT imaging is key for staging candidates for resection. The sensitivity and specificity of CT imaging for identifying lung cancer metastatic to the mediastinal lymph nodes are 57% (49–66%) and 82% (77–86%), respectively. Therefore, chest CT imaging alone does not provide definitive staging information. CT imaging helps determine where to biopsy, and how the mediastinum should be sampled.

The combination of PET using 2-[^{18}F] fluoro-2-deoxyglucose (FDG-PET) and CT is an important modality for identifying metastatic foci in the mediastinum or distant sites. The sensitivity and specificity of FDG-PET/CT for detecting mediastinal spread of primary lung cancer depend on the size of mediastinal nodes or masses. When mediastinal lymph nodes smaller than 1 cm are present, the sensitivity and specificity of FDG-PET/CT for tumor involvement of nodes are 74% and 96%, respectively. When CT shows lymph nodes larger than 1 cm, the sensitivity and specificity are 95% and 76%, respectively.

Obtaining an MRI of the brain is important to rule out brain metastases in all patients with SCLC and in patients with NSCLC with at least stage II disease or poorly differentiated histologies.

2. Preoperative assessment—See Chapter 3.

3. Pulmonary function testing—Many patients with NSCLC have moderate to severe chronic lung disease that increases the risk of perioperative complications as well as long-term pulmonary insufficiency following lung resection. All patients considered for surgery require spirometry. In the absence of other comorbidities, patients with good lung function (preoperative FEV_1 2 L or more) are at low risk for complications from lobectomy or pneumonectomy.

4. Screening—Screening with low-dose helical CT scans of the chest has been shown to improve lung cancer mortality rates. The National Lung Screening Trial, a multicenter randomized US trial involving over 53,000 current and former heavy smokers, showed that screening annually with low-dose helical CT for 3 years yielded a 20% relative reduction in lung cancer mortality and 6.7% reduction in all-cause mortality compared with chest radiography. Given these findings, US professional organizations have recommended annual screening with low-dose helical CT for lung cancer. The 2021 USPSTF recommendations specify annual low-dose CT for smokers aged 50–80 years who have at least a 20 pack-year smoking history and who either currently smoke or have quit within the last 15 years. Smoking cessation policies and efforts should be integrated with any screening program.

Treatment

A. Non–Small Cell Lung Carcinoma

Surgical resection offers the best chance for cure of NSCLC. Clinical features that preclude complete surgical resection include extrathoracic metastases or a malignant pleural effusion; or tumor involving the heart, pericardium, great vessels, esophagus, recurrent laryngeal or phrenic nerves, trachea, main carina, or contralateral mediastinal lymph nodes. Accordingly, stage I and stage II patients are treated with surgical resection where possible. Stage II and select cases of stage IB are additionally recommended to receive adjuvant chemotherapy. Stage IIIA patients have poor outcomes if treated with resection alone. They should undergo multimodality treatment that includes chemotherapy or radiotherapy, or both. Inoperable stage IIIA and stage IIIB patients are treated with concurrent chemotherapy and radiation therapy and have improved survival. Stage IV patients are treated with systemic therapy (targeted therapy, chemotherapy, or immunotherapy) or symptom-based palliative therapy, or both.

Surgical approach affects outcome. In 1994, the North American Lung Cancer Study Group conducted a prospective trial of stage IA patients randomized to lobectomy versus limited resection. They reported a threefold increased rate of local recurrence in the limited resection group ($P = 0.008$) and a trend toward an increase in overall death rate (increase of 30%, $P = 0.08$) and increase in cancer-related death rate (increase of 50%, $P = 0.09$), compared with patients receiving lobectomy. However, for patients who cannot tolerate lobectomy, a sublobar resection (wedge resection or segmentectomy) may be considered.

Patients with clinical stage I primary NSCLC, who are not candidates for surgery because of significant comorbidity or other surgical contraindication, are candidates for stereotactic body radiotherapy. Stereotactic body radiotherapy, which is composed of multiple non-parallel radiation beams that converge, allows the delivery of a relatively large dose of radiation to a small, well-defined target. For clinical stage I NSCLC, 3-year local control rates with stereotactic body radiotherapy exceed 90%, and large meta-analyses of nonrandomized data have shown 2-year survival of 70% and 5-year survival of 40%. Patients with locally advanced disease (stages IIIA and IIIB) who are not surgical candidates have improved survival when treated with concurrent chemotherapy and radiation therapy compared with no therapy, radiation alone, or even sequential chemotherapy and radiation.

Neoadjuvant chemotherapy consists of giving antineoplastic drugs in advance of surgery or radiation therapy. Neoadjuvant therapy can be used in select patients with stage IIIA or stage IIIB disease. Some studies suggest a survival advantage.

Adjuvant chemotherapy consists of administering antineoplastic drugs following surgery or radiation therapy. Cisplatin-containing regimens have been shown to confer an overall survival benefit in at least stage II disease and a subset of stage IB disease where primary tumor size exceeds 4 cm. The Lung Adjuvant Cisplatin Evaluation Collaborative Group, a meta-analysis of the five largest cisplatin-based adjuvant trials, reported a 5% absolute benefit in 5-year overall survival with a cisplatin-containing doublet regimen following surgery ($P = 0.005$) in patients with at least stage II disease.

For stage IIIB and stage IV NSCLC, options for therapy include targeted therapy, cytotoxic chemotherapy, and immunotherapy (checkpoint inhibitors) (Tables 39–2 and 39–3). The approach to therapy is individualized based on molecular profiling and PD-L1 testing. Molecular profiling is offered as next-generation sequencing multi-gene assays. The key driver mutations in lung cancer include *EGFR, ALK, BRAF, ROS1, NTRK, MET, RET*, and *KRAS* pathogenic variants, but only a minority of all lung cancer cases harbor these mutations. Difficulties in testing may arise when only small fine-needle aspirate biopsies are obtained; to have sufficient tissue for analysis, it is recommended that clinicians obtain core biopsies. PD-L1 expression is a flawed but actively used biomarker to assess possible response to checkpoint inhibitor therapy (specifically, programmed cell death protein-1 [PD-1] and PD-L1 inhibitors).

Targeted therapy has played a pivotal role in advanced NSCLC (Tables 39–2 and 39–3). Activating *EGFR* pathogenic variants are found in approximately 10–20% of the White population and 30–48% of the Asian population and are usually found among nonsmokers to light smokers, women, and persons with nonsquamous histologies (particularly adenocarcinomas). For patients with sensitizing *EGFR* variants, an EGFR tyrosine kinase inhibitor rather than platinum-based chemotherapy is the first-line treatment. Response rates with EGFR tyrosine kinase inhibitors in patients with *EGFR* variants are at least 70%, and median overall survival is estimated to be 21–33 months. Osimertinib (a third-generation irreversible EGFR tyrosine kinase inhibitor) is recommended as first-line treatment of *EGFR*-variant lung cancers. Phase 3 data show that osimertinib leads to a longer duration of response, longer progression-free survival, and lower rates of severe adverse events compared with earlier generation EGFR tyrosine kinase inhibitors.

Approximately 5% of all patients with NSCLC carry translocations of *ALK* resulting in novel fusion gene products with oncogenic activity. For patients with *ALK*-rearranged lung cancers, ALK tyrosine kinase inhibitors are recommended therapeutic agents. Alectinib, brigatinib, and lorlatinib are recommended as first-line agents in *ALK*-rearranged lung cancers with response rates ranging from 74% to 83%. For patients who have developed resistance to either first- or second-generation ALK inhibitors, lorlatinib (a third-generation ALK and ROS1 tyrosine kinase inhibitor) has shown a response rate of 47%. Approximately 1–2% of NSCLC harbor *ROS1* rearrangements and they are usually lung adenocarcinomas found among nonsmokers or light smokers. *ROS1*-rearranged lung cancers respond to crizotinib (*ALK, cMET*, and *ROS1* tyrosine kinase inhibitor) and entrectinib (multikinase inhibitor, including ROS-1) with response rates over 70%. MET exon 14 (METex14) skipping mutations are found in 3% of lung adenocarcinomas. Capmatinib or tepotinib (MET inhibitors) is recommended as first-line treatment for patients with METex14 skipping mutation. *BRAF* mutations have been found in 2% of NSCLC patients. The combination of dabrafenib (BRAF inhibitor) and trametinib (MEK inhibitor) has shown response rates of over 60% in patients with *BRAF V600E* pathogenic variants. Treatment with larotrectinib (TRKA/B/C inhibitor) or entrectinib (multikinase inhibitor, including TRKA/B/C) is recommended for patients whose tumors reveal NTRK 1/2/3 gene fusion. Selpercatinib and pralsetinib (RET inhibitors) are recommended first-line treatments for RET fusion–positive NSCLC. Finally, *KRAS* pathogenic variants are found among 30% of patients with adenocarcinomas, are associated with smoking, and indicate a poor prognosis. In May 2021, the FDA approved sotorasib (AMG 510) for treating *KRAS* G12C mutated lung cancers after progression on first-line treatment.

Immune checkpoint inhibition using PD-1 or PD-L1 inhibitors (nivolumab, pembrolizumab, atezolizumab, cemiplimab-rwlc, and durvalumab) has an important role in the treatment of NSCLC (Tables 39–2 and 39–3). Checkpoint inhibitors release T cells from the inhibitory signals they receive from tumor cells via the PD-1 pathway, restoring antitumor immunity. Atezolizumab (PD-L1 inhibitor) can be given for 1 year post adjuvant chemotherapy for resected stage II to IIIA NSCLC, based on a phase 3 trial showing improvement in disease-free survival compared with adjuvant chemotherapy without atezolizumab (P = 0.020). For stage III NSCLCs, a phase 3 trial has shown improved survival outcomes by adding durvalumab (PD-L1 inhibitor) as consolidation therapy post-definitive chemoradiation.

For stage IV NSCLC patients with tumors staining greater than 50% for PD-L1, PD-1 inhibitors (pembrolizumab and cemiplimab-rwlc) and PD-L1 inhibitors (atezolizumab) outperform first-line platinum-based chemotherapy, with response rates of 40–45% versus 20–30% and improvement in median progression-free survival. Five-year follow-up data for patients with 50% or greater PD-L1 expression show that patients who received pembrolizumab versus chemotherapy alone had improved median overall survival of 26 months versus 13 months. For patients with metastatic NSCLC regardless of PD-L1 status, phase 3 trials have shown improved survival outcomes with adding pembrolizumab to platinum-doublet chemotherapy as first-line therapy. One-year survival for pembrolizumab with platinum-doublet chemotherapy was 69% compared with 49% with chemotherapy alone ($P < 0.001$). If patients received chemotherapy alone as first-line treatment, PD-1 inhibitors are recommended as second-line treatment of NSCLC, regardless of PD-L1 staining intensity. Combined checkpoint inhibition with nivolumab (PD-1 inhibitor) and ipilimumab (monoclonal CTLA4 antibody) has also shown improved response rates and progression-free survival compared with chemotherapy in patients with metastatic NSCLC. However, significant side effects and toxicity have been reported with checkpoint inhibitors, especially autoimmune manifestations such as hepatitis, thyroiditis, hypophysitis, colitis, pneumonitis, and type 1 diabetes mellitus.

If no targetable mutations are found and there is inadequate PD-L1 expression on tumor cells, patients are either offered combination immunotherapy with cytotoxic chemotherapy or cytotoxic chemotherapy alone (Table 39–2). Although not curative, platinum-based chemotherapy has been shown in multiple clinical trials to provide a modest increase in overall survival in patients with stage IIIB and stage IV NSCLC compared with supportive care alone. Palliative chemotherapy also leads to improved quality of life and symptom control.

B. Small Cell Lung Carcinoma

Response rates of **SCLC** to cisplatin and etoposide (Table 39–2) are excellent with 80–90% response in limited-stage disease (50–60% complete response), and 60–80% response in extensive-stage disease (15–20% complete response). However, remissions tend to be short-lived with a median duration of 6–8 months. Once the disease has recurred, median survival is 3–4 months. Overall 2-year survival is 20–40% in limited-stage disease and 5% in extensive-stage disease (Table 39–5). Modest improvement in survival has been achieved with the addition of a checkpoint inhibitor (atezolizumab or durvalumab) to cisplatin or carboplatin and etoposide therapy in extensive-stage disease. Thoracic radiation therapy improves survival in patients with limited SCLC and is given concurrently with chemotherapy. There is a high rate of brain metastasis in patients with SCLC, even following a good response to chemotherapy.

Table 39–5. Median survival for small cell lung carcinoma following treatment.

Stage	Mean 2-Year Survival	Median Survival
Limited	20–40%	15–20 months
Extensive	5%	8–13 months

Data from multiple sources, including Van Meerbeeck JP et al. Small-cell lung cancer. Lancet. 2011;378:1741.

C. Palliative Therapy

Photoresection with the Nd:YAG laser is sometimes performed on central tumors to relieve endobronchial obstruction, improve dyspnea, and control hemoptysis. External beam radiation therapy is also used to control dyspnea, hemoptysis, endobronchial obstruction, pain from bony metastases, obstruction from superior vena cava syndrome, and symptomatic brain metastases. Resection of a *solitary* brain metastasis improves quality of life and survival when combined with radiation therapy if there is no evidence of other metastatic disease. Stereotactic radiation therapy is offered for limited brain metastases. Repeated thoracenteses, pleurodesis, and PleurX catheter tube placement are key interventions for palliation of symptomatic malignant pleural effusions. Pain is very common in advanced disease. Meticulous efforts at pain control are essential (see Chapter 5). In addition to standard oncologic care, early referral to a palliative care specialist is recommended in advanced disease to aid in pain and other symptom management. Such palliative care can modestly improve survival.

Prognosis

The overall 5-year survival rate for lung cancer is approximately 20%. Predictors of survival include the tumor type (SCLC versus NSCLC), molecular profiling, and stage, and the patient's performance status and weight loss in the prior 6 months. Patients with targetable mutations have better overall survival when compared with those without mutations due to superior efficacy of targeted drug therapy.

Felip E et al. Adjuvant atezolizumab after adjuvant chemotherapy in resected stage IB-IIIA non-small-cell lung cancer (IMpower010): a randomised, multicentre, open-label, phase 3 trial. Lancet. 2021;398:1344. [PMID: 34555333]

Reck M et al. Five-year outcomes with pembrolizumab versus chemotherapy for metastatic non-small-cell lung cancer with PD-L1 tumor proportion score ≥ 50. J Clin Oncol. 2021;39:2339. [PMID: 33872070]

Siegel RL et al. Cancer statistics, 2022. CA Cancer J Clin. 2022;72:7. [PMID: 35020204]

Skoulidis F et al. Sotorasib for lung cancers with *KRAS* p.G12C mutation. N Engl J Med. 2021;384:2371. [PMID: 34096690]
US Preventive Services Task Force. Screening for lung cancer: US Preventive Services Task Force Recommendation Statement. JAMA. 2021;325:962. [PMID: 33687470]

PULMONARY METASTASIS

Pulmonary metastasis results from the spread of an extrapulmonary malignant tumor through vascular or lymphatic channels or by direct extension. Metastases usually occur via the pulmonary artery and typically present as multiple nodules or masses on chest radiography. The radiographic differential diagnosis of multiple pulmonary nodules also includes pulmonary arteriovenous malformation, infections, sarcoidosis, rheumatoid nodules, and granulomatosis with polyangiitis. Metastases to the lungs are found in 20–55% of patients with various metastatic malignancies. Carcinomas of the kidney, breast, rectum, colon, and cervix and malignant melanoma are the most likely primary tumors.

Lymphangitic carcinomatosis denotes diffuse involvement of the pulmonary lymphatic network by primary or metastatic lung cancer, probably a result of extension of tumor from lung capillaries to the lymphatics. **Tumor embolization** from extrapulmonary cancer (renal cell carcinoma, hepatocellular carcinoma, choriocarcinoma) is an uncommon route for tumor spread to the lungs. Metastatic cancer may also present as a malignant pleural effusion.

Clinical Findings

A. Symptoms and Signs

Symptoms are uncommon but include cough, hemoptysis and, in advanced cases, dyspnea and hypoxemia. Symptoms are more often referable to the site of the primary tumor.

B. Laboratory Findings

The diagnosis of metastatic cancer involving the lungs is usually established by identifying a primary tumor. Appropriate studies should be ordered if there is a suspicion of any primary cancer, such as breast, thyroid, testis, colorectal, or prostate. If the history, physical examination, and initial studies fail to reveal the site of the primary tumor, attention is better focused on the lung, where tissue samples obtained by bronchoscopy, percutaneous needle biopsy, VATS, or thoracotomy may establish the histologic diagnosis and suggest the most likely primary cancer. Occasionally, cytologic studies of pleural fluid or pleural biopsy reveals the diagnosis.

C. Imaging

Chest radiographs usually show multiple spherical densities with sharp margins. The lesions are usually bilateral, pleural, or subpleural in location, and more common in lower lung zones. Lymphangitic spread and solitary pulmonary nodule are less common radiographic presentations of pulmonary metastasis. CT imaging of the chest, abdomen, and pelvis may reveal the site of a primary tumor and will help determine feasibility of surgical resection of the metastatic lung tumors. FDG-PET-CT scan is helpful in identifying the site of a primary cancer and identifying other areas of extrathoracic metastasis.

Treatment

Once the diagnosis has been established, management consists of treatment of the primary neoplasm, usually with systemic treatments, and treatment of any pulmonary complications. Surgical resection of a *solitary* pulmonary nodule can be considered in the patient with known current or previous extrapulmonary cancer. Local resection of one or more pulmonary metastases is feasible in a few carefully selected patients with various sarcomas and carcinomas (ie, testis, colorectal, and kidney). About 15–25% of metastatic solid tumor patients have metastases limited to the lungs and are surgical candidates. Surgical resection should be considered only if (1) the primary tumor is under control, (2) the patient has adequate cardiopulmonary reserve to tolerate resection, (3) all metastatic tumor can be resected, (4) effective nonsurgical approaches are not available, and (5) there is no evidence of extrathoracic metastases that are not controlled. Unfavorable prognostic factors also include shorter disease-free interval from primary tumor treatment to presentation of metastases and a larger number of metastases. However, to date, there have been no randomized data confirming the benefit of metastasectomy for pulmonary metastasis. For patients with unresectable disease or primary neoplasms for which pulmonary metastasectomy should not be considered, systemic treatment tailored to the primary tumor can be offered. Diligent attention to palliative care is essential (see Chapter 5).

Handy JR et al. Expert consensus document on pulmonary metastasectomy. Ann Thorac Surg. 2019;107:631. [PMID: 30476477]
Treasure T et al. Pulmonary metastasectomy versus continued active monitoring in colorectal cancer (PulMiCC): a multicentre randomised clinical trial. Trials. 2019;20:718. [PMID: 31831062]

MESOTHELIOMA

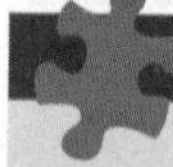

ESSENTIALS OF DIAGNOSIS

- Unilateral, nonpleuritic chest pain and dyspnea.
- Distant (> 20 years earlier) history of exposure to asbestos.
- Pleural effusion or pleural thickening or both on chest radiographs.
- Malignant cells in pleural fluid or tissue biopsy.

General Considerations

Mesotheliomas are primary tumors arising from the surface lining of the pleura (80% of cases) or peritoneum (20% of cases). Numerous studies have confirmed the association of **malignant pleural mesothelioma** with exposure to asbestos. The lifetime risk to asbestos workers of developing malignant pleural mesothelioma is as high as 10%. The latent period between exposure and onset of symptoms ranges from 20 to 40 years. The clinician should inquire about asbestos exposure through mining, milling, manufacturing, shipyard work, insulation, brake linings, building construction and demolition, roofing materials, and other asbestos products (pipes, textiles, paints, tiles, gaskets, panels).

Clinical Findings

A. Symptoms and Signs

The average interval between onset of symptoms and diagnosis is 2–3 months; the median age at diagnosis is 72–74 years in Western countries. Symptoms include the insidious onset of shortness of breath, nonpleuritic chest pain, and weight loss. Physical findings include dullness to percussion, diminished breath sounds and, in some cases, digital clubbing.

B. Laboratory Findings

Pleural fluid is exudative and often hemorrhagic. Cytologic tests of pleural fluid are often negative. VATS biopsy is usually necessary to obtain an adequate specimen for histologic diagnosis. The histologic variants of malignant pleural mesothelioma are epithelial (50–60%), sarcomatoid (10%), and biphasic (30–40%). Since distinction from benign inflammatory conditions and metastatic adenocarcinoma may be difficult, immunohistochemical stains are important to confirm the diagnosis.

C. Imaging

Radiographic abnormalities consist of nodular, irregular, unilateral pleural thickening and varying degrees of unilateral pleural effusion. Sixty percent of patients have right-sided disease, while only 5% have bilateral involvement. CT scans demonstrate the extent of pleural involvement. PET-CT is used to help differentiate benign from malignant pleural disease, improve staging accuracy, and identify candidates for aggressive surgical approaches.

Complications

Malignant pleural mesothelioma progresses rapidly as the tumor spreads along the pleural surface to involve the pericardium, mediastinum, and contralateral pleura. The tumor may eventually extend beyond the thorax to involve abdominal lymph nodes and organs. Progressive pain and dyspnea are characteristic. Local invasion of thoracic structures may cause superior vena cava syndrome, hoarseness, Horner syndrome, arrhythmias, and dysphagia.

Treatment

Chemotherapy is the mainstay of treatment (Tables 39–2 and 39–3), with cytoreductive surgery included in multimodality treatment only if there is localized disease that is amenable to complete macroscopic surgical resection. The optimal surgical approach is still under debate. For localized disease, surgical options include pleurectomy and decortication (surgical stripping of the pleura and pericardium from apex of the lung to diaphragm) or extrapleural pneumonectomy (a radical surgical procedure involving removal of the ipsilateral lung, parietal and visceral pleura, pericardium, and most of the hemidiaphragm). Surgical cytoreduction alone is not sufficient, and either chemotherapy or radiation therapy (or both) should be included in a multimodality approach. In advanced unresectable disease, palliative chemotherapy with cisplatin or carboplatin and pemetrexed can achieve response rates of 30–40%, can extend median overall survival to 12 months, and can improve quality of life. Adding bevacizumab (a monoclonal antibody to vascular endothelial growth factor [VEGF]) to cisplatin and pemetrexed has been shown to further improve overall survival. Nivolumab and ipilimumab (checkpoint inhibition therapy) can also be offered as first-line treatment, with improved outcomes among those with nonepithelioid tumors. Drainage of pleural effusions, pleurodesis, radiation therapy, and even surgical resection may offer palliative benefit to some patients.

Prognosis

Most patients die of respiratory failure and complications of local extension. Median survival time from diagnosis is 7–17 months. Five-year survival is 5–10%. Tumors that are predominantly sarcomatoid are more resistant to therapy and have a worse prognosis, with median survivals less than 1 year. Poor prognostic features include poor performance status, non-epithelioid histology, male sex, nodal involvement, elevated LD, high WBC, low hemoglobin, and high platelet count.

Banerji S et al. The role of immunotherapy in the treatment of malignant pleural mesothelioma. Curr Oncol. 2021;28:4542. [PMID: 34898559]

Scherpereel A et al; French Cooperative Thoracic Intergroup. Nivolumab or nivolumab plus ipilimumab in patients with relapsed malignant pleural mesothelioma (IFCT-1501 MAPS2): a multicentre, open-label, randomised, non-comparative, phase 2 trial. Lancet Oncol. 2019;20:239. [PMID: 30660609]

Scherpereel A et al. ERS/ESTS/EACTS/ESTRO guidelines for the management of malignant pleural mesothelioma. Eur Respir J. 2020;55:1900953. [PMID: 32451346]

HEPATOBILIARY CANCERS

Lawrence S. Friedman, MD

HEPATOCELLULAR CARCINOMA

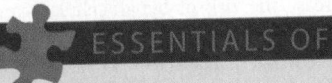

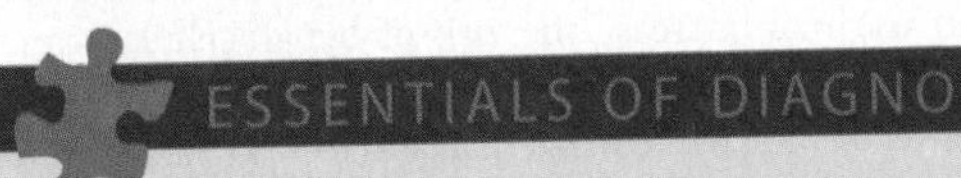

- Usually a complication of cirrhosis.
- Characteristic CT and MRI features may obviate the need for a confirmatory biopsy.

General Considerations

Malignant neoplasms of the liver that arise from parenchymal cells are called hepatocellular carcinomas (accounting for 85% of liver cancers); those that originate in the ductular cells are called cholangiocarcinomas (15% or less). Rare tumors of the liver include angiosarcoma, lymphoma, and combined hepatocellular carcinoma-cholangiocarcinoma.

Worldwide, hepatocellular carcinomas are the fourth most common cause of cancer-related deaths and the sixth most common in incidence. They are associated with cirrhosis in 85% of cases. In Africa and most of Asia, hepatitis B virus (HBV) infection (including "occult" HBV infection; see Chapter 16) is a major etiologic factor, and a family history of hepatocellular carcinoma increases the risk synergistically. In the United States and other Western countries, incidence rates rose over twofold after 1978, with slowing of the rate increase after 2006 except in men ages 55–64, presumably because of the increasing prevalence of cirrhosis caused by chronic hepatitis C virus (HCV) infection and nonalcoholic fatty liver disease (NAFLD). Rates appear to have plateaued since 2010 because of improved treatment of viral hepatitis. In Western countries, risk factors for hepatocellular carcinoma in patients known to have cirrhosis are male sex, age greater than 55 years (although there has been an increase in the number of younger cases), Hispanic or Asian ethnicity, family history in a first-degree relative, overweight, obesity (especially in early adulthood), alcohol use (especially in combination with obesity), tobacco use, diabetes mellitus, hypothyroidism (in women), a prolonged prothrombin time, a low platelet count, and an elevated serum transferrin saturation. The risk of hepatocellular carcinoma is higher in persons with a viral rather than nonviral cause of cirrhosis and may be increased in persons with autoimmune diseases. Other associations include high levels of HBV replication, high hepatitis B surface antigen levels, HBV genotype C, hepatitis D coinfection, elevated serum ALT and bilirubin and low serum albumin levels, and increased liver stiffness in persons with chronic hepatitis B (in whom antiviral therapy to suppress HBV replication appears to reduce the risk); HCV genotypes 1b and 3; lack of response to antiviral therapy for HCV infection; hemochromatosis (and possibly the C282Y carrier state); aflatoxin exposure (associated with pathogenic variant of the *TP53* gene); alpha-1-antiprotease (alpha-1-antitrypsin) deficiency; tyrosinemia; and radiation exposure. In patients with the metabolic syndrome and NAFLD, hepatocellular carcinoma may rarely arise from nonalcoholic steatohepatitis in the absence of cirrhosis. Hepatocellular adenoma may be a precursor for hepatocellular carcinoma (see Chapter 16). Evidence for an association with long-term use of oral contraceptives is inconclusive. Whereas sulfonylurea and insulin use may increase the risk of hepatocellular carcinoma, factors that appear protective include consumption of coffee, vegetables, white meat, fish, and n-3 polyunsaturated fatty acids; use of aspirin; and use of lipophilic HMG-CoA reductase inhibitors (statins) (eg, atorvastatin, simvastatin) and, in patients with diabetes, use of metformin.

The fibrolamellar variant of hepatocellular carcinoma generally occurs in young women with a second smaller peak in older persons; it is characterized by a distinctive histologic picture, absence of risk factors, unique genomic profiles, and an indolent course. Vinyl chloride exposure is associated with angiosarcoma of the liver. Hepatoblastoma, the most common malignant liver cancer in infants and young children, rarely occurs in adults.

Clinical Findings

A. Symptoms and Signs

The presence of a hepatocellular carcinoma may be unsuspected until there is deterioration in the condition of a cirrhotic patient who was formerly stable. Cachexia, weakness, and weight loss are associated symptoms. The sudden appearance of ascites, which may be bloody, suggests portal or hepatic vein thrombosis by cancer or bleeding from a necrotic cancer.

Physical examination may show tender enlargement of the liver, occasionally with a palpable mass. In Africa, the typical presentation in young patients is a rapidly expanding abdominal mass. Auscultation may reveal a bruit over the tumor or a friction rub when the tumor has extended to the surface of the liver.

B. Laboratory Findings

Laboratory tests may reveal leukocytosis, as opposed to the leukopenia that is frequently encountered in cirrhotic patients. Anemia is common, but a normal or elevated hematocrit value may be found in up to one-third of patients owing to elaboration of erythropoietin by the tumor. Sudden and sustained elevation of the serum alkaline phosphatase in a patient who was formerly stable is a common finding. HBsAg is present in most cases in endemic areas, whereas in the United States anti-HCV is found in up to 40% of cases. Serum **alpha-fetoprotein (AFP)** levels are elevated in up to 70% of patients with hepatocellular carcinoma in Western countries (although the sensitivity is lower in Blacks and levels are not elevated in patients with fibrolamellar hepatocellular carcinoma); however, mild elevations (10–200 ng/mL [10–200 mcg/L]) are also often seen in patients with chronic hepatitis. Serum levels of des-gamma-carboxy prothrombin are elevated in up to 90% of patients with hepatocellular carcinoma, but they may also be elevated in patients with vitamin K deficiency, chronic hepatitis, and metastatic cancer. Cytologic study of ascitic fluid rarely reveals malignant cells.

C. Imaging

Multiphasic helical CT and MRI with contrast enhancement are the preferred imaging studies for determining the location and vascularity of the tumor; MRI may be more sensitive than CT, and imaging with gadoxetic acid increases sensitivity. Lesions smaller than 1 cm may be difficult to characterize. Based on stringent criteria developed by the American College of Radiology through its Liver Imaging Reporting and Data System, the Organ Procurement and Transplantation Network, and the American Association for the Study of Liver Diseases, arterial phase enhancement of a lesion that is greater than or equal to 1 cm in diameter followed by delayed hypointensity ("washout") has a 90% specificity for hepatocellular carcinoma. Ultrasonography is less sensitive and more operator dependent but is used to screen for hepatic nodules in high-risk patients. Contrast-enhanced ultrasonography has a sensitivity and specificity approaching those of arterial phase helical CT but, unlike CT and MRI, cannot image the entire liver during the short duration of the arterial phase and is thus associated with false-positive results. In selected cases, endoscopic ultrasonography (EUS) may be useful. PET is under study and appears to improve detection of extrahepatic metastases.

D. Liver Biopsy and Staging

Liver biopsy is diagnostic, although seeding of the needle tract by cancer is a potential risk (1–3%). For lesions smaller than 1 cm, ultrasonography may be repeated every 3 months followed by further investigation of enlarging lesions. For lesions 1 cm or larger, biopsy can be deferred when characteristic arterial hypervascularity and delayed washout are demonstrated on either multiphasic helical CT or MRI with contrast enhancement in a patient with cirrhosis or if surgical resection is planned.

The TNM system is the commonly used classification to stage hepatocellular carcinoma. Staging is important not only because it correlates with the patient's long-term survival but also because it is used to determine which patients should receive adjuvant or neoadjuvant therapy.

The Barcelona Clinic Liver Cancer (BCLC) staging system is preferred and includes the Child-Pugh class, tumor stage, and liver function and has the advantage of linking overall stage with preferred treatment modalities and with an estimation of life expectancy.

Screening & Prevention

Surveillance (screening) for the development of hepatocellular carcinoma is recommended in patients with chronic hepatitis B (beginning as early as age 20 years in African persons, age 40 years in Asian men or Asian persons with a family history of hepatocellular carcinoma, and age 50 years in persons of other ethnicities) or cirrhosis caused by HCV, HBV, or alcohol. There is some evidence that screening for hepatocellular carcinoma leads to a survival advantage over clinical diagnosis, but only a minority of cases are detected by screening. The standard screening approach is performing ultrasonography and obtaining serum AFP level every 6 months, although AFP testing has low sensitivity. A serum AFP level of ≥ 20 ng/mL (20 mcg/L) is generally the cutoff value that should trigger further evaluation. CT and MRI are considered too expensive for screening. The sensitivity of ultrasonography alone for detecting early hepatocellular carcinoma is only 63%.

The risk of hepatocellular carcinoma developing in a patient with cirrhosis is 3–5% a year. Among patients with cirrhosis, over 60% of nodules smaller than 2 cm in diameter detected on a screening ultrasonography prove to be hepatocellular carcinoma. Patients with cancers detected by surveillance have a less advanced stage on average and greater likelihood that treatment will prolong survival than those whose cancers were not detected by surveillance. However, controversy persists about whether surveillance reduces cancer-related mortality.

Mass vaccination programs against HBV in developing countries are leading to reduced rates of hepatocellular carcinoma. Successful treatment of hepatitis B and of hepatitis C in patients with cirrhosis also reduces the subsequent risk of hepatocellular carcinoma, and thus hepatocellular carcinoma is considered a preventable neoplasm. However, hepatocellular carcinoma may still occur after clearance of hepatitis B surface antigen or cure of HCV infection, thereby reducing the benefit of treatment for HBV and HCV infection.

Treatment

If liver function is preserved (Child-Pugh class A or possibly B) and portal vein thrombosis is not present, surgical resection of a solitary hepatocellular carcinoma may result in cure. Laparoscopic liver resection has been performed in selected cases. Treatment of underlying chronic viral hepatitis, adjuvant chemotherapy, and adaptive immunotherapy may lower postsurgical recurrence rates.

Liver transplantation may be appropriate for small unresectable tumors in a patient with advanced cirrhosis, with reported 5-year survival rates of up to 75%. The recurrence-free survival may be better for liver transplantation than for resection in patients with well-compensated cirrhosis and small tumors (one tumor less than 5 cm or three or fewer tumors each less than 3 cm in diameter [Milan criteria]) and in those with expanded (University of California, San Francisco) criteria of one tumor less than or equal to 6.5 cm or three or fewer tumors less than or equal to 4.5 cm (or a combined tumor diameter of 8.5 cm) without vascular invasion. The Extended Toronto criteria include tumor differentiation, cancer-related symptoms, confinement of tumor to the liver, and absence of vascular invasion, without regard to tumor number or size, to determine candidacy for liver transplantation and appear to predict outcomes as well as the Milan criteria. After 6 months on the waiting list, patients with stage 2 hepatocellular carcinoma meeting the Milan criteria are awarded a fixed score of 3 points lower than the median Model for End-Stage Liver Disease (MELD) score for patients transplanted in the area where the candidate is listed (see Chapter 16), thereby increasing their chances of undergoing transplantation. However, orthotopic liver transplantation is often impractical because of the donor organ shortage, so living donor liver transplantation may be considered in these cases. Patients with larger tumors (3–5 cm), a serum AFP level of 1000 ng/mL (1000 mcg/L) or higher, or a MELD score of 20 or higher have poor posttransplantation survival. In patients with a serum AFP level greater than 1000 ng/mL (1000 mcg/L), downstaging by locoregional therapy to an AFP level less than 500 ng/mL (500 mcg/L) improves survival following subsequent liver transplantation.

Chemotherapy, hormonal therapy with tamoxifen, and long-acting octreotide have not been shown to prolong life, but transarterial chemoembolization (TACE), TACE with drug-eluting beads, transarterial chemoinfusion (TACI), and transarterial radioembolization (TARE) via the hepatic artery are not only palliative but may also prolong survival in patients with a large or multifocal tumor in the absence of extrahepatic spread. TACI and TARE are suitable for patients with portal vein thrombosis. TARE with yttrium-90 has been shown to result in a longer time to progression than TACE. Microwave ablation, radiofrequency ablation, cryotherapy, proton beam radiotherapy, or injection of absolute ethanol into tumors smaller than 2 cm may prolong survival in patients who are not candidates for resection and have tumors that are accessible; these interventions, as well as stereotactic body radiation therapy, may also provide a "bridge" to liver transplantation. Microwave ablation is becoming the preferred approach because it allows shorter treatment times and, like radiofrequency ablation, can be performed after TACE in select cases. Cryoablation may result in slower tumor progression than radiofrequency ablation for tumors that are 3.1–4 cm in diameter. Stereotactic body radiation therapy is also being used to treat unresectable hepatocellular carcinoma and may be effective in treating lesions larger than those treated with ablation techniques.

The combination of atezolizumab, an immune checkpoint inhibitor, and bevacizumab, an antibody to the VEGF receptor, is the preferred first-line therapy for advanced hepatocellular carcinoma and has been shown to be superior to sorafenib, an oral multikinase inhibitor of Raf kinase, the VEGF receptor, and the platelet-derived growth factor receptor (and others) that had been shown to prolong median survival as well as the time to radiologic progression by 3 months and had been the standard of care in these patients. Lenvatinib is another oral multikinase inhibitor that was approved by the FDA for the same indications as sorafenib. Regorafenib is an oral multikinase inhibitor that provides a survival benefit for patients whose disease progresses despite sorafenib therapy, and nivolumab and pembrolizumab are immune checkpoint inhibitors that have been approved for advanced hepatocellular carcinoma. The combination of nivolumab and ipilimumab has been recommended as second-line therapy after failure of sorafenib. Cabozantinib, another multikinase inhibitor, has been approved by the FDA for the treatment of hepatocellular carcinoma after prior treatment with sorafenib, as has ramucirumab, an antibody to the VEGF receptor, which is approved for patients with an AFP level greater than or equal to 400 ng/mL (400 mcg/L) and previous treatment with sorafenib. The modified Response Evaluation Criteria in Solid Tumors (mRECIST) are used to assess treatment response based on tumor shrinkage and viability after locoregional and antiangiogenic treatment. Meticulous efforts at palliative care are essential for patients in whom disease progresses despite treatment or in whom advanced tumors, vascular invasion, or extrahepatic spread are present. Severe pain may develop in such patients due to expansion of the liver capsule by the tumor and requires concerted efforts at pain management, including the use of opioids (see Chapter 5).

Prognosis

In the United States, overall 1- and 5-year survival rates for patients with hepatocellular carcinoma are 23% and 5%, respectively. Five-year survival rates rise to 56% for patients with localized resectable disease (T1, T2, selected T3 and T4; N0; M0) but are virtually nil for those with locally unresectable or advanced disease. In patients with HCV-related hepatocellular carcinoma, the serum AFP level at the time of diagnosis of cancer has been reported to be an independent predictor of mortality. A serum AFP level greater than or equal to 200 ng/mL (200 mcg/L) or increases of greater than 15 ng/mL/month predict worse outcomes in patients awaiting liver transplantation. In patients who are not eligible for surgery, an elevated serum CRP level is associated with poor survival. The fibrolamellar variant has been reported to have a higher recurrence rate but better survival than conventional hepatocellular carcinoma.

When to Refer

All patients with hepatocellular carcinoma should be referred to a specialist.

When to Admit

- Complications of cirrhosis.
- Severe pain.
- For surgery and other interventions.

Haber PK et al. Evidence-based management of hepatocellular carcinoma: systematic review and meta-analysis of randomized controlled trials (2002-2020). Gastroenterology. 2021; 161:879. [PMID: 34126063]

Kloeckner R et al. Local and regional therapies for hepatocellular carcinoma. Hepatology. 2021;73:137. [PMID: 32557715]

Ramai D et al. Fibrolamellar hepatocellular carcinoma: a population-based observational study. Dig Dis Sci. 2021; 66:308. [PMID: 32052215]

Rimassa L et al. Systemic treatment of HCC in special populations. J Hepatol. 2021;74:931. [PMID: 33248171]

Singal AG et al. Patient-reported barriers are associated with receipt of hepatocellular carcinoma surveillance in a multicenter cohort of patients with cirrhosis. Clin Gastroenterol Hepatol. 2021;19:987. [PMID: 32629122]

Thuluvath PJ et al. Role of locoregional therapies in patients with hepatocellular cancer awaiting liver transplantation. Am J Gastroenterol. 2021;116:57. [PMID: 33110015]

CARCINOMA OF THE BILIARY TRACT

ESSENTIALS OF DIAGNOSIS

- Presents with obstructive jaundice, usually painless, often with dilated biliary tract.
- Pain is more common in gallbladder carcinoma than cholangiocarcinoma.
- A dilated gallbladder may be palpable (Courvoisier sign).
- Diagnosis by cholangiography with biopsy and brushings for cytology.

General Considerations

Carcinoma of the gallbladder occurs in approximately 2% of all people operated on for biliary tract disease; the incidence, like that of carcinoma of the bile ducts, had been decreasing in the United States but may be increasing again in some Western countries because of lifestyle changes. The onset is notoriously insidious, and the diagnosis is often made unexpectedly at surgery. Cholelithiasis (often large, symptomatic stones) is usually present. Other risk factors are chronic infection of the gallbladder with *Salmonella typhi*, adenomatous gallbladder polyps over 1 cm in diameter (particularly with hypoechoic foci on EUS), mucosal calcification of the gallbladder (porcelain gallbladder), anomalous pancreaticobiliary ductal junction, high parity in women, increased BMI, and aflatoxin exposure. Spread of the cancer—by direct extension into the liver or to the peritoneal surface—may be seen on initial presentation.

Carcinoma of the bile ducts (cholangiocarcinoma) accounts for 10–25% of all hepatobiliary malignancies and 3% of all cancer deaths in the United States. It is more prevalent in persons aged 50–70 years, with a slight male predominance, and more common in Asia. About 50% arise at the confluence of the hepatic ducts (perihilar, or so-called Klatskin, tumors), and 40% arise in the distal extrahepatic bile duct (the incidence of which has risen since 1990); the remainder are intrahepatic (the incidence of which rose dramatically from the 1970s to the early 2000s and has continued to increase). Mortality from intrahepatic cholangiocarcinoma has been increasing. The frequency of carcinoma in persons with a choledochal cyst has been reported to be over 14% at 20 years, and surgical excision is recommended. Most cases of cholangiocarcinoma are sporadic. There is an increased incidence of cholangiocarcinoma in patients with bile duct adenoma; Caroli disease; a biliary-enteric anastomosis; ulcerative colitis, especially those with primary sclerosing cholangitis; biliary cirrhosis; diabetes mellitus; hyperthyroidism; chronic pancreatitis; heavy alcohol consumption; smoking; past exposure to Thorotrast, a contrast agent, and possibly PPI use. Premalignant lesions of the bile duct include biliary intraepithelial neoplasia and intraductal papillary neoplasia of the biliary system (biliary papillomatosis). Aspirin use and statin use are associated with a reduced risk of cholangiocarcinoma, and in patients with diabetes, metformin use is associated with a reduced risk of intrahepatic cholangiocarcinoma. In Southeast Asia, hepatolithiasis, chronic typhoid carriage, and infection of the bile ducts with helminths *(Clonorchis sinensis, Opisthorchis viverrini)* are associated with an increased risk of cholangiocarcinoma. HCV (and possibly HBV) infection, cirrhosis, HIV infection, nonalcoholic fatty liver disease, diabetes mellitus, obesity, and tobacco smoking are risk factors for intrahepatic cholangiocarcinoma.

The TNM system is the commonly used classification to stage carcinoma of the biliary tract, including gallbladder carcinomas and perihilar and intrahepatic cholangiocarcinomas. Staging is important not only because it correlates with the patient's long-term survival but also because it is used to determine which patients should receive adjuvant or neoadjuvant therapy.

Other staging systems consider the patient's age, performance status, tumor extent and form, perineural invasion, vascular encasement, hepatic lobe atrophy, underlying liver disease, and peritoneal metastasis.

Clinical Findings

A. Symptoms and Signs

Progressive jaundice is the most common and usually the first sign of obstruction of the extrahepatic biliary system. Pain in the right upper abdomen with radiation into the back is usually present early in the course of gallbladder carcinoma but occurs later in the course of bile duct carcinoma. Anorexia and weight loss are common and may be associated with fever and chills due to cholangitis. Rarely, hematemesis or melena results from erosion of cancer into a blood vessel (hemobilia). Fistula formation between the biliary system and adjacent organs may also occur. The course is usually one of rapid deterioration, with death occurring within a few months.

Physical examination reveals profound jaundice. Pruritus and skin excoriations are common. A palpable gallbladder with obstructive jaundice usually is said to signify malignant disease (Courvoisier sign); however, this clinical generalization has been proven to be accurate only about 50% of the time. Hepatomegaly due to hypertrophy of the unobstructed liver lobe is usually present and is associated with liver tenderness. Ascites may occur with peritoneal implants.

B. Laboratory Findings

With biliary obstruction, laboratory examination reveals predominantly conjugated hyperbilirubinemia, with total serum bilirubin values ranging from 5 to 30 mg/dL. There is usually concomitant elevation of the alkaline phosphatase and serum cholesterol. AST is normal or minimally elevated. The serum CA 19-9 level is elevated in up to 85% of patients and may help distinguish cholangiocarcinoma from a benign biliary stricture (in the absence of cholangitis), but this test is neither sensitive nor specific.

C. Imaging

Ultrasonography and contrast-enhanced, triple-phase, helical CT may show a gallbladder mass in gallbladder carcinoma and intrahepatic mass or biliary dilatation in carcinoma of the bile ducts. CT may also show involved regional lymph nodes and atrophy of a hepatic lobe because of vascular encasement with compensatory hypertrophy of the unaffected lobe. MRI with magnetic resonance cholangiopancreatography (MRCP) and gadolinium enhancement permits visualization of the entire biliary tract and detection of vascular invasion and obviates the need for angiography and, in some cases, direct cholangiography; it is the imaging procedure of choice but may understage malignant hilar strictures. The sensitivity and image quality can be increased with use of ferumoxide enhancement. The features of intrahepatic cholangiocarcinoma on MRI appear to differ from those of hepatocellular carcinoma, with contrast washout in the latter but not the former. In indeterminate cases, PET can detect cholangiocarcinomas as small as 1 cm and lymph node and distant metastases, but false-positive results occur. The most helpful diagnostic studies before surgery are either endoscopic retrograde cholangiography or percutaneous transhepatic cholangiography with biopsy and cytologic specimens, although false-negative biopsy and cytology results are common. Digital image analysis and fluorescent in situ hybridization of cytologic specimens for polysomy improve sensitivity. EUS with FNA of tumors, peroral cholangioscopy, confocal laser endomicroscopy, and intraductal ultrasonography may confirm a diagnosis of cholangiocarcinoma in a patient with bile duct stricture and an otherwise indeterminate evaluation, but FNA can result in cancer seeding and should be avoided if the cancer is potentially resectable.

Treatment

In young and fit patients, curative surgery for gallbladder carcinoma may be attempted if the cancer is well localized. The 5-year survival rate for carcinoma of the gallbladder invading the lamina propria or muscularis (stage 1, T1a or 1b, N0, M0) is as high as 85% with laparoscopic cholecystectomy but drops to 60%, even with a more extended open resection if there is perimuscular invasion (T2). The role of radical surgery for T3 and T4 tumors is debatable. If the cancer is unresectable at laparotomy, biliary-enteric bypass (eg, Roux-en-Y hepaticojejunostomy) can be performed. Carcinoma of the bile ducts is curable by surgery in less than 10% of cases. If resection margins are negative, the 5-year survival rate may be as high as 47% for intrahepatic cholangiocarcinomas, 41% for hilar cholangiocarcinoma, and 37% for distal cholangiocarcinomas, but the perioperative mortality rate may be as high as 10%. Factors predicting shorter survival for intrahepatic cholangiocarcinoma include large cancer size, multiple cancers, lymph node metastasis, and vascular invasion. Adjuvant chemotherapy with capecitabine has been shown to result in superior overall survival compared with no adjuvant therapy. Palliation can be achieved by placement of a self-expandable metal stent via an endoscopic or percutaneous transhepatic route. Covered metal stents may be more cost-effective than uncovered metal stents because of a longer duration of patency. However, they are associated with a higher rate of stent migration and cholecystitis due to occlusion of the cystic duct and are not associated with longer survival. For perihilar cancers, bilateral stents may be preferable to a unilateral stent when technically feasible. Plastic stents are less expensive initially, but not in the long term, because they are more prone to occlude than metal ones; they may be considered based on local expertise and physician preference. Photodynamic therapy in combination with stent placement prolongs survival when compared with stent placement alone in patients with nonresectable cholangiocarcinoma. Endoscopic retrograde cholangiopancreatography (ERCP)–directed radiofrequency ablation, TACE, and TARE are additional emerging options. Radiotherapy may relieve pain and contribute to biliary decompression. There is limited response to chemotherapy with gemcitabine alone, but the combination of cisplatin and gemcitabine or capecitabine and gemcitabine prolongs survival in patients with locally advanced or metastatic cholangiocarcinoma. Few patients survive for more than 24 months. Although cholangiocarcinoma is generally considered to be a contraindication to liver transplantation because of rapid cancer recurrence, a 5-year survival rate of 75% has been reported in patients with stage I and II perihilar cholangiocarcinoma undergoing chemoradiation and exploratory laparotomy followed by liver transplantation, and a 5-year survival rate of 67% has been reported in those with intrahepatic cholangiocarcinoma.

For those patients whose disease progresses despite treatment, meticulous efforts at palliative care are essential (see Chapter 5).

When to Refer

All patients with carcinoma of the biliary tract should be referred to a specialist.

When to Admit

- Biliary obstruction.
- Cholangitis.

Goyal L et al. Case 8-2021: a 34-year-old woman with cholangiocarcinoma. N Engl J Med. 2021;384:1054. [PMID: 33730458]

Kamal H et al. Association between proton pump inhibitor use and biliary tract cancer risk: a Swedish population-based cohort study. Hepatology. 2021;74:2021. [PMID: 34018229]

Kim D et al. Trends in the mortality of biliary tract cancers based on their anatomical site in the United States from 2009 to 2018. Am J Gastroenterol. 2021;116:1053. [PMID: 33929380]

Ponce CB et al. Gallstones, body mass index, C-reactive protein, and gallbladder cancer: Mendelian randomization analysis of Chilean and European genotype data. Hepatology. 2021; 73:1783. [PMID: 32893372]

Qumseya BJ et al. ASGE guideline on the role of endoscopy in the management of malignant hilar obstruction. Gastrointest Endosc. 2021;94:222. [PMID: 34023067]

CARCINOMA OF THE PANCREAS & AMPULLA OF VATER

ESSENTIALS OF DIAGNOSIS

- Obstructive jaundice (may be painless).
- Enlarged gallbladder (may be painful).
- Upper abdominal pain with radiation to back, weight loss, and thrombophlebitis are usually late manifestations.

General Considerations

Carcinoma is the most common neoplasm of the pancreas. About 75% are in the head and 25% in the body and tail of the organ. Pancreatic carcinomas account for 3% of all cancers and 7% of cancer deaths. The incidence is increasing. Ampullary carcinomas are much less common. Risk factors for pancreatic cancer include age, tobacco use (which is thought to cause 20–25% of cases), heavy alcohol use, obesity, chronic pancreatitis, diabetes mellitus, prior abdominal radiation, family history, and possibly gastric ulcer and exposure to arsenic and cadmium. New-onset diabetes mellitus after age 45 years occasionally heralds the onset of pancreatic cancer. In patients with diabetes, metformin use and possibly aspirin use may reduce the risk of pancreatic cancer slightly, but insulin use and glucagon-like peptide-1–based therapy (eg, sitagliptin) may increase the risk. About 7% of patients with pancreatic cancer have a family history of pancreatic cancer in a first-degree relative, compared with 0.6% of control patients. Most pancreatic cancers originate from pancreatic intraepithelial neoplasias, which measure less than 5 mm in diameter and can only be seen with a microscope.

In 5–10% of cases, pancreatic cancer occurs as part of a hereditary syndrome, including familial breast cancer (carriers of *BRCA2* have a 7% lifetime risk of pancreatic cancer), hereditary pancreatitis (*PSS1* mutation), familial atypical multiple mole melanoma (*p16/CDKN2A* mutation), Peutz-Jeghers syndrome (*STK11/LKB1* mutation), ataxia-telangiectasia (*ATM* mutation), and Lynch syndrome (hereditary nonpolyposis colorectal cancer [*MLH1*, *MSH2*, *MSH6* mutations]).

Neuroendocrine tumors account for 1–2% of pancreatic neoplasms and may be functional (producing gastrin, insulin, glucagon, vasoactive intestinal peptide, somatostatin, growth hormone–releasing hormone, adrenocorticotropic hormone, and others) or nonfunctional. Cystic neoplasms account for less than 10% of pancreatic neoplasms, but they are important because pancreatic cysts are common and may be mistaken for pseudocysts. A cystic neoplasm should be suspected when a cystic lesion in the pancreas is found in the absence of a history of pancreatitis or trauma. At least 15% of all pancreatic cysts are neoplasms. Serous cystadenomas (which account for 32–39% of cystic pancreatic neoplasms and also occur in patients with von Hippel-Lindau disease) are benign. However, mucinous cystic neoplasms (defined by the presence of ovarian stroma and accounting for 10–45% of cystic pancreatic neoplasms), intraductal papillary mucinous neoplasms (21–33% of cystic pancreatic neoplasms), solid pseudopapillary tumors (less than 5%, primarily in young women), and cystic islet cell tumors (3–5%) may be malignant. Their prognoses are better than the prognosis of pancreatic adenocarcinoma, unless the cystic neoplasm is at least locally advanced.

Clinical Findings

A. Symptoms and Signs

Pain is present in over 70% of cases and is often vague, diffuse, and located in the epigastrium or, when the lesion is in the tail, located in the left upper quadrant of the abdomen. Radiation of pain into the back is common and sometimes predominates. Sitting up and leaning forward may afford some relief, and this usually indicates that the lesion has spread beyond the pancreas and is inoperable. Diarrhea, perhaps due to maldigestion, is an occasional early symptom. Migratory thrombophlebitis is a rare sign. Weight loss is a common but late finding and may be associated with depression. Hyperglycemia and decreases in subcutaneous abdominal fat and serum lipid levels have been reported to precede a diagnosis of pancreatic cancer. Occasional patients (often aged 40 years or older) present with acute pancreatitis in the absence of an alternative cause. Jaundice is usually due to biliary obstruction by a cancer in the pancreatic head. A palpable gallbladder is also indicative of obstruction by a neoplasm (Courvoisier sign), but there are frequent exceptions. A hard, fixed, occasionally tender mass may be present. In advanced cases, a hard periumbilical (Sister Mary Joseph) nodule may be palpable.

B. Laboratory Findings

There may be mild anemia. Glycosuria, hyperglycemia, and impaired glucose tolerance or true diabetes mellitus are found in 10–20% of cases. The serum lipase or amylase level is occasionally elevated. Liver biochemical tests may suggest obstructive jaundice. Steatorrhea in the absence of jaundice is uncommon. Occult blood in the stool is suggestive of carcinoma of the ampulla of Vater (the combination of biliary obstruction and bleeding may give the stools a distinctive silver appearance). CA 19-9, with a sensitivity of 70% and a specificity of 87%, has generally not proven useful for early detection of pancreatic cancer but continues to be studied; increased values are also found in acute and chronic pancreatitis and cholangitis. Plasma chromogranin A levels are elevated in 88–100% of patients with pancreatic neuroendocrine tumors (NETs).

C. Imaging

Multiphase thin-cut helical CT is generally the initial diagnostic procedure and detects a mass in over 80% of cases. CT identifies metastases, delineates the extent of the tumor, and allows percutaneous FNA for cytologic studies and tumor markers. MRI is an alternative to CT. Ultrasonography is not reliable because of interference by intestinal gas. PET is a sensitive technique for detecting pancreatic cancer and metastases, but PET-CT is not a routine staging procedure. Selective celiac and superior mesenteric arteriography may demonstrate vessel invasion by cancer, a finding that would preclude attempts at surgical resection, but it is used uncommonly since the advent of multiphase helical CT. EUS is more sensitive than CT for detecting pancreatic cancer and is equivalent to CT for determining nodal involvement and resectability; contrast-enhanced EUS improves accuracy. A normal EUS excludes pancreatic cancer. EUS may also be used to guide FNA or biopsy for tissue diagnosis, tumor markers, and DNA analysis. ERCP may clarify an ambiguous CT or MRI study by delineating the pancreatic duct system or confirming an ampullary or biliary neoplasm. MRCP appears to be at least as sensitive as ERCP in diagnosing pancreatic cancer. In some centers, pancreatoscopy or intraductal ultrasonography is used to evaluate filling defects in the pancreatic duct and assess resectability of intraductal papillary mucinous cancers. With obstruction of the splenic vein, splenomegaly or gastric varices are present, the latter detected by endoscopy, EUS, or angiography.

Cystic neoplasms can be distinguished by their appearance on CT, EUS, and ERCP and features of the cyst fluid on gross, cytologic, and genetic analysis. For example, serous cystadenomas may have a central scar or honeycomb appearance; mucinous cystadenomas are unilocular or multilocular and contain mucin-rich fluid with high carcinoembryonic antigen levels (greater than 200 ng/mL [200 mcg/L]), low glucose levels, and *KRAS* pathogenic variants; and intraductal papillary mucinous neoplasms are associated with a dilated pancreatic duct and extrusion of gelatinous material from the ampulla.

Staging

The TNM system is the commonly used classification to stage pancreatic cancer. Staging is important not only because it correlates with the patient's long-term survival but also because it is used to determine which patients should receive adjuvant or neoadjuvant therapy. Localized pancreatic cancer includes resectable, borderline resectable (involving major vascular structures), and locally advanced (unresectable) disease. Over 30% of patients present with locally advanced disease and over 50% with metastatic disease.

Treatment

Abdominal exploration is usually necessary when cytologic diagnosis cannot be made or if resection is to be attempted (in up to 30% of patients with pancreatic carcinoma). In a patient with a localized mass in the head of the pancreas and without jaundice, laparoscopy may detect tiny peritoneal or liver metastases and thereby avoid resection in 4–13% of patients. Radical pancreaticoduodenal (Whipple) resection is indicated for cancers strictly limited to the head of the pancreas, periampullary area, and duodenum (T1, N0, M0). Five-year survival rate is 20–25% in this group and as high as 40% in those with negative resection margins and without lymph node involvement. Preoperative endoscopic decompression of an obstructed bile duct is often achieved with a plastic stent or short metal stent but does not reduce operative mortality and is associated with complications.

The best surgical results are achieved at centers that specialize in the multidisciplinary treatment of pancreatic cancer. Adjuvant chemotherapy with gemcitabine, 5-fluorouracil, or gemcitabine with capecitabine is superior to no adjuvant therapy. Gemcitabine with capecitabine and a modified FOLFIRINOX (5-fluorouracil, leucovorin, irinotecan, oxaliplatin) regimen have been found to be superior to gemcitabine alone. The role of adjuvant chemoradiation is controversial but often used in the United States. Neoadjuvant chemotherapy with or without radiation is increasingly being used to downstage patients and in those with resectable cancer. Common chemotherapy regimens for this purpose include FOLFIRINOX and gemcitabine with nanoparticle albumin-bound (nab)-paclitaxel. Chemoradiotherapy downstages about 30% of patients with locally advanced disease to allow resection.

When resection is not feasible, endoscopic stenting of the bile duct is performed to relieve jaundice. A plastic stent has generally been preferred if the patient's anticipated survival is less than 6 months (or if surgery is planned). A metal stent is preferred when anticipated survival is 6 months or greater. Whether covered metal stents designed to prevent cancer ingrowth offer an advantage over uncovered stents is uncertain because covered stents are associated with higher rates of migration and acute cholecystitis due to occlusion of the cystic duct. Surgical biliary bypass may be considered in patients expected to survive at least 6 months. Surgical duodenal bypass may be considered in patients in whom duodenal obstruction is expected to develop; alternatively, endoscopic placement of a self-expandable duodenal stent may be feasible. Chemoradiation may be used for palliation of unresectable cancer confined to the pancreas.

In metastatic pancreatic cancer, improved response rates have been reported with FOLFIRINOX and with the combination of gemcitabine and nab-paclitaxel. In patients who have received prior chemotherapy, a regimen of 5-fluorouracil and leucovorin in combination with nanoliposomal irinotecan has resulted in improved survival compared with 5-fluorouracil and leucovorin alone. Celiac plexus nerve block (see Chapter 5) done under CT or endoscopic ultrasound guidance or thoracoscopic splanchnicectomy may improve pain control.

Surgical resection is the treatment of choice for NETs, when feasible. Lesions that are less than 1 cm in diameter and nonfunctioning without evidence of local invasion or metastasis may be followed expectantly. Metastatic disease may be controlled with long-acting somatostatin analogs, interferon, chemotherapy, peptide-receptor radionuclide therapy (PRRT), and chemoembolization.

There is a consensus that asymptomatic incidental pancreatic cysts 2 cm or smaller are at low risk for harboring invasive carcinoma. The cysts may be monitored by imaging tests (MRI) in 1 year and then every 2 years for 5 years and probably longer if no changes are observed, with EUS and FNA performed if a cyst enlarges to 3 cm and another high-risk feature (dilated main pancreatic duct, presence of a solid component) develops. The optimal approach is uncertain, however, and other guidelines have been proposed. Surgical resection is indicated for mucinous cystic neoplasms, symptomatic serous cystadenomas, solid pseudopapillary tumors (which have a 15% risk of malignant transformation), and cystic tumors larger than 2 cm in diameter that remain undefined after helical CT, EUS, and diagnostic aspiration. All intraductal papillary mucinous neoplasms of the main pancreatic duct should be resected, but those of branch ducts may be monitored with serial imaging if they (1) are asymptomatic and exhibit benign features; (2) have a diameter less than 3 cm (some authorities recommend a diameter of 1.5 cm or smaller, but even lesions 3 cm or larger may be monitored in older adults with no other worrisome cyst features); and (3) lack nonenhancing mural nodules, a thick wall, or an abrupt change in the caliber of the pancreatic duct with distal pancreatic atrophy, or possibly bile duct dilatation and gallbladder adenomyomatosis. Most lesions with such benign features remain stable on follow-up, but a risk of malignancy persists for more than 10 years. Moreover, the risk of pancreatic ductal carcinoma and of nonpancreatic cancers is also increased in this group of patients. In the absence of locally advanced disease, survival is higher for malignant cystic neoplasms than for adenocarcinomas. The role of EUS-guided ablative treatment of potentially premalignant pancreatic cysts is under study. Endoscopic resection or ablation, with temporary placement of a pancreatic duct stent, may be feasible for ampullary adenomas, but patients must be followed for recurrence.

Prognosis

Carcinoma of the pancreas, especially in the body or tail, has a poor prognosis; 80–85% of patients present with advanced unresectable disease, and the reported 5-year survival rate is 2–5%. From 1980 to 2010, mortality from pancreatic cancer in the United States did not decrease, but it has since started to improve. Obesity may adversely affect mortality in Western countries. Metformin may improve survival in patients with diabetes and pancreatic adenocarcinoma, and use of statins preceding a diagnosis of pancreatic cancer may improve survival. Tumors of the ampulla have a better prognosis, with a reported 5-year survival rate of 20–40% after resection; jaundice and lymph node involvement are adverse prognostic factors. In carefully selected patients, resection of cancer of the pancreatic head is feasible and results in reasonable survival. In persons with a family history of pancreatic cancer in at least two first-degree relatives, or with a genetic syndrome associated with an increased risk of pancreatic cancer, screening with EUS and helical CT or MRI/MRCP should be considered beginning at age 50 years (age 40 years in *CKDN2A* or *PRSS1* mutation carriers and age 35 years in those with Peutz-Jeghers syndrome) or 10 years before the age at which pancreatic cancer was first diagnosed in a family member.

For those patients whose disease progresses despite treatment, meticulous efforts at palliative care are essential (see Chapter 5).

When to Refer

All patients with carcinoma involving the pancreas and the ampulla of Vater should be referred to a specialist.

When to Admit

Patients who require surgery and other interventions should be hospitalized.

Aslanian HR et al. AGA Clinical Practice Update on pancreas cancer screening in high-risk individuals: expert review. Gastroenterology. 2020;159:358. [PMID: 32416142]

Fahrmann JF et al. Lead-time trajectory of CA19-9 as an anchor marker for pancreatic cancer early detection. Gastroenterology. 2021;160:1373. [PMID: 33333055]

Huang J et al. Worldwide burden of risk factors for, and trends in pancreatic cancer. Gastroenterology. 2021;160:744. [PMID: 33058868]

Khalaf N et al. Burden of pancreatic cancer: from epidemiology to practice. Clin Gastroenterol Hepatol. 2021;19:876. [PMID: 32147593]

Park W et al. Pancreatic cancer: a review. JAMA. 2021;326:851. [PMID: 34547082]

ALIMENTARY TRACT CANCERS

Carling Ursem, MD

Kenneth R. McQuaid, MD

ESOPHAGEAL CANCER

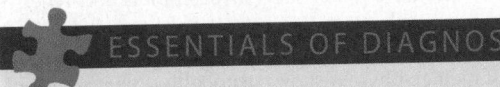

ESSENTIALS OF DIAGNOSIS

- Progressive dysphagia to solid food.
- Weight loss common.
- Endoscopy with biopsy establishes diagnosis.

General Considerations

Esophageal cancer usually develops in persons between 50 and 70 years of age. There were an estimated 19,260 new cases and 15,530 deaths from esophageal cancer in the United States in 2021. The ratio for new cases in men versus women is approximately 4:1. There are two histologic types: squamous cell carcinoma and adenocarcinoma, and their incidence has significant geographic variation. **Squamous cell carcinoma** is associated with low socioeconomic status; consumption of tobacco, alcohol, hot beverages, and nitrosamines; and poor nutritional status. It accounts for over 90% of cases of esophageal cancer in Eastern and Southeast Asia and sub-Saharan Africa. **Adenocarcinoma** is associated with age; obesity; smoking; and chronic GERD with Barrett metaplasia. Adenocarcinomas make up most new cases of esophageal cancer in North America and Northern and Western Europe. Most (90%) squamous cell carcinomas occur in the upper and middle third of the esophagus, whereas adenocarcinomas are more common in the distal esophagus and gastroesophageal junction.

Clinical Findings

A. Symptoms and Signs

Approximately 30-40% of patients with esophageal cancer present with stage IV, "incurable" disease. While early symptoms are nonspecific and subtle, over 90% eventually have solid food dysphagia, which progresses over weeks to months. Odynophagia is sometimes present. Significant weight loss is common. Local tumor extension into the tracheobronchial tree may result in a tracheo-esophageal fistula, characterized by coughing on swallowing or by pneumonia. Chest or back pain suggests mediastinal extension. Recurrent laryngeal nerve involvement may produce hoarseness. Physical examination is often unrevealing. The presence of supraclavicular or cervical lymphadenopathy or of hepatomegaly implies metastatic disease.

B. Laboratory Findings

Laboratory findings are nonspecific. Anemia related to chronic disease or occult blood loss is common. Elevated aminotransferase or alkaline phosphatase concentrations suggest hepatic or bony metastases. Hypoalbuminemia may result from malnutrition.

C. Imaging

A barium esophagogram may be the first study obtained to evaluate dysphagia. The appearance of a polypoid, obstructive, or ulcerative lesion suggests carcinoma and requires endoscopic evaluation. However, even lesions believed to be benign by radiography warrant endoscopic evaluation. Chest radiographs may show adenopathy, a widened mediastinum, pulmonary or bony metastases, or signs of tracheo-esophageal fistula such as pneumonia.

D. Upper Endoscopy

Endoscopy with biopsy establishes the diagnosis of esophageal carcinoma with a high degree of reliability. In some cases, significant submucosal spread of the tumor may yield nondiagnostic mucosal biopsies. Repeat biopsy may be necessary.

Staging

After confirmation of the diagnosis of esophageal carcinoma at esophagoscopy, the stage of the disease should be determined to guide the choice of therapy. Patients should undergo evaluation with contrast CT of the chest, abdomen, and pelvis to look for local tumor extension, lymphadenopathy, and metastases (eg, pulmonary or hepatic). If there is no evidence of extensive local spread or distant metastases on CT, then EUS with guided fine-needle biopsy of suspicious lymph nodes should be performed to evaluate the locoregional stage. PET with fluorodeoxyglucose or integrated PET-CT imaging is indicated to look for regional or distant spread prior to invasive surgery. Bronchoscopy is sometimes required in esophageal cancers above the carina to exclude tracheobronchial extension. Laparoscopy to exclude occult peritoneal carcinomatosis should be considered in patients with tumors at or near the gastroesophageal junction (see Gastric Adenocarcinoma).

Differential Diagnosis

Esophageal carcinoma must be distinguished from other causes of progressive dysphagia, including peptic stricture, achalasia, and adenocarcinoma of the gastric cardia with esophageal involvement. Benign-appearing peptic strictures should be biopsied at presentation to exclude occult malignancy.

Treatment

The approach to esophageal cancer treatment depends on the cancer stage and location, patient preference and functional status, and expertise of treating gastroenterologists, surgeons, oncologists, and radiation oncologists. It is helpful to classify patients into those with early stage ("curable") disease and those with advanced stage ("incurable") disease.

A. Therapy for "Curable" Disease

Superficial esophageal cancers confined to the epithelium (high-grade dysplasia or carcinoma in situ [Tis]), lamina propria (T1a), or submucosa (T1b) are increasingly recognized in endoscopic screening and surveillance programs. Esophagectomy achieves high cure rates for superficial tumors but is associated with mortality (2%) and morbidity. If performed by experienced clinicians, endoscopic mucosal resection of Tis and T1a cancers achieves equivalent long-term survival with less morbidity (see Barrett Esophagus, Chapter 15). Esophagectomy is recommended for superficial tumors that are invasive to the submucosa (T1b) because of higher rates of lymph node metastasis.

1. Surgery with or without neoadjuvant chemoradiation therapy—There are multiple surgical approaches to the resection of invasive but potentially "curable" esophageal cancers (stage IB, II, IIIA, or IIIB). Accepted techniques include en bloc transthoracic excision of the esophagus with extended lymph node dissection, transhiatal esophagogastrectomy (entailing laparotomy with cervical anastomosis), and minimally invasive esophagectomy techniques. Meta-analysis data suggest equivalent oncologic outcomes from minimally invasive esophagectomy and conventional open techniques, although there are fewer postoperative complications and shorter hospital stays with the laparoscopic approach. Multiple meta-analyses have shown that regardless of surgery type, surgery at a high-volume hospital is associated with decreased perioperative mortality.

Patients with stage I tumors have high cure rates with surgery alone and do not require radiation or chemotherapy. Whether radiation or chemotherapy or both are required in addition to surgery for T2N0 stage II tumors is a subject of ongoing debate. If regional lymph node metastases have occurred (stages IIB and III), the rate of cure with surgery alone is less than 20%. Meta-analysis of trials comparing neoadjuvant (preoperative) therapy followed by surgery with surgery alone suggests a 13% absolute improvement in 2-year survival with combined therapy. Neoadjuvant chemoradiation therapy is recommended for stage IIB and III tumors in fit patients. The preferred neoadjuvant chemotherapy regimen used with radiation is weekly carboplatin plus paclitaxel (Table 39–2). As an alternative, a combination of cisplatin plus 5-fluorouracil may be used along with radiation. When radiation therapy is considered, techniques that are less toxic such as intensity-modulated radiation therapy (IMRT) or proton beam therapy may be considered. For patients who complete neoadjuvant chemoradiation and undergo a complete resection but are found to have residual cancer in the resection specimen, a year of adjuvant immunotherapy with nivolumab is recommended.

2. Chemotherapy plus radiation therapy without surgery—Combined chemotherapy plus radiation therapy achieves long-term survival in up to 25% of patients and is superior to radiation alone. Chemoradiation alone should be considered in patients with localized disease (stage II or IIIA) who are poor surgical candidates due to serious medical illness or poor functional status (Eastern Cooperative Oncology Group score greater than 2). Patients with cervical esophageal cancers, which appear similar biologically to head and neck cancers and in whom surgery is highly morbid and typically not recommended, also should be considered for chemoradiation.

3. Supportive care during definitive therapy—Patients with significant tumor obstruction may require percutaneous gastric or jejunal tube placement to maintain adequate hydration and nutrition during neoadjuvant chemoradiation or chemotherapy. Multidisciplinary consultation is required to determine the optimal procedure and to optimize perioperative nutrition.

B. Therapy for "Incurable" Disease

More than half of patients have either locally extensive tumor spread (T4b) that is unresectable or distant metastases (M1) at the time of diagnosis. Surgery is not warranted in these patients. Since prolonged survival can be achieved in few patients, the primary goal is to provide relief from dysphagia and pain, to optimize quality of life, and to minimize treatment side effects. The optimal palliative approach depends on the presence or absence of metastatic disease, expected survival, patient preference, and institutional experience.

1. Chemotherapy or chemoradiation—Combined radiation therapy and chemotherapy may achieve palliation in two-thirds of patients but is associated with significant side effects. It should be considered for patients with locally advanced tumors without distant metastases who have good functional status and no significant medical problems, in whom prolonged survival may be achieved. Combination chemotherapy may be considered in patients with metastatic disease who still have good functional status and expected survival of at least several months.

The systemic therapy options are the same for metastatic esophageal, gastroesophageal junction, and gastric cancers (Table 39–2). Choice of treatment is increasingly influenced by the results of molecular testing, including PD-L1 expression, mismatch repair/microsatellite instability (MMR/MSI) and, for adenocarcinomas, *HER2* amplification testing. In patients with amplification of the *HER2* gene (approximately 15% of cases), addition of the monoclonal antibody trastuzumab (see Chapter 17) along with anti-PD-L1 therapy to chemotherapy is associated with prolonged survival. For patients without *HER2* amplification who have increased PD-L1 expression, the addition of a PD-1 or PD-L1 targeted antibody to chemotherapy improves overall survival. Immunotherapy should be considered for tumors with either microsatellite instability-high (MSI-H) or deficient mismatch repair (dMMR) protein expression. For the remainder of metastatic esophageal cancers, a PD-1 or PD-L1 targeted agent should be considered in the second-line or later setting. For patients with poor functional status, single-agent therapy with a fluoropyrimidine, a taxane, or irinotecan may be considered.

2. Local therapy for esophageal obstruction—Patients with advanced esophageal cancer often have a poor functional and nutritional status. Radiation therapy alone to the area of esophageal obstruction may afford short-term relief of pain and dysphagia. Rapid palliation of dysphagia may be achieved by peroral placement of permanent expandable wire stents (alone or followed by radiation). However, placement of these stents is complicated by perforation, migration, or tumor ingrowth in up to 40% of cases.

Prognosis

The overall 5-year survival rate of esophageal carcinoma is less than 20%. Apart from distant metastasis (M1b), the two most important predictors of poor survival are adjacent mediastinal spread (T4) and lymph node involvement. Whereas cure may be achieved in patients with regional lymph node involvement (stages IIB and III), involvement of nodes outside the chest (M1a) is indicative of metastatic disease (stage IV) that is incurable. For those patients whose disease progresses despite chemotherapy, meticulous efforts at palliative care are essential (see Chapter 5).

When to Refer

- Patients should be referred to a gastroenterologist for evaluation and staging (endoscopy with biopsy, EUS) and palliative endoscopic stenting.
- Patients with curable and resectable disease for whom neoadjuvant therapy may be appropriate (stage IIB or IIIA) should be referred to medical, radiation, and surgical oncologists for consideration of neoadjuvant chemotherapy, chemoradiotherapy, and surgical resection.
- Patients with metastatic disease should be referred to medical and radiation oncologists for consideration of palliative chemotherapy or chemoradiation.
- Patients with metastatic disease and obstructive tumors not amenable to or refractory to palliative radiation or stenting may require referral to an interventional radiologist, gastroenterologist, or surgeon for gastric or jejunal tube placement for hydration and liquid artificial nutrition. Early referral to palliative care may improve symptom management in patients with advanced or metastatic disease.

When to Admit

Patients with high-grade esophageal obstruction with inability to manage oral secretions or maintain hydration should be admitted. Acute complications such as perforation, bleeding, aspiration, or fistula also may require admission.

Ahmed O et al. AGA Clinical Practice Update on the optimal management of the malignant alimentary tract obstruction: expert review. Clin Gastroenterol Hepatol. 2021;19:1780. [PMID: 33813072]

American Cancer Society. Key statistics for esophageal cancer, 2022. https://www.cancer.org/cancer/esophagus-cancer/about/key-statistics.html

Boku N et al. Safety and efficacy of nivolumab in combination with S-1/capecitabine plus oxaliplatin in patients with previously untreated, unresectable, advanced, or recurrent gastric/gastroesophageal junction cancer: interim results of a randomized, phase II trial (ATTRACTION-4). Ann Oncol. 2019;30:250. [PMID: 30566590]

Gottlieb-Vedi E et al. Long-term survival in esophageal cancer after minimally invasive compared to open esophagectomy: a systematic review and meta-analysis. Ann Surg. 2019; 270:1005. [PMID: 30817355]

Mariette C et al; Fédération de Recherche en Chirurgie (FRENCH) and French Eso-Gastric Tumors (FREGAT) Working Group. Hybrid minimally invasive esophagectomy for esophageal cancer. N Engl J Med. 2019;380:152. [PMID: 30625052]

National Cancer Institute. SEER Cancer Statistics Factsheets: Esophageal Cancer, 2020. https://seer.cancer.gov/statfacts/html/esoph.html

National Comprehensive Cancer Network. Esophageal and esophagogastric junction cancers, Version5.2020, NCCN Clinical Practice Guidelines in Oncology. 2020 December 23. https://www.nccn.org/professionals/physician_gls/pdf/esophageal.pdf

GASTRIC ADENOCARCINOMA

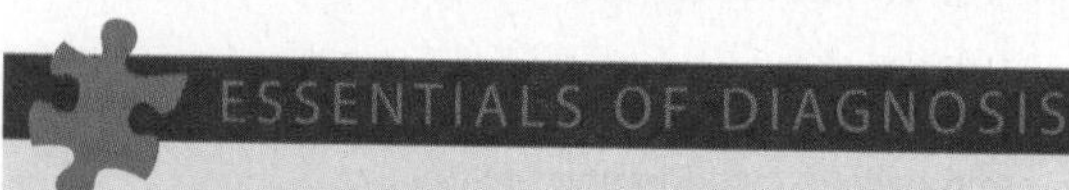

- Dyspeptic symptoms with weight loss in patients over age 40 years.
- Iron deficiency anemia: occult blood in stools.
- Abnormality detected on upper GI series, abdominal CT endoscopy; diagnosis established by endoscopic biopsy.

General Considerations

Gastric adenocarcinoma is the third most common cause of cancer death worldwide. Its main risk factors include increasing age, male gender, non-White race, smoking, and *Helicobacter pylori* infection. Chronic *H pylori* gastritis is the strongest risk factor, increasing the relative risk 3.5- to 20-fold.

The incidence of gastric adenocarcinoma has declined rapidly over the last 70 years, especially in Western countries, perhaps attributable to changes in diet (more fruits and vegetables), increased food refrigeration reduced toxic environmental exposures, and a decline in *H pylori* infections.

In the United States in 2022, gastric cancer will account for 1.5% of all new cancers (with an estimated 26,380 incident cases and an estimated 11,090 deaths). The incidence of gastric cancer remains high in Japan and many developing regions, including eastern Asia, Eastern Europe, Chile, Colombia, and Central America.

There are two main histologic variants of gastric cancer: "intestinal-type" (which resembles intestinal cancers in forming glandular structures) and "diffuse" (which is poorly differentiated and lacks glandular formation).

The incidence of **intestinal-type gastric cancer** has declined significantly, but it is still the more common type (70–80%); it occurs twice as often in men as women and primarily affects older people (mean age 68 years). It is estimated that 60–90% of cases may be attributable to *H pylori*. Other risk factors for intestinal-type gastric cancer include pernicious anemia, a history of partial gastric resection more than 15 years previously, smoking, and diets that are high in nitrates or salt and low in vitamin C.

Diffuse gastric cancer accounts for 20–30% of gastric cancer cases. In contrast to intestinal-type cancer, it affects men and women equally, occurs more commonly in young people, is not as strongly related to *H pylori* infection, and has a worse prognosis than intestinal-type cancer due to early metastasis. Diffuse gastric cancers are often attributable to acquired or hereditary mutations in the genes regulating the E-cadherin cell adhesion protein. Hereditary diffuse gastric cancer may arise at a young age, is often multifocal and infiltrating with signet ring cell histology and has a poor prognosis. These patients belong to families that have a germline mutation of E-cadherin *CDH1*, inherited in an autosomal dominant fashion and conferring a greater than 60% lifetime risk of gastric cancer. Prophylactic gastrectomy should be considered in patients known to carry this mutation.

Most gastric cancers arise in the body and antrum. These may occur in a variety of morphologic types: (1) polypoid or fungating intraluminal masses; (2) ulcerating masses; (3) diffusely spreading (**linitis plastica**), in which the cancer spreads through the submucosa, resulting in a rigid, atonic stomach with thickened folds (prognosis dismal); and (4) superficially spreading or "early" gastric cancer—confined to the mucosa or submucosa (with or without lymph node metastases) and associated with a favorable prognosis.

In contrast to the dramatic decline in cancers of the distal stomach, a rise in incidence of tumors of the gastric cardia has been noted. These tumors have demographic and pathologic features that resemble Barrett-associated esophageal adenocarcinomas (see Esophageal Cancer, above).

Clinical Findings

A. Symptoms and Signs

Gastric carcinoma is generally asymptomatic until quite advanced. Symptoms are nonspecific and are determined in part by the location of the tumor. Dyspepsia, vague epigastric pain, anorexia, early satiety, and weight loss are the presenting symptoms in most patients. Patients may derive initial symptomatic relief from over-the-counter remedies, further delaying diagnosis. Ulcerating lesions can lead to acute GI bleeding with hematemesis or melena. Pyloric obstruction results in postprandial vomiting. Lower esophageal obstruction causes progressive dysphagia. Physical examination is rarely helpful.

B. Laboratory Findings

Iron deficiency anemia due to chronic blood loss or anemia of chronic disease is common. Stool tests may be positive for occult blood. Circulating tumor markers do not have established clinical validity in screening or diagnosis of gastric cancer.

C. Endoscopy

Upper endoscopy should be obtained in all patients over age 60 years with new onset of epigastric symptoms (dyspepsia) and young patients with "alarm" symptoms (dysphagia, recurrent vomiting, significant weight loss), especially in immigrants from countries with a high prevalence of gastric cancer. Endoscopy with biopsies of suspicious lesions is highly sensitive for detecting gastric carcinoma. But it can be difficult to obtain adequate biopsy specimens in diffuse type gastric cancer.

D. Imaging

Once a gastric cancer is diagnosed, preoperative evaluation by contrast CT of chest, abdomen, and pelvis and by EUS is indicated to delineate the local extent of the primary tumor as well as to evaluate for nodal or distant metastases. EUS is superior to CT in determining the depth of tumor penetration and is useful for evaluation of early gastric cancers that may be removed by endoscopic mucosal resection. PET or combined PET-CT imaging is recommended for detection of distant metastasis.

Screening

In the United States and other countries with a relatively low incidence of gastric cancer, screening for gastric cancer is not recommended. Due to the higher incidence of gastric cancer in East Asia, population-based nationwide screening by upper endoscopy is implemented in South Korea and Japan. In Japan, approximately 40% of gastric cancers detected by screening are early stage, with a 5-year survival rate of almost 90%.

Because of its unproven efficacy and cost-effectiveness, screening and treating for *H pylori* infection is not recommended to prevent gastric cancer in asymptomatic US adults.

Staging

The TNM system used to stage gastric adenocarcinoma correlates with the patient's long-term survival and is used to determine which patients should receive adjuvant or neoadjuvant therapy.

Pathologic review should include (1) grade of tumor, (2) histologic subtype, (3) depth of invasion, (4) whether lymphatic or vascular invasion is present, and (5) if there is known metastatic disease, the status of human epidermal growth factor receptor 2 (HER2) protein expression by immunohistochemistry or fluorescent in situ hybridization or both, along with dMMR proteins or microsatellite instability-high (MSI-H) testing, and PD-1 and PD-L1 protein expression.

Differential Diagnosis

Ulcerating gastric adenocarcinomas are distinguished from benign gastric ulcers by biopsies. Approximately 3% of gastric ulcers initially believed to be benign later prove to be malignant. All gastric ulcers identified at endoscopy should be biopsied to exclude malignancy. Ulcers that are suspicious for malignancy to the endoscopist or that have atypia or dysplasia on histologic examination warrant repeat endoscopy in 2–3 months to verify healing and exclude malignancy. Nonhealing ulcers should be considered for resection. Infiltrative carcinoma with thickened gastric folds must be distinguished from lymphoma and other hypertrophic gastropathies.

Treatment

A. Curative Surgical Resection

Surgical resection is the primary treatment for nonmetastatic gastric adenocarcinoma and is the only therapy with curative potential. Laparoscopic resection achieves similar outcomes as, and lower overall complication rates than, open gastrectomy. In Japan and in specialized US centers, endoscopic mucosal resection is performed in selected patients with small (less than 1–2 cm), early (intramucosal or T1aN0) gastric cancers after careful staging with EUS. A staging laparoscopy prior to definitive surgery should be considered in patients with stage T1b or greater disease without radiographic evidence of distant metastases. Approximately 25% of patients undergoing surgery will be found to have locally unresectable tumors or peritoneal, hepatic, or distant lymph node metastases that are incurable. The remaining patients with confirmed localized disease should undergo radical surgical resection. For adenocarcinoma localized to the distal two-thirds of the stomach, a subtotal gastrectomy should be performed. For proximal gastric cancer or diffusely infiltrating disease, total gastrectomy is necessary. The goal of surgery is obtaining negative surgical margins. Vitamin B_{12} supplementation is required after gastrectomy. For patients with localized gastric cancer that is resectable, National Comprehensive Cancer Network (NCCN) treatment guidelines recommend gastrectomy with extended (D1), or modified regional (D2), lymph node dissection and sampling of 15 or more lymph nodes. D2 lymphadenectomy has been shown to improve disease-specific survival but is associated with increased postoperative mortality.

B. Perioperative Chemotherapy, Chemoradiation, or Radiation Therapy

Survival outcomes post-surgery alone remain poor (5-year survival of approximately 30%), particularly in those with node-positive disease. Multidisciplinary treatment decision-making involving the surgeon, radiation oncologist, and medical oncologist is imperative. The use of perioperative chemotherapy or adjuvant chemoradiation is associated with improved survival in patients with localized or locoregional gastric adenocarcinoma who undergo surgical resection. Triplet chemotherapy for resectable gastric cancer is recommended for patients who are fit but is associated with more toxicity than doublet chemotherapy.

Postoperative radiation therapy has not shown a clear benefit in the setting of aggressive surgical nodal dissection. Ongoing trials are assessing preoperative radiation therapy.

Tumors arising in the gastroesophageal junction are treated following algorithms for primary esophageal cancers (see Esophageal Cancer, above). When diagnosed as locally advanced or metastatic, they have a poor prognosis.

C. Immunotherapies and Targeted Therapies

The development of immunotherapy represents a promising strategy in a selected patients with locally advanced and metastatic gastric cancer. Testing for MSI-H, dMMR, PD-1, and PD-L1 is recommended in advanced disease to identify tumors that may respond to immunotherapy. Among gastric adenocarcinomas, MSI-H/dMMR is found in 8–16% and HER2 amplification in 22%. Systemic therapy regimens are generally the same as those used in esophageal adenocarcinomas.

D. Palliative Modalities

Many patients will be found to have advanced disease that is not amenable to curative intent surgery due to peritoneal or distant metastases or local invasion of other organs. In some of these cases, palliative resection of the tumor nonetheless may be indicated to alleviate pain, bleeding, or obstruction. For patients with unresectable disease and gastric outlet obstruction with good functional status, a surgical diversion with gastrojejunostomy may be indicated to prevent obstruction. Systemic therapy may be considered in patients with metastatic disease who still have good functional status and expected survival of at least several months. Patients with unresected tumors and limited life expectancy may be treated with endoscopic stent therapy, radiation therapy, or angiographic embolization to relieve bleeding or obstruction. The regimens used are the same as those for esophageal and gastroesophageal junction tumors discussed above (Table 39–2).

Prognosis

The 5-year survival for gastric cancer varies greatly by stage, location, and histologic features. Following surgery, the 5-year survival rates for stage IA and IB cancers treated with curative intent are between 60% and 80%, but for stage IIIC cancers, they are as low as 18%. Proximal gastric tumors have a 5-year survival of less than 15%, even with apparent localized disease. For those whose disease progresses despite therapy, palliative care is essential (see Chapter 5).

When to Refer

- Patients with dysphagia, weight loss, protracted vomiting, iron deficiency anemia, melena, or new-onset dyspepsia (especially if aged 60 years or older or associated with other alarm symptoms) in whom gastric cancer is suspected should be referred for endoscopy.
- Patients should be referred to a surgeon for attempt at curative resection of stage I, II, or III cancer, including staging laparoscopy if indicated.
- Prior to surgery, patients should be referred to an oncologist to determine the role for perioperative chemotherapy or adjuvant chemoradiation or chemotherapy.
- Patients who have undergone gastrectomy require consultation with a nutritionist due to propensity for malnutrition and complications, such as dumping syndrome and vitamin B_{12} deficiency, postoperatively.
- Patients with unresectable or metastatic disease should be referred to an oncologist for consideration of palliative chemotherapy or chemoradiation. Early referral to palliative care services may also be considered for symptom management in patients with advanced and metastatic disease.

When to Admit

Patients with acute bleeding, protracted vomiting, or inability to maintain hydration or nutrition.

ASGE Standards of Practice Committee; Jue TL et al. ASGE guideline on the role of endoscopy in the management of benign and malignant gastroduodenal obstruction. Gastrointest Endosc. 2021;93:309. [PMID: 33168194]

de Steur WO et al; CRITICS investigators. Adjuvant chemotherapy is superior to chemoradiation after D2 surgery for gastric cancer in the per-protocol analysis of the randomized CRITICS trial. Ann Oncol. 2021;32:360. [PMID: 33227408]

Joshi SS et al. Current treatment and recent progress in gastric cancer. CA Cancer J Clin. 2021;71:264. [PMID: 33592120]

Kawazoe A et al. Current status of immunotherapy for advanced gastric cancer. Jpn J Clin Oncol. 2021;51:20. [PMID: 33241322]

Ng SP et al. Role of radiation therapy in gastric cancer. Ann Surg Oncol. 2021;28:4151. [PMID: 33689079]

Shah SS et al. Population-based analysis of differences in gastric cancer incidence among races and ethnicities in individuals age 50 years and older. Gastroenterology. 2020;159:1705. [PMID: 32771406]

Zhu Y et al. HER2-targeted therapies in gastric cancer. Biochim Biophys Acta Rev Cancer. 2021;1876:188549. [PMID: 33894300]

GASTRIC LYMPHOMA

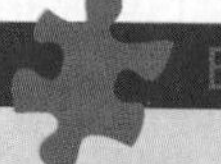

ESSENTIALS OF DIAGNOSIS

- Symptoms of dyspepsia, weight loss, or anemia.
- Distinguish **primary gastric lymphoma** with adjacent nodal spread from advanced systemic lymphoma with **secondary gastric lymphoma** involvement.
- Upper GI series or endoscopy shows thickened folds, ulcer, mass, or infiltrating lesions; diagnosis established by endoscopic biopsy.
- Abdominal CT and EUS required for staging.

General Considerations

Gastric lymphomas may be primary (arising from the gastric mucosa) or may represent a site of secondary involvement in patients with nodal lymphomas. Distinguishing advanced **primary gastric lymphoma** with adjacent nodal spread from **secondary gastric lymphoma** spread from advanced nodal lymphoma is essential because the prognosis and treatment of primary and secondary gastric lymphomas are different. **Primary gastric lymphoma** is the second most common gastric malignancy, accounting for 3–5% of gastric cancers. More than 95% of these are non-Hodgkin B-cell lymphomas mainly consisting of either **(1) mucosa-associated lymphoid tissue (MALT)-type lymphoma;** or **(2) diffuse large B-cell lymphoma.** Over 90% of low-grade primary gastric MALT-type lymphomas are associated with *H pylori* infection. *H pylori* leads to chronic inflammation, producing lymphoid tissue in the stomach mucosa (MALT) that can lead to malignant transformation.

Clinical Findings & Staging

The clinical presentation and endoscopic appearance of gastric lymphoma are like those of adenocarcinoma. Most patients have abdominal pain, weight loss, or bleeding. Patients with diffuse large B-cell lymphoma are more likely to have systemic symptoms.

At endoscopy, lymphoma may appear as an ulcer, mass, or diffusely infiltrating lesion. The diagnosis is established with endoscopic biopsy; FNA biopsy is not adequate. Since the disease can be multifocal, biopsies of both suspicious and normal-appearing areas are recommended. Biopsy specimens should be tested for *H pylori* and, if positive, for t(11;18) via PCR or FISH. EUS is the most sensitive test for determining the depth of invasion and presence of perigastric lymphadenopathy. All patients should undergo staging with CT scanning of chest, abdomen, and pelvis.

MALT-type lymphomas—For gastric MALT lymphomas, the Lugano staging system is most frequently used. Stage I is confined to the GI tract, stage II involves local or regional lymph nodes, stage IIE has invasion of adjacent organs or tissues, and stage IV has distant metastases. There is no stage III.

Diffuse large B-cell lymphomas—For patients with diffuse large B-cell lymphomas involving the stomach, combination PET-CT imaging, bone marrow biopsy with aspirate, tumor lysis laboratory tests, and hepatitis B and HIV serologies may be required for staging and treatment planning (see Chapter 13). Diffuse large B-cell lymphomas more likely present at an advanced stage.

Treatment

Treatment of primary gastric lymphomas depends on the tumor histology, grade, and stage.

A. MALT-Type Lymphomas

Those that are low-grade and localized to the stomach wall (stage I) or perigastric lymph nodes (stage IIE1) have an excellent prognosis. Patients with primary gastric MALT-lymphoma should be tested for *H pylori* infection and treated if positive. Complete lymphoma regression after successful *H pylori* eradication occurs in approximately 75% of cases of stage I and approximately 55% of stage IIE low-grade lymphoma. Remission may take as long as a year, and relapse occurs in about 2% of cases per year.

Failure of antibiotic treatment to achieve lymphoma regression may be due to genetic factors. Rates of remission after *H pylori* eradication are lower in patients whose tumors harbor specific gene translocations, including t(11;18) (API2-MALT1), t(1;14), or t(14;18). Of cancers positive for t(11;18), 95% do not respond to antibiotics. Patients with localized marginal zone MALT-type lymphomas who are not infected with *H pylori* or do not respond to *H pylori* antibiotic therapy may be treated with radiation therapy.

Endoscopic surveillance after antibiotic or radiation treatment is recommended every 3–6 months for 5 years to evaluate for recurrence. The long-term survival of low-grade MALT stage I lymphoma is over 90% and for stage II is 35–65%. Surgical resection is not recommended.

B. Diffuse Large B-Cell Lymphoma

Diffuse large B-cell lymphomas (or other higher-grade lymphomas with secondary GI involvement) usually present at an advanced stage with widely disseminated disease and are treated according to stage and subtype of lymphoma (see Chapter 13).

Surgery for diffuse large B-cell lymphoma (but not MALT) has been associated with a better prognosis than conservative treatment. Advanced stage disease can be treated with chemoimmunotherapy or radiation therapy for GI bleeding, threatened end-organ function, bulky disease, or progression. Diffuse large B-cell lymphoma has been successfully treated with two chemotherapeutic options (cyclophosphamide-doxorubicin-vincristine-prednisone [CHOP] or rituximab-CHOP). The presence of peri-gastric lymph nodes and the degree of tumor infiltration of the gastric wall are indications to treat with definitive radiotherapy.

Diamantidis MD et al. Primary gastric non-Hodgkin lymphomas: recent advances regarding disease pathogenesis and treatment. World J Gastroenterol. 2021;27:5932. [PMID: 34629810]

National Comprehensive Cancer Network. B-Cell Lymphomas, Version 1.2021, NCCN Clinical Practice Guidelines in Oncology. https://www.nccn.org/professionals/physician_gls/pdf/b-cell.pdf

Kim J et al. *Helicobacter pylori* and gastric cancer. Gastrointest Endosc Clin N Am. 2021;31:451. [PMID: 34053633]

Quéro L et al. Radiotherapy for gastric mucosa-associated lymphoid tissue lymphoma. World J Gastrointest Oncol. 2021;13:1453. [PMID: 34721777]

Vlăduţ C et al. Is mucosa-associated lymphoid tissue lymphoma an infectious disease? Role of *Helicobacter pylori* and eradication antibiotic therapy. Exp Ther Med. 2020;20:3546. [PMID: 32905014]

GASTRIC NEUROENDOCRINE TUMORS

Gastric NETs (gNETs) make up less than 1% of gastric neoplasms. They may occur sporadically or secondary to chronic hypergastrinemia that results in hyperplasia and transformation of enterochromaffin cells in the gastric fundus. gNETs have been classified into four types. Types 1 and 2 account for the majority and are caused by hypergastrinemia, type 1 in association with pernicious anemia (75%) and type 2 in association with Zollinger-Ellison syndrome (5%). Types 3 and 4 arise sporadically, are independent of gastrin production, and account for up to 20% of gNETs.

Type 1 gNETs are associated with chronic atrophic gastritis, gastric achlorhydria, and consequent secondary hypergastrinemia. Initial diagnostic workup includes CBC, serum vitamin B_{12} level, and intrinsic factor antibody to help diagnose pernicious anemia, followed by serum gastrin level. Staging involves upper endoscopy and EUS. For low-grade tumors (proliferation index of Ki-67 less than 3% or mitotic index of less than 2 mitoses/10 high-power fields [HPF] on histopathological analysis), somatostatin receptor–based imaging (somatostatin receptor scintigraphy or gallium-68 dotatate PET/CT) should be performed. For high-grade tumors (Ki-67 greater than 20% or greater than 20 mitoses/10 HPF), FDG-PET/CT is preferred to evaluate the extent of disease.

Type 2 gNETs are associated with Zollinger-Ellison syndrome caused by a gastrin-secreting NET (gastrinoma) most commonly located in the pancreas or duodenum. Although 75% of gastrinomas are sporadic, gNET caused by gastrinomas occur almost exclusively in patients with multiple endocrine neoplasia type 1 (MEN 1) in which chromosomal loss of 11q13 has been reported.

For types 1 and 2 gNETs, small lesions may be successfully treated with endoscopic resection followed by endoscopic surveillance every 6–12 months, or with observation. Antrectomy reduces serum gastrin levels and may lead to regression of small tumors. It can be considered in patients with type 1 gastric NETs to reduce recurrence risk and frequency of post-therapy monitoring. Patients with tumors larger than 2 cm should undergo endoscopic or surgical resection (see Small Intestinal Adenocarcinomas below). Type 2 gNETs with underlying gastrinoma and Zollinger-Ellison syndrome may be treated with somatostatin analog (octreotide) therapy.

Types 3 and **4 gNETs** are most often solitary, larger than 2 cm, and have a strong propensity for hepatic or pulmonary metastases and with associated carcinoid syndrome at initial presentation. In patients with type 3 or 4 gNETs, gallium-68 dotatate CT scan should be obtained to evaluate for metastatic disease.

Localized sporadic type 3 or type 4 gNETs should be treated with partial or total gastrectomy and regional lymphadenectomy. Advanced, low-grade gNETs can be monitored with serial scans, if asymptomatic. Octreotide may provide symptomatic relief for patients with gNETs that are functional (carcinoid syndrome). Advanced high-grade gastric neuroendocrine carcinomas are treated in a fashion similar to small cell lung cancers.

The prognosis of types 1 and 2 gNETs is good. The prognosis of types 3 and 4 gNETs is like the prognosis of gastric adenocarcinoma.

Hanna A et al. Gastric neuroendocrine tumors: reappraisal of type in predicting outcomes. Ann Surg Oncol. 2021;28:8838. [PMID: 34120268]

Köseoğlu H et al. Gastric neuroendocrine neoplasms: a review. World J Clin Cases. 2021;9:7973. [PMID: 34621854]

Mastracci L et al. Neuroendocrine neoplasms of the esophagus and stomach. Pathologica. 2021;113:5. [PMID: 33686305]

Shah MH et al. Neuroendocrine and Adrenal Tumors, Version 2. 2021, NCCN Clinical Practice Guidelines in Oncology. J Natl Compr Canc Netw. 2021;19:839. [PMID: 34340212]

GASTROINTESTINAL MESENCHYMAL TUMORS

Pathobiology & Diagnosis

GI mesenchymal tumors (stromal tumors, leiomyomas, and schwannomas) derive from mesenchymal stem cells. The most common are GI stromal tumors (GISTs), which originate from interstitial cells of Cajal. GISTs occur most commonly in the stomach (60%). Most cases are sporadic, but about 5% of cases are part of familial genetic syndromes. GISTs are potentially malignant and have an unpredictable evolution. Determination of the GIST molecular subtype upon diagnosis is important because it informs therapeutic decisions in both the adjuvant and metastatic setting. Approximately 80–90% of GISTs have gain-of-function mutations in *KIT*, a receptor tyrosine kinase or in PDGFRα, platelet-derived growth factor alpha.

Mesenchymal tumors may cause symptoms (most commonly bleeding, pain, or obstruction) or may be discovered incidentally on imaging studies or endoscopy. At endoscopy, they appear as a submucosal mass that may have central umbilication or ulceration. EUS with guided FNA biopsy is the optimal study for diagnosing gastric mesenchymal tumors and distinguishing them from other submucosal lesions. Percutaneous biopsy is not recommended due to risk of bleeding or intra-abdominal seeding. CT of the abdomen and pelvis with contrast, MRI, and PET imaging are useful in the diagnosis and staging. PET imaging also may be useful to monitor response to treatment.

It is difficult to distinguish benign from malignant tumors by EUS appearance or by FNA. In general, lesions are more likely benign if they are smaller than 2 cm, have a smooth border, and have a homogeneous echo pattern on EUS. But all GISTs have malignant potential, and the risk of developing metastasis is increased with tumor size greater than 2 cm, non-gastric location, and mitotic index greater than 5 mitoses per 50 HPF.

Treatment

A. Localized Treatment

Complete surgical resection, whether by laparotomy or laparoscopy, is the only potentially curative treatment of localized GISTs. Surgical resection is recommended for tumors that are 2 cm or larger, or are increasing in size, suspicious for malignancy on EUS, or symptomatic. The management of asymptomatic gastric lesions 2 cm or smaller depends on the EUS features. If no high-risk features are noted, endoscopic surveillance with serial EUS can be pursued. Because of the low but real long-term risk of malignancy, surgical resection should be considered in younger, otherwise healthy patients. Recurrences are common following surgical resection, occurring in 40–50% of patients within 3 years.

B. Systemic Treatment

The introduction of effective molecularly targeted therapies for GISTs has dramatically changed the clinical management and prognosis for patients with intermediate- and high-risk GISTs, as well as those with locally advanced and metastatic disease. Because the majority of GISTs are driven by pathogenic variants in *KIT* or *PDGFRα*, the tyrosine kinase inhibitor, imatinib, is now used across disease stages. Neoadjuvant therapy with imatinib may be considered for patients with localized GIST tumors who are deemed to be at high risk for resection because of comorbidities, tumor size, or tumor location. Adjuvant therapy with imatinib delays recurrence and prolongs survival, but it is not likely to be curative. For metastatic GISTs, imatinib has become the standard first-line treatment, inducing disease control in up to 80–85% of patients, with a median survival of almost 5 years. Patients who subsequently experience disease progression on imatinib therapy may be treated with second-, third-, and fourth-line therapy with sunitinib, regorafenib and ripretinib, respectively. Untreated metastatic GIST tumors are aggressive and carry a poor prognosis.

In the subset of tumors that have the PDGFRα D842V pathogenic variant, the KIT and PDGFRα inhibitor, avapritinib, results in an approximate 90% disease control rate. Finally, the role of immunotherapies for mesenchymal tumors is growing rapidly.

Arshad J et al. Immunotherapy strategies for gastrointestinal stromal tumor. Cancers (Basel). 2021;13:3525. [PMID: 34298737]
Heinrich MC et al. Avapritinib in advanced *PDGFRA D842V*-mutant gastrointestinal stromal tumour (NAVIGATOR): a multicentre, open-label, phase 1 trial. Lancet Oncol. 2020;21: 935. [PMID: 32615108]
Kelly CM et al. The management of metastatic GIST: current standard and investigational therapeutics. J Hematol Oncol. 2021;14:2. [PMID: 33402214]

MALIGNANCIES OF THE SMALL INTESTINE

The frequency of different tumor types varies by location within the small intestine. Adenocarcinomas are most common in the duodenum and jejunum and neuroendocrine tumors, in the ileum. Lymphomas and sarcomas each have similar incidences in the various segments of the small intestine.

1. Small Intestinal Adenocarcinomas

These cancers often present with abdominal pain and nausea. They are rare, with 11,790 new diagnoses estimated for 2022 in the United States. Adenocarcinomas are most often diagnosed at stage III or IV. The duodenum is the most common site of small bowel adenocarcinoma, specifically the periampullary region. **Ampullary carcinomas** may present with GI bleeding or jaundice due to bile duct obstruction. Surgical resection of early lesions is curative in up to 40% of patients.

Most cases of **nonampullary adenocarcinomas** present with symptoms of obstruction, acute or chronic GI bleeding, or weight loss. Resection is recommended for control of symptoms. For localized disease, the role of (neo)adjuvant chemotherapy is under investigation. The benefit of adjuvant therapy after resection of stage II or III tumors is unclear, but it is generally administered using chemotherapy agents active in colorectal cancer. For advanced/unresectable disease, first-line doublet chemotherapy is standard. Two trials suggest value from adding bevacizumab to chemotherapy. Pembrolizumab is an accepted treatment modality for mismatch repair-deficient tumors; more trials with immunotherapy are underway.

Mazlom H et al. Management of small bowel adenocarcinoma: making the most of the available evidence to inform routine practice. Curr Opin Oncol. 2021;33:368. [PMID: 33882527]
National Comprehensive Cancer Network. Small Bowel Adenocarcinoma, Version 1.2022, NCCN Clinical Practice Guidelines in Oncology. 2022 Mar 9. https://www.nccn.org/professionals/physician_gls/pdf/small_bowel.pdf

2. Small Intestinal Lymphomas

Lymphomas may arise primarily in the GI tract (see Gastric Lymphomas above) or may involve it secondarily in patients with disseminated lymphoma. In Western countries, primary GI lymphomas account for 5% of lymphomas and 20% of small bowel malignancies. There is an increased incidence of small intestinal lymphomas in patients with AIDS, Crohn disease, and those receiving immunosuppressive therapy. The most common histologic subtypes are non-Hodgkin extranodal marginal zone (MALT) B-cell lymphomas and diffuse large B-cell lymphomas. However, enteropathy-associated T-cell lymphoma (sometimes associated with celiac disease) appears to be increasing in incidence in the United States. In the Middle East, lymphomas may arise in the setting of immunoproliferative small intestinal disease. Other types of intestinal lymphomas include primary intestinal follicular cell lymphoma, mantle cell lymphoma, post-transplant lymphoproliferative disorder, and Burkitt lymphoma (see Chapter 13).

Presenting symptoms or signs of primary small bowel lymphoma include abdominal pain, weight loss, nausea and vomiting, distention, anemia, and occult blood in the stool. Fevers are unusual. Protein-losing enteropathy may result in hypoalbuminemia. CT enterography helps localize the site of the lesion. Diagnosis requires endoscopic, percutaneous, or laparoscopic biopsy. Imaging and possibly bone marrow biopsy are required to determine stage.

Treatment depends on the tumor histologic subtype and stage of disease (see Chapter 13). If feasible, surgical resection of localized primary intestinal lymphoma may be appropriate. Following resection with negative margins, the role of adjuvant chemotherapy in patients with limited disease (stage IE) is unclear. Locoregional radiation should be considered if surgical margins are positive. Patients with more extensive disease generally are treated according to the tumor histology.

Foukas PG et al. Recent advances upper gastrointestinal lymphomas: molecular updates and diagnostic implications. Histopathology. 2021;78:187. [PMID: 33382495]
National Comprehensive Cancer Network. B-Cell Lymphomas, Version 3.2022, NCCN Clinical Practice Guidelines in Oncology. 2022 Apr 25. https://www.nccn.org/professionals/physician_gls/pdf/b-cell.pdf
Small S et al. B cell lymphomas of the GI tract. Curr Gastroenterol Rep. 2021;23:9. [PMID: 33963950]

3. Intestinal Neuroendocrine Tumors

General Considerations

According to the 2019 WHO pathology grading system, high-grade gastroenteropancreatic neuroendocrine neoplasms can be divided into well-differentiated neuroendocrine tumors grade 3 (NETs G3) and poorly differentiated neuroendocrine carcinomas (NECs). The prognosis of NETs G3 is significantly better than that of NECs.

GI NETs (also called carcinoids) most commonly occur in the small intestine (45%) but are also found in the rectum (20%), appendix (17%), colon (11%), and stomach (less than 10%; see Gastric Neuroendocrine Tumors above). Carcinoid tumors are well-differentiated neuroendocrine tumors that may secrete a variety of hormones, including serotonin, somatostatin, gastrin, and substance P. Gastrin-secreting NETs (gastrinomas) are discussed in Chapter 14 (see Zollinger-Ellison syndrome).

Small intestinal carcinoids most commonly arise in the distal ileum within 60 cm of the ileocecal valve. Jejunal-ileal NETs are the second most frequent location. The risk of metastatic spread increases when the tumor is 1 cm or larger and when it is larger than 2 cm with invasion beyond the muscularis propria.

Appendiceal carcinoids are identified in 0.3% of appendectomies, usually as an incidental finding. Almost 80% of these tumors are smaller than 1 cm, and 90% are smaller than 2 cm. However, in patients with appendiceal carcinoid tumors larger than 2 cm, approximately 90% develop nodal and distant metastases; right hemicolectomy is recommended in these cases.

Rectal carcinoids are usually detected incidentally as submucosal nodules during proctoscopic examination and often locally excised by biopsy or snare polypectomy before the histologic diagnosis is known. Rectal carcinoids smaller than 1 cm virtually never metastasize and are treated effectively with local endoscopic or transanal excision. Larger tumors are associated with the development of metastasis in 10%. Hence, a more extensive cancer resection operation is warranted in fit patients with rectal carcinoid tumors larger than 1–2 cm or with high-risk features (such as invasion of muscularis propria or evidence of nodal involvement), or both.

Clinical Findings

A. Symptoms and Signs

Most intestinal carcinoids smaller than 1–2 cm are asymptomatic and difficult to detect by endoscopy or imaging studies. Such small intestinal carcinoids may present with intermittent abdominal pain, bowel obstruction, bleeding, or bowel infarction. Appendiceal and rectal carcinoids usually are small and asymptomatic, but large lesions can cause bleeding, obstruction, or altered bowel habits.

Carcinoid syndrome, which occurs in less than 10% of patients, is caused by tumor secretion of hormonal mediators. Manifestations include facial flushing, abdominal cramps and diarrhea, bronchospasm, cardiac lesions (pulmonary or tricuspid stenosis or regurgitation in 10–30%), and telangiectases. More than 90% of patients with carcinoid syndrome have hepatic metastases, usually from carcinoids of small bowel origin.

B. Laboratory Findings

Serum chromogranin A is elevated in most NETs. Although its sensitivity for small, localized carcinoids is unknown, serum chromogranin A is elevated in almost 90% of patients with advanced small bowel carcinoid. A variety of medications including PPIs can cause falsely elevated serum chromogranin A levels. Although it is less sensitive than serum chromogranin A, the urinary 5-hydroxyindoleacetic acid (5-HIAA) level is also elevated in patients with metastatic carcinoid and in carcinoid syndrome (symptomatic patients usually excrete more than 25 mg of 5-HIAA per day in the urine). Because certain foods and medications can interfere with 5-HIAA levels, these should be withheld for 48 hours before the 24-hour urine collection.

C. Imaging

Abdominal CT or MRI may demonstrate a mesenteric mass with tethering of the bowel, lymphadenopathy, and hepatic metastasis. (Most patients with carcinoid syndrome have liver metastasis on abdominal imaging.) Gallium 68 (^{68}Ga) DOTATATE PET scan has replaced somatostatin receptor scintigraphy as standard for staging; and may help identify disease that may benefit from treatment with somatostatin analogs (octreotide) or PRRT.

Treatment & Outcomes

Small intestinal carcinoids generally are indolent tumors with slow spread. Patients with disease confined to the small intestine should be treated with surgical excision. There is no proven role for adjuvant therapy after complete resection. Five-year survival rates for patients with stage I and II disease are 96% and 87%, respectively. In patients with resectable disease who have lymph node involvement (stage III), the 5-year survival rate is 74%; however, by 25 years, less than 25% remain disease-free. Across stages, prognosis is strongly associated with histologic differentiation and grade. Patients with grade 1 disease may not require treatment for many years even with metastatic disease. However, patients with grade 3 NET may have a clinical course more like a high-grade NEC.

In patients with advanced disease, therapy historically has been deferred until the patient is symptomatic, however, this is evolving as the number of available treatment options increases. Conventional cytotoxic chemotherapy agents do not achieve significant responses in carcinoid tumors and have not been associated with improved outcomes. For patients who are symptomatic from tumor bulk or carcinoid syndrome, the cornerstone of therapy is a long-acting somatostatin analog such as octreotide, which inhibits hormone secretion from the carcinoid tumor. In 90% of patients, this results in dramatic relief of carcinoid syndrome symptoms and may control tumor growth for a median period of 1 year. Options at disease progression include octreotide dose escalation, or addition of everolimus. For patients with somatostatin receptor–positive disease on imaging, another option after progression is treatment with PRRT, which consists of a somatostatin analog conjugated to a radioactive isotope such as yttrium-90 or lutetium-177. Studies of antiangiogenic kinase inhibitors, such as sunitinib and regorafenib, have shown some benefit. In selected patients with hepatic-dominant disease, resection of hepatic metastases or tumor debulking by liver-directed chemoembolization or radioembolization may provide dramatic improvement in carcinoid syndrome symptoms.

Patients with advanced, poorly differentiated intestinal NECs are treated in a similar fashion to those with small cell carcinomas. They have a poor prognosis.

Andreasi V et al. Update on gastroenteropancreatic neuroendocrine tumors. Dig Liver Dis. 2021;53:171. [PMID: 32912771]

Bonds M et al. Neuroendocrine tumors of the pancreaticobiliary and gastrointestinal tracts. Surg Clin North Am. 2020;100:635. [PMID: 32402306]

Milione M et al. Neuroendocrine neoplasms of the duodenum, ampullary region, jejunum and ileum. Pathologica. 2021; 113:12. [PMID: 33686306]

National Comprehensive Cancer Network. Neuroendocrine and Adrenal Tumors, Version 4.2021, NCCN Clinical Practice Guidelines in Oncology. 2021 Dec 14. https://www.nccn.org/professionals/physician_gls/pdf/neuroendocrine.pdf

Shi M et al. Gastroenteropancreatic neuroendocrine neoplasms G3: novel insights and unmet needs. Biochim Biophys Acta Rev Cancer. 2021;1876:188637. [PMID: 34678439]

4. Small Intestine Sarcoma

Sarcomas constitute approximately 10% of small bowel neoplasms and are commonly found in the jejunum and ileum. Most arise from stromal tumors (GISTs, see Gastrointestinal Mesenchymal Tumors, above); a minority arise from smooth muscle tumors (leiomyosarcomas). Common symptoms of small intestine sarcoma include pain, weight loss, bleeding, and perforation. As the lesions tend to enlarge extraluminally, obstruction is rare.

National Comprehensive Cancer Network. Soft Tissue Sarcoma, Version 1.2022, NCCN Clinical Practice Guidelines in Oncology. 2022 Mar 29. https://www.nccn.org/professionals/physician_gls/pdf/sarcoma.pdf

Zalcberg JR. Ripretinib for the treatment of advanced gastrointestinal stromal tumor. Therap Adv Gastroenterol. 2021; 14:17562848211008177. [PMID: 33948116]

COLORECTAL CANCER

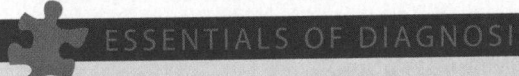

- Personal or family history of adenomatous or serrated polyps or colorectal cancer (CRC) is an important risk factor.
- Symptoms or signs depend on tumor location.
  - **Proximal colon:** fecal occult blood, anemia.
  - **Distal colon:** change in bowel habits, hematochezia.
- Diagnosis established with colonoscopy with biopsy.

General Considerations

CRC is the second leading cause of death due to malignancy in the United States. CRC will develop in approximately 4.2% of Americans and has a 5-year survival rate of 65%. In 2022, there will be an estimated 151,030 new CRC cases in the United States, with an estimated 53,200 deaths. Over the last 10 years, CRC incidence has declined by 1.7% per year and mortality by 3.2% per year, which is attributed to population-based CRC screening. The percentage of US adults aged 50–75 years who were up-to-date with recommended CRC screening was 67.1% in 2019.

CRCs are almost all adenocarcinomas, which tend to form bulky exophytic masses or annular constricting lesions. Most are thought to arise from malignant transformation of an adenomatous polyp (tubular, tubulovillous, or villous adenoma) or serrated polyp (hyperplastic polyp, traditional serrated adenoma, or sessile serrated adenoma). Polyps that are "advanced" (ie, polyps at least 1 cm in size, adenomas with villous features or high-grade dysplasia, or serrated polyps with dysplasia) are associated with a greater risk of cancer.

Approximately 85% of sporadic CRC arise from adenomatous polyps. They have loss of function of one or more tumor suppressor genes (eg, p53, APC, or DCC) due to a combination of spontaneous pathologic variants of one allele combined with chromosomal instability and aneuploidy (abnormal DNA content) that leads to deletion and loss of heterozygosity of the other allele (eg, 5q, 17q, or 18p deletion). Activation of oncogenes such as *KRAS* and *BRAF* is present in a subset of cancers with prognostic and therapeutic implications discussed further below.

Another 10–20% of CRC arise from serrated polyps, most of which have hypermethylation of CpG-rich promoter regions. This leads to inactivation of the DNA mismatch repair (MMR) gene *MLH1*, resulting in microsatellite instability (MSI-high [or MSI-H]) (the presence of a high number of insertions or deletions at repetitive DNA units) and activation of pathogenic variants of the *BRAF* gene. The vast majority of MSI-H tumors are due to loss of a mismatch repair (MMR) protein, which can be assess by IHC staining. Tumors lacking staining for an MMR protein are referred to as mismatch repair deficient (dMMR). Serrated CRC have distinct clinical and pathologic characteristics, including diploid DNA content, predominance in the proximal colon, poor differentiation, and more favorable prognosis.

Finally, up to 5% of CRC are caused by inherited pathogenic germline variants resulting in polyposis syndromes (eg, familial adenomatous polyposis) or hereditary nonpolyposis CRC (HNPCC or Lynch syndrome). These conditions are discussed further below and in Chapter 15.

Risk Factors

Several factors increase the risk of developing CRC, including smoking, consumption of red and processed meats, alcohol intake, diabetes mellitus, physical inactivity, obesity, and history of IBD or primary sclerosing cholangitis. However, 75% of all cases occur in people with no known predisposing factors.

A. Age

The incidence of CRC rises sharply after age 45 years, and 90% of cases occur in persons over the age of 50 years. The median age at diagnosis is 68 years for men and 72 years for women. Over the past two decades there has been a 20% decrease in incidence among adults over age 50 years (due to CRC screening programs) but a 50% increase in incidence among adults under age 50 years (especially in the distal colon and rectum). In the United States, the incidence of young adult–onset CRC is rising in all racial and ethnic groups. It is highest in Black adults, but the incidence is rising most quickly in non-Hispanic White adults. In the United States, the CRC incidence rate in adults over age 50 years is 40/100,000 and in adults younger than age 50 it is 13.1/100,000. It is estimated that by 2030, 10% of colon cancers and 20% of rectal cancers will occur in patients under age 50 years. The reason for the increase in incidence among adults under age 50 years is uncertain.

B. Family History of Neoplasia

A family history of CRC is present in approximately 20% of patients with colon cancer. Hereditary factors are believed to contribute to 20–30% of CRCs; however, the genes responsible for many of these cases have not yet been identified. Hereditary cancer syndromes (Lynch syndrome or polyposis syndromes) account for approximately 3–4% of CRC in patients 50 years or older but 10–15% of patients with young adult–onset CRC (see Chapter 15).

Lynch syndrome is the most common hereditary cancer syndrome responsible for CRC. Lynch syndrome is caused by pathogenic germline variants in one of four DNA mismatch repair genes (*MLH1*, *MSH2*, *MSH6*, or *PMS2*) or by a deletion in the *EPCAM* gene. Variants in the *MLH1* gene are correlated with the highest risk of CRC.

Approximately 6% of the Ashkenazi Jewish population has a missense pathologic variant in the *APC* gene *(APC I1307K)* that confers a modestly increased lifetime risk of developing CRC (OR 1.4–1.9) that phenotypically resembles sporadic CRC rather than familial adenomatous polyposis. Genetic screening is available, and patients harboring a variant in the *APC* gene merit more intensive colorectal screening.

A family history of CRC or adenomatous polyps is one of the most important risk factors for CRC. The risk of colon cancer is proportionate to the number and age of affected first-degree family members with colon neoplasia. People with one first-degree family member with CRC have an increased risk approximately two times that of the general population; however, the risk is almost four times if the family member was younger than 45 years when the cancer was diagnosed. Patients with two first-degree relatives have a fourfold increased, or 25–30% lifetime, risk of developing colon cancer. First-degree relatives of patients with adenomatous polyps also have a twofold increased risk for colorectal neoplasia, especially if they were younger than 60 years when the polyp was detected or if the polyp was 10 mm or larger.

C. Inflammatory Bowel Disease

The risk of adenocarcinoma of the colon begins to rise 8 years after disease onset in patients with ulcerative colitis and Crohn colitis (see Chapter 15). For this reason, initiation of surveillance with colonoscopy is recommended at 8–10 years after onset of IBD symptoms.

D. Dietary and Lifestyle Factors and Chemoprevention

In epidemiologic studies, diets rich in fats and red meat are associated with an increased risk of colorectal adenomas and cancer, whereas diets high in fruits, vegetables, and fiber are associated with a decreased risk. However, prospective studies have not shown a reduction in colon cancer or recurrence of adenomatous polyps with diets that are low in fat; that are high in fiber, fruits or vegetables; or that include calcium, folate, beta-carotene, or vitamin A, C, D, or E supplements.

Meta-analyses suggest that individuals with increased physical activity are up to 27% less likely to develop colon cancer. There also is a correlation between increasing BMI and cancer risk, such that for each increase of 5 in BMI, there is a 5% increased cancer risk. Patients with higher levels of pre- and post-diagnosis physical activity experience reduced CRC-specific mortality and all-cause mortality. Maintaining a healthy body weight, a healthy diet, and a physically active lifestyle are recommended in CRC survivors.

Low-dose aspirin has been controversial as a potential cancer chemotherapeutic agent. A draft 2021 USPSTF statement concluded that "the evidence is inadequate that low-dose aspirin use reduces CRC incidence or mortality." Because long-term aspirin use is associated with a low incidence of serious complications (GI hemorrhage, stroke), low-dose aspirin probably should not be routinely administered as a cancer chemopreventive agent without other medical indications.

E. Other Factors

The overall incidence of CRC is similar in men and women; however, similar incidence rates are reached in women about 4–6 years later than in men. A higher proportion of cancers are located in the proximal colon in women (46%) than men (37%). The incidence and mortality of colon adenocarcinoma is higher in Black and Native American persons than in White persons. It is unclear whether this is due to genetic or socioeconomic factors (eg, diet or reduced access to medical care).

Clinical Findings

A. Symptoms and Signs

Adenocarcinomas grow slowly and may be present for several years before symptoms appear. Many asymptomatic tumors may be detected by the presence of fecal occult blood (see Screening for Colorectal Neoplasms, below). Symptoms depend on the location of the carcinoma. Chronic blood loss from right-sided colonic cancers may cause iron deficiency anemia, manifested by fatigue and weakness. Obstruction, however, is uncommon because of the large diameter of the right colon and the liquid consistency of the fecal material. Lesions of the left colon often involve the bowel circumferentially. Because the left colon has a smaller diameter, and the fecal matter is solid, obstructive symptoms may develop with colicky abdominal pain and a change in bowel habits. Constipation may alternate with periods of increased frequency and loose stools. The stool may be streaked with blood, though marked bleeding is unusual. With rectal cancers, patients note tenesmus, urgency, and recurrent hematochezia. Physical examination is usually normal except in advanced disease. The liver should be examined for hepatomegaly, suggesting metastatic spread. For cancers of the distal rectum, digital examination is necessary to determine whether there is extension into the anal sphincter or fixation, suggesting extension to the pelvic floor.

B. Laboratory Findings

A CBC should be obtained to look for anemia. Elevated liver biochemical tests, particularly the serum alkaline phosphatase, raise suspicion of metastatic disease. The serum carcinoembryonic antigen (CEA) should be measured in all patients with proven CRC but is not appropriate for screening. The CEA is not elevated in many patients with confirmed CRC; conversely, the CEA may be elevated in active smokers and those with a variety of other nonmalignant conditions. That said, a preoperative CEA level greater than 5 ng/mL is a poor prognostic indicator. After complete surgical resection, CEA levels should normalize; persistently elevated levels suggest the presence of persistent disease and warrant further evaluation. CEA is routinely monitored at the time of adjuvant therapy and during postoperative surveillance for patients who had elevated levels before resection.

C. Colonoscopy

Colonoscopy is the required diagnostic procedure in patients with a clinical history suggestive of CRC or in patients with an abnormality suspicious for cancer detected on radiographic imaging. Colonoscopy and upper endoscopy should be considered in all adults with new-onset iron deficiency anemia. Colonoscopy permits biopsy for pathologic confirmation of malignancy.

D. Imaging

Chest, abdominal, and pelvic CT scans with contrast are required for preoperative staging of CRC. CT scans may demonstrate distant metastases but are less accurate in the determination of the level of local tumor extension (T stage) or lymphatic spread (N stage). Intraoperative assessment of the liver by direct palpation and ultrasonography can be performed to detect hepatic metastases (M stage). For rectal cancers (generally defined as tumors arising 12 cm or less proximal to the anal verge), pelvic MRI or endorectal ultrasonography is required to determine the depth of penetration of the cancer through the rectal wall (T stage) and perirectal lymph nodes (N stage), informing decisions about preoperative (neoadjuvant) chemoradiotherapy and operative management.

CT of the chest, abdomen, and pelvis is the best modality to assess for distant metastases of CRC. A combination of CT and MRI is the most reliable modality for detection of liver metastases. PET (with or without CT) is not routinely used for staging or surveillance since many CRCs are not highly PET avid and liver metastases may be inapparent amid high background liver activity.

Staging

The TNM system is the commonly used classification to stage CRC. Staging correlates with the patient's long-term survival and is used to determine which patients should receive neoadjuvant or adjuvant therapy.

Differential Diagnosis

The nonspecific symptoms of CRC may be confused with those of irritable bowel syndrome, diverticular disease, ischemic colitis, IBD, infectious colitis, and hemorrhoids. Neoplasm must be excluded in any patient over age 40 years who reports a change in bowel habits or hematochezia or who has an unexplained iron deficiency anemia or occult blood in stool samples.

Treatment

A. Colon Cancer

Surgical resection of the colonic tumor is the treatment of choice for almost all patients. It may be curative in patients with stage I, II, and III disease and even some patients with metastatic (stage IV) disease. Multiple studies demonstrate that minimally invasive, laparoscopically assisted colectomy results in similar outcomes and rates of recurrence to open colectomy. Regional dissection of at least 12 lymph nodes should be performed to determine staging, which guides decisions about adjuvant therapy. Following complete endoscopic removal of an adenomatous polyp (polypectomy) that is found on pathologic review to contain a focus of cancer invasion into the submucosa (T1 disease; "malignant polyp"), observation is a reasonable alternative to further surgical resection in carefully selected patients. Pathology review of CRCs should include testing for mismatch repair proteins for all patients. Tumors of patients with metastatic CRC should also be tested for extended *RAS* and *BRAF* pathogenic variant and, when feasible, comprehensive molecular profiling.

Following surgical resection, chemotherapy has been demonstrated to improve overall and tumor-free survival in select patients with colon cancer depending on stage (Table 39–2).

1. Stage I—Because of the excellent 5-year survival rate (approximately 92%), no adjuvant therapy is recommended for stage I colon cancer.

2. Stage II (node-negative disease)—The 5-year survival rate is approximately 87% for stage IIA disease and 63% for stage IIB disease. A significant survival benefit from adjuvant chemotherapy has not been demonstrated in most randomized clinical trials for stage II colon cancer (see discussion for stage III disease). However, otherwise healthy patients with stage II disease who are at higher risk for recurrence (perforation; obstruction; close or indeterminate margins; poorly differentiated histology; lymphatic, vascular, or perineural invasion; T4 tumors; or fewer than 12 lymph nodes sampled) may benefit from adjuvant chemotherapy. Patients whose tumors reveal MSI have a more favorable prognosis and do not benefit from 5-fluorouracil-based adjuvant therapy.

3. Stage III (node-positive disease)—With surgical resection alone, the expected 5-year survival rate is 30–50%. Postoperative adjuvant chemotherapy significantly increases disease-free survival as well as overall survival by up to 30% and is recommended for all fit patients (Table 39–2). Multiple large, well-designed studies of adjuvant therapy for stage III CRC have reported a higher rate of disease-free survival at 5 years for patients treated for 6 months postoperatively with a combination of oxaliplatin, 5-fluorouracil, and leucovorin (FOLFOX) (73.3%) than with 5-fluorouracil and leucovorin (FL) alone (67.4%). Similar benefit was reported for patients treated with oxaliplatin and capecitabine (orally active fluoropyrimidine). A large international randomized controlled trial comparing 3 months with 6 months of adjuvant therapy for colon cancer found that 3 months of adjuvant therapy resulted in equivalent disease-free survival for patients with earlier stage T1, T2, or T3, and N1 disease but not with more advanced T4 or N2 disease. For patients with high-risk disease (T4 or N2), 6 months of adjuvant chemotherapy are still recommended. The addition of a biologic agent (bevacizumab or cetuximab) to adjuvant chemotherapy does not improve outcomes.

4. Stage IV (metastatic disease)—Approximately 20% of patients have metastatic disease at the time of initial diagnosis, and another 25–30% eventually develop metastasis. Only 70–75% of patients with metastatic CRC survive beyond 1 year, 30–35% beyond 3 years, and fewer than 20% beyond 5 years from diagnosis.

A subset of patients with metastatic disease has limited disease that is potentially curable with surgical resection. Resection of isolated liver metastases may result in long-term (over 5 years) survival in 35–55% of cases. A subset of patients who have isolated pulmonary metastases may undergo resection (or radiation) with potential cure. In the absence of other treatment, the median survival is less than 12 months; however, with current therapies, median survival approaches 30 months. Surgery may also be warranted to provide palliation of tumor bleeding or obstruction.

Beyond surgical resection, radiation, and local ablative techniques for limited disease, the primary treatment for unresectable metastatic CRC is systemic therapy (cytotoxic chemotherapy, biologic therapy [eg, antibodies to cellular growth factors], immunotherapy, and combinations of these therapies). The goals of systemic therapy for patients with metastatic CRC are to slow tumor progression while maintaining a reasonable quality of life for as long as possible. Clinical trials completed in the past several years have demonstrated that tailoring treatment to the pathologic and molecular features of the cancer improves overall survival.

Cytotoxic chemotherapeutic options include either FOLFOX (the addition of oxaliplatin to 5-fluorouracil and folinic acid) or FOLFIRI (the addition of irinotecan to 5-fluorouracil and folinic acid) is the preferred first-line treatment regimen for fit patients. For convenience, oral capecitabine (instead of intravenous 5-fluorouracil and leucovorin) can be used in combination with oxaliplatin since it has similar efficacy to 5-fluorouracil; however, combination with irinotecan is not recommended due to increased toxicity (diarrhea).

Addition of biologic therapy to combination chemotherapy improves response rates and overall survival and is recommended in the first line of treatment in suitable patients. Genomic profiling to detect somatic variants (formerly, "mutations") identifies the treatments that may be most effective.

For the 50% of patients with metastatic CRC who have *KRAS/NRAS/BRAF* wild-type tumors, cetuximab and panitumumab (monoclonal antibodies to the epithelial growth factor receptor [EGFR]), in combination with chemotherapy, can extend median survival by 2 to 4 months compared with chemotherapy alone. However, for the 35% to 40% of patients with *KRAS* or *NRAS* sequence variations effective targeted therapies are not yet available. For the 5% to 10% with *BRAF* V600E sequence variations, targeted combination therapy with BRAF and EGFR inhibitors extend overall survival to 9.3 months, compared with 5.9 months for those receiving standard chemotherapy.

For the 5% with MSI or dMMR, immunotherapy may be used in first or subsequent line therapy; it has improved treatment outcomes with a median overall survival of 31.4 months in previously treated patients. Patients without a targetable sequence variation, or who have progressed on a targeted agent may be candidates for bevacizumab, a monoclonal antibody targeting VEGF. Combination of bevacizumab with FOLFOX or FOLFIRI prolongs mean survival by 2–5 months compared with either regimen alone.

When disease progresses despite treatment either with FOLFOX or with FOLFIRI (often in conjunction with bevacizumab or an EGFR-targeted antibody), therapy may be switched to the alternate regimen.

Clinical trial participation should be considered for eligible patients who are intolerant of or ineligible for standard therapies or in whom disease has progressed.

Up to 6.5% of stage IV CRC are dMMR or MSI-H. These cancers are susceptible to immune checkpoint blockade and have improved outcomes with the use of immunotherapy. Both pembrolizumab and nivolumab have been approved for the treatment of MSI-H or dMMR CRC. Additionally, both *TRK*-fusions and *HER2*-amplification can be seen in metastatic CRCs and such cancers have been shown to be responsive to targeted therapies.

Because the list of potentially actionable pathogenic variants continues to grow, extended molecular testing with a next-generation sequencing panel should be considered in all new diagnoses of metastatic CRC.

B. Rectal Cancer

The treatment approach to rectal cancer is guided by clinical staging as determined by colonoscopy and endorectal ultrasound or rectal MRI. In carefully selected patients with small (less than 4 cm), mobile, well-differentiated T1 rectal cancers that are less than 8 cm from the anal verge, transanal endoscopic or surgical excision may be considered. All other patients with rectal cancer require either a low anterior resection with a colorectal anastomosis or an abdominoperineal resection with a colostomy, depending on how far above the anal verge the cancer is located and the extent of local tumor spread.

For invasive rectal carcinoma, the combination of preoperative chemoradiation with either pre- or postoperative chemotherapy is generally recommended in all node-positive tumors and in T3 and greater tumors due to increased risk of local recurrence. The choice and timing of radiation and chemotherapy depend on a host of factors. Neoadjuvant chemoradiation has become the preferred standard in many centers because chemotherapy is more tolerable prior to surgery, leads to improved local control, and may result in improved long-term survival. For patients with clinical node-positive disease, a bulky primary cancer (T4), or a low-lying cancer that will require a permanent colostomy, giving all chemotherapy in the neoadjuvant setting (total neoadjuvant therapy) is now an option in NCCN guidelines and has become the preferred strategy for all T3 and greater tumors at many centers.

After neoadjuvant therapy, the operative approach (low anterior resection versus abdominoperineal resection with colostomy) depends on how far above the anal verge the cancer is located, its size and depth of penetration, and the patient's overall condition. Careful dissection of the entire mesorectum by either open or laparoscopic surgery reduces local recurrence to 5%. Although low anterior resections obviate a colostomy, they are associated with increased immediate postsurgical complications (eg, leak, dehiscence, stricture) and long-term defecatory complaints (eg, increased stool frequency, and incontinence). With unresectable rectal cancer, the patient may be palliated with a diverting colostomy.

Follow-Up After Surgery

Patients with CRC who have undergone resections for cure are monitored closely to look for evidence of symptomatic or asymptomatic tumor recurrence that may occasionally be amenable to curative resection. Patients should be evaluated every 3–6 months for 2 years and then every 6 months for a total of 5 years with history, physical examination, and laboratory surveillance, including serum CEA levels if baseline levels are elevated. The NCCN and American Society of Clinical Oncology guidelines recommend surveillance contrast CT scans of chest, abdomen, and pelvis up to every 6–12 months for up to 5 years postresection in high-risk stage II and all stage III patients. Patients who had a complete preoperative colonoscopy should undergo another colonoscopy 1 year after surgical resection. Patients who did not undergo full colonoscopy preoperatively should undergo a full colonoscopy after completion of all adjuvant therapy to exclude other synchronous colorectal neoplasms. If a colonoscopy does not detect new adenomatous polyps 1 year postoperatively, surveillance colonoscopy should be performed every 3–5 years thereafter to look for metachronous polyps or cancer. New onset of symptoms or a rising CEA warrants investigation with chest, abdominal, and pelvic CT and colonoscopy to look for a new primary tumor or recurrence, or metachronous metastatic disease that may be amenable to curative or palliative therapy. Most CRC recurrences occur within 3 years of the conclusion of treatment, and almost all (greater than 90%) occur within 5 years.

Prognosis

The stage of disease at presentation remains the most important determinant of 5-year survival in CRC, which is estimated in older registries as: stage I, greater than 90%; stage II, 70–85%; stage III with fewer than four positive lymph nodes, 67%; stage III with more than four positive lymph nodes, 33%; and stage IV, 5–7%. Long-term registry follow-up data from the modern chemotherapy era are not yet available. For each stage, rectal cancers have a worse prognosis. For those patients whose disease progresses despite therapy, meticulous efforts at palliative care are essential (see Chapter 5).

Screening for Colorectal Neoplasms

CRC is ideal for screening because it is a common disease that is fatal in almost 50% of cases and yet is curable if detected at an earlier stage. Furthermore, most cases arise from benign adenomatous or serrated polyps that progress over many years to cancer, and removal of these polyps has been shown to prevent the majority of cancers. CRC screening is endorsed by the USPSTF, the ACS, the NCCN, and every professional gastroenterology and colorectal surgery society. Although there is continued debate about the optimal cost-effective means of providing population screening, there is now almost unanimous consent that screening of some kind should be offered to all adults ages 45–75 years. The 2018 ACS and 2021 USPSTF recommendations for screening are listed in Table 39-6. Due to a rising incidence of CRC in adults younger than 50 years, the 2021 American College of Gastroenterology (ACG), 2021 USPSTF, and 2018 ACS guidelines all endorse consideration of screening in asymptomatic, average-risk adults beginning at age 45 years, and at younger ages for high-risk adults (such as those with a history of IBD or primary sclerosing cholangitis, or those with a family history of a first-degree relative with colorectal neoplasia [Table 39-6]).

The potential for harm from screening must be weighed against the likelihood of benefit, especially in older patients with comorbid illnesses and shorter life expectancy. Although routine screening is not recommended in adults above age 75 years, it may be considered on a case-by-case basis in adults aged 76–85 years, taking into account the patient's overall health and functional status and their prior screening history (Grade C recommendation).

Patients with first-degree relatives with colorectal neoplasms (cancer or adenomatous polyps) are at increased risk. Therefore, most guidelines recommend initiating screening at age 40–50 years (or 10 years younger than the familial diagnosis) in individuals with first-degree relatives with CRC or with advanced adenomas. Recommendations for screening in families with inherited cancer syndromes or IBD are provided in Chapter 15.

Table 39–6. Recommendations for colorectal cancer screening,[1] based on 2021 USPSTF and 2018 American Cancer Society recommendations.[2]

Average-risk individuals aged ≥ 45 years[2]
Annual fecal occult blood testing using higher sensitivity tests (Hemoccult SENSA)
Annual fecal immunochemical test (FIT)
Fecal DNA test (with FIT every 1–3 years)
Flexible sigmoidoscopy every 5 years
Colonoscopy every 10 years
CT colonography every 5 years
Individuals with a family history of a first-degree relative with colorectal neoplasia
Single first-degree relative with colorectal cancer diagnosed at age 60 years or older: Begin screening at age 40 years. Screening guidelines same as average-risk individual; however, preferred method is colonoscopy every 10 years.
Single first-degree relative with colorectal cancer or advanced adenoma diagnosed before age 60 years, or two first-degree relatives: Begin screening at age 40 years or at age 10 years younger than age at diagnosis of the youngest affected relative, whichever is first in time. Recommended screening: colonoscopy every 5 years.

[1]For recommendations for families with inherited polyposis syndromes or hereditary nonpolyposis colon cancer, see Chapter 15.
[2]The American Cancer Society recommends screening of average-risk adults aged 45–75 years; the USPSTF recommends screening of all adults aged 50–75 years (Grade A recommendation) and aged 45–49 years (Grade B). Both the American Cancer Society and USPSTF recommend screening in selected patients aged 76–85 years based on overall health, life expectancy, patient preferences, and prior screening results.

Screening tests may be classified into two broad categories: stool-based tests and examinations that visualize the structure of the colon by direct endoscopic inspection or radiographic imaging. The advantages and disadvantages of available tests are summarized below and should be discussed with patients prior to study selection. The US Multisociety Task Force and the 2021 ACG guidelines endorse the fecal immunochemical testing (FIT) and colonoscopy as the preferred stool-based and imaging-based screening modalities, respectively. However, the "best" test may be that which the patient agrees to do and then completes.

A. Stool-Based Tests

1. Fecal occult blood test—Most CRCs and some large adenomas result in increased chronic blood loss. A variety of tests for fecal occult blood are commercially available that have varying sensitivities and specificities for colorectal neoplasia. These include guaiac-based fecal occult blood testing (gFOBT) (eg, Hemoccult SENSA) that detects the pseudoperoxidase activity of heme or hemoglobin and testing that detects human globin (FIT). In clinical trials, FIT has proven superior to gFOBT in sensitivity for detection of CRC and advanced adenomas with similar specificity.

Because FIT is not affected by diet or medications and has superior accuracy, its use is preferred by many health care plans instead of gFOBT. FIT is also a suitable option for patients seeking a noninvasive screening test who are willing to undertake annual fecal testing. Patients with a positive FIT test must undergo further evaluation with colonoscopy. In 14 clinical studies (n = 45,403), the pooled sensitivity and specificity of FIT for CRC in average-risk patients were 74% and 94%, respectively, and in four studies (n = 12,424), FIT with stool DNA had pooled sensitivity of 93% and specificity of 85%. FIT testing is also the preferred option for population-based screening in various European and Australian programs.

2. Multitarget stool DNA assay—Stool DNA panel testing measures gene variants and methylated gene markers from exfoliated tumor cells. Fecal DNA panel testing is more sensitive but less specific than FIT, and as a result, has a higher false-positive rate. It is also more expensive than FIT.

The Cologuard test combines a fecal DNA panel with a FIT. In a prospective comparative trial conducted in persons at average risk for CRC undergoing colonoscopy, the sensitivity for CRC for Cologuard was 92.3% versus 73.8% for FIT alone and the sensitivity for adenomas larger than 1 cm or serrated polyps for Cologuard was 42.4% versus 23.8% for FIT alone. A positive stool DNA panel test requires colonoscopy evaluation.

B. Endoscopic Examinations of the Colon

1. Colonoscopy—Colonoscopy permits examination of the entire colon. In addition to detecting early cancers, colonoscopy allows removal of adenomatous polyps by biopsy or polypectomy, which is believed to reduce the risk of subsequent cancer. Over the past decade, there has been a dramatic increase in screening colonoscopy, with over 60% of US adults screened in the past 10 years. In asymptomatic individuals between 50 and 75 years of age undergoing screening colonoscopy, the prevalence of advanced colonic neoplasia is 4–11% and of colon cancer is 0.1–1%.

Although colonoscopy is believed to be the most sensitive test for detecting adenomas and cancer, it has several disadvantages. Adequate visualization of the entire colonic mucosa requires thorough bowel cleansing the evening and morning prior to the examination. To alleviate discomfort during the procedure, intravenous sedation is used for most patients, necessitating a companion to transport the patient home post-procedure. Serious complications occur uncommonly; they include perforation (0.1%), bleeding (0.25%), and death (2.9/100,000).

The skill of the operator has a major impact upon the quality of the colonoscopy examination. In several studies, the rate of CRC within 3 years of a screening colonoscopy was 0.7–0.9%, ie, approximately 1 in 110 patients. Population-based case-control and cohort studies suggest that colonoscopy is associated with greater reduction in CRC incidence and mortality in the distal colon (80%) than the proximal colon (40–60%). This may be attributable to incomplete examination of the proximal colon, and differences between the proximal and distal colon that include worse bowel preparation, suboptimal colonoscopic technique, and a higher prevalence of serrated polyps and flat adenomas, which are more difficult to identify than raised (sessile or pedunculated) polyps. To optimize diagnostic accuracy as well as patient safety and comfort, colonoscopy should be performed after optimal bowel preparation by a well-trained endoscopist who spends sufficient time (at least 7 minutes) carefully examining the colon (especially the proximal colon) while withdrawing the endoscope.

2. Flexible sigmoidoscopy—Use of a 60-cm flexible sigmoidoscope permits visualization of the rectosigmoid and descending colon. Adenomatous polyps are identified in 10–20% and CRCs in 1% of patients. The finding at sigmoidoscopy of an adenomatous polyp in the distal colon increases the likelihood at least twofold that an advanced neoplasm is present in the proximal colon. In four randomized clinical trials (n = 458,002), intention to screen with 1- or 2-time flexible sigmoidoscopy versus no screening was associated with a significant decrease in CRC-specific mortality (incidence rate ratio, 0.74 [95% CI, 0.68–0.80]).

The chief disadvantage of screening with flexible sigmoidoscopy is that it requires some bowel cleansing, it may be associated with some discomfort (since intravenous sedation is not used), and it does not examine the proximal colon. The prevalence of proximal versus distal neoplasia is higher in persons older than age 65 years, in Black adults, and in women.

C. Radiographic and Other Imaging of the Colon

1. CT colonography— CT colonography requires a similar bowel cleansing regimen as colonoscopy as well as insufflation of air into the colon through a rectal tube, which may be associated with discomfort.

Using imaging software with multidetector helical scanners, the sensitivity is greater than 95% for the detection of cancer and 86% for the detection of adenomatous polyps 6 mm or larger. CT colonography is less sensitive than colonoscopy for the detection of flat adenomas and serrated polyps.

The chief disadvantages of CT colonography are the need for a bowel preparation, limited availability in many health care systems, potential harms resulting from (repeated) low-dose ionizing radiation exposure, and the potential for finding incidental extracolonic findings that may lead to further evaluations. CT colonography is an excellent screening option in patients who do not wish to undergo or are unsuitable for colonoscopy and in patients in whom colonoscopy could not be completed.

2. Capsule colonoscopy—Imaging of the colon can be accomplished by oral ingestion of a capsule that captures video images of the colon. Compared with colonoscopy, the colon capsule has reduced sensitivity for polyps greater than 6 mm (64% versus 84%) and for CRCs (74% versus 100%). At present, it is approved by the FDA for evaluation in patients who are not suitable candidates for colonoscopy or in whom colonoscopy could not evaluate the proximal colon. In addition to its suboptimal sensitivity for neoplasia, the main disadvantages of capsule colonoscopy are its cost, need for extensive bowel preparation, varying reimbursement by insurance carriers, and small risk of small bowel obstruction.

When to Refer

- Patients with symptoms (change in bowel habits, hematochezia), signs (mass on abdominal examination or digital rectal examination [DRE]), or laboratory tests (iron deficiency anemia) suggestive of colorectal neoplasia should be referred for colonoscopy.
- Patients with suspected CRC or adenomatous polyps of any size should be referred for colonoscopy.
- Virtually all patients with proven CRC should be referred to a surgeon for resection. Patients with clinical stage T3 or node-positive rectal tumors (or both) also should be referred to medical and radiation oncologists preoperatively for neoadjuvant therapy. Patients with stage II, III, or IV colorectal tumors should be referred to a medical oncologist.

When to Admit

- Patients with complications of CRC (eg, obstruction, acute bleeding) requiring urgent evaluation and intervention.
- Patients with advanced metastatic disease requiring palliative care.

Biller LH et al. Diagnosis and treatment of metastatic colorectal cancer: a review. JAMA. 2021;325:669. [PMID: 33591350]

Burnett-Hartman AN et al. An update on the epidemiology, molecular characterization, diagnosis, and screening strategies for early-onset colorectal cancer. Gastroenterology. 2021;160:1041. [PMID: 33417940]

Lin JS et al. Screening for colorectal cancer: updated evidence report and systematic review for the US Preventive Services Task Force. JAMA. 2021;325:1978. [PMID: 34003220]

National Comprehensive Cancer Network. Colon Cancer, Version 1.2022, NCCN Clinical Practice Guidelines in Oncology. 2022 Feb 25. https://www.nccn.org/professionals/physician_gls/pdf/colon.pdf

National Comprehensive Cancer Network. Rectal Cancer, Version 1.2022, NCCN Clinical Practice Guidelines in Oncology. 2022 Feb 25. https://www.nccn.org/professionals/physician_gls/pdf/rectal.pdf

Shaukat A et al. ACG Clinical Guidelines: colorectal screening 2021. Am J Gastroenterol. 2021;116:458. [PMID: 33657038]

US Preventive Services Task Force. Colorectal Cancer: Screening 2021 May 18. https://www.uspreventiveservicestaskforce.org/uspstf/recommendation/colorectal-cancer-screening

CARCINOMA OF THE ANUS

Cancers arising from the mucosa of the anal canal are relatively rare, comprising only 2% of all GI malignancies. Anal carcinoma occurred in an estimated 8590 patients in the United States in 2020, more commonly in women than men (2:1 ratio). **Squamous cell carcinomas** (SCC) make up the majority of anal cancers; **adenocarcinomas** are uncommon.

Over 90% of anal cancers are associated with HPV infections (most commonly, HPV-16 and -18). Anal cancer is increased among women with HPV-associated cervical, vulvar or vaginal squamous intraepithelial lesions (CIN grade 3) or cancer, among men who are having sex with men, and among women and men who have HIV or have received a solid organ transplant.

Identification and screening of high-risk individuals with HPV testing and anal cytology facilitates detection of anal low- and high-grade squamous intraepithelial lesions (LSIL and HSIL, respectively) and early-stage cancers. Anoscopy (preferably high-resolution) with biopsy is warranted in patients with positive cytology. It is hypothesized that early detection and treatment of HSIL with either topical treatment or surgical ablation may reduce progression to advanced cancer. However, this has not yet been shown in prospective randomized studies and topical therapies are not yet FDA-approved.

The most common symptoms of anal carcinoma are bleeding, pain, and local mass. The lesion is often confused with hemorrhoids or other common anal disorders. These tumors tend to become annular, invade the sphincter, and spread upward via the lymphatics into the perirectal mesenteric lymphatic nodes. CT or MRI scans of the abdomen and pelvis are required to identify regional lymphadenopathy or metastatic disease at diagnosis; PET imaging may be used in conjunction.

Treatment depends on the tumor location, histology, and stage. Well-differentiated and small (less than 2 cm) superficial lesions of the perianal skin may be treated with wide local excision.

Squamous cell carcinoma of the anal canal as well as large perianal tumors invading the sphincter or rectum are treated with combined-modality external radiation with simultaneous chemotherapy (5-fluorouracil plus mitomycin). Local control is achieved in approximately 80% of patients. Radical surgery (abdominoperineal resection) is reserved for patients who fail chemotherapy and radiation therapy.

The 5-year survival rate is 81% for localized tumors and 30% for metastatic disease. No standard therapies beyond first line are established for advanced squamous cell anal carcinoma though metastatic disease is generally treated with carboplatin and paclitaxel. Checkpoint inhibitor therapy should be strongly considered in the second-line setting in patients with good performance status.

Treatment of **anal adenocarcinoma** is like that of rectal adenocarcinoma (see above), typically by trimodality therapy with chemoradiotherapy, chemotherapy and abdominoperineal resection.

Brogden DRL et al. Evaluating the efficacy of treatment options for anal intraepithelial neoplasia: a systematic review. Int J Colorectal Dis. 2021;36:213. [PMID: 32979069]

Lonardi S et al. Randomized phase II trial of avelumab alone or in combination with cetuximab for patients with previously treated, locally advanced, or metastatic squamous cell anal carcinoma: the CARACAS study. J Immunother Cancer. 2021;9:e002996. [PMID: 34815354]

National Cancer Institute. SEER Cancer Stat Facts: Anal Cancer, 2022. https://seer.cancer.gov/statfacts/html/anus.html

National Comprehensive Cancer Network. Anal Carcinoma, Version 1.2022, NCCN Clinical Practice Guidelines in Oncology. Version 1.2022. 2022 Mar 2. https://www.nccn.org/professionals/physician_gls/pdf/anal.pdf

CANCERS OF THE GENITOURINARY TRACT

Marc A. Dall'Era, MD

PROSTATE CANCER

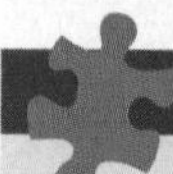

ESSENTIALS OF DIAGNOSIS

- Prostatic induration on DRE or elevation of PSA.
- Most often asymptomatic.
- Rarely: systemic symptoms (weight loss, bone pain).

General Considerations

Prostate cancer is the most common noncutaneous cancer and the second leading cause of cancer-related death in American men with an estimated 248,530 new prostate cancer diagnoses and 34,130 prostate cancer deaths in 2021. The clinical incidence, however, does not match the prevalence of the disease. Autopsy studies have demonstrated that more than 40% of men over age 50 years have prostate cancer, and its prevalence increases with age with 30% of men aged 60–69 years and 67% of men aged 80–89 years harboring the disease at autopsy. Prostate cancer is an extremely heterogenous disease and most of these occult cancers are small, indolent, and organ-confined cancers with few occult cancers having regional or metastatic disease. Although the global prevalence of prostatic cancer at autopsy is relatively consistent, the clinical incidence varies considerably (highest in North America, Europe, the Caribbean, Australia/New Zealand, and Southern Africa, and lowest in Northern Africa and Asia). In 2020, prostate cancer was the leading cause of cancer death among men in 48 countries. A 50-year-old American man has a lifetime risk of 40% for latent cancer, a 16% risk for developing clinically apparent cancer, and a 2.9% risk of death due to prostatic cancer. Black race, family history of prostatic cancer, and history of high dietary fat intake are risk factors for prostate cancer.

Clinical Findings

A. Symptoms and Signs

Presently, most prostate cancers are asymptomatic and are diagnosed because of elevations in serum PSA. However, some cases of prostate cancer are diagnosed based on discrete nodules or areas of induration within the prostate on a DRE. Obstructive voiding symptoms are most often due to benign prostatic hyperplasia, which occurs in the same age group. Nevertheless, large or locally extensive prostatic cancers can cause obstructive voiding symptoms, including urinary retention. Lymph node metastases can lead to lower extremity lymphedema, though this is extremely unusual. Because the axial skeleton is the most common site of metastases, patients may present with back pain, pathologic fractures, or rarely neurologic symptoms from epidural metastases and cord compression.

Table 39–7. Screening for prostate cancer: test performance.

Test	Sensitivity	Specificity	Positive Predictive Value
Abnormal PSA (> 4 ng/mL [mcg/L])	0.67	0.97	0.43
Abnormal DRE	0.50	0.94	0.24
Abnormal PSA or DRE	0.84	0.92	0.28
Abnormal PSA and DRE	0.34	0.995	0.49

DRE, digital rectal examination.
From Annals of Internal Medicine, Kramer BS et al.
Prostate cancer screening: what we know and what we need to know, 119(9): 914–23.

B. Laboratory Findings

1. Serum tumor markers—PSA is a glycoprotein produced only by prostatic cells, either benign or malignant. The serum level is typically low and correlates with the total volume of prostate tissue and tends to increase with age. Measurement of serum PSA is useful in detecting and staging prostate cancer, monitoring response to treatment, and identifying recurrence before it becomes clinically evident. As a screening test, PSA is elevated (greater than 4.0 ng/mL [4.0 mcg/L]) in 10–15% of men. PSA is not specific for cancer, and there is considerable overlap of values with men with benign prostate hyperplasia. The sensitivity, specificity, and positive predictive value of PSA and DRE are listed in Table 39–7. It is important to realize that a PSA reference range of less than or equal to 4.0 ng/mL is not appropriate for all men and that no PSA threshold excludes the diagnosis of prostate cancer (Table 39–8). More recent data suggest that a man's baseline PSA in his 50s is associated with long-term prostate cancer risk. Median PSA levels for men aged 40–49 years and 50–59 years are 0.7 ng/mL and 0.9 ng/mL, respectively. Baseline PSA level may assist with patient counseling regarding long-term prostate cancer risk and set appropriate screening intervals. Prostate cancer will be diagnosed in approximately 18–30% of men with PSA 4.1–10 ng/mL (4.1–10 mcg/L) and 50–70% of men with PSA greater than 10 ng/mL (10 mcg/L).

In untreated patients with prostate cancer, the level of PSA correlates with the volume and stage of disease. Patients with PSA levels less than 10 ng/mL (10 mcg/L) usually have localized and therefore potentially curable cancers with local therapy alone, while those with PSA levels greater than 40 ng/mL (40 mcg/L) are more likely to have advanced disease (seminal vesicle invasion, lymph node involvement, or occult distant metastases). Approximately 98% of patients with metastatic prostate cancer will have an elevated PSA level yet treatment decisions cannot be made based on PSA testing alone. A rising PSA after therapy is usually consistent with progressive disease, either locally recurrent or metastatic.

Table 39–8. Risk of prostate cancer in men with PSA ≤ 4.0 ng/mL (or mcg/L).

PSA Level (ng/mL [or mcg/L])	Percentage with Prostate Cancer	Percentage with High-Grade[1] Prostate Cancer
≤ 0.5	6.6	12.5
0.6–1.0	10.1	10.0
1.1–2.0	17.0	11.8
2.1–3.0	23.9	19.1
3.1–4.0	26.9	25.0

[1]High-grade cancer was defined as Gleason score ≥ 7.
Data from Thompson IM et al. Prevalence of prostate cancer among men with a prostate-specific antigen level ≤ 4.0 ng per milliliter. N Engl J Med. 2004;350:2239.

2. Miscellaneous laboratory testing—Patients with urinary retention or with ureteral obstruction due to locoregionally advanced prostate cancers may present with elevations in BUN or serum creatinine. Patients with bony metastases may have elevations in serum alkaline phosphatase or calcium. Laboratory and clinical evidence of disseminated intravascular coagulation can occur in patients with advanced prostate cancers.

3. Prostate biopsy—Ultrasound-guided biopsy is the standard method for detection of prostate cancer. A decision to recommend a prostate biopsy is generally not made on PSA levels alone but after careful prostate cancer risk assessment based on additional biomarker or imaging studies (Figure 39–2). The use of a spring-loaded, 18-gauge biopsy needle has allowed prostate biopsy to be performed with minimal patient discomfort and morbidity. Local anesthesia is standard and increases the tolerability of the procedure. While a transrectal approach is still most commonly practiced, rising rates of post-biopsy infection and sepsis have led to increasing utilization of transperineal biopsies. The specimen preserves glandular architecture and permits accurate grading. Prostate biopsy specimens are taken from all areas of the prostate including the apex, mid-portion, base and anterior gland. While extended-pattern biopsies, including a total of at least 10 biopsies, are associated with improved cancer detection and risk stratification of patients with newly diagnosed disease, suspicious hypoechoic prostatic lesions seen on transrectal ultrasound or pre-biopsy MRI may be targeted for biopsy. Patients with abnormalities of the seminal vesicles can have these structures specifically biopsied to identify local tumor invasion.

C. Imaging

Multiparametric MRI (mpMRI) has emerged as the imaging study of choice for localized prostate cancer detection and characterization. Prior to prostate cancer diagnosis, particularly among men with previous negative prostate biopsies, mpMRI is used to evaluate for suspicious

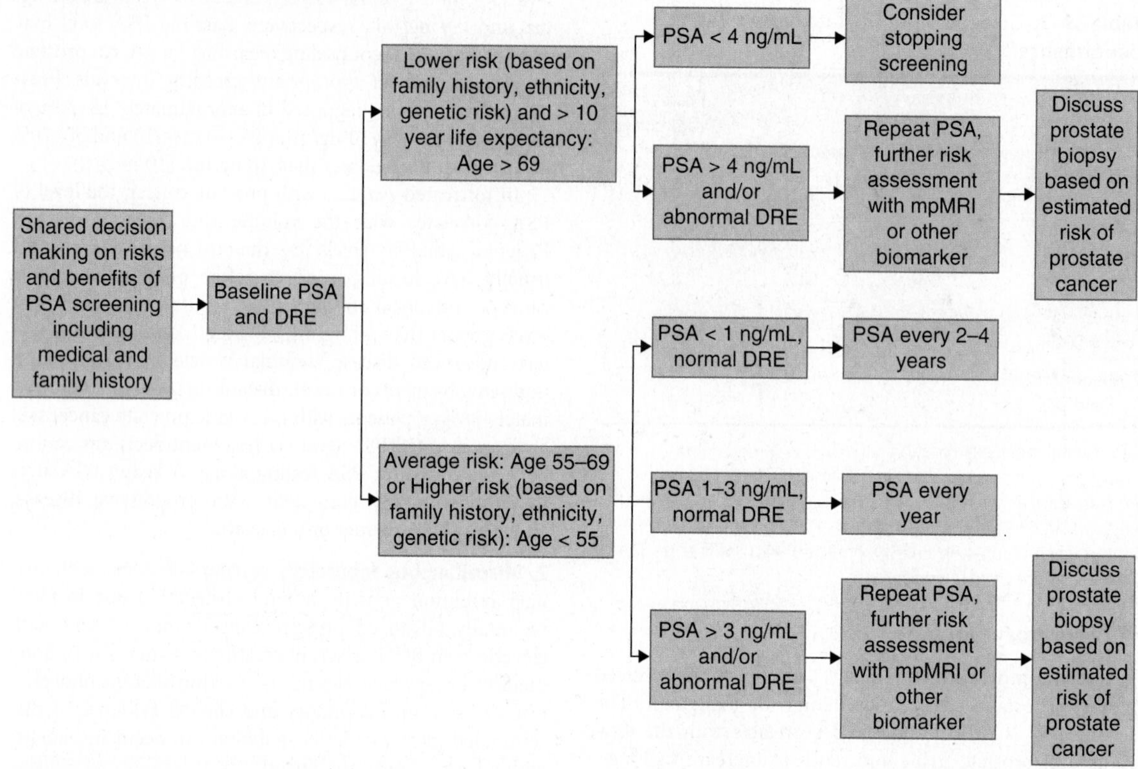

▲ **Figure 39–2.** An algorithm for prostate cancer early detection. DRE, digital rectal examination; mpMRI, multiparametric magnetic resonance imaging.

prostatic lesions and to aid in the decision to undergo prostate biopsy. Such lesions may then be sampled via MRI-guided needle biopsy or via MR Fusion (in which prostate MRI images are fused in real-time with images from an ultrasound-guided needle biopsy). Such an approach may improve not only overall cancer detection but discovery of potentially life-threatening disease while limiting overdetection of indolent prostate cancer or unnecessary prostate biopsies.

Use of imaging for staging should be tailored to the likelihood of advanced disease in newly diagnosed cases. Asymptomatic patients with low- to intermediate-grade cancers, thought to be localized to the prostate on DRE and **transrectal ultrasonography** and associated with modest elevations of PSA (ie, less than 10 ng/mL [10 mcg/L]), need no further imaging. Cross-sectional imaging with **CT or MRI** of the abdomen and pelvis and **radionuclide (99-technetium) bone scans** are generally the first-line staging studies performed, when indicated, to assess for nodal and bony metastases, respectively.

Conventional **radionuclide (99-technetium) bone scans** are superior to conventional plain skeletal radiographs in detecting bony metastases. Prostate cancer bony metastases tend to be multiple and most commonly occur in the axial skeleton. **Fluciclovine (Axumin) PET imaging** has been approved for suspected cancer recurrence based on elevated PSA after prior treatment and may also be useful in the early disease staging. **PSMA (prostate-specific membrane antigen) PET**, using small-molecule radiotracers targeting PSMA has shown significant promise as a next-generation imaging method and very likely will replace traditional imaging modalities in the near future. In 2021, the FDA approved both ^{68}Ga PSMA-11 and piflufolastat F 18 (Pylarify) injections, as PSMA–targeted PET imaging agents, to identify suspected metastasis or recurrence of prostate cancer. Both should be widely available for clinical use soon.

D. Genetic and Molecular Testing

The role of genetics and molecular testing in prostate cancer diagnosis and management is evolving. A family history of prostate cancer and certain other malignancies such as breast or ovarian cancer increases the risk of prostate cancer. Additionally, prostate cancer has been associated with several hereditary cancer syndromes (eg, Lynch syndrome, hereditary breast and ovarian cancer syndrome, etc.) with approximately 11% of patients with prostate cancer with at least one additional primary cancer carrying germline pathogenic variations. Consequently, some patients with prostate cancer and their families may have elevated risk for other cancers. Further, data suggest that some germline variations, such as *BRCA1/2*, are associated with lower PSA at diagnosis and increased risk of progression and death; approximately 12% of patients with metastatic prostate cancer have germline pathogenic variations in homologous

DNA repair genes. Finally, germline pathogenic variations in DNA repair genes can have implications for treatment and, as a result, play a role in personalized treatment. Patients with prostate cancer should have a thorough review of their family history and those with any concern, referred for genetic counseling and possible testing. Additionally, patients with high-risk disease or metastatic disease should undergo genetic evaluation as well. NCCN guidelines recommend considering germline genetic testing in men presenting with localized high-risk, regionally advanced, or metastatic disease. Commercially available cancer tissue RNA-based assays are available for further risk assessment after prostate cancer diagnosis; these may help determine the need for and timing of prostate cancer treatment as well as treatment intensity.

Screening for Prostate Cancer

The impact of prostate cancer screening on mortality remains controversial. However, screening can reduce the risk of prostate cancer–specific mortality when performed in an organized fashion. Two large, randomized trials have evaluated the benefit of PSA screening for early detection of prostate cancer. In the US Prostate, Lung, Colorectal, and Ovarian (PLCO) Cancer Screening Trial, no mortality benefit was observed after combined screening with PSA testing and DRE during 15-year follow-up. Although screening resulted in a 12% increase in prostate cancer detection, the cancer-specific mortality rate was similar in the screening and control arms (2.55 and 2.44 deaths per 10,000 person-years, respectively). However, an estimated 86% of control patients received at least one screening PSA test and 46% of control patients received yearly PSA screening (versus 99% and 84%, respectively for the intervention arm) during the trial. This high degree of crossover in the control arm likely impacted the ability of this trial to detect meaningful differences in cancer detection. Other criticisms of the negative PLCO study include use of a relatively high PSA threshold (4.0 ng/mL [4.0 mcg/L]) and significant screening of men in the 3 years prior to trial enrollment (44%).

Conversely, the European Randomized Study of Screening for Prostate Cancer trial demonstrated a significant 20% reduction in prostate cancer mortality with an absolute reduction of 1.75 deaths per 1000 men screened at 16 years. The number of men needed to be invited for screening to prevent one prostate cancer death was 570 at 16 years compared with 742 at 13 years, while the number of prostate cancers needing to be diagnosed to prevent one prostate cancer death was reduced from 26 to 18, underscoring the importance of adequate long-term follow-up for prostate cancer.

Multiple practice guidelines recommend discussion and shared decision-making regarding the risks and benefits of PSA screening and prostate cancer early detection. While PSA measurement is the most widely performed method of screening, DRE is still recommended. PSA testing increases the detection rate of prostate cancers compared with DRE alone. Approximately 2–2.5% of men older than 50 years of age will be found to have prostate cancer using PSA testing compared with a rate of approximately 1.5% using DRE alone. PSA is not specific for cancer, and there is considerable overlap of values with men with benign prostate hyperplasia. PSA-detected cancers are more likely to be localized compared with those detected by DRE alone. The Prostate Cancer Prevention Trial demonstrated a significant risk of prostate cancer even in men with PSA less than or equal to 4.0 ng/mL (4.0 mcg/L) (Table 39–8) and a web-based calculator has been developed to estimate the risk of harboring both prostate cancer and high-grade cancer (http://riskcalc.org/PBCG).

The frequency of PSA testing also remains a matter of debate. The traditional yearly screening approach may not be the most efficient; rather, earlier PSA testing at younger age may allow less frequent testing later and provide information regarding PSA velocity (changes in PSA over time). Men with PSA above the age-based median when tested between ages 40–60 years are at significantly increased risk for subsequent cancer detection over 25 years. Men aged 40–50 with PSA below 0.6 ng/mL (0.6 mcg/L) and aged 50–60 years with PSA below 0.71 ng/mL (0.71 mcg/L) may require less frequent PSA testing. In addition, men with PSA velocity greater than 0.35 ng/mL (0.35 mcg/L) per year measured 10–15 years before diagnosis had significantly worse cancer-specific survival compared with those with lower PSA velocity. A secondary data analysis from the PLCO trial also demonstrated that baseline PSA for younger men in their 50s can predict long-term risk of prostate cancer and can be used to tailor PSA screening intervals. Men with a baseline PSA of less than 1 ng/mL had a 1.5% incidence of prostate cancer at 13 years compared with 29.5% of men with baseline PSA levels greater than 4 ng/mL. The NCCN guidelines (https://www.nccn.org/professionals/physician_gls/pdf/prostate.pdf) for prostate cancer early detection incorporate many of these factors (Figure 39–2). The European Association of Urology recommends offering PSA screening to men beginning at age 40–50 years, dependent on risk factors, and subsequently initiating a risk-adapted strategy.

In 2018, the USPSTF issued a revised (Grade C) recommendation for men aged 55–69 years that the decision to undergo periodic PSA-based screening should be an individual one. Before deciding about screening, men should discuss its potential benefits and harms with their clinician, incorporating their own values and preferences in the decision. The revised recommendation acknowledges that, while screening offers some men a small potential benefit of reducing the chance of dying from prostate cancer, many other men will experience potential harms from screening. These include false-positive results that require additional testing and possible prostate biopsy; overdiagnosis and overtreatment of non–life-threatening disease; and treatment complications, such as incontinence and erectile dysfunction. In determining whether screening is appropriate in individual cases, the individual patient's family history, race/ethnicity, comorbid medical conditions, values about the benefits and harms of screening and treatment-specific outcomes, and other health needs should be considered. Clinicians should not screen men who do not express a preference for screening. For men aged 70 years or older, the USPSTF recommends against PSA-based screening (Grade D recommendation).

In general, PSA levels in isolation should not be used to guide decisions regarding the need for prostate biopsies. Additional biomarkers and imaging are now widely used to improve risk stratification for early detection of life-threatening prostate cancers. These also include establishment of age- and race-specific reference ranges, measurement of free serum and protein-bound levels of PSA (**percent free PSA**), and calculation of **PSA velocity**. Generally, men with PSA free fractions exceeding 25% are unlikely to have prostate cancer, whereas those with free fractions less than 10% have an approximately 50% chance of having prostate cancer. Additional commercially available serum- and urine-based tests, including the Select MDx, Prostate Health Index (PHI) and 4kscore, and ExoDx, may better identify not only men at greater risk for prostate cancer but those with more aggressive disease. mpMRI is also frequently used in the screening setting after a concerning PSA level is found. Multiple studies suggest that incorporating mpMRI into a prostate cancer screening and early detection pathway can lead to fewer negative prostate biopsies while improving overall detection of higher-grade prostate cancers. However, not all prostate cancers are visualized on mpMRI with its negative predictive value of 0.75. There is also variability in MRI quality and interpretation that must be considered when using MRI as a screening test prior to referral to a urologist.

Staging

Most prostate cancers are adenocarcinomas. Most arise in the peripheral zone of the prostate, though a small percentage arise in the central (5–10%) and transition zones (20%) of the gland. Pathologists utilize the Gleason grading system whereby a "primary" grade is applied to the architectural pattern of malignant glands occupying the largest area of the specimen and a "secondary" grade is assigned to the next largest area of cancer. Grading is based on architectural rather than histologic criteria, and five "grades" are possible. Adding the score of the primary and secondary grades gives a Gleason score from 2 to 10. In current practice, however, Gleason scores of 2–5 are no longer assigned. Gleason score correlates with tumor volume, pathologic stage, and prognosis. A simplified five-grade group system has been introduced by the International Society of Urological Pathologists; it is based on Gleason score and has gained clinical traction and may help patients better understand their disease.

Treatment

A. General Measures

The optimal management of localized prostate cancer remains controversial owing to the plethora of treatment options, side effects of the various options, and indolent nature of many prostate cancers. These factors have contributed to uncertainty regarding a definitive survival benefit of treating localized prostate cancer. To help guide treatment decision-making, patients are risk stratified (very low, low, intermediate, and high-risk) according to their PSA level at diagnosis, DRE, and prostate cancer grade (Gleason score). Additionally, patients should have an assessment of life expectancy prior to treatment decision-making since all patients with low-risk disease and many with intermediate-risk disease with less than 10-year life expectancy will not benefit from immediate treatment. Prognostic tissue-based risk biomarkers are also now available to help guide treatment decisions.

B. Active Surveillance

Active surveillance is now the preferred initial treatment recommendation for men with well-differentiated prostate cancer and low-risk clinical features. The goal of active surveillance is to avoid treatment in men who may never require it while recognizing and definitively treating men harboring higher-risk disease in order to balance cancer risk with the morbidity of treatment. Treatment decisions are made based on stage, PSA, and cancer grade (Gleason score) as well as the age and health of the patient. Active surveillance alone may be effective management for appropriately selected patients, typically those with low PSA, small volume, well-differentiated cancers, and life expectancy less than 10–15 years. For such patients, active surveillance involves serial PSA levels, DREs, periodic prostate mpMRI, and biopsies to reassess grade and extent of cancer. Different than watchful waiting, the goal of active surveillance is to identify early changes in the cancer when curative intervention can still be applied. Endpoints for intervention in patients on active surveillance, particularly PSA changes, have not been clearly defined and surveillance regimens remain an active area of research. Most men are offered definitive treatment when cancer grade changes are noted on surveillance biopsy. Contemporary series demonstrate freedom from definitive treatment in greater than half of patients at 5 years, and risk of developing metastases and suffering cancer-specific death in less than 3% and 2%, respectively, at 10 years. Delayed therapy for clinical signs of progression seems to have no negative impact on survival. Active surveillance is featured prominently in the AUA, NCCN and EAU guidelines and is the preferred management in most men with low- and some intermediate-risk prostate cancer. This approach is increasingly accepted and incorporated in routine clinical practice.

Watchful waiting is the preferred treatment for men with limited life expectancy who can be followed with PSA alone in the absence of any signs or symptoms of metastatic disease.

C. Radical Prostatectomy

During radical prostatectomy, the seminal vesicles, prostate, and ampullae of the vas deferens are removed. Refinements in technique have allowed preservation of urinary continence in most patients and erectile function in selected patients. Radical prostatectomy can be performed via open retropubic, transperineal, or laparoscopic (with or without robotic assistance) surgery. Local recurrence is uncommon after radical prostatectomy and related to pathologic stage. Organ-confined cancers rarely recur; however, cancers with adverse pathologic features (capsular penetration, seminal vesicle invasion) are associated with higher local (10–25%) and distant (20–50%) relapse rates.

Ideal candidates for radical prostatectomy include healthy patients with stages T1 and T2 prostate cancers. Patients with advanced local tumors (T4) or lymph node metastases are rarely candidates for prostatectomy alone, although surgery is sometimes used in combination with hormonal therapy and postoperative radiation therapy for select high-risk patients. Twenty-nine-year follow-up from the Scandinavian Prostate Cancer Group Study Number 4 randomized trial comparing radical prostatectomy to watchful waiting in men with localized prostate cancer demonstrated a prostate cancer survival advantage with surgery (RR 0.55, 95% CI 0.41–0.74) with an absolute difference in risk of 11.7%. The ProtecT trial randomized 1632 primarily low- and intermediate-risk men with clinically localized prostate cancer to either active monitoring, surgery, or radiotherapy. At 10 years follow-up, prostate cancer–specific mortality was low in all three groups and differences were not significant, though both surgery and radiotherapy were associated with lower rates of disease progression and metastases ($P < 0.001$ and $P = 0.004$, respectively). An undetectable PSA (less than 0.1 ng/mL) after surgery suggests no signs of residual or recurrent disease and no further imaging is required.

D. Radiation Therapy

Radiation can be delivered by a variety of techniques to the prostate and, when clinically indicated, to the pelvic lymph nodes. Conformal techniques, including three-dimensional conformal radiation, intensity-modulated radiotherapy, and image-guided radiotherapy, have become the standard of care for external photon-based radiotherapy, while proton beam therapy has gained acceptance as an alternative external beam therapy that theoretically may reduce toxicities. Additionally, hypofractionated and ultra-hypofractionated (ie, stereotactic radiotherapy) regimens have shown promising short- and intermediate-term outcomes versus conventionally dosed regimens. Low- and high-dose rate brachytherapy—the implantation of permanent or temporary radioactive sources (palladium, iodine, or iridium) into the prostate—can be used as monotherapy in those with low-grade or low-volume malignancies or combined with external beam radiation in patients with higher-grade or higher-volume disease. The PSA may initially rise after brachytherapy because of prostate inflammation and necrosis. This transient elevation ("PSA bounce") should not be mistaken for recurrence and may occur up to 20 months after treatment. Patients with intermediate- and high-risk disease benefit from concomitant androgen deprivation therapy for a specified period, which can be up to several years for men with high-grade, high-volume disease. As with surgery, the likelihood of local failure following radiation correlates with technique and cancer characteristics. The likelihood of a positive prostate biopsy more than 18 months after radiation varies between 20% and 60%. Patients with local recurrence are at an increased risk of cancer progression and cancer death compared with those who have negative biopsies. Survival of patients with localized cancers (T1, T2, and selected T3) approaches 65% at 10 years. Ambiguous target definitions, inadequate radiation doses, and understaging of the cancer may be responsible for the failure noted in some series.

E. Focal Therapy

To reduce the morbidity of localized prostate cancer treatment, there has been a growing interest in focal therapy. Focal therapy delivers energy to the prostate, destroying the tumor(s) and a margin of normal prostate tissue while avoiding collateral damage to the neurovascular bundles, external urinary sphincter, bladder, and rectum. To date, several energy sources (cryotherapy, high intensity focused ultrasound, lasers, etc) have been evaluated and several others are under development. The multifocal nature and the difficulty of localizing the prostate cancer with contemporary imaging techniques combined with the prolonged disease course, lack of clearly defined endpoints, and lack of randomized prospective data have limited the widespread adoption of focal therapies as well as a clear understanding of which are the ideal candidates.

F. Treatment for Locally and Regionally Advanced Disease

Those patients with high-risk or locally extensive cancers, including seminal vesicle and bladder neck invasion, are at increased risk for both local and distant relapse despite local therapy and often require multimodal approaches to treatment. Patients with advanced pathologic stage or positive surgical margins after prostatectomy are at an increased risk for local and distant tumor relapse. Due to these risks, such patients have been considered for adjuvant therapy (radiation for positive margins and seminal vesicle invasion or androgen deprivation or radiation, or both, for lymph node metastases). Two randomized clinical trials (EORTC 22911 and SWOG 8794) demonstrated improved progression-free and metastasis-free survival with early radiotherapy in these men, and subsequent analysis of SWOG 8794 showed improved overall survival in men receiving adjuvant radiation therapy. However, the publication of two trials comparing adjuvant radiotherapy with early-salvage therapy using contemporary radiotherapy techniques (GETUG-AFU17 and RAVES) demonstrated no difference in 5-year biochemical progression-free survival casting doubt on the benefit of adjuvant radiotherapy in the contemporary era.

A variety of investigational regimens are also being tested in an effort to improve cancer outcomes. Combination therapy (androgen deprivation combined with surgery or irradiation), newer forms of irradiation, and hormonal therapy alone are being tested, as is neoadjuvant and adjuvant chemotherapy. For patients with intermediate- and high-risk disease, neoadjuvant and adjuvant androgen deprivation therapy combined with external beam radiation therapy have demonstrated improved survival compared with external beam radiation therapy alone.

G. Metastatic Disease

Since death due to prostate carcinoma is almost invariably the result of failure to control metastatic disease, research has emphasized efforts to improve control of distant disease. Most prostate carcinomas are hormone dependent, and approximately 70–80% of men with metastatic prostate carcinoma will respond to various forms of androgen deprivation. **Androgen deprivation therapy** may be effective at several levels along the pituitary–gonadal axis using a variety of methods or agents (Table 39–9). Use of LH-releasing hormone (LHRH) agonists (leuprolide, goserelin) achieves medical castration without orchiectomy and is the most common method of reducing testosterone levels. A single LHRH antagonist (degarelix) is FDA-approved and has no short-term testosterone "flare" associated with LHRH agonists. Because of its rapid onset of action, **ketoconazole** should be considered in patients with advanced prostate cancer who present with spinal cord compression, bilateral ureteral obstruction, or disseminated intravascular coagulation. Although testosterone is the major circulating androgen, the adrenal gland secretes the androgens dehydroepiandrosterone, dehydroepiandrosterone sulfate, and androstenedione. This finding has led to the development of **abiraterone acetate** (an inhibitor of CYP17, a key enzyme in androgen synthesis) to block both testicular and adrenal androgens. Nonsteroidal antiandrogen agents act by competitively binding the receptor for dihydrotestosterone, the intracellular androgen responsible for prostate cell growth and development. In addition to immediate side effects of androgen deprivation (sexual dysfunction and hot flashes), the chronic suppression of testosterone leads to osteoporosis and risk of fractures, CVD and diabetes mellitus, and decreased muscle and increased fat. **Bisphosphonates** can prevent osteoporosis associated with androgen deprivation, decrease bone pain from metastases, and reduce skeletal-related events. **Denosumab**, a RANK ligand inhibitor, is approved for the

Table 39–9. Androgen deprivation for prostate cancer.

Level	Agent	Dose	Sequelae
Pituitary, hypothalamus	Diethylstilbestrol	1–3 mg orally daily	Gynecomastia, hot flushes, thromboembolic disease, erectile dysfunction
	LHRH agonists		
	Leuprolide	Daily subcutaneous injection	Erectile dysfunction, hot flushes, gynecomastia, rarely anemia
	Goserelin	Monthly to quarterly depot injection	
	Triptorelin	Monthly depot injection	
	Histrelin	Annual subcutaneous implant	
	LHRH antagonist		
	Degarelix	240 mg subcutaneously initial dose, then 80 mg subcutaneously monthly	Hot flushes, weight gain, erectile dysfunction, increased liver tests
Adrenal	Ketoconazole	400 mg three times orally daily	Adrenal insufficiency, nausea, rash, ataxia
	Aminoglutethimide	250 mg four times orally daily	Adrenal insufficiency, nausea, rash, ataxia
	Corticosteroid		
	Prednisone	20–40 mg orally daily	GI bleeding, fluid retention
	CYP17a1 inhibitor		
	Abiraterone	1000 mg orally daily (with prednisone 5 mg orally twice daily)	Weight gain, fluid retention, hypokalemia, hypertension
Testis	Orchiectomy		Gynecomastia, hot flushes, erectile dysfunction
Prostate cell	**Antiandrogens**		
	Flutamide	250 mg three times orally daily	No erectile dysfunction when used alone; nausea, diarrhea
	Bicalutamide	50 mg orally daily	Liver, cardiac, and pulmonary toxicity
	Enzalutamide	160 mg orally daily	Seizures, dizziness, asthenia
	Apalutamide	240 mg orally daily	Fatigue, leukopenia, hyperlipidemia, hyperglycemia, hyperkalemia, seizures (rare).
	Doralutamide	600 mg orally twice daily	Fatigue, extremity pain, rash
	Cytotoxic chemotherapeutic agents		
	Docetaxel	75 mg/m^2 intravenously once on day 1 of 21-day cycle (with prednisone 10 mg orally daily)	Bone marrow, skin, pulmonary, cardiac, GI, hepatic toxicities possible
	Cabazitaxel	20 mg/m^2 intravenously once on day 1 of 21-day cycle (with prednisone 10 mg orally daily)	

LHRH, LH-releasing hormone.

prevention of skeletal-related events in patients with bone metastases from prostate cancer and also appears to delay the development of these metastases in patients with castration-resistant prostate cancer. In addition, enzalutamide definitively improves metastasis-free survival in men with nonmetastatic castrate-resistant prostate cancer and rapidly rising PSAs.

The management of advanced prostate cancer is rapidly evolving. Contemporary management consists of initiating androgen deprivation therapy with orchiectomy, LHRH agonist, or LHRH antagonist. Patients at risk for disease-related symptoms (bone pain, obstructive voiding symptoms) should receive concurrent antiandrogens due to the initial elevation of serum testosterone that accompanies LHRH agonists. Further androgen manipulations, initiation of cytotoxic chemotherapy, and local therapy (eg, radiation) are defined by the cancer's castration sensitivity status. For patients with hormone-naïve metastatic prostate cancer, the addition of systemic cytotoxic chemotherapy with **docetaxel** to androgen deprivation therapy results in improved survival compared with androgen deprivation therapy alone, particularly in men with high-volume disease. Similarly, the addition of **abiraterone acetate** plus **prednisone** to androgen deprivation therapy results in superior survival compared with androgen deprivation therapy alone. Results from the PEACE-1 trial demonstrate that a three-drug regimen, with androgen deprivation therapy, docetaxel and abiraterone acetate used together, provides the best survival outcome for men with hormone-naïve metastatic cancer. With this regimen, the median survival for men with de novo metastatic prostate cancer is now expected to be 5 years. A benefit of local external beam radiation therapy to the prostate gland was demonstrated by STAMPEDE in which patients with low-volume metastatic disease who received external radiotherapy plus standard systemic therapy had improved overall survival compared with those who received only standard systemic therapy. Although under investigation, radical prostatectomy is not performed in patients with metastatic disease.

Patients with castrate-resistant disease or prostate cancer that demonstrates rising PSA or progression of disease despite castrate levels of serum testosterone (less than 50 ng/dL) should continue their LHRH agonist/antagonist regimen. Additional treatment options are stratified based on the presence of metastatic disease. Patients with nonmetastatic castrate-resistant disease and long PSA doubling time (longer than10 months) can simply be observed due to their relatively indolent disease. Conversely, nonmetastatic castrate-resistant patients with short doubling times (10 months or less) have demonstrated improved metastasis-free survival with the addition of one of the potent nonsteroidal androgen receptor antagonists, enzalutamide, apalutamide, or darolutamide, to androgen deprivation therapy. For patients with metastatic castrate-resistant prostate cancer, docetaxel was the first cytotoxic chemotherapy agent to improve survival. Enzalutamide and abiraterone improve overall survival in men with metastatic castrate-resistant prostate cancer in both the docetaxel-naïve and non-naïve setting. Cabazitaxel is a second-line taxane chemotherapy that improves overall survival in men who have received docetaxel. Sipuleucel-T, an autologous cellular immunotherapy, is FDA-approved in asymptomatic or minimally symptomatic men with metastatic castration-resistant prostate cancer. Radium-223 dichloride is approved for the treatment of men with castration-resistant, symptomatic bone metastases, with significant improvements in both overall survival and time to skeletal-related events (eg, fractures and spinal cord compression). Finally, patients who have undergone a genetics evaluation and are found to have specific germline or somatic pathogenic variants may benefit from personalized treatment strategies. Poly-ADP-ribose polymerase (PARP) inhibitors represent a novel class of anticancer agents with some activity against prostate cancer particularly in those patients harboring pathogenic variants in genes important for homologous recombination such as *BRCA1*, *BRCA2*, and *ATM*. There are two FDA-approved PARP inhibitors available for men with metastatic castrate-resistant prostate cancer with these genetic alterations.

Prognosis

The likelihood of success of active surveillance or treatment can be predicted using risk assessment tools that usually combine stage, grade, PSA level, and number and extent of positive prostate biopsies. Several web-based tools are available (eg, https://www.mskcc.org/nomograms/prostate). Widely used nomograms include the Kattan nomogram and the CAPRA nomogram. CAPRA uses serum PSA, Gleason score, clinical stage, percent positive biopsies, and patient age in a point system to risk stratify and predict the likelihood of PSA recurrence 3 and 5 years after radical prostatectomy as well as metastasis and prostate cancer–specific and overall survival. The CAPRA nomogram has been validated on large multicenter and international radical prostatectomy and radiation-treated cohorts.

The patterns of prostate cancer progression have been well defined. Small and well-differentiated cancers (Gleason grade 3) are usually confined within the prostate, whereas large-volume (greater than 4 mL) or poorly differentiated (Gleason grades 4 and 5) cancers are more often locally extensive or metastatic to regional lymph nodes or bone. Penetration of the prostate capsule by cancer is common and occurs along perineural spaces. Seminal vesicle invasion is associated with a high likelihood of regional or distant disease and disease recurrence. The most common sites of lymph node metastases are the obturator and internal iliac lymph node chains and of distant metastases, the axial skeleton.

When to Refer

- Refer all patients to a urologist for management of localized disease or for active surveillance.
- For metastatic disease, medical oncology should be consulted for consideration of systemic treatments.
- Active surveillance may be appropriate in selected patients with very low-volume, low-grade prostate cancer.
- Localized disease may be managed by active surveillance, surgery, or radiation therapy.
- Locally extensive, regionally advanced, and metastatic disease often require multimodal treatment strategies.

Gourd E. New advances in prostate cancer screening and monitoring. Lancet Oncol. 2020;21:887. [PMID: 32534632]

Hoffman KE et al. Patient-reported outcomes through 5 years for active surveillance, surgery, brachytherapy, or external beam radiation with or without androgen deprivation therapy for localized prostate cancer. JAMA. 2020;323:149. [PMID: 31935027]

Kneebone A et al. Adjuvant radiotherapy versus early salvage radiotherapy following radical prostatectomy (TROG 08 .03/ANZUP RAVES): a randomised, controlled, phase 3, non-inferiority trial. Lancet Oncol. 2020; 21:1331. [PMID: 33002437]

Kovac E et al. Association of baseline prostate specific antigen level with long-term diagnosis of clinically significant prostate cancer among patients aged 55 to 60 years: a secondary analysis of a cohort in the Prostate, Lung, Colorectal, and Ovarian (PLCO) Cancer Screening Trial. JAMA Netw Open. 2020;3:e1919284. [PMID: 31940039]

Sargos P et al. Adjuvant radiotherapy versus early salvage radiotherapy plus short-term androgen deprivation therapy in men with localised prostate cancer after radical prostatectomy (GETUG-AFU 17): a randomised, phase 3 trial. Lancet Oncol. 2020;21:1341. [PMID: 33002438]

Shoag JE et al. Reconsidering the trade-offs of prostate cancer screening. N Engl J Med. 2020;382:2465. [PMID: 32558473]

BLADDER CANCER

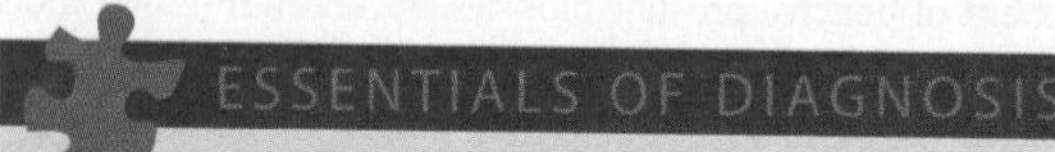

- Gross or microscopic hematuria.
- Irritative voiding symptoms.
- Positive urinary cytology in most patients.
- Filling defect within bladder noted on imaging.

General Considerations

Bladder cancer is the second most common urologic cancer; it occurs more commonly in men than women (3.1:1), and the mean age at diagnosis is 73 years. In 2022 in the United States, it is estimated that approximately 81,180 cases of bladder cancer will be diagnosed and 17,100 deaths will result. Cigarette smoking and exposure to industrial dyes or solvents are risk factors for the disease and account for approximately 60% and 15% of new cases, respectively. In the United States, almost all primary bladder cancers (98%) are epithelial malignancies, usually urothelial cell carcinomas (90%). Adenocarcinomas and squamous cell cancers account for approximately 2% and 7%, respectively. The latter is often associated with schistosomiasis, vesical calculi, or prolonged catheter use.

Clinical Findings

A. Symptoms and Signs

Hematuria—gross or microscopic, chronic or intermittent—is the presenting symptom in 85–90% of patients with bladder cancer (see Hematuria in Chapter 23). Irritative voiding symptoms (urinary frequency and urgency) occur in a small percentage of patients as a result of the location or size of the cancer. Most patients with bladder cancer do not have signs of the disease because of its superficial nature. Abdominal masses detected on bimanual examination may be present in patients with large-volume or deeply infiltrating cancers. Hepatomegaly or palpable lymphadenopathy may be present in patients with metastatic disease, and lymphedema of the lower extremities results from locally advanced cancers or metastases to pelvic lymph nodes.

B. Laboratory Findings

UA reveals microscopic or gross hematuria in the majority of cases. On occasion, hematuria is accompanied by pyuria. Azotemia may be present in a small number of cases associated with ureteral obstruction. Anemia may occasionally be due to chronic blood loss or to bone marrow metastases. Exfoliated cells from normal and abnormal urothelium can be readily detected in voided urine specimens. Cytology can be useful to detect the disease initially or to detect its recurrence. Cytology is sensitive in detecting cancers of higher grade and stage (80–90%), but less so in detecting noninvasive or well-differentiated lesions (50%). There are other novel urinary tumor markers under investigation for screening or assessing recurrence, progression, prognosis, or response to therapy.

C. Imaging

Bladder cancers may be identified as masses within the bladder using ultrasound, CT, or MRI. However, the presence of cancer is confirmed by cystoscopy and biopsy, with imaging primarily used to evaluate the upper urinary tract and to stage more advanced lesions.

D. Cystourethroscopy and Biopsy

The diagnosis and staging of bladder cancers are made by cystoscopy and transurethral resection. If cystoscopy—usually performed under local anesthesia—confirms the presence of a bladder tumor, the patient is scheduled for transurethral resection under general or regional anesthesia. Random bladder and transurethral prostate biopsies are occasionally performed to detect occult disease and potentially identify patients at greater risk for cancer recurrence and progression.

Pathology & Staging

Grading is based on cellular features: size, pleomorphism, mitotic rate, and hyperchromatism. Bladder cancer staging is based on the extent (depth) of bladder wall penetration and the presence of regional or distant metastases. Both cancer grade and stage influence the natural history of bladder cancer including local recurrence within the bladder and progression to higher-stage disease.

Treatment

Patients with non–muscle invasive cancers (Tis, Ta, T1) are treated with complete transurethral resection with selective use of a single dose intravesical chemotherapy immediately following resection. Patients with carcinoma in situ (Tis) and those with high-grade, non–muscle invasive lesions

(Ta or T1) are good candidates for additional intravesical therapy after resection due to a high risk for cancer recurrence and progression with surveillance alone. Patients with high-risk noninvasive cancers are often also treated with re-resection to confirm stage and grade prior to adjuvant intravesical therapy. Some patients with high-grade T1 (particularly recurrent) bladder cancers are recommended for radical cystectomy.

Patients with muscle invasive (T2+) but still localized cancers are at risk for both nodal metastases and progression and require more aggressive treatment. The gold standard treatment is neoadjuvant chemotherapy followed by radical cystectomy, which confers a survival advantage versus cystectomy alone. This is particularly important for higher-stage or bulky tumors to improve their surgical resectability. Trimodal bladder preservation therapy consisting of complete transurethral resection, sensitizing systemic chemotherapy, and external beam radiotherapy can offer similar outcomes in optimally selected patients.

A. Intravesical Therapy

Immunotherapeutic or chemotherapeutic agents delivered directly into the bladder via a urethral catheter can reduce the likelihood of recurrence in those who have undergone complete transurethral resection. Most agents are administered weekly for 6–12 weeks. Efficacy may be increased by prolonging contact time to 2 hours. The use of maintenance therapy after the initial induction regimen is beneficial. Common agents include gemcitabine, mitomycin, doxorubicin, valrubicin, and bacillus Calmette–Guérin (BCG), with the last being the only agent effective in reducing disease progression. Side effects of intravesical chemotherapy include irritative voiding symptoms and hemorrhagic cystitis. Patients in whom symptoms or infection develop from BCG may require antituberculosis therapy.

B. Surgical Treatment

Although transurethral resection is the initial form of treatment for all bladder tumors (since it is diagnostic, allows for proper staging, and controls superficial cancers), muscle-invasive cancers require more aggressive treatment. Partial cystectomy can be considered in selected patients with solitary lesions at the bladder dome or those with cancer in a bladder diverticulum. Radical cystectomy in men entails removal of the bladder, prostate, seminal vesicles, and surrounding fat and peritoneal attachments and in women removal of the bladder, uterus, cervix, urethra, anterior vaginal vault, and usually the ovaries. In women with anterior tumors, vaginal and reproductive organ-sparing surgery can be considered. Bilateral pelvic lymph node dissection is performed in all patients. Randomized trials have demonstrated similar oncologic outcomes and risks of complications with both open and robot-assisted laparoscopic cystectomy; however, robot-assisted techniques result in significantly less blood loss, lower need for blood transfusion, and slightly shorter convalescence. The most common method for urinary diversion involves creating a conduit of ileum or colon with a stoma that drains urine into an external appliance. However, in highly selected patients, continent forms of diversion can be performed that avoid the necessity of an external appliance.

C. Radiotherapy

External beam radiotherapy delivered in fractions over a 6- to 8-week period is generally well tolerated, but approximately 10–15% of patients will develop bladder, bowel, or rectal complications. Local recurrence is common after radiotherapy alone (30–70%) and it is therefore combined with radiosensitizing systemic chemotherapy to improve complete response and to decrease recurrence rates. Bladder-preserving chemoradiation can be offered to those patients seeking to keep their bladder and is best suited for selected patients with solitary T2 or limited T3 tumors without ureteral obstruction. Radiation with or without chemotherapy can be offered to patients with localized cancers and to patients who are poor candidates for radical cystectomy or to patients with metastatic disease seeking palliation of local symptoms. Salvage cystectomy following primary bladder radiotherapy is more challenging with greater risk of complications.

D. Chemotherapy

Metastatic disease is present in 15% of patients with newly diagnosed bladder cancer. Furthermore, metastases develop in up to 40% of patients within 2 years of cystectomy, including those patients who were believed to have localized disease at the time of treatment. Cisplatin-based combination chemotherapy results in partial or complete responses in 15–45% of patients (Table 39–2) and is the preferred approach.

Combination chemotherapy has been used to decrease recurrence rates in patients treated both with surgery and with radiotherapy. Neoadjuvant chemotherapy appears to benefit many patients with muscle-invasive disease prior to planned cystectomy. Molecular profiling may one day be able to predict better which patients are best candidates for this approach. Cisplatin-based chemotherapy is standard and patients who are not eligible for cisplatin should proceed with immediate cystectomy or consider enrollment in a clinical trial. Chemotherapy should also be considered before surgery in those with bulky lesions or those in whom regional metastases are suspected. Alternatively, adjuvant chemotherapy has been used after cystectomy in patients at high risk for recurrence, such as those who have lymph node involvement or extravesical local invasion. For patients with stage IIIB and stage IV disease, molecular/genetic testing should be considered to identify actionable pathogenic variants to target with second-line targeted therapies.

E. Immunotherapy

The FDA has now approved several checkpoint inhibitors as immunotherapy for patients with urothelial cancer at various stages. Approved anti–PDL-1 inhibitors include **atezolizumab**, **durvalumab**, and **avelumab** (Table 39–2). Approved anti-PD1 inhibitors include **nivolumab** and **pembrolizumab.** All are approved for second-line treatment of locally advanced or metastatic urothelial cancer that progressed during or after platinum-based chemotherapy. Additionally, atezolizumab and pembrolizumab are approved as first-line therapy in cisplatin-ineligible patients whose tumors express PD-L1 or in patients ineligible for any platinum-based chemotherapy regardless of PD-L1 expression status. Overall response rates of these agents are similar and range from 17% to 25% in locally advanced and metastatic urothelial bladder cancer. In many cases, responses to therapy are durable. Based on a single arm, phase 2 study, **pembrolizumab** is now FDA-approved for patients with high-risk, non–muscle invasive bladder cancers who have failed intravesical BCG therapy. Nivolumab has also been approved in the adjuvant setting after radical cystectomy or nephroureterectomy for patients with urothelial carcinoma who are considered at high risk for recurrence.

Ongoing trials are evaluating the role for neoadjuvant immunotherapy prior to cystectomy as multiple small studies demonstrate complete pathologic response rates of 31–46%.

F. Other Therapies

Activating pathogenic variants in the fibroblast growth factor receptor (FGFR) are common in urothelial carcinomas. The FGFR inhibitor **erdafitinib** is approved after initial therapy for patients with progressive metastatic urothelial carcinoma whose tumors harbor these mutations with expected response rates of up to 40%. **Enfortumab vedotin** is the first antibody-drug conjugate approved for advanced and metastatic urothelial carcinoma. The antibody targets Nectin-4 and demonstrates a 44% response rate (including 12% complete response) in patients who have progressed after multiple other lines of therapy.

Prognosis

The frequency of recurrence and progression are correlated with grade. Whereas progression may be noted in few low-grade cancers (19–37%), it is common with poorly differentiated lesions (33–67%). Carcinoma in situ is most often found in association with papillary bladder cancers. Its presence identifies patients at increased risk for recurrence and progression.

At initial presentation, approximately 50–80% of bladder cancers are non–muscle invasive: stage Ta, Tis, or T1. When properly treated, lymph node metastases and progression are uncommon in such patients and survival is excellent (81%). Five-year survival of patients with T2 and T3 disease ranges from 50% to 75% after radical cystectomy. Long-term survival for patients with metastatic disease at presentation is rare.

When to Refer

- Refer all patients to a urologist. Hematuria usually deserves evaluation with both upper urinary tract imaging and cystoscopy, particularly in a high-risk group (eg, older men).
- Refer when histologic diagnosis and staging require endoscopic resection of cancer.
- Muscle invasive and locally advanced tumors should be referred to a urologist and medical oncologist as treatment requires multidisciplinary care.
- Metastatic urothelial cancer should be managed by a medical oncologist.

Babjuk M et al. European Association of Urology guidelines on non-muscle-invasive bladder cancer (TaT1 and carcinoma in situ)–2019 update. Eur Urol. 2019;76:639. [PMID: 31443960]

Bajorin DF et al. Adjuvant nivolumab versus placebo in muscle-invasive urothelial carcinoma. N Engl J Med. 2021;384:2102. [PMID: 34077643]

Balar AV et al. Pembrolizumab monotherapy for the treatment of high-risk non-muscle-invasive bladder cancer unresponsive to BCG (KEYNOTE-057): an open-label, single-arm, multicentre, phase 2 study. Lancet Oncol. 2021;22:919. [PMID: 34051177]

Nadal R et al. Management of metastatic bladder cancer. Cancer Treat Rev. 2019;76:10. [PMID: 31030123]

National Comprehensive Cancer Network. Bladder Cancer, Version 1.2022, NCCN Clinical Practice Guidelines in Oncology. Version 1.2022. 2022 Feb 11. https://www.nccn.org/professionals/physician_gls/pdf/bladder.pdf

Rosenberg JE at al. Pivotal trial of enfortumab vedotin in urothelial carcinoma after platinum and anti-programmed death 1/programmed death ligand 1 therapy. J Clin Oncol. 2019; 37;2592. [PMID: 31356140]

CANCERS OF THE URETER & RENAL PELVIS

Cancers of the ureter and renal pelvis are rare and occur more commonly in patients who have bladder cancer, Balkan nephropathy, or Lynch syndrome, who smoke, or who have a long history of analgesic abuse. The majority are urothelial cell carcinomas. Gross or microscopic hematuria is present in most patients; flank pain secondary to bleeding and obstruction occurs less commonly. As with bladder cancers, urinary cytology is often positive in high-grade cancers. The most common signs identified at the time of CT or intravenous urography include an intraluminal filling defect, unilateral nonvisualization of the collecting system, and hydronephrosis. Ureteral and renal pelvic tumors must be differentiated from calculi, blood clots, papillary necrosis, or inflammatory and infectious lesions. Upper urinary tract lesions are accessible for diagnostic biopsy, fulguration, or resection using a ureteroscope. Treatment is based on the site, size, grade, depth of penetration, and number of cancers present. Endoscopic resection may be indicated in patients with limited renal function or focal, low-grade, cancers. Chemoablation with a mitomycin infused gel can be performed in very select patient with low-grade upper tract lesions. Most high-grade and high-volume cancers are excised with robotic, laparoscopic, or open nephroureterectomy (renal pelvic and upper ureteral lesions) or segmental excision of the ureter (distal ureteral lesions). A phase 3, randomized trial demonstrated significantly improved 3-year disease-free survival with dual agent adjuvant systemic chemotherapy after nephroureterectomy. Like with urothelial bladder cancers, use of chemotherapy prior to surgery may also improve outcomes and remains under investigation.

Birtle A et al. Adjuvant chemotherapy in upper tract urothelial carcinoma (the POUT trial): a phase 3, open-label, randomized controlled trial. Lancet. 2020;395:1268. [PMID: 32145825]

Kleinmann N et al. Primary chemoablation of low-grade upper tract urothelial carcinoma using UGN-101, a mitomycin-containing reverse thermal gel (OLYMPUS): an open-label, single-arm, phase 3 trial. Lancet Oncol. 2020; 21:776. [PMID: 32631491]

Leow JJ et al. Neoadjuvant and adjuvant chemotherapy for upper tract urothelial carcinoma: a 2020 systematic review and meta-analysis, and future perspectives on systemic therapy. Eur Urol. 2021;79:635. [PMID: 32798146]

Nazzani S et al. Survival effect of chemotherapy in metastatic upper urinary tract urothelial carcinoma. Clin Genitourin Cancer. 2019;17:e97. [PMID: 30337106]

Scotland KB et al. Long term outcomes of ureteroscopic management of upper tract urothelial carcinoma. Urol Oncol. 2020;38:850.e17. [PMID: 32773230]

RENAL CELL CARCINOMA

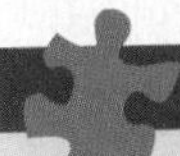

ESSENTIALS OF DIAGNOSIS

- Gross or microscopic hematuria.
- Flank pain or mass in some patients.
- Systemic symptoms such as fever, weight loss may be prominent.
- Solid renal mass on imaging.

General Considerations

Kidney (renal cell) and renal pelvis carcinomas account for 3.8% of all adult cancers. In 2022 in the United States, it is estimated that approximately 79,000 cases of renal cell carcinoma will be diagnosed and 13,920 deaths will result. Renal cell carcinoma has a peak incidence in the sixth decade of life and a male-to-female ratio of 2:1. It may be associated with several paraneoplastic syndromes.

Risk factors include physical inactivity, obesity, and diabetes mellitus. Cigarette smoking is the only known significant environmental risk factor. Familial causes of renal cell carcinoma have been identified (von Hippel-Lindau syndrome, hereditary papillary renal cell carcinoma, hereditary leiomyoma-renal cell carcinoma, and Birt-Hogg-Dubé syndrome). There is an association with dialysis-related acquired cystic disease and specific genetic aberrations (eg, Xp11.2 translocation). But sporadic carcinomas are far more common.

Renal cell carcinoma originates from the proximal tubule cells. Various histologic cell types are recognized (clear cell, papillary, chromophobe, collecting duct, and sarcomatoid).

Clinical Findings

A. Symptoms and Signs

Historically, 60% of patients presented with gross or microscopic hematuria. Flank pain or an abdominal mass was detected in approximately 30% of cases. The triad of flank pain, hematuria, and mass, found in only 10% of patients, is often a sign of advanced disease. Fever can occur as a paraneoplastic symptom. Symptoms of metastatic disease (cough, bone pain) occur in 20–30% of patients at presentation. Due to the widespread use of ultrasound and cross-sectional imaging, renal tumors are frequently detected incidentally in individuals with no urologic symptoms. Consequently, there has been profound stage migration toward lower stages of disease over the last 20 years with increased detection of small, indolent tumors. Population mortality rates have remained relatively stable.

B. Laboratory Findings

Contemporary studies suggest hematuria is present in less than 50% of patients. Erythrocytosis from increased erythropoietin production occurs in 5%, though anemia is more common; hypercalcemia may be present in up to 10% of patients. **Stauffer syndrome** is a reversible syndrome of hepatic dysfunction (with elevated liver tests) in the absence of metastatic disease.

C. Imaging

Solid renal masses are often first identified by abdominal ultrasonography or CT. CT and MRI scanning are the most valuable imaging tests for renal cell carcinoma. These scans confirm the character of the mass and provide valuable staging information with respect to regional lymph nodes, renal vein or vena cava tumor thrombus, and adrenal or liver metastases. CT and MRI also provide valuable information regarding the contralateral kidney (function, bilaterality of neoplasm). Chest radiographs or CT exclude pulmonary metastases. Bone scans should be performed for large tumors and in patients with bone pain or elevated serum alkaline phosphatase levels. Brain imaging should be obtained in patients with high metastatic burden or in those with neurologic deficits.

Differential Diagnosis

Solid renal masses are renal cell carcinoma until proven otherwise. Other solid masses include renal angiomyolipomas (fat density usually detectable by CT), renal pelvis urothelial cancers (more central location, involvement of the collecting system, positive urinary cytology), renal oncocytomas (indistinguishable from renal cell carcinoma preoperatively with standard imaging), renal abscesses, and adrenal tumors (anterosuperior to the kidney).

Treatment

Surgical extirpation is the primary treatment for localized renal cell carcinoma. Patients with a single kidney, bilateral lesions, or significant medical renal disease should be considered for partial nephrectomy. Patients harboring a small tumor with a normal contralateral kidney and good kidney function are also candidates for partial nephrectomy, while radical nephrectomy is indicated in patients with cancers larger than 7 cm and those in whom partial nephrectomy is not technically feasible. Radiofrequency and cryosurgical ablation are alternative options instead of surgery in select patients with tumors less than 3–4 cm with similar risk of metastatic progression but higher risk of local recurrence. Active surveillance is warranted in select patients (significant comorbidity, short life expectancy) and appears safe with low risk of 5-year systemic progression. Percutaneous biopsy can provide tumor histology and grade to help guide treatment decisions. For patients with von Hippel-Lindau disease and renal cell carcinoma, the recently approved HIF2a inhibitor, **belzutifan**, leads to dramatic size reductions in both renal and non-renal neoplasms and offers a new treatment option.

Cytotoxic chemotherapy has no role in the treatment of metastatic renal cell carcinoma. Historically, cytokine-based immunotherapies, such as interferon-alpha and interleukin-2, produced partial response rates of 15–20% and 15–35%, respectively (Table 39–2). Responders tended to have lower tumor burden, metastatic disease confined to the lung, and a high-performance status. Two randomized trials demonstrating a survival benefit of cytoreductive nephrectomy followed by systemic interferon-alpha compared with the use of systemic therapy alone led to the widespread adoption of cytoreductive nephrectomy. Patients most likely to benefit from cytoreduction were those with good performance status, lung only metastases, and good prognostic features.

The treatment of metastatic renal cell carcinoma has evolved rapidly over the last decade. Presently, management strategies are based on tumor histology and patient risk (favorable, intermediate, or poor). Several targeted medications, specifically VEGF, Raf kinase, and mTOR inhibitors, are effective (40–60% response rates) in patients with advanced kidney cancer (Table 39–2). These oral agents, which include **sunitinib, pazopanib, cabozantinib, axitinib, sorafenib** and **lenvatanib**, are generally well tolerated and particularly active for clear cell carcinoma. The optimal timing and combination of these agents remain to be determined. Sunitinib is approved for adjuvant use after complete surgical resection in patients with adverse pathologic features. The mTOR inhibitors **everolimus** and **temsirolimus** are approved for use in patients with prior anti-VEGF therapy, as is the combination of lenvatinib and everolimus. **Nivolumab** is an approved anti-PD-1 immunotherapy for treating metastatic disease that has progressed despite antiangiogenic therapy. Nivolumab in combination with the anti-CTLA4 immunotherapy **ipilimumab** (objective response rate 42%, complete response rate 9%) and **pembrolizumab** (anti-PD-1) in combination with the VEGF inhibitor **axitinib** (objective response rate 59%, complete response rate 5.8%) and **lenvatinib** in combination with **pembrolizumab** (objective response rate 71%, complete response rate 16.1%) have proved superior to **sunitinib** in previously untreated intermediate- and poor-risk metastatic clear cell renal cell carcinoma. These combinations are considered the standard first-line treatment (Table 39–2). Pembrolizumab is also now approved for adjuvant treatment after surgical resection of renal cell carcinoma in patients at high risk for disease recurrence.

The utilization of cytoreductive nephrectomy in combination with contemporary agents has decreased in response to the results of CARMENA in which patients with intermediate and poor-risk clear cell renal carcinoma had similar survival following cytoreductive nephrectomy with or without sunitinib and adoption of combination immunotherapy regimens (nivolumab plus ipilimumab, pembrolizumab plus axitinib). Still, there remains a role for cytoreductive surgery in select patients with intermediate-risk disease. The SURTIME randomized trial compared immediate versus deferred cytoreductive nephrectomy in patients with metastatic renal cell carcinoma treated with sunitinib and showed an overall survival advantage with the deferred approach. This may serve to identify patients who respond the best to systemic therapy prior to undergoing removal of the primary tumor.

Prognosis

After radical or partial nephrectomy, tumors confined to the renal capsule (T1–T2) demonstrate 5-year disease-free survival rate of 90–100%. Tumors extending beyond the renal capsule (T3 or T4) and node-positive tumors have 5-year disease-free survival rates of 50–60% and 0–15%, respectively. One subgroup of patients with nonlocalized disease has reasonable long-term survival, namely, those with solitary resectable metastases. In this setting, radical nephrectomy with resection of the solitary metastasis results in 5-year disease-free survival rate of 15–30%.

When to Refer

- Refer patients with solid renal masses or complex cysts to a urologist for further evaluation.
- Refer patients with renal cell carcinoma to a urologic surgeon for surgical excision.
- Refer patients with metastatic disease to an oncologist and urologist.

Bex A et al. Comparison of immediate vs deferred cytoreductive nephrectomy in patients with synchronous metastatic renal cell carcinoma receiving sunitinib: the SURTIME randomized clinical trial. JAMA Oncol. 2019;5:164. [PMID: 30543350]

Choueiri TK et al. Adjuvant pembrolizumab after nephrectomy in renal-cell carcinoma. N Engl J Med. 2021;385:683. [PMID: 34407342]

Jonasch E et al. Belzutifan for renal cell carcinoma in von Hippel-Lindau disease. N Engl J Med. 2021;385:2036. [PMID: 34818478]

Lalani AA et al. Systemic treatment of metastatic clear cell renal cell carcinoma in 2018: current paradigms, use of immunotherapy, and future directions. Eur Urol. 2019;75:100. [PMID: 30327274]

Motzer R et al; CLEAR Trial Investigators. Lenvatinib plus pembrolizumab or everolimus for advanced renal cell carcinoma. N Engl J Med. 2021;384:1289. [PMID: 33616314]

Rini BI et al; KEYNOTE-426 Investigators. Pembrolizumab plus axitinib versus sunitinib for advanced renal-cell carcinoma. N Engl J Med. 2019;380:1116. [PMID: 30779529]

OTHER PRIMARY TUMORS OF THE KIDNEY

Oncocytomas account for 3–5% of renal tumors, are usually benign, and are indistinguishable from renal cell carcinoma on preoperative imaging. These tumors are seen in other organs, including the adrenals, salivary glands, and thyroid and parathyroid glands.

Angiomyolipomas are rare benign tumors composed of fat, smooth muscle, and blood vessels. They are most commonly seen in patients with tuberous sclerosis (often multiple and bilateral) or in young to middle-aged women. CT scanning may identify the fat component, which is diagnostic for angiomyolipoma. Asymptomatic lesions less than 5 cm in diameter usually do not require intervention; large lesions can spontaneously bleed. Acute bleeding can be treated by angiographic embolization or, in rare cases, nephrectomy. Lesions over 5 cm are often prophylactically treated with angioembolization to reduce the risk of bleeding.

SECONDARY CANCERS OF THE KIDNEY

The kidney is not an infrequent site for metastatic disease. Of the solid tumors, lung cancer is the most common (20%), followed by breast (10%), stomach (10%), and the contralateral kidney (10%). Lymphoma, both Hodgkin and non-Hodgkin, may also involve the kidney, although it tends to appear as a diffusely infiltrative process resulting in renal enlargement rather than a discrete mass.

TESTICULAR CANCERS (Germ Cell Tumors)

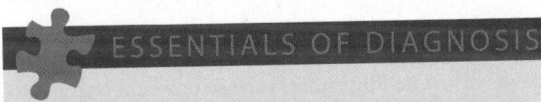

- Most common neoplasm in men aged 20–35 years.
- Patient typically discovers a painless nodule.
- Orchiectomy necessary for diagnosis.

General Considerations

Malignant tumors of the testis are rare, with approximately five to six cases per 100,000 males reported in the United States each year. Ninety to 95 percent of all primary testicular tumors are germ cell tumors and can be divided into two major categories: **nonseminomas**, including embryonal cell carcinoma (20%), teratoma (5%), choriocarcinoma (less than 1%), and mixed cell types (40%); and **seminomas** (35%). The remainder of primary testicular tumors are non-germ cell neoplasms (Leydig cell, Sertoli cell, gonadoblastoma). The lifetime probability of developing testicular cancer is 0.3% for an American male.

Approximately 5% of testicular cancers develop in a patient with a history of cryptorchism, with seminoma being the most common. However, 5–10% of these tumors occur in the contralateral, normally descended testis. The relative risk of development of malignancy is higher for the intra-abdominal testis (1:20) and lower for the inguinal testis (1:80). Placement of the cryptorchid testis into the scrotum (orchidopexy) does not alter its malignant potential but does facilitate routine examination and cancer detection.

Testicular cancer is slightly more common on the right than the left, paralleling the increased incidence of cryptorchidism on the right side. One to 2 percent of primary testicular cancers are bilateral and up to 50% of these men have a history of unilateral or bilateral cryptorchidism. Primary bilateral testicular cancers may occur synchronously or asynchronously but tend to be of the same histology. Seminoma is the most common histologic finding in bilateral *primary* testicular cancers, while malignant lymphoma is the most common bilateral testicular tumor overall.

In animal models, exogenous estrogen administration during pregnancy has been associated with an increased development of testicular tumors with relative risk ranging from 2.8 to 5.3. Other acquired factors such as trauma and infection-related testicular atrophy have been associated with testicular tumors; however, a causal relationship has not been established.

Clinical Findings

A. Symptoms and Signs

The most common symptom of testicular cancer is painless enlargement of the testis. Sensations of heaviness are not unusual. Patients are usually the first to recognize an abnormality, yet often delay in seeking medical attention ranges from 3 to 6 months. Acute testicular pain resulting from intratesticular hemorrhage occurs in approximately 10% of cases. Ten percent of patients are asymptomatic at presentation, and 10% manifest symptoms relating to metastatic disease such as back pain (retroperitoneal metastases), cough (pulmonary metastases), or lower extremity edema (vena cava obstruction).

A discrete mass or diffuse testicular enlargement is noted in most cases. Secondary hydroceles may be present in 5–10% of cases. In advanced disease, supraclavicular adenopathy may be present, and abdominal examination may reveal a mass. Gynecomastia is seen in 5% of germ cell tumors.

B. Laboratory Findings

Several serum markers are important in the diagnosis and monitoring of testicular carcinoma, including human chorionic gonadotropin (hCG), alpha-fetoprotein, and LD. Alpha-fetoprotein is never elevated with pure seminomas, and while hCG is occasionally elevated in seminomas, levels tend to be lower than those seen with nonseminomas. LD may be elevated with either type of tumor and is a marker for disease burden. Liver tests may be elevated in the presence of hepatic metastases, and anemia may be present in advanced disease.

C. Imaging

Scrotal ultrasound can readily determine whether a mass is intratesticular or extratesticular. Once the diagnosis of testicular cancer has been established by inguinal orchiectomy, clinical staging of the disease is accomplished by chest, abdominal, and pelvic CT scanning.

Staging

Testicular cancer is staged using the TNM system created based on extent of cancer in the testis, status of regional lymph nodes, the presence of metastases in distant lymph nodes or other viscera, and serum levels of tumor markers. Based on these features, germ cell tumors can be grouped to assign an overall stage: stage I lesion is confined to the testis; stage II demonstrates regional lymph node involvement in the retroperitoneum; and stage III indicates distant metastasis.

Differential Diagnosis

An incorrect diagnosis is made at the initial examination in up to 25% of patients with testicular tumors. Scrotal ultrasonography should be performed if any uncertainty exists with respect to the diagnosis. Although most intratesticular masses are malignant, a benign lesion—epidermoid cyst—may rarely be seen. Epidermoid cysts are usually very small benign nodules located just underneath the tunica albuginea; occasionally, however, they can be large. Testicular lymphoma is discussed below.

Treatment

Inguinal exploration with early vascular control of the spermatic cord structures is the initial intervention. If cancer cannot be excluded by examination of the testis, radical orchiectomy is warranted. Scrotal approaches and open testicular biopsies should be avoided. Further therapy depends on the histology of the tumor as well as the clinical stage. Men treated for testis cancer are at risk for infertility and fertility preservation should be offered to all men with early referral to a specialist.

Patients with clinical stage I **seminomas** are candidates for surveillance (preferred), single-agent carboplatin, or adjuvant radiotherapy. Stage IIA and IIB seminomas (retroperitoneal disease less than 2 cm diameter in IIA and 2–5 cm in IIB) are treated by radical orchiectomy plus retroperitoneal irradiation or primary systemic chemotherapy (etoposide and cisplatin or cisplatin, etoposide, and bleomycin) (Table 39–2). Seminomas of stage IIC (greater than 5-cm-diameter retroperitoneal nodes) and stage III receive primary systemic chemotherapy. After chemotherapy, surgical resection of residual retroperitoneal nodes is warranted if the node is greater than 3 cm in diameter and positive on PET scan, since 40% will harbor residual carcinoma.

Up to 75% of clinical stage I **nonseminomas** are cured by orchiectomy alone. Selected patients without specific risk factors have low-risk of recurrence and are generally offered surveillance after orchiectomy. These criteria include (1) cancer is confined within the tunica albuginea; (2) cancer does not demonstrate vascular invasion; (3) tumor markers normalize after orchiectomy; (4) radiographic imaging of the chest and abdomen shows no evidence of disease; and (5) the patient is reliable. Patients most likely to experience relapse on a surveillance regimen include those with predominantly embryonal cancer and those with vascular or lymphatic invasion identified in the orchiectomy specimen. Alternatives to surveillance for clinical stage I nonseminomas include adjuvant chemotherapy (bleomycin, etoposide, cisplatin) (Table 39–2) or retroperitoneal lymph node dissection.

Following orchiectomy, patients with bulky retroperitoneal disease (greater than 5-cm nodes) or metastatic nonseminomas are treated with combination chemotherapy (cisplatin and etoposide or cisplatin, etoposide, and bleomycin) (Table 39–2). If tumor markers normalize and a residual mass greater than 1 cm persists on imaging studies, it is resected because 15–20% will harbor residual cancer and 40% will harbor teratomas. Even if patients have a complete response to chemotherapy, some clinicians advocate retroperitoneal lymphadenectomy since 10% of patients may harbor residual carcinoma and 10%, retroperitoneal teratoma. If tumor markers fail to normalize following primary chemotherapy, salvage chemotherapy is required (cisplatin, etoposide, and ifosfamide).

Postoperative active surveillance by the clinician and patient means patients are followed up every 2–6 months for the first 2 years and every 4–6 months in the third year. For nonseminomas, tumor markers are obtained at each visit, and chest radiographs and abdominal and pelvic CT scans are obtained every 4–6 months. For seminomas, serum tumor markers may be obtained (optional), chest imaging is obtained only as clinically indicated, and abdominal and pelvic CT scans are performed every 3–6 months. Follow-up continues beyond the initial 3 years; however, 80% of relapses will occur within the first 2 years. With rare exceptions, patients who relapse can be cured by chemotherapy or surgery.

Prognosis

The 5-year disease-free survival rates for stage I and IIA **seminomas** (retroperitoneal disease less than 2 cm in diameter) treated by radical orchiectomy and retroperitoneal irradiation are 98% and 92–94%, respectively. Ninety-five percent of patients with stage III disease attain a complete response following orchiectomy and chemotherapy. The 5-year disease-free survival rate for patients with stage I **nonseminomas** (includes all treatments) ranges from 96–100%. For low-volume stage II disease, a 5-year disease-free survival of 90% is expected. Patients with bulky retroperitoneal or disseminated disease treated with primary chemotherapy followed by surgery have a 5-year disease-free survival rate of 55–80%.

When to Refer

Refer all patients with solid masses of the testis to a urologist and a medical oncologist if metastatic disease is suspected.

Goldberg H et al. Germ cell testicular tumors—contemporary diagnosis, staging and management of localized and advanced disease. Urology. 2019;125:8. [PMID: 30597167]

King J et al. Management of residual disease after chemotherapy in germ cell tumors. Curr Opin Oncol. 2020;32:250. [PMID: 32168037]

Pierorazio PM et al. Performance characteristics of clinical staging modalities for early-stage testicular germ cell tumors: a systematic review. J Urol. 2020;203:894. [PMID: 31609176]

Sineath RC et al. Preservation of fertility in testis cancer management. Urol Clin North Am. 2019;46:341. [PMID: 31277729]

SECONDARY CANCERS OF THE TESTIS

Secondary cancers of the testis are rare. In men over the age of 50 years, lymphoma is the most common. Overall, it is the most common secondary neoplasm of the testis, accounting for 5% of all testicular cancers. It may be seen in three clinical settings: (1) late manifestation of widespread lymphoma, (2) the initial presentation of clinically occult disease, and (3) primary extranodal disease. Radical orchiectomy is indicated to make the diagnosis. Prognosis is related to the stage of disease.

Metastasis to the testis is rare. The most common primary site of origin is the prostate, followed by the lung, GI tract, melanoma, and kidney.

CANCER COMPLICATIONS & EMERGENCIES

Sunny Wang, MD
Tiffany O. Dea, PharmD, BCOP

SPINAL CORD COMPRESSION

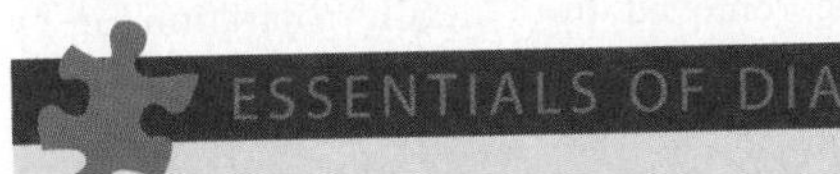

- Complication of metastatic solid tumor, lymphoma, or plasma cell myeloma.
- Back pain is most common presenting symptom.
- Prompt diagnosis is essential because once a severe neurologic deficit develops, it is often irreversible.
- Emergent treatment may prevent or potentially reverse paresis and urinary and bowel incontinence.

General Considerations

Cancers that cause spinal cord compression most commonly metastasize to the vertebral bodies, resulting in physical damage to the spinal cord from edema, hemorrhage, and pressure-induced ischemia to its vasculature. Persistent compression can result in irreversible changes to the myelin sheaths resulting in permanent neurologic impairment.

Prompt diagnosis and therapeutic intervention are essential. Patients who are treated promptly after symptoms appear may have partial or complete return of function and, depending on tumor sensitivity to specific treatment, may respond favorably to subsequent anticancer therapy.

Clinical Findings

A. Symptoms and Signs

Back pain at the level of the tumor mass occurs in over 80% of cases and may be aggravated by lying down, weight bearing, sneezing, or coughing; it usually precedes the development of neurologic symptoms or signs. Since involvement is usually epidural, a mixture of nerve root and spinal cord symptoms often develops. Progressive weakness and sensory changes commonly occur. Bowel and bladder symptoms progressing to incontinence are late findings.

The initial findings of impending cord compression may be quite subtle, and there should be a high index of suspicion when back pain or weakness of the lower extremities develops in a patient with cancer.

B. Imaging

MRI is usually the initial imaging procedure of choice in a patient with cancer and new-onset back pain. If the back pain symptom is nonspecific, a whole-body PET-CT scan with ^{18}F-2-deoxyglucose may be a useful screening procedure. Bone radiographs are neither sensitive nor specific for the evaluation of a patient with cancer and back pain. When neurologic findings suggest spinal cord compression, an emergent MRI should be obtained; the MRI should survey the entire spine to define all areas of tumor involvement for treatment planning purposes. MRI has a sensitivity of 93% and a specificity of 97% for diagnosis of metastatic spinal cord compression.

Treatment

Patients with a known cancer diagnosis found to have epidural impingement of the spinal cord should be given corticosteroids immediately. The initial dexamethasone dose is 10 mg intravenously followed by 4–6 mg every 6 hours intravenously or orally. Patients without a known diagnosis of cancer should have emergent surgery to relieve the impingement and obtain a pathologic specimen; preoperative corticosteroids should not be given since they might compromise the pathology results. Patients with solid tumors who have a single area of compression and who are considered candidates for surgery are best treated first with surgical decompression followed by radiation therapy. If multiple vertebral body levels are involved with cancer, fractionated radiation therapy is the preferred treatment option. Corticosteroids are generally tapered toward the end of radiation therapy.

Hoskin PJ et al. Effect of single-fraction vs multifraction radiotherapy on ambulatory status among patients with spinal canal compression from metastatic cancer: the SCORAD randomized clinical trial. JAMA. 2019;322:2084. [PMID: 31794625]

Lawton AJ et al. Assessment and management of patients with metastatic spinal cord compression: a multidisciplinary review. J Clin Oncol. 2019;37:61. [PMID: 30395488]

Terpos E et al. Treatment of multiple myeloma-related bone disease: recommendations from the Bone Working Group of the International Myeloma Working Group. Lancet Oncol. 2021;22:e119. [PMID: 33545067]

MALIGNANT EFFUSIONS

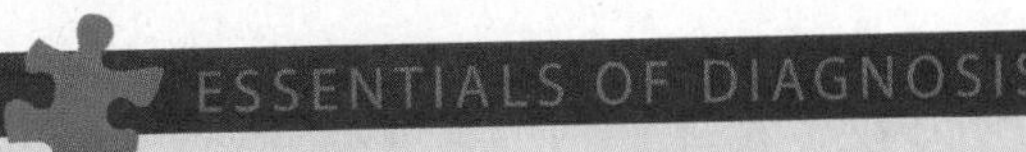

- Occur in pleural, pericardial, and peritoneal spaces.
- Caused by direct neoplastic involvement of serous surface or obstruction of lymphatic drainage.
- Half of undiagnosed effusions in patients not known to have cancer are malignant.

General Considerations

The development of an effusion in the pleural, pericardial, or peritoneal space may be the initial finding in a patient with cancer, or an effusion may appear during the course of disease progression. Direct involvement of the serous surface with tumor is the most frequent initiating cause of the accumulation of fluid. The most common malignancies causing pleural and pericardial effusions are lung and breast cancers; the most common malignancies associated with malignant ascites are ovarian, colorectal, stomach, and pancreatic cancers.

Clinical Findings

A. Symptoms and Signs

Patients with pleural and pericardial effusions complain of shortness of breath and orthopnea. Patients with ascites complain of abdominal distention and discomfort. Cardiac tamponade causing pressure equalization in the chambers impairs both filling and cardiac output and can be life-threatening. Signs of tamponade include tachycardia, muffled heart sounds, pulsus paradoxus, and hypotension. Signs of pleural effusions include decreased breath sounds, egophony, and percussion dullness.

B. Laboratory Findings

Malignancy is confirmed as the cause of an effusion when analysis of the fluid specimen shows malignant cells in either the cytology or cell block specimen.

C. Imaging

The presence of effusions can be confirmed with radiographic studies or ultrasonography.

Differential Diagnosis

The differential diagnosis of a malignant pleural or pericardial effusion includes nonmalignant processes, such as infection, PE, heart failure, and trauma. The differential diagnosis of malignant ascites includes similar benign processes, such as heart failure, cirrhosis, peritonitis, and pancreatic ascites. Bloody effusions are usually due to cancer, but a bloody pleural effusion can also be due to PE, trauma and, occasionally, infection. Chylous pleural or ascitic fluid is generally associated with obstruction of lymphatic drainage as might occur in lymphoma.

Treatment

The development of a malignant effusion is a late-stage manifestation of the cancer. Treatment is tailored to the underlying cancer, whether with targeted therapy, chemotherapy, or immunotherapy, depending on tumor testing results. Effective systemic treatment can lead to regression of the effusion. Acute symptoms related to the effusion often require urgent intervention with drainage of the effusion. Decisions regarding palliative management of malignant effusion are in large part dictated by the patient's symptoms and goals of care.

A. Pleural Effusion

A pleural effusion that is symptomatic may be managed initially with a **large-volume thoracentesis.** In some patients, the effusion slowly reaccumulates, which allows for periodic thoracentesis when the patient becomes symptomatic. However, in many patients, the effusion reaccumulates quickly, causing rapid return of shortness of breath. For those patients, two management options exist: pleurodesis or indwelling pleural catheter (eg, PleurX). In a meta-analysis of randomized controlled trials comparing indwelling pleural catheter with pleurodesis, indwelling pleural catheters resulted in shorter hospital stays and fewer repeat pleural interventions, but increased rates of cellulitis.

B. Pericardial Effusion

Fluid may be removed by a needle aspiration or by placement of a catheter for more thorough drainage. As with pleural effusions, most pericardial effusions will reaccumulate. Management options for recurrent, symptomatic effusions include prolonged catheter drainage or surgical intervention such as a pericardiotomy or pericardiectomy.

C. Malignant Ascites

Patients with malignant ascites not responsive to chemotherapy are generally treated with repeated large-volume paracenteses. Since the frequency of drainage to maintain comfort can compromise the patient's quality of life, other alternatives include placement of a catheter or port so that the patient, family member, or visiting nurse can drain fluid as needed at home. For patients with portal hypertension from large hepatic masses, diuretics may be useful to decrease the need for repeated paracentesis.

Lazaros G et al. New approaches to management of pericardial effusions. Curr Cardiol Rep. 2021;23:106. [PMID: 34196832]

Reddy CB et al. Summary for clinicians: clinical practice guideline for management of malignant pleural effusions. Ann Am Thorac Soc. 2019;16:17. [PMID: 30516394]

Walker S et al. Malignant pleural effusion management: keeping the flood gates shut. Lancet Respir Med. 2020;8:609. [PMID: 31669226]

HYPERCALCEMIA

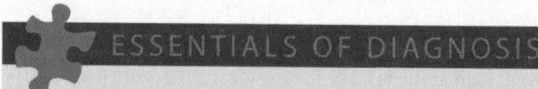

ESSENTIALS OF DIAGNOSIS

- Most common paraneoplastic endocrine syndrome.
- Usually symptomatic and severe (≥ 15 mg/dL [3.75 mmol/L]); accounts for most inpatients with hypercalcemia.
- The neoplasm is clinically apparent in nearly all cases when hypercalcemia is detected.

General Considerations

Hypercalcemia affects 20–30% of patients with cancer at some point during their illness. The most common cancers causing hypercalcemia are myeloma, breast carcinoma, and NSCLC. Hypercalcemia is caused by one of three mechanisms: systemic effects of tumor-released proteins, direct osteolysis of bone by tumor, or vitamin D–mediated osteoabsorption.

Clinical Findings

A. Symptoms and Signs

Symptoms and signs of hypercalcemia can be subtle; more severe symptoms occur with higher levels of hypercalcemia and with a rapidly rising calcium level. Early symptoms typically include anorexia, nausea, fatigue, constipation, and polyuria; later findings may include muscular weakness and hyporeflexia, confusion, psychosis, tremor, and lethargy.

B. Laboratory Findings

Symptoms and signs are caused by free calcium; as calcium is bound by protein in the serum, the measured serum calcium will underestimate the free or ionized calcium in patients with low albumin levels. Free ionized calcium can be measured. When the corrected serum calcium rises above 12 mg/dL (3 mmol/L), especially if the rise occurs rapidly, sudden death due to cardiac arrhythmia or asystole may occur. Initial workup for hypercalcemia includes obtaining serum PTH, PTHrP, and calcitriol (1,25-dihydroxycholecalciferol) levels.

C. ECG

ECG in hypercalcemia often shows a shortening of the QT interval.

Treatment

Emergency management should begin with the initiation of intravenous fluids with 0.9% saline at 100–300 mL/hour to ensure rehydration with brisk urinary output of the often volume-depleted patient. If kidney function is normal or only marginally impaired, a bisphosphonate should be given. Choices include pamidronate, 60–90 mg intravenously over 2–4 hours, or zoledronic acid, 4 mg intravenously over 15 minutes. Zoledronic acid is more potent than pamidronate and has the advantage of a shorter administration time as well as a longer duration of effect. Once hypercalcemia is controlled, treatment directed at the cancer should be initiated if possible. If hypercalcemia becomes refractory to repeated doses of bisphosphonates, other agents that can help control hypercalcemia (at least temporarily) include calcitonin and denosumab; corticosteroids can be useful in patients with myeloma and lymphoma. Salmon calcitonin, 4–8 IU/kg given subcutaneously or intramuscularly every 12 hours, can be used in patients with severe, symptomatic hypercalcemia; its onset of action is within hours but its hypocalcemic effect wanes in 2–3 days. Denosumab, 120 mg given subcutaneously weekly for 4 weeks followed by monthly administration, is a choice for long-term management of bisphosphonate-refractory hypercalcemia or for patients with kidney dysfunction that precludes use of a bisphosphonate.

Asonitis N et al. Diagnosis, pathophysiology, and management of hypercalcemia in malignancy: a review of the literature. Horm Metab Res. 2019;51:770. [PMID: 31826272]

Sheehan MT et al. Evaluation of diagnostic workup and etiology of hypercalcemia of malignancy in a cohort of 167 551 patients over 20 years. J Endocr Soc. 2021;5:bvab157. [PMID: 34703961]

HYPERURICEMIA & TUMOR LYSIS SYNDROME

ESSENTIALS OF DIAGNOSIS

- Complication of treatment-associated tumor lysis of hematologic and rapidly proliferating malignancies.
- May be worsened by thiazide diuretics.
- Rapid increase in serum uric acid can cause acute urate nephropathy from uric acid crystallization.
- Reducing pre-chemotherapy serum uric acid is fundamental to preventing urate nephropathy.

General Considerations

Tumor lysis syndrome (TLS) is seen most commonly following treatment of hematologic malignancies. However, TLS can develop from any tumor highly sensitive to chemotherapy. TLS is caused by the massive release of cellular material including nucleic acids, proteins, phosphorus, and potassium. If both the metabolism and excretion of these breakdown products are impaired, hyperuricemia, hyperphosphatemia, and hyperkalemia will develop abruptly. AKI may then develop from the crystallization and deposition of uric acid and calcium phosphate within the renal tubules, further exacerbating the hyperphosphatemia and hyperkalemia.

Clinical Findings

A. Symptoms and Signs

Symptoms of hyperphosphatemia include nausea, vomiting, anorexia, muscle cramps, tetany, and seizures. High levels of phosphorus and co-precipitation with calcium can cause renal tubule blockage, further exacerbating the kidney injury. Hyperkalemia, due to release of intracellular potassium and impaired kidney excretion, can cause arrhythmias and sudden death.

B. Laboratory Findings

The laboratory diagnosis of TLS include at least two of the following criteria observed within a 24-hour period: uric acid 8 mg/dL or higher (476 mcmol/L or higher), phosphate 4.5 mg/dL or higher (1.45 mmol/L or higher), potassium 6.0 mEq/L or more (6 mmol/L or more) (or a 25% increase from baseline for these parameters), and corrected serum calcium 7 mg/dL or lower (1.75 mmol/L or lower). A clinical diagnosis of TLS includes meeting the laboratory criteria and at least one clinical criterion: AKI (creatinine greater than or equal to 1.5 × upper limit of normal or increase greater than 0.3 g/dL or urinary output greater than 0.5 mL/kg/hour for 6 hours) or cardiac arrhythmia, sudden cardiac death, or seizure.

Treatment

Prevention is the most important factor in the management of TLS. Aggressive hydration at least 24 hours prior to chemotherapy as well as 24–48 hours after chemotherapy completion helps keep urine flowing and facilitates excretion of uric acid and phosphorus. It is recommended to maintain a urinary output of at least 100 mL/hour, and a daily urine volume of at least 3 L/day. If evidence of volume overload or inadequate urinary output develops, loop diuretics can be used. Thiazide diuretics are contraindicated because they increase uric acid levels and can interact with allopurinol. For patients at moderate risk of developing TLS, eg, those with intermediate-grade lymphomas and acute leukemias, allopurinol should be given before starting chemotherapy with dose reductions for impaired kidney function. Rasburicase is given intravenously to patients at high risk for developing TLS, eg, those with high-grade lymphomas or acute leukemias with markedly elevated WBC counts (acute myeloid leukemia, WBC count greater than 50,000/mcL [50×10^9/L] or acute lymphoblastic leukemia, WBC count greater than 100,000/mcL [100×10^9/L]). Rasburicase may also be considered for patients with baseline elevated uric acid who are being treated with venetoclax (Bcl-2 inhibitor) for chronic lymphocytic leukemia who have large lymph nodes (10 cm or larger) or nodes 5 cm or larger accompanied by WBC counts greater than 25,000/mcL (25×10^9/L); or in any patient in whom uric acid levels reach levels greater than 8 mg/dL despite treatment with allopurinol. Rasburicase cannot be given to patients with known glucose 6-phosphate dehydrogenase (G6PD) deficiency nor can it be given to pregnant or lactating women.

When to Refer

Should urinary output drop, serum creatinine or potassium levels rise, or hyperphosphatemia persist, a nephrologist should be immediately consulted to evaluate the need for dialysis.

Durani U et al. Emergencies in haematology: tumor lysis syndrome. Br J Haematol. 2020;188:494. [PMID: 31774551]

Matuszkiewicz-Rowinska J et al. Prevention and treatment of tumor lysis syndrome in the era of onco-nephrology progress. Kidney Blood Press Res. 2020;45:645. [PMID: 32998135]

INFECTIONS

Chapters 30 and 31 provide more detailed discussions of infections in the immunocompromised patient.

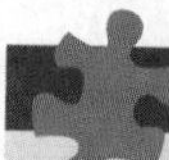

ESSENTIALS OF DIAGNOSIS

- In patients with neutropenia, infection is a medical emergency.
- Although sometimes attributable to other causes, the presence of fever, defined as a single temperature > 38.3°C (101°F) or a temperature of > 38°C (100.4°F) for > 1 hour, must be assumed to be due to an infection.

General Considerations

Many patients with disseminated neoplasms have increased susceptibility to infection. In some patients, this results from impaired defense mechanisms (eg, acute leukemia, Hodgkin lymphoma, myeloma, chronic lymphocytic leukemia); in others, it results from the myelosuppressive and immunosuppressive effects of cancer chemotherapy or a combination of these factors. Patients with cancer are at higher risk for infection with SARS-CoV-2, with more severe cases of COVID-19 infection and complications.

The source of a neutropenic febrile episode is determined in about 30% of cases through blood, urine, or sputum cultures. The bacterial organisms accounting for most infections in patients with cancer include gram-positive bacteria and gram-negative bacteria. Gram-positive organism infections are more common, but gram-negative infections are more serious and life-threatening. The risk of bacterial infections rises when the neutrophil count is below 500/mcL (0.5×10^9/L); the risk markedly increases when the count falls below 100/mcL (0.1×10^9/L) or when there is a prolonged duration of neutropenia, typically greater than 7 days.

Clinical Findings

A thorough physical examination should be performed. Appropriate cultures (eg, blood, sputum, urine and, if indicated, cerebrospinal fluid) and COVID-19 testing should always be obtained. Two sets of blood cultures should be drawn before starting antibiotics; if the patient has an indwelling catheter, one of the cultures should be drawn from the line. A chest radiograph should also be obtained.

Treatment

Empiric antibiotic therapy needs to be initiated within 1 hour of presentation and following the collection of blood cultures in the febrile neutropenic patient. The choice of antibiotics depends on a number of different factors including the patient's clinical status and any localizing source of infection. If the patient is clinically well, monotherapy with an intravenous beta-lactam with anti-*Pseudomonas* activity (cefepime, ceftazidime, imipenem/cilastatin, piperacillin/tazobactam) should be started (see Infections in the Immunocompromised Patient, Chapter 30). If the patient is clinically ill with hypotension or hypoxia, an intravenous aminoglycoside or fluoroquinolone should be added for "double" gram-negative bacteria coverage. If there is a strong suspicion of a gram-positive organism, such as from a *S aureus* catheter infection, intravenous vancomycin can be given empirically. Low-risk patients may be treated with oral antibiotics in the outpatient setting.

Antibiotics should be continued until the neutrophil count is rising and greater than 500/mcL (0.5×10^9/L) for at least 1 day and the patient has been afebrile for 2 days. If an organism is identified through the cultures, the antibiotics should be adjusted to the antibiotic sensitivities of the isolate; treatment should be continued for the appropriate period of time and at least until the neutrophil count recovers and fever resolves.

Braga CC et al. Clinical implications of febrile neutropenia guidelines in the cancer patient population. J Clin Oncol. 2019;15:25. [PMID: 30629901]

Cooksley T et al. Emerging challenges in the evaluation of fever in cancer patients at risk of febrile neutropenia in the era of COVID-19: a MASCC position paper. Support Care Cancer. 2021;29:1129. [PMID: 33230644]

PRIMARY CANCER TREATMENT

Sunny Wang, MD
Tiffany O. Dea, PharmD, BCOP

SYSTEMIC CANCER THERAPY

Detailed guidelines from the NCCN for cancer treatment can be found at www.nccn.org.

Use of cytotoxic drugs, hormones, antihormones, and biologic agents has become a highly specialized and increasingly effective means of treating cancer, with therapy administered and monitored by a medical oncologist or hematologist. Selection of specific drugs or protocols for various types of cancer is based on results of clinical trials. Increasingly, newer agents are being identified that target specific molecular pathways. Yet both initial and acquired drug resistance remains a challenge. Described mechanisms of drug resistance include impaired membrane transport of drugs, enhanced drug metabolism, mutated target proteins, and blockage of apoptosis due to mutations in cellular proteins (see Table 39–2 for suggested agents for various cancers).

TOXICITY & DOSE MODIFICATION OF CHEMOTHERAPEUTIC AGENTS

Use of chemotherapy to treat cancer is generally guided by results from clinical trials in individual tumor types. The complexity of treating cancer has increased over the last decade as more drugs, including those with targeted mechanisms of action, have been approved by the US FDA and introduced into general practice. Drug side effects and toxicities must be anticipated and carefully monitored. The short- and long-term toxicities of individual drugs are listed in Tables 39–3 and 39–10. Decisions on dose modifications for toxicities should be guided by the intent of therapy. In the palliative setting where the aim of therapy is to improve symptoms and quality of life, lowering doses to minimize toxicity is commonly done. However, when the goal of treatment is cure, dosing frequency and intensity should be maintained whenever possible.

Table 39–10. Commonly used supportive care agents.[1]

Agent	Indication	Usual Dose	Adverse Effects
Allopurinol (Xyloprim)	Prevent hyperuricemia from tumor lysis syndrome	600–800 mg/day orally	Acute: none Delayed: rash
Dexrazoxane (Zinecard)	Prevent cardiomyopathy secondary to doxorubicin; anthracycline-induced injection site extravasation	10 times the doxorubicin dose intravenously before doxorubicin; 1000 mg/m² intravenously on days 1 and 2, then 500 mg/m² intravenously on day 3	Acute: nausea Delayed: myelosuppression, elevated transaminases
Leucovorin	Rescue after high-dose methotrexate; in combination with 5-fluorouracil for colon cancer	10 mg/m² intravenously or orally every 6 hours; 20 mg/m² or 200–500 mg/m² intravenously before 5-fluorouracil; various doses	Acute: nausea, vomiting, diarrhea Delayed: stomatitis, fatigue
Mesna (Mesnex)	Prevent ifosfamide-induced hemorrhagic cystitis	20% of ifosfamide dose intravenously at 0, 4, and 8 hours; various doses	Acute: nausea, vomiting Delayed: fatigue
Palifermin (Kepivance)	Prevent mucositis following chemotherapy	60 mcg/kg/day intravenously for 3 days before and 3 days after chemotherapy	Acute: none Delayed: rash, fever, elevated serum amylase, erythema, edema
Radium (Ra)-223 dichloride (Xofigo)	Symptomatic bone metastases	50 kilobecquerel/kg (1.35 microCurie/kg) intravenously every 4 weeks for 6 cycles	Acute: nausea, vomiting, diarrhea, peripheral edema Delayed: myelosuppression
Rasburicase (Elitek)	Prevent hyperuricemia from tumor lysis syndrome	3–6 mg intravenously once	Acute: hypersensitivity, nausea, vomiting, diarrhea, fever, headache Delayed: rash, peripheral edema

(*continued*)

Table 39–10. Commonly used supportive care agents.[1] (continued)

Agent	Indication	Usual Dose	Adverse Effects
Bone-Modifying Agents			
Denosumab (Xgeva)	Osteolytic bone metastasis	120 mg subcutaneously every 4 weeks	Acute: nausea Delayed: hypocalcemia, hypophosphatemia, fatigue, osteonecrosis of the jaw
Pamidronate (Aredia)	Osteolytic bone metastasis, hypercalcemia of malignancy	90 mg intravenously every 3–4 weeks; 60–90 mg intravenously, may repeat after 7 days	Acute: nausea Delayed: dyspnea, arthralgia, bone pain, osteonecrosis of the jaw, nephrotoxicity, hypocalcemia
Zoledronic acid (Zometa)	Osteolytic bone metastasis, hypercalcemia of malignancy	4 mg intravenously every 3–4 weeks; 4 mg intravenously once, may repeat after 7 days	—
Growth Factors			
Darbepoetin alfa (Aranesp)	Chemotherapy-induced anemia	2.25 mcg/kg subcutaneously weekly; 500 mcg subcutaneously every 3 weeks	—
Epoetin alfa (Epogen, Procrit)	Chemotherapy-induced anemia	40,000 U subcutaneously once weekly; 150 U/kg subcutaneously three times a week	Acute: injection site reaction Delayed: hypertension, thromboembolic events, increased risk of tumor progression or recurrence
Filgrastim (Neupogen)	Febrile neutropenia prophylaxis, mobilization of peripheral stem cells	5–10 mcg/kg/day subcutaneously or intravenously once daily, treat past nadir	Acute: injection site reaction Delayed: bone pain
Pegfilgrastim (Neulasta)	Febrile neutropenia prophylaxis	6 mg subcutaneously once per chemotherapy cycle	—
Sargramostim (Leukine)	Myeloid reconstitution following bone marrow transplant, mobilization of peripheral blood stem cells	250 mcg/m^2 intravenously daily until the absolute neutrophil count is > 1500 cells/mcL (1.5 × 10^9/L) for 3 consecutive days	Acute: fever, rash, pruritus, nausea, vomiting, diarrhea, injection site reaction, dyspnea Delayed: asthenia, bone pain, mucositis, edema, arrhythmia

[1]For amifostine, levoleucovorin, pilocarpine, samarium, strontium, filgrastim-sndz, and tbo-filgrastim, see Table 39–10 in *CMDT Online* at www.accessmedicine.com.

A CBC including a differential count, with absolute neutrophil count and platelet count, and liver and kidney tests should be obtained before the initiation of chemotherapy. When the intent of chemotherapy is cure, including treatment in the adjuvant setting, every attempt should be made to schedule chemotherapy on time and at full dose. A CBC with differential may be checked at midcycle (to determine the nadir of the absolute neutrophil and platelet counts), and repeat CBC and liver and kidney function tests should be obtained immediately before the next cycle of chemotherapy.

Dose reductions may be necessary for patients with impaired kidney or liver function depending on the clearance mechanism of the drug. For patients receiving chemotherapy for palliation, bone marrow toxicity can be managed with dose reductions or delaying the next treatment cycle. A schema for dose modification is shown in Table 39–11.

Table 39–11. A common schema for dose modification of cancer chemotherapeutic agents.

Granulocyte Count	Platelet Count	Suggested Drug Dosage (% of Full Dose)
> 2000 cells/mcL (2 × 10^9/L)	> 100,000/mcL (100 × 10^9/L)	100%
1000–2000 cells/mcL (1–2 × 10^9/L)	75,000–100,000/mcL (75–100 × 10^9/L)	50%
< 1000 cells/mcL (1 × 10^9/L)	< 50,000/mcL (50 × 10^9/L)	0%

1. Bone Marrow Toxicity

A. Neutropenia

Granulocyte colony-stimulating factor (G-CSF), given as either daily subcutaneous injections (eg, filgrastim, 300 mcg or 480 mcg) or as a one-time dose (pegfilgrastim, 6 mg) beginning 24 hours after cytotoxic chemotherapy is completed, reduces the duration and severity of granulocytopenia following cytotoxic chemotherapy (Table 39–10). The American Society of Clinical Oncology and NCCN guidelines recommend primary prophylaxis with G-CSF when there is at least a 20% risk of febrile neutropenia or when age, medical history, and disease characteristics put the patient at high risk for complications related to myelosuppression.

B. Anemia

Erythropoiesis-stimulating agents ameliorate the anemia and its associated symptoms caused by cancer chemotherapy but these drugs have untoward effects, including an increased risk of thromboembolism, and possibly a decreased survival due to cancer-related deaths as well as a shortened time to tumor progression. The FDA recommends that these drugs should not be used when the intent of chemotherapy is curative. Administration of RBC transfusions is an alternative for managing symptomatic anemia in chemotherapy patients.

Erythropoiesis-stimulating agents can be an option in patients with cancer and symptomatic anemia undergoing palliative treatment; patient preference is important in determining when to use erythropoiesis-stimulating agents or transfusions. When using erythropoiesis-stimulating agents, treatment should not be initiated until the hemoglobin is less than 10 g/dL (100 g/L) and the agent held when the hemoglobin is greater than 12 g/dL (120 g/L). To have maximum therapeutic effect, patients need to be iron replete.

C. Thrombocytopenia

Drug management of chemotherapy-induced thrombocytopenia is more limited. Two drugs that activate the thrombopoietin receptor, romiplostim and eltrombopag, are FDA-approved for use in idiopathic thrombocytopenia, thrombocytopenia related to interferon therapy of hepatitis C, and thrombocytopenia in aplastic anemia. Trials to date have not demonstrated convincing efficacy in patients with chemotherapy-induced thrombocytopenia and neither agent is FDA-approved for this indication.

2. Chemotherapy-Induced Nausea & Vomiting

Several cytotoxic anticancer drugs can induce nausea and vomiting, which can be the most anticipated and stressful side effects for patients. Chemotherapy-induced nausea and vomiting is mediated in part by the stimulation of at least two CNS receptors, 5-hydroxytryptamine subtype 3 ($5HT_3$) and neurokinin subtype 1 (NK_1). Chemotherapy-induced nausea and vomiting can be anticipatory, occurring even before chemotherapy administration; acute, occurring within minutes to hours of chemotherapy administration; or delayed, lasting up to 7 days. Chemotherapy drugs are classified into high, moderate, low, and minimal likelihoods of causing emesis (90%, 30–90%, 10–30%, less than 10%, respectively). Highly emetogenic chemotherapy drugs include carmustine, cisplatin, or cyclophosphamide. Moderately emetogenic chemotherapy drugs include azacitidine, carboplatin, cyclophosphamide, cytarabine, doxorubicin, ifosfamide, oxaliplatin, and temozolomide. Low emetogenic drugs include bortezomib, capecitabine, docetaxel, erlotinib, etoposide, 5-fluorouracil, gemcitabine, lenalidomide, paclitaxel, and pemetrexed. Drugs with minimal risk of emesis include bevacizumab, bleomycin, cetuximab, rituximab, trastuzumab, and vincristine.

Major advances have occurred in the development of highly effective antiemetic drugs. **Antagonists to the $5HT_3$-receptor** include alosetron, granisetron, ondansetron, and palonosetron. Ondansetron can be given either intravenously (8 mg or 0.15 mg/kg) or orally (24 mg once before highly emetogenic chemotherapy, 8 mg twice daily for moderately emetogenic chemotherapy). Dosing of granisetron is 1 mg or 0.01 mg/kg intravenously or 1–2 mg orally.

Palonosetron, a long-acting $5HT_3$-receptor antagonist with high affinity for the receptor, is given once at a dose of 0.25 mg intravenously, both for acute and delayed emesis. As a class of drugs, the $5HT_3$-receptor antagonists have the potential to cause ECG changes, including QT prolongation.

Antagonists to the NK_1-receptor are aprepitant, fosaprepitant, and netupitant. Aprepitant is given as a 125-mg oral dose followed by an 80-mg dose on the second and third day along with a $5HT_3$-receptor antagonist and dexamethasone to increase its immediate and delayed protective effect for highly emetogenic chemotherapy. Fosaprepitant, the intravenous formulation of the prodrug to aprepitant, can be given at a dose of 115 mg if followed by 2 days of aprepitant or at a dose of 150 mg if given alone. NEPA is a single-dose capsule consisting of a combination of netupitant and palonosetron.

For highly emetogenic chemotherapy (eg, cisplatin), patients should be offered a four-drug regimen (a $5HT_3$-antagonist, dexamethasone, NK_1-receptor antagonist, and olanzapine), all given on the first day (and if used, aprepitant given again on the second and third days with dexamethasone and olanzapine continued on days 2–4. For moderately emetogenic chemotherapy, standard regimens include both three-drug regimens (an NK_1-antagonist, a $5HT_3$-antagonist, and dexamethasone) or a two-drug combination ($5HT_3$-antagonist and dexamethasone). Palonosetron is the preferred $5HT_3$-blocker due to its greater affinity for the $5HT_3$-receptor and its longer half-life. For low emetogenic chemotherapy drugs, a single agent such as a $5HT_3$-antagonist or prochlorperazine or dexamethasone can be given. Another medication that is helpful for anticipatory or refractory nausea and vomiting is olanzapine, 10 mg given orally once.

The importance of treating chemotherapy-induced nausea and vomiting expectantly and aggressively beginning with the first course of chemotherapy cannot be overemphasized. Patients being treated in the clinic setting should always be given antiemetics for home use with written instructions as well as contact numbers to call for advice.

3. Gastrointestinal Toxicity

Untoward effects of cancer chemotherapy include damage to the more rapidly growing cells of the body such as the mucosal lining from the mouth through the GI tract. Oral symptoms range from mild mouth soreness to frank ulcerations. Not uncommonly, mouth ulcerations will have superimposed candida or herpes simplex infections. In addition to receiving cytotoxic chemotherapy, a significant risk factor for development of oral mucositis is poor oral hygiene and existing caries or periodontal disease. Toxicity in the GI tract usually manifests as diarrhea. GI symptoms can range from mild symptoms of loose stools to life-threatening diarrhea leading to dehydration and electrolyte imbalances. Drugs most commonly associated with causing mucositis in the mouth and the GI tract are cytarabine, 5-fluorouracil, and methotrexate.

Patients undergoing treatment for head and neck cancer with concurrent chemotherapy and radiation therapy have a very high risk of developing severe mucositis.

Preventive strategies for oral mucositis include pretreatment dental care, particularly for all patients with head and neck cancer and any patient with cancer and poor dental hygiene who will be receiving chemotherapy. Once mucositis is encountered, superimposed fungal infections should be treated with topical antifungal medications or systemic therapy. Suspected herpetic infections can be treated with acyclovir or valacyclovir. Mucositis may also be managed with mouthwashes; it is also important to provide adequate pain medication.

Diarrhea is most associated with 5-fluorouracil, capecitabine, and irinotecan as well as the tyrosine kinase inhibitors (dasatinib, imatinib, nilotinib, regorafenib, sorafenib, sunitinib) and epithelial growth factor inhibitors (cetuximab, erlotinib, panitumumab). Mild to moderate diarrhea due to cytotoxic chemotherapy not related to immunotherapy, can be managed with oral antidiarrheal medication (loperamide, 4 mg initially followed by 2 mg every 2–4 hours until bowel movements are formed). Occasionally, severe diarrhea will cause dehydration, electrolyte imbalances, and AKI; these patients require inpatient management with aggressive intravenous hydration and electrolyte replacement. Diarrhea associated with checkpoint inhibitors is concerning for immune-related colitis and warrants workup to rule out infection. Consider a referral to a gastroenterologist for colonoscopy, an abdominal CT scan, and a trial of corticosteroids for grade 2 and higher diarrhea. Consider permanent discontinuation of the checkpoint inhibitor for grade 3 and higher diarrhea, especially any one of the CTLA-4 inhibitors.

4. Miscellaneous Drug-Specific Toxicities

The toxicities of individual drugs are summarized in Tables 39–3 and 39–10; however, several of these toxicities warrant additional mention, since they occur with frequently administered agents, and special measures are often indicated.

A. Hemorrhagic Cystitis Induced by Cyclophosphamide or Ifosfamide

Patients receiving cyclophosphamide must maintain a high fluid intake prior to and following the administration of the drug and be counseled to empty their bladders frequently. Early symptoms suggesting bladder toxicity include dysuria and increased frequency of urination. Should microscopic hematuria develop, it is advisable to stop the drug temporarily or switch to a different alkylating agent, to increase fluid intake, and to administer a urinary analgesic such as phenazopyridine. The neutralizing agent, mesna, can be used for patients in whom cystitis develops. With severe cystitis, large segments of bladder mucosa may be shed, resulting in prolonged gross hematuria. Such patients should be observed for signs of urinary obstruction and may require cystoscopy for removal of obstructing blood clots.

B. Neuropathy Due to Vinca Alkaloids and Other Chemotherapy Drugs

Neuropathy is caused by a number of different chemotherapy drugs, the most common being vincristine. The peripheral neuropathy can be sensory, motor, autonomic, or a combination of these types. In its mildest form, it consists of paresthesias of the fingers and toes. With continued vincristine therapy, the paresthesias extend to the proximal interphalangeal joints, hyporeflexia appears in the lower extremities, and significant weakness can develop. Other drugs in the vinca alkaloid class as well as the taxane drugs (docetaxel and paclitaxel) and agents to treat myeloma (bortezomib and thalidomide) cause similar toxicity.

Constipation is the most common symptom of autonomic neuropathy associated with the vinca alkaloids. Patients receiving these drugs should be started on mild cathartics (eg, senna and polyethylene glycol [Miralax]) and other agents (see Table 15–4); otherwise, severe impaction may result from an atonic bowel.

C. Methotrexate Toxicity

Methotrexate, a folate antagonist, is a commonly used component of regimens to treat patients with leptomeningeal disease, acute lymphoblastic leukemia, and sarcomas. Methotrexate is almost entirely eliminated by the kidney. Methotrexate toxicity affects cells with rapid turnover, including the bone marrow and mucosa resulting in myelosuppression and mucositis. High-dose methotrexate, usually defined as a dose of 500 mg/m^2 or more given over 4–36 hours, would be lethal without "rescue" of the normal tissues. Leucovorin, a form of folate, will reverse the toxic effects of methotrexate and is given until serum methotrexate levels are in the safe range (less than 0.05 mmol/L). It is crucial that high-dose methotrexate and leucovorin are given precisely according to protocol as deviations of the timing of methotrexate delivery or delay in rescue can result in death.

Vigorous hydration and bicarbonate loading can help prevent crystallization of high-dose methotrexate in the renal tubular epithelium and consequent nephrotoxicity. Daily monitoring of the serum creatinine is mandatory.

D. Cardiotoxicity from Anthracyclines and Other Chemotherapy Drugs

A number of cancer chemotherapy drugs are associated with cardiovascular complications including traditional drugs such as anthracyclines as well as new targeted agents. The anthracycline drugs can produce acute (during administration), subacute (days to months following administration), and delayed (years following administration) cardiac toxicity. The most feared complication is the delayed development of heart failure. Risk factors for this debilitating toxicity include the anthracycline cumulative dose, age over 70, previous or concurrent irradiation of the chest, preexisting cardiac disease, and concurrent administration of chemotherapy drugs such as trastuzumab. The problem is greatest with doxorubicin because it is the most commonly administered anthracycline due to its major role in the treatment of lymphomas, sarcomas, breast cancer, and certain other solid tumors. Patients receiving anthracyclines should have an assessment of LVEF. If the LVEF is greater than 50%, anthracyclines can be administered; if the LVEF is less than 30%, these drugs should not be given. For patients with intermediate values, anthracyclines can be cautiously given, if necessary, at lower doses with LVEF monitoring between doses. In general, patients should not receive total doses in excess of 450 mg/m^2; the dose should be lower if prior chest radiotherapy has been given. Unfortunately, toxicity may be irreversible and frequently fatal at total dosage levels above 550 mg/m^2. At lower total doses (eg, 350 mg/m^2), the symptoms and signs of heart failure generally respond well to medical therapy and discontinuation of the anthracycline.

As molecular mechanisms for cancer have been increasingly delineated, therapies have been developed that better target these mechanisms. Therapies targeting oncogenic pathways include (1) HER2 inhibitors; (2) VEGF signaling pathway inhibitors; (3) multitargeted tyrosine kinase inhibitors; (4) proteasome inhibitors; and (5) immune checkpoint inhibitors. Many of the pathways targeted by these drugs share a common biologic pathway in cardiac tissue. Untoward cardiac events are being increasingly reported with these agents, including arrhythmias, cardiac ischemia, myocarditis, thrombosis, and heart failure.

E. Cisplatin Nephrotoxicity and Neurotoxicity

Cisplatin is effective in treating testicular, bladder, head and neck, lung, and ovarian cancers. With cisplatin, the serious side effects of nephrotoxicity and neurotoxicity must be anticipated and aggressively managed. Patients must be vigorously hydrated prior to, during, and after cisplatin administration. Both kidney function and electrolytes must be monitored. The neurotoxicity is usually manifested as a peripheral neuropathy of mixed sensorimotor type and may be associated with painful paresthesias. Ototoxicity is a potentially serious manifestation of neurotoxicity and can progress to deafness. The second-generation platinum analog, carboplatin, is non-nephrotoxic, although it is myelosuppressive. In the setting of preexisting kidney disease or neuropathy, carboplatin can be substituted for cisplatin.

F. Immune Checkpoint Inhibitor–Associated Toxicity

Immune checkpoint inhibitors are widely used in the treatment of numerous cancers and include PD-1, PD-L1, and cytotoxic T lymphocyte antigen-4 (CTLA-4) inhibitors. Their main toxicities involve immune-related adverse events that occur via the same mechanisms for its antitumor effects (ie, self-reactive T cells escaping central tolerance). Common immune-related adverse events include thyroiditis, dermatitis, colitis, hepatitis, arthritis, arthralgias, and pneumonitis. Less common but serious immune-related adverse events include hypophysitis, myocarditis, myositis, Stevens-Johnson syndrome/toxic epidermal necrolysis, and type 1 diabetes mellitus. Many immune-related adverse events resolve by withholding the drugs or instituting immunosuppressive agents such as corticosteroids, or both options, but higher grade or persistent immune-related adverse events require specialty consultation, immune-modulating agents, and consideration of discontinuation of the immune checkpoint inhibitors. The combination of PD-1 or PD-L1 inhibitors with CTLA-4 inhibitors results in higher rates of grade 3 or higher and all grades of immune-related adverse events.

PROGNOSIS

Patients receiving chemotherapy for curative intent will often tolerate side effects with the knowledge that the treatment may result in eradication of their cancer. Patients receiving therapy for palliative intent often have their therapy tailored to improve quality of life while minimizing major side effects. A valuable sign of clinical improvement is the general well-being of the patient.

Brahmer JR et al. Society for Immunotherapy of Cancer (SITC) clinical practice guideline on immune checkpoint inhibitor-related adverse events. J Immunother Cancer. 2021;9:e002435. [PMID: 34172516]

Okada Y et al. One-day versus three-day dexamethasone in combination with palonosetron for the prevention of chemotherapy-induced nausea and vomiting: a systematic review and individual patient data-based meta-analysis. Oncologist. 2019;24:1593. [PMID: 31217343]

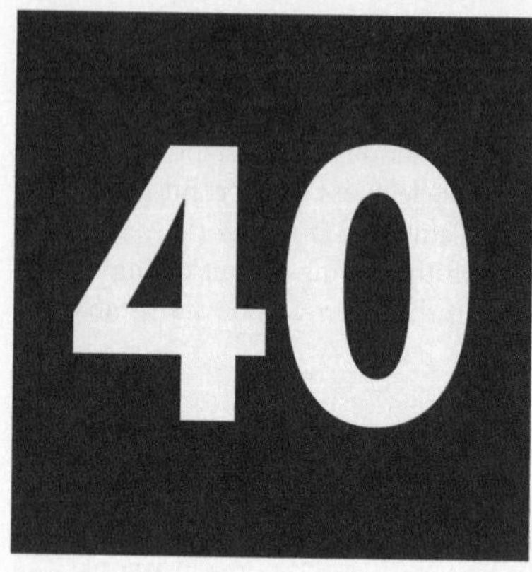

Genetic & Genomic Disorders

Reed E. Pyeritz, MD, PhD

ACUTE INTERMITTENT PORPHYRIA

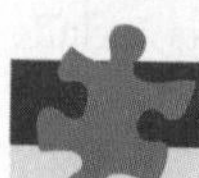

ESSENTIALS OF DIAGNOSIS

- Unexplained abdominal crisis, generally in young women.
- Acute peripheral or CNS dysfunction; recurrent psychiatric illnesses.
- Hyponatremia.
- Porphobilinogen in the urine during an attack.

General Considerations

Though there are several different types of porphyrias, the one with the most serious consequences and the one that usually presents in adulthood is acute intermittent porphyria (AIP), which is inherited as an autosomal dominant condition, though it remains clinically silent in most patients who carry a mutation in *HMBS*. Clinical illness usually develops in women. Symptoms begin in the teens or 20s, but onset can begin after menopause in rare cases. The disorder is caused by partial deficiency of hydroxymethylbilane synthase activity, leading to increased excretion of aminolevulinic acid and porphobilinogen in the urine. The diagnosis may be elusive if not specifically considered. The characteristic abdominal pain may be due to abnormalities in autonomic innervation in the gut. In contrast to other forms of porphyria, cutaneous photosensitivity is absent in AIP. Attacks are precipitated by numerous factors, including drugs and intercurrent infections. Harmful and relatively safe drugs for use in treatment are listed in Table 40–1. Hyponatremia may be seen, due in part to inappropriate release of ADH, although GI loss of sodium in some patients may be a contributing factor.

Clinical Findings

A. Symptoms and Signs

Patients show intermittent abdominal pain of varying severity, and in some instances, it may so simulate an acute abdomen as to lead to exploratory laparotomy. Because the origin of the abdominal pain is neurologic, there is an absence of fever and leukocytosis. Complete recovery between attacks is usual. Any part of the nervous system may be involved, with evidence for central, autonomic, and peripheral neuropathy. Peripheral neuropathy may be symmetric or asymmetric and mild or profound; in the latter instance, it can even lead to quadriplegia with respiratory paralysis. Other CNS manifestations include seizures, altered consciousness, psychosis, and abnormalities of the basal ganglia. Hyponatremia may further cause or exacerbate CNS manifestations.

B. Laboratory Findings

Often there is profound hyponatremia. The diagnosis can be confirmed by demonstrating an increased amount of porphobilinogen in the urine during an acute attack. Freshly voided urine is of normal color but may turn dark upon standing in light and air.

Most families have different mutations in *HMBS* causing AIP. Mutations can be detected in 90% of patients and used for presymptomatic and prenatal diagnosis.

Prevention

Avoidance of factors known to precipitate attacks of AIP—especially drugs—can reduce morbidity. Sulfonamides and barbiturates are the most common culprits; others are listed in Table 40–1 and online at https://porphyriafoundation.org/for-patients/about-porphyria/treatment-options/. Starvation diets and prolonged fasting also cause attacks and so must be avoided. Hormonal changes during pregnancy can precipitate crises.

Treatment

Treatment with a high-carbohydrate diet diminishes the number of attacks in some patients and is a reasonable empiric gesture considering its benignity. Acute attacks may be life-threatening and require prompt diagnosis, withdrawal of the inciting agent (if possible), and treatment with analgesics and intravenous glucose in saline and hemin. A minimum of 300 g of carbohydrates per day should be provided orally or intravenously. Electrolyte balance requires close attention. Hemin therapy has been used but with serious adverse effects, especially phlebitis and coagulopathy.

Table 40–1. Some of the "unsafe" and "probably safe" drugs used in the treatment of acute porphyrias.

Unsafe	Probably Safe
Alcohol	Acetaminophen
Alkylating agents	Amitriptyline
Barbiturates	Aspirin
Carbamazepine	Atropine
Chloroquine	Beta-adrenergic blockers
Chlorpropamide	Chloral hydrate
Clonidine	Chlordiazepoxide
Dapsone	Corticosteroids
Ergots	Diazepam
Erythromycin	Digoxin
Estrogens, synthetic	Diphenhydramine
Food additives	Guanethidine
Glutethimide	Hyoscine
Griseofulvin	Ibuprofen
Hydralazine	Imipramine
Ketamine	Insulin
Meprobamate	Lithium
Methyldopa	Naproxen
Metoclopramide	Nitrofurantoin
Nortriptyline	Opioid analgesics
Pentazocine	Penicillamine
Phenytoin	Penicillin and derivatives
Progestins	Phenothiazines
Pyrazinamide	Procaine
Rifampin	Streptomycin
Spironolactone	Succinylcholine
Succinimides	Tetracycline
Sulfonamides	Thiouracil
Theophylline	
Tolazamide	
Tolbutamide	
Valproic acid	

Givosiran, a delta aminolevulinic acid synthase-directed small interfering RNA, has become standard of care. This drug reduces attacks and the need for hemin use; it requires monthly subcutaneous administration. Liver transplantation is an option for patients with disease poorly controlled by medical therapy.

When to Refer

- For management of severe abdominal pain, seizures, or psychosis.
- For preventive management when a patient with porphyria considers becoming pregnant.
- For genetic counseling and molecular diagnosis.

When to Admit

The patient should be hospitalized for an acute attack when accompanied by mental status changes, seizure, or hyponatremia.

Gerischer LM et al. Acute porphyrias—a neurologic perspective. Brain Behav. 2021;11:e2389. [PMID: 34661997]

Lissing M et al. Liver transplantation for acute intermittent porphyria. Liver Transpl. 2021;27:491. [PMID: 33259654]

Pinto RJ et al. Porphyrias: a clinically based approach. Eur J Intern Med. 2019;67:24. [PMID: 31257150]

Stölzel U et al. Clinical guide and update on porphyrias. Gastroenterology. 2019;157:365. [PMID: 31085196]

Syed YY. Givosiran: a review in acute hepatic porphyria. Drugs. 2021;81:841. [PMID: 33871817]

Zhao L et al. Therapeutic strategies for acute intermittent porphyria. Intractable Rare Dis Res. 2020;9:205. [PMID: 33139979]

DOWN SYNDROME

ESSENTIALS OF DIAGNOSIS

- Typical craniofacial features (flat occiput, epicanthal folds, large tongue).
- Intellectual disability.
- Congenital heart disease (eg, atrioventricular canal defects) in 50% of patients.
- Three copies of chromosome 21 (trisomy 21) or a chromosome rearrangement that results in three copies of a region of the long arm of chromosome 21.

General Considerations

Nearly 0.5% of all human conceptions are trisomic for chromosome 21. Because of increased fetal mortality, birth incidence of Down syndrome is 1 per 700 but varies from 1 per 1000 in young mothers to more than three times as frequent in women of advanced maternal age. The presence of a fetus with Down syndrome can be detected in many pregnancies in the first or early second trimester through screening maternal serum for alpha-fetoprotein and other biomarkers ("multiple marker screening") and by detecting increased nuchal thickness and underdevelopment of the nasal bone on ultrasonography. Prenatal diagnosis with high sensitivity and specificity can be achieved by assaying fetal DNA that is circulating in maternal blood. The chance of bearing a child with Down syndrome increases exponentially with the age of the mother at conception and begins a marked rise after age 35 years. By age 45 years, the odds of having an affected child are as high as 1 in 40. The risk of other conditions associated with trisomy also increases, because of the predisposition of older oocytes to nondisjunction during meiosis. There is little risk of trisomy associated with increased paternal age. However, older men do have an increased risk of fathering a child with a new autosomal dominant condition. Because there are so many distinct conditions, however, the chance of fathering an offspring with any given one is extremely small.

Clinical Findings

A. Symptoms and Signs

Down syndrome is usually diagnosed at birth on the basis of the typical craniofacial features, hypotonia, and single palmar crease. Several serious problems that may be evident at birth or may develop early in childhood include duodenal atresia, congenital heart disease (especially atrioventricular canal defects), and hematologic malignancy. The intestinal and cardiac anomalies usually respond to surgery. A transient neonatal leukemia generally responds to conservative management. The incidences of both acute lymphoblastic and especially myeloid leukemias are increased in childhood. Leukemia typically responds to reduced-dose chemotherapy, but if relapse occurs, outcome is poor. Intelligence varies across a wide spectrum. Many people with Down syndrome do well in sheltered workshops and group homes, but few achieve full independence in adulthood. Other frequent complications include atlanto-axial instability, celiac disease, frequent infections due to immune deficiency, and hypothyroidism. An Alzheimer-like dementia usually becomes evident in the fourth or fifth decade of life. Patients with Down syndrome who survive childhood and who develop dementia have a reduced life expectancy; on average, they live to about age 55 years.

B. Laboratory Findings

Cytogenomic analysis should always be performed—even though most patients will have simple trisomy for chromosome 21—to detect unbalanced translocations; such patients may have a parent with a balanced translocation, and there will be a substantial recurrence risk of Down syndrome in future offspring of that parent and potentially that parent's relatives.

Treatment

Duodenal atresia should be treated surgically. Congenital heart disease should be treated as in any other patient. Effective treatment does no long-term harm to neurodevelopment. As yet, no medical treatment has been proven to affect the neurodevelopmental or the neurodegenerative aspects. Trials of supplementation with antioxidants have shown no benefit.

When to Refer

- For comprehensive evaluation of infants to investigate congenital heart disease, hematologic malignancy, and duodenal atresia.
- For genetic counseling of the parents.
- For signs of dementia in an adult patient.

When to Admit

A young patient should be hospitalized for failure to thrive, regurgitation, or breathlessness.

Badeau M et al. Genomics-based non-invasive prenatal testing for detection of fetal chromosomal aneuploidy in pregnant women. Cochrane Database Syst Rev. 2017;11:CD011767. [PMID: 29125628]

Boucher AC et al. Clinical and biological aspects of myeloid leukemia in Down syndrome. Leukemia 2021;35:3352. [PMID: 34518645]

Fortea J et al. Alzheimer's disease associated with Down syndrome: a genetic form of dementia. Lancet Neurol. 2021;20:930. [PMID: 34687637]

Gandy KC et al. The relationship between chronic health conditions and cognitive deficits in children, adolescents, and young adults with Down syndrome: a systematic review. PLoS One. 2020;15:e0239040. [PMID: 32915911]

Jafri SK et al. Use of antioxidants supplementation of developmental outcomes in children with Down syndrome—a systematic review and meta-analysis. Child Care Health Dev. 2022;48:177. [PMID: 34644809]

Neil N et al. Communication intervention for individuals with Down syndrome: systematic review and meta-analysis. Dev Neurorehabil. 2018;21:1. [PMID: 27537068]

Walpert M et al. A systematic review of unexplained early regression in adolescents and adults with Down syndrome. Brain Sci. 2021;11:1197. [PMID: 34573218]

FAMILIAL HYPERCHOLESTEROLEMIA

- Elevated serum total cholesterol and LDL cholesterol.
- Autosomal dominant inheritance.
- Mutation in *LRL, PCSK9*, or *APOB*.

General Considerations

Familial hypercholesterolemia (FH) is a group of autosomal dominant and recessive conditions that result in elevated LDL levels in the blood. High LDL predisposes to atherosclerosis, which in turn leads to premature MI and stroke. The incidence of these serious complications increases with age and when associated with the other common predispositions to atherosclerosis, such as smoking and hypertension. About 1 in 500 people in the United States have FH; worldwide, the prevalence is about 10 million. Only about 15% of FH cases are diagnosed and even fewer are treated effectively. Individuals who inherit two copies of a mutant gene that causes FH have a more severe disease that typically presents in childhood with severe hypercholesterolemia and early-onset arterial disease.

Clinical Findings

A. Symptoms and Signs

Yellow lipid deposits appear on tendons, especially the Achilles (tendon xanthoma).

B. Laboratory Findings

Total serum cholesterol with the LDL component is particularly high. A detailed family history and genetic testing should be obtained when individuals are younger than 40 years with an LDL level greater than 200 mg/mL and for individuals older than 40 years with a level greater than 250 mg/mL.

Prevention

In most instances, the elevated LDL is inherited as an autosomal dominant trait. An affected individual in all likelihood inherited FH from one parent, and each of his or her children has a 50/50 chance of inheriting FH. In uncommon cases, both parents have a mutation in the LDL receptor and one-quarter of their children, on average, will inherit two mutant alleles and have homozygous FH, which is a much more serious disease with manifestations in childhood.

Mutations in the following four genes can cause FH: (1) *LDLR*, which encodes the LDL receptor located on the surface of cells and responsible for moving LDL into the cell for metabolism is the most common mutant gene in FH; (2) *APOB*, which encodes a component of LDL and mutations inhibit binding to LDL receptor; (3) *PCSK9*, which encodes a protein that normally reduces production of LDL receptors, so mutations actually protect from hypercholesterolemia; and (4) *ARH*, which requires mutations in both alleles (autosomal recessive inheritance) to cause FH.

Treatment

Statins, usually at high doses, can reduce LDL levels, occasionally to acceptable levels (see Table 28–3). The earlier in life that treatment is begun, the better the outcome in reducing mortality from atherosclerosis. In homozygous FH, if high-dose statins do not reduce LDL sufficiently, treatment with a monoclonal antibody (eg, alirocumab and evolocumab) that blocks the action of the *PCSK9* enzyme (which inactivates hepatic receptors that transport LDL into the liver for metabolism) can be an expensive adjunct to standard therapy (see Chapter 28). If all else fails, then apheresis is needed to reduce LDL.

Another important need in effective management is to screen relatives who are at risk, certainly by measuring LDL levels, but increasingly by identifying the mutation in the family and utilizing that for screening.

When to Refer

- For comprehensive evaluation of infants for their lipid profile.
- For genetic counseling of the patient, his or her parents, siblings, and offspring.
- For signs of atherosclerotic CVD.

When to Admit

For signs or symptoms of acute arterial occlusive events.

Futema M et al. Genetic testing for familial hypercholesterolemia—past, present and future. J Lipid Res. 2021:62:100139. [PMID: 34666015]

Kramer AI et al. Estimating the prevalence of familial hypercholesterolemia in acute coronary syndrome: systematic review and meta-analysis. Can J Cardiol. 2019;35:1322. [PMID: 31500889]

Leonardi-Bee J et al. Effectiveness of cascade testing strategies in relatives for familial hypercholesterolemia: a systematic review and meta-analysis. Atherosclerosis. 2021;338:7. [PMID: 34753031]

Sabatine MS. PCSK9 inhibitors: clinical evidence and implementation. Nat Rev Cardiol. 2019;16:155. [PMID: 30420622]

Thompson GR. Use of apheresis in the age of new therapies for familial hypercholesterolemia. Curr Opin Lipidol. 2021;32: 363. [PMID: 34561311]

FRAGILE X SYNDROME

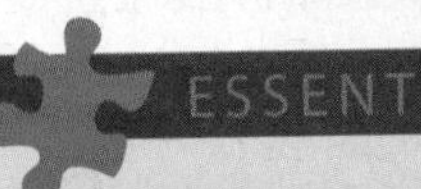

ESSENTIALS OF DIAGNOSIS

- Expanded trinucleotide repeat (> 200) in the *FMR1* gene.
- **Males:** mental impairment and autism; large testes after puberty.
- **Females:** learning disabilities or mental impairment; premature ovarian failure.
- Late-onset tremor and ataxia in males and females with moderate trinucleotide repeat (55–200) expansion (premutation carriers).

Clinical Findings

A. Symptoms and Signs

This X-linked condition accounts for more cases of mental impairment in males than any condition except Down syndrome; about 1 in 4000 males is affected. The CNS phenotype includes autism spectrum, impulsivity and aggressiveness, and repetitive behaviors. The condition also affects intellectual function in females, although less severely and about 50% less frequently than in males. Affected (heterozygous) young women show no physical signs other than early menopause, but they may have learning difficulties, anxiety, sensory issues, or frank impairment. Affected males show macro-orchidism (enlarged testes) after puberty, large ears and a prominent jaw, a high-pitched voice, autistic characteristics, and mental impairment. Some males show evidence of a mild connective tissue defect, with joint hypermobility and mitral valve prolapse.

Women who are premutation carriers (55–200 CGG repeats) are at increased risk for premature ovarian insufficiency (FXPOI) and mild cognitive abnormalities. Male and female premutation carriers are at risk for mood and anxiety disorders and the development of tremor and ataxia beyond middle age (fragile X-associated tremor/ataxia syndrome, FXTAS). Changes in the cerebellar white matter may be evident on MRI before symptoms appear. Because of the relatively high prevalence of premutation carriers in the general population (1/130–1/600), older people in whom any of these behavioral or neurologic problems develop should undergo testing of the *FMR1* locus.

B. Laboratory Findings

The first marker for this condition was a small gap, or fragile site, evident near the tip of the long arm of the X chromosome. Subsequently, the condition was found to be due to expansion of a trinucleotide repeat (CGG) near a gene called *FMR1*. All individuals have some CGG repeats in this location, but as the number increases beyond 52, the chances of further expansion during spermatogenesis or oogenesis increase.

Being born with one *FMR1* allele with 200 or more repeats results in mental impairment in most men and in about 60% of women. The more repeats, the greater the likelihood that further expansion will occur during gametogenesis; this results in anticipation, in which the disorder can worsen from one generation to the next.

Prevention

DNA diagnosis for the number of repeats has supplanted cytogenetic analysis for both clinical and prenatal diagnosis. This should be done on any male or female who has unexplained mental impairment. Newborn screening based on hypermethylation of the *FMR1* gene is being considered as a means of early detection and intervention.

Treatment

No treatment directly addresses the underlying genetic perturbation. Several treatments that address the imbalances in neurotransmission have been developed based on the mouse model and are in clinical trials. Valproic acid may reduce symptoms of hyperactivity and attention deficit, but standard therapies should be tried first.

When to Refer

- For otherwise unexplained mental impairment or learning difficulties in boys and girls.
- For otherwise unexplained tremor or ataxia in middle-aged individuals.
- For premature ovarian failure.
- For genetic counseling.

Fink DA et al. Fragile X associated primary ovarian insufficiency (FXPOI): case report and literature review. Front Genet. 2018;9:529. [PMID: 30542367]

Huang G et al. Long noncoding RNA can be a probable mechanism and novel target for diagnosis and therapy in fragile X syndrome. Front Genet. 2019;10:466. [PMID: 31191598]

Salcedo-Arellano MJ et al. Fragile X syndrome and associated disorders: clinical aspects and pathology. Neurobiol Dis. 2020;136:104740. [PMID: 31927143]

Spector E et al. Laboratory testing for fragile X, 2021 revision: a technical standard of the American College of Medical Genetics and Genomics (ACMG). Genet Med. 2021;23:799. [PMID: 33795824]

GAUCHER DISEASE

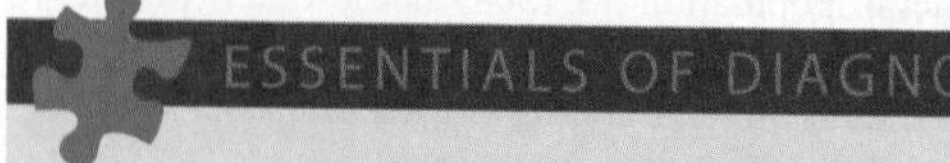

- Deficiency of beta-glucocerebrosidase.
- Anemia and thrombocytopenia.
- Hepatosplenomegaly.
- Pathologic fractures.

Clinical Findings

A. Symptoms and Signs

Gaucher disease has an autosomal recessive pattern of inheritance. A deficiency of beta-glucocerebrosidase causes an accumulation of sphingolipid within phagocytic cells throughout the body. Anemia and thrombocytopenia are common and may be symptomatic; both are due primarily to hypersplenism, but marrow infiltration with Gaucher cells may be a contributing factor. The abdomen can become painfully distended due to enlargement of the liver and spleen. Soft tissue masses, Gaucheromas, can occur anywhere in the body.

Cortical erosions of bones, especially the vertebrae and femur, are due to local infarctions, but the mechanism is unclear. Episodes of bone pain (termed "crises") are reminiscent of those in sickle cell disease. A hip fracture in a patient of any age with a palpable spleen—especially in a Jewish person of Eastern European origin—suggests the possibility of Gaucher disease. Peripheral neuropathy may develop in patients.

Patients with Gaucher disease and heterozygous carriers of a mutation in *GBA* are at increased risk for early-onset Parkinson disease and dementia with Lewy bodies.

Two uncommon forms of Gaucher disease, called type II and type III, involve neurologic accumulation of sphingolipid and a variety of neurologic problems. Type II is of infantile onset and has a poor prognosis. Heterozygotes for Gaucher disease are at increased risk for developing Parkinson disease.

B. Laboratory Findings

Bone marrow aspirates reveal typical Gaucher cells, which have an eccentric nucleus and periodic acid–Schiff (PAS)-positive inclusions, along with wrinkled cytoplasm and inclusion bodies of a fibrillar type. In addition, the serum acid phosphatase is elevated. Definitive diagnosis requires the demonstration of deficient glucocerebrosidase activity in leukocytes. Hundreds of pathogenic variants cause Gaucher disease and some are highly predictive of the neuronopathic forms. Thus, genetic testing especially in a young person, is of potential value. Only four pathogenic variants in glucocerebrosidase account for more than 90% of the disease among Ashkenazi Jews, in whom the carrier frequency is 1:15.

Prevention

Gaucher disease is the most common lysosomal storage disorder. Most clinical complications can be prevented by early institution of enzyme replacement therapy. Carrier screening, especially among of Ashkenazi Jewish descent, detects those couples at 25% risk of having an affected child. Prenatal diagnosis through mutation analysis is feasible. Because of an increased risk of malignancy, especially plasma cell myeloma and other hematologic cancers, regular screening of adults with Gaucher disease is warranted.

Treatment

Several recombinant forms of the enzyme glucocerebrosidase for intravenous administration on a regular basis reduces total body stores of glycolipid and improves orthopedic and hematologic manifestations. Unfortunately, the neurologic manifestations of types II and III have not improved with enzyme replacement therapy. The major drawback is the exceptional cost of enzyme replacement therapy. Eliglustat tartrate is an oral inhibitor of glucosylceramide synthase and reduces the compound that accumulates; while still quite expensive, this approach eliminates the need for frequent intravenous infusions. Early treatment of affected children normalizes growth and bone mineral density and improves liver and spleen size, anemia, and thrombocytopenia. In adults with thrombocytopenia due to splenic sequestration, enzyme replacement often obviates the need for splenectomy.

Biegstraaten M et al. Management goals for type 1 Gaucher disease: an expert consensus document from the European working group on Gaucher disease. Blood Cells Mol Dis. 2018;68:203. [PMID: 28274788]

Nabizadeh A et al. The clinical efficacy of imiglucerase versus eliglustat in patients with Gaucher's disease type 1: a systematic review. J Res Pharm Pract. 2018;7:171. [PMID: 30622983]

Roshan Lal T et al. The spectrum of neurological manifestations associated with Gaucher disease. Diseases. 2017;5:E10. [PMID: 28933363]

Starosta RT et al. Liver involvement in patients with Gaucher disease types I and III. Mol Genet Metab Rep. 2020;22:100564. [PMID: 32099816]

DISORDERS OF HOMOCYSTEINE METABOLISM

ESSENTIALS OF DIAGNOSIS

- Hyperhomocysteinemia: more vascular disease but lowering homocysteine levels is not helpful.
- Homocystinuria: Marfan-like habitus, ectopia lentis, mental impairment, thromboses.
- Elevated homocysteine in the urine or plasma.

General Considerations

Patients with clinical and angiographic evidence of CAD and cerebrovascular and peripheral vascular diseases tend to have higher levels of plasma homocysteine than persons without these vascular diseases. Elevated blood homocysteine also increases the risk of Alzheimer dementia in the older adults. Although these effects were initially thought to be due at least in part to heterozygotes for cystathionine beta-synthase deficiency, there is little supporting evidence. Rather, an important factor leading to hyperhomocysteinemia is folate deficiency. Pyridoxine (vitamin B_6) and vitamin B_{12} are also important in the metabolism of methionine, and deficiency of any of these vitamins can lead to accumulation of homocysteine. Several genes influence utilization of these vitamins and can predispose to deficiency. For example, having one copy—and especially two copies—of an allele that causes thermolability of methylene tetrahydrofolate reductase predisposes people to elevated fasting homocysteine levels. Both nutritional and most genetic deficiencies of these vitamins can be corrected by dietary supplementation of folic acid and, if serum levels are low, vitamins B_6 and B_{12}. In the United States, cereal grains are fortified with folic acid. However, therapy with B vitamins and folate lowers homocysteine levels significantly but does not reduce the risk of either venous thromboembolism or complications of CAD. The role of lowering homocysteine as primary prevention for CVD and stroke has received modest direct support in clinical trials. Hyperhomocysteinemia occurs with ESKD. In the general population, elevated homocysteine correlates with cognitive impairment.

Clinical Findings

A. Symptoms and Signs

Homocystinuria in its classic form is caused by cystathionine beta-synthase deficiency and exhibits autosomal recessive inheritance with a prevalence of 1 per 100,000. This results in extreme elevations of plasma and urinary homocystine levels, a basis for diagnosis of this disorder. Homocystinuria is similar in certain superficial aspects to Marfan syndrome, since patients may have a similar body habitus and ectopia lentis is almost always present. However, mental impairment is often present in homocystinuria, and the cardiovascular events are those of repeated venous and arterial thromboses whose precise cause remains obscure. Thus, the diagnosis should be suspected in patients in the second and third decades of life who have arterial or venous thromboses without other risk factors. Bone mineral density is reduced in untreated patients. Life expectancy is reduced, especially in untreated and pyridoxine-unresponsive patients; MI, stroke, and PE are the most common causes of death. This condition is diagnosed by newborn screening for hypermethioninemia; however, pyridoxine-responsive infants may not be detected. In addition, homozygotes for a common pathogenic allele, p.I278T, show marked clinical variability, with some unaffected as adults.

B. Laboratory Findings

Although many mutations have been identified in the cystathionine beta-synthase (*CBS*) gene, amino acid analysis of plasma remains the most appropriate diagnostic test. Patients should be studied after they have been off folate or pyridoxine supplementation for at least 1 week. Relatively few laboratories provide highly reliable assays for homocysteine. Processing of the specimen is crucial to obtain accurate results. The plasma must be separated within 30 minutes; otherwise, blood cells release the amino acid and the measurement will then be artificially elevated.

Prevention

Prenatal diagnosis and termination of the affected pregnancy are the only way to prevent the occurrence of *CBS*-deficient homocystinuria.

Treatment

About 50% of patients have a form of *CBS* deficiency that improves biochemically and clinically through pharmacologic doses of pyridoxine (50–500 mg orally daily) and folate (5–10 mg orally daily). For these patients, treatment that begins in infancy can prevent neurologic impairment and the other clinical problems. Patients who do not respond to pyridoxine must be treated with a dietary reduction in methionine and supplementation of cysteine, again beginning in infancy. The vitamin betaine is also useful in reducing plasma methionine levels by facilitating a metabolic pathway that bypasses the defective enzyme.

Patients with classic homocystinuria who have suffered venous thrombosis receive anticoagulation therapy, but there are no studies to support prophylactic use of warfarin or antiplatelet agents.

Bublil EM et al. Classical homocystinuria: from cystathionine beta-synthase deficiency to novel enzyme therapies. Biochimie. 2021;173:48. [PMID: 31857119]

Gales A et al. Adolescence/adult onset MTHFR deficiency may manifest as isolated and treatable distinct neuro-psychiatric syndromes. Orphanet J Rare Dis. 2018;13:29. [PMID: 29391032]

Poddar R. Hyperhomocysteinemia is an emerging comorbidity in ischemic stroke. Exp Neurol. 2021;336:113541. [PMID: 33278453]

Truitt C et al. Health functionalities of betaine in patients with homocystinuria. Front Nutr. 2021;8:690359. [PMID: 34568401]

Weber Hoss GR et al. Classical homocystinuria: a common inborn error of metabolism? An epidemiological study based on genetic databases. Mol Genet Genomic Med. 2020;8:e1214. [PMID: 32232970]

KLINEFELTER SYNDROME

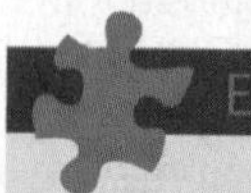

ESSENTIALS OF DIAGNOSIS

- Males with hypergonadotropic hypogonadism and small testes.
- 47,XXY karyotype.

Clinical Findings

A. Symptoms and Signs

Boys with an extra X chromosome are normal in appearance before puberty; thereafter, they have disproportionately long legs and arms, sparse body hair, a female escutcheon, gynecomastia, and small testes. Infertility is due to azoospermia; the seminiferous tubules are hyalinized. The incidence is 1 in 660 newborn male infants, but the diagnosis is often not made until a man is evaluated for inability to conceive. Intellectual disability is somewhat more common than in the general population. Many men with Klinefelter syndrome have language-based learning problems. However, their intelligence usually tests within the broad range of normal. In adulthood, detailed psychometric testing may reveal a deficiency in executive skills. The risk of osteoporosis, breast cancer, and diabetes mellitus is much higher in men with Klinefelter syndrome than in 46,XY men.

B. Laboratory Findings

Low serum testosterone is common. The karyotype is typically 47,XXY, but other sex chromosome anomalies cause variations of Klinefelter syndrome.

Prevention

Screening for cancer (especially of the breast), DVT, and glucose intolerance is indicated.

Treatment

Treatment with testosterone after puberty is advisable but will not restore fertility. However, men with Klinefelter syndrome have had mature sperm aspirated from their testes and injected into oocytes, resulting in fertilization. After the blastocysts have been implanted into the uterus of a partner, conception has resulted. But, men with Klinefelter syndrome do have an increased risk for aneuploidy in sperm, and therefore, genomic analysis of a blastocyst should be considered before implantation.

Akcan N et al. Klinefelter syndrome in childhood: variability in clinical and molecular findings. J Clin Res Pediatr Endocrinol. 2018;10:100. [PMID: 29022558]

Ross JL et al. Androgen treatment effects on motor function, cognition, and behavior in boys with Klinefelter syndrome. J Pediatr. 2017;185:193. [PMID: 28285751]

Skakkebæk A et al. Quality of life in men with Klinefelter syndrome: the impact of genotype, health, socioeconomics, and sexual function. Genet Med. 2018;20:214. [PMID: 28726803]

MARFAN SYNDROME

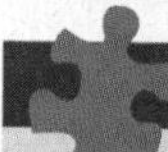

ESSENTIALS OF DIAGNOSIS

- Disproportionately tall stature, thoracic deformity, and joint laxity or contractures.
- Ectopia lentis and myopia.
- Aortic root dilation and dissection; mitral valve prolapse.
- Mutation in *FBN1*, the gene encoding fibrillin-1.

General Considerations

Marfan syndrome, a systemic connective tissue disease, has an autosomal dominant pattern of inheritance. It is characterized by abnormalities of the skeletal, ocular, and cardiovascular systems; spontaneous pneumothorax; dural ectasia; and striae atrophicae. Of most concern is disease of the ascending aorta, which begins as a dilated aortic root. Histology of the aorta shows diffuse medial degeneration. Mitral valve prolapse is common and frequently leads to regurgitation.

Clinical Findings

A. Symptoms and Signs

Affected patients are typically tall, with particularly long arms, legs, and digits (arachnodactyly). However, there can be wide variability in the clinical presentation. Commonly, scoliosis and anterior chest deformity, such as pectus excavatum, are present. Ectopia lentis is present in about half of patients; severe myopia is common and retinal detachment can occur. Mitral valve prolapse is seen in more than half of patients. Aortic root dilation is common and leads to aortic regurgitation or dissection with rupture. To diagnose Marfan syndrome, people with an affected relative need features in at least two systems. People with no family history need features in the skeletal system, two other systems, and one of the major criteria of ectopia lentis, dilation of the aortic root or aortic dissection or a pathogenic variant in *FBN1*.

B. Laboratory Findings

Pathogenic variants in the fibrillin gene (*FBN1*) on chromosome 15 cause Marfan syndrome. Nonetheless, no simple laboratory test is available to support the diagnosis in questionable cases because related conditions may also be due to defects in fibrillin. The pathogenesis of Marfan syndrome involves aberrant regulation of transforming growth factor (TGF)-beta activity. Pathogenic variants in either of two receptors for TGF-beta (TGFBR1 and TGFBR2) can cause conditions that resemble Marfan syndrome in terms of aortic aneurysm and dissection and autosomal dominant inheritance. Mutations in more than two dozen other genes can predispose adults to thoracic aortic aneurysm and dissection.

Prevention

There is prenatal and presymptomatic diagnosis for patients in whom the molecular defect in *FBN1* has been found.

Treatment

Children with Marfan syndrome require regular ophthalmologic surveillance to detect ectopia lentis, correct visual acuity and thus prevent amblyopia, and annual orthopedic consultation for diagnosis of scoliosis at an early enough stage so that bracing might delay progression. Patients of all ages require echocardiography at least annually to monitor aortic root diameter and mitral valve function. Long-term beta-adrenergic blockade, titrated to individual tolerance but enough to produce a negative inotropic effect (eg, atenolol, 1–2 mg/kg orally daily), retards the rate of aortic dilation. While inhibition of the TGF-beta signaling pathway through angiotensin receptor blockade (ARB) in mice with Marfan syndrome is highly effective, ARB treatment in humans is no more effective than beta-adrenergic blockade. Calcium channel blockers, once used as a substitute for beta-blockade, are detrimental to the aorta. Restriction from vigorous physical exertion protects from aortic dissection. Prophylactic replacement of the aortic root with a composite graft when the diameter reaches 45–50 mm in an adult (normal: less than 40 mm) prolongs life. Earlier prophylactic surgery should be considered when there is a strong family history of aortic dissection or when the diameter of the aortic root increases more than 3–4 mm per year. A valve-sparing procedure resuspends the patient's native aortic valve inside a graft that replaces the aneurysmal sinuses of Valsalva and ascending aorta, thus avoiding the need for lifelong anticoagulation. Women with Marfan syndrome are at heightened risk for aortic dissection in the peripartum and postpartum periods. Having an aortic root dimension greater than 40 mm should prompt consideration for prophylactic, valve-sparing aortic repair before undertaking a pregnancy.

Prognosis

People with Marfan syndrome who are untreated commonly die in the fourth or fifth decade from aortic dissection or heart failure secondary to aortic or mitral regurgitation. However, because of earlier diagnosis, lifestyle modifications, beta-adrenergic blockade, and prophylactic aortic and mitral valve surgery, life expectancy has increased by several decades. However, with the longer life expectancy, serious comorbidities that were previously infrequent are now more common. These comorbidities include obstructive sleep apnea, cardiomyopathy, aneurysms and dissections of the abdominal aorta and peripheral arteries, neurologic problems related to dural ectasia, and degenerative arthritis.

When to Refer

- For detailed ophthalmologic examination.
- For at least annual cardiologic evaluation.
- For moderate scoliosis.
- For pregnancy in a woman with Marfan syndrome.
- For genetic counseling.

When to Admit

Any patient with Marfan syndrome in whom severe or unusual chest pain develops should be hospitalized to exclude pneumothorax and aortic dissection.

Pyeritz RE. Etiology and pathogenesis of the Marfan syndrome: current understanding. Ann Cardiothorac Surg. 2017;6:595. [PMID: 29270371]

Pyeritz RE. Improved clinical history results in expanded natural history. Genet Med. 2019;21:1683. [PMID: 30573797]

Renner S et al. Next-generation sequencing of 32 genes associated with hereditary aortopathies and related disorders of connective tissue in a cohort of 199 patients. Genet Med. 2019;21:1832. [PMID: 30675029]

von Kodolitsch Y et al. Features of the Marfan syndrome not listed in the Ghent nosology—the dark side of the disease. Expert Rev Cardiovasc Ther. 2019;17:883. [PMID: 31829751]

HEREDITARY HEMORRHAGIC TELANGIECTASIA

ESSENTIALS OF DIAGNOSIS

- Recurrent epistaxis.
- Mucocutaneous telangiectases.
- Visceral arteriovenous malformations (especially lung, liver, brain, bowel).

Clinical Findings

A. Symptoms and Signs

Hereditary hemorrhagic telangiectasia (HHT), formerly termed "Osler-Weber-Rendu syndrome," is an autosomal dominant disorder of development of the vasculature. Epistaxis may begin in childhood or later in adolescence. Punctate telangiectases of the lips, tongue, fingers, and skin generally appear in later childhood and adolescence. Arteriovenous malformations (AVMs) can occur at any age in the brain, lungs, and liver. Bleeding from the GI tract is due to mucosal vascular malformations and usually is not a problem until mid-adult years or later. Pulmonary AVMs can cause hypoxemia (with peripheral cyanosis, dyspnea, and clubbing) and right-to-left shunting (with embolic stroke or brain abscess). The criteria for diagnosis require presence of three of the following four features: (1) recurrent epistaxis, (2) visceral AVMs, (3) mucocutaneous telangiectases, and (4) being the near relative of a clearly affected individual. Mutation analysis can be used for presymptomatic diagnosis or exclusion of the worry of HHT.

B. Laboratory Findings

MR or CT arteriography detects AVMs. Mutations in at least five genes can cause HHT. Three have been identified, and molecular analysis to identify them is available; these mutations in *ENG, ALK1*, and *SMAD4* account for about 87% of families with HHT. When the familial mutation is known, molecular testing is far more cost-effective than repeated clinical screening of relatives who are at risk.

Prevention

Embolization of pulmonary AVMs with wire coils or other occlusive devices reduces the risk of stroke and brain abscess. Treatment of brain AVMs reduces the risk of hemorrhagic stroke. All patients with HHT with evidence of a pulmonary shunt should practice routine endocarditis prophylaxis (see Table 33–5). All intravenous lines (except those for transfusion of RBCs and radiographic contrast) should have an air-filter to prevent embolization of an air bubble. Prenatal diagnosis through mutation detection is possible. All patients should be referred for genetic counseling.

Treatment

All patients in whom the diagnosis of HHT is considered should have an MRI of the brain with contrast. A contrast echocardiogram will detect most pulmonary AVMs when "bubbles" appear on the left side of the heart after 3–6 cardiac cycles. A positive contrast echocardiogram should be followed by a high-resolution CT angiogram for localization of pulmonary AVMs. Patients who have AVMs with a feeding artery of 2 mm diameter or greater should undergo embolization. After successful embolization of all treatable pulmonary AVMs, the CT angiogram should be repeated in 6 months and 3 years. A person with a negative contrast echocardiogram should have the test repeated every 5 years. Any person with a pulmonary AVM, even an embolized one, should utilize routine endocarditis prophylaxis. Several studies suggest that treatment with anti-estrogenic agents (eg, tamoxifen), thalidomide or its relatives, or anti-vascular endothelial growth factor agents (eg, bevacizumab) can reduce epistaxis and GI bleeding and improve hepatic shunting. However, two randomized, controlled clinical trials of intranasal bevacizumab therapy failed to show an improvement in epistaxis.

Anning R et al. Improvement in epistaxis management: the experience of a dedicated hereditary hemorrhagic telangiectasia clinic. ANZ J Surg. 2022;92:499. [PMID: 34724318]

Beckman JD et al. Integration of clinical parameters, genotype and epistaxis severity score to guide treatment for hereditary hemorrhagic telangiectasia associated bleeding. Orphanet J Rare Dis. 2020;15:185. [PMID: 32660636]

Beslow LA... Pyeritz RE et al. Cerebrovascular malformations in a pediatric hereditary hemorrhagic telangiectasia cohort. Pediatr Neurol. 2020;110:49. [PMID: 32718529]

Chick JFB et al. A survey of pulmonary arteriovenous malformation screening, management, and follow-up in Hereditary Hemorrhagic Telangiectasia Centers of Excellence. Cardiovasc Intervent Radiol. 2017;40:1003. [PMID: 28188364]

Faughnan ME et al. Second international guidelines for the diagnosis and management of hereditary hemorrhagic telangiectasia. Ann Intern Med. 2020;173:989. [PMID: 32894695]

Halderman AA et al. Bevacizumab for epistaxis in hereditary hemorrhagic telangiectasia: an evidence-based review. Am J Rhinol Allergy. 2018;32:258. [PMID: 29745243]

Kolarich AR et al. Imaging manifestations and interventional treatments for hereditary hemorrhagic telangiectasia. Radiographics. 2021;41:2157. [PMID: 34723698]

Lam S et al. Genetic counseling and testing for hereditary hemorrhagic telangiectasia. Clin Genet. 2022;101:275. [PMID: 34415050]

Pyeritz RE. Digital vascular lesions detected by transillumination. Am J Med Genet A. 2022;188:99. [PMID: 34529342]

Selected Pharmacogenetic Tests: Clinical Relevance

Chuanyi Mark Lu, MD

Genetic influences on drug response can be divided into several categories:

1. Altered pharmacokinetics (ie, drug absorption, distribution, tissue localization, biotransformation, and excretion). Examples include genetic polymorphisms in cytochrome P450 oxidase, dihydropyrimidine dehydrogenase, thiopurine methyltransferase enzyme, and uridine diphosphate glucuronosyltransferase enzyme.
2. Altered pharmacodynamics (ie, the effect of a drug at its therapeutic target and at other non-target sites). Genetic variations can modulate drug response by affecting the drug target itself or one of the downstream components in the target's mechanistic pathway. An example is the effect of polymorphisms in the gene encoding the vitamin K epoxide reductase complex on response to warfarin.
3. Effect on idiosyncratic drug reactions. An idiosyncratic reaction is an adverse drug reaction that cannot be anticipated based on the known drug target. Examples include the association of HLA-B*5701 with a hypersensitivity reaction to the antiretroviral nucleoside analog abacavir, and the association between HLA-B*5801 and life-threatening hypersensitivity reactions to allopurinol.
4. Effect on disease pathogenesis (ie, certain genetic variation or aberration [eg, somatic mutation]) can influence a disease pathogenesis by altering the disease severity or the response to specific or targeted therapy. For example, vemurafenib, an inhibitor of kinase BRAF, significantly improves survival in patients with unresectable or metastatic melanoma with the somatic V600E mutation in the *BRAF* gene. Most of the predictive biomarkers (eg, expression of PD-L1 or HER2, somatic mutations in *EGFR*, *KRAS*, or *IDH1/2*) for hematologic and oncologic drugs are regulatorily approved under ***companion diagnostics***. Another example is that patients who are deficient in glucose-6-phosphate dehydrogenase must avoid certain oxidizing drugs (eg, rasburicase) because they can cause severe hemolysis.

Pharmacogenetic testing can help in the selection of certain drugs and their dosages. Table 40–2 lists drugs for which genetic testing has been mandated or recommended.

Table 40–2. Selected pharmacogenetic tests: clinical relevance.[1]

Pharmacogenetic Biomarker	Selected Variants (variant allele, activity)	Allele Frequency	Drugs	Clinical Relevance
Inherited Variants				
CF transmembrane conductance regulator (CFTR)	CFTR G551D (defective)	Present in about 4% of patients with CF.	Ivacaftor	CFTR protein forms a channel that allows chloride ions to cross the membrane. In patients with CF and the pathogenic CFTR G551D variant, the channel fails to open. Ivacaftor corrects the effects of this variant and is approved for persons with CF age > 6 years who have at least one copy of the G551D variant.
Cytochrome P450 (CYP) 2C9 variants	2C9*2 (430C>T, ↓); 2C9*3 (1075A> C, ↓↓)	Present in 9–20% of White individuals, 1–3% of Black individuals, and < 1% of Asian individuals.	Warfarin	Hepatic CYP2C9 is responsible for the metabolic inactivation and clearance of warfarin. Patients carrying 2C9*2 or 2C9*3 (or both) (heterozygote, homozygote or compound heterozygote) require a reduced warfarin maintenance dose to reach a therapeutic INR. While INR remains the standard for monitoring warfarin therapy, CYP2C9 genotyping can be an important aid to the dosing strategy for warfarin-naïve patients, particularly White individuals.
CYP2C19 variants	2C19*2(681G>A, none); 2C19*3(636G>A, none); 2C19*4(1A>G, none); 2C19*5(1297C>T, none) 2C19*17 (g.-3402C>T and g.-806C>T, ↑)	Nonfunctional variants are present in 12–25% of Asian individuals, and 2–7% of White and Black individuals; 2C19*17 carrier status is present in about 25% of White individuals.	Clopidogrel	Clopidogrel must be metabolized in the liver by CYP isoenzymes, principally CYP2C19, to become active. When treated with clopidogrel at recommended dosages, patients with nonfunctional CYP2C19 variants have more cardiovascular events than do patients with normal CYP2C19 function. Alternative drug or intervention strategies should be considered for patients with 2C19 variants. The novel CYP2C19*17 carrier status is associated with increased enzyme activity and an increased risk of bleeding. CYP2C19 genotyping is recommended for patients who have had a cardiovascular event while taking clopidogrel or patients who are at high risk for poor outcomes.

(continued)

Table 40–2. Selected pharmacogenetic tests: clinical relevance.[1] (continued)

Pharmacogenetic Biomarker	Selected Variants (variant allele, activity)	Allele Frequency	Drugs	Clinical Relevance
Inherited Variants (cont.)				
CYP2D6 variants	2D6*1 (fully functional "wild-type"); 2D6*2 (2850C>T or 4180G>C; normal function variant); 2D6*3 (2549delA with or without 1749A>G), 2D6*4 (1846G>A, with or without 1858C>T, 2938C>T or 3877G>C), 2D6*5 (whole gene deletion) and 2D6*6 (1707delT) (nonfunctioning variants); 2D6*9 (1615-2617delAAG), 2D6*10 (100C>T), and 2D6*17 (1023C>T, 2850C>T) (partially functioning variants)	1–2% of the general population carry more than two copies of functional alleles (eg, *1/*1×N or *1/*2×N) and phenotypically *ultra rapidly* metabolize. 5–10% of the general population carry no functional alleles (eg, *4/*4, *4/*5, *5/*5, or *4/*6) and phenotypically *poorly* metabolize.	Codeine, nortriptyline	Both codeine and nortriptyline are metabolized in the liver by CYP2D6. Codeine is a prodrug and needs to be metabolized by CYP2D6, primarily to morphine, whereas nortriptyline is the active moiety and its metabolism results in inactivation of the drug. At conventional doses, patients who *poorly* metabolize codeine based upon CYP2D6 genotype will derive no therapeutic benefit from codeine but may be "overdosed" with for nortriptyline and are at increased risk for adverse effects. Conversely, at conventional doses of codeine, patients who *rapidly* metabolize codeine have higher than expected morphine levels (an initial "overdose"), with more adverse effects and a shorter than expected duration of pain control. On the other hand, patients may derive no therapeutic benefit from nortriptyline because of excessive metabolism of the drug.
CYP3A5 variants	3A5*1 (functional allele); 3A5*3 (6986A>G) (nonfunctional allele); 3A5*6 (14690G>A) and 3A5*7 (27131-27132ins T) (nonfunctional alleles)	3A5*3 is present in 82–95% of White individuals, 33% of Black individuals, and 65–85% of Asian individuals; 3A5*6 is present in 7–17% of Black individuals and 3A5*7 is present in 8% of Black individuals.	Tacrolimus	Individuals carrying two functional *1 alleles (*1/*1) *rapidly* metabolize. Individuals carrying one *1 allele and one nonfunctional allele (eg, *1/*3, *1/*6, *1/*7) *intermediate* metabolize. Individual carrying two nonfunctional alleles (*3/*3, etc.) poorly metabolize. Individuals carrying one or two functional alleles have decreased dose-adjusted trough levels of tacrolimus compared with those who carry only nonfunctional alleles. Accordingly, an increase of standard starting dose of 1.5–2× usual dose is needed for those who intermediately or rapidly metabolize tacrolimus.

Inherited Variants (cont.)				
Dihydropyrimidine dehydrogenase (DPD) variants	*DPYD**2A (1905+1G>A, none); *DPYD**13 (1679T>G, ↓↓); *DPYD* rs67376798 (2846A>T, ↓↓)	Nonfunctional variants are present in 0.1–1% of White individuals (eg, French descent).	5-Fluorouracil, capecitabine	Fluoropyrimidines (ie, 5-fluorouracil, capecitabine) are metabolized by the DPD enzyme, encoded by the *DPYD* gene. To avoid severe or even fatal drug toxicity, an alternative drug should be selected for patients who are homozygous for *DPYD* nonfunctional variants (*2A, *13, or rs67376798). Consider a 50% reduction in starting dose for heterozygous patients who have low DPD activity (30–70% of normal).
Glucose-6 phosphate dehydrogenase (*G6PD*) gene	G6PD A (p.Asn126Asp and p.Val68Met): ↓enzyme activity; G6PD Mediterranean (p.Ser218Phe): ↓↓ enzyme activity; G6PD Canton (p.Arg489Leu): ↓↓ enzyme activity	5% prevalence worldwide (> 25% in countries where malaria is or was endemic). G6PD A, G6PD Mediterranean, and G6PD Canton are most common in Black individuals, White individuals, and Asian individuals, respectively. Approximately 400 million people worldwide have G6PD deficiency.	Rasburicase, tafenoquine	RBCs that lack the enzyme G6PD are sensitive to oxidative damage due to a deficiency in NADPH. Those who have G6PD deficiency are at risk for life-threating hemolytic reactions and methemoglobinemia if given oxidizing drugs such as rasburicase, a uric oxidase used to treat high levels of uric acid. Rasburicase is contraindicated for individuals who are G6PD deficient (with or without hemolytic anemia); an alternative drug (eg, allopurinol) should be used. Similarly, G6PD testing must be performed before prescribing the anti-malaria drug tafenoquine.
HLA-B*1502 allele	HLA-B*1502	Present in 10–15% of Asian individuals and 1–2% of White individuals.	Carbamazepine	Carbamazepine is associated with serious or even fatal idiosyncratic skin reactions, eg, Stevens-Johnson syndrome and toxic epidermal necrolysis. The reactions are significantly more common in patients who carry the HLA-B*1502 allele. This allele occurs almost exclusively in patients with ancestry across broad areas of Asia, including South Asian Indians. HLA-B*1502 genotyping may be useful for risk stratification in patients of Asian descent. Patients carrying the HLA-B*1502 allele should not be given carbamazepine unless the expected benefit clearly outweighs the increased risk of serious skin reactions.

(*continued*)

Table 40–2. Selected pharmacogenetic tests: clinical relevance.[1] (continued)

Pharmacogenetic Biomarker	Selected Variants (variant allele, activity)	Allele Frequency	Drugs	Clinical Relevance
Inherited Variants (cont.)				
HLA-B*5701 allele	HLA-B*5701	Present in 6–8% of White individuals and selected Asian Indian individuals; present in 1–2% of Black and Asian individuals.	Abacavir	The major treatment-limiting toxicity for abacavir use is drug hypersensitivity, occurring in 5–8% of recipients within 6 weeks of commencing therapy. There is an established association between carriage of the HLA-B*5701 allele and abacavir hypersensitivity reactions. Patients who have the HLA-B*5701 allele should not be prescribed abacavir or an abacavir-containing regimen.
HLA-B*5801 allele	HLA-B*5801	Present in 6–8% of Southeast Asian individuals and < 1% in Western European individuals.	Allopurinol	Allopurinol can produce rare but severe hypersensitivity reactions (eg, toxic epidermal necrolysis and Stevens-Johnson syndrome), which are strongly associated with HLA-B*5801 alleles. Patients of Korean, Han Chinese, Japanese, or Thai origin should be screened for HLA-B*5801 allele, and if present, an alternative drug therapy is needed.
Solute carrier organic anion transporter family member 1B1 (*SLCO1B1*) gene	*SLCO1B1**5 (c.521T>C, ↓ for TC-allele and ↓↓ for CC-allele)	20–30% of the general population are heterozygous (TC-allele, moderate risk) and 2–4% are homozygous (CC-allele, high risk) for the c.521T>C variant.	Simvastatin	SLCO1B1 is an influx transporter that moves drugs into hepatocytes. Decrease in the activity of this transporter (SLCO1B1 c.521T>C variant) is associated with increased blood drug levels and increased risk of statin-induced myopathy and statin intolerance. Genotyping is recommended for patients beginning statins, especially simvastatin.
Thiopurine methyltransferase (TPMT) variants	TPMT*2 (238G>C, ↓); TPMT*3A (460G>A and 719A>G, ↓↓); TPMT*3B (460G>A, ↓); TPMT*3C (719A>G, ↓)	About 10–12% of White and Black individuals have reduced enzyme activity because they are heterozygous for one of the variant alleles. About 1 in 300 White individuals is homozygous for a variant allele.	AZA, 6-MP	AZA is a prodrug that is metabolized to 6-MP, which is then further metabolized to active 6-TG and inactive 6-MMP through hypoxanthine phosphoribosyltransferase and *TPMT*, respectively. Variation in the *TPMT* gene can result in functional inactivation of the enzyme and an increased risk of life-threatening, 6-TG-associated myelosuppression. TPMT genotyping before instituting AZA or 6-MP can help prevent toxicity by identifying individuals with low or absent TPMT enzyme activity. Patients with homozygous or compound heterozygous variant alleles should not be given AZA or 6-MP, while patients who are heterozygote with a single variant allele should be treated with lower doses.

Inherited Variants (cont.)				
Uridine diphosphoglucuronosyltransferase 1A1 (UGT1A1) variants	*UGT1A1**28 (7 TA repeats in promoter, ↓)	Homozygosity is present in 9–23% of White, Black, and South Asian Indian individuals, and in 1–2% of Eastern Asian individuals.	Irinotecan	Irinotecan is metabolized to active SN-38, a topoisomerase I inhibitor. SN-38 is further glucuronidated to inactive SN-38G by UGT1A1 and excreted. Heterozygous and homozygous UGT1A1*28 genotypes show a 25% and 70% decrease in enzyme activity, respectively. The presence of the UGT1A1*28 allele is a risk factor for the development of adverse reactions (eg, neutropenia, severe diarrhea). Testing for the allele can prevent drug toxicity at high doses of irinotecan.
Vitamin K epoxide reductase complex (VKORC1) variants	VKORC1 (–1639G>A)	The homozygous (–1639G>A) allele (–1639AA genotype) is present in approximately 15% of White and 80% of Chinese individuals.	Warfarin	The primary therapeutic target of warfarin is VKOR. Polymorphisms in the VKOR-encoding gene (*VKORC1*) explain about 30% of the phenotypic variability in drug effect. Patients carrying certain single nucleotide polymorphisms in the *VKORC1* gene (especially the –1639G>A allele) require a lower warfarin maintenance dose to reach a therapeutic INR.
Somatic Mutations				
BRAF gene	*BRAF* V600E or V600K mutation	40–60% of advanced melanomas; nearly all hairy cell leukemia.	Vemurafenib, encorafenib, dabrafenib, binimetinib, cobimetinib	Activating mutations in BRAF (a serine–threonine protein kinase) are present in 40–60% of advanced melanomas. Most (80–90%) mutations are the substitution of glutamic acid for valine at amino acid 600 (V600E mutation). These mutations are associated with a more aggressive clinical course. A BRAF inhibitor (eg, vemurafenib) has a high level of therapeutic activity against advanced melanomas containing the V600E/K mutation as well as relapsed/refractory hairy cell leukemia.

(continued)

Table 40–2. Selected pharmacogenetic tests: clinical relevance.[1] (continued)

Pharmacogenetic Biomarker	Selected Variants (variant allele, activity)	Allele Frequency	Drugs	Clinical Relevance
Somatic Mutations (cont.)				
Epidermal growth factor receptor (EGFR) (also known as human epidermal growth factor receptor [HER] 1 or erbB-1)	Activating mutation(s) in EGFR kinase (eg, S768I, L858R, L861Q, G719X, exon 19 deletions)	Mutations in the *EGFR* gene are observed in about 15% of NSCLC in the United States. In Asian populations, the incidence of *EGFR* mutations is 22–62%.	EGFR tyrosine kinase inhibitors (gefitinib, erlotinib, afatinib, osimertinib, dacomitinib)	Advanced NSCLC that is positive for activating EGFR mutation(s) is sensitive to EGFR-targeted TKIs. Analysis for the presence or absence of an activating mutation (eg, exon 19 deletions or exon 21 substitution mutations such as L858R) in EGFR is the standard approach to decide whether to use an EGFR TKI for the initial treatment of advanced NSCLC. Note that amplification of *EGFR* gene or EGFR overexpression by immunohistochemistry does not predict improved outcomes with EGFR TKI.
HER2 gene	*HER2* gene amplification	*HER2* gene amplification is present in about 20% of breast cancers and 11–25% of gastric cancers.	Trastuzumab, pertuzumab, ado-trastuzumab emtansine, fam-trastuzumab deruxtecan-nxki	Patients with *HER2* gene amplification are candidates for treatment with the HER2-directed antibody drug trastuzumab or pertuzumab. Patients without *HER2* amplification will not benefit from the treatment. FISH with labeled DNA probes to the pericentromeric region of chromosome 17 and to the HER2 locus is used to determine if a patient's breast cancer has *HER2* gene amplification. Immunohistochemistry stains are also used to determine if the tumor exhibits HER2 protein overexpression.
Isocitrate dehydrogenase-1/2 (*IDH1/2* gene)	*IDH1* mutations (R132 locus); *IDH2* mutations (R140 or R172 loci)	*IDH1/2* mutations are detected in 15–20% of AML and 4–5% of chronic myeloid neoplasms (MDS, MPN).	Enasidenib, ivosidenib	*IDH1* or *IDH2* mutations perturb DNA and histone methylation and lead to aberrant gene expression in hematopoietic stem cells through production of an abnormal metabolite, 2-hydroxyglutarate. The impact of *IDH1/2* mutations in AML is age- and context-dependent. Enasidenib and ivosidenib are selective mutation IDH2 and IDH1 inhibitors, respectively, and are indicated for the treatment of patients with relapsed or refractory and IDH-mutated AML.

Somatic Mutations (cont.)				
KRAS gene	*KRAS* mutations (in codons 12 and 13)	Present in 30–40% of CRC and 20–25% of NSCLC. *KRAS* G12C mutation is present in 12–14% of lung adenocarcinomas.	For CRC: Cetuximab Penitumumab For NSCLC: Gefitinib Erlotinib Sotorasib	The *KRAS* gene, a human proto-oncogene, encodes one of the proteins in the EGFR signaling pathway critical in the development and progression of cancer, particularly CRC and NSCLC. Cancer patients with mutated *KRAS* are not likely to respond to drugs targeting the EGFR pathway. To avoid unnecessary toxicity and cost, all patients being considered for anti-EGFR therapy should undergo *KRAS* mutation testing of their tumors. Sotorasib is approved for adult patients with *KRAS* G12C-mutated advanced or metastatic NSCLC.
Mcrosatellite instability-high (MSI-H) due to a deficiency in the mismatch repair (MMR) system because of mutations in MMR-specific proteins, including MLH1, MSH2, MSH6, PMS2, or EPCAM	MSI-H (high rate of variation in microsatellite length exists across the genome) indicates underlying deficiency in DNA MMR capability, which in turn is caused by mutations in one of the DNA MMR genes (*MLH1, MSH2, MSH6, PMS2, EPCAM*). MSI-H status is determined by PCR- or NGS-based tests, whereas deficient MMR is typically assessed by IHC.	Frequencies of MSI-H/deficient MMR in advanced/metastatic cancers: 16% endometrial, 9% colorectal, 3% gastric, 5% esophageal, 21% neuroendocrine (GI tract), 16% small bowel, 3% squamous (skin), 3% basal cell (skin), 3% bladder, 2% prostate, 1–2% small cell lung, biliary, pancreatic, thyroid, or unknown primary.	Pembrolizumab	Pembrolizumab (an immune checkpoint inhibitor) is approved for patients with unresectable or metastatic, MSI-H or deficient MMR solid tumors that have progressed following prior treatment and who have no satisfactory alternative treatment options or with MSI-H or deficient MMR CRC that has progressed following treatment with a fluoropyrimidine, oxaliplatin, and irinotecan.

(*continued*)

Table 40–2. Selected pharmacogenetic tests: clinical relevance.[1] (continued)

Pharmacogenetic Biomarker	Selected Variants (variant allele, activity)	Allele Frequency	Drugs	Clinical Relevance
Somatic Mutations (cont.)				
Programmed death ligand 1 (PD-L1)	PD-L1 protein expression as determined by qualitative IHC	PD-L1 expression level is measured using the tumor proportion score, the percentage of tumor cells staining for PD-L1 (0–100%). Approximately one-third of NSCLC cases have detectable PD-L1 expression by IHC. PD-L1 is expressed in 65–100% cHL and about 50% of PMBCL.	Pembrolizumab, cemiplimab-rwlc, nivolumab	PD-L1 is an immune-related biomarker that can be expressed on tumor cells. PD-L1 testing determines which patients are likely to benefit from treatment with an immune checkpoint inhibitor that targets PD-L1. Overexpression of PD-L1 is an approved companion diagnostic test for pembrolizumab and other immune checkpoint inhibitors in NSCLC with no EGFR or ALK aberrations, gastric/gastroesophageal junction cancer, squamous cell esophageal cancer, cervical cancer, urothelial cancer, triple-negative breast cancer, cHL, and PMBCL.

[1]Testing of these genetic biomarkers prior to instituting drug therapy is recommended or required per US FDA-approved drug labels. The predictive biomarkers for hematological and oncological drugs are regulatorily approved under companion diagnostics, which is a rapidly evolving area.

↓, decreased; ↓↓, markedly decreased; none, no activity; ↑, increased; >, single wild-type to variant nucleotide switch at the specific gene location.

6-MP, 6-mercaptopurine; 6-MMP, 6-methylmercaptopurine; 6-TG, 6-thioguanine; AML, acute myeloid leukemia; AZA, azathioprine; CF, cystic fibrosis; cHL, classic Hodgkin lymphoma; CRC, colorectal cancer; FISH, fluorescence in situ hybridization; IHC, immunohistochemistry; MDS, myelodysplastic syndrome; MPN, myeloproliferative neoplasm; NADPH, nicotinamide adenine dinucleotide phosphate; NGS, next-generation sequencing; NSCLC, non–small cell lung cancer; PMBLC, primary mediastinal B-cell lymphoma; TKI, tyrosine kinase inhibitor.

Table adapted and updated, from Nicoll D et al. *Guide to Diagnostic Tests*, 7th ed. McGraw-Hill; 2017.

Orthopedic Disorders & Sports Medicine

Anthony Luke, MD, MPH
C. Benjamin Ma, MD

Musculoskeletal problems account for about 10–20% of outpatient primary care clinical visits. Orthopedic problems can be classified as traumatic (ie, injury-related) or atraumatic (ie, degenerative or overuse syndromes) as well as acute or chronic. The history and physical examination are sufficient in most cases to establish the working diagnosis; the mechanism of injury is usually the most helpful part of the history in determining the diagnosis.

Laskowski ER et al. The telemedicine musculoskeletal examination. Mayo Clin Proc. 2020;95:1715. [PMID: 32753146]
Tanaka MJ et al. Telemedicine in the era of COVID-19: the virtual orthopaedic examination. J Bone Joint Surg Am. 2020;102:e57. Erratum in: J Bone Joint Surg Am. 2020;102:e121. [PMID: 32341311]

SHOULDER

1. Subacromial Impingement Syndrome

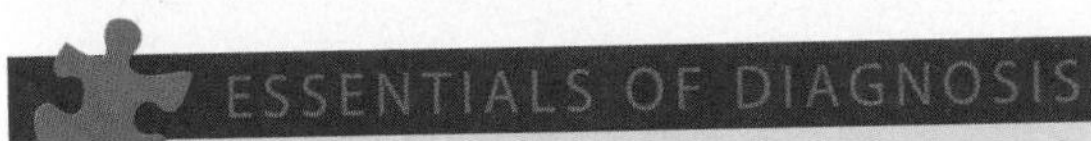

- Shoulder pain with overhead motion.
- Night pain with sleeping on shoulder.
- Numbness and pain radiation below the elbow are usually due to cervical spine disease.

General Considerations

The shoulder is a ball and socket joint. The socket is very shallow, however, which enables this joint to have the most motion of any joint. The shoulder, therefore, relies heavily on the surrounding muscles and ligaments to provide stability. The subacromial impingement syndrome describes a collection of diagnoses that cause mechanical inflammation in the subacromial space. Causes of impingement syndrome can be related to muscle strength imbalances, poor scapula control, rotator cuff tears, subacromial bursitis, and bone spurs.

With any shoulder problem, it is important to establish the patient's hand dominance, occupation, and recreational activities because shoulder injuries may present differently depending on the demands placed on the shoulder joint. Baseball pitchers with impingement syndrome may report pain while throwing, while older adults with even full-thickness rotator cuff tears may not report any pain because the demands on the joint are lower.

Clinical Findings

A. Symptoms and Signs

Subacromial impingement syndrome classically presents with one or more of the following: pain with overhead activities, nocturnal pain with sleeping on the shoulder, or pain on internal rotation (eg, putting on a jacket or bra). On inspection, there may be appreciable atrophy in the supraspinatus or infraspinatus fossa. The patient with impingement syndrome can have mild scapula winging or "dyskinesis." The patient often has a rolled-forward shoulder posture or head-forward posture. On palpation, the patient can have tenderness over the anterolateral shoulder at the edge of the greater tuberosity. The patient may lack full active range of motion but has preserved passive range of motion. Impingement symptoms can be elicited with the Neer and Hawkins impingement signs (Table 41–1).

B. Imaging

The following four radiographic views should be ordered to evaluate subacromial impingement syndrome: the anteroposterior (AP) scapula, the AP acromioclavicular joint, the lateral scapula (scapular Y), and the axillary lateral. The AP scapula view can rule out glenohumeral joint arthritis. The AP acromioclavicular view evaluates the acromioclavicular joint for inferior spurs. The scapula Y view evaluates the acromial shape, and the axillary lateral view visualizes the glenohumeral joint as well and for the presence of os acromiale.

MRI of the shoulder may demonstrate full- or partial-thickness tears or tendinosis. Ultrasound evaluation may demonstrate thickening of the rotator cuff tendons and tendinosis. Tears may also be visualized on ultrasound, although it is more difficult to identify partial tears from small full-thickness tears than on MRI.

Table 41–1. Shoulder examination.

Maneuver	Description
Inspection	Check the patient's posture and "SEADS" (*s*welling, *e*rythema, *a*trophy, *d*eformity, *s*urgical scars).
Palpation	Include important landmarks: acromioclavicular (AC) joint, long head of biceps tendon, coracoid, and greater tuberosity (supraspinatus insertion).
Range of motion testing: Check range of motion actively (patient performs) and passively (clinician performs).	
Flexion 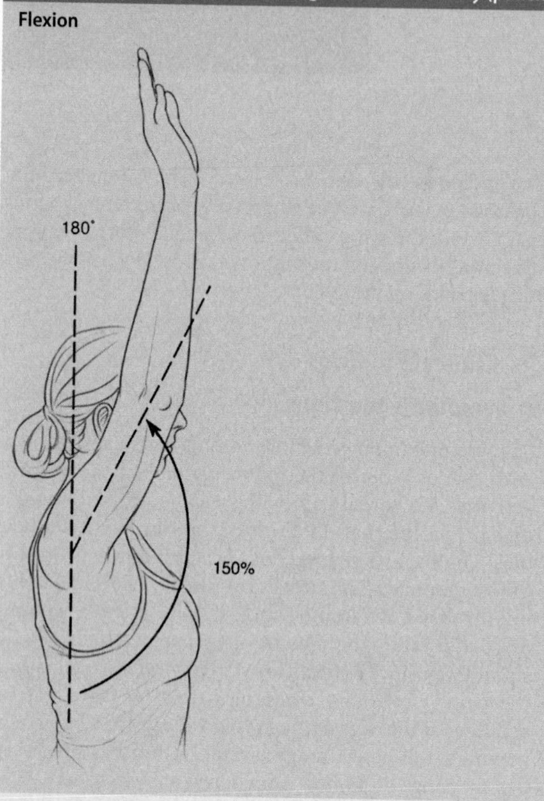 	Move the arm forward as high as possible in the sagittal plane.
External rotation 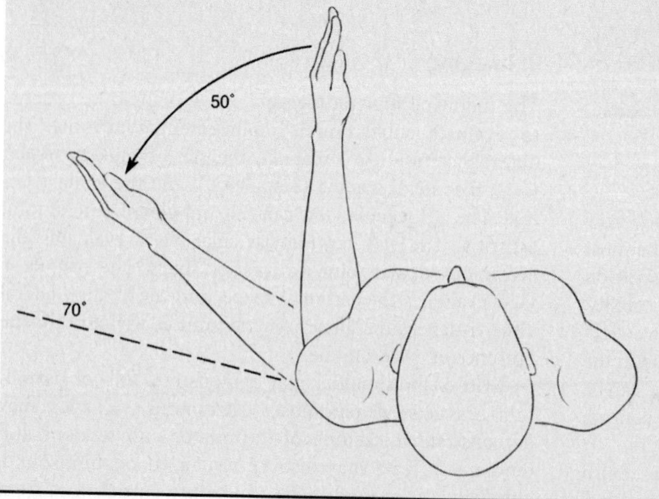 	Check with the patient's elbow touching their body so that external rotation occurs predominantly at the glenohumeral joint.

(*continued*)

Table 41–1. Shoulder examination. (continued)

Maneuver	Description
Internal rotation 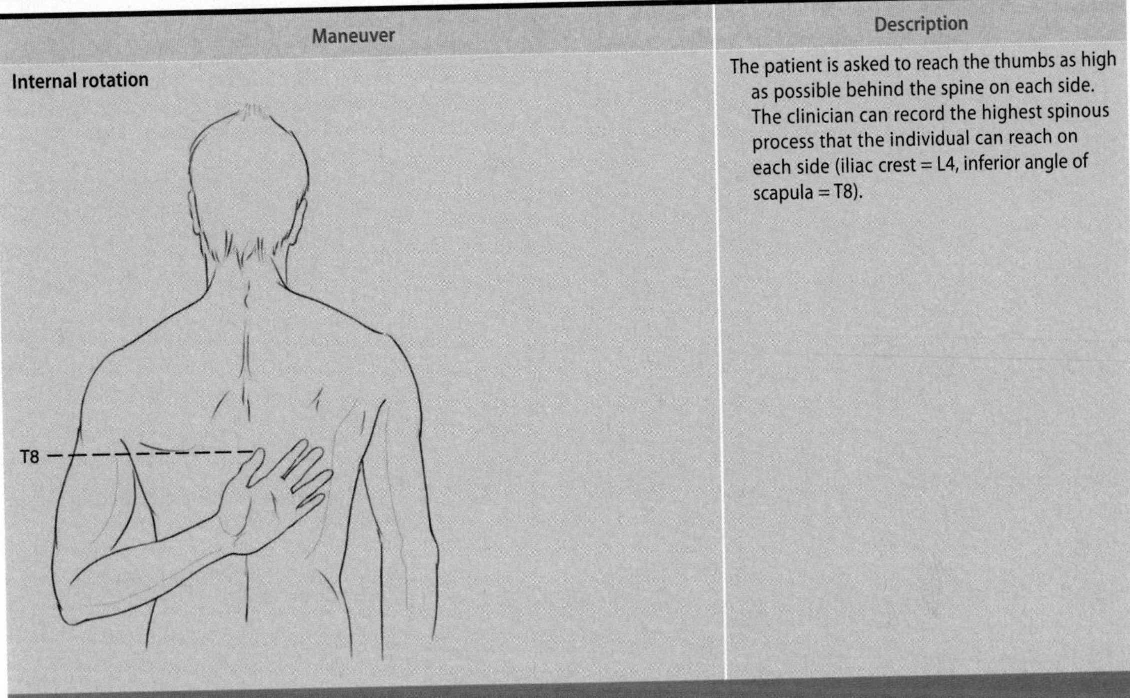	The patient is asked to reach the thumbs as high as possible behind the spine on each side. The clinician can record the highest spinous process that the individual can reach on each side (iliac crest = L4, inferior angle of scapula = T8).
Rotator Cuff Strength Testing	
Supraspinatus (open can) test 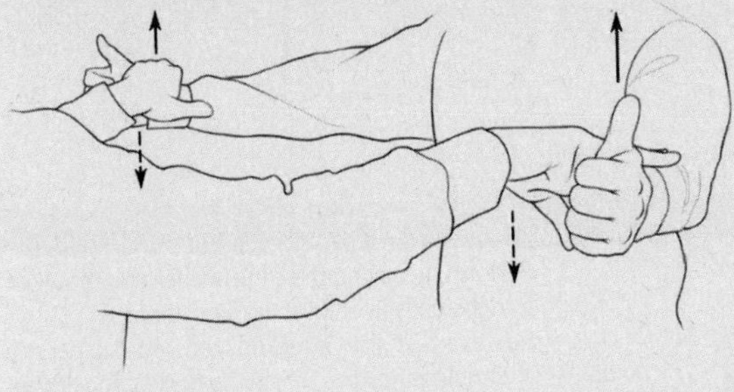	Perform resisted shoulder abduction at 90 degrees with slight forward flexion to around 45 degrees to test for supraspinatus tendon strength ("open can" test), or with shoulder abduction at 30 degrees and flexion to 30 degrees ("empty can" test).
External rotation 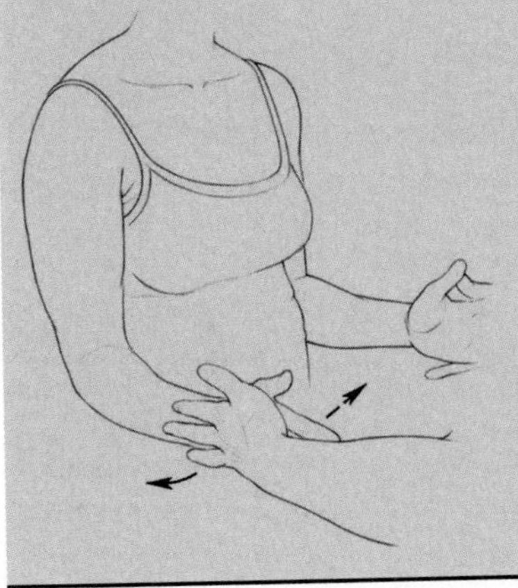	The patient resists by externally rotating the arms with elbows at his or her side.

(*continued*)

Table 41–1. Shoulder examination. (continued)

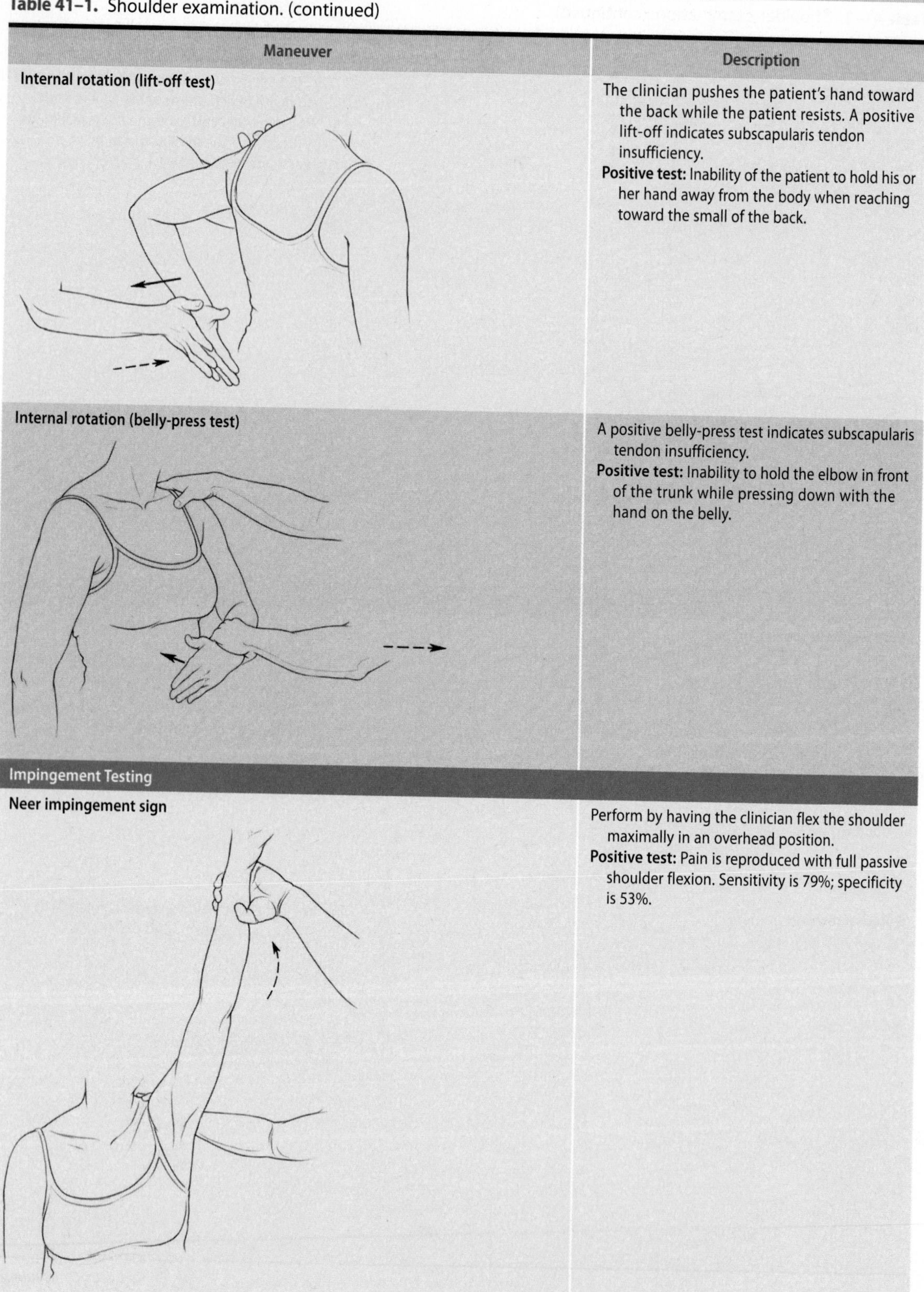

Maneuver	Description
Internal rotation (lift-off test)	The clinician pushes the patient's hand toward the back while the patient resists. A positive lift-off indicates subscapularis tendon insufficiency. **Positive test:** Inability of the patient to hold his or her hand away from the body when reaching toward the small of the back.
Internal rotation (belly-press test)	A positive belly-press test indicates subscapularis tendon insufficiency. **Positive test:** Inability to hold the elbow in front of the trunk while pressing down with the hand on the belly.
Impingement Testing	
Neer impingement sign	Perform by having the clinician flex the shoulder maximally in an overhead position. **Positive test:** Pain is reproduced with full passive shoulder flexion. Sensitivity is 79%; specificity is 53%.

(*continued*)

Table 41–1. Shoulder examination. (continued)

Maneuver	Description
Hawkins impingement sign 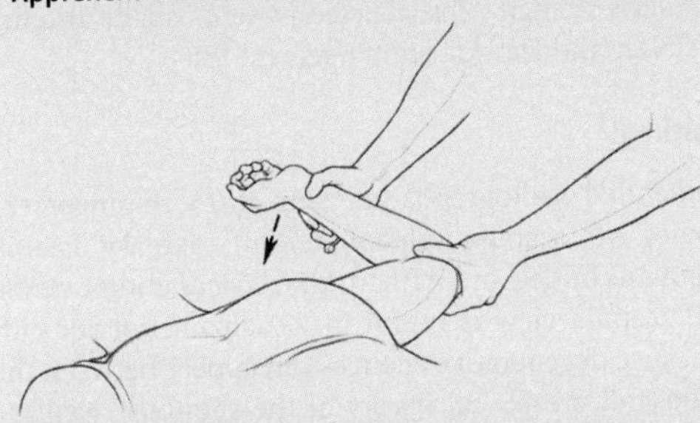	Perform with the shoulder forward flexed 90 degrees and the elbow flexed at 90 degrees. The shoulder is then maximally internally rotated to impinge the greater tuberosity on the undersurface of the acromion. **Positive test:** Pain is reproduced by this maneuver. Sensitivity is 79%; specificity is 59%.
Stability Testing	
Apprehension test 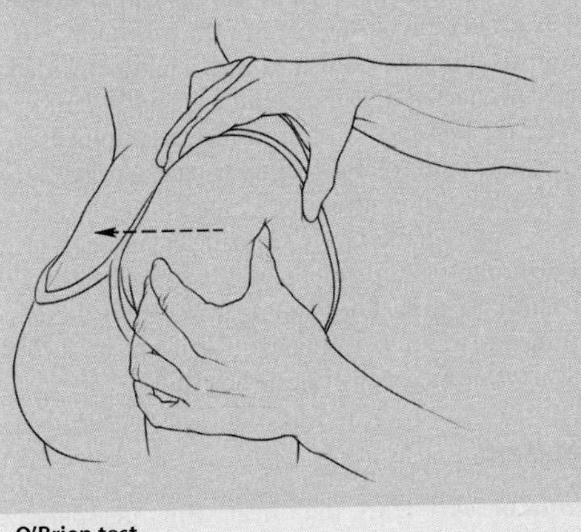	With persistent anterior instability or a recent dislocation, the patient feels pain or guards when the shoulder is abducted and externally rotated at 90 degrees. With posterior instability, the patient is apprehensive with the shoulder forward flexed and internally rotated to 90 degrees with a posteriorly directed force.
Load and shift test	Perform to determine shoulder instability by manually translating the humeral head anteriorly and posteriorly in relation to the glenoid. However, this test can be difficult to perform when the patient is not relaxed.
O'Brien test 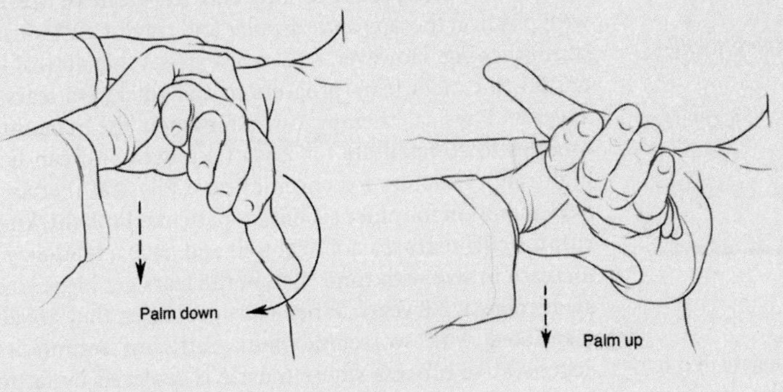	Performed to rule out labral cartilage tears that often occur following a shoulder subluxation or dislocation. The test involves flexing the patient's arm to 90 degrees, fully internally rotating the arm so the thumb is facing down (palm down), and adducting the arm to 10 degrees. Once positioned properly, the clinician applies downward force and asks the patient to resist. The test is then repeated in the same position except that the patient has his arm fully supinated (palm up). **Positive test:** There is pain deep in the shoulder with palm down more than the palm up. The O'Brien test can also be used to identify AC joint pathology. The patient would typically report pain equally directly over the AC joint with the palm down or up.

Treatment

A. Conservative

The first-line treatment for impingement syndrome is usually a conservative approach with education, activity modification, and physical therapy exercises.

Impingement syndrome can be caused by muscle weakness or tear. Rotator cuff muscle strengthening can alleviate weakness or pain, unless the tendons are seriously compromised, in which case exercises may cause more symptoms. Physical therapy is directed at rotator cuff muscle strengthening, scapula stabilization, and postural exercises. There is no strong evidence supporting the effectiveness of ice and NSAIDs as a prolonged therapy. In a Cochrane review, corticosteroid injections produced slightly better relief of symptoms in the short term when compared with placebo. Most patients respond well to conservative treatment.

B. Surgical

Procedures include arthroscopic acromioplasty with coracoacromial ligament release, bursectomy, or debridement or repair of rotator cuff tears. However, the value of acromioplasty alone for rotator cuff problems is not supported by evidence.

When to Refer

- Failure of conservative treatment over 3 months.
- Young and active patients with impingement due to full-thickness rotator cuff tears.

Consigliere P et al. Subacromial impingement syndrome: management challenges. Orthop Res Rev. 2018;10:83. [PMID: 30774463]

Saracoglu I et al. Does taping in addition to physiotherapy improve the outcomes in subacromial impingement syndrome? A systematic review. Physiother Theory Pract. 2018; 34:251. [PMID: 29111849]

2. Rotator Cuff Tears

ESSENTIALS OF DIAGNOSIS

- A common cause of shoulder impingement syndrome after age 40 years.
- Difficulty lifting the arm with limited active range of motion.
- Weakness with resisted strength testing suggests full-thickness tears.
- Tears can occur following trauma or can be more degenerative.

General Considerations

Rotator cuff tears can be caused by acute injuries related to falls on an outstretched arm or to pulling on the shoulder. They can also be related to chronic repetitive injuries with overhead movement and lifting. Partial rotator cuff tears are one of the most common reasons for impingement syndrome. Full-thickness rotator cuff tears are usually more symptomatic and may require surgical treatment. The most commonly torn tendon is the supraspinatus.

Clinical Findings

A. Symptoms and Signs

Most patients report weakness or pain with overhead movement. Night pain is also a common concern. The clinical findings with rotator cuff tears include those of the impingement syndrome except that with full-thickness rotator cuff tears there may be more obvious weakness noted with light resistance testing of specific rotator cuff muscles. Table 41–1 demonstrates tests for supraspinatus tendon strength test ("open can" test), infraspinatus/teres minor strength and subscapularis strength. The affected patient usually also has positive Neer and Hawkins impingement tests.

B. Imaging

Recommended radiographs are similar to impingement syndrome: AP scapula (glenohumeral), axillary lateral, supraspinatus outlet, and AP acromioclavicular joint views. The AP scapula view is useful in visualizing rotator cuff tears because degenerative changes can appear between the acromion and greater tuberosity of the shoulder. Axillary lateral views show superior elevation of the humeral head in relation to the center of the glenoid. Supraspinatus outlet views allow evaluation of the shape of the acromion. High-grade acromial spurs are associated with a higher incidence of rotator cuff tears. The AP acromioclavicular joint view evaluates for the presence of acromioclavicular joint arthritis, which can mimic rotator cuff tears, and for spurs that can cause rotator cuff injuries.

MRI is the best method for visualizing rotator cuff tears. The MR arthrogram can show partial or small (less than 1 cm) rotator cuff tears. For patients who cannot undergo MRI testing or when postoperative artifacts limit MRI evaluations, ultrasonography can be helpful.

Treatment

Partial rotator cuff tears may heal with nonoperative treatment. Most partial rotator cuff tears can be treated with physical therapy and scapular and rotator cuff muscle strengthening. However, research suggests that 40% of the partial-thickness tears progress to full-thickness tears in 2 years. Physical therapy can strengthen the remaining muscles to compensate for loss of strength and can have high rate of success for chronic tears. Physical therapy is also an option for older sedentary patients. **Full-thickness rotator cuff tears** do not heal well and have a tendency to increase in size with time; 49% of the tears get bigger over an average of 2.8 years. When tears get larger, they are also associated with worsening pain. Fatty infiltration is a degenerative process where muscle is replaced by fat following injury to the rotator cuff tendons. Fatty infiltration progresses in full-thickness rotator cuff tears, and it is a negative prognostic factor for successful surgical treatment. Fatty infiltration is an irreversible process so operative interventions are usually performed when the degree of infiltration is low. Most young active patients with acute, full-thickness tears should be treated with operative fixation. Full-thickness subscapularis tendon tears should undergo surgical repair since untreated tears usually lead to premature osteoarthritis (OA) of the shoulder. Nonetheless, physical therapy is indicated for atraumatic degenerative rotator cuff tears and success can be as high as 70%. That said, long-term (10-year) outcome studies show that surgical repair of rotator cuff tears can result in better outcomes than physical therapy alone.

When to Refer

- Young and active patients with full-thickness rotator cuff tears.
- Partial tears with greater than 50% involvement and with significant pain.
- Acute rotator cuff tears and loss of function.
- Older and sedentary patients with full-thickness rotator cuff tears who have not responded to nonoperative treatment.
- Full-thickness subscapularis tears.

Allen H et al. Overuse injuries of the shoulder. Radiol Clin North Am. 2019;57:897. [PMID: 31351540]

Amoo-Achampong K et al. Evaluating strategies and outcomes following rotator cuff tears. Shoulder Elbow. 2019;11:4. [PMID: 31019557]

Moosmayer S et al. At a 10-year follow-up, tendon repair is superior to physical therapy in the treatment of small and medium-sized rotator cuff tears. J Bone Joint Surg Am. 2019;101:1050. [PMID: 31220021]

Piper CC et al. Operative versus nonoperative treatment for the management of full-thickness rotator cuff tears: a systematic review and meta-analysis. J Shoulder Elbow Surg. 2018;27:572. [PMID: 29169957]

3. Shoulder Dislocation & Instability

ESSENTIALS OF DIAGNOSIS

- Most dislocations (95%) are in the anterior direction.
- Pain and apprehension with an unstable shoulder that is abducted and externally rotated.
- Acute shoulder dislocations should be reduced as quickly as possible, using manual relocation techniques if necessary.

General Considerations

The shoulder is a ball and socket joint, similar to the hip. However, the bony contours of the shoulder bones are much different than the hip. Overall, the joint has much less stability than the hip, allowing greater movement and action. Stabilizing the shoulder joint relies heavily on rotator cuff muscle strength and also scapular control. If patients have poor scapular control or weak rotator cuff tendons or tears, their shoulders are more likely to have instability. Ninety-five percent of the shoulder dislocations/instability occur in the anterior direction. Dislocations usually are caused by a fall on an outstretched and abducted arm. Patients report pain and feeling of instability when the arm is in the abducted and externally rotated position. Posterior dislocations are usually caused by falls from a height, epileptic seizures, or electric shocks. Traumatic shoulder dislocation can lead to instability. The rate of repeated dislocation is directly related to the patient's age: patients aged 21 years or younger have a 70–90% risk of redislocation, whereas patients aged 40 years or older have a much lower rate (20–30%). However, once the patient has a second dislocation, the recurrence rate is extremely high, up to 95%, regardless of age. Other risks include male sex and patients with hyperlaxity. Ninety percent of young active individuals who had traumatic shoulder dislocation have labral injuries often described as Bankart lesions when the anterior inferior labrum is torn, which can lead to continued instability. Older patients (over age 55 years) are more likely to have rotator cuff tears or fractures following dislocation. Atraumatic shoulder dislocations are usually caused by intrinsic ligament laxity or repetitive microtrauma leading to joint instability. This is often seen in athletes involved in overhead and throwing sports (eg, in swimmers, gymnasts, and pitchers).

Clinical Findings

A. Symptoms and Signs

For acute traumatic dislocations, patients usually have an obvious deformity with the humeral head dislocated anteriorly. The patient holds the shoulder and arm in an externally rotated position. The patient has acute pain and deformity. Even after reduction, the patient will continue to have limited range of motion and pain for 4–6 weeks, especially following a first-time shoulder dislocation.

Patients with recurrent dislocations can have less pain with subsequent dislocations. Posterior dislocations can be easily missed because the patient usually holds the shoulder and arm in an internally rotated position, which makes the shoulder deformity less obvious. Patients report difficulty pushing open a door.

Atraumatic shoulder instability is usually well tolerated with activities of daily living. Patients usually describe a "sliding" sensation during exercises or strenuous activities such as throwing. Such dislocations may be less symptomatic and can often undergo spontaneous reduction of the shoulder with pain resolving within days after onset. The clinical examination for shoulder instability includes the apprehension test, the load and shift test, and the O'Brien test (Table 41–1). Most patients with persistent shoulder instability have preserved range of motion.

B. Imaging

Radiographs for acute dislocations should include a standard trauma series of AP and axillary lateral scapula (glenohumeral) views to determine the relationship of the humerus and the glenoid and to rule out fractures. Orthogonal views are used to identify a posterior shoulder dislocation, which can be missed easily with one AP view of the shoulder. An axillary lateral view of the shoulder can be safely performed even in the acute setting of a patient with a painful shoulder dislocation. A scapula Y view in the acute setting is insufficient to diagnose dislocation. For chronic injuries or symptomatic instability, these recommended radiographic views are helpful to identify bony injuries and Hill-Sachs lesions (indented compression fractures at the posterior-superior part of the humeral head associated with anterior shoulder dislocation). MRI is commonly used to show soft tissue injuries to the labrum and to visualize associated rotator cuff tears. MRI arthrograms better identify labral tears and ligamentous structures. Three-dimensional CT scans are used to determine the significance of bone loss.

▶ Treatment

For **acute dislocations**, manual reductions are usually performed in the emergency department. The shoulder should be reduced as soon as possible. The Stimson procedure is the least traumatic method and is quite effective. The patient lies prone with the dislocated arm hanging off the examination table with a weight applied to the wrist to provide traction for 20–30 minutes. Afterward, gentle medial mobilization can be applied manually to assist the reduction. The shoulder can also be reduced with axial "traction" on the arm with "counter-traction" along the trunk. The patient should be sedated and relaxed. The shoulder can then be gently internally and externally rotated to guide it back into the socket.

Initial treatment of acute shoulder dislocations should include sling immobilization for 2–4 weeks along with pendulum exercises. Early physical therapy can be used to maintain range of motion and strengthening of rotator cuff muscles. Patients can also modify their activities to avoid active and risky sports. For patients with a traumatic incident and unilateral shoulder dislocation, a Bankart lesion is commonly present. Operative intervention is the only treatment that has been shown to decrease recurrence once a patient has a second dislocation. Open and arthroscopic stabilization have very similar outcomes. Repeated dislocations have been shown to increase the risk of arthritis and further bony deterioration.

The treatment of **atraumatic shoulder instability** is different than that of traumatic shoulder instability. Patients with chronic, recurrent shoulder dislocations should be managed with physical therapy and a regular maintenance program, consisting of scapular stabilization and postural and rotator cuff strengthening exercises. Activities may need to be modified. Surgical reconstructions are less successful for atraumatic shoulder instability than for traumatic shoulder instability. However, patients with recurrent dislocations have much higher incidence of bone loss or biceps pathology when compared with patients with first-time dislocations. They are also more likely to require open surgery with bone augmentation rather than arthroscopic stabilization.

▶ When to Refer

- Patients who are at risk for second dislocation, such as young patients and certain job holders (eg, police officers, firefighters, and rock climbers), to avoid recurrent dislocation or dislocation while at work.
- Patients who have not responded to a conservative approach or who have chronic instability.

Gottlieb M et al. Point-of-care ultrasound for the diagnosis of shoulder dislocation: a systematic review and meta-analysis. Am J Emerg Med. 2019;37:757. [PMID: 30797607]

Hasebroock AW et al. Management of primary anterior shoulder dislocations: a narrative review. Sports Med Open. 2019;5:31. [PMID: 31297678]

Kavaja L et al. Treatment after traumatic shoulder dislocation: a systematic review with a network meta-analysis. Br J Sports Med. 2018;52:1498. [PMID: 29936432]

4. Adhesive Capsulitis ("Frozen Shoulder")

ESSENTIALS OF DIAGNOSIS

- Very painful shoulder triggered by minimal or no trauma.
- Pain out of proportion to clinical findings during the inflammatory phase.
- Stiffness during the "freezing" phase and resolution during the "thawing" phase.

▶ General Considerations

Adhesive capsulitis ("frozen shoulder") is caused by acute inflammation of the shoulder capsule followed by scarring and remodeling. Injury to the shoulder likely triggers mast cell activation and release of growth factors and cytokines, which lead to metaplasia of fibroblasts into myofibroblasts, resulting in abnormal collagen deposition and fibrosis in the shoulder capsule. Adhesive capsulitis is seen commonly in patients aged 40–65 years old, and it occurs more often in women than men, especially in perimenopausal women or in patients with endocrine disorders, such as diabetes mellitus or thyroid disease. There is higher incidence of adhesive capsulitis following shoulder trauma (such as surgery) or breast cancer care (such as mastectomy), which may create a pro-inflammatory condition in the shoulder. Adhesive capsulitis is a self-limiting but very debilitating disease.

▶ Clinical Findings

A. Symptoms and Signs

Patients usually present with an extremely painful shoulder that has a limited range of motion with both passive and active movements. A useful clinical sign is limitation of movement of external rotation with the elbow by the side of the trunk (Table 41–1). Strength is usually normal but may appear diminished when the patient is in pain.

There are three phases: the inflammatory phase, the freezing phase, and the thawing phase. During the inflammatory phase, which usually lasts 4–6 months, patients report a very painful shoulder without obvious clinical findings to suggest trauma, fracture, or rotator cuff tear. During the "freezing" phase, which also usually lasts 4–6 months, the shoulder becomes stiffer and stiffer even though the pain is improving. The "thawing" phase can take up to a year as the shoulder slowly regains its motion. The total duration of an idiopathic frozen shoulder is usually about 24 months; it can be much longer for patients who have trauma or an endocrinopathy.

B. Imaging

Standard AP, axillary, and lateral glenohumeral radiographs are useful to rule out glenohumeral arthritis, which can also present with limited active and passive range of motion. Imaging can also rule out calcific tendinitis, which is an acute inflammatory process in which calcifications are visible in the soft tissue. However, adhesive capsulitis is usually a clinical diagnosis, and it does not need an extensive diagnostic workup.

Treatment

During the "acute inflammatory" and "freezing" phases, NSAIDs and physical therapy help to maintain motion. There is also evidence of short-term benefit from intra-articular corticosteroid injection or oral prednisone; a meta-analysis showed that intra-articular corticosteroid injection provided better pain relief than NSAIDs in the first 8 weeks. However, no difference was seen in range of motion or pain after 12 weeks, which is similar to other noncontrolled studies. One study demonstrated improvement at 6 weeks but not 12 weeks following 30 mg of daily prednisone for 3 weeks. During the "freezing" phase, the shoulder is less painful but remains stiff. Anti-inflammatory medication is not as helpful during the "thawing" phase as it is during the "freezing" phase, and the shoulder symptoms usually resolve with time. Surgical treatments, which are rarely indicated, include manipulation under anesthesia and arthroscopic release.

When to Refer

- When the patient does not respond after more than 6 months of conservative treatment.
- When there is no progress in or worsening of range of motion over 3 months.

Alsubheen SA et al. Effectiveness of nonsurgical interventions for managing adhesive capsulitis in patients with diabetes: a systematic review. Arch Phys Med Rehabil. 2019;100:350. [PMID: 30268804]

Cho CH et al. Treatment strategy for frozen shoulder. Clin Orthop Surg. 2019;11:249. [PMID: 31475043]

SPINE PROBLEMS

1. Low Back Pain

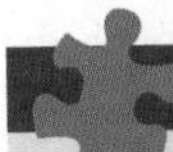

ESSENTIALS OF DIAGNOSIS

- Nerve root impingement is suspected when pain is leg-dominant rather than back-dominant.
- Alarming symptoms include unexplained weight loss, failure to improve with treatment, severe pain for > 6 weeks, and night or rest pain.
- Cauda equina syndrome is an emergency; often presents with bowel or bladder symptoms (or both).

General Considerations

Low back pain remains the number one cause of disability globally and is the second most common cause for primary care visits. The annual prevalence of low back pain is 15–45%. Annual health care spending for low back and neck pain is estimated to be $87.6 billion. Low back pain is the condition associated with the highest years lived with disability. Approximately 80% of episodes of low back pain resolve within 2 weeks and 90% resolve within 6 weeks. The exact cause of the low back pain is often difficult to diagnose; its cause is often multifactorial. There are usually degenerative changes in the lumbar spine involving the disks, facet joints, and vertebral endplates (Modic changes). The sacroiliac joint, muscles, and tendons also can cause pain.

Clinical Findings

A. Symptoms and Signs

Aggravating factors of flexion and prolonged sitting commonly suggest anterior spine disk problems, while extension pain suggests facet joint, stenosis, or sacroiliac joint problems. Alarming symptoms for back pain caused by cancer include unexplained weight loss, failure to improve with treatment, pain for more than 6 weeks, and pain at night or rest. History of cancer and age older than 50 years are other risk factors for malignancy. Alarming symptoms for infection include fever, rest pain, recent infection (UTI, cellulitis, pneumonia), or history of immunocompromise or injection drug use. The **cauda equina syndrome** is suggested by urinary retention or incontinence, saddle anesthesia, decreased anal sphincter tone or fecal incontinence, bilateral lower extremity weakness, and progressive neurologic deficits. Risk factors for back pain due to vertebral fracture include use of corticosteroids, age over 70 years, history of osteoporosis, severe trauma, and presence of a contusion or abrasion. Back pain may also be the presenting symptom in other serious medical problems, including AAA, peptic ulcer disease, kidney stones, or pancreatitis. Psychosocial factors and workplace factors should be assessed in cases where acute back pain becomes chronic. The patient's previous response to treatments and the results of risk prediction tools can help guide management. Most patients with persistent low back pain have co-occurring areas of pain, especially axial pain (18–58%), extremity pain (6–50%), and multisite musculoskeletal pain (10–89%).

The physical examination can be conducted with the patient in the standing, sitting, supine, and finally prone positions to avoid frequent repositioning of the patient. **In the standing position**, the patient's posture can be observed. Commonly encountered spinal asymmetries include scoliosis, thoracic kyphosis, and lumbar hyperlordosis. The active range of motion of the lumbar spine can be assessed while standing. The common directions include flexion, extension, rotation, and lateral bending. The one-leg standing extension test assesses for pain as the patient stands on one leg while extending the spine. A positive test can be caused by pars interarticularis fractures (spondylolysis or spondylolisthesis) or facet joint arthritis.

With the patient sitting, motor strength, reflexes, and sensation can be tested (Table 41–2). The major muscles in the lower extremities are assessed for weakness by eliciting a resisted isometric contraction for about 5 seconds. Comparing the strength bilaterally to detect subtle muscle weakness is important. Similarly, sensory testing to light touch can be checked in specific dermatomes for corresponding nerve root function. Knee, ankle, and Babinski reflexes can be checked.

In the supine position, the hip should be evaluated for range of motion, particularly internal rotation. The straight leg raise test puts traction and compression forces on the lower lumbar nerve roots.

In the prone position, the clinician can carefully palpate each vertebral level of the spine and sacroiliac joints for tenderness. A rectal examination is required if the cauda equina syndrome is suspected. Superficial skin tenderness to a light touch over the lumbar spine, overreaction to maneuvers in the regular back examination, low back pain on axial loading of spine in standing, and inconsistency in the straight leg raise test or on the neurologic examination suggest nonorthopedic causes for the pain or malingering.

Table 41–2. Neurologic testing of lumbosacral nerve disorders.

Nerve Root	Motor	Reflex	Sensory Area
L1	Hip flexion	None	Groin
L2	Hip flexion	None	Thigh
L3	Extension of knee	Knee jerk	Knee
L4	Dorsiflexion of ankle	Knee jerk	Medial calf
L5	Dorsiflexion of first toe	Babinski reflex	First dorsal web space between first and second toes
S1	Plantar flexion of foot, knee flexors, or hamstrings	Ankle jerk	Lateral foot
S2	Knee flexors or hamstrings	Knee flexor	Back of the thigh
S2–S4	External anal sphincter	Anal reflex, rectal tone	Perianal area

Table 41–3. AHRQ criteria for lumbar radiographs in patients with acute low back pain.

Possible fracture
Major trauma
Minor trauma in patients > 50 years of age
Long-term corticosteroid use
Osteoporosis
> 70 years of age
Possible tumor or infection
> 50 years of age
< 20 years of age
History of cancer
Constitutional symptoms
Recent bacterial infection
Injection drug use
Immunosuppression
Supine pain
Nocturnal pain

AHRQ, Agency for Healthcare Research and Quality.
Adapted from Bigos S et al. Acute Low Back Problems in Adults. Clinical Practice Guideline Quick Reference Guide No. 14. AHCPR Publication No. 95-0643. Rockville, MD: Agency for Health Care Policy and Research, Public Health Service, U.S. Department of Health and Human Services. December 1994.

B. Imaging

In the absence of alarming "red flag" symptoms suggesting infection, malignancy, or cauda equina syndrome, most patients do not need diagnostic imaging, including radiographs, in the first 6 weeks. The Agency for Healthcare Research and Quality guidelines for obtaining lumbar radiographs are summarized in Table 41–3. Most clinicians obtain radiographs for new back pain in patients older than 50 years. If done, radiographs of the lumbar spine should include AP and lateral views. Oblique views can be useful if the neuroforamina or bone lesions need to be visualized. MRI is the method of choice in the evaluation of symptoms not responding to conservative treatment or in the presence of red flags of serious conditions.

C. Special Tests

Electromyography or nerve conduction studies may be useful in assessing patients with possible nerve root symptoms lasting longer than 6 weeks; back pain may or may not also be present. These tests are usually not necessary if the diagnosis of radiculopathy is clear.

Treatment

A. Conservative

Nonpharmacologic treatments are key in the management of low back pain. Education alone improves patient satisfaction with recovery and recurrence. Patients require information and reassurance, especially when serious pathology is absent. Discussion must include reviewing safe and effective methods of symptom control as well as how to decrease the risk of recurrence with proper lifting techniques, abdominal wall/core strengthening, weight loss, and cigarette smoking cessation. Exercise, psychological therapies (eg, cognitive behavioral therapy), and multidisciplinary rehabilitation have been shown to be modestly effective for acute low back pain (strength of evidence, low). Complementary therapies, such as Tai Chi, mindfulness-based stress reduction, and yoga, have shown benefit for chronic low back pain patients.

Exercise, oral NSAIDs, and serotonin and norepinephrine reuptake inhibitors (duloxetine) were shown in a systematic review to produce a clinically meaningful reduction in pain, with exercise being the only intervention that demonstrated sustained benefit after the intervention ended. Aerobic exercise improves pain, disability, and mental health at short-term follow-up. Physical therapy exercise programs can be tailored to the patient's symptoms and pathology. A randomized controlled trial demonstrated that individualized physical therapy was clinically more beneficial than advice alone with sustained improvements at 6 months and 12 months. Strengthening and stabilization exercises effectively reduce pain and functional limitation compared with usual care. Heat and cold may be used for symptomatic treatment, with heat showing short-term benefits for acute low back pain. The efficacy of transcutaneous electrical nerve stimulation (TENS), back braces, massage and physical agents is unproven. There is good evidence that spinal manipulation and acupuncture provide short-term improvement compared with usual care. Improvements in posture including chair ergonomics or standing desks, core stability strengthening, physical conditioning, and modifications of activities to decrease physical strain are keys for ongoing management. A multidisciplinary approach to back pain care is beneficial to address the physical, psychological, and social aspects of low back pain, especially when pain is chronic, avoiding medication if possible.

If medications are needed, NSAIDs are effective in the early treatment of low back pain (see Chapter 20 and Table 5–5). Topical capsicum is effective short term (3 months or less). Acetaminophen and oral corticosteroids are relatively ineffective for chronic low back. There is limited evidence that muscle relaxants provide short-term relief; since these medications have addictive potential, they should be used with care. Muscle relaxants are best used if there is true muscle spasm that is painful rather than simply a protective response. Opioids alleviate pain in the short term but have the usual side effects and concerns of long-term opioid use (see Chapter 5). Treatment of more chronic neuropathic pain with alpha-2-delta ligands (eg, gabapentin), serotonin-norepinephrine reuptake inhibitors (eg, duloxetine), or tricyclic antidepressants (eg, nortriptyline) may be useful (see Table 5–8). Antidepressants are not recommended for the treatment of general low back pain.

Epidural injections may reduce pain in the short term and reduce the need for surgery in some patients within a 1-year period but not longer. Spinal injections are not recommended for initial care of patients with low back pain without radiculopathy. Intra-articular steroid injections and cooled radiofrequency ablation of the sacral lateral branch nerves and dorsal ramus of L5 can be considered for patients with persistent sacroiliac joint pain. There is fair evidence that thermal radiofrequency ablation of the facet joints improves pain for at least 6 months.

B. Surgical

Indications for back surgery include cauda equina syndrome, ongoing morbidity with no response to more than 6 months of conservative treatment, cancer, infection, or severe spinal deformity. Prognosis is improved when there is an anatomic lesion that can be corrected and symptoms are neurologic. Spinal surgery has limitations. Patient selection is very important; the specific surgery recommended should have very clear indications. Patients should understand that surgery can improve their pain but is unlikely to cure it. Surgery is not generally indicated for radiographic abnormalities alone when the patient is relatively asymptomatic. Depending on the surgery performed, possible complications include persistent pain; surgical site pain, especially if bone grafting is needed; infection; neurologic damage; non-union; cutaneous nerve damage; implant failure; DVT; and death.

▶ When to Refer

- Patients with the cauda equina syndrome.
- Patients with cancer, infection, fracture, or severe spinal deformity.
- Patients who have not responded to conservative treatment.

Galliker G et al. Low back pain in the emergency department: prevalence of serious spinal pathologies and diagnostic accuracy of red flags—a systematic review. Am J Med. 2020;133:60. [PMID: 31278933]

Kolber MR et al. PEER systematic review of randomized controlled trials: management of chronic low back pain in primary care. Can Fam Physician. 2021;67:e20. [PMID: 33483410]

Tucker HR et al. Harms and benefits of opioids for management of non-surgical acute and chronic low back pain: a systematic review. Br J Sports Med. 2020;54:664. [PMID: 30902816]

2. Spinal Stenosis

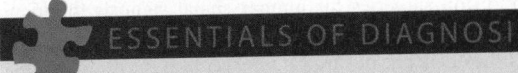

- ▶ Pain is usually worse with back extension and relieved by sitting.
- ▶ Occurs in older patients.
- ▶ May present with neurogenic claudication symptoms with walking.

▶ General Considerations

OA in the lumbar spine can cause narrowing of the spinal canal. A large disk herniation can also cause stenosis and compression of neural structures or the spinal artery resulting in "claudication" symptoms with ambulation. The condition usually affects patients aged 50 years or older.

Clinical Findings

Patients report pain that worsens with extension. They describe reproducible single or bilateral leg symptoms that are worse after walking several minutes and that are relieved by sitting ("neurogenic claudication"). On examination, patients often exhibit limited extension of the lumbar spine, which may reproduce the symptoms radiating down the legs. A thorough neurovascular examination is recommended (Table 41–2).

Treatment

Exercises, usually flexion-based as demonstrated by a physical therapist, can help relieve symptoms. Physical therapy showed similar results as surgical decompression in a randomized trial, though there was a 57% crossover rate from physical therapy to surgery. Facet joint corticosteroid injections can also reduce pain symptoms. While epidural corticosteroid injections have been shown to provide immediate improvements in pain and function for patients with radiculopathy, the benefits are small and only short term. Consequently, there is limited evidence to recommend epidural corticosteroids for spinal stenosis.

Surgical treatments for spinal stenosis include spinal decompression (widening the spinal canal or laminectomy), nerve root decompression (freeing a single nerve), and spinal fusion (joining the vertebra to eliminate motion and diminish pain from the arthritic joints). However, the role of surgery for spinal stenosis is limited. In one multicenter randomized trial, subgroups initially improved significantly more with surgery than with nonoperative treatment. Variables associated with greater treatment effects included lower baseline disability scores, not smoking, neuroforaminal stenosis, predominant leg pain rather than back pain, not lifting at work, and the presence of a neurologic deficit. However, long-term follow-up of the patients with symptomatic spinal stenosis who received surgery in the multicenter randomized trial showed less benefit of surgery between 4 and 8 years, suggesting that the advantage of surgery for spinal stenosis diminishes over time. A 2021 meta-analysis comparing fusion and nonfusion surgeries for lumbar spinal stenosis found no difference in clinical effects and complications, highlighting the challenge of surgical intervention for lumbar spinal stenosis.

When to Refer

- If a patient exhibits radicular or claudication symptoms for longer than 12 weeks.
- MRI or CT confirmation of significant, symptomatic spinal stenosis.
- However, surgery has not been shown to have clear benefit over nonsurgical treatment for lumbar spinal stenosis.

Cook CJ et al. Systematic review of diagnostic accuracy of patient history, clinical findings, and physical tests in the diagnosis of lumbar spinal stenosis. Eur Spine J. 2020;29:93. [PMID: 31312914]

Shen J et al. Comparison between fusion and non-fusion surgery for lumbar spinal stenosis: a meta-analysis. Adv Ther. 2021; 38:1404. [PMID: 33491158]

3. Lumbar Disk Herniation

ESSENTIALS OF DIAGNOSIS

- Pain with back flexion or prolonged sitting.
- Radicular pain into the leg due to compression of neural structures.
- Lower extremity numbness and weakness.

General Considerations

Lumbar disk herniation is usually due to bending or heavy loading (eg, lifting) with the back in flexion, causing herniation or extrusion of disk contents (nucleus pulposus) into the spinal cord area. However, there may not be an inciting incident. Disk herniations usually occur from degenerative disk disease (dessication of the annulus fibrosis) in patients between 30 and 50 years old. The L5–S1 disk is affected in 90% of cases. Compression of neural structures, such as the sciatic nerve, causes radicular pain. Severe compression of the spinal cord can cause the cauda equina syndrome, a surgical emergency.

Clinical Findings

A. Symptoms and Signs

Discogenic pain typically is localized in the low back at the level of the affected disk and is worse with activity. "Sciatica" causes electric shock-like pain radiating down the posterior aspect of the leg often to below the knee. Symptoms usually worsen with back flexion such as bending or sitting for long periods (eg, driving). A significant disk herniation can cause numbness and weakness, including weakness of plantar flexion of the foot (L5/S1) or dorsiflexion of the toes (L4/L5). The cauda equina syndrome should be ruled out if the patient reports perianal numbness or bowel or bladder incontinence.

B. Imaging

Plain radiographs are helpful to assess spinal alignment (scoliosis, lordosis), disk space narrowing, and OA changes. MRI is the best method to assess the level and morphology of the herniation and is recommended if surgery is planned. Provocative lumbar discography can be helpful for identifying the disc as the source of low back pain.

Treatment

For an acute exacerbation of pain symptoms, bed rest is appropriate for up to 48 hours. Otherwise, first-line treatments include modified activities; NSAIDs and other analgesics; and physical therapy, including core stabilization and

McKenzie back exercises. The McKenzie Method identifies the mechanical direction of motion in the back that causes more or less pain, using careful history and physical examination to guide the treatment approach. An exercise protocol is designed to centralize or alleviate the pain.

Following nonsurgical treatment for a lumbar disk for over 1 year, the incidence of low back pain recurrence is at least 40% and is predicted by longer time to initial resolution of pain. In a randomized trial, oral prednisone caused a modest improvement in function at 3 weeks, but there was no significant improvement in pain in patients with acute radiculopathy who were monitored for 1 year. The initial dose for oral prednisone is approximately 1 mg/kg once daily with tapering doses over 10–15 days. Analgesics for neuropathic pain, such as the calcium channel alpha-2-delta ligands (ie, gabapentin, pregabalin) or tricyclic antidepressants, may be helpful (see Chapter 5). Epidural and transforaminal corticosteroid injections can be beneficial. A 2020 Cochrane review of 25 placebo-controlled trials provides moderate-quality evidence that epidural corticosteroid injections are effective, although the treatment effects are small (mean difference less than 10%) and short-term for improving radicular pain for individuals. There is level I evidence for the use of transforaminal injections for radicular pain from disk herniation. Epidural injections have not shown any change in long-term surgery rates for disk herniations. Intradiscal electrothermal therapy has limited success in 40–50% of patients with reduction of pain up to 2 years.

The severity of pain and disability as well as failure of conservative therapy are the most important reasons for surgery. A large trial has shown that patients who underwent surgery for a lumbar disk herniation achieved greater improvement than conservatively treated patients in all primary and secondary outcomes except return-to-work status after 8-year follow-up. Patients with sequestered fragments, symptom duration greater than 6 months, higher levels of low back pain, or who were neither working nor disabled at baseline showed greater surgical treatment effects. Microdiskectomy is the standard treatment with a low rate of complications and satisfactory results in over 90% in the largest series. Minimally invasive percutaneous endoscopic spine surgery uses an endoscope to remove fragments of disk herniation (interlaminar or transforaminal approaches) under local anesthesia for the treatment of primary and recurrent disk disease. The most commonly reported complications of endoscopic lumbar surgery include dural tear, infection, and epidural hematoma. Percutaneous endoscopic diskectomy has promise, though there is lack of randomized controlled trials comparing it with open microdiskectomy. Recurrent disk herniations are treated with decompression surgeries and spinal fusion surgeries. Disk replacement surgery has shown benefits in short-term pain relief, disability, and quality of life compared with spine fusion surgery.

When to Refer

- Cauda equina syndrome.
- Progressive worsening of neurologic symptoms.
- Loss of motor function (sensory losses can be followed in the outpatient clinic).

Bailey CS et al. Surgery versus conservative care for persistent sciatica lasting 4 to 12 months. N Engl J Med. 2020;382:1093. [PMID: 32187469]

Butler AJ et al. Endoscopic lumbar surgery: the state of the art in 2019. Neurospine. 2019;16:15. [PMID: 30943703]

Carlson BB et al. Lumbar disc herniation: what has the Spine Patient Outcomes Research Trial taught us? Int Orthop. 2019;43:853. [PMID: 30767043]

Oliveira CB et al. Epidural corticosteroid injections for lumbosacral radicular pain. Cochrane Database Syst Rev. 2020;4: CD013577. [PMID: 32271952]

4. Neck Pain

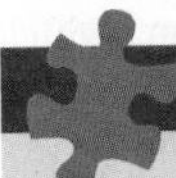

ESSENTIALS OF DIAGNOSIS

- Chronic neck pain is mostly caused by degenerative joint disease; whiplash often follows a traumatic neck injury.
- Poor posture is often a factor for persistent neck pain.

General Considerations

Most neck pain, especially in older patients, is due to mechanical degeneration involving the cervical disks, facet joints, and ligamentous structures and may occur in the setting of degenerative changes at other sites. Pain can also come from the supporting neck musculature, which often acts to protect the underlying neck structures. Posture is a very important factor, especially in younger patients. Many work-related neck symptoms are due to poor posture and repetitive motions over time. Acute injuries can also occur secondary to trauma. Whiplash occurs from rapid flexion and extension of the neck and affects 15–40% of people in motor vehicle accidents; chronic pain develops in 5–7%. Neck fractures are serious traumatic injuries acutely and can lead to OA in the long term. Ultimately, many degenerative conditions of the neck result in cervical canal stenosis or neural foraminal stenosis, sometimes affecting underlying neural structures.

Cervical radiculopathy can cause neurologic symptoms in the upper extremities usually involving the C5–C7 disks. Patients with neck pain may report associated headaches and shoulder pain. Both peripheral nerve entrapment and cervical radiculopathy, known as a "double crush" injury, may develop. Thoracic outlet syndrome, in which there is mechanical compression of the brachial plexus and neurovascular structures with overhead positioning of the arm, should be considered in the differential diagnosis of neck pain. Other causes of neck pain include rheumatoid arthritis, fibromyalgia, osteomyelitis, neoplasms, polymyalgia rheumatica, compression fractures, pain referred from visceral structures (eg, angina), and functional disorders. Amyotrophic lateral sclerosis, multiple sclerosis, syringomyelia, spinal cord tumors, and Parsonage-Turner syndrome can mimic myelopathy from cervical arthritis.

Clinical Findings

A. Symptoms and Signs

Neck pain may be limited to the posterior region or, depending on the level of the symptomatic joint, may radiate segmentally to the occiput, anterior chest, shoulder girdle, arm, forearm, and hand. It may be intensified by active or passive neck motions. The general distribution of pain and paresthesias corresponds roughly to the involved dermatome in the upper extremity.

The patient's posture should be assessed, checking for shoulder rolled-forward or head-forward posture as well as scoliosis in the thoracolumbar spine. Patients with discogenic neck pain often report pain with flexion, which causes cervical disks to herniate posteriorly. Extension of the neck usually affects the neural foraminal and facet joints of the neck. Rotation and lateral flexion of the cervical spine should be measured both to the left and the right. Limitation of cervical movements is the most common objective finding.

A detailed neurovascular examination of the upper extremities should be performed, including sensory input to light touch and temperature; motor strength testing, especially the hand intrinsic muscles (thumb extension strength [C6], opponens strength [thumb to pinky] [C7], and finger abductors and adductors strength [C8–T1]); and upper extremity reflexes (biceps, triceps, brachioradialis). True cervical radiculopathy symptoms should match an expected dermatomal or myotomal distribution. The Spurling test involves asking the patient to rotate and extend the neck to one side. The clinician can apply a gentle axial load to the neck. Reproduction of the cervical radiculopathy symptoms is a positive sign of nerve root compression. Palpation of the neck is best performed with the patient in the supine position where the clinician can palpate each level of the cervical spine with the muscles of the neck relaxed.

B. Imaging and Special Tests

Radiographs of the cervical spine include the AP and lateral view of the cervical spine. The odontoid view is usually added to rule out traumatic fractures and congenital abnormalities. Oblique views of the cervical spine can provide further information about arthritis changes and assess the neural foramina for narrowing. Plain radiographs can be normal in patients who have suffered an acute cervical strain. Comparative reduction in height of the involved disk space and osteophytes are frequent findings when there are degenerative changes in the cervical spine. Loss of cervical lordosis is commonly seen but is nonspecific.

MRI is the best method to assess the cervical spine since the soft tissue structures (such as the disks, spinal cord, and nerve roots) can be evaluated. If the patient has signs of cervical radiculopathy with motor weakness, these more sensitive imaging modalities should be obtained urgently. CT scanning is the most useful method if bony abnormalities, such as fractures, are suspected.

Electromyography is useful in differentiating peripheral nerve entrapment syndromes from cervical radiculopathy. However, sensitivity of electrodiagnostic testing for cervical radiculopathy ranges from only 50% to 71%, so a negative test does not rule out nerve root problems.

Treatment

In the absence of trauma or evidence of infection, malignancy, neurologic findings, or systemic inflammation, the patient can be treated conservatively. More frequent observation of patients in whom very severe symptoms are present early on after an injury is recommended because high pain-related disability is a predictor of poor outcome at 1 year even if individuals decline care. Ergonomics should be assessed at work and home. A course of specific neck exercises in physical therapy, including stretching, strengthening, and postural exercises, has been demonstrated to relieve symptoms with better short- to medium-term outcomes, although tailored programs were not clearly better than specific neck exercises. A soft cervical collar can be useful for short-term use (up to 1–2 weeks) in acute neck injuries. Chiropractic manual manipulation and mobilization can provide short-term benefit for mechanical neck pain. Although the rate of complications is low (5–10/million manipulations), care should be taken whenever there are neurologic symptoms present. Specific patients may respond to use of home cervical traction. NSAIDs are commonly used; opioids may be needed in cases of severe neck pain (Tables 5–5 and 5–6). Muscle relaxants (eg, cyclobenzaprine 5–10 mg orally three times daily) can be used short term if there is muscle spasm or as a sedative to aid in sleeping. Acute radicular symptoms can be treated with neuropathic medications (eg, gabapentin 300–1200 mg orally three times daily), and a short course of oral prednisone (5–10 days) can be considered (starting at 1 mg/kg). Cervical foraminal or facet joint injections can also reduce symptoms. Surgeries are successful in reducing neurologic symptoms in 80–90% of cases but are still considered as treatments of last resort. Common surgeries for cervical degenerative disk disease include anterior cervical diskectomy with fusion and cervical disk arthroplasty. A 2020 meta-analysis of 11 randomized controlled trials showed that beyond 5 years, cervical disk arthroplasty was superior to anterior diskectomy and fusion for the treatment of symptomatic cervical disk disease, with better success, lower reoperation rates, and superior longevity.

When to Refer

- Patients with severe symptoms with motor weakness.
- Surgical decompression surgery if the symptoms are severe and there is identifiable, correctable pathology.

Badhiwala JH et al. Cervical disc arthroplasty versus anterior cervical discectomy and fusion: a meta-analysis of rates of adjacent-level surgery to 7-year follow-up. J Spine Surg. 2020;6:217. [PMID: 32309660]

Martel JW et al. Evaluation and management of neck and back pain. Semin Neurol. 2019;39:41. [PMID: 30743291]

Sterling M. Best evidence rehabilitation for chronic pain part 4: neck pain. J Clin Med. 2019;8:E1219. [PMID: 31443149]

Villanueva-Ruiz I et al. Effectiveness of specific neck exercise for nonspecific neck pain; usefulness of strategies for patient selection and tailored exercise—a systematic review with meta-analysis. Phys Ther. 2022;102:pzab259. [PMID: 34935963]

UPPER EXTREMITY

1. Lateral & Medial Epicondylosis (Tendinopathy)

ESSENTIALS OF DIAGNOSIS

- Tenderness over the lateral or medial epicondyle.
- Diagnosis of tendinopathy is confirmed by pain with resisted strength testing and passive stretching of the affected tendon and muscle unit.
- Physical therapy and activity modification are more successful than anti-inflammatory treatments.

General Considerations

Tendinopathies involving the wrist extensors, flexors, and pronators are very common concerns. The underlying mechanism is chronic repetitive overuse causing microtrauma at the tendon insertion, although acute injuries can occur as well if the tendon is strained due to excessive loading. The traditional term "epicondylitis" is a misnomer because histologically tendinosis or degeneration in the tendon is seen rather than acute inflammation. Therefore, these entities should be referred to as "tendinopathy" or "tendinosis." Lateral epicondylosis involves the wrist extensors, especially the extensor carpi radialis brevis. This is usually caused be lifting with the wrist and the elbow extended. Medial epicondylosis involves the wrist flexors and most commonly the pronator teres tendon. Ulnar neuropathy and cervical radiculopathy should be considered in the differential diagnosis.

Clinical Findings

A. Symptoms and Signs

For lateral epicondylosis, the patient describes pain with the arm and wrist extended. For example, common concerns include pain while shaking hands, lifting objects, using a computer mouse, or hitting a backhand in tennis ("tennis elbow"). Medial epicondylosis presents with pain during motions in which the arm is repetitively pronated or the wrist is flexed. This is also known as "golfer's elbow" due to the motion of turning the hands over during the golf swing. For either, tenderness directly over the epicondyle is present, especially over the posterior aspect where the tendon insertion occurs. The proximal tendon and musculotendinous junction can also be sore. To confirm that the pain is due to tendinopathy, pain can be reproduced over the epicondyle with resisted wrist extension and third digit extension for lateral epicondylosis and resisted wrist pronation and wrist flexion for medial epicondylosis. The pain is also often reproduced with passive stretching of the affected muscle groups, which can be performed with the arm in extension. It is useful to check the ulnar nerve (located in a groove at the posteromedial elbow) for tenderness as well as to perform a Spurling test for cervical radiculopathy (see Neck Pain, above).

B. Imaging

Radiographs are often normal, although a small traction spur may be present in chronic cases (enthesopathy). Diagnostic investigations are usually unnecessary, unless the patient does not improve after up to 3 months of conservative treatment. At that point, a patient who demonstrates significant disability due to the pain should be assessed with an MRI or ultrasound. Ultrasound and MRI can visualize the tendon and confirm tendinosis or tears.

Treatment

Treatment is usually conservative, including patient education regarding activity modification and management of symptoms. Ice and NSAIDs can help with pain (Table 5–5). The mainstay of treatment is physical therapy exercises. The most important steps are to begin a good stretching program followed by strengthening exercises, particularly eccentric ones. Counterforce elbow braces might provide some symptomatic relief, although there is no published evidence to support their use. If the patient has severe or long-standing symptoms, injections can be considered. A randomized trial showed improvement with corticosteroid injection at 1 month as well as evidence of decreased tendon thickness and Doppler changes but no improvement at 3 months. Percutaneous needle tenotomy showed some positive results as an alternative to surgery but lacks demonstrated efficacy in a randomized control study.

Despite the increasing use of platelet-rich plasma (PRP) as a treatment for lateral epicondylitis, study results are inconsistent due to the varied methods of PRP preparations, varying post-injection recommendations, and improvement with placebo injections. However, a Cochrane review of 32 studies did not find that autologous blood or PRP injections provided significant improvement over placebo at 3 months or a clinical benefit for pain or function, especially at 6 or 12 months. A separate systematic review and meta-analysis of 11 studies showed better results for leukocyte-rich PRP than for leukocyte-poor PRP. Compared with ultrasound therapy, extracorporeal shock wave therapy has shown better efficacy for pain relief (as measured with visual analog scales) and better grip strength. However, it is used less commonly than injection treatments and is still considered second-line therapy.

When to Refer

Patients not responding to 6 months of conservative treatment should be referred for an injection procedure (PRP or tenotomy), surgical debridement, or repair of the tendon.

Karjalainen TV et al. Autologous blood and platelet-rich plasma injection therapy for lateral elbow pain. Cochrane Database Syst Rev. 2021;30;9:CD010951. [PMID: 34590307]

Kim GM et al. Current trends for treating lateral epicondylitis. Clin Shoulder Elb. 2019;22:227. [PMID: 33330224]

Shergill R et al. Ultrasound-guided interventions in lateral epicondylitis. J Clin Rheumatol. 2019;25:e27. [PMID: 30074911]

Shim JW et al. The effect of leucocyte concentration of platelet-rich plasma on outcomes in patients with lateral epicondylitis: a systematic review and meta-analysis. J Shoulder Elbow Surg. 2022;31:634. [PMID: 34861405]

2. Carpal Tunnel Syndrome

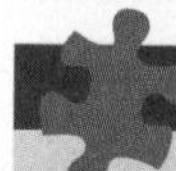

ESSENTIALS OF DIAGNOSIS

- Pain, burning, and tingling in the distribution of the median nerve.
- Initially, most bothersome during sleep.
- Late weakness or atrophy of the thenar eminence.
- Can be caused by repetitive wrist activities.
- Commonly seen during pregnancy and in patients with diabetes mellitus or rheumatoid arthritis.

General Considerations

An entrapment neuropathy, carpal tunnel syndrome is a painful disorder caused by compression of the median nerve between the carpal ligament and other structures within the carpal tunnel. The contents of the tunnel can be compressed by synovitis of the tendon sheaths or carpal joints, recent or malhealed fractures, tumors, tissue infiltration, and occasionally congenital syndromes (eg, mucopolysaccharidoses). The disorder may occur in fluid retention of pregnancy, in individuals with a history of repetitive use of the hands or following wrist injuries. Carpal tunnel syndrome can also be a feature of many systemic diseases, such as rheumatoid arthritis and other rheumatic disorders (inflammatory tenosynovitis), myxedema, amyloidosis, sarcoidosis, leukemia, acromegaly, and hyperparathyroidism. There is a familial type of carpal tunnel syndrome; the etiologic factor is unknown.

Clinical Findings

A. Symptoms and Signs

The initial symptoms are pain, burning, and tingling in the distribution of the median nerve (the palmar surfaces of the thumb, the index and long fingers, and the radial half of the ring finger). Aching pain may radiate proximally into the forearm and occasionally proximally to the shoulder and over the neck and chest. Pain is exacerbated by manual activity, particularly by extremes of volar flexion or dorsiflexion of the wrist. It is most bothersome at night. Impairment of sensation in the median nerve distribution may or may not be demonstrable. Subtle disparity between the affected and opposite sides can be shown by testing for two-point discrimination or by requiring the patient to identify different textures of cloth by rubbing them between the tips of the thumb and the index finger. A Tinel or Phalen sign may be positive. A **Tinel sign** is tingling or shock-like pain on volar wrist percussion. The **Phalen sign** is pain or paresthesia in the distribution of the median nerve when the patient flexes both wrists to 90 degrees for 60 seconds. The **carpal compression test**, in which numbness and tingling are induced by the direct application of pressure over the carpal tunnel, may be more sensitive and specific than the Tinel and Phalen tests. Muscle weakness or atrophy, especially of the thenar eminence, can appear later than sensory disturbances as compression of the nerve worsens.

B. Imaging

Ultrasound can demonstrate flattening of the median nerve beneath the flexor retinaculum. Sensitivity of ultrasound for carpal tunnel syndrome is variable but estimated between 54% and 98%.

C. Special Tests

Electromyography and nerve conduction studies show evidence of sensory conduction delay before motor delay, which can occur in severe cases and is most helpful when the diagnosis is unclear. Electrodiagnosis can provide information on focal median mononeuropathy at the wrist and can classify carpal tunnel syndrome from mild to severe, which may help in worker's compensation cases.

Treatment

Treatment is directed toward relief of pressure on the median nerve. When a causative lesion is discovered, it should be treated appropriately. Otherwise, patients in whom carpal tunnel syndrome is suspected should modify their hand activities. The affected wrist can be splinted in the neutral position for up to 3 months, but a series of Cochrane reviews show limited evidence for splinting, exercises, and ergonomic positioning. Moderate evidence supported benefit from several physical therapy and electrophysical modalities (eg, ultrasound therapy and radial extracorporeal shockwave therapy). These modalities provided short-term and mid-term relief of carpal tunnel syndrome symptoms in different studies. Oral corticosteroids or NSAIDs have also shown benefit for carpal tunnel syndrome. Methylprednisolone injections were found to have more effect at 10 weeks than placebo, but the benefits diminished by 1 year.

Compared with trigger finger management, which usually includes injections, as many as 71% of patients with carpal tunnel directly undergo surgery without first getting injections. There is strong evidence that a steroid injection to the carpal tunnel is more effective in the short term than surgery. Knowledge of pertinent anatomy and consistent technique are important to ensuring accurate needle placement during carpal tunnel injection; the accuracy of injection was only 76% in a 2020 study. A randomized, controlled trial showed both corticosteroid injection and surgery resolved symptoms, but only decompressive surgery led to resolution of neurophysiologic changes. Carpal tunnel release surgery can be beneficial if the patient has a positive electrodiagnostic test, at least moderate symptoms, high clinical probability, unsuccessful nonoperative treatment, and symptoms lasting longer than 12 months. Surgery can be done with an open approach or endoscopically, both yielding similar good improvements.

When to Refer

- If symptoms persist more than 3 months despite conservative treatment, including the use of a wrist splint.
- If thenar muscle (eg, abductor pollicis brevis) weakness or atrophy develops.

Billig JI et al. Utilization of diagnostic testing for carpal tunnel syndrome: a survey of the American Society for Surgery of the Hand. J Hand Surg Am. 2022;47:11. [PMID: 34991798]

Urits I et al. Recent advances in the understanding and management of carpal tunnel syndrome: a comprehensive review. Curr Pain Headache Rep. 2019;23:70. [PMID: 31372847]

3. Dupuytren Contracture

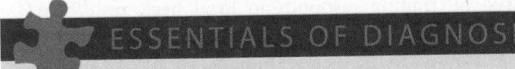

- Benign fibrosing disorder of the palmar fascia.
- Contracture of one or more fingers can lead to limited hand function.

General Considerations

This relatively common disorder is characterized by hyperplasia of the palmar fascia and related structures, with nodule formation and contracture of the palmar fascia. The cause is unknown, but the condition has a genetic predisposition and occurs primarily in White men over 50 years of age, particularly in those of Celtic descent. The incidence is higher among patients with alcohol use disorder and those with chronic systemic disorders (especially cirrhosis). It is also associated with systemic fibrosing syndrome, which includes plantar fibromatosis (10% of patients), Peyronie disease (1–2%), mediastinal and retroperitoneal fibrosis, and Riedel struma. The onset may be acute, but slowly progressive chronic disease is more common.

Clinical Findings

Dupuytren contracture manifests itself by nodular or cordlike thickening of one or both hands, with the fourth and fifth fingers most commonly affected. The patient may report tightness of the involved digits, with inability to satisfactorily extend the fingers, and on occasion there is tenderness. The resulting cosmetic problems may be unappealing, but in general the contracture is well tolerated since it exaggerates the normal position of function of the hand.

Treatment

Corticosteroid injections, percutaneous needle aponeurotomy, collagenase *Clostridium histolyticum* (CCH) injections, and open fasciectomy are common treatment options. If the palmar nodule is growing rapidly, injections of triamcinolone or collagenase into the nodule may be of benefit, while the CCH injection lyses collagen, thereby disrupting the contracted cords. Surgical options include open fasciectomy, partial fasciectomy, or percutaneous needle aponeurotomy and are indicated in patients with more severe flexion contractures. Splinting after surgery is beneficial. Recurrence and more adverse events are more likely to occur after surgery than with nonoperative treatments. Overall, treatment success is lower for proximal interphalangeal joints than for metacarpophalangeal joints. Fasciectomies are more successful for severe conditions involving multiple fingers, while percutaneous needle aponeurotomy is cost-effective and useful for milder cases and for single digit involvement. Some evidence suggests superior clinical outcomes of percutaneous needle aponeurotomy compared with CCH and a higher minor complication rate with CCH. Compared with placebo, tamoxifen therapy produced moderate evidence of improvement before or after a fasciectomy.

When to Refer

Referral can be considered when one or more digits are affected by severe contractures, which interfere with everyday activities and result in functional limitations.

Boe C et al. Dupuytren contractures: an update of recent literature. J Hand Surg Am. 2021;46:896. [PMID: 34452797]

Hirase T et al. Percutaneous needle fasciotomy versus collagenase injection for Dupuytren's contracture: a systematic review of comparative studies. J Hand Microsurg. 2021;13:150. [PMID: 34511831]

Yoon AP et al. Cost-effectiveness of recurrent Dupuytren contracture treatment. JAMA Netw Open. 2020;3:e2019861. [PMID: 33030553]

4. Bursitis

ESSENTIALS OF DIAGNOSIS

- Often occurs around bony prominences where it is important to reduce friction.
- Typically presents with local swelling that is painful acutely.
- Septic bursitis can present without fever or systemic signs.

General Considerations

Inflammation of bursae can lead to fluid accumulation in the synovial membranes overlying bony prominences. Predisposing factors include trauma, infection, or conditions such as rheumatoid arthritis, gout, pseudogout, rheumatoid arthritis, SLE, HIV, diabetes, or OA. The two common sites are the olecranon (Figure 41–1) and prepatellar bursae; however, others include subdeltoid, ischial, trochanteric, and semimembranosus-gastrocnemius (Baker cyst)

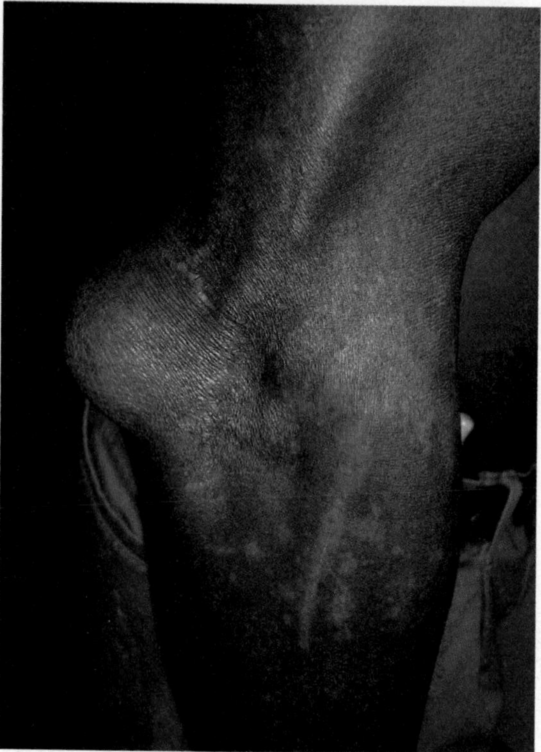

▲ **Figure 41–1.** Chronic aseptic olecranon bursitis without erythema or tenderness. (Reproduced with permission from Richard P. Usatine, MD, in Usatine RP, Smith MA, Mayeaux EJ Jr, Chumley H. *The Color Atlas of Family Medicine*, 2nd ed. McGraw-Hill, 2013.)

bursae. Septic bursitis can result from infection often preceded by direct trauma.

Clinical Findings

A. Symptoms and Signs

Bursitis presents with focal tenderness and swelling and is less likely to affect range of motion of the adjacent joint. Olecranon or prepatellar bursitis, for example, causes an oval (or, if chronic, bulbous) swelling at the tip of the elbow or knee and does not affect joint motion. Tenderness, erythema and warmth, cellulitis, a report of trauma, and evidence of a skin lesion are more common in septic bursitis but can be present in aseptic bursitis as well. Patients with septic bursitis can be febrile but the absence of fever does not exclude infection; one-third of those with septic olecranon bursitis are afebrile. A bursa can also become symptomatic when it ruptures. This is true for Baker cyst, the rupture of which can cause calf pain and swelling that mimic thrombophlebitis.

B. Imaging

Imaging is unnecessary unless there is concern for osteomyelitis, trauma, or other underlying pathology. Ruptured Baker cysts are imaged easily by sonography or MRI; imaging a presumed Baker cyst can exclude a DVT, which can be mimicked by a ruptured Baker cyst.

C. Special Tests

Acute swelling and redness at a bursal site call for aspiration to rule out infection especially if the patient is either febrile (temperature more than 37.8°C) or has prebursal warmth (temperature difference greater than 2.2°C) or both. A bursal fluid WBC count of greater than 1000/mcL (1.0×10^9/L) indicates inflammation from infection, rheumatoid arthritis, or gout. The bursal fluid of septic bursitis characteristically contains a purulent aspirate, fluid-to-serum glucose ratio less than 50%, WBC count more than 3000 cells/mcL (3.0×10^9/L), polymorphonuclear cells more than 50%, and a positive Gram stain for bacteria. Most cases are caused by *Staphylococcus aureus* or *Staphylococcus epidermidis;* the Gram stain is positive in two-thirds.

Treatment

In general, aspiration and corticosteroid injections in mild, nonseptic bursitis should be avoided to reduce complications of iatrogenic infection and skin atrophy. Bursitis caused by trauma responds to local heat, rest, NSAIDs (Table 5–5), and local corticosteroid injections. Repetitive minor trauma to the olecranon bursa should be eliminated by avoiding resting the elbow on a hard surface or by wearing an elbow pad. For chronic aseptic bursitis or when there are athletic or occupational demands, aspiration with intrabursal steroid injection can be performed. Ultrasound-guided aspiration and injection can improve the accuracy of the procedures. Treatment of a ruptured Baker cyst includes rest, leg elevation, and possibly injection of triamcinolone, 20–40 mg into the knee anteriorly (the knee compartment communicates with the cyst).

Treatment for septic bursitis involves incision and drainage and antibiotics usually delivered intravenously, especially against *S aureus* or *S epidermidis* (see Chapter 30).

When to Refer

- Septic bursitis requires immediate treatment with intravenous antibiotics and usually incision and draining.
- Elective surgical removal can be considered for chronic refractory cases with symptoms affecting activities of daily living.

Nchinda NN et al. Clinical management of olecranon bursitis: a review. J Hand Surg Am. 2021;46:501. [PMID: 33840568]

HIP

1. Hip Fractures

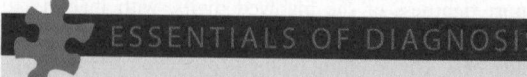

ESSENTIALS OF DIAGNOSIS

- Internal rotation of the hip is the best provocative diagnostic maneuver.
- Hip fractures should be surgically repaired as soon as possible (within 24 hours).
- Delayed treatment of hip fractures in older adults leads to increased complications and mortality.

General Considerations

Approximately 4% of the 7.9 million fractures that occur each year in the United States are hip fractures. There is a high mortality rate among older adult patients following hip fracture, with death occurring in 8–9% within 30 days and in approximately 25–30% within 1 year. Osteoporosis, female sex, height greater than 5-feet 8-inches, and age over 50 years are risk factors for hip fracture. Hip fractures usually occur after a fall. High-velocity trauma is needed in younger patients. Stress fractures can occur in athletes or individuals with poor bone mineral density following repetitive loading activities.

Clinical Findings

A. Symptoms and Signs

Patients typically report pain in the groin, though pain radiating to the lateral hip, buttock, or knee can also commonly occur. If a displaced fracture is present, the patient will not be able to bear weight and the leg may be externally rotated. Gentle logrolling of the leg with the patient supine helps rule out a fracture. Examination of the hip demonstrates pain with deep palpation in the area of the femoral triangle (similar to palpating the femoral artery). Provided the patient can tolerate it, the clinician can, with the patient supine, flex the hip to 90 degrees with the knee flexed to 90 degrees. The leg can then be internally and externally rotated to assess the range of motion on both sides. Pain with internal rotation of the hip is the most sensitive test to identify intra-articular hip pathology. Hip flexion, extension, abduction, and adduction strength can be tested.

Patients with hip stress fractures have less pain on physical examination than described previously but typically have pain with weight bearing. The Trendelenburg test can be performed to examine for weakness or instability of the hip abductors, primarily the gluteus medius muscle; the patient balances first on one leg, raising the non-standing knee toward the chest. The clinician can stand behind the patient and observe for dropping of the pelvis and buttock on the non-stance side. Another functional test is asking the patient to hop or jump during the examination. If the patient has a compatible clinical history of pain and is unable or unwilling to hop, then a stress fracture should be ruled out. The back should be carefully examined in patients who report hip discomfort, including examining for signs of sciatica.

Following displaced hip fractures, delay of operative intervention leads to an increased risk of perioperative morbidity and mortality. A thorough medical evaluation and treatment should be done to maximize the patient's ability to undergo operative intervention. A patient who was unable to get up after a fall may have been immobile for hours or even days. Her clinician must exclude rhabdomyolysis, hypothermia, DVT, PE, and other possible sequelae of prolonged immobilization.

B. Imaging

Useful radiographic imaging of the hip includes AP views of the pelvis and bilateral hips and frog-leg-lateral views of the painful hip. A CT scan or MRI may be necessary to identify the hip fracture pattern or to exclude non-displaced fractures. Hip fractures are generally described by location, including femoral neck, intertrochanteric, or subtrochanteric.

Treatment

Almost all patients with a hip fracture will require surgery and may need to be admitted to the hospital for pain control while they await surgery. Surgery is recommended within the first 24 hours because studies have shown that delaying surgery 48 hours results in at least twice the rate of major and minor medical complications, including pneumonia, pressure injuries (formerly pressure ulcers), and DVT. High-volume centers have multidisciplinary teams (including orthopedic surgeons, internists, social workers, and specialized physical therapists) to comanage these patients, which improves perioperative medical care and expedites preoperative evaluation leading to reduced costs. During the months of hip fracture recovery, prevention of pneumonia and functional decline and treatment of cardiac disease can reduce mortality.

Stress fractures in active patients require a period of protected weight bearing and a gradual return to activities, although it may take 4–6 months before a return to normal activities. Femoral neck fractures are commonly treated with hemiarthroplasty or total hip replacement. This allows the patient to begin weight bearing immediately postoperatively. Peritrochanteric hip fractures are treated with open reduction internal fixation, where plate and screw construct or intramedullary devices are used. The choice of implant will depend on the fracture pattern. Since fracture fixation requires the fracture to proceed to union, the patient may need to have protected weight bearing during the early postoperative period. Dislocation, periprosthetic fracture, and avascular necrosis of the hip are common complications after surgery. Patients should be mobilized as soon as possible postoperatively to avoid pulmonary complications and pressure injuries. Supervised physical therapy and rehabilitation are important for the patient to regain as much function as possible. Unfortunately, most patients following hip fractures will lose some degree of independence. Patients with hip fracture surgery when compared with elective total hip replacement have been shown to have higher risk of in-hospital mortality.

Prevention

Bone density screening can identify patients at risk for osteopenia or osteoporosis, and treatment can be planned accordingly (see Chapter 26). There is strong evidence that bisphosphonates, denosumab, and teriparatide reduce fractures compared with placebo, with relative risk reductions of 0.60–0.80 for nonvertebral fractures. There is an increase in atypical femoral fractures with bisphosphonate use (relative risk 1.7), especially in patients of an Asian race in North America, patients with femoral bowing, and patients who had used glucocorticoids. Consensus is that there is benefit in using bisphosphonates, particularly during the third through fifth years of therapy, with considerations for drug holidays. After 5 years of bisphosphonate use, there is an increased risk for atypical femur fractures. Nutrition and bone health (bone densitometry, serum calcium and 25-OH vitamin D levels) should be reviewed with the patient. However, there is no evidence that increasing calcium intake prevents hip fractures. For patients with decreased mobility, systemic anticoagulation should be considered to avoid DVT (see Table 14–14). Fall prevention exercise programs are available for older adult patients at risk for falls and hip fractures. Hip protectors are uncomfortable and have less use in preventing fractures.

When to Refer

- All patients in whom hip fracture is suspected.
- All patients with hip fracture or in whom the diagnosis is uncertain after radiographs.

Barceló M et al. Hip fracture and mortality: study of specific causes of death and risk factors. Arch Osteoporos. 2021;16:15. [PMID: 33452949]

Black DM et al. Atypical femur fracture risk versus fragility fracture prevention with bisphosphonates. N Engl J Med. 2020; 383:743. [PMID: 32813950]

Guyen O. Hemiarthroplasty or total hip arthroplasty in recent femoral neck fractures? Orthop Traumatol Surg Res. 2019; 105:S95. [PMID: 30449680]

Sobolev B et al; Canadian Collaborative Study of Hip Fractures. Mortality effects of timing alternatives for hip fracture surgery. CMAJ. 2018;190:E923. [PMID: 30087128]

Stirton JB et al. Total hip arthroplasty for the management of hip fracture: a review of the literature. J Orthop. 2019;16:141. [PMID: 30886461]

2. Hip Osteoarthritis

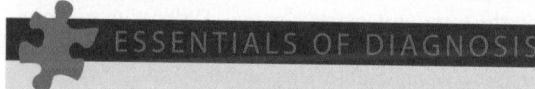

- Pain deep in the groin on the affected side.
- Swelling.
- Degeneration of joint cartilage.
- Loss of active and passive range of motion in severe OA.

General Considerations

In the United States, the prevalence of OA will grow as the number of persons over age 65 years doubles to more than 70 million by 2030. Cartilage loss and OA symptoms are preceded by damage to the collagen-proteoglycan matrix. The etiology of OA is often multifactorial, including previous trauma, prior high-impact activities, genetic factors, obesity, and rheumatologic or metabolic conditions. Femoroacetabular impingement, which affects younger active patients, is considered an early development of hip OA.

Clinical Findings

A. Symptoms and Signs

OA usually causes pain in the affected joint with loading of the joint or at the extremes of motion. Mechanical symptoms—such as swelling, grinding, catching, and locking—suggest internal derangement, which is indicated by damaged cartilage or bone fragments that affect the smooth range of motion expected at an articular joint. Pain can also produce the sensation of "buckling" or "giving way" due to muscle inhibition. As the joint degeneration becomes more advanced, the patient loses active range of motion and may lose passive range of motion as well.

Patients report pain deep in the groin on the affected side and have problems with weight-bearing activities such as walking, climbing stairs, and getting up from a chair. They may limp and develop a lurch during their gait, leaning toward the unaffected side as they walk to reduce pressure on the arthritic hip. The most specific findings to identify hip osteoarthritis were squat causing posterior pain, groin pain on passive abduction or adduction, abductor weakness, and decreased passive hip adduction or less passive internal rotation compared with the contralateral leg. The presence of normal passive hip adduction was most useful for suggesting the absence of OA (LR–, 0.25).

B. Imaging

An anterior-posterior weight-bearing radiograph of the pelvis with a lateral view of the symptomatic hip are preferred views for evaluation of hip OA. Joint space narrowing and sclerosis suggest early OA. Findings of femoroacetabular impingement are commonly reported on radiograph reports with arthritic changes and anatomic variations involving the acetabulum and femoral head neck junction. After age 35, MRI of the hips already shows labral changes in almost 70% of asymptomatic patients. Osteophytes near the femoral head or acetabulum and subchondral bone cysts (advanced Kellgren and Lawrence grade), superior or (supero) lateral femoral head migration, and subchondral sclerosis suggest the patient will more likely progress to total hip replacement. However, not all patients with radiographic hip OA have hip or groin pain; the converse is also true.

Treatment

A. Conservative

Changes in the articular cartilage are irreversible. Therefore, a cure for the diseased joint is not possible, although symptoms or structural issues can be managed to try to maintain activity level. Conservative treatment for patients with OA includes activity modification, proper footwear, therapeutic exercises, weight loss, and use of assistive devices (such as a cane). A 2014 randomized study found that physical therapy did not lead to greater improvement in pain or function compared with sham treatment in patients with hip OA. Analgesics may be effective in some cases. Corticosteroid injections can be considered for short-term relief of pain; however, hip injections are best performed under fluoroscopic, ultrasound, or CT guidance to ensure accurate injection in the joint. The risk of rapidly progressive degenerative changes following a single low-dose (40 mg or less) triamcinolone injection is low; the risk is higher following a high-dose (80 mg or higher) injection and multiple injections.

B. Surgical

Joint replacement surgeries are effective and cost-effective for patients with significant symptoms and functional limitations, providing improvements in pain, function, and quality of life. In considering surgery, racial and ethnic minority individuals are less willing to undergo total joint replacement, demonstrate worse surgical and functional outcomes, and have less access to hospital choices. Various surgical techniques and computer-assisted navigation during operation continue to be investigated. A review of nine randomized controlled trials concluded that a direct anterior approach for hip replacement was associated with a shorter incision, lower blood loss, lower pain scores, and earlier functional recovery. However, there was no significant difference in complication rates between groups for the direct anterior or posterior approaches nor were there any differences in patient-reported postoperative outcome measures at 1 year or beyond. There has not been clear clinical benefit of minimally invasive surgery compared with the standard invasive surgery, except for less total blood loss, shorter duration of surgery, and a shorter length of hospital stay.

Hip resurfacing surgery is an alternative for younger patients. Rather than use a traditional artificial joint implant of the whole neck and femur, only the femoral head is removed and replaced. Evidence to date suggests that hip resurfacing is comparable to total hip replacement. The cumulative survival rate of this implant at 10 years is estimated to be 94%. Concerns following resurfacing surgery include the risk of femoral neck fracture and collapse of the head. In a systematic review of national databases, the average time to revision was 3.0 years for metal-on-metal hip resurfacing versus 7.8 years for total hip arthroplasty. Dislocations were more frequent with total hip arthroplasty than metal-on-metal hip resurfacing: 4.4 versus 0.9 per 1000 person-years, respectively.

Guidelines recommend prophylaxis for venous thromboembolic disease for a minimum of 14 days after arthroplasty of the hip or knee using warfarin, low-molecular-weight heparin, fondaparinux, aspirin, rivaroxaban, dabigatran, apixaban, or portable mechanical compression (see Table 14–14). While bleeding risks are similar, patients taking warfarin are more likely to experience DVT and PE than patients taking rivaroxaban (see Chapter 14).

When to Refer

Patients with sufficient disability, limited benefit from conservative therapy, and evidence of severe OA on imaging can be referred for joint replacement surgery.

Hunter DJ et al. Osteoarthritis. Lancet. 2019;393:1745. [PMID: 31034380]

Metcalfe D et al. Does this patient have hip osteoarthritis? The Rational Clinical Examination Systematic Review. JAMA. 2019;322:2323. [PMID: 31846019]

Okike K et al. Rapidly destructive hip disease following intra-articular corticosteroid injection of the hip. J Bone Joint Surg Am. 2021;103:2070. [PMID: 34550909]

Usiskin I et al. Racial disparities in elective total joint arthroplasty for osteoarthritis. ACR Open Rheumatol. 2022;4:306. [PMID: 34989176]

KNEE

1. Knee Pain

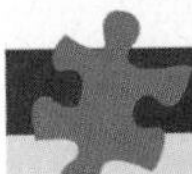

ESSENTIALS OF DIAGNOSIS

- Effusion can occur with intra-articular pathology (eg, OA, meniscus and cruciate ligament tears).
- Acute knee swelling (due to hemarthrosis) within 2 hours may indicate ligament injuries or patellar dislocation or fracture.

General Considerations

The knee is the largest joint in the body and is susceptible to injury from trauma, inflammation, infection, and degenerative changes. Table 41–4 shows the differential diagnosis of knee pain. OA of the knees is common after 50 years of age and can develop due to previous trauma, aging, activities, alignment issues, and genetic predisposition.

Acute hemarthrosis represents bloody swelling that usually occurs within the first 1–2 hours following trauma. In situations where the trauma may be activity-related and not a result of a fall or collision, the causes of the hemarthrosis most commonly include ACL tear (responsible for more than 70% in adults), fracture (patella, tibial plateau, femoral supracondylar, growth plate [physeal]), and patellar dislocation. Meniscal tears are unlikely to cause large hemarthrosis.

Clinical Findings

A. Symptoms and Signs

Evaluation of knee pain should begin with questions regarding duration and rapidity of symptom onset and the mechanism of injury or aggravating symptoms. Overuse or degenerative problems can occur with stress or compression from sports, hobbies, or occupation. A history of trauma or previous orthopedic problems with, or surgery to, the affected knee should also be specifically queried. Symptoms of infection (fever, recent bacterial infections, risk factors for sexually transmitted infections [such as gonorrhea] or other bacterial infections [such as staphylococcal infection]) should always be elicited.

Common symptoms include the following:

1. Grinding, clicking, or popping with bending may be indicative of OA or the patellofemoral syndrome.
2. "Locking" or "catching" when walking suggests an internal derangement, such as meniscal injury or a loose body in the knee.
3. Intra-articular swelling of the knee or an effusion indicates an internal derangement or a synovial pathology. Large swelling may cause a popliteal (Baker) cyst. Acute swelling within minutes to hours suggests a hemarthrosis, most likely due to an anterior cruciate ligament (ACL) injury, fracture, or patellar dislocation, especially if trauma is involved.

Table 41–4. Differential diagnosis of knee pain.

Mechanical dysfunction or disruption
Internal derangement of the knee: injury to the menisci or ligaments
Degenerative changes caused by osteoarthritis
Dynamic dysfunction or misalignment of the patella
Fracture as a result of trauma
Intra-articular inflammation or increased pressure
Internal derangement of the knee: injury to the menisci or ligaments
Inflammation or infection of the knee joint
Ruptured popliteal (Baker) cyst
Peri-articular inflammation
Internal derangement of the knee: injury to the menisci or ligaments
Prepatellar or anserine bursitis
Ligamentous sprain

4. Lateral "snapping" with flexion and extension of the knee may indicate inflammation of the iliotibial band.
5. Pain that is worsened with bending and walking down stairs suggests issues with the patellofemoral joint, usually degenerative such as chondromalacia of the patella or OA.
6. Pain that occurs when rising after prolonged sitting suggests a problem with tracking of the patella.

A knee joint effusion is characterized by swelling in the hollow or dimple around the patella and distention of the suprapatellar space.

The location of the knee pain combined with specific tests for anatomic structures are frequently sufficient to establish a diagnosis (Tables 41–5 and 41–6).

Table 41–5. Location of common causes of knee pain.

Medial knee pain
Medial compartment osteoarthritis
Medial collateral ligament strain
Medial meniscal injury
Anserine bursitis (pain over the proximal medial tibial plateau)
Anterior knee pain
Patellofemoral syndrome (often bilateral)
Osteoarthritis
Prepatellar bursitis (associated with swelling anterior to the patella)
"Jumper's knee" (pain at the inferior pole of the patella)
Septic arthritis
Gout or other inflammatory disorder
Lateral knee pain
Lateral meniscal injury
Iliotibial band syndrome (pain superficially along the distal iliotibial band near the lateral femoral condyle or lateral tibial insertion)
Lateral collateral ligament sprain (rare)
Posterior knee pain
Popliteal (Baker) cyst
Osteoarthritis
Meniscal tears
Hamstring or calf tendinopathy

B. Laboratory Findings

Laboratory testing of aspirated joint fluid, when indicated, can lead to a definitive diagnosis in most patients (see Tables 20–2 and 20–3).

C. Imaging

Knee pain is evaluated with plain (weight-bearing) radiographs and MRI most commonly, but CT and ultrasound are sometimes useful.

D. Treatment

Treatment of specific etiologies of knee pain is discussed below.

Bunt CW et al. Knee pain in adults and adolescents: the initial evaluation. Am Fam Physician. 2018;98:576. [PMID: 30325638]

2. Anterior Cruciate Ligament Injury

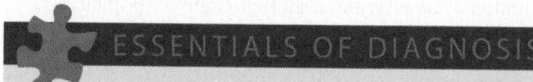

- An injury involving an audible pop when the knee buckles.
- Acute swelling immediately (or within 2 hours).
- Instability occurs with lateral movement activities and going down stairs.

General Considerations

The ACL connects the posterior aspect of the lateral femoral condyle to the anterior aspect of the tibia. Its main function is to control anterior translation of the tibia on the femur. It also provides rotational stability of the tibia on the femur. ACL tears are common with sporting injuries. They can result from both contact (valgus blow to the knee) and non-contact (jumping, pivoting, and deceleration) activities. The patient usually falls down following the injury and has acute swelling, difficulty with weight bearing, and instability. ACL injuries are common in skiing, soccer, football, and basketball among young adolescents and middle-aged patients. Prepubertal and older patients usually sustain fractures instead of ligamentous injuries.

Clinical Findings

A. Symptoms and Signs

Acute ACL injuries usually lead to acute swelling of the knee, causing difficulty with motion. After the swelling has resolved, the patient can walk with a "stiff-knee" gait or quadriceps avoidance gait because of the instability. Patients describe symptoms of instability while performing side-to-side maneuvers or descending stairs. Stability tests assess the amount of laxity of the knee while performing these maneuvers. The Lachman test (84–87% sensitivity and 93% specificity) is performed with the patient lying

Table 41–6. Knee examination.

Maneuver	Description
Inspection	Examine for the alignment of the lower extremities (varus, valgus, knee recurvatum), ankle eversion and foot pronation, gait, "SEADS" (*s*welling, *e*rythema, *a*trophy, *d*eformity, *s*urgical scars).
Palpation	Include important landmarks: patellofemoral joint, medial and lateral joint lines (especially posterior aspects), pes anserine bursa, distal iliotibial band and Gerdy tubercle (iliotibial band insertion).
Range of motion testing 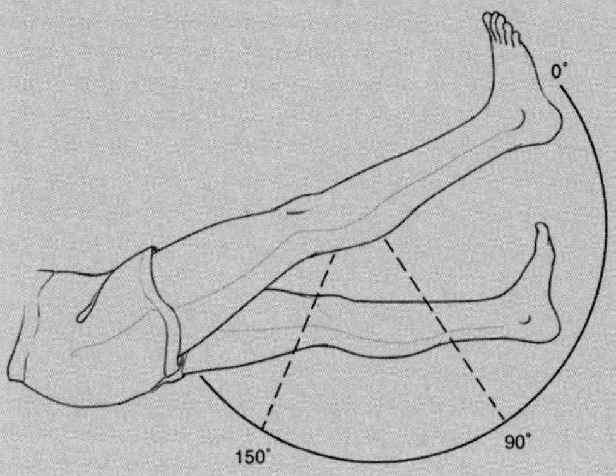 0° 90° 150°	Check range of motion actively (patient performs) and passively (clinician performs), especially with flexion and extension of the knee normally 0–10 degrees of extension and 120–150 degrees of flexion.
Knee strength testing	Test resisted knee extension and knee flexion strength manually.
Ligament Stress Testing	
Lachman test 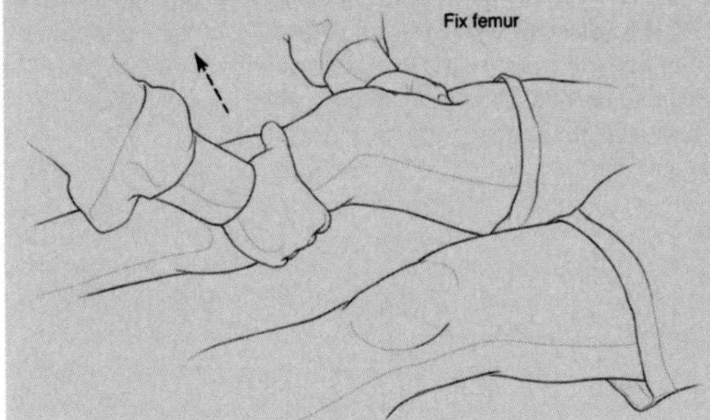 Fix femur	Performed with the patient lying supine and the knee flexed to 20–30 degrees. The examiner grasps the distal femur from the lateral side, and the proximal tibia with the other hand on the medial side. With the knee in neutral position, stabilize the femur, and pull the tibia anteriorly using a similar force to lift a 10- to 15-pound weight. **Positive test:** Excessive anterior translation of the tibia compared with the other side indicates injury to the anterior cruciate ligament.
Anterior drawer 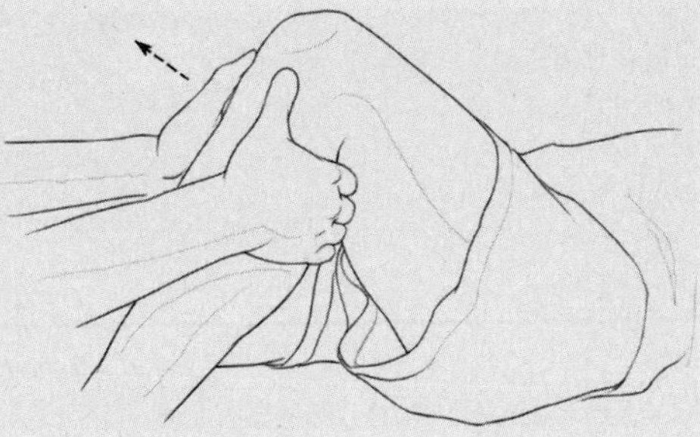	Performed with the patient lying supine and the knee flexed to 90 degrees. The clinician stabilizes the patient's foot by sitting on it and grasps the proximal tibia with both hands around the calf and pulls anteriorly. **Positive test:** There is anterior cruciate ligament laxity compared with the unaffected side.

(*continued*)

Table 41–6. Knee examination. (continued)

Maneuver	Description
Pivot shift 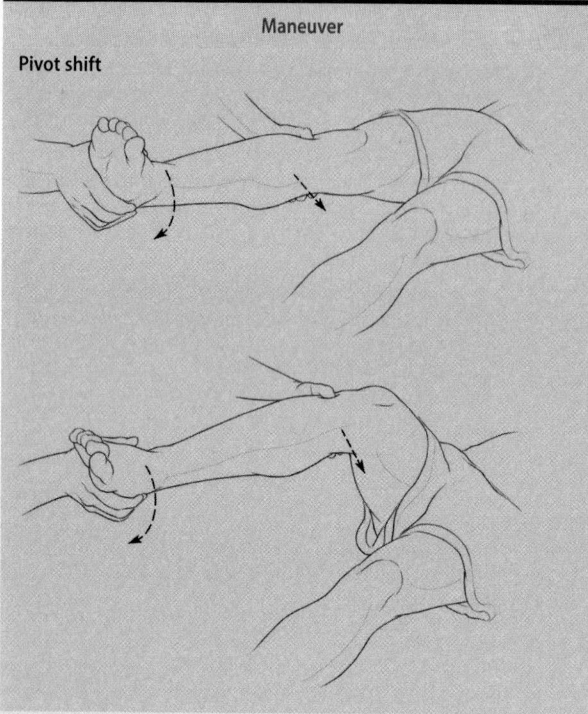	Used to determine the amount of rotational laxity of the knee. The patient is examined while lying supine with the knee in full extension. It is then slowly flexed while applying internal rotation and a valgus stress. **Positive test:** The clinician feels for a subluxation at 20–40 degrees of knee flexion. (The patient must remain very relaxed to have a positive test.)
Valgus stress 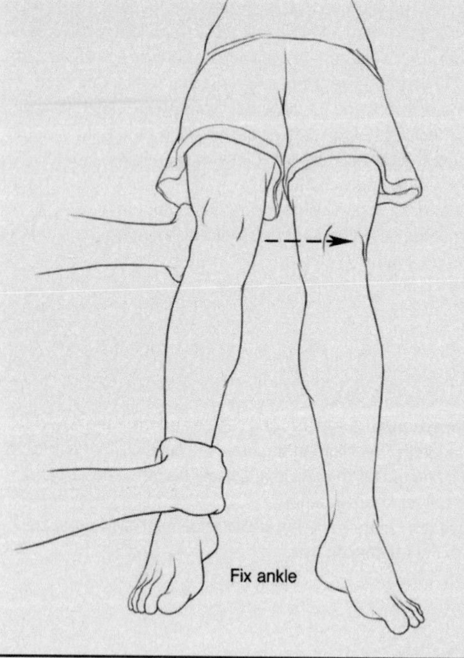	Performed with the patient lying supine. The clinician should stand on the outside of the patient's knee. With one hand, the clinician should hold the ankle while the other hand is supporting the leg at the level of the knee joint. A valgus stress is applied at the ankle to determine pain and laxity of the medial collateral ligament. The test should be performed at both 30 degrees and 0 degrees of knee extension. **Positive test:** Pain and laxity of the medial collateral ligament with valgus stress.

(*continued*)

Table 41–6. Knee examination. (continued)

Maneuver	Description
Varus stress	Performed with the patient lying supine. For the right knee, the clinician should be standing on the right side of the patient. The left hand of the examiner should be holding the ankle while the right hand is supporting the lateral thigh. A varus stress is applied at the ankle to determine pain and laxity of the lateral collateral ligament. The test should be performed at both 30 degrees and 0 degrees of knee flexion. **Positive test:** Pain and laxity of the lateral collateral ligament with varus stress.
Meniscal Signs	
McMurray test	Performed with the patient lying supine. The clinician flexes the knee until the patient reports pain. For this test to be valid, it must be flexed pain-free beyond 90 degrees. **Positive test:** The clinician externally rotates the patient's foot and then extends the knee while palpating the medial knee for "click" in the medial compartment of the knee or pain reproducing pain from a meniscus injury. To test the lateral meniscus, the same maneuver is repeated while rotating the foot internally (53% sensitivity and 59–97% specificity).
Modified McMurray 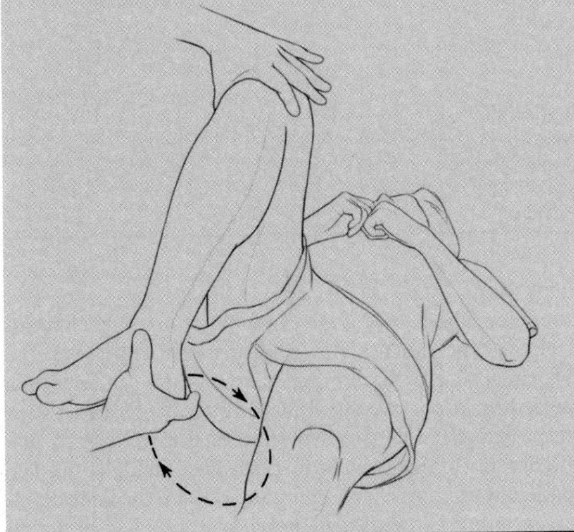	Performed with the patient lying supine and the hip flexed to 90 degrees. The knee is then flexed maximally with internal or external rotation of the lower leg. The knee can then be rotated with the lower leg in internal or external rotation to capture the torn meniscus underneath the condyles. **Positive test:** Pain over the joint line while the knee is being flexed and internally or externally rotated.

(*continued*)

Table 41–6. Knee examination. (continued)

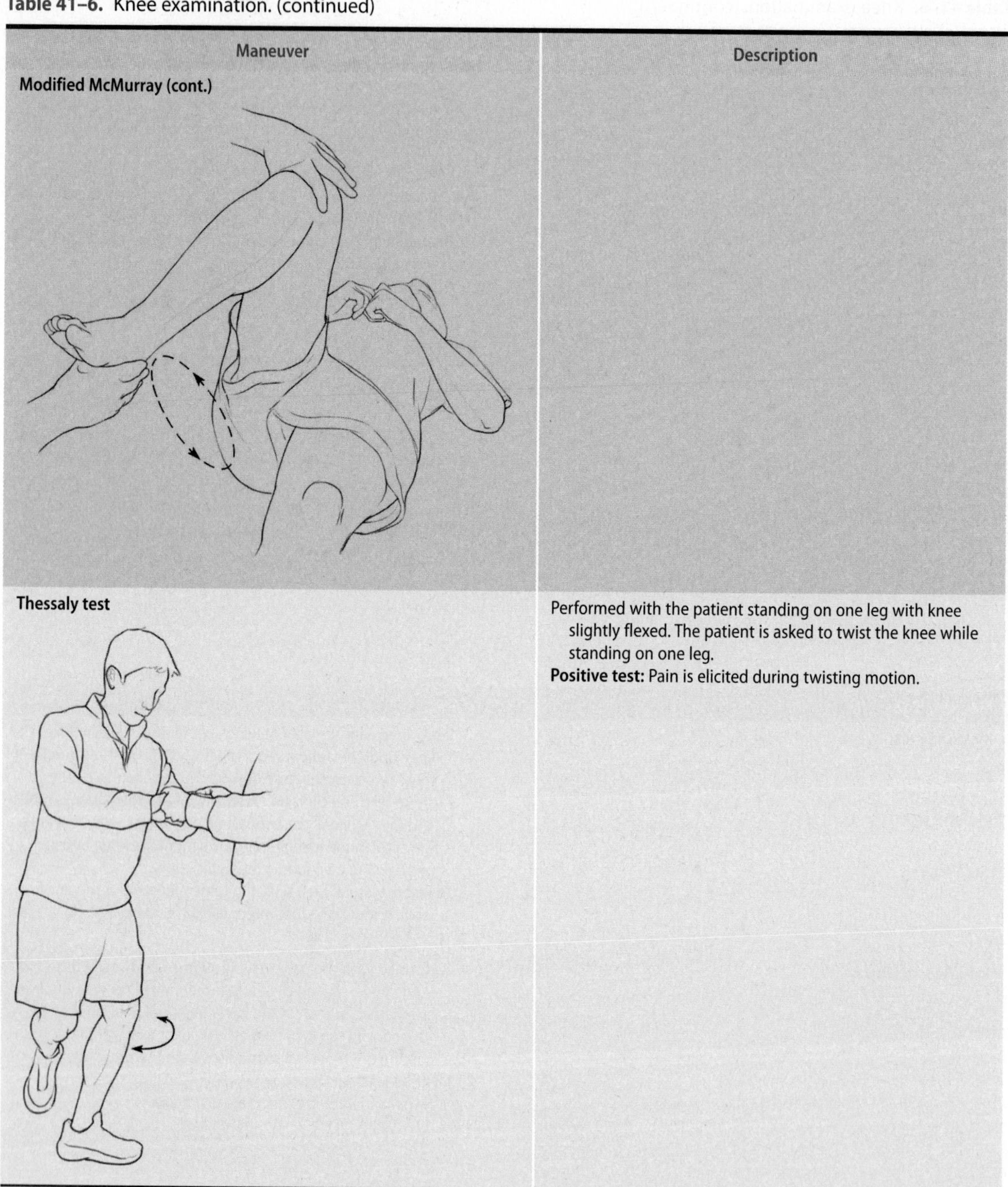

Maneuver	Description
Modified McMurray (cont.)	
Thessaly test	Performed with the patient standing on one leg with knee slightly flexed. The patient is asked to twist the knee while standing on one leg. **Positive test:** Pain is elicited during twisting motion.

supine and the knee flexed to 20–30 degrees (Table 41–6). The clinician grasps the distal femur from the lateral side and the proximal tibia with the other hand on the medial side. With the knee in neutral position, stabilize the femur, and pull the tibia anteriorly using a similar force to lift a 10- to 15-pound weight. Excessive anterior translation of the tibia compared with the other side indicates injury to the ACL. The anterior drawer test (48% sensitivity and 87% specificity) is performed with the patient lying supine and the knee flexed to 90 degrees (Table 41–6). The clinician stabilizes the patient's foot by sitting on it and grasps the proximal tibia with both hands around the calf and pulls anteriorly. A positive test finds ACL laxity compared with the unaffected side. The pivot shift test is used to determine the amount of rotational laxity of the knee (Table 41–6). The patient is examined while lying supine with the knee in full extension. It is then slowly flexed while applying internal rotation and a valgus stress. The clinician feels for a subluxation at 20–40 degrees of knee flexion. The patient must remain very relaxed to have a positive test.

B. Imaging

Plain radiographs are usually negative in ACL tears but are useful to rule out fractures. A small avulsion injury can sometimes be seen over the lateral compartment of the knee ("Segond" fracture) and is pathognomonic of an ACL injury. An ACL injury that avulsed the tibial spine can be seen in radiographs. MRI is the best tool to diagnose ACL tears and associated articular and meniscal cartilage issues. It has greater than 95% sensitivity and specificity for ACL tears.

Treatment

Most young and active patients will require surgical reconstruction of the ACL. Some data suggest that reconstruction within 5 months of the tear has better outcomes. However, a small, randomized trial suggested that acute ACL injuries can be treated nonoperatively and delayed ACL reconstruction had similar outcomes to acute ACL reconstructions. Patients for whom the reconstruction is delayed, however, have more cartilage or meniscus problems at the time of surgery. Common surgical techniques use the patient's own tissue, usually the patellar or hamstring tendons (autograft), or use a cadaver graft (allograft) to arthroscopically reconstruct the torn ACL. Different patient groups experienced improved results with specific surgical graft choices. However, allografts do have a higher failure rate when compared with autografts. Recovery from surgery usually requires 6 months.

Nonoperative treatments are usually reserved for older patients or those with a very sedentary lifestyle. Physical therapy can focus on hamstring strengthening and core stability. An ACL brace can help stability. Longitudinal studies have demonstrated that nonoperative management of an ACL tear can lead to a higher incidence of meniscus tears. Cost-analysis studies have shown that early ACL reconstruction can be more beneficial than nonoperative treatment and delayed subsequent surgeries.

When to Refer

- Almost all ACL tears should be referred to an orthopedic surgeon for evaluation.
- Individuals with instability in the setting of a chronic ACL tear (greater than 6 months) should be considered for surgical reconstruction.
- Patients with an ACL tear and associated meniscus or articular injuries may benefit from surgery to address the other injuries.

Filbay SR et al. Evidence-based recommendations for the management of anterior cruciate ligament (ACL) rupture. Best Pract Res Clin Rheumatol. 2019;33:33. [PMID: 31431274]

Webster KE et al. What is the evidence for and validity of return-to-sport testing after anterior cruciate ligament reconstruction surgery? A systematic review and meta-analysis. Sports Med. 2019;49:917. [PMID: 30905035]

3. Collateral Ligament Injury

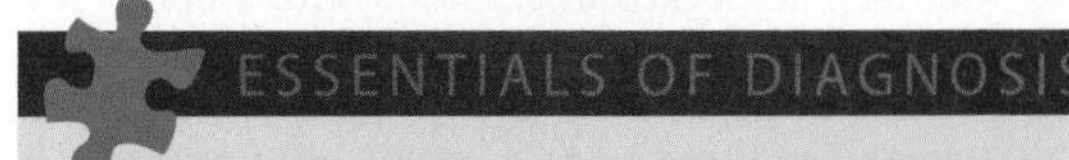

- Caused by a valgus or varus blow or stress to the knee.
- Pain and instability in the affected area.
- Limited range of motion.

General Considerations

The medial collateral ligament (MCL) is the most commonly injured ligament in the knee. It is usually injured with a valgus stress to the partially flexed knee. It can also occur with a blow to the lateral leg. The MCL is commonly injured with acute ACL injuries. The lateral collateral ligament (LCL) is less commonly injured, but this can occur with a medial blow to the knee. Since both collateral ligaments are extra-articular, injuries to these ligaments may not lead to any intra-articular effusion. Affected patients may have difficulty walking initially, but this can improve when the swelling decreases.

Clinical Findings

A. Symptoms and Signs

The main clinical findings for patients with collateral ligament injuries are pain along the course of the ligaments. The patient may have limited range of motion due to pain, especially during the first 2 weeks following the injury. The best tests to assess the collateral ligaments are the varus and valgus stress tests (Table 41–6). The test results can be graded from 1 to 3. Grade 1 is when the patient has pain with varus/valgus stress test but no instability. With grade 2 injuries, the patient has pain, and the knee shows instability at 30 degrees of knee flexion. In grade 3 injuries, the patient has marked instability but not much pain. The knee is often unstable at both 30 degrees and 0 degrees of knee flexion. The overall sensitivity of the tests is 86–96%.

B. Imaging

Radiographs are usually nondiagnostic except for avulsion injuries. However, radiographs should be used to rule out fractures that can occur with collateral ligament injuries. Isolated MCL injuries usually do not require evaluation by MRI, but MRI should be used to evaluate possible associated cruciate ligament injuries. LCL or posterolateral corner injuries should have MRI evaluation to exclude associated injuries and to determine their significance.

Treatment

Most MCL injuries can be treated with protected weight bearing and physical therapy. For grade 1 and 2 injuries, the patient can usually bear weight as tolerated with full range of motion. A hinged knee brace can be given to patients with grade 2 MCL tears to provide stability. Early physical therapy is recommended to protect range of motion and muscle strength. Grade 3 MCL injuries require long leg braces to provide stability. Patients can weight-bear, but only with the knee locked in extension with a brace. The motion can then be increased with the brace unlocked. Grade 3 injuries can take up to 6–8 weeks to heal. MCL injuries rarely need surgery. LCL injuries are less common but are usually associated with other ligament injuries (such as ACL and posterior cruciate ligament [PCL]). LCL injuries do not recover well with nonoperative treatment and usually require urgent surgical repair or reconstruction.

When to Refer

- Symptomatic instability with chronic MCL tears or acute MCL tears with other ligamentous injuries.
- LCL or posterolateral corner injuries require urgent surgical repair or reconstruction (within 1 week).

Elkin JL et al. Combined anterior cruciate ligament and medial collateral ligament knee injuries: anatomy, diagnosis, management recommendations, and return to sport. Curr Rev Musculoskelet Med. 2019;12:239. [PMID: 30929138]

Grawe B et al. Lateral collateral ligament injury about the knee: anatomy, evaluation, and management. J Am Acad Orthop Surg. 2018;26:e120. [PMID: 29443704]

4. Posterior Cruciate Ligament Injury

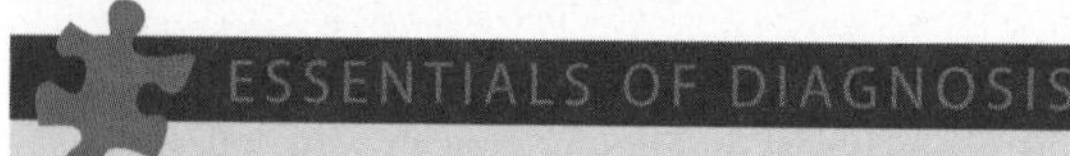

- Usually follows anterior trauma to the tibia, such as a dashboard injury from a motor vehicle accident.
- The knee may freely dislocate and reduce.
- One-third of multi-ligament injuries involving the PCL have neurovascular injuries.

General Considerations

The PCL is the strongest ligament in the knee. PCL injuries usually represent significant trauma and are highly associated with multi-ligament injuries and knee dislocations. More than 70–90% of PCL injuries have associated injuries to the posterolateral corner, MCL, and ACL. Neurovascular injuries occur in up to one-third of all knee dislocations or PCL injuries. There should be high suspicion for neurovascular injuries and a thorough neurovascular examination of the limb should be performed.

Clinical Findings

A. Symptoms and Signs

Most patients with acute injuries have difficulty with ambulation. Patients with chronic PCL injuries can ambulate without gross instability but may describe subjective "looseness" and often report pain and dysfunction, especially with bending. Clinical examinations of PCL injuries include the "sag sign"; the patient is placed supine and both hips and knees are flexed to 90 degrees. Because of gravity, the posterior cruciate ligament-injured knee will have an obvious set-off at the anterior tibia that is "sagging" posteriorly. The PCL ligament can also be examined using the posterior drawer test; the patient is placed supine with the knee flexed to 90 degrees. In a normal knee, the anterior tibia should be positioned about 10 mm anterior to the femoral condyle. The clinician can grasp the proximal tibia with both hands and push the tibia posteriorly. The movement, indicating laxity and possible tear of the PCL, is compared with the uninjured knee (90% sensitivity and 99% specificity). A PCL injury is sometimes mistaken for an ACL injury during the anterior drawer test since the tibia is subluxed posteriorly in a sagged position and can be abnormally translated forward, yielding a false-positive test for an ACL injury. Pain, swelling, pallor, and numbness in the affected extremity may suggest a knee dislocation with possible injury to the popliteal artery. If the lateral knee is unstable with varus stress testing (Table 41–6), the patient should be assessed for a posterolateral corner injury, which consists of injuries to the LCL, popliteus tendon, and popliteofibular ligament. Injuries to the posterolateral corner usually require urgent surgical treatment.

B. Imaging

Radiographs are often nondiagnostic but are required to diagnose any fractures. MRI is used to diagnose PCL and other associated injuries.

Treatment

Isolated PCL injuries can be treated nonoperatively. Acute injuries are usually immobilized using a knee brace with the knee extension; the patient uses crutches for ambulation. Physical therapy can help achieve increased range of motion and improved ambulation. Many PCL injuries are associated with other injuries and may require operative reconstruction.

When to Refer

- The patient should be seen urgently within 1–2 weeks.
- Posterolateral corner injury requires urgent surgical reconstruction.
- Isolated PCL tears may require surgery if the tear is complete (grade 3) and the patient is symptomatic.

Badri A et al. Clinical and radiologic evaluation of the posterior cruciate ligament-injured knee. Curr Rev Musculoskelet Med. 2018;11:515. [PMID: 29987531]

Devitt BM et al. Isolated posterior cruciate reconstruction results in improved functional outcome but low rates of return to preinjury level of sport: a systematic review and meta-analysis. Orthop J Sports Med. 2018;6:2325967118804478. [PMID: 30386804]

5. Meniscus Injuries

ESSENTIALS OF DIAGNOSIS

- Patient may or may not report an injury.
- Joint line pain and pain with deep squatting are the most sensitive signs.
- Difficulty with knee extension suggests an internal derangement that should be evaluated urgently with MRI.

General Considerations

The menisci act as shock absorbers within the knee. Injuries to a meniscus can lead to pain, clicking, and locking sensation. Most meniscus injuries occur with acute injuries (usually in younger patients) or repeated microtrauma, such as squatting or twisting (usually in older patients).

Clinical Findings

A. Symptoms and Signs

The patient may have an antalgic (painful) gait and difficulty with squatting. He or she may report catching or locking of the meniscal fragment. Physical findings can include effusion or joint line tenderness. Patients can usually point out the area of maximal tenderness along the joint line. Swelling usually occurs during the first 24 hours after the injury or later. Meniscus tears rarely lead to the immediate swelling that is commonly seen with fractures and ligament tears. Meniscus tears are commonly seen in arthritic knees. However, it is often unclear whether the pain is coming from the meniscus tear or the arthritis.

Provocative tests, including the McMurray test, the modified McMurray test, and the Thessaly test, can be performed to confirm the diagnosis (Table 41–6). Most symptomatic meniscus tears cause pain with deep squatting and when waddling (performing a "duck walk").

B. Imaging

Radiographs are usually normal but may show joint space narrowing, early OA changes, or loose bodies. MRI of the knee is the best diagnostic tool for meniscal injuries (93% sensitivity and 95% specificity). High signal through the meniscus (bright on T2 images) represents a meniscal tear.

Treatment

Conservative treatment can be used for degenerative tears in older patients. The treatment is similar for patients with mild knee OA, including analgesics and physical therapy for strengthening and core stability. A randomized controlled trial showed that physical therapy compared with arthroscopic partial meniscectomy had similar outcomes at 6 months. However, 30% of the patients who were assigned to physical therapy alone underwent surgery within 6 months.

Randomized studies have shown that arthroscopic surgery has no benefit over sham operations in patients who have degenerative meniscal tears, especially with imaging showing signs of osteoarthritis. Another randomized controlled trial found that patients with degenerative meniscus tears but no signs of arthritis on imaging treated conservatively with supervised exercise therapy had similar outcomes to those treated with arthroscopy at 2-year follow-up. There is crossover between the groups; patients can be treated with supervised exercise therapy first, and if they do not respond to nonoperative treatment, they can undergo meniscus surgeries. Acute tears in young and active patients with clinical signs of internal derangement (catching and swelling) and without signs of arthritis on imaging or patients with acute mechanical locking with a displaced meniscus can be best treated arthroscopically with meniscus repair or debridement. There is also evidence that untreated meniscus root tears can lead to accelerated osteoarthritic changes. Surgical treatment before cartilage breakdown is recommended for acute meniscus root injuries.

When to Refer

- If the patient has symptoms of internal derangement suspected as meniscus injury. The patient should receive an MRI to confirm the injury.
- If the patient cannot extend the knee due to a mechanical block, the patient should be evaluated as soon as possible. Certain shaped tears on MRI, such as bucket handle tears, meniscus root injuries, are amenable to meniscal repair surgery.
- If the patient has not responded to physical therapy and nonoperative treatment and continues to have symptoms related to the torn meniscus.
- If the patient has MRI confirmation of acute meniscus root injuries.

Driban JB et al. Accelerated knee osteoarthritis is characterized by destabilizing meniscal tears and pre-radiographic structural disease burden. Arthr Rheumatol. 2019;71:1089. [PMID: 30592385]

Karia M et al. Current concepts in the techniques, indications and outcomes of meniscal repairs. Eur J Orthop Surg Traumatol. 2019;29:509. [PMID: 30374643]

6. Patellofemoral Pain

ESSENTIALS OF DIAGNOSIS

- Pain experienced with bending activities (kneeling, squatting, climbing stairs).
- Lateral deviation or tilting of the patella in relation to the femoral groove.

General Considerations

Patellofemoral pain, also known as anterior knee pain, chondromalacia, or "runner's knee," describes any pain involving the patellofemoral joint. The pain affects any or all of the anterior knee structures, including the medial and lateral aspects of the patella as well as the quadriceps and patellar tendon insertions. The patella engages the femoral trochlear groove with approximately 30 degrees of knee flexion. Forces on the patellofemoral joint increase up to three times body weight as the knee flexes to 90 degrees (eg, climbing stairs), and five times body weight when going into full knee flexion (eg, squatting). Abnormal patellar tracking during flexion can lead to abnormal articular cartilage wear and pain. When the patient has ligamentous hyperlaxity, the patella can sublux out of the groove, usually laterally. Patellofemoral pain is also associated with muscle strength and flexibility imbalances as well as altered hip and ankle biomechanics.

Clinical Findings

A. Symptoms and Signs

Patients usually report pain in the anterior knee with bending movements and less commonly in full extension. Pain from this condition is localized under the kneecap but can sometimes be referred to the posterior knee or over the medial or lateral inferior patella. Symptoms may begin after a trauma or after repetitive physical activity, such as running and jumping. When maltracking, palpable and sometimes audible crepitus can occur.

Intra-articular swelling usually does not occur unless there are articular cartilage defects or if OA changes develop. On physical examination, it is important to palpate the articular surfaces of the patella. For example, the clinician can use one hand to move the patella laterally and use the fingertips of the other hand to palpate the lateral undersurface of the patella. Patellar mobility can be assessed by medially and laterally deviating the patella (deviation by one-quarter of the diameter of the kneecap is consider normal; greater than one-half the diameter suggests excessive mobility). The apprehension sign suggests instability of the patellofemoral joint and is positive when the patient becomes apprehensive when the patella is deviated laterally. The patellar grind test is performed by grasping the knee superior to the patella and pushing it downward with the patient supine and the knee extended, pushing the patella inferiorly. The patient is asked to contract the quadriceps muscle to oppose this downward translation, with reproduction of pain or grinding being the positive sign for chondromalacia of the patella. There are two common presentations: (1) patients whose ligaments and patella are too loose (hypermobility); and (2) patients who have soft tissues that are too tight, leading to excessive pressure on the joint.

Evaluation of the quadriceps strength and hip stabilizers can be accomplished by having the patient perform a one-leg squat without support. Normally, with a one-leg squat, the knee should align over the second metatarsal ray of the foot. Patients who are weak may display poor balance, with dropping of the pelvis (similar to a positive hip Trendelenburg sign) or excessive internal rotation of the knee medially.

B. Imaging

Diagnostic imaging has limited use in younger patients and is more helpful in older patients to assess for OA or to evaluate patients who do not respond to conservative treatment. Radiographs may show lateral deviation or tilting of the patella in relation to the femoral groove. MRI may show thinning of the articular cartilage but is not clinically necessary, except prior to surgery or to exclude other pathology.

Treatment

A. Conservative

For symptomatic relief, use of local modalities such as ice and anti-inflammatory medications can be beneficial. If the patient has signs of patellar hypermobility, physical therapy exercises are useful to strengthen the quadriceps (especially the vastus medialis obliquus muscle) to help stabilize the patella and improve tracking. There is consistent evidence that exercise therapy for patellofemoral pain syndrome may result in clinically important reduction in pain and improvement in functional ability. Lower quality research supports that hip and knee exercises are better than knee exercises alone. Strengthening the quadriceps and the posterolateral hip muscles such as the hip abductors that control rotation at the knee should be recommended. Support for the patellofemoral joint can be provided by use of a patellar stabilizer brace or special taping techniques. Correcting lower extremity alignment (with appropriate footwear or over-the-counter orthotics) can help improve symptoms, especially if the patient has pronation or high-arched feet. If the patient demonstrates tight peripatellar soft tissues, special focus should be put on stretching the hamstrings, iliotibial band, quadriceps, calves, and hip flexors.

B. Surgical

Surgery is rarely needed and is considered a last resort for patellofemoral pain. Procedures performed include lateral release or patellar realignment surgery. Surgery is indicated when patients have recurrent patella instability or dislocations.

When to Refer

Patients with persistent symptoms despite a course of conservative therapy.

Bolgla LA et al. National Athletic Trainers' Association Position Statement: management of individuals with patellofemoral pain. J Athl Train. 2018;53:820. [PMID: 30372640]

Crossley KM et al. Rethinking patellofemoral pain: prevention, management and long-term consequences. Best Pract Res Clin Rheumatol. 2019;33:48. [PMID: 31431275]

Saltychev M et al. Effectiveness of conservative treatment for patellofemoral pain syndrome: a systematic review and meta-analysis. J Rehabil Med. 2018;50:393. [PMID: 29392329]

7. Knee Osteoarthritis

ESSENTIALS OF DIAGNOSIS

- Degeneration of joint cartilage.
- Pain with bending or twisting activities.
- Swelling.
- Loss of active and passive range of motion in severe OA.

General Considerations

The incidence of knee OA in the United States is 240 per 100,000 person-years; the prevalence of OA will likely grow to 70 million persons by 2030 as the number of persons over age 65 increases.

Cartilage loss and OA symptoms are preceded by damage to the collagen-proteoglycan matrix. The etiology of

OA is often multifactorial including previous trauma, prior high-impact activities, genetic factors, obesity, and rheumatologic or metabolic conditions.

Clinical Findings

A. Symptoms and Signs

OA usually causes pain in the affected joint with loading of the joint or at the extremes of motion. Mechanical symptoms—such as swelling, grinding, catching, and locking—suggest internal derangement, which is indicated by damaged cartilage or bone fragments that affect the smooth range of motion expected at an articular joint. Pain can also produce the sensation of "buckling" or "giving way" due to muscle inhibition (Tables 41–4, 41–5, and 41–6). As the joint degeneration becomes more advanced, the patient loses active range of motion and may lose passive range of motion as well.

As the condition worsens, patients with knee OA have an increasingly limited ability to walk. Symptoms include pain with bending or twisting activities and going up and down stairs. Swelling, limping, and pain while sleeping are common symptoms of OA, especially as it progresses.

B. Imaging

The most commonly recommended radiographs include bilateral weight-bearing 45-degree bent knee posteroanterior, lateral, and patellofemoral joint views (Merchant view). Radiographic findings include diminished width of the articular cartilage causing joint space narrowing, subchondral sclerosis, presence of osteophytes, and cystic changes in the subchondral bone. MRI of the knee is most likely unnecessary unless other pathology is suspected, such as ischemic osteonecrosis of the knee.

Treatment

A. Conservative

Changes in the articular cartilage are irreversible. Therefore, a cure for the diseased joint is not possible, although symptoms or structural issues can be addressed to try to maintain activity level. Conservative treatment for all patients with OA includes activity modification, therapeutic exercises, and weight loss. Lifestyle modifications also include proper footwear and avoidance of high-impact activities. Optimal exercise programs for knee OA should focus on improving aerobic capacity, quadriceps muscle strength, or lower extremity performance; ideally, the programs should occur three times a week and be supervised.

Use of a cane in the hand opposite to the affected side is mechanically advantageous. Knee sleeves or braces provide some improvement in subjective pain symptoms most likely due to improvements in neuromuscular function. If patients have unicompartmental OA in the medial or lateral compartment, joint unloader braces are available to offload the degenerative compartment. Cushioning footwear and appropriate orthotics or shoe adjustments are useful for reducing impact to the lower extremities.

The first-line recommendation for pain management is topical nonsteroidal medication. Alternatively, topical capsaicin may be effective. Oral medications that have been shown to significantly improve pain include ibuprofen, naproxen, diclofenac, and celecoxib. If a traditional NSAID is indicated, the choice should be based on cost, side-effect profile, and adherence (Table 5–5). For patients with increased risk of GI bleeding, a cyclooxygenase (COX)-2 inhibitor (ie, celecoxib) or adding a PPI to the NSAID is recommended. A COX-2 inhibitor is no more effective than traditional NSAIDs; it may offer short-term, but probably not long-term, advantage in preventing GI complications. Acetaminophen has been shown to be less effective than NSAIDs but can be used in patients when NSAID use is contraindicated. Tramadol can be used appropriately in patients with severe OA as alternative to NSAIDs, while opioid use is discouraged. Turmeric supplements have shown some benefit for OA. Glucosamine and chondroitin sulfate are supplements that have been widely used and marketed for OA. Despite some initial promise, the best-controlled studies indicate these supplements are ineffective as analgesics in OA. However, they have minimal side effects and may be appropriate if the patient experiences subjective benefit.

Knee joint corticosteroid injections are options to help reduce pain and inflammation and can provide short-term pain relief, usually lasting about 6–12 weeks. While intra-articular triamcinolone is still commonly used in knee arthritis, a randomized controlled trial showed that 2 years of intra-articular triamcinolone every 3 months, compared with intra-articular saline, resulted in significantly greater quantitative cartilage volume loss by MRI and no significant difference in knee pain. This finding suggests that regular use of corticosteroid injections for long-term treatment of knee osteoarthritis should be avoided.

Viscosupplementation using injections of hyaluronic acid–based products is controversial. Because reviews suggested that viscosupplementation has a questionably clinically relevant effect size and an increased risk of non-threatening adverse events, the American Academy of Orthopedic Surgeons recommended that viscosupplementation should not be used in the treatment of knee OA. However, the American College of Rheumatology's 2012 OA guidelines still recommend the use of intra-articular hyaluronic acid injection for the treatment of OA of the knee in adults.

PRP injections contain high concentration of platelet-derived growth factors, which regulate some biologic processes in tissue repair. A meta-analysis of 10 studies demonstrated that PRP injections reduced pain in patients with knee OA more efficiently than placebo and hyaluronic acid injections. However, 9 of the 10 studies had a high risk of bias, and the underlying mechanism of biologic healing is unknown. An FDA safety and efficacy study showed that leukocyte-poor PRP autologous conditioned plasma improved overall Western Ontario and McMaster Universities Arthritis Index scores by 78% from the baseline score after 12 months, compared with 7% for the placebo group, although the sample size was small (30 patients).

B. Surgical

Two randomized trials demonstrated that arthroscopy does not improve outcomes at 1 year over placebo or routine conservative treatment of OA. Joint replacement surgeries are effective and cost-effective for patients with significant symptoms or functional limitations, providing improvements in pain, function, and quality of life. Minimally invasive surgeries and computer-assisted navigation during operation are being investigated as methods to improve techniques (eg, accurate placement of the hardware implant) and to reduce complication rates; however, major improvements have yet to be demonstrated.

Knee realignment surgery, such as high tibial osteotomy or partial knee replacement surgery, is indicated in patients younger than age 60 with unicompartmental OA who would benefit from delaying total knee replacement. Knee joint replacement surgery has been very successful in improving outcomes for patient with end-stage OA. Long-term series describe more than 95% survival rate of the implant at 15 years.

When to Refer

Patients with sufficient disability, limited benefit from conservative therapy, and evidence of severe OA can be referred for joint replacement surgery.

Bannuru RR et al. OARSI guidelines for the non-surgical management of knee, hip, and polyarticular osteoarthritis. Osteoarthritis Cartilage. 2019;27:1578 [PMID: 31278997]

O'Connell B et al. The use of PRP injections in the management of knee osteoarthritis. Cell Tissue Res. 2019;376:143. [PMID: 30758709]

Richardson C et al. Intra-articular hyaluronan therapy for symptomatic knee osteoarthritis. Rheum Dis Clin North Am. 2019;45:439. [PMID: 31277754]

Sharma L. Osteoarthritis of the knee. N Engl J Med. 2021;384:51. [PMID: 33406330]

Skou ST et al. Physical therapy for patients with knee and hip osteoarthritis: supervised, active treatment is current best practice. Clin Exp Rheumatol. 2019;37:112. [PMID: 31621559]

Vincent P. Intra-articular hyaluronic acid in the symptomatic treatment of knee osteoarthritis: a meta-analysis of single-injection products. Curr Ther Res Clin Exp. 2019;90:39. [PMID: 31289603]

ANKLE INJURIES

1. Inversion Ankle Sprains

ESSENTIALS OF DIAGNOSIS

- Localized pain and swelling.
- Most ankle injuries involve inversion injuries affecting the lateral ligaments.
- Consider chronic ankle instability or associated injuries if pain persists for > 3 months following an ankle sprain.

General Considerations

Ankle sprains are the most common sports injuries seen in outpatient clinics. Patients usually report "turning the ankle" during a fall or after landing on an irregular surface such as a hole or an opponent's foot. The most common mechanism of injury is an inversion and plantar flexion sprain, which injures the anterior talofibular (ATF) ligament rather than the calcaneofibular (CF) ligament. Other injuries that can occur with inversion ankle injuries are listed in Table 41–7. Women appear to sustain an inversion injury more frequently than men. Chronic ankle instability is defined as persistent pain, swelling, and "giving way" in combination with recurrent sprains for at least 12 months after the initial ankle sprain. Chronic ankle instability can occur in up to 43% of ankle sprains despite physical therapy, which makes appropriate attention to acute ankle sprains important.

Table 41–7. Injuries associated with ankle sprains.

Ligaments
Subtalar joint sprain
Sinus tarsi syndrome (ongoing anterolateral posttraumatic ankle pain)
Syndesmotic (distal tibiofibular ligamentous) sprain
Deltoid sprain
Lisfranc (tarsometatarsal bony or ligamentous) injury
Tendons
Posterior tibial tendon strain
Peroneal tendon subluxation
Bones
Osteochondral talus injury
Lateral talar process fracture
Posterior impingement (os trigonum)
Fracture at the base of the fifth metatarsal
Jones fracture (between base and middle of fifth metatarsal)
Salter (growth plate) fracture (fibula)
Ankle fractures

Clinical Findings

A. Symptoms and Signs

Symptoms following a sprain include localized pain and swelling over the lateral aspect of the ankle, difficulty weight bearing, and limping. On examination, there may be swelling or bruising over the lateral aspect of the ankle. The anterior, inferior aspect below the lateral malleolus is most often the point of maximal tenderness consistent with ATF and CF ligament injuries. The swelling may limit motion of the ankle.

Special stress tests for the ankle include the **anterior drawer test**; the clinician keeps the foot and ankle in the neutral position with the patient sitting, then uses one hand to fix the tibia and the other to hold the patient's heel and draw the ankle forward. Normally, there may be approximately 3 mm of translation until an endpoint is felt. A positive test includes increased translation of one foot compared with the other with loss of the endpoint of the ATF ligament.

Another stress test is the **subtalar tilt test**, which is performed with the foot in the neutral position with the patient sitting. The clinician uses one hand to fix the tibia and the other to hold and invert the calcaneus. Normal inversion at the subtalar joint is approximately 30 degrees. A positive test consists of increased subtalar joint inversion by greater than 10 degrees on the affected side with loss of endpoint for the CF ligament. To grade the severity of ankle sprains, no laxity on stress tests is considered a grade 1 injury, laxity of the ATF ligament on anterior drawer testing but a negative tilt test is a grade 2 injury, and both positive drawer and tilt tests signify a grade 3 injury. Difficulty jumping and landing within 2 weeks from the acute ankle sprain, abnormal postural or hip muscle control, or ligamentous laxity noted 8 weeks after injury are poor prognostic signs.

B. Imaging

Routine ankle radiographic views include the AP, lateral, and oblique (mortise) views. Less common views requested include the calcaneal view and subtalar view. The **Ottawa Ankle Rules** remain the best clinical prediction rules to guide the need for radiographs and have an 86–99% sensitivity and a 97–99% negative predictive value. If the patient is unable to bear weight immediately in the office setting or emergency department for four steps, then the clinician should check for (1) bony tenderness at the posterior edge of the medial or lateral malleolus and (2) bony tenderness over the navicular (medial midfoot) or at the base of the fifth metatarsal. If either malleolus demonstrates pain or deformity, then ankle radiographs should be obtained. If the foot has bony tenderness, obtain foot radiographs. An MRI is helpful when considering the associated injuries.

Treatment

Immediate treatment of an ankle sprain follows the MICE mnemonic: *m*odified activities, *i*ce, *c*ompression, and *e*levation. NSAIDs are useful in reducing pain and swelling in the first 72 hours following the ankle sprain. Subsequent treatment involves protected weight bearing with crutches and use of an ankle stabilizer brace, especially for grade 2 and 3 injuries. Early functional and dynamic rehabilitation exercises result in a shorter time to return to sport, increased functional performance, and decreased self-reported reinjury. Patients should be encouraged to do a program of exercises or physical therapy. Proprioception and balance exercises (eg, "wobble board") are useful to restore function to the ankle and prevent future ankle sprains. There is strong evidence for bracing and moderate evidence for neuromuscular training in preventing recurrence of an ankle sprain. Chronic instability can develop after acute ankle sprain in 10–20% of people and may require surgical stabilization with ligament reconstruction surgery.

When to Refer

- Ankle fractures.
- Recurrent ankle sprains or signs of chronic ligamentous ankle instability.
- No response after more than 3 months of conservative treatment.
- Suspicion of associated injuries.

Delahunt E et al. Risk factors for lateral ankle sprains and chronic ankle instability. J Athl Train. 2019;54:611. [PMID: 31161942]

Kaminski TW et al. Prevention of lateral ankle sprains. J Athl Train. 2019;54:650. [PMID: 31116041]

Tee E et al. Evidence for rehabilitation interventions after acute lateral ankle sprains in athletes: a scoping review. J Sport Rehabil. 2022:1. [PMID: 34969012]

2. Eversion ("High") Ankle Sprains

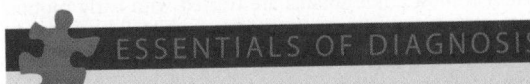

- Severe and prolonged pain.
- Limited range of motion.
- Mild swelling.
- Difficulty with weight bearing.

General Considerations

A syndesmotic injury or "high ankle" sprain involves the anterior *tibio*fibular ligament in the anterolateral aspect of the ankle, superior to the anterior *talo*fibular ligament. The injury mechanism often involves the foot being turned out or externally rotated and everted (eg, when being tackled). This injury is commonly missed or misdiagnosed as an ATF ligament sprain on initial visit.

Clinical Findings

A. Symptoms and Signs

Symptoms of a high ankle sprain include severe and prolonged pain over the anterior ankle at the anterior tibiofibular ligament, worse with weight bearing. This is often more painful than the typical ankle sprain. The point of maximal tenderness involves the anterior tibiofibular ligament, which is higher than the ATF ligament. It is also important to palpate the proximal fibula to rule out any proximal syndesmotic ligament injury and associated fracture known as a "maisonneuve fracture." There is often some mild swelling in this area, and the patient may or may not have an ankle effusion. The patient usually has limited range of motion in all directions. To perform the **external rotation stress test**, the clinician fixes the tibia with one hand and grasps the foot in the other with the ankle in the neutral position. The ankle is then dorsiflexed and externally rotated, reproducing the patient's pain. (**Note:** The patient's foot should have an intact neurovascular examination before undertaking this test.)

B. Imaging

Radiographs of the ankle should include the AP, mortise, and lateral views. The mortise view may demonstrate loss of the normal overlap between the tibia and fibula, which should be at least 1–2 mm. Asymmetry in the joint space around the tibiotalar joint suggests disruption of the syndesmotic ligaments. If there is proximal tenderness in the lower leg especially around the fibula, an AP and lateral view of the tibia and fibula should be obtained to rule out a proximal fibula fracture. Radiographs during an external rotation stress test may visualize instability at the distal tibiofibular joint. MRI is the best method to visualize injury to the tibiofibular ligament and to assess status of the other ligaments and the articular cartilage.

Treatment

Whereas most ankle sprains are treated with early motion and weight bearing, treatment for a high ankle sprain should be conservative with a cast or walking boot for 4–6 weeks. Thereafter, protected weight bearing with crutches is recommended until the patient can walk pain-free. Physical therapy can start early to regain range of motion and maintain strength with limited weight bearing initially.

When to Refer

If there is widening of the joint space and asymmetry at the tibiotalar joint, the patient should be referred urgently to a foot and ankle surgeon. Severe or prolonged persistent cases that do not heal may require internal fixation to avoid chronic instability at the tibiofibular joint.

Chen ET et al. Ankle sprains: evaluation, rehabilitation, and prevention. Curr Sports Med Rep. 2019;18:217. [PMID: 31385837]

Nickless JT et al. High ankle sprains: easy to miss, so follow these tips. J Fam Pract. 2019;68:E5. [PMID: 31039220]

Sexual & Gender Minority Health

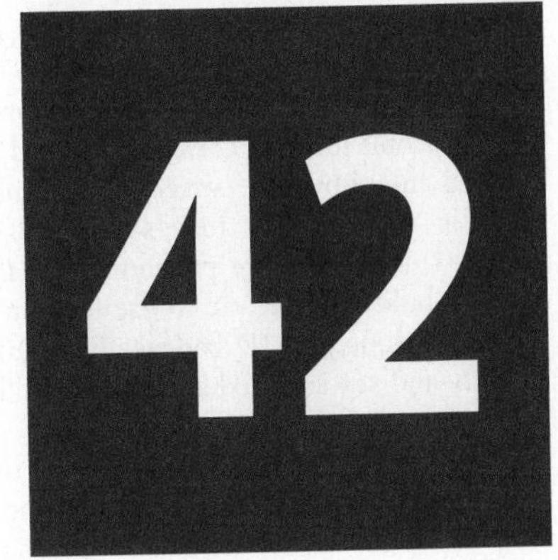

Patricia A. Robertson, MD
Nicole Rosendale, MD
Kevin L. Ard, MD, MPH
Kenneth H. Mayer, MD
Mitzi Hawkins, MD, MAS
Madeline B. Deutsch, MD, MPH

HEALTH CARE FOR SEXUAL & GENDER MINORITY PATIENTS

Definitions & Concepts

Gender identity is a person's internal sense of gender, which is independent from the sex assigned at birth. Gender is also independent from sexual orientation, which refers to a person's sexuality and encompasses three dimensions: identity, behavior, and desire. The term **sexual and gender minority (SGM)** refers to a broad group including lesbian women and gay men, bisexual, pansexual, and queer people, and transgender and gender nonbinary people—also commonly referred to as "LGBTQ" or "LGBTQ+." The plus sign is inclusive of individuals of other identities such as agender, genderqueer, and polysexual.

Population estimates of SGM adults in the United States range from 4.5% to 6.8%, depending on definitions; reliable population estimates, however, are lacking because there are no consistently applied federal and other administrative survey methodologies. Population estimates of SGM persons reach 20% if the definition of SGM includes gay or bisexual identity, any same-sex attraction, or same-sex sex in the last year

Transgender people have a gender identity that differs from the sex that was assigned at birth, including those who identify as nonbinary and those who have a gender identity that is neither man nor woman. **Transmasculine** refers to those who have a male- or masculine-spectrum gender identity but were assigned female at birth, and **transfeminine** refers to those who have a female- or feminine-spectrum gender identity but were assigned male at birth. Cisgender refers to people whose gender identity and birth assigned sex are the same (ie, they are not transgender). Transgender people may also be sexual minorities (ie, lesbian, gay, bisexual, etc) or straight/heterosexual. For the sake of expediency in this chapter, the sections on sexual minority (SM) men and women omit the term "cisgender"; however, readers of these sections should take into consideration that, for example, gay transmasculine persons may have vaginal receptive sex with cisgender men as sexual partners, and therefore should be screened for contraception needs, and cisgender lesbian women may have transfeminine partners who retain their penis.

Sexual identities include gay (those who are predominantly attracted to or sexually active with members of the same gender, or both), bisexual (those who are attracted to or sexually active with someone of the same gender and another gender, or both), and heterosexual or straight (someone who is attracted to or sexually active with people of another gender [historically the "opposite" gender], or both); however, other terms may be used, and terminology changes over time. A growing number of people identify as pansexual, which describes an attraction to people of any gender—man, woman, or along the spectrum between the two. The term "queer" has been reclaimed by many SGM people to represent someone with a sexual orientation, gender identity, or gender expression (the external manifestation of gender) that differs from that of a cisgender, heterosexual person. Because of the historical legacy of this term as derogatory, however, it should not be used unless someone specifies this as their identity. Studies have demonstrated that there is a broad diversity among those who identify as SGM and that many people have multiple gender identities or sexual orientations.

The three dimensions of sexual orientation—identity, behavior, and attraction—do not necessarily overlap. Health risk factors (eg, substance use) and outcomes have been found to be different among different dimensions. For example, one study found that gay and lesbian individuals with sexual identity-behavior discordance reported poorer psychological functioning and higher rates of alcohol binge drinking and suicidal ideation compared with those with identity-behavior concordance. The incomplete overlap of identity and behavior means that clinicians cannot rely upon self-reported identity to infer sexual behavior, and vice versa.

It is important to distinguish sexual orientation from gender identity. Knowing a person's gender identity does not identify their sexual orientation. Just as cisgender people may be sexually attracted to and have sex with people of any gender, so too can transmasculine, transfeminine, and nonbinary people have partners of any gender. Routinely asking about sexual orientation, and when relevant for the clinical issue at hand, sexual behavior, helps build trust between the patient and clinician, ensures appropriate medical care (for example, appropriate screening tests for sexually transmitted infections [STIs] and family planning), and contributes to better health outcomes. To ensure that people feel welcomed, the clinician can ask people for their correct name and pronouns by first offering the clinician's correct name and pronouns. For example, the clinician may say "Hello, I'm Dr. (insert name), I use they/them pronouns. What name and pronouns would you like me to use for you?" Pronouns can also be included on ID badges. To inquire about gender identity and sex assigned at birth, the following questions are recommended: "What is your current gender identity?" and "What sex were you assigned at birth?" The clinician needs to remember that name and pronouns may differ from what one thinks may "match" what people say are their gender identity or sex assigned at birth or what is on "official" documentation, but the clinician must always use the name and pronouns that people shared.

Sexual orientation and gender identity may also change over time or be situational (such as during incarceration, in educational settings, etc). People may also hide their sexual orientation and gender identity from others, including clinicians, to avoid stigma and discrimination. Revealing a person's sexual orientation, gender identity, or both is called "coming out." This process may occur at any point in life and may vary by context (eg, being "out" to family but not to coworkers).

Sexual orientation and gender identity can be fluid throughout a person's lifetime, and the binary concept of gender (that there are only girls and women or boys and men) is not evidence-based. Some legal policies are moving to reflect this fluidity. In the United States, fewer than half of the states have three genders on legal documents: female, male, or nonbinary (neither male nor female). These experiences and policies have implications for health screening for patients who receive care in health systems with pop-up reminders for sex-specific screening examinations such as mammography or prostate examinations.

Lunn MR et al. Using mobile technology to engage sexual and gender minorities in clinical research. PLoS One. 2019;14:e0216282. [PMID: 31048870]

Meyer IH et al. The Williams Institute, UCLA School of Law. LGBTQ people in the US: select findings from the Generations and TransPop Studies. 2021 Jun. https://williamsinstitute.law.ucla.edu/wp-content/uploads/Generations-TransPop-Toplines-Jun-2021.pdf

Health Disparities & The Minority Stress Model

Providing compassionate and informed health care for SGM patients, which include but are not limited to persons who identify as lesbian, gay, bisexual, transgender, and queer, involves the acknowledgment of the negative effects on health caused by discrimination and stigma. The theory of minority stress, first published by Virginia Brooks in 1981 and later expanded on by Ilan Meyer, proposes that individuals who identify as an SM experience chronic, additive, and unique stresses that stem from living in discriminatory social conditions; stressors include experiences of prejudice, expectations of rejection, the cognitive burden of deciding whether to come out in different circumstances, and internalized homophobia. SGM people are also underserved by the medical community and understudied, with worse health outcomes compared with the heterosexual and cisgender populations. These experiences differ also according to racial and ethnic backgrounds; SGM people of color often fare worse. One reason for these disparities is that a previous negative experience in a clinician's office influences whether the patient will repeat a visit even for an acute medical event, which can delay care and result in advanced disease. One in three transgender people report delays in seeking care due to prior discrimination, and one in five report being refused medical care due to their transgender identity. SGM adults are twice as likely to delay care than non-SGM adults. Some of the disparate health outcomes are related to limited access to the health care system due to financial issues and lack of federal anti-discrimination protection at times compounded by multiple marginalized identities. SGM people have higher rates of poverty, lower rates of home ownership, and higher rates of homelessness than non-SGM people. These structural issues will take time to change. However, clinicians can impact the health outcomes of SGM people by ensuring that the clinical space is welcoming to people of all genders and sexual orientations (see below), obtaining comprehensive data on sexual orientation and gender identity, and being aware of the specific health needs of SGM people in order to advance the health of SGM patients. A study from Norway found that sympathetic environments can counteract minority stress and support overall health.

The vast majority of SGM patients would like to come out to their clinician. Many clinicians, however, are concerned that their patients would be offended if asked about sexual orientation and gender identity. It is important that clinicians overcome any discomfort and ask appropriate questions of their patients. There are useful video resources to help clinicians with these issues; one example is the "Acknowledging Sex and Gender" online training video from the University of California San Francisco Center of Excellence for Transgender Health, available at https://prevention.ucsf.edu/transhealth/education/acknowledging-gender-sex. Specific populations have additional barriers to disclosure and thus shared decision-making, such as non-English language preference; a study of Latinx SGM patients and their clinicians found significant diversity among the Latinx SGM population and emphasized that providers need to be aware of patients' varying social support from family members and that professional interpreter services should be SGM competent. A study from South Africa found that discriminatory and prejudicial attitudes by health care providers, combined with their lack of competency and knowledge, are key reasons for SGM health disparities.

The number of adverse childhood experiences has been shown to be a predictor of future negative health outcomes; more SGM individuals have higher ACE scores (42% with four or more adverse childhood experiences) than heterosexual individuals (25% with four or more adverse childhood experiences). A broader study that included transgender persons found that adverse childhood experiences were responsible for 18% of mental health variances. Additionally, neglect the effect of being physically excluded from the family home due to sexual orientation or gender identity is a common experience that was not measured; many SGM youth are excluded from their home once they come out. A negative reaction of parents to their child's coming out is strongly associated with that child's future homelessness, depression, and substance use.

The SARS-CoV-2 pandemic has had a disproportionate effect on the SGM community, although data are limited as sexual orientation and gender identity data have not been routinely reported in prevalence or outcomes. SGM persons are more likely to be employed in workplaces highly impacted by the pandemic including food service, hospitals, education, and retail. One study found increased depression and anxiety coincident with the pandemic within the SGM community in persons who did not have preexisting anxiety or depression. Another study of young Swiss men found higher levels of psychological trauma, fear, isolation, and depression in SM men due to the pandemic. LGBT adults were more likely to be laid off or furloughed from jobs during the early pandemic when compared with non-LGBT adults. LGBT adults were also more likely to report difficulty affording household needs and rent or mortgage payments. A cross-sectional study of transgender individuals found higher odds of COVID-related medical care interruptions and housing instability compared with cisgender populations. Limited studies have suggested that the most common causes for vaccine hesitancy in the SGM population include concerns about the safety of the vaccine, efficacy, potential side effects, and previous negative experiences with health care providers. SGM persons have higher prevalence of comorbidities associated with severe COVID-19 infections, such as asthma and obesity. Persons of color (LGBT and non-LGBT) had higher positivity rates than non-LGBT White persons and were more likely to personally knowing someone who died of COVID-19.

Ayhan CHB et al. A systematic review of the discrimination against sexual and gender minority in health care settings. Int J Health Serv. 2020;50;44. [PMID: 31684808]

Flentje A et al. Depression and anxiety changes among sexual and gender minority people coinciding with onset of COVID-19 pandemic. J Gen Intern Med. 2020;35:2788. [PMID: 32556877]

Felt D et al. Instability in housing and medical care access: the inequitable impacts of the COVID-19 pandemic on U.S. transgender populations. Trans Health. 2021 Nov 30. https://doi.org/10.1089/trgh.2021.0129

Garg I et al. COVID-19 vaccine hesitancy in the LGBTQ+ population: a systematic review. Infect Dis Rep. 2021;13:872. [PMID: 34698208]

Heslin KC et al. Sexual orientation disparities in risk factors for adverse COVID-19-related outcomes, by race/ethnicity—behavioral risk factor surveillance system, United States, 2017-2019. MMWR Morb Mortal Wkly Rep. 2021;70:149. [PMID 33539330]

Ryan C et al. Family rejection as a predictor of negative health outcomes in white and Latino lesbian gay, and bisexual young adults. Pediatrics. 2009;123:346. [PMID: 19117902]

Sears B et al. The Williams Institute, UCLA School of Law. The impact of the fall 2020 surge of the COVID-19 pandemic on LGBT adults in the US. 2021 Feb. https://williamsinstitute.law.ucla.edu/wp-content/uploads/COVID-LGBT-Fall-Surge-Feb-2021.pdf

Making Clinical Environments Welcoming to All SGM Patients

Part of serving SGM patients is to create a welcoming clinical space where each person is cared for and respected for **all** of who they are—including their sexual orientation, gender identity, and gender expression while considering other key aspects of their identities and lived experience like race and ethnicity, age, educational level, geography and geo-political context, ability, and primary language. The use of people's correct names and pronouns throughout encounters is critical (see above). Implementation of comprehensive care including acknowledging, respecting, and specifying care as needed for someone based on their sexual orientation, gender identity, gender expression, and correct names and pronouns necessitates system change in many clinical settings. This includes making sure that (1) senior leadership is involved; (2) nondiscrimination policies are in place, are followed, and are prominently displayed; (3) open visitation policies are concordant with patients' choice of visitors; (4) outreach and engagement efforts are made for SGM patients; (5) staff receive culturally affirming training in the care of SGM people; (6) processes, forms, artwork, and reading materials reflect the diversity of SGM people; (7) data are collected about both sexual orientation and gender identity (including names and pronouns) in an open and nonjudgmental manner; (8) patients are routinely asked about their sexual health histories; (9) clinical care and services include prevention and wellness care with available family planning services and behavioral health services; (10) SGM staff are recruited and trained; (11) preventive care is concordant with clinical practice guidelines, where applicable; and (12) if all gender bathrooms are not available, a posting states that patients are welcome to use either the women's or men's bathroom and the patient can determine which bathroom to use. One exercise is to look at clinic materials (ie, signs, posters, brochures, magazines, intake forms, etc) and see if materials presume heterosexual behavior and gender conformity (heteronormative) and gender conformity (cisnormative). Often, materials discussing anatomy, sex, family planning, conception, pregnancy, and birth presume that everyone is cisgender, White, and primarily English-speaking. If so, find or create more broadly inclusive materials to replace them.

National LGBT Cancer Network. Cultural competency in-person trainings and on-line materials, updated 2017. https://cancer-network.org/programs/cultural-competency-training

National LGBT Education Center. https://www.lgbtqiahealth-education.org

Obtaining Sexual History From SGM Patients

The core history and physical examination is not different for SGM in comparison to other patients. Clinicians should approach each patient as an individual, using patients' correct pronouns, using appropriate terminology, respecting the diversity of gender identity as well as the differing desires for gender affirming treatments, and performing an appropriate physical examination for the clinical encounter. When relevant, anatomic changes from any prior gender affirming treatment should be noted. As with all adolescent or adult patients, a complete medical history should include a comprehensive sexual history. Clinicians may wish to preface discussion of the patient's sexual history with a statement indicating that this information is confidential and is important to provide optimal health care. However, patients should not be expected to discuss their gender identity or transition in detail unless it is relevant to the current visit. In addition, it is crucial that clinicians understand that transgender patients may have physical appearances (gender expression), names, and pronouns that do not reflect their legal names or sex marker, as listed on identity documents. Staff members must learn how to elicit patients' names and correct pronouns so that these can be used consistently.

Key data to gather in a relevant sexual history include sexual function and satisfaction; number of partners if the patient is sexually active; the gender(s) of the patient's sexual partner(s); and the potential to conceive an unplanned pregnancy with the sexual partner(s). It should be noted that "sex" means different things to different people. Therefore, clinicians should determine the types of sexual practices the patient engages in (eg, oral sex, penile insertive anal sex, receptive anal sex, penis-in-vagina sex, fingers-in-anus sex) acknowledging these may not line up with clinicians' assumptions based on a person's sexual orientation. Additional key questions include how often condoms are used, if at all, for the different sexual practices the patient engages in; and whether drugs or alcohol, or both, are consumed in conjunction with sex. Clinicians should also establish whether there is a history of STIs because a positive history may have implications for medical follow-up and sexual risk assessment (eg, frequency of screening, syphilis serologies, chlamydia and gonorrhea testing, and discussion about HIV preexposure prophylaxis [PrEP]). For example, a recent diagnosis of syphilis would indicate the need for rapid plasma reagin titer monitoring to ensure adequate treatment and would prompt consideration of PrEP due to the association of syphilis with HIV infection.

The Fenway Institute, which specializes in SGM health and health care, proposes using the following statement and follow-up questions:

"I am going to ask you some questions about your sexual health and sexuality that I ask all my patients. The answers to these questions are important for me to know how to help keep you healthy. Like the rest of this visit, this information is strictly confidential unless you tell me you are planning to harm yourself or someone else or describe someone else harming you."

Evidence suggests that most individuals are ready and willing to disclose to sensitive providers who make it clear the intent behind their questions. Additional questions include the following:

1. "Do you have a partner or a spouse?" or "Are you currently in a relationship?"
2. "When was the last time you had sex?"
3. "What is/are the gender(s) of your sexual partner(s)?"
4. "What body parts of yours touch which body parts of your partners?"
5. "How many people have you had sex with during the last year?"
6. "Do you have any desires regarding sexual intimacy that you would like to discuss?"

Rather than considering this a one-time intervention, it should be thought of as a process that is assessed over time and at critical junctures and changes in health status.

The Association of American Medical Colleges (AAMC) has created a series of online videos that highlight gender and sexual history taking (https://www.aamc.org/initiatives/diversity/450468/gender-and-sexual-history1.html and https://www.aamc.org/initiatives/diversity/450470/gender-and-sexual-history2.html); and ineffective history taking (https://www.aamc.org/initiatives/diversity/450472/ineffective-history-taking.html).

Centers for Disease Control and Prevention (CDC). A guide to taking a sexual history. https://www.cdc.gov/std/treatment/sexualhistory.pdf

The Electronic Health Record

Electronic health record (EHR) systems should include functionality for the recording of gender identity and sex assigned at birth as well as chosen name and pronouns. Chosen name and pronoun functionality should be displayed in all banners, schedules, and other viewing screens. Transgender persons can be identified within the EHR that supports the data collection of gender as separate from sex assigned at birth, by identifying those individuals whose entries for gender identity and birth sex differ. Collecting both gender identity and sex assigned at birth data are critical to understanding the population of people in care within a health system and their health needs, such as age-appropriate cancer screening and appropriate interpretation of laboratory values, which may differ from EHR-labeled normative values for those using gender affirming hormones.

Assessment and documentation in the EHR of a patient's sexual orientation and gender identity has been advocated in the United States by the National Academy of Medicine, the Joint Commission, and the Health Resources and Services Administration as fundamental to improving access to and quality of care for SGM people. However, there are risks for SGM people with having their sexual orientation and gender identity documented in the EHR. Examples of such risks include housing, child custody, and adoption discrimination. In 2020, the US Supreme Court determined that being fired on the basis of sexual orientation or transgender identity violated Title VII prohibition of discrimination on the basis of sex; however, there are still no federal protections against discrimination in housing, education, loans, or many other services. Further, same-sex relations are criminalized in 71 countries. Gender identity is likewise insufficiently protected. Therefore, although sexual orientation and gender identity are critical to caring for the whole person, discussing with patients before documenting in the EHR is best practice.

Davison K et al. Culturally competent gender, sex and sexual orientation information practices and electronic health records: rapid review. JMIR Med Inform. 2021;9:e25467. [PMID 33455901]

Rosendale N et al. Acute clinical care for transgender patients: a review. JAMA Intern Med. 2018;178:1535. [PMID: 30178031]

Family Planning

A. Pregnancy Prevention

Comprehensive family planning for SGM people is important to address, so that all people can decide when and how to build a family. Since a person's sexual orientation and gender identity do not determine sexual partners, all individuals should be asked about family-building intentions as well as contraception if pregnancy is undesired and their sexual activities that put them at risk for pregnancy.

Most lesbian women have been sexually active with men at some point in their lives (85–90%), and 30% of self-identified adult lesbians are currently sexually active with men as well as with women. Compared with young heterosexual women, fewer lesbian and bisexual youth use highly reliable contraception. On multiple surveys, one of the reasons that lesbians do not access gynecologic care is the assumption by clinicians that they are heterosexual, and the (insensitive) advocacy of birth control in that assumptive atmosphere about their sexuality (ie, heteronormative). On the other hand, multiple studies show that the unintended pregnancy rate of self-identified lesbian and bisexual youth is higher than that of the comparison heterosexual female youth. Lesbian and bisexual female adolescents were also more likely than their heterosexually identified peers to have engaged in sexual activity, have sex with cisgender boys at an earlier age, have had more frequent sex, and use a less effective contraceptive method.

Unintended pregnancy risk continues into adulthood with one sample from the Chicago Health and Life Experiences of Women survey reporting 24% of SM women having had unintended pregnancies. SM women also suffer higher rates of sexual assault compared with heterosexual women. If it has been determined that the patient self-identifies as a lesbian woman is having (penis-in-vagina) sex with men, one suggested question might be, "Are you planning to get pregnant this year?" If the answer is no, this is an opportunity to explain that studies show a higher unintended rate of pregnancy in lesbian youth and to review effective contraception options. It is also a good time to talk about protection from STIs when having sex with men (ie, discuss condoms). As with any person engaging in penis-in-vagina sex, experts recommend additional contraceptives to condoms. Condoms are only 80% reliable in preventing pregnancy with typical use. Long-acting reversible contraceptives, which are not patient or sexual act dependent and function effectively despite alcohol or other substance use, are especially important to consider. Long-acting reversible contraceptives such as an etonorgestrel subdermal implant in the arm (0.05% annual failure) or either the copper (0.3% annual failure) or levonorgestrel (0.2% annual failure) intrauterine devices are highly effective and typical use is generally equivalent to ideal use.

Importantly, patients should be counseled that gender affirming hormone therapy is not a reliable contraceptive method. Anyone with a vagina, uterus, ovaries, and fallopian tubes can potentially become pregnant if they engage in penis-in-vagina sex. Transfeminine persons (women who were assigned male sex at birth) and nonbinary individuals who have a penis and testes may still produce sperm capable of fertilizing an oocyte even if using gender affirming estrogen or testosterone blockers or both. Transmasculine persons and nonbinary individuals who were assigned female sex at birth can become pregnant, even in the setting of testosterone-induced amenorrhea. All patients at risk of pregnancy should be counseled on the importance of contraceptive use if they do not desire pregnancy. Any of the contraceptive methods available to cisgender people are appropriate for use by transgender people and those using gender affirming hormone therapy. Little is known about the contraceptive preferences of transgender people and clinical recommendations rely on expert opinion. Since testosterone is a teratogen, patients who become pregnant while using this therapy should be referred early in pregnancy for pregnancy options counseling by a clinician familiar with gender affirming care.

A 2021 study evaluated pregnancy termination for transgender, nonbinary, and gender expansive people and found that the majority preferred medication abortion, due to their belief that it was the least invasive, although most respondents had undergone a surgical abortion. The LGBTQIA Resource Center defines gender expansive as an "umbrella term used for individuals who broaden their own culture's commonly held definitions of gender, including expectations for its expression, identities, roles, and/or other perceived gender norms." Respondents most frequently recommended that clinics that provide abortions and many other services adopt gender-neutral or gender affirming intake forms, that providers use gender-neutral language, and that greater privacy be incorporated into the clinic.

The AAMC has produced a noteworthy video about family counseling and coming out (https://www.aamc.org/initiatives/diversity/450466/family-counseling.html).

Bonnington A...Hawkins M et al. Society of Family Planning clinical recommendations: contraceptive counseling for transgender and gender diverse people who were female sex assigned at birth. Contraception. 2020;102:70. [PMID: 32304766]

Krempasky C et al. Contraception across the transmasculine spectrum. Am J Obstet Gynecol. 2020:222:134. [PMID 31394072]

Moseson H et al. Abortion experiences and preferences of transgender, nonbinary, and gender-expansive people in the United States. Am J Obstet Gynecol. 2021;224:376.e1. [PMID: 32986990]

Porsch L et al. Contraceptive use by women across multiple components of sexual orientation: findings from the 2011–2017 National Survey of Family Growth. LGBT Health. 2020;7:321. [PMID: 32808867]

B. Family Building

Family building should be discussed with all patients, regardless of sexual orientation or gender identity. Options include foster-parenting or adoption (in some countries these options are not open to SGM persons), co-parenting partners' child or children, becoming pregnant, contracting with a surrogate, or step-parenting. Some fertility practices refuse to assist SGM people with conception even if it is legal. In 2021, the American College of Obstetricians and Gynecologists reaffirmed Committee Opinion No. 749, stating, "No matter how a child comes into a family, all children and parents deserve equitable protections and access to available resources to maximize the health of that family unit. Obstetricians-gynecologists should recognize the diversity in parenting desires that exists in the lesbian, gay, bisexual, transgender, queer, intersex, asexual and gender nonconforming communities and should take steps to ensure that clinical spaces are affirming and open to all parties, such that equitable and comprehensive, reproductive health care can meet the needs of these communities."[1]

Approximately 30% of SGM people are parents. There are many paths to family building, and each is dependent on personal desires, reproductive capacity of the person and those of a partner(s) if any; any biologic/medical constraints; and legal/political options. Many options exist for conception and clinicians should be prepared to counsel patients, provide resources and refer as appropriate. Patients may decide to have inseminations with an unknown donor from a sperm bank (some unknown donors sign a release so that the child may contact the donor when the child reaches 18 years old), and some may decide to involve a known sperm donor. Most sperm banks are regulated regarding the administration of medical history forms, testing for STIs, and genetic screening. Known donors may have risk factors but are not routinely screened. It is important for future parents to be as informed as they can be about the legal implications of each option. In some states and countries, unless the insemination with known donor sperm takes place in the office of a physician, the known donor has full legal rights as well as financial responsibilities for the offspring. In one study of 129 lesbian mothers with 77 index offspring, 77.5% of the mothers were satisfied with the type of donor chosen (36% had chosen known sperm donors, 25% open-identity donors, and 39% unknown donors). Donor access and custody concerns were the primary themes mentioned by lesbian mothers regarding their (dis)satisfaction with the type of sperm donor they had selected. When lesbian women seek donor insemination, there is no difference in pregnancy outcomes compared with heterosexual women. However, if there are fertility challenges, lesbian and single women often have more expense, as most insurance companies will not cover fertility costs unless there has been one year of well-timed intercourse without conception.

Some lesbian women and couples in whom both partners have a uterus and ovaries decide to do "co–in vitro fertilization (IVF)," which is also known as "reciprocal IVF" or in some cases "co-maternity" in which one partner provides an egg, it is fertilized in the laboratory with sperm of a known or unknown donor, and then the other partner carries the pregnancy. A report in 2021 demonstrated significantly better reproductive outcomes after reciprocal IVF, with a clinical pregnancy rate of 60% compared with 40% after autologous IVF, and live birth rate of 57.1% in reciprocal IVF versus 29.8% in autologous IVF (OR 3.05). However, both partners of the couple need to be willing to participate in reciprocal IVF.

Lactation for the non-gestational parent can sometimes be induced by using a protocol that stemmed originally from the experiences of adoptive mothers who were motivated to breastfeed. Lactation has been achieved for transmasculine and transfeminine persons as well. Many SGM people delay childbearing until later in life, with resultant issues of age-related infertility, increased pregnancy loss, and fetal chromosomal abnormalities. Pregnancy outcomes of bisexual and lesbian women compared with women who identify as heterosexual include increased risk of miscarriage (OR 1.77) and stillbirth (OR 2.85), as well as very preterm birth (OR 1.84).

There have been many studies on the overall outcomes of children of lesbian women, all of which have been favorable when comparing their children to children raised by heterosexual parents, despite the stigma the children may experience of having same-sex parents. A 2020 study using administrative data from the Netherlands, for example, found that children of same-sex parents performed better in both primary and secondary education compared with children of different-sex parents.

Biologic options for pregnancy for cisgender gay men or transfeminine persons include conceiving with someone who may or may not be interested in co-parenting with them, or contracting with a friend, relative, or surrogate to carry the pregnancy after the sperm and a donor egg are fertilized and placed in the uterus of the surrogate. For transgender people, there are other options based on the organs they currently have. Prior to initiation of any gender affirming hormones or gender affirming surgical procedures, a consultation with either an obstetrician/gynecologist or a reproductive endocrinologist to discuss fertility preservation and future genetic offspring is encouraged. Reproductive planning is often not a priority for a transitioning youth but may become a desire in the future and may also be a priority for potential grandparents. Options are limited for transgender youth who have not undergone endogenous puberty before either starting gender affirming hormones (with estrogen or testosterone) or puberty blockers and then going directly to estrogen or testosterone. The only future fertility option is either testicular or ovarian tissue cryopreservation, which is considered experimental. For transfeminine persons and gender nonbinary individuals who were male sex assigned at birth and who have reached adulthood after endogenous puberty, sperm can be stored ideally prior to the initiation of estrogen. Of note, though some transfeminine persons still produce sperm even after long-term estrogen exposure, it is recommended that sperm cryopreservation occur prior to hormone start because the effect on fertility is hard to quantify and coming off hormones can often be dysphoric. For transmasculine persons and nonbinary individuals who were female sex assigned at birth and have gone through endogenous puberty, next steps in genetic parentage will be based on the desire to carry a pregnancy and whether or not they have started gender affirming

[1]Reproduced with permission from ACOG Committee Opinion No. 749: Marriage and Family Building Equality for Lesbian, Gay, Bisexual, Transgender, Queer, Intersex, Asexual, and Gender Nonconforming Individuals. Obstet Gynecol. 2018;132(2):e82–e86.

hormones. Options include penis-in-vagina sex, intravaginal insemination, intrauterine insemination, and egg cryopreservation for the individual, a partner, or surrogate to carry. If a hysterectomy is planned as part of gender affirmation, discussion of whether ovaries are left in place should occur in light of consideration of future genetic parentage as well as future hormone regulation versus the risk of future ovarian cancer. In one study in Australia, however, only 7% of transgender and nonbinary adults had undertaken fertility preservation yet 95% said that fertility preservation should be offered to all transgender and nonbinary people. Participants who viewed genetic relatedness as important were more likely to have undertaken fertility preservation. Perinatal care providers should also ensure that all components of perinatal care are welcoming to SGM people. A 2019 case study of a 32-year-old man who came to the emergency department with abdominal pain and hypertension illustrates the limits of classification and gender that is taught to health professionals. Even though the patient explained that he was a transgender man and his human chorionic gonadotropic level was elevated, he did not receive immediate care as indicated for possible obstetrical complications, including preterm labor or placental abruption. He delivered a stillborn infant hours later.

All SGM persons planning a pregnancy should be encouraged to consult with a family attorney prior to conception, and if partnered, the partner needs to be aware of their rights and responsibilities. The law has not kept up with the variety of family constellations that are seen in SGM families. Examples of these constellations include two gay cisgender fathers parenting together, each using the same egg donor so that their children are half-siblings biologically; a lesbian couple composed of a transfeminine person and cisgender woman where one partner provides the sperm and another provides the egg and carries the pregnancy; a straight cisgender father parenting with a lesbian cisgender mother; a lesbian cisgender couple with the sperm donor being the brother of the parent who did not provide the egg so one mother is genetically related via the egg and the other mother is genetically related to the sperm (her brother's) thus being a biologic aunt; two cisgender lesbians each carrying a pregnancy conceived with their own eggs and using the same sperm donor so that their children are half-siblings; and two gay men where one is a cisgender man and provides the sperm and one is a transmasculine person and provides the egg and a surrogate carries the pregnancy.

Bos HM et al. Same-sex and different-sex parent households and child health outcomes: findings from the national survey of children's health. J Dev Behav Pediatr. 2016;37:179. [PMID: 27035692]

Kirubarajan A et al. Cultural competence in fertility care for lesbian, gay, bisexual, transgender and queer people: a systematic review of patient and provider perspectives. Fertil Steril. 2021;15:1294. [PMID 33610322]

Núñez A et al. Reproductive outcomes in lesbian couples undergoing reception of oocytes from partner versus autologous *in vitro* fertilization/intracytoplasmic sperm injection. LGBT Health. 2021;8:367. [PMID: 34061679]

Stroumsa D et al. The power and limits of classification—a 32-year-old man with abdominal pain. N Engl J Med. 2019;380:1885. [PMID: 31091369]

HEALTH CARE FOR LESBIAN & BISEXUAL WOMEN

Patricia A. Robertson, MD

Nicole Rosendale, MD

Cisgender lesbian and bisexual women are addressed together in this section since most medical literature does not delineate clearly enough between lesbian and bisexual cisgender women. Current medical literature also does not sufficiently consider the intersection of sexual orientation and gender identity to evaluate the specific health needs and concerns of lesbian and bisexual women who are of gender diverse experiences, nor is there sufficient research in the experiences of other SM women (ie, those who identify as pansexual, queer, asexual) to understand the current health needs of these individuals (although the few existing studies are included here). In the United States, women in same-sex couples are less likely to have primary care providers, get non-urgent medical care when needed, see a specialist, and feel that doctors spent enough time with them. Healthcare access is even more restricted at the intersection of sexual orientation, gender, race, and ethnicity. A 2021 study of Black and Latinx SM gender expansive women found that barriers to accessing care were linked to income and discrimination by providers. This is true worldwide with variability depending on the local sociopolitical climate. In countries with more restrictive laws and policies, health disparities are likely greater. Limited clinician training likely exacerbates the lack of preparedness to care for SM women.

Cerezo A et al. Healthcare access and health-related cultural norms in a community sample of Black and Latinx sexual minority gender expansive women. J Homosex. 2021 Nov 29. [Epub ahead of print] [PMID: 34842502]

Health Disparities Affecting Lesbian & Bisexual Women

Health disparities exist across the life span for lesbian and bisexual women compared with heterosexual women. The following are increased among lesbian and bisexual women: childhood physical abuse in the home, childhood sexual abuse, substance use including alcohol and tobacco, chlamydial infection as teens and young adults, sexual assault, depression, disabilities, increased BMI, intimate partner violence, threats and violence outside the home, asthma, migraine, back pain, dementia, and CVD. Sexual dysfunction for lesbian and bisexual women is seen less often or as often as heterosexual women but is understudied and likely assessed at rates lower than among heterosexual women. Concerns of sexual dysfunction can be detected by a single question in the medical history: "Do you have any questions or concerns about your sexuality or sexual health?"

As with other SGM individuals, aging and advanced care planning is of importance in lesbian and bisexual women. Studies of Irish SGM older adults reveal concerns about residential care outside of their own home as well as respect by health professionals; similarly, there are concerns about home services for lesbian and bisexual women in Canada and the United States. Lesbian and bisexual women have fewer children available to help them as they age compared with heterosexual women. Therefore, it is critical that health care providers identify health decision makers for all patients, including lesbian and bisexual women, who may find support in "family of choice" rather than "family of origin." This is especially important since same-sex/same-gender marriage is not allowed in many countries and is still considered socially unacceptable in many areas of the United States. To avoid conflict during critical decision-making moments, the health decision maker needs to be identified on the medical record after a private conversation with the patient. In one survey, only about 50% of same-sex couples who desired their partner to be the health decision maker had appropriate forms, and even if married, advance directives should be completed given past visitation denials. Many notable legal cases, including that of Sharon Kowalski and Karen Thompson, have documented the struggles that same-sex partners can face regarding visitation and appropriate recognition during end-of-life care or critical medical decision-making when these documents have not been completed. Elder abuse screening also needs to be done, since the incidence is unknown in this population.

Saunders CL et al. Long-term conditions among sexual minority adults in England: evidence from a cross-sectional analysis of responses to the English GP Patient Survey. BGJP Open. 2021;5:67. [PMID 34465579]

Cardiovascular Disease

The risk of CVD, including MI and stroke, appears to be higher in SM women compared with heterosexual peers; information on CVD outcomes is limited, however, and many studies rely on self-report rather than objective measures. Studies suggest that CVD risk is most influenced by psychosocial stress (ie, cumulative minority stress). In one study, lesbian and bisexual women were 14% older in vascular terms than their chronological age, which was 6% greater than that of their heterosexual counterparts; the risk was not fully explained by excessive smoking or alcohol use. Data from the Behavioral Risk Factor Surveillance System (2014–2016) showed that SM women, compared with their heterosexual counterparts, had increased modifiable CVD risk factors of mental distress (lesbian adjusted OR [AOR] 1.37; bisexual AOR 2.33), current smoking (lesbian AOR 1.65; bisexual AOR 1.29), heavy drinking (lesbian AOR 2.01; bisexual AOR 2.04), and obesity (lesbian AOR 1.50; bisexual AOR 1.29). SM women may have higher prevalence of hypertension compared with heterosexual counterparts. SMs, particularly bisexual women, were less likely than heterosexual peers to use statins for primary prevention but not secondary prevention, potentially highlighting a gap in access. Data from the Chicago Health and Life Experiences of Women study and the National Health Interview Survey found cardiometabolic risk factors (hypertension, diabetes, and obesity) and CVD outcomes, respectively, varied by sexual orientation and race/ethnicity highlighting the importance of intersectional assessments and interventions that account for sexual orientation, race, and ethnicity.

A 2020 American Heart Association scientific statement emphasizes the disparities across several cardiovascular risk factors compared with cisgender heterosexual peers, driven primarily by exposure to psychosocial stressors across the life span.

Caceres BA....Rosendale N et al. Assessing and addressing cardiovascular health in LGBTQ adults: a scientific statement from the American Heart Association. Circulation. 2020;142:e321. [PMID: 33028085]

Rosendale N et al. Sexual and gender minority health in neurology: a scoping review. JAMA Neurol. 2021;78:747. [PMID: 33616625]

Cigarette Smoking

Cigarette smoking is more common among lesbian and bisexual women than in heterosexual women. While estimates vary, a 2020 meta-analysis found that current cigarette use was most prevalent among bisexual women (37.7%) and lesbian women (31.7%) compared with heterosexual women (16.6%). The tobacco industry's well-documented targeted marketing to SGM groups and the use of cigarette smoking to cope with psychosocial stressors are contributing factors. A 2019 study found that early initiation of cigarette smoking (before age 15) accounts for 22–29% of the disparities in adult smoking rates. Rates of cigarette smoking, e-cigarette use, and hookah use in SM high school students are higher than heterosexual peers, particularly for bisexual youth. Protective factors against smoking behaviors for young LGB women included connections with other SGM people. Significant ethnic differences exist: Asian and Pacific Islander lesbian and bisexual women have four times higher odds of smoking than heterosexual Asian and Pacific Islander women.

Both traditional smoking cessation programs and targeted SGM programs are effective for SGM people. A review of smoking cessation programs for LGBTI (I = intersex) people found that with cultural modifications for LGBTI people, 61% had quit at the end of interventions and this stabilized to 39% at 3–6 months. In Canada, 24 focus groups in Toronto and Ottawa detailed eight overarching themes that would be important to them in a smoking intervention: (1) be LGBTQ+ specific; (2) be accessible in terms of location, time, availability, and cost; (3) be inclusive, relatable, and highlight diversity; (4) incorporate LGBTQ+ peer support and counseling services; (5) integrate other activities beyond smoking; (6) be positive, motivational, uplifting, and empowering; (7) provide concrete coping mechanisms; and (8) integrate rewards and incentives. Other studies have corroborated that both SGM-specific (such as relation to coming out, different norms and acceptability of smoking among SGM communities, or SGM-related minority stress) and previously identified factors seen in other populations (such as self-efficacy around quitting) are important to support SGM people in quitting smoking. Attention should be paid to messaging about cigarette smoking warnings because not all messages are perceived as equally effective by sexual minorities when compared with heterosexual people. Patients should be encouraged to check with community or online resources for smoking cessation programs and encourage participation in SGM tailored programs, if available.

Azagba S et al. Disparities in the frequency of tobacco products use by sexual identity status. Addict Behav. 2021;122:107032. [PMID: 34229134]

Li J et al. Tobacco use at the intersection of sex and sexual identity in the U.S., 2007-2020: a meta-analysis. Am J Prev Med. 2021;60:415. [PMID: 33218922]

Substance Use

Substance use is higher in lesbian and bisexual women compared with heterosexual women and is especially well-documented for cigarette smoking and alcohol use. A secondary analysis of alcohol, tobacco, and other drug use among lesbian and bisexual women in the American College Health Association's National College Health Assessment revealed that bisexual women had greater odds of using alcohol, tobacco, and marijuana than heterosexual women and lesbian women. Lesbian women had greater odds of using tobacco, marijuana, sedatives, hallucinogens, and other illicit drugs and misusing prescription drugs than heterosexual women. This increased rate of substance use persists for bisexual women over the age of 25 years but decreases for lesbian women at that time. Lesbian, gay, and bisexual women have an increased use of illicit opioids than do heterosexual adults. A study using 2015–2017 National Survey on Drug Use and Health data found the prevalence of opioid use in the preceding year was 5.9% in heterosexual women and 14.4 % in lesbian, gay and bisexual women. With the increase in the number of states allowing legal consumption of marijuana, marijuana use has increased in all communities, including the LGBTQ+ community. As with cigarette smoking, disparate substance use rates have been associated with psychosocial stress and mental health. Results from the longitudinal Chicago Health and Life Experiences of Women study showed that anxiety was prospectively associated with alcohol use, as were higher levels of perceived SM stigma. Alcohol use was prospectively associated with depression, suggesting a complex, multi-directional relationship between substance use, minority stress, and mental health.

Multiple interventions have been initiated to decrease alcohol and other substance use in lesbian and bisexual female youth. A 2020 study showed that greater LGBT supportive factors in a community (eg, PRIDE events) correlate with lower lifetime odds of marijuana use and smoking for girls. Although there are studies of substance use interventions in lesbian and bisexual women, more research is needed. Recommendations for improving substance use treatment for SM persons include providing interventionists with training in SGM cultural sensitivity. Another approach studied in the rural United States looked at training and deploying SGM peer-advocates to support mental health and substance use and "bridge the gap in culturally competent care." SM women, compared with heterosexual women, with lifetime alcohol use disorders are at heightened risk for concomitant psychiatric and drug use disorders, underscoring the need for substance abuse programs to provide access to individual counseling with mental health professionals.

Freitag TM et al. Variations in substance use and disorders among sexual minorities by race/ethnicity. Subst Use Misuse. 2021;56:921. [PMID: 33821743]

Gonzales G. Differences in 30-day marijuana use by sexual orientation identity: population-based evidence for seven states. LGBT Health. 2020;7:60. [PMID 31939720]

Hughes TL et al. Alcohol use among sexual minority women: methods used and lessons learned in the 20-Year Chicago Health and Life Experiences of Women Study. Int J Alcohol Drug Res. 2021;9:30. https://doi.org/10.7895/ijadr.289

Kidd JD et al. Risk and protective factors for substance use among sexual and gender minority youth: a scoping review. Curr Addict Rep. 2018;5:158. [PMID: 30393591]

López JD et al. Disparities in health behaviors and outcomes at the intersection of race and sexual identity among women: results from the 2011-2016 National Health and Nutrition Examination Survey. Prev Med. 2021;142:106379. [PMID: 33347873]

Body Weight

Most studies suggest higher prevalence of obesity and overweight in lesbians and bisexual women compared with heterosexual women. The prevalence of obesity may not be uniform across racial and ethnic groups, and SM women of color may experience higher rates of obesity compared with White SM women, although data are mixed. The reason for this difference is likely multifactorial and complex. Obesity and overweight may start at a young age in lesbian and bisexual youth, and they may conceptualize their weight differently than heterosexual peers.

A 2019 study found significant differences between bisexual women, lesbians, and heterosexual adults in body perception and ideals. Studies of physical activity have found that while there may be greater physical activity and fitness among some SM women, sedentary time is also increased in some. The Nurses Health Study III found that mostly heterosexual and lesbian women had healthier diets (as defined by the Dietary Approach to Stop Hypertension score and the American Heart Association 2020 Strategic Impact Goals) compared with exclusively heterosexual women. Psychosocial stress also plays a role. Bullying has been associated with high levels of unhealthy weight control behavior in SM youth. Lifetime trauma exposure has been associated with obesity in SM women, and a 2019 study of lesbian women showed an association between unhealthy eating patterns (binge eating, disordered eating and hazardous alcohol use, disordered eating, and high exercise) and higher rates of general discrimination, SM stress, social anxiety, negative affect, and lower social support.

Focus groups have identified themes related to weight for lesbian and bisexual women: aging, physical and mental health status, community norms, subgroup differences, family and partner support, and awareness and tracking of diet and physical activity. Findings from focus groups included (1) a preference for interventions focusing on promoting health and full life participation rather than on weight loss only, (2) cultural norms within the lesbian community that were accepting of larger body types, (3) an increased awareness in older age that the larger body size may exacerbate chronic health problems such as knee pain, and (4) the importance of social support and group structures in initiating and maintaining healthy behaviors. One study of 150 lesbian, bisexual, and queer women offered preliminary evidence that social support, resilience, and self-esteem help foster body appreciation, which might be protective against mental health concerns and disordered eating.

Burnette CB et al. Body appreciation in lesbian, bisexual and queer women: examining a model of social support, resilience, and self-esteem. Health Equity. 2019;3:238. [PMID 31289784]

Ingraham N. Perceptions of body size and health among older queer women of size following participation in a health programme. Cult Health Sex. 2019;21:636. [PMID: 30295146]

Pistella J et al. The role of peer victimization, sexual identity, and gender on unhealthy weight control behaviors in a representative sample of Texas youth. Int J Eat Disord. 2019;52:597. [PMID: 30805974]

Solazzo AL et al. Variation in diet quality across sexual orientation in a cohort of U.S. women. Cancer Causes Control. 2021;32:645. [PMID: 33846853]

VanKim NA et al. Sexual orientation and obesity: what do we know? Psych Issues. 2021;10:453. [PMID: 34595737]

Diabetes

There are limited studies examining diabetes and prediabetes in SM women and results are conflicting. In the Nurse's Health Study II, for example, lesbian and bisexual women had a 27% higher risk of developing type 2 diabetes than heterosexual women; however, this association was mediated by BMI. Data from the Behavioral Risk Factor Surveillance System (2017–2019) found slightly higher prevalence of diabetes in SM adults compared with heterosexual adults (12.5 versus 11.6); however, this difference varied by race or ethnicity. White SM adults had 1.12 higher prevalence compared with heterosexuals while differences in other racial or ethnic categories did not reach statistical significance. Given the association between obesity and diabetes, efforts to prevent obesity may also decrease disparities in diabetes and prediabetes.

Liu H et al. Sexual orientation and diabetes during the transition to adulthood. LGBT Health. 2019;6:227. [PMID: 31170023]

Pulmonary Disease

Pulmonary disease has not been rigorously studied in lesbian or bisexual women; most of the data come from studies of asthma, which generally find higher rates in SM women compared with heterosexual women. Older lesbian women have a higher prevalence of lifetime and current asthma, even when statistical models are used to correct for current and past cigarette smoking and obesity.

Increasingly, as this field of research matures, other findings of mediators on pulmonary health may help elucidate possible causative factors of pulmonary health. For example, one study of SGM persons found an association between shorter duration of sleep and outcomes, such as COPD prevalence. Further research is needed in this field, particularly considering disparate rates of smoking in SM women that may predispose to pulmonary disease.

Cabrera-Serrano A et al. Tobacco use and associated health conditions and risk factors in the lesbian, gay, bisexual, transgender, and transsexual populations of Puerto Rico, 2013–2015. PR Health Sci J. 2019;38:46. [PMID: 30924915]

Fredriksen-Goldsen KI et al. Chronic health conditions and key health indicators among lesbian, gay, and bisexual older US adults, 2013–2014. Am J Public Health. 2017;107:1332. [PMID: 28700299]

Veldhuis CB et al. Asthma status and risk among lesbian, gay, and bisexual adults in the United States: a scoping review. Ann Allergy Asthma Immunol. 2019;122:535. [PMID: 30721759]

Veliz P et al. LDCT lung cancer screening eligibility and use of CT scans for lung cancer among sexual minorities. Cancer Epidemiol. 2019;60:51. [PMID: 30909153]

Sexually Transmitted Infections

STIs occur in lesbian and bisexual women, but little population-based data are available to delineate precise risks. Asking about sexual *behaviors* in addition to sexual *identity* is key to identifying STI risk and advising appropriate testing, since risk may vary by specific sexual practice (eg, digital-vaginal, vaginal-vaginal, digital-anal, oral-vaginal, oral-anal contact) and the specific pathogen. Often data are mixed and inconsistent with respect to whether sources speak to infection risk by identity group or behavior. Delineating behavior-based risk and identity-based risk are important for research, assessments, and interventions. The CDC has found that women who have sex with women (WSW is identity-based) have diverse sexual practices (sexual practices are behavior-based); the CDC also noted that use of barrier protection in examined studies (eg, use of gloves, dental dams) was ubiquitously low.

Chlamydial infections were higher in 14- to 24-year-old women who reported same-sex behavior when attending family planning clinics in the US Pacific Northwest compared with women who reported exclusively heterosexual behavior. Possible explanations for this observation include differences in these groups' use of reproductive health care services, infrequent use of barrier methods to prevent STI transmission with female partners, trends toward higher-risk behaviors, and different social network characteristics. Regardless of sexual orientation, the CDC recommends annual *Chlamydia trachomatis* (and *Neisseria gonorrheae*) screening from the age of first sexual activity to the age of 25 years for all women.

It is important to ask lesbian and bisexual women about specific sexual practices, as some practices may carry a higher risk of STIs than others, although there has been little research on sexual practices and the risk of STIs in this population. Thus, inferences are drawn from heterosexual prevention of these infections. "Safer Sex Kits" have occasionally been distributed to WSW and women who have sex with women and men (WSWM) to decrease the risk of STIs, but intervention effectiveness has not been studied. These kits often include dental dams to prevent transmission of bacteria and viruses from oral sex, but the efficacy of dental dams for this function has not been studied. Female latex condoms and latex gloves may provide better protection against infectious transmission from oral sex since latex has been studied as a barrier for prevention of **HIV** and other STIs. Exchange of blood should be avoided as much as possible, especially in HIV-discordant lesbian couples, since viral genotype analysis has confirmed that HIV can be transmitted sexually between women. The clinician should encourage both partners in new lesbian couples to have comprehensive STI and HIV screening prior to sexual contact and recommend barrier protection for 6 months until the couple is again screened to verify that their HIV status is still negative. If the couple is consistently monogamous and HIV and other STI testing are negative, barrier precautions do not need to be continued. However, lesbian and bisexual women may not follow this advice, since many feel they are at low risk for HIV, which may be correct, but data are lacking. About 20–50% of lesbian women use sexual aids (eg, vibrators, dildos, or other sexual toys); these should not be shared with partners and should be cleaned after use. HPV can remain on these sexual aids for up to 24 hours after use, even after standard cleaning. Some lesbian and bisexual women are sex workers or have had sexual relationships with high-risk male sexual partners (sometimes gay male friends) and are at increased risk for STIs. CDC guidelines recommend that all women should be tested once in their lifetime for HIV, with testing repeated according to risk factors. If a lesbian or bisexual woman is in a high-risk relationship for HIV transmission (sex work, gay male partner), she should be educated about PrEP for HIV prevention and prescribed the appropriate medication.

The **herpes simplex virus (HSV)** can be transmitted sexually between women. The same precautions regarding the transmission of HSV should be provided to lesbian, bisexual, and heterosexual women; there should be no sexual contact during any prodromal symptoms that may precede a genital herpes outbreak or during the blister stage of the outbreak. Suppression of lesions can usually be accomplished with antiviral medications, such as acyclovir or valacyclovir, if the lesions are recurrent (see Chapter 6).

There is evidence of **HPV** transmission between female sexual partners. Certain strains of HPV are causally related to many precancerous and cancerous lesions, including cervical dysplasia and cervical cancer (see Chapter 18). Ten percent of lesbian women have never had sex with men, yet cervical dysplasia and cervical cancer develop in some of these women. All women (including lesbian women) need cervical cancer screening, which may include Papanicolaou smears, high-risk HPV strain testing, or both, according to timetables and risk factors provided by professional society guidelines. The rate of HPV vaccination in Black lesbian women was very low in one study; the OR for HPV vaccination was 0.16 for Black lesbian women compared with White heterosexual women, and 0.35 for White lesbian women compared with White heterosexual women. Bisexual women are vaccinated more frequently than either lesbian or heterosexual women. However, the overall HPV vaccination rate is low in adult women regardless of sexual orientation, so improvement in all groups should be the goal. Administration of the HPV vaccine is critical to the prevention of cervical cancer; the CDC recommends HPV vaccination for all persons through age 26 years; for unvaccinated adults ages 27 through 45 years, shared decision-making is recommended. Despite recommendations that cervical cancer screening, Papanicolaou testing or HPV testing, or both, be performed regardless of sexual orientation, this testing varies according to identity irrespective of behavior and some studies modify screening according to identity and behavior. In a national probability sample of who underwent Papanicolaou testing, WSWM had the same odds of testing as WSM only, whereas women with lifetime female partners had lower odds of testing. Those who identified as bisexual also had lower odds of testing.

Trichomonas vaginalis can be transmitted easily between female sexual partners. One study of women attending an STI clinic in the United States noted that *T vaginalis* was the most common curable STI found in this population with a prevalence of 17% in WSW and 24% in WSWM.

Bacterial vaginosis is common among women and, according to the CDC, even more common among WSW. It is unknown whether bacterial vaginosis can be transmitted between women. A study from Australia found a 27% prevalence of bacterial vaginosis in women and their female partners; risk factors for bacterial vaginosis were four or more lifetime female sexual partners, a female partner with bacterial vaginosis symptoms, and smoking at least 30 cigarettes weekly. Routine screening for bacterial vaginosis, however, is not recommended and testing should be based on symptoms. One approach for a WSW who has symptomatic bacterial vaginosis is to treat her and not her female sexual partners. If symptoms recur, her female sexual partners should be evaluated and treated with consideration of re-treating the index woman. This strategy may also be used for treatment of recurrent or hard to treat vulvovaginal candidiasis, which technically is not considered to be sexually transmitted, but anecdotally, improvement has occurred with treatment of the index patient and female partner.

Various strategies for making reproductive and sexual health clinics and providers more amenable to serving SGM people were studied by a group in the United States, but the findings (such as ensuring counseling involves inclusive safe sex discussions that are relevant to SGM people) have broad face validity and relevance for other regional and medical focus settings as well.

McCune KC et al. Clinical care of lesbian and bisexual women for the obstetrician gynecologist. Clin Obstet Gynecol. 2018;61:663. [PMID: 30285974]

Takemoto MLS et al. Prevalence of sexually transmitted infections and bacterial vaginosis among lesbian women: systematic review and recommendations to improve care. Cad Saude Publica. 2019;35:e00118118. [PMID: 30916178]

Cancer

Little is known about the incidence and prevalence of various cancers in lesbian and bisexual women, since sexual orientation has not been routinely included in cancer screening programs and cancer registries. However, some data suggest that SM women may be at a higher risk for cancer-related mortality than heterosexual counterparts.

Investigators from the Women's Health Study compared SM veterans and civilians to their heterosexual counterparts and found that SM women veterans had a higher risk of cancer-specific mortality. The National Health Interview Survey found bisexual women over age 65 years were 7.6% more likely to have a cancer diagnosis than a heterosexual woman of the same age, but the difference was not seen between lesbian and heterosexual women; the survey also found that lesbian and bisexual women have higher prevalence of cancer risk factors, such as tobacco use, underscoring the need for vigilant screening. Since lesbian and bisexual women have barriers to accessing health care and may not see a clinician on an annual basis, any visit to a health care provider is an opportunity to check on cancer screening status (eg, colonoscopy, mammography, cervical cancer screening). There is also recognition that upon receiving a cancer diagnosis, SGM people face challenges in receiving equitable care throughout the cancer care continuum and may experience cancer differently and have different needs during their care; heterosexual and SM cancer survivors in the UK reported receiving different care. One qualitative study with SGM breast cancer survivors underscored the challenges of disclosing sexual orientation during cancer care and the importance of provider recognition that varying social networks are critical to positive experiences of care provision. The 2017 American Society for Clinical Oncology position statement recommends five action steps to enhance SGM cancer care and reduce disparities: (1) patient education and support, (2) workforce development and diversity, (3) quality improvement strategies, (4) policy solutions, and (5) research strategies. All providers need to consider whether their prevention, screening, diagnostic, treatment, and palliative approaches will be equitably experienced by lesbian and bisexual women. The National Health Interview Survey from 2013–2018 showed differences in the quality of life for lesbian and bisexual women surviving cancer compared with heterosexual women; lesbian women reported higher odds of fair or poor self-rated health (OR 1.68), COPD (OR 1.98), and heart conditions (OR 1.90). Bisexual women reported higher odds of severe psychological distress (OR 3.03), heart conditions (OR 1.98), and food insecurity (OR 2.89) than did heterosexual women. Bisexual women had lower odds of receiving a recent mammogram (OR 0.42) than did heterosexual women.

Gonzales G et al. Cancer diagnoses among lesbian, gay, and bisexual adults: results from the 2013–2016 National Health Interview Survey. Cancer Causes Control. 2018;29:845. [PMID: 30043193]

Hudson J et al. Sexual and gender minority issues across NCCN Guidelines: results from a national survey. J Natl Compr Canc Netw. 2017;15:1379. [PMID: 29118229]

Webster R et al. How can we meet the support needs of LGBT cancer patients in oncology? A systematic review. Radiography (Lond). 2021;27:633. [PMID: 32800429]

A. Breast Cancer

The literature has been mixed on whether lesbian and bisexual women have a slight increased risk of breast cancer compared with heterosexual women; a 2013 systemic review found the few prevalence studies of breast cancer in lesbian women unreliable. Lesbian women, however, do have an increased prevalence of risk factors predisposing to breast cancer, including nulliparity (and decreased breastfeeding), alcohol use, obesity, and cigarette smoking. Vulnerability to inadequate screening, the development of cancer, or delayed diagnosis may further correlate with certain experiences such as a masculine gender presentation and practices like chest binding, as one study in China found. The literature is also inconsistent regarding the rate of mammography screening in lesbian women; however, a study done in Massachusetts showed that bisexual women were less likely than heterosexual women and lesbian women to adhere to mammography screening guidelines. Lesbian and bisexual women who have breast cancer may not want reconstruction at the same rate as heterosexual women and often find that breast cancer support groups focus on issues for heterosexual women (such as attractiveness to a male partner). Resilience and recovery factors vary in some ways between heterosexual and SM women.

Williams AD et al. Breast cancer risk, screening, and prevalence among sexual minority women: an analysis of the National Health Interview Survey. LGBT Health. 2020;7:109. [PMID: 32130086]

B. Cervical Cancer

Primary prevention of cervical cancer is essential. All persons between the ages of 9 and 45 years (routine recommended age is 11 to 12 years old) should receive the HPV vaccine series. HPV can be transmitted sexually between lesbian or heterosexual partners. Cervical cancer screening, with Papanicolaou smears, primary HPV testing, or both, should be part of lesbian and bisexual women's health care at the same intervals as for heterosexual women according to national and international guidelines. Lesbian and bisexual women, however, receive Papanicolaou smears at a lower rate than sexually active heterosexual women, in part because many of the Papanicolaou smears are done in reproductive health clinics; lesbians who are not interested in becoming pregnant or avoiding pregnancy may not access these clinical sites. In addition, some lesbian patients as well as their health care providers mistakenly think that lesbian women do not need Papanicolaou smears. *All lesbian and bisexual women need cervical cancer screening starting at the age of 21 years, consistent with recommendations for cervical cancer screening for all women.* Cancer prevention and control strategies for SM women that target provider education and policy intervention are needed to improve SM women's relationships with their providers and increase cervical cancer screening rates.

C. Lung Cancer

Compared with heterosexual women, lesbian and bisexual women are likely to have a higher rate of lung cancer due to their increased rate of cigarette smoking. The incidence and prevalence of lung cancer, however, have not been determined in this SM population. Nonetheless, gay men and lesbian women with significant use of cigarettes are at increased risk for lung cancer and are under-screened for early lung cancer detection with the use of low-dose helical computed tomography.

D. Endometrial and Ovarian Cancer

Endometrial and ovarian cancers are increased among those with nulliparity, which is more likely in SM women. Obesity, a known risk factor for both cancers, appears to be more prevalent among SM women. Conversely, the use of oral contraceptives, which is protective against the development of both of these cancers, is lower in lesbian women than in heterosexual women. Vigilance toward and education about presenting signs and symptoms (eg, postmenopausal bleeding, early satiety, unintended weight loss) are important to detect cancers as early as possible. Neither incidence nor prevalence of endometrial or ovarian cancer has been determined in this SM population. Lesbian women are less likely than heterosexual women to have had bilateral salpingectomies or bilateral tubal ligations for sterilization, procedures which decrease the risk for ovarian cancer, since about 70% of ovarian cancers start in the fallopian tubes.

Violence

Compared with heterosexual women, lesbian and bisexual women have higher exposures to violence throughout their lifetimes. Lifetime prevalence of sexual assault may be as high as 85%. A 2019 study concluded that sexual orientation clearly plays a role in victimization when they found that compared with heterosexual women, bisexual women had 3.7 times the odds of initial victimization and 7.3 times the odds of repeat victimization, and lesbian women had 3.2 times the odds of repeat victimization even after controlling for other sociodemographic factors. In a study of four countries in southern Africa, nearly one-third of lesbian and bisexual women experienced forced sex and assault including "corrective rape" by men as an attempt to change the women's sexual orientation. In a study from Brazil, qualitative interviews were done of youth coming out to their families: The family reactions were often violent, with persecution and even expulsion from the home, which impacted the youth's health and quality of life.

The CDC reports that 61% of bisexual women and 44% of lesbian women experience rape, physical violence, and stalking by an intimate partner. These rates are higher than similar trauma in heterosexual women (35%). Additionally, approximately 20% of bisexual women compared with 10% of heterosexual women have been raped by an intimate partner in their lifetimes. The rate of stalking experienced by bisexual women is twice that of heterosexual women and a higher percentage of bisexual women report being afraid of an intimate partner. A study of United States armed services veterans found that compared with heterosexual women veterans, lesbian, bisexual, and queer women veterans were twice as likely to report emotional mistreatment and physical intimate partner violence and three times as likely to report sexual intimate partner violence. Despite alarming rates for women of any identity, lesbian and bisexual women survivors of sexual assault and interpersonal violence may experience unique difficulties when seeking assistance. These problems include a limited understanding of interpersonal violence in the relationships of lesbian and bisexual women, stigma, and systemic inequities (such as shelters unwelcome to this population, perpetrating partners being allowed into the same shelters as the survivor of the domestic violence, "outing" someone as a psychological threat, and staff lacking cultural sensitivity and appropriate training in working with lesbian and bisexual women). Barriers to preventing SGM violence include stigma, systemic discrimination, and a lack of understanding of SGM intimate partner violence.

Community violence is experienced more frequently by SGM persons. In-depth interviews of Flemish SM persons who experienced anti-SGM violence revealed the use of four coping strategies: (1) avoidance, (2) assertiveness and confrontation, (3) cognitive change, and (4) social support. Applying these coping skills and actively attaching meaning to negative experiences helped these people overcome fear, embarrassment, or depressive feelings. The presence of a supportive network was important in facilitating the positive outcomes.

Swan LET et al. Discrimination and intimate partner violence victimization and perpetration among a convenience sample of LGBT individuals in Latin America. J Interpers Violence. 2021;36:8520. [PMID 31014171]

Mental Health

Lesbians and bisexual women have an increased risk of depression. Many of the health disparities and health risks faced by lesbians and bisexual women, such as depression and cardiovascular risk, have been attributed to minority stress. Therefore, rather than identifying mental health problems as synonymous with a SM identity or stemming from inborn association with minority sexual orientation, minority stress causes mental health challenges that stem from societal discrimination and stigma borne by individuals with minority identities (and behaviors). An examination of lesbian and bisexual women veterans from the US Behavioral Risk Factor Surveillance System found that SM women veterans were three times more likely than heterosexual women to experience "mental distress." Mortality risk from suicide is also elevated among women with same-sex partners. In the US National Epidemiologic Survey on Alcohol and Related Conditions–III, bisexual women had greater rates of specific psychiatric disorders than lesbians or heterosexual women. Resilience factors that are protective for mental distress and poorer mental health among lesbian, gay, bisexual, queer, and questioning youth and adults in Israel included family support as well as other community-level factors, such as friends' support, SGM connectedness, and having a steady partner. How parents react to an adolescent's coming out has a profound effect on their child's health outcomes. For those adolescents whose parents were supportive, there was less homelessness, depression, substance use, and unprotected sex. Interventions for building resilience can be important in achieving a reduction in anxiety and depression. There is some evidence that online friends can serve as a buffer and social support, especially for

SGM youth, although in-person social support appears to be more protective against victimization. However, social media can also be a place where SGM youth experience bullying.

Sexual orientation change efforts have now been outlawed in a few states in the United States, as well as in six countries (Germany, Malta, Ecuador, Brazil, Canada, and Taiwan). In a study in South Korea, participants who had undergone sexual orientation change efforts showed a 1.44–2.35 times higher prevalence of suicidal ideation and suicidal attempts than those without such an experience. Significant associations with suicidal observations and suicide attempts were also observed between having received advice to consider undergoing this experience.

There is evidence that being in a legally recognized same-sex relationship, particularly in marriage, diminishes mental health differences between heterosexual and lesbian, gay, and bisexual persons. In contrast, psychiatric disorders increased among lesbian, gay, and bisexual persons who lived in states in the United States that enacted constitutional amendments to ban same-sex marriage compared with states that did not. One study examined the mental health of individuals living in states before (wave 1, 2001–2002) and after (wave 2, 2004–2005) the enactment of same-sex marriage bans in 2004–2005. Among LGB respondents living in states that enacted the marriage bans, the National Epidemiologic Survey on Alcohol and Related Conditions (N = 34,653) revealed that there was a significantly increased prevalence of any mood disorder (36% increase), generalized anxiety disorder (248% increase), any alcohol use disorder (42% increase), and psychiatric comorbidity (36.3%) between wave 1 and wave 2 of the survey, suggesting that living in sociopolitical environments that do not legally recognize same-sex relationships can have deleterious effects on mental health.

Mental health inequities among bisexual and lesbian women are well documented. Compared with heterosexual women, bisexual and lesbian women are more likely to report lifetime depressive disorders, with bisexual women often faring the worst on mental health outcome. Risk factors for depression, such as victimization in childhood and adulthood, are more prevalent among bisexual women. One Chicago Health and Life Experiences study (an 18-year, community-based longitudinal study of SM women's health) compared Black bisexual and Black lesbian women with White lesbian women. The study found reports of victimization were higher in Black bisexual and Black lesbian women, but the odds of depression were significantly lower than in White lesbian women.

Internalized homophobia was significantly associated with depressive symptoms in a study in South Korea of LGB people. Only 22% had "come out" to their mother, and 11% to their father. Since the early 2000s, suicide rates in South Korea are among the highest of the Organization for Economic Co-operation and Development nations. The conclusion was that mental health interventions were needed for LGB adults who have high levels of internalized homophobia, as well as greater efforts are needed to enact protective legislation for SM individuals in South Korea.

Bostwick WB et al. Depression and victimization in a community sample of bisexual and lesbian women: an intersectional approach. Arch Sex Behav. 2019;48:131. [PMID: 29968037]

Lee H et al. Internalized homophobia, depressive symptoms, and suicidal ideation among lesbian, gay and bisexual adults in South Korea: an age-stratified analysis. LGBT Health. 2019;8:393. [PMID: 31746660]

Lee H et al. Sexual orientation change efforts, depressive symptoms and suicidality among lesbian, gay and bisexual adults: a cross sectional study in South Korea. LGBT Health. 2021;8:427. [PMID 34061676]

Schulman JK et al. Mental health in sexual minority and transgender women. Med Clin North Am. 2019;103:723. [PMID: 31078203]

HEALTH CARE FOR GAY & BISEXUAL MEN

Kevin L. Ard, MD, MPH

Kenneth H. Mayer, MD

This section is devoted to the primary care of cisgender gay, bisexual, and other men who have sex with men (MSM) regardless of their sexual identity. Most health-related research that focuses on MSM categorizes men based on their sexual behavior as MSM, rather than their self-reported identification as gay, bisexual, or other identities. Although sexual identity is not always congruent with sexual behavior, identity is important to recognize to optimize health and health care, especially when there is a difference on the basis of sexual identity (for example, gay- versus bisexual-identified men).

Demographics

The size of the MSM population in the United States is not known with certainty due to variability in the definition of sexual orientation used in surveys and the possibility that some survey respondents do not disclose gay or bisexual orientations because of concerns about discrimination. Nevertheless, based on available data, it is estimated that at least 2.2% of American adult men identify as gay, and an additional 1.4% of men identify as bisexual. The proportion of men who engage in sex with other men or experience sexual attraction to other men is estimated to be higher, with 7.3% and 6.2% of adult men reporting some same-sex attraction and sexual behavior, respectively, in one national survey.

Health Disparities

Gay, bisexual, and other MSM face health disparities stemming from the biologic aspects of their sexual behavior or from minority stress, or both. Because of these disparities, MSM have been identified as a priority population for health-related research and improvement in health care by both the National Academy of Medicine and the federal government's Healthy People 2020 initiative. These health disparities are exacerbated if MSM have experienced early life traumatic events, such as sexual abuse or familial rejection.

Makadon HJ, Mayer KH et al. *The Fenway Guide to Lesbian, Gay, Bisexual, and Transgender Health*, 2nd ed. American College of Physicians Press, 2015.

Office of Disease Prevention and Health Promotion (ODPHP). Healthy People 2020: lesbian, gay, bisexual, and transgender health. 2016. https://www.healthypeople.gov/2020/topics-objectives/topic/lesbian-gay-bisexual-and-transgender-health

A. HIV and Other STIs

MSM account for approximately 70% of all new **HIV infections** in the United States, despite representing a small proportion (less than 10% by any metric) of the country's male population. The high burden of HIV infection among MSM stems in part from the efficient transmission of the virus through receptive anal intercourse, which confers a higher risk of HIV infection than other sexual activities, such as penile-vaginal and oral intercourse. Role versatility can also uniquely potentiate HIV spread among MSM, since the same person can acquire HIV via receptive intercourse and then transmit by engaging in insertive anal intercourse with partners without HIV. The origin of disparate HIV rates between MSM and other populations is not solely biologic in origin, however, as societal stigma and psychosocial problems also contribute to sexual risk behavior among MSM. MSM of color face an increased risk of HIV; the CDC estimates that in the United States in 2019, 37% of new HIV diagnoses occurred among Black MSM, and 24% were among Hispanic/Latinx MSM. Racial and ethnic disparities in HIV infections among MSM are not because of differences in sexual behavior or substance use but rather such factors as lack of access to medical care, lower rates of recent HIV testing among non-White MSM, and assortative mixing (ie, being more likely to have sex with partners from one's own racial or ethnic group).

Beyond HIV, some STIs are more common among MSM. In 2019, at least 47% of primary and secondary syphilis diagnoses occurred in MSM or men who have sex with both men and women. **Syphilis** is associated with a high risk of subsequent HIV acquisition in MSM and may serve as a marker for individuals who could benefit from intensive HIV prevention efforts, such as PrEP. Increased cases of ocular syphilis, occasionally resulting in blindness, have been reported, with most cases occurring in MSM. The incidence of gonorrhea among MSM exceeds that among men who have sex with women (MSW) and has increased. MSM also are more likely than MSW to be infected with antibiotic-resistant gonorrhea. Most gonococcal infections in MSM occur at extragenital sites (ie, the pharynx or the rectum) where they may be asymptomatic, underscoring the importance of eliciting a comprehensive sexual history, including an inventory of potential anatomic exposures, to provide optimal STI screening for MSM.

MSM face increased risks of **viral hepatitis**. Outbreaks of hepatitis A infection have been documented in MSM, likely due to anal sexual contact, including oral-anal exposure ("rimming") as well as insertive and receptive practices. Likewise, hepatitis B is more common among MSM than the general population; approximately 20% of MSM have evidence of either current or prior infection with hepatitis B by age 30 years. This highlights the importance of universal hepatitis A and B vaccination for young MSM, preferably prior to the initiation of sexual contact. Finally, hepatitis C infection has been identified as prevalent among MSM with HIV and high-risk MSM without HIV; although hepatitis C is generally not efficiently transmitted via sexual contact, it is associated with condomless receptive anal sex, group sex, manual insertion of fingers into the rectum ("fisting"), and recent STIs, which make the rectal mucosa more susceptible to hepatitis C acquisition and transmission.

HPV infection, which can cause anogenital warts, anal dysplasia, and anal cancer, is more common among MSM than MSW. A meta-analysis estimated the prevalence of the oncogenic HPV type 16 in the anal canal to be 35.4% among MSM with HIV and 12.5% among MSM without HIV. Correspondingly, anal cancer incidence is higher among MSM with HIV than in MSM without HIV.

Enteric infections may be sexually transmitted among MSM engaging in anal sexual contact, especially oral-anal sexual contact, and should be considered in the differential diagnosis of GI concerns. These infections include giardiasis, amebiasis, and shigellosis. In addition, *Shigella* infections are more likely to be antibiotic-resistant among MSM than among other individuals.

Clusters of **meningococcal disease** among MSM in the United States and Europe have also been reported, particularly those frequenting sexualized environments, including saunas and bathhouses, prompting some jurisdictions to recommend meningococcal vaccination for high-risk MSM. Intimate contact with multiple partners has been identified as a risk factor for infection in some of these outbreaks.

Centers for Disease Control and Prevention (CDC). HIV and African American gay and bisexual men. 2022. https://www.cdc.gov/hiv/group/msm/bmsm.html

Centers for Disease Control and Prevention (CDC). HIV and gay and bisexual men. 2021. https://www.cdc.gov/hiv/group/msm/msm-content/incidence.html

Centers for Disease Control and Prevention (CDC). HIV and Hispanic/Latino gay and bisexual men: HIV incidence. 2021. https://www.cdc.gov/hiv/group/gay-bisexual-men/hispanic-latino/incidence.html

Mayer KH et al. The persistent and evolving HIV epidemic in American men who have sex with men. Lancet. 2021;397:1116. [PMID: 33617771]

Sullivan PS…Mayer KH et al. Epidemiology of HIV in the USA: epidemic burden, inequities, contexts, and responses. Lancet. 2021;397:1095. [PMID: 33617774]

B. Behavioral Health

Likely due to minority stress (ie, growing up in non-affirming societies), MSM experience mental health disorders more commonly than other men. Whether defined by self-reported identity as gay or bisexual or behaviorally by report of sexual activity with other men, MSM have a higher lifetime prevalence of depression and anxiety disorders than men who identify as heterosexual or those who report sexual activity only with women. Behaviorally bisexual men experience a higher burden of both depression and anxiety disorders, compared with men who engage in only same-gender sexual behavior, in part because bisexual men may have less access to defined communities of choice, like self-identified gay men. The increased prevalence of mental health disorders among behaviorally bisexual men may also stem from dual stigmatization by both the heterosexual and gay male communities, as well as internalized stigma. Among MSM overall, anti-gay violence, community alienation, and dissatisfaction with an idealized body image have all been associated with depression.

C. Substance Use

Compared with men who have only female sexual partners, MSM are more likely to report lifetime recreational drug use; they are specifically more likely to have used cocaine, hallucinogens, inhalants, analgesics, and tranquilizers. In addition, men who identify as gay or bisexual are more likely to smoke cigarettes than those who identify as heterosexual. Although it is not clear that MSM are more likely than others to use methamphetamines, methamphetamine use in MSM communities has been linked to increased sexual risk behavior and transmission of hepatitis C, HIV, and other STIs. Consistent with the minority stress model, experiences of discrimination have been independently associated with substance use among MSM.

Hoenigl M et al. Clear links between starting methamphetamine and increasing sexual risk behavior: a cohort study among men who have sex with men. J Acquir Immune Defic Syndr. 2016;71:551. [PMID: 26536321]

Preventive Care & Clinical Practice Guidelines

Clinicians can help address health disparities affecting MSM by following clinical practice guidelines that pertain to this population (Table 42–1). The CDC recommends that sexually active MSM undergo screening for HIV, syphilis, gonorrhea, and chlamydia annually and more often if the risk history warrants more frequent assessment. An HIV antibody-antigen assay is preferred for HIV screening because this test increases the sensitivity for detection of acute or recent HIV infection. Nucleic acid amplification testing (NAAT) provides optimal sensitivity for diagnosis of gonorrhea and chlamydia and can be performed on the oropharynx, rectum, urine, and urethra. MSM should be screened for these infections at any of the aforementioned sites that may have been exposed during sex, regardless of condom use. First-catch urine and urethral specimens for gonorrhea and chlamydia NAAT in men provide comparable accuracy; thus, there is no advantage to the urethral swab for routine screening. Rectal and pharyngeal swabs for NAAT can be self-collected. In the absence of an etiologic diagnosis, patients being treated for gonorrhea or chlamydia should receive therapy for both, since co-infections are common.

The CDC also recommends that MSM be screened for chronic hepatitis B infection at least once in their lives and that they be vaccinated against hepatitis A and B. Annual hepatitis C screening with a hepatitis C antibody test is recommended for MSM with HIV due to the elevated incidence of this infection in this population and the availability of well-tolerated, curative therapy. MSM without HIV who engage in sexual practices that may abrade the rectal mucosa (eg, group sex, fisting) may also benefit from annual hepatitis C screening.

The CDC, USPSTF, and the World Health Organization recommend **PrEP for HIV** for MSM at high risk for HIV

Table 42–1. Clinical practice guidelines pertaining to the care of men who have sex with men (MSM).

Recommendation	Comments
Immunizations	
HPV (quadri- or nonavalent)	Recommended up to age 26 years; the vaccine may be offered to those aged 27–45 years
Hepatitis A and B	Consider prevaccination serologic testing if the immunization history is uncertain; vaccinate if seronegative
Meningococcal	Recommended by some jurisdictions due to outbreaks of meningococcal disease among MSM
Medications	
Preexposure prophylaxis for HIV	For MSM at high, ongoing risk of HIV infection (eg, anal sex without a condom, recent STI diagnosis, sexual partner with HIV)
Postexposure prophylaxis for HIV	Consists of 28 days of antiretroviral medication following a discrete exposure to HIV
Screening Tests	
HIV serology	At least annually, more often if high risk
Syphilis serology	At least annually, more often if high risk
Nucleic acid amplification test for gonorrhea and chlamydia	At least annually, more often if high risk; all potentially exposed sites (oropharynx, urethra, rectum) should be screened, as indicated by the sexual history
Hepatitis C serology	Annually for MSM with HIV and MSM without HIV engaging in behaviors that might expose them to blood (eg, injection drug use or traumatic anal sexual practices)
Anal cytology	For MSM with HIV; the appropriateness of anal cytology for MSM without HIV is under study
Behavioral health (depression, substance use)	At the first clinical encounter, with follow-up screening for those who report behavioral health concerns

STI, sexually transmitted infection.

infection. FDA-approved options for MSM for PrEP include oral emtricitabine/tenofovir disoproxil fumarate, oral emtricitabine/tenofovir alafenamide, and long-acting injectable cabotegravir. Individuals at high risk include those who engage in condomless anal sex outside of a monogamous relationship with a man without HIV; those who have a recent diagnosis of a bacterial STI; and those who have sexual partners with HIV who are not consistently virologically suppressed on antiretroviral therapy. PrEP has been shown in randomized controlled trials to prevent HIV infection in MSM and is addressed in more detail in Chapter 31. The FDA has approved a condom to decrease transmission of STIs during anal intercourse (One Male Condom); condomless anal intercourse carries the greatest sexual exposure risk of HIV transmission. These condoms can also be used to reduce the rate of pregnancy and the transmission of STIs during vaginal intercourse.

Clinicians who care for MSM should also be aware of **postexposure prophylaxis (PEP)**, which consists of antiretrovirals started within 72 hours of a discrete exposure to HIV and taken for 28 days, and either provide PEP themselves or be able to rapidly link patients to PEP care (see Chapter 31).

HPV immunization with the quadrivalent or nonavalent vaccines is recommended for all boys and young men up to age 26 years. For unvaccinated adults aged 27–45 years, shared decision-making around HPV vaccination is recommended. The HIV Medicine Association recommends routinely screening MSM with HIV for anal cancer and cancer precursors with anal cytology; a randomized clinical trial, the ANCHOR study, showed that screening for and removing anal cancer precursors significantly reduced the risk of anal cancer compared with screening and monitoring alone. Patients with abnormal anal cytology are typically referred for high-resolution anoscopy with biopsy. Colonoscopy performed for colon cancer screening is not considered a substitute for anal cytology or high-resolution anoscopy because colonoscopy does not assess for cellular abnormalities in the anal canal. Anal cytology screening of MSM without HIV is not recommended in any national consensus guidelines, although some clinicians perform this screening due to the elevated risk of anal cancer in these men.

Finally, clinicians should ensure that MSM are offered preventive care recommended for all individuals, including smoking cessation counseling and pharmacotherapy, screening for depression, and assessment for and counseling about alcohol misuse (see Lesbian and Bisexual Women's Health, above). Some studies have found that behavioral health programs tailored specifically for MSM are more effective in promoting healthy behaviors than those that are not culturally sensitive.

Centers for Disease Control and Prevention (CDC). Updated guidelines for antiretroviral postexposure prophylaxis after sexual, injection-drug use, or other nonoccupational exposure to HIV—United States, 2016. MMWR Morb Mortal Wkly Rep. 2016;65:458. [PMID: 27149423]

Reback CJ et al. Development of an evidence-based, gay-specific cognitive behavioral therapy intervention for methamphetamine-abusing gay and bisexual men. Addict Behav. 2014;39:1286. [PMID: 22169619]

HEALTH CARE FOR TRANSGENDER & GENDER DIVERSE PEOPLE

Mitzi Hawkins, MD

Madeline B. Deutsch, MD, MPH

TERMINOLOGY

This section is dedicated to the unique health needs of transgender and gender diverse persons. The terms transgender and gender diverse as used in this text are inclusive of those who identify with the terms gender nonbinary, gender nonconforming, genderqueer, and transsexual. The umbrella term "transgender" incorporates a range of identities and experiences of individuals whose gender identities or expression, or both, differ from those associated with the sex assigned to them at birth. In contrast, the gender of cisgender individuals is concordant with the sex assigned to them at birth. The term transfeminine as used in this text refers to persons who identify along a female or feminine spectrum and transmasculine refers to people who identify along a male or masculine spectrum. Despite this simplification, a significant proportion of transgender people do not identify with a binary conception of gender. Transgender people may use any pronoun, including the gender-neutral singular pronoun "they." It is also important to note that sexual orientation is distinct from gender and transgender people, like cisgender people, have a diversity of sexual attraction and activity.

Demographics

Few well-designed, long-term, large studies describe the population and well-being of transgender people. Additionally, methodological challenges exist in the description of the transgender population; these limitations include inconsistent or incomplete collection of sexual orientation and gender identity information in the medical record, population databases, and health studies, and variable case definition (self-identification, clinical diagnosis, or receipt of gender affirming treatment). Survey-based studies that use self-identification report a prevalence of 0.5–4.5% transgender persons among adults and 2.5–8.4% among children and adolescents.

Deutsch MB et al. Electronic medical records and the transgender patient: recommendations from the World Professional Association for Transgender Health EMR Working Group. J Am Med Inform Assoc. 2013;20:700. [PMID: 23631835]

Zhang Q et al. Epidemiological considerations in transgender health: a systematic review with focus on higher quality data. Int J Transgend Health. 2020;21:125. [PMID: 33015664]

Disparities

Transgender people experience multiple structural barriers to health. High levels of societal stigma and discrimination, along with the lack of legal protections in education, the workplace, and housing, result in socioeconomic disadvantage and housing instability. Transgender people also face discrimination when seeking medical care. One in five transgender people reports delay in seeking medical care for fear of being mistreated based on their gender; among those who accessed a health care provider in the last year, 33% reported having a negative experience related to being transgender. These findings correlate with reports from healthcare professionals who state they lack the knowledge and skills necessary to provide care for transgender people.

James SE et al. Report of the 2015 U.S. Transgender Survey. Washington, DC: National Center for Transgender Equality. 2016. https://transequality.org/sites/default/files/docs/usts/USTS-Executive-Summary-Dec17.pdf

Stroumsa D et al. Transphobia rather than education predicts provider knowledge of transgender health care. Med Educ. 2019;53:398. [PMID: 30666699]

Gender Affirming Medical & Surgical Interventions

Many, but not all, transgender people will seek gender affirming medical or surgical treatments, or both, to align their physical appearance with their gender. Not all transgender people seek all interventions, and some may seek none; the standard of care is to allow each transgender person to seek only those interventions they desire to affirm their own gender identity. An individual's goals and expectations should be elicited before initiating treatment so that they can receive adequate counseling on options, expected outcomes, plan of care, and risks. When considering the risks of gender affirming treatment, the clinician must also consider the significant risks of withholding such treatment on the well-being of transgender patients, including detrimental effects on mental health, increased suicidality, and increased substance use.

Gender affirming treatments are recognized as medically necessary and essential services, shown to improve the well-being of transgender people in multiple psychosocial domains, including attendance at routine health maintenance. Gender affirming care is delivered in diverse settings by health professionals of many disciplines and specialties. Many treatments, including hormone therapy, can be provided in an informed-consent model by appropriately trained specialty and primary care clinicians competent in making the diagnosis of gender dysphoria. Mental health referral and treatment may be helpful for transgender people but is not a prerequisite for receiving gender affirming treatments. Referral to experienced providers or a multidisciplinary team may often be appropriate.

Many gender affirming treatments, including hormone therapy, impact the reproductive capacity of transgender people. Patients should be counseled on the reproductive implications of gender affirming treatments and options for fertility preservation.

Guidance on the management of gender affirming treatment is available from professional and specialty organizations along with publications from expert multidisciplinary clinics.

Bourns A. *Guidelines for Gender-Affirming Primary Care with Trans and Non-binary Patients*, 4th ed. Rainbow Health Ontario, 2019. https://www.rainbowhealthontario.ca/TransHealthGuide/

Coleman E et al. Standards of care for the health of transsexual, transgender, and gender-nonconforming people, version 7. Int J Transgenderism. 2012;13:165. https://doi.org/10.1080/15532739.2011.700873

Deutsch MB. *Guidelines for the Primary and Gender-Affirming Care of Transgender and Gender Nonbinary People*, 2nd ed. 2016. https://transcare.ucsf.edu/guidelines

Hembree WC et al. Endocrine treatment of gender-dysphoric/gender-incongruent persons: an Endocrine Society clinical practice guideline. J Clin Endocrinol Metab. 2017;102:3869. [PMID: 28945902]

Libman H et al. Caring for the transgender patient: grand rounds discussion from Beth Israel Deaconess Medical Center. Ann Intern Med. 2020;172:202. [PMID: 32016334]

T'Sjoen G et al. European Society for Sexual Medicine Position Statement: Assessment and hormonal management in adolescent and adult trans people, with attention for sexual function and satisfaction. J Sex Med. 2020;17:570. [PMID: 32111534]

A. Feminizing Hormone Therapy

The goals of feminizing hormone therapy include breast development, reduction of body hair, reduced muscle mass, and redistribution of body fat similar to that of cisgender women. The general approach of therapy is to obtain physiologic premenopausal cisgender female range estrogen and testosterone levels through the combined use of an estrogen with an androgen blocker, and in some cases a progestogen.

The most commonly used estrogen is 17-beta estradiol, in pill, patch, or injected form. The choice of route is based to some degree on patient preference (Table 42–2). Transdermal estradiol has a well-established safety profile based on studies in menopausal cisgender women. Injected estradiol is the least studied route and can be associated with both supratherapeutic levels as well as cyclical levels over the dosing interval. Estrogens should be continued after gonadectomy without reduction in dose. There is no direct evidence to guide decision-making regarding the discontinuation of estrogen once a patient arrives at a menopausal age, though most experts believe initiating or continuing hormone therapy in transfeminine persons after age 50 is appropriate. Ethinyl estradiol (found in hormonal contraceptives) should not be used due to excess thrombogenicity.

The most commonly used anti-androgen is spironolactone, a potassium-sparing diuretic that is frequently used for female hirsutism or adult acne. Spironolactone inhibits both the synthesis of and action of testosterone. In higher doses (100–200 mg orally daily), spironolactone can lead to suppression of androgen levels into the female physiologic range. Common side effects include orthostasis and polyuria. Monitoring should include periodic assessment of kidney function and serum potassium. Other options for those who cannot tolerate spironolactone include a gonadotropin-releasing hormone (GnRH) analog, orchiectomy, or the use of a progestogen. Finasteride and dutasteride (5-alpha-reductase inhibitors) are sometimes used as an alternative; however, they have limited effects. After gonadectomy, anti-androgens can be discontinued.

No studies have been conducted on the role of progestogens in transfeminine persons. Some believe there is benefit to breast development, mood, or libido. In cisgender women, progestins have been associated with an excess

Table 42–2. Feminizing hormone therapy.

Hormone Therapy	Dosage			Comments
	Initial, Low[1]	Initial, Typical	Maximum, Typical[2]	
Estrogen				
Estradiol oral/sublingual	1 mg/day	2–4 mg/day	8 mg/day	If > 2 mg is recommended, dose should be divided and taken twice daily.
Estradiol transdermal	50 mcg	100 mcg	100–400 mcg	Maximum available single patch dose is 100 mcg. Frequency of change is brand and product dependent. Patients may find that > 2 patches at a time are cumbersome.
Estradiol valerate, intramuscularly[3]	< 20 mg every 2 weeks	20 mg every 2 weeks	40 mg every 2 weeks	May divide dose into weekly injections for cyclical symptoms.
Estradiol cypionate, intramuscularly	< 2 mg every 2 weeks	2 mg every 2 weeks	5 mg every 2 weeks	May divide dose into weekly injections for cyclical symptoms.
Progestogen				
Medroxyprogesterone acetate (Provera)	2.5 mg orally each night at bedtime		5–10 mg orally each night at bedtime	
Micronized progesterone			100–200 mg orally each night at bedtime	
Androgen Blocker				
Spironolactone	25 mg orally daily	50 mg orally twice daily	200 mg orally twice daily	
Finasteride	1 mg orally daily		5 mg orally daily	
Dutasteride			0.5 mg orally daily	

[1]Initial low dosing for those who desire (or require due to medical history) a low dose or slow upward titration.
[2]Maximal effect does not necessarily require maximal dosing, as maximal doses do not necessarily represent a target or ideal dose. Dose increases should be based on patient response and monitored hormone levels.
[3]Available as standard US Pharmacopia (USP) as well as compounded products.

thromboembolism and breast cancer risk. Progestogens may be an effective anti-androgen, particularly cyproterone acetate, which is used widely outside the United States as the primary androgen blocker in feminizing regimens. If used, progestogens should be initiated after at least several months of estrogen plus anti-androgen as to mirror breast development in cisgender women.

The primary risk associated with estrogen therapy is venous thromboembolism (VTE). However, when using 17-beta estradiol at physiologic estrogen dosing, the risk is minimal. Prior studies showing 20- to 40-fold increased risk of VTE involved the use of ethinyl estradiol at doses of up to 200 mcg/day and did not control for tobacco use. More recent data found no increased risk of VTE in transfeminine persons using transdermal 17-beta estradiol. Thus, transdermal estradiol is the preferred route for those who use tobacco or with risk factors for or a personal history of VTE.

Totaro M et al. Risk of venous thromboembolism in transgender people undergoing hormone feminizing therapy: a prevalence meta-analysis and meta-regression study. Front Endocrinol (Lausanne). 2021;12:741866. [PMID: 34880832]

B. Masculinizing Hormone Therapy

The goals of masculinizing hormone therapy include facial and body hair growth, deepening of the voice, increased muscle mass, clitoral growth, induction of amenorrhea, and redistribution of body fat similar to that of cisgender men. The mainstay of therapy is administration of testosterone (Table 42–3). Blockade of estrogen is not needed; ovulation suppression, however, with or without progestogen treatment may be warranted to eliminate moliminal symptoms or in those with ongoing menses.

Testosterone may be injected (intramuscular or subcutaneous) or applied as a topical gel or patch. The use of daily topical testosterone or using a weekly (versus biweekly) injection interval can help maintain even hormone levels in those with cyclical mood symptoms or pelvic cramping.

Prior concerns of testosterone-induced hepatotoxicity were based on the use of oral methyltestosterone. There is no evidence to support a concern of hepatotoxicity in transmasculine persons using parenteral or topical testosterone.

Common side effects of testosterone therapy in transmasculine persons include acne and male pattern baldness, both of which can be approached as in cisgender men.

Table 42–3. Masculinizing hormone therapy.

Androgen	Dosage			Comment
	Initial, Low[1]	Initial, Typical	Maximum, Typical[2]	
Testosterone cypionate[3]	20 mg/week intramuscularly or subcutaneously	50 mg/week intramuscularly or subcutaneously	100 mg/week intramuscularly or subcutaneously	Double the dose for biweekly administration
Testosterone enthanate[3]	20 mg/week intramuscularly or subcutaneously	50 mg/week intramuscularly or subcutaneously	100 mg/week intramuscularly or subcutaneously	
Testosterone topical gel 1%	12.5–25 mg every morning	50 mg every morning	100 mg every morning	May come in pump or packet form
Testosterone topical gel 1.62%[4]	20.25 mg every morning	40.5–60.75 mg every morning	103.25 mg every morning	
Testosterone patch	1–2 mg every night	4 mg every night	8 mg every night	Patches come in 2-mg and 4-mg size. For lower doses, cut patch
Testosterone cream[5]	10 mg	50 mg	100 mg	
Testosterone axillary gel 2%	30 mg every morning	60 mg every morning	90–120 mg every morning	Comes in pump only; one pump = 30 mg
Testosterone undecanoate[6]	N/A	750 mg intramuscularly, repeat in 4 weeks, then every 10 weeks	N/A	Requires participation in manufacturer monitored program[6]

[1]Initial, low-dose regimen is recommended for genderqueer and nonbinary persons.
[2]Maximum dosing does not mean maximal effect. Furthermore, these dosage ranges do not necessarily represent a target or ideal dose. Dose increases or decreases should be based on patient response and monitored hormone levels.
[3]Available as standard US Pharmacopia (USP) as well as compounded products.
[4]Doses of less than 20.25 mg with 1.62% gel or less than 30 mg with 2% axillary gel may be difficult, since measuring one-half of a pump or packet can present a challenge. Patients requiring doses lower than 20.25 mg and whose insurance does not cover 1% gel may require prior authorization or an appeal.
[5]Testosterone creams are prepared by individual compounding pharmacies. Specific absorption and activity varies and consultation with the individual compounding pharmacist is recommended.
[6]Testosterone undecanoate has been associated with rare cases of pulmonary oil microembolism and anaphylaxis; in the United States, the drug is available only through the AVEED Risk Evaluation and Mitigation Strategy (REMS) Program (https://www.aveedrems.com/AveedUI/rems/preHome.action). All injections must be administered in an office or hospital setting by a trained and registered health care provider and monitored for 30 minutes afterward for adverse reactions.

Hemoglobin and hematocrit should be monitored, and if the levels are elevated, consider reducing testosterone dose or changing to a transdermal form or weekly injections to maintain more even levels. It is important to use cisgender male reference ranges for hemoglobin and hematocrit due to the erythropoietic effects of testosterone and frequent oligo- or amenorrheic status of transmasculine people. Polycystic ovarian syndrome and obesity have been found to be at an increased prevalence in transmasculine persons prior to beginning testosterone therapy. Testosterone is not contraindicated in the presence of these conditions; instead, related metabolic disorders can be managed concurrently.

C. Monitoring Hormone Therapy

Hormone effects should be monitored both by clinical results as well as hormone levels, if available. Patients should be reminded that results may vary and can take up to 5 years to reach maximal effect; supraphysiologic hormone levels are not likely to enhance results but may incur excess risk. Note that reported laboratory reference range values may differ depending on the recorded sex of the patient; in general, clinicians should use the reference ranges driven by the current hormonal status of the patient. For example, female reference ranges will be included on automated laboratory reports of a transmasculine person taking testosterone if still registered as female. The interpreting clinician should use the male reference ranges for any tests run on this patient that have sexually dimorphic reference ranges. Tables 42–4 and 42–5 describe general monitoring recommendations, rationales, and "sex-specific" laboratory values that may require individualized interpretation.

SoRelle JA et al. Impact of hormone therapy on laboratory values in transgender patients. Clin Chem. 2019;65:170. [PMID: 30518663]

D. Surgical Interventions

A wide range of surgical procedures are available to transgender people, including facial, chest, genital, and other procedures (Table 42–6). An increasing number of surgeries are being performed for gender affirmation;

Table 42–4. Laboratory monitoring for feminizing hormone therapy.

	Comments	Baseline	3 Months[1]	6 Months[1]	12 Months[1]	Yearly	As needed
BUN/creatinine/potassium	Only if spironolactone is used	X	X	X	X	X	
Lipids		X (if clinically indicated)		X	X		X
Hemoglobin A_{1C}		X		X	X	X	
Estradiol			X	X			X
Total testosterone			X	X	X		X
Sex hormone binding globulin (SHBG)[2]			X	X	X		X
Albumin[2]			X	X	X		X
Prolactin	Only if symptomatic						X

[1]In first year of therapy only.
[2]Used to calculate bioavailable testosterone (http://www.issam.ch/freetesto.htm).

complication rates are comparable to similar procedures performed for other indications.

Narayan SK et al. Gender confirmation surgery for the endocrinologist. Endocrinol Metab Clin North Am. 2019;48:403. [PMID: 31027548]

E. Long-Term Health Outcomes

The largest study of mortality among transgender people receiving gender affirming hormone therapy is a 2011 Dutch cohort of 966 transfeminine persons and 365 transmasculine persons. Importantly, this study did not control for a number of risk factors, including tobaccos use. All-cause as well as cardiovascular, cerebrovascular, and other disease-specific mortality among transmasculine persons did not differ from the general Dutch population of cisgender women. Among transfeminine persons, all-cause mortality was 51% higher than cisgender men in the general Dutch population, with the overwhelming majority of the difference due to HIV, drug overdose, and suicide; a 64% increased risk in cardiovascular mortality was seen; however, no significant difference was seen for cerebrovascular mortality. A retrospective cohort study of several thousand transmasculine and transfeminine persons enrolled in a large health plan in the United States found modest increases in cardiovascular, cerebrovascular, and venous thromboembolic events in transfeminine persons compared with a matched control group. Outcomes were not adjusted for dose or route of estrogen administration, however, and the absolute risk difference was low, with numbers needed to harm in the 80 to 120 range for various outcomes. No statistically significant difference was found in any of these outcomes in transmasculine persons compared with controls.

Asscheman H et al. A long-term follow-up study of mortality in transsexuals receiving treatment with cross-sex hormones. Eur J Endocrinol. 2011;164:635. [PMID: 21266549]
Getahun D et al. Cross-sex hormones and acute cardiovascular events in transgender persons: a cohort study. Ann Intern Med. 2018;169:205. [PMID: 29987313]

Table 42–5. Laboratory monitoring for masculinizing hormone therapy.

	Comments	Baseline[1]	3 Months[2]	6 Months[2]	12 Months[2]	Yearly	As Needed
Lipids	No evidence	X		X	X	X	X
Hemoglobin A_{1c} or fasting glucose		X		X	X	X	
Estradiol							X
Total testosterone			X	X	X		X
Albumin[3]			X	X	X		X
Hemoglobin and hematocrit		X	X	X	X	X	X

[1]Based on USPSTF guidelines.
[2]In first year of therapy only.
[3]Used to calculate bioavailable testosterone.

Table 42–6. Gender affirming procedures.

Surgical interventions
Voice surgery
Facial surgery (feminization/masculinization procedures)
Thyrochondroplasty (tracheal cartilage shave/augmentation)
Vulvoplasty, vaginoplasty
Phalloplasty, scrotoplasty, metoidioplasty, vaginectomy (including placement of penile/testicular prostheses)
Chest surgery (augmentation/mastectomy, also referred to as "top surgery")
Augmentation mammoplasty
Hysterectomy, salpingectomy
Gonadectomy (orchiectomy, oophorectomy)
Body contouring
Other interventions
Facial and body hair removal (laser hair removal and electrolysis)
Voice therapy and modification
Genital tucking and packing
Chest binding

Cancer Risk & Screening

Several retrospective studies have not identified an increased risk of cancer in transgender people compared with birth sex–matched controls. However, because of the numerous barriers to care as well as to identifying transgender people in clinical databases, underscreening and underreporting are likely. In general, an organ-based approach to screening should be taken. There are no modifications to screening recommendations (or recommendations not to screen) for ovarian, uterine, or cervical cancer in transmasculine persons. Breast cancer screening for transmasculine people who have not undergone mastectomy should be performed based on guidelines for cisgender women. The role of screening for breast cancer in transmasculine people who have undergone mastectomy is unknown and depends on the technique used as well as technical limitations on screening small amounts of residual breast tissue. In transfeminine people, breast cancer screening using guidelines for cisgender women is recommended, with the modifications starting at age 50 years and only after a minimum of 5 years of lifetime estrogen exposure. Screening for prostate cancer in transfeminine people is complicated beyond the current debate over the utility of prostate cancer screening in cisgender men by the effects of feminizing hormones on prostatic hypertrophy and interpretation of tests of prostate-specific antigen.

Cathcart-Rake EJ et al. Cancer in transgender patients: one case in 385,820 is indicative of a paucity of data. J Oncol Pract. 2018;14:270. [PMID: 29257720]

Deutsch MB. *Guidelines for the Primary and Gender-Affirming Care of Transgender and Gender Nonbinary People*, 2nd ed. 2016. https://transcare.ucsf.edu/guidelines

HIV

Disproportionately high rates of HIV infection among transgender people exist worldwide and the largest burden of these infections is among transfeminine people and transgender people of color; the lack of targeted HIV-prevention strategies for transgender communities may be one factor contributing to these disparities. Studies of pharmacologic PrEP demonstrate acceptability and efficacy among transgender people; compared with cisgender MSM, however, adherence to PrEP was lower in transgender women and uptake and knowledge was lower among all transgender people. Modest interactions may exist between antiretroviral drugs, including PrEP agents, and gender affirming hormone therapy; more research is needed to understand the possible clinical implications of these findings. Disparities also exist in treatment of HIV, with transfeminine persons less likely to report receiving antiretroviral treatment and to remain in care. Transgender people likely benefit from HIV prevention and treatment services integrated into other gender affirming care.

Poteat TC et al. HIV Antiretroviral treatment and pre-exposure prophylaxis in transgender individuals. Drugs. 2020;80:965. [PMID: 32451925]

Stutterheim SE et al. The worldwide burden of HIV in transgender individuals: an updated systematic review and meta-analysis. PLoS One. 2021;16:e0260063. [PMID: 34851961]

Index

NOTE: Page numbers in **boldface** type indicate a major discussion. A *t* following a page number indicates tabular material, and *f* following a page number indicates a figure. Drugs are listed under their generic names.

2-PAM, 1579, 1589
"3" sign, 325
4-Methylpyrazole, 1586
5-Alpha-reductase inhibitors, 966. *See also specific types*
5-FC. *See* Flucytosine
5-$HT_{1b/1d}$ receptor agonists, 971. *See also specific types*
5-HT_{1F} receptor agonist, 971
5-HT_3 receptor, 1655
5q loss, isolated, 526
6-MP, *TPMT* on metabolism of, 1670*t*
17-beta estradiol, feminizing hormone therapy, 1726
25-OH vitamin D, 1145. *See also* Vitamin D
45,XO/46,XX & 45,XO/35,XY mosaicism, **1193**
45,XO gonadal dysgenesis, **1191–1193**
46,X (abnormal X) karyotype, **1193**
46,XY disorders of sexual development, 1184

A
A3243G mutation, diabetes mellitus, 1197
Abacavir, **1339*t*, 1343**
- hepatotoxicity, 696
- HLA-B*5701 allele on toxicity of, 1670*t*
- myocardial infarction from, 1330

Abaloparatide, 1151, 1194
Abametapir, 131
Abatacept, 831, 860
ABCB4, 676*t*
ABCB11, 676*t*
ABCC2, 676*t*
ABCD, antihypertensive classes, 465
ABCD²I score, 987
ABCD² score, 987
ABCDE, skin cancer, 109*f*, 110
Abdominal abscess, initial antimicrobial therapy, 654, 1296*t*
Abdominal aortic aneurysm, 5*t*, 6, 42, **482–484**, 1465
Abdominal fistula, Crohn disease, 654
Abdominal infections, gram-negative, 1472
Abdominal pain, 80, 181. *See also specific disorders*
Abemaciclib, 752, 754, 757–758
Abeparvovec, hepatotoxicity, 696
Abetalipoproteinemia, vitamin E deficiency, 1262
Abiraterone (acetate), 1601*t*, 1640, 1640*t*, 1641
Abnormal illness disorder, **1053–1055**
Abnormal uterine bleeding, **763–765**, 764*t*
Abortion, **780**
- complete, 798
- incomplete, 798
- missed, 798
- prevalence, 773
- spontaneous, **797–799**
  - inevitable, 798
  - threatened, 798

Abortive poliomyelitis, 1374
Abscess. *See specific types*
Absence seizures, 979
Absidia, 221–222, 1544
Absorptive hypercalciuria, 956
Abuse
- elder, **67–68**, 68*t*
- opioid, 85, 86

Academy of Nutrition and Dietetics Criteria, 1250
Acalabrutinib, 531, 535, 1600*t*
Acalculous cholecystitis, 721
Acamprosate
- for alcohol-associated liver disease, 694
- for at-risk drinking, 1089

Acanthamoeba keratitis, **180**
Acanthosis nigricans, 1197, 1200, 1200*f*, 1216, 1237
Acarbose, 1204*t*, 1208, **1582**
Accelerated idioventricular rhythm, 379, 399
Acceptance and commitment therapy, 1052, 1057, 1068
Accessory atrioventricular pathways, paroxysmal supraventricular tachycardia from, **390–391**
Accidental systemic hypothermia, **1550–1552**, 1551*f*
Acclimatization, high-altitude, 1561, 1562
Accreta, 807
Accumulation, speed of, effusion, 429
Acebutolol, 461*t*, **1577–1578**
ACE inhibitors. *See* Angiotensin-converting enzyme inhibitors
Acellular pertussis vaccine, 1459
Acesulfame potassium, 1203
Acetaminophen
- adverse effects
  - anion gap elevation, 897
  - eosinophilic pulmonary syndromes, 297
  - hepatotoxicity, 82, 696
    - nomogram, 1572, 1572*f*
  - medication overuse headache, 974
  - tubulointerstitial disease, 937
- for low back pain, 1685
- mechanism of action, 79
- for migraine headache, 971
- number-needed-to-treat, 79
- for osteoarthritis, 821
- overdose
  - acetylcysteine for, 685
  - acute liver failure, **684–686**
  - anion gap elevation, 1570
- for pain, **82, 83*t***
- poisoning, 1568*t*, **1571–1573**, 1571*t*, 1572*f*, 1572*t*

Acetazolamide, 954, 1004
Acetohexamide, 1204*t*, 1206
Acetonitrile, 1579
Acetylcysteine, 685
Acetylsalicylic acid. *See* Aspirin
Achalasia, **618–619**
Acid
- eye injury, **198**
- poisoning, **1573**

Acid-base disorders, **894–902**. *See also specific types*
- anion gap acidosis
  - increased, **895–897**
  - normal, **897–899**, 897*t*
- chronic kidney disease, 918
- evaluation, 894, 894*b*
- ion gap, serum, 895
- metabolic acidosis, 895, 895*t*
- metabolic alkalosis, 895*t*, **899–901**, 900*t*, 901
  - chloride-responsive, 900–901, 900*t*
  - chloride-unresponsive, 900–901, 900*t*
- mixed, 894
- pathophysiology & analysis, 894–895, 894*b*, 895*t*
- primary, 894
- respiratory acidosis, 895*t***901**
- respiratory alkalosis, 895*t*, **901–902**, 901*t*

Acid maltase deficiency, **1044**
Acidosis
- anion gap
  - increased, **895–897**
  - normal, **897–899**, 897*t*
- hyperchloremic, normal anion gap, 896*t*, **897–898**
  - RTA type I, 897*t*, 898
  - RTA type II, 897*t*, 898
  - RTA type IV, hyporeninemic hypoaldosteronemic, 897*t*, 898
- metabolic, 895, 895*t*
  - acute kidney injury, 906
  - anion gap, 1570
  - drowning, 1554
  - hyperchloremic, normal anion gap, 896*t*, **897–898**, 897*t*
  - ketoacidosis, 896–897, 896*t*
  - lactic, 895–896, 896*t*
  - posthypercapneic, 900
- respiratory, 895*t*, **901**
- uremic, 897

Acinetobacter, 275, 1294*t*
Acitretin
- for lichen planus, 141
- for pityriasis rubra pilaris, 155
- for psoriasis, 137, 155

Aclidinium, 262
Acne
- female
  - contraception for, 774
  - danazol for, 768
  - polycystic ovary syndrome, 771
- steroid, 124

Acne vulgaris, **147–149**, 148*f*
Acoustic neuroma, 217–218
Acquired amegakaryocytic thrombocytopenia, 546
Acquired aplastic anemia, bone marrow failure, 546
Acquired immunodeficiency syndrome. *See* HIV/AIDS
Acquired platelet function disorders, **557**
Acquired protein C deficiency, portal vein thrombosis, 715
Acral lentiginous melanoma, 110
ACR Appropriateness Criteria, 1558–1559
Acromegaly, **1106–1107**, 1182
Acropachy, thyroid, 1121, 1127
ACTH-induced Cushing syndrome, 1182
Actinic dermatitis, chronic, 155

Actinic keratoses, **110–111,** 111*f*
Actinic prurigo, 155
Actinomyces (actinomycosis), 717, 1294*t*, **1473–1474**
Actinomyces israelii, **1473–1474**
Actinomycetoma, **1546**
Activated charcoal, 1568–1569
Active external rewarming, 1551
Active immunity, 1301
Activities of daily living assessment, older adult, 53
Acupuncture, 972*t*, 973, 1685
Acute adrenal crisis, 1157, 1158
Acute angle-closure crisis, 180
Acute angle-closure glaucoma, 170*t*, 177*t*–178*t*, **180–181**
Acute anterior uveitis, **183–184**
Acute bacterial prostatitis, **949–950,** 950*t*
Acute cardiogenic liver injury, **715**
Acute chest syndrome, sickle cell anemia, 512
Acute confusional state, 1095
Acute coronary syndrome, 22–25, 436–437
Acute coronary syndrome, without ST-segment elevation, **368–372**
  classification, 368
  clinical findings, 368–369
  treatment, 369–372
    anticoagulants, 370*t*, 371
    antiplatelet therapy, 369–371
      discontinuation for procedures, 371
    beta-blockers, 371, 461*t*–462*t*
    calcium channel blockers, 371–372
    coronary angiography, indications, 372, 372*t*
    general, 369
    initial, algorithm, 370*f*
    nitroglycerin, 371
    statins, 372
Acute eosinophilic pneumonia, 297
Acute fatty liver of pregnancy, 685, **817–818**
Acute generalized exanthematous pustulosis, **871–872**
Acute heart failure, **403–412.** *See also* Heart failure
  clinical findings, 404–406
  left, 403, 404
  pulmonary edema and, **413–414**
  right, 403, 404
  stages, 404
  treatment, **406–412,** 406*f*, 407*t*
    with preserved LVEF, 412
    with reduced LVEF, 406–412, 406*f*
    sodium restriction, 419
  ventricular septal defects, 329
Acute hemorrhagic necrotizing encephalopathy, COVID-19, 1404
Acute hypoxia, 1560
Acute idiopathic polyneuropathy, **1033–1034.** *See also* Guillain-Barré syndrome
Acute inflammatory pericarditis, **426–429**
Acute intermittent porphyria, 1031, **1658–1659,** 1659*t*
Acute interstitial pneumonia, 294*t*
Acute ischemic stroke, 469, 470*t*
Acute kidney injury, 903, **906–913**
  acute tubular necrosis, 907*t*, **908–910**
    ischemic, 908
    nephrotoxins, 908–909
  cardiorenal syndrome, **913**
  classification & differential diagnosis, 906–908, 907*t*
  clinical findings, 906
  COVID-19, **913,** 1404
  definition & stages, 906
  glomerulonephritis, 907*t*, **912–913**
  hyperkalemia, 885
  interstitial nephritis, 907*t*, **911–912**
  intrinsic, 907*t*, 908
  nephrogenic systemic fibrosis, **942**
  from peritonitis, spontaneous bacterial, 605
  postoperative, 50–51, 51*t*
  postrenal causes, 907*t*, 908
  prerenal azotemia, 906, 907–908, 907*t*
  rhabdomyolysis, 883, **910–911**
  uremia, 906, 908
Acute leukemia, **528–530**
Acute liver failure, **684–686,** 1368
Acute Liver Failure Early Dynamic model, 686
Acute Liver Failure Study Group index, 686
Acute lung injury, transfusion-related, 544
Acute lymphoblastic leukemia, **528–530,** 1595*t*
Acute mesenteric ischemia, **480–481**
Acute mesenteric vein occlusion, **481**
Acute motor and sensory axonal neuropathy, 1033
Acute motor axonal neuropathy, 1033
Acute mountain sickness, **1560–1562**
Acute myeloid leukemia, 510, **528–530,** 1595*t*
Acute myocardial infarction. *See* Myocardial infarction, acute
Acute-on-chronic liver failure, 700
Acute otitis media, **209,** 209*f*, 212
Acute pain, **79–80**
Acute pain syndromes, 1055
Acute Physiology and Chronic Health Evaluation, 729
Acute polymorphic ventricular tachycardia, 385*t*, 395–396, **399, 401**
Acute promyelocytic leukemia, **528–530**
Acute radiation syndrome, 1558–1559
Acute respiratory distress syndrome, **319–321**
  COVID-19–related, 1403
  disorders with, 320, 320*t*
  from gastric contents aspiration, 305
  pancreatitis, 731
Acute respiratory failure, **317–319**
Acute severe headache, 974
Acute tubular necrosis, 730, 904, 907*t*, **908–910**
Acyclovir, 1356*t*
  acute tubular necrosis from, 909
  for herpes simplex, 120–121, 1327
  for herpes zoster, 1327
  for trigeminal neuralgia, 978
  for varicella, 814, 1356*t*, 1360, 1361
Adalimumab
  for Crohn disease, 656–657
  infections with, 1273
  for inflammatory bowel disease, 651–652
  for psoriasis, 137
  for rheumatoid arthritis, 830–831
  for ulcerative colitis, 660–661
ADAMTS-13, thrombotic microangiopathy, 551
Adapalene, 148
Adaptive capacity, 1046
Addiction. *See* Substance use disorder; *specific substances*
Addison disease, **1156–1160**
  endocrine shock, 496
  hyperkalemia, 885–886
  hyperpigmentation, 163
  myopathy, 1045
Addisonian crisis, 1157, 1158
Adefovir, 687–688
Adenocarcinoma. *See also specific types*
  anus, 1633–1634
  bronchogenic, 1603
  endometrium, **791**
  esophageal, 1617
  gastric, **1620–1622**
  nasopharyngeal, 226
  small intestine, **1625**
  small intestine bleeding, 601
Adenocarcinoma in situ, bronchogenic, 1603
Adenoma, **665.** *See also specific types*
  adrenal, 1165–1167
  ear, **207**
  hepatocellular, **718**
  Islet of Langerhans, 1233
  pituitary, 998*t*
    anterior hypopituitarism, 1099
    nonfunctioning, **1110–1111**
Adenoma sebaceum, 1005
Adenomatous polyposis, familial, **667**
Adenomyomatosis, 720*t*, 721
Adenomyosis, pelvic pain, 769
Adenosine, 383, 385*t*
Adenovirus, **1418–1419.** *See also specific types and disorders*
  conjunctivitis/keratoconjunctivitis, 170
  diarrhea, 590
  hematopoietic cell transplant recipients, 1273
  pneumonia, community-acquired, 270
  serotypes & syndromes, 1418
  vectors, gene therapy, 1418
Adenovirus B14, 1418
Adherence, patient, 1–2
Adhesive capsulitis, 1225, 1677*t*, **1682–1683**
Adjustment disorders, **1046–1047,** 1069
Ado-trastuzumab, 1672*t*
Adrenal adenoma, unilateral, 1165–1167
Adrenal carcinomas, 1161, 1181
Adrenal cortex disorders, **1156–1166.** *See also specific types*
  adrenal insufficiency, primary, **1156–1160**
  aldosteronism, primary, **1164–1166**
  Cushing syndrome, **1160–1164**
Adrenal crisis, 496, 1157, 1158
Adrenal hyperplasia, bilateral, 1164, 1166
Adrenal incidentalomas, 1171
Adrenal infiltrative diseases, 1157
Adrenal insufficiency, **1156–1160**
  17-hydroxyprogesterone, low serum, 1184
  central, 1101
  endocrine shock, 496
  hypotonic hyponatremia, **878**
  primary, **1156–1160**
Adrenal masses, incidentally discovered, **1171**
Adrenal tumors, 1181. *See also specific types*
Adrenocorticotropic hormone, 1099
  Cushing syndrome from, 1182
  deficiency, 1101, **1156–1160**
Adrenoleukodystrophy, 1157
Adriamycin. *See* Doxorubicin
Aducanumab, 1016–1017
Advance care planning, **71–72,** 1715–1716
Advance directives, **71**
Advance financial planning, dementia, 57
Adverse children experiences, **1710**
Adverse drug reactions. *See also specific drugs and types*
  drug allergy, **870**
  non–IgE-mediated anaphylactic, **870**
  older adults, 66
  radiocontrast media reactions, **870**
  vancomycin flushing syndrome, **870**
Advisory Committee on Immunization Practices, 3, 4*t*
Adynamic bone disease, chronic kidney disease, 917, 917*f*
Aerobic exercise. *See also* Exercise/exercise therapy
  for dementia, 1017
  for menopausal symptoms, 1186
Aeromonas diarrhea, 1292
Aerophagia, 588
Afatinib, on non–small cell lung cancer, *EGFR* mutations, 1672*t*
Aflatoxin, gallbladder cancer, 1612

African Americans. *See also specific topics*
angiotensin II receptor blockers for, 454
hypertension treatment, drug, 466*t*, 467, 467*t*
African trypanosomiasis, **1496–1497,** 1497*t*
Afterload, 338, 348
Age-related hearing loss, 204, **212**
Age-related macular degeneration, 52, 67, **187**
Age-related refractive error, 67
Aggression disorders, **1084–1085**
Aggressive lymphomas, 534–535
Aging. *See* Older adults
Agitated delirium, 70–71
Agitation, 49, 70–71
Agoraphobia, 1049, 1051–1052
Agranulocytosis, from clozapine, 1066–1067
AGS Beers Criteria, 66
Aguesia, COVID-19, 1404
Aid in dying, 76
AIDS. *See* HIV/AIDS
AIDS myelopathy, **1026, 1323**
Aid to Capacity Evaluation, 68
Air pollution, 245, 259
Air swallowing, 588
Air trapping
asthma, 246
bronchial obstruction, 245
bronchiolitis, 268
COPD, 259
Air travel
barotrauma, **208**
lower extremity edema prevention, 29
safety & patient selection, **1562–1563**
Airways disorders, **244–268.** *See also specific types*
allergic bronchopulmonary aspergillosis, **265–266**
asthma, **245–258**
bronchiectasis, **265**
bronchiolitis, **267–268**
chronic obstructive pulmonary disease, **258–264,** 260*t*
cystic fibrosis, **266–267**
dyspnea, **18–20**
lower airways, **244–245**
bronchial obstruction, 245
tracheal obstruction, 244
tracheal stenosis, 244–245
upper airways, **244**
obstruction
acute, 244
chronic, 244
vocal fold dysfunction syndrome, 244
Akathisia, 1067, 1075
AL amyloidosis, 423–424, 936
Al-Anon, 1088
Albendazole
for angiostrongyliasis, 1529
for ascariasis, 1526
for clonorchiasis, 1522
for cutaneous larva migrans, 1530
for cysticercosis, 1524
for echinococcosis, 1525
for enterobiasis, 1529
for filariasis, lymphatic, 1531–1532
for giardiasis, 1519
for hookworm disease, 1527
for neurocysticercosis, 1524
for opisthorchiasis, 1522
for sarcocystosis, 1518
for strongyloidiasis, 1528
for trichuriasis, 1526–1527
+ ivermectin, 1526–1527
Albinism, 163
Albumin, glycated, 1201
Albuterol
for asthma, 249, 251, 252*t*
for COPD, 262, 263
for cystic fibrosis, 267
Alclometasone, 134, 139
Alclometasone dipropionate, 102*t*, 139
Alcohol-associated liver disease, **693–695**
Alcoholic hallucinosis, 1087, 1089, 1096
Alcoholic hepatitis, 47, 603
Alcoholic ketoacidosis, 896*t*, 897, 1570
Alcoholics Anonymous, 1078, 1088
Alcoholism. *See* Alcohol use/alcohol use disorder
Alcohols, sugar, 1203
Alcohol use/alcohol use disorder, **12,** 1086, **1086–1092,** 1090*t*
acute liver failure, 685
alcohol misuse, 1086
Alcohol Use Disorder Identification Test, 12–13, 13*t*, 1087
atrial fibrillation, 391, 392
at-risk drinking, 1086–1087
bone marrow failure, 546
cardiomyopathy, 404, 414, 418*t*, 419
classification, 1086
clinical findings
acute intoxication, 1087
alcoholic hallucinosis, 1087, 1096
chronic brain syndromes, 1087–1088
Korsakoff psychosis, 1087–1088
Wernicke encephalopathy, 1087
withdrawal & DTs, 1087, 1091
colorectal cancer and, 1627
complications, 1088
coronary heart disease, 355
differential diagnosis, 1088
drink, defined, 1086
Dupuytren contracture, 1691
epistaxis, 224
erosive gastritis/gastropathy, **620–622**
fibrocystic condition, 737
gout from, 823
gouty arthritis from, 826
hazardous, 12
heart failure, 404
hepatitis, 47, 603
hepatitis C, 689
hypertension, 444, 448*t*
hypoglycemia, 1091, 1233
hypoglycemia, with insulin therapy, 1220
hypokalemia, 893
hypomagnesemia, 893
hypophosphatemia, 1153
lesbian & bisexual women, 1716, 1717
lipid metabolism, 1241
lower esophageal sphincter, 306
Mallory-Weiss syndrome, 582, **613–614**
myocardial depression, 406
myocarditis, 417
myopathy, 1045
niacin deficiency, 1260
nutritional deficiency, polyneuropathy, **1032**
oral cancer, 227
osmotic demyelination, 880
osteonecrosis, 868
pancreatitis, 733
pregnancy, 795
prevention, **12–13,** 13*t*
salivary gland disorders, 235
screening, **12–13, 13*t***
seizures, 1567
sinus tachycardia, 355–356
thiamine deficiency, **1032,** 1259–1260
withdrawal, 1087, 1091
atrial fibrillation, 391
seizures, 1567
sinus tachycardia, 386
stress cardiomyopathy, 420
supraventricular arrhythmias, 387
syndrome, 1087
Alcohol use/alcohol use disorder, treatment
at-risk drinking
behavioral, 1089
medical, 1088–1089
psychological, 1088
social, 1088
hallucinosis, 1089
neuromodulatory therapy, 97*t*
psychological and social measures, 1092
upper GI bleeding, 596
withdrawal, 1089–1092, 1090*f*
benzodiazepines, 1050*t*, 1051
CIWA-Ar score based, 1089–1091
drying out, 1089
DTs, 1087, 1091
hospitalization, 1089
medications, 1089
other withdrawal-associated conditions, 1091–1092
seizures, 983
severity, assessing, 1089, 1090*f*
Alcohol Use Disorder Identification Test, 12–13, 13*t*, 1087
Aldicarb poisoning, **1588–1589**
Aldosterone, 468, 883
Aldosterone receptor antagonists, 378, **455,** 458*t*–459*t*. *See also specific types*
Aldosteronism
familial type 1, saccular aneurysm, 994
glucocorticoid-remediable, hypertension, 445
primary, **1164–1166**
Alectinib, 1600*t*, 1606
Alemtuzumab
hepatotoxicity, 696
for multiple sclerosis, 1025*t*
progressive multifocal leukoencephalopathy from, 1387
thyroiditis from, silent, 1115
Alendronate
for osteoporosis, 1150
peptic ulcer disease, 625
pill-induced esophagitis from, 613
Alfieri stitch, 422
Alfuzosin, 952, 965–966, 965*t*
Alimentary tract cancer, **1617–1634.** *See also specific types*
anus, carcinoma of, **1633–1634**
colorectal cancer, **1627–1633**
esophageal, **1617–1619**
gastric
adenocarcinoma, **1620–1622**
lymphoma, **1622–1623**
neuroendocrine tumors, **1623–1624**
gastrointestinal mesenchymal tumors, **1624–1625**
small intestine, **1625–1627**
adenocarcinomas, **1625**
intestinal neuroendocrine tumors, **1626–1627**
lymphomas, **1625**
sarcoma, **1627**
Alirocumab, 8, 358, 1245*t*, 1246–1247
Aliskiren, 451*t*, 454, **454**
ALK, lung cancer, 1606
Alkalies
eye injury, **198**
poisoning, **1573–1574**
Alkaline phosphatase, 675, 677*t*
Alkalosis
metabolic, 895*t*, **899–901,** 900*t*
chloride-responsive, 900–901, 900*t*
chloride-unresponsive, 900–901, 900*t*
respiratory, 895*t*, **901–902,** 901*t*

Alkhurma hemorrhagic fever, 1383
ALK tyrosine kinase inhibitors, 1606. *See also specific types*
Alkylating agents. *See also specific types*
leukemia from, 528
nitrogen mustards, 1598*t*
bendamustine, 1598*t*
cyclophosphamide, 1598*t*
ifosfamide, 1598*t*
platinum analogs, 1598*t*
carboplatin, 1598*t*
cisplatin, 1598*t*
oxaliplatin, 1598*t*
triazenes, 1598*t*
Allergen, 870. *See also specific disorders and allergens*
Allergic, 158*t*
Allergic asthma, 245
Allergic bronchopulmonary aspergillosis, **265–266, 1543–1544**
Allergic conjunctivitis, 172
Allergic disorders, **868–870**. *See also specific types*
adverse drug reactions
drug allergy, **870**
non–IgE-mediated anaphylactic, **870**
radiocontrast media, **870**
vancomycin flushing syndrome, **870**
delayed drug hypersensitivity, **30,** 157, 696, **871–872**
eye, **172**
corneal ulcer, 179
immediate hypersensitivity, **868–870,** 869*t*
rhinitis, 15, 16, **222–223**
vasculitis, 158*t*
Allergic & immunologic disorders, **868–874**
adverse drug reactions
drug allergy, **870**
non–IgE-mediated anaphylactic drug reactions, **870**
radiocontrast media reactions, **870**
vancomycin flushing syndrome, **870**
delayed drug hypersensitivity, **871–872**
acute generalized exanthematous pustulosis, **871–872**
aspirin- and NSAID-exacerbated respiratory disease, 245, **872**
drug exanthems, **871**
drug-induced hypersensitivity syndrome, **871**
drug reaction with eosinophilia and systemic symptoms, **30,** 157, 696, **871**
severe cutaneous adverse reactions, **871–872**
Stevens-Johnson syndrome/toxic epidermal necrolysis, 871
immediate hypersensitivity, **868–870**
anaphylaxis, **869–870,** 869*t*
food allergy, **868**
IgE-mediated, **870**
non–IgE-mediated, **870**
venom allergy, **868–869**
primary immunodeficiency disorders, adult, **872–874,** 872*t*
common variable immunodeficiency, **873–874**
complement disorders, 872*t*
Good syndrome, 872*t*
granulocyte disorders, 872*t*
hereditary angioedema, 872*t*
hypogammaglobulinemia, secondary, **874**
immunoglobulin subclass deficiency, **874**
selective IgA deficiency, **873**
specific (functional) antibody deficiency, **874**
Allodynia, 85
Allopregnanolone, 1077
Allopurinol
on azathioprine metabolism, 826
for cancer, 1653*t*
for cutaneous leishmaniasis, 1501
drug eruptions from, 157–158
drug interactions, 826
for gout, 942
for gouty arthritis, 825–826
HLA-B*5801 allele on toxicity of, 1670*t*
hypersensitivity, 825
for hyperuricemia, 1652
for hyperuricosuric calcium nephrolithiasis, 956
interstitial nephritis from, 911
Allow Natural Death, 72
Almotriptan, 971
Alogliptin, 1205*t,* 1210
Alopecia, **164–165**
androgenetic, 164–165
nonscarring, **164–165**
scarring, **165**
Alopecia areata, 165
Alopecia totalis, 165
Alopecia universalis, 165
Alosetron, 647, 1655
Alpelisib, 758, 1197
Alpha-1-antiprotease deficiency, COPD, 259
Alpha-1-antitrypsin
deficiency
bronchiectasis, **265**
COPD, 259
human, for COPD, 263
Alpha-adrenergic agonists. *See specific types*
Alpha-adrenergic antagonists (alpha blockers). *See also specific types*
for benign prostatic hyperplasia, 965–966, 965*t*
floppy iris syndrome from, 185, 199
for hypertension, **460,** 463*t*
ocular effects, adverse, 199, 200*t*
Alpha-fetoprotein, hepatocellular carcinomas, 1610, 1611
Alpha-gal hypersensitivity, 868
Alpha-globin gene, 504
Alpha-glucosidase, 1044
Alpha-glucosidase inhibitor poisoning, **1582**
5-Alpha-reductase inhibitors, 966. *See also specific types*
Alpha-thalassemia syndromes, **504–506,** 504*t*
Alpha-thalassemia trait, 505, 506
Alphavirus, 1379
Alprazolam, 1006, 1050*t,* 1051, **1581–1582**
Alprenolol poisoning, **1577–1578**
Alprostadil, 1223
Alteplase
for acute MI with ST-segment, 375–376, 376*t*
for pulmonary venous thromboembolism, 300
for stroke, 991
Alternaria, 1546–1547
Alternating current, 1557
Altitude disorders, **1559–1563**
air travel safety & patient selection, **1562–1563**
dysbarism & decompression sickness, 868, **1559–1560**
high-altitude illness, **1560–1562**
Altitude sickness, **1560–1562**
Aluminum, osteomalacia from, 917, 1153
Aluminum hydroxide, 917
Aluminum subacetate, 117
Alveolar hemorrhage syndromes, **303–304**
Alveolitis, 292, **307–308,** 307*t*
Alzheimer disease, 57, 446, 1015*t,* 1023
Amanita phalloides, 685, 696, 1565
Amantadine
for dyskinesia from antipsychotics, 1068
for echovirus, 1425
for Huntington disease, 1011
for Parkinson disease, 1007–1008
for parkinsonism, drug-induced, 1067
Amatoxin mushroom poisoning, 1587
Amaurosis fugax, 190, 478, 848, 989
Ambrisentan, 705, 841
Ambulatory ECG monitoring. *See* Electrocardiography, ambulatory monitoring
Amebiasis, 590, **716–717, 1513–1515,** 1515*t*
Amegakaryocytic thrombocytopenia, 546
Amegakaryocytic thrombocytopenia, acquired, 546
Amenorrhea
primary, **1184–1185**
secondary, **1185–1186**
American Indians, gallstones, 719
American Society for Parenteral and Enteral Nutrition, 1250
American trypanosomiasis, 25, 418, 619, **1498–1499**
Amifampridine, 1042
Amikacin, 145, 1475
Amiloride, 458*t,* 459*t,* 702, 886, 917
Aminocaproic acid, myopathy from, 1045
Aminoglutethimide, 1640*t*
Aminoglycosides. *See also specific types*
acute tubular necrosis from, 908–909
neuromuscular transmission disorders, **1042**
ototoxicity, 213
for prostatitis, 947*t,* 950
for pyelonephritis, 947*t,* 949
5-Aminosalicylic acid
for Crohn disease, 655
for inflammatory bowel disease, 649–650
for ulcerative colitis, 659–660
Amino transferase, serum, 675, 677*t*
Amiodarone, 383, 384*t*
for atrial fibrillation, 396
autoimmune thyroiditis from, 1112
goiter from, 1115
hepatotoxicity, 696
hyperthyroidism from, 1120
hypothyroidism from, 1115
myopathy from, 1045
thyroid storm from, 1120
Amitriptyline
for depression, 1073*t*
for diabetic neuropathy pain, 1222
for interstitial cystitis, 954
for migraine headache, 972*t*
for neuropathic pain, **91*t*,** 95
for tension-type headache prophylaxis, 973
for trigeminal neuralgia, 978
Amlodipine
for angina pectoris, 363
for hypertension, 451*t,* 452*t,* 453*t,* 457*t*
poisoning, **1578**
for Raynaud phenomenon, 839
Ammonia, hepatic encephalopathy, 704–705
Amnestic syndrome, 1096
Amniotomy, mothers with HIV/AIDS, 815
Amodiaquine, 1504*t,* 1506
Amoebic keratitis, **180**
Amoxapine, 1073*t*
Amoxicillin
for actinomycosis, 1474
for *Haemophilus,* 1461
for Lyme disease, 1494, 1495*t*
for peptic ulcer disease, 624*t*
for pneumococcal pneumonia, 1444
for rosacea, 150
for *Staphylococcus aureus,* 1441, 1441*t*

Amoxicillin/clavulanate
for animal bites, 1284
for cystitis, 947*t*
for diarrhea, diabetic, 1223
hepatotoxicity, 696
for *Moraxella catarrhalis,* 1461
Amoxicillin/clavulanic acid
for chest infections, anaerobic, 1472
for organ anaerobes, 1472
for peritonitis, spontaneous bacterial, 703
Amphetamines. *See also specific types*
abuse, **1093–1094**
for attention-deficit/hyperactivity disorders, 1081
chorea from, 1012
hypertension from, 1566
myocarditis from, 415*t*
poisoning, **1574**
on pregnancy, 795
pulmonary hypertension from, 432
sympathomimetic syndrome from, 1570
Amphotericin
for cryptococcal meningitis, 1318*t*, 1322
for fusarosis, 1546
Amphotericin B, 1539*t*
acute tubular necrosis from, 909
for candida endocarditis, 535
for *Candida glabrata,* 1535
for coccidioidomycosis, 1538, 1539*t*
for sporotrichosis, 1546
for visceral leishmaniasis, 1500–1501
Amphotericin B, liposomal, 1539*t*
for blastomycosis, 1545
for cryptococcosis, 1542–1543
for histoplasmosis, 1536
for mucormycosis, 1545
Amphotericin B lipid complex, 1539*t*
Ampicillin
for chorioamnionitis, 808
for enterococcus, 1443
eosinophilic pulmonary syndromes from, 297
for Group D streptococcus, endocarditis, 1457
hypersensitivity, 1300
for listeriosis, 1453
for prostatitis, 947*t*, 950, 951
for pyelonephritis, 947*t*, 949
for *Salmonella* carriers, 1464
for typhus, endemic, 1429
for UTI, pregnancy, 813
for *Vibrio,* 1467
Ampicillin-sulbactam
for *Bacteroides fragilis,* 1472
for chest infections, anaerobic, 1472
for cholangitis, community-acquired, 724
for *Moraxella catarrhalis,* 1461
for organ anaerobes, 1472
for peritonitis, spontaneous bacterial, 605
Amplification, hearing, 205
Ampulla of Vater carcinoma, **1614–1617**
Ampullary carcinomas, 1625
Amrinone, 499
Amyl nitrite, **1095, 1586–1587**
Amyloid, 423, **1031**
Amyloidosis, **540–542**
AL, 423–424
angina pectoris, 361
AV block, 387
cardiac, 423
cardiomyopathy
dilated, 404, 418, 418*t*, 419
restrictive, 423, **423–424,** 424
dialysis-related, 541
entrapment neuropathy, 1032
heart failure, 404, 405, 406, 407
hereditary, 541
LECT2, 541
localized, 541
nephrotic spectrum glomerular diseases, 931
primary, 541
renal, 924*t*, **935–936**
secondary, 541
senile, 423, 541
stress imaging, 361
systemic, 541
Amyotrophic lateral sclerosis, 1023, **1028**
Anabolic steroids, **1095,** 1179
Anaerobic bacterial infections. *See also specific types and infections*
gram-negative, **1471–1473**
bacteremia & endocarditis, 1473
chest, 1472
CNS, 1472
female genital tract & pelvis, 1473
head & neck, 1472
intra-abdominal, 1472, 1472*t*
skin & soft tissue, 1473, 1473*f*
Anaerobic pneumonia, 268, **276–278**
Anakinra
for gouty arthritis, 825, 827
for Kawasaki disease, 1438
for Still disease, adult, 831
Anal cancer/carcinoma, **1633–1634**. *See also* Colorectal cancer
anal fissures, 672
HIV/AIDS, squamous cell carcinoma, 1329–1330
treatment, 1597*t*
Analgesia. *See also* Pain/pain disorders, management; *specific types*
intrathecal, **96–97,** 97*t*
multimodal, 80
patient-controlled, 80
therapeutic window, 80
Analgesic nephropathy, 937
Analgesic rebound headache, **974**
Analgesics. *See also specific types*
Oxford League Table of Analgesics, 79
Polyanalgesic Conference Consensus, 97
WHO Analgesic Ladder, 80
Anal intercourse
condoms, 1723
epididymitis, **952–953**
hepatitis C, 682
HIV, 1311, 1332, 1723
proctitis, 590
STIs, 1723
Anaphylactoid reactions, 869
Anaphylaxis, **869–870**
definition & criteria, 869, 869*t*
IgE-dependent, 869
non–IgE-mediated anaphylactic drug reactions, **870**
Anaplasma capra, **1434**
Anaplasma phagocytophilum, 1427*t*, **1433–1434**
Anaplasmosis, 1427*t*, **1433–1434**
Anaplastic thyroid carcinoma, **1132–1133,** 1132*t*, 1135, 1137
Anastrozole, 1602*t*
for breast carcinoma, 754, 757, 757*t*
for gynecomastia, 1181
for hypogonadotropic hypogonadism, 962
for pelvic pain, 768
ANCAs
glomerulomatosis with polyangiitis, 851–853
glomerulonephritis, 852, 854, 855, 912, 923*t*, 925*f*, **928**
pauci-immune, 928–929
granulomatosis with polyangiitis, 852
eosinophilic, 854
levamisole-associated purpura, 855
microscopic polyangiitis, 853–854
nephritis spectrum glomerular disease, 926
polyarteritis nodosa, 850
primary sclerosing cholangitis, 726
relapsing polychondritis, 856
rheumatic diseases, 835*t*
vasculitides, 303, 847*t*, 851, 856 (*See also specific types*)
polyarteritis nodosa, 850
Ancyclostoma braziliense, cutaneous larva migrans, **1530**
Ancyclostoma caninum, 1527, **1530**
Ancyclostoma duodenale, 1527
Andes virus, 1395
Andexanet (alfa), 395, 1575
Androgenetic alopecia, 164–165
Androgen insensitivity (syndrome), 1176, 1184
Androgens. *See also specific types*
deprivation therapy, 1640, 1640*t*
for menopausal symptoms, 1190–1191
Anejaculation, 959
Anemia, **500–509**. *See also specific types*
aplastic, **516–518**
acquired, bone marrow failure, 546
causes, 516–517, 516*t*
from chloramphenicol, 1432
idiopathic, 516–517, 516*t*
from chemotherapy, **1655**
of chronic disease, **503–504**
pregnancy, 809
of chronic kidney disease, 918
classification
by mean RBC volume, 500, 501*t*
by RBC pathophysiology, 500, 501*t*
congenital, 500
Cooley, 505
definition, 500
folic acid deficiency, 500, **508–509,** 509*t*
pregnancy, 809
general approach, **500**
hemolytic, **509–519** (*See also* Hemolytic anemias)
aplastic, **516–518,** 516*t*, 517*t*
autoimmune, **514–515**
classification, 509–510, 509*t*
cold agglutinin disease, 500, **515–516**
glucose-6-phosphate dehydrogenase deficiency, **511**
neutropenia, **518–519,** 518*t*
paroxysmal nocturnal hemoglobinuria, **510–511**
sickle cell anemia & related syndromes, **512–513,** 513*t*
sickle cell trait, 513*t*, **514**
sickle thalassemia, 513*t*, **514**
of inflammation, **502**
iron deficiency, **500–502,** 501*t*
hookworm disease, 1527
pregnancy, 808–809
uterine leiomyoma, 766
macrocytic, 500
megaloblastic, 500, 501*t*
folic acid deficiency, **508–509,** 509*t*
pancytopenia, 517*t*
pregnancy, 809
subacute combined degeneration of spinal cord, 1027
vitamin B_{12} deficiency, **507–508,** 507*t*
microcytic, 500, 504
of older adults, **502**
of organ failure, **502**
parvovirus B19, 1420
pernicious, 507
pregnancy, **808–809**
preoperative evaluation/perioperative management, 47–48

Anemia (*Cont.*):
pyridoxine-responsive, 1261
retinal/choroidal hemorrhage, 193
sickle cell, **512–513,** 513*t* (*See also* Sickle cell disease)
pregnancy, 809
stroke, 512
thalassemias, **504–507,** 504*t,* 505*t*
vitamin B_{12} deficiency, **507–508,** 507*t*
Anesthesia/anesthetics. *See also specific types*
intrathecal, **96–97,** 97*t*
malignant hyperthermia from, 30
neuraxial, 80
regional, for acute pain, 79, 80
Aneurysm. *See specific types*
Angel dust. *See* Phencyclidine (PCP)
Angiitis, **481–482, 857.** *See also* Polyangiitis
Angina pectoris. *See also specific disorders*
aortic stenosis, 343
causes, 359
chest pain, 22–25
coronary angiography, 362
coronary artery disease, 359
coronary vasospasm and, normal coronary arteriogram, **367–368**
intestinal, **480–481**
jaw pain, 978
Ludwig, 233
Prinzmetal, 368
unstable, cardiac risk assessment/reduction, 42
vasospastic, 22
Vincent, **230**
Angina pectoris, chronic stable, **359–367,** 364*f,* 367*t*
causes, 359
clinical findings, 359–362
differential diagnosis, 362
prognosis, 367, 367*t*
referral & admission, 367
treatment, nitroglycerin, 362–363
treatment, preventing further attacks, 363–367, 364*f*
aggravating factors, 363
alternative & combination therapies, 363–365
beta-blockers, 363, 364*f*
calcium channel blocking agents, 363, 456*t*–457*t*
ivrabradine, 363
nitrates, long-acting, 363
nitroglycerin, 363
platelet-inhibiting agents, 365
ranolazine, 363
revascularization, 365–377
coronary artery bypass grafting, 366–367
extracorporeal counterpulsation, mechanical, 367
indications, 365–366
neuromodulation, 367
percutaneous coronary intervention/stenting, 365, 366
risk reduction, 365
Angiodysplasias, GI bleeding, 596, 599, 601
Angioectasias, GI bleeding, 596, 599, 601
Angioedema, **151–153,** 872*t*
Angiography
coronary
for acute coronary syndrome, without ST-segment elevation, 372, 372*t*
for acute MI, with ST-segment elevation, 378
after sudden cardiac arrest, 352
for angina pectoris, 362
left ventricular, 362
CT, multislice, for coronary artery disease, 361
digital subtraction
internal carotid artery ulceration, 479, 479*f*
tibial-popliteal artery occlusion, 476
radionuclide, 361
renal, for renal artery stenosis, 921
Angiomyolipomas, renal, 1647
Angioplasty
balloon, 366
carotid, 479
rescue, for acute MI with ST-segment elevation, 378
superficial femoral artery, 475
for tibial-pedal artery occlusive disease, 477
Angiosarcoma, liver, 1610
Angiostrongylus (angiostrongyliasis), **1529–1530**
Angiostrongylus cantonensis, 1529
Angiostrongylus costaricensis, 1529
Angiotensin-converting enzyme inhibitors. *See also specific types*
for acute MI, with ST-segment elevation, 377–378, 382
for cardiomyopathy, dilated, 419
for coronary heart disease prevention, 358
for diabetic nephropathy, 935
for focal segmental glomerulosclerosis, 933
for heart failure
with preserved LVEF, 412
with reduced LVEF, 407–408
hyperkalemia from, 886, 917
for hypertension, **450–454,** 451*t*–452*t*
hypoglycemia from, 1237
for IgA nephropathy, 927
on kidney, 907
for membranoproliferative glomerulonephritis, 929
for membranous nephropathy, 934
for nephrotic spectrum glomerular diseases, 932
preoperative evaluation/perioperative management, 45
Angiotensin II, 499
Angiotensin II receptor blockers. *See also specific types*
for African Americans, 454
for heart failure, 408
for hypertension, 452*t*–453*t,* **454**
preoperative evaluation/perioperative management, 45
Angiotensin receptor blockers. *See also specific types*
for acute MI, with ST-segment elevation, 378, 382
for cardiomyopathy, dilated, 419
for diabetic nephropathy, 935
for focal segmental glomerulosclerosis, 933
for heart failure, with preserved LVEF, 412
hyperkalemia from, 886, 917
for hypertension, 452*t*–453*t*
for IgA nephropathy, 927
for membranoproliferative glomerulonephritis, 929
for membranous nephropathy, 934
for nephrotic spectrum glomerular diseases, 932
Angiotensin receptor-neprilysin inhibitors. *See also specific types*
for cardiomyopathy, dilated, 419
for heart failure
with preserved ejection fraction, 406
with reduced LVEF, 408
Angle-closure glaucoma
acute, 170*t,* 177*t*–178*t,* **180–181**
chronic, 177*t*–178*t*
Angular cheilitis, HIV/AIDS, 1324
Anhedonia, 1069
Anhydrous ethyl alcohol with aluminum chloride, 125
Anidulafungin, 1540*t*
for candida endocarditis, 535
for candidiasis
esophageal, 1535
invasive, 1535
Anifrolumab, 835
Aniline poisoning, **1586–1587**
Animal wounds, **1283–1284**
Anion gap
formulas, 895
metabolic acidosis, 895, 896*t*
poisoning, 1570
urine, 898–899
Anion gap acidosis
increased anion gap, **895–897**
normal anion gap, **897–899,** 897*t*
Anisakis, dyspepsia, 579
Anisakis marina, gastritis, 624
Ankle-brachial index
aortoiliac disease, 473
femoro-popliteal disease, 475
tibial-pedal artery occlusive disease, 476
Ankle injuries, **1706–1708**
sprains, 1706*t*
eversion, **1707–1708**
inversion, **1706–1707**
Ankylosing spondylitis, **858–859,** 860
Annuloplasty
DeVega, 351
rings
anticoagulation management, 353
for mitral stenosis, 338
for tricuspid regurgitation, 351
Anogenital pruritus, **160–161,** 160*f*
Anorectal diseases, **669–673.** *See also specific types*
anal fissures, **672–673**
fecal incontinence, **671–672**
hemorrhoids, **669–670**
infections, **670–671**
lower GI bleeding, 599
perianal
abscess & fistula, **673**
pruritus, **673**
Anorectal infections, **670–671**
Chlamydia trachomatis, 671
condylomata acuminata, 671
herpes simplex type 2, 671
Neisseria gonorrhoeae, 670
Treponema pallidum, 670–671
Anorectal manometry, 586, 588, 645, 672
Anorexia-cachexia syndrome, 73
Anorexia nervosa, **1258–1259**
Anorgasmia, 1058, 1075
Anosmia, **223–224**
COVID-19, 1402, 1404
frontal lobe lesions, 999
Anosognosia, 999
Anovulation, 763, 771
Anterior cerebral artery occlusion, 988
Anterior chest wall syndrome, 362
Anterior cruciate ligament injury, **1696, 1700–1701**
Anterior drawer test, 1697*t*
ankle, 1697*t,* 1706–1707
knee, 1697*t,* 1700, 1702

Anterior hypopituitarism, **1099–1103**
acquired, 1100
aneurysmal subarachnoid hemorrhage, 994, 1100
bexarotene chemotherapy, 1100
ischemic stroke, 1100
Sheehan syndrome, 1100
traumatic brain injury, 1100
clinical findings, 1100–1102
complications, 1102
congenital, 1100
differential diagnosis, 1102
functional, 1100
gonadotropin deficiency, congenital, 1100
hormones, 1099
with mass lesions, 1099–1100
inflammatory/infiltrative lesions, 1099
other mass lesions, 1099
pituitary metastases, 1099
pituitary neuroendocrine tumors, 1099
pituitary stalk thickening, 1099–1100
vascular lesions, 1099
nonspecific, 1100
prognosis, 1103
treatment
corticosteroid, 1102
corticosteroid therapy, for lymphocytic hypophysitis, 1103
gonadotropin hormone, 1102–1103
human growth hormone, 1103
thyroid hormone, 1102
transsphenoidal surgery, 1103
without mass lesions
hypopituitarism, acquired, 1100
aneurysmal subarachnoid hemorrhage, 994, 1100
bexarotene chemotherapy, 1100
Sheehan syndrome, 1100
traumatic brain injury, 1100
hypopituitarism, congenital, 1100
hypopituitarism, functional, 1100
Anterior interosseous syndrome, **1035**
Anterior mediastinal mass, 292
Anterior pituitary hormones, 1099
Anterior uveitis, **183–184**
Anthracyclines, 1599*t*
for breast carcinoma, 752
cardiotoxicity, 1656
daunorubicin, 1599*t*
doxorubicin, 1599*t*
doxorubicin, liposomal, 1599*t*
idarubicin, 1599*t*
Anthrax, 1294*t*
Anti-amyloid therapy. *See also specific types*
for dementia, 1016–1017
Antiandrogens. *See also specific types*
apalutamide, 1602*t*
bicalutamide, 1602*t*
enzalutamide, 1602*t*
for prostate cancer, 1640, 1640*t*
Antiarrhythmics, **383, 384*t*–385*t***. *See also specific types*
beta-blockers, 383, 384*t*
for heart failure with reduced LVEF, 410–411
proarrhythmic effects, 383
sodium channel blockers, 383, 384*t*
tremor from, 1012
Vaughn-Williams classification, 383
class I, 383, 384*t*
class II, 383, 384*t*
class III, 383, 384*t*–385*t*
class IV, 383, 384*t*
Anti-beta-2-glycoprotein
antiphospholipid syndrome, 837
systemic lupus erythematosus, 834*t*, 835*t*
Antibiotic-associated colitis, **647–649**
Antibiotic lock therapy, 1279
Antibiotics, topical. *See also specific types*
acne, **104*t*–105*t***
impetigo, **105*t***
Antibody deficiency, specific, **874**
Anti-cardiolipin antibodies
antiphospholipid syndrome, 837
systemic lupus erythematosus, 832*t*, 834*t*, 835*t*
Anti-CCP antibodies
polymyositis/dermatomyositis, 835*t*
rheumatoid arthritis, 828, 835*t*, 864
systemic lupus erythematosus, 835t
systemic sclerosis
diffuse, 835*t*
limited, 835*t*
Anti-CD25 agents. *See also specific types*
for HTLV-1 adult T-cell leukemia, 1388
Anticholinergics. *See also specific types*
anticholinergic syndrome from, 1570
for asthma, 250*t*, 254
chorea from, 1012
hypertension from, 1566
for nausea, **584**
for Parkinson disease, 1009
poisoning, 1568*t*, **1577**
Anticholinergic syndrome, 1570
Anticholinesterase insecticide poisoning, **1588–1589**
Anticipatory anxiety, 1049
Anticoagulants/anticoagulation. *See also specific types*
for acute coronary syndrome, without ST-segment elevation, 370*t*, 371
for acute MI, 376, 376*t*, 377–378
for aortic valve stenosis, 345, 346*f*
for atrial fibrillation, 391, 392, **393–396, 393*t***
with hyperthyroidism, 1126–1127
for cardiomyopathy, dilated, 419
classes, **563–565**
direct-acting oral anticoagulants, **563–565,** 564*t*
fondaparinux, **563**
reversal agents, 563, **565*t***
unfractionated heparin & LMWHs, **563**
vitamin K antagonist (warfarin), **563**
for heart failure with reduced LVEF, 410
for left ventricular failure and reduced EF, 410
for pericarditis, 381
perioperative management, 43, 48–49, 48*t*
poisoning, **1575**
for postinfarction ischemia, 379
precardioversion, 397
pregnancy
for peripartum cardiomyopathy, 436
for valve disease, 437*t*
with prosthetic heart valves, **353–355,** 354*t*
for pulmonary hypertension, 433
for stroke, 991
for thrombus, mural, 381–382
for transient ischemic attacks, 987
Anticoagulants/anticoagulation, for venous thromboembolism, **563–565, 568–574**
before cardioversion, 397
classes, **563–565**
direct-acting oral, **563–565,** 564*t*
fondaparinux, **563**
reversal agents, 563, **565*t***
unfractionated heparin & LMWHs, **563**
vitamin K antagonist, **563**
duration, **571–573,** 574*t*
cancer-related VTE, 572–573
provoked *vs.* unprovoked VTE, 571–572
risk scoring systems, 572
thrombophilia workup, 573, 575*t*
initial, **568,** 569*t*–570*t*
initial, selecting, **568–571,** 571*t*
oral, direct-acting oral anticoagulants, 564*t*, 570–571
oral, warfarin, 571, 572*t*–574*t*
parenteral, heparins, 569–570
patient selection, 568, 571*t*
Simplified Pulmonary Embolism Severity Index, 568–569, 571*t*
secondary prevention, **573–574**
Anticonvulsants. *See also specific types*
drug eruptions from, 157
for personality disorders, 1061
poisoning, **1575–1576**
Anti-D (WinRho), 549
Antidepressants. *See also specific types*
for migraine headache, 972*t*
for personality disorders, 1060
poisoning, **1592–1593,** 1593*f*
for pruritis, 101–102, 107
on sleep, 1083
tricyclic (*See* Tricyclic antidepressants)
weight gain from, 1252, 1253*t*
Antidiabetics. *See also specific types*
weight gain from, 1252, 1253*t*
Antidiarrheal agents, **592**
Antidiuretic hormone. *See also* Sodium concentration disorders
cortisol on release of, 878
deficiency, central diabetes insipidus, **1104–1105**
Antidotes, poisoning, **1568,** 1568*t*
Antidromic reentrant tachycardia, 390
Antiemetics, 583–584, 583*t*. *See also specific types*
parkinsonism from, 1012
Antiepileptics. *See also specific types*
for migraine headache, 972*t*
weight gain from, 1252, 1253*t*
Antifungals, topical. *See also specific types*
imidazoles, **105*t***
other, **106*t***
Anti-GBM antibodies, 912
Anti-GBM antibody disease, 303
Anti-GBM glomerulonephritis, 912, 913, 923*t*, 925*f*, **928–929**
Antigenic drift
norovirus, 1423
seasonal influenza, 1410
Antigenic shift, seasonal influenza, 1410
Anti-glomerular basement membrane antibody disease, 303
Anti-HBc, 681
Anti-HBs, 680
Antihistamines. *See also specific types*
abuse, **1094**
anticholinergic syndrome from, 1570
for drug eruptions, 158
for insomnia, 1083
for nausea, **584**
poisoning, 1577
for pruritus, 101–102, 160
seizures from, 1567
weight gain from, 1252, 1253*t*
Antihypertensives, **450–464**. *See also specific types*
sympatholytic (*See also specific types*)
poisoning, **1579**
weight gain from, 1252, 1253*t*
Anti-IL-12/23 antibody. *See also specific types*
for Crohn disease, 657
for ulcerative colitis, 660
Anti-integrins. *See also specific types*
for inflammatory bowel disease, 652

Antilipidemic monoclonal antibody agents, 8
Antimalarials. *See also specific types*
for rheumatoid arthritis, 830
for systemic lupus erythematosus, 835
Antimetabolites, 1598*t*–1599*t*. *See also specific types*
folate antagonists, 1598*t*
methotrexate, 1598*t*
pemetrexed, 1598*t*
purine analogs, 1598*t*
fludarabine, 1598*t*
pyrimidine analogs, 1599*t*
azacitidine, 1599*t*
capecitabine, 1599*t*
cytarabine, 1599*t*
decitabine, 1599*t*
fluorouracil, 1599*t*
gemcitabine, 1599*t*
Antimicrobial therapy, **1293–1301**, 1293*t*–1298*t*. *See also specific types and infections*
adverse reactions and toxicity, 1299
"best guess," 1293
by clinical diagnosis, suspected
empiric, outpatient adults, 1297*t*–1298*t*
initial, hospitalized adults, 1296*t*
clinical response, 1298
cost, 1300
drug susceptibility tests, 1298–1299
duration, 1299
etiologic diagnosis, 1293, 1296*t*–1298*t*
hypersensitivity, penicillin allergy, 1300
initial, hospitalized adults, 1296*t*
laboratory control, 1298
by pathogen, medication of choice, 1293*t*–1295*t*
response, promptness, 1299
route of administration, 1299–1300
stewardship, 1300
Antimicrotubules. *See also specific types*
taxanes, 1599*t*
docetaxel, 1599*t*
paclitaxel, 1599*t*
paclitaxel protein-bound, 1599*t*
vinca alkaloids, vincristine, 1599*t*
Antineutrophil cytoplasmic autoantibody–associated vasculitides, 303, 851, 856. *See also* ANCAs
Anti-NMDA receptor–associated encephalitis, 1004*t*
Antinuclear antibody, autoimmune hepatitis, 692
Antiobesity medications, 1252–1257, 1254*t*–1256*t*. *See also specific types*
indications, 1252
liraglutide, 1253, 1255*t*, 1257
naltrexone ER + bupropion ER, 1253, 1255*t*
orlistat, 1252–1253, 1254*t*
phentermine, 1252, 1254*t*
phentermine + topiramate ER, 1253, 1254*t*
semaglutide, 1253, 1255*t*, 1257
Antioxidants, 1244. *See also specific types*
Antiphospholipid syndrome, **837–838**
pregnancy, **809**
pregnancy-associated, **837–838**
transient monocular visual loss, 190
Antiplatelet therapy. *See also specific types*
for acute coronary syndrome, without ST-segment elevation, 369–371
for acute MI with ST-segment elevation, after drug-eluting/bare metal stents, 375
for coronary heart disease prevention, 358
dual
for acute MI, with ST-segment elevation, 375
after discontinuation for procedures, 371
after transcatheter aortic valve replacement, 345
for angina pectoris, 365
for coronary heart disease prevention, 358
for myocardial infarction, 365
for prosthetic heart valves, 353
for stenting, 365
for stroke, 991
for transient ischemic attacks, 987
ulcer risk with, reducing, 628–629
Antipruritics. *See also specific types*
systemic, 101, 107
topical, 101, **106*t***
Antipsychotics. *See also specific types*
for aggression disorders, 1085
atypical
for dementia, 1017
diabetic ketoacidosis from, 1017
glucose intolerance from, 1197
poisoning, 1576
for behavioral dyscontrol, in autism, 1065
for bipolar disorder, 1078–1079
chorea from, 1012
diabetes mellitus from, 1066, 1066*t*, 1197
floppy iris syndrome from, 185
neuroleptic malignant syndrome from, 1567
for Parkinson disease, 1009
parkinsonism from, 1012
for personality disorders, 1060–1061
poisoning, **1576**
for psychedelic effects, 1093
for schizophreniform spectrum disorders, **1063–1068**
clinical indications, 1064–1065
dosage forms & patterns, 1063, 1064*t*, 1065–1066
potency and side effects, 1053, 1065*t*, 1066–1068, 1066*t*
for schizotypal personality, 1061
seizures from, 1567
for Tourette syndrome, 1065
tremor from, 1012
weight gain from, 1252, 1253*t*
Antiretroviral therapy. *See also specific types*
for cerebral lymphoma, 1001
for cytomegalovirus, 1367
Antiretroviral therapy, for HIV/AIDS, prevention, **1331–1334**
perinatal transmission, **1334**
postexposure prophylaxis, 4, 1286, **1333**
preexposure prophylaxis, 3–4, 1286, **1332**, 1333*t*
transmission risk/treatment as prevention, **1331**
Antiretroviral therapy, for HIV/AIDS, treatment, **1338–1351**, 1339*t*–1342*t*
adherence, patient, 1
combinations, fixed-dose, 1338, 1341–1343, **1342*t***
monitoring, 1349*f*, 1350–1351
goals, 1349*f*, 1350
medication adherence, 1350
medication resistance, 1350–1351
principles, 1338, 1341
regimen choice, 1341–1350
attachment inhibitor, **1341*t***, 1346–1347
fostemavir, **1341*t*, 1346–1347**
entry and fusion inhibitors, **1339*t***, 1341*t*, 1346
enfuvirtide, **1340*t*, 1341*t*, 1346**
ibalizumab, **1341*t*, 1346**
maraviroc, **1341*t*, 1346**
principles & overview, **1341*t***, 1346
entry inhibitors, **1340*t***
enfuvirtide, **1340*t***
initial, constructing, 1347–1350, 1347*t*–1348*t*, 1349*f*
integrase inhibitors, **1340*t*–1341*t***, 1345–1346
bictegravir, **1340*t*, 1346**
cabotegravir, **1341*t*, 1346**
dolutegravir, **1340*t*, 1346**
elvitegravir, **1340*t*, 1345–1346**
principles & overview, 1340*t*–1341*t*, 1345–1346
raltegravir, **1341*t*, 1345**
nonnucleoside reverse transcriptase inhibitors, **1339*t***, 1343–1344
doravirine, **1339*t*, 1344**
efavirenz, **1339*t*, 1343–1344**
etravirine, **1339*t*, 1344**
nevirapine, 696, **1339*t*, 1344**
principles & overview, **1339*t***, 1343
rilpivirine, **1339*t*, 1344**
nucleoside reverse transcriptase inhibitors, **1339*t***, 1341–1343
abacavir, **1339*t*, 1343**
combinations, fixed-dose, 1338, 1341–1343, **1342*t***
emtricitabine, **1339*t*, 1343**
lamivudine, **1339*t*, 1343**
principles & overview, **1339*t***, 1341–1343
zidovudine, **1339*t*, 1343**
nucleotide reverse transcriptase inhibitors, **1339*t***, 1341–1343
tenofovir, **1339*t*, 1343**
tenofovir alafenamide/emtricitabine, **1339*t*, 1343**
protease inhibitors, **1340*t***, 1344–1345
atazanavir, **1340*t*, 1345**
atazanavir/cobicistat, **1340*t*, 1345**
darunavir, **1340*t*, 1345**
lopinavir/r, **1340*t*, 1345**
principles & overview, **1340*t***, 1344–1345
ritonavir, **1340*t*, 1345**
resistance, regimens for, 1351
before resistance testing, 1338
Anti-SCL-70, 835*t*, 841
Antiseizure medications. *See also specific types*
chorea & tremor from, 1012
Antisocial personality disorder, **1059–1061**, 1060*t*
Antisynthetase syndrome, **843**
Antithrombotics, **563–578**. *See also specific types*
for acute MI, with ST-segment elevation, 378
anticoagulant classes, **563–565**
direct-acting oral, **563–565**, 564*t*
fondaparinux, **563**
reversal agents, 563, **565*t***
unfractionated heparin & LMWHs, **563**
vitamin K antagonist, **563**
for pulmonary embolism
contraindications, 575, 576*t*
high-risk, massive, 575, 577*t*
intermediate-risk, submassive, 575
for venous thromboembolism, **565–577** (*See also* Venous thromboembolism treatment, antithrombotic)
Anti-TNF therapies, 651–652. *See also specific types*
Anton syndrome, 999
Anus
dysplasia, HIV/AIDS, 1329–1330
fissures, 599, **672–673**
Anxiety
adjustment disorders, **1046–1047**
anticipatory, 1049
chest pain, 22, 23, 24

chronic pain syndromes, 1055–1056
COVID-19, 1404
hospitalization & illness, 1097
irritable bowel syndrome, 644
palpitations, 25
performance, 1049
postsurgical states, 1097
presurgical, 1097
Anxiety disorders, **1049–1052,** 1050*t*. *See also specific types*
gay & bisexual men, 1723
generalized, **1049, 1050**
lesbian & bisexual women, 1721–1722
panic, **1049, 1051**
phobic, **1049, 1051–1052**
psychological components, 1049
SARS-CoV-2 pandemic, sexual & gender minorities, 1711
self-generating, 1049
somatic components, 1049
triggers, 1049
Anxiety-panic-phobia-depression cycle, 1052
Anxiolytics, 1047, 1049, 1050–1051, 1050*t*. *See also specific types*
Aorta
ascending
aortic regurgitation, 349
aortic stenosis, 334*t*, 342, 343
coarctation, **325–326**
aortic dissection, 486
hypertension, 325, 445
intracranial aneurysm, 325
dilation
aortic regurgitation, 348
aortic stenosis, 342
coarctation of aorta, 325
pregnancy, 437*t*
dissection, **486–487**
acute, 469, 470*t*
aortic regurgitation, 347, 348
chest pain, 22, 23
coarctation of aorta, 325
hypertension, 446
pericardial tamponade, 429
pregnancy, 437, 437*t*
occlusion, **473–474**
pregnancy, vascular abnormalities, 436–437
ruptured, athletic deaths, 438
sclerosis, 342
stenosis, bicuspid, 333*t*
Aorta aneurysms
abdominal, 5*t*, 6, 42, **482–484,** 1465
mycotic, 1465
Salmonella, 1465
Aortic arch
aneurysm, superior vena cava obstruction, 492
coarctation of aorta, 325
emboli, 478
right-sided, tetralogy of Fallot, 330
Aortic regurgitation, 333*t*–335*t*, **347–349**
aortic stenosis, 343
cardiac risk assessment/reduction, 45
categories, 332
clinical findings, 348–349
coarctation of aorta, 325
giant cell arteritis, 848
hypertension, 447
reactive arthritis, 860
rheumatic fever, 425
Ross procedure, 345
tetralogy of Fallot, 330–332
treatment & prognosis, 348–349, 349*f*
Aortic root dilation, Marfan syndrome, labor, 438
Aortic (valve) stenosis, 333*t*–335*t*, **342–347**
athletic deaths, 438
cardiac risk assessment/reduction, 45
categories, 332
chest pain, 23
degenerative/calcific, 342
general considerations & clinical findings, 342–343
maternal mortality, pregnancy, 812
redefining, 342–343, 343*t*
treatment & prognosis, 343–347, 344*f*, 346*f*
Bentall procedure, 345
mechanical *vs.* prosthetic valve, 345
Ross procedure, 344
timing, algorithm, 343, 344*f*
valve replacement, surgical mortality, 344
valve replacement, transcatheter/surgical, 344–347, 346*f*
Wheat procedure, 345
tricuspid, **347**
unicuspid/bicuspid valve, 342
Aortic valve, unicuspid/bicuspid, 342
Aortic valve replacement
aortic regurgitation, 348–349
aortic stenosis, 344–345
classification, 349
Aortic vasculitis, 482
Aortoenteric fistula, upper GI bleeding, 596
Aorto-femoral bypass graft, 474
Aortoiliac occlusive disease, 473–474
Aortopathy, pregnancy, 435, 437*t*
Apalutamide, 1602*t*, 1640*t*, 1641
Apathetic hyperthyroidism, 1120, 1127
Apathy, 1015. *See also specific disorders*
APC, 665, **667,** 1628
Aphthous ulcers, **230,** 1324–1325
Apical ballooning syndrome, 373, 418, **420–421**
Apixaban, 563, 564*t*
for atrial fibrillation, **394–395,** 394*t*
for mitral stenosis, 336
poisoning, 1575
reversal agents, 563, 565*t*
for stroke prevention, 394, 394*t*
for venous thromboembolism
prophylaxis, 567*t*
treatment, 570–571, 570*t*
Aplastic anemia, **516–518**
acquired, bone marrow failure, 546
causes, 516–517, 516*t*
from chloramphenicol, 1432
idiopathic, 516–517, 516*t*
Aplastic crisis, 505
Apnea. *See also* Breathing/respiration; *specific types*
central, 316
mixed, 316
obstructive, 316
obstructive sleep, **316–317**
snoring, **233–234**
Apnea test, 1020
Apneustic breathing, 1019
APO1, focal segmental glomerulosclerosis, 933
APOE-e4 gene, 54
APOL1
chronic kidney disease, 914
COVID-19–associated nephropathy, 1404
HIV-associated nephropathy, 935
hypertensive kidney disease, 446
lupus nephritis, 930
Apophysomyces, 1544
Appendiceal carcinoids, 1626
Appendicitis, **641–642, 818**
Apprehension test, shoulder, 1679*t*
Apraclonidine overdose, **1579**
Apraxia, 999, 1015
Apremilast
for Behçet disease, 857
for lichen planus, 141
for psoriasis, 138
for psoriatic arthritis, 860
Aprepitant, 160, 583*t*, **584,** 1655
Aquablation, 968
Arbovirus encephalitides, **1379–1381**
mosquito-borne, 1379
tick-borne, 1379
Arcing burns, 1557
Arformoterol, 262
Arg133Trp, 1196
Argatroban, 553, 553*t*
Arginine, 1044
Arginine vasopressin, 498–499, 1099
Aripiprazole, 1066
adverse effects, 1065*t*
for aggression disorders, 1085
for bipolar disorder, 1078–1079
poisoning, 1576
for schizophreniform spectrum disorders, 1063–1064, 1064*t*, 1065*t*
Armodafinil, 1084
Arnold-Chiari malformation, 974, 1028
Aromatase inhibitors. *See also specific types*
anastrozole, 1602*t*
for breast carcinoma, 742, 754, 756, 757, 757*t*
exemestane, 1602*t*
for gynecomastia, 1181
letrozole, 1602*t*
Arousal, 1057
Arrhythmias, **383–403**. *See also* Heart rate & rhythm disorders; *specific types*
acute MI, with ST-segment elevation
conduction disturbances, 379–380
sinus bradycardia, 379
supraventricular tachyarrhythmias, 379
ventricular, 379
bigeminy, 398
cardiac risk assessment/reduction, 45
inherited syndromes, **401**
palpitations, 25
poisoning, **1566,** 1566*t*
retinal artery occlusion, 189
sinus, **386–387**
systemic lupus erythematosus, 834
tetralogy of Fallot, 330–332
Arrhythmogenic right ventricular cardiomyopathy, 399, 400, **401**
Arrhythmogenic right ventricular dysplasia, athletic deaths, 438, 440*t*
Arsenic
lung cancer and, 1603
poisoning, 1568*t*, **1576–1577**
ART. *See* Antiretroviral therapy
Artemether + amodiaquine, 1504*t*, 1505*t*, 1507
Artemether/artemisinin, 1504*t*, 1507–1508, 1521
Artemether-lumefantrine, 1504*t*
Artemether + lumefantrine, 1504*t*, 1507
Artemether + mefloquine, 1504*t*, 1507
Arterial aneurysm, **482–487**
abdominal aortic, 5*t*, 6, 42, **482–484,** 1465
aortic dissection, **486–487**
peripheral artery, **485–486**
thoracic aortic, **484–485**
Arterial blood gases
acid–base disorders, 894
asthma, 246
carbon monoxide poisoning, 1578
cough assessment, 15
drowning, 1554
dyspnea, 19–20
methemoglobinemia, 1586
non–lung resection surgery, 46
P. jirovecii pneumonia, 1312*t*, 1538
salicylate poisoning, 1590
shock, 497

Arterial occlusion of a limb, **477–478**
Arterial pulse pressure, wide, 347
Arteriography, coronary, 362
Arteriolar dilators, 463*t*, **464**. *See also specific types*
Arteriosclerosis, retinal vein occlusion, 188
Arteriovenous fistulae, spinal dural, **997**
Arteriovenous malformations
hereditary hemorrhagic telangiectasia, **1665–1666**
intracerebral hemorrhage, 992, 993
stroke, **995–996**
vertigo from, 217
Arteritis
giant cell, **848–849**
ischemic optic neuropathy, 193–194
retinal artery occlusion, 189–190
sixth nerve palsy, 196
third nerve palsy, 196
transient monocular visual loss, 190
Kawasaki disease, 1437
Takayasu, **849–850**
varicella, 1360
Artesunate, 1504*t*, 1505*t*, 1507–1508
Artesunate-amodiaquine, 1504*t*
Artesunate-mefloquine, 1504*t*
Artesunate-pyronaridine, 1504*t*
Artesunate-sulfadoxine-pyrimethamine, 1504*t*
Arthralgias, 80. *See also specific types*
lymphocytic choriomeningitis, 1384
rubella, 1373
Arthritis. *See also specific types*
infectious, **861–864**
gonococcal, **863–864,** 1469
Group A beta-hemolytic streptococcal, **1442**
HIV, **864,** 1323
nongonococcal, **861–863**
pneumococcal, 1444
rubella, 1373
tuberculous, **865**
viral, **864**
Lyme disease, 1492–1494, 1495*t*
polyarthritis
chronic inflammatory, 826
rheumatic fever/heart disease, 425, 425*t*
psoriatic, **859–860,** 1323
reactive, **860–861,** 861*f*
HIV/AIDS, 1323
uveitis, 183
rheumatoid, **827–831**
septic
antimicrobial therapy, initial, 1296*t*
injection drug abuse, 1287
nongonococcal acute, **861–863**
uveitis, 183
Arthritis, crystal deposition, **823–827**
calcium pyrophosphate deposition, **826–827**
degenerative joint disease, **819–823** (*See also* Degenerative joint disease)
gouty, **823–826** (*See also* Gout/gouty arthritis)
Arthritis-dermatitis syndrome, 863
Arthritis mutilans, 859
Arthrocentesis, joint fluid, 819, 820*t*
Arthropod lesions, **131–132**
bedbugs, **131**
caterpillars, urticating hair moths, **132**
chiggers/red bugs, **132**
fleas, **131**
mites
bird/rodent, **132**
stored products, **132**
ticks, **131**
tungiasis, **132**
Artifactual hypercalcemia, 1143
Artificial insemination, for azoospermia, 773
Artificial sweeteners, diabetes mellitus, 1203
Asbestos/asbestosis, 306*t*, **307,** 308, 430, 1603
Asboe-Hansen sign, 146
Ascarias (ascariasis), 297, **1526**
Ascaris lumbricoides, **1526**
Ascites
alcohol-associated liver disease, 694, 695
cirrhosis, 700–707, 706*t*
hepatic venous outflow obstruction, **713–714**
hyperbilirubinemia, conjugated, 674
malignant, **605–606**
pancreatic, 731
patient assessment, **602–604,** 602*t*
postoperative risk reduction, 47
treatment, with cirrhosis, 702–703
Ascorbic acid, **1261–1262**
Asenapine, 1063, **1064,** 1064*t*, 1065*t*
Aseptic meningitis. *See* Meningitis, aseptic
Aspartame, 1203
ASPEN/AND criteria, 1250
Aspergillus (aspergillosis), **1543–1544**
allergic bronchopulmonary, **265–266, 1543–1544**
chronic, 1543, 1544
COVID-19 pulmonary, 1405
with granulocytopenia, 1273
hematopoietic cell transplant recipients, 1273
household molds, **1547**
immunocompromised, pulmonary infiltrates, 279
invasive, 1543, 1544
neutropenia, 519
otitis externa, 206
prevention, 1544
sinusitis, invasive, 221–222
solid organ transplants, 1273
Aspergillus fumigatus, **1543–1544**
AIDS, otologic, 218
allergic bronchopulmonary, **265–266**
meningitis, health care–associated, 1281
Aspirated foreign body retention, **306**
Aspiration
enteric nutrition, 1268
pulmonary syndromes, **305–306** (*See also* Pulmonary aspiration syndromes)
Aspiration pneumonia, 276–278, 1287, 1297*t*
Aspirin
for acute coronary syndrome, without ST-segment elevation, 369, 371
for acute MI, ST-segment elevation, 374, 378
adverse effects
asthma, 245
GI bleeding, occult, 601
hepatic, 696
medication overuse headache, 974
peptic ulcer disease, **625–626**
renal, 822
respiratory alkalosis, 902
tubulointerstitial disease, 937
ulcer, reducing risk, 628–629
for angina pectoris, 364*f*
desensitization, **872**
for Kawasaki disease, 1438
for migraine headache, 971
for pain, **82, 83*t***
for pericarditis, 428
poisoning, **1589–1590**
on respiratory disease, 245, **872**
for stroke, 991
for thyroiditis, painful subacute, 1114
for transient ischemic attacks, 987
for VTE prophylaxis, 568*t*
Aspirin, low-dose
for acute coronary syndromes, without ST-segment elevation, 371
for acute MI, with ST-segment elevation, 378
after transcatheter aortic valve replacement, 345
for angina pectoris, 365
for antiphospholipid syndrome, pregnancy-associated, 838
for cardiovascular disease
on morbidity/mortality, 1224
prevention, 5*t*, 9
gout from, 823
for Kawasaki disease, 1438
for preeclampsia risk, pregnancy, 803
for prosthetic valves, 337, 345
pregnancy, 355
surgical risk assessment/reduction, 43
Assessment, physical. *See* Physical assessment; *specific topics*
Assisted reproductive technology, 773, 962–963
Assistive devices, older adults, 61
Astereognosis, 999
Asthma, **245–258**
air pollution, 245
allergic, 245
bronchoprovocation testing, 247
"cardiac," 246
catamenial, 246
combustion products, 245
complications, 247
control, assessing, 246, 246*t*
cough/cough-variant, 15, 17, 17*t*, 246
definition & pathogenesis, 245–246
differential diagnosis, 247
dyspnea, 18, 19
exercise-induced bronchoconstriction, 246
"functional," 247
general considerations, 245
laboratory findings, 246
late-onset T2-high, 245
from medications, 245–246
nonallergic, 245
with obesity, 245
occupational, 246
paradoxical vocal fold motion, 246
peak expiratory flow meters, 247
with persistent airflow limitation, 245
precipitants, 245–246
pregnancy, **812–813**
psychiatric causes, 247
pulmonary function testing, 246
referral, 258
symptoms and signs, 246
systemic vasculitis, 247
T2-high, 245
triad, 226
upper airway obstruction, 246
Asthma, treatment, 249–258
desensitization, 255
exacerbations, 255–258
acute care, 255, 257*f*
evaluation and classification, 255, 255*t*, 256*f*, 257*f*
mild to moderate, 255–257, 256*f*, 257*f*
primary care, 255, 256*f*
severe, 257–258
management approach, 247–249, 248*f*
control, assessment, 246*t*, 247
environmental factors, control, 249
personalized, 247, 248*f*
pharmacotherapy goals, 249
risk factors, treat modifiable, 249
self-management education & skills training, 249
severity, assessment, 247
uncontrolled *vs.* severe, 246*t*, 247–249

pharmacologic agents, 249–255, 250*t*–253*t*
add-on, 248*f*, 249
anticholinergics, 250*t*, 254
beta-adrenergic agonists, 249–254, 250*t*, 252*t*
corticosteroids
inhaled, 249, 250*t*, 253*t*
systemic, 250*t*, 252*t*–253*t*, 254, 256, 258
leukotriene modifiers, 251*t*, 254
long-term controllers, 249, 250*t*–251*t*
mediator inhibitors, 250*t*, 254
monoclonal antibody agents, 251*t*, 254
phosphodiesterase inhibitor, 251*t*, 254
reliever, 249, 252*t*–253*t*
vaccination, 255
Astrocytoma, 997*t*
Astrovirus, diarrhea, 590
ASXL1, 527, 528
Asymmetric septal hypertrophy, 418*t*, 421, 439
Atabecestat, hepatotoxicity, 696
Ataxia, **1031**. *See also specific types and disorders*
cerebellar, varicella, 1360
fragile X-associated tremor/ataxia syndrome, 1661
sensory, HIV/AIDS, 1323
Ataxia-telangiectasia, 1614, 1615
Atazanavir, **1340*t*, 1345**
Atazanavir/cobicistat, **1340*t*, 1345**
Atelectasis, postoperative risk reduction, 47
Atenolol, 461*t*, 796*t*
Atezolizumab, 1600*t*
for bladder cancer, 1643, 1644
for hepatocellular carcinoma, 1612
for non–small cell lung cancer, 1606–1607
for small cell lung cancer, 1606, 1607
thyroiditis from, silent, 1115
Atherosclerosis
acute MI, ST-segment elevation, 373
aneurysms, 483
thoracic artery, 484
angina pectoris, 359, 360, 361, 365
aortic stenosis, 342, 345
atrial fibrillation, 393
carotid artery, lipid disorders, 1241
chronic kidney disease, 916
cocaine on, 368
coronary calcium score, 361
coronary heart disease, **355,** 356*f*
prevention, 357–358
diabetes mellitus, 1224
electron beam CT, 361
familial hypercholesterolemia, 1660, 1661
femoral-popliteal, 474–475
flow-limiting stenoses, 473
hypertension, 140, 192, 446, 1660
hypertensive retinochoroidopathy, 192
intracranial, 478
LDL lowering on, 357
lipid disorders, 1240–1242, 1248
myocardial ischemia and, 358
normal coronary arteriograms, 368
patent foramen ovale, 987, 990
peripheral pulses, 447
pregnancy, 437
renal vascular hypertension, 445
smoking and, 1660
stroke, 988
superficial femoral artery, 474–475
systemic lupus erythematosus, 836
tibial-pedal artery occlusive disease, 476–477
transient ischemic attacks, 986
Atherosclerotic coronary artery disease, 26, **355–382**. *See also* Coronary heart disease
Atherosclerotic coronary vascular disease, lipid hypothesis, 1239
Atherosclerotic peripheral vascular disease, **473–481**. *See also specific types*
acute mesenteric vein occlusion, **481**
arterial occlusion of a limb, **477–478**
epidemiology, 473
intermittent claudication, 473
occlusive
aorta & iliac arteries, **473–474**
cerebrovascular disease, **478–480,** 479*t*
femoral & popliteal arteries, **474–476**
limb arterial, **477–478**
mesenteric vein, **481**
tibial & pedal arteries, **476–477**
visceral arterial insufficiency, **480–481**
Athletes/athlete screening, cardiovascular, **438–441**
12-element AHA recommendations, 438, 439*t*
COVID-19 myocarditis, 416, 416*t*, 439
sudden cardiac death, 439, 440*t*
Athlete's foot, **116–117**
Athletic hypertrophy, 421
Atlanta classification, revised, 729
ATM
breast cancer, 741
chronic lymphocytic leukemia, 531
Lynch syndrome, 1615
pancreas carcinoma, 1615
prostate cancer, 1641
Atogepant, 972*t*
Atonic seizure, 979
Atopic dermatitis, **133–135**
cataracts, 184
dyshidrotic, **144,** 144*f*
molluscum contagiosum, 1421
Atopic keratoconjunctivitis, 172
Atorvastatin, 357*t*
for cholesterol, high LDL, 1244, 1245*t*
for coronary heart disease, 357, 357*t*
for hypertension, 457*t*
Atovaquone, 1337*t*, 1510, 1541
Atovaquone-proguanil, 1504*t*, 1508
ATP7B, 711
Atrial ectopy, palpitations, 27
Atrial fibrillation, **391–396**
acute left ventricular failure, 380
acute MI, with ST-segment elevation, 379
from adenosine, 389
alcohol excess/withdrawal, 391
aortic valve replacement, bioprosthetic, 347
asymptomatic/"subclinical," 391
atrial septal defect, 326–328
AV block, 388
cardiac risk assessment/reduction, 45
cardiomyopathy
dilated, 419
hypertrophic, 421, 422
causes, 391
chronic kidney disease, 916
clinical findings, 391–392
ECG monitoring, 383, 391
echocardiography, 391–392
epidemiology, 391
heart failure, 404
incidence and prevalence, 391
lone, 393
mitral regurgitation, 333*t*, 338, 341, 341*f*
mitral stenosis, 336
paroxysmal, 389, 391
paroxysmal supraventricular tachycardia, accessory AV pathways, 390–391
pericarditis, 391, 392
constrictive, 427
postsurgical development, 45
retinal artery occlusion, 189, 190
stroke, **391–396,** 393*t*, 394*t*
prevention, 391
supraventricular tachyarrhythmias, 379, 386
tetralogy of Fallot, 332
thromboembolism, 392
transient, 393
transient monocular visual loss, 191
tricuspid regurgitation, 351
wearable device optic sensors, 383
Atrial fibrillation, treatment, **392–396,** 393*t*, 394*t*
ablation, pericarditis from, 427
amiodarone, 384*t*
catheter ablation, 383, 386
CHA_2DS_2-VASc Risk Score, 393, 393*t*
dofetilide, 385*t*
dronedarone, 385*t*
ibutilide, 385*t*
initial
hemodynamically stable, 392
hemodynamically unstable, 392
recurrent paroxysmal atrial fibrillation, 396
refractory, 396
sotalol, 385*t*
stroke prevention, DOACs, 393–394, 394*t*
subsequent, 392–396
anticoagulation/DOACs, 393–395, 393*t*, 394*t*
CHA_2DS_2-VASc score, 393, 393*t*
rate/rhythm control, 395–396
Atrial flutter, **396–397**
atrial tachycardia with, 398
stroke risk, 396
thromboembolism risk, 397
treatment
catheter ablation, 397
dofetilide, 385*t*
ibutilide, 385*t*
medications, 385*t*, 397
tricuspid regurgitation, 351
Atrial gallops, 373
Atrial myxoma, **433–434**
Atrial palpitations, 25, 26
Atrial premature beats, solitary, 397
Atrial septum
defects, **326–328,** 986
lipoma, 434
Atrial tachycardia, **397–398**
heart failure from, 412
multifocal, 397–398
paroxysmal, 383
solitary atrial premature beats, 397
Atrioventricular block, **387–388**
acute MI, with ST-segment elevation, 379–380
from adenosine, 385*t*
from beta-blockers, 384*t*
from catheter ablation, for preexcitation syndromes, 391
degrees, 387
from digoxin, 385*t*
myocarditis, 416*t*
from poisoning, 1566*t*
syncope, 343, 402, 403
Atrioventricular dissociation, **387**
Atrioventricular nodal reentrant tachycardia, 388
Atrioventricular pathways, accessory, PSVT from, **390–391**
Atrioventricular reciprocating tachycardia, 388
Atrioventricular synchrony, pacemaker, 388
At-risk drinking, 1086–1087
treatment
behavioral, 1089
medical, 1088–1089
psychological, 1088
social, 1088

Atrophic striae, from corticosteroids, 107
Atrophic urethritis, urinary incontinence, 62
Atrophie blanche, lower extremity edema, 28
Atropine
anticholinergic syndrome from, 1570
for beta-blocker poisoning, 1577
for calcium channel blocker poisoning, 1578
for cholinesterase inhibitor poisoning, 1589
for nerve agent poisoning, 1579
poisoning, **1577**
antidote, 1568*t*
Attachment inhibitor, HIV/AIDS, **1341*t*, 1346–1347**. *See also specific types*
Attention, complex, dementia, 53–54
Attention deficit hyperactivity disorders, 1013, **1081**
ATTR, 423
ATTR amyloid, 423
Atypical antipsychotics. *See under* Antipsychotics
Atypical nevi, **108,** 108*f*
Audiology, **204–205**
Auditory brainstem-evoked response screening, 205
Auditory diseases, central, vertigo from, 215*t*, 217–218
multiple sclerosis, 218
vascular compromise, 218
vestibular schwannoma, 217–218
Auer rod, acute myeloid leukemia, 529
Augmented breast disorders, **739–740**
Aura
brainstem, migraine with, 971
epilepsy, 980
migraine, 970
Auricle diseases, **205**
Austin Flint murmur, 347–348
Austrian triad, 1444
Autism spectrum disorders, **1082**
Autoantibodies, 834, 835*t*. *See also specific types and disorders*
Autoeczematization, 144
Autoimmune diseases, **827–847**. *See also specific types*
Addison disease, 1157
anemia, **514–515**
antiphospholipid syndrome, **837–838**
factor III antibodies, acquired, 561
hearing loss, **213**
hepatitis, **691–693**
HIV/AIDS, 1314, **1314** (*See also* HIV/AIDS)
hypoglycemia, **1237**
IgG_4-related disease, **846–847**
immune-mediated inflammatory myopathies, **842–844,** 843*f*
immune thrombocytopenia, 548
limbic encephalitis, seizures, 980
lupus, drug-induced, **836–837**
mixed connective tissue disease, overlap, & undifferentiated syndromes, **845**
myocarditis, 414, 415*t*
necrotizing myopathy, 1004*t*
pancreatitis, 733–735
paraneoplastic disorders, 1003, 1004*t*
polyendocrine syndrome type 2, 1112
Raynaud phenomenon, **838–839,** 839*f*, 840*t*
rheumatoid arthritis, **827–831**
seizures, 980
Sjögren syndrome, **845–846**
Still disease, adult, **831**
systemic lupus erythematosus, **832–836**
systemic sclerosis, **840–842**
Autoimmune thyroiditis, **1111–1114**
chronic lymphocytic, 1112
HHV-6, 1368
hyperthyroidism, 1119
hypothyroidism from, 1112, 1113, 1115
painless sporadic subacute, 1112, 1119, 1127
postpartum, 1112, 1119, 1127
pregnancy, 809
Autoinsufflation, 208
Autologous packed red blood cells transfusion, 542
Automated breast ultrasonography, 746
Automatisms, 979
Autonomic nervous system modulation, for hypertension, **464**
Autonomic neuropathy
diabetes mellitus, 1223–1224
paraneoplastic, 1004*t*
Autonomy, 76, 77
Autophony, 208
Autopsy, 78
Autosomal dominant polycystic kidney disease, 938*t*, **939–940,** 939*f*
Autosomal recessive trinucleotide repeat disease, **1031**
Avacopan, 853
Avalglucosidase alpha, acid maltase deficiency, 1044
Avanafil, 959–960
Avascular necrosis of bone, **868,** 1323
Avatrombopag, 549, 705
AV block. *See* Atrioventricular block
Avelumab, 1643
Avian influenza, **1414–1415**
AV nodal reentrant tachycardia, 388
Avoidant personality disorder, **1059–1061,** 1060*t*
a wave
pulmonary valve stenosis, 324
tetralogy of Fallot, 331
tricuspid stenosis, 350
Axial spondyloarthritis, **858–859**
Axillo-femoral bypass graft, 474
Axitinib, 1120, 1600*t*, 1646
Axonal degeneration, 1030
Axonal injury, diffuse, 1022*t*
AZA, *TPMT* on metabolism of, 1670*t*
Azacitidine, 1599*t*
Azarcon, toxicity, 1580*t*
Azathioprine
on allopurinol metabolism, 826
for autoimmune hepatitis, 692–693
for Behçet disease, 857
for bullous pemphigoid, 147
for Crohn disease, 656
for cytomegalovirus, in immunosuppressed, 1367
for eosinophilic granulomatosis with polyangiitis, 854
on febuxostat metabolism, 826
for immune-mediated inflammatory myopathies, 844
for inflammatory bowel disease, 650
for interstitial lung disease, scleroderma, 841
for lupus nephritis, 930
for microscopic polyangiitis, 854
for myasthenia gravis, 1041
for myasthenic syndrome, 1042
for neuromyelitis optica, 1026
nodular regenerative hyperplasia from, 715
for pancreatitis, 735
for pemphigus, 146
for photodermatitis, 156
progressive multifocal leukoencephalopathy from, 1387
for systemic lupus erythematosus, 835
for Takayasu arteritis, 850
for ulcerative colitis, 660
Azilsartan, 452*t*
Azithromycin
for babesiosis, 1510
for *Bordetella pertussis,* 1459
for chancroid, 1470
for chlamydial reactive arthritis, 861
for *Chlamydia trachomatis*
lymphogranuloma venereum, 1477
urethritis & cervicitis, 1478
for *Chlamydophila pneumoniae,* 1479
for cholera, 1466
for diarrhea
bloody, 1288
traveler's, 1293
for granuloma inguinale, 1471
for *Haemophilus,* 1461
hepatotoxicity, 696
for *Legionella,* 1462
for Lyme disease, 1494, 1495*t*
for *Mycobacterium abscessus, M. chelonae, M. fortuitum,* 1475
for *Mycobacterium avium* complex, 1475, 1476
prophylaxis, HIV/AIDS, 1337*t*
for pneumococcal pneumonia, 1444, 1445
for prostatitis, 948*t*
for psittacosis, 1478
for *Salmonella* gastroenteritis, 1464
for *Shigella,* 1465
for syphilis, 1483
for typhus
endemic, 1429
scrub, 1430
Azoospermia, 773, 962
Azotemia, 703–704, 903

B

Babesia divergens, 1510
Babesia duncani, 1510
Babesia microti (babesiosis), 1434, **1510**
Babesia venatorum, 1510
Babinski reflex, 1684, 1684*t*
Baby wipes allergy, 161
Bacillary angiomatosis, *Bartonella,* 1328, **1471**
Bacillus, 1272, 1294*t*
Bacillus Calmette-Guérin, 282, 287, 1643
Bacillus cereus diarrhea, 590, 1288, 1289*t*
Back fractures, from falls, 61
"Background" retinopathy, 191
Back pain
dysuria, 38
low, **1683–1685,** 1684*t*
cauda equina syndrome, 1682–1685
chronic, 80, 95
physical therapy for, 95
Baclofen
for alcohol-associated liver disease, 694
poisoning, **1581–1582**
for spasticity, 1026
for trigeminal neuralgia, 975
Bacteremia. *See also specific types*
anaerobic, 1473
Bartonella, 1471
Campylobacter, 1467
endocarditis, infectious, 1454, 1455
enterococcus, 1473
glomerulonephritis, 923*t*, **926–927**
gram-negative, **1462–1463**
listeriosis, 1453
Moraxella catarrhalis, 1461
pneumococcus pneumonia, 1473
salmonellosis, 1463, **1465**
bacteremia, 1465
enteric fever, 1463–1464
gastroenteritis, 1464
Staphylococcus, 1449

Staphylococcus aureus, **1449**
osteomyelitis, 1447
skin & soft tissue infections, 1447
Streptococcus
Group B, 1443
toxic shock syndrome, 1442
Vibrio, 1467
Bacterial infections, **1440–1473.** *See also specific types*
conjunctivitis, 170–171
endocarditis, infective (*See* Endocarditis, infective)
keratitis, **179**
rhinosinusitis, **218–221**
skin, **123–128** (*See also under* Skin infections)
cellulitis, **127–128,** 127*f*
erysipelas, **128**
erythema migrans, **128,** 129*f*
folliculitis & sycosis, **124–125,** 125*f*
furunculosis & carbuncles, **126–127**
impetigo, **123–124,** 124*f,* 1441, 1441*t*
Bacterial infections, gram-negative, **1458–1473.** *See also* Gram-negative bacilli
anaerobic, **1471–1473**
bacteremia & endocarditis, 1473
chest, 1472
CNS, 1472
female genital tract & pelvis, 1473
head & neck, 1472
intra-abdominal, 1472, 1472*t*
skin & soft tissue, 1473, 1473*f*
bacteremia & sepsis, **1462–1463**
Bartonella, **1471**
Bordetella bronchiseptica, **1459**
Bordetella pertussis, **1458–1459**
Campylobacter, 590, 1288, **1467**
chancroid, 1285, **1470**
cholera, 1288, 1290*t,* 1294*t,* **1466**
Escherichia coli gastroenteritis, **1465–1466**
gonococcal infections, **1469–1470**
granuloma inguinale, 1285–1286, **1470–1471**
Haemophilus, **1461**
Legionnaires disease, **1461–1462**
meningococcal meningitis, **1459–1461**
Moraxella catarrhalis, **1461**
plague, 1294*t,* **1468–1469**
Salmonellosis, **1463–1465**
bacteremia, **1465**
enteric fever, **1463–1464**
shigellosis, **1465**
tularemia, **1467–1468**
Vibrio, **1466–1467**
Bacterial infections, gram-positive, **1440–1453.** *See also* Pharyngitis; Tonsillitis
clostridial, **1450–1453**
botulism, **1042, 1452–1453**
myonecrosis, 1294*t,* **1450–1451,** 1473, 1473*f*
tetanus, **1451–1452,** 1452*t*
enterococcal, **1443**
listeriosis, **1453**
pneumococcal, **1444–1446**
meningitis, **1446**
pneumonia, **1444–1445**
Staphylococcus aureus, **1446–1450**
bacteremia, **1449**
coagulase-negative infections, **1449–1450**
coagulase-negative staphylococci, **1449–1450**
osteomyelitis, **1447–1448**
skin & soft tissue, **1446–1447,** 1447*f*
toxic shock syndrome, **1449,** 1449*f*
streptococcal, **1440–1443**
streptococcal, Group A beta-hemolytic streptococci, **1440–1443** (*See also Streptococcus,* Group A beta-hemolytic)
streptococcal, non–Group A, **1443**
Bacterial overgrowth, small intestine, **636**
Bacterial synergistic gangrene, 1473
Bacterial vaginosis, 784–785, 785*f,* 1285–1286, 1719
Bacteriuria, pregnancy, 813
Bacteroides
anaerobic pneumonia & lung abscess, 278
animal bites, 1283
medication of choice, 1294*t*
neck infections, deep, 233
nosocomial pneumonia, 275
Bacteroides fragilis, 1472
Bacteroides melaninogenicus, 1472
Bagassosis, 307*t*
Baker cyst
bursitis, 1691–1692
knee, 1695, 1696*t*
rupture, 28
BAL, 1583
Balance, 60, 61
Balanced crystalloid-like lactated Ringer solution, 902
Balanitis, 119, 860, 861*f*
Balanoposthitis, 1200
Balint syndrome, 999
Balkan nephropathy, 938, 1644
Balloon angioplasty, 366
Balloon atrial septostomy, 433
Balloon tube tamponade, for esophageal varices with portal hypertension, 616–617
Balloon valvuloplasty, percutaneous, for mitral stenosis, 337, 337*f*
Baloxavir, 1356*t,* 1412
Bankart lesion, 1681
Barbiturates, 1570, **1581–1582.** *See also specific types*
BARD1, breast cancer, 741
Bariatric surgery, 1218, 1257
Baricitinib, 830, 1405
Baritosis, 306*t*
Barium esophagography, 607, 609, 615, 618, 620
Barotrauma, **208,** 1560
Barrett esophagus, from GERD, **609–610**
Bartholin duct cysts & abscesses, **783,** 783*f*
Bartonella (bartonellosis), 1471, **1471**
Bartonella henselae, 493, **1471**
bacillary angiomatosis, 1328, 1471
lymphadenitis, 493
lymphadenopathy, reactive cervical, 242
Bartonella quintana, 1471
bacillary angiomatosis, 1328, 1471
lice, 130
Bartter syndrome, 884
hypokalemia, 882*t,* 883*f,* 884
metabolic alkalosis, 900, 900*t*
Basal cell carcinoma, **112–113,** 112*f,* 169
Basedow disease, **1119–1127.** *See also* Hyperthyroidism
Basilar artery occlusion, 990
Basilar skull fracture, vertigo, 216
"Bath salts" poisoning, 1574
Batteries, disc/button, poisoning, 1573–1574
Battle sign, 1021
Bazedoxifene, 1151
B-cell lymphomas
after Q fever, 1436
diffuse large, 534
HIV/AIDS, 1329
large, gastric, 1623
from methotrexate, 830
non-Hodgkin, hepatitis C, 682
B-cells, chronic lymphocytic leukemia, **530–532**
B-cells, pancreatic islet
diabetes mellitus
genetic defects, 1196*f,* 1236
type 1, 1195–1196, 1199
type 2, 1196
pancreatitis and subtotal pancreatectomy, 1197
sulfonylureas on, 1203
tumors, hypoglycemia from, **1233–1236,** 1233*t,* 1234*t*
BCG vaccine, 282, 287
BCL2, high-grade lymphoma, 534
bcl2 inhibitor, 531. *See also specific types*
BCL6, high-grade lymphoma, 534
bcr/abl fusion gene
absence, essential thrombocytosis, 522
chronic myeloid leukemia, 524, 525
leukemias & myeloproliferative neoplasms, 520
Beau lines, 166
Becaplermin, 162, 1221
Becker muscular dystrophy, 1043*t,* 1044
Beclomethasone dipropionate, 252*t*
Bedbugs, **131**
Bed rest, 59
Bedside Index for Severity in Acute Pancreatitis, 729
Beef tapeworm, **1523**
Beer, gouty arthritis from, 826
Beer potomania, 877
Bee stings, minimal change disease, 932
Behavior. *See also specific disorders and types*
activation, for depression, 1078
dementia problems, 56
health, gay & bisexual men, **1723–1724**
modification, for weight loss, 1252
sexual, 1709
Behçet syndrome/disease, 183, 482, **856–857**
Belantamab mafodotin, 538
Belching, **588**
Belimumab, 835–836
Belladonna poisoning, 1577
Bell palsy, **1036–1037,** 1036*f*
herpes simplex virus, 1026, 1354, 1355
varicella zoster, 1036, 1360
West Nile virus, 1380
Belly-press test, 1678*t*
Belzutifan, 1646
Bempedoic acid, 1245*t,* 1247
Benazepril, 451*t,* 1091
Bence Jones proteins, 904, 941
Bendamustine, 540, 1598*t*
Bendroflumethiazide, 458*t*
Beneficence, 77
Benign paroxysmal positioning vertigo, **216**
Benign prostatic hyperplasia, **963–969**
clinical findings, 963–964, 964*t*
differential diagnosis, 964
hematuria, microscopic, 943
incidence & prevalence, 963
risk factors, 963
treatment, 964–969
clinical practice guidelines, 964, 965*t*
enucleation, laser, 969
medical
5-alpha-reductase inhibitors, 966
alpha-blockers, 965–966, 965*t*
combination therapy, 966
phosphodiesterase-5 inhibitor, 966
mild symptoms, 964–965
minimally invasive therapies
aquablation, 968
prostate artery embolization, 968
prostatic urethral lift, 968
water vapor thermal therapy, 968

Benign prostatic hyperplasia, treatment (*Cont.*):
prostatectomy, simple, 968
transurethral surgical, **966–968,** 967*f*
laser vaporization of the prostate, 967–968
photoselective vaporization of the prostate, 968
transurethral electrovaporization of the prostate, 967
transurethral incision of the prostate, 966
transurethral resection of the prostate, 966
watchful waiting, 965
Benralizumab, 251*t*, 254
Bentall procedure, for aortic stenosis, 345
Benzathine penicillin, 426, 1336
Benzathine penicillin G, 1483, 1483*t*, 1487
Benzene, acute leukemia from, 528
Benznidazole, 1498–1499
Benzodiazepines. *See also specific types*
for aggression disorders, 1085
for akathisia, from antipsychotics, 1067
for alcohol withdrawal, 1050*t*, 1051, 1091
antipsychotics with, 1066
for bipolar disorder, 1078–1079
for dyskinesia from antipsychotics, 1068
for generalized anxiety disorder, 1050, 1050*t*
for insomnia, 1083
opioid overdose with, 84
overdose, 1051
for panic disorder, 1050*t*, 1051
poisoning, **1581–1582**
antidote, 1568*t*
flumazenil for, 1565
for serotonin syndrome, 1593
side effects, 1051
sympatholytic syndrome from, 1570
withdrawal symptoms, 1051
Benzolecgonine, 1574
Benzoyl peroxide, 148, 149
Benztropine (mesylate), 1009, 1067, 1576
Benzyl alcohol 5%, 131
Berger disease, 923*t*, **927**
Beriberi, **1032,** 1259–1260
Bernard-Soulier syndrome, **556–557**
Berry aneurysms, 325, 993, **994**
Berylliosis, 308
Beta-2 adrenergic agonists, 813, 1012. *See also specific types*
Beta-adrenergic agonists
for asthma, 249–254, 250*t*, 252*t*
atrial fibrillation from, 391
for bronchospasm, pulmonary edema, 414
for preterm birth, anticipated, 805–806
Beta-adrenergic blockers (beta-blockers), 383, 384*t*
for acute coronary syndrome, without ST-segment elevation, 371, 461*t*–462*t*
for acute MI, with ST-segment elevation, 377
for angina pectoris, 363, 364*f*
for atrial fibrillation, with hyperthyroidism, 1126
for cardiomyopathy
dilated, 419
hypertrophic, 422
on diabetes risk, 1197
for esophageal varices with portal hypertension, 617
for heart failure with reduced LVEF, 409
for hyperadrenergic postural orthostatic syndrome, 985
hyperkalemia from, 886, 917
for hypertension, **455, 460,** 461*t*
hypoglycemia from, 1237
for paroxysmal supraventricular tachycardia, 385*t*, 389
for performance anxiety, 1052
for pheochromocytoma, 460
poisoning, **1577–1578**
hypotension treatment, 1565
prophylactic perioperative, 43, 44*t*
for sinus tachycardia, with hyperthyroidism, 1126
surgical risk assessment/reduction, 43, 44*t*
for test anxiety, 1052
Beta cells, pentamidine on, 1237
(1,3)-Beta-D-glucan, 1534
aspergillosis, 1544
candida, 1534
coccidioidomycosis, 1537
pneumocystosis, 1538
17-beta estradiol, feminizing hormone therapy, 1726
Beta-globin gene cluster region, 504
Beta-glucocerebrosidase deficiency, 1662
Beta-hCG, 799–801
Betamethasone, 103*t*, 805
Beta^S gene, 512
Beta-thalassemia syndromes, **505–506,** 505*t*
intermedia, 506
major, 505, 506
minor, 506
Betazolol, 461*t*
Bethanechol, 1223
Bevacizumab, 1600*t*
for colorectal cancer, 1630
for glioma, 1000
for hepatocellular carcinoma, 1612
for mesothelioma, 1609
Bexarotene, 1100
cutaneous T-cell lymphoma, 114
Bezafibrate, 708, 1248
Bezold-Jarisch reflex, 360
Bicalutamide, 1183, 1597*t*, 1602*t*, 1640*t*
Bicarbonate
GI loss, hyperchloremic, normal anion gap metabolic acidosis, 896*t*, 897*t*, 898
Henderson-Hasselbach equation, 894
Bichloroacetic acid, 787
Bictegravir, **1340*t*, 1346**
Bictegravir/tenofovir alafenamide/emtricitabine, 1338
Bicuspid aortic stenosis, 333*t*
Bicuspid aortic valve, 335*t*
aortic dissection, 486
aortic regurgitation, 347
aortic root repair with, 348–349
ascending aortic aneurysm, 345
coarctation of aorta, 325
congenital, aortic stenosis, **342**
pregnancy management, 437*t*
Ross procedure for, 345
transcatheter aortic valve replacement with, 347
Bicuspid pulmonary valve, 330
Bigeminy, 398
Big toe, metatarsophalangeal joint osteoarthritis, 820, 824, 824*f*
Biguanide poisoning, **1582**
Bilateral adrenal hyperplasia, 1164, 1166
Bilateral vocal fold paralysis, 240
Bile acid–binding resins, 1245*t*, 1247–1248
Bile duct stones, 720*t*, **723–725**
Bile salt binders, 595
BiLE score, 686
Bilharziasis, **1520–1521**
Biliary obstruction, jaundice, 674–675
Biliary papillomatosis, 1613
Biliary stricture, **725–726**
Biliary tract carcinoma, **1612–1614**
Biliary tract diseases, **718–728,** 720*t*. *See also specific types*
biliary stricture, **725–726**
calcified gallbladder, 720*t*, 721, 1612
cholecystitis, **720–722,** 720*t*
choledocholithiasis & cholangitis, 720*t*, **723–725**
cholelithiasis (gallstones), **718–720,** 720*t*
dyspepsia, 579
HIV/AIDS, 1326
jaundice & abnormal liver biochemical test evaluation, **674–677,** 676*t*, 677*t*
pre- & postcholecystectomy syndromes, **722**
primary sclerosing cholangitis, **726–728**
Biloma, 725
Binge-eating disorder, obesity, 1251
Binimetinib, *BRAF* inhibitor action, 1671*t*
Biofeedback, 1055, 1057
Biologic therapies, 651–652, 1274. *See also specific types*
Biomarkers, cardiac. *See* Cardiac biomarkers
Biomass fuel cooking, COPD from, 259
Bipolar disorder
cyclothymic disorder, 1070
mania, 1070
prognosis, 1081
treatment, 1078–1081
antipsychotics, 1078–1079
carbamazepine, 1080
lamotrigine, 1080–1081
lithium, 1079–1080
valproic acid (divalproex), 1079
Bipolar I, 1070
Bipolar II, 1070
Bipolaris, 1546
Bird fancier's lung, 307*t*
Birth
preterm, 805
bacteriuria, 813
late, 805
prevention, 806
cervical cerclage for, 806
Birth control. *See* Contraception & family planning; *specific medications and procedures*
Birt-Hogg-Dubé syndrome, 1645
Bisacodyl, 586, 587*t*
Bisexual persons, 1709
Bisexual persons, health care
men, **1722–1725** (*See also* Gay & bisexual men, health care)
women, **1715–1722** (*See also* Lesbian & bisexual women, health care)
Bismuth, tubulointerstitial disease from, 937
Bismuth subcitrate, 591*f*, 624*t*
Bismuth subsalicylate, 624*t*, 627, **1589–1590**
Bismuth sucralfate, 627
Bisoprolol, 409, 461*t*
Bisphosphonates
for bone pain, metastatic, 95
for breast carcinoma, 754, 756
on hip fractures, 1693
for hypercalcemia, from bone respiration, 890
for hyperparathyroidism, 1145
for osteoporosis, 1149–1150, 1193–1194
side effects, 1150
Bite wounds, **1283–1284**
Bithionol, 1522, 1523
Bitolterol, 249
Bitot spots, vitamin A deficiency, 1262
Bivalirudin, 370*f*, 371, 553, 553*t*
Biventricular pacing
for dilated cardiomyopathy, 420
for heart failure
with preserved LVEF, 412
with reduced LVEF, 411
for mitral regurgitation, myocardial disease, 339
BK virus, 1385

Black cohosh, 1187
"Black eye," **197–198,** 225
Black-legged tick, 1434
Black licorice, 882*t*, 883*f*, 900
"Black" molds, 1546
Blacks. *See* African Americans
Black widow spiders, **1590–1591**
Bladder cancer, **1642–1644**
 hematuria, 39, 943, 1642
 treatment, 1597*t*, 1642–1644
Bladder training, 63
Blalock shunts, 330
Blastomycosis, **1545**
Bleeding. *See also* Hemorrhage; *specific types*
 3rd trimester, **806–807**
 diathesis, chronic kidney disease, 917
 GI, 502, **596–602**
  lower, acute, **598–600**
  occult, **601–602**
  suspected bowel, **601**
  upper, acute, **596–598**
 hemorrhoids, 599, 669
 menstrual, 501–502
 patient evaluation, 546, 547*t*
 risk, preoperative evaluation/perioperative management, 42, 42*t*, 48
 uterine, 501–502 (*See also* Menstruation)
  abnormal, reproductive age, **763–765,** 764*t*
  gestational trophoblastic disease, 801
  postmenopausal, **765**
Bleomycin, 123
Blepharitis, 139, **169,** 1353
Blepharospasm, 1011, 1012
Blind loop syndrome, vitamin B_{12} deficiency, 507
Blindness
 cataract, 184
 cortical, 999
 diabetic retinopathy, 67, 191, **191–192,** 1221
 "fleeting," 190
 giant cell arteritis, 848, 849
 glaucoma, chronic, 181, 183
 ocular trauma, 196
 onchocerciasis, 1532
 trachoma, 171
 trauma, ocular, 196
Blistering pemphigus foliaceus, 146
Bloating, **588**
Blood disorders, **500–545.** *See also specific types*
 anemias, **500–509**
 dyscrasias, retinal disorders, **193**
 hemolytic anemias, **509–519**
 leukemias
  acute, 510, **528–530,** 1595*t*
  chronic lymphocytic, **530–532**
  chronic myeloid, 520*t*, **524–526**
  classification, WHO, 519, 519*t*, 520*t*
  hairy cell, **532–533**
  Philadelphia chromosome, 520
 lymphomas, **533–542**
 myeloproliferative neoplasms
  classification, WHO, 519, 519*t*, 520*t*
  essential thrombocytosis, 520*t*, **522–523**
  myelodysplastic syndromes, **526–527**
  myelofibrosis, primary, 520*t*, **523–524**
  polycythemia vera, **520–521,** 520*t*, 521*t*
 transfusions, blood, **542–545** (*See also* Blood transfusions)
  cryoprecipitate, **545**
  fresh frozen plasma, **545**
  platelet, **544–545**
  RBC, **542–544**
Blood-filled cavities, 697
Blood gases, arterial. *See* Arterial blood gases
Blood pressure. *See also* Hypertension; Hypotension; *specific disorders*
 measurement & diagnosis, **442–444**
  definitions & guidelines, 365, 442, 443*f*
  labile hypertension, 444
  masked hypertension, 444
  measurement methods, times, and values, 442, 443*t*
  readings, number, 442
  sphygmomanometer, 442
  "white coat" hypertension, **442–444,** 468
 screening/cardiovascular disease prevention, 5*t*, 8–9
Blood transfusions, **542–545**
 compatibility testing, 542
 contaminated blood, 543–544
 cryoprecipitate, **545**
 fresh frozen plasma, **545**
 hemolytic transfusion reactions, 543
 HIV infection, 1313
 human T-cell lymphotropic virus, 1388
 hypersensitivity reactions, 543
 infectious disease transmission, 544
 leukoagglutinin reactions, 543
 platelet, **544–545**
 RBC, **542–544**
 transfusion graft-*versus*-host disease, 544
 transfusion-related acute lung injury, 544
 for upper GI bleeding, 597
Blood vessel disorders, **473–493.** *See also specific types*
 arterial aneurysms, **482–487**
  abdominal aortic, 5*t*, 6, 42, **482–484,** 1465
  aortic dissection, **486–487**
  peripheral artery, **485–486**
  thoracic aortic, **484–485**
 atherosclerotic peripheral vascular disease, **473–481**
 nonatherosclerotic vascular disease, **481–482**
 thromboangiitis obliterans, **481–482**
 venous diseases, **487–493**
  chronic venous insufficiency, **490–492,** 490*f*, 491*f*
  superficial venous thrombophlebitis, **489–490**
  superior vena caval obstruction, **492–493**
  varicose veins, **487–489**
"Blowout fracture," **197–198**
"Blue bloaters," 259, 260*t*
Blue nevi, **108,** 108*f*
B lymphocytes. *See* B-cells
BNP. *See* B-type natriuretic peptide
BODE index, 264
Body dysmorphic disorder, 1052
Body fat loss, subcutaneous, 1250
Body louse, 130
Body mass index, 10–11, **1251,** 1628
Body surface area estimation, 1554, 1555*f*
Body temperature. *See* Temperature, body
Body water, **875,** 875*t*
 fluid distribution, electrolyte disorders, **875,** 875*t*
 total, **875–876,** 875*t*, 881
  interstitial fluid, 875
  intracellular, 875
  plasma fluid, 875
  water deficit, calculation, 881–882
Boerhaave syndrome, 582
Boils, **126–127,** 1446
Bone/bone disorders. *See also specific types*
 alkaline phosphate deficiency, 1153
 avascular necrosis, **868,** 1323
 density/densitometry
  DXA, 1143, 1147, 1148, 1149, 1154
  hyperparathyroidism, 1142
  scanning, 1693
 diabetes mellitus on, 1225
 HIV/AIDS, 1323–1324
 ischemic necrosis, sickle cell anemia, 512
 overgrowths, ear canal, 207
 Paget disease of, **1155–1156**
 scans, radionuclide, for prostate cancer, 1636
 turnover, chronic kidney disease, 917, 917*f*
Bone-conducting hearing aids, 205
Bone marrow
 antipsychotics on, 1066
 chemotherapy on, **1655**
 failure, **546–548**
 infiltration, **548**
Bone mineral density, 1146, 1225
Bone-modifying agents, 754. *See also specific types*
Borderline personality disorder, **1059–1061,** 1060*t*
Bordetella bronchiseptica, **1459**
Bordetella pertussis, **1458–1459**
Boric acid, 785
Bornhold disease, 1423
Borrelia burgdorferi. *See* Lyme disease
Borrelia miyamotoi, 1434
Borrelia recurrentis, 1295*t*
Bortezomib, 1601*t*
 for amyloidosis, 541, 936
 neuropathy from, 1656
 for plasma cell myeloma, 538
 for Waldenström macroglobulinemia, 540
Bosentan, 705, 841
Bosutinib, 525, 1600*t*
Botulinum toxin, 619, 672–673, 1452
Botulinum toxin A, 972*t*, 973
Botulism, **1042, 1452–1453**
 diarrhea, 1289*t*
 dysautonomia, 984
 food-borne, 1042, 1452
 wound, injection drug use, 1286–1287
Bouchard nodes, 820, 821*f*
Bova score, 568–569
Bovine spongiform encephalopathy, 1385
Bowel obstruction, 70. *See also specific types*
Bowen disease, **114**
Boxelotor, 513
Brachial plexopathy, idiopathic, 1040
Brachial plexus neuropathy, **1040**
Brachiola, 1517
Bradycardia/bradyarrhythmias. *See also specific types*
 acquired long QT syndrome, 401
 acute MI, with ST-segment elevation, 373
 from adenosine, 385*t*
 angina pectoris, 360
 AV synchrony, 388
 from cold water, facial contact, 389
 from diltiazem, 385*t*
 from esmolol, 384*t*
 from ivabradine, 385*t*
 from metoprolol, 384*t*
 pacing for, 388
 from propranolol, 384*t*
 sinus, 379, **386–387,** 402, 403
 from sotalol, 385*t*
 tachy-brady syndrome, 386
Bradykinesia, Parkinson disease, 1007
BRAF, 665, 1671*t*
 colorectal cancer, 1630
 hairy cell leukemia, 532
 lung cancer, 1606
 malignant melanoma, 110
BRAF inhibitors, 533. *See also specific types*
BRAF V600E, 1671*t*
BRAF V600K, 1671*t*
Brain abscess, **1002,** 1281, 1282, 1296*t*
Brain death, **1020**
Brainstem
 aura, migraine with, 971
 glioma, 998*t*
 lesions, 999, 1020
 tumor, vertigo from, 217
 vascular disease, vertigo from, 217
 vomiting center, 581

Branchial cleft cysts, **241–242**
Branch retinal artery occlusion, **189–190**
Branch retinal vein occlusion, **188–189**
Brandt-Daroff exercises, 216
Brazilian spotted fever, 1427*t*, **1431**
BRCA, 754
BRCA1/2
breast carcinoma, 11, 741, 741*t*, 750
female, risk factor, 741
female, treatment
adjuvant systemic, 752
PARP inhibitors, 754
PARP targeting, 759
triple-negative cancer, 755
male, 762
colorectal cancer, 1636
ovarian cancer, 793
pancreas carcinoma, 1615
prostate cancer, 1641
Breakthrough pain, 81, 86
Breast
reconstruction, after breast carcinoma treatment, 761
self-examination, 743
Breast carcinoma, female, **737–761**
anatomic sites, frequency by, **743, 744*f***
bilateral, 749
BRCA 1/2 gene, 11, 741, 741*t*, 750
combined oral contraceptives and, 774
differential diagnosis, 747
ductal carcinoma in situ, **749**
early clinical findings, 743–747
evaluation
postmenopausal, 747*f*
premenopausal, 746*f*
imaging, 744–747
laboratory findings, 744
symptoms & signs, 743–744, 744*f*
early detection, 742–747
ER receptor-positive/-negative, 741
follow-up care, 760–761
incidence and risk factors, 740–741, 741*t*
inflammatory carcinoma, 748
Ki-67, 749, 752, 754
lesbian & bisexual women, **1720**
lobular carcinoma in situ, **749**
Paget carcinoma, 748
pathologic types, 748, 748*t*
pregnancy and lactation, 748–749
prevention, 742
prognosis, 759–760, 759*t*
screening, 742
screening/detection, 11
staging, 747–748, 747*t*
tumor biomarkers & gene expression profiling, 749–750
Breast carcinoma, female, treatment, 1597*t*
curative, 750–756
adjunctive systemic, 752–755
chemotherapy, anthracycline & cyclophosphamide regimens, 752
chemotherapy, taxanes, 752
duration & dose, 753
older women, 754–755
prognostic factors, 752
prognostic factors, node-negative, 750, 752*t*
side effects, 753
targeted therapy, aromatase inhibitors, 754
targeted therapy, bisphosphonates, 754
targeted therapy, bone-modifying agents, 754
targeted therapy, cyclin dependent kinase 4/6 inhibitors, 754
targeted therapy, HER2, 753
targeted therapy, PARP inhibitors, 754
targeted therapy, tamoxifen, 753
neoadjuvant
HER-2 positive, 755
hormone receptor–positive, HER-2 negative, 755
sentinel lymph node biopsy timing, 755–756
triple-negative, 755
primary, choice & timing, 747*t*, 750
radiotherapy, 751
sentinel node biopsy, 751, 751*f*
surgical resection
breast-conserving, 750–751, 751*f*
mastectomy, 751
palliative, 756–759
chemotherapy, 759
radiotherapy & bisphosphonates, 756
targeted, 756–759
HER2-targeted, 758
hormonally based, metastatic disease, 756–758, 757*t*
first-line, hormonally targeted, 757
first-line, hormonally targeted + CDK inhibition, 757–758
progression after hormonally based, 758
PARP, *BRCA1/2*-associated, 759
"triple-negative," 758–759
Breast carcinoma, male, **762**
Breast-conserving lumpectomy, 750–751, 751*f*
Breast-conserving therapy, breast carcinoma, 750–751, 751*f*
Breast disorders, **737–762**. *See also specific types*
abscess, **740** (*See also* Puerperal mastitis)
benign, **737–740**
augmented breast, **740**
breast abscess, **740** (*See also* Puerperal mastitis)
fat necrosis, **739–740**
fibroadenoma of breast, **738–739**
fibrocystic condition, **737–738**
nipple discharge, **739,** 739*t*
phyllodes tumor, 738–739
Paget disease, **114**, 744, 744*f*
Breastfeeding. *See* Lactation
Breathing/respiration
apneustic, 1019
central neurogenic hyperventilation, 1019
Cheyne-Stokes respiration, 1019
exercises, deep, postoperative risk reduction, 47
hyperventilation syndrome, **315**
intermittent positive-pressure, postoperative risk reduction, 47
obesity-hypoventilation syndrome, **315**
obstructive sleep apnea, **316–317**
sleep disorders, **1084** (*See also specific types*)
sleep-related, 33, **316**
Bremelanotide, 1059
Brentuximab vedotin, 535
Brief psychotic disorders, 1062
Brigatinib, 1606
Brill-Zinsser disease, 1426
Brimonidine, 150
Brimonidine overdose, **1579**
Brincidofovir, 1419, 1421
Brivaracetam, 975*t*
Broad waxy casts, 904*t*, 915, 937
Broca aphasia, 989
Brodalumab, 138
Brodifacoum poisoning, 1575
"Broken-heart syndrome," 373, 418, **420–421**
Bromine, inhalation poisoning, 1573
Bromocriptine
dystonia from, 1012
for hyperglycemia/diabetes mellitus, 1211
for hyperprolactinemia, 1109
for malignant hyperthermia, 1567
for neuroleptic malignant syndrome, 1576
serotonin syndrome from, 30
Bronchial carcinoid tumors, **291**
Bronchiectasis, **265,** 288
Bronchiolitis, **267–268**
Bronchiolitis obliterans, 268, 304
Bronchioloalveolar cell carcinoma, 1603
Bronchitis
Chlamydophila pneumoniae, 1479
wheezing and rhonchi, 16
Bronchoconstriction, 246. *See also specific disorders*
Bronchogenic carcinoma, **1603–1607**
cigarette smoking, 1603
clinical findings, 1603–1604, 1604*f*
cough, 16
hemoptysis, 21
histologic categories, 1603
paraneoplastic syndromes, 1603–1604
prognosis, 1607
risk factors, 1603
staging & survival, 1604–1605, 1605*t*
treatment
non–small cell lung carcinoma, 1605–1607
palliative, 1607
small cell lung carcinoma, 1607, 1607*t*
Bronchoprovocation testing, asthma, 247
Bronchus
foreign bodies, **241**
obstruction, 245
Brown recluse spider, **1590–1591**
Brown-Séquard syndrome, **1027**
Brucella, 1294*t*
Bruce protocol, 360, 367, 367*t*
Brudzinski sign, 36
Brugada syndrome, 26, 400, **401,** 439, 440*t*
Brugia malayi, 297, 1530–1531
Brugia timori, 1530–1531
Bruton tyrosine kinase inhibitors, 531. *See also specific types*
Bruxism, ear pain, 212
BTK inhibitors. *See also specific types*
for chronic lymphocytic leukemia, 531
for mantle cell lymphoma, 535
for Waldenström macroglobulinemia, 540
B-type natriuretic peptide (BNP)
aortic stenosis & left ventricular myocardial failure, 343, 344*f*
cardiomyopathy, restrictive, 424
heart failure, **405**
left ventricular dysfunction, 348
mitral regurgitation, 339
myocarditis, 415, 417
N-terminal proBNP
aortic stenosis & left ventricular myocardial failure, 343
cardiomyopathy, restrictive, 424
heart failure, **405**
mitral regurgitation, 339
myocarditis, 415, 417
preoperative evaluation, 43
tetralogy of Fallot, 331
traumatic heart disease, 434
pregnancy, 436
preoperative evaluation, 43
pulmonary edema, cardiogenic, 413
pulmonary venous thromboembolism, 298
recombinant, 413–414
Bubble contrast, 327
Budd-Chiari syndrome, 603, 685, **713–714**
Budesonide
clinical uses, 1193, 1194*t*
for Crohn disease, 655

for eosinophilic esophagitis, 614
for inflammatory bowel disease, 650
for microscopic colitis, 663
for ulcerative colitis, 659–660
Buerger disease, **481–482**
Bufotenin poisoning, 1581
Bulbar poliomyelitis, 1375
Bulimia nervosa, **1259**
Bullectomy, 264
Bullous, 102*t*
Bullous impetigo, HIV/AIDS, 1328
Bullous pemphigoid, **147**
Bumetanide, 458*t*, 470, 954
BUN, 905, 905*t*
BUN:creatinine ratio, 905, 907*t*
Bundle branch block
bilateral, 380
heart failure, reduced LVEF, 406*f*
left
acute MI, with ST-segment elevation, **373–375**, 380
angina pectoris, 361
AV block, 387–388
cardiomyopathy, dilated, 419, 420
heart failure, 411, 412
mitral regurgitation, 339
myocarditis, 415
paroxysmal supraventricular tachycardia, 388
accessory AV pathway, 390
syncope, 402
right
atrial septal defect, 327
AV block, 387
paroxysmal supraventricular tachycardia, 388
accessory AV pathway, 390
pulmonary valve regurgitation, 352
tetralogy of Fallot, 331
ventricular tachycardia, 399, 400
Bunyavirus hemorrhagic fevers, **1391–1392**
Bupivacaine, 97*t*, 1565
Buprenorphine, **87*t*,** 93–94, 1092, 1588
Bupropion
for attention-deficit/hyperactivity disorders, 1081
for depression, 1072, 1073*t*, 1074
for generalized anxiety disorder, 1051
poisoning, hypotension treatment, 1565
for psychotic depression, 1072, 1073*t*
seizures from, 1567
for sexual arousal disorder, from SSRIs, 1075
for tobacco dependence and smoking cessation, 7, 7*t*
toxicity, 1592
for weight loss, 1253, 1255*t*
Burkholderia cenocepacia, cystic fibrosis, 266
Burkholderia mallei, 1294*t*
Burkholderia pseudomallei, 1294*t*
Burkitt lymphoma, 535, 1364
Burning mouth syndrome, **230**
Burns
chemical, eye, **198**
clothing, 1557
electrical injury, 1557–1558
thermal, **1554–1557**, 1555*f*
body surface area estimation, 1554, 1555*f*
Bursitis, 1225, 1691, **1691–1692**, 1692*f*
Buruli ulcer, 1475
"Bush tea," sinusoidal obstruction syndrome from, 713
Buspirone, 1050*t*, 1051, 1085
Butalbital, 971, 974
Butanediol, 1582
Butenafine, 106*t*, 115
Butoconazole, 785
Button batteries, **241**, 1573–1574
Butyrophenones, 1012, 1576

C
C3 glomerulopathy, 912, 923*t*, **929**
C282Y, 695, 709–711
C481S, chronic lymphocytic leukemia, 531
CA 125, ovarian cancer, 793
Cabazitaxel, 1640*t*, 1641
Cabergoline, 1107, 1109, 1163
Cabotegravir, **1341*t*, 1346,** 1725
Cabozantinib, 1612, 1646
Cachexia, 1250
anorexia-cachexia syndrome, 73
cancer, 73
cardiac, exercise training on, 33
diabetic neuropathic, 1222
heart failure, 73
Cadmium, tubulointerstitial disease from, 937
Café au lait spots, 1005
Café coronary, **306**
Cafergot, 971
Caffeine
abuse, **1094**
fibrocystic condition, 738
lower esophageal sphincter, 306
for migraine headache, 971
poisoning, **1592**
tremor from, 1012
Calcific aortic stenosis, 342
Calcified gallbladder, 720*t*, 721
Calcineurin inhibitors. *See also specific types*
acute tubular necrosis from, 909
for focal segmental glomerulosclerosis, 933
for glomerulonephritis, 913
hyperkalemia from, 886
for lupus nephritis, 930, 931
for membranous nephropathy, 934
renal constriction from, 907
Calcipotriene, 137
Calcitonin
for hypercalcemia, 890, 1650
for hypercalcemia, salmon, 1651
in metastatic papillary and follicular tumors, 1133
for osteoporosis, 1151–1152
Calcitonin gene–related peptide antagonists, 971, 972*t*. *See also specific types*
Calcitriol, 137
Calcium
deficiency
osteomalacia from, 1153
rickets from, 1153
dietary, 1264
for osteoporosis, 1149
serum, normal, 886–890
Calcium carbonate, 917
hyperoxaluric calcium nephrolithiasis, 956
Calcium channel alpha2-delta ligands, 94, 94*t*. *See also specific types*
Calcium channel blockers. *See also specific types*
for acute coronary syndrome, without ST-segment elevation, 371–372
for acute MI, with ST-segment elevation, 378
for angina pectoris, 363, 364*f*, 456*t*–457*t*
for cardiomyopathy, hypertrophic, 422
for Cushing syndrome, 1163
for hypertension, **454–455**
dihydropyridine, **454–455,** 457*t*
nondihydropiridine, **454–455,** 456*t*
for interstitial cystitis, 954
lower extremity edema from, 28
parkinsonism from, 1012
for paroxysmal supraventricular tachycardia, 385*t*, 389
poisoning, **1578**
hypotension treatment, 1565
for preterm birth, anticipated, 805–806
for Raynaud phenomenon, 839
slow, 383, 385*t*
surgical risk assessment/reduction, 43
Calcium chloride, 894, 1578
Calcium citrate, 956, 1154
Calcium concentration disorders, **886–890**. *See also specific types*
hypercalcemia, **889–890**
hypocalcemia, **886–888,** 888*t*
Calcium gluconate, 1578
Calcium nephrolithiasis, medical treatment & prevention
hypercalciuria, 956
hyperoxaluria, 956–957
hyperuricosuria, 956
hypocitraturia, 957
Calcium oxalate stones, 954. *See also* Urinary stone disease
Calcium phosphate stones, 954. *See also* Urinary stone disease
Calcium polycarbophil, 586, 587*t*
Calcium pyrophosphate
crystals, pseudogout, 827
deposition, **826–827**
Calcium score, coronary, 361
Calcium therapy
kidney stones from, 954
for Paget disease of bone, 1156
Calcivirus, 1290*t*. *See also specific types*
Calculus
renal (*See* Kidney stones)
sialolithiasis, 235
Calf strain/trauma, lower extremity edema, 28
Calorimetry, indirect, 1266, 1269
CALR, 520, 522, 523
Calymmatobacterium granulomatis. *See Klebsiella granulomatis*
Camphor/menthol, 106*t*, 1567
Campylobacter, 590, 1288, **1467**
Campylobacter fetus subsp *fetus*, **1467**
Campylobacter jejuni, **1467**
diarrhea, 1289*t*, 1292
enteritis, Guillain-Barré syndrome and, 1033
medication of choice, 1294*t*
Campylobacter-like organisms, **1467**
Canagliflozin
for coronary heart disease prevention in diabetics, 358–359
for diabetes mellitus, 935, 1205*t*, 1210–1211, 1218
for hyperglycemia, 1205*t*, 1210–1211
for hypertension in elderly, 466
Canakinumab, 825, 831
c-ANCA, glomerulonephritis, 912
Cancer, **1594–1656**. *See also specific types*
common, by site, 1594, 1595*t*
complications & emergencies, **1649–1653**
hypercalcemia, **1650–1651**
hyperuricemia & tumor lysis syndrome, **1651–1652**
infections, **1652–1653**
malignant effusions, **1649–1650**
spinal cord compression, **1649**
death rates, 1594
etiology, 1594
fatigue, 70
gastrointestinal bleeding, lower, 599
hypercalcemia, 889
neuropathies, **1033**
obesity, 1251
pain, 79, **80**
prevention, **11–12**
prognosis, 72, **1657**

Cancer (*Cont.*):
radiation, CT, 1594
rheumatologic manifestations, **867**
risk factors
hypertension treatment, **464**
modifiable, 1594
sexual & gender minorities, **1730**
screening, 11–12 (*See also specific cancers*)
smoking & tobacco use, 1595
staging, **1595**
vitamin C deficiency, 1261
weight loss, involuntary, 32
Cancer, treatment, 1595. *See also specific cancers*
choices, 1595*t*–1598*t*
primary, **1653–1657**
systemic cancer therapy, 1595*t*–1598*t*, **1653**
toxicity & dose modifications, 1598*t*–1602*t*, **1653–1657,** 1653*t*–1654*t*
bone marrow, **1655**
cardiotoxicity, **1657**
chemotherapy-induced nausea & vomiting, **1655–1656**
cisplatin, **1657**
dose modifications, 1654*t*
gastrointestinal toxicity, **1656**
hemorrhagic cystitis, **1656**
immune checkpoint inhibitors, **1657**
methotrexate, **1656–1657**
neuropathy, **1656**
therapeutic agents, 1598*t*–1602*t*
venous thromboembolism, 572–573
Candesartan (cilexitil), 452*t*, 972*t*
Candida (candidiasis)
cervical, **784–785,** 784*f*
chorioretinitis, 193
endocarditis, 1534
esophageal, 1534, 1535
funguria, 1534, 1535
gastritis, 624
with granulocytopenia, 1273
hematopoietic cell transplant recipients, 1273
HIV/AIDS, 1324–1325, 1328
esophagitis, 1318*t*, 1325
skin infection, 1328
vaginal, 1318*t*, 1330
immunocompromised, pulmonary infiltrates, 279
invasive, 1534, 1535
liver abscess, 717
mucocutaneous, **118–119,** 119*f*
mucosal, 1534, 1535
neutropenia, 519
odynophagia, 607
oral, **229,** 229*f*
osteomyelitis/septic arthritis, 1287
paronychia, 166, 166*f*
solid organ transplant recipients, 1273
treatment, 1534–1535
uveitis, 183
vulvovaginal, **784–785,** 784*f*, 1255, 1534–1535
Candida albicans, 612, 1287, **1534–1535**
Candida antigen, 1421
Candida auris, 1535
Candida glabrata, 1535
Candida krusei, 1535
Candida parapsilosis, infective endocarditis, 1287
Candidiasis, **1534–1535**
Canine tapeworm, 1525–1526
Canker sore, **230**
Cannabidiol
for HIV/AIDS weight loss, 1316–1317
poisoning, 1585
for schizophrenia, **1064**
for seizures, 975*t*
Cannabinoids
hyperemesis syndrome, 584, 1585
for nausea, **584**
for neuropathic pain, 94*t*, 95
sympathomimetic syndrome from, 1570
synthetic, 1567, 1574, **1585**
Cannabis
on hepatitis C progression, 689
for HIV/AIDS weight loss, 1316–1317
for nausea & vomiting, 70
Cannabis sativa, 1093
"Cannon" A waves, palpitations, 26
Cantharidin, 121, 1421
Capecitabine, 1599*t*
for breast carcinoma, 759
for colorectal cancer, 1630
DPD variant metabolism of, 1669*t*
for gallbladder carcinoma, 1614
for pancreas carcinoma, 1616
Caplan syndrome, 306
Capmatinib, 1606
Capnocytophaga, cat and dog bites, 1283–1284
Caprini score, 566
Capsaicin
for diabetic peripheral neuropathy, 1222
for knee osteoarthritis, 83*t*, 821, 1705
for neuropathic pain, 94*t*, 95
for pruritus, anogenital/scrotal, 161
topical dermatologic, 106*t*
Capsicum, 1685
Capsule colonoscopy, for colorectal cancer screening, 1633
Captopril
for acute MI, with ST-segment elevation, 378
autoimmune hypoglycemia from, 1237
for heart failure with reduced LVEF, 407–408
for hypertension, 451*t*, 471*t*, 472
for hypertensive crises, systemic sclerosis, 841
membranous nephropathy, 934
Carbamate insecticides, 1570, **1588–1589**
Carbamazepine
for aggression disorders, 1085
for bipolar disorder, 1080
dystonia from, 1012
for facial pain, 978
for glossopharyngeal neuralgia, 978
hepatotoxicity, 696
for personality disorders, 1061
poisoning, 1571*t*, **1575–1576,** 1576
hemodialysis for, 1569*t*
repeat-dose charcoal for, 1569
for seizures, 975*t*
skin reactions, 1669*t*
teratogenicity, 813
for trigeminal neuralgia, 975
Carbapenems, 1442, 1467. *See also specific types*
Carbaryl poisoning, **1588–1589**
Carbohydrate-restricted diets, 1264
Carbonic anhydrase inhibitors, 954. *See also specific types*
Carbon monoxide
anion gap elevation from, 1570
diffusing capacity, pulmonary hypertension, 432
poisoning, 1571*t*, 1572*t*, **1578–1579**
antidote, 1568*t*
dyspnea, 18–20
headache, 35
parkinsonism from, 1006
Carboplatin, 759, 1598*t*, 1606, 1609
Carboxyhemoglobin complex, 1578
Carbuncles, **126–127,** 1447
Carcinogens. *See specific types*
Carcinoids/carcinoid disease, **1172**
appendiceal, 1626
bronchial, 291
GI, **1626–1627**
pulmonary valve regurgitation, 352
rectal, 1626
small intestinal, 1626
small intestine bleeding, 601
treatment, 1597*t*
tricuspid stenosis, 350
Carcinoid syndrome, 291, 1626
Carcinoma. *See* Cancer; *specific types*
Carcinomatous meningitis, **1001,** 1281
Cardiac. *See* Heart
Cardiac amyloidosis, 423
Cardiac arrest. *See* Sudden cardiac arrest/death
"Cardiac asthma," 246
Cardiac biomarkers. *See also specific types*
acute coronary syndromes, without ST-segment elevation, 368–369
angina pectoris, 367
cardiac risk assessment/reduction, 43
chest pain, 23, 24
heart failure, 412, 417
myocarditis, 412
preoperative evaluation & perioperative management, 43
traumatic heart disease, 434
ventricular fibrillation and sudden cardiac death, 400
Cardiac cachexia, exercise training on, 33
Cardiac catheterization
acute coronary syndrome, without ST-segment elevation, 372, 372*t*
acute heart failure & pulmonary edema, 414
acute MI with ST-segment elevation, 375, 378, 379, 380–381, 382
angina pectoris, 360, 362
aortic regurgitation, 348
aortic stenosis, 343
atrial fibrillation, 395
atrial septal defect, 327
cardiomyopathy, 418*t*
hypertrophic, 422
stress, 421
coarctation of aorta, 325
heart failure, 405–406
mitral regurgitation, 339
mitral stenosis, 336
myocardial ischemia, 372*t*
patent foramen ovale, 327
pericarditis, constrictive, 430–431
pulmonary valve regurgitation, 352
tetralogy of Fallot, 331
tricuspid stenosis, 350
ventricular septal defect, 329
Cardiac complications, perioperative, 42. *See also* Cardiac risk assessment/reduction, noncardiac surgery
Cardiac Disease in Pregnancy Investigation, 435
Cardiac glycosides, 1568*t*, 1581, **1581**. *See also specific types*
Cardiac output
acute MI, with ST-segment elevation, 373, 379–380
aortic regurgitation, 347
aortic stenosis, 342
cardiomyopathy, dilated, 418*t*
heart failure, 403
milrinone on, 414
mitral regurgitation, 339
mitral stenosis, 336
nesiritide on, 413–414
pregnancy, 812
pulmonary hypertension, 432, 433

rate & rhythm disorders on, 383
sinus bradycardia, 386
sinus tachycardia, 386
tricuspid regurgitation, 333*t*
Cardiac resynchronization. *See* Resynchronization, cardiac
Cardiac risk assessment/reduction, noncardiac surgery, **42–46**
arrhythmias, 45
cardiac biomarkers, 43
coronary artery disease, 43–44, 44*t*
coronary revascularization, 43–44
exercise capacity, 42
heart failure & left ventricular dysfunction, 44–45
hypertension, 45–46
ischemic testing, preoperative noninvasive, 42–43, 44*f*
myocardial infarction, postoperative, 45
Revised Cardiac Risk Index, 42, 43*t*
stress testing, 43
valvular heart disease, 45
Cardiac Risk Index, Revised, 42, 43*t*
Cardiac tumors, **433–434**
Cardiogenic liver injury, **715**
Cardiogenic pulmonary edema, **413–414**
Cardiogenic shock, **495–499,** 495*t*
Cardiogenic syncope, 402–403
Cardiomyopathy, **417–424**
acid maltase deficiency, 1044
alcoholic, 404, 414, 418*t*, 419
arrhythmogenic right ventricular, **401**
cirrhotic, 700–702
classification, 418*t*
cobalt, 419
cocaine, 415*t*, 417, 418*t*
congestive, 403–404
heart failure, 302–303
dilated, **417–420,** 418*t*
amyloidosis, 404, 418, 418*t*
athlete screening, 438.439*t*
athletic deaths, 438
atrial fibrillation, 391
causes, 40
clinical findings, 405
end-stage kidney disease, 418
heart failure, 302–303
HIV, 418, 420
jugular venous pulsations, 418
left bundle branch block, 419, 420
mitral regurgitation, 339, 341
myocarditis, 415, 416
palpitations, 26
perfusion defects, 361
pregnancy, 435, 436, 437*t*
sudden cardiac death, 400
ventricular tachycardia, 399
HIV, 417
hypertrophic, 404, 418*t*, **421–423**
asymmetric septal, 418*t*, 421, 439
athlete screening, 438–439, 439*t*, 440*t*
atrial fibrillation, 421, 422
heart failure, 404
interventions on, 336*t*
mitral regurgitation, 339
palpitations, 26
Valsalva maneuver, 336*t*, 421, 422
ischemic, heart failure, 302
palpitations, 25, 26
peripartum, 436, **436**
of pregnancy, **436**
restrictive, 418*t*, **423–424**
familial, 423
heart failure, 404
pulmonary capillary wedge pressure, 423
right ventricular, arrhythmogenic, 399, 400, **401**
stress, 373, 418, **420–421**
Cardiooncology, 417
Cardiorenal syndrome, **913**
Cardiotomy, 427, 428, 430
Cardiotoxicity, drug, 1656
Cardiovascular disease. *See also specific types*
chemoprevention, 5*t*, 9
chronic kidney disease and, 914
diabetes mellitus, 1224
heart disease, 1224
hypertension, 1224
peripheral vascular disease, 1224
hypertensive, 446
influenza, 1411
lesbian & bisexual women, **1716**
palpitations, 25
prevention, **4–9,** 5*t*
abdominal aortic aneurysm, 5*t*, 6, 42, **482–484,** 1465
aspirin, low-dose, 5*t*, 9
chemoprevention, 5*t*, 9
cigarette smoking & smoking cessation, 4, 5*t*, 6–8, 6*t*, 7*t*
hypertension, 4, 5*t*, 8–9
lipid disorders, 4, 5*t*, 8
risk factors, 4–6
risk prevention recommendations, 4, 5*t*
statins, 5*t*, 8, 355, 356*f*, 357–358, 357*t*
risk factors, 448, 449*t*, 450 (*See also specific types*)
Cardiovascular screening, athletes, **438–441,** 439*t*, 440*t*
Cardioversion
for acute MI, with ST-segment elevation, 379
anticoagulants before, 397
for atrial fibrillation, 392, 393, 395–396, 1126
for atrial flutter, 397
for paroxysmal supraventricular tachycardia, 389
for ventricular tachycardia, 399
Cardioverter defibrillator
implantable
for cardiomyopathy, dilated, 419
for heart failure with reduced LVEF, 411
for ventricular tachycardia, 398
wearable, 400
Carditis. *See also* Endocarditis; Myocarditis; Pericarditis
reactive arthritis, 860
rheumatic fever, 425
rheumatic fever/heart disease, 425, 425*t*
subclinical, 424
Carfilzomib, 538, 540
Cariprazine, 1063, **1064,** 1064*t*
Carisoprodol poisoning, **1581–1582**
Carney complex, acromegaly, 1106
Carnitine
deficiency, dilated cardiomyopathy, 418
for valproic acid–induced hyperammonemia, 1576
Carotid angioplasty, 479
Carotid artery
bruits, 478–479
dissection
headache, 974
retinal artery occlusion, 189–190
occlusion
headache, 974
transient monocular visual loss, 190
stenosis, **478–480,** 479*f*
on stroke risk, postsurgery, 49
Carotid circulation obstruction, **988–989,** 989*t*
Carotid endarterectomy, 479, 987
Carotid sinus
hypersensitivity, 402
massage, 389
Carotid stenting, 479
Carotidynia, 848
Carpal compression test, 1690
Carpal tunnel syndrome, 1225, **1690–1691**
Carpometacarpal joint osteoarthritis, 820
CARPREG I/II scoring systems, 435, 436*f*
Carvallo sign, 351
Carvedilol, 377, 409, 461*t*
Caspofungin (acetate), 1540*t*
for aspergillosis, 1544
for candida endocarditis, 535
for candidiasis, 1535
CaSR activators, 1145. *See also specific types*
Castleman disease, 1368
Cast nephropathy, 941
Casts, urinary. *See* Urinary casts; *specific types*
Cat
bites, **1283–1284**
feces/litter
pregnancy, 795
toxoplasmosis, **1511–1513**
Cataplexy, 1084
Cataract, 67, **184–185**
diabetic, 1221
surgery, 185, 200*t*, 201*t*
Catastrophic antiphospholipid syndrome, 837
Catatonia, 1063
from antipsychotics, 1067
malignant, **30**
"Catcher's mitt hand," 867
Catecholamine-*O*-methyltransferase inhibitors, 1009. *See also specific types*
Catecholaminergic polymorphic ventricular tachycardia, **401,** 440*t*
Catemenial asthma, 246
Caterpillars, urticating hair moths, **132**
Cat-flea typhus, 1433
Catheter ablation, for arrhythmias, **383–386**
atrial fibrillation, 395–396
atrial flutter, 397
atrial tachycardia, 398
paroxysmal supraventricular tachycardia, 388, 390–391
ventricular premature beats, 398
ventricular tachycardia, 400
Wolff-Parkinson-White syndrome, 390–391
Catheter-associated infections, 1278–1279
Catheterization, cardiac. *See* Cardiac catheterization
Catheter-related infections, **1276–1279**
Cathinones, 1567, 1570
Cat-scratch disease, 493, **1471**
bacillary angiomatosis, 1328, 1471
lymphadenitis, 493
lymphadenopathy, reactive cervical, 242
Cauda equina syndrome, 1682–1685, 1686–1687
"Cauliflower ear," 205
Cavernous hemangioma, **717–718**
Cavernous sinus thrombosis, 221
CBD. *See* Cannabidiol (CBD)
CCKomas, **1172**
CD3 complex, 1199
CD4 count
candidiasis, oral, 1324
COVID-19, 1321
cryptococcal meningitis, 1322
hairy leukoplakia, 1324
herpes zoster, 1327
HIV/AIDS, 1311, 1312*t*, 1314, 1314*f*, **1315–1316, 1315*t*,** 1335*t*
on HIV/AIDS complications
prophylaxis, 1337
treatment, 1338, 1341, 1344, 1346–1347, 1348*t*, 1349–1350
immune reconstitution, 1330–1331
immunizations, 1336

CD4 count (*Cont.*):
liver transplants, 1326
non-Hodgkin lymphoma, 1329
Pneumocystis pneumonia, 1320
progressive multifocal leukoencephalopathy, 1323
retinitis, CMV, 1324
syphilis, 1336
tuberculosis, 1311, 1312*t*, 1314, 1314*f*, **1315–1316, 1315*t***
prevention, 1336
CDKN1B, 1175
CEBPA, acute myeloid leukemia, 528
Cefadroxil, 149
Cefazolin
for Group A streptococcus
arthritis, 1442
endocarditis, 1457
for *Staphyloccocus*
bacteremia, 1449
coagulase-negative, endocarditis, 1457
for *Staphylococcus aureus*, 1441
methicillin-susceptible, cellulitis, 128
osteomyelitis, 1448
skin & soft tissue infections, 1447
for *Streptococcus pneumoniae*, endocarditis, 1457
Cefdinir, 1444
Cefepime, 1472, 1472*t*, 1652
Cefixime, 1470
Cefotaxime
for arthritis, nongonococcal acute, 862
for Lyme disease, 1494, 1495*t*
for peritonitis, spontaneous bacterial, 703
for pneumococcal meningitis, 1445
for *Streptococcus pneumoniae* endocarditis, 1457
Cefotetan, 786, 1470
Cefoxitin, 786, 1470, 1475
Cefpodoxime, 1444
Ceftazidime, 1472, 1472*t*, 1652
Ceftriaxone
for arthritis, nongonococcal, 862
for brain abscess, 1282
for *Campylobacter*, 1467
for chest infections, anaerobic, 1472, 1472*t*
for cholecystitis, 721
for CNS infections, anaerobic, 1472
for enterococcus, 1443
for epididymitis, 948*t*, 953
gallstones from, 719
for gonococcus, 863, 1470
for *Haemophilus* meningitis, 1461
for leptospirosis, 1491
for Lyme disease, 1494, 1495*t*
for meningococcus meningitis, 1461
for neurosyphilis, 1487
for pelvic inflammatory disease, 786
for peritonitis, spontaneous bacterial, 605, 703
for pneumococcus
meningitis, 1445
pneumonia, 1444
for pyelonephritis, 947*t*, 949
for *Salmonella*, 1464
for *Shigella*, 1465
for *Streptococcus*
Group A, endocarditis, 1457
Group D, endocarditis, 1457
for *Streptococcus pneumoniae* endocarditis, 1457
for syphilis, 1483, 1483*t*
for viridans streptococci
endocarditis, 1455, 1457
prosthetic valve, 1456
Cefuroxime, 732, 1494, 1495*t*
Cefuroxime axetil, 1461, 1494, 1495*t*
Ceiling effect, COX inhibitors, 79
Celecoxib
for dysmenorrhea, 767
for knee osteoarthritis, 1705
for pain, **82, 83*t***
peptic ulcer disease, **625–626**
renal toxicity, 822
ulcer risk with, reducing, 628
Celiac disease, **633–635**
cardiomyopathy, dilated, 418
collagenous colitis, 663
dermatitis herpetiformis, 633–634
iron deficiency, 501, 502
lactose intolerance, 634
myocarditis, 417
small intestine bleeding, 601
thyroiditis, 1112
Celiac plexus
block, 96, **98–99**
neurolysis, 80, **98–99**
Celiac sprue. *See* Celiac disease
Cellular immunity, impaired, infections, 1273
Cellulitis, **127–128,** 127*f*. *See also specific types*
edema, lower extremity, 27, 28, 29
eosinophilic, 1419
injection drug use, 1286
non-clostridial crepitant, 1473
orbital, **196**
peritonsillar, **232**
synergistic necrotizing, 1473
treatment, empiric antimicrobial therapy
nonpurulent, 1297*t*
surround furuncle, 1297*t*
variola/vaccinia, 1421
venous insufficiency ulcer, 162
Cemiplimab-rwlc, 1606, 1607, 1674*t*
Cenobamate, 975*t*
Centor criteria, 231
Central adrenal insufficiency, hypogonadotropic hypogonadism, 1101
Central apnea, 316
Central diabetes insipidus, **1104–1105**
primary, 1104
secondary, 1104
"Central fever," 30
Central hypothyroidism, 1101
Central monoamine depleting agents, 1012. *See also specific types*
Central nervous system disease, **1280–1283,** 1280*t*, 1281*t*. *See also* Nervous system disorders; *specific types*
angiitis, primary, **857**
HIV/AIDS, 1321–1323
cryptococcal meningitis, 1318*t*, 1322, 1331
dementia & neurocognitive disorders, 1322
lymphoma, 1311, 1322
meningitis & myelopathy, **1026, 1323**
meningococcal meningitis, 1323
progressive multifocal leukoencephalopathy, 1323
toxoplasmosis, 1319*t*, 1322
lymphoma
HIV/AIDS, 1311, 1322
primary, 535
neoplasm, olfactory dysfunction, 224
noninfectious meningeal irritation, 1281
Central nervous system infections
brain abscess, 1281
clinical findings, 1281–1282
CSF findings, 1280, 1280*t*
gram-negative, 1472
meningitis
aseptic, 1280, 1280*t*
bacterial, partially treated, 1281
chronic, 1280
cryptococcal, HIV/AIDS, 1318*t*, 1322, 1331
encephalitis, 1280–1281
granulomatous, 1280*t*
health care–associated, 1281
HIV/AIDS, **1026, 1323**
meningococcal, HIV/AIDS, 1323
purulent, 1280, 1280*t*, 1281*t*
spirochetal, 1280*t*
viral, 1280*t*
meningoencephalitis, 1280*t*
neighborhood reaction, 1280*t*, 1281
otitis media, chronic, **211**
treatment, 1282–1283
Central neurogenic hyperventilation, 1019
Central obesity, 1251
Central pontine myelinolysis, 879–880
Central retinal artery occlusion, 188*f*, **189–190,** 989
Central retinal vein occlusion, **188–189**
Central sleep apnea, **1084**
Central vein nutritional support, 1266
Centruroides stings, **1591–1592**
Cepfodoxime, 947*t*
Cephalexin
for acne vulgaris, 149
for cellulitis, 128
for cystitis, 947*t*
for furunculosis & carbuncles, 126
for impetigo, 124
for *Staphylococcus aureus*, 1441–1442, 1441*t*, 1447
for UTI, pregnancy, 813
Cephalosporins. *See also specific types*
for acne vulgaris, 149
acute tubular necrosis from, 909
drug eruptions from, 156
for erysipelas, 128
interstitial nephritis from, 911
for prostatitis, 051
Cercarial dermatitis, 1520
Cerclage, cervical, 798, 806
Cerdulatinib, 1388
Cerebellar artery occlusion, 990
Cerebellar disorders. *See also specific types*
ataxia, varicella, 1360
degeneration, 1004*t*
hemangioblastoma, 998*t*
lesions, 999
tumors, vertigo from, 217
Cerebellitis, 1360, 1363
Cerebral disorders. *See also specific types*
amyloid angiopathy, intracerebral hemorrhage, 992
aneurysms
autosomal dominant polycystic kidney disease, 940
berry, coarctation of aorta, 325
contusion, 1022*t*
edema
diabetic ketoacidosis, 1230
high-altitude, **1560–1562**
hemorrhage, 1022*t*
anticoagulation, 377, 394
coarctation of aorta, 325
fibrinolytics, 375–376
$P2Y_{12}$ inhibitor, 369
percutaneous coronary intervention, 375
platelet-inhibiting agents, 365
infarction, 327–328, **988–991,** 989*t* (*See also* Stroke)
laceration, 1022*t*
lymphoma, primary, 998*t*, **1001**
HIV/AIDS, 998*t*, **1001**
metastases, **1000–1001**
toxoplasmosis, **1001**
Cerebral salt wasting, 877–878, 994

Cerebrovascular disease. *See also specific types*
  combined oral contraceptives and, 774
  headache, 974
  hypertensive, 446
  malignant, 1003
  occlusive, **478–480,** 479*t*
Certolizumab, 651–652
  Crohn disease, 656
Certolizumab pegol, 830–831, 1273
Cerumen impaction, 204, **205–206**
Cervical adenitis
  adenovirus, 1418
  measles, 1370
Cervical biopsy, 788, 790
Cervical cancer, **789–790**
  HPV, HIV/AIDS, 1330
  human papillomavirus, 11
  lesbian & bisexual women, **1720**
  prevention
    HPV vaccine, 790
    Papanicolaou smear, 11, 788
  screening/testing, 11–12
  treatment, 1597*t*
Cervical candidiasis, **784–785,** 784*f*
Cervical cap, with contraceptive jelly, **778–779**
Cervical cerclage, 798, 806
Cervical degenerative disc disease, 1687–1688
Cervical disk protrusion, **1037,** 1038*f*–1039*f*
Cervical dysplasia, HIV/AIDS, 1330
Cervical dystonia, 1012
Cervical intraepithelial neoplasia, **787–789,** 787*t*, 788*f*
Cervical lymphadenopathy, reactive, 242
Cervical polyps, **767**
Cervical radiculopathy, 95
Cervical rib syndrome, **1040**
Cervical spine osteoarthritis, 820
Cervical spondylosis, 1037–1040
Cervicitis
  Chlamydia trachomatis, **1477–1478**
  gonococcus, 1469
  herpes simplex virus, 1353
  Mycoplasma genitalium, 1477
  Ureaplasma urealyticum, 1477
Cervicofacial actinomycosis, 1473–1474
Cervicogenic vertigo, **217**
Cervix, incompetent, 797–798
Cesarean delivery
  for HIV/AIDS mothers, 815
  puerperal infection, 808
Cestode infections, **1523–1526**. *See also specific types*
  invasive, **1524–1526**
    cysticercosis, **1524–1525**
    echinococcosis, **1525–1526**
  noninvasive
    beef tapeworm, **1523**
    dwarf tapeworm, **1523**
    fish tapeworm, 507, **1523**
    laboratory findings, 1523
    pork tapeworm, **1523**
    treatment, 1523–1524
Cetazolamide, kidney stones from, 954
Cetirizine, 152
Cetrorelix, 768
Cetuximab, 1600*t*, 1656, 1673*t*
  colorectal cancer, 1630
CFTR, 266, 733
CF transmembrane conductance regulator, 1667*t*
CFTR G551D, 1667*t*
CFTR gene, 266
CFTR modulators, 267
CHA_2DS_2-VASc Risk Score, 393, 393*t*
Chagas disease, 25, 418, 619, **1498–1499**
ChAglyCD3, on diabetes mellitus, 1199
Chalazion, **169**
Chancroid, 1285, **1470**
Channelopathies, 1045
Charcoal, activated, 1568–1569
Charcot arthropathy, 1222
Charcot joint, **867–868**
Charcot-Marie-Tooth disease, **1031**
Charcot triad, 723
Checkpoint inhibitors. *See* Immune checkpoint inhibitors; *specific types*
CHEK2, breast cancer, 741
Chemical conjunctivitis/keratitis, **198**
Chemical-induced reactions, photodermatitis, 155
Chemical meningitis, 1281
Chemical pneumonitis, 1277
Chemical warfare agents, organophosphate, 1588–1589
Chemiluminescence immunoassay–based screening algorithm, 1482
Chemo brain, 761
Chemoreceptor trigger zone, 581
Chemotherapy. *See also specific indications and types*
  emetogenic, treatment for, 1655
  leukemia from, 528
  nausea & vomiting from, **1655–1656**
  pain from, 80
  thrombocytopenia from, 547*t*, **548**
  tremor from, 1012
Chest pain, **22–25**. *See also* Heart disease; *specific disorders*
  clinical findings, 22–23
  diagnostic studies, 23–24
  dyspnea, 18
  esophageal motility disorder, **620**
  general considerations, 22
  physical examination, 23
  treatment, 24–25
Chewing, facial pain with, 978
Cheyne-Stokes respiration, 86, 1019–1020
Chickenpox. *See* Varicella-zoster virus (chickenpox)
Chiggers, **132**
Chikungunya fever, 864, 1357*t*, 1379, **1399–1400**
Chilblain, **1552**
Child-Pugh score, 47, 706, 706*t*
Chimeric antigen receptor T cells, infection risks, 1274
Chlamydia, **1477–1479**. *See also* Sexually transmitted diseases/infections
  gay & bisexual men, 1724
  keratoconjunctivitis, **171–172**
  lesbian & bisexual women, 1718
Chlamydia pneumoniae
  asthma exacerbations, 258
  medication of choice, 1295*t*
  pneumonia, community-acquired, 270, 272
Chlamydia trachomatis, **1477–1478**
  anorectal infections, 671
  Bartholin duct infection, 783
  cervicitis, **1477–1478**
  epididymitis, 952
  lesbian & bisexual women, 1718
  lymphogranuloma venereum, **1477**
  medication of choice, 1295*t*
  pelvic inflammatory disease, 786
  pharyngitis/tonsillitis, 231
  pregnancy, 814–815
  STDs, 1284–1286
  urethritis, 1285, **1477–1478**
  vaginal discharge, 1285
Chlamydophila pneumoniae, **1479**
  cholangitis, primary biliary, 707
  pneumonia, 269*t*
Chlamydophila psittacii, 1295*t*, **1478**
Chloasma, hyperpigmentation, 163
Chloramphenicol
  aplastic anemia from, 1432
  for *Bacteroides fragilis,* 1472
  for *Campylobacter,* 1467
  hepatotoxicity, 696
  for Rocky Mountain spotted fever, 1432
  for *Salmonella* carriers, 1464
  for typhus
    epidemic, 1428
    scrub, 1430
    tick, 1432
  for *Vibrio,* 1467
Chlordiazepoxide, 1091, **1581–1582**
Chlorhexidine
  for furunculosis & carbuncles, 126
  for gingival disease, 1325
  for staphylococcal folliculitis, 1328
Chloridazepoxide, 1050*t*
Chloride-responsive metabolic alkalosis, 900–901, 900*t*
Chloride-unresponsive metabolic alkalosis, 900–901, 900*t*
Chlorinated insecticides, seizures from, 1567
Chlorine poisoning, 1573
Chloroquine
  for arthritis, Chikungunya fever, 1400
  hyperpigmentation from, 163
  for malaria, 1504*t*, 1505–1506, 1505*t*
    prevention, 796, 1508*t*, 1509
  myopathy from, 1045
  ocular effects, adverse, 199, 202*t*
Chloroquine phosphate, 1505*t*
Chloroquine sulfate, 142
Chlorpromazine
  adverse effects, 1067
  drowsiness & orthostatic hypotension from, 1576
  drug-induced nephritis from, 837
  hyperpigmentation from, 163
  poisoning, 1576
  for schizophreniform spectrum disorders, 1063
  for serotonin syndrome, 1567, 1593
Chlorpropamide, 1204*t*, 1206
Chlorthalidone, 452*t*, 455, 458*t*, 461*t*, 463*t*, 956
Cholangiocarcinoma, 717, 1610, **1612–1614.** *See also* Hepatocellular carcinoma
  biliary obstruction, 674
  intrahepatic, cirrhosis, 710
  primary sclerosing cholangitis, 726–728
Cholangitis, 720*t*, **723–725**
  from biliary stricture, 725
  primary biliary, **707–709**
  sclerosing
    HIV/AIDS, 1326
    primary, **726–728**
Cholecystectomy
  bile duct stones after, 723
  biliary stricture after, 725
  for cholecystitis, 720*t*, 721–722
  for choledocholithiasis, 723–725
  for cholelithiasis, 719, 720*t*
  nonalcoholic fatty liver disease and, 698
  for pancreatitis, 731, 732
  postcholecystectomy syndrome, **722**
  precholecystectomy syndrome, **722**
  for primary sclerosing cholangitis, 727
Cholecystitis
  acalculous, 721
  acute, **720–722,** 720*t*
  chronic, 721
  HIV/AIDS, 1326
  pregnancy, **817**
  xanthogranulomatous, 721
Choledocholithiasis, 579, 720*t*, **723–725**
  vs. dyspepsia, 579
  pancreatitis from, 732

Cholelithiasis, **718–720,** 720*t*
vs. dyspepsia, 579
gallbladder cancer, 1612
pregnancy, **817**
Cholera, 1288, 1290*t*, 1294*t*, **1466**. *See also* *Vibrio*
Cholestatic jaundice
from antipsychotics, 1066
vitamin E deficiency, 1262
Cholesteatoma, **210,** 210*f*
Cholesterol. *See also* High-density lipoprotein (HDL) cholesterol; Hypercholesterolemia; Low-density lipoprotein (LDL) cholesterol
Friedewald equation, 1240
gallstones, 637, 719, 720*t*
lowering
on cardiovascular disease, 1239
primary prevention studies, 1240–1241
secondary prevention studies, 1241
therapeutic effects, **1240–1241**
pericardial effusions, 428, 430
screening/cardiovascular disease prevention, 5*t*, 8
total, 1239
Cholesterolosis, 721
Cholestyramine
for cholesterol, high LDL, 1245*t*, 1247–1248
for diarrhea, 595
for irritable bowel syndrome, 646
for pruritus, primary biliary cholangitis, 708
for secretory diarrhea, Crohn disease, 656
Choline, on hepatic steatosis from parenteral nutrition, 699
Cholinergic syndrome poisoning, 1570
Cholinergic urticaria, 151–153
Cholinesterase inhibitors, 1017, **1588–1589**. *See also specific types*
Chondrocalcinosis, 826
Chondroitin, 821, 1705
Chondromalacia, patella, 1696, 1703–1704
Chorea
Huntington disease, **1010–1011**
rheumatic fever/heart disease, 424, 425, 425*t*
Sydenham, 425, 425*t*
Chorioamnionitis, **808**
Choriocarcinoma, **801–802**
Chorioretinitis, toxoplasmosis, 1511
Choroidal hemorrhage, thrombocytopenia, 193
Chromium, 1267, 1603
Chronic actinic dermatitis, 155
Chronic angle-closure glaucoma, 177*t*–178*t*, **181–183**
Chronic bacterial prostatitis, **950–952,** 950*t*
Chronic coronary syndromes, **359–367,** 364*f*, 367*t*
Chronic cutaneous lupus erythematosus, **141–142**
Chronic disease. *See also specific types*
anemia of, **503–504**
vitamin C deficiency, 1261
Chronic eosinophilic pneumonia, 297
Chronic fatigue syndrome, **33–34,** 1435
Chronic glaucoma, 177*t*–178*t*, **181–183**
Chronic heart failure. *See* Heart failure
Chronic idiopathic orthostatic hypotension, 402
Chronic inflammatory polyarthritis, 826
Chronic inflammatory polyneuropathy, **1034**
Chronic intestinal pseudo-obstruction, **640–641**
Chronic kidney disease, 903, **913–922,** 919. *See also* End-stage kidney disease; *specific types*
cardiovascular disease risk, 915
causes, 914, 914*t*
reversible, 915, 915*t*
clinical findings, 914–915
gouty arthritis, 823–824
hypercalcemia, 917
hyperkalemia, 885
hypermagnesemia, 894
hyperphosphatemia, 892, 917
hypertension treatment, 466–467, 467*t*
hypocalcemia, 888
incidence & causes, 914
metabolic acidosis from, 917
nephrogenic systemic fibrosis, **942**
peptic ulcer disease, 625
pericarditis, uremic, 427
prognosis, end-stage kidney disease, 920–921
renal artery stenosis, **921–922**
renal glycosuria, 1200
stages, 914, 914*t*
surgical risk, 51
uremic syndrome, 915
vitamin C deficiency, 1261
Chronic kidney disease, complications, 915–919
acid-base disorders, 918
cardiovascular, 914, 915–916
atrial fibrillation, 916
coronary artery disease, 916
heart failure, 374, 916
hypertension, 451*t*–453*t*, 458*t*–459*t*, 915–916
pericarditis, 916
by stage & GFR, 916*f*
endocrine, 919
hematologic, 918
hyperkalemia, 918
metabolic bone disease, 917, 917*f*
neurologic, 919
Chronic kidney disease, treatment
dietary, 919
end-stage kidney disease, 920
medication, 919–920
progression, slowing, 919
Chronic low-back pain, 80, 95
Chronic lymphocytic leukemia, 514, 516, **530–532,** 1595*t*
Chronic lymphocytic thyroiditis, 1112
Chronic mesenteric ischemia, **480–481**
Chronic myeloid leukemia, 520*t*, **524–526,** 1595*t*
Chronic myelomonocytic leukemia, 526
Chronic obstructive pulmonary disease, **259–264**
clinical findings, 259–260
complications, 262
cough, 15, 16
definition and clinical syndrome, 259
differential diagnosis, 261–262
dyspnea, 18, 19, 20, 259, 260*t*, 264
etiology and epidemiology, 259
hemoptysis, 21
lung cancer and, 1603
multifocal atrial tachycardia, 397–398
patterns of disease, 259, 260*t*
postoperative pulmonary complications, 46
prevention, 262
prognosis, 264
referral and admission, 264
treatment, 261–265
ambulatory patients, 261–263
bullectomy, 264
hospitalized patients, 263–264
lung transplantation, 264
lung volume reduction surgery, 264
Chronic open-angle glaucoma, 177*t*–178*t*, **181–183**
Chronic otitis media, **209–211**
cholesteatoma, **210,** 210*f*
CNS infection, **211**
facial palsy/paralysis, **210**
mastoiditis, **210**
petrous apicitis, **210**
sigmoid sinus thrombosis, **211**
Chronic pain, **79**. *See also specific disorders*
definition, 82
disorders, **1055–1057,** 1056*f*
noncancer, **80**
prevalence, 82
temporal pattern, 86
Chronic pelvic pain syndrome, 950*t*, **951–952**
Chronic rheumatic heart disease, 424
Chronic systolic heart failure, 406
Chronic tophaceous arthritis, 826
Chronic traumatic encephalopathy, 1023
Chronic tubulointerstitial diseases, **936–938**
Chronic venous insufficiency, **490–492,** 490*f*, 491*f*
lower extremity edema, **27–29,** 28*t*
stasis dermatitis, 490, 490*f*
Chronic wasting disease, 1385
Chronification, pain, 79
Chronotropic incompetence, 386
Churg-Strauss syndrome. *See* Eosinophilic granulomatosis with polyangiitis
Chvostek sign, 888, 893
Chylomicronemia syndrome, familial, **1239**
Chylous effusion, 310
Cicatricial alopecia, **165**
Ciclopirox, 106*t*, 117
Cidofovir, 1356*t*
for adenovirus, 1419
for cytomegalovirus, 1367
for HHV-6, 1368
for molluscum contagiosum, 1421
for warts, 123
Cigarette smoking. *See* Smoking, cigarette
Ciguatera poisoning, **1590–1591,** 1590*t*
Cilostazol, 987
Cimetidine
for GERD, 610
for molluscum contagiosum, 1421
for peptic ulcer disease, 624*t*, 627
for stress gastritis, 621
for vancomycin flushing syndrome, 870
Cinacalcet, 917
Cinalcet, 890, 1145
Ciprofibrate, 1248, 1284
Ciprofloxacin
for acute bacterial cholangitis, 727
breastfeeding, 796*t*
for *Campylobacter,* 1467
for chancroid, 1470
for chest infections, anaerobic, 1472, 1472*t*
for cholangitis, community-acquired, 724
for cholecystitis, 721
for cyclosporiasis, 1518
for cystitis, 947*t*
for diarrhea, diabetic, 1223
for gonococcus, 1470
for granuloma inguinale, 1471
for *Haemophilus,* 1461
for *Moraxella catarrhalis,* 1461
for *Mycobacterium abscessus, M. chelonae, M. fortuitum,* 1475
for peritonitis, spontaneous bacterial, 703
for plague, 1469
for prostatitis
acute bacterial, 947*t*
chronic bacterial, 948*t*
for *Pseudomonas* folliculitis, 125
for pyelonephritis, 947*t*
for Q fever, 1436
for *Salmonella,* 1464
bacteremia, 1465
carriers, 1464
gastroenteritis, 1464

for *Shigella,* 1465
for *Staphylococcus aureus* osteomyelitis, 1448
for traveler's diarrhea, 1292–1293
for typhus, endemic, 1429
Circumcision, male
for HIV prevention, 1331
on HSV-2 infection, 1357
for STD prevention, 1286
Circumscribed neurodermatitis, **135–136,** 135*f*
Cirrhosis, **700–707**. *See also* Esophageal varices
acute-on-chronic liver failure, 700
alcohol-associated liver disease, 693
clinical findings, 700–701
complications, 701
differential diagnosis, 701
Dupuytren contracture, 1691
hepatitis C, chronic, 689
hepatitis D, 684
hepatocellular carcinomas, 1610
hypervolemic hyponatremia, 878
pathophysiology & progression, 700
peptic ulcer disease, 625
for peritonitis, spontaneous bacterial, 604
portal hypertension, 615
portal vein thrombosis, 715
preoperative evaluation/perioperative management, 47
prognosis, 706–707, 706*t*
treatment, 701–706
general measures, 701–702
liver transplantation, 705–706
treatment, for complications
ascites and edema, 702–703
coagulopathy, 705
hepatic encephalopathy, 704–705
hepatopulmonary syndrome, 705
hepatorenal syndrome, 703–704
peritonitis, spontaneous bacterial, 703
portopulmonary hypertension, 705
"Cirrhotic cardiomyopathy," 700–702
Cisgender
definition, 1715, 1725
females, 1709
males, 1722
Cisplatin, 1598*t*
for bladder cancer, 1643
for breast carcinoma, 759
for mesothelioma, 1609
nephrotoxicity, **1657**
neurotoxicity, **1657**
ototoxicity, 213, **1657**
for small cell lung cancer, 1606
Citalopram
for agitation, in dementia, 1017
for dementia, 1017
for depression, 1072, 1073*t*, 1074
hyponatremia from, 878
for irritable bowel syndrome, 646
safety, 1075
toxicity, 1592
CK-MBs
acute coronary syndromes, 360
with ST-segment elevation, 373–374
without ST-segment elevation, 369, 372
angina pectoris, 360, 366
myocarditis, 415
Cladophialophora, 1546
Cladosporium, 1546–1547
Cladribine, 532, 1025, 1025*t*
Clarithromycin
for *Bordetella pertussis,* 1459
for *Helicobacter pylori,* 627
hepatitis from, 1325
for *Legionella,* 1462
for *Mycobacterium abscessus, M. chelonae, M. fortuitum,* 1475
for *Mycobacterium avium* complex, 1337*t*, 1475
for *Mycobacterium marinum,* 1475
for peptic ulcer disease, 624*t*
for pneumococcal pneumonia, 1444
for prostatitis, 948*t*
Classic Blalock shunt, 330
Classic Kaposi sarcoma, **113**
Claudication, **476–477**
aortoiliac artery disease, 473–474
femoral-popliteal artery, 474–475
intermittent, 473
limb arterial occlusion, 477
neurogenic, 1686
Clavulanate, 1461
Clear liquid diet, 1263
Clevidipine, 470, 470*t*, 471*t*
Clindamycin
for animal bites, 1284
for babesiosis, 1510
for bacterial vaginosis, 785
for chest infections, anaerobic, 1472
for clostridial myonecrosis, 1451
for erysipelas, 128
for folliculitis, 125
for furunculosis & carbuncles, 126
for gonococcus, 1470
for malaria, 1505*t*
for metritis, 808
for MRSA
cellulitis, 128
necrotizing fasciitis, 1442
for organ anaerobes, 1472
pill-induced esophagitis from, 613
for rosacea, 150
for *Staphylococcus,* folliculitis, 1328
for *Staphylococcus aureus,* 1441–1442, 1441*t*
osteomyelitis, 1448
skin & soft tissue infections, 1447
toxic shock syndrome, 1449
for *Streptococcus,* toxic shock syndrome, 1443
Clindamycin/benzoyl peroxide, 104*t*
Clindamycin phosphate, 104*t*
Clinical Institute Withdrawal Assessment for Alcohol, Revised, 190*f*, 694, 1089, 1090*f*
Clinically isolated syndrome, 1024
Clinician self-care, end of life, 77
Clobazam, 975*t*
Clobetasol propionate, 104*t*
Clocortolone, 103*t*
Clofibrate, 719, 1045
Clomiphene, 771, 1103
Clomiphene citrate, 772–773, 1178
Clomipramine
for depression, 1073*t*, 1076
for obsessive-compulsive disorder, 1053
poisoning, hypotension treatment, 1565
Clonal cytopenias of undetermined significance, **502**
Clonal hematopoiesis of indeterminate potential, 526
Clonazepam, 1050*t*
for myoclonus, 1012
for panic disorder, 1050*t*, 1051
for periodic limb movement disorder, 1084
poisoning, **1581–1582**
for psychedelic effects, 1093
for seizures
absence, 977*t*
myoclonic, 977*t*
Clonic seizure, 979
Clonidine
for diarrhea, 595
for diarrhea, diabetic, 1223
for Gilles De La Tourette syndrome, 1013
for hyperadrenergic postural orthostatic syndrome, 985
for hypertension, 460, 463*t*, 471*t*, 472
neuromodulatory therapy, 97*t*
for opioid withdrawal, 1092
poisoning, **1579**
for PTSD, 1048
sympatholytic syndrome from, 1570
Clonorchiasis, **1522**
Clonorchis sinensis, 1522, 1613
Clopidogrel
for acute coronary syndrome, without ST-segment elevation, 369–370, 370*f*
for acute MI, ST-segment elevation, 374, 378
for angina pectoris, 364*f*, 365
for coronary heart disease prevention, 358
CYP isoenzyme metabolism of, 1667*t*
for transient ischemic attacks, 987
ulcer risk with, reducing, 628–629
Clorazepate, 1050*t*
Closed globe injury, **197–198**
Clostridial infections *(Clostridium),* **1450–1453**
botulism, 982, **1042,** 1286–1287, **1452–1453**
intra-abdominal, 1472
medication of choice, 1294*t*
myonecrosis, 1286, 1294*t*, **1450–1451,** 1473, 1473*f*
tetanus, **1451–1452,** 1452*t*
Clostridioides difficile diarrhea, 1288, 1289*t*
Clostridioides perfringens diarrhea, 1288
Clostridium bifermentans myonecrosis, 1450–1451
Clostridium botulinum, 1042, 1289*t*. *See also* Botulism
Clostridium difficile
antibiotic-associated colitis, **647–649**
colitis, 589–590
diarrhea, 590–591, 1288
Clostridium histolyticum, 960, 1450–1451
Clostridium novyi myonecrosis, 1450–1451
Clostridium perfringens
diarrhea, 590, 1288, 1289*t*
myonecrosis, 1450–1451
Clostridium ramosum myonecrosis, 1450–1451
Clostridium tetani, **1451–1452**
Clotrimazole
for candidiasis
mucocutaneous, 105*t*, 119
oral, 1325
vulvovaginal, 1535
for seborrheic dermatitis, 139
for tinea corporis, 105*t*, 115
for tinea versicolor, 105*t*, 118
topical dermatologic, 105*t*
for vulvovaginal candidiasis, 785
Clozapine
agranulocytosis from, 1066–1067
diabetic ketoacidosis from, 1197
for dyskinesia from antipsychotics, 1068
glucose intolerance from, 1197
for Huntington disease, 1011
for Parkinson disease, 1009
pericarditis from, 427
potency and side effects, 1065*t*
for schizophreniform spectrum disorders, 1063, 1064*t*, 1065*t*
for tardive dyskinesia, from antipsychotics, 1068
Clubbed fingers, 166, 166*f*, 266
Clue cells, 785, 785*f*
Cluster headache, **973**
CMV immune globulin, 1367
Coagulase-negative staphylococci, **1449–1450**

Coagulation disorders, 5*t*, 8, 355, 356*f*, 357–358, 357*t*, **557–563**. *See also specific types*
acquired, **561–562**
coagulopathy of liver disease, **562**
disseminated intravascular coagulation (*See* Disseminated intravascular coagulation)
factor II antibodies, **561**
factor V antibodies, **561**
factor VIII antibodies, **561**
heparin/fondaparinux/direct-acting oral anticoagulant use (*See* Anticoagulants; *specific agents*)
lupus anticoagulants, **562**
vitamin K deficiency, **562**
warfarin ingestion (*See* Warfarin)
congenital, **557–561**
factor II, V, VII, and X deficiencies, **561**
factor XI deficiency, 559*t*, **561**
factor XIII deficiency, **561**
hemophilia A & B, **557–559,** 559*t*
von Willebrand disease, **559–561,** 560*t*
other causes, **562**
Coagulopathy
chronic kidney disease hematologic, 918
COVID-19–associated, 1402, 1403
of liver disease, **562**
treatment, with cirrhosis, 705
Coal worker's pneumoconiosis, **306,** 306*t*, 308
Coarctation of aorta, **325–326**
aortic dissection, 486
hypertension, 325, 445
intracranial aneurysm, 325
Cobalt, 308, 419
Cobimetinib, 1601*t*, 1671*t*
Cocaine, **1093–1094**
acute MI, with ST-segment elevation, 373
atherosclerosis, 368
cardiotoxicity, 415*t*, 417, 418*t*
coronary vasospasm & myocardial ischemia/infarction, 368
crack, pulmonary syndromes, 309
epistaxis, 224
granulomatosis with polyangiitis, 853
hypertension from, 1566
levamisole adulteration, 856
myocardial ischemia/infarction, 368
myopathy from, 1045
poisoning, **1574**
on pregnancy, 795
primary angiitis of CNS, 857
pulmonary hypertension, 432
Raynaud phenomenon, 840*t*
seizures from, 1567
serotonin syndrome from, 30
sympathomimetic syndrome from, 1570
Coccidioides, with impaired cellular immunity, 1273
Coccidioidomycosis, **1537–1538**
Coccidioidomycosis immitis, 1537
Coccidioidomycosis posadasii, 1537
Coccidiosis, **1516–1518**
Cochlear implant, 67, 205
Cochlear otosclerosis, 211
Cockcroft-Gault formula, 905
Cocooning, 796
Codeine, 85, 85*t*, **89*t***
breastfeeding, 796*t*
CYP2D6 metabolism of, 1668*t*
for diarrhea, 595
for diarrhea, diabetic, 1223
morphine milligram equivalent doses, 85*t*
poisoning, **1587–1588**
Coenzyme Q10, 972*t*, 1044
Coffee, 719
Cogan syndrome, hearing loss, 213
Cognitive behavioral therapy
for attention-deficit/hyperactivity disorders, 1081
for chronic pain syndromes, 1057
for depression, 1078
for phobic disorders, 1052
for schizophrenia spectrum disorders, 1068
for somatic symptom disorders, 1054
for stress, 1047
Cognitive impairment. *See also* Dementia; *specific types*
delirium, 58
dementia, 54, 55–56
depression, 57
mild, 55, 1007, 1014
from opioids, 92
systemic exertion intolerance disease, 34
Cognitive processing therapy, 1048
Cognitive remediation therapy, 1068
Coin lesion, 290
Co–in vitro fertilization, 1714
Colchicine
for Behçet disease, 857
for calcium pyrophosphate deposition, 827
for cholangitis, primary biliary, 708–709
for gouty arthritis, 824–825
myopathy from, 1045
for pericarditis, 428
tamponade from, 428
Cold, common, **218–219**
Cold agglutinin, 515
Cold agglutinin disease, 500, **515–516**
"Cold" autoantibody, 516
Cold fever/sore, **120–121,** 120*f*
Cold urticaria, 151–153
Cold water, 389, 1550
Colecystokinin-producing tumors, **1172**
Colesevelam
for cholesterol, high LDL, 1245*t*, 1247–1248
for diarrhea, 595
for hyperglycemia/diabetes mellitus, 1211
for pruritus, primary biliary cholangitis, 708
for secretory diarrhea, Crohn disease, 656
Colestipol
for cholesterol, high LDL, 1245*t*, 1247–1248
for pruritus, primary biliary cholangitis, 708
for secretory diarrhea, Crohn disease, 656
Colitis
antibiotic-associated, **647–649**
Clostridium difficile, 589–590, **647–649**
collagenous, 663
herpes simplex virus, 1354
ischemic, **480–481,** 599
microscopic, **663**
pseudomembrane, 648
ulcerative, **658–662,** 658*t*
Collagenase *Clostridium histolyticum* injections, 1691
Collagen cross-linking, 168
Collagenous colitis, 663
Collateral ligament injury, **1701–1702**
Cologuard test, 1632
Colonic diverticulosis, **663**
Colonic pseudo-obstruction, **639–641**
Colonography, CT, for colorectal cancer screening, 1633
Colonoscopic polypectomy, 666
Colonoscopy, for colorectal cancer screening, 1632–1633
Colon polyps, **665**
Colon & rectum diseases, **643–669**. *See also specific types*
antibiotic-associated colitis, **647–649**
diverticular disease of colon, **663–665**
diverticulitis, **663–665**
diverticulosis, uncomplicated, **663**
hereditary colorectal cancer & polyposis syndromes, **666–669**
familial adenomatous polyposis, **667**
hamartomatous polyposis syndromes, **668**
Lynch syndrome, **668–669**
inflammatory bowel disease, **649–663**
Crohn disease, **653–658**
microscopic colitis, **663**
ulcerative colitis, **658–662,** 658*t*
irritable bowel syndrome, **643–647**
polyps
colon, **665**
nonfamilial adenomatous & serrated, **665–666**
Colorado tick fever, 1379, **1400–1401**
Colorectal cancer, **1627–1633**
from adenomas, 665
clinical findings, 1628–1629
Crohn disease, 654
flexible sigmoidoscopy, 1632–1633
hepatitis C, 11
hereditary nonpolyposis colon cancer, **668–669**
incidence & survival, 1627
inherited, 1627
polyp origins, 1627
postsurgical follow-up, 1631
prognosis, 1631
risk factors, 1627–1628
screening/detection, 11, **1631–1633,** 1632*t*
staging, 1629
treatment, 1597*t*, 1629–1631
colon cancer, by stage, 1629–1630
rectal cancer, 1630–1631
ulcerative colitis, 662
Colposcopy, 764*t*, 788
Columbia-Suicide Severity Risk Scale, Quick Inventory of Depressive Symptomatology, 1071
Coma. *See also* Stupor & coma
assessment & emergency measures, 1018–1019
causes, 1018
definition, 1018
diabetic, **1226,** 1226*t*
dysconjugate deviation, 1019
hyperglycemic, 1226, 1226*t*
hypoglycemic, 1226, 1226*t*
lactic acidosis, 1226
myxedema, 1115
poisoning, **1564–1565**
pupils, 1019
Co-maternity, 1714
Combined hepatocellular carcinoma-cholangiocarcinoma, 1610
Combined hormonal contraceptives, 768, 771
Combined oral contraceptives, **774–776,** 775*t*
for abnormal uterine bleeding, 764
for acne vulgaris, 149
breast carcinoma and, 774
cerebrovascular disease and, 774
contraindications & adverse effects, 774–776, 776*t*
headache and, 776
for hirsutism, female, 1183
hypertension and, 774
lactation and, 776
migraine headache and, 776
myocardial infarction and, 774
obesity and, 776
ovarian cancer and, 774
for pelvic pain, 768
retinal artery occlusion, 189
retinal vein occlusion, 188
stroke and, 774
thrombophilia and, 774
venous thromboembolism and, 774
weight gain from, 1252, 1253*t*

Combustion products
  asthma, 245
  inhalation, **304**
Comedones, 148
Comfrey, 713, 1580*t*
Common cold, **218–219,** 1418. *See also* Adenovirus
Common peroneal nerve palsy, **1036**
Common variable immunodeficiency, **873–874**
Commotio cordis, athlete screening, 438, 440*t*
Communication, patient, 66, 73, 73*t*
Community-acquired pneumonia, **268–274,** 272*t*. *See also* Pneumonia, community-acquired; *specific types*
Community-associated methicillin-resistant *Staphylococcus aureus* (CA-MRSA), 124
Compartment syndrome, 1553, 1556
Complement disorders, 872*t*
Complete abortion, 798
Complex attention, dementia, 53–54
Complex regional pain syndrome, **867**
Compound nevi, 107, 107*f*
Comprehensive behavior program, 1056–1057
Compulsions, 1052
Concussion, 216, 1021, 1022*t*, 1023
Condom, **779,** 1286, 1331, 1713
Conduction block
  AV, **387–388**
    acute MI, with ST-segment elevation, 379–380
  intraventricular, 387–388
Conduction velocity, motor/sensory, 1030
Conductive-based cooling, 1550
Conductive hearing loss, **204**
Conductive keratoplasty, 168
Condyloma acuminata, **121–123,** 122*f*, 671, **787,** 1284–1286
Condylomata lata, 671
Confidentiality, end of life, 77
Confusion assessment method, 58
Congenital adrenal hyperplasia, 1157
Congenital adrenal insufficiency, 1157
Congenital anemias, 500
Congenital disorders of platelet function, **556–557**
Congenital heart disease, adult, **323–332**
  atrial septal defect, **326–328**
  coarctation of aorta, **325–326**
  epidemiology & assessment, 323
  patent foramen ovale, **326–328**
  pregnancy, 435, 437*t*
  pulmonary valve stenosis, **323–324**
  tetralogy of Fallot, **330–332**
  ventricular septal defect, **328–330**
Congenital rubella syndrome, 1373
Congenital Zika syndrome, 1399
Congestive cardiomyopathy, 302–303, 403–404
Conization, cervical, 789, 790
Conjugal estrogen replacement, 1188
Conjugated hyperbilirubinemia, 674–675, 675*t*
Conjunctiva
  dryness, vitamin A deficiency, 1262
  foreign bodies, **197**
  Kaposi sarcoma, 193
  laceration, **198**
Conjunctivitis, **170–172,** 170*t*
  adenovirus, 1418
  allergic eye disease, **172**
  bacterial, **170–171**
  blepharitis, 169
  chemical, **198**
  chlamydial keratoconjunctivitis, **171–172**
  dry eyes, 16, **171–172,** 179
  enterovirus, 1424
  gonococcus, **171,** 1469
  hemorrhagic, contagious acute, 170
  inclusion, **171**
  onchocerciasis, 1532
  trachoma, **171**
  viral, **170,** 1356*t*
Connective tissue diseases. *See also* *specific types*
  cryoglobulinemia, **855**
  pericarditis, 427
  undifferentiated, **845**
Conn syndrome, 884, 1164, 1165, 1166
Constipation, **585–588**
  from autonomic neuropathy, chemotherapy, 1656
  clinical findings, 585–586
  etiology, 585, 585*t*
  from opioids, 70, 86, **91**
  postoperative, 47
  treatment, 586–588
    fecal impaction, 588
    palliative, 70
    pharmacologic, 586–588, 587*t*
  from vinca alkaloids, 1656
Constrictive bronchiolitis, 268
Constrictive pericarditis, **430–431**
  jugular venous pulsations, 429
  superior vena cava obstruction, 492
Contact dermatitis, **142–143**
  acute weeping, 143
  allergic, 142–143, 143*f*
  chronic, 143
  from dermatologic agents, 107
  irritant, 142–143, 143*f*
  subacute, 143
Contact lenses, 168
Contact ulcer, hoarseness, 238
Contagious pustular dermatitis, 1421
Continuous flow devices, for heart failure with reduced LVEF, 411–412
Continuous neuraxial drug delivery, 96*t*
Continuous positive airway pressure
  on hypertension, obesity, 444
  for obstructive sleep apnea, 317
  postoperative risk reduction, 47
Contraception & family planning, **773–780.** *See also specific topics*
  abortion, **780**
  cervical cap, with contraceptive jelly, **778–779**
  combined oral contraceptives, **774–776,** 775*t*, 776*t* (*See also* Combined oral contraceptives)
  condom, male/female, **779**
  contraceptive foam/cream/film/sponge/jelly/suppository, **779**
  diaphragm, with contraceptive jelly, **778**
  emergency, **779**
  fertile period awareness, **779**
  gender affirming hormone therapy, 1713
  intrauterine devices, **777–778,** 778*t*
  long-acting injections & implants, **777**
  postcoital, IUDs, 778
  progestin minipill, 775*t*, **776,** 776*t*
  sexual & gender minorities, 1713–1715
    family building, 1713–1715
    pregnancy prevention, 1713
  sterilization, **779–780**
  transdermal contraceptive patch, **777**
Contraceptive foam/cream/film/sponge/jelly/suppository, **779**
Contraceptive patch, transdermal, **777**
Contraceptive vaginal ring, **777**
Conversion disorder, 1053, 1054. *See also* Somatic symptom disorder
Cooley anemia, 505
Cooling, 1550
Coombs test
  autoimmune hemolytic anemia, 515
  cold agglutinin disease, 515
  Waldenström macroglobulinemia, 540
Copanlisib, 534
Copeptin, 881
Copper
  liver, Wilson disease, **711–713,** 712*f*, 1012
  nutritional support, 1267
Coral snake envenomation, **1590**
"Core-binding factor" leukemias, 528
Core body temperature, 1550, 1551
Core needle biopsy, for breast
  cancer, 745, 746, 746*f*, 747, 747*f*
    lobular carcinoma in situ, 749
    tumor biomarkers, 749
  fat necrosis, 740
  fibroadenoma, 738
  fibrocystic condition, 737
Core stabilization, for low-back pain, 95
Cornea
  abrasions, **197**
  foreign bodies, **197**
  infection, contact lenses, 168
  inflammation, HHV-6, 1368
  laceration, **198**
  ulcer, **172, 179**
Corneal reflex, stupor & coma, 1019
Coronary aneurysms, 1437. *See also* *specific types*
Coronary angiography. *See* Angiography, coronary
Coronary arteriography
  for coronary artery disease, selective, 362
  for coronary vasospasm & angina/MI, 368
  normal, coronary vasospasm and angina, **367–368**
Coronary artery anomalies
  congenital, athlete screening, 438–439, 440*t*
  pregnancy, 436–437
Coronary artery bypass grafting
  acute MI, with ST-segment elevation, 382
  for angina pectoris, 366–367
  cardiac risk assessment/reduction, 43–44
Coronary artery disease. *See also* Atherosclerosis; *specific types*
  angina pectoris, 359
  aortic stenosis, 343
  atherosclerotic, 26, **355–382**
  cardiac risk assessment/reduction, 43–44, 44*t*
    medications, 43, 44*t*
    revascularization, coronary, 43–44
  chronic kidney disease, 916
  HIV/AIDS, 1330
  imaging
    coronary arteriography, selective, 362
    CT angiography, multislice, 361
  risk factors, 355
Coronary calcium score, 361
Coronary heart disease, **355–382.** *See also* *specific types*
  acute coronary syndromes, without ST-segment elevation, **368–372**
  acute MI, with ST-segment elevation, **373–382**
  angina pectoris, **359–367,** 364*f*, 367*t*
  calcium supplements on, 1264
  chest pain, 22–25
  coronary vasospasm & angina/MI, normal coronary arteriograms, **367–368**
  epidemiology, 355
  lipid fractions & risk of, **1239–1240**
  morbidity & mortality, 355
  myocardial hibernation & stunning, **355–357,** 420
  prevention, **357–359**
    primary & secondary, 357–359
    statins, 5*t*, 8, 355, 356*f*, 357–358, 357*t*

Coronary heart disease (*Cont.*):
  risk factors, 4, 355
    family history, 355
    hypercholesterolemia, 355
    metabolic syndrome, 355
  sudden cardiac death, 400
Coronary revascularization. *See* Revascularization, coronary
Coronary sinus, atrial septal defect, 326
Coronary syndromes. *See also specific types*
  chronic, **359–367** (*See also* Angina pectoris, chronic stable)
Coronary vascular disease, lipid hypothesis, 1239
Coronary vasospasm
  angina, 359, **367–368**
  cocaine, 368
Coronaviruses, 590, 1401. *See also* SARS-CoV-1 (SARS); SARS-CoV-2
Corrigan pulse, 347
Corrosive acids, poisoning, 1573
Cortical blindness, 999
Cortical spreading depression, 970
Corticosteroids. *See also specific indications and types*
  cataracts from, 184
  clinical use, **1193–1194,** 1194*t*
  on fetus, 804
  infection risks, 1274
  integument thinning from, bleeding, 563
  kidney stones from, 954
  myopathy from, 1045
  ocular effects, adverse, 198–199, 201*t*
  osteonecrosis from, 868
  osteoporosis/osteoporotic fractures from, 1148, 1193–1194
  progressive multifocal leukoencephalopathy from, 1387
  weight gain from, 1252, 1253*t*
Corticotropin-releasing hormone (CRH), 1099
Cortisol
  on ADH release, 878
  deficiency, hyponatremia, 878
Cortisol withdrawal syndrome, 1163
Corynebacterium diphtheria, 231, 1294*t*
Corynebacterium haemolyticum pharyngitis/tonsillitis, 231
Corynebacterium jeikeium, 1272, 1294*t*
Cosyntropin stimulation test, 1111
Cough, **15–18**
  from ACE inhibitors, 408
  acute, 15–18
  acute MI, with ST-segment elevation, 373
  asthma, 15, 17, 17*t*
  bronchogenic carcinoma, 16
  COVID-19, 15
  diagnostic studies, 16–17, 16*t*
  differential diagnosis, 17
  effective, 15
  gastroesophageal reflux disease, 15–17, 17*t*
  headache from, 974
  heart failure, 404
  for paroxysmal supraventricular tachycardia, 389
  pericardial effusion, 429
  persistent and chronic, 15–18
  pertussis, 15–17
  physical examination, 16
  postnasal drip syndrome, 15–17, 17*t*
  subacute, 15
  symptoms, 15–16
  treatment, 17–18, 17*t*
Cough/cough-variant asthma, 15, 17, 17*t*, 246
Counterpressure maneuvers, 403
Courvoisier sign, 675–676, 1613, 1615
COVID-19. *See* SARS-CoV-2
COVID-19–associated collapsing glomerulopathy, 913
COVID-19–associated nephropathy, 1404
COVID-19–associated pulmonary aspergillosis, 1405
COVID-19–coagulopathy, 1402, 1403
COVID-19–related ARDS, 1403
Cowden disease, hamartomatous polyposis syndromes, 668
COX-1, 822
COX-2, 822
COX-2 inhibitors. *See specific types*
Coxibs. *See also* Celecoxib; *specific types*
  erosive gastritis/gastropathy, **620–622**
  peptic ulcer disease, **625–626**
  ulcer risk with, reducing, 628
Coxiella burnetii, 1427*t*, **1434–1436**
COX inhibitors, 79, **82, 83*t*–84*t***
Coxsackievirus, 170, **1423–1424,** 1424*f*
CPA1, 733
CPAP. *See* Continuous positive airway pressure
C-peptide
  autoimmune hypoglycemia, 1237
  factitious hypoglycemia, 1237
  maturity-onset diabetes of the young, 1196
Crabs, **130–131**
Crack cocaine inhalation, 309
Cranial nerve palsies. *See also specific types*
  eye and lid disorders, **195–196,** 195*f*
  sarcoidosis, 1032
  West Nile virus, 1380
Craniopharyngioma, 998*t*
Craving, 1086
Creatine, 1044, 1580*t*
Creatinine clearance, 905
Creeping eruption, **1530,** 1530*f*
CREST syndrome, 840
Creutzfeldt-Jakob disease, 1012, 1018, 1385–1386
Cricothyrotomy, **240,** 240–241
Crigler-Najjar syndrome, 675*t*
Crimean-Congo hemorrhagic fever, **1391–1392**
Crisaborole, 104*t*, 134
Critical illness
  myopathy, **1044**
  neuropathy, **1033**
Critical limb ischemia, 475
Crizanlizumab-tmca, 513
Crizotinib, 1606
Crohn disease, **653–658**
  anal fissures, 672
  bacterial overgrowth from, 636
  fistula in ano, 672
  gallstones, 719
  peptic ulcer disease, 625
  perianal abscess, 672
  primary sclerosing cholangitis, **726–728**
  short bowel syndrome, **637**
  small intestinal lymphoma and, 1625
  small intestine bleeding, 601
  vitamin B_{12} deficiency, 507
Cromolyn, 250*t*, 254, 813
Crowned dens syndrome, 826–827
CRT-P, 388
Cryoanalgesia, neuromodulatory therapy, 96, 97*t*
Cryoglobulin-associated glomerulonephritis, 923*t*, **929–930**
Cryoglobulinemia, **855**
  essential (mixed), 929
  hepatitis C, 682
  interstitial nephritis, 911
Cryoprecipitate transfusion, **545**
Cryptococcus (cryptococcosis), **1542–1543**
  with impaired cellular immunity, 1273
  meningitis, HIV/AIDS, **1001,** 1318*t*, 1322, 1331
  solid organ transplant recipients, 1273
  uveitis, 183
Cryptococcus gattii, **1542–1543**
Cryptococcus neoformans, **1542–1543**
Cryptogenic organizing pneumonia, 294*t*
Cryptogenic stroke, patent foramen ovale, 327–328, 987, 990
Cryptorchidism, **1179**
Cryptosporidium (cryptosporidiosis), 589, 1288, 1326, **1516–1518**
Cryptosporidium hominis, 1516
Cryptosporidium parvum, 1516
Crystal deposition arthritis, **823–827**. *See also* Arthritis, crystal deposition; Gout/gouty arthritis; *specific types*
  calcium pyrophosphate deposition, **826–827**
  degenerative joint disease, **819–823** (*See also* Degenerative joint disease)
  gouty arthritis, **823–826**
Crystalline lens
  cataract, 184
  glaucoma, acute angle-closure, 180
  opacities, cataract, 184
  surgery, 168
CSF3R, myeloproliferative neoplasms, 520
CT angiography, multislice, for coronary artery disease, 361
CT colonography, 666, 1633
CT-FFR, 361
CT-intravenous pyelogram (CT-IVP), for hematuria, 944–945
CTRC, 733
Cultural issues, 73, 74, 75, 81
Cunninghamella, 1544
Cupulolithiasis, 216
CURB-65, 273
Current, electrical, 1557
Curvularia, 1546
Cushing disease (syndrome), **1160–1164,** 1184
  ACTH, 1182
    elevation, 1161
    hirsutism & virilization, 1182
    normal/low, 1161
  clinical findings, 1161–1162
  cortisol withdrawal syndrome, 1163
  definition, 1160
  differential diagnosis, 1162
  hypertension, 445
  hypokalemia, 882*t*
  incidence, 1160
  myopathy, 1045
  obesity, 1251
  treatment, 1162–1163
Cutaneous larva migrans, **1530,** 1530*f*
Cutaneous leishmaniasis, **1499–1501,** 1500*f*
Cutaneous lupus erythematosus, **141–142,** 158*t*
Cutaneous T-cell lymphoma, **113–114**
Cutibacterium acnes, 147, 149
CVD risk calculator, 355
c-v wave, 324, 331
Cyanide
  anion gap elevation from, 1570
  antidote, 1580
  poisoning, 18–20, 1568*t*, **1579–1580**
Cyclic thrombocytopenia, **548**
Cyclin-dependent kinase 4/6 inhibitors. *See also specific types*
  for breast carcinoma, 754, 757–758
    + fulvestrant, 758
Cyclophosphamide, 1598*t*
  for amyloidosis, 541
  for Behçet disease, 857
  for breast carcinoma, 752, 755, 761
  breastfeeding, 796*t*
  chemical cystitis from, 943
  for glomerulonephritis, 913
  for granulomatosis with polyangiitis, 853

hemorrhagic cystitis from, **1656**
for hepatitis C, cryoglobulinemia in, 690
for IgA nephropathy, 927
for interstitial lung disease, scleroderma, 841
leukemia from, 528
for lupus nephritis, 836, 930
for membranoproliferative glomerulonephritis, 929
for membranous nephropathy, 934
for microscopic polyangiitis, 854
for pauci-immune glomerulonephritis, 928
for plasma cell myeloma, 538
for polyarteritis nodosa, 851
progressive multifocal leukoencephalopathy from, 1387
for systemic lupus erythematosus, 835
Cyclophosphamide-methotrexate-5-fluorouracil, 761
Cyclopropavir, 1367
Cyclospora (cyclosporiasis), 589, 1288, **1516–1518**
Cyclospora cayetanensis, 1516–1517
Cyclosporine
acute tubular necrosis from, 909
aplastic anemia, 517–518
for autoimmune hepatitis, 693
for Behçet disease, 857
gout from, 823
for HTLV1-associated myelopathy, 1389
hyperkalemia from, 886
on insulin secretion, 1197
for Kawasaki disease, 1438
for lichen planus, 141
for myasthenia gravis, 1041
myopathy from, 1045
for pityriasis rubra pilaris, 155
for psoriasis, 137
for psoriatic arthritis, 860
for psoriatic erythroderma, 155
for Sjögren syndrome, 845
for Stevens-Johnson syndrome, 154
for ulcerative colitis, 662
Cyclothymic disorder, 1070
CYP 2C9, 1667*t*
CYP 2C19, 1667*t*
CYP 2C19*2, 1667*t*
CYP 2C19*3, 1667*t*
CYP 2C19*4, 1667*t*
CYP 2C19*5, 1667*t*
CYP 2C19*17 carrier, 1667*t*
CYP 2D6, 1668*t*
CYP 3A5, 1668*t*
CYP2C9, 571
CYP2C9, 1667*t*
CYP3A inhibitors, 531. *See also specific types*
Cyproheptadine
for anorgasmia from SSRIs, 1075
for serotonin syndrome, 1567, 1593
for urticaria & angioedema, 152
Cyproterenone acetate, 1183
Cyst
Bartholin duct, **783,** 783*f*
branchial cleft, **241–242**
epidermal inclusion, **110**
renal, **938–939,** 938*t*
thyroglossal duct, **242**
vocal folds, **237**
Cystatin C, 905
Cystic, 102*t*
Cystic diseases of kidney, 824, 914, **938–941**
autosomal dominant polycystic kidney disease, 938*t*, **939–940,** 939*f*
cysts, simple/solitary, **938–939,** 938*t*
medullary sponge kidney, 938*t*, **940–941**
Cysticercosis, **1524–1525**
Cystic fibrosis, **266–267**
Cystic fibrosis transmembrane conductance regulator (CFTR) protein, 266, 733
Cystic hydatid disease, 1525–1526
Cystine calculi, 957
Cystine stones, 954. *See also* Urinary stone disease
Cystitis
acute, **945–946**
antimicrobial therapy, empiric, 1297*t*
chemical, 943
dacrocystitis, **169–170**
dysuria, **38–41,** 40*f*
hemorrhagic, from cyclophosphamide or ifosfamide, **1656**
interstitial, **953–954**
Cystocele, 769
Cystoisospora belli, 1516
Cytarabine, 1599*t*
Cytokines. *See specific types*
Cytokine storm, 414, 913
Cytomegalovirus disease, **1365–1368**. *See also specific types*
cataracts, 184
clinical findings, 1365–1366
CMV inclusion disease, 1365
diarrhea, 590
esophagitis, infectious, 612–613
gastritis, 624
hematopoietic cell transplant recipients, 1273
HIV/AIDS
pneumonia, 1321
polyradiculopathy, 1323
transverse myelitis, 1323
in immunocompetent, 1366
in immunocompromised, 1273, 1366
CMV retinitis, **193,** 1311, 1318*t*, 1324, 1324*f*, 1366
GI and hepatobiliary, 1366
neurologic, 1366
respiratory, 1366
interstitial nephritis, 911
odynophagia, 607
peptic ulcer disease, 625
perinatal, 1365
preemptive therapy, 1274–1275
prevention
antiretroviral therapy, 1367
vaccination, 1367
retinitis, **193,** 1311, 1318*t*, 1324, 1324*f*, 1366
HIV/AIDS, **193,** 1311, 1318*t*, 1324, 1324*f*
solid organ transplant recipients, 1273
treatment & prognosis, 1367
universal prophylaxis/preemptive therapy, 1274–1275
uveitis, 183

D

Dabigatran, 563, 564*t*
for acute MI, with ST-segment elevation, 378
for atrial fibrillation, stroke prevention, **393–395,** 394*t*
with hyperthyroidism, malabsorption, 1126
for intracranial venous thrombosis, 996
for mitral stenosis, 336
perioperative management, 48, 48*t*
poisoning, 1575
reversal agents, 563, 565*t*
for stroke prevention, 393–394, 394*t*
for transient ischemic attacks, 987
for venous thromboembolism, 567*t*, 570–571, 570*t*
Dabrafenib, 1601*t*, 1606, 1671*t*
Dacamitinib, 1672*t*
Daclatasvir, 690*t*
Dacrocystitis, **169–170**
Dactinomycin, 801
Dagliflozin, 409
Dairy allergy, 614, 1264
Dalfampridine, 1025*t*
Dalteparin, 567*t*
Danazol, 738, 768
Dantrolene, 1026, 1576
Dapagliflozin
for coronary heart disease prevention in diabetics, 358–359
for diabetes mellitus, 935, 1205*t*, 1210, 1218
Dapivirine, 1412
Dapsone
for bullous pemphigoid, 147
hepatotoxicity, 696
for *P. jirovecii* pneumonia, 1337*t*, 1541
poisoning, 1569, **1586–1587**
for relapsing polychondritis, 856
topical dermatologic, 104*t*
for toxoplasmosis, 1337*t*, 1513
Daptomycin
for MRSA
bacteremia, 1449
cellulitis, 128
endocarditis, 1457
necrotizing fasciitis, 1442
myopathy from, 1045
for peritonitis, spontaneous bacterial, 703
for staphylococcal bacteremia, 1449
Daratumumab, 538, 541, 936, 1600*t*
Darbepoetin, 504, 917
Darbepoetin alfa, 1654*t*
Darolutamide, 1640*t*, 1641
Darunavir, **1340*t*, 1345**
+ lamivudine, 1338
+ TDF/emtricitabine, 1338
+ tenofovir alafenamide/ emtricitabine, 1338
Dasabuvir, 689, 690*t*
Dasatinib, 525, 1601*t*, 1656
DASH diet, 448, 448*t*
Date-rape drug, 1582
Datura stramonium poisoning, 1577
Daunorubicin, 417, 1599*t*
Dawn phenomenon, 1217
DDAVP, 558, 559*t*, 560
D-dimer, pulmonary venous thromboembolism, 298
D-dimer test, 19, 28, 28*t*
Deafness
DID-MOAD, 1197
maternally inherited diabetes and deafness, 1197
Wolfram syndrome, 1197
Dean Ornish diet, 1243
Death
brain, **1020**
causes, 2–3, 2*t*
causes, preventable, 2, 3*t*
medical aid in dying, 76
sudden, **400–401** (*See also* Sudden cardiac arrest/death)
tasks after, **76–79**
Death certificate, 78
"Death rattle," 75
"Death with dignity," 76
Decerebrate posturing, 1019
Decision making
dementia, 54
end of life, 73
ethical, 2, 77
lesbian & bisexual women, 1716
serious illness, 71–72
advance care planning, 71–72
advance directives, 71
do not attempt resuscitation orders, 72
Physician (Medical) Orders for Life-Sustaining Treatment, 71–72
Physician (Medical) Orders for Scope of Treatment, 72

Decitabine, 1599*t*
Declaration of Montreal, 79
Decompression sickness, **1559–1560**
Deconditioning, from bed rest, 59
Decontamination
eyes, **1568**
gastrointestinal tract
activated charcoal, 1568–1569
general, 1568
hemodialysis, 1569, 1569*t*
repeat-dose charcoal, 1569
urinary manipulation, 1569
whole bowel irrigation, 1569
skin, **1568**
Decorticate posturing, 1019
De-efferented state, **1021**
Deep brain stimulation, 1006, 1011
Deep breathing exercises, postoperative risk reduction, 47
Deep inferior epigastric perforator flap, for breast reconstruction, 761
Deep neck infections, **233**
Deep vein thrombosis (DVT)
chronic venous insufficiency, **490–492,** 490*f*
edema, lower extremity, **27–29,** 28*t*
risk stratification
ruling out, 28, 28*t*
surgical inpatients, 566–568, 566*t*
superficial venous thrombophlebitis, 489
superior vena cava obstruction, 492
varicose veins and, 28
Deferasirox, 145, 711
Deferiprone, 711
Deferoxamine, 711
Defibrotide, 714
Deflazacort, 1193, 1194*t*
Degarelix, 1602*t*, 1640, 1640*t*
Degenerative aortic stenosis, 342
Degenerative joint disease, 83*t*–84*t*, **819–823,** 821*f*
Degenerative motor neuron diseases, **1028–1030**
amyotrophic lateral sclerosis, **1028**
primary lateral sclerosis, **1028**
progressive bulbar palsy, **1028**
progressive spinal muscular atrophy, **1028**
pseudobulbar palsy, **1028**
Degesterone acetate/ethinyl estradiol vaginal ring, 777
Dehydroepiandrosterone therapy, 1103, 1160
Dejerine-Sottas disease, **1031**
Delayed drug hypersensitivity, **871–872.** *See also* Drug-induced hypersensitivity syndrome
acute generalized exanthematous pustulosis, **871–872**
aspirin- and NSAID-exacerbated respiratory disease, 245, **872**
drug exanthems, **871**
drug-induced hypersensitivity syndrome, **871**
drug reaction with eosinophilia and systemic symptoms, **30,** 157, 696, **871**
severe cutaneous adverse reactions, **871–872**
acute generalized exanthematous pustulosis, **871–872**
drug-induced hypersensitivity syndrome, **871**
drug reaction with eosinophilia and systemic symptoms, **30,** 157, 696, **871**
Stevens-Johnson syndrome/toxic epidermal necrolysis, 871
Stevens-Johnson syndrome/toxic epidermal necrolysis, 871
Delayed pressure urticaria, 151–153
Delirium, 1095, 1096*t*
agitated, 70–71
from antipsychotics, 1066
cognitive impairment, 58
definition, 58, 70–71
vs. dementia, 1014
dementia and, 54, 55
hyperactive, 58
hypoactive, 58
incontinence, urinary, 62
medications and polypharmacy, 55, 58–59
older adults, 54, **58–59**
from opioids, 92
palliative care, 70–71
postoperative, 49
Delta-9-tetrahydrocannabinol (THC) poisoning, **1585**
Delta gap, 895
Delta wave, paroxysmal supraventricular tachycardia, 390
Delusional disorder, 1061
Delusions, 1062
Dementia, **1014–1018,** 1095–1096, 1096*t*. *See also* Cognitive impairment
age of onset, 1014
Alzheimer, hypertension, 446
clinical findings, 1014–1016
Creutzfeldt-Jakob disease, 1018
vs. delirium, 1014
differential diagnosis, 1015*t*, 1016
driving and, 1198
epidemiology, 1014
etiology & risk factors, 1014, 1015*t*
frontotemporal, 1015*t*
HIV/AIDS, 1311, 1322
Huntington disease, **1010–1011**
hypertension, 446
life expectancy, 57
mild cognitive impairment, 1014
older adults, **53–57**
Parkinson disease, 1007
pseudo-, 1014
rapidly progressive, 1017–1018
treatment, 1016–1018
vascular, 1015*t*
weight loss, involuntary, 32
Dementia with Lewy bodies, 1015*t*
Demodex folliculorum folliculitis, 124–125
Demyelination
paranodal, 1030
segmental, 1030
Dengue (fever), 1379, **1393–1395**
Dengue shock syndrome, 1393–1394
Dengvaxia (CYD-TDV), 1394–1395
Denileukin, silent thyroiditis from, 1115
Denosumab
for breast carcinoma, 754
for cancer, systemic, 1654*t*
on hip fractures, 1693
for hypercalcemia, 890, 1650, 1651
for hyperparathyroidism, 1145
for metastatic bone pain, 95
for osteoporosis, 1150–1151
for plasma cell myeloma, 538
for prostate cancer bone metastases, 1640–1641
Dentatorubral-pallidoluysian atrophy, 1010
Deoxyribonuclease, recombinant human, 267
Dependence
alcohol use disorder, 1086
opiate, 1092
opioid, 85, 86
physiologic, 1086
psychological, 1086
steroid, 1095
substance use, 1086
Dependency
depression, 1078
hospitalization & illness, 1097–1098
schizophrenia spectrum disorders, 1061
Dependent personality disorder, **1059–1061,** 1060*t*
Depersonalization, 999, 1062
Depigmentation, **163,** 163*f*. *See also* Hypopigmentation
Depo-medroxyprogesterone acetate, 767, 768, 777
Deprescribing, 61*t*, 66
Depression/depressive disorders, **1069–1081.** *See also* Major depressive disorder; *specific types*
adjustment disorders, **1046–1047**
alcohol use disorder, 1087
chronic pain syndromes, 1055–1056
clinical findings, 1069–1071
complications, 1071
COVID-19, 1404
dementia and, 54, 57
differential diagnosis, 1071
drug-induced, 1070–1071
end of life, 74
fatigue, 70
gay & bisexual men, 1723
hospitalization & illness related, 1097
illness, 1070–1071
incontinence, urinary, 62
irritable bowel syndrome, 644
lesbian & bisexual women, 1721–1722
major depressive disorder, **1069–1070**
melancholic depression, 1072
obesity, 1251
older adults, 54, **57–58**
Patient Health Questionnaire-2, 57
persistent depressive disorder, 1070
premenstrual dysphoric disorder, 1070
prenatal, postpartum effects, 1075
prevalence & factors, 1069
prognosis, 1081
schizophrenia, 1062
suicide risk, 1071
weight loss, involuntary, 32
Depression/depressive disorders, treatment, 1072–1078, 1074*f*
nonpharmacologic, 1077–1078
pharmacologic, 1072–1078
atypical antidepressants, 1072–1076, 1073*t*
classification, 1072, 1073*t*
cognitive issues, 1072
drug interactions, 1077
maintenance and tapering, 1077
major depression with atypical features, 1072
medication selection, 1072
melancholic depression, 1072
monoamine oxidase inhibitors, 1073*t*, 1076
psychotic depression, 1072
seasonal affective disorder, 1072
SNRIs, 1072–1075, 1073*t*
SSRIs, 1072–1075, 1073*t*
switching and combination therapy, 1077
tricyclic antidepressants, 1073*t*, 1076
postpartum, allopregnanolone for, 1077
Depressive episodes, 1078–1081
de Quervain thyroiditis, **1112–1114**
Dermacentor andersoni, 1400, 1431
Dermatitis. *See also specific types*
actinic, chronic, 155
atopic, **133–135**
cataracts, 184
dyshidrotic, **144,** 144*f*
molluscum contagiosum, 1421

cercarial, 1520
contact (*See* Contact dermatitis)
exfoliative, **154–155**
neurodermatitis, circumscribed, **135–136,** 135*f*
photodermatitis, 102*t,* **155–156**
seborrheic, **139–140,** 139*f*
stasis, 28, 490, 490*f*
vesiculobullous, of palms and soles, **144,** 144*f*
Dermatitis herpetiformis, **145**
celiac disease, 633–634
Dermatitis medicamentosa, **156–159,** 158*t*–159*t*
Dermatographism, 151–153
Dermatologic disorders, **101–165**. *See also specific types*
alopecia, **164–165**
nonscarring, **164–165**
scarring, **165**
drug eruption, **156–159,** 158*t*–159*t*
erythemas, **151–155**
exfoliative dermatitis, **154–155**
reactive erythemas, **151–154**
erythema multiforme/Stevens-Johnson syndrome/toxic epidermal necrolysis, **153–154,** 153*f,* 154*f*
urticaria & angioedema, **151–153,** 152*f*
HIV/AIDS
bacterial
bacillary angiomatosis, 1328
staphylococcal, 1327–1328
fungal
dermatophytes & *Candida,* 1328
seborrheic dermatitis, 1328
psoriasis, 1328
viral
herpes simplex, 1318*t,* 1327, 1327*f*
herpes zoster, 1318*t,* 1327
molluscum contagiosum, 1327, 1328*f*
xerosis, 1328
infections, **114–131** (*See also* Skin infections)
infestations & bites, **114–133**
arthropod lesions, **131–132**
bedbugs, **131**
caterpillars, urticating hair moths, **132**
chiggers/red bugs, **132**
fleas, **131**
mites, bird/rodent, **132**
mites, stored products, **132**
ticks, **131**
tungiasis, **132**
bacterial, **123–128**
inflammatory nodules, erythema nodosum, **132–133,** 133*f*
morphologic categorization, **102*t***
neoplastic lesions, **107–114** (*See also specific types*)
nonpigmented, **110–114**
benign lesions, epidermal inclusion cysts, **110**
malignant/premalignant lesions, **110–112**
actinic keratoses, **110–111**
basal cell carcinoma, **112–113,** 112*f*
Bowen disease, **114**
cutaneous T-cell lymphoma, **113–114**
Kaposi sarcoma, **113**
Paget disease, **114,** 744, 744*f*
squamous cell carcinoma, **111,** 111*f*
pigmented, **107–110**
benign pigmented, **107–109**
atypical nevi, **108,** 108*f*
blue nevi, **108,** 108*f*
freckles & lentigines, **108**
melanocytic nevi, **107,** 107*f*
seborrheic keratosis, **108,** 109*f*
malignant pigmented lesions, **109–110**
malignant melanoma, **109–110,** 109*f,* 169
nevi, 163
photodermatitis, 102*t,* **155–156**
pigmentary, **162–164**
primary
hyperpigmentation, **163**
hypopigmentation and depigmentation, **163,** 163*f*
secondary
hyperpigmentation, **163,** 163*f*
hypopigmentation, **163–164**
pruritus, **159–161**
anogenital, **160–161,** 160*f*
erythrasma, 160, 160*f*
pustular disorders, **147–151**
acne vulgaris, **147–149,** 148*f*
miliaria, **151**
rosacea, **149–150,** 150*f*
scaling disorders, **133–142**
atopic dermatitis, **133–135, 144,** 144*f,* 184, 1421
cutaneous lupus erythematosus, **141–142**
lichen planus, **140–141,** 140*f*
lichen simplex chronicus, **135–136,** 135*f*
pityriasis rosea, **138–139,** 138*f*
psoriasis, **136–138,** 136*f*
seborrheic dermatitis, **139–140,** 139*f*
ulcers, **161–162**
leg, venous insufficiency, **161–162,** 161*f*
vesicular & blistering dermatoses, **142–147**
bullous pemphigoid, **147**
contact dermatitis, **142–143**
acute weeping, 143
allergic, 142–143, 143*f*
chronic, 143
irritant, 142–143, 143*f*
subacute, 143
dermatitis herpetiformis, **145**
pemphigus, **145–147,** 146*f*
pompholyx, **144,** 144*f*
porphyria cutanea tarda, **144–145,** 145*f*
Dermatologic disorders, treatment, **101–107**
antipruritics, systemic, 101, 107
bathing, 101
complications, topical therapy, 107
corticosteroid, systemic (*See* Corticosteroids)
sunscreens, 107
topical therapy/agents, **101, 102*t*–106*t***
antibiotics, acne, **104*t*–105*t***
antibiotics, impetigo, **105*t***
antifungals, imidazoles, **105*t***
antifungals, other, **106*t***
antipruritics, 101, **106*t***
corticosteroids, 101, **102*t*–104*t***
drying agents, 101
emollients, 101
NSAIDs, **104*t***
Dermatomyositis, **842–844,** 843*f,* 1004*t*
Dermatophytes. *See specific types*
Desensitization
for asthma, 255
for phobias with depression, 1078
for phobic disorders, 1052
Designer drugs, **1095**
Desipramine
for attention-deficit/hyperactivity disorders, 1081
for depression, 1073*t,* 1076
for diabetic neuropathy pain, 1222
for irritable bowel syndrome, 646
for neuropathic pain, **91*t*,** 94*t,* 95
Desmopressin
for bleeding diathesis, CKD, 917
for hypernatremia, 881
for upper GI bleeding, 597
Desmopressin acetate, 880, 1105
Desogestrel, 775*t,* 776
Desonide, 102*t,* 139
Desoximetasone, 103*t*
Destination therapy, 419
Desvenlafaxine, 95, 1072, 1073*t,* 1075
Desynchronization sleep disorder, 1082
Detergent worker's lung, 307*t*
"Determinant-based" classification, 729–730
Detrusor
overactivity, 62, 63
underactivity, 63
Deutetrabenzine, 1010
DeVega annuloplasty, for tricuspid regurgitation, 352
Devic disease, **1026**
Dexamethasone
for adenoviral conjunctivitis, 1419
for amyloidosis, 541
for aphthous ulcers, 1325
for Behçet disease, 857
clinical uses, 1193, 1194*t*
for COVID-19, 1405
for *Haemophilus* meningitis, 1461
for nausea & vomiting, 583*t,* **584,** 1655
neuromodulatory therapy, 97*t*
for plasma cell myeloma, 538
for pneumococcal meningitis, 1282, 1445
for preeclampsia-eclampsia, 803–804
for preterm birth, anticipated, 805
for spinal metastases, epidural, 1002
for tuberculous meningitis, 1477
Dexlansoprazole
for GERD, 610
for NSAIDs, 622, 628
for peptic ulcer disease, 627
Dexmedetomidine, 97*t,* 1091
Dexrazoxane, 1653*t*
Dextroamphetamines, 1076–1077, **1093–1094**
Dextroamphetamine sulfate, 1084
Dextromethorphan, 30, **1584–1585**
Dextromethorphan/quinidine, 1029
Dextrose
for coma, poisoning, 1565
for stupor & coma, 1019
Diabetes Control and Complications Trial (DCCT), 1198
Diabetes insipidus
central, **1104–1105**
hypernatremia, 881
nephrogenic, 1105
vasopressinase-induced, 1105
Wolfram syndrome, 1197
Diabetes insipidus, diabetes mellitus, optic atrophy, and deafness (DIDMOAD), 1197
Diabetes mellitus, **1195–1203**
acanthosis nigricans, 1200, 1200*f,* 1216
from antipsychotics, 1066, 1066*t*
autoimmune markers, 1216, 1216*t*
cataracts, 184
classification & pathogenesis, **1195–1198**
autosomal recessive syndromes, **1197**
latent autoimmune diabetes of adulthood, 1195–1196
maturity-onset diabetes of the young, **1196–1197,** 1196*t*
mitochondrial DNA mutation, **1197**
secondary to other causes, **1197,** 1197*t*
type 1, **1195–1196**
type 1B, 1196

Diabetes mellitus, classification & pathogenesis (*Cont.*):
type 2, **1196**
Wolfram syndrome, **1197**
colorectal cancer and, 1627
coronary heart disease, 355
diabetes prevention trials, **1198**
endometrial adenocarcinoma from, 791
end-stage kidney disease, 914
epidemiology, 1195
gallstones, 719
glucose control, clinical trials, **1198–1199**
hematuria, 943
hypertension treatment, 466, 467*t*
laboratory findings, **1200–1203,** 1201*t*
lesbian & bisexual women, **1718**
on lipid metabolism, 1241
metabolic syndrome, **1197–1198**
nephrotic spectrum glomerular diseases, **931–932**
obesity, 1251
occult, postprandial hypoglycemia, **1236–1237**
pancreas carcinoma, 1615
peripheral artery disease, 473
polyneuropathy, **1031–1032**
pregnancy, **810–811**
gestational, **810–811,** 810*t*
overt, **811**
preoperative evaluation/perioperative management, 49–50
retinal artery occlusion, 189, **189–190**
retinopathy, 67, 191, **191–192**
salivary gland disorders, 235
screening/prevention, 4, 5*t*
stroke risk, 986
symptoms & signs, **1199–1200,** 1200*f*
Diabetes mellitus, treatment, **1203–1216**
complications, chronic, **1221–1226**
autonomic neuropathy
genitourinary system, 1223–1224
GI system, 1223
orthostatic hypotension, 1224
bone and joint, 1225
cardiovascular
heart disease, 1224
hypertension, 1224
peripheral vascular disease, 1224
nephropathy, 1221
neuropathy, 1221–1223
peripheral, 1221–1223
distal symmetric polyneuropathy, 1221–1222, 1222*f*
isolated peripheral neuropathy, 1222–1223
ocular
diabetic cataracts, 1221
diabetic retinopathy, 67, 191, **191–192,** 1221
glaucoma, 1221
skin and mucous membrane, 1224–1225
diet
fiber, 1203
general, 1203
glycemic index, 1203
sweeteners, artificial/other, 1203
hospital management, 1225–1226
insulin, **1211–1215,** 1212*t* (*See also* Insulin)
medications, for hyperglycemia, 1203–1211, 1204*t*
acarbose, 1204*t*, 1208
bromocriptine, 1211
colesevelam, 1211
combinations, 1211
D-phenylalanine derivatives, 1204*t*, 1206–1207
nateglinide, 1204*t*, 1206–1207, 1218, 1218*f*, 1220
repaglinide, 1204*t*, 1206, 1218, 1218*f*
DPP-4 inhibitors, 1205*t*, 1210
alogliptin, 1205*t*, 1210
linagliptin, 1205*t*, 1210
saxagliptin, 1205*t*, 1210
sitagliptin, 1205*t*, 1210
vildagliptin, 1205*t*, 1210
GLP-1 receptor agonists, 1204*t*–1205*t*, 1208–1210
dulaglutide, 1204*t*, 1209
exenatide, 1204*t*, 1209
liraglutide, 1205*t*, 1209
lixisenatide, 1205*t*, 1209
semaglutide, 1205*t*, 1209
incretins, 1204*t*, 1208–1210
meglitinide analogs
mitiglinide, 1204*t*, 1206
repaglinide, 1204*t*, 1206
metformin, 1204*t*, 1207
miglitol, 1204*t*, 1208
pramlintide, 1205*t*, 1211
sodium-glucose co-transporter 2 inhibitors, 1205*t*, 1210–1211
canagliflozin, 1205*t*, 1210–1211
dapagliflozin, 1205*t*, 1210
empagliflozin, 1205*t*, 1210
ertugliflozin, 1205*t*, 1210
sulfonylureas, 1203–1206, 1204*t*
glyburide, glipizide, gliclazide, and glimepiride, 1204*t*, 1206
tolazamide, acetohexamide, and chlorpropamide, 1204*t*, 1206
tolbutamide, 1204*t*, 1206
thiazolidinediones, 1204*t*, 1207–1208
rosiglitazone and pioglitazone, 1204*t*, 1207–1208
troglitazone, 1208
steps, management, 1216–1221
glycemic control, acceptable levels, 1219, 1219*t*
insulin therapy, complications, 1219–1221 (*See also under* Insulin therapy)
medications, 1216–1219
type 1, 1217, 1217*t*
type 2, 1217–1219, 1218*f*
type 2, glucose-lowering agents, 1218–1219, 1218*f*
type 2, weight reduction, 1217–1218
patient education, 1216
types, distinguishing, 1216, 1216*t*
transplantation
islet, 1215–1216
pancreas, 1215
Diabetes Prevention Program, 1199
Diabetic cataracts, 1221
Diabetic cheiroarthropathy, 1225
Diabetic coma, **1226,** 1226*t*
Diabetic dermopathy, 1225
Diabetic dyslipidemia, 1202
Diabetic ketoacidosis, 896*t*, 897, **1226–1230**
from atypical antipsychotics, 1197
causes, 1226
classification, 1228
clinical findings, 1227–1228
complications & prognosis, 1230
considerations, 1226
COVID-19, 1405
hyperphosphatemia, 892
laboratory finding, 1226*t*, 1227–1228
osmol gap, 1570
symptoms & signs, 1227
treatment, 1228–1230, 1296*t*
Diabetic nephropathy, 924*t*, **934–935,** 1221
Diabetic neuropathic cachexia, 1222
Diabetic neuropathy, 1221–1223
distal symmetric polyneuropathy, 1221–1222, 1222*f*
neurogenic arthropathy, 868
peripheral
distal symmetric polyneuropathy, 1221–1222, 1222*f*
isolated peripheral neuropathy, 1222–1223
Diabetic retinopathy, 67, 191, **191–192,** 1221
Diagnostic and Statistical Manual (DSM-5), 1046
Dialectical behavioral therapy, **1060**
Dialysis. *See also specific types*
amyloidosis from, 541
peritoneal, for end-stage kidney disease, 920
renal
amyloidosis from, 541
for end-stage kidney disease, 920
hypercalcemia, 890
hypocalcemia and hyperphosphatemia from, 890
surgical risk, 51
surgical risk, 51
Diaphragm, with contraceptive jelly, **778**
DIAPPERS, 62
Diarrhea, **589–595.** *See also specific pathogens and disorders*
from 5-fluorouracil, 1656
acute, **589–592**
etiology & clinical findings, 589–590, 589*t*, 1289*t*–1290*t*
evaluation, 591–592, 591*f*
infectious causes, 589–590, 589*t*
inflammatory, 590–591
noninflammatory, 590
treatment, 592
acute infectious, **1288–1290,** 1289*t*–1290*t* (*See also specific types*)
causes, 1288
food poisoning, 1288
inflammatory, 1288
noninflammatory, 1288
treatment, 1288, 1289*t*–1290*t*
antibiotic-associated, 647
from chemotherapy agents, 1656
chronic, **593–595**
clinical findings, 594–595, 594*f*
diagnosis, 594, 594*f*
etiology, 590*t*, 593
infections, 593
inflammatory conditions, 593
malabsorptive conditions, 593
medications, 593
motility disorders, 593
osmotic, 593
secretory conditions, 593
systemic conditions, 593
treatment, 595
coccidiosis & microsporidiosis, 1516–1517
cryptosporidiosis, 589, 1288, 1326, **1516–1518**
cyclosporiasis, 589, 1288, **1516–1518**
diabetic, 1223
enterotoxigenic *E. coli*, 590, 1289*t*, 1292, **1465–1466**
giardiasis, 589, 590, **1518–1519**
hypokalemia, 893
hypomagnesemia, 893
Isospora, 1288, **1516–1518**
measles, 1370
norovirus, **1422–1423**
pathophysiology, 589
severity, 589
traveler's, 590, **1292–1293**
treatment, antibiotic, 592
Diastolic rumble, tricuspid stenosis, 350

Diazepam, 1050*t*
for aggression disorders, 1085
for panic disorder, 1050*t*, 1051
poisoning, **1581–1582**
for seizures, from poisoning, 1567
for spasticity, 1026
Diazoxide, 1235
Diclofenac, 82, **83*t***
for gallstone pain, 719
hepatotoxicity, 696
for knee osteoarthritis, 1705
for neuropathic pain, **91*t***
for osteoarthritis, 83*t*, 821
Dicloxacillin
for cellulitis, 128, 162
for erysipelas, 128
for furunculosis & carbuncles, 126
for skin & soft tissue infections, 1447
for *Staphylococcus aureus*, 1441, 1441*t*
Dicyclomine, 646
Didanosine, 715, 1325
DID-MOAD, 1197
Diesel fuel, 245, 1603
Diet. *See also specific types*
for cardiovascular disease prevention, 5*t*
for constipation, 586
for gallstone prevention, 719
for heart failure with reduced LVEF, 411
for hypertension, 448
Dietary supplements/therapy. *See also* Supplements; *specific types*
acute liver failure from, 685
for diabetes mellitus
fiber, 1203
general, 1203
glycemic index, 1203
sweeteners, artificial/other, 1203
liver injury, 696
poisoning, **1580**, 1580*t*
Diethylcarbamazine, 1531–1532
Diethylene glycol poisoning, 1586
Diet therapy, **1262–1264**. *See also specific types*
consistency altering
clear liquids, 1263
full liquids, 1263
soft, 1263
food recall & tracking, 1262–1263
nutrient restrictions
carbohydrate, 1264
fat & low saturated fats, 1263–1264
protein, 1264
sodium, 1263
nutrient supplementation
calcium, 1264
fiber, 1264
potassium, 1264
types, 1262–1263
Dieulafoy lesion, upper GI bleeding, 596
Difenacoum poisoning, 1575
Differential time to positivity, 1278
Differentiated vulvar intraepithelial neoplasia, vulvar, 791
Diffuse alveolar hemorrhage, hemoptysis, 21
Diffuse axonal injury, 1022*t*
Diffuse idiopathic skeletal hyperostosis, 1225
Diffuse interstitial pneumonias, **292–294,** 293*t*, 294*t*
Diffuse large B-cell lymphoma, 534, 1623
Diffuse panbronchiolitis, 268
Diffuse paryenchymal lung disease, **292–297**. *See also* Interstitial lung disease
Diffuse stromal Leydig cell hyperplasia, 1182
Diflorasone diacetate, 103*t*
Diftitox, silent thyroiditis from, 1115
Digitalis glycosides. *See also specific types*
for heart failure with reduced LVEF, 409
Digitalis poisoning, 1568*t*, **1581**
Digital rectal examination, 1634
Digital subtraction angiography, 476, 479, 479*f*
Dignity, medical aid in dying, 76
Digoxin, 383, 385*t*
for atrial fibrillation, with hyperthyroidism, 1126
for heart failure with reduced LVEF, 409
poisoning, 1571*t*, 1572*t*
Digoxin immune Fab, 1581
Digoxin-specific antibodies, 1581
Dihydroartemisinin-piperaquine, 1504*t*, 1507
Dihydroergotamine, 973
Dihydroergotamine mesylate, 971
Dihydrofolate reductase, 1507
Dihydropteroate synthase, 1507
Dihydropyridines, 363, 372, 1163. *See also specific types*
Dihydropyrimidine dehydrogenase variants, 1669*t*
Dilated cardiomyopathy, **417–420,** 418*t*. *See also* Cardiomyopathy, dilated
Dilation & curettage, 764*t*
Diloxanide furoate, 1514–1515, 1515t
Diltiazem, 383, 385*t*
for anal fissures, 672
for angina pectoris, 363
for hypertension, 455, 456*t*
poisoning, **1578**
Dimercaprol, 1583
2,3-Dimercaptopropanesulfonic acid, 1577
Dimethicone, 131
Dimethyl fumarate, 1025, 1025*t*
Dimethyltryptamine derivatives, **1093**
Diphenhydramine
for antipsychotic poisoning, 1576
for atopic dermatitis, 135
breastfeeding, 796*t*
for dystonias, from antipsychotics, 1067
for insomnia, 1083
poisoning, 1577
for radiocontrast media reaction prevention, 870
seizures from, 1567
for vancomycin flushing syndrome, 870
Diphenoxylate with atropine, 595, 1223, 1326
Diphtheritic neuropathy, 1033
Diphyllobothrium latum, 507, 1523
Diplopia, 215, 848
Diptheria-tetanus-pertussis (DTaP) vaccine, 1459
Dipylidium caninum, 1523
Dipyridamole, 987
Direct-acting oral anticoagulants, **563–565,** 564*t*
for acute MI, with ST-segment elevation, 378
for atrial fibrillation, stroke prevention, **393–395,** 394*t*
for Kawasaki disease, 1438
perioperative management, 48, 48*t*
poisoning, 1575
with prosthetic heart valves, 353
for pulmonary venous thromboembolism, 300
reversal agents, 563, 565*t*
for stroke prevention, 393–395, 394*t*
for venous thromboembolism
prophylaxis, 567*t*, 573–574
treatment, 570–571, 570*t*
Direct antiglobulin test, 515, 540
Direct current, 1557
Direct factor Xa inhibitors, 358, 365. *See also specific types*
Directly observed therapy, pulmonary tuberculosis, 283, 284, 286
Direct thrombin inhibitors, 371, 553, 553*t*. *See also specific types*
Discogenic neck pain, **1037–1040**
cervical disk protrusion, **1037,** 1038*f*–1039*f*
cervical spondylosis, **1037–1040**
Discogenic pain, **1686–1687**
Discoid lupus erythematosus, **141–142**
Disease-modifying antirheumatic drugs
for Chikungunya fever, 864, 1400
for gonococcal arthritis, 861
for rheumatoid arthritis, **829–831**
biologic, 830–831
combination, 831
synthetic, 829–830
triple therapy, 831
Disease prevention & health promotion, **1–13**. *See also* Prevention, disease
adherence, 1–2
alcohol use disorder, 12–13, 13*t*
cancer, 11–12
exercise, 10
general approach, 1–2
guiding principles of care, 2
health maintenance & disease prevention, 2–9
injuries & violence, 12
overweight & obesity, 10–11
substance use disorder, 12–13, 13*t*
vaccination, 11–12
Disk batteries, poisoning, 1573–1574
Disk herniation, lumbar, **1686–1687**
Disopyramide, 383, 384*t*, 422
Disorders of sexual desire, **781, 1058**
Disseminated intravascular coagulation, **554–555,** 554*t*
acute leukemia, 529
drowning, 1553
Ebola viral disease, 1390
malignant disease, 1003
Distal interphalangeal joint osteoarthritis, 819, 820, 821
Distal muscular dystrophy, 1043*t*
Distal symmetric polyneuropathy, 1221–1222, 1222*f*
Distributive justice, 77
Distributive shock, **495–499,** 495*t*
endocrine, **496–497**
septic, **495–498**
Disulfiram, 696, 1089
Diuretics
for ascites and edema, from cirrhosis, 702
for cardiomyopathy, hypertrophic, 422
for focal segmental glomerulosclerosis, 933
gout from, 823
for heart failure
with preserved LVEF, 412
with reduced LVEF, 406–407
for hypertension, **455,** 458*t*–459*t*
hypokalemia from, 893
hypomagnesemia from, 893
kidney stones from, 954
loop
gout, 825
for heart failure with reduced LVEF, 407
for hypertension, **455,** 458*t*, 470, 471*t*
for hyponatremia, chronic, 879
ototoxicity, 213
potassium-sparing, for heart failure with reduced LVEF, 407
preoperative evaluation/perioperative management, 45–46
for pulmonary edema, 413
sulfonamide-containing, interstitial nephritis from, 911

Diuretics (*Cont.*):
thiazide
for calcium nephrolithiasis, 956
on diabetes risk, 1197
gout, 825
for heart failure with reduced LVEF, 407
for hypertension, **455,** 458*t*
for hyperuricemia, 1652
hyponatremia from, 878
hypotonic hyponatremia from, **878**
for renal hypercalciuria, 956
Divalproex, 1079
Diverticular disease of colon
diverticulitis, **663–665**
diverticulosis, uncomplicated, **663**
Diverticulitis, **663–665**
Diverticulosis
lower GI bleeding, 599
uncomplicated, **663**
Diving, **1559–1560**
perilymphatic fistula, 208, 217
underwater, barotrauma from, 208
Diving reflex, 389
Dix-Hallpike testing, 214–215
D-lactic acidosis, 896
DMPS, 1577
DNAR, 72
DNMT3A, myelodysplastic syndromes, 527
DNR, 72
DOACs. *See* Direct-acting oral anticoagulants
Dobrava-Belgrade virus, 1395
Dobutamine, 499
Docetaxel, 1599*t*
for breast carcinoma, 752, 758, 759
neuropathy from, 1656
for prostate cancer, 1640*t*, 1641
Doctor-patient relationship, on adherence, 2
Docusate sodium, 587*t*
Dofetilide, 383, 385*t*, 396
Dog bites, **1283–1284**
Dog hookworm, 1527
Dog tapeworm, 1523, 1525–1526
Dolutegravir, for HIV/AIDS, 1338, **1340*t*, 1346**
fixed-dose combinations, 1342*t*
integrase inhibitor class, 1345
+ lamivudine, 1338
for prevention, 1333, 1334
regimens, 1343, 1347*t*, 1348–1351
+ TDF/emtricitabine, 1338
+ tenofovir alafenamide/emtricitabine, 1338
with tuberculosis, 1320
Domestic violence
elder mistreatment, **67–68,** 68*t*
intimate partner, sexual, **782–783, 1721**
rape, **782–783**
Domperidone, 581
Donepezil, 1017
Do not attempt resuscitation orders, **72**
Dopamine, 498, 907, 1099
Dopamine agonists. *See also specific types*
chorea from, 1012
for hyperprolactinemia, 1109
for Parkinson disease, 1008
withdrawal syndrome, 1008
Dopamine antagonists, 583*t*, **584**. *See also specific types*
Doravirine, **1339*t*, 1344**
Double crush injury, 1687
"Double effect," 77
Double-hit lymphoma, 534
Double outlet right ventricle, 330
Double-protein expressors, 534
Down syndrome, **1659–1660**
Doxazosin, 460, 463*t*, 965–966, 965*t*, 966
Doxepin
for atopic dermatitis, 135
for depression, 1073*t*
for insomnia, 1083
for pruritus, 101, 161
topical dermatologic, 101, 106*t*
for urticaria & angioedema, 152
Doxorubicin (Adriamycin), 1599*t*
for bladder cancer, 1643
for breast carcinoma, 752, 761
cardiotoxicity, 417, 1656
for Kaposi sarcoma, 113
liposomal, 1599*t*
Doxycycline
for acne vulgaris, 149
for actinomycosis, 1474
for animal bites, 1284
for *Bartonella*, 1471
for bullous pemphigoid, 147
for CA-MRSA impetigo, 124
for chlamydial reactive arthritis, 861
for *Chlamydia trachomatis*
lymphogranuloma venereum, 1477
urethritis & cervicitis, 1478
for *Chlamydophila pneumoniae*, 1479
for diarrhea, diabetic, 1223
for epididymitis, 948*t*, 953
for furunculosis & carbuncles, 126
for gonococcus, 1470
for granuloma inguinale, 1471
for leptospirosis, 1491
for Lyme disease, 1494, 1495*t*
for malaria, 1504*t*, 1505*t*, 1508*t*, 1509
for MRSA, 128, 1328
for *Mycobacterium abscessus*, 1475
for *Mycobacterium chelonae*, 1475
for *Mycobacterium fortuitum*, 1475
for *Mycobacterium marinum*, 1475
for onchocerciasis, 1533
for pelvic inflammatory disease, 786
pill-induced esophagitis from, 613
for plague, 1469
for pneumococcal pneumonia, 1444
pregnancy, teratogenicity, 1432
for prostatitis, 948*t*
for psittacosis, 1478
for Q fever, 1436
for rickettsialpox, 1433
for Rocky Mountain spotted fever, 1432
for rosacea, 150
for spotted fever, 1433
for *Staphylococcus aureus*
osteomyelitis, 1448
skin & soft tissue infections, 1447
for syphilis, 1483*t*, 1484, 1488
for tularemia, 1468
for typhus
endemic, 1429
epidemic, 1428
scrub, 1430
tick, 1432
DPD variants, 1669*t*
D-penicillamine, 712–713
D-phenylalanine derivatives. *See also specific types*
for hyperglycemia/diabetes mellitus, 1204*t*, 1206–1207
nateglinide, 1204*t*, 1206–1207, 1218, 1218*f*, 1220
repaglinide, 1204*t*, 1206, 1218, 1218*f*
DPP-4 inhibitors. *See also specific types*
for hyperglycemia/diabetes mellitus, 1205*t*, 1210
alogliptin, 1205*t*, 1210
linagliptin, 1205*t*, 1210
saxagliptin, 1205*t*, 1210
sitagliptin, 1205*t*, 1210
vildagliptin, 1205*t*, 1210
DQA1*0301, 1237
DQB1, 707
DQB1*0302, 1237
*DRB1*08*, 707
DRB1*0406, 1237
Dream sleep, 1082
Dressler syndrome, 381, 427, 428
Drink, defined, 1086–1087
Drinking. *See also* Alcohol use disorder
at-risk, 1086–1087
Driving, dementia and, 56–57, 1018
Dronabinol, 1316
Dronedarone, 383, 385*t*, 396
Drop attacks, epileptic, 980
Droperidol poisoning, 1576
Drospirenone, 775*t*, 776
Drowning, **1553–1554**
Droxidopa, 985
Drug Addiction Treatment Act of 2000, 94
Drug allergy, **870**. *See also specific types*
Drug-eluting stents
for angina, 365
antiplatelet therapy after, 371, 375
pregnancy, 438
ST-segment elevation, 375
Drug eruptions, **156–159,** 158*t*–159*t*. *See also* Drug reactions; *specific types*
Drug exanthems, 158*t*, **871**
Drug fever, 1277
Drug-induced hypersensitivity syndrome, **871**. *See also* Delayed drug hypersensitivity; Hypersensitivity reactions
Drug-induced thrombocytopenia, **555,** 555*t*
Drug injection–related infections, **1286–1287**
aspiration pneumonia, 1287
hepatitis, 1287
HIV/AIDS, 1287
infective endocarditis, 1287
osteomyelitis, 1287
pulmonary septic emboli, 1287
septic arthritis, 1287
sexually transmitted diseases, 1287
skin, 1286–1287
tuberculosis, 1287
vascular infections, other, 1287
Drug reactions. *See also specific drugs and types*
acute liver failure, 685
drug allergy, **870**
non–IgE-mediated anaphylactic, **870**
older adults, 66
photodermatitis, 155
radiocontrast media, **870**
vancomycin flushing syndrome, **870**
Drug reaction with eosinophilia and systemic symptoms (DRESS) syndrome, **30,** 157, 696, **871**
liver injury, **30,** 157, 696, **871**
Drug-related illnesses. *See also specific types*
abnormal movements, **1012–1013**
asthma, 245–246
bone marrow failure, 546
cutaneous lupus erythematosus, subacute, 158*t*
delirium, 55, 58–59
depression, 1070–1071
drug-induced hypersensitivity syndrome, **871**
erosive gastritis/gastropathy, **620–622**
eye and lid, **198–203, 200*t*–202*t***
falls, 60
hemolytic anemia, 514
hepatotoxicity, **696–697**
hypersensitivity reactions, delayed, **871–872**
hypersensitivity syndrome, 157–158, 158*t*
hypoglycemia, **1237**
incontinence, urinary, 62
liver diseases, **696–697**
lung disease, 308–309, 308*t*

lupus, **836–837**
medication-assisted treatment, 13
older adults, 66
palpitations, 26
parkinsonism, 1012, 1067
parotid gland enlargement, 235
pemphigus, 146
peptic ulcer disease, 625
pericarditis, 427
phototoxicity, 155
pregnancy, teratogenicity/fetotoxicity, 794, 795*t*
prescribing cascade, 66
reconciliation, 66
thrombocytopenia, **555,** 555*t*
tremor, 1012
Drug-resistant tuberculosis, 280, 283, 285
Drugs
adherence, 1–2
discontinuation, 61*t*, 66
Drug use/abuse. *See* Substance use disorders
Drusen, retinal, 187
"Dry" age-related macular degeneration, **187**
Dry beriberi, 1260
Dry eyes
conjunctivitis, **171–172**
corneal ulcer, 179
Sjögren syndrome, 16
Drying agents, 101
Dry mouth, from antipsychotics, 1066
Dry powder inhalers, 249
D state sleep, 1082
DTs, 1087, 1091
Dual antiplatelet therapy. *See* Antiplatelet therapy, dual
Dual-chamber pacemaker, 387, 388
Dual orexin receptor antagonists, 1083–1084. *See also specific types*
Dual reverse transcriptase inhibitors. *See specific types*
Dubin-Johnson syndrome, conjugated hyperbilirubinemia, 674, 676*t*
Duchenne type muscular dystrophy, 1043–1044, 1043*t*
Ductal carcinoma in situ, 749. *See also* Breast carcinoma
Duke Treadmill Score, 367, 367*t*
Dulaglutide, 358–359, 1204*t*, 1209
Duloxetine
for chronic pain syndromes, 1057
for depression, 1072, 1073*t*
for diabetic peripheral neuropathy, 1222
for generalized anxiety disorder, 1050–1051
hepatotoxicity, 696
for low back pain, 1685
for neuropathic pain, **91*t*, 94–95,** 94*t*
for osteoarthritis, 821
Dumping syndrome, 1233, 1236
Duncan disease, 1364
Duodenum diseases, **620–632**. *See also* Stomach & duodenum diseases
Dupilumab
for asthma, 251*t*, 254
for atopic dermatitis, 135
for lichen simplex chronicus, 136
molluscum contagiosum from, 1421
Duplex ultrasonography
aortoiliac occlusive disease, 473
cerebrovascular disease, occlusive, 479
chronic venous insufficiency, 491
femoropopliteal occlusive disease, 475
post-thrombotic syndrome, 491
superficial venous thrombophlebitis, 489
varicose vein, 488
Dupuytren contracture, 1225, **1691**
Durable power of attorney for finance matters, 57
Durable power of attorney for health care, 71
Duroziez sign, 347
Durvalumab, 1606, 1643
Dutasteride, 966, 1726, 1727*t*
Duvelisib, 531, 534
Dwarf tapeworm, **1523**
DXA bone densitometry, 1143, 1147, 1148, 1149, 1154
Dyes, industrial, bladder cancer from, 1642
Dysautonomia, **984–985**
Dysbarism, 868, **1559–1560**
Dysconjugate deviation, 1019
Dyscrasias, **193,** 1237
Dysentery, 590–591
Shigella, 1465
Dysgerminomas, 1181
Dyshidrosis, **144,** 144*f*
Dyshidrotic eczema, **144,** 144*f*
Dyskeratosis congenita, 546
Dyslipidemia. *See* Cholesterol; Hypercholesterolemia; *specific disorders*
Dysmenorrhea, primary, **767**
Dyspareunia, **781–782**
Dyspepsia, **579–581**
Dysphagia, 606–607, **620**. *See also* Esophagus diseases
definition, 606
esophageal, 607, 607*t*
motility disorders, 620
webs, iron deficiency, 501
odynophagia, 607
oropharyngeal, 606, 606*t*
Dysplasia of cervix, **787–789,** 788*f*
Dyspnea, 15, **18–20**. *See also specific disorders*
bronchiectasis, 265
bronchiolitis, 267, 268
COPD, 18, 19, 20, 259, 260*t*, 264
COVID-19, 17, 19, 20, 70
cystic fibrosis, 266
definition, 69
palliative care, 69–70
Dyspnea, heart disease
acute coronary syndromes, without ST-segment elevation, 368
acute MI, with ST-segment elevation, 373
from adenosine, 385*t*
athlete, cardiovascular screening, 438, 439*t*
atrial flutter, 397
atrial tachycardia, 397
AV block, 387
cardiomyopathy
dilated, 419
hypertrophic, 418*t*, 421–422
restrictive, 418*t*
stress, 420
coronary artery disease, 362
exertional
aortic regurgitation, 347
atrial septal defect shunt, 327
heart failure, 404
mitral regurgitation, 338
mitral stenosis, 332
patent foramen ovale, 327
pulmonary hypertension, 432
heart failure, 403–406
\+ pulmonary edema, 413–414
left ventricular failure, 380
myocarditis, 415
paroxysmal supraventricular tachycardia, 388
pericardial effusion, 429
pericarditis
acute inflammatory, 427
constrictive, 430
pulmonary hypertension, 432
pulmonary valve stenosis, 323
sinus tachycardia, 387
ventricular tachycardia, 399
Dysthymia, 1070
Dystonias
from antipsychotics, 1067
torsion
focal, **1011–1012**
idiopathic, **1011**
Dysuria, **38–41**
clinical findings, 38–39, 40*f*
cystitis, 38–41
differential diagnosis, 39
herpes simplex virus, 1353
treatment, 39–41, 40*f*

E

EACA, 559*t*
Ear canal diseases, **205–207**
cerumen impaction, **205–206**
exostoses & osteomas, **207**
foreign bodies, **206**
neoplasia, **207**
otitis externa, **206–207,** 206*f*
pruritus, **207**
Ear diseases, **204–218**. *See also specific types*
AIDS, 218
auricle, **205**
central auditory & vestibular systems, 215*t*, 217–218
multiple sclerosis, 218
vascular compromise, 218
vestibular schwannoma, 217–218
earache, **212**
ear canal, **205–207**
cerumen impaction, **205–206**
exostoses & osteomas, **207**
foreign bodies, **206**
neoplasia, **207**
otitis externa, **206–207,** 206*f*
pruritus, **207**
eustachian tube, **207–208**
barotrauma, **208**
dysfunction, **207–208**
otitis media, serous, **208**
hearing loss, **204–205**
inner ear, **212–217**
hyperacusis, **214**
sensorineural hearing loss, 204, **212–213**
autoimmune, **213**
idiopathic sudden sensory hearing loss, 204, **212, 213**
noise trauma, **212**
ototoxicity, **213**
physical trauma, **212**
presbycusis, **212**
tinnitus, **213–214**
vertigo, **214–217,** 215*t*
vertigo syndromes, from central lesions, 215*t*, **217**
vertigo syndromes, from peripheral lesions, 215*t*, **216–217**
benign paroxysmal positioning vertigo, **216**
cervicogenic vertigo, **217**
labyrinthitis, **216**
Ménière disease, **216**
migrainous vertigo, **217**
perilymphatic fistula, **216–217**
superior semicircular canal dehiscence, **217**
traumatic vertigo, **216**
vestibular neuronitis, **216**
middle ear, **209–211**
neoplasia, **212**
otitis media
acute, **209,** 209*f*
chronic, **209–211,** 210*f*
otosclerosis, **211**
trauma, **211–212,** 211*f*

Ear infections. *See* Otitis externa; Otitis media; *specific types*
Early goal-directed therapy, for shock, 498
Ear trauma, middle ear, **211–212,** 211*f*
East African trypanosomiasis, **1496–1497,** 1497*t*
Eastern equine encephalitis, 1379
Eating disorders, **1258–1259**
  anorexia nervosa, **1258–1259**
  bulimia nervosa, **1259**
Ebanga, 1390
Ebola viral disease, **1389–1392,** 1391
Ebstein anomaly, tricuspid regurgitation, 351
Echinocandins, for *Candida,* 1540*t*
  Candida auris, 1535
  Candida glabrata, 1535
  Candida krusei, 1535
  endocarditis, 535
  invasive candidiasis, 1535
Echinococcosis, **1525–1526**
Echinococcus granulosus, 1525
Echinococcus multilocularis, 1525
Echocardiography, stress, for angina, 361
Echolalia, 1013, 1062
Echopraxia, 1013
Echovirus, **1424–1425**
e-cigarette or vaping product–associated lung injury, 261, **304–305**
Eclampsia, **802–804.** *See also* Preeclampsia-eclampsia
E. coli O104:H4, 1465–1466
E. coli O157:H7, 590, 1465–1466
Econazole, 105*t,* 115
Ecstasy. *See* Methylenedioxymethamphetamine (MDMA)
Ecthyma contagiosa, 1421
Ectopic ACTH-secreting tumors, 1163
Ectopic hormones, GEP-NETs, **1172**
Ectopic pregnancy, 794, **799–800**
Ectropion, **169**
Eculizumab
  for C3 glomerulopathies, 929
  infection risks, 1274
  for myasthenia gravis, 1041
  for neuromyelitis optica, 1026
  for paroxysmal nocturnal hemoglobinuria, 510
Eczema. *See* Atopic dermatitis
Eczema herpeticum, 135, 1354, 1357*t*
Edaravone, 1029
Edema. *See also specific types*
  cirrhosis, treatment, 702–703
  lower extremity, **27–29**
  refeeding, 1251
  tricuspid stenosis, 350
Edetate calcium disodium, 1583
Edge-to-edge MitraClip, mitral regurgitation, 339–340, 341*f*
Edoxaban, 563, 564*t*
  for atrial fibrillation, stroke prevention, **394,** 394*t*
  for mitral stenosis, 336
  poisoning, 1575
  for stroke prevention, 394, 394*t*
  for transient ischemic attacks, 987
  for venous thromboembolism, 570–571, 570*t*
Edwards SAPIEN XT valve, 324, 331, 347, 352
Efavirenz, **1339*t*, 1343–1344**
Effusive-constrictive pericarditis., 430
Efgartigimod, 1041
Efinaconazole
  for onychomycosis, 167
  topical dermatologic, 106*t*
Eflornithine, 771, 1497, 1497*t*
Egami score, 1438
EGFR, 1606, 1672*t*
EGFR tyrosine kinase inhibitors, 1672*t*. *See also specific types*
Egg allergies, 614, 868
Ehlers-Danlos syndrome
  bleeding from, 562
  diverticulosis, 663
  pregnancy risks, 435
  thoracic aortic aneurysm, 484
Ehrlichia chaffeensis, 1427*t,* **1433–1434**
Ehrlichia ewingii, 1427*t,* **1433–1434**
Ehrlichia muris euauclairensis, 1434
Ehrlichiosis, 1357*t,* 1427*t,* **1433–1434**
EIF2AK3, 1197
Eighth cranial nerve schwannoma, **217–218**
Eikenella corroden, animal bites, 1283
Eikenella injection drug skin infections, 1286
Eisenmenger physiology, 326, 432
Eisenmenger syndrome
  maternal mortality, pregnancy, 812
  pulmonary hypertension, 432, 433
  ventricular septal defect, 329
Ejaculation disturbances, 1058
  premature, 959
  retrograde, 959
Ejaculatory dysfunction therapy, 962
Elagolix, 768
Elapid envenomation, **1590**
Elbasvir, 1325
Elder abuse, **67–68,** 68*t*
Elderly. *See* Older adults
Elder mistreatment & self-neglect, **67–68,** 68*t*
Electrical alternans, 429
Electrical injury, **1557–1558**
Electrocardiography. *See also specific indications*
  ambulatory monitoring
    for angina pectoris, 361
    for athlete screening, COVID-19 myocarditis, 416*t*
    for commotio cordis, 440*t*
    for rate & rhythm disorders, 383
    for syncope, 402
    for ventricular arrhythmias, inherited, 401
    for ventricular premature beats, 398
    for ventricular tachycardia, 399
  for angina pectoris, 360–361
  antipsychotics on, 1066
Electroconvulsive therapy, for depression, 1077–1078
Electroencephalography. *See also specific indications*
  for epilepsy, 979, 981
  video electroencephalographic monitoring, 983
Electrolyte disorders, **875–894.** *See also specific types*
  calcium concentration disorders, **886–890**
    hypercalcemia, **889–890**
    hypocalcemia, **886–888,** 888*t*
  fluid management, **902,** 902*t*
  fractional excretion, electrolyte, 875
  magnesium concentration disorders, **892–894**
    hypermagnesemia, **894**
    hypomagnesemia, **893**
  patient assessment
    body water fluid distribution, **875,** 875*t*
    electrolytes, serum, **875**
    osmolality, serum, **875–876**
    urine, evaluation, **875**
  phosphorus concentration disorders, **890–892**
    hyperphosphatemia, **892,** 892*t*
    hypophosphatemia, **890–892,** 891*t*
  potassium concentration disorders, **882–886**
    hyperkalemia, **884–886,** 885*t,* 887*t*
    hypokalemia, **882–884,** 882*t,* 883*f*
  sodium concentration disorders, **876–882**
    hypernatremia, **880–882**
    hyponatremia, **876–880**
      diagnostic algorithm, 876, 877*f*
      etiology, 876–878, 877*f*
      hypotonic, **876–878,** 877*f,* 878*t,* 880
      isotonic & hypertonic, 876, 880
        hypertonic hyponatremia, 876
        pseudohyponatremia, 876, 880
      treatment, 879–880
Electrolyte free water clearance, 882
Electrolytes. *See also specific types and disorders*
  hot environments, water consumption, 1550
  nutritional support, 1266–1267
Electron beam CT, for angina pectoris, 361
Electronic directly observed therapy, for pulmonary tuberculosis, 283, 284
Elephantiasis, from filariasis, 1531, 1531*f*
Eletriptan, 971
Elexacaftor, 267
Elotuzumab, 538
Elsberg syndrome, herpes zoster, 1360
Eltrombopag, 517–518, 549, 1655
Eluxadoline, 646
Elvitegravir, **1340*t*, 1345–1346**
Emepronium bromide, pill-induced esophagitis from, 613
Emergency contraception, **779**
Emery-Dreifuss muscular dystrophy, 1043*t*
Emetine, myopathy from, 1045
Emetogenic drugs, 1655. *See also specific types*
Emicizumab, 558, 561
Emollients, 101
Emotional changes, temporal lobe lesions, 999
Emotional stress. *See* Stress, psychological/emotional
Emotive imagery, for phobic disorders, 1052
Empagliflozin
  for coronary heart disease prevention in diabetics, 358–359
  for diabetes mellitus, 935, 1218
  for heart failure with reduced LVEF, 409
  for hyperglycemia/diabetes mellitus, 1205*t,* 1210
Empathy, 2
Empyema, 278, 310, 313
  anaerobic pneumonia & lung abscess, 278
  Group A beta-hemolytic streptococci, **1442**
  middle ear, 209
  pleural effusions, 310, 310*t,* 311*t,* 313
  pneumococcal pneumonia, 1444
  pneumonia, 269*t,* 371
Emtansine, 1672*t*
Emtricitabine, 1325, 1333, **1339*t*, 1343,** 1725
Enalapril, 407–408, 451*t*
Enalaprilat, 470, 471*t*
Enasidenib, 1672*t*
Encephalitis, 1280–1281
  anti-NMDA receptor–associated, 1004*t*
  Chikungunya fever, 1400
  Colorado tick fever, 1401
  cytomegalovirus, 1366
  eastern equine, 1379
  Ebola viral disease, 1389–1390
  Epstein-Barr virus, 1363
  herpes simplex virus, 1354, 1355
  herpes zoster, 1360
  HHV-6, 1368
  HHV-7, 1358*t,* **1368**
  hyponatremia, 1354
  Japanese, 1379
  limbic, 1004*t*
  measles inclusion body, 1370
  Murray Valley, 1379
  parechovirus, 1426
  rubella, 1373

St. Louis, 1379
tick-borne, 1379, **1382–1384**
typhus, scrub, 1429
varicella, 1360
variola/vaccinia, 1421
Venezuelan equine, 1379
western equine, 1379
West Nile virus, 1380
Encephalitozoon, 1517
Encephalitozoon intestinalis, 1516–1517
Encephalomyelitis
limbic, 1004*t*
postinfectious, measles, 1369
Encephalopathy
acute hemorrhagic necrotizing, COVID-19, 1404
with esophageal varices, 616
hepatic, 704–705
HIV/AIDS, 1323
metabolic, 1003
Q fever, 1435
uremic, 918
Wernicke, 1014, **1018,** 1087
Encorafenib, *BRAF* inhibitor action, 1671*t*
Encrusted, 102*t*
End-diastolic pressure. *See* Ventricular end-diastolic pressure
Endemic goiter, **1137–1138**
Endemic Kaposi sarcoma, **113**
Endocarditis, infective, **1453–1457**
acute heart failure, 404
anaerobic bacteria, 1473
antimicrobial therapy, initial, 1296*t*
aortic regurgitation, 347, 348
aortic valve, 335*t*
candida, 1534–1535
clinical findings, 1454–1455, 1454*f*
complications, 1455
cryoglobulinemia, **855**
Duke criteria, modified, 1455
general considerations, 1454
gonococcus, 1470
Group A beta-hemolytic streptococci, **1443**
health care–associated infections, 1278
injection drug abuse, 1287, 1454
Janeway lesions, 1454
Libman-Sacks, systemic lupus erythematosus, 834
membranous nephropathy, 934
mitral regurgitation, 338, 339
native valve, 1454
Osler nodes, 1454
pneumococcal, 1444
prevention, 1455
dental procedures, 1456*t*
by procedure type, 1456*t*
prosthetic heart valves, 324, 332, 338
prosthetic heart valves, 1454
anticoagulation therapy, 354*t*
Melody valve, 329
percutaneous pulmonary valve replacement, 324
prophylaxis, 338, 1455, 1455*t*
pulmonary valve surgery, 324, 332
Q fever, 1435–1436
Roth spots, 1454
splinter hemorrhages, 1454, 1454*f*
Streptococcus gallolyticus, 1443
subacute bacterial, cryoglobulinemia, **855**
treatment, 1455–1458
anticoagulation, 1458
culture-negative, 1457–1458
empiric regimens, 1455
HACEK organisms, 1457
staphylococcus, 1457
streptococcus
Group D, 1457
other, 1457
viridans, 1455–1457
surgery, 1458
tricuspid valve, 351
ventricular septal defect, 329
Endocervical curettage, 764*t*
for cervical cancer, 790
for cervical intraepithelial neoplasia, 788
Endocrine disorders, **1099–1194**. *See also specific types*
adrenal cortex, **1156–1166**
adrenal insufficiency, primary, **1156–1160**
aldosteronism, primary, **1164–1166**
Cushing syndrome, **1160–1164**
adrenal masses, incidentally discovered, **1171**
amenorrhea & menopause
primary amenorrhea, **1184–1185**
secondary amenorrhea, **1185–1186**
corticosteroid, clinical use, **1193–1194,** 1194*t*
gastroenteropancreatic neuroendocrine tumors & carcinoid tumors, **1171–1173**
carcinoid tumors, **1172**
CCKomas, **1172**
ectopic hormones, **1172**
gastrinomas, **1171–1172**
glucagonomas, **1172**
insulinomas, **1171–1172**
somatostatinomas, **1172**
VIPomas, **1172**
gynecomastia, **1179–1181,** 1180*t*
hirsutism & virilization, **1181–1183**
acromegaly & ACTH-induced Cushing syndrome, 1182
adrenal carcinoma, 1181
diffuse stromal Leydig cell hyperplasia, 1182
dysgerminomas, 1181
hilar cell tumors, 1181
hyperreactio luteinalis, 1182
hypertrichosis lanuginosa, 1182
idiopathic & familial, 1181
luteoma of pregnancy, 1182
ovarian tumors, 1181
pharmacologic causes, 1182
polycystic ovary syndrome, **771, 1181,** 1182
porphyria cutanea tarda, 1182
pure androgen-secreting adrenal tumors, 1181
Sertoli-Leydig tumors, 1181
steroidogenic enzyme defects, **1181**
virilization, pregnancy, 1182
HIV/AIDS
hypogonadism, 1326–1327
mineralocorticoid, 1327
thyroid function, 1327
hypothalamus & pituitary gland, **1099–1111**
acromegaly & gigantism, **1106–1107**
anterior hypopituitarism, **1099–1103**
central diabetes insipidus, **1104–1105**
hyperprolactinemia, **1108–1110,** 1108*t*
pituitary adenomas, 998*t*, 1099, **1110–1111**
menarch, 1184
menopause, normal, **1186–1191**
metabolic bone disease, **1146–1156**
osteopenia, **1147**
osteoporosis, **1147–1152,** 1148*t*
Paget disease of bone, **1155–1156**
rickets & osteomalacia, **1152–1154,** 1152*t*
multiple endocrine neoplasia, **1173–1175**
acromegaly and gigantism, **1106–1107**
MEN 1, **1173–1174,** 1174*t*
MEN 2, **1174,** 1174*t*
MEN 3 (2B), **1174,** 1174*t*
MEN 4, **1174–1175,** 1174*t*
parathyroids, **1138–1146**
hyperparathyroidism, **1141–1146**
hypoparathyroidism & pseudohypoparathyroidism, **1138–1141,** 1140*t*
pheochromocytoma & paraganglioma, **1166–1171**
MEN 2 (MEN 2A), 1167
MEN 3 (MEN 2B), 1167
metastatic, 1170
pregnancy, pheochromocytoma, 1169–1170
von Hippel-Lindau disease type 2, 1167
von Recklinghausen neurofibromatosis type 1, 1167
preoperative evaluation/perioperative management, 49–50
diabetes mellitus, 49–50
glucocorticoid replacement, 50
thyroid disease, 50
testes & male breast, **1175–1179**
cryptorchidism, **1179**
gynecomastia, **1179–1181,** 1180*t*
hypogonadism, male, **1175–1179,** 1175*t*, 1177*t*
thyroid gland, **1111–1138**
hyperthyroidism, **1119–1127,** 1121*t*, 1123*t*
hypothyroidism & myxedema, **1114–1119,** 1117*t*
iodine deficiency disorder & endemic goiter, **1137–1138**
thyroid cancer, **1131–1137,** 1132*t*, 1134*t*
thyroid eye disease, **1128**
thyroiditis, **1111–1114**
thyroid nodules & multinodular goiter, **1129–1131,** 1129*t*
Turner syndrome, **1191–1193,** 1192*t*
45,XO/46,XX & 45,XO/35,XY mosaicism, **1193**
46,X (abnormal X) karyotype, **1193**
classic (45,XO gonadal dysgenesis), **1191–1193**
Endocrine myopathies, **1044**
Endocrine shock, **496–497**
End of life care, **72–77**
communication & care of patient, 73, 73*t*
cultural issues, 75
ethical & legal issues, 77
expectations, 73
family care, 77
hospice & other palliative care services, 75–76
lesbian & bisexual women, 1716
medical aid in dying, 76
nonabandonment, promise of, 73
nutrition & hydration, 73–74
pain, 79, **81**
prognosis, 72
psychological challenges, 74
self-care, clinician, 77
social challenges, 74, 74*t*
spiritual challenges, 74–75, 75*t*
withdrawal of curative efforts, 75
Endometrial biopsy, 764*t*
Endometrial carcinoma, **791, 1721**
Endometrial hyperplasia, 765
Endometrial intraepithelial neoplasia, 765
Endometriosis, **767–769**
Endometritis, **785–787**
Endometrium sampling, 763–764, 764*t*
Endophthalmitis, 185, 193, 198

Endoscopic retrograde cholangiopancreatography, 675–677
for bile duct
stones, 724–725
strictures, 675
for biliary strictures, 725
for cholecystitis, 722
for choledocholithiasis, 720*t*, 722, 723–725
for pancreatitis
acute, 728, 730, 732
chronic, 734, 735
pancreatitis after, 677, 732
pregnancy, 817
for primary sclerosing cholangitis, 726, 727
Endoscopic retrograde cholangiopancreatography-directed radiofrequency ablation, 1614
Endothelin-1 receptor antagonists, 841. *See also specific types*
Endothelin pathway, 302
Endotracheal intubation, 240
Endovascular mechanical embolectomy, for stroke, 991
End-stage kidney disease. *See also* Chronic kidney disease
autosomal dominant polycystic kidney disease, 939
cardiomyopathy, dilated, 418
causes & stages, 914, 914*t*
diabetes mellitus, 914
diabetic nephropathy, 934, 1221
glomerulonephritis, 914
hypertension, 446
mitral stenosis, prognosis, 338
prognosis, 920–921
treatment, 920
uremia, 917
Enemas, for constipation, 587*t*
Energy
deficiency, 1250
nutritional support, 1266
requirements, 1266
Enfortumab vedotin, 1644
Enfuvirtide, **1340*t*, 1341*t*, 1346**
Enoxaparin, 567*t*, 569*t*
Entacapone, 1009
Entamoeba dispar, **1513–1515,** 1515*t*
Entamoeba histolytica, **1513–1515,** 1515*t*
diarrhea, 1288, 1292
gastroenteritis, 1297*t*, 1298*t*
Entamoeba moshkovskii, **1513–1515,** 1515*t*
Entecavir, 687–688
Enteral nutritional support, 1267–1268, 1267*t*
Enteric fever, **1463–1464**
Enterobacter, 273, 275, 1294*t*
pyelonephritis, 948
Enterobacter aerogenes, liver abscess, 717
Enterobius vermicularis (enterobiasis), **1528–1529**
Enterocele, 769
Enterococcus, **1443**
cystitis, 945
peritonitis, 604
prostatitis, 950
Enterococcus faecalis, **1443**
infective endocarditis, 1287
medication of choice, 1293*t*
pyelonephritis, 948
Enterococcus faecium, 1293*t*, **1443**
Enterocolitis, 1326. *See also specific types*
Enterocytozoon, 1517
Enterocytozoon bieneusi, 1516–1517
Enterohemorrhagic *Escherichia coli* diarrhea, 590, 1289*t*, 1292, **1465–1466**
Enterotoxins
Clostridium difficile, 647–648
Staphylococcus aureus, 1449
Enteroviruses, **1423–1426**
aseptic meningitis & neurologic syndromes, 1423
conjunctivitis, epidemic, 1424
coxsackievirus, **1423–1424,** 1424*f*
diagnostic features, 1357*t*
echovirus, **1424–1425**
EV-A70, 170, **1425**
EV-A71, **1425**
EV-A72, **1425**
EV-A104, **1425**
EV-D68, **1425**
hand, foot, and mouth disease, 1424, 1424*f*
herpangina, 1423
human parechovirus, **1425–1426**
myocarditis, 1423
pericarditis, 1423
pleurodynia, epidemic, 1423
summer grippe, 1423
Enthesopathy
axial spondyloarthritis, 858
psoriatic arthritis, 860
seronegative spondyloarthropathies, 858
Entrapment neuropathy, 1032, 1034. *See also specific types*
Entrectinib, 1606
Entropion, **169**
Entry and fusion inhibitors, HIV/AIDS, **1339*t*,** 1341*t*, 1346. *See also specific types*
enfuvirtide, **1340*t*, 1341*t*, 1346**
ibalizumab, **1341*t*, 1346**
maraviroc, **1341*t*, 1346**
principles & overview, **1341*t*,** 1346
Entry inhibitors, **1340*t*.** *See also specific types*
Enucleation
laser, 969
prostatectomy, 968
Environmental emergencies, **1548–1563.** *See also specific types*
altitude disorders, **1559–1563**
air travel safety & patient selection, **1562–1563**
dysbarism & decompression sickness, 868, **1559–1560**
high-altitude illness, **1560–1562**
cold & heat, **1548–1553**
extreme temperature, 1548
heat disorders, **1548–1550**
heat exchange, body–environment, 1548
hypothermia
accidental systemic, **1550–1552,** 1551*f*
extremities, **1552–1553**
risk factors, 1548
drowning, **1553–1554**
electrical injury, **1557–1558**
radiation exposure, **1558–1559**
thermal burns, **1554–1557,** 1555*f*
Environmental lung disorders, **304–306.** *See also specific types*
e-cigarette or vaping product–associated lung injury, **304–305**
pulmonary aspiration syndromes, **305**
aspirated foreign body retention, **306**
café coronary, **306**
gastric contents
acute, **305**
chronic, **305–306**
smoke inhalation, **304**
Enzalutamide, 1602*t*, 1640*t*, 1641
Enzyme immunoassay-based screening algorithm, 1482
Enzyme inhibitors. *See also specific types*
anthracyclines, 1599*t*
daunorubicin, 1599*t*
doxorubicin, 1599*t*
doxorubicin, liposomal, 1599*t*
idarubicin, 1599*t*
topoisomerase inhibitors, 1599*t*
etoposide, 1599*t*
irinotecan, 1599*t*
Eosinophilia
drug reaction with eosinophilia and systemic symptoms, **30,** 157, 696, **871**
pulmonary, tropical, 1531
Eosinophilic cellulitis, 1419
Eosinophilic esophagitis, **614**
Eosinophilic folliculitis, 124–125
Eosinophilic granulomatosis with polyangiitis, 303, **854–855**
Eosinophilic meningoencephalitis, angiostrongyliasis, 1529
Eosinophilic myocarditis, 417
Eosinophilic pneumonia, 297
Eosinophilic pulmonary syndromes, **297**
EPCAM, 668, 1628, 1673*t*
Ependymoma, 998*t*, **1001–1002**
Ephedrine
hypertension from, treatment, 1566
kidney stones from, 954
poisoning, 1574
for postural hypotension & syncope, 985
sympathomimetic syndrome from, 1570
Epicondylosis, lateral & medial, **1689**
Epidemic Kaposi sarcoma, **113**
Epidemic keratoconjunctivitis, 170
Epidemic typhus, **1426–1429,** 1427*t*
Epidermal growth factor receptor, 1672*t*
Epidermal inclusion cysts, **110**
Epidermolysis bullosa, esophageal webs/rings, 614
Epididymitis
acute, **952–953**
antimicrobial therapy, empiric, 1298*t*
cytomegalovirus, 1366
Epidural hemorrhage, **997,** 1022*t*
Epigastric pain, 579
Epiglottitis, **237,** 1363, 1461
Epilepsia partialis continua, 1012
Epilepsy, **978–983**
after traumatic brain injury, 1023
classification, epilepsy syndromes, 980
classification, epilepsy types, 980
classification, seizure types, 979–980
focal-onset seizures, 979
generalized onset seizures, 979–980
clinical findings, 980–981
differential diagnosis, 981–982
etiology, 980–981
photosensitive, 981
pregnancy, **813**
prodromal symptoms, 980
seizures, 979
status epilepticus, 979, 983
temporal lobe, HHV-6, 1368
treatment, 976*t*–977*t*, 982–983
alcohol withdrawal seizures, 983
medications
discontinuance, 976*t*–977*t*, 982
monitoring, 982
medications & monitoring, **975*t*–977*t*, 982**
absence seizures, 977*t*
generalized or focal seizures, 975*t*–977*t*
myoclonic seizures, 977*t*
solitary seizures, 982–983
surgery, 982
tonic-clonic status epilepticus, 983
video electroencephalographic monitoring, 983
Epileptic drop attacks, 980
Epileptic spasms, 979, 980
Epinephrine
for anaphylaxis, 870
for beta-blocker poisoning, 1577

for calcium channel blocker poisoning, 1578
for drug eruptions, 158
for Mallory-Weiss syndrome, 613
renal constriction from, 907
Epirubicin, 417, 761
Epistaxis, **224–225**
Eplerenone
for acute MI, with ST-segment elevation, 378
for Cushing syndrome, 1163
for heart failure with reduced LVEF, 408
hyperkalemia from, 886, 917
for hypertension, 455, 458*t*
Epley maneuver, 216
Epoetin alfa (erythropoietin), 504, 917, 1338, 1654*t*
Epoetin beta, 917
Epoprostenol, 705, 841
Eprosartan, 452*t*
Epsilon-aminocaproic acid, 559*t*
Epstein-Barr virus
Burkitt lymphoma, 1364
hairy leukoplakia, **228,** 228*f*
HIV/AIDS, 1324
Hodgkin lymphoma, 1364
infection-related thrombocytopenia, 556
infectious mononucleosis, **1363–1364**
diagnostic features, 1357*t*
lymphoma, 1322
lymphomatoid granulomatosis, 1364
nasopharyngeal carcinoma, 1364
other conditions, **1364–1365**
post-transplant, 1364–1365
post-transplant lymphoproliferative disorders, 1365
T-cell lymphoproliferative disorder, 1364
T- & NK-cell lymphomas, 1364
X-linked lymphoproliferative syndrome, 1364
Eptifibatide, 371
Eptinezumab, 972*t*
Equianalgesic dosing, opioid, 85*t*, **87*t*–90*t***
Equine antithymocyte globulin, 517–518
Equine serum heptavalent botulism antitoxin, 1453
ER-2 negative breast cancer, 749–750
erbB-1 receptor, 1672*t*
Erb muscular dystrophy, 1043*t*
Erdafitinib, 1644
Erectile dysfunction, 919, **958–960,** 1058, 1223
Erection, 958–959
Erenumab, 972*t*
Ergocalciferol, 1154
Ergonovine, in pregnancy, 813
Ergotamines, 971, 974. *See also specific types*
Ergotamine tartrate, 973
Eribulin, 759
Erlotinib, 1601*t*
diarrhea from, 1656
for non–small cell lung cancer
EGFR, 1672*t*
KRAS, 1673*t*
Erosive, 102*t*
Erosive esophagitis
peptic stricture, 610
upper GI bleeding, 596
Erosive gastritis/gastropathy, **620–622**
ER receptor-negative breast cancer, 741
ER receptor-positive breast cancer, 741
Ertapenem, 1472, 1472*t*
Ertugliflozin, 1205*t*, 1210
Eructation, 588
Eruptive xanthomas
diabetes mellitus, 1200
lipid disorders, 1241, 1241*f*
Erysipelas, **128,** 1297*t*, 1441, 1441*f*, 1441*t*
Erythema, **151–155**
exfoliative dermatitis, **154–155**
figurate, 102*t*
reactive erythemas, **151–154**
erythema multiforme/Stevens-Johnson syndrome/toxic epidermal necrolysis, **153–154,** 153*f*, 154*f*
urticaria & angioedema, **151–153,** 152*f*
shaped, 102*t*
Erythema infectiosum, 1358*t*, **1419–1420**
Erythema marginatum, rheumatic fever, 425, 425*t*
Erythema migrans, **128,** 129*f*, 1492–1495, 1495*t*
Erythema multiforme, **153–154,** 153*f*, 1354, 1355
Erythema nodosum, **132–133,** 133*f*, 158*t*, 1537
Erythema pernio, **1552**
Erythrasma, pruritus, 160, 160*f*
Erythroderma, exfoliative, **154–155**
Erythromelalgia, 867, 1471
Erythromycin
for *Bordetella pertussis,* 1459
for cellulitis, 128
for chancroid, 1470
for *Chlamydia trachomatis,* lymphogranuloma venereum, 1477
for psittacosis, 1478
topical dermatologic, 105*t*
Erythromycin/benzoyl peroxide, 105*t*
Erythroparvovirus, 1358*t*, **1419–1420**
Erythroplakia, **227–229**
Erythropoiesis, iron-restricted, 503
Erythropoiesis-stimulating agents, for anemia, 917, 1655. *See also specific types*
Escharotomy, 1556
Escherichia coli
arthritis, nongonococcal acute, 862
cholangitis, primary biliary, 707
diarrhea
acute infectious, 1288
after foreign travel, 1288
enterohemorrhagic, 1289*t*
enterotoxigenic, 590, 1289*t*, 1292, **1465–1466**
Shiga-toxin, 590–592, 1288, 1289*t*
gastroenteritis, **1465–1466**
liver abscess, 717
medication of choice, 1294*t*
nosocomial pneumonia, 275
peritonitis, spontaneous bacterial, 604, 703
pneumonia, 269*t*
Shiga-toxin–producing, **1465–1466**
diarrhea, 590–592, 1288, 1289*t*
hemolytic-uremic syndrome, **550–552,** 551*t*, 590
urinary tract infections, 945
cystitis, 945
pregnancy, 813
prostatitis, 949
pyelonephritis, 948
Escitalopram, 1072, 1073*t*, 1186
Esketamine nasal spray, 1077
Eslicarbazepine, 975*t*
Esmolol, 383, 384*t*, 470, 470*t*, 471*t*, 1126
Esomeprazole
for GERD, 610
for GI hemorrhage from peptic ulcer disease, 630
for NSAIDs, 622, 628
for peptic ulcer disease, 627
for upper GI bleeding, 598
Esophageal cancer, **1617–1619**
Barrett esophagus, 609–610
dyspepsia, 579
treatment, 1596*t*
Esophageal candidiasis, 1534, 1535
Esophageal dysphagia, 607, 607*t*
Esophageal junction cancer, 1596*t*
Esophageal lesions, benign, **613–618**
eosinophilic esophagitis, **614**
esophageal varices, **615–618**
esophageal webs & rings, **614–615**
Mallory-Weiss syndrome, 582, **613–614**
Zenker diverticulum, **615**
Esophageal manometry, 607, 610, 619, 620
Esophageal motility disorders, **618–620**. *See also specific types*
achalasia, **618–619**
other primary, **620**
Esophageal perforation, 22, 23, 24
Esophageal pH-impedance, 607, 609, 611
Esophageal pH testing, 607, 609, 610
Esophageal reflux, from antipsychotics, 1066
Esophageal Schatzki rings, 614
Esophageal varices, **615–618**
Esophageal webs & rings, 501, **614–615**
Esophagitis
candidal, HIV/AIDS, 1318*t*, 1325
eosinophilic, **614**
erosive
peptic stricture, 610
upper GI bleeding, 596
GI bleeding, occult, 601
herpes simplex virus, 1354, 1355
infectious, **612–613**
pill-induced, 611, **613**
reflux, 608
Esophagography
barium, 607, 609, 615, 618, 620
video-, 607, 615
Esophagus diseases, **606–620**. *See also specific types*
esophageal lesions, benign, **613–618**
eosinophilic esophagitis, **614**
esophageal varices, **615–618**
esophageal webs & rings, **614–615**
Mallory-Weiss syndrome, 582, **613–614**
Zenker diverticulum, **615**
esophageal motility disorders, **618–620**
achalasia, **618–619**
other primary, **620**
gastroesophageal reflux disease, **608–612**
infectious esophagitis, **612–613**
pill-induced esophagitis, **613**
symptoms
dysphagia, 606–607, 606*t*, 607*t*
heartburn, 606
Esophagus foreign bodies, **241**
Espundia, **1500–1501**
Essential cryoglobulinemia, 929
Essential fatty acid deficiency, 1266, 1267, 1268
Essential hypertension, 444
Essential thrombocytosis, 520*t*, **522–523**
Essential tremor, **1006**
Estazolam, 1050*t*
Estimated glomerular filtration rate, 905
Estradiol
as feminizing hormone therapy, 1726–1727, 1727*t*, 1728, 1729*t*
for menopausal symptoms, 1188–1190
for uterine leiomyoma, 766
Estrogen
endometrial adenocarcinoma from, 791
fibrocystic condition, 737
for hot flushes, 1186
hypertension from, 446
lentigines from, 108
for menopausal symptoms, 1187–1189
nipple discharge, 739
oral conjugated, for abnormal uterine bleeding, 764
retinal vein occlusion, 188
venous thromboembolism risk, 1727
Estrogen-progestin contraceptives, 764
Estrogen receptor antagonist, pure, 1602*t*
Eszopiclone, 1050*t*, 1083

Etanercept
infections with, 1273
for psoriasis, 137–138
for rheumatoid arthritis, 830–831
for Stevens-Johnson syndrome, 154
Ethacrynic acid, 458*t*
Ethambutol, 284–285, 284*t*, 285*t*
for *Mycobacterium avium* complex, 1475
for *Mycobacterium kansasii*, 1475
for spinal tuberculosis, 865
for tuberculosis, pregnancy, 815
Ethanol
poisoning, 1571*t*, 1572*t*, **1581–1582**
sympatholytic syndrome from, 1570
Ethanol-induced hypoglycemia, **1237–1238**
Ethical issues/decision, 2, 77
Ethical principles, 2
Ethinyl estradiol, 764, 777, 1726
Ethmoiditis, 219
Ethosuximide, 977*t*
Ethyl alcohol. *See also* Alcohol
with aluminum chloride, for folliculitis, 125
Ethylenediaminetetraacetic acid, 556, 1583
Ethylene glycol
anion gap elevation from, 897, 1570
poisoning, 1568*t*, 1569*t*, 1571*t*, 1572*t*, **1586**
Ethynodiol diacetate, oral contraceptives, 775*t*
Etodolac, **83*t***
Etonogestrel subdermal implant, 767, 777, 1713
Etoposide, 528, 1599*t*, 1606
Etoposide, doxorubicin, cisplatin, and mitotane, 1163
Etravirine, **1339*t*, 1344**
Etretinate, 1328
ETV6, bone marrow failure, 546
Euglycemia, 811
Eumycetoma, **1546**
European Society for Parenteral and Enteral Nutrition Criteria, 1250
European Society of Cardiology 0/1-h algorithm, 24
Eustachian tube, 207
patulous, 208
Eustachian tube diseases, **207–208**
barotrauma, **208**
dysfunction, **207–208**
otitis media, serous, **208**
Euthyroid sick syndrome, 1116
Evaluation, preoperative, **42–51**
Evaporative cooling, 1550
Evening primrose oil, 738
Everolimus
for autoimmune hepatitis, 693
for breast carcinoma, 758
for renal cell carcinoma, 1646
for tuberous sclerosis, 1005
Eversion ankle sprains, **1707–1708**
Evinacumab, 1245*t*
Evolocumab, 8, 358, 1245*t*, 1246–1247
Exanthem, drug, 158*t*
Exanthema subitum, 1358*t*
Exanthematous viruses, **1419–1422**
acute, diagnostic features, 1357*t*–1358*t*
Erythroparvovirus, **1419–1420**
poxvirus, **1420–1422**
molluscum contagiosum, **1421**
monkeypox, **1421–1422**
Orf and paravaccinia, **1421**
orthopoxviruses, novel, **1422**
variola/vaccinia, **1420–1421**
Exanthems, 1357*t*–1358*t*. *See also specific types*
Exanthem subitum, 1358*t*, 1368
Excitement, 1057
Excoriation disorder, 1052
Executive function, 54, 1015. *See also specific disorders*
Exemestane for breast carcinoma, 754, 757, 757*t*, 758, 1602*t*
Exenatide, 1204*t*, 1209, **1582**
Exercise capacity, cardiac risk assessment/reduction, 33, 42
Exercise ECG, 360
Exercise/exercise therapy. *See also specific indications*
for adjustment disorder, 1047
for aortoiliac occlusive disease, 473–474
balance-focused, 61
on cardiac cachexia, 33
for dementia, 1017
for depression, 1078
for disease prevention, 5*t*, 10
for fall prevention, elderly, 61, 61*t*
for femoro-popliteal disease, 475
for gallstone prevention, 719
for heart failure with reduced LVEF, 411
on hypertension, 444, 448, 448*t*
hyponatremia from, **878**
for knee osteoarthritis, 821
for menopausal symptoms, 1186
migraine headache exacerbation from, 36, 36*t*
for nonalcoholic fatty liver disease, 699
older adults, 59
segmental wall motion abnormalities from, angina, 361
for systolic murmurs, 336*t*
for weight loss, 1252
Exercise-induced bronchoconstriction, 246
Exercise pressor response, hypertension, 448
Exertional chest pain, athlete cardiovascular screening, 438, 439*t*
Exertional dyspnea
aortic regurgitation, 347
atrial septal defect shunt, 327
heart failure, 404
mitral regurgitation, 338
mitral stenosis, 332
patent foramen ovale, 327
pulmonary hypertension, 432
Exertional heat stroke, **1549**
Exertion intolerance disease, systemic, **33–34**
Exfoliative dermatitis, **154–155**
Exfoliative erythroderma, **154–155**
Exhaustion, heat, **1549**
Existential review of systems, 74, 75*t*
Exophiala, 1546
Exostoses, **207**
Expectations, end of life care, 73
Exposure and response prevention, 1053
Exposure keratitis, 179
Exposure therapy, for PTSD, 1048
Exserohilum rostratum meningitis, 1281
Extensively drug-resistant tuberculosis, 280
Extensor posturing, 1019
External rotation
rotator cuff strength testing, 1677*t*
shoulder range of motion, 1676*t*
stress test, 1707
External vacuum therapy, for erectile dysfunction, 1223
Extracellular volume, 875
Extracorporeal counterpulsation, mechanical, for angina pectoris, 367
Extracorporeal life support, for hypothermia, 1551
Extracorporeal membrane oxygenation, 321, 1565
Extracorporeal shock wave lithotripsy, 957–958
Extramammary Paget disease, **114**
Extrapulmonary tuberculosis, 84–85, 280, 285–286, 865, 941, 1312*t*, 1320
Extrasystoles, ventricular, **398**
Extremities. *See also specific types*
hypothermia, **1552–1553**
lower
edema, **27–29**
venous pressure, normal, 27
upper, **1689–1692**
Extrinsic allergic alveolitis, **307–308,** 307*t*
Exudates, pleural, 310–311, 310*t*, 313
Eye and lid disorders, **168–203**. *See also specific types*
acid injury, **198**
age-related macular degeneration, 52, 67, **187**
alkali poisoning, 1574
cataract, **184–185**
cellulitis, orbital, **196**
conjunctivitis, **170–172,** 170*t*, **198,** 1356*t*
contusions, **197–198**
corneal ulcer, **172, 179**
cranial nerve palsies, **195–196,** 195*f*
decontamination, **1568**
drug effects, **198–203, 200*t*–202*t***
dry
conjunctivitis, **171–172**
corneal ulcer, 179
Sjögren syndrome, 16
glaucoma
acute angle-closure, 170*t*, 177*t*–178*t*, **180–181**
chronic, 177*t*–178*t*, **181–183**
HIV/AIDS
retinitis, cytomegalovirus, **193,** 1311, 1318*t*, 1324, 1324*f*
retinopathy, **193**
uveitis, 183
hypertension, ocular, **177*t*–178*t*,** 182, 183
inflammation, differential diagnosis, 170*t*
ischemic optic neuropathy, **193–194**
keratitis
chemical, **198**
infectious, **179–180**
laceration, eyelid, **198**
lids & lacrimal apparatus, **168–170**
management, ophthalmic agents, topical, **173*t*–178*t*** (*See also* Ophthalmic agents, topical)
management, precautions, **198–199,** 199*f*
anesthetics, local, 198
contaminated eye medications, 199
corticosteroid therapy, 198–199
pupillary dilation, 198
systemic effects, ocular drugs, **199–203, 200*t*–202*t***
topical therapy reactions, toxic & hypersensitivity, 199, 199*f*
movements, stupor & coma, 1019
neuritis, optic, **194–195**
optic disk swelling, **195**
pinguecula, **172**
pterygium, **172**
refractive errors, **168**
retinal, systemic diseases, **191–193**
blood dyscrasias, **193**
diabetic retinopathy, 67, 191, **191–192,** 1221
HIV/AIDS, **193**
hypertensive retinochoroidopathy, **192–193**
retinal artery occlusion, central & branch, 188*f*, **189–190**
retinal detachment, **185–186,** 186*f*
retinal vein occlusion, central & branch, **188–189,** 188*f*
thyroid eye disease (*See* Graves ophthalmopathy; Hyperthyroidism)
transient ischemic attack, ocular, **190–191**

transient monocular visual loss, **190–191**
trauma, ocular, **196–198**
contusions, **197–198**
corneal, 170*t*, **197**
foreign bodies, conjunctival & corneal, **197**
lacerations, **198**
uveitis after, 183
tumors, eyelid, **169**
uveitis, 170*t*, **183–184**
vitreous hemorrhage, **186**
Eyelid & lacrimal apparatus disorders, **168–170**
blepharitis, **169**
chalazion, **169**
dacrocystitis, **169–170**
entropion & ectropion, **169**
hordeolum, **168**
tumors, **169**
Ezetimibe, 696, 1245*t*, 1246
EZH2, myelodysplastic syndromes, 527
Ezogabine, 976*t*

F

Fabry disease, restrictive cardiomyopathy, 423
FACES Pain Rating Scale, 81, 81*t*
Facial grimacing, 1011
Facial pain, **974–978**
atypical, **978**
glossopharyngeal neuralgia, **978**
other causes, 978
postherpetic neuralgia, **978**
trigeminal neuralgia, **974–978**
Facial palsy/paralysis
AIDS, 218
Bell palsy, **1036–1037**, 1036*f*
otitis media, chronic, **210**
sarcoidosis, 1032
tick-borne encephalitis, 1383
Facioscapulohumeral muscular dystrophy, 1043*t*
Factitious disorder imposed on another, 1054
Factitious disorders, 1054
Factitious hypoglycemia, **1237**
Factor II
antibodies, acquired, **561**
deficiency, **561**
gene mutations, 432
Factor IX inhibitors, 558
Factor V
antibodies, acquired, **561**
bovine, 561
deficiency, **561**
Factor VIIa, recombinant activated, 705
Factor VIII
antibodies, acquired, **561**
concentrates, for factor VII antibodies, 561
inhibitors, 557, 558
Factor V Leiden mutation, 432, 713
Factor Xa inhibitors, poisoning, 1575
Factor X deficiency, **561**
Factor XI deficiency, 559*t*, **561**
Factor XIII deficiency, **561**
Failed back surgery syndrome, 80
Falls
assessment, 60, 60*t*
exercise, 61, 61*t*
older adults, **60–62**, 61*t*
risk factors, interventions, and prevention, 60–61, 61*t*
Faloxifene, 742
False beliefs, 1062
False localizing signs, 999
Famciclovir, 1356*t*
for herpes simplex, 120–121, 1327
for herpes zoster, 1327, 1356*t*, 1361
for varicella, 1356*t*, 1360
Familial adenomatous polyposis, **667**, 1627
Familial aldosteronism type 1, saccular aneurysm, 994
Familial amyloid polyneuropathy, **1031**
Familial chylomicronemia syndrome, **1239**
Familial Creutzfeldt-Jakob disease (fCJD), 1385–1386
Familial hemiplegic migraine, 970
Familial hypercholesterolemia, **1239**, **1660–1661**
Familial hypocalciuric hypercalcemia, 1144
Familial insomnia, fatal, 1385
Familial intrahepatic cholestasis syndromes, conjugated hyperbilirubinemia, 674, 676*t*
Familial juvenile polyposis, hamartomatous polyposis syndromes, 668
Familial Mediterranean fever, **606**
Familial tremor, **1006**
Family building, sexual & gender minorities, 1713–1715
Family care, end of life, 77
Family planning, **773–780**, 775*t*, 776*t*, 778*t*. *See also* Contraception & family planning
Family script, 1056
Famotidine
for GERD, 610
for pancreatic insufficiency, in chronic pancreatitis, 734
for peptic ulcer disease, 624*t*, 627
for stress gastritis, 621
Fam-trastuzumab deruxtecan-nxki, 1672*t*
Fanconi anemia, bone marrow failure, 546
Fanconi syndrome, 890, 898
fibroblast growth factor 23, 890
hypophosphatemia, 891, 891*t*
plasma cell myeloma, 941
renal glycosuria, 1200
tubular proteinuria, 904
Fansidar, 1517
Farmer's lung, 307*t*
Fasciola gigantica, 1521
Fasciola hepatica, 1521
Fascioliasis, **1521–1522**
Fasting, 719, 1233, 1233*t*
Fat, body, subcutaneous, 1250
Fatal familial insomnia, 1385
Fatigue, **33–34**, 70. *See also specific disorders*
Fat necrosis, breast, **739–740**
Fats, dietary
fat & low saturated fats, 1263–1264
fat-restricted diets, 1263–1264
nutritional support, 1266
restricted, 1263–1264
Fatty liver
acute fatty liver of pregnancy, 685, **817–818**
alcohol-associated, **693–695**
drug-/toxin-associated, 697
hemochromatosis with, 710
macrovesicular, 697
metabolic-associated fatty liver disease, 698
microvesicular, 697
nonalcoholic, **697–699**
5-FC. *See* Flucytosine
Febrile neutropenia, 519
Febrile nonhemolytic transfusion reaction, 30
Febuxostat, 825, 826, 942
Fecal immunochemical tests (FIT), 11
colorectal cancer, 1632
constipation, 585–586
GI bleeding, occult, 601
nonfamilial adenomatous & serrated polyps, 666
peptic ulcer disease, 626
suspected bowel bleeding, 601
Fecal impaction, 62, 588
Fecal incontinence, **671–672**
Fecal microbiota transplantation, for antibiotic-associated colitis, 649
Fecal occult blood test, 1632
constipation, 585–586
diarrhea, chronic, 594
GI bleeding, occult, 601
nonfamilial adenomatous & serrated polyps, 666
peptic ulcer disease, 626
suspected bowel bleeding, 601
FEIBA (factor eight inhibitor bypassing activity), 558
Felbamate, 976*t*, 1575–1576
Felodipine, 457*t*, 839, **1578**
Felty syndrome, 519, 828
Female hypogonadotropic hypogonadism, 1101
Female sexual dysfunction, **780–782**
orgasmic disorders, **781**
sexual arousal disorders, **781**
sexual desire disorders, **781**
sexual pain disorders, **781–782**
Feminizing hormone therapy, **1726–1727**, 1727*t*
Femoral artery
aneurysm, primary, **485–486**
pseudoaneurysm, 485, 486
Femoral cutaneous nerve, lateral, 1035
Femoral-femoral bypass graft, 474
Femoral nerve, 1035
Femoral neuropathy, **1035**
Femoral occlusion, **474–476**
Femoral-popliteal atherosclerosis, 474–475
Femoral-popliteal bypass, autologous saphenous vein, 475
Fenofibrate, 708, 1245*t*, 1248
Fenofibric acid, 1245*t*
Fenoldopam, 470, 470*t*, 471*t*
Fentanyl, **87*t***. *See also* Opioid overdose/poisoning
combination therapy, 97
intrathecal, 97, 97*t*
morphine milligram equivalent doses, 85*t*
neuromodulatory therapy, 97*t*
overdose deaths from, 84
poisoning, 1574, **1587–1588**
synthetic, 84–85, 85*t*
monitoring, 93
Ferric citrate, 917
Ferric pyrophosphate citrate, 502
Ferrous sulfate, 502, 917
Fertile period awareness contraception, **779**
Fertility preservation, 1714–1715
Fetal alcohol syndrome, **795**, 1088
Fetotoxic medications, 794, 795*t*
Fever, **29–31**. *See also specific disorders*
"central," 30
in children *vs.* adults, 30
dysuria, 38
episodic, 1271
neutropenic cancer chemotherapy patient, initial antimicrobial therapy, 1296*t*
pregnancy, 30
prolonged, 1271
recurrent, 1271
trauma, 30
Fever of unknown origin, 848, **1270–1272**
Fexinidazole, 1497, 1497*t*
Fexofenadine, 152
FGFR inhibitor, 1644. *See also specific types*
Fiber, dietary
on blood pressure, 448
on diabetes mellitus, 1203
high, 1264
on LDL cholesterol, 1244

Fiber laxatives, 586, 587*t*
Fibrates, 1045. *See also specific types*
Fibric acid derivatives, 1245*t*, 1248
Fibrin glue, factor V antibodies from, 561
Fibrinolytic therapy, 375–377, 376*t*. *See also specific types*
Fibroadenoma, breast, **738–739**
Fibroblast growth factor 23, 890, 1153
Fibrocystic condition, breast, **737–738,** 741
Fibrogenesis imperfecta ossium, 1153
Fibroid tumor, **765–766,** 769
Fibromuscular dysplasia
  renal artery, 466
  renal artery stenosis, **921–922**
  transient ischemic attacks, 986
Fibromyalgia, **865–866**
Fibrosis. *See specific types*
Fibrotic mediastinitis, superior vena cava obstruction, 492
Fibular nerve palsy, **1036**
Fidaxomicin, 648–649
Fifth disease, **1419–1420**
Figurate erythema, 102*t*
Filariasis, **1530–1533**
  lymphatic, **1530–1532,** 1531*f*
  onchocerciasis, **1532–1533**
Filgrastim, 519
  cancer, 1654*t*
Filociclovir, 1367
Finasteride
  for alopecia, 164
  for benign prostatic hyperplasia, 966
  as feminizing hormone therapy, 1726, 1727*t*
  for hirsutism, female, 1183
Fine-needle aspiration, 737, 745
Finerenone, hyperkalemia from, 917
Fingolimod, 1025*t*
Fire ant venom allergy, 868–869
Firearms deaths, 12
Fish allergies, 868
Fish oil supplements, 358
Fish tapeworm, 507, **1523**
Fistula
  aortoenteric, upper GI bleeding, 596
  Crohn disease, 654
  graft enteric, 483
  perianal, 654, **673**
  perilymphatic, 208, **216–217,** 217
  spinal dural arteriovenous, **997**
Fistula in ano, **672**
Fitz-Hugh-Curtis syndrome, 786
5-alpha-reductase inhibitors, 966. *See also specific types*
5-aminosalicylic acid
  for Crohn disease, 655
  for inflammatory bowel disease, 649–650
  for ulcerative colitis, 659–660
5-FC. *See* Flucytosine
5-$HT_{1b/1d}$ receptor agonists, 971. *See also specific types*
5-HT_{1F} receptor agonist, 971
5-HT_3 receptor, 1655
5q loss, isolated, 526
Fixed drug eruptions, 157, 158*t*
"Fixed" splitting, patent foramen ovale, 327
Flaccid myelitis, **1376**
  adenovirus, 1419
  coxsackievirus, 1423
  echovirus, 1424
  enterovirus 71, 1425
  enterovirus A70, 1425
  enterovirus D68, 1425
  nonpolio enteroviruses, 1376
  poliomyelitis, 1374, 1376
  West Nile virus, 1380
Flaccid paralysis, West Nile virus, 1380
Flail leaflet, 335*t*, 338
Flame burns, 1557
"Flap valve," 608
"Flashbacks," psychedelics, 1093
Flash burns, 1557
Flatulence, **588–589,** 645
Flat warts, 122
Flaviviruses, 1379
Flavocoxid, hepatotoxicity, 696
Fleas, **131**
Flecainide, 383, 384*t*, 396
"Fleeting blindness," 190
Flexible sigmoidoscopy, for colorectal cancer screening, 1632–1633
Flexion, shoulder range of motion, 1676*t*
Flexor posturing, 1019
FLI1, bone marrow failure, 546
Flibanserin, 1059
Flock worker's lung, 308
Floppy iris syndrome, 185, 200*t*, 201*t*
FLT3, acute myeloid leukemia, 528
FLT3-ITD, acute myeloid leukemia, 528
Fluciclovine PET imaging, 1636
Fluconazole, 1539*t*. *See also specific types*
  for *Candida*/candidiasis
    esophageal, 1325, 1535
    funguria, 1535
    invasive, 1535
    mucocutaneous, 119
    vulvovaginal, 785, 1535
  for *Candida glabrata*, 1535
  for coccidioidomycosis, 1537–1538, 1539*t*
  for cryptococcus, 1542–1543
    meningitis, 1318*t*, 1322
  for cutaneous leishmaniasis, 1501
  for onychomycosis, 167
  for tinea versicolor, 118
Flucytosine, 1318*t*, 1322, 1540*t*, 1542–1543
Fludarabine, 514, 1598*t*
Fludrocortisone, 985, 1159
Fludrocortisone acetate, 1160
Fluid management, **902,** 902*t*. *See also specific disorders*
Fluke infections, **1520–1523**
  liver & lung, **1521–1523**
    clonorchiasis & opisthorchiasis, **1522**
    fascioliasis, **1521–1522**
    paragonimiasis, **1522–1523**
  schistosomiasis, **1520–1521**
Flumazenil, 705, 1565, 1582
Flunisolide, 252*t*
Fluocinolone, 1127
Fluocinolone acetonide, 103*t*, 137
Fluocinonide, 103*t*, 1325
Fluorescent treponemal antibody absorption test, 1482
Fluorine inhalation poisoning, 1573
Fluoropyrimadines, DPD variant metabolism of, 1669*t*
Fluoroquinolones. *See also specific types*
  anaphylactic reactions, 870
  for animal bites, 1284
  for cystitis, 946
  for diarrhea, bloody, 1288
  for epididymitis, 953 (*See also specific types*)
  for genitourinary tract infections, 947*t*–948*t*
  hyperglycemia from, 1237
  hypoglycemia from, 1237
  for prostatitis, 948*t*, 951
  for traveler's diarrhea, 1293
Fluorouracil/5-fluorouracil, 1599*t*
  for actinic keratosis, 111
  for anal cancer, 1634
  for basal cell carcinoma, 112
  for Bowen disease, 114
  for colorectal cancer, 1630
  diarrhea from, 1656
  DPD variant metabolism of, 1669*t*
  nodular regenerative hyperplasia from, 715
  for pancreas carcinoma, 1616
  for squamous cell carcinoma, 111
  for warts, 123
Fluoxetine
  breastfeeding, 796*t*
  for depression, 1072, 1073*t*, 1074–1075
  hyponatremia from, 878
  for irritable bowel syndrome, 646
  for obsessive-compulsive disorder, 1053
  for panic disorder, 1051
  for paraphilias, 1058
  for personality disorders, 1060
  serotonin syndrome from, 1567
  toxicity, 1592
Fluphenazine, 1063, 1222
Fluphenazine decanoate, long-acting, 1066
Fluphenazine enanthate, long-acting, 1066
Flurandrenolide, 104*t*, 136
Flurazepam, 1050*t*, 1051, 1083
Flutamide, 696, 1183, 1597*t*, 1640*t*
Fluticasone, 614
Fluticasone propionate, 252*t*
Fluvastatin, 357*t*, 1245*t*
Fluvoxamine, 1053, 1072, 1073*t*, 1592
FMR1, 1661–1662
FOBT. *See* Fecal occult blood test
Focal nodular hyperplasia, **718**
Focal segmental glomerulosclerosis, 924*t*, 931, **933**
  COVID-19-associated collapsing glomerulopathy, 913
  nephrotic spectrum glomerular diseases, 931
Focal torsion dystonia, **1011–1012**
FODMAPs, 588–589, 645
Folate antagonists, 1598*t*. *See also specific types*
  methotrexate, 1598*t*
  pemetrexed, 1598*t*
Folate synthesis inhibitors, 1507. *See also specific types*
Folic acid
  deficiency, 500, **508–509,** 509*t*
  deficiency anemia, pregnancy, 809
  definition, 508
  dietary, 508
  for methotrexate-induced nausea, 137
  therapy, 509
Folinic acid, 1517, 1630
Follicle stimulating hormone, recombinant, 773, 962
Follicle stimulation hormone, 1099
Follicular bronchiolitis, 268
Follicular lymphoma, **243,** 534, 1436
Follicular thyroid cancer, 1132, 1132*t*, 1133–1135, 1134*t*, 1137
Folliculitis, **124–125,** 125*f*, 1328, 1446
Follow-up, after death, 78–79
Fomepizole (4-methylpyrazole), 1586
Fondaparinux, **563**
  for acute coronary syndrome, without ST-segment elevation, 370*f*, 371
  for heparin-induced thrombocytopenia, 553, 553*t*
  for venous thromboembolism, 567*t*, 569*t*
Food. *See also specific foods*
  allergies, **868**
    eosinophilic esophagitis, 614
    irritable bowel syndrome, 645
  challenge, 868
  intolerance, dyspepsia, 579
  poisoning, 1288, 1289*t*–1290*t*, 1449
  recall & tracking, 1262–1263
Food-borne botulism, 1452

Foot
- immersion, **1552**
- trench, **1552**
- ulcer, neuropathic, 1221–1222, 1222*f*

Foreign bodies
- aspirated, retention, **306**
- conjunctival & corneal, **197**
- ear canal, **206**
- intraocular, **197**
- trachea & bronchi, **241**
- upper aerodigestive tract, **241–243**
  - cancer metastases, 242–243, **242–243**
  - esophagus, **241**
  - lymphoma, **243**
  - neck masses, congenital, **241–242**
    - branchial cleft cysts, **241–242**
    - thyroglossal duct cysts, **242**
  - neck masses, diseases, **241**
  - neck masses, infectious & inflammatory, **242**
    - Lyme disease, 242
    - reactive cervical lymphadenopathy, 242
    - tuberculous & nontuberculous mycobacterial lymphadenitis, 242, **1475**
  - trachea & bronchi, **241**

Formoterol, 250*t*, 262
45,XO/46,XX & 45,XO/35,XY mosaicism, **1193**
45,XO gonadal dysgenesis, **1191–1193**
46,X (abnormal X) karyotype, **1193**
46,XY disorders of sexual development, 1184
Fosaprepitant, 583*t*, **584,** 1655
Foscarnet, 1356*t*, 1367, 1368
Fosfomycin, 946, 947*t*
Fosinopril, 451*t*
Fostamatinib, 549
Fostemavir, **1341*t*, 1346–1347**
4-methylpyrazole, 1586
Four factor prothrombin complex, 597
Four nerve palsy, 196
Foxglove, 1581
Fractional excretion
- electrolyte, 875
- of sodium, 907, 907*t*

Fractional flow reserve (FFR), 361, 362
Fracture Risk Assessment Tool (FRAX), **1147**
Fractures
- back, 61
- diabetes mellitus risk, 1225
- eye, "blowout," **197–198**
- hip, 61, **1692–1694**
- wrist, 61

Fragile X-associated tremor/ataxia syndrome (FXTAS), 1661
Fragile X syndrome, **1661–1662**
Frailty, 53, 64
Framingham risk score, 1198
Francisella tularensis, **1467–1468**
Freckles, **108**
- juvenile, 163
- senile, 163

Free-floating statoconia, 216
Fremanezumab, 972*t*
Freon poisoning, 1589
Fresh frozen plasma transfusion, **545**
- for anticoagulation reversal, 353
- for factor XI deficiency, 559*t*, 561
- for upper GI bleeding, 597

Fresh whole blood transfusion, 542
Friction rub
- chest pain, 23
- pericardial, 373, 381, 415, 427, 429
- pericarditis, 23

Friedewald equation, 1240
Friedreich ataxia, **1031**
Frontal lobe lesions, 999
Frontal sinusitis, 219
Frontotemporal dementia, 1015*t*
Frostbite, **552**
Frostnip, **552**
Frovatriptan, 971
Frozen shoulder, 1225, **1682–1683**
Fructosamine, serum, 1201
FTL, 710
Fukuda test, 215
Full liquid diet, 1263
Fulminant hepatitis, herpes simplex virus, 1354
Fulminant myocarditis, 415–416
Fulvestrant, 1602*t*
- for breast carcinoma, 756, 757, 757*t*
  - + CDK4/6 inhibitor, 758
  - + everolimus, 758

Fumagillin, 1517
Fumarate, 917
Functional alimentary hypoglycemia, **1236**
Functional antibody deficiency, **874**
Functional Assessment of Chronic Illness Therapy-Fatigue scale, 34
"Functional" asthma, 247
Functional dyspepsia, 579–581
Functional heartburn, 611
Functional neurologic disorder, 1054
Functional proteinuria, 904
Functional screening, older adult, 53
Function assessment, older adults, 52–53
Fundus abnormalities, hypertensive crisis with retinopathy, 193
Fungal infections. *See also specific types*
- keratitis, **180**
- otitis externa, 206
- sinusitis, invasive, **221–222**
- skin, **114–119** (*See also under* Dermatologic disorders)

Funguria, candidal, 1534, 1535
Furazolidone, 1519
Furosemide
- for ascites and edema, from cirrhosis, 702
- for hypertension, 458*t*, 470, 471*t*
- for idiopathic intracranial hypertension, 1004
- kidney stones from, 954

Furosemide stress test, 909–910
Furuncles
- with cellulitis, empiric antimicrobial therapy, 1297*t*
- *Staphylococcus,* HIV/AIDS, 1328
- *Staphylococcus aureus,* 1446

Furunculosis, **126–127**
Fusarium (fusariosis), 1273, 1546
Fusobacterium
- animal bites, 1283
- chest infections, 1472
- neck infections, deep, 233
- nosocomial pneumonia, 275
- skin infections, injection drug, 1286

Fusobacterium necrophorum, 233, 1472
Fusobacterium nucleatum, 278

G

G6PD, 1669*t*
G6PD gene, 1669*t*
G20210A, 713, 716
Gabapentin
- for chronic pain syndromes, 1057
- for diabetic neuropathy pain, 1222
- for hot flushes, 1187
- for neuropathic pain, **91*t*,** 94, 94*t*
- for peripheral neuropathy, HIV/AIDS, 1323
- for phobic disorders, 1051–1052
- poisoning, 1575–1576
- for pruritus, 159, 160
- for restless legs syndrome, 1013
- for seizures, 976*t*
- for social phobia, 1051
- for trigeminal neuralgia, 975, 977, 978

Gadolinium
- adverse effects, fatal, 361
- cardiac MRI, 361, 374, 415, 416*t*, 418*t*, 419, 422, 423, 428, 441
- necrotizing systemic fibrosis from, 361
- nephrogenic systemic fibrosis from, 942

Gait disorders. *See also specific types*
- evaluation, 60, 60*t*
- magnetic gait, 1016
- older adults, **60–62,** 60*t*

Galactomannan, aspergillosis, 1543–1544
Galactosemia, cataracts, 184
Galantamine, 1017
Galcanezumab, 972*t*, 973
Gallavardin phenomenon, 342
Gallbladder
- calcified, 720*t*, 721
- cholesterolosis, 720*t*
- episodic pain, 719
- gangrene, 722
- hydrops, 721

Gallbladder cancer, **1612–1614**
Gallop, 415
- atrial, 373
- right-sided, 331, 352
- S_3, 405, 418
- ventricular, 373

Gallstones, **718–720,** 720*t*. *See also* Cholelithiasis
- cholecystitis, **720–722,** 721*t*
- cholesterol, short bowel syndrome, 637
- *vs.* dyspepsia, 579
- pregnancy, 817

Gamma-butyrolactone, 1582
Gamma-hydroxybutyrate, 1570, **1582**
Gamolenic acid, 738
Ganciclovir, 1356*t*, 1367, 1368
Gangrene, 1473, 1473*f*
- bacterial synergistic, 1473
- foot, diabetes mellitus, 1224, 1294*t*
- gallbladder, 721
- gas, 1294*t*, **1450–1451,** 1473, 1473*f*

Gardnerella, bacterial vaginosis, 784–785, 785*f*
Gardnerella vaginalis, 1285
Gas, GI, **588–589**
- belching, **588**
- bloating, **588**
- flatulence, **588–589**

Gases, arterial blood. *See* Arterial blood gases
Gas gangrene, 1294*t*, **1450–1451,** 1473, 1473*f*
Gas sniffing/inhaling, **1095**
Gastrectomy
- sleeve, 1257
- vitamin B_{12} deficiency after, 507

Gastric adenocarcinoma, **1620–1622**
- diffuse gastric, 1620
- intestinal-type, 1620

Gastric band, laparoscopic adjustable, 1257
Gastric cancers, 622. *See also specific types*
- dyspepsia, 579
- treatment, 1597*t*
- upper GI bleeding, 596

Gastric contents aspiration, **305–306**
Gastric emptying
- antipsychotics on, 1066
- for poisoning, contraindications, 1568

Gastric lymphoma, **1622–1623**
Gastric metaplasia, 622
Gastric neuroendocrine tumors, **1623–1624**
Gastric outlet obstruction, 70, **631**
Gastrinomas, **1171–1173**
- with gastric acid hypersecretion, GERD, 611
- Zollinger-Ellison syndrome, 625, **631–632**

Gastrinoma triangle, 631
Gastritis & gastropathy, **620–624**
  Epstein-Barr virus gastritis, 1363
  erosive & hemorrhagic "gastritis," **620–622**
  gastritis types, infections, **624**
  nonerosive, nonspecific gastritis & intestinal metaplasia, **622–623**
    Helicobacter pylori gastritis, **622–623,** 624*t*
    pernicious anemia gastritis, **623**
  stress gastritis, **620–621**
Gastrocnemius tear/rupture, 28
Gastroenteritis
  antimicrobial therapy, empiric, 1297*t*
  E. coli, **1465–1466**
  viral, **1422–1423**
    norovirus, **1422–1423**
    rotavirus, **1422–1423**
Gastroenteropancreatic neuroendocrine tumors & carcinoid tumors, **1171–1173**
  carcinoid tumors, **1172**
  CCKomas, **1172**
  ectopic hormones, **1172**
  gastrinomas, **1171–1172**
  glucagonomas, **1172**
  insulinomas, **1171–1172**
  somatostatinomas, **1172**
Gastroesophageal junction
  dysfunction, 608
  laceration, upper GI bleeding, 596
  mucosal laceration of, 581, **613–614**
Gastroesophageal reflux disease (GERD), **608–612**
  Barrett esophagus from, **609–610**
  cough, 15–17, 17*t*
  dyspepsia, 579
  gastric contents aspiration, 305
  heartburn, 579
  hernia, hiatal, 588
  larynx, 236
  lower esophageal sphincter pressure, 608
  peptic stricture from, **610**
  prevalence, 608
Gastrointestinal bleeding, **596–602**
  acute lower, **598–600**
  acute upper, **596–598**
  occult, **601–602**
  suspected bowel bleeding, **601**
Gastrointestinal cytomegalovirus disease, 1366
Gastrointestinal disorders, **579–673.** *See also specific types*
  anorectal diseases, **669–673**
    anal fissures, **672–673**
    fecal incontinence, **671–672**
    hemorrhoids, **669–670**
    infections, **670–671**
    perianal abscess & fistula, **673**
    perianal pruritus, **673**
  colon & rectum diseases, **643–669**
    antibiotic-associated colitis, **647–649**
    diverticular disease of colon, **663–665**
      diverticulitis, **663–665**
      diverticulosis, uncomplicated, **663**
    hereditary colorectal cancer & polyposis syndromes, **666–669**
      familial adenomatous polyposis, **667**
      hamartomatous polyposis syndromes, **668**
      Lynch syndrome, **668–669**
    inflammatory bowel disease, **649–663**
      Crohn disease, **653–658**
      microscopic colitis, **663**
      ulcerative colitis, **658–662,** 658*t*
    irritable bowel syndrome, **643–647**
    polyps
      colon, **665**
      nonfamilial adenomatous & serrated, **665–666**
  esophagus diseases, **606–620**
    dysphagia, 606–607, 606*t*, 607*t*
    esophageal lesions, benign, **613–618**
      eosinophilic esophagitis, **614**
      esophageal varices, **615–618**
      esophageal webs & rings, **614–615**
      Mallory-Weiss syndrome, 582, **613–614**
      Zenker diverticulum, **615**
    esophageal motility disorders, **618–620**
      achalasia, **618–619**
      other primary, **620**
    gastroesophageal reflux disease, **608–612**
    heartburn, 606
    infectious esophagitis, **612–613**
    pill-induced esophagitis, **613**
  HIV/AIDS
    biliary disease, 1326
    enterocolitis, 1326
    esophagitis, candidal and other, 1318*t*, 1325
    gastropathy, 1326
    hepatic disease, 1325–1326
    malabsorption, 1326
  peritoneum diseases, **602–606**
    ascites, malignant, **605–606**
    ascites, patient assessment, **602–604,** 602*t*
    familial Mediterranean fever, **606**
    peritonitis, spontaneous bacterial, 602*t*, **604–605**
  small intestine diseases, **632–643**
    appendicitis, **641–642**
    intestinal motility disorders, **638–641**
      chronic intestinal pseudo-obstruction & gastroparesis, **640–641**
      colonic pseudo-obstruction, **639–641**
      paralytic ileus, **638–639**
    malabsorption, **632–638,** 633*t*
      bacterial overgrowth, **636**
      celiac disease, **633–635**
      lactase deficiency, **637–638**
      short bowel syndrome, **637**
      Whipple disease, **635–636**
    protein-losing enteropathy, **643**
    tuberculosis, intestinal, **643**
  stomach & duodenum diseases, **620–632**
    gastritis & gastropathy, **620–624**
      erosive & hemorrhagic "gastritis," **620–622**
      gastritis types, infections, **624**
      nonerosive, nonspecific gastritis & intestinal metaplasia, **622–623**
        Helicobacter pylori gastritis, **622–623,** 624*t*
      pernicious anemia gastritis, **623**
    peptic ulcer disease, **625–629**
    peptic ulcer disease complications, **629–632**
      gastric outlet obstruction, **631**
      hemorrhage, GI, **629–630**
      ulcer perforation, **631**
    Zollinger-Ellison syndrome, **631–632**
  symptoms & signs, **579–602**
    bleeding, GI, **596–602**
    constipation, **585–588**
    diarrhea, **589–595**
    dyspepsia, **579–581**
    gas, GI, **588–589**
    hiccups, **584–585**
    nausea & vomiting, **581–584**
  weight loss, involuntary, 32
Gastrointestinal mesenchymal tumors, **1624–1625**
Gastrointestinal tract decontamination
  activated charcoal, 1568–1569
  general, 1568
  hemodialysis, 1569, 1569*t*
  repeat-dose charcoal, 1569
  urinary manipulation, 1569
  whole bowel irrigation, 1569
Gastroparesis, 70, 579, **640–641,** 1223
Gastropathy, HIV/AIDS, 1326
GATA1, bone marrow failure, 546
Gatifloxacin, hypoglycemia from, 1237
Gaucher disease, 423, 868, 1662–1663
Gay & bisexual men, health care, **1722–1725**
  demographics, **1722**
  health disparities, **1722–1724**
Gay men, 1709
  cisgender, pregnancy options, 1714–1715
Gefitinib, 1601*t*, 1672*t*, 1673*t*
Gemcitabine, 1599*t*
  for bladder cancer, 1643
  for breast carcinoma, 759
  for gallbladder carcinoma, 1614
  myopathy from, 1045
  for pancreas carcinoma, 1616
Gemcitabine/carboplatin + pembrolizumab, 755, 758
Gemfibrozil, 1245*t*, 1248
Gender. *See also specific topics*
  assigned at birth, 1709
  on hypertension treatment, 466
  identity, 1709–1710
Gender affirming interventions, **1726–1729**
  hormone therapy, 1712
    contraception & family planning, 1713
    family building, 1714–1715
  medical & surgical, **1726–1730,** 1730*t*
    feminizing hormone therapy, **1726–1727,** 1727*t*
    fundamentals, 1726
    long-term health outcomes, **1729**
    masculinizing hormone therapy, **1727–1728,** 1728*t*
    monitoring hormone therapy, **1728,** 1729*t*
    surgical interventions, **1728–1729,** 1730*t*
  on reproductive capacity, 1726
Gender diverse, defined, 1725
Gender dysphoria, **1058–1059**
Gender identity, 1709–1710
Gender minority health, **1709–1730.** *See also* Sexual & gender minority health
Gender nonbinary, 1709
Gene expression profiling, breast carcinoma, 749–750
Generalized anxiety disorder, **1049, 1050**
General myoclonus, 1012
Gene therapy vectors, adenovirus, 1418
Genetic & genomic disorders, **1658–1674.** *See also specific types*
  acute intermittent porphyria, **1658–1659,** 1659*t*
  Down syndrome, **1659–1660**
  familial hypercholesterolemia, **1660–1661**
  fragile X syndrome, **1661–1662**
  Gaucher disease, **1662–1663**
  hereditary hemorrhagic telangiectasia, **1665–1666**
  homocysteine metabolism disorders, **1663–1664**
  Klinefelter syndrome, **1664**
  Marfan syndrome, **1664–1665**
  pharmacogenetic tests, clinical relevance, **1666, 1667*t*–1674*t***
Genital herpes, **120–121**
Genital tract infections, gram-negative, 1473
Genital ulcers. *See also specific types*
  adenovirus, 1418
  HSV-2, 1353
  from nonoxynol-9, 1331
  STDs, 1285
  typhus, endemic, 1428
Genital warts, 122, 122*f*
Genitourinary syndrome of menopause, 1186

Genitourinary tract cancers, **1634–1649**
bladder, **1642–1644**
kidney, **1646–1647**
prostate, **1634–1641,** 1635*t*, 1636*f*, 1640*t*
renal cell, **1645–1647**
testicular/germ cell, **1647–1649**
uterus & renal pelvis, **1644**
Genitourinary tract infections, **945–953**
chronic pelvic pain syndrome, 950*t*, **951–952**
cystitis, **945–946**
empiric therapy, **947*t*–948*t***
epididymitis, **952–953**
prostatitis
acute bacterial, **949–950,** 950*t*
chronic bacterial, **950–952,** 950*t*
nonbacterial chronic, 950*t*, **951–952**
pyelonephritis, **946–949**
renal infections, 945
Gentamicin
for *Bartonella,* 1471
for *Campylobacter,* 1467
for cholangitis, community-acquired, 724
for chorioamnionitis, 808
for enterococcus, 1443
for gonococcus, 1470
for Group B/C/G streptococcus endocarditis, 1457
for listeriosis, 1453
for metritis, 808
for plague, 1468
for prostatitis, 051
for pyelonephritis, 947*t*
for *Staphylococcus,* coagulase-negative, 1450, 1457
for tularemia, 1468
for viridans streptococci endocarditis, 1455
Gentian violet, 119
Geographic ulcers, herpes simplex keratitis, 179
Geriatric disorders, **52–68**. *See also* Older adults; *specific types*
adverse drug events, 66
assessment, older adult, 52–53, 53*f*
frailty, 53
function, 52–53
prognosis, 52
values & preferences, 52
delirium, **58–59**
dementia, **53–57**
depression, **57–58**
elder mistreatment & self-neglect, **67–68,** 68*t*
falls & gait disorders, **60–62,** 60*t*, 61*t*
general principles, 52
hearing impairment, **67**
immobility, **59–60**
incontinence, urinary, **62–64**
pharmacotherapy & polypharmacy, **66**
pressure injury, **64–65,** 65*t*
vision impairment, **67**
weight loss, involuntary, **64**
Germ cell tumors, 998*t*, **1647–1649**
Germinomas, 998*t*
Germinotropic lymphoproliferative disorder, 1368
Gerstmann-Sträussler-Scheinker syndrome, 1385
Gerstmann syndrome, 999
Gestational diabetes mellitus, **810–811,** 810*t*
Gestational hypertension, preeclampsia-eclampsia, **802–804,** 803*t*
Gestational thrombocytopenia, **556**
Gestational thyrotoxicosis, 1120
Gestational trophoblastic disease, **800–802**
Geste antagoniste, 1012
Giant cell arteritis, **848–849**
amaurosis fugax, 848
blindness, 848, 849
diplopia, 848
facial pain, 978
fever of unknown origin, 848
headache, **848–849**
herpes simplex virus, 1360
ischemic optic neuropathy, 193–194, 848
patient age, 1270
retinal artery occlusion, 189–190
sixth nerve palsy, 196
third nerve palsy, 196
transient monocular visual loss, 190
Giant cell granuloma, anterior hypopituitarism, 1099
Giant cell myocarditis, 414, 415*t*, 417
Giardia (giardiasis), 579, 589, 590, **1518–1519**
Giardia duodenalis, **1518–1519**
Giardia intestinalis, **1518–1519**
Giardia lamblia, 1292, **1518–1519**
Gigantism, **1106–1107**
Gilbert syndrome, 674, 675*t*, 676*t*, 697
Gilles De La Tourette syndrome, **1013–1014**
Gingival disease, HIV/AIDS, 1324–1325
Gingivitis, necrotizing ulcerative, **230**
Gingivostomatitis, **230,** 1353
Ginkgo, 1580*t*
Ginseng, 1580*t*
Gitelman syndrome, 882*t*, 883*f*, 884, 900
Glanders, 1294*t*
Glanzmann thrombasthenia, **556–557**
Glasgow Coma Scale, 1021, 1021*t*
Glatiramer acetate, 1025, 1025*t*
Glaucoma, **180–183**
acute angle-closure, 170*t*, 177*t*–178*t*, **180–181**
from antipsychotics, 1066
chronic, 177*t*–178*t*, 181–183, **181–183**
contusions and hyphema, 198
from corticosteroids, 198–199
diabetes mellitus, 1221
facial pain, 978
normal-tension, **181–183**
older adults, 67
from pupillary dilation, 198
retinal vein occlusions, 188–189
Gleason score, 1595, 1635*t*, 1638, 1641
Glecaprevir, 689, 690*t*, 691*t*
Gliclazide, 1204*t*, 1206
Glimepiride, 1204*t*, 1206
Glioblastoma, with methylated methylguanine-DNA methyltransferase promoter, 1000
Glioblastoma multiforme, 997*t*
Glioma
brainstem, 998*t*
intramedullary spinal, **1001–1002**
Glipizide, 1204*t*, 1206
GLI-similar 3 (GLIS3), 1197
Global Limb Anatomic Staging System (GLASS) vascular guidelines, 477
Global Registry of Acute Cardiac Events Risk Score, 24
Globe injury
closed, contusion, 197
ischemic optic neuropathy, 193–194
open, lesions, 198
Glomerular amyloidosis, plasma cell myeloma, 941
Glomerular diseases, **922–932**. *See also specific types*
classification, 922–923, 922*f*, 923*t*–924*t*
nephritic spectrum, 922–923, 922*f*, **924–932**
C3 glomerulopathies, 923*t*, **929**
classification & findings, 923, 923*t*
clinical findings, 922*f*, 924–926, 925*f*
glomerulonephritis
anti-GBM, 912, 913, 923*t*, 925*f*, **928–929**
cryoglobulin-associated, 923*t*, **929–930**
definition, 924
infection-related/postinfectious, 923*t*, **926–927**
membranoproliferative, 923*t*, **929**
pauci-immune, 923*t*, **928**
Goodpasture syndrome, 912, 913, 923*t*, 925*f*, **928–929**
hepatitis C virus–associated kidney disease, 923*t*, **930**
IgA nephropathy, 923*t*, **927**
IgA vasculitis, 923*t*, **927–928**
systemic IgA vasculitis, 923*t*
systemic lupus erythematosis, 923*t*, **930–931**
nephrotic spectrum, 922–923, 922*f*, 924*t*, **931–934**
causes, 932
classification & clinical findings, 923, 924*t*, 931–932
membranoproliferative glomerulonephropathy, 924*t*
primary renal disorders, 924*t*
focal segmental glomerulosclerosis, 924*t*, 931, **933**
membranous nephropathy, 924*t*, 926, 931, **933–934**
treatment, 932
Glomerular filtration rate
BUN, 905, 905*t*
BUN:creatinine ratio, 905, 907*t*
creatine clearance, 905
cystatin C, 905
estimated, 905
kidney disease, **904–905,** 905*t*
normal, 904
renal clearance, 904–905
Glomerular proteinuria, 904
Glomerulonephritis, 907*t*, **912–913**
anti-GBM, 912, 913, 923*t*, 925*f*, **928–929**
C3 glomerulopathy, 912, 923*t*, **929**
cryoglobulin-associated, 923*t*, **929–930**
cryoglobulinemia, 855
definition, 924
end-stage kidney disease, 914
eosinophilic granulomatosis with polyangiitis, 854
granulomatosis with polyangiitis, 851–853
Group A streptococci, 1440
IgA vasculitis, 855
immune complex, 912
infection-related/postinfectious, 923*t*, **926–927**
levamisole-associated purpura, 855
membranoproliferative, 923*t*, **929**
microscopic polyangiitis, 853–854
monoclonal immunoglobulin–mediated, 912
necrotizing, 852, 854
pauci-immune, 852, 854, 855, 912, 923*t*, **928**
relapsing polychondritis, 856
systemic lupus erythematosus, 834, 834*t*, 835, 856
vasculitis syndromes, 847*t*
Glomerulonephropathy, membranoproliferative, 924*t*
Glomerulopathy. *See also specific types*
C3, 912, 923*t*, **929**
COVID-19-associated collapsing, 913
sickle cell, 941
Glomus jugulare tumors, 212
Glomus tumors, middle ear, **212**
Glomus tympanicum, **212**
Glossitis, **229–230**
Glossodynia, **230**
Glossopharyngeal neuralgia, **978**
"Gloves and socks" syndrome, 1420
GLP-1. *See* Glucagon-like peptide 1

GLP-1 receptor agonists. *See* Glucagon-like peptide 1 receptor agonists; *specific types*
Glucagon, for beta-blocker poisoning, 1577
Glucagon-like peptide 1 (GLP-1), 1208, 1235, 1236
Glucagon-like peptide 1 receptor agonists. *See also specific types*
for hirsutism, female, 1183
for hyperglycemia/diabetes mellitus, 1204*t*–1205*t*, 1208–1210
coronary heart disease prevention, 358–359
dulaglutide, 1204*t*, 1209
exenatide, 1204*t*, 1209
liraglutide, 1205*t*, 1209
lixisenatide, 1205*t*, 1209
semaglutide, 1205*t*, 1209
type 2, 1218–1219, 1218*t*
weight loss, 1218
Glucagonomas, **1172**
Glucocorticoids. *See also specific indications and types*
tremor from, 1012
Glucokinase, mature-onset diabetes of young, 1196–1197, 1196*t*
Gluconate, 917
Glucosamine, 821, 1705
Glucose
blood, self-monitoring, 1202
intolerance
gallstones, 719
gestational diabetes mellitus, 810–811
monitoring systems
continuous, 1202
self-monitoring, 1202
plasma/serum, 1200
urine, 1200
Glucose-6-phosphate dehydrogenase deficiency, **511**
Glucose control, diabetes mellitus. *See also* Glycemic control
type 1, **1198**
type 2, **1198–1199**
Glucose-dehydrogenase pyrroloquinoline quinone systems, 1202
Glucose-dependent insulinotropic polypeptide, 1208
Glucose oxidase-based amperometric systems, 1202
Glucose tolerance test, oral, 1200–1201, 1201*t*
Gluten, 633
Gluten enteropathy. *See* Celiac disease
Gluten sensitivity, thyroiditis, 1112
Glyburide, 1204*t*, 1206
Glycated albumin, 1201
Glycated hemoglobin, 1201
Glycemic control. *See also* Glucose control, diabetes mellitus
for diabetes mellitus, acceptable levels, 1219, 1219*t*
for diabetic nephropathy, 935
Mediterranean-style eating pattern on, 1203
Glycemic index, 1203
Glycerol, neuromodulatory therapy, 97*t*
Glycolic acid, anion gap elevation from, 897
Glycoprotein Ib/IX receptor, 556
Glycoprotein II_B/III_A inhibitors, 371. *See also specific types*
Glycoprotein IIb/IIIa receptor, 556
Glycopyrrolate, 151, 262
Glycosuria, renal (nondiabetic), 1200
Gnathostomiasis, cutaneous larva migrans, 1530
Goiter
endemic, **1137–1138**
hypothyroidism, 1115
iodine deficiency disorder, **1137–1138**
multinodular, **1129–1131,** 1129*t*
toxic nodular/multinodular, 1119, 1125
Goldman Risk Score, modified, 24
Golfer's elbow, 1689
Golimumab
infections with, 1273
for inflammatory bowel disease, 651–652
for rheumatoid arthritis, 830–831
for ulcerative colitis, 660
Gonadal dysgenesis, **1191–1193,** 1192*t*
Gonadotropin. *See also specific types*
for anterior hypopituitarism, 1102–1103
deficiency
anterior hypopituitarism
acquired, 1100
congenital, 1100
Prader-Willi syndrome, 1100
hypogonadotropic hypogonadism, 1100–1101
for hypogonadism, male, 1178
Gonadotropin-releasing hormone, 1099, 1184, 1185
Gonadotropin-releasing hormone agonists. *See also specific types*
for female hirsutism, 1183
for pelvic pain, 768
for uterine leiomyoma, 766
Gonadotropin-releasing hormone analog, 1726, 1727*t*. *See also specific types*
Gonadotropin-releasing hormone antagonists, 766, 768
Gonococcus (gonorrhea), **1469–1470**. *See also* Sexually transmitted diseases/infections
animal bites, 1283
anorectal infections, 67
arthritis, **863–864**
Bartholin duct infection, 783
cervicitis, 1469
conjunctivitis, **171,** 1469
disseminated, 1469
epididymitis, 952
gay & bisexual men, 1723, 1724
lesbian & bisexual women, 1718
medication of choice, 1293*t*
pelvic inflammatory disease, 786
pharyngitis/tonsillitis, 231
pregnancy, 814
STDs, 1284–1286
urethritis, 1285, 1469
vaginal discharge, 1285
Gonorrhea. *See* Gonococcus (gonorrhea)
Goodpasture syndrome, 303, 912, 913, 923*t*, 925*f*, **928–929**
Good syndrome, 872*t*
Gordon syndrome, hypertension, 445
Goserelin (acetate), 757, 757*t*, 1602*t*, 1640, 1640*t*
Gottron papules, 842
Gout/gouty arthritis, **823–826**
chronic kidney disease, 823–824
diabetes mellitus, 1225
kidney and, **941–942**
MTP joint inflammation, 824, 824*f*
osteonecrosis, 868
primary/secondary, 823, 824*t*
prognosis, 826
tophus, 823
transplant patient, 826
treatment, 824–826
urate deposition & hyperuricemia, 823, 824*t*
uric acid kidney stones, 823
GRACE Risk Score, 372
Gradenigo syndrome, 210
Graft enteric fistula, 483
Graft-*versus*-host disease, 544, 614
Graham Steell murmur, 333*t*, 334*t*, 352
Gram-negative bacilli. *See also specific types*
hospital-/ventilator-acquired pneumonia, 276, 276*t*
immunocompromised, pulmonary infiltrates, 279
keratitis, 179
otitis externa, 206
Gram-negative bacterial infections, **1458–1473**. *See also* Bacterial infections, gram-negative
Gram-positive bacterial infections, **1440–1453**. *See also* Bacterial infections, gram-positive
Granisetron, **583–584,** 583*t*, 1655
Granular casts, 903, 904*t*, 907, 907*t*, 909
Granulocyte colony-stimulating factor, 1655
Granulocyte disorders, 872*t*
Granulocytopenia, in immunocompromised infections, 1273
Granuloma. *See also specific types*
giant cell, anterior hypopituitarism, 1099
hoarseness, 238
swimming pool, 1475
Granuloma inguinale, 1285–1286, **1470–1471**
Granulomatosis with polyangiitis, **851–853,** 852*f*
anterior hypopituitarism, 1099
hearing loss, 213
myocarditis, 415*t*, 417
patient age, 1270
pulmonary vasculitis, 303
sinonasal inflammatory disease, 226–227
Granulomatous disorders, 1144. *See also specific types*
hypercalcemia, 889
meningitis, 1280*t*
uveitis, **183–184**
Granulomatous infantisepticum, 1453
Graves dermopathy, 1121, 1127
Graves disease, 1113, **1119–1127,** 1405. *See also* Hyperthyroidism
Graves ophthalmopathy, **1128**
Grazoprevir, 1325
Great saphenous vein, varicose, **487–489**
Grieving, 78–79
Grimacing, facial, 1011
Grippe, summer, 1423
Griseofulvin, 167
Ground itch, 1527
Group A beta-hemolytic streptococci. *See Streptococcus,* Group A beta-hemolytic
Group B streptococci
metritis, postpartum, 814
pregnancy, **814**
Group D streptococci, 1443
endocarditis, 1457
Group psychotherapy, 1052, 1054, 1060
Growth hormone, 1099
acromegaly and gigantism, **1106–1107**
deficiency
anterior hypopituitarism, 1100
hypogonadotropic hypogonadism, 1101–1102
Growth hormone-releasing hormone, 1099
Guaiac-based fecal occult blood tests, 11, 1632
Guaifenesin, kidney stones from, 954
Guanabenz, 460, **1579**
Guanadrel, 460, 464
Guanethidine, 460, 464
Guanethidine hydrochloride, 1042
Guanfacine, 460, 463*t*, 972*t*, **1579**
Guanylate cyclase stimulant, 410, 841
Guanylcyclase C, 586

Guarana, 1580*t*
Guargum, 586, 587*t*
Guiding principles of care, 2
Guillain-Barré syndrome, 1030, **1033–1034**
  Campylobacter jejuni enteritis and, 1033
  Chikungunya fever, 1400
  COVID-19, 1404
  dysautonomia, 984
  Epstein-Barr virus, 1363
  lymphocytic choriomeningitis, 1384
  parechovirus, 1426
  West Nile virus, 1380
  Zika virus, 1399
Guselkumab, 138, 860
"Gut dialysis," 1569
Gynecologic disorders, **763–793**. *See also specific types*
  abnormal uterine bleeding, reproductive age, **763–765**, 764*t*
  Bartholin duct cysts & abscesses, **783**, 783*f*
  carcinoma
    cervix, **789–790**
    endometrium, **791**
    ovarian tumors & cancer, **792–793**
    vulva, **791–792**
  cervical intraepithelial neoplasia, **787–789,** 788*f*
  cervical polyps, **767**
  condyloma acuminata, **787**
  contraception & family planning, **773–780,** 775*t*, 776*t*, 778*t*
  diagnostic procedures, 764*t*
  endometrial sampling, 763–764, 764*t*
  HIV/AIDS
    cervical dysplasia, 1330
    pelvic inflammatory disease, 1330
    vaginal candidias, 1318*t*, 1330
  infertility, **772–773**
  leiomyoma of uterus, **765–766**
  pain, pelvic, **767–769**
    adenomyosis, fibroids, pelvic inflammatory disease, malpositioned IUD, **769**
    dysmenorrhea, primary, **767**
    endometriosis, **767–769**
  pelvic inflammatory disease, **785–787**
  pelvic organ prolapse, **769–770**
  polycystic ovary syndrome, **771, 1181**
  postmenopausal uterine bleeding, **765**
  premenstrual syndrome, **770**
  sexual dysfunction, female, **780–782**
  sexual violence, **782–783, 1721**
  vaginitis, **783–785,** 784*f*, 785*f*
Gynecomastia, 961, **1179–1181**
  from 5-alpha-reductase inhibitors, 966
  from ACTZ + triamterene, 459*t*
  Bantu men, 762
  causes, 1180*t*
  cirrhosis, 700
  hyperbilirubinemia, conjugated, 603
  liver disease, chronic, 603
  from spironolactone, 407, 455, 458*t*, 702
Gyromitra poisoning, 1587

H

H_1-antihistamines, 152, 880. *See also specific types*
H_2-receptor antagonists, 610–611, 622, 624*t*, 627. *See also specific types*
H5N1 virus, **1414–1415**
H7N7 virus, 1414
H63D, 710
H1069Q variant, Wilson disease, 711–712
HACEK organisms, 1457
Haemophilus, **1461**
  animal bites, 1283
  conjunctivitis, 170
  epiglottitis, 1461
  liver abscess, 717
  medication of choice, 1294*t*
  meningitis, 1461
Haemophilus ducreyi, 1285, **1470**
Haemophilus influenzae, **1461**
  bronchiectasis, 265
  cystic fibrosis, 266
  epiglottitis, 237
  immunocompromised, 1273
  laryngitis, 236
  orbital cellulitis, 196
  otitis media
    acute, 209, 209*f*, 211
    chronic, 210
  pelvic inflammatory disease, 786
  pneumonia, 269*t*
    community-acquired, 272, 273
    HIV/AIDS, 1320
  rhinosinusitis, 219
  vaccine, type b, 1302*t*–1303*t*, 1304*t*, 1308*t*
Hair pulling, 1052
Hairy cell leukemia, **532–533,** 867
Hairy leukoplakia, **228,** 228*f*, 1324
Hallucinations
  hypnagogic, 1084
  schizoaffective disorder, 1061
  schizophrenia, 1061
  temporal lobe lesions, 999
Hallucinogen poisoning, **1584–1585**
Hallucinosis, alcoholic, 1087, 1089, 1096
Halobetasol propionate, 104*t*
Haloperidol
  for aggression disorders, 1085
  for bipolar disorder, 1079
  for Gilles De La Tourette syndrome, 1013–1014
  for Huntington disease, 1010
  for hypertension, from poisoning, 1566
  IV, 1066
  for personality disorders, 1061
  poisoning, 1576
  for psychedelic effects, 1093
  for schizophreniform spectrum disorders, 1063, 1065
Haloperidol decanoate, long-acting, 1066
Halothane hepatotoxicity, 696
Hamartomatous polyposis syndromes, **668**
Hamilton, 1071
HAMP, 710
Hampton hump, 298
Hand
  bites, **1283–1284**
  immersion, **1552**
  squeezes, on blood pressure, 448, 448*t*
Hand, foot, and mouth disease, enterovirus, 1424, 1424*f*
Handgrip test, for systolic murmurs, 336*t*
Hand washing, prophylactic, 1274, 1278
Hantaan virus, 1395
Hantavirus cardiopulmonary syndrome, 1395
Hantaviruses, **1395–1396**
Hantavirus pulmonary syndrome, **1395–1396**
Haptoglobin, 510
Hard metal lung disease, 308
Harmless acute pancreatitis score (HAPS), 729
Harm reduction model, at-risk drinking, 1088
Harris-Benedict Equation, 1266
Hashimoto thyroiditis, **1112–1114**
  COVID-19, 1405
  HHV-6, 1368
  pregnancy, 809
  relapsing polychondritis, 856
Hashitoxicosis, 1113
Hawkins impingement sign, 1675, 1679*t*
Hay fever, 15, 16, **222–223**
Hazardous alcohol use, 12
HBeAg, hepatitis B, 681, 687
HBsAg, hepatitis B, 680, 687
hCG-secreting trophoblastic tumors, hyperthyroidism, 1120
HCV polymerase inhibitors, 689
HCV protease inhibitors, 689, 690*t*
Headache, **970–974**. *See also specific types*
  acute, **35–38**
    diagnostic studies, 37
    physical examination, 36–37
    symptoms, 35–36, 35*t*, 36*t*
    treatment, 37–38
  carotid artery occlusion/dissection, 974
  cerebrovascular disease, 974
  chronic, 80, 970
    daily, 974
  cluster, **973**
  combined oral contraceptives and, 776
  cough, primary, **974**
  dull/throbbing, 974
  giant cell arteritis, **848–849**
  idiopathic intracranial hypertension, 974, **1003–1005**
  intracranial mass lesion, **974**
  lumbar puncture, 974
  medication overuse, **974**
  migraine, 36, **970–973,** 972*t* (*See also* Migraine headache)
  posttraumatic, **973–974**
  prevalence & causes, 35
  primary syndromes, 970
  secondary causes, 970
    SNNOOP10 red flags, 36, 36*t*
  sentinel, 35
  severe, 35, 974, 993
  tension-type, **973**
Head injury, **1021–1023,** 1021*t*
  Battle sign, 1021
  chronic traumatic encephalopathy, 1023
  concussion, 1021
  Glasgow Coma Scale, 1021, 1021*t*
  injury mechanisms & acute cerebral sequelae, 1021, 1022*t*
  lucid interval, 1021
  posttraumatic headache, 973–974
  raccoon sign, 1021
  second impact syndrome, 1022
  traumatic brain injury, 1021
Head louse, 130
Head & neck cancer
  lymphoma, 243
  squamous cell carcinoma of larynx, **238–240**
  treatment, 1596*t*
Head & neck infections. *See specific types*
Head trauma
  inner ear damage, 212
  olfactory dysfunction, 224
  seizures from, 1567
Health care access
  lesbian & bisexual women, 1715, 1720
  transgender & gender diverse people, 1725–1726
Health care–associated infections, **1276–1279**. *See also specific types*
Health care–associated meningitis, 1281, 1282
Health disparities
  gay & bisexual men, **1722–1724**
  lesbian & bisexual women, **1715–1716**
  sexual & gender minority health, **1710–1711**
Health literacy, 1
Hearing aids, 67, 205
Hearing amplification, 67, 205
Hearing amplifiers, portable, 67

Hearing loss, **204–205**
age-related, 204, **212**
amplification for, 205
audiology, **204–205**
autoimmune, **213**
classification & epidemiology, 204, 205*t*
cochlear implant for, 205
conductive, **204**
hidden, 212
mass lesion, intracranial, 217–218
middle ear tumors, 212
multiple sclerosis, 218
older adults, **67**
sensorineural, 204, **212–213**
AIDS, 218
autoimmune, **213**
noise trauma, **212**
ototoxicity, **213**
physical trauma, **212**
presbycusis, **212**
Heart. *See also* Cardiac
emboli, 478
myxedema, 1115
Heart block. *See also specific types*
AV (*See* Atrioventricular block)
complete
acute MI, with ST-segment elevation, 379
atrial fibrillation, 391
atrial septal defect, 327
myocarditis, 415
pericarditis, 427
rate & rhythm disorders, 383
syncope, 403
Heartburn, 579, 606, 608, 611
Heart disease, **323–441**. *See also specific types*
athlete screening, cardiovascular, **438–441,** 439*t*, 440*t*
12-element AHA recommendations, 438, 439*t*
sudden cardiac death, potential causes, 439, 440*t*
cardiac tumors, **433–434**
primary, **433–434**
secondary, **434**
cardiomyopathy, **417–424**
dilated, **417–420,** 418*t*
hypertrophic, 404, 418*t*, **421–423**
restrictive, 404, 418*t*, **423–424**
stress, 373, 418, **420–421**
congenital, adult, **323–332** (*See also* Congenital heart disease, adult)
atrial septal defect, **326–328**
coarctation of aorta, **325–326**
epidemiology & assessment, 323
patent foramen ovale, **326–328**
pulmonary valve stenosis, **323–324**
tetralogy of Fallot, **330–332**
ventricular septal defect, **328–330**
coronary heart disease, **355–382**
acute coronary syndromes, without ST-segment elevation, **368–372** (*See also* Acute coronary syndrome, without ST-segment elevation)
acute MI, with ST-segment elevation, **373–382** (*See also under* Myocardial infarction, acute)
angina pectoris, **359–367,** 364*f*, 367*t*
coronary vasospasm & angina/MI, normal coronary arteriograms, **367–368**
epidemiology, 355
myocardial hibernation & stunning, **355–357,** 420
prevention
primary & secondary, 357–359
statins, 5*t*, 8, 355, 356*f*, 357–358, 357*t*
risk factors
family history, 355
hypercholesterolemia, 355
metabolic syndrome, 355
diabetes mellitus, 1224
heart failure, **403–414** (*See also* Heart failure)
myocarditis, **414–417**
infectious, **414–416,** 415*t*, 416*t*
noninfectious, **416–417**
obesity, 1251
pericardial diseases, **426–433**
pericardial effusion & tamponade, **429–430**
pericarditis
acute inflammatory, **426–429**
constrictive, 429, **430–431**
pulmonary hypertension, **431–433**
pregnancy, **435–438,** 812
cardiomyopathy of pregnancy, **436**
CARPREG I/II scoring systems, 435, 436*f*
coronary artery & aortic vascular abnormalities, **436–438**
management
labor, **438**
WHO guidelines, 435, 437*t*
rate & rhythm disorders, **383–403**
atrial fibrillation, **391–396**
atrial flutter, **396–397**
atrial tachycardia, **397–398**
AV block, **387–388**
classification & diagnosis, 383
inherited arrhythmia syndromes, **401**
management
antiarrhythmics, **383, 384*t*–385*t***
catheter ablation, 383–386
paroxysmal supraventricular tachycardia, 386, **388–389**
accessory AV pathway, **390–391**
sinus arrhythmia, **386–387**
sinus bradycardia, 379, **386–387**
sinus tachycardia, **386–387**
syncope, **402–403**
ventricular fibrillation & sudden death, **400–401**
ventricular premature beats, **398**
ventricular tachycardia, **398–400**
rheumatic fever, **424–426,** 425*t*
risk factors, 448, 449*t*
traumatic, **434–435**
valvular, **332–355,** 333*t*–335*t* (*See also* Valvular heart disease; *specific types*)
cardiac risk assessment/reduction, 45
interventions on, 336*t*
Heart failure, **403–414**
acute, **403–412** (*See also* Acute heart failure)
pulmonary edema and, **413–414**
cachexia, 73
cardiac risk assessment/reduction, 42, 44–45
chronic
atrial fibrillation, 391
digoxin for, 380
systolic, 406
chronic kidney disease, 374, 916
classification & causes, 403–404
clinical findings, 404–406
definition, 417
epidemiology, 403
hypervolemic hyponatremia, 878
left, 403–404
cardiomyopathy, restrictive, 418*t*, 423
right ventricle dilation, 351
liver in, **715**
mitral regurgitation, 338, 340
patent foramen ovale, 327
pregnancy, 812
prevention, 404
prognosis, referral, & admission, 412
renin–angiotensin system, 405
right, 350, 403–404, **403–404**
cardiomyopathy
dilated, 419
restrictive, 418*t*, 423, 424
mitral stenosis, 336
pericarditis, constrictive, 430, 431
pulmonary hypertension, 432
pulmonic stenosis, 324
tetralogy of Fallot, 330
tricuspid stenosis, 350
ventricular septal defect, 329
stages, 404
systemic lupus erythematosus, 834
from thyrotoxicosis, 1127
valvular heart diseases, 404
Heart failure, treatment, **406–412,** 406*f*
digoxin, 380
LVEF, preserved, **412**
nonpharmacologic, 412
pharmacologic
diuretics, 412
renin–angiotensin–aldosterone system inhibitors, 412
reversible causes, correction, 412
LVEF, reduced, **406–412,** 406*f*, 407*t*
dosing, evidence-based, 406, 407*t*
nonpharmacologic, 411–412
biventricular pacing, 411
case management, diet & exercise training, 411
continuous/pulsatile flow devices, 411–412
coronary revascularization, 411
implantable cardioverter defibrillator, 411
palliative care, 412
transplantation, 411
pharmacologic, 407–411
antiarrhythmics, 410–411
anticoagulation, 410
beta-blockers, 409
combined therapies, 410
digitalis glycosides, 409
diuretics, 406–407
harmful treatments, 410
ivabradine, 410
nitrates and hydralazine, 409–410
renin–angiotensin–aldosterone system inhibitors, 407–409
SGL2 inhibitors, 409
statins, 411
vericiguate, 410
phenotypic overview, 406, 406*f*
reversible causes, correction, 406
Heartland virus, **1392**
Heart murmurs. *See* Murmurs, heart
Heart rate & rhythm disorders, **383–403**. *See also specific types*
atrial fibrillation, **391–396**
atrial flutter, **396–397**
atrial tachycardia, **397–398**
AV block, **387–388**
classification & diagnosis, 383
inherited arrhythmia syndromes, **401**
management
antiarrhythmics, **383, 384*t*–385*t***
catheter ablation, 383–386
paroxysmal supraventricular tachycardia, 386, **388–389**
accessory AV pathway, **390–391**
sick sinus syndrome, **386–387**
sinus arrhythmia, **386–387**
sinus bradycardia, 379, **386–387**

sinus tachycardia, **386–387**
supraventricular tachycardia, 383
symptoms & diagnosis, 383
syncope, **402–403**
ventricular fibrillation & sudden death, **400–401**
ventricular premature beats, **398**
ventricular tachycardia, **398–400**
HEART Risk Score, 24
Heart sounds. *See also* Murmurs, heart
acute MI, with ST-segment elevation, 373
aortic regurgitation, 333*t*, 348
aortic stenosis, 333*t*
athlete cardiovascular screening, 438
heart failure, 405
mitral regurgitation, 333*t*, 338
mitral stenosis, 333*t*
myocardial infarction, acute, 23
pericardial effusion, 429
pulmonary valve regurgitation, 352
pulmonary valve stenosis, 327
tricuspid regurgitation, 333*t*
tricuspid stenosis, 333*t*
Heart transplantation, for heart failure with reduced LVEF, 411
Heart valves. *See also specific types and disorders*
for aortic stenosis, mechanical *vs.* prosthetic, 345
Heart valves, prosthetic
bioprosthetic
for atrial fibrillation, 347
direct-acting oral anticoagulants with, 353
endocarditis
anticoagulation therapy, 354*t*
Melody valve, 329
percutaneous pulmonary valve replacement, 324
prophylaxis, 338, 1455, 1455*t*
pulmonary valve surgery, 324, 332
management
anticoagulants, **353–355,** 354*t*
antiplatelet therapy, dual, 353
aspirin, low-dose, 337, 345
pregnancy, 355
heparin
low-molecular-weight, 353, 354*t*
unfractionated, 354*t*, 355, 370*f*
mitral, 337, 337*f*
Q fever, 1435–1436
tricuspid stenosis, 350
Heat cramps, **1549**
Heat disorders, **1548–1550**. *See also specific types*
heat cramps, **1549**
heat exhaustion, **1549**
heat stress, **1548–1549**
heat stroke, **1549**
exertional, **1549**
nonexertional, **1549**
heat syncope, **1549**
humidity on, 1548
hyperthermia, **1548**
metabolic rate, 1548
prevention & prognosis, 1550
risk factors, 1548–1549
treatment, 1549–1550
Heat exchange, body–environment, 1548
Heat exhaustion, **1549**
Heat rash, **151**
Heat stress, **1548–1549**
Heat stroke, 30, **1549**
Heat syncope, **1549**
Heavy metals, 937, 1568*t*, 1603. *See also specific types*
Heberden nodes, 820, 821*f*
Hedgehog pathway inhibitors. *See specific types*
Heinz bodies, 511
Helicobacter pylori
dyspepsia, 579, 580
gastric adenocarcinoma, 1620
gastric lymphoma, 1623
gastritis, **622–623,** 624*t*
immune thrombocytopenia, 548–549
peptic ulcer disease, **625–628**
testing, 626
treatment
eradication therapy, 627–628
medication of choice, 1294*t*
Heliotrope rash, 842, 843*f*
Heller cardiomyotomy, for achalasia, 619
HELLP syndrome, 555, 803
Helminthic infections, **1520–1533**. *See also specific types*
cestode, **1523–1526**
invasive, **1524–1526**
cysticercosis, **1524–1525**
echinococcosis, **1525–1526**
noninvasive
beef tapeworm, **1523**
dwarf tapeworm, **1523**
fish tapeworm, 507, **1523**
laboratory findings, 1523
pork tapeworm, **1523**
treatment, 1523–1524
filariasis, **1530–1533**
lymphatic, **1530–1532,** 1531*f*
onchocerciasis, **1532–1533**
nematode, intestinal, **1526–1529**
ascariasis, **1526**
enterobiasis, **1528–1529**
hookworm disease, **1527**
strongyloidiasis, **1527–1528**
trichuriasis, **1526–1527**
nematode, invasive, **1529–1530**
angiostrongyliasis, **1529–1530**
cutaneous larva migrans, **1530,** 1530*f*
trematode, **1520–1523**
liver & lung flukes, **1521–1523**
clonorchiasis & opisthorchiasis, **1522**
fascioliasis, **1521–1522**
paragonimiasis, **1522–1523**
schistosomiasis, **1520–1521**
Helvella poisoning, 1587
Hemarthrosis, knee, 1695
Hematemesis
GI hemorrhage, peptic ulcer disease, 629
Mallory-Weiss syndrome, 613
upper GI bleeding, 596
Hematochezia
anal fissures, 672
GI hemorrhage, peptic ulcer disease, 629–630
lower GI bleeding, 599
Hematological evaluation, preoperative, 47–49, 48*t*
Hematopoietic cell transplant recipients
immunizations, recommended, 1301
infections, 1273
prevention, 1275
Hematuria, **943–945,** 944*f*
autosomal dominant polycystic kidney disease, 940
bladder cancer, 39, 943, 1642
clinical findings, 943–945
follow-up, 945
with hemoptysis, 21
kidney disease, **904**
lower tract source, 943
risk stratification, 943, 944*f*
upper tract source, 943
Hemicrania continua, 973
Hemochromatosis, 163, **709–711**
Hemodialysis, 920, 1569, 1569*t*
Hemodynamic measurements, for shock, 497
Hemoglobin, glycated, 1201
Hemoglobin A_1, 1201
Hemoglobin A_{1c}, 1201
Hemoglobin A_2, 504–505, 909
Hemoglobin F, 504–505, 512, 514
Hemoglobin H, 505
Hemoglobin H disease, 505–506
Hemoglobinopathies, gout from, 823
Hemoglobin S, 512, 514
Hemoglobin SC disease, sickle cell retinopathy, 193
Hemoglobin SS, 512–513, 513*t*, 514
Hemoglobinuria, 502, 510, 904
Hemolysis, traumatic, 502
Hemolytic anemias, **509–519**
aplastic anemia, **516–518,** 516*t*, 517*t*
autoimmune, **514–515**
classification, 509–510, 509*t*
cold agglutinin disease, 500, **515–516**
drug-induced, 514
extrinsic, 509, 509*t*
G6PD deficiency, **511**
intrinsic, 509–510, 509*t*
neutropenia, **518–519,** 518*t*
paroxysmal nocturnal hemoglobinuria, **510–511**
sickle cell anemia & related syndromes, **512–513,** 513*t*
sickle cell trait, 513*t*, **514**
sickle thalassemia, 513*t*, **514**
Hemolytic crisis, 512
Hemolytic transfusion reactions, 543
Hemolytic-uremic syndrome
complement-mediated, **550–552,** 551*t*
Shiga toxin-mediated, **550–552,** 551*t*, 590
thrombotic microangiopathy, **550–552,** 551*t*
Hemopericardium, traumatic heart disease, 434
Hemophagocytosis, infection-related thrombocytopenia, 556
Hemophilia A, **557–559,** 559*t*, 561
Hemophilia B, **557–559,** 559*t*
Hemophilia C, 559*t*, **561**
Hemoptysis, **20–22**
Hemorrhage. *See also* Bleeding; *specific disorders*
alveolar, 21, **303–304**
Crohn disease, 654
gastrointestinal, peptic ulcer disease, **629–630**
immune, 303
intracerebral, 469, 470*t*
nonimmune causes, 303–304
retinal/choroidal, 193
subarachnoid (*See* Subarachnoid hemorrhage)
vitreous, **186**
Hemorrhagic conjunctivitis, 170
Hemorrhagic cystitis, from cyclophosphamide or ifosfamide, **1656**
Hemorrhagic fevers. *See also specific types*
Colorado tick fever, 1401
viral, **1389–1397**
Bunyavirus hemorrhagic fevers, **1391–1392**
Crimean-Congo hemorrhagic fever, **1391–1392**
Dengue, **1393–1395**
Ebola viral disease, **1389–1392**
hantaviruses, **1395–1396**
Heartland virus, **1392**
Lassa fever, **1391–1392**
Rift Valley fever, **1391–1393**
severe fever with thrombocytopenia syndrome, **1391–1392**
Songling virus, **1392**
yellow fever, **1396–1397**

Hemorrhagic fever with renal syndrome, **1395–1396**
Hemorrhagic "gastritis," **620–622**
Hemorrhagic shock, **497**
Hemorrhagic stroke, 446, 989*t*. *See also* Stroke
Hemorrhoids, 599, **669–670,** 670
Hemosiderin deposition, 163, 490
Hemosiderosis, 304, 505
Hemostasis and thrombosis disorders, **546–563.** *See also* Antithrombotics; Bleeding; Platelet disorders; *specific types*
  acquired, 546
  coagulation, **557–562**
    acquired, **561–562**
    congenital, **557–561**
    other causes, **562**
  heritable, 546
  patient evaluation, 546, 547*t*
  platelet, **546–557**
    count ranges, desired, 546, 547*t*
    qualitative, **556–557**
    thrombocytopenia, **546–556**
Hemothorax, 310, 311, **312**
Hemotympanum, 208, 211
Henderson-Hasselbalch equation, 894
Henoch-Schönlein purpura, **855–856**
  kidney disease, 923*t*, **927–928**
  typhus, scrub, 1429
Heparin. *See also* Low-molecular-weight heparin; Unfractionated heparin
  for acute coronary syndrome, without ST-segment elevation, 371
  hyperkalemia from, 886
  for intracranial venous thrombosis, 996
  for Kawasaki disease, 1438
  reversal agents, 563, 565*t*
Heparin-induced thrombocytopenia, **552–553,** 553*t*
Heparin-platelet factor 4, 552
Hepatic. *See also* Liver
Hepatic encephalopathy, 704–705
Hepatic failure, acute, **684–686**
Hepatic porphyria, dysautonomia, 984
Hepatic steatosis, 682
Hepatic venous outflow obstruction, **713–714**
Hepatitis, **677–684, 686–693.** *See also specific types*
  acute
    etiology, 677
    posttransfusion, 682
    vaccination, 678, 682
    viral, **686–691**
      acute liver failure, 685
      chronic, **686–691**
  alcoholic, 47, 603
  autoimmune, **691–693**
  chronic, 687
  clinical manifestations, 677–678
  Epstein-Barr virus, 1363
  herpes simplex virus, 1354
  hypoxic, **715**
  injection drug abuse, 1287
  ischemic, **715**
  pregnancy, **816**
  preoperative evaluation/perioperative management, 47
  Q fever, 1435
  rubella, 1373
  varicella, 1360
Hepatitis A
  acute, **677–679,** 678*f*
  screening, gay & bisexual men, 1724, 1724*f*
  vaccine, 796, 1304*t*, 1308*t*
Hepatitis B
  acute, **679–682,** 680*f*, 681*t*
  acute liver failure, 685
  arthritis, 864
  chronic, **687–688**
  cryoglobulinemia, 855
  gay & bisexual men, 1723
  hepatocellular carcinomas, 1610
  membranous nephropathy, 934
  polyarteritis nodosa, 850
  pregnancy, 816
  screening, gay & bisexual men, 1724, 1724*f*
  vaccine, 4*t*, 1304*t*–1305*t*, 1308*t*, 1336
Hepatitis B immune globulin, 68B
Hepatitis C
  acute, **682–684, 689–691,** 690*t*, 691*t*
  acute liver failure, 685
  arthritis, 864
  chronic, **689–690,** 690*t*, 691*t*, 1112
  colorectal cancer, 11
  cryoglobulinemia, **855**
  gay & bisexual men, 1723
  hepatocellular carcinomas, 1610
  immune thrombocytopenia, 548–549
  kidney disease, 923*t*, **930**
  lichen planus, 140
  membranous nephropathy, 934
  pregnancy, 816
  resistance testing, 1325
  screening, gay & bisexual men, 1724, 1724*f*
Hepatitis D
  acute, **684, 687–689**
  acute superimposed on chronic HBV, 687
  chronic, **687–688**
Hepatitis E, **684**
Hepatobiliary cancers, **1609–1617**
  carcinoma of biliary tract, **1612–1614**
  carcinoma of pancreas & ampulla of Vater, **1614–1617**
  hepatocellular adenoma, **718**
  hepatocellular carcinoma, **1609–1612**
Hepatobiliary cytomegalovirus disease, 1366
Hepatocellular adenoma, **718**
Hepatocellular carcinoma, **1609–1612**
  alcohol-associated cirrhosis, 695
  alpha-fetoprotein, 1610, 1611
  autoimmune hepatitis, 692
  cholangitis, primary biliary, 709
  cholelithiasis, 719
  cirrhosis, 701, 706–707
  clinical findings, 1610–1611
  epidemiology, 1610
  fibrolamellar variant, 1610
  hemochromatosis, 710
  hepatic abscess, pyogenic, 717
  hepatic venous outflow obstruction, 713, 714
  hepatitis B, chronic, 687–689
  hepatitis C, chronic, 691
  hepatitis D, 684, 687
  imaging, 675
  liver biopsy & staging, 1611
  non-alcoholic fatty liver disease, 699
  portal hypertension, noncirrhotic, 715
  risk factors, 1610
  screening & prevention, 1611
  treatment, 1598*t*, 1611–1612
Hepatocellular carcinoma-cholangiocarcinoma, combined, 1610
Hepatocellular injury, drugs and toxins, 696–697
Hepatocellular jaundice, liver biochemical tests, 676*t*
Hepatojugular reflux, heart failure, 404
Hepatolenticular degeneration, 163, **711–713**
Hepatomegaly
  alcohol-associated liver disease, 694
  bile duct obstruction, 723
  hemochromatosis, 710
  hepatitis, 678, 692
  jaundice, 675
  nonalcoholic fatty liver disease, 698
  tricuspid stenosis, 350
Hepatopulmonary syndrome, 705
Hepatorenal syndrome, with cirrhosis, 703–704
Hepatosplenomegaly
  beta-thalassemia intermedia, 506
  blood disorders, 500
  G6PD deficiency, 511
  thalassemias, 505
  Waldenström macroglobulinemia, 540
Hepatotoxins. *See also specific types*
  direct, 696
  drugs and toxins, 696–697
  histopathology, 696–697
  indirect, 696
Hepcidin, 501, 502
Heplisav-B, 682
HER1 receptor, 1672*t*
HER2, 1630, 1672*t*
HER2-negative breast cancer, 749–750
HER2-targeted therapy, 752, 753, 758
Herbal supplements. *See also specific types*
  acute liver failure, 685
  liver injury, 696
  poisoning, **1580,** 1580*t*
Herd immunity
  COVID-19 vaccine, 1407–1408
  hand, foot, and mouth disease, 1425
  measles, mumps, and rubella vaccine, 1370
  poliomyelitis vaccine, 1375
  rotavirus vaccine, 1422
HERDOO2 risk scoring system, 572
Hereditary amyloidosis, 541
Hereditary angioedema, 872*t*
Hereditary colorectal cancer & polyposis syndromes, **666–669**
  familial adenomatous polyposis, **667**
  hamartomatous polyposis syndromes, **668**
  Lynch syndrome, **668–669**
Hereditary hemorrhagic telangiectasia, 224, 562, **1665–1666**
Hereditary leiomyoma-renal cell carcinoma, 1645
Hereditary motor and sensory neuropathy (HMSN)
  type I, **1031**
  type II, **1031**
  type III, **1031**
  type IV, **1031**
Hereditary nonpolyposis colon cancer, **668–669,** 791, 1627
Hereditary ovarian cancer syndrome, 793
Hereditary papillary renal cell carcinoma, 1645
Hereditary syndrome neurofibromatosis type 2, **217–218**
Hernia
  hiatal, 588, 614
  vaginal, pelvic organ prolapse, 769
Herniation, lumbar disk, **1686–1687**
Herniation syndromes, 999
Heroin overdose/poisoning, **1587–1588**
Herpangina, enteroviruses, 1423
Herpes-associated erythema multiforme, 153, 1354
Herpes genitalis, pregnancy, **816**
Herpes gingivostomatitis, **230**
Herpes gladiatorum, 1353
Herpes labialis, 1353
Herpes simplex virus, **1353–1357,** 1354*f*, 1356*t*
  anorectal, 671
  Bell palsy, 1026, 1354, 1355
  clinical findings, 1353–1355
  cold fever/sore, **120–121,** 120*f*
  colitis, 1354
  congenital malformations, 1353–1354
  conjunctivitis/keratoconjunctivitis, 170
  disseminated disease, 1354, 1355

encephalitis, 1354, 1355
erythema multiforme, 1354, 1355
esophagitis, 612–613, 1354, 1355
genital, **120–121,** 1284–1286, 1353
gingivostomatitis, 1353
herpes gladiatorum, 1353
herpes labialis, 1353
HIV/AIDS, 1318*t,* 1327, 1327*f*
with impaired cellular immunity, 1273
keratitis, 172, 175*t,* **179,** 1353, 1354, 1355
lesbian & bisexual women, 1719
liver failure/fulminant hepatitis, 1354
meningitis, 1354, 1355
mucocutaneous disease, 1353
neonatal & congenital, 1353–1354, 1355
ocular, 1353, 1354
odynophagia, 607
pneumonia, 1354, 1355
pregnancy, 816
prevalence, 120
prevention, 1355–1357
proctitis, 1354, 1355
retinal necrosis, 1353
retinitis, HIV/AIDS, **193**
solid organ transplant recipients, 1273
stomatitis/gingivostomatitis, **230**
treatment & prophylaxis, 1355, 1356*t*
uveitis, 183, 1353, 1354, 1355
whitlow, 1353, 1354*f*
Herpesviruses, human. *See* Human herpesviruses; *specific types*
Herpes zoster (shingles), **1357–1363,** 1359*f*
clinical findings, 1359
complications, 1360
HIV/AIDS, 1318*t,* 1327
incidence, severity, & age, 1357
postherpetic neuralgia, **978,** 1360
prognosis, 1361
retinitis, 193
stroke, 1360
treatment, 1360–1361
uveitis, 183
vaccination, 4, 1362–1363
zoster sine herpete, 1360
Herpes zoster ophthalmicus, **179–180,** 1359, 1360
Herpes zoster oticus, 1359
Herpetic whitlow, 1353, 1354*f*
Heterosexual, 1709
Heterotypic immunity, 1422
Hexosaminidase deficiency, spinal muscular atrophy, 1029
HFE, 709, 710
HHV-6, **871,** 1358*t*
HHV-7, 1358*t,* 1368
HHV-8+ diffuse large cell lymphoma, 1368
Hiatal hernia, 588, 601, 614
Hiccups, **584–585**
Hidden hearing loss, 212
High-altitude cerebral edema, **1560–1562**
High-altitude illness, **1560–1562**
High-altitude pulmonary edema, **1560–1562**
"High" ankle sprains, **1707–1708**
High-density lipoprotein (HDL) cholesterol, 5*t,* 8, 355, **1202–1203**
High-grade lymphoma, 534
High-grade squamous intraepithelial lesions (HSIL), 788, 789, 792
Highly aggressive lymphoma, 535
Hilar cell tumors, 1181
Hill-Sachs lesions, 1682
Hill sign, 347
Hip, **1692–1695**
fractures, 61, **1692–1694**
osteoarthritis, 820, **1694–1695**
Hippocampal sclerosis, 980
Hirsutism & virilization, **1181–1183**
acromegaly & ACTH-induced Cushing syndrome, 1182
adrenal carcinoma, 1181
diffuse stromal Leydig cell hyperplasia, 1182
dysgerminomas, 1181
female hirsutism, **1181–1183**
contraception for, 774
danazol for, 768
polycystic ovary syndrome, **771, 1181**
hilar cell tumors, 1181
hyperreactio luteinalis, 1182
hypertrichosis lanuginosa, 1182
idiopathic & familial, 1181
luteoma of pregnancy, 1182
ovarian tumors, 1181
pharmacologic causes, 1182
polycystic ovary syndrome, **771, 1181,** 1182
porphyria cutanea tarda, 1182
pure androgen-secreting adrenal tumors, 1181
Sertoli-Leydig tumors, 1181
steroidogenic enzyme defects, **1181**
virilization, pregnancy, 1182
HISORt criteria, 734
Histoplasma (histoplasmosis), **1536–1537**
with impaired cellular immunity, 1273
interstitial nephritis, 911
progressive disseminated, 536
pulmonary, 536
Histoplasma capsulatum, 536
Histrelin, 1602*t,* 1640, 1640*t*
Histrionic personality disorder, **1059–1061,** 1060*t*
HIV/AIDS, **1311–1316.** *See also* Sexually transmitted diseases/infections
anal fissures, 672
aspergillosis, **1543–1544**
cancer, 1328–1330
anal dysplasia & squamous cell carcinoma, 1329–1330
Hodgkin disease, 1329
Kaposi sarcoma, **113,** 1319*t,* 1321, 1324, 1328–1329
non-Hodgkin lymphoma, 1319*t,* 1322, 1329
cardiomyopathy, 417
dilated, 418, 420
case definition, 1311, 1312*t*
CD4 counts, immunodeficiency and, 1311
cervical cancer, 790
children of HIV-positive mothers, 1313
clinical findings, 1314–1316
CD4 count and, 1311, 1314, 1314*f*
laboratory findings, 1315–1316, 1315*t*
symptoms & signs, 1314
course & prognosis, 1351
cryoglobulinemia, **855**
cryptococcal meningitis, **1001**
differential diagnosis, 1316
epidemiology, 1311–1313
eye and lid disorders
retinopathy, **193**
uveitis, 183
fever of unknown origin, 1270
gay & bisexual men, **1723**
hairy leukoplakia, oral, **228,** 228*f*
headache, acute, 35
herpes simplex retinitis, **193**
histoplasmosis, disseminated, **1536–1537**
HSV-2 seropositivity, 1353
HTLV-1/2 with, 1388
immune thrombocytopenia, 548–549
immunizations, recommended, 1301
injection drug abuse, 1287
intracranial mass lesions, **1001**
Kaposi sarcoma, **113**
Korsakoff syndrome, 1096
lesbian & bisexual women, 1719
lymphadenopathy, 242
molluscum contagiosum, 1421
myelopathy, **1026, 1323**
myocarditis, 414, 415*t*
nephropathy, 924*t,* **935**
otitis media, serous, 218
otologic manifestations, 218
pathophysiology, 1313–1315
autoimmunity and allergic & hypersensitivity reactions, **1314**
immunodeficiency, 1311, **1313–1314**
pericarditis, 427
peripheral neuropathies, 1323
P. jirovecii
otitis media, 218
pneumonia, **1538–1541**
polyneuropathy, 1032
pregnancy, **815–816**
prevalence, 1313
prognosis, 1311
progression, 1313
pulmonary hypertension, 432, 432*t,* 433
pulmonary tuberculosis treatment, 285 (*See also* Tuberculosis, pulmonary)
retinal disorders, **193**
rheumatic manifestations, **864**
screening, gay & bisexual men, 1724*f,* 1725
small intestinal lymphoma and, 1625
syphilis with, 1488
testing & counseling, 1331
toxoplasmosis, 1511
transgender & gender diverse people, 1730
transmission
bites, 1283
modes & risks, 1311–1313
uveitis, 183
HIV/AIDS, complications, 1316–1331
CD4 counts on
prophylaxis, 1337
treatment, 1338, 1341, 1344, 1346–1347, 1348*t,* 1349–1350
central nervous system disease, 1321–1323
cryptococcal meningitis, 1318*t,* 1322, 1331
dementia & neurocognitive disorders, 1322
lymphoma, 1322
meningitis & myelopathy, **1026, 1323**
meningococcal meningitis, 1323
progressive multifocal leukoencephalopathy, 1323
toxoplasmosis, 1319*t,* 1322
coronary artery disease, 1330
endocrinologic
hypogonadism, 1326–1327
mineralocorticoid, 1327
thyroid function, 1327
gastrointestinal
biliary disease, 1326
enterocolitis, 1326
esophagitis, candidal and other, 1318*t,* 1325
gastropathy, 1326
hepatic disease, 1325–1326
malabsorption, 1326
gynecologic
cervical dysplasia, 1330
pelvic inflammatory disease, 1330
vaginal candidias, 1318*t,* 1330
inflammatory reactions & immune reconstitution inflammatory syndromes, 1330–1331
malignancies, 1328–1330
anal dysplasia & squamous cell carcinoma, 1329–1330
Hodgkin disease, 1329
Kaposi sarcoma, **113,** 1319*t,* 1321, 1324, 1328–1329
non-Hodgkin lymphoma, 1319*t,* 1322, 1329

HIV/AIDS, complications (*Cont.*):
myopathy, 1324
opportunistic infections, 1318*t*–1319*t*
oral lesions
angular cheilitis, 1324
aphthous ulcers, 1324–1325
candidiasis, 1324–1325
gingival disease, 1324–1325
hairy leukoplakia, 1324
Kaposi sarcoma, 1319*t*, 1324, 1329
warts, 1324
peripheral nervous system disease
inflammatory demyelinating polyneuropathy, 1323
peripheral neuropathy, 1323
prophylaxis
Mycobacterium avium complex, 1337, 1337*t*
Pneumocystis pneumonia, 1337, 1337*t*
toxoplasmosis, 1337
pulmonary disease, 1317–1321
bacterial pneumonia, 1319*t*, 1320
CMV pneumonia, 1321
mycobacterial pneumonia, 1319*t*, 1320, 1320*f*
noninfectious, 1321
Pneumocystis pneumonia, 1274, 1311, 1316, 1317–1320, 1317*f*, 1319*t*
sinusitis, 1321
viral (SARS-CoV-2, etc.), 1321
retinitis, CMV, **193**, 1311, 1318*t*, 1324, 1324*f*
rheumatologic and bone, 1323–1324
arthritis, 1323
osteoporosis & osteopenia, 1323–1324
rheumatologic syndromes, 1323
skin
bacillary angiomatosis, 1328
dermatophytes & *Candida*, 1328
herpes simplex, 1318*t*, 1327, 1327*f*
herpes zoster, 1318*t*, 1327
molluscum contagiosum, 1327, 1328*f*
psoriasis, 1328
seborrheic dermatitis, 1328
staphylococcal, 1327–1328
xerosis, 1328
systemic, 1316–1317
nausea, 1317
weight loss, 1316–1317
treatment, 1337–1338
HIV/AIDS, prevention, **1331–1337**
primary, 1331–1334
ART, decreased transmission risk/ treatment as prevention, **1331**
ART, perinatal transmission, **1334**
ART, postexposure prophylaxis, **1333**
ART, preexposure prophylaxis, 3–4, 1286, **1332,** 1333*t*
blood/blood products, 1334
health care settings, 1334
HIV testing & counseling, 1331, 1334
postexposure prophylaxis, 4, 1286
vaccine, 1334
secondary, 1335–1337
health care maintenance & monitoring, 1335*t*
immunizations, 1335*t*, 1336
other measures, 1336–1337
syphilis, 1336
tuberculosis, 1335–1336
HIV/AIDS, treatment, **1337–1351**
adherence, patient, 1
antiretroviral therapy
as prevention, **1331–1334**
decreased transmission risk/treatment as prevention, **1331**
perinatal transmission, **1334**
postexposure prophylaxis, 4, 1286, **1333**
preexposure prophylaxis, 3–4, 1286, **1332,** 1333*t*
as treatment, **1338–1350,** 1339*t*–1342*t* (*See also* Antiretroviral therapy, for HIV/AIDS)
Hives, 151
HIV retinopathy, **193**
HLA-A3101, carbamazepine and, 1080
HLA-B27
axial spondyloarthritis, 858
IBD-associated spondyloarthritis, 861
psoriatic arthritis, 859
reactive arthritis, 860
seronegative spondyloarthropathies, 858
uveitis, 183
HLA-B1502, carbamazepine and, 1080
HLA-B*1502 allele, 1669*t*
HLA-B*5701 allele, 1670*t*
HLA-B*5801 allele, 1670*t*
HLADQB1, 1067
HLA-DR3, myasthenia gravis, 1040
HLA-DRB1 alleles, 827
HMG-CoA reductase inhibitors (statins)
for acute coronary syndrome, without ST-segment elevation, 372
adverse effects, 1244–1246
for cardiovascular/coronary heart disease, 5*t*, 8, 355, 356*f*, 357–358, 357*t*
for cholesterol, high LDL, 1244–1246, 1245*t*–1246*t*
for heart failure with reduced LVEF, 411
hepatotoxicity, 696
for hypercholesterolemia, 5*t*, 8, 355, 356*f*, 357–358, 357*t*
myopathy from, 1045
surgical risk assessment/reduction, 43
HNF1alpha, 718
Hoaglund sign, 1363
Hoarding, 1052
Hoarseness, **235–236**
Hodgkin disease, 932, 1029, 1329
Hodgkin lymphoma, **535–536,** 1364
Hog. *See* Phencyclidine (PCP)
Holiday heart, 391
Holmium laser enucleation of the prostate, 969
Home safety evaluation, 60
Homicide, 12
Homocysteine metabolism disorders, **1663–1664**
Homocystinuria, **1663–1664**
Homophobia, internalized, 1710, 1722
Honeybee venom allergy, 868–869
Hookworm, 1527, 1530
Hookworm disease, 297, 601, **1527**
Hordeolum, **168,** 169
Horner syndrome, 973, 1603
Hornet venom allergy, 868–869
Hospice, end of life care, 75–76
Hospital-acquired pneumonia, **274–276,** 276*t*, 277*t*
Hospital-associated fever of unknown origin, 1270
Hospital-associated infections, **1276–1279**
Hospital-associated sinusitis, 220
Hospitalization & illness-related disorders, **1096–1098**
Hot flushes, 1186
Hot tub folliculitis, 124–125
Household molds, **1546–1547**
HPV vaccine, 671
HR-positive breast cancer, HER-2 negative, 755
5-$HT_{1b/1d}$ receptor agonists, 971. *See also* *specific types*
5-HT_{1F} receptor agonist, 971
5-HT_3 receptor, 1655
HTLV-1 adult T-cell lymphoma/leukemia (ATL), 1388–1389
HTLV-1-associated myelopathy/tropical spastic paraparesis (HAM/TSP), 1388–1389
Human bites, 1283–1284
Human chorionic gonadotropin
beta-hCG
ectopic pregnancy, 799–800
hydatidiform moles, 800–801
gestational trophoblastic disease, 801
for hypogonadotropic hypogonadism, 962
for oligospermia, 1103
pregnancy, 794, 798, 800
Human epidermal growth factor receptor, 1672*t*
Human growth hormone, 1103
Human herpesviruses, **1353–1368**. *See also specific types*
areas affected, 1353
cytomegalovirus disease, **1365–1368**
Epstein-Barr virus
infectious mononucleosis, **1363–1364**
other conditions, **1364–1365**
HHV-1(HSV1)/HHV-2(HSV2), **1353–1357,** 1354*f*, 1356*t* (*See also* Herpes simplex virus (HSV-1 & HSV-2))
HHV-6, **1368**
HHV-7, 1358*t*, **1368**
HHV-8, **1368**
on HIV risk, 1353
varicella & herpes zoster, **1357–1363,** 1358*t*, 1359*f*
virus shedding, 1353
Human immunodeficiency virus. *See* HIV/AIDS
Human menopausal gonadotropin, 773
Human metapneumovirus, 1409
Human papillomavirus
anal cancers, **1633–1634**
anal dysplasia/squamous cell carcinoma, HIV/AIDS, 1329–1330
cervical cancer,1330, 790
cervical dysplasia, HIV/AIDS, 1330
cervical intraepithelial neoplasia, **787–789**
condylomata acuminata, **121–123,** 122*f*, 671, **787**
gay & bisexual men, 1723
inverted papillomas, 226
laryngeal cancer, 238–240
lesbian & bisexual women, 1719
neck masses, 241
oropharyngeal squamous cell carcinoma, 228–229
recurrent respiratory papillomatosis, 237
STDs, 1284–1286
vaccine, 4*t*, 671, 788–789, 1302*t*–1303*t*, 1305*t*, 1308*t*
cancer prevention, 11–12
gay & bisexual men, 1724*t*, 1725
lesbian & bisexual women, 1720
pregnancy, 796, 1302*t*–1303*t*
warts from, 122
Human parainfluenza viruses, 1409
Human parechovirus, **1425–1426**
Human RIG, 1378–1379
Human T-cell leukemia virus, **1026–1027**
Human T-cell lymphotropic virus, **1388–1389**
"Humidifier" lung, 307*t*
Humidity, on heat disorders, 1548
Humoral immunity, impaired, 1272–1273. *See also* Immunodeficiency disorders/immunocompromised
Hunter canal, 475
huntingin gene, 1010
Huntington disease, **1010–1011**

Huntington disease–like disorders, 1010
Hurler syndrome, restrictive cardiomyopathy, 423
Hutchinson sign, 1359, 1360
HVD DNA, hepatitis B, 681
Hyaline casts, 904*t*, 907, 907*t*
Hyaluronic acid, 1705
Hyaluronidase-fihj, 538
Hydatidiform mole, **800–802**
Hydralazine
  autoimmune hypoglycemia from, 1237
  drug-induced nephritis from, 837
  for heart failure with reduced LVEF, 409–410
  for hypertension, 463*t*, 464, 470–472, 471*t*
  for preeclampsia-eclampsia, 804
Hydrocarbon poisoning, 1589
Hydrocephalus, 994, 1016, 1384
Hydrochlorothiazide
  for hypertension, 451*t*, 453*t*, 455, 458*t*, 459*t*, 461*t*–462*t*
  for insulinoma, 1235
  photosensitivity from, 156
Hydrocodone, 85*t*, **89*t***, 93
Hydrocortisone
  for ACTH deficiency, adrenal insufficiency, 1159
  for adrenal insufficiency, 1159
  for anterior hypopituitarism, 1102
  for atopic dermatitis, 134
  for candidiasis, mucocutaneous, 119
  clinical uses, 1193, 1194*t*
  for pruritus, 101
  for seborrheic dermatitis, 139
  for thyrotoxic crisis/thyroid storm, 1127
  for ulcerative colitis, 659–660, 661
Hydrocortisone acetate, 102*t*
Hydrocortisone-pramoxine, 161
Hydrogenated starch hydrolysates, 1203
Hydrogen peroxide, 1421
Hydromorphone, **88*t***
  intrathecal, 97, 97*t*
  morphine milligram equivalent doses, 85*t*
  neuromodulatory therapy, 97*t*
  patient-controlled analgesia, 80
  poisoning, **1587–1588**
Hydrops, gallbladder, 721
Hydrops fetalis, 505
Hydroquinone, pigmentation changes from, 164
Hydroxocobalamin, 1580
Hydroxychloroquine
  for immune-mediated inflammatory myopathies, 844
  for lichen planus, 141
  for lupus nephritis, 930
  ocular effects, adverse, 199, 202*t*
  for palindromic rheumatism, 868
  for photodermatitis, 156
  for pompholyx, 145
  for Q fever, 1436
  for systemic lupus erythematosus, 835
Hydroxychloroquine sulfate
  for cutaneous lupus erythematosus, 142
  retinal toxicity, 830
  for rheumatoid arthritis, 830
  triple therapy, 830
Hydroxymethylglutaryl coenzyme A reductase inhibitors. *See* HMG-CoA reductase inhibitors (statins)
5-Hydroxytryptamine subtype 3, 1655
Hydroxyurea, 513
Hydroxyzine, 107, 135, 152, 1050*t*, 1083
Hymenolepis diminuta, 1523
Hymenolepis nana, 1523
Hyoscyamine, 646
Hyoscyamus niger poisoning, 1577
Hyperactive delirium, 58
Hyperacusis, **214**
Hyperadrenergic postural orthostatic syndrome, 985
Hyperaldosteronism, **1164–1166**
  diagnosis & workup, 445
  primary, 445, 884
Hyperalgesia, 85
Hyperandrogenism
  acne vulgaris, 147
  amenorrhea, 1184, 1185
  polycystic ovary syndrome, 771
Hyperbaric oxygen, 1578–1579
Hyperbilirubinemia
  autoimmune hepatitis, 693
  biliary stricture, 725
  conjugated/unconjugated, 674–675, 675*t*
  disorders, 675, 676*t*
  intrahepatic cholestasis of pregnancy, 674, 676*t*, **818**
  jaundice, **674, 675*t*, 676*t***
Hypercalcemia, **889–890**
  artifactual, 1143
  calcitriol-induced, 917
  cancer-related, 889, **1650–1651**
  chronic kidney disease, 917
  hyperparathyroidism, 1142
  plasma cell myeloma, 941
Hypercalcemia of malignancy, 1144
Hypercalciuria
  absorptive, 956
  calcium nephrolithiasis, 956
  renal calciuria, 956
  resorptive, 956
Hypercapnia, **901**
Hypercarotenoid, 1262
Hyperchloremic metabolic acidosis, normal anion gap, 896*t*, **897–898,** 897*t*
  RTA type I, 897*t*, 898
  RTA type II, 897*t*, 898
  RTA type IV, hyporeninemic hypoaldosteronemic, 897*t*, 898
Hypercholesterolemia. *See also* Lipid disorders
  aortic stenosis, 342
  coronary heart disease, 355, 356*f*
    prevention, 355, 356*f*, **357–358**
  familial, **1239, 1660–1661**
  high-fiber diets for, 1264
  niacin for, 1260
  screening & treatment, **1241–1243,** 1242*t*
    in older patients, 1243
  statins for, 5*t*, 8, 355, 356*f*, 357–358, 357*t*, 372
Hypercoagulable state, 190, 932
Hypercortisolism, **1160–1164**. *See also* Cushing disease (syndrome)
Hyperemesis gravidarum, **796–797,** 1096
Hyperemic stages, immersion foot/hand, 1552
Hypergammaglobulinemia, 538, 733
Hypergastrinemia, 632
Hyperglycemia. *See also* Diabetes mellitus; *specific disorders*
  diabetes, occult, 1236
  diabetic ketoacidosis, 896*t*, 897, **1226–1230,** 1226*t*, 1227, 1228, 1230 (*See also* Diabetic ketoacidosis)
  from fluoroquinolones, 1237
  hyperkalemia, 885
  medications for, 1203–1211, 1204*t*
    acarbose, 1204*t*, 1208
    bromocriptine, 1211
    colesevelam, 1211
    combinations, 1211
    D-phenylalanine derivatives, 1204*t*, 1206–1207
      nateglinide, 1204*t*, 1206–1207, 1218, 1218*f*, 1220
      repaglinide, 1204*t*, 1206, 1218, 1218*f*
    DPP-4 inhibitors, 1205*t*, 1210
      alogliptin, 1205*t*, 1210
      linagliptin, 1205*t*, 1210
      saxagliptin, 1205*t*, 1210
      sitagliptin, 1205*t*, 1210
      vildagliptin, 1205*t*, 1210
    GLP-1 receptor agonists, 1204*t*–1205*t*, 1208–1210
      dulaglutide, 1204*t*, 1209
      exenatide, 1204*t*, 1209
      liraglutide, 1205*t*, 1209
      lixisenatide, 1205*t*, 1209
      semaglutide, 1205*t*, 1209
    incretins, 1204*t*, 1208–1210
    meglitinide analogs
      mitiglinide, 1204*t*, 1206
      repaglinide, 1204*t*, 1206
    metformin, 1204*t*, 1207
    miglitol, 1204*t*, 1208
    pramlintide, 1205*t*, 1211
    sodium-glucose co-transporter 2 inhibitors, 1205*t*, 1210–1211
      canagliflozin, 1205*t*, 1210–1211
      dapagliflozin, 1205*t*, 1210
      empagliflozin, 1205*t*, 1210
      ertugliflozin, 1205*t*, 1210
    sulfonylureas, 1203–1206, 1204*t*
      glyburide, glipizide, gliclazide, and glimepiride, 1204*t*, 1206
      tolazamide, acetohexamide, and chlorpropamide, 1204*t*, 1206
      tolbutamide, 1204*t*, 1206
    thiazolidinediones, 1204*t*, 1207–1208
      rosiglitazone and pioglitazone, 1204*t*, 1207–1208
      troglitazone, 1208
  prebreakfast, on insulin therapy, 1217
Hyperglycemic coma, 1226
Hyperglycemic hyperosmolar coma, 1199
Hyperglycemic hyperosmolar state, **1230–1232**
Hypergonadotropic hypogonadism, 962, 1175–1176
Hyperhomocysteinemia, 189, **1663–1664**
Hyperinsulinemia. *See* Diabetes mellitus; *specific disorders*
Hyperkalemia, **884–886,** 885*t*, 887*t*
  acute kidney injury, 906
  acute tubular necrosis, 909
  chronic kidney disease, 918
  kidney diseases, 885
  postoperative, 51
  rhabdomyolysis, 885, 885*t*, 886
Hyperkalemic periodic paralysis, 885, 1045
Hyperkinetic seizure, 979
Hyperlactatemia, 880, 1232
Hyperlipidemia. *See also* Metabolic syndrome; *specific types*
  from antipsychotics, 1066, 1066*t*
  nephrotic spectrum glomerular diseases, 932
  retinal artery occlusion, **189–190**
Hypermagnesemia, **894**
Hypernatremia, **880–882**
Hyperoxaluric calcium nephrolithiasis, 956–957
Hyperparathyroidism, **1141–1146**
  "asymptomatic" primary, 1144
  classification, 1141–1142
  clinical findings, 1142–1143
  complications, 1143
  differential diagnosis, 1143–1144
  hypercalcemia, **889–890,** 889*t*, 890
  myopathy, 1045
  normocalcemic primary, 1142
  pancreatitis, chronic, 733
  pregnancy, 1142
  treatment, 1144–1146

Hyperphosphatemia, **892,** 892*t*
acute kidney injury, 906
acute tubular necrosis, 909
calcitriol-induced, 917
chronic kidney disease, 917, 917*f*
treatment, 917
Hyperpigmentation
from chlorpromazine, 1067
drug-induced, 158*t*
lower extremity edema, 28
mosaic, 163
nail, 166
post-inflammatory, 163
primary, **163**
secondary, **163,** 163*f*
from UV light, 164
Hyperprolactinemia, **1108–1110,** 1108*t*
hypogonadotropic hypogonadism, 1102–1103
Hyperproteinemia. *See also specific disorders*
pseudohyponatremia, 880
Hyperreactio luteinalis, 1182
Hypersensitivity disorders. *See also specific types*
minimal change disease, 932
penicillin allergy, 1300
pneumonitis, **307–308,** 307*t*
Hypersensitivity reactions, **870–872**
blood transfusions, 543
drug (*See also specific drugs; specific types*)
allopurinol, 825
HHV-6, 1368
ophthalmic, topical, 199, 199*f*
drug, delayed, **871–872**
acute generalized exanthematous pustulosis, **871–872**
aspirin- and NSAID-exacerbated respiratory disease, 245, **872**
drug exanthems, **871**
drug-induced hypersensitivity syndrome, **871**
drug reaction with eosinophilia and systemic symptoms, **30,** 157, 696, **871**
severe cutaneous adverse reactions, **871–872**
acute generalized exanthematous pustulosis, **871–872**
drug-induced hypersensitivity syndrome, **871**
drug reaction with eosinophilia and systemic symptoms, **30,** 157, 696, **871**
Stevens-Johnson syndrome/toxic epidermal necrolysis, 871
Stevens-Johnson syndrome/toxic epidermal necrolysis, 871
HIV/AIDS, 1314, **1314**
IgE-mediated immediate, **870**
immediate, **868–870**
anaphylaxis, **869–870,** 869*t*
food allergy, **868**
IgE-mediated, **870**
non–IgE-mediated, **870**
venom allergy, **868–869**
RBC transfusions, 543
Hypersomnias, **1084**
breathing-related sleep disorders, **1084**
Kleine-Levin syndrome, **1084**
narcolepsy syndrome, **1084**
periodic limb movement disorder, **1084**
shift work sleep disorder, **1084**
Hypertension, 182, 183, **442–472,** 447. *See also* Blood pressure
acute MI, with ST-segment elevation, 373
angina pectoris, 360, 363, 364*f*
aortic regurgitation, 347, 348
aortic stenosis, 342, 345
atrial fibrillation, stroke prevention, 391, 392, 393, 393*t*
autosomal dominant polycystic kidney disease, 940
blood pressure measurement & diagnosis, **442–444**
definitions & guidelines, 365, 442, 443*f*
labile hypertension, 444
masked hypertension, 444
measurement methods, times, and values, 442, 443*t*
readings, number, 442
sphygmomanometer, 442
"white coat" hypertension, **442–444,** 468
cardiomyopathy
dilated, 418
hypertrophic, 418*t*, 421
restrictive, 423
cardiovascular risk factors, 448, 449*t*
chronic kidney disease, 451*t*–453*t*, 458*t*–459*t*, 915–916
clinical findings, 446–448, 447*f*
coarctation of the aorta, **325–326**
combined oral contraceptives and, 774
complications
aortic dissection, 446
atherosclerosis, 446
cardiovascular disease, 446
cerebrovascular disease & dementia, 446
kidney disease, 446
coronary heart disease/prevention, 355, 357
definition, AHA, 365, 442, 443*f*
diabetes mellitus, 1224
drug-induced
amphetamines, 1566
anticholinergics, 1566
cocaine, 1566
MAO inhibitors, 1566
performance-enhancing products, 1566
Eisenmenger physiology, **326**
elderly, 442
end-stage kidney disease, 914
epidemiology, 8, 442
etiology & classification, **444–446**
primary essential, **444**
secondary, causes, **444–446,** 444*t*
coarctation of aorta, 325, 445
Cushing syndrome, 445
estrogen use, 446
genetic, 445
Gordon syndrome, 445
hyperaldosteronism, primary, 445
kidney disease, 445
Liddle syndrome, 445
metabolic syndrome, 444
other, 446
pheochromocytoma, 445
pregnancy, 445–446
pseudohypoaldosteronism type II, 445
renal vascular hypertension, 445
fibrinolytics with, risks, 375–376
heart failure, 403–407, 410, 412, 413
hemorrhagic stroke, 446
hypertensive urgencies & emergencies, **468–472** (*See also* Hypertensive urgencies & emergencies)
intracerebral hemorrhage, 992
intracranial, idiopathic, 974, **1003–1005**
ischemic stroke, 446
labile, 444
lesbian & bisexual women, 1716
malignant, headache, 35
masked, 444
morbidity & mortality, 442
NSAIDs and, 444
obesity, 444
ocular/ocular effects
age-related macular degeneration, 187
glaucoma, 182, 183
hypertensive retinochoroidopathy, 192–193
optic disc swelling, 195
retinal artery occlusion, 189
patent foramen ovale, 328
polycythemia and, 444
portal (*See* Portal hypertension)
portopulmonary, cirrhosis, 705
potassium on, dietary, 1264
pregnancy/gestational, **435,** 436*f*, 437*t*, 438, 445, **811–812** (*See also* Eclampsia; Preeclampsia-eclampsia)
preeclampsia-eclampsia, **802–804,** 803*t*
preeclampsia superimposed on, 811
preoperative evaluation/perioperative management, 45–46
pulmonary valve regurgitation, 352
renal artery stenosis, **921–922**
resistant hypertension, 468, 469*t*
retinal artery occlusion, 189
screening/prevention, 4, 5*t*, 8–9
secondary, 444–446, 444*t*
stress and, 444
supine, with orthostatic hypotension, 468
systemic lupus erythematosus, 834
treatment, nonpharmacologic, 444, 448, 448*t*, **464**
tricuspid valve regurgitation, 351
Hypertension, pulmonary, **301–303, 431–433**
atrial septal defect, 326–328
classification, 431–432, 432*t*
cocaine, 432
combined pre-/post-, 431
definition, 301
dyspnea, 18, 19, 20
Eisenmenger physiology/syndrome, 432, 433
hemoptysis, 21
left heart disease, 432
lung disease/hypoxemia, 301
mechanisms, unclear/multifactorial, 301
mitral regurgitation, 338, 339, 341
mitral stenosis, **332–338,** 333*t*–335*t*
myocarditis, 415
from obstruction, 301
pericardial diseases, **431–433**
pericardial fluid, 430
post-capillary, isolated, 431
precapillary, 431
pregnancy, 435, 437*t*, 812
pulmonary valve regurgitation, 352
sickle cell anemia, 512
syncope, cardiogenic, 402
venous, 405, 415
ventricular septal defect, **328–330**
Hypertension, treatment, **177*t*–178*t***
African Americans, 467, 467*t*
chronic kidney disease, 466–467, 467*t*
coexisting conditions, 467*t*
demographics on, 465, 466*t*
diabetes, 466, 467*t*
duration, 450
follow-up, 468
goals, 449–450, 449*t*
indications, 448, 449*t*
nocturnal, 468
nonadherence, 465–466
older adults, 467
other risk factors, 450
pharmacologic, **177*t*–178*t*, 450–464**
aldosterone receptor antagonists, **455,** 458*t*–459*t*
alpha-antagonists, **460,** 463*t*
angiotensin converting-enzyme inhibitors, 382, **450–454,** 451*t*–452*t*

angiotensin II receptor blockers, 452t–453t, **454**
arteriolar dilators, 463t, **464**
beta-blockers, **455, 460,** 461t–462t
calcium channel blockers, 378, **454–455,** 456t–457t
cancer risk, **464**
central sympatholytic action, **460,** 463t
diuretics, **455,** 458t–459t
peripheral sympathetic inhibitors, **460,** 463t, **464**
regimen development, **464–465,** 465t, 466t
renin inhibitors, **454**
risk reduction, 365
sex-specific considerations, 466
supine hypertension with orthostatic hypotension, 468
Hypertensive crisis, 193, 445
Hypertensive retinochoroidopathy, **192–193**
Hypertensive retinopathy, 447, 447f
Hypertensive urgencies & emergencies, **468–472**
acute aortic dissection, 469, 470t
definitions, 468–469
intracerebral hemorrhage, 469, 470t
stroke, acute ischemic, 469, 470t
treatment, approach, 469, 470t
treatment, pharmacologic, parenteral, **469–472**
bumetanide, 470
captopril, 471t, 472
clevidipine, 470, 470t, 471t
clonidine, 471t, 472
diuretics, loop, 470, 471t
enalaprilat, 470, 471t
esmolol, 470, 470t, 471t
fenoldopam, 470, 470t, 471t
furosemide, 470, 471t
hydralazine, 470–472, 471t
labetalol, 470, 470t, 471t
nicardipine, 469–470, 470t, 471t
nifedipine, 471t, 472
nitroglycerin, 471t, 472
nitroprusside sodium, 471t, 472
by site of end-organ damage, 469, 470t
Hyperthecosis, 1181, **1181**
Hyperthermia, **29–31, 1548**
definition and pathophysiology, 30
malignant, 30, 1277
from poisoning, **1567**
serotonin syndrome, 1567
Hyperthyroidism, **1119–1127,** 1121t, 1123t
from amiodarone, 384t, 1120
angina pectoris, 359
apathetic, 1120, 1127
classification, 1119–1120
complications, 1123
differential diagnosis, 1122
dyspnea, 19
endocrine shock, 496
Graves disease, 1119
hCG-secreting trophoblastic tumors, 1120
heart failure, 404, 419
hyperemesis gravidarum, 797
iodine-induced, 1120
laboratory findings, 1121–1122, 1121t
from levothyroxine, 1138
medication-induced, 1120
myopathy, 1045
overt, 810
palpitations, 25, 26
pregnancy, 810, 1120, 1122
preoperative evaluation/perioperative management, 50
prognosis, 1127
radioisotope uptaking/imaging, 1122
stress cardiomyopathy, 420
from struma ovarii, 1120
symptoms & signs, 1121
testicular choriocarcinoma, 1120
from thyroid cancer, 1133
thyroiditis, 1115
autoimmune, 1112, 1119, 1127
subacute, 1112, 1119, 1127
thyrotoxicosis factitia, 1120
toxic multinodular goiter & thyroid nodules, 1119
treatment, 1123–1127
amiodarone-induced thyrotoxicosis, 1126
complications, 1126–1127
apathetic hyperthyroidism, 1127
atrial fibrillation, 1126–1127
Graves dermopathy, 1127
heart failure, 1127
from postpartum thyroiditis, 1127
sinus tachycardia, 1126
thyroid acropachy, 1127
thyrotoxic crisis/thyroid storm, 1127
thyrotoxic hypokalemic periodic paralysis, 1127
Graves dermopathy, 1127
Graves disease, 1123–1125, 1123t
iodinated contrast agents, 1123t, 1124
iodine, radioactive, 1123t, 1124–1125
lithium carbonate, 1123t, 1124
pregnancy planning/pregnancy/lactation, 1126
propranolol, 1123, 1123t
thiourea drugs, 1123–1124, 1123t
with thyroiditis, 1125–1126
thyroid surgery, 1125
thyrotoxic hypokalemic periodic paralysis, 1127
toxic nodular goiter, 1125
toxic solitary thyroid nodules, 1125
from tyrosine kinase inhibitors, 1120
weight loss, 26
Hyperthyroiditis, thyrotoxicosis, 25
Hypertonic hyponatremia, 876, 880
Hypertrichosis lanuginosa, 1182
Hypertriglyceridemia, 1239, **1248–1249**
alcohol use, 1241
diabetes mellitus, 1241
eruptive xanthomas, 1241
gallstones, 719
lipemia retinalis, 1241
niacin for, 1260
pseudohyponatremia, 880
treatment
diet therapy, 1243
pharmacologic, 1244
algorithms, 1248, 1248f
bile acid–binding resins, 1245t, 1247–1248
fibric acid derivatives, 1245t, 1248
omega-3 fatty acids, 1245t, 1247
statins, 1244, 1245t–1246t
Hypertrophic cardiomyopathy, 404, 418t, **421–423**
asymmetrical septal, 418t, 421, 439
athlete screening, 438–439, 439t, 440t
atrial fibrillation, 421, 422
heart failure, 404
interventions on, 336t
mitral regurgitation, 339
palpitations, 26
Valsalva maneuver, 336t, 421, 422
Hypertrophy
athletic, 421
hypertension, 447
Hyperuricemia
acute tubular necrosis from, 909
cancer-related, **1651–1652**
diabetes mellitus, 1225
gouty arthritis, 823, 824t
plasma cell myeloma, 941
treatment, asymptomatic, 824
Hyperuricosuric calcium nephrolithiasis, 956
Hyperventilation, 315, **315,** 1232
Hyperviscosity (syndrome), 190, 537, 540
Hypervitaminosis. *See specific vitamins*
Hypervolemic hyponatremia, 877f, 878
Hyphema, eye contusion, **197–198**
Hypnagogic hallucinations, 1084
Hypnosis, 1054, 1057
Hypnotics, 1083. *See also specific types*
Hypoactive delirium, 58
Hypoactive sexual desire disorder, **1058**
Hypoalbunemia, 594
anasarca, 603
ascites, 602t
Crohn disease, 653
hypocalcemia, 888
protein-losing enteropathy, 635, 643
ulcerative colitis, 658–659
Hypoaldosteronism, 885t, 897t, 898
Hypobaric hypoxia
air travel, 1562
high-altitude illness, 1561
Hypocalcemia, **886–888**
chronic kidney disease, 917, 917f
rhabdomyolysis, 888t
seizures from, 1567
Hypochondriasis, 1053. *See also* Somatic symptom disorder
Hypochromic microcytic anemia, 504
Hypocitraturic calcium nephrolithiasis, 957
Hypogammaglobulinemia, secondary, **874**
Hypoglossal nerve stimulation, 317
Hypoglycemia
after gastric surgery, **1236**
alcohol-related, 1091, 1233
autoimmune, **1237**
ethanol-induced, **1237–1238**
factitious, **1237**
fasting, 1233, 1233t
functional alimentary, **1236**
immunopathologic, 1233
from insulin therapy, 1219
medication-induced, **1237**
nonislet cell tumor, **1236**
from pancreatic B cell tumor, **1233–1236,** 1234t
postprandial, 1233, 1233t, **1236–1237**
after gastric surgery, **1236**
autoimmune hypoglycemia, **1237**
diabetes, occult, **1236–1237**
functional alimentary hypoglycemia, **1236**
seizures from, 1567
Hypoglycemic agents, oral. *See also specific types*
poisoning, 1568t, **1582**
preoperative evaluation/perioperative management, 49–50
tremor from, 1012
Hypoglycemic coma, 1226
Hypoglycemic states, **1233–1238**
differential diagnosis, 1233, 1233t
factitious hypoglycemia, **1237**
hypoglycemia, from pancreatic B cell tumor, **1233–1236,** 1234t
insulin receptor antibodies, 1197, **1237**
medication- & ethanol-induced hypoglycemia, **1237–1238**
nonislet cell tumor hypoglycemia, **1236**
postprandial hypoglycemia, 1233, 1233t, **1236–1237**
after gastric surgery, **1236**
autoimmune hypoglycemia, **1237**
diabetes, occult, **1236–1237**
functional alimentary hypoglycemia, **1236**

Hypoglycemic unawareness, 1219–1220, 1233
Hypogonadism
HIV/AIDS, 1326–1327
hypergonadotropic, 962, 1175–1176
hypogonadotropic, 962, 1175, 1176
male, **1175–1179,** 1175*t*, 1177*t*
primary, 962
secondary, 962
Hypogonadotropic hypogonadism, 962, 1175, 1176
anterior hypopituitarism, 1100–1101
congenital, 1100
female, 1101
hyperprolactinemia, 1102–1103
male, 1101
Hypokalemia, **882–884,** 882*t*, 883*f*
Hypokalemic periodic paralysis, 1045, 1121, 1127
Hypomagnesemia, **893**
Hyponatremia, **876–880,** 877*f*
adrenal insufficiency, primary, 1156, 1159, 1160
after transsphenoidal pituitary surgery, 1110, 1162
anterior hypopituitarism, 1101, 1102
central diabetes insipidus, 1104
cosyntropin stimulation test, 1111
definition & development, 876
from desmopressin, 1105
encephalitis, 1354
hypothyroidism, 1116, 1117, 1118, **1118**
osteoporosis, 1148*t*
pituitary macroadenoma, 1111
seizures from, 1567
Sheehan syndrome, 1100
syndrome of inappropriate ADH secretion, 1116, 1153
treatment, 879–880
vasopressin deficiency, central diabetes insipidus, 1104–1105
Hyponatremia, hypotonic, 876–878, 880
ADH-dependent
adrenal insufficiency and hypothyroidism, **878**
exercise-associated hyponatremia, **878**
hypervolemic hyponatremia, 877*f*, 878
hypovolemic hyponatremia, 877–878, 877*f*
nausea, pain, and surgery, **878**
reset osmostat, **878**
syndrome of inappropriate ADH secretion, **878,** 878*t*, **879**
thiazide diuretics & other medications, **878**
ADH-independent
beer potomania and "tea and toast" diet, 877
psychogenic polydipsia, 876–877
renal impairment, 877
Hyponatremia, isotonic & hypertonic, 876, 880
hypertonic hyponatremia, 876
pseudohyponatremia, 876, 880
Hypoparathyroidism, **1138–1141,** 1140*t*
anterior, anterior pituitary hormones, 1099
myopathy, 1045
primary, hypocalcemia, 888
Hypophosphatasia, 1153
Hypophosphatemia, **890–892,** 891*t*, 1153
Hypophysitis, anterior hypopituitarism, 1099
Hypopigmentation, **163–164**
Hypopituitarism
acquired, 1100
anterior, **1099–1103** (*See also* Anterior hypopituitarism)
central, 1101
congenital, 1100
functional, 1100
ischemic stroke, 1100
spontaneous subarachnoid hemorrhage, 994, 1100
Hypopituitarism, anterior, **1099–1103**
Hypoprothrombinemia, from cirrhosis, 705
Hypopyon, 179, 180, 183
Hyporeninemic hypoaldosteronemic renal tubular acidosis, 897*t*, 898
Hyporeninemic hypoaldosteronism, 897*t*, 898
Hyposmia, **223–224**
Hypotension
acute MI with ST-segment elevation, 380–381
chronic idiopathic orthostatic, 402
definition, 496
orthostatic (*See* Orthostatic hypotension)
poisoning, **1565**
postprandial, 985
postural, 984, 985
shock, **495–499** (*See also* Shock)
Hypothalamus
arginine vasopressin synthesis, 1099
hormones (*See also specific hormones*)
pituitary regulatory, 1099
oxytocin synthesis, 1099
Hypothalamus disorders, **1099–1105**. *See also specific types*
central diabetes insipidus, **1104–1105**
hypogonadotropic hypogonadism, 1101
hypopituitarism, anterior, **1099–1103**
Hypothermia
accidental systemic, **1550–1552,** 1551*f*
ECG, 1551, 1551*f*
extremities, **1552–1553**
frostbite, **1552**
frostnip & chilblain, **1552**
immersion foot/hand, **1552**
poisoning, **1565**
stages, 1551
systemic, 1550
treatment, 1551–1552
Hypothyroidism, **878, 1114–1119,** 1117*t*
from amiodarone, 1115
from autoimmune thyroiditis, 1112, 1113, 1115
central, 1101
chronic kidney disease, 919
clinical findings, 1115–1116, 1116*t*, 1117*t*
complications, 1116–1117
differential diagnosis, 1116
endocrine shock, 496
goiter, 1115
gout, 823
hyponatremia, 878, 1118
hypotonic hyponatremia, **878**
on lipid metabolism, 1241
myopathy, 1045
obstructive sleep apnea, 316
overt, defined, 809
pregnancy, 1116
overt, 809–810
subclinical, 810
preoperative evaluation/perioperative management, 50
subclinical, 810, 1116
treatment
initial, 1117–1118
monitoring & optimizing, 1118–1119
TSH, elevated serum, 1118
TSH, low/suppressed serum, 1118–1119
TSH, normal serum, 1118
pregnancy, 1117, 1118
prognosis, 1119
Hypotonic hyponatremia, **876–878,** 880
ADH-dependent
adrenal insufficiency and hypothyroidism, **878**
exercise-associated hyponatremia, **878**
hypervolemic hyponatremia, 877*f*, 878
hypovolemic hyponatremia, 877–878, 877*f*
nausea, pain, and surgery, **878**
reset osmostat, **878**
syndrome of inappropriate ADH secretion, **878,** 878*t*, **879**
thiazide diuretics & other medications, **878**
ADH-independent
beer potomania and "tea and toast" diet, 877
psychogenic polydipsia, 876–877
renal impairment, 877
hypervolemic hyponatremia, 877*f*, 878
hypovolemic hyponatremia, 877–878, 877*f*
Hypoventilation, sleep-related, **1084**
Hypovitaminosis D. *See* Vitamin D, deficiency
Hypovolemia, prerenal azotemia, 906
Hypovolemic hyponatremia, 877–878, 877*f*
Hypovolemic shock, **495–499,** 495*t*
Hypoxemia
orthostatic, patent foramen ovale, 327
pulmonary hypertension, 301
Hypoxia
high-altitude illness, **1560–1562**
hypobaric
air travel, 1562
high-altitude illness, 1561
seizures from, 1567
shock, 495
Hypoxic hepatitis, **715**
Hypoxic lactic acidosis, 896
Hypoxic stress, 1561
Hysterical personality disorder, **1059–1061,** 1060*t*
Hysterosalpingography, 764*t*
Hysteroscopy, 764, 764*t*

I

Iatrogenic Creutzfeldt-Jakob disease, 1385–1386
Iatrogenic Kaposi sarcoma, **113**
Iatrogenic osmotic demyelination syndrome, 879–880
Iatrogenic pneumothorax, 313
Ibalizumab, **1341*t*, 1346**
Ibandronate, 1149
Ibandronate sodium, 1150
IBD-associated spondyloarthritis, **861**
Ibrexafungerp, 1535, 1540*t*
Ibrutinib, 531, 535, 540, 1601*t*
Ibuprofen, **83*t***
anion gap elevation from, 1570
for dysmenorrhea, 767
for knee osteoarthritis, 1705
for migraine headache, 971
Ibutilide, 383, 385*t*, 395, 397
"Ice," 1093
Ice water immersion, 1550
Icosapent ethyl, 358, 1245*t*, 1247, 1249
I COUGH, 47
Icterus, **674–677,** 676*t*, 677*t*. *See also* Jaundice
Idarubicin, 417, 1575, 1599*t*
Idarucizumab, 395
Idelalisib, 531, 534
Identity, sexual, 1709
IDH1/2, 1672*t*
Idiopathic aplastic anemia, 516–517, 516*t*
Idiopathic brachial plexopathy, 1040
Idiopathic duct-centric chronic pancreatitis, 733
Idiopathic interstitial pneumonias, 293, 294*t*

Idiopathic intracranial hypertension, 974, **1003–1005**
Idiopathic pulmonary fibrosis, 293, 295*f*
Idiopathic pulmonary hemosiderosis, 304
Idiopathic sudden sensory hearing loss, 204, **212, 213**
Idiopathic torsion dystonia, **1011**
Idioventricular rhythm, accelerated, acute MI with ST-segment elevation, 379
Idoxuridine, 1356*t*
Ifosfamide, 943, 1598*t*, **1656**
IgA
- deficiency, selective, **873**
- nephropathy, 923*t*, **927**
- vasculitis, **855–856**
  - kidney disease, 923*t*, **927–928**

IgE
- anaphylaxis, 869
- immediate hypersensitivity reactions, **870**

IgG_4
- disease, **846–847**
- thyroiditis, **1112–1114**

IgG-RT, 874
IgG subclasses, 874
IgM hypergammaglobulinemia, 538
IgVH, chronic lymphocytic leukemia, 531
Ileus, 638, **638–639**, 1066
Iliac artery occlusion, **473–474**
Iliac vein compression, 28
Iloperidone, 1063, 1064*t*, 1065*t*
Iloprost, 841
- portopulmonary hypertension, 705

Imatinib, 525, 1601*t*, 1625, 1656
Imidazoles. *See also specific types*
- hepatitis from, 1325
- for tinea manuum/pedis, 105*t*, 117
- for tinea versicolor, 105*t*, 118

Imipenem
- for *Bacteroides fragilis*, 1472
- for chest infections, anaerobic, 1472, 1472*t*
- for depression, 1076
- for *Mycobacterium abscessus, M. chelonae, M. fortuitum*, 1475
- for necrotizing fasciitis, 1442
- for nocardiosis, 1475
- for pancreatitis, sterile necrotizing, 732

Imipenem/cilastatin, 1652
Imipramine, 646, 1073*t*, 1084
Imiquimod
- for actinic keratosis, 111
- for basal cell carcinoma, 112
- for Bowen disease, 114
- for molluscum contagiosum, 121, 1421
- for squamous cell carcinoma, 111
- for warts
  - genital, 123
  - vulvar, 787

Immediate hypersensitivity reactions, **868–870**
- anaphylaxis, **869–870**, 869*t*
- food allergy, **868**
- IgE-mediated, **870**
- non–IgE-mediated, **870**
- venom allergy, **868–869**

Immersion foot/hand, **1552**
Immobility
- incontinence, urinary, 62
- older adults, **59–60**
- pressure injury, 64

Immune alveolar hemorrhage, 303
Immune checkpoint inhibitors, 758, 1387. *See also specific types*
- adverse effects/events, 867, 1607
- for anal cancer, 1634
- autoimmune thyroiditis from, 1112
- diabetes mellitus from, 1196
- diarrhea from, 1656
- hyperthyroidism from, 1120
- hypophysitis from, 1099
- infection risks, 1274
- interstitial nephritis from, 911
- for non–small cell lung cancer, 1606–1607
- for small cell lung cancer, 1606
- thyroiditis from, silent, 1115
- toxicity of, **1657**

Immune complex glomerulonephritis, 912
Immune insulin resistance, 1220, 1228
Immune-mediated inflammatory myopathies, **842–844**, 843*f*
- antibodies, 843, 843*t*
- antisynthetase syndrome, 843
- dermatomyositis, **842–844**
- heliotrope rash, 842, 843*f*
- immune-mediated necrotizing myopathy, 843
- inclusion body myositis, 843–844
- polymyositis, **842–844**

Immune-mediated necrotizing myopathy, **843**
Immune reconstitution inflammatory syndrome, 193, 1331, 1387
Immune thrombocytopenia, **548–550**, 550*f*
Immunity
- active, 1301
- herd (*See* Herd immunity)
- heterotypic, 1422
- impaired
  - cellular, infections, 1273
  - humoral, infections, 1272–1273
- passive, 1301

Immunization/vaccination, 3–4, 4*t*, **1301–1310**, 1302*t*–1309*t*. *See also specific types*
- active, 1301
- adverse effects, 1308*t*–1309*t*, 1310
- asthmatics, 255
- avian influenza, 1415
- Bacillus Calmette-Guérin, 282, 287
- Chikungunya fever, 1400
- cholera, 1466
- cocooning, 796
- contraindications, 1308*t*–1309*t*, 1310
- COVID-19, 3, 255, 261, 1304*t*, **1406–1408**
  - anaphylactic reactions, 869
  - asthmatics, 255
  - booster doses, 1407
  - breakthrough infections post vaccination, 1407
  - distribution, U.S., 1406
  - herd immunity and vaccine hesitancy, 1407–1408
  - immunocompromised, 1407
  - intracranial venous thrombosis, 996
  - mRNA, 870
  - myocarditis after, 414
  - pregnancy & lactation, 1407
  - rates, 1406
  - reactions & complications, 1406
  - "real world" efficacy & protective immunity duration, 1406–1407
  - storage, 1406
  - vaccine hesitancy, 1407–1408
- cytomegalovirus, 1367
- dengue, 1394–1395
- Ebola viral disease, 1391
- *Haemophilus influenzae*, type b, 1302*t*–1303*t*, 1304*t*, 1308*t*
- healthy adults, 1301
- hematopoietic cell transplant recipients, 1301
- hepatitis A, 678, 1302*t*–1304*t*, 1308*t*
  - gay & bisexual men, 1724, 1724*t*
- hepatitis B, 682, 1302*t*–1305*t*, 1308*t*
  - gay & bisexual men, 1724, 1724*t*
- HIV, 1301
- human papillomavirus, 4*t*, 11–12, 671, 788–789, 1302*t*–1303*t*, 1305*t*, 1308*t*
  - gay & bisexual men, 1724*t*, 1725
  - lesbian & bisexual women, 1720
  - pregnancy, 796, 1302*t*–1303*t*
- inactivated/killed vaccines, 1301
- inflammatory bowel disease, 652
- influenza, 4*t*, 273, 1302*t*–1303*t*, 1305*t*, 1308*t*, **1412–1413**
  - dose-sparing, 1413
  - pregnancy, 796, 1302*t*–1303*t*
- Japanese encephalitis, 1382
- Lassa virus, 1392–1393
- live attenuated vaccines, 1301
- measles, 1369, 1370–1371
- measles, mumps, and rubella, 1302*t*–1303*t*, 1306*t*, 1308*t*, 1370–1371, 1372, 1373
- measles-vectored Chikungunya virus vaccine, 1400
- meningococcal, 1460
  - gay & bisexual men, 1724*t*
  - group B (MenB), 1302*t*–1303*t*, 1306*t*, 1309*t*
  - oligosaccharide conjugate (MCV4, MenACWY), 1302*t*–1303*t*, 1306*t*, 1309*t*
  - polysaccharide conjugate (MPSV4), 1302*t*–1303*t*, 1306*t*, 1309*t*
- monkeypox, 1422
- passive, 1301
  - respiratory syncytial virus, 1410
- pneumococcal
  - conjugate (PCV13), 1302*t*–1303*t*, 1306*t*–1307*t*, 1309*t*
  - polysaccharide (PPSV23), 4*t*, 255, 273, 1302*t*–1303*t*, 1306*t*–1307*t*, 1309*t*
- poliomyelitis, 1374, 1375
- pregnancy, 796, 1301, 1302*t*–1303*t*
- rabies, 1378
- recommended adult, **1301, 1302*t*–1307*t***
- Rift Valley fever, 1392
- rotavirus, 1422
- safety, **1310**
- SARS-CoV-1, 1415
- solid organ transplant recipients, 1301
- tetanus, diphtheria, and pertussis (Tdap), 4*t*, 1302*t*–1303*t*, 1307*t*, 1309*t*, 1451, 1452*t*
  - pregnancy, 796, 1302*t*–1303*t*
- tetanus immune globulin, 1451, 1452*t*
- tick-borne encephalitis, 1383–1384
- for travelers, **1301, 1310**
- vaccine-preventable viral infections, **1368–1376** (*See also* Vaccine-preventable viral infections, major)
- varicella, 1302*t*–1303*t*, 1307*t*, 1309*t*
- variola/vaccinia, 1421
- West Nile virus, 1381
- whooping cough, 1459
- yellow fever, pregnancy, 795
- Zika virus, pregnancy, 795–796
- zoster, 1302*t*–1303*t*, 1306*t*, 1309*t*
  - recombinant, 978

Immunodeficiency disorders/immunocompromised. *See also specific disorders; specific types*
- cough, 17
- HIV/AIDS, 1311, 1312*t*, **1313–1314** (*See also* HIV/AIDS)
- humoral immunity, impaired, 1272–1273
- infections, **1272–1276**
  - biologics recipients, 1274
  - cellular immunity, impaired, 1273
  - clinical findings, 1274

Immunodeficiency disorders/immunocompromised, infections (*Cont.*):
- differential diagnosis, 1274
- granulocytopenia, 1273
- hematopoietic cell transplant recipients, 1273
- humoral immunity, impaired, 1272–1273
- other immunocompromised states, 1274
- prevention, 1274–1275
- solid organ transplant recipients, 1273
- treatment, 1275–1276
- tumor necrosis factor inhibitor recipients, 1273
- primary, adult, **872–874,** 872*t*
  - common variable immunodeficiency, **873–874**
  - complement disorders, 872*t*
  - Good syndrome, 872*t*
  - granulocyte disorders, 872*t*
  - hereditary angioedema, 872*t*
  - hypogammaglobulinemia, secondary, **874**
  - immunoglobulin subclass deficiency, **874**
  - selective IgA deficiency, **873**
  - specific antibody deficiency, **874**
- toxoplasmosis, **1511–1513**

Immunoglobulin subclass deficiency, **874**
Immunologic thrombocytopenia, HIV/AIDS, 1314
Immunopathologic hypoglycemia, 1233
Immunotherapy. *See specific types*
Impetigo, **105*t*, 123–124,** 124*f*, 1297*t*, 1441, 1441*t*
Impingement testing, shoulder
- Hawkins impingement sign, 1675, 1679*t*
- Neer impingement sign, 1675, 1678*t*

Implantable cardioverter defibrillator, 398, 411, 419
IMPROVE risk score, 566
Inactivated vaccines, 1301
Inactivated Vero cell culture-derived Japanese encephalitis vaccine, 1382
Inborn errors of metabolism, 184, 980
Incapacitated passenger, 1562
Incentive spirometry, for postoperative risk reduction, 46–47
Incident related pain, 86
Inclisiran, 358, 1245*t*, 1247
Inclusion body encephalitis, measles, 1370
Inclusion body myositis, 842, 843–844, **1044**
Inclusion conjunctivitis, **171**
Incompetent cervix, 797–798
Incomplete abortion, 798
Incontinence, fecal, **671–672**
Incontinence, urinary
- older adults, **62–64**
- overflow, 63–64
- stress, 63
- urge, 62, 63

Increased anion gap acidosis, **895–897**
Increta, 807
Incretins, 1204*t*, 1208–1210. *See also specific types*
Indacaterol, 262
Indapamide, 458*t*, 956
"Indigestion," 579
Indinavir, kidney stones from, 954
Indirect calorimetry, 1266, 1269
Indolent lymphomas, 534
Indomethacin, **83*t*,** 805–806, 974
Inevitable spontaneous abortion, 798
Infant. *See also specific topics*
- maternal effects, intrapartum fever, 30
- mortality, prematurity, 805
- shoulder dystocia, diabetic mothers, 810

Infarction. *See also* Myocardial infarction; *specific types*
- pain, 373
- painless, 373
- spinal cord, **996**

Infected pseudocyst, 731
Infections/infectious diseases, **1270–1293.** *See also* Antimicrobial therapy; *specific types*
- actinomycoses, 717, 1294*t*, **1473–1474**
- animal & bite wounds, **1283–1284**
- anorectal, **670–671**
- arthritis, **861–864**
  - gonococcal arthritis, **863–864**
  - HIV, rheumatic manifestations, **864,** 1323
  - nongonococcal acute bacterial arthritis, **861–863**
  - viral, **864**
- bacterial (*See also* Bacterial infections)
  - gram-negative, **1458–1473**
  - gram-positive, **1440–1458**
- blood transfusion transmission, 544
- cancer-related, **1652–1653**
- central nervous system, **1280–1283,** 1280*t*, 1281*t*
- *Chlamydiae,* **1477–1479**
  - *C. pneumoniae,* **1479**
  - *C. psittaci* & psittacosis, 1295*t*, **1478**
  - *C. trachomatis,* **1477–1478**
    - lymphogranuloma venereum, **1477**
    - urethritis & cervicitis, **1477–1478**
- diarrhea
  - acute infectious, **1288–1290,** 1289*t*–1290*t*
  - traveler's, **1292–1293**
- drug injection–related, **1286–1287**
- endocarditis (*See* Endocarditis, infective)
- esophagitis, **612–613**
- fever of unknown origin, **1270–1272**
- glomerulonephritis, 923*t*, **926–927**
- health care–associated, **1276–1279**
- immunization against, **1301–1310,** 1302*t*–1309*t* (*See also specific types*)
- immunocompromised, **1272–1276**
- incontinence, urinary, 62
- mycobacterial, **1475–1476**
  - *Mycobacterium tuberculosis,* 1476
  - nontuberculous
    - disseminated *Mycobacterium avium* complex, **1475–1476**
    - lymphadenitis, 242, **1475**
    - pulmonary, **287–289, 1475**
    - skin & soft tissue, **1475**
  - tuberculous meningitis, **1476–1477**
- myocarditis, **414–416,** 415*t*, 416*t*
  - COVID-19, 414, 416, 416*t*
- nocardiosis, 1295*t*, **1474–1475**
- prevention, 3–4, 4*t*
- pulmonary, **268–289**
- seizures, 980
- sexually transmitted diseases, **1284–1286**
- thrombocytopenia, **556**
- thyroiditis, **1112–1114**
- traveler, returning, **1291–1292**
- viral, **1353–1426** (*See also* Viral diseases)

Infectious mononucleosis, 1358*t*, **1363–1364**
Infertility
- definition, 960
- female, **772–773**
  - endometriosis, 767–768
  - pelvic inflammatory disease, 768
  - polycystic ovary syndrome, **771, 1181**
- from hypothyroidism, 1117
- male, 772, **960–963,** 961*f*

Inflammatory bowel disease, **649–663**
- colorectal cancer and, 1628
- Crohn disease, **653–658**
- immunizations, 652
- lifestyle & social support, 652
- lower GI bleeding, 599
- microscopic colitis, **663**
- pancreatitis, chronic, 733
- pharmacologic therapy, 649–652
  - 5-aminosalicylic acid, 649–650
  - anti-IL-12/23 antibody, 652
  - anti-integrins, 652
  - corticosteroids, 650
  - Janus kinase inhibitors, 650–651
  - methotrexate, 650
  - sphingosine 1-phosphate receptor modulators, 651
  - thiopurines (mercaptopurine, azathioprine), 650
- primary sclerosing cholangitis, **726–728**
- spondyloarthritis, **861**
- thyroiditis, 1112
- ulcerative colitis, **658–662,** 658*t*

Inflammatory diseases/disorders. *See also specific types*
- abdominal aortic aneurysm, 5*t*, 6, 42, **482–484,** 1465
- anterior hypopituitarism, 1099
- breast carcinoma, **748**
- diarrhea, 1288
- HIV/AIDS
  - demyelinating polyneuropathy, 1323
  - reactions, 1330–1331
- inflammatory power disease, occult GI bleeding, 601
- myopathies, immune-mediated, **842–844,** 843*f*
- nodules, erythema nodosum, **132–133,** 133*f*
- pericarditis, **426–429**
- vasculitis syndromes, **847–858** (*See also* Vasculitis syndromes)

Infliximab
- for autoimmune hepatitis, 693
- for Behçet disease, 857
- for Crohn disease, 656–657
- infections with, 1273
- for inflammatory bowel disease, 651–652
- for Kawasaki disease, 1438
- progressive multifocal leukoencephalopathy from, 1387
- for psoriasis, 137
- for rheumatoid arthritis, 830–831
- for ulcerative colitis, 660–661

Influenza
- avian, **1414–1415**
- community-acquired pneumonia, 270
- seasonal, **1410–1413** (*See also* Avian influenza; Seasonal influenza)
- vaccine, 4*t*, 273, 1302*t*–1303*t*, 1305*t*, 1308*t*
  - pregnancy, 796, 1302*t*–1303*t*
- zoonotic, 1414

Ingenol mebutate, 111
Inhalation chamber, 249
Inherited arrhythmia syndromes, **401**
Injection drug use. *See also* Substance use disorders; *specific drugs*
- endocarditis, 1454
- hepatitis C, 682
- hepatitis D, 684
- HIV infection, 1313
- human T-cell lymphotropic virus, 1388
- infections, **1286–1287**

Ink spot lentigines, 108
Inmazeb, 1390
Inner ear diseases, **212–217**. *See also specific types*
- hyperacusis, **214**
- sensorineural hearing loss, 204, **212–213**
  - autoimmune, **213**
  - idiopathic sudden, 204, **212, 213**
  - noise trauma, **212**
  - ototoxicity, **213**
  - physical trauma, **212**
  - presbycusis, **212**

tinnitus, **213–214**
vertigo, **214–217,** 215*t*
vertigo syndromes, from central lesions, 215*t*, **217**
vertigo syndromes, from peripheral lesions, 215*t*, **216–217**
benign paroxysmal positioning vertigo, **216**
cervicogenic vertigo, **217**
labyrinthitis, **216**
Ménière disease, **216**
migrainous vertigo, **217**
perilymphatic fistula, **216–217**
superior semicircular canal dehiscence, **217**
traumatic vertigo, **216**
vestibular neuronitis, **216**
Inotropic agents. *See specific types*
Insecticides, **1588–1589**
anticholinesterase, **1588–1589**
carbamate, 1570
chlorinated, 1567
organophosphorus, **1588–1589**
Insomnia, **1082–1084,** 1385
Instrumental activities of daily living assessment, 53
Insulin, **1211–1215,** 1212*t*
Insulin aspart, 121*t*, 1212–1213
Insulin degludec, 1212*t*, 1213, 1217, 1217*t*
Insulin detemir, 1212*t*, 1213, 1217, 1217*t*
Insulin glargine, 1212*t*, 1213, 1217, 1217*t*
Insulin glulisine, 121*t*, 1212–1213
Insulin icodec, 1212*t*, 1213
Insulin lispro, 121*t*, 1212–1213
Insulin neuritis, 1223
Insulinomas, **1171–1172, 1233–1236,** 1234*t*
Insulin pumps, 1214–1215
Insulin receptor antibodies, hypoglycemia from, 1197, **1237**
Insulin resistance, **1197–1198**. *See also* Metabolic syndrome
acanthosis nigricans, 1200, 1200*f*, 1216
corticosteroids on, 1197
diabetes mellitus, type 2, 1196, 1196*t*
diabetic dyslipidemia, 1202
diabetic ketoacidosis treatment, 1229–1230
drug-induced, 1197
gallstones, 719
immune, 1220, 1228
from infections, 1216
obesity, 1196
pioglitazone for, 1219
Insulin therapy
administration methods, 1214–1215
closed loop systems, 1215
inhaled, 1215
injection sites, 1214
pen injection devices, 1214
pumps, 1214–1215
syringes and needles, 1214
allergy, 1220
for beta-blocker poisoning, 1577
for calcium channel blocker poisoning, 1578
complications
hypoglycemia, 1219
hypoglycemic unawareness, 1219–1220
immunopathology
immune insulin resistance, 1220
insulin allergy, 1220
lipodystrophy, 1220–1221
dawn phenomenon, 1217
for diabetic ketoacidosis, 1228–1230
for hyperglycemic hyperosmolar state, 1230
poisoning, **1582**
hypotension treatment, 1565
preoperative/perioperative/postoperative, 50
preparations, 1212*t* (*See also specific types*)
available & bioavailability, 1212, 1212*t*
insulin lispro/aspart/glulisine, 121*t*, 1212–1213
long-acting, 1212*t*, 1213–1214
mixed, 1214
regular insulin, 1212
short-acting, 1212–1213, 1212*t*
Somogyi effect, 1217
Insulin therapy, for diabetes mellitus, 1211–1215, 1212*t*
administration methods, 1214–1215
closed loop systems, 1215
inhaled, 1215
injection sites, 1214
pen injection devices, 1214
pumps, 1214–1215
syringes and needles, 1214
available preparations & bioavailability, 1212, 1212*t*
bioavailability, 1212*t*
complications, 1219–1221
hypoglycemia, 1219
hypoglycemic unawareness, 1219–1220
immunopathology
immune insulin resistance, 1220
insulin allergy, 1220
lipodystrophy, 1220–1221
preparations, 1212*t*
available, 1212, 1212*t*
long-acting, 1212*t*, 1213–1214
mixed, 1214
short-acting, 1212–1213, 1212*t*
Integrase inhibitors, **1340*t*–1341*t*,** 1345–1346. *See also specific types*
bictegravir, **1340*t*, 1346**
cabotegravir, **1341*t*, 1346**
dolutegravir, **1340*t*, 1346**
elvitegravir, **1340*t*, 1345–1346**
principles & overview, **1340*t*–1341*t*,** 1345–1346
raltegravir, **1341*t*, 1345**
Integrase strand transfer inhibitors, dual. *See specific types*
"Intensive care unit psychosis," 1097
Interferon. *See also specific types*
for MERS-CoV, 1417
pegylated, for HTLV1-associated myelopathy, 1389
for SARS-CoV-1, 1415
Interferon gamma, fever from, 29
Interferon gamma release assays, 282–283, 1320, 1335–1336, 1335*t*
Interferon α
-2b, 1356*t*
goiter from, 1115
for HTLV1-associated myelopathy, 1389
-n3, 1356*t*
for renal cell carcinoma, 1646
thyroiditis from, silent, 1115
Interferon β
goiter from, 1115
pegylated, for multiple sclerosis, 1025*t*
Interferon β-1a, 1025*t*
Interferon β-1b, 1025*t*
Interleukin-1, fever, 29
Interleukin-1 inhibitors. *See also specific types*
for gouty arthritis, 825, 827
for Still disease, adult, 831
Interleukin-2
autoimmune thyroiditis from, 1112
goiter from, 1115
for renal cell carcinoma, 1646
thyroiditis from, silent, 1115
Interleukin-6, fever, 29
Intermittent claudication, 473
Intermittent explosive disorder, 1061
Intermittent positive-pressure breathing, postoperative risk reduction, 47
Internalized homophobia, 1710, 1722
Internal rotation
rotator cuff strength testing
belly-press test, 1678*t*
lift-off test, 1678*t*
shoulder range of motion, 1677*t*
International Normalized Ratio (INR), for warfarin
dosing adjustment, 571, 572*t*, 573*t*
supratherapeutic, 571, 574*t*
Interpersonal psychotherapy, for depression, 1078
Interstitial, defined, 292
Interstitial cystitis, **953–954**
Interstitial fluid volume, 875
Interstitial lung disease, **292–297,** 293*t*. *See also specific types*
diffuse interstitial pneumonias, **292–294,** 293*t*, 294*t*
eosinophilic pulmonary syndromes, 297
idiopathic interstitial pneumonias, 293, 294*t*
pulmonary alveolar proteinosis, 297
rheumatoid arthritis, 828
sarcoidosis, 295–296, 296*f*
Interstitial nephritis, 832, 907*t*, **911–912,** 1363
Interstitial pneumonia
acute, 294*t*
diffuse, **292–294,** 293*t*, 294*t*
idiopathic, 293, 294*t*, 308
Interstitial pneumonitis
Epstein-Barr virus, 1363
HIV/AIDS, 1314, 1321
from methotrexate, 830
Intertrigo, **119**
Interventricular septum rupture, 381
Interview, medical, 1
Intestinal angina, **480–481**
Intestinal motility disorders, **638–641**. *See also specific types*
chronic intestinal pseudo-obstruction & gastroparesis, **640–641**
colonic pseudo-obstruction, acute, **639–641**
paralytic ileus, acute, **638–639**
Intestinal nematode infections, **1526–1529**
ascariasis, **1526**
enterobiasis, **1528–1529**
hookworm disease, **1527**
strongyloidiasis, **1527–1528**
trichuriasis, **1526–1527**
Intestinal neuroendocrine tumors, **1626–1627**
Intestinal pseudo-obstruction, chronic, **640–641**
Intestinal tuberculosis, **643**
Intimate partner violence, sexual, **782–783, 1721**
Intra-abdominal infections, gram-negative, 1472, 1472*t*
Intra-aortic balloon counterpulsation, for acute MI with ST-segment elevation, 381
Intra-aortic balloon pump, for acute MI with ST-segment elevation, 380
Intra-arterial embolization, 598, 599
Intra-articular injections, for osteoarthritis, 821
Intracellular volume, 875
Intracerebral hemorrhage, 469, 470*t*, 989*t*, **992–993**
Intracranial aneurysm, 325, **994**
Intracranial hypertension, idiopathic, 974, **1003–1005**
Intracranial mass lesions, **997–1002**
AIDS, **1001**
brain abscess, **1002**
headache, **974**
metastatic tumors
cerebral metastases, **1000–1001**
leptomeningeal metastases, **1001**

Intracranial mass lesions (*Cont.*):
primary tumors, **997–1000,** 997*t*–998*t*
acoustic neurinoma, 998*t*
astrocytoma, 997*t*
brainstem and cerebellar lesions, 999
brainstem glioma, 998*t*
cerebellar hemangioblastoma, 998*t*
cerebral lymphoma, 998*t*, **1001**
craniopharyngioma, 998*t*
ependymoma, 998*t*
false localizing signs, 999
frontal lobe lesions, 999
germ cell tumors, 998*t*
glioblastoma multiforme, 997*t*
gliomas, 997
hemangioblastoma, 999
herniation syndromes, 999
medulloblastoma, 998*t*
meningioma, 997, 997*t*
mixed neuronal-glial tumors, 998*t*
neurofibromas, 997, 999
neuronal tumors, 998*t*
occipital lobe lesions, 999
oligodendroglioma, 998*t*
parietal lobe lesions, 999
pineal tumor, 998*t*
pituitary adenoma, 998*t*
retinoblastoma, 999
temporal lobe lesions, 999
Intracranial pressure, increased, 190, 195, 196
Intracranial venous thrombosis, stroke, **996**
Intraepidermal squamous cell carcinoma, **114**
Intrahepatic cholestasis of pregnancy, 674, 676*t*, **818**
Intralesional immunotherapy, for molluscum contagiosum, 121
Intralipid 20% lipid emulsion, 1578, 1593
Intraocular foreign bodies, **197**
Intraocular pressure, elevated
corticosteroids, ocular, 170*t*, 172
glaucoma
acute angle-closure, 181
chronic, 181–183
herpes zoster ophthalmicus, 179
retinal detachment, 186
Intraoral ulcerative lesions, **230**
Intrapartum fever, 30
Intrastromal corneal ring segments, 168
Intrathecal drug delivery system, 80, **96–97,** 97*t*
Intrauterine device, **777–778,** 778*t*, 1713
copper, 1713
hormonal
for dysmenorrhea, 767
levonorgestrel-releasing, for abnormal uterine bleeding, 764
for pelvic pain, 768
for polycystic ovary syndrome, 771
for uterine leiomyoma, 766
malpositioned, pelvic pain, 769
Intrauterine insemination, 962–963
Intravenous immunoglobulin
for adenovirus, 1419
factor III antibodies, acquired, 561
for immune-mediated inflammatory myopathies, 844
for immune thrombocytopenia, 549
for Kawasaki disease, 1438
for myasthenia gravis, 1041
for necrotizing fasciitis, 1442
parvovirus B19, 1420
for SARS-CoV-1, 1415
for *Staphylococcus aureus*, toxic shock syndrome, 1449
for Stevens-Johnson syndrome, 154
for toxic shock syndrome, streptococcal, 1443
Intravenous lipid emulsion. *See* Intralipid 20% lipid emulsion
Intraventricular conduction block, 387–388
Intrinsic acute kidney injury, 907*t*, 908
inv(16)(p13;q22), acute myeloid leukemia, 528
Invasive candidiasis, 1534, 1535
Invasive nematode infections, **1529–1530**
angiostrongyliasis, **1529–1530**
cutaneous larva migrans, **1530,** 1530*f*
Inverse psoriasis, 116
Inversion ankle sprains, **1706–1707**
Inverted papillomas, nasal, 226
In vitro fertilization, 962, 1714
Involuntary weight loss, **32–33, 64**. *See also* Weight, loss
Iodide, goiter from, 1115
Iodinated contrast agents. *See also* Iopanoic acid; Ipodate sodium
for hyperthyroidism, 1123*t*, 1124, 1125
for thyroiditis, painful subacute, 1114
for thyrotoxic crisis/thyroid storm, 1127
Iodine
deficiency disorder, **1137–1138**
hyperthyroidism from, 1120
inhalation poisoning, 1573
supplementation
autoimmune thyroiditis from, 1112
for iodine deficiency disorder, 1138
thyrotoxicosis from, 1138
Iodine, radioactive (^{131}I)
adverse effects, 1135
birth defects from, 1126
for hyperthyroidism, 1123*t*, 1124–1125
thyroid cancer, 1136
for thyroid cancers, 1134–1135
for toxic nodular goiter, 1125
Iodoquinol, 1514–1515, 1515t
Ionizing radiation, 1558, 1603. *See also* Radiation; Radiotherapy
Iopanoic acid
for hyperthyroidism, 1123*t*, 1124, 1125
for thyroiditis, painful subacute, 1114
Ipilimumab, 1600*t*
diabetes mellitus from, 1196
for hepatocellular carcinoma, 1612
hypophysitis from, 1099
for mesothelioma, 1609
for non–small cell lung cancer, 1607
for renal cell carcinoma, 1646
thyroiditis from, silent, 1115
Ipodate sodium
for hyperthyroidism, 1123*t*, 1124, 1125
for thyroiditis, painful subacute, 1114
for thyrotoxic crisis/thyroid storm, 1127
Ipratropium (bromide)
for asthma, 252*t*, 255, 257*f*, 258
with albuterol, 252*t*
for COPD, 262
Irbesartan, 452*t*
Iridodialysis, 197
Irinotecan, 1599*t*
for colorectal cancer, 1630
diarrhea from, 1656
for pancreas carcinoma, 1616
*UBT1A1*28* on metabolism/reactions, 1671*t*
Iron
anion gap elevation from, 1570
deficiency, 500
foreign body, eye, 197
overload, dilated cardiomyopathy, 418
poisoning, 1571*t*
antidote, 1568*t*
Iron deficiency anemia, **500–502,** 501*t*
causes, 500–501, 501*t*
esophageal webs/rings, 614
GI bleeding, occult, 601–602
hookworm disease, 1527
pregnancy, 808–809
uterine leiomyoma, 766
Iron oxide, lung cancer and, 1603
Iron-restricted erythropoiesis, 503
Iron therapy
for anemia of chronic kidney disease, 917
for iron deficiency, parenteral, 502
for iron deficiency anemia prevention, pregnancy, 809
pill-induced esophagitis from, 613
pregnancy, 808–809
refractoriness, 501
for restless legs syndrome, 1013
Irritable bowel syndrome, **643–647**
Isavuconazole, 1539*t*, 1544, 1545, 1546
Ischemia. *See also specific types*
postinfarction, 379
stress-induced, 361
testing, preoperative noninvasive, 42–43, 44*f*
Ischemic acute tubular necrosis, 908
Ischemic colitis, **480–481,** 599
Ischemic heart disease, 26, **355–382.** *See also* Coronary heart disease; *specific types*
Ischemic hepatitis, **715**
Ischemic hepatopathy, **715**
Ischemic optic neuropathy, **193–194,** 848
Ischemic rest pain, 476–477
Ischemic stroke. *See* Stroke
Islet cell carcinoma, **1233–1236,** 1234*t*
Islet of Langerhans adenoma, fasting hypoglycemia from, 1233
Islet transplantation, 1215–1216
Isoagglutinins, 542
Isobutyl nitrite poisoning, **1586–1587**
Isocitrate dehydrogenase-1/2 *(IDH1/2)* gene, 1672*t*
Isolated peripheral neuropathies, 1222–1223
Isolated post-capillary pulmonary hypertension, 431
Isomalt, 1203
Isoniazid, 284–285, 284*t*, 285*t*, 286
anion gap elevation from, 1570
autoimmune hypoglycemia from, 1237
hepatotoxicity, 696
for *Mycobacterium kansasii*, 1475
nephritis from, drug-induced, 837
poisoning, 1567*t*, 1568*t*, **1582–1583**
on pyridoxine metabolism, 1261
seizures from, 1567
for tuberculosis
HIV/AIDS, 1335–1336
meningitis, 1476
pregnancy, 815
spinal, 865
Isophane insulin, 1212*t*, 1213
Isopropanol, anion gap elevation from, 897
Isoproterenol, 1577, 1578
Isosorbide dinitrate, 363, 409
Isosorbide mononitrate, 363
Isospora (isosporiasis), 1288, **1516–1518**
Isospora belli, 1516
Isothenuria, 941
Isotonic hyponatremia, 876, 880
Isotretinoin, 142, 149
Isradipine, 457*t*, 839, **1578**
Istradefylline, 1009
Itraconazole, 1536, 1539*t*
for aspergillosis, 1544
for blastomycosis, 1545
for candidiasis, esophageal, 1535
for coccidioidomycosis, 1537
for eumycetoma, 1546
for histoplasmosis, 1536, 1539*t*
for onychomycosis, 167

for sporotrichosis, 1546
for tinea corporis, 115
for tinea cruris, 116
for tinea manuum/pedis, 117
Ivabradine, 383, 385*t*
for angina pectoris, **363**
for heart failure, 407*t*, **410**, 419
for sinus tachycardia, 387
for supraventricular tachycardia, 385*t*
Ivacaftor, 267, 1667*t*
Ivermectin
for ascariasis, 1526
for cutaneous larva migrans, 1530
for filariasis, lymphatic, 1531–1532
for onchocerciasis, 1533
for pediculosis capitis, 131
for rosacea, 150
for scabies, 130
for strongyloidiasis, 1528
toxicities, 1533
IVIG. *See* Intravenous immunoglobulin
Ivosidenib, 1672*t*
Ivrabradine, 363
Ixabepilone, 759
Ixazomib, 538
Ixekizumab, 138, 859, 860
Ixodes, 242
Ixodes pacificus, 1434
Ixodes persulcatus, 1434, 1492
Ixodes ricinus, 1434, 1492
Ixodes scapularis, 1434, 1492, 1509

J

JAK2
essential thrombocytosis, 522
myelofibrosis, primary, 523
myeloproliferative neoplasms, 520
polycythemia vera, 520–521
JAK inhibitors. *See* Janus kinase inhibitors
Jamestown Canyon virus, 1379
Janeway lesions, 1454
Janus kinase (JAK 1/3), 650
Janus kinase inhibitors. *See also specific types*
adverse effects, 830
for HTLV-1 adult T-cell leukemia, 1388
for inflammatory bowel disease, 650–651
for rheumatoid arthritis, 830
Japanese encephalitis, 1379, **1381–1382**
Jarisch-Herxheimer reaction, 1483, 1491
Jaundice, **674–677**, 676*t*, 677*t*
biliary obstruction, 674–675
biliary tract
carcinoma, 1613
diseases, **674–677**, 676*t*, 677*t*
cholestatic
from antipsychotics, 1066
vitamin E deficiency, 1262
classification, 674, 675*t*
clinical findings, 674–675
Crigler-Najjar syndrome, 675*t*
diagnostic studies, 675–677, 676*t*, 677*t*
Gilbert syndrome, 674, 675*t*, 676*t*, 697
hepatocellular, liver biochemical tests, 676*t*
hepatomegaly, 675
hyperbilirubinemia, **674–675*t*,** 675*t*, **676*t***
liver biopsy, 677
obstructive, evaluation, 675–677
pancreas carcinoma, 1615
pathophysiology & etiology, 674
Jaw
claudication, 978
pain, angina pectoris, 978
JC polyomavirus, 1323
JC virus, 1386–1387
JNJ-53718678, 1409
Jock itch, **115–116**
Joint fluid, 819, 820*t*, 821*t*
Jones criteria, 425, 425*t*
Jugular venous pressure
acute MI, with ST-segment elevation, 373
cardiomyopathy
constrictive, 430
dilated, 418*t*
restrictive, 418*t*
hepatojugular reflex, 404
Kussmaul sign, 373
pulmonary valve stenosis, 324
Jugular venous pulsations
acute MI with ST-segment elevation, 373
cardiomyopathy
dilated, 418
hypertrophic, 422
pericardial effusion, 428, 429
pericarditis, constrictive, 429
pulmonary hypertension, 431
tetralogy of Fallot, 331
tricuspid regurgitation, 351
tricuspid stenosis, 350
Junctional nevus, 107
Justice, distributive & procedural, 77
Juvenile freckles, 163
Juvenile idiopathic arthritis, uveitis, 183
Juvenile polyposis, familial, hamartomatous polyposis syndromes, 668
Juvenile rheumatoid arthritis, 1270

K

Kala azar, **1499–1501**
Kallmann syndrome, 1100, 1184
Kaolin pneumoconiosis, 306*t*
Kaposi sarcoma, **113**
conjunctiva, 193
HHV-8, 1368
HIV/AIDS, **113**, 1319*t*, 1321, 1324, 1328–1329
otologic manifestations, 218
Kaposi sarcoma inflammatory cytokine syndrome, 1368
Kaposi-Stemmer sign, 28
Katayama syndrome, 1520
Kato-Katz technique, 1521, 1522, 1526
Kava, 1580*t*
Kawasaki disease, 1358*t*, **1436–1439**
Kawasaki-like disease, 1437
Kawasaki shock syndrome, 1437
Kaysher-Fleischer ring, Wilson disease, 712, 712*f*
Kegel exercises, 63, 671, 672, 769
Kennedy syndrome, 1028–1029
Keratitis
chemical, **198**
exposure, 179
neurotrophic, 172, 180
Keratitis, infectious, **179–180**
Acanthamoeba, **180**
adenovirus, 1418
amoebic, **180**
bacterial, **179**
fungal, **180**
herpes simplex, 172, 175*t*, **179**, 1353, 1354
herpes zoster, 1360
herpes zoster ophthalmicus, **179–180**
variola/vaccinia, with corneal ulcerations, 1421
Keratoconjunctivitis
adenovirus, 170, 1418
atopic, 172
chlamydial, **171–172**
epidemic, 170
herpes simplex virus, 170, 1353
measles, 1370
molluscum contagiosum, 1421
vernal, 172
Keratoconjunctivitis sicca, 16, 170, 171, 832, 845
Keratoderma blennorrhagicum, 860
Keratolytics, 101. *See also specific types*
Keratomalacia, vitamin A deficiency, 1262
Keratoplasty, 168
Keratosis
actinic, **110–111**
seborrheic, **108**, 109*f*
Kernig sign, 36
Ketamine, 1077
Ketoacidosis, 896–897, 896*t*
alcoholic, 896*t*, 897
diabetic, 896*t*, 897
fasting/starvation, 896*t*, 897
Ketoconazole, 1539*t*
for angular cheilitis, 1325
for Cushing syndrome, 1163
hepatotoxicity, 696
for onychomycosis, 167
for prostate cancer, 1640, 1640*t*
for seborrheic dermatitis, 139
for tinea versicolor, 105*t*, 118
topical dermatologic, 105*t*
Ketoprofen, 767
Ketorolac, 79, **83*t***
Ketosis
diabetes mellitus, type 1, 1195
diabetic ketoacidosis, 1211
hyperglycemic coma, 1230
Keystone virus, 1379
Khorana risk score, 566
Ki-67, breast cancer, 749, 752, 754
Kidney. *See also* Renal
biopsy, 905–906
genitourinary tract infections, 945
impairment, hypotonic hyponatremia, 877
nephrogenic systemic fibrosis after, 942
perioperative management, 47, 51
Kidney cancers, 939, **1645–1647**
primary, **1646–1647**
secondary, **1647**
treatment, 1597*t*
Kidney disease, **903–942**. *See also specific types*
acute kidney injury, 903, **906–913**
assessment, **903–905**
duration, disease, **903**
glomerular filtration rate, **904–905**, 905*t*
hematuria, **904**
urinalysis, **903–905**
proteinuria, **903–904**
proteinuria, functional, 904
proteinuria, overload, 904
proteinuria, tubular, 904
urinary casts, 903, 904*t*
biopsy, **905–906**
cardiomyopathy, dilated, 418
chronic kidney disease, 903, **913–922**
cystic diseases of kidney, 824, **938–941**
autosomal dominant polycystic kidney disease, 938*t*, **939–940**, 939*f*
cysts, defined, 938
cysts, simple/solitary, **938–939**, 938*t*
medullary sponge kidney, 938*t*, **940–941**
glomerular diseases, **922–932**, 922*f*, 923*t*, 924*t* (*See also* Glomerular diseases)
nephrotic spectrum, 922*f*, 924*t*, **932–934**
hypertension, 445, 446
multisystem disease, variable kidney involvement, **941–942**
gout & kidney, **941–942**
nephrogenic systemic fibrosis, **942**
plasma cell myeloma, **941**
sickle cell disease, **941**
tuberculosis, **941**

Kidney disease (*Cont.*):
nephrotic spectrum, primary renal disorders, **932–934**
minimal change disease, 924*t*, 931, **932–933**
nephrotic spectrum, systemic disorders, **934–936**
diabetic nephropathy, 924*t*, **934–935**
HIV-associated nephropathy, 924*t*, **935**
renal amyloidosis, 924*t*, **935–936**
preoperative evaluation/perioperative management, 50–51, 51*t*
tubulointerstitial diseases, 834, **936–938,** 936*t*
uremia, 915, 917
urinary casts, 903, 904*t*
Kidney stones, 823, 943, 958
Kidney transplantation, 920, 927, 933
Kiesselbach plexus, 224
Killer vaccines, 1301
Killip classification, 372, 373
Kimmelstiel-Wilson nodules, 935
Kinase inhibitors, 1600*t*–1601*t*. *See also specific types*
acalabrutinib, 1600*t*
alectinib, 1600*t*
axitinib, 1600*t*
bosutinib, 1600*t*
cobimetinib, 1601*t*
dabrafenib, 1601*t*
dasatinib, 1601*t*
erlotinib, 1601*t*
gefitinib, 1601*t*
ibrutinib, 1601*t*
imatinib, 1601*t*
lenvatinib, 1601*t*
nilotinib, 1601*t*
osimertinib, 1601*t*
pazopanib, 1601*t*
regorafenib, 1601*t*
sunitinib, 1601*t*
trametinib, 1601*t*
vermurafenib, 1601*t*
Kindling, 1086
KIT, gastrointestinal mesenchymal tumors, 1624, 1625
Klatskin tumors, 1613
Klebsiella, 233, 948, 957, 1294*t*
Klebsiella granulomatis, granuloma inguinale, 1285–1286, **1470–1471**
Klebsiella pneumoniae
liver abscess, 717
peritonitis, spontaneous bacterial, 604
pneumonia, 269*t*
community-acquired, 270
nosocomial, 275
Kleine-Levin syndrome, **1084**
Klinefelter syndrome, 962, 1176, **1664**
Knee, **1695–1706**
anterior cruciate ligament injury, **1696, 1700–1701**
collateral ligament injury, **1701–1702**
hemarthrosis, 1695
meniscus injuries, **1702–1703**
osteoarthritis, 1695, 1696*t*, **1704–1706**
meniscus injuries, 1703
treatment, 83*t*, 820–821
pain, **1695–1696,** 1696*t*
patellofemoral pain, **1703–1704**
posterior cruciate ligament injury, **1701–1702**
Knee examination, 1695, 1697*t*–1700*t*
inspection & palpation, 1697*t*
ligament stress testing
anterior drawer, 1697*t*, 1700
Lachman test, 1696, 1697*t*, 1700
pivot shift, 1698*t*, 1700–1701
valgus stress, 1698*t*, 1701
varus stress, 1699*t*, 1702
meniscal signs
McMurray test, 1699*t*, 1703
McMurray test, modified, 1699*t*–1700*t*, 1703
Thessaly test, 1700*t*, 1703
range of motion testing, 1697*t*
Koebner phenomenon, 136, 140
KOH preparation, 114–115, 114*f*
Koplik spots, 1369, 1369*f*, 1370
Korsakoff syndrome, **1018,** 1087–1088, 1096
KRAS, 665, 1606, 1630, 1673*t*
Kratom poisoning, 1588
Kupffer cells, 514, 516, 701
Kuru, 1385
Kussmaul respiration, ketoacidosis, 1199
Kussmaul sign, 373, 430, 431
Kwashiorkor, 1250

L

L265P, Waldenström macroglobulinemia, 540
La belle indifférence, 1054
Labetalol
for hypertension, 461*t*, 470, 470*t*, 471*t*, 812, 1566
for preeclampsia-eclampsia, 804
for stroke, 991
Labile hypertension, 444
Labor
heart disease management, maternal, 435, **438**
preterm, **804–806**
Labyrinthine concussion, 216
Labyrinthitis, **216**
Lachman test, 1696, 1697*t*, 1700
Lacosamide, 976*t*, 1575–1576
Lacrimal apparatus disorders, **168–170**
Lacrimal sac infection, 169–170
La Crosse virus, 1379
Lactase deficiency, **637–638**
Lactation
antipsychotics on, 1066
breast cancer, 748
combined oral contraceptives and, 776
COVID-19 vaccine, 1407
drugs and, **795,** 796*t*
on iron balance, 501
non-gestational parent, 1714
tuberculosis treatment, 286
Lactic acid, anion gap elevation from, 897
Lactic acid-citric acid-potassium bitartrate, 779
Lactic acidosis, 895–896, **1232**
coma, 1226, 1226*t*
D-, 896
from metformin, 1207, 1232
shock, 495
type A, 896
type B, 896
Lactitol, 1203
Lactobacillus delbrueckii, primary biliary cholangitis, 707
Lactobacillus vaginitis, 784
Lactose intolerance, 634, 1264
Lactulose
for constipation, 586, 587*t*, 646
for encephalopathy with esophageal varices, 616
for hepatic encephalopathy, 704–705
Lacunar infarction, **988,** 989*t*. *See also* Stroke
Lambert-Eaton myasthenic syndrome, 984, 1004*t*, **1042**
Lamin A/C genotype, dilated cardiomyopathy, 418
Lamivudine, **1339*t*, 1343**
for hepatitis B, 687–688, 1325
for hepatitis D, 687–688
for HIV/AIDS, 1325, 1338
Lamotrigine
for bipolar disorder, 1080–1081
hepatotoxicity, 696
for personality disorders, 1061
poisoning, 1576
pregnancy, safety, 813
for seizures, 976*t*
for trigeminal neuralgia, 975
Langerhans cell histiocytosis, anterior hypopituitarism, 1099
Lanimavir, 1412
Lanreotide, 1107, 1173, 1235–1236
Lansoprazole
for GERD, 610
for NSAIDs
gastritis, 622
ulcer prevention, 628
for peptic ulcer disease, 627
Lanthanum carbonate, 917
Laparoscopic adjustable gastric band, 1257
Laparoscopy, gynecologic, 764*t*
Large B-cell lymphoma, diffuse, gastric, 1623
Large-cell lymphoma, from chronic lymphocytic leukemia, 530
Large needle biopsy. *See* Core needle biopsy
Larotrectinib, 1606
Laryngeal height, dyspnea, 19
Laryngeal leukoplakia, **238**
Laryngeal nerve, vocal fold paralysis, 240
Laryngeal stenosis, 244
Laryngitis, **236**
Laryngomalacia, 244
Laryngopharyngeal reflux, **236**
Larynx diseases, **235–241**. *See also specific types*
cricothyrotomy, **240**
epiglottitis, **237**
hoarseness & stridor, **235–236**
laryngitis, **236**
laryngopharyngeal reflux, **236**
masses
laryngeal leukoplakia, **238**
squamous cell carcinoma, **238–240**
vocal folds, traumatic lesions, **237–238**
recurrent respiratory papillomatosis, **237**
tracheostomy, **240–241**
vocal fold paralysis, **240**
Laser enucleation, 969
Laser thermal keratoplasty, 168
Laser vaporization of the prostate, 967–968
Lasmiditan, 971
Lassa fever, **1391–1392**
Lassitude, 33
Latent autoimmune diabetes of adulthood, 1195–1196, **1195–1196**
Latent tuberculosis infection, 279, 286–287
Late-onset T2-high asthma, 245
Late preterm birth, 805
Lateral collateral ligament, 1701
Lateral collateral ligament injury, **1701–1702**
Lateral epicondylosis, **1689**
Lateral femoral cutaneous nerve, 1035
Lateral medullary syndrome, 990
Lateral sclerosis, **1028**
Latrodectus mactans, **1590–1591**
Laxatives. *See also specific types*
abuse, **1094–1095**
for constipation, **586–588,** 587*t*, 646
hypermagnesemia, 894
LD-1 inhibitors, 1607. *See also specific types*
LDL. *See* Low-density lipoprotein cholesterol
Lead poisoning, **1583–1584**
antidote, 1568*t*
gout from, 823
tubulointerstitial disease from, 937
Learning, dementia, 54
LECT2 amyloidosis, 541
Ledipasvir, 683–684, 689, 690*t*

Lefluonomide
  adverse effects, 830
  pregnancy, contraindications, 830
  for psoriatic arthritis, 860
  for rheumatoid arthritis, 830
Left atrial appendage closure, 987–988
Left atrium enlargement, mitral regurgitation, 338
Left bundle branch block
  acute MI, with ST-segment elevation, **373–375,** 380
  angina pectoris, 361
  AV block, 387–388
  cardiomyopathy, dilated, 419, 420
  heart failure, 411, 412
  mitral regurgitation, 339
  myocarditis, 415
  paroxysmal supraventricular tachycardia, 388, 390
  syncope, 402
Left heart disease/failure, 403, **403–404,** 404. *See also* Heart failure
  bundle branch block, 411, 412
  cardiomyopathy, restrictive, 418*t*, 423
  pulmonary hypertension, 301, 432
  right ventricle dilation, 351
Left-to-right shunt
  atrial septal defect, 326–327
  Eisenmenger physiology, 432
  ventricular septal defect, 328–329
Left ventricle
  aneurysm, acute MI with ST-segment elevation, 381
  angiography, 362
  dilation, aortic regurgitation, 347
  dysfunction, cardiac risk assessment/reduction, 44–45
  enlargement, mitral regurgitation, 338
  heave, hypertension, 447
  hypertrophy, athletic deaths, 438
  Kawasaki disease, 1437
  systolic function, coarctation of aorta, 325
Left ventricular ejection fraction
  acute heart failure, 405
    preserved, 412
    reduced, **406–412,** 406*f*
  aortic regurgitation, 348, 349*f*
  aortic stenosis, 342–343, 343*t*, 344*f*, 346*f*
  bundle branch block, 406*f*
  cardiomyopathy
    dilated, 417–420
    peripartum, 436, 437*t*
    restrictive, 423, 424
    stress, 421
  CHA_2DS_2-VASc score, 393*t*
  coronary artery bypass grafting, operative mortality, 366
  mitral regurgitation, 339, 340, 340*f*, 341*f*
  myocarditis, noninfectious, 417
  postinfarction management, 382
  pregnancy, 435
  pulmonary hypertension, 432*t*
  radionuclide angiography, 361
Left ventricular end-diastolic pressure, 18, 19, 331
Left ventricular failure, 343, 348, 380
Leg
  lower extremity edema, **27–29,** 28*t*
  restless leg syndrome, **1084**
Legal issues, end of life care, 77
Legionella (Legionnaires disease), **1461–1462**
  immunocompromised, pulmonary infiltrates, 279
  with impaired cellular immunity, 1273
  medication of choice, 1294*t*
  pneumonia, 269*t*, 270, 272, 273
Legionella pneumophila pneumonia, community-acquired, 270, **1462**
Leiomyoma, **765–766,** 1624
Leiomyoma-renal cell carcinoma, hereditary, 1645
Leishmaniasis, **1499–1501,** 1500*f*
Lemborexant, 1050*t*, 1083–1084
Lemierre syndrome, 233, 1472
Lenalidomide, 1602*t*
  for amyloidosis, 541
  autoimmune thyroiditis from, 1112
  for cutaneous lupus erythematosus, 142
  for plasma cell myeloma, 538
  thyroiditis from, silent, 1115
Lens
  crystalline
    cataract, 184
    glaucoma, acute angle-closure, 180
    opacities, cataract, 184
    surgery, 168
  phakic intraocular, 168
Lentignes, **108,** 163
Lentigo melanoma, 109–110
Lenvatinib, 1601*t*, 1612, 1646
Leprosy
  polyneuropathy, 1032
  tuberculoid, polyneuropathy, 1032
Leptomeningeal metastases, **1001**
Leptospira (leptospirosis), **1490–1491**
  anicteric, 1491
  icteric, 1491
  interstitial nephritis, 911
  medication of choice, 1295*t*
Lesbian, 1709
Lesbian & bisexual women, health care, **1715–1722**
  aging & advance care planning, 1715–1716
  body weight, **1717–1718**
  cancer, **1719–1721**
    breast, **1720**
    cervical, **1720**
    endometrial & ovarian, **1721**
    lung, **1720–1721**
  cardiovascular disease, **1716**
  cisgender, 1715
  diabetes, **1718**
  family building, 1713–1715
  health care access, 1715, 1720
  health disparities, **1715–1716**
  mental health, **1721–1722**
  parents
    child outcomes, 1714
    pregnancy outcomes, 1714
  pregnancy prevention, 1713
  pulmonary disease, **1718**
  sexually transmitted infections, **1718–1719**
  smoking, cigarette, **1716–1717**
  substance use, **1717**
  violence, **1721**
Lesinurad, 826
Letrozole, 1602*t*
  for breast carcinoma, 754, 757, 757*t*
  for infertility, male, 773
  for pelvic pain, 768
  for pregnancy with polycystic ovary syndrome, 771
Leucovorin
  for cancer, 1653*t*
  for colorectal cancer, 1630
  on methotrexate toxicity, 1656
  for pancreas carcinoma, 1616
Leukemia
  acute, 510, **528–530**
    lymphoblastic, **528–530**
    mixed phenotype, **529**
    myeloid, **528–530**
    promyelocytic, **528–530**
  chronic
    lymphocytic, **530–532**
    myeloid, 520*t*, **524–526**
  classification, WHO, 519, 519*t*, 520*t*
  "core-binding factor," 528
  hairy cell, **532–533**
  immunocompromised, 1273
  Philadelphia chromosome, 520
  retinal/choroidal hemorrhage, 193
Leukoagglutinin reactions, 543
Leukocyte-depleted blood products, for cytomegalovirus, 1367
Leukoencephalopathy, non-determined, 1387
Leukoplakia, **227–229,** 227*f*
  hairy, **228,** 228*f*, 1324
  laryngeal masses, **238**
Leukotriene modifiers, 251*t*, 254. *See also specific types*
Leukotriene receptor antagonists, 813. *See also specific types*
Leuprolide (acetate), 1602*t*
  for breast carcinoma, 757, 757*t*
  for pelvic pain, 768
  for prostate cancer, 1602*t*, 1640, 1640*t*
Levalbuterol, 249, 252*t*
Levamisole-associated purpura, **855**
Levetiracetam
  poisoning, 1575–1576
  pregnancy, safety, 813
  for seizures, 976*t*, 977*t*
Levocarnitine, 1044
Levodopa
  chorea from, 1012
  dystonia from, 1012
  for idiopathic torsion dystonia, 1011
  for Parkinson disease, 1008
  for restless legs syndrome, 1013
Levofloxacin
  for cellulitis, venous insufficiency ulcer, 162
  for *Chlamydia trachomatis* urethritis/cervicitis, 1478
  for *Chlamydophila pneumoniae,* 1479
  for cystitis, 947*t*
  for epididymitis, 948*t*
  for *Haemophilus,* 1461
  hepatotoxicity, 696
  hypoglycemia from, 1237
  for *Legionella,* 1462
  for peritonitis, spontaneous bacterial, 703
  for plague, 1469
  for pneumococcal pneumonia, 1444, 1445
  for prostatitis, 948*t*
  for pyelonephritis, 947*t*
  for Q fever, 1436
  for *Salmonella,* 1464
  for *Shigella,* 1465
  for *Staphylococcus aureus* osteomyelitis, 1448
Levomilnacipran, 1072, 1073*t*, 1075
Levonorgestrel
  for hirsutism, female, 1183
  intrauterine devices, 777
  IUDS, for abnormal uterine bleeding & ovulatory dysfunction, 764
  oral contraceptives, low-dose, 775*t*
Levorphanol, **88*t***
Levothyroxine
  for anterior hypopituitarism, 1102
  for Hashimoto autoimmune thyroiditis, 1114
  hyperthyroidism from, 1138
  for hypothyroidism, 809–810, 1117
  for myxedema crisis, 1117
Levothyroxine suppression therapy
  for thyroid cancer, 1134, 1136
  for thyroid nodules, 1130–1131
Lewy bodies, dementia with, 1015*t*
Leydig cell hyperplasia, diffuse stromal, 1182

LHFH. *See* Luteinizing hormone–releasing hormone
Libido, decreased, 919, 958
Libman-Sacks endocarditis, systemic lupus erythematosus, 834
Lice, **130–131**
 STI, 1285
 typhus, **1426–1429,** 1427*t*
Lichenoid eruptions, drug, 158*t*
Lichen planus
 oral, **228**
 skin, **140–141,** 140*f*
Lichen planus–like eruptions, drug-related, 158*t*
Lichen simplex chronicus, **135–136,** 135*f*
Lichtheimia, 1544
Licorice, black, 882*t,* 883*f,* 900
Liddle syndrome, 882*t,* 900*t*
Liddle syndrome, hypertension, 445
Lidocaine, **91*t*,** 95, 97*t,* 383, 384*t*
Life expectancy, older adults, 52, 53*f*
Lift-off test, 1678*t*
Ligament stress testing, knee
 anterior drawer, 1697*t,* 1700
 Lachman test, 1696, 1697*t,* 1700
 pivot shift, 1698*t,* 1700–1701
 valgus stress, 1698*t,* 1701
 varus stress, 1699*t,* 1702
Lightning burn injury, 1557
Lily-of-the-valley, 1581
Limb. *See also* Extremities; *specific limbs*
 arterial occlusion, **477–478**
 ischemia threatening, 475, 476
Limb-girdle muscular dystrophy, 1043*t*
Limbic encephalitis/encephalomyelitis, 1004*t*
Linaclotide, 586, 587*t,* 646
Linagliptin, 1205*t,* 1210
Linezolid
 for enterococcus, 1443
 for furunculosis & carbuncles, 126
 for MRSA, 128, 1328, 1442
 for *Staphylococcus aureus* skin & soft tissue infections, 1447
Linitis plastica, 1620
Liothyronine, 1117
Lipase, for pancreatitis, 734, 735*t*
Lipemia retinalis, 1241
Lipid disorders, **1239–1243.** *See also* Hypercholesterolemia; Hypertriglyceridemia; *specific types*
 clinical presentations, **1241**
 eruptive xanthomas, 1241, 1241*f*
 familial chylomicronemia syndrome, **1239**
 familial hypercholesterolemia, **1239**
 Friedewald equation, 1240
 high blood cholesterol (*See also* Hypercholesterolemia)
  screening & treatment, **1241–1243,** 1242*t*
   in older patients, 1243
 lipemia retinalis, 1241
 lipid fractions & coronary heart disease risk, **1239–1240**
 lipid metabolism, secondary conditions on, **1241**
 lipoprotein(a), 1240
 Martin-Hopkins equation, 1240
 non-HDL cholesterol, 1240
 screening/prevention, 4, 5*t,* 8
 tendinous xanthomas, 1241
 triglycerides, high blood, **1248–1249**
Lipid disorders, treatment, **1240–1249**
 cholesterol lowering, therapeutic effects, **1240–1241**
 high LDL cholesterol, **1243–1249**
  algorithms, 1248, 1249*f*
  diet therapy, 1243–1244
  pharmacologic therapy, 1244–1248
   bempedoic acid, 1245*t,* 1247
   bile acid–binding resins, 1245*t,* 1247–1248
   ezetimibe, 1245*t,* 1246
   fibric acid derivatives, 1245*t,* 1248
   niacin, 1248
   omega-3 fatty acid preparations, 1245*t,* 1247
   proprotein convertase subtilisin/kexin type 9 inhibitors, 1245*t,* 1246–1247
   statins, 1244–1246, 1245*t*–1246*t*
Lipid emulsion, 1268
Lipid hypothesis, coronary vascular disease, 1239
Lipodermatosclerosis, lower extremity edema, 28
Lipodystrophy, 1220–1221, **1344–1345**
Lipoma, 434, 1647
Lipoprotein
 diabetes mellitus, 1202–1203
 high-density, 5*t,* 8, 355, **1202–1203**
 low-density (*See* Low-density lipoprotein cholesterol)
Lipoprotein(a), **1240**
Lipoprotein lipase, 1239
Lipschutz ulcers, 1428
Liquefaction necrosis, 1573
Liquid diet, 1263
Liquid nitrogen. *See* Nitrogen, liquid
Liraglutide, 358–359, 1205*t,* 1209, 1218, 1253, 1255*t,* 1257
Lisch nodules, 1005
Lisinopril, 407–408, 452*t,* 454, 796*t*
Listeria (listeriosis), **1453**
 with impaired cellular immunity, 1273
 liver abscess, 717
 medication of choice, 1294*t*
Listeria monocytogenes, **1453**
 diarrhea, 590
 hemochromatosis risk, 710
Literacy, health, 1
Lithium
 for aggression disorders, 1085
 autoimmune thyroiditis from, 1112
 for bipolar disorder, 1079–1080
 breastfeeding, 796*t*
 chorea from, 1012
 for dyskinesia from antipsychotics, 1068
 dystonia from, 1012
 goiter from, 1115
 minimal change disease, 932
 neuroleptic malignant syndrome from, 1067
 parkinsonism from, 1012
 poisoning, 1567*t,* 1569*t,* 1571*t,* 1572*t,* **1584**
 serotonin syndrome from, 30
 tremor from, 1012
Lithium carbonate, 973, 1123*t,* 1124
Live attenuated vaccines, 1301
Livedo racemosa, 850*t,* **857–858**
Livedo reticularis, 850, 850*f,* 850*t,* **857–858**
Liver. *See also* Hepatic
Liver cancers. *See* Hepatobiliary cancers; Hepatocellular carcinoma; *specific types*
Liver diseases, **677–718**. *See also specific types*
 abscess
  amebiasis, 1514
  pyogenic, **716–717**
 acute liver failure, **684–686**
 alcohol-associated, **693–695**
 biochemical tests, **675–677,** 676*t,* 677*t*
 cholangitis, primary biliary, **707–709**
 cirrhosis, **700–707**
 coagulopathy of, **562**
 drug- & toxin-induced injury, **696–697**
 heart failure, liver in, **715**
 hemochromatosis, **709–711**
 hepatic venous outflow obstruction, **713–714**
 hepatitis, **677–684, 686–693**
  A, acute, **677–679,** 678*f*
  autoimmune, **691–693**
  B
   acute, **679–682,** 680*f,* 681*t*
   chronic, **687–689**
  C
   acute, **682–684,** 683*f*
   chronic, **689–691,** 690*t,* 691*t*
  chronic, **686–691**
  D, **684**
   chronic, **687–689**
  E, **684**
 HIV/AIDS, 1325–1326
 jaundice & abnormal liver biochemical test evaluation, **674–677,** 676*t,* 677*t*
  biopsy, liver, 677
  imaging, 676–677
 neoplasms, benign, **717–718**
 nonalcoholic fatty liver disease, **697–699**
 porphyria, dysautonomia, 984
 portal hypertension, noncirrhotic, **715–716**
 preoperative evaluation/perioperative management, 47
 steatosis, 682
 Wilson disease, **711–713,** 712*f,* 1012
Liver failure
 acute, **684–686,** 1368
  HHV-6, 1368
 acute-on-chronic, 700
 herpes simplex virus, 1354
Liver flukes, **1521–1523**
 clonorchiasis, **1522**
 fascioliasis, **1521–1522**
 opisthorchiasis, **1522**
Liver transplantation. *See also specific indications*
 for acute liver failure, 686
 for alcohol-associated liver disease, 695
 for autoimmune hepatitis, 693
 biliary stricture from, 725
 for cholangitis
  primary biliary, 708–709
  primary sclerosing, 727, 728
 for cirrhosis, 705–707
 drug-/toxin-induced injury in, 696
 for esophageal varices with portal hypertension, 617
 for hemochromatosis, 711
 for hepatic disease, with HIV, 1326
 for hepatic venous outflow obstruction, 714
 for hepatitis B, 682
 for hepatitis C, 690, 691
 for hepatorenal syndrome, 704
 for liver neoplasms, benign, 718
 for nonalcoholic fatty liver disease, 699
 for portal hypertension, noncirrhotic, 716
 for pyogenic heart abscess, 717
 for Wilson disease, 713
Lixisenatide, 1205*t,* 1209
Load and shift test, shoulder, 1679*t*
Lobular carcinoma in situ, 749. *See also* Breast carcinoma
Localizing signs, false, 999
Locked-in syndrome, **1021**
Loeys-Dietz syndrome, pregnancy risks, 435
Löffler syndrome, 297
Lomitapide, 1245*t*
Lomustine, 1000
Lone Star tick *(Amblyomma americanum),* 1392, 1434

Long-acting beta-2-agonists. *See also specific types*
for asthma, 248*f*, 249–254, 250*t*
for COPD, 262, 263
Long-acting muscarinic antagonists. *See also specific types*
for asthma, 248*f*, 250*t*, 254
for COPD, 262, 263
Long-acting progestins, 771. *See also* Depo medroxyprogesterone acetate
Long-chain acyl coenzyme A dehydrogenase, acute fatty liver of pregnancy, 818
Long COVID, 19, 1405
Long QT syndrome, 26, **401**
acquired, **401**
athlete screening, 439, 439*t*, 440*t*
bradycardia, 401
hypercalcemia, acute kidney injury, 906
from ranolazine, 363
sudden cardiac arrest/death, 400, 401
treatment, beta-blocker, 384*t*
Long-term controller medications, for asthma, 249, 250*t*–251*t*. *See also specific types*
Loop diuretics
gout, 825
for heart failure with reduced LVEF, 407
for hypertension, **455**, 458*t*, 470, 471*t*
for hyponatremia, chronic, 879
ototoxicity, 213
Loop electrosurgical excision procedures, 789, 790
Loperamide, 592
for diarrhea, 595, 1223, 1288, 1292
for irritable bowel syndrome, 646
for short bowel syndrome, 637
Lopinavir/r, **1340*t*, 1345**
Lopinavir/ritonavir
for MERS-CoV, 1417, 1418
for SARS-CoV-1, 1415
Loratadine, 152
Lorazepam, 1050*t*
for adjustment disorder, 1047
for alcohol withdrawal, 1091
for hypertension, from poisoning, 1566
for insomnia, 1083
for panic disorder, insomnia, 1050*t*, 1051
for psychedelic effects, 1093
for seizures, from poisoning, 1567
Lorlatinib, 1606
Losartan, 453*t*, 454
Louse-borne typhus, **1426–1429**, 1427*t*
Lovastatin, 357*t*, 1245*t*
Low back pain, **1683–1685**, 1684*t*
cauda equina syndrome, 1682–1685
chronic, 80
physical therapy for, 95
Low-density lipoprotein cholesterol
coronary heart disease, 355
diabetes mellitus, 1202–1203, 1224
diet on, 1244–1245
estimation, 1240
high, treatment, **1243–1248**
algorithms, 1248, 1249*f*
diet therapy, 1243–1244
pharmacologic therapy, 1244–1248
bempedoic acid, 1245*t*, 1247
bile acid–binding resins, 1245*t*, 1247–1248
ezetimibe, 1245*t*, 1246
fibric acid derivatives, 1245*t*, 1248
niacin, 1248
omega-3 fatty acid preparations, 1245*t*, 1247
proprotein convertase subtilisin/kexin type 9 inhibitors, 1245*t*, 1246–1247
statins, 1244–1246, 1245*t*–1246*t*
screening/cardiovascular disease prevention, 5*t*, 8
very-low-density, 1240
Lower airways disorders. *See also specific types*
bronchial obstruction, 245
definition, 244
Lower esophageal sphincter
belching, 588
esophageal motility disorders, 618–619
GERD, 608
Lower extremity edema, **27–29**, 28*t*
Low-glycemic-index diet, 1252
Low-grade squamous intraepithelial lesions (LSIL), 788, 792
Low-molecular-weight heparin, **563**
for acute MI with ST-segment elevation, after drug-eluting/bare metal stents, 377
for antiphospholipid syndrome, pregnancy-associated, 838
for Budd-Chiari syndrome, 714
heparin-induced thrombocytopenia from, **552–553**, 553*t*
for intracranial venous thrombosis, 996
for Kawasaki disease, 1438
perioperative management, 48, 48*t*
with prosthetic heart valves, 353, 354*t*
for pulmonary venous thromboembolism, 300
reversal agents, 565*t*
for venous thromboembolism, 567*t*, 569–570, 569*t*
Loxapine, 1063, 1066
Loxosceles reclusa, **1590–1591**
Lp(a), PCSK9 on, 8
Lubiprostone, 586, 587*t*, 646
Lucid interval, 1021
Ludwig angina, 233
Lumacaftor, 267
Lumateperone, 1063, **1064**, 1064*t*
Lumbar disk herniation, **1686–1687**
Lumbar plexus neuropathy, 974, **1040**
Lumbar puncture headache, 35*t*, 37, 974
Lumbar spine
osteoarthritis, 820
surgery, post-laminectomy pain syndrome, 80
Lumbar sympathectomy, for hypertension, 464
Lumbosacral plexus lesions, **1040**
Lumefantrine, 1504*t*, 1505*t*, 1508–1509
Luminal GI tract dysfunction, 579
Lumpectomy, breast-conserving, 750–751, 751*f*
Lung. *See also* Pulmonary
abscess, **276–278**
evaluation, non–lung resection surgery, 46–47
Lung cancers, 11–12, **1603–1609**. *See also* Bronchogenic carcinoma; Pulmonary neoplasms; *specific types*
bronchogenic carcinoma, **1603–1607**
cerebral metastases, **1001**
hemoptysis, 21
HIV/AIDS, 1321
lesbian & bisexual women, **1720–1721**
mesothelioma, **1608–1609**
metastases, **1608**
screening, **289**
superior vena cava obstruction, 492
Lung flukes, paragonimiasis, **1523–1524**
Lung transplantation, 264, 267, **321–322**
Lung volume reduction surgery, for COPD, 264
Lungworm, rat, 1529
Lupus, drug-induced, **836–837**
Lupus anticoagulants, **562**
antiphospholipid syndrome, 837
levamisole-associated purpura, 855
systemic lupus erythematosus, 832*t*, 834*t*, 835*t*
Lupus nephritis, 833*t*–834*t*, 834–836, 923*t*, **930–931**
Lupus pernio, sarcoidosis, 295, 296*f*
Lupus profundus, 832
Lurasidone, 1063, **1064**, 1064*t*, 1065*t*
Luspatercept, 506
Lusutrombopag, 705
Luteinizing hormone, 1099
Luteinizing hormone–releasing hormone analogs/agonists. *See also specific types*
goserelin acetate, 1602*t*
leuprolide, 1602*t*
for paraphilias, 1058
for prostate cancer, 1602*t*, 1640, 1640*t*, 1641
triptorelin pamoate, 1602*t*
Luteinizing hormone–releasing hormone antagonists, 1602*t*, 1640, 1640*t*, 1641. *See also specific types*
Luteoma of pregnancy, 1182
Lyme borreliosis. *See* Lyme disease
Lyme disease, **1491–1495**
coinfections, 1494
erythema migrans, **128**, 129*f*, 1492–1495, 1495*t*
facial paralysis, 1036*f*
myopericarditis, 427
neck masses, 242
polyneuropathy, **1032**
post–Lyme disease syndrome, 1493
symptoms and signs, by stage, 1492–1493
tick vector & pathogenesis, 1493
treatment, 1295*t*, 1494, 1495*t*
Lymphadenitis, **493–494**. *See also specific disorders*
cat-scratch fever, 493
filariasis, 1531, 1531*f*
mycobacterial, 242, **1475**
Lymphangitic carcinomatosis, 1608
Lymphangitis, **493–494**, 1297*t*, 1531, 1531*f*
Lymphatic channel diseases, **493–494**
lymphangitis & lymphadenitis, **493–494**
lymphedema, **494**, 494*f*
Lymphatic filariasis, **1530–1532**, 1531*f*
Lymphedema, **494**, 494*f*
Lymphoblastic lymphoma, 535
Lymphocytic choriomeningitis, **1384–1385**
Lymphocytic hypophysitis, 1099, 1101, 1102, 1103
Lymphocytic interstitial pneumonitis, HIV/AIDS, 1314, 1321
Lymphocytic meningitis, 1354
Lymphocytosis, chronic lymphocytic leukemia, 530–531
Lymphoepithelioma, nasopharyngeal/paranasal, 226
Lymphogranuloma venereum, *Chlamydia trachomatis*, **1477**
Lymphomas, **533–542**. *See also specific types*
aggressive, 534–535
amyloidosis, **540–542**
autoimmune hemolytic anemia, 514
B-cell
after Q fever, 1436
diffuse large, 534
HIV/AIDS, 1329
large, gastric, 1623
from methotrexate, 830
non-Hodgkin, hepatitis C, 682
Burkitt, 535, 1364
cerebral, primary, 998*t*, **1001**
HIV/AIDS, 998*t*, **1001**
classification, 533, 533*t*
CNS, 535, 1311, 1322
cold agglutinin disease, 516
double-hit, 534

Lymphomas (*Cont.*):
Epstein-Barr virus, 1322, 1364
follicular, 534, 1436
gastric, **1622–1623**
head & neck, 243
HHV-8+ diffuse large cell, 1368
high-grade, 534
highly aggressive, 535
HIV/AIDS
CNS, 1311, 1322
non-Hodgkin, 1319*t*, 1322, 1329
primary effusion, 1321
Hodgkin, **535–536** (*See also* Hodgkin disease)
Epstein-Barr virus, 1364
immune thrombocytopenia, 548
indolent, 534
large-cell, 530
liver, 1610
lymphoblastic, 535
MALT-type, gastric, 1623
mantle cell, 535
marginal zone, 534, 682
hepatitis C, 682
monoclonal gammopathy of undetermined significance, **539**
neck, **243**
NK-cell, 227, 1363
non-Hodgkin, **533–535,** 533*t*
HIV/AIDS, 1319*t*, 1322, 1329
IgM hypergammaglobulinemia with, 538
nasopharyngeal, 226
treatment, 1595*t*, 1596*t*
peptic ulcer disease, 625
plasma cell myeloma, **536–539**
small intestine, 601, **1625**
small lymphocytic, 534
T-cell
cutaneous, **113–114**
drug-induced, 134
Epstein-Barr virus, 1364
HTLV-1 adult, 1388–1389
nasal, 227
peripheral, 535
from pimecrolimus, 134
from tacrolimus, 134
thyroid, 1132, 1137
thyroid mucosa-associated lymphoid tissue, 1135–1136
upper aerodigestive tract foreign bodies, **243**
Waldenström macroglobulinemia, **539–540**
Lymphomatoid granulomatosis, Epstein-Barr virus, 1364
Lymphoplasmacytic sclerosing pancreatitis, 733
Lymphoproliferative disease. *See also specific types*
immune thrombocytopenia, 548
Lynch syndrome, **668–669,** 791, 1615, 1627, 1644
Lysergic acid diethylamide (LSD), **1093, 1584–1585**

M

Macitentan, 705, 841
Macrocytic anemias, 500
Macrocytosis, myelodysplastic syndrome, 546
Macrophage activation syndrome, 831
Macropsia, 999
Macular degeneration, age-related, 52, 67, **187**
"Mad cow disease," 1385
Maddress discriminant function index, modified, 694
Maduromycosis, 1546
Magnesium
on calcium concentrations, 893
concentration disorders, **892–894**
hypermagnesemia, **894**
hypomagnesemia, **893**
deficiency
hypokalemia, 882*t*, 883, 883*f*, 884
hypophosphatemia, 883, 884
on nervous system, 892
normal plasma, 892
nutritional support, 1267
on parathyroid hormone, 893
Magnesium citrate, 587*t*, 883, 972*t*
Magnesium hydroxide, 586, 587*t*
Magnesium oxide, 893
Magnesium salicylate, **84*t***
Magnesium sulfate, 258, 804, 806
Magnetic gait, 1016
Magnetic resonance cholangiopancreatography, 726
for bile dilatation, 675
for biliary stricture, 675, 725
for choledocholithiasis, 675, 720*t*, 722
for pancreatitis, 730, 732, 734
pregnancy, 817
for primary sclerosing cholangitis, 726, 727
Magnetic resonance urogram, 944–945
Ma huang, 1580*t*
Major depressive disorder, **1069–1070**. *See also* Depression/depressive disorders
with atypical features, 1070, 1072
melancholic, 1070, 1072
older adults, 54, 57
with peripartum onset, 1070
psychotic, 072, 1070
with seasonal onset, 1070, 1072
Malabsorption (small intestine), **632–638,** 633*t*
bacterial overgrowth, **636**
celiac disease, **633–635**
clinical & laboratory manifestations, 632, 633*t*
Crohn disease, 654
HIV/AIDS, 1326
lactase deficiency, **637–638**
short bowel syndrome, **637**
systemic sclerosis, 841
Whipple disease, **635–636**
Malaria, **1502–1509**
clinical findings, **1502–1503,** 1503*f*
general considerations, **1502**
prevention, 1508*t*, 1509
prognosis, 1509
treatment, **1503–1509,** 1504*t*, 1505*t*, 1508*t*
antimalarial drugs, 1504*t*, 1505–1509, 1505*t*
amodiaquine, piperaquine, & pyronaridine, 1504*t*, 1506
antibiotics, 1504*t*, 1508
artemisins (qinghaosu), 1504*t*, 1505*t*, 1507–1508
atovaquone plus proguanil, 1504*t*, 1508
chloroquine, 1504*t*, 1505–1506, 1505*t*
folate synthesis inhibitors, 1507
lumefantrine, 1504*t*, 1508–1509
mefloquine, 1506
primaquine and tafenoquine, 1505*t*, 1507
quinine and quinidine, 1505*t*, 1506–1507
non-Falciparum, 1503–1504
severe, 1504–1505
uncomplicated Falciparum, 1504, 1504*t*, 1505*t*
Malarone, 1505*t*, 1508*t*, 1509
Malar rash, systemic lupus erythematosus, 834
Malassezia
seborrheic dermatitis, 139
tinea versicolor, 118
Malassezia furfur, seborrheic dermatitis, 1328
Malathion, 131, **1588–1589**
Males. *See also specific disorders*
hypogonadotropic hypogonadism, 1101
infertility, **960–963,** 961*f*
Peyronie disease, 959
Malignant ascites, **605–606**
Malignant catatonia, **30**
Malignant effusions, cancer-related, **1649–1650**
Malignant hypertension, 35, 192
Malignant hyperthermia, 30, 1277, 1567
Malignant melanoma, **109–110,** 109*f*, 169
Malignant otitis externa, **206–207,** 206*f*
Malignant pigmented lesions, **109–110,** 109*f*, 169
Malignant pleural effusion, 312–313
Malignant pleural mesothelioma, 1609
Mallory-Weiss syndrome, 582, **613–614**
Malnutrition
ASPEN/AND criteria, 1250
COVID-19, 1405
kwashiorkor, 1250
marasmus, 1250
protein–energy, **1250–1251**
Malocclusion, facial pain from, 978
Maltitol, 1203
MALT-type lymphoma, gastric, 1623
Mammalian target of rapamycin, 758. *See also specific types*
MammaPrint, 47, 51, 750, 752
Mammary Paget disease, **114,** 744, 744*f*
Mammography, breast cancer screening, 742–743
Manganese, nutritional support, 1267
Mania, **1069–1081**
Manic episodes, 1078–1081
Mannitol, 1203
Manometry
anorectal, 586, 588, 645, 672
esophageal, 607, 610, 619, 620
small intestine, 640
Mansonella, 1531
Mansonella perstans, 1532
Mantle cell lymphoma, 535
MAO inhibitors. *See* Monoamine oxidase inhibitors
Maple bark stripper's disease, 307*t*
Maprotiline, 1073*t*
Marasmus, 1250
Maraviroc, **1341*t*, 1346**
Marfan syndrome, **1664–1665**
aortic regurgitation, 347, 348
with aortic root dilatation, 438
pregnancy, 437–438, 437*t*, 812
athlete cardiovascular screening, 438, 439*tt*
bleeding from, 563
diverticulosis, 663
pregnancy risks, 435–436
thoracic aortic aneurysm, 484
Marginal blepharitis, 139
Marginal zone lymphomas, 534, 682
Marijuana use, **1093, 1585,** 1717
MARS, 704, 713
Marshall scoring system, modified, 729
Martin-Hopkins equation, 1240
MASCC score, 31
Masculinizing hormone therapy, **1727–1728,** 1728*t*
Masked hypertension, 444
Mastectomy, for breast carcinoma, 751
Masticatory claudication, facial pain from, 978
Mastitis, 119, **807–808**
Mastocytosis, systemic, peptic ulcer disease, 625
Mastoiditis, otitis media, 209, **210**
Maternally inherited diabetes and deafness (MIDD), 1197

Maturity-onset diabetes of the young, **1196–1197,** 1196*t*
Maxillary sinusitis, 219
Maxillary sinus tumors, 226
Mayaro virus, 1379
Mayer-Rokitansky-Küster-Hauser syndrome, 1184
May-Thurner syndrome, 28
Maze procedure, 337
MBX-400, 1367
McCune-Albright syndrome, acromegaly, 1106
McKenzie Method, 1687
McMurray test, 1699*t*, 1703
  modified, 1699*t*–1700*t*, 1703
MDMA. *See* Methylenedioxymethamphetamine (MDMA)
Meal replacement diets, 1252
Measles (rubeola), 1357*t*, 1358*t*, **1368–1371,** 1369*f*
Measles, mumps, and rubella (MMR) vaccine, 4*t*, 1306*t*, 1308*t*, 1370–1371, 1372, 1373
Measles inclusion body encephalitis, 1370
Measles-vectored Chikungunya virus vaccine (MV-CHIK), 1400
Mebendazole
  for ascariasis, 1526
  for echinococcosis, 1525, 1527
  for enterobiasis, 1529
  for hookworm disease, 1527
  for trichuriasis, 1526–1527
Mechanical extracorporeal counterpulsation, for angina pectoris, 367
Mechanical ventilation. *See* Ventilation, mechanical
Mechlorethamine, 114
Meckel diverticulum, small intestine bleeding, 601
Medial collateral ligament, 1701
Medial collateral ligament injury, **1701–1702**
Medial epicondylosis, **1689**
Median nerve, 1035
Mediastinal masses, **291–292**
Mediastinitis, fibrotic, superior vena cava obstruction, 492
Mediator inhibitors, 250*t*, 254. *See also specific types*
Medical aid in dying, 76
Medical collateral ligament injury, **1701–1702**
Medical interview, 1
Medical Orders for Life-Sustaining Treatment, 71–72
Medical Orders for Scope of Treatment, 72
Medication-assisted treatment, 13
Medication overuse headache, **974**
Medication reconciliation, 66
Medications. *See* Drug-related illnesses; Drugs; *specific types*
Mediterranean-style eating pattern/diet, 1243
  on cardiovascular events and stroke, 1203
  for gallstone prevention, 719
  on glycemic control and cardiovascular events, 1203
  for nonalcoholic fatty liver disease, 699
  for obesity, 1252
  omega-3 fatty acids, 1247
Medroxyprogesterone acetate, 764, 765, 1058. *See also* Depo-medroxyprogesterone acetate
Medtronic Melody valve, 324, 329, 331, 352
Medullary sponge kidney, 938*t*, **940–941**
Medullary thyroid cancer, 1132, 1132*t*, 1133, 1135, 1137
Medulloblastoma, 998*t*
Mefenamic acid, 767
Mefloquine, 1504*t*, 1506, 1508*t*, 1509
Megaloblastic anemias, 500, 501*t*
  folic acid deficiency, **508–509,** 509*t*
  pancytopenia, 517*t*
  pregnancy, 809
  subacute combined degeneration of spinal cord, 1027
  vitamin B_{12} deficiency, **507–508,** 507*t*
Megestrol acetate, 757*t*, 1316
Meglitinide analogs, for hyperglycemia/diabetes mellitus. *See also specific types*
  mitiglinide, 1204*t*, 1206
  repaglinide, 1204*t*, 1206
Meglumine antimonate, 1501
Meibomian gland
  carcinoma, 169
  infection
    blepharitis, 169
    chalazion, 170
    hordeolum, 168
MEK inhibitors, 199, 202*t*, 203. *See also specific types*
Melancholic depression, 1070, 1072
Melancholic major depression, 1070, 1072
Melanocytic nevi, **107,** 107*f*
Melanoma
  acral lentiginous, 110
  BRAF mutations, 1671*t*
  lentigo, 109–110
  malignant, **109–110,** 109*f*, 169
  superficial spreading, 109–110
  treatment, 1598*t*
Melarsoprol, 1497, 1497*t*
Melasma, hyperpigmentation, 163
MELAS syndrome, lactic acidosis from, 1232
Melatonin, 1083
Melena, 596, 599, 629
Melioidosis, 1294*t*
Melody valve, Medtronic, 324, 329, 331, 352
Meloxicam, **84*t***
Melphalan, 424, 528, 541, 936
Memantine, 972*t*, 1017
Membranoproliferative glomerulonephritis, hepatitis C, 682
Membranoproliferative glomerulonephropathy, 924*t*
Membranous nephropathy, 924*t*, 926, 931, **933–934**
Memory, 54, 1015
Menarch, 1184
Mendelson syndrome, **305,** 1277
Ménière disease, **216**
Meningeal irritation, noninfectious, 1281
Meningioma, 997, 997*t*
Meningitis. *See also specific pathogens and types*
  aseptic, 1280, 1280*t*
  carcinomatous, **1001,** 1281
  chemical, 1281
  chronic, 1280
  coccidioidomycosis, 1537
  Colorado tick fever, 1401
  COVID-19, 1404
  cryptococcus, **1542–1543**
    AIDS, **1001**
    HIV/AIDS, **1001,** 1318*t*, 1322, 1331
  echovirus, 1424
  encephalitis, 1280–1281
  enterovirus, 1423
  Epstein-Barr virus, 1363
  granulomatous, 1280*t*
  group B streptococcus, 1443
  Haemophilus, 1461
  health care–associated, 1281, 1282
  herpes simplex virus, 1354, 1355
  herpes zoster, 1360
  HIV/AIDS, 1323
  Kawasaki disease, 1438
  Listeria monocytogenes, 1453
  lymphocytic, benign recurrent, 1354
  meningococcus, 1323, **1459–1461**
  Mollaret, 1354
  Moraxella catarrhalis, 1461
  parechovirus, 1426
  partially treated, 1281
  Pneumococcus, 1282, **1446**
  purulent, 1280, 1280*t*, 1281*t*
  spirochetal, 1280*t*
  tick-borne encephalitis, 1383
  treatment
    antimicrobial therapy for, initial, 1296*t*
    postoperative, initial antimicrobial therapy, 1296*t*
  tuberculous, **1476–1477**
  viral, 1280*t*
  West Nile virus, 1380
Meningococcal, oligosaccharide conjugate (MCV4, MenACWY) vaccine, 1302*t*–1303*t*, 1306*t*, 1309*t*
Meningococcal group B vaccine (MenB), 1302*t*–1303*t*, 1306*t*, 1309*t*
Meningococcal polysaccharide conjugate vaccine (MPSV4), 1302*t*–1303*t*, 1306*t*, 1309*t*
Meningococcus
  gay & bisexual men, 1723
  medication of choice, 1293*t*
  meningitis, 1323, **1459–1461**
  meningococcemia, 1358*t*
  vaccines, 1460
Meningoencephalitis, 1280*t*, 1392
Meningomyelocele, 1028
Meniscus injuries, **1702–1703**
Menopause, 765
  normal, **1186–1191**
Menstruation
  anovulation, 763
  antipsychotics on, 1066
  asthma, catamenial, 246
  blood loss, 501–502, 763
  cessation, 1186
  frequency, 763
  iron loss, 601
Mentalization-based therapy, 1060
Menthol, 106*t*
Meperidine, 30, 85, **88*t***
Mepivacaine, neuromodulatory therapy, 97*t*
Mepolizumab, 251*t*, 254, 854–855
Meralgia paresthetica, **1035–1036**
Mercaptopurine/6-mercaptopurine
  for autoimmune hepatitis, 693
  for Crohn disease, 656
  for inflammatory bowel disease, 650
  for ulcerative colitis, 660
Mercury
  poisoning, 1568*t*, **1585–1586**
  tubulointerstitial disease from, 937
Meropenem
  for *Bacteroides fragilis*, 1472
  for *Campylobacter*, 1467
  for chest infections, anaerobic, 1472, 1472*t*
  for cholangitis, community-acquired, 724
  for peritonitis, spontaneous bacterial, 703
MERS-CoV, **1416–1418**
Mesalamine, 649–650, 659–660
Mescaline, **1093**
Mesenchymal tumors, gastrointestinal, **1624–1625**
Mesenteric ischemia
  acute, **480–481**
  chronic, **480–481**
  nonocclusive, **480–481**
Mesenteric vein occlusion, **481**
Mesial temporal lobe epilepsy, HHV-6, 1368

Mesial temporal sclerosis, 980, 1368
Mesna, 1653*t*
Mesoamerican nephropathy, 937–938
Mesothelioma, **1608–1609**
  malignant pleural, 1609
  treatment, 1596*t*
MET, lung cancer, 1606
Metabolic acidosis, 895
  acute kidney injury, 906
  anion gap, 1570
  chronic kidney disease, 917
  drowning, 1554
  hyperchloremic, normal ion gap, 897–898, 897*t*
  hyperkalemia, 885
  ketoacidosis, 896–897, 896*t*
  lactic, 895–896, 896*t*
  posthypercapneic, 900
Metabolic alkalosis, 895*t*, **899–901,** 900*t*
  chloride-responsive, 900–901, 900*t*
  chloride-unresponsive, 900–901, 900*t*
Metabolic-associated fatty liver disease, 698
Metabolic bone disease, **1146–1156.** *See also specific types*
  of chronic kidney disease, 917, 917*f*
  osteopenia, **1147**
  osteoporosis, **1147–1152,** 1148*t*
  Paget disease of bone, **1155–1156**
  rickets & osteomalacia, **1152–1154,** 1152*t*
Metabolic disturbances. *See specific types*
Metabolic dysfunction-associated fatty liver disease, 698
Metabolic encephalopathy, 1003, 1020
Metabolic syndrome, **1197–1198.** *See also* Insulin resistance
  angina, 365
  coronary heart disease, 355
  definition, 355
  hypertension, 444
  obesity, 355
Metacarpophalangeal joints, 821
Metals, heavy, 937, 1568*t*, 1603. *See also specific types*
Metapneumovirus, human, 1409
Metatarsophalangeal joint, big toe, 820, 824, 824*f*
Metatarsophalangeal joint inflammation, gouty arthritis, 824, 824*f*
Metered-dose inhalers, 249
MET exon 14 skipping mutations, lung cancer, 1606
Metformin
  anion gap elevation from, 1570
  on diabetes mellitus onset, in overweight, 1199
  for hirsutism, female, 1183
  for hyperglycemia/diabetes mellitus, 1204*t*, 1207
  lactic acidosis from, 1232
  for nonalcoholic fatty liver disease, 699
  poisoning, **1582**
  for polycystic ovary syndrome, 771
Methadone, **88*t*,** 92*t*, 93–94
  hypoglycemia from, 1237
  maintenance programs, 1092
  metabolism, 85
  morphine milligram equivalent doses, 85*t*
  for opioid poisoning, 1588
  for opioid withdrawal, 1092
Methamphetamines
  abuse, **1093–1094**
  combustion products, asthma, 245
  gay & bisexual men, 1724
  myopathy from, 1045
  poisoning, 1574
  serotonin syndrome from, 30
Methanol
  anion gap elevation from, 897, 1570
  poisoning, 1568*t*, 1569*t*, 1571*t*, 1572*t*, **1586**
Methcathinone poisoning, 1574
Methemoglobinemia
  agents inducing, poisoning, **1586–1587**
  dyspnea, 18, 19, 20
  headache, 35
  kidney dysfunction, 40
Methemoglobin poisoning, 1571*t*, 1572*t*
Methicillin-resistant *Staphylococcus aureus* (MRSA)
  for arthritis, nongonococcal acute, 862
  conjunctivitis, 170
  HIV/AIDS, 1328
  injection drug skin infections, 1286
  keratitis, 179
  nasal vestibulitis & colonization, 221
  osteomyelitis/septic arthritis, 1287, 1448
  pneumonia
    community-acquired, 273
    nosocomial, 275
  puerperal mastitis, 808
  risk factors, 276, 276*t*
  skin & soft tissue, **1446–1447,** 1447*f*
Methimazole
  birth defects from, 1126
  goiter from, 1115
  for hyperthyroidism, 1123*t*, 1124, 1237
  for thyrotoxic crisis/thyroid storm, 1127
Methotrexate, 1598*t*
  adverse effects, 830
  for autoimmune hepatitis, 693
  for bullous pemphigoid, 147
  for Chikungunya fever arthritis, 864, 1400
  for cholangitis, primary biliary, 709
  for Crohn disease, 656
  for ectopic pregnancy, 800
  for eosinophilic granulomatosis with polyangiitis, 854
  for gestational trophoblastic disease, 801
  hearing loss, 213
  for immune-mediated inflammatory myopathies, 844
  for inflammatory bowel disease, 650
  interstitial pneumonitis from, 830
  for Kawasaki disease, 1438
  for lymphoma
    cerebral, 1001
    CNS, 535
  for microscopic polyangiitis, 854
  for myasthenia gravis, 1041
  pregnancy, contraindication, 829
  for psoriasis, 137
  for psoriatic arthritis, 860
  for psoriatic erythroderma and pityriasis rubra pilaris, 155
  for rheumatoid arthritis, 829–830
  for scleroderma, 841
  for systemic lupus erythematosus, 835
  for Takayasu arteritis, 850
  toxicity, 1656, **1656–1657**
Methylated methylguanine-DNA methyltransferase promoter, glioblastoma with, 1000
Methylcellulose, 1264
Methylchloroisothiazolinone allergy, 161
Methylcobalamin, 507
Methyldopa
  drug-induced nephritis from, 837
  hepatotoxicity, 696
  for hypertension, 460, 463*t*, 812
  overdose, **1579**
Methylene blue, 1565, 1587
Methylenedioxymethamphetamine (MDMA), 1095
  hyponatremia from, 878
  poisoning, 1567*t*, 1574
  for PTSD, 1048
  serotonin syndrome from, 30
Methylenedioxypyrovalerone poisoning, 1574
Methylenetetrahydrofolate reductase *TT677* variant, hepatic venous outflow obstruction, 713
Methylisothiazolinone allergy, 161
Methylnaltrexone, 587–588
Methylphenidate
  abuse, **1093–1094**
  for attention-deficit/hyperactivity disorders, 1081
  for depression, 1076–1077
Methylprednisolone
  for adrenal insufficiency, 1158, 1159
  for alcohol-associated liver disease, 694
  for asthma, 250*t*, 252*t*
  clinical uses, 1193–1194, 1194*t*
  for congenital adrenal hyperplasia, 1183
  for Crohn disease, 656
  for hepatitis C, cryoglobulinemia, 690
  for lupus nephritis, 930
  for multiple sclerosis, 1024, 1025*t*
  neuromodulatory therapy, 97*t*
  for pauci-immune glomerulonephritis, 928
  for polyarteritis nodosa, 851
  for systemic lupus erythematosus, 835
  for thyroid eye disease, 1128
  for ulcerative colitis, 660, 661
Methylprednisolone acetate, 252*t*
4-Methylpyrazole, 1586
Methyl salicylate poisoning, **1589–1590**
Methyltestosterone, 1190–1191
Methylxanthine poisoning, **1592**
MET inhibitors, 1606. *See also specific types*
Metoclopramide
  for diabetic gastroparesis, 1223
  for dyspepsia, 581
  dystonia from, 1012
  for hyperemesis gravidarum, 797
  for nausea, 583*t*, **584**
  parkinsonism from, 1007
Metolazone, 458*t*
Metoprolol, 383, 384*t*
  for acute coronary syndrome, without ST-segment elevation, 371
  for hyperadrenergic postural orthostatic syndrome, 985
  for hypertension, 460, 461*t*–462*t*
Metoprolol succinate, 409
Metrifonate, 1521
Metritis, postpartum, **808,** 814
Metronidazole
  for amebiasis, 1514–1515, 1515t
  for bacterial vaginosis, 785
  for *Bacteroides fragilis,* 1472
  for brain abscess, 1282
  for *C. difficile* colitis, 648–649
  for chest infections, anaerobic, 1472, 1472*t*
  for cholangitis, community-acquired, 724
  for cholecystitis, 721
  for CNS infections, anaerobic, 1472
  for diarrhea, diabetic, 1223
  for giardiasis, 1519
  for gingival disease, 1325
  for gonococcus, 1470
  for *Helicobacter pylori,* 627
  for leg ulcers, venous insufficiency, 162
  for pelvic inflammatory disease, 786
  for peptic ulcer disease, 624*t*, 627
  for rosacea, 150
  for *Trichomonas vaginalis* vaginitis, 785
  for trichomoniasis, 1520
Metyrapone, 1163

Mexiletine, 383, 384*t*, 1044
Micafungin (sodium), 1540*t*
for aspergillosis, 1544
for candida endocarditis, 535
for candidiasis, 1535
MICE, 1707
Miconazole
for candidiasis, 105*t*, 119, 785, 1535
for tinea corporis, 105*t*, 115
for tinea versicolor, 105*t*, 118
topical dermatologic, 105*t*
Miconazole nitrate, 116
Microangiopathy, cardiac, from diabetes mellitus, 1224
Microcephaly, congenital, Zika virus, 1399
Microcytic anemias, 500, 504
Microlithiasis, 719
Micropsia, 999
Microsatellite instability-high, MMR system deficiency, 1673*t*
Microscopic colitis, **663**
Microscopic polyangiitis, **853–854**
Microsporidiosis, **1516–1518**
Microsporidium, 1517
Microsporum, 115
Midazolam, 1567
Middle cerebral artery occlusion, 988–989
Middle ear diseases, **209–211**
neoplasia, **212**
otitis media
acute, **209,** 209*f*
chronic, **209–211,** 210*f*
otosclerosis, **211**
trauma, **211–212,** 211*f*
Middle East respiratory–coronavirus (MERS-CoV), **1416–1418**
transmission and spread, 1401
Middle East respiratory syndrome (MERS), community-acquired pneumonia, 270
Middle mediastinal mass, 292
Midodrine, 704, 985
Mifepristone, 766, 780, 1072, 1419
Mifflin-St. Jeor Equation, 1266
Miglitol, 1204*t*, 1208, **1582**
Migraine aura, 970
Migraine headache, 36, **970–973,** 972*t*
aura without headache, 970
with brainstem aura, 971
clinical findings, 970–971
combined oral contraceptives and, 776
familial hemiplegic, 970
inheritance/familial/family history, 970–971
mitochondrial myopathies, 1044
pathophysiology, 970
photopsia, 970
recurrent painful ophthalmoplegic neuropathy, 971
retinal artery occlusion, 189
scotoma/scintillating scotomas, 970
treatment, 971–973, 972*t*
vertebrobasilar, vertigo from, 217
Migrainous vertigo, **217**
Mild cognitive impairment, 55, 1007, 1014
Miliaria, **151**
Miliaria crystallina, 151
Miliaria profunda, 151
Miliaria rubra, 151
Milk-alkali syndrome, 889, 889*t*, 900
Milker's nodules, 1421
Milk/milk products allergies, 614, 868
Milk thistle, 686
Miller Fisher syndrome, 1033
Milnacipran, 1057, 1072, 1073*t*, 1075
Milrinone, 499
Miltefosine, 1501
Mindfulness-based stress reduction, 1047
Mindfulness-based therapies, 1052, 1057, 1059
Mineralocorticoid receptor antagonists, 406, 932. *See also specific types*
Mineralocorticoids. *See specific types*
Mineral oil, 587*t*
Minerals. *See also specific types*
nutritional support, 1266–1267
Mini-cog, 54
Minilaparotomy sterilization, 779–780
Minimal change disease, 924*t*, 931, **932–933**
Minimally conscious state, **1020–1021**
Minipill, progestin, 776
Minocycline
for acne vulgaris, 149
drug-induced nephritis from, 837
hyperpigmentation from, 163, 163*f*
for *Mycobacterium marinum,* 1475
for nocardiosis, 1475
for rosacea, 150
for *Staphylococcus aureus,* skin & soft tissue infections, 1447
topical dermatologic, 105*t*
for typhus, scrub, 1430
Minority stress
gay & bisexual men, 1722–1724
lesbian & bisexual women, 1716, 1717, 1721
Minority stress model, **1710–1711,** 1724
Minoxidil
for alopecia, 164–165
for androgenic alopecia, 1182
for hypertension, 463*t*, 464
pericarditis from, 427
Mirizzi syndrome, 721
Mirtazapine, 160, 1072, 1073*t*, 1075
Mismatch repair system (MMR) mutations, MSI-H from, 1673*t*
Misoprostol, 627
Missed abortion, 798
Mistreatment. *See also specific types*
elder, **67–68,** 68*t*
Mitchell-Riley syndrome, 1197
Mites
bird/rodent, **132**
stored products, **132**
Mitiglinide, 1204*t*, 1206
Mitochondrial DNA mutation, diabetes mellitus, 1197
Mitochondrial myopathies, **1044**
Mitomycin, 1602*t*, 1634, 1643, 1644
Mitotane, 1163
Mitoxantrone, 417, 1025*t*
Mitragyna speciosa poisoning, 1588
Mitral clip (MitraClip), edge-to-edge, mitral regurgitation, 339–340, 341*f*
Mitral commissurotomy, 337, 337*f*
Mitral prosthetic valves, 337, 337*f*
Mitral regurgitation, 333*t*–335*t*, **338–341**
cardiac risk assessment/reduction, 45
categories, 332
general considerations & clinical findings, 338
rheumatic fever, 425
systemic lupus erythematosus, 834
treatment & prognosis, 339–341, 340*f*
Mitral stenosis, **332–338,** 333*t*–335*t*
cardiac risk assessment/reduction, 45
categories, 332
clinical findings, 336
DOACs for, 393–394, 394*t*
general considerations, 332
maternal mortality, pregnancy, 812
pulmonary edema from, 413
rheumatic, 350
treatment & prognosis, 336–338, 337*f*
vs. tricuspid stenosis, 350
vitamin K antagonist therapy for, 354*t*
Mitral valve
"clefts," 326
"parachute," 332
Mitral valve prolapse
angina, 360
mitral regurgitation, 334*t*–335*t*, 338, 339
palpitations, 25, 26
Mitral valve repair
annular ring, mitral stenosis, 332
mitral regurgitation, 339, 340, 341
Mitral valve replacement
anticoagulation after, 353, 353*t*
cardiomyopathy, hypertrophic, 422
mitral regurgitation, 338, 339, 340*f*, 341
mitral stenosis, 337*f*, 338
tricuspid annuloplasty with, 351
tricuspid valve replacement with, 350
Mixed acid-base disorders, 894
Mixed apnea, 316
Mixed connective tissue diseases, **845,** 934. *See also specific types*
Mixed cryoglobulinemia, 929
Mixed neuronal-glial tumors, 998*t*
Mixed phenotype acute leukemia, **529**
MLH1, 665, 668, 1615, 1628, 1673*t*
Mobitz type I AV block, 379, **387–388**
Mobitz type II AV block, 379–380, **387–388**
Modafinil, 708, 1025
Model for End-stage Liver Disease (MELD) score
acute liver failure, 685, 686
alcohol-associated liver disease, 694, 695
cirrhosis, 706–707, 706*t*
liver in heart failure, 715
surgical risk assessment, 47
Modified Blalock shunts, 330
Modified Goldman Risk Score, 24
Modified Marshall scoring system, 729
Modified Wells Score, 299*t*
Moexipril, 452*t*
Mogamulizumab, 1388, 1389
Mohs micrographic surgery, 111, 112
Moisturizers, skin, 101
Mole
atypical, **108,** 108*f*
changing, 110
hydatidiform, **800–802**
normal, **107,** 107*f*
Mollaret meningitis, 1354
Molluscipox virus, 1421
Molluscum contagiosum, **121,** 121*f*, 1327, 1328*f*, **1421**
Mometasone furoate, 103*t*, 252*t*
Mönckeberg medial calcific sclerosis, 476
Monkeypox, **1421–1422**
Monoamine oxidase inhibitors. *See also specific types*
for depression, 1072, 1073*t*, 1076
dietary limitations, 1076, 1076*t*
hypertension from, treatment, 1566
for melancholic depression, 1072, 1073*t*
for Parkinson disease, 1008–1009
for psychotic depression, 1072, 1073*t*
with serotonin reuptake inhibitor, serotonin syndrome from, 1567
serotonin syndrome from, 30
side effects, 1076
withdrawal symptoms, 1075
Monoclonal antibodies. *See also specific types*
for asthma, 251*t*, 254
Monoclonal antibodies, cancer, 1600*t*
atezolizumab, 1600*t*
bevacizumab, 1600*t*
cetuximab, 1600*t*

Monoclonal antibodies, cancer (*Cont.*):
daratumumab, 1600*t*
iplimumab, 1600*t*
nivolumab, 1600*t*
obinutuzumab, 1600*t*
panitumumab, 1600*t*
pertuzumab, 1600*t*
rituximab, 1600*t*
trastuzumab, 1600*t*
Monoclonal gammopathy
benign, 1032
of undetermined significance, **539,** 1032
Monoclonal immunoglobulin–mediated glomerulonephritis, 912
Monocular visual loss, transient, **190–191**
Monomethylhydrazine poisoning, 1587
Mononeuritis multiplex, 847*t*, 1032
complex regional pain syndrome, 867
eosinophilic granulomatosis with polyangiitis, 854
giant cell arteritis, 848
microscopic polyangiitis, 854
polyarteritis nodosa, 850
Mononeuropathies, **1034–1036**
carpal tunnel syndrome, **1690–1691**
chronic kidney disease, 919
diabetic, 1222–1223
entrapment neuropathy, 1034
Epstein-Barr virus, 1363
femoral neuropathy, **1035**
fibular nerve palsy, **1036**
meralgia paresthetica, **1035–1036**
pronator teres/anterior interosseous syndrome, **1035**
radial nerve lesions, **1035**
Saturday night palsy, 1034
sciatic nerve palsy, **1036**
tarsal tunnel syndrome, **1036**
ulnar nerve lesions, **1035**
Mononeuropathy multiplex, diabetic, 1222–1223
Montelukast, 251*t*, 254, 872
Montgomery-Asberg, 1071
Montreal Cognitive Assessment (MoCA), 54
Mood disorders, **1069–1081**. *See also specific types*
clinical findings, 1069–1071
adjustment disorder with depressed mood, 1069
bipolar disorder
cyclothymic disorder, 1070
mania, 1070
depressive disorders, 1069–1071
major depressive disorder, 1069–1070
persistent depressive disorder, 1070
premenstrual dysphoric disorder, 1070
secondary to illness/medications, 1070–1071
complications, 1071
differential diagnosis, 1071
prevalence & factors, 1069
prognosis, 1081
treatment, bipolar disorder/manic & depressive episodes, 1078–1081
treatment, depression, 1072–1078, 1074*f*
behavioral, 1078
medical, 1072–1078, 1073*t*, 1074*f*, 1076*t*
psychological, 1078
social, 1078
Moonshine, tubulointerstitial disease from, 937
Moraxella, 170, 179, 1283
Moraxella catarrhalis, **1461**
laryngitis, 236
medication of choice, 1293*t*
pneumonia, 269*t*, 270
rhinosinusitis, 219
Morbidly adherent placenta, **807**
Morbilliform, 102*t*
Morganella, 1294*t*
Morphine, **85–86,** 88*t*. *See also* Opioid overdose/poisoning
for acute MI, with ST-segment elevation, 377, 380
for dyspnea, 70
intrathecal, 97, 97*t*
neuromodulatory therapy, 97*t*
patient-controlled analgesia, 80
poisoning, **1587–1588**
for pulmonary edema, 413
Morphine milligram equivalent doses, 85–86, 85*t*
Mosaic hyperpigmentation, 163
Moths, urticating hair, **132**
Motility disorders. *See also specific types*
esophageal, **618–620**
achalasia, **618–619**
other primary, **620**
esophageal dysphagia, 607, 607*t*
intestinal, **638–641**
colonic pseudo-obstruction, acute, **639–641**
gastroparesis, **640–641**
intestinal pseudo-obstruction, chronic, **640–641**
paralytic ileus, **638–639**
irritable bowel syndrome, 644
Motor seizures, 979–980
Motor tics, 1013
Motor vehicle accidents, 12
Mourits clinical activity score, 1128
Movement disorders, nervous system, **1006–1014**. *See also specific types*
drug-induced abnormal movements, **1012–1013**
essential tremor, **1006**
Gilles De La Tourette syndrome, **1013–1014**
Huntington disease, **1010–1011**
myoclonus, **1012**
Parkinson disease, **1006–1010**
restless legs syndrome, **1013**
torsion dystonia
focal, **1011–1012**
idiopathic, **1011**
Wilson disease, **711–713,** 712*f*, 1012
Moxetumomab pasudotox, 533
Moxidectin, 1533
Moxifloxacin
for animal bites, 1284
for *Bacteroides fragilis*, 1472
for chest infections, anaerobic, 1472, 1472*t*
for *Chlamydophila pneumoniae*, 1479
for *Haemophilus*, 1461
hepatotoxicity, 696
for plague, 1469
for pneumococcal pneumonia, 1444, 1445
for Q fever, 1436
Moyamoya disease, saccular aneurysm, 994
6-MP, *TPMT* on metabolism of, 1670*t*
MPL, 520, 522, 523
MPO-ANCA, 852, 853
MRSA. *See* Methicillin-resistant *Staphylococcus aureus* (MRSA)
MSH2, 668, 1615, 1628, 1673*t*
MSH6, 668, 1615, 1628, 1673*t*
Mucocutaneous candidiasis, **118–119,** 119*f*
Mucocutaneous leishmaniasis, **1500–1501**
Mucocutaneous lymph node syndrome, **1436–1439**
Mucor (mucormycosis), 1544, **1544–1545**
gastritis, 624
with granulocytopenia, 1273
mucormycosis, 1544
sinusitis, invasive, 221–222
Mucosa-associated lymphoid tissue (MALT) tumors, stomach, 534
Mucosa-associated lymphoid tissue (MALT)-type lymphoma, gastric, 1623
Mucosal laceration of gastroesophageal junction, 581, **613–614**
Mucosal melanoma, nasopharyngeal, 226
Mucositis, preventing chemotherapy-related, 1656
Muddy brown casts, 903, 904*t*, 907, 907*t*, 909
Müllerian agenesis, 1184
Multicentric Castleman disease, HHV-8, 1368
Multidrug-resistant pathogens, risk factors, 276, 276*t*
Multidrug-resistant tuberculosis, 280
Multifocal atrial tachycardia, 397
Multifocal myoclonus, 1012
Multi-gated acquisition (MUGA) scan, 361
Multikinase inhibitors, 1606. *See also specific types*
Multinodular goiter, **1129–1131,** 1129*t*
Multiparametric MRI, for prostate cancer, 1635–1636
Multiple endocrine neoplasia
MEN 1, **1173–1174,** 1174*t*, 1233
MEN 2A, 1167, **1174,** 1174*t*
MEN 3 (2B), 1167, **1174,** 1174*t*
MEN 4, **1174–1175,** 1174*t*
Multiple mononeuropathy, sarcoidosis, 1032
Multiple myeloma. *See* Plasma cell myeloma
Multiple sclerosis, **1023–1026,** 1025*t*
vs. clinically isolated syndrome, 1024
diagnosis, 1023, 1024–1025
dissemination in space/time, 1024
hearing loss from, 218
primary progressive, 1023
relapsing-remitting, 1023
secondary progressive, 1023
treatment, 1024–1026, 1025*t*
vertigo from, 217, 218
Multislice CT angiography, for coronary artery disease, 361
Multisystem crisis, 1167
Multisystem immune-mediated diseases. *See also specific types*
patient age, 1270
Multisystem inflammatory syndrome
children, 1437
COVID-19, 1405
SARS-CoV-2, 1405
typhus, endemic, 1429
Multitarget stool DNA assay, 1632
Mumps vaccination, 1371, 1372
Munchausen by proxy, 1054
Munchausen syndrome, 1054
Mupirocin
for folliculitis, 125
for furunculosis, 126
for impetigo, 124
for MRSA impetigo, 124
for staphylococcal folliculitis, 1328
topical dermatologic, 105*t*
Mural thrombus, acute MI with ST-segment elevation, 381–382
Murmurs, heart. *See also* Heart sounds
Austin Flint, 347–348
coarctation of aorta, 325
Graham Steell, 333*t*, 334*t*, 352
mitral regurgitation, 338
mitral stenosis, 336
systolic
interventions on, 336*t*
patent foramen ovale, 327
valvular heart disease, interventions on, 336*t*
tricuspid regurgitation, 351
Muromonab, 1367

Muromonab-CD3, meningeal irritation from, 1281
Murphy sign, 720–721
Murray Valley encephalitis, 1379
Muscle mass depletion, 1250
Muscular dystrophies, **1043–1044,** 1043*t*
  Becker, 1043*t*, 1044
  distal, 1043*t*
  Duchenne type, 1043–1044, 1043*t*
  Emery-Dreifuss, 1043*t*
  facioscapulohumeral, 1043*t*
  limb-girdle, 1043*t*
  myotonic dystrophy, 1043*t*
  oculopharyngeal, 1043*t*
Mushroom picker's disease, 307*t*
Mushroom poisoning, 685–686, 696, **1587**
Musset sign, 333*t*, 347
MUTYH, 667
Myasthenia gravis, 1004*t*, **1040–1041**
Myasthenic crisis, 1041
Myasthenic syndrome, **1042**
MYC, high-grade lymphoma, 534
Mycetoma, **1546**
Mycobacteria *(Mycobacterium)*, **1475–1476.** *See also specific types and disorders*
  atypical, 287
    HIV/AIDS pulmonary disease, 1320
    with impaired cellular immunity, 1273
    lymphadenitis, 242, **1475**
    Mycobacterium tuberculosis, 1476–1477
    nontuberculous
      disseminated *Mycobacterium avium* complex, **1475–1476**
      lymphadenitis, 242, **1475**
      pulmonary, **287–289, 1475**
      skin & soft tissue, **1475**
    pneumonia, HIV/AIDS, 1319*t*, 1320, 1320*f*
    tuberculous (*See* Tuberculosis)
    tuberculous meningitis, **1476–1477**
    uveitis, 183
  Mycobacterium abscessus, 1475
    nontuberculous pulmonary disease, 288–289
  Mycobacterium avium complex, **1475**
    antiretroviral therapy, 1330–1331
    disseminated, **1475–1476**
    HIV/AIDS
      case definition, 1312*t*
      CD4 count and, 1314*f*
      hypogonadism, 1326
      liver disease, 1325
      malabsorption syndrome, 1326
      prophylaxis against, 1337, 1337*t*
      treatment, 1338
    nontuberculous pulmonary disease, 288
    treatment, 1295*t*, 1338
  Mycobacterium avium intracellulare, nontuberculous pulmonary disease, 288
  Mycobacterium bovis, intestinal, 643
  Mycobacterium chelonae, 288–289, 1475
  Mycobacterium fortuitum, 288–289, 1475
  Mycobacterium fortuitum-chelonei, 1295*t*
  Mycobacterium kansasii, 288, 1295*t*, **1475**
  Mycobacterium leprae, 1295*t*
  Mycobacterium malmoense, 288, 1475
  Mycobacterium marinum, 1475
  Mycobacterium szulgi, 1475
  Mycobacterium tuberculosis, 1476. *See also* Tuberculosis
    arthritis, **865**
    HIV/AIDS, 1320, 1320*f*
    intestinal, 643
    medication of choice, 1295*t*
    pleural effusion, 312
    pneumonia, community-acquired, 270
    pulmonary tuberculosis, **279–287**
    spinal tuberculosis, **864–865**
  Mycobacterium ulcerans, 1475
  Mycobacterium xenopi, 288, 1475
Mycophenolate mofetil
  for autoimmune hepatitis, 693
  for bullous pemphigoid, 147
  for C3 glomerulopathies, 929
  for cytomegalovirus, in immunosuppressed, 1367
  for focal segmental glomerulosclerosis, 933
  for glomerulonephritis, 913
  for immune-mediated inflammatory myopathies, 844
  for interstitial lung disease, scleroderma, 841
  for lichen planus, 141
  for lupus nephritis, 836, 930
  for membranoproliferative glomerulonephritis, 929
  for MERS-CoV, 1417
  for microscopic polyangiitis, 854
  for myasthenia gravis, 1041
  for neuromyelitis optica, 1026
  for pemphigus, 146
  progressive multifocal leukoencephalopathy from, 1387
  for systemic lupus erythematosus, 835
  for Takayasu arteritis, 850
Mycoplasma, 231, 957, 1295*t*
Mycoplasma genitalium, urethritis & cervicitis, 1477
Mycoplasma pneumoniae
  asthma exacerbations, 258
  mucocutaneous reaction, 153
  pneumonia, 269*t*
  pneumonia, community-acquired, 270, 272
Mycosis fungoides, **113–114**
Mycotic aneurysms, injection drug abuse, 1287
Mycotic infections, **1534–1547**
  agents for, 1539*t*–1540*t*
  aspergillosis, **1543–1544**
  "black" molds, 1546
  blastomycosis, **1545**
  candidiasis, **1534–1535**
  coccidioidomycosis, **1537–1538**
  cryptococcosis, **1542–1543**
  histoplasmosis, **1536–1537**
  household molds, **1546–1547**
  mucormycosis, **1544–1545**
  mycetoma, **1546**
  other opportunistic molds, 1546
  pneumocystis, **1538–1541**
  sporotrichosis, **1545–1546**
Mycotoxins, 1547
MYD88, Waldenström macroglobulinemia, 540
Myelin oligodendrocyte glycoprotein (MOG-IgG), 1026
Myelitis, 1004*t*
  acute flaccid, **1376**
  neuromyelitis optica, **1026**
  tick-borne encephalitis, 1383
Myelodysplastic syndromes, **526–527**. *See also specific types*
  bone marrow failure, 546
  from clonal cytopenias of undetermined significance, 502
  genetic abnormalities, 527
  International Prognostic Scoring System, 526
  relapsing polychondritis, 856
Myelofibrosis, primary, 520*t*, **523–524**
Myeloid growth factors, for neutropenia, 519
Myeloneuropathy, Chikungunya fever, 1400
Myelopathies
  AIDS, **1026, 1323**
  Chikungunya fever, 1400
  HIV/AIDS, **1026, 1323**
  human T-cell leukemia virus, **1026–1027**
Myeloproliferative disorders. *See also specific types*
  gout from, 823
  palpable purpura, 867
Myeloproliferative neoplasms
  causes & classifications, 519, 519*t*
  classification, WHO, 519, 519*t*, 520*t*
  essential thrombocytosis, 520*t*, **522–523**
  genes, 520
  laboratory features, 520*t*
  myelodysplastic syndromes, **526–527**
  myelofibrosis, primary, 520*t*, **523–524**
  polycythemia vera, **520–521,** 520*t*, 521*t*
Myerson sign, 1007
MYH9, bone marrow failure, 546
Myocardial fibrosis, cardiac MRI for, 361
Myocardial hibernation, **355**
Myocardial infarction
  cardiac risk assessment/reduction, 42
  combined oral contraceptives and, 774
  coronary vasospasm and, normal coronary arteriogram, **367–368**
  COVID-19, 1404
  diabetes mellitus, 1224
  Kawasaki disease, 1438
  lesbian & bisexual women, 1716
  palpitations, 25
  postoperative, 45
  silent, dyspnea, 18
Myocardial infarction, acute, with ST-segment elevation, **373–382**
  causes, 373
  clinical findings, 373–374
  complications, 379–381
    arrhythmias
      conduction disturbances, 379–380
      sinus bradycardia, 379
      supraventricular tachyarrhythmias, 379
      ventricular, 379
    ischemia, postinfarction, 379
    myocardial dysfunction
      acute left ventricular failure, 380
      hypotension & shock, 380–381
      left ventricular aneurysm, 381
      mechanical defects, 381
      mural thrombus, 381–382
      myocardial rupture, 381
      pericarditis, 381
      right ventricular infarction, 381
  fibrinolytic therapy, 375–377, 376*t*
  postinfarction management
    ACE inhibitors & ARBs, with left ventricular dysfunction, 382
    prevention, secondary, 382
    revascularization, 382
    risk stratification, 382
  treatment, 374–378
    ACE inhibitors, 377–378
    aldosterone antagonists, 378
    analgesia, 377
    angiotensin receptor blockers, 378
    aspirin, 374
    beta-adrenergic blockers, 377
    calcium channel blockers, 378
    coronary angiography, 378
    general measures, 377
    long-term antithrombotic therapy, 378
    nitrates, 377
    $P2Y_{12}$ inhibitors, 374
    reperfusion therapy, 375–377, 376*t*
      antiplatelet, after drug-eluting/bare metal stents, 375
      fibrinolytic, 375–377, 376*t*
      percutaneous coronary intervention, primary, 375
      stenting, 375

Myocardial ischemia. *See also* Myocardial infarction; *specific disorders*
acute, 22–23
acute coronary syndromes, without ST-segment elevation, 368–369
acute heart failure & pulmonary edema, 413
angina pectoris, 367
atrial fibrillation, 391
AV block, 387–388
cardiomyopathy, dilated, 419
catheterization & percutaneous coronary intervention for, 372*t*
coronary vasospasm, normal coronary arteriograms, **367–368**
heart failure, 405, 406
long QT syndrome, acquired, 401
mitral regurgitation, 339
rate & rhythm disorders, 383
ventricular tachycardia, 399
Myocardial perfusion scintigraphy, 361
Myocardial rupture, acute MI with ST-segment elevation, 381
Myocardial stress imaging, angina pectoris, 360–361
Myocardial stunning, **355–357,** 420
Myocarditis, **414–417**
adenovirus, 1419
athlete
cardiovascular screening, 438, 440*t*
deaths, 438
autoimmune, 414, 415*t*
AV block, 387
cardiomyopathy, dilated, 418*t,* 419
causes, 414, 415*t,* 416–417
from cocaine, 417
COVID-19
athletes, 416, 416*t,* 439–441
vaccine, 414, 1406
definition, 414
enteroviruses, 1423
eosinophilic, 417
fulminant, 415–416
genetic predisposition, 414
giant cell, 414, 415*t,* 417
granulomatosis with polyangiitis, 415*t,* 417
heart failure, 404
infectious, **414–416,** 415*t,* 416*t*
Kawasaki disease, 1437
mitral regurgitation, 339
noninfectious, **416–417**
parvovirus B19, 1419, 1420
pericarditis with, 427
primary/secondary, 414
systemic lupus erythematosus, 834
typhus, scrub, 1429
ventricular fibrillation & sudden death, 400
ventricular tachycardia, 399
Myoclonic-atonic seizures, 979
Myoclonic epilepsy, ragged red fiber syndrome (MERRF), 1044
Myoclonic seizure, 979
Myoclonic-tonic-clonic seizures, 979
Myoclonus, 1004*t,* **1012**
Myoglobin, 369, 909
Myoglobinuria, overload proteinemia, 904
Myomectomy, 766
Myonecrosis, 1286, **1450–1451**. *See also specific types*
Myopathic disorders/myopathies, **1042–1045.** *See also specific types*
acid maltase deficiency, **1044**
antisynthetase syndrome, **843**
autoimmune necrotizing, 1004*t*
Chikungunya fever, 1400
critical illness, **1044**
dermatomyositis, **842–844**
endocrine, **1044**
HIV/AIDS, 1324
immune-mediated inflammatory
antibodies, 843, 843*t*
antisynthetase syndrome, 843
dermatomyositis, **842–844**
heliotrope rash, 842, 843*f*
immune-mediated necrotizing, 843
inclusion body myositis, 843–844
polymyositis, **842–844**
immune-mediated necrotizing, **843**
inclusion body myositis, **1044**
inflammatory, immune-mediated, **842–844,** 843*f*
mitochondrial, **1044**
muscular dystrophies, **1043–1044,** 1043*t*
myotonia congenita, **1044**
myotonic dystrophy, **1044**
polymyositis, **842–844**
toxic, **1044**
Myopathy, encephalopathy, lactic acidosis, and stroke-like episodes (MELAS), 1044
Myopericarditis, 414, 427
Myositis, 843*t,* 1286
Myotomy-myomectomy, 422
Myotonia congenita, **1044**
Myotonic dystrophy, 184, 1043*t,* **1044**
Myringotomy
from barotrauma, ear, 208
for otitis media, 209, 210, 211
Myxedema, **1114–1119,** 1117*t*. *See also* Hypothyroidism
angina, 360
heart failure, 405
myocarditis, 416
pericarditis/pericardial effusions, 416, 417
Myxedema coma, 496, 1115
hyponatremia, 878
Myxedema crisis, 1117
Myxedema heart, 1115
Myxedema madness, 1115, 1116
Myxoma
atrial, **433–434**
cardiogenic syncope, 402

N
N9B2 virus, 1414
Nabumetone, **84*t***
N-acetylcysteine
for acetaminophen hepatotoxicity, 1572–1573
for alcohol-associated liver disease, 694–695
for trichotillomania, 165
Nadolol, 462*t,* 617, 622
Nafcillin
for MRSA, 128, 1457
for *Staphylococcus,* 1449, 1457
for *Staphylococcus aureus,* 1441, 1441*t,* 1447, 1448
Naftifine, 106*t*
Nail atrophy, 166
Nail disorders, **165–167**. *See also specific types*
morphologic, **165–167**
allergic reactions, 166
discoloration/crumbling, 166
local, 165–166, 166*f*
nail distortion/splitting, 165–166
onycholysis, 165
paronychia, 166–167, 166*f*
systemic/generalized skin diseases, 166, 166*f*
tinea unguium, **167**
Nail distortion, 165–166
Nail hyperpigmentation, 166
Nail pitting, 136, 136*f,* 166
Nail splitting, 165–166
Nail stippling, 166
Naldemedine, 587–588
Naloxegol, 587
Naloxone, 85, **86, 91,** 92, 92*t*
for clonidine overdose, 1579
monitoring, 93
for opiate/opioid poisoning, 1565, 1588
for opioid withdrawal, adverse effects, **86, 91**
for pruritus, primary biliary cholangitis, 708
for stupor & coma, 1019
Naltrexone, 93–94
for alcohol-associated liver disease, 694
for at-risk drinking, 1089
for opioid use disorder, 1092–1093
for pruritus, primary biliary cholangitis, 708
for weight loss, 1253, 1255*t*
Naphazoline overdose, **1579**
Naproxen, **84*t***
for complex regional pain syndrome, 867
for dysmenorrhea, 767
for knee osteoarthritis, 1705
for migraine headache, 971
Naratriptan, 971
Narcissistic disorder, **1059–1061,** 1060*t*
Narcolepsy syndrome, **1084**
Narcotics, 1092. *See also specific types*
Nasal decongestant overdose, **1579**
Nasal polyps, 224, **225–226**
Nasal pyramid fracture, 225
Nasal septoplasty, for obstructive sleep apnea, 317
Nasal trauma, **225**
Nasal tumors, benign, **225–226**
Nasal vestibulitis, **221**
Nasoduodenal tubes, 1265
Nasogastric tubes, 1265
Nasojejunal tubes, 1265
Nasolacrimal duct obstruction, congenital, 170
Nasopharyngeal carcinoma, 226, 1364
Natalizumab, 696, 1025*t,* 1274, 1387
Nateglinide, 1204*t,* 1206–1207, 1218, 1218*f,* 1220, 1237
National Lung Screening Trial, 289
National Surgical Quality Improvement Program (NSQIP) risk prediction tool, 42
Nausea & vomiting, 181, **581–584,** 582*t,* 583*t*
bowel obstruction, 70
causes, 581, 582*t*
chemotherapy-induced, **1655–1656**
complications, 582
definition, 581
dysuria, 38, 39
HIV/AIDS, 1317
hypotonic hyponatremia from, **878**
migraine headache, 36, 36*t*
from opioids, 86, 91–92
palliative care for, 70
in pregnancy, **796–797**
signs, symptoms & special examinations, 581
treatment, 582–584, 583*t*
Nearsightedness, 168, 185
Nebivolol, 460, 462*t*
Nebulizer therapy, 249
Necator americanus, 1527
Neck infections, deep, **233**
Neck masses. *See also specific types*
cancer metastases, **242–243**
congenital lesions, **241–242**
branchial cleft cysts, **241–242**
thyroglossal duct cysts, **242**
diseases, **241**
infectious & inflammatory, **242**
Lyme disease, 242
reactive cervical lymphadenopathy, 242
tuberculous & nontuberculous mycobacterial lymphadenitis, 242, **1475**
lymphoma, **243**

Neck pain, **1687–1688**
discogenic, **1037–1040**
cervical disk protrusion, **1037,** 1038*f*–1039*f*
cervical spondylosis, **1037–1040**
Neck pounding/pulsations, palpitations, 26
Necrobiosis lipoidica diabeticorum, 1225
Necrotizing arteritis, rheumatoid arthritis, 828
Necrotizing cellulitis, synergistic, 1473
Necrotizing fasciitis, 1473
injection drug use, 1286
Staphylococcus aureus, **1442,** 1447
Streptococcus pyogenes, **1442**
Necrotizing glomerulonephritis, 852, 854
Necrotizing pneumonia, 276–278
Necrotizing systemic fibrosis, from gadolinium, 361
Necrotizing ulcerative gingivitis, **230**
Nectin-4, 1644
Nedocromil, 250*t*, 254
Needle
sharing, HIV from, 1313
stick, HIV infection from, 1313
Neer impingement sign, 1675, 1678*t*
Nefazodone, 1072, 1073*t*, 1074, 1075
Negative symptoms, schizophrenia, 1061
Neglect, elder self-neglect, **67–68,** 68*t*
Neighborhood reaction, 1280*t*, 1281
Neisseria gonorrhoeae. *See* Gonococcus (gonorrhea)
Neisseria meningitidis
immunocompromised, 1273
medication of choice, 1293*t*
meningitis, 1323, **1459–1461**
vaccines, 1460
Nematode infections
GI bleeding, occult, 601
intestinal, **1526–1529**
ascariasis, **1526**
enterobiasis, **1528–1529**
hookworm disease, **1527**
strongyloidiasis, **1527–1528**
trichuriasis, **1526–1527**
invasive, **1529–1530**
angiostrongyliasis, **1529–1530**
cutaneous larva migrans, **1530,** 1530*f*
Neoadjuvant chemotherapy, 1606
Neologisms, 1062
Neonatal herpes, 1353–1354, 1355
Neostigmine, 1041
Nephritis. *See also* Glomerulonephritis; Pyelonephritis; *specific types*
interstitial, 907*t*, **911–912**
Epstein-Barr virus, 1363
systemic lupus erythematosus, 832
lupus, **911–912,** 923*t*
classification, 833*t*–834*t*, 834
laboratory findings, 834
treatment, 835–836
Nephrocalcinosis, medullary sponge kidney, 940
Nephrogenic diabetes insipidus, 1105
Nephrogenic systemic fibrosis, **942**
Nephrolithiasis
autosomal dominant polycystic kidney disease, 940
calcium, medical treatment & prevention
hypercalciuria, 956
hyperoxaluria, 956–957
hyperuricosuria, 956
hypocitraturia, 957
medullary sponge kidney, 940
uric acid, 942
Nephropathia epidemica, 1395
Nephropathy
COVID-19–associated, 1404
diabetic, 1221
Nephrosclerosis, hypertension, 446
Nephrosis, 2*t*. *See also specific disorders*
Nephrotic spectrum
glomerular diseases, 922*f*, 924*t*, **932–934**
primary renal disorders, **932–934**
minimal change disease, 924*t*, 931, **932–933**
systemic disorders, **934–936**
diabetic nephropathy, 924*t*, **934–935**
HIV-associated nephropathy, 924*t*, **935**
renal amyloidosis, 924*t*, **935–936**
Nephrotic syndrome, 878, 931
Nephrotoxins. *See also specific types*
acute kidney injury, 908–909
cisplatin, **1657**
Neratinib, 753
Nerve agents, 1570, **1579,** 1588–1589. *See also specific types*
Nerve blocks, 96
Nerve conduction velocity, motor/sensory, 1030
Nervous system disorders, **970–1045.** *See also specific types*
degenerative motor neuron diseases, **1028–1030**
amyotrophic lateral sclerosis, **1028**
primary lateral sclerosis, **1028**
progressive bulbar palsy, **1028**
progressive spinal muscular atrophy, **1028**
pseudobulbar palsy, **1028**
dementia, **1014–1018,** 1015*t*
dysautonomia, **984–985**
epilepsy, **978–983**
facial pain, **974–978**
atypical, **978**
glossopharyngeal neuralgia, **978**
other causes, 978
postherpetic neuralgia, **978**
trigeminal neuralgia, **974–978**
headache, **970–974** (*See also* Headache)
head injury, **1021–1023,** 1021*t*
cerebral sequelae, 1021, 1022*t*
Glasgow Coma Scale, 1021, 1021*t*
idiopathic intracranial hypertension, 974, **1003–1005**
intracranial & spinal mass lesions, **997–1002** (*See also* Intracranial mass lesions)
Korsakoff syndrome, **1018**
mononeuropathies, **1034–1036** (*See also* Mononeuropathies)
movement disorders, **1006–1014** (*See also* Movement disorders, nervous system)
multiple sclerosis, **1023–1026,** 1025*t*
myelopathies
AIDS, **1026, 1323**
human T-cell leukemia virus, **1026–1027**
neurocutaneous diseases
neurofibromatosis, **1005**
Sturge-Weber syndrome, **1005–1006**
tuberous sclerosis, **1005**
neuromyelitis optica, **1026**
nonmetastatic neurologic complications, malignant disease, **1003**
peripheral neuropathies, **1030–1045** (*See also* Peripheral neuropathies)
postural orthostatic tachycardia syndrome, **985**
spasticity, **1026**
spinal mass lesions
leptomeningeal metastases, **1001**
tumors, primary/metastatic, **1001**
spinal trauma, **1027**
stroke, **988–997** (*See also* Stroke)
stupor & coma, **1018–1021** (*See also* Coma; Stupor & coma)
subacute combined degeneration of spinal cord, **1027**
syringomelia, **1028**
transient ischemic attacks, **985–988**
vitamin E deficiency, **1026**
Wernicke encephalopathy, **1018**
Nesiritide, 413–414
Netupitant, 1655
Neuralgic amyotrophy, 1040
Neurally mediated syncope, 402–403
Neuraminadase inhibitors, 1412. *See also specific types*
Neuraxial anesthesia, 80, 96*t*
Neuritis. *See also* Mononeuritis multiplex
insulin, 1223
optic, **194–195, 1026,** 1363
peripheral, Epstein-Barr virus, 1363
Neurocognitive disorders, **1095–1096,** 1096*t*. *See also specific types*
amnestic syndrome, 1096
delirium, 1095, 1096*t*
dementia, **1095–1096,** 1096*t*
etiology, 1096*t*
HIV/AIDS, 1311, 1322
impaired thinking, 1095
organic problem, 1095
pseudodementia, 1096
substance-induced hallucinosis, 1087, 1089, 1096
Neurocutaneous diseases. *See also specific types*
neurofibromatosis, **1005**
Sturge-Weber syndrome, **1005–1006**
tuberous sclerosis, **1005**
Neurocysticercosis, 1524
Neurodermatitis, circumscribed, **135–136,** 135*f*
Neuroendocrine tumors. *See also specific types*
bronchial carcinoid, 291
gastric, **1623–1624**
gut, other, 632
intestinal, **1626–1627**
Neurofibromatosis, **1005**
NEUROG3, 1197
Neurogenic arthropathy, **867–868,** 868
Neurogenic claudication, 1686
Neurogenic shock, **496–497**
Neurokinin receptor antagonists, 583*t*, **584**
Neurokinin subtype 1 (NK1), 1655
Neuroleptic malignant syndrome, **31,** 1067, 1567, 1576
Neurolysis, celiac plexus, 80, **98–99**
Neuroma, 998*t*
Neuromodulation
for angina pectoris, 367
for migraine headache, 971
for pain, 97*t*
Neuromuscular transmission disorders, **1040–1042.** *See also specific types*
aminoglycoside, **1042**
botulism, 982, **1042,** 1286–1287, **1452–1453**
myasthenia gravis, 1004*t*, **1040–1041**
myasthenic syndrome, **1042**
Neuromyelitis optica, **1026**
Neuronal tumors, 998*t*
Neuropathic foot ulcer, 1221–1222, 1222*f*
Neuropathic pain
acute, 79
cancer, 80
chronic noncancer, **80**
management, **94–95**
corticosteroids, 95
dose lowering, 95
intrathecal drug delivery, **96–97,** 97*t*
opioids and, 86
pharmacologic, **91t, 94–95,** 94*t*
physical therapy, 95–96
psychological therapy, 95
spinal stimulation, **98**
management principles, 81–82
peripheral, medications for, 94–95, 94*t*

Neuropathic postural orthostatic syndrome, 985
Neuropathic pruritus, 159–160
Neuropathies, 1032, 1034, **1656**. *See also* Mononeuropathies; Polyneuropathies; *specific types*
Neuropathies, diabetes mellitus, **1221–1224**
- autonomic, **1223–1224**
  - diabetic, 1223–1224
  - genitourinary system, 1223–1224
  - GI system, 1223
  - orthostatic hypotension, 1224
  - paraneoplastic, 1004*t*
- peripheral, **1221–1223**
  - distal symmetric polyneuropathy, 1221–1222, 1222*f*
  - isolated peripheral neuropathy, 1222–1223
  - neurogenic arthropathy, 868

Neurostimulation, 96, 96*t*. *See also specific types and indications*
- for migraine headache, 973
- spinal, **98**

Neurosyphilis, empiric antimicrobial therapy, 1298*t*
Neurotoxins, 1590, **1657**. *See also specific types*
Neurotrophic keratitis, 172, 180
Neurotropic viruses, **1376–1389**. *See also specific types*
Neutral protamine Hagedorn insulin, 1212*t*, 1213
Neutropenia, **518–519**
- causes & classification, 518–519, 518*t*
- from chemotherapy, **1655**
- febrile, 519
- immunocompromised patient, infections, 1273
- normal and racial differences, 518

Neutropenic fever of unknown origin, 1270
Nevirapine, 696, **1339*t*, 1344**
Nevus
- atypical, **108,** 108*f*
- blue, **108,** 108*f*
- compound, 107, 107*f*
- junctional, 107
- melanocytic, **107,** 107*f*
- pigmented, 163

Newborn. *See also specific topics*
- maternal effects, intrapartum fever, 30
- persistent pulmonary hypertension of, 331, 432*t*

New World leishmaniasis, **1500**
Nexplanon, 777
NF1, 1005
NF-kappa-B (RANK), plasma cell myeloma, 537
NF-kappa-B ligand (RANKL) inhibitors, 95. *See also specific types*
Niacin (nicotinic acid)
- for cholesterol, high LDL, 1245*t*, 1248
- deficiency, **1260–1261**
- gout from, 823
- for hypercholesterolemia, 1260–1261
- for hypertriglyceridemia, 1260–1261
- toxicity, **1261**

Niacinamide, 1260
Nicardipine, 457*t*, 469–470, 470*t*, 471*t*, 991, **1578**
Nickel, lung cancer and, 1603
Niclosamide, 1523–1524
Nicotinamide, 111, 112, 147
Nicotine. *See also* Smoking
- cholinergic syndrome from, 1570
- replacement therapies, 7, 7*t*

Nicotinic acid. *See* Niacin (nicotinic acid)
Nifedipine
- for anal fissures, 672
- for angina pectoris, 363
- for high-altitude illness, 1561
- for hypertension, 457*t*, 471*t*, 472, 812
- for interstitial cystitis, 954
- poisoning, **1578**
- for preeclampsia-eclampsia, 804
- for preterm birth, anticipated, 806
- for Raynaud phenomenon, 839

Nifurtimox, 1498–1499
Night blindness, vitamin A deficiency, 1262
Night sweats, 1186
Nikolsky sign, 146
Nilotinib, 525, 1601*t*, 1656
Nimodipine poisoning, **1578**
Nipah virus, 1409
Nipple
- discharge, **739,** 739*t*
- Paget carcinoma, **748**
- Paget disease, **114,** 744, 744*f*

Nirsevimab, 1410
Nisoldipine, 457*t*, 839, **1578**
Nitazoxanide, 1517, 1519
Nithiodote, 1580
Nitrates
- for acute MI, with ST-segment elevation, 377
- for angina pectoris, 363, 364*f*
- for heart failure with reduced LVEF, 409–410
- for pulmonary edema, 413
- surgical risk assessment/reduction, 43
- tolerance, 363, 371, 410

Nitric oxide
- pathway, 302
- for pulmonary arterial hypertension, 433

Nitrite poisoning, **1586–1587**
Nitrobenzene poisoning, **1586–1587**
Nitrofurantoin, 297, 696, 813, 946, 947*t*
Nitrogen, liquid
- for actinic keratosis, 111
- hypopigmentation/depigmentation from, 163–164
- for warts
  - genital, 123
  - nongenital, 122

Nitrogen mustards, 1598*t*
- bendamustine, 1598*t*
- cyclophosphamide, 1598*t*
- ifosfamide, 1598*t*

Nitrogen oxide gas poisoning, **1586–1587**
Nitroglycerin
- for acute coronary syndrome, without ST-segment elevation, 371
- for acute MI, with ST-segment elevation, 377
- for anal fissures, 672
- for angina pectoris, 359, 362–363, 364*f*
- for heart failure with reduced LVEF, 409
- for hypertension, 471*t*, 472
- tolerance, 363, 371

Nitroprusside (sodium), 471*t*, 472, 1566
Nivolumab, 1600*t*
- for bladder cancer, 1643, 1644
- for colorectal cancer, 1630
- diabetes mellitus from, 1196
- for hepatocellular carcinoma, 1612
- for HTLV-1 adult T-cell leukemia, 1388
- hypophysitis from, 1099
- for mesothelioma, 1609
- for non–small cell lung cancer, 1606, 1607
- for PD-L1 cancers, 1674*t*
- for renal cell carcinoma, 1646

Nizatidine, 610, 624*t*, 627
NK_1-receptor antagonists, 1655
NK-cell lymphoma, 227, 1363
NMO-IgG, 1026
Nocardia (nocardiosis), 1273, 1295*t*, **1474–1475**
Nocardia asteroides complex, **1474**
Nocardia brasiliensis, **1474**
Nociceptive pain, 81
Nodular, 102*t*
Nodular regenerative hyperplasia, 697
Nodules
- inflammatory, erythema nodosum, **132–133,** 133*f*
- pulmonary, solitary, **290–291**
- "screamer's," 237
- "singer's," 237
- subcutaneous, 425, 425*t*
- thyroid, 1119, **1129–1131,** 1129*t*
- vocal folds, **237**

Noise trauma, **212**
Nonabandonment, promise of, 73
Nonalcoholic fatty liver disease, **697–699**
- aminotransferase, 675, 677*t*
- hepatocellular carcinomas, 1610
- HIV/AIDS, 1325
- surgical risk, 47

Nonalcoholic steatohepatitis with fibrosis, 1325
Nonallergic asthma, 245
Nonampullary adenocarcinomas, 1625
Nonasthmatic eosinophilic bronchitis, 15, 17
Nonatherosclerotic vascular disease, **481–482**
Nonbacterial chronic prostatitis, 950*t*, **951–952**
Nonbinary, 1709
Noncirrhotic portal hypertension, **715–716**
Non-clostridial crepitant cellulitis, 1473
Non-determined leukoencephalopathy, 1387
Nondiabetic glycosuria, 1200
Nondiabetic lumbosacral radiculoplexus neuropathy, 1040
Nonexertional heat stroke, **1549**
Nonfamilial adenomatous polyps, **665–666**
Nongeminomatous germ cell tumors, 998*t*
Nongonococcal acute bacterial arthritis, **861–863**
Nongranulomatous uveitis, **183–184**
Non-HDL cholesterol, 1240
Nonhemolytic transfusion reaction, 30
Non-Hodgkin lymphoma, **533–535,** 533*t*. *See also* B-cell lymphomas
- HIV/AIDS, 1319*t*, 1321, 1329
- IgM hypergammaglobulinemia with, 538
- nasopharyngeal, 226
- treatment, 1595*t*, 1596*t*

Non–IgE-mediated reactions, **870**
Noninfectious myocarditis, 415*t*, **416–417**
Noninflammatory diarrhea, 1288
Noninvasive positive-pressure ventilation (NIPPV), 264, 318
Noninvasive vagus nerve stimulation, for migraine headache, 971, 973
Nonionizing radiation, 1558
Nonislet cell tumor hypoglycemia, **1236**
Nonkeratinizing squamous cell carcinoma, nasopharyngeal/paranasal, 226
Nonmaleficence, medical aid in dying, 77
Nonmotor seizures, 979
Nonnucleoside reverse transcriptase inhibitors, HIV/AIDS, **1339*t*,** 1343–1344. *See also specific types*
- doravirine, **1339*t*, 1344**
- efavirenz, **1339*t*, 1343–1344**
- etravirine, **1339*t*, 1344**
- nevirapine, 696, **1339*t*, 1344**
- principles & overview, **1339*t*,** 1343
- rilpivirine, **1339*t*, 1344**

Nonocclusive mesenteric ischemia, **480–481**
Nonoxynol-9, **779**
- genital ulcers from, 1331

Nonparalytic poliomyelitis, 1374
Nonproliferative retinopathy, **191–192**
Non-rickettsiae–associated spotted fever, 1433
Nonscarring alopecia, **164–165**
Nonseminomas, **1647–1649**
Non–small cell lung carcinoma, 1596*t*, 1603, 1604–1607
Nonspecific interstitial pneumonia, 294*t*

Nonsteroidal antiinflammatory drugs. *See also specific types and disorders*
Nonsteroidal antiinflammatory drugs, adverse effects
anaphylactoid reactions, 869
asthma, 245
drug eruptions, 156–157
erosive gastritis/gastropathy, **620–622**
GI bleeding, occult, 601
GI toxicity, 822
hyperkalemia, 886, 917
hypertension, 444
hyponatremia, 878
interstitial nephritis, 911
mechanism of action, 822
medication overuse headache, 974
membranous nephropathy, 934
meningeal irritation, 1281
minimal change disease, 932
peptic ulcer disease, **625–629**
on renal perfusion, 907
renal toxicity, 822
on respiratory diseases, 245, **872**
tubulointerstitial disease, 937
ulcers, 601, 628–629
Nonsustained ventricular tachycardia, 398
Norelgestromin, transdermal contraceptive patch, 777
Norepinephrine
for acute liver failure, 685
for beta-blocker poisoning, 1577
for calcium channel blocker poisoning, 1578
for cardiogenic shock, 499
for distributive shock, 498
for hepatorenal syndrome, from cirrhosis, 704
renal constriction from, 907
Norethindrone, 775*t*, 776, 1183
Norethindrone acetate, 765, 766, 768, 775*t*
Norfloxacin, 703
Norgestimate, 775*t*, 1183
Normal anion gap acidosis, **897–899,** 897*t*
clinical findings & treatment, 899
urine anion gap, 898–899
urine osmolal gap, 899
Normal anion gap acidosis, hyperchloremic, 896*t*, **897–898**
RTA type I, 897–898, 897*t*
RTA type II, 897–898, 897*t*
RTA type IV, hyporeninemic hypoaldosteronemic, 897*t*, 898
Normal pressure hydrocephalus, 1016
Normal-tension glaucoma, **181–183**
Normocalcemic primary hyperparathyroidism, 1142
Normokalemic periodic paralysis, 1045
Norovirus, 589, 1290*t*, **1422–1423**
Nortriptyline
for chronic pain syndromes, 1057
for complex regional pain syndrome, 867
CYP2D6 metabolism of, 1668*t*
for depression, 1073*t*, 1076
for diabetic neuropathy pain, 1222
for irritable bowel syndrome, 646
for neuropathic pain, **91*t*,** 94*t*, 95
for trigeminal neuralgia, 978
Nose & paranasal sinus diseases, **218–227**. *See also specific types*
allergic rhinitis, **222–223**
epistaxis, **224–225**
infections, **218–222**
fungal sinusitis, invasive, **221–222**
nasal vestibulitis & *S. aureus* nasal colonization, **221**
rhinosinusitis, acute, **219–221**
viral rhinosinusitis (common cold), **218–219**
nasal trauma, **225**
olfactory dysfunction, **223–224**
tumors & granulomatous disease, **225–227**
benign nasal tumors, **225–226**
inverted papillomas, 226
nasal polyps, 225–226
malignant nasopharyngeal & paranasal sinus tumors, 226
sinonasal inflammatory disease, 226–227
Nosocomial pneumonia, **274–276,** 276*t*, 277*t*
Novichok poisoning, **1579**
Novosphingobium aromaticivorans, primary biliary cholangitis, 707
NPH insulin, 1212*t*, 1213
NPM1, acute myeloid leukemia, 528
NRAS, colorectal cancer, 1630
NREM sleep, 1082, 1083
NS5A inhibitors, 689. *See also specific types*
NSAIDs. *See* Nonsteroidal antiinflammatory drugs
N-terminal fragment of proBNP (NT-proBNP)
aortic stenosis & left ventricular myocardial failure, 343
cardiomyopathy, restrictive, 424
heart failure, **405**
mitral regurgitation, 339
myocarditis, 415, 417
preoperative evaluation, 43
tetralogy of Fallot, 331
traumatic heart disease, 434
NTRK, lung cancer, 1606
Nuclear factor kappa B ligand (RANK-L) receptor, 754
Nucleic acid amplification testing, TB, 280
Nucleoside analog. *See also specific types*
for hepatitis B & D, 687–688
for hepatitis C, 689
Nucleoside reverse transcriptase inhibitors, HIV/AIDS, **1339*t*,** 1341–1343. *See also specific types*
abacavir, **1339*t*, 1343**
combinations, fixed-dose, 1338, 1341–1343, **1342*t***
emtricitabine, **1339*t*, 1343**
lamivudine, **1339*t*, 1343**
myopathy from, 1045
principles & overview, **1339*t*,** 1341–1343
zidovudine, **1339*t*, 1343**
Nucleotide analogs. *See also specific types*
for hepatitis B & D, 687–688
for hepatitis C, 689
Nucleotide reverse transcriptase inhibitors, for HIV/AIDS, **1339*t*,** 1341–1343. *See also specific types*
tenofovir, **1339*t*, 1343**
tenofovir alafenamide/emtricitabine, **1339*t*, 1343**
Nusinersen, 1029
"Nutmeg liver," 715
Nutrient-restricted diets
carbohydrate, 1264
fat & low saturated fats, 1263–1264
protein, 1264
sodium, 1263
Nutrient supplementation
calcium, 1264
fiber, 1264
potassium, 1264
Nutrition
end of life care, 73–74
on frailty, 53
screening, 1251
Nutritional disorders, **1250–1269**. *See also specific types*
diet therapy, **1262–1264**
consistency altering
clear liquids, 1263
full liquids, 1263
soft, 1263
food recall & tracking, 1262–1263
nutrient restrictions
carbohydrate, 1264
fats & low saturated fats, 1263–1264
protein, 1264
sodium, 1263
nutrient supplementation
calcium, 1264
fiber, 1264
potassium, 1264
therapeutic diets, types, 1262–1263
eating disorders, **1258–1259**
anorexia nervosa, **1258–1259**
bulimia nervosa, **1259**
nutritional support, **1265–1269**
central vein, 1266
enteral, 1267–1268, 1267*t*
indications, 1265
methods, 1265–1266, 1265*f*
parenteral, 1265, 1266, 1268, 1269*t*
patient monitoring, 1269
requirements, 1266–1267
electrolytes, minerals, vitamins, & trace elements, 1266–1267
energy, 1266
fat, 1266
protein, 1266
water, 1266
obesity, **1251–1258** (*See also* Obesity)
polyneuropathy, alcohol use disorder, **1032**
protein–energy malnutrition, **1250–1251**
vitamin metabolism disorders, **1259–1262**
niacin deficiency, **1260–1261**
niacin toxicity, **1261**
riboflavin (B_2) deficiency, **1260**
riboflavin (B_2) toxicity, **1260**
thiamine (B_1) deficiency, **1259–1260**
thiamine (B_1) toxicity, **1260**
vitamin A deficiency, **1262**
vitamin A toxicity, **1262**
vitamin B_6 deficiency, **1261**
vitamin B_6 toxicity, **1261**
vitamin C (ascorbic acid) deficiency, **1261**
vitamin C (ascorbic acid) toxicity, **1261–1262**
vitamin E deficiency, **1262**
vitamin E toxicity, **1262**
Nutritional support, **1265–1269**
enteral
complications, 1267–1268
solutions, 1267, 1267*t*
indications, 1265
methods, 1265–1266, 1265*f*
oral supplements, 1265
parenteral, 1265, 1266
complications, 1268, 1269*t*
solutions, 1268
patient monitoring, 1269
peripheral vein, 1266
requirements, 1266–1267
electrolytes, minerals, vitamins, & trace elements, 1266–1267
energy, 1266
fat, 1266
protein, 1266
water, 1266
NYHA classification, heart failure, 404
Nystagmus, vertigo, 214–215, 216, 217
Nystatin, 119

O

Oat bran, on LDL cholesterol, 1244
Oatmeal, for irritable bowel syndrome, 645
OATP1B1, 676*t*
OATP1B3, 676*t*

Obesity. *See* Overweight/obesity; Weight, loss
Obesity-hypoventilation syndrome, **315**
Obeticholic acid, 696, 699, 708
Obinutuzumab, 531, 1600*t*
Obliterative bronchiolitis, 268
Obliterative portal venopathy, 715–716
O'Brien test, 1679*t*
Obsessions, 1052
Obsessive-compulsive disorders, 1013, **1052–1053**
Obsessive-compulsive personality disorder, **1059–1061,** 1060*t*
Obstetrics & obstetric disorders, **794–818**. *See also* Pregnancy; *specific types*
after breast carcinoma treatment, 761
air travel, 1562
alcohol, smoking, recreational drugs, **795**
amenorrhea, primary, 1184
aorta vascular abnormalities, 436–437
aortic dissection, 486
breast cancer, 748–749
cardiomyopathy, **436**
complications, **802–817**
2nd & 3rd trimesters, **802–807**
3rd trimester bleeding, **806–807**
preeclampsia-eclampsia, **802–804,** 803*t*
preterm labor, **804–806**
infectious conditions, **813–817**
chlamydia, 816–817
Group B streptococcus, **814**
hepatitis & carrier state, maternal, **816**
herpes genitalis, **816**
HIV/AIDS, **815–816**
syphilis & gonorrhea, 816
tuberculosis, **815**
urinary tract infection, **813–814**
varicella, **814**
medical conditions, **808–813**
anemia, **808–809**
antiphospholipid syndrome, **809**
asthma, **812–813**
diabetes mellitus, **810–811**
heart disease, **812**
hypertension, chronic, **811–812**
seizure disorders, **813**
thyroid disease, **809–810**
peripartum, **807–808**
chorioamnionitis & metritis, **808**
puerperal mastitis, **807–808**
coronary artery & aortic vascular abnormalities, **436–438**
diagnosis, **794**
drugs, contraindicated
leflunomide, 830
methotrexate, 829
Ebola viral disease, 1390
ectopic pregnancy, 794, **799–800**
fever, 30
gestational trophoblastic disease, **800–802**
GI, hepatic, & biliary disorders, **817–818**
acute fatty liver of pregnancy, 685, **817–818**
appendicitis, **818**
cholelithiasis & cholecystitis, **817**
intrahepatic cholestasis of pregnancy, **818**
heart disease, **435–438,** 812
CARPREG I/II scoring systems, 435, 436*f*
management, WHO guidelines, 435, 437*t*
strategies, 435, 437*t*
HHV-6, 1368
HHV-7, 1358*t*, **1368**
hypertension, 445–446
hyperthyroidism, 1121
hypothyroidism, 1116
immunizations, 1301, 1302*t*–1303*t*
COVID-19, 795, 1407
tetanus-diphtheria-pertussis, 1459
intrahepatic cholestasis of, conjugated hyperbilirubinemia, 674, 676*t*
on iron balance, 501
iron loss, 601
labor management, **438**
lactation, drugs, **795**, 796*t*
listeriosis, 1453
luteoma of, 1182
major depression, onset, 1070
mechanical heart valve, anticoagulation for, 353–355, 354*t*
meralgia paresthetica, **1035–1036**
mitral stenosis, 336, 812
moles, 107
parvovirus B19, 1420
pheochromocytoma in, 1169–1170
pregnancy diagnosis, **794**
pregnancy loss
recurrent, **799**
spontaneous, **797–799**
pregnancy tests, 794
prenatal care, **794–795,** 795*t*
alcohol, tobacco, recreational drugs, **795**
medications, teratogenicity/fetotoxicity, **794,** 795*t*
radiographs and noxious exposures, **795**
prosthetic heart valves, 355
pseudohyperparathyroidism of, 1144
radiographs, 795
recurrent pregnancy loss, **799**
renal glycosuria, 1200
Rocky Mountain spotted fever, 1427*t*, 1431
superficial venous thrombophlebitis, 489
symptoms & signs, 794
syphilis, 1488
thrombocytopenia, **556**
travel immunizations, **795–796**
tubal, **799–800**
tuberculosis treatment, 286
unintended, prevalence, 773
of unknown location, 794
vaccinations, **796**
valve disease, 437*t*
varicella, 1360
varicose veins, **487–489**
virilization, 1182
vomiting of pregnancy & hyperemesis gravidarum, **796–797**
Obstructive apnea, 316
Obstructive jaundice, 675–677, 676*t*
Obstructive shock, **495–499,** 495*t*
Obstructive sleep apnea, **316–317, 1084**
snoring, **233–234**
Obstructive uropathy, 936–937
Obturator sign, 640, 641
Occipital lobe lesions, 999
Occlusive cerebrovascular disease, **478–480,** 479*t*
Occult diabetes, postprandial hypoglycemia, **1236–1237**
Occult gastrointestinal bleeding, 601–602
Occupational asthma, 246
Occupational pulmonary diseases, **306–307.** *See also specific types*
hypersensitivity pneumonitis, **307–308,** 307*t*
other, 308
pneumoconiosis, **306–307,** 306*t*
asbestosis, 306*t*, **307,** 308
coal worker's pneumoconiosis, **306,** 306*t*, 308
silicosis, **306–307,** 306*t*, 308
talcosis, 306*t*, 308
Ocrelizumab, 1025, 1025*t*
Octreotide
for acromegaly, 1107
for *Cryptosporidium*, 1326
for Cushing syndrome, 1163
for diarrhea, 595
gallstones from, 719
for gastroenteropancreatic neuroendocrine tumors, 1173
for insulinoma, 1235–1236
for intestinal neuroendocrine tumors, 1626
for pain, in chronic pancreatitis, 734
for portal hypertension, esophageal varices from, 616
for short bowel syndrome, 637
for upper GI bleeding, 598
Ocular hypertension, **177*t*–178*t*,** 182, 183
Ocular transient ischemic attack, **190–191**
Ocular trauma, **196–198**
contusions, **197–198**
corneal, 170*t*
corneal abrasions, **197**
foreign bodies, conjunctival & corneal, **197**
lacerations, **198**
retinal detachment, 185
uveitis, 183
Oculocephalic reflex, 1019
Oculopharyngeal muscular dystrophy, 1043*t*
Oculovestibular reflex, 1019
Odynophagia, 607, 612
Ofatumumab, 1025, 1025*t*
Ofloxacin, 703, 1293
Ogilvie syndrome, **639–640**
Oil of evening primrose, 738
OKT3, meningeal irritation from, 1281
Olanzapine
for aggression disorders, 1085
for bipolar disorder, 1078–1079
diabetic ketoacidosis from, 1197
for dyskinesia from antipsychotics, 1068
glucose intolerance from, 1197
for hypertension, from poisoning, 1566
IV, 1066
for nausea, 583*t*, **584**
for personality disorders, 1060–1061
poisoning, 1576
potency and side effects, 1065*t*
for psychedelic effects, 1093
for schizophreniform spectrum disorders, 1063, 1064*t*, 1065, 1065*t*
Olaparib, 752, 754, 759
Older adults, **52–68**
abuse, **67–68,** 68*t*
adverse drug events, 66
anemia of, **502**
assessment, 52–53, 53*f*
breast carcinoma treatment, 754–755
delirium, 54, **58–59**
dementia, **53–57**
depression, 54, **57–58**
depressive symptoms, 57
falls & gait disorders, **60–62,** 60*t*, 61*t*
general principles, 52
hearing impairment, **67**
home safety evaluation, 60
hypertension, 442, 467
lesbian & bisexual women, 1715–1716
life expectancy, 52, 53*f*
macular degeneration, 52, 67, **187**
mistreatment & self-neglect, **67–68,** 68*t*
pharmacotherapy & polypharmacy, **66**
physical activity, 59
pressure injury, **64–65,** 65*t*
urinary incontinence, **62–64**
vision impairment, **67**
weight, body, 32
weight loss, involuntary, 32
Old World leishmaniasis, **1500**
Oleander, 1581
Olfactory dysfunction, **223–224**
Oligodendroglioma, 998*t*
Oligozoospermia, 961–962

Oliguria, 881
Olmesartan, 453*t*
Olodaterol, 262
Omalizumab, 152, 251*t*, 254
Ombitasvir, 690*t*
Omega-3 ethyl esters, 1245*t*, 1247
Omega-3 fatty acid preparations, 1245*t*, 1247
Omeprazole
  for GERD, 610
  for GI hemorrhage from peptic ulcer disease, 630
  for NSAIDs, 622, 628
  for pancreatic insufficiency, 734
  for peptic ulcer disease, 624*t*, 627
  for stress gastritis, 621
  for upper GI bleeding, 598
Onchocerca volvulus, 1532
Onchocerciasis, **1532–1533**
Oncocytoma, renal, 1646
Oncotype DX, 750, 752
Ondansetron, **583–584,** 583*t*, 708, 797, 1655
Onycholysis, 165
Onychomycosis, **167**
Oophoritis, measles, 1372
Open can test, 1677*t*
Opening snap, mitral stenosis, 336
Ophthalmic agents. *See also specific types*
  contaminated eye medications, 199
  corticosteroids, 198–199
  local anesthetics, 198
  pupillary dilation, 198
  systemic drugs, adverse ocular effects, **199–203, 200*t*–202*t***
  toxic & hypersensitivity reactions, 199, 199*f*
Ophthalmic agents, topical, **173*t*–178*t***
  antibiotic, **173*t*–175*t***
  antifungal, **175*t***
  anti-inflammatory, **175*t*–177*t***
    antihistamines, **175*t***
    antihistamines + mast cell stabilizers, **175*t***
    corticosteroids, **176*t***
    immunomodulators, **177*t***
    mast cell stabilizers, **175*t***
    NSAIDs, **176*t***
  antiviral, **175*t***
  glaucoma and ocular hypertension, **177*t*–178*t***
    beta-adrenergic blockers, **177*t***
    carbonic anhydrase inhibitors, **177*t***
    combined preparations, **178*t***
    miotics, **177*t***
    prostaglandin analogs, **178*t***
    Rho kinase inhibitor, **178*t***
    sympathomimetics, **177*t***
Ophthalmic artery occlusion, 989
Ophthalmoplegic migraine, 971
Ophthalmoplegic neuropathy, recurrent painful, 971
Opiate
  dependence, 1092
  poisoning, **1587–1588**
Opicapone, 1009
Opioid overdose/poisoning, 1568*t*, **1587–1588**
Opioid-receptor antagonists, 587–588, 901. *See also specific types*
Opioid Risk Tool, 93
Opioid use, for pain, **82–94, 87*t*–90*t*,** 92*t*–94*t*
  background, 82–84
  cancer pain, 80
  definition, 85
  indications, 82–84
  management principles, 85–86, 85*t*
    abuse, 85, 86
    addiction, 85
    adverse events, 86
    allodynia, 85
    CDC guidelines, 92, 92*t*
    dependence, 85, 86
    dosing
      initial, 86, 87*t*–90*t*
      pain control challenges, 86
    extended-release, 86
    hyperalgesia, 85
    monitoring, 93, 93*t*
    morphine milligram equivalent doses, 85–86, 85*t*
    mortality and dose, 86
    opioid use disorder, 93–94
    PEG scores, 93, 93*t*
    pseudoaddiction, 85
    rotation *vs.* dose escalation, 86
    temporal patterns of pain, 86
    weaning, 94
  metabolism, 85
  postoperative, reducing need for, 80
  prevalence, 84
  substance use disorder, 84
  tolerance, 86
  vomiting from, 70
  WHO Analgesic Ladder, 80
Opioid use/opioid use disorder
  addiction, 85
  adverse effects, 86, 91–92
  anaphylactic/anaphylactoid reactions, 869, 870
  cognitive impairment from, 92
  constipation from, 70, 86, **91**
  definition of, 1092
  delirium from, 92
  dependence, 1092
  for diarrhea, 592
  hypoglycemia from, 1237
  lesbian & bisexual women, 1717
  medication overuse headache from, 974
  nausea from, 86, 91–92
  for neuropathic pain, 94*t*
  opioid use disorder, 84, 85, 92*t*, **1092–1093**
    dose escalation, 86
    management, 93–94
    on pregnancy, 795
    prevention, 80
    tolerance, 86, 1092
    withdrawal, 1092
  for osteoarthritis, 821
  overdose
    benzodiazepines with, 84
    COVID-19 pandemic, 84
    deaths, 13, 84, 86
    mitigation strategies, 13
    prevalence and public health crisis, 84
  poisoning, naloxone for, 1565
  pruritus from, 92
  respiratory depression from, 86
  sedation from, 86, 92
  sympatholytic syndrome from, 1570
Opisthorchiasis, **1522**
Opisthorchis felineus, 1522
Opisthorchis viverrini, 1522, 1613
Opium, tincture of, 595
Opsoclonus, 1004*t*
Optic atrophy, Wolfram syndrome, 1197
Optic disc cupping, 181, 182
Optic disk swelling, 190, **195**
Optic neuritis, **194–195**
  Epstein-Barr virus, 1363
  neuromyelitis optica, **1026**
  varicella, 1360
Optic neuropathy, ischemic, **193–194**
Oral allergy syndrome, 868
Oral cancer, 227
Oral candidiasis, **229,** 229*f*, **1324**
Oral cavity & pharynx diseases, **227–234.** *See also specific types*
  candidiasis, oral, **229,** 229*f*, **1324**
  glossitis, glossodynia, & burning mouth syndrome, **229–230**
  HIV/AIDS lesions
    angular cheilitis, 1324
    aphthous ulcers, 1324–1325
    candidiasis, 1324–1325
    gingival disease, 1324–1325
    hairy leukoplakia, 1324
    Kaposi sarcoma, 1319*t*, 1324
    warts, 1324
  leukoplakia, erythroplakia, lichen planus, & oropharyngeal cancer, **227–229,** 227*f*, 228*f*
  neck infections, deep, **233**
  peritonsillar abscess & cellulitis, **232**
  pharyngitis & tonsillitis, **231–232,** 231*f*
  snoring, **233–234**
  ulcerative lesions, intraoral, **230**
Oral conjugated estrogens, 764
Oral contraceptives. *See also specific types*
  chorea from, 1012
  combined, **774–776,** 775*t* (*See also* Combined oral contraceptives)
  for dysmenorrhea, 767
  for hirsutism, female, 1183
  hypertension and, 446
  nipple discharge and, 739
  retinal artery occlusion from, 189
  retinal vein occlusion from, 188
  for uterine leiomyoma, 766
Oral glucose tolerance test, 1200–1201, 1201*t*
Oral hairy leukoplakia, **228,** 228*f*
Orbital cellulitis, **196**
Orchitis, measles, 1372
Orexin receptor antagonists, dual, 1083–1084. *See also specific types*
Orf virus, **1421**
Organ donation, 78
Organ failure
  anemia of, **502**
  pancreatitis, 731
Organic hallucinosis, 1087, 1089, 1096
Organizing pneumonia, 268
Organophosphates (organophosphorus)
  cholinergic syndrome from, 1570
  poisoning
    antidote, 1568*t*
    insecticide, **1588–1589**
    seizures, 1567*t*
Organosilanes, 1412. *See also specific types*
Organ preservation surgery, squamous cell carcinoma of larynx, 239
Orgasm, 1057
Orgasmic disorders/dysfunction, **781,** 1058
Orientia tsutsugamushi, 1427*t*, 1429
Orlistat, 1252–1253, 1254*t*
Ornithine aspartate, 705
Ornithosis, **1478**
Orogastric tubes, 1265
Oromandibular dystonia, 1011, 1012
Oropharyngeal cancer, 227, **227–229,** 228*f*
Oropharyngeal dysphagia, 606, 606*t*
Oropharyngeal squamous cell carcinoma, 228–229
Orthobunyavirus, 1379
Orthodromic reentrant tachycardia, 390
Orthokeratology, 168
Orthopedic disorders & sports medicine, **1675–1708.** *See also specific types*
  acute & chronic, 1675
  ankle, **1706–1708**
  hip, **1692–1695**
  knee, **1695–1706**
  shoulder, **1675–1683**
  spine, **1683–1688**
  traumatic & atraumatic, 1675
  upper extremities, **1689–1692**

Orthopoxviruses, novel, **1422**
Orthostatic hypotension
  from antipsychotics, 1066
  chronic idiopathic, 402
  diabetes mellitus, 1224
  hypertension with, supine, 468
  from phenothiazines, 1576
  from tricyclic antidepressants, 1076
Orthostatic hypoxemia, patent foramen ovale, 327
Orthostatic intolerance, systemic exertion intolerance disease, 34
"Orthostatic" proteinuria, 904
Orthostatic syncope, 402–403
Osborn waves, 1551, 1551*f*
Oseltamivir, 1356*t*, 1411, 1413–1415
Osilodrostat, 1163
Osimertinib, 1601*t*, 1672*t*
Osler nodes, 1454
Osler triad, 1444
Osler-Weber-Rendu syndrome, 224, 563, **1665–1666**
Osmolal gap, urine, 899
Osmolality
  plasma, 875–876
  serum, **875–876,** 1227
    estimating, 876, 1227
    hypernatremia, 880
    hyponatremia, 876, 877*f*
    hypovolemic hyponatremia, 877
Osmolarity, 875
Osmol gap
  calculation, 1570*t*
  poisoning, 1570, 1570*t*
Osmotic demyelination syndrome, iatrogenic, 879–880
Osmotic laxatives, 586, 587*t*
Ospemifene, 1190
Ossicular disruption, hearing loss, 204
Osteitis deformans, **1155–1156**
Osteitis fibrosa cystica, 1142
Osteoarthritis, **819–823,** 820
  Bouchard nodes, 820, 821*f*
  Heberden nodes, 820, 821*f*
  hip, 820, **1694–1695**
  knee, 1695, 1696*t*, **1704–1706**
    meniscus injuries, 1703
    treatment, 83*t*, 820–821
  lumbar disk herniation, 1686
  lumbar spine, 1685
  shoulder, rotator cuff tears, 1681
Osteogenesis imperfecta, bleeding from, 562–563
Osteomalacia, 917, 917*f*, **1152–1154,** 1152*t*
Osteomas, **207**
Osteomyelitis
  antimicrobial therapy, initial, 1296*t*
  cryoglobulinemia, 855
  injection drug abuse, 1287
  sickle cell anemia, 512
  Staphylococcus aureus, **1447–1448**
Osteonecrosis, **868**
Osteopenia, **1147,** 1323–1324, 1693
Osteoporosis, **1147–1152,** 1148*t*
  bone density scanning, 1693
  from corticosteroids, 1193–1194
  DXA bone densitometry, 1148
  fall risk, 61
  hip fractures, 1693
  HIV/AIDS, 1323–1324
  low back pain, 1683, 1684*t*
  prevention, 9
  from thyrotoxicosis, 1148
Ostium primum persistence, 326
Ostium secundum persistence, 326, 328
Otelixizumab, on diabetes mellitus, 1199
Otitis externa, **206–207,** 206*f*, 212
Otitis media
  acute, **209,** 209*f*, 212, 218
  antimicrobial therapy, empiric, 1297*t*
  chronic, **209–211**
    cholesteatoma, **210,** 210*f*
    CNS infection, **211**
    facial palsy/paralysis, **210**
    mastoiditis, **210**
    petrous apicitis, **210**
    sigmoid sinus thrombosis, **211**
  measles, 1370
  serous, **208,** 218
Otoconia, 216
Otolaryngology disorders, **204–243.** *See also specific types*
  ear diseases, **204–218**
  foreign bodies, upper aerodigestive tract, **241–243** (*See also* Foreign bodies, upper aerodigestive tract)
  larynx diseases, **235–241**
    cricothyrotomy, **240**
    epiglottitis, **237**
    hoarseness & stridor, **235–236**
    laryngitis, **236**
    laryngopharyngeal reflux, **236**
    masses
      laryngeal leukoplakia, **238**
      squamous cell carcinoma, **238–240**
      vocal folds, traumatic lesions, **237–238**
    recurrent respiratory papillomatosis, **237**
    tracheostomy, **240–241**
    vocal fold paralysis, **240**
  nose & paranasal sinus diseases, **218–227**
  oral cavity & pharynx diseases, **227–234**
  salivary gland diseases, **234–235**
    inflammatory & infiltrative disorders, chronic, **235**
    sialadenitis, **234–235**
    sialolithiasis, **234–235**
    tumors, **235**
Otosclerosis, 204, **211**
Ototoxicity. *See also specific drugs*
  of cisplatin, 213, **1657**
  hearing loss, sensorineural, **213**
Ottawa Ankle Rules, 1707
Ottawa clinical decision rule, subarachnoid hemorrhage, 37
Ovarian cancer, **792–793,** 1181
  combined oral contraceptives and, 774
  lesbian & bisexual women, **1721**
  palmar fasciitis, 867
  treatment, 1596*t*
Ovarian reserve, 772
Ovarian tumors, **792–793,** 1181
Overdose, **1564–1593.** *See also* Poisoning
  acetaminophen, **684–686,** 685, 1570
  antidepressants, 1592, 1593
  apraclonidine, **1579**
  benzodiazepines, 1051
  brimonidine, **1579**
  clonidine, 1579
  fentanyl, deaths, 84
  guanabenz, **1579**
  guanfacine, **1579**
  heroin, **1587–1588**
  initial evaluation, **1564**
  malignant hyperthermia from, 1567
  methyldopa, **1579**
  naphazoline, **1579**
  nasal decongestant, **1579**
  opioid, 13, 84, 86, 1568*t*, **1587–1588**
  tetrahydrozoline, **1579**
  tizanidine, **1579**
  tricyclic antidepressants, 1565–1567, 1567*t*, **1592–1593,** 1593*f*
Overflow incontinence, 63–64
Overlap syndrome, 842, **845**
Overload proteinuria, 904
Overt small intestine bleeding, 601
Overweight/obesity, **1251–1258.** *See also* Weight, loss
  asthma, 245
  binge-eating disorder, 1251
  body mass index, 10–11
  cancer, 1251
  central obesity, 1251
  colorectal cancer, 1627, 1628
  combined oral contraceptives and, 776
  coronary heart disease, 355
  Cushing syndrome, 1251
  definition & measurement, 1251
  degenerative joint disease, 820
  depression, 1251
  diabetes mellitus, 1251
  disease prevention, 10–11
  endometrial adenocarcinoma, 791
  etiology, 1251
  gallstones, 719
  GERD, 608
  health consequences, 1251
  heart disease, 1251
  hepatocellular carcinoma, 1610
  hypertension, 444
  insulin resistance, 1196
  lesbian & bisexual women, 1716, **1717–1718**
  medical evaluation, 1251–1252
  metabolic syndrome, 355
  osteoarthritis, 820
  pancreatic steatosis, 733
  prevention, 10–11
  psoriasis, 136
  stroke, 1251
  visceral, 1196
Overweight/obesity, treatment, **1252–1257**
  bariatric surgery, 1257
  dietary strategies, 1252
  eating behavior changes, 1252
  gastric band, laparoscopic adjustable, 1257
  lifestyle modification, 1252
  medications, **1252–1257,** 1254*t*–1256*t* (*See also specific types*)
    indications, 1252
    liraglutide, 1253, 1255*t*, 1257
    naltrexone ER + bupropion ER, 1253, 1255*t*
    orlistat, 1252–1253, 1254*t*
    phentermine, 1252, 1254*t*
    phentermine + topiramate ER, 1253, 1254*t*
    semaglutide, 1253, 1255*t*, 1257
  medications, on weight, 1252, 1253*t*
  physical activity, 1252
  Roux-en-Y gastric bypass, 1257
  sleeve gastrectomy, 1257
  "treatment gap," 1257
  weight loss, for risk factor improvement, 1252
Ovulation
  anovulation, 763
  dysfunction, 763
    polycystic ovary syndrome, **771, 1181**
Oxacillin
  hepatotoxicity, 696
  for MRSA endocarditis, 1457
  for *Staphylococcus*, 1449, 1457
  for *Staphylococcus aureus*, 1447, 1448
Oxalic acid, anion gap elevation from, 897
Oxaliplatin, 715, 1598*t*, 1616, 1630
Oxamniquine, 1521
Oxantel pamoate, 1526–1527
Oxazepam, 1050*t*
  poisoning, **1581–1582**
Oxcarbazepine
  for facial pain, 978
  for glossopharyngeal neuralgia, 978

pregnancy, safety, 813
for seizures, 976*t*
for trigeminal neuralgia, 975
Oxford League Table of Analgesics, 79
Oxiconazole, 105*t*
Oxitriptan, 1012
5-Oxoproline ingestion, 896*t*
Oxprenolol poisoning, **1577–1578**
Oxybenzone, photoallergic dermatitis from, 155
Oxycodone, **89*t***
breastfeeding, 796*t*
monitoring, 93
morphine milligram equivalent doses, 85*t*
poisoning, **1587–1588**
Oxycodone-naloxone, 1013
Oxygen
for COPD, 261–262, 261*t*, 264
hyperbaric, for carbon monoxide poisoning, 1578–1579
Oxymetazoline, 150, **1579**
Oxymorphone, 85*t*, **89*t***
Oxytocin, 804, 1099
Ozanimod, 651, 660–661, 1025, 1025*t*
Ozenoxacin, 105*t*, 124

P

$P2Y_{12}$ inhibitors, 365, 369–371, 370*f*, 374, 378. *See also specific types*
p16/CDKN2A, pancreas carcinoma, 1615
p53, breast cancer, 741
P450c17 deficiency, 1184
Pacemakers/pacing
for atrial fibrillation, 391
for AV block, 387–388
AV synchrony, 388
biventricular, for heart failure with reduced LVEF, 411
cardiac resynchronization therapy, for heart failure, 406*f*
CRT-P, 388
dual-chamber, 387, 388
for mitral regurgitation, 339
nomenclature, 388
prophylactic ventricular, 380
for sinus bradycardia, 386–387
tricuspid regurgitation from, 351
for tricuspid stenosis, 350
for vasovagal syncope, 403
for ventricular tachycardia, 399
Packed red blood cell transfusion, 542, 597
Paclitaxel, 113, 752, 759, 1599*t*, 1656
Padua Risk Assessment Model for VTE prophylaxis, 566, 566*t*
Paecilomyces, 1546
Paget carcinoma, **748**
Paget disease, **114**, 744, 744*f*
of bone, **1155–1156**
Pain disorder, psychological factors, 1053. *See also* Somatic symptom disorder
Painful bladder syndrome, **953–954**
Painful subacute thyroiditis, **1112–1114**
Painless sporadic subacute thyroiditis, **1112–1114**
Pain/pain disorders. *See also specific types*
acute, **79–80**, 86
syndromes, 1055
temporal, 86
assessment scales, 81, 81*t*
breakthrough, 81, 86
cancer, 79, **80**
chronic, 79, **82**, 86
noncancer, **80**
chronification, 79
definition, 79
end of life, 79, **81**
fatigue, 70
hypotonic hyponatremia from, **878**
incident related, 86
low-back, chronic, 80, 95, **1683–1685**, 1684*t*
nociceptive, 81
prevalence, 79
sexual, **781–782**
taxonomy, 79
Pain/pain disorders, management, **79–100**. *See also specific types*
acute, 79
barriers to good care, 82
Declaration of Montreal, 79
goals, 82
integrative medicine therapy, 96
interventional modalities, **96–100**
by anatomic location, 96*t*
cancer pain, 80
celiac plexus block & neurolysis, 80, 96, **98–99**
epidural corticosteroid injection, **99–100**
intrathecal drug delivery system, **96–97**, 97*t*
neuromodulatory therapies, 97*t*
spinal stimulation, **98**
patient-controlled analgesia, 80
pharmacologic strategies, **82–95** (*See also specific types*)
acetaminophen, aspirin, celecoxib, and NSAIDs, **82, 83*t*–84*t***
adjuvant medications & treatments, **95**
neuropathic pain, **91*t*, 94–95, 94*t***
opioids, **82–94, 87*t*–90*t***, 92*t*–94*t*
physical therapy, 95–96
principles, 81–82, 81*t*
psychological therapy, 95
therapeutic window, 80
Pain syndromes
acute, 1055
chronic, **1055–1057**, 1056*f* (*See also* Chronic pain)
PALB2, breast cancer, 741
Palbociclib, 757–758
Palifermin, 1653*t*
Palilalia, 1013
Palindromic rheumatism, **868**
Paliperidone, 1063, **1064**, 1064*t*, 1065*t*, 1066
Palivizumab, 1356*t*
Palliative care, **69–79**. *See also* Pain/pain disorders, management
after death tasks, 78–79
constipation, 70
decision making, serious illness, 71–72
definition & scope, 69
delirium & agitation, 70–71
"double effect," 77
dyspnea, 69–70
end of life, **72–77** (*See also* End of life care)
fatigue, 70
nausea & vomiting, 70
PALM-COEN, 764*t*
Palms
tinea, **116–117**
vesiculobullous dermatitis, **144**, 144*f*
Palonosetron, **583–584**, 583*t*, 1655
Palpable purpura, 855, 927
Palpitations, **25–27**, 27*t*
Palsy
progressive bulbar, **1028**
pseudobulbar, **1028**
2-PAM, 1579, 1589
Pamidronate, 95, 1150, 1651, 1654*t*
p-ANCA glomerulonephritis, 912
Pancreas carcinoma, **1614–1617**
Pancreas diseases, **728–736**. *See also specific types*
jaundice & abnormal liver biochemical test evaluation, **674–677**, 676*t*, 677*t*
pancreatitis, **728–736**
acute, **728–733**, 729*t*, 730*t*
chronic, **733–736**, 735*t*
Pancreas transplantation, 1215
Pancreatectomy, subtotal, on diabetes mellitus risk, 1197
Pancreatic abscess, 731
Pancreatic B cell tumor, hypoglycemia from, **1233–1236**, 1234*t*
Pancreatic carcinoma, 579, 1597*t*
Pancreatic enzyme replacement therapy, 734, 735*t*
Pancreatic insufficiency, 507, 734, 735*t*
Pancreatic islet B cells
diabetes mellitus
diabetes, occult, 1236
genetic defects, 1196*f*
type 1, 1195–1196, 1199
type 2, 1196
pancreatitis and subtotal pancreatectomy, 1197
sulfonylureas on, 1203
tumors, hypoglycemia from, **1233–1236**, 1233*t*, 1234*t*
Pancreatic neuroendocrine tumors, **1235–1236**
Pancreatitis
acute, **728–733**, 730*t*
necrotizing, 731–732
pregnancy, 817
severity assessment & mortality, 729–730, 729*t*, 730*t*
autoimmune, 733–735
B-cells, pancreatic islet, 1197
chronic, **733–736**, 735*t*
on diabetes mellitus risk, 1197
dyspepsia, 579
idiopathic duct-centric, 733
lymphoplasmacytic sclerosing, 733
severe necrotizing, 730–731
COVID-19, 1404
osteonecrosis, 868
prevalence and causes, 733
"tumefactive chronic," 734
Pancreatitis Activity Scoring System (PASS), 729
Pancytopenia
acute leukemia, 529
aplastic anemia, 516, 517, 517*t*, 546
causes, 517, 517*t*
hairy cell leukemia, 532
transfusion-associated graft-*versus*-host disease, 532
Panencephalitis, subacute sclerosing, 1370
Panhypopituitarism, hypogonadotropic hypogonadism, 1101, 1103
Panic-agoraphobia-depression, 1054
Panic attacks, 1049
Panic disorder, 25, 1049, **1049, 1051**
Panitumumab, 1600*t*, 1630, 1656
Panniculitis, erythema nodosum, 132
Pansexual, 1709
Pantoprazole
for GERD, 610
for GI hemorrhage from peptic ulcer disease, 630
for NSAIDs, 622, 628
for peptic ulcer disease, 627
for stress gastritis, 621
for upper GI bleeding, 598
Panuveitis, 183
Papain, 132, 241
Papanicolaou smear, 11, 788, 791
Papaverine, 1223
Papaverine with phentolamine, 1223
Papillary fibroelastoma, valvular, 434
Papillary & mixed papillary-follicular carcinoma, **1131–1132**, 1132*t*

Papillary muscle dysfunction/ rupture
acute MI, with ST-segment elevation, 373, 381
mitral regurgitation, 339, 360, 373
mitral stenosis, 332
tachycardias from, 383
tricuspid valve regurgitation, 351
Papillary renal cell carcinoma, hereditary, 1645
Papillary stenosis (biliary), HIV/AIDS, 1326
Papillary thyroid cancer, 1133–1135, 1134*t*, 1137
Papilledema, **195**
Papilloma
inverted, nasal, 226
Schneiderian, 226
Papillomatosis, recurrent respiratory, **237**
Papular, 102*t*
Paracetamol. *See* Acetaminophen
"Parachute mitral valve," 332
Paradoxical emboli, 986
Paradoxical vocal fold motion, asthma, 246
Paradoxic sleep, 1082
Paraganglioma, 26, **1166–1171**, 1167
Paragonimiasis, **1522–1523**
Paragonimus kellicotti, 1522
Paragonimus westermani, 1522
Parainfluenza virus, 270, 1409
Paralytic ileus, **638–639**
Paralytic poliomyelitis, 1375
Paralytic shellfish poisoning, **1590–1591**, 1590*t*
Paramalignant pleural effusion, 312
Paramyxoviruses, **1408–1410**. *See also specific types*
human metapneumovirus, 1409
human parainfluenza viruses, 1409
Nipah virus, 1409
respiratory syncytial virus, **1408–1410**
Paranasal sinus
diseases, **218–227** (*See also* Nose & paranasal sinus diseases)
endocrine syndrome, 889
pemphigus, 146
tumors, malignant, 226
Paraneoplastic disorders/syndromes. *See also specific types*
autoimmune, 1003, 1004*t*
bronchogenic carcinoma, 1603–1604
pain, 80
Paranodal demyelination, 1030
Paranoid ideation, 1062
Paranoid personality disorder, **1059–1061,** 1060*t*
Paraparesis, spastic. *See* Spastic paraparesis
Paraphilias, **1057–1058**
Parapneumonic pleural effusion, 313
Paraproteinemias, polyneuropathy, **1032**
Paraproteins, acute tubular necrosis from, 909
Parasitic infections. *See also specific types*
skin, **129–131**
pediculosis, **130–131**
scabies, **129–130,** 129*f*
Parasomnias, **1084**
Parasternal lift, 323, 405
Parathion poisoning, **1588–1589**
Parathyroid carcinoma, 1142, 1146
Parathyroidectomy, 1145–1146
Parathyroid gland disorders, **1138–1146**. *See also specific types*
hyperparathyroidism, **1141–1146**
hypoparathyroidism & pseudohypoparathyroidism, **1138–1141,** 1140*t*
Parathyroid hormone, magnesium on, 893
Paravaccinia, 1421, **1421**
Parechovirus, human, **1425–1426**
Paregoric, tincture of, 1223
Parenteral nutritional support, 1265, 1266, 1268, 1269*t*
Parietal lobe lesions, 999
Paritaprevir, 690*t*
Parkinson disease, **1006–1010**
bradykinesia, 1007
head trauma and, 1023
idiopathic, 1007
Myerson sign, 1007
postural instability, 1007
rigidity, 1007
treatment, 1007–1010
amantadine, 1007–1008
anticholinergic medications, 1009
antipsychotics, 1009
COMT inhibitors, 1009
dopamine agonists, 1008
istradefylline, 1009
levodopa, 1008
physical/occupation/speech therapies, 1009
rivastigmine, 1009
selective MAO inhibitors, 1008–1009
stimulation & ablative, 1009–1010
tremor, 1007
weight loss, involuntary, 32
Parkinsonism, **1006–1007**
carbon minoxide poisoning, 1006
drug-induced, 1007, 1012, 1067
postencephalitis, 1006
Parkland formula, 1555–1556
Parlivizumab, 1410
Paromomycin
for amebiasis, 1514–1515, 1515t
for cryptosporidiosis, 1326, 1517
for giardiasis, 1519
for visceral leishmaniasis, 1501
Paronychia, 166–167, 166*f*
Parotid gland
tenderness/swelling, measles, 1371–1372, 1371*f*
tumors, 235
Paroxetine
birth defects and, 1075
for depression, 1072, 1073*t*
for hot flushes, 1186–1187
hyponatremia from, 878
for irritable bowel syndrome, 646
for obsessive-compulsive disorder, 1053
for panic disorder, 1051
serotonin syndrome from, 1567
toxicity, 1592
Paroxysmal atrial fibrillation, 391
Paroxysmal hemicrania, 973
Paroxysmal nocturnal hemoglobinuria, **510–511**
Paroxysmal supraventricular tachycardia, 386, **388–389**
accessory AV pathway, **390–391**
vs. sinus tachycardia, 386
PARP inhibitors. *See also specific types*
for *BRCA1/2* breast cancer, 759
for breast carcinoma, 754
Parvovirus B19, 864, **1419–1420**
Pasireotide, 1163
Passenger, incapacitated, 1562
Passive congestion of liver, 715
Passive external rewarming, 1551
Passive immunity, 1301
Passive immunization, for respiratory syncytial virus, 1410
Pasteurella, cat and dog bites, 1283–1284
Patch, transdermal contraceptive, **777**
Patellofemoral pain, **1703–1704**
Patent foramen ovale, **326–328**
closure surgery, 987
cryptogenic stroke, 327–328, 987, 990
paradoxical emboli & TIA, 986
Pathergy phenomenon, 856
Patient adherence, 1–2
Patient care. *See specific types*
Patient-controlled analgesia, 80, 1098
Patient-delivered therapy, for STD prevention, 1286
Patient Health Questionnaire-2 (PHQ-2), 57
Patulous eustachian tube, 208
Pauci-immune glomerulonephritis, 852, 854, 855, 912, 923*t*, **928**
PAX-4, 1196
Pazopanib, 1601*t*, 1646
PCKS9, 1661
PD-1/immune checkpoint inhibitors, 1388. *See also specific types*
PDE-5 inhibitors, 959–960, 1223. *See also specific types*
PDGFRa, gastrointestinal mesenchymal tumors, 1625
PD-L1, 758, 1674*t*
PD-L1 inhibitors, 1607. *See also specific types*
PDX1 mutation, 1197
Peace pill. *See* Phencyclidine (PCP)
Peak expiratory flow meters, 247
Peanut allergies, 614, 868
Pedal artery occlusion, **476–477**
Pediculosis, **130–131**
Pediculus humanus var *capitis,* 130
Pediculus humanus var *corporis,* 130
Peer support groups, 1052, 1055, 1059
PEG 3350, 586, 587*t*, 646
Pegabalin, 1222
Pegcetacoplan, 510
Pegfilgrastim, 1654*t*
Peginterferon alfa-2a, 688
Pegloticase, 826
PEG scores, 93, 93*t*
Pegvisomant, 1107
Pegylated interferon. *See under* Interferon
Pelger-Huët abnormality, 527
Peliosis hepatitis, 697, 1471
Pellagra, 155, 1172, 1261
Pelvic floor muscle exercises, 63, 672
Pelvic infections. *See also specific types*
gram-negative, 1473
peripartum, **808**
Pelvic inflammatory disease, **785–787**
antimicrobial therapy, empiric, 1297*t*
gonococcus, 1470
HIV/AIDS, 1330
IUDs, 778
pelvic pain, 769
Pelvic organ prolapse, **769–770**
Pelvis pain, **767–769**
chronic, 80
dysmenorrhea, **767**
endometriosis, **767–769**
other, **769**
pelvic inflammatory disease, 769
pelvic pain syndrome, 950*t*, **951–952**
Pembrolizumab
for bladder cancer, 1643, 1644
for breast carcinoma, 752
triple-negative, 755, 758
diabetes mellitus from, 1196
for hepatocellular carcinoma, 1612
hypophysitis from, 1099
for MSI-H/deficient MMR solid tumors, 1673*t*
for non–small cell lung cancer, 1606, 1607
for PD-L1 cancers, 1674*t*
for renal cell carcinoma, 1646
for small intestinal adenocarcinomas, 1625
thyroiditis from, silent, 1115

Pemetrexed, 1598*t*, 1609
Pemphigoid, esophageal webs/rings, 614
Pemphigus, **145–147**, 146*f*
Pemphigus erythematosus, 146
Pemphigus vegetans, 146
Pemphigus vulgaris, 146, 614
Penciclovir, 1356*t*
Penicillamine
  autoimmune hypoglycemia from, 1237
  for Group B/C/G streptococcus endocarditis, 1457
  inflammation myopathy from, 1045
  for pneumococcal infections
    meningitis, 1445
    pneumonia, 1444
  for viridans streptococci, prosthetic valve, 1456
  for Wilson disease, 712–713
Penicillin. *See also specific types*
  allergy, 1300
  allergy testing, 870
  for clostridial myonecrosis, 1451
  cross-sensitizing & cross-reacting, 1300
  drug eruptions from, 156
  for enterococcus, 1443
  for gonococcus, 1470
  interstitial nephritis from, 911
  for leptospirosis, 1491
  for neurosyphilis, 1487
  pericarditis from, 427
  for rheumatic fever, 426
  for *Staphylococcus aureus,* 1441
  for streptococcus
    Group A pneumonia, 1442
    Group B, 1443
    Group D endocarditis, 1457
    toxic shock syndrome, 1443
    viridans streptococci endocarditis, 1455
  for *Streptococcus pneumoniae* endocarditis, 1457
  for *Vibrio,* 1467
Penicillin G
  for actinomycosis, 1474
  for Lyme disease, 1494, 1495*t*
  for meningococcus meningitis, 1460–1461
  for mushroom poisoning, 685–686
  for neurosyphilis, 1487
  for streptococcus endocarditis
    anaerobic/microaerophilic, 1473
    Group A, 1443
    Group D, 1457
    viridans, 1455, 1456–1457
  for streptococcus Group A arthritis, 1442
  for syphilis, 1483, 1483*t*
Penicillin V, 1474
Penicillin VK, 128
Penicillium, 1546–1547
Penile prosthetic surgery, 960
Penitumumab, 1673*t*
Penn State Equation, 1266
Pentalogy of Fallot, 330
Pentamidine
  on beta cells, 1237
  hepatitis from, 1325
  hyperinsulinemia & hyperglycemia from, 1237
  hypoglycemia from, 1237
  for *P. jirovecii* prophylaxis, HIV/AIDS, 1337*t*
Pentamidine isethionate, 1541
Pentavalent antimonials, 1501. *See also specific types*
Pentosan polysulfate (sodium), 199, 954
Pentostatin, 532
Pentoxifylline
  for alcohol-associated liver disease, 695
  for HTLV1-associated myelopathy, 1389
  for leg ulcers, venous insufficiency, 162
  for nonalcoholic fatty liver disease, 699
Peppermint oil, 646
Peptic stricture, from GERD, **610**
Peptic ulcer disease, **625–629**
  complications, **629–632**
    gastric outlet obstruction, **631**
    hemorrhage, GI, **629–630**
    ulcer perforation, **631**
  dyspepsia, 579
  epidemiology, 625
  fecal immunochemical tests, 626
  fecal occult blood tests, 626
  gastric outlet obstruction, **631**
  GI bleeding
    occult, 601
    upper, 596
  H. pylori, **625–629**
  NSAID, **625–630**
  treatment, 624*t*
    medical
      H. pylori ulcers, 627–628
      NSAID ulcers, 628–629
    pharmacologic
      acid-antisecretory agents, 627
      H. pylori eradication, 627
      mucosal defense enhancement, 627
PEP-to-PrEP, 1343
Peptostreptococcus
  anaerobic pneumonia & lung abscess, 278
  chest infections, 1472
  intra-abdominal infections, 1472
  skin infections, injection drug, 1286
Peramivir, 1356*t*, 1411, 1415
Perampanel, 976*t*
Perceptual-motor function, dementia, 54
Percreta, 807
PERC rule, pulmonary embolism, 21
Percutaneous balloon valvuloplasty, for mitral stenosis, 337, 337*f*
Percutaneous coronary intervention
  for acute coronary syndrome, without ST-segment elevation, 372, 372*t*
  for acute MI, with ST-segment elevation, 375
  for angina pectoris, 365, 366
  cardiac risk assessment/reduction, 43–44
  "facilitated," 375
  restenosis after, 366, 375
Percutaneous puncture, aspiration, injection, and re-aspiration (PAIR), 1525–1526
Percutaneous transcatheter valve replacement, 350
Percutaneous transhepatic cholangiography, 677
Perennial rhinitis, 222
Performance anxiety, 1049
Perianal abscess & fistula, 654, **673**
Perianal pruritus, **673**
Periaortic inflammation, 482
Pericardial effusion, **429–430**
Pericardial friction rub, 373, 381, 415, 427, 429
Pericardial stretch, 429
Pericardial tamponade, **429–430**
  cardiac tumors, 427, 434
  from colchicine, 428
  COVID-19, 427
  myocardial wall perforation, 386
  pericarditis
    constrictive, 430
    hemorrhagic, 380
  vs. pericarditis, 23
  traumatic heart disease, 434
Pericardial window, 428, 430
Pericarditis
  acute, 427
  acute inflammatory, **426–429**
  acute MI with ST-segment elevation, 381
  bacterial, 427
  chest pain, 22
  chronic, 427
  chronic kidney disease, 916
  constrictive, **430–431**
    jugular venous pulsations, 429
    superior vena caval obstruction, 492
  COVID-19, 427
    athlete screening, 439–441
    vaccine, 1406
  Dressler syndrome, 427
  drug-induced, 427
  enterovirus, acute nonspecific, 1423
  friction rub, 23
  incessant, 427
  myocarditis with, 427
  neoplastic, 427–428, 430
  Pneumococcus, 427, 1444
  postcardiotomy, 427
  post-myocardial infarction, 427
  radiation, 427
  recurrent, 427
  rheumatoid arthritis, 828
  stress cardiomyopathy, 420
  vs. tamponade, 23
  tuberculous, 427
  uremic, 427
  viral, 427
Pericardium diseases, **426–433**. *See also specific types*
  pericardial effusion & tamponade, **429–430**
  pericarditis, **426–431** (*See also* Pericardial effusion)
  pulmonary hypertension, **431–433**
  systemic lupus erythematosus, 834
Pericentesis, for ascites and edema, from cirrhosis, 702, 703
Perichondritis, 205
Perihilar tumors, 1613
Perilymphatic fistula
  diving, 208, 217
  vertigo, **216–217**
Perindopril, 452*t*
Periodic limb movement disorder, **1084**
Periodic limb movements of sleep, **1013**
Periodic paralysis syndromes, **1045**
Periodontitis
  HIV/AIDS, 1325
  sialadenitis, 234
Peripartum cardiomyopathy, **436**
Peripheral arterial disease, **473–481**
  arterial occlusion of a limb, **477–478**
  epidemiology, 473
  mesenteric vein occlusion, **481**
  occlusive
    aorta & iliac arteries, **473–474**
    cerebrovascular disease, **478–480**, 479*t*
    femoral & popliteal arteries, **474–476**
    tibial & pedal arteries, **476–477**
  visceral arterial insufficiency, **480–481**
Peripheral artery aneurysm, **485–486**
Peripherally inserted central catheter, superficial venous thrombophlebitis, **489–490**
Peripheral neuritis, Epstein-Barr virus, 1363
Peripheral neuropathies, 80, **1030–1045**. *See also specific types*
  axonal degeneration, 1030
  Bell palsy, **1036–1037**, 1036*f*
  brachial plexus neuropathy, **1040**
  cervical rib syndrome, **1040**
  Chikungunya fever, 1400
  chronic kidney disease, 919
  conduction velocity, motor/sensory, 1030

Peripheral neuropathies (*Cont.*):
  diabetic, 1221–1223
  discogenic neck pain, **1037–1040**
    cervical disk protrusion, **1037**, 1038*f*–1039*f*
    cervical spondylosis, **1037–1040**
    congenital abnormalities, 1037
  distal symmetric polyneuropathy, 1221–1222, 1222*f*
  HIV/AIDS, 1323
    inflammatory demyelinating polyneuropathy, 1323
    peripheral neuropathy, 1323
  isolated, 1222–1223
  lumbosacral plexus lesions, **1040**
  mononeuropathies, **1034–1036**
  myopathic disorders, **1042–1045** (*See also* Myopathic disorders/myopathies)
  neuromuscular transmission disorders, **1040–1042**
    aminoglycoside, **1042**
    botulism, 982, **1042**, 1286–1287, **1452–1453**
    myasthenia gravis, 1004*t*, **1040–1041**
    myasthenic syndrome, **1042**
  paranodal/segmental demyelination, 1030
  periodic paralysis syndromes, **1045**
  polyneuropathies, **1030–1034**
Peripheral sympathetic inhibitors, **460**, 463*t*, **464**. *See also specific types*
Peripheral T-cell lymphoma, 535
Peripheral thermometer, 29
Peripheral vascular disease, 1224. *See also specific types*
Peripheral vein nutritional support, 1266
Peripheral vestibular disease, 214–215. *See also specific types*
Peristalsis loss, achalasia, **618–619**
Peritoneal dialysis, for end-stage kidney disease, 920
Peritoneal diseases, **602–606**. *See also specific types*
  ascites, **602–604**, 602*t*
  familial Mediterranean fever, **606**
  malignant ascites, **605–606**
  peritonitis, spontaneous bacterial, 602*t*, **604–605**
    treatment, with cirrhosis, 703
Peritonitis
  spontaneous bacterial, 602*t*, **604–605**, 703
  tuberculous, ascites, 602
Peritonsillar abscess, **232**
Peritonsillar cellulitis, **232**
Periungual warts, 122
Permethrin, 130, 131
Pernicious anemia, 507, **623**, 1027, 1112
Per oral endoscopic myotomy, for achalasia, 619
Peroxisome proliferator-activated receptor-alpha agonists, 1245*t*, 1248. *See also specific types*
Peroxisome proliferator-activated receptor gamma, 1207
Perphenazine, 1063, 1064*t*, 1065, 1065*t*
Persistent depressive disorder, 1070
Persistent pulmonary hypertension of newborn, 331, 432*t*
Persistent vegetative state, **1020**
Personality disorders, **1059–1061**, 1060*t*. *See also specific types*
Pertussis, 15–17
Pertuzumab, 753, 755, 758, 1600*t*, 1672*t*
Pessaries, 63
Pesticide poisoning
  arsenic, 1577
  cholinesterase inhibitor, **1588–1589**
"Petit mal" seizures, 979
Petroleum distillate poisoning, **1589**
Petrous apicitis, **210**
Peutz-Jeghers syndrome, 668, 1615
Peyronie disease, 959, 1172
pH, esophageal
  impedance, 607, 609, 611
  recording, 607
  testing, 607, 609, 610
Phakic intraocular lens, 168
Phalen sign, 1690
Pharmacogenetic tests, clinical relevance, **1666**, **1667*t*–1674*t***
  BRAF gene, 1671*t*
  CF transmembrane conductance regulator, 1667*t*
  cytochrome P450 variants, 1667*t*–1668*t*
  dihydropyrimidine dehydrogenase variants, 1669*t*
  epidermal growth factor receptor, 1672*t*
  G6PD deficiency, 1669*t*
  HER2 gene, 1672*t*
  HLA-B*1502 allele, 1669*t*
  HLA-B*5701 allele, 1670*t*
  HLA-B*5801 allele, 1670*t*
  isocitrate dehydrogenase-1/2 gene, 1672*t*
  KRAS gene, 1673*t*
  microsatellite instability-high, MMR system deficiency, 1673*t*
  programmed death ligand 1, 1674*t*
  solute carrier organic anion transporter family member 1B1 gene, 1670*t*
  thiopurine methyltransferase variants, 1670*t*
  uridine diphosphoglucuronosyltransferase 1A1 variants, 1671*t*
  vitamin K epoxide reductase complex variants, 1671*t*
Pharmacomechanical thrombectomy catheters, for arterial occlusion of limb, acute, 478
Pharyngitis, **231–232**, 231*f*
  adenovirus, 1418
  antimicrobial therapy, empiric, 1297*t*
  Fusobacterium necrophorum, 233, 1472
  streptococcal, rheumatic fever, 424
Pharyngoconjunctival fever, 170, 1418
Pharynx diseases, **227–234**. *See also* Nose & paranasal sinus diseases
Phenazopyridine poisoning, **1586–1587**
Phencyclidine (PCP), 1063, 1084, **1093**, **1584–1585**
Phenelzine, 1073*t*
Phenibut poisoning, **1581–1582**
Phenobarbital, 1050*t*
  for alcohol withdrawal, 1091
  for hyperadrenergic postural orthostatic syndrome, 985
  poisoning, 1569*t*, **1581–1582**
  for seizures, 976*t*, 1567
Phenol, neuromodulatory therapy, 97*t*
Phenothiazines
  drowsiness & orthostatic hypotension from, 1576
  dystonia from, 1012
  for Huntington disease, 1010
  poisoning, 1576
Phentermine, 1252, 1253, 1254*t*
Phentolamine, 1566
Phenylephrine, 498, 1566
Phenytoin
  dystonia from, 1012
  eosinophilic pulmonary syndromes from, 297
  for facial pain, 978
  on folic acid absorption, 508
  hepatotoxicity, 696
  for myotonia congenita, 1044
  for myotonic dystrophy, 1044
  poisoning, 1569, **1575–1576**
  for seizures, 976*t*
  teratogenicity, 813
  for trigeminal neuralgia, 975
Pheochromocytoma
  beta-blockers for, 460
  headache, 35, 36*t*
  hypertension, 445
  hypertensive retinochoroidopathy, 192
  MEN 2 (MEN 2A), 1167
  MEN 3 (MEN 2B), 1167
  metastatic, 1167, 1170
  palpitations, 26
  pregnancy, 1169–1170
  pregnancy, pheochromocytoma, 1169–1170
  von Recklinghausen neurofibromatosis type 1, 1167
Philadelphia chromosome, 520
  absence, essential thrombocytosis, 522
  leukemia, 520
    acute lymphoblastic, 528
    chronic myeloid, 524, 525
Phlebotomy, for hemochromatosis, 711
Phobic disorders, **1049, 1051–1052**. *See also specific types*
Phonic tics, 1013
Phonophobia, migraine headache, 36, 36*t*
Phosphate
  deficiency, osteomalacia from, 1153
  for diabetic ketoacidosis, 1229
  fractional excretion, 891
  for hyperphosphatemia, hyperglycemic hyperosmolar state, 1230
Phosphatidylinositol-3-kinase (PI3K) inhibitors, 758. *See also specific types*
Phosphatonin, 1153
Phosphodiesterase inhibitors. *See also specific types*
  for asthma, 251*t*, 254
  for cardiogenic shock, 499
  for high-altitude illness prevention/treatment, 1561
  type 4, for COPD, 263
  type 5, for pulmonary hypertension, 841
Phosphorus, plasma, 890
Phosphorus concentration disorders, **890–892**. *See also specific types*
  hyperphosphatemia, **892**, 892*t*
  hypophosphatemia, **890–892**, 891*t*
Photoaging, lentigines, **108**
Photoallergy, 155
Photodermatitis, 102*t*, **155–156**
Photodynamic therapy, 111, 112, 114
Photophobia, 36, 36*t*, **197**
Photopsia, 969
Photoselective vaporization of the prostate, 968
Photosensitive epilepsy, 981
Photosensitivity, 155, 158*t*, 1067
Phototherapy, 114, 1078, 1328
Phototoxicity, 155
Phthirus pubis, 130
Phyllodes tumor, 738–739
Physical activity. *See* Exercise/exercise therapy
Physical assessment
  nutrition-focused, 1250
  older adults, 52–53
Physical therapy
  for osteoarthritis, 821
  for pain, 95–96
  for somatic symptom disorders, 1055
  for stroke, 991
Physician-assisted death, 76
Physician Orders for Life-Sustaining Treatment, 71–72
Physician Orders for Scope of Treatment, 72
Physiologic dependence, 1086

Physostigmine, cholinergic syndrome from, 1570
Phytanic acid metabolism, 1031
Phytonadione, 562, 705
PI3K, 1197
PI3 kinase delta inhibitors, 531, 534. *See also specific types*
PI3K inhibitors, 1197
Pibrentasvir, 689, 690*t*
Pickwickian syndrome, **315**
Piebaldism, 163
Pigmentary disorders, dermatologic, **162–164**. *See also specific types*
  drug-related, 158*t*–159*t*
  hyperpigmentation, lower extremity edema, 28
  primary
    hyperpigmentation, **163**
    hypopigmentation and depigmentation, **163,** 163*f*
  secondary
    hyperpigmentation, **163,** 163*f*
    hypopigmentation, **163–164**
Pigmented, 102*t*
Pigmented nevi, 163
PIK3CA, breast carcinoma, 758
Pill-induced esophagitis, 611, **613**
Pill-in-the-pocket treatment, 396
Pilocarpine, 845
Pimavanserin, 1009
Pimecrolimus
  for atopic dermatitis, 134
  for psoriasis, 137
  for seborrheic dermatitis, 139
  T cell lymphoma from, 134
  topical dermatologic, 104*t*
Pindolol, 462*t*
Pineal tumor, 998*t*
Pinguecula, **172**
Pingueculitis, 172
"Pink puffers," 259, 260*t*
Pinworm, **1528–1529**
Pioglitazone, 1204*t*, 1207–1208, **1582**
Piperacillin-tazobactam
  for anaerobic skin & soft tissue infections, 1473
  for *Bacteroides fragilis,* 1472
  for cancer, infections with, 1652
  for chest infections, anaerobic, 1472, 1472*t*
  for cholangitis, community-acquired, 724
  for necrotizing fasciitis, 1442
  for peritonitis, spontaneous bacterial, 703
Piperaquine, 1504*t*, 1506
Piperazines. *See also specific types*
  seizures from, 1567
Pirbuterol, 249, 252*t*
Pitavastatin, 1244, 1246*t*
Pitting edema, 490, 490*f*, 494
Pituitary adenomas, 998*t*, 1099, **1110–1111**
Pituitary gland disorders, **1099–1111**. *See also specific types*
  acromegaly & gigantism, **1106–1107**
  anterior hypopituitarism, **1099–1103**
  central diabetes insipidus, **1104–1105**
  hyperprolactinemia, **1108–1110,** 1108*t*
  macroadenomas, nonfunctioning, **1110–1111**
  metastases, anterior hypopituitarism, 1099
  microprolactinomas, hyperprolactinemia from, **1108–1110,** 1108*t*
  neuroendocrine tumors (*See also specific types*)
    acromegaly and gigantism, **1106–1107**
    anterior hypopituitarism, 1099
  pituitary adenomas, nonfunctioning, **1110–1111**
  thyrotrophe tumor, 1120
Pituitary gland hormones, 1099
Pituitary stalk thickening, anterior hypopituitarism, 1099–1100
Pit viper envenomation, **1590**
Pityriasis rosea, **138–139,** 138*f*
Pityriasis rosea–like eruptions, drug-related, 159*t*
Pityriasis versicolor, **117–118**
Pityrosporum folliculitis, hot tub, 124–125
Pityrosporum ovale, seborrheic dermatitis, 1328
Pivot shift test, 1698*t*, 1700–1701
PKD1, 939
PKD2, 939
PKR-like ER kinase, 1197
Placenta
  abruption, **807**
  morbidly adherent, **807**
Placenta previa, 807, **807**
Plague, 1294*t*, **1468–1469**
Plan B, **779**
Plantar warts, 122
Plant stanols/sterols, on LDL cholesterol, 1243
Plasma cell dyscrasias, 1237. *See also specific types*
Plasma cell myeloma, **536–539,** 941
  autoimmune hypoglycemia from, 1237
  benign monoclonal gammopathy, 1032
  gout from, 823
  kidney disease, **941**
  overload proteinemia, 904
  polyneuropathy, 1032
  relapsing polychondritis, 856
  treatment, 1596*t*
Plasmacytoma, 537
Plasma exchange
  for anti-GBM glomerulonephritis, 929
  for cryoglobulin-associated glomerulonephritis, 930
  for Goodpasture syndrome, 913, 929
  for hepatitis C, cryoglobulinemia, 690
  for IgA nephropathy, 927
  for IgA vasculitis, 928
  for membranoproliferative glomerulonephritis, 929
  for pauci-immune glomerulonephritis, 928
  for thrombotic thrombocytopenic purpura, 552
Plasma fluid volume, 875
Plasminogen activator, recombinant, 991
Platelet(s)
  counts, desired ranges, 546, 547*t*
  sequestration, **556**
  transfusion, **544–545**
Platelet-derived growth factor, myelofibrosis from, 523
Platelet disorders, **546–557**. *See also specific types*
  congenital, **556–557**
  count ranges, desired, 546, 547*t*
  patient evaluation, 546, 547*t*
  qualitative, **556–557**
    acquired disorders of platelet function, **557**
    congenital disorders of platelet function, **556–557**
  thrombocytopenia, **546–556**
    causes, 547*t*
    drug-induced, **555,** 555*t*
    infection/sepsis, **556**
    platelet destruction, increased, **548–555**
      disseminated intravascular coagulation, **554–555,** 554*t*
      heparin-induced thrombocytopenia, **552–553,** 553*t*
      immune thrombocytopenia, **548–550,** 550*f*
      thrombotic microangiopathy, **550–552,** 551*t*
    platelet production, decreased, **546–548**
      bone marrow failure, **546–548**
      bone marrow infiltration, **548**
      chemotherapy & irradiation, 547*t*, **548**
      cyclic thrombocytopenia, **548**
      nutritional deficiencies, **548**
    platelet sequestration, **556**
    posttransfusion purpura, **555–556**
    pregnancy, **556**
    pseudothrombocytopenia, **556**
    von Willebrand disease type 2B, **556,** 559*t*, 560
Platelet-inhibiting agents, 365. *See also specific types*
Platelet-rich plasma, 1689, 1705
Platinum analogs, 1598*t*. *See also specific types*
  carboplatin, 1598*t*
  cisplatin, 1598*t*
  oxaliplatin, 1598*t*
Platypnea orthodeoxia, patent foramen ovale, 327
Plecanatide, 586, 587*t*, 646
Pleistophora, 1517
Plenadren, 1159
Pleural diseases, **309–315**. *See also specific types*
  pleural effusion, **310–313,** 310*t*, 311*t*, 312*t*
  pleuritis, **309–310**
  pneumothorax, **313–315**
  rheumatoid arthritis, 828
Pleural effusion, **310–313,** 310*t*, 311*t*, 312*t*
  bronchogenic carcinoma, 1603
  exudates and transudates, 310–311, 310*t*, 312, 313
  hemothorax, 310, 311, **312**
  paramalignant, 312
Pleurisy, dyspnea, 18
Pleuritic pain, 309–310
Pleuritis, **309–310**
Pleurodynia, enterovirus, 1423
Plexiform neuromas, 1005
Plummer disease, 1119
Plummer-Vinson syndrome, 501, 614
PML-RAR-alpha, acute promyelocytic leukemia, 528
PMS2, 668, 1628, 1673*t*
Pneumatic dilation, for achalasia, 619
Pneumococcal conjugate (PCV13) vaccine, 1302*t*–1303*t*, 1306*t*–1307*t*, 1309*t*
Pneumococcal polysaccharide vaccine (PPSV23), 4*t*, 255, 273, 1302*t*–1303*t*, 1306*t*–1307*t*, 1309*t*
Pneumococcal polysaccharide (PPSV23) vaccine, 4*t*, 255, 273, 1306*t*–1307*t*, 1309*t*
Pneumococcus, **1444–1446**
  arthritis, 1444
  endocarditis, 1444
  meningitis, 1282, **1446**
  pericarditis, 427
  pneumonia, **1444–1445**
    bacteremia, 1473
    with influenza, 1411
Pneumoconiosis, **306–307,** 306*t*
  asbestosis, 306*t*, **307,** 308
  coal worker's pneumoconiosis, **306,** 306*t*, 308
  silicosis, **306–307,** 306*t*, 308
Pneumocystis. *See Pneumocystis jirovecii* pneumonia
Pneumocystis jirovecii pneumonia, **1538–1541,** 1539*t*–1540*t*
  hematopoietic cell transplant recipients, 1273
  HIV/AIDS, 1274, 1311, 1316, 1317–1320, 1317*f*, 1319*t*
  immunocompromised, 279, 1274
  with impaired cellular immunity, 1273
  otitis media, AIDS, 218
  pneumonia, 269*t*
  prevention, 1541

Pneumocystis jirovecii pneumonia (*Cont.*):
- prognosis, 1541
- solid organ transplant recipients, 1273
- treatment, 1338
  - atovaquone, 1541
  - dapsone, 1541
  - pentamidine isethionate, 1541
  - prednisone, 1541
  - primaquine/clindamycin, 1541
  - trimethoprim, 1541
  - trimethoprim-sulfamethoxazole, 1541

Pneumonia, **268–278**. *See also specific types*
- anaerobic, 268, **276–278**
- antimicrobial therapy, empiric, 1297*t*
- aspiration, 276–278
  - antimicrobial therapy, empiric, 1297*t*
  - injection drug abuse, 1287
- characteristics, 269*t*
- chest pain, 22
- *Chlamydophila pneumoniae,* 1479
- community-acquired
  - antimicrobial therapy, initial, 1296*t*
  - HIV/AIDS, 1320
- cough, 16, 16*t*
- diffuse interstitial, **292–294,** 293*t,* 294*t*
- dyspnea, 18, 19
- eosinophilic, 297
- fever, 31
- hemoptysis, 21
- herpes simplex virus, 1354, 1355
- HIV/AIDS
  - bacterial, 1319*t*, 1320
  - *Haemophilus influenza,* 1320
  - mycobacterial, 1319*t*, 1320, 1320*f*
  - *Pneumocystis,* 1274, 1311, 1316, 1317–1320, 1317*f,* 1319*t* (*See also Pneumocystis jirovecii* pneumonia)
- idiopathic interstitial, 293, 294*t*
- necrotizing, 276–278
- nosocomial, **274–276,** 276*t,* 277*t*
  - antimicrobial therapy, initial, 1296*t*
- organizing, 268
- perioperative, 45, 46, 47, 51
- *Pneumococcus,* **1444–1445**
  - with influenza, 1411
- *Pneumocystis jirovecii,* **1538–1541,** 1539*t*–1540*t* (*See also Pneumocystis jirovecii* pneumonia)
- postobstructive, bronchogenic carcinoma, 1603
- postoperative, 45, 46, 47, 51, 1296*t*
- Q fever, 1435
- *Streptococcus,* Group A beta-hemolytic, **1442**
- varicella, 1360
- variola/vaccinia, 1421
- ventilator-associated, **274–276,** 276*t,* 277*t,* 1277–1278

Pneumonia, community-acquired, **268–274,** 272*t*
- coccidioidomycosis, 1537
- HIV/AIDS, 1320
- prevention, 273
- treatment, 271–273, 272*t*

Pneumonia severity Index (PSI), 273

Pneumonitis
- chemical, 1277
- hypersensitivity, **307–308,** 307*t*
- interstitial, HIV/AIDS, 1321
- Q fever, 1435
- radiation, 309
- toxoplasmosis, 1511
- typhus, scrub, 1429

Pneumonococcus, medications for, 1293*t*

Pneumothorax, **313–315**
- dyspnea, 18
- iatrogenic, 313
- tension, 313
- traumatic, 313

Podagra, 824, 824*f*

Podofilox, 787

Podophyllotoxin, 121

Podophyllum resin, 123, 787

Poison control center, 1564

Poisoning, **1564–1593**. *See also specific types*
- acetaminophen, **1571–1573,** 1572*f,* 1572*t*
- acids, corrosive, **1573**
- alkalies, **1573–1574**
- amphetamines, **1574**
- anticoagulants, **1575**
- anticonvulsants, **1575–1576**
- antidepressants, **1592–1593,** 1593*f*
- antipsychotics, **1576**
- arsenic, **1576–1577**
- atropine & anticholinergics, **1577**
- benzodiazepines, **1581–1582**
- beta-blockers, **1577–1578**
- caffeine, **1592**
- calcium channel blockers, **1578**
- carbon monoxide, 1572*t*, **1578–1579**
- clonidine & sympatholytic antihypertensives, **1579**
- cocaine, **1574**
- cyanide, 18–20, **1579–1580**
- danger assessment, 1564
- diagnosis, 1569–1571, 1570*t*
- dietary supplements & herbal products, **1580,** 1580*t*
- digitalis & cardiac glycosides, **1581**
- digoxin, 1572*t*
- ethanol, 1572*t*, **1581–1582**
- ethylene glycol, 1572*t*
- gamma-hydroxybutyrate, **1582**
- hallucinogens, **1584–1585**
- hypoglycemic drugs, 1568*t*, **1582**
- initial evaluation, **1564**
- isoniazid, **1582–1583**
- lead, **1583–1584**
- lithium, 1572*t*, **1584**
- LSD, **1584–1585**
- marijuana & synthetic cannabinoids, **1585**
- mercury, **1585–1586**
- methanol & ethylene glycol, 1572*t*, **1586**
- methemoglobin, 1572*t*
- methemoglobinemia-inducing agents, **1586–1587**
- mushrooms, **1587**
- nerve agents, **1579**
- opiates & opioids, **1587–1588**
- patient observation, 1564
- pesticides, cholinesterase inhibitors, **1588–1589**
- petroleum distillates & solvents, **1589**
- salicylates, 1572*t*, **1589–1590**
- scorpion stings, **1591–1592**
- seafood, **1590–1591,** 1590*t*
- sedative-hypnotics, **1581–1582**
- snake bites, **1591**
- spider bites, **1591–1592**
- sulfonylureas, antidotes, 1568*t*
- symptomatic patient, **1564–1567**
  - arrhythmias, **1566,** 1566*t*
  - coma, **1564–1565**
  - hyperthermia, **1567**
  - hypotension, **1565**
  - hypothermia, **1565**
  - seizures, **1567,** 1567*t*
- theophylline, 1572*t*, **1592**
- valproic acid, 1572*t*

Poisoning, treatment
- antidotes, **1568,** 1568*t*
- decontamination, eyes, **1568**
- decontamination, GI
  - activated charcoal, 1568–1569
  - general, 1568
  - hemodialysis, 1569, 1569*t*
  - repeat-dose charcoal, 1569
  - urinary manipulation, 1569
  - whole bowel irrigation, 1569
- decontamination, skin, **1568**
- gastric emptying, contraindications, 1568

Poliomyelitis, **1374–1375**
- acute flaccid myelitis, **1376**
- vaccines, 1374, 1375

Pollen-associated food allergy syndrome, 868

Pollution, air, 245, 259

Poly-ADP-ribose polymerase inhibitors, 1641. *See also specific types*

Polyalcohol, 1203

Polyanalgesic Conference Consensus, 97

Polyangiitis
- eosinophilic granulomatosis with, 303, **854–855**
- granulomatosis with, **851–853,** 852*f*
  - hearing loss, 213
  - myocarditis, 415*t*, 417
  - pulmonary vasculitis, 303
  - sinonasal inflammatory disease, 226–227
- microscopic, **853–854**

Polyarteritis, polyneuropathy, **1032**

Polyarteritis nodosa, **850–851,** 850*f,* 1270

Polyarthritis, 425, 425*t*, 826

Polyarticular arthritis, rubella, 1373

Polychondritis, relapsing, 205

Polycystic kidney disease, saccular aneurysm, 994

Polycystic ovary syndrome, 147, **771,** 791, **1181,** 1182

Polycythemia, hypertension and, 444

Polycythemia vera, **520–521,** 520*t*, 521*t*

Polydipsia
- aldosteronism, 1165
- central diabetes insipidus, 1104–1105
- diabetes mellitus, 1227
- hypercalcemia, 1142
- hyperglycemic hyperosmolar states, 1230
- hyponatremia, 88, 877*f*, 879
- hypopituitarism, 1100
- from lithium, 1079
- MDMA, 878
- psychogenic, 876–877
- schizophreniform spectrum disorders, 1062

Polyethylene glycol, 586, 587*t*, 646

Polymorphic light eruption, 155

Polymorphic reticulosis, sinonasal inflammatory disease, 227

Polymorphous light eruption, 156

Polymyalgia rheumatica, **848–849,** 1270

Polymyositis, **842–844,** 1237

Polyneuropathies, **1030–1034**
- acute idiopathic, **1033–1034**
- Charcot-Marie-Tooth disease, **1031**
- chronic inflammatory, **1034**
- critical illness, **1033**
- Dejerine-Sottas disease, **1031**
- diptheritic neuropathy, 1033
- distal symmetric, 1221–1222, 1222*f*
- familial amyloid polyneuropathy, **1031**
- Friedreich ataxia, **1031**
- infectious & inflammatory diseases
  - AIDS, **1032**
  - leprosy, **1032**
  - Lyme borreliosis, **1032**
  - polyarteritis, **1032**
  - rheumatoid arteritis, **1032**
  - sarcoidosis, **1032**
- malignant disease, **1033**
- porphyria, **1031**
- Refsum disease, **1031**

systemic & metabolic diseases
alcohol use disorder, **1032**
diabetes mellitus, **1031–1032**
nutritional deficiency, **1032**
paraproteinemias, **1032**
uremia, **1032**
toxic, **1033**
treatment, 1030–1031
Polyols, 1203
Polypharmacy, 58–59, **66,** 1097
Polypoid corditis, **237**
Poly (adenosine diphosphate-ribose) polymerase (PARP), 759
Polyposis syndromes, **666–669,** 1627
familial adenomatous polyposis, **667**
hamartomatous, **668**
hamartomatous polyposis syndromes, **668**
Polyps
cervical, **767**
colon, **665**
excision, 764
nasal, 224, **225–226**
nonfamilial adenomatous & serrated, **665–666**
vocal folds, **237**
Polyradiculopathy, CMV, 1323
Polysomnography, obstructive sleep apnea, 316–317
Pomalidomide, 538
Pompe disease, **1044**
Pompholyx, **144,** 144*f*
Ponesimod, 1025, 1025*t*
Popcorn-worker's lung, 308
Popliteal artery aneurysm, **485–486**
Popliteal artery occlusion, **474–476,** 477
Porcelain gallbladder, 720*t*, 721, 1612
Pork tapeworm, **1523, 1524**
Porphyria, 984, **1031**
Porphyria cutanea tarda, **144–145,** 145*f*, 155, 710, 1182
Porphyromonas, animal bites, 1283
Portable hearing amplifiers, 67
Portal cavernoma, 715
Portal hypertension
ascites, 602, 602*t*
cirrhosis, 615
esophageal varices, 615
gastropathy, **620–622**
noncirrhotic, **715–716**
upper GI bleeding, 596
Portal vein thrombosis, cirrhosis, 715
Portopulmonary hypertension, 705
Portosystemic shunt surgery, for esophageal varices, 617
Posaconazole, 1535, 1539*t*, 1544, 1545, 1546
Positive reinforcement, for schizophrenia spectrum disorders, 1068
Positive symptoms, schizophrenia, 1061
Positivity, differential time to, 1278
Post-acute COVID-19 syndrome, 1405
Post-acute sequelae after SARS-CoV-2, 19, 1405
Post-capillary pulmonary hypertension, isolated, 431
Postcardiotomy pericarditis, 427
Postcholecystectomy syndromes, **722**
Postcoital contraception, IUDs, 778
Postconception therapy, 799
Postencephalitis parkinsonism, 1006
Postepileptic automatism, 979
Posterior cerebral artery occlusion, 990
Posterior cruciate ligament injury, **1701–1702**
Posterior drawer test, 1702
Posterior inferior cerebellar artery obstruction, 990
Posterior mediastinal mass, 292
Posterior uveitis, **183–184**
Postexposure prophylaxis, HIV, 4, 1286, **1333,** 1724*t*, 1725
Postherpetic neuralgia, 80, **978,** 1360, 1361
Posthospital adjustment, 1097
Postinfarction ischemia, 379
Postinfectious cold agglutinin disease, 516
Postinfectious encephalomyelitis, measles, 1369
Postinfectious glomerulonephritis, 923*t*, **926–927**
Post-inflammatory hyperpigmentation, 163
Post-laminectomy pain syndrome, 80
Postmenopausal uterine bleeding, **765**
Postmicturition syncope, 402–403
Post-myocardial infarction pericarditis, 427
Post-myocardial infarction syndrome, 381, 427, 428
Postnasal drip syndrome, 15–17, 17*t*
Postobstructive pneumonia, bronchogenic carcinoma, 1603
Postpartum depression, allopregnanolone for, 1077
Postpartum thyroiditis, 1112, 1119, 1127
Postphlebitic syndrome, 28
Post-poliomyelitis syndrome, 1375
Postpolypectomy surveillance, 666
Postprandial hypoglycemia, 1233, 1233*t*, **1236–1237**
after gastric surgery, **1236**
autoimmune hypoglycemia, **1237**
diabetes, occult, **1236–1237**
functional alimentary hypoglycemia, **1236**
Postprandial hypotension, 985
Postrenal acute kidney injury, 907*t*, 908
Postsurgical anxiety states, 1097
Post-thrombotic syndrome, 490–491
Posttransfusion purpura, **555–556**
Post-transplant lymphoproliferative disorders, Epstein-Barr virus, 1365
Posttraumatic headache, **973–974**
Post-traumatic stress disorder, **1047–1048,** 1086, 1404
Postural hypotension, 984, 985
Postural orthostatic tachycardia syndrome, 984, **985**
Postural syncope, 402–403
Potassium
for diabetic ketoacidosis, 1228–1229
dietary, 1264
nutritional support, 1267
Potassium chloride
for diabetic ketoacidosis, 1229
for hyperglycemic hyperosmolar state, 1230
pill-induced esophagitis from, 613
for thyrotoxic crisis/thyroid storm, 1127
Potassium citrate, 957
Potassium concentration disorders, **882–886.** *See also specific types*
hyperkalemia, **884–886,** 885*t*, 887*t*
hypokalemia, **882–884,** 882*t*, 883*f*
Potassium hydroxide, 121, 1421
Potassium iodide, 133, 1120
Potassium-sparing diuretics, 407. *See also* Diuretics; *specific types*
Pott disease, **864–865**
Pott puffy tumor, 221
Povidone-iodine eye drops, 1419
Powassan virus, 1379, 1383
Poxvirus, **1420–1422**
molluscum contagiosum, **1421**
monkeypox, **1421–1422**
Orf and paravaccinia, **1421**
orthopoxviruses, novel, **1422**
variola/vaccinia, **1420–1421**
PPSV23, 4*t*
PR-2 negative breast cancer, 749–750
PR3-ANCA, 852, 853
Prader-Willi syndrome, 1100, 1101
Pralidoxime, 1579, 1589
Pralsetinib, 1606
Pramipexole, 1008, 1013
Pramlintide, 1205*t*, 1211, **1582**
Pramoxine, 161
Pramoxine hydrochloride, 101, 106*t*
Prasugrel, 369–370, 370*f*, 374
Pravastatin, 357*t*, 1244, 1246*t*
Praziquantel
for clonorchiasis, 1522
for cysticercosis, 1524
for echinococcosis, 1525
for neurocysticercosis, 1524
for opisthorchiasis, 1522
for paragonimiasis, 1523
for schistosomiasis, 1521
for tapeworm, 1523
Prazosin, 460, 463*t*
Precapillary pulmonary hypertension, 431
Precholecystectomy syndrome, **722**
Preclosure, mitral valve, 348
Preconception therapy, 799
Prednicarbate, 103*t*
Prednisolone
for asthma, 250*t*, 252*t*
for Bell palsy, 1037
for Crohn disease, 655
for HTLV1-associated myelopathy, 1389
for immune thrombocytopenia, 549
Prednisone. *See also specific indications*
clinical uses, 1193–1194, 1194*t*
DEXA surveillance, 1147
kidney stones from, 954
Preeclampsia-eclampsia, **802–804,** 803*t*
gestational trophoblastic disease, 801
hypertensive retinochoroidopathy, 192
Preexcitation syndromes, **390–391**
Preexposure prophylaxis, HIV/AIDS, 3–4, 1286, **1332,** 1333*t*
gay & bisexual men, 1724–1725, 1724*t*
transgender & gender diverse people, 1730
Preformed toxins, 1288. *See also specific types*
Pregabalin
for chronic pain syndromes, 1057
for neuropathic pain, **91*t*,** 94, 94*t*
for pruritus, 159, 160
for restless legs syndrome, 1013
for seizures, 976*t*
for trigeminal neuralgia, 978
Pregnancy. *See* Obstetrics & obstetric disorders
Pregnancy-associated antiphospholipid syndrome, **837–838**
Pregnancy-associated immune thrombocytopenia, 549
Pregnancy loss
recurrent, **799**
spontaneous, **797–799**
Pregnancy tests, 794
Preload
aortic regurgitation, 348
mitral regurgitation, 338
Premature ejaculation, 959
Premature menopause, 1185–1186
Premature ovarian insufficiency, 1661
Premature ventricular contraction, 383, **398**
Premenstrual dysphoric disorder, **770,** 1070
Premenstrual syndrome, **770**
PREMM5 probability model, 668
Prenatal care, **794–795,** 795*t*
Preoccupations, obsessive-compulsive disorder, 1052

Preoperative evaluation & perioperative management, **42–51**
- asymptomatic patient evaluation, 42
- bleeding history, directed, 42, 42*t*
- cardiac complications, perioperative, 42
- cardiac risk assessment/reduction, noncardiac surgery, **42–46** (*See also* Cardiac risk assessment/reduction, noncardiac surgery)
  - arrhythmias, 45
  - cardiac biomarkers, 43
  - coronary artery disease, 43–44, 44*t*
  - coronary revascularization, 43–44
  - exercise capacity, 42
  - heart failure & left ventricular dysfunction, 44–45
  - hypertension, 45–46
  - ischemic testing, preoperative noninvasive, 42–43, 44*f*
  - myocardial infarction, postoperative, 45
  - Revised Cardiac Risk Index, 42, 43*t*
  - stress testing, 43
  - valvular heart disease, 45
- endocrine disease, 49–50
- hematological evaluation, 47–49, 48*t*
- kidney disease, 50–51, 51*t*
- liver disease, 47
- National Surgical Quality Improvement Program risk prediction tool, 42
- neurologic, 49
- pulmonary, non–lung resection surgery, 46–47, 46*t*
- surgical site infections, antibiotic prophylaxis, 51

Prerenal azotemia, 730, 906, 907–908, 907*t*
Presatovir, 1409
Presbycusis, **212**
"Presbyopia," older adults, 67
Prescribing cascade, 66
Pressure injury (ulcer), **64–65,** 65*t*
Pressure-natriuresis relationship, 444
Presurgical anxiety, 1097
Presyncope, palpitations, 26, 27*t*
Preterm birth, 805–806, 813
Preterm labor, **804–806**
Pretibial myxedema, 1121
Prevention, disease, **1–13**. *See also specific disorders*
- adherence, 1–2
- alcohol use disorder, 12–13, 13*t*
- cancer, 11–12
- cardiovascular disease, 4–9
  - abdominal aortic aneurysm, 5*t*, 6, 42, **482–484,** 1465
  - chemoprevention, 5*t*, 9
  - cigarette smoking & smoking cessation, 4, 5*t*, 6–8, 6*t*, 7*t*
  - hypertension, 4, 5*t*, 8–9
  - lipid disorders, 4, 5*t*, 8
  - risk factors, 4–6
  - risk prevention recommendations, 4, 5*t*
- death, 2, 2*t*
- exercise, 10
- gay & bisexual men, **1724–1725,** 1724*t*
- general approach, 1–2
- guiding principles of care, 2
- health maintenance & disease prevention, 2–9
- infectious diseases, 3–4, 4*t*
- injuries & violence, 12
- osteoporosis, 9
- overweight & obesity, 10–11
- primary, 2
- secondary, 2
- substance use disorder, 12–13, 13*t*
- tertiary, 2
- underutilization, 3
- vaccination, 11–12

Prevention bundles, 1279
Prevotella, 1281, 1283, 1294*t*
Prevotella melaninogenica, 278, 1472
Priapism, 959, 1083
Prickly heat, 151
Primaquine, 1504*t*, 1505*t*, 1508*t*, 1509
Primaquine/clindamycin, 1541
Primaquine phosphate, 1505*t*, 1507
Primary angiitis of the central nervous system, **857**
Primary biliary cholangitis, **707–709**
Primary Care-PTSD Screen, 1048
Primary effusion lymphoma, 1321, 1368
Primary essential hypertension, **444**
Primary hypogonadism, 962
Primary lateral sclerosis, **1028**
Primary prevention, 2
Primary progressive multiple sclerosis, 1023
Primary sclerosing cholangitis, **726–728**
Primidone, 976*t*, 1006
Primrose oil, evening, 738
Principles of care, guiding, 2
Prinzmetal angina, 368
Prion diseases, **1385–1386**
Prions, 1385
Pritelivir, 121
PRKAR1A, 1163
PRNP, 1018
Probenecid, 826, 954, 1483*t*
Probiotics, 647, 661. *See also specific types*
Procainamide, 383, 384*t*
- for atrial fibrillation, 395
- autoimmune hypoglycemia from, 1237
- drug-induced nephritis from, 837
- for myotonia congenita, 1044
- for myotonic dystrophy, 1044

Procaine penicillin, 1483*t*
Procalcitonin, 1445
- cough, 16
- dyspnea, 19
- fever, 30
- pneumonia, 19

Procarbazine, 1000
Procedural justice, 77
Prochlorperazine, 583*t*, **584,** 971, 1655
Proctitis
- herpes simplex virus, 1353, 1354, 1355
- *Treponema pallidum,* 671

Prodromal symptoms, epilepsy, 980
Progesterone therapy, 108, 1190. *See also specific types*
Progestins. *See also specific types*
- in cisgender women, 1726–1727
- IUDs, 1190
- long-acting, **777**
- for menopausal symptoms, 1187, 1188, 1190
- minipill, 775*t*, **776,** 776*t*
- for pelvic pain, 768
- in transfeminine persons, 1726

Progestogen, in transfeminine persons, 1726–1727, 1727*t*
Programmed cell death protein inhibitors, 1387. *See also* Immune checkpoint inhibitors; *specific types*
Programmed death ligand 1, 1674*t*
Programmed death ligand-1 inhibitors. *See also specific types*
- inflammation myopathy from, 1045

Progressive bulbar palsy, **1028**
Progressive disseminated histoplasmosis, 536
Progressive familial intrahepatic cholestasis syndromes, conjugated hyperbilirubinemia, 674, 676*t*
Progressive massive fibrosis, 306
Progressive multifocal leukoencephalopathy, 1323, 1331, **1386–1387**
Progressive multiple sclerosis, 1023
Progressive primary tuberculosis, 280
Progressive spinal muscular atrophy, **1028**
Prolactin, 1099
- deficiency, hypogonadotropic hypogonadism, 1101
- dopamine on secretion of, 1099

Prolactinomas, **1108–1110,** 1108*t*
Proliferative bronchiolitis, 268
Proliferative retinopathy, 185, **191–192**
Promethazine, 583*t*, **584,** 797
Promise of nonabandonment, 73
Promyelocytic leukemia
- acute, **528–530**
- lymphoblastic, **528–530**

Pronator teres syndrome, **1035**
Pronouncement, death, 78
Pronouns, gender identity, 1710, 1711, 1712, 1725
Propafenone, 383, 384*t*, 396
Propanil poisoning, **1586–1587**
Propionibacterium acnes, immunocompromised, 1272
Propofol, 1045, 1567
Propranolol, 383, 384*t*, 972*t*
- for aggression disorders, 1085
- for dyskinesia from antipsychotics, 1068
- for essential tremor, 1006
- for hyperadrenergic postural orthostatic syndrome, 985
- for hypertension, 462*t*
- for hyperthyroidism, 1123, 1123*t*, 1125, 1127
- for migraine headache, 972*t*
- for panic disorder, 1051
- for performance anxiety, 1052
- poisoning, **1577–1578**
- for portal hypertension, esophageal varices with, 617
- for portal hypertensive gastropathy, 622
- for sinus tachycardia, with hyperthyroidism, 1126
- for test anxiety, 1052
- for thyrotoxic crisis/thyroid storm, 1127
- for thyrotoxic hypokalemic periodic paralysis, 1127
- for toxic nodular goiter, 1123*t*, 1125

Proprotein convertase subtilisin/kexin type 9, 8, 358, 1239
Proprotein convertase subtilisin/kexin type 9 inhibitors, 8, 358, 1245*t*, 1246–1247
Propylene glycol, anion gap elevation from, 1570
Propylthiouracil, 1115, 1123*t*, 1124, 1126
Prospagnosia, 999
Prostacyclin pathway, 302
Prostaglandin E1, 1223
Prostaglandin E_2, 960
Prostaglandin F2, pregnancy contraindications, 813
Prostate, Lung, Colorectal and Ovarian Randomized Trial, 289
Prostate artery embolization, 968
Prostate cancer, **1634–1641,** 1635*t*, 1636*f*, 1640*t*
- clinical findings, 1634–1637, 1635*t*
- incidence, prevalence, & mortality, 1634
- prognosis, 1641
- screening/detection, 11, 1635, 1635*t*, 1636*f*, **1637–1638**
- staging/Gleason score, 1595, 1638, 1641
- treatment, 1597*t*, 1638–1641
  - active surveillance, 1638
  - androgen deprivation therapy, 1640, 1640*t*
  - antiandrogens, 1640, 1640*t*

focal therapy, 1639
general measures, 1638
LHRH agonist/antagonist, 1640, 1640*t*
locally/regionally advanced disease, 1639
metastatic disease, 1639–1641
prostatectomy, radical, 1638–1639
radiation therapy, 1639
Prostatectomy, simple, 968
Prostate-specific antigen (PSA), 1635, 1635*t*
Prostatic urethral lift, 968
Prostatitis
bacterial
acute, **949–950,** 950*t*
chronic, **950–952,** 950*t*
nonbacterial chronic, 950*t*, **951–952**
Prosthetic heart valves. *See* Heart valves, prosthetic
Protease-activated receptor-1 inhibitor, 365
Protease inhibitors, **1340*t*,** 1344–1345. *See also specific types*
atazanavir, **1340*t*, 1345**
atazanavir/cobicistat, **1340*t*, 1345**
darunavir, **1340*t*, 1345**
for hepatitis C, 689
kidney stones from, 954
lopinavir/r, **1340*t*, 1345**
principles & overview, **1340*t*,** 1344–1345
ritonavir, **1340*t*, 1345**
ritonavir-booster, pregnancy, 815
Proteasome inhibitors, 538, 540. *See also specific types*
Protein
deficiency, 1250
nutritional support, 1266
Protein C deficiency, portal vein thrombosis, 715
Protein–energy malnutrition, **1250–1251**
Protein-losing enteropathy, **643,** 1370
Protein-restricted diets, 1264
Proteinuria, **903–904**
autosomal dominant polycystic kidney disease, 939
chronic kidney disease, 915, 921
diabetic nephropathy, 934–935
focal segmental glomerulosclerosis, 933
functional, 904
glomerular, 904
glomerular diseases, 922*f*, 923
glomerulonephritis, 912, 930
anti-GBM glomerulonephritis & Goodpasture syndrome, 929
IgA nephropathy, 927
IgA vasculitis, 927
infection-related/postinfectious, 926
nephritic spectrum, 924–926
nephrotic spectrum, 924*t*, 931–932
pauci-immune, 928
systemic lupus erythematosus, 930
HIV-associated nephropathy, 935
interstitial nephritis, 911
membranous nephropathy, 934
minimal change disease, 933
"orthostatic," 904
overload, 904
plasma cell myeloma, 941
renal amyloidosis, 936
sickle cell disease, 941
tubular, 904
tubulointerstitial diseases, chronic, 937–938
Proteus
otitis externa, 206
otitis media
acute, AIDS, 218
chronic, 210
pyelonephritis, 948
struvite calculi, 957
Proteus mirabilis, 1294*t*
Proteus vulgaris, 717, 1294*t*
Prothrombin
antibodies, acquired, **561**
deficiency, **561**
gene mutations, 432
Prothrombin complex concentrate, 353, 395
Proton pump inhibitors. *See also specific types*
for alcoholic gastritis, 622
bacterial overgrowth from, 636
for Barrett esophagus, 610
for dyspepsia, 580–581
for eosinophilc esophagitis, 614
for GERD, 610–611
for GI bleeding, upper, 598
for *Helicobacter pylori,* 627
for hemochromatosis, 711
hypomagnesemia, 893
interstitial nephritis from, 911
for NSAIDs, 622, 628, 822
for peptic ulcer disease, 624*t*, 627–628, 630
for stress gastritis, 621
Protozoal infections, **1496–1520**. *See also specific types*
African trypanosomiasis, **1496–1497,** 1497*t*
amebiasis, **1513–1515,** 1515*t*
American trypanosomiasis, **1498–1499**
babesiosis, **1510**
coccidiosis & microsporidiosis, **1516–1518**
giardiasis, **1518–1519**
with impaired cellular immunity, 1273
leishmaniasis, **1499–1501,** 1500*f*
malaria, **1502–1509,** 1503*f*, 1504*t*, 1505*t*, 1508*t*
toxoplasmosis, **1511–1513**
trichomoniasis, **1519–1520**
Protriptyline, 1073*t*
Providencia, 957, 1294*t*
Proximal internal carotid artery emboli, strokes from, 478
Proximal interphalangeal joint osteoarthritis, 820, 821
Prozone phenomenon, 1482
Prucalopride, 586–587
Prurigo nodularis, 136
Pruritus, 102*t*, **159–161**
anogenital, **160–161,** 160*f*
ear canal, **207**
erythrasma, 160, 160*f*
from opioids, 92
perianal, **673**
Pruritus ani, tinea cruris, 116
PSC risk estimate tool (PREsTo), 727
Pseudallescheria boydii, 1546
Pseudoaddiction, opioid, 85
Pseudoallergy, complement activation, 870
Pseudoaneurysm, 381, 485, 486
Pseudobulbar palsy, **1028**
Pseudocyst, pancreatic, 730, 731
Pseudodementia, 1014, 1096
Pseudoephedrine, sympathomimetic syndrome from, 1570
Pseudofolliculitis, 124–125
Pseudogout, **826–827**
Pseudohermaphroditism, 1184
Pseudohyperkalemia, 885, 885*t*
Pseudohyperparathyroidism of pregnancy, 1144
Pseudohypoaldosteronism type II, hypertension, 445
Pseudohyponatremia, 876, 880
Pseudohypoparathyroidism, **1138–1141,** 1140*t*
Pseudomembrane colitis, 648
Pseudomonas
animal bites, 1283
arthritis, nongonococcal acute, 862
conjunctivitis, 170
endocarditis, infective, 1287
folliculitis, hot tub, 124–125
with granulocytopenia, 1273
meningitis, health care–associated, 1281
osteomyelitis/septic arthritis, 1287
otitis externa, 206
otitis media, acute, 218
pneumonia, community-acquired, 273
prostatitis, 949
pyelonephritis, 948
risk factors, 276, 276*t*
struvite calculi, 957
Pseudomonas aeruginosa
bronchiectasis, 265
cystic fibrosis, 266
keratitis, 179
medication of choice, 1294*t*
nosocomial pneumonia, 275
otitis externa, 206
otitis media, chronic, 210
pneumonia, 269*t*, 270
Pseudorheumatoid arthritis, **826–827**
Pseudothrombocytopenia, **556**
Pseudothrombophlebitis, 28
Pseudotumor cerebri, 974, **1003–1005**
Pseudoxanthoma elasticum, 423, 505
Psilocybin, **1093**
Psittacosis, **1478**
PSMA (prostate-specific membrane antigen) PET, 1636
Psoas sign, 640, 641
Psoriasiform eruptions, drug, 159*t*
Psoriasis, 116, **136–138,** 136*f*, 823, 1328
Psoriatic arthritis, 323, **859–860**
PSRR1, 733
PSS1, pancreas carcinoma, 1615
P & S solution, 137
PSTI, 733
Psychedelics, **1093**
Psychiatric disorders, **1046–1098**. *See also specific types*
adjustment, **1046–1047**
aggression, **1084–1085**
anxiety, **1049–1052,** 1050*t*
attention-deficit/hyperactivity, **1081**
autism, **1082–1084**
chronic pain, **1055–1057,** 1056*f*
depression, **1069–1081,** 1073*t*, 1074*f*, 1076*t*
Diagnostic and Statistical Manual, 1046
feeding & eating (*See* Nutritional disorders)
hospitalization & illness, **1096–1098**
lesbian & bisexual women, **1721–1722**
mania, **1069–1081,** 1073*t*, 1074*f*, 1076*t*
neurocognitive, **1095–1096,** 1096*t*
obsessive-compulsive & related, **1052–1053**
personality, **1059–1061,** 1060*t*
psychosexual, **1057–1059**
gender dysphoria, **1058–1059**
paraphilias, **1057–1058**
sexual dysfunction, **1058, 1059**
schizophrenia spectrum, **1061–1069,** 1064*t*, 1065*t*, 1066*t*
sleep-wake disorders, **1082–1084**
somatic symptom, **1053–1055**
factitious disorders, 1054
functional neurologic disorder/conversion disorder, 1054
somatic symptom disorder, 1054
substance use, **1086–1095**
alcohol use, **1086–1092,** 1090*t*
amyl nitrite, **1095**
anabolic steroids, **1095,** 1179
antihistamines, **1094**
caffeine, **1094**
designer drugs, **1095**
laxative abuse, **1094–1095**

Psychiatric disorders, substance use (*Cont.*):
marijuana, **1093**
opioid, **1092–1093**
phencyclidine, **1093**
psychedelics, **1093**
sedatives (anxiolytics), 1049, 1050–1051, 1050*t*
solvent/gas sniffing/inhaling, **1095**
stimulants: amphetamines & cocaine, **1093–1094**
trauma & stressor-related, **1047–1048**
Psychodynamic psychotherapy, 1060
Psychogenic nonepileptic seizures, 981–982, 1054
Psychogenic polydipsia, 876–877
Psychological dependence, 1086
Psychosexual disorders, **1057–1059**. *See also specific types*
gender dysphoria, **1058–1059**
paraphilias, **1057–1058**
sexual dysfunction, **1058, 1059**
Psychosis, 1061
drug-induced, 1063
"intensive care unit," 1097
myxedema madness, 1115, 1116
Psychotherapy, 95, 1048. *See also specific types*
Psychotic disorders, 1061, 1062. *See also specific types*
Psychotic major depression, 072, 1070
Psychotic resolution, 1062
Psyllium, 586, 587*t*, 645, 1244, 1264
Pteroylmonoglutamic acid, 508
Pterygium, **172**
PTF1A, 1197
PTH-related proteins, 889
PTSD Checklist, 1048
Pubic louse, 130
Puerperal mastitis, **807–808**
Puffer fish poisoning, **1590–1591**, 1590*t*
Pulmonary. *See also* Lung
Pulmonary alveolar proteinosis, **297**, 308–309, 308*t*
Pulmonary arterial hypertension, 301, 431–433
Pulmonary artery pressure, systolic, 301
Pulmonary aspiration syndromes, **305–306**
aspirated foreign body retention, **306**
café coronary, **306**
gastric contents, **305–306**
Pulmonary capillary wedge pressure
acute heart failure & pulmonary edema, 413
acute MI with ST-segment elevation, 380, 381
cardiomyopathy, restrictive, 423
heart failure, 404
mitral stenosis, 337*f*
pulmonary hypertension, 431, 433
Pulmonary circulation, 301
Pulmonary circulation disorders, **297–304**. *See also specific types*
alveolar hemorrhage syndromes, **303–304**
pulmonary hypertension, **301–303**
pulmonary vasculitis, **303**
pulmonary venous thromboembolism, **297–300**, 298*t*
Pulmonary disorders, **244–322**. *See also specific types*
acute respiratory distress syndrome, **319–321**, 320*t*
acute respiratory failure, **317–319**, 318*t*
airways, **244–268**
circulation, **297–304**
alveolar hemorrhage syndromes, **303–304**
pulmonary hypertension, **301–303**
pulmonary vasculitis, **303**
pulmonary venous thromboembolism, **297–300**, 298*t*
environmental, **304–306**
e-cigarette or vaping product–associated lung injury, **304–305**
pulmonary aspiration syndromes, **305**
aspirated foreign body retention, **306**
café coronary, **306**
gastric contents, **305**
gastric contents, chronic, **305–306**
smoke inhalation, **304**
environmental & occupational, **304–309**
eosinophilic pulmonary syndromes, **297**
HIV/AIDS, **1317–1321**
CMV pneumonia, 1321
mycobacteria, atypical, 1320
noninfectious, 1321
pneumonia
bacterial, 1319*t*, 1320
mycobacterial, 1319*t*, 1320, 1320*f*
Pneumocystis, 1274, 1311, 1316, 1317–1320, 1317*f*, 1319*t*
sinusitis, 1321
viral (SARS-CoV-2, etc.), 1321
infections, **268–289**
interstitial lung disease, **292–297**
differential diagnosis, 292, 293*t*
diffuse interstitial pneumonias, **292–294**, 293*t*, 294*t*
eosinophilic pulmonary syndromes, 297
idiopathic interstitial pneumonias, 293, 294*t*
pulmonary alveolar proteinosis, 297
sarcoidosis, 295–296, 296*f*
lesbian & bisexual women, **1718**
lung transplantation, **321–322**
neoplasms, **289–292**
bronchial carcinoid tumors, **291**
mediastinal masses, **291–292**
right middle lobe syndrome, **291**
screening, **289**
solitary pulmonary nodule, **290–291**
occupational, **306–307**
hypersensitivity pneumonitis, **307–308**, 307*t*
other, 308
pneumoconiosis, **306–307**, 306*t*
asbestosis, 306*t*, **307**, 308
coal worker's pneumoconiosis, **306**, 306*t*, 308
silicosis, **306–307**, 306*t*, 308
talcosis, 306*t*, 308
pleural, **309–315**
pleural effusion, **310–313**
pleuritis, **309–310**
pneumothorax, **313–315**
pneumonia, **268–278**
pulmonary alveolar proteinosis, **297**
pulmonary hypertension, 301
ventilation control, **315–317**
hyperventilation syndrome, **315**
obesity-hypoventilation syndrome, **315**
obstructive sleep apnea, **316–317**
sleep-related breathing disorders, **316**
Pulmonary edema
acute heart failure and, **413–414**
cardiogenic, **413–414**
drowning, 1554
high-altitude, **1560–1562**
noncardiac, 413
Pulmonary ejection click, 323, 324
Pulmonary embolism, **297–300**
chest pain, 22
dyspnea, 18
Fusobacterium necrophorum, 1472
massive, 568
submassive, 568
treatment, thrombolytic therapy, 575, 576*t*, 577*t*
Pulmonary Embolism Rule-Out Criteria, 299
Pulmonary Embolism Severity Score Index, 299, 568–569, 571*t*
Pulmonary eosinophilia, tropical, 1531
Pulmonary evaluation, non–lung resection surgery, 46–47, 46*t*
Pulmonary fibrosis, 293, 1603
Pulmonary function testing, 46, 246
Pulmonary hemosiderosis, idiopathic, 304
Pulmonary histoplasmosis, 536
Pulmonary hypertension, **301–303, 431–433**. *See also* Hypertension, pulmonary
Pulmonary infections, **268–289**. *See also specific types*
immunocompromised, pulmonary infiltrates, **278–279**
nontuberculous mycobacteria, **287–289**
pneumonia, **268–278**
characteristics, 269*t*
community-acquired, **268–274**, 272*t*
tuberculosis, **279–287** (*See also* Tuberculosis, pulmonary)
Pulmonary infiltrates, in immunocompromised, **278–279**
Pulmonary Kaposi sarcoma, **113**
Pulmonary Langerhans cell histiocytosis, 297
Pulmonary metastases, **1608**
Pulmonary neoplasms, **289–292**
bronchial carcinoid tumors, **291**
mediastinal masses, **291–292**
right middle lobe syndrome, **291**
screening, **289**
solitary pulmonary nodule, **290–291**
Pulmonary nodule, solitary, **290–291**
Pulmonary outflow tract obstruction, pulmonary valve stenosis, 324
Pulmonary radiation fibrosis, 309
Pulmonary rehabilitation, for COPD, 263
Pulmonary-renal syndrome, 853, 854
Pulmonary septic embolic, injection drug abuse, 1287
Pulmonary valve
endocarditis, 324
regurgitation, 331, **352–353**
categories, 332
pulmonary hypertension
pulmonary valve stenosis, 324
ventral septal defect, 330
tetralogy of Fallot, **330–331**
replacement
percutaneous, endocarditis after, 324
pulmonary valve regurgitation after, 352
stenosis, **323–324**
Pulmonary vascular resistance, atrial septal defect, 326
Pulmonary vasculitis, **303**
Pulmonary vasodilators, 302. *See also specific types*
Pulmonary venous hypertension, 301, 405, 415
Pulmonary venous thromboembolism, **298–300**, 298*t*
Pulsatile flow devices, for heart failure with reduced LVEF, 411–412
Pulsatile tinnitus, 212, 213–214
Pulsed dye laser, for molluscum contagiosum, 121
Pulse oximetry, 15, 16, 20, 23
Pulsus paradoxus, 23, 429, 430
Pupils, stupor & coma, 1019
Pure androgen-secreting adrenal tumors, 1181
Pure estrogen receptor antagonist, fulvestrant, 1602*t*
Purified protein derivative, 282
Purified protein derivative skin test, 643, 1320, 1335–1336, 1335*t*
Purine analogs, 1598*t*
Purpura fulminans, HHV-6, 1368
Purulent meningitis, 1280, 1280*t*, 1281*t*

Pustular, 102*t*
Pustular disorders, **147–151**. *See also specific types*
- acne vulgaris, **147–149**, 148*f*
- miliaria, **151**
- rosacea, **149–150**, 150*f*

Puumala virus, 1395
PUVA, 114, 141, 160
Pyelonephritis
- acute, **946–949**
- antimicrobial therapy
  - empiric, 1298*t*
  - nosocomial, initial, 1296*t*
- pregnancy, 813

Pylephlebitis, 715
Pyogenic hepatic abscess, **716–717**
Pyrantel pamoate, 1526, 1527, 1529
Pyrazinamide, 284–285, 284*t*, 285*t*
- hepatotoxicity, 696
- for spinal tuberculosis, 865
- for tuberculous meningitis, 1476

Pyrethroid, 1499
Pyridostigmine, 985, 1041
Pyridoxine, 712, 1583
Pyridoxine-responsive anemia, 1261
Pyrimethamine, 1001, 1337*t*, 1513, 1517–1518
Pyrimidine analogs, 1599*t*. *See also specific types*
- azacitidine, 1599*t*
- capecitabine, 1599*t*
- cytarabine, 1599*t*
- decitabine, 1599*t*
- fluorouracil, 1599*t*
- gemcitabine, 1599*t*

Pyrogenic cytokines, 29
Pyroglutamic acid ingestion, 896*t*
Pyronaridine, 1504*t*, 1506
Pyrosis, 606

Q

Q fever *(Coxiella burnetii)*, 1427*t*, **1434–1436**
Qinghaosu, 1504*t*, 1507–1508
5q loss, isolated, 526
QRS complex
- acute MI, with ST-segment elevation, 374, 379
- antiarrhythmics on, class III, 383
- aortic regurgitation, 335*t*
- atrial fibrillation, 391
- AV block, 387
- heart failure, 411, 412, 419, 420
- mitral regurgitation, 339
- paroxysmal supraventricular tachycardia, 388
  - accessory AV pathways, 390
- pericardial effusion/tamponade, 429
- pulmonary valve regurgitation, 352
- tetralogy of Fallot, 330, 331, 351
- ventricular premature beats, 398
- ventricular tachycardia, 398–399

QRS complex widening
- from antidepressants, 1593, 1593*f*
- from poisoning, 1566, 1566*t*
- tetralogy of Fallot, 331, 352

QTc prolongation, from antipsychotics, 1066, 1066*t*
QT prolongation, 1072, 1566, 1566*t*
Quadrantanopia, lower, 999
Quadruple therapy, 624*t*, 627
Quazepam, 1050*t*
Quebec beer-drinkers cardiomyopathy, 419
Queer, 1709
Quetiapine
- for bipolar disorder, 1079
- for Huntington disease, 1010
- for Parkinson disease, 1009
- poisoning, 1576
- potency and side effects, 1065*t*
- for schizophreniform spectrum disorders, 1063, 1064*t*, 1065*t*

Quick Inventory of Depressive Symptomatology, 1071
Quinagolide, 1109
Quinapril, 452*t*
Quincke sign, 333*t*, 347
Quinidine (gluconate), 383, 384*t*
- hepatotoxicity, 696
- for malaria, 1504*t*, 1505*t*, 1506–1507
- pill-induced esophagitis from, 613

Quinidine dihydrochloride, 1505*t*
Quinine, 1237, 1504*t*, 1510
Quinine dihydrochloride, 1505*t*, 1506–1507
Quinine sulfate, 1505*t*
Quinsy, 232
Quinupristin/dalfopristin, 1443

R

R_0, 1401
R 364D, 1432
Rabeprazole
- for GERD, 610
- for NSAIDs, 622, 628
- for peptic ulcer disease, 627

Rabies, **1376–1379**
- animal bites, 1283–1284
- encephalitic, 1377
- paralytic, 1377
- prevention, **1378–1379**

Rabies immune globulin, 1378
Raccoon sign, 1021
Racemose cysticercosis, 1524
RAD51D, breast cancer, 741
Radial nerve lesions, **1035**
Radiation. *See also* Radiotherapy
- exposure, **1558–1559**
  - cataracts, 185
  - leukemia from, 528
- ionizing, 1558, 1603
- nonionizing, 1558
- thrombocytopenia from, 547*t*, **548**

Radiation fibrosis, pulmonary, 309
Radiation lung injury, 309
Radiation pericarditis, 427
Radiation pneumonitis, 309
Radiation proctopathy, 599
"Radiation recall," 309
Radiocontrast media, 869, **870**, 909
Radiofrequency ablation/lesioning, neuromodulatory therapy, 96, 97*t*
Radionuclide imaging, 361, 1636
Radiotherapy. *See also specific disorders*
- for basal cell carcinoma, 112–113
- for breast carcinoma, 751, 756
- for cancer pain, 80

Radium (Ra)-223
- for cancer, 1653*t*
- for prostate cancer, 1641

Radon, lung cancer and, 1603
Rai classification, 531
Raloxifene
- for acromegaly, 1107
- for gynecomastia, 1181
- for hyperparathyroidism, 1145
- for menopausal symptoms, 1190
- for osteoporosis, 1151

Raltegravir, 1333, 1334, **1341*t*, 1345**, 1347*t*, 1349, 1351
Ramelteon, 1050*t*, 1083
Ramipril, 358, 407–408, 452*t*
Ramsay Hunt syndrome, 218, 1359, 1360
Ramucirumab, 1612
Range of motion testing
- knee, 1697*t*
- shoulder
  - external rotation, 1676*t*
  - flexion, 1676*t*
  - internal rotation, 1677*t*

RANK, plasma cell myeloma, 537
RANKL, plasma cell myeloma, 537
RANKL inhibitors, 95. *See also specific types*
Ranolazine, 363, 364*f*
Ranson criteria, 729, 729*t*, 732
Rape, **782–783**
Rape trauma syndrome, 782–783
Rapid cycling, bipolar disorder, 1070
Rapidly progressive dementia, 1017–1018
Rapid plasma reagin test, 1482
Rasagiline, 1008–1009
Rasburicase, 1652, 1653*t*, 1669*t*
Rashes, 156
Rat-bite fever, **1490**
Rate-dependent bypass tract, palpitations, 26
Ratelgravir, 1389
Rate & rhythm disorders, heart, **383–403**. *See also* Heart rate & rhythm disorders; *specific types*
Rat lungworm, 1529
Rattlesnake envenomation, **1590**
Ravulizumab, 510
Raynaud phenomenon, **838–839**, 839*f*, 840*t*
- from bleomycin, 123
- systemic lupus erythematosus, 832

RBC transfusions, **542–544**
Reactive arthritis, **860–861**, 861*f*
- HIV/AIDS, 1323
- HLA-B27, 860
- uveitis, 183

Reactive cervical lymphadenopathy, neck masses, 242
Reactive erythemas, **151–154**
- erythema multiforme/Stevens-Johnson syndrome/toxic epidermal necrolysis, **153–154**, 153*f*, 154*f*
- urticaria & angioedema, **151–153**, 152*f*

Reactive hypoglycemia. *See* Postprandial hypoglycemia
Real-time quaking induced conversion, 1018
Rebiana, 1203
Reciprocal IVF, 1714
Recklinghausen disease, 1005
Recombinant activated factor VIIa, 705
Recombinant human deoxyribonuclease, 267
Recombinant human TSH-stimulated ^{131}I therapy, 1135
Recombinant tissue plasminogen activator. *See* Tissue plasminogen activator
Recombinant vesicular stomatitis virus (rVSV)-based vaccine expressing Z ebolavirus (ZEBOV) glycoprotein, 1391
Rectal carcinoids, 1626
Rectocele, 769
Rectovaginal fistula, Crohn disease, 654
Rectum diseases, **643–669**. *See also* Colon & rectum diseases; *specific diseases*
Recurrent familial intrahepatic cholestasis syndromes, conjugated hyperbilirubinemia, 674, 676*t*
Recurrent laryngeal nerve, unilateral, vocal fold paralysis, 240
Recurrent painful ophthalmoplegic neuropathy, 971
Recurrent paroxysmal atrial fibrillation, 396
Recurrent pregnancy loss, **799**
Recurrent respiratory papillomatosis, **237**
Red blood cell
- casts, 903, 904*t*, 907*t*, 912, 922*f*, 926
- transfusions, **542–544**, 597

Red bugs, **132**
Reed-Sternberg cells, 535
Refeeding edema, 1251
Refeeding syndrome, 890, 891, 891*t*, 900*t*, 1250–1251
Reflex sympathetic dystrophy, **867**

Reflex syncope, 402–403
Reflux esophagitis, 608
Refractive errors, **168**
age-related, 67
contact lenses, 168
nearsightedness, reduced rate of progression, 168
surgery, 168
Refsum disease, **1031**
Regorafenib, 1601*t*
diarrhea from, 1656
for gastrointestinal mesenchymal tumors, 1625
for hepatocellular carcinoma, 1612
for intestinal neuroendocrine tumors, 1627
Reinke edema, **237**
Relapsing fever, 1295*t*, **1489–1490**
Relapsing polychondritis, 205, **856**
Relapsing-remitting multiple sclerosis, 1023
Relapsing symmetric seronegative synovitis with edema, 1420
Relaxation techniques, 1047, 1052. *See also specific types*
Reliever medications, for asthma, 249, 252*t*–253*t*. *See also specific types*
Relugolix, 766
Remdesivir, 696, 1356*t*, 1405
Remia, 906
Remitting seronegative synovitis with non-pitting edema, 867
REM sleep, 1082–1083
Renal. *See also* Kidney
Renal amyloidosis, 924*t*, **935–936**
Renal angiography, for renal artery stenosis, 921
Renal artery
fibromuscular dysplasia, 466
stenosis, **921–922**
Renal calciuria, 956
Renal calculi, 958
Renal calculus, 958
Renal cell carcinoma, 939, **1645–1647**
Renal clearance, 904–905
Renal cystic disease, 824, 914, **938–941,** 938*t*
autosomal dominant polycystic kidney disease, 938*t*, **939–940,** 939*f*
cysts
defined, 938
simple/solitary, **938–939,** 938*t*
medullary sponge kidney, 938*t*, **940–941**
Renal dialysis
amyloidosis from, 541
for end-stage kidney disease, 920
hypercalcemia, 890
hypocalcemia and hyperphosphatemia from, 890
surgical risk, 51
Renal glycosuria, 1200
Renal medulla, papillae infarction, sickle cell anemia, 512
Renal osteodystrophy, chronic kidney disease, 917, 917*f*
Renal parenchymal disease, hypertension, 445
Renal pelvis cancers, 939, **1644, 1645–1647**
Renal sympathetic denervation, for hypertension, 464
Renal tubular acidosis, 884
hyperkalemia, 917
hypokalemia, 884
type I (distal)
hyperchloremic, normal ion gap acidosis, 897–898, 897*t*
medullary sponge kidney, 940
type II (proximal), hyperchloremic, normal ion gap acidosis, 897–898, 897*t*
type IV, hyporeninemic hypoaldosteronemic, 896*t*, 897*t*, 898
Renal tubular cell casts, 904*t*, 907, 907*t*, 909
Renal tubulopathies, 884
Renal vascular hypertension, 445
Renal wasting, 884
Renin–angiotensin–aldosterone system inhibitors. *See also specific types*
for heart failure
with preserved LVEF, 412
with reduced LVEF, 407–409
for hypertension, essential, 444
Renin-angiotensin system, 325, 405
Renin inhibitors, **454**. *See also specific types*
Repaglinide, 1204*t*, 1206, 1218, 1218*f*, 1220, 1237
Reperfusion therapy, for acute MI with ST-segment elevation, 375–377, 376*t*. *See also specific types*
fibrinolytics, 375–377, 376*t*
percutaneous coronary intervention, 375
Repetitive transcranial magnetic stimulation, for depression, 1078
Rescue angioplasty, for acute MI with ST-segment elevation, 378
Reserpine, 460, 463*t*, 1007
Reset osmostat, hypotonic hyponatremia, **878**
Resilience building, lesbian & bisexual women, 1721–1722
Resistant hypertension, **468,** 469*t*
Reslizumab, 251*t*, 254
Resolution, 1057
Resorptive hypercalciuria, 956
Respiratory acidosis, 895*t*, **901**
Respiratory alkalosis, 895*t*, **901–902,** 901*t*
Respiratory bronchiolitis, 268
Respiratory bronchiolitis–associated interstitial lung disease, 268, 294*t*
Respiratory cytomegalovirus disease, 1366
Respiratory failure, 317, **317–319**. *See also specific disorders*
Respiratory syncytial virus (RSV), **1408–1410**
human metapneumovirus, 1409
human parainfluenza viruses, 1409
Nipah virus, 1409
pneumonia, community-acquired, 270
Respiratory tract infections. *See also specific types*
cough, 15
viral, **1401–1418** (*See also specific types*)
avian influenza, **1414–1415**
MERS-CoV, **1416–1418**
RSV & other paramyxoviruses, **1408–1410**
SARS-CoV-1, **1415–1416**
SARS-CoV-2, **1401–1408**
seasonal influenza, **1410–1413**
Restenosis
after balloon valvuloplasty, 345
after percutaneous coronary intervention/stenting, 366, 375
Restless legs syndrome, **1013, 1084**
Restlessness, terminal, 71
Restrictive cardiomyopathy, 404, 418*t*, 423, **423–424**
Resuscitation fluids, 902
Resynchronization, cardiac
for dilated cardiomyopathy, 420
for heart failure
with preserved LVEF, 412
with reduced LVEF, 406*f*, 411
for mitral regurgitation, 339
RET, lung cancer, 1606
Retapamulin, 105*t*, 124, 126
Retching, upper GI bleeding, 596
Reteplase, 375–376, 376*t*
Reticulocytopenia, 500, 501*t*, 517
Reticulocytosis, 500, 501*t*
Retina
degeneration, pigmentary, 1031
detachment, **185–186,** 186*f*
hemorrhage, thrombocytopenia, 193
hypertension, 447, 447*f*
necrosis
herpes simplex virus, 1353
herpes zoster, 1360
vasculitis, uveitis, 183–184
Retinal artery occlusion, central & branch, 188*f*, **189–190**
Retinal disorders, systemic diseases, **191–193**
blood dyscrasias, **193**
diabetic retinopathy, 67, 191, **191–192,** 1221
HIV/AIDS, **193**
hypertensive retinochoroidopathy, **192–193**
Retinal vein occlusion
central & branch, **188–189,** 188*f*
retinal detachment, 185
RET inhibitors, 1606. *See also specific types*
Retinitis
Bartonella, 1471
cytomegalovirus, **193,** 1311, 1318*t*, 1324, 1324*f*, 1366
herpes simplex virus, 193
herpes zoster virus, 193
Rift Valley fever disease, 1392
Retinochoroiditis, toxoplasmosis, 1511
Retinochoroidopathy, hypertensive, **192–193**
Retinoids. *See also specific types*
for acne vulgaris, 148, 149
for lichen planus, 141
for psoriasis, 137, 1328
for rosacea, 150
Retinopathy, 1004*t*
"background," 191
from chlorpromazine, 1067
diabetes mellitus, 67, 185, 191, **191–192**
HIV, **193**
hypertensive, 447, 447*f*
nonproliferative, **191–192**
proliferative, **191–192**
sickle cell, 193
toxic, 199
Retrobulbar inflammation, 1128
Retrograde ejaculation, 959
Retrosternal burning, 579
Returning traveler
fever of unknown origin, 1270
infections, **1291–1292**
Revascularization, coronary
for acute MI, with ST-segment elevation, 382
for angina pectoris, 365–377
coronary artery bypass grafting, 366–367
extracorporeal counterpulsation, 367
indications, 365–366
neuromodulation, 367
percutaneous coronary intervention/stenting, 365, 366
for heart failure with reduced LVEF, 411
preoperative evaluation & perioperative management, 43–44
Reversal agents, anticoagulation, 563, **565*t***
Reverse transcriptase inhibitors, dual. *See specific types*
Review of systems, existential, 74, 75*t*
Revised Atlanta classification, 729
Revised Cardiac Risk Index, 42, 43*t*
Rewarming, for hypothermia, **1551–1553**
Reye syndrome, 1360, 1411
Reynolds pentad, 723
RFX6, 1197
Rhabdomyolysis
acute kidney injury, 883, **910–911**
hyperkalemia, 885, 885*t*, 886
hyperphosphatemia, 892, 892*t*
hypocalcemia, 888*t*
hypophosphatemia, 891
Rhegmatogenous retinal detachment, 185–186

Rheumatic fever/heart disease, **424–426,** 425*t*, 842, **1440**. *See also specific types*
acute, 424
aortic regurgitation, 333*t*–335*t*, **347–349**
carditis, 425
chronic, 424
erythema marginatum, 425
Jones criteria, 425, 425*t*
mitral stenosis, **332–338,** 333*t*–335*t*
nodules, subcutaneous, 425
polyarthritis, 425
recurrence, prevention, 426
recurrent, prevention, 1440
subclinical carditis, 424
Sydenham chorea, 425
tricuspid stenosis, 350
Rheumatism, palindromic, **868**
Rheumatoid arthritis, **827–831,** 827*f*, 828*f*
autoimmune hypoglycemia from, 1237
HLA-DRB1 alleles, 827
inheritance, 827
juvenile, 1270
myasthenia gravis, 1040
patient age, 1270
pericarditis, 427
relapsing polychondritis, 856
treatment, 829–831
corticosteroids, 829
disease-modifying antirheumatic drugs, **829–831**
Rheumatoid nodules, 828, 828*f*
Rheumatologic, immunologic, & allergic disorders, **819–874**. *See also specific types*
allergic & immunologic disorders, **868–874**
arthritis, crystal deposition, **823–827**
arthritis, degenerative joint disease, **819–823**
arthritis, infectious, **861–864,** 1323
autoimmune diseases, **827–847**
autoimmune hemolytic anemia, 514
cancer, rheumatologic manifestations, **867**
complex regional pain syndrome, **867**
fibromyalgia, **865–866**
neurogenic arthropathy, **867–868**
osteonecrosis, **868**
palindromic rheumatism, **868**
rheumatologic disorders, **819–820,** 820*t*, 821*t*
seronegative spondyloarthropathies, **858–861**
thoracic outlet syndromes, **866–867**
tuberculosis, bones & joints, **864–865**
vasculitis syndromes, **847–858**
Rheumatologic disorders, **819–820,** 821*t*. *See also specific types*
HIV/AIDS, 1323–1324
arthritis, 1323
osteoporosis & osteopenia, 1323–1324
rheumatologic syndromes, 1323
joint fluid
examination, 819, 820*t*
groups, 819, 821*t*
joint pattern, 819, 820*t*
osteoarthritis, 820
Rhinitis
allergic, **222–223**
perennial, 222
senile, 222
vasomotor, 222
Rhinitis medicamentosa, 219
Rhinorrhea
allergic rhinitis, 222–223
pharyngitis & tonsillitis, 231
rhinosinusitis
CSF fluid, 220
viral, 218–219
sarcoidosis, 227
vasomotor rhinitis, 222
Rhinosinusitis, **218–221**
acute, **219–221**
classification, 226
viral, **218–219**
Rhizopus, 221–222, 1544
Rhodococcus equi, HIV/AIDS, 1320
Ribaroxaban, 394, 394*t*
Ribavirin, 1356*t*
for adenovirus, 1419
for Crimean-Congo hemorrhagic fever, 1392
for echovirus, 1425
for hemorrhagic fever with renal syndrome, 1396
for hepatitis E, 677
for MERS-CoV, 1417, 1418
for respiratory syncytial virus, 1405
for SARS-CoV-1, 1415
Rib notching, 325
Ribociclib, 757–758
Riboflavin (vitamin B_2)
deficiency, **1260**
for migraine headache, 1323
toxicity, **1260**
Richter syndrome, 530
Rickets, **1152–1154**
Rickettsia aeschlimannii, 1432
Rickettsia africae, 1432
Rickettsia akari, 1427*t*, 1433
Rickettsia australis, 1432
Rickettsia candidatus, 1432
Rickettsia conorii, 1432
Rickettsia elis, 1427*t*, 1428
Rickettsia felis, 1433
Rickettsia helvetica, 1432
Rickettsia japonica, 1432
Rickettsial diseases, **1426–1436,** 1427*t*. *See also specific types*
other Rickettsial & rickettsial-like, 1427*t*, **1433–1436**
ehrlichiosis & anaplasmosis, 1427*t*, **1433–1434**
Q fever, 1427*t*, **1434–1436**
spotted fevers, 1427*t*, **1430–1433**
rickettsialpox, 1427*t*, **1433**
Rocky Mountain spotted fever, 1427*t*, **1430–1432,** 1431*f*
tick typhus, 1427*t*, **1432–1433**
typhus group, **1426–1430,** 1427*t*
epidemic typhus, **1426–1429,** 1427*t*
scrub typhus, 1427*t*, **1429–1430**
Rickettsial fever, 1427*t*, **1432–1433**
Rickettsialpox, 1427*t*, **1433**
Rickettsia massiliae, 1432
Rickettsia monacensis, 1432
Rickettsia parkeri, 1432
Rickettsia prowazekii, 1426, 1427*t*
Rickettsia raoultii, 1432
Rickettsia rickettsi, 1427*t*, 1430–1431
Rickettsia rioja, 1432
Rickettsia sibirica, 1432
Rickettsia slovaca, 1432
Rickettsia typhi, 1427*t*, 1428
Riedel thyroiditis, 846, **1112–1114**
Rifabutin
for *Mycobacterium avium* complex, 1475, 1476
for peptic ulcer disease, 624*t*, 627
for *Streptococcus pneumoniae* endocarditis, 1457
for tuberculosis, HIV/AIDS, 1320
Rifampin, 284–285, 284*t*, 285*t*, 286
for anaplasmosis, 1434
for *Bartonella*, 1471
for biliary cholangitis, primary, 708
for chlamydial reactive arthritis, 861
for ehrlichiosis, 1434
for folliculitis, 125
for furunculosis & carbuncles, 126
interstitial nephritis from, 911
for *Mycobacterium avium* complex, 1475
for *Mycobacterium kansasii*, 1475
for spinal tuberculosis, 865
for *Staphylococcus*, coagulase-negative endocarditis, 1457
for *Staphylococcus aureus*
impetigo, 124
osteomyelitis, 1448
for tuberculosis
HIV/AIDS, 1336
pregnancy, 815
for tuberculous meningitis, 1476
for typhus, scrub, 1430
Rifapentin, 284*t*, 286, 1336
Rifaximin
for diarrhea, diabetic, 1223
for irritable bowel syndrome, 647
for rosacea, 150
for traveler's diarrhea, 1293
Rift Valley fever, **1391–1393,** 1434
Right bundle branch block
atrial septal defect, 327
AV block, 387
paroxysmal supraventricular tachycardia, 388
with accessory AV pathway, 390
pulmonary valve regurgitation, 352
tetralogy of Fallot, 331
ventricular tachycardia, 399, 400
Right heart failure, **403–404**. *See also* Heart failure
cardiomyopathy
dilated, 419
restrictive, 418*t*, 423, 424
mitral stenosis, 336
pericarditis, constrictive, 430, 431
pulmonary hypertension, 432
pulmonic stenosis, 324
tetralogy of Fallot, 330
tricuspid stenosis, 350
ventricular septal defect, 329
Right middle lobe syndrome, **291**
Right-to-left shunt
atrial septal defect, 326–328
pulmonary hypertension, 433
pulmonary valve stenosis, 324
syncope, 402
ventricular septal defect, 329–330
Right ventricle
arrhythmogenic dysplasia, athletic deaths, 438, 440*t*
cardiomyopathy, arrhythmogenic, 399, 400, 401
dilation, tricuspid regurgitation, 351
hypertrophy
atrial septal defect, 327
pulmonary valve regurgitation, 352
pulmonary valve stenosis, 323–324
tetralogy of Fallot, 330, **330–331**
infarction, acute MI with ST-segment elevation, 381
infundibulum, stenosis, 323
outflow obstructions, 323
tetralogy of Fallot, 330, 332
ventricular septal defect, 329
Right ventricular end-diastolic pressure, constrictive pericarditis, 431
Right ventricular infundibulum stenosis, tetralogy of Fallot, **330–331**
Right ventricular lift, 352
Rigidity, Parkinson disease, 1007
Rilpivirine, **1339*t*, 1344**
Riluzole, 1029
Rimegepant, 972*t*
Rimegepant sulfate, 971
Ringed sideroblasts, 526, 546–547

Ringer solution, balanced crystalloid-like lactated, 902
Rinne test, 205
Riociguat, 841
Ripretinib, 1625
Risankizumab, 138
Risdiplam, 1029
Risedronate, 613, 1150
Risperidone
  for aggression disorders, 1085
  for bipolar disorder, 1078–1079
  IV, 1066
  for personality disorders, 1061
  poisoning, 1576
  potency and side effects, 1065*t*
  for psychedelic effects, 1093
  for schizophreniform spectrum disorders, 1063, 1064*t*, 1065, 1065*t*
Ritonavir, **1340*t*, 1345,** 1415, 1417, 1418
Rituals, obsessive-compulsive disorder, 1052
Rituximab, 1600*t*
  for autoimmune hepatitis, 693
  for chronic lymphocytic leukemia, 531–532
  COVID-19 use, caution, 831
  for glomerulonephritis, 913, 928
  for granulomatosis with polyangiitis, 853
  for hepatitis C, cryoglobulinemia in, 690
  for histoplasmosis, 1537
  for IgA vasculitis, 928
  for immune-mediated inflammatory myopathies, 844
  for immune thrombocytopenia, 549
  on influenza vaccination, 1413
  for lymphoma
    cerebral, 1001
    CNS, 535
    indolent, 534
  for membranous nephropathy, 934
  for microscopic polyangiitis, 854
  for myasthenia gravis, 1041
  for neuromyelitis optica, 1026
  for pancreatitis, 735
  for pemphigus, 146
  progressive multifocal leukoencephalopathy from, 1387
  for rheumatoid arthritis, 831
  for Riedel thyroiditis, 1114
  for thyroid eye disease, 1128
  for Waldenström macroglobulinemia, 540
Rivaroxaban, 563, 564*t*
  for acute MI, with ST-segment elevation, 378
  for angina pectoris, 365
  for atrial fibrillation, stroke prevention, 393, **394–395,** 394*t*
  for coronary heart disease prevention, 358
  hepatotoxicity, 696
  for mitral stenosis, 336
  poisoning, 1575
  reversal agents, 563, 565*t*
  for transient ischemic attacks, 987
  for venous thromboembolism, 567*t*, 570–571, 570*t*
Rivastigmine, 1009, 1017
Rizatriptan, 971
Rocio virus, 1379
Rocky Mountain spotted fever, 911, 1358*t*, 1427*t*, **1430–1432,** 1431*f*
Rodent tapeworm, 1523
Roe v. Wade, 780
Roflumilast, 263
Rolapreptitant, 583*t*, **584**
Romberg test, 214
Romiplostim, 549, 1655
Romosozumab, 1152
Ropinrole, 1008, 1013
Ropivacaine, neuromodulatory therapy, 97*t*
ROS1, lung cancer, 1606
Rosacea, 107, **149–150,** 150*f*
Rosemont criteria, 734
Roseola, 1358*t*, **1368**
Roseola infantum, 1368
Rosiglitazone, 1204*t*, 1207–1208, **1582**
Ross procedure
  aortic stenosis, 345
  pulmonary regurgitation after, 352
  pulmonary valve stenosis after, 323
Rosuvastatin, 357*t*, 1244, 1246*t*
Rotarix, 1422
RotaSiil, 1422
RotaTeq, 1422
Rotation
  external
    rotator cuff strength testing, 1677*t*
    shoulder range of motion, 1676*t*
  internal
    rotator cuff strength testing
      belly-press test, 1678*t*
      lift-off test, 1678*t*
    shoulder range of motion, 1677*t*
Rotator cuff strength testing
  external rotation, 1677*t*
  internal rotation
    belly-press test, 1678*t*
    lift-off test, 1678*t*
  supraspinatus test, 1677*t*
Rotator cuff tears, 1677*t*, 1678*t*, 1679*t*, **1680–1681**
Rotavac, 1422
Rotavirus, 590, 1290*t*, **1422–1423**
Roth spots, 193, 1454
Rotigotine, 1008, 1013
Rotor syndrome, 675*t*, 676*t*
Rotterdam Criteria, 771
Roundworm infections, **1529–1530**
  intestinal, **1526–1529**
    ascariasis, **1526**
    enterobiasis, **1528–1529**
    hookworm disease, **1527**
    strongyloidiasis, **1527–1528**
    trichuriasis, **1526–1527**
  invasive, **1529–1530**
    angiostrongyliasis, **1529–1530**
    cutaneous larva migrans, **1530,** 1530*f*
Roux-en-Y gastric bypass surgery
  for obesity, 1257
  postprandial hypoglycemia, 1233
RS3PE, 867
RU 486, 780
Rubella, **1373–1374**
  cataracts, 184
  congenital rubella syndrome, 323, 1373
  diagnostic features, 1358*t*
  postnatal, 1373
Rubeola. *See* Measles (rubeola)
Rufinamide, 976*t*
Rule of nines, adult, 1554, 1555*f*
Runner's knee, 1703
RUNX1, 527, 528
RUNX1/ RUNX1T1 protein, acute myeloid leukemia, 527
Ruxolitinib, 165, 1388

S

S_3 gallop, 405, 418
S_4 gallop, hypertension, 447
S65C, 710
Saccharin, 1203
Saccular aneurysm, 325, 993, **994**
Sacituzumab govitecan, 758–759
Sacral meningoradiculitis, herpes zoster, 1360
Sacroiliitis, reactive arthritis, 860
Sacubitril, 406
Sacubitril + valsartan, 408
Safety evaluation, home, older adults, 60
Safinamide, 1009
Sag sign, 1702
Saksenaea, 1544
Salicylates. *See also specific types*
  anion gap elevation from, 897, 1570
  hypoglycemia from, 1237
  poisoning, 1569*t*, 1571*t*, 1572*t*, **1589–1590**
  respiratory alkalosis from, 902
  for rheumatic fever, 426
Salicylic acid
  anion gap elevation from, 897
  for molluscum contagiosum, 121
  for psoriasis, 137
  for warts, 122
Saline infusion sonohysterography, 764*t*
Salivary gland diseases, **234–235**. *See also specific types*
  infiltrative, chronic, **235**
  inflammatory, acute
    sialadenitis, **234–235**
    sialolithiasis, **235**
  inflammatory, chronic, **235**
  tumors, **235**
Salmeterol, 250*t*, 262
Salmon calcitonin, 1651
Salmonella (salmonellosis), **1463–1465**
  bacteremia, **1465**
  diarrhea, 590
    acute infectious, 1288, 1290*t*
    after foreign travel, 1288
    traveler's, 1292
  enteric fever, **1463–1464**
  with impaired cellular immunity, 1273
  liver abscess, 717
  medication of choice, 1294*t*
Salmonella enterica subsp *enterica*, 1463
Salmonella enteriditis, 1463
Salmonella paratyphi, 1463
Salmonella typhi, 1463
Salmonella typhimurium, 1463
Salpingectomy, 779–780
Salpingitis, **785–787,** 1473
Salt-restricted diets, 1263
Salt wasting, cerebral, 877–878
Salt-wasting congenital adrenal hyperplasia, 1158
Salvia divinorum, **1584–1585**
Same-sex marriage, on mental health, 1722
Samter's triad, 226, 872
Saphenous veins, varicose veins, **487–489**
SAPIEN XT valve, Edwards, 324, 331, 347, 352
Sarcocystis (sarcocystosis), 1516, **1516–1518**
Sarcoidosis, 295–296, 1144
  age, patient, 1270
  angina pectoris, 361
  anterior hypopituitarism, 1099
  AV block, 387
  cardiomyopathy
    dilated, 418, 418*t*, 419
    restrictive, 423, 424
  gout, 823
  heart failure, 404, 406
  hypercalcemia, 889
  interstitial lung disease, 295–296, 296*f*
  interstitial nephritis, 911
  lung cancer and, 1603
  meningeal irritation, 1281
  myocarditis, 415*t*, 417
  pericarditis, constrictive, 430
  rhinorrhea, 227
  right ventricle, tricuspid valve regurgitation, 351
  salivary gland disorders, 235
  sinonasal inflammatory disease, 227
  skin, 295, 296*f*
  uveitis, 183

Sarcoma
  Kaposi, **113,** 1319*t,* 1321, 1324, 1328–1329
  nasopharyngeal, 226
  small intestine, **1627**
  soft tissue, 1598*t*
Sarcoptes scabiei, 129
Sargramostim, 519, 1654*t*
Sarilumab, 831
Sarin poisoning, **1579**
SARS-CoV-1 (SARS), **1415–1416**
SARS-CoV-2 (COVID-19), 3, **1401–1408**
  acute kidney injury, **913**
  acute respiratory distress syndrome, 321
  aminotransferase, 675, 677*t*
  ARDS, 1403
  aspergillosis, **1543–1544**
  with cancer, 1652
  clinical findings, 1402–1403
  clinical self-care, 77
  coagulopathy, 1402, 1403
  collapsing glomerulopathy, 913
  complications, 1403–1405
    aguesia, 1404
    anosmia, 1402, 1404
    ARDS, 1403
    cardiac, 1404
    coagulopathy, 1402, 1403–1404
    dermatologic, 1404
    endocrine, 1405
    immune activation, 1403
    infectious, 1404–1405
    long COVID, 19, 1405
    multisystem inflammatory syndrome, 1405
    neurologic, 1404
    pancreatitis, 1404
    post-acute COVID-19 syndrome, 1405
    postoperative, 1405
    psychiatric, 1404
    pulmonary, 1403
    pulmonary aspergillosis, 1405
    renal, 1404
  cough, 15, 17
  death, 2, 2*t*
  death from, 72, 78
  diarrhea, 589
  differential diagnosis, 1403
  Durable Power of Attorney for Health Care, 71
  dyspnea, 17, 19, 20, 70
  end of life care, 72
  epidemiology, clinical, 1401
  ethical issues of care, 1408
  focal segmental glomerulosclerosis, 933
  hemoptysis, 21
  HIV/AIDS, 1321
  illness spectrum, 1321
  immune thrombocytopenia, 548
  immunity, naturally acquired, 1408
  mucormycosis, 1545
  myocarditis, 414, 416, 416*t*
    athletes, 416, 416*t,* 439–441
  myopericarditis, 414
  nephropathy, 1404
  palpitations, 25
  pandemic
    depression, 1069
    opioid overdoses, 84
    tracheal intubation practices, 318
  pericarditis, 427
  pneumonia, 269*t*
  pregnancy, 795
  prognosis, 72
  PTSD, frontline worker, 1047
  public health concerns, 1402
  pulmonary aspergillosis, 1405
  referral, 1408
  risk factors, 1402
  on sexual & gender minorities, 1711
  smell & taste, loss of, 15
  social distancing, 79
  stroke, 1404
  surgical mortality after, 46
  tamponade, cardiac, 427
  transmission, 1401–1402
  treatment, 1405
  treatment, severe disease
    primary VTE prevention, **577–578**
    thrombotic complications & hypercoagulability, 577–578
SARS-CoV-2 (COVID-19), prevention, 1405–1408
  personal & public health measures, 1405–1406
  vaccines, 3, 255, 261, 273, 1304*t,* 1406–1408
    anaphylactic reactions, 869
    asthmatics, 255
    booster doses, 1407
    breakthrough infections, 1407
    distribution, U.S., 1406
    herd immunity and vaccine hesitancy, 1407–1408
    HIV/AIDS, 1336
    immunocompromised, 1407
    intracranial venous thrombosis, 996
    mRNA, 870
    myocarditis after, 414
    pregnancy & lactation, 795, 1407
    rates, 1406
    reactions & complications, 1406
    "real world" efficacy & protective immunity duration, 1406–1407
    storage, 1406
  variants, 1402
  visitation restrictions, family, 77
Satralizumab, 1026
Saturated fats, low, dietary, 1263–1264
Saturday night palsy, 1034
Saxagliptin, 1205*t,* 1210
Scabies, **129–130,** 129*f,* 1285
Scalded skin syndrome, *Staphylococcus aureus,* 1449, 1449*f*
Scaling disorders, **133–142.** *See also specific types*
  atopic dermatitis, **133–135, 144,** 144*f,* 184, 1421
  cutaneous lupus erythematosus, **141–142**
  lichen planus, **140–141,** 140*f*
  lichen simplex chronicus, **135–136,** 135*f*
  pityriasis rosea, **138–139,** 138*f*
  psoriasis, **136–138,** 136*f*
  seborrheic dermatitis, **139–140,** 139*f*
Scalp lacerations, 1022
Scaly, 102*t*
Scapular winging, 1675
Scarlatina, 1440
Scarlet fever, 1358*t,* **1440**
Scarring alopecia, **165**
Scedosporium, with granulocytopenia, 1273
Scedosporium apiospermum, 1546
Schatzki rings, esophageal, 614
Schema-focused therapy, 1060
Schistosoma guineensis, 1520
Schistosoma haematobium, 1520–1521
Schistosoma intercalatum, 1520
Schistosoma japonicum, 1520–1521
Schistosoma mansoni, 1520–1521
Schistosoma mekongi, 1520
Schistosomiasis, **1520–1521**
Schizoaffective disorder, 1061–1062
Schizoid personality disorder, **1059–1061,** 1060*t*
Schizophrenia, 1061, 1071
Schizophrenia spectrum disorders, **1061–1069**
  classification, 1061–1062
    brief psychotic disorders, 1062
    delusional disorder, 1061
    schizoaffective disorder, 1061–1062
    schizophrenia, 1061
    schizophreniform disorders, 1062
  hallucinations, 1061, 1062
  treatment, nonpharmacologic, 1068
  treatment, pharmacologic, **1063–1068**
    clinical indications, 1064–1065
    dosage forms & patterns, 1063, 1064*t,* 1065–1066
    potency and side effects, 1065*t*
    side effects, **1066–1068,** 1066*t*
      akathisia, 1067
      common, 1066–1067, 1066*t*
      dystonia, 1067
      neuroleptic malignant syndrome, 1067
      parkinsonism, drug-induced, 1067
      tardive dyskinesia, 1067–1068
Schizophreniform disorders, 1062
Schizotypal personality disorder, **1059–1061,** 1060*t*
Schneiderian papillomas, 226
Schwannoma
  GI, 1624
  vestibular, **217–218**
Sciatica, 1686
Sciatic nerve palsy, **1036**
Scintillating scotomas, 36, 970
Sclera
  foreign bodies, 197
  laceration, **198**
Scleritis, granulomatosis with polyangiitis, 852, 852*f*
Scleroderma, **840–842.** *See also* Systemic sclerosis
Scleroderma renal crisis, 841
Sclerosing cholangitis, **726–728,** 1326
Sclerotherapy, varicose vein, 488
Scombroid poisoning, **1590–1591,** 1590*t*
Scopolamine, 1570, 1577
Scorpion stings, **1591–1592**
Scotoma, scintillating, 36, 970
"Screamer's nodules," 237
Screening. *See specific types*
Scrub typhus, 1427*t,* **1429–1430**
Scuba diving, dysbarism & decompression sickness, **1559–1560**
Scurvy, 1261
SDHB, 1170
Seafood poisoning, **1590–1591,** 1590*t*
Seasonal affective disorder, 1070, 1072
Seasonal influenza, **1410–1413**
  antigenic drift, 1410
  prevention/vaccination, 4*t,* 273, 1302*t*–1303*t,* 1305*t,* 1308*t,* **1412–1413**
  Reye syndrome, 1411
Seborrheic dermatitis, **139–140,** 139*f,* 1328
Seborrheic keratosis, **108,** 109*f*
Secnidazole, 785
Secondary hypogonadism, 962
Secondary prevention, 2
Secondary progressive multiple sclerosis, 1023
Second impact syndrome, 1022
Secretagogues, 586. *See also specific types*
Secukinumab, 138, 859, 860
Sedative-hypnotics. *See also specific types*
  for insomnia, 1083
  poisoning, **1581–1582**
  sympatholytic syndrome from, 1570
  withdrawal, seizures in, 1567
Sedatives, 1047, 1049, 1050–1051, 1050*t.* *See also specific types*
Segmental demyelination, 1030
Segmental myoclonus, 1012

Segmental wall motion abnormalities, exercise-induced, 361
Segond fracture, 1701
Seizures/seizure disorders. *See also* Epilepsy; *specific types*
  absence, 979
  alcohol withdrawal, 1087, 1091
  from antidepressant overdose, 1592, 1593
  atonic, 979
  atypical absence, 979
  automatisms, 979
  clonic, 979
  clonic/myoclonic, 979
  COVID-19, 1404
  definition, 979
  epileptic spasms, 979
  generalized onset, 979–980
  hyperkinetic, 979
  medications for, 975*t*–977*t*
    absence seizures, 977*t*
    generalized or focal seizures, 975*t*–977*t*
    myoclonic seizures, 977*t*
  motor, 979–980
  myoclonic, 979
  myoclonic-atonic, 979
  myoclonic-tonic-clonic, 979
  nonmotor, 979
  poisoning, **1567,** 1567*t*
  pregnancy, **813**
  psychogenic nonepileptic, 981–982, 1054
  recurrent unprovoked, 979
  serial, 979
  tonic, 979
  tonic-clonic, focal to bilateral, 979
  from tricyclic antidepressants, 1076
Selective estrogen receptor modulators (SERMs). *See also specific types*
  for breast cancer prevention, 742
  for gynecomastia, 1181
  for menopausal symptoms, 1190
  for osteoporosis, 1151
  tamoxifen, 1602*t*
Selective IgA deficiency, **873**
Selective progesterone receptor modulators, 766. *See also specific types*
Selective serotonin reuptake inhibitors. *See also specific types*
  for adjustment disorder, 1047
  adverse effects
    akathisia, 1075
    extrapyramidal symptoms, 1075
    serotonin syndrome, 1075
    sexual, 1075
  for aggression disorders, 1085
  for anxiety disorder, generalized, 1050, 1050*t*
  for dementia, 1017
  for depression, 1072–1075, 1073*t*
  erectile dysfunction from, 1059
  for hot flushes, 1186–1187
  hyponatremia from, 878
  for irritable bowel syndrome, 646
  with MAO inhibitor, serotonin syndrome from, 1567
  for neuropathic pain, 94*t*
  for obsessive-compulsive disorder, 1052–1053
  for panic disorder, 1050*t*, 1051
  for paraphilias, 1058
  for personality disorders, 1060
  for phobic disorders, 1051–1052
  for psychotic depression, 1072, 1073*t*
  for PTSD, 1047
  serotonin syndrome from, 30
  withdrawal symptoms, 1075
Selegiline, 1009, 1073*t*
Selenium
  deficiency, dilated cardiomyopathy, 418
  for Hashimoto autoimmune thyroiditis, 1114
  nutritional support, 1267
  for seborrheic dermatitis, 139
Selenium sulfide, 118
Selexipag, 705, 841
Self-hypnosis, 1055
Self-neglect
  definition, 67
  elder, **67–68,** 68*t*
Self-respect, medical aid in dying, 76
Selinexor, 538
Selpercatinib, 1606
Semaglutide, 1253, 1255*t*, 1257
  for coronary heart disease prevention in diabetics, 358–359
  for diabetes mellitus, cardiovascular outcomes, 1218
  for hyperglycemia/diabetes mellitus, 1205*t*, 1209
Semen analysis, 960–961, 961*f*
Semicircular canal dehiscence, superior, **217**
Seminomas, **1647–1649**
Senile amyloidosis, 541
Senile freckles, 163
Senile rhinitis, 222
Senile systemic amyloidosis, 423
Senna, 586, 587*t*
Sensorimotor neuropathy, 1004*t*
Sensorineural hearing loss, 204, **212–213,** 218
Sensory ataxia, HIV/AIDS, 1323
Sensory neuronopathy, 1004*t*
Sentinel headache, 35
Sentinel lymph node biopsy
  after neoadjuvant therapy, false-negatives, 755–756
  breast carcinoma, timing, 755–756
  malignant melanoma, 110
Seoul virus, 1395
Sepsis
  definition, 495–496
  gram-negative bacterial, **1462–1463**
  Group B streptococcus, 1443
  identification, clinical tools, 496
  thrombocytopenia, **556**
Septic arthritis. *See also specific types*
  antimicrobial therapy, initial, 1296*t*
  injection drug abuse, 1287
  nongonococcal acute, **861–863**
Septic shock, **495–498**
Septic thrombophlebitis
  antimicrobial therapy, initial, 1296*t*
  health care–associated infections, 1278
  otitis media, chronic, 211
Sequential Organ Failure Assessment, 496, 685, 729, 731
Sequoiosis, 307*t*
Serial seizures, 979
Seronegative spondyloarthropathies, **858–861**
  axial spondyloarthritis, **858–859**
  IBD-associated spondyloarthritis, **861**
  psoriatic arthritis, **859–860**
  reactive arthritis, **860–861,** 861*f*
Serotonergic agents. *See specific types*
Serotonin 5-HT_3-receptor agonists, 586–587, 971. *See also specific types*
Serotonin 5-HT_3-receptor antagonists, **583–584,** 583*t*, 647. *See also specific types*
Serotonin and norepinephrine reuptake inhibitors. *See also specific types*
  for chronic pain syndromes, 1057
  for depression, 1072–1075, 1073*t*
  for generalized anxiety disorder, 1050–1051, 1050*t*
  for neuropathic pain, 94–95, 94*t*
  for panic disorder, 1051
  for phobic disorders, 1051
Serotonin syndrome, **30,** 31, 95, 1567
  from antidepressant overdose, 1592, 1593
  from SSRIs, 1075, 1567
Serous otitis media, **208,** 218
Serrated polyps, **665–666**
Serratia, 1287, 1294*t*
Serratia marcescens infective endocarditis, 1287
Sertaconazole, 105*t*
Sertoli-Leydig tumors, 1181
Sertraline
  for depression, 1072, 1073*t*, 1074
  for irritable bowel syndrome, 646
  for obsessive-compulsive disorder, 1053
  for panic disorder, 1051
  for personality disorders, 1060
  safety, 1075
  serotonin syndrome from, 1567
  toxicity, 1592
Serum aminotransferase elevation, 675, 677*t*
Sevelamer carbonate, 917
17-beta estradiol, feminizing hormone therapy, 1726
Severe acute respiratory syndrome (SARS-CoV-1), **1415–1416**
Severe acute respiratory syndrome–coronavirus 2019 (SARS-CoV-2), **1401–1408.** *See also* SARS-CoV-2
Severe cutaneous adverse reactions, **871–872**
  acute generalized exanthematous pustulosis, **871–872**
  drug-induced hypersensitivity syndrome, **871**
  drug reaction with eosinophilia and systemic symptoms, **30,** 157, 696, **871**
  Stevens-Johnson syndrome/toxic epidermal necrolysis, 871
Severe fever with thrombocytopenia syndrome, **1391–1392**
Sex hormone replacement, 1149
Sexual activity, stages, 1057
Sexual and gender minority, 1709
Sexual arousal disorders, **781**
Sexual assault, **782–783**
  lesbian & bisexual women, 1721
  sexual & gender minorities, 1713
  STD risk after, 1285–1286
Sexual desire disorders, **781, 1058**
Sexual dysfunction, **1058, 1059,** 1066, 1066*t*. *See also specific types*
  female, **780–782**
    orgasmic disorders, **781**
    sexual arousal disorders, **781**
    sexual desire disorders, **781**
    sexual pain disorders, **781–782**
  lesbian & bisexual women, 1715
  male, **958–960**
    anejaculation, 959
    erectile dysfunction, **958–959**
    Peyronie disease, 959
    premature ejaculation, 959
    priapism, 959
    retrograde ejaculation, 959
Sexual & gender minority health, **1709–1730**
  cancer risk & screening, **1730**
  clinical environments, welcoming, 1711
  comprehensive care, 1711
  definitions & concepts, **1709–1710**
    cisgender, 1709
    gender identity, 1709–1710
    pronouns, 1710
    sexual & gender minority, 1709
    transgender, 1709
    transmasculine/transfeminine, 1709

electronic health record, **1712**
family planning, **1713–1715**
family building, 1713–1715
pregnancy prevention, 1713
gender affirming interventions, **1726–1729**
hormone therapy, 1712
contraception & family planning, 1713
family building, 1714–1715
health care, gay & bisexual men, **1722–1725**
demographics, **1722**
health disparities, **1722–1724**
behavioral health, **1723–1724**
HIV and other STIs, **1723**
substance use, **1724**
health care, lesbian & bisexual women, **1715–1722** (*See also* Lesbian & bisexual women, health care)
health care, transgender & diverse people, **1725–1730**
demographics, **1725**
disparities, **1725–1726**
gender affirming medical & surgical interventions, **1726–1730,** 1730*t*
feminizing hormone therapy, **1726–1727,** 1727*t*
fundamentals, 1726
long-term health outcomes, **1729**
masculinizing hormone therapy, **1727–1728,** 1728*t*
monitoring hormone therapy, **1728,** 1729*t*
surgical interventions, **1728–1729,** 1730*t*
terminology, **1725**
health disparities & minority stress model, **1710–1711**
HIV, **1730**
parents, 1714
preventive care & clinical practice guidelines, **1724–1725,** 1724*t*
SARS-CoV-1 pandemic, 1711
sexual history, 1711–1712
unintended pregnancy risk, 1713
Sexual history, 1711–1712
Sexual identities, defined, 1709
Sexual identity-behavior discordance, 1709
Sexual intercourse, unlawful, 782
Sexually transmitted diseases/infections, **1284–1286**. *See also specific types*
adenovirus, 1418
Chlamydia, **171–172, 1477–1479,** 1718, 1724
common, 1284–1285
epididymitis, **952–953**
gay & bisexual men, **1723**
gender identity, 1710
genital ulcers, 1285
gonococcus, **1469–1470** (*See also* Gonococcus (gonorrhea))
hepatitis C, 682
history, 1712
HIV/AIDS, **1311–1316** (*See also* HIV/AIDS)
immunization, 3–4, 4*t*
injection drug abuse, 1287
lesbian & bisexual women, **1718–1719**
pregnancy, **814–815**
screening & prevention, 1285–1286
sexual & gender minorities, 1713
syphilis, **1480–1488** (*See also* Syphilis)
urethritis, 1285
vaginal discharge, 1285
Sexual orientation, 1709–1710
Sexual pain disorders, **781–782**
Sexual violence, **782–783, 1721**
Sézary syndrome, from cutaneous T-cell lymphoma, 113
SF3B1, myelodysplastic syndromes, 527
SGLT2, 1200
SGLT2 inhibitors. *See* Sodium-glucose co-transporter 2 inhibitors; *specific types*
Shagreen patches, 1005
Shaped erythema, 102*t*
Shaver disease, 306*t*
Sheehan syndrome, hypopituitarism, 1100
Sheep liver fluke, 1521
Shellfish
allergies, 614, 868
paralytic poisoning, **1590–1591,** 1590*t*
Shift work sleep disorder, **1084**
Shiga-toxin–producing *Escherichia coli,* **1465–1466**
diarrhea, 590–592, 1288, 1289*t*
hemolytic-uremic syndrome, **550–552,** 551*t*, 590
Shigella (shigellosis), **1465**
diarrhea, 590, 1288, 1290*t*, 1292
medication of choice, 1294*t*
Shigella dysenteriae, 1465
Shigella flexneri, 1465
Shigella sonnei, 1465
Shingles. *See* Herpes zoster (shingles)
"Shin spots," 1225
Shivering, 1550
Shock, **495–499,** 495*t*
acute MI with ST-segment elevation, 380–381
cardiogenic, **495–499,** 495*t*
distributive, **495–499,** 495*t*
endocrine, **496–497**
septic, **495–498**
hemorrhagic, **497**
hypovolemic, **495–499,** 495*t*
neurogenic, **496–497**
obstructive, **495–499,** 495*t*
treatment, 497–499
early goal-directed therapy, 498
general, 497
hemodynamic measurements, 497
medications, 498–499
other modalities, 499
vasoactive therapy, 498–499
volume replacement, 497–498
Shock liver, **715**
Short-acting beta-2-agonists. *See also specific types*
for asthma, 247, 248*f*, 249–254, 252*t*, 255–258, 256*f*, 257*f*
for COPD, 252*t*, 255–258, 256*f*, 257*f*, 262
Short-acting muscarinic antagonists. *See also specific types*
for asthma, 250*t*, 254
for COPD, 262
Short bowel syndrome, **637**
Short-lasting neuralgiform headache, 973
Short saphenous vein, varicose veins, **487–489**
Shoulder, **1675–1683**
adhesive capsulitis, 1225, 1677*t*, 1682, **1682–1683**
dislocation & instability, 1679*t*, **1681–1682**
apprehension, 1679*t*
load and shift test, 1679*t*
O'Brien test, 1679*t*
dystocia, infants of diabetic mothers, 810
impingement testing
Hawkins impingement sign, 1675, 1679*t*
Neer impingement sign, 1675, 1678*t*
rotator cuff tears, 1677*t*, 1678*t*, 1679*t*, **1680–1681**
subacromial impingement syndrome, **1675–1680,** 1678*t*, 1679*t*
Neer and Hawkins impingement signs, 1675, 1678*t*, 1679*t*
Shoulder examination, 1675, 1676*t*–1679*t*
inspection, 1676*t*
palpation, 1676*t*
range of motion testing
external rotation, 1676*t*
flexion, 1676*t*
internal rotation, 1677*t*
rotator cuff strength testing
external rotation, 1677*t*
internal rotation
belly-press test, 1678*t*
lift-off test, 1678*t*
supraspinatus test, 1677*t*
stability testing
apprehension test, 1679*t*
load and shift test, 1679*t*
O'Brien test, 1679*t*
"Shoulder-hand syndrome," 867
Sialadenitis, **234–235**
Sialolithiasis, **235**
Sicca symptoms, 16, 171, 845–846
Sicca syndrome, 323, 984
Sickle beta^0-thalassemia, 513*t*, 514
Sickle beta$^+$-thalassemia, 513*t*, 514
Sickle cell anemia, **512–513,** 513*t*, 809
Sickle cell disease
hematuria & papillary necrosis, 943
kidney disease, **941**
osteonecrosis, 868
preoperative evaluation, 47
Sickle cell glomerulopathy, 941
Sickle cell retinopathy, 193
Sickle cell trait, 513*t*, **514,** 943
Sickle thalassemia, 513*t*, **514**
Sick sinus syndrome, **386–387**
Sideroblasts, ringed, 526
Siderosis, 307*t*
Sigmoidoscopy, flexible, for colorectal cancer screening, 1632–1633
Sigmoid sinus thrombosis, **211**
Sildenafil
for erectile dysfunction, 959–960, 1059, 1075, 1223
for portopulmonary hypertension, 705
for pulmonary hypertension, scleroderma, 841
Silent sporadic subacute thyroiditis, 1112
Silent thyroiditis, from hyperthyroidism, 1112, 1119, 1127
Silibinin, 685–686, 1587
Silicone gel, breast augmentation, 740
Silicosis, **306–307,** 306*t*, 308
Silodosin, 952, 965–966, 965*t*
Silymarin, 686, 1587
Simple phobias, 1049
Simplified Pulmonary Embolism Severity Index (PESI), 299, 568–569, 571*t*
Simultagnosia, 999
Simvastatin, 357*t*
for cholesterol, high LDL, 1244, 1246, 1246*t*
for hirsutism, female, 1183
SLCO1B1 on metabolisms of, 1670*t*
Sinecatechins, 123, 787
Sinequan, 160
"Singer's nodules," 237
Sin Nombre virus, 1395–1396
Sinonasal inflammatory disease, 226–227
Sinus, coronary, atrial septal defect, 326
Sinus arrhythmia, **386–387**
Sinus bradycardia, **386–387**
acute MI, with ST-segment elevation, 379
from poisoning, 1566*t*
syncope, 402, 403

Sinusitis
antimicrobial therapy, empiric, 1297*t*
chronic, cough, 16
facial pain, 978
frontal, acute, 219
fungal, invasive, **221–222**
HIV/AIDS, 1321
hospital-associated, 220
maxillary, acute, 219
sphenoid, 219
Sinusoidal obstruction syndrome, 697, 713
Sinus tachycardia, **386–387**
acute MI, with ST-segment elevation, 379
from poisoning, 1566*t*
Sinus thrombosis, **211,** 221
Sinus venosus defect, 326
Siponimod, 1025, 1025*t*
Sipuleucel-T, 1641
Sirolimus, 693, 1197
Sisunatovir, 1409
Sitagliptin, 1205*t*, 1210, **1582**
6-MP, *TPMT* on metabolism of, 1670*t*
Sixth disease, 1368
Sixth nerve palsy, 196
Sjögren syndrome, **845–846**
cryoglobulinemia, **855**
interstitial nephritis, 911
salivary gland disorders, 234, 235
sialadenitis, 234
sicca symptoms, 16, 171, 845–846
thyroiditis, 1112
Skin. *See also* Dermatologic disorders
innervation, **1038*f*–1039*f***
Skin decontamination, **1568,** 1574
Skin infections, **114–131**
bacterial, **123–128**
cellulitis, **127–128,** 127*f*
erysipelas, **128**
erythema migrans, **128,** 129*f*
folliculitis & sycosis, **124–125,** 125*f*
furunculosis & carbuncles, **126–127**
impetigo, 1, **123–124,** 124*f*
fungal, **114–119**
candidiasis, mucocutaneous, **118–119,** 119*f*
general measures & prevention, 115
intertrigo, **119**
KOH preparation, 114–115, 114*f*
tinea circinata, **115**
tinea corporis, **115**
tinea cruris, **115–116**
tinea manuum/tinea pedis, **116–117,** 117*f*
tinea versicolor, **117–118**
treatment principles, 115
Group A beta-hemolytic streptococci, **1440–1442,** 1441*f*, 1441*t*
erysipelas, 1441, 1441*f*, 1441*t*
impetigo, 1441, 1441*t*
injection drug abuse, 1286–1287
parasitic, **129–131**
pediculosis, **130–131**
scabies, **129–130,** 129*f*
viral, **119–123**
herpes simplex, **120–121,** 120*f*
herpes zoster (*See* Herpes zoster)
molluscum contagiosum, **121,** 121*f*
warts, **121–123,** 122*f*
Skin picking, 1052
Skin-popping, 1286
Skin prick allergen testing, 870
Skin & soft tissue infections. *See also specific types*
gram-negative bacteria, 1473, 1473*f*
mycobacterial, 1475
Staphylococcus, 1441*t*
Staphylococcus aureus, **1446–1447,** 1447*f*
Streptococcus, 1441–1442, 1441*t*
treatment, 1441–1442, 1441*t*
Skin ulcers, 27, 28, **64–65,** 65*t*
Skull fracture, 216, 1022
"Slapped cheek fever," 864
SLC40A1, 710
SLCO1B1, 1670*t*
Sleep, 1082
Sleep apnea
cardiomyopathy, dilated, 418, 419
central, **1084**
obstructive, **233–234, 316–317, 1084**
patent foramen ovale, 327
pulmonary hypertension, 432
Sleep-disordered breathing, obstructive sleep apnea, **316–317**
Sleep hygiene, 1083
Sleeping sickness, **1496–1497**
Sleep panic attacks, 1049
Sleep paralysis, 1084
Sleep-related breathing disorders, 33, **316.** *See also specific types*
fatigue & systemic intolerance disease, 33
obstructive sleep apnea, **233–234, 316–317, 1084**
Sleep-related hypoventilation, **1084**
Sleep-wake disorders, **1082–1084**
desynchronization sleep disorder, 1082
hypersomnia, **1084**
insomnia, **1082–1084**
parasomnias, **1084**
Sleeve gastrectomy, 1257
SLGT2 inhibitors, 1205*t*, **1210–1211.** *See also* Sodium-glucose co-transporter 2 (SGLT2) inhibitors
Small bowel. *See* Small intestine
Small cell carcinoma, myasthenic syndrome, **1042**
Small cell lung cancer/carcinoma, 1596*t*, 1603–1605, 1607, 1607*t*
Small intestine cancers, **1625–1627**
adenocarcinomas, **1625**
carcinoids, 1626
intestinal neuroendocrine tumors, **1626–1627**
lymphomas, **1625**
sarcoma, **1627**
Small intestine disorders, **632–643.** *See also specific types*
appendicitis, **641–642**
bleeding
overt, 601
suspected, 601
malabsorption, **632–638,** 633*t*
bacterial overgrowth, **636**
celiac disease, **633–635**
lactase deficiency, **637–638**
short bowel syndrome, **637**
Whipple disease, **635–636**
manometry, 640
motility disorders, **638–641**
colonic pseudo-obstruction, **639–641**
gastroparesis, **640–641**
intestinal pseudo-obstruction, chronic, **640–641**
paralytic ileus, **638–639**
obstruction, Crohn disease, 654
protein-losing enteropathy, **643**
tuberculosis, intestinal, **643**
Small lymphocytic lymphoma, 534
Smallpox, 1358*t*, **1420–1421.** *See also* Variola/vaccinia (smallpox)
Small-vessel vasculitis, rheumatoid arthritis, 828
Smell disorders
COVID-19, 15
olfactory dysfunction, **223–224**
Smithburn vaccine, 1393
SMN1, 1028, 1029
SMN2, 1029
Smoke inhalation, **304**
Smoking, cigarette, **6–8**
abdominal aortic aneurysm, 5*t*, 6, 42, **482–484,** 1465
aortoiliac artery occlusive disease, 473
asbestos workers, 307
biliary cholangitis, primary, 707
bladder cancer, 1642
bronchogenic carcinoma, 1603
cataracts, 185
cervical cancer, 790
cessation, **6–8**
cardiovascular risk prevention, 4, 5*t*
counseling strategies, 6–7, 7*t*
medications, 7, 7*t*
colorectal cancer and, 1627
COPD from, **258–264**
coronary artery disease, 355
gay & bisexual men, 1724
hypertension, essential, 444
laryngeal leukoplakia, 238
lesbian & bisexual women, **1716–1717**
lower esophageal sphincter, 305–306
lung cancer screening, 12
morbidity, 6
neck masses, 241
obstructive sleep apnea, 316
pancreatitis, chronic, 733
polypoid corditis, 237
on pregnancy, 795
Raynaud phenomenon, 839
reactive cervical lymphadenopathy, 242
renal cell carcinoma, 1645
respiratory bronchiolitis, 268
retinal vein occlusion, 188
on sleep, 1083
smoke inhalation, **304**
squamous cell carcinoma of larynx, 238–240
thromboangiitis obliterans, **481–482**
on thyroid eye disease, 1128
undertreatment, 6
ureter & renal pelvis cancers, 1644
vitamin C deficiency, 1261
Smoking, tobacco. *See also* Smoking, cigarette
cancer risk, 1595
cholangiocarcinoma, intrahepatic, 1613
environmental smoke, lung cancer and, 1603
hepatitis C progression, chronic, 689
lesbian & bisexual women, 1716, 1717
pancreatitis, chronic, 733
on pregnancy, 795
Smoking cessation, **6–8**
after acute MI with ST-segment elevation, 382
for angina pectoris, 364*f*, 367
cardiovascular risk prevention, 4, 5*t*
on COPD, 261
for coronary heart disease prevention, 355, 357
counseling strategies, 6, 6*t*
gay & bisexual men, 1725
lesbian & bisexual women, 1716–1717
medications, 7, 7*t*
preoperative, 46
Smoldering myeloma, 537–538
Snake bites, 1568*t*, **1591**
Sneddon syndrome, 858
SNNOOP10 red flags, 36, 36*t*
Snoring, **233–234**
Soap, 101
Social phobias, 1049, 1051–1052
Sodium
correction, hypernatremia, 882

dietary
diets restricting, 1263
on hypertension, 448, 448*t*
nutritional support, 1267
Sodium benzoate, 705
Sodium bicarbonate
for beta-blocker poisoning, 1577
for diabetic ketoacidosis, 1229
for D-lactic acidosis, 896*t*
for hyperkalemia, 886, 887*t*
in hypokalemia diagnosis, 883*f*
for kidney failure, anion gap metabolic acidosis, 896*t*
for lactic acidosis, 1232
for pancreatic insufficiency, in chronic pancreatitis, 734
for pyroglutamic acid ingestion, 896*t*
for tricyclic antidepressant poisoning, 1593
Sodium channel blockers, 383, 384*t*, 1565
Sodium concentration disorders, **876–882**. *See also specific types*
hypernatremia, **880–882**
hyponatremia, **876–880**
diagnostic algorithm, 877*f*
hypotonic, 876–878, 880
isotonic & hypertonic, 876, 880
hypertonic hyponatremia, 876
pseudohyponatremia, 876, 880
treatment, 879–880
Sodium-glucose co-transporter 2 (SGLT2) inhibitors, 932, 1236, **1582**
Sodium-glucose co-transporter 2 inhibitors, for hyperglycemia/diabetes mellitus, 1205*t*, 1210–1211, 1218, 1218*f*, 1219, 1221
canagliflozin, 1205*t*, 1210–1211
coronary heart disease prevention, 358–359
dapagliflozin, 1205*t*, 1210
diabetic ketoacidosis from, 1227
diabetic nephropathy, 935
empagliflozin, 1205*t*, 1210
ertugliflozin, 1205*t*, 1210
focal segmental glomerulosclerosis, 933
heart failure
with preserved ejection fraction, 406
with reduced LVEF, 409
in hospital, 1225
Sodium phosphate enema, 587*t*
Sodium stibogluconate, 1501
Sodium valproate, 1389
Sofosbuvir, 683–684, 689, 690*t*, 691*t*
Soft diets, 1263
Soft tissue sarcomas, 1598*t*
Solar urticaria, 151–153
Soles
tinea, **116–117**, 117*f*
vesiculobullous dermatitis, **144**, 144*f*
Solid organ transplant recipients. *See also specific types*
fever of unknown origin, 1270
immunizations, recommended, 1301
infections, 1273
prevention, 1275
Solitary atrial premature beats, 397
Solitary pulmonary nodule, **290–291**, 1608
Soluble guanylate cyclase stimulator, 410
Solute carrier organic anion transporter family member 1B1 *(SLCO1B1)* gene, 1670*t*
Solvents. *See also specific types*
bladder cancer, 1642
poisoning, **1589**
sniffing/inhaling, **1095**
Soman poisoning, **1579**
Somatic pain, **79–81**
Somatic symptom disorders, **1053–1055**
factitious, 1054
functional neurologic disorder/conversion, 1054
occupational therapy for, 1055
somatic symptom, 1054
Somatization
disorder, 1053 (*See also* Somatic symptom disorder)
irritable bowel syndrome, 644
Somatostatin, 616, 1099
Somatostatinomas, **1172**
Somatotropin. *See* Growth hormone
Somogyi effect, 1217
Songling virus, **1392**
SONIC (spectrum of neurocognitive impairment in cirrhosis), 704
Sonidegib, 113
Sonohysterography, saline infusion, 764*t*
Sorafenib
diarrhea from, 1656
for hepatocellular carcinoma, 1612
hyperthyroidism from, 1120
for renal cell carcinoma, 1646
for Rift Valley fever, 1392
Sorbitol, 586, 587*t*, 1203
Sotalol, 383, 385*t*, 396
Sotorasib, 1606, 1673*t*
Soy allergies, 614, 868
Spacer, 249
Spasms, epileptic, 979, 980
Spasticity, **1026**. *See also specific disorders*
Spastic paraparesis
cervical disk protrusion, 1037
cervical spondylosis, 1037
HIV/AIDS, 1323
HTLV-1-associated myelopathy, 1388–1389
multiple sclerosis, 1023
Specific antibody deficiency, **874**
Speech discrimination, 205
"Speed," 1093
Speed of accumulation, effusion, 429
Sperm
cryopreservation, 1714
motility, antipsychotics on, 1066
Sphenoid sinusitis, 219
Sphenopalatine ganglion stimulation, for cluster headache prevention, 973
Sphingosine 1-phosphate receptor modulators, 651. *See also specific types*
Sphingosine 1-phosphate receptors, 651
Sphygmomanometer, 442
Spider bites, **1591–1592**
Spinal cord
compression, **1649**
injury
fever, 30
traumatic, neurogenic shock, 496
vascular diseases
arteriovenous fistulae, **997**
epidural/subdural hemorrhage, **997**
infarction, **996**
Spinal muscular atrophies, **1028–1029**
Spinal stimulation, **98**, 367
Spine, **1683–1688**
low back pain, 80, 95, **1683–1685**, 1684*t*
lumbar disk herniation, **1686–1687**
mass lesions
leptomeningeal metastases, **1001**
tumors, primary/metastatic, **1001**
neck pain, **1687–1688**
paralysis, tick-borne encephalitis, 1383
poliomyelitis, 1375
stenosis, **1685–1686**
trauma, **1027**
tuberculosis, **864–865**
tumors, primary & metastatic, **1001–1002**
SPINK1, 733
Spinocerebellar degeneration, vitamin E deficiency, 1026
Spinosad, 131
Spiritual challenges, end of life care, 74–75, 75*t*
Spirochetal infections, **1480–1495**. *See also specific types*
Leptospira, 911, 1295*t*, **1490–1491**
Lyme disease, 1295*t*, **1491–1495**, 1495*t*
meningitis, 1280*t*
rat-bite fever, **1490**
relapsing fever, 1295*t*, **1489–1490**
syphilis, **1480–1488**
treponematoses, non-sexually transmitted, **1488**
Spirometry, asthma, 246
Spironolactone
for acne vulgaris, 149
for acute MI, with ST-segment elevation, 378
for alopecia, 164–165
for ascites and edema, 702
for Cushing syndrome, 1163
as feminizing hormone therapy, 1726
for heart failure with reduced LVEF, 408
for hirsutism, female, 771, 1183
hyperkalemia from, 886, 917
for hypertension, 455, 458*t*, 459*t*
Spirulina, 1580*t*
Spleen tyrosine kinase, 1388
Splenic vein obstruction, 715
Splenomegaly
alcohol-associated liver disease, 694
aplastic anemia, 517
beta-thalassemia intermedia, 506
blood disorders, 500
cholangitis, primary biliary, 709
chronic myeloid leukemia, 525
cirrhosis, 700
Epstein-Barr virus, 1363
essential thrombocytosis, 522
Felty syndrome, 519
G6PD deficiency, 511
hairy cell leukemia, 532
hepatic venous outflow obstruction, 713
hepatitis A, 678
jaundice, 674
myelodysplastic syndromes, 526
myelofibrosis, primary, 520*t*, **523–524**
nonalcoholic fatty liver disease, 698
platelet sequestration, 556
polycythemia vera, 520, 521
portal hypertension, noncirrhotic, 716
sickle cell anemia, 512
sickle thalassemia, 514
thalassemias, 505
Waldenström macroglobulinemia, 540
Wilson disease, 712
Splenorenal shunts, portal vein thrombosis, 715
Splinter hemorrhages, endocarditis, 1454, 1454*f*
Spondyloarthritis
axial, **858–859**
IBD-associated, **861**
Spontaneous abortion, **797–799**
Spontaneous bacterial peritonitis, 602*t*, **604–605**, 703
Spontaneous pneumothorax, 18, 313–314
Spontaneous pregnancy loss, **797–799**
Spontaneous subarachnoid hemorrhage, **993–994**
Spoon nails, 166
Sporadic Creutzfeldt-Jakob disease, 1385–1386
Sporothrix schenckii, 1545–1546
Sporotrichosis, **1545–1546**
Sports medicine, **1675–1708**. *See also* Orthopedic disorders & sports medicine

Spotted fevers, 1427*t*, **1430–1433**
non-rickettsiae, 1433
rickettsialpox, 1427*t*, **1433**
Rocky Mountain spotted fever, 1427*t*, **1430–1432,** 1431*f*
tick typhus, 1427*t*, **1432–1433**
Sprains, ankle, 1706*t*
eversion, **1707–1708**
inversion, **1706–1707**
Sprue. *See* Celiac disease
Sputum/sputum examination
blood, 21
cough, 16
hemoptysis, 21
nonasthmatic eosinophilic bronchitis, 17
Squamous cell carcinoma, **111,** 111*f*
anus, 1633–1634
bronchogenic, 1603, 1604*f*
cervical, 790
ear canal, 207
from erosive lichen planus, 140
esophageal, 1617
eyelid, 169
intraepidermal, **114**
larynx, **238–240**
nasopharyngeal/paranasal, 226
oral cavity, **227,** 228*f*
oropharyngeal, 228–229
"Square root" sign, 418*t*, 431
Squaric acid dibutylester, 122
Squatting
for cardiomyopathy, hypertrophic, 336*t*, 422
for syncope, 403
for systolic murmurs, 336*t*
SRSF2, myelodysplastic syndromes, 527
SSRIs. *See* Selective serotonin reuptake inhibitors
S stage sleep, 1082
Stability testing, shoulder
apprehension test, 1679*t*
load and shift test, 1679*t*
O'Brien test, 1679*t*
Stalevo, 1009
Standing, for systolic murmurs, 336*t*
Stannosis, 307*t*
Stanols, plant, on LDL cholesterol, 1243–1244
Stapedectomy, 211
Staphylococcus
arthritis, nongonococcal acute, 862
diarrhea, 1290*t*
glomerulonephritis, 923*t*, **926–927**
keratitis, 179
methicillin-resistant, 1293*t*
methicillin-susceptible, 1293*t*
otitis media, HIV/AIDS, 218
perianal pruritus, 672
skin infections, HIV/AIDS, 1327–1328
struvite calculi, 957
Staphylococcus aureus, **1446–1450**
animal bites, 1283
bacteremia, **1449**
brain abscess, 1281
breast abscess, 740
bronchiectasis, 265
cellulitis, 127
coagulase-negative, **1449–1450**
cystic fibrosis, 266
dacrocystitis, 169
diarrhea, 590
acute infectious, 1288
endocarditis, infective, 1453–1455, 1457
with granulocytopenia, 1273
hordeolum, 168
immunocompromised, pulmonary infiltrates, 279
impetigo, 124
infective endocarditis, 1287
liver abscess, 717
lymphangitis & lymphadenitis, 493
meningitis, health care–associated, 1281
nasal colonization, **221**
nasal vestibulitis & colonization, 221
necrotizing fasciitis, **1442**
osteomyelitis/septic arthritis, 1287, **1447–1448**
otitis media, chronic, 210, 211
paronychia, 166, 166*f*
pneumonia, 269*t*
community-acquired, 270, 273
nosocomial, 275
puerperal mastitis, 807
pyelonephritis, 948
rhinosinusitis, 219
sialadenitis, 234–235
sialadenitis, 234–235
skin & soft tissue, **1446–1447,** 1447*f*
HIV/AIDS, 1327–1328
injection drug use, 1286
toxic shock syndrome, **1449,** 1449*f*
venous thrombophlebitis, superficial, **489–490**
Staphylococcus cohnii, 1450
Staphylococcus epidermidis, 1450
dacrocystitis, 169
immunocompromised, 1272
Staphylococcus haemolyticus, 1450
Staphylococcus hominis, 1450
Staphylococcus saccharolyticus, 1450
Staphylococcus saprophyticus, 1450
Staphylococcus warnerii, 1450
Starch hydrolysates, hydrogenated, 1203
Starvation, ketoacidosis, 896*t*, 897
Stasis dermatitis, 28, 490, 490*f*
Statins. *See* HMG-CoA reductase inhibitors (statins)
Status epilepticus, 979
from antidepressants, 1593, 1593*f*
from theophylline/caffeine poisoning, 1592
treatment, 983
Statutory rape, 782. *See also* Sexual violence
Stauffer syndrome, renal cell carcinoma, 1645
Stavudine, 715, 1325
Steatosis, hepatic
acute liver failure, 685
alcohol-associated fatty liver disease, 694–695
aminotransferase elevation, 677*t*
hemochromatosis, 710
hepatitis C, 683, 689
macrovesicular, 698
microvesicular, 685, 697, 698
nonalcoholic fatty liver disease, 698–699
Steatosis, pancreatic, obesity, 733
STEC. *See* Shiga-toxin-producing *Escherichia coli*
Stein-Leventhal syndrome, 1181, **1181**
STEMI. *See* ST-segment elevation
STEMI equivalent, 374
Stenosis. *See specific types*
Stenotrophomonas maltophilia pneumonia, 275
Stensen duct, 235
Stents/stenting
for acute MI, with ST-segment elevation, 375
after acute MI, 375, 378
aspirin after, 369
for coarctation of the aorta, 325–326
for coronary artery disease, 382
drug-eluting
for angina, 365
antiplatelet therapy after, 371, 375
pregnancy, 438
ST-segment elevation, 375
dual antiplatelet therapy after, 358, 365
intravascular ultrasound of, 362
$P2Y_{12}$ inhibitor after, 372
percutaneous coronary intervention with, **366**
percutaneous/transcatheter
for angina pectoris, 366
mitral regurgitation, 340
mitral stenosis, 337
tetralogy of Fallot, 366
tricuspid stenosis, 350
for pulmonary stenosis, branch, 332
restenosis after, 366, 375
superficial femoral artery, 475
Sterilization, **779–780**
Steroid acne, 124
Steroidogenic enzyme defects, **1181**
Steroid rosacea, 107
Steroids. *See also* Corticosteroids; *specific types*
anabolic, **1095,** 1179
weight gain from, 1252, 1253*t*
Sterols, plant, on LDL cholesterol, 1243–1244
Stevens-Johnson syndrome/toxic epidermal necrolysis, **153–154,** 154*f*, 871, **871**
from allopurinol, 1670*t*
carbamazepine, 1669*t*
drug-related, 159*t*
from lamotrigine, 1080
Stiff person syndrome, 1004*t*
Still disease, adult, **831,** 1270
Stimulant laxatives, for constipation, 586, 587*t*
Stimulants. *See also specific types*
abuse, **1093–1094**
STK11/LKB1, pancreas carcinoma, 1615
St. Louis encephalitis, 1379
Stomach cancers, 579, 596, 622, 1597*t*. *See also specific types*
Stomach & duodenum diseases, **620–632.** *See also specific types*
gastritis & gastropathy, **620–624**
erosive & hemorrhagic "gastritis," **620–622**
gastritis types, infections, **624**
nonerosive, nonspecific gastritis & intestinal metaplasia, **622–623**
Helicobacter pylori gastritis, **622–623,** 624*t*
pernicious anemia gastritis, **623**
peptic ulcer disease, **625–629**
peptic ulcer disease complications, **629–632**
gastric outlet obstruction, **631**
hemorrhage, GI, **629–630**
ulcer perforation, **631**
Zollinger-Ellison syndrome, 625, **631–632**
Stomatitis
herpes, **230**
neutropenia, 519
ulcerative, **230**
Stone disease. *See also specific types*
urinary, **954–958**
Stool surfactants, 587*t*. *See also specific types*
Storage pool disease, **557**
Strawberry cervix, **784–785,** 784*f*
"Strawberry gallbladder," 721
Strawberry tongue, 1440
Streptococcus, **1440–1443**
arthritis, 862
Group A beta-hemolytic, **1440–1443**
acute rheumatic fever & scarlet fever, **1440**
arthritis, **1442**
endocarditis, **1443**
erysipelas, 1441, 1441*f*, 1441*t*
impetigo, 1441, 1441*t*
necrotizing fasciitis, **1442**
otitis media
acute, 209, 209*f*
chronic, 210, **211**